MW00713806

Drug Information Handbook *for* Dentistry

Oral Medicine for Medically-Compromised Patients & Specific Oral Conditions

10th Edition

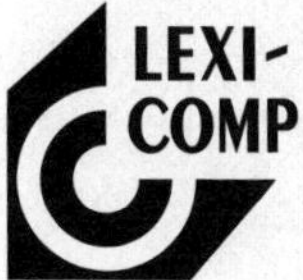

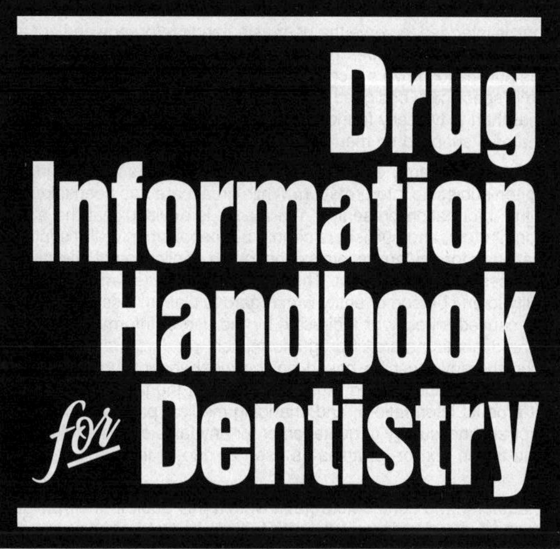

Oral Medicine for Medically-Compromised Patients & Specific Oral Conditions

10th Edition

Richard L. Wynn, BSPharm, PhD
Professor of Pharmacology
Baltimore College of Dental Surgery
Dental School
University of Maryland Baltimore
Baltimore, Maryland

Timothy F. Meiller, DDS, PhD
Professor
Diagnostic Sciences and Pathology
Baltimore College of Dental Surgery
Professor of Oncology
Greenebaum Cancer Center
University of Maryland Baltimore
Baltimore, Maryland

Harold L. Crossley, DDS, PhD
Professor Emeritus
Baltimore College of Dental Surgery
Dental School
University of Maryland Baltimore
Baltimore, Maryland

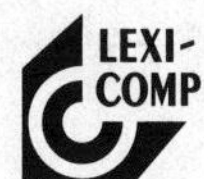

NOTICE

This handbook is intended to serve the user as a handy reference and not as a complete drug information resource. It does not include information on every therapeutic agent available. The publication covers a combination of commonly used drugs in dentistry and medicine and is specifically designed to present important aspects of drug data in a more concise format than is typically found in medical literature, exhaustive drug compendia, or product material supplied by manufacturers.

Drug information is constantly evolving because of ongoing research and clinical experience and is often subject to interpretation. While great care has been taken to ensure the accuracy of the information presented, the reader is advised that the authors, editors, reviewers, contributors, and publishers cannot be responsible for the continued currency of the information or for any errors, omissions, or the application of this information, or for any consequences arising therefrom. Therefore, the author(s) and/or the publisher shall have no liability to any person or entity with regard to claims, loss, or damage caused, or alleged to be caused, directly or indirectly, by the use of information contained herein. Because of the dynamic nature of drug information, readers are advised that decisions regarding drug therapy must be based on the independent judgment of the clinician, changing information about a drug (eg, as reflected in the literature and manufacturer's most current product information), and changing medical practices. The editors are not responsible for any inaccuracy of quotation or for any false or misleading implication that may arise due to the text or formulas as used or due to the quotation of revisions no longer official.

The editors, authors, and contributors have written this book in their private capacities. No official support or endorsement by any federal or state agency or pharmaceutical company is intended or inferred.

The publishers have made every effort to trace the copyright holders for borrowed material. If they have inadvertently overlooked any, they will be pleased to make the necessary arrangements at the first opportunity.

If you have any suggestions or questions regarding any information presented in this handbook, please contact our drug information pharmacist at (330) 650-6506.

Copyright © 2005 by Lexi-Comp, Inc. All rights reserved.

Copyright © 2003, 9th Edition; 2002, 8th Edition; 2001, 7th Edition; 2000, 6th Edition; 1999, 5th Edition; 1998, 4th Edition; 1997, 3rd Edition; 1997, 2nd Edition; 1996, 1st Edition.

Printed in Canada. No part of this publication may be reproduced, stored in a retrieval system, or transmitted, in any form or by any means, electronic, mechanical, photocopying, recording, or otherwise, without the prior written permission of the publisher.

This manual was produced using the FormuLex™ Program — a complete publishing service of Lexi-Comp, Inc.

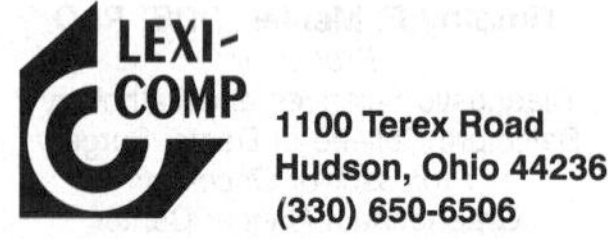

1100 Terex Road
Hudson, Ohio 44236
(330) 650-6506

ISBN 1-59195-102-X North American edition

ISBN 1-59195-103-8 Delta Dental® edition (not for sale)

TABLE OF CONTENTS

About the Authors ... 3
Editorial Advisory Panel ... 4
Preface to the Tenth Edition ... 10
Acknowledgments ... 11
Description of Sections and Fields ... 12
FDA Pregnancy Categories ... 15
FDA Name Differentiation Project – The Use of Tall-Man Letters ... 16
Controlled Substances ... 17
Prescription Writing ... 18
Abbreviations, Acronyms, and Symbols ... 18
Safe Writing Practices ... 23
Pharmacology of Drug Metabolism and Interactions ... 24

ALPHABETICAL LISTING OF DRUGS ... 41

NATURAL PRODUCTS: HERBAL AND DIETARY SUPPLEMENTS ... 1409
ALPHABETICAL LISTING OF NATURAL PRODUCTS ... 1411
Effects on Various Systems ... 1453

ORAL MEDICINE TOPICS

Part I: Dental Management and Therapeutic Considerations in Medically-Compromised Patients
Table of Contents ... 1457
Cardiovascular Diseases ... 1458
Gastrointestinal Disorders ... 1476
Respiratory Diseases ... 1478
Endocrine Disorders and Pregnancy ... 1481
HIV Infection and AIDS ... 1484
Rheumatoid Arthritis, Osteoarthritis, and Osteoporosis ... 1490
Nonviral Infectious Diseases ... 1495
Antibiotic Prophylaxis - Preprocedural Guidelines for Dental Patients ... 1509
Systemic Viral Diseases ... 1519

Part II: Dental Management and Therapeutic Considerations in Patients With Specific Oral Conditions and Other Medicine Topics
Table of Contents ... 1525
Oral Pain ... 1526
Oral Bacterial Infections ... 1533
Periodontal Diseases ... 1542
Oral Fungal Infections ... 1544
Oral Viral Infections ... 1547
Oral Nonviral Soft Tissue Ulcerations or Erosions ... 1551
Dentin Hypersensitivity, High Caries Index, and Xerostomia ... 1555
Management of Sialorrhea ... 1557
Temporomandibular Dysfunction (TMD) ... 1564
Patients Requiring Sedation ... 1567
Management of Patients Undergoing Cancer Therapy ... 1569

Part III: Other Oral Medicine Topics
Table of Contents ... 1573
Dentist's Role in Recognizing Domestic Violence ... 1574
Chemical Dependency and Smoking Cessation ... 1576
Animal and Human Bites Guidelines ... 1582
Dental Office Emergencies ... 1584
Suggested Readings ... 1589

TABLE OF CONTENTS *(Continued)*

APPENDIX

Standard Conversions

Apothecary / Metric Conversions 1598
Pounds / Kilograms Conversion 1599

Calcium Channel Blockers and Gingival Hyperplasia

Some General Observations of CCB-Induced GH 1600
Calcium Channel Blockers 1602

Infectious Disease Information

Occupational Exposure to Bloodborne Pathogens (Standard / Universal Precautions) 1603
Immunizations (Vaccines) 1614

Laboratory Values

Normal Blood Values 1620

Over-the-Counter Dental Products

Dentifrice Products 1621
Mouth Pain, Cold Sore, and Canker Sore Products 1633
Oral Rinse Products 1638

Miscellaneous

Top 200 Prescribed Drugs in 2003 1642
Multivitamin Products 1644
Dental Drug Use in Pregnancy and Breast-Feeding 1657

INDEXES

Pharmacologic Category Index 1659
Alphabetical Index 1681

ABOUT THE AUTHORS

Richard L. Wynn, BSPharm, PhD

Richard L. Wynn, PhD, is Professor of Pharmacology at the Baltimore College of Dental Surgery, Dental School, University of Maryland Baltimore. Dr Wynn has served as a dental educator, researcher, and teacher of dental pharmacology and dental hygiene pharmacology for his entire professional career. He holds a BS (pharmacy; registered pharmacist, Maryland), an MS (physiology) and a PhD (pharmacology) from the University of Maryland. Dr Wynn chaired the Department of Pharmacology at the University of Maryland Dental School from 1980 to 1995. Previously, he chaired the Department of Oral Biology at the University of Kentucky College of Dentistry.

Dr Wynn has to his credit over 300 publications including original research articles, textbooks, textbook chapters, monographs, and articles in continuing education journals. He has given over 500 continuing education seminars to dental professionals in the U.S., Canada, and Europe. Dr Wynn has been a consultant to the drug industry for 22 years and his research laboratories have contributed to the development of new analgesics and anesthetics. He is a consultant to the U.S. Pharmacopeia, Dental Drugs and Products section, the Academy of General Dentistry, the American Dental Association, and a former consultant to the Council on Dental Education, Commission on Accreditation. He is a featured columnist and his drug review articles, entitled *Pharmacology Today*, appear in each issue of *General Dentistry*, a journal published by the Academy. One of his primary interests continues to be keeping dental professionals informed on all aspects of drug use in dental practice.

Timothy F. Meiller, DDS, PhD

Dr Meiller is Professor of Diagnostic Sciences and Pathology at the Baltimore College of Dental Surgery and Professor of Oncology in the Program of Oncology at the Greenebaum Cancer Center, University of Maryland Baltimore. He has held his position in Diagnostic Sciences at the Dental School for 26 years and serves as an attending faculty at the Greenebaum Cancer Center.

Dr Meiller is a Diplomate of the American Board of Oral Medicine and a graduate of Johns Hopkins University and the University of Maryland Dental and Graduate Schools, holding a DDS and a PhD in Immunology/Virology. He has over 200 publications to his credit, maintains an active general dental practice, and is a consultant to the National Institutes of Health. He is currently engaged in ongoing investigations into cellular immune dysfunction in oral diseases associated with AIDS, in cancer patients, and in other medically-compromised patients.

Harold L. Crossley, DDS, PhD

Dr Crossley is Professor Emeritus at the Baltimore College of Dental Surgery, Dental School, University of Maryland Baltimore. A native of Rhode Island, he received a Bachelor of Science degree in Pharmacy from the University of Rhode Island in 1964. He later was awarded the Master of Science (1970) and Doctorate degrees (1972) in the area of Pharmacology. The University of Maryland Dental School in Baltimore awarded Dr Crossley the DDS degree in 1980. He is the Director of Conjoint Sciences and Preclinical Studies at the School of Dentistry and maintains an intramural part-time private dental practice.

Dr Crossley has coauthored a number of articles dealing with law enforcement on both a local and federal level. This liaison with law enforcement agencies keeps him well-acquainted with the "drug culture." He has been appointed to the Governor's Commission on Prescription Drug Abuse and the Maryland State Dental Association's Well-Being Committee. Drawing on this unique background, Dr Crossley has become nationally and internationally recognized as an expert on street drugs and chemical dependency, as well as the clinical pharmacology of dental drugs.

EDITORIAL ADVISORY PANEL

Judith A. Aberg, MD
Director of HIV Services
Washington University School of Medicine
St Louis, Missouri

Lora Armstrong, RPh, PharmD, BCPS
Director, Pharmacy & Therapeutics Committee Formulary Process
Caremark, Inc.
Northbrook, Illinois

William Alvarez Jr., PharmD
Clinical Specialist, Cardiology
Johns Hopkins Hospital
Baltimore, Maryland

David Au, MD
Assistant Professor of Medicine
University of Washington
Seattle, Washington

Kenneth A. Bachmann, PhD, FCP
Distinguished University Professor of Pharmacology
Codirector, Center for Applied Pharmacology
University of Toledo
Toledo, Ohio

Verna L. Baughman, MD
Professor
Anesthesiology and Neurosurgery
University of Illinois
Chicago, Illinois

Judith L. Beizer, PharmD, FASCP
Chair and Clinical Professor
Department of Clinical Pharmacy Practice
St John's University College of Pharmacy and Allied Health Professions
Jamaica, New York

Mark F. Bonfiglio, BS, PharmD, RPh
Director of Pharmacotherapy Resources
Lexi-Comp, Inc
Hudson, Ohio

Debbie Bramble, PharmD
Clinical Specialist, Medical Oncology
Johns Hopkins Hospital
Baltimore, Maryland

Larisa Humma Cavallari, PharmD, BCPS
Assistant Professor, Section of Cardiology
University of Illinois
Chicago, Illinois

Harold L. Crossley, DDS, PhD
Associate Professor of Pharmacology
Baltimore College of Dental Surgery
Dental School
University of Maryland Baltimore
Baltimore, Maryland

Francesca E. Cunningham, PharmD
Program Director for Pharmacoepidemiologic Research
Veterans Affairs
PBM/SHG
Associate Professor
Pharmacy Practice/Anesthesiology
University of Illinois
Chicago, Illinois

Wayne R. DeMott, MD
Consultant in Pathology and Laboratory Medicine
Shawnee Mission, Kansas

Samir Desai, MD
Assistant Professor of Medicine
Department of Medicine
Baylor College of Medicine
Houston, Texas
Staff Physician
Veterans Affairs Medical Center
Houston, Texas

Andrew J. Donnelly, PharmD, MBA
Director of Pharmacy
and
Clinical Professor of Pharmacy Practice
University of Illinois Medical Center at Chicago
Chicago, Illinois

Kimberly Duggan, BScPharm
School of Pharmacy
Memorial University of Newfoundland
St John's, Newfoundland

Thom C. Dumsha, DDS
Associate Professor and Chair
Dental School
University of Maryland Baltimore
Baltimore, Maryland

Michael S. Edwards, PharmD, MBA
Assistant Director, Weinberg Pharmacy
Johns Hopkins Hospital
Baltimore, Maryland

Vicki L. Ellingrod-Ringold, PharmD, BCPP
Assistant Professor
University of Iowa
Iowa City, Iowa

Margaret A. Fitzgerald, MS, APRN, BC, NP-C, FAANP
President, Principal Lecturer
Fitzgerald Health Education Associates
Andover, Massachusetts
Nurse Practitioner
Greater Lawrence Family Health Center
Lawrence, Massachusetts
Visiting Professor
Husson College
Bangor, Maine
Visiting Professor
Simmons College
Boston, Massachusetts

Matthew A. Fuller, PharmD, BCPS, BCPP, FASHP
Clinical Pharmacy Specialist, Psychiatry
Cleveland Department of Veterans Affairs Medical Center
Brecksville, Ohio
Associate Clinical Professor of Psychiatry
Clinical Instructor of Psychology
Case Western Reserve University
Cleveland, Ohio
Adjunct Associate Professor of Clinical Pharmacy
University of Toledo
Toledo, Ohio

Morton P. Goldman, PharmD
Assistant Director, Pharmacotherapy Services
The Cleveland Clinic Foundation
Cleveland, Ohio

Jeffrey P. Gonzales, PharmD
Critical Care Pharmacy Specialist
The Cleveland Clinic Foundation
Cleveland, Ohio

Barbara L. Gracious, MD
Assistant Professor of Psychiatry and Pediatrics
Case Western Reserve University
Director of Child Psychiatry and Training & Education
University Hospitals of Cleveland
Cleveland, Ohio

EDITORIAL ADVISORY PANEL *(Continued)*

Larry D. Gray, PhD, ABMM
TriHealth Clinical Microbiology Laboratory
Bethesda and Good Samaritan Hospitals
Cincinnati, Ohio

James L. Gutmann, DDS
Professor and Director of Graduate Endodontics
The Texas A & M University System
Baylor College of Dentistry
Dallas, Texas

Tracey Hagemann, PharmD
Associate Professor
College of Pharmacy
The University of Oklahoma
Oklahoma City, Oklahoma

Charles E. Hawley, DDS, PhD
Professor Emeritus
Department of Periodontics
University of Maryland
Consultant on Periodontics
Commission on Dental Accreditation of the American Dental Association

Martin D. Higbee, PharmD, CGP
Associate Professor
Department of Pharmacy Practice and Science
The University of Arizona
Tucson, Arizona

Jane Hurlburt Hodding, PharmD
Director, Pharmacy
Miller Children's Hospital
Long Beach, California

Rebecca T. Horvat, PhD
Assistant Professor of Pathology and Laboratory Medicine
University of Kansas Medical Center
Kansas City, Kansas

Collin A. Hovinga, PharmD
Neuropharmacologist
Miami Children's Hospital
Miami, Florida

Darrell T. Hulisz, PharmD
Department of Family Medicine
Case Western Reserve University
Cleveland, Ohio

Sana Isa-Pratt, MD
Attending Physician
Department of Medicine
Overlake Hospital
Bellevue, Washington

David S. Jacobs, MD
President, Pathologists Chartered
Consultant in Pathology and Laboratory Medicine
Overland Park, Kansas

Bernard L. Kasten, Jr, MD, FCAP
Vice-President/Chief Medical Officer
Quest Diagnostics Inc
Teteroboro, New Jersey

Polly E. Kintzel, PharmD, BCPS, BCOP
Clinical Specialist for Stem Cell Transplantation
Detroit Medical Center
Harper Hospital
Detroit, Michigan

Jill Kolesar, PharmD, FCCP, BCPS
Associate Professor of Pharmacy
University of Wisconsin
Madison, Wisconsin

Donna M. Kraus, PharmD, FAPhA
Associate Professor of Pharmacy Practice
Departments of Pharmacy Practice and Pediatrics
Pediatric Clinical Pharmacist
University of Illinois
Chicago, Illinois

Daniel L. Krinsky, RPh, MS
Director, Pharmacotherapy Sales and Marketing
Lexi-Comp, Inc
Hudson, Ohio

Kay Kyllonen, PharmD
Clinical Specialist
The Cleveland Clinic Children's Hospital
Cleveland, Ohio

Charles Lacy, RPh, PharmD, FCSHP
Facilitative Officer, Clinical Programs
Nevada College of Pharmacy
Las Vegas, Nevada

Brenda R. Lance, RN, MSN
Manager of Service Integration
Ritzman Infusion Services
Akron, Ohio

Leonard L. Lance, RPh, BSPharm
Clinical Pharmacist
Lexi-Comp Inc
Hudson, Ohio

Jerrold B. Leikin, MD, FACP, FACEP, FACMT, FAACT
Director, Medical Toxicology
Evanston Northwestern Healthcare-OMEGA
Glenbrook Hospital
Glenview, Illinois
Associate Director
Toxikon Consortium at Cook County Hospital
Chicago, Illinois
Professor of Medicine
Pharmacology and Health Systems Management
Rush Medical College
Chicago, Ilinois
Professor of Medicine
Feinberg School of Medicine
Northwestern University
Chicago, Ilinois

Jeffrey D. Lewis, PharmD
Pharmacotherapy Specialist
Lexi-Comp, Inc
Hudson, Ohio

Timothy F. Meiller, DDS, PhD
Professor
Diagnostic Sciences and Pathology
Baltimore College of Dental Surgery
Professor of Oncology
Greenebaum Cancer Center
University of Maryland Baltimore
Baltimore, Maryland

Franklin A. Michota, Jr, MD
Head, Section of Hospital and Preoperative Medicine
Department of General Internal Medicine
The Cleveland Clinic Foundation
Cleveland, Ohio

Michael A. Militello, PharmD, BCPS
Clinical Cardiology Specialist
Department of Pharmacy
The Cleveland Clinic Foundation
Cleveland, Ohio

J. Robert Newland, DDS, MS
Professor
Department of Diagnostic Sciences
University of Texas Health Science Center
Houston, Texas

EDITORIAL ADVISORY PANEL *(Continued)*

Eugene S. Olsowka, MD, PhD
Pathologist
Institute of Pathology PC
Saginaw, Michigan

Dwight K. Oxley, MD
Consultant in Pathology and Laboratory Medicine
Wichita, Kansas

Frank P. Paloucek, PharmD, DABAT
Clinical Associate Professor in Pharmacy Practice
Director, Residency Programs
University of Illinois
Chicago, Illinois

Christopher J. Papasian, PhD
Director of Diagnostic Microbiology and Immunology Laboratories
Truman Medical Center
Kansas City, Missouri

Alpa Patel, PharmD
Clinical Specialist, Infectious Diseases
Johns Hopkins Hospital
Baltimore, Maryland

Laura-Lynn Pollack, BScPharm, NARTC
Pharmacist / Health Educator
Victoria, British Columbia

Luis F. Ramirez, MD
Adjunct Associate Professor of Psychiatry
Case Western Reserve University
Cleveland, Ohio

James B. Ray, PharmD
Coordinator, Palliative Care Consult Service
Hamot Medical Center
Erie, Pennsylvania

A.J. (Fred) Remillard, PharmD
Assistant Dean, Research and Graduate Affairs
College of Pharmacy and Nutrition
University of Saskatchewan
Saskatoon, Saskatchewan

Martha Sajatovic, MD
Associate Professor of Psychiatry
Case Western Reserve University
Cleveland, Ohio

Todd P. Semla, PharmD
Associate Professor of Clinical Psychiatry
Feinberg School of Medicine
Northwestern University
Evanston, Illinois

Francis G. Serio, DMD, MS
Professor & Chairman
Department of Periodontics
University of Mississippi
Jackson, Mississippi

Stephen Shalansky, PharmD, FCSHP
Research Coordinator, Pharmacy Department
St Paul's Hospital
Vancouver, British Columbia

Dominic A. Solimando, Jr, MA
Oncology Pharmacist
President, Oncology Pharmacy Services, Inc
Arlington, VA

Joni Lombardi Stahura, BS, PharmD, RPh
Pharmacotherapy Specialist
Lexi-Comp, Inc
Hudson, Ohio

Carol K. Taketomo, PharmD
Pharmacy Manager
Children's Hospital Los Angeles
Los Angeles, California

Mary Temple, PharmD
Pediatric Clinical Research Specialist
Hillcrest Hospital
Mayfield Heights, Ohio

Liz Tomsik, PharmD, BCPS
Pharmacotherapy Specialist
Lexi-Comp, Inc
Hudson, Ohio

Beatrice B. Turkoski, RN, PhD
Associate Professor, Graduate Faculty,
Advanced Pharmacology
College of Nursing
Kent State University
Kent, Ohio

Anne Marie Whelan, PharmD
College of Pharmacy
Dalhouise University
Halifax, Nova Scotia

Richard L. Wynn, PhD
Professor of Pharmacology
Baltimore College of Dental Surgery
Dental School
University of Maryland Baltimore
Baltimore, Maryland

PREFACE TO THE TENTH EDITION

The philosophy of the *Drug Information Handbook for Dentistry* remains the same as in all previous editions. Complete cross-referencing of generic and brand names, medical and oral conditions, along with foreign brands as well, makes the text an easy to use reference. We are confident that dental practitioners and staff members can easily access needed information and clinicians can cross-reference between an oral medicine problem, a suggested drug regimen, and the important pharmacologic information necessary to move ahead with a treatment selection.

The alphabetical index contains over 7,500 entries including generic drug names, natural products, synonyms, and U.S., Canadian, and Mexican brand names. The authors of the *Drug Information Handbook for Dentistry* are extremely happy that the text has continued to receive indicators of success. We wish to thank all the practitioners and students that have made each of the previous editions widely successful. In this new 10th edition, we have tried to respond to all the comments and creative suggestions that come from our readership each year.

The monographs for over 1,500 drugs have been updated and the fields made easier to identify for all the drugs. The expanded monographs include additional information on dosing for drugs of particular dental interest and appropriate dosing of medical drugs to use as a reference in patient evaluation. In addition, the adverse reactions sections and the important use and effects on dental treatment have been updated throughout. As in each previous edition, the Oral Medicine section has been updated thoroughly to include new drug formulations and prescribing information useful in managing common oral conditions.

We know that our text remains an excellent companion to oral medicine and medical reference libraries that every clinician must have available. We are sincerely hopeful that the dental practitioner and dental student find this reference text to be an important compliment to the information needed to practice dentistry. The active general practitioner, the specialist, the dental hygienist, and the advanced student of dentistry or dental hygiene will be better prepared for patient care while using this new 10th edition.

Richard L. Wynn

Timothy F. Meiller

Harold L. Crossley

ACKNOWLEDGMENTS

This handbook exists in its present form as a result of the concerted efforts of many individuals, including Jack D. Bolinski, DDS, and Brad F. Bolinski, who recognized the need for a comprehensive dental and medical drug compendium; the publisher and president of Lexi-Comp, Inc, Robert D. Kerscher; Mark F. Bonfiglio, BS, PharmD, RPh, director of pharmacotherapy resources; Stacy S. Robinson, editorial manager; Ginger Stein, project manager; Barbara F. Kerscher, production manager; Jeanne Wilson, production systems liaison; David C. Marcus, director of information systems; Tracey J. Henterly, graphic designer; Alexandra Hart, composition specialist; and Brad F. Bolinski, product manager.

Much of the material contained in this book was a result of contributions by pharmacists throughout the United States and Canada. Lexi-Comp has assisted many medical institutions in developing hospital-specific formulary manuals that contain clinical drug information, as well as dosing. Working with these clinical pharmacists, hospital pharmacy and therapeutics committees, and hospital drug information centers, Lexi-Comp has developed an evolutionary drug database that reflects the practice of pharmacy in these major institutions.

Special acknowledgment goes out to all Lexi-Comp staff members for their contributions to this handbook. In addition, the authors wish to thank their families, friends, and colleagues who supported them in their efforts to complete this handbook.

DESCRIPTION OF SECTIONS AND FIELDS

The *Drug Information Handbook for Dentistry, 10th Edition* is organized into six sections: Introductory text; alphabetical listing of drug monographs; natural products; oral medicine topics; appendix; and indexes which include pharmacologic categories and alphabetical listings containing generic product names and synonyms, as well as U.S., Canadian, and Mexican brand names.

INTRODUCTORY TEXT

Helpful guides to understanding the organization and format of the information in this handbook.

DRUG MONOGRAPHS

This alphabetical listing of drugs contains comprehensive monographs for medications commonly prescribed in dentistry and concise monographs for other popular drugs which dental patients may be taking. Monographs may contain the following fields:

Generic Name	U.S. adopted name
Pronunciation	Phonetic pronunciation guide
Related Information	Cross-reference(s) to pertinent information in other sections of this handbook
U.S. Brand Names	Trade name(s) (manufacturer-specific) found in the United States. The symbol [DSC] appears after trade names that have been recently discontinued.
Canadian Brand Names	Trade name(s) found in Canada
Mexican Brand Names	Trade name(s) found in Mexico
Generic Available	Indicated by a "yes" or "no" if information available
Synonyms	Other names or accepted abbreviations of the generic drug
Pharmacologic Category	Indicates one or more systematic classifications of the drug
Dental Use	Information pertaining to appropriate dental-specific indications of the drug
Use	Information pertaining to appropriate FDA-approved indications of the drug
Unlabeled/Investigational Use	Information pertaining to non-FDA approved and investigational indications of the drug
Local Anesthetic/Vasoconstrictor Precautions	Specific information to prevent potential drug interactions related to anesthesia
Effects on Dental Treatment	Includes significant side effects of drug therapy which may directly or indirectly affect dental treatment or diagnosis; may also contain suggested management approaches and patient handling or care.
Significant Adverse Effects	Side effects are grouped by percentage of incidence (if known) and/or body system; in the interest of saving space, <1% effects are grouped only by percentage **Note:** For nondental-specific drugs, this field includes only the most **Common Adverse Effects** and does not include <1% effects.
Restrictions	The controlled substance classification from the Drug Enforcement Agency (DEA). U.S. schedules are I-V. Schedules vary by country and sometimes state (ie, Massachusetts uses I-VI)
Dosage	The amount of the drug to be typically given or taken during therapy for children and adults; also includes any dosing adjustment/comments for renal impairment or hepatic failure
Mechanism of Action	How the drug works in the body to elicit a response
Contraindications	Information pertaining to inappropriate use of the drug
Warnings/Precautions	Precautionary considerations, hazardous conditions related to use of the drug, and disease states or patient populations in which the drug should be cautiously used
Drug Interactions	If a drug has demonstrated involvement with cytochrome P450 enzymes, the initial line of this field will identify the drug as an inhibitor, inducer, or substrate of specific isoenzymes (ie, CYP1A2). Isoenzymes are identified as substrates (minor or major), inhibitors (weak or moderate or strong), and inducers (weak or strong). A summary of this information can also be found in a tabular format within the introductory section. The remainder of the field presents a description of the interaction between the drug listed in the monograph and other drugs or drug classes. May include possible mechanisms and effect of combined therapy. May also include a strategy to manage the patient on combined therapy (ie, quinidine). **Note:** For nondental-specific drugs, the Drug Interactions field is abbreviated and broken down into 3 subcategories: **Cytochrome P450 Effect, Increased Effect/Toxicity, and Decreased Effect**

Ethanol/Nutrition/Herb Interactions	Information regarding potential interactions with food, nutritionals, herbal products, vitamins, or ethanol
Dietary Considerations	Includes information on how the medication should be taken relative to meals or food
Pharmacodynamics/Kinetics	The magnitude of a drug's effect depends on the drug concentration at the site of action. The pharmacodynamics are expressed in terms of onset of action and duration of action. Pharmacokinetics are expressed in terms of absorption, distribution (including appearance in breast milk and crossing of the placenta), protein binding, metabolism, bioavailability, half-life, time to peak serum concentration, and elimination.
Pregnancy Risk Factor	Five categories established by the FDA to indicate the potential of a systemically absorbed drug for causing birth defects
Lactation	Information describing characteristics of using the drug listed in the monograph while breast-feeding (where recommendation of American Academy of Pediatrics differs, notation is made).
Breast-Feeding Considerations	Further information relating to taking the drug while nursing
Dosage Forms	Information with regard to form, strength, and availability of the drug **Note:** For nondental-specific drugs, the information is strung with the forms in all caps and bolded and uses the following abbreviations: AERO = aerosol; CAP = capsule; CONC = concentrate; CRM = cream; CRYST = crystals; ELIX = elixir; GRAN = granules; INF = infusion; INJ = injection; LIQ = liquid; LOZ = lozenge; OINT = ointment; SHAMP = shampoo; SOLN = solution; SUPP = suppository; SUSP = suspension; SYR = syrup; TAB = tablet.
Comments	Additional pertinent information
Selected Readings	Sources and literature where the user may find additional information

NATURAL PRODUCTS: HERBAL AND DIETARY SUPPLEMENTS

This section is divided into three parts. First, is a brief introduction to popular natural products, followed by an alphabetical listing of herbal and dietary supplements commonly purchased over-the-counter which patients may be taking. The third section contains a description of the known effects of natural products on various body systems. Monographs may contain the following:

NATURAL PRODUCT MONOGRAPHS

Name	Common name
Related Information	Cross-reference(s) to related monographs
Synonyms	Other names (scientific or slang) and accepted abbreviations
Use	Information pertaining to appropriate medical indications for the product; some include recommendations from Commission E.
Local Anesthetic/Vasoconstrictor Precautions	Specific information to prevent potential interactions related to anesthesia
Effects on Bleeding	How the product affects bleeding during dental procedures
Adverse Reactions	Side effects grouped according to body systems
Dosage	The amount of the product to be typically given or taken during therapy
Mechanism of Action/Effect	How the product works in the body to elicit a response
Contraindications	Information pertaining to inappropriate use of the product
Warnings	Cautions and hazardous conditions related to use
Potential/Suspected Interactions	Drugs and other natural products that may affect therapy

DESCRIPTION OF SECTIONS AND FIELDS *(Continued)*

ORAL MEDICINE TOPICS

This section is divided into three major parts and contains text on Oral Medicine topics. In each subsection, the systemic condition or the oral disease state is described briefly, followed by the pharmacologic considerations with which the dentist must be familiar.

Part I: **Dental Management and Therapeutic Considerations in Medically-Compromised Patients:** Focuses on common medical conditions and their associated drug therapies with which the dentist must be familiar. Patient profiles with commonly associated drug regimens are described.

Part II: **Dental Management and Therapeutic Considerations in Patients With Specific Oral Conditions:** Focuses on therapies the dentist may choose to prescribe for patients suffering from oral disease or who are in need of special care. Some overlap between these sections has resulted from systemic conditions that have oral manifestations and vice-versa. Cross-references to the descriptions and the monographs for individual drugs described elsewhere in this handbook allow for easy retrieval of information. Example prescriptions of selected drug therapies for each condition are presented so that the clinician can evaluate alternate approaches to treatment. Seldom is there a single drug of choice.

Those drug prescriptions listed represent prototype drugs and popular prescriptions and are examples only. The pharmacologic category index is available for cross-referencing if alternatives or additional drugs are sought.

Part III: **Other Oral Medicine Topics:** Includes protocol for office emergencies, domestic violence, chemical dependency, and animal/human bites, in addition to suggested readings.

APPENDIX

The appendix is broken down into various sections for easy use and offers a compilation of tables and guidelines which can often be helpful when considering patient care. It includes descriptions of most over-the-counter oral care products and dental drug interactions, in addition to, infectious disease information and the top 200 drugs prescribed in 2003.

INDEXES

This section includes a pharmacologic category index with an easy-to-use classification system in alphabetical order and an alphabetical index which provides a quick reference for major topics within the sections, generic names, synonyms, U.S., Canadian, and Mexican brand names. From this index, the reader can cross-reference to the monographs, oral medicine topics, and appendix information.

FDA PREGNANCY CATEGORIES

Throughout this book there is a field labeled Pregnancy Risk Factor (PRF) and the letter A, B, C, D, or X immediately following which signifies a category. The FDA has established these five categories to indicate the potential of a systemically absorbed drug for causing birth defects. The key differentiation among the categories rests upon the reliability of documentation and the risk:benefit ratio. Pregnancy Category X is particularly notable in that if any data exists that may implicate a drug as a teratogen and the risk:benefit ratio is clearly negative, the drug is contraindicated during pregnancy.

These categories are summarized as follows:

- A Controlled studies in pregnant women fail to demonstrate a risk to the fetus in the first trimester with no evidence of risk in later trimesters. The possibility of fetal harm appears remote.
- B Either animal-reproduction studies have not demonstrated a fetal risk but there are no controlled studies in pregnant women, or animal-reproduction studies have shown an adverse effect (other than a decrease in fertility) that was not confirmed in controlled studies in women in the first trimester and there is no evidence of a risk in later trimesters.
- C Either studies in animals have revealed adverse effects on the fetus (teratogenic or embryocidal effects or other) and there are no controlled studies in women, or studies in women and animals are not available. Drugs should be given only if the potential benefits justify the potential risk to the fetus.
- D There is positive evidence of human fetal risk, but the benefits from use in pregnant women may be acceptable despite the risk (eg, if the drug is needed in a life-threatening situation or for a serious disease for which safer drugs cannot be used or are ineffective).
- X Studies in animals or human beings have demonstrated fetal abnormalities or there is evidence of fetal risk based on human experience, or both, and the risk of the use of the drug in pregnant women clearly outweighs any possible benefit. The drug is contraindicated in women who are or may become pregnant.

FDA NAME DIFFERENTIATION PROJECT: THE USE OF TALL-MAN LETTERS

Confusion between similar drug names is an important cause of medication errors. For years, The Institute For Safe Medication Practices (ISMP), has urged generic manufacturers to use a combination of large and small letters as well as bolding (ie, chlorpro**MAZINE** and chlorpro**PAMIDE**) to help distinguish drugs with look-alike names, especially when they share similar strengths. Recently the FDA's Division of Generic Drugs began to issue recommendation letters to manufacturers suggesting this novel way to label their products to help reduce this drug name confusion. Although this project has had marginal success, the method has successfully eliminated problems with products such as diphenhydr**AMINE** and dimenhy**DRINATE**. Hospitals should also follow suit by making similar changes in their own labels, preprinted order forms, computer screens and printouts, and drug storage location labels.

The following is a list of product names and recommended FDA revisions you will find in this book:

Drug Product	Recommended Revision
acetazolamide	aceta**ZOLAMIDE**
acetohexamide	aceto**HEXAMIDE**
bupropion	bu**PROP**ion
buspirone	bus**PIR**one
chlorpromazine	chlorpro**MAZINE**
chlorpropamide	chlorpro**PAMIDE**
clomiphene	clomi**PHENE**
clomipramine	clomi**PRAMINE**
cycloserine	cyclo**SERINE**
cyclosporine	cyclo**SPORINE**
daunorubicin	**DAUNO**rubicin
dimenhydrinate	dimenhy**DRINATE**
diphenhydramine	diphenhydr**AMINE**
dobutamine	**DOBUT**amine
dopamine	**DOP**amine
doxorubicin	**DOXO**rubicin
glipizide	glipi**ZIDE**
glyburide	gly**BURIDE**
hydralazine	hydr**ALAZINE**
hydroxyzine	hydr**OXY**zine
medroxyprogesterone	medroxy**PROGESTER**one
methylprednisolone	methyl**PREDNIS**olone
methyltestosterone	methyl**TESTOSTER**one
nicardipine	ni**CAR**dipine
nifedipine	**NIFE**dipine
prednisolone	predniso**LONE**
prednisone	predni**SONE**
sulfadiazine	sulfa**DIAZINE**
sulfisoxazole	sulfi**SOXAZOLE**
tolazamide	**TOLAZ**amide
tolbutamide	**TOLBUT**amide
vinblastine	vin**BLAS**tine
vincristine	vin**CRIS**tine

Institute for Safe Medication Practices. "New Tall-Man Lettering Will Reduce Mix-Ups Due to Generic Drug Name Confusion," *ISMP Medication Safety Alert*, September 19, 2001. Available at: http://www.ismp.org.

Institute for Safe Medication Practices. "Prescription Mapping, Can Improve Efficiency While Minimizing Errors With Look-Alike Products," *ISMP Medication Safety Alert*, October 6, 1999. Available at: http://www.ismp.org.

U.S. Pharmacopeia, "USP Quality Review: Use Caution-Avoid Confusion," March 2001, No. 76. Available at: http://www.usp.org.

CONTROLLED SUBSTANCES

Schedule I = C-I

The drugs and other substances in this schedule have no legal medical uses except research. They have a **high** potential for abuse. They include selected opiates such as heroin, opium derivatives, and hallucinogens.

Schedule II = C-II

The drugs and other substances in this schedule have legal medical uses and a **high** abuse potential which may lead to severe dependence. They include former "Class A" narcotics, amphetamines, barbiturates, and other drugs.

Schedule III = C-III

The drugs and other substances in this schedule have legal medical uses and a **lesser** degree of abuse potential which may lead to **moderate** dependence. They include former "Class B" narcotics and other drugs.

Schedule IV = C-IV

The drugs and other substances in this schedule have legal medial uses and **low** abuse potential which may lead to **moderate** dependence. They include barbiturates, benzodiazepines, propoxyphenes, and other drugs.

Schedule V = C-V

The drugs and other substances in this schedule have legal medical uses and **low** abuse potential which may lead to **moderate** dependence. They include narcotic cough preparations, diarrhea preparations, and other drugs.

Note: These are federal classifications. Your individual state may place a substance into a more restricted category. When this occurs, the more restricted category applies. Consult your state law.

PRESCRIPTION WRITING

Doctor's Name
Address
Phone Number

Patient's Name/Date

Patient's Address/Age

Rx

Drug Name/Dosage Size

Disp: Number of tablets, capsules, ounces to be dispensed (roman numerals added as precaution for abused drugs)

Sig: Direction on how drug is to be taken

Doctor's signature

State license number

DEA number (if required)

PRESCRIPTION REQUIREMENTS

1. Date
2. Full name and address of patient
3. Name and address of prescriber
4. Signature of prescriber

If Class II drug, Drug Enforcement Agency (DEA) number necessary.

If Class II and Class III narcotic, a triplicate prescription form (in the state of California) is necessary and it must be handwritten by the prescriber.

Please turn to appropriate oral medicine chapters for examples of prescriptions.

ABBREVIATIONS, ACRONYMS, AND SYMBOLS

Abbreviation	Meaning
$\overline{aa}$, aa	of each
AA	Alcoholics Anonymous
ABG	arterial blood gases
ac	before meals or food
ACA	Adult Children of Alcoholics
ACLS	advanced cardiac life support
ad	to, up to
a.d.	right ear
ADHD	attention-deficit/hyperactivity disorder
ADLs	activities of daily living
ad lib	at pleasure
AIDS	acquired immune deficiency syndrome
AIMS	Abnormal Involuntary Movement Scale
a.l.	left ear
ALS	amyotrophic lateral sclerosis
AM	morning
AMA	against medical advice
amp	ampul
amt	amount
aq	water
aq. dest.	distilled water
ARC	AIDS-related complex
ARDS	adult respiratory distress syndrome
ARF	acute renal failure
a.s.	left ear
ASAP	as soon as possible
a.u.	each ear
AUC	area under the curve
BDI	Beck Depression Inventory
bid	twice daily
BLS	basic life support

ABBREVIATIONS, ACRONYMS, AND SYMBOLS

Abbreviation	Meaning
bm	bowel movement
BMI	body mass index
bp	blood pressure
BPH	benign prostatic hyperplasia
BPRS	Brief Psychiatric Rating Scale
BSA	body surface area
c	a gallon
c̄	with
CA	cancer
CABG	coronary artery bypass graft
CAD	coronary artery disease
cal	calorie
cap	capsule
CBT	cognitive behavioral therapy
cc	cubic centimeter
CCL	creatinine clearance
CF	cystic fibrosis
CGI	Clinical Global Impression
CIE	chemotherapy-induced emesis
cm	centimeter
CIV	continuous I.V. infusion
CNS	central nervous system
comp	compound
cont	continue
COPD	chronic obstructive pulmonary disease
CRF	chronic renal failure
CT	computed tomography
d	day
DBP	diastolic blood pressure
d/c	discontinue
dil	dilute
disp	dispense
div	divide
DOE	dyspnea on exertion
DSM-IV	Diagnostic and Statistical Manual
DTs	delirium tremens
dtd	give of such a dose
DVT	deep vein thrombosis
Dx	diagnosis
ECT	electroconvulsive therapy
EEG	electroencephalogram
EKG	electrocardiogram
elix, el	elixir
emp	as directed
EPS	extrapyramidal side effects
ESRD	end stage renal disease
et	and
EtOH	alcohol
ex aq	in water
f, ft	make, let be made
FDA	Food and Drug Administration
FMS	fibromyalgia syndrome
g	gram
GA	Gamblers Anonymous
GAD	generalized anxiety disorder
GAF	Global Assessment of Functioning Scale
GABA	gamma-aminobutyric acid
GERD	gastroesophageal reflux disease
GFR	glomerular filtration rate
GITS	gastrointestinal therapeutic system
gr	grain
gtt	a drop

PRESCRIPTION WRITING *(Continued)*

ABBREVIATIONS, ACRONYMS, AND SYMBOLS

Abbreviation	Meaning
GVHD	graft versus host disease
h	hour
HAM-A	Hamilton Anxiety Scale
HAM-D	Hamilton Depression Scale
hs	at bedtime
HSV	herpes simplex virus
HTN	hypertension
IBD	inflammatory bowel disease
IBS	irritable bowel syndrome
ICH	intracranial hemorrhage
IHSS	idiopathic hypertrophic subaortic stenosis
I.M.	intramuscular
IOP	intraocular pressure
IU	international unit
I.V.	intravenous
kcal	kilocalorie
kg	kilogram
KIU	kallikrein inhibitor unit
L	liter
LAMM	L-α-acetyl methadol
liq	a liquor, solution
LVH	left ventricular hypertrophy
M	mix; Molar
MADRS	Montgomery Asbery Depression Rating Scale
MAOIs	monamine oxidase inhibitors
mcg	microgram
MDEA	3,4-methylene-dioxy amphetamine
m. dict	as directed
MDMA	3,4 methylene-dioxy methamphetamine
mEq	milliequivalent
mg	milligram
mixt	a mixture
mL	milliliter
mm	millimeter
mM	millimolar
MMSE	mini mental status examination
MPPP	l-methyl-4-proprionoxy-4-phenyl pyridine
MR	mental retardation
MRI	magnetic resonance imaging
MS	multiple sclerosis
NF	National Formulary
NKA	no known allergies
NMS	neuroleptic malignant syndrome
no.	number
noc	in the night
non rep	do not repeat, no refills
NPO	nothing by mouth
NSAID	nonsteroidal anti-inflammatory drug
NV	nausea and vomiting
O, Oct	a pint
OA	osteoarthritis
OCD	obsessive-compulsive disorder
o.d.	right eye
o.l.	left eye
o.s.	left eye
o.u.	each eye
PANSS	Positive and Negative Symptom Scale
PAT	paroxysmal artrial tachycardia
pc, post cib	after meals
PCP	phencyclidine

ABBREVIATIONS, ACRONYMS, AND SYMBOLS

Abbreviation	Meaning
PD	Parkinson's disease
PE	pulmonary embolus
per	through or by
PID	pelvic inflammatory disease
PM	afternoon or evening
P.O.	by mouth
PONV	postoperative nausea and vomiting
P.R.	rectally
prn	as needed
PSVT	paroxysmal superventricular tachycardia
PTA	prior to admission
PTSD	post-traumatic stress disorder
PUD	peptic ulcer disease
pulv	a powder
PVD	peripheral vascular disease
q	every
qad	every other day
qd	every day
qh	every hour
qid	four times a day
qod	every other day
qs	a sufficient quantity
qs ad	a sufficient quantity to make
qty	quantity
qv	as much as you wish
RA	rheumatoid arthritis
REM	rapid eye movement
Rx	take, a recipe
rep	let it be repeated
$\bar{s}$	without
sa	according to art
SAH	subarachnoid hemorrhage
sat	saturated
SBE	subacute bacterial endocarditis
SBP	systolic blood pressure
SIADH	syndrome of inappropriate antidiuretic hormone secretion
sig	label, or let it be printed
SL	sublingual
SLE	systemic lupus erythematosus
SOB	shortness of breath
sol	solution
solv	dissolve
$\overline{ss}$	one-half
sos	if there is need
SSKI	saturated solution of potassium iodide
SSRIs	selective serotonin reuptake inhibitors
stat	at once, immediately
STD	sexually transmitted disease
SubQ	subcutaneous
supp	suppository
SVT	supraventricular tachycardia
Sx	symptom
syr	syrup
tab	tablet
tal	such
TCA	tricyclic antidepressant
TD	tardive dyskinesia
tid	three times a day
TKO	to keep open
TPN	total parenteral nutrition
tr, tinct	tincture
trit	triturate

PRESCRIPTION WRITING *(Continued)*

ABBREVIATIONS, ACRONYMS, AND SYMBOLS

Abbreviation	Meaning
tsp	teaspoonful
Tx	treatment
ULN	upper limits of normal
ung	ointment
URI	upper respiratory infection
USAN	United States Adopted Names
USP	United States Pharmacopeia
UTI	urinary tract infection
u.d., ut dict	as directed
v.o.	verbal order
VTE	venous thromboembolism
VZV	varicella zoster virus
w.a.	while awake
x3	3 times
x4	4 times
YBOC	Yale Brown Obsessive-Compulsive Scale
YMRS	Young Mania Rating Scale

SAFE WRITING PRACTICES

Health professionals and their support personnel frequently produce handwritten copies of information they see in print; therefore, such information is subjected to even greater possibilities for error or misinterpretation on the part of others. Thus, particular care must be given to how drug names and strengths are expressed when creating written healthcare documents. The following are a few examples of safe writing rules suggested by the Institute for Safe Medication Practices, Inc.*

1. There should be a space between a number and its units as it is easier to read. There should be no periods after the abbreviations mg or mL.

Correct	Incorrect
10 mg	10mg
100 mg	100mg

2. Never place a decimal and a zero after a whole number (2 mg is correct and 2.0 mg is **incorrect**). If the decimal point is not seen because it falls on a line or because individuals are working from copies where the decimal point is not seen, this causes a tenfold overdose.
3. Just the opposite is true for numbers less than one. Always place a zero before a naked decimal (0.5 mL is correct, .5 mL is **incorrect**).
4. Never abbreviate the word unit. The handwritten U or u, looks like a 0 (zero), and may cause a tenfold overdose error to be made.
5. IU is not a safe abbreviation for international units. The handwritten IU looks like IV. Write out international units or use int. units.
6. Q.D. is not a safe abbreviation for once daily, as when the Q is followed by a sloppy dot, it looks like QID which means four times daily.
7. O.D. is not a safe abbreviation for once daily, as it is properly interpreted as meaning "right eye" and has caused liquid medications such as saturated solution of potassium iodide and Lugol's solution to be administered incorrectly. There is no safe abbreviation for once daily. It must be written out in full.
8. Do not use chemical names such as 6-mercaptopurine or 6-thioguanine, as sixfold overdoses have been given when these were not recognized as chemical names. The proper names of these drugs are mercaptopurine or thioguanine.
9. Do not abbreviate drug names (5FC, 6MP, 5-ASA, MTX, HCTZ, CPZ, PBZ, etc) as they are misinterpreted and cause error.
10. Do not use the apothecary system or symbols.
11. Do not abbreviate microgram as µg; instead use mcg as there is less likelihood of misinterpretation.
12. When writing an outpatient prescription, write a complete prescription. A complete prescription can prevent the prescriber, the pharmacist, and/or the patient from making a mistake and can eliminate the need for further clarification. The legible prescriptions should contain:
    a. patient's full name
    b. for pediatric or geriatric patients: their age (or weight where applicable)
    c. drug name, dosage form and strength; if a drug is new or rarely prescribed, print this information
    d. number or amount to be dispensed
    e. complete instructions for the patient, including the purpose of the medication
    f. when there are recognized contraindications for a prescribed drug, indicate to the pharmacist that you are aware of this fact (ie, when prescribing a potassium salt for a patient receiving an ACE inhibitor, write "K serum leveling being monitored")

*From "Safe Writing" by Davis NM, PharmD and Cohen MR, MS, Lecturers and Consultants for Safe Medication Practices, 1143 Wright Drive, Huntington Valley, PA 19006. Phone: (215) 947-7566.

PHARMACOLOGY OF DRUG METABOLISM AND INTERACTIONS

Most drugs are eliminated from the body, at least in part, by being chemically altered to less lipid-soluble products (ie, metabolized), and thus are more likely to be excreted via the kidneys or the bile. Phase I metabolism includes drug hydrolysis, oxidation, and reduction, and results in drugs that are more polar in their chemical structure, while Phase II metabolism involves the attachment of an additional molecule onto the drug (or partially metabolized drug) in order to create an inactive and/or more water soluble compound. Phase II processes include (primarily) glucuronidation, sulfation, glutathione conjugation, acetylation, and methylation.

Virtually any of the Phase I and II enzymes can be inhibited by some xenobiotic or drug. Some of the Phase I and II enzymes can be induced. Inhibition of the activity of metabolic enzymes will result in increased concentrations of the substrate (drug), whereas induction of the activity of metabolic enzymes will result in decreased concentrations of the substrate. For example, the well-documented enzyme-inducing effects of phenobarbital may include a combination of Phase I and II enzymes. Phase II glucuronidation may be increased via induced UDP-glucuronosyltransferase (UGT) activity, whereas Phase I oxidation may be increased via induced cytochrome P450 (CYP) activity. However, for most drugs, the primary route of metabolism (and the primary focus of drug-drug interaction) is Phase I oxidation, and specifically, metabolism.

CYP enzymes may be responsible for the metabolism (at least partial metabolism) of approximately 75% of all drugs, with the CYP3A subfamily responsible for nearly half of this activity. Found throughout plant, animal, and bacterial species, CYP enzymes represent a superfamily of xenobiotic metabolizing proteins. There have been several hundred CYP enzymes identified in nature, each of which has been assigned to a family (1, 2, 3, etc), subfamily (A, B, C, etc), and given a specific enzyme number (1, 2, 3, etc) according to the similarity in amino acid sequence that it shares with other enzymes. Of these many enzymes, only a few are found in humans, and even fewer appear to be involved in the metabolism of xenobiotics (eg, drugs). The key human enzyme subfamilies include CYP1A, CYP2A, CYP2B, CYP2C, CYP2D, CYP2E, and CYP3A.

CYP enzymes are found in the endoplasmic reticulum of cells in a variety of human tissues (eg, skin, kidneys, brain, lungs), but their predominant sites of concentration and activity are the liver and intestine. Though the abundance of CYP enzymes throughout the body is relatively equally distributed among the various subfamilies, the relative contribution to drug metabolism is (in decreasing order of magnitude) CYP3A4 (nearly 50%), CYP2D6 (nearly 25%), CYP2C8/9 (nearly 15%), then CYP1A2, CYP2C19, CYP2A6, and CYP2E1. Owing to their potential for numerous drug-drug interactions, those drugs that are identified in preclinical studies as substrates of CYP3A enzymes are often given a lower priority for continued research and development in favor of drugs that appear to be less affected by (or less likely to affect) this enzyme subfamily.

Each enzyme subfamily possesses unique selectivity toward potential substrates. For example, CYP1A2 preferentially binds medium-sized, planar, lipophilic molecules, while CYP2D6 preferentially binds molecules that possess a basic nitrogen atom. Some CYP subfamilies exhibit polymorphism (ie, multiple allelic variants that manifest differing catalytic properties). The best described polymorphisms involve CYP2C9, CYP2C19, and CYP2D6. Individuals possessing "wild type" gene alleles exhibit normal functioning CYP capacity. Others, however, possess allelic variants that leave the person with a subnormal level of catalytic potential (so called "poor metabolizers"). Poor metabolizers would be more likely to experience toxicity from drugs metabolized by the affected enzymes (or less effects if the enzyme is responsible for converting a prodrug to it's active form as in the case of codeine). The percentage of people classified as poor metabolizers varies by enzyme and population group. As an example, approximately 7% of Caucasians and only about 1% of Orientals appear to be CYP2D6 poor metabolizers.

CYP enzymes can be both inhibited and induced by other drugs, leading to increased or decreased serum concentrations (along with the associated effects), respectively. Induction occurs when a drug causes an increase in the amount of smooth endoplasmic reticulum, secondary to increasing the amount of the affected CYP enzymes in the tissues. This "revving up" of the CYP enzyme system may take several days to reach peak activity, and likewise, may take several days, even months, to return to normal following discontinuation of the inducing agent.

CYP inhibition occurs via several potential mechanisms. Most commonly, a CYP inhibitor competitively (and reversibly) binds to the active site on the enzyme, thus preventing the substrate from binding to the same site, and preventing the substrate from being metabolized. The affinity of an inhibitor for an enzyme may be expressed by an inhibition constant (Ki) or IC50 (defined as the concentration of the inhibitor required to cause 50% inhibition under a given set of conditions). In addition to reversible competition for an enzyme site, drugs may inhibit enzyme activity by binding to sites on the enzyme other than that to which the substrate would bind, and thereby cause a change in the functionality or physical structure of the enzyme. A drug may also bind to the enzyme in an irreversible (ie, "suicide") fashion. In such a case, it is not the concentration of drug at the enzyme site that is important (constantly binding and releasing), but the number of molecules available for binding (once bound, always bound).

Although an inhibitor or inducer may be known to affect a variety of CYP subfamilies, it may only inhibit one or two in a clinically important fashion. Likewise, although a substrate is known to be at least partially metabolized by a variety of CYP enzymes, only one or two enzymes may contribute significantly enough to its overall metabolism to warrant concern when used with potential inducers or inhibitors. Therefore, when attempting to predict the level of risk of using two drugs that may affect each other via altered CYP function, it is important to identify the relative effectiveness of the inhibiting/inducing drug on the CYP subfamilies that significantly contribute to the metabolism of the substrate. The contribution of a specific CYP pathway to substrate metabolism should be considered not only in light of other known CYP pathways, but also other nonoxidative pathways for substrate metabolism (eg, glucuronidation) and transporter proteins (eg, P-glycoprotein) that may affect the presentation of a substrate to a metabolic pathway.

SMOKING AND DRUG METABOLISM

Another area of intense interest involves smoking effects on drug metabolism, as well as, the effects of smoking cessation drugs. A review of the literature suggests that at least a dozen drugs interact with cigarette smoke in a clinically significant manner. Polycyclic aromatic hydrocarbons (PAHs) are largely responsible for enhancing drug metabolism. Cigarette smoke induces an increase in the concentration of CYP1A2, the isoenzyme responsible for metabolism of theophylline. Theophylline is, therefore, eliminated more quickly in smokers than in nonsmokers. As a result of hepatic induction of CYP1A2, serum concentrations of theophylline have been shown to be reduced in smokers. Cigarette smoking may substantially reduce tacrine plasma concentrations. The manufacturer states that mean plasma tacrine concentrations in smokers are about one-third of the concentration in nonsmokers (presumably after multiple doses of tacrine).

Patients with insulin-dependent diabetes who smoke heavily may require a higher dosage of insulin than nonsmokers. Cigarette smoking may also reduce serum concentrations of flecainide. Although the mechanism of this interaction is unknown, enhanced hepatic metabolism is possible. Propoxyphene, a pain reliever, has been found to be less effective in heavy smokers than in nonsmokers. The mechanism for the inefficacy of propoxyphene in smokers compared with nonsmokers may be enhanced biotransformation.

Frankl and Soloff reported in a study of five young, healthy, chronic smokers that propranolol, followed by smoking, significantly decreased cardiac output and significantly increased blood pressure and peripheral resistance compared with smoking alone. Steady-state concentrations of propranolol were found to be lower in smokers than in nonsmokers. Lastly, the incidence of drowsiness associated with the use of diazepam and chlordiazepoxide showed that drowsiness was less likely to occur in smokers than in nonsmokers. Smoking probably acts by producing arousal of the central nervous system rather than by accelerating metabolism and reducing concentrations of these drugs in the brain. Finally, the interaction between smoking and oral contraceptives is complex and may be deadly. Women >35 years of age who smoke >15 cigarettes daily may be at increased risk of myocardial infarction.

The norepinephrine and serotonin reuptake inhibitors, as a new class of smoking cessation drugs, have also received attention relative to metabolic interactions. *In vitro* studies indicate that bupropion is primarily metabolized to hydroxybupropion by the CYP2B6 isoenzyme. Therefore, the potential exists for a drug interaction between Zyban® and drugs that affect the CYP2B6 isoenzyme metabolism (eg, orphenadrine and cyclophosphamide). The hydroxybupropion metabolite of bupropion does not appear to be metabolized by the cytochrome P450 isoenzymes. No systemic data have been collected on the metabolism of Zyban® following concomitant administration with other drugs, or alternatively, the effect of concomitant administration of Zyban® on the metabolism of other drugs.

Animal data, however, indicated that bupropion may be an inducer of drug-metabolizing enzymes in humans. However, following chronic administration of bupropion, 100 mg 3 times/day, to 8 healthy male volunteers for 14 days, there was no evidence of induction of its own metabolism. Because bupropion is extensively metabolized, coadministration of other drugs may affect its clinical activity. Certain drugs may induce the metabolism of bupropion (eg, carbamazepine, phenobarbital, phenytoin), while other drugs may inhibit its metabolism (eg, cimetidine). Studies in animals demonstrated that the acute toxicity of bupropion is enhanced by the MAO inhibitor, phenelzine.

Limited clinical data suggest a higher incidence of adverse experiences in patients receiving concurrent administration of bupropion and levodopa. Administration of Zyban® to patients receiving levodopa concurrently should be undertaken with caution, using small initial doses and gradual dosage increases. Concurrent administration of Zyban® and agents that lower the seizure threshold should be undertaken only with extreme caution. Physiological changes resulting from smoking cessation itself, with or without treatment with Zyban®, may alter the pharmacokinetics of some concomitant medications, which may require dosage adjustment.

PHARMACOLOGY OF DRUG METABOLISM AND INTERACTIONS *(Continued)*

INTERACTIONS BETWEEN CIGARETTE SMOKE AND DRUGS

Drug	Mechanism	Effect on Cigarette Smokers
Theophylline	Induction of the CYP1A2 isoenzyme	May lead to reduced theophylline serum concentrations and decreased clinical effect; elimination of theophylline is considerably more rapid
Tacrine	Induction of the CYP1A2 isoenzyme	Effectiveness of tacrine may be decreased
Insulin	Decreased insulin absorption; may be related to peripheral vasoconstriction	Insulin-dependent diabetics who smoke heavily may require a 15% to 30% higher dose of insulin than nonsmokers
Flecainide	Unknown	May reduce flecainide serum concentrations
Propoxyphene	Unknown	May require higher dosage of propoxyphene to achieve analgesic effects
Propranolol	Increased release of catacholamines (eg, epinephrine) in smokers	May have increased blood pressure and heart rate relative to nonsmokers; consider effects on prevention of angina pectoris and stroke
Diazepam	Unclear as to whether pharmacokinetics are altered or end-organ responsiveness is decreased	May require larger doses of diazepam and chlordiazepoxide to achieve sedative effects

Adapted from Schein, JR, "Cigarette Smoking and Clinically Significant Drug Interactions," *Ann Pharmacother*, 1995, 29(11):1139-47.

SUMMARY

Once a drug has been metabolized in the liver, it is eliminated through several different mechanisms. One is directly through bile, into the intestine, and eventually excreted in feces. More commonly, the metabolites and the original drug pass back into the liver from the general circulation and are carried to other organs and tissues. Eventually, these metabolites are excreted through the kidney. In the kidney, the drug and its metabolites may be filtered by the glomerulus or secreted by the renal tubules into the urine. From the kidney, some of the drug may be reabsorbed and pass back into the blood. The drug may also be carried to the lung. If the drug or its metabolite is volatile, it can pass from the blood into the alveolar air and be eliminated in the breath. To a minor extent, drugs and metabolites can be excreted by sweat and saliva. In nursing mothers, drugs are also excreted in mother's milk.

The clinical considerations of drug metabolism may affect which other drugs can and should be administered. Drug tolerance may be a consideration, in that larger doses of a drug may be necessary to obtain effect in patients in which the metabolism is extremely rapid. These interactions, via cytochrome P450 or its isoforms, can occasionally be used beneficially to increase/maintain blood levels of one drug by administering a second drug. Dental clinicians should attempt to stay current on this topic of drug interactions as knowledge evolves.

HOW TO USE THE TABLES

The following CYP SUBSTRATES, INHIBITORS, and INDUCERS tables provide a clinically relevant perspective on drugs that are affected by, or affect, cytochrome P450 (CYP) enzymes. Not all human, drug-metabolizing CYP enzymes are specifically (or separately) included in the tables. Some enzymes have been excluded because they do not appear to significantly contribute to the metabolism of marketed drugs (eg, CYP2C18). Others have been combined in recognition of the difficulty in distinguishing their metabolic activity one from another, or the clinical practicality of doing so (eg, CYP2C8/9, CYP3A4). In the case of CYP3A4, the industry routinely uses this single enzyme designation to represent all enzymes in the CYP3A subfamily. CYP3A7 is present in fetal livers. It is effectively absent from adult livers. CYP3A4 (adult) and CYP3A7 (fetal) appear to share similar properties in their respective hosts. The impact of CYP3A7 in fetal and neonatal drug interactions has not been investigated.

The **CYP Substrates table** contains a list of drugs reported to be metabolized, at least in part, by one or more CYP enzymes. An enzyme that appears to play a clinically significant (major) role in a drug's metabolism is indicated by "●", and an enzyme whose role appears to be clinically insignificant (minor) is indicated by "○". A clinically significant designation is the result of a two-phase review. The first phase considered the contribution of each CYP enzyme to the overall metabolism of the drug. The enzyme pathway was considered potentially clinically relevant if it was responsible for at least 30% of the metabolism of the drug. If so, the drug was subjected to a second phase. The second phase considered the clinical relevance of a substrate's concentration being increased twofold, or decreased by one-half (such as might be observed if combined with an effective CYP inhibitor or inducer, respectively). If either of these changes was considered to present a clinically significant concern, the CYP pathway for the drug was designated "major." If neither change would appear to present a clinically significant concern, or if the CYP enzyme was responsible for a smaller portion of the overall metabolism (ie, <30%), the pathway was designated "minor."

The **CYP Inhibitors table** contains a list of drugs that are reported to inhibit one or more CYP enzymes. Enzymes that are strongly inhibited by a drug are indicated by "●". Enzymes that are moderately inhibited are indicated by "◑". Enzymes that are weakly inhibited are indicated by "○". The designations are the result of a review of published clinical reports, available Ki data, and assessments published by other experts in the field. As it pertains to Ki values set in a ratio with achievable serum drug concentrations ([I]) under normal dosing conditions, the following parameters were employed: [I]/Ki ≥1 = strong; [I]/Ki 0.1-1 = moderate; [I]/Ki <0.1 = weak.

The **CYP Inducers table** contains a list of drugs that are reported to induce one or more CYP enzymes. Enzymes that appear to be effectively induced by a drug are indicated by "●", and enzymes that do not appear to be effectively induced are indicated by "○". The designations are the result of a review of published clinical reports and assessments published by experts in the field.

In general, clinically significant interactions are more likely to occur between substrates and either inhibitors or inducers of the same enzyme(s), all of which have been indicated by "●". However, these assessments possess a degree of subjectivity, at times based on limited indications regarding the significance of CYP effects of particular agents. An attempt has been made to balance a conservative, clinically-sensitive presentation of the data with a desire to avoid the numbing effect of a "beware of everything" approach. Even so, other potential interactions (ie, those involving enzymes indicated by "○") may warrant consideration in some cases. It is important to note that information related to CYP metabolism of drugs is expanding at a rapid pace, and thus, the contents of this table should only be considered to represent a "snapshot" of the information available at the time of publication.

Selected Readings

Bjornsson TD, Callaghan JT, Einolf HJ, et al, "The Conduct of *in vitro* and *in vivo* Drug-Drug Interaction Studies: A PhRMA Perspective," *J Clin Pharmacol*, 2003, 43(5):443-69.

Drug-Drug Interactions, Rodrigues AD, ed, New York, NY: Marcel Dekker, Inc, 2002.

Hersh EV and Moore PA, "Drug Interactions in Dentistry: The Importance of Knowing Your CYP's," *J Am Dent Assoc*, 2004, 135(3):298-311.

Levy RH, Thummel KE, Trager WF, et al, eds, *Metabolic Drug Interactions*, Philadelphia, PA: Lippincott Williams & Wilkins, 2000.

Michalets EL, "Update: Clinically Significant Cytochrome P-450 Drug Interactions," *Pharmacotherapy*, 1998, 18(1):84-112.

Thummel KE and Wilkinson GR, "*In vitro* and *in vivo* Drug Interactions Involving Human CYP3A," *Annu Rev Pharmacol Toxicol*, 1998, 38:389-430.

Wynn RL and Meiller TF, "CYP Enzymes and Adverse Drug Reactions," *Gen Dent*, 1998, 46(5):436-8.

Zhang Y and Benet LZ, "The Gut as a Barrier to Drug Absorption: Combined Role of Cytochrome P450 3A and P-Glycoprotein," *Clin Pharmacokinet*, 2001, 40(3):159-68.

Selected Websites

http://www.gentest.com

http://www.imm.ki.se/CYPalleles

http://medicine.iupui.edu/flockhart

http://www.mhc.com/Cytochromes

PHARMACOLOGY OF DRUG METABOLISM AND INTERACTIONS *(Continued)*

CYP Substrates

● = major substrate
○ = minor substrate

Drug	1A2	2A6	2B6	2C8/9	2C19	2D6	2E1	3A4
Acetaminophen	○	○		○		○	○	○
Albendazole	○							○
Albuterol								●
Alfentanil								●
Almotriptan						○		○
Alosetron	○			●				○
Alprazolam								●
Aminophylline	●						○	○
Amiodarone	○			●	○	○		●
Amitriptyline	○		○	○	○	●		○
Amlodipine								●
Amoxapine						●		
Amphetamine						○		
Amprenavir				○				●
Aprepitant	○				○			●
Argatroban								○
Aripiprazole						●		●
Aspirin				○				
Atazanavir								●
Atomoxetine					○	●		
Atorvastatin								●
Azelastine	○				○	○		○
Azithromycin								○
Benzphetamine			○					●
Benztropine						○		
Betaxolol	●					●		
Dexarolene								○
Bezafibrate								○
Bisoprolol						○		●
Bortezomib	○			○	○	○		●
Bosentan				●				●
Brinzolamide								○
Bromazepam								●
Bromocriptine								●
Budesonide								●
Bupivacaine	○				○	○		○
Buprenorphine								●
BuPROPion	○	○	●	○		○	○	○
BusPIRone						○		●
Busulfan								●
Caffeine	●			○		○	○	○
Candesartan				○				
Capsaicin							○	
Captopril						●		
Carbamazepine				○				●
Carisoprodol					●			
Carteolol						○		
Carvedilol	○			●		●	○	○
Celecoxib				○				○
Cerivastatin								●
Cetirizine								○
Cevimeline						○		○
Chlordiazepoxide								●
Chloroquine						●		●
Chlorpheniramine						○		●
ChlorproMAZINE	○					●		○
ChlorproPAMIDE				○				
Chlorzoxazone	○	○				○	●	○
Cilostazol	○				○	○		○
Cinacalcet	○					○		○

CYP Substrates *(continued)*

Drug	1A2	2A6	2B6	2C8/9	2C19	2D6	2E1	3A4
Cisapride	○	○	○	○	○			●
Citalopram					●	○		●
Clarithromycin								●
Clobazam								●
Clofibrate								○
ClomiPRAMINE	●				●	●		○
Clonazepam								●
Clopidogrel	○							○
Clorazepate								●
Clozapine	●	○		○	○	○		○
Cocaine								●
Codeine[1]						●		○
Colchicine								●
Cyclobenzaprine	●					○		○
Cyclophosphamide[2]		○	●	○	○			●
CycloSPORINE								●
Dacarbazine	●						●	
Dantrolene								●
Dapsone				○	○		○	●
Delavirdine						○		●
Desipramine	○					●		
Desogestrel					●			
Dexamethasone								○
Dexmedetomidine		●						
Dextroamphetamine						●		
Dextromethorphan		○		○	○	●	○	○
Diazepam	○		○	○	●			●
Diclofenac	○		○	○	○	○		○
Digitoxin								●
Digoxin								○
Dihydrocodeine[1]						●		
Dihydroergotamine								●
Diltiazem				○		○		●
Dirithromycin								○
Disopyramide								●
Disulfiram	○	○	○			○	○	○
Docetaxel								●
Dofetilide								○
Dolasetron				○				○
Domperidone								○
Donepezil						○		○
Dorzolamide				○				○
Doxepin	●					●		●
DOXOrubicin						●		●
Doxycycline								●
Drospirenone								○
Dutasteride								○
Efavirenz			●					●
Eletriptan								●
Enalapril								●
Enflurane							●	
Eplerenone								●
Ergoloid mesylates								●
Ergonovine								●
Ergotamine								●
Erythromycin			○					●
Escitalopram					●			●
Esomeprazole					●			○
Estazolam								○
Estradiol	●	○	○	○	○	○	○	●
Estrogens, conjugated A/synthetic	●	○	○	○	○	○	○	●
Estrogens, conjugated equine	●	○	○	○	○	○	○	●
Estrogens, conjugated esterified	●		○	○			○	●
Estrone	●		○	○			○	●

PHARMACOLOGY OF DRUG METABOLISM AND INTERACTIONS *(Continued)*

CYP Substrates *(continued)*

Drug	1A2	2A6	2B6	2C8/9	2C19	2D6	2E1	3A4
Estropipate	●		○	○			○	●
Ethinyl estradiol								●
Ethosuximide								●
Etonogestrel								○
Etoposide	○						○	●
Exemestane								○
Felbamate							○	●
Felodipine								●
Fenofibrate								○
Fentanyl								●
Fexofenadine								○
Finasteride								○
Flecainide	○					●		
Fluoxetine	○		○	●	○	●	○	○
Fluphenazine						●		
Flurazepam								●
Flurbiprofen				○				
Flutamide	●							●
Fluticasone								●
Fluvastatin				○		○		○
Fluvoxamine	●					●		
Formoterol		○		○	○	○		
Fosamprenavir (as amprenavir)				○				●
Fosphenytoin (as phenytoin)				●	●			○
Frovatriptan	○							
Fulvestrant								○
Galantamine						○		○
Gefitinib								●
Gemfibrozil								○
Glimepiride				●				
GlipiZIDE				●				
Granisetron								○
Guanabenz	●							
Halazepam								○
Halofantrine				○		○		●
Haloperidol	○					●		●
Halothane		○	○	○		○	●	○
Hydrocodone[1]						●		
Hydrocortisone								○
Ibuprofen				○	○			
Ifosfamide[3]		○	○	○	○			●
Imatinib	○			○	○	○		●
Imipramine	○		○		●	●		○
Imiquimod	○							○
Indinavir						○		●
Indomethacin				○	○			
Irbesartan				○				
Irinotecan			●					●
Isoflurane							●	
Isoniazid							●	
Isosorbide								●
Isosorbide dinitrate								●
Isosorbide mononitrate								●
Isradipine								●
Itraconazole								●
Ivermectin								○
Ketamine			●	●				●
Ketoconazole								●
Labetalol						●		
Lansoprazole				○	●			●
Letrozole		○						●
Levobupivacaine	○							○

CYP Substrates *(continued)*

Drug	1A2	2A6	2B6	2C8/9	2C19	2D6	2E1	3A4
Levomethadyl acetate hydrochloride			○					●
Levonorgestrel								●
Lidocaine	○	○	○	○		●		●
Lomustine						●		
Lopinavir								○
Loratadine						○		○
Losartan				●				●
Lovastatin								●
Maprotiline						●		
MedroxyPROGESTERone								●
Mefenamic acid				○				
Mefloquine								●
Meloxicam				○				○
Mephenytoin			○	●	●			
Mephobarbital			○	○	●			
Mestranol[4]				●				●
Methadone				○	○	○		●
Methamphetamine						●		
Methoxsalen		○						
Methsuximide					●			
Methylergonovine								●
Methylphenidate						●		
MethylPREDNISolone								○
Methysergide								●
Metoclopramide	○					○		
Metoprolol					○	●		
Mexiletine	●					●		
Miconazole								●
Midazolam			○					●
Mifepristone								○
Miglustat								●
Mirtazapine	●			○		●		●
Moclobemide					●	●		
Modafinil								●
Mometasone furoate								○
Montelukast				●				●
Moricizine								●
Morphine sulfate						○		
Naproxen	○			○				
Nateglinide				●				●
Nefazodone						●		●
Nelfinavir				○	●	○		●
Nevirapine			○			○		●
NiCARdipine	○			○		○	○	●
Nicotine	○	○	○	○	○	○	○	○
NIFEdipine						○		●
Nilutamide					●			
Nimodipine								●
Nisoldipine								●
Nitrendipine								●
Norelgestromin								○
Norethindrone								●
Norgestrel								●
Nortriptyline	○				○	●		○
Olanzapine	○					○		
Omeprazole		○		○	●	○		○
Ondansetron	○			○		○	○	●
Orphenadrine	○		○			○		○
Oxybutynin								○
Oxycodone[1]						●		
Paclitaxel				●				●
Palonosetron	○					○		○
Pantoprazole					●			○
Paroxetine						●		
Pentamidine					●			

PHARMACOLOGY OF DRUG METABOLISM AND INTERACTIONS *(Continued)*

CYP Substrates *(continued)*

Drug	1A2	2A6	2B6	2C8/9	2C19	2D6	2E1	3A4
Pergolide								●
Perphenazine	○			○	○	●		○
Phencyclidine								●
Phenobarbital				○	●		○	●
Phenytoin				●	●			○
Pimecrolimus								○
Pimozide	●							●
Pindolol						●		
Pioglitazone				●				●
Pipecuronium				○				
Pipotiazine						●		●
Piroxicam				○				
Pravastatin								○
Prazepam								○
PrednisoLONE								○
PredniSONE								○
Primaquine								●
Procainamide						●		
Progesterone	○	○		○	●	○		●
Proguanil	○				○			○
Promethazine			●			●		
Propafenone	○					●		○
Propofol	○	○	●	●	○	○	○	○
Propranolol	●				○	●		○
Protriptyline						●		
Quazepam								○
Quetiapine						○		●
Quinidine				○			○	●
Quinine	○				○			○
Rabeprazolo					●			●
Ranitidine	○				○	○		
Repaglinide				○				●
Rifabutin	●							●
Rifampin		●		●				●
Riluzole	●							
Risperidone						●		○
Ritonavir	○		○			○		●
Rofecoxib				○				
Ropinirole	●							○
Ropivacaine	○		○			○		○
Rosiglitazone				●				
Rosuvastatin				○				○
Saquinavir						○		●
Selegiline	○	○	●	●		○		○
Sertraline			○	○	●	●		○
Sevoflurane		○	○				●	○
Sibutramine								●
Sildenafil				○				●
Simvastatin								●
Sirolimus								●
Spiramycin								●
Sufentanil								●
SulfaDIAZINE				●			○	○
Sulfamethoxazole				●				○
Sulfinpyrazone				●				○
SulfiSOXAZOLE				●				
Suprofen				○				
Tacrine	●							
Tacrolimus								●
Tamoxifen		○	○	●		●	○	●
Tamsulosin						●		●
Telithromycin	○							●
Temazepam			○	○	○			○

CYP Substrates *(continued)*

Drug	1A2	2A6	2B6	2C8/9	2C19	2D6	2E1	3A4
Teniposide								●
Terbinafine	○			○	○			○
Testosterone			○	○	○			○
Tetracycline								●
Theophylline	●			○		○	●	●
Thiabendazole	○							
Thioridazine					○	●		
Thiothixene	●							
Tiagabine								●
Ticlopidine								●
Timolol						●		
Tiotropium						○		○
TOLBUTamide				●	○			
Tolcapone		○						○
Tolterodine				○	○	●		●
Toremifene	○							●
Torsemide				●				
Tramadol[1]						●		○
Trazodone						○		●
Tretinoin		○	○	○				
Triazolam								●
Trifluoperazine	●							
Trimethadione				○	○		●	○
Trimethoprim				●				●
Trimipramine					●	●		●
Troleandomycin								●
Valdecoxib				○				○
Valproic acid		○	○	○	○		○	
Vardenafil								●
Venlafaxine				○	○	●		●
Verapamil	○		○	○			○	●
VinBLAStine						○		●
VinCRIStine								●
Vinorelbine						○		●
Voriconazole				●	●			○
Warfarin	○			●	○			○
Yohimbine						○		
Zafirlukast				●				
Zaleplon								○
Zidovudine		○		○	○			○
Zileuton	○			○				○
Ziprasidone	○							○
Zolmitriptan	○							
Zolpidem	○			○	○	○		●
Zonisamide					○			●
Zopiclone				●				●
Zuclopenthixol						●		

[1]This opioid analgesic is bioactivated *in vivo* via CYP2D6. Inhibiting this enzyme would decrease the effects of the analgesic. The active metabolite might also affect, or be affected by, CYP enzymes.
[2]Cyclophosphamide is bioactivated *in vivo* to acrolein via CYP2B6 and 3A4. Inhibiting these enzymes would decrease the effects of cyclophosphamide.
[3]Ifosfamide is bioactivated *in vivo* to acrolein via CYP3A4. Inhibiting this enzyme would decrease the effects of ifosfamide.
[4]Mestranol is bioactivated *in vivo* to ethinyl estradiol via CYP2C8/9. See Ethinyl Estradiol for additional CYP information.

PHARMACOLOGY OF DRUG METABOLISM AND INTERACTIONS *(Continued)*

CYP Inhibitors

● = strong inhibitor
◑ = moderate inhibitor
○ = weak inhibitor

Drug	1A2	2A6	2B6	2C8/9	2C19	2D6	2E1	3A4
Acebutolol						○		
Acetaminophen								○
AcetaZOLAMIDE								○
Albendazole	○							
Alosetron	○						○	
Amiodarone	●	◑	○	◑	○	◑		◑
Amitriptyline	○			○	○	○	○	
Amlodipine	◑	○	○	○		○		○
Amphetamine						○		
Amprenavir					○			●
Anastrozole	○			○				○
Aprepitant				○				○
Atazanavir	○			○				●
Atorvastatin								○
Azelastine			○	○	○	○		○
Azithromycin								○
Bepridil						○		
Betamethasone								○
Betaxolol						○		
Biperiden						○		
Bortezomib	○			○	◑	○		○
Bromazepam							○	
Bromocriptine	○							○
Buprenorphine	○	○			○	○		
BuPROPion						○		
Caffeine	●							◑
Candesartan				○				
Celecoxib						○		
Cerivastatin								○
Chloramphenicol				○				○
Chloroquine						◑		
Chlorpheniramine						○		
ChlorproMAZINE						●	○	
Chlorzoxazone							○	○
Cholecalciferol				○	○	○		
Cimetidine	◑			○	◑	◑	○	◑
Cinacalcet						○		
Ciprofloxacin	●							○
Cisapride						○		○
Citalopram	○		○		○	○		
Clarithromycin	○							●
Clemastine						○		○
Clofazimine								○
Clofibrate		○						
ClomiPRAMINE						◑		
Clopidogrel				○				
Clotrimazole	○	○	○	○	○	○	○	◑
Clozapine	○			○	○	◑	○	○
Cocaine						●		○
Codeine						○		
Cyclophosphamide								○
CycloSPORINE				○				◑
Danazol								○
Delavirdine	○			●	●	●		●
Desipramine		◑	◑			◑	○	◑
Dexmedetomidine	○			○		●		○
Dextromethorphan						○		
Diazepam					○			○
Diclofenac	◑			○			○	●

CYP Inhibitors *(continued)*

Drug	1A2	2A6	2B6	2C8/9	2C19	2D6	2E1	3A4
Dihydroergotamine								○
Diltiazem				○		○		◑
Dimethyl sulfoxide				○	○			
DiphenhydrAMINE						◑		
Disulfiram	○	○	○	○		○	●	○
Docetaxel								○
Dolasetron						○		
DOXOrubicin			◑			○		○
Doxycycline								●
Drospirenone	○			○	○			○
Econazole							○	
Efavirenz				○	○			○
Enoxacin	●							●
Entacapone	○	○		○	○	○	○	○
Eprosartan				○				
Ergotamine								○
Erythromycin	○							◑
Escitalopram						○		
Estradiol	○							
Estrogens, conjugated A/synthetic	○							
Estrogens, conjugated equine	○							
Ethinyl estradiol	○		○		○			○
Ethotoin					○			
Etoposide				○				○
Felbamate					○			
Felodipine				○		○		○
Fentanyl								○
Fexofenadine						○		
Flecainide						○		
Fluconazole	○			●	●			◑
Fluoxetine	◑		○	○	◑	●		○
Fluphenazine	○			○		○	○	
Flurazepam							○	
Flurbiprofen				●				
Flutamide	○							
Fluvastatin	○			◑		○		○
Fluvoxamine	●		○	○	●	○		○
Fosamprenavir (as amprenavir)					○			●
Gefitinib					○	○		
Gemfibrozil	◑			●	●			
Glyburide								○
Grapefruit juice								◑
Halofantrine						○		
Haloperidol						◑		◑
HydrALAZINE								○
HydrOXYzine						○		
Ibuprofen				●				
Ifosfamide								○
Imatinib				○		○		●
Imipramine	○				○	◑	○	
Indinavir				○	○	○		●
Indomethacin				●	○			
Interferon alfa-2a	○							
Interferon alfa-2b	○							
Interferon gamma-1b	○						○	
Irbesartan				◑		○		○
Isoflurane			○					
Isoniazid	○	◑		◑	●	◑	◑	●
Isradipine								○
Itraconazole								●
Ketoconazole	●	◑	○	●	◑	◑		●
Ketoprofen				○				
Labetalol						○		
Lansoprazole				○	◑	○		○

PHARMACOLOGY OF DRUG METABOLISM AND INTERACTIONS *(Continued)*

CYP Inhibitors *(continued)*

Drug	1A2	2A6	2B6	2C8/9	2C19	2D6	2E1	3A4
Leflunomide				○				
Letrozole		○			○			
Lidocaine	●					◑		◑
Lomefloxacin	●							
Lomustine						○		○
Loratadine					◑	○		
Losartan	○			◑	○			○
Lovastatin				○		○		○
Mefenamic acid				●				
Mefloquine						○		○
Meloxicam				○				
Mephobarbital					○			
Mestranol	○		○		○			○
Methadone						◑		○
Methimazole	○	○	○	○	○	◑	○	○
Methotrimeprazine						○		
Methoxsalen	●	●		○	○	○	○	○
Methsuximide					○			
Methylphenidate						○		
MethylPREDNISolone								○
Metoclopramide						○		
Metoprolol						○		
Metronidazole				○				◑
Metyrapone		○						
Mexiletine	●							
Miconazole	◑	●	○	●	●	●	◑	●
Midazolam				○				○
Mifepristone						○		○
Mirtazapine	○							○
Mitoxantrone								○
Moclobemide	○				○	○		
Modafinil	○	○		○	●		○	○
Montelukast				○				
Nalidixic acid	●							
Nateglinide				○				
Nefazodone	○		○			○		●
Nelfinavir	○		○	○	○	○		●
Nevirapine	○					○		○
NiCARdipine				●	◑	◑		●
Nicotine		○					○	
NIFEdipine	◑			○		○		○
Nilutamide					○			
Nisoldipine	○							○
Nitrendipine								○
Nizatidine								○
Norfloxacin	●							◑
Nortriptyline						○	○	
Ofloxacin	●							
Olanzapine	○			○	○	○		○
Omeprazole	○			◑	●	○		○
Ondansetron	○			○		○		
Orphenadrine	○	○	○	○	○	○	○	○
Oxcarbazepine					○			
Oxprenolol						○		
Oxybutynin						○		○
Pantoprazole				◑				
Paroxetine	○		◑	○	○	●		○
Peginterferon alfa-2a	○							
Peginterferon alfa-2b	○							
Pentamidine				○	○	○		○
Pentoxifylline	○							
Pergolide						●		○
Perphenazine	○					○		

CYP Inhibitors *(continued)*

Drug	1A2	2A6	2B6	2C8/9	2C19	2D6	2E1	3A4
Phencyclidine								○
Pilocarpine		○					○	○
Pimozide					○	○	○	○
Pindolol						○		
Pioglitazone				●	○	◑		
Piroxicam				●				
Pravastatin				○		○		○
Praziquantel						○		
PrednisoLONE								○
Primaquine	●					○		○
Probenecid					○			
Progesterone				○	○			○
Promethazine						○		
Propafenone	○			○		○		
Propofol	◑			○	◑	○	○	●
Propoxyphene				○		○		○
Propranolol	○					○		
Pyrimethamine				◑		◑		
Quinidine				○		●		●
Quinine				◑		●		○
Quinupristin								○
Rabeprazole					◑	○		○
Ranitidine	○					○		
Risperidone						○		○
Ritonavir				○	○	●	○	●
Rofecoxib	○							
Ropinirole	○					●		
Rosiglitazone				◑	○	○		
Saquinavir				○	○	○		◑
Selegiline	○	○		○	○	○	○	○
Sertraline	○		◑	○	◑	◑		◑
Sildenafil	○			○	○	○	○	○
Simvastatin				○		○		
Sirolimus								○
Sulconazole	○	○		○	○	○	○	○
SulfaDIAZINE				●				
Sulfamethoxazole				◑				
Sulfinpyrazone				◑				
SulfiSOXAZOLE				●				
Tacrine	○							
Tacrolimus								○
Tamoxifen			○	○				○
Telithromycin						○		●
Telmisartan					○			
Teniposide				○				○
Tenofovir	○							
Terbinafine						●		
Testosterone								○
Tetracycline								◑
Theophylline	○							
Thiabendazole	●							
Thioridazine	○			○		◑	○	
Thiotepa			○					
Thiothixene						○		
Ticlopidine	○			○	●	◑	○	○
Timolol						○		
Tioconazole	○	○		○	○	○	○	
Tocainide	○							
TOLBUTamide				●				
Tolcapone				○				
Topiramate					○			
Torsemide					○			
Tranylcypromine	◑	●		○	◑	◑	○	○
Trazodone						◑		○
Tretinoin				○				
Triazolam				○				

PHARMACOLOGY OF DRUG METABOLISM AND INTERACTIONS *(Continued)*

CYP Inhibitors *(continued)*

Drug	1A2	2A6	2B6	2C8/9	2C19	2D6	2E1	3A4
Trimethoprim				◑				
Tripelennamine						◑		
Triprolidine						○		
Troleandomycin								◑
Valdecoxib				○	○			
Valproic acid				○	○	○		○
Valsartan				○				
Venlafaxine			○			○		○
Verapamil	○			○		○		◑
VinBLAStine						○		○
VinCRIStine								○
Vinorelbine						○		○
Voriconazole				○	○			◑
Warfarin				◑	○			
Yohimbine						○		
Zafirlukast	○			◑	○	○		○
Zileuton	○							
Ziprasidone						○		○

CYP Inducers

● = effectively induced
○ = not effectively induced

Drug	1A2	2A6	2B6	2C8/9	2C19	2D6	2E1	3A4
Aminoglutethimide	●				●			●
Amobarbital		●						
Aprepitant				○				○
Bexarotene								○
Bosentan				○				○
Calcitriol								○
Carbamazepine	●		●	●	●			●
Clofibrate			○				○	○
Colchicine				○			○	○
Cyclophosphamide			○	○				
Dexamethasone		○	○	○				○
Dicloxacillin								○
Efavirenz (in liver only)			○					○
Estradiol								○
Estrogens, conjugated A/synthetic								○
Estrogens, conjugated equine								○
Felbamate								○
Fosphenytoin (as phenytoin)			●	●	●			●
Griseofulvin	○			○				○
Hydrocortisone								○
Ifosfamide				○				
Insulin preparations	○							
Isoniazid (after D/C)							○	
Lansoprazole	○							
MedroxyPROGESTERone								○
Mephobarbital		○						
Metyrapone								○
Modafinil	○		○					○
Moricizine	○							○
Nafcillin								●
Nevirapine			●					●
Norethindrone					○			
Omeprazole	○							
Oxcarbazepine								●
Paclitaxel								○
Pantoprazole	○							○
Pentobarbital		●						●
Phenobarbital	●	●	●	●				●
Phenytoin			●	●	●			●
Pioglitazone								○
PredniSONE					○			○
Primaquine	○							
Primidone[1]	●		●	●				●
Rifabutin								●
Rifampin	●	●	●	●	●			●
Rifapentine				●				●
Ritonavir (long-term)	○			○				○
Rofecoxib								○
Secobarbital		●		●				
Sulfinpyrazone								○
Terbinafine								○
Topiramate								○
Tretinoin							○	
Troglitazone								○
Valproic acid		○						

[1]Primidone is partially metabolized to phenobarbital. See Phenobarbital for additional CYP information.

ALPHABETICAL LISTING OF DRUGS

1370-999-397 *see* Anagrelide *on page 130*

A_1-PI *see* Alpha$_1$-Proteinase Inhibitor *on page 84*

A200® Lice [OTC] *see* Permethrin *on page 1070*

A-200® Maximum Strength [OTC] *see* Pyrethrins and Piperonyl Butoxide *on page 1153*

A and D® Ointment [OTC] *see* Vitamin A and Vitamin D *on page 1382*

Abacavir (a BAK a veer)

Related Information

HIV Infection and AIDS *on page 1484*

U.S. Brand Names Ziagen®

Canadian Brand Names Ziagen®

Generic Available No

Synonyms Abacavir Sulfate; ABC

Pharmacologic Category Antiretroviral Agent, Reverse Transcriptase Inhibitor (Nucleoside)

Use Treatment of HIV infections in combination with other antiretroviral agents

Local Anesthetic/Vasoconstrictor Precautions No information available to require special precautions

Effects on Dental Treatment No significant effects or complications reported

Common Adverse Effects Hypersensitivity reactions (which may be fatal) occur in ~5% of patients. Symptoms may include anaphylaxis, fever, rash (including erythema multiforme), fatigue, diarrhea, abdominal pain; respiratory symptoms (eg, pharyngitis, dyspnea, cough, adult respiratory distress syndrome, or respiratory failure); headache, malaise, lethargy, myalgia, myolysis, arthralgia, edema, paresthesia, nausea and vomiting, mouth ulcerations, conjunctivitis, lymphadenopathy, hepatic failure, and renal failure.

Note: Rates of adverse reactions were defined during combination therapy with other antiretrovirals (lamivudine and efavirenz **or** lamivudine and zidovudine). Only reactions which occurred at a higher frequency than in the comparator group are noted. Adverse reaction rates attributable to abacavir alone are not available.

>10%:

- Central nervous system: Headache (13%)
- Gastrointestinal: Nausea (19%, children 9%)

1% to 10%:

- Central nervous system: Depression (6%), dizziness (6%), fever (6%, children 9%), anxiety (5%)
- Dermatologic; Rash (5%, children 7%)
- Gastrointestinal: Diarrhea (7%), vomiting (children 9%)
- Hematologic: Thrombocytopenia (1%)
- Hepatic: AST increased (6%)
- Neuromuscular and skeletal: Musculoskeletal pain (5% to 6%)
- Miscellaneous: Hypersensitivity reactions (9%; may include reactions to other components of antiretroviral regimen), infection (EENT 5%)

Mechanism of Action Nucleoside reverse transcriptase inhibitor. Abacavir is a guanosine analogue which is phosphorylated to carbovir triphosphate which interferes with HIV viral RNA dependent DNA polymerase resulting in inhibition of viral replication.

Drug Interactions

Increased Effect/Toxicity: Abacavir increases the blood levels of amprenavir. Abacavir may decrease the serum concentration of methadone in some patients. Concomitant use of ribavirin and nucleoside analogues may increase the risk of developing lactic acidosis (includes adefovir, didanosine, lamivudine, stavudine, zalcitabine, zidovudine).

Pharmacodynamics/Kinetics

- Absorption: Rapid and extensive absorption
- Distribution: V_d: 0.86 L/kg
- Protein binding: 50%
- Metabolism: Hepatic via alcohol dehydrogenase and glucuronyl transferase to inactive carboxylate and glucuronide metabolites
- Bioavailability: 83%
- Half-life elimination: 1.5 hours
- Time to peak: 0.7-1.7 hours
- Excretion: Primarily urine (as metabolites, 1.2% as unchanged drug); feces (16% total dose)

Pregnancy Risk Factor C

Abacavir, Lamivudine, and Zidovudine

(a BAK a veer, la MI vyoo deen, & zye DOE vyoo deen)

Related Information

Abacavir *on page 42*
Lamivudine *on page 794*
Zidovudine *on page 1398*

U.S. Brand Names Trizivir®

Generic Available No

Synonyms Azidothymidine, Abacavir, and Lamivudine; AZT, Abacavir, and Lamivudine; Compound S, Abacavir, and Lamivudine; Lamivudine, Abacavir, and Zidovudine; 3TC, Abacavir, and Zidovudine; ZDV, Abacavir, and Lamivudine; Zidovudine, Abacavir, and Lamivudine

Pharmacologic Category Antiretroviral Agent, Reverse Transcriptase Inhibitor (Nucleoside)

Use Treatment of HIV infection (either alone or in combination with other antiretroviral agents) in patients whose regimen would otherwise contain the components of Trizivir®

Local Anesthetic/Vasoconstrictor Precautions No information available to require special precautions

Effects on Dental Treatment No significant effects or complications reported

Common Adverse Effects Fatal hypersensitivity reactions have occurred in patients taking abacavir (in Trizivir®). If Trizivir® is to be restarted following an interruption in therapy, first evaluate the patient for previously unsuspected symptoms of hypersensitivity. Do not restart if hypersensitivity is suspected or if hypersensitivity cannot be ruled out.

The following information is based on CNAAB3003 study data concerning effects noted in patients receiving abacavir, lamivudine, and zidovudine. See individual agent monographs for additional information.

>10%:

Endocrine & metabolic: Increased triglycerides (25%)

Gastrointestinal: Nausea (47%), nausea and vomiting (16%), diarrhea (12%), loss of appetite/anorexia (11%)

1% to 10%:

Central nervous system: Insomnia (7%)

Miscellaneous: Hypersensitivity (5% based on abacavir component)

Other (frequency unknown): Pancreatitis, increased GGT

Mechanism of Action The combination of abacavir, lamivudine, and zidovudine is believed to act synergistically to inhibit reverse transcriptase via DNA chain termination after incorporation of the nucleoside analogue as well as to delay the emergence of mutations conferring resistance

Drug Interactions

Increased Effect/Toxicity: See individual agents.

Decreased Effect: See individual agents.

Pharmacodynamics/Kinetics Bioavailability studies of Trizivir® show no difference in AUC or C_{max} when compared to abacavir, lamivudine, and zidovudine given together as individual agents. See individual agents.

Pregnancy Risk Factor C

Abacavir Sulfate *see* Abacavir *on page 42*

Abarelix

(a ba REL iks)

U.S. Brand Names Plenaxis™

Generic Available No

Synonyms PPI-149; R-3827

Pharmacologic Category Gonadotropin Releasing Hormone Antagonist

Use Palliative treatment of advanced symptomatic prostate cancer; treatment is limited to men who are not candidates for LHRH therapy, refuse surgical castration, and have one or more of the following complications due to metastases or local encroachment: 1) risk of neurological compromise, 2) ureteral or bladder outlet obstruction, or 3) severe bone pain (persisting despite narcotic analgesia)

Local Anesthetic/Vasoconstrictor Precautions No information available to require special precautions

Effects on Dental Treatment No significant effects or complications reported

Common Adverse Effects

>10%:

Cardiovascular: Hot flushes (79%), peripheral edema (15%)

Central nervous system: Sleep disturbance (44%), pain (31%), dizziness (12%), headache (12%)

Endocrine & metabolic: Breast enlargement (30%), nipple discharge/tenderness (20%)

(Continued)

Abarelix *(Continued)*

Gastrointestinal: Constipation (15%), diarrhea (11%)
Neuromuscular & skeletal: Back pain (17%)
Respiratory: Upper respiratory infection (12%)

1% to 10%:
Central nervous system: Fatigue (10%)
Endocrine & metabolic: Serum triglycerides increased (10%)
Gastrointestinal: Nausea (10%)
Genitourinary: Dysuria (10%), micturition frequency (10%), urinary retention (10%), urinary tract infection (10%)
Hepatic: Transaminase levels increased (2% to 8%)
Miscellaneous: Allergic reactions (urticaria, pruritus, syncope, hypotension): risk increases with prolonged treatment (in clinical trials, cumulative risk increased from 0.5% at 56 days to 2.9% at 676 days of therapy)

Restrictions Abarelix is not distributed through retail pharmacies. Prescribing and distribution of abarelix is limited to physicians and hospital pharmacies participating in the Plenaxis™ PLUS program. Contact Praecis Pharmaceuticals at www.plenaxisplus.com or by calling 1-877-772-3247.

Mechanism of Action Competes with naturally occurring GnRH for binding on receptors of the pituitary. Suppresses LH and FSH, resulting in decreased testosterone. Unlike LHRH agonists, does not induce an initial rise in serum testosterone.

Drug Interactions

Increased Effect/Toxicity: When used with other QT_c-prolonging agents, additive effects QT_c prolongation may occur with concurrent therapy. Life-threatening ventricular arrhythmias may result; example drugs include class Ia and class III antiarrhythmics, cisapride, selected quinolones, erythromycin, pimozide, mesoridazine, and thioridazine.

Pharmacodynamics/Kinetics

Distribution: V_d: 4040 L (± 1607)
Metabolism: Hepatic, via peptide hydrolysis
Half-life elimination: 13 days
Time to peak, serum: 3 days (following I.M. administration)
Excretion: Urine (13% unchanged drug)

Pregnancy Risk Factor X

Abbott-43818 *see* Leuprolide *on page 805*
Abbreviations, Acronyms, and Symbols *see page 18*
ABC *see* Abacavir *on page 42*
ABCD *see* Amphotericin B Cholesteryl Sulfate Complex *on page 119*

Abciximab (ab SIK si mab)

Related Information

Cardiovascular Diseases *on page 1458*

U.S. Brand Names ReoPro®
Canadian Brand Names Reopro™
Generic Available No
Synonyms C7E3; 7E3
Pharmacologic Category Antiplatelet Agent, Glycoprotein IIb/IIIa Inhibitor

Use Prevention of acute cardiac ischemic complications in patients at high risk for abrupt closure of the treated coronary vessel and patients at risk of restenosis; an adjunct with heparin to prevent cardiac ischemic complications in patients with unstable angina not responding to conventional therapy when a percutaneous coronary intervention is scheduled within 24 hours

Local Anesthetic/Vasoconstrictor Precautions No information available to require special precautions

Effects on Dental Treatment Key adverse event(s) related to dental treatment: As with all anticoagulants, bleeding is a potential adverse effect of abciximab during dental surgery; risk is dependent on multiple variables, including the intensity of anticoagulation and patient susceptibility. Medical consult is suggested. It is unlikely that ambulatory patients presenting for dental treatment will be taking intravenous anticoagulant therapy.

Common Adverse Effects As with all drugs which may affect hemostasis, bleeding is associated with abciximab. Hemorrhage may occur at virtually any site. Risk is dependent on multiple variables, including the concurrent use of multiple agents which alter hemostasis and patient susceptibility.

>10%:
Cardiovascular: Hypotension (14%), chest pain (11%)
Gastrointestinal: Nausea (14%)
Hematologic: Minor bleeding (4% to 17%)

Neuromuscular & skeletal: Back pain (18%)

1% to 10%:

Cardiovascular: Bradycardia (5%), peripheral edema (2%)

Central nervous system: Headache (7%)

Gastrointestinal: Vomiting (7%), abdominal pain (3%)

Hematologic: Major bleeding (1% to 14%), thrombocytopenia: <100,000 cells/mm^3 (3% to 6%); <50,000 cells/mm^3 (0.4% to 2%)

Local: Injection site pain (4%)

Mechanism of Action Fab antibody fragment of the chimeric human-murine monoclonal antibody 7E3; this agent binds to platelet IIb/IIIa receptors, resulting in steric hindrance, thus inhibiting platelet aggregation

Drug Interactions

Increased Effect/Toxicity: The risk of bleeding is increased when abciximab is given with heparin, other anticoagulants, thrombolytics, or antiplatelet drugs. However, aspirin and heparin were used concurrently in the majority of patients in the major clinical studies of abciximab. Allergic reactions may be increased in patients who have received diagnostic or therapeutic monoclonal antibodies due to the presence of HACA antibodies. Concomitant use of other glycoprotein IIb/IIIa antagonists is contraindicated.

Pharmacodynamics/Kinetics Half-life elimination: ~30 minutes

Pregnancy Risk Factor C

Abelcet® *see* Amphotericin B (Lipid Complex) *on page 121*

Abilify™ *see* Aripiprazole *on page 142*

ABLC *see* Amphotericin B (Lipid Complex) *on page 121*

A/B Otic *see* Antipyrine and Benzocaine *on page 135*

Abreva® [OTC] *see* Docosanol *on page 459*

Absorbable Cotton *see* Cellulose (Oxidized/Regenerated) *on page 293*

Absorbable Gelatin Sponge *see* Gelatin (Absorbable) *on page 650*

Absorbine Jr.® Antifungal [OTC] *see* Tolnaftate *on page 1312*

9-AC *see* Aminocamptothecin *on page 96*

Acarbose (AY car bose)

Related Information

Endocrine Disorders and Pregnancy *on page 1481*

U.S. Brand Names Precose®

Canadian Brand Names Prandase®

Mexican Brand Names Glucobay®

Generic Available No

Pharmacologic Category Antidiabetic Agent, Alpha-Glucosidase Inhibitor

Use

Monotherapy, as indicated as an adjunct to diet to lower blood glucose in patients with type 2 diabetes mellitus (noninsulin dependent, NIDDM) whose hyperglycemia cannot be managed on diet alone

Combination with a sulfonylurea, metformin, or insulin in patients with type 2 diabetes mellitus (noninsulin dependent, NIDDM) when diet plus acarbose do not result in adequate glycemic control. The effect of acarbose to enhance glycemic control is additive to that of other hypoglycemic agents when used in combination.

Local Anesthetic/Vasoconstrictor Precautions No information available to require special precautions

Effects on Dental Treatment No significant effects or complications reported

Common Adverse Effects >10%:

Gastrointestinal: Abdominal pain (21%) and diarrhea (33%) tend to return to pretreatment levels over time, and the frequency and intensity of flatulence (77%) tend to abate with time

Hepatic: Elevated liver transaminases

Mechanism of Action Competitive inhibitor of pancreatic α-amylase and intestinal brush border α-glucosidases, resulting in delayed hydrolysis of ingested complex carbohydrates and disaccharides and absorption of glucose; dose-dependent reduction in postprandial serum insulin and glucose peaks; inhibits the metabolism of sucrose to glucose and fructose

Drug Interactions

Increased Effect/Toxicity: Acarbose may increase the risk of hypoglycemia when used with oral hypoglycemics.

Decreased Effect: The effect of acarbose is antagonized/decreased by thiazide and related diuretics, corticosteroids, phenothiazines, thyroid products, estrogens, oral contraceptives, phenytoin, nicotinic acid, sympathomimetics,

(Continued)

Acarbose *(Continued)*

calcium channel-blocking drugs, isoniazid, intestinal adsorbents (eg, charcoal), and digestive enzyme preparations (eg, amylase, pancreatin). Acarbose decreases the absorption/serum concentration of digoxin.

Pharmacodynamics/Kinetics

Absorption: <2% as active drug

Metabolism: Exclusively via GI tract, principally by intestinal bacteria and digestive enzymes; 13 metabolites identified

Bioavailability: Low systemic bioavailability of parent compound; acts locally in GI tract

Excretion: Urine (~34%)

Pregnancy Risk Factor B

A-Caro-25® *see* Beta-Carotene *on page 198*

Accolate® *see* Zafirlukast *on page 1394*

AccuHist® Pediatric [DSC] *see* Brompheniramine and Pseudoephedrine *on page 220*

AccuNeb™ *see* Albuterol *on page 71*

Accupril® *see* Quinapril *on page 1158*

Accuretic™ *see* Quinapril and Hydrochlorothiazide *on page 1160*

Accutane® *see* Isotretinoin *on page 773*

ACE *see* Captopril *on page 252*

Acebutolol (a se BYOO toe lole)

Related Information

Cardiovascular Diseases *on page 1458*

U.S. Brand Names Sectral®

Canadian Brand Names Apo-Acebutolol®; Gen-Acebutolol; Monitan®; Novo-Acebutolol; Nu-Acebutolol; Rhotral; Sectral®

Generic Available Yes

Synonyms Acebutolol Hydrochloride

Pharmacologic Category Antiarrhythmic Agent, Class II; Beta Blocker With Intrinsic Sympathomimetic Activity

Use Treatment of hypertension, ventricular arrhythmias, angina

Local Anesthetic/Vasoconstrictor Precautions No information available to require special precautions

Effects on Dental Treatment Acebutolol is a cardioselective beta-blocker. Local anesthetic with vasoconstrictor can be safely used in patients medicated with acebutolol. Nonselective beta-blockers (ie, propranolol, nadolol) enhance the pressor response to epinephrine, resulting in hypertension and bradycardia; this has not been reported for acebutolol. Many nonsteroidal anti-inflammatory drugs, such as ibuprofen and indomethacin, can reduce the hypotensive effect of beta-blockers after 3 or more weeks of therapy with the NSAID. Short-term NSAID use (ie, 3 days) requires no special precautions in patients taking beta-blockers.

Common Adverse Effects

>10%: Central nervous system: Fatigue (11%)

1% to 10%:

- Cardiovascular: Chest pain (2%), edema (2%), bradycardia, hypotension, CHF
- Central nervous system: Headache (6%), dizziness (6%), insomnia (3%), depression (2%), abnormal dreams (2%), anxiety, hyperesthesia, hypoesthesia, impotence
- Dermatologic: Rash (2%), pruritus
- Gastrointestinal: Constipation (4%), diarrhea (4%), dyspepsia (4%), nausea (4%), flatulence (3%), vomiting, abdominal pain
- Genitourinary: Micturition frequency (3%), dysuria, nocturia, impotence (2%)
- Neuromuscular & skeletal: Arthralgia (2%), myalgia (2%), back pain, joint pain
- Ocular: Abnormal vision (2%), conjunctivitis, dry eyes, eye pain
- Respiratory: Dyspnea (4%), rhinitis (2%), cough (1%), pharyngitis, wheezing

Potential adverse effects (based on experience with other beta-blocking agents) include reversible mental depression, disorientation, catatonia, short-term memory loss, emotional lability, slightly clouded sensorium, laryngospasm, respiratory distress, allergic reactions, erythematous rash, agranulocytosis, purpura, thrombocytopenia, mesenteric artery thrombosis, ischemic colitis, alopecia, Peyronie's disease, claudication

Mechanism of Action Competitively blocks $beta_1$-adrenergic receptors with little or no effect on $beta_2$-receptors except at high doses; exhibits membrane stabilizing and intrinsic sympathomimetic activity

Drug Interactions

Cytochrome P450 Effect: Inhibits CYP2D6 (weak)

Increased Effect/Toxicity: Acebutolol may increase the effects of other drugs which slow AV conduction (digoxin, verapamil, diltiazem), alpha-blockers (prazosin, terazosin), and alpha-adrenergic stimulants (epinephrine, phenylephrine). Acebutolol may mask the tachycardia from hypoglycemia caused by insulin and oral hypoglycemics. In patients receiving concurrent therapy, the risk of hypertensive crisis is increased when either clonidine or the beta-blocker is withdrawn. Reserpine has been shown to enhance the effect of acebutolol. Beta-blockers may increase the action or levels of ethanol, disopyramide, nondepolarizing muscle relaxants, and theophylline although the effects are difficult to predict.

Decreased Effect: Decreased effect of acebutolol with aluminum salts, barbiturates, calcium salts, cholestyramine, colestipol, NSAIDs, penicillins (ampicillin), rifampin, and salicylates due to decreased bioavailability and plasma levels. The effect of sulfonylureas may be decreased by beta-blockers; however, the decreased effect has not been shown with tolbutamide.

Pharmacodynamics/Kinetics

Onset of action: 1-2 hours

Duration: 12-24 hours

Absorption: Oral: 40%

Protein binding: 5% to 15%

Metabolism: Extensive first-pass effect

Half-life elimination: 6-7 hours

Time to peak: 2-4 hours

Excretion: Feces (~55%); urine (35%)

Pregnancy Risk Factor B (manufacturer); D (2nd and 3rd trimesters - expert analysis)

Acebutolol Hydrochloride *see* Acebutolol *on page 46*

Aceon® *see* Perindopril Erbumine *on page 1068*

Acephen® [OTC] *see* Acetaminophen *on page 47*

Acetadote® *see* Acetylcysteine *on page 61*

Acetaminophen (a seet a MIN oh fen)

Related Information

Oral Pain *on page 1526*

Oxycodone and Acetaminophen *on page 1029*

U.S. Brand Names Acephen® [OTC]; Aspirin Free Anacin® Maximum Strength [OTC]; Cetafen® [OTC]; Cetafen Extra® [OTC]; Comtrex® Sore Throat Maximum Strength [OTC]; ElixSure™ Fever/Pain [OTC]; Feverall® [OTC]; Genapap® [OTC]; Genapap® Children [OTC]; Genapap® Extra Strength [OTC]; Genapap® Infant [OTC]; Genebs® [OTC]; Genebs® Extra Strength [OTC]; Mapap® [OTC]; Mapap® Arthritis [OTC]; Mapap® Children's [OTC]; Mapap® Extra Strength [OTC]; Mapap® Infants [OTC]; Redutemp® [OTC]; Silapap® Children's [OTC]; Silapap® Infants [OTC]; Tylenol® [OTC]; Tylenol® 8 Hour [OTC]; Tylenol® Arthritis Pain [OTC]; Tylenol® Children's [OTC]; Tylenol® Extra Strength [OTC]; Tylenol® Infants [OTC]; Tylenol® Junior Strength [OTC]; Tylenol® Sore Throat [OTC]; Valorin [OTC]; Valorin Extra [OTC]

Canadian Brand Names Abenol®; Apo-Acetaminophen®; Atasol®; Pediatrix; Tempra®; Tylenol®

Mexican Brand Names Andox®; Datril®; Magnidol®; Neodol®; Neodolito®; Sedalito®; Sinedol®; Temperal®; Tempra®; Tylex®

Generic Available Yes

Synonyms APAP; N-Acetyl-P-Aminophenol; Paracetamol

Pharmacologic Category Analgesic, Miscellaneous

Dental Use Treatment of postoperative pain

Use Treatment of mild to moderate pain and fever (antipyretic/analgesic); does not have antirheumatic or anti-inflammatory effects

Local Anesthetic/Vasoconstrictor Precautions No information available to require special precautions

Effects on Dental Treatment No significant effects or complications reported

Significant Adverse Effects Frequency not defined.

Dermatologic: Rash

Endocrine & metabolic: May increase chloride, uric acid, glucose; may decrease sodium, bicarbonate, calcium

Hematologic: Anemia; blood dyscrasias (neutropenia, pancytopenia, leukopenia)

Hepatic: May increase bilirubin, alkaline phosphatase

(Continued)

Acetaminophen *(Continued)*

Renal: May increase ammonia, nephrotoxicity with chronic overdose, analgesic nephropathy

Miscellaneous: Hypersensitivity reactions (rare)

Dosage Oral, rectal:

Children <12 years: 10-15 mg/kg/dose every 4-6 hours as needed; do **not** exceed 5 doses (2.6 g) in 24 hours; alternatively, the following age-based doses may be used; see table.

Acetaminophen Dosing

Age	Dosage (mg)	Age	Dosage (mg)
0-3 mo	40	4-5 y	240
4-11 mo	80	6-8 y	320
1-2 y	120	9-10 y	400
2-3 y	160	11 y	480

Note: Higher rectal doses have been studied for use in preoperative pain control in children. However, specific guidelines are not available and dosing may be product dependent. The safety and efficacy of alternating acetaminophen and ibuprofen dosing has not been established.

Adults: 325-650 mg every 4-6 hours or 1000 mg 3-4 times/day; do **not** exceed 4 g/day

Dosing interval in renal impairment:

Cl_{cr} 10-50 mL/minute: Administer every 6 hours

Cl_{cr} <10 mL/minute: Administer every 8 hours (metabolites accumulate)

Hemodialysis: Moderately dialyzable (20% to 50%)

Dosing adjustment/comments in hepatic impairment: Use with caution. Limited, low-dose therapy usually well tolerated in hepatic disease/cirrhosis. However, cases of hepatotoxicity at daily acetaminophen dosages <4 g/day have been reported. Avoid chronic use in hepatic impairment.

Mechanism of Action Inhibits the synthesis of prostaglandins in the central nervous system and peripherally blocks pain impulse generation; produces antipyresis from inhibition of hypothalamic heat-regulating center

Contraindications Hypersensitivity to acetaminophen or any component of the formulation

Warnings/Precautions Limit dose to <4 g/day. May cause severe hepatic toxicity on acute overdose; in addition, chronic daily dosing in adults has resulted in liver damage in some patients. Use with caution in patients with alcoholic liver disease; consuming ≥3 alcoholic drinks/day may increase the risk of liver damage. Use caution in patients with known G6PD deficiency.

OTC labeling: When used for self-medication, patients should be instructed to contact healthcare provider if used for fever lasting >3 days or for pain lasting >10 days in adults or >5 days in children.

Drug Interactions Substrate (minor) of CYP1A2, 2A6, 2C8/9, 2D6, 2E1, 3A4; **Inhibits** CYP3A4 (weak)

Decreased effect: Barbiturates, carbamazepine, hydantoins, rifampin, sulfinpyrazone may decrease the analgesic effect of acetaminophen; cholestyramine may decrease acetaminophen absorption (separate dosing by at least 1 hour)

Increased toxicity: Barbiturates, carbamazepine, hydantoins, isoniazid, rifampin, sulfinpyrazone may increase the hepatotoxic potential of acetaminophen; chronic ethanol abuse increases risk for acetaminophen toxicity; effect of warfarin may be enhanced

Ethanol/Nutrition/Herb Interactions

Ethanol: Excessive intake of ethanol may increase the risk of acetaminophen-induced hepatotoxicity. Avoid ethanol or limit to <3 drinks/day.

Food: Rate of absorption may be decreased when given with food.

Herb/Nutraceutical: St John's wort may decrease acetaminophen levels.

Dietary Considerations Chewable tablets may contain phenylalanine (amount varies, ranges between 3-12 mg/tablet); consult individual product labeling.

Pharmacodynamics/Kinetics

Onset of action: <1 hour

Duration: 4-6 hours

Absorption: Incomplete; varies by dosage form

Protein binding: 8% to 43% at toxic doses

Metabolism: At normal therapeutic dosages, hepatic to sulfate and glucuronide metabolites, while a small amount is metabolized by CYP to a highly reactive intermediate (acetylimidoquinone) which is conjugated with glutathione and inactivated; at toxic doses (as little as 4 g daily) glutathione conjugation becomes insufficient to meet the metabolic demand causing an increase in acetylimidoquinone concentration, which may cause hepatic cell necrosis

Half-life elimination: Prolonged following toxic doses

Neonates: 2-5 hours

Adults: 1-3 hours (may be increased in elderly; however, this should not affect dosing)

Time to peak, serum: Oral: 10-60 minutes; may be delayed in acute overdoses

Excretion: Urine (2% to 5% unchanged; 55% as glucuronide metabolites; 30% as sulphate metabolites)

Pregnancy Risk Factor B

Lactation Enters breast milk/compatible

Dosage Forms

Caplet (Cefaten® Extra Strength, Genapap® Extra Strength, Genebs® Extra Strength, Mapap® Extra Strength, Tylenol® Extra Strength): 500 mg

Caplet, extended release (Mapap® Arthritis, Tylenol® Arthritis Pain): 650 mg

Capsule (Mapap® Extra Strength): 500 mg

Elixir: 160 mg/5 mL (120 mL, 480 mL, 3780 mL)

Mapap® Children's: 160 mg/5 mL (120 mL) [alcohol free; contains benzoic acid and sodium benzoate; cherry flavor]

Gelcap (Mapap® Extra Strength, Tylenol® Extra Strength): 500 mg

Geltab (Mapap® Extra Strength, Tylenol® Extra Strength): 500 mg

Geltab, extended release (Tylenol® 8 Hour): 650 mg

Liquid, oral: 500 mg/15 mL (240 mL)

Comtrex® Sore Throat Maximum Strength: 500 mg/15 mL (240 mL) [contains sodium benzoate; honey lemon flavor]

Genapap® Children: 160 mg/5 mL (120 mL) [contains sodium benzoate; cherry and grape flavors]

Silapap®: 160 mg/5 mL (120 mL, 240 mL, 480 mL) [sugar free; contains sodium benzoate; cherry flavor]

Tylenol® Extra Strength: 500 mg/15 mL (240 mL) [contains sodium benzoate; cherry flavor]

Tylenol® Sore Throat: 500 mg/15 mL (240 mL) [contains sodium benzoate; cherry and honey-lemon flavors]

Solution, oral drops: 80 mg/0.8 mL (15 mL) [droppers are marked at 0.4 mL (40 mg) and at 0.8 mL (80 mg)]

Genapap® Infant: 80 mg/0.8 mL (15 mL) [fruit flavor]

Silapap® Infant's: 80 mg/0.8 mL (15 mL, 30 mL) [contains sodium benzoate; cherry flavor]

Solution, oral: 160 mg/5 mL (120 mL, 480 mL)

Suppository, rectal: 120 mg, 325 mg, 650 mg

Acephen®: 120 mg, 325 mg, 650 mg

Feverall®: 80 mg, 120 mg, 325 mg, 650 mg

Mapap®: 125 mg, 650 mg

Suspension, oral:

Mapap® Children's: 160 mg/5 mL (120 mL) [contains sodium benzoate; cherry flavor]

Tylenol® Children's: 160 mg/5 mL (120 mL, 240 mL) [contains sodium benzoate; bubblegum, cherry, and grape flavors]

Suspension, oral drops:

Mapap® Infants 80 mg/0.8 mL (15 mL, 30 mL) [contains sodium benzoate; cherry flavor]

Tylenol® Infants: 80 mg/0.8 mL (15 mL, 30 mL) [contains sodium benzoate; cherry and grape flavors]

Syrup, oral (ElixSure™ Fever/Pain): 160 mg/5 mL (120 mL) [bubblegum, cherry, and grape flavors]

Tablet: 325 mg, 500 mg

Aspirin Free Anacin® Extra Strength, Genapap® Extra Strength, Genebs® Extra Strength, Mapap® Extra Strength, Redutemp®, Tylenol® Extra Strength, Valorin Extra: 500 mg

Cetafen®, Genapap®, Genebs®, Mapap®, Tylenol®, Valorin: 325 mg

Tablet, chewable: 80 mg

Genapap® Children: 80 mg [contains phenylalanine 6 mg/tablet; fruit and grape flavors]

Mapap® Children's: 80 mg [contains phenylalanine 3 mg/tablet; bubblegum, fruit, and grape flavors]

Mapap® Junior Strength: 160 mg [contains phenylalanine 12 mg/tablet; grape flavor]

Tylenol® Children's: 80 mg [fruit and grape flavors contain phenylalanine 3 mg/tablet; bubblegum flavor contains phenylalanine 6 mg/tablet]

(Continued)

Acetaminophen *(Continued)*

Tylenol® Junior Strength: 160 mg [contains phenylalanine 6 mg/tablet; fruit and grape flavors]

Comments Doses of acetaminophen >5 g/day for several weeks can produce severe, often fatal liver damage. Hepatotoxicity caused by acetaminophen is potentiated by chronic ethanol consumption. It has been reported that a combination of two quarts of whiskey a day with 8-10 acetaminophen tablets daily resulted in severe liver toxicity. People who consume ethanol at the same time that they use acetaminophen, even in therapeutic doses, are at risk of developing hepatotoxicity.

A study by Hylek, et al, suggested that the combination of acetaminophen with warfarin (Coumadin®) may cause enhanced anticoagulation. The following recommendations have been made by Hylek, et al, and supported by an editorial in *JAMA* by Bell.

Dose and duration of acetaminophen should be as low as possible, individualized and monitored.

The study by Hylek reported the following:

For patients who reported taking the equivalent of at least 4 regular strength (325 mg) tablets for longer than a week, the odds of having an INR >6.0 were increased 10-fold above those not taking acetaminophen. Risk decreased with lower intakes of acetaminophen reaching a background level of risk at a dose of 6 or fewer 325 mg tablets per week.

Selected Readings

Ahmad N, Grad HA, Haas DA, et al, "The Efficacy of Nonopioid Analgesics for Postoperative Dental Pain: A Meta-Analysis," *Anesth Prog*, 1997, 44(4):119-26.

Bell WR, "Acetaminophen and Warfarin: Undesirable Synergy," *JAMA*, 1998, 279(9):702-3.

Botting RM, "Mechanism of Action of Acetaminophen: Is There a Cyclooxygenase 3?" *Clin Infect Dis*, 2000, Suppl 5:S202-10.

Chandrasekharan NV, Dai H, Roos KL, et al, "COX-3, a Cyclooxygenase-1 Variant Inhibited by Acetaminophen and Other Analgesic/Antipyretic Drugs: Cloning, Structure, and Expression," *Proc Natl Acad Sci U S A*, 2002, 99(21):13926-31.

Dart RC, Kuffner EK, and Rumack BH, "Treatment of Pain or Fever With Paracetamol (Acetaminophen) in the Alcoholic Patient: A Systematic Review," *Am J Ther*, 2000, 7(2):123-34.

Dionne R, "Additive Analgesia Without Opioid Side Effects," *Compend Contin Educ Dent*, 2000, 21(7):572-4, 576-7.

Dionne RA and Berthold CW, "Therapeutic Uses of Nonsteroidal Anti-inflammatory Drugs in Dentistry," *Crit Rev Oral Biol Med*, 2001, 12(4):315-30.

Graham GG and Scott KF, "Mechanisms of Action of Paracetamol and Related Analgesics," *Inflammopharmacology*, 2003, 11(4):401-13.

Grant JA and Weiler JM, "A Report of a Rare Immediate Reaction After Ingestion of Acetaminophen," *Ann Allergy Asthma Immunol*, 2001, 87(3):227-9.

Hylek EM, Heiman H, Skates SJ, et al, "Acetaminophen and Other Risk Factors for Excessive Warfarin Anticoagulation," *JAMA*, 1998, 279(9):657-62.

Kwan D, Bartle WR, and Walker SE, "The Effects of Acetaminophen on Pharmacokinetics and Pharmacodynamics of Warfarin," *J Clin Pharmacol*, 1999, 39(1):68-75.

Lee WM, "Drug-Induced Hepatotoxicity," *N Engl J Med*, 1995, 333(17):1118-27.

Licht H, Seeff LB, and Zimmerman HJ, "Apparent Potentiation of Acetaminophen Hepatotoxicity by Alcohol," *Ann Intern Med*, 1980, 92(4):511.

McClain CJ, Price S, Barve S, et al, "Acetaminophen Hepatotoxicity: An Update," *Curr Gastroenterol Rep*, 1999, 1(1):42-9.

Nguyen AM, Graham DY, Gage T, et al, "Nonsteroidal Anti-Inflammatory Drug Use in Dentistry: Gastrointestinal Implications," *Gen Dent*, 1999, 47(6):590-6.

Schwab JM, Schluesener HJ, and Laufer S, "COX-3: Just Another COX or the Solitary Elusive Target of Paracetamol?" *Lancet*, 2003, 361(9362):981-2.

Shek KL, Chan LN, and Nutescu E, "Warfarin-Acetaminophen Drug Interaction Revisited," *Pharmacotherapy*, 1999, 19(10):1153-8.

Tanaka E, Yamazaki K, and Misawa S, "Update: The Clinical Importance of Acetaminophen Hepatotoxicity in Nonalcoholic and Alcoholic Subjects," *J Clin Pharm Ther*, 2000, 25(5):325-32.

Wynn RL, "Update on Nonprescription Pain Relievers for Dental Pain," *Gen Dent*, 2004, 52(2):94-8.

Acetaminophen and Chlorpheniramine *see* Chlorpheniramine and Acetaminophen *on page 314*

Acetaminophen and Codeine (a seet a MIN oh fen & KOE deen)

Related Information

Acetaminophen *on page 47*

Codeine *on page 369*

U.S. Brand Names Capital® and Codeine; Tylenol® With Codeine

Canadian Brand Names ratio-Emtec; ratio-Lenoltec; Triatec-8; Triatec-8 Strong; Triatec-30; Tylenol Elixir with Codeine; Tylenol No. 1; Tylenol No. 1 Forte; Tylenol No. 2 with Codeine; Tylenol No. 3 with Codeine; Tylenol No. 4 with Codeine

Generic Available Yes

Synonyms Codeine and Acetaminophen

Pharmacologic Category Analgesic, Narcotic

Dental Use Treatment of postoperative pain

Use Relief of mild to moderate pain

Local Anesthetic/Vasoconstrictor Precautions No information available to require special precautions

Effects on Dental Treatment No significant effects or complications reported

Significant Adverse Effects

>10%:

Central nervous system: Lightheadedness, dizziness, sedation
Gastrointestinal: Nausea, vomiting
Respiratory: Dyspnea

1% to 10%:

Central nervous system: Euphoria, dysphoria
Dermatologic: Pruritus
Gastrointestinal: Constipation, abdominal pain
Miscellaneous: Histamine release

<1% (Limited to important or life-threatening): Antidiuretic hormone release, biliary tract spasm, bradycardia, hypotension, increased intracranial pressure, physical and psychological dependence, respiratory depression, urinary retention

Restrictions C-III; C-V

Note: In countries outside of the U.S., some formulations of Tylenol® with Codeine (eg, Tylenol® No.3) include caffeine.

Dosage Doses should be adjusted according to severity of pain and response of the patient. Adult doses ≥60 mg codeine fail to give commensurate relief of pain but merely prolong analgesia and are associated with an appreciably increased incidence of side effects. Oral:

Children: Analgesic:

Codeine: 0.5-1 mg codeine/kg/dose every 4-6 hours

Acetaminophen: 10-15 mg/kg/dose every 4 hours up to a maximum of 2.6 g/24 hours for children <12 years; **alternatively, the following can be used:**

3-6 years: 5 mL 3-4 times/day as needed of elixir
7-12 years: 10 mL 3-4 times/day as needed of elixir
>12 years: 15 mL every 4 hours as needed of elixir

Adults:

Antitussive: Based on codeine (15-30 mg/dose) every 4-6 hours (maximum: 360 mg/24 hours based on codeine component)

Analgesic: Based on codeine (30-60 mg/dose) every 4-6 hours (maximum: 4000 mg/24 hours based on acetaminophen component)

Dosing adjustment in renal impairment: See individual monographs for Acetaminophen and Codeine

Mechanism of Action Inhibits the synthesis of prostaglandins in the central nervous system and peripherally blocks pain impulse generation; produces antipyresis from inhibition of hypothalamic heat-regulating center; binds to opiate receptors in the CNS, causing inhibition of ascending pain pathways, altering the perception of and response to pain; causes cough supression by direct central action in the medulla; produces generalized CNS depression. Caffeine (contained in some non-U.S. formulations) is a CNS stimulant; use with acetaminophen and codeine increases the level of analgesia provided by each agent.

Contraindications Hypersensitivity to acetaminophen, codeine, or any component of the formulation; significant respiratory depression (in unmonitored settings); acute or severe bronchial asthma; hypercapnia; paralytic ileus

Warnings/Precautions Use with caution in patients with hypersensitivity reactions to other phenanthrene derivative opioid agonists (morphine, hydrocodone, hydromorphone, levorphanol, oxycodone, oxymorphone); tablets contain metabisulfite which may cause allergic reactions. Tolerance or drug dependence may result from extended use.

Limit total acetaminophen dose to <4 g/day. May cause severe hepatic toxicity on acute overdose; in addition, chronic daily dosing in adults has resulted in liver damage in some patients. Use with caution in patients with alcoholic liver disease; consuming 3 alcoholic drinks/day may increase the risk of liver damage. Use caution in patients with known G6PD deficiency.

This combination should be used with caution in elderly or debilitated patients, hypotension, adrenocortical insufficiency, thyroid disorders, prostatic hyperplasia, urethral stricture, seizure disorder, CNS depression, head injury or increased intracranial pressure. Causes sedation; caution must be used in performing tasks which require alertness (eg, operating machinery or driving). Safety and efficacy in pediatric patients have not been established.

Note: Some non-U.S. formulations (including most Canadian formulations) may contain caffeine as an additional ingredient. Caffeine may cause CNS and

(Continued)

Acetaminophen and Codeine *(Continued)*

cardiovascular stimulation, as well as GI irritation in high doses. Use with caution in patients with a history of peptic ulcer or GERD; avoid in patients with symptomatic cardiac arrhythmias.

Drug Interactions Acetaminophen: **Substrate** (minor) of CYP1A2, 2A6, 2C8/9, 2D6, 2E1, 3A4; **Inhibits** CYP3A4 (weak)

Increased toxicity: CNS depressants, phenothiazines, tricyclic antidepressants, guanabenz, MAO inhibitors (may also decrease blood pressure); effect of warfarin may be enhanced

Ethanol/Nutrition/Herb Interactions Ethanol: Excessive intake of ethanol may increase the risk of acetaminophen-induced hepatotoxicity. Avoid ethanol or limit to <3 drinks/day.

Dietary Considerations May be taken with food.

Pharmacodynamics/Kinetics See individual agents.

Pregnancy Risk Factor C

Lactation Enters breast milk/use caution

Dosage Forms [DSC] = Discontinued product; [CAN] = Canadian brand name

Caplet:

ratio-Lenoltec No. 1 [CAN], Tylenol No. 1 [CAN]: Acetaminophen 300 mg, codeine phosphate, 8 mg and caffeine 15 mg [not available in the U.S.]

Tylenol No. 1 Forte [CAN]: Acetaminophen 500 mg, codeine phosphate 8 mg, and caffeine 15 mg [not available in the U.S.]

Elixir, oral [C-V]: Acetaminophen 120 mg and codeine phosphate 12 mg per 5 mL (5 mL, 10 mL, 12.5 mL, 15 mL, 120 mL, 480 mL) [contains alcohol 7%]

Tylenol® with Codeine [DSC]: Acetaminophen 120 mg and codeine phosphate 12 mg per 5 mL (480 mL) [contains alcohol 7%; cherry flavor]

Tylenol Elixir with Codeine [CAN]: Acetaminophen 160 mg and codeine phosphate 8 mg per 5 mL (500 mL) [contains alcohol 7%, sucrose 31%; cherry flavor; not available in the U.S.]

Suspension, oral [C-V] (Capital® and Codeine): Acetaminophen 120 mg and codeine phosphate 12 mg per 5 mL (480 mL) [alcohol free; fruit punch flavor]

Tablet [C-III]: Acetaminophen 300 mg and codeine phosphate 15 mg; acetaminophen 300 mg and codeine phosphate 30 mg; acetaminophen 300 mg and codeine phosphate 60 mg

ratio-Emtec [CAN], Triatec-30 [CAN]: Acetaminophen 300 mg and codeine phosphate 30 mg [not available in the U.S.]

ratio-Lenoltec No. 1 [CAN]: Acetaminophen 300 mg, codeine phosphate 8 mg, and caffeine 15 mg [Not available in the U. S.]

ratio-Lenoltec No. 2 [CAN], Tylenol No. 2 with Codeine [CAN]: Acetaminophen 300 mg, codeine phosphate 15 mg, and caffeine 15 mg [not available in the U.S.]

ratio-Lenoltec No. 3 [CAN], Tylenol No. 3 with Codeine [CAN]: Acetaminophen 300 mg, codeine phosphate 30 mg, and caffeine 15 mg [not available in the U.S.]

ratio-Lenoltec No. 4 [CAN], Tylenol No. 4 with Codeine [CAN]: Acetaminophen 300 mg and codeine phosphate 60 mg [not available in the U.S.]

Triatec-8 [CAN]: Acetaminophen 325 mg, codeine phosphate 8 mg, and caffeine 30 mg [not available in the U.S.]

Triatec-8 Strong [CAN]: Acetaminophen 500 mg, codeine phosphate 8 mg, and caffeine 30 mg [not available in the U.S.]

Tylenol® with Codeine No. 3: Acetaminophen 300 mg and codeine phosphate 30 mg [contains sodium metabisulfite]

Tylenol® with Codeine No. 4: Acetaminophen 300 mg and codeine phosphate 60 mg [contains sodium metabisulfite]

Comments Codeine products, as with other narcotic analgesics, are recommended only for acute dosing (ie, 3 days or less). The most common adverse effect you will see in your dental patients from codeine is nausea, followed by sedation and constipation. Codeine has narcotic addiction liability, especially when given long-term. Because of the acetaminophen component, this product should be used with caution in patients with alcoholic liver disease.

A study by Hylek, et al, suggested that the combination of acetaminophen with warfarin (Coumadin®) may cause enhanced anticoagulation. The following recommendations have been made by Hylek, et al, and supported by an editorial in *JAMA* by Bell.

Dose and duration of acetaminophen should be as low as possible, individualized and monitored.

The study by Hylek reported the following:

For patients who reported taking the equivalent of at least 4 regular strength (325 mg) tablets for longer than a week, the odds of having an INR >6.0 were increased 10-fold above those not taking acetaminophen. Risk decreased with lower intakes of acetaminophen reaching a background level of risk at a dose of 6 or fewer 325 mg tablets per week.

Selected Readings

Change DJ, Fricke JR, Bird SR, et al, "Rofecoxib Versus Codeine/Acetaminophen in Postoperative Dental Pain: A Double-Blind, Randomized, Placebo- and Active Comparator-Controlled Clinical Trial," *Clin Ther*, 2001, 23(9):1446-55.

Dionne RA, "New Approaches to Preventing and Treating Postoperative Pain," *J Am Dent Assoc*, 1992, 123(6):26-34.

Forbes JA, Butterworth GA, Burchfield WH, et al, "Evaluation of Ketorolac, Aspirin, and an Acetaminophen-Codeine Combination in Postoperative Oral Surgery Pain," *Pharmacotherapy*, 1990, 10(6 Pt 2):77S-93S.

Gobetti JP, "Controlling Dental Pain," *J Am Dent Assoc*, 1992, 123(6):47-52.

Mullican WS and Lacy JR, "Tramadol/Acetaminophen Combination Tablets and Codeine/Acetaminophen Combination Capsules for the Management of Chronic Pain: A Comparative Trial," *Clin Ther*, 2001, 23(9):1429-45.

Wynn RL, "Narcotic Analgesics for Dental Pain: Available Products, Strengths, and Formulations," *Gen Dent*, 2001, 49(2):126-8, 130, 132 passim.

Acetaminophen and Diphenhydramine

(a seet a MIN oh fen & dye fen HYE dra meen)

Related Information

Acetaminophen *on page 47*

DiphenhydrAMINE *on page 448*

U.S. Brand Names Anacin PM Aspirin Free [OTC] [DSC]; Excedrin® P.M. [OTC]; Goody's PM® Powder; Legatrin PM® [OTC]; Percogesic® Extra Strength [OTC]; Tylenol® PM Extra Strength [OTC]; Tylenol® Severe Allergy [OTC]

Generic Available Yes: Excludes powder

Synonyms Diphenhydramine and Acetaminophen

Pharmacologic Category Analgesic, Miscellaneous

Use Aid in the relief of insomnia accompanied by minor pain

Local Anesthetic/Vasoconstrictor Precautions No information available to require special precautions

Effects on Dental Treatment Key adverse event(s) related to dental treatment: Xerostomia (normal salivary flow resumes upon discontinuation).

Common Adverse Effects See individual agents.

Drug Interactions

Cytochrome P450 Effect:

Acetaminophen: **Substrate** (minor) of CYP1A2, 2A6, 2C8/9, 2D6, 2E1, 3A4; **Inhibits** CYP3A4 (weak)

Diphenhydramine: **Inhibits** CYP2D6 (moderate)

Pharmacodynamics/Kinetics See individual agents.

Acetaminophen and Hydrocodone *see* Hydrocodone and Acetaminophen *on page 702*

Acetaminophen and Oxycodone *see* Oxycodone and Acetaminophen *on page 1029*

Acetaminophen and Pentazocine *see* Pentazocine and Acetaminophen *on page 1064*

Acetaminophen and Phenyltoloxamine

(a seet a MIN oh fen & fen il to LOKS a meen)

Related Information

Acetaminophen *on page 47*

U.S. Brand Names Genesec® [OTC]; Percogesic® [OTC]; Phenylgesic® [OTC]

Generic Available Yes

Synonyms Phenyltoloxamine and Acetaminophen

Pharmacologic Category Analgesic, Non-narcotic

Use Relief of mild to moderate pain

Local Anesthetic/Vasoconstrictor Precautions No information available to require special precautions

Effects on Dental Treatment No significant effects or complications reported

Drug Interactions

Cytochrome P450 Effect: Acetaminophen: **Substrate** (minor) of CYP1A2, 2A6, 2C8/9, 2D6, 2E1, 3A4; **Inhibits** CYP3A4 (weak)

Pregnancy Risk Factor B

Acetaminophen and Pseudoephedrine

(a seet a MIN oh fen & soo doe e FED rin)

Related Information

Acetaminophen *on page 47*

Pseudoephedrine *on page 1147*

U.S. Brand Names Alka-Seltzer Plus® Cold and Sinus Liquigels [OTC]; Cetafen Cold® [OTC]; Genapap™ Sinus Maximum Strength [OTC]; Mapap

(Continued)

Acetaminophen and Pseudoephedrine *(Continued)*

Sinus Maximum Strength [OTC]; Medi-Synal [OTC]; Ornex® [OTC]; Ornex® Maximum Strength [OTC]; Sinus-Relief® [OTC]; Sinutab® Sinus [OTC]; Sudafed® Sinus and Cold [OTC]; Sudafed® Sinus Headache [OTC]; SudoGest Sinus [OTC]; Tylenol® Cold, Infants [OTC]; Tylenol® Sinus, Children's [OTC]; Tylenol® Sinus Day Non-Drowsy [OTC]

Canadian Brand Names Dristan® N.D.; Dristan® N.D., Extra Strength; Sinutab® Non Drowsy; Sudafed® Head Cold and Sinus Extra Strength; Tylenol® Decongestant; Tylenol® Sinus

Generic Available Yes

Synonyms Pseudoephedrine and Acetaminophen

Pharmacologic Category Alpha/Beta Agonist; Analgesic, Miscellaneous

Use Relief of mild to moderate pain; relief of congestion

Local Anesthetic/Vasoconstrictor Precautions Use with caution since pseudoephedrine is a sympathomimetic amine which could interact with epinephrine to cause a pressor response

Effects on Dental Treatment Key adverse event(s) related to dental treatment: Pseudoephedrine: Xerostomia (normal salivary flow resumes upon discontinuation).

Common Adverse Effects See individual agents.

Drug Interactions

Cytochrome P450 Effect: Acetaminophen: **Substrate** (minor) of CYP1A2, 2A6, 2C8/9, 2D6, 2E1, 3A4; **Inhibits** CYP3A4 (weak)

Pharmacodynamics/Kinetics See individual agents.

Acetaminophen and Tramadol

(a seet a MIN oh fen & TRA ma dole)

Related Information

Acetaminophen *on page 47*

U.S. Brand Names Ultracet™

Generic Available No

Synonyms APAP and Tramadol; Tramadol Hydrochloride and Acetaminophen

Pharmacologic Category Analgesic, Non-narcotic; Analgesic, Miscellaneous

Dental Use Treatment of postoperative pain (≤5 days)

Use Short-term (≤5 days) management of acute pain

Local Anesthetic/Vasoconstrictor Precautions No information available to require special precautions

Effects on Dental Treatment Key adverse event(s) related to dental treatment: Xerostomia and changes in salivation (normal salivary flow resumes upon discontinuation).

Significant Adverse Effects

1% to 10%:

Central nervous system: Somnolence (6%), dizziness (3%), insomnia (2%), anxiety, confusion, euphoria, fatigue, headache, nervousness, somnolence, tremor

Dermatologic: Pruritus (2%), rash

Endocrine & metabolic: Hot flashes

Gastrointestinal: Constipation (6%), anorexia (3%), diarrhea (3%), nausea (3%), dry mouth (2%), abdominal pain, dyspepsia, flatulence, vomiting

Genitourinary: Prostatic disorder (2%)

Neuromuscular & skeletal: Weakness

Miscellaneous: Diaphoresis increased (4%)

<1% (Limited to important or life-threatening): Allergic reactions, amnesia, anaphylactoid reactions, anaphylaxis, arrhythmia, coma, depersonalization, drug abuse, dysphagia, dyspnea, emotional lability, hallucination, hepatitis, hypertonia, impotence, liver failure, migraine, muscle contractions (involuntary), oliguria, paresthesia, paroniria, pulmonary edema, rigors, seizures, serotonin syndrome, shivering, Stevens-Johnson syndrome, suicidal tendency, stupor, syncope, tinnitus, tongue edema, toxic epidermal necrolysis, urinary retention, urticaria, vertigo

A withdrawal syndrome may occur with abrupt discontinuation; includes anxiety, diarrhea, hallucinations (rare), nausea, pain, piloerection, rigors, sweating, and tremors. Uncommon discontinuation symptoms may include severe anxiety, panic attacks, or paresthesia.

Dosage Oral: Adults: Acute pain: Two tablets every 4-6 hours as needed for pain relief (maximum: 8 tablets/day); treatment should not exceed 5 days

Dosage adjustment in renal impairment: Cl_{cr} <30 mL/minute: Maximum of 2 tablets every 12 hours; treatment should not exceed 5 days

Dosage adjustment in hepatic impairment: Use is not recommended.

Mechanism of Action

Based on **acetaminophen** component: Inhibits the synthesis of prostaglandins in the central nervous system and peripherally blocks pain impulse generation; produces antipyresis from inhibition of hypothalamic heat-regulating center

Based on **tramadol** component: Binds to μ-opiate receptors in the CNS causing inhibition of ascending pain pathways, altering the perception of and response to pain; also inhibits the reuptake of norepinephrine and serotonin, which also modifies the ascending pain pathway

Contraindications Hypersensitivity to acetaminophen, tramadol, opioids, or any component of the formulation; opioid-dependent patients; acute intoxication with ethanol, hypnotics, narcotics, centrally-acting analgesics, opioids, or psychotropic drugs; hepatic dysfunction

Warnings/Precautions Should be used only with extreme caution in patients receiving MAO inhibitors. Use with caution and reduce dosage when administering to patients receiving other CNS depressants. Seizures may occur when taken within the recommended dosage; risk is increased in patients receiving serotonin reuptake inhibitors (SSRIs or anorectics), tricyclic antidepressants, other cyclic compounds (including cyclobenzaprine, promethazine), neuroleptics, MAO inhibitors, or drugs which may lower seizure threshold. Patients with a history of seizures, or with a risk of seizures (head trauma, metabolic disorders, CNS infection, or malignancy, or during alcohol/drug withdrawal) are also at increased risk. Do not use with ethanol or other acetaminophen- or tramadol-containing products.

Limit acetaminophen to <4 g/day. May cause severe hepatic toxicity in acute overdose; in addition, chronic daily dosing in adults has resulted in liver damage in some patients. Use with caution in patients with alcoholic liver disease; consuming ≥3 alcoholic drinks/day may increase the risk of liver damage. Use caution in patients with known G6PD deficiency.

Elderly patients and patients with chronic respiratory disorders may be at greater risk of adverse events. Use with caution in patients with increased intracranial pressure or head injury. Use tramadol with caution and reduce dosage in patients with renal dysfunction and in patients with myxedema, hypothyroidism, or hypoadrenalism. Tolerance or drug dependence may result from extended use (withdrawal symptoms have been reported); abrupt discontinuation should be avoided. Tapering of dose at the time of discontinuation limits the risk of withdrawal symptoms. Safety and efficacy in pediatric patients have not been established.

Drug Interactions

Acetaminophen: **Substrate** (minor) of CYP1A2, 2A6, 2C8/9, 2D6, 2E1, 3A4; **Inhibits** CYP3A4 (weak)

Tramadol: **Substrate** of CYP2D6 (major), 3A4 (minor)

Amphetamines: May increase the risk of seizures with tramadol.

Anesthetic agents: May increase risk of CNS and respiratory depression; use together with caution and in reduced dosage.

Barbiturates: Barbiturates may increase the hepatotoxic effects of acetaminophen; in addition, acetaminophen levels may be lowered.

Carbamazepine: Carbamazepine decreases half-life of tramadol by 33% to 50%; also have increase risk of seizures; in addition, carbamazepine may increase the hepatotoxic effects and lower serum levels of acetaminophen; concomitant use is not recommended.

CYP2D6 inhibitors: May decrease the effects of tramadol. Example inhibitors include chlorpromazine, delavirdine, fluoxetine, miconazole, paroxetine, pergolide, quinidine, quinine, ritonavir, and ropinirole.

Digoxin: Rare reports of digoxin toxicity with concomitant tramadol use.

Hydantoin anticonvulsants: Phenytoin may increase the hepatotoxic effects of acetaminophen; in addition, acetaminophen levels may be lowered.

MAO inhibitors: May increase the risk of seizures. Use extreme caution.

Naloxone: May increase the risk of seizures (if administered in tramadol overdose).

Neuroleptic agents: May increase the risk of tramadol-associated seizures and may have additive CNS depressant effects.

Narcotics: May increase risk of CNS and respiratory depression; use together with caution and in reduced dosage.

Opioids: May increase the risk of seizures, and may have additive CNS depressant effects. Use together with caution and in reduced dosage.

Phenothiazines: May increase risk of CNS and respiratory depression; use together with caution and in reduced dosage.

Rifampin: Rifampin may increase the clearance of acetaminophen.

Quinidine: May increase the tramadol serum concentrations by inhibiting CYP metabolism.

(Continued)

Acetaminophen and Tramadol *(Continued)*

SSRIs: May increase the risk of seizures with tramadol by inhibiting CYP metabolism (citalopram, fluoxetine, paroxetine, sertraline).

Sulfinpyrazone: Sulfinpyrazone may increase the hepatotoxic effects of acetaminophen; in addition, acetaminophen levels may be lowered.

Tricyclic antidepressants: May increase the risk of seizures.

Warfarin: Acetaminophen and tramadol may lead to an elevation of prothrombin times; monitor.

Ethanol/Nutrition/Herb Interactions

Ethanol: Avoid ethanol (increased liver toxicity with concomitant use).

Food: May delay time to peak plasma levels, however, the extent of absorption is not affected.

Herb/Nutraceutical:

Acetaminophen: Avoid St John's wort (may decrease acetaminophen levels).

Tramadol: Avoid valerian, St John's wort, kava kava, gotu kola (may increase CNS depression).

Dietary Considerations May be taken with or without food. Avoid use of ethanol and ethanol-containing products.

Pharmacodynamics/Kinetics See individual agents.

Pregnancy Risk Factor C

Lactation Tramadol: Enters breast milk/contraindicated

Breast-Feeding Considerations Not recommended for post-delivery analgesia in nursing mothers.

Dosage Forms Tablet: Acetaminophen 325 mg and tramadol hydrochloride 37.5 mg

Selected Readings

Fricke JR Jr, Hewitt DJ, Jordan DM, et al, "A Double-Blind Placebo-Controlled Comparison of Tramadol/Acetaminophen and Tramadol in Patients With Postoperative Dental Pain," *Pain*, 2004, 109(3):250-7.

Fricke JR Jr, Karim R, Jordan D, et al, "A Double-Blind, Single-Dose Comparison of the Analgesic Efficacy of Tramadol/Acetaminophen Combination Tablets, Hydrocodone/Acetaminophen Combination Tablets, and Placebo After Oral Surgery," *Clin Ther*, 2002, 24(6):953-68.

Hiller B and Rosenberg M, "Ultracet: A New Combination Analgesic," *J Mass Dent Soc*, 2003, 52(2):38-40.

Medve RA, Wang J, and Karim R, "Tramadol and Acetaminophen Tablets for Dental Pain," *Anesth Prog*, 2001, 48(3):79-81.

Smith AB, Ravikumar TS, Kamin M, et al, "Combination Tramadol Plus Acetaminophen for Postsurgical Pain," *Am J Surg*, 2004, 187(4):521-7.

Wynn RL, "NSAIDS and Cardiovascular Effects, Celecoxib for Dental Pain, and a New Analgesic - Tramadol with Acetaminophen," *Gen Dent*, 2002, 50(3):218-222.

Acetaminophen, Aspirin, and Caffeine

(a seet a MIN oh fen, AS pir in, & KAF een)

Related Information

Acetaminophen *on page 47*

Aspirin *on page 151*

U.S. Brand Names Excedrin® Extra Strength [OTC]; Excedrin® Migraine [OTC]; Fem-Prin® [OTC]; Genaced™ [OTC]; Goody's® Extra Strength Headache Powder [OTC]; Goody's® Extra Strength Pain Relief [OTC]; Pain-Off [OTC]; Vanquish® Extra Strength Pain Reliever [OTC]

Generic Available Yes

Synonyms Aspirin, Acetaminophen, and Caffeine; Aspirin, Caffeine and Acetaminophen; Caffeine, Acetaminophen, and Aspirin; Caffeine, Aspirin, and Acetaminophen

Pharmacologic Category Analgesic, Miscellaneous

Use Relief of mild to moderate pain; mild to moderate pain associated with migraine headache

Local Anesthetic/Vasoconstrictor Precautions No information available to require special precautions

Effects on Dental Treatment No significant effects or complications reported

Common Adverse Effects See individual agents.

Drug Interactions

Cytochrome P450 Effect:

Acetaminophen: **Substrate** (minor) of CYP1A2, 2A6, 2C8/9, 2D6, 2E1, 3A4; **Inhibits** CYP3A4 (weak)

Aspirin: **Substrate** (minor) of CYP2C8/9

Caffeine: **Substrate** of CYP1A2 (major), 2C8/9 (minor), 2D6 (minor), 2E1 (minor), 3A4 (minor); **Inhibits** CYP1A2 (weak), 3A4 (moderate)

Pharmacodynamics/Kinetics See individual agents.

Pregnancy Risk Factor D

Acetaminophen, Butalbital, and Caffeine *see* Butalbital, Acetaminophen, and Caffeine *on page 236*

Acetaminophen, Caffeine, and Dihydrocodeine

(a seet a MIN oh fen, KAF een, & dye hye droe KOE deen)

U.S. Brand Names Panlor® DC; Panlor® SS

Generic Available No

Synonyms Caffeine, Dihydrocodeine, and Acetaminophen; Dihydrocodeine Bitartrate, Acetaminophen, and Caffeine

Pharmacologic Category Analgesic Combination (Narcotic)

Use Relief of moderate to moderately-severe pain

Local Anesthetic/Vasoconstrictor Precautions No information available to require special precautions

Effects on Dental Treatment No significant effects or complications reported

Significant Adverse Effects Frequency not defined. Most common reactions with this combination include:

Central nervous system: Dizziness, drowsiness, lightheadedness, sedation

Dermatologic: Pruritus, skin reactions

Gastrointestinal: Constipation, nausea, vomiting

Restrictions C-III

Dosage Oral: Adults: Relief of pain:

Panlor® DC: 2 capsules every 4 hours as needed; adjust dose based on severity of pain (maximum dose: 10 capsules/24 hours)

Panlor® SS: 1 tablet every 4 hours as needed; adjust dose based on severity of pain (maximum dose: 5 tablets/24 hours)

Mechanism of Action

Acetaminophen inhibits the synthesis of prostaglandins in the central nervous system and peripherally blocks pain impulse generation; produces antipyresis from inhibition of hypothalamic heat-regulating center.

Caffeine is a CNS stimulant; use with acetaminophen and dihydrocodeine increases the level of analgesia provided by each agent.

Dihydrocodeine binds to opiate receptors in the CNS, causing inhibition of ascending pain pathways, altering the perception of and response to pain; produces generalized CNS depression.

Contraindications Hypersensitivity to acetaminophen, caffeine, dihydrocodeine, codeine, or any component of the formulation; significant respiratory depression (in unmonitored settings); acute or severe bronchial asthma; hypercapnia; paralytic ileus

Warnings/Precautions Acetaminophen may cause severe hepatotoxicity in acute overdose; limit acetaminophen to <4 g/day; in addition, chronic daily dosing in adults has resulted in liver damage in some patients. Use with caution in patients with alcoholic liver disease; consuming ≥3 alcoholic drinks/day may increase the risk of liver damage. Use caution in patients with known G6PD deficiency. Caffeine may cause CNS and cardiovascular stimulation as well as GI irritation in high doses. Dihydrocodeine should be used with caution in patients with hypersensitivity reactions to other phenanthrene derivative opioid agonists (morphine, hydrocodone, hydromorphone, levorphanol, oxycodone, oxymorphone), respiratory diseases including asthma, emphysema, COPD, or severe hepatic or renal insufficiency. Use caution with MAO inhibitors.

This combination should be used with caution in elderly or debilitated patients, hypotension, adrenocortical insufficiency, thyroid disorders, prostatic hyperplasia, urethral stricture, seizure disorder, CNS depression, head injury or increased intracranial pressure. Causes sedation; caution must be used in performing tasks which require alertness (eg, operating machinery or driving). Safety and efficacy in pediatric patients have not been established.

Drug Interactions

Acetaminophen: **Substrate** (minor) of CYP1A2, 2A6, 2C8/9, 2D6, 2E1, 3A4; **Inhibits** CYP3A4 (weak)

Caffeine: **Substrate** of CYP1A2 (major), 2C8/9 (minor), 2D6 (minor), 2E1 (minor), 3A4 (minor); **Inhibits** CYP1A2 (weak), 3A4 (moderate)

Dihydrocodeine: **Substrate** of CYP2D6 (major)

Acetaminophen: See individual monograph for associated interactions.

Caffeine:

CYP1A2 inhibitors: May increase the levels/effects of caffeine. Example inhibitors include amiodarone, fluvoxamine, ketoconazole, quinolone antibiotics, and rofecoxib.

CYP3A4 substrates: Caffeine may increase the levels/effects of CYP3A4 substrates. Example substrates include benzodiazepines, calcium channel blockers, ergot derivatives, mirtazapine, nateglinide, nefazodone, tacrolimus, and venlafaxine.

Quinolone antibiotics: Quinolones may increase the level/effects of caffeine.

(Continued)

Acetaminophen, Caffeine, and Dihydrocodeine *(Continued)*

Dihydrocodeine:

CYP2D6 inhibitors: May decrease the effects of dihydrocodeine. Example inhibitors include chlorpromazine, delavirdine, fluoxetine, miconazole, paroxetine, pergolide, quinidine, quinine, ritonavir, and ropinirole.

Quinidine: Quinidine may decrease the effects of dihydrocodeine.

Ethanol/Nutrition/Herb Interactions

Ethanol: Excessive intake of ethanol may increase the risk of acetaminophen-induced toxicity. Ethanol may also increase CNS depression.

Pregnancy Risk Factor C

Lactation Enters breast milk/not recommended

Breast-Feeding Considerations Acetaminophen and caffeine are both excreted in breast milk. Specific information for dihydrocodeine is not available; however, similar agents (eg, codeine, morphine) are excreted in breast milk.

Dosage Forms

Capsule (Panlor® DC): Acetaminophen 356.4 mg, caffeine 30 mg, and dihydrocodeine bitartrate 16 mg

Tablet (Panlor® SS): Acetaminophen 712.8 mg, caffeine 60 mg, and dihydrocodeine bitartrate 32 mg

Acetaminophen, Caffeine, Codeine, and Butalbital *see* Butalbital, Acetaminophen, Caffeine, and Codeine *on page 236*

Acetaminophen, Caffeine, Hydrocodone, Chlorpheniramine, and Phenylephrine *see* Hydrocodone, Chlorpheniramine, Phenylephrine, Acetaminophen, and Caffeine *on page 712*

Acetaminophen, Chlorpheniramine, and Pseudoephedrine

(a seet a MIN oh fen, klor fen IR a meen, & soo doe e FED rin)

Related Information

Acetaminophen *on page 47*

Pseudoephedrine *on page 1147*

U.S. Brand Names Actifed® Cold and Sinus [OTC]; Alka-Seltzer® Plus Cold Liqui-Gels® [OTC]; Children's Tylenol® Plus Cold [OTC]; Comtrex® Maximum Strength Sinus and Nasal Decongestant [OTC]; Sinutab® Sinus Allergy Maximum Strength [OTC]; Thera-Flu® Cold and Sore Throat Night Time [OTC]; Tylenol® Allergy Sinus [OTC]

Canadian Brand Names Sinutab® Sinus & Allergy; Tylenol® Allergy Sinus

Generic Available Yes

Synonyms Acetaminophen, Pseudoephedrine, and Chlorpheniramine; Chlorpheniramine, Acetaminophen, and Pseudoephedrine; Chlorpheniramine, Pseudoephedrine, and Acetaminophen; Pseudoephedrine, Acetaminophen, and Chlorpheniramine; Pseudoephedrine, Chlorpheniramine, and Acetaminophen

Pharmacologic Category Analgesic, Miscellaneous; Antihistamine

Use Temporary relief of sinus symptoms

Local Anesthetic/Vasoconstrictor Precautions Use with caution since pseudoephedrine is a sympathomimetic amine which could interact with epinephrine to cause a pressor response

Effects on Dental Treatment Key adverse event(s) related to dental treatment:

Chlorpheniramine: Significant xerostomia with prolonged use (normal salivary flow resumes upon discontinuation).

Pseudoephedrine: Xerostomia (normal salivary flow resumes upon discontinuation).

Common Adverse Effects See individual agents.

Drug Interactions

Cytochrome P450 Effect:

Acetaminophen: **Substrate** (minor) of CYP1A2, 2A6, 2C8/9, 2D6, 2E1, 3A4; **Inhibits** CYP3A4 (weak)

Chlorpheniramine: **Substrate** of CYP2D6 (minor), 3A4 (major); **Inhibits** CYP2D6 (weak)

Pharmacodynamics/Kinetics See individual agents.

Pregnancy Risk Factor B

Acetaminophen, Dextromethorphan, and Pseudoephedrine

(a seet a MIN oh fen, deks troe meth OR fan, & soo doe e FED rin)

Related Information

Acetaminophen *on page 47*
Dextromethorphan *on page 421*
Pseudoephedrine *on page 1147*

U.S. Brand Names Alka-Seltzer® Plus Flu Liqui-Gels® [OTC]; Comtrex® Non-Drowsy Cold and Cough Relief [OTC]; Contac® Severe Cold and Flu/ Non-Drowsy [OTC]; Infants' Tylenol® Cold Plus Cough Concentrated Drops [OTC]; Sudafed® Severe Cold [OTC]; Thera-Flu® Severe Cold Non-Drowsy [OTC] [DSC]; Triaminic® Cough and Sore Throat Formula [OTC]; Tylenol® Cold Day Non-Drowsy [OTC]; Tylenol® Flu Non-Drowsy Maximum Strength [OTC]; Vicks® DayQuil® Multi-Symptom Cold and Flu [OTC]

Canadian Brand Names Contac® Cough, Cold and Flu Day & Night™; Sudafed® Cold & Cough Extra Strength; Tylenol® Cold Daytime

Generic Available Yes

Synonyms Dextromethorphan, Acetaminophen, and Pseudoephedrine; Pseudoephedrine, Acetaminophen, and Dextromethorphan; Pseudoephedrine, Dextromethorphan, and Acetaminophen

Pharmacologic Category Antihistamine; Antitussive

Use Treatment of mild to moderate pain and fever; symptomatic relief of cough and congestion

Local Anesthetic/Vasoconstrictor Precautions Use with caution since pseudoephedrine is a sympathomimetic amine which could interact with epinephrine to cause a pressor response

Effects on Dental Treatment Key adverse event(s) related to dental treatment: Pseudoephedrine: Xerostomia (normal salivary flow resumes upon discontinuation).

Common Adverse Effects See individual agents.

Drug Interactions

Cytochrome P450 Effect:

Acetaminophen: **Substrate** (minor) of CYP1A2, 2A6, 2C8/9, 2D6, 2E1, 3A4; **Inhibits** CYP3A4 (weak)

Dextromethorphan: **Substrate** of CYP2B6 (minor), 2C8/9 (minor), 2C19 (minor), 2D6 (major), 2E1 (minor), 3A4 (minor); **Inhibits** CYP2D6 (weak)

Pharmacodynamics/Kinetics See individual agents.

Acetaminophen, Dichloralphenazone, and Isometheptene *see* Acetaminophen, Isometheptene, and Dichloralphenazone *on page 59*

Acetaminophen, Isometheptene, and Dichloralphenazone

(a seet a MIN oh fen, eye soe me THEP teen, & dye KLOR al FEN a zone)

Related Information

Acetaminophen *on page 47*

U.S. Brand Names I.D.A.; Midrin®; Migrin-A

Generic Available Yes

Synonyms Acetaminophen, Dichloralphenazone, and Isometheptene; Dichloralphenazone, Acetaminophen, and Isometheptene; Dichloralphenazone, Isometheptene, and Acetaminophen; Isometheptene, Acetaminophen, and Dichloralphenazone; Isometheptene, Dichloralphenazone, and Acetaminophen

Pharmacologic Category Analgesic, Miscellaneous

Use Relief of migraine and tension headache

Local Anesthetic/Vasoconstrictor Precautions No information available to require special precautions

Effects on Dental Treatment No significant effects or complications reported

Common Adverse Effects Frequency not defined.

Central nervous system: Transient dizziness
Dermatological: Rash

Restrictions C-IV

Drug Interactions

Cytochrome P450 Effect: Acetaminophen: **Substrate** (minor) of CYP1A2, 2A6, 2C8/9, 2D6, 2E1, 3A4; **Inhibits** CYP3A4 (weak)

Pregnancy Risk Factor B

Acetaminophen, Pseudoephedrine, and Chlorpheniramine *see* Acetaminophen, Chlorpheniramine, and Pseudoephedrine *on page 58*

Acetasol® HC *see* Acetic Acid, Propylene Glycol Diacetate, and Hydrocortisone *on page 60*

AcetaZOLAMIDE (a set a ZOLE a mide)

U.S. Brand Names Diamox® Sequels®

Canadian Brand Names Apo-Acetazolamide®; Diamox®

Mexican Brand Names Acetadiazol®

Generic Available Yes: Injection, tablet

Pharmacologic Category Anticonvulsant, Miscellaneous; Carbonic Anhydrase Inhibitor; Diuretic, Carbonic Anhydrase Inhibitor; Ophthalmic Agent, Antiglaucoma

Use Treatment of glaucoma (chronic simple open-angle, secondary glaucoma, preoperatively in acute angle-closure); drug-induced edema or edema due to congestive heart failure (adjunctive therapy); centrencephalic epilepsies (immediate release dosage form); prevention or amelioration of symptoms associated with acute mountain sickness

Unlabeled/Investigational Use Urine alkalinization; respiratory stimulant in COPD

Local Anesthetic/Vasoconstrictor Precautions No information available to require special precautions

Effects on Dental Treatment Key adverse event(s) related to dental treatment: Metallic taste (resolves upon discontinuation).

Mechanism of Action Reversible inhibition of the enzyme carbonic anhydrase resulting in reduction of hydrogen ion secretion at renal tubule and an increased renal excretion of sodium, potassium, bicarbonate, and water to decrease production of aqueous humor; also inhibits carbonic anhydrase in central nervous system to retard abnormal and excessive discharge from CNS neurons

Pregnancy Risk Factor C

Acetic Acid, Hydrocortisone, and Propylene Glycol Diacetate *see* Acetic Acid, Propylene Glycol Diacetate, and Hydrocortisone *on page 60*

Acetic Acid, Propylene Glycol Diacetate, and Hydrocortisone

(a SEE tik AS id, PRO pa leen GLY kole dye AS e tate, & hye droe KOR ti sone)

Related Information

Hydrocortisone *on page 714*

U.S. Brand Names Acetasol® HC; VōSoL® HC

Canadian Brand Names VōSoL® HC

Generic Available Yes

Synonyms Acetic Acid, Hydrocortisone, and Propylene Glycol Diacetate; Hydrocortisone, Acetic Acid, and Propylene Glycol Diacetate; Hydrocortisone, Propylene Glycol Diacetate, and Acetic Acid; Propylene Glycol Diacetate, Acetic Acid, and Hydrocortisone; Propylene Glycol Diacetate, Hydrocortisone, and Acetic Acid

Pharmacologic Category Otic Agent, Anti-infective

Use Treatment of superficial infections of the external auditory canal caused by organisms susceptible to the action of the antimicrobial, complicated by swelling

Local Anesthetic/Vasoconstrictor Precautions No information available to require special precautions

Effects on Dental Treatment No significant effects or complications reported

AcetoHEXAMIDE (a set oh HEKS a mide)

Related Information

Endocrine Disorders and Pregnancy *on page 1481*

Generic Available Yes

Synonyms Dymelor [DSC]

Pharmacologic Category Antidiabetic Agent, Sulfonylurea

Use Adjunct to diet for the management of mild to moderately severe, stable, type 2 diabetes mellitus (noninsulin dependent, NIDDM)

Local Anesthetic/Vasoconstrictor Precautions No information available to require special precautions

Effects on Dental Treatment Key adverse event(s) related to dental treatment: Use salicylates with caution in patients taking acetohexamide due to potential increased hypoglycemia. NSAIDs such as ibuprofen, naproxen, and others may be safely used. Acetohexamide-dependent diabetics (noninsulin-dependent, type 1) should be appointed for dental treatment in mornings to minimize chance of stress-induced hypoglycemia.

Mechanism of Action Believed to cause hypoglycemia by stimulating insulin release from the pancreatic beta cells; reduces glucose output from the liver (decreases gluconeogenesis); insulin sensitivity is increased at peripheral target sites (alters receptor sensitivity/receptor density); potentiates effects of ADH; may produce mild diuresis and significant uricosuric activity

Pregnancy Risk Factor D

Acetohydroxamic Acid (a SEE toe hye droks am ik AS id)

U.S. Brand Names Lithostat®

Canadian Brand Names Lithostat®

Generic Available No

Synonyms AHA

Pharmacologic Category Urinary Tract Product

Use Adjunctive therapy in chronic urea-splitting urinary infection

Local Anesthetic/Vasoconstrictor Precautions No information available to require special precautions

Effects on Dental Treatment No significant effects or complications reported

Pregnancy Risk Factor X

Acetoxymethylprogesterone *see* MedroxyPROGESTERone *on page 862*

Acetylcholine (a se teel KOE leen)

U.S. Brand Names Miochol-E®

Canadian Brand Names Miochol-E®

Generic Available No

Synonyms Acetylcholine Chloride

Pharmacologic Category Cholinergic Agonist; Ophthalmic Agent, Miotic

Use Produces complete miosis in cataract surgery, keratoplasty, iridectomy and other anterior segment surgery where rapid miosis is required

Local Anesthetic/Vasoconstrictor Precautions No information available to require special precautions

Effects on Dental Treatment No significant effects or complications reported

Mechanism of Action Causes contraction of the sphincter muscles of the iris, resulting in miosis and contraction of the ciliary muscle, leading to accommodation spasm

Pregnancy Risk Factor C

Acetylcholine Chloride *see* Acetylcholine *on page 61*

Acetylcysteine (a se teel SIS teen)

U.S. Brand Names Acetadote®; Mucomyst®

Canadian Brand Names Mucomyst®; Parvolex®

Generic Available Yes: Solution for inhalation

Synonyms Acetylcysteine Sodium; Mercapturic Acid; NAC; *N*-Acetylcysteine; *N*-Acetyl-L-cysteine

Pharmacologic Category Antidote; Mucolytic Agent

Use Adjunctive mucolytic therapy in patients with abnormal or viscid mucous secretions in acute and chronic bronchopulmonary diseases; pulmonary complications of surgery and cystic fibrosis; diagnostic bronchial studies; antidote for acute acetaminophen toxicity

Unlabeled/Investigational Use Prevention of radiocontrast-induced renal dysfunction (oral); distal intestinal obstruction syndrome (DIOS, previously referred to as meconium ileus equivalent)

Local Anesthetic/Vasoconstrictor Precautions No information available to require special precautions

Effects on Dental Treatment Key adverse event(s) related to dental treatment: Stomatitis, drowsiness, fever, vomiting, nausea, bronchospasm, rhinorrhea, hemoptysis, and dizziness.

Common Adverse Effects

Inhalation: Frequency not defined.

Central nervous system: Drowsiness, chills, fever

Gastrointestinal: Vomiting, nausea, stomatitis

Local: Irritation, stickiness on face following nebulization

Respiratory: Bronchospasm, rhinorrhea, hemoptysis

Miscellaneous: Acquired sensitization (rare), clamminess, unpleasant odor during administration

Intravenous:

>10%: Miscellaneous: Anaphylactoid reaction (~17%; reported as severe in 1% or moderate in 10% of patients within 15 minutes of first infusion; severe in 1% or mild-to-moderate in 6% to 7% of patients after 60 minute-infusion)

(Continued)

Acetylcysteine *(Continued)*

1% to 10%:

Cardiovascular: Angioedema (2% to 8%), vasodilation (1% to 6%), hypotension (1% to 4%), tachycardia (1% to 4%), syncope (1% to 3%), chest tightness (1%), flushing (1%)

Central nervous system: Dysphoria (<1% to 2%)

Dermatologic: Urticaria (2% to 7%), rash (1% to 5%), facial erythema (≤1%), palmar erythema (≤1%), pruritus (≤1% to 3%), pruritus with rash and vasodilation (2% to 9%)

Gastrointestinal: Vomiting (<1% to 10%), nausea (1% to 10%), dyspepsia (≤1%)

Neuromuscular & skeletal: Gait disturbance (<1% to 2%)

Ocular: Eye pain (<1% to 3%)

Otic: Ear pain (1%)

Respiratory: Bronchospasm (1% to 6%), cough (1% to 4%), dyspnea (<1% to 3%), pharyngitis (1%), rhinorrhea (1%), rhonchi (1%), throat tightness (1%)

Miscellaneous: Diaphoresis (≤1%)

Mechanism of Action Exerts mucolytic action through its free sulfhydryl group which opens up the disulfide bonds in the mucoproteins thus lowering mucous viscosity. The exact mechanism of action in acetaminophen toxicity is unknown; thought to act by providing substrate for conjugation with the toxic metabolite.

Drug Interactions

Decreased Effect: Adsorbed by activated charcoal; clinical significance is minimal, though, once a pure acetaminophen ingestion requiring N-acetylcysteine is established; further charcoal dosing is unnecessary once the appropriate initial charcoal dose is achieved (5-10 g:g acetaminophen)

Pharmacodynamics/Kinetics

Onset of action: Inhalation: 5-10 minutes

Duration: Inhalation: >1 hour

Distribution: 0.47 L/kg

Protein binding, plasma: 83%

Half-life elimination:

Reduced acetylcysteine: 2 hours

Total acetylcysteine: Adults: 5.5 hours; Newborns: 11 hours

Time to peak, plasma: Oral: 1-2 hours

Excretion: Urine

Pregnancy Risk Factor B

Acetylcysteine Sodium *see* Acetylcysteine *on page 61*

Acetylsalicylic Acid *see* Aspirin *on page 151*

Achromycin *see* Tetracycline *on page 1280*

Aciclovir *see* Acyclovir *on page 64*

Acidulated Phosphate Fluoride *see* Fluoride *on page 603*

Aciphex® *see* Rabeprazole *on page 1164*

Aclovate® *see* Alclometasone *on page 74*

4-(9-Acridinylamino) Methanesulfon-m-Anisidide *see* Amsacrine *on page 129*

Acridinyl Anisidide *see* Amsacrine *on page 129*

Acrivastine and Pseudoephedrine

(AK ri vas teen & soo doe e FED rin)

Related Information

Pseudoephedrine *on page 1147*

U.S. Brand Names Semprex®-D

Generic Available No

Synonyms Pseudoephedrine and Acrivastine

Pharmacologic Category Antihistamine

Use Temporary relief of nasal congestion, decongest sinus openings, running nose, itching of nose or throat, and itchy, watery eyes due to hay fever or other upper respiratory allergies

Local Anesthetic/Vasoconstrictor Precautions Use with caution since pseudoephedrine is a sympathomimetic amine which could interact with epinephrine to cause a pressor response

Effects on Dental Treatment Key adverse event(s) related to dental treatment: Pseudoephedrine: Xerostomia (normal salivary flow resumes upon discontinuation).

Common Adverse Effects

>10%: Central nervous system: Drowsiness, headache

1% to 10%:

Cardiovascular: Tachycardia, palpitations

Central nervous system: Nervousness, dizziness, insomnia, vertigo, lightheadedness, fatigue

Gastrointestinal: Nausea, vomiting, xerostomia, diarrhea

Genitourinary: Dysuria

Neuromuscular & skeletal: Weakness

Respiratory: Pharyngitis, cough increase

Miscellaneous: Diaphoresis

Mechanism of Action Refer to Pseudoephedrine monograph; acrivastine is an analogue of triprolidine and it is considered to be relatively less sedating than traditional antihistamines; believed to involve competitive blockade of H_1-receptor sites resulting in the inability of histamine to combine with its receptor sites and exert its usual effects on target cells

Drug Interactions

Increased Effect/Toxicity: Increased risk of hypertensive crisis when acrivastine and pseudoephedrine are given with MAO inhibitors or sympathomimetics. Increased risk of severe CNS depression when given with CNS depressants and ethanol.

Decreased Effect: Decreased effect of guanethidine, reserpine, methyldopa, and beta-blockers when given in conjunction with acrivastine and pseudoephedrine.

Pharmacodynamics/Kinetics

Pseudoephedrine: See Pseudoephedrine monograph.

Acrivastine:

Metabolism: Minimally hepatic

Time to peak: ~1.1 hours

Excretion: Urine (84%); feces (13%)

Pregnancy Risk Factor B

ACT *see* Dactinomycin *on page 394*

ACT® [OTC] *see* Fluoride *on page 603*

Act-D *see* Dactinomycin *on page 394*

ACTH *see* Corticotropin *on page 376*

ActHIB® *see* *Haemophilus* b Conjugate Vaccine *on page 680*

Acticin® *see* Permethrin *on page 1070*

Actidose-Aqua® [OTC] *see* Charcoal *on page 303*

Actidose® with Sorbitol [OTC] *see* Charcoal *on page 303*

Actifed® Cold and Allergy [OTC] *see* Triprolidine and Pseudoephedrine *on page 1345*

Actifed® Cold and Sinus [OTC] *see* Acetaminophen, Chlorpheniramine, and Pseudoephedrine *on page 58*

Actigall® *see* Ursodiol *on page 1354*

Actimmune® *see* Interferon Gamma-1b *on page 758*

Actinomycin *see* Dactinomycin *on page 394*

Actinomycin Cl *see* Dactinomycin *on page 394*

Actinomycin D *see* Dactinomycin *on page 394*

Actiq® *see* Fentanyl *on page 581*

Actisite® *see* Tetracycline (Periodontal) *on page 1282*

Activase® *see* Alteplase *on page 88*

Activated Carbon *see* Charcoal *on page 303*

Activated Charcoal *see* Charcoal *on page 303*

Activated Dimethicone *see* Simethicone *on page 1222*

Activated Ergosterol *see* Ergocalciferol *on page 503*

Activated Methylpolysiloxane *see* Simethicone *on page 1222*

Activated Protein C, Human, Recombinant *see* Drotrecogin Alfa *on page 478*

Activella™ *see* Estradiol and Norethindrone *on page 521*

Actonel® *see* Risedronate *on page 1185*

Actos® *see* Pioglitazone *on page 1091*

ACU-dyne® [OTC] *see* Povidone-Iodine *on page 1107*

Acular® *see* Ketorolac *on page 787*

Acular LS™ *see* Ketorolac *on page 787*

Acular® PF *see* Ketorolac *on page 787*

ACV *see* Acyclovir *on page 64*

Acycloguanosine *see* Acyclovir *on page 64*

Acyclovir (ay SYE kloe veer)

Related Information

Oral Viral Infections *on page 1547*
Sexually-Transmitted Diseases *on page 1504*
Systemic Viral Diseases *on page 1519*
Valacyclovir *on page 1354*

U.S. Brand Names Zovirax®

Canadian Brand Names Alti-Acyclovir; Apo-Acyclovir®; Gen-Acyclovir; Nu-Acyclovir; ratio-Acyclovir; Zovirax®

Mexican Brand Names Acifur®; Cicloferon®; Isavir®; Laciken®; Opthavir®; Zovirax®

Generic Available Yes: Excludes cream, ointment

Synonyms Aciclovir; ACV; Acycloguanosine

Pharmacologic Category Antiviral Agent

Dental Use Treatment of initial and prophylaxis of recurrent mucosal and cutaneous herpes simplex (HSV-1 and HSV-2) infections

Use Treatment of genital herpes simplex virus (HSV), herpes labialis (cold sores), herpes zoster (shingles), HSV encephalitis, neonatal HSV, mucocutaneous HSV, varicella-zoster (chickenpox)

Unlabeled/Investigational Use Prevention of HSV reactivation in HIV positive patients; prevention of HSV reactivation in hematopoietic stem cell transplant (HSCT); prevention of CMV infection after bone marrow transplants in HSV and CMV seropositive individuals

Local Anesthetic/Vasoconstrictor Precautions No information available to require special precautions

Effects on Dental Treatment Key adverse event(s) related to dental treatment: Topical (Zovirax® cream): Dry/cracked lips and dry/flaky skin were reported in fewer than 1 in 100 patients in clinical studies.

Significant Adverse Effects

Systemic: Oral:

1% to 10%:

- Central nervous system: Lightheadedness, headache
- Gastrointestinal: Diarrhea, nausea, vomiting, abdominal pain

Systemic: Parenteral:

>10%:

- Central nervous system: Lightheadedness
- Gastrointestinal: Anorexia

1% to 10%:

- Dermatologic: Hives, itching, rash
- Gastrointestinal: Nausea, vomiting
- Hepatic: Liver function tests increased
- Local: Inflammation at injection site or phlebitis
- Renal: Acute renal failure, BUN increased, creatinine increased

Topical:

>10%: Mild pain, burning, or stinging

1% to 10%: Itching

All forms: <1% (Limited to important or life-threatening): Abdominal pain, aggression, alopecia, anaphylaxis, anemia, angioedema, ataxia, coma, confusion, consciousness decreased, delirium, dizziness, dysarthria, encephalopathy, erythema multiforme, fatigue, fever, gastrointestinal distress, hallucinations, hepatitis, hyperbilirubinemia, jaundice, leukocytoclastic vasculitis, leukopenia, local tissue necrosis (following extravasation), mental depression, paresthesia, peripheral edema, photosensitization, pruritus, psychosis, renal failure, seizures, somnolence, Stevens-Johnson syndrome, thrombocytopenia, thrombocytopenic purpura/hemolytic uremic syndrome (TTP/HUS), toxic epidermal necrolysis, tremors, urticaria

Dosage Note: Obese patients should be dosed using ideal body weight

Genital HSV:

I.V.: Children ≥12 years and Adults (immunocompetent): Initial episode, severe: 5 mg/kg every 8 hours for 5-7 days

Oral:

Children:

Initial episode (unlabeled use): 40-80 mg/kg/day divided into 3-4 doses for 5-10 days (maximum: 1 g/day)

Chronic suppression (unlabeled use; limited data): 80 mg/kg/day in 3 divided doses (maximum: 1 g/day), re-evaluate after 12 months of treatment

Adults:

Initial episode: 200 mg every 4 hours while awake (5 times/day) for 10 days (per manufacturer's labeling); 400 mg 3 times/day for 5-10 days has also been reported

Recurrence: 200 mg every 4 hours while awake (5 times/day) for 5 days (per manufacturer's labeling; begin at earliest signs of disease); 400 mg 3 times/day for 5 days has also been reported

Chronic suppression: 400 mg twice daily or 200 mg 3-5 times/day, for up to 12 months followed by re-evaluation (per manufacturer's labeling); 400-1200 mg/day in 2-3 divided doses has also been reported

Topical: Adults (immunocompromised): Ointment: Initial episode: $^1/_2$" ribbon of ointment for a 4" square surface area every 3 hours (6 times/day) for 7 days

Herpes labialis (cold sores): Topical: Children ≥12 years and Adults: Cream: Apply 5 times/day for 4 days

Herpes zoster (shingles):

Oral: Adults (immunocompetent): 800 mg every 4 hours (5 times/day) for 7-10 days

I.V.:

Children <12 years (immunocompromised): 20 mg/kg/dose every 8 hours for 7 days

Children ≥12 years and Adults (immunocompromised): 10 mg/kg/dose or 500 mg/m^2/dose every 8 hours for 7 days

HSV encephalitis: I.V.:

Children 3 months to 12 years: 20 mg/kg/dose every 8 hours for 10 days (per manufacturer's labeling); dosing for 14-21 days also reported

Children ≥12 years and Adults: 10 mg/kg/dose every 8 hours for 10 days (per manufacturer's labeling); 10-15 mg/kg/dose every 8 hours for 14-21 days also reported

Mucocutaneous HSV:

I.V.:

Children <12 years (immunocompromised): 10 mg/kg/dose every 8 hours for 7 days

Children ≥12 years and Adults (immunocompromised): 5 mg/kg/dose every 8 hours for 7 days (per manufacturer's labeling); dosing for up to 14 days also reported

Oral: Adults (immunocompromised, unlabeled use): 400 mg 5 times a day for 7-14 days

Topical: Ointment: Adults (nonlife-threatening, immunocompromised): $^1/_2$" ribbon of ointment for a 4" square surface area every 3 hours (6 times/day) for 7 days

Neonatal HSV: I.V.: Neonate: Birth to 3 months: 10 mg/kg/dose every 8 hours for 10 days (manufacturer's labeling); 15 mg/kg/dose or 20 mg/kg/dose every 8 hours for 14-21 days has also been reported

Varicella-zoster (chickenpox): Begin treatment within the first 24 hours of rash onset:

Oral:

Children ≥2 years and ≤40 kg (immunocompetent): 20 mg/kg/dose (up to 800 mg/dose) 4 times/day for 5 days

Children >40 kg and Adults (immunocompetent): 800 mg/dose 4 times a day for 5 days

I.V.:

Children <1 year (immunocompromised, unlabeled use): 10 mg/kg/dose every 8 hours for 7-10 days

Children ≥1 year and Adults (immunocompromised, unlabeled use): 1500 mg/m^2/day divided every 8 hours or 10 mg/kg/dose every 8 hours for 7-10 days

Prevention of HSV reactivation in HIV-positive patients, for use only when recurrences are frequent or severe (unlabeled use): Oral:

Children: 80 mg/kg/day in 3-4 divided doses

Adults: 200 mg 3 times/day or 400 mg 2 times/day

Prevention of HSV reactivation in HSCT (unlabeled use): Note: Start at the beginning of conditioning therapy and continue until engraftment or until mucositis resolves (~30 days)

Oral: Adults: 200 mg 3 times/day

I.V.:

Children: 250 mg/m^2/dose every 8 hours or 125 mg/m^2/dose every 6 hours

Adults: 250 mg/m^2/dose every 12 hours

(Continued)

Acyclovir *(Continued)*

Bone marrow transplant recipients (unlabeled use): I.V.: Children and Adults: Allogeneic patients who are HSV and CMV seropositive: 500 mg/m^2/dose (10 mg/kg) every 8 hours; for clinically-symptomatic CMV infection, consider replacing acyclovir with ganciclovir

Dosing adjustment in renal impairment:

Oral:

Cl_{cr} 10-25 mL/minute: Normal dosing regimen 800 mg every 4 hours: Administer 800 mg every 8 hours

Cl_{cr} <10 mL/minute:

Normal dosing regimen 200 mg every 4 hours, 200 mg every 8 hours, or 400 mg every 12 hours: Administer 200 mg every 12 hours

Normal dosing regimen 800 mg every 4 hours: Administer 800 mg every 12 hours

I.V.:

Cl_{cr} 25-50 mL/minute: Administer recommended dose every 12 hours

Cl_{cr} 10-25 mL/minute: Administer recommended dose every 24 hours

Cl_{cr} <10 mL/minute: Administer 50% of recommended dose every 24 hours

Hemodialysis: Administer dose after dialysis

Peritoneal dialysis: No supplemental dose needed

CAVH: 3.5 mg/kg/day

CVVHD/CVVH: Adjust dose based upon Cl_{cr} 30 mL/minute

Mechanism of Action Acyclovir is converted to acyclovir monophosphate by virus-specific thymidine kinase then further converted to acyclovir triphosphate by other cellular enzymes. Acyclovir triphosphate inhibits DNA synthesis and viral replication by competing with deoxyguanosine triphosphate for viral DNA polymerase and being incorporated into viral DNA.

Contraindications Hypersensitivity to acyclovir, valacyclovir, or any component of the formulation

Warnings/Precautions Use with caution in immunocompromised patients; thrombocytopenic purpura/hemolytic uremic syndrome (TTP/HUS) has been reported. Use caution in the elderly, pre-existing renal disease or in those receiving other nephrotoxic drugs. Maintain adequate hydration during I.V. therapy. Use I.V. preparation with caution in patients with underlying neurologic abnormalities, serious hepatic or electrolyte abnormalities, or substantial hypoxia.

Chickenpox: Treatment should begin within 24 hours of appearance of rash; oral route not recommended for routine use in otherwise healthy children with varicella, but may be effective in patients at increased risk of moderate to severe infection (>12 years of age, chronic cutaneous or pulmonary disorders, long-term salicylate therapy, corticosteroid therapy).

Genital herpes: Physical contact should be avoided when lesions are present; transmission may also occur in the absence of symptoms. Treatment should begin with the first signs or symptoms.

Herpes labialis: For external use only to the lips and face; do not apply to eye or inside the mouth or nose. Treatment should begin with the first signs or symptoms.

Herpes zoster: Acyclovir should be started within 72 hours of appearance of rash to be effective.

Drug Interactions Increased CNS side effects with zidovudine and probenecid

Ethanol/Nutrition/Herb Interactions Food: Does not appear to affect absorption of acyclovir.

Dietary Considerations May be taken with or without food. Acyclovir 500 mg injection contains sodium ~50 mg (~2 mEq).

Pharmacodynamics/Kinetics

Absorption: Oral: 15% to 30%

Distribution: Widely (ie, brain, kidney, lungs, liver, spleen, muscle, uterus, vagina, CSF)

Protein binding: 9% to 33%

Metabolism: Converted by viral enzymes to acyclovir monophosphate, and further converted to diphosphate then triphosphate (active form) by cellular enzymes

Bioavailability: Oral: 10% to 20% with normal renal function (bioavailability decreases with increased dose)

Half-life elimination: Terminal: Neonates: 4 hours; Children 1-12 years: 2-3 hours; Adults: 3 hours

Time to peak, serum: Oral: Within 1.5-2 hours

Excretion: Urine (62% to 90% as unchanged drug and metabolite)

Pregnancy Risk Factor B

Lactation Enters breast milk/use with caution (AAP rates "compatible")

Breast-Feeding Considerations Nursing mothers with herpetic lesions near or on the breast should avoid breast-feeding.

Dosage Forms

Capsule: 200 mg
Cream, topical: 5% (2 g)
Injection, powder for reconstitution, as sodium: 500 mg, 1000 mg
Injection, solution, as sodium [preservative free]: 25 mg/mL (20 mL, 40 mL); 50 mg/mL (10 mL, 20 mL)
Ointment, topical: 5% (3 g, 15 g)
Suspension, oral: 200 mg/5 mL (480 mL) [banana flavor]
Tablet: 400 mg, 800 mg

AD3L *see* Valrubicin *on page 1362*

Adagen® *see* Pegademase Bovine *on page 1050*

Adalat® CC *see* NIFEdipine *on page 984*

Adalimumab (a da LIM yoo mab)

Related Information

Rheumatoid Arthritis, Osteoarthritis, and Osteoporosis *on page 1490*

U.S. Brand Names Humira™

Generic Available No

Synonyms Antitumor Necrosis Factor Apha (Human); D2E7; Human Antitumor Necrosis Factor-alpha

Pharmacologic Category Antirheumatic, Disease Modifying; Monoclonal Antibody

Use Treatment of active rheumatoid arthritis (moderate to severe) in patients with inadequate response to one or more disease-modifying antirheumatic drugs (DMARDs)

Local Anesthetic/Vasoconstrictor Precautions No information available to require special precautions

Effects on Dental Treatment No significant effects or complications reported

Common Adverse Effects

>10%:
- Central nervous system: Headache (12%)
- Dermatologic: Rash (12%)
- Respiratory: Upper respiratory tract infection (17%), sinusitis (11%)

5% to 10%:
- Cardiovascular: Hypertension (5%)
- Endocrine & metabolic: Hyperlipidemia (7%), hypercholesterolemia (6%)
- Gastrointestinal: Nausea (9%), abdominal pain (7%)
- Genitourinary: Urinary tract infection (8%)
- Local: Injection site reaction (8%)
- Neuromuscular & skeletal: Back pain (6%)
- Renal: Hematuria (5%)
- Miscellaneous: Accidental injury (10%), flu-like syndrome (7%)

Mechanism of Action Adalimumab is a recombinant monoclonal antibody that binds to human tumor necrosis factor alpha (TNF-alpha) receptor sites, thereby interfering with endogenous TNF-alpha activity. Elevated TNF levels in the synovial fluid are involved in the pathologic pain and joint destruction in rheumatoid arthritis. Adalimumab decreases signs and symptoms of rheumatoid arthritis and inhibits progression of structural damage.

Pharmacodynamics/Kinetics

Distribution: V_d: 4.7-6 L; Synovial fluid concentrations: 31% to 95% of serum
Bioavailability: Absolute: 64%
Half-life elimination: Terminal: ~2 weeks (range 10-20 days)
Time to peak, serum: SubQ: 131 ± 56 hours
Excretion: Clearance increased in the presence of anti-adalimumab antibodies; decreased in patients 40 to >75 years

Pregnancy Risk Factor B

Adamantanamine Hydrochloride *see* Amantadine *on page 92*

Adapalene (a DAP a leen)

U.S. Brand Names Differin®

Canadian Brand Names Differin®

Mexican Brand Names Adaferin®

Generic Available No

Pharmacologic Category Acne Products

Use Treatment of acne vulgaris

Local Anesthetic/Vasoconstrictor Precautions No information available to require special precautions

(Continued)

Adapalene *(Continued)*

Effects on Dental Treatment No significant effects or complications reported

Common Adverse Effects >10%: Dermatologic: Erythema, scaling, dryness, pruritus, burning, pruritus or burning immediately after application

Mechanism of Action Retinoid-like compound which is a modulator of cellular differentiation, keratinization and inflammatory processes, all of which represent important features in the pathology of acne vulgaris

Pharmacodynamics/Kinetics

Absorption: Topical: Minimal

Excretion: Bile

Pregnancy Risk Factor C

Adderall® *see* Dextroamphetamine and Amphetamine *on page 419*

Adderall XR™ *see* Dextroamphetamine and Amphetamine *on page 419*

Adefovir (a DEF o veer)

Related Information

HIV Infection and AIDS *on page 1484*

U.S. Brand Names Hepsera™

Generic Available No

Synonyms Adefovir Dipivoxil

Pharmacologic Category Antiretroviral Agent, Reverse Transcriptase Inhibitor (Nucleoside)

Use Treatment of chronic hepatitis B with evidence of active viral replication (based on persistent elevation of ALT/AST or histologic evidence), including patients with lamivudine-resistant hepatitis B

Local Anesthetic/Vasoconstrictor Precautions No information available to require special precautions

Effects on Dental Treatment No significant effects or complications reported

Common Adverse Effects

>10%: Renal: Hematuria (11% vs. 10% in placebo-treated)

1% to 10%:

Central nervous system: Fever, headache,

Dermatologic: Rash, pruritus

Gastrointestinal: Dyspepsia (3%), nausea, vomiting, flatulence, diarrhea, abdominal pain

Hepatic: AST/ALT increased, abnormal liver function, hepatic failure

Neuromuscular & skeletal: Weakness

Renal: Serum creatinine increased (4%), renal failure, renal insufficiency

Note: In patients with baseline renal dysfunction, frequency of increased serum creatinine has been observed to be as high as 26% to 37%; the role of adefovir in these changes could not be established.

Respiratory: Cough increased, sinusitis, pharyngitis

Mechanism of Action Acyclic nucleotide reverse transcriptase inhibitor (adenosine analog) which interferes with HBV viral RNA dependent DNA polymerase resulting in inhibition of viral replication.

Drug Interactions

Increased Effect/Toxicity: Ibuprofen increases the bioavailability of adefovir. Concurrent use of nephrotoxic agents (including aminoglycosides, cyclosporine, NSAIDs, tacrolimus, vancomycin) may increase the risk of nephrotoxicity.

Pharmacodynamics/Kinetics

Distribution: 0.35-0.39 L/kg

Protein binding: ≤4%

Metabolism: Prodrug; rapidly converted to adefovir (active metabolite) in intestine

Bioavailability: 59%

Half-life elimination: 7.5 hours; prolonged in renal impairment

Time to peak: 1.75 hours

Excretion: Urine (45% as active metabolite within 24 hours)

Pregnancy Risk Factor C

Adefovir Dipivoxil *see* Adefovir *on page 68*

Adenine Arabinoside *see* Vidarabine *on page 1376*

Adenocard® *see* Adenosine *on page 68*

Adenoscan® *see* Adenosine *on page 68*

Adenosine (a DEN oh seen)

U.S. Brand Names Adenocard®; Adenoscan®

Canadian Brand Names Adenocard®

Generic Available No

Synonyms 9-Beta-D-ribofuranosyladenine

Pharmacologic Category Antiarrhythmic Agent, Class IV; Diagnostic Agent

Use

Adenocard®: Treatment of paroxysmal supraventricular tachycardia (PSVT) including that associated with accessory bypass tracts (Wolff-Parkinson-White syndrome); when clinically advisable, appropriate vagal maneuvers should be attempted prior to adenosine administration; **not effective in atrial flutter, atrial fibrillation, or ventricular tachycardia**

Adenoscan®: Pharmacologic stress agent used in myocardial perfusion thallium-201 scintigraphy

Local Anesthetic/Vasoconstrictor Precautions No information available to require special precautions

Effects on Dental Treatment No significant effects or complications reported

Mechanism of Action Slows conduction time through the AV node, interrupting the re-entry pathways through the AV node, restoring normal sinus rhythm

Pregnancy Risk Factor C

ADH *see* Vasopressin *on page 1369*

Adipex-P® *see* Phentermine *on page 1076*

Adoxa™ *see* Doxycycline *on page 471*

ADR *see* DOXOrubicin *on page 469*

Adrenalin® (Dental) *see* Epinephrine *on page 496*

Adrenocorticotropic Hormone *see* Corticotropin *on page 376*

Adria *see* DOXOrubicin *on page 469*

Adriamycin PFS® *see* DOXOrubicin *on page 469*

Adriamycin RDF® *see* DOXOrubicin *on page 469*

Adrucil® *see* Fluorouracil *on page 605*

Adsorbent Charcoal *see* Charcoal *on page 303*

Advair Diskus® *see* Fluticasone and Salmeterol *on page 619*

Advantage-S™ [OTC] *see* Nonoxynol 9 *on page 995*

Advate *see* Antihemophilic Factor (Recombinant) *on page 135*

Advicor™ *see* Niacin and Lovastatin *on page 979*

Advil® [OTC] *see* Ibuprofen *on page 728*

Advil® Children's [OTC] *see* Ibuprofen *on page 728*

Advil® Cold, Children's [OTC] *see* Pseudoephedrine and Ibuprofen *on page 1149*

Advil® Cold & Sinus [OTC] *see* Pseudoephedrine and Ibuprofen *on page 1149*

Advil® Infants' [OTC] *see* Ibuprofen *on page 728*

Advil® Junior [OTC] *see* Ibuprofen *on page 728*

Advil® Migraine [OTC] *see* Ibuprofen *on page 728*

AeroBid® *see* Flunisolide *on page 599*

AeroBid®-M *see* Flunisolide *on page 599*

Afrin® [OTC] *see* Oxymetazoline *on page 1034*

Afrin® Extra Moisturizing [OTC] *see* Oxymetazoline *on page 1034*

Afrin® Original [OTC] *see* Oxymetazoline *on page 1034*

Afrin® Severe Congestion [OTC] *see* Oxymetazoline *on page 1034*

Afrin® Sinus [OTC] *see* Oxymetazoline *on page 1034*

Aftate® Antifungal [OTC] *see* Tolnaftate *on page 1312*

AG *see* Aminoglutethimide *on page 98*

Agalsidase Beta (aye GAL si days BAY ta)

U.S. Brand Names Fabrazyme®

Generic Available No

Synonyms Alpha-Galactosidase-A (Human, Recombinant); r-h α-GAL

Pharmacologic Category Enzyme

Use Replacement therapy for Fabry disease

Local Anesthetic/Vasoconstrictor Precautions No information available to require special precautions

Effects on Dental Treatment No significant effects or complications reported

Common Adverse Effects Note: The most common and serious adverse reactions are infusion reactions (symptoms may include fever, tachycardia, hypertension, throat tightness, dyspnea, chills, abdominal pain, pruritus, urticaria, vomiting).

>10%:

Cardiovascular: Edema (21%), chest pain (17%), hypotension (14%)

Central nervous system: Fever (48%), headache (45%), anxiety (28%), pain (21%), dizziness (14%), paresthesia (14%)

(Continued)

Agalsidase Beta *(Continued)*

Dermatologic: Pallor (14%)
Gastrointestinal: Nausea (28%)
Miscellaneous: Infusion reactions (alteration of temperature sensation 17%)
Neuromuscular & skeletal: Rigors (52%), skeletal pain (21%)
Respiratory: Rhinitis (38%), pharyngitis (28%)

1% to 10%:
Cardiovascular: Cardiomegaly (10%), hypertension (10%)
Central nervous system: Depression (10%)
Gastrointestinal: Dyspepsia (10%)
Genitourinary: Testicular pain (7%)
Neuromuscular & skeletal: Arthrosis (10%)
Respiratory: Bronchitis (10%), bronchospasm (7%), laryngitis (7%), sinusitis (7%)

Other reported severe reactions (frequency not established): Arrhythmia, ataxia, bradycardia, cardiac arrest, cardiac output decreased, nephritic syndrome, stroke, vertigo

Mechanism of Action Agalsidase beta is a recombinant form of the enzyme alpha-galactosidase-A, which is required for the hydrolysis of GL-3 and other glycosphingolipids. The compounds may accumulate (over many years) within the tissues of patients with Fabry disease, leading to renal and cardiovascular complications. In clinical trials of limited duration, agalsidase been noted to reduce tissue inclusions of a key sphingolipid (GL-3). It is believed that long-term enzyme replacement may reduce clinical manifestations of renal failure, cardiomyopathy, and stroke. However, the relationship to a reduction in clinical manifestations has not been established.

Pharmacodynamics/Kinetics Half-life elimination: 42-102 minutes (nonlinear)

Pregnancy Risk Factor B

Agenerase® *see* Amprenavir *on page 128*
Aggrastat® *see* Tirofiban *on page 1304*
Aggrenox® *see* Aspirin and Dipyridamole *on page 156*
$AgNO_3$ *see* Silver Nitrate *on page 1221*
Agoral® Maximum Strength Laxative [OTC] *see* Senna *on page 1213*
Agrylin® *see* Anagrelide *on page 130*
AGT *see* Aminoglutethimide *on page 98*
AHA *see* Acetohydroxamic Acid *on page 61*
AH-Chew® *see* Chlorpheniramine, Phenylephrine, and Methscopolamine *on page 317*
AHF (Human) *see* Antihemophilic Factor (Human) *on page 134*
AHF (Porcine) *see* Antihemophilic Factor (Porcine) *on page 134*
AHF (Recombinant) *see* Antihemophilic Factor (Recombinant) *on page 135*
A-hydroCort® *see* Hydrocortisone *on page 714*
AK-Con™ *see* Naphazoline *on page 964*
AK-Dilate® *see* Phenylephrine *on page 1078*
Akineton® *see* Biperiden *on page 207*
AK-Nefrin® *see* Phenylephrine *on page 1078*
Akne-Mycin® *see* Erythromycin *on page 508*
AK-Pentolate® *see* Cyclopentolate *on page 383*
AK-Poly-Bac® *see* Bacitracin and Polymyxin B *on page 178*
AK-Pred® *see* PrednisoLONE *on page 1113*
AK-Rinse™ *see* Balanced Salt Solution *on page 181*
AK-Spore® H.C. [DSC] *see* Bacitracin, Neomycin, Polymyxin B, and Hydrocortisone *on page 179*
AK-Sulf® *see* Sulfacetamide *on page 1244*
AK-T-Caine™ *see* Tetracaine *on page 1278*
AKTob® *see* Tobramycin *on page 1306*
AK-Tracin® [DSC] *see* Bacitracin *on page 178*
AK-Trol® *see* Neomycin, Polymyxin B, and Dexamethasone *on page 974*
Akwa Tears® [OTC] *see* Artificial Tears *on page 148*
Alamag [OTC] *see* Aluminum Hydroxide and Magnesium Hydroxide *on page 91*
Alamag Plus [OTC] *see* Aluminum Hydroxide, Magnesium Hydroxide, and Simethicone *on page 92*
Alamast™ *see* Pemirolast *on page 1055*
Alatrofloxacin Mesylate *see* Trovafloxacin *on page 1348*
Alavert™ [OTC] *see* Loratadine *on page 841*

Alavert™ Allergy and Sinus [OTC] *see* Loratadine and Pseudoephedrine *on page 842*

Albalon® *see* Naphazoline *on page 964*

Albendazole (al BEN da zole)

U.S. Brand Names Albenza®

Mexican Brand Names Bendapar®; Digezanol®; Endoplus®; Eskazole®; Gascop®; Lurdex®; Zentel®

Generic Available No

Pharmacologic Category Anthelmintic

Use Treatment of parenchymal neurocysticercosis caused by *Taenia solium* and cystic hydatid disease of the liver, lung, and peritoneum caused by *Echinococcus granulosus*

Unlabeled/Investigational Use Albendazole has activity against *Ascaris lumbricoides* (roundworm); *Ancylostoma caninum*; *Ancylostoma duodenale* and *Necator americanus* (hookworms); cutaneous larva migrans; *Enterobius vermicularis* (pinworm); *Gnathostoma spinigerum; Gongylonema* sp; *Hymenolepis nana* sp (tapeworms); *Mansonella perstans* (filariasis); *Opisthorchis sinensis* and *Opisthorchis viverrini* (liver flukes); *Strongyloides stercoralis* and *Trichuris trichiura* (whipworm); visceral larva migrans (toxocariasis); activity has also been shown against the liver fluke *Clonorchis sinensis, Giardia lamblia, Cysticercus cellulosae,* and *Echinococcus multilocularis.* Albendazole has also been used for the treatment of intestinal microsporidiosis (*Encephalitozoon intestinalis*), disseminated microsporidiosis (*E. hellem, E. cuniculi, E. intestinalis, Pleistophora* sp, *Trachipleistophora* sp, *Brachiola vesicularum*), and ocular microsporidiosis (*E. hellem, E. cuniculi, Vittaforma corneae*).

Local Anesthetic/Vasoconstrictor Precautions No information available to require special precautions

Effects on Dental Treatment No significant effects or complications reported

Common Adverse Effects

N = Neurocysticercosis; H = Hydatid disease

>10:

- Central nervous system: Headache (11% - N; 1% - H)
- Hepatic: LFTs Increased (~15% - H; <1% - N)

1% to 10%:

- Central nervous system: Dizziness, vertigo, fever (≤1%); intracranial pressure increased (1% - N), meningeal signs (1% - N)
- Dermatologic: Alopecia (2% - H; <1% - N)
- Gastrointestinal: Abdominal pain (6% - H; 0% - N); nausea/vomiting (3% to 6%)
- Hematologic: Leukopenia (reversible) (<1%)
- Miscellaneous: Allergic reactions (<1%)

Mechanism of Action Active metabolite, albendazole, causes selective degeneration of cytoplasmic microtubules in intestinal and tegmental cells of intestinal helminths and larvae; glycogen is depleted, glucose uptake and cholinesterase secretion are impaired, and desecratory substances accumulate intracellulary. ATP production decreases causing energy depletion, immobilization, and worm death.

Drug Interactions

Cytochrome P450 Effect: Substrate (minor) of CYP1A2, 3A4; **Inhibits** CYP1A2 (weak)

Pharmacodynamics/Kinetics

Absorption: <5%; may increase up to 4-5 times when administered with a fatty meal

Distribution: Well inside hydatid cysts and CSF

Protein binding: 70%

Metabolism: Hepatic; extensive first-pass effect; pathways include rapid sulfoxidation (major), hydrolysis, and oxidation

Half-life elimination: 8-12 hours

Time to peak, serum: 2-2.4 hours

Excretion: Urine (<1% as active metabolite); feces

Pregnancy Risk Factor C

Albenza® *see* Albendazole *on page 71*

Albuterol (al BYOO ter ole)

Related Information

Dental Office Emergencies *on page 1584*

Ipratropium and Albuterol *on page 761*

Respiratory Diseases *on page 1478*

(Continued)

Albuterol *(Continued)*

U.S. Brand Names AccuNeb™; Proventil®; Proventil® HFA; Proventil® Repetabs®; Ventolin® [DSC]; Ventolin® HFA; Volmax®; VoSpire ER™

Canadian Brand Names Airomir; Alti-Salbutamol; Apo-Salvent®; Gen-Salbutamol; PMS-Salbutamol; ratio-Inspra-Sal; ratio-Salbutamol; Rhoxal-salbutamol; Salbu-2; Salbu-4; Ventolin®; Ventolin® Diskus; Ventolin® HFA; Ventrodisk

Mexican Brand Names Inspiryl®; Salbulin Autohaler®; Ventolin®; Volmax®

Generic Available Yes: Excludes extended release

Synonyms Albuterol Sulfate; Salbutamol

Pharmacologic Category Beta$_2$-Adrenergic Agonist

Use Bronchodilator in reversible airway obstruction due to asthma or COPD; prevention of exercise-induced bronchospasm

Local Anesthetic/Vasoconstrictor Precautions No information available to require special precautions

Effects on Dental Treatment Key adverse event(s) related to dental treatment: Xerostomia (normal salivary flow resumes upon discontinuation).

Common Adverse Effects Incidence of adverse effects is dependent upon age of patient, dose, and route of administration.

Cardiovascular: Angina, atrial fibrillation, chest discomfort, extrasystoles, flushing, hypertension, palpitations, tachycardia

Central nervous system: CNS stimulation, dizziness, drowsiness, headache, insomnia, irritability, lightheadedness, migraine, nervousness, nightmares, restlessness, sleeplessness, tremor

Dermatologic: Angioedema, erythema multiforme, rash, Stevens-Johnson syndrome, urticaria

Endocrine & metabolic: Hypokalemia, serum glucose increased, serum potassium decreased

Gastrointestinal: Diarrhea, dry mouth, gastroenteritis, nausea, unusual taste, vomiting, tooth discoloration

Genitourinary: Micturition difficulty

Neuromuscular & skeletal: Muscle cramps, weakness

Otic: Otitis media, vertigo

Respiratory: Asthma exacerbation, bronchospasm, cough, epistaxis, laryngitis, oropharyngeal drying/irritation, oropharyngeal edema

Miscellaneous: Allergic reaction, lymphadenopathy

Dosage

Oral:

- Children: Bronchospasm (treatment):
  - 2-6 years: 0.1-0.2 mg/kg/dose 3 times/day; maximum dose not to exceed 12 mg/day (divided doses)
  - 6-12 years: 2 mg/dose 3-4 times/day; maximum dose not to exceed 24 mg/day (divided doses)
    - Extended release: 4 mg every 12 hours; maximum dose not to exceed 24 mg/day (divided doses)
- Children >12 years and Adults: Bronchospasm (treatment): 2-4 mg/dose 3-4 times/day; maximum dose not to exceed 32 mg/day (divided doses)
  - Extended release: 8 mg every 12 hours; maximum dose not to exceed 32 mg/day (divided doses). A 4 mg dose every 12 hours may be sufficient in some patients, such as adults of low body weight.
- Elderly: Bronchospasm (treatment): 2 mg 3-4 times/day; maximum: 8 mg 4 times/day

Inhalation: MDI 90 mcg/puff:

- Children ≤12 years:
  - Bronchospasm (acute): 4-8 puffs every 20 minutes for 3 doses, then every 1-4 hours; spacer/holding-chamber device should be used
  - Exercise-induced bronchospasm (prophylaxis): 1-2 puffs 5 minutes prior to exercise
- Children >12 years and Adults:
  - Bronchospasm (acute): 4-8 puffs every 20 minutes for up to 4 hours, then every 1-4 hours as needed
  - Exercise-induced bronchospasm (prophylaxis): 2 puffs 5-30 minutes prior to exercise
- Children ≥4 years and Adults: Bronchospasm (chronic treatment): 1-2 inhalations every 4-6 hours; maximum: 12 inhalations/day
  - NIH guidelines: 2 puffs 3-4 times a day as needed; may double dose for mild exacerbations

Nebulization:

Children ≤12 years:

Bronchospasm (treatment): 0.05 mg/kg every 4-6 hours; minimum dose: 1.25 mg, maximum dose: 2.5 mg

2-12 years: AccuNeb™: 0.63 mg or 1.25 mg 3-4 times/day, as needed, delivered over 5-15 minutes

Children >40 kg, patients with more severe asthma, or children 11-12 years: May respond better with a 1.25 mg dose

Bronchospasm (acute): Solution 0.5%: 0.15 mg/kg (minimum dose: 2.5 mg) every 20 minutes for 3 doses, then 0.15-0.3 mg/kg (up to 10 mg) every 1-4 hours as needed; may also use 0.5 mg/kg/hour by continuous infusion. Continuous nebulized albuterol at 0.3 mg/kg/hour has been used safely in the treatment of severe status asthmaticus in children; continuous nebulized doses of 3 mg/kg/hour ± 2.2 mg/kg/hour in children whose mean age was 20.7 months resulted in no cardiac toxicity; the optimal dosage for continuous nebulization remains to be determined.

Note: Use of the 0.5% solution should be used for bronchospasm (acute or treatment) in children <15 kg. AccuNeb™ has not been studied for the treatment of acute bronchospasm; use of the 0.5% concentrated solution may be more appropriate.

Children >12 years and Adults:

Bronchospasm (treatment): 2.5 mg, diluted to a total of 3 mL, 3-4 times/day over 5-15 minutes

NIH guidelines: 1.25-5 mg every 4-8 hours

Bronchospasm (acute) in intensive care patients: 2.5-5 mg every 20 minutes for 3 doses, then 2.5-10 mg every 1-4 hours as needed, **or** 10-15 mg/hour continuously

Hemodialysis: Not removed

Peritoneal dialysis: Significant drug removal is unlikely based on physiochemical characteristics

Mechanism of Action Relaxes bronchial smooth muscle by action on beta$_2$-receptors with little effect on heart rate

Contraindications Hypersensitivity to albuterol, adrenergic amines, or any component of the formulation

Warnings/Precautions Optimize anti-inflammatory treatment before initiating maintenance treatment with albuterol. Do not use as a component of chronic therapy without an anti-inflammatory agent. Only the mildest forms of asthma (Step 1 and/or exercise-induced) would not require concurrent use based upon asthma guidelines. Patient must be instructed to seek medical attention in cases where acute symptoms are not relieved or a previous level of response is diminished. The need to increase frequency of use may indicate deterioration of asthma, and treatment must not be delayed.

Use caution in patients with cardiovascular disease (arrhythmia or hypertension or CHF), convulsive disorders, diabetes, glaucoma, hyperthyroidism, or hypokalemia. Beta agonists may cause elevation in blood pressure, heart rate, and result in CNS stimulation/excitation. Beta$_2$ agonists may increase risk of arrhythmia, increase serum glucose, or decrease serum potassium.

Do not exceed recommended dose; serious adverse events including fatalities, have been associated with excessive use of inhaled sympathomimetics. Rarely, paradoxical bronchospasm may occur with use of inhaled bronchodilating agents; this should be distinguished from inadequate response. All patients should utilize a spacer device when using a metered-dose inhaler; in addition, face masks should be used in children <4 years of age.

Because of its minimal effect on beta$_1$-receptors and its relatively long duration of action, albuterol is a rational choice in the elderly when an inhaled beta agonist is indicated. Oral use should be avoided in the elderly due to adverse effects. Patient response may vary between inhalers that contain chlorofluorocarbons and those which are chlorofluorocarbon-free.

Drug Interactions

Cytochrome P450 Effect: Substrate of CYP3A4 (major)

Increased Effect/Toxicity: When used with inhaled ipratropium, an increased duration of bronchodilation may occur. Cardiovascular effects are potentiated in patients also receiving MAO inhibitors, tricyclic antidepressants, and sympathomimetic agents (eg, amphetamine, dopamine, dobutamine). Albuterol may increase the risk of malignant arrhythmias with inhaled anesthetics (eg, enflurane, halothane).

Decreased Effect: When used with nonselective beta-adrenergic blockers (eg, propranolol) the effect of albuterol is decreased. Levels/effects of albuterol may be decreased by aminoglutethimide, carbamazepine, nafcillin,

(Continued)

Albuterol *(Continued)*

nevirapine, phenobarbital, phenytoin, rifamycins, and other CYP3A4 inducers.

Ethanol/Nutrition/Herb Interactions

Food: Avoid or limit caffeine (may cause CNS stimulation).

Herb/Nutraceutical: Avoid ephedra, yohimbe (may cause CNS stimulation).

Dietary Considerations Oral forms should be administered with water 1 hour before or 2 hours after meals.

Pharmacodynamics/Kinetics

Onset of action: Peak effect: Nebulization/oral inhalation: 0.5-2 hours; Oral: 2-3 hours

Duration: Nebulization/oral inhalation: 3-4 hours; Oral: 4-6 hours

Metabolism: Hepatic to an inactive sulfate

Half-life elimination: Inhalation: 3.8 hours; Oral: 3.7-5 hours

Excretion: Urine (30% as unchanged drug)

Pregnancy Risk Factor C

Dosage Forms AERO, oral: 90 mcg/dose (17 g); (Proventil®): 90 mcg/dose (17 g). **AERO, oral** [chlorofluorocarbon free]: (Proventil® HFA): 90 mcg/dose (6.7 g); (Ventolin® HFA): 90 mcg/dose (18 g). **SOLN, oral inhalation**: 0.083% (3 mL); 0.5% (20 mL); (AccuNeb™): 0.63 mg/3 mL (3 mL), 1.25 mg/3 mL (3 mL); (Proventil®): 0.083% (3 mL), 0.5% (20 mL). **SYR:** 2 mg/5 mL (480 mL). **TAB:** 2 mg, 4 mg. **TAB, extended release:** (Proventil® Repetabs®): 4 mg; (Volmax®, VoSpire™): 4 mg, 8 mg

Albuterol and Ipratropium *see* Ipratropium and Albuterol *on page 761*

Albuterol Sulfate *see* Albuterol *on page 71*

Alcaine® *see* Proparacaine *on page 1134*

Alcalak [OTC] *see* Calcium Carbonate *on page 245*

Alclometasone (al kloe MET a sone)

U.S. Brand Names Aclovate®

Generic Available No

Synonyms Alclometasone Dipropionate

Pharmacologic Category Corticosteroid, Topical

Use Treatment of inflammation of corticosteroid-responsive dermatosis (low potency topical corticosteroid)

Local Anesthetic/Vasoconstrictor Precautions No information available to require special precautions

Effects on Dental Treatment No significant effects or complications reported

Common Adverse Effects 1% to 10%:

Dermatologic: Itching, erythema, dryness papular rashes

Local: Burning, irritation

Mechanism of Action Stimulates the synthesis of enzymes needed to decrease inflammation, suppress mitotic activity, and cause vasoconstriction

Pregnancy Risk Factor C

Alclometasone Dipropionate *see* Alclometasone *on page 74*

Aldactazide® *see* Hydrochlorothiazide and Spironolactone *on page 701*

Aldactone® *see* Spironolactone *on page 1235*

Aldara™ *see* Imiquimod *on page 738*

Aldesleukin (al des LOO kin)

U.S. Brand Names Proleukin®

Canadian Brand Names Proleukin®

Mexican Brand Names Proleukin®

Generic Available No

Synonyms Epidermal Thymocyte Activating Factor; ETAF; IL-2; Interleukin-2; Lymphocyte Mitogenic Factor; NSC-373364; T-Cell Growth Factor; TCGF; Thymocyte Stimulating Factor

Pharmacologic Category Biological Response Modulator

Use Treatment of metastatic renal cell cancer, melanoma

Unlabeled/Investigational Use Investigational: Multiple myeloma, HIV infection, and AIDS; may be used in conjunction with lymphokine-activated killer (LAK) cells, tumor-infiltrating lymphocyte (TIL) cells, interleukin-1, and interferons; colorectal cancer; non-Hodgkin's lymphoma

Local Anesthetic/Vasoconstrictor Precautions No information available to require special precautions

Effects on Dental Treatment Key adverse event(s) related to dental treatment: Stomatitis.

Common Adverse Effects

>10%:

Cardiovascular: Hypotension (85%), dose-limiting, possibly fatal; sinus tachycardia (70%); arrhythmias (22%); edema (47%); angina

Central nervous system: Mental status changes (transient memory loss, confusion, drowsiness) (73%); dizziness (17%); cognitive changes, fatigue, malaise, somnolence and disorientation (25%); headaches, insomnia, paranoid delusion

Dermatologic: Macular erythematous rash (100% of patients on high-dose therapy); pruritus (48%); erythema (41%); rash (26%); exfoliative dermatitis (14%); dry skin (15%)

Endocrine & metabolic: Fever and chills (89%); low electrolyte levels (magnesium, calcium, phosphate, potassium, sodium) (1% to 15%)

Gastrointestinal: Nausea and vomiting (87%); diarrhea (76%); stomatitis (32%); GI bleeding (13%); weight gain (23%), anorexia (27%)

Hematologic: Anemia (77%); thrombocytopenia (64%); leukopenia (34%) - may be dose-limiting; coagulation disorders (10%)

Hepatic: Transient elevations of bilirubin (64%) and enzymes (56%); jaundice (11%)

Neuromuscular & skeletal: Weakness; rigors - respond to acetaminophen, diphenhydramine, an NSAID, or meperidine

Renal: Oliguria/anuria (63%, severe in 5% to 6%), proteinuria (12%); renal failure (dose-limiting toxicity) manifested as oliguria noted within 24-48 hours of initiation of therapy; marked fluid retention, azotemia, and increased serum creatinine seen, which may return to baseline within 7 days of discontinuation of therapy; hypophosphatemia

Respiratory: Congestion (54%); dyspnea (27% to 52%)

Miscellaneous: Pain (54%), infection (including sepsis and endocarditis) due to neutrophil impairment (23%)

1% to 10%:

Cardiovascular: Capillary leak syndrome, including peripheral edema, ascites, pulmonary infiltration, and pleural effusion (2% to 4%), may be dose-limiting and potentially fatal; myocardial infarction (2%)

Central nervous system: Seizures (1%)

Endocrine & metabolic: Hypo- and hyperglycemia (2%); increased electrolyte levels (magnesium, calcium, phosphate, potassium, sodium) (1%), hypothyroidism

Hepatic: Ascites (4%)

Neuromuscular & skeletal: Arthralgia (6%), myalgia (6%)

Renal: Hematuria (9%), increased creatinine (5%)

Respiratory: Pleural effusions, edema (10%)

Mechanism of Action Aldesleukin promotes proliferation, differentiation, and recruitment of T and B cells, natural killer (NK) cells, and thymocytes; aldesleukin also causes cytolytic activity in a subset of lymphocytes and subsequent interactions between the immune system and malignant cells; aldesleukin can stimulate lymphokine-activated killer (LAK) cells and tumor-infiltrating lymphocytes (TIL) cells. LAK cells (which are derived from lymphocytes from a patient and incubated in aldesleukin) have the ability to lyse cells which are resistant to NK cells; TIL cells (which are derived from cancerous tissue from a patient and incubated in aldesleukin) have been shown to be 50% more effective than LAK cells in experimental studies.

Drug Interactions

Increased Effect/Toxicity: Aldesleukin may affect central nervous function; therefore, interactions could occur following concomitant administration of psychotropic drugs (eg, narcotics, analgesics, antiemetics, sedatives, tranquilizers).

Concomitant administration of drugs possessing nephrotoxic (eg, aminoglycosides, indomethacin), myelotoxic (eg, cytotoxic chemotherapy), cardiotoxic (eg, doxorubicin), or hepatotoxic (eg, methotrexate, asparaginase) effects with aldesleukin may increase toxicity in these organ systems. The safety and efficacy of aldesleukin in combination with chemotherapies has not been established.

Beta-blockers and other antihypertensives may potentiate the hypotension seen with aldesleukin.

Decreased Effect: Corticosteroids have been shown to decrease toxicity of aldesleukin, but have not been used since there is concern that they may reduce the efficacy of the lymphokine.

Pharmacodynamics/Kinetics

Distribution: V_d: 4-7 L; primarily in plasma and then in the lymphocytes

Bioavailability: I.M.: 37%

Half-life elimination: Initial: 6-13 minutes; Terminal: 80-120 minutes

Pregnancy Risk Factor C

Aldomet *see* Methyldopa *on page 906*

Aldoril® *see* Methyldopa and Hydrochlorothiazide *on page 906*

Aldoril® D *see* Methyldopa and Hydrochlorothiazide *on page 906*

Aldroxicon I [OTC] *see* Aluminum Hydroxide, Magnesium Hydroxide, and Simethicone *on page 92*

Aldroxicon II [OTC] *see* Aluminum Hydroxide, Magnesium Hydroxide, and Simethicone *on page 92*

Aldurazyme® *see* Laronidase *on page 800*

Alefacept (a LE fa sept)

U.S. Brand Names Amevive®

Generic Available No

Synonyms B 9273; BG 9273; Human LFA-3/IgG(1) Fusion Protein; LFA-3/IgG(1) Fusion Protein, Human

Pharmacologic Category Monoclonal Antibody

Use Treatment of moderate to severe plaque psoriasis in adults who are candidates for systemic therapy or phototherapy

Local Anesthetic/Vasoconstrictor Precautions No information available to require special precautions

Effects on Dental Treatment No significant effects or complications reported

Common Adverse Effects

≥10%:

Hematologic: Lymphopenia (up to 10% of patients required temporary discontinuation, up to 17% during a second course of therapy)

Local: Injection site reactions (up to 16% of patients; includes pain, inflammation, bleeding, edema, or other reaction)

1% to 10%:

Central nervous system: Chills (6%; primarily during intravenous administration), dizziness

Dermatologic: Pruritus

Gastrointestinal: Nausea

Neuromuscular & skeletal: Myalgia

Respiratory: Pharyngitis, cough increased

Miscellaneous: Malignancies (1% vs 0.2% in placebo), antibodies to alefacept (3%; significance unknown), infections (1% to 2% requiring hospitalization)

Restrictions Alefacept will be distributed directly to physician offices or to a specialty pharmacy; injections are intended to be administered in the physician's office

Mechanism of Action Binds to CD2, a receptor on the surface of lymphocytes, inhibiting their interaction with leukocyte functional antigen 3 (LFA-3). Interaction between CD2 and LFA-3 is important for the activation of T-lymphocytes in psoriasis. Activated T-lymphocytes secrete a number of inflammatory mediators, including interferon gamma, which are involved in psoriasis. Since CD2 is primarily expressed on T-lymphocytes, treatment results in a reduction in $CD4^+$ and $CD8^+$ T-lymphocytes, with lesser effects on other cell populations (NK- and B-lymphocytes).

Drug Interactions

Increased Effect/Toxicity: No formal drug interaction studies have been completed.

Decreased Effect: No formal drug interaction studies have been completed.

Pharmacodynamics/Kinetics

Distribution: V_d: 0.094 L/kg

Bioavailability: 63% (following I.M. administration)

Half-life: 270 hours (following I.V. administration)

Excretion: Clearance: 0.25 mL/hour/kg

Pregnancy Risk Factor B

Alemtuzumab (ay lem TU zoo mab)

U.S. Brand Names Campath®

Generic Available No

Synonyms Campath-1H; DNA-derived Humanized Monoclonal Antibody; Humanized IgG1 Anti-CD52 Monoclonal Antibody

Pharmacologic Category Antineoplastic Agent, Monoclonal Antibody

Use Treatment of B-cell chronic lymphocytic leukemia (B-CLL)

Unlabeled/Investigational Use Treatment of refractory T-cell prolymphocytic leukemia (T-PLL); rheumatoid arthritis; graft versus host disease; multiple myeloma

Local Anesthetic/Vasoconstrictor Precautions No information available to require special precautions

Effects on Dental Treatment Key adverse event(s) related to dental treatment: Stomatitis and mucositis.

Common Adverse Effects

>10%:

Cardiovascular: Hypotension (15% to 32%, infusion-related), peripheral edema (13%), hypertension (11%), tachycardia/SVT (11%)

Central nervous system: Drug-related fever (83%, infusion-related), fatigue (22% to 34%, infusion-related), headache (13% to 24%), dysthesias (15%), dizziness (12%), neutropenic fever (10%)

Dermatologic: Rash (30% to 40%, infusion-related), urticaria (22% to 30%, infusion-related), pruritus (14% to 24%, infusion-related)

Gastrointestinal: Nausea (47% to 54%), vomiting (33% to 41%), anorexia (20%), diarrhea (13% to 22%), stomatitis/mucositis (14%), abdominal pain (11%)

Hematologic: Lymphopenia, severe neutropenia (64% to 70%); severe anemia (38% to 47%) and severe thrombocytopenia (50% to 52%) may be prolonged and dose-limiting

Neuromuscular & skeletal: Rigors (89%, infusion-related), skeletal muscle pain (24%), weakness (13%), myalgia (11%)

Respiratory: Dyspnea (17% to 26%, infusion-related), cough (25%), bronchitis/pneumonitis (21%), pharyngitis (12%)

Miscellaneous: Infection (43% including sepsis, pneumonia, opportunistic infections; received PCP pneumonia and herpes prophylaxis); diaphoresis (19%)

1% to 10%:

Cardiovascular: Chest pain (10%)

Central nervous system: Insomnia (10%), malaise (9%), depression (7%), temperature change sensation (5%), somnolence (5%)

Dermatologic: Purpura (8%)

Gastrointestinal: Dyspepsia (10%), constipation (9%)

Hematologic: Pancytopenia /marrow hypoplasia (6%), positive Coombs' test without hemolysis (2%), autoimmune thrombocytopenia (2%), antibodies to alemtuzumab (2%), autoimmune hemolytic anemia (1%)

Neuromuscular & skeletal: Back pain (10%), tremor (7%)

Respiratory: Bronchospasm (9%), epistaxis (7%), rhinitis (7%)

Mechanism of Action Recombinant monoclonal antibody binds to CD52, a nonmodulating antigen present on the surface of B and T lymphocytes, a majority of monocytes, macrophages, NK cells and a subpopulation of granulocytes. After binding to $CD52^+$ cells, an antibody-dependent lysis occurs.

Pharmacodynamics/Kinetics Half-life elimination: 12 days

Pregnancy Risk Factor C

Alendronate (a LEN droe nate)

Related Information

Rheumatoid Arthritis, Osteoarthritis, and Osteoporosis *on page 1490*

U.S. Brand Names Fosamax®

Canadian Brand Names Fosamax®; Novo-Alendronate

Generic Available No

Synonyms Alendronate Sodium

Pharmacologic Category Bisphosphonate Derivative

Use Treatment and prevention of osteoporosis in postmenopausal females; treatment of osteoporosis in males; Paget's disease of the bone in patients who are symptomatic, at risk for future complications, or with alkaline phosphatase ≥2 times the upper limit of normal; treatment of glucocorticoid-induced osteoporosis in males and females with low bone mineral density who are receiving a daily dosage ≥7.5 mg of prednisone (or equivalent)

Local Anesthetic/Vasoconstrictor Precautions No information available to require special precautions

Effects on Dental Treatment No significant effects or complications reported

Common Adverse Effects Note: Incidence of adverse effects increases significantly in patients treated for Paget's disease at 40 mg/day, mostly GI adverse effects.

>10%: Endocrine & metabolic: Hypocalcemia (transient, mild, 18%); hypophosphatemia (transient, mild, 10%)

(Continued)

Alendronate *(Continued)*

1% to 10%:

Central nervous system: Headache (0.2% to 3%)

Gastrointestinal: Abdominal pain (1% to 7%), acid reflux (1% to 5%), dyspepsia (1% to 4%), nausea (1% to 4%), flatulence (0.2% to 4%), diarrhea (0.6% to 3%), constipation (0.3% to 3%), esophageal ulcer (0.1% to 2%), abdominal distension (0.2% to 1%), gastritis (0.2% to 1%), vomiting (0.2% to 1%), dysphagia (0.1% to 1%), gastric ulcer (1%), melena (1%)

Neuromuscular & skeletal: Musculoskeletal pain (0.4% to 4%), muscle cramps (0.2% to 1%)

Dosage Oral: Adults: **Note:** Patients treated with glucocorticoids and those with Paget's disease should receive adequate amounts of calcium and vitamin D.

Osteoporosis in postmenopausal females:

Prophylaxis: 5 mg once daily **or** 35 mg once weekly

Treatment: 10 mg once daily **or** 70 mg once weekly

Osteoporosis in males: 10 mg once daily **or** 70 mg once weekly

Osteoporosis secondary to glucocorticoids in males and females: Treatment: 5 mg once daily; a dose of 10 mg once daily should be used in postmenopausal females who are not receiving estrogen.

Paget's disease of bone in males and females: 40 mg once daily for 6 months

Retreatment: Relapses during the 12 months following therapy occurred in 9% of patients who responded to treatment. Specific retreatment data are not available. Retreatment with alendronate may be considered, following a 6-month post-treatment evaluation period, in patients who have relapsed based on increases in serum alkaline phosphatase, which should be measured periodically. Retreatment may also be considered in those who failed to normalize their serum alkaline phosphatase.

Elderly: No dosage adjustment is necessary

Dosage adjustment in renal impairment:

Cl_{cr} 35-60 mL/minute: None necessary

Cl_{cr} <35 mL/minute: Alendronate is not recommended due to lack of experience

Dosage adjustment in hepatic impairment: None necessary

Mechanism of Action A bisphosphonate which inhibits bone resorption via actions on osteoclasts or on osteoclast precursors; decreases the rate of bone resorption direction, leading to an indirect decrease in bone formation

Contraindications Hypersensitivity to alendronate, other bisphosphonates, or any component of the formulation; hypocalcemia; abnormalities of the esophagus which delay esophageal emptying such as stricture or achalasia; inability to stand or sit upright for at least 30 minutes; oral solution should not be used in patients at risk of aspiration

Warnings/Precautions Use caution in patients with renal impairment; hypocalcemia must be corrected before therapy initiation; ensure adequate calcium and vitamin D intake. May cause irritation to upper gastrointestinal mucosa. Esophagitis, esophageal ulcers, esophageal erosions, and esophageal stricture (rare) have been reported; risk increases in patients unable to comply with dosing instructions. Use with caution in patients with dysphagia, esophageal disease, gastritis, duodenitis, or ulcers (may worsen underlying condition).

Drug Interactions

Increased Effect/Toxicity: I.V. ranitidine has been shown to double the bioavailability of alendronate. Estrogen replacement therapy, in combination with alendronate, may enhance the therapeutic effects of both agents on the maintenance of bone mineralization. An increased incidence of adverse GI effects has been noted when >10 mg alendronate is used in patients taking aspirin-containing products.

Decreased Effect: Oral medications (especially those containing multivalent cations, including calcium and antacids): May interfere with alendronate absorption; wait at least 30 minutes after taking alendronate before taking any oral medications

Ethanol/Nutrition/Herb Interactions Food: All food and beverages interfere with absorption. Coadministration with caffeine may reduce alendronate efficacy. Coadministration with dairy products may decrease alendronate absorption. Beverages (especially orange juice and coffee), food, and medications (eg, antacids, calcium, iron, and multivalent cations) may reduce the absorption of alendronate as much as 60%.

Dietary Considerations Ensure adequate calcium and vitamin D intake; however, wait at least 30 minutes after taking alendronate before taking any supplement. Must be taken with plain water first thing in the morning and at least 30 minutes before the first food or beverage of the day.

Pharmacodynamics/Kinetics

Distribution: 28 L (exclusive of bone)

Protein binding: ~78%

Metabolism: None

Bioavailability: Fasting: Female: 0.7%; Male: 0.6%; reduced 60% with food or drink

Half-life elimination: Exceeds 10 years

Excretion: Urine; feces (as unabsorbed drug)

Pregnancy Risk Factor C

Dosage Forms SOLN, oral, as monosodium trihydrate: 70 mg/75 mL. **TAB:** 5 mg, 10 mg, 35 mg, 40 mg, 70 mg

Alendronate Sodium *see* Alendronate *on page 77*

Alenic Alka Tablet [OTC] *see* Aluminum Hydroxide and Magnesium Trisilicate *on page 91*

Aler-Dryl [OTC] *see* DiphenhydrAMINE *on page 448*

Alesse® *see* Ethinyl Estradiol and Levonorgestrel *on page 545*

Aleve® [OTC] *see* Naproxen *on page 965*

Alfenta® *see* Alfentanil *on page 79*

Alfentanil (al FEN ta nil)

U.S. Brand Names Alfenta®

Canadian Brand Names Alfenta®

Generic Available Yes

Synonyms Alfentanil Hydrochloride

Pharmacologic Category Analgesic, Narcotic

Use Analgesic adjunct given by continuous infusion or in incremental doses in maintenance of anesthesia with barbiturate or N_2O or a primary anesthetic agent for the induction of anesthesia in patients undergoing general surgery in which endotracheal intubation and mechanical ventilation are required

Local Anesthetic/Vasoconstrictor Precautions No information available to require special precautions

Effects on Dental Treatment Key adverse event(s) related to dental treatment: Orthostatic hypotension.

Erythromycin inhibits the liver metabolism of alfentanil resulting in increased sedation and prolonged respiratory depression.

Common Adverse Effects

>10%:

- Cardiovascular: Bradycardia, peripheral vasodilation
- Central nervous system: Drowsiness, sedation, increased intracranial pressure
- Gastrointestinal: Nausea, vomiting, constipation
- Endocrine & metabolic: Antidiuretic hormone release
- Ocular: Miosis

1% to 10%:

- Cardiovascular: Cardiac arrhythmias, orthostatic hypotension
- Central nervous system: Confusion, CNS depression
- Ocular: Blurred vision

Restrictions C-II

Mechanism of Action Binds with stereospecific receptors at many sites within the CNS, increases pain threshold, alters pain perception, inhibits ascending pain pathways; is an ultra short-acting narcotic

Drug Interactions

Cytochrome P450 Effect: Substrate of CYP3A4 (major)

Increased Effect/Toxicity: Dextroamphetamine may enhance the analgesic effect of morphine and other opiate agonists. CNS depressants (eg, benzodiazepines, barbiturates, tricyclic antidepressants), erythromycin, reserpine, beta-blockers may increase the toxic effects of alfentanil. Alfentanil levels/effects may be increased by azole antifungals, ciprofloxacin, clarithromycin, diclofenac, doxycycline, erythromycin, imatinib, isoniazid, nefazodone, nicardipine, propofol, protease inhibitors, quinidine, verapamil, and other inhibitors of CYP3A4.

Pharmacodynamics/Kinetics

Onset of action: Rapid

Duration (dose dependent): 30-60 minutes

Distribution: V_d: Newborns, premature: 1 L/kg; Children: 0.163-0.48 L/kg; Adults: 0.46 L/kg

Half-life elimination: Newborns, premature: 5.33-8.75 hours; Children: 40-60 minutes; Adults: 83-97 minutes

Pregnancy Risk Factor C

Alfentanil Hydrochloride *see* Alfentanil *on page 79*
Alferon® N *see* Interferon Alfa-n3 *on page 755*

Alfuzosin (al FYOO zoe sin)

U.S. Brand Names Uroxatral™
Generic Available No
Synonyms Alfuzosin Hydrochloride
Pharmacologic Category $Alpha_1$ Blocker
Use Treatment of the functional symptoms of benign prostatic hyperplasia (BPH)
Local Anesthetic/Vasoconstrictor Precautions No information available to require special precautions
Effects on Dental Treatment No significant effects or complications reported
Common Adverse Effects

1% to 10%:

Central nervous system: Dizziness (6%), fatigue (3%), headache (3%), pain (1% to 2%)
Gastrointestinal: Abdominal pain (1% to 2%), constipation (1% to 2%), dyspepsia (1% to 2%), nausea (1% to 2%)
Genitourinary: Impotence (1% to 2%)
Respiratory: Upper respiratory tract infection (3%), bronchitis (1% to 2%), pharyngitis (1% to 2%), sinusitis (1% to 2%)

Mechanism of Action An antagonist of $alpha_1$ adrenoreceptors in the lower urinary tract. Smooth muscle tone is mediated by the sympathetic nervous stimulation of $alpha_1$ adrenoreceptors, which are abundant in the prostate, prostatic capsule, prostatic urethra, and bladder neck. Blockade of these adrenoreceptors can cause smooth muscles in the bladder neck and prostate to relax, resulting in an improvement in urine flow rate and a reduction in symptoms of BPH.

Drug Interactions

Cytochrome P450 Effect: Substrate of CYP3A4 (major)

Increased Effect/Toxicity: Alfuzosin levels/effects may be increased by azole antifungals, ciprofloxacin, clarithromycin, diclofenac, doxycycline, erythromycin, imatinib, isoniazid, nefazodone, nicardipine, propofol, protease inhibitors, quinidine, verapamil, and other CYP3A4 inhibitors. Concurrent use of itraconazole, ketoconazole, or ritonavir is contraindicated.

Decreased Effect: Levels/effects of alfuzosin may be decreased by aminoglutethimide, carbamazepine, nafcillin, nevirapine, phenobarbital, phenytoin, rifamycins, and other CYP3A4 inducers.

Pharmacodynamics/Kinetics

Absorption: Decreased 50% under fasting conditions
Distribution: V_d: 3.2 L/kg
Protein binding: 82% to 90%
Metabolism: Hepatic, primarily via CYP3A4; metabolism includes oxidation, O-demethylation and N-dealkylation; forms metabolites (inactive)
Bioavailability: 49% following a meal
Half-life elimination: 10 hours
Time to peak, plasma: 8 hours following a meal
Excretion: Feces (69%); urine (24%)

Pregnancy Risk Factor B

Alfuzosin Hydrochloride *see* Alfuzosin *on page 80*

Alglucerase (al GLOO ser ase)

U.S. Brand Names Ceredase®
Generic Available No
Synonyms Glucocerebrosidase
Pharmacologic Category Enzyme
Use Replacement therapy for Gaucher's disease (type 1)
Local Anesthetic/Vasoconstrictor Precautions No information available to require special precautions
Effects on Dental Treatment No significant effects or complications reported
Common Adverse Effects Frequency not defined.

Cardiovascular: Peripheral edema
Central nervous system: Chills, fatigue, fever, headache, lightheadedness
Endocrine & metabolic: Hot flashes, menstrual abnormalities
Gastrointestinal: Abdominal discomfort, diarrhea, nausea, oral ulcerations, vomiting
Local: Injection site: Abscess, burning, discomfort, pruritus, swelling
Neuromuscular & skeletal: Backache, weakness

Miscellaneous: Dysosmia; hypersensitivity reactions (abdominal cramping, angioedema, chest discomfort, flushing, hypotension, nausea, pruritus, respiratory symptoms, urticaria); IgG antibody formation (~13%)

Mechanism of Action Alglucerase is a modified form of glucocerebrosidase; it is prepared from human placental tissue. Glucocerebrosidase is an enzyme deficient in Gaucher's disease. It is needed to catalyze the hydrolysis of glucocerebroside to glucose and ceramide.

Pharmacodynamics/Kinetics Half-life elimination: ~3-11 minutes

Pregnancy Risk Factor C

Alimta® *see* Pemetrexed *on page 1054*

Alinia™ *see* Nitazoxanide *on page 989*

Alitretinoin (a li TRET i noyn)

U.S. Brand Names Panretin®

Canadian Brand Names Panretin™

Generic Available No

Pharmacologic Category Antineoplastic Agent, Miscellaneous

Use Orphan drug: Topical treatment of cutaneous lesions in AIDS-related Kaposi's sarcoma

Unlabeled/Investigational Use Cutaneous T-cell lymphomas

Local Anesthetic/Vasoconstrictor Precautions No information available to require special precautions

Effects on Dental Treatment No significant effects or complications reported

Common Adverse Effects

>10%:

Central nervous system: Pain (0% to 34%)

Dermatologic: Rash (25% to 77%), pruritus (8% to 11%)

Neuromuscular & skeletal: Paresthesia (3% to 22%)

5% to 10%:

Cardiovascular: Edema (3% to 8%)

Dermatologic: Exfoliative dermatitis (3% to 9%), skin disorder (0% to 8%)

Mechanism of Action Binds to retinoid receptors to inhibit growth of Kaposi's sarcoma

Drug Interactions

Increased Effect/Toxicity: Increased toxicity of DEET may occur if products containing this compound are used concurrently with alitretinoin. Due to limited absorption after topical application, interaction with systemic medications is unlikely.

Pharmacodynamics/Kinetics Absorption: Not extensive

Pregnancy Risk Factor D

Alka-Mints® [OTC] *see* Calcium Carbonate *on page 245*

Alka-Seltzer® Gas Relief [OTC] *see* Simethicone *on page 1222*

Alka-Seltzer® Plus Cold and Cough [OTC] *see* Chlorpheniramine, Phenylephrine, and Dextromethorphan *on page 316*

Alka-Seltzer® Plus Cold and Sinus Liquigels [OTC] *see* Acetaminophen and Pseudoephedrine *on page 53*

Alka-Seltzer® Plus Cold Liqui-Gels® [OTC] *see* Acetaminophen, Chlorpheniramine, and Pseudoephedrine *on page 58*

Alka-Seltzer® Plus Flu Liqui-Gels® [OTC] *see* Acetaminophen, Dextromethorphan, and Pseudoephedrine *on page 59*

Alkeran® *see* Melphalan *on page 866*

Allbee® C-800 [OTC] *see* Vitamin B Complex Combinations *on page 1382*

Allbee® C-800 + Iron [OTC] *see* Vitamin B Complex Combinations *on page 1382*

Allbee® with C [OTC] *see* Vitamin B Complex Combinations *on page 1382*

Allegra® *see* Fexofenadine *on page 587*

Allegra-D® *see* Fexofenadine and Pseudoephedrine *on page 588*

Aller-Chlor® [OTC] *see* Chlorpheniramine *on page 313*

Allerest® Maximum Strength Allergy and Hay Fever [OTC] *see* Chlorpheniramine and Pseudoephedrine *on page 315*

Allerfrim® [OTC] *see* Triprolidine and Pseudoephedrine *on page 1345*

Allergen® *see* Antipyrine and Benzocaine *on page 135*

AllerMax® [OTC] *see* DiphenhydrAMINE *on page 448*

Allerphed® [OTC] *see* Triprolidine and Pseudoephedrine *on page 1345*

Allersol® *see* Naphazoline *on page 964*

Allfen Jr *see* Guaifenesin *on page 672*

Allfen *(reformulation)* *see* Guaifenesin and Potassium Guaiacolsulfonate *on page 675*

Allopurinol (al oh PURE i nole)

U.S. Brand Names Aloprim™; Zyloprim®

Canadian Brand Names Apo-Allopurinol®; Zyloprim®

Mexican Brand Names Atisuril®; Zyloprim®

Generic Available Yes: Tablet

Synonyms Allopurinol Sodium

Pharmacologic Category Xanthine Oxidase Inhibitor

Use

Oral: Prevention of attack of gouty arthritis and nephropathy; treatment of secondary hyperuricemia which may occur during treatment of tumors or leukemia; prevention of recurrent calcium oxalate calculi

I.V.: Treatment of elevated serum and urinary uric acid levels when oral therapy is not tolerated in patients with leukemia, lymphoma, and solid tumor malignancies who are receiving cancer chemotherapy

Local Anesthetic/Vasoconstrictor Precautions No information available to require special precautions

Effects on Dental Treatment No significant effects or complications reported

Common Adverse Effects The most common adverse reaction to allopurinol is a skin rash (usually maculopapular; however, more severe reactions, including Stevens-Johnson syndrome, have also been reported). While some studies cite an incidence of these reactions as high as >10% of cases (often in association with ampicillin or amoxicillin), the product labeling cites a much lower incidence, reflected below. Allopurinol should be discontinued at the first appearance of a rash or other sign of hypersensitivity.

>1%:

Dermatologic: Rash (1.5%)

Gastrointestinal: Nausea (1.3%), vomiting (1.2%)

Renal: Renal failure/impairment (1.2%)

Mechanism of Action Allopurinol inhibits xanthine oxidase, the enzyme responsible for the conversion of hypoxanthine to xanthine to uric acid. Allopurinol is metabolized to oxypurinol which is also an inhibitor of xanthine oxidase; allopurinol acts on purine catabolism, reducing the production of uric acid without disrupting the biosynthesis of vital purines.

Drug Interactions

Increased Effect/Toxicity: Allopurinol may increase the effects of azathioprine, chlorpropamide, mercaptopurine, theophylline, and oral anticoagulants. An increased risk of bone marrow suppression may occur when given with myelosuppressive agents (cyclophosphamide, possibly other alkylating agents). Amoxicillin/ampicillin, ACE inhibitors, and thiazide diuretics have been associated with hypersensitivity reactions when combined with allopurinol (rare), and the incidence of rash may be increased with penicillins (ampicillin, amoxicillin). Urinary acidification with large amounts of vitamin C may increase kidney stone formation.

Decreased Effect: Ethanol decreases effectiveness.

Pharmacodynamics/Kinetics

Onset of action: Peak effect: 1-2 weeks

Absorption: Oral: ~80%; Rectal: Poor and erratic

Distribution: V_d: ~1.6 L/kg; V_{ss}: 0.84-0.87 L/kg; enters breast milk

Protein binding: <1%

Metabolism: ~75% to active metabolites, chiefly oxypurinol

Bioavailability: 49% to 53%

Half-life elimination:

Normal renal function: Parent drug: 1-3 hours; Oxypurinol: 18-30 hours

End-stage renal disease: Prolonged

Time to peak, plasma: Oral: 30-120 minutes

Excretion: Urine (76% as oxypurinol, 12% as unchanged drug)

Allopurinol and oxypurinol are dialyzable

Pregnancy Risk Factor C

Allopurinol Sodium *see* Allopurinol *on page 82*

All-*trans*-Retinoic Acid *see* Tretinoin (Oral) *on page 1328*

Almacone® [OTC] *see* Aluminum Hydroxide, Magnesium Hydroxide, and Simethicone *on page 92*

Almacone Double Strength® [OTC] *see* Aluminum Hydroxide, Magnesium Hydroxide, and Simethicone *on page 92*

Almora® [OTC] *see* Magnesium Gluconate *on page 853*

Almotriptan (al moh TRIP tan)

U.S. Brand Names Axert™

Canadian Brand Names Axert™

Generic Available No
Synonyms Almotriptan Malate
Pharmacologic Category Serotonin 5-HT_{1D} Receptor Agonist
Use Acute treatment of migraine with or without aura
Local Anesthetic/Vasoconstrictor Precautions No information available to require special precautions
Effects on Dental Treatment Key adverse effect(s) related to dental treatment: Xerostomia (normal salivary flow resumes upon discontinuation).
Common Adverse Effects 1% to 10%:
Central nervous system: Headache (>1%), dizziness (>1%), somnolence (>1%)
Gastrointestinal: Nausea (1% to 2%), xerostomia (1%)
Neuromuscular & skeletal: Paresthesia (1%)
Mechanism of Action Selective agonist for serotonin (5-HT_{1B}, 5-HT_{1D}, 5-HT_{1F} receptors) in cranial arteries; causes vasoconstriction and reduce sterile inflammation associated with antidromic neuronal transmission correlating with relief of migraine
Drug Interactions
Cytochrome P450 Effect: Substrate (minor) of CYP2D6, 3A4
Increased Effect/Toxicity: Ergot-containing drugs prolong vasospastic reactions; ketoconazole increases almotriptan serum concentration; select serotonin reuptake inhibitors may increase symptoms of hyper-reflexia, weakness, and incoordination; MAO inhibitors may increase toxicity
Pharmacodynamics/Kinetics
Absorption: Well absorbed
Distribution: V_d: 180-200 L
Protein binding: ~35%
Metabolism: MAO type A oxidative deamination (~27% of dose); via CYP3A4 and 2D6 (~12% of dose) to inactive metabolites
Bioavailability: 70%
Half-life elimination: 3-4 hours
Time to peak: 1-3 hours
Excretion: Urine (40% as unchanged drug); feces (13% unchanged and metabolized)
Pregnancy Risk Factor C

Almotriptan Malate *see* Almotriptan *on page 82*
Alocril™ *see* Nedocromil *on page 970*
Aloe Vesta® 2-n-1 Antifungal [OTC] *see* Miconazole *on page 922*
Alomide® *see* Lodoxamide *on page 836*
Alophen® [OTC] *see* Bisacodyl *on page 208*
Aloprim™ *see* Allopurinol *on page 82*
Alora® *see* Estradiol *on page 518*

Alosetron (a LOE se tron)

U.S. Brand Names Lotronex®
Mexican Brand Names Lotronex®
Generic Available No
Pharmacologic Category Selective 5-HT_3 Receptor Antagonist
Use Treatment of irritable bowel syndrome (IBS) in women with severe diarrhea-predominant IBS who have failed to respond to conventional therapy
Unlabeled/Investigational Use Investigational: Alosetron has demonstrated effectiveness as an antiemetic for a wide variety of causes of emesis.
Local Anesthetic/Vasoconstrictor Precautions No information available to require special precautions
Effects on Dental Treatment Key adverse event(s) related to dental treatment: Throat and tonsil discomfort and pain.
Common Adverse Effects
>10%: Gastrointestinal: Constipation (29%)
1% to 10%: Gastrointestinal: Nausea (6%), gastrointestinal discomfort and pain (6%), abdominal discomfort and pain (7%), abdominal distention (2%), hemorrhoids (2%)
Restrictions Only physicians enrolled in GlaxoSmithKline's Prescribing Program for Lotronex® may prescribe this medication. Program stickers must be affixed to all prescriptions; no phone, fax or computerized prescriptions are permitted with this program.
Mechanism of Action Alosetron is a potent and selective antagonist of a subtype of the serotonin receptor, 5-HT_3 receptor. 5-HT_3 receptors are extensively distributed on enteric neurons in the human gastrointestinal tract, as well as other peripheral and central locations. Activation of these channels affect
(Continued)

Alosetron *(Continued)*

the regulation of visceral pain, colonic transit, and gastrointestinal secretions. In patients with irritable bowel syndrome, improvement in pain, abdominal discomfort, urgency, and diarrhea may occur.

Drug Interactions

Cytochrome P450 Effect: Substrate of CYP1A2 (minor), 2C8/9 (major), 3A4 (minor); **Inhibits** CYP1A2 (weak), 2E1 (weak)

Increased Effect/Toxicity: CYP2C8/9 inhibitors may increase the levels/effects of alosetron; example inhibitors include delavirdine, fluconazole, gemfibrozil, ketoconazole, nicardipine, NSAIDs, pioglitazone, and sulfonamides.

Pharmacodynamics/Kinetics

Distribution: V_d: 65-95 L

Protein binding: 82%

Metabolism: Extensive hepatic metabolism. Alosetron is metabolized by CYP2C9, 3A4, and 1A2. Thirteen metabolites have been detected in the urine. Biological activity of these metabolites in unknown.

Bioavailability: Mean: 50% to 60% (range: 30% to >90%)

Half-life elimination: 1.5 hours for alosetron

Time to peak: 1 hour after oral administration

Excretion: Urine (73%) and feces (24%); 7% as unchanged drug (1% feces, 6% urine)

Pregnancy Risk Factor B

Aloxi™ *see* Palonosetron *on page 1040*

Alpha$_1$-Antitrypsin *see* Alpha$_1$-Proteinase Inhibitor *on page 84*

Alpha$_1$-PI *see* Alpha$_1$-Proteinase Inhibitor *on page 84*

Alpha$_1$-Proteinase Inhibitor (al fa won PRO tee in ase in HI bi tor)

U.S. Brand Names Aralast™; Prolastin®; Zemaira™

Canadian Brand Names Prolastin®

Generic Available No

Synonyms A$_1$-PI; Alpha$_1$-Antitrypsin; Alpha$_1$-PI; Alpha$_1$-Proteinase Inhibitor, Human; α_1-PI

Pharmacologic Category Antitrypsin Deficiency Agent

Use Replacement therapy in congenital alpha$_1$-antitrypsin deficiency with clinical emphysema

Local Anesthetic/Vasoconstrictor Precautions No information available to require special precautions

Effects on Dental Treatment Key adverse event(s) related to dental treatment: Pharyngitis.

Common Adverse Effects

>10%: Hepatic: ALT/AST increased (11%; ~4 times ULN)

1% to 10%: Respiratory: Pharyngitis (2%)

Mechanism of Action Alpha$_1$-antitrypsin (AAT) is the principle protease inhibitor in the serum. Its major physiologic role is to render proteolytic enzymes (secreted during inflammation) inactive. A decrease in AAT, as seen in congenital AAT deficiency, leads to increased elastic damage in the lung, causing emphysema.

Pharmacodynamics/Kinetics

Half-life elimination: Metabolic: 5.9 days (Aralast™)

Time to peak, serum: Threshold levels achieved after 3 weeks

Pregnancy Risk Factor C

Alpha$_1$-Proteinase Inhibitor, Human *see* Alpha$_1$-Proteinase Inhibitor *on page 84*

Alpha-Galactosidase-A (Human, Recombinant) *see* Agalsidase Beta *on page 69*

Alphagan® P *see* Brimonidine *on page 218*

Alphanate® *see* Antihemophilic Factor (Human) *on page 134*

AlphaNine® SD *see* Factor IX *on page 571*

Alphaquin HP *see* Hydroquinone *on page 719*

Alprazolam (al PRAY zoe lam)

Related Information

Patients Requiring Sedation *on page 1567*

Temporomandibular Dysfunction (TMD) *on page 1564*

U.S. Brand Names Alprazolam Intensol®; Xanax®; Xanax XR®

Canadian Brand Names Alti-Alprazolam; Apo-Alpraz®; Gen-Alprazolam; Novo-Alprazol; Nu-Alprax; Xanax®; Xanax TS™

Mexican Brand Names Tafil®

Generic Available Yes: Immediate release tablet

Pharmacologic Category Benzodiazepine

Use Treatment of anxiety disorder (GAD); panic disorder, with or without agoraphobia; anxiety associated with depression

Unlabeled/Investigational Use Anxiety in children

Local Anesthetic/Vasoconstrictor Precautions No information available to require special precautions

Effects on Dental Treatment Key adverse event(s) related to dental treatment: Significant xerostomia and changes in salivation (normal salivary flow resumes upon discontinuation).

Significant Adverse Effects

>10%:

Central nervous system: Depression, drowsiness, dysarthria, fatigue, headache, irritability, lightheadedness, memory impairment, sedation

Endocrine & metabolic: Libido decreased, menstrual disorders

Gastrointestinal: Appetite increased/decreased, salivation decreased, weight gain/loss, xerostomia

1% to 10%:

Cardiovascular: Hypotension

Central nervous system: Abnormal coordination, akathisia, attention disturbance, confusion, derealization, disorientation, disinhibition, dizziness, hypersomnia, nightmares, vertigo

Dermatologic: Dermatitis, pruritus, rash

Endocrine & metabolic: Libido increased

Gastrointestinal: Diarrhea, dyspepsia, salivation increased, vomiting

Genitourinary: Incontinence, micturation difficulty, sexual dysfunction

Neuromuscular & skeletal: Arthralgia, ataxia, muscle cramps, muscle twitching, myalgia, paresthesia, rigidity, tremor

Ophthalmic: Blurred vision

Otic: Tinnitus

Respiratory: Allergic rhinitis, dyspnea, nasal congestion

Miscellaneous: Diaphoresis

<1% (Limited to important or life-threatening): Amnesia, falls, gynecomastia, hepatic failure, hepatitis, hyperprolactinemia, hypotension, seizures, Stevens-Johnson syndrome, syncope, tachycardia, urticaria

Restrictions C-IV

Dosage Oral: **Note:** Treatment >4 months should be re-evaluated to determine the patient's continued need for the drug

Children: Anxiety (unlabeled use): Immediate release: Initial: 0.005 mg/kg/dose or 0.125 mg/dose 3 times/day; increase in increments of 0.125-0.25 mg, up to a maximum of 0.02 mg/kg/dose or 0.06 mg/kg/day (0.375-3 mg/day)

Adults:

Anxiety: Immediate release: Effective doses are 0.5-4 mg/day in divided doses; the manufacturer recommends starting at 0.25-0.5 mg 3 times/day; titrate dose upward; maximum: 4 mg/day

Anxiety associated with depression: Immediate release: Average dose required: 2.5-3 mg/day in divided doses

Ethanol withdrawal (unlabeled use): Immediate release: Usual dose: 2-2.5 mg/day in divided doses

Panic disorder:

Immediate release: Initial: 0.5 mg 3 times/day; dose may be increased every 3-4 days in increments ≤1 mg/day; many patients obtain relief at 2 mg/day, as much as 10 mg/day may be required

Extended release: 0.5-1 mg once daily; may increase dose every 3-4 days in increments ≤1 mg/day (range: 3-6 mg/day)

Switching from immediate release to extended release: Patients may be switched to extended release tablets by taking the total daily dose of the immediate release tablets and giving it once daily using the extended release preparation.

Dose reduction: Abrupt discontinuation should be avoided. Daily dose may be decreased by 0.5 mg every 3 days, however, some patients may require a slower reduction. If withdrawal symptoms occur, resume previous dose and discontinue on a less rapid schedule.

Elderly: Elderly patients may be more sensitive to the effects of alprazolam including ataxia and oversedation. The elderly may also have impaired renal function leading to decreased clearance. The smallest effective dose should be used. Titrate gradually, if needed.

Immediate release: Initial 0.25 mg 2-3 times/day

Extended release: Initial: 0.5 mg once daily

(Continued)

Alprazolam *(Continued)*

Dosing adjustment in hepatic impairment: Reduce dose by 50% to 60% or avoid in cirrhosis

Mechanism of Action Binds to stereospecific benzodiazepine receptors on the postsynaptic GABA neuron at several sites within the central nervous system, including the limbic system, reticular formation. Enhancement of the inhibitory effect of GABA on neuronal excitability results by increased neuronal membrane permeability to chloride ions. This shift in chloride ions results in hyperpolarization (a less excitable state) and stabilization.

Contraindications Hypersensitivity to alprazolam or any component of the formulation (cross-sensitivity with other benzodiazepines may exist); narrow-angle glaucoma; concurrent use with ketoconazole or itraconazole; pregnancy

Warnings/Precautions Rebound or withdrawal symptoms, including seizures may occur 18 hours to 3 days following abrupt discontinuation or large decreases in dose (more common in patients receiving >4 mg/day or prolonged treatment). Dose reductions or tapering must be approached with extreme caution. Breakthrough anxiety may occur at the end of dosing interval. Use with caution in patients receiving concurrent CYP3A4 inhibitors, particularly when these agents are added to therapy. Has weak uricosuric properties, use with caution in renal impairment or predisposition to urate nephropathy. Use with caution in elderly or debilitated patients, patients with hepatic disease (including alcoholics), renal impairment, or obese patients.

Causes CNS depression (dose-related) resulting in sedation, dizziness, confusion, or ataxia which may impair physical and mental capabilities. Patients must be cautioned about performing tasks which require mental alertness (eg, operating machinery or driving). Use with caution in patients receiving other CNS depressants or psychoactive agents. Effects with other sedative drugs or ethanol may be potentiated. Benzodiazepines have been associated with falls and traumatic injury and should be used with extreme caution in patients who are at risk of these events (especially the elderly). Use with caution in patients with respiratory disease or impaired gag reflex.

Use caution in patients with depression, particularly if suicidal risk may be present. Episodes of mania or hypomania have occurred in depressed patients treated with alprazolam. May cause physical or psychological dependence - use with caution in patients with a history of drug dependence. Acute withdrawal, including seizures, may be precipitated in patients after administration of flumazenil to patients receiving long-term benzodiazepine therapy.

Benzodiazepines have been associated with anterograde amnesia. Paradoxical reactions, including hyperactive or aggressive behavior, have been reported with benzodiazepines, particularly in adolescent/pediatric or psychiatric patients. Does not have analgesic, antidepressant, or antipsychotic properties.

Benzodiazepines have the potential to cause harm to the fetus, particularly when administered during the first trimester. In addition, withdrawal symptoms may occur in the neonate following *in utero* exposure. Use of alprazolam during pregnancy should be avoided. In addition, symptoms of withdrawal, lethargy, and loss of body weight have been reported in infants exposed to alprazolam and/or benzodiazepines while nursing; use during breast-feeding is not recommended.

Drug Interactions Substrate of CYP3A4 (major)

CNS depressants: Sedative effects and/or respiratory depression may be additive with CNS depressants. Includes ethanol, barbiturates, narcotic analgesics, and other sedative agents; monitor for increased effect

CYP3A4 inducers: CYP3A4 inducers may decrease the levels/effects of alprazolam. Example inducers include aminoglutethimide, carbamazepine, nafcillin, nevirapine, phenobarbital, phenytoin, and rifamycins.

CYP3A4 inhibitors: May increase the levels/effects of alprazolam. Example inhibitors include azole antifungals, ciprofloxacin, clarithromycin, diclofenac, doxycycline, erythromycin, imatinib, isoniazid, nefazodone, nicardipine, propofol, protease inhibitors, quinidine, and verapamil. Contraindicated with itraconazole and ketoconazole.

Levodopa: Therapeutic effects may be diminished in some patients following the addition of a benzodiazepine; limited/inconsistent data.

Oral contraceptives: May decrease the clearance of some benzodiazepines (those which undergo oxidative metabolism); monitor for increased benzodiazepine effect.

Theophylline: May partially antagonize some of the effects of benzodiazepines; monitor for decreased response; may require higher doses for sedation.

Tricyclic antidepressants: Plasma concentrations of imipramine and desipramine have been reported to be increased 31% and 20%, respectively, by concomitant administration; monitor.

Ethanol/Nutrition/Herb Interactions

Cigarette smoking: May decrease alprazolam concentrations up to 50%.

Ethanol: Avoid ethanol (may increase CNS depression).

Food: Alprazolam serum concentration is unlikely to be increased by grapefruit juice because of alprazolam's high oral bioavailability. The C_{max} of the extended release formulation is increased by 25% when a high-fat meal is given 2 hours before dosing. T_{max} is decreased 30% when food given immediately prior to dose. T_{max} is increased by 30% when food is given ≥1 hour after dose.

Herb/Nutraceutical: St John's wort may decrease alprazolam levels. Avoid valerian, St John's wort, kava kava, gotu kola (may increase CNS depression).

Pharmacodynamics/Kinetics

Distribution: V_d: 0.9-1.2 L/kg; enters breast milk

Protein binding: 80%

Metabolism: Hepatic via CYP3A4; forms 2 active metabolites (4-hydroxyalprazolam and α-hydroxyalprazolam)

Bioavailability: 90%

Half-life elimination:

- Adults: 11.2 hours (range: 6.3-26.9)
- Elderly: 16.3 hours (range: 9-26.9 hours)
- Alcoholic liver disease: 19.7 hours (range: 5.8-65.3 hours)
- Obesity: 21.8 hours (range: 9.9-40.4 hours)

Time to peak, serum: 1-2 hours

Excretion: Urine (as unchanged drug and metabolites)

Pregnancy Risk Factor D

Lactation Enters breast milk/not recommended (AAP rates "of concern")

Breast-Feeding Considerations Symptoms of withdrawal, lethargy, and loss of body weight have been reported in infants exposed to alprazolam and/or benzodiazepines while nursing. Breast-feeding is not recommended.

Dosage Forms

Solution, oral (Alprazolam Intensol®): 1 mg/mL (30 mL)

Tablet (Xanax®): 0.25 mg, 0.5 mg, 1 mg, 2 mg

Tablet, extended release (Xanax XR®): 0.5 mg, 1 mg, 2 mg, 3 mg

Alprazolam Intensol® *see* Alprazolam *on page 84*

Alprostadil (al PROS ta dill)

U.S. Brand Names Caverject®; Caverject® Impulse™; Edex®; Muse®; Prostin VR Pediatric®

Canadian Brand Names Caverject®; Muse® Pellet; Prostin® VR

Mexican Brand Names Caverject®; Muse®

Generic Available Yes

Synonyms PGE_1; Prostaglandin E_1

Pharmacologic Category Prostaglandin

Use

Prostin VR Pediatric®: Temporary maintenance of patency of ductus arteriosus in neonates with ductal-dependent congenital heart disease until surgery can be performed. These defects include cyanotic (eg, pulmonary atresia, pulmonary stenosis, tricuspid atresia, Fallot's tetralogy, transposition of the great vessels) and acyanotic (eg, interruption of aortic arch, coarctation of aorta, hypoplastic left ventricle) heart disease

Caverject®: Treatment of erectile dysfunction of vasculogenic, psychogenic, or neurogenic etiology; adjunct in the diagnosis of erectile dysfunction

Edex®, Muse®: Treatment of erectile dysfunction of vasculogenic, psychogenic, or neurogenic etiology

Unlabeled/Investigational Use Investigational: Treatment of pulmonary hypertension in infants and children with congenital heart defects with left-to-right shunts

Local Anesthetic/Vasoconstrictor Precautions No information available to require special precautions

Effects on Dental Treatment No significant effects or complications reported

Mechanism of Action Causes vasodilation by means of direct effect on vascular and ductus arteriosus smooth muscle; relaxes trabecular smooth muscle by dilation of cavernosal arteries when injected along the penile shaft,

(Continued)

Alprostadil *(Continued)*

allowing blood flow to and entrapment in the lacunar spaces of the penis (ie, corporeal veno-occlusive mechanism)

Pregnancy Risk Factor X/C (Muse®)

Alrex® *see* Loteprednol *on page 847*
Altace® *see* Ramipril *on page 1167*
Altamist [OTC] *see* Sodium Chloride *on page 1227*

Alteplase (AL te plase)

Related Information

Cardiovascular Diseases *on page 1458*

U.S. Brand Names Activase®; Cathflo™ Activase®

Canadian Brand Names Activase® rt-PA; Cathflo™ Activase®

Mexican Brand Names Actilyse®

Generic Available No

Synonyms Alteplase, Recombinant; Alteplase, Tissue Plasminogen Activator, Recombinant; tPA

Pharmacologic Category Thrombolytic Agent

Use Management of acute myocardial infarction for the lysis of thrombi in coronary arteries; management of acute massive pulmonary embolism (PE) in adults

Acute myocardial infarction (AMI): Chest pain ≥20 minutes, ≤12-24 hours; S-T elevation ≥0.1 mV in at least two ECG leads

Acute pulmonary embolism (APE): Age ≤75 years: As soon as possible within 5 days of thrombotic event. Documented massive pulmonary embolism by pulmonary angiography or echocardiography or high probability lung scan with clinical shock.

Cathflo™ Activase®: Restoration of central venous catheter function

Unlabeled/Investigational Use Acute peripheral arterial occlusive disease

Local Anesthetic/Vasoconstrictor Precautions No information available to require special precautions

Effects on Dental Treatment Key adverse event(s) related to dental treatment: As with all drugs which may affect hemostasis, bleeding is the major adverse effect associated with alteplase. Hemorrhage may occur at virtually any site; risk is dependent on multiple variables, including the dosage administered, concurrent use of multiple agents which alter hemostasis, and patient predisposition. Rapid lysis of coronary artery thrombi by thrombolytic agents may be associated with reperfusion-related atrial and/or ventricular arrhythmias.

Common Adverse Effects As with all drugs which may affect hemostasis, bleeding is the major adverse effect associated with alteplase. Hemorrhage may occur at virtually any site. Risk is dependent on multiple variables, including the dosage administered, concurrent use of multiple agents which alter hemostasis, and patient predisposition. Rapid lysis of coronary artery thrombi by thrombolytic agents may be associated with reperfusion-related atrial and/or ventricular arrhythmias. **Note:** Lowest rate of bleeding complications expected with dose used to restore catheter function.

1% to 10%:

- Cardiovascular: Hypotension
- Central nervous system: Fever
- Dermatologic: Bruising (1%)
- Gastrointestinal: GI hemorrhage (5%), nausea, vomiting
- Genitourinary: GU hemorrhage (4%)
- Local: Bleeding at catheter puncture site (15.3%, accelerated administration)
- Hematologic: Bleeding (0.5% major, 7% minor: GUSTO trial)

Additional cardiovascular events associated **with use in myocardial infarction:** AV block, cardiogenic shock, heart failure, cardiac arrest, recurrent ischemia/infarction, myocardial rupture, electromechanical dissociation, pericardial effusion, pericarditis, mitral regurgitation, cardiac tamponade, thromboembolism, pulmonary edema, asystole, ventricular tachycardia, bradycardia, ruptured intracranial AV malformation, seizure, hemorrhagic bursitis, cholesterol crystal embolization

Additional events associated **with use in pulmonary embolism:** Pulmonary re-embolization, pulmonary edema, pleural effusion, thromboembolism

Additional events associated **with use in stroke:** Cerebral edema, cerebral herniation, seizure, new ischemic stroke

Mechanism of Action Initiates local fibrinolysis by binding to fibrin in a thrombus (clot) and converts entrapped plasminogen to plasmin

Drug Interactions

Increased Effect/Toxicity: The potential for hemorrhage with alteplase is increased by oral anticoagulants (warfarin), heparin, low molecular weight heparins, and drugs which affect platelet function (eg, NSAIDs, dipyridamole, ticlopidine, clopidogrel, IIb/IIIa antagonists). Concurrent use with aspirin and heparin may increase the risk of bleeding. However, aspirin and heparin were used concomitantly with alteplase in the majority of patients in clinical studies.

Decreased Effect: Aminocaproic acid (an antifibrinolytic agent) may decrease the effectiveness of thrombolytic therapy. Nitroglycerin may increase the hepatic clearance of alteplase, potentially reducing lytic activity (limited clinical information).

Pharmacodynamics/Kinetics

Duration: >50% present in plasma cleared ~5 minutes after infusion terminated, ~80% cleared within 10 minutes

Excretion: Clearance: Rapidly from circulating plasma (550-650 mL/minute), primarily hepatic; >50% present in plasma is cleared within 5 minutes after the infusion is terminated, ~80% cleared within 10 minutes

Pregnancy Risk Factor C

Alteplase, Recombinant *see* Alteplase *on page 88*

Alteplase, Tissue Plasminogen Activator, Recombinant *see* Alteplase *on page 88*

ALternaGel® [OTC] *see* Aluminum Hydroxide *on page 90*

Altinac™ *see* Tretinoin (Topical) *on page 1329*

Altocor™ [DSC] *see* Lovastatin *on page 848*

Altoprev™ *see* Lovastatin *on page 848*

Altretamine (al TRET a meen)

U.S. Brand Names Hexalen®

Canadian Brand Names Hexalen®

Generic Available No

Synonyms Hexamethylmelamine; HEXM; HMM; HXM; NSC-13875

Pharmacologic Category Antineoplastic Agent, Miscellaneous

Use Palliative treatment of persistent or recurrent ovarian cancer

Local Anesthetic/Vasoconstrictor Precautions No information available to require special precautions

Effects on Dental Treatment No significant effects or complications reported

Common Adverse Effects

>10%:

Central nervous system: Peripheral sensory neuropathy, neurotoxicity (21%; may be progressive and dose-limiting)

Gastrointestinal: Nausea/vomiting (50% to 70%), anorexia (48%), diarrhea (48%)

Hematologic: Anemia, thrombocytopenia (31%), leukopenia (62%), neutropenia

1% to 10%:

Central nervous system: Seizures

Gastrointestinal: Stomach cramps

Hepatic: Alkaline phosphatase increased

Mechanism of Action Although altretamine clinical antitumor spectrum resembles that of alkylating agents, the drug has demonstrated activity in alkylator-resistant patients. The drug selectively inhibits the incorporation of radioactive thymidine and uridine into DNA and RNA, inhibiting DNA and RNA synthesis; reactive intermediates covalently bind to microsomal proteins and DNA; can spontaneously degrade to demethylated melamines and formaldehyde which are also cytotoxic.

Drug Interactions

Increased Effect/Toxicity: Altretamine may cause severe orthostatic hypotension when administered with MAO inhibitors. Cimetidine may decrease metabolism of altretamine.

Decreased Effect: Phenobarbital may increase metabolism of altretamine which may decrease the effect.

Pharmacodynamics/Kinetics

Absorption: Well absorbed (75% to 89%)

Distribution: Highly concentrated hepatically and renally; low in other organs

Metabolism: Hepatic; rapid and extensive demethylation; active metabolites

Half-life elimination: 13 hours

Time to peak, plasma: 0.5-3 hours

Excretion: Urine (<1% as unchanged drug)

Pregnancy Risk Factor D

Alu-Cap® [OTC] *see* Aluminum Hydroxide *on page 90*

Aluminum Chloride (a LOO mi num KLOR ide)

U.S. Brand Names Gingi-Aid® Gingival Retraction Cord; Gingi-Aid® Solution; Hemodent® Gingival Retraction Cord

Generic Available Yes

Pharmacologic Category Astringent; Hemostatic Agent

Dental Use Hemostatic; gingival retraction; to control bleeding created during a dental procedure

Use Hemostatic

Local Anesthetic/Vasoconstrictor Precautions No information available to require special precautions

Effects on Dental Treatment No significant effects or complications reported

Significant Adverse Effects No data reported

Mechanism of Action Precipitates tissue and blood proteins causing a mechanical obstruction to hemorrhage from injured blood vessels

Contraindications No data reported

Warnings/Precautions Since large amounts of astringents may cause tissue irritation and possible damage, only small amounts should be applied

Drug Interactions No data reported

Dosage Forms

Retraction cord [impregnated with aqueous solution]: 1 mg/inch (72 inches); 2 mg/inch (72 inches)

Retraction cord [impregnated with aqueous 10% solution and dried]: 0.9 mg/inch (84 inches); 1.8 mg/inch (84 inches)

Solution, aqueous: 10 g/100 mL water (15 mL, 30 mL)

Aluminum Hydroxide (a LOO mi num hye DROKS ide)

U.S. Brand Names ALternaGel® [OTC]; Alu-Cap® [OTC]

Canadian Brand Names Amphojel®; Basaljel®

Generic Available Yes: Suspension

Pharmacologic Category Antacid; Antidote

Use Treatment of hyperacidity; hyperphosphatemia

Local Anesthetic/Vasoconstrictor Precautions No information available to require special precautions

Effects on Dental Treatment Key adverse event(s) related to dental treatment: Chalky taste. Aluminum and magnesium ions prevent GI absorption of tetracycline by forming a large ionized chelated molecule with the aluminum ion and tetracyclines in the stomach. Aluminum hydroxide prevents GI absorption of ketoconazole and itraconazole by increasing the pH in the GI tract. Any of these drugs should be administered at least 1 hour before $Al(OH)_3$.

Common Adverse Effects Frequency not defined.

Gastrointestinal: Constipation, stomach cramps, fecal impaction, nausea, vomiting, discoloration of feces (white speckles)

Endocrine & metabolic: Hypophosphatemia, hypomagnesemia

Mechanism of Action Neutralizes hydrochloride in stomach to form $Al(Cl)_3$ salt + H_2O

Drug Interactions

Decreased Effect: Aluminum hydroxide may decrease the absorption of allopurinol, antibiotics (tetracyclines, quinolones, some cephalosporins), bisphosphonate derivatives, corticosteroids, cyclosporine, delavirdine, iron salts, imidazole antifungals, isoniazid, mycophenolate, penicillamine, phosphate supplements, phenytoin, phenothiazines, trientine. Absorption of aluminum hydroxide may be decreased by citric acid derivatives.

Pregnancy Risk Factor C

Aluminum Hydroxide and Magnesium Carbonate

(a LOO mi num hye DROKS ide & mag NEE zhum KAR bun nate)

Related Information

Aluminum Hydroxide *on page 90*

U.S. Brand Names Gaviscon® Extra Strength [OTC]; Gaviscon® Liquid [OTC]

Generic Available Yes

Synonyms Magnesium Carbonate and Aluminum Hydroxide

Pharmacologic Category Antacid

Use Temporary relief of symptoms associated with gastric acidity

Local Anesthetic/Vasoconstrictor Precautions No information available to require special precautions

Effects on Dental Treatment Key adverse event(s) related to dental treatment: Chalky taste. Aluminum and magnesium ions prevent GI absorption of tetracycline by forming a large ionized chelated molecule with the tetracyclines in the stomach. Aluminum hydroxide prevents GI absorption of ketoconazole and itraconazole by increasing the pH in the GI tract. Any of these drugs should be administered at least 1 hour before aluminum hydroxide.

Common Adverse Effects 1% to 10%:

Endocrine & metabolic: Hypermagnesemia, aluminum intoxication (prolonged use and concomitant renal failure), hypophosphatemia

Gastrointestinal: Constipation, diarrhea

Neuromuscular & skeletal: Osteomalacia

Drug Interactions

Decreased Effect: Tetracyclines, digoxin, indomethacin, or iron salts, isoniazid, allopurinol, benzodiazepines, corticosteroids, penicillamine, phenothiazines, ranitidine, ketoconazole, itraconazole

Aluminum Hydroxide and Magnesium Hydroxide

(a LOO mi num hye DROKS ide & mag NEE zhum hye DROK side)

Related Information

Aluminum Hydroxide *on page 90*

Magnesium Hydroxide *on page 853*

U.S. Brand Names Alamag [OTC]; Maalox® TC (Therapeutic Concentrate) [OTC] [DSC]; Rulox; Rulox No. 1

Canadian Brand Names Diovol®; Diovol® Ex; Gelusil®; Gelusil® Extra Strength; Mylanta™; Univol®

Generic Available Yes

Synonyms Magnesium Hydroxide and Aluminum Hydroxide

Pharmacologic Category Antacid

Use Antacid, hyperphosphatemia in renal failure

Local Anesthetic/Vasoconstrictor Precautions No information available to require special precautions

Effects on Dental Treatment Key adverse event(s) related to dental treatment: Chalky taste. Aluminum and magnesium ions prevent GI absorption of tetracycline by forming a large ionized chelated molecule with the tetracyclines in the stomach. Aluminum hydroxide prevents GI absorption of ketoconazole and itraconazole by increasing the pH in the GI tract. Any of these drugs should be administered at least 1 hour before aluminum hydroxide.

Common Adverse Effects

>10%: Gastrointestinal: Constipation, chalky taste, stomach cramps, fecal impaction

1% to 10%: Gastrointestinal: Nausea, vomiting, discoloration of feces (white speckles)

Drug Interactions

Decreased Effect: Tetracyclines, digoxin, indomethacin, or iron salts, isoniazid, allopurinol, benzodiazepines, corticosteroids, penicillamine, phenothiazines, ranitidine, ketoconazole, itraconazole

Pregnancy Risk Factor C

Aluminum Hydroxide and Magnesium Trisilicate

(a LOO mi num hye DROKS ide & mag NEE zhum trye SIL i kate)

Related Information

Aluminum Hydroxide *on page 90*

U.S. Brand Names Alenic Alka Tablet [OTC]; Gaviscon® Tablet [OTC]; Genaton Tablet [OTC]

Generic Available Yes

Synonyms Magnesium Trisilicate and Aluminum Hydroxide

Pharmacologic Category Antacid

Use Temporary relief of hyperacidity

Local Anesthetic/Vasoconstrictor Precautions No information available to require special precautions

Effects on Dental Treatment Key adverse event(s) related to dental treatment: Chalky taste. Aluminum and magnesium ions prevent GI absorption of tetracycline by forming a large ionized chelated molecule with the tetracyclines in the stomach. Aluminum hydroxide prevents GI absorption of ketoconazole and itraconazole by increasing the pH in the GI tract. Any of these drugs should be administered at least 1 hour before aluminum hydroxide.

Drug Interactions

Decreased Effect: Tetracyclines, digoxin, indomethacin, or iron salts, isoniazid, allopurinol, benzodiazepines, corticosteroids, penicillamine, phenothiazines, ranitidine, ketoconazole, itraconazole

Pregnancy Risk Factor C

Aluminum Hydroxide, Magnesium Hydroxide, and Simethicone

(a LOO mi num hye DROKS ide, mag NEE zhum hye DROKS ide, & sye METH i kone)

Related Information

Aluminum Hydroxide *on page 90*

Magnesium Hydroxide *on page 853*

U.S. Brand Names Alamag Plus [OTC]; Aldroxicon I [OTC]; Aldroxicon II [OTC]; Almacone® [OTC]; Almacone Double Strength® [OTC]; Maalox® [OTC]; Maalox® Max [OTC]; Mylanta® Liquid [OTC]; Mylanta® Maximum Strength Liquid [OTC]

Canadian Brand Names Diovol Plus®; Mylanta™ Double Strength; Mylanta™ Extra Strength; Mylanta™ regular Strength

Generic Available Yes

Synonyms Magnesium Hydroxide, Aluminum Hydroxide, and Simethicone; Simethicone, Aluminum Hydroxide, and Magnesium Hydroxide

Pharmacologic Category Antacid; Antiflatulent

Use Temporary relief of hyperacidity associated with gas; may also be used for indications associated with other antacids

Local Anesthetic/Vasoconstrictor Precautions No information available to require special precautions

Effects on Dental Treatment Key adverse event(s) related to dental treatment: Chalky taste. Aluminum and magnesium ions prevent GI absorption of tetracycline by forming a large ionized chelated molecule with the tetracyclines in the stomach. Aluminum hydroxide prevents GI absorption of ketoconazole and itraconazole by increasing the pH in the GI tract. Any of these drugs should be administered at least 1 hour before aluminum hydroxide.

Common Adverse Effects

>10%: Gastrointestinal: Chalky taste, stomach cramps, constipation, decreased bowel motility, fecal impaction, hemorrhoids

1% to 10%: Gastrointestinal: Nausea, vomiting, discoloration of feces (white speckles)

Drug Interactions

Decreased Effect: Tetracyclines, digoxin, indomethacin, or iron salts, isoniazid, allopurinol, benzodiazepines, corticosteroids, penicillamine, phenothiazines, ranitidine, ketoconazole, itraconazole

Pregnancy Risk Factor C

Aluminum Potassium Sulfate and Epinephrine (Racemic) (Dental) *see* Epinephrine (Racemic) and Aluminum Potassium Sulfate *on page 497*

Aluminum Sucrose Sulfate, Basic *see* Sucralfate *on page 1242*

Aluminum Sulfate and Calcium Acetate

(a LOO mi num SUL fate & KAL see um AS e tate)

U.S. Brand Names Domeboro® [OTC]; Pedi-Boro® [OTC]

Generic Available No

Synonyms Calcium Acetate and Aluminum Sulfate

Pharmacologic Category Topical Skin Product

Use Astringent wet dressing for relief of inflammatory conditions of the skin and to reduce weeping that may occur in dermatitis

Local Anesthetic/Vasoconstrictor Precautions No information available to require special precautions

Effects on Dental Treatment No significant effects or complications reported

Alupent® *see* Metaproterenol *on page 885*

Alustra™ *see* Hydroquinone *on page 719*

Amantadine (a MAN ta deen)

Related Information

Respiratory Diseases *on page 1478*

Systemic Viral Diseases *on page 1519*

U.S. Brand Names Symmetrel®

Canadian Brand Names Endantadine®; PMS-Amantadine; Symmetrel®

Generic Available Yes

Synonyms Adamantanamine Hydrochloride; Amantadine Hydrochloride

Pharmacologic Category Anti-Parkinson's Agent, Dopamine Agonist; Antiviral Agent

Use Prophylaxis and treatment of influenza A viral infection; treatment of parkinsonism; treatment of drug-induced extrapyramidal symptoms

Unlabeled/Investigational Use Creutzfeldt-Jakob disease

Local Anesthetic/Vasoconstrictor Precautions No information available to require special precautions

Effects on Dental Treatment Key adverse event(s) related to dental treatment: Xerostomia (prolonged use may cause significant xerostomia; normal salivary flow resumes upon discontinuation) and orthostatic hypotension.

Common Adverse Effects 1% to 10%:

Cardiovascular: Orthostatic hypotension, peripheral edema

Central nervous system: Insomnia, depression, anxiety, irritability, dizziness, hallucinations, ataxia, headache, somnolence, nervousness, dream abnormality, agitation, fatigue, confusion

Dermatologic: Livedo reticularis

Gastrointestinal: Nausea, anorexia, constipation, diarrhea, xerostomia

Respiratory: Dry nose

Mechanism of Action As an antiviral, blocks the uncoating of influenza A virus preventing penetration of virus into host; antiparkinsonian activity may be due to its blocking the reuptake of dopamine into presynaptic neurons or by increasing dopamine release from presynaptic fibers

Drug Interactions

Increased Effect/Toxicity: Anticholinergics (benztropine and trihexyphenidyl) may potentiate CNS side effects of amantadine. Hydrochlorothiazide, triamterene, and/or trimethoprim may increase toxicity of amantadine; monitor for altered response.

Pharmacodynamics/Kinetics

Onset of action: Antidyskinetic: Within 48 hours

Absorption: Well absorbed

Distribution: V_d: Normal: 1.5-6.1 L/kg; Renal failure: 5.1 ± 0.2 L/kg; in saliva, tear film, and nasal secretions; in animals, tissue (especially lung) concentrations higher than serum concentrations; crosses blood-brain barrier

Protein binding: Normal renal function: ~67%; Hemodialysis: ~59%

Metabolism: Not appreciable; small amounts of an acetyl metabolite identified

Bioavailability: 86% to 90%

Half-life elimination: Normal renal function: 16 ± 6 hours (9-31 hours); End-stage renal disease: 7-10 days

Excretion: Urine (80% to 90% unchanged) by glomerular filtration and tubular secretion

Total clearance: 2.5-10.5 L/hour

Pregnancy Risk Factor C

Amantadine Hydrochloride *see* Amantadine *on page 92*

Amaryl® *see* Glimepiride *on page 659*

Ambenonium (am be NOE nee um)

U.S. Brand Names Mytelase®

Canadian Brand Names Mytelase®

Generic Available No

Synonyms Ambenonium Chloride

Pharmacologic Category Cholinergic Agonist

Use Treatment of myasthenia gravis

Local Anesthetic/Vasoconstrictor Precautions No information available to require special precautions

Effects on Dental Treatment No significant effects or complications reported

Pregnancy Risk Factor C

Ambenonium Chloride *see* Ambenonium *on page 93*

Ambien® *see* Zolpidem *on page 1404*

Ambifed-G DM *see* Guaifenesin, Pseudoephedrine, and Dextromethorphan *on page 676*

AmBisome® *see* Amphotericin B (Liposomal) *on page 122*

Amcinonide (am SIN oh nide)

U.S. Brand Names Cyclocort®

Canadian Brand Names Amcort®; Cyclocort®

Generic Available Yes

Pharmacologic Category Corticosteroid, Topical

Use Relief of the inflammatory and pruritic manifestations of corticosteroid-responsive dermatoses (high potency corticosteroid)

Local Anesthetic/Vasoconstrictor Precautions No information available to require special precautions

Effects on Dental Treatment No significant effects or complications reported

(Continued)

Amcinonide *(Continued)*

Common Adverse Effects Frequency not defined.

Dermatologic: Acne, hypopigmentation, allergic dermatitis, maceration of the skin, skin atrophy, striae, miliaria, telangiectasia

Endocrine & metabolic: HPA suppression, Cushing's syndrome, growth retardation

Local: Burning, itching, irritation, dryness, folliculitis, hypertrichosis

Systemic: Suppression of HPA axis, Cushing's syndrome, hyperglycemia; these reactions occur more frequently with occlusive dressings

Miscellaneous: Secondary infection

Mechanism of Action Stimulates the synthesis of enzymes needed to decrease inflammation, suppress mitotic activity, and cause vasoconstriction

Pharmacodynamics/Kinetics

Absorption: Adequate through intact skin; increases with skin inflammation or occlusion

Metabolism: Hepatic

Excretion: Urine and feces

Pregnancy Risk Factor C

Amerge® *see* Naratriptan *on page 967*

Americaine® [OTC] *see* Benzocaine *on page 191*

Americaine® Anesthetic Lubricant *see* Benzocaine *on page 191*

A-Methapred® *see* MethylPREDNISolone *on page 910*

Amethocaine Hydrochloride *see* Tetracaine *on page 1278*

Amethopterin *see* Methotrexate *on page 897*

Amevive® *see* Alefacept *on page 76*

Amfepramone *see* Diethylpropion *on page 434*

AMG 073 *see* Cinacalcet *on page 331*

Amibid LA [DSC] *see* Guaifenesin *on page 672*

Amicar® *see* Aminocaproic Acid *on page 97*

Amidate® *see* Etomidate *on page 566*

Amifostine (am i FOS teen)

U.S. Brand Names Ethyol®

Canadian Brand Names Ethyol®

Mexican Brand Names Ethyol®

Generic Available No

Synonyms Ethiofos; Gammaphos; WR2721; YM-08310

Pharmacologic Category Adjuvant, Chemoprotective Agent (Cytoprotective); Antidote

Use Reduce the incidence of moderate to severe xerostomia in patients undergoing postoperative radiation treatment for head and neck cancer, where the radiation port includes a substantial portion of the parotid glands. Reduce the cumulative renal toxicity associated with repeated administration of cisplatin in patients with advanced ovarian cancer or nonsmall cell lung cancer.

Local Anesthetic/Vasoconstrictor Precautions No information available to require special precautions

Effects on Dental Treatment No significant effects or complications reported

Common Adverse Effects >10%:

Cardiovascular: Flushing; hypotension (62%)

Central nervous system: Chills, dizziness, somnolence

Gastrointestinal: Nausea/vomiting (may be severe)

Respiratory: Sneezing

Miscellaneous: Feeling of warmth/coldness, hiccups

Mechanism of Action Prodrug that is dephosphorylated by alkaline phosphatase in tissues to a pharmacologically active free thiol metabolite. The free thiol is available to bind to, and detoxify, reactive metabolites of cisplatin; and can also act as a scavenger of free radicals that may be generated in tissues.

Drug Interactions

Increased Effect/Toxicity: Special consideration should be given to patients receiving antihypertensive medications or other drugs that could potentiate hypotension.

Pharmacodynamics/Kinetics

Distribution: V_d: 3.5 L

Metabolism: Hepatic dephosphorylation to two metabolites (active-free thiol and disulfide)

Half-life elimination: 9 minutes

Excretion: Urine

Clearance, plasma: 2.17 L/minute

Pregnancy Risk Factor C

Amigesic® *see* Salsalate *on page 1207*

Amikacin (am i KAY sin)

Related Information

Tuberculosis *on page 1495*

U.S. Brand Names Amikin®

Canadian Brand Names Amikin®

Mexican Brand Names Akacin®; Amikafur®; Amikalem®; Amikason's® [inj.]; Amikayect®; Amikin®; A.M.K.®; Biclin®; Gamikal® [inj.]; Oprad®; Yectamid®

Generic Available Yes

Synonyms Amikacin Sulfate

Pharmacologic Category Antibiotic, Aminoglycoside

Use Treatment of serious infections due to organisms resistant to gentamicin and tobramycin including *Pseudomonas*, *Proteus*, *Serratia*, and other gram-positive bacilli (bone infections, respiratory tract infections, endocarditis, and septicemia); documented infection of mycobacterial organisms susceptible to amikacin

Local Anesthetic/Vasoconstrictor Precautions No information available to require special precautions

Effects on Dental Treatment No significant effects or complications reported

Common Adverse Effects 1% to 10%:

Central nervous system: Neurotoxicity

Otic: Ototoxicity (auditory), ototoxicity (vestibular)

Renal: Nephrotoxicity

Mechanism of Action Inhibits protein synthesis in susceptible bacteria by binding to 30S ribosomal subunits

Drug Interactions

Increased Effect/Toxicity: Amikacin may increase or prolong the effect of neuromuscular blocking agents. Concurrent use of amphotericin (or other nephrotoxic drugs) may increase the risk of amikacin-induced nephrotoxicity. The risk of ototoxicity from amikacin may be increased with other ototoxic drugs.

Pharmacodynamics/Kinetics

Absorption: I.M.: May be delayed in the bedridden patient

Distribution: Primarily into extracellular fluid (highly hydrophilic); penetrates blood-brain barrier when meninges inflamed; crosses placenta

Relative diffusion of antimicrobial agents from blood into CSF: Good only with inflammation (exceeds usual MICs)

CSF:blood level ratio: Normal meninges: 10% to 20%; Inflamed meninges: 15% to 24%

Half-life elimination (renal function and age dependent):

Infants: Low birth weight (1-3 days): 7-9 hours; Full-term >7 days: 4-5 hours

Children: 1.6-2.5 hours

Adults: Normal renal function: 1.4-2.3 hours; Anuria/end-stage renal disease: 28-86 hours

Time to peak, serum: I.M.: 45-120 minutes

Excretion: Urine (94% to 98%)

Pregnancy Risk Factor D

Amikacin Sulfate *see* Amikacin *on page 95*

Amikin® *see* Amikacin *on page 95*

Amiloride (a MIL oh ride)

Related Information

Cardiovascular Diseases *on page 1458*

U.S. Brand Names Midamor® [DSC]

Canadian Brand Names Midamor®

Generic Available Yes

Synonyms Amiloride Hydrochloride

Pharmacologic Category Diuretic, Potassium-Sparing

Use Counteracts potassium loss induced by other diuretics in the treatment of hypertension or edematous conditions including CHF, hepatic cirrhosis, and hypoaldosteronism; usually used in conjunction with more potent diuretics such as thiazides or loop diuretics

Unlabeled/Investigational Use Investigational: Cystic fibrosis; reduction of lithium-induced polyuria

Local Anesthetic/Vasoconstrictor Precautions No information available to require special precautions

Effects on Dental Treatment No significant effects or complications reported

Common Adverse Effects 1% to 10%:

Central nervous system: Headache, fatigue, dizziness

(Continued)

Amiloride *(Continued)*

Endocrine & metabolic: Hyperkalemia (up to 10%; risk reduced in patients receiving kaliuretic diuretics), hyperchloremic metabolic acidosis, dehydration, hyponatremia, gynecomastia

Gastrointestinal: Nausea, diarrhea, vomiting, abdominal pain, gas pain, appetite changes, constipation

Genitourinary: Impotence

Neuromuscular & skeletal: Muscle cramps, weakness

Respiratory: Cough, dyspnea

Mechanism of Action Interferes with potassium/sodium exchange (active transport) in the distal tubule, cortical collecting tubule and collecting duct by inhibiting sodium, potassium-ATPase; decreases calcium excretion; increases magnesium loss

Drug Interactions

Increased Effect/Toxicity: Increased risk of amiloride-associated hyperkalemia with triamterene, spironolactone, ACE inhibitors or angiotensin receptor antagonists, potassium preparations, cyclosporine, tacrolimus, and indomethacin. Amiloride may increase the toxicity of amantadine and lithium by reduction of renal excretion. Quinidine and amiloride together may increase risk of malignant arrhythmias.

Decreased Effect: Decreased effect of amiloride with use of NSAIDs. Amoxicillin's absorption may be reduced with concurrent use.

Pharmacodynamics/Kinetics

Onset of action: 2 hours

Duration: 24 hours

Absorption: ~15% to 25%

Distribution: V_d: 350-380 L

Protein binding: 23%

Metabolism: No active metabolites

Half-life elimination: Normal renal function: 6-9 hours; End-stage renal disease: 8-144 hours

Time to peak, serum: 6-10 hours

Excretion: Urine and feces (equal amounts as unchanged drug)

Pregnancy Risk Factor B

Amiloride and Hydrochlorothiazide

(a MIL oh ride & hye droe klor oh THYE a zide)

Related Information

Amiloride *on page 95*

Hydrochlorothiazide *on page 699*

U.S. Brand Names Moduretic® [DSC]

Canadian Brand Names Apo-Amilzide®; Moduret®; Moduretic®; Novamilor; Nu-Amilzide

Generic Available Yes

Synonyms Hydrochlorothiazide and Amiloride

Pharmacologic Category Diuretic, Combination

Use Potassium-sparing diuretic; antihypertensive

Local Anesthetic/Vasoconstrictor Precautions No information available to require special precautions

Effects on Dental Treatment No significant effects or complications reported

Common Adverse Effects See individual agents.

Drug Interactions

Increased Effect/Toxicity: See individual agents.

Decreased Effect: See individual agents.

Pharmacodynamics/Kinetics See individual agents.

Pregnancy Risk Factor B

Amiloride Hydrochloride *see* Amiloride *on page 95*

2-Amino-6-Mercaptopurine *see* Thioguanine *on page 1288*

2-Amino-6-Trifluoromethoxy-benzothiazole *see* Riluzole *on page 1183*

Aminobenzylpenicillin *see* Ampicillin *on page 124*

Aminocamptothecin (a min o camp to THE sin)

Generic Available No

Synonyms 9-AC; 9-Aminocamptothecin; NSC-603071

Pharmacologic Category Antineoplastic Agent, DNA Binding Agent; Enzyme Inhibitor, Topoisomerase I Inhibitor

Unlabeled/Investigational Use Phase II trials: Relapsed lymphoma, refractory breast cancer, nonsmall cell lung cancer, untreated colorectal carcinoma

Local Anesthetic/Vasoconstrictor Precautions No information available to require special precautions

Effects on Dental Treatment No significant effects or complications reported

Common Adverse Effects Frequency not defined.

Central nervous system: Fatigue
Dermatologic: Alopecia
Gastrointestinal: Nausea, vomiting, diarrhea, mucositis, anorexia
Hematologic: Neutropenia (may be dose-limiting), thrombocytopenia (reversible, but may be dose-limiting depending on administration schedule), anemia

Mechanism of Action Aminocamptothecin binds to topoisomerase I, stabilizing the cleavable DNA-topoisomerase I complex, resulting in arrest of the replication fork and inhibition of DNA synthesis.

Drug Interactions

Decreased Effect: Anticonvulsants may decrease aminocamptothecin levels.

Pharmacodynamics/Kinetics Ratio of lactone to total drug is 8.7 ± 4.7% because of instability of aminocamptothecin lactone in plasma.

Distribution: V_d: 46-92 L
Metabolism: None identified
Half-life elimination: Terminal: 8-17 hours for total aminocamptothecin
Excretion: Urine (32% of total drug delivered)

9-Aminocamptothecin *see* Aminocamptothecin *on page 96*

Aminocaproic Acid (a mee noe ka PROE ik AS id)

U.S. Brand Names Amicar®

Canadian Brand Names Amicar®

Generic Available Yes: Syrup, tablet

Synonyms Epsilon Aminocaproic Acid

Pharmacologic Category Hemostatic Agent

Use Treatment of excessive bleeding from fibrinolysis

Unlabeled/Investigational Use Treatment of traumatic hyphema

Local Anesthetic/Vasoconstrictor Precautions No information available to require special precautions

Effects on Dental Treatment No significant effects or complications reported

Common Adverse Effects Frequency not defined.

Cardiovascular: Arrhythmia, bradycardia, hypotension, peripheral ischemia, syncope, thrombosis
Central nervous system: Confusion, delirium, dizziness, fatigue, hallucinations, headache, intracranial hypertension, malaise, seizures, stroke
Dermatologic: Rash, pruritus
Gastrointestinal: Abdominal pain, anorexia, cramps, diarrhea, GI irritation, nausea
Genitourinary: Dry ejaculation
Hematologic: Agranulocytosis, bleeding time increased, leukopenia, thrombocytopenia
Neuromuscular & skeletal: CPK increased, myalgias, myositis, myopathy, rhabdomyolysis (rare), weakness
Ophthalmic: Watery eyes, vision decreased
Otic: Tinnitus
Renal: Failure (rare), myoglobinuria (rare)
Respiratory: Dyspnea, nasal congestion, pulmonary embolism

Mechanism of Action Competitively inhibits activation of plasminogen to plasmin, also, a lesser antiplasmin effect

Drug Interactions

Increased Effect/Toxicity: Increased risk of hypercoagulability with oral contraceptives, estrogens. Should not be administered with factor IX complex concentrated or anti-inhibitor complex concentrates due to an increased risk of thrombosis.

Pharmacodynamics/Kinetics

Onset of action: ~1-72 hours
Distribution: Widely through intravascular and extravascular compartments; V_d: Oral: 23 L, I.V.: 30 L
Metabolism: Minimally hepatic
Half-life elimination: 2 hours
Time to peak: Oral: Within 2 hours
Excretion: Urine (65% as unchanged drug, 11% as metabolite)

Pregnancy Risk Factor C

(Continued)

Aminocaproic Acid *(Continued)*

Comments Antifibrinolytic drugs are useful to control bleeding after dental extractions in patients with hemophilia. A clinical trial reported that aminocaproic acid or tranexamic acid reduces both recurrent bleeding and the amount of clotting factor replacement therapy required. In adults, the oral dose was 50-60 mg aminocaproic acid per kg every 4 hours until dental sockets were completely healed.

Extemporaneous solutions incorporating 100 mg aminocaproic acid per 5 mL of oral solution have been used as an oral rinse with some success. Use, however, must be carefully considered since they may not show efficacy in all patients with either drug-induced or hereditary coagulation problems. Studies are ongoing and commercial products may be available in the future.

Amino-Cerv™ *see* Urea *on page 1353*

Aminoglutethimide (a mee noe gloo TETH i mide)

U.S. Brand Names Cytadren®

Generic Available No

Synonyms AG; AGT; BA-16038; Elipten

Pharmacologic Category Aromatase Inhibitor; Enzyme Inhibitor; Hormone Antagonist, Anti-Adrenal; Nonsteroidal Aromatase Inhibitor

Use Suppression of adrenal function in selected patients with Cushing's syndrome

Unlabeled/Investigational Use Treatment of prostate cancer (androgen synthesis inhibitor)

Local Anesthetic/Vasoconstrictor Precautions No information available to require special precautions

Effects on Dental Treatment Key adverse event(s) related to dental treatment: Nausea and orthostatic hypotension.

Common Adverse Effects Most adverse effects will diminish in incidence and severity after the first 2-6 weeks

>10%:
- Central nervous system: Headache, dizziness, drowsiness, lethargy, clumsiness
- Dermatologic: Skin rash
- Gastrointestinal: Nausea, anorexia
- Hepatic: Cholestatic jaundice
- Neuromuscular & skeletal: Myalgia
- Renal: Nephrotoxicity
- Respiratory: Pulmonary alveolar damage

1% to 10%:
- Cardiovascular: Hypotension, tachycardia, orthostasis
- Dermatologic: Hirsutism, pruritus
- Endocrine & metabolic: Adrenocortical insufficiency
- Gastrointestinal: Vomiting

Mechanism of Action Blocks the enzymatic conversion of cholesterol to delta-5-pregnenolone, thereby reducing the synthesis of adrenal glucocorticoids, mineralocorticoids, estrogens, aldosterone, and androgens

Drug Interactions

Cytochrome P450 Effect: Induces CYP1A2 (strong), 2C19 (strong), 3A4 (strong)

Decreased Effect: Aminoglutethimide may decrease therapeutic effect of dexamethasone, digitoxin (after 3-8 weeks), warfarin, medroxyprogesterone, megestrol, and tamoxifen. Aminoglutethimide may decrease the levels/effects of aminophylline, benzodiazepines, calcium channel blockers, citalopram, clarithromycin, cyclosporine, diazepam, erythromycin, estrogens, fluvoxamine, methsuximide, mirtazapine, nateglinide, nefazodone, nevirapine, phenytoin, proton pump inhibitors, protease inhibitors, ropinirole, sertraline, tacrolimus, theophylline, venlafaxine, voriconazole and other drugs metabolized by CYP1A2, 2C19, or 3A4.

Pharmacodynamics/Kinetics

Onset of action: Adrenal suppression: 3-5 days; following withdrawal of therapy, adrenal function returns within 72 hours

Absorption: 90%

Distribution: Crosses placenta

Protein binding, plasma: 20% to 25%

Metabolism: Major metabolite is N-acetylaminoglutethimide; induces its own metabolism

Half-life elimination: 7-15 hours; shorter following multiple doses

Excretion: Urine (34% to 50% as unchanged drug, 25% as metabolites)

Pregnancy Risk Factor D

Aminolevulinic Acid (a MEE noh lev yoo lin ik AS id)

U.S. Brand Names Levulan® Kerastick®

Canadian Brand Names Levulan®

Generic Available No

Synonyms Aminolevulinic Acid Hydrochloride

Pharmacologic Category Photosensitizing Agent, Topical; Topical Skin Product

Use Treatment of minimally to moderately thick actinic keratoses (grade 1 or 2) of the face or scalp; to be used in conjunction with blue light illumination

Local Anesthetic/Vasoconstrictor Precautions No information available to require special precautions

Effects on Dental Treatment Key adverse event(s) related to dental treatment: Bleeding/hemorrhage.

Common Adverse Effects

Transient stinging, burning, itching, erythema, and edema result from the photosensitizing properties of this agent. Symptoms subside between 1 minute and 24 hours after turning off the blue light illuminator. Severe stinging or burning was reported in at least 50% of patients from at least 1 lesional site treatment.

>10%: Dermatologic: Severe stinging or burning (50%), scaling of the skin/crusted skin (64% to 71%), hyperpigmentation/hypopigmentation (22% to 36%), itching (14% to 25%), erosion (2% to 14%)

1% to 10%:

Central nervous system: Dysesthesia (up to 2%)

Dermatologic: Skin ulceration (2% to 4%), vesiculation (4% to 5%), pustular drug eruption (up to 4%), skin disorder (5% to 12%)

Hematologic: Bleeding/hemorrhage (2% to 4%)

Local: Wheal/flare (2% to 7%), local pain (1%), tenderness (1% to 2%), edema (1%), scabbing (up to 2%), ulceration (2% to 4%), excoriation (1%)

Mechanism of Action Aminolevulinic acid is a metabolic precursor of protoporphyrin IX (PpIX), which is a photosensitizer. Photosensitization following application of aminolevulinic acid topical solution occurs through the metabolic conversion to PpIX. When exposed to light of appropriate wavelength and energy, accumulated PpIX produces a photodynamic reaction.

Drug Interactions

Increased Effect/Toxicity: Photosensitizing agents such as griseofulvin, thiazide diuretics, sulfonamides, sulfonylureas, phenothiazines, and tetracyclines theoretically may increase the photosensitizing potential of aminolevulinic acid.

Pharmacodynamics/Kinetics

PpIX:

Peak fluorescence intensity: 11 hours ± 1 hour

Half-life, mean clearance for lesions: 30 ± 10 hours

Pregnancy Risk Factor C

Aminolevulinic Acid Hydrochloride *see* Aminolevulinic Acid *on page 99*

Aminophylline (am in OFF i lin)

Related Information

Respiratory Diseases *on page 1478*

Theophylline *on page 1285*

Canadian Brand Names Phyllocontin®; Phyllocontin®-350

Mexican Brand Names Drafilyn®

Generic Available Yes

Synonyms Theophylline Ethylenediamine

Pharmacologic Category Theophylline Derivative

Use Bronchodilator in reversible airway obstruction due to asthma or COPD; increase diaphragmatic contractility

Local Anesthetic/Vasoconstrictor Precautions No information available to require special precautions

Effects on Dental Treatment Prescribe erythromycin products with caution to patients taking theophylline products. Erythromycin will delay the normal metabolic inactivation of theophyllines leading to increased blood levels; this has resulted in nausea, vomiting, and CNS restlessness.

Common Adverse Effects

Uncommon at serum theophylline concentrations ≤15 mcg/mL

1% to 10%:

Cardiovascular: Tachycardia

Central nervous system: Nervousness, restlessness

Gastrointestinal: Nausea, vomiting

(Continued)

Aminophylline *(Continued)*

Mechanism of Action Causes bronchodilatation, diuresis, CNS and cardiac stimulation, and gastric acid secretion by blocking phosphodiesterase which increases tissue concentrations of cyclic adenine monophosphate (cAMP) which in turn promotes catecholamine stimulation of lipolysis, glycogenolysis, and gluconeogenesis and induces release of epinephrine from adrenal medulla cells

Drug Interactions

Cytochrome P450 Effect: Substrate of CYP1A2 (major), 2E1 (minor), 3A4 (minor)

Increased Effect/Toxicity: Levels/effects of aminophylline may be increased by amiodarone, ciprofloxacin, fluvoxamine, ketoconazole, lomefloxacin, ofloxacin, and rofecoxib and other CYP1A2 inhibitors.

Decreased Effect: Levels/effects of aminophylline may be decreased by aminoglutethimide, carbamazepine, phenobarbital, rifampin, and other CYP1A2 inducers.

Pharmacodynamics/Kinetics

Theophylline:

Absorption: Oral: Dosage form dependent

Distribution: 0.45 L/kg based on ideal body weight

Protein binding: 40%, primarily to albumin

Metabolism: Children >1 year and Adults: Hepatic; involves CYP1A2, 2E1 and 3A4; forms active metabolites (caffeine and 3-methylxanthine)

Half-life elimination: Highly variable and dependent upon age, liver function, cardiac function, lung disease, and smoking history

Time to peak, serum:

Oral: Immediate release: 1-2 hours

I.V.: Within 30 minutes

Excretion: Urine Children >3 months and Adults: 10% unchanged

Pregnancy Risk Factor C

Aminosalicylate Sodium *see* Aminosalicylic Acid *on page 100*

Aminosalicylic Acid (a mee noe sal i SIL ik AS id)

Related Information

Rheumatoid Arthritis, Osteoarthritis, and Osteoporosis *on page 1490*

Tuberculosis *on page 1495*

U.S. Brand Names Paser®

Canadian Brand Names Nemasol® Sodium

Generic Available No

Synonyms Aminosalicylate Sodium; 4-Aminosalicylic Acid; Para-Aminosalicylate Sodium; PAS; Sodium PAS

Pharmacologic Category Salicylate

Use Adjunctive treatment of tuberculosis used in combination with other antitubercular agents

Unlabeled/Investigational Use Crohn's disease

Local Anesthetic/Vasoconstrictor Precautions No information available to require special precautions

Effects on Dental Treatment NSAID formulations are known to reversibly decrease platelet aggregation via mechanisms different than observed with aspirin. The dentist should be aware of the potential of abnormal coagulation. Caution should also be exercised in the use of NSAIDs in patients already on anticoagulant therapy with drugs such as warfarin (Coumadin®).

Common Adverse Effects Frequency not defined.

Cardiovascular: Pericarditis, vasculitis

Central nervous system: Encephalopathy, fever

Dermatologic: Skin eruptions

Endocrine & metabolic: Goiter (with or without myxedema), hypoglycemia

Gastrointestinal: Abdominal pain, diarrhea, nausea, vomiting

Hematologic: Agranulocytosis, anemia (hemolytic), leukopenia, thrombocytopenia

Hepatic: Hepatitis, jaundice

Ocular: Optic neuritis

Respiratory: Eosinophilic pneumonia

Mechanism of Action Aminosalicylic acid (PAS) is a highly specific bacteriostatic agent active against *M. tuberculosis*. Structurally related to para-aminobenzoic acid (PABA) and its mechanism of action is thought to be similar to the sulfonamides, a competitive antagonism with PABA; disrupts plate biosynthesis in sensitive organisms.

Drug Interactions

Decreased Effect: Aminosalicylic acid may decrease serum levels of digoxin and vitamin B_{12}.

Pharmacodynamics/Kinetics

Absorption: Readily, >90%

Protein binding: 50% to 60%

Metabolism: Hepatic (>50%) via acetylation

Half-life elimination: Reduced with renal impairment

Time to peak, serum: 6 hours

Excretion: Urine (>80% as unchanged drug and metabolites)

Pregnancy Risk Factor C

4-Aminosalicylic Acid *see* Aminosalicylic Acid *on page 100*

5-Aminosalicylic Acid *see* Mesalamine *on page 882*

Aminoxin® [OTC] *see* Pyridoxine *on page 1154*

Amiodarone (a MEE oh da rone)

Related Information

Cardiovascular Diseases *on page 1458*

U.S. Brand Names Cordarone®; Pacerone®

Canadian Brand Names Alti-Amiodarone; Cordarone®; Gen-Amiodarone; Novo-Amiodarone; Rhoxal-amiodarone

Mexican Brand Names Braxan®; Cordarone®

Generic Available Yes

Synonyms Amiodarone Hydrochloride

Pharmacologic Category Antiarrhythmic Agent, Class III

Use

Oral: Management of life-threatening recurrent ventricular fibrillation (VF) or hemodynamically unstable ventricular tachycardia (VT)

I.V.: Initiation of treatment and prophylaxis of frequency recurring VF and unstable VT in patients refractory to other therapy. Also, used for patients when oral amiodarone is indicated, but who are unable to take oral medication.

Unlabeled/Investigational Use

Conversion of atrial fibrillation to normal sinus rhythm; maintenance of normal sinus rhythm

Prevention of postoperative atrial fibrillation during cardiothoracic surgery

Paroxysmal supraventricular tachycardia (SVT)

Control of rapid ventricular rate due to accessory pathway conduction in pre-excited atrial arrhythmias [ACLS guidelines]

After defibrillation and epinephrine in cardiac arrest with persistent ventricular tachycardia (VT) or ventricular fibrillation (VF) [ACLS guidelines]

Control of hemodynamically stable VT, polymorphic VT or wide-complex tachycardia of uncertain origin [ACLS guidelines]

Local Anesthetic/Vasoconstrictor Precautions No information available to require special precautions

Effects on Dental Treatment Key adverse event(s) related to dental treatment: Oral: Abnormal salivation and taste.

Common Adverse Effects In a recent meta-analysis, patients taking lower doses of amiodarone (152-330 mg daily for at least 12 months) were more likely to develop thyroid, neurologic, skin, ocular, and bradycardic abnormalities than those taking placebo (Vorperian, 1997). Pulmonary toxicity was similar in both the low dose amiodarone group and in the placebo group but there was a trend towards increased toxicity in the amiodarone group. Gastrointestinal and hepatic events were seen to a similar extent in both the low dose amiodarone group and placebo group.

>10%:

- Cardiovascular: Hypotension (I.V. 16%, refractory in rare cases)
- Central nervous system (3% to 40%): Abnormal gait/ataxia, dizziness, fatigue, headache, malaise, impaired memory, involuntary movement, insomnia, poor coordination, peripheral neuropathy, sleep disturbances, tremor
- Dermatologic: Photosensitivity (10% to 75%)
- Endocrine & Metabolic: Hypothyroidism (1% to 22%)
- Gastrointestinal: Nausea, vomiting, anorexia and constipation (10% to 33%), AST or ALT level >2X normal (15% to 50%)

1% to 10%:

- Cardiovascular: Congestive heart failure (3%), bradycardia (3% to 5%), AV block (5%), conduction abnormalities, SA node dysfunction (1% to 3%), cardiac arrhythmias, flushing, edema. Additional effects associated with

(Continued)

Amiodarone *(Continued)*

I.V. administration include asystole, cardiac arrest, electromechanical dissociation, ventricular tachycardia, and cardiogenic shock.

Dermatologic: Slate blue skin discoloration (<10%)

Endocrine & metabolic: Hyperthyroidism (<3%), libido decreased

Gastrointestinal: Abdominal pain, abnormal salivation, abnormal taste (oral)

Hematologic: Coagulation abnormalities

Hepatic: Hepatitis and cirrhosis (<3%)

Local: Phlebitis (I.V., with concentrations >3 mg/mL)

Ocular: Visual disturbances (2% to 9%), corneal microdeposits (occur in a majority of patients and lead to visual disturbance in ~10%), halo vision (<5% occurring especially at night), optic neuritis (1%)

Respiratory: Pulmonary toxicity has been estimated to occur at a frequency between 2% and 7% of patients (some reports indicate a frequency as high as 17%). Toxicity may present as hypersensitivity pneumonitis; pulmonary fibrosis (cough, fever, malaise); pulmonary inflammation; interstitial pneumonitis; or alveolar pneumonitis. ARDS has been reported in up to 2% of patients receiving I. V. amiodarone, and postoperatively in patients receiving oral amiodarone.

Miscellaneous: Abnormal smell (oral)

Mechanism of Action Class III antiarrhythmic agent which inhibits adrenergic stimulation, prolongs the action potential and refractory period in myocardial tissue; decreases AV conduction and sinus node function

Drug Interactions

Cytochrome P450 Effect: Substrate of CYP1A2 (minor), 2C8/9 (major at low concentration), 2C19 (minor), 2D6 (minor), 3A4 (major); **Inhibits** CYP1A2 (strong), 2A6 (moderate), 2B6 (weak), 2C8/9 (moderate), 2C19 (weak), 2D6 (moderate), 3A4 (moderate)

Increased Effect/Toxicity: Note: Due to the long half-life of amiodarone, drug interactions may take 1 or more weeks to develop. The effect of drugs which prolong the QT interval, including amitriptyline, bepridil, cisapride, disopyramide, erythromycin, gatifloxacin, haloperidol, imipramine, moxifloxacin, quinidine, pimozide, procainamide, sotalol, sparfloxacin, theophylline, and thioridazine may be increased. Cisapride, gatifloxacin, moxifloxacin, and sparfloxacin are contraindicated. Use of amiodarone with diltiazem, verapamil, digoxin, beta-blockers, and other drugs which delay AV conduction may cause excessive AV block (amiodarone may also decrease the metabolism of some of these agents - see below).

Amiodarone may increase the levels of digoxin (reduce dose by 50% on initiation), flecainide (decrease dose up to 33%), phenothiazines, procainamide (reduce dose), and quinidine. Amiodarone may increase the levels/effects of aminophylline, amphetamines, selected benzodiazepines, selected beta-blockers, calcium channel blockers, cyclosporine, dexmedetomidine, dextromethorphan, fluoxetine, fluvoxamine, glimepiride, glipizide, ifosfamide, lidocaine, mexiletine, mirtazapine, nateglinide, nefazodone, paroxetine, phenytoin, pioglitazone, risperidone, ritonavir, ropinirole, rosiglitazone, sildenafil (and other PDE-5 inhibitors), sertraline, tacrolimus, theophylline, thioridazine, tricyclic antidepressants, trifluoperazine, venlafaxine, warfarin, and other CYP1A2, 2A6, 2C8/9, CYP2D6, and/or CYP3A4 substrates. Selected benzodiazepines (midazolam, triazolam), cisapride, ergot alkaloids, selected HMG-CoA reductase inhibitors (lovastatin and simvastatin), mesoridazine, pimozide, and thioridazine are generally contraindicated with strong CYP3A4 inhibitors. When used with strong CYP3A4 inhibitors, dosage adjustment/limits are recommended for sildenafil and other PDE-5 inhibitors; consult individual monographs.

The levels/effects of amiodarone may be increased by amprenavir, cimetidine, delavirdine, fluconazole, gemfibrozil, indinavir, ketoconazole, nelfinavir, nicardipine, NSAIDs, pioglitazone, ritonavir, sulfonamides, and other CYP2C8/9 inhibitors.

Concurrent use of fentanyl may lead to bradycardia, sinus arrest, and hypotension. Amiodarone may alter thyroid function and response to thyroid supplements. Amiodarone enhances the myocardial depressant and conduction defects of inhalation anesthetics (monitor).

Decreased Effect: Levels/effects of amiodarone may be decreased by carbamazepine, phenobarbital, phenytoin, rifampin, rifapentine, secobarbital, and other CYP2C8/9 inducers. Amiodarone may decrease the levels/effects of codeine, hydrocodone, oxycodone, tramadol, and other prodrug substrates of CYP2D6. Amiodarone may alter thyroid function and response to thyroid supplements; monitor closely.

Pharmacodynamics/Kinetics

Onset of action: Oral: 3 days to 3 weeks; I.V.: May be more rapid

Peak effect: 1 week to 5 months

Duration after discontinuing therapy: 7-50 days

Note: Mean onset of effect and duration after discontinuation may be shorter in children than adults

Distribution: V_d: 66 L/kg (range: 18-148 L/kg); crosses placenta; enters breast milk in concentrations higher than maternal plasma concentrations

Protein binding: 96%

Metabolism: Hepatic via CYP2C8 and 3A4, major metabolite active; possible enterohepatic recirculation

Bioavailability: Oral: ~50%

Half-life elimination: Terminal: 40-55 days (range: 26-107 days); shorter in children than adults

Excretion: Feces; urine (<1% as unchanged drug)

Pregnancy Risk Factor D

Amiodarone Hydrochloride *see* Amiodarone *on page 101*

Amipaque® [DSC] *see* Radiological/Contrast Media (Nonionic) *on page 1166*

Ami-Tex PSE *see* Guaifenesin and Pseudoephedrine *on page 675*

Amitone® [OTC] *see* Calcium Carbonate *on page 245*

Amitriptyline (a mee TRIP ti leen)

Related Information

Temporomandibular Dysfunction (TMD) *on page 1564*

U.S. Brand Names Elavil® [DSC]

Canadian Brand Names Apo-Amitriptyline®; Levate®; PMS-Amitriptyline

Mexican Brand Names Anapsique®; Tryptanol®

Generic Available Yes

Synonyms Amitriptyline Hydrochloride

Pharmacologic Category Antidepressant, Tricyclic (Tertiary Amine)

Use Relief of symptoms of depression

Unlabeled/Investigational Use Analgesic for certain chronic and neuropathic pain; prophylaxis against migraine headaches; treatment of depressive disorders in children

Local Anesthetic/Vasoconstrictor Precautions Use with caution; epinephrine, norepinephrine and levonordefrin have been shown to have an increased pressor response in combination with TCAs

Effects on Dental Treatment Key adverse event(s) related to dental treatment: Xerostomia and changes in salivation (normal salivary flow resumes upon discontinuation), and orthostatic hypotension. Amitriptyline is the most anticholinergic and sedating of the antidepressants; pronounced effects on the cardiovascular system; long-term treatment with TCAs such as amitriptyline increases the risk of caries by reducing salivation and salivary buffer capacity. In a study by Rundergren, et al, pathological alterations were observed in the oral mucosa of 72% of 58 patients; 55% had new carious lesions after taking TCAs for a median of 5½ years. Current research is investigating the use of the salivary stimulant pilocarpine (Salagen®) to overcome the xerostomia from amitriptyline.

Common Adverse Effects Anticholinergic effects may be pronounced; moderate to marked sedation can occur (tolerance to these effects usually occurs).

Frequency not defined.

Cardiovascular: Orthostatic hypotension, tachycardia, nonspecific ECG changes, changes in AV conduction, cardiomyopathy (rare), MI, stroke, heart block, arrhythmias, syncope, hypertension, palpitation

Central nervous system: Restlessness, dizziness, insomnia, sedation, fatigue, anxiety, impaired cognitive function, seizures, extrapyramidal symptoms, coma, hallucinations, confusion, disorientation, impaired coordination, ataxia, headache, nightmares, hyperpyrexia

Dermatologic: Allergic rash, urticaria, photosensitivity, alopecia

Endocrine & metabolic: Syndrome of inappropriate ADH secretion

Gastrointestinal: Weight gain, xerostomia, constipation, paralytic ileus, nausea, vomiting, anorexia, stomatitis, peculiar taste, diarrhea, black tongue

Genitourinary: Urinary retention

Hematologic: Bone marrow depression, purpura, eosinophilia

Ocular: Blurred vision, mydriasis, ocular pressure increased

Otic: Tinnitus

Neuromuscular & skeletal: Numbness, paresthesia, peripheral neuropathy, tremor, weakness

(Continued)

Amitriptyline *(Continued)*

Miscellaneous: Diaphoresis; withdrawal reactions (nausea, headache, malaise)

Dosage

Children:

Chronic pain management (unlabeled use): Oral: Initial: 0.1 mg/kg at bedtime, may advance as tolerated over 2-3 weeks to 0.5-2 mg/kg at bedtime

Depressive disorders (unlabeled use): Oral: Initial doses of 1 mg/kg/day given in 3 divided doses with increases to 1.5 mg/kg/day have been reported in a small number of children (n=9) 9-12 years of age; clinically, doses up to 3 mg/kg/day (5 mg/kg/day if monitored closely) have been proposed

Migraine prophylaxis (unlabeled use): Oral: Initial: 0.25 mg/kg/day, given at bedtime; increase dose by 0.25 mg/kg/day to maximum 1 mg/kg/day. Reported dosing ranges: 0.1-2 mg/kg/day; maximum suggested dose: 10 mg

Adolescents: Depressive disorders: Oral: Initial: 25-50 mg/day; may administer in divided doses; increase gradually to 100 mg/day in divided doses

Adults:

Depression:

Oral: 50-150 mg/day single dose at bedtime or in divided doses; dose may be gradually increased up to 300 mg/day

I.M.: 20-30 mg 4 times/day

Migraine prophylaxis (unlabeled use): Oral: Initial: 10-25 mg at bedtime; usual dose: 150 mg; reported dosing ranges: 10-400 mg/day

Pain management (unlabeled use): Oral: Initial: 25 mg at bedtime; may increase as tolerated to 100 mg/day

Elderly: Depression: Oral: Initial: 10-25 mg at bedtime; dose should be increased in 10-25 mg increments every week if tolerated; dose range: 25-150 mg/day

Dosing interval in hepatic impairment: Use with caution and monitor plasma levels and patient response

Hemodialysis: Nondialyzable

Mechanism of Action Increases the synaptic concentration of serotonin and/or norepinephrine in the central nervous system by inhibition of their reuptake by the presynaptic neuronal membrane

Contraindications Hypersensitivity to amitriptyline or any component of the formulation (cross-sensitivity with other tricyclics may occur); use of MAO inhibitors within past 14 days; acute recovery phase following myocardial infarction; concurrent use of cisapride

Warnings/Precautions Often causes drowsiness/sedation, resulting in impaired performance of tasks requiring alertness (eg, operating machinery or driving). Sedative effects may be additive with other CNS depressants and/or ethanol. The degree of sedation is very high relative to other antidepressants. May worsen psychosis in some patients or precipitate a shift to mania or hypomania in patients with bipolar disease. May cause hyponatremia/SIADH. May increase the risks associated with electroconvulsive therapy. This agent should be discontinued, when possible, prior to elective surgery. Therapy should not be abruptly discontinued in patients receiving high doses for prolonged periods.

May cause orthostatic hypotension; the risk of this problem is very high relative to other antidepressants. Use with caution in patients at risk of hypotension or in patients where transient hypotensive episodes would be poorly tolerated (cardiovascular disease or cerebrovascular disease). The degree of anticholinergic blockade produced by this agent is very high relative to other cyclic antidepressants; use with caution in patients with urinary retention, benign prostatic hyperplasia, narrow-angle glaucoma, xerostomia, visual problems, constipation, or a history of bowel obstruction. May alter glucose control - use with caution in patients with diabetes.

The possibility of a suicide attempt is inherent in major depression and may persist until remission occurs. Use caution in high-risk patients during initiation of therapy. Prescriptions should be written for the smallest quantity consistent with good patient care. Use with caution in patients with a history of cardiovascular disease (including previous MI, stroke, tachycardia, or conduction abnormalities). The risk of conduction abnormalities with this agent is high relative to other antidepressants. May lower seizure threshold - use caution in patients with a previous seizure disorder or condition predisposing to seizures such as brain damage, alcoholism, or concurrent therapy with other drugs which lower the seizure threshold. Use with caution in hyperthyroid patients or those receiving thyroid supplementation. Use with caution in patients with hepatic or renal dysfunction and in elderly patients. Not recommended for use in patients <12 years of age.

Drug Interactions

Cytochrome P450 Effect: Substrate of CYP1A2 (minor), 2B6 (minor), 2C8/9 (minor), 2C19 (minor), 2D6 (major), 3A4 (minor); **Inhibits** CYP1A2 (weak), 2C8/9 (weak), 2C19 (weak), 2D6 (weak), 2E1 (weak)

Increased Effect/Toxicity: Amitriptyline increases the effects of amphetamines, anticholinergics, other CNS depressants (sedatives, hypnotics, or ethanol), carbamazepine, tolazamide, chlorpropamide, and warfarin. When used with MAO inhibitors, hyperpyrexia, hypertension, tachycardia, confusion, seizures, and **deaths have been reported** (serotonin syndrome). Serotonin syndrome has also been reported with ritonavir (rare). Levels/effects of amitriptyline may be increased by chlorpromazine, delavirdine, fluoxetine, miconazole, paroxetine, pergolide, quinidine, quinine, ritonavir, ropinirole, and other CYP2D6 inhibitors. Cimetidine, fenfluramine, grapefruit juice, indinavir, methylphenidate, diltiazem, valproate, and verapamil may increase the serum concentrations of tricyclic antidepressants (TCAs). Use of lithium with a TCA may increase the risk for neurotoxicity. Phenothiazines may increase concentration of some TCAs and TCAs may increase the concentration of phenothiazines. Pressor response to I.V. epinephrine, norepinephrine, and phenylephrine may be enhanced in patients receiving TCAs (**Note:** Effect is unlikely with epinephrine or levonordefrin dosages typically administered as infiltration in combination with local anesthetics). Combined use of beta-agonists or drugs which prolong QT_c (including quinidine, procainamide, disopyramide, cisapride, sparfloxacin, gatifloxacin, moxifloxacin) with TCAs may predispose patients to cardiac arrhythmias.

Decreased Effect: Amitriptyline inhibits the antihypertensive response to bethanidine, clonidine, debrisoquin, guanadrel, guanethidine, guanabenz, or guanfacine. Cholestyramine and colestipol may bind TCAs and reduce their absorption.

Ethanol/Nutrition/Herb Interactions

Ethanol: Avoid ethanol (may increase CNS depression).

Food: Grapefruit juice may inhibit the metabolism of some TCAs and clinical toxicity may result.

Herb/Nutraceutical: St John's wort may decrease amitriptyline levels. Avoid valerian, St John's wort, kava kava, gotu kola (may increase CNS depression).

Pharmacodynamics/Kinetics

Onset of action: Migraine prophylaxis: 6 weeks, higher dosage may be required in heavy smokers because of increased metabolism; Depression: 4-6 weeks, reduce dosage to lowest effective level

Distribution: Crosses placenta; enters breast milk

Metabolism: Hepatic to nortriptyline (active), hydroxy and conjugated derivatives; may be impaired in the elderly

Half-life elimination: Adults: 9-27 hours (average: 15 hours)

Time to peak, serum: ~4 hours

Excretion: Urine (18% as unchanged drug); feces (small amounts)

Pregnancy Risk Factor C

Dosage Forms TAB: 10 mg, 25 mg, 50 mg, 75 mg, 100 mg, 150 mg

Selected Readings

Boakes AJ, Laurence DR, Teoh PC, et al, "Interactions Between Sympathomimetic Amines and Antidepressant Agents in Man," *Br Med J*, 1973, 1(849):311-5.

Friedlander AH and Mahler ME, "Major Depressive Disorder. Psychopathology, Medical Management, and Dental Implications," *J Am Dent Assoc*, 2001, 132(5):629-38.

Ganzberg S, "Psychoactive Drugs," *ADA Guide to Dental Therapeutics*, 2nd ed, Chicago, IL: ADA Publishing, a Division of ADA Business Enterprises, Inc, 2000, 376-405.

Jastak JT and Yagiela JA, "Vasoconstrictors and Local Anesthesia: A Review and Rationale for Use," *J Am Dent Assoc*, 1983, 107(4):623-30.

Rundegren J, van Dijken J, Mörnstad H, et al, "Oral Conditions in Patients Receiving Long-Term Treatment With Cyclic Antidepressant Drugs," *Swed Dent J*, 1985, 9(2):55-64.

Yagiela JA, "Adverse Drug Interactions in Dental Practice: Interactions Associated With Vasoconstrictors. Part V of a Series," *J Am Dent Assoc*, 1999, 130(5):701-9.

Amitriptyline and Chlordiazepoxide

(a mee TRIP ti leen & klor dye az e POKS ide)

Related Information

Amitriptyline *on page 103*

Chlordiazepoxide *on page 307*

U.S. Brand Names Limbitrol®; Limbitrol® DS

Canadian Brand Names Limbitrol®

Generic Available Yes

Synonyms Chlordiazepoxide and Amitriptyline

(Continued)

Amitriptyline and Chlordiazepoxide *(Continued)*

Pharmacologic Category Antidepressant, Tricyclic (Tertiary Amine); Benzodiazepine

Use Treatment of moderate to severe anxiety and/or agitation and depression

Local Anesthetic/Vasoconstrictor Precautions Use with caution; epinephrine, norepinephrine and levonordefrin have been shown to have an increased pressor response in combination with TCAs

Effects on Dental Treatment

Amitriptyline: The most anticholinergic and sedating of the antidepressants; pronounced effects on the cardiovascular system; long-term treatment with TCAs such as amitriptyline increases the risk of caries by reducing salivation and salivary buffer capacity. In a study by Rundergren, et al, pathological alterations were observed in the oral mucosa of 72% of 58 patients; 55% had new carious lesions after taking TCAs for a median of 5½ years. Current research is investigating the use of the salivary stimulant pilocarpine (Salagen®) to overcome the xerostomia from amitriptyline.

Chlordiazepoxide: Over 10% of patients will experience xerostomia which disappears with cessation of drug therapy.

Common Adverse Effects See individual agents.

Restrictions C-IV

Drug Interactions

Cytochrome P450 Effect:

Amitriptyline: **Substrate** of CYP1A2 (minor), 2B6 (minor), 2C8/9 (minor), 2C19 (minor), 2D6 (major), 3A4 (minor); **Inhibits** CYP1A2 (weak), 2C8/9 (weak), 2C19 (weak), 2D6 (weak), 2E1 (weak)

Chlordiazepoxide: **Substrate** of CYP3A4 (major)

Increased Effect/Toxicity: See individual agents.

Decreased Effect: See individual agents.

Pharmacodynamics/Kinetics See individual agents.

Pregnancy Risk Factor D

Amitriptyline and Perphenazine

(a mee TRIP ti leen & per FEN a zeen)

Related Information

Amitriptyline *on page 103*

Perphenazine *on page 1070*

U.S. Brand Names Triavil®

Canadian Brand Names Etrafon®; Triavil®

Generic Available Yes

Synonyms Perphenazine and Amitriptyline

Pharmacologic Category Antidepressant, Tricyclic (Tertiary Amine); Antipsychotic Agent, Phenothiazine, Piperazine

Use Treatment of patients with moderate to severe anxiety and depression

Unlabeled/Investigational Use Depression with psychotic features

Local Anesthetic/Vasoconstrictor Precautions

Amitriptyline: Use with caution; epinephrine, norepinephrine and levonordefrin have been shown to have an increased pressor response in combination with TCAs

Perphenazine: No information available to require special precautions

Effects on Dental Treatment Key adverse event(s) related to dental treatment:

Amitriptyline: Xerostomia (normal salivary flow resumes upon discontinuation). The most anticholinergic and sedating of the antidepressants; pronounced effects on the cardiovascular system; long-term treatment with TCAs such as amitriptyline increases the risk of caries by reducing salivation and salivary buffer capacity. In a study by Rundergren, et al, pathological alterations were observed in the oral mucosa of 72% of 58 patients; 55% had new carious lesions after taking TCAs for a median of 5½ years. Current research is investigating the use of the salivary stimulant pilocarpine (Salagen®) to overcome the xerostomia from amitriptyline.

Perphenazine: Extrapyramidal symptoms (pseudoparkinsonism, akathisia, dystonias, tardive dyskinesia), dizziness, seizures, headache, drowsiness, paradoxical excitement, restlessness, and hyperactivity.

Tardive dyskinesia: Prevalence rate may be 40% in elderly; development of the syndrome and the irreversible nature are proportional to duration and total cumulative dose over time. Extrapyramidal reactions are more common in elderly with up to 50% developing these reactions after 60 years of age. Drug-induced Parkinson's syndrome occurs often; akathisia is the most common extrapyramidal reaction in elderly.

Increased confusion, memory loss, psychotic behavior, and agitation frequently occur as a consequence of anticholinergic effects. Antipsychotic associated sedation in nonpsychotic patients is extremely unpleasant due to feelings of depersonalization, derealization, and dysphoria.

Common Adverse Effects Frequency not defined.

Based on **amitriptyline** component: Anticholinergic effects may be pronounced; moderate to marked sedation can occur (tolerance to these effects usually occurs).

Cardiovascular: Orthostatic hypotension, tachycardia, nonspecific ECG changes, changes in AV conduction

Central nervous system: Restlessness, dizziness, insomnia, sedation, fatigue, anxiety, impaired cognitive function, seizures, extrapyramidal symptoms

Dermatologic: Allergic rash, urticaria, photosensitivity

Gastrointestinal: Weight gain, xerostomia, constipation

Genitourinary: Urinary retention

Ocular: Blurred vision, mydriasis

Miscellaneous: Diaphoresis

Based on **perphenazine** component:

Cardiovascular: Hypotension, orthostatic hypotension, hypertension, tachycardia, bradycardia, dizziness, cardiac arrest

Central nervous system: Extrapyramidal symptoms (pseudoparkinsonism, akathisia, dystonias, tardive dyskinesia), dizziness, cerebral edema, seizures, headache, drowsiness, paradoxical excitement, restlessness, hyperactivity, insomnia, neuroleptic malignant syndrome (NMS), impairment of temperature regulation

Dermatologic: Increased sensitivity to sun, rash, discoloration of skin (blue-gray)

Endocrine & metabolic: Hypoglycemia, hyperglycemia, galactorrhea, lactation, breast enlargement, gynecomastia, menstrual irregularity, amenorrhea, SIADH, changes in libido

Gastrointestinal: Constipation, weight gain, vomiting, stomach pain, nausea, xerostomia, salivation, diarrhea, anorexia, ileus

Genitourinary: Difficulty in urination, ejaculatory disturbances, incontinence, polyuria, ejaculating dysfunction, priapism

Hematologic: Agranulocytosis, leukopenia, eosinophilia, hemolytic anemia, thrombocytopenic purpura, pancytopenia

Hepatic: Cholestatic jaundice, hepatotoxicity

Neuromuscular & skeletal: Tremor

Ocular: Pigmentary retinopathy, blurred vision, cornea and lens changes

Respiratory: Nasal congestion

Miscellaneous: Diaphoresis

Drug Interactions

Cytochrome P450 Effect:

Amitriptyline: **Substrate** of CYP1A2 (minor), 2B6 (minor), 2C8/9 (minor), 2C19 (minor), 2D6 (major), 3A4 (minor); **Inhibits** CYP1A2 (weak), 2C8/9 (weak), 2C19 (weak), 2D6 (weak), 2E1 (weak)

Perphenazine: **Substrate** of CYP1A2 (minor), 2C8/9 (minor), 2C19 (minor), 2D6 (major), 3A4 (minor); **Inhibits** CYP1A2 (weak), 2D6 (weak)

Increased Effect/Toxicity: See individual agents.

Decreased Effect: See individual agents.

Pharmacodynamics/Kinetics See individual agents.

Pregnancy Risk Factor D

Amitriptyline Hydrochloride *see* Amitriptyline *on page 103*

AmLactin® [OTC] *see* Lactic Acid and Ammonium Hydroxide *on page 793*

Amlexanox (am LEKS an oks)

Related Information

Oral Nonviral Soft Tissue Ulcerations or Erosions *on page 1551*

U.S. Brand Names Aphthasol®

Generic Available No

Pharmacologic Category Anti-inflammatory, Locally Applied

Use Treatment of aphthous ulcers (ie, canker sores)

Unlabeled/Investigational Use Allergic disorders

Local Anesthetic/Vasoconstrictor Precautions No information available to require special precautions

Effects on Dental Treatment Key adverse event(s) related to dental treatment: Allergic contact dermatitis and oral irritation. Discontinue therapy if rash or contact mucositis develops.

(Continued)

Amlexanox *(Continued)*

Significant Adverse Effects

1% to 2%:

Dermatologic: Allergic contact dermatitis

Gastrointestinal: Oral irritation

<1% (Limited to important or life-threatening): Contact mucositis

Dosage Administer (0.5 cm - ¼") directly on ulcers 4 times/day following oral hygiene, after meals, and at bedtime

Mechanism of Action As a benzopyrano-bipyridine carboxylic acid derivative, amlexanox has anti-inflammatory and antiallergic properties; it inhibits chemical mediatory release of the slow-reacting substance of anaphylaxis (SRS-A) and may have antagonistic effects on interleukin-3

Contraindications Hypersensitivity to amlexanox or any component of the formulation

Warnings/Precautions Discontinue therapy if rash or contact mucositis develops.

Pharmacodynamics/Kinetics

Absorption: Some from swallowed paste

Metabolism: Hydroxylated and conjugated metabolites

Half-life elimination: 3.5 hours

Time to peak, serum: 2 hours

Excretion: Urine (17% as unchanged drug)

Pregnancy Risk Factor B

Lactation Excretion in breast milk unknown/use caution

Dosage Forms Paste: 5% (5 g) [contains benzyl alcohol]

Comments Treatment of canker sores with amlexanox showed a 76% median reduction in ulcer size compared to a 40% reduction with placebo. Greer, et al, reported an overall mean reduction in ulcer size of 1.82 mm^2 for patients treated with 5% amlexanox versus an average reduction of 0.52 mm^2 for the control group. Recent studies in over thousands of patients have confirmed that amlexanox accelerates the resolution of pain and healing of aphthous ulcers more significantly than vehicle and no treatment.

Selected Readings

Barrons RW, "Treatment Strategies for Recurrent Oral Aphthous Ulcers," *Am J Health Syst Pharm*, 2001, 58(1):41-50.

Binnie WH, Curro FA, Khandwala A, et al, "Amlexanox Oral Paste: A Novel Treatment That Accelerates the Healing of Aphthous Ulcers," *Compend Contin Educ Dent*, 1997, 18(11):1116-8, 1120-2, 1124.

Eisen D and Lynch DP, "Selecting Topical and Systemic Agents for Recurrent Aphthous Stomatitis," *Cutis*, 2001, 68(3):201-6.

Greer RO Jr, Lindenmuth JE, Juarez T, et al, "A Double-Blind Study of Topically Applied 5% Amlexanox in the Treatment of Aphthous Ulcers," *J Oral Maxillofac Surg*, 1993, 51(3):243-8.

Khandwala A, Van Inwegen RG, and Alfano MC, "5% Amlexanox Oral Paste, A New Treatment for Recurrent Minor Aphthous Ulcers: I. Clinical Demonstration of Acceleration of Healing and Resolution of Pain," *Oral Surg Oral Med Oral Pathol Oral Radiol Endod*, 1997, 83(2):222-30.

Khandwala A, Van Inwegen RG, Charney MR, et al, "5% Amlexanox Oral Paste, A New Treatment for Recurrent Minor Aphthous Ulcers: II. Pharmacokinetics and Demonstration of Clinical Safety," *Oral Surg Oral Med Oral Pathol Oral Radiol Endod*, 1997, 83(2):231-8.

Amlodipine (am LOE di peen)

Related Information

Calcium Channel Blockers and Gingival Hyperplasia *on page 1600*

Calcium Channel Blockers, Comparative Pharmacokinetics *on page 1602*

Cardiovascular Diseases *on page 1458*

U.S. Brand Names Norvasc®

Canadian Brand Names Norvasc®

Mexican Brand Names Norvas®

Generic Available No

Synonyms Amlodipine Besylate

Pharmacologic Category Calcium Channel Blocker

Use Treatment of hypertension and angina

Local Anesthetic/Vasoconstrictor Precautions No information available to require special precautions

Effects on Dental Treatment Fewer reports of gingival hyperplasia with amlodipine than with other CCBs (usually resolves upon discontinuation); consultation with physician is suggested.

Common Adverse Effects

>10%: Cardiovascular: Peripheral edema (2% to 15% dose-related)

1% to 10%:

Cardiovascular: Flushing (1% to 3%), palpitations (1% to 4%)

Central nervous system: Headache (7%; similar to placebo 8%), dizziness (1% to 3%), fatigue (4%), somnolence (1% to 2%)

Dermatologic: Rash (1% to 2%), pruritus (1% to 2%)
Endocrine & metabolic: Male sexual dysfunction (1% to 2%)
Gastrointestinal: Nausea (3%), abdominal pain (1% to 2%), dyspepsia (1% to 2%), gingival hyperplasia
Neuromuscular & skeletal: Muscle cramps (1% to 2%), weakness (1% to 2%)
Respiratory: Dyspnea (1% to 2%), pulmonary edema (15% from PRAISE trial, CHF population)

Dosage Oral:
Children 6-17 years: Hypertension: 2.5-5 mg once daily
Adults:
Hypertension: Initial dose: 5 mg once daily; maximum dose: 10 mg once daily. In general, titrate in 2.5 mg increments over 7-14 days. Usual dosage range (JNC 7): 2.5-10 mg once daily.
Angina: Usual dose: 5-10 mg
Elderly: Dosing should start at the lower end of dosing range due to possible increased incidence of hepatic, renal, or cardiac impairment. Elderly patients also show decreased clearance of amlodipine.
Hypertension: 2.5 mg once daily
Angina: 5 mg once daily
Dialysis: Hemodialysis and peritoneal dialysis does not enhance elimination. Supplemental dose is not necessary.
Dosage adjustment in hepatic impairment:
Angina: Administer 5 mg once daily.
Hypertension: Administer 2.5 mg once daily.

Mechanism of Action Inhibits calcium ion from entering the "slow channels" or select voltage-sensitive areas of vascular smooth muscle and myocardium during depolarization, producing a relaxation of coronary vascular smooth muscle and coronary vasodilation; increases myocardial oxygen delivery in patients with vasospastic angina

Contraindications Hypersensitivity to amlodipine or any component of the formulation

Warnings/Precautions Use with caution and titrate dosages for patients with impaired renal or hepatic function; use caution when treating patients with CHF, sick-sinus syndrome, severe left ventricular dysfunction, hypertrophic cardiomyopathy (especially obstructive), concomitant therapy with beta-blockers or digoxin, edema, or increased intracranial pressure with cranial tumors; do not abruptly withdraw (may cause chest pain); elderly may experience hypotension and constipation more readily.

Drug Interactions
Cytochrome P450 Effect: Substrate of CYP3A4 (major); **Inhibits** CYP1A2 (moderate), 2A6 (weak), 2B6 (weak), 2C8/9 (weak), 2D6 (weak), 3A4 (weak)
Increased Effect/Toxicity: Amlodipine may increase the levels/effects of aminophylline, fluvoxamine, mexiletine, mirtazapine, ropinirole, theophylline, trifluoperazine and other CYP1A2 substrates. Levels/effects of amlodipine may be increased by azole antifungals, ciprofloxacin, clarithromycin, diclofenac, doxycycline, erythromycin, imatinib, isoniazid, nefazodone, nicardipine, propofol, protease inhibitors, quinidine, telithromycin, verapamil, and other CYP3A4 inhibitors. Cyclosporine levels may be increased by amlodipine. Blood pressure-lowering effects of sildenafil, tadalafil, and vardenafil are additive with amlodipine (use caution).
Decreased Effect: Calcium may reduce the calcium channel blocker's hypotensive effects. Levels/effects of amlodipine may be decreased by aminoglutethimide, carbamazepine, nafcillin, nevirapine, phenobarbital, phenytoin, rifamycins, and other CYP3A4 inducers.

Ethanol/Nutrition/Herb Interactions
Food: Grapefruit juice may modestly increase amlodipine levels.
Herb/Nutraceutical: St John's wort may decrease amlodipine levels. Avoid dong quai if using for hypertension (has estrogenic activity). Avoid ephedra, yohimbe, ginseng (may worsen hypertension). Avoid garlic (may have increased antihypertensive effects).

Dietary Considerations May be taken without regard to meals.

Pharmacodynamics/Kinetics
Onset of action: 30-50 minutes
Peak effect: 6-12 hours
Duration: 24 hours
Absorption: Oral: Well absorbed
Protein binding: 93%
Metabolism: Hepatic (>90%) to inactive metabolite
Bioavailability: 64% to 90%
Half-life elimination: 30-50 hours
(Continued)

Amlodipine *(Continued)*

Excretion: Urine

Pregnancy Risk Factor C

Dosage Forms TAB [equivalent to amlodipine base] 2.5 mg, 5 mg, 10 mg

Selected Readings

Jorgensen MG, "Prevalence of Amlodipine-Related Gingival Hyperplasia," *J Periodontol*, 1997, 68(7):676-8.

Wynn RL, "An Update on Calcium Channel Blocker-Induced Gingival Hyperplasia," *Gen Dent*, 1995, 43(3):218-22.

Wynn RL, "Calcium Channel Blockers and Gingival Hyperplasia," *Gen Dent*, 1991, 39(4):240-3.

Amlodipine and Atorvastatin

(am LOW di peen & a TORE va sta tin)

U.S. Brand Names Caduet®

Generic Available No

Synonyms Atorvastatin Calcium and Amlodipine Besylate

Pharmacologic Category Antilipemic Agent, HMG-CoA Reductase Inhibitor; Calcium Channel Blocker

Use For use when treatment with both agents is appropriate:

Amlodipine is used for the treatment of hypertension and angina.

Atorvastatin is used with dietary therapy for the following:

Hyperlipidemias: To reduce elevations in total cholesterol, LDL-C, apolipoprotein B, and triglycerides in patients with primary hypercholesterolemia (elevations of 1 or more components are present in Fredrickson type IIa, IIb, III, and IV hyperlipidemias); treatment of homozygous familial hypercholesterolemia

Heterozygous familial hypercholesterolemia (HeFH): In adolescent patients (10-17 years of age, females >1 year postmenarche) with HeFH having LDL-C ≥190 mg/dL **or** LDL ≥160 mg/dL with positive family history of premature cardiovascular disease (CVD) or with 2 or more CVD risk factors in the adolescent patient

Local Anesthetic/Vasoconstrictor Precautions No information available to require special precautions

Effects on Dental Treatment No significant effects or complications reported

Common Adverse Effects See individual agents.

Mechanism of Action

Amlodipine: Inhibits calcium ion from entering the "slow channels" or select voltage-sensitive areas of vascular smooth muscle and myocardium during depolarization, producing a relaxation of coronary vascular smooth muscle and coronary vasodilation; increases myocardial oxygen delivery in patients with vasospastic angina

Atorvastatin: Inhibitor of 3-hydroxy-3-methylglutaryl coenzyme A (HMG-CoA) reductase, the rate limiting enzyme in cholesterol synthesis (reduces the production of mevalonic acid from HMG-CoA); this then results in a compensatory increase in the expression of LDL receptors on hepatocyte membranes and a stimulation of LDL catabolism

Drug Interactions

Cytochrome P450 Effect:

Amlodipine: **Substrate** of CYP3A4 (major); **Inhibits** CYP1A2 (moderate), 2A6 (weak), 2B6 (weak), 2C8/9 (weak), 2D6 (weak), 3A4 (weak)

Atorvastatin: **Substrate** of CYP3A4 (major); **Inhibits** CYP3A4 (weak)

Pharmacodynamics/Kinetics See individual agents.

Pregnancy Risk Factor X

Amlodipine and Benazepril (am LOE di peen & ben AY ze pril)

Related Information

Amlodipine *on page 108*

Benazepril *on page 187*

U.S. Brand Names Lotrel®

Generic Available No

Synonyms Benazepril and Amlodipine

Pharmacologic Category Antihypertensive Agent, Combination

Use Treatment of hypertension

Local Anesthetic/Vasoconstrictor Precautions No information available to require special precautions

Effects on Dental Treatment Fewer reports of gingival hyperplasia with amlodipine than with other CCBs (usually resolves upon discontinuation); consultation with physician is suggested.

Common Adverse Effects See individual agents.

Dosage Oral:

Adults: Dose is individualized, given once daily

Elderly: Initial dose: 2.5 mg based on amlodipine component

Dosage adjustment in renal impairment: Cl_{cr} ≤30 mL/minute: Use of combination product is not recommended.

Dosage adjustment in hepatic impairment: Initial dose: 2.5 mg based on amlodipine component

Mechanism of Action The mechanism through which benazepril lowers blood pressure is believed to be primarily suppression of the renin-angiotensin-aldosterone system, benazepril has an antihypertensive effect even in patients with low-renin hypertension; amlodipine is a dihydropyridine calcium antagonist that inhibits the transmembrane influx of calcium ions into vascular smooth muscle and cardiac muscle; amlodipine is a peripheral arterial vasodilator that acts directly on vascular smooth muscle to cause a reduction in peripheral vascular resistance and reduction in blood pressure

Contraindications Hypersensitivity to amlodipine, benazepril, other ACE inhibitors, or any component of the formulation; pregnancy (2nd and 3rd trimesters)

Warnings/Precautions Used as a replacement for separate dosing of components or combination when response to single agent is suboptimal; the fixed combination is not indicated for initial treatment of hypertension; see individual monographs for additional warnings/precautions

Drug Interactions

Cytochrome P450 Effect: Amlodipine: **Substrate** of CYP3A4 (major); **Inhibits** CYP1A2 (moderate), 2A6 (weak), 2B6 (weak), 2C8/9 (weak), 2D6 (weak), 3A4 (weak)

Increased Effect/Toxicity: See individual agents.

Decreased Effect: See individual agents.

Pharmacodynamics/Kinetics See individual agents.

Pregnancy Risk Factor C/D (2nd and 3rd trimesters)

Dosage Forms CAP: Amlodipine 2.5 mg and benazepril 10 mg; amlodipine 5 mg and benazepril 10 mg; amlodipine 5 mg and benazepril 20 mg; amlodipine 10 mg and benazepril 20 mg

Selected Readings

Wynn RL, "An Update on Calcium Channel Blocker-Induced Gingival Hyperplasia," *Gen Dent*, 1995, 43(3):218-22.

Wynn RL, "Calcium Channel Blockers and Gingival Hyperplasia," *Gen Dent*, 1991, 39(4):240-3.

Amlodipine Besylate *see* Amlodipine *on page 108*

Ammens® Medicated Deodorant [OTC] *see* Zinc Oxide *on page 1400*

Ammonapse *see* Sodium Phenylbutyrate *on page 1230*

Ammonia Spirit (Aromatic)

(a MOE nee ah SPEAR it, air oh MAT ik)

Related Information

Dental Office Emergencies *on page 1584*

Generic Available Yes

Synonyms Smelling Salts

Pharmacologic Category Respiratory Stimulant

Use Respiratory and circulatory stimulant, treatment of fainting

Local Anesthetic/Vasoconstrictor Precautions No information available to require special precautions

Effects on Dental Treatment No significant effects or complications reported

Significant Adverse Effects 1% to 10%:

Gastrointestinal: Nausea, vomiting

Respiratory: Irritation to nasal mucosa, coughing

Dosage Used as "smelling salts" to treat or prevent fainting

Contraindications Hypersensitivity to ammonia or any component of the formulation

Drug Interactions No data reported

Pregnancy Risk Factor C

Dosage Forms Solution for inhalation [ampul]: 1.7% to 2.1% (0.33 mL)

Ammonium Chloride (a MOE nee um KLOR ide)

Generic Available Yes

Pharmacologic Category Electrolyte Supplement, Parenteral

Use Treatment of hypochloremic states or metabolic alkalosis

Local Anesthetic/Vasoconstrictor Precautions No information available to require special precautions

Effects on Dental Treatment No significant effects or complications reported

Common Adverse Effects Frequency not defined.

Central nervous system: Headache, coma, drowsiness, EEG abnormalities, mental confusion, seizures

(Continued)

Ammonium Chloride *(Continued)*

Dermatologic: Rash
Endocrine & metabolic: Calcium-deficient tetany, hyperchloremia, hypokalemia, metabolic acidosis, potassium and sodium may be decreased
Gastrointestinal: Abdominal pain, gastric irritation, nausea, vomiting
Hepatic: Ammonia may be increased
Local: Pain at site of injection
Neuromuscular & skeletal: Twitching
Respiratory: Hyperventilation

Mechanism of Action Increases acidity by increasing free hydrogen ion concentration

Pharmacodynamics/Kinetics
Metabolism: Hepatic; forms urea and hydrochloric acid
Excretion: Urine

Pregnancy Risk Factor C

Ammonium Lactate *see* Lactic Acid and Ammonium Hydroxide *on page 793*

Amnesteem™ *see* Isotretinoin *on page 773*

Amobarbital (am oh BAR bi tal)

U.S. Brand Names Amytal®

Canadian Brand Names Amytal®

Generic Available No

Synonyms Amylobarbitone

Pharmacologic Category Barbiturate

Use Hypnotic in short-term treatment of insomnia; reduce anxiety and provide sedation preoperatively

Unlabeled/Investigational Use Therapeutic or diagnostic "Amytal® Interviewing"; Wada test

Local Anesthetic/Vasoconstrictor Precautions No information available to require special precautions

Effects on Dental Treatment No significant effects or complications reported

Mechanism of Action Interferes with transmission of impulses from the thalamus to the cortex of the brain resulting in an imbalance in central inhibitory and facilitatory mechanisms

Pregnancy Risk Factor D

Amobarbital and Secobarbital

(am oh BAR bi tal & see koe BAR bi tal)

Related Information
Amobarbital *on page 112*

U.S. Brand Names Tuinal® [DSC]

Generic Available No

Synonyms Secobarbital and Amobarbital

Pharmacologic Category Barbiturate

Use Short-term treatment of insomnia

Local Anesthetic/Vasoconstrictor Precautions No information available to require special precautions

Effects on Dental Treatment No significant effects or complications reported

Pregnancy Risk Factor D

Amonafide (a MON a fide)

Generic Available No

Synonyms Amonafide Hydrochloride; Benzisoquinolinedione; BIDA; M-FA-142; Nafidimide; NSC-308847

Pharmacologic Category Antineoplastic Agent, DNA Binding Agent; Enzyme Inhibitor, Topoisomerase II Inhibitor

Unlabeled/Investigational Use Has shown some activity against breast, prostate, renal cell, ovarian, pancreatic, and nonsmall cell lung cancers

Local Anesthetic/Vasoconstrictor Precautions No information available to require special precautions

Effects on Dental Treatment No significant effects or complications reported

Common Adverse Effects
>10%:
Gastrointestinal: Nausea and vomiting (mild)
Hematologic: Granulocytopenia, possibly dose-limiting; nadir occurs at days 12-15, recovery by day 21
1% to 10%:
Cardiovascular: Chest pain
Central nervous system: Dizziness, fatigue, headache

Dermatologic: Skin rash, exfoliative dermatitis, alopecia
Local: Inflammatory reactions
Otic: Tinnitus
Neuromuscular & skeletal: Myoclonic jerking, weakness

Mechanism of Action Amonafide acts as a DNA intercalator, stabilizing DNA to thermal denaturation and producing single-strand DNA breaks.

Pharmacodynamics/Kinetics

Distribution: V_d: 370-530 L/m^2
Protein binding: High
Half-life:
Elimination: 3.5-11 hours
Terminal: 3-6 hours
Metabolism: Hepatic, primarily by oxidation and N-acetylation. N-acetylamonafide (active) and amonafide-N′-oxide are the major metabolites. Clearance depends on whether the patient is a fast or slow acetylator. Fast acetylators may experience greater toxicity from the drug.
Excretion: Urine (3% to 22% as unchanged drug)

Amonafide Hydrochloride *see* Amonafide *on page 112*

Amoxapine (a MOKS a peen)

Generic Available Yes

Synonyms Asendin [DSC]

Pharmacologic Category Antidepressant, Tricyclic (Secondary Amine)

Use Treatment of depression, psychotic depression, depression accompanied by anxiety or agitation

Local Anesthetic/Vasoconstrictor Precautions Use with caution; epinephrine, norepinephrine and levonordefrin have been shown to have an increased pressor response in combination with TCAs

Effects on Dental Treatment Key adverse event(s) related to dental treatment: Xerostomia and changes in salivation (normal salivary flow resumes upon discontinuation). Long-term treatment with TCAs, such as amoxapine, increases the risk of caries by reducing salivation and salivary buffer capacity.

Common Adverse Effects

>10%:
Central nervous system: Drowsiness
Gastrointestinal: Xerostomia, constipation

1% to 10%:
Central nervous system: Dizziness, headache, confusion, nervousness, restlessness, insomnia, ataxia, excitement, anxiety
Dermatologic: Edema, skin rash
Endocrine: Elevated prolactin levels
Gastrointestinal: Nausea
Neuromuscular & skeletal: Tremor, weakness
Ocular: Blurred vision
Miscellaneous: Diaphoresis

Mechanism of Action Reduces the reuptake of serotonin and norepinephrine. The metabolite, 7-OH-amoxapine has significant dopamine receptor blocking activity similar to haloperidol.

Drug Interactions

Cytochrome P450 Effect: Substrate of CYP2D6 (major)

Increased Effect/Toxicity: Amoxapine increases the effects of amphetamines, anticholinergics, other CNS depressants (sedatives, hypnotics, or ethanol), chlorpropamide, tolazamide, and warfarin. When used with MAO inhibitors, hyperpyrexia, hypertension, tachycardia, confusion, seizures, and **deaths have been reported** (serotonin syndrome). Serotonin syndrome has also been reported with ritonavir (rare). CYP2D6 inhibitors may increase the levels/effects of amoxapine; example inhibitors include chlorpromazine, delavirdine, fluoxetine, miconazole, paroxetine, pergolide, quinidine, quinine, ritonavir, and ropinirole. Use of lithium with a TCA may increase the risk for neurotoxicity. Phenothiazines may increase concentration of some TCAs and TCAs may increase the concentration of phenothiazines. Pressor response to I.V. epinephrine, norepinephrine, and phenylephrine may be enhanced in patients receiving TCAs (**Note:** Effect is unlikely with epinephrine or levonordefrin dosages typically administered as infiltration in combination with local anesthetics). Combined use of beta-agonists or drugs which prolong QT_c (including quinidine, procainamide, disopyramide, cisapride, sparfloxacin, gatifloxacin, moxifloxacin) with TCAs may predispose patients to cardiac arrhythmias.

Decreased Effect: Amoxapine inhibits the antihypertensive effects of bethanidine, clonidine, debrisoquin, guanadrel, guanethidine, guanabenz, or

(Continued)

Amoxapine *(Continued)*

guanfacine. Cholestyramine and colestipol may bind TCAs and reduce their absorption.

Pharmacodynamics/Kinetics

Onset of antidepressant effect: Usually occurs after 1-2 weeks, but may require 4-6 weeks

Absorption: Rapid and well absorbed

Distribution: V_d: 0.9-1.2 L/kg; enters breast milk

Protein binding: 80%

Metabolism: Primarily hepatic

Half-life elimination: Parent drug: 11-16 hours; Active metabolite (8-hydroxy): Adults: 30 hours

Time to peak, serum: 1-2 hours

Excretion: Urine (as unchanged drug and metabolites)

Pregnancy Risk Factor C

Amoxicillin (a moks i SIL in)

Related Information

Animal and Human Bites Guidelines *on page 1582*
Antibiotic Prophylaxis, Preprocedural Guidelines for Dental Patients *on page 1509*
Cardiovascular Diseases *on page 1458*
Gastrointestinal Disorders *on page 1476*
Oral Bacterial Infections *on page 1533*
Periodontal Diseases *on page 1542*
Sexually-Transmitted Diseases *on page 1504*

U.S. Brand Names Amoxil®; DisperMox™; Moxilin®; Trimox®

Canadian Brand Names Amoxil®; Apo-Amoxi®; Gen-Amoxicillin; Lin-Amox; Novamoxin®; Nu-Amoxi; PMS-Amoxicillin

Mexican Brand Names Acimox®; Aclimafel®; Acroxil®; Amoxifur®; Amoxil®; Amoxinovag®; Amoxisol®; Ampliron®; Ardine®; Flemoxon®; Gimalxina®; Grunicina®; Hidramox®; Moxlin® Penamox®; Polymox®; Servamox®; Solciclina®; Xalyn-Or®

Generic Available Yes

Synonyms Amoxicillin Trihydrate; Amoxycillin; *p*-Hydroxyampicillin

Pharmacologic Category Antibiotic, Penicillin

Dental Use Antibiotic for standard prophylactic regimen for dental patients who are at risk for endocarditis

Use Treatment of otitis media, sinusitis, and infections caused by susceptible organisms involving the respiratory tract, skin, and urinary tract; prophylaxis of bacterial endocarditis in patients undergoing surgical or dental procedures; as part of a multidrug regimen for *H. pylori* eradication

Unlabeled/Investigational Use Postexposure prophylaxis for anthrax exposure with documented susceptible organisms

Local Anesthetic/Vasoconstrictor Precautions No information available to require special precautions

Effects on Dental Treatment Prolonged use of penicillins may lead to development of oral candidiasis.

Significant Adverse Effects Frequency not defined.

Central nervous system: Hyperactivity, agitation, anxiety, insomnia, confusion, convulsions, behavioral changes, dizziness

Dermatologic: Acute exanthematous pustulosis, erythematous maculopapular rashes, erythema multiforme, Stevens-Johnson syndrome, exfoliative dermatitis, toxic epidermal necrolysis, hypersensitivity vasculitis, urticaria

Gastrointestinal: Nausea, vomiting, diarrhea, hemorrhagic colitis, pseudomembranous colitis, tooth discoloration (brown, yellow, or gray; rare)

Hematologic: Anemia, hemolytic anemia, thrombocytopenia, thrombocytopenia purpura, eosinophilia, leukopenia, agranulocytosis

Hepatic: Elevated AST (SGOT) and ALT (SGPT), cholestatic jaundice, hepatic cholestasis, acute cytolytic hepatitis

Dosage Oral:

Children ≤3 months: 20-30 mg/kg/day divided every 12 hours

Children: >3 months and <40 kg: Dosing range: 20-50 mg/kg/day in divided doses every 8-12 hours

Ear, nose, throat, genitourinary tract, or skin/skin structure infections:

Mild to moderate: 25 mg/kg/day in divided doses every 12 hours **or** 20 mg/kg/day in divided doses every 8 hours

Severe: 45 mg/kg/day in divided doses every 12 hours **or** 40 mg/kg/day in divided doses every 8 hours

Acute otitis media due to highly resistant strains of *S. pneumoniae:* Doses as high as 80-90 mg/kg/day divided every 12 hours have been used

Lower respiratory tract infections: 45 mg/kg/day in divided doses every 12 hours **or** 40 mg/kg/day in divided doses every 8 hours

Subacute bacterial endocarditis prophylaxis: 50 mg/kg 1 hour before procedure

Anthrax exposure (unlabeled use): **Note:** Postexposure prophylaxis only with documented susceptible organisms:

<40 kg: 15 mg/kg every 8 hours

≥40 kg: 500 mg every 8 hours

Adults: Dosing range: 250-500 mg every 8 hours or 500-875 mg twice daily; maximum dose: 2-3 g/day

Ear, nose, throat, genitourinary tract or skin/skin structure infections:

Mild to moderate: 500 mg every 12 hours **or** 250 mg every 8 hours

Severe: 875 mg every 12 hours **or** 500 mg every 8 hours

Lower respiratory tract infections: 875 mg every 12 hours **or** 500 mg every 8 hours

Endocarditis prophylaxis: 2 g 1 hour before procedure

Helicobacter pylori eradication: 1000 mg twice daily; requires combination therapy with at least one other antibiotic and an acid-suppressing agent (proton pump inhibitor or H_2 blocker)

Anthrax exposure (unlabeled use): **Note:** Postexposure prophylaxis only with documented susceptible organisms: 500 mg every 8 hours

Dosing interval in renal impairment: The 875 mg tablet should not be used in patients with Cl_{cr} <30 mL/minute.

Cl_{cr} 10-30 mL/minute: 250-500 mg every 12 hours

Cl_{cr} <10 mL/minute: 250-500 mg every 24 hours

Dialysis: Moderately dialyzable (20% to 50%) by hemo- or peritoneal dialysis; approximately 50 mg of amoxicillin per liter of filtrate is removed by continuous arteriovenous or venovenous hemofiltration; dose as per Cl_{cr} <10 mL/minute guidelines

Mechanism of Action Inhibits bacterial cell wall synthesis by binding to one or more of the penicillin binding proteins (PBPs); which in turn inhibits the final transpeptidation step of peptidoglycan synthesis in bacterial cell walls, thus inhibiting cell wall biosynthesis. Bacteria eventually lyse due to ongoing activity of cell wall autolytic enzymes (autolysins and murein hydrolases) while cell wall assembly is arrested.

Contraindications Hypersensitivity to amoxicillin, penicillin, or any component of the formulation

Warnings/Precautions In patients with renal impairment, doses and/or frequency of administration should be modified in response to the degree of renal impairment; a high percentage of patients with infectious mononucleosis have developed rash during therapy with amoxicillin; a low incidence of cross-allergy with other beta-lactams and cephalosporins exists

Drug Interactions

Allopurinol: Theoretically has an additive potential for amoxicillin rash

Aminoglycosides: May be synergistic against selected organisms

Methotrexate: Penicillins may increase the exposure to methotrexate during concurrent therapy; monitor.

Oral contraceptives: Anecdotal reports suggesting decreased contraceptive efficacy with penicillins have been refuted by more rigorous scientific and clinical data.

Probenecid, disulfiram: May increase levels of penicillins (amoxicillin)

Warfarin: Effects of warfarin may be increased

Dietary Considerations May be taken with food. Amoxil® chewable contains phenylalanine 1.82 mg per 200 mg tablet, phenylalanine 3.64 mg per 400 mg tablet. DisperMox™ contains phenylalanine 5.6 mg in each 200 mg and 400 mg tablet.

Pharmacodynamics/Kinetics

Absorption: Oral: Rapid and nearly complete; food does not interfere

Distribution: Widely to most body fluids and bone; poor penetration into cells, eyes, and across normal meninges

Pleural fluids, lungs, and peritoneal fluid; high urine concentrations are attained; also into synovial fluid, liver, prostate, muscle, and gallbladder; penetrates into middle ear effusions, maxillary sinus secretions, tonsils, sputum, and bronchial secretions; crosses placenta; low concentrations enter breast milk

CSF:blood level ratio: Normal meninges: <1%; Inflamed meninges: 8% to 90%

Protein binding: 17% to 20%

Metabolism: Partially hepatic

(Continued)

Amoxicillin *(Continued)*

Half-life elimination:
Neonates, full-term: 3.7 hours
Infants and Children: 1-2 hours
Adults: Normal renal function: 0.7-1.4 hours
Cl_{cr} <10 mL/minute: 7-21 hours
Time to peak: Capsule: 2 hours; Suspension: 1 hour
Excretion: Urine (80% as unchanged drug); lower in neonates

Pregnancy Risk Factor B

Lactation Enters breast milk/compatible

Dosage Forms [DSC] = Discontinued product
Capsule, as trihydrate: 250 mg, 500 mg
Amoxil®, Moxilin®, Trimox®: 250 mg, 500 mg
Powder for oral suspension, as trihydrate: 125 mg/5 mL (80 mL, 100 mL, 150 mL); 200 mg/5 mL (50 mL, 75 mL, 100 mL); 250 mg/5 mL (80 mL, 100 mL, 150 mL); 400 mg/5 mL (50 mL, 75 mL, 100 mL)
Amoxil®: 125 mg/5 mL (150 mL) [contains sodium benzoate; strawberry flavor] [DSC]; 200 mg/5 mL (5 mL, 50 mL, 75 mL, 100 mL) [contains sodium benzoate; bubblegum flavor]; 250 mg/5 mL (100 mL, 150 mL) [contains sodium benzoate; bubblegum flavor]; 400 mg/5 mL (5 mL, 50 mL, 75 mL, 100 mL) [contains sodium benzoate; bubblegum flavor]
Moxilin®: 250 mg/5 mL (100 mL, 150 mL)
Trimox®: 125 mg/5 mL (80 mL, 100 mL, 150 mL); 250 mg/5 mL (80 mL, 100 mL, 150 mL) [contains sodium benzoate; raspberry-strawberry flavor]
Powder for oral suspension, as trihydrate [drops] (Amoxil®): 50 mg/mL (15 mL [DSC], 30 mL) [bubblegum flavor]
Tablet, as trihydrate [film coated] (Amoxil®): 500 mg, 875 mg
Tablet, chewable, as trihydrate: 125 mg, 200 mg, 250 mg, 400 mg
Amoxil®: 200 mg [contains phenylalanine 1.82 mg/tablet; cherry banana peppermint flavor]; 400 mg [contains phenylalanine 3.64 mg/tablet; cherry banana peppermint flavor]
Tablet, for oral suspension, as trihydrate (DisperMox™): 200 mg [contains phenylalanine 5.6 mg; strawberry flavor]; 400 mg [contains phenylalanine 5.6 mg; strawberry flavor]; 600 mg [contains phenylalanine 11.23 mg; strawberry flavor]

Selected Readings

ADA Division of Legal Affairs, "A Legal Perspective on Antibiotic Prophylaxis," *J Am Dent Assoc*, 2003, 134(9):1260.

American Dental Association; American Academy of Orthopedic Surgeons, "Antibiotic Prophylaxis for Dental Patients With Total Joint Replacements," *J Am Dent Assoc*, 2003, 134(7):895-9.

American Dental Association Council on Scientific Affairs, "Combating Antibiotic Resistance," *J Am Dent Assoc*, 2004, 135(4):484-7.

Dajani AS, Taubert KA, Wilson W, et al, "Prevention of Bacterial Endocarditis. Recommendations by the American Heart Association," *JAMA*, 1997, 277(22):1794-801.

Dajani AS, Taubert KA, Wilson W, et al, "Prevention of Bacterial Endocarditis: Recommendations by the American Heart Association," *J Am Dent Assoc*, 1997, 128(8):1142-51.

Wynn RL, Bergman SA, Meiller TF, et al, "Antibiotics in Treating Oral-Facial Infections of Odontogenic Origin: An Update", *Gen Dent*, 2001, 49(3):238-40, 242, 244 passim.

Amoxicillin and Clavulanate Potassium

(a moks i SIL in & klav yoo LAN ate poe TASS ee um)

Related Information
Amoxicillin *on page 114*
Animal and Human Bites Guidelines *on page 1582*
Oral Bacterial Infections *on page 1533*

U.S. Brand Names Augmentin®; Augmentin ES-600®; Augmentin XR™

Canadian Brand Names Alti-Amoxi-Clav; Apo-Amoxi-Clav®; Augmentin®; Clavulin®; ratio-AmoxiClav

Generic Available Yes: Excludes extended release

Synonyms Amoxicillin and Clavulanic Acid

Pharmacologic Category Antibiotic, Penicillin

Dental Use Treatment of orofacial infections when beta-lactamase-producing staphylococci and beta-lactamase-producing *Bacteroides* are present

Use Treatment of otitis media, sinusitis, and infections caused by susceptible organisms involving the lower respiratory tract, skin and skin structure, and urinary tract; spectrum same as amoxicillin with additional coverage of beta-lactamase producing *B. catarrhalis*, *H. influenzae*, *N. gonorrhoeae*, and *S. aureus* (not MRSA). The expanded coverage of this combination makes it a useful alternative when amoxicillin resistance is present and patients cannot tolerate alternative treatments.

Local Anesthetic/Vasoconstrictor Precautions No information available to require special precautions

Effects on Dental Treatment Prolonged use of penicillins may lead to development of oral candidiasis.

Significant Adverse Effects

>10%: Gastrointestinal: Diarrhea (3% to 34%; incidence varies upon dose and regimen used)

1% to 10%:

Dermatologic: Diaper rash, skin rash, urticaria

Gastrointestinal: Abdominal discomfort, loose stools, nausea, vomiting

Genitourinary: Vaginitis

Miscellaneous: Moniliasis

<1% (Limited to important or life-threatening): Cholestatic jaundice, flatulence, headache, hepatic dysfunction, prothrombin time increased, thrombocytosis

Additional adverse reactions seen with **ampicillin-class antibiotics:** Agitation, agranulocytosis, ALT elevated, anaphylaxis, anemia, angioedema, anxiety, AST elevated, behavioral changes, black "hairy" tongue, confusion, convulsions, crystalluria, dizziness, enterocolitis, eosinophilia, erythema multiforme, exanthematous pustulosis, exfoliative dermatitis, gastritis, glossitis, hematuria, hemolytic anemia, hemorrhagic colitis, indigestion, insomnia, hyperactivity, interstitial nephritis, leukopenia, mucocutaneous candidiasis, pruritus, pseudomembranous colitis, serum sickness-like reaction, Stevens-Johnson syndrome, stomatitis, thrombocytopenia, thrombocytopenic purpura, tooth discoloration, toxic epidermal necrolysis

Dosage Note: Dose is based on the amoxicillin component; see "Augmentin® Product-Specific Considerations" table.

Augmentin® Product-Specific Considerations

Strength	Form	Consideration
125 mg	CT, S	q8h dosing
	S	For adults having difficulty swallowing tablets, 125 mg/5 mL suspension may be substituted for 500 mg tablet.
200 mg	CT, S	q12h dosing
	CT	Contains phenylalanine
	S	For adults having difficulty swallowing tablets, 200 mg/5 mL suspension may be substituted for 875 mg tablet.
250 mg	CT, S, T	q8h dosing
	CT	Contains phenylalanine
	T	Not for use in patients <40 kg
	CT, T	Tablet and chewable tablet are not interchangeable due to differences in clavulanic acid.
	S	For adults having difficulty swallowing tablets, 250 mg/5 mL suspension may be substituted for 500 mg tablet.
400 mg	CT, S	q12h dosing
	CT	Contains phenylalanine
	S	For adults having difficulty swallowing tablets, 400 mg/5 mL suspension may be substituted for 875 mg tablet.
500 mg	T	q8h or q12h dosing
600 mg	S	q12 h dosing
		Contains phenylalanine
		Not for use in adults or children ≥40 kg
		600 mg/5 mL suspension is not equivalent to or interchangeable with 200 mg/5 mL or 400 mg/5 mL due to differences in clavulanic acid.
875 mg	T	q12 h dosing; not for use in Cl_{cr} <30 mL/minute
1000 mg	XR	q12h dosing
		Not for use in children <16 years of age
		Not interchangeable with two 500 mg tablets
		Not for use in Cl_{cr} <30 mL/minute or hemodialysis

Legend: CT = chewable tablet, S = suspension, T = tablet, XR = extended release.

Infants <3 months: 30 mg/kg/day divided every 12 hours using the 125 mg/5 mL suspension

Children ≥3 months and <40 kg:

Otitis media: 90 mg/kg/day divided every 12 hours for 10 days

Lower respiratory tract infections, severe infections, sinusitis: 45 mg/kg/day divided every 12 hours **or** 40 mg/kg/day divided every 8 hours

Less severe infections: 25 mg/kg/day divided every 12 hours or 20 mg/kg/day divided every 8 hours

Children >40 kg and Adults: 250-500 mg every 8 hours or 875 mg every 12 hours

(Continued)

Amoxicillin and Clavulanate Potassium *(Continued)*

Children ≥16 years and Adults:

Acute bacterial sinusitis: Extended release tablet: Two 1000 mg tablets every 12 hours for 10 days

Community-acquired pneumonia: Extended release tablet: Two 1000 mg tablets every 12 hours for 7-10 days

Dosing interval in renal impairment:

Cl_{cr} <30 mL/minute: Do not use 875 mg tablet or extended release tablets

Cl_{cr} 10-30 mL/minute: 250-500 mg every 12 hours

Cl_{cr} <10 mL/minute: 250-500 every 24 hours

Hemodialysis: Moderately dialyzable (20% to 50%)

250-500 mg every 24 hours; administer dose during and after dialysis. Do not use extended release tablets.

Peritoneal dialysis: Moderately dialyzable (20% to 50%)

Amoxicillin: Administer 250 mg every 12 hours

Clavulanic acid: Dose for Cl_{cr} <10 mL/minute

Continuous arteriovenous or venovenous hemofiltration effects:

Amoxicillin: ~50 mg of amoxicillin/L of filtrate is removed

Clavulanic acid: Dose for Cl_{cr} <10 mL/minute

Mechanism of Action Clavulanic acid binds and inhibits beta-lactamases that inactivate amoxicillin resulting in amoxicillin having an expanded spectrum of activity. Amoxicillin inhibits bacterial cell wall synthesis by binding to one or more of the penicillin binding proteins (PBPs); which in turn inhibits the final transpeptidation step of peptidoglycan synthesis in bacterial cell walls, thus inhibiting cell wall biosynthesis. Bacteria eventually lyse due to ongoing activity of cell wall autolytic enzymes (autolysins and murein hydrolases) while cell wall assembly is arrested.

Contraindications Hypersensitivity to amoxicillin, clavulanic acid, penicillin, or any component of the formulation; history of cholestatic jaundice or hepatic dysfunction with amoxicillin/clavulanate potassium therapy

Warnings/Precautions Prolonged use may result in superinfection; in patients with renal impairment, doses and/or frequency of administration should be modified in response to the degree of renal impairment; high percentage of patients with infectious mononucleosis have developed rash during therapy; a low incidence of cross-allergy with cephalosporins exists; incidence of diarrhea is higher than with amoxicillin alone. Use caution in patients with hepatic dysfunction. Hepatic dysfunction, although rare, is more common in elderly and/or males, and occurs more frequently with prolonged treatment, and may occur after therapy is complete. Due to differing content of clavulanic acid, not all formulations are interchangeable. Some products contain phenylalanine.

Drug Interactions

Allopurinol: Additive potential for amoxicillin rash

Aminoglycosides: May be synergistic against selected organisms

Methotrexate: Penicillins may increase the exposure to methotrexate during concurrent therapy; monitor.

Oral contraceptives: Anecdotal reports suggesting decreased contraceptive efficacy with penicillins have been refuted by more rigorous scientific and clinical data.

Probenecid: May increase levels of penicillins (amoxicillin)

Warfarin: Effects of warfarin may be increased

Dietary Considerations May be taken with meals or on an empty stomach; take with meals to increase absorption and decrease GI intolerance; may mix with milk, formula, or juice. Extended release tablets should be taken with food. Some products contain phenylalanine; avoid use in phenylketonurics. All dosage forms contain potassium.

Pharmacodynamics/Kinetics Amoxicillin pharmacokinetics are not affected by clavulanic acid.

Amoxicillin: See Amoxicillin monograph.

Clavulanic acid:

Metabolism: Hepatic

Excretion: Urine (30% to 40% as unchanged drug)

Pregnancy Risk Factor B

Lactation Enters breast milk/use caution (AAP rates "compatible")

Breast-Feeding Considerations The AAP considers amoxicillin to be "compatible" with breast-feeding.

Dosage Forms

Powder for oral suspension: 200: Amoxicillin 200 mg and clavulanate potassium 28.5 mg per 5 mL (100 mL) [contains phenylalanine]; 400: Amoxicillin 400 mg and clavulanate potassium 57 mg per 5 mL (100 mL) [contains phenylalanine]

Augmentin®:

125: Amoxicillin 125 mg and clavulanate potassium 31.25 mg per 5 mL (75 mL, 100 mL, 150 mL) [banana flavor]

200: Amoxicillin 200 mg and clavulanate potassium 28.5 mg per 5 mL (50 mL, 75 mL, 100 mL) [contains phenylalanine 7 mg/5 mL; orange-raspberry flavor]

250: Amoxicillin 250 mg and clavulanate potassium 62.5 mg per 5 mL (75 mL, 100 mL, 150 mL) [orange flavor]

400: Amoxicillin 400 mg and clavulanate potassium 57 mg per 5 mL (50 mL, 75 mL, 100 mL) [contains phenylalanine 7 mg/5 mL; orange-raspberry flavor]

Augmentin ES-600®: Amoxicillin 600 mg and clavulanic potassium 42.9 mg per 5 mL (75 mL, 125 mL, 200 mL) [contains phenylalanine 7 mg/5 mL; orange flavor]

Tablet: 500: Amoxicillin trihydrate 500 mg and clavulanate potassium 125 mg; 875: Amoxicillin trihydrate 875 mg and clavulanate potassium 125 mg

Augmentin®:

250: Amoxicillin trihydrate 250 mg and clavulanate potassium 125 mg

500: Amoxicillin trihydrate 500 mg and clavulanate potassium 125 mg

875: Amoxicillin trihydrate 875 mg and clavulanate potassium 125 mg

Tablet, chewable: 200: Amoxicillin trihydrate 200 mg and clavulanate potassium 28.5 mg [contains phenylalanine]; 400: Amoxicillin trihydrate 400 mg and clavulanate potassium 57 mg [contains phenylalanine]

Augmentin®:

125: Amoxicillin trihydrate 125 mg and clavulanate potassium 31.25 mg [lemon-lime flavor]

200: Amoxicillin trihydrate 200 mg and clavulanate potassium 28.5 mg [contains phenylalanine 2.1 mg/tablet; cherry-banana flavor]

250: Amoxicillin trihydrate 250 mg and clavulanate potassium 62.5 mg [lemon-lime flavor]

400: Amoxicillin trihydrate 400 mg and clavulanate potassium 57 mg [contains phenylalanine 4.2 mg/tablet; cherry-banana flavor]

Tablet, extended release (Augmentin XR™): Amoxicillin 1000 mg and clavulanic acid 62.5 mg

Comments In maxillary sinus, anterior nasal cavity, and deep neck infections, beta-lactamase-producing staphylococci and beta-lactamase-producing *Bacteroides* usually are present. In these situations, antibiotics that resist the beta-lactamase enzyme are indicated. Amoxicillin and clavulanic acid is administered orally for moderate infections. Ampicillin sodium and sulbactam sodium (Unasyn®) is administered parenterally for more severe infections.

Selected Readings

American Dental Association Council on Scientific Affairs, "Combating Antibiotic Resistance," *J Am Dent Assoc*, 2004, 135(4):484-7.

Wynn RL, Bergman SA, Meiller TF, et al, "Antibiotics in Treating Oral-Facial Infections of Odontogenic Origin: An Update," *Gen Dent*, 2001, 49(3):238-40, 242, 244 passim.

Amoxicillin and Clavulanic Acid *see* Amoxicillin and Clavulanate Potassium *on page 116*

Amoxicillin, Lansoprazole, and Clarithromycin *see* Lansoprazole, Amoxicillin, and Clarithromycin *on page 798*

Amoxicillin Trihydrate *see* Amoxicillin *on page 114*

Amoxil® *see* Amoxicillin *on page 114*

Amoxycillin *see* Amoxicillin *on page 114*

Amphetamine and Dextroamphetamine *see* Dextroamphetamine and Amphetamine *on page 419*

Amphocin® *see* Amphotericin B (Conventional) *on page 120*

Amphotec® *see* Amphotericin B Cholesteryl Sulfate Complex *on page 119*

Amphotericin B Cholesteryl Sulfate Complex

(am foe TER i sin bee kole LES te ril SUL fate KOM plecks)

Related Information

Amphotericin B (Conventional) *on page 120*

U.S. Brand Names Amphotec®

Canadian Brand Names Amphotec®

Generic Available No

Synonyms ABCD; Amphotericin B Colloidal Dispersion

Pharmacologic Category Antifungal Agent, Parenteral

Use Treatment of invasive aspergillosis in patients who have failed amphotericin B deoxycholate treatment, or who have renal impairment or experience unacceptable toxicity which precludes treatment with amphotericin B deoxycholate in effective doses.

(Continued)

Amphotericin B Cholesteryl Sulfate Complex *(Continued)*

Unlabeled/Investigational Use Effective in patients with serious *Candida* species infections

Local Anesthetic/Vasoconstrictor Precautions No information available to require special precautions

Effects on Dental Treatment No significant effects or complications reported

Common Adverse Effects

>10%: Central nervous system: Chills, fever

1% to 10%:

Cardiovascular: Hypotension, tachycardia
Central nervous system: Headache
Dermatologic: Rash
Endocrine & metabolic: Hypokalemia, hypomagnesemia
Gastrointestinal: Nausea, diarrhea, abdominal pain
Hematologic: Thrombocytopenia
Hepatic: LFT change
Neuromuscular & skeletal: Rigors
Renal: Elevated creatinine
Respiratory: Dyspnea

Note: Amphotericin B colloidal dispersion has an improved therapeutic index compared to conventional amphotericin B, and has been used safely in patients with amphotericin B-related nephrotoxicity; however, continued decline of renal function has occurred in some patients.

Mechanism of Action Binds to ergosterol altering cell membrane permeability in susceptible fungi and causing leakage of cell components with subsequent cell death. Proposed mechanism suggests that amphotericin causes an oxidation-dependent stimulation of macrophages (Lyman, 1992).

Drug Interactions

Increased Effect/Toxicity: Toxic effect with other nephrotoxic drugs (eg, cyclosporine and aminoglycosides) may be additive. Corticosteroids may increase potassium depletion caused by amphotericin. Amphotericin B may predispose patients receiving digitalis glycosides or neuromuscular blocking agents to toxicity secondary to hypokalemia.

Decreased Effect: Pharmacologic antagonism may occur with azole antifungals (eg, ketoconazole, miconazole).

Pharmacodynamics/Kinetics

Distribution: V_d: Total volume increases with higher doses, reflects increasing uptake by tissues (with 4 mg/kg/day = 4 L/kg); predominantly distributed in the liver; concentrations in kidneys and other tissues are lower than observed with conventional amphotericin B

Half-life elimination: 28-29 hours; prolonged with higher doses

Pregnancy Risk Factor B

Amphotericin B Colloidal Dispersion *see* Amphotericin B Cholesteryl Sulfate Complex *on page 119*

Amphotericin B (Conventional)

(am foe TER i sin bee con VEN sha nal)

Related Information

Oral Fungal Infections *on page 1544*

U.S. Brand Names Amphocin®; Fungizone®

Canadian Brand Names Fungizone®

Generic Available Yes: Powder for reconstitution

Synonyms Amphotericin B Desoxycholate

Pharmacologic Category Antifungal Agent, Parenteral; Antifungal Agent, Topical

Use Treatment of severe systemic and central nervous system infections caused by susceptible fungi such as *Candida* species, *Histoplasma capsulatum, Cryptococcus neoformans, Aspergillus* species, *Blastomyces dermatitidis, Torulopsis glabrata,* and *Coccidioides immitis*; fungal peritonitis; irrigant for bladder fungal infections; and topically for cutaneous and mucocutaneous candidal infections; used in fungal infection in patients with bone marrow transplantation, amebic meningoencephalitis, ocular aspergillosis (intraocular injection), candidal cystitis (bladder irrigation), chemoprophylaxis (low-dose I.V.), immunocompromised patients at risk of aspergillosis (intranasal/nebulized), refractory meningitis (intrathecal), coccidioidal arthritis (intra-articular/I.M.).

Low-dose amphotericin B 0.1-0.25 mg/kg/day has been administered after bone marrow transplantation to reduce the risk of invasive fungal disease.

Alternative routes of administration and extemporaneous preparations have been used when standard antifungal therapy is not available (eg, inhalation, intraocular injection, subconjunctival application, intracavitary administration into various joints and the pleural space).

Local Anesthetic/Vasoconstrictor Precautions No information available to require special precautions

Effects on Dental Treatment No significant effects or complications reported

Common Adverse Effects

>10%:

Central nervous system: Fever, chills, headache, malaise, generalized pain
Endocrine & metabolic: Hypokalemia, hypomagnesemia
Gastrointestinal: Anorexia
Hematologic: Anemia
Renal: Nephrotoxicity

1% to 10%:

Cardiovascular: Hypotension, hypertension, flushing
Central nervous system: Delirium, arachnoiditis, pain along lumbar nerves
Gastrointestinal: Nausea, vomiting
Genitourinary: Urinary retention
Hematologic: Leukocytosis
Local: Thrombophlebitis
Neuromuscular & skeletal: Paresthesia (especially with I.T. therapy)
Renal: Renal tubular acidosis, renal failure

Mechanism of Action Binds to ergosterol altering cell membrane permeability in susceptible fungi and causing leakage of cell components with subsequent cell death. Proposed mechanism suggests that amphotericin causes an oxidation-dependent stimulation of macrophages (Lyman, 1992).

Drug Interactions

Increased Effect/Toxicity: Use of amphotericin with other nephrotoxic drugs (eg, cyclosporine and aminoglycosides) may result in additive toxicity. Amphotericin may increase the toxicity of flucytosine. Antineoplastic agents may increase the risk of amphotericin-induced nephrotoxicity, bronchospasms, and hypotension. Corticosteroids may increase potassium depletion caused by amphotericin. Amphotericin B may predispose patients receiving digitalis glycosides or neuromuscular-blocking agents to toxicity secondary to hypokalemia.

Decreased Effect: Pharmacologic antagonism may occur with azole antifungal agents (ketoconazole, miconazole).

Pharmacodynamics/Kinetics

Distribution: Minimal amounts enter the aqueous humor, bile, CSF (inflamed or noninflamed meninges), amniotic fluid, pericardial fluid, pleural fluid, and synovial fluid

Protein binding, plasma: 90%

Half-life elimination: Biphasic: Initial: 15-48 hours; Terminal: 15 days

Time to peak: Within 1 hour following a 4- to 6-hour dose

Excretion: Urine (2% to 5% as biologically active form); ~40% eliminated over a 7-day period and may be detected in urine for at least 7 weeks after discontinued use

Pregnancy Risk Factor B

Amphotericin B Desoxycholate *see* Amphotericin B (Conventional) *on page 120*

Amphotericin B (Lipid Complex)

(am foe TER i sin bee LIP id KOM pleks)

Related Information

Amphotericin B (Conventional) *on page 120*

U.S. Brand Names Abelcet®

Canadian Brand Names Abelcet®

Generic Available No

Synonyms ABLC

Pharmacologic Category Antifungal Agent, Parenteral

Use Treatment of aspergillosis or any type of progressive fungal infection in patients who are refractory to or intolerant of conventional amphotericin B therapy

Unlabeled/Investigational Use Effective in patients with serious *Candida* species infections

Local Anesthetic/Vasoconstrictor Precautions No information available to require special precautions

Effects on Dental Treatment No significant effects or complications reported

(Continued)

Amphotericin B (Lipid Complex) *(Continued)*

Common Adverse Effects Nephrotoxicity and infusion-related hyperpyrexia, rigor, and chilling are reduced relative to amphotericin deoxycholate.

>10%:

Central nervous system: Chills, fever

Renal: Increased serum creatinine

1% to 10%:

Cardiovascular: Hypotension, cardiac arrest

Central nervous system: Headache, pain

Dermatologic: Rash

Endocrine & metabolic: Bilirubinemia, hypokalemia, acidosis

Gastrointestinal: Nausea, vomiting, diarrhea, gastrointestinal hemorrhage, abdominal pain

Renal: Renal failure

Respiratory: Respiratory failure, dyspnea, pneumonia

Mechanism of Action Binds to ergosterol altering cell membrane permeability in susceptible fungi and causing leakage of cell components with subsequent cell death. Proposed mechanism suggests that amphotericin causes an oxidation-dependent stimulation of macrophages (Lyman, 1992).

Drug Interactions

Increased Effect/Toxicity: See Drug Interactions - Increased Effect/Toxicity in Amphotericin B (Conventional) *on page 120.*

Decreased Effect: See Drug Interactions - Decreased Effect in Amphotericin B (Conventional) *on page 120.*

Pharmacodynamics/Kinetics

Distribution: V_d: Increases with higher doses; reflects increased uptake by tissues (131 L/kg with 5 mg/kg/day)

Half-life elimination: ~24 hours

Excretion: Clearance: Increases with higher doses (5 mg/kg/day): 400 mL/hour/kg

Pregnancy Risk Factor B

Amphotericin B (Liposomal)

(am foe TER i sin bee lye po SO mal)

Related Information

Amphotericin B (Conventional) *on page 120*

U.S. Brand Names AmBisome®

Canadian Brand Names AmBisome®

Generic Available No

Synonyms L-AmB

Pharmacologic Category Antifungal Agent, Parenteral

Use Empirical therapy for presumed fungal infection in febrile, neutropenic patients. Treatment of patients with *Aspergillus* species, *Candida* species and/or *Cryptococcus* species infections refractory to amphotericin B desoxycholate, or in patients where renal impairment or unacceptable toxicity precludes the use of amphotericin B desoxycholate. Treatment of cryptococcal meningitis in HIV-infected patients. Treatment of visceral leishmaniasis.

Unlabeled/Investigational Use Effective in patients with serious *Candida* species infections

Local Anesthetic/Vasoconstrictor Precautions No information available to require special precautions

Effects on Dental Treatment Key adverse event(s) related to dental treatment: Facial swelling, postural hypotension, mucositis, stomatitis, and ulcerative stomatitis.

Common Adverse Effects Percentage of adverse reactions is dependent upon population studied and may vary with respect to premedications and underlying illness. Incidence of decreased renal function and infusion-related events are lower than rates observed with amphotericin B deoxycholate.

>10%:

Cardiovascular: Peripheral edema (15%), edema (12% to 14%), tachycardia (9% to 18%), hypotension (7% to 14%), hypertension (8% to 20%), chest pain (8% to 12%), hypervolemia (8% to 12%)

Central nervous system: Chills (29% to 48%), insomnia (17% to 22%), headache (9% to 20%), anxiety (7% to 14%), pain (14%), confusion (9% to 13%)

Dermatologic: Rash (5% to 25%), pruritus (11%)

Endocrine & metabolic: Hypokalemia (31% to 51%), hypomagnesemia (15% to 50%), hyperglycemia (8% to 23%), hypocalcemia (5% to 18%), hyponatremia (8% to 12%)

Gastrointestinal: Nausea (16% to 40%), vomiting (10% to 32%), diarrhea (11% to 30%), abdominal pain (7% to 20%), constipation (15%), anorexia (10% to 14%)
Hematologic: Anemia (27% to 48%), blood transfusion reaction (9% to 18%), leukopenia (15% to 17%), thrombocytopenia (6% to 13%)
Hepatic: Increased alkaline phosphatase (7% to 22%), increased BUN (7% to 21%), bilirubinemia (9% to 18%), increased ALT (15%), increased AST (13%), abnormal liver function tests (not specified) (4% to 13%)
Local: Phlebitis (9% to 11%)
Neuromuscular & skeletal: Weakness (6% to 13%), back pain (12%)
Renal: Increased creatinine (18% to 40%), hematuria (14%)
Respiratory: Dyspnea (18% to 23%), lung disorder (14% to 18%), increased cough (2% to 18%), epistaxis (8% to 15%), pleural effusion (12%), rhinitis (11%)
Miscellaneous: Sepsis (7% to 14%), infection (11% to 12%)

2% to 10%:
Cardiovascular: Arrhythmia, atrial fibrillation, bradycardia, cardiac arrest, cardiomegaly, facial swelling, flushing, postural hypotension, valvular heart disease, vascular disorder
Central nervous system: Agitation, abnormal thinking, coma, convulsion, depression, dysesthesia, dizziness (7% to 8%), hallucinations, malaise, nervousness, somnolence
Dermatologic: Alopecia, bruising, cellulitis, dry skin, maculopapular rash, petechia, purpura, skin discoloration, skin disorder, skin ulcer, urticaria, vesiculobullous rash
Endocrine & metabolic: Acidosis, increased amylase, fluid overload, hypernatremia (4%), hyperchloremia, hyperkalemia, hypermagnesemia, hyperphosphatemia, hypophosphatemia, hypoproteinemia, increased lactate dehydrogenase, increased nonprotein nitrogen
Gastrointestinal: Constipation, dry mouth, dyspepsia, enlarged abdomen, eructation, fecal incontinence, flatulence, gastrointestinal hemorrhage (10%), hematemesis, hemorrhoids, gum/oral hemorrhage, ileus, mucositis, rectal disorder, stomatitis, ulcerative stomatitis
Genitourinary: Vaginal hemorrhage
Hematologic: Coagulation disorder, hemorrhage, decreased prothrombin, thrombocytopenia
Hepatic: Hepatocellular damage, hepatomegaly, veno-occlusive liver disease
Local: Injection site inflammation
Neuromuscular & skeletal: Arthralgia, bone pain, dystonia, myalgia, neck pain, paresthesia, rigors, tremor
Ocular: Conjunctivitis, dry eyes, eye hemorrhage
Renal: Abnormal renal function, acute kidney failure, dysuria, kidney failure, toxic nephropathy, urinary incontinence
Respiratory: Asthma, atelectasis, cough, dry nose, hemoptysis, hyperventilation, lung edema, pharyngitis, pneumonia, respiratory alkalosis, respiratory insufficiency, respiratory failure, sinusitis, hypoxia (6% to 8%)
Miscellaneous: Allergic reaction, cell-mediated immunological reaction, flu-like syndrome, graft versus host disease, herpes simplex, hiccup, procedural complication (8% to 10%), diaphoresis (7%)

Mechanism of Action Binds to ergosterol altering cell membrane permeability in susceptible fungi and causing leakage of cell components with subsequent cell death. Proposed mechanism suggests that amphotericin causes an oxidation-dependent stimulation of macrophages (Lyman, 1992).

Drug Interactions

Increased Effect/Toxicity: Drug interactions have not been studied in a controlled manner; however, drugs that interact with conventional amphotericin B may also interact with amphotericin B liposome for injection. See Drug Interactions - Increased Effect/Toxicity in Amphotericin B (Conventional) monograph.

Pharmacodynamics/Kinetics

Distribution: V_d: 131 L/kg
Half-life elimination: Terminal: 174 hours

Pregnancy Risk Factor B

Comments Amphotericin B, liposomal is a true single bilayer liposomal drug delivery system. Liposomes are closed, spherical vesicles created by mixing specific proportions of amphophilic substances such as phospholipids and cholesterol so that they arrange themselves into multiple concentric bilayer membranes when hydrated in aqueous solutions. Single bilayer liposomes are then formed by microemulsification of multilamellar vesicles using a homogenizer. Amphotericin B, liposomal consists of these unilamellar bilayer liposomes
(Continued)

Amphotericin B (Liposomal) *(Continued)*

with amphotericin B intercalated within the membrane. Due to the nature and quantity of amphophilic substances used, and the lipophilic moiety in the amphotericin B molecule, the drug is an integral part of the overall structure of the amphotericin B liposomes. Amphotericin B, liposomal contains true liposomes that are <100 nm in diameter.

Ampicillin (am pi SIL in)

Related Information

Antibiotic Prophylaxis, Preprocedural Guidelines for Dental Patients *on page 1509*

Cardiovascular Diseases *on page 1458*

U.S. Brand Names Principen®

Canadian Brand Names Apo-Ampi®; Novo-Ampicillin; Nu-Ampi

Mexican Brand Names Anglopen®; Flamicina®; Lampicin®

Generic Available Yes

Synonyms Aminobenzylpenicillin; Ampicillin Sodium; Ampicillin Trihydrate

Pharmacologic Category Antibiotic, Penicillin

Dental Use I.V. or I.M. administration for the prevention of bacterial endocarditis in patients unable to take oral amoxicillin

Use Treatment of susceptible bacterial infections (nonbeta-lactamase-producing organisms); susceptible bacterial infections caused by streptococci, pneumococci, nonpenicillinase-producing staphylococci, *Listeria*, meningococci; some strains of *H. influenzae*, *Salmonella*, *Shigella*, *E. coli*, *Enterobacter*, and *Klebsiella*

Local Anesthetic/Vasoconstrictor Precautions No information available to require special precautions

Effects on Dental Treatment Key adverse event(s) related to dental treatment: Oral candidiasis.

Significant Adverse Effects Frequency not defined.

Central nervous system: Fever, penicillin encephalopathy, seizures

Dermatologic: Erythema multiforme, exfoliative dermatitis, rash, urticaria

Note: Appearance of a rash should be carefully evaluated to differentiate (if possible) nonallergic ampicillin rash from hypersensitivity reaction. Incidence is higher in patients with viral infections, *Salmonella* infections, lymphocytic leukemia, or patients that have hyperuricemia.

Gastrointestinal: Black hairy tongue, diarrhea, enterocolitis, glossitis, nausea, pseudomembranous colitis, sore mouth or tongue, stomatitis, vomiting

Hematologic: Agranulocytosis, anemia, hemolytic anemia, eosinophilia, leukopenia, thrombocytopenia purpura

Hepatic: AST increased

Renal: Interstitial nephritis (rare)

Respiratory: Laryngeal stridor

Miscellaneous: Anaphylaxis, serum sickness-like reaction

Dosage

Infants and Children:

- Mild-to-moderate infections:
  - I.M., I.V.: 100-150 mg/kg/day in divided doses every 6 hours (maximum: 2-4 g/day)
  - Oral: 50-100 mg/kg/day in doses divided every 6 hours (maximum: 2-4 g/day)
- Severe infections/meningitis: I.M., I.V.: 200-400 mg/kg/day in divided doses every 6 hours (maximum: 6-12 g/day)
- **Endocarditis prophylaxis:** I.M., I.V.:
  - Dental, oral, respiratory tract, or esophageal procedures: 50 mg/kg within 30 minutes prior to procedure in patients unable to take oral amoxicillin
  - Genitourinary and gastrointestinal tract (except esophageal) procedures:
    - High-risk patients: 50 mg/kg (maximum: 2 g) within 30 minutes prior to procedure, followed by ampicillin 25 mg/kg (or amoxicillin 25 mg/kg orally) 6 hours later; must be used in combination with gentamicin.
    - Moderate-risk patients: 50 mg/kg within 30 minutes prior to procedure

Adults:

- Susceptible infections:
  - Oral: 250-500 mg every 6 hours
  - I.M., I.V.: 250-500 mg every 6 hours
- Sepsis/meningitis: I.M., I.V.: 150-250 mg/kg/24 hours divided every 3-4 hours (range: 6-12 g/day)
- **Endocarditis prophylaxis:** I.M., I.V.:
  - Dental, oral, respiratory tract, or esophageal procedures: 2 g within 30 minutes prior to procedure in patients unable to take oral amoxicillin

Genitourinary and gastrointestinal tract (except esophageal) procedures:
High-risk patients: 2 g within 30 minutes prior to procedure, followed by ampicillin 1 g (or amoxicillin 1 g orally) 6 hours later; must be used in combination with gentamicin
Moderate-risk patients: 2 g within 30 minutes prior to procedure

Dosing interval in renal impairment:
Cl_{cr} >50 mL/minute: Administer every 6 hours
Cl_{cr} 10-50 mL/minute: Administer every 6-12 hours
Cl_{cr} <10 mL/minute: Administer every 12-24 hours

Hemodialysis: Moderately dialyzable (20% to 50%); administer dose after dialysis

Peritoneal dialysis: Moderately dialyzable (20% to 50%)
Administer 250 mg every 12 hours

Continuous arteriovenous or venovenous hemofiltration effects: Dose as for Cl_{cr} 10-50 mL/minute; ~50 mg of ampicillin per liter of filtrate is removed

Mechanism of Action Inhibits bacterial cell wall synthesis by binding to one or more of the penicillin binding proteins (PBPs); which in turn inhibits the final transpeptidation step of peptidoglycan synthesis in bacterial cell walls, thus inhibiting cell wall biosynthesis. Bacteria eventually lyse due to ongoing activity of cell wall autolytic enzymes (autolysins and murein hydrolases) while cell wall assembly is arrested.

Contraindications Hypersensitivity to ampicillin, any component of the formulation, or other penicillins

Warnings/Precautions Dosage adjustment may be necessary in patients with renal impairment; a low incidence of cross-allergy with other beta-lactams exists; high percentage of patients with infectious mononucleosis have developed rash during therapy with ampicillin. Appearance of a rash should be carefully evaluated to differentiate a nonallergic ampicillin rash from a hypersensitivity reaction. Ampicillin rash occurs in 5% to 10% of children receiving ampicillin and is a generalized dull red, maculopapular rash, generally appearing 3-14 days after the start of therapy. It normally begins on the trunk and spreads over most of the body. It may be most intense at pressure areas, elbows, and knees.

Drug Interactions

Allopurinol: Theoretically has an additive potential for ampicillin/amoxicillin rash

Aminoglycosides: May be synergistic against selected organisms

Methotrexate: Penicillins may increase the exposure to methotrexate during concurrent therapy; monitor.

Oral contraceptives: Anecdotal reports suggesting decreased contraceptive efficacy with penicillins have been refuted by more rigorous scientific and clinical data.

Probenecid, disulfiram: May increase levels of penicillins (ampicillin)

Warfarin: Effects of warfarin may be increased

Ethanol/Nutrition/Herb Interactions Food: Food decreases ampicillin absorption rate; may decrease ampicillin serum concentration.

Dietary Considerations Take on an empty stomach 1 hour before or 2 hours after meals.

Sodium content of 5 mL suspension (250 mg/5 mL): 10 mg (0.4 mEq)

Sodium content of 1 g: 66.7 mg (3 mEq)

Pharmacodynamics/Kinetics

Absorption: Oral: 50%

Distribution: Bile, blister, and tissue fluids; penetration into CSF occurs with inflamed meninges only, good only with inflammation (exceeds usual MICs)
Normal meninges: Nil; Inflamed meninges: 5% to 10%

Protein binding: 15% to 25%

Half-life elimination:
Children and Adults: 1-1.8 hours
Anuria/end-stage renal disease: 7-20 hours

Time to peak: Oral: Within 1-2 hours

Excretion: Urine (~90% as unchanged drug) within 24 hours

Pregnancy Risk Factor B

Lactation Enters breast milk/use caution

Dosage Forms

Capsule (Principen®): 250 mg, 500 mg

Injection, powder for reconstitution, as sodium: 125 mg, 250 mg, 500 mg, 1 g, 2 g, 10 g

Powder for oral suspension (Principen®): 125 mg/5 mL (100 mL, 200 mL); 250 mg/5 mL (100 mL, 200 mL)

(Continued)

Ampicillin *(Continued)*

Selected Readings

ADA Division of Legal Affairs, "A Legal Perspective on Antibiotic Prophylaxis," *J Am Dent Assoc*, 2003, 134(9):1260.

American Dental Association; American Academy of Orthopedic Surgeons, "Antibiotic Prophylaxis for Dental Patients With Total Joint Replacements," *J Am Dent Assoc*, 2003, 134(7):895-9.

American Dental Association Council on Scientific Affairs, "Combating Antibiotic Resistance," *J Am Dent Assoc*, 2004, 135(4):484-7.

Dajani AS, Taubert KA, Wilson W, et al, "Prevention of Bacterial Endocarditis. Recommendations by the American Heart Association," *JAMA*, 1997, 277(22):1794-801.

Dajani AS, Taubert KA, Wilson W, et al, "Prevention of Bacterial Endocarditis: Recommendations by the American Heart Association," *J Am Dent Assoc*, 1997, 128(8):1142-51.

Wynn RL, Bergman SA, Meiller TF, et al, "Antibiotics in Treating Oral-Facial Infections of Odontogenic Origin: An Update", *Gen Dent*, 2001, 49(3):238-40, 242, 244 passim.

Ampicillin and Probenecid (am pi SIL in & proe BEN e sid)

U.S. Brand Names Probampacin®

Generic Available No

Synonyms Probenecid and Ampicillin (Dental)

Pharmacologic Category Antibiotic, Penicillin

Use Uncomplicated infections caused by susceptible strains of *Neisseria gonorrhoeae* in adults

Local Anesthetic/Vasoconstrictor Precautions No information available to require special precautions

Effects on Dental Treatment Key adverse event(s) related to dental treatment: Oral candidiasis (after chronic dosing), facial flushing, and sore gums.

Common Adverse Effects

>10%:
- Central nervous system: Headache
- Dermatologic: Rash
- Gastrointestinal: Anorexia, nausea, vomiting, diarrhea, oral candidiasis
- Neuromuscular & skeletal: Gouty arthritis (acute)

1% to 10%:
- Cardiovascular: Flushing of face
- Central nervous system: Dizziness
- Dermatologic: Skin rash, itching
- Gastrointestinal: Sore gums, severe abdominal or stomach cramps and pain
- Genitourinary: Dysuria
- Renal: Renal calculi

Drug Interactions

Cytochrome P450 Effect: Probenecid: **Inhibits** CYP2C19 (weak)

Increased Effect/Toxicity: Although anecdotal reports suggest oral contraceptive efficacy could be reduced by penicillins, this has been refuted by more rigorous scientific and clinical data. Penicillins may increase the exposure to methotrexate during concurrent therapy; monitor.

Pharmacodynamics/Kinetics See individual agents.

Pregnancy Risk Factor B

Ampicillin and Sulbactam (am pi SIL in & SUL bak tam)

Related Information

Ampicillin *on page 124*

Sexually-Transmitted Diseases *on page 1504*

U.S. Brand Names Unasyn®

Canadian Brand Names Unasyn®

Generic Available Yes

Synonyms Sulbactam and Ampicillin

Pharmacologic Category Antibiotic, Penicillin

Dental Use Parenteral beta-lactamase-resistant antibiotic combination to treat more severe orofacial infections where beta-lactamase-producing staphylococci and beta-lactamase-producing *Bacteroides* are present

Use Treatment of susceptible bacterial infections involved with skin and skin structure, intra-abdominal infections, gynecological infections; spectrum is that of ampicillin plus organisms producing beta-lactamases such as *S. aureus*, *H. influenzae*, *E. coli*, *Klebsiella*, *Acinetobacter*, *Enterobacter*, and anaerobes

Local Anesthetic/Vasoconstrictor Precautions No information available to require special precautions

Effects on Dental Treatment Prolonged use of penicillins may lead to development of oral candidiasis.

Significant Adverse Effects Also see Ampicillin monograph

>10%: Local: Pain at injection site (I.M.)

1% to 10%:
- Dermatologic: Rash

Gastrointestinal: Diarrhea
Local: Pain at injection site (I.V.), thrombophlebitis
Miscellaneous: Allergic reaction (may include serum sickness, urticaria, bronchospasm, hypotension, etc)
<1% (Limited to important or life-threatening): Abdominal distension, candidiasis, chest pain, chills, dysuria, edema, epistaxis, erythema, facial swelling, fatigue, flatulence, glossitis, hairy tongue, headache, interstitial nephritis, itching, liver enzymes increased, malaise, mucosal bleeding, nausea, pseudomembranous colitis, seizures, substernal pain, throat tightness, thrombocytopenia, urine retention, vomiting

Dosage Unasyn® (ampicillin/sulbactam) is a combination product. Dosage recommendations for Unasyn® are based on the ampicillin component.

Children ≥1 year: I.V.:
Mild-to-moderate infections: 100-150 mg ampicillin/kg/day (150-300 mg Unasyn®) divided every 6 hours; maximum: 8 g ampicillin/day (12 g Unasyn®)
Severe infections: 200-400 mg ampicillin/kg/day divided every 6 hours; maximum: 8 g ampicillin/day (12 g Unasyn®)

Adults: I.M., I.V.: 1-2 g ampicillin (1.5-3 g Unasyn®) every 6 hours; maximum: 8 g ampicillin/day (12 g Unasyn®)

Dosing interval in renal impairment:
Cl_{cr} 15-29 mL/minute: Administer every 12 hours
Cl_{cr} 5-14 mL/minute: Administer every 24 hours

Mechanism of Action The addition of sulbactam, a beta-lactamase inhibitor, to ampicillin extends the spectrum of ampicillin to include some beta-lactamase producing organisms; inhibits bacterial cell wall synthesis by binding to one or more of the penicillin binding proteins (PBPs); which in turn inhibits the final transpeptidation step of peptidoglycan synthesis in bacterial cell walls, thus inhibiting cell wall biosynthesis. Bacteria eventually lyse due to ongoing activity of cell wall autolytic enzymes (autolysins and murein hydrolases) while cell wall assembly is arrested.

Contraindications Hypersensitivity to ampicillin, sulbactam, penicillins, or any component of the formulations

Warnings/Precautions Dosage adjustment may be necessary in patients with renal impairment; a low incidence of cross-allergy with other beta-lactams exists; high percentage of patients with infectious mononucleosis have developed rash during therapy with ampicillin. Appearance of a rash should be carefully evaluated to differentiate a nonallergic ampicillin rash from a hypersensitivity reaction. Ampicillin rash occurs in 5% to 10% of children receiving ampicillin and is a generalized dull red, maculopapular rash, generally appearing 3-14 days after the start of therapy. It normally begins on the trunk and spreads over most of the body. It may be most intense at pressure areas, elbows, and knees.

Drug Interactions
Allopurinol: Theoretically has an additive potential for ampicillin/amoxicillin rash
Aminoglycosides: May be synergistic against selected organisms
Methotrexate: Penicillins may increase the exposure to methotrexate during concurrent therapy; monitor.
Oral contraceptives: Anecdotal reports suggesting decreased contraceptive efficacy with penicillins have been refuted by more rigorous scientific and clinical data.
Probenecid, disulfiram: May increase levels of penicillins (ampicillin)
Warfarin: Effects of warfarin may be increased

Dietary Considerations Sodium content of 1.5 g injection: 115 mg (5 mEq)

Pharmacodynamics/Kinetics
Ampicillin: See Ampicillin monograph.
Sulbactam:
Distribution: Bile, blister, and tissue fluids
Protein binding: 38%
Half-life elimination: Normal renal function: 1-1.3 hours
Excretion: Urine (~75% to 85% as unchanged drug) within 8 hours

Pregnancy Risk Factor B

Lactation Enters breast milk/use caution

Dosage Forms Injection, powder for reconstitution: 3 g [ampicillin sodium 2 g and sulbactam sodium 1 g]; 15 g [ampicillin sodium 10 g and sulbactam sodium 5 g] [bulk package]
Unasyn®: 1.5 g [ampicillin sodium 1 g and sulbactam sodium 0.5 g]; 3 g [ampicillin sodium 2 g and sulbactam sodium 1 g]; 15 g [ampicillin sodium 10 g and sulbactam sodium 5 g] [bulk package]

(Continued)

Ampicillin and Sulbactam *(Continued)*

Comments In maxillary sinus, anterior nasal cavity, and deep neck infections, beta-lactamase-producing staphylococci and beta-lactamase-producing *Bacteroides* usually are present. In these situations, antibiotics that resist the beta-lactamase enzyme should be administered. Amoxicillin and clavulanic acid is administered orally for moderate infections. Ampicillin sodium and sulbactam sodium (Unasyn®) is administered parenterally for more severe infections.

Ampicillin Sodium *see* Ampicillin *on page 124*

Ampicillin Trihydrate *see* Ampicillin *on page 124*

Amprenavir (am PREN a veer)

Related Information

HIV Infection and AIDS *on page 1484*
Tuberculosis *on page 1495*

U.S. Brand Names Agenerase®

Canadian Brand Names Agenerase®

Generic Available No

Pharmacologic Category Antiretroviral Agent, Protease Inhibitor

Use Treatment of HIV infections in combination with at least two other antiretroviral agents; oral solution should only be used when capsules or other protease inhibitors are not therapeutic options

Local Anesthetic/Vasoconstrictor Precautions No information available to require special precautions

Effects on Dental Treatment Key adverse event(s) related to dental treatment: Perioral tingling/numbness and taste disorder.

Common Adverse Effects Protease inhibitors cause dyslipidemia which includes elevated cholesterol and triglycerides and a redistribution of body fat centrally to cause increased abdominal girth, buffalo hump, facial atrophy, and breast enlargement. These agents also cause hyperglycemia.

>10%:

- Central nervous system: Paresthesia (peripheral 10% to 14%)
- Dermatologic: Rash (22%)
- Endocrine & metabolic: Hyperglycemia (>160 mg/dL: 37% to 41%), hypertriglyceridemia (>399 mg/dL: 36% to 47%; >750 mg/dL: 8% to 13%)
- Gastrointestinal: Nausea (43% to 74%), vomiting (24% to 34%), diarrhea (39% to 60%), abdominal symptoms
- Miscellaneous: Perioral tingling/numbness (26% to 31%)

1% to 10%:

- Central nervous system: Depression (4% to 15%), headache, fatigue, depression, mood disorder
- Dermatologic: Stevens-Johnson syndrome (1% of total, 4% of patients who develop a rash)
- Endocrine & metabolic: Hyperglycemia (>251 mg/dL: 2% to 3%)
- Gastrointestinal: Taste disorders (2% to 10%)
- Hepatic: AST increased (3% to 5%), ALT increased (4%), amylase increased (3% to 4%)

Mechanism of Action Binds to the protease activity site and inhibits the activity of the enzyme. HIV protease is required for the cleavage of viral polyprotein precursors into individual functional proteins found in infectious HIV. Inhibition prevents cleavage of these polyproteins, resulting in the formation of immature, noninfectious viral particles.

Drug Interactions

Cytochrome P450 Effect: Substrate of CYP2C8/9 (minor), 3A4 (major); **Inhibits** CYP2C19 (weak), 3A4 (strong)

Increased Effect/Toxicity: Concurrent use of cisapride, midazolam, pimozide, quinidine, or triazolam is contraindicated. Concurrent use of ergot alkaloids (dihydroergotamine, ergotamine, ergonovine, methylergonovine) with amprenavir is also contraindicated (may cause vasospasm and peripheral ischemia). Concurrent use of oral solution with disulfiram or metronidazole is contraindicated, due to the risk of propylene glycol toxicity.

Serum concentrations of amiodarone, bepridil, lidocaine, quinidine and other antiarrhythmics may be increased, potentially leading to toxicity; when amprenavir is coadministered with ritonavir, flecainide and propafenone are contraindicated. HMG-CoA reductase inhibitors serum concentrations may be increased by amprenavir, increasing the risk of myopathy/rhabdomyolysis; lovastatin and simvastatin are not recommended; fluvastatin and pravastatin may be safer alternatives.

Amprenavir may increase the levels/effects of selected benzodiazepines (midazolam and triazolam are contraindicated), calcium channel blockers, cyclosporine, mirtazapine, nateglinide, nefazodone, quinidine, sildenafil (and other PDE-5 inhibitors), tacrolimus, venlafaxine, and other CYP3A4 substrates. When used with strong CYP3A4 inhibitors, dosage adjustment/ limits are recommended for sildenafil and other PDE-5 inhibitors; refer to individual monographs.

Concurrent therapy with ritonavir may result in increased serum concentrations: dosage adjustment is recommended; avoid concurrent use of amprenavir and ritonavir oral solutions due to metabolic competition between formulation components. Clarithromycin, indinavir, nelfinavir may increase serum concentrations of amprenavir.

Decreased Effect: Serum concentrations of estrogen (oral contraceptives) may be decreased, use alternative (nonhormonal) forms of contraception. Dexamethasone may decrease the therapeutic effect of amprenavir. Serum concentrations of delavirdine may be decreased; may lead to loss of virologic response and possible resistance to delavirdine; concomitant use is not recommended. Efavirenz and nevirapine may decrease serum concentrations of amprenavir (dosing for combinations not established). Avoid St John's wort (may lead to subtherapeutic concentrations of amprenavir). Effect of amprenavir may be diminished when administered with methadone (consider alternative antiretroviral); in addition, effect of methadone may be reduced (dosage increase may be required). The levels/effects of amprenavir may be decreased by include aminoglutethimide, carbamazepine, nafcillin, nevirapine, phenobarbital, phenytoin, rifamycins, and other CYP3A4 inducers. The administration of didanosine (buffered formulation) should be separated from amprenavir by 1 hour to limit interaction between formulations.

Pharmacodynamics/Kinetics

Absorption: 63%
Distribution: 430 L
Protein binding: 90%
Metabolism: Hepatic via CYP (primarily CYP3A4)
Bioavailability: Not established; increased sixfold with high-fat meal
Half-life elimination: 7.1-10.6 hours
Time to peak: 1-2 hours
Excretion: Feces (75%); urine (14% as metabolites)

Pregnancy Risk Factor C

AMPT *see* Metyrosine *on page 920*
Amrinone Lactate *see* Inamrinone *on page 743*
AMSA *see* Amsacrine *on page 129*

Amsacrine (AM sah kreen)

Generic Available No

Synonyms 4-(9-Acridinylamino) Methanesulfon-m-Anisidide; Acridinyl Anisidide; AMSA; m-AMSA; NSC-249992

Pharmacologic Category Antineoplastic Agent

Unlabeled/Investigational Use Investigational: Refractory acute lymphocytic and nonlymphocytic leukemias, Hodgkin's disease, and non-Hodgkin's lymphomas; possibly some activity against head and neck tumors

Local Anesthetic/Vasoconstrictor Precautions No information available to require special precautions

Effects on Dental Treatment Key adverse event(s) related to dental treatment: Oral ulcerations and stomatitis.

Common Adverse Effects

>10%:

Cardiovascular: ECG changes (T-wave flattening, S-T wave alterations) consistent with anterolateral ischemia, ventricular fibrillation, ventricular extrasystoles, atrial tachycardia and fibrillation, congestive heart failure, cardiac arrest. Patients with hypokalemia, who have received >400 mg/m^2 of doxorubicin or daunorubicin (or the equivalent), >200 mg/m^2 of amsacrine within 48 hours, or a total dose of anthracycline + amsacrine >900 mg/m^2 have an increased risk of cardiac toxicity.

Dermatologic: Alopecia

Gastrointestinal: Nausea and vomiting (30%), diarrhea (30%), dose-limiting stomatitis (32%), oral ulceration (10%)

Genitourinary: Orange-red discoloration of the urine

Hematologic: Leukopenia (nadir at 10 days); thrombocytopenia (nadir at 12-14 days), with recovery at 21-25 days

Hepatic: Hyperbilirubinemia (30%), increased liver enzymes (10%)

(Continued)

Amsacrine *(Continued)*

Local: Phlebitis

1% to 10%:

Central nervous system: Headache, dizziness, confusion, convulsions

Hematologic: Anemia

Neuromuscular & skeletal: Paresthesias

Ocular: Blurred vision

Mechanism of Action Amsacrine has been shown to inhibit DNA synthesis by binding to, and intercalating with, DNA and inhibition of topoisomerase II activity.

Pharmacodynamics/Kinetics

Distribution: V_d: 1.67 L/kg; minimal CNS penetration

Protein binding: 96% to 98%

Metabolism: Hepatic, to inactive metabolites (major metabolite is 5′ glutathione conjugate)

Half-life elimination: 1.4-5 hours; Terminal: 5.6-7.8 hours

Excretion: Bile; urine (2% to 10% as unchanged drug)

Amyl Nitrite (AM il NYE trite)

Generic Available Yes

Synonyms Isoamyl Nitrite

Pharmacologic Category Antidote; Vasodilator

Use Coronary vasodilator in angina pectoris; adjunct in treatment of cyanide poisoning; produce changes in the intensity of heart murmurs

Local Anesthetic/Vasoconstrictor Precautions No information available to require special precautions

Effects on Dental Treatment Key adverse event(s) related to dental treatment: Postural hypotension.

Common Adverse Effects 1% to 10%:

Cardiovascular: Postural hypotension, cutaneous flushing of head, neck, and clavicular area, tachycardia

Central nervous system: Headache, restlessness

Gastrointestinal: Nausea, vomiting

Drug Interactions

Increased Effect/Toxicity: Ethanol taken with amyl nitrite may have additive side effects. Avoid concurrent use of sildenafil - severe reactions may result.

Pharmacodynamics/Kinetics

Onset of action: Angina: Within 30 seconds

Duration: 3-15 minutes

Pregnancy Risk Factor X

Amylobarbitone *see* Amobarbital *on page 112*

Amytal® *see* Amobarbital *on page 112*

Anacin PM Aspirin Free [OTC] [DSC] *see* Acetaminophen and Diphenhydramine *on page 53*

Anadrol® *see* Oxymetholone *on page 1035*

Anafranil® *see* ClomiPRAMINE *on page 355*

Anagrelide (an AG gre lide)

U.S. Brand Names Agrylin®

Canadian Brand Names Agrylin®

Generic Available No

Synonyms 1370-999-397; Anagrelide Hydrochloride; BL4162A; 6,7-Dichloro-1,5-Dihydroimidazo [2,1b] quinazolin-2(3H)-one Monohydrochloride

Pharmacologic Category Phospholipase A_2 Inhibitor

Use Treatment of essential thrombocythemia (ET) and thrombocythemia associated with chronic myelogenous leukemia (CML), polycythemia vera, and other myeloproliferative disorders

Local Anesthetic/Vasoconstrictor Precautions No information available to require special precautions

Effects on Dental Treatment Key adverse event(s) related to dental treatment: Orthostatic hypotension.

Common Adverse Effects Frequency not defined.

Cardiovascular: Palpitations (27%), chest pain (8%), tachycardia (7%), orthostatic hypotension, CHF, cardiomyopathy, myocardial infarction (rare), complete heart block, angina, and atrial fibrillation, hypertension, pericardial perfusion (rare)

Central nervous system: Headache (44%), dizziness (15%), bad dreams, impaired concentration ability

Hematologic: Anemia, thrombocytopenia, ecchymosis and lymphadenoma have been reported rarely

Respiratory: Pleural effusion

Mechanism of Action Anagrelide appears to inhibit cyclic nucleotide phosphodiesterase and the release of arachidonic acid from phospholipase, possibly by inhibiting phospholipase A_2. It also causes a dose-related reduction in platelet production, which results from decreased megakaryocyte hypermaturation. The drug disrupts the postmitotic phase of maturation.

Drug Interactions

Decreased Effect: There is a single case report that suggests sucralfate may interfere with anagrelide absorption.

Pharmacodynamics/Kinetics

Duration: 6-24 hours

Metabolism: Hepatic

Half-life elimination, plasma: 1.3 hours

Time to peak, serum: 1 hour

Excretion: Urine (<1% as unchanged drug)

Pregnancy Risk Factor C

Anagrelide Hydrochloride *see* Anagrelide *on page 130*

Anakinra (an a KIN ra)

U.S. Brand Names Kineret®

Canadian Brand Names Kineret®

Generic Available No

Synonyms IL-1Ra; Interleukin-1 Receptor antagonist

Pharmacologic Category Antirheumatic, Disease Modifying; Interleukin-1 Receptor Antagonist

Use Reduction of signs and symptoms of moderately- to severely-active rheumatoid arthritis in adult patients who have failed one or more disease-modifying antirheumatic drugs (DMARDs); may be used alone or in combination with DMARDs (other than tumor necrosis factor-blocking agents)

Local Anesthetic/Vasoconstrictor Precautions No information available to require special precautions

Effects on Dental Treatment No significant effects or complications reported

Common Adverse Effects

>10%:

Central nervous system: Headache (12%)

Local: Injection site reaction (majority mild, typically lasting 14-28 days, characterized by erythema, ecchymosis, inflammation and pain; up to 71%)

Miscellaneous: Infection (40% versus 35% in placebo; serious infections in 2% to 7%)

1% to 10%:

Gastrointestinal: Nausea (8%), diarrhea (7%), abdominal pain (5%)

Hematologic: Decreased WBCs (8%)

Respiratory: Sinusitis (7%)

Miscellaneous: Flu-like symptoms (6%)

Mechanism of Action Binds to the interleukin-1 (IL-1) receptor. IL-1 is induced by inflammatory stimuli and mediates a variety of immunological responses, including degradation of cartilage (loss of proteoglycans) and stimulation of bone resorption.

Drug Interactions

Increased Effect/Toxicity: Concurrent use of anakinra and etanercept has been associated with an increased risk of serious infection while American College of Rheumatology (ACR) response rates were not improved, as compared to etanercept alone. Use caution with other drugs known to block or decrease the activity of tumor necrosis factor (TNF); includes infliximab and thalidomide.

Pharmacodynamics/Kinetics

Bioavailability: SubQ: 95%

Half-life elimination: Terminal: 4-6 hours

Time to peak: SubQ: 3-7 hours

Pregnancy Risk Factor B

Ana-Kit® *see* Epinephrine and Chlorpheniramine *on page 497*

Analpram-HC® *see* Pramoxine and Hydrocortisone *on page 1109*

AnaMantle® HC *see* Lidocaine and Hydrocortisone *on page 826*

Anaprox® *see* Naproxen *on page 965*

Anaprox® DS *see* Naproxen *on page 965*

Anaspaz® *see* Hyoscyamine *on page 724*

Anastrozole (an AS troe zole)

U.S. Brand Names Arimidex®

Canadian Brand Names Arimidex®

Mexican Brand Names Arimidex®

Generic Available No

Synonyms ICI-D1033; ZD1033

Pharmacologic Category Antineoplastic Agent, Miscellaneous

Use Treatment of locally-advanced or metastatic breast cancer (ER-positive or hormone receptor unknown) in postmenopausal women; treatment of advanced breast cancer in postmenopausal women with disease progression following tamoxifen therapy; adjuvant treatment of early ER-positive breast cancer in postmenopausal women

Local Anesthetic/Vasoconstrictor Precautions No information available to require special precautions

Effects on Dental Treatment Key adverse event(s) related to dental treatment: Xerostomia (normal salivary flow resumes upon discontinuation).

Common Adverse Effects

>10%:

Cardiovascular: Vasodilatation (25% to 35%)

Central nervous system: Pain (11% to 15%), headache (9% to 13%), depression (5% to 11%)

Endocrine & metabolic: Hot flashes (12% to 35%)

Neuromuscular & skeletal: Weakness (16% to 17%), arthritis (14%), arthralgia (13%), back pain (8% to 12%), bone pain (5% to 11%)

Respiratory: Cough increased (7% to 11%), pharyngitis (6% to 12%)

1% to 10%:

Cardiovascular: Peripheral edema (5% to 10%), hypertension (5% to 9%), chest pain (5% to 7%)

Central nervous system: Insomnia (6% to 9%), dizziness (6%), anxiety (5%), lethargy (1%), fever, malaise, confusion, nervousness, somnolence

Dermatologic: Rash (6% to 10%), alopecia, pruritus

Endocrine & metabolic: Hypercholesteremia (7%)

Gastrointestinal: Vomiting (8% to 9%), constipation (7% to 9%), abdominal pain (7% to 8%), diarrhea (7% to 8%), anorexia (5% to 7%), xerostomia (6%), dyspepsia (5%), weight gain (2% to 8%), weight loss

Genitourinary: Urinary tract infection (6%), vulvovaginitis (6%), vaginal bleeding (5%) leukorrhea (2%), vaginal hemorrhage (2%), vaginal dryness (2%)

Hematologic: Anemia, leukopenia

Hepatic: Liver function tests increased, alkaline phosphatase increased

Local: Deep vein thrombosis, thrombophlebitis

Neuromuscular & skeletal: Osteoporosis (7%), fracture (7%), arthrosis (6%), paresthesia (5% to 6%), hypertonia (3%), myalgia, arthralgia

Ocular: Cataracts (4%)

Respiratory: Dyspnea (6% to 10%), sinusitis, bronchitis, rhinitis

Miscellaneous: Lymph edema (9%), infection (7%), flu-syndrome (5% to 7%), diaphoresis (2% to 4%)

Mechanism of Action Potent and selective nonsteroidal aromatase inhibitor. By inhibiting aromatase, the conversion of androstenedione to estrone, and testosterone to estradiol, is prevented. Anastrozole causes an 85% decrease in estrone sulfate levels.

Drug Interactions

Cytochrome P450 Effect: Inhibits CYP1A2 (weak), 2C8/9 (weak), 3A4 (weak)

Decreased Effect:

Estrogens: Concurrent use may decrease efficacy of anastrozole.

Tamoxifen: Decreased plasma concentration of anastrozole; avoid concurrent use.

Pharmacodynamics/Kinetics

Onset of estradiol reduction: 24 hours

Duration of estradiol reduction: 6 days

Absorption: Well absorbed (80%); not affected by food

Protein binding, plasma: 40%

Metabolism: Extensively hepatic (85%) via N-dealkylation, hydroxylation, and glucuronidation; primary metabolite inactive

Half-life elimination: 50 hours

Excretion: Urine (10% as unchanged drug; 60% as metabolites)

Pregnancy Risk Factor D

Anatuss LA *see* Guaifenesin and Pseudoephedrine *on page 675*

Anbesol® [OTC] *see* Benzocaine *on page 191*

Anbesol® Baby [OTC] *see* Benzocaine *on page 191*
Anbesol® Maximum Strength [OTC] *see* Benzocaine *on page 191*
Ancef® *see* Cefazolin *on page 278*
Ancobon® *see* Flucytosine *on page 596*
Andehist DM NR Drops *see* Carbinoxamine, Pseudoephedrine, and Dextromethorphan *on page 263*
Andehist NR Drops *see* Carbinoxamine and Pseudoephedrine *on page 262*
Andehist NR Syrup *see* Brompheniramine and Pseudoephedrine *on page 220*
Androderm® *see* Testosterone *on page 1276*
AndroGel® *see* Testosterone *on page 1276*
Android® *see* MethylTESTOSTERone *on page 912*
Anectine® [DSC] *see* Succinylcholine *on page 1241*
Anestacon® *see* Lidocaine *on page 819*
Aneurine Hydrochloride *see* Thiamine *on page 1287*
Anexsia® *see* Hydrocodone and Acetaminophen *on page 702*
Angiomax® *see* Bivalirudin *on page 212*
Animal and Human Bites Guidelines *see page 1582*
Anolor 300 *see* Butalbital, Acetaminophen, and Caffeine *on page 236*
Ansaid® *see* Flurbiprofen *on page 613*
Ansamycin *see* Rifabutin *on page 1179*
Antabuse® *see* Disulfiram *on page 456*
Antagon® *see* Ganirelix *on page 647*
Antazoline and Naphazoline *see* Naphazoline and Antazoline *on page 964*

Anthralin (AN thra lin)

U.S. Brand Names Drithocreme®; Dritho-Scalp®; Psoriatec™
Canadian Brand Names Anthraforte®; Anthranol®; Anthrascalp®; Micanol®
Mexican Brand Names Anthranol®
Generic Available No
Synonyms Dithranol
Pharmacologic Category Antipsoriatic Agent; Keratolytic Agent
Use Treatment of psoriasis (quiescent or chronic psoriasis)
Local Anesthetic/Vasoconstrictor Precautions No information available to require special precautions
Effects on Dental Treatment No significant effects or complications reported
Mechanism of Action Reduction of the mitotic rate and proliferation of epidermal cells in psoriasis by inhibiting synthesis of nucleic protein from inhibition of DNA synthesis to affected areas
Pregnancy Risk Factor C

Anthrax Vaccine (Adsorbed) (AN thraks vak SEEN ad SORBED)

Related Information
Immunizations (Vaccines) *on page 1614*
U.S. Brand Names BioThrax™
Generic Available No
Synonyms AVA
Pharmacologic Category Vaccine
Use Immunization against *Bacillus anthracis*. Recommended for individuals who may come in contact with animal products which come from anthrax endemic areas and may be contaminated with *Bacillus anthracis* spores; recommended for high-risk persons such as veterinarians and other handling potentially infected animals. Routine immunization for the general population is not recommended.

The Department of Defense is implementing an anthrax vaccination program against the biological warfare agent anthrax, which will be administered to all active duty and reserve personnel.

Unlabeled/Investigational Use Postexposure prophylaxis in combination with antibiotics
Local Anesthetic/Vasoconstrictor Precautions No information available to require special precautions
Effects on Dental Treatment No significant effects or complications reported
Common Adverse Effects (Includes pre- and post-licensure data; systemic reactions reported more often in women than in men)

>10%:

Central nervous system: Malaise (4% to 11%)

Local: Tenderness (58% to 71%), erythema (12% to 43%), subcutaneous nodule (4% to 39%), induration (8% to 21%), warmth (11% to 19%), local pruritus (7% to 19%)

(Continued)

Anthrax Vaccine (Adsorbed) *(Continued)*

Neuromuscular & skeletal: Arm motion limitation (7% to 12%)

1% to 10%:

Central nervous system: Headache (4% to 7%), fever (<1% to 7%)
Gastrointestinal: Anorexia (4%), vomiting (4%), nausea (<1% to 4%)
Local: Mild local reactions (edema/induration <30mm) (9%), edema (8%)
Neuromuscular & skeletal: Myalgia (4% to 7%)
Respiratory: Respiratory difficulty (4%)

Restrictions Not commercially available in the U.S.; presently, all anthrax vaccine lots are owned by the U.S. Department of Defense. The Centers for Disease Control (CDC) does not currently recommend routine vaccination of the general public.

Mechanism of Action Active immunization against *Bacillus anthracis.* The vaccine is prepared from a cell-free filtrate of *B. anthracis*, but no dead or live bacteria.

Drug Interactions

Decreased Effect: Effect of vaccine may be decreased with chemotherapy, corticosteroids (high doses, ≥14 days), immunosuppressant agents and radiation therapy; consider waiting at least 3 months between discontinuing therapy and administering vaccine.

Pharmacodynamics/Kinetics Duration: Unknown; may be 1-2 years following two inoculations based on animal data

Pregnancy Risk Factor D

AntibiOtic® Ear *see* Neomycin, Polymyxin B, and Hydrocortisone *on page 975*

Antibiotic Prophylaxis, Preprocedural Guidelines for Dental Patients *see page 1509*

Anti-CD11a *see* Efalizumab *on page 483*

Anti-CD20 Monoclonal Antibody *see* Rituximab *on page 1191*

Antidigoxin Fab Fragments, Ovine *see* Digoxin Immune Fab *on page 440*

Antidiuretic Hormone *see* Vasopressin *on page 1369*

Antihemophilic Factor (Human)

(an tee hee moe FIL ik FAK tor HYU man)

U.S. Brand Names Alphanate®; Hemofil® M; Humate-P®; Koāte®-DVI; Monarc® M; Monoclate-P®

Canadian Brand Names Hemofil® M; Humate-P®

Generic Available Yes

Synonyms AHF (Human); Factor VIII (Human)

Pharmacologic Category Antihemophilic Agent; Blood Product Derivative

Use Management of hemophilia A for patients in whom a deficiency in factor VIII has been demonstrated; can be of significant therapeutic value in patients with acquired factor VIII inhibitors not exceeding 10 Bethesda units/mL

Humate-P®: In addition, indicated as treatment of spontaneous bleeding in patients with severe von Willebrand disease and in mild and moderate von Willebrand disease where desmopressin is known or suspected to be inadequate

Orphan status: Alphanate®: Management of von Willebrand disease

Local Anesthetic/Vasoconstrictor Precautions No information available to require special precautions

Effects on Dental Treatment No significant effects or complications reported

Mechanism of Action Protein (factor VIII) in normal plasma which is necessary for clot formation and maintenance of hemostasis; activates factor X in conjunction with activated factor IX; activated factor X converts prothrombin to thrombin, which converts fibrinogen to fibrin, and with factor XIII forms a stable clot

Pharmacodynamics/Kinetics Half-life elimination: Mean: 12-17 hours with hemophilia A; consult specific product labeling

Pregnancy Risk Factor C

Antihemophilic Factor (Porcine)

(an tee hee moe FIL ik FAK ter POR seen)

U.S. Brand Names Hyate:C®

Generic Available No

Synonyms AHF (Porcine); Factor VIII (Porcine)

Pharmacologic Category Antihemophilic Agent

Use Management of hemophilia A in patients with antibodies to human factor VIII (consider use of human factor VIII in patients with antibody titer of <5 Bethesda units/mL); management of previously nonhemophilic patients with spontaneously-acquired inhibitors to human factor VIII, regardless of initial antihuman inhibitor titer

Local Anesthetic/Vasoconstrictor Precautions No information available to require special precautions

Effects on Dental Treatment No significant effects or complications reported

Common Adverse Effects Reactions tend to lessen in frequency and severity as further infusions are given; hydrocortisone and/or antihistamines may help to prevent or alleviate side effects and may be prescribed as precautionary measures.

1% to 10%:

Central nervous system: Fever, headache, chills
Dermatologic: Rashes
Gastrointestinal: Nausea, vomiting

Mechanism of Action Factor VIII is the coagulation portion of the factor VIII complex in plasma. Factor VIII acts as a cofactor for factor IX to activate factor X in the intrinsic pathway of blood coagulation.

Pharmacodynamics/Kinetics Half-life elimination: 10-11 hours (patients without detectable inhibitors)

Pregnancy Risk Factor C

Antihemophilic Factor (Recombinant)

(an tee hee moe FIL ik FAK tor ree KOM be nant)

U.S. Brand Names Advate; Helixate® FS; Kogenate® FS; Recombinate™; ReFacto®

Canadian Brand Names Helixate® FS; Kogenate®; Kogenate® FS; Recombinate™; ReFacto®

Generic Available No

Synonyms AHF (Recombinant); Factor VIII (Recombinant); rAHF

Pharmacologic Category Antihemophilic Agent

Use Management of hemophilia A (classic hemophilia) for patients in whom a deficiency in factor VIII has been demonstrated; prevention and control of bleeding episodes; perioperative management of hemophilia A; can be of significant therapeutic value in patients with acquired factor VIII inhibitors not exceeding 10 Bethesda units/mL

Local Anesthetic/Vasoconstrictor Precautions No information available to require special precautions

Effects on Dental Treatment No significant effects or complications reported

Mechanism of Action Protein (factor VIII) in normal plasma which is necessary for clot formation and maintenance of hemostasis; activates factor X in conjunction with activated factor IX; activated factor X converts prothrombin to thrombin, which converts fibrinogen to fibrin, and with factor XIII forms a stable clot

Pharmacodynamics/Kinetics Half-life elimination: Mean: 14-16 hours

Pregnancy Risk Factor C

Anti-inhibitor Coagulant Complex

(an tee-in HI bi tor coe AG yoo lant KOM pleks)

U.S. Brand Names Autoplex® T; Feiba VH®

Canadian Brand Names Feiba® VH Immuno

Generic Available No

Synonyms Coagulant Complex Inhibitor

Pharmacologic Category Antihemophilic Agent; Blood Product Derivative

Use Patients with factor VIII inhibitors who are to undergo surgery or those who are bleeding

Local Anesthetic/Vasoconstrictor Precautions No information available to require special precautions

Effects on Dental Treatment No significant effects or complications reported

Pregnancy Risk Factor C

Antiplaque Agents *see page 1556*

Antipyrine and Benzocaine (an tee PYE reen & BEN zoe kane)

Related Information

Benzocaine *on page 191*

U.S. Brand Names A/B Otic; Allergen®; Aurodex; Auroto

Canadian Brand Names Auralgan®

Generic Available Yes

Synonyms Benzocaine and Antipyrine

Pharmacologic Category Otic Agent, Analgesic; Otic Agent, Cerumenolytic

(Continued)

Antipyrine and Benzocaine *(Continued)*

Use Temporary relief of pain and reduction of swelling associated with acute congestive and serous otitis media, swimmer's ear, otitis externa; facilitates ear wax removal

Local Anesthetic/Vasoconstrictor Precautions No information available to require special precautions

Effects on Dental Treatment No significant effects or complications reported

Pregnancy Risk Factor C

Antiseptic Mouthwash *see* Mouthwash (Antiseptic) *on page 948*

Antithrombin III (an tee THROM bin three)

U.S. Brand Names Thrombate III®

Canadian Brand Names Thrombate III®

Generic Available No

Synonyms AT III; Heparin Cofactor I

Pharmacologic Category Anticoagulant; Blood Product Derivative

Use Treatment of hereditary antithrombin III deficiency in connection with surgical or obstetrical procedures; thromboembolism

Unlabeled/Investigational Use Acquired antithrombin III deficiencies related to disseminated intravascular coagulation (DIC)

Local Anesthetic/Vasoconstrictor Precautions No information available to require special precautions

Effects on Dental Treatment No significant effects or complications reported

Common Adverse Effects 1% to 10%: Central nervous system: Dizziness (2%)

Mechanism of Action Antithrombin III is the primary physiologic inhibitor of *in vivo* coagulation. It is an alpha$_2$-globulin. Its principal actions are the inactivation of thrombin, plasmin, and other active serine proteases of coagulation, including factors IXa, Xa, XIa, XIIa, and VIIa. The inactivation of proteases is a major step in the normal clotting process. The strong activation of clotting enzymes at the site of every bleeding injury facilitates fibrin formation and maintains normal hemostasis. Thrombosis in the circulation would be caused by active serine proteases if they were not inhibited by antithrombin III after the localized clotting process. Patients with congenital deficiency are in a prethrombotic state, even if asymptomatic, as evidenced by elevated plasma levels of prothrombin activation fragment, which are normalized following infusions of antithrombin III concentrate.

Drug Interactions

Increased Effect/Toxicity: Heparin's anticoagulant effects are potentiated by antithrombin III (half-life of antithrombin III is decreased by heparin). Risk of hemorrhage with antithrombin III may be increased by drotrecogin, thrombolytic agents, oral anticoagulants (warfarin), and drugs which affect platelet function (eg, aspirin, NSAIDs, dipyridamole, ticlopidine, clopidogrel, and IIb/IIIa antagonists).

Pharmacodynamics/Kinetics Half-life elimination: Biologic: 2.5 days (immunologic assay); 3.8 days (functional AT-III assay)

Pregnancy Risk Factor B

Antithymocyte Globulin (Equine)

(an te THY moe site GLOB yu lin, E kwine)

U.S. Brand Names Atgam®

Canadian Brand Names Atgam®

Generic Available No

Synonyms Antithymocyte Immunoglobulin; ATG; Horse Antihuman Thymocyte Gamma Globulin; Lymphocyte Immune Globulin

Pharmacologic Category Immunosuppressant Agent

Use Prevention and treatment of acute renal allograft rejection; treatment of moderate to severe aplastic anemia in patients not considered suitable candidates for bone marrow transplantation

Unlabeled/Investigational Use Prevention and treatment of other solid organ allograft rejection; prevention of graft-versus-host disease following bone marrow transplantation

Local Anesthetic/Vasoconstrictor Precautions No information available to require special precautions

Effects on Dental Treatment Key adverse event(s) related to dental treatment: Stomatitis.

Common Adverse Effects

>10%:

Central nervous system: Fever, chills

Dermatologic: Pruritus, rash, urticaria
Hematologic: Leukopenia, thrombocytopenia

1% to 10%:

Cardiovascular: Bradycardia, chest pain, CHF, edema, encephalitis, hypotension, hypertension, myocarditis, tachycardia
Central nervous system: Agitation, headache, lethargy, lightheadedness, listlessness, seizures
Gastrointestinal: Diarrhea, nausea, stomatitis, vomiting
Hepatic: Hepatosplenomegaly, liver function tests abnormal
Local: Pain at injection site, phlebitis, thrombophlebitis, burning soles/palms
Neuromuscular & skeletal: Myalgia, back pain, arthralgia
Ocular: Periorbital edema
Renal: Abnormal renal function tests
Respiratory: Dyspnea, respiratory distress
Miscellaneous: Anaphylaxis, serum sickness, viral infection, night sweats, diaphoresis, lymphadenopathy

Mechanism of Action May involve elimination of antigen-reactive T-lymphocytes (killer cells) in peripheral blood or alteration of T-cell function

Pharmacodynamics/Kinetics

Distribution: Poorly into lymphoid tissues; binds to circulating lymphocytes, granulocytes, platelets, bone marrow cells
Half-life elimination, plasma: 1.5-12 days
Excretion: Urine (~1%)

Pregnancy Risk Factor C

Antithymocyte Immunoglobulin *see* Antithymocyte Globulin (Equine) *on page 136*

Antitumor Necrosis Factor Apha (Human) *see* Adalimumab *on page 67*

Anti-VEGF Monoclonal Antibody *see* Bevacizumab *on page 204*

Antivert® *see* Meclizine *on page 859*

Antizol® *see* Fomepizole *on page 627*

Anturane *see* Sulfinpyrazone *on page 1249*

Anucort-HC® *see* Hydrocortisone *on page 714*

Anusol-HC® *see* Hydrocortisone *on page 714*

Anusol® HC-1 [OTC] *see* Hydrocortisone *on page 714*

Anusol® Ointment [OTC] *see* Pramoxine *on page 1109*

Anzemet® *see* Dolasetron *on page 461*

APAP *see* Acetaminophen *on page 47*

APAP and Tramadol *see* Acetaminophen and Tramadol *on page 54*

Apatate® [OTC] *see* Vitamin B Complex Combinations *on page 1382*

ApexiCon™ *see* Diflorasone *on page 435*

ApexiCon™ E *see* Diflorasone *on page 435*

Aphedrid™ [OTC] *see* Triprolidine and Pseudoephedrine *on page 1345*

Aphrodyne® *see* Yohimbine *on page 1393*

Aphthasol® *see* Amlexanox *on page 107*

Apidra™ *see* Insulin Preparations *on page 749*

Aplisol® *see* Tuberculin Tests *on page 1349*

Aplonidine *see* Apraclonidine *on page 138*

Apokyn™ *see* Apomorphine *on page 137*

Apomorphine (a poe MOR feen)

U.S. Brand Names Apokyn™

Generic Available No

Synonyms Apomorphine Hydrochloride; Apomorphine Hydrochloride Hemihydrate

Pharmacologic Category Anti-Parkinson's Agent, Dopamine Agonist

Use Treatment of hypomobility, "off" episodes with Parkinson's disease

Unlabeled/Investigational Use Treatment of erectile dysfunction

Local Anesthetic/Vasoconstrictor Precautions No information available to require special precautions

Effects on Dental Treatment Key adverse event(s) related to dental treatment: Orthostatic hypotension has been reported in significant numbers of patients.

Common Adverse Effects

>10%:

Cardiovascular: Chest pain/pressure or angina (15%)
Central nervous system: Drowsiness or somnolence (35%), dizziness or orthostatic hypotension (20%)
Gastrointestinal: Nausea and/or vomiting (30%)

(Continued)

Apomorphine *(Continued)*

Neuromuscular & skeletal: Falls (30%), dyskinesias (24% to 35%)
Respiratory: Yawning (40%), rhinorrhea (20%)

1% to 10%:

Cardiovascular: Edema (10%), vasodilation (3%), hypotension (2%), syncope (2%), congestive heart failure
Central nervous system: Hallucinations or confusion (10%), anxiety, depression, fatigue, headache, insomnia, pain
Dermatologic: Bruising
Endocrine & metabolic: Dehydration
Gastrointestinal: Constipation, diarrhea
Local: Injection site reactions
Neuromuscular & skeletal: Arthralgias, weakness
Miscellaneous: Diaphoresis increased

Mechanism of Action Stimulates postsynaptic D2-type receptors within the caudate-putamen in the brain.

Drug Interactions

Cytochrome P450 Effect: Substrate (minor) of CYP1A2, 3A4, 2C19; **Inhibits** CYP1A2 (weak), 3A (weak), 2C19 (weak)

Increased Effect/Toxicity: Antihypertensives, vasodilators, and $5HT_3$ antagonists may increase risk of hypotension. QT_c prolongation may rarely occur with concurrent use of QT_c-prolonging agents. Effects of concomitant levodopa may be increased.

Decreased Effect: Typical antipsychotics may decrease the efficacy of apomorphine.

Pharmacodynamics/Kinetics

Onset: SubQ: Rapid
Duration: V_d (mean): 218 L
Metabolism: Not established; potential routes of metabolism include sulfation, N-demethylation, glucuronidation, and oxidation; catechol-O methyltranferase and nonenzymatic oxidation. CYP isoenzymes do not appear to play a significant role.
Half-life elimination: Terminal: 40 minutes
Time to peak, plasma: Improved motor scores: 20 minutes
Excretion: Urine 93% (as metabolites); feces 16%

Pregnancy Risk Factor C

Apomorphine Hydrochloride *see* Apomorphine *on page 137*
Apomorphine Hydrochloride Hemihydrate *see* Apomorphine *on page 137*
APPG *see* Penicillin G Procaine *on page 1060*

Apraclonidine (a pra KLOE ni deen)

U.S. Brand Names Iopidine®
Canadian Brand Names Iopidine®
Generic Available No
Synonyms Aplonidine; Apraclonidine Hydrochloride; p-Aminoclonidine
Pharmacologic Category $Alpha_2$ Agonist, Ophthalmic

Use Prevention and treatment of postsurgical intraocular pressure (IOP) elevation; short-term, adjunctive therapy in patients who require additional reduction of IOP

Local Anesthetic/Vasoconstrictor Precautions No information available to require special precautions

Effects on Dental Treatment Key adverse event(s) related to dental treatment: Xerostomia (normal salivary flow resumes upon discontinuation).

Mechanism of Action Apraclonidine is a potent alpha-adrenergic agent similar to clonidine; relatively selective for $alpha_2$-receptors but does retain some binding to $alpha_1$-receptors; appears to result in reduction of aqueous humor formation; its penetration through the blood-brain barrier is more polar than clonidine which reduces its penetration through the blood-brain barrier and suggests that its pharmacological profile is characterized by peripheral rather than central effects.

Pregnancy Risk Factor C

Apraclonidine Hydrochloride *see* Apraclonidine *on page 138*

Aprepitant (ap RE pi tant)

U.S. Brand Names Emend®
Generic Available No
Synonyms L 754030; MK 869
Pharmacologic Category Antiemetic; Substance P/Neurokinin 1 Receptor Antagonist

Use Prevention of acute and delayed nausea and vomiting associated with highly-emetogenic chemotherapy in combination with a corticosteroid and 5-HT_3 receptor antagonist

Local Anesthetic/Vasoconstrictor Precautions No information available to require special precautions

Effects on Dental Treatment Key adverse event(s) related to dental treatment: Hiccups.

Common Adverse Effects Percentages reported as part of combination therapy.

>10%:

Central nervous system: Fatigue (18%)
Gastrointestinal: Nausea (13%)
Neuromuscular & skeletal: Weakness (18%)
Miscellaneous: Hiccups (11%)

1% to 10%:

Central nervous system: Dizziness (7%)
Endocrine & metabolic: Dehydration (6%)
Gastrointestinal: Diarrhea (10%), abdominal pain (5%), epigastric discomfort (4%), gastritis (4%)
Hepatic: ALT increased (6%), AST increased (3%)
Renal: BUN increased (5%), proteinuria (7%), serum creatinine increased (4%)

Mechanism of Action Prevents acute and delayed vomiting by selectively inhibiting the substance P/neurokinin 1 (NK_1) receptor.

Drug Interactions

Cytochrome P450 Effect: Substrate of CYP1A2 (minor), 2C19 (minor), 3A4 (major); **Inhibits** CYP2C8/9 (weak), 3A4 (weak); **Induces** CYP2C9 (weak), 3A4 (weak)

Increased Effect/Toxicity: Use with cisapride or pimozide is contraindicated. CYP3A4 inhibitors may increase the levels/effects of aprepitant; example inhibitors include azole antifungals, ciprofloxacin, clarithromycin, diclofenac, doxycycline, erythromycin, imatinib, isoniazid, nefazodone, nicardipine, propofol, protease inhibitors, quinidine, and verapamil. Aprepitant may increase the bioavailability of corticosteroids; dose adjustment of dexamethasone and methylprednisolone is needed.

Decreased Effect: CYP3A4 inducers may decrease the levels/effects of aprepitant; example inducers include aminoglutethimide, carbamazepine, nafcillin, nevirapine, phenobarbital, phenytoin, and rifamycins. Metabolism of warfarin may be induced; monitor INR following the start of each cycle. Efficacy of oral contraceptives may be decreased (plasma levels of ethinyl estradiol and norethindrone decreased with concomitant use). Plasma levels of both paroxetine and aprepitant are decreased with concomitant use.

Pharmacodynamics/Kinetics

Distribution: V_d: 70 L; crosses the blood brain barrier
Protein binding: >95%
Metabolism: Extensively hepatic via CYP3A4 (major); CYP1A2 and CYP2C19 (minor); forms seven metabolites (weakly active)
Bioavailability: 60% to 65%
Half-life elimination: Terminal: 9-13 hours
Time to peak, plasma: 4 hours

Pregnancy Risk Factor B

Apresazide [DSC] *see* Hydralazine and Hydrochlorothiazide *on page 698*
Apresoline [DSC] *see* HydrALAZINE *on page 697*
Apri® *see* Ethinyl Estradiol and Desogestrel *on page 536*
Aprodine® [OTC] *see* Triprolidine and Pseudoephedrine *on page 1345*

Aprotinin (a proe TYE nin)

U.S. Brand Names Trasylol®
Canadian Brand Names Trasylol®
Mexican Brand Names Trasylol®
Generic Available No
Pharmacologic Category Blood Product Derivative; Hemostatic Agent

Use Reduction or prevention of blood loss in patients undergoing coronary artery bypass surgery when a high risk of excessive bleeding exists, including open heart reoperation, pre-existing coagulopathies, operations on the great vessels, and when a patient's beliefs prohibit blood transfusions

Local Anesthetic/Vasoconstrictor Precautions No information available to require special precautions

Effects on Dental Treatment No significant effects or complications reported

(Continued)

Aprotinin *(Continued)*

Common Adverse Effects 1% to 10%: Atrial fibrillation, atrial flutter, bronchoconstriction, dyspnea, fever, heart failure, hypotension, increased potential for postoperative renal dysfunction, mental confusion, myocardial infarction, phlebitis, supraventricular tachycardia, ventricular tachycardia

Mechanism of Action Serine protease inhibitor; inhibits plasmin, kallikrein, and platelet activation producing antifibrinolytic effects; a weak inhibitor of plasma pseudocholinesterase. It also inhibits the contact phase activation of coagulation and preserves adhesive platelet glycoproteins making them resistant to damage from increased circulating plasmin or mechanical injury occurring during bypass

Drug Interactions

Increased Effect/Toxicity: Heparin and aprotinin prolong ACT; the ACT becomes a poor measure of adequate anticoagulation with the concurrent use of these drugs. Use with succinylcholine or tubocurarine may produce prolonged or recurring apnea.

Decreased Effect: Aprotinin blocks the fibrinolytic activity of thrombolytic agents (alteplase, streptokinase). The antihypertensive effects of captopril (and other ACE inhibitors) may be blocked; avoid concurrent use.

Pharmacodynamics/Kinetics

Half-life elimination: 2.5 hours

Excretion: Urine

Pregnancy Risk Factor B

Aquacare® [OTC] *see* Urea *on page 1353*
Aquachloral® Supprettes® *see* Chloral Hydrate *on page 304*
Aqua Gem E® [OTC] *see* Vitamin E *on page 1383*
AquaLase™ *see* Balanced Salt Solution *on page 181*
Aqua Lube Plus [OTC] *see* Nonoxynol 9 *on page 995*
AquaMEPHYTON® [DSC] *see* Phytonadione *on page 1084*
Aquanil™ HC [OTC] *see* Hydrocortisone *on page 714*
Aquaphilic® With Carbamide [OTC] *see* Urea *on page 1353*
AquaSite® [OTC] *see* Artificial Tears *on page 148*
Aquasol A® *see* Vitamin A *on page 1382*
Aquasol E® [OTC] *see* Vitamin E *on page 1383*
Aquatab® *see* Guaifenesin and Pseudoephedrine *on page 675*
Aquatab® C *see* Guaifenesin, Pseudoephedrine, and Dextromethorphan *on page 676*
Aquatab® D Dose Pack *see* Guaifenesin and Pseudoephedrine *on page 675*
Aquatab® DM *see* Guaifenesin and Dextromethorphan *on page 673*
Aquatensen® *see* Methyclothiazide *on page 905*
Aquazide® H *see* Hydrochlorothiazide *on page 699*
Aqueous Procaine Penicillin G *see* Penicillin G Procaine *on page 1060*
Ara-A *see* Vidarabine *on page 1376*
Arabinofuranosyladenine *see* Vidarabine *on page 1376*
Arabinosylcytosine *see* Cytarabine *on page 390*
Ara-C *see* Cytarabine *on page 390*
Aralast™ *see* Alpha$_1$-Proteinase Inhibitor *on page 84*
Aralen® *see* Chloroquine *on page 311*
Aranesp® *see* Darbepoetin Alfa *on page 399*
Arava® *see* Leflunomide *on page 801*
Aredia® *see* Pamidronate *on page 1041*
Arestin™ *see* Minocycline Hydrochloride (Periodontal) *on page 933*

Argatroban (ar GA troh ban)

Related Information

Cardiovascular Diseases *on page 1458*

Generic Available No

Pharmacologic Category Anticoagulant, Thrombin Inhibitor

Use Prophylaxis or treatment of thrombosis in adults with heparin-induced thrombocytopenia; adjunct to percutaneous coronary intervention (PCI) in patients who have or are at risk of thrombosis associated with heparin-induced thrombocytopenia

Local Anesthetic/Vasoconstrictor Precautions No information available to require special precautions

Effects on Dental Treatment Key adverse event(s) related to dental treatment: As with all anticoagulants, bleeding is a potential adverse effect of argatroban during dental surgery; risk is dependent on multiple variables, including the intensity of anticoagulation and patient susceptibility. Medical consult is suggested. It is unlikely that ambulatory patients presenting for dental treatment will be taking intravenous anticoagulant therapy.

Common Adverse Effects As with all anticoagulants, bleeding is the major adverse effect of argatroban. Hemorrhage may occur at virtually any site. Risk is dependent on multiple variables, including the intensity of anticoagulation and patient susceptibility.

>10%:

Gastrointestinal: Gastrointestinal bleed (minor, 14%; <1% in PCI)

Genitourinary: Genitourinary bleed and hematuria (minor, 12%)

1% to 10%:

Cardiovascular: Hypotension (7%), cardiac arrest (6%), ventricular tachycardia (5%), atrial fibrillation (3%), cerebrovascular disorder (2%)

Central nervous system: Fever (7%), pain (5%), intracranial bleeding (1%, only observed in patients also receiving streptokinase or tissue plasminogen activator)

Gastrointestinal: Diarrhea (6%), nausea (5%), vomiting (4%), abdominal pain (3%), bleeding (major, 2%)

Genitourinary: Urinary tract infection (5%)

Hematologic: Decreased hemoglobin <2 g/dL and hematocrit (minor, 10%)

Local: Bleeding at the injection site (minor, 2% to 5%)

Renal: Abnormal renal function (3%)

Respiratory: Dyspnea (8% to 10%), coughing (3% to 10%), hemoptysis (minor, 3%), pneumonia (3%)

Miscellaneous: Sepsis (6%), infection (4%)

Mechanism of Action A direct, highly selective thrombin inhibitor. Reversibly binds to the active thrombin site of free and clot-associated thrombin. Inhibits fibrin formation; activation of coagulation factors V, VIII, and XIII; protein C; and platelet aggregation.

Drug Interactions

Cytochrome P450 Effect: Substrate of CYP3A4 (minor)

Increased Effect/Toxicity: Drugs which affect platelet function (eg, aspirin, NSAIDs, dipyridamole, ticlopidine, clopidogrel), anticoagulants, or thrombolytics may potentiate the risk of hemorrhage. Sufficient time must pass after heparin therapy is discontinued; allow heparin's effect on the aPTT to decrease

Concomitant use of argatroban with warfarin increases PT and INR greater than that of warfarin alone. Argatroban is commonly continued during the initiation of warfarin therapy to assure anticoagulation and to protect against possible transient hypercoagulability.

Pharmacodynamics/Kinetics

Onset of action: Immediate

Distribution: 174 mL/kg

Protein binding: Albumin: 20%; α_1-acid glycoprotein: 35%

Metabolism: Hepatic via hydroxylation and aromatization. Metabolism via CYP3A4/5 to four known metabolites plays a minor role. Unchanged argatroban is the major plasma component. Plasma concentration of metabolite M1 is 0% to 20% of the parent drug and is three- to fivefold weaker.

Half-life elimination: 39-51 minutes; Hepatic impairment: ≤181 minutes

Time to peak: Steady-state: 1-3 hours

Excretion: Feces (65%); urine (22%); low quantities of metabolites M2-4 in urine

Pregnancy Risk Factor B

Arginine (AR ji neen)

U.S. Brand Names R-Gene®

Generic Available No

Synonyms Arginine Hydrochloride

Pharmacologic Category Diagnostic Agent

Use Pituitary function test (growth hormone)

Unlabeled/Investigational Use Management of severe, uncompensated, metabolic alkalosis (pH ≥7.55) **after** optimizing therapy with sodium and potassium supplements

Local Anesthetic/Vasoconstrictor Precautions No information available to require special precautions

Effects on Dental Treatment No significant effects or complications reported

Mechanism of Action

Stimulates pituitary release of growth hormone and prolactin through origins in the hypothalamus; patients with impaired pituitary function have lower or no increase in plasma concentrations of growth hormone after administration of

(Continued)

Arginine *(Continued)*

arginine. Arginine hydrochloride has been used for severe metabolic alkalosis due to its high chloride content.

Arginine hydrochloride has been used investigationally to treat metabolic alkalosis. Arginine contains 475 mEq of hydrogen ions and 475 mEq of chloride ions/L. Arginine is metabolized by the liver to produce hydrogen ions. It may be used in patients with relative hepatic insufficiency because arginine combines with ammonia in the body to produce urea.

Pregnancy Risk Factor B

Arginine Hydrochloride *see* Arginine *on page 141*

8-Arginine Vasopressin *see* Vasopressin *on page 1369*

Aricept® *see* Donepezil *on page 462*

Arimidex® *see* Anastrozole *on page 132*

Aripiprazole (ay ri PIP ray zole)

U.S. Brand Names Abilify™

Mexican Brand Names Abilify™

Generic Available No

Synonyms BMS 337039; OPC-14597

Pharmacologic Category Antipsychotic Agent, Quinolinone

Use Treatment of schizophrenia

Unlabeled/Investigational Use Psychosis, bipolar disorder

Local Anesthetic/Vasoconstrictor Precautions No information available to require special precautions

Effects on Dental Treatment Key adverse event(s) related to dental treatment: Extrapyramidal symptoms (similar to placebo).

Common Adverse Effects

>10%:

Central nervous system: Headache (32%), anxiety (25%), insomnia (24%), lightheadedness (11%), somnolence (11%)

Endocrine & metabolic: Weight gain (8% to 30%; highest frequency in patients with BMI <23)

Gastrointestinal: Nausea (14%), vomiting (12%)

1% to 10%:

Cardiovascular: Edema (peripheral, 1%), chest pain (1%), hypertension (1%), tachycardia (1%), hypotension (1%), bradycardia (1%)

Central nervous system: Akathisia (10%), extrapyramidal symptoms (6%; similar to placebo), fever (2%), depression (1%), nervousness (1%), mania (1%), confusion (1%)

Dermatologic: Rash (6%), ecchymosis (1%), pruritus (1%)

Endocrine & metabolic: Hypothyroidism (1%), weight loss (1%)

Gastrointestinal: Constipation (10%), anorexia (1%)

Genitourinary: Urinary incontinence (1%)

Hematologic: Anemia (1%)

Neuromuscular & skeletal: Weakness (7%), tremor (3%), neck pain (1%), neck rigidity (1%), muscle cramp (1%), cogwheel rigidity (1%), CPK increased (1%)

Ocular: Blurred vision (3%), conjunctivitis (1%)

Respiratory: Rhinitis (4%), cough (3%), dyspnea (1%), pneumonia (1%)

Miscellaneous: Flu-like syndrome (1%)

Mechanism of Action Aripiprazole exhibits high affinity for D_2, D_3, 5-HT_{1A}, and 5-HT_{2A} receptors; moderate affinity for D_4, 5-HT_{2C}, 5-HT_7, alpha, and H_1 receptors. It also possesses moderate affinity for the serotonin reuptake transporter; has no affinity for muscarinic receptors. Aripiprazole functions as a partial agonist at the D_2 and 5-HT_{1A} receptors, and as an antagonist at the 5-HT_{2A} receptor.

Drug Interactions

Cytochrome P450 Effect: Substrate (major) of CYP2D6, 3A4

Increased Effect/Toxicity: CYP2D6 inhibitors may increase the levels/effects of aripiprazole; example inhibitors include chlorpromazine, delavirdine, fluoxetine, miconazole, paroxetine, pergolide, quinidine, quinine, ritonavir, and ropinirole. CYP3A4 inhibitors may increase the levels/effects of aripiprazole; example inhibitors include azole antifungals, ciprofloxacin, clarithromycin, diclofenac, doxycycline, erythromycin, imatinib, isoniazid, nefazodone, nicardipine, propofol, protease inhibitors, quinidine, and verapamil. Manufacturer recommends a 50% reduction in dose during concurrent ketoconazole therapy. Similar reductions in dose may be required with other potent inhibitors.

Decreased Effect: CYP3A4 inducers may decrease the levels/effects of aripiprazole; example inducers include aminoglutethimide, carbamazepine, nafcillin, nevirapine, phenobarbital, phenytoin, and rifamycins. Manufacturer recommends a doubling of the aripiprazole dose when carbamazepine is added. Similar increases may be required with other inducers.

Pharmacodynamics/Kinetics

Onset: Initial: 1-3 weeks

Absorption: Well absorbed

Distribution: V_d: 4.9 L/kg

Protein binding: 99%, primarily to albumin

Metabolism: Hepatic, via CYP2D6, CYP3A4 (dehydro-aripiprazole metabolite has affinity for D2 receptors similar to the parent drug and represents 40% of the parent drug exposure in plasma)

Bioavailability: 87%

Half-life: Aripiprazole: 75 hours; dehydro-aripiprazole: 94 hours

Time to peak, plasma: 3-5 hours; delayed 3 hours with high-fat meal

Excretion: Feces (55%), urine (25%); primarily as metabolites

Pregnancy Risk Factor C

Comments Aripiprazole works differently from the classic antipsychotics, such as chlorpromazine, in that it does not appear to block central dopaminergic receptors, but rather seems to be a stabilizer of dopamine-serotonin central systems. The risk of extrapyramidal reactions such as pseudoparkinsonism, acute dystonic reactions, akathisia and tardive dyskinesia are low and the frequencies reported are similar to placebo. Aripiprazole may be associated with neuroleptic malignant syndrme (NMS).

Aristocort® *see* Triamcinolone *on page 1330*

Aristocort® A *see* Triamcinolone *on page 1330*

Aristocort® Forte *see* Triamcinolone *on page 1330*

Aristospan® *see* Triamcinolone *on page 1330*

Arixtra® *see* Fondaparinux *on page 628*

Arlidin® *see* Nylidrin *on page 1002*

A.R.M® [OTC] *see* Chlorpheniramine and Pseudoephedrine *on page 315*

Armour® Thyroid *see* Thyroid *on page 1293*

Aromasin® *see* Exemestane *on page 569*

Artane *see* Trihexyphenidyl *on page 1340*

ArthriCare® for Women Extra Moisturizing [OTC] *see* Capsaicin *on page 252*

ArthriCare® for Women Silky Dry [OTC] *see* Capsaicin *on page 252*

Arthropan® [OTC] [DSC] *see* Choline Salicylate *on page 325*

Arthrotec® *see* Diclofenac and Misoprostol *on page 430*

Articaine Hydrochloride and Epinephrine [Dental] *see* Articaine Hydrochloride and Epinephrine (Canada) *on page 143*

Articaine Hydrochloride and Epinephrine [Dental] *see* Articaine Hydrochloride and Epinephrine (U.S.) *on page 145*

Articaine Hydrochloride and Epinephrine (Canada)

(AR ti kane hye droe KLOR ide & ep i NEF rin)

Related Information

Articaine Hydrochloride and Epinephrine (U.S.) *on page 145*

Epinephrine *on page 496*

Oral Pain *on page 1526*

Canadian Brand Names Astracaine®; Astracaine® Forte; Septanest® N; Septanest® SP; Ultracaine® D-S; Ultracaine® D-S Forte

Synonyms Articaine Hydrochloride and Epinephrine [Dental]

Pharmacologic Category Local Anesthetic

Use Anesthesia for infiltration and nerve block anesthesia in clinical dentistry

Local Anesthetic/Vasoconstrictor Precautions No information available to require special precautions

Effects on Dental Treatment No significant effects or complications reported

Significant Adverse Effects Frequency not defined.

Cardiovascular: Myocardial depression, arrhythmias, tachycardia, bradycardia, blood pressure changes, edema

Central nervous system: Excitation, depression, nervousness, dizziness, headache, somnolence, unconsciousness, convulsions, chills

Dermatologic: Allergic reactions include cutaneous lesions, urticaria, itching, reddening of skin

Gastrointestinal: Vomiting, allergic reactions include nausea and diarrhea

Local: Reactions at the site of injection, swelling, burning, ischemia, tissue necrosis

(Continued)

Articaine Hydrochloride and Epinephrine (Canada) *(Continued)*

Neuromuscular & skeletal: Tremors

Ocular: Visual disturbances, blurred vision, blindness, diplopia, pupillary constriction

Otic: Tinnitus

Respiratory: Allergic reactions include wheezing, acute asthmatic attacks

Dosage Adults:

Ultracaine DS® Forte:

- Infiltration:
  - Volume: 0.5-2.5 mL
  - Total dose: 20-100 mg
- Nerve block:
  - Volume: 0.5-3.4 mL
  - Total dose: 20-136 mg
- Oral surgery:
  - Volume: 1-5.1 mL
  - Total dose: 40-204 mg

Ultracaine DS®:

- Infiltration:
  - Volume: 0.5-2.5 mL
  - Total dose: 20-100 mg
- Nerve block:
  - Volume: 0.5-3.4 mL
  - Total dose: 20-136 mg
- Oral surgery:
  - Volume: 1-5.1 mL
  - Total dose: 40-204 mg

Maximum dose: 7 mg/kg

To date, Ultracaine® has not been administered to children <4 years of age, nor in doses >5 mg/kg in children between the ages of 4 and 12

Mechanism of Action Blocks nerve conduction by interfering with the permeability of the nerve axonal membrane to sodium ions; this results in the loss of the generation of the nerve axon potential

Contraindications Hypersensitivity to any components of the formulation and/or local anesthetics of the amide group; in the presence of inflammation and/or sepsis near the injection site; in patients with severe shock, any degree of heart block, paroxysmal tachycardia, known arrhythmia with rapid heart rate, narrow-angle glaucoma, cholinesterase deficiency, existing neurologic disease, severe hypertension; when articaine with epinephrine is used, the caution required of any vasopressor drug should be followed

Warnings/Precautions Articaine should be used cautiously in persons with known drug allergies or sensitivities, or suspected sensitivity to the amide-type local anesthetics. Avoid excessive premedications with sedatives, tranquilizers, and antiemetic agents. Inject slowly with frequent aspirations and if blood is aspirated, relocate needle. Articaine should be used with extreme caution in patients having a history of thyrotoxicosis or diabetes. Due to the sulfite component of the articaine preparation, hypersensitivity reactions may occur occasionally in patients with bronchial asthma.

Drug Interactions

MAO inhibitors: Administration of local anesthetic solutions containing epinephrine may produce severe, prolonged hypertension

Tricyclic antidepressants: Pressor response to I.V. epinephrine, norepinephrine, and phenylephrine may be enhanced in patients receiving TCAs (**Note:** Effect is unlikely with epinephrine or levonordefrin dosages typically administered as infiltration in combination with local anesthetics)

Dosage Forms Injection:

Ultracaine DS®: Articaine hydrochloride with epinephrine [1:200,000] and sodium metabisulfite [0.5 mg/mL] and an antioxidant and water for injection (1.7 mL) [50s]

Ultracaine DS Forte®: Articaine hydrochloride 4% with epinephrine [1:100,000] and sodium metabisulfite [0.5 mg/mL] and an antioxidant and water for injection (1.7 mL) [50s]

Selected Readings

Budenz AW, "Local Anesthetics in Dentistry: Then and Now," *J Calif Dent Assoc*, 2003, 31(5):388-96.

Dower JS Jr, "A Review of Paresthesia in Association With Administration of Local Anesthesia," *Dent Today*, 2003, 22(2):64-9.

Finder RL and Moore PA, "Adverse Drug Reactions to Local Anesthesia," *Dent Clin North Am*, 2002, 46(4):747-57, x.

Haas DA, "An Update on Local Anesthetics in Dentistry," *J Can Dent Assoc*, 2002, 68(9):546-51.

Hawkins JM and Moore PA, "Local Anesthesia: Advances in Agents and Techniques," *Dent Clin North Am*, 2002, 46(4):719-32, ix.

"Injectable Local Anesthetics," *J Am Dent Assoc*, 2003, 134(5):628-9.

Malamed SF, "Allergy and Toxic Reactions to Local Anesthetics," *Dent Today*, 2003, 22(4):114-6, 118-21.

Weaver JM, "Articaine, A New Local Anesthetic for American Dentists: Will It Supersede Lidocaine?" *Anesth Prog*, 1999, 46(4):111-2.

Wynn RL, Bergman SA, and Meiller TF, "Paresthesia Associated With Local Anesthetics: A Perspective on Articaine," *Gen Dent*, 2003, 51(6):498-501.

Articaine Hydrochloride and Epinephrine (U.S.)

(AR ti kane hye droe KLOR ide & ep i NEF rin)

Related Information

Articaine Hydrochloride and Epinephrine (Canada) *on page 143*

Epinephrine *on page 496*

Oral Pain *on page 1526*

U.S. Brand Names Septocaine™

Generic Available No

Synonyms Articaine Hydrochloride and Epinephrine [Dental]

Pharmacologic Category Local Anesthetic

Dental Use Anesthesia agent for infiltration and nerve block anesthesia in clinical dentistry; Septocaine™ is indicated for local, infiltrative, or conductive anesthesia in both simple and complex dental and periodontal procedures

Local Anesthetic/Vasoconstrictor Precautions No information available to require special precautions

Effects on Dental Treatment No significant effects or complications reported

Significant Adverse Effects Adverse reactions to Septocaine™ are characteristic of those associated with other amide-type local anesthetics; adverse reactions to this group of drugs may also result from excessive plasma levels which may be due to overdosage, unintentional intravascular injection, or slow metabolic degradation.

≥1% (in controlled trial of 882 patients):

- Central nervous system: Headache (4%), paresthesia (1%)
- Gastrointestinal: Gingivitis (1%)
- Miscellaneous: Pain (body as a whole 13%), facial edema (1%)

<1% (adverse and intercurrent events recorded in 1 or more patients in controlled trials, occurring at an overall rate of <1%, and considered clinically significant): Abdominal pain, accidental injury, arthralgia, asthenia, back pain, constipation, diarrhea, dizziness, dry mouth, dysmenorrhea, dyspepsia, ear pain, ecchymosis, edema, facial paralysis, glossitis, gum hemorrhage, hemorrhage, hyperesthesia, increased salivation, injection site pain, lymphadenopathy, malaise, migraine, mouth ulceration, myalgia, nausea, neck pain, nervousness, neuropathy, osteomyelitis, paresthesia, pharyngitis, pruritus, rhinitis, skin disorder, somnolence, stomatitis, syncope, tachycardia, taste perversion, thirst, tongue edema, tooth disorder, vomiting

Dosage Summary of recommended volumes and concentrations for various types of anesthetic procedures; dosages (administered by submucosal injection and/or nerve block) apply to normal healthy adults:

Infiltration: Injection volume of 4% solution: 0.5-2.5 mL; total dose of Septocaine™: 20-100 mg

Nerve block: Injection volume of 4% solution: 0.5-3.4 mL; total dose of Septocaine™: 20-136 mg

Oral surgery: Injection volume of 4% solution: 1-5.1 mL; total dose of Septocaine™: 40-204 mg

Note: These dosages are guides only; other dosages may be used; however, do not exceed maximum recommended dose

The clinician is reminded that these doses serve only as a guide to the amount of anesthetic required for most routine procedures. The actual volumes to be used depend upon a number of factors, such as type and extent of surgical procedure, depth of anesthesia, degree of muscular relaxation, and condition of the patient. In all cases, the smallest dose that will produce the desired result should be given. Dosages should be reduced for pediatric patients, elderly patients, and patients with cardiac and/or liver disease.

Children <4 years: Safety and efficacy have not been established

Children 4-16 years (dosages in a clinical trial of 61 patients):

- Simple procedures: 0.76-5.65 mg/kg (0.9-5.1 mL) was administered safely to 51 patients
- Complex procedures: 0.37-7.48 mg/kg (0.7-3.9 mL) was administered safely to 10 patients
- **Note:** Approximately 13% of the pediatric patients required additional injections for complete anesthesia

(Continued)

Articaine Hydrochloride and Epinephrine (U.S.) *(Continued)*

Geriatric patients (dosages in a clinical trial):

65-75 years:

Simple procedures: 0.43-4.76 mg/kg (0.9-11.9 mL) was administered safely to 35 patients

Complex procedures: 1.05-4.27 mg/kg (1.3-6.8 mL) was administered safely to 19 patients

≥75 years:

Simple procedures: 0.78-4.76 mg/kg (1.3-11.9 mL) was administered safely to 7 patients

Complex procedures: 1.12-2.17 mg/kg (1.3-5.1 mL) was administered safely to 4 patients

Note: Approximately 6% of the patients 65-75 years of age (none of the patients ≥75 years of age) required additional injections for complete anesthesia, compared to 11% of the patients 17-65 years of age who required additional injections.

Maximum recommended dosages:

Children (use in pediatric patients <4 years is not recommended): Not to exceed 7 mg/kg (0.175 mL/kg) **or** 3.2 mg/lb (0.0795 mL/lb) of body weight

Adults (normal, healthy): Submucosal infiltration and/or nerve block: Not to exceed 7 mg/kg (0.175 mL/kg) **or** 3.2 mg/lb (0.0795 mL/lb) of body weight

The following numbers of dental cartridges (1.7 mL) provide the indicated amounts of articaine hydrochloride 4% and epinephrine 1:100,000:

1 cartridge provides 68 mg articaine HCl (4%) and 0.017 mg vasoconstrictor (epinephrine 1:100,000)

2 cartridges provides 136 mg articaine HCl (4%) and 0.034 mg vasoconstrictor (epinephrine 1:100,000)

3 cartridges provides 204 mg articaine HCl (4%) and 0.051 mg vasoconstrictor (epinephrine 1:100,000)

4 cartridges provides 272 mg articaine HCl (4%) and 0.068 mg vasoconstrictor (epinephrine 1:100,000)

5 cartridges provides 340 mg articaine HCl (4%) and 0.085 mg vasoconstrictor (epinephrine 1:100,000)

6 cartridges provides 408 mg articaine HCl (4%) and 0.102 mg vasoconstrictor (epinephrine 1:100,000)

7 cartridges provides 476 mg articaine HCl (4%) and 0.119 mg vasoconstrictor (epinephrine 1:100,000)

8 cartridges provides 544 mg articaine HCl (4%) and 0.136 mg vasoconstrictor (epinephrine 1:100,000)

Mechanism of Action Local anesthetics block the generation and conduction of nerve impulses, presumably by increasing the threshold for electrical excitation in the nerve, by slowing the propagation of the nerve impulse, and by reducing the rate of rise of the action potential. In general, the progression of anesthesia is related to the diameter, myelination, and conduction velocity of the affected nerve fibers. Clinically, the order of loss of nerve function is as follows: 1) pain, 2) temperature, 3) touch, 4) proprioception, and 5) skeletal muscle tone.

Contraindications Hypersensitivity to local anesthetics of the amide type or to sodium metabisulfite

Warnings/Precautions Intravascular injections should be avoided; aspiration should be performed prior to administration of Septocaine™; the needle must be repositioned until no return of blood can be elicited by aspiration; however, absence of blood in the syringe does not guarantee that intravascular injection has been avoided. **Accidental intravascular injection may be associated with convulsions, followed by CNS or cardiorespiratory depression and coma, ultimately progressing to respiratory arrest.** Dental practitioners and/or clinicians using local anesthetic agents should be well trained in diagnosis and management of emergencies that may arise from the use of these agents. Resuscitative equipment, oxygen, and other resuscitative drugs should be available for immediate use.

Because Septocaine™ contains epinephrine, which can cause local tissue necrosis or systemic toxicity, usual precautions for epinephrine administration should be observed. Administration of articaine HCl with epinephrine results in a three- to fivefold increase in plasma epinephrine concentrations compared to baseline; however, in healthy adults, it does not appear to be associated with marked increases in blood pressure or heart rate, except in the case of accidental intravascular injection.

Also contains sodium metabisulfite, which may cause allergic-type reactions (including anaphylactic symptoms, and life-threatening or less severe asthmatic episodes) in certain susceptible patients. The overall prevalence of the sulfite sensitivity in the general population is unknown, and is seen more frequently in asthmatic than in nonasthmatic persons.

To avoid serious adverse effects and high plasma levels, the lowest dosage resulting in effective anesthesia should be administered. Repeated doses may cause significant increases in blood levels with each repeated dose due to the possibility of accumulation of the drug or its metabolites. Tolerance to elevated blood levels varies with patient status. Reduced dosages, commensurate with age and physical condition, should be given to debilitated patients, elderly patients, acutely-ill patients, and pediatric patients. Septocaine™ should also be used with caution in patients with heart block.

Local anesthetic solutions containing a vasoconstrictor (such as Septocaine™) should be used cautiously. Patients with peripheral vascular disease or hypertensive vascular disease may exhibit exaggerated vasoconstrictor response, possibly resulting in ischemic injury or necrosis. It should also be used cautiously in patients during or following the administration of a potent general anesthetic agent, since cardiac arrhythmias may occur under these conditions.

Systemic absorption of local anesthetics may produce CNS and cardiovascular effects. Changes in cardiac conduction, excitability, refractoriness, contractility, and peripheral vascular resistance are minimal at blood concentrations produced by therapeutic doses. However, toxic blood concentrations depress cardiac conduction and excitability, which may lead to AV block, ventricular arrhythmias, and cardiac arrest (sometimes resulting in death). In addition, myocardial contractility is depressed and peripheral vasodilation occurs, leading to decreased cardiac output and arterial blood pressure.

Careful and constant monitoring of cardiovascular and respiratory (adequacy of ventilation) vital signs and the patient's state of consciousness should be done following each local anesthetic injection; at such times, restlessness, anxiety, tinnitus, dizziness, blurred vision, tremors, depression, or drowsiness may be early warning signs of CNS toxicity.

In vitro studies show that ~5% to 10% of articaine is metabolized by the human liver microsomal P450 isoenzyme system; however, no studies have been performed in patient with liver dysfunction, and caution should be used in patients with severe hepatic disease. Use with caution in patients with impaired cardiovascular function, since they may be less able to compensate for function changes associated with prolonged AV conduction produced by these drugs.

Small doses of local anesthetics injected into dental blocks may produce adverse reactions similar to systemic toxicity seen in unintentional intravascular injections at larger doses. Confusion, convulsions, respiratory depression and/or respiratory arrest, and cardiovascular stimulation or depression have been reported. These reactions may be due to intra-arterial injection of the local anesthetic with retrograde flow to the cerebral circulation. Patients receiving such blocks should be observed constantly with resuscitative equipment and personnel trained in treatment of adverse reactions immediately available. Dosage recommendations should not be exceeded.

Drug Interactions

MAO inhibitors: Administration of local anesthetic solutions containing epinephrine may produce severe, prolonged hypertension

Phenothiazines, butyrophenones: May reduce or reverse the pressor effects of epinephrine; concurrent use of these agents should be avoided; in situations when concurrent therapy is necessary, careful patient monitoring is essential

Tricyclic antidepressants: Pressor response to I.V. epinephrine, norepinephrine, and phenylephrine may be enhanced in patients receiving TCAs (**Note:** Effect is unlikely with epinephrine or levonordefrin dosages typically administered as infiltration in combination with local anesthetics)

Pharmacodynamics/Kinetics

Onset of action: 1-6 minutes

Duration: Complete anesthesia: ~1 hour

Metabolism: Hepatic via plasma carboxyesterase to articainic acid (inactive)

Half-life elimination: Articaine: 1.8 hours; Articainic acid: 1.5 hours

Excretion: Urine (primarily as metabolites)

Pregnancy Risk Factor C

Breast-Feeding Considerations It is not known whether articaine is excreted in human milk. Because many drugs are excreted in human milk, caution should be exercised when Septocaine™ is administered to a nursing woman.

(Continued)

Articaine Hydrochloride and Epinephrine (U.S.) *(Continued)*

Dosage Forms Injection, solution (Septocaine™): Articaine hydrochloride 4% and epinephrine bitartrate 1:100,000 (1.7 mL) [contains sodium metabisulfite]

Comments Septocaine™ (articaine hydrochloride 4% and epinephrine 1:100,000) is the first FDA approval in 30 years of a new local dental anesthetic providing complete pulpal anesthesia for approximately 1 hour. Chemically, articaine contains both an amide linkage and an ester linkage, making it chemically unique in the class of local anesthetics. Since it contains the ester linkage, articaine HCl is rapidly metabolized by plasma carboxyesterase to its primary metabolite, articainic acid, which is an inactive product of this metabolism. According to the manufacturer, *in vitro* studies show that the human liver microsomal P450 isoenzyme system metabolizes approximately 5% to 10% of available articaine with nearly quantitative conversion to articainic acid. The elimination half-life of articaine is about 1.8 hours, and that of articainic acid is about 1.5 hours. Articaine is excreted primarily through urine with 53% to 57% of the administered dose eliminated in the first 24 hours following submucosal administration. Articainic acid is the primary metabolite in urine. A minor metabolite, articainic acid glucuronide, is also excreted in the urine. Articaine constitutes only 2% of the total dose excreted in urine.

Selected Readings

Budenz AW, "Local Anesthetics in Dentistry: Then and Now," *J Calif Dent Assoc*, 2003, 31(5):388-96.

Dower JS Jr, "A Review of Paresthesia in Association With Administration of Local Anesthesia," *Dent Today*, 2003, 22(2):64-9.

Finder RL and Moore PA, "Adverse Drug Reactions to Local Anesthesia," *Dent Clin North Am*, 2002, 46(4):747-57, x.

Haas DA, "An Update on Local Anesthetics in Dentistry," *J Can Dent Assoc*, 2002, 68(9):546-51.

Hawkins JM and Moore PA, "Local Anesthesia: Advances in Agents and Techniques," *Dent Clin North Am*, 2002, 46(4):719-32, ix.

"Injectable Local Anesthetics," *J Am Dent Assoc*, 2003, 134(5):628-9.

Malamed SF, Gagnon S, Leblanc D, "A Comparison Between Articaine HCl and Lidocaine HCl in Pediatric Dental Patients," *Pediatr Dent*, 2000, 22(4):307-11.

Malamed SF, "Allergy and Toxic Reactions to Local Anesthetics," *Dent Today*, 2003, 22(4):114-6, 118-21.

Malamed SF, Gagnon S, Leblanc D, "Articaine Hydrochloride: A Study of the Safety of a New Amide Local Anesthetic," *J Am Dent Assoc*, 2001, 132(2):177-85.

Malamed SF, Gagnon S, Leblanc D, "Efficacy of Articaine: A New Amide Local Anesthetic," *J Am Dent Assoc*, 2000, 131(5):635-42.

Schertzer ER Jr, "Articaine vs lidocaine," *J Am Dent Assoc*, 2000, 131(9):1248, 1250.

Weaver JM, "Articaine, A New Local Anesthetic for American Dentists: Will It Supersede Lidocaine?" *Anesth Prog*, 1999, 46(4):111-2.

Wynn RL, Bergman SA, and Meiller TF, "Paresthesia Associated With Local Anesthetics: A Perspective on Articaine," *Gen Dent*, 2003, 51(6):498-501.

Artificial Tears (ar ti FISH il tears)

U.S. Brand Names Akwa Tears® [OTC]; AquaSite® [OTC]; Bion® Tears [OTC]; HypoTears [OTC]; HypoTears PF [OTC]; Isopto® Tears [OTC]; Liquifilm® Tears [OTC]; Moisture® Eyes [OTC]; Moisture® Eyes PM [OTC]; Murine® Tears [OTC]; Murocel® [OTC]; Nature's Tears® [OTC]; Nu-Tears® [OTC]; Nu-Tears® II [OTC]; OcuCoat® [OTC]; OcuCoat® PF [OTC]; Puralube® Tears [OTC]; Refresh® [OTC]; Refresh® Plus [OTC]; Refresh® Tears [OTC]; Teargen® [OTC]; Teargen® II [OTC]; Tearisol® [OTC]; Tears Again® [OTC]; Tears Naturale® [OTC]; Tears Naturale® Free [OTC]; Tears Naturale® II [OTC]; Tears Plus® [OTC]; Tears Renewed® [OTC]; Ultra Tears® [OTC]; Viva-Drops® [OTC]

Canadian Brand Names Teardrops®

Generic Available Yes

Synonyms Hydroxyethylcellulose; Polyvinyl Alcohol

Pharmacologic Category Ophthalmic Agent, Miscellaneous

Use Ophthalmic lubricant; for relief of dry eyes and eye irritation

Local Anesthetic/Vasoconstrictor Precautions No information available to require special precautions

Effects on Dental Treatment No significant effects or complications reported

Pregnancy Risk Factor C

ASA *see* Aspirin *on page 151*

5-ASA *see* Mesalamine *on page 882*

Asacol® *see* Mesalamine *on page 882*

Ascorbic Acid (a SKOR bik AS id)

U.S. Brand Names C-500-GR™ [OTC]; Cecon® [OTC]; Cevi-Bid® [OTC]; C-Gram [OTC]; Dull-C® [OTC]; Vita-C® [OTC]

Canadian Brand Names Proflavanol C™; Revitalose C-1000®

Mexican Brand Names Cevalin®; Redoxon®

Generic Available Yes

Synonyms Vitamin C

Pharmacologic Category Vitamin, Water Soluble

Use Prevention and treatment of scurvy and to acidify the urine

Unlabeled/Investigational Use Investigational: In large doses to decrease the severity of "colds"; dietary supplementation; a 20-year study was recently completed involving 730 individuals which indicates a possible decreased risk of death by stroke when ascorbic acid at doses ≥45 mg/day was administered

Local Anesthetic/Vasoconstrictor Precautions No information available to require special precautions

Effects on Dental Treatment No significant effects or complications reported

Significant Adverse Effects

1% to 10%: Renal: Hyperoxaluria (incidence dose-related)

<1% (Limited to important or life-threatening): Dizziness, faintness, fatigue, flank pain, headache

Dosage Oral, I.M., I.V., SubQ:

Recommended daily allowance (RDA):
- <6 months: 30 mg
- 6 months to 1 year: 35 mg
- 1-3 years: 15 mg; upper limit of intake should not exceed 400 mg/day
- 4-8 years: 25 mg; upper limit of intake should not exceed 650 mg/day
- 9-13 years: 45 mg; upper limit of intake should not exceed 1200 mg/day
- 14-18 years: Upper limit of intake should not exceed 1800 mg/day
  - Male: 75 mg
  - Female: 65 mg
- Adults: Upper limit of intake should not exceed 2000 mg/day
  - Male: 90 mg
  - Female: 75 mg;
- Pregnant female:
  - ≤18 years: 80 mg; upper limit of intake should not exceed 1800 mg/day
  - 19-50 years: 85 mg; upper limit of intake should not exceed 2000 mg/day
- Lactating female:
  - ≤18 years: 15 mg; upper limit of intake should not exceed 1800 mg/day
  - 19-50 years: 20 mg; upper limit of intake should not exceed 2000 mg/day
- Adult smoker: Add an additional 35 mg/day

Children:
- Scurvy: 100-300 mg/day in divided doses for at least 2 weeks
- Urinary acidification: 500 mg every 6-8 hours
- Dietary supplement: 35-100 mg/day

Adults:
- Scurvy: 100-250 mg 1-2 times/day for at least 2 weeks
- Urinary acidification: 4-12 g/day in 3-4 divided doses
- Prevention and treatment of colds: 1-3 g/day
- Dietary supplement: 50-200 mg/day

Mechanism of Action Not fully understood; necessary for collagen formation and tissue repair; involved in some oxidation-reduction reactions as well as other metabolic pathways, such as synthesis of carnitine, steroids, and catecholamines and conversion of folic acid to folinic acid

Warnings/Precautions Diabetics and patients prone to recurrent renal calculi (eg, dialysis patients) should not take excessive doses for extended periods of time

Drug Interactions

Decreased effect:
- Aspirin (decreases ascorbate levels, increases aspirin)
- Fluphenazine (decreases fluphenazine levels)
- Warfarin (decreased effect)

Increased effect:
- Iron (absorption enhanced)
- Oral contraceptives (increased contraceptive effect)

Dietary Considerations Sodium content of 1 g: ~5 mEq

Pharmacodynamics/Kinetics

Absorption: Oral: Readily absorbed; an active process thought to be dose dependent

Distribution: Large

Metabolism: Hepatic via oxidation and sulfation

Excretion: Urine (with high blood levels)

Pregnancy Risk Factor A/C (dose exceeding RDA recommendation)

Lactation Enters breast milk/compatible

Dosage Forms

Capsule: 500 mg, 1000 mg

(Continued)

Ascorbic Acid *(Continued)*

C-500-GR™: 500 mg
Capsule, timed release: 500 mg
Crystal (Vita-C®): 4 g/teaspoonful (100 g)
Injection, solution: 250 mg/mL (2 mL, 30 mL); 500 mg/mL (50 mL)
Cenolate®: 500 mg/mL (1 mL, 2 mL) [contains sodium hydrosulfite]
Powder, solution (Dull-C®): 4 g/teaspoonful (100 g, 500 g)
Solution, oral (Cecon®): 90 mg/mL (50 mL)
Tablet: 100 mg, 250 mg, 500 mg, 1000 mg
C-Gram: 1000 mg
Tablet, chewable: 100 mg, 250 mg, 500 mg [some products may contain aspartame]
Tablet, timed release: 500 mg, 1000 mg, 1500 mg
Cevi-Bid®: 500 mg

Ascorbic Acid and Ferrous Sulfate *see* Ferrous Sulfate and Ascorbic Acid *on page 587*

Ascriptin® [OTC] *see* Aspirin *on page 151*

Ascriptin® Extra Strength [OTC] *see* Aspirin *on page 151*

Asendin [DSC] *see* Amoxapine *on page 113*

Asparaginase (a SPEAR a ji nase)

U.S. Brand Names Elspar®

Canadian Brand Names Elspar®; Kidrolase®

Mexican Brand Names Leunase®

Generic Available No

Synonyms *E. coli* Asparaginase; *Erwinia* Asparaginase; L-asparaginase; NSC-106977 (*Erwinia*); NSC-109229 (*E. coli*)

Pharmacologic Category Antineoplastic Agent, Miscellaneous

Use Treatment of acute lymphocytic leukemia, lymphoma

Local Anesthetic/Vasoconstrictor Precautions No information available to require special precautions

Effects on Dental Treatment Key adverse event(s) related to dental treatment: Stomatitis.

Common Adverse Effects Note: Immediate effects: Fever, chills, nausea, and vomiting occur in 50% to 60% of patients.

>10%:

Central nervous system: Fatigue, somnolence, depression, hallucinations, agitation, disorientation or convulsions (10% to 60%), stupor, confusion, coma (25%)
Endocrine & metabolic: Fever, chills (50% to 60%), hyperglycemia (10%)
Gastrointestinal: Nausea, vomiting (50% to 60%), anorexia, abdominal cramps (70%), acute pancreatitis (15%, may be severe in some patients)
Hematologic: Hypofibrinogenemia and depression of clotting factors V and VIII, variable decreased in factors VII and IX, severe protein C deficiency and decrease in antithrombin III (may be dose-limiting or fatal)
Hepatic: Transient elevations of transaminases, bilirubin, and alkaline phosphatase
Hypersensitivity: Acute allergic reactions (fever, rash, urticaria, arthralgia, hypotension, angioedema, bronchospasm, anaphylaxis (15% to 35%); may be dose-limiting in some patients, may be fatal)
Renal: Azotemia (66%)

1% to 10%:

Endocrine & metabolic: Hyperuricemia
Gastrointestinal: Stomatitis

Mechanism of Action Asparaginase inhibits protein synthesis by hydrolyzing asparagine to aspartic acid and ammonia. Leukemia cells, specially lymphoblasts, require exogenous asparagine; normal cells can synthesize asparagine. Asparaginase is cycle-specific for the G_1 phase.

Drug Interactions

Increased Effect/Toxicity: Increased toxicity has been noticed when asparaginase is administered with vincristine (neuropathy) and prednisone (hyperglycemia). Decreased metabolism when used with cyclophosphamide. Increased hepatotoxicity when used with mercaptopurine.

Decreased Effect: Asparaginase terminates methotrexate action.

Pharmacodynamics/Kinetics

Absorption: I.M.: Produces peak blood levels 50% lower than those from I.V. administration
Distribution: V_d: 4-5 L/kg; 70% to 80% of plasma volume; does not penetrate CSF

Metabolism: Systemically degraded
Half-life elimination: 8-30 hours
Excretion: Urine (trace amounts)
Clearance: Unaffected by age, renal or hepatic function

Pregnancy Risk Factor C

Aspart, Insulin *see* Insulin Preparations *on page 749*

Aspercin [OTC] *see* Aspirin *on page 151*

Aspercin Extra [OTC] *see* Aspirin *on page 151*

Aspergum® [OTC] *see* Aspirin *on page 151*

Aspirin (AS pir in)

Related Information

Butalbital, Aspirin, and Caffeine *on page 238*
Cardiovascular Diseases *on page 1458*
Carisoprodol and Aspirin *on page 266*
Carisoprodol, Aspirin, and Codeine *on page 267*
Oral Pain *on page 1526*
Oxycodone and Aspirin *on page 1032*
Rheumatoid Arthritis, Osteoarthritis, and Osteoporosis *on page 1490*

U.S. Brand Names Ascriptin® [OTC]; Ascriptin® Extra Strength [OTC]; Aspercin [OTC]; Aspercin Extra [OTC]; Aspergum® [OTC]; Bayer® Aspirin [OTC]; Bayer® Aspirin Extra Strength [OTC]; Bayer® Aspirin Regimen Adult Low Strength [OTC]; Bayer® Aspirin Regimen Children's [OTC]; Bayer® Aspirin Regimen Regular Strength [OTC]; Bayer® Extra Strength Arthritis Pain Regimen [OTC]; Bayer® Plus Extra Strength [OTC]; Bayer® Women's Aspirin Plus Calcium [OTC]; Bufferin® [OTC]; Bufferin® Extra Strength [OTC]; Buffinol [OTC]; Buffinol Extra [OTC]; Easprin®; Ecotrin® [OTC]; Ecotrin® Low Strength [OTC]; Ecotrin® Maximum Strength [OTC]; Halfprin® [OTC]; St. Joseph® Adult Aspirin [OTC]; Sureprin 81™ [OTC]; ZORprin®

Canadian Brand Names Asaphen; Asaphen E.C.; Entrophen®; Novasen

Mexican Brand Names ASA 500®; Aspirina Protect®; Coraspir®; Ecotrin®

Generic Available Yes: Excludes gum

Synonyms Acetylsalicylic Acid; ASA

Pharmacologic Category Salicylate

Dental Use Treatment of postoperative pain

Use Treatment of mild to moderate pain, inflammation, and fever; may be used as prophylaxis of myocardial infarction; prophylaxis of stroke and/or transient ischemic episodes; management of rheumatoid arthritis, rheumatic fever, osteoarthritis, and gout (high dose); adjunctive therapy in revascularization procedures (coronary artery bypass graft [CABG], percutaneous transluminal coronary angioplasty [PTCA], carotid endarterectomy)

Unlabeled/Investigational Use Low doses have been used in the prevention of pre-eclampsia, recurrent spontaneous abortions, prematurity, fetal growth retardation (including complications associated with autoimmune disorders such as lupus or antiphospholipid syndrome)

Local Anesthetic/Vasoconstrictor Precautions No information available to require special precautions

Effects on Dental Treatment Key adverse event(s) related to dental treatment: As with all drugs which may affect hemostasis, bleeding is associated with aspirin. Hemorrhage may occur at virtually any site; risk is dependent on multiple variables including dosage, concurrent use of multiple agents which alter hemostasis, and patient susceptibility. Many adverse effects of aspirin are dose-related, and are rare at low dosages. Other serious reactions are idiosyncratic, related to allergy or individual sensitivity.

Significant Adverse Effects As with all drugs which may affect hemostasis, bleeding is associated with aspirin. Hemorrhage may occur at virtually any site. Risk is dependent on multiple variables including dosage, concurrent use of multiple agents which alter hemostasis, and patient susceptibility. Many adverse effects of aspirin are dose-related, and are extremely rare at low dosages. Other serious reactions are idiosyncratic, related to allergy or individual sensitivity. Accurate estimation of frequencies is not possible.

Central nervous system: Fatigue, insomnia, nervousness, agitation, confusion, dizziness, headache, lethargy, cerebral edema, hyperthermia, coma

Cardiovascular: Hypotension, tachycardia, dysrhythmias, edema

Dermatologic: Rash, angioedema, urticaria

Endocrine & metabolic: Acidosis, hyperkalemia, dehydration, hypoglycemia (children), hyperglycemia, hypernatremia (buffered forms)

Gastrointestinal: Nausea, vomiting, dyspepsia, epigastric discomfort, heartburn, stomach pains, gastrointestinal ulceration (6% to 31%), gastric erosions, gastric erythema, duodenal ulcers

(Continued)

Aspirin *(Continued)*

Hematologic: Anemia, disseminated intravascular coagulation, prolongation of prothrombin times, coagulopathy, thrombocytopenia, hemolytic anemia, bleeding, iron-deficiency anemia

Hepatic: Hepatotoxicity, increased transaminases, hepatitis (reversible)

Neuromuscular & skeletal: Rhabdomyolysis, weakness, acetabular bone destruction (OA)

Otic: Hearing loss, tinnitus

Renal: Interstitial nephritis, papillary necrosis, proteinuria, renal failure (including cases caused by rhabdomyolysis), increased BUN, increased serum creatinine

Respiratory: Asthma, bronchospasm, dyspnea, laryngeal edema, hyperpnea, tachypnea, respiratory alkalosis, noncardiogenic pulmonary edema

Miscellaneous: Anaphylaxis, prolonged pregnancy and labor, stillbirths, low birth weight, peripartum bleeding, Reye's syndrome

Postmarketing and/or case reports: Colonic ulceration, esophageal stricture, esophagitis with esophageal ulcer, esophageal hematoma, oral mucosal ulcers (aspirin-containing chewing gum), coronary artery spasm, conduction defect and atrial fibrillation (toxicity), delirium, ischemic brain infarction, colitis, rectal stenosis (suppository), cholestatic jaundice, periorbital edema, rhinosinusitis

Dosage

Children:

Analgesic and antipyretic: Oral, rectal: 10-15 mg/kg/dose every 4-6 hours, up to a total of 4 g/day

Anti-inflammatory: Oral: Initial: 60-90 mg/kg/day in divided doses; usual maintenance: 80-100 mg/kg/day divided every 6-8 hours; monitor serum concentrations

Antiplatelet effects: Adequate pediatric studies have not been performed; pediatric dosage is derived from adult studies and clinical experience and is not well established; suggested doses have ranged from 3-5 mg/kg/day to 5-10 mg/kg/day given as a single daily dose. Doses are rounded to a convenient amount (eg, ½ of 80 mg tablet).

Mechanical prosthetic heart valves: 6-20 mg/kg/day given as a single daily dose (used in combination with an oral anticoagulant in children who have systemic embolism despite adequate oral anticoagulation therapy (INR 2.5-3.5) and used in combination with low-dose anticoagulation (INR 2-3) and dipyridamole when full-dose oral anticoagulation is contraindicated)

Blalock-Taussig shunts: 3-5 mg/kg/day given as a single daily dose

Kawasaki disease: Oral: 80-100 mg/kg/day divided every 6 hours; monitor serum concentrations; after fever resolves: 3-5 mg/kg/day once daily; in patients without coronary artery abnormalities, give lower dose for at least 6-8 weeks or until ESR and platelet count are normal; in patients with coronary artery abnormalities, low-dose aspirin should be continued indefinitely

Antirheumatic: Oral: 60-100 mg/kg/day in divided doses every 4 hours

Adults:

Analgesic and antipyretic: Oral, rectal: 325-650 mg every 4-6 hours up to 4 g/day

Anti-inflammatory: Oral: Initial: 2.4-3.6 g/day in divided doses; usual maintenance: 3.6-5.4 g/day; monitor serum concentrations

Myocardial infarction prophylaxis: 75-325 mg/day; use of a lower aspirin dosage has been recommended in patients receiving ACE inhibitors

Acute myocardial infarction: 160-325 mg/day

CABG: 325 mg/day starting 6 hours following procedure

PTCA: Initial: 80-325 mg/day starting 2 hours before procedure; longer pretreatment durations (up to 24 hours) should be considered if lower dosages (80-100 mg) are used

Carotid endarterectomy: 81-325 mg/day preoperatively and daily thereafter

Acute stroke : 160-325 mg/day, initiated within 48 hours (in patients who are not candidates for thrombolytics and are not receiving systemic anticoagulation)

Stroke prevention/TIA: 30-325 mg/day (dosages up to 1300 mg/day in 2-4 divided doses have been used in clinical trials)

Pre-eclampsia prevention (unlabeled use): 60-80 mg/day during gestational weeks 13-26 (patient selection criteria not established)

Dosing adjustment in renal impairment: Cl_{cr} <10 mL/minute: Avoid use.

Hemodialysis: Dialyzable (50% to 100%)

Dosing adjustment in hepatic disease: Avoid use in severe liver disease.

Mechanism of Action Inhibits prostaglandin synthesis, acts on the hypothalamus heat-regulating center to reduce fever, blocks prostaglandin synthetase action which prevents formation of the platelet-aggregating substance thromboxane A_2

Contraindications Hypersensitivity to salicylates, other NSAIDs, or any component of the formulation; asthma; rhinitis; nasal polyps; inherited or acquired bleeding disorders (including factor VII and factor IX deficiency); do not use in children (<16 years of age) for viral infections (chickenpox or flu symptoms), with or without fever, due to a potential association with Reye's syndrome; pregnancy (3rd trimester especially)

Warnings/Precautions Use with caution in patients with platelet and bleeding disorders, renal dysfunction, dehydration, erosive gastritis, or peptic ulcer disease. Heavy ethanol use (>3 drinks/day) can increase bleeding risks. Avoid use in severe renal failure or in severe hepatic failure. Discontinue use if tinnitus or impaired hearing occurs. Caution in mild-moderate renal failure (only at high dosages). Patients with sensitivity to tartrazine dyes, nasal polyps and asthma may have an increased risk of salicylate sensitivity. Surgical patients should avoid ASA if possible, for 1-2 weeks prior to surgery, to reduce the risk of excessive bleeding.

When used for self-medication (OTC labeling): Children and teenagers who have or are recovering from chickenpox or flu-like symptoms should not use this product. Changes in behavior (along with nausea and vomiting) may be an early sign of Reye's syndrome; patients should be instructed to contact their healthcare provider if these occur.

Drug Interactions Substrate of CYP2C8/9 (minor)

ACE inhibitors: The effects of ACE inhibitors may be blunted by aspirin administration, particularly at higher dosages.

Buspirone increases aspirin's free % *in vitro.*

Carbonic anhydrase inhibitors and corticosteroids have been associated with alteration in salicylate serum concentrations.

Heparin and low molecular weight heparins: Concurrent use may increase the risk of bleeding.

Methotrexate serum levels may be increased; consider discontinuing aspirin 2-3 days before high-dose methotrexate treatment or avoid concurrent use.

NSAIDs may increase the risk of gastrointestinal adverse effects and bleeding. Serum concentrations of some NSAIDs may be decreased by aspirin.

Platelet inhibitors (IIb/IIIa antagonists): Risk of bleeding may be increased.

Probenecid effects may be antagonized by aspirin.

Sulfonylureas: The effects of older sulfonylurea agents (tolazamide, tolbutamide) may be potentiated due to displacement from plasma proteins. This effect does not appear to be clinically significant for newer sulfonylurea agents (glyburide, glipizide, glimepiride).

Valproic acid may be displaced from its binding sites which can result in toxicity.

Verapamil may potentiate the prolongation of bleeding time associated with aspirin.

Warfarin and oral anticoagulants may increase the risk of bleeding.

Ethanol/Nutrition/Herb Interactions

Ethanol: Avoid ethanol (may enhance gastric mucosal damage).

Food: Food may decrease the rate but not the extent of oral absorption.

Folic acid: Hyperexcretion of folate; folic acid deficiency may result, leading to macrocytic anemia.

Iron: With chronic aspirin use and at doses of 3-4 g/day, iron-deficiency anemia may result.

Sodium: Hypernatremia resulting from buffered aspirin solutions or sodium salicylate containing high sodium content. Avoid or use with caution in CHF or any condition where hypernatremia would be detrimental.

Benedictine liqueur, prunes, raisins, tea, and gherkins: Potential salicylate accumulation.

Fresh fruits containing vitamin C: Displace drug from binding sites, resulting in increased urinary excretion of aspirin.

Herb/Nutraceutical: Avoid cat's claw, dong quai, evening primrose, feverfew, garlic, ginger, ginkgo, red clover, horse chestnut, green tea, ginseng (all have additional antiplatelet activity). Limit curry powder, paprika, licorice; may cause salicylate accumulation. These foods contain 6 mg salicylate/100 g. An ordinarily American diet contains 10-200 mg/day of salicylate.

Dietary Considerations Take with food or large volume of water or milk to minimize GI upset.

Pharmacodynamics/Kinetics

Duration: 4-6 hours

Absorption: Rapid

(Continued)

Aspirin *(Continued)*

Distribution: V_d: 10 L; readily into most body fluids and tissues

Metabolism: Hydrolyzed to salicylate (active) by esterases in GI mucosa, red blood cells, synovial fluid, and blood; metabolism of salicylate occurs primarily by hepatic conjugation; metabolic pathways are saturable

Bioavailability: 50% to 75% reaches systemic circulation

Half-life elimination: Parent drug: 15-20 minutes; Salicylates (dose dependent): 3 hours at lower doses (300-600 mg), 5-6 hours (after 1 g), 10 hours with higher doses

Time to peak, serum: ~1-2 hours

Excretion: Urine (75% as salicyluric acid, 10% as salicylic acid)

Pregnancy Risk Factor C/D (full-dose aspirin in 3rd trimester - expert analysis)

Lactation Enters breast milk/use caution

Dosage Forms

Caplet:
- Bayer® Aspirin: 325 mg [film coated]
- Bayer® Aspirin Extra Strength: 500 mg [film coated]
- Bayer® Extra Strength Arthritis Pain Regimen: 500 mg [enteric coated]
- Bayer® Women's Aspirin Plus Calcium: 81 mg [contains elemental calcium 300 mg]

Caplet, buffered (Ascriptin® Extra Strength): 500 mg [contains aluminum hydroxide, calcium carbonate, and magnesium hydroxide]

Gelcap (Bayer® Aspirin Extra Strength): 500 mg

Gum (Aspergum®): 227 mg [cherry or orange flavor]

Suppository, rectal: 300 mg, 600 mg

Tablet: 325 mg
- Aspercin: 325 mg
- Aspercin Extra: 500 mg
- Bayer® Aspirin: 325 mg [film coated]

Tablet, buffered: 325 mg
- Ascriptin®: 325 mg [contains aluminum hydroxide, calcium carbonate, and magnesium hydroxide]
- Bayer® Plus Extra Strength: 500 mg [contains calcium carbonate]
- Bufferin®: 325 mg [contains citric acid]
- Bufferin® Extra Strength: 500 mg [contains citric acid]
- Buffinol: 325 mg [contains magnesium oxide]
- Buffinol Extra: 500 mg [contains magnesium oxide]

Tablet, chewable: 81 mg
- Bayer® Aspirin Regimen Children's Chewable: 81 mg [cherry, mint or orange flavor]
- St. Joseph® Adult Aspirin: 81 mg [orange flavor]

Tablet, controlled release (ZORprin®): 800 mg

Tablet, enteric coated: 81 mg, 325 mg, 500 mg, 650 mg
- Bayer® Aspirin Regimen Adult Low Strength, Ecotrin® Low Strength, St. Joseph Adult Aspirin: 81 mg
- Bayer® Aspirin Regimen Regular Strength, Ecotrin®: 325 mg
- Easprin®: 975 mg
- Ecotrin® Maximum Strength: 500 mg
- Halfprin: 81 mg, 162 mg
- Sureprin 81™: 81 mg

Comments There is no scientific evidence to warrant discontinuance of aspirin prior to dental surgery. Patients taking one aspirin tablet daily as an antithrombotic and who require dental surgery should be given special consideration in consultation with the physician before removal of the aspirin relative to prevention of postoperative bleeding.

Selected Readings

Daniel NG, Goulet J, Bergeron M, et al, "Antiplatelet Drugs: Is There a Surgical Risk?" *J Can Dent Assoc*, 2002, 68(11):683-7.

Forbes JA, Butterworth GA, Burchfield WH, et al, "Evaluation of Ketorolac, Aspirin, and an Acetaminophen-Codeine Combination in Postoperative Oral Surgery Pain," *Pharmacotherapy*, 1990, 10(6 Pt 2):77S-93S.

Hurlen M, Erikssen J, Smith P, et al, "Comparison of Bleeding Complications of Warfarin and Warfarin Plus Acetylsalicylic Acid: A Study in 3166 Outpatients," *J Intern Med*, 1994, 236(3):299-304.

Jeske AH, Suchko GD, ADA Council on Scientific Affairs and Division of Science, et al, "Lack of a Scientific Basis for Routine Discontinuation of Oral Anticoagulation Therapy Before Dental Treatment," *J Am Dent Assoc*, 2003, 134(11):1492-7.

Little JW, Miller CS, Henry RG, et al, "Antithrombotic Agents: Implications in Dentistry," *Oral Surg Oral Med Oral Pathol Oral Radiol Endod*, 2002, 93(5):544-51.

Schrodi J, Recio L, Fiorellini J, et al, "The Effect of Aspirin on the Periodontal Parameter Bleeding on Probing," *J Periodontol*, 2002, 73(8):871-6.

Scully C and Wolff A, "Oral Surgery in Patients on Anticoagulant Therapy," *Oral Surg Oral Med Oral Pathol Oral Radiol Endod*, 2002, 94(1):57-64.

Aspirin, Acetaminophen, and Caffeine *see* Acetaminophen, Aspirin, and Caffeine *on page 56*

Aspirin and Carisoprodol *see* Carisoprodol and Aspirin *on page 266*

Aspirin and Codeine (AS pir in & KOE deen)

Related Information

Aspirin *on page 151*
Codeine *on page 369*
Oral Pain *on page 1526*

Canadian Brand Names Coryphen® Codeine

Generic Available Yes

Synonyms Codeine and Aspirin

Pharmacologic Category Analgesic, Narcotic

Dental Use Treatment of postoperative pain

Use Relief of mild to moderate pain

Local Anesthetic/Vasoconstrictor Precautions No information available to require special precautions

Effects on Dental Treatment Key adverse event(s) related to dental treatment: Elderly are a high-risk population for adverse effects from nonsteroidal anti-inflammatory agents. As many as 60% of elderly patients with GI complications from NSAIDs can develop peptic ulceration and/or hemorrhage asymptomatically. Concomitant disease and drug use contribute to the risk of GI adverse effects. Use lowest effective dose for shortest period possible. Consider renal function decline with age.

Significant Adverse Effects Frequency not defined.

Cardiovascular: Palpitations, hypotension, bradycardia, peripheral vasodilation
Central nervous system: CNS depression, increased intracranial pressure
Dermatologic: Pruritus, rash, urticaria
Endocrine & metabolic: Antidiuretic hormone release
Gastrointestinal: Nausea, vomiting, constipation
Hematologic: Occult bleeding
Hepatic: Hepatotoxicity
Respiratory: Respiratory depression, bronchospasm
Ocular: Miosis
Miscellaneous: Physical and psychological dependence, biliary or urinary tract spasm, histamine release, anaphylaxis

Restrictions C-III

Dosage Oral:

Children:
  Aspirin: 10 mg/kg/dose every 4 hours
  Codeine: 0.5-1 mg/kg/dose every 4 hours
Adults: 1-2 tablets every 4-6 hours as needed for pain

Dosing adjustment in renal impairment:
  Cl_{cr} 10-50 mL/minute: Administer 75% of dose
  Cl_{cr} <10 mL/minute: Avoid use

Dosing interval in hepatic disease: Avoid use in severe liver disease

Mechanism of Action Aspirin inhibits prostaglandin synthesis, acts on the hypothalamus heat-regulating center to reduce fever, blocks prostaglandin synthetase action which prevents formation of the platelet-aggregating substance thromboxane A_2; codeine binds to opiate receptors (mu and kappa subtypes) in the CNS causing inhibition of ascending pain pathways, altering the perception of and response to pain

Contraindications Hypersensitivity to aspirin, codeine, or any component of the formulation; premature infants or during labor for delivery of a premature infant; pregnancy

Warnings/Precautions Use with caution in patients with impaired renal function, erosive gastritis, or peptic ulcer disease

Enhanced analgesia has been seen in elderly patients on therapeutic doses of narcotics; duration of action may be increased in the elderly; the elderly may be particularly susceptible to the CNS depressant and constipating effects of narcotics

Drug Interactions Aspirin: **Substrate** of CYP2C8/9 (minor)

Also see individual agents.

Ethanol/Nutrition/Herb Interactions Food: Food decreases rate but not extent of absorption (oral).

Dietary Considerations May be taken with food or milk to minimize GI distress.

Pharmacodynamics/Kinetics See individual agents.

Pregnancy Risk Factor D

Lactation Enters breast milk/use caution

(Continued)

Aspirin and Codeine *(Continued)*

Dosage Forms Tablet:

#3: Aspirin 325 mg and codeine phosphate 30 mg

#4: Aspirin 325 mg and codeine phosphate 60 mg

Comments Codeine products, as with other narcotic analgesics, are recommended only for limited acute dosing (ie, 3 days or less). The most common adverse effect you will see in your dental patients from codeine is nausea, followed by sedation and constipation. Codeine has narcotic addiction liability, especially when given long-term. The aspirin component has anticoagulant effects and can affect bleeding times.

Selected Readings

Dionne RA, "New Approaches to Preventing and Treating Postoperative Pain," *J Am Dent Assoc*, 1992, 123(6):26-34.

Gobetti JP, "Controlling Dental Pain," *J Am Dent Assoc*, 1992, 123(6):47-52.

Aspirin and Dipyridamole (AS pir in & dye peer ID a mole)

Related Information

Aspirin *on page 151*

Cardiovascular Diseases *on page 1458*

Dipyridamole *on page 453*

U.S. Brand Names Aggrenox®

Canadian Brand Names Aggrenox®

Generic Available No

Synonyms Aspirin and Extended-Release Dipyridamole; Dipyridamole and Aspirin

Pharmacologic Category Antiplatelet Agent

Use Reduction in the risk of stroke in patients who have had transient ischemia of the brain or completed ischemic stroke due to thrombosis

Local Anesthetic/Vasoconstrictor Precautions No information available to require special precautions

Effects on Dental Treatment No significant effects or complications reported

Common Adverse Effects

>10%:

- Central nervous system: Headache (38%)
- Gastrointestinal: Dyspepsia, abdominal pain (18%), nausea (16%), diarrhea (13%)

1% to 10%:

- Cardiovascular: Cardiac failure (2%)
- Central nervous system: Pain (6%), seizures (2%), fatigue (6%), malaise (2%), syncope (1%), amnesia (2%), confusion (1%), somnolence (1%)
- Dermatologic: Purpura (1%)
- Gastrointestinal: Vomiting (8%), bleeding (4%), rectal bleeding (2%), hemorrhoids (1%), hemorrhage (1%), anorexia (1%)
- Hematologic: Anemia (2%)
- Neuromuscular & skeletal: Back pain (5%), weakness (2%), arthralgia (6%), arthritis (2%), arthrosis (1%), myalgia (1%)
- Respiratory: Cough (2%), upper respiratory tract infections (1%), epistaxis (2%)

Mechanism of Action The antithrombotic action results from additive antiplatelet effects. Dipyridamole inhibits the uptake of adenosine into platelets, endothelial cells, and erythrocytes. Aspirin inhibits platelet aggregation by irreversible inhibition of platelet cyclooxygenase and thus inhibits the generation of thromboxane A2.

Drug Interactions

Cytochrome P450 Effect: Aspirin: **Substrate** of CYP2C8/9 (minor)

Increased Effect/Toxicity: See individual agents.

Decreased Effect: See individual agents.

Pharmacodynamics/Kinetics See individual agents.

Pregnancy Risk Factor D

Aspirin and Extended-Release Dipyridamole *see* Aspirin and Dipyridamole *on page 156*

Aspirin and Hydrocodone *see* Hydrocodone and Aspirin *on page 705*

Aspirin and Meprobamate (AS pir in & me proe BA mate)

Related Information

Aspirin *on page 151*

Meprobamate *on page 878*

U.S. Brand Names Equagesic®

Canadian Brand Names 292 MEP®

Generic Available No

Synonyms Meprobamate and Aspirin
Pharmacologic Category Antianxiety Agent, Miscellaneous
Use Adjunct to treatment of skeletal muscular disease in patients exhibiting tension and/or anxiety
Local Anesthetic/Vasoconstrictor Precautions No information available to require special precautions
Effects on Dental Treatment Key adverse event(s) related to dental treatment: Elderly are a high-risk population for adverse effects from nonsteroidal anti-inflammatory agents. As many as 60% of elderly patients with GI complications from NSAIDs can develop peptic ulceration and/or hemorrhage asymptomatically. Concomitant disease and drug use contribute to the risk of GI adverse effects. Use lowest effective dose for shortest period possible. Consider renal function decline with age.
Common Adverse Effects See individual agents.
Restrictions C-IV
Drug Interactions
Cytochrome P450 Effect: Aspirin: **Substrate** of CYP2C8/9 (minor)
Increased Effect/Toxicity: See individual agents.
Decreased Effect: See individual agents.
Pharmacodynamics/Kinetics See individual agents.
Pregnancy Risk Factor D

Aspirin and Oxycodone *see* Oxycodone and Aspirin *on page 1032*

Aspirin and Pravastatin (AS pir in & PRA va stat in)

Related Information
Aspirin *on page 151*
Pravastatin *on page 1109*

U.S. Brand Names Pravigard™ PAC
Generic Available No
Synonyms Buffered Aspirin and Pravastatin Sodium; Pravastatin and Aspirin
Pharmacologic Category Antilipemic Agent, HMG-CoA Reductase Inhibitor; Salicylate
Use Combination therapy in patients who need treatment with aspirin and pravastatin to reduce the incidence of cardiovascular events, including myocardial infarction, stroke, and death.
Local Anesthetic/Vasoconstrictor Precautions No information available to require special precautions
Effects on Dental Treatment See aspirin monograph.
Common Adverse Effects Clinical studies of this combination product have not been conducted. See individual agents.
Mechanism of Action
Aspirin: Inhibits prostaglandin synthesis, acts on the hypothalamus heat-regulating center to reduce fever, blocks prostaglandin synthetase action which prevents formation of the platelet-aggregating substance thromboxane A_2
Pravastatin: Competitive inhibitor of 3-hydroxy-3-methylglutaryl coenzyme A (HMG-CoA) reductase, which is the rate-limiting enzyme involved in *de novo* cholesterol synthesis.
Drug Interactions
Cytochrome P450 Effect:
Aspirin: **Substrate** of CYP2C8/9 (minor)
Pravastatin: **Substrate** of CYP3A4 (minor); **Inhibits** CYP2C8/9 (weak), 2D6 (weak), 3A4 (weak)
Increased Effect/Toxicity: See individual agents.
Decreased Effect: See individual agents.
Pharmacodynamics/Kinetics See individual agents.
Pregnancy Risk Factor X

Aspirin, Caffeine and Acetaminophen *see* Acetaminophen, Aspirin, and Caffeine *on page 56*
Aspirin, Caffeine, and Butalbital *see* Butalbital, Aspirin, and Caffeine *on page 238*
Aspirin, Caffeine, and Propoxyphene *see* Propoxyphene, Aspirin, and Caffeine *on page 1138*
Aspirin, Carisoprodol, and Codeine *see* Carisoprodol, Aspirin, and Codeine *on page 267*
Aspirin Free Anacin® Maximum Strength [OTC] *see* Acetaminophen *on page 47*
Aspirin, Orphenadrine, and Caffeine *see* Orphenadrine, Aspirin, and Caffeine *on page 1018*

Astelin® *see* Azelastine *on page 173*
AsthmaNefrin® *see* Epinephrine (Racemic) *on page 497*
Astramorph/PF™ *see* Morphine Sulfate *on page 947*
Atacand® *see* Candesartan *on page 248*
Atacand HCT™ *see* Candesartan and Hydrochlorothiazide *on page 249*
Atarax® *see* HydrOXYzine *on page 723*

Atazanavir (at a za NA veer)

U.S. Brand Names Reyataz®

Generic Available No

Synonyms Atazanavir Sulfate; BMS-232632

Pharmacologic Category Antiretroviral Agent, Protease Inhibitor

Use Treatment of HIV-1 infections in combination with at least two other antiretroviral agents

Note: In patients with prior virologic failure, coadministration with ritonavir is recommended.

Local Anesthetic/Vasoconstrictor Precautions No information available to require special precautions

Effects on Dental Treatment No significant effects or complications reported

Common Adverse Effects Protease inhibitors cause dyslipidemia which includes elevated cholesterol and triglycerides and a redistribution of body fat centrally to cause increased abdominal girth, buffalo hump, facial atrophy, and breast enlargement. These agents also cause hyperglycemia.

>10%:

Dermatologic: Rash (21%; median onset 8 weeks)
Gastrointestinal: Nausea (6% to 14%)
Hepatic: Bilirubin increased (>2.6 times ULN: 35% to 47%), amylase increased (14%)

3% to 10%:

Central nervous system: Depression (4% to 8%), dizziness (1% to 2%), fatigue (2% to 5%), fever (4% to 5%), headache (1% to 6%), insomnia (1% to 3%), pain (1% to 3%), peripheral neuropathy (1% to 4%)
Endocrine & metabolic: Lipodystrophy (1% to 8%)
Gastrointestinal: Abdominal pain (4%), vomiting (3% to 4%), diarrhea (1% to 11%)
Hepatic: Jaundice (7% to 8%), transaminases increased (2% to 9%)
Neuromuscular & skeletal: Myalgia (4%)
Respiratory: Cough increased (3% to 5%)

Mechanism of Action Inhibits the HIV-1 protease; inhibition of the viral protease prevents cleavage of the gag-pol polyprotein resulting in the production of immature, noninfectious virus

Drug Interactions

Cytochrome P450 Effect: Substrate of CYP3A4 (major); **Inhibits** CYP1A2 (weak), 2C9 (weak), 3A4 (strong)

Increased Effect/Toxicity: Serum concentrations of medications significantly metabolized by CYP3A4 or UGT1A1 may be elevated by atazanavir. Concurrent therapy with bepridil, cisapride, ergot derivatives (dihydroergotamine, ergonovine, ergotamine, methylergonovine), indinavir, irinotecan, lovastatin, midazolam, pimozide, simvastatin or triazolam is contraindicated (or not recommended, per manufacturer).

Atazanavir may increase the levels/effects of selected benzodiazepines, calcium channel blockers, cyclosporine, mirtazapine, nateglinide, nefazodone, quinidine, sildenafil (and other PDE-5 inhibitors), tacrolimus, tenofovir, venlafaxine, and other CYP3A4 substrates. When used with strong CYP3A4 inhibitors, dosage adjustment/limits are recommended for sildenafil and other PDE-5 inhibitors; consult individual monographs. Serum concentrations of antiarrhythmics (amiodarone, lidocaine, and quinidine) may be increased; monitor serum concentrations of these agents.

The levels/effects of atazanavir may be increased by azole antifungals, ciprofloxacin, clarithromycin, diclofenac, doxycycline, erythromycin, imatinib, isoniazid, nefazodone, nicardipine, propofol, protease inhibitors, quinidine, telithromycin, verapamil, and other CYP3A4 inhibitors. When used with strong Serum concentrations of atazanavir are increased by ritonavir. Specific dosing adjustment of atazanavir in combination with ritonavir and efavirenz has been established. Serum concentrations of saquinavir may be increased by atazanavir. Dosing recommendations for the combination have not been established. Tenofovir concentrations are increased by atazanavir. Concurrent use of indinavir may increase the risk of hyperbilirubinemia. Concurrent administration is not recommended.

Atazanavir may increase warfarin's hypoprothrombinemic effect; monitor INR closely. Serum levels of the hormones in oral contraceptives may increase significantly with administration of atazanavir; use with caution at lowest effective dose. Atazanavir may increase serum concentrations of clarithromycin, potentially increasing the risk of QT_c prolongation. A 50% reduction in clarithromycin dose or an alternative agent (except in *M. avium* complex infections) should be considered. An increase in rifabutin plasma AUC (>200%) has been observed when coadministered with atazanavir (decrease rifabutin's dose by up to 75%).

Decreased Effect: Concurrent use of proton pump inhibitors may reduce atazanavir absorption; avoid concurrent use. Antacids and buffered formulations (ie, didanosine buffered tablets) may reduce the serum concentrations of atazanavir. Administer atazanavir 2 hours before or 1 hour after these medications. H_2 antagonists may reduce the absorption of atazanavir; avoid concurrent use or administer at least 12 hours apart.

The levels/effects of atazanavir may be decreased by aminoglutethimide, carbamazepine, nafcillin, nevirapine, phenobarbital, phenytoin, rifamycins, and other CYP3A4 inducers. Rifampin decreases bioavailability of protease inhibitors by ~90%; loss of virologic response and resistance may occur; the two drugs should not be administered together. St John's wort (*Hypericum perforatum*) decreases serum concentrations of protease inhibitors and may lead to treatment failures; concurrent use is contraindicated. Tenofovir may decrease serum concentrations of atazanavir, resulting in a loss of virologic response (specific atazanavir dosing recommendations provided by manufacturer).

Pharmacodynamics/Kinetics

Protein binding: 86%

Metabolism: Hepatic, via multiple pathways including CYP3A4

Half-life elimination: ~7 hours

Time to peak, plasma: 2.5 hours

Excretion: Feces (79% as metabolites, 20% as unchanged drug); urine (13% as metabolites, 7% as unchanged drug)

Pregnancy Risk Factor B

Atazanavir Sulfate *see* Atazanavir *on page 158*

Atenolol (a TEN oh lole)

Related Information

Cardiovascular Diseases *on page 1458*

U.S. Brand Names Tenormin®

Canadian Brand Names Apo-Atenol®; Gen-Atenolol; Novo-Atenol; Nu-Atenol; PMS-Atenolol; Rhoxal-atenolol; Tenolin; Tenormin®

Mexican Brand Names Blokium®; Tenormin®

Generic Available Yes: Tablet

Pharmacologic Category Beta Blocker, $Beta_1$ Selective

Use Treatment of hypertension, alone or in combination with other agents; management of angina pectoris, postmyocardial infarction patients

Unlabeled/Investigational Use Acute ethanol withdrawal, supraventricular and ventricular arrhythmias, and migraine headache prophylaxis

Local Anesthetic/Vasoconstrictor Precautions No information available to require special precautions

Effects on Dental Treatment Atenolol is a cardioselective beta-blocker. Local anesthetic with vasoconstrictor can be safely used in patients medicated with atenolol. Nonselective beta-blockers (ie, propranolol, nadolol) enhance the pressor response to epinephrine, resulting in hypertension and bradycardia; this has not been reported for atenolol. Many nonsteroidal anti-inflammatory drugs, such as ibuprofen and indomethacin, can reduce the hypotensive effect of beta-blockers after 3 or more weeks of therapy with the NSAID. Short-term NSAID use (ie, 3 days) requires no special precautions in patients taking beta-blockers.

Common Adverse Effects 1% to 10%:

Cardiovascular: Persistent bradycardia, hypotension, chest pain, edema, heart failure, second- or third-degree AV block, Raynaud's phenomenon

Central nervous system: Dizziness, fatigue, insomnia, lethargy, confusion, mental impairment, depression, headache, nightmares

Gastrointestinal: Constipation, diarrhea, nausea

Genitourinary: Impotence

Miscellaneous: Cold extremities

(Continued)

Atenolol *(Continued)*

Dosage

Oral:

Children: 0.8-1 mg/kg/dose given daily; range of 0.8-1.5 mg/kg/day; maximum dose: 2 mg/kg/day

Adults:

Hypertension: 25-50 mg once daily, may increase to 100 mg/day. Doses >100 mg are unlikely to produce any further benefit.

Angina pectoris: 50 mg once daily, may increase to 100 mg/day. Some patients may require 200 mg/day.

Postmyocardial infarction: Follow I.V. dose with 100 mg/day or 50 mg twice daily for 6-9 days postmyocardial infarction.

I.V.:

Hypertension: Dosages of 1.25-5 mg every 6-12 hours have been used in short-term management of patients unable to take oral enteral beta-blockers

Postmyocardial infarction: Early treatment: 5 mg slow I.V. over 5 minutes; may repeat in 10 minutes. If both doses are tolerated, may start oral atenolol 50 mg every 12 hours or 100 mg/day for 6-9 days postmyocardial infarction.

Dosing interval for oral atenolol in renal impairment:

Cl_{cr} 15-35 mL/minute: Administer 50 mg/day maximum.

Cl_{cr} <15 mL/minute: Administer 50 mg every other day maximum.

Hemodialysis: Moderately dialyzable (20% to 50%) via hemodialysis; administer dose postdialysis or administer 25-50 mg supplemental dose.

Peritoneal dialysis: Elimination is not enhanced; supplemental dose is not necessary.

Mechanism of Action Competitively blocks response to beta-adrenergic stimulation, selectively blocks $beta_1$-receptors with little or no effect on $beta_2$-receptors except at high doses

Contraindications Hypersensitivity to atenolol or any component of the formulation; sinus bradycardia; sinus node dysfunction; heart block greater than first-degree (except in patients with a functioning artificial pacemaker); cardiogenic shock; uncompensated cardiac failure; pulmonary edema; pregnancy

Warnings/Precautions Safety and efficacy in children have not been established. Administer cautiously in compensated heart failure and monitor for a worsening of the condition (efficacy of atenolol in heart failure has not been established). Beta-blocker therapy should not be withdrawn abruptly (particularly in patients with CAD), but gradually tapered to avoid acute tachycardia, hypertension, and/or ischemia. Use caution with concurrent use of beta-blockers and either verapamil or diltiazem; bradycardia or heart block can occur. Avoid concurrent I.V. use of both agents. Beta-blockers should be avoided in patients with bronchospastic disease (asthma) and peripheral vascular disease (may aggravate arterial insufficiency). Atenolol, with B1 selectivity, has been used cautiously in bronchospastic disease with close monitoring. Use cautiously in diabetics - may mask hypoglycemic symptoms. May mask signs of thyrotoxicosis. May cause fetal harm when administered in pregnancy. Use cautiously in the renally impaired (dosage adjustment required). Use care with anesthetic agents which decrease myocardial function. Caution in myasthenia gravis.

Drug Interactions

Increased Effect/Toxicity: Atenolol may increase the effects of other drugs which slow AV conduction (digoxin, verapamil, diltiazem), alpha-blockers (prazosin, terazosin), and alpha-adrenergic stimulants (epinephrine, phenylephrine). Atenolol may mask the tachycardia from hypoglycemia caused by insulin and oral hypoglycemics. In patients receiving concurrent therapy, the risk of hypertensive crisis is increased when either clonidine or the beta-blocker is withdrawn. Reserpine has been shown to enhance the effect of atenolol. Beta-blockers may increase the action or levels of ethanol, disopyramide, nondepolarizing muscle relaxants, and theophylline although the effects are difficult to predict.

Decreased Effect: Decreased effect of atenolol with aluminum salts, barbiturates, calcium salts, cholestyramine, colestipol, NSAIDs, penicillins (ampicillin), rifampin, salicylates, and sulfinpyrazone due to decreased bioavailability and plasma levels. Beta-blockers may decrease the effect of sulfonylureas.

Ethanol/Nutrition/Herb Interactions

Food: Atenolol serum concentrations may be decreased if taken with food.

Herb/Nutraceutical: Avoid dong quai if using for hypertension (has estrogenic activity). Avoid ephedra, yohimbe, ginseng (may worsen hypertension). Avoid garlic (may have increased antihypertensive effect).

Dietary Considerations May be taken without regard to meals.

Pharmacodynamics/Kinetics

Onset of action: Peak effect: Oral: 2-4 hours

Duration: Normal renal function: 12-24 hours

Absorption: Incomplete

Distribution: Low lipophilicity; does not cross blood-brain barrier

Protein binding: 3% to 15%

Metabolism: Limited hepatic

Half-life elimination: Beta:

Neonates: ≤35 hours; Mean: 16 hours

Children: 4.6 hours; children >10 years may have longer half-life (>5 hours) compared to children 5-10 years (<5 hours)

Adults: Normal renal function: 6-9 hours, prolonged with renal impairment; End-stage renal disease: 15-35 hours

Excretion: Feces (50%); urine (40% as unchanged drug)

Pregnancy Risk Factor D

Dosage Forms INJ, solution: 0.5 mg/mL (10 mL). **TAB:** 25 mg, 50 mg, 100 mg

Selected Readings

Foster CA and Aston SJ, "Propranolol-Epinephrine Interaction: A Potential Disaster," *Plast Reconstr Surg*, 1983, 72(1):74-8.

Wong DG, Spence JD, Lamki L, et al, "Effect of Nonsteroidal Anti-inflammatory Drugs on Control of Hypertension of Beta-Blockers and Diuretics," *Lancet*, 1986, 1(8488):997-1001.

Wynn RL, "Dental Nonsteroidal Anti-inflammatory Drugs and Prostaglandin-Based Drug Interactions-Part Two," *Gen Dent*, 1992, 40(2):104, 106, 108.

Wynn RL, "Epinephrine Interactions With Beta-Blockers," *Gen Dent*, 1994, 42(1):16, 18.

Atenolol and Chlorthalidone (a TEN oh lole & klor THAL i done)

Related Information

Atenolol *on page 159*

Chlorthalidone *on page 321*

U.S. Brand Names Tenoretic®

Canadian Brand Names Tenoretic®

Generic Available Yes

Synonyms Chlorthalidone and Atenolol

Pharmacologic Category Antihypertensive Agent, Combination

Use Treatment of hypertension with a cardioselective beta-blocker and a diuretic

Local Anesthetic/Vasoconstrictor Precautions No information available to require special precautions

Effects on Dental Treatment Atenolol is a cardioselective beta-blocker. Local anesthetic with vasoconstrictor can be safely used in patients medicated with atenolol. Nonselective beta-blockers (ie, propranolol, nadolol) enhance the pressor response to epinephrine, resulting in hypertension and bradycardia; this has not been reported for atenolol. Many nonsteroidal anti-inflammatory drugs, such as ibuprofen and indomethacin, can reduce the hypotensive effect of beta-blockers after 3 or more weeks of therapy with the NSAID. Short-term NSAID use (ie, 3 days) requires no special precautions in patients taking beta-blockers.

Common Adverse Effects See individual agents.

Pharmacodynamics/Kinetics See individual agents.

Pregnancy Risk Factor D

ATG *see* Antithymocyte Globulin (Equine) *on page 136*

Atgam® *see* Antithymocyte Globulin (Equine) *on page 136*

AT III *see* Antithrombin III *on page 136*

Ativan® *see* Lorazepam *on page 842*

Atomoxetine (AT oh mox e teen)

U.S. Brand Names Strattera™

Generic Available No

Synonyms Atomoxetine Hydrochloride; LY139603; Methylphenoxy-Benzene Propanamine; Tomoxetine

Pharmacologic Category Norepinephrine Reuptake Inhibitor, Selective

Use Treatment of attention deficit/hyperactivity disorder (ADHD)

Unlabeled/Investigational Use Treatment of depression

Local Anesthetic/Vasoconstrictor Precautions Use vasoconstrictor with caution. Atomoxetine may increase heart rate or blood pressure in the presence of pressor agents. Pressor agents include the vasoconstrictors epinephrine and levonordefrin (Neo-Cobefrin®)

Effects on Dental Treatment Key adverse event(s) related to dental treatment: Xerostomia (normal salivary flow resumes upon discontinuation).

(Continued)

Atomoxetine *(Continued)*

Common Adverse Effects Percentages as reported in children and adults; some adverse reactions may be increased in "poor metabolizers" (CYP2D6).

>10%:

Central nervous system: Headache (17% to 27%), insomnia (16%)

Gastrointestinal: Xerostomia (4% to 21%), abdominal pain (20%), vomiting (15%), appetite decreased (10% to 14%), nausea (12%)

Respiratory: Cough (11%)

1% to 10%:

Cardiovascular: Palpitations (4%), systolic blood pressure increased (2% to 9%), orthostatic hypotension (2%), tachycardia (2%)

Central nervous system: Fatigue/lethargy (7% to 9%), irritability (8%), somnolence (7%), dizziness (6%), mood swings (5%), abnormal dreams (4%), sleep disturbance (4%), pyrexia (3%), rigors (3%), crying (2%)

Dermatologic: Dermatitis (2% to 4%)

Endocrine & metabolic: Dysmenorrhea (7%), libido decreased (6%), menstruation disturbance (3%), orgasm abnormal (2%), weight loss (2%)

Gastrointestinal: Dyspepsia (6% to 8%), diarrhea (4%), flatulence (2%), constipation (3% to 10%)

Genitourinary: Erectile disturbance (7%), ejaculatory disturbance (5%), prostatitis (3%), impotence (3%)

Neuromuscular & skeletal: Paresthesia (4%), myalgia (3%)

Otic: Ear infection (3%)

Renal: Urinary retention/hesitation (8%)

Respiratory: Rhinorrhea (4%), sinus headache (3%), sinusitis (6%)

Miscellaneous: Diaphoresis increased (4%), influenza (3%)

Mechanism of Action Selectively inhibits the reuptake of norepinephrine (Ki 4.5nM) with little to no activity at the other neuronal reuptake pumps or receptor sites.

Drug Interactions

Cytochrome P450 Effect: Substrate of CYP2C19 (minor), 2D6 (major)

Increased Effect/Toxicity: MAO inhibitors may increase risk of CNS toxicity (combined use is contraindicated). CYP2D6 inhibitors may increase the levels/effects of atomoxetine; example inhibitors include chlorpromazine, delavirdine, fluoxetine, miconazole, paroxetine, pergolide, quinidine, quinine, ritonavir, and ropinirole. Albuterol may increase risk of cardiovascular toxicity.

Pharmacodynamics/Kinetics

Absorption: Rapid

Distribution: V_d: I.V.: 0.85 L/kg

Protein binding: 98%, primarily albumin

Metabolism: Hepatic, via CYP2D6 and CYP2C19; forms metabolites (4-hydroxyatomoxetine, active, equipotent to atomoxetine; N-desmethylatomoxetine in poor metabolizers, limited activity)

Bioavailability: 63% in extensive metabolizers; 94% in poor metabolizers

Half-life elimination: Atomoxetine: 5 hours (up to 24 hours in poor metabolizers); Active metabolites: 4-hydroxyatomoxetine: 6-8 hours; N-desmethylatomoxetine: 6-8 hours (34-40 hours in poor metabolizers)

Time to peak, plasma: 1-2 hours

Excretion: Urine (80%, as conjugated 4-hydroxy metabolite); feces (17%)

Pregnancy Risk Factor C

Atomoxetine Hydrochloride *see* Atomoxetine *on page 161*

Atorvastatin (a TORE va sta tin)

Related Information

Cardiovascular Diseases *on page 1458*

U.S. Brand Names Lipitor®

Canadian Brand Names Lipitor®

Mexican Brand Names Lipitor®

Generic Available No

Pharmacologic Category Antilipemic Agent, HMG-CoA Reductase Inhibitor

Use Used with dietary therapy for the following:

Hyperlipidemias: To reduce elevations in total cholesterol, LDL-C, apolipoprotein B, and triglycerides in patients with primary hypercholesterolemia (elevations of 1 or more components are present in Fredrickson type IIa, IIb, III, and IV hyperlipidemias); treatment of homozygous familial hypercholesterolemia

Heterozygous familial hypercholesterolemia (HeFH): In adolescent patients (10-17 years of age, females >1 year postmenarche) with HeFH having LDL-C ≥190 mg/dL **or** LDL ≥160 mg/dL with positive family history of premature cardiovascular disease (CVD) or with 2 or more CVD risk factors in the adolescent patient

Local Anesthetic/Vasoconstrictor Precautions No information available to require special precautions

Effects on Dental Treatment No significant effects or complications reported

Common Adverse Effects

>10%: Central nervous system: Headache (3% to 17%)

2% to 10%:

Cardiovascular: Chest pain, peripheral edema

Central nervous system: Weakness (0% to 4%), insomnia, dizziness

Dermatologic: Rash (1% to 4%)

Gastrointestinal: Abdominal pain (0% to 4%), constipation (0% to 3%), diarrhea (0% to 4%), dyspepsia (1% to 3%), flatulence (1% to 3%), nausea

Genitourinary: Urinary tract infection

Neuromuscular & skeletal: Arthralgia (0% to 5%), myalgia (0% to 6%), back pain (0% to 4%), arthritis

Respiratory: Sinusitis (0% to 6%), pharyngitis (0% to 3%), bronchitis, rhinitis

Miscellaneous: Infection (2% to 10%), flu-like syndrome (0% to 3%), allergic reaction (0% to 3%)

<2% (Limited to important or life-threatening symptoms): Pneumonia, dyspnea, epistaxis, face edema, fever, photosensitivity, malaise, edema, gastroenteritis, elevated transaminases, colitis, vomiting, gastritis, xerostomia, rectal hemorrhage, esophagitis, eructation, glossitis, stomatitis, anorexia, increased appetite, biliary pain, cheilitis, duodenal ulcer, dysphagia, enteritis, melena, gingival hemorrhage, tenesmus, hepatitis, pancreatitis, cholestatic jaundice, paresthesia, somnolence, abnormal dreams, decreased libido, emotional lability, incoordination, peripheral neuropathy, torticollis, facial paralysis, hyperkinesia, depression, hypesthesia, hypertonia, leg cramps, bursitis, myasthenia, myositis, tendinous contracture, pruritus, alopecia, dry skin, urticaria, acne, eczema, seborrhea, skin ulcer, cystitis, hematuria, impotence, dysuria, nocturia, epididymitis, fibrocystic breast disease, vaginal hemorrhage, nephritis, abnormal urination, amblyopia, tinnitus, deafness, glaucoma, taste loss, taste perversion, palpitation, vasodilation, syncope, migraine, postural hypotension, phlebitis, arrhythmia, angina, hypertension, hyperglycemia, gout, weight gain, hypoglycemia, ecchymosis, anemia, lymphadenopathy, thrombocytopenia, petechiae, pharyngitis, rhinitis, myopathy

Dosage Oral: **Note:** Doses should be individualized according to the baseline LDL-cholesterol levels, the recommended goal of therapy, and patient response; adjustments should be made at intervals of 2-4 weeks

Children 10-17 years (females >1 year postmenarche): HeFH: 10 mg once daily (maximum: 20 mg/day)

Adults: Hyperlipidemias: Initial: 10-20 mg once daily; patients requiring >45% reduction in LDL-C may be started at 40 mg once daily; range: 10-80 mg once daily

Dosing adjustment in renal impairment: No dosage adjustment is necessary.

Dosing adjustment in hepatic impairment: Do not use in active liver disease.

Mechanism of Action Inhibitor of 3-hydroxy-3-methylglutaryl coenzyme A (HMG-CoA) reductase, the rate limiting enzyme in cholesterol synthesis (reduces the production of mevalonic acid from HMG-CoA); this then results in a compensatory increase in the expression of LDL receptors on hepatocyte membranes and a stimulation of LDL catabolism

Contraindications Hypersensitivity to atorvastatin or any component of the formulation; active liver disease; unexplained persistent elevations of serum transaminases; pregnancy; breast-feeding

Warnings/Precautions Secondary causes of hyperlipidemia should be ruled out prior to therapy. Liver function must be monitored by periodic laboratory assessment. Rhabdomyolysis with acute renal failure has occurred. Risk is increased with concurrent use of clarithromycin, danazol, diltiazem, fluvoxamine, indinavir, nefazodone, nelfinavir, ritonavir, verapamil, troleandomycin, cyclosporine, fibric acid derivatives, erythromycin, niacin, or azole antifungals. Weigh the risk versus benefit when combining any of these drugs with atorvastatin. Discontinue in any patient experiencing an acute or serious condition predisposing to renal failure secondary to rhabdomyolysis. Use with caution in patients who consume large amounts of ethanol or have a history of liver disease. Safety and efficacy have not been established in patients <10 years or in premenarcheal girls.

(Continued)

Atorvastatin *(Continued)*

Drug Interactions

Cytochrome P450 Effect: Substrate of CYP3A4 (major); **Inhibits** CYP3A4 (weak)

Increased Effect/Toxicity: CYP3A4 inhibitors may increase the levels/effects of atorvastatin; example inhibitors include azole antifungals, ciprofloxacin, clarithromycin, diclofenac, doxycycline, erythromycin, imatinib, isoniazid, nefazodone, nicardipine, propofol, protease inhibitors, quinidine, and verapamil. The risk of myopathy and rhabdomyolysis due to concurrent use of a CYP3A4 inhibitor with atorvastatin is probably less than lovastatin or simvastatin. Cyclosporine, clofibrate, fenofibrate, gemfibrozil, and niacin also may increase the risk of myopathy and rhabdomyolysis. The effect/toxicity of levothyroxine may be increased by atorvastatin. Levels of digoxin and ethinyl estradiol may be increased by atorvastatin.

Decreased Effect: Colestipol, antacids decreased plasma concentrations but effect on LDL-cholesterol was not altered. Cholestyramine may decrease absorption of atorvastatin when administered concurrently.

Ethanol/Nutrition/Herb Interactions

Ethanol: Avoid excessive ethanol consumption (due to potential hepatic effects).

Food: Atorvastatin serum concentrations may be increased by grapefruit juice; avoid concurrent intake of large quantities (>1 quart/day).

Herb/Nutraceutical: St John's wort may decrease atorvastatin levels.

Dietary Considerations May take with food if desired; may take without regard to time of day. Before initiation of therapy, patients should be placed on a standard cholesterol-lowering diet for 3-6 months and the diet should be continued during drug therapy.

Pharmacodynamics/Kinetics

Onset of action: Initial changes: 3-5 days; Maximal reduction in plasma cholesterol and triglycerides: 2 weeks

Absorption: Rapid

Protein binding: 98%

Metabolism: Hepatic; forms active ortho- and parahydroxylated derivates and an inactive beta-oxidation product

Half-life elimination: Parent drug: 14 hours

Time to peak, serum: 1-2 hours

Excretion: Bile; urine (2% as unchanged drug)

Pregnancy Risk Factor X

Dosage Forms TAB: 10 mg, 20 mg, 40 mg, 80 mg

Selected Readings

Siedlik PH, Olson, SC, Yang BB, et al, "Erythromycin Coadministration Increases Plasma Atorvastatin Concentrations," *J Clin Pharmacol*, 1999, 39(5):501-4.

Atorvastatin Calcium and Amlodipine Besylate *see* Amlodipine and Atorvastatin *on page 110*

Atovaquone (a TOE va kwone)

Related Information

Systemic Viral Diseases *on page 1519*

U.S. Brand Names Mepron®

Canadian Brand Names Mepron®

Generic Available No

Pharmacologic Category Antiprotozoal

Use Acute oral treatment of mild to moderate *Pneumocystis carinii* pneumonia (PCP) in patients who are intolerant to co-trimoxazole; prophylaxis of PCP in patients intolerant to co-trimoxazole; treatment/suppression of *Toxoplasma gondii* encephalitis, primary prophylaxis of HIV-infected persons at high risk for developing *Toxoplasma gondii* encephalitis

Local Anesthetic/Vasoconstrictor Precautions No information available to require special precautions

Effects on Dental Treatment Key adverse event(s) related to dental treatment: Oral moniliasis.

Common Adverse Effects Note: Adverse reaction statistics have been compiled from studies including patients with advanced HIV disease; consequently, it is difficult to distinguish reactions attributed to atovaquone from those caused by the underlying disease or a combination, thereof.

>10%:

- Central nervous system: Headache, fever, insomnia, anxiety
- Dermatologic: Rash
- Gastrointestinal: Nausea, diarrhea, vomiting
- Respiratory: Cough

1% to 10%:
Central nervous system: Dizziness
Dermatologic: Pruritus
Endocrine & metabolic: Hypoglycemia, hyponatremia
Gastrointestinal: Abdominal pain, constipation, anorexia, dyspepsia, increased amylase
Hematologic: Anemia, neutropenia, leukopenia
Hepatic: Elevated liver enzymes
Neuromuscular & skeletal: Weakness
Renal: Elevated BUN/creatinine
Miscellaneous: Oral moniliasis

Mechanism of Action Has not been fully elucidated; may inhibit electron transport in mitochondria inhibiting metabolic enzymes

Drug Interactions

Increased Effect/Toxicity: Possible increased toxicity with other highly protein-bound drugs.

Decreased Effect: Rifamycins (rifampin) used concurrently decrease the steady-state plasma concentrations of atovaquone.

Pharmacodynamics/Kinetics
Absorption: Significantly increased with a high-fat meal
Distribution: 3.5 L/kg
Protein binding: >99%
Metabolism: Undergoes enterohepatic recirculation
Bioavailability: Tablet: 23%; Suspension: 47%
Half-life elimination: 2-3 days
Excretion: Feces (94% as unchanged drug)

Pregnancy Risk Factor C

Atovaquone and Proguanil (a TOE va kwone & pro GWA nil)

Related Information
Atovaquone *on page 164*

U.S. Brand Names Malarone™

Canadian Brand Names Malarone™

Generic Available No

Synonyms Proguanil and Atovaquone

Pharmacologic Category Antimalarial Agent

Use Prevention or treatment of acute, uncomplicated *P. falciparum* malaria

Local Anesthetic/Vasoconstrictor Precautions No information available to require special precautions

Effects on Dental Treatment No significant effects or complications reported

Common Adverse Effects The following adverse reactions were reported in ≥5% of adults taking atovaquone/proguanil in treatment doses.

>10%: Gastrointestinal: Abdominal pain (17%), nausea (12%), vomiting (12% adults, 10% to 13% children)

1% to 10%:
Central nervous system: Headache (10%), dizziness (5%)
Dermatologic: Pruritus (6% children)
Gastrointestinal: Diarrhea (8%), anorexia (5%)
Neuromuscular & skeletal: Weakness (8%)

Adverse reactions reported in placebo-controlled clinical trials when used for prophylaxis. In general, reactions were similar to (or lower than) those seen with placebo:

>10%:
Central nervous system: Headache (22% adults, 19% children)
Gastrointestinal: Abdominal pain (33% children)
Neuromuscular & skeletal: Myalgia (12% adults)

1% to 10%:
Central nervous system: Fever (5% adults, 6% children), vivid dreams (2%)
Gastrointestinal: Abdominal pain (9% adults), diarrhea (6% adults, 2% children), dyspepsia (3% adults), gastritis (3% adults), oral ulceration (2%), vomiting (1% adults, 7% children)
Neuromuscular & skeletal: Back pain (8% adults)
Respiratory: Upper respiratory tract infection (8% adults), cough (6% adults, 9% children)
Miscellaneous: Flu-like syndrome (2% adults, 9% children)

In addition, 54% of adults in the placebo-controlled trials reported any adverse event (65% for placebo) and 60% of children reported adverse events (62% for placebo).

Mechanism of Action
Atovaquone: Selectively inhibits parasite mitochondrial electron transport.

(Continued)

Atovaquone and Proguanil *(Continued)*

Proguanil: The metabolite cycloguanil inhibits dihydrofolate reductase, disrupting deoxythymidylate synthesis. Together, atovaquone/cycloguanil affect the erythrocytic and exoerythrocytic stages of development.

Drug Interactions

Cytochrome P450 Effect: Proguanil: **Substrate** (minor) of 1A2, 2C19, 3A4

Decreased Effect: Metoclopramide decreases bioavailability of atovaquone. Rifabutin decreases atovaquone levels by 34%. Rifampin decreases atovaquone levels by 50%. Tetracycline decreases plasma concentrations of atovaquone by 40%.

Pharmacodynamics/Kinetics

Atovaquone: See Atovaquone monograph.

Proguanil:

Absorption: Extensive
Distribution: 42 L/kg
Protein binding: 75%
Metabolism: Hepatic to active metabolites, cycloguanil (via CYP2C19) and 4-chlorophenylbiguanide
Half-life elimination: 12-21 hours
Excretion: Urine (40% to 60%)

Pregnancy Risk Factor C

ATRA *see* Tretinoin (Oral) *on page 1328*
Atridox™ *see* Doxycycline Hyclate (Periodontal) *on page 475*
AtroPen® *see* Atropine *on page 166*

Atropine (A troe peen)

Related Information

Cardiovascular Diseases *on page 1458*

U.S. Brand Names AtroPen®; Atropine-Care®; Isopto® Atropine; Sal-Tropine™

Canadian Brand Names Dioptic's Atropine Solution; Isopto® Atropine; Minim's Atropine Solution

Mexican Brand Names Tropyn Z®

Generic Available Yes: Excludes tablet

Synonyms Atropine Sulfate

Pharmacologic Category Anticholinergic Agent; Anticholinergic Agent, Ophthalmic; Antidote; Antispasmodic Agent, Gastrointestinal; Ophthalmic Agent, Mydriatic

Use

Injection: Preoperative medication to inhibit salivation and secretions; treatment of symptomatic sinus bradycardia; AV block (nodal level); ventricular asystole; antidote for organophosphate pesticide poisoning
Ophthalmic: Produce mydriasis and cycloplegia for examination of the retina and optic disc and accurate measurement of refractive errors; uveitis
Oral: Inhibit salivation and secretions

Unlabeled/Investigational Use Pulseless electric activity, asystole, neuromuscular blockade reversal; treatment of nerve agent toxicity (chemical warfare) in combination with pralidoxime

Local Anesthetic/Vasoconstrictor Precautions No information available to require special precautions

Effects on Dental Treatment Key adverse event(s) related to dental treatment: Xerostomia and changes in salivation (normal salivary flow resumes upon discontinuation), dry throat, and nasal dryness.

Significant Adverse Effects Severity and frequency of adverse reactions are dose related and vary greatly; listed reactions are limited to significant and/or life-threatening.

Cardiovascular: Arrhythmia, flushing, hypotension, palpitation, tachycardia
Central nervous system: Ataxia, coma, delirium, disorientation, dizziness, drowsiness, excitement, fever, hallucinations, headache, insomnia, nervousness, weakness
Dermatologic: Anhidrosis, urticaria, rash, scarlatiniform rash
Gastrointestinal: Bloating, constipation, delayed gastric emptying, loss of taste, nausea, paralytic ileus, vomiting, xerostomia
Genitourinary: Urinary hesitancy, urinary retention
Ocular: Angle-closure glaucoma, blurred vision, cycloplegia, dry eyes, mydriasis, ocular tension increased
Respiratory: Dyspnea, laryngospasm, pulmonary edema
Miscellaneous: Anaphylaxis

Restrictions The AtroPen® formulation is available for use primarily by the Department of Defense.

Dosage

Neonates, Infants, and Children: Doses <0.1 mg have been associated with paradoxical bradycardia.

Inhibit salivation and secretions (preanesthesia): Oral, I.M., I.V., SubQ:

<5 kg: 0.02 mg/kg/dose 30-60 minutes preop then every 4-6 hours as needed. Use of a minimum dosage of 0.1 mg in neonates <5 kg will result in dosages >0.02 mg/kg. There is no documented minimum dosage in this age group.

>5 kg: 0.01-0.02 mg/kg/dose to a maximum 0.4 mg/dose 30-60 minutes preop; minimum dose: 0.1 mg

Alternate dosing:

3-7 kg (7-16 lb): 0.1 mg
8-11 kg (17-24 lb): 0.15 mg
11-18 kg (24-40 lb): 0.2 mg
18-29 kg (40-65 lb): 0.3 mg
>30 kg (>65 lb): 0.4 mg

Bradycardia: I.V., intratracheal: 0.02 mg/kg, minimum dose 0.1 mg, maximum single dose: 0.5 mg in children and 1 mg in adolescents; may repeat in 5-minute intervals to a maximum total dose of 1 mg in children or 2 mg in adolescents. (**Note:** For intratracheal administration, the dosage must be diluted with normal saline to a total volume of 1-5 mL). When treating bradycardia in neonates, reserve use for those patients unresponsive to improved oxygenation and epinephrine.

Infants and Children: Nerve agent toxicity management (unlabeled use): See "**Note**" in Adults dosing.

Prehospital ("in the field"): I.M.:

Birth to <2 years: Mild-to-moderate symptoms: 0.05 mg/kg; severe symptoms: 0.1 mg/kg
2-10 years: Mild-to-moderate symptoms: 1 mg; severe symptoms: 2 mg
>10 years: Mild-to-moderate symptoms: 2 mg; severe symptoms: 4 mg

Hospital/emergency department: I.M.:

Birth to <2 years: Mild-to-moderate symptoms: 0.05 mg/kg I.M. **or** 0.02 mg/kg I.V.; severe symptoms: 0.1 mg/kg I.M. **or** 0.02 mg/kg I.V.
2-10 years: Mild-to-moderate symptoms: 1 mg; severe symptoms: 2 mg
>10 years: Mild-to-moderate symptoms: 2 mg; severe symptoms: 4 mg

Children: Organophosphate or carbamate poisoning:

I.V.: 0.03-0.05 mg/kg every 10-20 minutes until atropine effect, then every 1-4 hours for at least 24 hours

I.M. (AtroPen®): Mild symptoms: Administer dose listed below as soon as exposure is known or suspected. If severe symptoms develop after first dose, 2 additional doses should be repeated in 10 minutes; do not administer more than 3 doses. Severe symptoms: Immediately administer 3 doses as follows:

<6.8 kg (15 lbs): Use of **AtroPen® formulation not recommended;** administer atropine 0.05 mg/kg
6.8-18 kg (15-40 lbs): 0.5 mg/dose
18-41 kg (40-90 lbs): 1 mg/dose
>41 kg (>90 lbs): 2 mg/dose

Adults (doses <0.5 mg have been associated with paradoxical bradycardia):

Asystole or pulseless electrical activity: I.V.: 1 mg; repeat in 3-5 minutes if asystole persists; total dose of 0.04 mg/kg; may give intratracheally in 10 mL NS (intratracheal dose should be 2-2.5 times the I.V. dose)

Inhibit salivation and secretions (preanesthesia):

I.M., I.V., SubQ: 0.4-0.6 mg 30-60 minutes preop and repeat every 4-6 hours as needed

Bradycardia: I.V.: 0.5-1 mg every 5 minutes, not to exceed a total of 3 mg or 0.04 mg/kg; may give intratracheally in 10 mL NS (intratracheal dose should be 2-2.5 times the I.V. dose)

Neuromuscular blockade reversal: I.V.: 25-30 mcg/kg 60 seconds before neostigmine or 7-10 mcg/kg in combination with edrophonium

Organophosphate or carbamate poisoning:

I.V.: 2 mg, followed by 2 mg every 5-60 minutes until adequate atropinization has occurred; initial doses of up to 6 mg may be used in life-threatening cases

I.M. (AtroPen®): Mild symptoms: Administer 2 mg as soon as exposure is known or suspected. If severe symptoms develop after first dose, 2 additional doses should be repeated in 10 minutes; do not administer more than 3 doses. Severe symptoms: Immediately administer three 2 mg doses.

Nerve agent toxicity management (unlabeled use): I.M.: See **Note**. Prehospital ("in the field") or hospital/emergency department: Mild-to-moderate symptoms: 2-4 mg; severe symptoms: 6 mg

(Continued)

Atropine *(Continued)*

Note: Pralidoxime is a component of the management of nerve agent toxicity; consult pralidoxime monograph for specific route and dose. For prehospital ("in the field") management, repeat atropine I.M. (children: 0.05-0.1 mg/kg; adults: 2 mg) at 5-10 minute intervals until secretions have diminished and breathing is comfortable or airway resistance has returned to near normal. For hospital management, repeat atropine I.M. (infants 1 mg; all others: 2 mg) at 5-10 minute intervals until secretions have diminished and breathing is comfortable or airway resistance has returned to near normal.

Mydriasis, cycloplegia (preprocedure): Ophthalmic (1% solution): Instill 1-2 drops 1 hour before procedure.

Uveitis: Ophthalmic:

1% solution: Instill 1-2 drops 4 times/day

Ointment: Apply a small amount in the conjunctival sac up to 3 times/day; compress the lacrimal sac by digital pressure for 1-3 minutes after instillation

Elderly, frail patients: Nerve agent toxicity management (unlabeled use): I.M.: See **"Note"** in Adults dosing.

Prehospital ("in the field"): Mild-to-moderate symptoms: 1 mg; severe symptoms: 2-4 mg

Hospital/emergency department: Mild-to-moderate symptoms: 1 mg; severe symptoms: 2 mg

Mechanism of Action Blocks the action of acetylcholine at parasympathetic sites in smooth muscle, secretory glands and the CNS; increases cardiac output, dries secretions, antagonizes histamine and serotonin

Contraindications Hypersensitivity to atropine or any component of the formulation; narrow-angle glaucoma; adhesions between the iris and lens; tachycardia; obstructive GI disease; paralytic ileus; intestinal atony of the elderly or debilitated patient; severe ulcerative colitis; toxic megacolon complicating ulcerative colitis; hepatic disease; obstructive uropathy; renal disease; myasthenia gravis (unless used to treat side effects of acetylcholinesterase inhibitor); asthma; thyrotoxicosis; Mobitz type II block

Warnings/Precautions Heat prostration can occur in the presence of a high environmental temperature. Psychosis can occur in sensitive individuals. The elderly may be sensitive to side effects. Use caution in patients with myocardial ischemia. Use caution in hyperthyroidism, autonomic neuropathy, BPH, CHF, tachyarrhythmias, hypertension, and hiatal hernia associated with reflux esophagitis. Use with caution in children with spastic paralysis.

AtroPen®: There are no absolute contraindications for the use of atropine in organophosphate poisonings, however, use caution in those patients where the use of atropine would be otherwise contraindicated. Formulation for use by trained personnel only.

Drug Interactions

Drugs with anticholinergic activity (including phenothiazines and TCAs) may increase anticholinergic effects when used concurrently.

Sympathomimetic amines may cause tachyarrhythmias; avoid concurrent use.

Pharmacodynamics/Kinetics

Onset of action: I.V.: Rapid

Absorption: Complete

Distribution: Widely throughout the body; crosses placenta; trace amounts enter breast milk; crosses blood-brain barrier

Metabolism: Hepatic

Half-life elimination: 2-3 hours

Excretion: Urine (30% to 50% as unchanged drug and metabolites)

Pregnancy Risk Factor C

Lactation Enters breast milk (trace amounts)/use caution (AAP rates "compatible")

Breast-Feeding Considerations Anticholinergic agents may suppress lactation.

Dosage Forms

Injection, solution, as sulfate: 0.05 mg/mL (5 mL); 0.1 mg/mL (5 mL, 10 mL); 0.4 mg/mL (0.5 mL, 1 mL, 20 mL); 0.5 mg/mL (1 mL); 1 mg/mL (1 mL)

AtroPen® [prefilled auto-injector]: 2 mg/0.7 mL (0.7 mL)

Ointment, ophthalmic, as sulfate: 1% (3.5 g)

Solution, ophthalmic, as sulfate: 1% (5 mL, 15 mL)

Atropine-Care®: 1% (2 mL)

Isopto® Atropine: 1% (5 mL, 15 mL)

Tablet, as sulfate (Sal-Tropine™): 0.4 mg

Atropine and Difenoxin *see* Difenoxin and Atropine *on page 434*

Atropine and Diphenoxylate *see* Diphenoxylate and Atropine *on page 451*

Atropine-Care® *see* Atropine *on page 166*

Atropine, Hyoscyamine, Scopolamine, and Phenobarbital *see* Hyoscyamine, Atropine, Scopolamine, and Phenobarbital *on page 725*

Atropine, Hyoscyamine, Scopolamine, Kaolin, and Pectin *see* Hyoscyamine, Atropine, Scopolamine, Kaolin, and Pectin *on page 726*

Atropine, Hyoscyamine, Scopolamine, Kaolin, Pectin, and Opium *see* Hyoscyamine, Atropine, Scopolamine, Kaolin, Pectin, and Opium *on page 726*

Atropine Sulfate *see* Atropine *on page 166*

Atropine Sulfate (Dental Tablets)

(A troe peen SUL fate DEN tal TAB lets)

Related Information

Atropine *on page 166*

Management of Sialorrhea *on page 1557*

U.S. Brand Names Sal-Tropine™

Generic Available No

Pharmacologic Category Anticholinergic Agent

Dental Use Reduction of salivation and bronchial secretions

Use Treatment of GI disorders (eg, peptic ulcer disease, irritable bowel syndrome, hypermotility of colon)

Local Anesthetic/Vasoconstrictor Precautions No information available to require special precautions

Effects on Dental Treatment

Key adverse event(s) related to dental treatment:

Doses <0.1 mg have been associated with paradoxical bradycardia

Children: May produce fever (by inhibiting heat loss by evaporation), scarlitiniform rash

Causes significant xerostomia when used in therapeutic doses (normal salivary flow resumes upon discontinuation):

- 0.5 mg: Slight dryness of nose and mouth; bradycardia
- 1 mg: Increased dryness of nose and mouth; thirst; slowing then acceleration of heart rate; mydriasis
- 2 mg: Significant xerostomia; tachycardia with palpitations; mydriasis; slight blurring of vision; flushing, dry skin
- 5 mg: Increase in above symptoms plus disturbance of speech; difficulty swallowing; headache; hot, dry skin; restlessness with asthenia
- 10 mg: Above symptoms to extreme degree plus ataxia, excitement, disorientation, hallucinations, delirium, coma

Dosage

Inhibition of salivation and secretions (preanesthesia): Oral:

Neonates, Infants, and Children (no documented minimum dosage):

- 3-7 kg (7-16 lb): 0.1 mg
- 8-11 kg (17-24 lb): 0.15 mg
- 11-18 kg (24-40 lb): 0.2 mg
- 18-29 kg (40-65 lb): 0.3 mg
- >30 kg (>65 lb): 0.4 mg

Adults: 0.4 mg; may repeat in 4 hours, if necessary.

Mechanism of Action Refer to Atropine monograph.

Contraindications Refer to Atropine monograph.

Warnings/Precautions Lower doses (<0.5 mg) may have vagalmimetic effects (ie, increase vagal tone causing paradoxical bradycardia). A total dose of 3 mg (0.04 mg/kg) results in full vagal blockade in humans. Doses of 0.5-1 mg of atropine are mildly stimulating to the CNS. Geriatric patients may be sensitive to side effects; anticholinergic agents are generally not well tolerated in the elderly and their use should be avoided when possible. Larger doses may produce mental disturbances; psychosis can occur in sensitive individuals. Heat prostration can occur in the presence of a high environmental temperature. Use caution in CHF, tachyarrhythmias, hypertension, and hiatal hernia associated with reflux esophagitis. Lower doses (<0.5 mg) may have vagalmimetic effects (ie, increase vagal tone causing paradoxical bradycardia). A total dose of 3 mg (0.04 mg/kg) results in full vagal blockade in humans.

Drug Interactions

Increased Effect: Atropine-induced mouth dryness may be increased if it is given with other drugs that have anticholinergic actions, such as tricyclic antidepressants, antipsychotics, some antihistamines, and antiparkinsonism drugs.

Decreased Effect: May interfere with absorption of other medications.

(Continued)

Atropine Sulfate (Dental Tablets) *(Continued)*

Breast-Feeding Considerations Although atropine enters breast milk (trace amounts), the AAP rates this drug as "compatible" with breast-feeding; should be used with caution; anticholinergic agents may suppress lactation

Dosage Forms Tablet, as sulfate (Sal-Tropine™): 0.4 mg

Atrovent® *see* Ipratropium *on page 761*

A/T/S® *see* Erythromycin *on page 508*

Attapulgite (at a PULL gite)

Related Information

Oral Nonviral Soft Tissue Ulcerations or Erosions *on page 1551*

U.S. Brand Names Children's Kaopectate® [DSC] [OTC]; Diasorb® [OTC]; Kaopectate® Advanced Formula [DSC] [OTC]; Kaopectate® Maximum Strength Caplets [DSC] [OTC]

Canadian Brand Names Kaopectate®

Generic Available Yes

Pharmacologic Category Antidiarrheal

Use Symptomatic treatment of diarrhea

Local Anesthetic/Vasoconstrictor Precautions No information available to require special precautions

Effects on Dental Treatment No significant effects or complications reported

Mechanism of Action Controls diarrhea because of its absorbent action

Pregnancy Risk Factor B

Attenuvax® *see* Measles Virus Vaccine (Live) *on page 858*

Augmentin® *see* Amoxicillin and Clavulanate Potassium *on page 116*

Augmentin ES-600® *see* Amoxicillin and Clavulanate Potassium *on page 116*

Augmentin XR™ *see* Amoxicillin and Clavulanate Potassium *on page 116*

Auranofin (au RANE oh fin)

Related Information

Rheumatoid Arthritis, Osteoarthritis, and Osteoporosis *on page 1490*

U.S. Brand Names Ridaura®

Canadian Brand Names Ridaura®

Generic Available No

Pharmacologic Category Gold Compound

Use Management of active stage of classic or definite rheumatoid arthritis in patients that do not respond to or tolerate other agents; psoriatic arthritis; adjunctive or alternative therapy for pemphigus

Local Anesthetic/Vasoconstrictor Precautions No information available to require special precautions

Effects on Dental Treatment Key adverse event(s) related to dental treatment: Glossitis and stomatitis.

Common Adverse Effects

>10%:

- Dermatologic: Itching, rash
- Gastrointestinal: Stomatitis
- Ocular: Conjunctivitis
- Renal: Proteinuria

1% to 10%:

- Dermatologic: Urticaria, alopecia
- Gastrointestinal: Glossitis
- Hematologic: Eosinophilia, leukopenia, thrombocytopenia
- Renal: Hematuria

Mechanism of Action The exact mechanism of action of gold is unknown; gold is taken up by macrophages which results in inhibition of phagocytosis and lysosomal membrane stabilization; other actions observed are decreased serum rheumatoid factor and alterations in immunoglobulins. Additionally, complement activation is decreased, prostaglandin synthesis is inhibited, and lysosomal enzyme activity is decreased.

Drug Interactions

Increased Effect/Toxicity: Toxicity of penicillamine, antimalarials, hydroxychloroquine, cytotoxic agents, and immunosuppressants may be increased.

Pharmacodynamics/Kinetics

Onset of action: Delayed; therapeutic response may require as long as 3-4 months

Duration: Prolonged

Absorption: Oral: ~20% gold in dose is absorbed

Protein binding: 60%

Half-life elimination (single or multiple dose dependent): 21-31 days

Time to peak, serum: ~2 hours
Excretion: Urine (60% of absorbed gold); remainder in feces

Pregnancy Risk Factor C

Aurodex *see* Antipyrine and Benzocaine *on page 135*
Aurolate® *see* Gold Sodium Thiomalate *on page 668*
Auroto *see* Antipyrine and Benzocaine *on page 135*
Autoplex® T *see* Anti-inhibitor Coagulant Complex *on page 135*
AVA *see* Anthrax Vaccine (Adsorbed) *on page 133*
Avagard™ [OTC] *see* Chlorhexidine Gluconate *on page 308*
Avage™ *see* Tazarotene *on page 1262*
Avalide® *see* Irbesartan and Hydrochlorothiazide *on page 764*
Avandamet™ *see* Rosiglitazone and Metformin *on page 1201*
Avandia® *see* Rosiglitazone *on page 1199*
Avapro® *see* Irbesartan *on page 763*
Avapro® HCT *see* Irbesartan and Hydrochlorothiazide *on page 764*
Avastin™ *see* Bevacizumab *on page 204*
Avelox® *see* Moxifloxacin *on page 949*
Avelox® I.V. *see* Moxifloxacin *on page 949*
Aventyl® HCl *see* Nortriptyline *on page 999*
Aviane™ *see* Ethinyl Estradiol and Levonorgestrel *on page 545*
Avinza™ *see* Morphine Sulfate *on page 947*
Avita® *see* Tretinoin (Topical) *on page 1329*
Avitene® *see* Microfibrillar Collagen Hemostat *on page 923*
Avodart™ *see* Dutasteride *on page 479*
Avonex® *see* Interferon Beta-1a *on page 756*
Axert™ *see* Almotriptan *on page 82*
Axid® *see* Nizatidine *on page 995*
Axid® AR [OTC] *see* Nizatidine *on page 995*
AY-25650 *see* Triptorelin *on page 1346*
Aygestin® *see* Norethindrone *on page 996*
Ayr® Baby Saline [OTC] *see* Sodium Chloride *on page 1227*
Ayr® Saline [OTC] *see* Sodium Chloride *on page 1227*
Ayr® Saline Mist [OTC] *see* Sodium Chloride *on page 1227*

Azacitidine (ay za SYE ti deen)

Generic Available No

Synonyms AZA-CR; 5-Azacytidine; 5-AZC; Ladakamycin; NSC-102816

Pharmacologic Category Antineoplastic Agent, Miscellaneous

Unlabeled/Investigational Use Investigational: Refractory acute lymphocytic and myelogenous leukemia; myelodysplastic syndrome

Local Anesthetic/Vasoconstrictor Precautions No information available to require special precautions

Effects on Dental Treatment Key adverse event(s) related to dental treatment: Mucositis.

Common Adverse Effects

>10%:
- Central nervous system: Coma (9% to 22% at doses of 300-750 mg/m²/day)
- Gastrointestinal: Nausea/vomiting (50% to 85%), diarrhea (50%), mucositis
- Hematologic: Leukopenia, thrombocytopenia (34%; nadirs at ~20-30 days)
- Local: Injection site reaction: Redness, irritation, discomfort

1% to 10%:
- Cardiovascular: Hypotension (6%)
- Central nervous system: Coma (5% at doses of 150-200 mg/m²/day)
- Dermatologic: Rash (2%)
- Hematologic: Anemia (4%)
- Hepatic: Hepatic abnormalities (7%; increased enzyme levels up to coma)
- Renal: Renal toxicity (azotemia, hypophosphatemia, tubular acidosis)

Restrictions Available through NCI

Mechanism of Action No precise mechanism of action has been established. The drug appears to interfere with nucleic acid metabolism prior to the steps involving cytidine and uridine, with its major activity in the S phase of the cell cycle. Postulated mechanisms include:
- Phosphorylation to a triphosphate and direct incorporation into DNA
- Phosphorylation to a triphosphate, competition with cytosine triphosphate, and incorporation into RNA, producing defective messenger and transfer RNA
- Competition with uridine and cytidine for uridine kinase

(Continued)

Azacitidine *(Continued)*

Inhibition of orotidylic acid decarboxylase, inhibiting pyrimidine synthesis

Pharmacodynamics/Kinetics

Absorption: SubQ: Rapid and complete
Distribution: Does not cross blood-brain barrier
Metabolism: Hepatic; hydrolysis to several metabolites
Half-life elimination: ~4 hours
Excretion: Urine (50% to 85%); feces (minor)

Pregnancy Risk Factor C

AZA-CR *see* Azacitidine *on page 171*
Azactam® *see* Aztreonam *on page 177*
5-Azacytidine *see* Azacitidine *on page 171*
Azasan® *see* Azathioprine *on page 172*

Azathioprine (ay za THYE oh preen)

U.S. Brand Names Azasan®; Imuran®

Canadian Brand Names Alti-Azathioprine; Apo-Azathioprine®; Gen-Azathioprine; Imuran®

Mexican Brand Names Azatrilem®; Imuran®

Generic Available Yes

Synonyms Azathioprine Sodium

Pharmacologic Category Immunosuppressant Agent

Use Adjunct with other agents in prevention of rejection of kidney transplants; also used in severe active rheumatoid arthritis unresponsive to other agents; other autoimmune diseases (ITP, SLE, MS, Crohn's disease)

Unlabeled/Investigational Use Adjunct in prevention of rejection of solid organ (nonrenal) transplants

Local Anesthetic/Vasoconstrictor Precautions No information available to require special precautions

Effects on Dental Treatment Key adverse event(s) related to dental treatment: Aphthous stomatitis.

Common Adverse Effects Frequency not defined.

Central nervous system: Fever, chills
Dermatologic: Alopecia, erythematous or maculopapular rash
Gastrointestinal: Nausea, vomiting, anorexia, diarrhea, aphthous stomatitis, pancreatitis
Hematologic: Leukopenia, thrombocytopenia, anemia, pancytopenia (bone marrow suppression may be determined, in part, by genetic factors, ie, patients with TPMT deficiency are at higher risk)
Hepatic: Hepatotoxicity, jaundice, hepatic veno-occlusive disease
Neuromuscular & skeletal: Arthralgias
Ocular: Retinopathy
Miscellaneous: Rare hypersensitivity reactions which include myalgias, rigors, dyspnea, hypotension, serum sickness, rash; secondary infections may occur secondary to immunosuppression

Mechanism of Action Azathioprine is an imidazolyl derivative of mercaptopurine; antagonizes purine metabolism and may inhibit synthesis of DNA, RNA, and proteins; may also interfere with cellular metabolism and inhibit mitosis

Drug Interactions

Increased Effect/Toxicity: Allopurinol may increase serum levels of azathioprine's active metabolite (mercaptopurine). Decrease azathioprine dose to $^1/_3$ to $^1/_4$ of normal dose. Azathioprine and ACE inhibitors may induce severe leukopenia. Aminosalicylates (olsalazine, mesalamine, sulfasalazine) may inhibit TPMT, increasing toxicity/myelosuppression of azathioprine.

Decreased Effect: Azathioprine may result in decreased action of warfarin.

Pharmacodynamics/Kinetics

Distribution: Crosses placenta
Protein binding: ~30%
Metabolism: Extensively hepatic via xanthine oxidase to mercaptopurine (active); mercaptopurine requires detoxification by thiopurine methyltransferase (TPMT)
Half-life elimination: Parent drug: 12 minutes; mercaptopurine: 0.7-3 hours; End-stage renal disease: Slightly prolonged
Excretion: Urine (primarily as metabolites)

Pregnancy Risk Factor D

Azathioprine Sodium *see* Azathioprine *on page 172*
5-AZC *see* Azacitidine *on page 171*

Azelaic Acid (a zeh LAY ik AS id)

U.S. Brand Names Azelex®; Finacea™

Mexican Brand Names Cutacelan®

Generic Available No

Pharmacologic Category Topical Skin Product, Acne

Use Topical treatment of mild to moderate inflammatory acne vulgaris; treatment of mild to moderate rosacea

Finacea™: Not FDA-approved for the treatment of acne

Local Anesthetic/Vasoconstrictor Precautions No information available to require special precautions

Effects on Dental Treatment No significant effects or complications reported

Common Adverse Effects Frequency not defined.

Dermatologic: Pruritus, stinging, edema, seborrhea, erythema, dryness, rash, peeling, dermatitis, contact dermatitis, irritation

Local: Burning, tingling

Neuromuscular & skeletal: Paresthesia

Mechanism of Action Azelaic acid is a dietary constituent normally found in whole grain cereals, can be formed endogenously. Exact mechanism is not known; *in vitro*, azelaic acid possesses antimicrobial activity against *Propionibacterium acnes* and *Staphylococcus epidermidis*; may decrease microcomedo formation

Pharmacodynamics/Kinetics

Absorption: ~3% to 5% penetrates stratum corneum; up to 10% found in epidermis and dermis; 4% systemic

Half-life elimination: Topical: Healthy subjects: 12 hours

Excretion: Urine (as unchanged drug)

Pregnancy Risk Factor B

Azelastine (a ZEL as teen)

U.S. Brand Names Astelin®; Optivar®

Canadian Brand Names Astelin®

Mexican Brand Names Astelin®; Az®

Generic Available No

Synonyms Azelastine Hydrochloride

Pharmacologic Category Antihistamine

Use

Nasal spray: Treatment of the symptoms of seasonal allergic rhinitis such as rhinorrhea, sneezing, and nasal pruritus in children ≥5 years of age and adults; treatment of the symptoms of vasomotor rhinitis in children ≥12 years of age and adults

Ophthalmic: Treatment of itching of the eye associated with seasonal allergic conjunctivitis in children ≥3 years of age and adults

Local Anesthetic/Vasoconstrictor Precautions No information available to require special precautions

Effects on Dental Treatment Key adverse event(s) related to dental treatment: Bitter taste, xerostomia (normal salivary flow resumes upon discontinuation), aphthous stomatitis, glossitis, and burning sensation in throat. Chronic use of antihistamines will inhibit salivary flow, particularly in elderly patients; may contribute to periodontal disease and oral discomfort.

Common Adverse Effects

Nasal spray:

>10%:

Central nervous system: Headache (15%), somnolence (12%)

Gastrointestinal: Bitter taste (20%)

2% to 10%:

Central nervous system: Dizziness (2%), fatigue (2%)

Gastrointestinal: Nausea (3%), weight gain (2%), dry mouth (3%)

Respiratory: Nasal burning (4%), pharyngitis (4%), paroxysmal sneezing (3%), rhinitis (2%), epistaxis (2%)

<2%:

Cardiovascular: Flushing, hypertension, tachycardia

Central nervous system: Drowsiness, fatigue, vertigo, depression, nervousness, hypoesthesia, anxiety, depersonalization, sleep disorder, abnormal thinking, malaise

Dermatologic: Contact dermatitis, eczema, hair and follicle infection, furunculosis

Gastrointestinal: Constipation, gastroenteritis, glossitis, increased appetite, ulcerative stomatitis, vomiting, increased ALT, aphthous stomatitis, abdominal pain

Genitourinary: Urinary frequency, hematuria, albuminuria, amenorrhea

(Continued)

Azelastine *(Continued)*

Neuromuscular & skeletal: Myalgia, vertigo, temporomandibular dislocation, hypoesthesia, hyperkinesia, back pain, extremity pain
Ocular: Conjunctivitis, watery eyes, eye pain
Respiratory: Bronchospasm, coughing, throat burning, laryngitis
Miscellaneous: Allergic reactions, viral infections

Ophthalmic:
>10%:
Central nervous system: Headache (15%)
Ocular: Transient burning/stinging (30%)
1% to 10%:
Central nervous system: Fatigue
Genitourinary: Bitter taste (10%)
Ocular: Conjunctivitis, eye pain, blurred vision (temporary)
Respiratory: Asthma, dyspnea, pharyngitis
Miscellaneous: Flu-like syndrome

Mechanism of Action Competes with histamine for H_1-receptor sites on effector cells and inhibits the release of histamine and other mediators involved in the allergic response. When used intranasally, reduces hyper-reactivity of the airways; increases the motility of bronchial epithelial cilia, improving mucociliary transport

Drug Interactions

Cytochrome P450 Effect: Substrate (minor) of CYP1A2, 2C19, 2D6, 3A4; **Inhibits** CYP2B6 (weak), 2C8/9 (weak), 2C19 (weak), 2D6 (weak), 3A4 (weak)

Increased Effect/Toxicity: May cause additive sedation when concomitantly administered with other CNS depressant medications. Cimetidine can increase the AUC and C_{max} of azelastine by as much as 65%.

Pharmacodynamics/Kinetics

Onset of action: Peak effect: Nasal spray: 3 hours; Ophthalmic solution: 3 minutes
Duration: Nasal spray: 12 hours; Ophthalmic solution: 8 hours
Protein binding: 88%
Metabolism: Hepatic via CYP; active metabolite, desmethylazelastine
Bioavailability: Intranasal: 40%
Half-life elimination: 22 hours
Time to peak, serum: 2-3 hours

Pregnancy Risk Factor C

Azelastine Hydrochloride *see* Azelastine *on page 173*

Azelex® *see* Azelaic Acid *on page 173*

Azidothymidine *see* Zidovudine *on page 1398*

Azidothymidine, Abacavir, and Lamivudine *see* Abacavir, Lamivudine, and Zidovudine *on page 43*

Azithromycin (az ith roe MYE sin)

Related Information

Antibiotic Prophylaxis, Preprocedural Guidelines for Dental Patients *on page 1509*
Sexually-Transmitted Diseases *on page 1504*

U.S. Brand Names Zithromax®

Canadian Brand Names Zithromax®

Mexican Brand Names Azitrocin®

Generic Available No

Synonyms Azithromycin Dihydrate; Zithromax® TRI-PAK™; Zithromax® Z-PAK®

Pharmacologic Category Antibiotic, Macrolide

Dental Use Alternate antibiotic in the treatment of common orofacial infections caused by aerobic gram-positive cocci and susceptible anaerobes alternate antibiotic for the prevention of bacterial endocarditis in patients undergoing dental procedures

Use Treatment of acute otitis media due to *H. influenzae, M. catarrhalis*, or *S. pneumoniae*; pharyngitis/tonsillitis due to *S. pyogenes*; treatment of mild-to-moderate upper and lower respiratory tract infections, infections of the skin and skin structure, community-acquired pneumonia, pelvic inflammatory disease (PID), sexually-transmitted diseases (urethritis/cervicitis), pharyngitis/tonsillitis (alternative to first-line therapy), and genital ulcer disease (chancroid) due to susceptible strains of *C. trachomatis, M. catarrhalis, H. influenzae, S. aureus, S. pneumoniae, Mycoplasma pneumoniae*, and *C. psittaci*; acute bacterial exacerbations of chronic obstructive pulmonary disease (COPD) due to *H. influenzae, M. catarrhalis,* or *S. pneumoniae*; acute bacterial sinusitis

Unlabeled/Investigational Use Prevention of (or to delay onset of) or treatment of MAC in patients with advanced HIV infection; prophylaxis of bacterial endocarditis in patients who are allergic to penicillin and undergoing surgical or dental procedures

Local Anesthetic/Vasoconstrictor Precautions No information available to require special precautions

Effects on Dental Treatment No significant effects or complications reported

Significant Adverse Effects

1% to 10%: Gastrointestinal: Diarrhea, nausea, abdominal pain, cramping, vomiting (especially with high single-dose regimens)

<1% (Limited to important or life-threatening): Acute renal failure, allergic reaction, aggressive behavior, anaphylaxis, angioedema, arrhythmias (including ventricular tachycardia), cholestatic jaundice, deafness, enteritis, erythema multiforme (rare), headache (especially with high-dose), hearing loss, hepatic necrosis (rare), hepatitis, hypertrophic pyloric stenosis, hypotension, interstitial nephritis, leukopenia, pancreatitis, paresthesia, pruritus, pseudomembranous colitis, QT_c prolongation (rare), seizures, somnolence, Stevens-Johnson syndrome (rare), syncope, taste abnormality, thrombocytopenia, tinnitus, tongue discoloration (rare), torsade de pointes (rare), urticaria, vertigo

Dosage

Oral:

Children ≥6 months:

Community-acquired pneumonia: 10 mg/kg on day 1 (maximum: 500 mg/day) followed by 5 mg/kg/day once daily on days 2-5 (maximum: 250 mg/day)

Bacterial sinusitis: 10 mg/kg once daily for 3 days (maximum: 500 mg/day)

Otitis media:

1-day regimen: 30 mg/kg as a single dose (maximum dose: 1500 mg)

3-day regimen: 10 mg/kg once daily for 3 days (maximum: 500 mg/day)

5-day regimen: 10 mg/kg on day 1 (maximum: 500 mg/day) followed by 5 mg/kg/day once daily on days 2-5 (maximum: 250 mg/day)

Children ≥2 years: Pharyngitis, tonsillitis: 12 mg/kg/day once daily for 5 days (maximum: 500 mg/day)

Children:

M. avium-infected patients with acquired immunodeficiency syndrome (unlabeled use): 5 mg/kg/day once daily (maximum dose: 250 mg/day) or 20 mg/kg (maximum dose: 1200 mg) once weekly given alone or in combination with rifabutin

Treatment and secondary prevention of disseminated MAC (unlabeled use): 5 mg/kg/day once daily (maximum dose: 250 mg/day) in combination with ethambutol, with or without rifabutin

Prophylaxis for bacterial endocarditis (unlabeled use): 15 mg/kg 1 hour before procedure

Uncomplicated chlamydial urethritis or cervicitis (unlabeled use): Children ≥45 kg: 1 g as a single dose

Adolescents ≥16 years and Adults:

Respiratory tract, skin and soft tissue infections: 500 mg on day 1 followed by 250 mg/day on days 2-5 (maximum: 500 mg/day)

Alternative regimen: Bacterial exacerbation of COPD: 500 mg/day for a total of 3 days

Bacterial sinusitis: 500 mg/day for a total of 3 days

Urethritis/cervicitis:

Due to *C. trachomatis*: 1 g as a single dose

Due to *N. gonorrhoeae*: 2 g as a single dose

Chancroid due to *H. ducreyi*: 1 g as a single dose

Prophylaxis of disseminated *M. avium* complex disease in patient with advanced HIV infection (unlabeled use): 1200 mg once weekly (may be combined with rifabutin)

Treatment of disseminated *M. avium* complex disease in patient with advanced HIV infection (unlabeled use): 600 mg daily (in combination with ethambutol 15 mg/kg)

Prophylaxis for bacterial endocarditis (unlabeled use): 500 mg 1 hour prior to the procedure

I.V.: Adults:

Community-acquired pneumonia: 500 mg as a single dose for at least 2 days, follow I.V. therapy by the oral route with a single daily dose of 500 mg to complete a 7-10 day course of therapy

(Continued)

Azithromycin *(Continued)*

Pelvic inflammatory disease (PID): 500 mg as a single dose for 1-2 days, follow I.V. therapy by the oral route with a single daily dose of 250 mg to complete a 7-day course of therapy

Dosage adjustment in renal impairment: Use caution in patients with Cl_{cr} <10 mL/minute

Mechanism of Action Inhibits RNA-dependent protein synthesis at the chain elongation step; binds to the 50S ribosomal subunit resulting in blockage of transpeptidation

Contraindications Hypersensitivity to azithromycin, other macrolide antibiotics, or any component of the formulation

Warnings/Precautions Use with caution in patients with hepatic dysfunction; hepatic impairment with or without jaundice has occurred chiefly in older children and adults; it may be accompanied by malaise, nausea, vomiting, abdominal colic, and fever; discontinue use if these occur. May mask or delay symptoms of incubating gonorrhea or syphilis, so appropriate culture and susceptibility tests should be performed prior to initiating azithromycin. Pseudomembranous colitis has been reported with use of macrolide antibiotics; use caution with renal dysfunction. Prolongation of the QT_c interval has been reported with macrolide antibiotics; use caution in patients at risk of prolonged cardiac repolarization. Safety and efficacy have not been established in children <6 months of age with acute otitis media, acute bacterial sinusitis, or community-acquired pneumonia, or in children <2 years of age with pharyngitis/tonsillitis.

Drug Interactions Substrate of CYP3A4 (minor); **Inhibits** CYP3A4 (weak)

Decreased peak serum levels: Aluminum- and magnesium-containing antacids by 24% but not total absorption

Increased effect/toxicity: Azithromycin may increase levels of tacrolimus, phenytoin, ergot alkaloids, alfentanil, bromocriptine, carbamazepine, cyclosporine, digoxin, disopyramide, and triazolam; azithromycin did not affect the response to warfarin or theophylline although caution is advised when administered together; nelfinavir may increase azithromycin serum levels (monitor for adverse effects)

Avoid use with pimozide due to significant risk of cardiotoxicity

Ethanol/Nutrition/Herb Interactions Food: Rate and extent of GI absorption may be altered depending upon the formulation. Azithromycin suspension, not tablet form, has significantly increased absorption (46%) with food.

Dietary Considerations

Powder for oral suspension may be administered with or without food.

Tablet may be administered with food to decrease GI effects.

Sodium content:

Injection: 114 mg (4.96 mEq) per vial

Powder: 3.7 mg per 100 mg/5 mL of constituted solution; 7.4 mg per 200 mg/5 mL of constituted solution; 37 mg per 1 g single-dose packet

Tablet: 0.9 mg/250 mg tablet; 1.8 mg/500 mg tablet; 2.1 mg/600 mg tablet

Pharmacodynamics/Kinetics

Absorption: Rapid

Distribution: Extensive tissue; distributes well into skin, lungs, sputum, tonsils, and cervix; penetration into CSF is poor

Protein binding (concentration dependent): 7% to 50%

Metabolism: Hepatic

Bioavailability: 37%; variable effect with food (increased with oral suspension, unchanged with tablet)

Half-life elimination: Terminal: 68 hours

Time to peak, serum: 2.3-4 hours

Excretion: Feces (50% as unchanged drug); urine (~5% to 12%)

Pregnancy Risk Factor B

Lactation Enters breast milk/use caution

Breast-Feeding Considerations Based on one case report, azithromycin has been shown to accumulate in breast milk.

Dosage Forms

Injection, powder for reconstitution, as dihydrate: 500 mg

Powder for oral suspension, as dihydrate: 100 mg/5 mL (15 mL); 200 mg/5 mL (15 mL, 22.5 mL, 30 mL) [cherry creme de vanilla and banana flavor]; 1 g [single-dose packet; cherry creme de vanilla and banana flavor]

Tablet, as dihydrate: 250 mg, 500 mg, 600 mg

Zithromax® TRI-PAK™ [unit-dose pack]: 500 mg (3s)

Zithromax® Z-PAK® [unit-dose pack]: 250 mg (6s)

Selected Readings

ADA Division of Legal Affairs, "A Legal Perspective on Antibiotic Prophylaxis," *J Am Dent Assoc*, 2003, 134(9):1260.

American Dental Association Council on Scientific Affairs, "Combating Antibiotic Resistance," *J Am Dent Assoc*, 2004, 135(4):484-7.

Cotter CJ and Bierne JC, "Azithromycin for Odontogenic Infection," *J Oral Maxillofac Surg*, 2003, 61(10):1238.

Dajani AS, Taubert KA, Wilson W, et al, "Prevention of Bacterial Endocarditis. Recommendations by the American Heart Association," *JAMA*, 1997, 277(22):1794-801.

Dajani AS, Taubert KA, Wilson W, et al, "Prevention of Bacterial Endocarditis: Recommendations by the American Heart Association," *J Am Dent Assoc*, 1997, 128(8):1142-51.

Moore PA, "Dental Therapeutic Indications for the Newer Long-Acting Macrolide Antibiotics," *J Am Dent Assoc*, 1999, 130(9):1341-3.

Williams JD, Maskell JP, Shain H, et al, "Comparative *In Vitro* Activity of Azithromycin, Macrolides (Erythromycin, Clarithromycin and Spiramycin) and Streptogramin RP 59500 Against Oral Organisms," *J Antimicrob Chemother*, 1992, 30(1):27-37.

Wynn RL, "New Erythromycins," *Gen Dent*, 1996, 44(4):304-7.

Wynn RL, Bergman SA, Meiller TF, et al, "Antibiotics in Treating Oral-Facial Infections of Odontogenic Origin: An Update", *Gen Dent*, 2001, 49(3):238-40, 242, 244 passim.

Azithromycin Dihydrate *see* Azithromycin *on page 174*

Azmacort® *see* Triamcinolone *on page 1330*

Azo-Gesic® [OTC] *see* Phenazopyridine *on page 1072*

Azopt® *see* Brinzolamide *on page 218*

Azo-Standard® [OTC] *see* Phenazopyridine *on page 1072*

AZT *see* Zidovudine *on page 1398*

AZT + 3TC *see* Zidovudine and Lamivudine *on page 1399*

AZT, Abacavir, and Lamivudine *see* Abacavir, Lamivudine, and Zidovudine *on page 43*

Azthreonam *see* Aztreonam *on page 177*

Aztreonam (AZ tree oh nam)

U.S. Brand Names Azactam®

Canadian Brand Names Azactam®

Generic Available No

Synonyms Azthreonam

Pharmacologic Category Antibiotic, Miscellaneous

Use Treatment of patients with urinary tract infections, lower respiratory tract infections, septicemia, skin/skin structure infections, intra-abdominal infections, and gynecological infections caused by susceptible gram-negative bacilli

Local Anesthetic/Vasoconstrictor Precautions No information available to require special precautions

Effects on Dental Treatment No significant effects or complications reported

Common Adverse Effects As reported in adults:

1% to 10%:

- Dermatologic: Rash
- Gastrointestinal: Diarrhea, nausea, vomiting
- Local: Thrombophlebitis, pain at injection site

Mechanism of Action Inhibits bacterial cell wall synthesis by binding to one or more of the penicillin binding proteins (PBPs); which in turn inhibits the final transpeptidation step of peptidoglycan synthesis in bacterial cell walls, thus inhibiting cell wall biosynthesis. Bacteria eventually lyse due to ongoing activity of cell wall autolytic enzymes (autolysins and murein hydrolases) while cell wall assembly is arrested. Monobactam structure makes cross-allergenicity with beta-lactams unlikely.

Drug Interactions

Decreased Effect: Avoid antibiotics that induce beta-lactamase production (cefoxitin, imipenem).

Pharmacodynamics/Kinetics

Absorption: I.M.: Well absorbed; I.M. and I.V. doses produce comparable serum concentrations

Distribution: Widely to most body fluids and tissues; crosses placenta; enters breast milk

- V_d: Children: 0.2-0.29 L/kg; Adults: 0.2 L/kg
- Relative diffusion of antimicrobial agents from blood into CSF: Good only with inflammation (exceeds usual MICs)
- CSF:blood level ratio: Meninges: Inflamed: 8% to 40%; Normal: ~1%

Protein binding: 56%

Metabolism: Hepatic (minor %)

Half-life elimination:

- Children 2 months to 12 years: 1.7 hours
- Adults: Normal renal function: 1.7-2.9 hours
- End-stage renal disease: 6-8 hours

Time to peak: I.M., I.V. push: Within 60 minutes; I.V. infusion: 1.5 hours

(Continued)

Aztreonam *(Continued)*

Excretion: Urine (60% to 70% as unchanged drug); feces (~13% to 15%)

Pregnancy Risk Factor B

Azulfidine® *see* Sulfasalazine *on page 1249*
Azulfidine® EN-tabs® *see* Sulfasalazine *on page 1249*
B 9273 *see* Alefacept *on page 76*
BA-16038 *see* Aminoglutethimide *on page 98*
Babee® Cof Syrup [OTC] *see* Dextromethorphan *on page 421*
Babee® Teething® [OTC] *see* Benzocaine *on page 191*
Baby Gasz [OTC] *see* Simethicone *on page 1222*
BAC *see* Benzalkonium Chloride *on page 190*
Bacid® [OTC] *see Lactobacillus on page 793*
Baciguent® [OTC] *see* Bacitracin *on page 178*
BaciiM® *see* Bacitracin *on page 178*
Bacillus Calmette-Guérin (BCG) Live *see* BCG Vaccine *on page 183*

Bacitracin (bas i TRAY sin)

U.S. Brand Names AK-Tracin® [DSC]; Baciguent® [OTC]; BaciiM®

Canadian Brand Names Baciguent®

Generic Available Yes

Pharmacologic Category Antibiotic, Ophthalmic; Antibiotic, Topical; Antibiotic, Miscellaneous

Use Treatment of susceptible bacterial infections mainly; has activity against gram-positive bacilli; due to toxicity risks, systemic and irrigant uses of bacitracin should be limited to situations where less toxic alternatives would not be effective

Unlabeled/Investigational Use Oral administration: Successful in antibiotic-associated colitis; has been used for enteric eradication of vancomycin-resistant enterococci (VRE)

Local Anesthetic/Vasoconstrictor Precautions No information available to require special precautions

Effects on Dental Treatment No significant effects or complications reported

Common Adverse Effects 1% to 10%:
- Cardiovascular: Hypotension, edema of the face/lips, tightness of chest
- Central nervous system: Pain
- Dermatologic: Rash, itching
- Gastrointestinal: Anorexia, nausea, vomiting, diarrhea, rectal itching
- Hematologic: Blood dyscrasias
- Miscellaneous: Diaphoresis

Mechanism of Action Inhibits bacterial cell wall synthesis by preventing transfer of mucopeptides into the growing cell wall

Drug Interactions

Increased Effect/Toxicity: Nephrotoxic drugs, neuromuscular blocking agents, and anesthetics (increased neuromuscular blockade).

Pharmacodynamics/Kinetics
- Duration: 6-8 hours
- Absorption: Poor from mucous membranes and intact or denuded skin; rapidly following I.M. administration; not absorbed by bladder irrigation, but absorption can occur from peritoneal or mediastinal lavage
- Distribution: CSF: Nil even with inflammation
- Protein binding, plasma: Minimal
- Time to peak, serum: I.M.: 1-2 hours
- Excretion: Urine (10% to 40%) within 24 hours

Pregnancy Risk Factor C

Bacitracin and Polymyxin B (bas i TRAY sin & pol i MIKS in bee)

Related Information

Bacitracin *on page 178*
Polymyxin B *on page 1100*

U.S. Brand Names AK-Poly-Bac®; Betadine® First Aid Antibiotics + Moisturizer [OTC]; Polysporin® Ophthalmic; Polysporin® Topical [OTC]

Canadian Brand Names LID-Pack®; Optimyxin®; Polycidin® Ophthalmic Ointment

Generic Available Yes

Synonyms Polymyxin B and Bacitracin

Pharmacologic Category Antibiotic, Ophthalmic; Antibiotic, Topical

Use Treatment of superficial infections caused by susceptible organisms

Local Anesthetic/Vasoconstrictor Precautions No information available to require special precautions

Effects on Dental Treatment No significant effects or complications reported

Common Adverse Effects 1% to 10%: Local: Rash, itching, burning, anaphylactoid reactions, swelling, conjunctival erythema

Mechanism of Action See individual monographs for Bacitracin and Polymyxin B

Pharmacodynamics/Kinetics See individual agents.

Pregnancy Risk Factor C

Bacitracin, Neomycin, and Polymyxin B

(bas i TRAY sin, nee oh MYE sin, & pol i MIKS in bee)

Related Information

Bacitracin *on page 178*

Neomycin *on page 973*

Polymyxin B *on page 1100*

U.S. Brand Names Neosporin® Neo To Go® [OTC]; Neosporin® Ophthalmic Ointment; Neosporin® Topical [OTC]

Canadian Brand Names Neosporin® Ophthalmic Ointment; Neotopic®

Generic Available Yes

Synonyms Neomycin, Bacitracin, and Polymyxin B; Polymyxin B, Bacitracin, and Neomycin; Triple Antibiotic

Pharmacologic Category Antibiotic, Ophthalmic; Antibiotic, Topical

Use Helps prevent infection in minor cuts, scrapes and burns; short-term treatment of superficial external ocular infections caused by susceptible organisms

Local Anesthetic/Vasoconstrictor Precautions No information available to require special precautions

Effects on Dental Treatment No significant effects or complications reported

Common Adverse Effects Frequency not defined.

Dermatologic: Reddening, allergic contact dermatitis

Local: Itching, failure to heal, swelling, irritation

Ophthalmic: Conjunctival edema

Miscellaneous: Anaphylaxis

Mechanism of Action Refer to individual monographs for Bacitracin; Neomycin Sulfate; and Polymyxin B Sulfate

Pharmacodynamics/Kinetics See individual agents.

Pregnancy Risk Factor C

Bacitracin, Neomycin, Polymyxin B, and Hydrocortisone

(bas i TRAY sin, nee oh MYE sin, pol i MIKS in bee, & hye droe KOR ti sone)

Related Information

Bacitracin *on page 178*

Hydrocortisone *on page 714*

Neomycin *on page 973*

Polymyxin B *on page 1100*

U.S. Brand Names AK-Spore® H.C. [DSC]; Cortisporin® Ointment

Canadian Brand Names Cortisporin® Topical Ointment

Generic Available Yes: Ophthalmic ointment

Synonyms Hydrocortisone, Bacitracin, Neomycin, and Polymyxin B; Neomycin, Bacitracin, Polymyxin B, and Hydrocortisone; Polymyxin B, Bacitracin, Neomycin, and Hydrocortisone

Pharmacologic Category Antibiotic, Ophthalmic; Antibiotic, Otic; Antibiotic, Topical; Corticosteroid, Ophthalmic; Corticosteroid, Otic; Corticosteroid, Topical

Use Prevention and treatment of susceptible inflammatory conditions where bacterial infection (or risk of infection) is present

Local Anesthetic/Vasoconstrictor Precautions No information available to require special precautions

Effects on Dental Treatment No significant effects or complications reported

Common Adverse Effects Frequency not defined.

Dermatologic: Rash, generalized itching

Ocular: Irritation

Respiratory: Apnea

Miscellaneous: Secondary infection

Mechanism of Action Refer to individual monographs for Bacitracin, Neomycin, Polymyxin B, and Hydrocortisone

(Continued)

Bacitracin, Neomycin, Polymyxin B, and Hydrocortisone *(Continued)*

Drug Interactions

Cytochrome P450 Effect: Hydrocortisone: **Substrate** of CYP3A4 (minor); **Induces** CYP3A4 (weak)

Pharmacodynamics/Kinetics See individual agents.

Pregnancy Risk Factor C

Bacitracin, Neomycin, Polymyxin B, and Pramoxine

(bas i TRAY sin, nee oh MYE sin, pol i MIKS in bee, & pra MOKS een)

U.S. Brand Names Neosporin® + Pain Ointment [OTC]; Spectrocin Plus™ [OTC]

Generic Available Yes

Synonyms Neomycin, Bacitracin, Polymyxin B, and Pramoxine; Polymyxin B, Neomycin, Bacitracin, and Pramoxine; Pramoxine, Neomycin, Bacitracin, and Polymyxin B

Pharmacologic Category Antibiotic, Topical

Use Prevention and treatment of susceptible superficial topical infections and provide temporary relief of pain or discomfort

Local Anesthetic/Vasoconstrictor Precautions No information available to require special precautions

Effects on Dental Treatment No significant effects or complications reported

Baclofen (BAK loe fen)

U.S. Brand Names Lioresal®

Canadian Brand Names Apo-Baclofen®; Gen-Baclofen; Lioresal®; Liotec; Nu-Baclo; PMS-Baclofen

Generic Available Yes: Tablets only

Pharmacologic Category Skeletal Muscle Relaxant

Use Treatment of reversible spasticity associated with multiple sclerosis or spinal cord lesions

Orphan drug: Intrathecal: Treatment of intractable spasticity caused by spinal cord injury, multiple sclerosis, and other spinal disease (spinal ischemia or tumor, transverse myelitis, cervical spondylosis, degenerative myelopathy)

Unlabeled/Investigational Use Intractable hiccups, intractable pain relief, bladder spasticity, trigeminal neuralgia, cerebral palsy, Huntington's chorea

Local Anesthetic/Vasoconstrictor Precautions No information available to require special precautions

Effects on Dental Treatment No significant effects or complications reported

Common Adverse Effects

>10%:

- Central nervous system: Drowsiness, vertigo, psychiatric disturbances, insomnia, slurred speech, ataxia, hypotonia
- Neuromuscular & skeletal: Weakness

1% to 10%:

- Cardiovascular: Hypotension
- Central nervous system: Fatigue, confusion, headache
- Dermatologic: Rash
- Gastrointestinal: Nausea, constipation
- Genitourinary: Polyuria

Mechanism of Action Inhibits the transmission of both monosynaptic and polysynaptic reflexes at the spinal cord level, possibly by hyperpolarization of primary afferent fiber terminals, with resultant relief of muscle spasticity

Drug Interactions

Increased Effect/Toxicity: Baclofen may decrease the clearance of ibuprofen or other NSAIDs and increase the potential for renal toxicity. Effects may be additive with CNS depressants.

Pharmacodynamics/Kinetics

Onset of action: 3-4 days

Peak effect: 5-10 days

Absorption (dose dependent): Oral: Rapid

Protein binding: 30%

Metabolism: Hepatic (15% of dose)

Half-life elimination: 3.5 hours

Time to peak, serum: Oral: Within 2-3 hours

Excretion: Urine and feces (85% as unchanged drug)

Pregnancy Risk Factor C

BactoShield® CHG [OTC] *see* Chlorhexidine Gluconate *on page 308*

Bactrim™ *see* Sulfamethoxazole and Trimethoprim *on page 1246*

Bactrim™ DS *see* Sulfamethoxazole and Trimethoprim *on page 1246*
Bactroban® *see* Mupirocin *on page 951*
Bactroban® Nasal *see* Mupirocin *on page 951*
Baking Soda *see* Sodium Bicarbonate *on page 1226*
BAL *see* Dimercaprol *on page 447*

Balanced Salt Solution (BAL anced salt soe LOO shun)

U.S. Brand Names AK-Rinse™; AquaLase™; BSS®; BSS Plus®
Canadian Brand Names BSS®; BSS® Plus; Eye-Stream®
Generic Available Yes
Pharmacologic Category Ophthalmic Agent, Miscellaneous
Use Intraocular irrigating solution; also used to soothe and cleanse the eye in conjunction with hard contact lenses
Local Anesthetic/Vasoconstrictor Precautions No information available to require special precautions
Effects on Dental Treatment No significant effects or complications reported

BAL in Oil® *see* Dimercaprol *on page 447*
Balmex® [OTC] *see* Zinc Oxide *on page 1400*
Balnetar® [OTC] *see* Coal Tar *on page 367*

Balsalazide (bal SAL a zide)

U.S. Brand Names Colazal®
Generic Available No
Synonyms Balsalazide Disodium
Pharmacologic Category 5-Aminosalicylic Acid Derivative; Anti-inflammatory Agent
Use Treatment of mild to moderate active ulcerative colitis
Local Anesthetic/Vasoconstrictor Precautions No information available to require special precautions
Effects on Dental Treatment No significant effects or complications reported
Common Adverse Effects 1% to 10%:

Central nervous system: Headache (8%), insomnia (2%), fatigue (2%), fever (2%), pain (2%), dizziness (1%)

Gastrointestinal: Abdominal pain (6%), diarrhea (5%), nausea (5%), vomiting (4%), anorexia (2%), dyspepsia (2%), flatulence (2%), rectal bleeding (2%), cramps (1%), constipation (1%), dry mouth (1%), frequent stools (1%)

Genitourinary: Urinary tract infection (1%)

Neuromuscular & skeletal: Arthralgia (4%), back pain (2%), myalgia (1%)

Respiratory: Respiratory infection (4%), cough (2%), pharyngitis (2%), rhinitis (2%), sinusitis (1%)

Miscellaneous: Flu-like syndrome (1%)

Additional adverse reactions reported with mesalamine products (limited to important or life-threatening symptoms): Acute intolerance syndrome (cramping, abdominal pain, bloody diarrhea, fever, headache, pruritus, rash), alopecia, cholestatic jaundice, cirrhosis, elevated liver function tests, eosinophilic pneumonitis, hepatocellular damage, hepatotoxicity, jaundice, Kawasaki-like syndrome, liver failure, liver necrosis, nephrotic syndrome, pancreatitis, pericarditis, and renal dysfunction

Mechanism of Action Balsalazide is a prodrug, converted by bacterial azoreduction to 5-aminosalicylic acid (active), 4-aminobenzoyl-β-alanine (inert), and their metabolites. 5-aminosalicylic acid may decrease inflammation by blocking the production of arachidonic acid metabolites topically in the colon mucosa.

Drug Interactions

Decreased Effect: No studies have been conducted. Oral antibiotics may potentially interfere with 5-aminosalicylic acid release in the colon.

Pharmacodynamics/Kinetics

Onset of action: Delayed; may require several days to weeks

Absorption: Very low and variable

Protein binding: ≥99%

Metabolism: Azoreduced in the colon to 5-aminosalicylic acid (active), 4-aminobenzoyl-β-alanine (inert), and N-acetylated metabolites

Half-life elimination: Primary effect is topical (colonic mucosa); systemic half-life not determined

Time to peak: 1-2 hours

Excretion: Feces (65% as 5-aminosalicylic acid, 4-aminobenzoyl-β-alanine, and N-acetylated metabolites); urine (25% as N-acetylated metabolites); Parent drug: Urine or feces (<1%)

Pregnancy Risk Factor B

Balsalazide Disodium *see* Balsalazide *on page 181*

Balsam Peru, Trypsin, and Castor Oil *see* Trypsin, Balsam Peru, and Castor Oil *on page 1349*

Bancap HC® *see* Hydrocodone and Acetaminophen *on page 702*

Band-Aid® Hurt-Free™ Antiseptic Wash [OTC] *see* Lidocaine *on page 819*

Banophen® [OTC] *see* DiphenhydrAMINE *on page 448*

Base Ointment *see* Zinc Oxide *on page 1400*

Basiliximab (ba si LIK si mab)

U.S. Brand Names Simulect®

Canadian Brand Names Simulect®

Mexican Brand Names Simulect®

Generic Available No

Pharmacologic Category Monoclonal Antibody

Use Prophylaxis of acute organ rejection in renal transplantation

Local Anesthetic/Vasoconstrictor Precautions No information available to require special precautions

Effects on Dental Treatment Key adverse event(s) related to dental treatment: Facial edema and ulcerative stomatitis. Causes gingival hypertrophy (GH) similar to that caused by cyclosporine; early reports indicate that frequency/incidence of basiliximab-induced GH not as high as cyclosporine-induced GH.

Common Adverse Effects Administration of basiliximab did not appear to increase the incidence or severity of adverse effects in clinical trials. Adverse events were reported in 96% of both the placebo and basiliximab groups.

>10%:

- Cardiovascular: Peripheral edema, hypertension, atrial fibrillation
- Central nervous system: Fever, headache, insomnia, pain
- Dermatologic: Wound complications, acne
- Endocrine & metabolic: Hypokalemia, hyperkalemia, hyperglycemia, hyperuricemia, hypophosphatemia, hypercholesterolemia
- Gastrointestinal: Constipation, nausea, diarrhea, abdominal pain, vomiting, dyspepsia
- Genitourinary: Urinary tract infection
- Hematologic: Anemia
- Neuromuscular & skeletal: Tremor
- Respiratory: Dyspnea, infection (upper respiratory)
- Miscellaneous: Viral infection

3% to 10%:

- Cardiovascular: Chest pain, cardiac failure, hypotension, arrhythmia, tachycardia, generalized edema, abnormal heart sounds, angina pectoris
- Central nervous system: Hypoesthesia, neuropathy, agitation, anxiety, depression, malaise, fatigue, rigors, dizziness
- Dermatologic: Cyst, hypertrichosis, pruritus, rash, skin disorder, skin ulceration
- Endocrine & metabolic: Dehydration, diabetes mellitus, fluid overload, hypercalcemia, hyperlipidemia, hypoglycemia, hypomagnesemia, acidosis, hypertriglyceridemia, hypocalcemia, hyponatremia
- Gastrointestinal: Flatulence, gastroenteritis, GI hemorrhage, gingival hyperplasia, melena, esophagitis, stomatitis, enlarged abdomen, moniliasis, ulcerative stomatitis, weight gain
- Genitourinary: Impotence, genital edema, albuminuria, bladder disorder, hematuria, urinary frequency, oliguria, abnormal renal function, renal tubular necrosis, ureteral disorder, urinary retention, dysuria
- Hematologic: Hematoma, hemorrhage, purpura, thrombocytopenia, thrombosis, polycythemia, leukopenia
- Neuromuscular & skeletal: Arthralgia, arthropathy, cramps, fracture, hernia, myalgia, paresthesia, weakness, back pain, leg pain
- Ocular: Cataract, conjunctivitis, abnormal vision
- Respiratory: Bronchitis, bronchospasm, pneumonia, pulmonary edema, sinusitis, rhinitis, coughing, pharyngitis
- Miscellaneous: Accidental trauma, facial edema, sepsis, infection, increased glucocorticoids, herpes infection

Mechanism of Action Chimeric (murine/human) monoclonal antibody which blocks the alpha-chain of the interleukin-2 (IL-2) receptor complex; this receptor is expressed on activated T lymphocytes and is a critical pathway for activating cell-mediated allograft rejection

Drug Interactions

Increased Effect/Toxicity: Basiliximab is an immunoglobulin; specific drug interactions have not been evaluated, but are not anticipated.

Decreased Effect: Basiliximab is an immunoglobulin; specific drug interactions have not been evaluated, but are not anticipated. It is not known if the immune response to vaccines will be impaired during or following basiliximab therapy.

Pharmacodynamics/Kinetics

Duration: Mean: 36 days (determined by IL-2R alpha saturation)

Distribution: Mean: V_d: Children: 5.2 ± 2.8 L; Adults: 8.6 ± 4.1 L

Half-life elimination: Children: 9.4 days; Adults: Mean: 7.2 days

Excretion: Clearance: Children: 20 mL/hour; Adults: Mean: 41 mL/hour

Pregnancy Risk Factor B (manufacturer)

Bausch & Lomb® Computer Eye Drops [OTC] *see* Glycerin *on page 667*

Bausch & Lomb Earwax Removal [OTC] *see* Carbamide Peroxide *on page 259*

Bayer® Aspirin [OTC] *see* Aspirin *on page 151*

Bayer® Aspirin Extra Strength [OTC] *see* Aspirin *on page 151*

Bayer® Aspirin Regimen Adult Low Strength [OTC] *see* Aspirin *on page 151*

Bayer® Aspirin Regimen Children's [OTC] *see* Aspirin *on page 151*

Bayer® Aspirin Regimen Regular Strength [OTC] *see* Aspirin *on page 151*

Bayer® Extra Strength Arthritis Pain Regimen [OTC] *see* Aspirin *on page 151*

Bayer® Plus Extra Strength [OTC] *see* Aspirin *on page 151*

Bayer® Women's Aspirin Plus Calcium [OTC] *see* Aspirin *on page 151*

BayGam® *see* Immune Globulin (Intramuscular) *on page 739*

BayHep B™ *see* Hepatitis B Immune Globulin *on page 688*

BayRab® *see* Rabies Immune Globulin (Human) *on page 1165*

BayRho-D® Full-Dose *see* Rh_o(D) Immune Globulin *on page 1176*

BayRho-D® Mini-Dose *see* Rh_o(D) Immune Globulin *on page 1176*

BayTet™ *see* Tetanus Immune Globulin (Human) *on page 1277*

Baza® Antifungal [OTC] *see* Miconazole *on page 922*

Baza® Clear [OTC] *see* Vitamin A and Vitamin D *on page 1382*

B-Caro-T™ *see* Beta-Carotene *on page 198*

BCG, Live *see* BCG Vaccine *on page 183*

BCG Vaccine (bee see jee vak SEEN)

Related Information

Immunizations (Vaccines) *on page 1614*

U.S. Brand Names TheraCys®; TICE® BCG

Canadian Brand Names ImmuCyst®; Oncotice™; Pacis™

Generic Available No

Synonyms Bacillus Calmette-Guérin (BCG) Live; BCG, Live

Pharmacologic Category Biological Response Modulator; Vaccine

Use Immunization against tuberculosis and immunotherapy for cancer; treatment of bladder cancer

BCG vaccine is not routinely recommended for use in the U.S. for prevention of tuberculosis

BCG vaccine is strongly recommended for infants and children with negative tuberculin skin tests who:

- are at high risk of intimate and prolonged exposure to persistently untreated or ineffectively treated patients with infectious pulmonary tuberculosis, and
- cannot be removed from the source of exposure, and
- cannot be placed on long-term preventive therapy
- are continuously exposed with tuberculosis who have bacilli resistant to isoniazid and rifampin

BCG is also recommended for tuberculin-negative infants and children in groups in which the rate of new infections exceeds 1% per year and for whom the usual surveillance and treatment programs have been attempted but are not operationally feasible

Local Anesthetic/Vasoconstrictor Precautions No information available to require special precautions

Effects on Dental Treatment No significant effects or complications reported

Common Adverse Effects All serious adverse reactions must be reported to the U.S. Department of Health and Human Services (DHHS) Vaccine Adverse Event Reporting System (VAERS) 1-800-822-7967.

>10%:

Gastrointestinal: Nausea and vomiting (3% to 16%)

Genitourinary: Dysuria (62%), polyuria (42%), hematuria (26% to 40%), cystitis (6% to 30%), urinary urgency (6% to 18%)

(Continued)

BCG Vaccine *(Continued)*

Miscellaneous: Flu-like syndrome including fever, chills (42%)

1% to 10%:

Central nervous system: Fatigue, headache, dizziness

Gastrointestinal: Anorexia, diarrhea

Genitourinary: Urinary incontinence (2% to 6%)

Mechanism of Action BCG live is an attenuated strain of bacillus Calmette-Guérin used as a biological response modifier; BCG live, when used intravesicular for treatment of bladder carcinoma *in situ*, is thought to cause a local, chronic inflammatory response involving macrophage and leukocyte infiltration of the bladder. By a mechanism not fully understood, this local inflammatory response leads to destruction of superficial tumor cells of the urothelium. Evidence of systemic immune response is also commonly seen, manifested by a positive PPD tuberculin skin test reaction, however, its relationship to clinical efficacy is not well-established. BCG is active immunotherapy which stimulates the host's immune mechanism to reject the tumor.

Pregnancy Risk Factor C

BCNU *see* Carmustine *on page 268*

B Complex Combinations *see* Vitamin B Complex Combinations *on page 1382*

B-D™ Glucose [OTC] *see* Glucose (Instant) *on page 663*

Bebulin® VH *see* Factor IX Complex (Human) *on page 572*

Becaplermin (be KAP ler min)

U.S. Brand Names Regranex®

Canadian Brand Names Regranex®

Generic Available No

Synonyms Recombinant Human Platelet-Derived Growth Factor B; rPDGF-BB

Pharmacologic Category Growth Factor, Platelet-Derived; Topical Skin Product

Use Debridement adjunct for the treatment of diabetic ulcers that occur on the lower limbs and feet

Local Anesthetic/Vasoconstrictor Precautions No information available to require special precautions

Effects on Dental Treatment No significant effects or complications reported

Mechanism of Action Recombinant B-isoform homodimer of human platelet-derived growth factor (rPDGF-BB) which enhances formation of new granulation tissue, induces fibroblast proliferation, and differentiation to promote wound healing

Pharmacodynamics/Kinetics

Onset of action: Complete healing: 15% of patients within 8 weeks, 25% at 10 weeks

Absorption: Minimal

Distribution: Binds to PDGF-beta receptors in normal skin and granulation tissue

Pregnancy Risk Factor C

Beclomethasone (be kloe METH a sone)

Related Information

Respiratory Diseases *on page 1478*

U.S. Brand Names Beconase® [DSC]; Beconase® AQ; QVAR®

Canadian Brand Names Apo-Beclomethasone®; Gen-Beclo; Nu-Beclomethasone; Propaderm®; QVAR®; Rivanase AQ; Vanceril® AEM

Generic Available No

Synonyms Beclomethasone Dipropionate

Pharmacologic Category Corticosteroid, Inhalant (Oral); Corticosteroid, Nasal

Use

Oral inhalation: Maintenance and prophylactic treatment of asthma; includes those who require corticosteroids and those who may benefit from a dose reduction/elimination of systemically administered corticosteroids. Not for relief of acute bronchospasm

Nasal aerosol: Symptomatic treatment of seasonal or perennial rhinitis and to prevent recurrence of nasal polyps following surgery

Local Anesthetic/Vasoconstrictor Precautions No information available to require special precautions

Effects on Dental Treatment Key adverse event(s) related to dental treatment: Oral candidiasis, xerostomia (normal salivary flow resumes upon discontinuation), nasal dryness, and dry throat. Localized infections with *Candida*

albicans or *Aspergillus niger* occur frequently in the mouth and pharynx with repetitive use of oral inhaler; may require treatment with appropriate antifungal therapy or discontinuance of inhaler use.

Common Adverse Effects Frequency not defined.

Central nervous system: Agitation, depression, dizziness, dysphonia, headache, lightheadedness, mental disturbances

Dermatologic: Acneiform lesions, angioedema, atrophy, bruising, pruritus, purpura, striae, rash, urticaria

Endocrine & metabolic: Cushingoid features, growth velocity reduction in children and adolescents, HPA function suppression, weight gain

Gastrointestinal: Dry/irritated nose, throat and mouth, hoarseness, localized *Candida* or *Aspergillus* infections, loss of smell, loss of taste, nausea, unpleasant smell, unpleasant taste, vomiting

Local: Nasal spray: Burning, epistaxis, localized *Candida* infections, nasal septum perforation (rare), nasal stuffiness, nosebleeds, rhinorrhea, sneezing, transient irritation, ulceration of nasal mucosa (rare)

Ocular: Cataracts, glaucoma, increased intraocular pressure

Respiratory: Cough, paradoxical bronchospasm, pharyngitis, sinusitis, wheezing

Miscellaneous: Anaphylactic/anaphylactoid reactions, death (due to adrenal insufficiency, reported during and after transfer from systemic corticosteroids to aerosol in asthmatic patients), immediate and delayed hypersensitivity reactions

Dosage Nasal inhalation and oral inhalation dosage forms are not to be used interchangeably

Aqueous inhalation, nasal (Beconase® AQ): Children ≥6 years and Adults: 1-2 inhalations each nostril twice daily; total dose 168-336 mcg/day

Intranasal (Beconase®):

Children 6-12 years: 1 inhalation in each nostril 3 times/day; total dose 252 mcg/day

Children ≥12 years and Adults: 1 inhalation in each nostril 2-4 times/day or 2 inhalations each nostril twice daily (total dose 168-336 mcg/day); usual maximum maintenance: 1 inhalation in each nostril 3 times/day (252 mcg/day)

Oral inhalation (doses should be titrated to the lowest effective dose once asthma is controlled) (QVAR®):

Children 5-11 years: Initial: 40 mcg twice daily; maximum dose: 80 mcg twice daily

Children ≥12 years and Adults:

Patients previously on bronchodilators only: Initial dose 40-80 mcg twice daily; maximum dose: 320 mcg twice day

Patients previously on inhaled corticosteroids: Initial dose 40-160 mcg twice daily; maximum dose: 320 mcg twice daily

Mechanism of Action Controls the rate of protein synthesis, depresses the migration of polymorphonuclear leukocytes, fibroblasts, reverses capillary permeability, and lysosomal stabilization at the cellular level to prevent or control inflammation

Contraindications Hypersensitivity to beclomethasone or any component of the formulation; status asthmaticus

Warnings/Precautions Not to be used in status asthmaticus or for the relief of acute bronchospasm; safety and efficacy in children <6 years of age have not been established. May cause suppression of hypothalamic-pituitary-adrenal (HPA) axis, particularly in younger children or in patients receiving high doses for prolonged periods. Particular care is required when patients are transferred from systemic corticosteroids to inhaled products due to possible adrenal insufficiency or withdrawal from steroids, including an increase in allergic symptoms. Patients receiving 20 mg per day of prednisone (or equivalent) may be most susceptible. Fatalities have occurred due to adrenal insufficiency in asthmatic patients during and after transfer from systemic corticosteroids to aerosol steroids; aerosol steroids do **not** provide the systemic steroid needed to treat patients having trauma, surgery, or infections. Withdrawal and discontinuation of the corticosteroid should be done slowly and carefully.

Controlled clinical studies have shown that orally-inhaled and intranasal corticosteroids may cause a reduction in growth velocity in pediatric patients. (In studies of orally-inhaled corticosteroids, the mean reduction in growth velocity was approximately 1 centimeter per year [range 0.3-1.8 cm per year] and appears to be related to dose and duration of exposure.) The growth of pediatric patients receiving inhaled corticosteroids, should be monitored routinely (eg, via stadiometry). To minimize the systemic effects of orally-inhaled and intranasal corticosteroids, each patient should be titrated to the lowest effective dose.

(Continued)

Beclomethasone *(Continued)*

May suppress the immune system, patients may be more susceptible to infection. Use with caution in patients with systemic infections or ocular herpes simplex. Avoid exposure to chickenpox and measles. Corticosteroids should be used with caution in patients with diabetes, hypertension, osteoporosis, peptic ulcer, glaucoma, cataracts, or tuberculosis. Use caution in hepatic impairment.

Drug Interactions

Increased Effect/Toxicity: The addition of salmeterol has been demonstrated to improve response to inhaled corticosteroids (as compared to increasing steroid dosage).

Pharmacodynamics/Kinetics

Onset of action: Therapeutic effect: 1-4 weeks

Absorption: Readily; quickly hydrolyzed by pulmonary esterases prior to absorption

Distribution: Beclomethasone: 20 L; active metabolite: 424 L

Protein binding: 87%

Metabolism: Hepatic via CYP3A4 to active metabolites

Bioavailability: Of active metabolite, 44% following nasal inhalation (43% from swallowed portion)

Half-life elimination: Initial: 3 hours

Excretion: Feces (60%); urine (12%)

Pregnancy Risk Factor C

Dosage Forms AERO, oral inhalation (QVAR®): 40 mcg/inhalation [100 metered doses] (7.3 g); 80 mcg/inhalation [100 metered doses] (7.3 g). **SUSP, intranasal, aqueous** [spray] (Beconase® AQ): 42 mcg/inhalation [180 metered doses] (25 g)

Beclomethasone Dipropionate *see* Beclomethasone *on page 184*

Beconase® [DSC] *see* Beclomethasone *on page 184*

Beconase® AQ *see* Beclomethasone *on page 184*

Behenyl Alcohol *see* Docosanol *on page 459*

Belladonna and Opium (bel a DON a & OH pee um)

Related Information

Opium Tincture *on page 1015*

U.S. Brand Names B&O Supprettes®

Generic Available Yes

Synonyms Opium and Belladonna

Pharmacologic Category Analgesic Combination (Narcotic); Antispasmodic Agent, Urinary

Use Relief of moderate to severe pain associated with rectal or bladder tenesmus that may occur in postoperative states and neoplastic situations; pain associated with ureteral spasms not responsive to non-narcotic analgesics and to space intervals between injections of opiates

Local Anesthetic/Vasoconstrictor Precautions No information available to require special precautions

Effects on Dental Treatment Key adverse event(s) related to dental treatment: Xerostomia and changes in salivation (normal salivary flow resumes upon discontinuation), and dry throat and nose.

Mechanism of Action Anticholinergic alkaloids act primarily by competitive inhibition of the muscarinic actions of acetylcholine on structures innervated by postganglionic cholinergic neurons and on smooth muscle; resulting effects include antisecretory activity on exocrine glands and intestinal mucosa and smooth muscle relaxation. Contains many narcotic alkaloids including morphine; its mechanism for gastric motility inhibition is primarily due to this morphine content; it results in a decrease in digestive secretions, an increase in GI muscle tone, and therefore a reduction in GI propulsion.

Pregnancy Risk Factor C

Belladonna, Phenobarbital, and Ergotamine

(bel a DON a, fee noe BAR bi tal, & er GOT a meen)

Related Information

Ergotamine *on page 505*

Phenobarbital *on page 1073*

U.S. Brand Names Bellamine S; Bel-Tabs

Canadian Brand Names Bellergal® Spacetabs®

Generic Available Yes

Synonyms Belladonna, Phenobarbital, and Ergotamine Tartrate; Ergotamine Tartrate, Belladonna, and Phenobarbital; Phenobarbital, Belladonna, and Ergotamine Tartrate

Pharmacologic Category Ergot Derivative

Use Management and treatment of menopausal disorders, GI disorders, and recurrent throbbing headache

Local Anesthetic/Vasoconstrictor Precautions No information available to require special precautions

Effects on Dental Treatment Key adverse event(s) related to dental treatment: Xerostomia (normal salivary flow resumes upon discontinuation), dry throat, nasal dryness, and difficulty swallowing.

Pregnancy Risk Factor X

Belladonna, Phenobarbital, and Ergotamine Tartrate *see* Belladonna, Phenobarbital, and Ergotamine *on page 186*

Bellamine S *see* Belladonna, Phenobarbital, and Ergotamine *on page 186*

Bel-Tabs *see* Belladonna, Phenobarbital, and Ergotamine *on page 186*

Benadryl® Allergy [OTC] *see* DiphenhydrAMINE *on page 448*

Benadryl® Allergy and Sinus Fastmelt™ [OTC] *see* Diphenhydramine and Pseudoephedrine *on page 451*

Benadryl® Allergy/Sinus [OTC] *see* Diphenhydramine and Pseudoephedrine *on page 451*

Benadryl® Children's Allergy and Cold Fastmelt™ [OTC] *see* Diphenhydramine and Pseudoephedrine *on page 451*

Benadryl® Children's Allergy and Sinus [OTC] *see* Diphenhydramine and Pseudoephedrine *on page 451*

Benadryl® Dye-Free Allergy [OTC] *see* DiphenhydrAMINE *on page 448*

Benadryl® Gel [OTC] *see* DiphenhydrAMINE *on page 448*

Benadryl® Gel Extra Strength [OTC] *see* DiphenhydrAMINE *on page 448*

Benadryl® Injection *see* DiphenhydrAMINE *on page 448*

Benazepril (ben AY ze pril)

Related Information

Cardiovascular Diseases *on page 1458*

U.S. Brand Names Lotensin®

Canadian Brand Names Lotensin®

Mexican Brand Names Lotensin®

Generic Available Yes

Synonyms Benazepril Hydrochloride

Pharmacologic Category Angiotensin-Converting Enzyme (ACE) Inhibitor

Use Treatment of hypertension, either alone or in combination with other antihypertensive agents

Unlabeled/Investigational Use Treatment of left ventricular dysfunction after myocardial infarction

Local Anesthetic/Vasoconstrictor Precautions No information available to require special precautions

Effects on Dental Treatment No significant effects or complications reported

Common Adverse Effects 1% to 10%:

Cardiovascular: Postural dizziness (2%)

Central nervous system: Headache (6%), dizziness (4%), fatigue (3%), somnolence (2%)

Endocrine & metabolic: Hyperkalemia (1%), increased uric acid

Gastrointestinal: Nausea (2%)

Renal: Increased serum creatinine (2%), worsening of renal function may occur in patients with bilateral renal artery stenosis or hypovolemia

Respiratory: Cough (1% to 10%)

Dosage Oral: Hypertension:

Children ≥6 years: Initial: 0.2 mg/kg/day as monotherapy; dosing range: 0.1-0.6 mg/kg/day (maximum dose: 40 mg/day)

Adults: Initial: 10 mg/day in patients not receiving a diuretic; 20-40 mg/day as a single dose or 2 divided doses; the need for twice-daily dosing should be assessed by monitoring peak (2-6 hours after dosing) and trough responses.

Note: Patients taking diuretics should have them discontinued 2-3 days prior to starting benazepril. If they cannot be discontinued, then initial dose should be 5 mg; restart after blood pressure is stabilized if needed.

Elderly: Oral: Initial: 5-10 mg/day in single or divided doses; usual range: 20-40 mg/day; adjust for renal function; also see "Note" in Adults dosing.

Dosing interval in renal impairment: Cl_{cr} <30 mL/minute:

Children: Use is not recommended.

Adults: Administer 5 mg/day initially; maximum daily dose: 40 mg.

(Continued)

Benazepril *(Continued)*

Hemodialysis: Moderately dialyzable (20% to 50%); administer dose postdialysis or administer 25% to 35% supplemental dose.

Peritoneal dialysis: Supplemental dose is not necessary.

Mechanism of Action Competitive inhibition of angiotensin I being converted to angiotensin II, a potent vasoconstrictor, through the angiotensin I-converting enzyme (ACE) activity, with resultant lower levels of angiotensin II which causes an increase in plasma renin activity and a reduction in aldosterone secretion

Contraindications Hypersensitivity to benazepril or any component of the formulation; angioedema or serious hypersensitivity related to previous treatment with an ACE inhibitor; bilateral renal artery stenosis; patients with idiopathic or hereditary angioedema; pregnancy (2nd and 3rd trimesters)

Warnings/Precautions Anaphylactic reactions can occur. Angioedema can occur at any time during treatment (especially following first dose). Angioedema may involve head and neck (potentially affecting the airway) or the intestine (presenting with abdominal pain). Careful blood pressure monitoring with first dose (hypotension can occur especially in volume depleted patients). Dosage adjustment needed in renal impairment. Use with caution in hypovolemia; collagen vascular diseases; valvular stenosis (particularly aortic stenosis); hyperkalemia; or before, during, or immediately after anesthesia. Avoid rapid dosage escalation which may lead to renal insufficiency. Hypersensitivity reactions may be seen during hemodialysis with high-flux dialysis membranes (eg, AN69). Deterioration in renal function can occur with initiation. Use with caution in unilateral renal artery stenosis and pre-existing renal insufficiency.

Drug Interactions

Increased Effect/Toxicity: Potassium supplements, co-trimoxazole (high dose), angiotensin II receptor antagonists (eg, candesartan, losartan, irbesartan) or potassium-sparing diuretics (amiloride, spironolactone, triamterene) may result in elevated serum potassium levels when combined with benazepril. ACE inhibitor effects may be increased by phenothiazines or probenecid (increases levels of captopril). ACE inhibitors may increase serum concentrations/effects of digoxin, lithium, and sulfonlyureas. Diuretics have additive hypotensive effects with ACE inhibitors, and hypovolemia increases the potential for adverse renal effects of ACE inhibitors. In patients with compromised renal function, coadministration with NSAIDs may result in further deterioration of renal function. Allopurinol and ACE inhibitors may cause a higher risk of hypersensitivity reaction when taken concurrently.

Decreased Effect: Aspirin (high dose) may reduce the therapeutic effects of ACE inhibitors; at low dosages this does not appear to be significant. Rifampin may decrease the effect of ACE inhibitors. Antacids may decrease the bioavailability of ACE inhibitors (may be more likely to occur with captopril); separate administration times by 1-2 hours. NSAIDs, specifically indomethacin, may reduce the hypotensive effects of ACE inhibitors.

Ethanol/Nutrition/Herb Interactions Herb/Nutraceutical: Avoid dong quai if using for hypertension (has estrogenic activity). Avoid ephedra, yohimbe, ginseng (may worsen hypertension). Avoid garlic (may have increased antihypertensive effect).

Pharmacodynamics/Kinetics

Reduction in plasma angiotensin-converting enzyme (ACE) activity:

Onset of action: Peak effect: 1-2 hours after 2-20 mg dose

Duration: >90% inhibition for 24 hours after 5-20 mg dose

Reduction in blood pressure:

Peak effect: Single dose: 2-4 hours; Continuous therapy: 2 weeks

Absorption: Rapid (37%); food does not alter significantly; metabolite (benazeprilat) itself unsuitable for oral administration due to poor absorption

Distribution: V_d: ~8.7 L

Metabolism: Rapidly and extensively hepatic to its active metabolite, benazeprilat, via enzymatic hydrolysis; extensive first-pass effect

Half-life elimination: Benazeprilat: Effective: 10-11 hours; Terminal: Children: 5 hours, Adults: 22 hours

Time to peak: Parent drug: 0.5-1 hour

Excretion: Clearance: Nonrenal clearance (ie, biliary, metabolic) appears to contribute to the elimination of benazeprilat (11% to 12%), particularly patients with severe renal impairment; hepatic clearance is the main elimination route of unchanged benazepril

Dialysis: ~6% of metabolite removed in 4 hours of dialysis following 10 mg of benazepril administered 2 hours prior to procedure; parent compound not found in dialysate

Pregnancy Risk Factor C/D (2nd and 3rd trimesters)

Dosage Forms TAB: 5 mg, 10 mg, 20 mg, 40 mg

Benazepril and Amlodipine *see* Amlodipine and Benazepril *on page 110*

Benazepril and Hydrochlorothiazide

(ben AY ze pril & hye droe klor oh THYE a zide)

Related Information

Benazepril *on page 187*

Hydrochlorothiazide *on page 699*

U.S. Brand Names Lotensin® HCT

Generic Available Yes

Synonyms Hydrochlorothiazide and Benazepril

Pharmacologic Category Antihypertensive Agent, Combination

Use Treatment of hypertension

Local Anesthetic/Vasoconstrictor Precautions No information available to require special precautions

Effects on Dental Treatment No significant effects or complications reported

Common Adverse Effects See individual agents.

Pharmacodynamics/Kinetics See individual agents.

Pregnancy Risk Factor C/D (2nd and 3rd trimesters)

Benazepril Hydrochloride *see* Benazepril *on page 187*

Bendroflumethiazide

(ben droe floo meth EYE a zide)

Related Information

Cardiovascular Diseases *on page 1458*

U.S. Brand Names Naturetin® [DSC]

Generic Available No

Pharmacologic Category Diuretic, Thiazide

Use Management of mild to moderate hypertension, edema associated with congestive heart failure, pregnancy, or nephrotic syndrome; reportedly does not alter serum electrolyte concentrations appreciably at recommended doses

Local Anesthetic/Vasoconstrictor Precautions No information available to require special precautions

Effects on Dental Treatment Key adverse event(s) related to dental treatment: Orthostatic hypotension.

Common Adverse Effects 1% to 10%:

Cardiovascular: Orthostatic hypotension

Endocrine & metabolic: Hyponatremia, hypokalemia

Gastrointestinal: Anorexia, upset stomach, diarrhea

Mechanism of Action Like other thiazide diuretics, it inhibits sodium, chloride, and water reabsorption in the renal distal tubules, thereby producing diuresis with a resultant reduction in plasma volume; hypothetically may reduce peripheral resistance through increased prostacyclin synthesis

Drug Interactions

Increased Effect/Toxicity: Increased effect of thiazides with furosemide and other loop diuretics. Increased hypotension and/or renal adverse effects of ACE inhibitors may result in aggressively diuresed patients. Beta-blockers increase hyperglycemic effects of thiazides in type 2 diabetes mellitus. Cyclosporine and thiazides can increase the risk of gout or renal toxicity. Digoxin toxicity can be exacerbated if a thiazide induces hypokalemia or hypomagnesemia. Lithium toxicity can occur with thiazides due to reduced renal excretion of lithium. Thiazides may prolong the duration of action with neuromuscular blocking agents.

Decreased Effect: Effects of oral hypoglycemics may be decreased. Decreased absorption of hydrochlorothiazide with cholestyramine and colestipol. NSAIDs can decrease the efficacy of thiazides, reducing the diuretic and antihypertensive effects.

Pregnancy Risk Factor D

Bendroflumethiazide and Nadolol *see* Nadolol and Bendroflumethiazide *on page 957*

BeneFix® *see* Factor IX *on page 571*

Benemid [DSC] *see* Probenecid *on page 1124*

Benicar™ *see* Olmesartan *on page 1010*

Benicar HCT™ *see* Olmesartan and Hydrochlorothiazide *on page 1010*

Benoquin® *see* Monobenzone *on page 944*

Bentoquatam

(BEN toe kwa tam)

U.S. Brand Names IvyBlock® [OTC]

Generic Available No

Synonyms Quaternium-18 Bentonite

(Continued)

Bentoquatam *(Continued)*

Pharmacologic Category Topical Skin Product

Use Skin protectant for the prevention of allergic contact dermatitis to poison oak, ivy, and sumac

Local Anesthetic/Vasoconstrictor Precautions No information available to require special precautions

Effects on Dental Treatment No significant effects or complications reported

Mechanism of Action An organoclay substance which is capable of absorbing or binding to urushiol, the active principle in poison oak, ivy, and sumac. Bentoquatam serves as a barrier, blocking urushiol skin contact/absorption.

Bentyl® *see* Dicyclomine *on page 432*

Benylin® Adult [OTC] *see* Dextromethorphan *on page 421*

Benylin® Expectorant [OTC] *see* Guaifenesin and Dextromethorphan *on page 673*

Benylin® Pediatric [OTC] *see* Dextromethorphan *on page 421*

Benza® [OTC] *see* Benzalkonium Chloride *on page 190*

Benzac® *see* Benzoyl Peroxide *on page 194*

Benzac® AC *see* Benzoyl Peroxide *on page 194*

Benzac® AC Wash *see* Benzoyl Peroxide *on page 194*

BenzaClin® *see* Clindamycin and Benzoyl Peroxide *on page 350*

Benzac® W *see* Benzoyl Peroxide *on page 194*

Benzac® W Wash *see* Benzoyl Peroxide *on page 194*

Benzagel® *see* Benzoyl Peroxide *on page 194*

Benzagel® Wash *see* Benzoyl Peroxide *on page 194*

Benzalkonium Chloride (benz al KOE nee um KLOR ide)

Related Information

Periodontal Diseases *on page 1542*

U.S. Brand Names Benza® [OTC]; HandClens® [OTC]; 3M™ Cavilon™ Skin Cleanser [OTC]; Ony-Clear [OTC] [DSC]; Zephiran® [OTC]

Generic Available Yes

Synonyms BAC

Pharmacologic Category Antibiotic, Topical

Use Surface antiseptic and germicidal preservative

Local Anesthetic/Vasoconstrictor Precautions No information available to require special precautions

Effects on Dental Treatment No significant effects or complications reported

Common Adverse Effects 1% to 10%: Hypersensitivity

Pregnancy Risk Factor C

Benzalkonium Chloride and Isopropyl Alcohol

(benz al KOE nee um KLOR ide & eye so PRO pil AL koe hol)

Related Information

Oral Viral Infections *on page 1547*

U.S. Brand Names Viroxyn® [OTC]

Generic Available No

Synonyms Isopropyl Alcohol Tincture of Benzylkonium Chloride

Pharmacologic Category Antiseptic, Topical

Dental Use Topical: Germicidal for the treatment of cold sores/fever blisters

Local Anesthetic/Vasoconstrictor Precautions No information available to require special precautions

Effects on Dental Treatment No significant effects or complications reported

Significant Adverse Effects Frequency not defined

Ocular: Irritation (following inadvertent contact)

Respiratory: Vapors may cause coughing, dyspnea

Dosage Topical: One single application treatment to affected area. Secondary events (new viral load in the initial lesion, which may occur 12-72 hours after initial symptoms) or additional sore presentations will require additional treatment with a new vial. See Comments for application instructions.

Manufacturer states medication should not be used >3 times/day; however, instructions indicate that a single application is generally effective if instructions are followed.

Mechanism of Action Germicidal due to disruption of the viral capsid coat by the quaternary ammonium benzalkonium chloride ingredient

Contraindications Hypersensitivity to benzalkonium chloride, isopropyl alcohol, or any component of the formulation

Warnings/Precautions For topical use only; ingestion may lead to gastric irritation or distress. Avoid contact with eyes; flush with eye bath if inadvertent contact occurs. Avoid use of anionic cleansers or acidic products for at least 1 hour following application (active ingredient will be neutralized); avoid the use of soap, toothpaste, cleansers, or drinks containing citric acid (including lemonade and orange juice). Should not be used >3 times/day. Avoid use in pregnant or lactating women. Avoid use in children <2 years of age. Formulation in isopropyl alcohol is flammable; avoid use near sparks, flames, or high temperatures.

Drug Interactions No specific drug interactions have been reported

Dietary Considerations Avoid citric acid-containing beverages (eg, lemonade or orange juice) for at least 1 hour following application

Dosage Forms Solution, topical (Viroxyn®): Benzalkonium 0.13% in isopropyl alcohol [kit includes 3 single-dose applicators]

Comments Use this product according to the following directions from the manufacturer. 1) Prior to treatment, clean area to be treated of all other preparations (ointments, treatments, lipstick). Do not use soap or other cleansers. A dry wipe may be sufficient, or you may use water or alcohol if necessary. 2) Remove cap from vial and replace on the other end over the clear plastic tube. Hold vial between thumb and index finger, applicator end up. Pinch vial in the center at top of cap until the inner ampoule of medication breaks. 3) Hold white applicator down and allow medication to saturate the swab. If necessary, pinch vial gently until a drop of medication just appears. 4) Place the applicator against the area of skin to be treated so that the tip of the applicator is held flat against the skin. The key is to massage medication into the sore and the surrounding area by rubbing. Do not rub so hard that you cause damage to the skin. For best results, the patient should massage drug into the sore by rubbing. The rubbing should proceed for about 10 minutes or until all the drug has been massaged into the sore. The application may sting. This is normal and should subside quickly. For best results, medication must penetrate the subepidermal layers of the skin to site of infection. The ingredients facilitate penetration, but mechanical action is critical. Simply dabbing the drug onto the sore is not likely to give best results. 5) If treating at prodrome (tingling sensation before lesion erupts), a more vigorous rubbing is easily tolerated and gives best results. If the lesion has progressed to vesicle or ulcerated lesion, the patient may prefer to rub less vigorously but for a longer time period. 6) Keep applicator saturated at all times. If necessary, pause and hold vial so as to allow medication to flow into applicator. When finished recap vial. Dispose of immediately. Do not disassemble. Store at room temperature. Flammable; do not expose to high heat or flame. Keep out of reach of children.

Benzamycin® *see* Erythromycin and Benzoyl Peroxide *on page 512*

Benzamycin® Pak *see* Erythromycin and Benzoyl Peroxide *on page 512*

Benzashave® *see* Benzoyl Peroxide *on page 194*

Benzathine Benzylpenicillin *see* Penicillin G Benzathine *on page 1058*

Benzathine Penicillin G *see* Penicillin G Benzathine *on page 1058*

Benzazoline Hydrochloride *see* Tolazoline *on page 1309*

Benzedrex® [OTC] *see* Propylhexedrine *on page 1144*

Benzene Hexachloride *see* Lindane *on page 829*

Benzhexol Hydrochloride *see* Trihexyphenidyl *on page 1340*

Benzisoquinolinedione *see* Amonafide *on page 112*

Benzmethyzin *see* Procarbazine *on page 1125*

Benzocaine (BEN zoe kane)

Related Information

Mouth Pain, Cold Sore, and Canker Sore Products *on page 1633*
Oral Pain *on page 1526*

U.S. Brand Names Americaine® [OTC]; Americaine® Anesthetic Lubricant; Anbesol® [OTC]; Anbesol® Baby [OTC]; Anbesol® Maximum Strength [OTC]; Babee® Teething® [OTC]; Benzodent® [OTC]; Chiggerex® [OTC]; Chiggertox® [OTC]; Cylex® [OTC]; Detane® [OTC]; Foille® [OTC]; Foille® Medicated First Aid [OTC]; Foille® Plus [OTC]; HDA® Toothache [OTC]; Hurricaine®; Lanacane® [OTC]; Mycinettes® [OTC]; Orabase®-B [OTC]; Orajel® [OTC]; Orajel® Baby [OTC]; Orajel® Baby Nighttime [OTC]; Orajel® Maximum Strength [OTC]; Orasol® [OTC]; Solarcaine® [OTC]; Trocaine® [OTC]; Zilactin®-B [OTC]; Zilactin® Baby [OTC]

Canadian Brand Names Anbesol® Baby; Zilactin-B®; Zilactin Baby®

Generic Available Yes

Synonyms Ethyl Aminobenzoate

Pharmacologic Category Local Anesthetic

Dental Use Ester-type topical local anesthetic for temporary relief of pain associated with toothache, minor sore throat pain, and canker sore

(Continued)

Benzocaine *(Continued)*

Use Temporary relief of pain associated with local anesthetic for pruritic dermatosis, pruritus, minor burns, acute congestive and serous otitis media, swimmer's ear, otitis externa, toothache, minor sore throat pain, canker sores, hemorrhoids, rectal fissures, anesthetic lubricant for passage of catheters and endoscopic tubes; nonprescription diet aid

Local Anesthetic/Vasoconstrictor Precautions No information available to require special precautions

Effects on Dental Treatment No significant effects or complications reported

Significant Adverse Effects Dose-related and may result in high plasma levels

1% to 10%:

Dermatologic: Angioedema, contact dermatitis

Local: Burning, stinging

<1% (Limited to important or life-threatening): Edema, methemoglobinemia in infants, urethritis, urticaria

Dosage Children and Adults:

Mucous membranes: Dosage varies depending on area to be anesthetized and vascularity of tissues

Oral mouth/throat preparations: Refer to specific package labeling or as directed by physician. **Note:** Do not administer for >2 days or use in children <2 years of age, unless directed by physician.

Topical: Apply to affected area as needed

Mechanism of Action Ester local anesthetic blocks both the initiation and conduction of nerve impulses by decreasing the neuronal membrane's permeability to sodium ions, which results in inhibition of depolarization with resultant blockade of conduction

Contraindications Hypersensitivity to benzocaine, other ester-type local anesthetics, or any component of the formulation; secondary bacterial infection of area; ophthalmic use; see package labeling for specific contraindications

Warnings/Precautions Not intended for use when infections are present

Drug Interactions May antagonize actions of sulfonamides

Dietary Considerations When used as a nonprescription diet aid, take just prior to food consumption.

Pharmacodynamics/Kinetics

Absorption: Topical: Poor to intact skin; well absorbed from mucous membranes and traumatized skin

Metabolism: Hepatic (to a lesser extent) and plasma via hydrolysis by cholinesterase

Excretion: Urine (as metabolites)

Pregnancy Risk Factor C

Lactation Excretion in breast milk unknown

Dosage Forms

Aerosol, oral spray (Hurricaine®): 20% (60 mL) [cherry flavor]

Aerosol, topical spray:

- Americaine®: 20% (20 mL, 120 mL)
- Foille®: 5% (97.5 mL) [contains chloroxylenol 0.63%]
- Foille® Plus: 5% (105 mL) [contains chloroxylenol 0.63% and alcohol 57.33%]
- Solarcaine®: 20% (90 mL, 120 mL, 135 mL) [contains triclosan, alcohol 0.13%]

Cream, topical: 5% (30 g, 454 g)

- Lanacane®: 20% (30g)

Gel, oral:

- Anbesol® 6.3% (7.5 g)
- Anbesol® Baby, Detane®, Orajel® Baby: 7.5% (7.5 g, 10 g, 15 g)
- Anbesol® Maximum Strength, Orajel® Maximum Strength: 20% (6 g, 7.5 g, 10 g)
- HDA® Toothache: 6.5% (15 mL) [contains benzyl alcohol]
- Hurricaine®: 20% (5 g, 30 g) [mint, pina colada, watermelon, and wild cherry flavors]
- Orabase-B®: 20% (7 g)
- Orajel®, Orajel® Baby Nighttime, Zilactin®-B, Zilactin® Baby: 10% (6 g, 7.5 g, 10 g)

Gel, topical (Americaine® Anesthetic Lubricant): 20% (2.5 g, 28 g) [contains 0.1% benzethonium chloride

Liquid, oral:

- Anbesol®, Orasol®: 6.3% (9 mL, 15 mL, 30 mL)
- Anbesol® Maximum Strength: 20% (9 mL, 14 mL)

Hurricaine®: 20% (30 mL) [pina colada and wild cherry flavors]
Orajel®: 10% (13 mL) [contains tartrazine]
Orajel® Baby: 7.5% (13 mL)
Liquid, topical (Chiggertox®): 2% (30 mL)
Lotion, oral (Babee® Teething): 2.5% (15 mL)
Lozenge:
Cylex®, Mycinettes®: 15 mg [Cylex® contains cetylpyridinium chloride 5 mg]
Trocaine®: 10 mg
Ointment, oral (Benzodent®): 20% (30 g)
Ointment, topical:
Chiggerex®: 2% (52 g)
Foille® Medicated First Aid: 5% (3.5 g, 28 g) [contains chloroxylenol 0.1%, benzyl alcohol; corn oil base]
Paste, oral (Orabase®-B): 20% (7 g)

Benzocaine and Antipyrine *see* Antipyrine and Benzocaine *on page 135*

Benzocaine and Cetylpyridinium Chloride *see* Cetylpyridinium and Benzocaine *on page 301*

Benzocaine, Butyl Aminobenzoate, Tetracaine, and Benzalkonium Chloride

(BEN zoe kane, BYOO til a meen oh BENZ oh ate, TET ra kane, & benz al KOE nee um KLOR ide)

Related Information
Benzalkonium Chloride *on page 190*
Benzocaine *on page 191*
Tetracaine *on page 1278*

U.S. Brand Names Cetacaine®

Generic Available No

Synonyms Tetracaine Hydrochloride, Benzocaine Butyl Aminobenzoate, and Benzalkonium Chloride

Pharmacologic Category Local Anesthetic

Use Topical anesthetic to control pain or gagging

Local Anesthetic/Vasoconstrictor Precautions No information available to require special precautions

Effects on Dental Treatment No significant effects or complications reported

Significant Adverse Effects Dose related and may result from high plasma levels

1% to 10%:
Dermatologic: Contact dermatitis, angioedema
Local: Burning, stinging

<1% (Limited to important or life-threatening): Edema, methemoglobinemia (risk may be increased in infants), tenderness, urethritis, urticaria,

Dosage Apply to affected area for approximately 1 second or less

Pregnancy Risk Factor C

Lactation For topical use

Dosage Forms
Aerosol, topical: Benzocaine 14%, butyl aminobenzoate 2%, tetracaine 2%, and benzalkonium chloride 0.5% (56 g)
Gel, topical: Benzocaine 14%, butyl aminobenzoate 2%, tetracaine 2%, and benzalkonium chloride 0.5% (29 g)
Liquid, topical: Benzocaine 14%, butyl aminobenzoate 2%, tetracaine 2%, and benzalkonium chloride 0.5% (56 mL)

Benzodent® [OTC] *see* Benzocaine *on page 191*

Benzoin (BEN zoin)

U.S. Brand Names TinBen® [OTC] [DSC]

Generic Available Yes

Synonyms Gum Benjamin

Pharmacologic Category Antibiotic, Topical; Topical Skin Product

Use Protective application for irritations of the skin; sometimes used in boiling water as steam inhalants for their expectorant and soothing action

Local Anesthetic/Vasoconstrictor Precautions No information available to require special precautions

Effects on Dental Treatment No significant effects or complications reported

Benzonatate (ben ZOE na tate)

Related Information
Management of Patients Undergoing Cancer Therapy *on page 1569*

U.S. Brand Names Tessalon®

(Continued)

Benzonatate *(Continued)*

Canadian Brand Names Tessalon®

Mexican Brand Names Tesalon®; Tusical®; Tusitato®

Generic Available Yes

Pharmacologic Category Antitussive

Use Symptomatic relief of nonproductive cough

Local Anesthetic/Vasoconstrictor Precautions No information available to require special precautions

Effects on Dental Treatment No significant effects or complications reported

Common Adverse Effects 1% to 10%:

Central nervous system: Sedation, headache, dizziness
Dermatologic: Rash
Gastrointestinal: GI upset
Neuromuscular & skeletal: Numbness in chest
Ocular: Burning sensation in eyes
Respiratory: Nasal congestion

Dosage Children >10 years and Adults: Oral: 100 mg 3 times/day or every 4 hours up to 600 mg/day

Mechanism of Action Tetracaine congener with antitussive properties; suppresses cough by topical anesthetic action on the respiratory stretch receptors

Contraindications Hypersensitivity to benzonatate, related compounds (such as tetracaine), or any component of the formulation

Pharmacodynamics/Kinetics

Onset of action: Therapeutic: 15-20 minutes
Duration: 3-8 hours

Pregnancy Risk Factor C

Dosage Forms CAP: 100 mg; (Tessalon®): 100 mg, 200 mg

Benzoyl Peroxide (BEN zoe il peer OKS ide)

U.S. Brand Names Benzac®; Benzac® AC; Benzac® AC Wash; Benzac® W; Benzac® W Wash; Benzagel®; Benzagel® Wash; Benzashave®; Brevoxyl®; Brevoxyl® Cleansing; Brevoxyl® Wash; Clearplex [OTC]; Clinac™ BPO; Del Aqua®; Desquam-E™; Desquam-X®; Exact® Acne Medication [OTC]; Fostex® 10% BPO [OTC]; Loroxide® [OTC]; Neutrogena® Acne Mask [OTC]; Neutrogena® On The Spot® Acne Treatment [OTC]; Oxy 10® Balanced Medicated Face Wash [OTC]; Oxy 10® Balance Spot Treatment [OTC]; Palmer's® Skin Success Acne [OTC]; PanOxyl®; PanOxyl®-AQ; PanOxyl® Aqua Gel; PanOxyl® Bar [OTC]; Seba-Gel™; Triaz®; Triaz® Cleanser; Zapzyt® [OTC]

Canadian Brand Names Acetoxyl®; Benoxyl®; Benzac AC®; Benzac W® Gel; Benzac W® Wash; Desquam-X®; Oxyderm™; PanOxyl®; PanOxyl®-AQ; Solugel®

Mexican Brand Names Benoxyl®; Benzac®; Benzaderm®; Solugel®

Generic Available Yes: Excludes cream and soap

Pharmacologic Category Topical Skin Product; Topical Skin Product, Acne

Use Adjunctive treatment of mild to moderate acne vulgaris and acne rosacea

Local Anesthetic/Vasoconstrictor Precautions No information available to require special precautions

Effects on Dental Treatment No significant effects or complications reported

Common Adverse Effects 1% to 10%: Dermatologic: Irritation, contact dermatitis, dryness, erythema, peeling, stinging

Mechanism of Action Releases free-radical oxygen which oxidizes bacterial proteins in the sebaceous follicles decreasing the number of anaerobic bacteria and decreasing irritating-type free fatty acids

Pharmacodynamics/Kinetics

Absorption: ~5% via skin; gel more penetrating than cream
Metabolism: Converted to benzoic acid in skin

Pregnancy Risk Factor C

Benzoyl Peroxide and Clindamycin *see* Clindamycin and Benzoyl Peroxide *on page 350*

Benzoyl Peroxide and Erythromycin *see* Erythromycin and Benzoyl Peroxide *on page 512*

Benzoyl Peroxide and Hydrocortisone

(BEN zoe il peer OKS ide & hye droe KOR ti sone)

Related Information

Benzoyl Peroxide *on page 194*
Hydrocortisone *on page 714*

U.S. Brand Names Vanoxide-HC®

Canadian Brand Names Vanoxide-HC
Generic Available No
Synonyms Hydrocortisone and Benzoyl Peroxide
Pharmacologic Category Topical Skin Product; Topical Skin Product, Acne
Use Treatment of acne vulgaris and oily skin
Local Anesthetic/Vasoconstrictor Precautions No information available to require special precautions
Effects on Dental Treatment No significant effects or complications reported
Common Adverse Effects See individual agents.
Drug Interactions
Cytochrome P450 Effect: Hydrocortisone: **Substrate** of CYP3A4 (minor); **Induces** CYP3A4 (weak)
Pharmacodynamics/Kinetics See individual agents.
Pregnancy Risk Factor C

Benzphetamine (benz FET a meen)

U.S. Brand Names Didrex®
Canadian Brand Names Didrex®
Generic Available No
Synonyms Benzphetamine Hydrochloride
Pharmacologic Category Anorexiant
Use Short-term adjunct in exogenous obesity
Local Anesthetic/Vasoconstrictor Precautions Use with caution since amphetamines have actions similar to epinephrine and norepinephrine
Effects on Dental Treatment Key adverse event(s) related to dental treatment: Xerostomia (normal salivary flow resumes upon discontinuation) and metallic taste.
Common Adverse Effects Frequency not defined.

Cardiovascular: Hypertension, palpitations, tachycardia, chest pain, T-wave changes, arrhythmias, pulmonary hypertension, valvulopathy

Central nervous system: Euphoria, nervousness, insomnia, restlessness, dizziness, anxiety, headache, agitation, confusion, mental depression, psychosis, CVA, seizure

Dermatologic: Alopecia, urticaria, skin rash, ecchymosis, erythema

Endocrine & metabolic: Changes in libido, gynecomastia, menstrual irregularities, porphyria

Gastrointestinal: Nausea, vomiting, abdominal cramps, constipation, xerostomia, metallic taste

Genitourinary: Impotence

Hematologic: Bone marrow depression, agranulocytosis, leukopenia

Neuromuscular & skeletal: Tremor

Ocular: Blurred vision, mydriasis

Restrictions C-III
Mechanism of Action Noncatechol sympathomimetic amines with pharmacologic actions similar to ephedrine; require breakdown by monoamine oxidase for inactivation; produce central nervous system and respiratory stimulation, a pressor response, mydriasis, bronchodilation, and contraction of the urinary sphincter; thought to have a direct effect on both alpha- and beta-receptor sites in the peripheral system, as well as release stores of norepinephrine in adrenergic nerve terminals; central nervous system action is thought to occur in the cerebral cortex and reticular activating system; anorexigenic effect is probably secondary to the CNS-stimulating effect; the site of action is probably the hypothalamic feeding center.
Drug Interactions
Cytochrome P450 Effect: Substrate of CYP2B6 (minor), 3A4 (major)
Increased Effect/Toxicity: Amphetamines may precipitate hypertensive crisis or serotonin syndrome in patients receiving MAO inhibitors (selegiline >10 mg/day, isocarboxazid, phenelzine, tranylcypromine, furazolidone). Serotonin syndrome has also been associated with combinations of amphetamines and SSRIs; these combinations should be avoided. TCAs may enhance the effects of amphetamines, potentially leading to hypertensive crisis. Large doses of antacids or urinary alkalinizers increase the half-life and duration of action of amphetamines. May precipitate arrhythmias in patients receiving general anesthetics. Inhibitors of CYP2D6 may increase the effects of amphetamines (includes amiodarone, cimetidine, delavirdine, fluoxetine, paroxetine, propafenone, quinidine, and ritonavir). CYP3A4 inhibitors may increase the levels/effects of benzphetamine; example inhibitors include azole antifungals, ciprofloxacin, clarithromycin, diclofenac, doxycycline, erythromycin, imatinib, isoniazid, nefazodone, nicardipine, propofol, protease inhibitors, quinidine, and verapamil.

(Continued)

Benzphetamine *(Continued)*

Decreased Effect: Amphetamines inhibit the antihypertensive response to guanethidine and guanadrel. Urinary acidifiers decrease the half-life and duration of action of amphetamines. CYP3A4 inducers may decrease the levels/effects of benzphetamine; example inducers include aminoglutethimide, carbamazepine, nafcillin, nevirapine, phenobarbital, phenytoin, and rifamycins.

Pregnancy Risk Factor X

Benzphetamine Hydrochloride *see* Benzphetamine *on page 195*

Benztropine (BENZ troe peen)

U.S. Brand Names Cogentin®

Canadian Brand Names Apo-Benztropine®; Cogentin®

Generic Available Yes: Tablet

Synonyms Benztropine Mesylate

Pharmacologic Category Anticholinergic Agent; Anti-Parkinson's Agent, Anticholinergic

Use Adjunctive treatment of Parkinson's disease; treatment of drug-induced extrapyramidal symptoms (except tardive dyskinesia)

Local Anesthetic/Vasoconstrictor Precautions No information available to require special precautions

Effects on Dental Treatment Key adverse event(s) related to dental treatment: Xerostomia and changes in salivation (normal salivary flow resumes upon discontinuation), dry throat, and nasal dryness (very prevalent).

Common Adverse Effects Frequency not defined.

Cardiovascular: Tachycardia

Central nervous system: Confusion, disorientation, memory impairment, toxic psychosis, visual hallucinations

Dermatologic: Rash

Endocrine & metabolic: Heat stroke, hyperthermia

Gastrointestinal: Xerostomia, nausea, vomiting, constipation, ileus

Genitourinary: Urinary retention, dysuria

Ocular: Blurred vision, mydriasis

Miscellaneous: Fever

Mechanism of Action Possesses both anticholinergic and antihistaminic effects. *In vitro* anticholinergic activity approximates that of atropine; *in vivo* it is only about half as active as atropine. Animal data suggest its antihistaminic activity and duration of action approach that of pyrilamine maleate. May also inhibit the reuptake and storage of dopamine and thereby, prolong the action of dopamine.

Drug Interactions

Cytochrome P450 Effect: Substrate of CYP2D6 (minor)

Increased Effect/Toxicity: Central and/or peripheral anticholinergic syndrome can occur when benztropine is administered with amantadine, rimantadine, narcotic analgesics, phenothiazines and other antipsychotics (especially with high anticholinergic activity), tricyclic antidepressants, quinidine and some other antiarrhythmics, and antihistamines. Benztropine may increase the absorption of digoxin.

Decreased Effect: May increase gastric degradation of levodopa and decrease the amount of levodopa absorbed by delaying gastric emptying. Therapeutic effects of cholinergic agents (tacrine, donepezil) and neuroleptics may be antagonized.

Pharmacodynamics/Kinetics

Onset of action: Oral: Within 1 hour; Parenteral: Within 15 minutes

Duration: 6-48 hours

Metabolism: Hepatic (N-oxidation, N-dealkylation, and ring hydroxylation)

Bioavailability: 29%

Pregnancy Risk Factor C

Benztropine Mesylate *see* Benztropine *on page 196*

Benzylpenicillin Benzathine *see* Penicillin G Benzathine *on page 1058*

Benzylpenicillin Potassium *see* Penicillin G (Parenteral/Aqueous) *on page 1059*

Benzylpenicillin Sodium *see* Penicillin G (Parenteral/Aqueous) *on page 1059*

Benzylpenicilloyl-polylysine (BEN zil pen i SIL oyl pol i LIE seen)

U.S. Brand Names Pre-Pen®

Generic Available No

Synonyms Penicilloyl-polylysine; PPL

Pharmacologic Category Diagnostic Agent

Use Adjunct in assessing the risk of administering penicillin (penicillin or benzylpenicillin) in adults with a history of clinical penicillin hypersensitivity

Local Anesthetic/Vasoconstrictor Precautions No information available to require special precautions

Effects on Dental Treatment No significant effects or complications reported

Common Adverse Effects Frequency not defined.

Cardiovascular: Hypotension

Dermatologic: Angioneurotic edema, pruritus, erythema, urticaria

Local: Intense local inflammatory response at skin test site, wheal (locally)

Respiratory: Dyspnea

Miscellaneous: Systemic allergic reactions occur rarely

Mechanism of Action Elicits IgE antibodies which produce type I accelerate urticarial reactions to penicillins

Drug Interactions

Decreased Effect: Corticosteroids and other immunosuppressive agents may inhibit the immune response to the skin test.

Pregnancy Risk Factor C

Bepridil (BE pri dil)

Related Information

Calcium Channel Blockers and Gingival Hyperplasia *on page 1600*

Calcium Channel Blockers, Comparative Pharmacokinetics *on page 1602*

Cardiovascular Diseases *on page 1458*

U.S. Brand Names Vascor® [DSC]

Canadian Brand Names Vascor®

Generic Available No

Synonyms Bepridil Hydrochloride

Pharmacologic Category Calcium Channel Blocker

Use Treatment of chronic stable angina; due to side effect profile, reserve for patients who have been intolerant of other antianginal therapy; bepridil may be used alone or in combination with nitrates or beta-blockers

Local Anesthetic/Vasoconstrictor Precautions No information available to require special precautions

Effects on Dental Treatment Key adverse event(s) related to dental treatment: Xerostomia (normal salivary flow resumes upon discontinuation). Other drugs of this class can cause gingival hyperplasia (ie, nifedipine) but there have been no reports for bepridil.

Common Adverse Effects

>10%:

Central nervous system: Dizziness

Gastrointestinal: Nausea, dyspepsia

1% to 10%:

Cardiovascular: Bradycardia, edema, palpitations, QT prolongation (dose-related; up to 5% with prolongation of ≥25%), CHF (1%)

Central nervous system: Nervousness, headache (7% to 13%), drowsiness, psychiatric disturbances (<2%), insomnia (2% to 3%)

Dermatologic: Rash (≤2%)

Endocrine & metabolic: Sexual dysfunction

Gastrointestinal: Diarrhea, anorexia, xerostomia, constipation, abdominal pain, dyspepsia, flatulence

Neuromuscular & skeletal: Weakness (7% to 14%), tremor (<9%), paresthesia (3%)

Ocular: Blurred vision

Otic: Tinnitus

Respiratory: Rhinitis, dyspnea (≤9%), cough (≤2%)

Miscellaneous (≤2%): Flu syndrome, diaphoresis

Mechanism of Action Bepridil, a type 4 calcium antagonist, possesses characteristics of the traditional calcium antagonists, inhibiting calcium ion from entering the "slow channels" or select voltage-sensitive areas of vascular smooth muscle and myocardium during depolarization and producing a relaxation of coronary vascular smooth muscle and coronary vasodilation. However, bepridil may also inhibit fast sodium channels (inward), which may account for some of its side effects (eg, arrhythmias); a direct bradycardia effect of bepridil has been postulated via direct action on the S-A node.

Drug Interactions

Cytochrome P450 Effect: Inhibits CYP2D6 (weak)

Increased Effect/Toxicity: Use with H_2 blockers may increase bioavailability of bepridil. Use of bepridil with beta-blockers may increase cardiac depressant effects on AV conduction. Bepridil may increase serum levels/effects of carbamazepine, cyclosporine, digitalis, quinidine, and theophylline. Concurrent use of fentanyl with bepridil may increase hypotension. Use with

(Continued)

Bepridil *(Continued)*

amprenavir, atazanavir, ritonavir, sparfloxacin (possibly also gatifloxacin and moxifloxacin) may increase risk of bepridil toxicity, especially its cardiotoxicity. Use with cisapride may increase the risk of malignant arrhythmias, concurrent use is contraindicated. Blood pressure-lowering effects may be additive with sildenafil, tadalafil, and vardenafil (use caution).

Pharmacodynamics/Kinetics

Onset of action: 1 hour
Absorption: 100%
Protein binding: >99%
Metabolism: Hepatic
Bioavailability: 60%
Half-life elimination: 24 hours
Time to peak: 2-3 hours
Excretion: Urine (as metabolites)

Pregnancy Risk Factor C

Bepridil Hydrochloride *see* Bepridil *on page 197*

Beractant (ber AKT ant)

U.S. Brand Names Survanta®

Canadian Brand Names Survanta®

Mexican Brand Names Survanta®

Generic Available No

Synonyms Bovine Lung Surfactant; Natural Lung Surfactant

Pharmacologic Category Lung Surfactant

Use Prevention and treatment of respiratory distress syndrome (RDS) in premature infants

Prophylactic therapy: Body weight <1250 g in infants at risk for developing or with evidence of surfactant deficiency (administer within 15 minutes of birth)

Rescue therapy: Treatment of infants with RDS confirmed by x-ray and requiring mechanical ventilation (administer as soon as possible - within 8 hours of age)

Local Anesthetic/Vasoconstrictor Precautions No information available to require special precautions

Effects on Dental Treatment No significant effects or complications reported

Common Adverse Effects During the dosing procedure:

>10%: Cardiovascular: Transient bradycardia
1% to 10%: Respiratory: Oxygen desaturation

Mechanism of Action Replaces deficient or ineffective endogenous lung surfactant in neonates with respiratory distress syndrome (RDS) or in neonates at risk of developing RDS. Surfactant prevents the alveoli from collapsing during expiration by lowering surface tension between air and alveolar surfaces.

Pharmacodynamics/Kinetics Excretion: Clearance: Alveolar clearance is rapid

Beta-Carotene (BAY ta KARE oh teen)

U.S. Brand Names A-Caro-25®; B-Caro-T™; Lumitene™

Generic Available Yes

Pharmacologic Category Vitamin, Fat Soluble

Unlabeled/Investigational Use Prophylaxis and treatment of polymorphous light eruption; prophylaxis against photosensitivity reactions in erythropoietic protoporphyria

Local Anesthetic/Vasoconstrictor Precautions No information available to require special precautions

Effects on Dental Treatment No significant effects or complications reported

Common Adverse Effects >10%: Dermatologic: Carotenodermia (yellowing of palms, hands, or soles of feet, and to a lesser extent the face)

Mechanism of Action The exact mechanism of action in erythropoietic protoporphyria has not as yet been elucidated; although patient must become carotenemic before effects are observed, there appears to be more than a simple internal light screen responsible for the drug's action. A protective effect was achieved when beta-carotene was added to blood samples. The concentrations of solutions used were similar to those achieved in treated patients. Topically applied beta-carotene is considerably less effective than systemic therapy.

Pharmacodynamics/Kinetics

Metabolism: Prior to absorption, converted to vitamin A in the wall of the small intestine, then oxidized to retinoic acid and retinol in the presence of fat and bile acids; small amounts are then stored in the liver; retinol (active) is conjugated with glucuronic acid

Excretion: Urine and feces

Pregnancy Risk Factor C

Betadine® [OTC] *see* Povidone-Iodine *on page 1107*

Betadine® First Aid Antibiotics + Moisturizer [OTC] *see* Bacitracin and Polymyxin B *on page 178*

Betadine® Ophthalmic *see* Povidone-Iodine *on page 1107*

9-Beta-D-ribofuranosyladenine *see* Adenosine *on page 68*

Betagan® *see* Levobunolol *on page 808*

Betaine Anhydrous (BAY ta een an HY drus)

U.S. Brand Names Cystadane®

Canadian Brand Names Cystadane™

Generic Available No

Pharmacologic Category Homocystinuria, Treatment Agent

Use Orphan drug: Treatment of homocystinuria to decrease elevated homocysteine blood levels; included within the category of homocystinuria are deficiencies or defects in cystathionine beta-synthase (CBS), 5,10-methylenetetrahydrofolate reductase (MTHFR), and cobalamin cofactor metabolism (CBL).

Local Anesthetic/Vasoconstrictor Precautions No information available to require special precautions

Effects on Dental Treatment No significant effects or complications reported

Common Adverse Effects Minimal; have included nausea, GI distress, and diarrhea

Pregnancy Risk Factor C

Betamethasone (bay ta METH a sone)

Related Information

Respiratory Diseases *on page 1478*

U.S. Brand Names Beta-Val®; Celestone®; Celestone® Soluspan®; Diprolene®; Diprolene® AF; Luxiq®; Maxivate®

Canadian Brand Names Betaderm; Betaject™; Betnesol®; Betnovate®; Celestoderm®-EV/2; Celestoderm®-V; Celestone® Soluspan®; Diprolene® Glycol; Diprosone®; Ectosone; Prevex® B; Taro-Sone®; Topilene®; Topisone®; Valisone® Scalp Lotion

Mexican Brand Names Celestone®

Generic Available Yes: Excludes foam

Synonyms Betamethasone Dipropionate; Betamethasone Dipropionate, Augmented; Betamethasone Sodium Phosphate; Betamethasone Valerate; Flubenisolone

Pharmacologic Category Corticosteroid, Systemic; Corticosteroid, Topical

Dental Use Treatment of a variety of oral diseases of allergic, inflammatory, or autoimmune origin

Use Inflammatory dermatoses such as seborrheic or atopic dermatitis, neurodermatitis, anogenital pruritus, psoriasis, inflammatory phase of xerosis

Local Anesthetic/Vasoconstrictor Precautions No information available to require special precautions

Effects on Dental Treatment No significant effects or complications reported

Significant Adverse Effects

Systemic:

>10%:

Central nervous system: Insomnia, nervousness

Gastrointestinal: Increased appetite, indigestion

1% to 10%:

Central nervous system: Dizziness or lightheadedness, headache

Dermatologic: Hirsutism, hypopigmentation

Endocrine & metabolic: Diabetes mellitus

Neuromuscular & skeletal: Arthralgia

Ocular: Cataracts, glaucoma

Respiratory: Epistaxis

Miscellaneous: Diaphoresis

<1% (Limited to important or life-threatening): Alkalosis, amenorrhea, Cushing's syndrome, delirium, euphoria, glucose intolerance, growth suppression, hallucinations, hyperglycemia, hypokalemia, pituitary-adrenal (HPA) axis suppression, pseudotumor cerebri, psychoses, seizures, sodium and water retention, vertigo

(Continued)

Betamethasone *(Continued)*

Topical:

1% to 10%:

Dermatologic: Itching, allergic contact dermatitis, erythema, dryness papular rashes, folliculitis, furunculosis, pustules, pyoderma, vesiculation, hyperesthesia, skin infection (secondary)

Local: Burning, irritation

<1% (Limited to important or life-threatening): Cataracts (posterior subcapsular), Cushing's syndrome, glaucoma, hypokalemic syndrome

Dosage Base dosage on severity of disease and patient response

Children: Use lowest dose listed as initial dose for adrenocortical insufficiency (physiologic replacement)

I.M.: 0.0175-0.125 mg base/kg/day divided every 6-12 hours **or** 0.5-7.5 mg base/m^2/day divided every 6-12 hours

Oral: 0.0175-0.25 mg/kg/day divided every 6-8 hours **or** 0.5-7.5 mg/m^2/day divided every 6-8 hours

Topical:

≤12 years: Use is not recommended.

>12 years: Apply a thin film twice daily; use minimal amount for shortest period of time to avoid HPA axis suppression

Adolescents and Adults:

Oral: 2.4-4.8 mg/day in 2-4 doses; range: 0.6-7.2 mg/day

I.M.: Betamethasone sodium phosphate and betamethasone acetate: 0.6-9 mg/day (generally, $^1/_3$ to $^1/_2$ of oral dose) divided every 12-24 hours

Foam: Apply twice daily, once in the morning and once at night to scalp

Adults:

Intrabursal, intra-articular, intradermal: 0.25-2 mL

Intralesional: Rheumatoid arthritis/osteoarthritis:

Very large joints: 1-2 mL

Large joints: 1 mL

Medium joints: 0.5-1 mL

Small joints: 0.25-0.5 mL

Topical: Apply thin film 2-4 times/day. Therapy should be discontinued when control is achieved; if no improvement is seen, reassessment of diagnosis may be necessary.

Dosing adjustment in hepatic impairment: Adjustments may be necessary in patients with liver failure because betamethasone is extensively metabolized in the liver

Mechanism of Action Controls the rate of protein synthesis, depresses the migration of polymorphonuclear leukocytes, fibroblasts, reverses capillary permeability, and lysosomal stabilization at the cellular level to prevent or control inflammation

Contraindications Hypersensitivity to betamethasone or any component of the formulation; systemic fungal infections

Warnings/Precautions Not to be used in status asthmaticus or for the relief of acute bronchospasm; topical use in patients ≤12 years of age is not recommended. May cause suppression of hypothalamic-pituitary-adrenal (HPA) axis, particularly in younger children or in patients receiving high doses for prolonged periods. Particular care is required when patients are transferred from systemic corticosteroids to inhaled products due to possible adrenal insufficiency or withdrawal from steroids, including an increase in allergic symptoms. Patients receiving 20 mg per day of prednisone (or equivalent) may be most susceptible. Fatalities have occurred due to adrenal insufficiency in asthmatic patients during and after transfer from systemic corticosteroids to aerosol steroids; aerosol steroids do **not** provide the systemic steroid needed to treat patients having trauma, surgery, or infections. Withdrawal and discontinuation of the corticosteroid should be done slowly and carefully

Controlled clinical studies have shown that orally-inhaled and intranasal corticosteroids may cause a reduction in growth velocity in pediatric patients. (In studies of orally-inhaled corticosteroids, the mean reduction in growth velocity was approximately 1 centimeter per year [range 0.3-1.8 cm per year] and appears to be related to dose and duration of exposure.) The growth of pediatric patients receiving inhaled corticosteroids, should be monitored routinely (eg, via stadiometry). To minimize the systemic effects of orally-inhaled and intranasal corticosteroids, each patient should be titrated to the lowest effective dose.

May suppress the immune system, patients may be more susceptible to infection. Use with caution in patients with systemic infections or ocular herpes simplex. Avoid exposure to chickenpox and measles.

Use with caution in patients with hypothyroidism, cirrhosis, ulcerative colitis; do not use occlusive dressings on weeping or exudative lesions and general caution with occlusive dressings should be observed; discontinue if skin irritation or contact dermatitis should occur; do not use in patients with decreased skin circulation

Drug Interactions Inhibits CYP3A4 (weak)

Phenytoin, phenobarbital, rifampin increase clearance of betamethasone.

Potassium-depleting diuretics increase potassium loss.

Skin test antigens, immunizations: Betamethasone may decrease response and increase potential infections.

Insulin or oral hypoglycemics: Betamethasone may increase blood glucose.

Ethanol/Nutrition/Herb Interactions

Ethanol: Avoid ethanol (may enhance gastric mucosal irritation).

Food: Betamethasone interferes with calcium absorption.

Herb/Nutraceutical: Avoid cat's claw, echinacea (have immunostimulant properties).

Dietary Considerations May be taken with food to decrease GI distress.

Pharmacodynamics/Kinetics

Protein binding: 64%

Metabolism: Hepatic

Half-life elimination: 6.5 hours

Time to peak, serum: I.V.: 10-36 minutes

Excretion: Urine (<5% as unchanged drug)

Pregnancy Risk Factor C

Lactation Excretion in breast milk unknown/use caution

Breast-Feeding Considerations Systemic corticosteroids are excreted in human milk. The extent of topical absorption is variable. Use with caution while breast-feeding; do not apply to nipples.

Dosage Forms [DSC] = Discontinued product

Note: Potency expressed as betamethasone base.

Cream, topical, as dipropionate: 0.05% (15 g, 45 g)
 Maxivate®: 0.05% (45 g)

Cream, topical, as dipropionate augmented (Diprolene® AF): 0.05% (15 g, 50 g)

Cream, topical, as valerate: 0.1% (15 g, 45 g)
 Beta-Val®: 0.1% (15 g, 45 g)

Foam, topical, as valerate (Luxiq®): 0.12% (50 g, 100 g) [contains alcohol 60.4%]

Gel, topical, as dipropionate augmented: 0.05% (15 g, 50 g)
 Diprolene® [DSC]: 0.05% (15 g, 50 g)

Injection, suspension (Celestone® Soluspan®): Betamethasone sodium phosphate 3 mg/mL and betamethasone acetate 3 mg/mL [6 mg/mL] (5 mL)

Lotion, topical, as dipropionate: 0.05% (60 mL)
 Maxivate®: 0.05% (60 mL)

Lotion, topical, as dipropionate augmented (Diprolene®): 0.05% (30 mL, 60 mL)

Lotion, topical, as valerate (Beta-Val®): 0.1% (60 mL)

Ointment, topical, as dipropionate: 0.05% (15 g, 45 g)
 Maxivate®: 0.05% (45 g)

Ointment, topical, as dipropionate augmented: 0.05% (15 g, 45 g, 50 g)
 Diprolene®: 0.05% (15 g, 50 g)

Ointment, topical, as valerate: 0.1% (15 g, 45 g)

Syrup, as base (Celestone®): 0.6 mg/5 mL (118 mL)

Betamethasone and Clotrimazole

(bay ta METH a sone & kloe TRIM a zole)

Related Information

Betamethasone *on page 199*

Clotrimazole *on page 363*

U.S. Brand Names Lotrisone®

Canadian Brand Names Lotriderm®

Generic Available Yes: Cream

Synonyms Clotrimazole and Betamethasone

Pharmacologic Category Antifungal Agent, Topical; Corticosteroid, Topical

Use Topical treatment of various dermal fungal infections (including tinea pedis, cruris, and corpora in patients ≥17 years of age)

Local Anesthetic/Vasoconstrictor Precautions No information available to require special precautions

Effects on Dental Treatment No significant effects or complications reported

(Continued)

Betamethasone and Clotrimazole *(Continued)*

Common Adverse Effects Also see individual agents.

1% to 10%:

Dermatologic: Dry skin (2%)

Local: Burning (2%)

Neuromuscular & skeletal: Paresthesia (2%)

Mechanism of Action Betamethasone dipropionate is a corticosteroid. Clotrimazole is an antifungal agent.

Drug Interactions

Cytochrome P450 Effect:

Betamethasone: **Inhibits** CYP3A4 (weak)

Clotrimazole: **Inhibits** CYP1A2 (weak), 2A6 (weak), 2B6 (weak), 2C8/9 (weak), 2C19 (weak), 2D6 (weak), 2E1 (weak), 3A4 (moderate)

Pharmacodynamics/Kinetics See individual agents.

Pregnancy Risk Factor C

Betamethasone Dipropionate *see* Betamethasone *on page 199*

Betamethasone Dipropionate, Augmented *see* Betamethasone *on page 199*

Betamethasone Sodium Phosphate *see* Betamethasone *on page 199*

Betamethasone Valerate *see* Betamethasone *on page 199*

Betapace® *see* Sotalol *on page 1231*

Betapace AF® *see* Sotalol *on page 1231*

Betasept® [OTC] *see* Chlorhexidine Gluconate *on page 308*

Betaseron® *see* Interferon Beta-1b *on page 757*

Betatar® [OTC] *see* Coal Tar *on page 367*

Beta-Val® *see* Betamethasone *on page 199*

Betaxolol (be TAKS oh lol)

Related Information

Cardiovascular Diseases *on page 1458*

U.S. Brand Names Betoptic® S; Kerlone®

Canadian Brand Names Betoptic® S

Generic Available Yes: Solution, tablet

Synonyms Betaxolol Hydrochloride

Pharmacologic Category Beta Blocker, $Beta_1$ Selective

Use Treatment of chronic open-angle glaucoma and ocular hypertension; management of hypertension

Local Anesthetic/Vasoconstrictor Precautions No information available to require special precautions

Effects on Dental Treatment Betaxolol is a cardioselective beta-blocker. Local anesthetic with vasoconstrictor can be safely used in patients medicated with betaxolol. Nonselective beta-blockers (ie, propranolol, nadolol) enhance the pressor response to epinephrine, resulting in hypertension and bradycardia; this has not been reported for betaxolol. Many nonsteroidal anti-inflammatory drugs, such as ibuprofen and indomethacin, can reduce the hypotensive effect of beta-blockers after 3 or more weeks of therapy with the NSAID. Short-term NSAID use (ie, 3 days) requires no special precautions in patients taking beta-blockers.

Common Adverse Effects

Ophthalmic:

>10%: Ocular: Conjunctival hyperemia

1% to 10%:

Ocular: Anisocoria, corneal punctate keratitis, keratitis, corneal staining, decreased corneal sensitivity, eye pain, vision disturbances

Systemic:

>10%:

Central nervous system: Drowsiness, insomnia

Endocrine & metabolic: Decreased sexual ability

1% to 10%:

Cardiovascular: Bradycardia, palpitations, edema, CHF, reduced peripheral circulation

Central nervous system: Mental depression

Gastrointestinal: Diarrhea or constipation, nausea, vomiting, stomach discomfort

Respiratory: Bronchospasm

Miscellaneous: Cold extremities

Mechanism of Action Competitively blocks $beta_1$-receptors, with little or no effect on $beta_2$-receptors; ophthalmic reduces intraocular pressure by reducing the production of aqueous humor

Drug Interactions

Cytochrome P450 Effect: Substrate (major) of CYP1A2, 2D6; **Inhibits** CYP2D6 (weak)

Increased Effect/Toxicity: CYP1A2 inhibitors may increase the levels/effects of betaxolol; example inhibitors include amiodarone, ciprofloxacin, fluvoxamine, ketoconazole, lomefloxacin, ofloxacin, and rofecoxib. CYP2D6 inhibitors may increase the levels/effects of betaxolol; example inhibitors include chlorpromazine, delavirdine, fluoxetine, miconazole, paroxetine, pergolide, quinidine, quinine, ritonavir, and ropinirole. The heart rate-lowering effects of betaxolol are additive with other drugs which slow AV conduction (digoxin, verapamil, diltiazem). Reserpine increases the effects of betaxolol. Concurrent use of betaxolol may increase the effects of alpha-blockers (prazosin, terazosin), alpha-adrenergic stimulants (epinephrine, phenylephrine), and the vasoconstrictive effects of ergot alkaloids. Betaxolol may mask the tachycardia from hypoglycemia caused by insulin and oral hypoglycemics. In patients receiving concurrent therapy, the risk of hypertensive crisis is increased when either clonidine or the beta-blocker is withdrawn. Beta-blockers may increase the action or levels of ethanol, disopyramide, nondepolarizing muscle relaxants, and theophylline although the effects are difficult to predict.

Decreased Effect: CYP1A2 inducers may decrease the levels/effects of betaxolol; example inducers include aminoglutethimide, carbamazepine, phenobarbital, and rifampin. Decreased effect of betaxolol with aluminum salts, barbiturates, calcium salts, cholestyramine, colestipol, NSAIDs, penicillins (ampicillin), rifampin, salicylates, and sulfinpyrazone due to decreased bioavailability and plasma levels. Beta-blockers may decrease the effect of sulfonylureas.

Pharmacodynamics/Kinetics

Onset of action: Ophthalmic: 30 minutes; Oral: 1-1.5 hours
Duration: Ophthalmic: ≥12 hours
Absorption: Ophthalmic: Some systemic; Oral: ~100%
Metabolism: Hepatic to multiple metabolites
Protein binding: Oral: 50%
Bioavailability: Oral: 89%
Half-life elimination: Oral: 12-22 hours
Time to peak: Ophthalmic: ~2 hours; Oral: 1.5-6 hours
Excretion: Urine

Pregnancy Risk Factor C (manufacturer); D (2nd and 3rd trimesters - expert analysis)

Betaxolol Hydrochloride *see* Betaxolol *on page 202*

Betaxon® *see* Levobetaxolol *on page 808*

Bethanechol (be THAN e kole)

U.S. Brand Names Urecholine®

Canadian Brand Names Duvoid®; Myotonachol®; PMS-Bethanechol

Generic Available Yes

Synonyms Bethanechol Chloride

Pharmacologic Category Cholinergic Agonist

Use Nonobstructive urinary retention and retention due to neurogenic bladder

Unlabeled/Investigational Use Treatment and prevention of bladder dysfunction caused by phenothiazines; diagnosis of flaccid or atonic neurogenic bladder; gastroesophageal reflux

Local Anesthetic/Vasoconstrictor Precautions No information available to require special precautions

Effects on Dental Treatment This is a cholinergic agent similar to pilocarpine; expect to see salivation and sweating in patients.

Common Adverse Effects Frequency not defined.

Cardiovascular: Hypotension, tachycardia, flushed skin
Central nervous system: Headache, malaise
Gastrointestinal: Abdominal cramps, diarrhea, nausea, vomiting, salivation, eructation
Genitourinary: Urinary urgency
Ocular: Lacrimation, miosis
Respiratory: Asthmatic attacks, bronchial constriction
Miscellaneous: Diaphoresis

Mechanism of Action Stimulates cholinergic receptors in the smooth muscle of the urinary bladder and gastrointestinal tract resulting in increased peristalsis, increased GI and pancreatic secretions, bladder muscle contraction, and increased ureteral peristaltic waves

(Continued)

Bethanechol *(Continued)*

Drug Interactions

Increased Effect/Toxicity: Bethanechol and ganglionic blockers may cause a critical fall in blood pressure. Cholinergic drugs or anticholinesterase agents may have additive effects with bethanechol.

Decreased Effect: Procainamide, quinidine may decrease the effects of bethanechol. Anticholinergic agents (atropine, antihistamines, TCAs, phenothiazines) may decrease effects.

Pharmacodynamics/Kinetics

Onset of action: 30-90 minutes

Duration: Up to 6 hours

Absorption: Variable

Pregnancy Risk Factor C

Bethanechol Chloride *see* Bethanechol *on page 203*

Betimol® *see* Timolol *on page 1299*

Betoptic® S *see* Betaxolol *on page 202*

Bevacizumab (be vuh SIZ uh mab)

U.S. Brand Names Avastin™

Generic Available No

Synonyms Anti-VEGF Monoclonal Antibody; rhuMAb-VEGF

Pharmacologic Category Antineoplastic Agent, Monoclonal Antibody; Vascular Endothelial Growth Factor (VEGF) Inhibitor

Use Treatment of metastatic colorectal cancer as a component of multidrug therapy

Unlabeled/Investigational Use Breast cancer, malignant mesothelioma, prostate cancer

Local Anesthetic/Vasoconstrictor Precautions No information available to require special precautions

Effects on Dental Treatment No significant effects or complications reported

Common Adverse Effects No data are available concerning the frequency of adverse reactions to bevacizumab alone. The frequencies noted below are from two controlled clinical trials of bevacizumab in combination with irinotecan, fluorouracil, and leucovorin (IFL). These frequencies, where noted, are compared to the incidence in the placebo-controlled arms of the trials.

>10%:

Cardiovascular: Hypertension (23% to 34% vs 14%, severe/life-threatening 12% vs 2%); hypotension (7% to 15% vs 7%); thromboembolism (18% vs 15%)

Central nervous system: Pain (61% to 62% vs 55%, severe 8% vs 5%); abdominal pain (50% to 61% vs 55%, severe/life-threatening 8% vs 5%); headache (26% vs 19%); dizziness (19% to 26% vs 20%)

Dermatologic: Alopecia (6% to 32% vs 26%), dry skin (7% to 20% vs 7%), exfoliative dermatitis (3% to 19% vs 3%), skin discoloration (2% to 16% vs 3%)

Endocrine & metabolic: Weight loss (15% to 16% vs 10%), hypokalemia (12% to 16% vs 11%)

Gastrointestinal: Diarrhea (severe/life-threatening 34% vs 25%); vomiting (47% to 52% vs 47%); anorexia (35% to 43% vs 30%); constipation (29% to 40% vs 29%, severe/life-threatening 4% vs 2%); stomatitis (30% to 32% vs 18%); dyspepsia (17% to 24% vs 15%); flatulence (11% to 19% vs 10%); taste disorder (14% to 21% vs 9%)

Hematologic: Leukopenia (severe/life-threatening 37% vs 31%), epistaxis (32% to 35% vs 10%), gastrointestinal hemorrhage (19% to 24% vs 6%), neutropenia (severe/life-threatening 21% vs 14%)

Neuromuscular & skeletal: Weakness (73% to 74% vs 70%, severe/life-threatening 10% vs 7%); myalgia (8% to 15% vs 7%)

Ocular: Tearing increased (6% to 18% vs 2%)

Renal: Proteinuria includes nephrotic syndrome in some patients (36% vs 24%)

Respiratory: Upper respiratory infection (40% to 47% vs 39%), dyspnea (25% to 26% vs 15%)

1% to 10%:

Cardiovascular: DVT (6% to 9% vs 3%, severe/life-threatening 9% vs 5%); intra-arterial thrombosis (severe/life-threatening 3% vs 1%)

Central nervous system: Confusion (1% to 6% vs 1%), syncope (severe/life-threatening 3% vs 1%), abnormal gait (1% to 5% vs 0%)

Dermatologic: Skin ulcer (6% vs 1%), nail disorders (2% to 8% vs 3%)

Endocrine & metabolic: Infusion reactions (<3%)

Gastrointestinal: Dry mouth (4% to 7% vs 2%), colitis (1% to 6% vs 1%)
Hematologic: Thrombocytopenia (5% vs 0%)
Hepatic: Bilirubinemia (1% to 6% vs 0%)
Renal: Urinary frequency/urgency (3% to 6% vs 1%)
Respiratory: Voice alteration (6% to 9% vs 2%)

Mechanism of Action Bevacizumab is a recombinant, humanized monoclonal antibody which binds to (and neutralizes) vascular endothelial growth factor (VEGF), preventing its association with endothelial receptors. VEGF binding initiates angiogenesis (endothelial proliferation and the formation of new blood vessels). The inhibition of microvascular growth is believed to retard the growth of all tissues (including metastatic tissue).

Drug Interactions

Increased Effect/Toxicity: Bevacizumab may potentiate the cardiotoxic effects of anthracyclines. Serum concentrations of irinotecan's active metabolite may be increased by bevacizumab; an approximate 33% increase has been observed.

Pharmacodynamics/Kinetics

Distribution: V_d: 46 mL/kg
Half-life elimination: 20 days (range: 11-50 days)
Excretion: Clearance: 2.75-5 mL/kg/day

Pregnancy Risk Factor C

Bexarotene (beks AIR oh teen)

U.S. Brand Names Targretin®

Canadian Brand Names Targretin®

Generic Available No

Pharmacologic Category Antineoplastic Agent, Miscellaneous

Use

Oral: Treatment of cutaneous manifestations of cutaneous T-cell lymphoma in patients who are refractory to at least one prior systemic therapy

Topical: Treatment of cutaneous lesions in patients with refractory cutaneous T-cell lymphoma (stage 1A and 1B) or who have not tolerated other therapies

Local Anesthetic/Vasoconstrictor Precautions No information available to require special precautions

Effects on Dental Treatment Key adverse event(s) related to dental treatment: Xerostomia (normal salivary flow resumes upon discontinuation) and gingivitis.

Common Adverse Effects First percentage is at a dose of 300 mg/m²/day; the second percentage is at a dose >300 mg/m²/day.

>10%:

Cardiovascular: Peripheral edema (13% to 11%)
Central nervous system: Headache (30% to 42%), chills (10% to 13%)
Dermatologic: Rash (17% to 23%), exfoliative dermatitis (10% to 28%)
Endocrine & metabolic: Hyperlipidemia (about 79% in both dosing ranges), hypercholesteremia (32% to 62%), hypothyroidism (29% to 53%)
Hematologic: Leukopenia (17% to 47%)
Neuromuscular & skeletal: Weakness (20% to 45%)
Miscellaneous: Infection (13% to 23%)

<10%:

Cardiovascular: Hemorrhage, hypertension, angina pectoris, right heart failure, tachycardia, cerebrovascular accident
Central nervous system: Fever (5% to 17%), insomnia (5% to 11%), subdural hematoma, syncope, depression, agitation, ataxia, confusion, dizziness, hyperesthesia
Dermatologic: Dry skin (about 10% for both dosing ranges), alopecia (4% to 11%), skin ulceration, acne, skin nodule, maculopapular rash, serous drainage, vesicular bullous rash, cheilitis
Endocrine & metabolic: Hypoproteinemia, hyperglycemia, weight loss/gain, serum amylase (elevated), breast pain
Gastrointestinal: Abdominal pain (11% to 4%), nausea (16% to 8%), diarrhea (7% to 42%), vomiting (4% to 13%), anorexia (2% to 23%), constipation, xerostomia, flatulence, colitis, dyspepsia, gastroenteritis, gingivitis, melena, pancreatitis,
Genitourinary: Albuminuria, hematuria, urinary incontinence, urinary tract infection, urinary urgency, dysuria, kidney function abnormality
Hematologic: Hypochromic anemia (4% to 13%), anemia (6% to 25%), eosinophilia, thrombocythemia, coagulation time increased, lymphocytosis, thrombocytopenia
Hepatic: LDH increase (7% to 13%), hepatic failure

(Continued)

Bexarotene *(Continued)*

Neuromuscular & skeletal: Back pain (2% to 11%), arthralgia, myalgia, bone pain, myasthenia, arthrosis, neuropathy
Ocular: Dry eyes, conjunctivitis, blepharitis, corneal lesion, visual field defects, keratitis
Otic: Ear pain, otitis externa
Renal: Creatinine (elevated)
Respiratory: Pharyngitis, rhinitis, dyspnea, pleural effusion, bronchitis, increased cough, lung edema, hemoptysis, hypoxia
Miscellaneous: Flu-like syndrome (4% to 13%), bacterial infection (1% to 13%)

Topical:
Cardiovascular: Edema (10%)
Central nervous system: Headache (14%), weakness (6%), pain (30%)
Dermatologic: Rash (14% to 72%), pruritus (6% to 40%), contact dermatitis (14%), exfoliative dermatitis (6%)
Hematologic: Leukopenia (6%), lymphadenopathy (6%)
Neuromuscular & skeletal: Paresthesia (6%)
Respiratory: Cough (6%), pharyngitis (6%)
Miscellaneous: Diaphoresis (6%), infection (18%)

Mechanism of Action The exact mechanism is unknown. Binds and activates retinoid X receptor subtypes. Once activated, these receptors function as transcription factors that regulate the expression of genes which control cellular differentiation and proliferation. Bexarotene inhibits the growth *in vitro* of some tumor cell lines of hematopoietic and squamous cell origin.

Drug Interactions

Cytochrome P450 Effect: Substrate of CYP3A4 (minor); **Induces** CYP3A4 (weak)

Increased Effect/Toxicity: Bexarotene plasma concentrations may be increased by gemfibrozil. Bexarotene may increase the toxicity of DEET.

Decreased Effect: Bexarotene may decrease the plasma levels of hormonal contraceptives and tamoxifen.

Pharmacodynamics/Kinetics
Absorption: Significantly improved by a fat-containing meal
Protein binding: >99%
Metabolism: Hepatic via CYP3A4 isoenzyme; four metabolites identified; further metabolized by glucuronidation
Half-life elimination: 7 hours
Time to peak: 2 hours
Excretion: Primarily feces; urine (<1% as unchanged drug and metabolites)

Pregnancy Risk Factor X

Bextra® *see* Valdecoxib *on page 1356*
BG 9273 *see* Alefacept *on page 76*
Biaxin® *see* Clarithromycin *on page 343*
Biaxin® XL *see* Clarithromycin *on page 343*

Bicalutamide (bye ka LOO ta mide)

U.S. Brand Names Casodex®
Canadian Brand Names Casodex®
Mexican Brand Names Casodex®
Generic Available No
Synonyms CDX; ICI-176334
Pharmacologic Category Antineoplastic Agent, Antiandrogen
Use In combination therapy with LHRH agonist analogues in treatment of advanced prostatic carcinoma
Local Anesthetic/Vasoconstrictor Precautions No information available to require special precautions
Effects on Dental Treatment Key adverse event(s) related to dental treatment: Xerostomia (normal salivary flow resumes upon discontinuation).
Common Adverse Effects Endocrine & metabolic: Hot flashes (8% to 24% in combination with LHRH agonists), gynecomastia (23% to 62%), breast tenderness (25% to 60%)

≥2% to <5%:
Cardiovascular: Angina pectoris, CHF, edema
Central nervous system: Anxiety, depression, confusion, somnolence, nervousness, fever, chills
Dermatologic: Dry skin, pruritus, alopecia
Endocrine & metabolic: Breast pain, diabetes mellitus, decreased libido, dehydration, gout

Gastrointestinal: Anorexia, dyspepsia, rectal hemorrhage, xerostomia, melena, weight gain
Genitourinary: Polyuria, urinary impairment, dysuria, urinary retention, urinary urgency
Hepatic: Alkaline phosphatase increased
Neuromuscular & skeletal: Myasthenia, arthritis, myalgia, leg cramps, pathological fracture, neck pain, hypertonia, neuropathy
Renal: Creatinine increased
Respiratory: Cough increased, pharyngitis, bronchitis, pneumonia, rhinitis, lung disorder
Miscellaneous: Sepsis, neoplasma

Mechanism of Action Pure nonsteroidal antiandrogen that binds to androgen receptors; specifically a competitive inhibitor for the binding of dihydrotestosterone and testosterone; prevents testosterone stimulation of cell growth in prostate cancer

Drug Interactions

Increased Effect/Toxicity: Bicalutamide may displace warfarin from protein binding sites which may result in an increased anticoagulant effect, especially when bicalutamide therapy is started after the patient is already on warfarin.

Pharmacodynamics/Kinetics

Absorption: Rapid and complete
Protein binding: 96%
Metabolism: Extensively hepatic; stereospecific metabolism
Half-life elimination: Up to 10 days; active enantiomer 5.8 days
Excretion: Urine and feces (as unchanged drug and metabolites)

Pregnancy Risk Factor X

Bicillin® C-R *see* Penicillin G Benzathine and Penicillin G Procaine *on page 1058*

Bicillin® C-R 900/300 *see* Penicillin G Benzathine and Penicillin G Procaine *on page 1058*

Bicillin® L-A *see* Penicillin G Benzathine *on page 1058*

Bicitra® *see* Sodium Citrate and Citric Acid *on page 1228*

BiCNu® *see* Carmustine *on page 268*

BIDA *see* Amonafide *on page 112*

Biltricide® *see* Praziquantel *on page 1111*

Bimatoprost (bi MAT oh prost)

U.S. Brand Names Lumigan®

Canadian Brand Names Lumigan®

Mexican Brand Names Lumigan®

Generic Available No

Pharmacologic Category Ophthalmic Agent, Miscellaneous

Use Reduction of intraocular pressure (IOP) in patients with open-angle glaucoma or ocular hypertension; should be used in patients who are intolerant of other IOP-lowering medications or failed treatment with another IOP-lowering medication

Local Anesthetic/Vasoconstrictor Precautions No information available to require special precautions

Effects on Dental Treatment No significant effects or complications reported

Mechanism of Action As a synthetic analog of prostaglandin with ocular hypotensive activity, bimatoprost decreases intraocular pressure by increasing the outflow of aqueous humor.

Pregnancy Risk Factor C

Biocef® *see* Cephalexin *on page 294*

Biofed [OTC] *see* Pseudoephedrine *on page 1147*

Biolon™ *see* Hyaluronate and Derivatives *on page 696*

Bion® Tears [OTC] *see* Artificial Tears *on page 148*

Bio-Statin® *see* Nystatin *on page 1003*

BioThrax™ *see* Anthrax Vaccine (Adsorbed) *on page 133*

Biperiden (bye PER i den)

U.S. Brand Names Akineton®

Canadian Brand Names Akineton®

Mexican Brand Names Akineton®

Generic Available No

Synonyms Biperiden Hydrochloride; Biperiden Lactate

Pharmacologic Category Anticholinergic Agent; Anti-Parkinson's Agent, Anticholinergic

(Continued)

Biperiden *(Continued)*

Use Adjunct in the therapy of all forms of Parkinsonism; control of extrapyramidal symptoms secondary to antipsychotics

Local Anesthetic/Vasoconstrictor Precautions No information available to require special precautions

Effects on Dental Treatment Key adverse event(s) related to dental treatment: Xerostomia (normal salivary flow resumes upon discontinuation), nasal dryness, dry throat (very prevalent), and orthostatic hypotension.

Common Adverse Effects Frequency not defined.

Cardiovascular: Orthostatic hypotension, bradycardia

Central nervous system: Drowsiness, euphoria, disorientation, agitation, sleep disorder (decreased REM sleep and increased REM latency)

Gastrointestinal: Constipation, xerostomia

Genitourinary: Urinary retention

Neuromuscular & skeletal: Choreic movements

Ocular: Blurred vision

Mechanism of Action Biperiden is a weak peripheral anticholinergic agent with nicotinolytic activity. The beneficial effects in Parkinson's disease and neuroleptic-induced extrapyramidal symptoms are believed to be due to the inhibition of striatal cholinergic receptors.

Drug Interactions

Cytochrome P450 Effect: Inhibits CYP2D6 (weak)

Increased Effect/Toxicity: Central and/or peripheral anticholinergic syndrome can occur when administered with amantadine (or rimantadine), narcotic analgesics, phenothiazines and other antipsychotics (especially with high anticholinergic activity), tricyclic antidepressants, quinidine and some other antiarrhythmics, and antihistamines. Anticholinergics may increase the bioavailability of atenolol (and possibly other beta-blockers). Anticholinergics may decrease gastric degradation and increase the amount of digoxin or levodopa absorbed by delaying gastric emptying.

Decreased Effect: Anticholinergics may antagonize the therapeutic effect of neuroleptics and cholinergic agents (includes tacrine and donepezil).

Pharmacodynamics/Kinetics

Bioavailability: 29%

Half-life elimination, serum: 18.4-24.3 hours

Time to peak, serum: 1-1.5 hours

Pregnancy Risk Factor C

Biperiden Hydrochloride *see* Biperiden *on page 207*

Biperiden Lactate *see* Biperiden *on page 207*

Bisac-Evac™ [OTC] *see* Bisacodyl *on page 208*

Bisacodyl (bis a KOE dil)

U.S. Brand Names Alophen® [OTC]; Bisac-Evac™ [OTC]; Bisacodyl Uniserts® [OTC]; Correctol® Tablets [OTC]; Doxidan® *(reformulation)* [OTC]; Dulcolax® [OTC]; Femilax™ [OTC]; Fleet® Bisacodyl Enema [OTC]; Fleet® Stimulant Laxative [OTC]; Gentlax® [OTC]; Modane Tablets® [OTC]; Veracolate [OTC]

Canadian Brand Names Apo-Bisacodyl®; Carter's Little Pills®; Dulcolax®

Mexican Brand Names Dulcolan®

Generic Available Yes: Excludes enema

Pharmacologic Category Laxative, Stimulant

Use Treatment of constipation; colonic evacuation prior to procedures or examination

Local Anesthetic/Vasoconstrictor Precautions No information available to require special precautions

Effects on Dental Treatment No significant effects or complications reported

Mechanism of Action Stimulates peristalsis by directly irritating the smooth muscle of the intestine, possibly the colonic intramural plexus; alters water and electrolyte secretion producing net intestinal fluid accumulation and laxation

Drug Interactions

Decreased Effect: Milk or antacids may decrease the effect of bisacodyl. Bisacodyl may decrease the effect of warfarin.

Pharmacodynamics/Kinetics

Onset of action: Oral: 6-10 hours; Rectal: 0.25-1 hour

Absorption: Oral, rectal: Systemic, <5%

Pregnancy Risk Factor C

Bisacodyl Uniserts® [OTC] *see* Bisacodyl *on page 208*

bis-chloronitrosourea *see* Carmustine *on page 268*

Bismatrol *see* Bismuth *on page 209*

Bismuth (BIZ muth)

Related Information

Gastrointestinal Disorders *on page 1476*

U.S. Brand Names Children's Kaopectate® *(reformulation)* [OTC]; Diotame® [OTC]; Kaopectate® [OTC]; Kaopectate® Extra Strength [OTC]; Pepto-Bismol® [OTC]; Pepto-Bismol® Maximum Strength [OTC]

Generic Available Yes

Synonyms Bismatrol; Bismuth Subgallate; Bismuth Subsalicylate; Pink Bismuth

Pharmacologic Category Antidiarrheal

Use

Subsalicylate formulation: Symptomatic treatment of mild, nonspecific diarrhea; control of traveler's diarrhea (enterotoxigenic *Escherichia coli*); as part of a multidrug regimen for *H. pylori* eradication to reduce the risk of duodenal ulcer recurrence

Subgallate formulation: An aid to reduce fecal odors from a colostomy or ileostomy

Local Anesthetic/Vasoconstrictor Precautions No information available to require special precautions

Effects on Dental Treatment Key adverse event(s) related to dental treatment: Darkening of tongue.

Common Adverse Effects Frequency not defined; subsalicylate formulation:

Central nervous system: Anxiety, confusion, headache, mental depression, slurred speech

Gastrointestinal: Discoloration of the tongue (darkening), grayish black stools, impaction may occur in infants and debilitated patients

Neuromuscular & skeletal: Muscle spasms, weakness

Ocular: Hearing loss, tinnitus

Mechanism of Action Bismuth subsalicylate exhibits both antisecretory and antimicrobial action. This agent may provide some anti-inflammatory action as well. The salicylate moiety provides antisecretory effect and the bismuth exhibits antimicrobial directly against bacterial and viral gastrointestinal pathogens.

Drug Interactions

Increased Effect/Toxicity: Toxicity of aspirin, warfarin, and/or hypoglycemics may be increased.

Decreased Effect: The effects of tetracyclines and uricosurics may be decreased.

Pharmacodynamics/Kinetics

Absorption: Bismuth: <1%; Subsalicylate: >90%

Metabolism: Bismuth subsalicylate is converted to salicylic acid and insoluble bismuth salts in the GI tract.

Half-life elimination: Terminal: Bismuth: Highly variable

Excretion: Bismuth: Urine and feces; Salicylate: Urine

Pregnancy Risk Factor C/D (3rd trimester)

Bismuth Subgallate *see* Bismuth *on page 209*

Bismuth Subsalicylate *see* Bismuth *on page 209*

Bismuth Subsalicylate, Metronidazole, and Tetracycline

(BIZ muth sub sa LIS i late, me troe NI da zole, & tet ra SYE kleen)

Related Information

Bismuth *on page 209*

Metronidazole *on page 917*

Tetracycline *on page 1280*

U.S. Brand Names Helidac®

Generic Available No

Synonyms Bismuth Subsalicylate, Tetracycline, and Metronidazole; Metronidazole, Bismuth Subsalicylate, and Tetracycline; Metronidazole, Tetracycline, and Bismuth Subsalicylate; Tetracycline, Bismuth Subsalicylate, and Metronidazole; Tetracycline, Metronidazole, and Bismuth Subsalicylate

Pharmacologic Category Antibiotic, Tetracycline Derivative; Antidiarrheal

Use In combination with an H_2 antagonist, as part of a multidrug regimen for *H. pylori* eradication to reduce the risk of duodenal ulcer recurrence

Local Anesthetic/Vasoconstrictor Precautions No information available to require special precautions

Effects on Dental Treatment Tetracyclines are not recommended for use during pregnancy since they can cause enamel hypoplasia and permanent teeth discoloration; long-term use associated with oral candidiasis.

(Continued)

Bismuth Subsalicylate, Metronidazole, and Tetracycline *(Continued)*

Common Adverse Effects Also see individual agents.

>1%:

Central nervous system: Dizziness

Gastrointestinal: Nausea, diarrhea, abdominal pain, vomiting, anal discomfort, anorexia

Neuromuscular & skeletal: Paresthesia

Mechanism of Action Bismuth subsalicylate, metronidazole, and tetracycline individually have demonstrated *in vitro* activity against most susceptible strains of *H. pylori* isolated from patients with duodenal ulcers. Resistance to metronidazole is increasing in the U.S.; an alternative regimen, not containing metronidazole, if *H. pylori* is not eradicated follow therapy.

Drug Interactions

Cytochrome P450 Effect:

Metronidazole: **Inhibits** CYP2C8/9 (weak), 3A4 (moderate)

Tetracycline: **Substrate** of CYP3A4 (major); **Inhibits** CYP3A4 (moderate)

Increased Effect/Toxicity: See individual agents.

Decreased Effect: See individual agents.

Pharmacodynamics/Kinetics See individual agents.

Pregnancy Risk Factor D (tetracycline); B (metronidazole)

Bismuth Subsalicylate, Tetracycline, and Metronidazole *see* Bismuth Subsalicylate, Metronidazole, and Tetracycline *on page 209*

Bisoprolol (bis OH proe lol)

Related Information

Cardiovascular Diseases *on page 1458*

U.S. Brand Names Zebeta®

Canadian Brand Names Monocor®; Zebeta®

Generic Available Yes

Synonyms Bisoprolol Fumarate

Pharmacologic Category Beta Blocker, $Beta_1$ Selective

Use Treatment of hypertension, alone or in combination with other agents

Unlabeled/Investigational Use Angina pectoris, supraventricular arrhythmias, PVCs

Local Anesthetic/Vasoconstrictor Precautions No information available to require special precautions

Effects on Dental Treatment Bisoprolol is a cardioselective beta-blocker. Local anesthetic with vasoconstrictor can be safely used in patients medicated with bisoprolol. Nonselective beta-blockers (ie, propranolol, nadolol) enhance the pressor response to epinephrine, resulting in hypertension and bradycardia; this has not been reported for bisoprolol. Many nonsteroidal anti-inflammatory drugs, such as ibuprofen and indomethacin, can reduce the hypotensive effect of beta-blockers after 3 or more weeks of therapy with the NSAID. Short-term NSAID use (ie, 3 days) requires no special precautions in patients taking beta-blockers.

Common Adverse Effects

>10%:

Central nervous system: Drowsiness, insomnia

Endocrine & metabolic: Decreased sexual ability

1% to 10%:

Cardiovascular: Bradycardia, palpitations, edema, CHF, reduced peripheral circulation

Central nervous system: Mental depression

Gastrointestinal: Diarrhea or constipation, nausea, vomiting, stomach discomfort

Ocular: Mild ocular stinging and discomfort, tearing, photophobia, decreased corneal sensitivity, keratitis

Respiratory: Bronchospasm

Miscellaneous: Cold extremities

Mechanism of Action Selective inhibitor of $beta_1$-adrenergic receptors; competitively blocks $beta_1$-receptors, with little or no effect on $beta_2$-receptors at doses <10 mg

Drug Interactions

Cytochrome P450 Effect: Substrate of CYP2D6 (minor), 3A4 (major)

Increased Effect/Toxicity: Bisoprolol may increase the effects of other drugs which slow AV conduction (digoxin, verapamil, diltiazem), alpha-blockers (prazosin, terazosin), and alpha-adrenergic stimulants (epinephrine, phenylephrine). Bisoprolol may mask the tachycardia from hypoglycemia caused by insulin and oral hypoglycemics. In patients receiving concurrent therapy, the risk of hypertensive crisis is increased when either clonidine or the beta-blocker is withdrawn. Reserpine has been shown to enhance the effect of beta-blockers. Beta-blockers may increase the action or levels of ethanol, disopyramide, nondepolarizing muscle relaxants, and theophylline although the effects are difficult to predict. CYP3A4 inhibitors may increase the levels/effects of bisoprolol; example inhibitors include azole antifungals, ciprofloxacin, clarithromycin, diclofenac, doxycycline, erythromycin, imatinib, isoniazid, nefazodone, nicardipine, propofol, protease inhibitors, quinidine, and verapamil.

Decreased Effect: Decreased effect of bisoprolol with aluminum salts, calcium salts, cholestyramine, colestipol, NSAIDs, penicillins (ampicillin), and salicylates due to decreased bioavailability and plasma levels. The effect of sulfonylureas may be decreased by beta-blockers. CYP3A4 inducers may decrease the levels/effects of bisoprolol; example inducers include aminoglutethimide, carbamazepine, nafcillin, nevirapine, phenobarbital, phenytoin, and rifamycins.

Pharmacodynamics/Kinetics

Onset of action: 1-2 hours

Absorption: Rapid and almost complete

Distribution: Widely; highest concentrations in heart, liver, lungs, and saliva; crosses blood-brain barrier; enters breast milk

Protein binding: 26% to 33%

Metabolism: Extensively hepatic; significant first-pass effect

Half-life elimination: 9-12 hours

Time to peak: 1.7-3 hours

Excretion: Urine (3% to 10% as unchanged drug); feces (<2%)

Pregnancy Risk Factor C (manufacturer); D (2nd and 3rd trimesters - expert analysis)

Bisoprolol and Hydrochlorothiazide

(bis OH proe lol & hye droe klor oh THYE a zide)

Related Information

Bisoprolol *on page 210*

Hydrochlorothiazide *on page 699*

U.S. Brand Names Ziac®

Canadian Brand Names Ziac®

Generic Available Yes

Synonyms Hydrochlorothiazide and Bisoprolol

Pharmacologic Category Antihypertensive Agent, Combination

Use Treatment of hypertension

Local Anesthetic/Vasoconstrictor Precautions No information available to require special precautions

Effects on Dental Treatment Bisoprolol is a cardioselective beta-blocker. Local anesthetic with vasoconstrictor can be safely used in patients medicated with bisoprolol. Nonselective beta-blockers (ie, propranolol, nadolol) enhance the pressor response to epinephrine, resulting in hypertension and bradycardia; this has not been reported for bisoprolol. Many nonsteroidal anti-inflammatory drugs, such as ibuprofen and indomethacin, can reduce the hypotensive effect of beta-blockers after 3 or more weeks of therapy with the NSAID. Short-term NSAID use (ie, 3 days) requires no special precautions in patients taking beta-blockers.

Common Adverse Effects

>10%: Central nervous system: Fatigue

1% to 10%:

- Cardiovascular: Chest pain, edema, bradycardia, hypotension
- Central nervous system: Headache, dizziness, depression, abnormal dreams
- Dermatologic: Rash, photosensitivity
- Endocrine & metabolic: Hypokalemia, fluid and electrolyte imbalances (hypocalcemia, hypomagnesemia, hyponatremia), hyperglycemia
- Gastrointestinal: Constipation, diarrhea, dyspepsia, nausea, insomnia, flatulence
- Genitourinary: Micturition (frequency)
- Hematologic: Rarely blood dyscrasias
- Neuromuscular & skeletal: Arthralgia, myalgia
- Ocular: Abnormal vision
- Renal: Prerenal azotemia
- Respiratory: Rhinitis, cough, dyspnea

(Continued)

Bisoprolol and Hydrochlorothiazide *(Continued)*

Drug Interactions

Cytochrome P450 Effect: Bisoprolol: **Substrate** of CYP2D6 (minor), 3A4 (major)

Increased Effect/Toxicity: See individual agents.

Decreased Effect: See individual agents.

Pharmacodynamics/Kinetics See individual agents.

Pregnancy Risk Factor C/D (2nd and 3rd trimesters)

Bisoprolol Fumarate *see* Bisoprolol *on page 210*
Bistropamide *see* Tropicamide *on page 1348*

Bivalirudin (bye VAL i roo din)

U.S. Brand Names Angiomax®

Canadian Brand Names Angiomax®

Generic Available No

Synonyms Hirulog

Pharmacologic Category Anticoagulant, Thrombin Inhibitor

Use Anticoagulant used in conjunction with aspirin for patients with unstable angina undergoing percutaneous transluminal coronary angioplasty (PTCA)

Local Anesthetic/Vasoconstrictor Precautions No information available to require special precautions

Effects on Dental Treatment No significant effects or complications reported

Common Adverse Effects As with all anticoagulants, bleeding is the major adverse effect of bivalirudin. Hemorrhage may occur at virtually any site. Risk is dependent on multiple variables, including the intensity of anticoagulation and patient susceptibility. Additional adverse effects are often related to idiosyncratic reactions, and the frequency is difficult to estimate.

Adverse reactions reported were generally less than those seen with heparin.

>10%:

- Cardiovascular: Hypotension (12% bivalirudin vs 17% heparin)
- Central nervous system: Pain (15%), headache (12%)
- Gastrointestinal: Nausea (15%)
- Neuromuscular & skeletal: Back pain (42% vs 44% heparin)

1% to 10%:

- Cardiovascular: Hypertension (6%), bradycardia (5%)
- Central nervous system: Insomnia (7%), anxiety (6%), fever (5%), nervousness (5%)
- Gastrointestinal: Vomiting (6%), dyspepsia (5%), abdominal pain (5%)
- Genitourinary: Urinary retention (4%)
- Hematologic: Major hemorrhage (4% bivalirudin vs 9% heparin), transfusion required (2% bivalirudin vs 6% heparin)
- Local: Injection site pain (8%)
- Neuromuscular & skeletal: Pelvic pain (6%)

Mechanism of Action Bivalirudin acts as a specific and reversible direct thrombin inhibitor, binding to circulating and clot-bound thrombin. Shows linear dose- and concentration-dependent prolongation of ACT, aPTT, PT and TT.

Drug Interactions

Increased Effect/Toxicity: Aspirin may increase anticoagulant effect of bivalirudin (Note: All clinical trials included coadministration of aspirin). Limited drug interaction studies have not yet shown pharmacodynamic interactions between bivalirudin and ticlopidine, abciximab, or low molecular weight heparin (low molecular weight heparin was discontinued at least 8 hours prior to bivalirudin administration).

Pharmacodynamics/Kinetics

Onset of action: Immediate

Duration: Coagulation times return to baseline ~1 hour following discontinuation of infusion

Distribution: 0.2 L/kg

Protein binding, plasma: Does not bind other than thrombin

Half-life elimination: Normal renal function: 25 minutes; Cl_{cr} 10-29 mL/minute: 57 minutes

Excretion: Urine, proteolytic cleavage

Pregnancy Risk Factor B

BL4162A *see* Anagrelide *on page 130*
Blenoxane® *see* Bleomycin *on page 213*
Bleo *see* Bleomycin *on page 213*

Bleomycin (blee oh MYE sin)

U.S. Brand Names Blenoxane®
Canadian Brand Names Blenoxane®
Mexican Brand Names Blanoxan®; Bleolem®
Generic Available Yes
Synonyms Bleo; Bleomycin Sulfate; BLM; NSC-125066
Pharmacologic Category Antineoplastic Agent, Antibiotic
Use Treatment of squamous cell carcinomas, melanomas, sarcomas, testicular carcinoma, Hodgkin's lymphoma, and non-Hodgkin's lymphoma

Orphan drug: Sclerosing agent for malignant pleural effusion

Local Anesthetic/Vasoconstrictor Precautions No information available to require special precautions

Effects on Dental Treatment Key adverse event(s) related to dental treatment: Stomatitis.

Common Adverse Effects

>10%:

Cardiovascular: Raynaud's phenomenon

Dermatologic: Pain at the tumor site, phlebitis. About 50% of patients develop erythema, induration, hyperkeratosis, and peeling of the skin, particularly on the palmar and plantar surfaces of the hands and feet. Hyperpigmentation (50%), alopecia, nailbed changes may also occur. These effects appear dose-related and reversible with discontinuation of the drug.

Gastrointestinal: Stomatitis and mucositis (30%), anorexia, weight loss

Respiratory: Tachypnea, rales, acute or chronic interstitial pneumonitis and pulmonary fibrosis (5% to 10%), hypoxia and death (1%). Symptoms include cough, dyspnea, and bilateral pulmonary infiltrates. The pathogenesis is not certain, but may be due to damage of pulmonary, vascular, or connective tissue. Response to steroid therapy is variable and somewhat controversial.

Miscellaneous: Acute febrile reactions (25% to 50%); anaphylactoid reactions characterized by hypotension, confusion, fever, chills, and wheezing. Onset may be immediate or delayed for several hours.

1% to 10%:

Dermatologic: Rash (8%), skin thickening, diffuse scleroderma, onycholysis

Miscellaneous: Acute anaphylactoid reactions

Mechanism of Action Inhibits synthesis of DNA; binds to DNA leading to single- and double-strand breaks

Drug Interactions

Increased Effect/Toxicity: Lomustine increases severity of leukopenia. Cisplatin may decrease bleomycin elimination.

Decreased Effect: Bleomycin may decrease plasma levels of digoxin. Concomitant therapy with phenytoin results in decreased phenytoin levels.

Pharmacodynamics/Kinetics

Absorption: I.M. and intrapleural administration: 30% to 50% of I.V. serum concentrations; intraperitoneal and SubQ routes produce serum concentrations equal to those of I.V.

Distribution: V_d: 22 L/m^2; highest concentrations in skin, kidney, lung, heart tissues; lowest in testes and GI tract; does not cross blood-brain barrier

Protein binding: 1%

Metabolism: Via several tissues including hepatic, GI tract, skin, pulmonary, renal, and serum

Half-life elimination: Biphasic (renal function dependent):

Normal renal function: Initial: 1.3 hours; Terminal: 9 hours

End-stage renal disease: Initial: 2 hours; Terminal: 30 hours

Time to peak, serum: I.M.: Within 30 minutes

Excretion: Urine (50% to 70% as active drug)

Pregnancy Risk Factor D

Bleomycin Sulfate *see* Bleomycin *on page 213*
Bleph®-10 *see* Sulfacetamide *on page 1244*
Blephamide® *see* Sulfacetamide and Prednisolone *on page 1245*
Blis-To-Sol® [OTC] *see* Tolnaftate *on page 1312*
BLM *see* Bleomycin *on page 213*
Blocadren® *see* Timolol *on page 1299*
BMS-232632 *see* Atazanavir *on page 158*
BMS 337039 *see* Aripiprazole *on page 142*
Bonine® [OTC] *see* Meclizine *on page 859*
Bontril PDM® *see* Phendimetrazine *on page 1072*
Bontril® Slow-Release *see* Phendimetrazine *on page 1072*

Bortezomib (bore TEZ oh mib)

U.S. Brand Names Velcade™

Generic Available No

Synonyms LDP-341; MLN341; PS-341

Pharmacologic Category Proteasome Inhibitor

Use Treatment of multiple myeloma in patients who have had two prior therapies and had disease progression during the previous therapy

Local Anesthetic/Vasoconstrictor Precautions No information available to require special precautions

Effects on Dental Treatment Key adverse event(s) related to dental treatment: Abnormal taste and stomatitis.

Common Adverse Effects

>10%:

Cardiovascular: Edema (25%), hypotension (12%)

Central nervous system: Pyrexia (36%), headache (28%), insomnia (27%), dizziness (21%, excludes vertigo), anxiety (14%)

Dermatologic: Rash (21%), pruritus (11%)

Endocrine & metabolic: Dehydration (18%)

Gastrointestinal: Nausea (64%), diarrhea (51%), appetite decreased (43%), constipation (43%), vomiting (36%), abdominal pain (13%), abnormal taste (13%), dyspepsia (13%)

Hematologic: Thrombocytopenia (43%, Grade 3: 27%, Grade 4: 3%); anemia (32%, Grade 3: 9%); neutropenia (24%, Grade 3: 13%, Grade 4: 3%)

Neuromuscular & skeletal: Asthenic conditions (65%, Grade 3: 18% - includes fatigue, malaise, weakness); peripheral neuropathy (37%, Grade 3: 14%); arthralgia (26%); limb pain (26%); paresthesia and dysesthesia (23%), back pain (14%); bone pain (14%); muscle cramps (14%); myalgia (14%); rigors (12%)

Ocular: Blurred vision (11%)

Respiratory: Dyspnea (22%), upper respiratory tract infection (18%), cough (17%)

Miscellaneous: Herpes zoster (11%)

1% to 10%: Respiratory: Pneumonia (10%)

Mechanism of Action Bortezomib inhibits proteasomes, enzyme complexes which regulate protein homeostasis within the cell. Specifically, it reversibly inhibits chymotrypsin-like activity at the 26S proteasome, leading to activation of signaling cascades, cell-cycle arrest and apoptosis.

Drug Interactions

Cytochrome P450 Effect: Substrate of CYP1A2 (minor), 2C8/9 (minor), 2C19 (minor), 2D6 (minor), 3A4 (major); **Inhibits** CYP1A2 (weak), 2C8/9 (weak), 2C19 (moderate), 2D6 (weak), 3A4 (weak)

Increased Effect/Toxicity: Bortezomib may increase the levels/effects citalopram, diazepam, methsuximide, phenytoin, propranolol, sertraline, and other CYP2C19 substrates. Levels/effects of bortezomib may be increased by azole antifungals, ciprofloxacin, clarithromycin, diclofenac, doxycycline, erythromycin, imatinib, isoniazid, nefazodone, nicardipine, propofol, protease inhibitors, quinidine, telithromycin, verapamil, and other CYP3A4 inhibitors.

Decreased Effect: Levels/effects of bortezomib may be decreased by aminoglutethimide, carbamazepine, nafcillin, nevirapine, phenobarbital, phenytoin, rifamycins, and other CYP3A4 inducers.

Pharmacodynamics/Kinetics

Protein binding: ~83%

Metabolism: Hepatic via CYP 1A2, 2C9, 2C19, 2D6, 3A4; forms metabolites (inactive)

Half-life elimination: 9-15 hours

Pregnancy Risk Factor D

Bosentan (boe SEN tan)

U.S. Brand Names Tracleer®

Canadian Brand Names Tracleer®

Generic Available No

Pharmacologic Category Endothelin Antagonist

Use Treatment of pulmonary artery hypertension (PAH) in patients with World Health Organization (WHO) Class III or IV symptoms to improve exercise capacity and decrease the rate of clinical deterioration

Unlabeled/Investigational Use Investigational: Congestive heart failure

Local Anesthetic/Vasoconstrictor Precautions No information available to require special precautions

Effects on Dental Treatment No significant effects or complications reported

Common Adverse Effects

>10%:

Central nervous system: Headache (16% to 22%)

Hematologic: Hemoglobin decreased (≥1 g/dL in up to 57%; typically in first 6 weeks of therapy)

Hepatic: Serum transaminases increased (>3 times upper limit of normal; up to 11%)

Respiratory: Nasopharyngitis (11%)

1% to 10%:

Cardiovascular: Flushing (7% to 9%), edema (lower limb, 8%; generalized 4%), hypotension (7%), palpitations (5%)

Central nervous system: Fatigue (4%)

Dermatologic: Pruritus (4%)

Gastrointestinal: Dyspepsia (4%)

Hematologic: Anemia (3%)

Hepatic: Abnormal hepatic function (6% to 8%)

Restrictions Bosentan (Tracleer®) is available only through a limited distribution program directly from the manufacturer (Actelion Pharmaceuticals 1-866-228-3546). It will not be available through wholesalers or individual pharmacies.

Mechanism of Action Blocks endothelin receptors on vascular endothelium and smooth muscle. Stimulation of these receptors is associated with vasoconstriction. Although bosentan blocks both ET_A and ET_B receptors, the affinity is higher for the A subtype. Improvement in symptoms of pulmonary artery hypertension and a decrease in the rate of clinical deterioration have been demonstrated in clinical trials.

Drug Interactions

Cytochrome P450 Effect: Substrate (major) of CYP2C8/9, 3A4; **Induces** CYP2C8/9 (weak), 3A4 (weak)

Increased Effect/Toxicity: An increased risk of serum transaminase elevations was observed during concurrent therapy with glyburide; concurrent use is contraindicated. Cyclosporine increases serum concentrations of bosentan (approximately 3-4 times baseline). Concurrent use of cyclosporine is contraindicated.

CYP2C8/9 inhibitors may increase the levels/effects of bosentan; example inhibitors include delavirdine, fluconazole, gemfibrozil, ketoconazole, nicardipine, NSAIDs, pioglitazone, and sulfonamides. CYP3A4 inhibitors may increase the levels/effects of bosentan; example inhibitors include azole antifungals, ciprofloxacin, clarithromycin, diclofenac, doxycycline, erythromycin, imatinib, isoniazid, nefazodone, nicardipine, propofol, protease inhibitors, quinidine, and verapamil.

Decreased Effect: Bosentan may enhance the metabolism of cyclosporine, decreasing its serum concentrations by ~50%; effect on sirolimus and/or tacrolimus has not been specifically evaluated, but may be similar. Concurrent use of cyclosporine is contraindicated. Bosentan is a weak inducer, but may increase the metabolism of drugs metabolized by CYP2C8/9. CYP2C8/9 inducers may decrease the levels/effects of bosentan; example inducers include carbamazepine, phenobarbital, phenytoin, rifampin, rifapentine, and secobarbital. CYP3A4 inducers may decrease the levels/effects of bosentan; example inducers include aminoglutethimide, carbamazepine, nafcillin, nevirapine, phenobarbital, phenytoin, and rifamycins. Bosentan may enhance the metabolism of methadone resulting in methadone withdrawal.

Pharmacodynamics/Kinetics

Distribution: V_d: 18 L

Protein binding, plasma: >98% to albumin

Metabolism: Hepatic via CYP2C9 and 3A4 to three primary metabolites (one having pharmacologic activity)

Bioavailability: 50%

Half-life elimination: 5 hours; prolonged with heart failure, possibly in PAH

Excretion: Feces (as metabolites); urine (<3% as unchanged drug)

Pregnancy Risk Factor X

B&O Supprettes® *see* Belladonna and Opium *on page 186*

Botox® *see* Botulinum Toxin Type A *on page 215*

Botox® Cosmetic *see* Botulinum Toxin Type A *on page 215*

Botulinum Toxin Type A (BOT yoo lin num TOKS in type aye)

U.S. Brand Names Botox®; Botox® Cosmetic

Canadian Brand Names Botox®; Botox® Cosmetic

Generic Available No

(Continued)

Botulinum Toxin Type A *(Continued)*

Pharmacologic Category Neuromuscular Blocker Agent, Toxin; Ophthalmic Agent, Toxin

Use Treatment of strabismus and blepharospasm associated with dystonia (including benign essential blepharospasm or VII nerve disorders in patients ≥12 years of age); cervical dystonia (spasmodic torticollis) in patients ≥16 years of age; temporary improvement in the appearance of lines/wrinkles of the face (moderate to severe glabellar lines associated with corrugator and/or procerus muscle activity) in adult patients ≤65 years of age

Orphan drug: Treatment of dynamic muscle contracture in pediatric cerebral palsy patients

Unlabeled/Investigational Use Treatment of oromandibular dystonia, spasmodic dysphonia (laryngeal dystonia) and other dystonias (ie, writer's cramp, focal task-specific dystonias); migraine treatment and prophylaxis

Local Anesthetic/Vasoconstrictor Precautions No information available to require special precautions

Effects on Dental Treatment Key adverse event(s) related to dental treatment: Xerostomia (normal salivary flow resumes upon discontinuation), facial pain, and facial weakness. Affects occur in ~1 week and may last up to several months.

Common Adverse Effects Adverse effects usually occur in 1 week and may last up to several months

>10% :

- Central nervous system: Headache (cervical dystonia up to 11%, reduction of glabellar lines up to 13%; can occur with other uses)
- Gastrointestinal: Dysphagia (cervical dystonia 19%)
- Neuromuscular & skeletal: Neck pain (cervical dystonia 11%)
- Ocular: Ptosis (blepharospasm 10% to 40%, strabismus 1% to 38%, reduction of glabellar lines 1% to 5%); vertical deviation (strabismus 17%)
- Respiratory: Upper respiratory infection (cervical dystonia 12%),

2% to 10%:

- Central nervous system: Dizziness (cervical dystonia, reduction of glabellar lines); speech disorder (cervical dystonia), fever (cervical dystonia), drowsiness (cervical dystonia)
- Gastrointestinal: Xerostomia (cervical dystonia), nausea (cervical dystonia, reduction of glabellar lines)
- Local: Injection site reaction
- Neuromuscular & skeletal: Back pain (cervical dystonia); hypertonia (cervical dystonia); weakness (cervical dystonia, reduction of glabellar lines); facial pain (reduction of glabellar lines)
- Ocular: Dry eyes (blepharospasm 6%), superficial punctate keratitis (blepharospasm 6%)
- Respiratory: Cough (cervical dystonia), rhinitis (cervical dystonia), infection (reduction of glabellar lines)
- Miscellaneous: Flu syndrome (cervical dystonia, reduction of glabellar lines)

Mechanism of Action Botulinum A toxin is a neurotoxin produced by *Clostridium botulinum*, spore-forming anaerobic bacillus, which appears to affect only the presynaptic membrane of the neuromuscular junction in humans, where it prevents calcium-dependent release of acetylcholine and produces a state of denervation. Muscle inactivation persists until new fibrils grow from the nerve and form junction plates on new areas of the muscle-cell walls.

Drug Interactions

Increased Effect/Toxicity: Aminoglycosides, neuromuscular-blocking agents

Pharmacodynamics/Kinetics

Onset of action (improvement):

- Blepharospasm: ~3 days
- Cervical dystonia: ~2 weeks
- Strabismus: ~1-2 days
- Reduction of glabellar lines (Botox® Cosmetic): 1-2 days, increasing in intensity during first week

Duration:

- Blepharospasm: ~3 months
- Cervical dystonia: <3 months
- Strabismus: ~2-6 weeks
- Reduction of glabellar lines (Botox® Cosmetic): Up to 3 months

Absorption: Not expected to be present in peripheral blood at recommended doses

Time to peak:

- Blepharospasm: 1-2 weeks
- Cervical dystonia: ~6 weeks

Strabismus: Within first week

Pregnancy Risk Factor C (manufacturer)

Botulinum Toxin Type B (BOT yoo lin num TOKS in type bee)

U.S. Brand Names Myobloc®

Generic Available No

Pharmacologic Category Neuromuscular Blocker Agent, Toxin

Use Treatment of cervical dystonia (spasmodic torticollis)

Unlabeled/Investigational Use Treatment of cervical dystonia in patients who have developed resistance to botulinum toxin type A

Local Anesthetic/Vasoconstrictor Precautions No information available to require special precautions

Effects on Dental Treatment Key adverse event(s) related to dental treatment: Xerostomia (normal salivary flow resumes upon discontinuation), stomatitis, and abnormal taste.

Common Adverse Effects

>10%:

Central nervous system: Headache (10% to 16%), pain (6% to 13%; placebo 10%)

Gastrointestinal: Dysphagia (10% to 25%), xerostomia (3% to 34%)

Local: Injection site pain (12% to 16%)

Neuromuscular & skeletal: Neck pain (up to 17%; placebo: 16%)

Miscellaneous: Infection (13% to 19%; placebo: 15%)

1% to 10%:

Cardiovascular: Chest pain, vasodilation, peripheral edema

Central nervous system: Dizziness (3% to 6%), fever, malaise, migraine, anxiety, tremor, hyperesthesia, somnolence, confusion, vertigo

Dermatologic: Pruritus, bruising

Gastrointestinal: Nausea (3% to 10%; placebo: 5%), dyspepsia (up to 10%; placebo: 5%), vomiting, stomatitis, taste perversion

Genitourinary: Urinary tract infection, cystitis, vaginal moniliasis

Hematologic: Serum neutralizing activity

Neuromuscular & skeletal: Torticollis (up to 8%; placebo: 7%), arthralgia (up to 7%; placebo: 5%), back pain (3% to 7%; placebo: 3%), myasthenia (3% to 6%; placebo: 3%), weakness (up to 6%; placebo: 4%), arthritis

Ocular: Amblyopia, abnormal vision

Otic: Otitis media, tinnitus

Respiratory: Cough (3% to 7%; placebo: 3%), rhinitis (1% to 5%; placebo: 6%), dyspnea, pneumonia

Miscellaneous: Flu-syndrome (6% to 9%), allergic reaction, viral infection, abscess, cyst

Mechanism of Action Botulinum B toxin is a neurotoxin produced by *Clostridium botulinum,* spore-forming anaerobic bacillus. It cleaves synaptic Vesicle Association Membrane Protein (VAMP; synaptobrevin) which is a component of the protein complex responsible for docking and fusion of the synaptic vesicle to the presynaptic membrane. By blocking neurotransmitter release, botulinum B toxin paralyzes the muscle.

Drug Interactions

Increased Effect/Toxicity: Aminoglycosides, neuromuscular-blocking agents, botulinum toxin type A, other agents which may block neuromuscular transmission

Pharmacodynamics/Kinetics

Duration: 12-16 weeks

Absorption: Not expected to be present in peripheral blood at recommended doses

Pregnancy Risk Factor C (manufacturer)

Boudreaux's® Butt Paste [OTC] *see* Zinc Oxide *on page 1400*

Bovine Lung Surfactant *see* Beractant *on page 198*

Bravelle™ *see* Follitropins *on page 626*

Breathe Right® Saline [OTC] *see* Sodium Chloride *on page 1227*

Brethaire [DSC] *see* Terbutaline *on page 1273*

Brethine® *see* Terbutaline *on page 1273*

Bretylium (bre TIL ee um)

Related Information

Cardiovascular Diseases *on page 1458*

Generic Available Yes

Synonyms Bretylium Tosylate

Pharmacologic Category Antiarrhythmic Agent, Class III

(Continued)

Bretylium *(Continued)*

Use Treatment of ventricular tachycardia and fibrillation; treatment of other serious ventricular arrhythmias resistant to lidocaine

Local Anesthetic/Vasoconstrictor Precautions No information available to require special precautions

Effects on Dental Treatment No significant effects or complications reported

Mechanism of Action Class III antiarrhythmic; after an initial release of norepinephrine at the peripheral adrenergic nerve terminals, inhibits further release by postganglionic nerve endings in response to sympathetic nerve stimulation

Pregnancy Risk Factor C

Bretylium Tosylate *see* Bretylium *on page 217*

Brevibloc® *see* Esmolol *on page 515*

Brevicon® *see* Ethinyl Estradiol and Norethindrone *on page 550*

Brevital® Sodium *see* Methohexital *on page 895*

Brevoxyl® *see* Benzoyl Peroxide *on page 194*

Brevoxyl® Cleansing *see* Benzoyl Peroxide *on page 194*

Brevoxyl® Wash *see* Benzoyl Peroxide *on page 194*

Bricanyl [DSC] *see* Terbutaline *on page 1273*

Brimonidine (bri MOE ni deen)

U.S. Brand Names Alphagan® P

Canadian Brand Names Alphagan™; PMS-Brimonidine Tartrate; ratio-Brimonidine

Mexican Brand Names Alphagan®

Generic Available Yes

Synonyms Brimonidine Tartrate

Pharmacologic Category $Alpha_2$ Agonist, Ophthalmic; Ophthalmic Agent, Antiglaucoma

Use Lowering of intraocular pressure (IOP) in patients with open-angle glaucoma or ocular hypertension

Local Anesthetic/Vasoconstrictor Precautions No information available to require special precautions

Effects on Dental Treatment Key adverse event(s) related to dental treatment: Xerostomia (normal salivary flow resumes upon discontinuation).

Mechanism of Action Selective for $alpha_2$-receptors; appears to result in reduction of aqueous humor formation and increase uveoscleral outflow

Pregnancy Risk Factor B

Brimonidine Tartrate *see* Brimonidine *on page 218*

Brinzolamide (brin ZOH la mide)

U.S. Brand Names Azopt®

Canadian Brand Names Azopt®

Generic Available No

Pharmacologic Category Carbonic Anhydrase Inhibitor; Ophthalmic Agent, Antiglaucoma

Use Lowers intraocular pressure in patients with ocular hypertension or open-angle glaucoma

Local Anesthetic/Vasoconstrictor Precautions No information available to require special precautions

Effects on Dental Treatment Key adverse event(s) related to dental treatment: Taste disturbances.

Mechanism of Action Brinzolamide inhibits carbonic anhydrase, leading to decreased aqueous humor secretion. This results in a reduction of intraocular pressure.

Pregnancy Risk Factor C

Brioschi® [OTC] *see* Sodium Bicarbonate *on page 1226*

British Anti-Lewisite *see* Dimercaprol *on page 447*

BRL 43694 *see* Granisetron *on page 671*

Brofed® *see* Brompheniramine and Pseudoephedrine *on page 220*

Bromaline® [OTC] *see* Brompheniramine and Pseudoephedrine *on page 220*

Bromaxefed RF *see* Brompheniramine and Pseudoephedrine *on page 220*

Bromazepam (broe MA ze pam)

Canadian Brand Names Apo-Bromazepam®; Gen-Bromazepam; Lectopam®; Novo-Bromazepam; Nu-Bromazepam

Mexican Brand Names Lexotan®

Generic Available Yes

Pharmacologic Category Benzodiazepine

Use Short-term, symptomatic treatment of anxiety

Local Anesthetic/Vasoconstrictor Precautions No information available to require special precautions

Effects on Dental Treatment Key adverse event(s) related to dental treatment: Xerostomia (normal salivary flow resumes upon discontinuation).

Common Adverse Effects Frequency not defined.

Cardiovascular: Hypotension, palpitations, tachycardia

Central nervous system: Drowsiness, ataxia, dizziness, confusion, depression, euphoria, lethargy, slurred speech, stupor, headache, seizures, anterograde amnesia. In addition, paradoxical reactions (including excitation, agitation, hallucinations, and psychosis) are known to occur with benzodiazepines.

Dermatologic: Rash, pruritus

Endocrine & metabolic: Hyperglycemia, hypoglycemia

Gastrointestinal: Xerostomia, nausea, vomiting

Genitourinary: Incontinence, libido decreased

Hematologic: Hemoglobin decreased, hematocrit decreased, WBCs increased/decreased

Hepatic: Transaminases increased, alkaline phosphatase increased, bilirubin increased

Neuromuscular & skeletal: Weakness, muscle spasm

Ocular: Blurred vision, depth perception decreased

Restrictions CDSA IV; Not available in U.S.

Mechanism of Action Binds to stereospecific benzodiazepine receptors on the postsynaptic GABA neuron at several sites within the central nervous system, including the limbic system, reticular formation. Enhancement of the inhibitory effect of GABA on neuronal excitability results by increased neuronal membrane permeability to chloride ions. This shift in chloride ions results in hyperpolarization (a less excitable state) and stabilization.

Drug Interactions

Cytochrome P450 Effect: Substrate of CYP3A4 (major); **Inhibits** CYP2E1 (weak)

Increased Effect/Toxicity: Benzodiazepines potentiate the CNS depressant effects of narcotic analgesics, barbiturates, phenothiazines, ethanol, antihistamines, MAO inhibitors, sedative-hypnotics, and cyclic antidepressants. CYP3A4 inhibitors may increase the levels/effects of bromazepam; example inhibitors include azole antifungals, ciprofloxacin, clarithromycin, diclofenac, doxycycline, erythromycin, imatinib, isoniazid, nefazodone, nicardipine, propofol, protease inhibitors, quinidine, and verapamil.

Decreased Effect: CYP3A4 inducers may decrease the levels/effects of bromazepam; example inducers include aminoglutethimide, carbamazepine, nafcillin, nevirapine, phenobarbital, phenytoin, and rifamycins.

Pharmacodynamics/Kinetics

Protein binding: 70%

Metabolism: Hepatic

Bioavailability: 60%

Half-life elimination: 20 hours

Excretion: Urine (69%), as metabolites

Pregnancy Risk Factor D (based on other benzodiazepines)

Bromfed® [OTC] [DSC] *see* Brompheniramine and Pseudoephedrine *on page 220*

Bromfed-PD® [OTC] [DSC] *see* Brompheniramine and Pseudoephedrine *on page 220*

Bromfenex® *see* Brompheniramine and Pseudoephedrine *on page 220*

Bromfenex® PD *see* Brompheniramine and Pseudoephedrine *on page 220*

Bromhist Pediatric *see* Brompheniramine and Pseudoephedrine *on page 220*

Bromocriptine (broe moe KRIP teen)

U.S. Brand Names Parlodel®

Canadian Brand Names Apo-Bromocriptine®; Parlodel®; PMS-Bromocriptine

Mexican Brand Names Parlodel®; Serocryptin®

Generic Available Yes: Tablet

Synonyms Bromocriptine Mesylate

Pharmacologic Category Anti-Parkinson's Agent, Dopamine Agonist; Ergot Derivative

Use

Amenorrhea with or without galactorrhea; infertility or hypogonadism; prolactin-secreting adenomas; acromegaly; Parkinson's disease

A previous indication for prevention of postpartum lactation was withdrawn voluntarily by Sandoz Pharmaceuticals Corporation.

(Continued)

Bromocriptine *(Continued)*

Unlabeled/Investigational Use Neuroleptic malignant syndrome

Local Anesthetic/Vasoconstrictor Precautions No information available to require special precautions

Effects on Dental Treatment Key adverse event(s) related to dental treatment: Orthostatic hypotension.

Common Adverse Effects

>10%:

Central nervous system: Headache, dizziness

Gastrointestinal: Nausea

1% to 10%:

Cardiovascular: Orthostatic hypotension

Central nervous system: Fatigue, lightheadedness, drowsiness

Gastrointestinal: Anorexia, vomiting, abdominal cramps, constipation

Respiratory: Nasal congestion

Mechanism of Action Semisynthetic ergot alkaloid derivative and a dopamine receptor agonist which activates postsynaptic dopamine receptors in the tuberoinfundibular and nigrostriatal pathways

Drug Interactions

Cytochrome P450 Effect: Substrate of CYP3A4 (major); **Inhibits** CYP1A2 (weak), 3A4 (weak)

Increased Effect/Toxicity: Effects of bromocriptine may be increased by antifungals (azole derivatives); macrolide antibiotics; protease inhibitors; MAO inhibitors. Bromocriptine may increase the effects of sibutramine and other serotonin agonists (serotonin syndrome). CYP3A4 inhibitors may increase the levels/effects of bromocriptine; example inhibitors include azole antifungals, ciprofloxacin, clarithromycin, diclofenac, doxycycline, erythromycin, imatinib, isoniazid, nefazodone, nicardipine, propofol, protease inhibitors, quinidine, and verapamil.

Decreased Effect: Effects of bromocriptine may be diminished by antipsychotics, metoclopramide.

Pharmacodynamics/Kinetics

Protein binding: 90% to 96%

Metabolism: Primarily hepatic

Half-life elimination: Biphasic: Initial: 6-8 hours; Terminal: 50 hours

Time to peak, serum: 1-2 hours

Excretion: Feces; urine (2% to 6% as unchanged drug)

Pregnancy Risk Factor B

Bromocriptine Mesylate *see* Bromocriptine *on page 219*

Bromodiphenhydramine and Codeine

(brome oh dye fen HYE dra meen & KOE deen)

Related Information

Codeine *on page 369*

Generic Available Yes

Synonyms Codeine and Bromodiphenhydramine

Pharmacologic Category Antihistamine/Antitussive

Use Relief of upper respiratory symptoms and cough associated with allergies or common cold

Local Anesthetic/Vasoconstrictor Precautions No information available to require special precautions

Effects on Dental Treatment Key adverse event(s) related to dental treatment: Bromodiphenhydramine: Xerostomia (normal salivary flow resumes upon discontinuation).

Restrictions C-V

Pregnancy Risk Factor C

Brompheniramine and Pseudoephedrine

(brome fen IR a meen & soo doe e FED rin)

Related Information

Pseudoephedrine *on page 1147*

U.S. Brand Names AccuHist® Pediatric [DSC]; Andehist NR Syrup; Brofed®; Bromaline® [OTC]; Bromaxefed RF; Bromfed® [OTC] [DSC]; Bromfed-PD® [OTC] [DSC]; Bromfenex®; Bromfenex® PD; Bromhist Pediatric; Children's Dimetapp® Elixir Cold & Allergy [OTC]; Histex™ SR; Lodrane®; Lodrane® 12D; Lodrane® LD; Rondec® Syrup; Touro™ Allergy

Generic Available Yes: Excludes capsule (sustained release), liquid, tablet (extended release)

Synonyms Brompheniramine Maleate and Pseudoephedrine Hydrochloride; Brompheniramine Maleate and Pseudoephedrine Sulfate; Pseudoephedrine and Brompheniramine

Pharmacologic Category Antihistamine/Decongestant Combination

Use Temporary relief of symptoms of seasonal and perennial allergic rhinitis, and vasomotor rhinitis, including nasal obstruction

Local Anesthetic/Vasoconstrictor Precautions Use with caution since pseudoephedrine is a sympathomimetic amine which could interact with epinephrine to cause a pressor response

Effects on Dental Treatment Key adverse event(s) related to dental treatment:

Brompheniramine: Prolonged use may decrease salivary flow.

Pseudoephedrine: Xerostomia (normal salivary flow resumes upon discontinuation).

Common Adverse Effects Frequency not defined.

Cardiovascular: Arrhythmias, flushing, hypertension, pallor, palpitations, tachycardia

Central nervous system: Convulsions, CNS stimulation, dizziness, excitability (children; rare), giddiness, hallucinations, headache, insomnia, irritability, lassitude, nervousness, sedation

Gastrointestinal: Anorexia, diarrhea, dyspepsia, nausea, vomiting, xerostomia

Neuromuscular skeletal: Tremors, weakness

Ocular: Diplopia

Renal: Dysuria, polyuria, urinary retention (with BPH)

Respiratory: Respiratory difficulty

Mechanism of Action Brompheniramine maleate is an antihistamine with H_1-receptor activity; pseudoephedrine, a sympathomimetic amine and isomer of ephedrine, acts as a decongestant in respiratory tract mucous membranes with less vasoconstrictor action than ephedrine in normotensive individuals.

Pharmacodynamics/Kinetics

See Pseudoephedrine monograph.

Brompheniramine:

Metabolism: Hepatic

Time to peak: Syrup: 5 hours

Excretion: Urine

Pregnancy Risk Factor C

Brompheniramine Maleate and Pseudoephedrine Hydrochloride *see* Brompheniramine and Pseudoephedrine *on page 220*

Brompheniramine Maleate and Pseudoephedrine Sulfate *see* Brompheniramine and Pseudoephedrine *on page 220*

Broncho Saline® [OTC] *see* Sodium Chloride *on page 1227*

Brontex® *see* Guaifenesin and Codeine *on page 673*

BSS® *see* Balanced Salt Solution *on page 181*

BSS Plus® *see* Balanced Salt Solution *on page 181*

B-type Natriuretic Peptide (Human) *see* Nesiritide *on page 976*

Budesonide (byoo DES oh nide)

U.S. Brand Names Entocort™ EC; Pulmicort Respules®; Pulmicort Turbuhaler®; Rhinocort® Aqua®

Canadian Brand Names Entocort®; Gen-Budesonide AQ; Pulmicort®; Rhinocort® Turbuhaler®

Mexican Brand Names Pulmicort®; Rhinocort®

Generic Available No

Pharmacologic Category Corticosteroid, Inhalant (Oral); Corticosteroid, Nasal; Corticosteroid, Systemic

Use

Intranasal: Children ≥6 years of age and Adults: Management of symptoms of seasonal or perennial rhinitis

Nebulization: Children 12 months to 8 years: Maintenance and prophylactic treatment of asthma

Oral capsule: Treatment of active Crohn's disease (mild to moderate) involving the ileum and/or ascending colon

Oral inhalation: Maintenance and prophylactic treatment of asthma; includes patients who require corticosteroids and those who may benefit from systemic dose reduction/elimination

Local Anesthetic/Vasoconstrictor Precautions No information available to require special precautions

Effects on Dental Treatment Key adverse event(s) related to dental treatment: Xerostomia (normal salivary flow resumes upon discontinuation), dry throat, abnormal taste, and herpes simplex. Localized infections with *Candida*
(Continued)

Budesonide *(Continued)*

albicans or *Aspergillus niger* have occurred frequently in the mouth and pharynx with repetitive use of oral inhaler of corticosteroids. These infections may require treatment with appropriate antifungal therapy or discontinuance of treatment with corticosteroid inhaler.

Common Adverse Effects Reaction severity varies by dose and duration; not all adverse reactions have been reported with each dosage form.

>10%:

Central nervous system: Oral capsule: Headache (up to 21%)

Gastrointestinal: Oral capsule: Nausea (up to 11%)

Respiratory: Respiratory infection, rhinitis

Miscellaneous: Symptoms of HPA axis suppression and/or hypercorticism (acne, easy bruising, fat redistribution, striae, edema) may occur in >10% of patients following administration of dosage forms which result in higher systemic exposure (ie, oral capsule), but may be less frequent than rates observed with comparator drugs (prednisolone). These symptoms may be rare (<1%) following administration via methods which result in lower exposures (topical).

1% to 10%:

Cardiovascular: Syncope, edema, hypertension

Central nervous system: Chest pain, dysphonia, emotional lability, fatigue, fever, insomnia, migraine, nervousness, pain, dizziness, vertigo

Dermatologic: Bruising, contact dermatitis, eczema, pruritus, pustular rash, rash

Endocrine & metabolic: Hypokalemia, adrenal insufficiency

Gastrointestinal: Abdominal pain, anorexia, diarrhea, dry mouth, dyspepsia, gastroenteritis, oral candidiasis, taste perversion, vomiting, weight gain, flatulence

Hematologic: Cervical lymphadenopathy, purpura, leukocytosis

Neuromuscular & skeletal: Arthralgia, fracture, hyperkinesis, hypertonia, myalgia, neck pain, weakness, paresthesia, back pain

Ocular: Conjunctivitis, eye infection

Otic: Earache, ear infection, external ear infection

Respiratory: Bronchitis, bronchospasm, cough, epistaxis, nasal irritation, pharyngitis, sinusitis, stridor

Miscellaneous: Allergic reaction, flu-like syndrome, herpes simplex, infection, moniliasis, viral infection, voice alteration

Dosage

Nasal inhalation: (Rhinocort® Aqua®): Children ≥6 years and Adults: 64 mcg/day as a single 32 mcg spray in each nostril. Some patients who do not achieve adequate control may benefit from increased dosage. A reduced dosage may be effective after initial control is achieved.

Maximum dose: Children <12 years: 128 mcg/day; Adults: 256 mcg/day

Nebulization: Children 12 months to 8 years: Pulmicort Respules®: Titrate to lowest effective dose once patient is stable; start at 0.25 mg/day or use as follows:

Previous therapy of bronchodilators alone: 0.5 mg/day administered as a single dose or divided twice daily (maximum daily dose: 0.5 mg)

Previous therapy of inhaled corticosteroids: 0.5 mg/day administered as a single dose or divided twice daily (maximum daily dose: 1 mg)

Previous therapy of oral corticosteroids: 1 mg/day administered as a single dose or divided twice daily (maximum daily dose: 1 mg)

Oral inhalation:

Children ≥6 years:

Previous therapy of bronchodilators alone: 200 mcg twice initially which may be increased up to 400 mcg twice daily

Previous therapy of inhaled corticosteroids: 200 mcg twice initially which may be increased up to 400 mcg twice daily

Previous therapy of oral corticosteroids: The highest recommended dose in children is 400 mcg twice daily

Adults:

Previous therapy of bronchodilators alone: 200-400 mcg twice initially which may be increased up to 400 mcg twice daily

Previous therapy of inhaled corticosteroids: 200-400 mcg twice initially which may be increased up to 800 mcg twice daily

Previous therapy of oral corticosteroids: 400-800 mcg twice daily which may be increased up to 800 mcg twice daily

NIH Guidelines (NIH, 1997) (give in divided doses twice daily):

Children:

"Low" dose: 100-200 mcg/day

"Medium" dose: 200-400 mcg/day (1-2 inhalations/day)
"High" dose: >400 mcg/day (>2 inhalation/day)
Adults:
"Low" dose: 200-400 mcg/day (1-2 inhalations/day)
"Medium" dose: 400-600 mcg/day (2-3 inhalations/day)
"High" dose: >600 mcg/day (>3 inhalation/day)

Oral: Adults: Crohn's disease: 9 mg once daily in the morning; safety and efficacy have not been established for therapy duration >8 weeks; recurring episodes may be treated with a repeat 8-week course of treatment

Note: Treatment may be tapered to 6 mg once daily for 2 weeks prior to complete cessation. Patients receiving CYP3A4 inhibitors should be monitored closely for signs and symptoms of hypercorticism; dosage reduction may be required.

Dosage adjustment in hepatic impairment: Monitor closely for signs and symptoms of hypercorticism; dosage reduction may be required.

Mechanism of Action Controls the rate of protein synthesis, depresses the migration of polymorphonuclear leukocytes, fibroblasts, reverses capillary permeability, and lysosomal stabilization at the cellular level to prevent or control inflammation

Contraindications Hypersensitivity to budesonide or any component of the formulation

Inhalation: Contraindicated in primary treatment of status asthmaticus, acute episodes of asthma; not for relief of acute bronchospasm

Warnings/Precautions May cause hypercorticism and/or suppression of hypothalamic-pituitary-adrenal (HPA) axis, particularly in younger children or in patients receiving high doses for prolonged periods. Particular care is required when patients are transferred from systemic corticosteroids to products with lower systemic bioavailability (ie, inhalation). May lead to possible adrenal insufficiency or withdrawal from steroids, including an increase in allergic symptoms. Patients receiving prolonged therapy of ≥20 mg per day of prednisone (or equivalent) may be most susceptible. Aerosol steroids do **not** provide the systemic steroid needed to treat patients having trauma, surgery, or infections.

Controlled clinical studies have shown that orally-inhaled and intranasal corticosteroids may cause a reduction in growth velocity in pediatric patients. (In studies of orally-inhaled corticosteroids, the mean reduction in growth velocity was approximately 1 centimeter per year [range 0.3-1.8 cm per year] and appears to be related to dose and duration of exposure.) To minimize the systemic effects of orally-inhaled and intranasal corticosteroids, each patient should be titrated to the lowest effective dose. Growth should be routinely monitored in pediatric patients.

May suppress the immune system, patients may be more susceptible to infection. Use with caution in patients with systemic infections or ocular herpes simplex. Avoid exposure to chickenpox and measles. Corticosteroids should be used with caution in patients with diabetes, hypertension, osteoporosis, peptic ulcer, glaucoma, cataracts, or tuberculosis. Use caution in hepatic impairment. Enteric-coated capsules should not be crushed or chewed.

Drug Interactions

Cytochrome P450 Effect: Substrate of CYP3A4 (major)

Increased Effect/Toxicity: Cimetidine may decrease the clearance and increase the bioavailability of budesonide, increasing its serum concentrations. In addition, CYP3A4 inhibitors may increase the serum level and/or toxicity of budesonide this effect was shown with ketoconazole, but not erythromycin. Other potential inhibitors include amiodarone, cimetidine, clarithromycin, delavirdine, diltiazem, dirithromycin, disulfiram, fluoxetine, fluvoxamine, grapefruit juice, indinavir, itraconazole, ketoconazole, nefazodone, nevirapine, propoxyphene, quinupristin-dalfopristin, ritonavir, saquinavir, verapamil, zafirlukast, zileuton. The addition of salmeterol has been demonstrated to improve response to inhaled corticosteroids (as compared to increasing steroid dosage).

Decreased Effect: Theoretically, proton pump inhibitors (omeprazole, pantoprazole) alter gastric pH may affect the rate of dissolution of enteric-coated capsules. Administration with omeprazole did not alter kinetics of budesonide capsules.

Ethanol/Nutrition/Herb Interactions

Food: Grapefruit juice may double systemic exposure of orally-administered budesonide. Administration of capsules with a high-fat meal delays peak concentration, but does not alter the extent of absorption.

Herb/Nutraceutical: St John's wort may decrease budesonide levels.

Dietary Considerations Avoid grapefruit juice when using oral capsules.

(Continued)

Budesonide *(Continued)*

Pharmacodynamics/Kinetics

Onset of action: Respules®: 2-8 days; Rhinocort® Aqua®: ~10 hours; Turbuhaler®: 24 hours

Peak effect: Respules®: 4-6 weeks; Rhinocort® Aqua®: ~2 weeks; Turbuhaler®: 1-2 weeks

Absorption: Capsule: Rapid and complete

Distribution: 2.2-3.9 L/kg

Protein binding: 85% to 90%

Metabolism: Hepatic via CYP3A4 to two metabolites: 16 alpha-hydroxyprednisolone and 6 beta-hydroxybudesonide; minor activity

Bioavailability: Limited by high first-pass effect; Capsule: 9% to 21%; Respules®: 6%; Turbuhaler®: 6% to 13%; Nasal: 34%

Half-life elimination: 2-3.6 hours

Time to peak: Capsule: 30-600 minutes (variable in Crohn's disease); Respules®: 10-30 minutes; Turbuhaler®: 1-2 hours; Nasal: 1 hour

Excretion: Urine (60%) and feces as metabolites

Pregnancy Risk Factor C/B (Pulmicort Respules® and Turbuhaler®)

Dosage Forms CAP, enteric coated (Entocort™ EC): 3 mg. **POWDER, oral inhalation** (Pulmicort Turbuhaler®): 200 mcg/inhalation (104 g); (additional dosage strengths available in Canada: 100 mcg/inhalation, 400 mcg/inhalation). **SPRAY, nasal** (Rhinocort® Aqua®): 32 mcg/inhalation (8.6 g). **SUSP, oral inhalation** (Pulmicort Respules®): 0.25 mg/2 mL (30s), 0.5 mg/2 mL (30s)

Buffered Aspirin and Pravastatin Sodium *see* Aspirin and Pravastatin *on page 157*

Bufferin® [OTC] *see* Aspirin *on page 151*

Bufferin® Extra Strength [OTC] *see* Aspirin *on page 151*

Buffinol [OTC] *see* Aspirin *on page 151*

Buffinol Extra [OTC] *see* Aspirin *on page 151*

Bumetanide (byoo MET a nide)

Related Information

Cardiovascular Diseases *on page 1458*

U.S. Brand Names Bumex®

Canadian Brand Names Bumex®; Burinex®

Mexican Brand Names Bumedyl®; Drenural®; Miccil®

Generic Available Yes

Pharmacologic Category Diuretic, Loop

Use Management of edema secondary to congestive heart failure or hepatic or renal disease including nephrotic syndrome; may be used alone or in combination with antihypertensives in the treatment of hypertension; can be used in furosemide-allergic patients

Local Anesthetic/Vasoconstrictor Precautions No information available to require special precautions

Effects on Dental Treatment No significant effects or complications reported

Common Adverse Effects

>10%:

Endocrine & metabolic: Hyperuricemia (18%), hypochloremia (15%), hypokalemia (15%)

Renal: Azotemia (11%)

1% to 10%:

Central nervous system: Dizziness (1%)

Endocrine & metabolic: Hyponatremia (9%), hyperglycemia (7%), variations in phosphorus (5%), CO_2 content (4%), bicarbonate (3%), and calcium (2%)

Neuromuscular & skeletal: Muscle cramps (1%)

Otic: Ototoxicity (1%)

Renal: Increased serum creatinine (7%)

Mechanism of Action Inhibits reabsorption of sodium and chloride in the ascending loop of Henle and proximal renal tubule, interfering with the chloride-binding cotransport system, thus causing increased excretion of water, sodium, chloride, magnesium, phosphate and calcium; it does not appear to act on the distal tubule

Drug Interactions

Increased Effect/Toxicity: Bumetanide-induced hypokalemia may predispose to digoxin toxicity and may increase the risk of arrhythmia with drugs which may prolong QT interval, including type Ia and type III antiarrhythmic agents, cisapride, and some quinolones (sparfloxacin, gatifloxacin, and moxifloxacin). The risk of toxicity from lithium and salicylates (high dose) may be increased by loop diuretics. Hypotensive effects and/or adverse renal effects of ACE inhibitors and NSAIDs are potentiated by bumetanide-induced hypovolemia. The effects of peripheral adrenergic-blocking drugs or ganglionic blockers may be increased by bumetanide.

Bumetanide may increase the risk of ototoxicity with other ototoxic agents (aminoglycosides, cis-platinum), especially in patients with renal dysfunction. Synergistic diuretic effects occur with thiazide-type diuretics. Diuretics tend to be synergistic with other antihypertensive agents, and hypotension may occur.

Decreased Effect: Glucose tolerance may be decreased by loop diuretics, requiring adjustment of hypoglycemic agents. Cholestyramine or colestipol may reduce bioavailability of bumetanide. Indomethacin (and other NSAIDs) may reduce natriuretic and hypotensive effects of diuretics. Hypokalemia may reduce the efficacy of some antiarrhythmics.

Pharmacodynamics/Kinetics

Onset of action: Oral, I.M.: 0.5-1 hour; I.V.: 2-3 minutes

Duration: 6 hours

Distribution: V_d: 13-25 L/kg

Protein binding: 95%

Metabolism: Partially hepatic

Half-life elimination: Neonates: ~6 hours; Infants (1 month): ~2.4 hours; Adults: 1-1.5 hours

Excretion: Primarily urine (as unchanged drug and metabolites)

Pregnancy Risk Factor C (manufacturer); D (expert analysis)

Bumex® *see* Bumetanide *on page 224*

Buphenyl® *see* Sodium Phenylbutyrate *on page 1230*

Bupivacaine (byoo PIV a kane)

Related Information

Oral Pain *on page 1526*

U.S. Brand Names Marcaine®; Marcaine® Spinal; Sensorcaine®; Sensorcaine®-MPF

Canadian Brand Names Marcaine®; Sensorcaine®

Mexican Brand Names Buvacaina®

Generic Available Yes

Synonyms Bupivacaine Hydrochloride

Pharmacologic Category Local Anesthetic

Use Local anesthetic (injectable) for peripheral nerve block, infiltration, sympathetic block, caudal or epidural block, retrobulbar block

Local Anesthetic/Vasoconstrictor Precautions No information available to require special precautions

Effects on Dental Treatment No significant effects or complications reported

Significant Adverse Effects Frequency not defined.

Cardiovascular: Cardiac arrest, hypotension, bradycardia, palpitations

Central nervous system: Seizures, restlessness, anxiety, dizziness

Gastrointestinal: Nausea, vomiting

Neuromuscular & skeletal: Weakness

Ocular: Blurred vision

Otic: Tinnitus

Respiratory: Apnea

Dosage Dose varies with procedure, depth of anesthesia, vascularity of tissues, duration of anesthesia and condition of patient. Some formulations contain metabisulfites (in epinephrine-containing injection); do not use solutions containing preservatives for caudal or epidural block.

Local anesthesia: Infiltration: 0.25% infiltrated locally; maximum: 175 mg

Caudal block (with or without epinephrine, preservative free):
- Children: 1-3.7 mg/kg
- Adults: 15-30 mL of 0.25% or 0.5%

Epidural block (other than caudal block - with or without epinephrine, preservative free):
- Administer in 3-5 mL increments, allowing sufficient time to detect toxic manifestations of inadvertent I.V. or I.T. administration:
  - Children: 1.25 mg/kg/dose
  - Adults: 10-20 mL of 0.25% or 0.5%
  - Surgical procedures requiring a high degree of muscle relaxation and prolonged effects **only**: 10-20 mL of 0.75% (**Note:** Not to be used in obstetrical cases)

Maxillary and mandibular infiltration and nerve block: 9 mg (1.8 mL) of 0.5% (with epinephrine) per injection site; a second dose may be administered if

(Continued)

Bupivacaine *(Continued)*

necessary to produce adequate anesthesia after allowing up to 10 minutes for onset, up to a maximum of 90 mg per dental appointment

Obstetrical anesthesia: Incremental dose: 3-5 mL of 0.5% (not exceeding 50-100 mg in any dosing interval); allow sufficient time to detect toxic manifestations or inadvertent I.V. or I.T. injection

Peripheral nerve block: 5 mL of 0.25 or 0.5%; maximum: 400 mg/day

Sympathetic nerve block: 20-50 mL of 0.25%

Retrobulbar anesthesia: 2-4 mL of 0.75%

Spinal anesthesia: Solution of 0.75% bupivacaine in 8.25% dextrose is used:

- Lower extremity and perineal procedures: 1 mL
- Lower abdominal procedures: 1.6 mL
- Obstetrical:
  - Normal vaginal delivery: 0.8 mL (higher doses may be required in some patients)
  - Cesarean section: 1-1.4 mL

Mechanism of Action Blocks both the initiation and conduction of nerve impulses by decreasing the neuronal membrane's permeability to sodium ions, which results in inhibition of depolarization with resultant blockade of conduction

Contraindications Hypersensitivity to bupivacaine hydrochloride, amide-type local anesthetics (etidocaine, lidocaine, mepivacaine, prilocaine, ropivacaine) or any component of the formulation (para-aminobenzoic acid or parabens in specific formulations); not to be used for obstetrical paracervical block anesthesia

Warnings/Precautions Use with caution in patients with hepatic impairment. Some commercially available formulations contain sodium metabisulfite, which may cause allergic-type reactions; not recommended for use in children <12 years of age. The solution for spinal anesthesia should not be used in children <18 years of age. **Do not use solutions containing preservatives for caudal or epidural block**. Local anesthetics have been associated with rare occurrences of sudden respiratory arrest; convulsions due to systemic toxicity leading to cardiac arrest have also been reported, presumably following unintentional intravascular injection. The 0.75% is **not** recommended for obstetrical anesthesia. A test dose is recommended prior to epidural administration (prior to initial dose) and all reinforcing doses with continuous catheter technique.

Drug Interactions Substrate (minor) of CYP1A2, 2C19, 2D6, 3A4

Increased effect: Hyaluronidase

Increased toxicity: Beta-blockers, ergot-type oxytocics, MAO inhibitors, TCAs, phenothiazines, vasopressors

Pharmacodynamics/Kinetics

Onset of action: Anesthesia (route dependent): 4-10 minutes

Duration: 1.5-8.5 hours

Metabolism: Hepatic

Half-life elimination (age dependent): Neonates: 8.1 hours; Adults: 1.5-5.5 hours

Excretion: Urine (~6%)

Pregnancy Risk Factor C

Lactation Enters breast milk/contraindicated

Dosage Forms

Injection, solution, as hydrochloride [preservative free]: 0.25% [2.5 mg/mL] (10 mL, 20 mL, 30 mL, 50 mL); 0.5% [5 mg/mL] (10 mL, 20 mL, 30 mL); 0.75% [7.5 mg/mL] (10 mL, 20 mL, 30 mL)

- Marcaine®: 0.25% [2.5 mg/mL] (10 mL, 30 mL, 50 mL); 0.5% [5 mg/mL] (10 mL, 30 mL); 0.75% [7.5 mg/mL] (10 mL, 30 mL)
- Marcaine® Spinal: 0.75% [7.5 mg/mL] (2 mL) [in dextrose 8.25%]
- Sensorcaine®-MPF: 0.25% [2.5 mg/mL] (10 mL, 30 mL); 0.5% [5 mg/mL] (10 mL, 30 mL); 0.75% [7.5 mg/mL] (10 mL, 30 mL)

Injection, solution, as hydrochloride (Marcaine®, Sensorcaine®): 0.25% [2.5 mg/mL] (50 mL); 0.5% [5 mg/mL] (50 mL) [contains methylparaben]

Injection, solution, with epinephrine 1:200,000, as hydrochloride [preservative free]: 0.25% [2.5 mg/mL] (10 mL, 30 mL); 0.5 % [5 mg/mL] (30 mL)

- Marcaine®: 0.25% [2.5 mg/mL] (10 mL, 30 mL); 0.5% [5 mg/mL] (3 mL, 10 mL, 30 mL); 0.75% [7.5 mg/mL] (30 mL) [contains sodium metabisulfite]
- Sensorcaine®-MPF: 0.25% [2.5 mg/mL] (10 mL, 30 mL); 0.5% [5 mg/mL] (10 mL, 30 mL); 0.75% [7.5 mg/mL] (30 mL) [contains sodium metabisulfite]

Injection, solution, with epinephrine 1:200,000, as hydrochloride [with preservative] (Marcaine®, Sensorcaine®): 0.25% [2.5 mg/mL] (50 mL); 0.5% [5 mg/mL] (50 mL) [contains methylparaben and sodium metabisulfite]

Bupivacaine and Epinephrine (byoo PIV a kane & ep i NEF rin)

Related Information

Bupivacaine *on page 225*
Epinephrine *on page 496*
Oral Pain *on page 1526*

U.S. Brand Names Marcaine® with Epinephrine

Canadian Brand Names Sensorcaine® With Epinephrine

Generic Available Yes

Synonyms Epinephrine and Bupivacaine (Dental)

Pharmacologic Category Local Anesthetic

Dental Use Local anesthesia

Local Anesthetic/Vasoconstrictor Precautions No information available to require special precautions

Effects on Dental Treatment It is common to misinterpret psychogenic responses to local anesthetic injection as an allergic reaction. Intraoral injections are perceived by many patients as a stressful procedure in dentistry. Common symptoms to this stress are diaphoresis, palpitations, hyperventilation. Patients may exhibit hypersensitivity to bisulfites contained in local anesthetic solution to prevent oxidation of epinephrine. In general, patients reacting to bisulfites have a history of asthma and their airways are hyper-reactive to asthmatic syndrome.

Degree of adverse effects in the CNS and cardiovascular system is directly related to the blood levels of bupivacaine. Bradycardia, hypersensitivity reactions (rare; may be manifest as dermatologic reactions and edema at injection site), asthmatic syndromes

High blood levels: Anxiety, restlessness, disorientation, confusion, dizziness, tremors, seizures, CNS depression (resulting in somnolence, unconsciousness and possible respiratory arrest), nausea, and vomiting.

Significant Adverse Effects Degree of adverse effects in the central nervous system and cardiovascular system are directly related to the blood levels of bupivacaine

Cardiovascular: Myocardial effects include a decrease in contraction force as well as a decrease in electrical excitability and myocardial conduction rate resulting in bradycardia and reduction in cardiac output.

Central nervous system: High blood levels result in anxiety, restlessness, disorientation, confusion, dizziness, tremors and seizures. This is followed by depression of CNS resulting in somnolence, unconsciousness and possible respiratory arrest. Nausea and vomiting may also occur. In some cases, symptoms of CNS stimulation may be absent and the primary CNS effects are somnolence and unconsciousness.

Hypersensitivity reactions: Extremely rare, but may be manifest as dermatologic reactions and edema at injection site. Asthmatic syndromes have occurred. Patients may exhibit hypersensitivity to bisulfites contained in local anesthetic solution to prevent oxidation of epinephrine. In general, patients reacting to bisulfites have a history of asthma and their airways are hyper-reactive to asthmatic syndrome.

Psychogenic reactions: It is common to misinterpret psychogenic responses to local anesthetic injection as an allergic reaction. Intraoral injections are perceived by many patients as a stressful procedure in dentistry. Common symptoms to this stress are diaphoresis, palpitations, hyperventilation, generalized pallor and a fainting feeling.

Dosage

# of Cartridges (1.8 mL)	Mg Bupivacaine (0.5%)	Mg Vasoconstrictor (Epinephrine 1:200,000)
1	9	0.009
2	18	0.018
3	27	0.027
4	36	0.036
5	45	0.045
6	54	0.054
7	63	0.063
8	72	0.072
9	81	0.081
10	90	0.090

(Continued)

Bupivacaine and Epinephrine *(Continued)*

Children <10 years: Dosage has not been established

Children >10 years and Adults: Infiltration and nerve block in maxillary and mandibular area: 9 mg (1.8 mL) of bupivacaine as a 0.5% solution with epinephrine 1:200,000 per injection site. A second dose may be administered if necessary to produce adequate anesthesia after allowing up to 10 minutes for onset. Up to a maximum of 90 mg of bupivacaine hydrochloride per dental appointment. The effective anesthetic dose varies with procedure, intensity of anesthesia needed, duration of anesthesia required, and physical condition of the patient; always use the lowest effective dose along with careful aspiration.

The following numbers of dental carpules (1.8 mL) provide the indicated amounts of bupivacaine hydrochloride 0.5% and vasoconstrictor (epinephrine 1:200,000): See table on previous page.

Note: Adult and children doses of bupivacaine hydrochloride with epinephrine cited from USP Dispensing Information (USP DI), 17th ed, The United States Pharmacopeial Convention, Inc, Rockville, MD, 1997, 134.

Mechanism of Action Local anesthetics bind selectively to the intracellular surface of sodium channels to block influx of sodium into the axon. As a result, depolarization necessary for action potential propagation and subsequent nerve function is prevented. The block at the sodium channel is reversible. When drug diffuses away from the axon, sodium channel function is restored and nerve propagation returns.

Epinephrine prolongs the duration of the anesthetic actions of bupivacaine by causing vasoconstriction (alpha adrenergic receptor agonist) of the vasculature surrounding the nerve axons. This prevents the diffusion of bupivacaine away from the nerves resulting in a longer retention in the axon

Contraindications Hypersensitivity to bupivacaine or any component of the formulation

Warnings/Precautions Should be avoided in patients with uncontrolled hyperthyroidism

Drug Interactions Bupivacaine: **Substrate** (minor) of CYP1A2, 2C19, 2D6, 3A4

Also see individual agents.

Pharmacodynamics/Kinetics

Onset of action: Infiltration and nerve block: 2-20 minutes

Duration: Infiltration: 1 hour; Nerve block: 5-7 hours

Half-life elimination, serum: Adults: 1.5-5.5 hours

Pregnancy Risk Factor C

Dosage Forms Injection: Bupivacaine hydrochloride 0.5% with epinephrine 1:200,000 (1.8 mL cartridges in boxes of 50)

Selected Readings

Ayoub ST and Coleman AE, "A Review of Local Anesthetics," *Gen Dent*, 1992, 40(4):285-7, 289-90.

Budenz AW, "Local Anesthetics in Dentistry: Then and Now," *J Calif Dent Assoc*, 2003, 31(5):388-96.

Dower JS Jr, "A Review of Paresthesia in Association With Administration of Local Anesthesia," *Dent Today*, 2003, 22(2):64-9.

Finder RL and Moore PA, "Adverse Drug Reactions to Local Anesthesia," *Dent Clin North Am*, 2002, 46(4):747-57, x.

Haas DA, "An Update on Local Anesthetics in Dentistry," *J Can Dent Assoc*, 2002, 68(9):546-51.

Hawkins JM and Moore PA, "Local Anesthesia: Advances in Agents and Techniques," *Dent Clin North Am*, 2002, 46(4):719-32, ix.

"Injectable Local Anesthetics," *J Am Dent Assoc*, 2003, 134(5):628-9.

Jastak JT and Yagiela JA, "Vasoconstrictors and Local Anesthesia: A Review and Rationale for Use," *J Am Dent Assoc*, 1983, 107(4):623-30.

MacKenzie TA and Young ER, "Local Anesthetic Update," *Anesth Prog*, 1993, 40(2):29-34.

Malamed SF, "Allergy and Toxic Reactions to Local Anesthetics," *Dent Today*, 2003, 22(4):114-6, 118-21.

Wahl MJ, Schmitt MM, Overton DA, et al, "Injection Pain of Bupivacaine With Epinephrine vs. Prilocaine Plain," *J Am Dent Assoc*, 2002, 133(12):1652-6.

Wynn RL, "Epinephrine Interactions With Beta-Blockers," *Gen Dent*, 1994, 42(1):16, 18.

Yagiela JA, "Local Anesthetics," *Anesth Prog*, 1991, 38(4-5):128-41.

Bupivacaine and Lidocaine *see* Lidocaine and Bupivacaine *on page 822*

Bupivacaine Hydrochloride *see* Bupivacaine *on page 225*

Buprenex® *see* Buprenorphine *on page 228*

Buprenorphine (byoo pre NOR feen)

U.S. Brand Names Buprenex®; Subutex®

Canadian Brand Names Buprenex®

Mexican Brand Names Temgesic®

Generic Available Yes: Injection

Synonyms Buprenorphine Hydrochloride

Pharmacologic Category Analgesic, Narcotic

Use

Injection: Management of moderate to severe pain

Tablet: Treatment of opioid dependence

Unlabeled/Investigational Use Injection: Heroin and opioid withdrawal

Local Anesthetic/Vasoconstrictor Precautions No information available to require special precautions

Effects on Dental Treatment No significant effects or complications reported

Common Adverse Effects

Injection:

>10%: Central nervous system: Sedation

1% to 10%:

Cardiovascular: Hypotension

Central nervous system: Respiratory depression, dizziness, headache

Gastrointestinal: Vomiting, nausea

Ocular: Miosis

Otic: Vertigo

Miscellaneous: Diaphoresis

Tablet:

>10:

Central nervous system: Headache (30%), pain (24%), insomnia (21% to 25%), Oralety (12%), depression (11%)

Gastrointestinal: Nausea (10% to 14%), abdominal pain (12%), constipation (8% to 11%)

Neuromuscular & skeletal: Back pain (14%), weakness (14%)

Respiratory: Rhinitis (11%)

Miscellaneous: Withdrawal syndrome (19%; placebo 37%), infection (12% to 20%), diaphoresis (12% to 13%)

1% to 10%:

Central nervous system: Chills (6%), nervousness (6%), somnolence (5%), dizziness (4%), fever (3%)

Gastrointestinal: Vomiting (5% to 8%), diarrhea (5%), dyspepsia (3%)

Ocular: Lacrimation (5%)

Respiratory: Cough (4%), pharyngitis (4%)

Miscellaneous: Flu-like syndrome (6%)

Restrictions Injection: C-V; Tablet: C-III

Prescribing of tablets for opioid dependence is limited to physicians who have met the qualification criteria and have received a DEA number specific to prescribing this product. Tablets will be available through pharmacies and wholesalers which normally provide controlled substances.

Mechanism of Action Buprenorphine exerts its analgesic effect via high affinity binding to μ opiate receptors in the CNS; displays both agonist and antagonist activity

Drug Interactions

Cytochrome P450 Effect: Substrate of CYP3A4 (major); **Inhibits** CYP1A2 (weak), 2A6 (weak), 2C19 (weak), 2D6 (weak)

Increased Effect/Toxicity: Barbiturate anesthetics and other CNS depressants may produce additive respiratory and CNS depression. Respiratory and CV collapse was reported in a patient who received diazepam and buprenorphine. Effects may be additive with other CNS depressants. CYP3A4 inhibitors may increase the levels/effects of buprenorphine; example inhibitors include azole antifungals, ciprofloxacin, clarithromycin, diclofenac, doxycycline, erythromycin, imatinib, isoniazid, nefazodone, nicardipine, propofol, protease inhibitors, quinidine, and verapamil.

Decreased Effect: CYP3A4 inducers may decrease the levels/effects of buprenorphine; example inducers include aminoglutethimide, carbamazepine, nafcillin, nevirapine, phenobarbital, phenytoin, and rifamycins. Naltrexone may antagonize the effect of narcotic analgesics; concurrent use or use within 7-10 days of injection for pain relief is contraindicated.

Pharmacodynamics/Kinetics

Onset of action: Analgesic: 10-30 minutes

Duration: 6-8 hours

Absorption: I.M., SubQ: 30% to 40%

Distribution: V_d: 97-187 L/kg

Protein binding: High

Metabolism: Primarily hepatic; extensive first-pass effect

Half-life elimination: 2.2-3 hours

Excretion: Feces (70%); urine (20% as unchanged drug)

Pregnancy Risk Factor C

Buprenorphine and Naloxone

(byoo pre NOR feen & nal OKS one)

U.S. Brand Names Suboxone®

Generic Available No

Synonyms Buprenorphine Hydrochloride and Naloxone Hydrochloride Dihydrate; Naloxone and Buprenorphine; Naloxone Hydrochloride Dihydrate and Buprenorphine Hydrochloride

Pharmacologic Category Analgesic, Narcotic

Use Treatment of opioid dependence

Local Anesthetic/Vasoconstrictor Precautions No information available to require special precautions

Effects on Dental Treatment No significant effects or complications reported

Common Adverse Effects Also see individual agents.

>10%:

Central nervous system: Headache (36%), pain (22%)
Gastrointestinal: Nausea (15%), constipation (12%), abdominal pain (11%)
Miscellaneous: Withdrawal syndrome (25%; placebo 37%), diaphoresis (14%)

1% to 10%:

Cardiovascular: Vasodilation (9%)
Gastrointestinal: Vomiting (7%)

Restrictions C-III; Prescribing of tablets for opioid dependence is limited to physicians who have met the qualification criteria and have received a DEA number specific to prescribing this product. Tablets will be available through pharmacies and wholesalers which normally provide controlled substances.

Mechanism of Action See individual agents.

Drug Interactions

Decreased Effect: See individual agents.

Pharmacodynamics/Kinetics See individual agents.

Absorption: Absorption of the combination product is variable among patients following sublingual use, but variability within each individual patient is low.

Pregnancy Risk Factor C

Buprenorphine Hydrochloride *see* Buprenorphine *on page 228*

Buprenorphine Hydrochloride and Naloxone Hydrochloride Dihydrate *see* Buprenorphine and Naloxone *on page 230*

BuPROPion (byoo PROE pee on)

Related Information

Chemical Dependency and Smoking Cessation *on page 1576*

U.S. Brand Names Wellbutrin®; Wellbutrin SR®; Wellbutrin XL™; Zyban®

Canadian Brand Names Wellbutrin®; Zyban®

Mexican Brand Names Wellbutrin®

Generic Available Yes: Excludes Wellbutrin XL™

Pharmacologic Category Antidepressant, Dopamine-Reuptake Inhibitor; Smoking Cessation Aid

Use Treatment of depression; adjunct in smoking cessation

Unlabeled/Investigational Use Attention-deficit/hyperactivity disorder (ADHD)

Local Anesthetic/Vasoconstrictor Precautions Although this is not a tricyclic antidepressant, it can cause hypertensive episodes and should be used with caution in the presence of a vasoconstrictor.

Effects on Dental Treatment Key adverse event(s) related to dental treatment: Abnormal taste, significant xerostomia (normal salivary flow resumes with discontinuation).

Common Adverse Effects Frequencies, when reported, reflect highest incidence reported with sustained release product.

>10%:

Central nervous system: Dizziness (11%), headache (25%), insomnia (16%)
Gastrointestinal: Nausea (18%), xerostomia (24%)
Respiratory: Pharyngitis (11%)

1% to 10%:

Cardiovascular: Arrhythmias, chest pain (4%), flushing, hypertension (may be severe), hypotension, palpitation (5%), syncope, tachycardia
Central nervous system: Agitation (9%), anxiety (6%), confusion, depression, euphoria, hostility, irritability (2%), memory decreased (3%), migraine, nervousness (3%), sleep disturbance, somnolence (3%)
Dermatologic: Pruritus (4%), rash (4%), sweating increased (5%), urticaria (1%)
Endocrine & metabolic: Hot flashes, libido decreased, menstrual complaints

Gastrointestinal: Abdominal pain, anorexia (3%), appetite increased, constipation (5%), diarrhea (7%), dyspepsia, dysphagia (2%), taste perversion (4%), vomiting (2%)

Genitourinary: Urinary frequency (5%)

Neuromuscular & skeletal: Arthralgia (4%), arthritis (2%), myalgia (6%), neck pain, paresthesia (2%), tremor (3%), twitching (2%)

Ocular: Amblyopia (2%), blurred vision

Otic: Auditory disturbance, tinnitus (6%)

Respiratory: Cough increased (2%), sinusitis (1%)

Miscellaneous: Allergic reaction (including anaphylaxis, pruritus, urticaria), infection

Dosage Oral:

Children and Adolescents: ADHD (unlabeled use): 1.4-6 mg/kg/day

Adults:

Depression:

Immediate release: 100 mg 3 times/day; begin at 100 mg twice daily; may increase to a maximum dose of 450 mg/day

Sustained release: Initial: 150 mg/day in the morning; may increase to 150 mg twice daily by day 4 if tolerated; target dose: 300 mg/day given as 150 mg twice daily; maximum dose: 400 mg/day given as 200 mg twice daily

Extended release: Initial: 150 mg/day in the morning; may increase as early as day 4 of dosing to 300 mg/day; maximum dose: 450 mg/day

Smoking cessation (Zyban®): Initiate with 150 mg once daily for 3 days; increase to 150 mg twice daily; treatment should continue for 7-12 weeks

Elderly: Depression: 50-100 mg/day, increase by 50-100 mg every 3-4 days as tolerated; there is evidence that the elderly respond at 150 mg/day in divided doses, but some may require a higher dose

Dosing adjustment/comments in renal impairment: Effect of renal disease on bupropion's pharmacokinetics has not been studied; elimination of the major metabolites of bupropion may be affected by reduced renal function. Patients with renal failure should receive a reduced dosage initially and be closely monitored.

Dosing adjustment in hepatic impairment:

Note: The mean AUC increased by ~1.5-fold for hydroxybupropion and ~2.5-fold for erythro/threohydrobupropion; median T_{max} was observed 19 hours later for hydroxybupropion, 31 hours later for erythro/threohydrobupropion; mean half-life for hydroxybupropion increased fivefold, and increased twofold for erythro/threohydrobupropion in patients with severe hepatic cirrhosis compared to healthy volunteers.

Mild to moderate hepatic impairment: Use with caution and/or reduced dose/frequency

Severe hepatic cirrhosis: Use with extreme caution; maximum dose:

Wellbutrin®: 75 mg/day

Wellbutrin SR®: 100 mg/day or 150 mg every other day

Wellbutrin XL™: 150 mg every other day

Zyban®: 150 mg every other day

Mechanism of Action Aminoketone antidepressant structurally different from all other marketed antidepressants; like other antidepressants the mechanism of bupropion's activity is not fully understood. Bupropion is a relatively weak inhibitor of the neuronal uptake of serotonin, norepinephrine, and dopamine, and does not inhibit monoamine oxidase. Metabolite inhibits the reuptake of norepinephrine. The primary mechanism of action is thought to be dopaminergic and/or noradrenergic.

Contraindications Hypersensitivity to bupropion or any component of the formulation; seizure disorder; anorexia/bulimia; use of MAO inhibitors within 14 days; patients undergoing abrupt discontinuation of ethanol or sedatives (including benzodiazepines); patients receiving other dosage forms of bupropion

Warnings/Precautions When using immediate release tablets, seizure risk is increased at total daily dosage >450 mg, individual dosages >150 mg, or by sudden, large increments in dose. The risk of seizures is increased in patients with a history of seizures, anorexia/bulimia, head trauma, CNS tumor, severe hepatic cirrhosis, abrupt discontinuation of sedative-hypnotics or ethanol, medications which lower seizure threshold (antipsychotics, antidepressants, theophyllines, systemic steroids), stimulants, or hypoglycemic agents. Discontinue and do not restart in patients experiencing a seizure. May cause CNS stimulation (restlessness, anxiety, insomnia) or anorexia. May cause weight loss; use caution in patients where weight loss is not desirable. The incidence of sexual dysfunction with bupropion is generally lower than with SSRIs.

(Continued)

BuPROPion *(Continued)*

Use caution in patients with cardiovascular disease, history of hypertension, or coronary artery disease; treatment-emergent hypertension (including some severe cases) has been reported, both with bupropion alone and in combination with nicotine transdermal systems.

Use with caution in patients with hepatic or renal dysfunction and in elderly patients. Elderly patients may be at greater risk of accumulation during chronic dosing. May cause motor or cognitive impairment in some patients, use with caution if tasks requiring alertness such as operating machinery or driving are undertaken. May worsen psychosis in some patients or precipitate a shift to mania or hypomania in patients with bipolar disorder. Monotherapy in patients with bipolar disorder should be avoided. The possibility of a suicide attempt is inherent in major depression and may persist until remission occurs. Monitor for worsening of depression or suicidality, especially during initiation of therapy or with dose increases or decreases. Worsening depression and severe abrupt suicidality that are not part of the presenting symptoms may require discontinuation or modification of drug therapy. Use caution in high-risk patients during initiation of therapy. Prescriptions should be written for the smallest quantity consistent with good patient care. The patient's family or caregiver should be alerted to monitor patients for the emergence of suicidality and associated behaviors such as anxiety, agitation, panic attacks, insomnia, irritability, hostility, impulsivity, akathisia, hypomania, and mania; patients should be instructed to notify their healthcare provider if any of these symptoms or worsening depression occur.

Arthralgia, myalgia, and fever with rash and other symptoms suggestive of delayed hypersensitivity resembling serum sickness reported.

Drug Interactions

Cytochrome P450 Effect: Substrate of CYP1A2 (minor), 2A6 (minor), 2B6 (major), 2C8/9 (minor), 2D6 (minor), 2E1 (minor), 3A4 (minor); **Inhibits** CYP2D6 (weak)

Increased Effect/Toxicity: Treatment-emergent hypertension may occur in patients treated with bupropion and nicotine patch. Cimetidine may inhibit the metabolism (increase clinical/adverse effects) of bupropion. Toxicity of bupropion is enhanced by levodopa and phenelzine (MAO inhibitors). Risk of seizures may be increased with agents that may lower seizure threshold (antipsychotics, antidepressants, theophylline, abrupt discontinuation of benzodiazepines, systemic steroids). Effect of warfarin may be altered by bupropion. Concurrent use with amantadine appears to result in a higher incidence of adverse effects; use caution. CYP2B6 inhibitors may increase the levels/effects of bupropion; example inhibitors include desipramine, paroxetine, and sertraline. Combined use of CYP2B6 inhibitors (orphenadrine, thiotepa, cyclophosphamide) with bupropion may increase serum concentrations and may result in seizures.

Decreased Effect: CYP2B6 inducers may decrease the levels/effects of bupropion; example inducers include carbamazepine, nevirapine, phenobarbital, phenytoin, and rifampin. Effect of warfarin may be altered by bupropion.

Ethanol/Nutrition/Herb Interactions

Ethanol: Ethanol (may increase CNS depression).

Herb/Nutraceutical: Avoid valerian, St John's wort, SAMe, gotu kola, kava kava (may increase CNS depression).

Pharmacodynamics/Kinetics

Absorption: Rapid

Distribution: V_d: 19-21 L/kg

Protein binding: 82% to 88%

Metabolism: Extensively hepatic to 3 active metabolites: Hydroxybupropion, erythrohydrobupropion, threohydrobupropion (metabolite activity ranges from $^1/_5$ to $^1/_2$ potency of bupropion)

Bioavailability: 5% to 20% in animals

Half-life:

- Distribution: 3-4 hours
- Elimination: 21 ± 9 hours; Metabolites: Hydroxybupropion: 20 ± 5 hours; Erythrohydrobupropion: 33 ± 10 hours; Threohydrobupropion: 37 ± 13 hours

Time to peak, serum: Bupropion: ~3 hours; bupropion extended release: ~5 hours

- Metabolites: Hydroxybupropion, erythrohydrobupropion, threohydrobupropion: 6 hours

Excretion: Urine (87%); feces (10%)

Pregnancy Risk Factor B

Dosage Forms TAB (Wellbutrin®): 75 mg, 100 mg. **TAB, extended release** (Wellbutrin XL™): 150 mg, 300 mg. **TAB, sustained release:** 100 mg, 150 mg [equivalent to Wellbutrin® SR], 150 mg [equivalent to Zyban®]; (Wellbutrin® SR): 100 mg, 150 mg, 200 mg; (Zyban®): 150 mg

Selected Readings

Tonstad S and Johnston JA, "Does Bupropion Have Advantages Over Other Medical Therapies in the Cessation of Smoking?" *Expert Opin Pharmacother*, 2004, 5(4):727-34.

Burnamycin [OTC] *see* Lidocaine *on page 819*

Burn Jel [OTC] *see* Lidocaine *on page 819*

Burn-O-Jel [OTC] *see* Lidocaine *on page 819*

BuSpar® *see* BusPIRone *on page 233*

BusPIRone (byoo SPYE rone)

Related Information

Patients Requiring Sedation *on page 1567*

U.S. Brand Names BuSpar®

Canadian Brand Names Apo-Buspirone®; BuSpar®; Buspirex; Gen-Buspirone; Lin-Buspirone; Novo-Buspirone; Nu-Buspirone; PMS-Buspirone

Mexican Brand Names Neurosine®

Generic Available Yes

Synonyms Buspirone Hydrochloride

Pharmacologic Category Antianxiety Agent, Miscellaneous

Use Management of generalized anxiety disorder (GAD)

Unlabeled/Investigational Use Management of aggression in mental retardation and secondary mental disorders; major depression; potential augmenting agent for antidepressants; premenstrual syndrome

Local Anesthetic/Vasoconstrictor Precautions No information available to require special precautions

Effects on Dental Treatment Key adverse event(s) related to dental treatment: Xerostomia (normal salivary flow resumes upon discontinuation).

Common Adverse Effects

>10%: Central nervous system: Dizziness

1% to 10%:

- Central nervous system: Drowsiness, EPS, serotonin syndrome, confusion, nervousness, lightheadedness, excitement, anger, hostility, headache
- Dermatologic: Rash
- Gastrointestinal: Diarrhea, nausea
- Neuromuscular & skeletal: Muscle weakness, numbness, paresthesia, incoordination, tremor
- Ocular: Blurred vision, tunnel vision
- Miscellaneous: Diaphoresis, allergic reactions

Dosage Oral:

Generalized anxiety disorder:

- Children and Adolescents: Initial: 5 mg daily; increase in increments of 5 mg/day at weekly intervals as needed, to a maximum dose of 60 mg/day divided into 2-3 doses
- Adults: 15 mg/day (7.5 mg twice daily); may increase in increments of 5 mg/day every 2-4 days to a maximum of 60 mg/day; target dose for most people is 30 mg/day (15 mg twice daily)

Dosing adjustment in renal or hepatic impairment: Buspirone is metabolized by the liver and excreted by the kidneys. Patients with impaired hepatic or renal function demonstrated increased plasma levels and a prolonged half-life of buspirone. Therefore, use in patients with severe hepatic or renal impairment cannot be recommended.

Mechanism of Action The mechanism of action of buspirone is unknown. Buspirone has a high affinity for serotonin 5-HT_{1A} and 5-HT_2 receptors, without affecting benzodiazepine-GABA receptors; buspirone has moderate affinity for dopamine D_2 receptors

Contraindications Hypersensitivity to buspirone or any component of the formulation

Warnings/Precautions Safety and efficacy not established in children <18 years of age; use in hepatic or renal impairment is not recommended; does not prevent or treat withdrawal from benzodiazepines. Low potential for cognitive or motor impairment. Use with MAO inhibitors may result in hypertensive reactions.

Drug Interactions

Cytochrome P450 Effect: Substrate of CYP2D6 (minor), 3A4 (major)

Increased Effect/Toxicity: Concurrent use of buspirone with SSRIs or trazodone may cause serotonin syndrome. Buspirone should not be used

(Continued)

BusPIRone *(Continued)*

concurrently with an MAO inhibitor due to reports of increased blood pressure; theoretically, a selective MAO type B inhibitors (selegiline) has a lower risk of this reaction. Concurrent use of buspirone with nefazodone may increase risk of CNS adverse events; limit buspirone initial dose (eg, 2.5 mg/day). CYP3A4 inhibitors may increase the levels/effects of buspirone; example inhibitors include azole antifungals, ciprofloxacin, clarithromycin, diclofenac, doxycycline, erythromycin, imatinib, isoniazid, nefazodone, nicardipine, propofol, protease inhibitors, quinidine, and verapamil.

Decreased Effect: CYP3A4 inducers may decrease the levels/effects of buspirone; example inducers include aminoglutethimide, carbamazepine, nafcillin, nevirapine, phenobarbital, phenytoin, and rifamycins.

Ethanol/Nutrition/Herb Interactions

Ethanol: Ethanol (may increase CNS depression).

Food: Food may decrease the absorption of buspirone, but it may also decrease the first-pass metabolism, thereby increasing the bioavailability of buspirone. Grapefruit juice may cause increased buspirone concentrations; avoid concurrent use.

Herb/Nutraceutical: St John's wort may decrease buspirone levels or increase CNS depression. Avoid valerian, gotu kola, kava kava (may increase CNS depression).

Pharmacodynamics/Kinetics

Absorption: Oral: ~100%

Distribution: V_d: 5.3 L/kg

Protein binding: 95%

Metabolism: Hepatic via oxidation; extensive first-pass effect

Bioavailability: ~4%

Half-life elimination: Mean: 2.4 hours (range: 2-11 hours)

Time to peak, serum: Within 0.7-1.5 hours

Excretion: Urine: 65%; feces: 35%; ~1% dose excreted unchanged

Pregnancy Risk Factor B

Dosage Forms TAB: 5 mg, 7.5 mg, 10 mg, 15 mg, 30 mg; (BuSpar®): 5 mg, 10 mg, 15 mg, 30 mg

Buspirone Hydrochloride *see* BusPIRone *on page 233*

Busulfan (byoo SUL fan)

U.S. Brand Names Busulfex®; Myleran®

Canadian Brand Names Busulfex®; Myleran®

Mexican Brand Names Myleran®

Generic Available No

Pharmacologic Category Antineoplastic Agent, Alkylating Agent

Use

Oral: Chronic myelogenous leukemia and bone marrow disorders, such as polycythemia vera and myeloid metaplasia, conditioning regimens for bone marrow transplantation

I.V.: Combination therapy with cyclophosphamide as a conditioning regimen prior to allogeneic hematopoietic progenitor cell transplantation for chronic myelogenous leukemia

Local Anesthetic/Vasoconstrictor Precautions No information available to require special precautions

Effects on Dental Treatment No significant effects or complications reported

Common Adverse Effects

Fertility/carcinogenesis: Sterility, ovarian suppression, amenorrhea, azoospermia, and testicular atrophy; malignant tumors have been reported in patients on busulfan therapy.

>10%: Hematologic: Severe pancytopenia, leukopenia, thrombocytopenia, anemia, and bone marrow suppression are common and patients should be monitored closely while on therapy. Since this is a delayed effect (busulfan affects the stem cells), the drug should be discontinued temporarily at the first sign of a large or rapid fall in any blood element. Some patients may develop bone marrow fibrosis or chronic aplasia which is probably due to the busulfan toxicity. In large doses, busulfan is myeloablative and is used for this reason in BMT. Myelosuppressive:

WBC: Moderate

Platelets: Moderate

Onset: 7-10 days

Nadir: 14-21 days

Recovery: 28 days

1% to 10%:

Dermatologic: Hyperpigmentation skin (busulfan tan), urticaria, erythema, alopecia

Endocrine & metabolic: Amenorrhea

Gastrointestinal: Nausea, vomiting, diarrhea; drug has little effect on the GI mucosal lining

Neuromuscular & skeletal: Weakness

Mechanism of Action Reacts with N-7 position of guanosine and interferes with DNA replication and transcription of RNA. Busulfan has a more marked effect on myeloid cells (and is, therefore, useful in the treatment of CML) than on lymphoid cells. The drug is also very toxic to hematopoietic stem cells (thus its usefulness in high doses in BMT preparative regimens). Busulfan exhibits little immunosuppressive activity. Interferes with the normal function of DNA by alkylation and cross-linking the strands of DNA.

Drug Interactions

Cytochrome P450 Effect: Substrate of CYP3A4 (major)

Increased Effect/Toxicity: CYP3A4 inhibitors may increase the levels/effects of busulfan; example inhibitors include azole antifungals, ciprofloxacin, clarithromycin, diclofenac, doxycycline, erythromycin, imatinib, isoniazid, nefazodone, nicardipine, propofol, protease inhibitors, quinidine, and verapamil. Metronidazole may increase busulfan plasma levels.

Decreased Effect: CYP3A4 inducers may decrease the levels/effects of busulfan; example inducers include aminoglutethimide, carbamazepine, nafcillin, nevirapine, phenobarbital, phenytoin, and rifamycins.

Pharmacodynamics/Kinetics

Duration: 28 days

Absorption: Rapid and complete

Distribution: V_d: ~1 L/kg; into CSF and saliva with levels similar to plasma

Protein binding: ~14%

Metabolism: Extensively hepatic (may increase with multiple doses)

Half-life elimination: After first dose: 3.4 hours; After last dose: 2.3 hours

Time to peak, serum: Oral: Within 4 hours; I.V.: Within 5 minutes

Excretion: Urine (10% to 50% as metabolites) within 24 hours (<2% as unchanged drug)

Pregnancy Risk Factor D

Busulfex® *see* Busulfan *on page 234*

Butabarbital (byoo ta BAR bi tal)

U.S. Brand Names Butisol Sodium®

Generic Available No

Pharmacologic Category Barbiturate

Use Sedative; hypnotic

Local Anesthetic/Vasoconstrictor Precautions No information available to require special precautions

Effects on Dental Treatment No significant effects or complications reported

Common Adverse Effects

>10%: Central nervous system: Dizziness, lightheadedness, drowsiness, "hangover" effect

1% to 10%:

Central nervous system: Confusion, mental depression, unusual excitement, nervousness, faint feeling, headache, insomnia, nightmares

Gastrointestinal: Constipation, nausea, vomiting

Restrictions C-III

Mechanism of Action Interferes with transmission of impulses from the thalamus to the cortex of the brain resulting in an imbalance in central inhibitory and facilitatory mechanisms

Drug Interactions

Increased Effect/Toxicity: When butabarbital is combined with other CNS depressants, ethanol, narcotic analgesics, antidepressants, or benzodiazepines, additive respiratory and CNS depression may occur. Barbiturates may enhance the hepatotoxic potential of acetaminophen overdoses. Chloramphenicol, MAO inhibitors, valproic acid, and felbamate may inhibit barbiturate metabolism. Barbiturates may impair the absorption of griseofulvin, and may enhance the nephrotoxic effects of methoxyflurane.

Decreased Effect: Barbiturates such as butabarbital are hepatic enzyme inducers, and may increase the metabolism of antipsychotics, some beta-blockers (unlikely with atenolol and nadolol), calcium channel blockers, chloramphenicol, cimetidine, corticosteroids, cyclosporine, disopyramide, doxycycline, ethosuximide, felbamate, furosemide, griseofulvin, lamotrigine, phenytoin, propafenone, quinidine, tacrolimus, TCAs, and theophylline.

(Continued)

Butabarbital *(Continued)*

Barbiturates may increase the metabolism of estrogens and reduce the efficacy of oral contraceptives; an alternative method of contraception should be considered. Barbiturates inhibit the hypoprothrombinemic effects of oral anticoagulants via increased metabolism. Barbiturates may enhance the metabolism of methadone resulting in methadone withdrawal.

Pharmacodynamics/Kinetics

Distribution: V_d: 0.8 L/kg
Protein binding: 26%
Metabolism: Hepatic
Half-life elimination: 1.6 days to 5.8 days
Time to peak, serum: 40-60 minutes
Excretion: Urine (as metabolites)

Pregnancy Risk Factor D

Butalbital, Acetaminophen, and Caffeine

(byoo TAL bi tal, a seet a MIN oh fen, & KAF een)

Related Information

Acetaminophen *on page 47*

U.S. Brand Names Anolor 300; Esgic®; Esgic-Plus™; Fioricet®; Repan®; Zebutal™

Generic Available Yes

Synonyms Acetaminophen, Butalbital, and Caffeine

Pharmacologic Category Barbiturate

Use Relief of the symptomatic complex of tension or muscle contraction headache

Local Anesthetic/Vasoconstrictor Precautions No information available to require special precautions

Effects on Dental Treatment No significant effects or complications reported

Common Adverse Effects

>10%:

- Central nervous system: Dizziness, lightheadedness, drowsiness, "hangover" effect
- Gastrointestinal: Nausea, heartburn, stomach pains, dyspepsia, epigastric discomfort

1% to 10%:

- Central nervous system: Confusion, mental depression, unusual excitement, nervousness, faint feeling, headache, insomnia, nightmares, fatigue
- Dermatologic: Skin rash
- Gastrointestinal: Constipation, vomiting, gastrointestinal ulceration
- Hematologic: Hemolytic anemia
- Neuromuscular & skeletal: Weakness
- Respiratory: Troubled breathing
- Miscellaneous: Anaphylactic shock

Drug Interactions

Cytochrome P450 Effect:

Acetaminophen: **Substrate** (minor) of CYP1A2, 2A6, 2C8/9, 2D6, 2E1, 3A4; **Inhibits** CYP3A4 (weak)

Caffeine: **Substrate** of CYP1A2 (major), 2C8/9 (minor), 2D6 (minor), 2E1 (minor), 3A4 (minor); **Inhibits** CYP1A2 (weak), 3A4 (moderate)

Increased Effect/Toxicity: MAO inhibitors may enhance CNS effects of butalbital. Increased effect (CNS depression) with narcotic analgesics, ethanol, general anesthetics, tranquilizers such as chlordiazepoxide, sedative hypnotics, or other CNS depressants.

Decreased Effect: Butalbital may diminish effects of uricosuric agents such as probenecid and sulfinpyrazone.

Pregnancy Risk Factor D

Butalbital, Acetaminophen, Caffeine, and Codeine

(byoo TAL bi tal, a seet a MIN oh fen, KAF een, & KOE deen)

Related Information

Acetaminophen *on page 47*
Codeine *on page 369*

U.S. Brand Names Fioricet® with Codeine

Generic Available Yes

Synonyms Acetaminophen, Caffeine, Codeine, and Butalbital; Caffeine, Acetaminophen, Butalbital, and Codeine; Codeine, Acetaminophen, Butalbital, and Caffeine

Pharmacologic Category Analgesic Combination (Narcotic); Barbiturate

Use Relief of symptoms of complex tension (muscle contraction) headache

Local Anesthetic/Vasoconstrictor Precautions No information available to require special precautions

Effects on Dental Treatment Key adverse event(s) related to dental treatment: Xerostomia (normal salivary flow resumes upon discontinuation).

Significant Adverse Effects Frequency not defined.

Cardiovascular: Tachycardia, palpitation, hypotension, edema, syncope

Central nervous system: Drowsiness, fatigue, mental confusion, disorientation, nervousness, hallucination, euphoria, depression, seizure, headache, agitation, fainting, excitement, fever

Dermatologic: Rash, erythema, pruritus, urticaria, erythema multiforme, exfoliative dermatitis, toxic epidermal necrolysis

Gastrointestinal: Nausea, xerostomia, constipation, gastrointestinal spasm, heartburn, flatulence

Genitourinary: Urinary retention, diuresis

Neuromuscular & skeletal: Leg pain, weakness, numbness

Otic: Tinnitus

Miscellaneous: Allergic reaction, anaphylaxis

Note: Potential reactions associated with components of Fioricet® with Codeine include agranulocytosis, irritability, nausea, thrombocytopenia, tremor, vomiting

Restrictions C-III

Dosage Oral: Adults: 1-2 capsules every 4 hours. Total daily dosage should not exceed 6 capsules.

Dosing adjustment/comments in hepatic impairment: Use with caution. Limited, low-dose therapy usually well tolerated in hepatic disease/cirrhosis. However, cases of hepatotoxicity at daily acetaminophen dosages <4 g/day have been reported. Avoid chronic use in hepatic impairment.

Mechanism of Action Combination product for the treatment of tension headache. Contains codeine (narcotic analgesic), butalbital (barbiturate), caffeine (CNS stimulant), and acetaminophen (nonopiate, nonsalicylate analgesic).

Contraindications Hypersensitivity to butalbital, codeine, caffeine, acetaminophen, or any component of the formulation; porphyria; known G6PD deficiency; pregnancy (prolonged use or high doses at term)

Warnings/Precautions Limit acetaminophen to <4 g/day. May cause severe hepatic toxicity in acute overdose; in addition, chronic daily dosing in adults has resulted in liver damage in some patients. Use with caution in patients with hypersensitivity reactions to other phenanthrene derivative opioid agonists (eg, morphine, hydrocodone, oxycodone). Use caution with Addison's disease, severe renal or hepatic impairment. Use caution in patients with head injury or other intracranial lesions, acute abdominal conditions, urethral stricture of BPH, or in patients with respiratory diseases. Elderly and/or debilitated patients may be more susceptible to CNS depressants, as well as constipating effects of narcotics. Tolerance or drug dependence may result from extended use. Safety and efficacy in pediatric patients have not been established.

Drug Interactions

Acetaminophen: **Substrate** of (minor) CYP1A2, 2A6, 2C8/9, 2D6, 2E1, 3A4; **Inhibits** CYP3A4 (weak)

Caffeine: **Substrate** of CYP1A2 (major), 2C8/9 (minor), 2D6 (minor), 2E1 (minor), 3A4 (minor); **Inhibits** CYP1A2 (weak), 3A4 (moderate)

Also see individual monographs for Acetaminophen and Codeine.

Butalbital: Refer to Phenobarbital monograph.

Ethanol/Nutrition/Herb Interactions Ethanol: Avoid ethanol (may increase CNS depression).

Pregnancy Risk Factor C (per manufacturer); D (prolonged use or high doses at term)

Lactation Enters breast milk/not recommended

Breast-Feeding Considerations Codeine, caffeine, barbiturates, and acetaminophen are excreted in breast milk in small amounts. Discontinuation of breast-feeding or discontinuation of the drug should be considered.

Dosage Forms Capsule: Butalbital 50 mg, caffeine 40 mg, acetaminophen 325 mg, and codeine phosphate 30 mg

Selected Readings

Botting RM, "Mechanism of Action of Acetaminophen: Is There a Cyclooxygenase 3?" *Clin Infect Dis*, 2000, Suppl 5:S202-10.

Dart RC, Kuffner EK, and Rumack BH, "Treatment of Pain or Fever With Paracetamol (Acetaminophen) in the Alcoholic Patient: A Systematic Review," *Am J Ther*, 2000, 7(2):123-34.

Grant JA and Weiler JM, "A Report of a Rare Immediate Reaction After Ingestion of Acetaminophen," *Ann Allergy Asthma Immunol*, 2001, 87(3):227-9.

Kwan D, Bartle WR, and Walker SE, "The Effects of Acetaminophen on Pharmacokinetics and Pharmacodynamics of Warfarin," *J Clin Pharmacol*, 1999, 39(1):68-75.

McClain CJ, Price S, Barve S, et al, "Acetaminophen Hepatotoxicity: An Update," *Curr Gastroenterol Rep*, 1999, 1(1):42-9.

(Continued)

Butalbital, Acetaminophen, Caffeine, and Codeine *(Continued)*

Shek KL, Chan LN, and Nutescu E, "Warfarin-Acetaminophen Drug Interaction Revisited," *Pharmacotherapy*, 1999, 19(10):1153-8.

Tanaka E, Yamazaki K, and Misawa S, "Update: The Clinical Importance of Acetaminophen Hepatotoxicity in Nonalcoholic and Alcoholic Subjects," *J Clin Pharm Ther*, 2000, 25(5):325-32.

Butalbital, Aspirin, and Caffeine

(byoo TAL bi tal, AS pir in, & KAF een)

Related Information

Aspirin *on page 151*

U.S. Brand Names Fiorinal®

Canadian Brand Names Fiorinal®

Generic Available Yes

Synonyms Aspirin, Caffeine, and Butalbital; Butalbital Compound

Pharmacologic Category Barbiturate

Use Relief of the symptomatic complex of tension or muscle contraction headache

Local Anesthetic/Vasoconstrictor Precautions No information available to require special precautions

Effects on Dental Treatment No significant effects or complications reported

Common Adverse Effects

>10%:

- Central nervous system: Dizziness, lightheadedness, drowsiness, "hangover" effect
- Gastrointestinal: Heartburn, stomach pains, dyspepsia, epigastric discomfort, nausea

1% to 10%:

- Central nervous system: Confusion, mental depression, unusual excitement, nervousness, faint feeling, headache, insomnia, nightmares, fatigue
- Dermatologic: Skin rash
- Gastrointestinal: Constipation, vomiting, gastrointestinal ulceration
- Hematologic: Hemolytic anemia
- Neuromuscular & skeletal: Weakness
- Respiratory: Troubled breathing
- Miscellaneous: Anaphylactic shock

Restrictions C-III

Drug Interactions

Cytochrome P450 Effect:

Aspirin: **Substrate** of CYP2C8/9 (minor)

Caffeine: **Substrate** of CYP1A2 (major), 2C8/9 (minor), 2D6 (minor), 2E1 (minor), 3A4 (minor); **Inhibits** CYP1A2 (weak), 3A4 (moderate)

Increased Effect/Toxicity: Enhanced effect/toxicity with oral anticoagulants (warfarin), oral antidiabetic agents, insulin, mercaptopurine, methotrexate, NSAIDs, narcotic analgesics (propoxyphene, meperidine, etc), benzodiazepines, sedative-hypnotics, other CNS depressants. The CNS effects of butalbital may be enhanced by MAO inhibitors.

Decreased Effect: May decrease the effect of uricosuric agents (probenecid and sulfinpyrazone) reducing their effect on gout.

Pregnancy Risk Factor C/D (prolonged use or high doses at term)

Butalbital, Aspirin, Caffeine, and Codeine

(byoo TAL bi tal, AS pir in, KAF een, & KOE deen)

Related Information

Aspirin *on page 151*

Codeine *on page 369*

U.S. Brand Names Fiorinal® With Codeine; Phrenilin® with Caffeine and Codeine

Canadian Brand Names Fiorinal®-C 1/2; Fiorinal®-C 1/4; Tecnal C 1/2; Tecnal C 1/4

Generic Available Yes

Synonyms Butalbital Compound and Codeine; Codeine and Butalbital Compound; Codeine, Butalbital, Aspirin, and Caffeine

Pharmacologic Category Analgesic Combination (Narcotic); Barbiturate

Use Mild to moderate pain when sedation is needed

Local Anesthetic/Vasoconstrictor Precautions No information available to require special precautions

Effects on Dental Treatment No significant effects or complications reported

Common Adverse Effects

>10%:

Central nervous system: Dizziness, lightheadedness, drowsiness

Gastrointestinal: Nausea, heartburn, stomach pains, dyspepsia, epigastric discomfort

1% to 10%:

Central nervous system: Confusion, mental depression, unusual excitement, nervousness, faint feeling, insomnia, nightmares, intoxicated feeling

Dermatologic: Rash

Gastrointestinal: Constipation, GI ulceration

Restrictions C-III

Drug Interactions

Cytochrome P450 Effect:

Aspirin: **Substrate** of CYP2C8/9 (minor)

Caffeine: **Substrate** of CYP1A2 (major), 2C8/9 (minor), 2D6 (minor), 2E1 (minor), 3A4 (minor); **Inhibits** CYP1A2 (weak), 3A4 (moderate)

Increased Effect/Toxicity: MAO inhibitors may enhance the CNS effects of butalbital. In patients receiving concomitant corticosteroids during the chronic use of ASA, withdrawal of corticosteroids may result in salicylism. Butalbital compound and codeine may enhance effects of oral anticoagulants. Increased effect with oral antidiabetic agents and insulin, mercaptopurine and methotrexate, NSAIDs, other narcotic analgesics, ethanol, general anesthetics, tranquilizers such as chlordiazepoxide, sedative hypnotics, or other CNS depressants.

Decreased Effect: Aspirin, butalbital, caffeine, and codeine may diminish effects of uricosuric agents such as probenecid and sulfinpyrazone.

Pregnancy Risk Factor C/D (prolonged use or high doses at term)

Butalbital Compound *see* Butalbital, Aspirin, and Caffeine *on page 238*

Butalbital Compound and Codeine *see* Butalbital, Aspirin, Caffeine, and Codeine *on page 238*

Butenafine (byoo TEN a feen)

U.S. Brand Names Lotrimin® Ultra™ [OTC]; Mentax®

Generic Available No

Synonyms Butenafine Hydrochloride

Pharmacologic Category Antifungal Agent, Topical

Use Topical treatment of tinea pedis (athlete's foot), tinea cruris (jock itch), tinea corporis (ringworm), and tinea versicolor

Local Anesthetic/Vasoconstrictor Precautions No information available to require special precautions

Effects on Dental Treatment No significant effects or complications reported

Common Adverse Effects >1%: Dermatologic: Burning, stinging, irritation, erythema, pruritus (2%)

Mechanism of Action Butenafine exerts antifungal activity by blocking squalene epoxidation, resulting in inhibition of ergosterol synthesis (antidermatophyte and *Sporothrix schenckii* activity). In higher concentrations, the drug disrupts fungal cell membranes (anticandidal activity).

Pharmacodynamics/Kinetics

Absorption: Minimal systemic

Metabolism: Hepatic via hydroxylation

Half-life elimination: 35 hours

Time to peak, serum: 6 hours

Pregnancy Risk Factor B

Butenafine Hydrochloride *see* Butenafine *on page 239*

Butisol Sodium® *see* Butabarbital *on page 235*

Butoconazole (byoo toe KOE na zole)

Related Information

Sexually-Transmitted Diseases *on page 1504*

U.S. Brand Names Gynazole-1®; Mycelex®-3 [OTC]

Canadian Brand Names Femstat® One

Mexican Brand Names Femstal®

Generic Available No

Synonyms Butoconazole Nitrate

Pharmacologic Category Antifungal Agent, Vaginal

Use Local treatment of vulvovaginal candidiasis

Local Anesthetic/Vasoconstrictor Precautions No information available to require special precautions

Effects on Dental Treatment No significant effects or complications reported

(Continued)

Butoconazole *(Continued)*

Common Adverse Effects Frequency not defined.

Gastrointestinal: Abdominal pain or cramping

Genitourinary: Pelvic pain; vulvar/vaginal burning, itching, soreness, and swelling

Mechanism of Action Increases cell membrane permeability in susceptible fungi (*Candida*)

Pharmacodynamics/Kinetics

Absorption: 2%

Metabolism: Not reported

Time to peak: 12-24 hours

Pregnancy Risk Factor C (use only in 2nd or 3rd trimester)

Butoconazole Nitrate *see* Butoconazole *on page 239*

Butorphanol (byoo TOR fa nole)

U.S. Brand Names Stadol®; Stadol® NS [DSC]

Canadian Brand Names Apo-Butorphanol®; PMS-Butorphanol; Stadol NS™

Generic Available Yes

Synonyms Butorphanol Tartrate

Pharmacologic Category Analgesic, Narcotic

Use

Parenteral: Management of moderate to severe pain; preoperative medication; supplement to balanced anesthesia; management of pain during labor

Nasal spray: Management of moderate to severe pain, including migraine headache pain

Local Anesthetic/Vasoconstrictor Precautions No information available to require special precautions

Effects on Dental Treatment Key adverse event(s) related to dental treatment: Xerostomia (normal salivary flow resumes upon discontinuation) and unpleasant aftertaste.

Common Adverse Effects

>10%:

Central nervous system: Drowsiness (43%), dizziness (19%), insomnia (Stadol® NS)

Gastrointestinal: Nausea/vomiting (13%)

Respiratory: Nasal congestion (Stadol® NS)

1% to 10%:

Cardiovascular: Vasodilation, palpitations

Central nervous system: Lightheadedness, headache, lethargy, anxiety, confusion, euphoria, somnolence

Dermatologic: Pruritus

Gastrointestinal: Anorexia, constipation, xerostomia, stomach pain, unpleasant aftertaste

Neuromuscular & skeletal: Tremor, paresthesia, weakness

Ocular: Blurred vision

Otic: Ear pain, tinnitus

Respiratory: Bronchitis, cough, dyspnea, epistaxis, nasal irritation, pharyngitis, rhinitis, sinus congestion, sinusitis, upper respiratory infection

Miscellaneous: Diaphoresis (increased)

Restrictions C-IV

Mechanism of Action Mixed narcotic agonist-antagonist with central analgesic actions; binds to opiate receptors in the CNS, causing inhibition of ascending pain pathways, altering the perception of and response to pain; produces generalized CNS depression

Drug Interactions

Increased Effect/Toxicity: Increased toxicity with CNS depressants, phenothiazines, barbiturates, skeletal muscle relaxants, alfentanil, guanabenz, and MAO inhibitors.

Pharmacodynamics/Kinetics

Onset of action: I.M.: 5-10 minutes; I.V.: <10 minutes; Nasal: Within 15 minutes

Peak effect: I.M.: 0.5-1 hour; I.V.: 4-5 minutes

Duration: I.M., I.V.: 3-4 hours; Nasal: 4-5 hours

Absorption: Rapid and well absorbed

Protein binding: 80%

Metabolism: Hepatic

Bioavailability: Nasal: 60% to 70%

Half-life elimination: 2.5-4 hours

Excretion: Primarily urine

Pregnancy Risk Factor C/D (prolonged use or high doses at term)

Butorphanol Tartrate *see* Butorphanol *on page 240*

B Vitamin Combinations *see* Vitamin B Complex Combinations *on page 1382*

BW-430C *see* Lamotrigine *on page 795*

BW524W91 *see* Emtricitabine *on page 487*

C2B8 *see* Rituximab *on page 1191*

C2B8 Monoclonal Antibody *see* Rituximab *on page 1191*

C7E3 *see* Abciximab *on page 44*

C8-CCK *see* Sincalide *on page 1224*

311C90 *see* Zolmitriptan *on page 1403*

C225 *see* Cetuximab *on page 300*

C-500-GR™ [OTC] *see* Ascorbic Acid *on page 148*

Cabergoline (ca BER goe leen)

U.S. Brand Names Dostinex®

Canadian Brand Names Dostinex®

Generic Available No

Pharmacologic Category Ergot Derivative

Use Treatment of hyperprolactinemic disorders, either idiopathic or due to pituitary adenomas

Unlabeled/Investigational Use Adjunct for the treatment of Parkinson's disease

Local Anesthetic/Vasoconstrictor Precautions No information available to require special precautions

Effects on Dental Treatment Key adverse event(s) related to dental treatment: Xerostomia (normal salivary flow resumes upon discontinuation), throat irritation, and toothache.

Common Adverse Effects

>10%:

- Central nervous system: Headache (26%), dizziness (17%)
- Gastrointestinal: Nausea (29%)

1% to 10%:

- Body as whole: Asthenia (6%), fatigue (5%), syncope (1%), influenza-like symptoms (1%), malaise (1%), periorbital edema (1%), peripheral edema (1%)
- Cardiovascular: Hot flashes (3%), hypotension (1%), dependent edema (1%), palpitations (1%)
- Central nervous system: Vertigo (4%), depression (3%), somnolence (2%), anxiety (1%), insomnia (1%), impaired concentration (1%), nervousness (1%)
- Dermatologic: Acne (1%), pruritus (1%)
- Endocrine: Breast pain (2%), dysmenorrhea (1%)
- Gastrointestinal: Constipation (7%), abdominal pain (5%), dyspepsia (5%), vomiting (4%), xerostomia (2%), diarrhea (2%), flatulence (2%), throat irritation (1%), toothache (1%), anorexia (1%)
- Neuromuscular & skeletal: Pain (2%), arthralgia (1%), paresthesias (2%)
- Ocular: Abnormal vision (1%)
- Respiratory: Rhinitis (1%)

Mechanism of Action Cabergoline is a long acting dopamine receptor agonist with a high affinity for D_2 receptors; prolactin secretion by the anterior pituitary is predominantly under hypothalamic inhibitory control exerted through the release of dopamine

Drug Interactions

Increased Effect/Toxicity: Cabergoline may increase the effects of sibutramine and other serotonin agonists (serotonin syndrome).

Decreased Effect: Effects of cabergoline may be diminished by antipsychotics, metoclopramide.

Pharmacodynamics/Kinetics

- Distribution: Extensive, particularly to the pituitary
- Protein binding: 40% to 42%
- Metabolism: Extensively hepatic; minimal CYP
- Half-life elimination: 63-69 hours
- Time to peak: 2-3 hours

Pregnancy Risk Factor B

Caduet® *see* Amlodipine and Atorvastatin *on page 110*

Cafergot® *see* Ergotamine and Caffeine *on page 506*

Caffeine, Acetaminophen, and Aspirin *see* Acetaminophen, Aspirin, and Caffeine *on page 56*

Caffeine, Acetaminophen, Butalbital, and Codeine *see* Butalbital, Acetaminophen, Caffeine, and Codeine *on page 236*

Caffeine and Ergotamine *see* Ergotamine and Caffeine *on page 506*

Caffeine and Sodium Benzoate

(KAF een & SOW dee um BEN zoe ate)

Generic Available Yes

Synonyms Sodium Benzoate and Caffeine

Pharmacologic Category Diuretic, Miscellaneous

Use Emergency stimulant in acute circulatory failure, diuretic

Unlabeled/Investigational Use Relief of spinal puncture headache

Local Anesthetic/Vasoconstrictor Precautions No information available to require special precautions

Effects on Dental Treatment No significant effects or complications reported

Common Adverse Effects Frequency not defined.

Cardiovascular: Tachycardia, extrasystoles, palpitations

Central nervous system: Insomnia, restlessness, nervousness, mild delirium, headache, anxiety

Gastrointestinal: Nausea, vomiting, gastric irritation

Neuromuscular & skeletal: Muscle tension following abrupt cessation of drug after regular consumption of 500-600 mg/day

Renal: Diuresis

Drug Interactions

Cytochrome P450 Effect: Caffeine: **Substrate** of CYP1A2 (major), 2C8/9 (minor), 2D6 (minor), 2E1 (minor), 3A4 (minor); **Inhibits** CYP1A2 (weak), 3A4 (moderate)

Pregnancy Risk Factor C

Caffeine, Aspirin, and Acetaminophen *see* Acetaminophen, Aspirin, and Caffeine *on page 56*

Caffeine, Dihydrocodeine, and Acetaminophen *see* Acetaminophen, Caffeine, and Dihydrocodeine *on page 57*

Caffeine, Hydrocodone, Chlorpheniramine, Phenylephrine, and Acetaminophen *see* Hydrocodone, Chlorpheniramine, Phenylephrine, Acetaminophen, and Caffeine *on page 712*

Caffeine, Orphenadrine, and Aspirin *see* Orphenadrine, Aspirin, and Caffeine *on page 1018*

Caffeine, Propoxyphene, and Aspirin *see* Propoxyphene, Aspirin, and Caffeine *on page 1138*

Calan® *see* Verapamil *on page 1373*

Calan® SR *see* Verapamil *on page 1373*

Calcarb 600 [OTC] *see* Calcium Carbonate *on page 245*

Calcibind® *see* Cellulose Sodium Phosphate *on page 294*

Calci-Chew® [OTC] *see* Calcium Carbonate *on page 245*

Calcifediol (kal si fe DYE ole)

U.S. Brand Names Calderol® [DSC]

Canadian Brand Names Calderol®

Generic Available No

Synonyms 25-HCC; 25-Hydroxycholecalciferol; 25-Hydroxyvitamin D_3

Pharmacologic Category Vitamin D Analog

Use Treatment and management of metabolic bone disease associated with chronic renal failure or hypocalcemia in patients on chronic renal dialysis

Local Anesthetic/Vasoconstrictor Precautions No information available to require special precautions

Effects on Dental Treatment Key adverse event(s) related to dental treatment: Metallic taste and xerostomia (normal salivary flow resumes upon discontinuation).

Common Adverse Effects Frequency not defined.

Cardiovascular: Hypotension, cardiac arrhythmias, hypertension

Central nervous system: Irritability, headache, somnolence, seizures (rare)

Dermatologic: Pruritus

Endocrine & metabolic: Hypercalcemia, polydipsia, hypermagnesemia

Gastrointestinal: Nausea, vomiting, constipation, anorexia, pancreatitis, metallic taste, xerostomia

Hepatic: Elevated LFTs

Neuromuscular & skeletal: Myalgia, bone pain

Ocular: Conjunctivitis, photophobia

Renal: Polyuria

Mechanism of Action Vitamin D analog that (along with calcitonin and parathyroid hormone) regulates serum calcium homeostasis by promoting absorption of calcium and phosphorus in the small intestine; promotes renal tubule resorption of phosphate; increases rate of accretion and resorption in bone minerals

Drug Interactions

Increased Effect/Toxicity: The effect of calcifediol is increased with thiazide diuretics. Additive effect with antacids (magnesium).

Decreased Effect: The effect of calcifediol is decreased when taken with cholestyramine or colestipol.

Pharmacodynamics/Kinetics

Absorption: Rapid from small intestines

Distribution: Activated in kidneys; stored in liver and fat depots

Half-life elimination: 12-22 days

Time to peak: Within 4 hours

Excretion: Feces

Pregnancy Risk Factor C (manufacturer); A/D (dose exceeding RDA recommendation) (expert analysis)

Calciferol™ *see* Ergocalciferol *on page 503*

Calcijex® *see* Calcitriol *on page 244*

Calci-Mix®[OTC] *see* Calcium Carbonate *on page 245*

Calcipotriene (kal si POE try een)

U.S. Brand Names Dovonex®

Generic Available No

Pharmacologic Category Topical Skin Product; Vitamin D Analog

Use Treatment of moderate plaque psoriasis

Local Anesthetic/Vasoconstrictor Precautions No information available to require special precautions

Effects on Dental Treatment No significant effects or complications reported

Common Adverse Effects

>10%: Dermatologic: Burning, itching, skin irritation, erythema, dry skin, peeling, rash, worsening of psoriasis

1% to 10%: Dermatologic: Dermatitis

Mechanism of Action Synthetic vitamin D_3 analog which regulates skin cell production and proliferation

Pregnancy Risk Factor C

Calcitonin (kal si TOE nin)

Related Information

Rheumatoid Arthritis, Osteoarthritis, and Osteoporosis *on page 1490*

U.S. Brand Names Miacalcin®

Canadian Brand Names Calcimar®; Caltine®; Miacalcin® NS

Mexican Brand Names Miacalcic® [salmon]; Oseum® [salmon]; Tonocalcin® [salmon]

Generic Available No

Synonyms Calcitonin (Salmon)

Pharmacologic Category Antidote

Use Calcitonin (salmon): Treatment of Paget's disease of bone (osteitis deformans); adjunctive therapy for hypercalcemia; used in postmenopausal osteoporosis and osteogenesis imperfecta

Local Anesthetic/Vasoconstrictor Precautions No information available to require special precautions

Effects on Dental Treatment No significant effects or complications reported

Common Adverse Effects

>10%:

Cardiovascular: Facial flushing

Gastrointestinal: Nausea, diarrhea, anorexia

Local: Edema at injection site

1% to 10%:

Genitourinary: Polyuria

Neuromuscular & skeletal: Back/joint pain

Respiratory: Nasal bleeding/crusting (following intranasal administration)

Mechanism of Action Structurally similar to human calcitonin; it directly inhibits osteoclastic bone resorption; promotes the renal excretion of calcium, phosphate, sodium, magnesium and potassium by decreasing tubular reabsorption; increases the jejunal secretion of water, sodium, potassium, and chloride

Drug Interactions

Decreased Effect: Calcitonin may be antagonized by calcium and vitamin D in treating hypercalcemia.

(Continued)

Calcitonin *(Continued)*

Pharmacodynamics/Kinetics

Hypercalcemia:

Onset of action: ~2 hours

Duration: 6-8 hours

Distribution: Does not cross placenta

Half-life elimination: SubQ: 1.2 hours

Excretion: Urine (as inactive metabolites)

Pregnancy Risk Factor C

Calcitonin (Salmon) *see* Calcitonin *on page 243*

Cal-Citrate® 250 [OTC] *see* Calcium Citrate *on page 246*

Calcitriol (kal si TRYE ole)

U.S. Brand Names Calcijex®; Rocaltrol®

Canadian Brand Names Rocaltrol®

Mexican Brand Names Rocaltrol®; Tirocal®

Generic Available Yes

Synonyms 1,25 Dihydroxycholecalciferol

Pharmacologic Category Vitamin D Analog

Use Management of hypocalcemia in patients on chronic renal dialysis; management of secondary hyperparathyroidism in moderate to severe chronic renal failure; management of hypocalcemia in hypoparathyroidism and pseudohypoparathyroidism

Unlabeled/Investigational Use Decrease severity of psoriatic lesions in psoriatic vulgaris; vitamin D resistant rickets

Local Anesthetic/Vasoconstrictor Precautions No information available to require special precautions

Effects on Dental Treatment Key adverse event(s) related to dental treatment: Metallic taste and xerostomia (normal salivary flow resumes upon discontinuation).

Common Adverse Effects

>10%: Endocrine & metabolic: Hypercalcemia (33%)

Frequency not defined:

Cardiovascular: Cardiac arrhythmias, hypertension, hypotension

Central nervous system: Headache, irritability, seizures (rare), somnolence, psychosis

Dermatologic: Pruritus, erythema multiforme

Endocrine & metabolic: Hypermagnesemia, polydipsia

Gastrointestinal: Anorexia, constipation, metallic taste, nausea, pancreatitis, vomiting, xerostomia

Hepatic: Elevated LFTs

Neuromuscular & skeletal: Bone pain, myalgia, dystrophy, soft tissue calcification

Ocular: Conjunctivitis, photophobia

Renal: Polyuria

Mechanism of Action Promotes absorption of calcium in the intestines and retention at the kidneys thereby increasing calcium levels in the serum; decreases excessive serum phosphatase levels, parathyroid hormone levels, and decreases bone resorption; increases renal tubule phosphate resorption

Drug Interactions

Cytochrome P450 Effect: Induces CYP3A4 (weak)

Increased Effect/Toxicity: Risk of hypercalcemia with thiazide diuretics. Risk of hypermagnesemia with magnesium-containing antacids. Risk of digoxin toxicity may be increased (if hypercalcemia occurs).

Decreased Effect: Cholestyramine and colestipol decrease absorption/effect of calcitriol. Thiazide diuretics and corticosteroids may reduce the effect of calcitriol.

Pharmacodynamics/Kinetics

Onset of action: ~2-6 hours

Duration: 3-5 days

Absorption: Oral: Rapid

Protein binding: 99.9%

Metabolism: Primarily to 1,24,25-trihydroxycholecalciferol and 1,24,25-trihydroxy ergocalciferol

Half-life elimination: 3-8 hours

Excretion: Primarily feces; urine (4% to 6%)

Pregnancy Risk Factor C (manufacturer); A/D (dose exceeding RDA recommendation) (expert analysis)

Calcium Acetate (KAL see um AS e tate)

Related Information

Rheumatoid Arthritis, Osteoarthritis, and Osteoporosis *on page 1490*

U.S. Brand Names PhosLo®

Generic Available Yes: Solution for injection

Pharmacologic Category Antidote; Calcium Salt; Electrolyte Supplement, Parenteral

Use

Oral: Control of hyperphosphatemia in end-stage renal failure; does not promote aluminum absorption

I.V.: Calcium supplementation in parenteral nutrition therapy

Local Anesthetic/Vasoconstrictor Precautions No information available to require special precautions

Effects on Dental Treatment No significant effects or complications reported

Mechanism of Action Combines with dietary phosphate to form insoluble calcium phosphate which is excreted in feces

Pregnancy Risk Factor C

Calcium Acetate and Aluminum Sulfate *see* Aluminum Sulfate and Calcium Acetate *on page 92*

Calcium Carbonate (KAL see um KAR bun ate)

Related Information

Rheumatoid Arthritis, Osteoarthritis, and Osteoporosis *on page 1490*

U.S. Brand Names Alcalak [OTC]; Alka-Mints® [OTC]; Amitone® [OTC]; Calcarb 600 [OTC]; Calci-Chew® [OTC]; Calci-Mix®[OTC]; Cal-Gest [OTC]; Cal-Mint [OTC]; Caltrate® 600 [OTC]; Chooz® [OTC]; Florical® [OTC]; Mylanta® Children's [OTC]; Nephro-Calci® [OTC]; Os-Cal® 500 [OTC]; Oysco 500 [OTC]; Oyst-Cal 500 [OTC]; Titralac ™ [OTC]; Titralac™ Extra Strength [OTC]; Tums® [OTC]; Tums® 500 [OTC]; Tums® E-X [OTC]; Tums® Extra Strength Sugar Free [OTC]; Tums® Smooth Dissolve [OTC]; Tums® Ultra [OTC]

Canadian Brand Names Apo-Cal®; Calcite-500; Caltrate®; Os-Cal®

Mexican Brand Names Calsan®; Caltrate®; Osteomin®

Generic Available Yes: Excludes capsule

Pharmacologic Category Antacid; Antidote; Calcium Salt; Electrolyte Supplement, Oral

Use As an antacid, and treatment and prevention of calcium deficiency or hyperphosphatemia (eg, osteoporosis, osteomalacia, mild/moderate renal insufficiency, hypoparathyroidism, postmenopausal osteoporosis, rickets); has been used to bind phosphate

Local Anesthetic/Vasoconstrictor Precautions No information available to require special precautions

Effects on Dental Treatment Key adverse event(s) related to dental treatment: Xerostomia (normal salivary flow resumes upon discontinuation).

Mechanism of Action As dietary supplement, used to prevent or treat negative calcium balance; in osteoporosis, it helps to prevent or decrease the rate of bone loss. The calcium in calcium salts moderates nerve and muscle performance and allows normal cardiac function. Also used to treat hyperphosphatemia in patients with advanced renal insufficiency by combining with dietary phosphate to form insoluble calcium phosphate, which is excreted in feces. Calcium salts as antacids neutralize gastric acidity resulting in increased gastric an duodenal bulb pH; they additionally inhibit proteolytic activity of peptic if the pH is increased >4 and increase lower esophageal sphincter tone.

Calcium Carbonate and Magnesium Hydroxide

(KAL see um KAR bun ate & mag NEE zhum hye DROKS ide)

U.S. Brand Names Mylanta® Gelcaps® [OTC]; Mylanta® Supreme [OTC]; Mylanta® Ultra [OTC]; Rolaids® [OTC]; Rolaids® Extra Strength [OTC]

Generic Available No

Synonyms Magnesium Hydroxide and Calcium Carbonate

Pharmacologic Category Antacid

Use Hyperacidity

Local Anesthetic/Vasoconstrictor Precautions No information available to require special precautions

Effects on Dental Treatment No significant effects or complications reported

Calcium Carbonate and Simethicone

(KAL see um KAR bun ate & sye METH i kone)

Related Information

Calcium Carbonate *on page 245*

U.S. Brand Names Titralac® Plus [OTC]

(Continued)

Calcium Carbonate and Simethicone *(Continued)*

Generic Available No

Synonyms Simethicone and Calcium Carbonate

Pharmacologic Category Antacid; Antiflatulent

Use Relief of acid indigestion, heartburn

Local Anesthetic/Vasoconstrictor Precautions No information available to require special precautions

Effects on Dental Treatment Do not give tetracyclines concomitantly.

Pharmacodynamics/Kinetics See individual agents.

Pregnancy Risk Factor C

Calcium Carbonate, Magnesium Hydroxide, and Famotidine *see* Famotidine, Calcium Carbonate, and Magnesium Hydroxide *on page 574*

Calcium Channel Blockers and Gingival Hyperplasia *see page 1600*

Calcium Channel Blockers, Comparative Pharmacokinetics *see page 1602*

Calcium Chloride (KAL see um KLOR ide)

Generic Available Yes

Pharmacologic Category Calcium Salt; Electrolyte Supplement, Parenteral

Use Cardiac resuscitation when epinephrine fails to improve myocardial contractions, cardiac disturbances of hyperkalemia, hypocalcemia, or calcium channel blocking agent toxicity; emergent treatment of hypocalcemic tetany, treatment of hypermagnesemia

Local Anesthetic/Vasoconstrictor Precautions No information available to require special precautions

Effects on Dental Treatment No significant effects or complications reported

Mechanism of Action Moderates nerve and muscle performance via action potential excitation threshold regulation

Pregnancy Risk Factor C

Calcium Citrate (KAL see um SIT rate)

Related Information

Rheumatoid Arthritis, Osteoarthritis, and Osteoporosis *on page 1490*

U.S. Brand Names Cal-Citrate® 250 [OTC]; Citracal® [OTC]

Canadian Brand Names Osteocit®

Generic Available Yes

Pharmacologic Category Calcium Salt

Use Antacid; treatment and prevention of calcium deficiency or hyperphosphatemia (eg, osteoporosis, osteomalacia, mild/moderate renal insufficiency, hypoparathyroidism, postmenopausal osteoporosis, rickets)

Local Anesthetic/Vasoconstrictor Precautions No information available to require special precautions

Effects on Dental Treatment No significant effects or complications reported

Mechanism of Action Moderates nerve and muscle performance via action potential excitation threshold regulation

Pregnancy Risk Factor C

Calcium Disodium Edetate *see* Edetate Calcium Disodium *on page 482*

Calcium Disodium Versenate® *see* Edetate Calcium Disodium *on page 482*

Calcium EDTA *see* Edetate Calcium Disodium *on page 482*

Calcium Glubionate (KAL see um gloo BYE oh nate)

Related Information

Rheumatoid Arthritis, Osteoarthritis, and Osteoporosis *on page 1490*

Mexican Brand Names Calcium-Sandoz®

Generic Available Yes

Pharmacologic Category Calcium Salt

Use Adjunct in treatment and prevention of postmenopausal osteoporosis; treatment and prevention of calcium depletion or hyperphosphatemia (eg, osteoporosis, osteomalacia, mild/moderate renal insufficiency, hypoparathyroidism, rickets)

Local Anesthetic/Vasoconstrictor Precautions No information available to require special precautions

Effects on Dental Treatment No significant effects or complications reported

Mechanism of Action As dietary supplement, used to prevent or treat negative calcium balance; in osteoporosis, it helps to prevent or decrease the rate of bone loss. The calcium in calcium salts moderates nerve and muscle performance and allows normal cardiac function.

Pregnancy Risk Factor C

Calcium Gluconate (KAL see um GLOO koe nate)

Related Information

Rheumatoid Arthritis, Osteoarthritis, and Osteoporosis *on page 1490*

Generic Available Yes

Pharmacologic Category Calcium Salt; Electrolyte Supplement, Oral; Electrolyte Supplement, Parenteral

Use Treatment and prevention of hypocalcemia; treatment of tetany, cardiac disturbances of hyperkalemia, cardiac resuscitation when epinephrine fails to improve myocardial contractions, hypocalcemia, or calcium channel blocker toxicity; calcium supplementation

Local Anesthetic/Vasoconstrictor Precautions No information available to require special precautions

Effects on Dental Treatment No significant effects or complications reported

Mechanism of Action As dietary supplement, used to prevent or treat negative calcium balance; in osteoporosis, it helps to prevent or decrease the rate of bone loss. The calcium in calcium salts moderates nerve and muscle performance and allows normal cardiac function.

Pregnancy Risk Factor C

Calcium Lactate (KAL see um LAK tate)

Related Information

Rheumatoid Arthritis, Osteoarthritis, and Osteoporosis *on page 1490*

Generic Available Yes

Pharmacologic Category Calcium Salt

Use Adjunct in prevention of postmenopausal osteoporosis; treatment and prevention of calcium depletion

Local Anesthetic/Vasoconstrictor Precautions No information available to require special precautions

Effects on Dental Treatment No significant effects or complications reported

Mechanism of Action As dietary supplement, used to prevent or treat negative calcium balance; in osteoporosis, it helps to prevent or decrease the rate of bone loss. The calcium in calcium salts moderates nerve and muscle performance and allows normal cardiac function.

Pregnancy Risk Factor C

Calcium Leucovorin *see* Leucovorin *on page 804*

Calcium Pantothenate *see* Pantothenic Acid *on page 1044*

Calcium Phosphate (Tribasic) (KAL see um FOS fate tri BAY sik)

Related Information

Rheumatoid Arthritis, Osteoarthritis, and Osteoporosis *on page 1490*

U.S. Brand Names Posture® [OTC]

Generic Available No

Synonyms Tricalcium Phosphate

Pharmacologic Category Calcium Salt

Use Adjunct in prevention of postmenopausal osteoporosis; treatment and prevention of calcium depletion

Local Anesthetic/Vasoconstrictor Precautions No information available to require special precautions

Effects on Dental Treatment No significant effects or complications reported

Mechanism of Action As dietary supplement, used to prevent or treat negative calcium balance; in osteoporosis, it helps to prevent or decrease the rate of bone loss. The calcium in calcium salts moderates nerve and muscle performance and allows normal cardiac function.

Pregnancy Risk Factor C

CaldeCORT® [OTC] *see* Hydrocortisone *on page 714*

Calderol® [DSC] *see* Calcifediol *on page 242*

Calfactant (kaf AKT ant)

U.S. Brand Names Infasurf®

Generic Available No

Pharmacologic Category Lung Surfactant

Use Prevention of respiratory distress syndrome (RDS) in premature infants at high risk for RDS and for the treatment ("rescue") of premature infants who develop RDS

Prophylaxis: Therapy at birth with calfactant is indicated for premature infants <29 weeks of gestational age at significant risk for RDS. Should be administered as soon as possible, preferably within 30 minutes after birth.

(Continued)

Calfactant *(Continued)*

Treatment: For infants ≤72 hours of age with RDS (confirmed by clinical and radiologic findings) and requiring endotracheal intubation.

Local Anesthetic/Vasoconstrictor Precautions No information available to require special precautions

Effects on Dental Treatment No significant effects or complications reported

Common Adverse Effects

Cardiovascular: Bradycardia (34%), cyanosis (65%)

Respiratory: Airway obstruction (39%), reflux (21%), requirement for manual ventilation (16%), reintubation (1% to 10%)

Mechanism of Action Endogenous lung surfactant is essential for effective ventilation because it modifies alveolar surface tension, thereby stabilizing the alveoli. Lung surfactant deficiency is the cause of respiratory distress syndrome (RDS) in premature infants and lung surfactant restores surface activity to the lungs of these infants.

Pharmacodynamics/Kinetics No human studies of absorption, biotransformation, or excretion have been performed

Cal-Gest [OTC] *see* Calcium Carbonate *on page 245*

Cal-Mint [OTC] *see* Calcium Carbonate *on page 245*

Caltrate® 600 [OTC] *see* Calcium Carbonate *on page 245*

Camila™ *see* Norethindrone *on page 996*

Campath® *see* Alemtuzumab *on page 76*

Campath-1H *see* Alemtuzumab *on page 76*

Campho-Phenique® [OTC] *see* Camphor and Phenol *on page 248*

Camphor and Phenol (KAM for & FEE nole)

U.S. Brand Names Campho-Phenique® [OTC]

Generic Available No

Synonyms Phenol and Camphor

Pharmacologic Category Topical Skin Product

Use Relief of pain and for minor infections

Local Anesthetic/Vasoconstrictor Precautions No information available to require special precautions

Effects on Dental Treatment No significant effects or complications reported

Pregnancy Risk Factor C

Camphorated Tincture of Opium *see* Paregoric *on page 1045*

Camptosar® *see* Irinotecan *on page 764*

Camptothecin-11 *see* Irinotecan *on page 764*

Canasa™ *see* Mesalamine *on page 882*

Cancidas® *see* Caspofungin *on page 272*

Candesartan (kan de SAR tan)

Related Information

Cardiovascular Diseases *on page 1458*

U.S. Brand Names Atacand®

Canadian Brand Names Atacand®

Mexican Brand Names Atacand®

Generic Available No

Synonyms Candesartan Cilexetil

Pharmacologic Category Angiotensin II Receptor Blocker

Use Alone or in combination with other antihypertensive agents in treating essential hypertension

Unlabeled/Investigational Use Congestive heart failure

Local Anesthetic/Vasoconstrictor Precautions No information available to require special precautions

Effects on Dental Treatment No significant effects or complications reported

Common Adverse Effects May be associated with worsening of renal function in patients dependent on renin-angiotensin-aldosterone system.

Cardiovascular: Flushing, tachycardia, palpitations, angina, MI

Central nervous system: Dizziness, lightheadedness, drowsiness, headache, vertigo, anxiety, depression, somnolence, fever

Dermatologic: Angioedema, rash

Endocrine & metabolic: Hyperglycemia, hypertriglyceridemia, hyperuricemia

Genitourinary: Hematuria

Neuromuscular & skeletal: Back pain, increased CPK, weakness

Respiratory: Upper respiratory tract infection, bronchitis, epistaxis

Miscellaneous: Diaphoresis (increased)

Mechanism of Action Candesartan is an angiotensin receptor antagonist. Angiotensin II acts as a vasoconstrictor. In addition to causing direct vasoconstriction, angiotensin II also stimulates the release of aldosterone. Once aldosterone is released, sodium as well as water are reabsorbed. The end result is an elevation in blood pressure. Candesartan binds to the AT1 angiotensin II receptor. This binding prevents angiotensin II from binding to the receptor thereby blocking the vasoconstriction and the aldosterone secreting effects of angiotensin II.

Drug Interactions

Cytochrome P450 Effect: Substrate of CYP2C8/9 (minor); **Inhibits** CYP2C8/9 (weak)

Increased Effect/Toxicity: The risk of lithium toxicity may be increased by candesartan; monitor lithium levels. Concurrent use with potassium-sparing diuretics (amiloride, spironolactone, triamterene), potassium supplements, or trimethoprim (high-dose) may increase the risk of hyperkalemia.

Pharmacodynamics/Kinetics

Onset of action: 2-3 hours

Peak effect: 6-8 hours

Duration: >24 hours

Distribution: V_d: 0.13 L/kg

Protein binding: 99%

Metabolism: To candesartan by the intestinal wall cells

Bioavailability: 15%

Half-life elimination (dose dependent): 5-9 hours

Time to peak: 3-4 hours

Excretion: Urine (26%)

Clearance: Total body: 0.37 mL/kg/minute; Renal: 0.19 mL/kg/minute

Pregnancy Risk Factor C/D (2nd and 3rd trimesters)

Candesartan and Hydrochlorothiazide

(kan de SAR tan & hye droe klor oh THYE a zide)

Related Information

Candesartan *on page 248*

Cardiovascular Diseases *on page 1458*

Hydrochlorothiazide *on page 699*

U.S. Brand Names Atacand HCT™

Canadian Brand Names Atacand® Plus

Generic Available No

Synonyms Candesartan Cilexetil and Hydrochlorothiazide

Pharmacologic Category Angiotensin II Receptor Blocker Combination

Use Treatment of hypertension; combination product should not be used for initial therapy

Local Anesthetic/Vasoconstrictor Precautions No information available to require special precautions

Effects on Dental Treatment No significant effects or complications reported

Common Adverse Effects Reactions which follow have been reported with the combination product; see individual drug monographs for additional adverse reactions that may be expected from each agent.

1% to 10%:

Central nervous system: Dizziness (3%), headache (3%, placebo 5%)

Neuromuscular & skeletal: Back pain (3%)

Respiratory: Upper respiratory tract infection (4%)

Miscellaneous: Flu-like symptoms (2%)

Mechanism of Action

Candesartan: Candesartan is an angiotensin receptor antagonist. Angiotensin II acts as a vasoconstrictor. In addition to causing direct vasoconstriction, angiotensin II also stimulates the release of aldosterone. Once aldosterone is released, sodium as well as water are reabsorbed. The end result is an elevation in blood pressure. Candesartan binds to the AT1 angiotensin II receptor. This binding prevents angiotensin II from binding to the receptor, thereby blocking the vasoconstriction and the aldosterone-secreting effects of angiotensin II.

Hydrochlorothiazide: Inhibits sodium reabsorption in the distal tubules causing increased excretion of sodium and water as well as potassium and hydrogen ions

Drug Interactions

Cytochrome P450 Effect: Candesartan: **Substrate** of CYP2C8/9 (minor); **Inhibits** CYP2C8/9 (weak)

Increased Effect/Toxicity: See individual agents.

Decreased Effect: See individual agents.

Pharmacodynamics/Kinetics See individual agents.

Pregnancy Risk Factor C/D (2nd and 3rd trimesters)

Candesartan Cilexetil *see* Candesartan *on page 248*

Candesartan Cilexetil and Hydrochlorothiazide *see* Candesartan and Hydrochlorothiazide *on page 249*

Cankaid® [OTC] *see* Carbamide Peroxide *on page 259*

Cantharidin (kan THAR e din)

Canadian Brand Names Canthacur®; Cantharone®

Generic Available No

Pharmacologic Category Keratolytic Agent

Use Removal of ordinary and periungual warts

Local Anesthetic/Vasoconstrictor Precautions No information available to require special precautions

Effects on Dental Treatment No significant effects or complications reported

Common Adverse Effects 1% to 10%:

Cardiovascular: Syncope
Central nervous system: Delirium, ataxia
Dermatologic: Dermal irritation, dermal burns, acantholysis
Gastrointestinal: GI hemorrhage, rectal bleeding, dysphagia
Genitourinary: Priapism
Hepatic: Fatty degeneration
Neuromuscular & skeletal: Hyper-reflexia
Ocular: Conjunctivitis, iritis, keratitis
Renal: Proteinuria, hematuria
Respiratory: Burning of oropharynx

Pregnancy Risk Factor C

Cantil® *see* Mepenzolate *on page 869*

Capastat® Sulfate *see* Capreomycin *on page 251*

Capecitabine (ka pe SITE a been)

Related Information

Fluorouracil *on page 605*

U.S. Brand Names Xeloda®

Canadian Brand Names Xeloda®

Mexican Brand Names Xeloda®

Generic Available No

Pharmacologic Category Antineoplastic Agent, Antimetabolite

Use Treatment of metastatic colorectal cancer, metastatic breast cancer

Local Anesthetic/Vasoconstrictor Precautions No information available to require special precautions

Effects on Dental Treatment Key adverse event(s) related to dental treatment: Stomatitis, abnormal taste, and taste disturbance.

Common Adverse Effects Frequency listed derived from monotherapy trials.

>10%:

Cardiovascular: Edema (9% to 15%)
Central nervous system: Fatigue (~40%), fever (12% to 18%), pain (colorectal cancer: 12%)
Dermatologic: Palmar-plantar erythrodysesthesia (hand-and-foot syndrome) (~55%, may be dose limiting), dermatitis (27% to 37%)
Gastrointestinal: Diarrhea (~55%, may be dose limiting), mild to moderate nausea (43% to 53%), vomiting (27% to 37%), stomatitis (~25%), decreased appetite (colorectal cancer: 26%), anorexia (23%), abdominal pain (20% to 35%), constipation (~15%)
Hematologic: Lymphopenia (94%), anemia (72% to 80%; Grade 3/4: <1% to 3%), neutropenia (13% to 26%; Grade 3/4: 1% to 2%), thrombocytopenia (24%; Grade 3/4: 1% to 3%)
Hepatic: Increased bilirubin (22% to 48%)
Neuromuscular & skeletal: Paresthesia (21%)
Ocular: Eye irritation (~15%)
Respiratory: Dyspnea (colorectal cancer: 14%)

5% to 10%:

Cardiovascular: Venous thrombosis (colorectal cancer: 8%), chest pain (colorectal cancer: 6%)
Central nervous system: Headache (~10%), dizziness (~8%), insomnia (8%), mood alteration (colorectal cancer: 5%), depression (colorectal cancer: 5%)
Dermatologic: Nail disorders (7%), skin discoloration (colorectal cancer: 7%), alopecia (colorectal cancer: 6%)

Endocrine & metabolic: Dehydration (7%)

Gastrointestinal: Motility disorder (colorectal cancer: 10%), oral discomfort (colorectal cancer: 10%), dyspepsia (8%), upper GI inflammatory disorders (colorectal cancer: 8%), hemorrhage (colorectal cancer: 6%), ileus (colorectal cancer: 6%), taste disturbance (colorectal cancer: 6%)

Neuromuscular & skeletal: Back pain (colorectal cancer: 10%), myalgia (9%), neuropathy (colorectal cancer: 10%), arthralgia (colorectal cancer: 8%), limb pain (colorectal cancer: 6%)

Respiratory: Cough (7%), sore throat (2%), epistaxis (3%)

Ocular: Abnormal vision (colorectal cancer: 5%)

Miscellaneous: Viral infection (colorectal cancer: 5%)

Mechanism of Action Capecitabine is a prodrug of fluorouracil. It undergoes hydrolysis in the liver and tissues to form fluorouracil which is the active moiety. Fluorouracil is a fluorinated pyrimidine antimetabolite that inhibits thymidylate synthetase, blocking the methylation of deoxyuridylic acid to thymidylic acid, interfering with DNA, and to a lesser degree, RNA synthesis. Fluorouracil appears to be phase specific for the G_1 and S phases of the cell cycle.

Drug Interactions

Increased Effect/Toxicity: Response to warfarin may be increased by capecitabine.

Pharmacodynamics/Kinetics

Absorption: Rapid and extensive

Protein binding: <60%; 35% to albumin

Metabolism: Hepatic: Inactive metabolites: 5′-deoxy-5-fluorocytidine, 5′-deoxy-5-fluorouridine; Tissue: Active metabolite: Fluorouracil

Half-life elimination: 0.5-1 hour

Time to peak: 1.5 hours; Fluorouracil: 2 hours

Excretion: Urine (96%, 50% as α-fluoro-β-alanine)

Pregnancy Risk Factor D

Capex™ *see* Fluocinolone *on page 601*

Capital® and Codeine *see* Acetaminophen and Codeine *on page 50*

Capitrol® *see* Chloroxine *on page 313*

Capoten® *see* Captopril *on page 252*

Capozide® *see* Captopril and Hydrochlorothiazide *on page 255*

Capreomycin (kap ree oh MYE sin)

Related Information

Tuberculosis *on page 1495*

U.S. Brand Names Capastat® Sulfate

Generic Available No

Synonyms Capreomycin Sulfate

Pharmacologic Category Antibiotic, Miscellaneous; Antitubercular Agent

Use Treatment of tuberculosis in conjunction with at least one other antituberculosis agent

Local Anesthetic/Vasoconstrictor Precautions No information available to require special precautions

Effects on Dental Treatment No significant effects or complications reported

Common Adverse Effects

>10%:

Otic: Ototoxicity [subclinical hearing loss (11%), clinical loss (3%)], tinnitus

Renal: Nephrotoxicity (36%, increased BUN)

1% to 10%: Hematologic: Eosinophilia (dose-related, mild)

Mechanism of Action Capreomycin is a cyclic polypeptide antimicrobial. It is administered as a mixture of capreomycin IA and capreomycin IB. The mechanism of action of capreomycin is not well understood. Mycobacterial species that have become resistant to other agents are usually still sensitive to the action of capreomycin. However, significant cross-resistance with viomycin, kanamycin, and neomycin occurs.

Drug Interactions

Increased Effect/Toxicity: May increase effect/duration of nondepolarizing neuromuscular blocking agents. Additive toxicity (nephrotoxicity and ototoxicity), respiratory paralysis may occur with aminoglycosides (eg, streptomycin).

Pharmacodynamics/Kinetics

Half-life elimination: Normal renal function: 4-6 hours

Time to peak, serum: I.M.: ~1 hour

Excretion: Urine (as unchanged drug)

Pregnancy Risk Factor C

Capreomycin Sulfate *see* Capreomycin *on page 251*

Capsagel® [OTC] *see* Capsaicin *on page 252*

Capsaicin (kap SAY sin)

Related Information

Cayenne *on page 1418*

U.S. Brand Names ArthriCare® for Women Extra Moisturizing [OTC]; ArthriCare® for Women Silky Dry [OTC]; Capsagel® [OTC]; Capzasin-HP® [OTC]; Capzasin-P® [OTC]; TheraPatch® Warm [OTC]; Zostrix® [OTC]; Zostrix®-HP [OTC]

Canadian Brand Names Antiphogistine Rub A-535 Capsaicin; Zostrix®; Zostrix® H.P.

Generic Available Yes: Cream

Pharmacologic Category Analgesic, Topical; Topical Skin Product

Use Topical treatment of pain associated with postherpetic neuralgia, rheumatoid arthritis, osteoarthritis, diabetic neuropathy; postsurgical pain

Unlabeled/Investigational Use Treatment of pain associated with psoriasis, chronic neuralgias unresponsive to other forms of therapy, and intractable pruritus

Local Anesthetic/Vasoconstrictor Precautions No information available to require special precautions

Effects on Dental Treatment No significant effects or complications reported

Common Adverse Effects Frequency not defined.

Dermatologic: Itching, stinging sensation, erythema

Local: Transient burning on application which usually diminishes with repeated use

Respiratory: Cough

Mechanism of Action Induces release of substance P, the principal chemomediator of pain impulses from the periphery to the CNS, from peripheral sensory neurons; after repeated application, capsaicin depletes the neuron of substance P and prevents reaccumulation

Drug Interactions

Cytochrome P450 Effect: Substrate of CYP2E1 (minor)

Pharmacodynamics/Kinetics

Onset of action: 14-28 days

Peak effect: 4-6 weeks of continuous therapy

Duration: Several hours

Pregnancy Risk Factor C

Captopril (KAP toe pril)

Related Information

Cardiovascular Diseases *on page 1458*

U.S. Brand Names Capoten®

Canadian Brand Names Alti-Captopril; Apo-Capto®; Capoten™; Gen-Captopril; Novo-Captopril; Nu-Capto; PMS-Captopril

Mexican Brand Names Capoten®; Captral®; Cardipril®; Cryopril®; Ecaten®; Kenolan®; Lenpryl®; Romir®

Generic Available Yes

Synonyms ACE

Pharmacologic Category Angiotensin-Converting Enzyme (ACE) Inhibitor

Use Management of hypertension; treatment of congestive heart failure, left ventricular dysfunction after myocardial infarction, diabetic nephropathy

Unlabeled/Investigational Use Treatment of hypertensive crisis, rheumatoid arthritis; diagnosis of anatomic renal artery stenosis, hypertension secondary to scleroderma renal crisis; diagnosis of aldosteronism, idiopathic edema, Bartter's syndrome, postmyocardial infarction for prevention of ventricular failure; increase circulation in Raynaud's phenomenon, hypertension secondary to Takayasu's disease

Local Anesthetic/Vasoconstrictor Precautions No information available to require special precautions

Effects on Dental Treatment Key adverse event(s) related to dental treatment: Loss or diminished perception of taste and orthostatic hypotension.

Common Adverse Effects

1% to 10%:

Cardiovascular: Hypotension (1% to 3%), tachycardia (1%), chest pain (1%), palpitation (1%)

Dermatologic: Rash (maculopapular or urticarial) (4% to 7%), pruritus (2%); in patients with rash, a positive ANA and/or eosinophilia has been noted in 7% to 10%.

Endocrine & metabolic: Hyperkalemia (1% to 11%)

Hematologic: Neutropenia may occur in up to 4% of patients with renal insufficiency or or collagen-vascular disease.

Renal: Proteinuria (1%), increased serum creatinine, worsening of renal function (may occur in patients with bilateral renal artery stenosis or hypovolemia)

Respiratory: Cough (<1% to 2%)

Miscellaneous: Hypersensitivity reactions (rash, pruritus, fever, arthralgia, and eosinophilia) have occurred in 4% to 7% of patients (depending on dose and renal function); dysgeusia - loss of taste or diminished perception (2% to 4%)

Frequency not defined:

Cardiovascular: Angioedema, cardiac arrest, cerebrovascular insufficiency, rhythm disturbances, orthostatic hypotension, syncope, flushing, pallor, angina, myocardial infarction, Raynaud's syndrome, CHF

Central nervous system: Ataxia, confusion, depression, nervousness, somnolence

Dermatologic: Bullous pemphigus, erythema multiforme, Stevens-Johnson syndrome, exfoliative dermatitis

Endocrine & metabolic: Increased serum transaminases, increased serum bilirubin, increased alkaline phosphatase, gynecomastia

Gastrointestinal: Pancreatitis, glossitis, dyspepsia

Genitourinary: Urinary frequency, impotence

Hematologic: Anemia, thrombocytopenia, pancytopenia, agranulocytosis, anemia

Hepatic: Jaundice, hepatitis, hepatic necrosis (rare), cholestasis, hyponatremia (symptomatic)

Neuromuscular & skeletal: Asthenia, myalgia, myasthenia

Ocular: Blurred vision

Renal: Renal insufficiency, renal failure, nephrotic syndrome, polyuria, oliguria

Respiratory: Bronchospasm, eosinophilic pneumonitis, rhinitis

Miscellaneous: Anaphylactoid reactions

Dosage Note: Dosage must be titrated according to patient's response; use lowest effective dose. Oral:

Infants: Initial: 0.15-0.3 mg/kg/dose; titrate dose upward to maximum of 6 mg/kg/day in 1-4 divided doses; usual required dose: 2.5-6 mg/kg/day

Children: Initial: 0.5 mg/kg/dose; titrate upward to maximum of 6 mg/kg/day in 2-4 divided doses

Older Children: Initial: 6.25-12.5 mg/dose every 12-24 hours; titrate upward to maximum of 6 mg/kg/day

Adolescents: Initial: 12.5-25 mg/dose given every 8-12 hours; increase by 25 mg/dose to maximum of 450 mg/day

Adults:

Acute hypertension (urgency/emergency): 12.5-25 mg, may repeat as needed (may be given sublingually, but no therapeutic advantage demonstrated)

Hypertension:

Initial dose: 12.5-25 mg 2-3 times/day; may increase by 12.5-25 mg/dose at 1- to 2-week intervals up to 50 mg 3 times/day; maximum dose: 150 mg 3 times/day; add diuretic before further dosage increases

Usual dose range (JNC 7): 25-100 mg/day in 2 divided doses

Congestive heart failure:

Initial dose: 6.25-12.5 mg 3 times/day in conjunction with cardiac glycoside and diuretic therapy; initial dose depends upon patient's fluid/electrolyte status

Target dose: 50 mg 3 times/day

Maximum dose: 150 mg 3 times/day

LVD after MI: Initial dose: 6.25 mg followed by 12.5 mg 3 times/day; then increase to 25 mg 3 times/day during next several days and then over next several weeks to target dose of 50 mg 3 times/day

Diabetic nephropathy: 25 mg 3 times/day; other antihypertensives often given concurrently

Dosing adjustment in renal impairment:

Cl_{cr} 10-50 mL/minute: Administer at 75% of normal dose.

Cl_{cr} <10 mL/minute: Administer at 50% of normal dose.

Note: Smaller dosages given every 8-12 hours are indicated in patients with renal dysfunction; renal function and leukocyte count should be carefully monitored during therapy.

Hemodialysis: Moderately dialyzable (20% to 50%); administer dose postdialysis or administer 25% to 35% supplemental dose.

Peritoneal dialysis: Supplemental dose is not necessary.

(Continued)

Captopril *(Continued)*

Mechanism of Action Competitive inhibitor of angiotensin-converting enzyme (ACE); prevents conversion of angiotensin I to angiotensin II, a potent vasoconstrictor; results in lower levels of angiotensin II which causes an increase in plasma renin activity and a reduction in aldosterone secretion

Contraindications Hypersensitivity to captopril or any component of the formulation; angioedema related to previous treatment with an ACE inhibitor; idiopathic or hereditary angioedema; bilateral renal artery stenosis; pregnancy (2nd or 3rd trimester)

Warnings/Precautions Anaphylactic reactions can occur. Angioedema can occur at any time during treatment (especially following first dose). Angioedema may involve head and neck (potentially affecting the airway) or the intestine (presenting with abdominal pain). Careful blood pressure monitoring with first dose (hypotension can occur especially in volume depleted patients). Use with caution in collagen vascular diseases; valvular stenosis (particularly aortic stenosis); hyperkalemia; or before, during, or immediately after anesthesia. Avoid rapid dosage escalation which may lead to renal insufficiency. Neutropenia/agranulocytosis with myeloid hyperplasia can rarely occur. If patient has renal impairment then a baseline WBC with differential and serum creatinine should be evaluated and monitored closely during the first 3 months of therapy. Hypersensitivity reactions may be seen during hemodialysis with high-flux dialysis membranes (eg, AN69). Deterioration in renal function can occur with initiation.

Use with caution and decrease dosage in patients with renal impairment (especially renal artery stenosis), severe CHF, or with coadministered diuretic therapy; experience in children is limited. Severe hypotension may occur in patients who are sodium and/or volume depleted, initiate lower doses and monitor closely when starting therapy in these patients; ACE inhibitors may be preferred agents in elderly patients with CHF and diabetes mellitus (diabetic proteinuria is reduced, minimal CNS effects, and enhanced insulin sensitivity); however, due to decreased renal function, tolerance must be carefully monitored.

Drug Interactions

Cytochrome P450 Effect: Substrate of CYP2D6 (major)

Increased Effect/Toxicity: Potassium supplements, co-trimoxazole (high dose), angiotensin II receptor antagonists (candesartan, losartan, irbesartan, etc), or potassium-sparing diuretics (amiloride, spironolactone, triamterene) may result in elevated serum potassium levels when combined with captopril. CYP2D6 inhibitors may increase the levels/effects of captopril; example inhibitors include chlorpromazine, delavirdine, fluoxetine, miconazole, paroxetine, pergolide, quinidine, quinine, ritonavir, and ropinirole. ACE inhibitor effects may be increased by phenothiazines or probenecid (increases levels of captopril). ACE inhibitors may increase serum concentrations/effects of digoxin, lithium, and sulfonlyureas.

Diuretics have additive hypotensive effects with ACE inhibitors, and hypovolemia increases the potential for adverse renal effects of ACE inhibitors. In patients with compromised renal function, coadministration with NSAIDs may result in further deterioration of renal function. Allopurinol and ACE inhibitors may cause a higher risk of hypersensitivity reaction when taken concurrently.

Decreased Effect: Aspirin (high dose) may reduce the therapeutic effects of ACE inhibitors; at low dosages this does not appear to be significant. Rifampin may decrease the effect of ACE inhibitors. Antacids may decrease the bioavailability of ACE inhibitors (may be more likely to occur with captopril); separate administration times by 1-2 hours. NSAIDs, specifically indomethacin, may reduce the hypotensive effects of ACE inhibitors. More likely to occur in low renin or volume dependent hypertensive patients.

Ethanol/Nutrition/Herb Interactions

Food: Captopril serum concentrations may be decreased if taken with food. Long-term use of captopril may result in a zinc deficiency which can result in a decrease in taste perception.

Herb/Nutraceutical: Avoid dong quai if using for hypertension (has estrogenic activity). Avoid ephedra, yohimbe, ginseng (may worsen hypertension). Avoid garlic (may have increased antihypertensive effect).

Dietary Considerations Should be taken at least 1 hour before or 2 hours after eating.

Pharmacodynamics/Kinetics

Onset of action: Peak effect: Blood pressure reduction: 1-1.5 hours after dose

Duration: Dose related, may require several weeks of therapy before full hypotensive effect

Absorption: 60% to 75%; reduced 30% to 40% by food

Protein binding: 25% to 30%
Metabolism: 50%
Half-life elimination (renal and cardiac function dependent):
Adults, healthy volunteers: 1.9 hours; Congestive heart failure: 2.06 hours; Anuria: 20-40 hours
Excretion: Urine (95%) within 24 hours

Pregnancy Risk Factor C/D (2nd and 3rd trimesters)

Dosage Forms TAB: 12.5 mg, 25 mg, 50 mg, 100 mg

Captopril and Hydrochlorothiazide

(KAP toe pril & hye droe klor oh THYE a zide)

Related Information

Captopril *on page 252*
Cardiovascular Diseases *on page 1458*
Hydrochlorothiazide *on page 699*

U.S. Brand Names Capozide®

Canadian Brand Names Capozide®

Generic Available Yes

Synonyms Hydrochlorothiazide and Captopril

Pharmacologic Category Antihypertensive Agent, Combination

Use Management of hypertension and treatment of congestive heart failure

Local Anesthetic/Vasoconstrictor Precautions No information available to require special precautions

Effects on Dental Treatment No significant effects or complications reported

Common Adverse Effects See individual agents.

Mechanism of Action Captopril is a competitive inhibitor of angiotensin-converting enzyme (ACE); prevents conversion of angiotensin I to angiotensin II, a potent vasoconstrictor. This results in lower levels of angiotensin II which causes an increase in plasma renin activity and a reduction in aldosterone secretion. Hydrochlorothiazide inhibits sodium reabsorption in the distal tubules causing increased excretion of sodium and water as well as potassium and hydrogen ions.

Drug Interactions

Cytochrome P450 Effect: Captopril: **Substrate** of CYP2D6 (major)

Increased Effect/Toxicity: See individual agents.

Decreased Effect: See individual agents.

Pharmacodynamics/Kinetics See individual agents.

Pregnancy Risk Factor C/D (2nd and 3rd trimesters)

Capzasin-HP® [OTC] *see* Capsaicin *on page 252*
Capzasin-P® [OTC] *see* Capsaicin *on page 252*
Carac™ *see* Fluorouracil *on page 605*
Carafate® *see* Sucralfate *on page 1242*

Carbachol (KAR ba kole)

U.S. Brand Names Carbastat® [DSC]; Isopto® Carbachol; Miostat®

Canadian Brand Names Carbastat®; Isopto® Carbachol; Miostat®

Generic Available No

Synonyms Carbacholine; Carbamylcholine Chloride

Pharmacologic Category Cholinergic Agonist; Ophthalmic Agent, Antiglaucoma; Ophthalmic Agent, Miotic

Use Lowers intraocular pressure in the treatment of glaucoma; cause miosis during surgery

Local Anesthetic/Vasoconstrictor Precautions No information available to require special precautions

Effects on Dental Treatment Key adverse event(s) related to dental treatment: Increased salivation.

Mechanism of Action Synthetic direct-acting cholinergic agent that causes miosis by stimulating muscarinic receptors in the eye

Pregnancy Risk Factor C

Carbacholine *see* Carbachol *on page 255*

Carbamazepine (kar ba MAZ e peen)

U.S. Brand Names Carbatrol®; Epitol®; Tegretol®; Tegretol®-XR

Canadian Brand Names Apo-Carbamazepine®; Gen-Carbamazepine CR; Novo-Carbamaz; Nu-Carbamazepine; PMS-Carbamazepine; Taro-Carbamazepine Chewable; Tegretol®

Mexican Brand Names Carbazep®; Carbazina®; Clostedal® [tabs]; Neugeron®; Tegretol®

(Continued)

Carbamazepine *(Continued)*

Generic Available Yes: Excludes capsule (extended release), tablet (extended release)

Synonyms CBZ

Pharmacologic Category Anticonvulsant, Miscellaneous

Dental Use Pain relief of trigeminal or glossopharyngeal neuralgia

Use Partial seizures with complex symptomatology (psychomotor, temporal lobe), generalized tonic-clonic seizures (grand mal), mixed seizure patterns

Unlabeled/Investigational Use Treatment of bipolar disorders and other affective disorders, resistant schizophrenia, ethanol withdrawal, restless leg syndrome, psychotic behavior associated with dementia, post-traumatic stress disorders

Local Anesthetic/Vasoconstrictor Precautions No information available to require special precautions

Effects on Dental Treatment Key adverse event(s) related to dental treatment: Oral ulceration.

Significant Adverse Effects Frequency not defined.

Cardiovascular: Edema, CHF, syncope, bradycardia, hypertension or hypotension, AV block, arrhythmias, thrombophlebitis, thromboembolism, lymphadenopathy

Central nervous system: Sedation, dizziness, fatigue, ataxia, confusion, headache, slurred speech, aseptic meningitis (case report)

Dermatologic: Rash, urticaria, toxic epidermal necrolysis, Stevens-Johnson syndrome, photosensitivity reaction, alterations in skin pigmentation, exfoliative dermatitis, erythema multiforme, purpura, alopecia

Endocrine & metabolic: Hyponatremia, SIADH, fever, chills

Gastrointestinal: Nausea, vomiting, gastric distress, abdominal pain, diarrhea, constipation, anorexia, pancreatitis

Genitourinary: Urinary retention, urinary frequency, azotemia, renal failure, impotence

Hematologic: Aplastic anemia, agranulocytosis, eosinophilia, leukopenia, pancytopenia, thrombocytopenia, bone marrow suppression, acute intermittent porphyria, leukocytosis

Hepatic: Hepatitis, abnormal liver function tests, jaundice, hepatic failure

Neuromuscular & skeletal: Peripheral neuritis

Ocular: Blurred vision, nystagmus, lens opacities, conjunctivitis

Otic: Tinnitus, hyperacusis

Miscellaneous: Hypersensitivity (including multiorgan reactions, may include vasculitis, disorders mimicking lymphoma, eosinophilia, hepatosplenomegaly), diaphoresis

Dosage Oral (dosage must be adjusted according to patient's response and serum concentrations):

Children:

<6 years: Initial: 5 mg/kg/day; dosage may be increased every 5-7 days to 10 mg/kg/day; then up to 20 mg/kg/day if necessary; administer in 2-4 divided doses

6-12 years: Initial: 100 mg twice daily or 10 mg/kg/day in 2 divided doses; increase by 100 mg/day at weekly intervals depending upon response; usual maintenance: 20-30 mg/kg/day in 2-4 divided doses (maximum dose: 1000 mg/day)

Children >12 years and Adults: 200 mg twice daily to start, increase by 200 mg/day at weekly intervals until therapeutic levels achieved; usual dose: 400-1200 mg/day in 2-4 divided doses; maximum dose: 12-15 years: 1000 mg/day, >15 years: 1200 mg/day; some patients have required up to 1.6-2.4 g/day

Trigeminal or glossopharyngeal neuralgia: Initial: 100 mg twice daily with food, gradually increasing in increments of 100 mg twice daily as needed; usual maintenance: 400-800 mg daily in 2 divided doses; maximum dose: 1200 mg/day

Elderly: 100 mg 1-2 times daily, increase in increments of 100 mg/day at weekly intervals until therapeutic level is achieved; usual dose: 400-1000 mg/day

Dosing adjustment in renal impairment: Cl_{cr} <10 mL/minute: Administer 75% of dose

Mechanism of Action In addition to anticonvulsant effects, carbamazepine has anticholinergic, antineuralgic, antidiuretic, muscle relaxant and antiarrhythmic properties; may depress activity in the nucleus ventralis of the thalamus or decrease synaptic transmission or decrease summation of temporal stimulation leading to neural discharge by limiting influx of sodium ions across cell membrane or other unknown mechanisms; stimulates the release of ADH and potentiates its action in promoting reabsorption of water; chemically related to tricyclic antidepressants

Contraindications Hypersensitivity to carbamazepine or any component of the formulation; may have cross-sensitivity with tricyclic antidepressants; marrow depression; MAO inhibitor use; pregnancy (may harm fetus)

Warnings/Precautions MAO inhibitors should be discontinued for a minimum of 14 days before carbamazepine is begun; administer with caution to patients with history of cardiac damage, hepatic or renal disease; potentially fatal blood cell abnormalities have been reported following treatment; patients with a previous history of adverse hematologic reaction to any drug may be at increased risk; early detection of hematologic change is important; advise patients of early signs and symptoms including fever, sore throat, mouth ulcers, infections, easy bruising, petechial or purpuric hemorrhage; carbamazepine is not effective in absence, myoclonic or akinetic seizures; exacerbation of certain seizure types have been seen after initiation of carbamazepine therapy in children with mixed seizure disorders. Elderly may have increased risk of SIADH-like syndrome. Carbamazepine has mild anticholinergic activity; use with caution in patients with increased intraocular pressure (monitor closely), or sensitivity to anticholinergic effects (urinary retention, constipation). Drug should be discontinued if there are any signs of hypersensitivity.

Drug Interactions **Substrate** of CYP2C8/9 (minor), 3A4 (major); **Induces** CYP1A2 (strong), 2B6 (strong), 2C8/9 (strong), 2C19 (strong), 3A4 (strong)

Acetaminophen: Carbamazepine may enhance hepatotoxic potential of acetaminophen; risk is greater in acetaminophen overdose

Antipsychotics: Carbamazepine may enhance the metabolism (decrease the efficacy) of antipsychotics; monitor for altered response; dose adjustment may be needed

Barbiturates: May reduce serum concentrations of carbamazepine; monitor

Benzodiazepines: Serum concentrations and effect of benzodiazepines may be reduced by carbamazepine; monitor for decreased effect

Calcium channel blockers: Diltiazem and verapamil may increase carbamazepine levels, due to enzyme inhibition (see below); other calcium channel blockers (felodipine) may be decreased by carbamazepine due to enzyme induction

Chlorpromazine: **Note:** Carbamazepine suspension is incompatible with chlorpromazine solution. Schedule carbamazepine suspension at least 1-2 hours apart from other liquid medicinals.

Corticosteroids: Metabolism may be increased by carbamazepine

Cyclosporine (and other immunosuppressants): Carbamazepine may enhance the metabolism of immunosuppressants, decreasing its clinical effect; includes both cyclosporine and tacrolimus.

CYP1A2 substrates: Carbamazepine may decrease the levels/effects of CYP1A2 substrates. Example substrates include aminophylline, estrogens, fluvoxamine, mirtazapine, ropinirole, and theophylline.

CYP2B6 substrates: Carbamazepine may decrease the levels/effects of CYP2B6 substrates. Example substrates include bupropion, efavirenz, promethazine, selegiline, and sertraline.

CYP2C8/9 substrates: Carbamazepine may decrease the levels/effects of CYP2C8/9 substrates. Example substrates include amiodarone, fluoxetine, glimepiride, glipizide, losartan, nateglinide, phenytoin, pioglitazone, rosiglitazone, sertraline, sulfonamides, warfarin, and zafirlukast.

CYP2C19 substrates: Carbamazepine may decrease the levels/effects of CYP2C19 substrates. Example substrates include citalopram, diazepam, methsuximide, phenytoin, propranolol, proton pump inhibitors, sertraline, and voriconazole.

CYP3A4 inducers: CYP3A4 inducers may decrease the levels/effects of carbamazepine. Example inducers include aminoglutethimide, nafcillin, nevirapine, phenobarbital, phenytoin, and rifamycins. Carbamazepine may induce its own metabolism.

CYP3A4 inhibitors: May increase the levels/effects of carbamazepine. Example inhibitors include azole antifungals, ciprofloxacin, clarithromycin, diclofenac, doxycycline, erythromycin, imatinib, isoniazid, nefazodone, nicardipine, propofol, protease inhibitors, quinidine, and verapamil.

CYP3A4 substrates: Carbamazepine may decrease the levels/effects of CYP3A4 substrates. Example substrates include benzodiazepines, calcium channel blockers, clarithromycin, cyclosporine, erythromycin, estrogens, mirtazapine, nateglinide, nefazodone, nevirapine, protease inhibitors, tacrolimus, and venlafaxine.

Danazol: May increase serum concentrations of carbamazepine; monitor

Doxycycline: Carbamazepine may enhance the metabolism of doxycycline, decreasing its clinical effect

Ethosuximide: Serum levels may be reduced by carbamazepine

(Continued)

Carbamazepine *(Continued)*

Felbamate: May increase carbamazepine levels and toxicity (increased epoxide metabolite concentrations); carbamazepine may decrease felbamate levels due to enzyme induction
Immunosuppressants: Carbamazepine may enhance the metabolism of immunosuppressants, decreasing its clinical effect; includes both cyclosporine and tacrolimus
Isoniazid: May increase the serum concentrations and toxicity of carbamazepine; in addition, carbamazepine may increase the hepatic toxicity of isoniazid (INH)
Isotretinoin: May decrease the effect of carbamazepine
Lamotrigine: Increases the epoxide metabolite of carbamazepine resulting in toxicity; carbamazepine increases the metabolism of lamotrigine
Lithium: Neurotoxicity may result in patients receiving concurrent carbamazepine
Loxapine: May increase concentrations of epoxide metabolite and toxicity of carbamazepine
Mefloquine: Concomitant use with carbamazepine may reduce seizure control by lowering plasma levels. Monitor.
Methadone: Carbamazepine may enhance the metabolism of methadone resulting in methadone withdrawal
Methylphenidate: concurrent use of carbamazepine may reduce the therapeutic effect of methylphenidate; limited documentation; monitor for decreased effect
Neuromuscular blocking agents, nondepolarizing: Effects may be of shorter duration when administered to patients receiving carbamazepine
Oral contraceptives: Metabolism may be increased by carbamazepine, resulting in a loss of efficacy
Phenytoin: Carbamazepine levels may be decreased by phenytoin; metabolism may be altered by carbamazepine
SSRIs: Metabolism may be increased by carbamazepine (due to enzyme induction)
Theophylline: Serum levels may be reduced by carbamazepine
Thioridazine: **Note:** Carbamazepine suspension is incompatible with thioridazine liquid. Schedule carbamazepine suspension at least 1-2 hours apart from other liquid medicinals.
Thyroid: Serum levels may be reduced by carbamazepine
Tramadol: Tramadol's risk of seizures may be increased with TCAs (carbamazepine may be associated with similar risk due to chemical similarity to TCAs)
Tricyclic antidepressants: May increase serum concentrations of carbamazepine; carbamazepine may decrease concentrations of tricyclics due to enzyme induction
Valproic acid: Serum levels may be reduced by carbamazepine; carbamazepine levels may also be altered by valproic acid
Warfarin: Carbamazepine may inhibit the hypoprothrombinemic effects of oral anticoagulants via increased metabolism; this combination should generally be avoided

Ethanol/Nutrition/Herb Interactions

Ethanol: Avoid ethanol (may increase CNS depression).
Food: Carbamazepine serum levels may be increased if taken with food. Carbamazepine serum concentration may be increased if taken with grapefruit juice; avoid concurrent use.
Herb/Nutraceutical: Avoid evening primrose (seizure threshold decreased). Avoid valerian, St John's wort, kava kava, gotu kola (may increase CNS depression).

Dietary Considerations Drug may cause GI upset, take with large amount of water or food to decrease GI upset. May need to split doses to avoid GI upset.

Pharmacodynamics/Kinetics

Absorption: Slow
Distribution: V_d: Neonates: 1.5 L/kg; Children: 1.9 L/kg; Adults: 0.59-2 L/kg
Protein binding: 75% to 90%; may be decreased in newborns
Metabolism: Hepatic to active epoxide metabolite; induces hepatic enzymes to increase metabolism
Bioavailability: 85%
Half-life elimination: Initial: 18-55 hours; Multiple doses: Children: 8-14 hours; Adults: 12-17 hours
Time to peak, serum: Unpredictable, 4-8 hours
Excretion: Urine (1% to 3% as unchanged drug)

Pregnancy Risk Factor D

Lactation Enters breast milk/compatible

Breast-Feeding Considerations Crosses into breast milk. AAP considers **compatible** with breast-feeding.

Dosage Forms

Capsule, extended release (Carbatrol®): 100 mg, 200 mg, 300 mg
Suspension, oral: 100 mg/5 mL (10 mL, 450 mL)
Tegretol®: 100 mg/5 mL (450 mL) [citrus vanilla flavor]
Tablet (Epitol®, Tegretol®): 200 mg
Tablet, chewable (Tegretol®): 100 mg
Tablet, extended release (Tegretol®-XR): 100 mg, 200 mg, 400 mg

Carbamide *see* Urea *on page 1353*

Carbamide Peroxide (KAR ba mide per OKS ide)

Related Information

Oral Rinse Products *on page 1638*

U.S. Brand Names Bausch & Lomb Earwax Removal [OTC]; Cankaid® [OTC]; Debrox® [OTC]; Dent's Ear Wax [OTC]; E•R•O [OTC]; Gly-Oxide® [OTC]; Murine® Ear [OTC]; Orajel® Perioseptic® Spot Treatment [OTC]

Generic Available Yes

Synonyms Urea Peroxide

Pharmacologic Category Anti-inflammatory, Locally Applied; Otic Agent, Cerumenolytic

Use Relief of minor inflammation of gums, oral mucosal surfaces and lips including canker sores and dental irritation; emulsify and disperse ear wax

Local Anesthetic/Vasoconstrictor Precautions No information available to require special precautions

Effects on Dental Treatment No significant effects or complications reported

Significant Adverse Effects Frequency not defined.

Dermatologic: Rash
Local: Irritation, redness
Miscellaneous: Superinfections

Dosage Children and Adults:

Oral solution (should not be used for >7 days): Oral preparation should not be used in children <2 years of age; apply several drops undiluted on affected area 4 times/day after meals and at bedtime; expectorate after 2-3 minutes **or** place 10 drops onto tongue, mix with saliva, swish for several minutes, expectorate

Otic:

Children <12 years: Tilt head sideways and individualize the dose according to patient size; 3 drops (range: 1-5 drops) twice daily for up to 4 days, tip of applicator should not enter ear canal; keep drops in ear for several minutes by keeping head tilted and placing cotton in ear

Children ≥12 years and Adults: Tilt head sideways and instill 5-10 drops twice daily up to 4 days, tip of applicator should not enter ear canal; keep drops in ear for several minutes by keeping head tilted and placing cotton in ear

Mechanism of Action Carbamide peroxide releases hydrogen peroxide which serves as a source of nascent oxygen upon contact with catalase; deodorant action is probably due to inhibition of odor-causing bacteria; softens impacted cerumen due to its foaming action

Contraindications Hypersensitivity to carbamide peroxide or any component of the formulation; otic preparation should not be used in patients with a perforated tympanic membrane; ear drainage, ear pain or rash in the ear

Warnings/Precautions

Oral: With prolonged use of oral carbamide peroxide, there is a potential for overgrowth of opportunistic organisms; damage to periodontal tissues; delayed wound healing; should not be used for longer than 7 days; not for OTC use in children <2 years of age

Otic: Do not use if ear drainage or discharge, ear pain, irritation, or rash in ear; should not be used for longer than 4 days; not for OTC use in children <12 years of age

Drug Interactions No data reported

Pharmacodynamics/Kinetics Onset of action: ~24 hours

Pregnancy Risk Factor C

Dosage Forms

Solution, oral: 10% (60 mL)
Cankaid®: 10% (22 mL) [in anhydrous glycerol]
Gly-Oxide®: 10% (15 mL, 60 mL) [contains glycerin]
Orajel® Perioseptic® Spot Treatment: 15% (13.3 mL) [contains anhydrous glycerin]

(Continued)

Carbamide Peroxide *(Continued)*

Solution, otic: 6.5% (15 mL)

Debrox®: 6.5% (15 mL, 30 mL) [contains propylene glycol]

Bausch & Lomb Earwax Removal, Dent's Ear Wax, E•R•O, Murine® Ear: 6.5% (15 mL)

Carbamylcholine Chloride *see* Carbachol *on page 255*

Carbastat® [DSC] *see* Carbachol *on page 255*

Carbatrol® *see* Carbamazepine *on page 255*

Carbaxefed DM RF *see* Carbinoxamine, Pseudoephedrine, and Dextromethorphan *on page 263*

Carbaxefed RF *see* Carbinoxamine and Pseudoephedrine *on page 262*

Carbenicillin (kar ben i SIL in)

U.S. Brand Names Geocillin®

Generic Available No

Synonyms Carbenicillin Indanyl Sodium; Carindacillin

Pharmacologic Category Antibiotic, Penicillin

Use Treatment of serious urinary tract infections and prostatitis caused by susceptible gram-negative aerobic bacilli

Local Anesthetic/Vasoconstrictor Precautions No information available to require special precautions

Effects on Dental Treatment Key adverse event(s) related to dental treatment: Unpleasant taste and glossitis. Prolonged use of penicillins may lead to development of oral candidiasis.

Common Adverse Effects

>10%: Gastrointestinal: Diarrhea

1% to 10%: Gastrointestinal: Nausea, bad taste, vomiting, flatulence, glossitis

Mechanism of Action Inhibits bacterial cell wall synthesis by binding to one or more of the penicillin binding proteins (PBPs); which in turn inhibits the final transpeptidation step of peptidoglycan synthesis in bacterial cell walls, thus inhibiting cell wall biosynthesis. Bacteria eventually lyse due to ongoing activity of cell wall autolytic enzymes (autolysins and murein hydrolases) while cell wall assembly is arrested.

Drug Interactions

Increased Effect/Toxicity: Increased bleeding effects if taken with high doses of heparin or oral anticoagulants. Aminoglycosides may be synergistic against selected organisms. Penicillins may increase the exposure to methotrexate during concurrent therapy; monitor. Probenecid and disulfiram may increase levels of penicillins (carbenicillin).

Decreased Effect: Decreased effectiveness with tetracyclines. Although anecdotal reports suggest oral contraceptive efficacy could be reduced by penicillins, this has been refuted by more rigorous scientific and clinical data.

Pharmacodynamics/Kinetics

Absorption: 30% to 40%

Distribution: Crosses placenta; small amounts enter breast milk; distributes into bile; low concentrations attained in CSF

Protein binding: ~50%

Half-life elimination: Children: 0.8-1.8 hours; Adults: 1-1.5 hours, prolonged to 10-20 hours with renal insufficiency

Time to peak, serum: Normal renal function: 0.5-2 hours; concentrations are inadequate for treatment of systemic infections

Excretion: Urine (~80% to 99% as unchanged drug)

Pregnancy Risk Factor B

Carbenicillin Indanyl Sodium *see* Carbenicillin *on page 260*

Carbetapentane and Chlorpheniramine

(kar bay ta PEN tane & klor fen IR a meen)

Related Information

Chlorpheniramine *on page 313*

U.S. Brand Names Tannate 12 S; Tannic-12; Tannic-12 S; Tannihist-12 RF; Tussi-12®; Tussi-12 S™; Tussizone-12 RF™

Generic Available Yes

Synonyms Carbetapentane Tannate and Chlorpheniramine Tannate; Chlorpheniramine and Carbetapentane

Pharmacologic Category Antihistamine/Antitussive

Use Symptomatic relief of cough associated with upper respiratory tract conditions, such as the common cold, bronchitis, bronchial asthma

Local Anesthetic/Vasoconstrictor Precautions No information available to require special precautions

Effects on Dental Treatment Key adverse event(s) related to dental treatment: Dry mucous membranes. Chronic use of antihistamines will inhibit salivary flow, particularly in elderly patients; this may contribute to periodontal disease and oral discomfort.

Common Adverse Effects Frequency not defined.

Central nervous system: Drowsiness, excitation (children), sedation

Gastrointestinal: GI motility decreased, dry mucous membranes

Mechanism of Action Carbetapentane is a nonopiod cough suppressant; chlorpheniramine, is an H_1-receptor antagonist

Drug Interactions

Increased Effect/Toxicity: Sedative effects of CNS depressants may be potentiated; MAO inhibitors may increase and prolong anticholinergic effects; avoid use with and within 14 days of treatment with MAO inhibitors

Pharmacodynamics/Kinetics

Carbetapentane: Data not available

Chlorpheniramine: See individual monograph

Pregnancy Risk Factor C

Carbetapentane, Ephedrine, Phenylephrine, and Chlorpheniramine *see* Chlorpheniramine, Ephedrine, Phenylephrine, and Carbetapentane *on page 316*

Carbetapentane, Phenylephrine, and Pyrilamine

(kay bay ta PEN tane, fen il EF rin, & peer Il a meen)

U.S. Brand Names Tussi-12® D; Tussi-12® DS

Generic Available Yes: Suspension

Synonyms Phenylephrine Tannate, Carbetapentane Tannate, and Pyrilamine Tannate; Pyrilamine, Phenylephrine, and Carbetapentane

Pharmacologic Category Antihistamine; Antihistamine/Decongestant/Antitussive; Antitussive; Decongestant

Use Symptomatic relief of cough associated with respiratory tract conditions such as the common cold, bronchial asthma, acute and chronic bronchitis

Local Anesthetic/Vasoconstrictor Precautions Use with caution since phenylephrine is a sympathomimetic amine which could interact with epinephrine to cause a pressor response

Effects on Dental Treatment Key adverse event(s) related to dental treatment: Tachycardia, palpitations (use vasoconstrictor with caution), and xerostomia (normal salivary flow resumes upon discontinuation).

Mechanism of Action

Carbetapentane is a nonopioid cough suppressant

Phenylephrine hydrochloride is a sympathomimetic agent (primarily alpha), decongestant.

Pyrilamine is an H_1-receptor antagonist.

Pregnancy Risk Factor C

Carbetapentane Tannate and Chlorpheniramine Tannate *see* Carbetapentane and Chlorpheniramine *on page 260*

Carbidopa (kar bi DOE pa)

U.S. Brand Names Lodosyn®

Generic Available No

Pharmacologic Category Anti-Parkinson's Agent, Dopamine Agonist

Use Given with levodopa in the treatment of parkinsonism to enable a lower dosage of levodopa to be used and a more rapid response to be obtained and to decrease side-effects; for details of administration and dosage; has no effect without levodopa

Local Anesthetic/Vasoconstrictor Precautions No information available to require special precautions

Effects on Dental Treatment Key adverse event(s) related to dental treatment: Orthostatic hypotension. Dopaminergic therapy in Parkinson's disease includes the use of carbidopa in combination with levodopa. Carbidopa/levodopa combination is associated with orthostatic hypotension. Patients medicated with this drug combination should be carefully assisted from the chair and observed for signs of orthostatic hypotension.

Common Adverse Effects Adverse reactions are associated with concomitant administration with levodopa

>10%: Central nervous system: Anxiety, confusion, nervousness, mental depression

1% to 10%:

Cardiovascular: Orthostatic hypotension, palpitations, cardiac arrhythmias

Central nervous system: Memory loss, nervousness, insomnia, fatigue, hallucinations, ataxia, dystonic movements

(Continued)

Carbidopa *(Continued)*

Gastrointestinal: Nausea, vomiting, GI bleeding
Ocular: Blurred vision

Mechanism of Action Carbidopa is a peripheral decarboxylase inhibitor with little or no pharmacological activity when given alone in usual doses. It inhibits the peripheral decarboxylation of levodopa to dopamine; and as it does not cross the blood-brain barrier, unlike levodopa, effective brain concentrations of dopamine are produced with lower doses of levodopa. At the same time, reduced peripheral formation of dopamine reduces peripheral side-effects, notably nausea and vomiting, and cardiac arrhythmias, although the dyskinesias and adverse mental effects associated with levodopa therapy tend to develop earlier.

Pharmacodynamics/Kinetics

Absorption: 40% to 70%
Distribution: Does not cross the blood-brain barrier; in rats, reported to cross placenta and be excreted in milk
Protein binding: 36%
Half-life elimination: 1-2 hours
Excretion: Urine (as unchanged drug and metabolites)

Pregnancy Risk Factor C

Carbidopa and Levodopa *see* Levodopa and Carbidopa *on page 811*

Carbidopa, Levodopa, and Entacapone *see* Levodopa, Carbidopa, and Entacapone *on page 812*

Carbihist *see* Carbinoxamine *on page 262*

Carbinoxamine (kar bi NOKS a meen)

U.S. Brand Names Carbihist; Carbinoxamine PD; Carboxine; Histex™ CT; Histex™ I/E; Histex™ PD; Palgic; Pediatex™

Generic Available Yes: Liquid

Synonyms Carbinoxamine Maleate

Pharmacologic Category Antihistamine

Use Seasonal and perennial allergic rhinitis; urticaria

Local Anesthetic/Vasoconstrictor Precautions No information available to require special precautions

Effects on Dental Treatment Key adverse event(s) related to dental treatment: Xerostomia (normal salivary flow resumes upon discontinuation).

Common Adverse Effects Frequency not defined.

Central nervous system: Dizziness, excitability (children), headache, nervousness, sedation
Gastrointestinal: Anorexia, diarrhea, heartburn, nausea, vomiting, xerostomia
Neuromuscular & skeletal: Weakness
Ocular: Diplopia
Renal: Polyuria

Mechanism of Action Carbinoxamine competes with histamine for H_1-receptor sites on effector cells in the gastrointestinal tract, blood vessels, and respiratory tract.

Drug Interactions

Increased Effect/Toxicity: Increased sedation/CNS depression with barbiturates, other CNS depressants and tricyclic antidepressants; anticholinergic effects may be increased by MAO inhibitors

Pharmacodynamics/Kinetics Half-life elimination: 10-20 hours

Pregnancy Risk Factor C

Carbinoxamine and Pseudoephedrine

(kar bi NOKS a meen & soo doe e FED rin)

Related Information

Pseudoephedrine *on page 1147*

U.S. Brand Names Andehist NR Drops; Carbaxefed RF; Carboxine-PSE; Hydro-Tussin™-CBX; Palgic®-D; Palgic®-DS; Pediatex™-D; Rondec® Drops; Rondec® Tablets; Rondec-TR®; Sildec

Generic Available Yes

Synonyms Pseudoephedrine and Carbinoxamine

Pharmacologic Category Adrenergic Agonist Agent; Antihistamine, H_1 Blocker; Decongestant

Use Seasonal and perennial allergic rhinitis; vasomotor rhinitis

Local Anesthetic/Vasoconstrictor Precautions Use with caution since pseudoephedrine is a sympathomimetic amine which could interact with epinephrine to cause a pressor response

Effects on Dental Treatment Key adverse event(s) related to dental treatment: Pseudoephedrine: Xerostomia (normal salivary flow resumes upon discontinuation).

Common Adverse Effects Frequency not defined.

Cardiovascular: Arrhythmias, cardiovascular collapse, hypertension, pallor, tachycardia

Central nervous system: Anxiety, convulsions, CNS stimulation, dizziness, excitability (children; rare), fear, hallucinations, headache, insomnia, nervousness, restlessness, sedation

Gastrointestinal: Anorexia, diarrhea, dyspepsia, nausea, vomiting, xerostomia

Neuromuscular skeletal: Tremors, weakness

Ocular: Diplopia

Renal: Dysuria, polyuria, urinary retention (with BPH)

Respiratory: Respiratory difficulty

Mechanism of Action Carbinoxamine competes with histamine for H_1-receptor sites on effector cells in the gastrointestinal tract, blood vessels, and respiratory tract; pseudoephedrine, a sympathomimetic amine and isomer of ephedrine, acts as a decongestant in respiratory tract mucous membranes with less vasoconstrictor action than ephedrine in normotensive individuals

Drug Interactions

Increased Effect/Toxicity: Increased sedation/CNS depression with barbiturates and other CNS depressants; anticholinergic effects may be increased by MAO inhibitors, tricyclic antidepressants

Decreased Effect: May decrease effects of antihypertensive agents.

Pregnancy Risk Factor C

Carbinoxamine, Dextromethorphan, and Pseudoephedrine *see* Carbinoxamine, Pseudoephedrine, and Dextromethorphan *on page 263*

Carbinoxamine Maleate *see* Carbinoxamine *on page 262*

Carbinoxamine PD *see* Carbinoxamine *on page 262*

Carbinoxamine, Pseudoephedrine, and Dextromethorphan

(kar bi NOKS a meen, soo doe e FED rin, & deks troe meth OR fan)

Related Information

Dextromethorphan *on page 421*

Pseudoephedrine *on page 1147*

U.S. Brand Names Andehist DM NR Drops; Carbaxefed DM RF; Decahist-DM; Pediatex™-DM; Rondec®-DM Drops; Sildec-DM; Tussafed®

Generic Available Yes

Synonyms Carbinoxamine, Dextromethorphan, and Pseudoephedrine; Dextromethorphan, Carbinoxamine, and Pseudoephedrine; Dextromethorphan, Pseudoephedrine, and Carbinoxamine; Pseudoephedrine, Carbinoxamine, and Dextromethorphan; Pseudoephedrine, Dextromethorphan, and Carbinoxamine

Pharmacologic Category Antihistamine/Decongestant/Antitussive

Use Relief of coughs and upper respiratory symptoms, including nasal congestion, associated with allergy or the common cold

Local Anesthetic/Vasoconstrictor Precautions Use with caution since pseudoephedrine is a sympathomimetic amine which could interact with epinephrine to cause a pressor response

Effects on Dental Treatment Key adverse event(s) related to dental treatment: Pseudoephedrine: Xerostomia (normal salivary flow resumes upon discontinuation).

Common Adverse Effects Frequency not defined.

Cardiovascular: Arrhythmias, cardiovascular collapse, hypertension, pallor, tachycardia

Central nervous system: Anxiety, convulsions, CNS stimulation, dizziness, drowsiness, excitability (children; rare), fear, hallucinations, headache, insomnia, nervousness, restlessness, sedation

Gastrointestinal: Anorexia, diarrhea, dyspepsia, GI upset, nausea, vomiting, xerostomia

Neuromuscular skeletal: Tremors, weakness

Ocular: Diplopia

Renal: Dysuria, polyuria, urinary retention (with BPH)

Respiratory: Respiratory difficulty

Mechanism of Action Carbinoxamine competes with histamine for H_1-receptor sites on effector cells in the gastrointestinal tract, blood vessels, and respiratory tract; pseudoephedrine, a sympathomimetic amine and isomer of ephedrine, acts as a decongestant in respiratory tract mucous membranes with less vasoconstrictor action than ephedrine in normotensive individuals;

(Continued)

Carbinoxamine, Pseudoephedrine, and Dextromethorphan *(Continued)*

dextromethorphan, a non-narcotic antitussive, increases cough threshold by its activity on the medulla oblongata.

Drug Interactions

Cytochrome P450 Effect: Dextromethorphan: **Substrate** of CYP2B6 (minor), 2C8/9 (minor), 2C19 (minor), 2D6 (major), 2E1 (minor), 3A4 (minor); **Inhibits** CYP2D6 (weak)

Pregnancy Risk Factor C

Carbinoxamine, Pseudoephedrine, and Hydrocodone *see* Hydrocodone, Carbinoxamine, and Pseudoephedrine *on page 712*

Carbocaine® [DSC] *see* Mepivacaine *on page 873*

Carbocaine® 2% with Neo-Cobefrin® [DSC] *see* Mepivacaine and Levonordefrin *(WITHDRAWN FROM MARKET) on page 875*

Carbocaine® 3% *see* Mepivacaine (Dental Anesthetic) *on page 877*

Carbol-Fuchsin Solution (kar bol-FOOK sin soe LOO shun)

U.S. Brand Names Castellani Paint Modified

Generic Available No

Pharmacologic Category Antifungal Agent, Topical

Use Treatment of superficial mycotic infections

Local Anesthetic/Vasoconstrictor Precautions No information available to require special precautions

Effects on Dental Treatment No significant effects or complications reported

Carbolic Acid *see* Phenol *on page 1075*

Carboplatin (KAR boe pla tin)

U.S. Brand Names Paraplatin®

Canadian Brand Names Paraplatin-AQ

Mexican Brand Names Blastocarb®; Carbotec®; Paraplatin®

Generic Available No

Synonyms CBDCA

Pharmacologic Category Antineoplastic Agent, Alkylating Agent

Use Treatment of ovarian cancer

Unlabeled/Investigational Use Lung cancer, head and neck cancer, endometrial cancer, esophageal cancer, bladder cancer, breast cancer, cervical cancer, CNS tumors, germ cell tumors, osteogenic sarcoma, and high-dose therapy with stem cell/bone marrow support

Local Anesthetic/Vasoconstrictor Precautions No information available to require special precautions

Effects on Dental Treatment Key adverse event(s) related to dental treatment: Stomatitis.

Common Adverse Effects

>10%:

- Dermatologic: Alopecia (includes other agents in combination with carboplatin)
- Endocrine & metabolic: Hypomagnesemia, hypokalemia, hyponatremia, hypocalcemia; less severe than those seen after cisplatin (usually asymptomatic)
- Gastrointestinal: Nausea, vomiting, stomatitis
- Hematologic: Myelosuppression is dose-related and is the dose-limiting toxicity; thrombocytopenia is the predominant manifestation, with a reported incidence of 37% in patients receiving 400 mg/m^2 as a single agent and 80% in patients receiving 520 mg/m^2; leukopenia has been reported in 27% to 38% of patients receiving carboplatin as a single agent
  Nadir: ~21 days following a single dose
- Hepatic: Alkaline phosphatase increased, AST increased (usually mild and reversible)
- Otic: Hearing loss at high tones (above speech ranges, up to 19%); clinically-important ototoxicity is not usually seen
- Renal: Increases in creatinine and BUN have been reported; most of them are mild and they are commonly reversible; considerably less nephrotoxic than cisplatin

1% to 10%:

- Gastrointestinal: Diarrhea, anorexia
- Hematologic: Hemorrhagic complications
- Local: Pain at injection site
- Neuromuscular & skeletal: Peripheral neuropathy (4% to 6%; up to 10% in older and/or previously-treated patients)
- Otic: Ototoxicity

Mechanism of Action Carboplatin is an alkylating agent which covalently binds to DNA; possible cross-linking and interference with the function of DNA

Drug Interactions

Increased Effect/Toxicity: Nephrotoxic drugs; aminoglycosides increase risk of ototoxicity. When administered as sequential infusions, observational studies indicate a potential for increased toxicity when platinum derivatives (carboplatin, cisplatin) are administered before taxane derivatives (docetaxel, paclitaxel).

Pharmacodynamics/Kinetics

Distribution: V_d: 16 L/kg; Into liver, kidney, skin, and tumor tissue

Protein binding: 0%; platinum is 30% irreversibly bound

Metabolism: Minimally hepatic to aquated and hydroxylated compounds

Half-life elimination: Terminal: 22-40 hours; Cl_{cr} >60 mL/minute: 2.5-5.9 hours

Excretion: Urine (~60% to 90%) within 24 hours

Pregnancy Risk Factor D

Carboprost *see* Carboprost Tromethamine *on page 265*

Carboprost Tromethamine (KAR boe prost tro METH a meen)

U.S. Brand Names Hemabate®

Canadian Brand Names Hemabate®

Generic Available No

Synonyms Carboprost

Pharmacologic Category Abortifacient; Prostaglandin

Use Termination of pregnancy and refractory postpartum uterine bleeding

Unlabeled/Investigational Use Investigational: Hemorrhagic cystitis

Local Anesthetic/Vasoconstrictor Precautions No information available to require special precautions

Effects on Dental Treatment No significant effects or complications reported

Common Adverse Effects

>10%: Gastrointestinal: Nausea (33%)

1% to 10%: Cardiovascular: Flushing (7%)

Mechanism of Action Carboprost tromethamine is a prostaglandin similar to prostaglandin F_2 alpha (dinoprost) except for the addition of a methyl group at the C-15 position. This substitution produces longer duration of activity than dinoprost; carboprost stimulates uterine contractility which usually results in expulsion of the products of conception and is used to induce abortion between 13-20 weeks of pregnancy. Hemostasis at the placentation site is achieved through the myometrial contractions produced by carboprost.

Drug Interactions

Increased Effect/Toxicity: Toxicity may be increased by oxytocic agents.

Pregnancy Risk Factor X

Carbose D *see* Carboxymethylcellulose *on page 265*

Carboxine *see* Carbinoxamine *on page 262*

Carboxine-PSE *see* Carbinoxamine and Pseudoephedrine *on page 262*

Carboxymethylcellulose (kar boks ee meth il SEL yoo lose)

U.S. Brand Names Refresh Liquigel™ [OTC]; Refresh Plus® [OTC]; Refresh Tears® [OTC]; Tears Again® Gel Drops™ [OTC]; Tears Again® Night and Day™ [OTC]; Theratears®

Canadian Brand Names Celluvisc™; Refresh Plus™; Refresh Tears™

Generic Available Yes

Synonyms Carbose D; Carboxymethylcellulose Sodium

Pharmacologic Category Ophthalmic Agent, Miscellaneous

Use Artificial tear substitute

Local Anesthetic/Vasoconstrictor Precautions No information available to require special precautions

Effects on Dental Treatment No significant effects or complications reported

Carboxymethylcellulose Sodium *see* Carboxymethylcellulose *on page 265*

Cardene® *see* NiCARdipine *on page 980*

Cardene® I.V. *see* NiCARdipine *on page 980*

Cardene® SR *see* NiCARdipine *on page 980*

Cardiovascular Diseases *see page 1458*

Cardizem® *see* Diltiazem *on page 444*

Cardizem® CD *see* Diltiazem *on page 444*

Cardizem® LA *see* Diltiazem *on page 444*

Cardizem® SR *see* Diltiazem *on page 444*

Cardura® *see* Doxazosin *on page 465*

Carimune™ *see* Immune Globulin (Intravenous) *on page 740*
Carindacillin *see* Carbenicillin *on page 260*
Carisoprodate *see* Carisoprodol *on page 266*

Carisoprodol (kar eye soe PROE dole)

Related Information

Carisoprodol and Aspirin *on page 266*
Carisoprodol, Aspirin, and Codeine *on page 267*

U.S. Brand Names Soma®

Canadian Brand Names Soma®

Generic Available Yes

Synonyms Carisoprodate; Isobamate

Pharmacologic Category Skeletal Muscle Relaxant

Dental Use Treatment of muscle spasms and pain assosicated with acute temporomandibular joint pain

Use Skeletal muscle relaxant

Local Anesthetic/Vasoconstrictor Precautions No information available to require special precautions

Effects on Dental Treatment No significant effects or complications reported

Significant Adverse Effects

>10%: Central nervous system: Drowsiness

1% to 10%:
- Cardiovascular: Tachycardia, tightness in chest, flushing of face, syncope
- Central nervous system: Mental depression, allergic fever, dizziness, lightheadedness, headache, paradoxical CNS stimulation
- Dermatologic: Angioedema, dermatitis (allergic)
- Gastrointestinal: Nausea, vomiting, stomach cramps
- Neuromuscular & skeletal: Trembling
- Ocular: Burning eyes
- Respiratory: Dyspnea
- Miscellaneous: Hiccups

<1% (Limited to important or life-threatening): Aplastic anemia, clumsiness, eosinophilia, erythema multiforme, leukopenia, rash, urticaria

Dosage Oral: Adults: 350 mg 3-4 times/day; take last dose at bedtime; compound: 1-2 tablets 4 times/day

Mechanism of Action Precise mechanism is not yet clear, but many effects have been ascribed to its central depressant actions

Contraindications Hypersensitivity to carisoprodol, meprobamate or any component of the formulation; acute intermittent porphyria

Warnings/Precautions May cause CNS depression, which may impair physical or mental abilities. Effects with other sedative drugs or ethanol may be potentiated. Use with caution in patients with hepatic/renal dysfunction. Tolerance or drug dependence may result from extended use.

Drug Interactions Substrate of CYP2C19 (major)

Increased toxicity: Ethanol, CNS depressants, phenothiazines

CYP2C19 inhibitors: May increase the levels/effects of carisoprodol. Example inhibitors include delavirdine, fluconazole, fluvoxamine, gemfibrozil, isoniazid, omeprazole, and ticlopidine.

Ethanol/Nutrition/Herb Interactions Ethanol: Avoid ethanol (may increase CNS depression).

Pharmacodynamics/Kinetics

Onset of action: ~30 minutes
Duration: 4-6 hours
Distribution: Crosses placenta; high concentrations enter breast milk
Metabolism: Hepatic
Half-life elimination: 8 hours
Excretion: Urine

Pregnancy Risk Factor C

Lactation Enters breast milk (high concentrations)/not recommended

Dosage Forms Tablet: 350 mg

Carisoprodol and Aspirin (kar eye soe PROE dole & AS pir in)

Related Information

Aspirin *on page 151*
Carisoprodol *on page 266*

U.S. Brand Names Soma® Compound

Generic Available Yes

Synonyms Aspirin and Carisoprodol

Pharmacologic Category Skeletal Muscle Relaxant

Dental Use Treatment of muscle spasms and pain associated with acute temporomandibular joint pain

Use Skeletal muscle relaxant

Local Anesthetic/Vasoconstrictor Precautions No information available to require special precautions

Effects on Dental Treatment Key adverse event(s) related to dental treatment: Elderly are a high-risk population for adverse effects from nonsteroidal anti-inflammatory agents. As many as 60% of elderly patients with GI complications from NSAIDs can develop peptic ulceration and/or hemorrhage asymptomatically. Concomitant disease and drug use contribute to the risk of GI adverse effects. Use lowest effective dose for shortest period possible. Consider renal function decline with age.

Dosage Oral: Adults: 1-2 tablets 4 times/day

Drug Interactions

Carisoprodol: **Substrate** of CYP2C19 (major)

Aspirin: **Substrate** of CYP2C8/9 (minor)

Also see individual agents.

Ethanol/Nutrition/Herb Interactions Ethanol: Avoid ethanol (may increase CNS depression).

Pharmacodynamics/Kinetics See individual agents.

Pregnancy Risk Factor C/D (full-dose aspirin in 3rd trimester)

Lactation Enters breast milk/contraindicated

Dosage Forms Tablet: Carisoprodol 200 mg and aspirin 325 mg

Carisoprodol, Aspirin, and Codeine

(kar eye soe PROE dole, AS pir in, and KOE deen)

Related Information

Aspirin *on page 151*

Carisoprodol *on page 266*

Codeine *on page 369*

U.S. Brand Names Soma® Compound w/Codeine

Generic Available Yes

Synonyms Aspirin, Carisoprodol, and Codeine; Codeine, Aspirin, and Carisoprodol

Pharmacologic Category Skeletal Muscle Relaxant

Dental Use Treatment of muscle spasms and pain associated with acute temporomandibular joint pain

Use Skeletal muscle relaxant

Local Anesthetic/Vasoconstrictor Precautions No information available to require special precautions

Effects on Dental Treatment Key adverse event(s) related to dental treatment: Elderly are a high-risk population for adverse effects from nonsteroidal anti-inflammatory agents. As many as 60% of elderly patients with GI complications from NSAIDs can develop peptic ulceration and/or hemorrhage asymptomatically. Concomitant disease and drug use contribute to the risk of GI adverse effects. Use lowest effective dose for shortest period possible. Consider renal function decline with age.

Restrictions C-III

Dosage Oral: Adults: 1 or 2 tablets 4 times/day

Drug Interactions

Carisoprodol: **Substrate** of CYP2C19 (major)

Aspirin: **Substrate** of CYP2C8/9 (minor)

Also see individual agents.

Ethanol/Nutrition/Herb Interactions Ethanol: Avoid ethanol (may increase CNS depression).

Pharmacodynamics/Kinetics See individual agents.

Pregnancy Risk Factor C/D (full-dose aspirin in 3rd trimester)

Lactation Enters breast milk/contraindicated

Dosage Forms Tablet: Carisoprodol 200 mg, aspirin 325 mg, and codeine phosphate 16 mg

Carmol® 10 [OTC] *see* Urea *on page 1353*

Carmol® 20 [OTC] *see* Urea *on page 1353*

Carmol® 40 *see* Urea *on page 1353*

Carmol® Deep Cleaning *see* Urea *on page 1353*

Carmol-HC® *see* Urea and Hydrocortisone *on page 1353*

Carmol® Scalp *see* Sulfacetamide *on page 1244*

Carmustine (kar MUS teen)

U.S. Brand Names BiCNu®; Gliadel®

Canadian Brand Names BiCNu®

Mexican Brand Names Bicnu®

Generic Available No

Synonyms BCNU; bis-chloronitrosourea; Carmustinum; NSC-409962; WR-139021

Pharmacologic Category Antineoplastic Agent; Antineoplastic Agent, Alkylating Agent (Nitrosourea); Antineoplastic Agent, DNA Adduct-Forming Agent; Antineoplastic Agent, DNA Binding Agent

Use

Injection: Treatment of brain tumors (glioblastoma, brainstem glioma, medulloblastoma, astrocytoma, ependymoma, and metastatic brain tumors), multiple myeloma, Hodgkin's disease, non-Hodgkin's lymphomas, melanoma, lung cancer, colon cancer

Wafer (implant): Adjunct to surgery in patients with recurrent glioblastoma multiforme; adjunct to surgery and radiation in patients with high-grade malignant glioma

Local Anesthetic/Vasoconstrictor Precautions No information available to require special precautions

Effects on Dental Treatment Key adverse event(s) related to dental treatment: Stomatitis.

Common Adverse Effects

>10%:

Cardiovascular: Hypotension with high dose therapy, due to the alcohol content of the diluent

Central nervous system: Dizziness, ataxia; Wafers: Seizures (54%) postoperatively

Dermatologic: Pain and burning at the injection site (may be relieved by diluting the drug and infusing it through a fast-running dextrose or saline infusion); phlebitis

Gastrointestinal: Severe nausea and vomiting, usually begins within 2-4 hours of drug administration and lasts for 4-6 hours. Patients should receive a prophylactic antiemetic regimen including a serotonin (5-HT_3) antagonist and dexamethasone

Hematologic: Myelosuppression - cumulative, dose-related, delayed, thrombocytopenia is usually more common and more severe than leukopenia

Onset: 7-14 days

Nadir: 21-35 days

Recovery: 42-56 days

Hepatic: Reversible increases in bilirubin, alkaline phosphatase, and SGOT occur in 20% to 25% of patients

Ocular: Ocular toxicities (transient conjunctival flushing and blurred vision), retinal hemorrhages

Respiratory: Interstitial fibrosis occurs in up to 50% of patients receiving a cumulative dose >1400 mg/m^2, or bone marrow transplantation doses; may be delayed up to 3 years; rare in patients receiving lower doses. A history of lung disease or concomitant bleomycin therapy may increase the risk of this reaction. Patients should have baseline and periodic pulmonary function tests, patients with forced vital capacity (FVC) or carbon monoxide diffusing capacity of the lungs (DLCO) <70% of predicted are at higher risk.

1% to 10%:

Central nervous system: Wafers: Amnesia, aphasia, ataxia, cerebral edema, confusion, convulsion, depression, diplopia, dizziness, headache, hemiplegia, hydrocephalus, insomnia, meningitis, somnolence, stupor

Dermatologic: Facial flushing, probably due to the alcohol diluent; alopecia

Gastrointestinal: Anorexia, constipation, diarrhea, stomatitis

Hematologic: Anemia

Mechanism of Action Interferes with the normal function of DNA by alkylation and cross-linking the strands of DNA, and by possible protein modification

Drug Interactions

Increased Effect/Toxicity: Carmustine given in combination with cimetidine is reported to cause bone marrow depression. Carmustine given in combination with etoposide is reported to cause severe hepatic dysfunction with hyperbilirubinemia, ascites, and thrombocytopenia. Diluent for infusion contains alcohol; avoid concurrent use of medications that inhibit aldehyde dehydrogenase-2 or cause disulfiram-like reactions.

Pharmacodynamics/Kinetics

Distribution: Readily crosses blood-brain barrier producing CSF levels equal to 15% to 70% of blood plasma levels; enters breast milk; highly lipid soluble

Metabolism: Rapidly hepatic
Half-life elimination: Biphasic: Initial: 1.4 minutes; Secondary: 20 minutes (active metabolites: plasma half-life of 67 hours)
Excretion: Urine (~60% to 70%) within 96 hours; lungs (6% to 10% as CO_2)

Pregnancy Risk Factor D

Carmustinum *see* Carmustine *on page 268*
Carnitor® *see* Levocarnitine *on page 810*
Carrington Antifungal [OTC] *see* Miconazole *on page 922*

Carteolol (KAR tee oh lole)

Related Information
Cardiovascular Diseases *on page 1458*

U.S. Brand Names Cartrol®; Ocupress® [DSC]

Canadian Brand Names Cartrol® Oral; Ocupress® Ophthalmic

Generic Available Yes: Ophthalmic solution

Synonyms Carteolol Hydrochloride

Pharmacologic Category Beta Blocker With Intrinsic Sympathomimetic Activity; Ophthalmic Agent, Antiglaucoma

Use Management of hypertension; treatment of chronic open-angle glaucoma and intraocular hypertension

Local Anesthetic/Vasoconstrictor Precautions No information available to require special precautions

Effects on Dental Treatment Carteolol is a nonselective beta-blocker and may enhance the pressor response to epinephrine, resulting in hypertension and bradycardia. Many nonsteroidal anti-inflammatory drugs, such as ibuprofen and indomethacin, can reduce the hypotensive effect of beta-blockers after 3 or more weeks of therapy with the NSAID. Short-term NSAID use (ie, 3 days) requires no special precautions in patients taking beta-blockers.

Common Adverse Effects

Ophthalmic:
>10%: Ocular: Conjunctival hyperemia
1% to 10%: Ocular: Anisocoria, corneal punctate keratitis, corneal staining, decreased corneal sensitivity, eye pain, vision disturbances

Systemic:
>10%:
Central nervous system: Drowsiness, insomnia
Endocrine & metabolic: Decreased sexual ability
1% to 10%:
Cardiovascular: Bradycardia, palpitations, edema, CHF, reduced peripheral circulation
Central nervous system: Mental depression
Gastrointestinal: Diarrhea or constipation, nausea, vomiting, stomach discomfort
Respiratory: Bronchospasm
Miscellaneous: Cold extremities

Mechanism of Action Blocks both $beta_1$- and $beta_2$-receptors and has mild intrinsic sympathomimetic activity; has negative inotropic and chronotropic effects and can significantly slow AV nodal conduction

Drug Interactions

Cytochrome P450 Effect: Substrate of CYP2D6 (minor)

Increased Effect/Toxicity: Carteolol may increase the effects of other drugs which slow AV conduction (digoxin, verapamil, diltiazem), alpha-blockers (prazosin, terazosin), and alpha-adrenergic stimulants (epinephrine, phenylephrine). Carteolol may mask the tachycardia from hypoglycemia caused by insulin and oral hypoglycemics. In patients receiving concurrent therapy, the risk of hypertensive crisis is increased when either clonidine or the beta-blocker is withdrawn. Reserpine has been shown to enhance the effect of beta-blockers. Beta-blockers may increase the action or levels of ethanol, disopyramide, nondepolarizing muscle relaxants, and theophylline although the effects are difficult to predict.

Decreased Effect: Decreased effect of beta-blockers with aluminum salts, barbiturates, calcium salts, cholestyramine, colestipol, NSAIDs, penicillins (ampicillin), rifampin, salicylates, and sulfinpyrazone due to decreased bioavailability and plasma levels. Beta-blockers may decrease the effect of sulfonylureas (possibly hyperglycemia). Nonselective beta-blockers blunt the effect of beta-2 adrenergic agonists (albuterol).

Pharmacodynamics/Kinetics
Onset of action: Oral: 1-1.5 hours
Peak effect: 2 hours

(Continued)

Carteolol *(Continued)*

Duration: 12 hours
Absorption: Oral: 80%
Protein binding: 23% to 30%
Metabolism: 30% to 50%
Half-life elimination: 6 hours
Excretion: Urine (as metabolites)

Pregnancy Risk Factor C (manufacturer); D (2nd and 3rd trimesters - expert analysis)

Carteolol Hydrochloride *see* Carteolol *on page 269*
Cartia XT™ *see* Diltiazem *on page 444*
Cartrol® *see* Carteolol *on page 269*

Carvedilol (KAR ve dil ole)

Related Information
Cardiovascular Diseases *on page 1458*

U.S. Brand Names Coreg®
Canadian Brand Names Coreg®
Mexican Brand Names Dilatrend®
Generic Available No
Pharmacologic Category Beta Blocker With Alpha-Blocking Activity

Use Mild to severe heart failure of ischemic or cardiomyopathic origin (usually in addition to standardized therapy); left ventricular dysfunction following myocardial infarction (MI); management of hypertension

Unlabeled/Investigational Use Angina pectoris

Local Anesthetic/Vasoconstrictor Precautions Use with caution, epinephrine has interacted with noncardioselective beta-blockers to result in initial hypertensive episode followed by bradycardia

Effects on Dental Treatment Key adverse event(s) related to dental treatment: Postural hypotension and periodontitis. Noncardioselective beta-blockers enhance the pressor response to epinephrine, resulting in hypertension and bradycardia. Many nonsteroidal anti-inflammatory drugs, such as ibuprofen and indomethacin, can reduce the hypotensive effect of beta-blockers after 3 or more weeks of therapy with the NSAID. Short-term NSAID use (ie, 3 days) requires no special precautions in patients taking beta-blockers.

Common Adverse Effects Note: Frequency ranges include data from hypertension and heart failure trials. Higher rates of adverse reactions have generally been noted in patients with CHF. However, the frequency of adverse effects associated with placebo is also increased in this population. Events occurring at a frequency > placebo in clinical trials.

>10%:
- Cardiovascular: Hypotension (9% to 14%)
- Central nervous system: Dizziness (6% to 32%), fatigue (4% to 24%)
- Endocrine & metabolic: Hyperglycemia (5% to 12%), weight gain (10% to 12%)
- Gastrointestinal: Diarrhea (2% to 12%)
- Neuromuscular & skeletal: Weakness (11%)

1% to 10%:
- Cardiovascular: Bradycardia (2% to 10%), hypertension (3%), AV block (3%), angina (2% to 6%), postural hypotension (2%), syncope (3% to 8%), dependent edema (4%), palpitations, peripheral edema (1% to 7%), generalized edema (5% to 6%)
- Central nervous system: Headache (5% to 8%), fever (3%), paresthesia (2%), somnolence (2%), insomnia (2%), malaise, hypesthesia, vertigo
- Endocrine & metabolic: Gout (6%), hypercholesterolemia (4%), dehydration (2%), hyperkalemia (3%), hypervolemia (2%), hypertriglyceridemia (1%), hyperuricemia, hypoglycemia, hyponatremia
- Gastrointestinal: Nausea (4% to 9%), vomiting (6%), melena, periodontitis
- Genitourinary: Hematuria (3%), impotence
- Hematologic: Thrombocytopenia (1% to 2%), decreased prothrombin, purpura
- Hepatic: Increased transaminases, increased alkaline phosphatase
- Neuromuscular & skeletal: Back pain (2% to 7%), arthralgia (6%), myalgia (3%), muscle cramps
- Ocular: Blurred vision (3% to 5%)
- Renal: Increased BUN (6%), abnormal renal function, albuminuria, glycosuria, increased creatinine (3%), kidney failure
- Respiratory: Rhinitis (2%), increased cough (5%)

Miscellaneous: Injury (3% to 6%), allergy, sudden death

Dosage Oral: Adults: Reduce dosage if heart rate drops to <55 beats/minute.

Hypertension: 6.25 mg twice daily; if tolerated, dose should be maintained for 1-2 weeks, then increased to 12.5 mg twice daily. Dosage may be increased to a maximum of 25 mg twice daily after 1-2 weeks. Maximum dose: 50 mg/day

Congestive heart failure: 3.125 mg twice daily for 2 weeks; if this dose is tolerated, may increase to 6.25 mg twice daily. Double the dose every 2 weeks to the highest dose tolerated by patient. (Prior to initiating therapy, other heart failure medications should be stabilized and fluid retention minimized.)

Maximum recommended dose:

Mild to moderate heart failure:

<85 kg: 25 mg twice daily

>85 kg: 50 mg twice daily

Severe heart failure: 25 mg twice daily

Left ventricular dysfunction following MI: Initial 3.125-6.25 mg twice daily; increase dosage incrementally (ie, from 6.25 to 12.5 mg twice daily) at intervals of 3-10 days, based on tolerance, to a target dose of 25 mg twice daily. **Note**: Should be initiated only after patient is hemodynamically stable and fluid retention has been minimized.

Angina pectoris (unlabeled use): 25-50 mg twice daily

Dosing adjustment in renal impairment: None necessary

Dosing adjustment in hepatic impairment: Use is contraindicated in severe liver dysfunction.

Mechanism of Action As a racemic mixture, carvedilol has nonselective beta-adrenoreceptor and alpha-adrenergic blocking activity. No intrinsic sympathomimetic activity has been documented. Associated effects in hypertensive patients include reduction of cardiac output, exercise- or beta agonist-induced tachycardia, reduction of reflex orthostatic tachycardia, vasodilation, decreased peripheral vascular resistance (especially in standing position), decreased renal vascular resistance, reduced plasma renin activity, and increased levels of atrial natriuretic peptide. In CHF, associated effects include decreased pulmonary capillary wedge pressure, decreased pulmonary artery pressure, decreased heart rate, decreased systemic vascular resistance, increased stroke volume index, and decreased right arterial pressure (RAP).

Contraindications Hypersensitivity to carvedilol or any component of the formulation; patients with decompensated cardiac failure requiring intravenous inotropic therapy; bronchial asthma or related bronchospastic conditions; second- or third-degree AV block, sick sinus syndrome, and severe bradycardia (except in patients with a functioning artificial pacemaker); cardiogenic shock; severe hepatic impairment; pregnancy (2nd and 3rd trimesters)

Warnings/Precautions Initiate cautiously and monitor for possible deterioration in patient status (including symptoms of CHF). Adjustment of other medications (ACE inhibitors and/or diuretics) may be required. In severe chronic heart failure, trial patients were excluded if they had cardiac-related rales, ascites, or a serum creatinine >2.8 mg/dL. Patients should be advised to avoid driving or other hazardous tasks during initiation of therapy due to the risk of syncope. Avoid abrupt discontinuation (may be associated with angina, arrhythmia, or myocardial infarction), particularly in patients with coronary artery disease; dose should be tapered over 1-2 weeks with close monitoring. Manufacturer recommends discontinuation of therapy if liver injury occurs (confirmed by laboratory testing). Use caution in patients with PVD (can aggravate arterial insufficiency). Use caution with concurrent use of verapamil or diltiazem; bradycardia or heart block can occur. Patients with bronchospastic disease should not receive beta-blockers. Use cautiously in diabetics because it can mask prominent hypoglycemic symptoms. May mask signs of thyrotoxicosis. Use care with anesthetic agents that decrease myocardial function. Safety and efficacy in children <18 years of age have not been established.

Drug Interactions

Cytochrome P450 Effect: Substrate of CYP1A2 (minor), 2C8/9 (major), 2D6 (major), 2E1 (minor), 3A4 (minor)

Increased Effect/Toxicity: CYP2C8/9 inhibitors may increase the levels/effects of carvedilol; example inhibitors include delavirdine, fluconazole, gemfibrozil, ketoconazole, nicardipine, NSAIDs, pioglitazone, and sulfonamides. CYP2D6 inhibitors may increase the levels/effects of carvedilol; example inhibitors include chlorpromazine, delavirdine, fluoxetine, miconazole, paroxetine, pergolide, quinidine, quinine, ritonavir, and ropinirole. Clonidine and cimetidine increase the serum levels and effects of carvedilol. Carvedilol may increase the levels of cyclosporine. Carvedilol may increase the effects of other drugs which slow AV conduction (digoxin, verapamil,

(Continued)

Carvedilol *(Continued)*

diltiazem), alpha-blockers (prazosin, terazosin), and alpha-adrenergic stimulants (epinephrine, phenylephrine). Carvedilol may mask the tachycardia from hypoglycemia caused by insulin and oral hypoglycemics. In patients receiving concurrent therapy, the risk of hypertensive crisis is increased when either clonidine or the beta-blocker is withdrawn. Reserpine has been shown to enhance the effect of beta-blockers. Beta-blockers may increase the action or levels of disopyramide, and theophylline although the effects are difficult to predict.

Decreased Effect: CYP2C8/9 inducers may decrease the levels/effects of carvedilol; example inducers include carbamazepine, phenobarbital, phenytoin, rifampin, rifapentine, and secobarbital. Decreased effect of beta-blockers has also occurred with antacids, barbiturates, calcium channel blockers, cholestyramine, colestipol, NSAIDs, penicillins (ampicillin), and salicylates due to decreased bioavailability and plasma levels. Beta-blockers may decrease the effect of sulfonylureas. Nonselective beta-blockers blunt the effect of beta-2 adrenergic agonists (albuterol).

Ethanol/Nutrition/Herb Interactions Herb/Nutraceutical: Avoid dong quai if using for hypertension (has estrogenic activity). Avoid ephedra, yohimbe, ginseng (may worsen hypertension). Avoid garlic (may have increased antihypertensive effect).

Dietary Considerations Should be taken with food to minimize the risk of orthostatic hypotension.

Pharmacodynamics/Kinetics

Onset of action: 1-2 hours

Peak antihypertensive effect: ~1-2 hours

Absorption: Rapid; food decreases rate but not extent of absorption; administration with food minimizes risks of orthostatic hypotension

Distribution: V_d: 115 L

Protein binding: >98%, primarily to albumin

Metabolism: Extensively hepatic, via **CYP2C9, 2D6,** 3A4, and 2C19 (2% excreted unchanged); three active metabolites (4-hydroxyphenyl metabolite is 13 times more potent than parent drug for beta-blockade); first-pass effect; plasma concentrations in the elderly and those with cirrhotic liver disease are 50% and 4-7 times higher, respectively

Bioavailability: 25% to 35%

Half-life elimination: 7-10 hours

Excretion: Primarily feces

Pregnancy Risk Factor C (manufacturer); D (2nd and 3rd trimesters - expert analysis)

Dosage Forms TAB: 3.125 mg, 6.25 mg, 12.5 mg, 25 mg

Selected Readings

Foster CA and Aston SJ, "Propranolol-Epinephrine Interaction: A Potential Disaster," *Plast Reconstr Surg*, 1983, 72(1):74-8.

Wong DG, Spence JD, Lamki L, et al, "Effect of Nonsteroidal Anti-inflammatory Drugs on Control of Hypertension of Beta-Blockers and Diuretics," *Lancet*, 1986, 1(8488):997-1001.

Wynn RL, "Dental Nonsteroidal Anti-inflammatory Drugs and Prostaglandin-Based Drug Interactions, Part Two," *Gen Dent*, 1992, 40(2):104, 106, 108.

Wynn RL, "Epinephrine Interactions With Beta-Blockers," *Gen Dent*, 1994, 42(1):16, 18.

Casanthranol and Docusate *see* Docusate and Casanthranol *on page 460*

Casodex® *see* Bicalutamide *on page 206*

Caspofungin (kas poe FUN jin)

U.S. Brand Names Cancidas®

Canadian Brand Names Cancidas®

Mexican Brand Names Cancidas®

Generic Available No

Synonyms Caspofungin Acetate

Pharmacologic Category Antifungal Agent, Parenteral

Use Treatment of invasive *Aspergillus* infections; treatment of candidemia and other *Candida* infections (abscesses, esophageal, intra-abdominal, peritonitis, pleural space)

Local Anesthetic/Vasoconstrictor Precautions No information available to require special precautions

Effects on Dental Treatment No significant effects or complications reported

Common Adverse Effects

>10%:

Central nervous system: Headache (up to 11%), fever (3% to 26%)

Hematologic: Hemoglobin decreased (3% to 12%)

Hepatic: Serum alkaline phosphatase (3% to 11%) increased, transaminases increased (up to 13%)

Local: Infusion site reactions (2% to 12%), phlebitis (up to 16%)

1% to 10%:

Cardiovascular: Flushing (3%), facial edema (up to 3%), hypertension (2%), tachycardia (1% to 2%), hypotension (1%)

Central nervous system: Dizziness (2%), chills (up to 5%), pain (1% to 5%), insomnia (1%)

Dermatologic: Rash (<1% to 5%), pruritus (1% to 3%), erythema (1% to 2%)

Endocrine & metabolic: Hypokalemia (10%)

Gastrointestinal: Nausea (2% to 6%), vomiting (1% to 4%), abdominal pain (2% to 4%), diarrhea (1% to 4%), anorexia (1%)

Hematologic: Eosinophils increased (3%), neutrophils decreased (2% to 3%), WBC decreased (5% to 6%), anemia (up to 4%), platelet count decreased (2% to 3%)

Hepatic: Bilirubin increased (3%)

Local: Phlebitis/thrombophlebitis (4% to 6%), induration (up to 3%)

Neuromuscular & skeletal: Myalgia (up to 3%), paresthesia (1% to 3%), tremor (2%)

Renal: Nephrotoxicity (8%)*, proteinuria (5%), hematuria (2%), serum creatinine increased (<1% to 4%), urinary WBCs increased (up to 8%), urinary RBCs increased (1% to 4%), blood urea nitrogen increased (1%)

*Nephrotoxicity defined as serum creatinine ≥2X baseline value or ≥1 mg/dL in patients with serum creatinine above ULN range (patients with Cl_{cr} <30 mL/minute were excluded)

Miscellaneous: Flu-like syndrome (3%), diaphoresis (up to 1%)

Mechanism of Action Inhibits synthesis of β(1,3)-D-glucan, an essential component of the cell wall of susceptible fungi. Highest activity in regions of active cell growth. Mammalian cells do not require β(1,3)-D-glucan, limiting potential toxicity.

Drug Interactions

Increased Effect/Toxicity: Concurrent administration of cyclosporine may increase caspofungin concentrations; hepatic serum transaminases may be observed.

Decreased Effect: Caspofungin may decrease blood concentrations of tacrolimus. Dosage adjustment of caspofungin to 70 mg is required for patients on rifampin.

Pharmacodynamics/Kinetics

Protein binding: 97% to albumin

Metabolism: Slowly, via hydrolysis and *N*-acetylation as well as by spontaneous degradation, with subsequent metabolism to component amino acids. Overall metabolism is extensive.

Half-life elimination: Beta (distribution): 9-11 hours; Terminal: 40-50 hours

Excretion: Urine (41% as metabolites, 1% to 9% unchanged) and feces (35% as metabolites)

Pregnancy Risk Factor C

Caspofungin Acetate *see* Caspofungin *on page 272*

Castellani Paint Modified *see* Carbol-Fuchsin Solution *on page 264*

Castor Oil (KAS tor oyl)

U.S. Brand Names Emulsoil® [OTC] [DSC]; Purge® [OTC]

Generic Available Yes: Oil

Synonyms Oleum Ricini

Pharmacologic Category Laxative, Miscellaneous

Use Preparation for rectal or bowel examination or surgery; rarely used to relieve constipation; also applied to skin as emollient and protectant

Local Anesthetic/Vasoconstrictor Precautions No information available to require special precautions

Effects on Dental Treatment No significant effects or complications reported

Mechanism of Action Acts primarily in the small intestine; hydrolyzed to ricinoleic acid which reduces net absorption of fluid and electrolytes and stimulates peristalsis

Pregnancy Risk Factor X

Castor Oil, Trypsin, and Balsam Peru *see* Trypsin, Balsam Peru, and Castor Oil *on page 1349*

Cataflam® *see* Diclofenac *on page 427*

Catapres® *see* Clonidine *on page 358*

Catapres-TTS® *see* Clonidine *on page 358*

Cathflo™ Activase® *see* Alteplase *on page 88*

Caverject® *see* Alprostadil *on page 87*

Caverject® Impulse™ *see* Alprostadil *on page 87*

CB-1348 *see* Chlorambucil *on page 305*
CBDCA *see* Carboplatin *on page 264*
CBZ *see* Carbamazepine *on page 255*
CCNU *see* Lomustine *on page 838*
2-CdA *see* Cladribine *on page 342*
CDDP *see* Cisplatin *on page 337*
CDX *see* Bicalutamide *on page 206*
Ceclor® *see* Cefaclor *on page 274*
Ceclor® CD *see* Cefaclor *on page 274*
Cecon® [OTC] *see* Ascorbic Acid *on page 148*
Cedax® *see* Ceftibuten *on page 287*
CEE *see* Estrogens (Conjugated/Equine) *on page 525*
CeeNU® *see* Lomustine *on page 838*

Cefaclor (SEF a klor)

U.S. Brand Names Ceclor®; Ceclor® CD; Raniclor™

Canadian Brand Names Apo-Cefaclor®; Ceclor®; Novo-Cefaclor; Nu-Cefaclor; PMS-Cefaclor

Mexican Brand Names Ceclor®

Generic Available Yes

Pharmacologic Category Antibiotic, Cephalosporin (Second Generation)

Dental Use Alternative antibiotic for treatment of orofacial infections in patients allergic to penicillins; susceptible bacteria including aerobic gram-positive bacteria and anaerobes

Use Treatment of susceptible bacterial infections including otitis media, lower respiratory tract infections, acute exacerbations of chronic bronchitis, pharyngitis and tonsillitis, urinary tract infections, skin and skin structure infections

Local Anesthetic/Vasoconstrictor Precautions No information available to require special precautions

Effects on Dental Treatment No significant effects or complications reported

Significant Adverse Effects

1% to 10%:

- Dermatologic: Rash (maculopapular, erythematous, or morbilliform) (1% to 2%)
- Gastrointestinal: Diarrhea (3%)
- Genitourinary: Vaginitis (2%)
- Hematologic: Eosinophilia (2%)
- Hepatic: Transaminases increased (3%)
- Miscellaneous: Moniliasis (2%)

<1% (Limited to important or life-threatening): Agitation, agranulocytosis, anaphylaxis, angioedema, aplastic anemia, arthralgia, cholestatic jaundice, CNS irritability, confusion, dizziness, hallucinations, hemolytic anemia, hepatitis, hyperactivity, insomnia, interstitial nephritis, nausea, nervousness, neutropenia, paresthesia, PT prolonged, pruritus, pseudomembranous colitis, seizures, serum-sickness, somnolence, Stevens-Johnson syndrome, thrombocytopenia, toxic epidermal necrolysis, urticaria, vomiting

Reactions reported with other cephalosporins include abdominal pain, cholestasis, fever, hemorrhage, renal dysfunction, superinfection, toxic nephropathy

Dosage Oral:

Children >1 month: Dosing range: 20-40 mg/kg/day divided every 8-12 hours; maximum dose: 1 g/day
- Otitis media: 40 mg/kg/day divided every 12 hours
- Pharyngitis: 20 mg/kg/day divided every 12 hours

Adults: Dosing range: 250-500 mg every 8 hours
- Extended release tablets:
  - Acute bacterial exacerbations of or secondary infections with chronic bronchitis: 500 mg every 12 hours for 7 days
  - Pharyngitis, tonsillitis, uncomplicated skin and skin structure infections: 375 mg every 12 hours for 10 days

Dosing adjustment in renal impairment:
- Cl_{cr} 10-50 mL/minute: Administer 50% to 100% of dose
- Cl_{cr} <10 mL/minute: Administer 50% of dose

Hemodialysis: Moderately dialyzable (20% to 50%)

Mechanism of Action Inhibits bacterial cell wall synthesis by binding to one or more of the penicillin-binding proteins (PBPs) which in turn inhibits the final transpeptidation step of peptidoglycan synthesis in bacterial cell walls, thus inhibiting cell wall biosynthesis. Bacteria eventually lyse due to ongoing activity of cell wall autolytic enzymes (autolysins and murein hydrolases) while cell wall assembly is arrested.

Contraindications Hypersensitivity to cefaclor, any component of the formulation, or other cephalosporins

Warnings/Precautions Modify dosage in patients with severe renal impairment. Prolonged use may result in superinfection. Use with caution in patients with a history of penicillin allergy especially IgE-mediated reactions (eg, anaphylaxis, urticaria). Beta-lacatamase-negative, ampicillin-resistant (BLNAR) strains of *H. influenzae* should be considered resistant to cefaclor. Extended release tablets are not approved for use in children <16 years of age.

Drug Interactions

Aminoglycosides: May be additive to nephrotoxicity.

Furosemide: May be additive to nephrotoxicity.

Probenecid: May decrease cephalosporin elimination.

Ethanol/Nutrition/Herb Interactions

Food: Cefaclor serum levels may be decreased slightly if taken with food. The bioavailability of cefaclor extended release tablets is decreased 23% and the maximum concentration is decreased 67% when taken on an empty stomach.

Dietary Considerations Capsule, chewable tablet, and suspension may be taken with or without food. Extended release tablet should be taken with food. Raniclor™ contains phenylalanine 2.8 mg/cefaclor 125 mg.

Pharmacodynamics/Kinetics

Absorption: Well absorbed, acid stable

Distribution: Widely throughout the body and reaches therapeutic concentration in most tissues and body fluids, including synovial, pericardial, pleural, peritoneal fluids; bile, sputum, and urine; bone, myocardium, gallbladder, skin and soft tissue; crosses placenta; enters breast milk

Protein binding: 25%

Metabolism: Partially hepatic

Half-life elimination: 0.5-1 hour; prolonged with renal impairment

Time to peak: Capsule: 60 minutes; Suspension: 45 minutes

Excretion: Urine (80% as unchanged drug)

Pregnancy Risk Factor B

Lactation Enters breast milk/use caution

Breast-Feeding Considerations Theoretically, drug absorbed by nursing infant may change bowel flora or affect fever work-up result. Small amounts can be detected in breast milk (trace amounts after 1 hour, increasing to 0.16 mcg/mL at 5 hours). **Note:** As a class, cephalosporins are used to treat bacterial infections in infants.

Dosage Forms

Capsule (Ceclor®): 250 mg, 500 mg

Powder for oral suspension: 125 mg/5 mL (75 mL, 150 mL); 187 mg/5 mL (50 mL, 100 mL); 250 mg/5 mL (75 mL, 150 mL); 375 mg/5 mL (50 mL, 100 mL)

Ceclor®: 125 mg/5 mL (150 mL); 187 mg/5 mL (100 mL); 250 mg/5 mL (75 mL, 150 mL); 375 mg/5 mL (100 mL)

Tablet, chewable (Raniclor™): 125 mg [contains phenylalanine 2.8 mg; fruity flavor], 187 mg [contains phenylalanine 4.2 mg; fruity flavor], 250 mg [contains phenylalanine 5.6 mg; fruity flavor], 375 mg [contains phenylalanine 8.4 mg; fruity flavor]

Tablet, extended release (Ceclor® CD): 375 mg, 500 mg

Comments Patients allergic to penicillins can use a cephalosporin; the incidence of cross-reactivity between penicillins and cephalosporins is 1% when the allergic reaction to penicillin is delayed. Cefaclor is effective against anaerobic bacteria, but the sensitivity of alpha-hemolytic *Streptococcus* vary; approximately 10% of strains are resistant. Nearly 70% are intermediately sensitive. If the patient has a history of immediate reaction to penicillin, the incidence of cross-reactivity is 20%; cephalosporins are contraindicated in these patients.

Cefadroxil (sef a DROKS il)

Related Information

Antibiotic Prophylaxis, Preprocedural Guidelines for Dental Patients *on page 1509*

U.S. Brand Names Duricef®

Canadian Brand Names Apo-Cefadroxil®; Duricef™; Novo-Cefadroxil

Mexican Brand Names Cefamox®; Duracef®

Generic Available Yes: Capsule, tablet

Synonyms Cefadroxil Monohydrate

Pharmacologic Category Antibiotic, Cephalosporin (First Generation)

(Continued)

Cefadroxil *(Continued)*

Dental Use Alternative antibiotic for prevention of bacterial endocarditis. Individuals allergic to amoxicillin (penicillins) may receive cefadroxil provided they have not had an immediate, local, or systemic IgE-mediated anaphylactic allergic reaction to penicillin.

Use Treatment of susceptible bacterial infections, including those caused by group A beta-hemolytic *Streptococcus*; prophylaxis against bacterial endocarditis in patients who are allergic to penicillin and undergoing surgical or dental procedures

Local Anesthetic/Vasoconstrictor Precautions No information available to require special precautions

Effects on Dental Treatment No significant effects or complications reported

Significant Adverse Effects

1% to 10%: Gastrointestinal: Diarrhea

<1% (Limited to important or life-threatening): Abdominal pain, agranulocytosis, anaphylaxis, angioedema, arthralgia, cholestasis, dyspepsia, erythema multiforme, fever, nausea, neutropenia, pruritus, pseudomembranous colitis, rash (maculopapular and erythematous), serum sickness, Stevens-Johnson syndrome, thrombocytopenia, transaminases increased, urticaria, vaginitis, vomiting

Reactions reported with other cephalosporins include abdominal pain, aplastic anemia, BUN increased, creatinine increased, eosinophilia, hemolytic anemia, hemorrhage, pancytopenia, prolonged prothrombin time, renal dysfunction, seizures, superinfection, toxic epidermal necrolysis, toxic nephropathy

Dosage Oral:

Children: 30 mg/kg/day divided twice daily up to a maximum of 2 g/day

Adults: 1-2 g/day in 2 divided doses

Prophylaxis against bacterial endocarditis:

Children: 50 mg/kg 1 hour prior to the procedure

Adults: 2 g 1 hour prior to the procedure

Dosing interval in renal impairment:

Cl_{cr} 10-25 mL/minute: Administer every 24 hours

Cl_{cr} <10 mL/minute: Administer every 36 hours

Mechanism of Action Inhibits bacterial cell wall synthesis by binding to one or more of the penicillin-binding proteins (PBPs) which in turn inhibits the final transpeptidation step of peptidoglycan synthesis in bacterial cell walls, thus inhibiting cell wall biosynthesis. Bacteria eventually lyse due to ongoing activity of cell wall autolytic enzymes (autolysins and murein hydrolases) while cell wall assembly is arrested.

Contraindications Hypersensitivity to cefadroxil, other cephalosporins, or any component of the formulation

Warnings/Precautions Modify dosage in patients with severe renal impairment; prolonged use may result in superinfection; use with caution in patients with a history of penicillin allergy especially IgE-mediated reactions (eg, anaphylaxis, angioedema, urticaria). May cause antibiotic-associated colitis or colitis secondary to *C. difficile.*

Drug Interactions

Increased effect: Probenecid may decrease cephalosporin elimination

Increased toxicity: Furosemide, aminoglycosides may be a possible additive to nephrotoxicity

Ethanol/Nutrition/Herb Interactions Food: Concomitant administration with food, infant formula, or cow's milk does **not** significantly affect absorption.

Pharmacodynamics/Kinetics

Absorption: Rapid and well absorbed

Distribution: Widely throughout the body and reaches therapeutic concentrations in most tissues and body fluids, including synovial, pericardial, pleural, and peritoneal fluids; bile, sputum, and urine; bone, myocardium, gallbladder, skin and soft tissue; crosses placenta; enters breast milk

Protein binding: 20%

Half-life elimination: 1-2 hours; Renal failure: 20-24 hours

Time to peak, serum: 70-90 minutes

Excretion: Urine (>90% as unchanged drug)

Pregnancy Risk Factor B

Lactation Enters breast milk (small amounts)/use caution (AAP rates "compatible")

Breast-Feeding Considerations Theoretically, drug absorbed by nursing infant may change bowel flora or affect fever work-up result. **Note:** As a class, cephalosporins are used to treat infections in infants.

Dosage Forms

Capsule, as monohydrate: 500 mg

Powder for oral suspension, as monohydrate: 250 mg/5 mL (50 mL, 100 mL); 500 mg/5 mL (75 mL, 100 mL) [contains sodium benzoate; orange-pineapple flavor]

Tablet, as monohydrate: 1 g

Selected Readings

ADA Division of Legal Affairs, "A Legal Perspective on Antibiotic Prophylaxis," *J Am Dent Assoc*, 2003, 134(9):1260.

"Advisory Statement. Antibiotic Prophylaxis for Dental Patients With Total Joint Replacements. American Dental Association; American Academy of Orthopedic Surgeons," *J Am Dent Assoc*, 1997, 128(7):1004-8.

American Dental Association Council on Scientific Affairs, "Combating Antibiotic Resistance," *J Am Dent Assoc*, 2004, 135(4):484-7.

Dajani AS, Taubert KA, Wilson W, et al, "Prevention of Bacterial Endocarditis. Recommendations by the American Heart Association," *JAMA*, 1997, 277(22):1794-801.

Dajani AS, Taubert KA, Wilson W, et al, "Prevention of Bacterial Endocarditis: Recommendations by the American Heart Association," *J Am Dent Assoc*, 1997, 128(8):1142-51.

Donowitz GR and Mandell GL, "Drug Therapy. Beta-Lactam Antibiotics (1)," *N Engl J Med*, 1988, 318(7):419-26.

Donowitz GR and Mandell GL, "Drug Therapy. Beta-Lactam Antibiotics (2)," *N Engl J Med*, 1988, 318(8):490-500.

Gustaferro CA and Steckelberg JM, "Cephalosporin Antimicrobial Agents and Related Compounds," *Mayo Clin Proc*, 1991, 66(10):1064-73.

Cefadroxil Monohydrate *see* Cefadroxil *on page 275*

Cefamandole (sef a MAN dole)

U.S. Brand Names Mandol® [DSC]

Generic Available No

Synonyms Cefamandole Nafate

Pharmacologic Category Antibiotic, Cephalosporin (Second Generation)

Use Treatment of susceptible bacterial infection; mainly respiratory tract, skin and skin structure, bone and joint, urinary tract and gynecologic, septicemia; surgical prophylaxis. Active against methicillin-sensitive staphylococci, many streptococci, and various gram-negative bacilli including *E. coli*, some *Klebsiella*, *P. mirabilis*, *H. influenzae*, and *Moraxella*.

Local Anesthetic/Vasoconstrictor Precautions No information available to require special precautions

Effects on Dental Treatment No significant effects or complications reported

Common Adverse Effects Contains MTT side chain which may lead to increased risk of hypoprothrombinemia and bleeding.

1% to 10%:

Gastrointestinal: Diarrhea

Local: Thrombophlebitis

Reactions reported with other cephalosporins include toxic epidermal necrolysis, Stevens-Johnson syndrome, abdominal pain, superinfection, renal dysfunction, toxic nephropathy, aplastic anemia, hemolytic anemia, hemorrhage, pancytopenia, vaginitis, seizures

Mechanism of Action Inhibits bacterial cell wall synthesis by binding to one or more of the penicillin-binding proteins (PBPs) which in turn inhibits the final transpeptidation step of peptidoglycan synthesis in bacterial cell walls, thus inhibiting cell wall biosynthesis. Bacteria eventually lyse due to ongoing activity of cell wall autolytic enzymes (autolysins and murein hydrolases) while cell wall assembly is arrested.

Drug Interactions

Increased Effect/Toxicity: Disulfiram-like reaction has been reported when taken within 72 hours of ethanol consumption. Increased cefamandole plasma levels when taken with probenecid. Aminoglycosides, furosemide when taken with cefamandole may increase nephrotoxicity. Increase in hypoprothrombinemic effect with warfarin or heparin and cefamandole.

Pharmacodynamics/Kinetics

Distribution: Well throughout the body, except CSF; poor penetration even with inflamed meninges

Protein binding: 56% to 78%

Metabolism: Extensive enterohepatic recirculation

Half-life elimination: 30-60 minutes

Time to peak, serum: I.M.: 1-2 hours

Excretion: Primarily urine (as unchanged drug); feces (high concentrations)

Pregnancy Risk Factor B

Cefamandole Nafate *see* Cefamandole *on page 277*

Cefazolin (sef A zoe lin)

Related Information

Animal and Human Bites Guidelines *on page 1582*

Antibiotic Prophylaxis, Preprocedural Guidelines for Dental Patients *on page 1509*

U.S. Brand Names Ancef®

Generic Available Yes

Synonyms Cefazolin Sodium

Pharmacologic Category Antibiotic, Cephalosporin (First Generation)

Dental Use Alternative antibiotic for prevention of bacterial endocarditis when parenteral administration is needed. Individuals allergic to amoxicillin (penicillins) may receive cefazolin provided they have not had an immediate, local, or systemic IgE-mediated anaphylactic allergic reaction to penicillin. Alternate antibiotic for premedication in patients not allergic to penicillin who may be at potential increased risk of hematogenous total joint infection when parenteral administration is needed.

Use Treatment of respiratory tract, skin and skin structure, genital, urinary tract, biliary tract, bone and joint infections, and septicemia due to susceptible gram-positive cocci (except enterococcus); some gram-negative bacilli including *E. coli*, *Proteus*, and *Klebsiella* may be susceptible; perioperative prophylaxis

Unlabeled/Investigational Use Prophylaxis against bacterial endocarditis

Local Anesthetic/Vasoconstrictor Precautions No information available to require special precautions

Effects on Dental Treatment No significant effects or complications reported

Significant Adverse Effects Frequency not defined.

Central nervous system: Fever, seizures

Dermatologic: Rash, pruritus, Stevens-Johnson syndrome

Gastrointestinal: Diarrhea. nausea, vomiting, abdominal cramps, anorexia, pseudomembranous colitis, oral candidiasis

Genitourinary: Vaginitis

Hepatic: Transaminases increased, hepatitis

Hematologic: Eosinophilia, neutropenia, leukopenia, thrombocytopenia, thrombocytosis

Local: Pain at injection site, phlebitis

Renal: BUN increased, serum creatinine increased, renal failure

Miscellaneous: Anaphylaxis

Reactions reported with other cephalosporins include toxic epidermal necrolysis, abdominal pain, cholestasis, superinfection, toxic nephropathy, aplastic anemia, hemolytic anemia, hemorrhage, prolonged prothrombin time, pancytopenia

Dosage I.M., I.V.:

Children >1 month: 25-100 mg/kg/day divided every 6-8 hours; maximum: 6 g/day

Adults: 250 mg to 2 g every 6-12 (usually 8) hours, depending on severity of infection; maximum dose: 12 g/day

Prophylaxis against bacterial endocarditis (unlabeled use):

Infants and Children: 25 mg/kg 30 minutes before procedure; maximum dose: 1 g

Adults: 1 g 30 minutes before procedure

Dosing adjustment in renal impairment:

Cl_{cr} 10-30 mL/minute: Administer every 12 hours

Cl_{cr} <10 mL/minute: Administer every 24 hours

Hemodialysis: Moderately dialyzable (20% to 50%); administer dose postdialysis or administer supplemental dose of 0.5-1 g after dialysis

Peritoneal dialysis: Administer 0.5 g every 12 hours

Continuous arteriovenous or venovenous hemofiltration: Dose as for Cl_{cr} 10-30 mL/minute; removes 30 mg of cefazolin per liter of filtrate per day

Mechanism of Action Inhibits bacterial cell wall synthesis by binding to one or more of the penicillin-binding proteins (PBPs) which in turn inhibits the final transpeptidation step of peptidoglycan synthesis in bacterial cell walls, thus inhibiting cell wall biosynthesis. Bacteria eventually lyse due to ongoing activity of cell wall autolytic enzymes (autolysins and murein hydrolases) while cell wall assembly is arrested.

Contraindications Hypersensitivity to cefazolin sodium, any component of the formulation, or other cephalosporins

Warnings/Precautions Modify dosage in patients with severe renal impairment; prolonged use may result in superinfection; use with caution in patients with a history of penicillin allergy especially IgE-mediated reactions (eg, anaphylaxis, angioedema, urticaria). May cause antibiotic-associated colitis or colitis secondary to *C. difficile*.

Drug Interactions

Aminoglycosides: Aminoglycosides increase nephrotoxic potential.

Probenecid: High-dose probenecid decreases clearance.

Warfarin: Cefazolin may increase the hypothrombinemic response to warfarin (due to alteration of GI microbial flora).

Dietary Considerations Sodium content of 1 g: 48 mg (2 mEq)

Pharmacodynamics/Kinetics

Distribution: Widely into most body tissues and fluids including gallbladder, liver, kidneys, bone, sputum, bile, pleural, and synovial; CSF penetration is poor; crosses placenta; enters breast milk

Protein binding: 74% to 86%

Metabolism: Minimally hepatic

Half-life elimination: 90-150 minutes; prolonged with renal impairment

Time to peak, serum: I.M.: 0.5-2 hours

Excretion: Urine (80% to 100% as unchanged drug)

Pregnancy Risk Factor B

Lactation Enters breast milk (small amounts)/use caution (AAP rates "compatible")

Breast-Feeding Considerations Theoretically, drug absorbed by nursing infant may change bowel flora or affect fever work-up result. **Note:** As a class, cephalosporins are used to treat infections in infants.

Dosage Forms

Infusion [premixed in D_5W]: 500 mg (50 mL); 1 g (50 mL)

Injection, powder for reconstitution: 500 mg, 1 g, 10 g, 20 g

Ancef®: 1 g, 10 g

Selected Readings

ADA Division of Legal Affairs, "A Legal Perspective on Antibiotic Prophylaxis," *J Am Dent Assoc*, 2003, 134(9):1260.

"Advisory Statement. Antibiotic Prophylaxis for Dental Patients With Total Joint Replacements. American Dental Association; American Academy of Orthopedic Surgeons," *J Am Dent Assoc*, 1997, 128(7):1004-8.

American Dental Association; American Academy of Orthopedic Surgeons, "Antibiotic Prophylaxis for Dental Patients With Total Joint Replacements," *J Am Dent Assoc*, 2003, 134(7):895-9.

American Dental Association Council on Scientific Affairs, "Combating Antibiotic Resistance," *J Am Dent Assoc*, 2004, 135(4):484-7.

Dajani AS, Taubert KA, Wilson W, et al, "Prevention of Bacterial Endocarditis. Recommendations by the American Heart Association," *JAMA*, 1997, 277(22):1794-801.

Dajani AS, Taubert KA, Wilson W, et al, "Prevention of Bacterial Endocarditis: Recommendations by the American Heart Association," *J Am Dent Assoc*, 1997, 128(8):1142-51.

Donowitz GR and Mandell GL, "Drug Therapy. Beta-Lactam Antibiotics (1)," *N Engl J Med*, 1988, 318(7):419-26.

Donowitz GR and Mandell GL, "Drug Therapy. Beta-Lactam Antibiotics (2)," *N Engl J Med*, 1988, 318(8):490-500.

Gustaferro CA and Steckelberg JM, "Cephalosporin Antimicrobial Agents and Related Compounds," *Mayo Clin Proc*, 1991, 66(10):1064-73.

Cefazolin Sodium *see* Cefazolin *on page 278*

Cefdinir (SEF di ner)

U.S. Brand Names Omnicef®

Canadian Brand Names Omnicef®

Generic Available No

Synonyms CFDN

Pharmacologic Category Antibiotic, Cephalosporin (Third Generation)

Use Treatment of community-acquired pneumonia, acute exacerbations of chronic bronchitis, acute bacterial otitis media, acute maxillary sinusitis, pharyngitis/tonsillitis, and uncomplicated skin and skin structure infections.

Local Anesthetic/Vasoconstrictor Precautions No information available to require special precautions

Effects on Dental Treatment No significant effects or complications reported

Common Adverse Effects

1% to 10%

Dermatologic: Cutaneous moniliasis (1%)

Gastrointestinal: Diarrhea (8%), rash (3%), vomiting (1%), increased GGT (1%)

Reactions reported with other cephalosporins include dizziness, fever, headache, encephalopathy, asterixis, neuromuscular excitability, seizures, aplastic anemia, interstitial nephritis, toxic nephropathy, angioedema, hemorrhage, prolonged PT, serum-sickness reactions, and superinfection

Mechanism of Action Inhibits bacterial cell wall synthesis by binding to one or more of the penicillin-binding proteins (PBPs) which in turn inhibits the final transpeptidation step of peptidoglycan synthesis in bacterial cell walls, thus inhibiting cell wall biosynthesis. Bacteria eventually lyse due to ongoing activity

(Continued)

Cefdinir *(Continued)*

of cell wall autolytic enzymes (autolysins and murein hydrolases) while cell wall assembly is arrested.

Drug Interactions

Increased Effect/Toxicity: Probenecid increases the effects of cephalosporins by decreasing the renal elimination in those which are secreted by tubular secretion. Anticoagulant effects may be increased when administered with cephalosporins.

Decreased Effect: Coadministration with iron or antacids reduces the rate and extent of cefdinir absorption.

Pharmacodynamics/Kinetics

Protein binding: 60% to 70%
Metabolism: Minimally hepatic
Bioavailability: Capsule: 16% to 21%; suspension 25%
Half-life elimination: 100 minutes
Excretion: Primarily urine

Pregnancy Risk Factor B

Cefditoren (sef de TOR en)

U.S. Brand Names Spectracef™

Generic Available No

Synonyms Cefditoren Pivoxil

Pharmacologic Category Antibiotic, Cephalosporin

Use Treatment of acute bacterial exacerbation of chronic bronchitis or community-acquired pneumonia (due to susceptible organisms including *Haemophilus influenzae, Haemophilus parainfluenzae, Streptococcus pneumoniae*-penicillin susceptible only, *Moraxella catarrhalis*); pharyngitis or tonsillitis (*Streptococcus pyogenes*); and uncomplicated skin and skin-structure infections (*Staphylococcus aureus*-not MRSA, *Streptococcus pyogenes*)

Local Anesthetic/Vasoconstrictor Precautions No information available to require special precautions

Effects on Dental Treatment No significant effects or complications reported

Significant Adverse Effects

>10%: Gastrointestinal: Diarrhea (11% to 15%)

1% to 10%:

- Central nervous system: Headache (2% to 3%)
- Endocrine & metabolic: Glucose increased (1%)
- Gastrointestinal: Nausea (4% to 6%), abdominal pain (2%), dyspepsia (1% to 2%), vomiting (1%)
- Genitourinary: Vaginal moniliasis (3% to 6%)
- Hematologic: Hematocrit decreased (2%)
- Renal: Hematuria (3%), urinary white blood cells increased (2%)

<1% (Limited to important or life-threatening): Acute renal failure, allergic reaction, arthralgia, BUN increased, coagulation time increased, eosinophilic pneumonia, interstitial pneumonia, positive direct Coombs' test, pseudomembranous colitis, rash, thrombocytopenia

Additional adverse effects seen with cephalosporin antibiotics: Anaphylaxis, aplastic anemia, cholestasis, erythema multiforme, hemorrhage, hemolytic anemia, renal dysfunction, reversible hyperactivity, serum sickness-like reaction, Stevens-Johnson syndrome, toxic epidermal necrolysis, toxic nephropathy

Dosage Oral: Children ≥12 years and Adults:

Acute bacterial exacerbation of chronic bronchitis: 400 mg twice daily for 10 days

Community-acquired pneumonia: 400 mg twice daily for 14 days

Pharyngitis, tonsillitis, uncomplicated skin and skin structure infections: 200 mg twice daily for 10 days

Elderly: Refer to adult dosing

Dosage adjustment in renal impairment:

Cl_{cr} 30-49 mL/minute: Maximum dose: 200 mg twice daily
Cl_{cr} <30 mL/minute: Maximum dose: 200 mg once daily
End-stage renal disease: Appropriate dosing not established

Dosage adjustment in hepatic impairment:

Mild or moderate impairment: Adjustment not required
Severe impairment (Child-Pugh Class C): Specific guidelines not available

Mechanism of Action Inhibits bacterial cell wall synthesis by binding to one or more of the penicillin binding proteins (PBPs); which in turn inhibits the final transpeptidation step of peptidoglycan synthesis in bacterial cell walls, thus inhibiting cell wall biosynthesis. Bacteria eventually lyse due to ongoing activity of cell wall autolytic enzymes (autolysins and murein hydrolases) while cell wall assembly is arrested.

Contraindications Hypersensitivity to cefditoren, other cephalosporins, milk protein, or any component of the formulation; carnitine deficiency

Warnings/Precautions Use with caution in patients with a history of penicillin allergy, especially IgE-mediated reactions (eg, anaphylaxis, urticaria). May cause antibiotic-associated colitis or colitis secondary to *C. difficile.* Modify dosage in patients with severe renal impairment. Caution in individuals with seizure disorders. Prolonged use may result in superinfection. Use caution in patients with renal or hepatic impairment. Cefditoren causes renal excretion of carnitine, do not use in patients with carnitine deficiency; not for long-term therapy due to the possible development of carnitine deficiency over time. Cefditoren tablets contain sodium caseinate, which may cause hypersensitivity reactions in patients with milk protein hypersensitivity; this does not affect patients with lactose intolerance. Safety and efficacy have not been established in children <12 years of age.

Drug Interactions

Antacids: Aluminum- and magnesium-containing antacids decrease oral absorption; concomitant use should be avoided.

Histamine H_2 antagonists: Famotidine decreases oral absorption; concomitant use should be avoided.

Probenecid: Serum concentration of cefditoren may be increased.

Ethanol/Nutrition/Herb Interactions Food: Moderate- to high-fat meals increase bioavailability and maximum plasma concentration.

Dietary Considerations Cefditoren should be taken with meals. Plasma carnitine levels are decreased during therapy (39% with 200 mg dosing, 63% with 400 mg dosing); normal concentrations return within 7-10 days after treatment is discontinued.

Pharmacodynamics/Kinetics

Distribution: 9.3 ± 1.6 L

Protein binding: 88% (*in vitro*), primarily to albumin

Metabolism: Cefditoren pivoxil is hydrolyzed to cefditoren (active) and pivalate

Bioavailability: ~14% to 16%, increased by moderate to high-fat meal

Half-life elimination: 1.6 ± 0.4 hours

Time to peak: 1.5-3 hours

Excretion: Urine (as cefditoren and pivaloylcarnitine)

Pregnancy Risk Factor B

Lactation Excretion in breast milk unknown/use caution

Dosage Forms Tablet, as pivoxil: 200 mg [equivalent to cefditoren; contains sodium caseinate]

Cefditoren Pivoxil *see* Cefditoren *on page 280*

Cefepime (SEF e pim)

U.S. Brand Names Maxipime®

Canadian Brand Names Maxipime®

Mexican Brand Names Maxipime®

Generic Available No

Synonyms Cefepime Hydrochloride

Pharmacologic Category Antibiotic, Cephalosporin (Fourth Generation)

Use Treatment of uncomplicated and complicated urinary tract infections, including pyelonephritis caused by typical urinary tract pathogens; monotherapy for febrile neutropenia; uncomplicated skin and skin structure infections caused by *Streptococcus pyogenes*; moderate to severe pneumonia caused by pneumococcus, *Pseudomonas aeruginosa*, and other gram-negative organisms; complicated intra-abdominal infections (in combination with metronidazole). Also active against methicillin-susceptible staphylococci, *Enterobacter* sp, and many other gram-negative bacilli.

Children 2 months to 16 years: Empiric therapy of febrile neutropenia patients, uncomplicated skin/soft tissue infections, pneumonia, and uncomplicated/complicated urinary tract infections.

Local Anesthetic/Vasoconstrictor Precautions No information available to require special precautions

Effects on Dental Treatment No significant effects or complications reported

Common Adverse Effects

>10%: Hematologic: Positive Coombs' test without hemolysis

1% to 10%:

Central nervous system: Fever (1%), headache (1%)

Dermatologic: Rash, pruritus

Gastrointestinal: Diarrhea, nausea, vomiting

Local: Pain, erythema at injection site

(Continued)

Cefepime *(Continued)*

Reactions reported with other cephalosporins include aplastic anemia, erythema multiforme, hemolytic anemia, hemorrhage, pancytopenia, prolonged PT, renal dysfunction, Stevens-Johnson syndrome, superinfection, toxic epidermal necrolysis, toxic nephropathy, vaginitis

Mechanism of Action Inhibits bacterial cell wall synthesis by binding to one or more of the penicillin-binding proteins (PBPs) which in turn inhibits the final transpeptidation step of peptidoglycan synthesis in bacterial cell walls, thus inhibiting cell wall biosynthesis. Bacteria eventually lyse due to ongoing activity of cell wall autolytic enzymes (autolysis and murein hydrolases) while cell wall assembly is arrested.

Drug Interactions

Increased Effect/Toxicity: High-dose probenecid decreases clearance and increases effect of cefepime. Aminoglycosides increase nephrotoxic potential when taken with cefepime.

Pharmacodynamics/Kinetics

Absorption: I.M.: Rapid and complete

Distribution: V_d: Adults: 14-20 L; penetrates into inflammatory fluid at concentrations ~80% of serum levels and into bronchial mucosa at levels ~60% of those reached in the plasma; crosses blood-brain barrier

Protein binding, plasma: 16% to 19%

Metabolism: Minimally hepatic

Half-life elimination: 2 hours

Time to peak: 0.5-1.5 hours

Excretion: Urine (85% as unchanged drug)

Pregnancy Risk Factor B

Cefepime Hydrochloride *see* Cefepime *on page 281*

Cefixime (sef IKS eem)

Related Information

Sexually-Transmitted Diseases *on page 1504*

U.S. Brand Names Suprax®

Canadian Brand Names Suprax®

Mexican Brand Names Denvar®

Generic Available No

Pharmacologic Category Antibiotic, Cephalosporin (Third Generation)

Use Treatment of urinary tract infections, otitis media, respiratory infections due to susceptible organisms including *S. pneumoniae* and *S. pyogenes*, *H. influenzae* and many Enterobacteriaceae; uncomplicated cervical/urethral gonorrhea due to *N. gonorrhoeae*

Local Anesthetic/Vasoconstrictor Precautions No information available to require special precautions

Effects on Dental Treatment No significant effects or complications reported

Common Adverse Effects

>10%: Gastrointestinal: Diarrhea (16%)

2% to 10%: Gastrointestinal: Abdominal pain, nausea, dyspepsia, flatulence, loose stools

Reactions reported with other cephalosporins include interstitial nephritis, aplastic anemia, hemolytic anemia, hemorrhage, pancytopenia, agranulocytosis, colitis, superinfection

Mechanism of Action Inhibits bacterial cell wall synthesis by binding to one or more of the penicillin binding proteins (PBPs); which in turn inhibits the final transpeptidation step of peptidoglycan synthesis in bacterial cell walls, thus inhibiting cell wall biosynthesis. Bacteria eventually lyse due to ongoing activity of cell wall autolytic enzymes (autolysins and murein hydrolases) while cell wall assembly is arrested.

Drug Interactions

Increased Effect/Toxicity: Aminoglycosides and furosemide may be possible additives to nephrotoxicity. Probenecid increases cefixime concentration. Cefixime may increase carbamazepine. Cefixime may increase prothrombin time when administered with warfarin.

Pharmacodynamics/Kinetics

Absorption: 40% to 50%

Distribution: Widely throughout the body and reaches therapeutic concentration in most tissues and body fluids, including synovial, pericardial, pleural, peritoneal; bile, sputum, and urine; bone, myocardium, gallbladder, and skin and soft tissue

Protein binding: 65%

Bioavailability: Bioavailability of suspension is higher than that of the tablet.

Half-life elimination: Normal renal function: 3-4 hours; Renal failure: Up to 11.5 hours
Time to peak, serum: 2-6 hours; delayed with food
Excretion: Urine (50% of absorbed dose as active drug); feces (10%)
Pregnancy Risk Factor B

Cefizox® *see* Ceftizoxime *on page 288*
Cefotan® *see* Cefotetan *on page 283*

Cefotaxime (sef oh TAKS eem)

Related Information
Sexually-Transmitted Diseases *on page 1504*
U.S. Brand Names Claforan®
Canadian Brand Names Claforan®
Mexican Brand Names Benaxima®; Biosint®; Cefradil® [inj.]; Claforan®; Fotexina®; Taporin® [inj.]; Viken®
Generic Available Yes: Powder
Synonyms Cefotaxime Sodium
Pharmacologic Category Antibiotic, Cephalosporin (Third Generation)
Use Treatment of susceptible infection in respiratory tract, skin and skin structure, bone and joint, urinary tract, gynecologic as well as septicemia, and documented or suspected meningitis. Active against most gram-negative bacilli (not *Pseudomonas*) and gram-positive cocci (not enterococcus). Active against many penicillin-resistant pneumococci.
Local Anesthetic/Vasoconstrictor Precautions No information available to require special precautions
Effects on Dental Treatment No significant effects or complications reported
Common Adverse Effects
1% to 10%:
Dermatologic: Rash, pruritus
Gastrointestinal: Diarrhea, nausea, vomiting, colitis
Local: Pain at injection site
Reactions reported with other cephalosporins include agranulocytosis, aplastic anemia, cholestasis, hemolytic anemia, hemorrhage, nephropathy, pancytopenia, renal dysfunction, seizures, superinfection.
Mechanism of Action Inhibits bacterial cell wall synthesis by binding to one or more of the penicillin-binding proteins (PBPs) which in turn inhibits the final transpeptidation step of peptidoglycan synthesis in bacterial cell walls, thus inhibiting cell wall biosynthesis. Bacteria eventually lyse due to ongoing activity of cell wall autolytic enzymes (autolysins and murein hydrolases) while cell wall assembly is arrested.
Drug Interactions
Increased Effect/Toxicity: Probenecid may decrease cephalosporin elimination resulting in increased levels. Furosemide, aminoglycosides in combination with cefotaxime may result in additive nephrotoxicity.
Pharmacodynamics/Kinetics
Distribution: Widely to body tissues and fluids including aqueous humor, ascitic and prostatic fluids, bone; penetrates CSF best when meninges are inflamed; crosses placenta; enters breast milk
Metabolism: Partially hepatic to active metabolite, desacetylcefotaxime
Half-life elimination:
Cefotaxime: Premature neonates <1 week: 5-6 hours; Full-term neonates <1 week: 2-3.4 hours; Adults: 1-1.5 hours; prolonged with renal and/or hepatic impairment
Desacetylcefotaxime: 1.5-1.9 hours; prolonged with renal impairment
Time to peak, serum: I.M.: Within 30 minutes
Excretion: Urine (as unchanged drug and metabolites)
Pregnancy Risk Factor B

Cefotaxime Sodium *see* Cefotaxime *on page 283*

Cefotetan (SEF oh tee tan)

Related Information
Animal and Human Bites Guidelines *on page 1582*
Sexually-Transmitted Diseases *on page 1504*
U.S. Brand Names Cefotan®
Canadian Brand Names Cefotan®
Generic Available No
Synonyms Cefotetan Disodium
Pharmacologic Category Antibiotic, Cephalosporin (Second Generation)
Use Less active against staphylococci and streptococci than first generation cephalosporins, but active against anaerobes including *Bacteroides fragilis*;
(Continued)

Cefotetan *(Continued)*

active against gram-negative enteric bacilli including *E. coli*, *Klebsiella*, and *Proteus*; used predominantly for respiratory tract, skin and skin structure, bone and joint, urinary tract and gynecologic as well as septicemia; surgical prophylaxis; intra-abdominal infections and other mixed infections

Local Anesthetic/Vasoconstrictor Precautions No information available to require special precautions

Effects on Dental Treatment No significant effects or complications reported

Common Adverse Effects Contains MTT side chain which may lead to increased risk of hypoprothrombinemia and bleeding.

1% to 10%:
- Gastrointestinal: Diarrhea (1.3%)
- Hepatic: Increased transaminases (1.2%)
- Miscellaneous: Hypersensitivity reactions (1.2%)

Reactions reported with other cephalosporins include seizures, Stevens-Johnson syndrome, toxic epidermal necrolysis, renal dysfunction, toxic nephropathy, cholestasis, aplastic anemia, hemolytic anemia, hemorrhage, pancytopenia, agranulocytosis, colitis, superinfection

Mechanism of Action Inhibits bacterial cell wall synthesis by binding to one or more of the penicillin-binding proteins (PBPs) which in turn inhibits the final transpeptidation step of peptidoglycan synthesis in bacterial cell walls, thus inhibiting cell wall biosynthesis. Bacteria eventually lyse due to ongoing activity of cell wall autolytic enzymes (autolysins and murein hydrolases) while cell wall assembly is arrested.

Drug Interactions

Increased Effect/Toxicity: Probenecid may decrease cephalosporin elimination. Furosemide, aminoglycosides in combination with cefotetan may result in additive nephrotoxicity. May cause disulfiram-like reaction with concomitant ethanol use. Effects of warfarin may be enhanced by cefotetan (due to effects on gastrointestinal flora).

Pharmacodynamics/Kinetics

Distribution: Widely to body tissues and fluids including bile, sputum, prostatic, peritoneal; low concentrations enter CSF; crosses placenta; enters breast milk

Protein binding: 76% to 90%

Half-life elimination: 3-5 hours

Time to peak, serum: I.M.: 1.5-3 hours

Excretion: Primarily urine (as unchanged drug); feces (20%)

Pregnancy Risk Factor B

Cefotetan Disodium *see* Cefotetan *on page 283*

Cefoxitin (se FOKS i tin)

Related Information

Sexually-Transmitted Diseases *on page 1504*

U.S. Brand Names Mefoxin®

Canadian Brand Names Mefoxin®

Generic Available Yes: Powder for injection

Synonyms Cefoxitin Sodium

Pharmacologic Category Antibiotic, Cephalosporin (Second Generation)

Use Less active against staphylococci and streptococci than first generation cephalosporins, but active against anaerobes including *Bacteroides fragilis*; active against gram-negative enteric bacilli including *E. coli*, *Klebsiella*, and *Proteus*; used predominantly for respiratory tract, skin and skin structure, bone and joint, urinary tract and gynecologic as well as septicemia; surgical prophylaxis; intra-abdominal infections and other mixed infections; indicated for bacterial *Eikenella corrodens* infections

Local Anesthetic/Vasoconstrictor Precautions No information available to require special precautions

Effects on Dental Treatment No significant effects or complications reported

Common Adverse Effects

1% to 10%: Gastrointestinal: Diarrhea

Reactions reported with other cephalosporins include seizures, Stevens-Johnson syndrome, toxic epidermal necrolysis, erythema multiforme, urticaria, serum-sickness reactions, renal dysfunction, toxic nephropathy, cholestasis, aplastic anemia, hemolytic anemia, hemorrhage, pancytopenia, agranulocytosis, colitis, vaginitis, superinfection

Mechanism of Action Inhibits bacterial cell wall synthesis by binding to one or more of the penicillin-binding proteins (PBPs) which in turn inhibits the final transpeptidation step of peptidoglycan synthesis in bacterial cell walls, thus inhibiting cell wall biosynthesis. Bacteria eventually lyse due to ongoing activity of cell wall autolytic enzymes (autolysins and murein hydrolases) while cell wall assembly is arrested.

Drug Interactions

Increased Effect/Toxicity: Probenecid may decrease cephalosporin elimination. Furosemide, aminoglycosides in combination with cefoxitin may result in additive nephrotoxicity.

Pharmacodynamics/Kinetics

Distribution: Widely to body tissues and fluids including pleural, synovial, ascitic, bile; poorly penetrates into CSF even with inflammation of the meninges; crosses placenta; small amounts enter breast milk

Protein binding: 65% to 79%

Half-life elimination: 45-60 minutes; significantly prolonged with renal impairment

Time to peak, serum: I.M.: 20-30 minutes

Excretion: Urine (85% as unchanged drug)

Pregnancy Risk Factor B

Cefoxitin Sodium *see* Cefoxitin *on page 284*

Cefpodoxime (sef pode OKS eem)

U.S. Brand Names Vantin®

Canadian Brand Names Vantin®

Mexican Brand Names Orelox®

Generic Available No

Synonyms Cefpodoxime Proxetil

Pharmacologic Category Antibiotic, Cephalosporin (Third Generation)

Use Treatment of susceptible acute, community-acquired pneumonia caused by *S. pneumoniae* or nonbeta-lactamase producing *H. influenzae*; acute uncomplicated gonorrhea caused by *N. gonorrhoeae*; uncomplicated skin and skin structure infections caused by *S. aureus* or *S. pyogenes*; acute otitis media caused by *S. pneumoniae*, *H. influenzae*, or *M. catarrhalis*; pharyngitis or tonsillitis; and uncomplicated urinary tract infections caused by *E. coli*, *Klebsiella*, and *Proteus*

Local Anesthetic/Vasoconstrictor Precautions No information available to require special precautions

Effects on Dental Treatment No significant effects or complications reported

Common Adverse Effects

>10%:

Dermatologic: Diaper rash (12%)

Gastrointestinal: Diarrhea in infants and toddlers (15%)

1% to 10%:

Central nervous system: Headache (1%)

Dermatologic: Rash (1%)

Gastrointestinal: Diarrhea (7%), nausea (4%), abdominal pain (2%), vomiting (1% to 2%)

Genitourinary: Vaginal infections (3%)

Reactions reported with other cephalosporins include seizures, Stevens-Johnson syndrome, toxic epidermal necrolysis, erythema multiforme, urticaria, serum-sickness reactions, renal dysfunction, interstitial nephritis toxic nephropathy, cholestasis, aplastic anemia, hemolytic anemia, hemorrhage, pancytopenia, agranulocytosis, colitis, vaginitis, superinfection

Mechanism of Action Inhibits bacterial cell wall synthesis by binding to one or more of the penicillin-binding proteins (PBPs) which in turn inhibits the final transpeptidation step of peptidoglycan synthesis in bacterial cell walls, thus inhibiting cell wall biosynthesis. Bacteria eventually lyse due to ongoing activity of cell wall autolytic enzymes (autolysins and murein hydrolases) while cell wall assembly is arrested.

Drug Interactions

Increased Effect/Toxicity: Probenecid may decrease cephalosporin elimination. Furosemide, aminoglycosides in combination with cefpodoxime may result in additive nephrotoxicity.

Decreased Effect: Antacids and H_2-receptor antagonists reduce absorption and serum concentration of cefpodoxime.

Pharmacodynamics/Kinetics

Absorption: Rapid and well absorbed (50%), acid stable; enhanced in the presence of food or low gastric pH

Distribution: Good tissue penetration, including lung and tonsils; penetrates into pleural fluid

Protein binding: 18% to 23%

Metabolism: De-esterified in GI tract to active metabolite, cefpodoxime

(Continued)

Cefpodoxime *(Continued)*

Half-life elimination: 2.2 hours; prolonged with renal impairment
Time to peak: Within 1 hour
Excretion: Urine (80% as unchanged drug) in 24 hours

Pregnancy Risk Factor B

Cefpodoxime Proxetil *see* Cefpodoxime *on page 285*

Cefprozil (sef PROE zil)

U.S. Brand Names Cefzil®

Canadian Brand Names Cefzil®

Mexican Brand Names Procef®

Generic Available No

Pharmacologic Category Antibiotic, Cephalosporin (Second Generation)

Use Treatment of otitis media and infections involving the respiratory tract and skin and skin structure; active against methicillin-sensitive staphylococci, many streptococci, and various gram-negative bacilli including *E. coli*, some *Klebsiella*, *P. mirabilis*, *H. influenzae*, and *Moraxella*.

Local Anesthetic/Vasoconstrictor Precautions No information available to require special precautions

Effects on Dental Treatment No significant effects or complications reported

Common Adverse Effects

1% to 10%:

Central nervous system: Dizziness (1%)
Dermatologic: Diaper rash (2%)
Gastrointestinal: Diarrhea (3%), nausea (4%), vomiting (1%), abdominal pain (1%)
Genitourinary: Vaginitis, genital pruritus (2%)
Hepatic: Increased transaminases (2%)
Miscellaneous: Superinfection

Reactions reported with other cephalosporins include seizures, toxic epidermal necrolysis, renal dysfunction, interstitial nephritis, toxic nephropathy, aplastic anemia, hemolytic anemia, hemorrhage, pancytopenia, agranulocytosis, colitis, vaginitis, superinfection

Mechanism of Action Inhibits bacterial cell wall synthesis by binding to one or more of the penicillin-binding proteins (PBPs) which in turn inhibits the final transpeptidation step of peptidoglycan synthesis in bacterial cell walls, thus inhibiting cell wall biosynthesis. Bacteria eventually lyse due to ongoing activity of cell wall autolytic enzymes (autolysins and murein hydrolases) while cell wall assembly is arrested.

Drug Interactions

Increased Effect/Toxicity: Probenecid may decrease cephalosporin elimination. Furosemide, aminoglycosides in combination with cefprozil may result in additive nephrotoxicity.

Pharmacodynamics/Kinetics

Absorption: Well absorbed (94%)
Distribution: Low amounts enter breast milk
Protein binding: 35% to 45%
Half-life elimination: Normal renal function: 1.3 hours
Time to peak, serum: Fasting: 1.5 hours
Excretion: Urine (61% as unchanged drug)

Pregnancy Risk Factor B

Ceftazidime (SEF tay zi deem)

U.S. Brand Names Ceptaz® [DSC]; Fortaz®; Tazicef®

Canadian Brand Names Fortaz®

Mexican Brand Names Fortum®; Izadima®; Tagal® [inj.]; Taxifur® [inj.]

Generic Available No

Pharmacologic Category Antibiotic, Cephalosporin (Third Generation)

Use Treatment of documented susceptible *Pseudomonas aeruginosa* infection and infections due to other susceptible aerobic gram-negative organisms; empiric therapy of a febrile, granulocytopenic patient

Local Anesthetic/Vasoconstrictor Precautions No information available to require special precautions

Effects on Dental Treatment No significant effects or complications reported

Common Adverse Effects

1% to 10%:

Gastrointestinal: Diarrhea (1%)
Local: Pain at injection site (1%)
Miscellaneous: Hypersensitivity reactions (2%)

Reactions reported with other cephalosporins include seizures, urticaria, serum-sickness reactions, renal dysfunction, interstitial nephritis, toxic nephropathy, elevated BUN, elevated creatinine, cholestasis, aplastic anemia, hemolytic anemia, pancytopenia, agranulocytosis, colitis, prolonged PT, hemorrhage, superinfection

Mechanism of Action Inhibits bacterial cell wall synthesis by binding to one or more of the penicillin-binding proteins (PBPs) which in turn inhibits the final transpeptidation step of peptidoglycan synthesis in bacterial cell walls, thus inhibiting cell wall biosynthesis. Bacteria eventually lyse due to ongoing activity of cell wall autolytic enzymes (autolysins and murein hydrolases) while cell wall assembly is arrested.

Drug Interactions

Increased Effect/Toxicity: Probenecid may decrease cephalosporin elimination. Aminoglycosides: *in vitro* studies indicate additive or synergistic effect against some strains of Enterobacteriaceae and *Pseudomonas aeruginosa*. Furosemide, aminoglycosides in combination with ceftazidime may result in additive nephrotoxicity.

Pharmacodynamics/Kinetics

Distribution: Widely throughout the body including bone, bile, skin, CSF (higher concentrations achieved when meninges are inflamed), endometrium, heart, pleural and lymphatic fluids

Protein binding: 17%

Half-life elimination: 1-2 hours, prolonged with renal impairment; Neonates <23 days: 2.2-4.7 hours

Time to peak, serum: I.M.: ~1 hour

Excretion: Urine (80% to 90% as unchanged drug)

Pregnancy Risk Factor B

Ceftibuten (sef TYE byoo ten)

Related Information

Oral Bacterial Infections *on page 1533*

U.S. Brand Names Cedax®

Mexican Brand Names Cedax®

Generic Available No

Pharmacologic Category Antibiotic, Cephalosporin (Third Generation)

Use Oral cephalosporin for treatment of bronchitis, otitis media, and pharyngitis/tonsillitis due to *H. influenzae* and *M. catarrhalis*, both beta-lactamase-producing and nonproducing strains, as well as *S. pneumoniae* (weak) and *S. pyogenes*

Local Anesthetic/Vasoconstrictor Precautions No information available to require special precautions

Effects on Dental Treatment No significant effects or complications reported

Common Adverse Effects

1% to 10%:

- Central nervous system: Headache (3%), dizziness (1%)
- Gastrointestinal: Nausea (4%), diarrhea (3%), dyspepsia (2%), vomiting (1%), abdominal pain (1%)
- Hematologic: Increased eosinophils (3%), decreased hemoglobin (2%), thrombocytosis
- Hepatic: Increased ALT (1%), increased bilirubin (1%)
- Renal: Increased BUN (4%)

Reactions reported with other cephalosporins include anaphylaxis, fever, paresthesia, pruritus, Stevens-Johnson syndrome, toxic epidermal necrolysis, erythema multiforme, angioedema, pseudomembranous colitis, hemolytic anemia, candidiasis, vaginitis, encephalopathy, asterixis, neuromuscular excitability, seizures, serum-sickness reactions, renal dysfunction, interstitial nephritis, toxic nephropathy, cholestasis, aplastic anemia, hemolytic anemia, pancytopenia, agranulocytosis, colitis, prolonged PT, hemorrhage, superinfection

Mechanism of Action Inhibits bacterial cell wall synthesis by binding to one or more of the penicillin-binding proteins (PBPs) which in turn inhibits the final transpeptidation step of peptidoglycan synthesis in bacterial cell walls, thus inhibiting cell wall biosynthesis. Bacteria eventually lyse due to ongoing activity of cell wall autolytic enzymes (autolysins and murein hydrolases) while cell wall assembly is arrested.

Drug Interactions

Increased Effect/Toxicity: High-dose probenecid decreases clearance. Aminoglycosides in combination with ceftibuten may increase nephrotoxic potential.

(Continued)

Ceftibuten *(Continued)*

Pharmacodynamics/Kinetics

Absorption: Rapid; food decreases peak concentrations, delays T_{max}, and lowers AUC

Distribution: V_d: Children: 0.5 L/kg; Adults: 0.21 L/kg

Half-life elimination: 2 hours

Time to peak: 2-3 hours

Excretion: Urine

Pregnancy Risk Factor B

Ceftin® *see* Cefuroxime *on page 289*

Ceftizoxime (sef ti ZOKS eem)

Related Information

Sexually-Transmitted Diseases *on page 1504*

U.S. Brand Names Cefizox®

Canadian Brand Names Cefizox®

Generic Available No

Synonyms Ceftizoxime Sodium

Pharmacologic Category Antibiotic, Cephalosporin (Third Generation)

Use Treatment of susceptible bacterial infection, mainly respiratory tract, skin and skin structure, bone and joint, urinary tract and gynecologic, as well as septicemia; active against many gram-negative bacilli (not *Pseudomonas*), some gram-positive cocci (not *Enterococcus*), and some anaerobes

Local Anesthetic/Vasoconstrictor Precautions No information available to require special precautions

Effects on Dental Treatment No significant effects or complications reported

Common Adverse Effects

1% to 10%:

Central nervous system: Fever

Dermatologic: Rash, pruritus

Hematologic: Eosinophilia, thrombocytosis

Hepatic: Elevated transaminases, alkaline phosphatase

Local: Pain, burning at injection site

Other reactions reported with cephalosporins include Stevens-Johnson syndrome, toxic epidermal necrolysis, erythema multiforme, pseudomembranous colitis, angioedema, hemolytic anemia, candidiasis, encephalopathy, asterixis, neuromuscular excitability, seizures, serum-sickness reactions, renal dysfunction, interstitial nephritis, toxic nephropathy, cholestasis, aplastic anemia, hemolytic anemia, pancytopenia, agranulocytosis, colitis, prolonged PT, hemorrhage, superinfection

Mechanism of Action Inhibits bacterial cell wall synthesis by binding to one or more of the penicillin-binding proteins (PBPs) which in turn inhibits the final transpeptidation step of peptidoglycan synthesis in bacterial cell walls, thus inhibiting cell wall biosynthesis. Bacteria eventually lyse due to ongoing activity of cell wall autolytic enzymes (autolysins and murein hydrolases) while cell wall assembly is arrested.

Drug Interactions

Increased Effect/Toxicity: Probenecid may decrease cephalosporin elimination. Furosemide, aminoglycosides in combination with ceftizoxime may result in additive nephrotoxicity.

Pharmacodynamics/Kinetics

Distribution: V_d: 0.35-0.5 L/kg; widely into most body tissues and fluids including gallbladder, liver, kidneys, bone, sputum, bile, pleural and synovial fluids; has good CSF penetration; crosses placenta; small amounts enter breast milk

Protein binding: 30%

Half-life elimination: 1.6 hours; Cl_{cr} <10 mL/minute: 25 hours

Time to peak, serum: I.M.: 0.5-1 hour

Excretion: Urine (as unchanged drug)

Pregnancy Risk Factor B

Ceftizoxime Sodium *see* Ceftizoxime *on page 288*

Ceftriaxone (sef trye AKS one)

Related Information

Animal and Human Bites Guidelines *on page 1582*

Sexually-Transmitted Diseases *on page 1504*

U.S. Brand Names Rocephin®

Canadian Brand Names Rocephin®

Mexican Brand Names Benaxona®; Cefaxona® [inj.]; Ceftrex® [inj.]; Rocephin®; Tacex® [inj.]; Terbac® [inj.]; Triakon® [inj.]

Generic Available No

Synonyms Ceftriaxone Sodium

Pharmacologic Category Antibiotic, Cephalosporin (Third Generation)

Use Treatment of lower respiratory tract infections, acute bacterial otitis media, skin and skin structure infections, bone and joint infections, intra-abdominal and urinary tract infections, sepsis and meningitis due to susceptible organisms; documented or suspected infection due to susceptible organisms in home care patients and patients without I.V. line access; treatment of documented or suspected gonococcal infection or chancroid; emergency room management of patients at high risk for bacteremia, periorbital or buccal cellulitis, salmonellosis or shigellosis, and pneumonia of unestablished etiology (<5 years of age); treatment of Lyme disease, depends on the stage of the disease (used in Stage II and Stage III, but not stage I; doxycycline is the drug of choice for Stage I)

Local Anesthetic/Vasoconstrictor Precautions No information available to require special precautions

Effects on Dental Treatment No significant effects or complications reported

Common Adverse Effects

1% to 10%:

- Dermatologic: Rash (2%)
- Gastrointestinal: Diarrhea (3%)
- Hematologic: Eosinophilia (6%), thrombocytosis (5%), leukopenia (2%)
- Hepatic: Elevated transaminases (3.1% to 3.3%)
- Local: Pain, induration at injection site (I.V. 1%); warmth, tightness, induration (5% to 17%) following I.M. injection
- Renal: Increased BUN (1%)

Mechanism of Action Inhibits bacterial cell wall synthesis by binding to one or more of the penicillin-binding proteins (PBPs) which in turn inhibits the final transpeptidation step of peptidoglycan synthesis in bacterial cell walls, thus inhibiting cell wall biosynthesis. Bacteria eventually lyse due to ongoing activity of cell wall autolytic enzymes (autolysins and murein hydrolases) while cell wall assembly is arrested.

Drug Interactions

Increased Effect/Toxicity: Aminoglycosides may result in synergistic antibacterial activity. High-dose probenecid decreases clearance. Aminoglycosides increase nephrotoxic potential.

Pharmacodynamics/Kinetics

Absorption: I.M.: Well absorbed

Distribution: Widely throughout the body including gallbladder, lungs, bone, bile, CSF (higher concentrations achieved when meninges are inflamed); crosses placenta; enters amniotic fluid and breast milk

Protein binding: 85% to 95%

Half-life elimination: Normal renal and hepatic function: 5-9 hours

Neonates: Postnatal: 1-4 days old: 16 hours; 9-30 days old: 9 hours

Time to peak, serum: I.M.: 1-2 hours

Excretion: Urine (33% to 65% as unchanged drug); feces

Pregnancy Risk Factor B

Ceftriaxone Sodium *see* Ceftriaxone *on page 288*

Cefuroxime (se fyoor OKS eem)

U.S. Brand Names Ceftin®; Zinacef®

Canadian Brand Names Apo-Cefuroxime®; Ceftin®; Kefurox®; ratio-Cefuroxime; Zinacef®

Mexican Brand Names Cefuracet®; Cetoxil® [tabs]; Cetoxil® [inj.]; Froxal® [inj.]; Zinnat®; Zinnat® [inj.]

Generic Available Yes

Synonyms Cefuroxime Axetil; Cefuroxime Sodium

Pharmacologic Category Antibiotic, Cephalosporin (Second Generation)

Use Treatment of infections caused by staphylococci, group B streptococci, *H. influenzae* (type A and B), *E. coli*, *Enterobacter*, *Salmonella*, and *Klebsiella*; treatment of susceptible infections of the lower respiratory tract, otitis media, urinary tract, skin and soft tissue, bone and joint, sepsis and gonorrhea

Local Anesthetic/Vasoconstrictor Precautions No information available to require special precautions

Effects on Dental Treatment No significant effects or complications reported

(Continued)

Cefuroxime *(Continued)*

Common Adverse Effects

1% to 10%:

Hematologic: Eosinophilia (7%), decreased hemoglobin and hematocrit (10%)

Hepatic: Increased transaminases (4%), increased alkaline phosphatase (2%)

Local: Thrombophlebitis (2%)

Reactions reported with other cephalosporins include agranulocytosis, aplastic anemia, asterixis, encephalopathy, hemorrhage, neuromuscular excitability, serum-sickness reactions, superinfection, toxic nephropathy

Mechanism of Action Inhibits bacterial cell wall synthesis by binding to one or more of the penicillin-binding proteins (PBPs) which in turn inhibits the final transpeptidation step of peptidoglycan synthesis in bacterial cell walls, thus inhibiting cell wall biosynthesis. Bacteria eventually lyse due to ongoing activity of cell wall autolytic enzymes (autolysins and murein hydrolases) while cell wall assembly is arrested.

Drug Interactions

Increased Effect/Toxicity: High-dose probenecid decreases clearance. Aminoglycosides in combination with cefuroxime may result in additive nephrotoxicity.

Pharmacodynamics/Kinetics

Absorption: Oral (cefuroxime axetil): Increases with food

Distribution: Widely to body tissues and fluids; crosses blood-brain barrier; therapeutic concentrations achieved in CSF even when meninges are not inflamed; crosses placenta; enters breast milk

Protein binding: 33% to 50%

Bioavailability: Tablet: Fasting: 37%; Following food: 52%

Half-life elimination: Adults: 1-2 hours; prolonged with renal impairment

Time to peak, serum: I.M.: ~15-60 minutes; I.V.: 2-3 minutes

Excretion: Urine (66% to 100% as unchanged drug)

Pregnancy Risk Factor B

Cefuroxime Axetil *see* Cefuroxime *on page 289*

Cefuroxime Sodium *see* Cefuroxime *on page 289*

Cefzil® *see* Cefprozil *on page 286*

Celebrex® *see* Celecoxib *on page 290*

Celecoxib (se le KOKS ib)

Related Information

Rheumatoid Arthritis, Osteoarthritis, and Osteoporosis *on page 1490*

U.S. Brand Names Celebrex®

Canadian Brand Names Celebrex®

Mexican Brand Names Celebrex®

Generic Available No

Pharmacologic Category Nonsteroidal Anti-inflammatory Drug (NSAID), COX-2 Selective

Use Relief of the signs and symptoms of osteoarthritis; relief of the signs and symptoms of rheumatoid arthritis in adults; decreasing intestinal polyps in familial adenomatous polyposis (FAP); management of acute pain; treatment of primary dysmenorrhea

Local Anesthetic/Vasoconstrictor Precautions No information available to require special precautions

Effects on Dental Treatment Key adverse event(s) related to dental treatment: Stomatitis, abnormal taste, xerostomia (normal salivary flow resumes upon discontinuation), and tooth disorder. Nonselective NSAIDs are known to reversibly decrease platelet aggregation via mechanisms different than observed with aspirin. According to the manufacturer, celecoxib, at single doses up to 800 mg and multiple doses of 600 mg twice daily, had no effect on platelet aggregation or bleeding time. Comparative NSAIDs (naproxen 500 mg twice daily, ibuprofen 800 mg three times daily or diclofenac 75 mg twice daily) significantly reduced platelet aggregation and prolonged the bleeding times.

Significant Adverse Effects

>10%: Central nervous system: Headache (15.8%)

2% to 10%:

Cardiovascular: Peripheral edema (2.1%)

Central nervous system: Insomnia (2.3%), dizziness (2%)

Dermatologic : Skin rash (2.2%)

Gastrointestinal: Dyspepsia (8.8%), diarrhea (5.6%), abdominal pain (4.1%), nausea (3.5%), flatulence (2.2%)

Neuromuscular & skeletal: Back pain (2.8%)
Respiratory: Upper respiratory tract infection (8.1%), sinusitis (5%), pharyngitis (2.3%), rhinitis (2%)
Miscellaneous: Accidental injury (2.9%)

<2%, postmarketing, and/or case reports (limited to important or life-threatening): Acute renal failure, agranulocytosis, albuminuria, allergic reactions, alopecia, anaphylactoid reactions, angioedema, aplastic anemia, arthralgia, aseptic meningitis, ataxia, bronchospasm, cerebrovascular accident, CHF, colitis, conjunctivitis, cystitis, deafness, diabetes mellitus, dyspnea, dysuria, ecchymosis, erythema multiforme, esophageal perforation, esophagitis, exfoliative dermatitis, flu-like syndrome, gangrene, gastroenteritis, gastroesophageal reflux, gastrointestinal bleeding, glaucoma, hematuria, hepatic failure, hepatitis, hypertension, hypoglycemia, hypokalemia, hyponatremia, interstitial nephritis, intestinal perforation, jaundice, leukopenia, melena, migraine, myalgia, myocardial infarction, neuralgia, neuropathy, pancreatitis, pancytopenia, paresthesia, photosensitivity, prostate disorder, pulmonary embolism, rash, renal calculi, sepsis, Stevens-Johnson syndrome, stomatitis, sudden death, syncope, thrombophlebitis, tinnitus, toxic epidermal necrolysis, urticaria, vaginal bleeding, vaginitis, vasculitis, ventricular fibrillation, vertigo, vomiting

Dosage Adults: Oral:

Acute pain or primary dysmenorrhea: Initial dose: 400 mg, followed by an additional 200 mg if needed on day 1; maintenance dose: 200 mg twice daily as needed

Familial adenomatous polyposis (FAP): 400 mg twice daily

Osteoarthritis: 200 mg/day as a single dose or in divided dose twice daily

Rheumatoid arthritis: 100-200 mg twice daily

Elderly: No specific adjustment is recommended. However, the AUC in elderly patients may be increased by 50% as compared to younger subjects. Use the lowest recommended dose in patients weighing <50 kg.

Dosing adjustment in renal impairment: No specific dosage adjustment is recommended; not recommended in patients with advanced renal disease

Dosing adjustment in hepatic impairment: Reduced dosage is recommended (AUC may be increased by 40% to 180%); decrease dose by 50% in patients with moderate hepatic impairment (Child-Pugh Class II)

Mechanism of Action Inhibits prostaglandin synthesis by decreasing the activity of the enzyme, cyclooxygenase-2 (COX-2), which results in decreased formation of prostaglandin precursors. Celecoxib does not inhibit cyclooxygenase-1 (COX-1) at therapeutic concentrations.

Contraindications Hypersensitivity to celecoxib, any component of the formulation, sulfonamides, aspirin, or other NSAIDs; pregnancy (3rd trimester)

Warnings/Precautions Gastrointestinal irritation, ulceration, bleeding, and perforation may occur with NSAIDs (it is unclear whether celecoxib is associated with rates of these events which are similar to nonselective NSAIDs). Use with caution in patients with a history of GI disease (bleeding or ulcers), use lowest dose for shortest time possible. Use with caution in patients with decreased renal function, hepatic disease, CHF, hypertension, or asthma. Anaphylactoid reactions may occur, even with no prior exposure to celecoxib. Use caution in patients with known or suspected deficiency of cytochrome P450 isoenzyme 2C9. Safety and efficacy have not been established in patients <18 years of age.

Drug Interactions **Substrate** (minor) of CYP2C8/9, 3A4; **Inhibits** CYP2D6 (weak)

ACE inhibitors: Antihypertensive effect may be diminished by celecoxib.

Aspirin: Low-dose aspirin may be used with celecoxib, however, monitor for GI complications.

Fluconazole: Fluconazole increases celecoxib concentrations twofold. Lowest dose of celecoxib should be used.

Lithium: Plasma levels of lithium are increased by ~17% when used with celecoxib. Monitor lithium levels closely when treatment with celecoxib is started or withdrawn.

Loop diuretics (bumetanide, furosemide, torsemide): Natriuretic effect of furosemide and other loop diuretics may be decreased by celecoxib.

Methotrexate: Severe bone marrow suppression, aplastic anemia, and GI toxicity have been reported with concomitant NSAID therapy. Selective COX-2 inhibitors appear to have a lower risk of this toxicity, however, caution is warranted.

Thiazide diuretics: Natriuretic effects of thiazide diuretics may be decreased by celecoxib.

Warfarin: Bleeding events and increased prothrombin time have been reported with concomitant use. Monitor closely, especially in the elderly.

(Continued)

Celecoxib *(Continued)*

Ethanol/Nutrition/Herb Interactions

Ethanol: Avoid ethanol (increased GI irritation).

Food: Peak concentrations are delayed and AUC is increased by 10% to 20% when taken with a high-fat meal.

Dietary Considerations Lower doses (200 mg twice daily) may be taken without regard to meals. Larger doses should be taken with food to improve absorption.

Pharmacodynamics/Kinetics

Distribution: V_d (apparent): 400 L

Protein binding: 97% to albumin

Metabolism: Hepatic via CYP2C9; forms inactive metabolites

Bioavailability: Absolute: Unknown

Half-life elimination: 11 hours

Time to peak: 3 hours

Excretion: Urine (as metabolites, <3% as unchanged drug)

Pregnancy Risk Factor C/D (3rd trimester)

Lactation Enters breast milk/not recommended

Breast-Feeding Considerations Based on limited data, celecoxib has been found to be excreted in milk; a decision should be made whether to discontinue nursing or discontinue the drug, taking into account the importance of the drug to the mother.

Dosage Forms Capsule: 100 mg, 200 mg, 400 mg

Comments According to the manufacturer, two out of 5,285 patients (0.04%) experienced significant upper GI bleeding, at 14 and 32 days after initiation of dosing. Approximately 40% of the 5,285 patients were in studies that required them to be free of ulcers by endoscopy at entry into the study. As a result, the manufacturer stressed that it is unclear if the study population is representative of the general population. As of this printing, long-term studies comparing the incidence of serious upper GI adverse effects in patients taking celecoxib compared to other nonselective NSAIDs had not been reported. Celecoxib does not appear to inhibit platelet aggregation at recommended doses. Reports have shown that celecoxib does not generally affect platelet counts, prothrombin time or partial thromboplastin time (PTT).

Cross-reactivity, including bronchospasm, between aspirin and other NSAIDs has been reported in aspirin-sensitive patients. The manufacturer suggests that celecoxib should not be administered to patients with this type of aspirin sensitivity and should be used with caution in patients with pre-existing asthma.

The manufacturer studied the effect of celecoxib on the anticoagulant effect of warfarin and found no alteration of anticoagulant effect, as determined by prothrombin time, in patients taking 2 mg to 5 mg daily. However, the manufacturer has issued a caution when using celecoxib with warfarin since those patients are at increased risk of bleeding complications.

A literature report suggested that the enzyme COX-2 (cyclo-oxygenase type 2) is a major source of systemic prostacyclin biosynthesis in humans. Prostacyclin is involved in blood vessel dilation and inhibition of blood clotting. In view of the fact that celecoxib inhibits the COX-2 enzyme, prostacyclin production could be suppressed. The resultant effects on hemostasis are unknown at this time.

Recent news reports have noted an association between selective COX-2 inhibitors and increased cardiovascular risk. This was prompted by publication of a meta-analysis entitled "Risk of Cardiovascular Events Associated With Selective COX-2 Inhibitors" in the August 22, 2001, edition of the *Journal of the American Medical Association* (JAMA), viewable at http://jama.ama-assn.org/issues/v286n8/rfull/jsc10193.html. The researchers reanalyzed four previously published trials, assessing cardiovascular events in patients receiving either celecoxib or rofecoxib. They found an association between the use of COX-2 inhibitors and cardiovascular events (including MI and ischemic stroke). The annualized MI rate was found to be significantly higher in patients receiving celecoxib or rofecoxib than in the control (placebo) group from a recent meta-analysis of primary prevention trials. Although cause and effect cannot be established (these trials were originally designed to assess GI effects, not cardiovascular ones), the authors believe the available data raise a cautionary flag concerning the risk of cardiovascular events with the use of COX-2 inhibitors. The manufacturers of these agents, as well as other healthcare professionals, dispute the methods and validity of the study's conclusions. To date, the FDA has not required any change in the labeling of these agents. Further study is required before any potential risk may be defined.

Selected Readings

Dionne R, "COX-2 Inhibitors: Better Than Ibuprofen for Dental Pain?" *Compend Contin Educ Dent*, 1999, 20(6):518-20, 522-4.

Doyle G, Jayawardena S, Ashraf E, et al, "Efficacy and Tolerability of Nonprescription Ibuprofen Versus Celecoxib for Dental Pain," *J Clin Pharmacol*, 2002, 42(8):912-9.

Everts B, Wahrborg P, Hedner T, "COX-2 Specific Inhibitors - The Emergence of a New Class of Analgesic and Anti-inflammatory Drugs," *Clin Rheumatol*, 2000, 19(5):331-43.

Jeske AH, "COX-2 Inhibitors and Dental Pain Control," *J Gt Houst Dent Soc*, 1999, 71(4):39-40.

Jeske AH, "Selecting New Drugs for Pain Control: Evidence-Based Decisions or Clinical Impressions?" *J Am Dent Assoc*, 2002, 133(8):1052-6.

Jouzeau JY, Terlain B, Abid A, et al, "Cyclo-oxygenase Isoenzymes. How Recent Findings Affect Thinking About Nonsteroidal Anti-inflammatory Drugs," *Drugs*, 1997, 53(4):563-82.

Kaplan-Machlis B and Klostermeyer BS, "The Cyclo-oxygenase-2 Inhibitors: Safety and Effectiveness," *Ann Pharmacother*, 1999, 33(9):979-88.

Kellstein D, Ott D, Jayawardene S, et al, "Analgesic Efficacy of a Single Dose of Lumiracoxib Compared With Rofecoxib, Celecoxib and Placebo in the Treatment of Post-Operative Dental Pain," *Int J Clin Pract*, 2004, 58(3):244-50.

Kurumbail RG, Stevens AM, Gierse JK, et al, "Structural Basis for Selective Inhibition of Cyclo-oxygenase-2 By Anti-inflammatory Agents," *Nature*, 1996, 384(6610):644-8.

Malmstrom K, Daniels S, Kotey P, et al, "Comparison of Rofecoxib and Celecoxib, Two Cyclooxygenase-2 Inhibitors, in Postoperative Dental Pain: A Randomized Placebo- and Active-Comparator-Controlled Clinical Trial," *Clin Ther*, 1999, 21(10):1653-63.

McAdam BF, Catella-Lawson F, Mardini IA, et al, "Systemic Biosynthesis of Prostacyclin by Cyclo-oxygenase (COX)-2: The Human Pharmacology of a Selective Inhibitor of COX-2," *Proc Natl Acad Sci U S A*, 1999, 96(1):272-7.

Moore PA and Hersh EV, "Celecoxib and Rofecoxib. The Role of COX-2 Inhibitors in Dental Practice," *J Am Dent Assoc*, 2001, 132(4):451-6.

Needleman P and Isakson PC, "The Discovery and Function of COX-2," *J Rheumatol*, 1997, 24(S49):6-8.

Whelton A, Maurath CJ, Verburg KM, et al, "Renal Safety and Tolerability of Celecoxib, a Novel Cyclo-oxygenase-2 Inhibitor," *Am J Ther*, 2000, 7(3):159-75.

Wynn RL, "The New COX-2 Inhibitors: Celecoxib and Rofecoxib," *Home Health Care Consultant*, 2001, 8(10):24-31.

Wynn RL, "The New COX-2 Inhibitors: Rofecoxib (Vioxx®) and Celecoxib (Celebrex™)," *Gen Dent*, 2000, 48(1):16-20.

Wynn RL, "NSAIDS and Cardiovascular Effects, Celecoxib for Dental Pain, and a New Analgesic - Tramadol With Acetaminophen," *Gen Dent*, 2002, 50(3):218-222.

Celestone® *see* Betamethasone *on page 199*

Celestone® Soluspan® *see* Betamethasone *on page 199*

Celexa™ *see* Citalopram *on page 339*

CellCept® *see* Mycophenolate *on page 952*

Cellulose (Oxidized/Regenerated)

(SEL yoo lose, OKS i dyzed re JEN er aye ted)

U.S. Brand Names Surgicel®

Generic Available No

Synonyms Absorbable Cotton; Oxidized Regenerated Cellulose

Pharmacologic Category Hemostatic Agent

Dental Use To control bleeding created during a dental procedure

Use Hemostatic; temporary packing for the control of capillary, venous, or small arterial hemorrhage

Local Anesthetic/Vasoconstrictor Precautions No information available to require special precautions

Effects on Dental Treatment No significant effects or complications reported

Significant Adverse Effects 1% to 10%:

Central nervous system: Headache

Respiratory: Nasal burning or stinging, sneezing (rhinological procedures)

Miscellaneous: Encapsulation of fluid, foreign body reactions (with or without) infection

Dosage Minimal amounts of the fabric strip are laid on the bleeding site or held firmly against the tissues until hemostasis occurs

Mechanism of Action Cellulose, oxidized regenerated is saturated with blood at the bleeding site and swells into a brownish or black gelatinous mass which aids in the formation of a clot. When used in small amounts, it is absorbed from the sites of implantation with little or no tissue reaction.

Warnings/Precautions Autoclaving causes physical breakdown of the product. Closing the material in a contaminated wound without drainage may lead to complications. The material should not be moistened before insertion since the hemostatic effect is greater when applied dry. The material should not be impregnated with anti-infective agents. Its hemostatic effect is not enhanced by the addition of thrombin. The material may be left *in situ* when necessary but it is advisable to remove it once hemostasis is achieved.

Drug Interactions No data reported

Pregnancy Risk Factor No data reported

(Continued)

Cellulose (Oxidized/Regenerated) *(Continued)*

Dosage Forms

Strip, oxidized regenerated cellulose [absorbable hemostat]:
- Surgicel®:
  - 1/2" x 2" (24s)
  - 2" x 3" (24s)
  - 2" x 14" (24s)
  - 4" x 8" (24s)
- Surgicel® NU-KNIT:
  - 1" x 1" (24s)
  - 1" x 3 1/2" (10s)
  - 3" x 4" (24s)
  - 6" x 9" (10s)
- Surgicel® Fibrillar:
  - 1" x 2" (10s)
  - 2" x 4" (10s)
  - 4" x 4" (10s)

Cellulose Sodium Phosphate

(sel yoo lose SOW dee um FOS fate)

U.S. Brand Names Calcibind®

Canadian Brand Names Calcibind®

Generic Available No

Synonyms CSP; Sodium Cellulose Phosphate

Pharmacologic Category Urinary Tract Product

Use Adjunct to dietary restriction to reduce renal calculi formation in absorptive hypercalciuria type I

Local Anesthetic/Vasoconstrictor Precautions No information available to require special precautions

Effects on Dental Treatment No significant effects or complications reported

Pregnancy Risk Factor C

Celontin® *see* Methsuximide *on page 904*

Cenestin® *see* Estrogens (Conjugated A/Synthetic) *on page 524*

Centrum® [OTC] *see* Vitamins (Multiple/Oral) *on page 1384*

Centrum® Performance™ [OTC] *see* Vitamins (Multiple/Oral) *on page 1384*

Centrum® Silver® [OTC] *see* Vitamins (Multiple/Oral) *on page 1384*

Cēpacol® Gold [OTC] *see* Cetylpyridinium *on page 301*

Cēpacol® Maximum Strength [OTC] *see* Dyclonine *on page 480*

Cēpacol Viractin® [OTC] *see* Tetracaine *on page 1278*

Cēpastat® [OTC] *see* Phenol *on page 1075*

Cēpastat® Extra Strength [OTC] *see* Phenol *on page 1075*

Cephalexin (sef a LEKS in)

Related Information

Antibiotic Prophylaxis, Preprocedural Guidelines for Dental Patients *on page 1509*

Oral Bacterial Infections *on page 1533*

U.S. Brand Names Biocef®; Keflex®; Panixine DisperDose™

Canadian Brand Names Apo-Cephalex®; Keftab®; Novo-Lexin®; Nu-Cephalex

Generic Available Yes

Synonyms Cephalexin Monohydrate

Pharmacologic Category Antibiotic, Cephalosporin (First Generation)

Dental Use Prophylaxis in total joint replacement patients undergoing dental procedures which produce bacteremia; alternative antibiotic for prevention of bacterial endocarditis

Note: Individuals allergic to amoxicillin (penicillins) may receive cephalexin provided they have not had an immediate, local, or systemic IgE-mediated anaphylactic allergic reaction to penicillin.

Use Treatment of susceptible bacterial infections including respiratory tract infections, otitis media, skin and skin structure infections, bone infections and genitourinary tract infections, including acute prostatitis; alternative therapy for acute bacterial endocarditis prophylaxis

Local Anesthetic/Vasoconstrictor Precautions No information available to require special precautions

Effects on Dental Treatment No significant effects or complications reported

Significant Adverse Effects Frequency not defined.

Central nervous system: Agitation, confusion, dizziness, fatigue, hallucinations, headache

Dermatologic: Angioedema, erythema multiforme (rare), rash, Stevens-Johnson syndrome (rare), toxic epidermal necrolysis (rare), urticaria
Gastrointestinal: Abdominal pain, diarrhea, dyspepsia, gastritis, nausea (rare), pseudomembranous colitis, vomiting (rare)
Genitourinary: Genital pruritus, genital moniliasis, vaginitis, vaginal discharge
Hematologic: Eosinophilia, neutropenia, thrombocytopenia
Hepatic: AST/ALT increased, cholestatic jaundice (rare), transient hepatitis (rare)
Neuromuscular & skeletal: Arthralgia, arthritis, joint disorder
Renal: Interstitial nephritis (rare)
Miscellaneous: Allergic reactions

Dosage Oral:

Children >1 year: Dosing range: 25-50 mg/kg/day every 6-8 hours; more severe infections: 50-100 mg/kg/day in divided doses every 6-8 hours; maximum: 4 g/24 hours
Otitis media: 75-100 mg/kg/day in 4 divided doses
Streptococcal pharyngitis, skin and skin structure infections: 25-50 mg/kg/day divided every 12 hours
Uncomplicated cystitis: Children >15 years: Refer to Adults dosing
Prophylaxis of bacterial endocarditis (dental, oral, respiratory tract, or esophageal procedures): 50 mg/kg 1 hour prior to procedure (maximum: 2 g)

Adults: Dosing range: 250-1000 mg every 6 hours; maximum: 4 g/day
Streptococcal pharyngitis, skin and skin structure infections: 500 mg every 12 hours
Uncomplicated cystitis: 500 mg every 12 hours for 7-14 days
Prophylaxis of bacterial endocarditis (dental, oral, respiratory tract, or esophageal procedures): 2 g 1 hour prior to procedure

Dosing adjustment in renal impairment: Adults: Cl_{cr} <10 mL/minute: 250-500 mg every 12 hours
Hemodialysis: Moderately dialyzable (20% to 50%)

Mechanism of Action Inhibits bacterial cell wall synthesis by binding to one or more of the penicillin-binding proteins (PBPs) which in turn inhibits the final transpeptidation step of peptidoglycan synthesis in bacterial cell walls, thus inhibiting cell wall biosynthesis. Bacteria eventually lyse due to ongoing activity of cell wall autolytic enzymes (autolysins and murein hydrolases) while cell wall assembly is arrested.

Contraindications Hypersensitivity to cephalexin, any component of the formulation, or other cephalosporins

Warnings/Precautions Modify dosage in patients with severe renal impairment, prolonged use may result in superinfection; use with caution in patients with a history of penicillin allergy, especially IgE-mediated reactions (eg, anaphylaxis, urticaria). May cause antibiotic-associated colitis or colitis secondary to *C. difficile*.

Drug Interactions

Aminoglycosides: Increase nephrotoxic potential.
Probenecid: High-dose probenecid decreases clearance of cephalexin.

Ethanol/Nutrition/Herb Interactions Food: Peak antibiotic serum concentration is lowered and delayed, but total drug absorbed is not affected. Cephalexin serum levels may be decreased if taken with food.

Dietary Considerations Take without regard to food. If GI distress, take with food. Panixine DisperDose™ contains phenylalanine 2.8 mg/cephalexin 125 mg.

Pharmacodynamics/Kinetics

Absorption: Delayed in young children
Distribution: Widely into most body tissues and fluids, including gallbladder, liver, kidneys, bone, sputum, bile, and pleural and synovial fluids; CSF penetration is poor; crosses placenta; enters breast milk
Protein binding: 6% to 15%
Half-life elimination: Adults: 0.5-1.2 hours; prolonged with renal impairment
Time to peak, serum: ~1 hour
Excretion: Urine (80% to 100% as unchanged drug) within 8 hours

Pregnancy Risk Factor B

Lactation Enters breast milk (small amounts)/use caution

Breast-Feeding Considerations Theoretically, drug absorbed by nursing infant may change bowel flora or affect fever work-up result. Cephalexin levels can be detected in breast milk, reaching a maximum concentration 4 hours after a single oral dose and gradually decreasing by 8 hours after administration. **Note:** As a class, cephalosporins are used to treat bacterial infections in infants.

Dosage Forms

Capsule: 250 mg, 500 mg
(Continued)

Cephalexin *(Continued)*

Biocef®: 500 mg
Keflex®: 250 mg, 500 mg

Powder for oral suspension: 125 mg/5 mL (100 mL, 200 mL); 250 mg/5 mL (100 mL, 200 mL)
Biocef®: 125 mg/5 mL (100 mL); 250 mg/5 mL (100 mL)

Tablet, for oral suspension (Panixine DisperDose™): 125 mg [contains phenylalanine 2.8 mg; peppermint flavor], 250 mg [contains phenylalanine 5.6 mg; peppermint flavor]

Selected Readings

ADA Division of Legal Affairs, "A Legal Perspective on Antibiotic Prophylaxis," *J Am Dent Assoc*, 2003, 134(9):1260.

"Advisory Statement. Antibiotic Prophylaxis for Dental Patients With Total Joint Replacements. American Dental Association; American Academy of Orthopedic Surgeons," *J Am Dent Assoc*, 1997, 128(7):1004-8.

American Dental Association; American Academy of Orthopedic Surgeons, "Antibiotic Prophylaxis for Dental Patients With Total Joint Replacements," *J Am Dent Assoc*, 2003, 134(7):895-9.

American Dental Association Council on Scientific Affairs, "Combating Antibiotic Resistance," *J Am Dent Assoc*, 2004, 135(4):484-7.

Dajani AS, Taubert KA, Wilson W, et al, "Prevention of Bacterial Endocarditis. Recommendations by the American Heart Association," *JAMA*, 1997, 277(22):1794-801.

Dajani AS, Taubert KA, Wilson W, et al, "Prevention of Bacterial Endocarditis: Recommendations by the American Heart Association," *J Am Dent Assoc*, 1997, 128(8):1142-51.

Saxon A, Beall GN, Rohr AS, et al, "Immediate Hypersensitivity Reactions to Beta-Lactam Antibiotics," *Ann Intern Med*, 1987, 107(2):204-15.

Wynn RL, Bergman SA, Meiller TF, et al, "Antibiotics in Treating Oral-Facial Infections of Odontogenic Origin: An Update," *Gen Dent*, 2001, 49(3):238-40, 242, 244 passim.

Cephalexin Monohydrate *see* Cephalexin *on page 294*

Cephalothin (sef A loe thin)

Generic Available Yes

Synonyms Cephalothin Sodium

Pharmacologic Category Antibiotic, Cephalosporin (First Generation)

Use Treatment of infections when caused by susceptible strains in respiratory, genitourinary, gastrointestinal, skin and soft tissue, bone and joint infections; septicemia; treatment of susceptible gram-positive bacilli and cocci (never enterococcus); some gram-negative bacilli including *E. coli*, *Proteus*, and *Klebsiella* may be susceptible

Local Anesthetic/Vasoconstrictor Precautions No information available to require special precautions

Effects on Dental Treatment No significant effects or complications reported

Common Adverse Effects Frequency not defined.

Dermatologic: Maculopapular and erythematous rash
Gastrointestinal: Diarrhea, nausea, vomiting, dyspepsia, pseudomembranous colitis
Local: Bleeding, pain and induration at injection site

Reactions reported with other cephalosporins include anaphylaxis, erythema multiforme, toxic epidermal necrolysis, Stevens-Johnson syndrome, dizziness, fever, headache, CNS irritability, seizures, decreased hemoglobin, neutropenia, leukopenia, agranulocytosis, pancytopenia, aplastic anemia, hemolytic anemia, interstitial nephritis, toxic nephropathy, vaginitis, angioedema, cholestasis, hemorrhage, prolonged PT, serum-sickness reactions, superinfection

Mechanism of Action Inhibits bacterial cell wall synthesis by binding to one or more of the penicillin-binding proteins (PBPs) which in turn inhibits the final transpeptidation step of peptidoglycan synthesis in bacterial cell walls, thus inhibiting cell wall biosynthesis. Bacteria eventually lyse due to ongoing activity of cell wall autolytic enzymes (autolysins and murein hydrolases) while cell wall assembly is arrested.

Pharmacodynamics/Kinetics

Distribution: Does not penetrate CSF unless meninges are inflamed; crosses placenta; small amounts enter breast milk
Protein binding: 65% to 80%
Metabolism: Partially hepatic and renal via deacetylation
Half-life elimination: 30-60 minutes
Excretion: Urine (50% to 75% as unchanged drug)

Pregnancy Risk Factor B

Cephalothin Sodium *see* Cephalothin *on page 296*

Cephradine (SEF ra deen)

Related Information

Antibiotic Prophylaxis, Preprocedural Guidelines for Dental Patients *on page 1509*

U.S. Brand Names Velosef®

Generic Available No

Pharmacologic Category Antibiotic, Cephalosporin (First Generation)

Dental Use Prophylaxis in total joint replacement patients undergoing dental procedures which produce bacteremia

Use Treatment of infections when caused by susceptible strains in respiratory, genitourinary, gastrointestinal, skin and soft tissue, bone and joint infections; treatment of susceptible gram-positive bacilli and cocci (never enterococcus); some gram-negative bacilli including *E. coli*, *Proteus*, and *Klebsiella* may be susceptible

Local Anesthetic/Vasoconstrictor Precautions No information available to require special precautions

Effects on Dental Treatment No significant effects or complications reported

Significant Adverse Effects Frequency not defined.

Central nervous system: Dizziness
Dermatologic: Rash, pruritus
Gastrointestinal: Diarrhea, nausea, vomiting, pseudomembranous colitis
Hematologic: Leukopenia, neutropenia, eosinophilia
Neuromuscular & skeletal: Joint pain
Renal: BUN increased, creatinine increased

Reactions reported with other cephalosporins include anaphylaxis, erythema multiforme, toxic epidermal necrolysis, Stevens-Johnson syndrome, fever, headache, encephalopathy, asterixis, neuromuscular excitability, seizures, agranulocytosis, pancytopenia, aplastic anemia, hemolytic anemia, interstitial nephritis, toxic nephropathy, vaginitis, angioedema, cholestasis, hemorrhage, prolonged PT, serum-sickness reactions, superinfection

Dosage Oral:

Children ≥9 months: Usual dose: 25-50 mg/kg/day in divided doses every 6 hours
  Otitis media: 75-100 mg/kg/day in divided doses every 6 or 12 hours (maximum: 4 g/day)
Adults: 250-500 mg every 6-12 hours
Dosing adjustment in renal impairment: Adults:
  Cl_{cr} 10-50 mL/minute: 250 mg every 6 hours
  Cl_{cr} <10 mL/minute: 125 mg every 6 hours

Mechanism of Action Inhibits bacterial cell wall synthesis by binding to one or more of the penicillin-binding proteins (PBPs) which in turn inhibits the final transpeptidation step of peptidoglycan synthesis in bacterial cell walls, thus inhibiting cell wall biosynthesis. Bacteria eventually lyse due to ongoing activity of cell wall autolytic enzymes (autolysins and murein hydrolases) while cell wall assembly is arrested.

Contraindications Hypersensitivity to cephradine, any component of the formulation, or cephalosporins

Warnings/Precautions Use caution with renal impairment; dose adjustment required. Prolonged use may result in superinfection; use with caution in patients with a history of penicillin allergy, especially IgE-mediated reactions (eg, anaphylaxis, urticaria). May cause antibiotic-associated colitis or colitis secondary to *C. difficile*.

Drug Interactions

Increased effect: High-dose probenecid decreases clearance
Increased toxicity: Aminoglycosides may increase nephrotoxic potential

Ethanol/Nutrition/Herb Interactions Food: Food delays cephradine absorption but does not decrease extent.

Dietary Considerations May administer with food to decrease GI distress.

Pharmacodynamics/Kinetics

Absorption: Well absorbed
Distribution: Widely into most body tissues and fluids including gallbladder, liver, kidneys, bone, sputum, bile, and pleural and synovial fluids; CSF penetration is poor; crosses placenta; enters breast milk
Protein binding: 18% to 20%
Half-life elimination: 1-2 hours; prolonged with renal impairment
Time to peak, serum: 1-2 hours
Excretion: Urine (~80% to 90% as unchanged drug) within 6 hours

Pregnancy Risk Factor B

Lactation Enters breast milk/use caution

Breast-Feeding Considerations Theoretically, drug absorbed by nursing infant may change bowel flora or affect fever work-up result. **Note:** As a class, cephalosporins are used to treat infections in infants.

Dosage Forms [DSC] = Discontinued product

Capsule: 250 mg, 500 mg [DSC]

(Continued)

Cephradine *(Continued)*

Powder for oral suspension: 250 mg/5 mL (100 mL) [fruit flavor]

Selected Readings

ADA Division of Legal Affairs, "A Legal Perspective on Antibiotic Prophylaxis," *J Am Dent Assoc*, 2003, 134(9):1260.

"Advisory Statement. Antibiotic Prophylaxis for Dental Patients With Total Joint Replacements. American Dental Association; American Academy of Orthopedic Surgeons," *J Am Dent Assoc*, 1997, 128(7):1004-8.

American Dental Association; American Academy of Orthopedic Surgeons, "Antibiotic Prophylaxis for Dental Patients With Total Joint Replacements," *J Am Dent Assoc*, 2003, 134(7):895-9.

American Dental Association Council on Scientific Affairs, "Combating Antibiotic Resistance," *J Am Dent Assoc*, 2004, 135(4):484-7.

Donowitz GR and Mandell GL, "Drug Therapy. Beta-Lactam Antibiotics (1)," *N Engl J Med*, 1988, 318(7):419-26.

Donowitz GR and Mandell GL, "Drug Therapy. Beta-Lactam Antibiotics (2)," *N Engl J Med*, 1988, 318(8):490-500.

Gustaferro CA and Steckelberg JM, "Cephalosporin Antimicrobial Agents and Related Compounds," *Mayo Clin Proc*, 1991, 66(10):1064-73.

Ceptaz® [DSC] *see* Ceftazidime *on page 286*

Cerebyx® *see* Fosphenytoin *on page 635*

Ceredase® *see* Alglucerase *on page 80*

Cerezyme® *see* Imiglucerase *on page 736*

Cerubidine® *see* DAUNOrubicin Hydrochloride *on page 401*

Cerumenex® *see* Triethanolamine Polypeptide Oleate-Condensate *on page 1338*

Cervidil® *see* Dinoprostone *on page 447*

C.E.S. *see* Estrogens (Conjugated/Equine) *on page 525*

Cetacaine® *see* Benzocaine, Butyl Aminobenzoate, Tetracaine, and Benzalkonium Chloride *on page 193*

Cetacort® *see* Hydrocortisone *on page 714*

Cetafen® [OTC] *see* Acetaminophen *on page 47*

Cetafen Cold® [OTC] *see* Acetaminophen and Pseudoephedrine *on page 53*

Cetafen Extra® [OTC] *see* Acetaminophen *on page 47*

Ceta-Plus® *see* Hydrocodone and Acetaminophen *on page 702*

Cetirizine (se TI ra zeen)

U.S. Brand Names Zyrtec®

Canadian Brand Names Apo-Cetirizine®; Reactine™

Mexican Brand Names Virlix®; Zyrtec®

Generic Available No

Synonyms Cetirizine Hydrochloride; P-071; UCB-P071

Pharmacologic Category Antihistamine

Use Perennial and seasonal allergic rhinitis and other allergic symptoms including urticaria; chronic idiopathic urticaria

Local Anesthetic/Vasoconstrictor Precautions No information available to require special precautions

Effects on Dental Treatment Key adverse event(s) related to dental treatment: Xerostomia and increased salivation (normal salivary flow resumes upon discontinuation), stomatitis, loss of taste, abnormal taste, tongue discoloration, and ulcerative stomatitis.

Common Adverse Effects

>10%: Central nervous system: Headache (children 11% to 14%, placebo 12%), somnolence (adults 14%, children 2% to 4%)

2% to 10%:

- Central nervous system: Insomnia (children 9%, adults <2%), fatigue (adults 6%), malaise (4%), dizziness (adults 2%)
- Gastrointestinal: Abdominal pain (children 4% to 6%), dry mouth (adults 5%), diarrhea (children 2% to 3%), nausea (children 2% to 3%, placebo 2%), vomiting (children 2% to 3%)
- Respiratory: Epistaxis (children 2% to 4%, placebo 3%), pharyngitis (children 3% to 6%, placebo 3%), bronchospasm (children 2% to 3%, placebo 2%)

Dosage Oral:

Children:

- 6-12 months: Chronic urticaria, perennial allergic rhinitis: 2.5 mg once daily
- 12 months to <2 years: Chronic urticaria, perennial allergic rhinitis: 2.5 mg once daily; may increase to 2.5 mg every 12 hours if needed
- 2-5 years: Chronic urticaria, perennial or seasonal allergic rhinitis: Initial: 2.5 mg once daily; may be increased to 2.5 mg every 12 hours **or** 5 mg once daily

Children ≥6 years and Adults: Chronic urticaria, perennial or seasonal allergic rhinitis: 5-10 mg once daily, depending upon symptom severity

Elderly Initial: 5 mg once daily; may increase to 10 mg/day. **Note:** Manufacturer recommends 5 mg/day in patients ≥77 years of age.

Dosage adjustment in renal/hepatic impairment:

Children <6 years: Cetirizine use not recommended

Children 6-11 years: <2.5 mg once daily

Children ≥12 and Adults:

Cl_{cr} 11-31 mL/minute, hemodialysis, or hepatic impairment: Administer 5 mg once daily

Cl_{cr} <11 mL/minute, not on dialysis: Cetirizine use not recommended

Mechanism of Action Competes with histamine for H_1-receptor sites on effector cells in the gastrointestinal tract, blood vessels, and respiratory tract

Contraindications Hypersensitivity to cetirizine, hydroxyzine, or any component of the formulation

Warnings/Precautions Cetirizine should be used cautiously in patients with hepatic or renal dysfunction, the elderly and in nursing mothers. May cause drowsiness, use caution performing tasks which require alertness (eg, operating machinery or driving). Safety and efficacy in pediatric patients <6 months have not been established.

Drug Interactions

Cytochrome P450 Effect: Substrate of CYP3A4 (minor)

Increased Effect/Toxicity: Increased toxicity with CNS depressants and anticholinergics.

Ethanol/Nutrition/Herb Interactions Ethanol: Avoid ethanol (may increase CNS depression).

Dietary Considerations May be taken with or without food.

Pharmacodynamics/Kinetics

Onset of action: 15-30 minutes

Absorption: Rapid

Protein binding, plasma: Mean: 93%

Metabolism: Limited hepatic

Half-life elimination: 8 hours

Time to peak, serum: 1 hour

Excretion: Urine (70%); feces (10%)

Pregnancy Risk Factor B

Dosage Forms SYR: 5 mg/5 mL (120 mL, 480 mL). **TAB:** 5 mg, 10 mg. **TAB, chewable:** 5 mg, 10 mg

Cetirizine and Pseudoephedrine

(se TI ra zeen & soo doe e FED rin)

Related Information

Cetirizine *on page 298*

Pseudoephedrine *on page 1147*

U.S. Brand Names Zyrtec-D 12 Hour™

Canadian Brand Names Reactine® Allergy and Sinus

Generic Available No

Synonyms Cetirizine Hydrochloride and Pseudoephedrine Hydrochloride; Pseudoephedrine Hydrochloride and Cetirizine Hydrochloride

Pharmacologic Category Antihistamine/Decongestant Combination

Use Treatment of symptoms of seasonal or perennial allergic rhinitis

Local Anesthetic/Vasoconstrictor Precautions Use with caution since pseudoephedrine is a sympathomimetic amine which could interact with epinephrine to cause a pressor response

Effects on Dental Treatment Key adverse event(s) related to dental treatment: Pseudoephedrine: Xerostomia (normal salivary flow resumes upon discontinuation).

Common Adverse Effects Percentages reported with combination product. Additional adverse effects reported; refer to individual monographs.

1% to 10%:

Central nervous system: Insomnia (4%), fatigue (2%), somnolence (2%), dizziness (1%)

Gastrointestinal: Xerostomia (4%)

Respiratory: Pharyngitis (2%), epistaxis (1%)

Mechanism of Action Cetirizine is an antihistamine; exhibits selective inhibition of H_1 receptors. Pseudoephedrine is a sympathomimetic and exerts a decongestant action on nasal mucosa.

(Continued)

Cetirizine and Pseudoephedrine *(Continued)*

Drug Interactions

Cytochrome P450 Effect: Cetirizine: **Substrate** of CYP3A4 (minor)

Increased Effect/Toxicity: See individual agents.

Decreased Effect: See individual agents.

Pharmacodynamics/Kinetics

Zyrtec-D 12 Hour™:

Half-life elimination: Cetirizine: 7.9 hours; Pseudoephedrine: 6 hours

Time to peak: Cetirizine: 2.2 hours; Pseudoephedrine: 4.4 hours

Excretion: Urine (70%); feces (10%)

See individual Cetirizine and Pseudoephedrine monographs.

Pregnancy Risk Factor C

Cetirizine Hydrochloride *see* Cetirizine *on page 298*

Cetirizine Hydrochloride and Pseudoephedrine Hydrochloride *see* Cetirizine and Pseudoephedrine *on page 299*

Cetrorelix (set roe REL iks)

U.S. Brand Names Cetrotide®

Canadian Brand Names Cetrotide®

Generic Available No

Synonyms Cetrorelix Acetate

Pharmacologic Category Gonadotropin Releasing Hormone Antagonist

Use Inhibits premature luteinizing hormone (LH) surges in women undergoing controlled ovarian stimulation

Local Anesthetic/Vasoconstrictor Precautions No information available to require special precautions

Effects on Dental Treatment No significant effects or complications reported

Common Adverse Effects

1% to 10%:

Central nervous system: Headache (1%)

Endocrine & metabolic: Ovarian hyperstimulation syndrome, WHO grade II or III (4%)

Gastrointestinal: Nausea (1%)

Hepatic: Increased ALT, AST, GGT, and alkaline phosphatase (1% to 2%)

Mechanism of Action Competes with naturally occurring GnRH for binding on receptors of the pituitary. This delays luteinizing hormone surge, preventing ovulation until the follicles are of adequate size.

Drug Interactions

Increased Effect/Toxicity: No formal studies have been performed.

Decreased Effect: No formal studies have been performed.

Pharmacodynamics/Kinetics

Onset of action: 0.25 mg dose: 2 hours; 3 mg dose: 1 hour

Duration: 3 mg dose (single dose): 4 days

Absorption: Rapid

Protein binding: 86%

Metabolism: Transformed by peptidases; cetrorelix and peptides (1-9), (1-7), (1-6), and (1-4) are found in the bile; peptide (1-4) is the predominant metabolite

Bioavailability: 85%

Half-life elimination: 0.25 mg dose: 5 hours; 0.25 mg multiple doses: 20.6 hours; 3 mg dose: 62.8 hours

Time to peak: 0.25 mg dose: 1 hour; 3 mg dose: 1.5 hours

Excretion: Feces (5% to 10% as unchanged drug and metabolites); urine (2% to 4% as unchanged drug); within 24 hours

Pregnancy Risk Factor X

Cetrorelix Acetate *see* Cetrorelix *on page 300*

Cetrotide® *see* Cetrorelix *on page 300*

Cetuximab (se TUK see mab)

U.S. Brand Names Erbitux™

Generic Available No

Synonyms C225; IMC-C225

Pharmacologic Category Antineoplastic Agent, Monoclonal Antibody; Epidermal Growth Factor Receptor (EGFR) Inhibitor

Use Treatment of epidermal growth factor receptor (EGFR) expressing, metastatic colorectal carcinoma; may be used in combination with irinotecan in patients who are refractory to irinotecan-based chemotherapy or as a single agent in patients who are intolerant to irinotecan-based chemotherapy.

Unlabeled/Investigational Use Breast cancer, head and neck cancer, tumors overexpressing EGFR

Local Anesthetic/Vasoconstrictor Precautions No information available to require special precautions

Effects on Dental Treatment No significant effects or complications reported

Common Adverse Effects

>10%:

Central nervous system: Weakness/malaise (49%), fever (33%), headache (25%), pain (19%)

Dermatologic: Acneform rash (90%; ~10% severe), nail disorder (16%)

Gastrointestinal: Nausea (mild-to-moderate 29%), constipation (28%), diarrhea (28%), abdominal pain (25%), vomiting (25%), anorexia (25%), stomatitis (11%)

Neuromuscular & skeletal: Back pain (11%)

Respiratory: Dyspnea (20%)

Miscellaneous: Infusion reaction (25%; ~3% severe; ~90% with first infusion), infection (11%)

1% to 10%:

Cardiovascular: Peripheral edema (10%)

Central nervous system: Insomnia (10%), depression (9%)

Dermatologic: Pruritus (10%), alopecia (5%), skin disorder (5%)

Endocrine & metabolic: Dehydration (9%)

Gastrointestinal: Weight loss (9%), dyspepsia (7%)

Hematologic: Anemia (10%), leukopenia (1%)

Hepatic: Alkaline phosphatase increased (5% to 10%), transaminases increased (5% to 10%)

Ocular: Conjunctivitis (7%)

Renal: Kidney failure (2%)

Respiratory: Cough increased (10%), pulmonary embolus (1%)

Miscellaneous: Sepsis (3%)

Mechanism of Action Recombinant human/mouse chimeric monoclonal antibody which binds specifically to the epidermal growth factor receptor (EGFR, HER1, c-ErbB-1) and competitively inhibits the binding of epidermal growth factor (EGF) and other ligands. Binding to the EGFR blocks phosphorylation and activation of receptor-associated kinases, resulting in inhibition of cell growth, induction of apoptosis, and decreased matrix metalloproteinase and vascular endothelial growth factor production.

Drug Interactions

Increased Effect/Toxicity: Interactions have not been evaluated in clinical trials.

Pharmacodynamics/Kinetics

Distribution: V_d: ~2-3 L/m^2

Half-life elimination: 114 hours (range: 75-188 hours)

Pregnancy Risk Factor C

Cetylpyridinium (SEE til peer i DI nee um)

U.S. Brand Names Cēpacol® Gold [OTC]

Generic Available No

Synonyms Cetylpyridinium Chloride; CPC

Pharmacologic Category Antiseptic, Oral Mouthwash

Use Antiseptic to aid in the prevention and reduction of plaque and gingivitis, and to freshen breath

Local Anesthetic/Vasoconstrictor Precautions No information available to require special precautions

Effects on Dental Treatment Key adverse event(s) related to dental treatment: Tooth and tongue staining and oral irritation.

Significant Adverse Effects Frequency not defined: Gastrointestinal: Tooth and tongue staining, oral irritation

Dosage Children ≥6 years and Adults: Oral (OTC labeling): Rinse or gargle to freshen mouth; may be used before or after brushing

Contraindications Hypersensitivity to cetylpyridinium or any component of the formulation

Warnings/Precautions Not labeled for OTC use in children <6 years of age.

Pregnancy Risk Factor C

Dosage Forms Liquid, as chloride [mouthwash/gargle]: 0.05% (120 mL, 360 mL, 720 mL, 960 mL) [contains alcohol 14% and tartrazine]

Cetylpyridinium and Benzocaine

(SEE til peer i DI nee um & BEN zoe kane)

Related Information

Cetylpyridinium *on page 301*

(Continued)

Cetylpyridinium and Benzocaine *(Continued)*

Canadian Brand Names Cēpacol®; Kank-A®

Synonyms Benzocaine and Cetylpyridinium Chloride; Cetylpyridinium Chloride and Benzocaine

Pharmacologic Category Local Anesthetic

Use Symptomatic relief of sore throat

Local Anesthetic/Vasoconstrictor Precautions No information available to require special precautions

Effects on Dental Treatment No significant effects or complications reported

Restrictions Not available in U.S.

Dosage Antiseptic/anesthetic: Oral: Dissolve in mouth as needed for sore throat

Drug Interactions See individual agents.

Pregnancy Risk Factor C

Cetylpyridinium Chloride *see* Cetylpyridinium *on page 301*

Cetylpyridinium Chloride and Benzocaine *see* Cetylpyridinium and Benzocaine *on page 301*

Cevi-Bid® [OTC] *see* Ascorbic Acid *on page 148*

Cevimeline (se vi ME leen)

Related Information

Management of Patients Undergoing Cancer Therapy *on page 1569*

U.S. Brand Names Evoxac®

Canadian Brand Names Evoxac®

Generic Available No

Synonyms Cevimeline Hydrochloride

Pharmacologic Category Cholinergic Agonist

Use Treatment of symptoms of dry mouth in patients with Sjögren's syndrome

Local Anesthetic/Vasoconstrictor Precautions No information available to require special precautions

Effects on Dental Treatment Key adverse event(s) related to dental treatment: Excessive salivation, salivary gland pain, xerostomia (normal salivary flow resumes upon discontinuation), ulcerative stomatitis, and tooth disorder.

Significant Adverse Effects

>10%:

- Central nervous system: Headache (14%; placebo 20%)
- Gastrointestinal: Nausea (14%), diarrhea (10%)
- Respiratory: Rhinitis (11%), sinusitis (12%), upper respiratory infection (11%)
- Miscellaneous: Increased diaphoresis (19%)

1% to 10%:

- Cardiovascular: Peripheral edema, chest pain, edema, palpitation
- Central nervous system: Dizziness (4%), fatigue (3%), pain (3%), insomnia (2%), anxiety (1%), fever, depression, migraine, vertigo
- Dermatologic: Rash (4%; placebo 6%), pruritus, skin disorder, erythematous rash
- Endocrine & metabolic: Hot flashes (2%)
- Gastrointestinal: Dyspepsia (8%; placebo 9%), abdominal pain (8%), vomiting (5%), excessive salivation (2%), constipation, salivary gland pain, dry mouth, sialoadenitis, ulcerative stomatitis
- Genitourinary: Urinary tract infection (6%), vaginitis, cystitis
- Hematologic: Anemia
- Local: Abscess
- Neuromuscular & skeletal: Back pain (5%), arthralgia (4%), skeletal pain (3%), rigors (1%), hypertonia, tremor, myalgia
- Ocular: Conjunctivitis (4%), abnormal vision, eye pain, eye abnormality, xerophthalmia
- Otic: Earache, otitis media
- Respiratory: Coughing (6%), bronchitis (4%), pneumonia, epistaxis
- Miscellaneous: Flu-like syndrome, infection, fungal infection, allergy, hiccups

<1% (Limited to important or life-threatening): Aggravated multiple sclerosis, aggressive behavior, alopecia, angina, anterior chamber hemorrhage, aphasia, apnea, arrhythmia, arthropathy, avascular necrosis (femoral head), bronchospasm, bullous eruption, bundle branch block, cholelithiasis, coma, deafness, delirium, depersonalization, dyskinesia, eosinophilia, esophageal stricture, esophagitis, fall, gastric ulcer, gastrointestinal hemorrhage, gingival hyperplasia, glaucoma, granulocytopenia, hallucination, hematuria, hypothyroidism, ileus, impotence, intestinal obstruction, leukopenia, lymphocytosis, manic reaction, myocardial infarction, neuropathy, paralysis, paranoia, paresthesia, peptic ulcer, pericarditis, peripheral ischemia, photosensitivity reaction, pleural effusion, pulmonary embolism, pulmonary fibrosis, renal

calculus, seizure, sepsis, somnolence, syncope, systemic lupus erythematosus, tenosynovltls, thrombocytopenia, thrombocytopenic purpura, thrombophlebitis, T-wave inversion, urinary retention, vasculitis

Dosage Adults: Oral: 30 mg 3 times/day

Dosage adjustment in renal/hepatic impairment: Not studied; no specific dosage adjustment is recommended

Elderly: No specific dosage adjustment is recommended; however, use caution when initiating due to potential for increased sensitivity

Mechanism of Action Binds to muscarinic (cholinergic) receptors, causing an increase in secretion of exocrine glands (including salivary glands)

Contraindications Hypersensitivity to cevimeline or any component of the formulation; uncontrolled asthma; narrow-angle glaucoma; acute iritis; other conditions where miosis is undesirable

Warnings/Precautions May alter cardiac conduction and/or heart rate; use caution in patients with significant cardiovascular disease, including angina, myocardial infarction, or conduction disturbances. Cevimeline has the potential to increase bronchial smooth muscle tone, airway resistance, and bronchial secretions; use with caution in patients with controlled asthma, COPD, or chronic bronchitis. May cause decreased visual acuity (particularly at night and in patients with central lens changes) and impaired depth perception. Patients should be cautioned about driving at night or performing hazardous activities in reduced lighting. May cause a variety of parasympathomimetic effects, which may be particularly dangerous in elderly patients; excessive sweating may lead to dehydration in some patients.

Use with caution in patients with a history of biliary stones or nephrolithiasis; cevimeline may induce smooth muscle spasms, precipitating cholangitis, cholecystitis, biliary obstruction, renal colic, or ureteral reflux in susceptible patients. Patients with a known or suspected deficiency of CYP2D6 may be at higher risk of adverse effects. Safety and efficacy has not been established in pediatric patients.

Drug Interactions Substrate (minor) of CYP2D6, CYP3A4

Increased effect: The effects of other cholinergic agents may be increased during concurrent administration with cevimeline. Concurrent use of cevimeline and beta-blockers may increase the potential for conduction disturbances.

Decreased effect: Anticholinergic agents (atropine, TCAs, phenothiazines) may antagonize the effects of cevimeline

Dietary Considerations Take with or without food.

Pharmacodynamics/Kinetics

Distribution: V_d: 6 L/kg

Protein binding: <20%

Metabolism: Hepatic via CYP2D6 and CYP3A4

Half-life elimination: 5 hours

Time to peak: 1.5-2 hours

Excretion: Urine (as metabolites and unchanged drug)

Pregnancy Risk Factor C

Lactation Excretion in breast milk unknown/not recommended

Dosage Forms Capsule, as hydrochloride: 30 mg

Cevimeline Hydrochloride *see* Cevimeline *on page 302*

CFDN *see* Cefdinir *on page 279*

CG *see* Chorionic Gonadotropin (Human) *on page 326*

CGP-42446 *see* Zoledronic Acid *on page 1402*

CGP 57148B *see* Imatinib *on page 734*

C-Gram [OTC] *see* Ascorbic Acid *on page 148*

CharcoAid G® [OTC] *see* Charcoal *on page 303*

Charcoal (CHAR kole)

U.S. Brand Names Actidose-Aqua® [OTC]; Actidose® with Sorbitol [OTC]; CharcoAid G® [OTC]; Charcoal Plus® DS [OTC]; Charcocaps® [OTC]; EZ-Char™ [OTC]; Kerr Insta-Char® [OTC]; Liqui-Char® [OTC] [DSC]

Canadian Brand Names Charcadole®; Charcadole®, Aqueous; Charcadole® TFS

Generic Available Yes

Synonyms Activated Carbon; Activated Charcoal; Adsorbent Charcoal; Liquid Antidote; Medicinal Carbon; Medicinal Charcoal

Pharmacologic Category Antidote

Use Emergency treatment in poisoning by drugs and chemicals; aids the elimination of certain drugs and improves decontamination of excessive ingestions of sustained-release products or in the presence of bezoars; repetitive doses

(Continued)

Charcoal *(Continued)*

have proven useful to enhance the elimination of certain drugs (eg, theophylline, phenobarbital, and aspirin); repetitive doses for gastric dialysis in uremia to adsorb various waste products; dietary supplement (digestive aid)

Local Anesthetic/Vasoconstrictor Precautions No information available to require special precautions

Effects on Dental Treatment No significant effects or complications reported

Mechanism of Action Adsorbs toxic substances or irritants, thus inhibiting GI absorption; adsorbs intestinal gas; the addition of sorbitol results in hyperosmotic laxative action causing catharsis

Pregnancy Risk Factor C

Charcoal Plus® DS [OTC] *see* Charcoal *on page 303*

Charcocaps® [OTC] *see* Charcoal *on page 303*

Chemical Dependency and Smoking Cessation *see page 1576*

Cheracol® *see* Guaifenesin and Codeine *on page 673*

Cheracol® D [OTC] *see* Guaifenesin and Dextromethorphan *on page 673*

Cheracol® Plus [OTC] *see* Guaifenesin and Dextromethorphan *on page 673*

Cheratussin DAC *see* Guaifenesin, Pseudoephedrine, and Codeine *on page 676*

CHG *see* Chlorhexidine Gluconate *on page 308*

Chiggerex® [OTC] *see* Benzocaine *on page 191*

Chiggertox® [OTC] *see* Benzocaine *on page 191*

Children's Dimetapp® Elixir Cold & Allergy [OTC] *see* Brompheniramine and Pseudoephedrine *on page 220*

Children's Kaopectate® [DSC] [OTC] *see* Attapulgite *on page 170*

Children's Kaopectate® *(reformulation)* [OTC] *see* Bismuth *on page 209*

Children's Sudafed® Cough & Cold [OTC] *see* Pseudoephedrine and Dextromethorphan *on page 1148*

Children's Tylenol® Plus Cold [OTC] *see* Acetaminophen, Chlorpheniramine, and Pseudoephedrine *on page 58*

Chirocaine® *see* Levobupivacaine *on page 809*

Chloral *see* Chloral Hydrate *on page 304*

Chloral Hydrate (KLOR al HYE drate)

U.S. Brand Names Aquachloral® Supprettes®; Somnote™

Canadian Brand Names PMS-Chloral Hydrate

Generic Available Yes: Syrup

Synonyms Chloral; Hydrated Chloral; Trichloroacetaldehyde Monohydrate

Pharmacologic Category Hypnotic, Miscellaneous

Dental Use Short-term sedative/hypnotic for dental procedures

Use Short-term sedative and hypnotic (<2 weeks), sedative/hypnotic for diagnostic procedures; sedative prior to EEG evaluations

Local Anesthetic/Vasoconstrictor Precautions No information available to require special precautions

Effects on Dental Treatment No significant effects or complications reported

Significant Adverse Effects Frequency not defined.

- Central nervous system: Ataxia, disorientation, sedation, excitement (paradoxical), dizziness, fever, headache, confusion, lightheadedness, nightmares, hallucinations, drowsiness, "hangover" effect
- Dermatologic: Rash, urticaria
- Gastrointestinal: Gastric irritation, nausea, vomiting, diarrhea, flatulence
- Hematologic: Leukopenia, eosinophilia, acute intermittent porphyria
- Miscellaneous: Physical and psychological dependence may occur with prolonged use of large doses

Restrictions C-IV

Dosage

Children:

- Sedation or anxiety: Oral, rectal: 5-15 mg/kg/dose every 8 hours (maximum: 500 mg/dose)
- Prior to EEG: Oral, rectal: 20-25 mg/kg/dose, 30-60 minutes prior to EEG; may repeat in 30 minutes to maximum of 100 mg/kg or 2 g total
- Hypnotic: Oral, rectal: 20-40 mg/kg/dose up to a maximum of 50 mg/kg/24 hours or 1 g/dose or 2 g/24 hours
- Conscious sedation: Oral: 50-75 mg/kg/dose 30-60 minutes prior to procedure; may repeat 30 minutes after initial dose if needed, to a total maximum dose of 120 mg/kg or 1 g total

Adults: Oral, rectal:

- Sedation, anxiety: 250 mg 3 times/day

Hypnotic: 500-1000 mg at bedtime or 30 minutes prior to procedure, not to exceed 2 g/24 hours

Dosing adjustment/comments in renal impairment: Cl_{cr} <50 mL/minute: Avoid use

Hemodialysis: Dialyzable (50% to 100%); supplemental dose is not necessary

Dosing adjustment/comments in hepatic impairment: Avoid use in patients with severe hepatic impairment

Mechanism of Action Central nervous system depressant effects are due to its active metabolite trichloroethanol, mechanism unknown

Contraindications Hypersensitivity to chloral hydrate or any component of the formulation; hepatic or renal impairment; gastritis or ulcers; severe cardiac disease

Warnings/Precautions Use with caution in patients with porphyria; use with caution in neonates, drug may accumulate with repeated use, prolonged use in neonates associated with hyperbilirubinemia; tolerance to hypnotic effect develops, therefore, not recommended for use >2 weeks; taper dosage to avoid withdrawal with prolonged use; trichloroethanol (TCE), a metabolite of chloral hydrate, is a carcinogen in mice; there is no data in humans. Chloral hydrate is considered a second line hypnotic agent in the elderly. Recent interpretive guidelines from the Centers for Medicare and Medicaid Services (CMS) discourage the use of chloral hydrate in residents of long-term care facilities.

Drug Interactions

CNS depressants: Sedative effects and/or respiratory depression with chloral hydrate may be additive with other CNS depressants; monitor for increased effect; includes ethanol, sedatives, antidepressants, narcotic analgesics, and benzodiazepines

Furosemide: Diaphoresis, flushing, and hypertension have occurred in patients who received I.V. furosemide within 24 hours after administration of chloral hydrate; consider using a benzodiazepine

Phenytoin: Half-life may be decreased by chloral hydrate; limited documentation (small, single-dose study); monitor

Warfarin: Effect of oral anticoagulants may be increased by chloral hydrate; monitor INR; warfarin dosage may require adjustment. Chloral hydrate's metabolite may displace warfarin from its protein binding sites resulting in an increase in the hypoprothrombinemic response to warfarin.

Ethanol/Nutrition/Herb Interactions

Ethanol: Avoid ethanol (may increase CNS depression).

Herb/Nutraceutical: Avoid valerian, St John's wort, kava kava, gotu kola (may increase CNS depression).

Pharmacodynamics/Kinetics

Onset of action: Peak effect: 0.5-1 hour

Duration: 4-8 hours

Absorption: Oral, rectal: Well absorbed

Distribution: Crosses placenta; negligible amounts enter breast milk

Metabolism: Rapidly hepatic to trichloroethanol (active metabolite); variable amounts hepatically and renally to trichloroacetic acid (inactive)

Half-life elimination: Active metabolite: 8-11 hours

Excretion: Urine (as metabolites); feces (small amounts)

Pregnancy Risk Factor C

Lactation Enters breast milk/compatible

Dosage Forms

Capsule (Somnote™): 500 mg

Suppository, rectal (Aquachloral® Supprettes®): 325 mg [contains tartrazine], 650 mg

Syrup: 500 mg/5 mL (480 mL) [contains sodium benzoate]

Chlorambucil (klor AM byoo sil)

U.S. Brand Names Leukeran®

Canadian Brand Names Leukeran®

Mexican Brand Names Leukeran®

Generic Available No

Synonyms CB-1348; Chlorambucilum; Chloraminophene; Chlorbutinum; NSC-3088; WR-139013

Pharmacologic Category Antineoplastic Agent, Alkylating Agent

Use Management of chronic lymphocytic leukemia, Hodgkin's and non-Hodgkin's lymphoma; breast and ovarian carcinoma; Waldenström's macroglobulinemia, testicular carcinoma, thrombocythemia, choriocarcinoma

Local Anesthetic/Vasoconstrictor Precautions No information available to require special precautions

(Continued)

Chlorambucil *(Continued)*

Effects on Dental Treatment Key adverse event(s) related to dental treatment: Stomatitis.

Common Adverse Effects

>10%:

Dermatologic: Skin rashes

Hematologic: Myelosuppression (common, dose-limiting)

Onset (days): 7

Nadir (days): 14

Recovery (days): 28; may be prolonged to 6-8 weeks in some patients

Hepatic: Transient elevations in liver enzymes

1% to 10%:

Endocrine & metabolic: Hyperuricemia, menstrual cramps

Gastrointestinal: Mild nausea or vomiting, diarrhea, stomatitis

Mechanism of Action Interferes with DNA replication and RNA transcription by alkylation and cross-linking the strands of DNA

Drug Interactions

Decreased Effect: Patients may experience impaired immune response to vaccines; possible infection after administration of live vaccines in patients receiving immunosuppressants.

Pharmacodynamics/Kinetics

Absorption: 70% to 80% with meals

Distribution: V_d: 0.14-0.24 L/kg

Protein binding: ~99%

Metabolism: Hepatic; active metabolite, phenylacetic acid mustard

Bioavailability: Reduced 10% to 20% with food

Half-life elimination: 1.5 hours; Phenylacetic acid mustard: 2.5 hours

Excretion: Urine (60% primarily as metabolites, <1% as unchanged drug)

Pregnancy Risk Factor D

Chlorambucilum *see* Chlorambucil *on page 305*

Chloraminophene *see* Chlorambucil *on page 305*

Chloramphenicol (klor am FEN i kole)

U.S. Brand Names Chloromycetin® Sodium Succinate

Canadian Brand Names Chloromycetin®; Diochloram®; Pentamycetin®

Mexican Brand Names Chloromycetin®; Clorafen® [caps]; Cloramfeni®; Cloran®; Clordil® [caps]; Quemicetina®

Generic Available Yes

Pharmacologic Category Antibiotic, Miscellaneous

Use Treatment of serious infections due to organisms resistant to other less toxic antibiotics or when its penetrability into the site of infection is clinically superior to other antibiotics to which the organism is sensitive; useful in infections caused by *Bacteroides*, *H. influenzae*, *Neisseria meningitidis*, *Salmonella*, and *Rickettsia*; active against many vancomycin-resistant enterococci

Local Anesthetic/Vasoconstrictor Precautions No information available to require special precautions

Effects on Dental Treatment No significant effects or complications reported

Common Adverse Effects

Three (3) major toxicities associated with chloramphenicol include:

Aplastic anemia, an idiosyncratic reaction which can occur with any route of administration; usually occurs 3 weeks to 12 months after initial exposure to chloramphenicol

Bone marrow suppression is thought to be dose-related with serum concentrations >25 mcg/mL and reversible once chloramphenicol is discontinued; anemia and neutropenia may occur during the first week of therapy

Gray syndrome is characterized by circulatory collapse, cyanosis, acidosis, abdominal distention, myocardial depression, coma, and death; reaction appears to be associated with serum levels ≥50 mcg/mL; may result from drug accumulation in patients with impaired hepatic or renal function

Additional adverse reactions, frequency not defined:

Central nervous system: Confusion, delirium, depression, fever, headache

Dermatologic: Angioedema, rash, urticaria

Gastrointestinal: Diarrhea, enterocolitis, glossitis, nausea, stomatitis, vomiting

Hematologic: Granulocytopenia, hypoplastic anemia, pancytopenia, thrombocytopenia

Ocular: Optic neuritis

Miscellaneous: Anaphylaxis, hypersensitivity reactions

Mechanism of Action Reversibly binds to 50S ribosomal subunits of susceptible organisms preventing amino acids from being transferred to growing peptide chains thus inhibiting protein synthesis

Drug Interactions

Cytochrome P450 Effect: Inhibits CYP2C8/9 (weak), 3A4 (weak)

Increased Effect/Toxicity: Chloramphenicol increases serum concentrations of chlorpropamide, phenytoin, and oral anticoagulants.

Decreased Effect: Phenobarbital and rifampin may decrease serum concentrations of chloramphenicol.

Pharmacodynamics/Kinetics

Distribution: To most tissues and body fluids; readily crosses placenta; enters breast milk

CSF:blood level ratio: Normal meninges: 66%; Inflamed meninges: >66%

Protein binding: 60%

Metabolism: Extensively hepatic (90%) to inactive metabolites, principally by glucuronidation; chloramphenicol sodium succinate is hydrolyzed by esterases to active base

Half-life elimination

Normal renal function: 1.6-3.3 hours

End-stage renal disease: 3-7 hours

Cirrhosis: 10-12 hours

Excretion: Urine (5% to 15%)

Pregnancy Risk Factor C

ChloraPrep® [OTC] *see* Chlorhexidine Gluconate *on page 308*

Chloraseptic® Gargle [OTC] *see* Phenol *on page 1075*

Chloraseptic® Mouth Pain Spray [OTC] *see* Phenol *on page 1075*

Chloraseptic® Rinse [OTC] *see* Phenol *on page 1075*

Chloraseptic® Spray [OTC] *see* Phenol *on page 1075*

Chloraseptic® Spray for Kids [OTC] *see* Phenol *on page 1075*

Chlorbutinum *see* Chlorambucil *on page 305*

Chlordiazepoxide (klor dye az e POKS ide)

U.S. Brand Names Librium®

Canadian Brand Names Apo-Chlordiazepoxide®

Generic Available Yes: Capsule

Synonyms Methaminodiazepoxide Hydrochloride

Pharmacologic Category Benzodiazepine

Use Management of anxiety disorder or for the short-term relief of symptoms of anxiety; withdrawal symptoms of acute alcoholism; preoperative apprehension and anxiety

Local Anesthetic/Vasoconstrictor Precautions No information available to require special precautions

Effects on Dental Treatment Key adverse event(s) related to dental treatment: Xerostomia (normal salivary flow resumes upon discontinuation).

Common Adverse Effects

>10%:

Central nervous system: Drowsiness, fatigue, ataxia, lightheadedness, memory impairment, dysarthria, irritability

Dermatologic: Rash

Endocrine & metabolic: Decreased libido, menstrual disorders

Gastrointestinal: Xerostomia, decreased salivation, increased or decreased appetite, weight gain/loss

Genitourinary: Micturition difficulties

1% to 10%:

Cardiovascular: Hypotension

Central nervous system: Confusion, dizziness, disinhibition, akathisia, increased libido

Dermatologic: Dermatitis

Gastrointestinal: Increased salivation

Genitourinary: Sexual dysfunction, incontinence

Neuromuscular & skeletal: Rigidity, tremor, muscle cramps

Otic: Tinnitus

Respiratory: Nasal congestion

Restrictions C-IV

Mechanism of Action Binds to stereospecific benzodiazepine receptors on the postsynaptic GABA neuron at several sites within the central nervous system, including the limbic system, reticular formation. Enhancement of the inhibitory effect of GABA on neuronal excitability results by increased neuronal membrane permeability to chloride ions. This shift in chloride ions results in hyperpolarization (a less excitable state) and stabilization.

(Continued)

Chlordiazepoxide *(Continued)*

Drug Interactions

Cytochrome P450 Effect: Substrate of CYP3A4 (major)

Increased Effect/Toxicity: Chlordiazepoxide potentiates the CNS depressant effects of narcotic analgesics, barbiturates, phenothiazines, ethanol, antihistamines, MAO inhibitors, sedative-hypnotics, and cyclic antidepressants. CYP3A4 inhibitors may increase the levels/effects of chlordiazepoxide; example inhibitors include azole antifungals, ciprofloxacin, clarithromycin, diclofenac, doxycycline, erythromycin, imatinib, isoniazid, nefazodone, nicardipine, propofol, protease inhibitors, quinidine, and verapamil.

Decreased Effect: CYP3A4 inducers may decrease the levels/effects of chlordiazepoxide; example inducers include aminoglutethimide, carbamazepine, nafcillin, nevirapine, phenobarbital, phenytoin, and rifamycins.

Pharmacodynamics/Kinetics

Distribution: V_d: 3.3 L/kg; crosses placenta; enters breast milk

Protein binding: 90% to 98%

Metabolism: Extensively hepatic to desmethyldiazepam (active and long-acting)

Half-life elimination: 6.6-25 hours; End-stage renal disease: 5-30 hours; Cirrhosis: 30-63 hours

Time to peak, serum: Oral: Within 2 hours; I.M.: Results in lower peak plasma levels than oral

Excretion: Urine (minimal as unchanged drug)

Pregnancy Risk Factor D

Chlordiazepoxide and Amitriptyline *see* Amitriptyline and Chlordiazepoxide *on page 105*

Chlordiazepoxide and Clidinium *see* Clidinium and Chlordiazepoxide *on page 347*

Chlorhexidine Gluconate (klor HEKS i deen GLOO koe nate)

Related Information

Antiplaque Agents *on page 1556*

Dentin Hypersensitivity, High Caries Index, and Xerostomia *on page 1555*

Management of Patients Undergoing Cancer Therapy *on page 1569*

Oral Bacterial Infections *on page 1533*

Oral Nonviral Soft Tissue Ulcerations or Erosions *on page 1551*

Periodontal Diseases *on page 1542*

U.S. Brand Names Avagard™ [OTC]; BactoShield® CHG [OTC]; Betasept® [OTC]; ChloraPrep® [OTC]; Chlorostat® [OTC]; Dyna-Hex® [OTC]; Hibiclens® [OTC]; Hibistat® [OTC]; Operand® Chlorhexidine Gluconate [OTC]; Peridex®; PerioChip®; PerioGard®

Canadian Brand Names Apo-Chlorhexadine®; Hibidil® 1:2000; ORO-Clense; SpectroGram 2™

Generic Available Yes: Oral liquid

Synonyms CHG; 3M™ Avagard™ [OTC]

Pharmacologic Category Antibiotic, Oral Rinse; Antibiotic, Topical

Dental Use

Antibacterial dental rinse; chlorhexidine is active against gram-positive and gram-negative organisms, facultative anaerobes, aerobes, and yeast

Chip, for periodontal pocket insertion: Indicated as an adjunct to scaling and root planing procedures for reduction of pocket depth in patients with adult periodontitis; may be used as part of a periodontal maintenance program

Use Skin cleanser for surgical scrub, cleanser for skin wounds, preoperative skin preparation, germicidal hand rinse, and as antibacterial dental rinse. Chlorhexidine is active against gram-positive and gram-negative organisms, facultative anaerobes, aerobes, and yeast.

Orphan drug: Peridex®: Oral mucositis with cytoreductive therapy when used for patients undergoing bone marrow transplant

Local Anesthetic/Vasoconstrictor Precautions No information available to require special precautions

Effects on Dental Treatment Key adverse event(s) related to dental treatment: Increased tartar on teeth, altered taste perception, staining of oral surfaces (mucosa, teeth, dorsum of tongue), and oral/tongue irritation. Staining may be visible as soon as 1 week after therapy begins and is more pronounced when there is a heavy accumulation of unremoved plaque and when teeth fillings have rough surfaces. Stain does not have a clinically adverse effect but because removal may not be possible, patient with frontal restoration should be advised of the potential permanency of the stain.

Significant Adverse Effects

Oral:

>10%: Increase of tartar on teeth, changes in taste. Staining of oral surfaces (mucosa, teeth, dorsum of tongue) may be visible as soon as 1 week after therapy begins and is more pronounced when there is a heavy accumulation of unremoved plaque and when teeth fillings have rough surfaces. Stain does not have a clinically adverse effect but because removal may not be possible, patient with frontal restoration should be advised of the potential permanency of the stain.

1% to 10%: Gastrointestinal: Tongue irritation, oral irritation

<1% (Limited to important or life-threatening): Dyspnea, facial edema, nasal congestion

Topical: Skin erythema and roughness, dryness, sensitization, allergic reactions

Dosage Adults:

Oral rinse (Peridex®, PerioGard®):

Floss and brush teeth, completely rinse toothpaste from mouth and swish 15 mL (one capful) undiluted oral rinse around in mouth for 30 seconds, then expectorate. Caution patient not to swallow the medicine and instruct not to eat for 2-3 hours after treatment. (Cap on bottle measures 15 mL.)

Treatment of gingivitis: Oral prophylaxis: Swish for 30 seconds with 15 mL chlorhexidine, then expectorate; repeat twice daily (morning and evening). Patient should have a re-evaluation followed by a dental prophylaxis every 6 months.

Periodontal chip: One chip is inserted into a periodontal pocket with a probing pocket depth ≥5 mm. Up to 8 chips may be inserted in a single visit. Treatment is recommended every 3 months in pockets with a remaining depth ≥5 mm. If dislodgment occurs 7 days or more after placement, the subject is considered to have had the full course of treatment. If dislodgment occurs within 48 hours, a new chip should be inserted. The chip biodegrades completely and does not need to be removed. Patients should avoid dental floss at the site of PerioChip® insertion for 10 days after placement because flossing might dislodge the chip.

Insertion of periodontal chip: Pocket should be isolated and surrounding area dried prior to chip insertion. The chip should be grasped using forceps with the rounded edges away from the forceps. The chip should be inserted into the periodontal pocket to its maximum depth. It may be maneuvered into position using the tips of the forceps or a flat instrument.

Cleanser:

Surgical scrub: Scrub 3 minutes and rinse thoroughly, wash for an additional 3 minutes

Hand sanitizer (Avagard™): Dispense 1 pumpful in palm of one hand; dip fingertips of opposite hand into solution and work it under nails. Spread remainder evenly over hand and just above elbow, covering all surfaces. Repeat on other hand. Dispense another pumpful in each hand and reapply to each hand up to the wrist. Allow to dry before gloving.

Hand wash: Wash for 15 seconds and rinse

Hand rinse: Rub 15 seconds and rinse

Mechanism of Action The bactericidal effect of chlorhexidine is a result of the binding of this cationic molecule to negatively charged bacterial cell walls and extramicrobial complexes. At low concentrations, this causes an alteration of bacterial cell osmotic equilibrium and leakage of potassium and phosphorous resulting in a bacteriostatic effect. At high concentrations of chlorhexidine, the cytoplasmic contents of the bacterial cell precipitate and result in cell death.

Contraindications Hypersensitivity to chlorhexidine gluconate or any component of the formulation

Warnings/Precautions

Oral: Staining of oral surfaces (mucosa, teeth, tooth restorations, dorsum of tongue) may occur; may be visible as soon as 1 week after therapy begins and is more pronounced when there is a heavy accumulation of unremoved plaque and when teeth fillings have rough surfaces. Stain does not have a clinically adverse effect, but because removal may not be possible, patient with frontal restoration should be advised of the potential permanency of the stain.

Topical: For topical use only. Keep out of eyes and ears. May stain fabric. There have been case reports of anaphylaxis following chlorhexidine disinfection. Not for preoperative preparation of face or head; avoid contact with meninges.

Drug Interactions No data reported

Pharmacodynamics/Kinetics

Topical hand sanitizer (Avagard™): Duration of antimicrobial protection: 6 hours

(Continued)

Chlorhexidine Gluconate *(Continued)*

Oral rinse (Peridex®, PerioGard®):

Absorption: ~30% retained in the oral cavity following rinsing and slowly released into oral fluids; poorly absorbed

Time to peak, plasma: Oral rinse: Detectable levels not present after 12 hours

Excretion: Feces (~90%); urine (<1%)

Pregnancy Risk Factor B

Dosage Forms

Chip, for periodontal pocket insertion (PerioChip®): 2.5 mg

Liquid, topical [surgical scrub]:

Avagard™: 1% (500 mL) [contains ethyl alcohol and moisturizers]

BactoShield® CHG: 2% (120 mL, 480 mL, 750 mL, 1000 mL, 3800 mL); 4% (120 mL, 480 mL, 750 mL, 1000 mL, 3800 mL) [contains isopropyl alcohol]

Betasept®: 4% (120 mL, 240 mL, 480 mL, 960 mL, 3840 mL) [contains isopropyl alcohol]

ChloraPrep®: 2% (0.67 mL, 1.5 mL, 3 mL, 10.5 mL) [contains isopropyl alcohol 70%; prefilled applicator]

Chlorostat®: 2% (360 mL, 3840 mL) [contains isopropyl alcohol]

Dyna-Hex: 2% (120 mL, 960 mL, 3840 mL); 4% (120 mL, 960 mL, 3840 mL)

Hibiclens®: 4% (15 mL, 120 mL, 240 mL, 480 mL, 960 mL, 3840 mL) [contains isopropyl alcohol]

Operand® Chlorhexidine Gluconate: 2% (120 mL); 4% (120 mL, 240 mL, 480 mL, 960 mL, 3840 mL) [contains isopropyl alcohol]

Liquid, oral rinse: 0.12% (480 mL)

Peridex®: 0.12% (480 mL) [contains alcohol 11.6%]

PerioGard®: 0.12% (480 mL) [contains alcohol 11.6%; mint flavor]

Liquid, topical: Hibistat®: 0.5% (240 mL, 480 mL) [contains isopropyl alcohol]

Pad [prep pad]: Hibistat®: 0.5% (50s) [contains isopropyl alcohol]

Sponge/Brush (BactoShield® CHG, Hibiclens®): 4% per sponge/brush [contains isopropyl alcohol]

Selected Readings

al-Tannir MA and Goodman HS, "A Review of Chlorhexidine and Its Use in Special Populations," *Spec Care Dentist*, 1994, 14(3):116-22.

Ercan E, Ozekinci T, Atakul F, et al, "Antibacterial Activity of 2% Chlorhexidine Gluconate and 5.25% Sodium Hypochlorite in Infected Root Canal: *In Vivo* Study," *J Endod*, 2004, 30(2):84-7.

Ferretti GA, Brown AT, Raybould TP, et al, "Oral Antimicrobial Agents - Chlorhexidine," *NCI Monogr*, 1990, 9:51-5.

Greenstein G, Berman C, and Jaffin R, "Chlorhexidine. An Adjunct to Periodontal Therapy," *J Periodontol*, 1986, 57(6):370-7.

Johnson BT, "Uses of Chlorhexidine in Dentistry," *Gen Dent*, 1995, 43(2):126-32, 134-40.

Noiri Y, Okami Y, Narimatsu M, et al, "Effects of Chlorhexidine, Minocycline, and Metronidazole on Porphyromonas Gingivalis Strain 381 in Biofilms," *J Periodontol*, 2003, 74(11):1647-51.

Reddy MS, Jeffcoat MK, Geurs NC, et al, "Efficacy of Controlled-Release Subgingival Chlorhexidine to Enhance Periodontal Regeneration," *J Periodontol*, 2003, 74(4):411-9.

Soskolne WA, Proskin HM, and Stabholz A, "Probing Depth Changes Following 2 Years of Periodontal Maintenance Therapy Including Adjunctive Controlled Release of Chlorhexidine," *J Periodontol*, 2003, 74(4):420-7.

Yusof ZA, "Chlorhexidine Mouthwash: A Review of Its Pharmacological Activity, Clinical Effects, Uses and Abuses," *Dent J Malays*, 1988, 10(1):9-16.

Chlormeprazine *see* Prochlorperazine *on page 1126*

2-Chlorodeoxyadenosine *see* Cladribine *on page 342*

Chloroethane *see* Ethyl Chloride *on page 561*

Chloromag® *see* Magnesium Chloride *on page 852*

Chloromycetin® Sodium Succinate *see* Chloramphenicol *on page 306*

Chlorophyll (KLOR oh fil)

U.S. Brand Names Nullo® [OTC]

Generic Available Yes

Synonyms Chlorophyllin

Pharmacologic Category Gastrointestinal Agent, Miscellaneous

Use Control fecal and urinary odors in colostomy, ileostomy, or incontinence

Local Anesthetic/Vasoconstrictor Precautions No information available to require special precautions

Effects on Dental Treatment No significant effects or complications reported

Common Adverse Effects Frequency not defined: Gastrointestinal: Mild diarrhea, green stools, abdominal cramping

Chlorophyllin *see* Chlorophyll *on page 310*

Chloroprocaine (klor oh PROE kane)

Related Information

Oral Pain *on page 1526*

U.S. Brand Names Nesacaine®; Nesacaine®-MPF

Canadian Brand Names Nesacaine®-CE

Generic Available Yes

Synonyms Chloroprocaine Hydrochloride

Pharmacologic Category Local Anesthetic

Use Infiltration anesthesia and peripheral and epidural anesthesia

Local Anesthetic/Vasoconstrictor Precautions No information available to require special precautions

Effects on Dental Treatment No significant effects or complications reported

Mechanism of Action Chloroprocaine HCl is benzoic acid, 4-amino-2-chloro-2-(diethylamino) ethyl ester monohydrochloride. Chloroprocaine is an ester-type local anesthetic, which stabilizes the neuronal membranes and prevents initiation and transmission of nerve impulses thereby affecting local anesthetic actions. Local anesthetics including chloroprocaine, reversibly prevent generation and conduction of electrical impulses in neurons by decreasing the transient increase in permeability to sodium. The differential sensitivity generally depends on the size of the fiber; small fibers are more sensitive than larger fibers and require a longer period for recovery. Sensory pain fibers are usually blocked first, followed by fibers that transmit sensations of temperature, touch, and deep pressure. High concentrations block sympathetic somatic sensory and somatic motor fibers. The spread of anesthesia depends upon the distribution of the solution. This is primarily dependent on the volume of drug injected.

Drug Interactions

Increased Effect/Toxicity: Avoid concurrent use of bupivacaine due to safety and efficacy concerns.

Decreased Effect: The para-aminobenzoic acid metabolite of chloroprocaine may decrease the efficacy of sulfonamide antibiotics.

Pharmacodynamics/Kinetics

Onset of action: 6-12 minutes

Duration: 30-60 minutes

Metabolism: Plasma cholinesterases

Excretion: Urine

Pregnancy Risk Factor C

Chloroprocaine Hydrochloride *see* Chloroprocaine *on page 310*

Chloroquine (KLOR oh kwin)

U.S. Brand Names Aralen®

Canadian Brand Names Aralen®

Generic Available Yes

Synonyms Chloroquine Phosphate

Pharmacologic Category Aminoquinoline (Antimalarial)

Use Suppression or chemoprophylaxis of malaria; treatment of uncomplicated or mild to moderate malaria; extraintestinal amebiasis

Unlabeled/Investigational Use Rheumatoid arthritis; discoid lupus erythematosus

Local Anesthetic/Vasoconstrictor Precautions No information available to require special precautions

Effects on Dental Treatment Key adverse event(s) related to dental treatment: Stomatitis.

Common Adverse Effects Frequency not defined.

Cardiovascular: Hypotension (rare), ECG changes (rare; including T-wave inversion), cardiomyopathy

Central nervous system: Fatigue, personality changes, headache, psychosis, seizures, delirium, depression

Dermatologic: Pruritus, hair bleaching, pleomorphic skin eruptions, alopecia, lichen planus eruptions, alopecia, mucosal pigmentary changes (blue-black), photosensitivity

Gastrointestinal: Nausea, diarrhea, vomiting, anorexia, stomatitis, abdominal cramps

Hematologic: Aplastic anemia, agranulocytosis (reversible), neutropenia, thrombocytopenia

Neuromuscular & skeletal: Rare cases of myopathy, neuromyopathy, proximal muscle atrophy, and depression of deep tendon reflexes have been reported

Ocular: Retinopathy (including irreversible changes in some patients long-term or high-dose therapy), blurred vision

Otic: Nerve deafness, tinnitus, reduced hearing (risk increased in patients with pre-existing auditory damage)

(Continued)

Chloroquine *(Continued)*

Mechanism of Action Binds to and inhibits DNA and RNA polymerase; interferes with metabolism and hemoglobin utilization by parasites; inhibits prostaglandin effects; chloroquine concentrates within parasite acid vesicles and raises internal pH resulting in inhibition of parasite growth; may involve aggregates of ferriprotoporphyrin IX acting as chloroquine receptors causing membrane damage; may also interfere with nucleoprotein synthesis

Drug Interactions

Cytochrome P450 Effect: Substrate (major) of CYP2D6, 3A4; **Inhibits** CYP2D6 (moderate)

Increased Effect/Toxicity: Chloroquine may increase the levels/effects of dextromethorphan, fluoxetine, lidocaine, mirtazapine, nefazodone, paroxetine, risperidone, ritonavir, thioridazine, tricyclic antidepressants, venlafaxine, and other CYP2D6 substrates. Chloroquine may increase the levels/effects of cyclosporine. The levels/effects of chloroquine may be increased by azole antifungals, chlorpromazine, cimetidine, ciprofloxacin, clarithromycin, delavirdine, diclofenac, doxycycline, erythromycin, fluoxetine, imatinib, isoniazid, miconazole, nefazodone, nicardipine, paroxetine, pergolide, propofol, protease inhibitors, quinidine, quinine, ritonavir, ropinirole, telithromycin, verapamil, and other CYP2D6 or 3A4 inhibitors.

Decreased Effect: Chloroquine levels may be decreased by antacids or kaolin. Chloroquine may decrease ampicillin and/or praziquantel levels. Chloroquine may decrease the levels/effects of CYP2D6 prodrug substrates; example prodrug substrates include codeine, hydrocodone, oxycodone, and tramadol. The levels/effects of chloroquine may be decreased by aminoglutethimide, carbamazepine, nafcillin, nevirapine, phenobarbital, phenytoin, rifamycins, and other CYP3A4 inducers.

Pharmacodynamics/Kinetics

Duration: Small amounts may be present in urine months following discontinuation of therapy

Absorption: Oral: Rapid (~89%)

Distribution: Widely in body tissues (eg, eyes, heart, kidneys, liver, lungs) where retention prolonged; crosses placenta; enters breast milk

Metabolism: Partially hepatic

Half-life elimination: 3-5 days

Time to peak, serum: 1-2 hours

Excretion: Urine (~70% as unchanged drug); acidification of urine increases elimination

Pregnancy Risk Factor C

Chloroquine Phosphate *see* Chloroquine *on page 311*

Chlorostat® [OTC] *see* Chlorhexidine Gluconate *on page 308*

Chlorothiazide (klor oh THYE a zide)

Related Information

Cardiovascular Diseases *on page 1458*

U.S. Brand Names Diuril®

Canadian Brand Names Diuril®

Generic Available Yes: Tablet

Pharmacologic Category Diuretic, Thiazide

Use Management of mild to moderate hypertension; adjunctive treatment of edema

Local Anesthetic/Vasoconstrictor Precautions No information available to require special precautions

Effects on Dental Treatment Key adverse event(s) related to dental treatment: Orthostatic hypotension.

Common Adverse Effects Frequency not defined.

Cardiovascular: Hypotension, orthostatic hypotension, necrotizing angiitis

Central nervous system: Dizziness, headache, restlessness, vertigo

Dermatologic: Alopecia, erythema multiforme, exfoliative dermatitis, photosensitivity, Stevens-Johnson syndrome, toxic epidermal necrolysis

Endocrine & metabolic: Cholesterol increased, hypokalemia, hypomagnesemia, triglycerides increased

Gastrointestinal: Abdominal cramping, anorexia, constipation, diarrhea, gastric irritation, nausea, pancreatitis, sialadenitis, vomiting

Genitourinary: Impotence

Hematologic: Agranulocytosis, aplastic anemia, hemolytic anemia, leukopenia, thrombocytopenia

Hepatic: Jaundice

Neuromuscular & skeletal: Muscle spasm, paresthesias, weakness

Ocular: Blurred vision, xanthopsia

Renal: Azotemia, hematuria, interstitial nephritis, renal failure, renal dysfunction
Respiratory: Pneumonitis, pulmonary edema, respiratory distress
Miscellaneous: Anaphylactic reactions, systemic lupus erythematosus

Mechanism of Action Inhibits sodium reabsorption in the distal tubules causing increased excretion of sodium and water as well as potassium and hydrogen ions, magnesium, phosphate, calcium

Drug Interactions

Increased Effect/Toxicity: Increased effect of chlorothiazide with furosemide and other loop diuretics. Increased hypotension and/or renal adverse effects of ACE inhibitors may result in aggressively diuresed patients. Beta-blockers increase hyperglycemic effects of thiazides in Type 2 diabetes mellitus. Cyclosporine and thiazides can increase the risk of gout or renal toxicity. Digoxin toxicity can be exacerbated if a thiazide induces hypokalemia or hypomagnesemia. Lithium toxicity can occur with thiazides due to reduced renal excretion of lithium. Thiazides may prolong the duration of action with neuromuscular-blocking agents. Corticosteroids may increase electrolyte-depletion effects of chlorothiazide.

Decreased Effect: Effects of oral hypoglycemics may be decreased. Decreased absorption of chlorothiazide with cholestyramine and colestipol. NSAIDs can decrease the efficacy of thiazides, reducing the diuretic and antihypertensive effects.

Pharmacodynamics/Kinetics

Onset of action: Diuresis: Oral: 2 hours; I.V.: 15 minutes
Duration of diuretic action: Oral: 6-12 hours; I.V.: ~2 hours
Absorption: Oral: Poor
Half-life elimination: 1-2 hours
Time to peak, serum: Oral: ~4 hours; I.V.: 30 minutes
Excretion: Urine (as unchanged drug)

Pregnancy Risk Factor C (manufacturer); D (expert analysis)

Chloroxine (klor OKS een)

U.S. Brand Names Capitrol®
Canadian Brand Names Capitrol®
Generic Available No
Pharmacologic Category Topical Skin Product
Use Treatment of dandruff or seborrheic dermatitis of the scalp
Local Anesthetic/Vasoconstrictor Precautions No information available to require special precautions
Effects on Dental Treatment No significant effects or complications reported
Pregnancy Risk Factor C

Chlorphen [OTC] *see* Chlorpheniramine *on page 313*

Chlorpheniramine (klor fen IR a meen)

Related Information

Oral Bacterial Infections *on page 1533*

U.S. Brand Names Aller-Chlor® [OTC]; Chlorphen [OTC]; Chlor-Trimeton® [OTC]; Diabetic Tussin® Allergy Relief [OTC]
Canadian Brand Names Chlor-Tripolon®; Novo-Pheniram
Generic Available Yes: Tablet
Synonyms Chlorpheniramine Maleate; CTM
Pharmacologic Category Antihistamine
Use Perennial and seasonal allergic rhinitis and other allergic symptoms including urticaria
Local Anesthetic/Vasoconstrictor Precautions No information available to require special precautions
Effects on Dental Treatment Key adverse event(s) related to dental treatment: Xerostomia (normal salivary flow resumes upon discontinuation). Chronic use of antihistamines will inhibit salivary flow, particularly in elderly patients; this may contribute to periodontal disease and oral discomfort.

Common Adverse Effects

>10%:
Central nervous system: Slight to moderate drowsiness
Respiratory: Thickening of bronchial secretions

1% to 10%:
Central nervous system: Headache, excitability, fatigue, nervousness, dizziness
Gastrointestinal: Nausea, xerostomia, diarrhea, abdominal pain, appetite increase, weight gain
Genitourinary: Urinary retention

(Continued)

Chlorpheniramine *(Continued)*

Neuromuscular & skeletal: Arthralgia, weakness
Ocular: Diplopia
Renal: Polyuria
Respiratory: Pharyngitis

Mechanism of Action Competes with histamine for H_1-receptor sites on effector cells in the gastrointestinal tract, blood vessels, and respiratory tract

Drug Interactions

Cytochrome P450 Effect: Substrate of CYP2D6 (minor), 3A4 (major); **Inhibits** CYP2D6 (weak)

Increased Effect/Toxicity: CNS depressants may increase the degree of sedation and respiratory depression with antihistamines. May increase the absorption of digoxin. Central and/or peripheral anticholinergic syndrome can occur when administered with amantadine, rimantadine, narcotic analgesics, phenothiazines and other antipsychotics (especially with high anticholinergic activity), tricyclic antidepressants, quinidine, disopyramide, procainamide, and antihistamines. CYP3A4 inhibitors may increase the levels/effects of chlorpheniramine; example inhibitors include azole antifungals, ciprofloxacin, clarithromycin, diclofenac, doxycycline, erythromycin, imatinib, isoniazid, nefazodone, nicardipine, propofol, protease inhibitors, quinidine, and verapamil.

Decreased Effect: May increase gastric degradation of levodopa and decrease the amount of levodopa absorbed by delaying gastric emptying. Therapeutic effects of cholinergic agents (tacrine, donepezil) and neuroleptics may be antagonized.

Pharmacodynamics/Kinetics Half-life elimination, serum: 20-24 hours

Pregnancy Risk Factor B

Chlorpheniramine, Acetaminophen, and Pseudoephedrine *see* Acetaminophen, Chlorpheniramine, and Pseudoephedrine *on page 58*

Chlorpheniramine and Acetaminophen

(klor fen IR a meen & a seet a MIN oh fen)

Related Information

Acetaminophen *on page 47*
Chlorpheniramine *on page 313*

U.S. Brand Names Coricidin HBP® Cold and Flu [OTC]

Generic Available No

Synonyms Acetaminophen and Chlorpheniramine

Pharmacologic Category Antihistamine/Analgesic

Use Symptomatic relief of congestion, headache, aches and pains of colds and flu

Local Anesthetic/Vasoconstrictor Precautions No information available to require special precautions

Effects on Dental Treatment Key adverse event(s) related to dental treatment: Chronic use of antihistamines will inhibit salivary flow, particularly in elderly patients; this may contribute to periodontal disease and oral discomfort.

Common Adverse Effects See individual agents.

Drug Interactions

Cytochrome P450 Effect:

Acetaminophen: **Substrate** (minor) of CYP1A2, 2A6, 2C8/9, 2D6, 2E1, 3A4; **Inhibits** CYP3A4 (weak)

Chlorpheniramine: **Substrate** of CYP2D6 (minor), 3A4 (major); **Inhibits** CYP2D6 (weak)

Pharmacodynamics/Kinetics See individual agents.

Chlorpheniramine and Carbetapentane *see* Carbetapentane and Chlorpheniramine *on page 260*

Chlorpheniramine and Hydrocodone *see* Hydrocodone and Chlorpheniramine *on page 707*

Chlorpheniramine and Phenylephrine

(klor fen IR a meen & fen il EF rin)

Related Information

Chlorpheniramine *on page 313*

U.S. Brand Names Dallergy-JR®; Ed A-Hist®; Histatab® Plus [OTC]; Rynatan®; Rynatan® Pediatric Suspension

Generic Available No

Synonyms Chlorpheniramine Maleate and Phenylephrine Hydrochloride; Chlorpheniramine Tannate and Phenylephrine Tannate; Phenylephrine and Chlorpheniramine

Pharmacologic Category Antihistamine/Decongestant Combination

Use Temporary relief of nasal congestion and eustachian tube congestion as well as runny nose, sneezing, itching of nose or throat, itchy and watery eyes

Local Anesthetic/Vasoconstrictor Precautions Use with caution since phenylephrine is a sympathomimetic amine which could interact with epinephrine to cause a pressor response

Effects on Dental Treatment Key adverse event(s) related to dental treatment:

Chlorpheniramine: Prolonged use will cause significant xerostomia (normal salivary flow resumes upon discontinuation).

Phenylephrine: Up to 10% of patients could experience tachycardia, palpitations, and xerostomia (prolonged use worsens); use vasoconstrictor with caution.

Common Adverse Effects See individual agents.

Drug Interactions

Cytochrome P450 Effect: Chlorpheniramine: **Substrate** of CYP2D6 (minor), 3A4 (major); **Inhibits** CYP2D6 (weak)

Increased Effect/Toxicity: See individual agents.

Decreased Effect: See individual agents.

Pharmacodynamics/Kinetics See individual agents.

Pregnancy Risk Factor C

Chlorpheniramine and Pseudoephedrine

(klor fen IR a meen & soo doe e FED rin)

Related Information

Chlorpheniramine *on page 313*

Pseudoephedrine *on page 1147*

U.S. Brand Names Allerest® Maximum Strength Allergy and Hay Fever [OTC]; A.R.M® [OTC]; Chlor-Trimeton® Allergy D [OTC]; C-Phed Tannate; Deconamine®; Deconamine® SR; Genaphed Plus [OTC]; Hayfebrol® [OTC]; Histex™; Kronofed-A®; Kronofed-A®-Jr; PediaCare® Cold and Allergy [OTC]; Rhinosyn® [OTC]; Rhinosyn-PD® [OTC]; Ryna® [OTC] [DSC]; Sudafed® Sinus & Allergy [OTC]; Tanafed®; Tanafed DP™; Triaminic® Cold and Allergy [OTC]

Canadian Brand Names Triaminic® Cold & Allergy

Generic Available Yes: Tablet, extended release capsule, suspension

Synonyms Chlorpheniramine Maleate and Pseudoephedrine Hydrochloride; Chlorpheniramine Tannate and Pseudoephedrine Tannate; Dexchlorpheniramine Tannate and Pseudoephedrine Tannate; Pseudoephedrine and Chlorpheniramine

Pharmacologic Category Antihistamine/Decongestant Combination

Use Relief of nasal congestion associated with the common cold, hay fever, and other allergies, sinusitis, eustachian tube blockage, and vasomotor and allergic rhinitis

Local Anesthetic/Vasoconstrictor Precautions Use with caution since pseudoephedrine is a sympathomimetic amine which could interact with epinephrine to cause a pressor response

Effects on Dental Treatment Key adverse event(s) related to dental treatment:

Chlorpheniramine: Prolonged use will cause significant xerostomia (normal salivary flow resumes upon discontinuation).

Pseudoephedrine: Xerostomia (prolonged use worsens; normal salivary flow resumes upon discontinuation).

Common Adverse Effects See individual agents.

Mechanism of Action

Chlorpheniramine competes with histamine for H_1-receptor sites on effector cells in the gastrointestinal tract, blood vessels, and respiratory tract. Dexchlorpheniramine is the predominant active isomer of chlorpheniramine and is approximately twice as active as the racemic compound.

Pseudoephedrine is a sympathomimetic amine and isomer of ephedrine; acts as a decongestant in respiratory tract mucous membranes with less vasoconstrictor action than ephedrine in normotensive individuals.

Drug Interactions

Cytochrome P450 Effect: Chlorpheniramine: **Substrate** of CYP2D6 (minor), 3A4 (major); **Inhibits** CYP2D6 (weak)

Increased Effect/Toxicity: See individual agents.

Decreased Effect: See individual agents.

Pharmacodynamics/Kinetics See individual agents.

Pregnancy Risk Factor C

Chlorpheniramine, Ephedrine, Phenylephrine, and Carbetapentane

(klor fen IR a meen, e FED rin, fen il EF rin, & kar bay ta PEN tane)

Related Information

Chlorpheniramine *on page 313*

U.S. Brand Names Rynatuss®; Rynatuss® Pediatric; Tetra Tannate Pediatric

Generic Available No

Synonyms Carbetapentane, Ephedrine, Phenylephrine, and Chlorpheniramine; Ephedrine, Chlorpheniramine, Phenylephrine, and Carbetapentane; Phenylephrine, Ephedrine, Chlorpheniramine, and Carbetapentane

Pharmacologic Category Antihistamine/Decongestant/Antitussive

Use Symptomatic relief of cough with a decongestant and an antihistamine

Local Anesthetic/Vasoconstrictor Precautions

Ephedrine: Use vasoconstrictor with caution since ephedrine may enhance cardiostimulation and vasopressor effects of sympathomimetics

Phenylephrine: Use with caution since phenylephrine is a sympathomimetic amine which could interact with epinephrine to cause a pressor response

Effects on Dental Treatment Key adverse event(s) related to dental treatment:

Chlorpheniramine: Prolonged use will cause significant xerostomia (normal salivary flow resumes upon discontinuation).

Ephedrine: No significant effects or complications reported.

Phenylephrine: Up to 10% of patients could experience tachycardia, palpitations, and xerostomia; use vasoconstrictor with caution.

Drug Interactions

Cytochrome P450 Effect: Chlorpheniramine: **Substrate** of CYP2D6 (minor), 3A4 (major); **Inhibits** CYP2D6 (weak)

Increased Effect/Toxicity: See individual agents.

Decreased Effect: See individual agents.

Pregnancy Risk Factor C

Chlorpheniramine, Hydrocodone, Phenylephrine, Acetaminophen, and Caffeine *see* Hydrocodone, Chlorpheniramine, Phenylephrine, Acetaminophen, and Caffeine *on page 712*

Chlorpheniramine Maleate *see* Chlorpheniramine *on page 313*

Chlorpheniramine Maleate and Phenylephrine Hydrochloride *see* Chlorpheniramine and Phenylephrine *on page 314*

Chlorpheniramine Maleate and Pseudoephedrine Hydrochloride *see* Chlorpheniramine and Pseudoephedrine *on page 315*

Chlorpheniramine, Phenylephrine, and Dextromethorphan

(klor fen IR a meen, fen il EF rin, & deks troe meth OR fan)

Related Information

Chlorpheniramine *on page 313*

Dextromethorphan *on page 421*

U.S. Brand Names Alka-Seltzer Plus® Cold and Cough [OTC]

Generic Available No

Synonyms Dextromethorphan, Chlorpheniramine, and Phenylephrine; Phenylephrine, Chlorpheniramine, and Dextromethorphan

Pharmacologic Category Antihistamine/Decongestant/Antitussive

Use Temporary relief of cough due to minor throat and bronchial irritation; relieves nasal congestion, runny nose and sneezing

Local Anesthetic/Vasoconstrictor Precautions

Chlorpheniramine, Dextromethorphan: No information available to require special precautions

Phenylephrine: Use with caution since phenylephrine is a sympathomimetic amine which could interact with epinephrine to cause a pressor response

Effects on Dental Treatment Key adverse event(s) related to dental treatment:

Chlorpheniramine: Prolonged use will cause significant xerostomia (normal salivary flow resumes upon discontinuation).

Dextromethorphan: No significant effects or complications reported

Phenylephrine: Up to 10% of patients could experience tachycardia, palpitations, and xerostomia (prolonged use worsens); use vasoconstrictor with caution.

Drug Interactions

Cytochrome P450 Effect:

Chlorpheniramine: **Substrate** of CYP2D6 (minor), 3A4 (major); **Inhibits** CYP2D6 (weak)

Dextromethorphan: **Substrate** of CYP2B6 (minor), 2C8/9 (minor), 2C19 (minor), 2D6 (major), 2E1 (minor), 3A4 (minor); **Inhibits** CYP2D6 (weak)

Increased Effect/Toxicity: See individual agents.

Decreased Effect: See individual agents.

Pharmacodynamics/Kinetics See individual agents.

Chlorpheniramine, Phenylephrine, and Methscopolamine

(klor fen IR a meen, fen il EF rin, & meth skoe POL a meen)

Related Information

Chlorpheniramine *on page 313*

U.S. Brand Names AH-Chew®; D.A.II™ [DSC]; Dallergy®; Dehistine; Drize®-R; Dura-Vent®/DA [DSC]; Extendryl; Extendryl JR; Extendryl SR; Hista-Vent® DA; Vanex Forte™-D

Generic Available No

Synonyms Methscopolamine, Chlorpheniramine, and Phenylephrine; Phenylephrine, Chlorpheniramine, and Methscopolamine

Pharmacologic Category Antihistamine/Decongestant/Anticholinergic

Use Treatment of upper respiratory symptoms such as respiratory congestion, allergic rhinitis, vasomotor rhinitis, sinusitis, and allergic skin reactions of urticaria and angioedema

Local Anesthetic/Vasoconstrictor Precautions Use with caution since phenylephrine is a sympathomimetic amine which could interact with epinephrine to cause a pressor response

Effects on Dental Treatment Key adverse event(s) related to dental treatment:

Chlorpheniramine: Significant xerostomia with prolonged use (normal salivary flow resumes upon discontinuation).

Methscopolamine: Anticholinergic side effects can cause a reduction of saliva production or secretion contributes to discomfort and dental disease (ie, caries, oral candidiasis and periodontal disease).

Phenylephrine: Tachycardia, palpitations, and xerostomia; use vasoconstrictor with caution.

Common Adverse Effects Frequency not defined.

Cardiovascular: Arrhythmias, bradycardia, cardiovascular collapse, flushing, hypotension, pallor, palpitation, tachycardia

Central nervous system: Anxiety, convulsions, CNS depression, dizziness, drowsiness, excitability, fear, giddiness, hallucinations, headache, insomnia, irritability, lassitude, restlessness, tenseness, tremor

Gastrointestinal: Constipation, dysphagia, gastric irritation, nausea, xerostomia

Genitourinary: Dysuria, urinary retention

Neuromuscular & skeletal: Weakness

Ocular: Blurred vision, mydriasis

Respiratory: Dry nose, dry throat, respiratory difficulty

Mechanism of Action

Chlorpheniramine maleate: Antihistamine

Phenylephrine hydrochloride: Sympathomimetic agent (primarily alpha), decongestant

Methscopolamine nitrate: Derivative of scopolamine, antisecretory effects

Drug Interactions

Cytochrome P450 Effect: Chlorpheniramine: **Substrate** of CYP2D6 (minor), 3A4 (major); **Inhibits** CYP2D6 (weak)

Increased Effect/Toxicity: Increased effects/toxicity seen with concomitant use of antihistamines, beta-adrenergic blockers, CNS depressants, and MAO inhibitors

Decreased Effect: Decreased effects of antihypertensive agents seen with concomitant use

Pharmacodynamics/Kinetics See individual agents.

Pregnancy Risk Factor C

Chlorpheniramine, Phenylephrine, and Phenyltoloxamine

(klor fen IR a meen, fen il EF rin, & fen il tole LOKS a meen)

Related Information

Chlorpheniramine *on page 313*

U.S. Brand Names Comhist®; Nalex®-A

Generic Available No

Synonyms Phenylephrine, Chlorpheniramine, and Phenyltoloxamine; Phenyltoloxamine, Chlorpheniramine, and Phenylephrine

Pharmacologic Category Antihistamine/Decongestant Combination

(Continued)

Chlorpheniramine, Phenylephrine, and Phenyltoloxamine *(Continued)*

Use Symptomatic relief of rhinitis and nasal congestion due to colds or allergy

Local Anesthetic/Vasoconstrictor Precautions Use with caution since phenylephrine is a sympathomimetic amine which could interact with epinephrine to cause a pressor response

Effects on Dental Treatment Key adverse event(s) related to dental treatment:

Chlorpheniramine: Prolonged use will cause significant xerostomia (normal salivary flow resumes upon discontinuation).

Phenylephrine: Up to 10% of patients could experience tachycardia, palpitations, and xerostomia; use vasoconstrictor with caution.

Common Adverse Effects Frequency not defined.

Cardiovascular: Hypotension, palpitations

Central nervous system: Headache, dizziness, sedation, excitation (children), nervousness, seizures

Dermatologic: Urticaria, drug rash

Gastrointestinal: Dry mouth, anorexia, nausea, vomiting, diarrhea, constipation, GI upset

Genitourinary: Urinary frequency, urinary retention

Hematologic: Agranulocytosis, leukopenia, thrombocytopenia

Ocular: Blurred vision

Respiratory: Dry nose/throat, thickening of bronchial secretions, wheezing, stuffy nose, tightness of chest

Drug Interactions

Cytochrome P450 Effect: Chlorpheniramine: **Substrate** of CYP2D6 (minor), 3A4 (major); **Inhibits** CYP2D6 (weak)

Increased Effect/Toxicity: See individual agents.

Decreased Effect: See individual agents.

Pregnancy Risk Factor C

Chlorpheniramine, Phenylephrine, Codeine, and Potassium Iodide

(klor fen IR a meen, fen il EF rin, KOE deen, & poe TASS ee um EYE oh dide)

Related Information

Chlorpheniramine *on page 313*

Codeine *on page 369*

U.S. Brand Names Pediacof®

Generic Available No

Synonyms Codeine, Chlorpheniramine, Phenylephrine, and Potassium Iodide; Phenylephrine, Chlorpheniramine, Codeine, and Potassium Iodide; Potassium Iodide, Chlorpheniramine, Phenylephrine, and Codeine

Pharmacologic Category Antihistamine/Decongestant/Antitussive/Expectorant

Use Symptomatic relief of rhinitis, nasal congestion and cough due to colds or allergy

Local Anesthetic/Vasoconstrictor Precautions Use with caution since phenylephrine is a sympathomimetic amine which could interact with epinephrine to cause a pressor response

Effects on Dental Treatment Key adverse event(s) related to dental treatment:

Chlorpheniramine: Prolonged use will cause significant xerostomia (normal salivary flow resumes upon discontinuation).

Phenylephrine: Up to 10% of patients could experience tachycardia, palpitations, and xerostomia (prolonged use worsens); use vasoconstrictor with caution.

Restrictions C-V

Drug Interactions

Cytochrome P450 Effect: Chlorpheniramine: **Substrate** of CYP2D6 (minor), 3A4 (major); **Inhibits** CYP2D6 (weak)

Increased Effect/Toxicity: See individual agents.

Decreased Effect: See individual agents.

Chlorpheniramine, Pseudoephedrine, and Acetaminophen *see* Acetaminophen, Chlorpheniramine, and Pseudoephedrine *on page 58*

Chlorpheniramine, Pseudoephedrine, and Codeine

(klor fen IR a meen, soo doe e FED rin, & KOE deen)

Related Information

Chlorpheniramine *on page 313*

Pseudoephedrine *on page 1147*

U.S. Brand Names Dihistine® DH

Generic Available Yes

Synonyms Codeine, Chlorpheniramine, and Pseudoephedrine; Pseudoephedrine, Chlorpheniramine, and Codeine

Pharmacologic Category Antihistamine/Decongestant/Antitussive

Use Temporary relief of cough associated with minor throat or bronchial irritation or nasal congestion due to common cold, allergic rhinitis, or sinusitis

Local Anesthetic/Vasoconstrictor Precautions Use with caution since pseudoephedrine is a sympathomimetic amine which could interact with epinephrine to cause a pressor response

Effects on Dental Treatment Key adverse event(s) related to dental treatment:

Chlorpheniramine: Significant xerostomia with prolonged use (normal salivary flow resumes upon discontinuation).

Pseudoephedrine: Xerostomia (normal salivary flow resumes upon discontinuation).

Common Adverse Effects See individual agents.

Restrictions C-V

Drug Interactions

Cytochrome P450 Effect: Chlorpheniramine: **Substrate** of CYP2D6 (minor), 3A4 (major); **Inhibits** CYP2D6 (weak)

Increased Effect/Toxicity: See individual agents.

Decreased Effect: See individual agents.

Pharmacodynamics/Kinetics See individual agents.

Pregnancy Risk Factor C

Chlorpheniramine, Pseudoephedrine, and Dihydrocodeine *see* Pseudoephedrine, Dihydrocodeine, and Chlorpheniramine *on page 1150*

Chlorpheniramine Tannate and Phenylephrine Tannate *see* Chlorpheniramine and Phenylephrine *on page 314*

Chlorpheniramine Tannate and Pseudoephedrine Tannate *see* Chlorpheniramine and Pseudoephedrine *on page 315*

ChlorproMAZINE (klor PROE ma zeen)

U.S. Brand Names Thorazine® [DSC]

Canadian Brand Names Apo-Chlorpromazine®; Largactil®; Novo-Chlorpromazine

Mexican Brand Names Largactil®

Generic Available Yes: Tablet

Synonyms Chlorpromazine Hydrochloride; CPZ

Pharmacologic Category Antipsychotic Agent, Phenothiazine, Aliphatic

Use Control of mania; treatment of schizophrenia; control of nausea and vomiting; relief of restlessness and apprehension before surgery; acute intermittent porphyria; adjunct in the treatment of tetanus; intractable hiccups; combativeness and/or explosive hyperexcitable behavior in children 1-12 years of age and in short-term treatment of hyperactive children

Unlabeled/Investigational Use Management of psychotic disorders

Local Anesthetic/Vasoconstrictor Precautions Most pharmacology textbooks state that in presence of phenothiazines, systemic doses of epinephrine paradoxically decrease the blood pressure. This is the so called "epinephrine reversal" phenomenon. This has never been observed when epinephrine is given by infiltration as part of the anesthesia procedure.

Effects on Dental Treatment Key adverse event(s) related to dental treatment:

Significant hypotension may occur, especially when the drug is administered parenterally. Orthostatic hypotension is due to alpha-receptor blockade; elderly are at greater risk.

Tardive dyskinesia: Prevalence rate may be 40% in elderly; development of the syndrome and the irreversible nature are proportional to duration and total cumulative dose over time. Extrapyramidal reactions are more common in elderly with up to 50% developing these reactions after 60 years of age. Drug-induced Parkinson's syndrome occurs often; akathisia is the most common extrapyramidal reaction in elderly.

(Continued)

ChlorproMAZINE *(Continued)*

Increased confusion, memory loss, psychotic behavior, and agitation frequently occur as a consequence of anticholinergic effects. Antipsychotic-associated sedation in nonpsychotic patients is extremely unpleasant due to feelings of depersonalization, derealization, and dysphoria.

Common Adverse Effects Frequency not defined.

Cardiovascular: Postural hypotension, tachycardia, dizziness, nonspecific QT changes

Central nervous system: Drowsiness, dystonias, akathisia, pseudoparkinsonism, tardive dyskinesia, neuroleptic malignant syndrome, seizures

Dermatologic: Photosensitivity, dermatitis, skin pigmentation (slate gray)

Endocrine & metabolic: Lactation, breast engorgement, false-positive pregnancy test, amenorrhea, gynecomastia, hyper- or hypoglycemia

Gastrointestinal: Xerostomia, constipation, nausea

Genitourinary: Urinary retention, ejaculatory disorder, impotence

Hematologic: Agranulocytosis, eosinophilia, leukopenia, hemolytic anemia, aplastic anemia, thrombocytopenic purpura

Hepatic: Jaundice

Ocular: Blurred vision, corneal and lenticular changes, epithelial keratopathy, pigmentary retinopathy

Mechanism of Action Blocks postsynaptic mesolimbic dopaminergic receptors in the brain; exhibits a strong alpha-adrenergic blocking effect and depresses the release of hypothalamic and hypophyseal hormones; believed to depress the reticular activating system, thus affecting basal metabolism, body temperature, wakefulness, vasomotor tone, and emesis

Drug Interactions

Cytochrome P450 Effect: Substrate of CYP1A2 (minor), 2D6 (major), 3A4 (minor); **Inhibits** CYP2D6 (strong), 2E1 (weak)

Increased Effect/Toxicity: The levels/effects of chlorpromazine may be increased by delavirdine, fluoxetine, miconazole, paroxetine, pergolide, quinidine, quinine, ritonavir, ropinirole, and other CYP2D6 inhibitors. Effects on CNS depression may be additive when chlorpromazine is combined with CNS depressants (narcotic analgesics, ethanol, barbiturates, cyclic antidepressants, antihistamines, or sedative-hypnotics). Chlorpromazine may increase the levels/effects of amphetamines, selected beta-blockers, dextromethorphan, fluoxetine, lidocaine, mirtazapine, nefazodone, paroxetine, risperidone, ritonavir, thioridazine, tricyclic antidepressants, and venlafaxine and other CYP2D6 substrates. Chlorpromazine may increase the effects/toxicity of anticholinergics, antihypertensives, lithium (rare neurotoxicity), trazodone, or valproic acid. Concurrent use with TCA may produce increased toxicity or altered therapeutic response. Chloroquine and propranolol may increase chlorpromazine concentrations. Hypotension may occur when chlorpromazine is combined with epinephrine. May increase the risk of arrhythmia when combined with antiarrhythmics, cisapride, pimozide, sparfloxacin, or other drugs which prolong QT interval. Metoclopramide may increase risk of extrapyramidal symptoms (EPS).

Decreased Effect: Chlorpromazine may decrease the levels/effects of CYP2D6 prodrug substrates; example prodrug substrates include codeine, hydrocodone, oxycodone, and tramadol. Phenothiazines inhibit the ability of bromocriptine to lower serum prolactin concentrations. Benztropine (and other anticholinergics) may inhibit the therapeutic response to chlorpromazine and excess anticholinergic effects may occur. Antihypertensive effects of guanethidine and guanadrel may be inhibited by chlorpromazine. Chlorpromazine may inhibit the antiparkinsonian effect of levodopa. Chlorpromazine and possibly other low potency antipsychotics may reverse the pressor effects of epinephrine.

Pharmacodynamics/Kinetics

Onset of action: I.M.: 15 minutes; Oral: 30-60 minutes

Absorption: Rapid

Distribution: V_d: 20 L/kg; crosses the placenta; enters breast milk

Protein binding: 92% to 97%

Metabolism: Extensively hepatic to active and inactive metabolites

Bioavailability: 20%

Half-life, biphasic: Initial: 2 hours; Terminal: 30 hours

Excretion: Urine (<1% as unchanged drug) within 24 hours

Pregnancy Risk Factor C

Chlorpromazine Hydrochloride *see* ChlorproMAZINE *on page 319*

ChlorproPAMIDE (klor PROE pa mide)

Related Information

Endocrine Disorders and Pregnancy *on page 1481*

U.S. Brand Names Diabinese®

Canadian Brand Names Apo-Chlorpropamide®; Novo-Propamide

Mexican Brand Names Diabinese®; Insogen®

Generic Available Yes

Pharmacologic Category Antidiabetic Agent, Sulfonylurea

Use Management of blood sugar in type 2 diabetes mellitus (noninsulin dependent, NIDDM)

Unlabeled/Investigational Use Neurogenic diabetes insipidus

Local Anesthetic/Vasoconstrictor Precautions No information available to require special precautions

Effects on Dental Treatment Chlorpropamide-dependent diabetics (noninsulin dependent, Type 2) should be appointed for dental treatment in morning in order to minimize chance of stress-induced hypoglycemia.

Common Adverse Effects

>10%:

Central nervous system: Headache, dizziness

Gastrointestinal: Anorexia, constipation, heartburn, epigastric fullness, nausea, vomiting, diarrhea

1% to 10%: Dermatologic: Skin rash, urticaria, photosensitivity

Mechanism of Action Stimulates insulin release from the pancreatic beta cells; reduces glucose output from the liver; insulin sensitivity is increased at peripheral target sites

Drug Interactions

Cytochrome P450 Effect: Substrate of CYP2C8/9 (minor)

Increased Effect/Toxicity: A possible interaction between chlorpropamide and fluoroquinolone antibiotics has been reported resulting in a potentiation of hypoglycemic action of chlorpropamide. Toxic potential is increased when given concomitantly with other highly protein bound drugs (ie, phenylbutazone, oral anticoagulants, hydantoins, salicylates, NSAIDs, beta-blockers, sulfonamides) - increase hypoglycemic effect. Ethanol may be associated with disulfiram reactions. Phenylbutazone may increase hypoglycemic effects. Possible interactions between chlorpropamide and coumarin derivatives have been reported that may either potentiate or weaken the effects of coumarin derivatives.

Decreased Effect: Certain drugs tend to produce hyperglycemia and may lead to loss of control (ie, thiazides and other diuretics, corticosteroids, phenothiazines, thyroid products, estrogens, oral contraceptives, phenytoin, nicotinic acid, sympathomimetics, calcium channel blocking drugs, and isoniazid). Possible interactions between chlorpropamide and coumarin derivatives have been reported that may either potentiate or weaken the effects of coumarin derivatives.

Pharmacodynamics/Kinetics

Onset of action: Peak effect: ~6-8 hours

Distribution: V_d: 0.13-0.23 L/kg; enters breast milk

Protein binding: 60% to 90%

Metabolism: Extensively hepatic (~80%)

Half-life elimination: 30-42 hours; prolonged in elderly or with renal impairment

End-stage renal disease: 50-200 hours

Time to peak, serum: 3-4 hours

Excretion: Urine (10% to 30% as unchanged drug)

Pregnancy Risk Factor C

Chlorthalidone (klor THAL i done)

Related Information

Cardiovascular Diseases *on page 1458*

U.S. Brand Names Thalitone®

Canadian Brand Names Apo-Chlorthalidone®

Generic Available Yes

Synonyms Hygroton

Pharmacologic Category Diuretic, Thiazide

Use Management of mild to moderate hypertension when used alone or in combination with other agents; treatment of edema associated with congestive heart failure or nephrotic syndrome. Recent studies have found chlorthalidone effective in the treatment of isolated systolic hypertension in the elderly.

Local Anesthetic/Vasoconstrictor Precautions No information available to require special precautions

Effects on Dental Treatment No significant effects or complications reported

(Continued)

Chlorthalidone *(Continued)*

Common Adverse Effects 1% to 10%:

Dermatologic: Photosensitivity
Endocrine & metabolic: Hypokalemia
Gastrointestinal: Anorexia, epigastric distress

Mechanism of Action Sulfonamide-derived diuretic that inhibits sodium and chloride reabsorption in the cortical-diluting segment of the ascending loop of Henle

Drug Interactions

Increased Effect/Toxicity: Increased effect of chlorthalidone with furosemide and other loop diuretics. Increased hypotension and/or renal adverse effects of ACE inhibitors may result in aggressively diuresed patients. Beta-blockers increase hyperglycemic effects of thiazides in Type 2 diabetes mellitus. Cyclosporine and thiazides can increase the risk of gout or renal toxicity. Digoxin toxicity can be exacerbated if a thiazide induces hypokalemia or hypomagnesemia. Lithium toxicity can occur with thiazides due to reduced renal excretion of lithium. Thiazides may prolong the duration of action with neuromuscular blocking agents.

Decreased Effect: Effects of oral hypoglycemics may be decreased. Decreased absorption of chlorthalidone with cholestyramine and colestipol. NSAIDs can decrease the efficacy of chlorthalidone, reducing the diuretic and antihypertensive effects.

Pharmacodynamics/Kinetics

Onset of action: Peak effect: 2-6 hours
Absorption: 65%
Distribution: Crosses placenta; enters breast milk
Metabolism: Hepatic
Half-life elimination: 35-55 hours; may be prolonged with renal impairment; Anuria: 81 hours
Excretion: Urine (~50% to 65% as unchanged drug)

Pregnancy Risk Factor B (manufacturer); D (expert analysis)

Chlorthalidone and Atenolol *see* Atenolol and Chlorthalidone *on page 161*
Chlorthalidone and Clonidine *see* Clonidine and Chlorthalidone *on page 360*
Chlor-Trimeton® [OTC] *see* Chlorpheniramine *on page 313*
Chlor-Trimeton® Allergy D [OTC] *see* Chlorpheniramine and Pseudoephedrine *on page 315*

Chlorzoxazone (klor ZOKS a zone)

Related Information

Temporomandibular Dysfunction (TMD) *on page 1564*

U.S. Brand Names Parafon Forte® DSC

Canadian Brand Names Parafon Forte®; Strifon Forte®

Generic Available Yes

Pharmacologic Category Skeletal Muscle Relaxant

Dental Use Treatment of muscle spasm and pain associated with acute temporomandibular joint pain

Use Symptomatic treatment of muscle spasm and pain associated with acute musculoskeletal conditions

Local Anesthetic/Vasoconstrictor Precautions No information available to require special precautions

Effects on Dental Treatment No significant effects or complications reported

Significant Adverse Effects Frequency not defined.

Central nervous system: Dizziness, drowsiness, lightheadedness, paradoxical stimulation, malaise
Dermatologic: Rash, petechiae, ecchymoses (rare), angioneurotic edema
Gastrointestinal: Nausea, vomiting, stomach cramps
Genitourinary: Urine discoloration
Hepatic: Liver dysfunction
Miscellaneous: Anaphylaxis (very rare)

Dosage Oral:

Children: 20 mg/kg/day or 600 mg/m^2/day in 3-4 divided doses
Adults: 250-500 mg 3-4 times/day up to 750 mg 3-4 times/day

Mechanism of Action Acts on the spinal cord and subcortical levels by depressing polysynaptic reflexes

Contraindications Hypersensitivity to chlorzoxazone or any component of the formulation; impaired liver function

Drug Interactions Substrate of CYP1A2 (minor), 2A6 (minor), 2D6 (minor), 2E1 (major), 3A4 (minor); **Inhibits** CYP2E1 (weak), 3A4 (weak)

CNS depressants: Effects may be increased by chlorzoxazone.

CYP2E1 inhibitors: May increase the levels/effects of chlorzoxazone. Example inhibitors include disulfiram, isoniazid, and miconazole.
Disulfiram: May increase chlorzoxazone concentration; monitor.
Isoniazid: May increase chlorzoxazone concentration; monitor.

Ethanol/Nutrition/Herb Interactions Ethanol: Avoid ethanol (may increase CNS depression).

Pharmacodynamics/Kinetics
Onset of action: ~1 hour
Duration: 6-12 hours
Absorption: Readily absorbed
Metabolism: Extensively hepatic via glucuronidation
Excretion: Urine (as conjugates)

Pregnancy Risk Factor C

Lactation Excretion in breast milk unknown/not recommended

Dosage Forms
Caplet (Parafon Forte® DSC): 500 mg
Tablet: 250 mg, 500 mg

Cholac® *see* Lactulose *on page 794*

Cholecalciferol (kole e kal SI fer ole)

U.S. Brand Names Delta-D®

Canadian Brand Names D-Vi-Sol®

Generic Available Yes

Synonyms D_3

Pharmacologic Category Vitamin D Analog

Use Dietary supplement, treatment of vitamin D deficiency, or prophylaxis of deficiency

Local Anesthetic/Vasoconstrictor Precautions No information available to require special precautions

Effects on Dental Treatment Key adverse event(s) related to dental treatment: Metallic taste and xerostomia (normal salivary flow resumes upon discontinuation).

Common Adverse Effects Frequency not defined.
Cardiovascular: Hypotension, cardiac arrhythmias, hypertension, arrhythmia
Central nervous system: Irritability, headache, somnolence, overt psychosis (rare)
Dermatologic: Pruritus
Endocrine & metabolic: Polydipsia
Gastrointestinal: Nausea, vomiting, anorexia, pancreatitis, metallic taste, dry mouth, constipation, weight loss
Genitourinary: Albuminuria, polyuria
Hepatic: Increased liver function test
Neuromuscular & skeletal: Bone pain, myalgia, weakness, muscle pain
Ocular: Conjunctivitis, photophobia
Renal: Azotemia, nephrocalcinosis

Drug Interactions
Cytochrome P450 Effect: Inhibits CYP2C8/9 (weak), 2C19 (weak), 2D6 (weak)

Pregnancy Risk Factor C

Cholestyramine Resin (koe LES teer a meen REZ in)

Related Information
Cardiovascular Diseases *on page 1458*

U.S. Brand Names Prevalite®; Questran®; Questran® Light

Canadian Brand Names Novo-Cholamine; Novo-Cholamine Light; PMS-Cholestyramine; Questran®; Questran® Light Sugar Free

Generic Available Yes

Pharmacologic Category Antilipemic Agent, Bile Acid Sequestrant

Use Adjunct in the management of primary hypercholesterolemia; pruritus associated with elevated levels of bile acids; diarrhea associated with excess fecal bile acids; binding toxicologic agents; pseudomembraneous colitis

Local Anesthetic/Vasoconstrictor Precautions No information available to require special precautions

Effects on Dental Treatment No significant effects or complications reported

Common Adverse Effects
>10%: Gastrointestinal: Constipation, heartburn, nausea, vomiting, stomach pain
1% to 10%:
Central nervous system: Headache
Gastrointestinal: Belching, bloating, diarrhea

(Continued)

Cholestyramine Resin *(Continued)*

Mechanism of Action Forms a nonabsorbable complex with bile acids in the intestine, releasing chloride ions in the process; inhibits enterohepatic reuptake of intestinal bile salts and thereby increases the fecal loss of bile salt-bound low density lipoprotein cholesterol

Drug Interactions

Decreased Effect:

Cholestyramine can reduce the absorption of numerous medications when used concurrently. Give other medications 1 hour before or 4-6 hours after giving cholestyramine. Medications which may be affected include HMG-CoA reductase inhibitors, thiazide diuretics, propranolol (and potentially other beta-blockers), corticosteroids, thyroid hormones, digoxin, valproic acid, NSAIDs, loop diuretics, sulfonylureas, troglitazone (and potentially other agents in this class).

Warfarin and other oral anticoagulants: Hypoprothrombinemic effects may be reduced by cholestyramine. Separate administration times (as detailed above) and monitor INR closely when initiating or discontinuing.

Pharmacodynamics/Kinetics

Onset of action: Peak effect: 21 days

Absorption: None

Excretion: Feces (as insoluble complex with bile acids)

Pregnancy Risk Factor C

Choline Magnesium Trisalicylate

(KOE leen mag NEE zhum trye sa LIS i late)

Related Information

Rheumatoid Arthritis, Osteoarthritis, and Osteoporosis *on page 1490*

Temporomandibular Dysfunction (TMD) *on page 1564*

U.S. Brand Names Trilisate® [DSC]

Generic Available Yes

Synonyms Tricosal

Pharmacologic Category Salicylate

Use Management of osteoarthritis, rheumatoid arthritis, and other arthritis; acute painful shoulder

Local Anesthetic/Vasoconstrictor Precautions No information available to require special precautions

Effects on Dental Treatment NSAID formulations are known to reversibly decrease platelet aggregation via mechanisms different than observed with aspirin. The dentist should be aware of the potential of abnormal coagulation. Caution should also be exercised in the use of NSAIDs in patients already on anticoagulant therapy with drugs such as warfarin (Coumadin®).

Common Adverse Effects

<20%:

Gastrointestinal: Nausea, vomiting, diarrhea, heartburn, dyspepsia, epigastric pain, constipation

Otic: Tinnitus

<2%:

Central nervous system: Headache, lightheadedness, dizziness, drowsiness, lethargy

Otic: Hearing impairment

Mechanism of Action Inhibits prostaglandin synthesis; acts on the hypothalamus heat-regulating center to reduce fever; blocks the generation of pain impulses

Drug Interactions

Increased Effect/Toxicity: Choline magnesium trisalicylate may increase the hypoprothrombinemic effect of warfarin.

Decreased Effect: Antacids may decrease choline magnesium trisalicylate absorption/ salicylate concentrations.

Pharmacodynamics/Kinetics

Onset of action: Peak effect: ~2 hours

Absorption: Stomach and small intestines

Distribution: Readily into most body fluids and tissues; crosses placenta; enters breast milk

Half-life elimination (dose dependent): Low dose: 2-3 hours; High dose: 30 hours

Time to peak, serum: ~2 hours

Pregnancy Risk Factor C/D (3rd trimester)

Choline Salicylate (KOE leen sa LIS i late)

Related Information

Rheumatoid Arthritis, Osteoarthritis, and Osteoporosis *on page 1490*

Temporomandibular Dysfunction (TMD) *on page 1564*

U.S. Brand Names Arthropan® [OTC] [DSC]

Canadian Brand Names Teejel®

Generic Available No

Pharmacologic Category Salicylate

Use Temporary relief of pain of rheumatoid arthritis, rheumatic fever, osteoarthritis, and other conditions for which oral salicylates are recommended; useful in patients in which there is difficulty in administering doses in a tablet or capsule dosage form, because of the liquid dosage form

Local Anesthetic/Vasoconstrictor Precautions No information available to require special precautions

Effects on Dental Treatment NSAID formulations are known to reversibly decrease platelet aggregation via mechanisms different than observed with aspirin. The dentist should be aware of the potential of abnormal coagulation. Caution should also be exercised in the use of NSAIDs in patients already on anticoagulant therapy with drugs such as warfarin (Coumadin®).

Common Adverse Effects

>10%: Gastrointestinal: Nausea, heartburn, stomach pains, dyspepsia, epigastric discomfort

1% to 10%:

- Central nervous system: Fatigue
- Dermatologic: Rash
- Gastrointestinal: Gastrointestinal ulceration
- Hematologic: Hemolytic anemia
- Neuromuscular & skeletal: Weakness
- Respiratory: Dyspnea
- Miscellaneous: Anaphylactic shock

Mechanism of Action Inhibits prostaglandin synthesis; acts on the hypothalamus heat-regulating center to reduce fever; blocks the generation of pain impulses

Drug Interactions

Increased Effect/Toxicity: Effect of warfarin may be increased.

Decreased Effect: Decreased effect of salicylates with antacids. Effect of ACE inhibitors and diuretics may be decreased by concurrent therapy with NSAIDs.

Pharmacodynamics/Kinetics

Absorption: Stomach and small intestines in ~2 hours

Distribution: Readily into most body fluids and tissues; crosses placenta; enters breast milk

Protein binding: 75% to 90%

Metabolism: Hepatically hydrolyzed to salicylate

Half-life elimination (dose dependent): Low dose: 2-3 hours; High dose: 30 hours

Time to peak, serum: 1-2 hours

Excretion: Urine

Pregnancy Risk Factor C/D (3rd trimester)

Chondroitin Sulfate and Sodium Hyaluronate

(kon DROY tin SUL fate & SOW de um hye al yoor ON ate)

U.S. Brand Names Viscoat®

Generic Available No

Synonyms Sodium Hyaluronate-Chrondroitin Sulfate

Pharmacologic Category Ophthalmic Agent, Viscoelastic

Use Surgical aid in anterior segment procedures, protects corneal endothelium and coats intraocular lens thus protecting it

Local Anesthetic/Vasoconstrictor Precautions No information available to require special precautions

Effects on Dental Treatment No significant effects or complications reported

Mechanism of Action Functions as a tissue lubricant and is thought to play an important role in modulating the interactions between adjacent tissues

Pregnancy Risk Factor C

Chooz® [OTC] *see* Calcium Carbonate *on page 245*

Choriogonadotropin Alfa *see* Chorionic Gonadotropin (Recombinant) *on page 326*

Chorionic Gonadotropin (Human)

(kor ee ON ik goe NAD oh troe pin, HYU man)

Related Information

Chorionic Gonadotropin (Recombinant) *on page 326*

U.S. Brand Names Novarel™; Pregnyl®

Canadian Brand Names Humegon®; Pregnyl®; Profasi® HP

Generic Available Yes

Synonyms CG; hCG

Pharmacologic Category Ovulation Stimulator

Use Induces ovulation and pregnancy in anovulatory, infertile females; treatment of hypogonadotropic hypogonadism, prepubertal cryptorchidism; spermatogenesis induction with follitropin alfa or follitropin beta

Local Anesthetic/Vasoconstrictor Precautions No information available to require special precautions

Effects on Dental Treatment No significant effects or complications reported

Common Adverse Effects

1% to 10%:

- Central nervous system: Mental depression, fatigue
- Endocrine & metabolic: Pelvic pain, ovarian cysts, enlargement of breasts, precocious puberty
- Local: Pain at the injection site
- Neuromuscular & skeletal: Premature closure of epiphyses

Mechanism of Action Stimulates production of gonadal steroid hormones by causing production of androgen by the testis; as a substitute for luteinizing hormone (LH) to stimulate ovulation

Pharmacodynamics/Kinetics

Half-life elimination: Biphasic: Initial: 11 hours; Terminal: 23 hours

Excretion: Urine (as unchanged drug) within 3-4 days

Pregnancy Risk Factor C

Chorionic Gonadotropin (Recombinant)

(kor ee ON ik goe NAD oh troe pin ree KOM be nant)

Related Information

Chorionic Gonadotropin (Human) *on page 326*

U.S. Brand Names Ovidrel®

Generic Available No

Synonyms Choriogonadotropin Alfa; r-hCG

Pharmacologic Category Gonadotropin; Ovulation Stimulator

Use As part of an assisted reproductive technology (ART) program, induces ovulation in infertile females who have been pretreated with follicle stimulating hormones (FSH); induces ovulation and pregnancy in infertile females when the cause of infertility is functional

Local Anesthetic/Vasoconstrictor Precautions No information available to require special precautions

Effects on Dental Treatment No significant effects or complications reported

Common Adverse Effects

2% to 10%:

- Endocrine & metabolic: Ovarian cyst (3%), ovarian hyperstimulation (<2% to 3%)
- Gastrointestinal: Abdominal pain (3% to 4%), nausea (3%), vomiting (3%)
- Local: Injection site: Pain (8%), bruising (3% to 5%), reaction (<2% to 3%), inflammation (<2% to 2%)
- Miscellaneous: Postoperative pain (5%)

<2%:

- Cardiovascular: Cardiac arrhythmia, heart murmur
- Central nervous system: Dizziness, emotional lability, fever, headache, insomnia, malaise
- Dermatologic: Pruritus, rash
- Endocrine & metabolic: Breast pain, hot flashes, hyperglycemia, intermenstrual bleeding, vaginal hemorrhage
- Gastrointestinal: Abdominal enlargement, diarrhea, flatulence
- Genitourinary: Cervical carcinoma, cervical lesion, dysuria, genital herpes, genital moniliasis, leukorrhea, urinary incontinence, urinary tract infection, vaginitis
- Hematologic: Leukocytosis
- Neuromuscular & skeletal: Back pain, paresthesias
- Renal: Albuminuria
- Respiratory: Cough, pharyngitis, upper respiratory tract infection
- Miscellaneous: Ectopic pregnancy, hiccups

In addition, the following have been reported with menotropin therapy: Adnexal torsion, hemoperitoneum, mild to moderate ovarian enlargement, pulmonary and vascular complications. Ovarian neoplasms have also been reported (rare) with multiple drug regimens used for ovarian induction (relationship not established).

Mechanism of Action Luteinizing hormone analogue produced by recombinant DNA techniques; stimulates rupture of the ovarian follicle once follicular development has occurred.

Drug Interactions

Increased Effect/Toxicity: Specific drug interaction studies have not been conducted.

Pharmacodynamics/Kinetics

Distribution: V_d: 5.9 ± 1 L

Bioavailability: 40%

Half-life elimination: Initial: 4 hours; Terminal: 29 hours

Time to peak: 12-24 hours

Excretion: Urine (10% of dose)

Pregnancy Risk Factor X

Chromium *see* Trace Metals *on page 1319*

Cialis® *see* Tadalafil *on page 1257*

Ciclopirox (sye kloe PEER oks)

Related Information

Oral Fungal Infections *on page 1544*

U.S. Brand Names Loprox®; Penlac™

Canadian Brand Names Loprox®; Penlac™

Mexican Brand Names Loprox®

Generic Available No

Synonyms Ciclopirox Olamine

Pharmacologic Category Antifungal Agent, Topical

Use

Cream/suspension: Treatment of tinea pedis (athlete's foot), tinea cruris (jock itch), tinea corporis (ringworm), cutaneous candidiasis, and tinea versicolor (pityriasis)

Gel: Treatment of tinea pedis (athlete's foot), tinea corporis (ringworm); seborrheic dermatitis of the scalp

Lacquer: Topical treatment of mild to moderate onychomycosis of the fingernails and toenails

Shampoo: Treatment of seborrheic dermatitis of the scalp

Local Anesthetic/Vasoconstrictor Precautions No information available to require special precautions

Effects on Dental Treatment No significant effects or complications reported

Common Adverse Effects

>10%: Local: Burning sensation (gel: 34%; ≤1% with other forms)

1% to 10%:

Central nervous system: Headache

Dermatologic: Pruritus, rash

Local: Irritation, redness, or pain

Mechanism of Action Inhibiting transport of essential elements in the fungal cell disrupting the synthesis of DNA, RNA, and protein

Pharmacodynamics/Kinetics

Absorption: Cream, solution: <2% through intact skin; increased with gel; <5% with lacquer

Distribution: Scalp application: To epidermis, corium (dermis), including hair, hair follicles, and sebaceous glands

Protein binding: 94% to 98%

Half-life elimination: Biologic: 1.7 hours (solution); elimination: 5.5 hours (gel)

Excretion: Urine (gel: 3% to 10%); feces (small amounts)

Pregnancy Risk Factor B

Ciclopirox Olamine *see* Ciclopirox *on page 327*

Cidecin *see* Daptomycin *on page 399*

Cidofovir (si DOF o veer)

Related Information

Systemic Viral Diseases *on page 1519*

U.S. Brand Names Vistide®

Generic Available No

Pharmacologic Category Antiviral Agent

(Continued)

Cidofovir *(Continued)*

Use Treatment of cytomegalovirus (CMV) retinitis in patients with acquired immunodeficiency syndrome (AIDS). **Note:** Should be administered with probenecid.

Local Anesthetic/Vasoconstrictor Precautions No information available to require special precautions

Effects on Dental Treatment Key adverse event(s) related to dental treatment: Stomatitis and abnormal taste.

Common Adverse Effects

>10%:

Central nervous system: Infection, chills, fever, headache, amnesia, anxiety, confusion, seizures, insomnia

Dermatologic: Alopecia, rash, acne, skin discoloration

Gastrointestinal: Nausea, vomiting, diarrhea, anorexia, abdominal pain, constipation, dyspepsia, gastritis

Hematologic: Thrombocytopenia, neutropenia, anemia

Neuromuscular & skeletal: Weakness, paresthesia

Ocular: Amblyopia, conjunctivitis, ocular hypotony

Renal: Tubular damage, proteinuria, elevated creatinine

Respiratory: Asthma, bronchitis, coughing, dyspnea, pharyngitis

1% to 10%:

Cardiovascular: Hypotension, pallor, syncope, tachycardia

Central nervous system: Dizziness, hallucinations, depression, somnolence, malaise

Dermatologic: Pruritus, urticaria

Endocrine & metabolic: Hyperglycemia, hyperlipidemia, hypocalcemia, hypokalemia, dehydration

Gastrointestinal: Abnormal taste, stomatitis

Genitourinary: Glycosuria, urinary incontinence, urinary tract infections

Neuromuscular & skeletal: Skeletal pain

Ocular: Retinal detachment, iritis, uveitis, abnormal vision

Renal: Hematuria

Respiratory: Pneumonia, rhinitis, sinusitis

Miscellaneous: Diaphoresis, allergic reactions

Mechanism of Action Cidofovir is converted to cidofovir diphosphate which is the active intracellular metabolite; cidofovir diphosphate suppresses CMV replication by selective inhibition of viral DNA synthesis. Incorporation of cidofovir into growing viral DNA chain results in reductions in the rate of viral DNA synthesis.

Drug Interactions

Increased Effect/Toxicity: Drugs with nephrotoxic potential (eg, amphotericin B, aminoglycosides, foscarnet, and I.V. pentamidine) should be avoided during cidofovir therapy.

Pharmacodynamics/Kinetics The following pharmacokinetic data is based on a combination of cidofovir administered with probenecid:

Distribution: V_d: 0.54 L/kg; does not cross significantly into CSF

Protein binding: <6%

Metabolism: Minimal; phosphorylation occurs intracellularly

Half-life elimination, plasma: ~2.6 hours

Excretion: Urine

Pregnancy Risk Factor C

Cilazapril (sye LAY za pril)

Canadian Brand Names Inhibace®

Mexican Brand Names Inibace®

Synonyms Cilazapril Monohydrate

Pharmacologic Category Angiotensin-Converting Enzyme (ACE) Inhibitor

Use Management of hypertension; treatment of congestive heart failure

Local Anesthetic/Vasoconstrictor Precautions No information available to require special precautions

Effects on Dental Treatment Key adverse event(s) related to dental treatment: Orthostatic hypotension.

Common Adverse Effects 1% to 10%

Cardiovascular: Palpitation (up to 1%), hypotension (symptomatic, up to 1% in CHF patients), orthostatic hypotension (2%)

Central nervous system: Headache (3% to 5%), dizziness (3% to 8%), fatigue (2% to 3%)

Gastrointestinal: Nausea (1% to 3%)

Neuromuscular & skeletal: Weakness (0.3% to 2%)

Renal: Increased serum creatinine

Respiratory: Cough (2% in hypertension, up to 7.5% in CHF patients)

Restrictions Not available in U.S.

Mechanism of Action Competitive inhibitor of angiotensin-converting enzyme (ACE); prevents conversion of angiotensin I to angiotensin II, a potent vasoconstrictor; results in lower levels of angiotensin II which causes an increase in plasma renin activity and a reduction in aldosterone secretion.

Drug Interactions

Increased Effect/Toxicity: Potassium supplements, sulfamethoxazole/trimethoprim (high dose), angiotensin II receptor antagonists (eg, candesartan, losartan, irbesartan), or potassium-sparing diuretics (amiloride, spironolactone, triamterene) may result in elevated serum potassium levels when combined with cilazapril. ACE inhibitor effects may be increased by phenothiazines or probenecid (increases levels of other ACE inhibitors). ACE inhibitors may increase serum concentrations/effects of digoxin, lithium, and sulfonlyureas.

Diuretics have additive hypotensive effects with ACE inhibitors, and hypovolemia increases the potential for adverse renal effects of ACE inhibitors. In patients with compromised renal function, coadministration with nonsteroidal anti-inflammatory drugs may result in further deterioration of renal function. Allopurinol and ACE inhibitors may cause a higher risk of hypersensitivity reaction when taken concurrently

Decreased Effect: Aspirin (high dose) may reduce the therapeutic effects of ACE inhibitors; at low dosages this does not appear to be significant. Rifampin may decrease the effect of ACE inhibitors. Antacids may decrease the bioavailability of ACE inhibitors (may be more likely to occur with captopril); separate administration times by 1-2 hours. NSAIDs, specifically indomethacin, may reduce the hypotensive effects of ACE inhibitors. More likely to occur in low renin or volume-dependent hypertensive patients.

Pharmacodynamics/Kinetics

Onset: Antihypertensive: ~1 hour

Duration: Therapeutic effect: 24 hours

Absorption: Rapid

Metabolism: To active form (cilazaprilat)

Bioavailability: 57%

Half-life elimination: Cilazaprilat: Terminal: 36-49 hours

Time to peak: 3-7 hours

Excretion: In urine (91%)

Pregnancy Risk Factor Not assigned; C/D (2nd and 3rd trimesters) based on other ACE inhibitors

Cilazapril Monohydrate *see* Cilazapril *on page 328*

Cilostazol (sil OH sta zol)

U.S. Brand Names Pletal®

Canadian Brand Names Pletal®

Generic Available No

Synonyms OPC-13013

Pharmacologic Category Antiplatelet Agent; Phosphodiesterase Enzyme Inhibitor

Use Symptomatic management of peripheral vascular disease, primarily intermittent claudication; currently being investigated for the treatment of acute coronary syndromes and for graft patency improvement in percutaneous coronary interventions with or without stenting

Unlabeled/Investigational Use Investigational: Treatment of acute coronary syndromes and for graft patency improvement in percutaneous coronary interventions with or without stenting

Local Anesthetic/Vasoconstrictor Precautions No information available to require special precautions

Effects on Dental Treatment Key adverse event(s) related to dental treatment: Postural hypotension and tongue edema (per manufacturer). If a patient is to undergo elective surgery and an antiplatelet effect is not desired, a medical consult is suggested to consider reduction or discontinuation of cilostazol dose prior to surgery.

Common Adverse Effects

>10%:

Central nervous system: Headache (27% to 34%)

Gastrointestinal: Abnormal stools (12% to 15%), diarrhea (12% to 19%)

Miscellaneous: Infection (10% to 14%)

2% to 10%:

Cardiovascular: Peripheral edema (7% to 9%), palpitation (5% to 10%), tachycardia (4%)

(Continued)

Cilostazol *(Continued)*

Central nervous system: Dizziness (9% to 10%)
Gastrointestinal: Dyspepsia (6%), nausea (6% to 7%), abdominal pain (4% to 5%), flatulence (2% to 3%)
Neuromuscular & skeletal: Back pain (6% to 7%), myalgia (2% to 3%)
Respiratory: Rhinitis (7% to 12%), pharyngitis (7% to 10%), cough (3% to 4%)

Mechanism of Action Cilostazol and its metabolites are inhibitors of phosphodiesterase III. As a result cyclic AMP is increased leading to inhibition of platelet aggregation and vasodilation. Other effects of phosphodiesterase III inhibition include increased cardiac contractility, accelerated AV nodal conduction, increased ventricular automaticity, heart rate, and coronary blood flow.

Drug Interactions

Cytochrome P450 Effect: Substrate (minor) of CYP1A2, 2C19, 2D6, 3A4

Increased Effect/Toxicity: Cilostazol serum concentrations may be increased by erythromycin, diltiazem, and omeprazole. Increased concentrations of cilostazol may be anticipated during concurrent therapy with other inhibitors of CYP3A4 (ie, clarithromycin, ketoconazole, itraconazole, fluconazole, miconazole, fluvoxamine, fluoxetine, nefazodone, and sertraline) or inhibitors of CYP2C19. Aspirin-induced inhibition of platelet aggregation is potentiated by concurrent cilostazol. The effect on platelet aggregation with other antiplatelet drugs is unknown.

Pharmacodynamics/Kinetics

Onset of action: 2-4 weeks; may require up to 12 weeks
Protein binding: 97% to 98%
Metabolism: Hepatic via CYP3A4 (primarily), 1A2, 2C19, and 2D6; at least one metabolite has significant activity
Half-life elimination: 11-13 hours
Excretion: Urine (74%) and feces (20%) as metabolites

Pregnancy Risk Factor C

Ciloxan® *see* Ciprofloxacin *on page 331*

Cimetidine (sye MET i deen)

Related Information

Gastrointestinal Disorders *on page 1476*

U.S. Brand Names Tagamet®; Tagamet® HB 200 [OTC]

Canadian Brand Names Apo-Cimetidine®; Gen-Cimetidine; Novo-Cimetidine; Nu-Cimet; PMS-Cimetidine; Tagamet® HB

Mexican Brand Names Cimetase®; Tagamet®

Generic Available Yes

Pharmacologic Category Histamine H_2 Antagonist

Use Short-term treatment of active duodenal ulcers and benign gastric ulcers; long-term prophylaxis of duodenal ulcer; gastric hypersecretory states; gastroesophageal reflux; prevention of upper GI bleeding in critically-ill patients; labeled for OTC use for prevention or relief of heartburn, acid indigestion, or sour stomach

Unlabeled/Investigational Use Part of a multidrug regimen for *H. pylori* eradication to reduce the risk of duodenal ulcer recurrence

Local Anesthetic/Vasoconstrictor Precautions No information available to require special precautions

Effects on Dental Treatment No significant effects or complications reported

Common Adverse Effects 1% to 10%:

Central nervous system: Dizziness, agitation, headache, drowsiness
Gastrointestinal: Diarrhea, nausea, vomiting

Mechanism of Action Competitive inhibition of histamine at H_2-receptors of the gastric parietal cells resulting in reduced gastric acid secretion, gastric volume and hydrogen ion concentration reduced

Drug Interactions

Cytochrome P450 Effect: Inhibits CYP1A2 (moderate), 2C8/9 (weak), 2C19 (moderate), 2D6 (moderate), 2E1 (weak), 3A4 (moderate)

Increased Effect/Toxicity: Cimetidine may increase the levels/effects of aminophylline, amphetamines, selected beta-blockers, selected benzodiazepines, calcium channel blockers, citalopram, cyclosporine, dextromethorphan, diazepam, ergot derivatives, fluoxetine, fluvoxamine, lidocaine, methsuximide, mexiletine, mirtazapine, nateglinide, nefazodone, paroxetine, phenytoin, propranolol, risperidone, ritonavir, ropinirole, sertraline, sildenafil (and other PDE-5 inhibitors), tacrolimus, theophylline, thioridazine, tricyclic antidepressants, trifluoperazine, venlafaxine, and other CYP1A2, 2C19, or 2D6 substrates.

Cimetidine increases warfarin's effect in a dose-related manner, and may increase levels/effects of meperidine, metronidazole, moricizine, procainamide, propafenone, quinidine, quinolone antibiotics, tacrine, and triamterene. Cimetidine increases carmustine's myelotoxicity; avoid concurrent use.

Decreased Effect: Cimetidine may decrease the levels/effects of CYP2D6 prodrug substrates (eg, codeine, hydrocodone, oxycodone, and tramadol). Ketoconazole, fluconazole, itraconazole (especially capsule) decrease serum concentration; avoid concurrent use with H_2 antagonists. Delavirdine's absorption is decreased; avoid concurrent use with H_2 antagonists.

Pharmacodynamics/Kinetics

Onset of action: 1 hour
Duration: 6 hours
Distribution: Crosses placenta; enters breast milk
Protein binding: 20%
Metabolism: Partially hepatic
Bioavailability: 60% to 70%
Half-life elimination: Neonates: 3.6 hours; Children: 1.4 hours; Adults: Normal renal function: 2 hours
Time to peak, serum: Oral: 1-2 hours
Excretion: Primarily urine (as unchanged drug); feces (some)

Pregnancy Risk Factor B

Cinacalcet (sin a KAL cet)

U.S. Brand Names Sensipar™

Generic Available No

Synonyms AMG 073; Cinacalcet Hydrochloride

Pharmacologic Category Calcimimetic

Use Treatment of secondary hyperparathyroidism in dialysis patients; treatment of hypercalcemia in patients with parathyroid carcinoma

Unlabeled/Investigational Use Primary hyperthyroidism

Local Anesthetic/Vasoconstrictor Precautions No information available to require special precautions

Effects on Dental Treatment No significant effects or complications reported

Common Adverse Effects

>10%:

Endocrine & metabolic: Hypocalcemia
Gastrointestinal: Nausea (31%), vomiting (27%), diarrhea (21%)
Neuromuscular & skeletal: Myalgia (15%)

1% to 10%:

Cardiovascular: Hypertension (7%)
Central nervous system: Dizziness (10%), seizure (1%)
Endocrine & metabolic: Testosterone decreased
Gastrointestinal: Anorexia (6%)
Neuromuscular & skeletal: Weakness (7%), chest pain (6%)

Mechanism of Action Increases the sensitivity of the calcium-sensing receptor on the parathyroid gland.

Drug Interactions

Cytochrome P450 Effect: Substrate of CYP1A2, 2D6, 3A4; **Inhibits** CYP2D6

Increased Effect/Toxicity: Cinacalcet increases levels of amitriptyline and nortriptyline. Ketoconazole may increase cinacalcet levels.

Pharmacodynamics/Kinetics

Distribution: V_d: 1000 L
Protein binding: 93% to 97%
Metabolism: Hepatic via CYP3A4, 2D6, 1A2; forms inactive metabolites
Half-life elimination: Terminal: 30-40 hours
Time to peak, plasma: Nadir in iPTH levels: 2-6 hours postdose
Excretion: Urine 80% (as metabolites); feces 15%

Pregnancy Risk Factor C

Cinacalcet Hydrochloride *see* Cinacalcet *on page 331*

Cipro® *see* Ciprofloxacin *on page 331*

Ciprodex® *see* Ciprofloxacin and Dexamethasone *on page 336*

Ciprofloxacin (sip roe FLOKS a sin)

Related Information

Sexually-Transmitted Diseases *on page 1504*
Tuberculosis *on page 1495*

U.S. Brand Names Ciloxan®; Cipro®; Cipro® XR

Canadian Brand Names Ciloxan®; Cipro®; Cipro® XL

(Continued)

Ciprofloxacin *(Continued)*

Mexican Brand Names Cimogal®; Ciprobiotic® [tabs]; Ciproflox®; Ciproflox® [inj.]; Ciprofur® [tabs]; Ciproxina®; Ciproxina® [inj.]; Eni®; Kenzoflex®; Microrgan® [caps]; Mitroken® [tabs]; Nivoflox® [tabs]; Nivoflox® [inj.]; Novoquin®; Opthaflox®; Quinoflox®; Sophixin®; Suiflox® [tabs]; Zipra®

Generic Available Yes: Suspension, tablet

Synonyms Ciprofloxacin Hydrochloride

Pharmacologic Category Antibiotic, Ophthalmic; Antibiotic, Quinolone

Dental Use Useful as a single agent or in combination with metronidazole in the treatment of periodontitis associated with the presence of *Actinobacillus actinomycetemcomitans* (AA), as well as enteric rods/pseudomonads

Use

Children: Complicated urinary tract infections and pyelonephritis due to *E. coli*. **Note:** Although effective, ciprofloxacin is not the drug of first choice in children.

Children and adults: To reduce incidence or progression of disease following exposure to aerolized *Bacillus anthracis*. Ophthalmologically, for superficial ocular infections (corneal ulcers, conjunctivitis) due to susceptible strains

Adults: Treatment of the following infections when caused by susceptible bacteria: Urinary tract infections; acute uncomplicated cystitis in females; chronic bacterial prostatitis; lower respiratory tract infections (including acute exacerbations of chronic bronchitis); acute sinusitis; skin and skin structure infections; bone and joint infections; complicated intra-abdominal infections (in combination with metronidazole); infectious diarrhea; typhoid fever due to *Salmonella typhi* (eradication of chronic typhoid carrier state has not been proven); uncomplicated cervical and urethra gonorrhea (due to *N. gonorrhoeae*); nosocomial pneumonia; empirical therapy for febrile neutropenic patients (in combination with piperacillin)

Unlabeled/Investigational Use Acute pulmonary exacerbations in cystic fibrosis (children); cutaneous/gastrointestinal/oropharyngeal anthrax (treatment, children and adults); disseminated gonococcal infection (adults); chancroid (adults); prophylaxis to *Neisseria meningitidis* following close contact with an infected person

Local Anesthetic/Vasoconstrictor Precautions No information available to require special precautions

Effects on Dental Treatment No significant effects or complications reported

Significant Adverse Effects

1% to 10%:

Central nervous system: Neurologic events (children 2%, includes dizziness, insomnia, nervousness, somnolence); fever (children 2%)

Dermatologic: Rash (children 2%, adults 1%)

Gastrointestinal: Nausea (children/adults 3%); diarrhea (children 5%, adults 2%); vomiting (children 5%, adults 1%); abdominal pain (children 3%, adults <1%); dyspepsia (children 3%)

Hepatic: ALT/AST increased (adults 2%)

Respiratory: Rhinitis (children 3%)

<1% (Limited to important or life-threatening): Abnormal gait, acute renal failure, agitation, agranulocytosis, allergic reactions, anaphylaxis, anemia, angina pectoris, arthralgia, bone marrow depression (life-threatening), cardiopulmonary arrest, cerebral thrombosis, cholestatic jaundice, confusion, crystalluria, delirium, dizziness, drowsiness, dyspnea, edema, eosinophilia, erythema multiforme, erythema nodosum, gastrointestinal bleeding, hallucinations, headache, hemolytic anemia, hepatic necrosis, hypertension, hypotension, injection site reactions, insomnia, interstitial nephritis, intestinal perforation, laryngeal edema, lightheadedness, methemoglobinemia, migraine, myasthenia gravis (exacerbation), myocardial infarction, nightmares, palpitations, pancreatitis, paranoia, photosensitivity, prolongation of PT, pseudomembranous colitis, psychosis, renal calculi, seizures, serum sickness-like reaction, Stevens-Johnson syndrome, syncope, tachycardia, tendon rupture, toxic epidermal necrolysis, tremor, vasculitis, visual disturbance, weakness

Dosage Note: Extended release tablets and immediate release formulations are not interchangeable. Unless otherwise specified, oral dosing reflects the use of immediate release formulations.

Children (see Warnings/Precautions):

Oral:

Complicated urinary tract infection or pyelonephritis: Children 1-17 years: 20-30 mg/kg/day in 2 divided doses (every 12 hours) for 10-21 days; maximum: 1.5 g/day

Cystic fibrosis (unlabeled use): Children 5-17 years: 40 mg/kg/day divided every 12 hours administered following 1 week of I.V. therapy has been reported in a clinical trial; total duration of therapy: 10-21 days

Anthrax:

Inhalational (postexposure prophylaxis): 15 mg/kg/dose every 12 hours for 60 days; maximum: 500 mg/dose

Cutaneous (treatment, CDC guidelines): 10-15 mg/kg every 12 hours for 60 days (maximum: 1 g/day); amoxicillin 80 mg/kg/day divided every 8 hours is an option for completion of treatment after clinical improvement. **Note:** In the presence of systemic involvement, extensive edema, lesions on head/neck, refer to I.V. dosing for treatment of inhalational/gastrointestinal/oropharyngeal anthrax

I.V.:

Complicated urinary tract infection or pyelonephritis: Children 1-17 years: 6-10 mg/kg every 8 hours for 10-21 days (maximum: 400 mg/dose)

Cystic fibrosis (unlabeled use): Children 5-17 years: 30 mg/kg/day divided every 8 hours for 1 week, followed by oral therapy, has been reported in a clinical trial

Anthrax:

Inhalational (postexposure prophylaxis): 10 mg/kg/dose every 12 hours for 60 days; do **not** exceed 400 mg/dose (800 mg/day)

Inhalational/gastrointestinal/oropharyngeal (treatment, CDC guidelines): Initial: 10-15 mg/kg every 12 hours for 60 days (maximum: 500 mg/dose); switch to oral therapy when clinically appropriate; refer to Adults dosing for notes on combined therapy and duration

Adults: Oral:

Periodontitis: Ciprofloxacin and metronidazole 500 mg each twice daily for 8 days

Urinary tract infection:

Acute uncomplicated: Immediate release formulation: 100 mg or 250 mg every 12 hours for 3 days

Acute uncomplicated pyelonephritis: Extended release formulation: 1000 mg every 24 hours for 7-14 days

Uncomplicated/acute cystitis: Extended release formulation: 500 mg every 24 hours for 3 days

Mild/moderate: Immediate release formulation: 250 mg every 12 hours for 7-14 days

Severe/complicated:

Immediate release formulation: 500 mg every 12 hours for 7-14 days

Extended release formulation: 1000 mg every 24 hours for 7-14 days

Lower respiratory tract, skin/skin structure infections: 500-750 mg twice daily for 7-14 days depending on severity and susceptibility

Bone/joint infections: 500-750 mg twice daily for 4-6 weeks, depending on severity and susceptibility

Infectious diarrhea: 500 mg every 12 hours for 5-7 days

Intra-abdominal (in combination with metronidazole): 500 mg every 12 hours for 7-14 days

Typhoid fever: 500 mg every 12 hours for 10 days

Urethral/cervical gonococcal infections: 250-500 mg as a single dose (CDC recommends concomitant doxycycline or azithromycin due to developing resistance; avoid use in Asian or Western Pacific travelers)

Disseminated gonococcal infection (CDC guidelines): 500 mg twice daily to complete 7 days of therapy (initial treatment with ceftriaxone 1 g I.M./I.V. daily for 24-48 hours after improvement begins)

Chancroid (CDC guidelines): 500 mg twice daily for 3 days

Sinusitis (acute): 500 mg every 12 hours for 10 days

Chronic bacterial prostatitis: 500 mg every 12 hours for 28 days

Anthrax:

Inhalational (postexposure prophylaxis): 500 mg every 12 hours for 60 days

Cutaneous (treatment, CDC guidelines): Immediate release formulation: 500 mg every 12 hours for 60 days. **Note:** In the presence of systemic involvement, extensive edema, lesions on head/neck, refer to I.V. dosing for treatment of inhalational/gastrointestinal/oropharyngeal anthrax

Adults: I.V.:

Bone/joint infections:

Mild to moderate: 400 mg every 12 hours for 4-6 weeks

Severe or complicated: 400 mg every 8 hours for 4-6 weeks

Lower respiratory tract, skin/skin structure infections:

Mild to moderate: 400 mg every 12 hours for 7-14 days

Severe or complicated: 400 mg every 8 hours for 7-14 days

Nosocomial pneumonia (mild to moderate to severe): 400 mg every 8 hours for 10-14 days

Prostatitis (chronic, bacterial): 400 mg every 12 hours for 28 days

(Continued)

Ciprofloxacin *(Continued)*

Sinusitis (acute): 400 mg every 12 hours for 10 days
Urinary tract infection:
Mild to moderate: 200 mg every 12 hours for 7-14 days
Severe or complicated: 400 mg every 12 hours for 7-14 days
Febrile neutropenia (with piperacillin): 400 mg every 8 hours for 7-14 days
Intra-abdominal infection (with metronidazole): 400 mg every 12 hours for 7-14 days
Anthrax:
Inhalational (postexposure prophylaxis): 400 mg every 12 hours for 60 days
Inhalational/gastrointestinal/oropharyngeal (treatment, CDC guidelines): 400 mg every 12 hours. **Note:** Initial treatment should include two or more agents predicted to be effective (per CDC recommendations). Agents suggested for use in conjunction with ciprofloxacin or doxycycline include rifampin, vancomycin, imipenem, penicillin, ampicillin, chloramphenicol, clindamycin, and clarithromycin. May switch to oral antimicrobial therapy when clinically appropriate. Continue combined therapy for 60 days.

Elderly: No adjustment needed in patients with normal renal function

Ophthalmic:
Solution: Children >1 year and Adults:
Bacterial conjunctivitis: Instill 1-2 drops in eye(s) every 2 hours while awake for 2 days and 1-2 drops every 4 hours while awake for the next 5 days
Corneal ulcer: Instill 2 drops into affected eye every 15 minutes for the first 6 hours, then 2 drops into the affected eye every 30 minutes for the remainder of the first day. On day 2, instill 2 drops into the affected eye hourly. On days 3-14, instill 2 drops into affected eye every 4 hours. Treatment may continue after day 14 if re-epithelialization has not occurred.
Ointment: Children >2 years and Adults: Bacterial conjunctivitis: Apply a 1/2" ribbon into the conjunctival sac 3 times/day for the first 2 days, followed by a 1/2" ribbon applied twice daily for the next 5 days

Dosing adjustment in renal impairment: Adults:
Cl_{cr} 30-50 mL/minute: Oral: 250-500 mg every 12 hours
Cl_{cr} <30 mL/minute: Acute uncomplicated pyelonephritis or complicated UTI: Oral: Extended release formulation: 500 mg every 24 hours
Cl_{cr} 5-29 mL/minute:
Oral: 250-500 mg every 18 hours
I.V.: 200-400 mg every 18-24 hours

Dialysis: Only small amounts of ciprofloxacin are removed by hemo- or peritoneal dialysis (<10%); usual dose: Oral: 250-500 mg every 24 hours following dialysis

Continuous arteriovenous or venovenous hemodiafiltration effects: Administer 200-400 mg I.V. every 12 hours

Mechanism of Action Inhibits DNA-gyrase in susceptible organisms; inhibits relaxation of supercoiled DNA and promotes breakage of double-stranded DNA

Contraindications Hypersensitivity to ciprofloxacin, any component of the formulation, or other quinolones

Warnings/Precautions CNS stimulation may occur (tremor, restlessness, confusion, and very rarely hallucinations or seizures). Use with caution in patients with known or suspected CNS disorder. Prolonged use may result in superinfection. Tendon inflammation and/or rupture have been reported with ciprofloxacin and other quinolone antibiotics. Risk may be increased with concurrent corticosteroids, particularly in the elderly. Discontinue at first sign of tendon inflammation or pain. Adverse effects, including those related to joints and/or surrounding tissues, are increased in pediatric patients.

Severe hypersensitivity reactions, including anaphylaxis, have occurred with quinolone therapy. Quinolones may exacerbate myasthenia gravis, use with caution (rare, potentially life-threatening weakness of respiratory muscles may occur). Use caution in renal impairment. Avoid excessive sunlight; may cause moderate-to-severe phototoxicity reactions.

Drug Interactions Inhibits CYP1A2 (strong), 3A4 (weak)

Aluminum/magnesium products, didanosine, quinapril, and sucralfate may decrease absorption of ciprofloxacin by ≥90% if administered concurrently. Administer ciprofloxacin at least 4 hours and preferably 6 hours after the dose of these agents or change to an H_2 antagonist or omeprazole.

Antineoplastic agents may decrease the absorption of quinolones.

Calcium, iron, zinc, and multivitamins with minerals products may decrease absorption of ciprofloxacin significantly if administered concurrently. Administer ciprofloxacin 2 hours before dose or at least 6 hours after the dose of these agents.

Cimetidine, and other H_2 antagonists may inhibit renal elimination of quinolones. No effect on bioavailability demonstrated with ciprofloxacin.

Corticosteroids: Concurrent use may increase the risk of tendon rupture, particularly in elderly patients (overall incidence rare).

Cyclosporine: Ciprofloxacin may increase serum levels.

CYP1A2 substrates: Ciprofloxacin may increase the levels/effects of CYP1A2 substrates. Example substrates include aminophylline, fluvoxamine, mexiletine, mirtazapine, ropinirole, theophylline, and trifluoperazine.

Foscarnet has been associated with an increased risk of seizures with some quinolones.

Loop diuretics: Serum levels of some quinolones are increased by loop diuretic administration. May diminish renal excretion.

Methotrexate: Quinolones may block renal secretion of methotrexate; monitor.

NSAIDs: The CNS stimulating effect of some quinolones may be enhanced, resulting in neuroexcitation and/or seizures.

Probenecid: Blocks renal secretion of quinolones, increasing concentrations.

Theophylline (and caffeine): Serum levels may be increased by ciprofloxacin; in addition, CNS stimulation/seizures may occur at lower theophylline serum levels due to additive CNS effects.

Warfarin: The hypoprothrombinemic effect of warfarin is enhanced by ciprofloxacin; monitor INR closely during therapy.

Ethanol/Nutrition/Herb Interactions

Food: Food decreases rate, but not extent, of absorption. Ciprofloxacin serum levels may be decreased if taken with dairy products or calcium-fortified juices. Ciprofloxacin may increase serum caffeine levels if taken with caffeine.

Enteral feedings may decrease plasma concentrations of ciprofloxacin probably by >30% inhibition of absorption. Ciprofloxacin should not be administered with enteral feedings. The feeding would need to be discontinued for 1-2 hours prior to and after ciprofloxacin administration. Nasogastric administration produces a greater loss of ciprofloxacin bioavailability than does nasoduodenal administration.

Herb/Nutraceutical: Avoid dong quai, St John's wort (may also cause photosensitization).

Dietary Considerations

Food: Drug may cause GI upset; take without regard to meals (manufacturer prefers that immediate release tablet is taken 2 hours after meals). Extended release tablet may be taken with meals that contain dairy products (calcium content <800 mg), but not with dairy products alone.

Dairy products, calcium-fortified juices, oral multivitamins, and mineral supplements: Absorption of ciprofloxacin is decreased by divalent and trivalent cations. The manufacturer states that the usual dietary intake of calcium (including meals which include dairy products) has not been shown to interfere with ciprofloxacin absorption. Ciprofloxacin may be taken 2 hours before or 6 hours after any of these products.

Caffeine: Patients consuming regular large quantities of caffeinated beverages may need to restrict caffeine intake if excessive cardiac or CNS stimulation occurs.

Pharmacodynamics/Kinetics

Absorption: Oral: Immediate release tablet: Rapid (~50% to 85%)

Distribution: V_d: 2.1-2.7 L/kg; tissue concentrations often exceed serum concentrations especially in kidneys, gallbladder, liver, lungs, gynecological tissue, and prostatic tissue; CSF concentrations: 10% of serum concentrations (noninflamed meninges), 14% to 37% (inflamed meninges); crosses placenta; enters breast milk

Protein binding: 20% to 40%

Metabolism: Partially hepatic; forms 4 metabolites (limited activity)

Half-life elimination: Children: 2.5 hours; Adults: Normal renal function: 3-5 hours

Time to peak: Oral: Immediate release tablet: 0.5-2 hours; Extended release tablet: 1-2.5 hours

Excretion: Urine (30% to 50% as unchanged drug); feces (20% to 40%)

Pregnancy Risk Factor C

Lactation Enters breast milk/contraindicated (AAP rates "compatible")

Breast-Feeding Considerations Ciprofloxacin is excreted in breast milk; however, the exposure to the infant is considered small and one source suggests that the decision to breast-feed be independent of the need for the

(Continued)

Ciprofloxacin *(Continued)*

antibiotic in the mother. Another source recommends the mother wait 48 hours after the last dose of ciprofloxacin to continue nursing.

Dosage Forms

Infusion, [premixed in D_5W] (Cipro®): 200 mg (100 mL); 400 mg (200 mL) [latex free]

Injection, solution (Cipro®): 10 mg/mL (20 mL, 40 mL, 120 mL)

Ointment, ophthalmic, as hydrochloride (Ciloxan®): 3.33 mg/g [0.3% base] (3.5 g)

Solution, ophthalmic, as hydrochloride (Ciloxan®): 3.5 mg/mL [0.3% base] (2.5 mL, 5 mL, 10 mL) [contains benzalkonium chloride]

Microcapsules for oral suspension (Cipro®): 250 mg/5 mL (100 mL); 500 mg/5 mL (100 mL) [strawberry flavor]

Tablet [film coated]: 250 mg, 500 mg, 750 mg
Cipro®: 100 mg, 250 mg, 500 mg, 750 mg

Tablet, extended release [film coated] (Cipro® XR): 500 mg [equivalent to ciprofloxacin hydrochloride 287.5 mg and ciprofloxacin base 212.6 mg]; 1000 mg [equivalent to ciprofloxacin hydrochloride 574.9 mg and ciprofloxacin base 425.2 mg]

Selected Readings

Rams TE and Slots J, "Antibiotics in Periodontal Therapy: An Update," *Compendium*, 1992, 13(12):1130, 1132, 1134.

Wynn RL, Bergman SA, Meiller TF, et al, "Antibiotics in Treating Oral-Facial Infections of Odontogenic Origin: An Update," *Gen Dent*, 2001, 49(3):238-40, 242, 244 passim.

Ciprofloxacin and Dexamethasone

(sip roe FLOKS a sin & deks a METH a sone)

Related Information

Ciprofloxacin *on page 331*
Dexamethasone *on page 411*

U.S. Brand Names Ciprodex®

Generic Available No

Synonyms Ciprofloxacin Hydrochloride and Dexamethasone; Dexamethasone and Ciprofloxacin

Pharmacologic Category Antibiotic/Corticosteroid, Otic

Use Treatment of acute otitis media in pediatric patients with tympanostomy tubes or acute otitis externa in children and adults

Local Anesthetic/Vasoconstrictor Precautions No information available to require special precautions

Effects on Dental Treatment No significant effects or complications reported

Mechanism of Action Ciprofloxacin is a quinolone antibiotic; dexamethasone is a corticosteroid used to decrease inflammation accompanying bacterial infections

Pregnancy Risk Factor C

Ciprofloxacin and Hydrocortisone

(sip roe FLOKS a sin & hye droe KOR ti sone)

Related Information

Hydrocortisone *on page 714*

U.S. Brand Names Cipro® HC

Canadian Brand Names Cipro® HC

Generic Available No

Synonyms Hydrocortisone and Ciprofloxacin

Pharmacologic Category Antibiotic/Corticosteroid, Otic

Use Treatment of acute otitis externa, sometimes known as "swimmer's ear"

Local Anesthetic/Vasoconstrictor Precautions No information available to require special precautions

Effects on Dental Treatment No significant effects or complications reported

Ciprofloxacin Hydrochloride *see* Ciprofloxacin *on page 331*

Ciprofloxacin Hydrochloride and Dexamethasone *see* Ciprofloxacin and Dexamethasone *on page 336*

Cipro® HC *see* Ciprofloxacin and Hydrocortisone *on page 336*

Cipro® XR *see* Ciprofloxacin *on page 331*

Cisapride (SIS a pride)

U.S. Brand Names Propulsid®

Mexican Brand Names Enteropride®; Kinestase®; Prepulsid®; Unamol®

Generic Available No

Pharmacologic Category Gastrointestinal Agent, Prokinetic

Use Treatment of nocturnal symptoms of gastroesophageal reflux disease (GERD); has demonstrated effectiveness for gastroparesis, refractory constipation, and nonulcer dyspepsia

Local Anesthetic/Vasoconstrictor Precautions No information available to require special precautions

Effects on Dental Treatment Key adverse event(s) related to dental treatment: Xerostomia (normal salivary flow resumes upon discontinuation).

Common Adverse Effects

>5%:

Central nervous system: Headache

Dermatologic: Rash

Gastrointestinal: Diarrhea, GI cramping, dyspepsia, flatulence, nausea, xerostomia

Respiratory: Rhinitis

<5%:

Cardiovascular: Tachycardia

Central nervous system: Extrapyramidal effects, somnolence, fatigue, seizures, insomnia, anxiety

Hematologic: Thrombocytopenia, increased LFTs, pancytopenia, leukopenia, granulocytopenia, aplastic anemia

Respiratory: Sinusitis, coughing, upper respiratory tract infection, increased incidence of viral infection

Restrictions In U.S., available via limited-access protocol only (1-800-JANSSEN).

Mechanism of Action Enhances the release of acetylcholine at the myenteric plexus. *In vitro* studies have shown cisapride to have serotonin-4 receptor agonistic properties which may increase gastrointestinal motility and cardiac rate; increases lower esophageal sphincter pressure and lower esophageal peristalsis; accelerates gastric emptying of both liquids and solids.

Drug Interactions

Cytochrome P450 Effect: Substrate of CYP1A2 (minor), 2A6 (minor), 2B6 (minor), 2C8/9 (minor), 2C19 (minor), 3A4 (major); **Inhibits** CYP2D6 (weak), 3A4 (weak)

Increased Effect/Toxicity: Cisapride may increase blood levels of warfarin, diazepam, cimetidine, ranitidine, and CNS depressants. The risk of cisapride-induced malignant arrhythmias may be increased by azole antifungals (fluconazole, itraconazole, ketoconazole, miconazole), antiarrhythmics (Class Ia; quinidine, procainamide, and Class III; amiodarone, sotalol), bepridil, cimetidine, maprotiline, macrolide antibiotics (erythromycin, clarithromycin, troleandomycin), molindone, nefazodone, protease inhibitors (amprenavir, atazanavir, indinavir, nelfinavir, ritonavir), phenothiazines (eg, prochlorperazine, promethazine), sertindole, tricyclic antidepressants (eg amitriptyline), and some quinolone antibiotics (sparfloxacin, gatifloxacin, moxifloxacin). Other strong inhibitors of CYP3A4 (including diclofenac, doxycycline, imatinib, isoniazid, nefazodone, nicardipine, propofol, and verapamil) should be avoided. Cardiovascular disease or electrolyte imbalances (potentially due to diuretic therapy) increase the risk of malignant arrhythmias.

Decreased Effect: Cisapride may decrease the effect of atropine and digoxin.

Pharmacodynamics/Kinetics

Onset of action: 0.5-1 hour

Protein binding: 97.5% to 98%

Metabolism: Extensively hepatic to norcisapride

Bioavailability: 35% to 40%

Half-life elimination: 6-12 hours

Excretion: Urine and feces (<10%)

Pregnancy Risk Factor C

Cisplatin (SIS pla tin)

U.S. Brand Names Platinol®-AQ

Mexican Brand Names Blastolem®; Platinol®; Tecnoplatin® [inj.]

Generic Available Yes

Synonyms CDDP

Pharmacologic Category Antineoplastic Agent, Alkylating Agent

Use Treatment of head and neck, breast, testicular, and ovarian cancer; Hodgkin's and non-Hodgkin's lymphoma; neuroblastoma; sarcomas, bladder, gastric, lung, esophageal, cervical, and prostate cancer; myeloma, melanoma, mesothelioma, small cell lung cancer, and osteosarcoma

Local Anesthetic/Vasoconstrictor Precautions No information available to require special precautions

(Continued)

Cisplatin *(Continued)*

Effects on Dental Treatment No significant effects or complications reported

Common Adverse Effects

>10%:

Central nervous system: Neurotoxicity: Peripheral neuropathy is dose- and duration-dependent. The mechanism is through axonal degeneration with subsequent damage to the long sensory nerves. Toxicity can first be noted at cumulative doses of 200 mg/m^2, with measurable toxicity at cumulative doses >350 mg/m^2. This process is irreversible and progressive with continued therapy.

Dermatologic: Mild alopecia

Gastrointestinal: Cisplatin is one of the most emetogenic agents used in cancer chemotherapy; nausea and vomiting occur in 76% to 100% of patients and is dose-related. Prophylactic antiemetics should always be prescribed; nausea and vomiting may last up to 1 week after therapy.

Hematologic: Myelosuppressive: Mild with moderate doses, mild to moderate with high-dose therapy

WBC: Mild

Platelets: Mild

Onset: 10 days

Nadir: 14-23 days

Recovery: 21-39 days

Hepatic: Elevation of liver enzymes

Renal: Nephrotoxicity: Related to elimination, protein binding, and uptake of cisplatin. Two types of nephrotoxicity: Acute renal failure and chronic renal insufficiency.

Acute renal failure and azotemia is a dose-dependent process and can be minimized with proper administration and prophylaxis. Damage to the proximal tubules by unbound cisplatin is suspected to cause the toxicity. It is manifested as increased BUN/creatinine, oliguria, protein wasting, and potassium, calcium, and magnesium wasting.

Chronic renal dysfunction can develop in patients receiving multiple courses of cisplatin. Slow release of tissue-bound cisplatin may contribute to chronic nephrotoxicity. Manifestations of this toxicity are varied, and can include sodium and water wasting, nephropathy, hyperuricemia, decreased Cl_{cr}, and magnesium wasting.

Recommendations for minimizing nephrotoxicity include:

Prepare cisplatin in saline-containing vehicles

Infuse dose over 24 hours

Vigorous hydration (125-150 mL/hour) before, during, and after cisplatin administration

Simultaneous administration of either mannitol or furosemide

Pretreatment with amifostine

Avoid other nephrotoxic agents (aminoglycosides, amphotericin, etc)

Otic: Ototoxicity: Ototoxicity occurs in 10% to 30%, and is manifested as high frequency hearing loss. Baseline audiography should be performed. Ototoxicity is especially pronounced in children.

1% to 10%: Local: Extravasation: May cause thrombophlebitis and tissue damage if infiltrated; may use sodium thiosulfate as antidote, but consult hospital policy for guidelines.

Irritant chemotherapy

Mechanism of Action Inhibits DNA synthesis by the formation of DNA cross-links; denatures the double helix; covalently binds to DNA bases and disrupts DNA function; may also bind to proteins; the *cis*-isomer is 14 times more cytotoxic than the *trans*-isomer; both forms cross-link DNA but cis-platinum is less easily recognized by cell enzymes and, therefore, not repaired. Cisplatin can also bind two adjacent guanines on the same strand of DNA producing intrastrand cross-linking and breakage.

Drug Interactions

Increased Effect/Toxicity: Cisplatin and ethacrynic acid have resulted in severe ototoxicity in animals. Delayed bleomycin elimination with decreased glomerular filtration rate. When administered as sequential infusions, observational studies indicate a potential for increased toxicity when platinum derivatives (carboplatin, cisplatin) are administered before taxane derivatives (docetaxel, paclitaxel).

Decreased Effect: Sodium thiosulfate theoretically inactivates drug systemically; has been used clinically to reduce systemic toxicity with intraperitoneal administration of cisplatin.

Pharmacodynamics/Kinetics

Distribution: I.V.: Rapidly into tissue; high concentrations in kidneys, liver, ovaries, uterus, and lungs

Protein binding: >90%

Metabolism: Nonenzymatic; inactivated (in both cell and bloodstream) by sulfhydryl groups; covalently binds to glutathione and thiosulfate

Half-life elimination: Initial: 20-30 minutes; Beta: 60 minutes; Terminal: ~24 hours; Secondary half-life: 44-73 hours

Excretion: Urine (>90%); feces (10%)

Pregnancy Risk Factor D

13-*cis*-Retinoic Acid *see* Isotretinoin *on page 773*

Citalopram (sye TAL oh pram)

Related Information

Escitalopram *on page 513*

U.S. Brand Names Celexa™

Canadian Brand Names Celexa™

Mexican Brand Names Seropram® [tabs]

Generic Available No

Synonyms Citalopram Hydrobromide; Nitalapram

Pharmacologic Category Antidepressant, Selective Serotonin Reuptake Inhibitor

Use Treatment of depression

Unlabeled/Investigational Use Treatment of dementia, smoking cessation, ethanol abuse, obsessive-compulsive disorder (OCD) in children, diabetic neuropathy

Local Anesthetic/Vasoconstrictor Precautions Although caution should be used in patients taking tricyclic antidepressants, no interactions have been reported with vasoconstrictors and citalopram, a nontricyclic antidepressant which acts to increase serotonin

Effects on Dental Treatment Key adverse event(s) related to dental treatment: Xerostomia (normal salivary flow resumes upon discontinuation). Premarketing trials reported abnormal taste.

Common Adverse Effects

>10%:

Central nervous system: Somnolence, insomnia

Gastrointestinal: Nausea, xerostomia

Miscellaneous: Diaphoresis

<10%:

Central nervous system: Anxiety, anorexia, agitation, yawning

Dermatologic: Rash, pruritus

Endocrine & metabolic: Sexual dysfunction

Gastrointestinal: Diarrhea, dyspepsia, vomiting, abdominal pain, weight gain

Neuromuscular & skeletal: Tremor, arthralgia, myalgia

Respiratory: Cough, rhinitis, sinusitis

Dosage Oral:

Children and Adolescents: OCD (unlabeled use): 10-40 mg/day

Adults: Depression: Initial: 20 mg/day, generally with an increase to 40 mg/day; doses of more than 40 mg are not usually necessary. Should a dose increase be necessary, it should occur in 20 mg increments at intervals of no less than 1 week. Maximum dose: 60 mg/day; reduce dosage in elderly or those with hepatic impairment.

Mechanism of Action A bicyclic phthalane derivative, citalopram selectively inhibits serotonin reuptake in the presynaptic neurons

Contraindications Hypersensitivity to citalopram or any component of the formulation; hypersensitivity or other adverse sequelae during therapy with other SSRIs; concomitant use with MAO inhibitors or within 2 weeks of discontinuing MAO inhibitors.

Warnings/Precautions As with all antidepressants, use with caution in patients with a history of mania (may activate hypomania/mania). Monotherapy in patients with bipolar disorder should be avoided. Patients should be screened for bipolar disorder, since using antidepressants alone may induce manic episodes with this condition. Has a low potential to impair cognitive or motor performance; caution operating hazardous machinery or driving. The possibility of a suicide attempt is inherent in major depression and may persist until remission occurs. Monitor for worsening of depression or suicidality, especially during initiation of therapy or with dose increases or decreases. Worsening depression and severe abrupt suicidality that are not part of the presenting symptoms may require discontinuation or modification of drug therapy. Use with caution in patients with a history of seizures. Use caution in high-risk patients during initiation of therapy. Prescriptions should be written for the smallest quantity consistent with good patient care.

(Continued)

Citalopram *(Continued)*

Use with caution in patients with hepatic or renal dysfunction, in elderly patients, concomitant CNS depressants, and pregnancy (high doses of citalopram has been associated with teratogenicity in animals). Use caution with concomitant use of NSAIDs, ASA, or other drugs that affect coagulation; the risk of bleeding is potentiated. May cause hyponatremia/SIADH. May cause or exacerbate sexual dysfunction. Upon discontinuation of citalopram therapy, gradually taper dose. If intolerable symptoms occur following a decrease in dosage or upon discontinuation of therapy, then resuming the previous dose with a more gradual taper should be considered. The patient's family or caregiver should be alerted to monitor patients for the emergence of suicidality and associated behaviors such as anxiety, agitation, panic attacks, insomnia, irritability, hostility, impulsivity, akathisia, hypomania, and mania; patients should be instructed not to abruptly discontinue this medication, but notify their healthcare provider if any of these symptoms or worsening depression occur.

Drug Interactions

Cytochrome P450 Effect: Substrate of CYP2C19 (major), 2D6 (minor), 3A4 (major); **Inhibits** CYP1A2 (weak), 2B6 (weak), 2C19 (weak), 2D6 (weak)

Increased Effect/Toxicity: Citalopram should not be used with nonselective MAO inhibitors (phenelzine, isocarboxazid) or other drugs with MAO inhibition (linezolid); fatal reactions have been reported. Wait 5 weeks after stopping citalopram before starting a nonselective MAO inhibitor and 2 weeks after stopping an MAO inhibitor before starting citalopram. Concurrent selegiline has been associated with mania, hypertension, or serotonin syndrome (risk may be reduced relative to nonselective MAO inhibitors).

CYP2C19 inhibitors may increase the levels/effects of citalopram; example inhibitors include delavirdine, fluconazole, fluvoxamine, gemfibrozil, isoniazid, omeprazole, and ticlopidine. CYP3A4 inhibitors may increase the levels/effects of citalopram; example inhibitors include azole antifungals, ciprofloxacin, clarithromycin, diclofenac, doxycycline, erythromycin, imatinib, isoniazid, nefazodone, nicardipine, propofol, protease inhibitors, quinidine, and verapamil.

Combined use of SSRIs and amphetamines, buspirone, meperidine, nefazodone, serotonin agonists (such as sumatriptan), sibutramine, other SSRIs, sympathomimetics, ritonavir, tramadol, and venlafaxine may increase the risk of serotonin syndrome. Risk of hyponatremia may increase with concurrent use of loop diuretics (bumetanide, furosemide, torsemide). Citalopram may increase the hypoprothrombinemic response to warfarin. Concomitant use of citalopram and NSAIDs, aspirin, or other drugs affecting coagulation has been associated with an increased risk of bleeding; monitor.

Combined use of sumatriptan (and other serotonin agonists) may result in toxicity; weakness, hyper-reflexia, and incoordination have been observed with sumatriptan and SSRIs. In addition, concurrent use may theoretically increase the risk of serotonin syndrome; includes sumatriptan, naratriptan, rizatriptan, and zolmitriptan.

Decreased Effect: CYP2C19 inducers may decrease the levels/effects of citalopram; example inducers include aminoglutethimide, carbamazepine, phenytoin, and rifampin. Cyproheptadine may inhibit the effects of serotonin reuptake inhibitors. CYP3A4 inducers may decrease the levels/effects of citalopram; example inducers include aminoglutethimide, carbamazepine, nafcillin, nevirapine, phenobarbital, phenytoin, and rifamycins.

Ethanol/Nutrition/Herb Interactions

Ethanol: Avoid ethanol (may increase CNS depression).

Herb/Nutraceutical: Avoid valerian, St John's wort, SAMe, kava kava, and gotu kola (may increase CNS depression).

Dietary Considerations May be taken without regard to food.

Pharmacodynamics/Kinetics

Distribution: V_d: 12 L/kg

Protein binding, plasma: ~80%

Metabolism: Extensively hepatic, including CYP, to N-demethylated, N-oxide, and deaminated metabolites

Bioavailability: 80%

Half-life elimination: 24-48 hours; average 35 hours (doubled with hepatic impairment)

Time to peak, serum: 1-6 hours, average within 4 hours

Excretion: Urine (10% as unchanged drug)

Note: Clearance was decreased, while AUC and half-life were significantly increased in elderly patients and in patients with hepatic impairment. Mild to moderate renal impairment may reduce clearance (17%) and prolong half-life of citalopram. No pharmacokinetic information is available concerning patients with severe renal impairment.

Pregnancy Risk Factor C

Dosage Forms SOLN, oral: 10 mg/5 mL (240 mL). **TAB:** 10 mg, 20 mg, 40 mg

Comments Problems with SSRI-induced bruxism have been reported and may preclude their use; clinicians attempting to evaluate any patient with bruxism or involuntary muscle movement, who is simultaneously being treated with an SSRI drug, should be aware of the potential association.

Citalopram Hydrobromide *see* Citalopram *on page 339*

Citanest® Forte *see* Prilocaine and Epinephrine *on page 1120*

Citanest® Plain *see* Prilocaine *on page 1118*

Citracal® [OTC] *see* Calcium Citrate *on page 246*

Citrate of Magnesia *see* Magnesium Citrate *on page 853*

Citric Acid and d-gluconic Acid Irrigant *see* Citric Acid, Magnesium Carbonate, and Glucono-Delta-Lactone *on page 341*

Citric Acid and Potassium Citrate *see* Potassium Citrate and Citric Acid *on page 1106*

Citric Acid Bladder Mixture *see* Citric Acid, Magnesium Carbonate, and Glucono-Delta-Lactone *on page 341*

Citric Acid, Magnesium Carbonate, and Glucono-Delta-Lactone

(SI trik AS id, mag NEE see um KAR bo nate, and GLOO kon o DEL ta LAK tone)

U.S. Brand Names Renacidin®

Generic Available No

Synonyms Citric Acid and d-gluconic Acid Irrigant; Citric Acid Bladder Mixture; Citric Acid, Magnesium Hydroxycarbonate, D-Gluconic Acid, Magnesium Acid Citrate, and Calcium Carbonate; Hemiacidrin

Pharmacologic Category Urinary Tract Product

Use Prevention of formation of calcifications of indwelling urinary tract cathoters; treatment of renal and bladder calculi of the apatite or struvite type

Local Anesthetic/Vasoconstrictor Precautions No information available to require special precautions

Effects on Dental Treatment No significant effects or complications reported

Common Adverse Effects

>10%:

Central nervous system: Fever (20% to 40%)

Genitourinary: Urothelial ulceration with or without edema (13%)

Miscellaneous: Transient flank pain

1% to 10%:

Endocrine & metabolic: Hypermagnesemia, hyperphosphatemia

Genitourinary: Urinary tract infection, dysuria, hematuria, bladder irritability

Neuromuscular & skeletal: Back pain

Renal: Creatinine increased

Mechanism of Action Magnesium from the irrigating solution is exchanged for calcium in the stone matrix. The magnesium stones are soluble and are able to dissolve in the acidic pH of the solution.

Pregnancy Risk Factor C

Citric Acid, Magnesium Hydroxycarbonate, D-Gluconic Acid, Magnesium Acid Citrate, and Calcium Carbonate *see* Citric Acid, Magnesium Carbonate, and Glucono-Delta-Lactone *on page 341*

Citric Acid, Sodium Citrate, and Potassium Citrate

(SIT rik AS id, SOW dee um SIT rate, & poe TASS ee um SIT rate)

U.S. Brand Names Cytra-3; Polycitra®; Polycitra®-LC

Generic Available Yes

Synonyms Potassium Citrate, Citric Acid, and Sodium Citrate; Sodium Citrate, Citric Acid, and Potassium Citrate

Pharmacologic Category Alkalinizing Agent, Oral

Use Conditions where long-term maintenance of an alkaline urine is desirable as in control and dissolution of uric acid and cystine calculi of the urinary tract

Local Anesthetic/Vasoconstrictor Precautions No information available to require special precautions

Effects on Dental Treatment No significant effects or complications reported

Common Adverse Effects Frequency not defined.

(Continued)

Citric Acid, Sodium Citrate, and Potassium Citrate *(Continued)*

Cardiovascular: Cardiac abnormalities

Endocrine & metabolic: Metabolic alkalosis, calcium levels, hyperkalemia, hypernatremia

Gastrointestinal: Diarrhea

Neuromuscular & skeletal: Tetany

Drug Interactions

Increased Effect/Toxicity: Increased toxicity/levels of amphetamines, ephedrine, pseudoephedrine, flecainide, quinidine, and quinine due to urinary alkalinization.

Decreased Effect: Decreased effect/levels of lithium, chlorpropamide, and salicylates due to urinary alkalinization.

Pregnancy Risk Factor Not established

Citrovorum Factor *see* Leucovorin *on page 804*
Citrucel® [OTC] *see* Methylcellulose *on page 905*
CL-118,532 *see* Triptorelin *on page 1346*
CI-719 *see* Gemfibrozil *on page 651*
CL-825 *see* Pentostatin *on page 1065*
CL-184116 *see* Porfimer *on page 1103*
Cla *see* Clarithromycin *on page 343*

Cladribine (KLA dri been)

U.S. Brand Names Leustatin®

Canadian Brand Names Leustatin®

Generic Available Yes

Synonyms 2-CdA; 2-Chlorodeoxyadenosine

Pharmacologic Category Adjuvant, Radiosensitizing Agent; Antineoplastic Agent, Antimetabolite (Purine Antagonist); Antineoplastic Agent, Antimetabolite

Use Treatment of hairy cell leukemia, chronic lymphocytic leukemia (CLL), chronic myelogenous leukemia (CML)

Unlabeled/Investigational Use Non-Hodgkin's lymphomas, progressive multiple sclerosis

Local Anesthetic/Vasoconstrictor Precautions No information available to require special precautions

Effects on Dental Treatment No significant effects or complications reported

Common Adverse Effects

>10%:

Allergic: Fever (70%), chills (18%); skin reactions (erythema, itching) at the catheter site (18%)

Central nervous system: Fatigue (17%), headache (13%)

Dermatologic: Rash

Hematologic: Myelosuppression, common, dose-limiting; leukopenia (70%); anemia (37%); thrombocytopenia (12%)

Nadir: 5-10 days

Recovery: 4-8 weeks

1% to 10%:

Cardiovascular: Edema, tachycardia

Central nervous system: Dizziness; pains; chills; malaise; severe infections, possibly related to thrombocytopenia

Dermatologic: Pruritus, erythema

Gastrointestinal: Nausea, mild to moderate, usually not seen at doses <0.3 mg/kg/day; constipation; abdominal pain

Neuromuscular & skeletal: Myalgia, arthralgia, weakness

Renal: Renal failure at high (>0.3 mg/kg/day) doses

Miscellaneous: Diaphoresis, delayed herpes zoster infections, tumor lysis syndrome

Mechanism of Action A purine nucleoside analogue; prodrug which is activated via phosphorylation by deoxycytidine kinase to a 5'-triphosphate derivative. This active form incorporates into DNA to result in the breakage of DNA strand and shutdown of DNA synthesis. This also results in a depletion of nicotinamide adenine dinucleotide and adenosine triphosphate (ATP). Cladribine is cell-cycle nonspecific.

Pharmacodynamics/Kinetics

Absorption: Oral: 55%; SubQ: 100%; Rectal: 20%

Distribution: V_d: 4.52 ± 2.82 L/kg

Protein binding, plasma: 20%

Metabolism: Hepatic; 5'-triphosphate moiety-active

Half-life elimination: Biphasic: Alpha: 25 minutes; Beta: 6.7 hours; Terminal, mean: Normal renal function: 5.4 hours

Excretion: Urine (21% to 44%)

Clearance: Estimated systemic: 640 mL/hour/kg

Pregnancy Risk Factor D

Claforan® *see* Cefotaxime *on page 283*

Claravis™ *see* Isotretinoin *on page 773*

Clarinex® *see* Desloratadine *on page 408*

Claripel™ *see* Hydroquinone *on page 719*

Clarithromycin (kla RITH roe mye sin)

Related Information

Antibiotic Prophylaxis, Preprocedural Guidelines for Dental Patients *on page 1509*

Gastrointestinal Disorders *on page 1476*

Oral Bacterial Infections *on page 1533*

Respiratory Diseases *on page 1478*

U.S. Brand Names Biaxin®; Biaxin® XL

Canadian Brand Names Biaxin®; Biaxin® XL; ratio-Clarithromycin

Mexican Brand Names Adel®; Klaricid®; Mabicrol®

Generic Available No

Synonyms Cla

Pharmacologic Category Antibiotic, Macrolide

Dental Use Alternate antibiotic in the treatment of common orofacial infections caused by aerobic gram-positive cocci and susceptible anaerobes alternate antibiotic for the prevention of bacterial endocarditis in patients undergoing dental procedures

Use

Children:

- Pharyngitis/tonsillitis, acute maxillary sinusitis, uncomplicated skin/skin structure infections, and mycobacterial infections due to the above organisms
- Acute otitis media (*H. influenzae*, *M. catarrhalis*, or *S. pneumoniae*)
- Prevention of disseminated mycobacterial infections due to MAC disease in patients with advanced HIV infection

Adults:

- Pharyngitis/tonsillitis due to susceptible *S. pyogenes*
- Acute maxillary sinusitis and acute exacerbation of chronic bronchitis due to susceptible *H. influenzae*, *M. catarrhalis*, or *S. pneumoniae*
- Pneumonia due to susceptible *H. influenzae*, *Mycoplasma pneumoniae*, *S. pneumoniae*, or *Chlamydia pneumoniae* (TWAR);
- Uncomplicated skin/skin structure infections due to susceptible *S. aureus*, *S. pyogenes*
- Disseminated mycobacterial infections due to *M. avium* or *M. intracellulare*
- Prevention of disseminated mycobacterial infections due to *M. avium* complex (MAC) disease (eg, patients with advanced HIV infection)
- Duodenal ulcer disease due to *H. pylori* in regimens with other drugs including amoxicillin and lansoprazole or omeprazole, ranitidine bismuth citrate, bismuth subsalicylate, tetracycline, and/or an H_2 antagonist
- Alternate antibiotic for prophylaxis of bacterial endocarditis in patients who are allergic to penicillin and undergoing surgical or dental procedures

Local Anesthetic/Vasoconstrictor Precautions No information available to require special precautions

Effects on Dental Treatment Key adverse event(s) related to dental treatment: Abnormal taste.

Significant Adverse Effects

1% to 10%:

- Central nervous system: Headache (adults and children 2%)
- Dermatologic: Rash (children 3%)
- Gastrointestinal: Diarrhea (adults 6%, children 6%); vomiting (children 6%); nausea (adults 3%); abnormal taste (adults 7%); heartburn (adults 2%); abdominal pain (adults 2%, children 3%)
- Hepatic: Prothrombin time increased (1%)
- Renal: BUN increased (4%)

<1% (Limited to important or life-threatening): Anaphylaxis, *Clostridium difficile* colitis, dyspnea, hallucinations, hearing loss (reversible), hepatic failure, hepatitis, hypoglycemia, jaundice, leukopenia, manic behavior, neuromuscular blockade (case reports), neutropenia, pancreatitis, psychosis, QT prolongation, seizures, Stevens-Johnson syndrome, thrombocytopenia, tooth discoloration, torsade de pointes, toxic epidermal necrolysis, tremor, ventricular tachycardia, vertigo

(Continued)

Clarithromycin *(Continued)*

Dosage Oral:

Children ≥6 months: 15 mg/kg/day divided every 12 hours for 10 days

Mycobacterial infection (prevention and treatment): 7.5 mg/kg twice daily, up to 500 mg twice daily

Prophylaxis of bacterial endocarditis: 15 mg/kg 1 hour before procedure (maximum dose: 500 mg)

Adults:

Usual dose: 250-500 mg every 12 hours **or** 1000 mg (two 500 mg extended release tablets) once daily for for 7-14 days

Upper respiratory tract: 250-500 mg every 12 hours for 10-14 days

Pharyngitis/tonsillitis: 250 mg every 12 hours for 10 days

Acute maxillary sinusitis: 500 mg every 12 hours **or** 1000 mg (two 500 mg extended release tablets) once daily for 14 days

Lower respiratory tract: 250-500 mg every 12 hours for 7-14 days

Acute exacerbation of chronic bronchitis due to:

M. catarrhalis and *S. pneumoniae*: 250 mg every 12 hours **or** 1000 mg (two 500 mg extended release tablets) once daily for 7-14 days

H. influenzae: 500 mg every 12 hours for 7-14 days

Pneumonia due to:

C. pneumoniae, *M. pneumoniae*, and *S. pneumoniae*: 250 mg every 12 hours for 7-14 days **or** 1000 mg (two 500 mg extended release tablets) once daily for 7 days

H. influenzae: 250 mg every 12 hours for 7 days **or** 1000 mg (two 500 mg extended release tablets) once daily for 7 days

Mycobacterial infection (prevention and treatment): 500 mg twice daily (use with other antimycobacterial drugs, eg, ethambutol, clofazimine, or rifampin)

Prophylaxis of bacterial endocarditis: 500 mg 1 hour prior to procedure

Uncomplicated skin and skin structure: 250 mg every 12 hours for 7-14 days

Helicobacter pylori: Combination regimen with bismuth subsalicylate, tetracycline, clarithromycin, and an H_2-receptor antagonist; or combination of omeprazole and clarithromycin; 250 mg twice daily to 500 mg 3 times/day

Dosing adjustment in renal impairment:

Cl_{cr} <30 mL/minute: Half the normal dose or double the dosing interval

In combination with ritonavir:

Cl_{cr} 30-60 mL/minute: Decrease clarithromycin dose by 50%

Cl_{cr} <30 mL/minute: Decrease clarithromycin dose by 75%

Dosing adjustment in hepatic impairment: No dosing adjustment is needed as long as renal function is normal

Elderly: Pharmacokinetics are similar to those in younger adults; may have age-related reductions in renal function; monitor and adjust dose if necessary

Mechanism of Action Exerts its antibacterial action by binding to 50S ribosomal subunit resulting in inhibition of protein synthesis. The 14-OH metabolite of clarithromycin is twice as active as the parent compound against certain organisms.

Contraindications Hypersensitivity to clarithromycin, erythromycin, or any macrolide antibiotic; use with ergot derivatives, pimozide, cisapride; combination with ranitidine bismuth citrate should not be used in patients with history of acute porphyria or Cl_{cr} <25 mL/minute

Warnings/Precautions Dosage adjustment required with severe renal impairment, decreased dosage or prolonged dosing interval may be appropriate; antibiotic-associated colitis has been reported with use of clarithromycin. Macrolides (including clarithromycin) have been associated with rare QT prolongation and ventricular arrhythmias, including torsade de pointes. Safety and efficacy in children <6 months of age have not been established.

Drug Interactions Substrate of CYP3A4 (major); **Inhibits** CYP1A2 (weak), 3A4 (strong)

Alfentanil (and possibly other narcotic analgesics): Serum levels may be increased by clarithromycin; monitor for increased effect.

Antipsychotic agents (particularly mesoridazine and thioridazine): Risk of QT_c prolongation and malignant arrhythmias may be increased.

Benzodiazepines (those metabolized by CYP3A4, including alprazolam, midazolam, triazolam): Serum levels may be increased by clarithromycin; somnolence and confusion have been reported.

Bromocriptine: Serum levels may be increased by clarithromycin; monitor for increased effect.

Buspirone: Serum levels may be increased by clarithromycin; monitor.

Calcium channel blockers (felodipine, verapamil, and potentially others metabolized by CYP3A4): Serum levels may be increased by clarithromycin; monitor.

Carbamazepine: Serum levels may be increased by clarithromycin; monitor.

Cilostazol: Serum levels may be increased by clarithromycin; monitor.

Cisapride: Serum levels may be increased by clarithromycin; serious arrhythmias have occurred; concurrent use contraindicated.

Clindamycin (and lincomycin): Use with clarithromycin may result in pharmacologic antagonism; manufacturer recommends avoiding this combination.

Clozapine: Serum levels may be increased by clarithromycin; monitor.

Colchicine: serum levels/toxicity may be increased by clarithromycin; monitor.

Cyclosporine: Serum levels may be increased by clarithromycin; monitor serum levels.

CYP3A4 inducers: CYP3A4 inducers may decrease the levels/effects of clarithromycin. Example inducers include aminoglutethimide, carbamazepine, nafcillin, nevirapine, phenobarbital, phenytoin, and rifamycins.

CYP3A4 inhibitors: May increase the levels/effects of clarithromycin. Example inhibitors include azole antifungals, ciprofloxacin, diclofenac, doxycycline, erythromycin, imatinib, isoniazid, nefazodone, nicardipine, propofol, protease inhibitors, quinidine, and verapamil.

CYP3A4 substrates: Clarithromycin may increase the levels/effects of CYP3A4 substrates. Example substrates include benzodiazepines, calcium channel blockers, mirtazapine, nateglinide, nefazodone, tacrolimus, and venlafaxine. Selected benzodiazepines (midazolam and triazolam), cisapride, ergot alkaloids, selected HMG-CoA reductase inhibitors (lovastatin and simvastatin), and pimozide are generally contraindicated with strong CYP3A4 inhibitors.

Delavirdine: Serum levels may be increased by clarithromycin; monitor.

Digoxin: Serum levels may be increased by clarithromycin; digoxin toxicity and potentially fatal arrhythmias have been reported; monitor digoxin levels.

Disopyramide: Serum levels may be increased by clarithromycin; in addition, QT_c prolongation and risk of malignant arrhythmia may be increased; avoid combination.

Ergot alkaloids: Concurrent use may lead to acute ergot toxicity (severe peripheral vasospasm and dysesthesia).

Fluconazole: Increases clarithromycin levels and AUC by ~25%

HMG-CoA reductase inhibitors (atorvastatin, lovastatin, and simvastatin); Clarithromycin may increase serum levels of "statins" metabolized by CYP3A4, increasing the risk of myopathy/rhabdomyolysis (does not include fluvastatin and pravastatin). Switch to pravastatin/fluvastatin or suspend treatment during course of clarithromycin therapy.

Loratadine: Serum levels may be increased by clarithromycin; monitor.

Methylprednisolone: Serum levels may be increased by clarithromycin; monitor.

Neuromuscular-blocking agents: May be potentiated by clarithromycin (case reports).

Phenytoin: Serum levels may be increased by clarithromycin; other evidence suggested phenytoin levels may be decreased in some patients; monitor.

Pimozide: Serum levels may be increased, leading to malignant arrhythmias; concomitant use is contraindicated.

Protease inhibitors (amprenavir, nelfinavir, and ritonavir): May increase serum levels of clarithromycin.

QT_c-prolonging agents: Concomitant use may increase the risk of malignant arrhythmias.

Quinidine: Serum levels may be increased by clarithromycin; in addition, the risk of QT_c prolongation and malignant arrhythmias may be increased during concurrent use.

Quinolone antibiotics (sparfloxacin, gatifloxacin, or moxifloxacin): Concurrent use may increase the risk of malignant arrhythmias.

Rifabutin: Serum levels may be increased by clarithromycin; monitor.

Sildenafil, tadalafil, vardenafil: Serum levels may be increased by clarithromycin. Do not exceed single sildenafil doses of 25 mg in 48 hours, a single tadalafil dose of 10 mg in 72 hours, or a single vardenafil dose of 2.5 mg in 24 hours.

Tacrolimus: Serum levels may be increased by clarithromycin; monitor serum concentration.

Theophylline: Serum levels may be increased by clarithromycin; monitor.

Valproic acid (and derivatives): Serum levels may be increased by clarithromycin; monitor.

Vinblastine (and vincristine): Serum levels may be increased by clarithromycin.

Warfarin: Effects may be potentiated; monitor INR closely and adjust warfarin dose as needed or choose another antibiotic

Zafirlukast: Serum levels may be decreased by clarithromycin; monitor.

(Continued)

Clarithromycin *(Continued)*

Zidovudine: Peak levels (but not AUC) of zidovudine may be increased; other studies suggest levels may be decreased.

Zopiclone: Serum levels may be increased by clarithromycin; monitor.

Ethanol/Nutrition/Herb Interactions

Food: Delays absorption; total absorption remains unchanged.

Herb/Nutraceutical: St John's wort may decrease clarithromycin levels.

Dietary Considerations May be taken with or without meals; may be taken with milk. Biaxin® XL should be taken with food.

Pharmacodynamics/Kinetics

Absorption: Highly stable in presence of gastric acid (unlike erythromycin); food delays but does not affect extent of absorption

Distribution: Widely into most body tissues except CNS

Metabolism: Partially hepatic; converted to 14-OH clarithromycin (active metabolite)

Bioavailability: 50%

Half-life elimination: 5-7 hours

Time to peak: 2-4 hours

Excretion: Primarily urine

Clearance: Approximates normal GFR

Pregnancy Risk Factor C

Lactation Excretion in breast milk unknown/use caution

Breast-Feeding Considerations Erythromycins may be taken while breast-feeding. Use caution.

Dosage Forms

Granules for oral suspension (Biaxin®): 125 mg/5 mL (50 mL, 100 mL); 250 mg/5 mL (50 mL, 100 mL) [fruit punch flavor]

Tablet [film coated] (Biaxin®): 250 mg, 500 mg

Tablet, extended release [film coated] (Biaxin® XL): 500 mg

Selected Readings

ADA Division of Legal Affairs, "A Legal Perspective on Antibiotic Prophylaxis," *J Am Dent Assoc*, 2003, 134(9):1260.

American Dental Association Council on Scientific Affairs, "Combating Antibiotic Resistance," *J Am Dent Assoc*, 2004, 135(4):484-7.

Amsden GW, "Erythromycin, Clarithromycin, and Azithromycin: Are the Differences Real?" *Clin Ther*, 1996, 18(1):56-72.

Dajani AS, Taubert KA, Wilson W, et al, "Prevention of Bacterial Endocarditis. Recommendations by the American Heart Association," *JAMA*, 1997, 277(22):1794-801.

Dajani AS, Taubert KA, Wilson W, et al, "Prevention of Bacterial Endocarditis: Recommendations by the American Heart Association," *J Am Dent Assoc*, 1997, 128(8):1142-51.

Moore PA, "Dental Therapeutic Indications for the Newer Long-Acting Macrolide Antibiotics," *J Am Dent Assoc*, 1999, 130(9):1341-3.

"Pimozide (Orap) Contraindicated With Clarithromycin (Biaxin®) and Other Macrolide Antibiotics," *FDA Medical Bulletin*, October 1996, 26 (3).

Wynn RL, "New Erythromycins," *Gen Dent*, 1996, 44(4):304-7.

Wynn RL, Bergman SA, Meiller TF, et al, "Antibiotics in Treating Oral-Facial Infections of Odontogenic Origin: An Update," *Gen Dent*, 2001, 49(3):238-40, 242, 244 passim.

Clarithromycin, Lansoprazole, and Amoxicillin *see* Lansoprazole, Amoxicillin, and Clarithromycin *on page 798*

Claritin® [OTC] *see* Loratadine *on page 841*

Claritin-D® 12-Hour [OTC] *see* Loratadine and Pseudoephedrine *on page 842*

Claritin-D® 24-Hour [OTC] *see* Loratadine and Pseudoephedrine *on page 842*

Claritin® Hives Relief [OTC] *see* Loratadine *on page 841*

Clear Eyes® [OTC] *see* Naphazoline *on page 964*

Clear Eyes® ACR [OTC] *see* Naphazoline *on page 964*

Clearplex [OTC] *see* Benzoyl Peroxide *on page 194*

Clemastine (KLEM as teen)

U.S. Brand Names Dayhist® Allergy [OTC]; Tavist® Allergy [OTC]

Mexican Brand Names Tavist®

Generic Available Yes

Synonyms Clemastine Fumarate

Pharmacologic Category Antihistamine

Use Perennial and seasonal allergic rhinitis and other allergic symptoms including urticaria

Local Anesthetic/Vasoconstrictor Precautions No information available to require special precautions

Effects on Dental Treatment Key adverse event(s) related to dental treatment: Xerostomia (normal salivary flow resumes upon discontinuation).

Common Adverse Effects Frequency not defined.

Cardiovascular: Palpitations, hypotension, tachycardia

Central nervous system: Dyscoordination, sedation, slight to moderate somnolence, sleepiness, confusion, restlessness, nervousness, insomnia, irritability, fatigue, headache, increased dizziness

Dermatologic: Rash, photosensitivity

Gastrointestinal: Diarrhea, nausea, xerostomia, epigastric distress, vomiting, constipation

Genitourinary: Urinary frequency, difficult urination, urinary retention

Hematologic: Hemolytic anemia, thrombocytopenia, agranulocytosis

Ocular: Blurred vision

Otic: Tinnitus

Respiratory: Thickening of bronchial secretions

Miscellaneous: Anaphylaxis

Mechanism of Action Competes with histamine for H_1-receptor sites on effector cells in the gastrointestinal tract, blood vessels, and respiratory tract

Drug Interactions

Cytochrome P450 Effect: Inhibits CYP2D6 (weak), 3A4 (weak)

Increased Effect/Toxicity: CNS depressants may increase the degree of sedation and respiratory depression with antihistamines. May increase the absorption of digoxin. Central and/or peripheral anticholinergic syndrome can occur when administered with amantadine, rimantadine, narcotic analgesics, phenothiazines and other antipsychotics (especially with high anticholinergic activity), tricyclic antidepressants, quinidine, disopyramide, procainamide, and antihistamines.

Decreased Effect: May increase gastric degradation of levodopa and decrease the amount of levodopa absorbed by delaying gastric emptying. Therapeutic effects of cholinergic agents (tacrine, donepezil) and neuroleptics may be antagonized.

Pharmacodynamics/Kinetics

Onset of action: Peak effect: Therapeutic: 5-7 hours

Duration: 8-16 hours

Absorption: Almost complete

Metabolism: Hepatic

Excretion: Urine

Pregnancy Risk Factor B

Clemastine Fumarate *see* Clemastine *on page 346*

Cleocin® *see* Clindamycin *on page 348*

Cleocin HCl® *see* Clindamycin *on page 348*

Cleocin Pediatric® *see* Clindamycin *on page 348*

Cleocin Phosphate® *see* Clindamycin *on page 348*

Cleocin T® *see* Clindamycin *on page 348*

Clidinium and Chlordiazepoxide

(kli DI nee um & klor dye az e POKS ide)

U.S. Brand Names Librax®

Canadian Brand Names Apo-Chlorax®; Librax®

Generic Available Yes

Synonyms Chlordiazepoxide and Clidinium

Pharmacologic Category Antispasmodic Agent, Gastrointestinal; Benzodiazepine

Use Adjunct treatment of peptic ulcer; treatment of irritable bowel syndrome

Local Anesthetic/Vasoconstrictor Precautions No information available to require special precautions

Effects on Dental Treatment Key adverse event(s) related to dental treatment: Xerostomia and changes in salivation (normal salivary flow resumes upon discontinuation).

Common Adverse Effects 1% to 10%:

Central nervous system: Drowsiness, ataxia, confusion, anticholinergic side effects

Gastrointestinal: Dry mouth, constipation, nausea

Drug Interactions

Cytochrome P450 Effect: Chlordiazepoxide: **Substrate** of CYP3A4 (major)

Increased Effect/Toxicity: Additive effects may result from concomitant benzodiazepine and/or anticholinergic therapy.

Pregnancy Risk Factor D

Climara® *see* Estradiol *on page 518*

Clinac™ BPO *see* Benzoyl Peroxide *on page 194*

Clindagel® *see* Clindamycin *on page 348*

ClindaMax™ *see* Clindamycin *on page 348*

Clindamycin (klin da MYE sin)

Related Information

Animal and Human Bites Guidelines *on page 1582*

Antibiotic Prophylaxis, Preprocedural Guidelines for Dental Patients *on page 1509*

Cardiovascular Diseases *on page 1458*

Oral Bacterial Infections *on page 1533*

Periodontal Diseases *on page 1542*

Sexually-Transmitted Diseases *on page 1504*

U.S. Brand Names Cleocin®; Cleocin HCl®; Cleocin Pediatric®; Cleocin Phosphate®; Cleocin T®; Clindagel®; ClindaMax™; Clindets®

Canadian Brand Names Alti-Clindamycin; Apo-Clindamycin®; Clindoxyl®; Dalacin® C; Dalacin® T; Dalacin® Vaginal; Novo-Clindamycin

Mexican Brand Names Clindazyn® [inj.]; Cutaclin® [gel]; Dalacin C®; Dalacin C® [inj.]; Dalacin T®; Dalacin V®; Galecin® [inj.]; Klyndaken®

Generic Available Yes: Excludes vaginal suppositories, vaginal cream

Synonyms Clindamycin Hydrochloride; Clindamycin Palmitate; Clindamycin Phosphate

Pharmacologic Category Antibiotic, Miscellaneous

Dental Use Alternate antibiotic, when amoxicillin cannot be used, for the standard regimen for prevention of bacterial endocarditis in patients undergoing dental procedures; alternate antibiotic in the treatment of common orofacial infections caused by aerobic gram-positive cocci and susceptible anaerobes; alternate antibiotic for prophylaxis for dental patients with total joint replacement

Use Treatment against aerobic and anaerobic streptococci (except enterococci), most staphylococci, *Bacteroides* sp and *Actinomyces*; pelvic inflammatory disease (I.V.); topically in treatment of severe acne; vaginally for *Gardnerella vaginalis*

Unlabeled/Investigational Use Bacterial vaginosis; may be useful in PCP; alternate treatment for toxoplasmosis

Local Anesthetic/Vasoconstrictor Precautions No information available to require special precautions

Effects on Dental Treatment No significant effects or complications reported

Significant Adverse Effects

Systemic:

>10%: Gastrointestinal: Diarrhea, abdominal pain

1% to 10%:

Cardiovascular: Hypotension

Dermatologic: Urticaria, rashes, Stevens-Johnson syndrome

Gastrointestinal: Pseudomembranous colitis, nausea, vomiting

Local: Thrombophlebitis, sterile abscess at I.M. injection site

Miscellaneous: Fungal overgrowth, hypersensitivity

<1% (Limited to important or life-threatening): Granulocytopenia, neutropenia, polyarthritis, renal dysfunction (rare), thrombocytopenia

Topical:

>10%: Dermatologic: Dryness, burning, itching, scaliness, erythema, or peeling of skin (lotion, solution); oiliness (gel, lotion)

<1% (Limited to important or life-threatening): Pseudomembranous colitis, nausea, vomiting, diarrhea (severe), abdominal pain, folliculitis, hypersensitivity reactions

Vaginal:

>10%: Genitourinary: Vaginitis or vulvovaginal pruritus (from *Candida albicans*), painful intercourse

1% to 10%:

Central nervous system: Dizziness, headache

Gastrointestinal: Diarrhea, nausea, vomiting, stomach cramps

Dosage Avoid in neonates (contains benzyl alcohol)

Infants and Children:

Oral: 8-20 mg/kg/day as hydrochloride; 8-25 mg/kg/day as palmitate in 3-4 divided doses; minimum dose of palmitate: 37.5 mg 3 times/day

I.M., I.V.:

<1 month: 15-20 mg/kg/day

>1 month: 20-40 mg/kg/day in 3-4 divided doses

Children: **Prevention of bacterial endocarditis** (unlabeled use): Oral: 20 mg/kg 1 hour before procedure with no follow-up dose needed; for patients allergic to penicillin and unable to take oral medications: 20 mg/kg I.V. within 30 minutes before procedure

Children ≥12 years and Adults: Topical: Apply a thin film twice daily

Adults:

Oral: 150-450 mg/dose every 6-8 hours; maximum dose: 1.8 g/day

Prevention of bacterial endocarditis in patients unable to take amoxicillin (unlabeled use): Oral: 600 mg 1 hour before procedure with no follow-up dose needed; for patients allergic to penicillin and unable to take oral medications: 600 mg I.V. within 30 minutes before procedure

I.M., I.V.: 1.2-1.8 g/day in 2-4 divided doses; maximum dose: 4.8 g/day

Pelvic inflammatory disease: I.V.: 900 mg every 8 hours with gentamicin 2 mg/kg, then 1.5 mg/kg every 8 hours; continue after discharge with doxycycline 100 mg twice daily to complete 14 days of total therapy

Pneumocystis carinii pneumonia (unlabeled use):
- Oral: 300-450 mg 4 times/day with primaquine
- I.M., I.V.: 1200-2400 mg/day with pyrimethamine
- I.V.: 600 mg 4 times/day with primaquine

Bacterial vaginosis (unlabeled use):
- Oral: 300 mg twice daily for 7 days
- Intravaginal:
  - Suppositories: Insert one ovule (100 mg clindamycin) daily into vagina at bedtime for 3 days
  - Cream: One full applicator inserted intravaginally once daily before bedtime for 3 or 7 consecutive days

Dosing adjustment in hepatic impairment: Adjustment recommended in patients with severe hepatic disease

Mechanism of Action Reversibly binds to 50S ribosomal subunits preventing peptide bond formation thus inhibiting bacterial protein synthesis; bacteriostatic or bactericidal depending on drug concentration, infection site, and organism

Contraindications Hypersensitivity to clindamycin or any component of the formulation; previous pseudomembranous colitis; hepatic impairment

Warnings/Precautions Dosage adjustment may be necessary in patients with severe hepatic dysfunction; can cause severe and possibly fatal colitis; use with caution in patients with a history of pseudomembranous colitis; discontinue drug if significant diarrhea, abdominal cramps, or passage of blood and mucus occurs. Avoid in neonates (contains benzyl alcohol).

Drug Interactions Increased duration of neuromuscular blockade from tubocurarine, pancuronium

Ethanol/Nutrition/Herb Interactions

Food: Peak concentrations may be delayed with food.

Herb/Nutraceutical: St John's wort may decrease clindamycin levels.

Dietary Considerations May be taken with food.

Pharmacodynamics/Kinetics

Absorption: Topical: ~10%; Oral: Rapid (90%)

Distribution: High concentrations in bone and urine; no significant levels in CSF, even with inflamed meninges; crosses placenta; enters breast milk

Metabolism: Hepatic

Bioavailability: Topical: <1%

Half-life elimination: Neonates: Premature: 8.7 hours; Full-term: 3.6 hours; Adults: 1.6-5.3 hours (average: 2-3 hours)

Time to peak, serum: Oral: Within 60 minutes; I.M.: 1-3 hours

Excretion: Urine (10%) and feces (~4%) as active drug and metabolites

Pregnancy Risk Factor B

Lactation Enters breast milk/compatible

Dosage Forms Note: Strength is expressed as base

Capsule, as hydrochloride: 150 mg, 300 mg
- Cleocin HCl®: 75 mg [contains tartrazine], 150 mg [contains tartrazine], 300 mg

Cream, vaginal, as phosphate (Cleocin®): 2% (40 g) [contains benzyl alcohol; packaged with 7 disposable applicators]

Gel, topical, as phosphate: 1% [10 mg/g] (30 g, 60 g)
- Cleocin T®: 1% [10 mg/g] (30 g, 60 g)
- Clindagel®: 1% [10 mg/g] (40 mL, 75 mL)
- ClindaMax™: 1% (30 g, 60 g)

Granules for oral solution, as palmitate (Cleocin Pediatric®): 75 mg/5 mL (100 mL) [cherry flavor]

Infusion, as phosphate [premixed in D_5W] (Cleocin Phosphate®): 300 mg (50 mL); 600 mg (50 mL); 900 mg (50 mL)

Injection, solution, as phosphate (Cleocin Phosphate®): 150 mg/mL (2 mL, 4 mL, 6 mL, 60 mL) [contains benzyl alcohol and disodium edetate 0.5 mg]

Lotion, as phosphate (Cleocin T®, ClindaMax™): 1% [10 mg/mL] (60 mL)

Pledgets, topical: 1% (60s) [contains alcohol]
- Clindets®: 1% (69s) [contains isopropyl alcohol 52%]
- Cleocin T®: 1% (60s) [contains isopropyl alcohol 50%]

(Continued)

Clindamycin *(Continued)*

Solution, topical, as phosphate (Cleocin T®): 1% [10 mg/mL] (30 mL, 60 mL) [contains isopropyl alcohol 50%]

Suppository, vaginal, as phosphate (Cleocin®): 100 mg (3s)

Selected Readings

ADA Division of Legal Affairs, "A Legal Perspective on Antibiotic Prophylaxis," *J Am Dent Assoc*, 2003, 134(9):1260.

"Advisory Statement. Antibiotic Prophylaxis for Dental Patients With Total Joint Replacements. American Dental Association; American Academy of Orthopedic Surgeons," *J Am Dent Assoc*, 1997, 128(7):1004-8.

American Dental Association; American Academy of Orthopedic Surgeons, "Antibiotic Prophylaxis for Dental Patients With Total Joint Replacements," *J Am Dent Assoc*, 2003, 134(7):895-9.

American Dental Association Council on Scientific Affairs, "Combating Antibiotic Resistance," *J Am Dent Assoc*, 2004, 135(4):484-7.

Dajani AS, Taubert KA, Wilson W, et al, "Prevention of Bacterial Endocarditis. Recommendations by the American Heart Association," *JAMA*, 1997, 277(22):1794-801.

Dajani AS, Taubert KA, Wilson W, et al, "Prevention of Bacterial Endocarditis: Recommendations by the American Heart Association," *J Am Dent Assoc*, 1997, 128(8):1142-51.

Sandor GK, Low DE, Judd PL, et al, "Antimicrobial Treatment Options in the Management of Odontogenic Infections," *J Can Dent Assoc*, 1998, 64(7):508-14.

Wynn RL, "Clindamycin: An Often Forgotten But Important Antibiotic," *AGD Impact*, 1994, 22:10.

Wynn RL and Bergman SA, "Antibiotics and Their Use in the Treatment of Orofacial Infections, Part I," *Gen Dent*, 1994, 42(5):398, 400, 402.

Wynn RL and Bergman SA, "Antibiotics and Their Use in the Treatment of Orofacial Infections, Part II," *Gen Dent*, 1994, 42(6):498-502.

Wynn RL, Bergman SA, Meiller TF, et al, "Antibiotics in Treating Oral-Facial Infections of Odontogenic Origin: An Update," *Gen Dent*, 2001, 49(3):238-40, 242, 244 passim.

Clindamycin and Benzoyl Peroxide

(klin da MYE sin & BEN zoe il peer OKS ide)

Related Information

Benzoyl Peroxide *on page 194*

Clindamycin *on page 348*

U.S. Brand Names BenzaClin®; Duac™

Generic Available No

Synonyms Benzoyl Peroxide and Clindamycin; Clindamycin Phosphate and Benzoyl Peroxide

Pharmacologic Category Topical Skin Product; Topical Skin Product, Acne

Use Topical treatment of acne vulgaris

Local Anesthetic/Vasoconstrictor Precautions No information available to require special precautions

Effects on Dental Treatment No significant effects or complications reported

Common Adverse Effects Frequency not defined: Dermatologic: Dry skin, pruritus, peeling, erythema, sunburn, redness, burning

Mechanism of Action Clindamycin and benzoyl peroxide have activity against *Propionibacterium acnes in vitro*. This organism has been associated with acne vulgaris. Benzoyl peroxide releases free-radical oxygen which oxidizes bacterial proteins in the sebaceous follicles decreasing the number of anaerobic bacteria and decreasing irritating-type free fatty acids. Clindamycin reversibly binds to 50S ribosomal subunits preventing peptide bond formation thus inhibiting bacterial protein synthesis; bacteriostatic or bactericidal depending on drug concentration, infection site, and organism.

Drug Interactions

Increased Effect/Toxicity: Tretinoin may cause increased adverse events with concurrent use.

Decreased Effect: Erythromycin may antagonize clindamycin's effects.

Pharmacodynamics/Kinetics See individual agents.

Absorption: Benzoyl peroxide: <2% systemically absorbed

Metabolism: Benzoyl peroxide: Converted to benzoic acid in the skin

Pregnancy Risk Factor C

Clindamycin Hydrochloride *see* Clindamycin *on page 348*

Clindamycin Palmitate *see* Clindamycin *on page 348*

Clindamycin Phosphate *see* Clindamycin *on page 348*

Clindamycin Phosphate and Benzoyl Peroxide *see* Clindamycin and Benzoyl Peroxide *on page 350*

Clindets® *see* Clindamycin *on page 348*

Clinoril® *see* Sulindac *on page 1251*

Clobazam (KLOE ba zam)

Canadian Brand Names Alti-Clobazam; Apo-Clobazam®; Frisium®; Novo-Clobazam; PMS-Clobazam

Mexican Brand Names Frisium®

Generic Available Yes

Pharmacologic Category Benzodiazepine

Use Adjunctive treatment of epilepsy

Unlabeled/Investigational Use Monotherapy for epilepsy or intermittent seizures

Local Anesthetic/Vasoconstrictor Precautions No information available to require special precautions

Effects on Dental Treatment Key adverse event(s) related to dental treatment: Xerostomia (normal salivary flow resumes upon discontinuation). Paradoxical reactions (including excitation, agitation, hallucinations, and psychosis) are known to occur with benzodiazepines.

Common Adverse Effects

Central nervous system: Drowsiness (17%), ataxia (4%), dizziness (2%), behavior disorder (1%), confusion, depression, lethargy, slurred speech, tremor, anterograde amnesia. In addition, paradoxical reactions (including excitation, agitation, hallucinations, and psychosis) are known to occur with benzodiazepines.

Dermatologic: Rash, pruritus, urticaria

Gastrointestinal: Weight gain (2%); dose-related: Xerostomia, constipation, nausea

Hematologic: Decreased WBCs and other hematologic abnormalities have been rarely associated with benzodiazepines

Neuromuscular & skeletal: Muscle spasm

Ocular: Blurred vision (1%)

Restrictions Not available in U.S.

Mechanism of Action Clobazam is a 1,5 benzodiazepine which binds to stereospecific benzodiazepine receptors on the postsynaptic GABA neuron at several sites within the central nervous system, including the limbic system, reticular formation. Enhancement of the inhibitory effect of GABA on neuronal excitability results by increased neuronal membrane permeability to chloride ions. This shift in chloride ions results in hyperpolarization (a less excitable state) and stabilization.

Drug Interactions

Cytochrome P450 Effect: Substrate of CYP3A4 (major)

Increased Effect/Toxicity: Benzodiazepines potentiate the CNS depressant effects of narcotic analgesics, barbiturates, phenothiazines, ethanol, antihistamines, MAO inhibitors, sedative-hypnotics, and cyclic antidepressants. CYP3A4 inhibitors may increase the levels/effects of clobazam; example inhibitors include azole antifungals, ciprofloxacin, clarithromycin, diclofenac, doxycycline, erythromycin, imatinib, isoniazid, nefazodone, nicardipine, propofol, protease inhibitors, quinidine, and verapamil.

Decreased Effect: CYP3A4 inducers may decrease the levels/effects of clobazam; example inducers include aminoglutethimide, carbamazepine, nafcillin, nevirapine, phenobarbital, phenytoin, and rifamycins.

Pharmacodynamics/Kinetics

Absorption: Rapid

Protein binding: 85% to 91%

Metabolism: Hepatic via N-dealkylation (likely via CYP) to active metabolite (N-desmethyl), and glucuronidation

Bioavailability: 87%

Half-life elimination: 18 hours; N-desmethyl (active): 42 hours

Time to peak: 15 minutes to 4 hours

Excretion: Urine (90%), as metabolites

Pregnancy Risk Factor Not assigned; similar agents rated D. Contraindicated in 1st trimester (per manufacturer).

Clobetasol (kloe BAY ta sol)

Related Information

Oral Nonviral Soft Tissue Ulcerations or Erosions *on page 1551*

U.S. Brand Names Clobex™; Cormax®; Embeline™ E; Olux®; Temovate®; Temovate E®

Canadian Brand Names Dermovate®; Gen-Clobetasol; Novo-Clobetasol®

Generic Available Yes: Excludes foam

Synonyms Clobetasol Propionate

Pharmacologic Category Corticosteroid, Topical

Use Short-term relief of inflammation of moderate to severe corticosteroid-responsive dermatoses (very high potency topical corticosteroid)

Local Anesthetic/Vasoconstrictor Precautions No information available to require special precautions

Effects on Dental Treatment No significant effects or complications reported

(Continued)

Clobetasol *(Continued)*

Common Adverse Effects Frequency not defined; may depend upon formulation used, length of application, surface area covered, and the use of occlusive dressings.

Endocrine & metabolic: Adrenal suppression, Cushing's syndrome, hyperglycemia

Local: Application site: Burning, cracking/fissuring of the skin, dryness, erythema, folliculitis, irritation, numbness, pruritus, skin atrophy, stinging, telangiectasia

Renal: Glucosuria

Effects reported with other high-potency topical steroids: Acneiform eruptions, allergic contact dermatitis, hypertrichosis, hypopigmentation, maceration of the skin, miliaria, perioral dermatitis, secondary infection

Mechanism of Action Stimulates the synthesis of enzymes needed to decrease inflammation, suppress mitotic activity, and cause vasoconstriction

Pharmacodynamics/Kinetics

Absorption: Percutaneous absorption is variable and dependent upon many factors including vehicle used, integrity of epidermis, dose, and use of occlusive dressings

Metabolism: Hepatic

Excretion: Urine and feces

Pregnancy Risk Factor C

Clobetasol Propionate *see* Clobetasol *on page 351*

Clobex™ *see* Clobetasol *on page 351*

Clocortolone (kloe KOR toe lone)

U.S. Brand Names Cloderm®

Canadian Brand Names Cloderm®

Generic Available No

Synonyms Clocortolone Pivalate

Pharmacologic Category Corticosteroid, Topical

Use Inflammation of corticosteroid-responsive dermatoses (intermediate-potency topical corticosteroid)

Local Anesthetic/Vasoconstrictor Precautions No information available to require special precautions

Effects on Dental Treatment No significant effects or complications reported

Common Adverse Effects

1% to 10%:

Dermatologic: Itching, erythema

Local: Burning, dryness, irritation, papular rashes

Mechanism of Action Stimulates the synthesis of enzymes needed to decrease inflammation, suppress mitotic activity, and cause vasoconstriction

Pharmacodynamics/Kinetics

Absorption: Percutaneous absorption is variable and dependent upon many factors including vehicle used, integrity of epidermis, dose, and use of occlusive dressings; small amounts enter circulatory system via skin

Metabolism: Hepatic

Excretion: Urine and feces

Pregnancy Risk Factor C

Clocortolone Pivalate *see* Clocortolone *on page 352*

Clocream® [OTC] *see* Vitamin A and Vitamin D *on page 1382*

Cloderm® *see* Clocortolone *on page 352*

Clofazimine (kloe FA zi meen)

Related Information

Tuberculosis *on page 1495*

U.S. Brand Names Lamprene®

Canadian Brand Names Lamprene®

Generic Available No

Synonyms Clofazimine Palmitate

Pharmacologic Category Leprostatic Agent

Use Treatment of lepromatous leprosy including dapsone-resistant leprosy and lepromatous leprosy with erythema nodosum leprosum; multibacillary leprosy

Unlabeled/Investigational Use Investigational: Multidrug-resistant tuberculosis

Local Anesthetic/Vasoconstrictor Precautions No information available to require special precautions

Effects on Dental Treatment No significant effects or complications reported

Common Adverse Effects
>10%:
Dermatologic: Dry skin
Gastrointestinal: Abdominal pain, nausea, vomiting, diarrhea
Miscellaneous: Pink to brownish-black discoloration of the skin
1% to 10%:
Dermatologic: Rash, pruritus
Endocrine & metabolic: Elevated blood sugar
Gastrointestinal: Fecal discoloration
Genitourinary: Discoloration of urine
Ocular: Discoloration of conjunctiva; irritation, burning, and itching of the eyes
Miscellaneous: Discoloration of sputum, sweat

Restrictions Clofazimine is no longer available through most US pharmacies. Requests for clofazimine to treat leprosy should be directed to the National Hansen's Disease Program (a division of the U.S. Department of Health and Human Services), which holds the IND for this indication. The Administrative Officer may be contacted at 225-578-9861 (phone) or 225-578-9856 (fax). Requests for clofazimine to treat MDRTB must be directed to the Division of Special Pathogen and Immunologic Drug Products (HFD-590) at 301-827-2127 (phone). These requests will be distributed by single-patient INDs administered by the FDA. Physicians must register as an investigator for this indication.

Mechanism of Action Binds preferentially to mycobacterial DNA to inhibit mycobacterial growth; also has some anti-inflammatory activity through an unknown mechanism

Drug Interactions
Cytochrome P450 Effect: Inhibits CYP3A4 (weak)
Decreased Effect: Combined use may decrease effect with dapsone (unconfirmed).

Pharmacodynamics/Kinetics
Absorption: Variable (45% to 62%)
Distribution: Highly lipophilic; deposited primarily in fatty tissue and cells of the reticuloendothelial system; taken up by macrophages throughout the body; distributed to breast milk, mesenteric lymph nodes, adrenal glands, subcutaneous fat, liver, bile, gallbladder, spleen, small intestine, muscles, bones, and skin; does not appear to cross blood-brain barrier; remains in tissues for prolonged periods
Metabolism: Partially hepatic to two metabolites
Half-life elimination: Terminal: 8 days; Tissue: 70 days
Time to peak, serum: Chronic therapy: 1-6 hours
Excretion: Primarily feces; urine (negligible amounts as unchanged drug); sputum, saliva, and sweat (small amounts)

Pregnancy Risk Factor C

Clofazimine Palmitate *see* Clofazimine *on page 352*

Clofibrate (kloe FYE brate)

Related Information
Cardiovascular Diseases *on page 1458*

Canadian Brand Names Claripex; Novo-Fibrate

Generic Available Yes

Pharmacologic Category Antilipemic Agent, Fibric Acid

Use Adjunct to dietary therapy in the management of hyperlipidemias associated with high triglyceride levels (types III, IV, V); primarily lowers triglycerides and very low density lipoprotein

Local Anesthetic/Vasoconstrictor Precautions No information available to require special precautions

Effects on Dental Treatment Key adverse event(s) related to dental treatment: Stomatitis.

Common Adverse Effects Frequency not defined.
Common: Gastrointestinal: Nausea, diarrhea
Less common:
Central nervous system: Headache, dizziness, fatigue
Gastrointestinal: Vomiting, loose stools, heartburn, flatulence, abdominal distress, epigastric pain
Neuromuscular & skeletal: Muscle cramping, aching, weakness, myalgia
Frequency unknown:
Central nervous system: Fever
Cardiovascular: Chest pain, cardiac arrhythmias
Dermatologic: Rash, urticaria, pruritus, alopecia, toxic epidermal necrolysis, erythema multiforme, Stevens-Johnson syndrome; dry, brittle hair
(Continued)

Clofibrate *(Continued)*

Endocrine & metabolic: Polyphagia, gynecomastia, hyperkalemia
Gastrointestinal: Stomatitis, gallstones, pancreatitis, gastritis, peptic ulcer, weight gain
Genitourinary: Impotence, decreased libido
Hematologic: Leukopenia, anemia, eosinophilia, agranulocytosis, thrombocytopenic purpura
Hepatic: Increased liver function test, hepatomegaly, jaundice
Local: Thrombophlebitis
Neuromuscular & skeletal: Myalgia, myopathy, myositis, arthralgia, rhabdomyolysis, increased creatinine phosphokinase (CPK), rheumatoid arthritis, tremor
Ocular: Photophobic
Renal: Dysuria, hematuria, proteinuria, renal toxicity (allergic), rhabdomyolysis-induced renal failure
Miscellaneous: Flu-like syndrome, increased diaphoresis, systemic lupus erythematosus

Restrictions Not available in U.S.

Mechanism of Action Mechanism is unclear but thought to reduce cholesterol synthesis and triglyceride hepatic-vascular transference

Drug Interactions

Cytochrome P450 Effect: Substrate of CYP3A4 (minor); **Inhibits** CYP2A6 (weak); **Induces** CYP2B6 (weak), 2E1 (weak), 3A4 (weak)

Increased Effect/Toxicity: Clofibrate may increase effects of warfarin, insulin, and sulfonylureas. Clofibrate's levels may be increased with probenecid. HMG-CoA reductase inhibitors (atorvastatin, cerivastatin, fluvastatin, lovastatin, pravastatin, simvastatin) may increase the risk of myopathy and rhabdomyolysis. The manufacturer warns against the concomitant use. However, combination therapy with statins has been used in some patients with resistant hyperlipidemias (with great caution).

Decreased Effect: Rifampin (and potentially other inducers of CYP3A4) may reduce blood levels of clofibrate.

Pharmacodynamics/Kinetics

Absorption: Complete
Distribution: V_d: 5.5 L/kg; crosses placenta
Protein binding: 95%
Metabolism: Hepatic to an inactive glucuronide ester; intestinal transformation required to activate drug
Half-life elimination: 6-24 hours, significantly prolonged with renal impairment; Anuria: 110 hours
Time to peak, serum: 3-6 hours
Excretion: Urine (40% to 70%)

Pregnancy Risk Factor C

Clomid® *see* ClomiPHENE *on page 354*

ClomiPHENE (KLOE mi feen)

U.S. Brand Names Clomid®; Serophene®

Canadian Brand Names Clomid®; Milophene®; Serophene®

Generic Available Yes

Synonyms Clomiphene Citrate

Pharmacologic Category Ovulation Stimulator

Use Treatment of ovulatory failure in patients desiring pregnancy

Unlabeled/Investigational Use Male infertility

Local Anesthetic/Vasoconstrictor Precautions No information available to require special precautions

Effects on Dental Treatment No significant effects or complications reported

Common Adverse Effects

>10%: Endocrine & metabolic: Hot flashes, ovarian enlargement

1% to 10%:

Cardiovascular: Thromboembolism
Central nervous system: Mental depression, headache
Endocrine & metabolic: Breast enlargement (males), breast discomfort (females), abnormal menstrual flow
Gastrointestinal: Distention, bloating, nausea, vomiting, hepatotoxicity
Ocular: Blurring of vision, diplopia, floaters, after-images, phosphenes, photophobia

Mechanism of Action Induces ovulation by stimulating the release of pituitary gonadotropins

Drug Interactions

Decreased Effect: Decreased response when used with danazol. Decreased estradiol response when used with clomiphene.

Pharmacodynamics/Kinetics

Metabolism: Undergoes enterohepatic recirculation

Half-life elimination: 5-7 days

Excretion: Primarily feces; urine (small amounts)

Pregnancy Risk Factor X

Clomiphene Citrate *see* ClomiPHENE *on page 354*

ClomiPRAMINE (kloe MI pra meen)

U.S. Brand Names Anafranil®

Canadian Brand Names Anafranil®; Apo-Clomipramine®; CO Clomipramine; Gen-Clomipramine; Novo-Clopramine

Mexican Brand Names Anafranil®

Generic Available Yes

Synonyms Clomipramine Hydrochloride

Pharmacologic Category Antidepressant, Tricyclic (Tertiary Amine)

Use Treatment of obsessive-compulsive disorder (OCD)

Unlabeled/Investigational Use Depression, panic attacks, chronic pain

Local Anesthetic/Vasoconstrictor Precautions Use with caution; epinephrine, norepinephrine and levonordefrin have been shown to have an increased pressor response in combination with TCAs

Effects on Dental Treatment Key adverse event(s) related to dental treatment: Xerostomia and changes in salivation (normal salivary flow resumes upon discontinuation). Long-term treatment with TCAs, such as clomipramine, increases the risk of caries by reducing salivation and salivary buffer capacity.

Common Adverse Effects

>10%:

Central nervous system: Dizziness, drowsiness, headache, insomnia, nervousness

Endocrine & metabolic: Libido changes

Gastrointestinal: Xerostomia, constipation, increased appetite, nausea, weight gain, dyspepsia, anorexia, abdominal pain

Neuromuscular & skeletal: Fatigue, tremor, myoclonus

Miscellaneous: Increased diaphoresis

1% to 10%:

Cardiovascular: Hypotension, palpitations, tachycardia

Central nervous system: Confusion, hypertonia, sleep disorder, yawning, speech disorder, abnormal dreaming, paresthesia, memory impairment, anxiety, twitching, impaired coordination, agitation, migraine, depersonalization, emotional lability, flushing, fever

Dermatologic: Rash, pruritus, dermatitis

Gastrointestinal: Diarrhea, vomiting

Genitourinary: Difficult urination

Ocular: Blurred vision, eye pain

Mechanism of Action Clomipramine appears to affect serotonin uptake while its active metabolite, desmethylclomipramine, affects norepinephrine uptake

Drug Interactions

Cytochrome P450 Effect: Substrate of CYP1A2 (major), 2C19 (major), 2D6 (major), 3A4 (minor); **Inhibits** CYP2D6 (moderate)

Increased Effect/Toxicity: The levels/effects of clomipramine may be increased by amiodarone, chlorpromazine, ciprofloxacin, delavirdine, fluconazole, fluoxetine, fluvoxamine, gemfibrozil, isoniazid, ketoconazole, lomefloxacin, miconazole, ofloxacin, omeprazole, paroxetine, pergolide, quinidine, quinine, ritonavir, rofecoxib, ropinirole, ticlopidine, and other CYP1A2, 2C19, or 2D6 inhibitors. Clomipramine may increase the levels/effects of amphetamines, selected beta-blockers, dextromethorphan, fluoxetine, lidocaine, mirtazapine, nefazodone, paroxetine, risperidone, ritonavir, thioridazine, tricyclic antidepressants, venlafaxine, and other CYP2D6 substrates.

Clomipramine increases the effects of amphetamines, anticholinergics, lithium, other CNS depressants (sedatives, hypnotics, ethanol), chlorpropamide, tolazamide, phenothiazines, and warfarin. When used with MAO inhibitors or other serotonergic drugs, serotonin syndrome may occur. Serotonin syndrome has also been reported with ritonavir (rare). Pressor response to I.V. epinephrine, norepinephrine, and phenylephrine may be enhanced in patients receiving TCAs (**Note:** Effect is unlikely with epinephrine or levonordefrin dosages typically administered as infiltration in combination with local anesthetics). Combined use of beta-agonists or drugs which prolong QT_c

(Continued)

ClomiPRAMINE *(Continued)*

(including quinidine, procainamide, disopyramide, cisapride, sparfloxacin, gatifloxacin, moxifloxacin) with TCAs may predispose patients to cardiac arrhythmias.

Decreased Effect: The levels/effects of clomipramine may be decreased by aminoglutethimide, carbamazepine, phenobarbital, phenytoin, rifampin, and other CYP1A2 or 2C19 inducers. Clomipramine may decrease the levels/effects of CYP2D6 prodrug substrates (eg, codeine, hydrocodone, oxycodone, tramadol). Clomipramine inhibits the antihypertensive response to bethanidine, clonidine, debrisoquin, guanadrel, guanethidine, guanabenz, and guanfacine. Cholestyramine and colestipol may decrease the absorption of clomipramine.

Pharmacodynamics/Kinetics

Absorption: Rapid

Metabolism: Hepatic to desmethylclomipramine (active); extensive first-pass effect

Half-life elimination: 20-30 hours

Pregnancy Risk Factor C

Clomipramine Hydrochloride *see* ClomiPRAMINE *on page 355*

Clonazepam (kloe NA ze pam)

U.S. Brand Names Klonopin®

Canadian Brand Names Alti-Clonazepam; Apo-Clonazepam®; Clonapam; Gen-Clonazepam; Klonopin®; Novo-Clonazepam; Nu-Clonazepam; PMS-Clonazepam; Rho-Clonazepam; Rivotril®

Mexican Brand Names Kenoket®; Rivotril®

Generic Available Yes: Tablet

Pharmacologic Category Benzodiazepine

Use Alone or as an adjunct in the treatment of petit mal variant (Lennox-Gastaut), akinetic, and myoclonic seizures; petit mal (absence) seizures unresponsive to succimides; panic disorder with or without agoraphobia

Unlabeled/Investigational Use Restless legs syndrome; neuralgia; multifocal tic disorder; parkinsonian dysarthria; bipolar disorder; adjunct therapy for schizophrenia

Local Anesthetic/Vasoconstrictor Precautions No information available to require special precautions

Effects on Dental Treatment Key adverse event(s) related to dental treatment: Xerostomia and changes in salivation (normal salivary flow resumes upon discontinuation).

Significant Adverse Effects Reactions reported in patients with seizure and/or panic disorder. Frequency not defined.

Cardiovascular: Edema (ankle or facial), palpitations

Central nervous system: Amnesia, ataxia (seizure disorder ~30%; panic disorder 5%), behavior problems (seizure disorder ~25%), coma, confusion, depression, dizziness, drowsiness (seizure disorder ~50%), emotional lability, fatigue, fever, hallucinations, headache, hypotonia, hysteria, insomnia, intellectual ability reduced, memory disturbance, nervousness; paradoxical reactions (including aggressive behavior, agitation, anxiety, excitability, hostility, irritability, nervousness, nightmares, sleep disturbance, vivid dreams); psychosis, slurred speech, somnolence (panic disorder 37%), suicidal attempt, vertigo

Dermatologic: Hair loss, hirsutism, skin rash

Endocrine & metabolic: Dysmenorrhea, libido increased/decreased

Gastrointestinal: Abdominal pain, anorexia, appetite increased/decreased, coated tongue, constipation, dehydration, diarrhea, gastritis, gum soreness, nausea, weight changes (loss/gain), xerostomia

Genitourinary: Colpitis, dysuria, ejaculation delayed, enuresis, impotence, micturition frequency, nocturia, urinary retention, urinary tract infection

Hematologic: Anemia, eosinophilia, leukopenia, thrombocytopenia

Hepatic: Alkaline phosphatase increased (transient), hepatomegaly, serum transaminases increased (transient)

Neuromuscular & skeletal: Choreiform movements, coordination abnormal, dysarthria, muscle pain, muscle weakness, myalgia, tremor

Ocular: Blurred vision, eye movements abnormal, diplopia, nystagmus

Respiratory: Chest congestion, cough, bronchitis, hypersecretions, pharyngitis, respiratory depression, respiratory tract infection, rhinitis, rhinorrhea, shortness of breath, sinusitis

Miscellaneous: Allergic reaction, aphonia, dysdiadochokinesis, encopresis, "glassy-eyed" appearance, hemiparesis, lymphadenopathy

Restrictions C-IV

Dosage Oral:

Children <10 years or 30 kg: Seizure disorders:

Initial daily dose: 0.01-0.03 mg/kg/day (maximum: 0.05 mg/kg/day) given in 2-3 divided doses; increase by no more than 0.5 mg every third day until seizures are controlled or adverse effects seen

Usual maintenance dose: 0.1-0.2 mg/kg/day divided 3 times/day, not to exceed 0.2 mg/kg/day

Adults:

Seizure disorders:

Initial daily dose not to exceed 1.5 mg given in 3 divided doses; may increase by 0.5-1 mg every third day until seizures are controlled or adverse effects seen (maximum: 20 mg/day)

Usual maintenance dose: 0.05-0.2 mg/kg; do not exceed 20 mg/day

Panic disorder: 0.25 mg twice daily; increase in increments of 0.125-0.25 mg twice daily every 3 days; target dose: 1 mg/day (maximum: 4 mg/day)

Discontinuation of treatment: To discontinue, treatment should be withdrawn gradually. Decrease dose by 0.125 mg twice daily every 3 days until medication is completely withdrawn.

Elderly: Initiate with low doses and observe closely

Hemodialysis: Supplemental dose is not necessary

Mechanism of Action The exact mechanism is unknown, but believed to be related to its ability to enhance the activity of GABA; suppresses the spike-and-wave discharge in absence seizures by depressing nerve transmission in the motor cortex

Contraindications Hypersensitivity to clonazepam or any component of the formulation (cross-sensitivity with other benzodiazepines may exist); significant liver disease; narrow-angle glaucoma; pregnancy

Warnings/Precautions Use with caution in elderly or debilitated patients, patients with hepatic disease (including alcoholics), or renal impairment. Use with caution in patients with respiratory disease or impaired gag reflex or ability to protect the airway from secretions (salivation may be increased). Worsening of seizures may occur when added to patients with multiple seizure types. Concurrent use with valproic acid may result in absence status. Monitoring of CBC and liver function tests has been recommended during prolonged therapy.

Causes CNS depression (dose-related) resulting in sedation, dizziness, confusion, or ataxia which may impair physical and mental capabilities. Patients must be cautioned about performing tasks which require mental alertness (eg, operating machinery or driving). Use with caution in patients receiving other CNS depressants or psychoactive agents. Effects with other sedative drugs or ethanol may be potentiated. Benzodiazepines have been associated with falls and traumatic injury and should be used with extreme caution in patients who are at risk of these events (especially the elderly).

Use caution in patients with depression, particularly if suicidal risk may be present. Use with caution in patients with a history of drug dependence. Benzodiazepines have been associated with dependence and acute withdrawal symptoms, including seizures, on discontinuation or reduction in dose. Acute withdrawal, including seizures, may be precipitated in patients after administration of flumazenil to patients receiving long-term benzodiazepine therapy.

Benzodiazepines have been associated with anterograde amnesia. Paradoxical reactions, including hyperactive or aggressive behavior, have been reported with benzodiazepines, particularly in adolescent/pediatric or psychiatric patients. Does not have analgesic, antidepressant, or antipsychotic properties.

Drug Interactions Substrate of CYP3A4 (major)

CNS depressants: Sedative effects and/or respiratory depression may be additive with CNS depressants; includes ethanol, barbiturates, narcotic analgesics, and other sedative agents; monitor for increased effect

CYP3A4 inducers: CYP3A4 inducers may decrease the levels/effects of clonazepam. Example inducers include aminoglutethimide, carbamazepine, nafcillin, nevirapine, phenobarbital, phenytoin, and rifamycins.

CYP3A4 inhibitors: May increase the levels/effects of clonazepam. Example inhibitors include azole antifungals, ciprofloxacin, clarithromycin, diclofenac, doxycycline, erythromycin, imatinib, isoniazid, nefazodone, nicardipine, propofol, protease inhibitors, quinidine, and verapamil.

Disulfiram: Disulfiram may inhibit the metabolism of clonazepam; monitor for increased benzodiazepine effect

(Continued)

Clonazepam *(Continued)*

Levodopa: Therapeutic effects may be diminished in some patients following the addition of a benzodiazepine; limited/inconsistent data

Oral contraceptives: May decrease the clearance of some benzodiazepines (those which undergo oxidative metabolism); monitor for increased benzodiazepine effect

Theophylline: May partially antagonize some of the effects of benzodiazepines; monitor for decreased response; may require higher doses for sedation

Valproic acid: The combined use of clonazepam and valproic acid has been associated with absence seizures

Ethanol/Nutrition/Herb Interactions

Ethanol: Avoid ethanol (may increase CNS depression).

Food: Clonazepam serum concentration is unlikely to be increased by grapefruit juice because of clonazepam's high oral bioavailability.

Herb/Nutraceutical: St John's wort may decrease clonazepam levels. Avoid valerian, St John's wort, kava kava, gotu kola (may increase CNS depression).

Pharmacodynamics/Kinetics

Onset of action: 20-60 minutes

Duration: Infants and young children: 6-8 hours; Adults: ≤12 hours

Absorption: Well absorbed

Distribution: Adults: V_d: 1.5-4.4 L/kg

Protein binding: 85%

Metabolism: Extensively hepatic via glucuronide and sulfate conjugation

Half-life elimination: Children: 22-33 hours; Adults: 19-50 hours

Time to peak, serum: 1-3 hours; Steady-state: 5-7 days

Excretion: Urine (<2% as unchanged drug); metabolites excreted as glucuronide or sulfate conjugates

Pregnancy Risk Factor D

Lactation Enters breast milk/not recommended

Breast-Feeding Considerations Clonazepam enters breast milk; clinical effects on the infant include CNS depression, respiratory depression reported (no recommendation from the AAP).

Dosage Forms

Tablet: 0.5 mg, 1 mg, 2 mg

Tablet, orally-disintegrating [wafer]: 0.125 mg, 0.25 mg, 0.5 mg, 1 mg, 2 mg

Clonidine (KLON i deen)

Related Information

Cardiovascular Diseases *on page 1458*

U.S. Brand Names Catapres®; Catapres-TTS®; Duraclon™

Canadian Brand Names Apo-Clonidine®; Carapres®; Dixarit®; Novo-Clonidine; Nu-Clonidine

Generic Available Yes: Tablet

Synonyms Clonidine Hydrochloride

Pharmacologic Category Alpha$_2$-Adrenergic Agonist

Use Management of mild to moderate hypertension; either used alone or in combination with other antihypertensives

Orphan drug: Duraclon™: For continuous epidural administration as adjunctive therapy with intraspinal opiates for treatment of cancer pain in patients tolerant to or unresponsive to intraspinal opiates

Unlabeled/Investigational Use Heroin or nicotine withdrawal; severe pain; dysmenorrhea; vasomotor symptoms associated with menopause; ethanol dependence; prophylaxis of migraines; glaucoma; diabetes-associated diarrhea; impulse control disorder, attention-deficit/hyperactivity disorder (ADHD), clozapine-induced sialorrhea

Local Anesthetic/Vasoconstrictor Precautions No information available to require special precautions

Effects on Dental Treatment Key adverse event(s) related to dental treatment: Significant xerostomia (normal salivary flow resumes upon discontinuation), orthostatic hypotension, and abnormal taste.

Common Adverse Effects Incidence of adverse events is not always reported.

>10%:

Central nervous system: Drowsiness (35% oral, 12% transdermal), dizziness (16% oral, 2% transdermal)

Dermatologic: Transient localized skin reactions characterized by pruritus, and erythema (15% to 50% transdermal)

Gastrointestinal: Dry mouth (40% oral, 25% transdermal)

1% to 10%:

Cardiovascular: Orthostatic hypotension (3% oral)

Central nervous system: Headache (1% oral, 5% transdermal), sedation (3% transdermal), fatigue (6% transdermal), lethargy (3% transdermal), insomnia (2% transdermal), nervousness (3% oral, 1% transdermal), mental depression (1% oral)

Dermatologic: Rash (1% oral), allergic contact sensitivity (5% transdermal), localized vesiculation (7%), hyperpigmentation (5% at application site), edema (3%), excoriation (3%), burning (3%), throbbing, blanching (1%), papules (1%), and generalized macular rash (1%) has occurred in patients receiving transdermal clonidine.

Endocrine & metabolic: Sodium and water retention, sexual dysfunction (3% oral, 2% transdermal), impotence (3% oral, 2% transdermal), weakness (10% transdermal)

Gastrointestinal: Nausea (5% oral, 1% transdermal), vomiting (5% oral), anorexia and malaise (1% oral), constipation (10% oral, 1% transdermal), dry throat (2% transdermal), taste disturbance (1% transdermal), weight gain (1% oral)

Genitourinary: Nocturia (1% oral)

Hepatic: Liver function test (mild abnormalities, 1% oral)

Miscellaneous: Withdrawal syndrome (1% oral)

Dosage

Children:

Oral:

Hypertension: Initial: 5-10 mcg/kg/day in divided doses every 8-12 hours; increase gradually at 5- to 7-day intervals to 25 mcg/kg/day in divided doses every 6 hours; maximum: 0.9 mg/day

Clonidine tolerance test (test of growth hormone release from pituitary): 0.15 mg/m^2 or 4 mcg/kg as single dose

ADHD (unlabeled use): Initial: 0.05 mg/day; increase every 3-7 days by 0.05 mg/day to 3-5 mcg/kg/day given in divided doses 3-4 times/day (maximum dose: 0.3-0.4 mg/day)

Epidural infusion: Pain management: Reserved for patients with severe intractable pain, unresponsive to other analgesics or epidural or spinal opiates: Initial: 0.5 mcg/kg/hour; adjust with caution, based on clinical effect

Adults:

Oral:

Acute hypertension (urgency): Initial 0.1-0.2 mg; may be followed by additional doses of 0.1 mg every hour, if necessary, to a maximum total dose of 0.6 mg

Hypertension: Initial dose: 0.1 mg twice daily (maximum recommended dose: 2.4 mg/day); usual dose range (JNC 7): 0.1-0.8 mg/day in 2 divided doses

Nicotine withdrawal symptoms: 0.1 mg twice daily to maximum of 0.4 mg/day for 3-4 weeks

Transdermal: Hypertension: Apply once every 7 days; for initial therapy start with 0.1 mg and increase by 0.1 mg at 1- to 2-week intervals (dosages >0.6 mg do not improve efficacy); usual dose range (JNC 7): 0.1-0.3 mg once weekly

Epidural infusion: Pain management: Starting dose: 30 mcg/hour; titrate as required for relief of pain or presence of side effects; minimal experience with doses >40 mcg/hour; should be considered an adjunct to intraspinal opiate therapy

Elderly: Initial: 0.1 mg once daily at bedtime, increase gradually as needed

Dosing adjustment in renal impairment: Cl_{cr} <10 mL/minute: Administer 50% to 75% of normal dose initially

Dialysis: Not dialyzable (0% to 5%) via hemo- or peritoneal dialysis; supplemental dose not necessary

Mechanism of Action Stimulates alpha$_2$-adrenoceptors in the brain stem, thus activating an inhibitory neuron, resulting in reduced sympathetic outflow from the CNS, producing a decrease in peripheral resistance, renal vascular resistance, heart rate, and blood pressure; epidural clonidine may produce pain relief at spinal presynaptic and postjunctional alpha$_2$-adrenoceptors by preventing pain signal transmission; pain relief occurs only for the body regions innervated by the spinal segments where analgesic concentrations of clonidine exist

Contraindications Hypersensitivity to clonidine hydrochloride or any component of the formulation

Warnings/Precautions Gradual withdrawal is needed (over 1 week for oral, 2-4 days with epidural) if drug needs to be stopped. Patients should be instructed about abrupt discontinuation (causes rapid increase in BP and

(Continued)

Clonidine *(Continued)*

symptoms of sympathetic overactivity). In patients on both a beta-blocker and clonidine where withdrawal of clonidine is necessary, withdraw the beta-blocker first and several days before clonidine. Then slowly decrease clonidine.

Use with caution in patients with severe coronary insufficiency; conduction disturbances; recent MI, CVA, or chronic renal insufficiency. Caution in sinus node dysfunction. Discontinue within 4 hours of surgery then restart as soon as possible after. Clonidine injection should be administered via a continuous epidural infusion device. Epidural clonidine is not recommended for perioperative, obstetrical, or postpartum pain. It is not recommended for use in patients with severe cardiovascular disease or hemodynamic instability. In all cases, the epidural may lead to cardiovascular instability (hypotension, bradycardia). May cause significant CNS depression and xerostomia. Caution in patients with pre-existing CNS disease or depression. Elderly may be at greater risk for CNS depressive effects, favoring other agents in this population.

Drug Interactions

Increased Effect/Toxicity: Concurrent use with antipsychotics (especially low potency), narcotic analgesics, or nitroprusside may produce additive hypotensive effects. Clonidine may decrease the symptoms of hypoglycemia with oral hypoglycemic agents or insulin. Alcohol, barbiturates, and other CNS depressants may have additive CNS effects when combined with clonidine. Epidural clonidine may prolong the sensory and motor blockade of local anesthetics. Clonidine may increase cyclosporine (and perhaps tacrolimus) serum concentrations. Beta-blockers may potentiate bradycardia in patients receiving clonidine and may increase the rebound hypertension of withdrawal. Tricyclic antidepressants may also enhance the hypertensive response associated with abrupt clonidine withdrawal.

Decreased Effect: Tricyclic antidepressants (TCAs) antagonize the hypotensive effects of clonidine.

Ethanol/Nutrition/Herb Interactions

Ethanol: Avoid ethanol (may increase CNS depression).

Herb/Nutraceutical: Avoid dong quai if using for hypertension (has estrogenic activity). Avoid ephedra, yohimbe, ginseng (may worsen hypertension). Avoid valerian, St John's wort, kava kava, gotu kola (may increase CNS depression).

Dietary Considerations Hypertensive patients may need to decrease sodium and calories in diet.

Pharmacodynamics/Kinetics

Onset of action: Oral: 0.5-1 hour

Duration: 6-10 hours

Distribution: V_d: Adults: 2.1 L/kg; highly lipid soluble; distributes readily into extravascular sites

Protein binding: 20% to 40%

Metabolism: Extensively hepatic to inactive metabolites; undergoes enterohepatic recirculation

Bioavailability: 75% to 95%

Half-life elimination: Adults: Normal renal function: 6-20 hours; Renal impairment: 18-41 hours

Time to peak: 2-4 hours

Excretion: Urine (65%, 32% as unchanged drug); feces (22%)

Pregnancy Risk Factor C

Dosage Forms INJ, epidural solution [preservative free] (Duraclon™): 100 mcg/mL (10 mL); 500 mcg/mL (10 mL). **PATCH, transdermal** [once-weekly patch]: (Catapres-TTS®-1): 0.1 mg/24 hours (4s); (Catapres-TTS®-2): 0.2 mg/24 hours (4s); (Catapres-TTS®-3): 0.3 mg/24 hours (4s). **TAB** (Catapres®): 0.1 mg, 0.2 mg, 0.3 mg

Clonidine and Chlorthalidone (KLON i deen & klor THAL i done)

Related Information

Chlorthalidone *on page 321*

Clonidine *on page 358*

U.S. Brand Names Clorpres®; Combipres® [DSC]

Generic Available No

Synonyms Chlorthalidone and Clonidine

Pharmacologic Category Antihypertensive Agent, Combination

Use Management of mild to moderate hypertension

Local Anesthetic/Vasoconstrictor Precautions No information available to require special precautions

Effects on Dental Treatment No significant effects or complications reported

Common Adverse Effects See individual agents.

Pharmacodynamics/Kinetics See individual agents.

Pregnancy Risk Factor C

Clonidine Hydrochloride *see* Clonidine *on page 358*

Clopidogrel (kloh PID oh grel)

Related Information

Cardiovascular Diseases *on page 1458*

U.S. Brand Names Plavix®

Canadian Brand Names Plavix®

Generic Available No

Synonyms Clopidogrel Bisulfate

Pharmacologic Category Antiplatelet Agent

Use Reduce atherosclerotic events (myocardial infarction, stroke, vascular deaths) in patients with atherosclerosis documented by recent myocardial infarction (MI), recent stroke, or established peripheral arterial disease; prevention of thrombotic complications after coronary stenting; acute coronary syndrome (unstable angina or non-Q-wave MI)

Unlabeled/Investigational Use In aspirin-allergic patients, prevention of coronary artery bypass graft closure (saphenous vein)

Local Anesthetic/Vasoconstrictor Precautions No information available to require special precautions

Effects on Dental Treatment If a patient is to undergo elective surgery and an antiplatelet effect is not desired, clopidogrel should be discontinued 7 days prior to surgery only upon approval via a medical consult with prescribing physician. As with all drugs which may affect hemostasis, bleeding is associated with clopidogrel. Hemorrhage may occur at virtually any site; risk is dependent on multiple variables, including the concurrent use of multiple agents which alter hemostasis and patient susceptibility.

Common Adverse Effects As with all drugs which may affect hemostasis, bleeding is associated with clopidogrel. Hemorrhage may occur at virtually any site. Risk is dependent on multiple variables, including the concurrent use of multiple agents which alter hemostasis and patient susceptibility.

>10%: Gastrointestinal: The overall incidence of gastrointestinal events (including abdominal pain, vomiting, dyspepsia, gastritis and constipation) has been documented to be 27% compared to 30% in patients receiving aspirin.

3% to 10%:

- Cardiovascular: Chest pain (8%), edema (4%), hypertension (4%)
- Central nervous system: Headache (3% to 8%), dizziness (2% to 6%), depression (4%), fatigue (3%), general pain (6%)
- Dermatologic: Rash (4%), pruritus (3%)
- Endocrine & metabolic: Hypercholesterolemia (4%)
- Gastrointestinal: Abdominal pain (2% to 6%), dyspepsia (2% to 5%), diarrhea (2% to 5%), nausea (3%)
- Genitourinary: Urinary tract infection (3%)
- Hematologic: Purpura (5%), epistaxis (3%)
- Hepatic: Liver function test abnormalities (<3%; discontinued in 0.11%)
- Neuromuscular & skeletal: Arthralgia (6%), back pain (6%)
- Respiratory: Dyspnea (5%), rhinitis (4%), bronchitis (4%), coughing (3%), upper respiratory infections (9%)
- Miscellaneous: Flu-like syndrome (8%)

1% to 3%:

- Cardiovascular: Atrial fibrillation, cardiac failure, palpitation, syncope
- Central nervous system: Fever, insomnia, vertigo, anxiety
- Dermatologic: Eczema
- Endocrine & metabolic: Gout, hyperuricemia
- Gastrointestinal: Constipation, GI hemorrhage, vomiting
- Genitourinary: Cystitis
- Hematologic: Hematoma, anemia
- Neuromuscular & skeletal: Arthritis, leg cramps, neuralgia, paresthesia, weakness
- Ocular: Cataract, conjunctivitis

Dosage Oral: Adults:

Recent MI, recent stroke, or established arterial disease: 75 mg once daily

Acute coronary syndrome: Initial: 300 mg loading dose, followed by 75 mg once daily (in combination with aspirin 75-325 mg once daily). **Note:** A loading dose of 600 mg has been used in some investigations; limited research exists comparing the two doses.

(Continued)

Clopidogrel *(Continued)*

Prevention of coronary artery bypass graft closure (saphenous vein): Aspirin-allergic patients (unlabeled use): Loading dose: 300 mg 6 hours following procedure; maintenance: 50-100 mg/day

Dosing adjustment in renal impairment and elderly: None necessary

Mechanism of Action Blocks the ADP receptors, which prevent fibrinogen binding at that site and thereby reduce the possibility of platelet adhesion and aggregation

Contraindications Hypersensitivity to clopidogrel or any component of the formulation; active pathological bleeding such as PUD or intracranial hemorrhage; coagulation disorders

Warnings/Precautions Cases of thrombotic thrombocytopenic purpura (TTP) have been reported, usually within the first 2 weeks of therapy. Patients receiving anticoagulants or other antiplatelet drugs concurrently, liver disease, patients having a previous hypersensitivity or other untoward effects related to ticlopidine, hypertension, renal impairment, history of bleeding or hemostatic disorders or drug-related hematologic disorders, and in patients scheduled for major surgery consider discontinuing 5 days prior to that surgery

Drug Interactions

Cytochrome P450 Effect: Substrate (minor) of CYP1A2, 3A4; **Inhibits** CYP2C8/9 (weak)

Increased Effect/Toxicity: At high concentrations, clopidogrel may interfere with the metabolism of amiodarone, cisapride, cyclosporine, diltiazem, fluvastatin, irbesartan, losartan, oral hypoglycemics, paclitaxel, phenytoin, quinidine, sildenafil, tamoxifen, torsemide, verapamil, and some NSAIDs which may result in toxicity. Clopidogrel and naproxen resulted in an increase of GI occult blood loss. Anticoagulants (warfarin, thrombolytics, drotrecogin alfa) or other antiplatelet agents may increase the risk of bleeding. Rifampin may increase the effects of clopidogrel (monitor).

Decreased Effect: Atorvastatin may attenuate the effects of clopidogrel; monitor. CYP3A4-inhibiting macrolide antibiotics may attenuate the effects of clopidogrel (including clarithromycin, erythromycin, and troleandomycin); monitor.

Ethanol/Nutrition/Herb Interactions Herb/Nutraceutical: Avoid cat's claw, dong quai, evening primrose, feverfew, garlic, ginger, ginkgo, red clover, horse chestnut, green tea, ginseng (all have additional antiplatelet activity).

Dietary Considerations May be taken without regard to meals.

Pharmacodynamics/Kinetics

Onset of action: Inhibition of platelet aggregation detected: 2 hours after 300 mg administered; after second day of treatment with 50-100 mg/day

Peak effect: 50-100 mg/day: Bleeding time: 5-6 days; Platelet function: 3-7 days

Absorption: Well absorbed

Metabolism: Extensively hepatic via hydrolysis; biotransformation primarily to carboxyl acid derivative (inactive). The active metabolite that inhibits platelet aggregation has not been isolated.

Half-life elimination: ~8 hours

Time to peak, serum: ~1 hour

Excretion: Urine

Pregnancy Risk Factor B

Dosage Forms TAB, film coated: 75 mg

Selected Readings

Daniel NG, Goulet J, Bergeron M, et al, "Antiplatelet Drugs: Is There a Surgical Risk?" *J Can Dent Assoc*, 2002, 68(11):683-7.

Jeske AH, Suchko GD, ADA Council on Scientific Affairs and Division of Science, et al, "Lack of a Scientific Basis for Routine Discontinuation of Oral Anticoagulation Therapy Before Dental Treatment," *J Am Dent Assoc*, 2003, 134(11):1492-7.

Little JW, Miller CS, Henry RG, et al, "Antithrombotic Agents: Implications in Dentistry," *Oral Surg Oral Med Oral Pathol Oral Radiol Endod*, 2002, 93(5):544-51.

Scully C and Wolff A, "Oral Surgery in Patients on Anticoagulant Therapy," *Oral Surg Oral Med Oral Pathol Oral Radiol Endod*, 2002, 94(1):57-64.

Wynn RL, "Clopidogrel (Plavix): Dental Considerations of an Antiplatelet Drug," *Gen Dent*, 2001, 49(6):564-8.

Clopidogrel Bisulfate *see* Clopidogrel *on page 361*

Clorazepate (klor AZ e pate)

U.S. Brand Names Tranxene®; Tranxene® SD™; Tranxene® SD™-Half Strength; T-Tab®

Canadian Brand Names Apo-Clorazepate®; Novo-Clopate

Mexican Brand Names Tranxene®

Generic Available Yes

Synonyms Clorazepate Dipotassium; Tranxene T-Tab®

Pharmacologic Category Benzodiazepine

Use Treatment of generalized anxiety disorder; management of ethanol withdrawal; adjunct anticonvulsant in management of partial seizures

Local Anesthetic/Vasoconstrictor Precautions No information available to require special precautions

Effects on Dental Treatment Key adverse event(s) related to dental treatment: Xerostomia (normal salivary flow resumes upon discontinuation). Many patients will experience drowsiness; orthostatic hypotension is possible. It is suggested that narcotic analgesics not be given for pain control to patients taking clorazepate due to enhanced sedation.

Common Adverse Effects Frequency not defined.

Cardiovascular: Hypotension

Central nervous system: Drowsiness, fatigue, ataxia, lightheadedness, memory impairment, insomnia, anxiety, headache, depression, slurred speech, confusion, nervousness, dizziness, irritability

Dermatologic: Rash

Endocrine & metabolic: Decreased libido

Gastrointestinal: Xerostomia, constipation, diarrhea, decreased salivation, nausea, vomiting, increased or decreased appetite

Neuromuscular & skeletal: Dysarthria, tremor

Ocular: Blurred vision, diplopia

Restrictions C-IV

Mechanism of Action Binds to stereospecific benzodiazepine receptors on the postsynaptic GABA neuron at several sites within the central nervous system, including the limbic system, reticular formation. Enhancement of the inhibitory effect of GABA on neuronal excitability results by increased neuronal membrane permeability to chloride ions. This shift in chloride ions results in hyperpolarization (a less excitable state) and stabilization.

Drug Interactions

Cytochrome P450 Effect: Substrate of CYP3A4 (major)

Increased Effect/Toxicity: Clorazepate potentiates the CNS depressant effects of narcotic analgesics, barbiturates, phenothiazines, ethanol, antihistamines, MAO inhibitors, sedative-hypnotics, and cyclic antidepressants. CYP3A4 inhibitors may increase the levels/effects of clorazepate; example inhibitors include azole antifungals, ciprofloxacin, clarithromycin, diclofenac, doxycycline, erythromycin, imatinib, isoniazid, nefazodone, nicardipine, propofol, protease inhibitors, quinidine, and verapamil.

Decreased Effect: CYP3A4 inducers may decrease the levels/effects of clorazepate; example inducers include aminoglutethimide, carbamazepine, nafcillin, nevirapine, phenobarbital, phenytoin, and rifamycins.

Pharmacodynamics/Kinetics

Onset of action: 1-2 hours

Duration: Variable, 8-24 hours

Distribution: Crosses placenta; appears in urine

Metabolism: Rapidly decarboxylated to desmethyldiazepam (active) in acidic stomach prior to absorption; hepatically to oxazepam (active)

Half-life elimination: Adults: Desmethyldiazepam: 48-96 hours; Oxazepam: 6-8 hours

Time to peak, serum: ~1 hour

Excretion: Primarily urine

Pregnancy Risk Factor D

Clorazepate Dipotassium *see* Clorazepate *on page 362*

Clorpactin® WCS-90 [OTC] *see* Oxychlorosene *on page 1027*

Clorpres® *see* Clonidine and Chlorthalidone *on page 360*

Clotrimazole (kloe TRIM a zole)

Related Information

Oral Fungal Infections *on page 1544*

Sexually-Transmitted Diseases *on page 1504*

U.S. Brand Names Cruex® Cream [OTC]; Gyne-Lotrimin® 3 [OTC]; Lotrimin® AF Athlete's Foot Cream [OTC]; Lotrimin® AF Athlete's Foot Solution [OTC]; Lotrimin® AF Jock Itch Cream [OTC]; Mycelex®; Mycelex®-7 [OTC]; Mycelex® Twin Pack [OTC]

Canadian Brand Names Canesten® Topical; Canesten® Vaginal; Clotrimaderm; Trivagizole-3®

Mexican Brand Names Candimon®; Lotrimin®

Generic Available Yes: Cream, solution

Pharmacologic Category Antifungal Agent, Oral Nonabsorbed; Antifungal Agent, Topical; Antifungal Agent, Vaginal

(Continued)

Clotrimazole *(Continued)*

Dental Use Treatment of susceptible fungal infections, including oropharyngeal candidiasis; limited data suggests that the use of clotrimazole troches may be effective for prophylaxis against oropharyngeal candidiasis in neutropenic patients

Use Treatment of susceptible fungal infections, including oropharyngeal candidiasis, dermatophytoses, superficial mycoses, and cutaneous candidiasis, as well as vulvovaginal candidiasis; limited data suggest that clotrimazole troches may be effective for prophylaxis against oropharyngeal candidiasis in neutropenic patients

Local Anesthetic/Vasoconstrictor Precautions No information available to require special precautions

Effects on Dental Treatment No significant effects or complications reported

Significant Adverse Effects

Oral:

>10%: Hepatic: Abnormal liver function tests

1% to 10%:

Gastrointestinal: Nausea and vomiting may occur in patients on clotrimazole troches

Local: Mild burning, irritation, stinging to skin or vaginal area

Vaginal:

1% to 10%: Genitourinary: Vulvar/vaginal burning

<1% (Limited to important or life-threatening): Burning or itching of penis of sexual partner; polyuria; vulvar itching, soreness, edema, or discharge

Dosage

Children >3 years and Adults:

Oral:

Prophylaxis: 10 mg troche dissolved 3 times/day for the duration of chemotherapy or until steroids are reduced to maintenance levels

Treatment: 10 mg troche dissolved slowly 5 times/day for 14 consecutive days

Topical (cream, solution): Apply twice daily; if no improvement occurs after 4 weeks of therapy, re-evaluate diagnosis

Children >12 years and Adults:

Vaginal:

Cream:

1%: Insert 1 applicatorful vaginal cream daily (preferably at bedtime) for 7 consecutive days

2%: Insert 1 applicatorful vaginal cream daily (preferably at bedtime) for 3 consecutive days

Tablet: Insert 100 mg/day for 7 days or 500 mg single dose

Topical (cream, solution): Apply to affected area twice daily (morning and evening) for 7 consecutive days

Mechanism of Action Binds to phospholipids in the fungal cell membrane altering cell wall permeability resulting in loss of essential intracellular elements

Contraindications Hypersensitivity to clotrimazole or any component of the formulation

Warnings/Precautions Clotrimazole should not be used for treatment of systemic fungal infection; safety and effectiveness of clotrimazole lozenges (troches) in children <3 years of age have not been established; when using topical formulation, avoid contact with eyes

Drug Interactions **Inhibits** CYP1A2 (weak), 2A6 (weak), 2B6 (weak), 2C8/9 (weak), 2C19 (weak), 2D6 (weak), 2E1 (weak), 3A4 (moderate)

CYP3A4 substrates: Clotrimazole may increase the levels/effects of CYP3A4 substrates. Example substrates include benzodiazepines, calcium channel blockers, cyclosporine, mirtazapine, nateglinide, nefazodone, sildenafil (and other PDE-5 inhibitors), tacrolimus, and venlafaxine. Selected benzodiazepines (midazolam and triazolam), cisapride, ergot alkaloids, selected HMG-CoA reductase inhibitors (lovastatin and simvastatin), and pimozide are generally contraindicated with strong CYP3A4 inhibitors.

Pharmacodynamics/Kinetics

Absorption: Topical: Negligible through intact skin

Time to peak, serum:

Oral topical: Salivary levels occur within 3 hours following 30 minutes of dissolution time

Vaginal cream: High vaginal levels: 8-24 hours

Vaginal tablet: High vaginal levels: 1-2 days

Excretion: Feces (as metabolites)

Pregnancy Risk Factor B (topical); C (troches)

Lactation Excretion in breast milk unknown

Dosage Forms

Combination pack (Mycelex®-7): Vaginal tablet 100 mg (7s) and vaginal cream 1% (7 g)

Cream, topical: 1% (15 g, 30 g, 45 g)

Cruex®: 1% (15 g)

Lotrimin® AF Athlete's Foot: 1% (12 g, 24 g)

Lotrimin® AF Jock Itch: 1% (12 g)

Cream, vaginal: 2% (21 g)

Mycelex®-7: 1% (45 g)

Solution, topical: 1% (10 mL, 30 mL)

Lotrimin® AF Athlete's Foot: 1% (10 mL)

Tablet, vaginal (Gyne-Lotrimin® 3): 200 mg (3s)

Troche (Mycelex®): 10 mg

Clotrimazole and Betamethasone *see* Betamethasone and Clotrimazole *on page 201*

Cloxacillin (kloks a SIL in)

Canadian Brand Names Apo-Cloxi®; Novo-Cloxin; Nu-Cloxi; Riva-Cloxacillin

Generic Available Yes

Synonyms Cloxacillin Sodium

Pharmacologic Category Antibiotic, Penicillin

Dental Use Treatment of susceptible orofacial infections (notably penicillinase-producing staphylococci)

Use Treatment of susceptible bacterial infections, notably penicillinase-producing staphylococci causing respiratory tract, skin and skin structure, bone and joint, urinary tract infections

Local Anesthetic/Vasoconstrictor Precautions No information available to require special precautions

Effects on Dental Treatment Key adverse event(s) related to dental treatment: Prolonged use of penicillins may lead to development of oral candidiasis.

Significant Adverse Effects

1% to 10%: Gastrointestinal: Nausea, diarrhea, abdominal pain

<1% (Limited to important or life-threatening): Agranulocytosis, anemia, BUN increased, creatinine increased, eosinophilia, fever, hematuria, hemolytic anemia, hepatotoxicity, hypersensitivity, interstitial nephritis, leukopenia, neutropenia, prolonged PT, pseudomembranous colitis, rash (maculopapular to exfoliative), seizures with extremely high doses and/or renal failure, serum sickness-like reactions, thrombocytopenia, transient elevated LFTs, vaginitis, vomiting

Restrictions Not available in U.S.

Dosage Oral:

Children >1 month (<20 kg): 50-100 mg/kg/day in divided doses every 6 hours; up to a maximum of 4 g/day

Children (>20 kg) and Adults: 250-500 mg every 6 hours

Hemodialysis: Not dialyzable (0% to 5%)

Mechanism of Action Inhibits bacterial cell wall synthesis by binding to one or more of the penicillin-binding proteins (PBPs) which in turn inhibits the final transpeptidation step of peptidoglycan synthesis in bacterial cell walls, thus inhibiting cell wall biosynthesis. Bacteria eventually lyse due to ongoing activity of cell wall autolytic enzymes (autolysins and murein hydrolases) while cell wall assembly is arrested.

Contraindications Hypersensitivity to cloxacillin, any component of the formulation, or penicillins

Warnings/Precautions Monitor PT if patient concurrently on warfarin, elimination of drug is slow in renally impaired; use with caution in patients allergic to cephalosporins due to a low incidence of cross-hypersensitivity

Drug Interactions

Methotrexate: Penicillins may increase the exposure to methotrexate during concurrent therapy; monitor.

Oral contraceptives: Anecdotal reports suggesting decreased contraceptive efficacy with penicillins have been refuted by more rigorous scientific and clinical data.

Probenecid, disulfiram: May increase levels of penicillins (cloxacillin)

Warfarin: Effects of warfarin may be increased

Dietary Considerations Should be taken 1 hour before or 2 hours after meals with water.

Sodium content of 250 mg capsule: 13.8 mg (0.6 mEq)

Sodium content of suspension 5 mL of 125 mg/5 mL: 11 mg (0.48 mEq)

(Continued)

Cloxacillin *(Continued)*

Pharmacodynamics/Kinetics

Absorption: Oral: ~50%

Distribution: Widely to most body fluids and bone; penetration into cells, into eye, and across normal meninges is poor; crosses placenta; enters breast milk; inflammation increases amount that crosses blood-brain barrier

Protein binding: 90% to 98%

Metabolism: Extensively hepatic to active and inactive metabolites

Half-life elimination: 0.5-1.5 hours; prolonged with renal impairment and in neonates

Time to peak, serum: 0.5-2 hours

Excretion: Urine and feces

Pregnancy Risk Factor B

Lactation Excretion in breast milk unknown

Breast-Feeding Considerations No data reported; however, other penicillins may be taken while breast-feeding.

Dosage Forms

Capsule, as sodium: 250 mg, 500 mg

Powder for oral suspension, as sodium: 125 mg/5 mL (100 mL, 200 mL)

Cloxacillin Sodium *see* Cloxacillin *on page 365*

Clozapine (KLOE za peen)

U.S. Brand Names Clozaril®; Fazaclo™

Canadian Brand Names Clozaril®; Gen-Clozapine; Rhoxal-clozapine

Mexican Brand Names Clopsine®; Leponex®

Generic Available Yes

Pharmacologic Category Antipsychotic Agent, Dibenzodiazepine

Use Treatment-refractory schizophrenia; to reduce risk of recurrent suicidal behavior in schizophrenia or schizoaffective disorder

Unlabeled/Investigational Use Schizoaffective disorder, bipolar disorder, childhood psychosis, severe obsessive-compulsive disorder

Local Anesthetic/Vasoconstrictor Precautions Most pharmacology textbooks state that in presence of phenothiazines, systemic doses of epinephrine paradoxically decrease the blood pressure. This is the so called "epinephrine reversal" phenomenon. This has never been observed when epinephrine is given by infiltration as part of the anesthesia procedure.

Effects on Dental Treatment Key adverse event(s) related to dental treatment: Sialorrhea and xerostomia (normal salivary flow resumes upon discontinuation). Many patients may experience orthostatic hypotension with clozapine; precautions should be taken; do not use atropine-like drugs for xerostomia in patients taking clozapine due to significant potentiation.

Common Adverse Effects

>10%:

- Cardiovascular: Tachycardia
- Central nervous system: Drowsiness, dizziness
- Gastrointestinal: Constipation, weight gain, sialorrhea
- Genitourinary: Urinary incontinence

1% to 10%:

- Cardiovascular: Angina, ECG changes, hypertension, hypotension, syncope
- Central nervous system: Akathisia, seizures, headache, nightmares, akinesia, confusion, insomnia, fatigue, myoclonic jerks, restlessness, agitation, lethargy, ataxia, slurred speech, depression, anxiety
- Dermatologic: Rash
- Gastrointestinal: Abdominal discomfort, anorexia, diarrhea, heartburn, xerostomia, nausea, vomiting
- Hematologic: Eosinophilia, leukopenia, leukocytosis
- Hepatic: Liver function tests abnormal
- Neuromuscular & skeletal: Tremor, rigidity, hyperkinesia, weakness
- Ocular: Visual disturbances
- Respiratory: Rhinorrhea
- Miscellaneous: Diaphoresis (increased), fever

Restrictions Patient-specific registration is required to dispense clozapine. Monitoring systems for individual clozapine manufacturers are independent. If a patient is switched from one brand/manufacturer of clozapine to another, the patient must be entered into a new registry (must be completed by the prescriber and delivered to the dispensing pharmacy). Healthcare providers, including pharmacists dispensing clozapine, are encouraged to verify the patient's hematological status and qualification to receive clozapine with all existing registries.

Mechanism of Action Clozapine is a weak $dopamine_1$ and $dopamine_2$ receptor blocker, but blocks D_1-D_5 receptors; in addition, it blocks the $serotonin_2$, alpha-adrenergic, histamine H_1, and cholinergic receptors

Drug Interactions

Cytochrome P450 Effect: Substrate of CYP1A2 (major), 2A6 (minor), 2C8/9 (minor), 2C19 (minor), 2D6 (minor), 3A4 (minor); **Inhibits** CYP1A2 (weak), 2C8/9 (weak), 2C19 (weak), 2D6 (moderate), 2E1 (weak), 3A4 (weak)

Increased Effect/Toxicity: May potentiate anticholinergic and hypotensive effects of other drugs. Benzodiazepines in combination with clozapine may produce respiratory depression and hypotension, especially during the first few weeks of therapy. May potentiate effect/toxicity of risperidone. Clozapine serum concentrations may be increased by inhibitors of CYP1A2 (list of inhibitors is extensive, but includes amiodarone, ciprofloxacin, fluvoxamine, ketoconazole, lomefloxacin, ofloxacin, and rofecoxib). Clozapine may increase the levels/effects of amphetamines, selected beta-blockers, substrates; example substrates include dextromethorphan, fluoxetine, lidocaine, mirtazapine, nefazodone, paroxetine, risperidone, ritonavir, thioridazine, tricyclic antidepressants, venlafaxine, and other CYP2D6 substrates. Metoclopramide may increase risk of extrapyramidal symptoms (EPS).

Decreased Effect: Clozapine may decrease the levels/effects of CYP2D6 prodrug substrates; example prodrug substrates include codeine, hydrocodone, oxycodone, and tramadol. The levels/effects of clozapine may be decreased by carbamazepine, phenobarbital, primidone, rifampin, and other CYP1A2 inducers. Cigarette smoking (nicotine) may enhance the metabolism of clozapine. Clozapine may reverse the pressor effect of epinephrine (avoid in treatment of drug-induced hypotension).

Pharmacodynamics/Kinetics

Protein binding: 97% to serum proteins

Metabolism: Extensively hepatic

Bioavailability: 12% to 81%

Half-life elimination: 12 hours (range: 4-66 hours)

Time to peak: 2.5 hours

Excretion: Urine (~50%) and feces (30%) with trace amounts of unchanged drug

Pregnancy Risk Factor B

Clozaril® *see* Clozapine *on page 366*

Coagulant Complex Inhibitor *see* Anti-inhibitor Coagulant Complex *on page 135*

Coagulation Factor VIIa *see* Factor VIIa (Recombinant) *on page 571*

Coal Tar (KOLE tar)

U.S. Brand Names Balnetar® [OTC]; Betatar® [OTC]; Cutar® [OTC]; DHS™ Tar [OTC]; DHS™ Targel [OTC]; Doak® Tar [OTC]; Estar® [OTC]; Exorex®; Ionil T® [OTC]; Ionil T® Plus [OTC]; MG 217® [OTC]; MG 217® Medicated Tar [OTC]; Neutrogena® T/Gel [OTC]; Neutrogena® T/Gel Extra Strength [OTC]; Oxipor® VHC [OTC]; Pentrax® [OTC]; Polytar® [OTC]; PsoriGel® [OTC]; Reme-t™ [OTC]; Tegrin® [OTC]; Zetar® [OTC]

Canadian Brand Names Balnetar®; Estar®; SpectroTar Skin Wash™; Targel®; Zetar®

Generic Available No

Synonyms Crude Coal Tar; LCD; Pix Carbonis

Pharmacologic Category Topical Skin Product

Use Topically for controlling dandruff, seborrheic dermatitis, or psoriasis

Local Anesthetic/Vasoconstrictor Precautions No information available to require special precautions

Effects on Dental Treatment No significant effects or complications reported

Pregnancy Risk Factor C

Coal Tar and Salicylic Acid (KOLE tar & sal i SIL ik AS id)

Related Information

Coal Tar *on page 367*

Salicylic Acid *on page 1205*

U.S. Brand Names Tarsum® [OTC]; X-Seb™ T [OTC]

Canadian Brand Names Sebcur/T®

Generic Available Yes

Synonyms Salicylic Acid and Coal Tar

Pharmacologic Category Topical Skin Product

Use Seborrheal dermatitis, dandruff, psoriasis

Local Anesthetic/Vasoconstrictor Precautions No information available to require special precautions

(Continued)

Coal Tar and Salicylic Acid *(Continued)*

Effects on Dental Treatment No significant effects or complications reported

Pregnancy Risk Factor C

Cocaine (koe KANE)

Generic Available Yes

Synonyms Cocaine Hydrochloride

Pharmacologic Category Local Anesthetic

Use Topical anesthesia for mucous membranes

Local Anesthetic/Vasoconstrictor Precautions Although plain local anesthetic is not contraindicated, vasoconstrictor is absolutely contraindicated in any patient under the influence of or within 2 hours of cocaine use

Effects on Dental Treatment Key adverse event(s) related to dental treatment: Loss of taste perception. See Comments.

Common Adverse Effects

>10%:

Central nervous system: CNS stimulation

Gastrointestinal: Loss of taste perception

Respiratory: Rhinitis, nasal congestion

Miscellaneous: Loss of smell

1% to 10%:

Cardiovascular: Heart rate (decreased) with low doses, tachycardia with moderate doses, hypertension, cardiomyopathy, cardiac arrhythmias, myocarditis, QRS prolongation, Raynaud's phenomenon, cerebral vasculitis, thrombosis, fibrillation (atrial), flutter (atrial), sinus bradycardia, CHF, pulmonary hypertension, sinus tachycardia, tachycardia (supraventricular), arrhythmias (ventricular), vasoconstriction

Central nervous system: Fever, nervousness, restlessness, euphoria, excitation, headache, psychosis, hallucinations, agitation, seizures, slurred speech, hyperthermia, dystonic reactions, cerebral vascular accident, vasculitis, clonic-tonic reactions, paranoia, sympathetic storm

Dermatologic: Skin infarction, pruritus, madarosis

Gastrointestinal: Nausea, anorexia, colonic ischemia, spontaneous bowel perforation

Genitourinary: Priapism, uterine rupture

Hematologic: Thrombocytopenia

Neuromuscular & skeletal: Chorea (extrapyramidal), paresthesia, tremors, fasciculations

Ocular: Mydriasis (peak effect at 45 minutes; may last up to 12 hours), sloughing of the corneal epithelium, ulceration of the cornea, iritis, mydriasis, chemosis

Renal: Myoglobinuria, necrotizing vasculitis

Respiratory: Tachypnea, nasal mucosa damage (when snorting), hyposmia, bronchiolitis obliterans organizing pneumonia

Miscellaneous: "Washed-out" syndrome

Restrictions C-II

Mechanism of Action Ester local anesthetic blocks both the initiation and conduction of nerve impulses by decreasing the neuronal membrane's permeability to sodium ions, which results in inhibition of depolarization with resultant blockade of conduction; interferes with the uptake of norepinephrine by adrenergic nerve terminals producing vasoconstriction

Drug Interactions

Cytochrome P450 Effect: Substrate of CYP3A4 (major); **Inhibits** CYP2D6 (strong), 3A4 (weak)

Increased Effect/Toxicity: Cocaine may increase the levels/effects of CYP2D6 substrates (eg, amphetamines, selected beta-blockers, dextromethorphan, fluoxetine, lidocaine, mirtazapine, nefazodone, paroxetine, risperidone, ritonavir, thioridazine, tricyclic antidepressants, venlafaxine). Increased toxicity with MAO inhibitors. Use with epinephrine may cause extreme hypertension and/or cardiac arrhythmias. CYP3A4 inhibitors may increase the levels/effects of cocaine (eg, azole antifungals, ciprofloxacin, clarithromycin, diclofenac, doxycycline, erythromycin, imatinib, isoniazid, nefazodone, nicardipine, propofol, protease inhibitors, quinidine, verapamil).

Pharmacodynamics/Kinetics Following topical administration to mucosa:

Onset of action: ~1 minute

Peak effect: ~5 minutes

Duration (dose dependent): ≥30 minutes; cocaine metabolites may appear in urine of neonates up to 5 days after birth due to maternal cocaine use shortly before birth

Absorption: Well absorbed through mucous membranes; limited by drug-induced vasoconstriction; enhanced by inflammation

Distribution: Enters breast milk

Metabolism: Hepatic; major metabolites are ecgonine methyl ester and benzoyl ecgonine

Half-life elimination: 75 minutes

Excretion: Primarily urine (<10% as unchanged drug and metabolites)

Pregnancy Risk Factor C/X (nonmedicinal use)

Comments The cocaine user, regardless of how the cocaine was administered, presents a potential life-threatening situation in the dental operatory. A patient under the influence of cocaine could be compared to a car going 100 mph. Blood pressure is elevated, heart rate is likely increased, and the use of a local anesthetic with epinephrine may result in a medical emergency. Such patients can be identified by their jitteriness, irritability, talkativeness, tremors, and short, abrupt speech patterns. These same signs and symptoms may also be seen in a normal dental patient with preoperative dental anxiety; therefore, the dentist must be particularly alert in order to identify the potential cocaine abuser. If cocaine use is suspected, the patient should never be given a local anesthetic with vasoconstrictor, for fear of exacerbating the cocaine-induced sympathetic response. Life-threatening episodes of cardiac arrhythmias and hypertensive crises have been reported when local anesthetic with vasoconstrictor was administered to a patient under the influence of cocaine. No local anesthetic, used by any dentist, can interfere with, nor test positive by cocaine in any urine testing screen. Therefore, the dentist does not need to be concerned with any false drug-use accusations associated with dental anesthesia.

Cocaine Hydrochloride *see* Cocaine *on page 368*

Codafed® Expectorant *see* Guaifenesin, Pseudoephedrine, and Codeine *on page 676*

Codafed® Pediatric Expectorant *see* Guaifenesin, Pseudoephedrine, and Codeine *on page 676*

Codeine (KOE deen)

Related Information

Carisoprodol, Aspirin, and Codeine *on page 267*

Oral Pain *on page 1526*

Canadian Brand Names Codeine Contin®

Generic Available Yes

Synonyms Codeine Phosphate; Codeine Sulfate; Methylmorphine

Pharmacologic Category Analgesic, Narcotic; Antitussive

Dental Use Treatment of postoperative pain

Use Treatment of mild to moderate pain; antitussive in lower doses; dextromethorphan has equivalent antitussive activity but has much lower toxicity in accidental overdose

Local Anesthetic/Vasoconstrictor Precautions No information available to require special precautions

Effects on Dental Treatment No significant effects or complications reported

Significant Adverse Effects

>10%:

Central nervous system: Drowsiness

Gastrointestinal: Constipation

1% to 10%:

Cardiovascular: Tachycardia or bradycardia, hypotension

Central nervous system: Dizziness, lightheadedness, false feeling of well being, malaise, headache, restlessness, paradoxical CNS stimulation, confusion

Dermatologic: Rash, urticaria

Gastrointestinal: Dry mouth, anorexia, nausea, vomiting

Hepatic: Increased transaminases

Genitourinary: Decreased urination, ureteral spasm

Local: Burning at injection site

Neuromuscular & skeletal: Weakness

Ocular: Blurred vision

Respiratory: Dyspnea

Miscellaneous: Physical and psychological dependence, histamine release

<1% (Limited to important or life-threatening): Convulsions, hallucinations, insomnia, mental depression, nightmares

Restrictions C-II

Dosage Note: These are guidelines and do not represent the maximum doses that may be required in all patients. Doses should be titrated to pain relief/ prevention. Doses >1.5 mg/kg body weight are not recommended.

(Continued)

Codeine *(Continued)*

Analgesic:

Children: Oral, I.M., SubQ: 0.5-1 mg/kg/dose every 4-6 hours as needed; maximum: 60 mg/dose

Adults:

Oral: 30 mg every 4-6 hours as needed; patients with prior opiate exposure may require higher initial doses. Usual range: 15-120 mg every 4-6 hours as needed

Oral, controlled release formulation (Codeine Contin®, not available in U.S.): 50-300 mg every 12 hours. **Note:** A patient's codeine requirement should be established using prompt release formulations; conversion to long acting products may be considered when chronic, continuous treatment is required. Higher dosages should be reserved for use only in opioid-tolerant patients.

I.M., SubQ: 30 mg every 4-6 hours as needed; patients with prior opiate exposure may require higher initial doses. Usual range: 15-120 mg every 4-6 hours as needed; more frequent dosing may be needed

Antitussive: Oral (for nonproductive cough):

Children: 1-1.5 mg/kg/day in divided doses every 4-6 hours as needed: Alternative dose according to age:

2-6 years: 2.5-5 mg every 4-6 hours as needed; maximum: 30 mg/day

6-12 years: 5-10 mg every 4-6 hours as needed; maximum: 60 mg/day

Adults: 10-20 mg/dose every 4-6 hours as needed; maximum: 120 mg/day

Dosing adjustment in renal impairment:

Cl_{cr} 10-50 mL/minute: Administer 75% of dose

Cl_{cr} <10 mL/minute: Administer 50% of dose

Dosing adjustment in hepatic impairment: Probably necessary in hepatic insufficiency

Mechanism of Action Binds to opiate receptors in the CNS, causing inhibition of ascending pain pathways, altering the perception of and response to pain; causes cough supression by direct central action in the medulla; produces generalized CNS depression

Contraindications Hypersensitivity to codeine or any component of the formulation; pregnancy (prolonged use or high doses at term)

Warnings/Precautions An opioid-containing analgesic regimen should be tailored to each patient's needs and based upon the type of pain being treated (acute versus chronic), the route of administration, degree of tolerance for opioids (naive versus chronic user), age, weight, and medical condition. The optimal analgesic dose varies widely among patients. Doses should be titrated to pain relief/prevention.

Use with caution in patients with hypersensitivity reactions to other phenanthrene derivative opioid agonists (morphine, hydrocodone, hydromorphone, levorphanol, oxycodone, oxymorphone); respiratory diseases including asthma, emphysema, COPD, or severe liver or renal insufficiency; some preparations contain sulfites which may cause allergic reactions; tolerance or drug dependence may result from extended use

Not recommended for use for cough control in patients with a productive cough; not recommended as an antitussive for children <2 years of age; the elderly may be particularly susceptible to the CNS depressant and confusion as well as constipating effects of narcotics

Not approved for I.V. administration (although this route has been used clinically). If given intravenously, must be given slowly and the patient should be lying down. Rapid intravenous administration of narcotics may increase the incidence of serious adverse effects, in part due to limited opportunity to assess response prior to administration of the full dose. Access to respiratory support should be immediately available

Drug Interactions **Substrate** of CYP2D6 (major), 3A4 (minor); **Inhibits** CYP2D6 (weak)

CYP2D6 inhibitors: May decrease the effects of codeine. Example inhibitors include chlorpromazine, delavirdine, fluoxetine, miconazole, paroxetine, pergolide, quinidine, quinine, ritonavir, and ropinirole.

Decreased effect with cigarette smoking

Increased toxicity: CNS depressants, phenothiazines, TCAs, other narcotic analgesics, guanabenz, MAO inhibitors, neuromuscular blockers

Ethanol/Nutrition/Herb Interactions

Ethanol: Avoid or limit ethanol (may increase CNS depression). Watch for sedation.

Herb/Nutraceutical: St John's wort may decrease codeine levels. Avoid valerian, St John's wort, kava kava, gotu kola (may increase CNS depression).

Pharmacodynamics/Kinetics

Onset of action: Oral: 0.5-1 hour; I.M.: 10-30 minutes

Peak effect: Oral: 1-1.5 hours; I.M.: 0.5-1 hour

Duration: 4-6 hours

Absorption: Oral: Adequate

Distribution: Crosses placenta; enters breast milk

Protein binding: 7%

Metabolism: Hepatic to morphine (active)

Half-life elimination: 2.5-3.5 hours

Excretion: Urine (3% to 16% as unchanged drug, norcodeine, and free and conjugated morphine)

Pregnancy Risk Factor C/D (prolonged use or high doses at term)

Lactation Enters breast milk/use caution (AAP rates "compatible")

Dosage Forms

Injection, as phosphate: 15 mg/mL (2 mL); 30 mg/mL (2 mL) [contains sodium metabisulfite]

Solution, oral, as phosphate: 15 mg/5 mL (5 mL, 500 mL) [strawberry flavor]

Tablet, controlled release (Codeine Contin®) [not available in U.S.]: 50 mg, 100 mg, 150 mg, 200 mg

Tablet, as phosphate: 30 mg, 60 mg

Tablet, as sulfate: 15 mg, 30 mg, 60 mg

Comments It is recommended that codeine not be used as the sole entity for analgesia because of moderate efficacy along with relatively high incidence of nausea, sedation, and constipation. In addition, codeine has some narcotic addiction liability. Codeine in combination with acetaminophen or aspirin is recommended. Maximum effective analgesic dose of codeine is 60 mg (1 grain). Beyond 60 mg increases respiratory depression only. Sodium thiosulfate is an effective chemical antidote for codeine poisoning.

Selected Readings

Desjardins PJ, Cooper SA, Gallegos TL, et al, "The Relative Analgesic Efficacy of Propiram Fumarate, Codeine, Aspirin, and Placebo in Postimpaction Dental Pain," *J Clin Pharmacol*, 1984, 24(1):35-42.

Forbes JA, Keller CK, Smith JW, et al, "Analgesic Effect of Naproxen Sodium, Codeine, a Naproxen-Codeine Combination and Aspirin on the Postoperative Pain of Oral Surgery," *Pharmacotherapy*, 1986, 6(5):211-8.

Codeine, Acetaminophen, Butalbital, and Caffeine *see* Butalbital, Acetaminophen, Caffeine, and Codeine *on page 236*

Codeine and Acetaminophen *see* Acetaminophen and Codeine *on page 50*

Codeine and Aspirin *see* Aspirin and Codeine *on page 155*

Codeine and Bromodiphenhydramine *see* Bromodiphenhydramine and Codeine *on page 220*

Codeine and Butalbital Compound *see* Butalbital, Aspirin, Caffeine, and Codeine *on page 238*

Codeine and Guaifenesin *see* Guaifenesin and Codeine *on page 673*

Codeine and Promethazine *see* Promethazine and Codeine *on page 1131*

Codeine, Aspirin, and Carisoprodol *see* Carisoprodol, Aspirin, and Codeine *on page 267*

Codeine, Butalbital, Aspirin, and Caffeine *see* Butalbital, Aspirin, Caffeine, and Codeine *on page 238*

Codeine, Chlorpheniramine, and Pseudoephedrine *see* Chlorpheniramine, Pseudoephedrine, and Codeine *on page 319*

Codeine, Chlorpheniramine, Phenylephrine, and Potassium Iodide *see* Chlorpheniramine, Phenylephrine, Codeine, and Potassium Iodide *on page 318*

Codeine, Guaifenesin, and Pseudoephedrine *see* Guaifenesin, Pseudoephedrine, and Codeine *on page 676*

Codeine Phosphate *see* Codeine *on page 369*

Codeine, Promethazine, and Phenylephrine *see* Promethazine, Phenylephrine, and Codeine *on page 1132*

Codeine, Pseudoephedrine, and Triprolidine *see* Triprolidine, Pseudoephedrine, and Codeine *on page 1346*

Codeine Sulfate *see* Codeine *on page 369*

Codiclear® DH *see* Hydrocodone and Guaifenesin *on page 708*

Cod Liver Oil *see* Vitamin A and Vitamin D *on page 1382*

Cogentin® *see* Benztropine *on page 196*

Co-Gesic® *see* Hydrocodone and Acetaminophen *on page 702*

Cognex® *see* Tacrine *on page 1254*

Colace® [OTC] *see* Docusate *on page 459*

Colazal® *see* Balsalazide *on page 181*

ColBenemid *see* Colchicine and Probenecid *on page 372*

Colchicine (KOL chi seen)

Canadian Brand Names ratio-Colchicine

Mexican Brand Names Colchiquim®

Generic Available Yes

Pharmacologic Category Colchicine

Use Treatment of acute gouty arthritis attacks and prevention of recurrences of such attacks

Unlabeled/Investigational Use Primary biliary cirrhosis; management of familial Mediterranean fever

Local Anesthetic/Vasoconstrictor Precautions No information available to require special precautions

Effects on Dental Treatment No significant effects or complications reported

Common Adverse Effects

>10%: Gastrointestinal: Nausea, vomiting, diarrhea, abdominal pain

1% to 10%:

Dermatologic: Alopecia

Gastrointestinal: Anorexia

Mechanism of Action Decreases leukocyte motility, decreases phagocytosis in joints and lactic acid production, thereby reducing the deposition of urate crystals that perpetuates the inflammatory response

Drug Interactions

Cytochrome P450 Effect: Substrate of CYP3A4 (major); **Induces** CYP2C8/9 (weak), 2E1 (weak), 3A4 (weak)

Increased Effect/Toxicity: Alkalizing agents potentiate effects of colchicine. CYP3A4 inhibitors may increase the levels/effects of colchicine; example inhibitors include azole antifungals, ciprofloxacin, clarithromycin, diclofenac, doxycycline, erythromycin, imatinib, isoniazid, nefazodone, nicardipine, propofol, protease inhibitors, quinidine, and verapamil. Concurrent use of cyclosporine with colchicine may increase toxicity of colchicine.

CYP3A4 inhibitors: May increase the levels/effects of colchicine. Example inhibitors include azole antifungals, ciprofloxacin, clarithromycin, diclofenac, doxycycline, erythromycin, imatinib, isoniazid, nefazodone, nicardipine, propofol, protease inhibitors, quinidine, and verapamil.

Pharmacodynamics/Kinetics

Onset of action: Oral: Pain relief: ~12 hours if adequately dosed

Distribution: Concentrates in leukocytes, kidney, spleen, and liver; does not distribute in heart, skeletal muscle, and brain

Protein binding: 10% to 31%

Metabolism: Partially hepatic via deacetylation

Half-life elimination: 12-30 minutes; End-stage renal disease: 45 minutes

Time to peak, serum: Oral: 0.5-2 hours, declining for the next 2 hours before increasing again due to enterohepatic recycling

Excretion: Primarily feces; urine (10% to 20%)

Pregnancy Risk Factor C (oral); D (parenteral)

Colchicine and Probenecid (KOL chi seen & proe BEN e sid)

Related Information

Colchicine *on page 372*

Generic Available Yes

Synonyms ColBenemid; Probenecid and Colchicine

Pharmacologic Category Antigout Agent; Anti-inflammatory Agent; Uricosuric Agent

Use Treatment of chronic gouty arthritis when complicated by frequent, recurrent acute attacks of gout

Local Anesthetic/Vasoconstrictor Precautions No information available to require special precautions

Effects on Dental Treatment No significant effects or complications reported

Common Adverse Effects 1% to 10%:

Cardiovascular: Flushing

Central nervous system: Headache, dizziness

Dermatologic: Rash, alopecia

Gastrointestinal: Anorexia, nausea, vomiting, diarrhea, abdominal pain

Hematologic: Anemia, leukopenia, aplastic anemia, agranulocytosis

Hepatic: Hepatic necrosis, hepatotoxicity

Neuromuscular & skeletal: Peripheral neuritis, myopathy

Renal: Nephrotic syndrome, uric acid stones, polyuria

Miscellaneous: Hypersensitivity reactions

Drug Interactions
Cytochrome P450 Effect:
Colchicine: **Substrate** of CYP3A4 (major); **Induces** CYP2C8/9 (weak), 2E1 (weak), 3A4 (weak)
Probenecid: **Inhibits** CYP2C19 (weak)
Pharmacodynamics/Kinetics See individual agents.
Pregnancy Risk Factor C

Colesevelam (koh le SEV a lam)

Related Information
Cardiovascular Diseases *on page 1458*
U.S. Brand Names WelChol®
Canadian Brand Names WelChol®
Generic Available No
Pharmacologic Category Antilipemic Agent, Bile Acid Sequestrant
Use Adjunctive therapy to diet and exercise in the management of elevated LDL in primary hypercholesterolemia (Fredrickson type IIa) when used alone or in combination with an HMG-CoA reductase inhibitor
Local Anesthetic/Vasoconstrictor Precautions No information available to require special precautions
Effects on Dental Treatment No significant effects or complications reported
Significant Adverse Effects
>10%: Gastrointestinal: Constipation (11%)
2% to 10%:
Gastrointestinal: Dyspepsia (8%)
Neuromuscular & skeletal: Weakness (4%), myalgia (2%)
Respiratory: Pharyngitis (3%)
Dosage Adult: Oral:
Monotherapy: 3 tablets twice daily with meals or 6 tablets once daily with a meal; maximum dose: 7 tablets/day
Combination therapy with an HMG-CoA reductase inhibitor: 4-6 tablets daily; maximum dose: 6 tablets/day
Dosage adjustment in renal impairment: No recommendations made
Dosage adjustment in hepatic impairment: No recommendations made
Elderly: No recommendations made
Mechanism of Action Colesevelam binds bile acids including glycocholic acid in the intestine, impeding their reabsorption. Increases the fecal loss of bile salt-bound LDL-C
Contraindications Hypersensitivity to colesevelam or any component of the formulation; bowel obstruction
Warnings/Precautions Use caution in treating patients with serum triglyceride levels >300 mg/dL (excluded from trials). Safety and efficacy has not been established in pediatric patients. Use caution in dysphagia, swallowing disorders, severe GI motility disorders, major GI tract surgery, and in patients susceptible to fat-soluble vitamin deficiencies. Minimal effects are seen on HDL-C and triglyceride levels. Secondary causes of hypercholesterolemia should be excluded before initiation.
Drug Interactions
Sustained-release verapamil AUC and C_{max} were reduced. Clinical significance unknown.
Digoxin, lovastatin, metoprolol, quinidine, valproic acid, or warfarin absorption was not significantly affected with concurrent administration.
Clinical effects of atorvastatin, lovastatin, and simvastatin were not changed by concurrent administration.
Dietary Considerations Should be taken with meal(s). Follow dietary guidelines.
Pharmacodynamics/Kinetics
Onset of action: Peak effect: Therapeutic: ~2 weeks
Absorption: Insignificant
Excretion: Urine (0.05%) after 1 month of chronic dosing
Pregnancy Risk Factor B
Lactation Excretion in breast milk unknown
Dosage Forms Tablet, as hydrochloride [film coated]: 625 mg

Colestid® *see* Colestipol *on page 373*

Colestipol (koe LES ti pole)

Related Information
Cardiovascular Diseases *on page 1458*
U.S. Brand Names Colestid®
Canadian Brand Names Colestid®
(Continued)

Colestipol *(Continued)*

Generic Available No

Synonyms Colestipol Hydrochloride

Pharmacologic Category Antilipemic Agent, Bile Acid Sequestrant

Use Adjunct in management of primary hypercholesterolemia; regression of arteriolosclerosis; relief of pruritus associated with elevated levels of bile acids; possibly used to decrease plasma half-life of digoxin in toxicity

Local Anesthetic/Vasoconstrictor Precautions No information available to require special precautions

Effects on Dental Treatment No significant effects or complications reported

Common Adverse Effects

>10%: Gastrointestinal: Constipation

1% to 10%:

Central nervous system: Headache, dizziness, anxiety, vertigo, drowsiness, fatigue

Gastrointestinal: Abdominal pain and distention, belching, flatulence, nausea, vomiting, diarrhea

Mechanism of Action Binds with bile acids to form an insoluble complex that is eliminated in feces; it thereby increases the fecal loss of bile acid-bound low density lipoprotein cholesterol

Drug Interactions

Decreased Effect: Colestipol can reduce the absorption of numerous medications when used concurrently. Give other medications 1 hour before or 4 hours after giving colestipol. Medications which may be affected include HMG-CoA reductase inhibitors, thiazide diuretics, propranolol (and potentially other beta-blockers), corticosteroids, thyroid hormones, digoxin, valproic acid, NSAIDs, loop diuretics, sulfonylureas, troglitazone (and potentially other agents in this class - pioglitazone and rosiglitazone).

Warfarin and other oral anticoagulants: Absorption is reduced by cholestyramine and may also be reduced by colestipol. Separate administration times (as detailed above).

Pharmacodynamics/Kinetics

Absorption: None

Excretion: Feces

Pregnancy Risk Factor C

Colestipol Hydrochloride *see* Colestipol *on page 373*

Colgate Total® Toothpaste *see* Triclosan and Fluoride *on page 1337*

Colistimethate (koe lis ti METH ate)

U.S. Brand Names Coly-Mycin® M

Canadian Brand Names Coly-Mycin® M

Generic Available Yes

Synonyms Colistimethate Sodium

Pharmacologic Category Antibiotic, Miscellaneous

Use Treatment of infections due to sensitive strains of certain gram-negative bacilli which are resistant to other antibacterials or in patients allergic to other antibacterials

Unlabeled/Investigational Use Used as inhalation in the prevention of *Pseudomonas aeruginosa* respiratory tract infections in immunocompromised patients, and used as inhalation adjunct agent for the treatment of *P. aeruginosa* infections in patients with cystic fibrosis and other seriously ill or chronically ill patients

Local Anesthetic/Vasoconstrictor Precautions No information available to require special precautions

Effects on Dental Treatment No significant effects or complications reported

Common Adverse Effects 1% to 10%:

Central nervous system: Vertigo, slurring of speech

Dermatologic: Urticaria

Gastrointestinal: GI upset

Respiratory: Respiratory arrest

Renal: Nephrotoxicity

Mechanism of Action Hydrolyzed to colistin, which acts as a cationic detergent which damages the bacterial cytoplasmic membrane causing leaking of intracellular substances and cell death

Drug Interactions

Increased Effect/Toxicity: Other nephrotoxic drugs, neuromuscular blocking agents.

Pharmacodynamics/Kinetics

Distribution: Widely, except for CNS, synovial, pleural, and pericardial fluids

Half-life elimination: 1.5-8 hours; Anuria: ≤2-3 days
Time to peak: ~2 hours
Excretion: Primarily urine (as unchanged drug)

Pregnancy Risk Factor C

Colistimethate Sodium *see* Colistimethate *on page 374*

CollaCote® *see* Collagen (Absorbable) *on page 375*

Collagen *see* Microfibrillar Collagen Hemostat *on page 923*

Collagen (Absorbable) (KOL la jen, ab SORB able)

U.S. Brand Names CollaCote®; CollaPlug®; CollaTape®

Generic Available Yes

Pharmacologic Category Hemostatic Agent

Dental Use To control bleeding created during dental surgery

Use Hemostatic

Local Anesthetic/Vasoconstrictor Precautions No information available to require special precautions

Effects on Dental Treatment No significant effects or complications reported

Significant Adverse Effects No data reported

Dosage Children and Adults: A sufficiently large dressing should be selected so as to completely cover the oral wound

Mechanism of Action The highly porous sponge structure absorbs blood and wound exudate. The collagen component causes aggregation of platelets which bind to collagen fibrils. The aggregated platelets degranulate, releasing coagulation factors that promote the formation of fibrin.

Contraindications No data reported

Warnings/Precautions Should not be used on infected or contaminated wounds

Drug Interactions No data reported

Lactation Compatible

Dosage Forms

Wound dressing:
- 3/8" x 3/4"
- 3/4" x 1 1/2"
- 1" x 3"

Collagenase (KOL la je nase)

U.S. Brand Names Santyl®

Canadian Brand Names Santyl®

Generic Available No

Pharmacologic Category Enzyme, Topical Debridement

Use Promotes debridement of necrotic tissue in dermal ulcers and severe burns

Orphan drug: Injection: Treatment of Peyronie's disease; treatment of Dupytren's disease

Local Anesthetic/Vasoconstrictor Precautions No information available to require special precautions

Effects on Dental Treatment No significant effects or complications reported

Common Adverse Effects Frequency not defined.

Local: Irritation, Pain and burning may occur at site of application

Mechanism of Action Collagenase is an enzyme derived from the fermentation of *Clostridium histolyticum* and differs from other proteolytic enzymes in that its enzymatic action has a high specificity for native and denatured collagen. Collagenase will not attack collagen in healthy tissue or newly formed granulation tissue. In addition, it does not act on fat, fibrin, keratin, or muscle.

Drug Interactions

Decreased Effect: Enzymatic activity is inhibited by detergents, benzalkonium chloride, hexachlorophene, nitrofurazone, tincture of iodine, and heavy metal ions (silver and mercury).

Pregnancy Risk Factor C

CollaPlug® *see* Collagen (Absorbable) *on page 375*

CollaTape® *see* Collagen (Absorbable) *on page 375*

Colocort™ *see* Hydrocortisone *on page 714*

Coly-Mycin® M *see* Colistimethate *on page 374*

Colyte® *see* Polyethylene Glycol-Electrolyte Solution *on page 1100*

CombiPatch® *see* Estradiol and Norethindrone *on page 521*

Combipres® [DSC] *see* Clonidine and Chlorthalidone *on page 360*

Combivent® *see* Ipratropium and Albuterol *on page 761*

Combivir® *see* Zidovudine and Lamivudine *on page 1399*

Comhist® *see* Chlorpheniramine, Phenylephrine, and Phenyltoloxamine *on page 317*
Commit™ [OTC] *see* Nicotine *on page 981*
Compazine® [DSC] *see* Prochlorperazine *on page 1126*
Compound E *see* Cortisone *on page 377*
Compound F *see* Hydrocortisone *on page 714*
Compound S *see* Zidovudine *on page 1398*
Compound S, Abacavir, and Lamivudine *see* Abacavir, Lamivudine, and Zidovudine *on page 43*
Compound W® [OTC] *see* Salicylic Acid *on page 1205*
Compound W® One Step Wart Remover [OTC] *see* Salicylic Acid *on page 1205*
Compoz® Nighttime Sleep Aid [OTC] *see* DiphenhydrAMINE *on page 448*
Compro™ *see* Prochlorperazine *on page 1126*
Comtan® *see* Entacapone *on page 494*
Comtrex® Maximum Strength Sinus and Nasal Decongestant [OTC] *see* Acetaminophen, Chlorpheniramine, and Pseudoephedrine *on page 58*
Comtrex® Non-Drowsy Cold and Cough Relief [OTC] *see* Acetaminophen, Dextromethorphan, and Pseudoephedrine *on page 59*
Comtrex® Sore Throat Maximum Strength [OTC] *see* Acetaminophen *on page 47*
Conceptrol® [OTC] *see* Nonoxynol 9 *on page 995*
Concerta® *see* Methylphenidate *on page 908*
Condylox® *see* Podofilox *on page 1099*
Congestac® *see* Guaifenesin and Pseudoephedrine *on page 675*
Conjugated Estrogen and Methyltestosterone *see* Estrogens (Esterified) and Methyltestosterone *on page 530*
Constilac® *see* Lactulose *on page 794*
Constulose® *see* Lactulose *on page 794*
Contac® Severe Cold and Flu/Non-Drowsy [OTC] *see* Acetaminophen, Dextromethorphan, and Pseudoephedrine *on page 59*
Copaxone® *see* Glatiramer Acetate *on page 658*
Copegus® *see* Ribavirin *on page 1177*
Copolymer-1 *see* Glatiramer Acetate *on page 658*
Copper *see* Trace Metals *on page 1319*
Cordarone® *see* Amiodarone *on page 101*
Cordran® *see* Flurandrenolide *on page 611*
Cordran® SP *see* Flurandrenolide *on page 611*
Coreg® *see* Carvedilol *on page 270*
Corgard® *see* Nadolol *on page 956*
Coricidin HBP® Cold and Flu [OTC] *see* Chlorpheniramine and Acetaminophen *on page 314*
Corlopam® *see* Fenoldopam *on page 579*
Cormax® *see* Clobetasol *on page 351*
Correctol® Tablets [OTC] *see* Bisacodyl *on page 208*
CortaGel® Maximum Strength [OTC] *see* Hydrocortisone *on page 714*
Cortaid® Intensive Therapy [OTC] *see* Hydrocortisone *on page 714*
Cortaid® Maximum Strength [OTC] *see* Hydrocortisone *on page 714*
Cortaid® Sensitive Skin With Aloe [OTC] *see* Hydrocortisone *on page 714*
Cortef® *see* Hydrocortisone *on page 714*
Corticool® [OTC] *see* Hydrocortisone *on page 714*

Corticotropin (kor ti koe TROE pin)

U.S. Brand Names H.P. Acthar® Gel

Generic Available No

Synonyms ACTH; Adrenocorticotropic Hormone; Corticotropin, Repository

Pharmacologic Category Corticosteroid, Systemic

Use Acute exacerbations of multiple sclerosis; diagnostic aid in adrenocortical insufficiency, severe muscle weakness in myasthenia gravis

Cosyntropin is preferred over corticotropin for diagnostic test of adrenocortical insufficiency (cosyntropin is less allergenic and test is shorter in duration)

Local Anesthetic/Vasoconstrictor Precautions No information available to require special precautions

Effects on Dental Treatment No significant effects or complications reported

Common Adverse Effects Frequency not defined.

Central nervous system: Insomnia, nervousness
Dermatologic: Hirsutism

Endocrine & metabolic: Diabetes mellitus
Gastrointestinal: Increased appetite, indigestion
Neuromuscular & skeletal: Arthralgia
Ocular: Cataracts
Respiratory: Epistaxis

Mechanism of Action Stimulates the adrenal cortex to secrete adrenal steroids (including hydrocortisone, cortisone), androgenic substances, and a small amount of aldosterone

Pregnancy Risk Factor C

Corticotropin, Repository *see* Corticotropin *on page 376*

Cortifoam® *see* Hydrocortisone *on page 714*

Cortisol *see* Hydrocortisone *on page 714*

Cortisone (KOR ti sone)

Related Information

Respiratory Diseases *on page 1478*
Triamcinolone *on page 1330*

Canadian Brand Names Cortone®

Generic Available Yes

Synonyms Compound E; Cortisone Acetate

Pharmacologic Category Corticosteroid, Systemic

Use Management of adrenocortical insufficiency

Local Anesthetic/Vasoconstrictor Precautions No information available to require special precautions

Effects on Dental Treatment A compromised immune response may occur if patient has been taking systemic cortisone. The need for corticosteroid coverage in these patients should be considered before any dental treatment; consult with physician.

Common Adverse Effects

>10%:
Central nervous system: Insomnia, nervousness
Gastrointestinal: Increased appetite, indigestion

1% to 10%:
Dermatologic: Hirsutism
Endocrine & metabolic: Diabetes mellitus
Neuromuscular & skeletal: Arthralgia
Ocular: Cataracts, glaucoma
Respiratory: Epistaxis

Mechanism of Action Decreases inflammation by suppression of migration of polymorphonuclear leukocytes and reversal of increased capillary permeability

Drug Interactions

Increased Effect/Toxicity: Estrogens may increase cortisone effects. Cortisone may increase ulcerogenic potential of NSAIDs, and may increase potassium deletion due to diuretics.

Decreased Effect: Enzyme inducers (barbiturates, phenytoin, rifampin) may decrease cortisone effects. Effect of live virus vaccines may be decreased. Anticholinesterase agents may decrease effect of cortisone.
Cortisone may decrease effects of warfarin and salicylates.

Pharmacodynamics/Kinetics

Onset of action: Peak effect: Oral: ~2 hours; I.M.: 20-48 hours
Duration: 30-36 hours
Absorption: Slow
Distribution: Muscles, liver, skin, intestines, and kidneys; crosses placenta; enters breast milk
Metabolism: Hepatic to inactive metabolites
Half-life elimination: 0.5-2 hours; End-stage renal disease: 3.5 hours
Excretion: Urine and feces

Pregnancy Risk Factor D

Cortisone Acetate *see* Cortisone *on page 377*

Cortisporin® Cream *see* Neomycin, Polymyxin B, and Hydrocortisone *on page 975*

Cortisporin® Ointment *see* Bacitracin, Neomycin, Polymyxin B, and Hydrocortisone *on page 179*

Cortisporin® Ophthalmic *see* Neomycin, Polymyxin B, and Hydrocortisone *on page 975*

Cortisporin® Otic *see* Neomycin, Polymyxin B, and Hydrocortisone *on page 975*

Cortizone®-5 [OTC] *see* Hydrocortisone *on page 714*

Cortizone®-10 Maximum Strength [OTC] *see* Hydrocortisone *on page 714*

Cortizone®-10 Plus Maximum Strength [OTC] *see* Hydrocortisone *on page 714*
Cortizone® 10 Quick Shot [OTC] *see* Hydrocortisone *on page 714*
Cortizone® for Kids [OTC] *see* Hydrocortisone *on page 714*
Cortrosyn® *see* Cosyntropin *on page 378*
Corvert® *see* Ibutilide *on page 731*
Corzide® *see* Nadolol and Bendroflumethiazide *on page 957*
Cosmegen® *see* Dactinomycin *on page 394*
Cosopt® *see* Dorzolamide and Timolol *on page 464*

Cosyntropin (koe sin TROE pin)

U.S. Brand Names Cortrosyn®
Canadian Brand Names Cortrosyn®
Generic Available No
Synonyms Synacthen; Tetracosactide
Pharmacologic Category Diagnostic Agent
Use Diagnostic test to differentiate primary adrenal from secondary (pituitary) adrenocortical insufficiency
Local Anesthetic/Vasoconstrictor Precautions No information available to require special precautions
Effects on Dental Treatment No significant effects or complications reported
Common Adverse Effects Frequency not defined.
Cardiovascular: Bradycardia, hypertension, peripheral edema, tachycardia
Dermatologic: Rash
Local: Whealing with redness at the injection site
Miscellaneous: Anaphylaxis, hypersensitivity reaction
Mechanism of Action Stimulates the adrenal cortex to secrete adrenal steroids (including hydrocortisone, cortisone), androgenic substances, and a small amount of aldosterone
Pharmacodynamics/Kinetics Time to peak, serum: I.M., IVP: ~1 hour; plasma cortisol levels rise in healthy individuals within 5 minutes
Pregnancy Risk Factor C

Co-Trimoxazole *see* Sulfamethoxazole and Trimethoprim *on page 1246*
Coumadin® *see* Warfarin *on page 1389*
Covera-HS® *see* Verapamil *on page 1373*
Co-Vidarabine *see* Pentostatin *on page 1065*
Coviracil *see* Emtricitabine *on page 487*
Cozaar® *see* Losartan *on page 845*
CP-99,219-27 *see* Trovafloxacin *on page 1348*
CPC *see* Cetylpyridinium *on page 301*
C-Phed Tannate *see* Chlorpheniramine and Pseudoephedrine *on page 315*
CPM *see* Cyclophosphamide *on page 384*
CPT-11 *see* Irinotecan *on page 764*
CPZ *see* ChlorproMAZINE *on page 319*
Creomulsion® Cough [OTC] *see* Dextromethorphan *on page 421*
Creomulsion® for Children [OTC] *see* Dextromethorphan *on page 421*
Creon® *see* Pancrelipase *on page 1042*
Creo-Terpin® [OTC] *see* Dextromethorphan *on page 421*
Crestor® *see* Rosuvastatin *on page 1202*
Cresylate® *see* m-Cresyl Acetate *on page 857*
Crinone® *see* Progesterone *on page 1128*
Critic-Aid Skin Care® [OTC] *see* Zinc Oxide *on page 1400*
Crixivan® *see* Indinavir *on page 744*
Crolom® *see* Cromolyn *on page 378*
Cromoglycic Acid *see* Cromolyn *on page 378*

Cromolyn (KROE moe lin)

Related Information
Respiratory Diseases *on page 1478*
U.S. Brand Names Crolom®; Gastrocrom®; Intal®; Nasalcrom® [OTC]; Opticrom®
Canadian Brand Names Apo-Cromolyn®; Intal®; Nalcrom®; Nu-Cromolyn; Opticrom®
Generic Available Yes: Excludes oral spray, oral solution
Synonyms Cromoglycic Acid; Cromolyn Sodium; Disodium Cromoglycate; DSCG
Pharmacologic Category Mast Cell Stabilizer

Use

Inhalation: May be used as an adjunct in the prophylaxis of allergic disorders, including asthma; prevention of exercise-induced bronchospasm

Nasal: Prevention and treatment of seasonal and perennial allergic rhinitis

Oral: Systemic mastocytosis

Ophthalmic: Treatment of vernal keratoconjunctivitis, vernal conjunctivitis, and vernal keratitis

Unlabeled/Investigational Use Oral: Food allergy, treatment of inflammatory bowel disease

Local Anesthetic/Vasoconstrictor Precautions No information available to require special precautions

Effects on Dental Treatment Key adverse event(s) related to dental treatment:

Inhalation: Unpleasant taste.

Intranasal: Xerostomia (normal salivary flow resumes upon discontinuation).

Systemic: Glossitis, stomatitis, and unpleasant taste.

Common Adverse Effects

Inhalation: >10%: Gastrointestinal: Unpleasant taste in mouth

Nasal:

>10%: Respiratory: Increase in sneezing, burning, stinging, or irritation inside of nose

1% to 10%:

Central nervous system: Headache

Gastrointestinal: Unpleasant taste

Respiratory: Hoarseness, coughing, postnasal drip

<1% (Limited to important or life-threatening): Anaphylactic reactions, epistaxis

Ophthalmic: Frequency not defined:

Ocular: Conjunctival injection, dryness around the eye, edema, eye irritation, immediate hypersensitivity reactions, itchy eyes, puffy eyes, styes, rash, watery eyes

Respiratory: Dyspnea

Systemic: Frequency not defined:

Cardiovascular: Angioedema, chest pain, edema, flushing, palpitations, premature ventricular contractions, tachycardia

Central nervous system: Anxiety, behavior changes, convulsions, depression, dizziness, fatigue, hallucinations, headache, irritability, insomnia, lethargy, migraine, nervousness, hypoesthesia, postprandial lightheadedness, psychosis

Dermatologic: Erythema, photosensitivity, pruritus, purpura, rash, urticaria

Gastrointestinal: Abdominal pain, constipation, diarrhea, dyspepsia, dysphagia, esophagospasm, flatulence, glossitis, nausea, stomatitis, unpleasant taste, vomiting

Genitourinary: Dysuria, urinary frequency

Hematologic: Neutropenia, pancytopenia, polycythemia

Hepatic: Liver function test abnormal

Local: Burning

Neuromuscular & skeletal: Arthralgia, leg stiffness, leg weakness, myalgia, paresthesia

Otic: Tinnitus

Respiratory: Dyspnea, pharyngitis

Miscellaneous: Lupus erythematosus

Mechanism of Action Prevents the mast cell release of histamine, leukotrienes and slow-reacting substance of anaphylaxis by inhibiting degranulation after contact with antigens

Pharmacodynamics/Kinetics

Onset: Response to treatment:

Nasal spray: May occur at 1-2 weeks

Ophthalmic: May be seen within a few days; treatment for up to 6 weeks is often required

Oral: May occur within 2-6 weeks

Absorption:

Inhalation: ~8% reaches lungs upon inhalation; well absorbed

Oral: <1% of dose absorbed

Half-life elimination: 80-90 minutes

Time to peak, serum: Inhalation: ~15 minutes

Excretion: Urine and feces (equal amounts as unchanged drug); exhaled gases (small amounts)

Pregnancy Risk Factor B

Cromolyn Sodium *see* Cromolyn *on page 378*

Crosseal™ *see* Fibrin Sealant Kit *on page 589*

Crotamiton (kroe TAM i tonn)

U.S. Brand Names Eurax®

Mexican Brand Names Eurax®

Generic Available No

Pharmacologic Category Scabicidal Agent

Use Treatment of scabies (*Sarcoptes scabiei*) and symptomatic treatment of pruritus

Local Anesthetic/Vasoconstrictor Precautions No information available to require special precautions

Effects on Dental Treatment No significant effects or complications reported

Common Adverse Effects Frequency not defined. Topical:

Dermatologic: Pruritus, contact dermatitis, rash

Local: Local irritation

Miscellaneous: Allergic sensitivity reactions, warm sensation

Mechanism of Action Crotamiton has scabicidal activity against *Sarcoptes scabiei*; mechanism of action unknown

Pregnancy Risk Factor C

Crude Coal Tar *see* Coal Tar *on page 367*

Cruex® Cream [OTC] *see* Clotrimazole *on page 363*

Cryselle™ *see* Ethinyl Estradiol and Norgestrel *on page 557*

Crystalline Penicillin *see* Penicillin G (Parenteral/Aqueous) *on page 1059*

Crystal Violet *see* Gentian Violet *on page 657*

Crystodigin *see* Digitoxin *on page 437*

CsA *see* CycloSPORINE *on page 386*

CSP *see* Cellulose Sodium Phosphate *on page 294*

CTM *see* Chlorpheniramine *on page 313*

CTX *see* Cyclophosphamide *on page 384*

Cubicin™ *see* Daptomycin *on page 399*

Cuprimine® *see* Penicillamine *on page 1057*

Curosurf® *see* Poractant Alfa *on page 1102*

Cutar® [OTC] *see* Coal Tar *on page 367*

Cutivate® *see* Fluticasone *on page 616*

CyA *see* CycloSPORINE *on page 386*

Cyanocobalamin (sye an oh koe BAL a min)

U.S. Brand Names Nascobal®

Canadian Brand Names Scheinpharm B12

Generic Available Yes

Synonyms Vitamin B_{12}

Pharmacologic Category Vitamin, Water Soluble

Use Treatment of pernicious anemia; vitamin B_{12} deficiency; increased B_{12} requirements due to pregnancy, thyrotoxicosis, hemorrhage, malignancy, liver or kidney disease

Local Anesthetic/Vasoconstrictor Precautions No information available to require special precautions

Effects on Dental Treatment No significant effects or complications reported

Significant Adverse Effects

1% to 10%:

- Central nervous system: Headache (2% to 11%), anxiety, dizziness, pain, nervousness, hypoesthesia
- Dermatologic: Itching
- Gastrointestinal: Sore throat, nausea and vomiting, dyspepsia, diarrhea
- Neuromuscular & skeletal: Weakness (1% to 4%), back pain, arthritis, myalgia, paresthesia, abnormal gait
- Respiratory: Dyspnea, rhinitis

<1% (Limited to important or life-threatening): Anaphylaxis, CHF, peripheral vascular thrombosis, pulmonary edema, urticaria

Dosage

Recommended daily allowance (RDA):
- Children: 0.3-2 mcg
- Adults: 2 mcg

Nutritional deficiency:
- Intranasal gel: 500 mcg once weekly
- Oral: 25-250 mcg/day

Anemias: I.M. or deep SubQ (oral is not generally recommended due to poor absorption and I.V. is not recommended due to more rapid elimination):
- Pernicious anemia, congenital (if evidence of neurologic involvement): 1000 mcg/day for at least 2 weeks; maintenance: 50-100 mcg/month or 100 mcg

for 6-7 days; if there is clinical improvement, give 100 mcg every other day for 7 doses, then every 3-4 days for 2-3 weeks; follow with 100 mcg/month for life. Administer with folic acid if needed.

Children: 30-50 mcg/day for 2 or more weeks (to a total dose of 1000-5000 mcg), then follow with 100 mcg/month as maintenance dosage

Adults: 100 mcg/day for 6-7 days; if improvement, administer same dose on alternate days for 7 doses; then every 3-4 days for 2-3 weeks; once hematologic values have returned to normal, maintenance dosage: 100 mcg/month. **Note:** Use only parenteral therapy as oral therapy is not dependable.

Hematologic remission (without evidence of nervous system involvement): Intranasal gel: 500 mcg once weekly

Vitamin B_{12} deficiency:

Children:

Neurologic signs: 100 mcg/day for 10-15 days (total dose of 1-1.5 mg), then once or twice weekly for several months; may taper to 60 mcg every month

Hematologic signs: 10-50 mcg/day for 5-10 days, followed by 100-250 mcg/dose every 2-4 weeks

Adults: Initial: 30 mcg/day for 5-10 days; maintenance: 100-200 mcg/month

Schilling test: I.M.: 1000 mcg

Mechanism of Action Coenzyme for various metabolic functions, including fat and carbohydrate metabolism and protein synthesis, used in cell replication and hematopoiesis

Contraindications Hypersensitivity to cyanocobalamin or any component of the formulation, cobalt; hereditary optic nerve atrophy, Leber's disease

Warnings/Precautions I.M. route used to treat pernicious anemia; vitamin B_{12} deficiency for >3 months results in irreversible degenerative CNS lesions; treatment of vitamin B_{12} megaloblastic anemia may result in severe hypokalemia, sometimes, fatal, when anemia corrects due to cellular potassium requirements. B_{12} deficiency masks signs of polycythemia vera; vegetarian diets may result in B_{12} deficiency; pernicious anemia occurs more often in gastric carcinoma than in general population. Patients with Leber's disease may suffer rapid optic atrophy when treated with vitamin B_{12}.

Drug Interactions Neomycin, colchicine, anticonvulsants may decrease absorption, chloramphenicol may decrease B_{12} effects

Pharmacodynamics/Kinetics

Absorption: From the terminal ileum in presence of calcium; gastric "intrinsic factor" must be present to transfer the compound across the intestinal mucosa

Distribution: Principally stored in the liver, also stored in the kidneys and adrenals

Protein binding: To transcobalamin II

Metabolism: Converted in tissues to active coenzymes, methylcobalamin and deoxyadenosylcobalamin

Pregnancy Risk Factor A/C (dose exceeding RDA recommendation); C (nasal gel)

Lactation Enters breast milk/compatible

Dosage Forms

Gel, intranasal (Nascobal®): 500 mcg/0.1 mL (2.3 mL)

Injection, solution: 1000 mcg/mL (1 mL, 10 mL, 30 mL) [products may contain benzyl alcohol]

Lozenge [OTC]: 100 mcg, 250 mcg, 500 mcg

Tablet [OTC]: 50 mcg, 100 mcg, 250 mcg, 500 mcg, 1000 mcg, 5000 mcg

Tablet, extended release [OTC]: 1500 mcg

Tablet, sublingual [OTC]: 2500 mcg

Cyanocobalamin, Folic Acid, and Pyridoxine *see* Folic Acid, Cyanocobalamin, and Pyridoxine *on page 626*

Cyclessa® *see* Ethinyl Estradiol and Desogestrel *on page 536*

Cyclizine (SYE kli zeen)

U.S. Brand Names Marezine® [OTC]

Generic Available No

Synonyms Cyclizine Hydrochloride; Cyclizine Lactate

Pharmacologic Category Antihistamine

Use Prevention and treatment of nausea, vomiting, and vertigo associated with motion sickness; control of postoperative nausea and vomiting

Local Anesthetic/Vasoconstrictor Precautions No information available to require special precautions

(Continued)

Cyclizine *(Continued)*

Effects on Dental Treatment Key adverse event(s) related to dental treatment: Xerostomia (normal salivary flow resumes upon discontinuation).

Common Adverse Effects

>10%:

Central nervous system: Drowsiness
Gastrointestinal: Xerostomia

1% to 10%:

Central nervous system: Headache
Dermatologic: Dermatitis
Gastrointestinal: Nausea
Genitourinary: Urinary retention
Ocular: Diplopia
Renal: Polyuria

Mechanism of Action Cyclizine is a piperazine derivative with properties of histamines. The precise mechanism of action in inhibiting the symptoms of motion sickness is not known. It may have effects directly on the labyrinthine apparatus and central actions on the labyrinthine apparatus and on the chemoreceptor trigger zone. Cyclizine exerts a central anticholinergic action.

Drug Interactions

Increased Effect/Toxicity: Increased effect/toxicity with CNS depressants, alcohol.

Pregnancy Risk Factor B

Cyclizine Hydrochloride *see* Cyclizine *on page 381*
Cyclizine Lactate *see* Cyclizine *on page 381*

Cyclobenzaprine (sye kloe BEN za preen)

Related Information

Temporomandibular Dysfunction (TMD) *on page 1564*

U.S. Brand Names Flexeril®

Canadian Brand Names Apo-Cyclobenzaprine®; Flexeril®; Flexitec; Gen-Cyclobenzaprine; Novo-Cycloprine; Nu-Cyclobenzaprine

Generic Available Yes

Synonyms Cyclobenzaprine Hydrochloride

Pharmacologic Category Skeletal Muscle Relaxant

Dental Use Treatment of muscle spasm associated with acute temporomandibular joint pain

Use Treatment of muscle spasm associated with acute painful musculoskeletal conditions

Local Anesthetic/Vasoconstrictor Precautions No information available to require special precautions

Effects on Dental Treatment Key adverse event(s) related to dental treatment: Xerostomia and changes in salivation (normal salivary flow resumes upon discontinuation).

Significant Adverse Effects

>10%:

Central nervous system: Drowsiness (29% to 39%), dizziness (1% to 11%)
Gastrointestinal: Xerostomia (21% to 32%)

1% to 10%:

Central nervous system: Fatigue (1% to 6%), confusion (1% to 3%), headache (1% to 3%), irritability (1% to 3%), mental acuity decreased (1% to 3%), nervousness (1% to 3%)
Gastrointestinal: Abdominal pain (1% to 3%), constipation (1% to 3%), diarrhea (1% to 3%), dyspepsia (1% to 3%), nausea (1% to 3%)
Neuromuscular & skeletal: Muscle weakness (1% to 3%)
Ocular: Blurred vision (1% to 3%)
Respiratory: Pharyngitis (1% to 3%)

<1% (Limited to important or life-threatening): Ageusia, agitation, anaphylaxis, angioedema, anorexia, arrhythmia, cholestasis, diplopia, facial edema, gastritis, hallucinations, hepatitis (rare), hypertonia, hypotension, insomnia, jaundice, liver function tests abnormal, malaise, palpitation, paresthesia, pruritus, psychosis, rash, seizures, tachycardia, thinking abnormal, tinnitus, tongue edema, tremors, urinary frequency, urinary retention, urticaria, vertigo, vomiting

Dosage Oral: **Note:** Do not use longer than 2-3 weeks

Adults: Initial: 5 mg 3 times/day; may increase to 10 mg 3 times/day if needed
Elderly: 5 mg 3 times/day; plasma concentration and incidence of adverse effects are increased in the elderly; dose should be titrated slowly

Dosage adjustment in hepatic impairment:

Mild: 5 mg 3 times/day; use with caution and titrate slowly
Moderate to severe: Use not recommended

Mechanism of Action Centrally-acting skeletal muscle relaxant pharmacologically related to tricyclic antidepressants; reduces tonic somatic motor activity influencing both alpha and gamma motor neurons

Contraindications Hypersensitivity to cyclobenzaprine or any component of the formulation; do not use concomitantly or within 14 days of MAO inhibitors; hyperthyroidism; congestive heart failure; arrhythmias; acute recovery phase of MI

Warnings/Precautions Cyclobenzaprine shares the toxic potentials of the tricyclic antidepressants and the usual precautions of tricyclic antidepressant therapy should be observed; use with caution in patients with urinary hesitancy, angle-closure glaucoma, hepatic impairment, or in the elderly. Do not use concomitantly or within 14 days after MAO inhibitors; combination may cause hypertensive crisis, severe convulsions. Safety and efficacy have not been established in patients <15 years of age.

Drug Interactions Substrate of CYP1A2 (major), 2D6 (minor), 3A4 (minor)

Anticholinergics: Because of cyclobenzaprine's anticholinergic action, use with caution in patients receiving these agents.

CNS depressants: Effects may be enhanced by cyclobenzaprine.

CYP1A2 inhibitors: May increase the levels/effects of cyclobenzaprine. Example inhibitors include amiodarone, ciprofloxacin, fluvoxamine, ketoconazole, lomefloxacin, ofloxacin, and rofecoxib.

Guanethidine: Antihypertensive effect of guanethidine may be decreased; effect seen with tricyclic antidepressants.

MAO inhibitors: Do not use concomitantly or within 14 days after MAO inhibitors.

Tramadol: May increase risk of seizure; effect seen with tricyclic antidepressants and tramadol.

Ethanol/Nutrition/Herb Interactions

Ethanol: Avoid ethanol (may increase CNS depression).

Herb/Nutraceutical: Avoid valerian, kava kava, gotu kola (may increase CNS depression).

Pharmacodynamics/Kinetics

Onset of action: ~1 hour

Duration: 12-24 hours

Absorption: Complete

Metabolism: Hepatic via CYP3A4, 1A2, and 2D6; may undergo enterohepatic recirculation

Bioavailability: 33% to 55%

Half-life elimination: 18 hours (range: 8-37 hours)

Time to peak, serum: 3-8 hours

Excretion: Urine (as inactive metabolites); feces (as unchanged drug)

Pregnancy Risk Factor B

Lactation Excretion in breast milk unknown/not recommended

Dosage Forms

Tablet, as hydrochloride: 10 mg

Flexeril®: 5 mg, 10 mg [film coated]

Cyclobenzaprine Hydrochloride *see* Cyclobenzaprine *on page 382*

Cyclocort® *see* Amcinonide *on page 93*

Cyclogyl® *see* Cyclopentolate *on page 383*

Cyclomydril® *see* Cyclopentolate and Phenylephrine *on page 384*

Cyclopentolate (sye kloe PEN toe late)

U.S. Brand Names AK-Pentolate®; Cyclogyl®; Cylate®

Canadian Brand Names Cyclogyl®; Diopentolate®

Generic Available Yes

Synonyms Cyclopentolate Hydrochloride

Pharmacologic Category Anticholinergic Agent, Ophthalmic

Use Diagnostic procedures requiring mydriasis and cycloplegia

Local Anesthetic/Vasoconstrictor Precautions No information available to require special precautions

Effects on Dental Treatment No significant effects or complications reported

Mechanism of Action Prevents the muscle of the ciliary body and the sphincter muscle of the iris from responding to cholinergic stimulation, causing mydriasis and cycloplegia

Pregnancy Risk Factor C

Cyclopentolate and Phenylephrine

(sye kloe PEN toe late & fen il EF rin)

Related Information

Cyclopentolate *on page 383*

U.S. Brand Names Cyclomydril®

Generic Available No

Synonyms Phenylephrine and Cyclopentolate

Pharmacologic Category Ophthalmic Agent, Antiglaucoma

Use Induce mydriasis greater than that produced with cyclopentolate HCl alone

Local Anesthetic/Vasoconstrictor Precautions No information available to require special precautions

Effects on Dental Treatment No significant effects or complications reported

Pregnancy Risk Factor C

Cyclopentolate Hydrochloride *see* Cyclopentolate *on page 383*

Cyclophosphamide (sye kloe FOS fa mide)

U.S. Brand Names Cytoxan®

Canadian Brand Names Cytoxan®; Procytox®

Mexican Brand Names Genoxal®; Ledoxina®

Generic Available Yes: Tablet

Synonyms CPM; CTX; CYT; NSC-26271

Pharmacologic Category Antineoplastic Agent, Alkylating Agent

Use

Oncologic: Treatment of Hodgkin's and non-Hodgkin's lymphoma, Burkitt's lymphoma, chronic lymphocytic leukemia (CLL), chronic myelocytic leukemia (CML), acute myelocytic leukemia (AML), acute lymphocytic leukemia (ALL), mycosis fungoides, multiple myeloma, neuroblastoma, retinoblastoma, rhabdomyosarcoma, Ewing's sarcoma; breast, testicular, endometrial, ovarian, and lung cancers, and in conditioning regimens for bone marrow transplantation

Nononcologic: Prophylaxis of rejection for kidney, heart, liver, and bone marrow transplants, severe rheumatoid disorders, nephrotic syndrome, Wegener's granulomatosis, idiopathic pulmonary hemosideroses, myasthenia gravis, multiple sclerosis, systemic lupus erythematosus, lupus nephritis, autoimmune hemolytic anemia, idiopathic thrombocytic purpura (ITP), macroglobulinemia, and antibody-induced pure red cell aplasia

Local Anesthetic/Vasoconstrictor Precautions No information available to require special precautions

Effects on Dental Treatment Key adverse event(s) related to dental treatment: Mucositis and stomatitis.

Common Adverse Effects

>10%:

Dermatologic: Alopecia (40% to 60%) but hair will usually regrow although it may be a different color and/or texture. Hair loss usually begins 3-6 weeks after the start of therapy.

Endocrine & metabolic: Fertility: May cause sterility; interferes with oogenesis and spermatogenesis; may be irreversible in some patients; gonadal suppression (amenorrhea)

Gastrointestinal: Nausea and vomiting occur more frequently with larger doses, usually beginning 6-10 hours after administration; anorexia, diarrhea, mucositis, and stomatitis are also seen

Genitourinary: Severe, potentially fatal acute hemorrhagic cystitis, believed to be a result of chemical irritation of the bladder by acrolein, a cyclophosphamide metabolite, occurs in 7% to 12% of patients and has been reported in up to 40% of patients in some series. Patients should be encouraged to drink plenty of fluids during therapy (most adults will require at least 2 L/day), void frequently, and avoid taking the drug at night. With large I.V. doses, I.V. hydration is usually recommended. The use of mesna and/or continuous bladder irrigation is rarely needed for doses <2 g/m^2.

Hematologic: Thrombocytopenia and anemia are less common than leukopenia

Onset: 7 days

Nadir: 10-14 days

Recovery: 21 days

1% to 10%:

Cardiovascular: Facial flushing

Central nervous system: Headache

Dermatologic: Skin rash

Renal: SIADH may occur, usually with doses >50 mg/kg (or 1 g/m^2); renal tubular necrosis, which usually resolves with discontinuation of the drug, is also reported

Respiratory: Nasal congestion occurs when I.V. doses are administered too rapidly (large doses via 30-60 minute infusion); patients experience runny eyes, rhinorrhea, sinus congestion, and sneezing during or immediately after the infusion. If needed, a decongestant or decongestant/antihistamine (eg, pseudoephedrine or pseudoephedrine/triprolidine) can be used to prevent or relieve these symptoms.

Mechanism of Action Cyclophosphamide is an alkylating agent that prevents cell division by cross-linking DNA strands and decreasing DNA synthesis. It is a cell cycle phase nonspecific agent. Cyclophosphamide also possesses potent immunosuppressive activity. Cyclophosphamide is a prodrug that must be metabolized to active metabolites in the liver.

Drug Interactions

Cytochrome P450 Effect: Substrate of CYP2A6 (minor), 2B6 (major), 2C8/9 (minor), 2C19 (minor), 3A4 (major); **Inhibits** CYP3A4 (weak); **Induces** CYP2B6 (weak), 2C8/9 (weak)

Increased Effect/Toxicity: Allopurinol may cause an increase in bone marrow depression and may result in significant elevations of cyclophosphamide cytotoxic metabolites.

Anesthetic agents: Cyclophosphamide reduces serum pseudocholinesterase concentrations and may prolong the neuromuscular blocking activity of succinylcholine. Use with caution with halothane, nitrous oxide, and succinylcholine.

Chloramphenicol causes prolonged cyclophosphamide half-life and increased toxicity.

CYP2B6 inducers: CYP2B6 inducers may increase the levels/effects of acrolein (the active metabolite of cyclophosphamide). Example inducers include carbamazepine, nevirapine, phenobarbital, phenytoin, and rifampin.

CYP3A4 inducers: CYP3A4 inducers may increase the levels/effects of acrolein (the active metabolite of cyclophosphamide). Example inducers include aminoglutethimide, carbamazepine, nafcillin, nevirapine, phenobarbital, phenytoin, and rifamycins.

Doxorubicin: Cyclophosphamide may enhance cardiac toxicity of anthracyclines.

Tetrahydrocannabinol results in enhanced immunosuppression in animal studies.

Thiazide diuretics: Leukopenia may be prolonged.

Decreased Effect: Cyclophosphamide may decrease digoxin serum levels. CYP2B6 inhibitors may decrease the levels/effects of acrolein (the active metabolite of cyclophosphamide); example inhibitors include desipramine, paroxetine, and sertraline. CYP3A4 inhibitors may decrease the levels/effects of acrolein (the active metabolite of cyclophosphamide); example inhibitors include azole antifungals, ciprofloxacin, clarithromycin, diclofenac, doxycycline, erythromycin, imatinib, isoniazid, nefazodone, nicardipine, propofol, protease inhibitors, quinidine, and verapamil.

Pharmacodynamics/Kinetics

Absorption: Oral: Well absorbed

Distribution: V_d: 0.48-0.71 L/kg; crosses placenta; crosses into CSF (not in high enough concentrations to treat meningeal leukemia)

Protein binding: 10% to 56%

Metabolism: Hepatic to active metabolites acrolein, 4-aldophosphamide, 4-hydroperoxycyclophosphamide, and nor-nitrogen mustard

Bioavailability: >75%

Half-life elimination: 4-8 hours

Time to peak, serum: Oral: ~1 hour

Excretion: Urine (<30% as unchanged drug, 85% to 90% as metabolites)

Pregnancy Risk Factor D

CycloSERINE (sye kloe SER een)

Related Information

Tuberculosis *on page 1495*

U.S. Brand Names Seromycin®

Generic Available No

Pharmacologic Category Antibiotic, Miscellaneous; Antitubercular Agent

Use Adjunctive treatment in pulmonary or extrapulmonary tuberculosis

Unlabeled/Investigational Use Treatment of Gaucher's disease

Local Anesthetic/Vasoconstrictor Precautions No information available to require special precautions

(Continued)

CycloSERINE *(Continued)*

Effects on Dental Treatment No significant effects or complications reported

Common Adverse Effects Frequency not defined.

Cardiovascular: Cardiac arrhythmias

Central nervous system: Drowsiness, headache, dizziness, vertigo, seizures, confusion, psychosis, paresis, coma

Dermatologic: Rash

Endocrine & metabolic: Vitamin B_{12} deficiency

Hematologic: Folate deficiency

Hepatic: Liver enzymes increased

Neuromuscular & skeletal: Tremor

Mechanism of Action Inhibits bacterial cell wall synthesis by competing with amino acid (D-alanine) for incorporation into the bacterial cell wall; bacteriostatic or bactericidal

Drug Interactions

Increased Effect/Toxicity: Alcohol, isoniazid, and ethionamide increase toxicity of cycloserine. Cycloserine inhibits the hepatic metabolism of phenytoin and may increase risk of epileptic seizures.

Pharmacodynamics/Kinetics

Absorption: ~70% to 90%

Distribution: Widely to most body fluids and tissues including CSF, breast milk, bile, sputum, lymph tissue, lungs, and ascitic, pleural, and synovial fluids; crosses placenta

Half-life elimination: Normal renal function: 10 hours

Metabolism: Hepatic

Time to peak, serum: 3-4 hours

Excretion: Urine (60% to 70% as unchanged drug) within 72 hours; feces (small amounts); remainder metabolized

Pregnancy Risk Factor C

Cyclosporin A *see* CycloSPORINE *on page 386*

CycloSPORINE (SYE kloe spor een)

U.S. Brand Names Gengraf®; Neoral®; Restasis™; Sandimmune®

Canadian Brand Names Apo-Cyclosporine®; Neoral®; Rhoxal-cyclosporine; Sandimmune® I.V.

Generic Available Yes

Synonyms CsA; CyA; Cyclosporin A

Pharmacologic Category Immunosuppressant Agent

Use Prophylaxis of organ rejection in kidney, liver, and heart transplants, has been used with azathioprine and/or corticosteroids; severe, active rheumatoid arthritis (RA) not responsive to methotrexate alone; severe, recalcitrant plaque psoriasis in nonimmunocompromised adults unresponsive to or unable to tolerate other systemic therapy

Ophthalmic emulsion (Restasis™): Increase tear production when suppressed tear production is presumed to be due to keratoconjunctivitis sicca-associated ocular inflammation (in patients not already using topical anti-inflammatory drugs or punctal plugs)

Unlabeled/Investigational Use Short-term, high-dose cyclosporine as a modulator of multidrug resistance in cancer treatment; allogenic bone marrow transplants for prevention and treatment of graft-versus-host disease; also used in some cases of severe autoimmune disease (ie, SLE, myasthenia gravis) that are resistant to corticosteroids and other therapy; focal segmental glomerulosclerosis

Local Anesthetic/Vasoconstrictor Precautions No information available to require special precautions

Effects on Dental Treatment Key adverse event(s) related to dental treatment: Gingival hypertrophy, mouth sores, swallowing difficulty, gingivitis, gum hyperplasia, xerostomia (normal salivary flow resumes upon discontinuation), abnormal taste, tongue disorder, tooth disorder, gum hyperplasia, and gingival bleeding.

Common Adverse Effects Note: Adverse reactions reported with kidney, liver, and heart transplantation, unless otherwise noted. Although percentage is reported for specific condition, reaction may occur in anyone taking cyclosporine. [Reactions reported for rheumatoid arthritis (RA) are based on cyclosporine (modified) 2.5 mg/kg/day versus placebo.]

>10%:

Cardiovascular: Hypertension (13% to 53%; psoriasis 25% to 27%)

Central nervous system: Headache (2% to 15%; RA 17%, psoriasis 14% to 16%)

Dermatologic: Hirsutism (21% to 45%), hypertrichosis (RA 19%)
Endocrine & metabolic: Increased triglycerides (psoriasis 15%), female reproductive disorder (psoriasis 8% to 11%)
Gastrointestinal: Nausea (RA 23%), diarrhea (RA 12%), gum hyperplasia (4% to 16%), abdominal discomfort (RA 15%), dyspepsia (RA 12%)
Neuromuscular & skeletal: Tremor (12% to 55%)
Renal: Renal dysfunction/nephropathy (25% to 38%; RA 10%, psoriasis 21%), creatinine elevation ≥50% (RA 24%), increased creatinine (psoriasis 16% to 20%)
Respiratory: Upper respiratory infection (psoriasis 8% to 11%)
Miscellaneous: Infection (psoriasis 24% to 25%)

Kidney, liver, and heart transplant only (≤2% unless otherwise noted):
Cardiovascular: Flushes (<1% to 4%), myocardial infarction
Central nervous system: Convulsions (1% to 5%), anxiety, confusion, fever, lethargy
Dermatologic: Acne (1% to 6%), brittle fingernails, hair breaking, pruritus
Endocrine & metabolic: Gynecomastia (<1% to 4%), hyperglycemia
Gastrointestinal: Nausea (2% to 10%), vomiting (2% to 10%), diarrhea (3% to 8%), abdominal discomfort (<1% to 7%), cramps (0% to 4%), anorexia, constipation, gastritis, mouth sores, pancreatitis, swallowing difficulty, upper GI bleed, weight loss
Hematologic: Leukopenia (<1% to 6%), anemia, thrombocytopenia
Hepatic: Hepatotoxicity (<1% to 7%)
Neuromuscular & skeletal: Paresthesia (1% to 3%), joint pain, muscle pain, tingling, weakness
Ocular: Conjunctivitis, visual disturbance
Otic: Hearing loss, tinnitus
Renal: Hematuria
Respiratory: Sinusitis (<1% to 7%)
Miscellaneous: Lymphoma (<1% to 6%), allergic reactions, hiccups, night sweats

Rheumatoid arthritis only (1% to <3% unless otherwise noted):
Cardiovascular: Hypertension (8%), edema (5%), chest pain (4%), arrhythmia (2%), abnormal heart sounds, cardiac failure, myocardial infarction, peripheral ischemia
Central nervous system: Dizziness (8%), pain (6%), insomnia (4%), depression (3%), migraine (2%), anxiety, hypoesthesia, emotional lability, impaired concentration, malaise, nervousness, paranoia, somnolence, vertigo
Dermatologic: Purpura (3%), abnormal pigmentation, angioedema, cellulitis, dermatitis, dry skin, eczema, folliculitis, nail disorder, pruritus, skin disorder, urticaria
Endocrine & metabolic: Menstrual disorder (3%), breast fibroadenosis, breast pain, diabetes mellitus, goiter, hot flashes, hyperkalemia, hyperuricemia, hypoglycemia, libido increased/decreased
Gastrointestinal: Vomiting (9%), flatulence (5%), gingivitis (4%), gum hyperplasia (2%), constipation, dry mouth, dysphagia, enanthema, eructation, esophagitis, gastric ulcer, gastritis, gastroenteritis, gingival bleeding, glossitis, peptic ulcer, salivary gland enlargement, taste perversion, tongue disorder, tooth disorder, weight loss/gain
Genitourinary: Leukorrhea (1%), abnormal urine, micturition urgency, nocturia, polyuria, pyelonephritis, urinary incontinence, uterine hemorrhage
Hematologic: Anemia, leukopenia
Hepatic: Bilirubinemia
Neuromuscular & skeletal: Paresthesia (8%), tremor (8%), leg cramps/muscle contractions (2%), arthralgia, bone fracture, joint dislocation, myalgia, neuropathy, stiffness, synovial cyst, tendon disorder, weakness
Ocular: Abnormal vision, cataract, conjunctivitis, eye pain
Otic: Tinnitus, deafness, vestibular disorder
Renal: Increased BUN, hematuria, renal abscess
Respiratory: Cough (5%), dyspnea (5%), sinusitis (4%), abnormal chest sounds, bronchospasm, epistaxis
Miscellaneous: Infection (9%), abscess, allergy, bacterial infection, carcinoma, fungal infection, herpes simplex, herpes zoster, lymphadenopathy, moniliasis, diaphoresis increased, tonsillitis, viral infection

Psoriasis only (1% to <3% unless otherwise noted):
Cardiovascular: Chest pain, flushes
Central nervous system: Psychiatric events (4% to 5%), pain (3% to 4%), dizziness, fever, insomnia, nervousness, vertigo
Dermatologic: Hypertrichosis (5% to 7%), acne, dry skin, folliculitis, keratosis, pruritus, rash, skin malignancies

(Continued)

CycloSPORINE *(Continued)*

Endocrine & metabolic: Hot flashes

Gastrointestinal: Nausea (5% to 6%), diarrhea (5% to 6%), gum hyperplasia (4% to 6%), abdominal discomfort (3% to 6%), dyspepsia (2% to 3%), abdominal distention, appetite increased, constipation, gingival bleeding

Genitourinary: Micturition increased

Hematologic: Bleeding disorder, clotting disorder, platelet disorder, red blood cell disorder

Hepatic: Hyperbilirubinemia

Neuromuscular & skeletal: Paresthesia (5% to 7%), arthralgia (1% to 6%)

Ocular: Abnormal vision

Respiratory: Bronchospasm (5%), cough (5%), dyspnea (5%), rhinitis (5%), respiratory infection

Miscellaneous: Flu-like symptoms (8% to 10%)

Ophthalmic emulsion (Restasis™):

>10%: Ocular: Burning (17%)

1% to 10%: Ocular: Hyperemia (conjunctival 5%), eye pain, pruritus, stinging

Mechanism of Action Inhibition of production and release of interleukin II and inhibits interleukin II-induced activation of resting T-lymphocytes.

Drug Interactions

Cytochrome P450 Effect: Substrate of CYP3A4 (major); **Inhibits** CYP2C8/9 (weak), 3A4 (moderate)

Increased Effect/Toxicity: The levels/effects of cyclosporine may be increased by allopurinol, azole antifungals, ciprofloxacin, clarithromycin, diclofenac, doxycycline, erythromycin, imatinib, isoniazid, metoclopramide, nefazodone, nicardipine, octreotide, propofol, protease inhibitors, quinidine, telithromycin, verapamil, and other CYP3A4 inhibitors. Cyclosporine may increase the levels/effects of selected benzodiazepines, calcium channel blockers, cisapride, cyclosporine, ergot alkaloids, selected HMG-CoA reductase inhibitors, mesoridazine, mirtazapine, nateglinide, nefazodone, pimozide, prednisolone (dosage adjustment may be required), quinidine, sildenafil (and other PDE-5 inhibitors), tacrolimus, thioridazine, venlafaxine, and other CYP3A4 substrates. Drugs that enhance nephrotoxicity of cyclosporine include aminoglycosides, amphotericin B, acyclovir, cimetidine, ketoconazole, lovastatin, melphalan, NSAIDs, ranitidine, and trimethoprim and sulfamethoxazole, Cyclosporine increases toxicity of digoxin, diuretics, methotrexate, nifedipine.

Decreased Effect: Isoniazid and ticlopidine decrease cyclosporine concentrations. The levels/effects of cyclosporine may be decreased by aminoglutethimide, carbamazepine, nafcillin, nevirapine, phenobarbital, phenytoin, rifamycins, and other CYP3A4 inducers. Orlistat may decrease absorption of cyclosporine; avoid concomitant use. Vaccination may be less effective; avoid use of live vaccines during therapy.

Pharmacodynamics/Kinetics

Absorption:

Ophthalmic emulsion: Serum concentrations not detectable.

Oral:

Cyclosporine (non-modified): Erratic and incomplete; dependent on presence of food, bile acids, and GI motility; larger oral doses are needed in pediatrics due to shorter bowel length and limited intestinal absorption

Cyclosporine (modified): Erratic and incomplete; increased absorption, up to 30% when compared to cyclosporine (non-modified); less dependent on food, bile acids, or GI motility when compared to cyclosporine (non-modified)

Distribution: Widely in tissues and body fluids including the liver, pancreas, and lungs; crosses placenta; enters breast milk

V_{dss}: 4-6 L/kg in renal, liver, and marrow transplant recipients (slightly lower values in cardiac transplant patients; children <10 years have higher values)

Protein binding: 90% to 98% to lipoproteins

Metabolism: Extensively hepatic via CYP; forms at least 25 metabolites; extensive first-pass effect following oral administration

Bioavailability: Oral:

Cyclosporine (non-modified): Dependent on patient population and transplant type (<10% in adult liver transplant patients and as high as 89% in renal transplant patients); bioavailability of Sandimmune® capsules and oral solution are equivalent; bioavailability of oral solution is ~30% of the I.V. solution

Children: 28% (range: 17% to 42%); gut dysfunction common in BMT patients and oral bioavailability is further reduced

Cyclosporine (modified): Bioavailability of Neoral® capsules and oral solution are equivalent:
Children: 43% (range: 30% to 68%)
Adults: 23% greater than with cyclosporine (non-modified) in renal transplant patients; 50% greater in liver transplant patients
Half-life elimination: Oral: May be prolonged in patients with hepatic impairment and shorter in pediatric patients due to the higher metabolism rate
Cyclosporine (non-modified): Biphasic: Alpha: 1.4 hours; Terminal: 19 hours (range: 10-27 hours)
Cyclosporine (modified): Biphasic: Terminal: 8.4 hours (range: 5-18 hours)
Time to peak, serum: Oral:
Cyclosporine (non-modified): 2-6 hours; some patients have a second peak at 5-6 hours
Cyclosporine (modified): Renal transplant: 1.5-2 hours
Excretion: Primarily feces; urine (6%, 0.1% as unchanged drug and metabolites)

Pregnancy Risk Factor C

Cyklokapron® *see* Tranexamic Acid *on page 1323*
Cylate® *see* Cyclopentolate *on page 383*
Cylert® *see* Pemoline *on page 1055*
Cylex® [OTC] *see* Benzocaine *on page 191*

Cyproheptadine (si proe HEP ta deen)

Canadian Brand Names Periactin®
Mexican Brand Names Viternum®
Generic Available Yes
Synonyms Cyproheptadine Hydrochloride; Periactin
Pharmacologic Category Antihistamine
Use Perennial and seasonal allergic rhinitis and other allergic symptoms including urticaria
Unlabeled/Investigational Use Appetite stimulation, blepharospasm, cluster headaches, migraine headaches, Nelson's syndrome, pruritus, schizophrenia, spinal cord damage associated spasticity, and tardive dyskinesia
Local Anesthetic/Vasoconstrictor Precautions No information available to require special precautions
Effects on Dental Treatment Key adverse event(s) related to dental treatment: Xerostomia (normal salivary flow resumes upon discontinuation).
Common Adverse Effects
>10%:
Central nervous system: Slight to moderate drowsiness
Respiratory: Thickening of bronchial secretions
1% to 10%:
Central nervous system: Headache, fatigue, nervousness, dizziness
Gastrointestinal: Appetite stimulation, nausea, diarrhea, abdominal pain, xerostomia
Neuromuscular & skeletal: Arthralgia
Respiratory: Pharyngitis
Mechanism of Action A potent antihistamine and serotonin antagonist, competes with histamine for H_1-receptor sites on effector cells in the gastrointestinal tract, blood vessels, and respiratory tract
Drug Interactions
Increased Effect/Toxicity: Cyproheptadine may potentiate the effect of CNS depressants. MAO inhibitors may cause hallucinations when taken with cyproheptadine.
Pharmacodynamics/Kinetics
Absorption: Completely
Metabolism: Almost completely hepatic
Excretion: Urine (>50% primarily as metabolites); feces (~25%)
Pregnancy Risk Factor B

Cyproheptadine Hydrochloride *see* Cyproheptadine *on page 389*
Cystadane® *see* Betaine Anhydrous *on page 199*
Cystagon® *see* Cysteamine *on page 389*

Cysteamine (sis TEE a meen)

U.S. Brand Names Cystagon®
Generic Available No
Synonyms Cysteamine Bitartrate
Pharmacologic Category Anticystine Agent; Urinary Tract Product
(Continued)

Cysteamine *(Continued)*

Use Orphan drug: Treatment of nephropathic cystinosis

Local Anesthetic/Vasoconstrictor Precautions No information available to require special precautions

Effects on Dental Treatment No significant effects or complications reported

Mechanism of Action Reacts with cystine in the lysosome to convert it to cysteine and to a cysteine-cysteamine mixed disulfide, both of which can then exit the lysosome in patients with cystinosis, an inherited defect of lysosomal transport

Pregnancy Risk Factor C

Cysteamine Bitartrate *see* Cysteamine *on page 389*

Cysteine (SIS te een)

Generic Available Yes

Synonyms Cysteine Hydrochloride

Pharmacologic Category Nutritional Supplement

Use Supplement to crystalline amino acid solutions, in particular the specialized pediatric formulas (eg, Aminosyn® PF, TrophAmine®) to meet the intravenous amino acid nutritional requirements of infants receiving parenteral nutrition (PN)

Local Anesthetic/Vasoconstrictor Precautions No information available to require special precautions

Effects on Dental Treatment No significant effects or complications reported

Mechanism of Action Cysteine is a sulfur-containing amino acid synthesized from methionine via the transulfuration pathway. It is a precursor of the tripeptide glutathione and also of taurine. Newborn infants have a relative deficiency of the enzyme necessary to affect this conversion. Cysteine may be considered an essential amino acid in infants.

Cysteine Hydrochloride *see* Cysteine *on page 390*

Cystospaz® *see* Hyoscyamine *on page 724*

Cystospaz-M® *see* Hyoscyamine *on page 724*

CYT *see* Cyclophosphamide *on page 384*

Cytadren® *see* Aminoglutethimide *on page 98*

Cytarabine (sye TARE a been)

U.S. Brand Names Cytosar-U®

Canadian Brand Names Cytosar®

Mexican Brand Names Laracit®

Generic Available Yes

Synonyms Arabinosylcytosine; Ara-C; Cytarabine Hydrochloride; Cytosine Arabinosine Hydrochloride; NSC-63878

Pharmacologic Category Antineoplastic Agent, Antimetabolite

Use Cytarabine is one of the most active agents in leukemia; also active against lymphoma, meningeal leukemia, and meningeal lymphoma; has little use in the treatment of solid tumors

Local Anesthetic/Vasoconstrictor Precautions No information available to require special precautions

Effects on Dental Treatment Key adverse event(s) related to dental treatment: Mucositis.

Common Adverse Effects

>10%:

- Central nervous system: Fever (>80%)
- Dermatologic: Alopecia
- Gastrointestinal: Nausea, vomiting, diarrhea, and mucositis which subside quickly after discontinuing the drug; GI effects may be more pronounced with divided I.V. bolus doses than with continuous infusion
- Hematologic: Myelosuppression; neutropenia and thrombocytopenia are severe, anemia may also occur
  - Onset: 4-7 days
  - Nadir: 14-18 days
  - Recovery: 21-28 days
- Hepatic: Hepatic dysfunction, mild jaundice, and acute increases in transaminases can be produced
- Ocular: Tearing, ocular pain, foreign body sensation, photophobia, and blurred vision may occur with high-dose therapy; ophthalmic corticosteroids usually prevent or relieve the condition

1% to 10%:

- Cardiovascular: Thrombophlebitis, cardiomegaly

Central nervous system: Dizziness, headache, somnolence, confusion, malaise; a severe cerebellar toxicity occurs in about 8% of patients receiving a high dose (>36-48 g/m^2/cycle); it is irreversible or fatal in about 1%

Dermatologic: Skin freckling, itching, cellulitis at injection site; rash, pain, erythema, and skin sloughing of the palmar and plantar surfaces may occur with high-dose therapy. Prophylactic topical steroids and/or skin moisturizers may be useful.

Genitourinary: Urinary retention

Neuromuscular & skeletal: Myalgia, bone pain

Respiratory: Syndrome of sudden respiratory distress, including tachypnea, hypoxemia, interstitial and alveolar infiltrates progressing to pulmonary edema, pneumonia

Mechanism of Action Inhibition of DNA synthesis. Cytosine gains entry into cells by a carrier process, and then must be converted to its active compound, aracytidine triphosphate. Cytosine is a purine analog and is incorporated into DNA; however, the primary action is inhibition of DNA polymerase resulting in decreased DNA synthesis and repair. The degree of cytotoxicity correlates linearly with incorporation into DNA; therefore, incorporation into the DNA is responsible for drug activity and toxicity. Cytarabine is specific for the S phase of the cell cycle.

Drug Interactions

Increased Effect/Toxicity: Alkylating agents and radiation and purine analogs when coadministered with cytarabine may result in increased toxic effects. Methotrexate, when administered prior to cytarabine, may enhance the efficacy and toxicity of cytarabine; some combination treatment regimens (eg, hyper-CVAD) have been designed to take advantage of this interaction.

Decreased Effect: Decreased effect of gentamicin, flucytosine. Decreased digoxin oral tablet absorption.

Pharmacodynamics/Kinetics

Distribution: V_d: Total body water; widely and rapidly since it enters the cells readily; crosses blood-brain barrier with CSF levels of 40% to 50% of plasma level

Metabolism: Primarily hepatic; aracytidine triphosphate is the active moiety; about 86% to 96% of dose is metabolized to inactive uracil arabinoside

Half-life elimination: Initial: 7-20 minutes; Terminal: 0.5-2.6 hours

Excretion: Urine (~80% as metabolites) within 24-36 hours

Pregnancy Risk Factor D

Cytarabine Hydrochloride *see* Cytarabine *on page 390*

Cytarabine (Liposomal) (sye TARE a been lip po SOE mal)

U.S. Brand Names DepoCyt™

Canadian Brand Names DepoCyt™

Generic Available No

Pharmacologic Category Antineoplastic Agent, Antimetabolite

Use Treatment of neoplastic (lymphomatous) meningitis

Local Anesthetic/Vasoconstrictor Precautions No information available to require special precautions

Effects on Dental Treatment No significant effects or complications reported

Common Adverse Effects Chemical arachnoiditis is commonly observed, and may include neck pain, neck rigidity, headache, fever, nausea, vomiting, and back pain. It may occur in up to 100% of cycles without dexamethasone prophylaxis. The incidence is reduced to 33% when dexamethasone is used concurrently.

>10%:

Central nervous system: Headache (28%), confusion (14%), somnolence (12%), fever (11%), pain (11%)

Gastrointestinal: Vomiting (12%), nausea (11%)

1% to 10%:

Cardiovascular: Peripheral edema (7%)

Gastrointestinal: Constipation (7%)

Genitourinary: Incontinence (3%)

Hematologic: Neutropenia (9%), thrombocytopenia (8%), anemia (1%)

Neuromuscular & skeletal: Back pain (7%), weakness (19%), abnormal gait (4%)

Mechanism of Action This is a sustained-release formulation of the active ingredient cytarabine, which acts through inhibition of DNA synthesis; cell cycle-specific for the S phase of cell division; cytosine gains entry into cells by a carrier process, and then must be converted to its active compound; cytosine acts as an analog and is incorporated into DNA; however, the primary action is

(Continued)

Cytarabine (Liposomal) *(Continued)*

inhibition of DNA polymerase resulting in decreased DNA synthesis and repair; degree of its cytotoxicity correlates linearly with its incorporation into DNA; therefore, incorporation into the DNA is responsible for drug activity and toxicity

Drug Interactions

Increased Effect/Toxicity: No formal studies of interactions with other medications have been conducted. The limited systemic exposure minimizes the potential for interaction between liposomal cytarabine and other medications.

Decreased Effect: No formal studies of interactions with other medications have been conducted. The limited systemic exposure minimizes the potential for interaction between liposomal cytarabine and other medications.

Pharmacodynamics/Kinetics

Absorption: Systemic exposure following intrathecal administration is negligible since transfer rate from CSF to plasma is slow
Metabolism: In plasma to ara-U (inactive)
Half-life elimination, CSF: 100-263 hours
Time to peak, CSF: Intrathecal: ~5 hours
Excretion: Primarily urine (as metabolites - ara-U)

Pregnancy Risk Factor D

Cytomel® *see* Liothyronine *on page 831*
Cytosar-U® *see* Cytarabine *on page 390*
Cytosine Arabinosine Hydrochloride *see* Cytarabine *on page 390*
Cytotec® *see* Misoprostol *on page 936*
Cytovene® *see* Ganciclovir *on page 646*
Cytoxan® *see* Cyclophosphamide *on page 384*
Cytra-2 *see* Sodium Citrate and Citric Acid *on page 1228*
Cytra-3 *see* Citric Acid, Sodium Citrate, and Potassium Citrate *on page 341*
Cytra-K *see* Potassium Citrate and Citric Acid *on page 1106*
D2E7 *see* Adalimumab *on page 67*
D_3 *see* Cholecalciferol *on page 323*
D-3-Mercaptovaline *see* Penicillamine *on page 1057*
d4T *see* Stavudine *on page 1238*

Dacarbazine (da KAR ba zeen)

U.S. Brand Names DTIC-Dome®

Canadian Brand Names DTIC®

Generic Available Yes

Synonyms DIC; Dimethyl Triazeno Imidazol Carboxamide; DTIC; Imidazol Carboxamide Dimethyltriazene; Imidazole Carboxamide; WR-139007

Pharmacologic Category Antineoplastic Agent, Alkylating Agent (Triazene)

Use Treatment of malignant melanoma, Hodgkin's disease, soft-tissue sarcomas, fibrosarcomas, rhabdomyosarcoma, islet cell carcinoma, medullary carcinoma of the thyroid, and neuroblastoma

Local Anesthetic/Vasoconstrictor Precautions No information available to require special precautions

Effects on Dental Treatment Key adverse event(s) related to dental treatment: Metallic taste.

Common Adverse Effects

>10%:

Gastrointestinal: Nausea and vomiting (>90%), can be severe and dose-limiting; nausea and vomiting decrease on successive days when dacarbazine is given daily for 5 days; diarrhea

Hematologic: Myelosuppression, leukopenia, thrombocytopenia - dose-limiting
Onset: 5-7 days
Nadir: 7-10 days
Recovery: 21-28 days

Local: Pain on infusion, may be minimized by administration through a central line, or by administration as a short infusion (eg, 1-2 hours as opposed to bolus injection)

1% to 10%:

Dermatologic: Alopecia, rash, photosensitivity
Gastrointestinal: Anorexia, metallic taste
Miscellaneous: Flu-like syndrome (fever, myalgias, malaise)

Mechanism of Action Alkylating agent which appears to form methyl-carbonium ions that attack nucleophilic groups in DNA; cross-links strands of

DNA resulting in the inhibition of DNA, RNA, and protein synthesis, the exact mechanism of action is still unclear.

Drug Interactions

Cytochrome P450 Effect: Substrate (major) of CYP1A2, 2E1

Increased Effect/Toxicity: CYP1A2 inhibitors may increase the levels/effects of dacarbazine; example inhibitors include amiodarone, ciprofloxacin, fluvoxamine, ketoconazole, lomefloxacin, ofloxacin, and rofecoxib. CYP2E1 inhibitors may increase the levels/effects of dacarbazine; example inhibitors include disulfiram, isoniazid, and miconazole.

Decreased Effect: CYP1A2 inducers may decrease the levels/effects of dacarbazine; example inducers include aminoglutethimide, carbamazepine, phenobarbital, and rifampin. Patients may experience impaired immune response to vaccines; possible infection after administration of live vaccines in patients receiving immunosuppressants.

Pharmacodynamics/Kinetics

Onset of action: I.V.: 18-24 days

Distribution: V_d: 0.6 L/kg, exceeding total body water; suggesting binding to some tissue (probably liver)

Protein binding: 5%

Metabolism: Extensively hepatic; hepatobiliary excretion is probably of some importance; metabolites may also have an antineoplastic effect

Half-life elimination: Biphasic: Initial: 20-40 minutes; Terminal: 5 hours

Excretion: Urine (~30% to 50% as unchanged drug)

Pregnancy Risk Factor C

Daclizumab (dac KLYE zue mab)

U.S. Brand Names Zenapax®

Canadian Brand Names Zenapax®

Generic Available No

Pharmacologic Category Immunosuppressant Agent

Use Part of an immunosuppressive regimen (including cyclosporine and corticosteroids) for the prophylaxis of acute organ rejection in patients receiving renal transplant

Unlabeled/Investigational Use Graft-versus-host disease

Local Anesthetic/Vasoconstrictor Precautions No information available to require special precautions

Effects on Dental Treatment No significant effects or complications reported

Common Adverse Effects Although reported adverse events are frequent, when daclizumab is compared with placebo the incidence of adverse effects is similar between the two groups. Many of the adverse effects reported during clinical trial use of daclizumab may be related to the patient population, transplant procedure, and concurrent transplant medications. Diarrhea, fever, postoperative pain, pruritus, respiratory tract infections, urinary tract infections, and vomiting occurred more often in children than adults.

≥5%:

Cardiovascular: Chest pain, edema, hypertension, hypotension, tachycardia, thrombosis

Central nervous system: Dizziness, fatigue, fever, headache, insomnia, pain, post-traumatic pain, tremor

Dermatologic: Acne, cellulitis, wound healing impaired

Gastrointestinal: Abdominal distention, abdominal pain, constipation, diarrhea, dyspepsia, epigastric pain, nausea, pyrosis, vomiting

Genitourinary: Dysuria

Hematologic: Bleeding

Neuromuscular & skeletal: Back pain, musculoskeletal pain

Renal: Oliguria, renal tubular necrosis

Respiratory: Cough, dyspnea, pulmonary edema,

Miscellaneous: Lymphocele, wound infection

≥2% to <5%:

Central nervous system: Anxiety, depression, shivering

Dermatologic: Hirsutism, pruritus, rash

Endocrine & metabolic: Dehydration, diabetes mellitus, fluid overload

Gastrointestinal: Flatulence, gastritis, hemorrhoids

Genitourinary: Urinary retention, urinary tract bleeding

Local: Application site reaction

Neuromuscular & skeletal: Arthralgia, leg cramps, myalgia, weakness

Ocular: Vision blurred

Renal: Hydronephrosis, renal damage, renal insufficiency

Respiratory: Atelectasis, congestion, hypoxia, pharyngitis, pleural effusion, rales, rhinitis

Miscellaneous: Night sweats, prickly sensation, diaphoresis

(Continued)

Daclizumab *(Continued)*

Mechanism of Action Daclizumab is a chimeric (90% human, 10% murine) monoclonal IgG antibody produced by recombinant DNA technology. Daclizumab inhibits immune reactions by binding and blocking the alpha-chain of the interleukin-2 receptor (CD25) located on the surface of activated lymphocytes.

Drug Interactions

Increased Effect/Toxicity: The combined use of daclizumab, cyclosporine, mycophenolate mofetil, and corticosteroids has been associated with an increased mortality in a population of cardiac transplant recipients, particularly in patients who received antilymphocyte globulin and in patients with severe infections.

Pharmacodynamics/Kinetics

Distribution: V_d:

Adults: Central compartment: 0.031 L/kg; Peripheral compartment: 0.043 L/kg

Children: Central compartment: 0.067 L/kg; Peripheral compartment: 0.047 L/kg

Half-life elimination (estimated): Adults: Terminal: 20 days; Children: 13 days

Pregnancy Risk Factor C

DACT *see* Dactinomycin *on page 394*

Dactinomycin (dak ti noe MYE sin)

U.S. Brand Names Cosmegen®

Canadian Brand Names Cosmegen®

Mexican Brand Names Ac-De®

Generic Available No

Synonyms ACT; Act-D; Actinomycin; Actinomycin Cl; Actinomycin D; DACT; NSC-3053

Pharmacologic Category Antineoplastic Agent, Antibiotic

Use Treatment of testicular tumors, melanoma, choriocarcinoma, Wilms' tumor, neuroblastoma, retinoblastoma, rhabdomyosarcoma, uterine sarcomas, Ewing's sarcoma, Kaposi's sarcoma, sarcoma botryoides, and soft tissue sarcoma

Local Anesthetic/Vasoconstrictor Precautions No information available to require special precautions

Effects on Dental Treatment Key adverse event(s) related to dental treatment: Stomatitis and mucositis.

Common Adverse Effects

>10%:

Central nervous system: Fatigue, malaise, fever, lethargy

Dermatologic: Alopecia (reversible), skin eruptions, acne, increased pigmentation or sloughing of previously irradiated skin, maculopapular rash

Endocrine & metabolic: Hypocalcemia

Gastrointestinal: Severe nausea, vomiting, anorexia

Hematologic: Myelosuppression, anemia

Onset: 7 days

Nadir: 14-21 days

Recovery: 21-28 days

Local: Extravasation: An irritant and should be administered through a rapidly running I.V. line; extravasation can lead to tissue necrosis, pain, and ulceration

1% to 10%: Gastrointestinal: Mucositis, stomatitis, diarrhea, abdominal pain

Mechanism of Action Binds to the guanine portion of DNA intercalating between guanine and cytosine base pairs inhibiting DNA and RNA synthesis and protein synthesis

Drug Interactions

Increased Effect/Toxicity: Dactinomycin potentiates the effects of radiation therapy.

Pharmacodynamics/Kinetics

Distribution: High concentrations found in bone marrow and tumor cells, submaxillary gland, liver, and kidney; crosses placenta; poor CSF penetration

Metabolism: Hepatic, minimal

Half-life elimination: 36 hours

Time to peak, serum: I.V.: 2-5 minutes

Excretion: Bile (50%); feces (14%); urine (~10% as unchanged drug)

Pregnancy Risk Factor C

DAD *see* Mitoxantrone *on page 938*

D.A.II™ [DSC] *see* Chlorpheniramine, Phenylephrine, and Methscopolamine *on page 317*

Dakin's Solution *see* Sodium Hypochlorite Solution *on page 1228*

Dallergy® *see* Chlorpheniramine, Phenylephrine, and Methscopolamine *on page 317*

Dallergy-JR® *see* Chlorpheniramine and Phenylephrine *on page 314*

Dalmane® *see* Flurazepam *on page 612*

***d*-Alpha Tocopherol** *see* Vitamin E *on page 1383*

Dalteparin (dal TE pa rin)

Related Information

Cardiovascular Diseases *on page 1458*

U.S. Brand Names Fragmin®

Canadian Brand Names Fragmin®

Generic Available No

Pharmacologic Category Low Molecular Weight Heparin

Use Prevention of deep vein thrombosis which may lead to pulmonary embolism, in patients requiring abdominal surgery who are at risk for thromboembolism complications (eg, patients >40 years of age, obesity, patients with malignancy, history of deep vein thrombosis or pulmonary embolism, and surgical procedures requiring general anesthesia and lasting >30 minutes); prevention of DVT in patients undergoing hip-replacement surgery; patients immobile during an acute illness; acute treatment of unstable angina or non-Q-wave myocardial infarction; prevention of ischemic complications in patients on concurrent aspirin therapy

Unlabeled/Investigational Use Active treatment of deep vein thrombosis

Local Anesthetic/Vasoconstrictor Precautions No information available to require special precautions

Effects on Dental Treatment No significant effects or complications reported

Common Adverse Effects 1% to 10%

Hematologic: Bleeding (3% to 5%), wound hematoma (0.1% to 3%)

Local: Pain at injection site (up to 12%), injection site hematoma (0.2% to 7%)

Mechanism of Action Low molecular weight heparin analog with a molecular weight of 4000-6000 daltons; the commercial product contains 3% to 15% heparin with a molecular weight <3000 daltons, 65% to 78% with a molecular weight of 3000-8000 daltons and 14% to 26% with a molecular weight >8000 daltons; while dalteparin has been shown to inhibit both factor Xa and factor IIa (thrombin), the antithrombotic effect of dalteparin is characterized by a higher ratio of antifactor Xa to antifactor IIa activity (ratio = 4)

Drug Interactions

Increased Effect/Toxicity: The risk of bleeding with dalteparin may be increased by drugs which affect platelet function (eg, aspirin, NSAIDs, dipyridamole, ticlopidine, clopidogrel), oral anticoagulants, and thrombolytic agents. Although the risk of bleeding may be increased during concurrent warfarin therapy, dalteparin is commonly continued during the initiation of warfarin therapy to assure anticoagulation and to protect against possible transient hypercoagulability.

Pharmacodynamics/Kinetics

Onset of action: 1-2 hours

Duration: >12 hours

Half-life elimination (route dependent): 2-5 hours

Time to peak, serum: 4 hours

Pregnancy Risk Factor B

Damason-P® *see* Hydrocodone and Aspirin *on page 705*

Danaparoid (da NAP a roid)

U.S. Brand Names Orgaran® [DSC]

Canadian Brand Names Orgaran®

Generic Available No

Synonyms Danaparoid Sodium

Pharmacologic Category Anticoagulant

Use Prevention of postoperative deep vein thrombosis following elective hip replacement surgery

Unlabeled/Investigational Use Systemic anticoagulation for patients with heparin-induced thrombocytopenia: factor Xa inhibition is used to monitor degree of anticoagulation if necessary

Local Anesthetic/Vasoconstrictor Precautions No information available to require special precautions

Effects on Dental Treatment Key adverse event(s) related to dental treatment: As with all anticoagulants, bleeding is the major adverse effect of

(Continued)

Danaparoid *(Continued)*

danaparoid. Hemorrhage may occur at virtually any site; risk is dependent on multiple variables.

Common Adverse Effects As with all anticoagulants, bleeding is the major adverse effect of danaparoid. Hemorrhage may occur at virtually any site. Risk is dependent on multiple variables.

>10%:

Central nervous system: Fever (22%)

Gastrointestinal: Nausea (4% to 14%), constipation (4% to 11%)

1% to 10%:

Cardiovascular: Peripheral edema (3%), edema (3%)

Central nervous system: Insomnia (3%), headache (3%), asthenia (2%), dizziness (2%), pain (9%)

Dermatologic: Rash (2% to 5%), pruritus (4%)

Gastrointestinal: Vomiting (3%)

Genitourinary: Urinary tract infection (3% to 4%), urinary retention (2%)

Hematologic: Anemia (2%)

Local: Injection site pain (8% to 14%), injection site hematoma (5%)

Neuromuscular & skeletal: Joint disorder (3%)

Miscellaneous: Infection (2%)

Mechanism of Action Prevents fibrin formation in coagulation pathway via thrombin generation inhibition by anti-Xa and anti-IIa effects.

Drug Interactions

Increased Effect/Toxicity: The risk of hemorrhage associated with danaparoid may be increased with thrombolytic agents, oral anticoagulants (warfarin) and drugs which affect platelet function (eg, aspirin, NSAIDs, dipyridamole, ticlopidine, clopidogrel).

Pharmacodynamics/Kinetics

Onset of action: Peak effect: SubQ: Maximum antifactor Xa and antithrombin (antifactor IIa) activities occur in 2-5 hours

Half-life elimination, plasma: Mean: Terminal: ~24 hours

Excretion: Primarily urine

Pregnancy Risk Factor B

Danaparoid Sodium *see* Danaparoid *on page 395*

Danazol (DA na zole)

U.S. Brand Names Danocrine®

Canadian Brand Names Cyclomen®; Danocrine®

Mexican Brand Names Ladogal®; Norciden®

Generic Available Yes

Pharmacologic Category Androgen

Use Treatment of endometriosis, fibrocystic breast disease, and hereditary angioedema

Local Anesthetic/Vasoconstrictor Precautions No information available to require special precautions

Effects on Dental Treatment No significant effects or complications reported

Common Adverse Effects Frequency not defined.

Cardiovascular: Benign intracranial hypertension (rare), edema, flushing, hypertension

Central nervous system: Anxiety (rare), chills (rare), convulsions (rare), depression, dizziness, emotional lability, fainting, fever (rare), Guillain-Barré syndrome, headache, nervousness, sleep disorders, tremor

Dermatologic: Acne, hair loss, mild hirsutism, maculopapular rash, papular rash, petechial rash, pruritus, purpuric rash, seborrhea, Stevens-Johnson syndrome (rare), photosensitivity (rare), urticaria, vesicular rash

Endocrine & metabolic: Amenorrhea (which may continue post therapy), breast size reduction, clitoris hypertrophy, glucose intolerance, HDL decreased, LDL increased, libido changes, nipple discharge, menstrual disturbances (spotting, altered timing of cycle), semen abnormalities (changes in volume, viscosity, sperm count/motility), spermatogenesis reduction

Gastrointestinal: Appetite changes (rare), bleeding gums (rare), constipation, gastroenteritis, nausea, pancreatitis (rare), vomiting, weight gain

Genitourinary: Vaginal dryness, vaginal irritation, pelvic pain

Hematologic: Eosinophilia, erythrocytosis (reversible), leukocytosis, leukopenia, platelet count increased, polycythemia, RBC increased, thrombocytopenia

Hepatic: Cholestatic jaundice, hepatic adenoma, jaundice, liver enzymes (elevated), malignant tumors (after prolonged use), peliosis hepatis

Neuromuscular & skeletal: Back pain, carpal tunnel syndrome (rare), extremity pain, joint lockup, joint pain, joint swelling, muscle cramps, neck pain, paresthesias, spasms, weakness
Ocular: Cataracts (rare), visual disturbances
Renal: Hematuria
Respiratory: Nasal congestion (rare)
Miscellaneous: Voice change (hoarseness, sore throat, instability, deepening of pitch), diaphoresis

Mechanism of Action Suppresses pituitary output of follicle-stimulating hormone and luteinizing hormone that causes regression and atrophy of normal and ectopic endometrial tissue; decreases rate of growth of abnormal breast tissue; reduces attacks associated with hereditary angioedema by increasing levels of C4 component of complement

Drug Interactions

Cytochrome P450 Effect: Inhibits CYP3A4 (weak)

Increased Effect/Toxicity: Danazol may increase serum levels of carbamazepine, cyclosporine, tacrolimus, and warfarin leading to toxicity; dosage adjustment may be needed; monitor. Concomitant use of danazol and HMG-CoA reductase inhibitors may lead to severe myopathy or rhabdomyolysis. Danazol may enhance the glucose-lowering effect of hypoglycemic agents.

Decreased Effect: Danazol may decrease effectiveness of hormonal contraceptives. Nonhormonal birth control methods are recommended.

Pharmacodynamics/Kinetics

Onset of action: Therapeutic: ~4 weeks
Metabolism: Extensively hepatic, primarily to 2-hydroxymethylethisterone
Half-life elimination: 4.5 hours (variable)
Time to peak, serum: Within 2 hours
Excretion: Urine

Pregnancy Risk Factor X

Danocrine® *see* Danazol *on page 396*
Dantrium® *see* Dantrolene *on page 397*

Dantrolene (DAN troe leen)

U.S. Brand Names Dantrium®

Canadian Brand Names Dantrium®

Generic Available No

Synonyms Dantrolene Sodium

Pharmacologic Category Skeletal Muscle Relaxant

Use Treatment of spasticity associated with spinal cord injury, stroke, cerebral palsy, or multiple sclerosis; treatment of malignant hyperthermia

Unlabeled/Investigational Use Neuroleptic malignant syndrome (NMS)

Local Anesthetic/Vasoconstrictor Precautions No information available to require special precautions

Effects on Dental Treatment No significant effects or complications reported

Common Adverse Effects

>10%:
Central nervous system: Drowsiness, dizziness, lightheadedness, fatigue
Dermatologic: Rash
Gastrointestinal: Diarrhea (mild), nausea, vomiting
Neuromuscular & skeletal: Muscle weakness

1% to 10%:
Cardiovascular: Pleural effusion with pericarditis
Central nervous system: Chills, fever, headache, insomnia, nervousness, mental depression
Gastrointestinal: Diarrhea (severe), constipation, anorexia, stomach cramps
Ocular: Blurred vision
Respiratory: Respiratory depression

Mechanism of Action Acts directly on skeletal muscle by interfering with release of calcium ion from the sarcoplasmic reticulum; prevents or reduces the increase in myoplasmic calcium ion concentration that activates the acute catabolic processes associated with malignant hyperthermia

Drug Interactions

Cytochrome P450 Effect: Substrate of CYP3A4 (major)

Increased Effect/Toxicity: Increased toxicity with estrogens (hepatotoxicity), CNS depressants (sedation), MAO inhibitors, phenothiazines, clindamycin (increased neuromuscular blockade), verapamil (hyperkalemia and cardiac depression), warfarin, clofibrate, and tolbutamide. CYP3A4 inhibitors may increase the levels/effects of dantrolene; example inhibitors include azole antifungals, ciprofloxacin, clarithromycin, diclofenac, doxycycline,

(Continued)

Dantrolene *(Continued)*

erythromycin, imatinib, isoniazid, nefazodone, nicardipine, propofol, protease inhibitors, quinidine, and verapamil.

Decreased Effect: CYP3A4 inducers may decrease the levels/effects of dantrolene; example inducers include aminoglutethimide, carbamazepine, nafcillin, nevirapine, phenobarbital, phenytoin, and rifamycins.

Pharmacodynamics/Kinetics

Absorption: Oral: Slow and incomplete

Metabolism: Hepatic

Half-life elimination: 8.7 hours

Excretion: Feces (45% to 50%); urine (25% as unchanged drug and metabolites)

Pregnancy Risk Factor C

Dantrolene Sodium *see* Dantrolene *on page 397*

Dapcin *see* Daptomycin *on page 399*

Dapiprazole (DA pi pray zole)

U.S. Brand Names Rēv-Eyes™

Generic Available No

Synonyms Dapiprazole Hydrochloride

Pharmacologic Category Alpha$_1$ Blocker, Ophthalmic

Use Reverse dilation due to drugs (adrenergic or parasympathomimetic) after eye exams

Local Anesthetic/Vasoconstrictor Precautions No information available to require special precautions

Effects on Dental Treatment No significant effects or complications reported

Mechanism of Action Dapiprazole is a selective alpha-adrenergic blocking agent, exerting effects primarily on alpha$_1$-adrenoreceptors. It induces miosis via relaxation of the smooth dilator (radial) muscle of the iris, which causes pupillary constriction. It is devoid of cholinergic effects. Dapiprazole also partially reverses the cycloplegia induced with parasympatholytic agents such as tropicamide. Although the drug has no significant effect on the ciliary muscle *per se*, it may increase accommodative amplitude, therefore relieving the symptoms of paralysis of accommodation.

Pregnancy Risk Factor B

Dapiprazole Hydrochloride *see* Dapiprazole *on page 398*

Dapsone (DAP sone)

Related Information

HIV Infection and AIDS *on page 1484*

Mexican Brand Names Dapsoderm-X®

Generic Available Yes

Synonyms Diaminodiphenylsulfone

Pharmacologic Category Antibiotic, Miscellaneous

Use Treatment of leprosy and dermatitis herpetiformis (infections caused by *Mycobacterium leprae*)

Unlabeled/Investigational Use Prophylaxis of toxoplasmosis in severely-immunocompromised patients; alternative agent for *Pneumocystis carinii* pneumonia prophylaxis (monotherapy) and treatment (in combination with trimethoprim)

Local Anesthetic/Vasoconstrictor Precautions No information available to require special precautions

Effects on Dental Treatment No significant effects or complications reported

Common Adverse Effects 1% to 10%: Hematologic: Hemolysis, methemoglobinemia

Mechanism of Action Competitive antagonist of para-aminobenzoic acid (PABA) and prevents normal bacterial utilization of PABA for the synthesis of folic acid

Drug Interactions

Cytochrome P450 Effect: Substrate of CYP2C8/9 (minor), 2C19 (minor), 2E1 (minor), 3A4 (major)

Increased Effect/Toxicity: Folic acid antagonists (methotrexate) may increase the risk of hematologic reactions of dapsone; probenecid decreases dapsone excretion; trimethoprim with dapsone may increase toxic effects of both drugs. CYP3A4 inhibitors may increase the levels/effects of dapsone; example inhibitors include azole antifungals, ciprofloxacin, clarithromycin, diclofenac, doxycycline, erythromycin, imatinib, isoniazid, nefazodone, nicardipine, propofol, protease inhibitors, quinidine, and verapamil.

Decreased Effect: Para-aminobenzoic acid and rifampin levels are decreased when given with dapsone. CYP3A4 inducers may decrease the levels/effects of dapsone; example inducers include aminoglutethimide, carbamazepine, nafcillin, nevirapine, phenobarbital, phenytoin, and rifamycins.

Pharmacodynamics/Kinetics

Absorption: Well absorbed

Distribution: V_d: 1.5 L/kg; throughout total body water and present in all tissues, especially liver and kidney

Metabolism: Hepatic

Half-life elimination: 30 hours (range: 10-50 hours)

Excretion: Urine

Pregnancy Risk Factor C

Daptomycin (DAP toe mye sin)

U.S. Brand Names Cubicin™

Generic Available No

Synonyms Cidecin; Dapcin; LY146032

Pharmacologic Category Antibiotic, Cyclic Lipopeptide

Use Treatment of complicated skin and skin structure infections caused by susceptible aerobic Gram-positive organisms

Unlabeled/Investigational Use Treatment of MRSA, VRE, bacteremia, and endocarditis

Local Anesthetic/Vasoconstrictor Precautions No information available to require special precautions

Effects on Dental Treatment No significant effects or complications reported

Common Adverse Effects

1% to 10%:

Cardiovascular: Hypotension (2%), hypertension (1%)

Central nervous system: Headache (5%), insomnia (5%), dizziness (2%), fever (2%)

Dermatologic: Rash (4%), pruritus (3%)

Gastrointestinal: Constipation (6%), nausea (6%), diarrhea (5%), vomiting (3%), dyspepsia (1%)

Genitourinary: Urinary tract infection (2%)

Hematologic: Anemia (2%)

Hepatic: Transaminases increased (3%)

Local: Injection site reaction (6%)

Neuromuscular & skeletal: CPK increased (3%), limb pain (2%), arthralgia (1%)

Renal: Renal failure (2%)

Respiratory: Dyspnea (2%)

Miscellaneous: Infection (fungal, 3%)

Mechanism of Action Daptomycin binds to components of the cell membrane of susceptible organisms and causes rapid depolarization, inhibiting intracellular synthesis of DNA, RNA, and protein. Daptomycin is bactericidal and bacterial killing is concentration-dependent.

Drug Interactions

Increased Effect/Toxicity: No clinically-significant interactions have been identified. Theoretically, concurrent use of drugs which may cause myopathy may increase the risk of these reactions. Limited clinical studies with HMG-CoA reductase inhibitors have not demonstrated an increase in adverse effects.

Pharmacodynamics/Kinetics

Distribution: 0.09 L/kg

Protein binding: 92%

Half-life elimination: 8-9 hours (up to 28 hours in renal impairment)

Excretion: Urine (78%; primarily as unchanged drug); feces (6%)

Pregnancy Risk Factor B

Daranide® *see* Dichlorphenamide *on page 427*

Daraprim® *see* Pyrimethamine *on page 1154*

Darbepoetin Alfa (dar be POE e tin AL fa)

U.S. Brand Names Aranesp®

Canadian Brand Names Aranesp®

Generic Available No

Synonyms Erythropoiesis Stimulating Protein

Pharmacologic Category Colony Stimulating Factor; Growth Factor; Recombinant Human Erythropoietin

(Continued)

Darbepoetin Alfa *(Continued)*

Use Treatment of anemia associated with chronic renal failure (CRF), including patients on dialysis (ESRD) and patients not on dialysis; anemia associated with chemotherapy for nonmyeloid malignancies

Local Anesthetic/Vasoconstrictor Precautions No information available to require special precautions

Effects on Dental Treatment No significant effects or complications reported

Common Adverse Effects **Note:** Frequency of adverse events cited in patients with CRF or cancer and may be, in part, a reflection of population in which the drug is used and/or associated with dialysis procedures.

>10%:

Cardiovascular: Hypertension (4% to 23%), hypotension (22%), edema (21%), peripheral edema (11%), arrhythmia (10%)

Central nervous system: Fatigue (9% to 33%), fever (9% to 19%), headache (12% to 16%), dizziness (8% to 14%)

Gastrointestinal: Diarrhea (16% to 22%), constipation (5% to 18%) vomiting (15%), nausea (14%), abdominal pain (12%)

Neuromuscular & skeletal: Myalgia (21%), arthralgia (11% to 13%), limb pain (10%)

Respiratory: Upper respiratory infection (14%), dyspnea (12%), cough (10%)

Miscellaneous: Infection (27%)

1% to 10%:

Cardiovascular: Angina/chest pain (6% to 8%), fluid overload (6%), CHF (6%), thrombosis (6%), MI (2%)

Central nervous system: Seizure (<1% to 1%), stroke (1%), TIA (1%)

Dermatologic: Pruritus (8%), rash (7%)

Endocrine & metabolic: Dehydration (5%)

Local: Injection site pain (7%)

Neuromuscular & skeletal: Back pain (8%), weakness (5%)

Respiratory: Bronchitis (6%), pulmonary embolism (1%)

Miscellaneous: Vascular access thrombosis (8%, annualized rate 0.22 events per patient year), vascular access infection (6%), influenza-like symptoms (6%), vascular access hemorrhage (6%)

Mechanism of Action Induces erythropoiesis by stimulating the division and differentiation of committed erythroid progenitor cells; induces the release of reticulocytes from the bone marrow into the bloodstream, where they mature to erythrocytes. There is a dose response relationship with this effect. This results in an increase in reticulocyte counts followed by a rise in hematocrit and hemoglobin levels. When administered SubQ or I.V., darbepoetin's half-life is ~3 times that of epoetin alfa concentrations.

Pharmacodynamics/Kinetics

Onset of action: Increased hemoglobin levels not generally observed until 2-6 weeks after initiating treatment

Absorption: SubQ: Slow

Distribution: V_d: 0.06 L/kg

Bioavailability: CRF: SubQ: ~37% (range: 30% to 50%)

Half-life elimination: CRF: Terminal: I.V.: 21 hours, SubQ: 49 hours; **Note:** Half-life is ~3 times as long as epoetin alfa

Time to peak: SubQ: CRF: 34 hours (range: 24-72 hours); Cancer: 90 hours (range: 71-123 hours)

Pregnancy Risk Factor C

Darvocet A500™ *see* Propoxyphene and Acetaminophen *on page 1137*

Darvocet-N® 50 *see* Propoxyphene and Acetaminophen *on page 1137*

Darvocet-N® 100 *see* Propoxyphene and Acetaminophen *on page 1137*

Darvon® *see* Propoxyphene *on page 1136*

Darvon® Compound *see* Propoxyphene, Aspirin, and Caffeine *on page 1138*

Darvon-N® *see* Propoxyphene *on page 1136*

Daunomycin *see* DAUNOrubicin Hydrochloride *on page 401*

DAUNOrubicin Citrate (Liposomal)

(daw noe ROO bi sin SI trate lip po SOE mal)

U.S. Brand Names DaunoXome®

Generic Available No

Pharmacologic Category Antineoplastic Agent, Anthracycline

Use First-line cytotoxic therapy for advanced HIV-associated Kaposi's sarcoma

Local Anesthetic/Vasoconstrictor Precautions No information available to require special precautions

Effects on Dental Treatment Key adverse event(s) related to dental treatment: Stomatitis.

Common Adverse Effects

>10%:

Central nervous system: Fatigue (51%), headache (28%), neuropathy (13%)

Hematologic: Myelosuppression, neutropenia (51%), thrombocytopenia, anemia

Onset: 7 days

Nadir: 14 days

Recovery: 21 days

Gastrointestinal: Abdominal pain, vomiting, anorexia (23%); diarrhea (38%); nausea (55%)

Respiratory: Cough (28%), dyspnea (26%), rhinitis

Miscellaneous: Allergic reactions (24%)

1% to 10%:

Cardiovascular: Hypertension, palpitations, syncope, tachycardia, chest pain, edema

Dermatologic: Alopecia (8%), pruritus (7%)

Endocrine & metabolic: Hot flashes

Gastrointestinal: Constipation (7%), stomatitis (10%)

Neuromuscular & skeletal: Arthralgia (7%), myalgia (7%)

Ocular: Conjunctivitis, eye pain (5%)

Respiratory: Sinusitis

Mechanism of Action Liposomes have been shown to penetrate solid tumors more effectively, possibly because of their small size and longer circulation time. Once in tissues, daunorubicin is released. Daunorubicin inhibits DNA and RNA synthesis by intercalation between DNA base pairs and by steric obstruction; and intercalates at points of local uncoiling of the double helix. Although the exact mechanism is unclear, it appears that direct binding to DNA (intercalation) and inhibition of DNA repair (topoisomerase II inhibition) result in blockade of DNA and RNA synthesis and fragmentation of DNA.

Drug Interactions

Decreased Effect: Patients may experience impaired immune response to vaccines; possible infection after administration of live vaccines in patients receiving immunosuppressants.

Pharmacodynamics/Kinetics

Distribution: V_d: 3-6.4 L

Metabolism: Similar to daunorubicin, but metabolite plasma levels are low

Half-life elimination: Distribution: 4.4 hours; Terminal: 3-5 hours

Excretion: Primarily feces; some urine

Clearance, plasma: 17.3 mL/minute

Pregnancy Risk Factor D

DAUNOrubicin Hydrochloride

(daw noe ROO bi sin hye droe KLOR ide)

U.S. Brand Names Cerubidine®

Canadian Brand Names Cerubidine®

Mexican Brand Names Rubilem® [inj.]

Generic Available Yes

Synonyms Daunomycin; DNR; NSC-82151; Rubidomycin Hydrochloride

Pharmacologic Category Antineoplastic Agent, Anthracycline

Use Treatment of acute lymphocytic (ALL) and nonlymphocytic (ANLL) leukemias

Local Anesthetic/Vasoconstrictor Precautions No information available to require special precautions

Effects on Dental Treatment Key adverse event(s) related to dental treatment: Stomatitis and discoloration of saliva.

Common Adverse Effects

>10%:

Cardiovascular: Transient ECG abnormalities (supraventricular tachycardia, S-T wave changes, atrial or ventricular extrasystoles); generally asymptomatic and self-limiting. Congestive heart failure, dose-related, may be delayed for 7-8 years after treatment. Cumulative dose, radiation therapy, age, and use of cyclophosphamide all increase the risk. Recommended maximum cumulative doses:

No risk factors: 550-600 mg/m^2

Concurrent radiation: 450 mg/m^2

Regardless of cumulative dose, if the left ventricular ejection fraction is <30% to 40%, the drug is usually not given

Dermatologic: Alopecia, radiation recall

Gastrointestinal: Mild nausea or vomiting, stomatitis

Genitourinary: Discoloration of urine (red)

(Continued)

DAUNOrubicin Hydrochloride *(Continued)*

Hematologic: Myelosuppression, primarily leukopenia; thrombocytopenia and anemia
Onset: 7 days
Nadir: 10-14 days
Recovery: 21-28 days

1% to 10%:
Dermatologic: Skin "flare" at injection site; discoloration of saliva, sweat, or tears
Endocrine & metabolic: Hyperuricemia
Gastrointestinal: GI ulceration, diarrhea

Mechanism of Action Inhibition of DNA and RNA synthesis by intercalation between DNA base pairs and by steric obstruction. Daunomycin intercalates at points of local uncoiling of the double helix. Although the exact mechanism is unclear, it appears that direct binding to DNA (intercalation) and inhibition of DNA repair (topoisomerase II inhibition) result in blockade of DNA and RNA synthesis and fragmentation of DNA.

Drug Interactions

Decreased Effect: Patients may experience impaired immune response to vaccines; possible infection after administration of live vaccines in patients receiving immunosuppressants.

Pharmacodynamics/Kinetics

Distribution: Many body tissues, particularly the liver, kidneys, lung, spleen, and heart; not into CNS; crosses placenta; V_d: 40 L/kg
Metabolism: Primarily hepatic to daunorubicinol (active), then to inactive aglycones, conjugated sulfates, and glucuronides
Half-life elimination: Distribution: 2 minutes; Elimination: 14-20 hours; Terminal: 18.5 hours; Daunorubicinol plasma half-life: 24-48 hours
Excretion: Feces (40%); urine (~25% as unchanged drug and metabolites)

Pregnancy Risk Factor D

DaunoXome® *see* DAUNOrubicin Citrate (Liposomal) *on page 400*
DAVA *see* Vindesine *on page 1379*
1-Day™ [OTC] *see* Tioconazole *on page 1302*
Dayhist® Allergy [OTC] *see* Clemastine *on page 346*
Daypro® *see* Oxaprozin *on page 1022*
dCF *see* Pentostatin *on page 1065*
DDAVP® *see* Desmopressin *on page 409*
ddC *see* Zalcitabine *on page 1395*
ddI *see* Didanosine *on page 433*
Deacetyl Vinblastine Carboxamide *see* Vindesine *on page 1379*
1-Deamino-8-D-Arginine Vasopressin *see* Desmopressin *on page 409*
Debacterol® *see* Sulfonated Phenolics in Aqueous Solution *on page 1250*
Debrox® [OTC] *see* Carbamide Peroxide *on page 259*
Decadron® *see* Dexamethasone *on page 411*
Decadron® Phosphate [DSC] *see* Dexamethasone *on page 411*
Deca-Durabolin® [DSC] *see* Nandrolone *on page 963*
Decahist-DM *see* Carbinoxamine, Pseudoephedrine, and Dextromethorphan *on page 263*
Declomycin® *see* Demeclocycline *on page 404*
Decofed® [OTC] *see* Pseudoephedrine *on page 1147*
Deconamine® *see* Chlorpheniramine and Pseudoephedrine *on page 315*
Deconamine® SR *see* Chlorpheniramine and Pseudoephedrine *on page 315*
Deconsal® II *see* Guaifenesin and Pseudoephedrine *on page 675*
Defen-LA® *see* Guaifenesin and Pseudoephedrine *on page 675*

Deferoxamine (de fer OKS a meen)

U.S. Brand Names Desferal®

Canadian Brand Names Desferal®; PMS-Deferoxamine

Generic Available Yes

Synonyms Deferoxamine Mesylate

Pharmacologic Category Antidote

Use Acute iron intoxication when serum iron is >450-500 mcg/dL or when clinical signs of significant iron toxicity exist; chronic iron overload secondary to multiple transfusions; iron overload secondary to congenital anemias; hemochromatosis

Unlabeled/Investigational Use Removal of corneal rust rings following surgical removal of foreign bodies; diagnostic test for iron and aluminum overload

Investigational: Treatment of aluminum accumulation in renal failure; treatment of aluminum-induced bone disease

Local Anesthetic/Vasoconstrictor Precautions No information available to require special precautions

Effects on Dental Treatment No significant effects or complications reported

Common Adverse Effects Frequency not defined.

Cardiovascular: Flushing, hypotension, tachycardia, shock, edema

Central nervous system: Convulsions, fever, dizziness, neuropathy, paresthesia, seizures, exacerbation of aluminum-related encephalopathy (dialysis), headache, CNS depression, coma, aphasia, agitation

Dermatologic: Erythema, urticaria, pruritus, rash, cutaneous wheal formation

Endocrine & metabolic: Hypocalcemia

Gastrointestinal: Abdominal discomfort, diarrhea, nausea

Genitourinary: Dysuria

Hematologic: Thrombocytopenia, leukopenia

Local: Pain and induration at injection site

Neuromuscular & skeletal: Leg cramps

Ocular: Blurred vision, visual loss, scotoma, visual field defects, impaired vision, optic neuritis, cataracts, retinal pigmentary abnormalities

Otic: Hearing loss, tinnitus

Renal: Renal impairment, acute renal failure

Respiratory: Acute respiratory distress syndrome (with dyspnea, cyanosis)

Miscellaneous: Anaphylaxis

Mechanism of Action Complexes with trivalent ions (ferric ions) to form ferrioxamine, which are removed by the kidneys

Drug Interactions

Increased Effect/Toxicity: May cause loss of consciousness when administered with prochlorperazine. Concomitant treatment with vitamin C (>500 mg/day) has been associated with cardiac impairment.

Pharmacodynamics/Kinetics

Absorption: Oral: <15%

Metabolism: Hepatic to ferrioxamine

Half-life elimination: Parent drug: 6.1 hours; Ferrioxamine: 5.8 hours

Excretion: Urine (as unchanged drug and metabolites)

Pregnancy Risk Factor C

Deferoxamine Mesylate *see* Deferoxamine *on page 402*

Dehistine *see* Chlorpheniramine, Phenylephrine, and Methscopolamine *on page 317*

Dehydrobenzperidol *see* Droperidol *on page 477*

Del Aqua® *see* Benzoyl Peroxide *on page 194*

Delatestryl® *see* Testosterone *on page 1276*

Delavirdine (de la VIR deen)

Related Information

HIV Infection and AIDS *on page 1484*

Tuberculosis *on page 1495*

U.S. Brand Names Rescriptor®

Canadian Brand Names Rescriptor®

Mexican Brand Names Rescriptor®

Generic Available No

Synonyms U-90152S

Pharmacologic Category Antiretroviral Agent, Reverse Transcriptase Inhibitor (Non-nucleoside)

Use Treatment of HIV-1 infection in combination with at least two additional antiretroviral agents

Local Anesthetic/Vasoconstrictor Precautions No information available to require special precautions

Effects on Dental Treatment No significant effects or complications reported

Common Adverse Effects

>10%: Dermatologic: Rash (3.2% required discontinuation)

1% to 10%:

Central nervous system: Headache, fatigue

Dermatologic: Pruritus

Gastrointestinal: Nausea, diarrhea, vomiting

Metabolic: Increased ALT (SGPT), increased AST (SGOT)

Mechanism of Action Delavirdine binds directly to reverse transcriptase, blocking RNA-dependent and DNA-dependent DNA polymerase activities

(Continued)

Delavirdine *(Continued)*

Drug Interactions

Cytochrome P450 Effect: Substrate of CYP2D6 (minor), 3A4 (major); **Inhibits** CYP1A2 (weak), 2C8/9 (strong), 2C19 (strong), 2D6 (strong), 3A4 (strong)

Increased Effect/Toxicity: Concurrent therapy with selected benzodiazepines (alprazolam, midazolam, triazolam), ergot derivatives, cisapride, and pimozide is contraindicated. Concurrent therapy with lovastatin or simvastatin is not recommended (per manufacturer). Delavirdine may alter the levels/effects of lopinavir, ritonavir, and saquinavir (dosage adjustments may be required). Delavirdine may increase the levels/effects of amiodarone, amphetamines, selected benzodiazepines, selected beta-blockers, calcium channel blockers, citalopram, cyclosporine, dextromethorphan, diazepam, fluoxetine, glimepiride, glipizide, lidocaine, methsuximide, mirtazapine, nateglinide, nefazodone, paroxetine, phenytoin, pioglitazone, quinidine, risperidone, rosiglitazone, sertraline, sildenafil (and other PDE-5 inhibitors), tacrolimus, thioridazine, tricyclic antidepressants, venlafaxine, warfarin, and other CYP2C8/9, 2C19, or 2D6 substrates. When used with strong CYP3A4 inhibitors, dosage adjustment/limits are recommended for sildenafil and other PDE-5 inhibitors; refer to individual monographs. Dosage adjustment is recommended with clarithromycin.

Decreased Effect: The levels/effects of delavirdine may be decreased by aminoglutethimide, carbamazepine, nafcillin, nevirapine, phenobarbital, phenytoin, rifamycins, and other CYP3A4 inducers; concurrent therapy may lead to resistance and/or loss of efficacy. Decreased plasma concentrations of delavirdine with amprenavir, dexamethasone, didanosine, and saquinavir. Decreased absorption of delavirdine with antacids, histamine-2 receptor antagonists, proton pump inhibitors (omeprazole, lansoprazole), and didanosine. Delavirdine decreases plasma concentrations of didanosine. Delavirdine may decrease the levels/effects of CYP2D6 prodrug substrates (eg, codeine, hydrocodone, oxycodone, tramadol).

Pharmacodynamics/Kinetics

Absorption: Rapid

Distribution: Low concentration in saliva and semen; CSF 0.4% concurrent plasma concentration

Protein binding: ~98%, primarily albumin

Metabolism: Hepatic via CYP3A4 and 2D6 (**Note:** May reduce CYP3A activity and inhibit its own metabolism.)

Bioavailability: 85%

Half-life elimination: 2-11 hours

Time to peak, plasma: 1 hour

Excretion: Urine (51%, <5% as unchanged drug); feces (44%); nonlinear kinetics exhibited

Pregnancy Risk Factor C

Delestrogen® *see* Estradiol *on page 518*

Delfen® [OTC] *see* Nonoxynol 9 *on page 995*

Delsym® [OTC] *see* Dextromethorphan *on page 421*

Delta-9-tetrahydro-cannabinol *see* Dronabinol *on page 477*

Delta-9 THC *see* Dronabinol *on page 477*

Deltacortisone *see* PredniSONE *on page 1115*

Delta-D® *see* Cholecalciferol *on page 323*

Deltadehydrocortisone *see* PredniSONE *on page 1115*

Deltahydrocortisone *see* PrednisoLONE *on page 1113*

Deltasone® *see* PredniSONE *on page 1115*

Demadex® *see* Torsemide *on page 1317*

Demeclocycline (dem e kloe SYE kleen)

U.S. Brand Names Declomycin®

Canadian Brand Names Declomycin®

Generic Available Yes

Synonyms Demeclocycline Hydrochloride; Demethylchlortetracycline

Pharmacologic Category Antibiotic, Tetracycline Derivative

Use Treatment of susceptible bacterial infections (acne, gonorrhea, pertussis and urinary tract infections) caused by both gram-negative and gram-positive organisms

Unlabeled/Investigational Use Treatment of chronic syndrome of inappropriate secretion of antidiuretic hormone (SIADH)

Local Anesthetic/Vasoconstrictor Precautions No information available to require special precautions

Effects on Dental Treatment Tetracyclines are not recommended for use during pregnancy or in children ≤8 years of age since they have been reported to cause enamel hypoplasia and permanent teeth discoloration. Tetracyclines should only be used in these patients if other agents are contraindicated or alternative antimicrobials will not eradicate the organism. Long-term use associated with oral candidiasis.

Common Adverse Effects Frequency not defined.

Cardiovascular: Pericarditis

Central nervous system: Bulging fontanels (infants), dizziness, headache, pseudotumor cerebri (adults)

Dermatologic: Angioneurotic edema, erythema multiforme, erythematous rash, maculopapular rash, photosensitivity, pigmentation of skin, Stevens-Johnson syndrome (rare), urticaria

Endocrine & metabolic: Discoloration of thyroid gland (brown/black), nephrogenic diabetes insipidus

Gastrointestinal: Anorexia, diarrhea, dysphagia, enterocolitis, esophageal ulcerations, glossitis, nausea, pancreatitis, vomiting

Genitourinary: Balanitis

Hematologic: Eosinophilia, neutropenia, hemolytic anemia, thrombocytopenia

Hepatic: Hepatitis (rare), hepatotoxicity (rare), liver enzymes increased, liver failure (rare)

Neuromuscular & skeletal: Myasthenic syndrome, polyarthralgia, tooth discoloration (children < 8 years, rarely in adults)

Ocular: Visual disturbances

Otic: Tinnitus

Renal: Acute renal failure

Respiratory: Pulmonary infiltrates

Miscellaneous: Anaphylaxis, anaphylactoid purpura, lupus-like syndrome, systemic lupus erythematosus exacerbation

Mechanism of Action Inhibits protein synthesis by binding with the 30S and possibly the 50S ribosomal subunit(s) of susceptible bacteria; may also cause alterations in the cytoplasmic membrane; inhibits the action of ADH in patients with chronic SIADH

Drug Interactions

Increased Effect/Toxicity: Methoxyflurane anesthesia may cause fatal nephrotoxicity; retinoic acid derivatives may increase adverse and toxic effects; warfarin may result in increased anticoagulation; methotrexate levels may be increased

Decreased Effect: Antacid preparations containing calcium, magnesium, aluminum bismuth, or sodium bicarbonate may decrease tetracycline absorption; bile acid sequestrants, quinapril (magnesium-containing formulation), iron, or zinc may also decrease absorption; penicillin decrease therapeutic effect of tetracyclines. Although anecdotal reports suggest oral contraceptive efficacy could be reduced by tetracyclines, this has been refuted by more rigorous scientific and clinical data.

Pharmacodynamics/Kinetics

Onset of action: SIADH: Several days

Absorption: ~50% to 80%; reduced by food and dairy products

Protein binding: 41% to 50%

Metabolism: Hepatic (small amounts) to inactive metabolites; undergoes enterohepatic recirculation

Half-life elimination: 10-17 hours

Time to peak, serum: 3-6 hours

Excretion: Urine (42% to 50% as unchanged drug)

Pregnancy Risk Factor D

Demeclocycline Hydrochloride *see* Demeclocycline *on page 404*

Demerol® *see* Meperidine *on page 870*

4-Demethoxydaunorubicin *see* Idarubicin *on page 732*

Demethylchlortetracycline *see* Demeclocycline *on page 404*

Demser® *see* Metyrosine *on page 920*

Demulen® *see* Ethinyl Estradiol and Ethynodiol Diacetate *on page 540*

Denavir® *see* Penciclovir *on page 1056*

Denileukin Diftitox (de ni LOO kin DIF ti toks)

U.S. Brand Names ONTAK®

Generic Available No

Pharmacologic Category Antineoplastic Agent, Miscellaneous

Use Treatment of persistent or recurrent cutaneous T-cell lymphoma whose malignant cells express the CD25 component of the IL-2 receptor

(Continued)

Denileukin Diftitox *(Continued)*

Local Anesthetic/Vasoconstrictor Precautions No information available to require special precautions

Effects on Dental Treatment No significant effects or complications reported

Common Adverse Effects

The occurrence of adverse events diminishes after the first two treatment courses. Infusion-related hypersensitivity reactions have been reported in 69% of patients. Reactions are variable, but may include hypotension, back pain, dyspnea, vasodilation, rash, chest pain, tachycardia, dysphagia, syncope or anaphylaxis. In addition, a flu-like syndrome, beginning several hours to days following infusion, occurred in 91% of patients.

In 27% of patients a vascular leak syndrome occurred, characterized by hypotension, edema, or hypoalbuminemia. The syndrome usually developed within the first 2 weeks of infusion. Six percent of patients who developed this syndrome required hospitalization. The symptoms may persist or even worsen despite cessation of denileukin diftitox.

Severe (Grade 3 and 4) reactions which occurred with an incidence over 10% included: Chills/fever (22%), asthenia (22%), infection (24%), pain (13%), nausea/vomiting (14%), hypoalbuminemia (14%), transaminase elevation (15%), edema (15%), dyspnea (14%), and rash (13%).

The following list of symptoms reported during treatment includes all levels of severity:

>10%:

Cardiovascular: Edema (47%), hypotension (36%), chest pain (24%), vasodilation (22%), tachycardia (12%)

Central nervous system: Fever/chills (81%), headache (26%), pain (48%), dizziness (22%), nervousness (11%)

Dermatologic: Rash (34%), pruritus (20%)

Endocrine & metabolic: Hypoalbuminemia (83%), hypocalcemia (17%), weight loss (14%)

Gastrointestinal: Nausea/vomiting (64%), anorexia (36%), diarrhea (29%)

Hematologic: Decreased lymphocyte count (34%), anemia (18%)

Hepatic: Increased transaminases (61%)

Neuromuscular & skeletal: Asthenia (66%), myalgia (17%)

Respiratory: Dyspnea (29%), increased cough (26%), pharyngitis (17%), rhinitis (13%)

Miscellaneous: Hypersensitivity (69%), infection (48%), vascular leak syndrome (27%), increased diaphoresis (10%), paresthesia (13%)

1% to 10%:

Cardiovascular: Hypertension (6%), arrhythmias (6%), myocardial infarction (1%)

Central nervous system: Insomnia (9%), confusion (8%)

Endocrine & metabolic: Dehydration (9%), hypokalemia (6%), hyperthyroidism (<5%), hypothyroidism (<5%)

Gastrointestinal: Constipation (9%), dyspepsia (7%), dysphagia (6%), pancreatitis (<5%)

Genitourinary: Hematuria (10%), albuminuria (10%), pyuria (10%)

Hematologic: Thrombotic events (7%), thrombocytopenia (8%), leukopenia (6%)

Local: Injection site reaction (8%), anaphylaxis (1%)

Neuromuscular & skeletal: Arthralgia (8%)

Renal: Increased creatinine (7%), acute renal insufficiency (<5%), microscopic hematuria (<5%)

Respiratory: Lung disorder (8%)

Mechanism of Action Denileukin diftitox is a fusion protein (a combination of amino acid sequences from diphtheria toxin and interleukin-2) which selectively delivers the cytotoxic activity of diphtheria toxin to targeted cells. It interacts with the high-affinity IL-2 receptor on the surface of malignant cells to inhibit intracellular protein synthesis, rapidly leading to cell death.

Pharmacodynamics/Kinetics

Distribution: V_d: 0.06-0.08 L/kg

Metabolism: Hepatic via proteolytic degradation (animal studies)

Half-life elimination: Distribution: 2-5 minutes; Terminal: 70-80 minutes

Pregnancy Risk Factor C

Dental Office Emergencies *see page 1584*

Dentifrice Products *see page 1621*

Dentin Hypersensitivity, High Caries Index, and Xerostomia *see page 1555*

DentiPatch® *see* Lidocaine (Transoral) *on page 828*

Dentist's Role in Recognizing Domestic Violence *see page 1574*

Dent's Ear Wax [OTC] *see* Carbamide Peroxide *on page 259*
Deoxycoformycin *see* Pentostatin *on page 1065*
2'-Deoxycoformycin *see* Pentostatin *on page 1065*
Depacon® *see* Valproic Acid and Derivatives *on page 1359*
Depakene® *see* Valproic Acid and Derivatives *on page 1359*
Depakote® Delayed Release *see* Valproic Acid and Derivatives *on page 1359*
Depakote® ER *see* Valproic Acid and Derivatives *on page 1359*
Depakote® Sprinkle® *see* Valproic Acid and Derivatives *on page 1359*
Depen® *see* Penicillamine *on page 1057*
DepoCyt™ *see* Cytarabine (Liposomal) *on page 391*
DepoDur™ *see* Morphine Sulfate *on page 947*
Depo®-Estradiol *see* Estradiol *on page 518*
Depo-Medrol® *see* MethylPREDNISolone *on page 910*
Depo-Provera® *see* MedroxyPROGESTERone *on page 862*
Depo-Provera® Contraceptive *see* MedroxyPROGESTERone *on page 862*
Depo®-Testosterone *see* Testosterone *on page 1276*
Deprenyl *see* Selegiline *on page 1212*
Dermarest Dricort® [OTC] *see* Hydrocortisone *on page 714*
Dermasept Antifungal [OTC] *see* Tolnaftate *on page 1312*
Derma-Smoothe/FS® *see* Fluocinolone *on page 601*
Dermatop® *see* Prednicarbate *on page 1113*
Dermazene® *see* Iodoquinol and Hydrocortisone *on page 759*
Dermtex® HC [OTC] *see* Hydrocortisone *on page 714*
Desacetyl Vinblastine Amide Sulfate *see* Vindesine *on page 1379*
Deserpidine and Methyclothiazide *see* Methyclothiazide and Deserpidine *on page 905*
Desferal® *see* Deferoxamine *on page 402*
Desiccated Thyroid *see* Thyroid *on page 1293*

Desipramine (des IP ra meen)

U.S. Brand Names Norpramin®

Canadian Brand Names Alti-Desipramine; Apo-Desipramine®; Norpramin®; Novo-Desipramine; Nu-Desipramine; PMS-Desipramine

Generic Available Yes

Synonyms Desipramine Hydrochloride; Desmethylimipramine Hydrochloride

Pharmacologic Category Antidepressant, Tricyclic (Secondary Amine)

Use Treatment of depression

Unlabeled/Investigational Use Analgesic adjunct in chronic pain; peripheral neuropathies; substance-related disorders; attention-deficit/hyperactivity disorder (ADHD)

Local Anesthetic/Vasoconstrictor Precautions Use with caution; epinephrine, norepinephrine and levonordefrin have been shown to have an increased pressor response in combination with TCAs

Effects on Dental Treatment Key adverse event(s) related to dental treatment: Xerostomia and changes in salivation (normal salivary flow resumes upon discontinuation), and unpleasant taste. Long-term treatment with TCAs increases the risk of caries by reducing salivation and salivary buffer capacity.

Common Adverse Effects Frequency not defined.

Cardiovascular: Arrhythmias, hypotension, hypertension, palpitations, heart block, tachycardia

Central nervous system: Dizziness, drowsiness, headache, confusion, delirium, hallucinations, nervousness, restlessness, parkinsonian syndrome, insomnia, disorientation, anxiety, agitation, hypomania, exacerbation of psychosis, incoordination, seizures, extrapyramidal symptoms

Dermatologic: Alopecia, photosensitivity, skin rash, urticaria

Endocrine & metabolic: Breast enlargement, galactorrhea, SIADH

Gastrointestinal: Xerostomia, decreased lower esophageal sphincter tone may cause GE reflux, constipation, nausea, unpleasant taste, weight gain/loss, anorexia, abdominal cramps, diarrhea, heartburn

Genitourinary: Difficult urination, sexual dysfunction, testicular edema

Hematologic: Agranulocytosis, eosinophilia, purpura, thrombocytopenia

Hepatic: Cholestatic jaundice, increased liver enzyme

Neuromuscular & skeletal: Fine muscle tremors, weakness, numbness, tingling, paresthesia of extremities, ataxia

Ocular: Blurred vision, disturbances of accommodation, mydriasis, increased intraocular pressure

Miscellaneous: Diaphoresis (excessive), allergic reactions

(Continued)

Desipramine *(Continued)*

Mechanism of Action Traditionally believed to increase the synaptic concentration of norepinephrine (and to a lesser extent, serotonin) in the central nervous system by inhibition of its reuptake by the presynaptic neuronal membrane. However, additional receptor effects have been found including desensitization of adenyl cyclase, down regulation of beta-adrenergic receptors, and down regulation of serotonin receptors.

Drug Interactions

Cytochrome P450 Effect: Substrate of CYP1A2 (minor), 2D6 (major); **Inhibits** CYP2A6 (moderate), 2B6 (moderate), 2D6 (moderate), 2E1 (weak), 3A4 (moderate)

Increased Effect/Toxicity: Desipramine increases the effects of amphetamines, anticholinergics, other CNS depressants (sedatives, hypnotics, or ethanol), chlorpropamide, tolazamide, and warfarin. When used with MAO inhibitors, serotonin syndrome may occur. Serotonin syndrome has also been reported with ritonavir (rare). The levels/effects of desipramine may be increased by chlorpromazine, delavirdine, fluoxetine, miconazole, paroxetine, pergolide, quinidine, quinine, ritonavir, ropinirole, and other CYP2D6 inhibitors.

Cimetidine, grapefruit juice, indinavir, methylphenidate, diltiazem, and verapamil may increase the serum concentration of TCAs. Use of lithium with a TCA may increase the risk for neurotoxicity. Phenothiazines may increase concentration of some TCAs and TCAs may increase concentration of phenothiazines. Pressor response to I.V. epinephrine, norepinephrine, and phenylephrine may be enhanced in patients receiving TCAs (**Note:** Effect is unlikely with epinephrine or levonordefrin dosages typically administered as infiltration in combination with local anesthetics). Combined use of beta-agonists or drugs which prolong QT_c (including quinidine, procainamide, disopyramide, cisapride, sparfloxacin, gatifloxacin, moxifloxacin) with TCAs may predispose patients to cardiac arrhythmias.

Desipramine may increase the levels/effects of selected benzodiazepines, bupropion, calcium channel blockers, cisapride, dexmedetomidine, dextromethorphan, ergot derivatives, ifosfamide, fluoxetine, selected HMG-CoA reductase inhibitors, lidocaine, mesoridazine, mirtazapine, nateglinide, nefazodone, paroxetine, pimozide, promethazine, propofol, quinidine, risperidone, ritonavir, selegiline, sertraline, sildenafil (and other PDE-5 inhibitors), tacrolimus, thioridazine, tricyclic antidepressants, venlafaxine, and other CYP2A6, 2B6, 2D6, or 3A4 substrates.

Decreased Effect: Desipramine may decrease the levels/effects of CYP2D6 prodrug substrates (eg, codeine, hydrocodone, oxycodone, tramadol). Desipramine's serum levels/effect may be decreased by carbamazepine, cholestyramine, colestipol, phenobarbital, and rifampin. Desipramine inhibits the antihypertensive effect of to bethanidine, clonidine, debrisoquin, guanadrel, guanethidine, guanabenz, or guanfacine.

Pharmacodynamics/Kinetics

Onset of action: 1-3 weeks; Maximum antidepressant effect: >2 weeks
Absorption: Well absorbed
Metabolism: Hepatic
Half-life elimination: Adults: 7-60 hours
Time to peak, plasma: 4-6 hours
Excretion: Urine (70%)

Pregnancy Risk Factor C

Desipramine Hydrochloride *see* Desipramine *on page 407*
Desitin® [OTC] *see* Zinc Oxide *on page 1400*
Desitin® Creamy [OTC] *see* Zinc Oxide *on page 1400*

Desloratadine (des lor AT a deen)

U.S. Brand Names Clarinex®

Canadian Brand Names Aerius®

Generic Available No

Pharmacologic Category Antihistamine, Nonsedating

Use Relief of nasal and non-nasal symptoms of seasonal allergic rhinitis (SAR) and perennial allergic rhinitis (PAR); treatment of chronic idiopathic urticaria (CIU)

Local Anesthetic/Vasoconstrictor Precautions No information available to require special precautions

Effects on Dental Treatment Key adverse event(s) related to dental treatment: Xerostomia (normal salivary flow resumes upon discontinuation).

Common Adverse Effects

>10%: Central nervous system: Headache (14%)

1% to 10%:

Central nervous system: Fatigue (2% to 5%), somnolence (2%), dizziness (4%)

Endocrine & metabolic: Dysmenorrhea (2%)

Gastrointestinal: Xerostomia (3%), nausea (5%), dyspepsia (3%)

Neuromuscular & skeletal: Myalgia (2% to 3%)

Respiratory: Pharyngitis (3% to 4%)

Dosage Oral: Adults and Children ≥12 years: 5 mg once daily

Dosage adjustment in renal/hepatic impairment: 5 mg every other day

Mechanism of Action Desloratadine, a major metabolite of loratadine, is a long-acting tricyclic antihistamine with selective peripheral histamine H_1 receptor antagonistic activity and additional anti-inflammatory properties.

Contraindications Hypersensitivity to desloratadine, loratadine, or any component of the formulation

Warnings/Precautions Dose should be adjusted in patients with liver or renal impairment. Use with caution in patients known to be slow metabolizers of desloratadine (incidence of side effects may be increased). RediTabs® contain phenylalanine. Safety and efficacy have not been established for children <12 years of age.

Drug Interactions

Increased Effect/Toxicity: With concurrent use of desloratadine and erythromycin or ketoconazole, the C_{max} and AUC of desloratadine and its metabolite are increased; however, no clinically-significant changes in the safety profile of desloratadine were observed in clinical studies.

Ethanol/Nutrition/Herb Interactions Food: Does not affect bioavailability.

Dietary Considerations May be taken with or without food. Orally-disintegrating tablets contain phenylalanine 1.75 mg/tablet.

Pharmacodynamics/Kinetics

Protein binding: Desloratadine: 82% to 87%; 3-hydroxydesloratadine: 85% to 89%

Metabolism: Hepatic to active metabolite, 3-hydroxydesloratadine (specific enzymes not identified); undergoes glucuronidation. Decreased in slow metabolizers of desloratadine. Not expected to affect or be affected by medications metabolized by CYP with normal doses.

Half-life elimination: 27 hours

Time to peak: 3 hours

Excretion: Urine and feces (as metabolites)

Pregnancy Risk Factor C

Dosage Forms TAB (Clarinex®): 5 mg. **TAB, orally-disintegrating** (Clarinex® RediTabs®): 5 mg

Desmethylimipramine Hydrochloride *see* Desipramine *on page 407*

Desmopressin (des moe PRES in)

U.S. Brand Names DDAVP®; Stimate™

Canadian Brand Names Apo-Desmopressin®; DDAVP®; Minirin®; Octostim®

Mexican Brand Names Minirin®

Generic Available Yes: Injection only

Synonyms 1-Deamino-8-D-Arginine Vasopressin; Desmopressin Acetate

Pharmacologic Category Antihemophilic Agent; Hemostatic Agent; Vasopressin Analog, Synthetic

Use Treatment of diabetes insipidus; control of bleeding in hemophilia A, and mild-to-moderate classic von Willebrand disease (type I); primary nocturnal enuresis

Local Anesthetic/Vasoconstrictor Precautions No information available to require special precautions

Effects on Dental Treatment No significant effects or complications reported

Common Adverse Effects Frequency not defined (may be dose or route related).

Cardiovascular: Acute cerebrovascular thrombosis, acute MI, blood pressure increased/decreased, chest pain, edema, facial flushing, palpitations

Central nervous system: Agitation, chills, coma, dizziness, headache, insomnia, somnolence

Endocrine & metabolic: Hyponatremia, water intoxication

Gastrointestinal: Abdominal cramps, dyspepsia, nausea, sore throat, vomiting

Genitourinary: Balanitis, vulval pain

Local: Injection: Burning pain, erythema, and swelling at the injection site

Respiratory: Cough, nasal congestion, epistaxis

Miscellaneous: Allergic reactions (rare), anaphylaxis (rare)

(Continued)

Desmopressin *(Continued)*

Mechanism of Action Enhances reabsorption of water in the kidneys by increasing cellular permeability of the collecting ducts; possibly causes smooth muscle constriction with resultant vasoconstriction; raises plasma levels of von Willebrand factor and factor VIII

Drug Interactions

Increased Effect/Toxicity: Chlorpropamide, fludrocortisone may increase ADH response.

Decreased Effect: Demeclocycline and lithium may decrease ADH response.

Pharmacodynamics/Kinetics

Intranasal administration: Onset of increased factor VIII activity: 30 minutes (dose related)
Peak effect 1.5 hours

I.V. infusion:
Onset of increased factor VIII activity: 30 minutes (dose related)
Peak effect: 1.5-2 hours
Half-life elimination: Terminal: 75 minutes

Oral tablets:
Onset of action: ADH: ~1 hour
Peak effect: 4-7 hours
Half-life elimination: 1.5-2.5 hours
Bioavailability: 5% compared to intranasal; 0.16% compared to I.V.

Pregnancy Risk Factor B

Desmopressin Acetate *see* Desmopressin *on page 409*

Desogen® *see* Ethinyl Estradiol and Desogestrel *on page 536*

Desogestrel and Ethinyl Estradiol *see* Ethinyl Estradiol and Desogestrel *on page 536*

Desonide (DES oh nide)

U.S. Brand Names DesOwen®; LoKara™; Tridesilon®

Canadian Brand Names Desocort®; PMS-Desonide

Mexican Brand Names Desowen®

Generic Available Yes

Pharmacologic Category Corticosteroid, Topical

Use Adjunctive therapy for inflammation in acute and chronic corticosteroid responsive dermatosis (low potency corticosteroid)

Local Anesthetic/Vasoconstrictor Precautions No information available to require special precautions

Effects on Dental Treatment No significant effects or complications reported

Mechanism of Action Stimulates the synthesis of enzymes needed to decrease inflammation, suppress mitotic activity, and cause vasoconstriction

Pharmacodynamics/Kinetics

Onset of action: ~7 days
Absorption: Extensive from scalp, face, axilla, and scrotum; adequate through epidermis on appendages; may be increased with occlusion or addition of penetrants (eg, urea, DMSO)
Metabolism: Hepatic
Excretion: Primarily urine

Pregnancy Risk Factor C

DesOwen® *see* Desonide *on page 410*

Desoximetasone (des oks i MET a sone)

U.S. Brand Names Topicort®; Topicort®-LP

Canadian Brand Names Desoxi®; Taro-Desoximetasone; Topicort®

Generic Available Yes

Pharmacologic Category Corticosteroid, Topical

Use Relieves inflammation and pruritic symptoms of corticosteroid-responsive dermatosis (intermediate- to high-potency topical corticosteroid)

Local Anesthetic/Vasoconstrictor Precautions No information available to require special precautions

Effects on Dental Treatment No significant effects or complications reported

Mechanism of Action Stimulates the synthesis of enzymes needed to decrease inflammation, suppress mitotic activity, and cause vasoconstriction

Pharmacodynamics/Kinetics

Absorption: May be increased with occlusion, inflammation, or vary with site of application
Ointment: Systemic absorption with occlusion: 7%
Metabolism: Hepatic

Half-life elimination: Emollient cream: 15-17 hours
Excretion: Urine, feces

Pregnancy Risk Factor C

Desoxyephedrine Hydrochloride *see* Methamphetamine *on page 891*

Desoxyn® *see* Methamphetamine *on page 891*

Desoxyphenobarbital *see* Primidone *on page 1122*

Desquam-E™ *see* Benzoyl Peroxide *on page 194*

Desquam-X® *see* Benzoyl Peroxide *on page 194*

Desyrel® *see* Trazodone *on page 1326*

Detane® [OTC] *see* Benzocaine *on page 191*

Detrol® *see* Tolterodine *on page 1312*

Detrol® LA *see* Tolterodine *on page 1312*

Detussin® *see* Hydrocodone and Pseudoephedrine *on page 711*

Dex4 Glucose [OTC] *see* Glucose (Instant) *on page 663*

Dexacidin® *see* Neomycin, Polymyxin B, and Dexamethasone *on page 974*

Dexacine™ *see* Neomycin, Polymyxin B, and Dexamethasone *on page 974*

Dexalone® [OTC] *see* Dextromethorphan *on page 421*

Dexamethasone (deks a METH a sone)

Related Information

Dental Office Emergencies *on page 1584*
Neomycin, Polymyxin B, and Dexamethasone *on page 974*
Oral Nonviral Soft Tissue Ulcerations or Erosions *on page 1551*
Respiratory Diseases *on page 1478*

U.S. Brand Names Decadron®; Decadron® Phosphate [DSC]; Dexamethasone Intensol®; DexPak® TaperPak®; Maxidex®

Canadian Brand Names Decadron®; Dexasone®; Diodex®; Maxidex®; PMS-Dexamethasone

Mexican Brand Names Alin®; Decadron®; Dexagrin®; Indarzona®

Generic Available Yes

Synonyms Dexamethasone Sodium Phosphate

Pharmacologic Category Antiemetic; Anti-inflammatory Agent; Anti-inflammatory Agent, Ophthalmic; Corticosteroid, Ophthalmic; Corticosteroid, Systemic; Corticosteroid, Topical

Dental Use Treatment of a variety of oral diseases of allergic, inflammatory or autoimmune origin

Use Systemically and locally for chronic swelling; allergic, hematologic, neoplastic, and autoimmune diseases; may be used in management of cerebral edema, septic shock, as a diagnostic agent, antiemetic

Unlabeled/Investigational Use General indicator consistent with depression; diagnosis of Cushing's syndrome

Local Anesthetic/Vasoconstrictor Precautions No information available to require special precautions

Effects on Dental Treatment No significant effects or complications reported

Significant Adverse Effects

Systemic:

>10%:

Central nervous system: Insomnia, nervousness
Gastrointestinal: Increased appetite, indigestion

1% to 10%:

Dermatologic: Hirsutism
Endocrine & metabolic: Diabetes mellitus
Neuromuscular & skeletal: Arthralgia
Ocular: Cataracts
Respiratory: Epistaxis

<1% (Limited to important or life-threatening): Abdominal distention, acne, amenorrhea, bone growth suppression, bruising, Cushing's syndrome, delirium, euphoria, hallucinations, headache, hyperglycemia, hyperpigmentation, hypersensitivity reactions, mood swings, muscle wasting, pancreatitis, seizures, skin atrophy, sodium and water retention, ulcerative esophagitis

Topical: <1% (Limited to important or life-threatening): Acneiform eruptions, allergic contact dermatitis, burning, dryness, folliculitis, hypertrichosis, hypopigmentation, irritation, itching, miliaria, perioral dermatitis, secondary infection, skin atrophy, skin maceration, striae

Dosage

Children:

Antiemetic (prior to chemotherapy): I.V. (should be given as sodium phosphate): 5-20 mg given 15-30 minutes before treatment

(Continued)

Dexamethasone *(Continued)*

Anti-inflammatory immunosuppressant: Oral, I.M., I.V. (injections should be given as sodium phosphate): 0.08-0.3 mg/kg/day **or** 2.5-10 mg/m²/day in divided doses every 6-12 hours

Extubation or airway edema: Oral, I.M., I.V. (injections should be given as sodium phosphate): 0.5-2 mg/kg/day in divided doses every 6 hours beginning 24 hours prior to extubation and continuing for 4-6 doses afterwards

Cerebral edema: I.V. (should be given as sodium phosphate): Loading dose: 1-2 mg/kg/dose as a single dose; maintenance: 1-1.5 mg/kg/day (maximum: 16 mg/day) in divided doses every 4-6 hours for 5 days then taper for 5 days, then discontinue

Bacterial meningitis in infants and children >2 months: I.V. (should be given as sodium phosphate): 0.6 mg/kg/day in 4 divided doses every 6 hours for the first 4 days of antibiotic treatment; start dexamethasone at the time of the first dose of antibiotic

Physiologic replacement: Oral, I.M., I.V.: 0.03-0.15 mg/kg/day **or** 0.6-0.75 mg/m²/day in divided doses every 6-12 hours

Adults:

Antiemetic:

Prophylaxis: Oral, I.V.: 10-20 mg 15-30 minutes before treatment on each treatment day

Continuous infusion regimen: Oral or I.V.: 10 mg every 12 hours on each treatment day

Mildly emetogenic therapy: Oral, I.M., I.V.: 4 mg every 4-6 hours

Delayed nausea/vomiting: Oral: 4-10 mg 1-2 times/day for 2-4 days **or**
8 mg every 12 hours for 2 days; then
4 mg every 12 hours for 2 days **or**
20 mg 1 hour before chemotherapy; then
10 mg 12 hours after chemotherapy; then
8 mg every 12 hours for 4 doses; then
4 mg every 12 hours for 4 doses

Anti-inflammatory:

Oral, I.M., I.V. (injections should be given as sodium phosphate): 0.75-9 mg/day in divided doses every 6-12 hours

I.M. (as acetate): 8-16 mg; may repeat in 1-3 weeks

Intralesional (as acetate): 0.8-1.6 mg

Intra-articular/soft tissue (as acetate): 4-16 mg; may repeat in 1-3 weeks

Intra-articular, intralesional, or soft tissue (as sodium phosphate): 0.4-6 mg/day

Ophthalmic:

Ointment: Apply thin coating into conjunctival sac 3-4 times/day; gradually taper dose to discontinue

Suspension: Instill 2 drops into conjunctival sac every hour during the day and every other hour during the night; gradually reduce dose to every 3-4 hours, then to 3-4 times/day

Topical: Apply 1-4 times/day. Therapy should be discontinued when control is achieved; if no improvement is seen, reassessment of diagnosis may be necessary.

Chemotherapy: Oral, I.V.: 40 mg every day for 4 days, repeated every 4 weeks (VAD regimen)

Cerebral edema: I.V. 10 mg stat, 4 mg I.M./I.V. (should be given as sodium phosphate) every 6 hours until response is maximized, then switch to oral regimen, then taper off if appropriate; dosage may be reduced after 24 days and gradually discontinued over 5-7 days

Dexamethasone suppression test (depression indicator) or diagnosis for Cushing's syndrome (unlabeled uses): Oral: 1 mg at 11 PM, draw blood at 8 AM the following day for plasma cortisol determination

Physiological replacement: Oral, I.M., I.V. (should be given as sodium phosphate): 0.03-0.15 mg/kg/day **or** 0.6-0.75 mg/m²/day in divided doses every 6-12 hours

Treatment of shock:

Addisonian crisis/shock (ie, adrenal insufficiency/responsive to steroid therapy): I.V. (given as sodium phosphate): 4-10 mg as a single dose, which may be repeated if necessary

Unresponsive shock (ie, unresponsive to steroid therapy): I.V. (given as sodium phosphate): 1-6 mg/kg as a single I.V. dose or up to 40 mg initially followed by repeat doses every 2-6 hours while shock persists

Hemodialysis: Supplemental dose is not necessary

Peritoneal dialysis: Supplemental dose is not necessary

Mechanism of Action Decreases inflammation by suppression of migration of polymorphonuclear leukocytes and reversal of increased capillary permeability; suppresses normal immune response. Dexamethasone's mechanism of antiemetic activity is unknown.

Contraindications Hypersensitivity to dexamethasone or any component of the formulation; active untreated infections; ophthalmic use in viral, fungal, or tuberculosis diseases of the eye

Warnings/Precautions Use with caution in patients with hypothyroidism, cirrhosis, hypertension, CHF, ulcerative colitis, thromboembolic disorders. Corticosteroids should be used with caution in patients with diabetes, osteoporosis, peptic ulcer, glaucoma, cataracts, or tuberculosis. Use caution in hepatic impairment. Because of the risk of adverse effects, systemic corticosteroids should be used cautiously in the elderly in the smallest possible dose and for the shortest possible time.

May cause suppression of hypothalamic-pituitary-adrenal (HPA) axis, particularly in younger children or in patients receiving high doses for prolonged periods. Particular care is required when patients are transferred from systemic corticosteroids to inhaled products due to possible adrenal insufficiency or withdrawal from steroids, including an increase in allergic symptoms. Patients receiving 20 mg per day of prednisone (or equivalent) may be most susceptible. Fatalities have occurred due to adrenal insufficiency in asthmatic patients during and after transfer from systemic corticosteroids to aerosol steroids; aerosol steroids do **not** provide the systemic steroid needed to treat patients having trauma, surgery, or infections

Controlled clinical studies have shown that orally-inhaled and intranasal corticosteroids may cause a reduction in growth velocity in pediatric patients. (In studies of orally-inhaled corticosteroids, the mean reduction in growth velocity was approximately 1 centimeter per year [range 0.3-1.8 cm per year] and appears to be related to dose and duration of exposure.) The growth of pediatric patients receiving inhaled corticosteroids, should be monitored routinely (eg, via stadiometry). To minimize the systemic effects of orally-inhaled and intranasal corticosteroids, each patient should be titrated to the lowest effective dose.

May suppress the immune system, patients may be more susceptible to infection. Use with caution in patients with systemic infections or ocular herpes simplex. Avoid exposure to chickenpox and measles.

Drug Interactions Substrate of CYP3A4 (minor); **Induces** CYP2A6 (weak), 2B6 (weak), 2C8/9 (weak), 3A4 (weak)

Decreased effect: Barbiturates, phenytoin, rifampin may decrease dexamethasone effects; dexamethasone decreases effect of salicylates, vaccines, toxoids

Increased effect: Salmeterol: The addition of salmeterol has been demonstrated to improve response to inhaled corticosteroids (as compared to increasing steroid dosage).

Ethanol/Nutrition/Herb Interactions

Ethanol: Avoid ethanol (may enhance gastric mucosal irritation).

Food: Dexamethasone interferes with calcium absorption. Limit caffeine.

Herb/Nutraceutical: Avoid cat's claw, echinacea (have immunostimulant properties).

Dietary Considerations May be taken with meals to decrease GI upset. May need diet with increased potassium, pyridoxine, vitamin C, vitamin D, folate, calcium, and phosphorus.

Pharmacodynamics/Kinetics

Onset of action: Acetate: Prompt

Duration of metabolic effect: 72 hours; acetate is a long-acting repository preparation

Metabolism: Hepatic

Half-life elimination: Normal renal function: 1.8-3.5 hours; Biological half-life: 36-54 hours

Time to peak, serum: Oral: 1-2 hours; I.M.: ~8 hours

Excretion: Urine and feces

Pregnancy Risk Factor C

Lactation Excretion in breast milk unknown

Dosage Forms [DSC] = Discontinued product

Elixir, as base: 0.5 mg/5 mL (240 mL) [contains alcohol 5%; raspberry flavor]

Injection, solution, as sodium phosphate: 4 mg/mL (1 mL, 5 mL, 10 mL, 25 mL, 30 mL); 10 mg/mL (1 mL, 10 mL)

Decadron® Phosphate: 4 mg/mL (5 mL, 25 mL); 24 mg/mL (5 mL) [contains sodium bisulfite] [DSC]

Ointment, ophthalmic, as sodium phosphate: 0.05% (3.5 g)

(Continued)

Dexamethasone *(Continued)*

Solution, ophthalmic, as sodium phosphate: 0.1% (5 mL)
Solution, oral: 0.5 mg/5 mL (500 mL) [cherry flavor]
Solution, oral concentrate (Dexamethasone Intensol®): 1 mg/mL (30 mL) [contains alcohol 30%]
Suspension, ophthalmic (Maxidex®): 0.1% (5 mL, 15 mL)
Tablet: 0.25 mg, 0.5 mg, 0.75 mg, 1 mg, 1.5 mg, 2 mg, 4 mg, 6 mg [some 0.5 mg tablets may contain tartrazine]
Decadron®: 0.5 mg, 0.75 mg, 4 mg
DexPak® TaperPak®: 1.5 mg [51 tablets on taper dose card]

Dexamethasone and Ciprofloxacin *see* Ciprofloxacin and Dexamethasone *on page 336*

Dexamethasone and Neomycin *see* Neomycin and Dexamethasone *on page 973*

Dexamethasone and Tobramycin *see* Tobramycin and Dexamethasone *on page 1307*

Dexamethasone Intensol® *see* Dexamethasone *on page 411*

Dexamethasone, Neomycin, and Polymyxin B *see* Neomycin, Polymyxin B, and Dexamethasone *on page 974*

Dexamethasone Sodium Phosphate *see* Dexamethasone *on page 411*

Dexbrompheniramine and Pseudoephedrine

(deks brom fen EER a meen & soo doe e FED rin)

Related Information

Pseudoephedrine *on page 1147*

U.S. Brand Names Drixoral® Cold & Allergy [OTC]

Canadian Brand Names Drixoral®

Generic Available Yes

Synonyms Pseudoephedrine and Dexbrompheniramine

Pharmacologic Category Antihistamine/Decongestant Combination

Use Relief of symptoms of upper respiratory mucosal congestion in seasonal and perennial nasal allergies, acute rhinitis, rhinosinusitis and eustachian tube blockage

Local Anesthetic/Vasoconstrictor Precautions Use with caution since pseudoephedrine is a sympathomimetic amine which could interact with epinephrine to cause a pressor response

Effects on Dental Treatment Key adverse event(s) related to dental treatment: Pseudoephedrine: Xerostomia (normal salivary flow resumes upon discontinuation).

Pregnancy Risk Factor B

Dexchlorpheniramine (deks klor fen EER a meen)

Generic Available Yes

Synonyms Dexchlorpheniramine Maleate

Pharmacologic Category Antihistamine

Use Perennial and seasonal allergic rhinitis and other allergic symptoms including urticaria

Local Anesthetic/Vasoconstrictor Precautions No information available to require special precautions

Effects on Dental Treatment Key adverse event(s) related to dental treatment: Significant xerostomia (normal salivary flow resumes upon discontinuation).

Common Adverse Effects

>10%:
Central nervous system: Slight to moderate drowsiness
Respiratory: Thickening of bronchial secretions

1% to 10%:
Central nervous system: Headache, fatigue, nervousness, dizziness
Gastrointestinal: Appetite increase, weight gain, nausea, diarrhea, abdominal pain, xerostomia
Neuromuscular & skeletal: Arthralgia
Respiratory: Pharyngitis

Mechanism of Action Competes with histamine for H_1-receptor sites on effector cells in the gastrointestinal tract, blood vessels, and respiratory tract

Drug Interactions

Increased Effect/Toxicity: CNS depressants may increase the degree of sedation and respiratory depression with antihistamines. May increase the absorption of digoxin. Central and/or peripheral anticholinergic syndrome can occur when administered with amantadine, rimantadine, narcotic analgesics, phenothiazines and other antipsychotics (especially with high anticholinergic activity), tricyclic antidepressants, quinidine, disopyramide, procainamide, and antihistamines.

Decreased Effect: May increase gastric degradation of levodopa and decrease the amount of levodopa absorbed by delaying gastric emptying. Therapeutic effects of cholinergic agents (tacrine, donepezil) and neuroleptics may be antagonized.

Pharmacodynamics/Kinetics

Onset of action: ~1 hour
Duration: 3-6 hours
Absorption: Well absorbed
Metabolism: Hepatic

Pregnancy Risk Factor B

Dexchlorpheniramine Maleate *see* Dexchlorpheniramine *on page 414*

Dexchlorpheniramine Tannate and Pseudoephedrine Tannate *see* Chlorpheniramine and Pseudoephedrine *on page 315*

Dexedrine® *see* Dextroamphetamine *on page 418*

Dexferrum® *see* Iron Dextran Complex *on page 766*

Dexmedetomidine (deks MED e toe mi deen)

U.S. Brand Names Precedex™

Canadian Brand Names Precedex™

Generic Available No

Synonyms Dexmedetomidine Hydrochloride

Pharmacologic Category $Alpha_2$-Adrenergic Agonist; Sedative

Use Sedation of initially intubated and mechanically ventilated patients during treatment in an intensive care setting; duration of infusion should not exceed 24 hours

Unlabeled/Investigational Use Unlabeled uses include premedication prior to anesthesia induction with thiopental; relief of pain and reduction of opioid dose following laparoscopic tubal ligation; as an adjunct anesthetic in ophthalmic surgery; treatment of shivering; premedication to attenuate the cardiostimulatory and postanesthetic delirium of ketamine

Local Anesthetic/Vasoconstrictor Precautions No information available to require special precautions

Effects on Dental Treatment Key adverse event(s) related to dental treatment: Xerostomia and changes in salivation (normal salivary flow resumes upon discontinuation).

Common Adverse Effects

>10%:
- Cardiovascular: Hypotension (30%)
- Gastrointestinal: Nausea (11%)

1% to 10%:
- Cardiovascular: Bradycardia (8%), atrial fibrillation (7%)
- Central nervous system: Pain (3%)
- Hematologic: Anemia (3%), leukocytosis (2%)
- Renal: Oliguria (2%)
- Respiratory: Hypoxia (6%), pulmonary edema (2%), pleural effusion (3%)
- Miscellaneous: Infection (2%), thirst (2%)

Mechanism of Action Selective $alpha_2$-adrenoceptor agonist with sedative properties; $alpha_1$ activity was observed at high doses or after rapid infusions

Drug Interactions

Cytochrome P450 Effect: Substrate of CYP2A6 (major); **Inhibits** CYP1A2 (weak), 2C8/9 (weak), 2D6 (strong), 3A4 (weak)

Increased Effect/Toxicity: The levels/effects of dexmedetomidine may be increased by isoniazid, methoxsalen, miconazole, and other CYP2A6 inhibitors. Dexmedetomidine may increase the levels/effects of amphetamines, selected beta-blockers, dextromethorphan, fluoxetine, lidocaine, mirtazapine, nefazodone, paroxetine, risperidone, ritonavir, thioridazine, tricyclic antidepressants, venlafaxine, and other CYP2D6 substrates. Hypotension and/or bradycardia may be increased by vasodilators and heart rate-lowering agents.

Decreased Effect: Dexmedetomidine may decrease the levels/effects of CYP2D6 prodrug substrates; example prodrug substrates include codeine, hydrocodone, oxycodone, and tramadol.

Pharmacodynamics/Kinetics

Onset of action: Rapid
Distribution: V_{ss}: Approximately 118 L; rapid
Protein binding: 94%

(Continued)

Dexmedetomidine *(Continued)*

Metabolism: Hepatic via glucuronidation and CYP2A6
Half-life elimination: 6 minutes; Terminal: 2 hours
Excretion: Urine (95%); feces (4%)

Pregnancy Risk Factor C

Dexmedetomidine Hydrochloride *see* Dexmedetomidine *on page 415*

Dexmethylphenidate (dex meth il FEN i date)

U.S. Brand Names Focalin™

Generic Available No

Synonyms Dexmethylphenidate Hydrochloride

Pharmacologic Category Central Nervous System Stimulant

Use Treatment of attention-deficit/hyperactivity disorder (ADHD)

Local Anesthetic/Vasoconstrictor Precautions No information available to require special precautions

Effects on Dental Treatment No significant effects or complications reported

Common Adverse Effects

>10%: Gastrointestinal: Abdominal pain (15%)

1% to 10%:
- Central nervous system: Fever (5%)
- Gastrointestinal: Nausea (9%), anorexia (6%)

Adverse effects seen with **methylphenidate** (frequency not defined):
- Cardiovascular: Angina, cardiac arrhythmias, cerebral arteritis, cerebral occlusion, hypertension, hypotension, palpitations, pulse increase/ decrease, tachycardia
- Central nervous system: Depression, dizziness, drowsiness, fever, headache, insomnia, nervousness, neuroleptic malignant syndrome (NMS), Tourette's syndrome, toxic psychosis
- Dermatologic: Erythema multiforme, exfoliative dermatitis, hair loss, rash, urticaria
- Endocrine & metabolic: Growth retardation
- Gastrointestinal: Abdominal pain, anorexia, nausea, vomiting, weight loss
- Hematologic: Anemia, leukopenia, thrombocytopenic purpura
- Hepatic: Abnormal liver function tests, hepatic coma, transaminase elevation
- Neuromuscular & skeletal: Arthralgia, dyskinesia
- Ocular: Blurred vision
- Renal: Necrotizing vasculitis
- Respiratory: Cough increased, pharyngitis, sinusitis, upper respiratory tract infection
- Miscellaneous: Hypersensitivity reactions

Restrictions C-II

Mechanism of Action Dexmethylphenidate is the more active, *d-threo*-enantiomer, of racemic methylphenidate. It is a CNS stimulant; blocks the reuptake of norepinephrine and dopamine, and increases their release into the extraneuronal space.

Drug Interactions

Increased Effect/Toxicity: Methylphenidate may cause hypertensive effects when used in combination with MAO inhibitors or drugs with MAO-inhibiting activity (linezolid). Risk may be less with selegiline (MAO type B selective at low doses); it is best to avoid this combination. NMS has been reported in a patient receiving methylphenidate and venlafaxine. Methylphenidate may increase levels of phenytoin, phenobarbital, TCAs, and warfarin. Increased toxicity with clonidine and sibutramine.

Decreased Effect: Effectiveness of antihypertensive agents may be decreased. Carbamazepine may decrease the effect of methylphenidate.

Pharmacodynamics/Kinetics

Absorption: Rapid
Metabolism: Via de-esterification to inactive metabolite, *d*-α-phenyl-piperidine acetate (*d*-ritalinic acid)
Half-life elimination: 2.2 hours
Time to peak: Fasting: 1-1.5 hours
Excretion: Urine (90%)

Pregnancy Risk Factor C

Dexmethylphenidate Hydrochloride *see* Dexmethylphenidate *on page 416*

DexPak® TaperPak® *see* Dexamethasone *on page 411*

Dexpanthenol (deks PAN the nole)

U.S. Brand Names Panthoderm® [OTC]

Generic Available Yes: Injection

Synonyms Pantothenyl Alcohol

Pharmacologic Category Gastrointestinal Agent, Stimulant; Topical Skin Product

Use Prophylactic use to minimize paralytic ileus; treatment of postoperative distention; topical to relieve itching and to aid healing of minor dermatoses

Local Anesthetic/Vasoconstrictor Precautions No information available to require special precautions

Effects on Dental Treatment No significant effects or complications reported

Common Adverse Effects Frequency not defined.

Cardiovascular: Slight drop in blood pressure
Central nervous system: Agitation
Dermatologic: Dermatitis, irritation, itching, urticaria
Gastrointestinal: Diarrhea, hyperperistalsis, vomiting
Neuromuscular & skeletal: Paresthesia
Respiratory: Dyspnea
Miscellaneous: Allergic reactions

Mechanism of Action A pantothenic acid B vitamin analog that is converted to coenzyme A internally; coenzyme A is essential to normal fatty acid synthesis, amino acid synthesis and acetylation of choline in the production of the neurotransmitter, acetylcholine

Drug Interactions

Increased Effect/Toxicity: Increased/prolonged effect when dexpanthenol injection is given with succinylcholine; do not give dexpanthenol within 1 hour of succinylcholine.

Pregnancy Risk Factor C

Dexrazoxane (deks ray ZOKS ane)

U.S. Brand Names Zinecard®

Canadian Brand Names Zinecard®

Generic Available No

Synonyms ICRF-187

Pharmacologic Category Cardioprotectant

Use Reduction of the incidence and severity of cardiomyopathy associated with doxorubicin administration in women with metastatic breast cancer who have received a cumulative doxorubicin dose of 300 mg/m^2 and who would benefit from continuing therapy with doxorubicin. It is not recommended for use with the initiation of doxorubicin therapy.

Local Anesthetic/Vasoconstrictor Precautions No information available to require special precautions

Effects on Dental Treatment No significant effects or complications reported

Common Adverse Effects Unless specified, frequency not defined.

Dermatologic: Alopecia, urticaria, recall skin reaction, extravasation
Endocrine & metabolic: Serum amylase increased, serum calcium decreased, serum triglycerides increased
Gastrointestinal: Nausea, vomiting (mild)
Hematologic: Myelosuppression, neutropenia (~12%), thrombocytopenia (~4%)
Hepatic: AST/ALT increased, bilirubin increased

Mechanism of Action Derivative of EDTA; potent intracellular chelating agent. The mechanism of cardioprotectant activity is not fully understood. Appears to be converted intracellularly to a ring-opened chelating agent that interferes with iron-mediated oxygen free radical generation thought to be responsible, in part, for anthracycline-induced cardiomyopathy.

Pharmacodynamics/Kinetics

Distribution: V_d: 22-22.4 L/m^2
Protein binding: None
Half-life elimination: 2.1-2.5 hours
Excretion: Urine (42%)
Clearance, renal: 3.35 L/hour/m^2; Plasma: 6.25-7.88 L/hour/m^2

Pregnancy Risk Factor C

Dextran (DEKS tran)

Related Information

Dextran 1 *on page 418*

U.S. Brand Names Gentran®; LMD®

Canadian Brand Names Gentran®

Mexican Brand Names Rheomacrodex®

Generic Available Yes

Synonyms Dextran 40; Dextran 70; Dextran, High Molecular Weight; Dextran, Low Molecular Weight

(Continued)

Dextran *(Continued)*

Pharmacologic Category Plasma Volume Expander

Use Blood volume expander used in treatment of shock or impending shock when blood or blood products are not available; dextran 40 is also used as a priming fluid in cardiopulmonary bypass and for prophylaxis of venous thrombosis and pulmonary embolism in surgical procedures associated with a high risk of thromboembolic complications

Local Anesthetic/Vasoconstrictor Precautions No information available to require special precautions

Effects on Dental Treatment No significant effects or complications reported

Mechanism of Action Produces plasma volume expansion by virtue of its highly colloidal starch structure, similar to albumin

Pharmacodynamics/Kinetics

Onset of action: Minutes to 1 hour (depending upon the molecular weight polysaccharide administered)

Excretion: Urine (~75%) within 24 hours

Pregnancy Risk Factor C

Dextran 1 (DEKS tran won)

Related Information

Dextran *on page 417*

U.S. Brand Names Promit®

Generic Available No

Pharmacologic Category Plasma Volume Expander

Use Prophylaxis of serious anaphylactic reactions to I.V. infusion of dextran

Local Anesthetic/Vasoconstrictor Precautions No information available to require special precautions

Effects on Dental Treatment No significant effects or complications reported

Mechanism of Action Binds to dextran-reactive immunoglobulin without bridge formation and no formation of large immune complexes

Pregnancy Risk Factor C

Dextran 40 *see* Dextran *on page 417*

Dextran 70 *see* Dextran *on page 417*

Dextran, High Molecular Weight *see* Dextran *on page 417*

Dextran, Low Molecular Weight *see* Dextran *on page 417*

Dextroamphetamine (deks troe am FET a meen)

Related Information

Dextroamphetamine and Amphetamine *on page 419*

U.S. Brand Names Dexedrine®; Dextrostat®

Canadian Brand Names Dexedrine®

Generic Available Yes

Synonyms Dextroamphetamine Sulfate

Pharmacologic Category Stimulant

Use Narcolepsy; attention-deficit/hyperactivity disorder (ADHD)

Unlabeled/Investigational Use Exogenous obesity; depression; abnormal behavioral syndrome in children (minimal brain dysfunction)

Local Anesthetic/Vasoconstrictor Precautions Use vasoconstrictor with caution in patients taking dextroamphetamine. Amphetamines enhance the sympathomimetic response of epinephrine and norepinephrine leading to potential hypertension and cardiotoxicity.

Effects on Dental Treatment Key adverse event(s) related to dental treatment: Xerostomia (normal salivary flow resumes upon discontinuation). Up to 10% of patients taking dextroamphetamines may present with hypertension. The use of local anesthetic without vasoconstrictor is recommended in these patients.

Common Adverse Effects Frequency not defined.

Cardiovascular: Palpitations, tachycardia, hypertension, cardiomyopathy

Central nervous system: Overstimulation, euphoria, dyskinesia, dysphoria, exacerbation of motor and phonic tics, restlessness, insomnia, dizziness, headache, psychosis, Tourette's syndrome

Dermatologic: Rash, urticaria

Endocrine & metabolic: Changes in libido

Gastrointestinal: Diarrhea, constipation, anorexia, weight loss, xerostomia, unpleasant taste

Genitourinary: Impotence

Neuromuscular & skeletal: Tremor

Restrictions C-II

Mechanism of Action Blocks reuptake of dopamine and norepinephrine from the synapse, thus increases the amount of circulating dopamine and norepinephrine in cerebral cortex to reticular activating system; inhibits the action of monoamine oxidase and causes catecholamines to be released. Peripheral actions include elevated blood pressure, weak bronchodilator, and respiratory stimulant action.

Drug Interactions

Cytochrome P450 Effect: Substrate of CYP2D6 (major)

Increased Effect/Toxicity: CYP2D6 inhibitors may increase the levels/effects of dextroamphetamine; example inhibitors include chlorpromazine, delavirdine, fluoxetine, miconazole, paroxetine, pergolide, quinidine, quinine, ritonavir, and ropinirole. Dextroamphetamine may precipitate hypertensive crisis or serotonin syndrome in patients receiving MAO inhibitors (selegiline >10 mg/day, isocarboxazid, phenelzine, tranylcypromine, furazolidone). Serotonin syndrome has also been associated with combinations of amphetamines and SSRIs; these combinations should be avoided. TCAs may enhance the effects of amphetamines. Large doses of antacids or urinary alkalinizers increase the half-life and duration of action of amphetamines. May precipitate arrhythmias in patients receiving general anesthetics.

Decreased Effect: Amphetamines inhibit the antihypertensive response to guanethidine and guanadrel. Urinary acidifiers decrease the half-life and duration of action of amphetamines.

Pharmacodynamics/Kinetics

Onset of action: 1-1.5 hours

Distribution: V_d: Adults: 3.5-4.6 L/kg; distributes into CNS; mean CSF concentrations are 80% of plasma; enters breast milk

Metabolism: Hepatic via CYP monooxygenase and glucuronidation

Half-life elimination: Adults: 10-13 hours

Time to peak, serum: T_{max}: Immediate release: 3 hours; sustained release: 8 hours

Excretion: Urine (as unchanged drug and inactive metabolites)

Pregnancy Risk Factor C

Dextroamphetamine and Amphetamine

(deks troe am FET a meen & am FET a meen)

Related Information

Dextroamphetamine *on page 418*

U.S. Brand Names Adderall®; Adderall XR™

Generic Available Yes: Tablet

Synonyms Amphetamine and Dextroamphetamine

Pharmacologic Category Stimulant

Use Attention-deficit/hyperactivity disorder (ADHD); narcolepsy

Local Anesthetic/Vasoconstrictor Precautions Use vasoconstrictor with caution in patients taking dextroamphetamine. Amphetamines enhance the sympathomimetic response of epinephrine and norepinephrine leading to potential hypertension and cardiotoxicity.

Effects on Dental Treatment Key adverse event(s) related to dental treatment: Up to 10% of patients taking dextroamphetamines may present with hypertension. The use of local anesthetic without vasoconstrictor is recommended in these patients.

Common Adverse Effects

As reported with Adderall XR™:

>10%:

Central nervous system: Insomnia (1% to 17%)

Gastrointestinal: Appetite decreased (22%), abdominal pain (14%)

1% to 10%:

Central nervous system: Emotional lability (1% to 9%), nervousness (6%), fever (4%), dizziness (2%), weakness (2%)

Gastrointestinal: Vomiting (7%), nausea (5%), anorexia (3%), diarrhea (2%), dyspepsia (2%), weight loss (1%)

Miscellaneous: Infection (2% to 4%)

In addition, the following have been reported with amphetamine use:

Frequency not defined:

Cardiovascular: Palpitations, tachycardia, hypertension, cardiomyopathy

Central nervous system: Overstimulation, euphoria, dyskinesia, dysphoria, exacerbation of motor and phonic tics, restlessness, insomnia, headache, psychosis, exacerbation of Tourette's syndrome

Dermatologic: Rash, urticaria

Endocrine & metabolic: Changes in libido

Gastrointestinal: Constipation, xerostomia, unpleasant taste

Genitourinary: Impotence

Neuromuscular & skeletal: Tremor

(Continued)

Dextroamphetamine and Amphetamine *(Continued)*

Restrictions C-II

Dosage Oral: **Note:** Use lowest effective individualized dose; administer first dose as soon as awake

ADHD:

Children: <3 years: Not recommended

Children: 3-5 years (Adderall®): Initial 2.5 mg/day given every morning; increase daily dose in 2.5 mg increments at weekly intervals until optimal response is obtained (maximum dose: 40 mg/day given in 1-3 divided doses); use intervals of 4-6 hours between additional doses

Children: ≥6 years:

Adderall®: Initial: 5 mg 1-2 times/day; increase daily dose in 5 mg increments at weekly intervals until optimal response is obtained (usual maximum dose: 40 mg/day given in 1-3 divided doses); use intervals of 4-6 hours between additional doses

Adderall XR™: 5-10 mg once daily in the morning; if needed, may increase daily dose in 5-10 mg increments at weekly intervals (maximum dose: 30 mg/day)

Narcolepsy: Adderall®:

Children: 6-12 years: Initial: 5 mg/day; increase daily dose in 5 mg at weekly intervals until optimal response is obtained (maximum dose: 60 mg/day given in 1-3 divided doses)

Children >12 years and Adults: Initial: 10 mg/day; increase daily dose in 10 mg increments at weekly intervals until optimal response is obtained (maximum dose: 60 mg/day given in 1-3 divided doses)

Mechanism of Action Blocks reuptake of dopamine and norepinephrine from the synapse, thus increases the amount of circulating dopamine and norepinephrine in cerebral cortex to reticular activating system; inhibits the action of monoamine oxidase and causes catecholamines to be released. Peripheral actions include elevated blood pressure, weak bronchodilator, and respiratory stimulant action.

Contraindications Hypersensitivity to dextroamphetamine, amphetamine, or any component of the formulation; advanced arteriosclerosis; symptomatic cardiovascular disease; moderate to severe hypertension; hyperthyroidism; hypersensitivity or idiosyncrasy to the sympathomimetic amines; glaucoma; agitated states; patients with a history of drug abuse; during or within 14 days following MAO inhibitor (hypertensive crisis)

Drug Interactions

Cytochrome P450 Effect:

Dextroamphetamine: **Substrate** of CYP2D6 (major)

Amphetamine: **Substrate** of CYP2D6 (major); **Inhibits** CYP2D6 (weak)

Increased Effect/Toxicity: CYP2D6 inhibitors may increase the levels/effects of amphetamine and dextroamphetamine; example inhibitors include chlorpromazine, delavirdine, fluoxetine, miconazole, paroxetine, pergolide, quinidine, quinine, ritonavir, and ropinirole. Dextroamphetamine and amphetamine may precipitate hypertensive crisis or serotonin syndrome in patients receiving MAO inhibitors (selegiline >10 mg/day, isocarboxazid, phenelzine, tranylcypromine, furazolidone). Serotonin syndrome has also been associated with combinations of amphetamines and SSRIs; these combinations should be avoided. TCAs may enhance the effects of amphetamines, potentially leading to hypertensive crisis. Large doses of antacids or urinary alkalinizers increase the half-life and duration of action of amphetamines. May precipitate arrhythmias in patients receiving general anesthetics.

Decreased Effect: Amphetamines inhibit the antihypertensive response to guanethidine and guanadrel. Urinary acidifiers decrease the half-life and duration of action of amphetamines.

Ethanol/Nutrition/Herb Interactions

Ethanol: Avoid ethanol (may increase CNS depression).

Food: Dextroamphetamine serum levels may be altered if taken with acidic food, juices, or vitamin C. Avoid caffeine.

Herb/Nutraceutical: Avoid ephedra (may cause hypertension or arrhythmias).

Pharmacodynamics/Kinetics

Onset: 30-60 minutes

Duration: 4-6 hours

Absorption: Well-absorbed

Distribution: V_d: Adults: 3.5-4.6 L/kg; concentrates in breast milk (avoid breast-feeding); distributes into CNS, mean CSF concentrations are 80% of plasma

Half-life elimination:

Children: D-amphetamine: 9 hours; L-amphetamine: 11 hours

Adults: D-amphetamine: 10 hours; L-amphetamine: 13 hours

Metabolism: Hepatic via cytochrome P450 monooxygenase and glucuronidation

Time to peak: T_{max}: Adderall®: 3 hours; Adderall XR™: 7 hours

Excretion: 70% of a single dose is eliminated within 24 hours; excreted as unchanged amphetamine (30%), benzoic acid, hydroxyamphetamine, hippuric acid, norephedrine, and *p*-hydroxynorephedrine

Pregnancy Risk Factor C

Dosage Forms CAP, extended release (Adderall XR™): 5 mg [dextroamphetamine sulfate 1.25 mg, dextroamphetamine saccharate 1.25 mg, amphetamine aspartate monohydrate 1.25 mg, amphetamine sulfate 1.25 mg] (equivalent to amphetamine base 3.1 mg); 10 mg [dextroamphetamine sulfate 2.5 mg, dextroamphetamine saccharate 2.5 mg, amphetamine aspartate monohydrate 2.5 mg, amphetamine sulfate 2.5 mg] (equivalent to amphetamine base 6.3 mg); 15 mg [dextroamphetamine sulfate 3.75 mg, dextroamphetamine saccharate 3.75 mg, amphetamine aspartate monohydrate 3.75 mg, amphetamine sulfate 3.75 mg] (equivalent to amphetamine base 9.4 mg); 20 mg [dextroamphetamine sulfate 5 mg, dextroamphetamine saccharate 5 mg, amphetamine aspartate monohydrate 5 mg, amphetamine sulfate 5 mg] (equivalent to amphetamine base 12.5 mg); 25 mg [dextroamphetamine sulfate 6.25 mg, dextroamphetamine saccharate 6.25 mg, amphetamine aspartate monohydrate 6.25 mg, amphetamine sulfate 6.25 mg] (equivalent to amphetamine base 15.6 mg); 30 mg [dextroamphetamine sulfate 7.5 mg, dextroamphetamine saccharate 7.5 mg, amphetamine aspartate monohydrate 7.5 mg, amphetamine sulfate 7.5 mg] (equivalent to amphetamine base 18.8 mg). **TAB** (Adderall®): 5 mg [dextroamphetamine sulfate 1.25 mg, dextroamphetamine saccharate 1.25 mg, amphetamine aspartate 1.25 mg, amphetamine sulfate 1.25 mg] (equivalent to amphetamine base 3.13 mg); 7.5 mg [dextroamphetamine 1.875 mg, dextroamphetamine saccharate 1.875 mg, amphetamine aspartate 1.875 mg, amphetamine sulfate 1.875 mg] (equivalent to amphetamine base 4.7 mg); 10 mg [dextroamphetamine sulfate 2.5 mg, dextroamphetamine saccharate 2.5 mg, amphetamine aspartate 2.5 mg, amphetamine sulfate 2.5 mg] (equivalent to amphetamine base 6.3 mg); 12.5 mg [dextroamphetamine sulfate 3.125 mg, dextroamphetamine saccharate 3.125 mg, amphetamine aspartate 3.125 mg, amphetamine sulfate 3.125 mg] (equivalent to amphetamine base 7.8 mg); 15 mg [dextroamphetamine sulfate 3.75 mg, dextroamphetamine saccharate 3.75 mg, amphetamine aspartate 3.75 mg, amphetamine sulfate 3.75 mg] (equivalent to amphetamine base 9.4 mg); 20 mg [dextroamphetamine sulfate 5 mg, dextroamphetamine saccharate 5 mg, amphetamine aspartate 5 mg, amphetamine sulfate 5 mg] (equivalent to amphetamine base 12.6 mg); 30 mg [dextroamphetamine sulfate 7.5 mg, dextroamphetamine saccharate 7.5 mg, amphetamine aspartate 7.5 mg, amphetamine sulfate 7.5 mg] (equivalent to amphetamine base 18.8 mg)

Dextroamphetamine Sulfate *see* Dextroamphetamine *on page 418*

Dextromethorphan (deks troe meth OR fan)

Related Information

Codeine *on page 369*

Guaifenesin, Pseudoephedrine, and Dextromethorphan *on page 676*

U.S. Brand Names Babee® Cof Syrup [OTC]; Benylin® Adult [OTC]; Benylin® Pediatric [OTC]; Creomulsion® Cough [OTC]; Creomulsion® for Children [OTC]; Creo-Terpin® [OTC]; Delsym® [OTC]; Dexalone® [OTC]; ElixSure™ Cough [OTC]; Hold® DM [OTC]; PediaCare® Infants' Long-Acting Cough [OTC]; Pertussin® DM [OTC]; Robitussin® CoughGels™[OTC]; Robitussin® Honey Cough [OTC]; Robitussin® Maximum Strength Cough [OTC]; Robitussin® Pediatric Cough [OTC]; Scot-Tussin DM® Cough Chasers [OTC]; Silphen DM® [OTC]; Simply Cough® [OTC]; Vicks® 44® Cough Relief [OTC]

Mexican Brand Names Athos®; Bekidiba Dex®; Neopulmonier®; Romilar®

Generic Available Yes

Pharmacologic Category Antitussive

Use Symptomatic relief of coughs caused by minor viral upper respiratory tract infections or inhaled irritants; most effective for a chronic nonproductive cough

Unlabeled/Investigational Use *N*-methyl-D-aspartate (NMDA) antagonist in cerebral injury

Local Anesthetic/Vasoconstrictor Precautions No information available to require special precautions

Effects on Dental Treatment No significant effects or complications reported

(Continued)

Dextromethorphan *(Continued)*

Mechanism of Action Chemical relative of morphine lacking narcotic properties except in overdose; controls cough by depressing the medullary cough center

Drug Interactions

Cytochrome P450 Effect: Substrate of CYP2B6 (minor), 2C8/9 (minor), 2C19 (minor), 2D6 (major), 2E1 (minor), 3A4 (minor); **Inhibits** CYP2D6 (weak)

Increased Effect/Toxicity: CYP2D6 inhibitors may increase the levels/effects of dextromethorphan; example inhibitors include chlorpromazine, delavirdine, fluoxetine, miconazole, paroxetine, pergolide, quinidine, quinine, ritonavir, and ropinirole. Dextromethorphan may increase effect/toxicity of MAO inhibitors.

Pharmacodynamics/Kinetics

Onset of action: Antitussive: 15-30 minutes

Duration: ≤6 hours

Pregnancy Risk Factor C

Dextromethorphan, Acetaminophen, and Pseudoephedrine *see* Acetaminophen, Dextromethorphan, and Pseudoephedrine *on page 59*

Dextromethorphan and Guaifenesin *see* Guaifenesin and Dextromethorphan *on page 673*

Dextromethorphan and Promethazine *see* Promethazine and Dextromethorphan *on page 1131*

Dextromethorphan and Pseudoephedrine *see* Pseudoephedrine and Dextromethorphan *on page 1148*

Dextromethorphan, Carbinoxamine, and Pseudoephedrine *see* Carbinoxamine, Pseudoephedrine, and Dextromethorphan *on page 263*

Dextromethorphan, Chlorpheniramine, and Phenylephrine *see* Chlorpheniramine, Phenylephrine, and Dextromethorphan *on page 316*

Dextromethorphan, Guaifenesin, and Potassium Guaiacolsulfonate *see* Guaifenesin, Potassium Guaiacolsulfonate, and Dextromethorphan *on page 675*

Dextromethorphan, Guaifenesin, and Pseudoephedrine *see* Guaifenesin, Pseudoephedrine, and Dextromethorphan *on page 676*

Dextromethorphan, Pseudoephedrine, and Carbinoxamine *see* Carbinoxamine, Pseudoephedrine, and Dextromethorphan *on page 263*

Dextropropoxyphene *see* Propoxyphene *on page 1136*

Dextrose and Tetracaine *see* Tetracaine and Dextrose *on page 1279*

Dextrose, Levulose and Phosphoric Acid *see* Fructose, Dextrose, and Phosphoric Acid *on page 638*

Dextrostat® *see* Dextroamphetamine *on page 418*

DFMO *see* Eflornithine *on page 485*

DHAD *see* Mitoxantrone *on page 938*

DHAQ *see* Mitoxantrone *on page 938*

DHE *see* Dihydroergotamine *on page 442*

D.H.E. 45® *see* Dihydroergotamine *on page 442*

DHPG Sodium *see* Ganciclovir *on page 646*

DHS™ Sal [OTC] *see* Salicylic Acid *on page 1205*

DHS™ Tar [OTC] *see* Coal Tar *on page 367*

DHS™ Targel [OTC] *see* Coal Tar *on page 367*

DHS™ Zinc [OTC] *see* Pyrithione Zinc *on page 1155*

DHT™ *see* Dihydrotachysterol *on page 443*

DHT™ Intensol™ *see* Dihydrotachysterol *on page 443*

Diaβeta® *see* GlyBURIDE *on page 664*

Diabetic Tussin® Allergy Relief [OTC] *see* Chlorpheniramine *on page 313*

Diabetic Tussin C® *see* Guaifenesin and Codeine *on page 673*

Diabetic Tussin® DM [OTC] *see* Guaifenesin and Dextromethorphan *on page 673*

Diabetic Tussin® DM Maximum Strength [OTC] *see* Guaifenesin and Dextromethorphan *on page 673*

Diabetic Tussin® EX [OTC] *see* Guaifenesin *on page 672*

Diabinese® *see* ChlorproPAMIDE *on page 321*

Diaminocyclohexane Oxalatoplatinum *see* Oxaliplatin *on page 1020*

Diaminodiphenylsulfone *see* Dapsone *on page 398*

Diamox® Sequels® *see* AcetaZOLAMIDE *on page 60*

Diasorb® [OTC] *see* Attapulgite *on page 170*

Diastat® *see* Diazepam *on page 423*

Diatx™ *see* Vitamin B Complex Combinations *on page 1382*
DiatxFe™ *see* Vitamin B Complex Combinations *on page 1382*

Diazepam (dye AZ e pam)

Related Information

Dental Office Emergencies *on page 1584*
Patients Requiring Sedation *on page 1567*
Temporomandibular Dysfunction (TMD) *on page 1564*

U.S. Brand Names Diastat®; Diazepam Intensol®; Valium®

Canadian Brand Names Apo-Diazepam®; Diastat®; Diazemuls®; Valium®

Mexican Brand Names Alboral®; Ortopsique®; Pacitran®; Valium®

Generic Available Yes: Injection, tablet, solution only

Pharmacologic Category Benzodiazepine

Dental Use Oral medication for preoperative dental anxiety; sedative component in I.V. conscious sedation in oral surgery patients; skeletal muscle relaxant

Use Management of anxiety disorders, ethanol withdrawal symptoms; skeletal muscle relaxant; treatment of convulsive disorders

Orphan drug: Viscous solution for rectal administration: Management of selected, refractory epilepsy patients on stable regimens of antiepileptic drugs (AEDs) requiring intermittent use of diazepam to control episodes of increased seizure activity

Unlabeled/Investigational Use Panic disorders; preoperative sedation, light anesthesia, amnesia

Local Anesthetic/Vasoconstrictor Precautions No information available to require special precautions

Effects on Dental Treatment Key adverse event(s) related to dental treatment: Xerostomia and changes in salivation (normal salivary flow resumes upon discontinuation).

Significant Adverse Effects Frequency not defined.

Cardiovascular: Hypotension
Central nervous system: Drowsiness, ataxia, amnesia, slurred speech, paradoxical excitement or rage, fatigue, insomnia, memory impairment, headache, anxiety, depression, vertigo, confusion
Dermatologic: Rash
Endocrine & metabolic: Changes in libido
Gastrointestinal: Changes in salivation, constipation, nausea
Genitourinary: Incontinence, urinary retention
Hepatic: Jaundice
Local: Phlebitis, pain with injection
Neuromuscular & skeletal: Dysarthria, tremor
Ocular: Blurred vision, diplopia
Respiratory: Decrease in respiratory rate, apnea

Restrictions C-IV

Dosage Oral absorption is more reliable than I.M.

Children:
- Conscious sedation for procedures: Oral: 0.2-0.3 mg/kg (maximum: 10 mg) 45-60 minutes prior to procedure
- Sedation/muscle relaxant/anxiety:
  - Oral: 0.12-0.8 mg/kg/day in divided doses every 6-8 hours
  - I.M., I.V.: 0.04-0.3 mg/kg/dose every 2-4 hours to a maximum of 0.6 mg/kg within an 8-hour period if needed
- Status epilepticus:
  - Infants 30 days to 5 years: I.V.: 0.05-0.3 mg/kg/dose given over 2-3 minutes, every 15-30 minutes to a maximum total dose of 5 mg; repeat in 2-4 hours as needed **or** 0.2-0.5 mg/dose every 2-5 minutes to a maximum total dose of 5 mg
  - >5 years: I.V.: 0.05-0.3 mg/kg/dose given over 2-3 minutes every 15-30 minutes to a maximum total dose of 10 mg; repeat in 2-4 hours as needed **or** 1 mg/dose given over 2-3 minutes, every 2-5 minutes to a maximum total dose of 10 mg
  - Rectal: 0.5 mg/kg, then 0.25 mg/kg in 10 minutes if needed

Anticonvulsant (acute treatment): Rectal gel formulation:
- Infants <6 months: Not recommended
- Children <2 years: Safety and efficacy have not been studied
- Children 2-5 years: 0.5 mg/kg
- Children 6-11 years: 0.3 mg/kg
- Children ≥12 years and Adults: 0.2 mg/kg
- **Note:** Dosage should be rounded upward to the next available dose, 2.5, 5, 10, 15, and 20 mg/dose; dose may be repeated in 4-12 hours if needed; do not use more than 5 times per month or more than once every 5 days

(Continued)

Diazepam *(Continued)*

Adolescents: Conscious sedation for procedures:
Oral: 10 mg
I.V.: 5 mg, may repeat with 1/2 dose if needed
Adults:
Anxiety/sedation/skeletal muscle relaxant:
Oral: 2-10 mg 2-4 times/day
I.M., I.V.: 2-10 mg, may repeat in 3-4 hours if needed
Sedation in the ICU patient: I.V.: 0.03-0.1 mg/kg every 30 minutes to 6 hours
Status epilepticus: I.V.: 5-10 mg every 10-20 minutes, up to 30 mg in an 8-hour period; may repeat in 2-4 hours if necessary
Rapid tranquilization of agitated patient (administer every 30-60 minutes):
Oral: 5-10 mg; average total dose for tranquilization: 20-60 mg
Elderly: Oral: Initial:
Anxiety: 1-2 mg 1-2 times/day; increase gradually as needed, rarely need to use >10 mg/day (watch for hypotension and excessive sedation)
Skeletal muscle relaxant: 2-5 mg 2-4 times/day
Hemodialysis: Not dialyzable (0% to 5%); supplemental dose is not necessary
Dosing adjustment in hepatic impairment: Reduce dose by 50% in cirrhosis and avoid in severe/acute liver disease

Mechanism of Action Binds to stereospecific benzodiazepine receptors on the postsynaptic GABA neuron at several sites within the central nervous system, including the limbic system, reticular formation. Enhancement of the inhibitory effect of GABA on neuronal excitability results by increased neuronal membrane permeability to chloride ions. This shift in chloride ions results in hyperpolarization (a less excitable state) and stabilization.

Contraindications Hypersensitivity to diazepam or any component of the formulation (cross-sensitivity with other benzodiazepines may exist); narrow-angle glaucoma; not for use in children <6 months of age (oral) or <30 days of age (parenteral); pregnancy

Warnings/Precautions Diazepam has been associated with increasing the frequency of grand mal seizures. Withdrawal has also been associated with an increase in the seizure frequency. Use with caution with drugs which may decrease diazepam metabolism. Use with caution in elderly or debilitated patients, patients with hepatic disease (including alcoholics), or renal impairment. Active metabolites with extended half-lives may lead to delayed accumulation and adverse effects. Use with caution in patients with respiratory disease or impaired gag reflex.

Acute hypotension, muscle weakness, apnea, and cardiac arrest have occurred with parenteral administration. Acute effects may be more prevalent in patients receiving concurrent barbiturates, narcotics, or ethanol. Appropriate resuscitative equipment and qualified personnel should be available during administration and monitoring. Avoid use of the injection in patients with shock, coma, or acute ethanol intoxication. Intra-arterial injection or extravasation of the parenteral formulation should be avoided. Parenteral formulation contains propylene glycol, which has been associated with toxicity when administered in high dosages.

Causes CNS depression (dose-related) resulting in sedation, dizziness, confusion, or ataxia which may impair physical and mental capabilities. Patients must be cautioned about performing tasks which require mental alertness (eg, operating machinery or driving). Use with caution in patients receiving other CNS depressants or psychoactive agents. Effects with other sedative drugs or ethanol may be potentiated. The dosage of narcotics should be reduced by approximately 1/3 when diazepam is added. Benzodiazepines have been associated with falls and traumatic injury and should be used with extreme caution in patients who are at risk of these events (especially the elderly).

Use caution in patients with depression, particularly if suicidal risk may be present. Use with caution in patients with a history of drug dependence. Benzodiazepines have been associated with dependence and acute withdrawal symptoms on discontinuation or reduction in dose. Acute withdrawal, including seizures, may be precipitated in patients after administration of flumazenil to patients receiving long-term benzodiazepine therapy.

Diazepam has been associated with anterograde amnesia. Paradoxical reactions, including hyperactive or aggressive behavior, have been reported with benzodiazepines, particularly in adolescent/pediatric or psychiatric patients. Does not have analgesic, antidepressant, or antipsychotic properties.

Drug Interactions **Substrate** of CYP1A2 (minor), 2B6 (minor), 2C8/9 (minor), 2C19 (major), 3A4 (major); **Inhibits** CYP2C19 (weak), 3A4 (weak)

CNS depressants: Sedative effects and/or respiratory depression may be additive with CNS depressants; includes ethanol, barbiturates, narcotic analgesics, and other sedative agents; monitor for increased effect

CYP2C19 inducers: May decrease the levels/effects of diazepam. Example inducers include aminoglutethimide, carbamazepine, phenytoin, and rifampin.

CYP2C19 inhibitors: May increase the levels/effects of diazepam. Example inhibitors include delavirdine, fluconazole, fluvoxamine, gemfibrozil, isoniazid, omeprazole, and ticlopidine.

CYP3A4 inducers: CYP3A4 inducers may decrease the levels/effects of diazepam. Example inducers include aminoglutethimide, carbamazepine, nafcillin, nevirapine, phenobarbital, phenytoin, and rifamycins.

CYP3A4 inhibitors: May increase the levels/effects of diazepam. Example inhibitors include azole antifungals, ciprofloxacin, clarithromycin, diclofenac, doxycycline, erythromycin, imatinib, isoniazid, nefazodone, nicardipine, propofol, protease inhibitors, quinidine, and verapamil.

Levodopa: Therapeutic effects may be diminished in some patients following the addition of a benzodiazepine; limited/inconsistent data

Oral contraceptives: May decrease the clearance of some benzodiazepines (those which undergo oxidative metabolism); monitor for increased benzodiazepine effect

Theophylline: May partially antagonize some of the effects of benzodiazepines; monitor for decreased response; may require higher doses for sedation

Ethanol/Nutrition/Herb Interactions

Ethanol: Avoid ethanol (may increase CNS depression).

Food: Diazepam serum levels may be increased if taken with food. Diazepam effect/toxicity may be increased by grapefruit juice; avoid concurrent use.

Herb/Nutraceutical: St John's wort may decrease diazepam levels. Avoid valerian, St John's wort, kava kava, gotu kola (may increase CNS depression).

Pharmacodynamics/Kinetics

I.V.: Status epilepticus:

Onset of action: Almost immediate

Duration: 20-30 minutes

Absorption: Oral: 85% to 100%, more reliable than I.M.

Protein binding: 98%

Metabolism: Hepatic

Half-life elimination: Parent drug: Adults: 20-50 hours; increased half-life in neonates, elderly, and those with severe hepatic disorders; Active major metabolite (desmethyldiazepam): 50-100 hours; may be prolonged in neonates

Pregnancy Risk Factor D

Lactation Enters breast milk/contraindicated (AAP rates "of concern")

Breast-Feeding Considerations Clinical effects on the infant include sedation; AAP reports that USE MAY BE OF CONCERN.

Dosage Forms

Gel, rectal (Diastat®):

Adult rectal tip [6 cm]: 5 mg/mL (15 mg, 20 mg) [contains ethyl alcohol, sodium benzoate, benzyl alcohol; twin pack]

Pediatric rectal tip [4.4 cm]: 5 mg/mL (2.5 mg, 5 mg) [contains ethyl alcohol, sodium benzoate, benzyl alcohol; twin pack]

Universal rectal tip [for pediatric and adult use; 4.4 cm]: 5 mg/mL (10 mg) [contains ethyl alcohol, sodium benzoate, benzyl alcohol; twin pack]

Injection, solution: 5 mg/mL (2 mL, 10 mL) [may contain benzyl alcohol, sodium benzoate, benzoic acid]

Solution, oral: 5 mg/5 mL (5 mL, 500 mL) [wintergreen-spice flavor]

Solution, oral concentrate (Diazepam Intensol®): 5 mg/mL (30 mL)

Tablet (Valium®): 2 mg, 5 mg, 10 mg

Diazepam Intensol® *see* Diazepam *on page 423*

Diazoxide (dye az OKS ide)

U.S. Brand Names Hyperstat®; Proglycem®

Canadian Brand Names Hyperstat® I.V.; Proglycem®

Mexican Brand Names Sefulken® [inj.]

Generic Available No

Pharmacologic Category Antihypertensive; Antihypoglycemic Agent

Use

Oral: Hypoglycemia related to islet cell adenoma, carcinoma, hyperplasia, or adenomatosis, nesidioblastosis, leucine sensitivity, or extrapancreatic malignancy

I.V.: Severe hypertension

(Continued)

Diazoxide *(Continued)*

Local Anesthetic/Vasoconstrictor Precautions No information available to require special precautions

Effects on Dental Treatment No significant effects or complications reported

Common Adverse Effects 1% to 10%:

Cardiovascular: Hypotension

Central nervous system: Dizziness

Gastrointestinal: Nausea, vomiting

Neuromuscular & skeletal: Weakness

Mechanism of Action Inhibits insulin release from the pancreas; produces direct smooth muscle relaxation of the peripheral arterioles which results in decrease in blood pressure and reflex increase in heart rate and cardiac output

Drug Interactions

Increased Effect/Toxicity: Diuretics and hypotensive agents may potentiate diazoxide adverse effects. Diazoxide may decrease warfarin protein binding.

Decreased Effect: Diazoxide may increase phenytoin metabolism or free fraction.

Pharmacodynamics/Kinetics

Onset of action: Hyperglycemic: Oral: ~1 hour

Peak effect: Hypotensive: I.V.: ~5 minutes

Duration: Hyperglycemic: Oral: Normal renal function: 8 hours; Hypotensive: I.V.: Usually 3-12 hours

Protein binding: 90%

Half-life elimination: Children: 9-24 hours; Adults: 20-36 hours; End-stage renal disease: >30 hours

Excretion: Urine (50% as unchanged drug)

Pregnancy Risk Factor C

Dibenzyline® *see* Phenoxybenzamine *on page 1075*

Dibucaine (DYE byoo kane)

U.S. Brand Names Nupercainal® [OTC]

Generic Available Yes

Pharmacologic Category Local Anesthetic

Dental Use Amide derivative local anesthetic for minor skin conditions

Use Fast, temporary relief of pain and itching due to hemorrhoids, minor burns

Local Anesthetic/Vasoconstrictor Precautions No information available to require special precautions

Effects on Dental Treatment No significant effects or complications reported

Significant Adverse Effects 1% to 10%:

Dermatologic: Angioedema, contact dermatitis

Local: Burning

Dosage Children and Adults: Topical: Apply gently to the affected areas; no more than 30 g for adults or 7.5 g for children should be used in any 24-hour period

Mechanism of Action Local anesthetics bind selectively to the intracellular surface of sodium channels to block influx of sodium into the axon. As a result, depolarization necessary for action potential propagation and subsequent nerve function is prevented. The block at the sodium channel is reversible. When drug diffuses away from the axon, sodium channel function is restored and nerve propagation returns.

Contraindications Hypersensitivity to amide-type anesthetics, ophthalmic use

Drug Interactions No data reported

Pharmacodynamics/Kinetics

Onset of action: ~15 minutes

Duration: 2-4 hours

Absorption: Poor through intact skin; well absorbed through mucous membranes and excoriated skin

Pregnancy Risk Factor C

Breast-Feeding Considerations No data reported; however, topical administration is probably compatible.

Dosage Forms Ointment: 1% (30 g, 454 g)

Nupercainal®: 1% (30 g, 60g) [contains sodium bisulfite]

DIC *see* Dacarbazine *on page 392*

Dichloralphenazone, Acetaminophen, and Isometheptene *see* Acetaminophen, Isometheptene, and Dichloralphenazone *on page 59*

Dichloralphenazone, Isometheptene, and Acetaminophen *see* Acetaminophen, Isometheptene, and Dichloralphenazone *on page 59*

6,7-Dichloro-1,5-Dihydroimidazo [2,1b] quinazolin-2(3H)-one Monohydrochloride *see* Anagrelide *on page 130*

Dichlorodifluoromethane and Trichloromonofluoromethane

(dye klor oh dye flor oh METH ane & tri klor oh mon oh flor oh METH ane)

Related Information

Temporomandibular Dysfunction (TMD) *on page 1564*

U.S. Brand Names Fluori-Methane®

Generic Available No

Synonyms Trichloromonofluoromethane and Dichlorodifluoromethane

Pharmacologic Category Analgesic, Topical

Dental Use Topical application in the management of myofascial pain, restricted motion, and muscle spasm

Use Management of pain associated with injections

Local Anesthetic/Vasoconstrictor Precautions No information available to require special precautions

Effects on Dental Treatment No significant effects or complications reported

Significant Adverse Effects No data reported

Dosage Invert bottle over treatment area approximately 12" away from site of application; open dispenseal spring valve completely, allowing liquid to flow in a stream from the bottle. The rate of spraying is approximately 10 cm/second and should be continued until entire muscle has been covered.

Contraindications Hypersensitivity to dichlorofluoromethane and/or trichloromonofluoromethane, or any component of the formulation; patients having vascular impairment of the extremities

Warnings/Precautions For external use only; care should be taken to minimize inhalation of vapors, especially with application to head and neck; avoid contact with eyes; should not be applied to the point of frost formation

Drug Interactions No data reported

Pharmacodynamics/Kinetics No data reported

Dosage Forms Aerosol, topical: Dichlorodifluoromethane 15% and trichloromonofluoromethane 85% (103 mL) [contains chlorofluorocarbons]

Dichlorotetrafluoroethane and Ethyl Chloride *see* Ethyl Chloride and Dichlorotetrafluoroethane *on page 562*

Dichlorphenamide (dye klor FEN a mide)

U.S. Brand Names Daranide®

Canadian Brand Names Daranide®

Generic Available No

Synonyms Diclofenamide

Pharmacologic Category Carbonic Anhydrase Inhibitor; Diuretic, Carbonic Anhydrase Inhibitor; Ophthalmic Agent, Antiglaucoma

Use Adjunct in treatment of open-angle glaucoma and perioperative treatment for angle-closure glaucoma

Local Anesthetic/Vasoconstrictor Precautions No information available to require special precautions

Effects on Dental Treatment Key adverse event(s) related to dental treatment: Metallic taste.

Pregnancy Risk Factor C

Dichysterol *see* Dihydrotachysterol *on page 443*

Diclofenac (dye KLOE fen ak)

Related Information

Rheumatoid Arthritis, Osteoarthritis, and Osteoporosis *on page 1490*

Temporomandibular Dysfunction (TMD) *on page 1564*

U.S. Brand Names Cataflam®; Solaraze™; Voltaren®; Voltaren Ophthalmic®; Voltaren®-XR

Canadian Brand Names Apo-Diclo®; Apo-Diclo Rapide®; Apo-Diclo SR®; Cataflam®; Diclotec; Novo-Difenac; Novo-Difenac K; Novo-Difenac-SR; Nu-Diclo; Nu-Diclo-SR; Pennsaid®; PMS-Diclofenac; PMS-Diclofenac SR; Riva-Diclofenac; Riva-Diclofenac-K; Voltaren®; Voltaren Ophtha®; Voltaren Rapide®

Mexican Brand Names 3-A Ofteno®; Artrenac®; Cataflam®; Cataflam Dispersible®; Deflox®; Deflox® [suspension]; Dicloran®; Dolaren®; Dolflam®; Fustaren®; Galedol®; Lifenac®; Liroken®; Logesic®; Merxil®; Selectofen®; Volfenac Gel®; Volfenac Retard®; Voltaren®; Voltaren Emulgel®

Generic Available Yes

Synonyms Diclofenac Potassium; Diclofenac Sodium

(Continued)

Diclofenac *(Continued)*

Pharmacologic Category Nonsteroidal Anti-inflammatory Drug (NSAID); Nonsteroidal Anti-inflammatory Drug (NSAID), Ophthalmic; Nonsteroidal Anti-inflammatory Drug (NSAID), Oral

Dental Use Immediate-release tablets: Acute treatment of mild to moderate pain

Use

Immediate release: Ankylosing spondylitis; primary dysmenorrhea; acute and chronic treatment of rheumatoid arthritis, osteoarthritis

Delayed-release tablets: Acute and chronic treatment of rheumatoid arthritis, osteoarthritis, ankylosing spondylitis

Extended-release tablets: Chronic treatment of osteoarthritis, rheumatoid arthritis

Ophthalmic solution: Postoperative inflammation following cataract extraction; temporary relief of pain and photophobia in patients undergoing corneal refractive surgery

Topical gel: Actinic keratosis (AK) in conjunction with sun avoidance

Unlabeled/Investigational Use Juvenile rheumatoid arthritis

Local Anesthetic/Vasoconstrictor Precautions No information available to require special precautions

Effects on Dental Treatment NSAID formulations are known to reversibly decrease platelet aggregation via mechanisms different than observed with aspirin. The dentist should be aware of the potential of abnormal coagulation. Caution should also be exercised in the use of NSAIDs in patients already on anticoagulant therapy with drugs such as warfarin (Coumadin®).

Significant Adverse Effects

>10%:

Local: Application site reactions (gel): Pruritus (31% to 52%), rash (35% to 46%), contact dermatitis (19% to 33%), dry skin (25% to 27%), pain (15% to 26%), exfoliation (6% to 24%), paresthesia (8% to 20%)

Ocular: Ophthalmic drops (incidence may be dependent upon indication): Lacrimation (30%), keratitis (28%), elevated IOP (15%), transient burning/stinging (15%)

1% to 10%:

Central nervous system: Headache (7%), dizziness (3%)

Dermatologic: Pruritus (1% to 3%), rash (1% to 3%)

Endocrine & metabolic: Fluid retention (1% to 3%)

Gastrointestinal: Abdominal cramps (3% to 9%), abdominal pain (3% to 9%), constipation (3% to 9%), diarrhea (3% to 9%), flatulence (3% to 9%), indigestion (3% to 9%), nausea (3% to 9%), abdominal distention (1% to 3%), peptic ulcer/GI bleed (0.6% to 2%)

Hepatic: Increased ALT/AST (2%)

Local: Application site reactions (gel): Edema (4%)

Ocular: Ophthalmic drops: Abnormal vision, acute elevated IOP, blurred vision, conjunctivitis, corneal deposits, corneal edema, corneal opacity, corneal lesions, discharge, eyelid swelling, injection, iritis, irritation, itching, lacrimation disorder, ocular allergy

Otic: Tinnitus (1% to 3%)

<1% (Limited to important or life-threatening): Oral dosage forms: Acute renal failure, agranulocytosis, allergic purpura, alopecia, anaphylactoid reactions, anaphylaxis, angioedema, aplastic anemia, aseptic meningitis, asthma, bullous eruption, cirrhosis, CHF, eosinophilia, erythema multiforme major, GI hemorrhage, hearing loss, hemolytic anemia, hepatic necrosis, hepatitis, hepatorenal syndrome, interstitial nephritis, jaundice, laryngeal edema, leukopenia, nephrotic syndrome, pancreatitis, papillary necrosis, photosensitivity, purpura, Stevens-Johnson syndrome, swelling of lips and tongue, thrombocytopenia, urticaria, visual changes, vomiting

Dosage Adults:

Oral:

Analgesia/primary dysmenorrhea: Starting dose: 50 mg 3 times/day; maximum dose: 150 mg/day

Rheumatoid arthritis: 150-200 mg/day in 2-4 divided doses (100 mg/day of sustained release product)

Osteoarthritis: 100-150 mg/day in 2-3 divided doses (100-200 mg/day of sustained release product)

Ankylosing spondylitis: 100-125 mg/day in 4-5 divided doses

Ophthalmic:

Cataract surgery: Instill 1 drop into affected eye 4 times/day beginning 24 hours after cataract surgery and continuing for 2 weeks

Corneal refractive surgery: Instill 1-2 drops into affected eye within the hour prior to surgery, within 15 minutes following surgery, and then continue for 4 times/day, up to 3 days

Topical: Apply gel to lesion area twice daily for 60-90 days

Dosage adjustment in renal impairment: Monitor closely in patients with significant renal impairment

Dosage adjustment in hepatic impairment: No specific dosing recommendations

Elderly: No specific dosing recommendations; elderly may demonstrate adverse effects at lower doses than younger adults, and >60% may develop asymptomatic peptic ulceration with or without hemorrhage; monitor renal function

Mechanism of Action Inhibits prostaglandin synthesis by decreasing the activity of the enzyme, cyclooxygenase, which results in decreased formation of prostaglandin precursors. Mechanism of action for the treatment of AK has not been established.

Contraindications Hypersensitivity to diclofenac, any component of the formulation, aspirin or other NSAIDs, including patients who experience bronchospasm, asthma, rhinitis, or urticaria following NSAID or aspirin; porphyria; pregnancy (3rd trimester)

Warnings/Precautions Use with caution in patients with CHF, dehydration, hypertension, decreased renal or hepatic function, history of GI disease, active gastrointestinal ulceration or bleeding, or those receiving anticoagulants. Anaphylactoid reactions have been reported with NSAID use, even without prior exposure; may be more common in patients with the aspirin triad. Use with caution in patients with pre-existing asthma. Rare cases of severe hepatic reactions (including necrosis, jaundice, fulminant hepatitis) have been reported. Vision changes (including changes in color) have been rarely reported with oral diclofenac. Topical gel should not be applied to the eyes, open wounds, infected areas, or to exfoliative dermatitis. Monitor patients for 1 year following application of ophthalmic drops for corneal refractive procedures. Patients using ophthalmic drops should not wear soft contact lenses. Ophthalmic drops may slow/delay healing or prolong bleeding time following surgery. Elderly are at a high risk for adverse effects from NSAIDs. As many as 60% of elderly can develop peptic ulceration and/or hemorrhage asymptomatically.

Use lowest effective dose for shortest period possible. Use of NSAIDs can compromise existing renal function especially when Cl_{cr} is <30 mL/minute. CNS adverse effects such as confusion, agitation, and hallucination are generally seen in overdose or high-dose situations; however, elderly may demonstrate these adverse effects at lower doses than younger adults. Withhold for at least 4-6 half-lives prior to surgical or dental procedures.

Drug Interactions Substrate (minor) of CYP1A2, 2B6, 2C8/9, 2C19, 2D6, 3A4; **Inhibits** CYP1A2 (moderate), 2C8/9 (weak), 2E1 (weak), 3A4 (strong)

ACE inhibitors: Antihypertensive effects may be decreased by concurrent therapy with NSAIDs; monitor blood pressure

Angiotensin II antagonists: Antihypertensive effects may be decreased by concurrent therapy with NSAIDs; monitor blood pressure

Anticoagulants (warfarin, heparin, LMWHs) in combination with NSAIDs can cause increased risk of bleeding.

Other antiplatelet drugs (ticlopidine, clopidogrel, aspirin, abciximab, dipyridamole, eptifibatide, tirofiban) can cause an increased risk of bleeding.

Cholestyramine and colestipol reduce the bioavailability of diclofenac; separate administration times.

Corticosteroids may increase the risk of GI ulceration; avoid concurrent use.

Cyclosporine: NSAIDs may increase serum creatinine, potassium, blood pressure, and cyclosporine levels; monitor cyclosporine levels and renal function carefully.

CYP1A2 substrates: Diclofenac may increase the levels/effects of CYP1A2 substrates. Example substrates include aminophylline, fluvoxamine, mexiletine, mirtazapine, ropinirole, theophylline, and trifluoperazine.

CYP3A4 substrates: Diclofenac may increase the levels/effects of CYP3A4 substrates. Example substrates include benzodiazepines, calcium channel blockers, mirtazapine, nateglinide, nefazodone, tacrolimus, and venlafaxine. Selected benzodiazepines (midazolam and triazolam), cisapride, ergot alkaloids, selected HMG-CoA reductase inhibitors (lovastatin and simvastatin), and pimozide are generally contraindicated with strong CYP3A4 inhibitors.

Gentamicin and amikacin serum concentrations are increased by indomethacin in premature infants. Results may apply to other aminoglycosides and NSAIDs.

Hydralazine's antihypertensive effect is decreased; avoid concurrent use.

(Continued)

Diclofenac *(Continued)*

Lithium levels can be increased; avoid concurrent use if possible or monitor lithium levels and adjust dose. Sulindac may have the least effect. When NSAID is stopped, lithium will need adjustment again.

Loop diuretics efficacy (diuretic and antihypertensive effect) is reduced. Indomethacin reduces this efficacy, however, it may be anticipated with any NSAID.

Methotrexate: Severe bone marrow suppression, aplastic anemia, and GI toxicity have been reported with concomitant NSAID therapy. Avoid use during moderate or high-dose methotrexate (increased and prolonged methotrexate levels). NSAID use during low-dose treatment of rheumatoid arthritis has not been fully evaluated; extreme caution is warranted.

Thiazides antihypertensive effects are decreased; avoid concurrent use.

Verapamil plasma concentration is decreased by diclofenac; avoid concurrent use.

Warfarin's INRs may be increased by piroxicam. Other NSAIDs may have the same effect depending on dose and duration. Monitor INR closely. Use the lowest dose of NSAIDs possible and for the briefest duration.

Ethanol/Nutrition/Herb Interactions

Ethanol: Avoid ethanol (may enhance gastric mucosal irritation).

Herb/Nutraceutical: Avoid cat's claw, dong quai, evening primrose, feverfew, garlic, ginger, ginkgo, red clover, horse chestnut, green tea, ginseng (all have additional antiplatelet activity).

Dietary Considerations May be taken with food to decrease GI distress.

Diclofenac potassium = Cataflam®; potassium content: 5.8 mg (0.15 mEq) per 50 mg tablet

Pharmacodynamics/Kinetics

Onset of action: Cataflam® is more rapid than sodium salt (Voltaren®) because it dissolves in the stomach instead of the duodenum

Absorption: Topical gel: 10%

Protein binding: 99% to albumin

Metabolism: Hepatic to several metabolites

Half-life elimination: 2 hours

Time to peak, serum: Cataflam®: ~1 hour; Voltaren®: ~2 hours

Excretion: Urine (65%); feces (35%)

Pregnancy Risk Factor B/D (3rd trimester)

Lactation Enters breast milk/use caution

Dosage Forms

Gel, as sodium (Solaraze™): 30 mg/g (50 g)

Solution, ophthalmic, as sodium (Voltaren Ophthalmic®): 0.1% (2.5 mL, 5 mL)

Tablet, as potassium (Cataflam®): 50 mg

Tablet, delayed release, enteric coated, as sodium (Voltaren®): 25 mg, 50 mg, 75 mg

Tablet, extended release, as sodium (Voltaren®-XR): 100 mg

Selected Readings

Kubitzek F, Ziegler G, Gold MS, et al, "Analgesic Efficacy of Low-Dose Diclofenac Versus Paracetamol and Placebo in Postoperative Dental Pain," *J Orofac Pain*, 2003, 17(3):237-44.

Diclofenac and Misoprostol

(dye KLOE fen ak & mye soe PROST ole)

Related Information

Diclofenac *on page 427*

Rheumatoid Arthritis, Osteoarthritis, and Osteoporosis *on page 1490*

U.S. Brand Names Arthrotec®

Canadian Brand Names Arthrotec®

Generic Available No

Synonyms Misoprostol and Diclofenac

Pharmacologic Category Nonsteroidal Anti-inflammatory Drug (NSAID), Oral; Prostaglandin

Use The diclofenac component is indicated for the treatment of osteoarthritis and rheumatoid arthritis; the misoprostol component is indicated for the prophylaxis of NSAID-induced gastric and duodenal ulceration

Local Anesthetic/Vasoconstrictor Precautions No information available to require special precautions

Effects on Dental Treatment No significant effects or complications reported

Common Adverse Effects Also see individual agents.

>10%: Gastrointestinal: Abdominal pain (21%), diarrhea (19%), nausea (11%), dyspepsia (14%)

1% to 10%:

Endocrine & metabolic: Elevated transaminase levels

Gastrointestinal: Flatulence (9%)
Hematologic: Anemia
Miscellaneous: Anaphylactic reactions

Mechanism of Action See individual agents.

Drug Interactions

Cytochrome P450 Effect: Diclofenac: **Substrate** (minor) of CYP1A2, 2B6, 2C8/9, 2C19, 2D6, 3A4; **Inhibits** CYP1A2 (moderate), 2C8/9 (weak), 2E1 (weak), 3A4 (strong)

Increased Effect/Toxicity: Aspirin (shared toxicity), digoxin (elevated digoxin levels), warfarin (synergistic bleeding potential), methotrexate (increased methotrexate levels), cyclosporine (increased nephrotoxicity), lithium (increased lithium levels). Diclofenac may increase the levels/effects of CYP3A4 substrates (eg, benzodiazepines, calcium channel blockers, mirtazapine, nateglinide, nefazodone, tacrolimus, and venlafaxine). Selected benzodiazepines (midazolam and triazolam), cisapride, ergot alkaloids, selected HMG-CoA reductase inhibitors (lovastatin and simvastatin), and pimozide are generally contraindicated with strong CYP3A4 inhibitors.

Decreased Effect: Aspirin (displaces diclofenac from binding sites), antihypertensive agents (decreased blood pressure control), antacids (may decrease absorption). Antihypertensive effects of ACE inhibitors and angiotensin antagonists may be decreased by concurrent therapy with NSAIDs.

Pharmacodynamics/Kinetics See individual agents.

Pregnancy Risk Factor X

Diclofenac Potassium *see* Diclofenac *on page 427*
Diclofenac Sodium *see* Diclofenac *on page 427*
Diclofenamide *see* Dichlorphenamide *on page 427*

Dicloxacillin (dye kloks a SIL in)

Related Information

Oral Bacterial Infections *on page 1533*

Canadian Brand Names Dycill®; Pathocil®

Mexican Brand Names Cilpen® [inj.]; Ditterolina®; Posipen®

Generic Available Yes

Synonyms Dicloxacillin Sodium

Pharmacologic Category Antibiotic, Penicillin

Dental Use Treatment of susceptible orofacial infections (notably penicillinase-producing staphylococci)

Use Treatment of systemic infections such as pneumonia, skin and soft tissue infections, and osteomyelitis caused by penicillinase-producing staphylococci

Local Anesthetic/Vasoconstrictor Precautions No information available to require special precautions

Effects on Dental Treatment Key adverse event(s) related to dental treatment: Prolonged use of penicillins may lead to development of oral candidiasis.

Significant Adverse Effects

1% to 10%: Gastrointestinal: Nausea, diarrhea, abdominal pain

<1% (Limited to important or life-threatening): Agranulocytosis, eosinophilia, hemolytic anemia, hepatotoxicity, hypersensitivity, interstitial nephritis, leukopenia, neutropenia, prolonged PT, pseudomembranous colitis, rash (maculopapular to exfoliative), seizures with extremely high doses and/or renal failure, serum sickness-like reactions, thrombocytopenia, vaginitis, vomiting

Dosage Oral:

Use in newborns not recommended

Children <40 kg: 12.5-25 mg/kg/day divided every 6 hours; doses of 50-100 mg/kg/day in divided doses every 6 hours have been used for therapy of osteomyelitis

Children >40 kg and Adults: 125-250 mg every 6 hours

Dosage adjustment in renal impairment: Not necessary

Hemodialysis: Not dialyzable (0% to 5%); supplemental dosage not necessary

Peritoneal dialysis: Supplemental dosage not necessary

Continuous arteriovenous or venovenous hemofiltration: Supplemental dosage not necessary

Mechanism of Action Inhibits bacterial cell wall synthesis by binding to one or more of the penicillin binding proteins (PBPs); which in turn inhibits the final transpeptidation step of peptidoglycan synthesis in bacterial cell walls, thus inhibiting cell wall biosynthesis. Bacteria eventually lyse due to ongoing activity of cell wall autolytic enzymes (autolysins and murein hydrolases) while cell wall assembly is arrested.

Contraindications Hypersensitivity to dicloxacillin, penicillin, or any component of the formulation

(Continued)

Dicloxacillin *(Continued)*

Warnings/Precautions Monitor PT if patient concurrently on warfarin; elimination of drug is slow in neonates; use with caution in patients allergic to cephalosporins

Drug Interactions Induces CYP3A4 (weak)

Methotrexate: Penicillins may increase the exposure to methotrexate during concurrent therapy; monitor.

Oral contraceptives: Anecdotal reports suggesting decreased contraceptive efficacy with penicillins have been refuted by more rigorous scientific and clinical data.

Probenecid, disulfiram: May increase levels of penicillins (dicloxacillin)

Warfarin: Concurrent use may decrease effect of warfarin

Ethanol/Nutrition/Herb Interactions Food: Decreases drug absorption rate; decreases drug serum concentration.

Dietary Considerations Administer on an empty stomach 1 hour before or 2 hours after meals. Sodium content of 250 mg capsule: 13 mg (0.6 mEq)

Pharmacodynamics/Kinetics

Absorption: 35% to 76%; rate and extent reduced by food

Distribution: Throughout body with highest concentrations in kidney and liver; CSF penetration is low; crosses placenta; enters breast milk

Protein binding: 96%

Half-life elimination: 0.6-0.8 hour; slightly prolonged with renal impairment

Time to peak, serum: 0.5-2 hours

Excretion: Feces; urine (56% to 70% as unchanged drug); prolonged in neonates

Pregnancy Risk Factor B

Lactation Excretion in breast milk unknown (probably similar to penicillin G)

Breast-Feeding Considerations No data reported; however, other penicillins may be taken while breast-feeding.

Dosage Forms Capsule: 250 mg, 500 mg

Dicloxacillin Sodium *see* Dicloxacillin *on page 431*

Dicyclomine (dye SYE kloe meen)

U.S. Brand Names Bentyl®

Canadian Brand Names Bentylol®; Formulex®; Lomine

Generic Available Yes: Excludes syrup

Synonyms Dicyclomine Hydrochloride; Dicycloverine Hydrochloride

Pharmacologic Category Anticholinergic Agent

Use Treatment of functional disturbances of GI motility such as irritable bowel syndrome

Unlabeled/Investigational Use Urinary incontinence

Local Anesthetic/Vasoconstrictor Precautions No information available to require special precautions

Effects on Dental Treatment Key adverse event(s) related to dental treatment: Xerostomia and changes in salivation (normal salivary flow resumes upon discontinuation).

Common Adverse Effects Adverse reactions are included here that have been reported for pharmacologically similar drugs with anticholinergic/antispasmodic action; frequency not defined.

Cardiovascular: Syncope, tachycardia, palpitations

Central nervous system: Dizziness, lightheadedness, tingling, headache, drowsiness, nervousness, numbness, mental confusion and/or excitement, dyskinesia, lethargy, speech disturbance, insomnia

Dermatologic: Rash, urticaria, itching, and other dermal manifestations; severe allergic reaction or drug idiosyncrasies including anaphylaxis

Endocrine & metabolic: Suppression of lactation

Gastrointestinal: Xerostomia, nausea, vomiting, constipation, bloated feeling, abdominal pain, taste loss, anorexia

Genitourinary: Urinary hesitancy, urinary retention, impotence

Neuromuscular & skeletal: Weakness

Ocular: Blurred vision, diplopia, mydriasis, cycloplegia, increased ocular tension

Respiratory: Dyspnea, apnea, asphyxia, nasal stuffiness or congestion, sneezing, throat congestion

Miscellaneous: Decreased diaphoresis

Mechanism of Action Blocks the action of acetylcholine at parasympathetic sites in smooth muscle, secretory glands and the CNS

Drug Interactions

Increased Effect/Toxicity: Dicyclomine taken with anticholinergics, amantadine, narcotic analgesics, Type I antiarrhythmics, antihistamines, phenothiazines, tricyclic antidepressants may result in increased toxicity.

Decreased Effect: Decreased effect with phenothiazines, anti-Parkinson's drugs, haloperidol, sustained release dosage forms, and with antacids.

Pharmacodynamics/Kinetics

Onset of action: 1-2 hours

Duration: ≤4 hours

Absorption: Oral: Well absorbed

Metabolism: Extensive

Half-life elimination: Initial: 1.8 hours; Terminal: 9-10 hours

Excretion: Urine (small amounts as unchanged drug)

Pregnancy Risk Factor B

Dicyclomine Hydrochloride *see* Dicyclomine *on page 432*

Dicycloverine Hydrochloride *see* Dicyclomine *on page 432*

Didanosine (dye DAN oh seen)

Related Information

HIV Infection and AIDS *on page 1484*

U.S. Brand Names Videx®; Videx® EC

Canadian Brand Names Videx®; Videx® EC

Mexican Brand Names Videx®

Generic Available No

Synonyms ddI; Dideoxyinosine

Pharmacologic Category Antiretroviral Agent, Reverse Transcriptase Inhibitor (Nucleoside)

Use Treatment of HIV infection; always to be used in combination with at least two other antiretroviral agents

Local Anesthetic/Vasoconstrictor Precautions No information available to require special precautions

Effects on Dental Treatment Key adverse event(s) related to dental treatment: Xerostomia (normal salivary flow resumes upon discontinuation).

Common Adverse Effects As reported in monotherapy studies; risk of toxicity may increase when combined with other agents.

>10%:

Gastrointestinal: Increased amylase (15% to 17%), abdominal pain (7% to 13%), diarrhea (19% to 28%)

Neuromuscular & skeletal: Peripheral neuropathy (17% to 20%)

1% to 10%:

Dermatologic: Rash, pruritus

Endocrine & metabolic: Increased uric acid

Gastrointestinal: Pancreatitis; patients >65 years of age had a higher frequency of pancreatitis than younger patients

Hepatic: Increased SGOT, increased SGPT, increased alkaline phosphatase

Mechanism of Action Didanosine, a purine nucleoside (adenosine) analog and the deamination product of dideoxyadenosine (ddA), inhibits HIV replication *in vitro* in both T cells and monocytes. Didanosine is converted within the cell to the mono-, di-, and triphosphates of ddA. These ddA triphosphates act as substrate and inhibitor of HIV reverse transcriptase substrate and inhibitor of HIV reverse transcriptase thereby blocking viral DNA synthesis and suppressing HIV replication.

Drug Interactions

Increased Effect/Toxicity: Concomitant administration of other drugs which have the potential to cause peripheral neuropathy or pancreatitis may increase the risk of these toxicities Allopurinol may increase didanosine concentration; avoid concurrent use. Concomitant use of antacids with buffered tablet or pediatric didanosine solution may potentiate adverse effects of aluminum- or magnesium-containing antacids. Ganciclovir may increase didanosine concentration; monitor. Hydroxyurea may precipitate didanosine-induced pancreatitis if added to therapy; concomitant use is not recommended. Coadministration with ribavirin or tenofovir may increase exposure to didanosine and/or its active metabolite increasing the risk or severity of didanosine toxicities, including pancreatitis, lactic acidosis, and peripheral neuropathy; monitor closely and suspend therapy if signs or symptoms of toxicity are noted.

Decreased Effect: Didanosine buffered tablets and pediatric oral solution may decrease absorption of quinolones or tetracyclines (administer 2 hours prior to didanosine buffered formulations). Didanosine should be held during PCP treatment with pentamidine. Didanosine may decrease levels of

(Continued)

Didanosine *(Continued)*

indinavir. Drugs whose absorption depends on the level of acidity in the stomach such as ketoconazole, itraconazole, and dapsone should be administered at least 2 hours prior to the buffered formulations of didanosine (not affected by delayed release capsules). Methadone may decrease didanosine concentrations.

Pharmacodynamics/Kinetics

Absorption: Subject to degradation by acidic pH of stomach; some formulations are buffered to resist acidic pH; ≤50% reduction in peak plasma concentration is observed in presence of food. Delayed release capsules contain enteric-coated beadlets which dissolve in the small intestine.

Distribution: V_d: Children: 35.6 L/m²; Adults: 1.08 L/kg

Protein binding: <5%

Metabolism: Has not been evaluated in humans; studies conducted in dogs show extensive metabolism with allantoin, hypoxanthine, xanthine, and uric acid being the major metabolites found in urine

Bioavailability: 42%

Half-life elimination:

Children and Adolescents: 0.8 hour

Adults: Normal renal function: 1.5 hours; active metabolite, ddATP, has an intracellular half-life >12 hours *in vitro*; Renal impairment: 2.5-5 hours

Time to peak: Buffered tablets: 0.67 hours; Delayed release capsules: 2 hours

Excretion: Urine (~55% as unchanged drug)

Clearance: Total body: Averages 800 mL/minute

Pregnancy Risk Factor B

Dideoxycytidine *see* Zalcitabine *on page 1395*

Dideoxyinosine *see* Didanosine *on page 433*

Didrex® *see* Benzphetamine *on page 195*

Didronel® *see* Etidronate Disodium *on page 563*

Diethylpropion (dye eth il PROE pee on)

U.S. Brand Names Tenuate®; Tenuate® Dospan®

Canadian Brand Names Tenuate®; Tenuate® Dospan®

Mexican Brand Names Ifa Norex®; Neobes®

Generic Available Yes

Synonyms Amfepramone; Diethylpropion Hydrochloride

Pharmacologic Category Anorexiant

Use Short-term adjunct in a regimen of weight reduction based on exercise, behavioral modification, and caloric reduction in the management of exogenous obesity for patients with an initial body mass index ≥30 kg/m² or ≥27 kg/m² in the presence of other risk factors (diabetes, hypertension)

Unlabeled/Investigational Use Migraine

Local Anesthetic/Vasoconstrictor Precautions Use vasoconstrictor with caution in patients taking diethylpropion. Amphetamine-like drugs such as diethylpropion enhance the sympathomimetic response of epinephrine and norepinephrine leading to potential hypertension and cardiotoxicity.

Effects on Dental Treatment Key adverse event(s) related to dental treatment: Xerostomia and changes in salivation (normal salivary flow resumes upon discontinuation), and metallic taste (the use of local anesthetic without vasoconstrictor is recommended in these patients).

Mechanism of Action Diethylpropion is used as an anorexiant agent possessing pharmacological and chemical properties similar to those of amphetamines. The mechanism of action of diethylpropion in reducing appetite appears to be secondary to CNS effects, specifically stimulation of the hypothalamus to release catecholamines into the central nervous system; anorexiant effects are mediated via norepinephrine and dopamine metabolism. An increase in physical activity and metabolic effects (inhibition of lipogenesis and enhancement of lipolysis) may also contribute to weight loss.

Pregnancy Risk Factor B

Diethylpropion Hydrochloride *see* Diethylpropion *on page 434*

Difenoxin and Atropine (dye fen OKS in & A troe peen)

Related Information

Atropine *on page 166*

U.S. Brand Names Motofen®

Generic Available No

Synonyms Atropine and Difenoxin

Pharmacologic Category Antidiarrheal

Use Treatment of diarrhea

Local Anesthetic/Vasoconstrictor Precautions No information available to require special precautions

Effects on Dental Treatment Key adverse event(s) related to dental treatment: Xerostomia (normal salivary flow resumes upon discontinuation).

Common Adverse Effects 1% to 10%:

Central nervous system: Dizziness, drowsiness, lightheadedness, headache

Gastrointestinal: Nausea, vomiting, xerostomia, epigastric distress

Restrictions C-IV

Drug Interactions

Increased Effect/Toxicity: Concurrent use with MAO inhibitors may precipitate hypertensive crisis. May potentiate action of barbiturates, tranquilizers, narcotics, and alcohol. Difenoxin has the potential to prolong biological half-life of drugs for which the rate of elimination is dependent on the microsomal drug metabolizing enzyme system.

Pharmacodynamics/Kinetics

Absorption: Rapid and well absorbed

Metabolism: To inactive hydroxylated metabolite

Time to peak, plasma: Within 40-60 minutes

Excretion: Urine and feces (primarily as conjugates)

Pregnancy Risk Factor C

Differin® *see* Adapalene *on page 67*

Diflorasone (dye FLOR a sone)

U.S. Brand Names ApexiCon™; ApexiCon™ E; Florone®; Maxiflor® [DSC]; Psorcon®; Psorcon® e™

Canadian Brand Names Florone®; Psorcon®

Generic Available Yes

Synonyms Diflorasone Diacetate

Pharmacologic Category Corticosteroid, Topical

Use Relieves inflammation and pruritic symptoms of corticosteroid-responsive dermatosis (high to very high potency topical corticosteroid)

Maxiflor®: High potency topical corticosteroid

Psorcon™: Very high potency topical corticosteroid

Local Anesthetic/Vasoconstrictor Precautions No information available to require special precautions

Effects on Dental Treatment No significant effects or complications reported

Mechanism of Action Decreases inflammation by suppression of migration of polymorphonuclear leukocytes and reversal of increased capillary permeability

Pharmacodynamics/Kinetics

Absorption: Negligible, around 1% reaches dermal layers or systemic circulation; occlusive dressings increase absorption percutaneously

Metabolism: Primarily hepatic

Pregnancy Risk Factor C

Diflorasone Diacetate *see* Diflorasone *on page 435*

Diflucan® *see* Fluconazole *on page 594*

Diflunisal (dye FLOO ni sal)

Related Information

Oral Pain *on page 1526*

Rheumatoid Arthritis, Osteoarthritis, and Osteoporosis *on page 1490*

Temporomandibular Dysfunction (TMD) *on page 1564*

U.S. Brand Names Dolobid®

Canadian Brand Names Apo-Diflunisal®; Novo-Diflunisal; Nu-Diflunisal

Mexican Brand Names Dolobid®

Generic Available Yes

Pharmacologic Category Nonsteroidal Anti-inflammatory Drug (NSAID), Oral

Dental Use Treatment of postoperative pain

Use Management of inflammatory disorders usually including rheumatoid arthritis and osteoarthritis; can be used as an analgesic for treatment of mild to moderate pain

Local Anesthetic/Vasoconstrictor Precautions No information available to require special precautions

Effects on Dental Treatment NSAID formulations are known to reversibly decrease platelet aggregation via mechanisms different than observed with aspirin. The dentist should be aware of the potential of abnormal coagulation. Caution should also be exercised in the use of NSAIDs in patients already on anticoagulant therapy with drugs such as warfarin (Coumadin®).

(Continued)

Diflunisal *(Continued)*

Significant Adverse Effects

1% to 10%:

Cardiovascular: Chest pain, arrhythmias

Central nervous system: Dizziness, headache

Dermatologic: Rash

Endocrine & metabolic: Fluid retention

Gastrointestinal: Abdominal cramps, bloated feeling, constipation, diarrhea, indigestion, nausea, vomiting, mouth soreness

Genitourinary: Vaginal bleeding

Otic: Tinnitus

<1% (Limited to important or life-threatening): Agranulocytosis, angioedema, chest pain, dyspnea, edema, erythema multiforme, exfoliative dermatitis, hallucinations, hearing loss, hemolytic anemia, hepatitis, interstitial nephritis, itching, mental depression, nephrotic syndrome, renal impairment, seizures, Stevens-Johnson syndrome, thrombocytopenia, toxic epidermal necrolysis, urticaria, vasculitis, wheezing

Dosage Adults: Oral:

Pain: Initial: 500-1000 mg followed by 250-500 mg every 8-12 hours; maximum daily dose: 1.5 g

Inflammatory condition: 500-1000 mg/day in 2 divided doses; maximum daily dose: 1.5 g

Dosing adjustment in renal impairment: Cl_{cr} <50 mL/minute: Administer 50% of normal dose

Mechanism of Action Inhibits prostaglandin synthesis by decreasing the activity of the enzyme, cyclooxygenase, which results in decreased formation of prostaglandin precursors

Contraindications Hypersensitivity to diflunisal or any component of the formulation; may be a cross-sensitivity with other NSAIDs including aspirin; should not be used in patients with active GI bleeding; pregnancy (3rd trimester)

Warnings/Precautions Peptic ulceration and GI bleeding have been reported; platelet function and bleeding time are inhibited; ophthalmologic effects; impaired renal function, use lower dosage; dehydration; peripheral edema; possibility of Reye's syndrome; elevation in liver tests. Withhold for at least 4-6 half-lives prior to surgical or dental procedures.

Drug Interactions

ACE inhibitors: Antihypertensive effects may be decreased by concurrent therapy with NSAIDs; monitor blood pressure

Angiotensin II antagonists: Antihypertensive effects may be decreased by concurrent therapy with NSAIDs; monitor blood pressure

Antacids: Decreased effect (may decrease absorption)

Increased effect/toxicity: Digoxin, anticoagulants, phenytoin, sulfonylureas, sulfonamides, lithium, hydrochlorothiazide, acetaminophen (levels)

Methotrexate: Severe bone marrow suppression, aplastic anemia, and GI toxicity have been reported with concomitant NSAID therapy. Avoid use during moderate or high-dose methotrexate (increased and prolonged methotrexate levels). NSAID use during low-dose treatment of rheumatoid arthritis has not been fully evaluated; extreme caution is warranted.

Ethanol/Nutrition/Herb Interactions

Ethanol: Avoid ethanol (may enhance gastric mucosal irritation).

Herb/Nutraceutical: Avoid cat's claw, dong quai, evening primrose, feverfew, garlic, ginger, ginkgo, red clover, horse chestnut, green tea, ginseng (all have additional antiplatelet activity).

Dietary Considerations Should be taken with food to decrease GI distress.

Pharmacodynamics/Kinetics

Onset of action: Analgesic: ~1 hour

Duration: 8-12 hours

Absorption: Well absorbed

Distribution: Enters breast milk

Metabolism: Extensively hepatic

Half-life elimination: 8-12 hours; prolonged with renal impairment

Time to peak, serum: 2-3 hours

Excretion: Urine (~3% as unchanged drug, 90% as glucuronide conjugates) within 72-96 hours

Pregnancy Risk Factor C (1st and 2nd trimesters); D (3rd trimester)

Lactation Enters breast milk/use caution

Dosage Forms Tablet: 250 mg, 500 mg

Selected Readings

Ahmad N, Grad HA, Haas DA, et al, "The Efficacy of Nonopioid Analgesics for Postoperative Dental Pain: A Meta-Analysis," *Anesth Prog*, 1997, 44(4):119-26.

Brooks PM and Day RO, "Nonsteroidal Anti-inflammatory Drugs - Differences and Similarities," *N Engl J Med*, 1991, 324(24):1716-25.

Dionne R, "Additive Analgesia Without Opioid Side Effects," *Compend Contin Educ Dent*, 2000, 21(7):572-4, 576-7.

Dionne RA, "New Approaches to Preventing and Treating Postoperative Pain," *J Am Dent Assoc*, 1992, 123(6):26-34.

Dionne RA and Berthold CW, "Therapeutic Uses of Nonsteroidal Anti-inflammatory Drugs in Dentistry," *Crit Rev Oral Biol Med*, 2001, 12(4):315-30.

Forbes JA, Calderazzo JP, Bowser MW, et al, "A 12-Hour Evaluation of the Analgesic Efficacy of Diflunisal, Aspirin, and Placebo in Postoperative Dental Pain," *J Clin Pharmacol*, 1982, 22(2-3):89-96.

Gobetti JP, "Controlling Dental Pain," *J Am Dent Assoc*, 1992, 123(6):47-52.

Nguyen AM, Graham DY, Gage T, et al, "Nonsteroidal Anti-inflammatory Drug Use in Dentistry: Gastrointestinal Implications," *Gen Dent*, 1999, 47(6):590-6.

Selcuk E, Gomel M, Bellibas SE, et al, "Comparison of the Analgesic Effects of Diflunisal and Paracetamol in the Treatment of Postoperative Dental Pain," *Int J Clin Pharmacol Res*, 1996, 16(2-3):57-65.

Digibind® *see* Digoxin Immune Fab *on page 440*

DigiFab™ *see* Digoxin Immune Fab *on page 440*

Digitek® *see* Digoxin *on page 437*

Digitoxin (di ji TOKS in)

Related Information

Cardiovascular Diseases *on page 1458*

Digoxin *on page 437*

Digoxin Immune Fab *on page 440*

Generic Available No

Synonyms Crystodigin

Pharmacologic Category Antiarrhythmic Agent, Class IV

Use Treatment of congestive heart failure, atrial fibrillation, atrial flutter, paroxysmal atrial tachycardia, and cardiogenic shock

Local Anesthetic/Vasoconstrictor Precautions Use vasoconstrictor with caution due to risk of cardiac arrhythmias with digitoxin.

Effects on Dental Treatment Sensitive gag reflex may cause difficulty in taking a dental impression.

Common Adverse Effects 1% to 10%: Gastrointestinal: Anorexia, nausea, vomiting

Restrictions Not available in U.S.

Mechanism of Action Digitalis binds to and inhibits magnesium and adenosine triphosphate dependent sodium and potassium ATPase thereby increasing the influx of calcium ions, from extracellular to intracellular cytoplasm due to the inhibition of sodium and potassium ion movement across the myocardial membranes; this increase in calcium ions results in a potentiation of the activity of the contractile heart muscle fibers and an increase in the force of myocardial contraction (positive inotropic effect); digitalis may also increase intracellular entry of calcium via slow calcium channel influx; stimulates release and blocks re-uptake of norepinephrine; decreases conduction through the SA and AV nodes

Drug Interactions

Cytochrome P450 Effect: Substrate of CYP3A4 (major)

Increased Effect/Toxicity: CYP3A4 inhibitors may increase the levels/effects of digitoxin; example inhibitors include azole antifungals, ciprofloxacin, clarithromycin, diclofenac, doxycycline, erythromycin, imatinib, isoniazid, nefazodone, nicardipine, propofol, protease inhibitors, quinidine, and verapamil.

Decreased Effect: CYP3A4 inducers may decrease the levels/effects of digitoxin (eg, aminoglutethimide, carbamazepine, nafcillin, nevirapine, phenobarbital, phenytoin, and rifamycins).

Pharmacodynamics/Kinetics

Absorption: 90% to 100%

Distribution: V_d: 7 L/kg

Protein binding: 90% to 97%

Metabolism: Hepatic (50% to 70%)

Half-life elimination: 7-8 days

Time to peak: 8-12 hours

Excretion: Urine and feces (30% to 50% as unchanged drug)

Pregnancy Risk Factor C

Digoxin (di JOKS in)

Related Information

Cardiovascular Diseases *on page 1458*

Digitoxin *on page 437*

Digoxin Immune Fab *on page 440*

(Continued)

Digoxin *(Continued)*

U.S. Brand Names Digitek®; Lanoxicaps®; Lanoxin®

Canadian Brand Names Digoxin CSD; Lanoxicaps®; Lanoxin®; Novo-Digoxin

Mexican Brand Names Lanoxin®; Mapluxin®

Generic Available Yes; Excludes capsule

Pharmacologic Category Antiarrhythmic Agent, Class IV; Cardiac Glycoside

Use Treatment of congestive heart failure and to slow the ventricular rate in tachyarrhythmias such as atrial fibrillation, atrial flutter, and supraventricular tachycardia (paroxysmal atrial tachycardia); cardiogenic shock

Local Anesthetic/Vasoconstrictor Precautions Use vasoconstrictor with caution due to risk of cardiac arrhythmias with digoxin

Effects on Dental Treatment Sensitive gag reflex may cause difficulty in taking a dental impression.

Common Adverse Effects Incidence of reactions are not always reported.

Cardiovascular: Heart block; first-, second- (Wenckebach), or third-degree heart block; asystole; atrial tachycardia with block; AV dissociation; accelerated junctional rhythm; ventricular tachycardia or ventricular fibrillation; PR prolongation; ST segment depression

Central nervous system: Visual disturbances (blurred or yellow vision), headache (3%), weakness, dizziness (5%), apathy, confusion, mental disturbances (4%), anxiety, depression, delirium, hallucinations, fever

Dermatologic: Maculopapular rash (2%), erythematous, scarlatiniform, papular, vesicular or bullous rashes, urticaria, pruritus, facial, angioneurotic or laryngeal edema, shedding of fingernails or toenails, alopecia

Gastrointestinal: Nausea (3%), vomiting (2%), diarrhea (3%), abdominal pain

Children are more likely to experience cardiac arrhythmias as a sign of excessive dosing. The most common are conduction disturbances or tachyarrhythmias (atrial tachycardia with or without block) and junctional tachycardia. Ventricular tachyarrhythmias are less common. In infants, sinus bradycardia may be a sign of digoxin toxicity. Any arrhythmia seen in a child on digoxin should be considered as digoxin toxicity. The gastrointestinal and central nervous system symptoms are not frequently seen in children.

Dosage When changing from oral (tablets or liquid) or I.M. to I.V. therapy, dosage should be reduced by 20% to 25%. Refer to the following: See table.

Dosage Recommendations for Digoxin

Age	Total Digitalizing Dose[2] (mcg/kg[1])		Daily Maintenance Dose[3] (mcg/kg[1])	
	P.O.	I.V. or I.M.	P.O.	I.V. or I.M.
Preterm infant[1]	20-30	15-25	5-7.5	4-6
Full-term infant[1]	25-35	20-30	6-10	5-8
1 mo - 2 y[1]	35-60	30-50	10-15	7.5-12
2-5 y[1]	30-40	25-35	7.5-10	6-9
5-10 y[1]	20-35	15-30	5-10	4-8
>10 y[1]	10-15	8-12	2.5-5	2-3
Adults	0.75-1.5 mg	0.5-1 mg	0.125-0.5 mg	0.1-0.4 mg

[1]Based on lean body weight and normal renal function for age. Decrease dose in patients with ↓ renal function; digitalizing dose often not recommended in infants and children.

[2]Give one-half of the total digitalizing dose (TDD) in the initial dose, then give one-quarter of the TDD in each of two subsequent doses at 8- to 12-hour intervals. Obtain EKG 6 hours after each dose to assess potential toxicity.

[3]Divided every 12 hours in infants and children <10 years of age. Given once daily to children >10 years of age and adults.

Dosing adjustment/interval in renal impairment:

Cl_{cr} 10-50 mL/minute: Administer 25% to 75% of dose or every 36 hours

Cl_{cr} <10 mL/minute: Administer 10% to 25% of dose or every 48 hours

Reduce loading dose by 50% in ESRD

Hemodialysis: Not dialyzable (0% to 5%)

Mechanism of Action

Congestive heart failure: Inhibition of the sodium/potassium ATPase pump which acts to increase the intracellular sodium-calcium exchange to increase intracellular calcium leading to increased contractility

Supraventricular arrhythmias: Direct suppression of the AV node conduction to increase effective refractory period and decrease conduction velocity - positive inotropic effect, enhanced vagal tone, and decreased ventricular rate to fast atrial arrhythmias. Atrial fibrillation may decrease sensitivity and increase tolerance to higher serum digoxin concentrations.

Contraindications Hypersensitivity to digoxin or any component of the formulation; hypersensitivity to cardiac glycosides (another may be tried); history of toxicity; ventricular tachycardia or fibrillation; idiopathic hypertrophic subaortic stenosis; constrictive pericarditis; amyloid disease; second- or third-degree heart block (except in patients with a functioning artificial pacemaker); Wolff-Parkinson-White syndrome and atrial fibrillation concurrently

Warnings/Precautions Use with caution in patients with hypoxia, myxedema, hypothyroidism, acute myocarditis; patients with incomplete AV block (Stokes-Adams attack) may progress to complete block with digitalis drug administration; use with caution in patients with acute myocardial infarction, severe pulmonary disease, advanced heart failure, idiopathic hypertrophic subaortic stenosis, Wolff-Parkinson-White syndrome, sick-sinus syndrome (bradyarrhythmias), amyloid heart disease, and constrictive cardiomyopathies; adjust dose with renal impairment and when verapamil, quinidine or amiodarone are added to a patient on digoxin; elderly and neonates may develop exaggerated serum/tissue concentrations due to age-related alterations in clearance and pharmacodynamic differences; exercise will reduce serum concentrations of digoxin due to increased skeletal muscle uptake; recent studies indicate photopsia, chromatopsia and decreased visual acuity may occur even with therapeutic serum drug levels; reduce or hold dose 1-2 days before elective electrical cardioversion

Drug Interactions

Cytochrome P450 Effect: Substrate of CYP3A4 (minor)

Increased Effect/Toxicity: Beta-blocking agents (propranolol), verapamil, and diltiazem may have additive effects on heart rate. Carvedilol has additive effects on heart rate and inhibits the metabolism of digoxin. Digoxin levels may be increased by amiodarone (reduce digoxin dose 50%), bepridil, cyclosporine, diltiazem, indomethacin, itraconazole, some macrolides (erythromycin, clarithromycin), methimazole, nitrendipine, propafenone, propylthiouracil, quinidine (reduce digoxin dose 33% to 50% on initiation), tetracyclines, and verapamil. Moricizine may increase the toxicity of digoxin (mechanism undefined). Spironolactone may interfere with some digoxin assays, but may also increase blood levels directly. Succinylcholine administration to patients on digoxin has been associated with an increased risk of arrhythmias. Rare cases of acute digoxin toxicity have been associated with parenteral calcium (bolus) administration. The following medications have been associated with increased digoxin blood levels which appear to be of limited clinical significance: Famciclovir, flecainide, ibuprofen, fluoxetine, nefazodone, cimetidine, famotidine, ranitidine, omeprazole, trimethoprim.

Decreased Effect: Amiloride and spironolactone may reduce the inotropic response to digoxin. Cholestyramine, colestipol, kaolin-pectin, and metoclopramide may reduce digoxin absorption. Levothyroxine (and other thyroid supplements) may decrease digoxin blood levels. Penicillamine has been associated with reductions in digoxin blood levels The following reported interactions appear to be of limited clinical significance: Aminoglutethimide, aminosalicylic acid, aluminum-containing antacids, sucralfate, sulfasalazine, neomycin, ticlopidine.

Ethanol/Nutrition/Herb Interactions

Food: Digoxin peak serum levels may be decreased if taken with food. Meals containing increased fiber (bran) or foods high in pectin may decrease oral absorption of digoxin.

Herb/Nutraceutical: Avoid ephedra (risk of cardiac stimulation). Avoid natural licorice (causes sodium and water retention and increases potassium loss).

Dietary Considerations Maintain adequate amounts of potassium in diet to decrease risk of hypokalemia (hypokalemia may increase risk of digoxin toxicity).

Pharmacodynamics/Kinetics

Onset of action: Oral: 1-2 hours; I.V.: 5-30 minutes

Peak effect: Oral: 2-8 hours; I.V.: 1-4 hours

Duration: Adults: 3-4 days both forms

Absorption: By passive nonsaturable diffusion in the upper small intestine; food may delay, but does not affect extent of absorption

Distribution:

Normal renal function: 6-7 L/kg

V_d: Extensive to peripheral tissues, with a distinct distribution phase which lasts 6-8 hours; concentrates in heart, liver, kidney, skeletal muscle, and intestines. Heart/serum concentration is 70:1. Pharmacologic effects are delayed and do not correlate well with serum concentrations during distribution phase.

Hyperthyroidism: Increased V_d

(Continued)

Digoxin *(Continued)*

Hyperkalemia, hyponatremia: Decreased digoxin distribution to heart and muscle
Hypokalemia: Increased digoxin distribution to heart and muscles
Concomitant quinidine therapy: Decreased V_d
Chronic renal failure: 4-6 L/kg
Decreased sodium/potassium ATPase activity - decreased tissue binding
Neonates, full-term: 7.5-10 L/kg
Children: 16 L/kg
Adults: 7 L/kg, decreased with renal disease

Protein binding: 30%; in uremic patients, digoxin is displaced from plasma protein binding sites

Metabolism: Via sequential sugar hydrolysis in the stomach or by reduction of lactone ring by intestinal bacteria (in ~10% of population, gut bacteria may metabolize up to 40% of digoxin dose); metabolites may contribute to therapeutic and toxic effects of digoxin; metabolism is reduced with CHF

Bioavailability: Oral (formulation dependent): Elixir: 75% to 85%; Tablet: 70% to 80%

Half-life elimination (age, renal and cardiac function dependent):
Neonates: Premature: 61-170 hours; Full-term: 35-45 hours
Infants: 18-25 hours
Children: 35 hours
Adults: 38-48 hours
Adults, anephric: 4-6 days

Half-life elimination: Parent drug: 38 hours; Metabolites: Digoxigenin: 4 hours; Monodigitoxoside: 3-12 hours

Time to peak, serum: Oral: ~1 hour

Excretion: Urine (50% to 70% as unchanged drug)

Pregnancy Risk Factor C

Dosage Forms CAP (Lanoxicaps®): 50 mcg, 100 mcg, 200 mcg. **ELIX:** 50 mcg/mL (2.5 mL, 5 mL, 60 mL); (Lanoxin® [pediatric]): 50 mcg/mL (60 mL). **INJ:** 250 mcg/mL (1 mL, 2 mL); (Lanoxin®): 250 mcg/mL (2 mL). **INJ, pediatric:** 100 mcg/mL (1 mL). **TAB:** 125 mcg, 250 mcg, 500 mcg; (Digitek®, Lanoxin®): 125 mcg, 250 mcg

Digoxin Immune Fab (di JOKS in i MYUN fab)

Related Information

Digitoxin *on page 437*
Digoxin *on page 437*

U.S. Brand Names Digibind®; DigiFab™

Canadian Brand Names Digibind®

Generic Available No

Synonyms Antidigoxin Fab Fragments, Ovine

Pharmacologic Category Antidote

Use Treatment of life-threatening or potentially life-threatening digoxin intoxication, including:

- acute digoxin ingestion (ie, >10 mg in adults or >4 mg in children)
- chronic ingestions leading to steady-state digoxin concentrations > 6 ng/mL in adults or >4 ng/mL in children
- manifestations of digoxin toxicity due to overdose (life-threatening ventricular arrhythmias, progressive bradycardia, second- or third-degree heart block not responsive to atropine, serum potassium >5 mEq/L in adults or >6 mEq in children)

Local Anesthetic/Vasoconstrictor Precautions No information available to require special precautions

Effects on Dental Treatment No significant effects or complications reported

Common Adverse Effects Frequency not defined.

Cardiovascular: Effects (due to withdrawal of digitalis) include exacerbation of low cardiac output states and CHF, rapid ventricular response in patients with atrial fibrillation; postural hypotension
Endocrine & metabolic: Hypokalemia
Local: Phlebitis
Miscellaneous: Allergic reactions, serum sickness

Mechanism of Action Digoxin immune antigen-binding fragments (Fab) are specific antibodies for the treatment of digitalis intoxication in carefully selected patients; binds with molecules of digoxin or digitoxin and then is excreted by the kidneys and removed from the body

Drug Interactions

Increased Effect/Toxicity: Digoxin: Following administration of digoxin immune Fab, serum digoxin levels are markedly increased due to bound complexes (may be clinically misleading, since bound complex cannot interact with receptors).

Pharmacodynamics/Kinetics

Onset of action: I.V.: Improvement in 2-30 minutes for toxicity

Half-life elimination: 15-20 hours; prolonged with renal impairment

Excretion: Urine; undetectable amounts within 5-7 days

Pregnancy Risk Factor C

Dihematoporphyrin Ether *see* Porfimer *on page 1103*

Dihistine® DH *see* Chlorpheniramine, Pseudoephedrine, and Codeine *on page 319*

Dihistine® Expectorant *see* Guaifenesin, Pseudoephedrine, and Codeine *on page 676*

Dihydrocodeine, Aspirin, and Caffeine

(dye hye droe KOE deen, AS pir in, & KAF een)

Related Information

Aspirin *on page 151*

Oral Pain *on page 1526*

U.S. Brand Names Synalgos®-DC

Generic Available No

Synonyms Dihydrocodeine Compound

Pharmacologic Category Analgesic, Narcotic

Dental Use Management of postoperative pain

Use Management of mild to moderate pain that requires relaxation

Local Anesthetic/Vasoconstrictor Precautions No information available to require special precautions

Effects on Dental Treatment Key adverse event(s) related to dental treatment: Dihydrocodeine: nausea, followed by sedation and constipation. Elderly are a high-risk population for adverse effects from nonsteroidal anti-inflammatory agents. As many as 60% of elderly patients with GI complications from NSAIDs can develop peptic ulceration and/or hemorrhage asymptomatically. Concomitant disease and drug use contribute to the risk of GI adverse effects. Use lowest effective dose for shortest period possible. Consider renal function decline with age.

Significant Adverse Effects

>10%:

- Central nervous system: Lightheadedness, dizziness, drowsiness, sedation
- Dermatologic: Pruritus, skin reactions
- Gastrointestinal: Nausea, vomiting, constipation

1% to 10%:

- Cardiovascular: Hypotension, palpitations, bradycardia, peripheral vasodilation
- Central nervous system: Increased intracranial pressure
- Endocrine & metabolic: Antidiuretic hormone release
- Gastrointestinal: Biliary tract spasm
- Genitourinary: Urinary tract spasm
- Ocular: Miosis
- Respiratory: Respiratory depression
- Miscellaneous: Histamine release, physical and psychological dependence with prolonged use

Restrictions C-III

Dosage

Adults: Oral: 1-2 capsules every 4-6 hours as needed for pain

Elderly: Initial dosing should be cautious (low end of adult dosing range)

Mechanism of Action Binds to opiate receptors in the CNS, causing inhibition of ascending pain pathways, altering the perception of and response to pain; causes cough suppression by direct central action in the medulla; produces generalized CNS depression

Contraindications Hypersensitivity to dihydrocodeine or any component of the formulation; pregnancy (prolonged use or high doses at term)

Warnings/Precautions Use with caution in patients with hypersensitivity reactions to other phenanthrene derivative opioid agonists (morphine, hydrocodone, hydromorphone, levorphanol, oxycodone, oxymorphone); respiratory diseases including asthma, emphysema, COPD, or severe liver or renal insufficiency; some preparations contain sulfites which may cause allergic reactions; dextromethorphan has equivalent antitussive activity but has much lower toxicity in accidental overdose; tolerance of drug dependence may result from extended use

(Continued)

Dihydrocodeine, Aspirin, and Caffeine *(Continued)*

Drug Interactions Substrate of CYP2D6 (major) based on dihydrocodeine

CYP2D6 inhibitors: May decrease the effects of dihydrocodeine. Example inhibitors include chlorpromazine, delavirdine, fluoxetine, miconazole, paroxetine, pergolide, quinidine, quinine, ritonavir, and ropinirole.

MAO inhibitors may increase adverse symptoms

Ethanol/Nutrition/Herb Interactions Ethanol: Avoid ethanol (may increase CNS depression).

Pharmacodynamics/Kinetics

Onset of action: 10-30 minutes

Duration: 4-6 hours

Metabolism: Hepatic

Half-life elimination, serum: 3.8 hours

Time to peak, serum: 30-60 minutes

Pregnancy Risk Factor B/D (prolonged use or high doses at term)

Lactation Excretion in breast milk unknown/use caution

Breast-Feeding Considerations

Acetaminophen: May be taken while breast-feeding.

Aspirin: Use cautiously due to potential adverse effects in nursing infants.

Dihydrocodeine: No data reported.

Dosage Forms Capsule (Synalgos®-DC): Dihydrocodeine bitartrate 16 mg, aspirin 356.4 mg, and caffeine 30 mg

Dihydrocodeine Bitartrate, Acetaminophen, and Caffeine *see* Acetaminophen, Caffeine, and Dihydrocodeine *on page 57*

Dihydrocodeine Bitartrate, Pseudoephedrine Hydrochloride, and Chlorpheniramine Maleate *see* Pseudoephedrine, Dihydrocodeine, and Chlorpheniramine *on page 1150*

Dihydrocodeine Compound *see* Dihydrocodeine, Aspirin, and Caffeine *on page 441*

DiHydro-CP *see* Pseudoephedrine, Dihydrocodeine, and Chlorpheniramine *on page 1150*

Dihydroergotamine (dye hye droe er GOT a meen)

U.S. Brand Names D.H.E. 45®; Migranal®

Canadian Brand Names Migranal®

Generic Available Yes: Injection

Synonyms DHE; Dihydroergotamine Mesylate

Pharmacologic Category Ergot Derivative

Use Treatment of migraine headache with or without aura; injection also indicated for treatment of cluster headaches

Unlabeled/Investigational Use Adjunct for DVT prophylaxis for hip surgery, for orthostatic hypotension, xerostomia secondary to antidepressant use, and pelvic congestion with pain

Local Anesthetic/Vasoconstrictor Precautions No information available to require special precautions

Effects on Dental Treatment Key adverse event(s) related to dental treatment: Rhinitis and abnormal taste.

Common Adverse Effects

>10%: Nasal spray: Respiratory: Rhinitis (26%)

1% to 10%: Nasal spray:

Central nervous system: Dizziness (4%), somnolence (3%)

Endocrine & metabolic: Hot flashes (1%)

Gastrointestinal: Nausea (10%), taste disturbance (8%), vomiting (4%), diarrhea (2%)

Local: Application site reaction (6%)

Neuromuscular & skeletal: Weakness (1%), stiffness (1%)

Respiratory: Pharyngitis (3%)

Mechanism of Action Ergot alkaloid alpha-adrenergic blocker directly stimulates vascular smooth muscle to vasoconstrict peripheral and cerebral vessels; also has effects on serotonin receptors

Drug Interactions

Cytochrome P450 Effect: Substrate of CYP3A4 (major); **Inhibits** CYP3A4 (weak)

Increased Effect/Toxicity: CYP3A4 inhibitors may increase the levels/effects of dihydroergotamine; example inhibitors include azole antifungals, ciprofloxacin, clarithromycin, diclofenac, doxycycline, erythromycin, imatinib, isoniazid, nefazodone, nicardipine, propofol, protease inhibitors, quinidine, and verapamil. Ergot alkaloids are contraindicated with potent CYP3A4 inhibitors. Dihydroergotamine may increase the effects of 5-HT_1 agonists (eg, sumatriptan), MAO inhibitors, sibutramine, and other serotonin agonists (serotonin syndrome). Severe vasoconstriction may occur when peripheral vasoconstrictors or beta-blockers are used in patients receiving ergot alkaloids; concurrent use is contraindicated.

Decreased Effect: Effects of dihydroergotamine may be diminished by antipsychotics, metoclopramide. Antianginal effects of nitrates may be reduced by ergot alkaloids.

Pharmacodynamics/Kinetics

Onset of action: 15-30 minutes
Duration: 3-4 hours
Distribution: V_d: 14.5 L/kg
Protein binding: 93%
Metabolism: Extensively hepatic
Half-life elimination: 1.3-3.9 hours
Time to peak, serum: I.M.: 15-30 minutes
Excretion: Primarily feces; urine (10% mostly as metabolites)

Pregnancy Risk Factor X

Dihydroergotamine Mesylate *see* Dihydroergotamine *on page 442*

Dihydroergotoxine *see* Ergoloid Mesylates *on page 504*

Dihydrogenated Ergot Alkaloids *see* Ergoloid Mesylates *on page 504*

Dihydrohydroxycodeinone *see* Oxycodone *on page 1027*

Dihydromorphinone *see* Hydromorphone *on page 718*

Dihydrotachysterol (dye hye droe tak ISS ter ole)

U.S. Brand Names DHT™; DHT™ Intensol™; Hytakerol®

Canadian Brand Names Hytakerol®

Generic Available No

Synonyms Dichysterol

Pharmacologic Category Vitamin D Analog

Use Treatment of hypocalcemia associated with hypoparathyroidism; prophylaxis of hypocalcemic tetany following thyroid surgery

Local Anesthetic/Vasoconstrictor Precautions No information available to require special precautions

Effects on Dental Treatment No significant effects or complications reported

Common Adverse Effects >10%:

Endocrine & metabolic: Hypercalcemia
Renal: Elevated serum creatinine, hypercalciuria

Mechanism of Action Synthetic analogue of vitamin D with a faster onset of action; stimulates calcium and phosphate absorption from the small intestine, promotes secretion of calcium from bone to blood; promotes renal tubule resorption of phosphate

Drug Interactions

Increased Effect/Toxicity: Thiazide diuretics may increase calcium levels.

Decreased Effect: Decreased effect/levels of vitamin D if taken with cholestyramine, colestipol, or mineral oil. Phenytoin and phenobarbital may inhibit activation leading to decreased effectiveness.

Pharmacodynamics/Kinetics

Onset of action: Peak effect: Calcium: 2-4 weeks
Duration: ≤9 weeks
Absorption: Well absorbed
Distribution: Stored in liver, fat, skin, muscle, and bone
Excretion: Feces

Pregnancy Risk Factor A/D (dose exceeding RDA recommendation)

Dihydroxyanthracenedione Dihydrochloride *see* Mitoxantrone *on page 938*

1,25 Dihydroxycholecalciferol *see* Calcitriol *on page 244*

Dihydroxydeoxynorvinkaleukoblastine *see* Vinorelbine *on page 1380*

Dihydroxypropyl Theophylline *see* Dyphylline *on page 480*

Diiodohydroxyquin *see* Iodoquinol *on page 759*

Dilacor® XR *see* Diltiazem *on page 444*

Dilantin® *see* Phenytoin *on page 1080*

Dilatrate®-SR *see* Isosorbide Dinitrate *on page 770*

Dilaudid® *see* Hydromorphone *on page 718*

Dilaudid-HP® *see* Hydromorphone *on page 718*

Dilor® *see* Dyphylline *on page 480*

Diltia XT® *see* Diltiazem *on page 444*

Diltiazem (dil TYE a zem)

Related Information

Calcium Channel Blockers and Gingival Hyperplasia *on page 1600*
Calcium Channel Blockers, Comparative Pharmacokinetics *on page 1602*
Cardiovascular Diseases *on page 1458*

U.S. Brand Names Cardizem®; Cardizem® CD; Cardizem® LA; Cardizem® SR; Cartia XT™; Dilacor® XR; Diltia XT®; Taztia XT™; Tiazac®

Canadian Brand Names Alti-Diltiazem CD; Apo-Diltiaz®; Apo-Diltiaz CD®; Apo-Diltiaz SR®; Cardizem®; Cardizem® CD; Cardizem® SR; Gen-Diltiazem; Gen-Diltiazem SR; Med-Diltiazem; Novo-Diltazem; Novo-Diltazem-CD; Novo-Diltazem SR; Nu-Diltiaz; Nu-Diltiaz-CD; ratio-Diltiazem CD; Rhoxal-diltiazem CD; Rhoxal-diltiazem SR; Syn-Diltiazem®; Tiazac®

Mexican Brand Names Angiotrofin®; Tilazem®

Generic Available Yes

Synonyms Diltiazem Hydrochloride

Pharmacologic Category Calcium Channel Blocker

Use

Oral: Essential hypertension; chronic stable angina or angina from coronary artery spasm

Injection: Atrial fibrillation or atrial flutter; paroxysmal supraventricular tachycardia (PSVT)

Unlabeled/Investigational Use Investigational: Therapy of Duchenne muscular dystrophy

Local Anesthetic/Vasoconstrictor Precautions No information available to require special precautions

Effects on Dental Treatment Key adverse event(s) related to dental treatment: Diltiazem has been reported to cause >10% incidence of gingival hyperplasia; usually disappears with discontinuation (consultation with physician is suggested).

Common Adverse Effects Note: Frequencies represent ranges for various dosage forms. Patients with impaired ventricular function and/or conduction abnormalities may have higher incidence of adverse reactions.

>10%:

- Cardiovascular: Edema (2% to 15%)
- Central nervous system: Headache (5% to 12%)

2% to 10%:

- Cardiovascular: AV block (first degree 2% to 8%), edema (lower limb 2% to 8%), pain (6%), bradycardia (2% to 6%), hypotension (<2% to 4%), vasodilation (2% to 3%), extrasystoles (2%), flushing (1% to 2%), palpitations (1% to 2%)
- Central nervous system: Dizziness (3% to 10%), nervousness (2%)
- Dermatologic: Rash (1% to 4%)
- Endocrine & metabolic: Gout (1% to 2%)
- Gastrointestinal: Dyspepsia (1% to 6%), constipation (<2% to 4%), vomiting (2%), diarrhea (1% to 2%)
- Local: Injection site reactions: Burning, itching (4%)
- Neuromuscular & skeletal: Weakness (1% to 4%), myalgia (2%)
- Respiratory: Rhinitis (<2% to 10%), pharyngitis (2% to 6%), dyspnea (1% to 6%), bronchitis (1% to 4%), sinus congestion (1% to 2%)

Dosage Adults:

Oral:

Angina:

- Capsule, extended release (Cardizem® CD, Cartia XT™, Dilacor XR®, Diltia XT™, Tiazac®): Initial: 120-180 mg once daily (maximum dose: 480 mg/day)
- Tablet, extended release (Cardizem® LA): 180 mg once daily; may increase at 7- to 14-day intervals (maximum recommended dose: 360 mg/day)
- Tablet, immediate release (Cardizem®): Usual starting dose: 30 mg 4 times/day; usual range: 180-360 mg/day

Hypertension:

- Capsule, extended release (Cardizem® CD, Cartia XT™, Dilacor XR®, Diltia XT™, Tiazac®): Initial: 180-240 mg once daily; dose adjustment may be made after 14 days; usual dose range (JNC 7): 180-420 mg/day; Tiazac®: usual dose range: 120-540 mg/day
- Capsule, sustained release (Cardizem® SR): Initial: 60-120 mg twice daily; dose adjustment may be made after 14 days; usual range: 240-360 mg/day
- Tablet, extended release (Cardizem® LA): Initial: 180-240 mg once daily; dose adjustment may be made after 14 days; usual dose range (JNC 7): 120-540 mg/day

Note: Elderly: Patients ≥60 years may respond to a lower initial dose (ie, 120 mg once daily using extended release capsule)

I.V.: Atrial fibrillation, atrial flutter, PSVT:

Initial bolus dose: 0.25 mg/kg actual body weight over 2 minutes (average adult dose: 20 mg)

Repeat bolus dose (may be administered after 15 minutes if the response is inadequate.): 0.35 mg/kg actual body weight over 2 minutes (average adult dose: 25 mg)

Continuous infusion (requires an infusion pump; infusions >24 hours or infusion rates >15 mg/hour are not recommended.): Initial infusion rate of 10 mg/hour; rate may be increased in 5 mg/hour increments up to 15 mg/hour as needed; some patients may respond to an initial rate of 5 mg/hour.

If diltiazem injection is administered by continuous infusion for >24 hours, the possibility of decreased diltiazem clearance, prolonged elimination half-life, and increased diltiazem and/or diltiazem metabolite plasma concentrations should be considered.

Conversion from I.V. diltiazem to oral diltiazem: Start oral approximately 3 hours after bolus dose.

Oral dose (mg/day) is approximately equal to [rate (mg/hour) x 3 + 3] x 10.

3 mg/hour = 120 mg/day
5 mg/hour = 180 mg/day
7 mg/hour = 240 mg/day
11 mg/hour = 360 mg/day

Dosing comments in renal/hepatic impairment: Use with caution as extensively metabolized by the liver and excreted in the kidneys and bile.

Dialysis: Not removed by hemo- or peritoneal dialysis; supplemental dose is not necessary.

Mechanism of Action Inhibits calcium ion from entering the "slow channels" or select voltage-sensitive areas of vascular smooth muscle and myocardium during depolarization, producing a relaxation of coronary vascular smooth muscle and coronary vasodilation; increases myocardial oxygen delivery in patients with vasospastic angina

Contraindications Hypersensitivity to diltiazem or any component of the formulation; sick sinus syndrome; second- or third-degree AV block (except in patients with a functioning artificial pacemaker); hypotension (systolic <90 mm Hg); acute MI and pulmonary congestion

Warnings/Precautions Use with caution and titrate dosages for patients with hypotension or patients taking antihypertensives, impaired renal or hepatic function, or when treating patients with CHF. Use caution with concomitant therapy with beta-blockers or digoxin. Monitor LFTs during therapy since these enzymes may rarely be increased and symptoms of hepatic injury may occur; usually reverses with drug discontinuation; avoid abrupt withdrawal of calcium blockers since rebound angina is theoretically possible.

Drug Interactions

Cytochrome P450 Effect: Substrate of CYP2C8/9 (minor), 2D6 (minor), 3A4 (major); **Inhibits** CYP2C8/9 (weak), 2D6 (weak), 3A4 (moderate)

Increased Effect/Toxicity: Diltiazem effects may be additive with amiodarone, beta-blockers, or digoxin, which may lead to bradycardia, other conduction delays, and decreased cardiac output. The levels/effects of diltiazem may be increased by azole antifungals, ciprofloxacin, clarithromycin, diclofenac, doxycycline, erythromycin, imatinib, isoniazid, nefazodone, nicardipine, propofol, protease inhibitors, quinidine, telithromycin, verapamil, and other CYP3A4 inhibitors.

Diltiazem may increase the levels/effects of selected benzodiazepines, calcium channel blockers, cisapride, cyclosporine, ergot alkaloids, selected HMG-CoA reductase inhibitors, mesoridazine, mirtazapine, nateglinide, nefazodone, pimozide, quinidine, sildenafil (and other PDE-5 inhibitors), tacrolimus, thioridazine, venlafaxine, and other CYP3A4 substrates. Blood pressure-lowering effects may be additive with sildenafil, tadalafil, and vardenafil (use caution).

Decreased Effect: Levels/effects of diltiazem may be decreased by aminoglutethimide, carbamazepine, nafcillin, nevirapine, phenobarbital, phenytoin, rifamycins, and other CYP3A4 inducers.

Ethanol/Nutrition/Herb Interactions

Ethanol: Avoid ethanol (may increase risk of hypotension or vasodilation).

Food: Diltiazem serum levels may be elevated if taken with food. Serum concentrations were not altered by grapefruit juice in small clinical trials.

(Continued)

Diltiazem *(Continued)*

Herb/Nutraceutical: St John's wort may decrease diltiazem levels. Avoid dong quai if using for hypertension (has estrogenic activity). Avoid ephedra (may worsen arrhythmia or hypertension). Avoid yohimbe, ginseng (may worsen hypertension). Avoid garlic (may have increased antihypertensive effect).

Pharmacodynamics/Kinetics

Onset of action: Oral: Immediate release tablet: 30-60 minutes

Absorption: 70% to 80%

Distribution: V_d: 3-13 L/kg; enters breast milk

Protein binding: 77% to 85%

Metabolism: Hepatic; extensive first-pass effect; following single I.V. injection, plasma concentrations of N-monodesmethyldiltiazem and desacetyldiltiazem are typically undetectable; however, these metabolites accumulate to detectable concentrations following 24-hour constant rate infusion. N-monodesmethyldiltiazem appears to have 20% of the potency of diltiazem; desacetyldiltiazem is about 50% as potent as the parent compound.

Bioavailability: Oral: ~40% to 60%

Half-life elimination: Immediate release tablet: 3-4.5 hours, may be prolonged with renal impairment

Time to peak, serum: Immediate release tablet: 2-3 hours

Excretion: Urine and feces (primarily as metabolites)

Pregnancy Risk Factor C

Dosage Forms CAP, extended release [once-daily dosing]: 120 mg, 180 mg, 240 mg, 300 mg; (Cardizem® CD, Taztia XT™): 120 mg, 180 mg, 240 mg, 300 mg, 360 mg; (Cartia XT™): 120 mg, 180 mg, 240 mg, 300 mg; (Dilacor® XR, Diltia XT®): 120 mg, 180 mg, 240 mg; (Tiazac®): 120 mg, 180 mg, 240 mg, 300 mg, 360 mg, 420 mg. **CAP, sustained release** [twice-daily dosing] (Cardizem® SR): 60 mg, 90 mg, 120 mg. **INJ, solution:** 5 mg/mL (5 mL, 10 mL, 25 mL). **INJ, powder for reconstitution** (Cardizem®): 25 mg, 100 mg. **TAB** (Cardizem®): 30 mg, 60 mg, 90 mg, 120 mg **TAB, extended release** (Cardizem® LA): 120 mg, 180 mg, 240 mg, 300 mg, 360 mg, 420 mg

Diltiazem Hydrochloride *see* Diltiazem *on page 444*

DimenhyDRINATE (dye men HYE dri nate)

U.S. Brand Names Dramamine® [OTC]; Hydrate® [DSC]; TripTone® [OTC]

Canadian Brand Names Apo-Dimenhydrinate®; Gravol®; Novo-Dimenate

Mexican Brand Names Dramamine®; Vomisin®

Generic Available Yes

Pharmacologic Category Antihistamine

Use Treatment and prevention of nausea, vertigo, and vomiting associated with motion sickness

Local Anesthetic/Vasoconstrictor Precautions No information available to require special precautions

Effects on Dental Treatment Key adverse event(s) related to dental treatment: Significant xerostomia (normal salivary flow resumes upon discontinuation).

Common Adverse Effects

>10%:

- Central nervous system: Slight to moderate drowsiness
- Respiratory: Thickening of bronchial secretions

1% to 10%:

- Central nervous system: Headache, fatigue, nervousness, dizziness
- Gastrointestinal: Appetite increase, weight gain, nausea, diarrhea, abdominal pain, xerostomia
- Neuromuscular & skeletal: Arthralgia
- Respiratory: Pharyngitis

Mechanism of Action Competes with histamine for H_1-receptor sites on effector cells in the gastrointestinal tract, blood vessels, and respiratory tract; blocks chemoreceptor trigger zone, diminishes vestibular stimulation, and depresses labyrinthine function through its central anticholinergic activity

Drug Interactions

Increased Effect/Toxicity: CNS depressants may increase the degree of sedation and respiratory depression with antihistamines. May increase the absorption of digoxin. Central and/or peripheral anticholinergic syndrome can occur when administered with amantadine, rimantadine, narcotic analgesics, phenothiazines and other antipsychotics (especially with high anticholinergic activity), tricyclic antidepressants, quinidine, disopyramide, procainamide, and antihistamines.

Decreased Effect: May increase gastric degradation of levodopa and decrease the amount of levodopa absorbed by delaying gastric emptying.

Therapeutic effects of cholinergic agents (tacrine, donepezil) and neuroleptics may be antagonized.

Pharmacodynamics/Kinetics

Onset of action: Oral: ~15-30 minutes

Absorption: Oral: Well absorbed

Pregnancy Risk Factor B

Dimercaprol (dye mer KAP role)

U.S. Brand Names BAL in Oil®

Generic Available No

Synonyms BAL; British Anti-Lewisite; Dithioglycerol

Pharmacologic Category Antidote

Use Antidote to gold, arsenic (except arsine), and mercury poisoning (except nonalkyl mercury); adjunct to edetate calcium disodium in lead poisoning; possibly effective for antimony, bismuth, chromium, copper, nickel, tungsten, or zinc

Local Anesthetic/Vasoconstrictor Precautions No information available to require special precautions

Effects on Dental Treatment No significant effects or complications reported

Common Adverse Effects

>10%:

Cardiovascular: Hypertension, tachycardia (dose-related)

Central nervous system: Headache

1% to 10%: Gastrointestinal: Nausea, vomiting

Mechanism of Action Sulfhydryl group combines with ions of various heavy metals to form relatively stable, nontoxic, soluble chelates which are excreted in urine

Drug Interactions

Increased Effect/Toxicity: Toxic complexes with iron, cadmium, selenium, or uranium.

Pharmacodynamics/Kinetics

Distribution: To all tissues including the brain

Metabolism: Rapidly hepatic to inactive metabolites

Time to peak, serum: 0.5-1 hour

Excretion: Urine

Pregnancy Risk Factor C

Dimetapp® 12-Hour Non-Drowsy Extentabs® [OTC] *see* Pseudoephedrine *on page 1147*

Dimetapp® Children's ND [OTC] *see* Loratadine *on page 841*

Dimetapp® Cold and Congestion [OTC] *see* Guaifenesin, Pseudoephedrine, and Dextromethorphan *on page 676*

Dimetapp® Decongestant [OTC] *see* Pseudoephedrine *on page 1147*

β,β-Dimethylcysteine *see* Penicillamine *on page 1057*

Dimethyl Triazeno Imidazol Carboxamide *see* Dacarbazine *on page 392*

Dinoprostone (dye noe PROST one)

U.S. Brand Names Cervidil®; Prepidil®; Prostin E_2®

Canadian Brand Names Cervidil®; Prepidil®; Prostin E2®

Mexican Brand Names Prepidil®; Propess®

Generic Available No

Synonyms PGE_2; Prostaglandin E_2

Pharmacologic Category Abortifacient; Prostaglandin

Use

Gel: Promote cervical ripening prior to labor induction; usage for gel include any patient undergoing induction of labor with an unripe cervix, most commonly for pre-eclampsia, eclampsia, postdates, diabetes, intrauterine growth retardation, and chronic hypertension

Suppositories: Terminate pregnancy from 12th through 28th week of gestation; evacuate uterus in cases of missed abortion or intrauterine fetal death; manage benign hydatidiform mole

Vaginal insert: Initiation and/or cervical ripening in patients at or near term in whom there is a medical or obstetrical indication for the induction of labor

Local Anesthetic/Vasoconstrictor Precautions No information available to require special precautions

Effects on Dental Treatment No significant effects or complications reported

Common Adverse Effects

>10%:

Central nervous system: Headache

Gastrointestinal: Vomiting, diarrhea, nausea

(Continued)

Dinoprostone *(Continued)*

1% to 10%:

Cardiovascular: Bradycardia

Central nervous system: Fever

Neuromuscular & skeletal: Back pain

Mechanism of Action A synthetic prostaglandin E_2 abortifacient that stimulates uterine contractions similar to those seen during natural labor

Drug Interactions

Increased Effect/Toxicity: Increased effect of oxytocics.

Pharmacodynamics/Kinetics

Onset of action (uterine contractions): Within 10 minutes

Duration: Up to 2-3 hours

Absorption: Vaginal: Slow

Metabolism: In many tissues including renal, pulmonary, and splenic systems

Excretion: Primarily urine; feces (small amounts)

Pregnancy Risk Factor C

Diocto® [OTC] *see* Docusate *on page 459*

Diocto C® [DSC] [OTC] *see* Docusate and Casanthranol *on page 460*

Dioctyl Calcium Sulfosuccinate *see* Docusate *on page 459*

Dioctyl Sodium Sulfosuccinate *see* Docusate *on page 459*

Diotame® [OTC] *see* Bismuth *on page 209*

Diovan® *see* Valsartan *on page 1363*

Diovan HCT® *see* Valsartan and Hydrochlorothiazide *on page 1364*

Dipentum® *see* Olsalazine *on page 1011*

Diphen® [OTC] *see* DiphenhydrAMINE *on page 448*

Diphen® AF [OTC] *see* DiphenhydrAMINE *on page 448*

Diphen® Cough [OTC] *see* DiphenhydrAMINE *on page 448*

Diphenhist [OTC] *see* DiphenhydrAMINE *on page 448*

DiphenhydrAMINE (dye fen HYE dra meen)

Related Information

Dental Office Emergencies *on page 1584*

Diphenhydramine and Pseudoephedrine *on page 451*

Management of Patients Undergoing Cancer Therapy *on page 1569*

Oral Nonviral Soft Tissue Ulcerations or Erosions *on page 1551*

Oral Viral Infections *on page 1547*

U.S. Brand Names Aler-Dryl [OTC]; AllerMax® [OTC]; Banophen® [OTC]; Benadryl® Allergy [OTC]; Benadryl® Dye-Free Allergy [OTC]; Benadryl® Gel [OTC]; Benadryl® Gel Extra Strength [OTC]; Benadryl® Injection; Compoz® Nighttime Sleep Aid [OTC]; Diphen® [OTC]; Diphen® AF [OTC]; Diphen® Cough [OTC]; Diphenhist [OTC]; Genahist® [OTC]; Hydramine® [OTC]; Hydramine® Cough [OTC]; Hyrexin-50®; Nytol® [OTC]; Nytol® Maximum Strength [OTC]; Siladryl® Allergy [OTC]; Silphen® [OTC]; Sleepinal® [OTC]; Sominex® [OTC]; Sominex® Maximum Strength [OTC]; Tusstat®; Twilite® [OTC]; Unisom® Maximum Strength SleepGels® [OTC]

Canadian Brand Names Allerdryl®; Allernix; Benadryl®; Nytol®; Nytol® Extra Strength; PMS-Diphenhydramine; Simply Sleep®

Mexican Brand Names Tzoali®

Generic Available Yes

Synonyms Diphenhydramine Hydrochloride

Pharmacologic Category Antihistamine

Dental Use Symptomatic relief of nasal mucosal congestion

Use Symptomatic relief of allergic symptoms caused by histamine release which include nasal allergies and allergic dermatosis; can be used for mild nighttime sedation; prevention of motion sickness and as an antitussive; has antinauseant and topical anesthetic properties; treatment of antipsychotic-induced extrapyramidal symptoms

Local Anesthetic/Vasoconstrictor Precautions No information available to require special precautions

Effects on Dental Treatment Key adverse event(s) related to dental treatment: Xerostomia (normal salivary flow resumes upon discontinuation) and dry mucous membranes. Chronic use of antihistamines will inhibit salivary flow, particularly in elderly patients; may contribute to periodontal disease and oral discomfort.

Significant Adverse Effects Frequency not defined.

Cardiovascular: Hypotension, palpitations, tachycardia

Central nervous system: Sedation, sleepiness, dizziness, disturbed coordination, headache, fatigue, nervousness, paradoxical excitement, insomnia, euphoria, confusion

Dermatologic: Photosensitivity, rash, angioedema, urticaria

Gastrointestinal: Nausea, vomiting, diarrhea, abdominal pain, xerostomia, appetite increase, weight gain, dry mucous membranes, anorexia

Genitourinary: Urinary retention, urinary frequency, difficult urination

Hematologic: Hemolytic anemia, thrombocytopenia, agranulocytosis

Neuromuscular & skeletal: Tremor, paresthesia

Ocular: Blurred vision

Respiratory: Thickening of bronchial secretions

Dosage

Children:

Oral, I.M., I.V.:

Treatment of moderate to severe allergic reactions: 5 mg/kg/day or 150 mg/m^2/day in divided doses every 6-8 hours, not to exceed 300 mg/day

Minor allergic rhinitis or motion sickness:

2 to <6 years: 6.25 mg every 4-6 hours; maximum: 37.5 mg/day

6 to <12 years: 12.5-25 mg every 4-6 hours; maximum: 150 mg/day

≥12 years: 25-50 mg every 4-6 hours; maximum: 300 mg/day

Night-time sleep aid: 30 minutes before bedtime:

2 to <12 years: 1 mg/kg/dose; maximum: 50 mg/dose

≥12 years: 50 mg

Oral: Antitussive:

2 to <6 years: 6.25 mg every 4 hours; maximum 37.5 mg/day

6 to <12 years: 12.5 mg every 4 hours; maximum 75 mg/day

≥12 years: 25 mg every 4 hours; maximum 150 mg/day

I.M., I.V.: Treatment of dystonic reactions: 0.5-1 mg/kg/dose

Adults:

Oral: 25-50 mg every 6-8 hours

Minor allergic rhinitis or motion sickness: 25-50 mg every 4-6 hours; maximum: 300 mg/day

Moderate to severe allergic reactions: 25-50 mg every 4 hours, not to exceed 400 mg/day

Nighttime sleep aid: 50 mg at bedtime

I.M., I.V.: 10-50 mg in a single dose every 2-4 hours, not to exceed 400 mg/day

Dystonic reaction: 50 mg in a single dose; may repeat in 20-30 minutes if necessary

Topical: For external application, not longer than 7 days

Mechanism of Action Competes with histamine for H_1-receptor sites on effector cells in the gastrointestinal tract, blood vessels, and respiratory tract; anticholinergic and sedative effects are also seen

Contraindications Hypersensitivity to diphenhydramine or any component of the formulation; acute asthma; not for use in neonates

Warnings/Precautions Causes sedation, caution must be used in performing tasks which require alertness (eg, operating machinery or driving). Sedative effects of CNS depressants or ethanol are potentiated. Use with caution in patients with angle-closure glaucoma, pyloroduodenal obstruction (including stenotic peptic ulcer), urinary tract obstruction (including bladder neck obstruction and symptomatic prostatic hyperplasia), hyperthyroidism, increased intraocular pressure, and cardiovascular disease (including hypertension and tachycardia). Diphenhydramine has high sedative and anticholinergic properties, so it may not be considered the antihistamine of choice for prolonged use in the elderly. May cause paradoxical excitation in pediatric patients, and can result in hallucinations, coma, and death in overdose. Some preparations contain sodium bisulfite; syrup formulations may contain alcohol.

Drug Interactions Inhibits CYP2D6 (moderate)

Amantadine, rimantadine: Central and/or peripheral anticholinergic syndrome can occur when administered with amantadine or rimantadine

Anticholinergic agents: Central and/or peripheral anticholinergic syndrome can occur when administered with narcotic analgesics, phenothiazines and other antipsychotics (especially with high anticholinergic activity), tricyclic antidepressants, quinidine and some other antiarrhythmics, and antihistamines

Atenolol: Drugs with high anticholinergic activity may increase the bioavailability of atenolol (and possibly other beta-blockers); monitor for increased effect

Cholinergic agents: Drugs with high anticholinergic activity may antagonize the therapeutic effect of cholinergic agents; includes donepezil, rivastigmine, and tacrine

(Continued)

DiphenhydrAMINE *(Continued)*

CNS depressants: Sedative effects may be additive with CNS depressants; includes ethanol, benzodiazepines, barbiturates, narcotic analgesics, and other sedative agents; monitor for increased effect

CYP2D6 substrates: Diphenhydramine may increase the levels/effects of CYP2D6 substrates. Example substrates include amphetamines, selected beta-blockers, dextromethorphan, fluoxetine, lidocaine, mirtazapine, nefazodone, paroxetine, risperidone, ritonavir, thioridazine, tricyclic antidepressants, and venlafaxine.

CYP2D6 prodrug substrates: Diphenhydramine may decrease the levels/effects of CYP2D6 prodrug substrates. Example prodrug substrates include codeine, hydrocodone, oxycodone, and tramadol.

Digoxin: Drugs with high anticholinergic activity may decrease gastric degradation and increase the amount of digoxin absorbed by delaying gastric emptying

Ethanol: Syrup should not be given to patients taking drugs that can cause disulfiram reactions (ie, metronidazole, chlorpropamide) due to high alcohol content

Levodopa: Drugs with high anticholinergic activity may increase gastric degradation and decrease the amount of levodopa absorbed by delaying gastric emptying

Neuroleptics: Drugs with high anticholinergic activity may antagonize the therapeutic effects of neuroleptics

Ethanol/Nutrition/Herb Interactions

Ethanol: Avoid ethanol (may increase CNS depression).

Herb/Nutraceutical: Avoid valerian, St John's wort, kava kava, gotu kola (may increase CNS depression).

Pharmacodynamics/Kinetics

Onset of action: Maximum sedative effect: 1-3 hours

Duration: 4-7 hours

Protein binding: 78%

Metabolism: Extensively hepatic; smaller degrees in pulmonary and renal systems; significant first-pass effect

Bioavailability: Oral: 40% to 60%

Half-life elimination: 2-8 hours; Elderly: 13.5 hours

Time to peak, serum: 2-4 hours

Excretion: Urine (as unchanged drug)

Pregnancy Risk Factor B

Lactation Enters breast milk/contraindicated

Breast-Feeding Considerations Infants may be more sensitive to the effects of antihistamines.

Dosage Forms

Capsule, as hydrochloride: 25 mg, 50 mg
- Banophen®, Diphen®, Diphenhist®, Genahist®: 25 mg
- Nytol® Maximum Strength, Sleepinal®: 50 mg

Elixir, as hydrochloride: 12.5 mg/5 mL (5 mL, 10 mL, 20 mL, 120 mL, 480 mL, 3780 mL)
- Banophen®: 12.5 mg/5 mL (120 mL, 480 mL, 3840 mL)
- Diphen AF: 12.5 mg/5 mL (120 mL, 240 mL, 480 mL, 3840 mL) [alcohol free; cherry flavor]
- Genahist®: 12.5 mg/5 mL (120 mL)
- Hydramine®: 12.5 mg/5 mL (120 mL) [alcohol free; cherry flavor]

Gel, topical, as hydrochloride:
- Benadryl®: 1% (120 mL)
- Benadryl® Extra Strength: 2% (120 mL)

Injection, solution, as hydrochloride: 10 mg/mL (30 mL); 50 mg/mL (1 mL, 10 mL)
- Benadryl®: 50 mg/mL (1 mL, 10 mL)
- Hyrexin®: 50 mg/mL (10 mL)

Liquid, as hydrochloride:
- Benadryl® Allergy: 12.5 mg/5 mL (120 mL, 240 mL) [alcohol free; cherry flavor]
- Benadryl® Dye-Free Allergy: 12.5 mg/5 mL (120 mL) [alcohol free, dye free, sugar free; bubblegum flavor]

Softgel, as hydrochloride:
- Benadryl® Dye-Free Allergy: 25 mg [dye-free]
- Unisom® Maximum Strength SleepGels®: 50 mg

Solution, oral, as hydrochloride:
- AllerMax®: 12.5 mg/5 mL (120 mL)
- Diphenhist®: 12.5 mg/5 mL (120 mL, 480 mL)

Solution, topical, as hydrochloride [spray]: 1% (60 mL); 2% (60 mL)

Syrup, as hydrochloride: 12.5 mg/5 mL (120 mL, 240 mL, 480 mL)
Diphen® Cough: 12.5 mg/5 mL (120 mL, 240 mL, 480 mL) [contains alcohol 5.1%; raspberry flavor]
Diphenhist®: 12.5 mg/5 mL (120 mL)
Hydramine® Cough: 12.5 mg/5 mL (120 mL, 480 mL) [contains alcohol 5%; fruit flavor]
Siladryl® Allergy, Silphen® Cough: 12.5 mg/5 mL (120 mL, 240 mL, 480 mL)
Tusstat®: 12.5 mg/5 mL (120 mL, 240 mL, 3840 mL)
Tablet, as hydrochloride: 25 mg, 50 mg
Aler-Dryl, AllerMax®, Compoz® Nighttime Sleep Aid, Sominex® Maximum Strength, Twilite®: 50 mg
Banophen®, Benadryl® Allergy, Diphenhist®, Genahist®, Nytol®, Sominex®: 25 mg
Tablet, chewable, as hydrochloride (Benadryl® Allergy): 12.5 mg [contains phenylalanine 4.2 mg/tablet; grape flavor]

Comments 25-50 mg of diphenhydramine orally every 4-6 hours can be used to treat mild dermatologic manifestations of allergic reactions to penicillin and other antibiotics. Diphenhydramine is not recommended as local anesthetic for either infiltration route or nerve block since the vehicle has caused local necrosis upon injection. A 50:50 mixture of diphenhydramine liquid (12.5 mg/5 mL) in Kaopectate® or Maalox® is used as a local application for recurrent aphthous ulcers; swish 1 tablespoonful for 2 minutes 4 times/day.

Diphenhydramine and Acetaminophen *see* Acetaminophen and Diphenhydramine *on page 53*

Diphenhydramine and Pseudoephedrine

(dye fen HYE dra meen & soo doe e FED rin)

Related Information

DiphenhydrAMINE *on page 448*
Pseudoephedrine *on page 1147*

U.S. Brand Names Benadryl® Allergy and Sinus Fastmelt™ [OTC]; Benadryl® Allergy/Sinus [OTC]; Benadryl® Children's Allergy and Cold Fastmelt™ [OTC]; Benadryl® Children's Allergy and Sinus [OTC]

Generic Available No

Synonyms Pseudoephedrine and Diphenhydramine

Pharmacologic Category Antihistamine/Decongestant Combination

Use Relief of symptoms of upper respiratory mucosal congestion in seasonal and perennial nasal allergies, acute rhinitis, rhinosinusitis, and eustachian tube blockage

Local Anesthetic/Vasoconstrictor Precautions Use with caution since pseudoephedrine is a sympathomimetic amine which could interact with epinephrine to cause a pressor response

Effects on Dental Treatment Key adverse event(s) related to dental treatment: Pseudoephedrine: Xerostomia (normal salivary flow resumes upon discontinuation). Chronic use of antihistamines will inhibit salivary flow, particularly in elderly patients; this may contribute to periodontal disease and oral discomfort.

Common Adverse Effects See individual agents.

Drug Interactions

Cytochrome P450 Effect: Diphenhydramine: **Inhibits** CYP2D6 (moderate)
Increased Effect/Toxicity: See individual agents.
Decreased Effect: See individual agents.

Diphenhydramine Hydrochloride *see* DiphenhydrAMINE *on page 448*
Diphenhydramine, Hydrocodone, and Phenylephrine *see* Hydrocodone, Phenylephrine, and Diphenhydramine *on page 713*

Diphenoxylate and Atropine

(dye fen OKS i late & A troe peen)

Related Information

Atropine *on page 166*

U.S. Brand Names Lomotil®; Lonox®

Canadian Brand Names Lomotil®

Generic Available Yes

Synonyms Atropine and Diphenoxylate

Pharmacologic Category Antidiarrheal

Use Treatment of diarrhea

Local Anesthetic/Vasoconstrictor Precautions No information available to require special precautions

Effects on Dental Treatment Key adverse event(s) related to dental treatment: Significant xerostomia (normal salivary flow resumes upon discontinuation).

(Continued)

Diphenoxylate and Atropine *(Continued)*

Common Adverse Effects 1% to 10%:

Central nervous system: Nervousness, restlessness, dizziness, drowsiness, headache, mental depression

Gastrointestinal: Paralytic ileus, xerostomia

Genitourinary: Urinary retention and dysuria

Ocular: Blurred vision

Respiratory: Respiratory depression

Restrictions C-V

Mechanism of Action Diphenoxylate inhibits excessive GI motility and GI propulsion; commercial preparations contain a subtherapeutic amount of atropine to discourage abuse

Drug Interactions

Increased Effect/Toxicity: MAO inhibitors (hypertensive crisis), CNS depressants when taken with diphenoxylate may result in increased adverse effects, antimuscarinics (paralytic ileus). May prolong half-life of drugs metabolized in liver.

Pharmacodynamics/Kinetics

Atropine: See Atropine monograph.

Diphenoxylate:

Onset of action: Antidiarrheal: 45-60 minutes

Peak effect: Antidiarrheal: ~2 hours

Duration: Antidiarrheal: 3-4 hours

Absorption: Well absorbed

Metabolism: Extensively hepatic to diphenoxylic acid (active)

Half-life elimination: 2.5 hours

Time to peak, serum: 2 hours

Excretion: Primarily feces (as metabolites); urine (~14%, <1% as unchanged drug)

Pregnancy Risk Factor C

Diphenylhydantoin *see* Phenytoin *on page 1080*

Diphtheria and Tetanus Toxoids and Acellular Pertussis Adsorbed, Hepatitis B (Recombinant) and Inactivated Poliovirus Vaccine Combined *see* Diphtheria, Tetanus Toxoids, Acellular Pertussis, Hepatitis B (Recombinant), and Poliovirus (Inactivated) Vaccine *on page 452*

Diphtheria CRM_{197} Protein *see* Pneumococcal Conjugate Vaccine (7-Valent) *on page 1098*

Diphtheria CRM_{197} Protein Conjugate *see Haemophilus* b Conjugate Vaccine *on page 680*

Diphtheria, Tetanus Toxoids, Acellular Pertussis, Hepatitis B (Recombinant), and Poliovirus (Inactivated) Vaccine

(dif THEER ee a, TET a nus TOKS oyds, ay CEL yoo lar per TUS sis, hep a TYE tis bee ree KOM be nant, & POE lee oh VYE rus vak SEEN, in ak ti VAY ted vak SEEN)

Related Information

Immunizations (Vaccines) *on page 1614*

Poliovirus Vaccine (Inactivated) *on page 1099*

Tetanus Toxoid (Adsorbed) *on page 1277*

Tetanus Toxoid (Fluid) *on page 1278*

U.S. Brand Names Pediarix™

Generic Available No

Synonyms Diphtheria and Tetanus Toxoids and Acellular Pertussis Adsorbed, Hepatitis B (Recombinant) and Inactivated Poliovirus Vaccine Combined

Pharmacologic Category Vaccine

Use Combination vaccine for the active immunization against diphtheria, tetanus, pertussis, hepatitis B virus (all known subtypes), and poliomyelitis (caused by poliovirus types 1, 2, and 3)

Local Anesthetic/Vasoconstrictor Precautions No information available to require special precautions

Effects on Dental Treatment No significant effects or complications reported

Common Adverse Effects All serious adverse reactions must be reported to the U.S. Department of Health and Human Services (DHHS) Vaccine Adverse Event Reporting System (VAERS) 1-800-822-7967.

As reported in a U.S. lot Consistency Study:

>10%:

Central nervous system:

Sleeping increased (28% to 47%, grade 3: <1% to 2%)

Restlessness (28% to 30%, grade 3: ≤1%)

Fever ≥100.4°F (26% to 31%); >103.1°F (<1%); incidence of fever is higher than reported with separately administered vaccines

Gastrointestinal: Appetite decreased (19% to 22%, grade 3: <1%)

Local: Injection site:

Redness (25% to 36%, >20 mm: ≤1%)

Pain (23% to 30%, grade 3: ≤1%)

Swelling (15% to 22%; >20 mm: 1%)

Miscellaneous: Fussiness (57% to 64%; grade 3: 2% to 3%)

Refer to individual product monographs for additional adverse reactions, including postmarketing and case reports.

Mechanism of Action Promotes active immunity to diphtheria, tetanus, pertussis, hepatitis B and poliovirus (types 1, 2 and 3) by inducing production of specific antibodies and antitoxins.

Drug Interactions

Decreased Effect: Immunosuppressant medications or therapies (antimetabolites, alkylating agents, cytotoxic drugs, corticosteroids, irradiation) may decrease vaccine effectiveness, consider deferring vaccination for 3 months after immunosuppressant therapy is discontinued.

Pharmacodynamics/Kinetics Onset of action: Immune response observed to all components 1 month following the 3-dose series

Pregnancy Risk Factor C

Diphtheria, Tetanus Toxoids, and Acellular Pertussis Vaccine *see page 1614*

Diphtheria, Tetanus Toxoids, and Acellular Pertussis Vaccine and *Haemophilus influenzae* b Conjugate Vaccine (Combined) *see page 1614*

Diphtheria Toxoid Conjugate *see Haemophilus* b Conjugate Vaccine *on page 680*

Dipivalyl Epinephrine *see* Dipivefrin *on page 453*

Dipivefrin (dye PI ve frin)

U.S. Brand Names Propine®

Canadian Brand Names Apo-Dipivefrin®; Ophtho-Dipivefrin™; PMS-Dipivefrin; Propine®

Generic Available Yes

Synonyms Dipivalyl Epinephrine; Dipivefrin Hydrochloride; DPE

Pharmacologic Category Alpha/Beta Agonist; Ophthalmic Agent, Antiglaucoma; Ophthalmic Agent, Vasoconstrictor

Use Reduces elevated intraocular pressure in chronic open-angle glaucoma; also used to treat ocular hypertension, low tension, and secondary glaucomas

Local Anesthetic/Vasoconstrictor Precautions No information available to require special precautions

Effects on Dental Treatment No significant effects or complications reported

Mechanism of Action Dipivefrin is a prodrug of epinephrine which is the active agent that stimulates alpha- and/or beta-adrenergic receptors increasing aqueous humor outflow

Pregnancy Risk Factor B

Dipivefrin Hydrochloride *see* Dipivefrin *on page 453*

Diprivan® *see* Propofol *on page 1135*

Diprolene® *see* Betamethasone *on page 199*

Diprolene® AF *see* Betamethasone *on page 199*

Dipropylacetic Acid *see* Valproic Acid and Derivatives *on page 1359*

Dipyridamole (dye peer ID a mole)

U.S. Brand Names Persantine®

Canadian Brand Names Apo-Dipyridamole FC®; Novo-Dipiradol; Persantine®

Generic Available Yes

Pharmacologic Category Antiplatelet Agent; Vasodilator

Use Maintains patency after surgical grafting procedures including coronary artery bypass; used with warfarin to decrease thrombosis in patients after artificial heart valve replacement; used with aspirin to prevent coronary artery thrombosis; in combination with aspirin or warfarin to prevent other thromboembolic disorders. Dipyridamole may also be given 2 days prior to open heart

(Continued)

Dipyridamole *(Continued)*

surgery to prevent platelet activation by extracorporeal bypass pump and as a diagnostic agent in CAD.

Unlabeled/Investigational Use Treatment of proteinuria in pediatric renal disease

Local Anesthetic/Vasoconstrictor Precautions No information available to require special precautions

Effects on Dental Treatment No significant effects or complications reported

Common Adverse Effects

>10%:

Cardiovascular: Exacerbation of angina pectoris (20% I.V.)

Central nervous system: Dizziness (14% oral), headache (12% I.V.)

1% to 10%:

Cardiovascular: Hypotension (5%), hypertension (2%), blood pressure lability (2%), ECG abnormalities (ST-T changes, extrasystoles), chest pain, tachycardia (3% I.V.)

Central nervous system: Headache (2% I.V.), flushing (3% I.V.), fatigue (1% I.V.)

Dermatologic: Rash (2% oral)

Gastrointestinal: Abdominal distress (6% oral), nausea (5% I.V.)

Neuromuscular & skeletal: Paresthesia (1% I.V.)

Respiratory: Dyspnea (3% I.V.)

Mechanism of Action Inhibits the activity of adenosine deaminase and phosphodiesterase, which causes an accumulation of adenosine, adenine nucleotides, and cyclic AMP; these mediators then inhibit platelet aggregation and may cause vasodilation; may also stimulate release of prostacyclin or PGD_2; causes coronary vasodilation

Drug Interactions

Increased Effect/Toxicity: Dipyridamole enhances the risk of bleeding with aspirin (and other antiplatelet agents), heparin, low-molecular weight heparins, and warfarin. Adenosine blood levels and pharmacologic effects are increased with dipyridamole; consider reduced doses of adenosine.

Decreased Effect: Decreased vasodilation from I.V. dipyridamole when given to patients taking theophylline. Theophylline may reduce the pharmacologic effects of dipyridamole (hold theophylline preparations for 36-48 hours before dipyridamole facilitated stress test).

Pharmacodynamics/Kinetics

Absorption: Readily, but variable

Distribution: Adults: V_d: 2-3 L/kg

Protein binding: 91% to 99%

Metabolism: Hepatic

Half-life elimination: Terminal: 10-12 hours

Time to peak, serum: 2-2.5 hours

Excretion: Feces (as glucuronide conjugates and unchanged drug)

Pregnancy Risk Factor B

Dipyridamole and Aspirin *see* Aspirin and Dipyridamole *on page 156*

Dirithromycin (dye RITH roe mye sin)

U.S. Brand Names Dynabac®

Generic Available No

Pharmacologic Category Antibiotic, Macrolide

Use Treatment of mild to moderate upper and lower respiratory tract infections due to *Moraxella catarrhalis*, *Streptococcus pneumoniae*, *Legionella pneumophila*, *H. influenzae*, or *S. pyogenes*, ie, acute exacerbation of chronic bronchitis, secondary bacterial infection of acute bronchitis, community-acquired pneumonia, pharyngitis/tonsillitis, and uncomplicated infections of the skin and skin structure due to *Staphylococcus aureus*

Local Anesthetic/Vasoconstrictor Precautions No information available to require special precautions

Effects on Dental Treatment No significant effects or complications reported

Common Adverse Effects 1% to 10%:

Central nervous system: Headache, dizziness, vertigo, insomnia

Dermatologic: Rash, pruritus, urticaria

Endocrine & metabolic: Hyperkalemia

Gastrointestinal: Abdominal pain, nausea, diarrhea, vomiting, dyspepsia, flatulence

Hematologic: Thrombocytosis, eosinophilia, segmented neutrophils

Neuromuscular & skeletal: Weakness, pain, increased CPK

Respiratory: Increased cough, dyspnea

Mechanism of Action After being converted during intestinal absorption to its active form, erythromycylamine, dirithromycin inhibits protein synthesis by binding to the 50S ribosomal subunits of susceptible microorganisms

Drug Interactions

Cytochrome P450 Effect: Substrate of CYP3A4 (minor)

Increased Effect/Toxicity: Absorption of dirithromycin is slightly enhanced with concomitant antacids and H_2 antagonists. Dirithromycin may, like erythromycin, increase the effect of alfentanil, anticoagulants, bromocriptine, carbamazepine, cyclosporine, digoxin, disopyramide, ergots, methylprednisolone, cisapride, and triazolam.

Note: Interactions with nonsedating antihistamines (eg, astemizole) or theophylline are not known to occur; however, caution is advised with coadministration.

Pharmacodynamics/Kinetics

Absorption: Rapid
Distribution: V_d: 800 L; rapidly and widely (higher levels in tissues than plasma)
Protein binding: 14% to 30%
Metabolism: Hydrolyzed to erythromycylamine
Bioavailability: 10%
Half-life elimination: 8 hours (range: 2-36 hours)
Time to peak: 4 hours
Excretion: Feces (81% to 97%)

Pregnancy Risk Factor C

Disalcid® [DSC] *see* Salsalate *on page 1207*
Disalicylic Acid *see* Salsalate *on page 1207*
Disodium Cromoglycate *see* Cromolyn *on page 378*
Disodium Thiosulfate Pentahydrate *see* Sodium Thiosulfate *on page 1230*
***d*-Isoephedrine Hydrochloride** *see* Pseudoephedrine *on page 1147*

Disopyramide (dye soe PEER a mide)

Related Information

Cardiovascular Diseases *on page 1458*

U.S. Brand Names Norpace®; Norpace® CR

Canadian Brand Names Norpace®; Rythmodan®; Rythmodan®-LA

Generic Available Yes

Synonyms Disopyramide Phosphate

Pharmacologic Category Antiarrhythmic Agent, Class Ia

Use Suppression and prevention of unifocal and multifocal atrial and premature, ventricular premature complexes, coupled ventricular tachycardia; effective in the conversion of atrial fibrillation, atrial flutter, and paroxysmal atrial tachycardia to normal sinus rhythm and prevention of the recurrence of these arrhythmias after conversion by other methods

Local Anesthetic/Vasoconstrictor Precautions No information available to require special precautions

Effects on Dental Treatment Key adverse event(s) related to dental treatment: Xerostomia (normal salivary flow resumes upon discontinuation).

Common Adverse Effects The most common adverse effects are related to cholinergic blockade. The most serious adverse effects of disopyramide are hypotension and CHF.

>10%:
Gastrointestinal: Xerostomia (32%), constipation (11%)
Genitourinary: Urinary hesitancy (14% to 23%)

1% to 10%:
Cardiovascular: Congestive heart failure, hypotension, cardiac conduction disturbance, edema, syncope, chest pain
Central nervous system: Fatigue, headache, malaise, dizziness, nervousness
Dermatologic: Rash, generalized dermatoses, pruritus
Endocrine & metabolic: Hypokalemia, elevated cholesterol, elevated triglycerides
Gastrointestinal: Dry throat, nausea, abdominal distension, flatulence, abdominal bloating, anorexia, diarrhea, vomiting, weight gain
Genitourinary: Urinary retention, urinary frequency, urinary urgency, impotence (1% to 3%)
Neuromuscular & skeletal: Muscle weakness, muscular pain
Ocular: Blurred vision, dry eyes
Respiratory: Dyspnea

Mechanism of Action Class Ia antiarrhythmic: Decreases myocardial excitability and conduction velocity; reduces disparity in refractory between normal

(Continued)

Disopyramide *(Continued)*

and infarcted myocardium; possesses anticholinergic, peripheral vasoconstrictive, and negative inotropic effects

Drug Interactions

Cytochrome P450 Effect: Substrate of CYP3A4 (major)

Increased Effect/Toxicity: Disopyramide may increase the effects/toxicity of anticholinergics, beta-blockers, flecainide, procainamide, quinidine, or propafenone. Digoxin and quinidine serum concentrations may be increased by disopyramide.

CYP3A4 inhibitors may increase the levels/effects of disopyramide. Example inhibitors include azole antifungals, ciprofloxacin, clarithromycin, diclofenac, doxycycline, erythromycin, imatinib, isoniazid, nefazodone, nicardipine, propofol, protease inhibitors, quinidine, and verapamil.

Disopyramide effect/toxicity may be additive with drugs which may prolong the QT interval - amiodarone, amitriptyline, bepridil, cisapride (use is contraindicated), disopyramide, erythromycin, haloperidol, imipramine, pimozide, quinidine, sotalol, and thioridazine. In addition concurrent use with sparfloxacin, gatifloxacin, and moxifloxacin may result in additional prolongation of the QT interval; concurrent use is contraindicated.

Decreased Effect: CYP3A4 inducers may decrease the levels/effects of disopyramide; example inducers include aminoglutethimide, carbamazepine, nafcillin, nevirapine, phenobarbital, phenytoin, and rifamycins.

Pharmacodynamics/Kinetics

Onset of action: 0.5-3.5 hours

Duration: 1.5-8.5 hours

Absorption: 60% to 83%

Protein binding (concentration dependent): 20% to 60%

Metabolism: Hepatic to inactive metabolites

Half-life elimination: Adults: 4-10 hours; prolonged with hepatic or renal impairment

Excretion: Urine (40% to 60% as unchanged drug); feces (10% to 15%)

Pregnancy Risk Factor C

Disopyramide Phosphate *see* Disopyramide *on page 455*

DisperMox™ *see* Amoxicillin *on page 114*

Disulfiram (dye SUL fi ram)

U.S. Brand Names Antabuse®

Generic Available No

Pharmacologic Category Aldehyde Dehydrogenase Inhibitor

Use Management of chronic alcoholism

Local Anesthetic/Vasoconstrictor Precautions No information available to require special precautions

Effects on Dental Treatment No significant effects or complications reported

Common Adverse Effects Frequency not defined.

Central nervous system: Drowsiness, headache, fatigue, psychosis

Dermatologic: Rash, acneiform eruptions, allergic dermatitis

Gastrointestinal: Metallic or garlic-like aftertaste

Genitourinary: Impotence

Hepatic: Hepatitis (cholestatic and fulminant), hepatic failure (multiple case reports)

Neuromuscular & skeletal: Peripheral neuritis, polyneuritis, peripheral neuropathy

Ocular: Optic neuritis

Mechanism of Action Disulfiram is a thiuram derivative which interferes with aldehyde dehydrogenase. When taken concomitantly with alcohol, there is an increase in serum acetaldehyde levels. High acetaldehyde causes uncomfortable symptoms including flushing, nausea, thirst, palpitations, chest pain, vertigo, and hypotension. This reaction is the basis for disulfiram use in postwithdrawal long-term care of alcoholism.

Drug Interactions

Cytochrome P450 Effect: Substrate (minor) of CYP1A2, 2A6, 2B6, 2D6, 2E1, 3A4; **Inhibits** CYP1A2 (weak), 2A6 (weak), 2B6 (weak), 2C8/9 (weak), 2D6 (weak), 2E1 (strong), 3A4 (weak)

Increased Effect/Toxicity: Disulfiram results in severe ethanol intolerance (disulfiram reaction) secondary to disulfiram's ability to inhibit aldehyde dehydrogenase; this combination should be avoided. Combined use with isoniazid, metronidazole, or MAO inhibitors may result in adverse CNS effects; this combination should be avoided. Some pharmaceutic dosage forms include ethanol, including elixirs and intravenous trimethoprim-sulfamethoxazole (contains 10% ethanol as a solubilizing agent); these may inadvertently provoke a disulfiram reaction. Disulfiram may increase the levels/effects of inhalational anesthetics, trimethadione, and other CYP2E1 substrates. Disulfiram may increase serum concentrations of benzodiazepines that undergo oxidative metabolism (all but oxazepam, lorazepam, temazepam). Disulfiram increases phenytoin and theophylline serum concentrations; toxicity may occur. Disulfiram inhibits the metabolism of warfarin resulting in an increased hypoprothrombinemic response.

Pharmacodynamics/Kinetics

Onset of action: Full effect: 12 hours

Duration: ~1-2 weeks after last dose

Absorption: Rapid

Metabolism: To diethylthiocarbamate

Excretion: Feces and exhaled gases (as metabolites)

Pregnancy Risk Factor C

Dithioglycerol *see* Dimercaprol *on page 447*

Dithranol *see* Anthralin *on page 133*

Ditropan® *see* Oxybutynin *on page 1026*

Ditropan® XL *see* Oxybutynin *on page 1026*

Diuril® *see* Chlorothiazide *on page 312*

Divalproex Sodium *see* Valproic Acid and Derivatives *on page 1359*

5071-1DL(6) *see* Megestrol *on page 865*

***dl*-Alpha Tocopherol** *see* Vitamin E *on page 1383*

4-DMDR *see* Idarubicin *on page 732*

DNA-derived Humanized Monoclonal Antibody *see* Alemtuzumab *on page 76*

DNase *see* Dornase Alfa *on page 463*

DNR *see* DAUNOrubicin Hydrochloride *on page 401*

Doak® Tar [OTC] *see* Coal Tar *on page 367*

Doan's® [OTC] *see* Magnesium Salicylate *on page 854*

Doan's® Extra Strength [OTC] *see* Magnesium Salicylate *on page 854*

DOBUTamine (doe BYOO ta meen)

Related Information

Cardiovascular Diseases *on page 1458*

U.S. Brand Names Dobutrex®

Canadian Brand Names Dobutrex®

Mexican Brand Names Dobuject®; Dobutrex®; Oxiken®

Generic Available Yes

Synonyms Dobutamine Hydrochloride

Pharmacologic Category Adrenergic Agonist Agent

Use Short-term management of patients with cardiac decompensation

Unlabeled/Investigational Use Positive inotropic agent for use in myocardial dysfunction of sepsis

Local Anesthetic/Vasoconstrictor Precautions No information available to require special precautions

Effects on Dental Treatment No significant effects or complications reported

Common Adverse Effects Incidence of adverse events is not always reported.

Cardiovascular: Increased heart rate, increased blood pressure, increased ventricular ectopic activity, hypotension, premature ventricular beats (5%, dose-related), anginal pain (1% to 3%), nonspecific chest pain (1% to 3%), palpitations (1% to 3%)

Central nervous system: Fever (1% to 3%), headache (1% to 3%), paresthesia

Endocrine & metabolic: Slight decrease in serum potassium

Gastrointestinal: Nausea (1% to 3%)

Hematologic: Thrombocytopenia (isolated cases)

Local: Phlebitis, local inflammatory changes and pain from infiltration, cutaneous necrosis (isolated cases)

Neuromuscular & skeletal: Mild leg cramps

Respiratory: Dyspnea (1% to 3%)

Mechanism of Action Stimulates $beta_1$-adrenergic receptors, causing increased contractility and heart rate, with little effect on $beta_2$- or alpha-receptors

Drug Interactions

Increased Effect/Toxicity: General anesthetics (eg, halothane or cyclopropane) and usual doses of dobutamine have resulted in ventricular arrhythmias in animals. Bretylium and may potentiate dobutamine's effects.

(Continued)

DOBUTamine *(Continued)*

Beta-blockers (nonselective ones) may increase hypertensive effect; avoid concurrent use. Cocaine may cause malignant arrhythmias. Guanethidine, MAO inhibitors, methyldopa, reserpine, and tricyclic antidepressants can increase the pressor response to sympathomimetics.

Decreased Effect: Beta-adrenergic blockers may decrease effect of dobutamine and increase risk of severe hypotension.

Pharmacodynamics/Kinetics

Onset of action: I.V.: 1-10 minutes

Peak effect: 10-20 minutes

Metabolism: In tissues and hepatically to inactive metabolites

Half-life elimination: 2 minutes

Excretion: Urine (as metabolites)

Pregnancy Risk Factor B

Dobutamine Hydrochloride *see* DOBUTamine *on page 457*

Dobutrex® *see* DOBUTamine *on page 457*

Docetaxel (doe se TAKS el)

U.S. Brand Names Taxotere®

Canadian Brand Names Taxotere®

Mexican Brand Names Taxotere®

Generic Available No

Synonyms NSC-628503; RP-6976

Pharmacologic Category Antineoplastic Agent, Natural Source (Plant) Derivative

Use Treatment of locally-advanced or metastatic breast cancer; treatment of locally-advanced or metastatic nonsmall cell lung cancer (NSCLC) in combination with cisplatin in treatment of patients who have not previously received chemotherapy for unresected NSCLC; treatment of prostate cancer (hormone refractory, metastatic)

Unlabeled/Investigational Use Investigational: Treatment of gastric, pancreatic, head and neck, and ovarian cancers, soft tissue sarcoma, and melanoma

Local Anesthetic/Vasoconstrictor Precautions No information available to require special precautions

Effects on Dental Treatment Key adverse event(s) related to dental treatment: Mucositis, stomatitis, and taste perversion.

Common Adverse Effects Note: Frequencies cited for nonsmall cell lung cancer and breast cancer treatment. Exact frequency may vary based on tumor type, prior treatment, premedication, and dosage of docetaxel.

>10%:

Cardiovascular: Fluid retention, including peripheral edema, pleural effusions, and ascites (33% to 47%); may be more common at cumulative doses ≥400 mg/m^2. Up to 64% in breast cancer patients with dexamethasone premedication.

Dermatologic: Alopecia (56% to 76%); nail disorder (11% to 31%, banding, onycholysis, hypo- or hyperpigmentation)

Gastrointestinal: Mucositis/stomatitis (26% to 42%, severe in 6% to 7%), may be dose-limiting (premedication may reduce frequency and severity); nausea and vomiting (40% to 80%, severe in 1% to 5%); diarrhea (33% to 43%)

Hematologic: Myelosuppression, neutropenia (75% to 85%), thrombocytopenia, anemia

Onset: 4-7 days

Nadir: 5-9 days

Recovery: 21 days

Hepatic: Transaminase levels increased (18%)

Neuromuscular & skeletal: Myalgia (3% to 21%); neurosensory changes (paresthesia, dysesthesia, pain) noted in 23% to 49% (severe in up to 6%). Motor neuropathy (including weakness) noted in as many as 16% of lung cancer patients (severe in up to 5%). Neuropathy may be more common at higher cumulative docetaxel dosages or with prior cisplatin therapy.

Miscellaneous: Hypersensitivity reactions (6% to 13%; angioedema, rash, flushing, fever, hypotension); frequency substantially reduced by premedication with dexamethasone starting one day prior to docetaxel administration.

1% to 10%:

Cardiovascular: Hypotension (3%)

Dermatologic: Rash and skin eruptions (6%)

Gastrointestinal: Taste perversion (6%)

Hepatic: Bilirubin increased (9%)

Neuromuscular & skeletal: Arthralgia (3% to 9%)
Miscellaneous: Infusion site reactions (up to 4%)

Mechanism of Action Docetaxel promotes the assembly of microtubules from tubulin dimers, and inhibits the depolymerization of tubulin which stabilizes microtubules in the cell. This results in inhibition of DNA, RNA, and protein synthesis. Most activity occurs during the M phase of the cell cycle.

Drug Interactions

Cytochrome P450 Effect: Substrate of CYP3A4 (major); **Inhibits** CYP3A4 (weak)

Increased Effect/Toxicity: CYP3A4 inhibitors may increase the levels/effects of docetaxel; example inhibitors include azole antifungals, ciprofloxacin, clarithromycin, diclofenac, doxycycline, erythromycin, imatinib, isoniazid, nefazodone, nicardipine, propofol, protease inhibitors, quinidine, and verapamil. When administered as sequential infusions, observational studies indicate a potential for increased toxicity when platinum derivatives (carboplatin, cisplatin) are administered before taxane derivatives (docetaxel, paclitaxel).

Decreased Effect: CYP3A4 inducers may decrease the levels/effects of docetaxel; example inducers include aminoglutethimide, carbamazepine, nafcillin, nevirapine, phenobarbital, phenytoin, and rifamycins.

Pharmacodynamics/Kinetics Exhibits linear pharmacokinetics at the recommended dosage range

Distribution: Extensive extravascular distribution and/or tissue binding; V_d: 80-90 L/m^2, V_{dss}: 113 L (mean steady state)

Protein binding: 94%, primarily to alpha$_1$-acid glycoprotein, albumin, and lipoproteins

Metabolism: Hepatic; oxidation via CYP3A4 to metabolites

Half-life elimination: Alpha, beta, gamma: 4 minutes, 36 minutes, and 10-18 hours, respectively

Excretion: Feces (75%); urine (6%); ~80% within 48 hours

Clearance: Total body: Mean: 21 L/hour/m^2

Pregnancy Risk Factor D

Docosanol (doe KOE san ole)

U.S. Brand Names Abreva® [OTC]

Generic Available No

Synonyms Behenyl Alcohol; *n*-Docosanol

Pharmacologic Category Antiviral Agent, Topical

Use Treatment of herpes simplex of the face or lips

Local Anesthetic/Vasoconstrictor Precautions No information available to require special precautions

Effects on Dental Treatment No significant effects or complications reported

Significant Adverse Effects Limited information; headache reported (frequency similar to placebo)

Dosage Children ≥12 years and Adults: Topical: Apply 5 times/day to affected area of face or lips. Start at first sign of cold sore or fever blister and continue until healed.

Mechanism of Action Prevents viral entry and replication at the cellular level

Contraindications Hypersensitivity to docosanol or any component of the formulation

Warnings/Precautions For external use only. Do not apply to inside of mouth or around eyes. Not for use in children <12 years of age.

Dosage Forms Cream: 10% (2 g)

Comments Wash hands before and after applying cream. Begin treatment at first tingle of cold sore or fever blister. Rub into area gently, but completely. Do not apply directly to inside of mouth or around eyes. Contact healthcare provider if sore gets worse or does not heal within 10 days. Do not share this product with others, may spread infection. Notify healthcare professional if pregnant or breast-feeding.

Docusate (DOK yoo sate)

U.S. Brand Names Colace® [OTC]; Diocto® [OTC]; Docusoft-S™ [OTC]; DOS® [OTC]; D-S-S® [OTC]; ex-lax® Stool Softener [OTC]; Fleet® Sof-Lax® [OTC]; Genasoft® [OTC]; Phillips'® Stool Softener Laxative [OTC]; Surfak® [OTC]

Canadian Brand Names Albert® Docusate; Apo-Docusate-Calcium®; Apo-Docusate-Sodium®; Colace®; Colax-C®; Novo-Docusate Calcium; Novo-Docusate Sodium; PMS-Docusate Calcium; PMS-Docusate Sodium; Regulex®; Selax®; Soflax™

Generic Available Yes

(Continued)

Docusate *(Continued)*

Synonyms Dioctyl Calcium Sulfosuccinate; Dioctyl Sodium Sulfosuccinate; Docusate Calcium; Docusate Potassium; Docusate Sodium; DOSS; DSS

Pharmacologic Category Stool Softener

Use Stool softener in patients who should avoid straining during defecation and constipation associated with hard, dry stools; prophylaxis for straining (Valsalva) following myocardial infarction. A safe agent to be used in elderly; some evidence that doses <200 mg are ineffective; stool softeners are unnecessary if stool is well hydrated or "mushy" and soft; shown to be ineffective used long-term.

Unlabeled/Investigational Use Ceruminolytic

Local Anesthetic/Vasoconstrictor Precautions No information available to require special precautions

Effects on Dental Treatment Key adverse event(s) related to dental treatment: Throat irritation.

Common Adverse Effects 1% to 10%:

Gastrointestinal: Intestinal obstruction, diarrhea, abdominal cramping

Miscellaneous: Throat irritation

Mechanism of Action Reduces surface tension of the oil-water interface of the stool resulting in enhanced incorporation of water and fat allowing for stool softening

Drug Interactions

Increased Effect/Toxicity: Increased toxicity with mineral oil, phenolphthalein.

Decreased Effect: Decreased effect of warfarin with high doses of docusate.

Pharmacodynamics/Kinetics

Onset of action: 12-72 hours

Excretion: Feces

Pregnancy Risk Factor C

Docusate and Casanthranol (DOK yoo sate & ka SAN thra nole)

Related Information

Docusate *on page 459*

U.S. Brand Names Diocto C® [DSC] [OTC]; Docusoft Plus™ [DSC] [OTC]; Doxidan® [DSC] [OTC]; Fleet® Sof-Lax® Overnight [DSC] [OTC]; Genasoft® Plus [DSC] [OTC]; Peri-Colace® [DSC] [OTC]

Canadian Brand Names Peri-Colace®

Generic Available No

Synonyms Casanthranol and Docusate; DSS With Casanthranol

Pharmacologic Category Laxative/Stool Softener

Use Treatment of constipation generally associated with dry, hard stools and decreased intestinal motility

Local Anesthetic/Vasoconstrictor Precautions No information available to require special precautions

Effects on Dental Treatment Key adverse event(s) related to dental treatment: Throat irritation.

Common Adverse Effects 1% to 10%:

Dermatologic: Rash

Gastrointestinal: Intestinal obstruction, diarrhea, abdominal cramping, throat irritation

Pregnancy Risk Factor C

Docusate Calcium *see* Docusate *on page 459*

Docusate Potassium *see* Docusate *on page 459*

Docusate Sodium *see* Docusate *on page 459*

Docusoft Plus™ [DSC] [OTC] *see* Docusate and Casanthranol *on page 460*

Docusoft-S™ [OTC] *see* Docusate *on page 459*

Dofetilide (doe FET il ide)

Related Information

Cardiovascular Diseases *on page 1458*

U.S. Brand Names Tikosyn™

Canadian Brand Names Tikosyn™

Generic Available No

Pharmacologic Category Antiarrhythmic Agent, Class III

Use Maintenance of normal sinus rhythm in patients with chronic atrial fibrillation/atrial flutter of longer than 1-week duration who have been converted to normal sinus rhythm; conversion of atrial fibrillation and atrial flutter to normal sinus rhythm

Local Anesthetic/Vasoconstrictor Precautions No information available to require special precautions

Effects on Dental Treatment No significant effects or complications reported

Common Adverse Effects

Supraventricular arrhythmia patients (incidence > placebo)

>10%: Central nervous system: Headache (11%)

2% to 10%:

Central nervous system: Dizziness (8%), insomnia (4%)

Cardiovascular: Ventricular tachycardia (2.6% to 3.7%), chest pain (10%), torsade de pointes (3.3% in CHF patients and 0.9% in patients with a recent MI; up to 10.5% in patients receiving doses in excess of those recommended). Torsade de pointes occurs most frequently within the first 3 days of therapy.

Dermatologic: Rash (3%)

Gastrointestinal: Nausea (5%), diarrhea (3%), abdominal pain (3%)

Neuromuscular & skeletal: Back pain (3%)

Respiratory: Dyspnea (6%), respiratory tract infection (7%)

Miscellaneous: Flu syndrome (4%)

<2%:

Central nervous system: CVA, facial paralysis, flaccid paralysis, migraine, paralysis

Cardiovascular: AV block (0.4% to 1.5%), ventricular fibrillation (0% to 0.4%), bundle branch block, heart block, edema, heart arrest, myocardial infarct, sudden death, syncope

Dermatologic: Angioedema

Gastrointestinal: Liver damage

Neuromuscular & skeletal: Paresthesia

Respiratory: Cough

>2% (incidence ≤ placebo): Anxiety, pain, angina, atrial fibrillation, hypertension, palpitation, supraventricular tachycardia, peripheral edema, urinary tract infection, weakness, arthralgia, diaphoresis

Mechanism of Action Vaughan Williams Class III antiarrhythmic activity. Blockade of the cardiac ion channel carrying the rapid component of the delayed rectifier potassium current. Dofetilide has no effect on sodium channels, adrenergic alpha-receptors, or adrenergic beta-receptors. It increases the monophasic action potential duration due to delayed repolarization. The increase in the QT interval is a function of prolongation of both effective and functional refractory periods in the His-Purkinje system and the ventricles. Changes in cardiac conduction velocity and sinus node function have not been observed in patients with or without structural heart disease. PR and QRS width remain the same in patients with pre-existing heart block and or sick sinus syndrome.

Drug Interactions

Cytochrome P450 Effect: Substrate of CYP3A4 (minor)

Increased Effect/Toxicity: Dofetilide concentrations are increased by cimetidine, verapamil, ketoconazole, and trimethoprim (concurrent use of these agents is contraindicated). Dofetilide levels may also be increased by renal cationic transport inhibitors (including triamterene, metformin, amiloride, and megestrol). Diuretics and other drugs which may deplete potassium and/or magnesium (aminoglycoside antibiotics, amphotericin, cyclosporine) may increase dofetilide's toxicity (torsade de pointes). Use of QT_c-prolonging agents (including bepridil, cisapride, erythromycin, tricyclic antidepressants, phenothiazines, sparfloxacin, gatifloxacin, moxifloxacin) is contraindicated.

Pharmacodynamics/Kinetics

Absorption: >90%

Distribution: V_d: 3 L/kg

Protein binding: 60% to 70%

Metabolism: Hepatic via CYP3A4, but low affinity for it; metabolites formed by N-dealkylation and N-oxidation

Bioavailability: >90%

Half-life elimination: 10 hours

Time to peak: Fasting: 2-3 hours

Excretion: Urine (80%, 80% as unchanged drug, 20% as inactive or minimally active metabolites); renal elimination consists of glomerular filtration and active tubular secretion via cationic transport system

Pregnancy Risk Factor C

Dolasetron (dol A se tron)

U.S. Brand Names Anzemet®

Canadian Brand Names Anzemet®

Mexican Brand Names Anzemet®

(Continued)

Dolasetron *(Continued)*

Generic Available No

Synonyms Dolasetron Mesylate; MDL 73,147EF

Pharmacologic Category Antiemetic; Selective 5-HT_3 Receptor Antagonist

Use Prevention of nausea and vomiting associated with emetogenic cancer chemotherapy, including initial and repeat courses; prevention of postoperative nausea and vomiting and treatment of postoperative nausea and vomiting (injectable form only)

Generally **not** recommended for treatment of existing chemotherapy-induced emesis (CIE) or for prophylaxis of nausea from agents with a low emetogenic potential.

Local Anesthetic/Vasoconstrictor Precautions No information available to require special precautions

Effects on Dental Treatment Key adverse event(s) related to dental treatment: Taste alterations.

Common Adverse Effects

>10%:

Central nervous system: Headache (31%), dizziness, lightheadedness (23%)

Gastrointestinal: Loose stools/diarrhea (50%); increased appetite (27%); taste alterations (12%)

1% to 10%:

Cardiovascular: Hypertension, hypotension (6%), ECG abnormalities, prolonged P-R, QRS, and QT_c intervals

Central nervous system: Sedation (8%), slow movement (3%), nervousness (3%), fatigue (2%), listlessness, grogginess

Gastrointestinal: Nausea (6%), constipation (3%), diarrhea, abdominal pain, flatulence

Hepatic: Mild elevations of serum aminotransferases (7%)

Local: Pain at injection site (1%)

Neuromuscular & skeletal: Paresthesia

Ocular: Visual disturbances (mostly blurred vision) (9%); photosensitivity (2%)

Mechanism of Action Selective serotonin receptor (5-HT_3) antagonist, blocking serotonin both peripherally (primary site of action) and centrally at the chemoreceptor trigger zone

Drug Interactions

Cytochrome P450 Effect: Substrate (minor) of CYP2C8/9, 3A4; **Inhibits** CYP2D6 (weak)

Increased Effect/Toxicity: Increased blood levels of active metabolite may occur during concurrent administration of cimetidine and atenolol. Inhibitors of this isoenzyme may increase blood levels of active metabolite. Due to the potential to potentiate QT_c prolongation, drugs which may prolong QT interval directly (eg, antiarrhythmics) or by causing alterations in electrolytes (eg, diuretics) should be used with caution.

Decreased Effect: Blood levels of active metabolite are decreased during coadministration of rifampin.

Pharmacodynamics/Kinetics

Metabolism: Hepatic to a reduced alcohol (active metabolite MDL 74,156)

Half-life elimination: Dolasetron: 10 minutes; MDL 74,156: 8 hours

Excretion: Urine (as unchanged drug)

Pregnancy Risk Factor B

Dolasetron Mesylate *see* Dolasetron *on page 461*

Dolobid® *see* Diflunisal *on page 435*

Dolophine® *see* Methadone *on page 889*

Domeboro® [OTC] *see* Aluminum Sulfate and Calcium Acetate *on page 92*

Dome Paste Bandage *see* Zinc Gelatin *on page 1400*

Donepezil (doh NEP e zil)

U.S. Brand Names Aricept®

Canadian Brand Names Aricept®

Mexican Brand Names Eranz®

Generic Available No

Synonyms E2020

Pharmacologic Category Acetylcholinesterase Inhibitor (Central)

Use Treatment of mild to moderate dementia of the Alzheimer's type

Unlabeled/Investigational Use Attention-deficit/hyperactivity disorder (ADHD), behavioral syndromes in dementia

Local Anesthetic/Vasoconstrictor Precautions No information available to require special precautions

Effects on Dental Treatment No significant effects or complications reported

Common Adverse Effects

>10%:

Central nervous system: Headache

Gastrointestinal: Nausea, diarrhea

1% to 10%:

Cardiovascular: Syncope, chest pain, hypertension, atrial fibrillation, hypotension, hot flashes

Central nervous system: Abnormal dreams, depression, dizziness, fatigue, insomnia, somnolence

Dermatologic: Bruising

Gastrointestinal: Anorexia, vomiting, weight loss, fecal incontinence, GI bleeding, bloating, epigastric pain

Genitourinary: Frequent urination

Neuromuscular & skeletal: Muscle cramps, arthritis, body pain

Mechanism of Action Alzheimer's disease is characterized by cholinergic deficiency in the cortex and basal forebrain, which contributes to cognitive deficits. Donepezil reversibly and noncompetitively inhibits centrally-active acetylcholinesterase, the enzyme responsible for hydrolysis of acetylcholine. This appears to result in increased concentrations of acetylcholine available for synaptic transmission in the central nervous system.

Drug Interactions

Cytochrome P450 Effect: Substrate (minor) of CYP2D6, 3A4

Increased Effect/Toxicity: A synergistic effect may be seen with concurrent administration of succinylcholine or cholinergic agonists (bethanechol).

Decreased Effect: Anticholinergic agents (benztropine) may inhibit the effects of donepezil.

Pharmacodynamics/Kinetics

Absorption: Well absorbed

Protein binding: 96%, primarily to albumin (75%) and α_1-acid glycoprotein (21%)

Metabolism: Extensively to four major metabolites (two are active) via CYP2D6 and 3A4; undergoes glucuronidation

Bioavailability: 100%

Half-life elimination: 70 hours; time to steady-state: 15 days

Time to peak, plasma: 3-4 hours

Excretion: Urine (as unchanged drug)

Pregnancy Risk Factor C

Donnapectolin-PG® *see* Hyoscyamine, Atropine, Scopolamine, Kaolin, Pectin, and Opium *on page 726*

Donnatal® *see* Hyoscyamine, Atropine, Scopolamine, and Phenobarbital *on page 725*

Donnatal Extentabs® *see* Hyoscyamine, Atropine, Scopolamine, and Phenobarbital *on page 725*

Dopamine *see page 1458*

Dopram® *see* Doxapram *on page 465*

Doral® *see* Quazepam *on page 1155*

Dornase Alfa (DOOR nase AL fa)

U.S. Brand Names Pulmozyme®

Canadian Brand Names Pulmozyme™

Mexican Brand Names Pulmozyme®

Generic Available No

Synonyms DNase; Recombinant Human Deoxyribonuclease

Pharmacologic Category Enzyme

Use Management of cystic fibrosis patients to reduce the frequency of respiratory infections that require parenteral antibiotics, and to improve pulmonary function

Unlabeled/Investigational Use Treatment of chronic bronchitis

Local Anesthetic/Vasoconstrictor Precautions No information available to require special precautions

Effects on Dental Treatment Key adverse event(s) related to dental treatment: Pharyngitis.

Common Adverse Effects

>10%:

Respiratory: Pharyngitis

Miscellaneous: Voice alteration

(Continued)

Dornase Alfa *(Continued)*

1% to 10%:
- Cardiovascular: Chest pain
- Dermatologic: Rash
- Ocular: Conjunctivitis
- Respiratory: Laryngitis, cough, dyspnea, hemoptysis, rhinitis, hoarse throat, wheezing

Mechanism of Action The hallmark of cystic fibrosis lung disease is the presence of abundant, purulent airway secretions composed primarily of highly polymerized DNA. The principal source of this DNA is the nuclei of degenerating neutrophils, which is present in large concentrations in infected lung secretions. The presence of this DNA produces a viscous mucous that may contribute to the decreased mucociliary transport and persistent infections that are commonly seen in this population. Dornase alfa is a deoxyribonuclease (DNA) enzyme produced by recombinant gene technology. Dornase selectively cleaves DNA, thus reducing mucous viscosity and as a result, airflow in the lung is improved and the risk of bacterial infection may be decreased.

Pharmacodynamics/Kinetics

Onset of action: Nebulization: Enzyme levels are measured in sputum in ~15 minutes

Duration: Rapidly declines

Pregnancy Risk Factor B

Doryx® *see* Doxycycline *on page 471*

Dorzolamide (dor ZOLE a mide)

U.S. Brand Names Trusopt®

Canadian Brand Names Trusopt®

Mexican Brand Names Trusopt®

Generic Available No

Synonyms Dorzolamide Hydrochloride

Pharmacologic Category Carbonic Anhydrase Inhibitor; Ophthalmic Agent, Antiglaucoma

Use Lowers intraocular pressure in patients with ocular hypertension or open-angle glaucoma

Local Anesthetic/Vasoconstrictor Precautions No information available to require special precautions

Effects on Dental Treatment No significant effects or complications reported

Mechanism of Action Reversible inhibition of the enzyme carbonic anhydrase resulting in reduction of hydrogen ion secretion at renal tubule and an increased renal excretion of sodium, potassium, bicarbonate, and water to decrease production of aqueous humor; also inhibits carbonic anhydrase in central nervous system to retard abnormal and excessive discharge from CNS neurons

Pregnancy Risk Factor C

Dorzolamide and Timolol (dor ZOLE a mide & TYE moe lole)

U.S. Brand Names Cosopt®

Canadian Brand Names Cosopt®

Generic Available No

Synonyms Timolol and Dorzolamide

Pharmacologic Category Beta-Adrenergic Blocker; Carbonic Anhydrase Inhibitor

Use Lowers intraocular pressure to treat glaucoma in patients with ocular hypertension or open-angle glaucoma

Local Anesthetic/Vasoconstrictor Precautions No information available to require special precautions

Effects on Dental Treatment No significant effects or complications reported

Common Adverse Effects See individual agents.

Drug Interactions

Cytochrome P450 Effect:

Dorzolamide: **Substrate** (minor) of CYP2C8/9, 3A4

Timolol: **Substrate** of CYP2D6 (major); **Inhibits** CYP2D6 (weak)

Increased Effect/Toxicity: See individual agents.

Decreased Effect: See individual agents.

Pharmacodynamics/Kinetics See individual agents.

Dorzolamide Hydrochloride *see* Dorzolamide *on page 464*

DOS® [OTC] *see* Docusate *on page 459*

DOSS *see* Docusate *on page 459*

Dostinex® *see* Cabergoline *on page 241*

Dovonex® *see* Calcipotriene *on page 243*

Doxapram (DOKS a pram)

U.S. Brand Names Dopram®

Generic Available Yes

Synonyms Doxapram Hydrochloride

Pharmacologic Category Respiratory Stimulant; Stimulant

Use Respiratory and CNS stimulant for respiratory depression secondary to anesthesia, drug-induced CNS depression; acute hypercapnia secondary to COPD

Local Anesthetic/Vasoconstrictor Precautions No information available to require special precautions

Effects on Dental Treatment No significant effects or complications reported

Common Adverse Effects Frequency not defined.

Cardiovascular: Arrhythmia, blood pressure increased, chest pain, chest tightness, flushing, heart rate changes, T waves lowered, ventricular tachycardia, ventricular fibrillation

Central nervous system: Apprehension, Babinski turns positive, disorientation, dizziness, hallucinations, headache, hyperactivity, pyrexia, seizures

Derm: Pruritus

Gastrointestinal: Diarrhea, nausea, vomiting

Genitourinary: Urinary retention

Hematologic: Hematocrit decreased, hemoglobin decreased, hemolysis, red blood cell count decreased

Local: Phlebitis

Neuromuscular & skeletal: Clonus, deep tendon reflexes increase, fasciculations, involuntary muscle movement, muscle spasm, paresthesia

Ophthalmic: Pupillary dilatation

Renal: Albuminuria, BUN increased, spontaneous voiding

Respiratory: Bronchospasm, cough, dyspnea, hiccups, hyperventilation, laryngospasm, rebound hypoventilation, tachypnea

Miscellaneous: Diaphoresis

Mechanism of Action Stimulates respiration through action on respiratory center in medulla or indirectly on peripheral carotid chemoreceptors

Drug Interactions

Increased Effect/Toxicity: Increased blood pressure with sympathomimetics, MAO inhibitors. Halothane, cyclopropane, and enflurane may sensitize the myocardium to catecholamine and epinephrine which is released at the initiation of doxapram, hence, separate discontinuation of anesthetics and start of doxapram until the volatile agent has been excreted.

Pharmacodynamics/Kinetics

Onset of action: Respiratory stimulation: I.V.: 20-40 seconds

Peak effect: 1-2 minutes

Duration: 5-12 minutes

Half-life elimination, serum: Adults: Mean: 3.4 hours

Pregnancy Risk Factor B

Doxapram Hydrochloride *see* Doxapram *on page 465*

Doxazosin (doks AY zoe sin)

Related Information

Cardiovascular Diseases *on page 1458*

U.S. Brand Names Cardura®

Canadian Brand Names Alti-Doxazosin; Apo-Doxazosin®; Cardura-1™; Cardura-2™; Cardura-4™; Gen-Doxazosin; Novo-Doxazosin

Mexican Brand Names Cardura®

Generic Available Yes

Synonyms Doxazosin Mesylate

Pharmacologic Category Alpha$_1$ Blocker

Use Treatment of hypertension alone or in conjunction with diuretics, cardiac glycosides, ACE inhibitors, or calcium antagonists (particularly appropriate for those with hypertension and other cardiovascular risk factors such as hypercholesterolemia and diabetes mellitus); treatment of urinary outflow obstruction and/or obstructive and irritative symptoms associated with benign prostatic hyperplasia (BPH), particularly useful in patients with troublesome symptoms who are unable or unwilling to undergo invasive procedures, but who require rapid symptomatic relief; can be used in combination with finasteride

Local Anesthetic/Vasoconstrictor Precautions No information available to require special precautions

(Continued)

Doxazosin *(Continued)*

Effects on Dental Treatment Key adverse event(s) related to dental treatment: Xerostomia (normal salivary flow resumes upon discontinuation) and orthostatic hypotension.

Common Adverse Effects Note: "Combination therapy" refers to doxazosin and finasteride.

>10%:

Cardiovascular: Postural hypotension (combination therapy 18%)

Central nervous system: Dizziness (16% to 19%; combination therapy 23%), headache (10% to 14%)

Endocrine & metabolic: Impotence (combination therapy 23%), libido decreased (combination therapy 12%)

Genitourinary: Ejaculation disturbances (combination therapy 14%)

Neuromuscular & skeletal: Weakness (combination therapy 17%)

1% to 10%:

Cardiovascular: Orthostatic hypotension (dose-related; 0.3% up to 10%), edema (3% to 4%), hypotension (2%), palpitation (1% to 2%), chest pain (1% to 2%), arrhythmia (1%), syncope (2%), flushing (1%)

Central nervous system: Fatigue (8% to 12%), somnolence (3% to 5%), nervousness (2%), pain (2%), vertigo (2%), insomnia (1%), anxiety (1%), paresthesia (1%), movement disorder (1%), ataxia (1%), hypertonia (1%), depression (1%), weakness (1%)

Dermatologic: Rash (1%), pruritus (1%)

Endocrine & metabolic: Sexual dysfunction (2%)

Gastrointestinal: Abdominal pain (2%), diarrhea (2%), dyspepsia (1% to 2%), nausea (2% to 3%), xerostomia (1% to 2%), constipation (1%), flatulence (1%)

Genitourinary: Urinary tract infection (1%), impotence (1%), polyuria (2%), incontinence (1%)

Neuromuscular & skeletal: Back pain (2%), arthritis (1%), muscle weakness (1%), myalgia (1%), muscle cramps (1%)

Ocular: Abnormal vision (1% to 2%), conjunctivitis (1%)

Otic: Tinnitus (1%)

Respiratory: Rhinitis (3%), dyspnea (1% to 3%), respiratory disorder (1%), epistaxis (1%)

Miscellaneous: Flu-like syndrome (1%), increased diaphoresis (1%)

Dosage Oral:

Adults: 1 mg once daily in morning or evening; may be increased to 2 mg once daily. Thereafter titrate upwards, if needed, over several weeks, balancing therapeutic benefit with doxazosin-induced postural hypotension

Hypertension: Maximum dose: 16 mg/day

BPH: Goal: 4-8 mg/day; maximum dose: 8 mg/day

Elderly: Initial: 0.5 mg once daily

Mechanism of Action Competitively inhibits postsynaptic alpha-adrenergic receptors which results in vasodilation of veins and arterioles and a decrease in total peripheral resistance and blood pressure; approximately 50% as potent on a weight by weight basis as prazosin

Contraindications Hypersensitivity to quinazolines (prazosin, terazosin), doxazosin, or any component of the formulation; concurrent use with phosphodiesterase-5 (PDE-5) inhibitors including sildenafil (>25 mg), tadalafil, or vardenafil

Warnings/Precautions Use with caution in patients with renal impairment. Can cause marked hypotension and syncope with sudden loss of consciousness with the first dose. Prostate cancer should be ruled out before starting for BPH. Anticipate a similar effect if therapy is interrupted for a few days, if dosage is increased rapidly, or if another antihypertensive drug is introduced.

Drug Interactions

Increased Effect/Toxicity: Increased hypotensive effect with beta-blockers, diuretics, ACE inhibitors, calcium channel blockers, other antihypertensive medications, sildenafil (use with extreme caution at a dose ≤25 mg), tadalafil (contraindicated by the manufacturer), and vardenafil (contraindicated by the manufacturer).

Decreased Effect: Decreased hypotensive effect with NSAIDs.

Ethanol/Nutrition/Herb Interactions Herb/Nutraceutical: Avoid dong quai if using for hypertension (has estrogenic activity). Avoid ephedra, yohimbe, ginseng (may worsen hypertension). Avoid saw palmetto when used for BPH (due to limited experience with this combination). Avoid garlic (may have increased antihypertensive effect).

Pharmacodynamics/Kinetics Not significantly affected by increased age

Duration: >24 hours

Metabolism: Extensively hepatic
Half-life elimination: 22 hours
Time to peak, serum: 2-3 hours
Excretion: Feces (63%); urine (9%)

Pregnancy Risk Factor C

Dosage Forms TAB: 1 mg, 2 mg, 4 mg, 8 mg

Doxazosin Mesylate *see* Doxazosin *on page 465*

Doxepin (DOKS e pin)

U.S. Brand Names Prudoxin™; Sinequan®; Zonalon®

Canadian Brand Names Apo-Doxepin®; Novo-Doxepin; Sinequan®; Zonalon

Generic Available Yes: Capsule, solution

Synonyms Doxepin Hydrochloride

Pharmacologic Category Antidepressant, Tricyclic (Tertiary Amine); Topical Skin Product

Use

Oral: Depression

Topical: Short-term (<8 days) management of moderate pruritus in adults with atopic dermatitis or lichen simplex chronicus

Unlabeled/Investigational Use Analgesic for certain chronic and neuropathic pain; anxiety

Local Anesthetic/Vasoconstrictor Precautions Use with caution; epinephrine, norepinephrine and levonordefrin have been shown to have an increased pressor response in combination with TCAs

Effects on Dental Treatment Key adverse event(s) related to dental treatment: Xerostomia and changes in salivation (normal salivary flow resumes upon discontinuation).

Oral: Aphthous stomatitis, unpleasant taste, trouble with gums.
Topical: Taste alteration

Long-term treatment with TCAs increases the risk of caries by reducing salivation and salivary buffer capacity.

Common Adverse Effects

Oral: Frequency not defined.

Cardiovascular: Hypotension, hypertension, tachycardia
Central nervous system: Drowsiness, dizziness, headache, disorientation, ataxia, confusion, seizure
Dermatologic: Alopecia, photosensitivity, rash, pruritus
Endocrine & metabolic: Breast enlargement, galactorrhea, SIADH, increase or decrease in blood sugar, increased or decreased libido
Gastrointestinal: Xerostomia, constipation, vomiting, indigestion, anorexia, aphthous stomatitis, nausea, unpleasant taste, weight gain, diarrhea, trouble with gums, decreased lower esophageal sphincter tone may cause GE reflux
Genitourinary: Urinary retention, testicular edema
Hematologic: Agranulocytosis, leukopenia, eosinophilia, thrombocytopenia, purpura
Neuromuscular & skeletal: Weakness, tremors, numbness, paresthesia, extrapyramidal symptoms, tardive dyskinesia
Ocular: Blurred vision
Otic: Tinnitus
Miscellaneous: Diaphoresis (excessive), allergic reactions

Topical:

>10%:
Central nervous system: Drowsiness (22%)
Dermatologic: Stinging/burning (23%)

1% to 10%:
Cardiovascular: Edema: (1%)
Central nervous system: Dizziness (2%), emotional changes (2%)
Gastrointestinal: Xerostomia (10%), taste alteration (2%)

Mechanism of Action Increases the synaptic concentration of serotonin and norepinephrine in the central nervous system by inhibition of their reuptake by the presynaptic neuronal membrane

Drug Interactions

Cytochrome P450 Effect: Substrate (major) of CYP1A2, 2D6, 3A4

Increased Effect/Toxicity: Doxepin increases the effects of amphetamines, anticholinergics, other CNS depressants (sedatives, hypnotics, or ethanol), chlorpropamide, tolazamide, and warfarin. When used with MAO inhibitors, hyperpyrexia, hypertension, tachycardia, confusion, seizures, and **deaths**

(Continued)

Doxepin *(Continued)*

have been reported (serotonin syndrome). Serotonin syndrome has also been reported with ritonavir (rare).

CYP1A2 inhibitors may increase the levels/effects of doxepin; example inhibitors include amiodarone, fluvoxamine, ketoconazole, quinolone antibiotics, and rofecoxib. CYP2D6 inhibitors may increase the levels/effects of doxepin; example inhibitors include chlorpromazine, delavirdine, fluoxetine, miconazole, paroxetine, pergolide, quinidine, quinine, ritonavir, and ropinirole. CYP3A4 inhibitors may increase the levels/effects of doxepin. Example inhibitors include azole antifungals, ciprofloxacin, clarithromycin, diclofenac, doxycycline, erythromycin, imatinib, isoniazid, nefazodone, nicardipine, propofol, protease inhibitors, quinidine, and verapamil. Cimetidine, grapefruit juice, indinavir, methylphenidate, diltiazem, and verapamil may increase the serum concentrations of TCAs. Use of lithium with a TCA may increase the risk for neurotoxicity. Phenothiazines may increase concentration of some TCAs and TCAs may increase concentration of phenothiazines.

Pressor response to I.V. epinephrine, norepinephrine, and phenylephrine may be enhanced in patients receiving TCAs (**Note:** Effect is unlikely with epinephrine or levonordefrin dosages typically administered as infiltration in combination with local anesthetics). Combined use of beta-agonists or drugs which prolong QT_c (including quinidine, procainamide, disopyramide, cisapride, sparfloxacin, gatifloxacin, moxifloxacin) with TCAs may predispose patients to cardiac arrhythmias.

Decreased Effect: CYP1A2 inducers may decrease the levels/effects of doxepin; example inducers include aminoglutethimide, carbamazepine, phenobarbital, and rifampin. Doxepin inhibits the antihypertensive response to bethanidine, clonidine, debrisoquin, guanadrel, guanethidine, guanabenz, and guanfacine. Cholestyramine and colestipol may bind TCAs and reduce their absorption. CYP3A4 inducers may decrease the levels/effects of doxepin; example inducers include aminoglutethimide, carbamazepine, nafcillin, nevirapine, phenobarbital, phenytoin, and rifamycins.

Pharmacodynamics/Kinetics

Onset of action: Peak effect: Antidepressant: Usually >2 weeks; Anxiolytic: may occur sooner

Absorption: Following topical application, plasma levels may be similar to those achieved with oral administration

Distribution: Crosses placenta; enters breast milk

Protein binding: 80% to 85%

Metabolism: Hepatic; metabolites include desmethyldoxepin (active)

Half-life elimination: Adults: 6-8 hours

Excretion: Urine

Pregnancy Risk Factor B (cream); C (all other forms)

Doxepin Hydrochloride *see* Doxepin *on page 467*

Doxercalciferol (doks er kal si fe FEER ole)

U.S. Brand Names Hectorol®

Canadian Brand Names Hectorol®

Generic Available No

Synonyms 1α-Hydroxyergocalciferol

Pharmacologic Category Vitamin D Analog

Use Treatment of secondary hyperparathyroidism in patients with chronic kidney disease

Local Anesthetic/Vasoconstrictor Precautions No information available to require special precautions

Effects on Dental Treatment No significant effects or complications reported

Common Adverse Effects

Note: As reported in dialysis patients.

>10%:

Cardiovascular: Edema (34%)

Central nervous system: Headache (28%), malaise (28%), dizziness (12%)

Gastrointestinal: Nausea/vomiting (24%)

Respiratory: Dyspnea (12%)

1% to 10%:

Cardiovascular: Bradycardia (7%)

Central nervous system: Sleep disorder (3%)

Dermatologic: Pruritus (8%)

Gastrointestinal: Anorexia (5%), constipation (3%), dyspepsia (5%), weight gain (5%)

Neuromuscular & skeletal: Arthralgia (5%)

Miscellaneous: Abscess (3%)

Mechanism of Action Doxercalciferol is metabolized to the active form of vitamin D. The active form of vitamin D controls the intestinal absorption of dietary calcium, the tubular reabsorption of calcium by the kidneys, and in conjunction with PTH, the mobilization of calcium from the skeleton.

Drug Interactions

Increased Effect/Toxicity: Doxercalciferol toxicity may be increased by concurrent use of other vitamin D supplements or magnesium-containing antacids and supplements.

Decreased Effect: Absorption of doxercalciferol is reduced with mineral oil and cholestyramine.

Pharmacodynamics/Kinetics

Metabolism: Hepatic via CYP27

Half-life elimination: Active metabolite: 32-37 hours; up to 96 hours

Pregnancy Risk Factor B

Doxidan® [DSC] [OTC] *see* Docusate and Casanthranol *on page 460*

Doxidan® ***(reformulation)*** **[OTC]** *see* Bisacodyl *on page 208*

Doxil® *see* DOXOrubicin (Liposomal) *on page 470*

DOXOrubicin (doks oh ROO bi sin)

Related Information

DOXOrubicin (Liposomal) *on page 470*

U.S. Brand Names Adriamycin PFS®; Adriamycin RDF®; Rubex®

Canadian Brand Names Adriamycin®

Mexican Brand Names Adriblastina®; Caelyx®; Doxolem®; Doxotec®

Generic Available Yes

Synonyms ADR; Adria; Doxorubicin Hydrochloride; Hydroxydaunomycin Hydrochloride; Hydroxyldaunorubicin Hydrochloride; NSC-123127

Pharmacologic Category Antineoplastic Agent, Anthracycline

Use Treatment of leukemias, lymphomas, multiple myeloma, osseous and nonosseous sarcomas, mesotheliomas, germ cell tumors of the ovary or testis, and carcinomas of the head and neck, thyroid, lung, breast, stomach, pancreas, liver, ovary, bladder, prostate, uterus, and neuroblastoma

Local Anesthetic/Vasoconstrictor Precautions No information available to require special precautions

Effects on Dental Treatment Key adverse event(s) related to dental treatment: Stomatitis.

Common Adverse Effects

>10%:

Dermatologic: Alopecia, radiation recall

Gastrointestinal: Nausea, vomiting, stomatitis, GI ulceration, anorexia, diarrhea

Genitourinary: Discoloration of urine, mild dysuria, urinary frequency, hematuria, bladder spasms, cystitis following bladder instillation

Hematologic: Myelosuppression, primarily leukopenia (75%); thrombocytopenia and anemia

Onset: 7 days

Nadir: 10-14 days

Recovery: 21-28 days

1% to 10%:

Cardiovascular: Transient ECG abnormalities (supraventricular tachycardia, S-T wave changes, atrial or ventricular extrasystoles); generally asymptomatic and self-limiting. Congestive heart failure, dose-related, may be delayed for 7-8 years after treatment. Cumulative dose, mediastinal/pericardial radiation therapy, cardiovascular disease, age, and use of cyclophosphamide (or other cardiotoxic agents) all increase the risk.

Recommended maximum cumulative doses:

No risk factors: 550 mg/m^2

Concurrent radiation: 450 mg/m^2

Note: Regardless of cumulative dose, if the left ventricular ejection fraction is <30% to 40%, the drug is usually not given.

Dermatologic: Skin "flare" at injection site; discoloration of saliva, sweat, or tears

Endocrine & metabolic: Hyperuricemia

Mechanism of Action Inhibition of DNA and RNA synthesis by intercalation between DNA base pairs by inhibition of topoisomerase II and by steric obstruction. Doxorubicin intercalates at points of local uncoiling of the double helix. Although the exact mechanism is unclear, it appears that direct binding to DNA (intercalation) and inhibition of DNA repair (topoisomerase II inhibition) result in blockade of DNA and RNA synthesis and fragmentation of DNA.

(Continued)

DOXOrubicin *(Continued)*

Doxorubicin is also a powerful iron chelator; the iron-doxorubicin complex can bind DNA and cell membranes and produce free radicals that immediately cleave the DNA and cell membranes.

Drug Interactions

Cytochrome P450 Effect: Substrate (major) of CYP2D6, 3A4; **Inhibits** CYP2B6 (moderate), 2D6 (weak), 3A4 (weak)

Increased Effect/Toxicity: Allopurinol may enhance the antitumor activity of doxorubicin (animal data only). Cyclosporine may increase doxorubicin levels, enhancing hematologic toxicity or may induce coma or seizures. Cyclophosphamide enhances the cardiac toxicity of doxorubicin by producing additional myocardial cell damage. Mercaptopurine increases doxorubicin toxicities. Streptozocin greatly enhances leukopenia and thrombocytopenia. Verapamil alters the cellular distribution of doxorubicin and may result in increased cell toxicity by inhibition of the P-glycoprotein pump. Paclitaxel reduces doxorubicin clearance and increases toxicity if administered prior to doxorubicin. High doses of progesterone enhance toxicity (neutropenia and thrombocytopenia).

Doxorubicin may increase the levels/effects of bupropion, promethazine, propofol, selegiline, sertraline, and other CYP2B6 substrates. The levels/effects of doxorubicin may be increased by azole antifungals, chlorpromazine, ciprofloxacin, clarithromycin, delavirdine, diclofenac, doxycycline, erythromycin, fluoxetine, imatinib, isoniazid, miconazole, nefazodone, nicardipine, paroxetine, pergolide, propofol, protease inhibitors, quinidine, quinine, ritonavir, ropinirole, telithromycin, verapamil and other inhibitors of CYP2D6 or 3A4. Based on mouse studies, cardiotoxicity may be enhanced by verapamil. Concurrent therapy with actinomycin-D may result in recall pneumonitis following radiation.

Decreased Effect: The levels/effects of doxorubicin may be decreased by aminoglutethimide, carbamazepine, nafcillin, nevirapine, phenobarbital, phenytoin, rifamycins, and other CYP3A4 inducers. Doxorubicin may decrease plasma levels and effectiveness of digoxin. Doxorubicin may decrease the antiviral activity of zidovudine.

Pharmacodynamics/Kinetics

Absorption: Oral: Poor (<50%)

Distribution: V_d: 25 L/kg; to many body tissues, particularly liver, spleen, kidney, lung, heart; does not distribute into the CNS; crosses placenta

Protein binding, plasma: 70%

Metabolism: Primarily hepatic to doxorubicinol (active), then to inactive aglycones, conjugated sulfates, and glucuronides

Half-life elimination:

Distribution: 10 minutes

Elimination: Doxorubicin: 1-3 hours; Metabolites: 3-3.5 hours

Terminal: 17-30 hours

Male: 54 hours; Female: 35 hours

Excretion: Feces (~40% to 50% as unchanged drug); urine (~3% to 10% as metabolites, 1% doxorubicinol, <1% adrimycine aglycones, and unchanged drug)

Clearance: Male: 113 L/hour; Female: 44 L/hour

Pregnancy Risk Factor D

Doxorubicin Hydrochloride *see* DOXOrubicin *on page 469*

Doxorubicin Hydrochloride (Liposomal) *see* DOXOrubicin (Liposomal) *on page 470*

DOXOrubicin (Liposomal) (doks oh ROO bi sin lip pah SOW mal)

Related Information

DOXOrubicin *on page 469*

U.S. Brand Names Doxil®

Canadian Brand Names Caelyx®

Generic Available No

Synonyms Doxorubicin Hydrochloride (Liposomal)

Pharmacologic Category Antineoplastic Agent, Anthracycline

Use Treatment of AIDS-related Kaposi's sarcoma, breast cancer, ovarian cancer, solid tumors

Local Anesthetic/Vasoconstrictor Precautions No information available to require special precautions

Effects on Dental Treatment Key adverse event(s) related to dental treatment: Mucositis.

Common Adverse Effects

>10%:

Gastrointestinal: Nausea (18%)

Hematologic: Myelosuppression, leukopenia (60% to 80%), thrombocytopenia (6% to 24%), anemia (6% to 53%)

Onset: 7 days

Nadir: 10-14 days

Recovery: 21-28 days

1% to 10%:

Cardiovascular: Arrhythmias, pericardial effusion, tachycardia, cardiomyopathy, CHF (1%)

Dermatologic: Hyperpigmentation of nail beds; erythematous streaking of vein; alopecia (9%)

Gastrointestinal: Vomiting (8%), mucositis (7%)

Miscellaneous: Infusion-related reactions (bronchospasm, chest tightness, chills, dyspnea, facial edema, flushing, headache, hypotension, pruritus) have occurred (up to 10%)

Mechanism of Action Doxil® is doxorubicin hydrochloride encapsulated in long-circulating STEALTH® liposomes. Liposomes are microscopic vesicles composed of a phospholipid bilayer that are capable of encapsulating active drugs. Doxorubicin works through inhibition of topoisomerase-II at the point of DNA cleavage. A second mechanism of action is the production of free radicals (the hydroxy radical OH) by doxorubicin, which in turn can destroy DNA and cancerous cells. Doxorubicin is also a very powerful iron chelator, equal to deferoxamine. The iron-doxorubicin complex can bind DNA and cell membranes rapidly and produce free radicals that immediately cleave the DNA and cell membranes. Inhibits DNA and RNA synthesis by intercalating between DNA base pairs and by steric obstruction; active throughout entire cell cycle.

Drug Interactions

Cytochrome P450 Effect: Substrate (major) of CYP2D6, 3A4; **Inhibits** CYP2B6 (moderate), 2D6 (weak), 3A4 (weak)

Increased Effect/Toxicity: Allopurinol may enhance the antitumor activity of doxorubicin (animal data only). Cyclosporine may increase doxorubicin levels, enhancing hematologic toxicity or may induce coma or seizures. Cyclophosphamide enhances the cardiac toxicity of doxorubicin by producing additional myocardial cell damage. Mercaptopurine increases doxorubicin toxicities. Streptozocin greatly enhances leukopenia and thrombocytopenia. Verapamil alters the cellular distribution of doxorubicin and may result in increased cell toxicity by inhibition of the P-glycoprotein pump. Paclitaxel reduces doxorubicin clearance and increases toxicity if administered prior to doxorubicin. High doses of progesterone enhance toxicity (neutropenia and thrombocytopenia).

Doxorubicin may increase the levels/effects of bupropion, promethazine, propofol, selegiline, sertraline, and other CYP2B6 substrates. The levels/effects of doxorubicin may be increased by azole antifungals, chlorpromazine, ciprofloxacin, clarithromycin, delavirdine, diclofenac, doxycycline, erythromycin, fluoxetine, imatinib, isoniazid, miconazole, nefazodone, nicardipine, paroxetine, pergolide, propofol, protease inhibitors, quinidine, quinine, ritonavir, ropinirole, telithromycin, verapamil and other inhibitors of CYP2D6 or 3A4. Based on mouse studies, cardiotoxicity may be enhanced by verapamil. Concurrent therapy with actinomycin-D may result in recall pneumonitis following radiation.

Decreased Effect: The levels/effects of doxorubicin may be decreased by aminoglutethimide, carbamazepine, nafcillin, nevirapine, phenobarbital, phenytoin, rifamycins, and other CYP3A4 inducers. Doxorubicin may decrease plasma levels and effectiveness of digoxin. Doxorubicin may decrease the antiviral activity of zidovudine.

Pharmacodynamics/Kinetics

Distribution: V_{dss}: Confined mostly to the vascular fluid volume

Protein binding, plasma: Doxorubicin: 70%

Metabolism: Hepatic and in plasma to both active and inactive metabolites

Excretion: Urine (5% as doxorubicin or doxorubicinol)

Clearance: Mean: 0.041 L/hour/m^2

Pregnancy Risk Factor D

Doxy-100® *see* Doxycycline *on page 471*

Doxycycline (doks i SYE kleen)

Related Information

Animal and Human Bites Guidelines *on page 1582*

Periodontal Diseases *on page 1542*

(Continued)

Doxycycline *(Continued)*

Sexually-Transmitted Diseases *on page 1504*

U.S. Brand Names Adoxa™; Doryx®; Doxy-100®; Monodox®; Vibramycin®; Vibra-Tabs®

Canadian Brand Names Apo-Doxy®; Apo-Doxy Tabs®; Doxycin; Doxytec; Novo-Doxylin; Nu-Doxycycline; Vibra-Tabs®

Mexican Brand Names Vibramicina®

Generic Available Yes: Excludes powder for oral solution, syrup

Synonyms Doxycycline Calcium; Doxycycline Hyclate; Doxycycline Monohydrate

Pharmacologic Category Antibiotic, Tetracycline Derivative

Dental Use See Dental Use in Doxycycline Hyclate (Periodontal) *on page 475* and Doxycycline (Subantimicrobial) *on page 476.*

Use Principally in the treatment of infections caused by susceptible *Rickettsia*, *Chlamydia*, and *Mycoplasma*; alternative to mefloquine for malaria prophylaxis; treatment for syphilis, uncomplicated *Neisseria gonorrhoeae*, *Listeria*, *Actinomyces israelii*, and *Clostridium* infections in penicillin-allergic patients; for community-acquired pneumonia and other common infections due to susceptible organisms; anthrax due to *Bacillus anthracis,* including inhalational anthrax (postexposure); treatment of infections caused by uncommon susceptible gram-negative and gram-positive organisms including *Borrelia recurrentis*, *Ureaplasma urealyticum*, *Haemophilus ducreyi*, *Yersinia pestis*, *Francisella tularensis*, *Vibrio cholerae*, *Campylobacter fetus*, *Brucella* spp, *Bartonella bacilliformis*, and *Calymmatobacterium granulomatis*

Unlabeled/Investigational Use Sclerosing agent for pleural effusion injection; treatment of vancomycin-resistant enterococci (VRE)

Local Anesthetic/Vasoconstrictor Precautions No information available to require special precautions

Effects on Dental Treatment Key adverse event(s) related to dental treatment: Glossitis and tooth discoloration (children). Opportunistic "superinfection" with *Candida albicans*; tetracyclines are not recommended for use during pregnancy or in children ≤8 years of age since they have been reported to cause enamel hypoplasia and permanent teeth discoloration. The use of tetracyclines should only be used in these patients if other agents are contraindicated or alternative antimicrobials will not eradicate the organism.

Significant Adverse Effects Frequency not defined:

Cardiovascular: Intracranial hypertension, pericarditis

Dermatologic: Angioneurotic edema, exfoliative dermatitis (rare), photosensitivity, rash, urticaria

Endocrine & metabolic: Brown/black discoloration of thyroid gland (no dysfunction reported)

Gastrointestinal: Anorexia, diarrhea, enterocolitis, inflammatory lesions in anogenital region

Hematologic: Eosinophilia, hemolytic anemia, neutropenia, thrombocytopenia

Renal: Increased BUN

Miscellaneous: Anaphylactoid purpura, bulging fontanels (infants), SLE exacerbation

Dosage

Children:

Anthrax: Doxycycline should be used in children if antibiotic susceptibility testing, exhaustion of drug supplies, or allergic reaction preclude use of penicillin or ciprofloxacin. For treatment, the consensus recommendation does not include a loading dose for doxycycline.

Inhalational (postexposure prophylaxis) (*MMWR*, 2001, 50:889-893): Oral, I.V. (use oral route when possible):

≤8 years: 2.2 mg/kg every 12 hours for 60 days

>8 years and ≤45 kg: 2.2 mg/kg every 12 hours for 60 days

>8 years and >45 kg: 100 mg every 12 hours for 60 days

Cutaneous (treatment): Oral: See dosing for "Inhalational (postexposure prophylaxis)"

Note: In the presence of systemic involvement, extensive edema, and/or lesions on head/neck, doxycycline should initially be administered I.V.

Inhalational/GI/oropharyngeal (treatment): I.V.: Refer to dosing for inhalational anthrax (postexposure prophylaxis). Switch to oral therapy when clinically appropriate; refer to "Note" on combined therapy and duration under Adult dosing.

Note: If liquid doxycycline is unavailable for the treatment of anthrax, emergency doses may be prepared for children using the tablets: Crush one 100 mg tablet and grind into a fine powder. Mix with 4 teaspoons of food or drink (lowfat milk, chocolate milk, chocolate pudding, or apple juice). Appropriate dose may be taken from this mixture. Mixture may be stored for up to 24 hours. Dairy mixtures should be refrigerated; apple juice may be stored at room temperature.

U.S. Food and Drug Administration, Center for Drug Evaluation and Research, "How to Prepare Emergency Dosages of Doxycycline at Home for Infants and Children," April 25, 2003, viewable at http://www.fda.gov/cder/drug/infopage/penG_doxy/doxycyclinePeds.htm, last accessed May 8, 2003.

Children ≥8 years (<45 kg): Susceptible infections: Oral, I.V.: 2-5 mg/kg/day in 1-2 divided doses, not to exceed 200 mg/day

Children >8 years (>45 kg) and Adults: Susceptible infections: Oral, I.V.: 100-200 mg/day in 1-2 divided doses

Acute gonococcal infection (PID) in combination with another antibiotic: 100 mg every 12 hours until improved, followed by 100 mg orally twice daily to complete 14 days

Community-acquired pneumonia: 100 mg twice daily

Lyme disease: Oral: 100 mg twice daily for 14-21 days

Early syphilis: 200 mg/day in divided doses for 14 days

Late syphilis: 200 mg/day in divided doses for 28 days

Uncomplicated chlamydial infections: 100 mg twice daily for ≥7 days

Endometritis, salpingitis, parametritis, or peritonitis: 100 mg I.V. twice daily with cefoxitin 2 g every 6 hours for 4 days and for ≥48 hours after patient improves; then continue with oral therapy 100 mg twice daily to complete a 10- to 14-day course of therapy

Sclerosing agent for pleural effusion injection (unlabeled use): 500 mg as a single dose in 30-50 mL of NS or SWI

Adults:

Anthrax:

Inhalational (postexposure prophylaxis): Oral, I.V. (use oral route when possible): 100 mg every 12 hours for 60 days (*MMWR*, 2001, 50:889-93); **Note:** Preliminary recommendation, FDA review and update is anticipated.

Cutaneous (treatment): Oral: 100 mg every 12 hours for 60 days. **Note:** In the presence of systemic involvement, extensive edema, lesions on head/neck, refer to I.V. dosing for treatment of inhalational/GI/oropharyngeal anthrax

Inhalational/GI/oropharyngeal (treatment): I.V.: Initial: 100 mg every 12 hours; switch to oral therapy when clinically appropriate; some recommend initial loading dose of 200 mg, followed by 100 mg every 8-12 hours (*JAMA*, 1997, 278:399-411). **Note:** Initial treatment should include two or more agents predicted to be effective (per CDC recommendations). Agents suggested for use in conjunction with doxycycline or ciprofloxacin include rifampin, vancomycin, imipenem, penicillin, ampicillin, chloramphenicol, clindamycin, and clarithromycin. May switch to oral antimicrobial therapy when clinically appropriate. Continue combined therapy for 60 days

Dialysis: Not dialyzable; 0% to 5% by hemo- and peritoneal methods or by continuous arteriovenous or venovenous hemofiltration. Supplemental dosage unnecessary.

Mechanism of Action Inhibits protein synthesis by binding with the 30S and possibly the 50S ribosomal subunit(s) of susceptible bacteria; may also cause alterations in the cytoplasmic membrane

Doxycycline inhibits collagenase *in vitro* and has been shown to inhibit collagenase in the gingival crevicular fluid in adults with periodontitis

Contraindications Hypersensitivity to doxycycline, tetracycline or any component of the formulation; children <8 years of age, except in treatment of anthrax (including inhalational anthrax postexposure prophylaxis); severe hepatic dysfunction; pregnancy

Warnings/Precautions Do not use during pregnancy; use of tetracyclines during tooth development may cause permanent discoloration of the teeth and enamel hypoplasia. Prolonged use may result in superinfection, including oral or vaginal candidiasis. Photosensitivity reaction may occur with this drug; avoid prolonged exposure to sunlight or tanning equipment. Avoid in children ≤8 years of age.

Drug Interactions Substrate of CYP3A4 (major); **Inhibits** CYP3A4 (strong)

Antacids (containing aluminum, calcium, or magnesium): Decreased absorption of tetracyclines

Anticoagulants: Tetracyclines may decrease plasma thrombin activity; monitor

Barbiturates: Decreased half-life of doxycycline

Carbamazepine: Decreased half-life of doxycycline

(Continued)

Doxycycline *(Continued)*

CYP3A4 inducers: CYP3A4 inducers may decrease the levels/effects of doxycycline. Example inducers include aminoglutethimide, carbamazepine, nafcillin, nevirapine, phenobarbital, phenytoin, and rifamycins.

CYP3A4 substrates: Doxycycline may increase the levels/effects of CYP3A4 substrates. Example substrates include benzodiazepines, calcium channel blockers, mirtazapine, nateglinide, nefazodone, tacrolimus, and venlafaxine. Selected benzodiazepines (midazolam and triazolam), cisapride, ergot alkaloids, selected HMG-CoA reductase inhibitors (lovastatin and simvastatin), and pimozide are generally contraindicated with strong CYP3A4 inhibitors.

Iron-containing products: Decreased absorption of tetracyclines

Methoxyflurane: Concomitant use may cause fatal renal toxicity.

Oral contraceptives: Anecdotal reports suggesting decreased contraceptive efficacy with tetracyclines have been refuted by more rigorous scientific and clinical data.

Phenytoin: Decreased half-life of doxycycline

Ethanol/Nutrition/Herb Interactions

Ethanol: Avoid or limit use (<3 drinks/day); chronic ingestion may decrease serum concentration.

Food: Administer with food or milk due to GI intolerance; may decrease absorption up to 20%. Of currently available tetracyclines, doxycycline has the least affinity for calcium; may decrease absorption of amino acids, calcium, iron, magnesium, and zinc. Administration with calcium or iron may decrease doxycycline absorption. Boiled milk, buttermilk, or yogurt may reduce diarrhea.

Crushed tablets may be mixed with 4 teaspoons of food or drink (lowfat milk, chocolate milk, chocolate pudding, or apple juice) for emergency pediatric dosing if liquid unavailable for treatment of anthrax (see Dosage).

Herb/Nutraceutical: Avoid dong quai; may cause additional photosensitization. Avoid St John's wort; may decrease serum concentration and cause additional photosensitization.

Dietary Considerations Take with food if gastric irritation occurs. While administration with food may decrease GI absorption of doxycycline by up to 20%, administration on an empty stomach is not recommended due to GI intolerance. Of currently available tetracyclines, doxycycline has the least affinity for calcium.

Pharmacodynamics/Kinetics

Absorption: Oral: Almost complete; reduced by food or milk by 20%

Distribution: Widely into body tissues and fluids including synovial, pleural, prostatic, seminal fluids, and bronchial secretions; saliva, aqueous humor, and CSF penetration is poor; readily crosses placenta; enters breast milk

Protein binding: 90%

Metabolism: Not hepatic; partially inactivated in GI tract by chelate formation

Half-life elimination: 12-15 hours (usually increases to 22-24 hours with multiple doses); End-stage renal disease: 18-25 hours

Time to peak, serum: 1.5-4 hours

Excretion: Feces (30%); urine (23%)

Pregnancy Risk Factor D

Lactation Enters breast milk/not recommended

Breast-Feeding Considerations Tetracyclines enter breast milk and breast-feeding is not recommended. Use of tetracyclines during tooth development may cause permanent discoloration of the teeth and enamel hypoplasia. Tetracyclines also form a complex in bone-forming tissue, leading to a decreased fibula growth rate when given to premature infants.

Dosage Forms

Capsule, as hyclate: 50 mg, 100 mg
  Vibramycin®: 100 mg

Capsule, as monohydrate (Monodox®): 50 mg, 100 mg

Capsule, coated pellets, as hyclate (Doryx®): 75 mg, 100 mg

Injection, powder for reconstitution, as hyclate (Doxy-100®): 100 mg

Powder for oral suspension, as monohydrate (Vibramycin®): 25 mg/5 mL (60 mL) [raspberry flavor]

Syrup, as calcium (Vibramycin®): 50 mg/5 mL (480 mL) [contains sodium metabisulfite; raspberry-apple flavor]

Tablet, as hyclate: 100 mg
  Vibra-Tabs®: 100 mg

Tablet, as monohydrate (Adoxa™): 50 mg, 75 mg, 100 mg

Doxycycline Calcium *see* Doxycycline *on page 471*

Doxycycline Hyclate *see* Doxycycline *on page 471*

Doxycycline Hyclate (Periodontal)

(doks i SYE kleen HI klayt pair ee oh DON tol)

Related Information

Doxycycline *on page 471*

U.S. Brand Names Atridox™

Generic Available No

Pharmacologic Category Antibiotic, Tetracycline Derivative

Dental Use Treatment of chronic adult periodontitis for gain in clinical attachment, reduction in probing depth, and reduction in bleeding upon probing

Use Used exclusively in dental applications

Local Anesthetic/Vasoconstrictor Precautions No information available to require special precautions

Effects on Dental Treatment Key adverse event(s) related to dental treatment: Discoloration of teeth (in children), gum discomfort, toothache, periodontal abscess, tooth sensitivity, broken tooth, tooth mobility, endodontic abscess, and jaw pain

Mechanical oral hygiene procedures (ie, tooth brushing, flossing) should be avoided in any treated area for 7 days.

Effects reported in clinical trials were similar in incidence between doxycycline-containing product and vehicle alone; comparable to standard therapies including scaling and root planing or oral hygiene. Although there is no known relationship between doxycycline and hypertension, unspecified essential hypertension was noted in 1.6% of the doxycycline gel group, as compared to 0.2% in the vehicle group (allergic reactions to the vehicle were also reported in two patients).

Significant Adverse Effects Systemic: Gastrointestinal: Diarrhea (3%)

Dosage Oral, subgingival: Dose depends on size, shape and number of pockets treated. Application may be repeated four months after initial treatment. The delivery system consists of 2 separate syringes in a single pouch. Syringe A contains 450 mg of a bioabsorbable polymer gel; syringe B contains doxycycline hyclate 50 mg. To prepare for instillation, couple syringe A to syringe B. Inject contents of syringe A (purple stripe) into syringe B, then push contents back into syringe A. Repeat this mixing cycle at a rate of one cycle per second for 100 cycles. If syringes are stored prior to use (a maximum of 3 days), repeat mixing cycle 10 times before use. After appropriate mixing, contents should be in syringe A. Holding syringes vertically, with syringe A at the bottom, pull back on the syringe A plunger, allowing contents to flow down barrel for several seconds. Uncouple syringes and attach enclosed blunt cannula to syringe A. Local anesthesia is not required for placement. Cannula tip may be bent to resemble periodontal probe and used to explore pocket. Express product from syringe until pocket is filled. To separate tip from formulation, turn tip towards the tooth and press against tooth surface to achieve separation. An appropriate dental instrument may be used to pack gel into the pocket. Pockets may be covered with either Coe-pak™ or Octyldent™ dental adhesive.

Mechanism of Action Inhibits protein synthesis by binding with the 30S and possibly the 50S ribosomal subunit(s) of susceptible bacteria; may also cause alterations in the cytoplasmic membrane

Doxycycline inhibits collagenase *in vitro* and has been shown to inhibit collagenase in the gingival crevicular fluid in adults with periodontitis

Contraindications Hypersensitivity to doxycycline, tetracycline or any component of the formulation; children <8 years of age; severe hepatic dysfunction; pregnancy

Warnings/Precautions Do not use during pregnancy; use of tetracyclines during tooth development may cause permanent discoloration of the teeth and enamel hypoplasia. Prolonged use may result in superinfection, including oral or vaginal candidiasis. Photosensitivity may occur; avoid prolonged exposure to sunlight or tanning equipment. Atridox™ has not been evaluated or tested in immunocompromised patients, those with oral candidiasis, or conditions characterized by severe periodontal defects with little remaining periodontium. May result in overgrowth of nonsusceptible organisms, including fungi. Effects of treatment >6 months have not been evaluated; has not been evaluated for use in regeneration of alveolar bone.

Drug Interactions Iron and bismuth subsalicylate may decrease doxycycline bioavailability; barbiturates, phenytoin, and carbamazepine decrease doxycycline's half-life; increased effect of warfarin. Concurrent use of tetracycline and Penthrane® has been reported to result in fatal renal toxicity.

Dietary Considerations May be taken with food, milk, or water.

(Continued)

Doxycycline Hyclate (Periodontal) *(Continued)*

Pharmacodynamics/Kinetics Systemic absorption from dental subgingival gel may occur, but is limited by the slow rate of dissolution from this formulation over 7 days.

Pregnancy Risk Factor D

Breast-Feeding Considerations Tetracyclines enter breast milk and breast-feeding is not recommended. Use of tetracyclines during tooth development may cause permanent discoloration of the teeth and enamel hypoplasia. Tetracyclines also form a complex in bone-forming tissue, leading to a decreased fibula growth rate when given to premature infants.

Dosage Forms Gel, subgingival (Atridox™): 50 mg in each 500 mg of blended formulation [2-syringe system includes doxycycline syringe (50 mg) and delivery system syringe (450 mg) with a blunt cannula]

Doxycycline Monohydrate *see* Doxycycline *on page 471*

Doxycycline (Subantimicrobial)

(doks i SYE kleen, sub an tee mye KROE bee ul)

Related Information

Doxycycline *on page 471*

U.S. Brand Names Periostat®

Generic Available No

Pharmacologic Category Antibiotic, Tetracycline Derivative

Dental Use Adjunct to scaling and root planing to promote attachment level gain and to reduce pocket depth in adult periodontitis (systemic levels are subinhibitory against bacteria)

Local Anesthetic/Vasoconstrictor Precautions No information available to require special precautions

Effects on Dental Treatment No significant effects or complications reported

Dosage Adults: **Adjunctive treatment for periodontitis:** Oral: 20 mg twice daily at least 1 hour before or 2 hours after morning and evening meals for up to 9 months

Mechanism of Action Has been shown to inhibit collagenase activity *in vitro*; has been noted to reduce elevated collagenase activity in the gingival crevicular fluid of patients with periodontal disease; systemic levels do not reach inhibitory concentrations against bacteria

Contraindications Hypersensitivity to doxycycline, tetracycline or any component of the formulation; children <8 years of age; pregnancy

Warnings/Precautions Do not use during pregnancy; use of tetracyclines during tooth development may cause permanent discoloration of the teeth and enamel hypoplasia. Prolonged use may result in superinfection, including oral or vaginal candidiasis. Photosensitivity may occur; avoid prolonged exposure to sunlight or tanning equipment. Effectiveness has not been established in patients with coexisting oral candidiasis; use with caution in patients with a history or predisposition to oral candidiasis.

Breast-Feeding Considerations Tetracyclines enter breast milk and breast-feeding is not recommended. Use of tetracyclines during tooth development may cause permanent discoloration of the teeth and enamel hypoplasia. Tetracyclines also form a complex in bone-forming tissue, leading to a decreased fibula growth rate when given to premature infants.

Dosage Forms Tablet (Periostat®): 20 mg

Selected Readings

Lee HM, Ciancio SG, Tuter G, et al, "Subantimicrobial Dose Doxycycline Efficacy as a Matrix Metalloproteinase Inhibitor in Chronic Periodontitis Patients is Enhanced When Combined With a Non-Steroidal Anti-inflammatory Drug," *J Periodontol*, 2004, 75(3):453-63.

DPA *see* Valproic Acid and Derivatives *on page 1359*

DPE *see* Dipivefrin *on page 453*

D-Penicillamine *see* Penicillamine *on page 1057*

DPH *see* Phenytoin *on page 1080*

DPM™ [OTC] *see* Urea *on page 1353*

Dramamine® [OTC] *see* DimenhyDRINATE *on page 446*

Dramamine® Less Drowsy Formula [OTC] *see* Meclizine *on page 859*

Drisdol® *see* Ergocalciferol *on page 503*

Dristan® Sinus [OTC] *see* Pseudoephedrine and Ibuprofen *on page 1149*

Drithocreme® *see* Anthralin *on page 133*

Dritho-Scalp® *see* Anthralin *on page 133*

Drixoral® Cold & Allergy [OTC] *see* Dexbrompheniramine and Pseudoephedrine *on page 414*

Drize®-R *see* Chlorpheniramine, Phenylephrine, and Methscopolamine *on page 317*

Dronabinol (droe NAB i nol)

Related Information

Chemical Dependency and Smoking Cessation *on page 1576*

U.S. Brand Names Marinol®

Canadian Brand Names Marinol®

Generic Available No

Synonyms Delta-9-tetrahydro-cannabinol; Delta-9 THC; Tetrahydrocannabinol; THC

Pharmacologic Category Antiemetic; Appetite Stimulant

Use Chemotherapy-associated nausea and vomiting refractory to other antiemetic; AIDS- and cancer-related anorexia

Local Anesthetic/Vasoconstrictor Precautions No information available to require special precautions

Effects on Dental Treatment Key adverse event(s) related to dental treatment: Xerostomia (normal salivary flow resumes upon discontinuation) and orthostatic hypotension.

Common Adverse Effects

>10%:

Central nervous system: Drowsiness (48%), sedation (53%), confusion (30%), dizziness (21%), detachment, anxiety, difficulty concentrating, mood change

Gastrointestinal: Appetite increased (when used as an antiemetic), xerostomia (38% to 50%)

1% to 10%:

Cardiovascular: Orthostatic hypotension, tachycardia

Central nervous system: Ataxia (4%), depression (7%), headache, vertigo, hallucinations (5%), memory lapse (4%)

Neuromuscular & skeletal: Paresthesia, weakness

Restrictions C-III

Mechanism of Action Unknown, may inhibit endorphins in the emetic center, suppress prostaglandin synthesis, and/or inhibit medullary activity through an unspecified cortical action

Drug Interactions

Increased Effect/Toxicity: Increased toxicity (drowsiness) with alcohol, barbiturates, and benzodiazepines.

Pharmacodynamics/Kinetics

Onset of action: Within 1 hour

Absorption: Oral: 90% to 95%; ~5% to 10% of dose gets into systemic circulation

Distribution: V_d: 2.5-6.4 L; tetrahydrocannabinol is highly lipophilic and distributes to adipose tissue

Protein binding: 97% to 99%

Metabolism: Hepatic to at least 50 metabolites, some of which are active; 11-hydroxytetrahydrocannabinol (11-OH-THC) is the major metabolite; extensive first-pass effect

Half-life elimination: THC: 19-24 hours; THC metabolites: 49-53 hours

Time to peak, serum: 2-3 hours

Excretion: Feces (35% as unconjugated metabolites); urine (10% to 15% as acid metabolites and conjugates)

Pregnancy Risk Factor C

Droperidol (droe PER i dole)

U.S. Brand Names Inapsine®

Mexican Brand Names Dehydrobenzperidol®

Generic Available Yes

Synonyms Dehydrobenzperidol

Pharmacologic Category Antiemetic; Antipsychotic Agent, Butyrophenone

Use Antiemetic in surgical and diagnostic procedures; preoperative medication in patients when other treatments are ineffective or inappropriate

Local Anesthetic/Vasoconstrictor Precautions Manufacturer's information states that droperidol may block vasopressor activity of epinephrine. This has not been observed during use of epinephrine as a vasoconstrictor in local anesthesia.

Effects on Dental Treatment Key adverse event(s) related to dental treatment: Orthostatic hypotension.

Common Adverse Effects

>10%:

Cardiovascular: QT_c prolongation (dose dependent)

Central nervous system: Restlessness, anxiety, extrapyramidal symptoms, dystonic reactions, pseudoparkinsonian signs and symptoms, tardive

(Continued)

Droperidol *(Continued)*

dyskinesia, seizures, altered central temperature regulation, sedation, drowsiness

Endocrine & metabolic: Swelling of breasts

Gastrointestinal: Weight gain, constipation

1% to 10%:

Cardiovascular: Hypotension (especially orthostatic), tachycardia, abnormal T waves with prolonged ventricular repolarization, hypertension

Central nervous system: Hallucinations, persistent tardive dyskinesia, akathisia

Gastrointestinal: Nausea, vomiting

Genitourinary: Dysuria

Mechanism of Action Antiemetic effect is a result of blockade of dopamine stimulation of the chemoreceptor trigger zone. Other effects include alpha-adrenergic blockade, peripheral vascular dilation, and reduction of the pressor effect of epinephrine resulting in hypotension and decreased peripheral vascular resistance; may also reduce pulmonary artery pressure

Drug Interactions

Increased Effect/Toxicity: Droperidol in combination with certain forms of conduction anesthesia may produce peripheral vasodilitation and hypotension. Droperidol and CNS depressants will likely have additive CNS effects. Droperidol and cyclobenzaprine may have an additive effect on prolonging the QT interval. Use caution with other agents known to prolong QT interval (Class I or Class III antiarrhythmics, some quinolone antibiotics, cisapride, some phenothiazines, pimozide, tricyclic antidepressants). Potassium- or magnesium-depleting agents (diuretics, aminoglycosides, amphotericin B, cyclosporine) may increase risk of arrhythmias. Metoclopramide may increase risk of extrapyramidal symptoms (EPS).

Pharmacodynamics/Kinetics

Onset of action: Peak effect: Parenteral: ~30 minutes

Duration: Parenteral: 2-4 hours, may extend to 12 hours

Absorption: I.M.: Rapid

Distribution: Crosses blood-brain barrier and placenta

V_d: Children: ~0.25-0.9 L/kg; Adults: ~2 L/kg

Protein binding: Extensive

Metabolism: Hepatic, to *p*-fluorophenylacetic acid, benzimidazolone, *p*-hydroxypiperidine

Half-life elimination: Adults: 2.3 hours

Excretion: Urine (75%, <1% as unchanged drug); feces (22%, 11% to 50% as unchanged drug)

Pregnancy Risk Factor C

Drospirenone and Ethinyl Estradiol *see* Ethinyl Estradiol and Drospirenone *on page 538*

Drotrecogin Alfa (dro TRE coe jin AL fa)

U.S. Brand Names Xigris®

Canadian Brand Names Xigris®

Generic Available No

Synonyms Activated Protein C, Human, Recombinant; Drotrecogin Alfa, Activated; Protein C (Activated), Human, Recombinant

Pharmacologic Category Protein C (Activated)

Use Reduction of mortality from severe sepsis (associated with organ dysfunction) in adults at high risk of death (eg, APACHE II score ≥25)

Local Anesthetic/Vasoconstrictor Precautions No information available to require special precautions

Effects on Dental Treatment Key adverse event(s) related to dental treatment: As with all drugs which may affect hemostasis, bleeding is the major adverse effect associated with drotrecogin alfa. Hemorrhage may occur at virtually any site; risk is dependent on multiple variables, including the dosage administered, concurrent use of multiple agents which alter hemostasis, and patient predisposition.

Common Adverse Effects As with all drugs which may affect hemostasis, bleeding is the major adverse effect associated with drotrecogin alfa. Hemorrhage may occur at virtually any site. Risk is dependent on multiple variables, including the dosage administered, concurrent use of multiple agents which alter hemostasis, and patient predisposition.

>10%

Dermatologic: Bruising

Gastrointestinal: Gastrointestinal bleeding

1% to 10%: Hematologic: Bleeding (serious 2.4% during infusion vs 3.5% during 28-day study period; individual events listed as <1%)

Mechanism of Action Inhibits factors Va and VIIIa, limiting thrombotic effects. Additional *in vitro* data suggest inhibition of plasminogen activator inhibitor-1 (PAF-1) resulting in profibrinolytic activity, inhibition of macrophage production of tumor necrosis factor, blocking of leukocyte adhesion, and limitation of thrombin-induced inflammatory responses. Relative contribution of effects on the reduction of mortality from sepsis is not completely understood.

Drug Interactions

Increased Effect/Toxicity: Concurrent use of antiplatelet agents, including aspirin (>650 mg/day, recent use within 7 days), cilostazol, clopidogrel, dipyridamole, ticlopidine, NSAIDs, or glycoprotein IIb/IIIa antagonists (recent use within 7 days) may increase risk of bleeding. Concurrent use of low molecular weight heparins or heparin at therapeutic rates of infusion may increase the risk of bleeding. However, the use of low-dose prophylactic heparin does not appear to affect safety. Recent use of thrombolytic agents (within 3 days) may increase the risk of bleeding. Recent use of warfarin (within 7 days or elevation of INR ≥3) may increase the risk of bleeding. Other drugs which interfere with coagulation may increase risk of bleeding (including antithrombin III, danaparoid, direct thrombin inhibitors)

Pharmacodynamics/Kinetics

Duration: Plasma nondetectable within 2 hours of discontinuation

Metabolism: Inactivated by endogenous plasma protease inhibitors; mean clearance: 40 L/hour; increased with severe sepsis (~50%)

Half-life elimination: 1.6 hours

Pregnancy Risk Factor C

Drotrecogin Alfa, Activated *see* Drotrecogin Alfa *on page 478*

Droxia™ *see* Hydroxyurea *on page 722*

Dr. Scholl's® Callus Remover [OTC] *see* Salicylic Acid *on page 1205*

Dr. Scholl's® Clear Away [OTC] *see* Salicylic Acid *on page 1205*

DSCG *see* Cromolyn *on page 378*

D-Ser(Bu^t)^6,Azgly^{10}-LHRH *see* Goserelin *on page 670*

D-S-S® [OTC] *see* Docusate *on page 459*

DSS With Casanthranol *see* Docusate and Casanthranol *on page 460*

DTIC *see* Dacarbazine *on page 392*

DTIC-Dome® *see* Dacarbazine *on page 392*

DTO *see* Opium Tincture *on page 1015*

D-Trp(6)-LHRH *see* Triptorelin *on page 1346*

Duac™ *see* Clindamycin and Benzoyl Peroxide *on page 350*

Dulcolax® [OTC] *see* Bisacodyl *on page 208*

Dulcolax® Milk of Magnesia [OTC] *see* Magnesium Hydroxide *on page 853*

Dull-C® [OTC] *see* Ascorbic Acid *on page 148*

Duocaine™ *see* Lidocaine and Bupivacaine *on page 822*

DuoFilm® [OTC] *see* Salicylic Acid *on page 1205*

DuoNeb™ *see* Ipratropium and Albuterol *on page 761*

DuoPlant® [DSC] [OTC] *see* Salicylic Acid *on page 1205*

DuP 753 *see* Losartan *on page 845*

Duraclon™ *see* Clonidine *on page 358*

Duragesic® *see* Fentanyl *on page 581*

Duramist® Plus [OTC] *see* Oxymetazoline *on page 1034*

Duramorph® *see* Morphine Sulfate *on page 947*

Duranest® [DSC] *see* Etidocaine and Epinephrine *on page 562*

Duration® [OTC] *see* Oxymetazoline *on page 1034*

Duratuss™ *see* Guaifenesin and Pseudoephedrine *on page 675*

Duratuss® DM *see* Guaifenesin and Dextromethorphan *on page 673*

Duratuss™ GP *see* Guaifenesin and Pseudoephedrine *on page 675*

Duratuss® HD *see* Hydrocodone, Pseudoephedrine, and Guaifenesin *on page 713*

Dura-Vent®/DA [DSC] *see* Chlorpheniramine, Phenylephrine, and Methscopolamine *on page 317*

Duricef® *see* Cefadroxil *on page 275*

Dutasteride (doo TAS teer ide)

U.S. Brand Names Avodart™

Generic Available No

Pharmacologic Category 5 Alpha-Reductase Inhibitor

Use Treatment of symptomatic benign prostatic hyperplasia (BPH)

(Continued)

Dutasteride *(Continued)*

Unlabeled/Investigational Use Treatment of male patterned baldness

Local Anesthetic/Vasoconstrictor Precautions No information available to require special precautions

Effects on Dental Treatment No significant effects or complications reported

Common Adverse Effects

>10%: Endocrine & metabolic: Serum testosterone increased, thyroid-stimulating hormone increased

1% to 10%: Endocrine & metabolic: Impotence (1% to 5%), libido decreased (1% to 3%), ejaculation disorders (1%), gynecomastia (including breast tenderness, breast enlargement) (1%)

Note: Frequency of adverse events (except gynecomastia) tends to decrease with continued use (>6 months).

Mechanism of Action Dutasteride is a 4-azo analog of testosterone and is a competitive, selective inhibitor of both reproductive tissues (type 2) and skin and hepatic (type 1) 5α-reductase. This results in inhibition of the conversion of testosterone to dihydrotestosterone and markedly suppresses serum dihydrotestosterone levels.

Drug Interactions

Cytochrome P450 Effect: Substrate of CYP3A4 (minor)

Increased Effect/Toxicity: Calcium channel blockers, nondihydropyridine (diltiazem, verapamil) increase dutasteride levels with concurrent use.

Pharmacodynamics/Kinetics

Absorption: Via skin when handling capsules

Distribution: ~12% of serum concentrations partitioned into semen

Protein binding: 99% to albumin; ~97% to α_1-acid glycoprotein; >96% to semen protein

Metabolism: Hepatic via CYP3A4 isoenzyme; forms metabolites: 6-hydroxydutasteride has activity similar to parent compound, 4′-hydroxydutasteride and 1,2-dihydrodutasteride are much less potent than parent *in vitro*

Bioavailability: 60% (range: 40% to 94%)

Half-life elimination: Terminal: ~5 weeks

Time to peak: 2-3 hours

Excretion: Feces (40% as metabolites, 5% as unchanged drug); urine (<1% as unchanged drug); 55% of dose unaccounted for

Pregnancy Risk Factor X

DVA *see* Vindesine *on page 1379*

DW286 *see* Gemifloxacin *on page 653*

Dyazide® *see* Hydrochlorothiazide and Triamterene *on page 701*

Dyclonine (DYE kloe neen)

U.S. Brand Names Cēpacol® Maximum Strength [OTC]; Sucrets® [OTC]

Generic Available No

Synonyms Dyclonine Hydrochloride

Pharmacologic Category Local Anesthetic; Local Anesthetic, Oral

Use Local anesthetic prior to laryngoscopy, bronchoscopy, or endotracheal intubation; use topically for temporary relief of pain associated with oral mucosa or anogenital lesions

Local Anesthetic/Vasoconstrictor Precautions No information available to require special precautions

Effects on Dental Treatment No significant effects or complications reported

Mechanism of Action Blocks impulses at peripheral nerve endings in skin and mucous membranes by altering cell membrane permeability to ionic transfer

Pharmacodynamics/Kinetics

Onset of action: Local anesthetic: 2-10 minutes

Duration: 30-60 minutes

Pregnancy Risk Factor C

Dyclonine Hydrochloride *see* Dyclonine *on page 480*

Dymelor [DSC] *see* AcetoHEXAMIDE *on page 60*

Dynabac® *see* Dirithromycin *on page 454*

Dynacin® *see* Minocycline *on page 931*

DynaCirc® *see* Isradipine *on page 774*

DynaCirc® CR *see* Isradipine *on page 774*

Dyna-Hex® [OTC] *see* Chlorhexidine Gluconate *on page 308*

Dyphylline (DYE fi lin)

U.S. Brand Names Dilor®; Lufyllin®

Canadian Brand Names Dilor®; Lufyllin®

Generic Available No
Synonyms Dihydroxypropyl Theophylline
Pharmacologic Category Theophylline Derivative
Use Bronchodilator in reversible airway obstruction due to asthma or COPD
Local Anesthetic/Vasoconstrictor Precautions No information available to require special precautions
Effects on Dental Treatment Do not prescribe any erythromycin product to patients taking theophylline products. Erythromycin will delay the normal metabolic inactivation of theophyllines leading to increased blood levels; this has resulted in nausea, vomiting and CNS restlessness.
Pregnancy Risk Factor C

Dyrenium® *see* Triamterene *on page 1334*
E_2C and MPA *see* Estradiol and Medroxyprogesterone *on page 520*
7E3 *see* Abciximab *on page 44*
E2020 *see* Donepezil *on page 462*
EarSol® HC *see* Hydrocortisone *on page 714*
Easprin® *see* Aspirin *on page 151*

Echothiophate Iodide (ek oh THYE oh fate EYE oh dide)

U.S. Brand Names Phospholine Iodide®
Generic Available No
Synonyms Ecostigmine Iodide
Pharmacologic Category Ophthalmic Agent, Antiglaucoma; Ophthalmic Agent, Miotic
Use Used as miotic in treatment of open-angle glaucoma; may be useful in specific case of narrow-angle glaucoma; accommodative esotropia
Local Anesthetic/Vasoconstrictor Precautions No information available to require special precautions
Effects on Dental Treatment No significant effects or complications reported
Mechanism of Action Produces miosis and changes in accommodation by inhibiting cholinesterase, thereby preventing the breakdown of acetylcholine; acetylcholine is, therefore, allowed to continuously stimulate the iris and ciliary muscles of the eye
Pregnancy Risk Factor C

EC-Naprosyn® *see* Naproxen *on page 965*
***E. coli* Asparaginase** *see* Asparaginase *on page 150*

Econazole (e KONE a zole)

U.S. Brand Names Spectazole®
Canadian Brand Names Ecostatin®; Spectazole™
Mexican Brand Names Micostyl®; Pevaryl Lipogel®
Generic Available Yes
Synonyms Econazole Nitrate
Pharmacologic Category Antifungal Agent, Topical
Use Topical treatment of tinea pedis (athlete's foot), tinea cruris (jock itch), tinea corporis (ringworm), tinea versicolor, and cutaneous candidiasis
Local Anesthetic/Vasoconstrictor Precautions No information available to require special precautions
Effects on Dental Treatment No significant effects or complications reported
Common Adverse Effects 1% to 10%: Genitourinary: Vulvar/vaginal burning
Mechanism of Action Alters fungal cell wall membrane permeability; may interfere with RNA and protein synthesis, and lipid metabolism
Drug Interactions
Cytochrome P450 Effect: Inhibits CYP2E1 (weak)
Pharmacodynamics/Kinetics
Absorption: <10%
Metabolism: Hepatic to more than 20 metabolites
Excretion: Urine; feces (<1%)
Pregnancy Risk Factor C

Econazole Nitrate *see* Econazole *on page 481*
Econopred® *see* PrednisoLONE *on page 1113*
Econopred® Plus *see* PrednisoLONE *on page 1113*
Ecostigmine Iodide *see* Echothiophate Iodide *on page 481*
Ecotrin® [OTC] *see* Aspirin *on page 151*
Ecotrin® Low Strength [OTC] *see* Aspirin *on page 151*
Ecotrin® Maximum Strength [OTC] *see* Aspirin *on page 151*
Ed A-Hist® *see* Chlorpheniramine and Phenylephrine *on page 314*

Edathamil Disodium *see* Edetate Disodium *on page 482*
Edecrin® *see* Ethacrynic Acid *on page 533*

Edetate Calcium Disodium

(ED e tate KAL see um dye SOW dee um)

U.S. Brand Names Calcium Disodium Versenate®

Generic Available No

Synonyms Calcium Disodium Edetate; Calcium EDTA

Pharmacologic Category Chelating Agent

Use Treatment of symptomatic acute and chronic lead poisoning or for symptomatic patients with high blood lead levels; used as an aid in the diagnosis of lead poisoning; possibly useful in poisoning by zinc, manganese, and certain heavy radioisotopes

Local Anesthetic/Vasoconstrictor Precautions No information available to require special precautions

Effects on Dental Treatment No significant effects or complications reported

Common Adverse Effects Frequency not defined.

Cardiovascular: Arrhythmias, ECG changes, hypotension
Central nervous system: Chills, fever, headache
Dermatologic: Cheilosis, skin lesions
Endocrine & metabolic: Hypercalcemia
Gastrointestinal: Anorexia, GI upset, nausea, vomiting
Hematologic: Anemia, bone marrow suppression (transient)
Hepatic: Liver function test increased (mild)
Local: Thrombophlebitis following I.V. infusion (when concentration >5 mg/mL), pain at injection site following I.M. injection
Neuromuscular & skeletal: Arthralgia, numbness, tremor, paresthesia
Ocular: Lacrimation
Renal: Renal tubular necrosis, microscopic hematuria, proteinuria
Respiratory: Nasal congestion, sneezing
Miscellaneous: Zinc deficiency

Mechanism of Action Calcium is displaced by divalent and trivalent heavy metals, forming a nonionizing soluble complex that is excreted in urine

Drug Interactions

Decreased Effect: Do not use simultaneously with zinc insulin preparations; do not mix in the same syringe with dimercaprol.

Pharmacodynamics/Kinetics

Onset of action: Chelation of lead: I.V.: 1 hour
Absorption: I.M., SubQ: Well absorbed
Distribution: Into extracellular fluid; minimal CSF penetration
Half-life elimination, plasma: I.M.: 1.5 hours; I.V.: 20 minutes
Excretion: Urine (as metal chelates or unchanged drug); decreased GFR decreases elimination

Pregnancy Risk Factor B

Edetate Disodium

(ED e tate dye SOW dee um)

U.S. Brand Names Endrate®

Generic Available Yes

Synonyms Edathamil Disodium; EDTA; Sodium Edetate

Pharmacologic Category Chelating Agent

Use Emergency treatment of hypercalcemia; control digitalis-induced cardiac dysrhythmias (ventricular arrhythmias)

Local Anesthetic/Vasoconstrictor Precautions No information available to require special precautions

Effects on Dental Treatment No significant effects or complications reported

Common Adverse Effects Rapid I.V. administration or excessive doses may cause a sudden drop in serum calcium concentration which may lead to hypocalcemic tetany, seizures, arrhythmias, and death from respiratory arrest. Do **not** exceed recommended dosage and rate of administration.

1% to 10%: Gastrointestinal: Nausea, vomiting, abdominal cramps, diarrhea

Mechanism of Action Chelates with divalent or trivalent metals to form a soluble complex that is then eliminated in urine

Drug Interactions

Increased Effect/Toxicity: Increased effect of insulin (edetate disodium may decrease blood glucose concentrations and reduce insulin requirements in diabetic patients treated with insulin).

Pharmacodynamics/Kinetics

Metabolism: None
Half-life elimination: 20-60 minutes
Time to peak: I.V.: 24-48 hours

Excretion: Following chelation: Urine (95%); chelates within 24-48 hours

Pregnancy Risk Factor C

Edex® *see* Alprostadil *on page 87*

Edrophonium (ed roe FOE nee um)

U.S. Brand Names Enlon®; Reversol®

Canadian Brand Names Enlon®

Generic Available Yes

Synonyms Edrophonium Chloride

Pharmacologic Category Antidote; Cholinergic Agonist; Diagnostic Agent

Use Diagnosis of myasthenia gravis; differentiation of cholinergic crises from myasthenia crises; reversal of nondepolarizing neuromuscular blockers; adjunct treatment of respiratory depression caused by curare overdose

Local Anesthetic/Vasoconstrictor Precautions No information available to require special precautions

Effects on Dental Treatment No significant effects or complications reported

Common Adverse Effects Frequency not defined.

Cardiovascular: Arrhythmias (especially bradycardia), hypotension, decreased carbon monoxide, tachycardia, AV block, nodal rhythm, nonspecific ECG changes, cardiac arrest, syncope, flushing

Central nervous system: Convulsions, dysarthria, dysphonia, dizziness, loss of consciousness, drowsiness, headache

Dermatologic: Skin rash, thrombophlebitis (I.V.), urticaria

Gastrointestinal: Hyperperistalsis, nausea, vomiting, salivation, diarrhea, stomach cramps, dysphagia, flatulence

Genitourinary: Urinary urgency

Neuromuscular & skeletal: Weakness, fasciculations, muscle cramps, spasms, arthralgias

Ocular: Small pupils, lacrimation

Respiratory: Increased bronchial secretions, laryngospasm, bronchiolar constriction, respiratory muscle paralysis, dyspnea, respiratory depression, respiratory arrest, bronchospasm

Miscellaneous: Diaphoresis (increased), anaphylaxis, allergic reactions

Mechanism of Action Inhibits destruction of acetylcholine by acetylcholinesterase. This facilitates transmission of impulses across myoneural junction and results in increased cholinergic responses such as miosis, increased tonus of intestinal and skeletal muscles, bronchial and ureteral constriction, bradycardia, and increased salivary and sweat gland secretions.

Drug Interactions

Increased Effect/Toxicity: Digoxin may enhance bradycardia potential of edrophonium. Effects of succinylcholine, decamethonium, nondepolarizing muscle relaxants (eg, pancuronium, vecuronium) are prolonged by edrophonium. I.V. acetazolamide, neostigmine, physostigmine, and acute muscle weakness may increase the effects of edrophonium.

Decreased Effect: Atropine, nondepolarizing muscle relaxants, procainamide, and quinidine may antagonize the effects of edrophonium.

Pharmacodynamics/Kinetics

Onset of action: I.M.: 2-10 minutes; I.V.: 30-60 seconds

Duration: I.M.: 5-30 minutes: I.V.: 10 minutes

Distribution: V_d: 1.1 L/kg

Half-life elimination: 1.8 hours

Pregnancy Risk Factor C

Edrophonium Chloride *see* Edrophonium *on page 483*

EDTA *see* Edetate Disodium *on page 482*

E.E.S.® *see* Erythromycin *on page 508*

Efalizumab (e fa li ZOO mab)

U.S. Brand Names Raptiva™

Generic Available No

Synonyms Anti-CD11a; hu1124

Pharmacologic Category Immunosuppressant Agent; Monoclonal Antibody

Use Treatment of chronic moderate-to-severe plaque psoriasis in patients who are candidates for systemic therapy or phototherapy

Local Anesthetic/Vasoconstrictor Precautions No information available to require special precautions

Effects on Dental Treatment No significant effects or complications reported

Common Adverse Effects

>10%:

Central nervous system: Headache (32%), chills (13%)

(Continued)

Efalizumab *(Continued)*

Gastrointestinal: Nausea (11%)
Hematologic: Lymphocytosis (40%), leukocytosis (26%)
Miscellaneous: First-dose reaction (29%, described as chills, fever, headache, myalgia, and nausea occurring within 2 days of the first injection; percent reported in patients receiving a 1 mg/kg dose; severity decreased with 0.7 mg/kg dose); infection (29%, serious infection <1%)

1% to 10%:
Cardiovascular: Peripheral edema (1% to 2%)
Central nervous system: Pain (10%), fever (7%)
Dermatologic: Acne (4%), psoriasis (1% to 2%), urticaria (1%)
Hepatic: Alkaline phosphatase elevated (4%)
Neuromuscular & skeletal: Myalgia (8%), back pain (4%), arthralgia (1% to 2%), weakness (1% to 2%)
Miscellaneous: Antibodies to efalizumab (6%), hypersensitivity reaction (8%), flu-like syndrome (7%)

Mechanism of Action Efalizumab is a recombinant monoclonal antibody which binds to CD11a, a subunit of leukocyte function antigen-1 (LFA-1) found on leukocytes. By binding to CD11a, efalizumab blocks multiple T-cell mediated responses involved in the pathogenesis of psoriatic plaques.

Drug Interactions

Decreased Effect: Note: Formal drug interaction studies have not been conducted. Acellular, live, and live-attenuated vaccines should not be administered during therapy.

Pharmacodynamics/Kinetics

Onset: Reduction of CD11a expression and free CD11a-binding sites seen 1-2 days after the first dose; time to steady state serum concentration: 4 weeks
Response to therapy (75% reduction from baseline of PASI score): Observed after 12 weeks

Duration: CD11a expression was ~74% of baseline at 5-13 weeks after discontinuing dose; free CD11a binding sites were at ~85% of baseline at 8-13 weeks following discontinuation; response to therapy (75% reduction from baseline PASI score) continued 1-2 months after discontinuation

Bioavailability: SubQ: 50%

Excretion: Time to eliminate (at steady state): 25 days

Pregnancy Risk Factor C

Efavirenz (e FAV e renz)

Related Information

HIV Infection and AIDS *on page 1484*
Tuberculosis *on page 1495*

U.S. Brand Names Sustiva®

Canadian Brand Names Sustiva®

Generic Available No

Pharmacologic Category Antiretroviral Agent, Reverse Transcriptase Inhibitor (Non-nucleoside)

Use Treatment of HIV-1 infections in combination with at least two other antiretroviral agents

Local Anesthetic/Vasoconstrictor Precautions No information available to require special precautions

Effects on Dental Treatment Key adverse event(s) related to dental treatment: Xerostomia (normal salivary flow resumes upon discontinuation) and abnormal taste.

Common Adverse Effects

>10%:
Central nervous system: Dizziness* (2% to 28%), depression (1% to 16%), insomnia (6% to 16%), anxiety (1% to 11%), pain* (1% to 13%)
Dermatologic: Rash* (NCI grade 1: 9% to 11%, NCI grade 2: 15% to 32%, NCI grade 3 or 4: <1%); 26% experienced new rash vs 17% in control groups; up to 46% of pediatric patients experience rash (median onset: 8 days)
Endocrine & metabolic: HDL increased (25% to 35%), total cholesterol increased (20% to 40%)
Gastrointestinal: Diarrhea* (3% to 14%), nausea* (2% to 12%)

1% to 10%:
Central nervous system: Impaired concentration (2% to 8%), headache* (2% to 7%), somnolence (2% to 7%), fatigue (2% to 7%), abnormal dreams (1% to 6%), nervousness (2% to 6%), severe depression (2%), hallucinations (1%)
Dermatologic: Pruritus (1% to 9%), diaphoresis increased (1% to 2%)

Gastrointestinal: Vomiting* (6% to 7%), dyspepsia (3%), abdominal pain (1% to 3%), anorexia (1% to 2%)

*Adverse effect reported in ≥10% of patients 3-16 years of age

Mechanism of Action As a non-nucleoside reverse transcriptase inhibitor, efavirenz has activity against HIV-1 by binding to reverse transcriptase. It consequently blocks the RNA-dependent and DNA-dependent DNA polymerase activities including HIV-1 replication. It does not require intracellular phosphorylation for antiviral activity.

Drug Interactions

Cytochrome P450 Effect: Substrate (major) of CYP2B6, 3A4; **Inhibits** CYP2C8/9 (weak), 2C19 (weak), 3A4 (weak); **Induces** CYP2B6 (weak), 3A4 (weak)

Increased Effect/Toxicity: Coadministration with medications metabolized by these enzymes may lead to increased concentration-related effects. Cisapride, midazolam, triazolam, and ergot alkaloids may result in life-threatening toxicities; concurrent use is contraindicated. May increase (or decrease) effect of warfarin.

Decreased Effect: CYP2B6 inducers may decrease the levels/effects of efavirenz; example inducers include carbamazepine, nevirapine, phenobarbital, phenytoin, and rifampin. St John's wort may decrease serum concentrations of efavirenz. Concentrations of indinavir and/or lopinavir may be reduced; dosage adjustments required. Concentrations of saquinavir may be decreased (use as sole protease inhibitor is not recommended). Serum concentrations of methadone may be decreased; monitor for withdrawal. May decrease (or increase) effect of warfarin. Serum concentrations of sertraline may be decreased by efavirenz. CYP3A4 inducers may decrease the levels/effects of efavirenz; example inducers include aminoglutethimide, carbamazepine, nafcillin, nevirapine, phenobarbital, phenytoin, and rifamycins. Voriconazole serum levels may be reduced by efavirenz (concurrent use is contraindicated).

Pharmacodynamics/Kinetics

Absorption: Increased by fatty meals

Distribution: CSF concentrations exceed free fraction in serum

Protein binding: >99%, primarily to albumin

Metabolism: Hepatic via CYP3A4 and 2B6; may induce its own metabolism

Half-life elimination: Single dose: 52-76 hours; Multiple doses: 40-55 hours

Time to peak: 3-8 hours

Excretion: Feces (16% to 41% primarily as unchanged drug); urine (14% to 34% as metabolites)

Pregnancy Risk Factor C

Effer-K™ *see* Potassium Bicarbonate and Potassium Citrate *on page 1105*

Effexor® *see* Venlafaxine *on page 1370*

Effexor® XR *see* Venlafaxine *on page 1370*

Eflone® *see* Fluorometholone *on page 605*

Eflornithine (ee FLOR ni theen)

U.S. Brand Names Vaniqa™

Generic Available No

Synonyms DFMO; Eflornithine Hydrochloride

Pharmacologic Category Antiprotozoal; Topical Skin Product

Use Cream: Females ≥12 years: Reduce unwanted hair from face and adjacent areas under the chin

Orphan status: Injection: Treatment of meningoencephalitic stage of *Trypanosoma brucei gambiense* infection (sleeping sickness)

Local Anesthetic/Vasoconstrictor Precautions No information available to require special precautions

Effects on Dental Treatment No significant effects or complications reported

Common Adverse Effects

Injection:

>10%: Hematologic (reversible): Anemia (55%), leukopenia (37%), thrombocytopenia (14%)

1% to 10%:

Central nervous system: Seizures (may be due to the disease) (8%), dizziness

Dermatologic: Alopecia

Gastrointestinal: Vomiting, diarrhea

Hematologic: Eosinophilia

Otic: Hearing impairment

(Continued)

Eflornithine *(Continued)*

Topical:

>10%: Dermatologic: Acne (11% to 21%), pseudofolliculitis barbae (5% to 15%)

1% to 10%:

Central nervous system: Headache (4% to 5%), dizziness (1%), vertigo (0.3% to 1%)

Dermatologic: Pruritus (3% to 4%), burning skin (2% to 4%), tingling skin (1% to 4%), dry skin (2% to 3%), rash (1% to 3%), facial edema (0.3% to 3%), alopecia (1% to 2%), skin irritation (1% to 2%), erythema (0% to 2%), ingrown hair (0.3% to 2%), folliculitis (0% to 1%)

Gastrointestinal: Dyspepsia (2%), anorexia (0.7% to 2%)

Mechanism of Action Eflornithine exerts antitumor and antiprotozoal effects through specific, irreversible ("suicide") inhibition of the enzyme ornithine decarboxylase (ODC). ODC is the rate-limiting enzyme in the biosynthesis of putrescine, spermine, and spermidine, the major polyamines in nucleated cells. Polyamines are necessary for the synthesis of DNA, RNA, and proteins and are, therefore, necessary for cell growth and differentiation. Although many microorganisms and higher plants are able to produce polyamines from alternate biochemical pathways, all mammalian cells depend on ornithine decarboxylase to produce polyamines. Eflornithine inhibits ODC and rapidly depletes animal cells of putrescine and spermidine; the concentration of spermine remains the same or may even increase. Rapidly dividing cells appear to be most susceptible to the effects of eflornithine. Topically, the inhibition of ODC in the skin leads to a decreased rate of hair growth.

Drug Interactions

Increased Effect/Toxicity: Cream: Possible interactions with other topical products have not been studied.

Decreased Effect: Cream: Possible interactions with other topical products have not been studied.

Pharmacodynamics/Kinetics

Absorption: Topical: <1%

Half-life elimination: I.V.: 3-3.5 hours; Topical: 8 hours

Excretion: Primarily urine (as unchanged drug)

Pregnancy Risk Factor C

Eflornithine Hydrochloride *see* Eflornithine *on page 485*

Efudex® *see* Fluorouracil *on page 605*

E-Gems® [OTC] *see* Vitamin E *on page 1383*

EHDP *see* Etidronate Disodium *on page 563*

Elavil® [DSC] *see* Amitriptyline *on page 103*

Eldepryl® *see* Selegiline *on page 1212*

Eldisine Lilly 99094 *see* Vindesine *on page 1379*

Eldopaque® [OTC] *see* Hydroquinone *on page 719*

Eldopaque Forte® *see* Hydroquinone *on page 719*

Eldoquin® [OTC] *see* Hydroquinone *on page 719*

Eldoquin Forte® *see* Hydroquinone *on page 719*

Electrolyte Lavage Solution *see* Polyethylene Glycol-Electrolyte Solution *on page 1100*

Elestat™ *see* Epinastine *on page 496*

Eletriptan (el e TRIP tan)

U.S. Brand Names Relpax®

Mexican Brand Names Relpax®

Generic Available No

Synonyms Eletriptan Hydrobromide

Pharmacologic Category Serotonin 5-$HT_{1B, 1D}$ Receptor Agonist

Use Acute treatment of migraine, with or without aura

Local Anesthetic/Vasoconstrictor Precautions No information available to require special precautions

Effects on Dental Treatment Key adverse event(s) related to dental treatment: Xerostomia (normal salivary flow resumes upon discontinuation).

Common Adverse Effects 1% to 10%:

Cardiovascular: Chest pain/tightness (1% to 4%; placebo 1%), palpitation

Central nervous system: Dizziness (3% to 7%; placebo 3%), somnolence (3% to 7%; placebo 4%), headache (3% to 4%; placebo 3%), chills, pain, vertigo

Gastrointestinal: Nausea (4% to 8%; placebo 5%), xerostomia (2% to 4%, placebo 2%), dysphagia (1% to 2%), abdominal pain/discomfort (1% to 2%; placebo 1%), dyspepsia (1% to 2%; placebo 1%)

Neuromuscular & skeletal: Weakness (4% to 10%), paresthesia (3% to 4%), back pain, hypertonia, hypesthesia
Respiratory: Pharyngitis
Miscellaneous: Diaphoresis

Mechanism of Action Selective agonist for serotonin ($5\text{-}HT_{1B}$, $5\text{-}HT_{1D}$, $5\text{-}HT_{1F}$ receptors) in cranial arteries; causes vasoconstriction and reduce sterile inflammation associated with antidromic neuronal transmission correlating with relief of migraine

Drug Interactions

Cytochrome P450 Effect: Substrate of CYP3A4 (major)

Increased Effect/Toxicity: CYP3A4 inhibitors increase serum concentration and half-life of eletriptan; do not use eletriptan within 72 hours of potent CYP3A4 inhibitors (eg, azole antifungals, ciprofloxacin, clarithromycin, diclofenac, doxycycline, erythromycin, imatinib, isoniazid, nefazodone, nicardipine, propofol, protease inhibitors, quinidine, verapamil). Ergot-containing drugs prolong vasospastic reactions; do not use within 24 hours of eletriptan.

Pharmacodynamics/Kinetics

Absorption: Well absorbed
Distribution: V_d: 138 L
Protein binding: ~85%
Metabolism: Hepatic via CYP3A4; forms one metabolite (active)
Bioavailability: ~50%, increased with high-fat meal
Half-life elimination: 4 hours (Elderly: 4.4-5.7 hours); Metabolite: ~13 hours
Time to peak, plasma: 1.5-2 hours

Pregnancy Risk Factor C

Eletriptan Hydrobromide *see* Eletriptan *on page 486*
Elidel® *see* Pimecrolimus *on page 1088*
Eligard™ *see* Leuprolide *on page 805*
Elimite® *see* Permethrin *on page 1070*
Elipten *see* Aminoglutethimide *on page 98*
Elitek™ *see* Rasburicase *on page 1171*
Elixophyllin® *see* Theophylline *on page 1285*
Elixophyllin-GG® *see* Theophylline and Guaifenesin *on page 1286*
ElixSure™ Cough [OTC] *see* Dextromethorphan *on page 421*
ElixSure™ Fever/Pain [OTC] *see* Acetaminophen *on page 47*
Ellence® *see* Epirubicin *on page 498*
Elmiron® *see* Pentosan Polysulfate Sodium *on page 1065*
Elocon® *see* Mometasone Furoate *on page 943*
Eloxatin™ *see* Oxaliplatin *on page 1020*
Elspar® *see* Asparaginase *on page 150*
Emadine® *see* Emedastine *on page 487*
Embeline™ E *see* Clobetasol *on page 351*
Emcyt® *see* Estramustine *on page 523*

Emedastine (em e DAS teen)

U.S. Brand Names Emadine®

Synonyms Emedastine Difumarate

Pharmacologic Category Antihistamine, H_1 Blocker, Ophthalmic

Use Treatment of allergic conjunctivitis

Local Anesthetic/Vasoconstrictor Precautions No information available to require special precautions

Effects on Dental Treatment No significant effects or complications reported

Mechanism of Action Selective histamine H_1-receptor antagonist for topical ophthalmic use

Pregnancy Risk Factor B

Emedastine Difumarate *see* Emedastine *on page 487*
Emend® *see* Aprepitant *on page 138*
Emetrol® [OTC] *see* Fructose, Dextrose, and Phosphoric Acid *on page 638*
Emgel® *see* Erythromycin *on page 508*
Emko® [OTC] *see* Nonoxynol 9 *on page 995*
EMLA® *see* Lidocaine and Prilocaine *on page 826*

Emtricitabine (em trye SYE ta been)

U.S. Brand Names Emtriva™

Generic Available No

Synonyms BW524W91; Coviracil; FTC

(Continued)

Emtricitabine *(Continued)*

Pharmacologic Category Antiretroviral Agent, Reverse Transcriptase Inhibitor (Nucleoside)

Use Treatment of HIV infection in combination with at least two other antiretroviral agents

Unlabeled/Investigational Use Investigational: Hepatitis B

Local Anesthetic/Vasoconstrictor Precautions No information available to require special precautions

Effects on Dental Treatment No significant effects or complications reported

Common Adverse Effects Clinical trials were conducted in patients receiving other antiretroviral agents, and it is not possible to correlate frequency of adverse events with emtricitabine alone. The range of frequencies of adverse events is generally comparable to comparator groups, with the exception of hyperpigmentation, which occurred more frequently in patients receiving emtricitabine.

>10%:

- Central nervous system: Headache (13% to 22%), dizziness (4% to 25%), insomnia (7% to 16%)
- Dermatologic: Rash (17% to 30%; includes rash, pruritus, maculopapular rash, vesiculobullous rash, pustular rash, and allergic reaction)
- Gastrointestinal: Diarrhea (23%), nausea (13% to 18%), abdominal pain (8% to 14%)
- Neuromuscular & skeletal: Weakness (12% to 16%), CPK increased (11% to 12%)
- Respiratory: Cough (14%), rhinitis (12% to 18%)

1% to 10%:

- Central nervous system: Abnormal dreams (2% to 11%), depression (6% to 9%), neuropathy/neuritis (4%)
- Dermatologic: Hyperpigmentation (2% to 6%; primarily of palms and/or soles but may include tongue, arms, lip and nails; generally mild and nonprogressive without associated local reactions such as pruritus or rash)
- Endocrine & metabolic: Serum triglycerides increased (9% to 10%), disordered glucose homeostasis (2% to 3%), serum amylase increased (2% to 5%)
- Gastrointestinal: Dyspepsia (4% to 8%), vomiting (9%)
- Hepatic: Transaminases increased (2% to 6%), bilirubin increased (1%)
- Neuromuscular & skeletal: Myalgia (4% to 6%), arthralgia (3% to 5%), paresthesia (5% to 6%)

Mechanism of Action Nucleoside reverse transcriptase inhibitor; emtricitabine is a cytosine analogue which is phosphorylated intracellularly to emtricitabine 5'-triphosphate which interferes with HIV viral RNA dependent DNA polymerase resulting in inhibition of viral replication.

Drug Interactions

Increased Effect/Toxicity: Concomitant use of ribavirin and nucleoside analogues may increase the risk of developing lactic acidosis.

Pharmacodynamics/Kinetics

Absorption: Rapid, extensive
Protein binding: <4%
Metabolism: Limited, via oxidation and conjugation (not via CYP isoenzymes)
Bioavailability: 93%
Half-life elimination: Normal renal function: 10 hours
Time to peak, plasma: 1-2 hours
Excretion: Urine (86% primarily as unchanged drug, 13% as metabolites); feces (14%)

Pregnancy Risk Factor B

Emtriva™ *see* Emtricitabine *on page 487*

Emulsoil® [OTC] [DSC] *see* Castor Oil *on page 273*

ENA 713 *see* Rivastigmine *on page 1192*

Enalapril (e NAL a pril)

Related Information

Cardiovascular Diseases *on page 1458*
Enalapril and Felodipine *on page 491*

U.S. Brand Names Vasotec®

Canadian Brand Names Vasotec®

Mexican Brand Names Enaladil®; Feliberal®; Glioten®; Kenopril®; Norpril®; Palane®; Pulsol® [tabs]; Renitec®

Generic Available Yes

Synonyms Enalaprilat; Enalapril Maleate

Pharmacologic Category Angiotensin-Converting Enzyme (ACE) Inhibitor

Use Management of mild to severe hypertension; treatment of congestive heart failure, left ventricular dysfunction after myocardial infarction

Unlabeled/Investigational Use

Unlabeled: Hypertensive crisis, diabetic nephropathy, rheumatoid arthritis, diagnosis of anatomic renal artery stenosis, hypertension secondary to scleroderma renal crisis, diagnosis of aldosteronism, idiopathic edema, Bartter's syndrome, postmyocardial infarction for prevention of ventricular failure

Investigational: Severe congestive heart failure in infants, neonatal hypertension, acute pulmonary edema

Local Anesthetic/Vasoconstrictor Precautions No information available to require special precautions

Effects on Dental Treatment Key adverse event(s) related to dental treatment: Abnormal taste and orthostatic hypotension.

Common Adverse Effects Note: Frequency ranges include data from hypertension and heart failure trials. Higher rates of adverse reactions have generally been noted in patients with CHF. However, the frequency of adverse effects associated with placebo is also increased in this population.

1% to 10%:

Cardiovascular: Hypotension (0.9% to 7%), chest pain (2%), syncope (0.5% to 2%), orthostasis (2%), orthostatic hypotension (2%)

Central nervous system: Headache (2% to 5%), dizziness (4% to 8%), fatigue (2% to 3%), weakness (2%)

Dermatologic: Rash (2%)

Gastrointestinal: Abnormal taste, abdominal pain, vomiting, nausea, diarrhea, anorexia, constipation

Neuromuscular & skeletal: Weakness

Renal: Increased serum creatinine (0.2% to 20%), worsening of renal function (in patients with bilateral renal artery stenosis or hypovolemia)

Respiratory (1% to 2%): Bronchitis, cough, dyspnea

Dosage Use lower listed initial dose in patients with hyponatremia, hypovolemia, severe congestive heart failure, decreased renal function, or in those receiving diuretics.

Oral: **Enalapril**: Children 1 month to 16 years: Hypertension: Initial: 0.08 mg/kg (up to 5 mg) once daily; adjust dosage based on patient response; doses >0.58 mg/kg (40 mg) have not been evaluated in pediatric patients

Investigational: Congestive heart failure: Initial oral doses of **enalapril**: 0.1 mg/kg/day increasing as needed over 2 weeks to 0.5 mg/kg/day have been used in infants

Investigational: Neonatal hypertension: I.V. doses of **enalaprilat**: 5-10 mcg/kg/dose administered every 8-24 hours have been used; monitor patients carefully; select patients may require higher doses

Adults:

Oral: **Enalapril:**

Hypertension: 2.5-5 mg/day then increase as required; usual dose range (JNC 7): 2.5-40 mg/day in 1-2 divided doses. **Note:** Initiate with 2.5 mg if patient is taking a diuretic which cannot be discontinued. May add a diuretic if blood pressure cannot be controlled with enalapril alone.

Heart failure: As standard therapy alone or with diuretics, beta-blockers, and digoxin, initiate with 2.5 mg once or twice daily (usual range: 5-20 mg/day in 2 divided doses; target: 40 mg)

Asymptomatic left ventricular dysfunction: 2.5 mg twice daily, titrated as tolerated to 20 mg/day

I.V.: **Enalaprilat:**

Hypertension: 1.25 mg/dose, given over 5 minutes every 6 hours; doses as high as 5 mg/dose every 6 hours have been tolerated for up to 36 hours. **Note:** If patients are concomitantly receiving diuretic therapy, begin with 0.625 mg I.V. over 5 minutes; if the effect is not adequate after 1 hour, repeat the dose and administer 1.25 mg at 6-hour intervals thereafter; if adequate, administer 0.625 mg I.V. every 6 hours.

Heart failure: Avoid I.V. administration in patients with unstable heart failure or those suffering acute myocardial infarction.

Conversion from I.V. to oral therapy if not concurrently on diuretics: 5 mg once daily; subsequent titration as needed; if concurrently receiving diuretics and responding to 0.625 mg I.V. every 6 hours, initiate with 2.5 mg/day.

Dosing adjustment in renal impairment:

Oral: Enalapril:

Cl_{cr} 30-80 mL/minute: Administer 5 mg/day titrated upwards to maximum of 40 mg.

(Continued)

Enalapril *(Continued)*

Cl_{cr} <30 mL/minute: Administer 2.5 mg day; titrated upward until blood pressure is controlled.

For heart failure patients with sodium <130 mEq/L or serum creatinine >1.6 mg/dL, initiate dosage with 2.5 mg/day, increasing to twice daily as needed. Increase further in increments of 2.5 mg/dose at >4-day intervals to a maximum daily dose of 40 mg.

I.V.: Enalaprilat:

Cl_{cr} >30 mL/minute: Initiate with 1.25 mg every 6 hours and increase dose based on response.

Cl_{cr} <30 mL/minute: Initiate with 0.625 mg every 6 hours and increase dose based on response.

Hemodialysis: Moderately dialyzable (20% to 50%); administer dose postdialysis (eg, 0.625 mg I.V. every 6 hours) or administer 20% to 25% supplemental dose following dialysis; Clearance: 62 mL/minute.

Peritoneal dialysis: Supplemental dose is not necessary, although some removal of drug occurs.

Dosing adjustment in hepatic impairment: Hydrolysis of enalapril to enalaprilat may be delayed and/or impaired in patients with severe hepatic impairment, but the pharmacodynamic effects of the drug do not appear to be significantly altered; no dosage adjustment.

Mechanism of Action Competitive inhibitor of angiotensin-converting enzyme (ACE); prevents conversion of angiotensin I to angiotensin II, a potent vasoconstrictor; results in lower levels of angiotensin II which causes an increase in plasma renin activity and a reduction in aldosterone secretion

Contraindications Hypersensitivity to enalapril or enalaprilat; angioedema related to previous treatment with an ACE inhibitor; patients with idiopathic or hereditary angioedema; bilateral renal artery stenosis; pregnancy (2nd and 3rd trimesters)

Warnings/Precautions Anaphylactic reactions can occur. Angioedema can occur at any time during treatment (especially following first dose). Angioedema may involve head and neck (potentially affecting the airway) or the intestine (presenting with abdominal pain). Careful blood pressure monitoring with first dose (hypotension can occur especially in volume depleted patients). Dosage adjustment needed in renal impairment. Use with caution in hypovolemia; collagen vascular diseases; valvular stenosis (particularly aortic stenosis); hyperkalemia; or before, during, or immediately after anesthesia. Avoid rapid dosage escalation which may lead to renal insufficiency. Hypersensitivity reactions may be seen during hemodialysis with high-flux dialysis membranes (eg, AN69). Hyperkalemia may rarely occur. Neutropenia/agranulocytosis with myeloid hyperplasia can rarely occur. If patient has renal impairment then a baseline WBC with differential and serum creatinine should be evaluated and monitored closely during the first 3 months of therapy. Use with caution in unilateral renal artery stenosis and pre-existing renal insufficiency. Experience in children is limited.

Drug Interactions

Cytochrome P450 Effect: Substrate of CYP3A4 (major)

Increased Effect/Toxicity: Potassium supplements, co-trimoxazole (high dose), angiotensin II receptor antagonists (eg, candesartan, losartan, irbesartan), or potassium-sparing diuretics (amiloride, spironolactone, triamterene) may result in elevated serum potassium levels when combined with enalapril. ACE inhibitor effects may be increased by phenothiazines or probenecid (increases levels of captopril). ACE inhibitors may increase serum concentrations/effects of digoxin, lithium, and sulfonlyureas.

Diuretics have additive hypotensive effects with ACE inhibitors, and hypovolemia increases the potential for adverse renal effects of ACE inhibitors. In patients with compromised renal function, coadministration with NSAIDs may result in further deterioration of renal function. Allopurinol and ACE inhibitors may cause a higher risk of hypersensitivity reaction when taken concurrently.

Decreased Effect: Aspirin (high dose) may reduce the therapeutic effects of ACE inhibitors; at low dosages this does not appear to be significant. Antacids may decrease the bioavailability of ACE inhibitors (may be more likely to occur with captopril); separate administration times by 1-2 hours. NSAIDs may reduce the hypotensive effects of ACE inhibitors. More likely to occur in low renin or volume-dependent hypertensive patients. CYP3A4 inducers may decrease the levels/effects of enalapril; example inducers include aminoglutethimide, carbamazepine, nafcillin, nevirapine, phenobarbital, phenytoin, and rifamycins.

Ethanol/Nutrition/Herb Interactions Herb/Nutraceutical: St John's wort may decrease enalapril levels. Avoid dong quai if using for hypertension (has estrogenic activity). Avoid ephedra, yohimbe, ginseng (may worsen hypertension). Avoid natural licorice (causes sodium and water retention and increases potassium loss). Avoid garlic (may have increased antihypertensive effect).

Dietary Considerations Limit salt substitutes or potassium-rich diet.

Pharmacodynamics/Kinetics

Onset of action: Oral: ~1 hour

Duration: Oral: 12-24 hours

Absorption: Oral: 55% to 75%

Protein binding: 50% to 60%

Metabolism: Prodrug, undergoes hepatic biotransformation to enalaprilat

Half-life elimination:

Enalapril: Adults: Healthy: 2 hours; Congestive heart failure: 3.4-5.8 hours

Enalaprilat: Infants 6 weeks to 8 months old: 6-10 hours; Adults: 35-38 hours

Time to peak, serum: Oral: Enalapril: 0.5-1.5 hours; Enalaprilat (active): 3-4.5 hours

Excretion: Urine (60% to 80%); some feces

Pregnancy Risk Factor C/D (2nd and 3rd trimesters)

Dosage Forms INJ, solution, as enalaprilat 1.25 mg/mL (1 mL, 2 mL). **TAB, as maleate** (Vasotec®): 2.5 mg, 5 mg, 10 mg, 20 mg

Enalapril and Felodipine (e NAL a pril & fe LOE di peen)

Related Information

Enalapril *on page 488*

Felodipine *on page 576*

U.S. Brand Names Lexxel®

Canadian Brand Names Lexxel®

Generic Available No

Synonyms Felodipine and Enalapril

Pharmacologic Category Antihypertensive Agent, Combination

Use Treatment of hypertension, however, not indicated for initial treatment of hypertension; replacement therapy in patients receiving separate dosage forms (for patient convenience); when monotherapy with one component fails to achieve desired antihypertensive effect, or when dose-limiting adverse effects limit upward titration of monotherapy

Local Anesthetic/Vasoconstrictor Precautions No information available to require special precautions

Effects on Dental Treatment Key adverse event(s) related to dental treatment: Gingival hyperplasia (fewer reports with felodipine than with other CCBs); resolves upon discontinuation (consultation with physician is suggested).

Common Adverse Effects See individual agents.

Mechanism of Action See individual agents.

Drug Interactions

Cytochrome P450 Effect:

Enalapril: **Substrate** of CYP3A4 (major)

Felodipine: **Substrate** of CYP3A4 (major); **Inhibits** CYP2C8/9 (weak), 2D6 (weak), 3A4 (weak)

Increased Effect/Toxicity: See individual agents.

Decreased Effect: See individual agents.

Pharmacodynamics/Kinetics See individual agents.

Pregnancy Risk Factor C/D (2nd and 3rd trimesters)

Enalapril and Hydrochlorothiazide

(e NAL a pril & hye droe klor oh THYE a zide)

Related Information

Cardiovascular Diseases *on page 1458*

Enalapril *on page 488*

Hydrochlorothiazide *on page 699*

U.S. Brand Names Vaseretic®

Canadian Brand Names Vaseretic®

Generic Available Yes

Synonyms Hydrochlorothiazide and Enalapril

Pharmacologic Category Antihypertensive Agent, Combination

Use Treatment of hypertension

Local Anesthetic/Vasoconstrictor Precautions No information available to require special precautions

Effects on Dental Treatment No significant effects or complications reported

Common Adverse Effects See individual agents.

(Continued)

Enalapril and Hydrochlorothiazide *(Continued)*

Drug Interactions

Cytochrome P450 Effect: Enalapril: **Substrate** of CYP3A4 (major)

Pharmacodynamics/Kinetics See individual agents.

Pregnancy Risk Factor C/D (2nd and 3rd trimesters)

Enalaprilat *see* Enalapril *on page 488*

Enalapril Maleate *see* Enalapril *on page 488*

Enbrel® *see* Etanercept *on page 532*

Encare® [OTC] *see* Nonoxynol 9 *on page 995*

Endal® *see* Guaifenesin and Phenylephrine *on page 674*

Endal® HD *see* Hydrocodone, Phenylephrine, and Diphenhydramine *on page 713*

Endocet® *see* Oxycodone and Acetaminophen *on page 1029*

Endocrine Disorders and Pregnancy *see page 1481*

Endodan® *see* Oxycodone and Aspirin *on page 1032*

Endrate® *see* Edetate Disodium *on page 482*

Enduron® *see* Methyclothiazide *on page 905*

Enduronyl® *see* Methyclothiazide and Deserpidine *on page 905*

Enduronyl® Forte *see* Methyclothiazide and Deserpidine *on page 905*

Enfuvirtide (en FYOO vir tide)

U.S. Brand Names Fuzeon™

Canadian Brand Names Fuzeon™

Generic Available No

Synonyms T-20

Pharmacologic Category Antiretroviral Agent, Fusion Protein Inhibitor

Use Treatment of HIV-1 infection in combination with other antiretroviral agents in treatment-experienced patients with evidence of HIV-1 replication despite ongoing antiretroviral therapy

Local Anesthetic/Vasoconstrictor Precautions No information available to require special precautions

Effects on Dental Treatment Key adverse event(s) related to dental treatment: Taste disturbance.

Common Adverse Effects

>10%:

- Central nervous system: Insomnia (11%)
- Local: Injection site reactions (98%; may include pain, erythema, induration, pruritus, ecchymosis, nodule or cyst formation)

1% to 10%:

- Central nervous system: Depression (9%), anxiety (6%)
- Dermatologic: Pruritus (5%)
- Endocrine & metabolic: Weight loss (7%), anorexia (3%)
- Gastrointestinal: Triglycerides increased (9%), appetite decreased (6%), constipation (4%), abdominal pain (3%), pancreatitis (2%), taste disturbance (2%), serum amylase increased (6%)
- Hematologic: Eosinophilia (8%), anemia (2%)
- Hepatic: Serum transaminases increased (4%)
- Local: Injection site infection (1%)
- Neuromuscular & skeletal: Neuropathy (9%), weakness (6%), myalgia (5%)
- Ocular: Conjunctivitis (2%)
- Respiratory: Cough (7%), pneumonia (4.7 events per 100 patient years vs 0.61 events per 100 patient years in control group), sinusitis (6%)
- Miscellaneous: Infections (4% to 6%), flu-like symptoms (2%), lymphadenopathy (2%)

Mechanism of Action Binds to the first heptad-repeat (HR1) in the gp41 subunit of the viral envelope glycoprotein. Inhibits the fusion of HIV-1 virus with CD4 cells by blocking the conformational change in gp41 required for membrane fusion and entry into CD4 cells

Drug Interactions

Increased Effect/Toxicity: No significant interactions identified.

Decreased Effect: No significant interactions identified.

Pharmacodynamics/Kinetics

Distribution: V_d: 5.5 L

Protein binding: 92%

Metabolism: Proteolytic hydrolysis (CYP isoenzymes do not appear to contribute to metabolism); clearance: 24.8 mL/hour/kg

Half-life elimination: 3.8 hours

Time to peak: 8 hours

Pregnancy Risk Factor B

Engerix-B® *see* Hepatitis B Vaccine *on page 689*

Engerix-B® and Havrix® *see* Hepatitis A (Inactivated) and Hepatitis B (Recombinant) Vaccine *on page 686*

Enhanced-potency Inactivated Poliovirus Vaccine *see* Poliovirus Vaccine (Inactivated) *on page 1099*

Enlon® *see* Edrophonium *on page 483*

Enoxaparin (ee noks a PA rin)

Related Information

Cardiovascular Diseases *on page 1458*

U.S. Brand Names Lovenox®

Canadian Brand Names Lovenox®; Lovenox® HP

Mexican Brand Names Clexane®

Generic Available No

Synonyms Enoxaparin Sodium

Pharmacologic Category Low Molecular Weight Heparin

Use

DVT Treatment (acute): Inpatient treatment (patients with and without pulmonary embolism) and outpatient treatment (patients without pulmonary embolism)

DVT prophylaxis: Following hip or knee replacement surgery, abdominal surgery, or in medical patients with severely-restricted mobility during acute illness in patients at risk of thromboembolic complications

Note: High-risk patients include those with one or more of the following risk factors: >40 years of age, obesity, general anesthesia lasting >30 minutes, malignancy, history of deep vein thrombosis or pulmonary embolism

Unstable angina and non-Q-wave myocardial infarction (to prevent ischemic complications)

Unlabeled/Investigational Use Prophylaxis and treatment of thromboembolism in children

Local Anesthetic/Vasoconstrictor Precautions No information available to require special precautions

Effects on Dental Treatment Key adverse event(s) related to dental treatment: As with all anticoagulants, bleeding is the major adverse effect of enoxaparin. Hemorrhage may occur at virtually any site; risk is dependent on multiple variables. At the recommended doses, single injections of enoxaparin do not significantly influence platelet aggregation or affect global clotting time (ie, PT or aPTT).

Common Adverse Effects As with all anticoagulants, bleeding is the major adverse effect of enoxaparin. Hemorrhage may occur at virtually any site. Risk is dependent on multiple variables. At the recommended doses, single injections of enoxaparin do not significantly influence platelet aggregation or affect global clotting time (ie, PT or aPTT).

1% to 10%:

Central nervous system: Fever (5% to 8%), confusion, pain

Dermatologic: Erythema, bruising

Gastrointestinal: Nausea (3%), diarrhea

Hematologic: Hemorrhage (5% to 13%), thrombocytopenia (2%), hypochromic anemia (2%)

Hepatic: Increased ALT/AST

Local: Injection site hematoma (9%), local reactions (irritation, pain, ecchymosis, erythema)

Thrombocytopenia with thrombosis: Cases of heparin-induced thrombocytopenia (some complicated by organ infarction, limb ischemia, or death) have been reported.

Mechanism of Action Standard heparin consists of components with molecular weights ranging from 4000-30,000 daltons with a mean of 16,000 daltons. Heparin acts as an anticoagulant by enhancing the inhibition rate of clotting proteases by antithrombin III impairing normal hemostasis and inhibition of factor Xa. Low molecular weight heparins have a small effect on the activated partial thromboplastin time and strongly inhibit factor Xa. Enoxaparin is derived from porcine heparin that undergoes benzylation followed by alkaline depolymerization. The average molecular weight of enoxaparin is 4500 daltons which is distributed as (≤20%) 2000 daltons (≥68%) 2000-8000 daltons, and (≤15%) >8000 daltons. Enoxaparin has a higher ratio of antifactor Xa to antifactor IIa activity than unfractionated heparin.

Drug Interactions

Increased Effect/Toxicity: Risk of bleeding with enoxaparin may be increased with thrombolytic agents, oral anticoagulants (warfarin), drugs

(Continued)

Enoxaparin *(Continued)*

which affect platelet function (eg, aspirin, NSAIDs, dipyridamole, ticlopidine, clopidogrel, and IIb/IIIa antagonists). Although the risk of bleeding may be increased during concurrent therapy with warfarin, enoxaparin is commonly continued during the initiation of warfarin therapy to assure anticoagulation and to protect against possible transient hypercoagulability. Some cephalosporins and penicillins may block platelet aggregation, theoretically increasing the risk of bleeding.

Pharmacodynamics/Kinetics

Onset of action: Peak effect: SubQ: Antifactor Xa and antithrombin (antifactor IIa): 3-5 hours

Duration: 40 mg dose: Antifactor Xa activity: ~12 hours

Protein binding: Does not bind to heparin binding proteins

Half-life elimination, plasma: 2-4 times longer than standard heparin, independent of dose

Excretion: Urine

Pregnancy Risk Factor B

Enoxaparin Sodium *see* Enoxaparin *on page 493*

Enpresse™ *see* Ethinyl Estradiol and Levonorgestrel *on page 545*

Entacapone (en TA ka pone)

U.S. Brand Names Comtan®

Canadian Brand Names Comtan®

Generic Available No

Pharmacologic Category Anti-Parkinson's Agent, COMT Inhibitor

Use Adjunct to levodopa/carbidopa therapy in patients with idiopathic Parkinson's disease who experience "wearing-off" symptoms at the end of a dosing interval

Local Anesthetic/Vasoconstrictor Precautions No information available to require special precautions

Effects on Dental Treatment Key adverse event(s) related to dental treatment: Orthostatic hypotension and abnormal taste. Dopaminergic therapy in Parkinson's disease (ie, treatment with levodopa) is associated with orthostatic hypotension. Entacapone enhances levodopa bioavailability and may increase the occurrence of hypotension/syncope in the dental patient. The patient should be carefully assisted from the chair and observed for signs of orthostatic hypotension.

Common Adverse Effects

>10%:

Gastrointestinal: Nausea (14%)

Neuromuscular & skeletal: Dyskinesia (25%), placebo (15%)

1% to 10%:

Cardiovascular: Orthostatic hypotension (4%), syncope (1%)

Central nervous system: Dizziness (8%), fatigue (6%), hallucinations (4%), anxiety (2%), somnolence (2%), agitation (1%)

Dermatologic: Purpura (2%)

Gastrointestinal: Diarrhea (10%), abdominal pain (8%), constipation (6%), vomiting (4%), dry mouth (3%), dyspepsia (2%), flatulence (2%), gastritis (1%), taste perversion (1%)

Genitourinary: Brown-orange urine discoloration (10%)

Neuromuscular & skeletal: Hyperkinesia (10%), hypokinesia (9%), back pain (4%), weakness (2%)

Respiratory: Dyspnea (3%)

Miscellaneous: Increased diaphoresis (2%), bacterial infection (1%)

Mechanism of Action Entacapone is a reversible and selective inhibitor of catechol-O-methyltransferase (COMT). When entacapone is taken with levodopa, the pharmacokinetics are altered, resulting in more sustained levodopa serum levels compared to levodopa taken alone. The resulting levels of levodopa provide for increased concentrations available for absorption across the blood-brain barrier, thereby providing for increased CNS levels of dopamine, the active metabolite of levodopa.

Drug Interactions

Cytochrome P450 Effect: Inhibits CYP1A2 (weak), 2A6 (weak), 2C8/9 (weak), 2C19 (weak), 2D6 (weak), 2E1 (weak), 3A4 (weak)

Increased Effect/Toxicity: Cardiac effects with drugs metabolized by COMT (eg, epinephrine, isoproterenol, dopamine, apomorphine, bitolterol, dobutamine, methyldopa) increased other CNS depressants; nonselective MAO inhibitors are not recommended; chelates iron. Caution with drugs that interfere with glucuronidation, intestinal, biliary excretion, intestinal beta-glucuronidase (eg, probenecid, cholestyramine, erythromycin, chloramphenicol, rifampicin, ampicillin).

Decreased Effect: Entacapone is an iron chelator and an iron supplement should not be administered concurrently with this medicine.

Pharmacodynamics/Kinetics

Onset of action: Rapid

Peak effect: 1 hour

Absorption: Rapid

Distribution: I.V.: V_{dss}: 20 L

Protein binding: 98%, primarily to albumin

Metabolism: Isomerization to the *cis*-isomer, followed by direct glucuronidation of the parent and *cis*-isomer

Bioavailability: 35%

Half-life elimination: Β phase: 0.4-0.7 hours; Υ phase: 2.4 hours

Time to peak, serum: 1 hour

Excretion: Feces (90%); urine (10%)

Pregnancy Risk Factor C

Entacapone, Carbidopa, and Levodopa *see* Levodopa, Carbidopa, and Entacapone *on page 812*

Entertainer's Secret® [OTC] *see* Saliva Substitute *on page 1205*

Entex® LA *see* Guaifenesin and Phenylephrine *on page 674*

Entex® PSE *see* Guaifenesin and Pseudoephedrine *on page 675*

Entocort™ EC *see* Budesonide *on page 221*

Entsol® [OTC] *see* Sodium Chloride *on page 1227*

Enulose® *see* Lactulose *on page 794*

Enzone® *see* Pramoxine and Hydrocortisone *on page 1109*

Ephedrine (e FED rin)

Related Information

Ephedra *on page 1424*

U.S. Brand Names Pretz-D® [OTC]

Generic Available Yes

Synonyms Ephedrine Sulfate

Pharmacologic Category Alpha/Beta Agonist

Use Treatment of bronchial asthma, nasal congestion, acute bronchospasm, idiopathic orthostatic hypotension

Local Anesthetic/Vasoconstrictor Precautions Use vasoconstrictor with caution since ephedrine may enhance cardiostimulation and vasopressor effects of sympathomimetics such as epinephrine

Effects on Dental Treatment Key adverse event(s) related to dental treatment: Xerostomia (normal salivary flow resumes upon discontinuation).

Common Adverse Effects Frequency not defined.

Cardiovascular: Hypertension, tachycardia, palpitations, elevation or depression of blood pressure, unusual pallor, chest pain, arrhythmias

Central nervous system: CNS stimulating effects, nervousness, anxiety, apprehension, fear, tension, agitation, excitation, restlessness, irritability, insomnia, hyperactivity, dizziness, headache

Gastrointestinal: Xerostomia, nausea, anorexia, GI upset, vomiting

Genitourinary: Painful urination

Neuromuscular & skeletal: Trembling, tremor (more common in the elderly), weakness

Respiratory: Dyspnea

Miscellaneous: Diaphoresis (increased)

Mechanism of Action Releases tissue stores of epinephrine and thereby produces an alpha- and beta-adrenergic stimulation; longer-acting and less potent than epinephrine

Drug Interactions

Increased Effect/Toxicity: Increased (toxic) cardiac stimulation with other sympathomimetic agents, theophylline, cardiac glycosides, or general anesthetics. Increased blood pressure with atropine or MAO inhibitors.

Decreased Effect: Alpha- and beta-adrenergic blocking agents decrease ephedrine vasopressor effects.

Pharmacodynamics/Kinetics

Onset of action: Oral: Bronchodilation: 0.25-1 hour

Duration: Oral: 3-6 hours

Distribution: Crosses placenta; enters breast milk

Metabolism: Minimally hepatic

Half-life elimination: 2.5-3.6 hours

Excretion: Urine (60% to 77% as unchanged drug) within 24 hours

Pregnancy Risk Factor C

Ephedrine, Chlorpheniramine, Phenylephrine, and Carbetapentane *see* Chlorpheniramine, Ephedrine, Phenylephrine, and Carbetapentane *on page 316*

Ephedrine Sulfate *see* Ephedrine *on page 495*

Epidermal Thymocyte Activating Factor *see* Aldesleukin *on page 74*

Epifoam® *see* Pramoxine and Hydrocortisone *on page 1109*

Epinastine (ep i NAS teen)

U.S. Brand Names Elestat™

Mexican Brand Names Flurinol®

Generic Available No

Synonyms Epinastine Hydrochloride

Pharmacologic Category Antihistamine, H_1 Blocker, Ophthalmic

Use Treatment of allergic conjunctivitis

Local Anesthetic/Vasoconstrictor Precautions No information available to require special precautions

Effects on Dental Treatment No significant effects or complications reported

Mechanism of Action Selective H_1-receptor antagonist; inhibits release of histamine from the mast cell

Pregnancy Risk Factor C

Epinastine Hydrochloride *see* Epinastine *on page 496*

Epinephrine (ep i NEF rin)

Related Information

Dental Office Emergencies *on page 1584*
Respiratory Diseases *on page 1478*

U.S. Brand Names Adrenalin® (Dental); Sus-Phrine® (Dental)

Generic Available Yes

Pharmacologic Category Adrenergic Agonist Agent; Alpha/Beta Agonist; Antidote; Bronchodilator; Vasoconstrictor

Dental Use Emergency drug for treatment of anaphylactic reactions; used as vasoconstrictor to prolong local anesthesia

Local Anesthetic/Vasoconstrictor Precautions No information available to require special precautions

Effects on Dental Treatment No significant effects or complications reported

Significant Adverse Effects No data reported

Dosage Hypersensitivity reaction:

Children: SubQ: 0.01 mg/kg every 15 minutes for 2 doses then every 4 hours as needed (single doses not to exceed 0.5 mg)

Adults: I.M., SubQ: 0.2-0.5 mg every 20 minutes to 4 hours (single dose maximum: 1 mg)

Mechanism of Action Stimulates alpha-, beta$_1$-, and beta$_2$-adrenergic receptors resulting in relaxation of smooth muscle of the bronchial tree, cardiac stimulation, and dilation of skeletal muscle vasculature; small doses can cause vasodilation via beta$_2$-vascular receptors; large doses may produce constriction of skeletal and vascular smooth muscle; decreases production of aqueous humor and increases aqueous outflow; dilates the pupil by contracting the dilator muscle

Contraindications Hypersensitivity to epinephrine or any component of the formulation; cardiac arrhythmias, angle-closure glaucoma

Warnings/Precautions Use with caution in elderly patients, patients with diabetes mellitus, cardiovascular diseases (angina, tachycardia, myocardial infarction), thyroid disease, or cerebral arteriosclerosis, Parkinson's; some products contain sulfites as antioxidants. Rapid I.V. infusion may cause death from cerebrovascular hemorrhage or cardiac arrhythmias. Oral inhalation of epinephrine is **not** the preferred route of administration.

Drug Interactions Increased cardiac irritability if administered concurrently with halogenated inhalational anesthetics, beta-blocking agents, alpha-blocking agents

Pharmacodynamics/Kinetics Absorption: None

Pregnancy Risk Factor C

Breast-Feeding Considerations Usual infiltration doses of epinephrine given to nursing mothers has not been shown to affect the health of the nursing infant.

Dosage Forms

Injection (Adrenalin®): 1 mg/mL [1:1000] (1 mL, 30 mL)
Injection for suspension (Sus-Phrine®): 5 mg/mL [1:200] (0.3 mL, 5 mL)

Epinephrine and Bupivacaine (Dental) *see* Bupivacaine and Epinephrine *on page 227*

Epinephrine and Chlorpheniramine

(ep i NEF rin & klor fen IR a meen)

U.S. Brand Names Ana-Kit®

Generic Available No

Synonyms Insect Sting Kit

Pharmacologic Category Antidote

Use Anaphylaxis emergency treatment of insect bites or stings by the sensitive patient that may occur within minutes of insect sting or exposure to an allergic substance

Local Anesthetic/Vasoconstrictor Precautions No information available to require special precautions

Effects on Dental Treatment No significant effects or complications reported

Drug Interactions

Cytochrome P450 Effect: Chlorpheniramine: **Substrate** of CYP2D6 (minor), 3A4 (major); **Inhibits** CYP2D6 (weak)

Epinephrine and Lidocaine *see* Lidocaine and Epinephrine *on page 823*

Epinephrine and Prilocaine (Dental) *see* Prilocaine and Epinephrine *on page 1120*

Epinephrine (Racemic) (ep i NEF rin, ra SEE mik)

U.S. Brand Names AsthmaNefrin®; microNefrin®; S-2®; Vaponefrin®

Generic Available Yes

Pharmacologic Category Alpha/Beta Agonist; Vasoconstrictor

Dental Use Emergency drug for treatment of bronchoconstriction

Local Anesthetic/Vasoconstrictor Precautions No information available to require special precautions

Effects on Dental Treatment No significant effects or complications reported

Significant Adverse Effects No data reported

Drug Interactions No data reported

Pharmacodynamics/Kinetics

Onset of action: Bronchodilation: SubQ: 5-10 minutes; Inhalation: ~1 minute

Absorption: Oral: None

Dosage Forms Solution for oral inhalation (AsthmaNefrin®, microNefrin®, S-2®): Racepinephrine 2.25% [epinephrine base 1.125%] (7.5 mL, 15 mL, 30 mL)

Epinephrine (Racemic) and Aluminum Potassium Sulfate

(ep i NEF rin, ra SEE mik and a LOO mi num poe TASS ee um SUL fate)

Related Information

Epinephrine (Racemic) *on page 497*

U.S. Brand Names Van R Gingibraid®

Generic Available No

Synonyms Aluminum Potassium Sulfate and Epinephrine (Racemic) (Dental)

Pharmacologic Category Adrenergic Agonist Agent; Alpha/Beta Agonist; Astringent; Vasoconstrictor

Dental Use Gingival retraction

Local Anesthetic/Vasoconstrictor Precautions No information available to require special precautions

Effects on Dental Treatment Key adverse event(s) related to dental treatment: Tissue retraction around base of the tooth (therapeutic effect).

Significant Adverse Effects No data reported

Dosage Pass the impregnated yarn around the neck of the tooth and place into gingival sulcus; normal tissue moisture, water, or gingival retraction solutions activate impregnated yarn. Limit use to one quadrant of the mouth at a time; recommended use is for 3-8 minutes in the mouth.

Mechanism of Action Epinephrine stimulates alpha, adrenergic receptors to cause vasoconstriction in blood vessels in gingiva; aluminum potassium sulfate, precipitates tissue and blood proteins

Contraindications Hypersensitivity to epinephrine or any component of the formulation; cardiovascular disease, hyperthyroidism, or diabetes; do not apply to areas of heavy or deep bleeding or over exposed bone

Warnings/Precautions Caution should be exercised whenever using gingival retraction cords with epinephrine since it delivers vasoconstrictor doses of racemic epinephrine to patients; the general medical history should be thoroughly evaluated before using in any patient

Drug Interactions No data reported

Pharmacodynamics/Kinetics No data reported

(Continued)

Epinephrine (Racemic) and Aluminum Potassium Sulfate *(Continued)*

Dosage Forms

Yarn, saturated in solution of 8% racemic epinephrine and 7% aluminum potassium sulfate:

Type "0e": 0.20 ± 0.10 mg epinephrine/inch
Type "1e": 0.40 ± 0.20 mg epinephrine/inch
Type "2e": 0.60 ± 0.20 mg epinephrine/inch

Epipodophyllotoxin *see* Etoposide *on page 567*
EpiQuin™ Micro *see* Hydroquinone *on page 719*

Epirubicin (ep i ROO bi sin)

U.S. Brand Names Ellence®
Canadian Brand Names Ellence®; Pharmorubicin®
Mexican Brand Names Epilem® [inj.]; Farmorubicin®
Generic Available No
Synonyms Pidorubicin; Pidorubicin Hydrochloride
Pharmacologic Category Antineoplastic Agent, Anthracycline
Use Adjuvant therapy for primary breast cancer
Local Anesthetic/Vasoconstrictor Precautions No information available to require special precautions
Effects on Dental Treatment Key adverse event(s) related to dental treatment: Mucositis.

Common Adverse Effects

>10%:

Central nervous system: Lethargy (1% to 46%)
Dermatologic: Alopecia (69% to 95%)
Endocrine & metabolic: Amenorrhea (69% to 72%), hot flashes (5% to 39%)
Gastrointestinal: Nausea, vomiting (83% to 92%), mucositis (9% to 59%), diarrhea (7% to 25%)
Hematologic: Leukopenia (49% to 80%; Grade 3 and 4: 1.5% to 58.6%), neutropenia (54% to 80%), anemia (13% to 72%), thrombocytopenia (5% to 49%)
Local: Injection site reactions (3% to 20%)
Ocular: Conjunctivitis (1% to 15%)
Miscellaneous: Infection (15% to 21%)

1% to 10%:

Cardiovascular: Congestive heart failure (0.4% to 1.5%), decreased LVEF (asymptomatic) (1.4% to 1.8%); recommended maximum cumulative dose: 900 mg/m^2
Central nervous system: Fever (1% to 5%)
Dermatologic: Rash (1% to 9%), skin changes (0.7% to 5%)
Gastrointestinal: Anorexia (2% to 3%)

Other reactions (percentage not specified): Acute myelogenous leukemia (0.2% at 3 years), acute lymphoid leukemia, increased transaminases, radiation recall, skin and nail hyperpigmentation, photosensitivity reaction, hypersensitivity, anaphylaxis, urticaria, premature menopause in women

Mechanism of Action Epirubicin is an anthracycline antibiotic. Epirubicin is known to inhibit DNA and RNA synthesis by steric obstruction after intercalating between DNA base pairs; active throughout entire cell cycle. Intercalation triggers DNA cleavage by topoisomerase II, resulting in cytocidal activity. Epirubicin also inhibits DNA helicase, and generates cytotoxic free radicals.

Drug Interactions

Increased Effect/Toxicity: Cimetidine increased the blood levels of epirubicin (AUC increased by 50%).

Pharmacodynamics/Kinetics

Distribution: V_{ss} 21-27 L/kg
Protein binding: 77% to albumin
Metabolism: Extensively via hepatic and extrahepatic (including RBCs) routes
Half-life elimination: Triphasic; Mean terminal: 33 hours
Excretion: Feces; urine (lesser extent)

Pregnancy Risk Factor D

Epitol® *see* Carbamazepine *on page 255*
Epivir® *see* Lamivudine *on page 794*
Epivir-HBV® *see* Lamivudine *on page 794*

Eplerenone (e PLER en one)

U.S. Brand Names Inspra™
Generic Available No

Pharmacologic Category Antihypertensive; Selective Aldosterone Blocker

Use Treatment of hypertension (may be used alone or in combination with other antihypertensive agents); treatment of CHF following acute MI

Local Anesthetic/Vasoconstrictor Precautions No information available to require special precautions

Effects on Dental Treatment No significant effects or complications reported

Common Adverse Effects

>10%: Endocrine & metabolic: Hypertriglyceridemia (1% to 15%, dose related); hypokalemia (16% in CHF)

1% to 10%:

Central nervous system: Dizziness (3%), fatigue (2%)

Endocrine & metabolic: Breast pain (males <1% to 1%), serum creatinine increased (6% in CHF), gynecomastia (males <1% to 1%), hyponatremia (2%, dose related), hypercholesterolemia (<1% to 1%); hyperkalemia (dose related, <1%; 6% in left ventricular dysfunction)

Gastrointestinal: Diarrhea (2%), abdominal pain (1%)

Genitourinary: Abnormal vaginal bleeding (<1% to 2%)

Renal: Albuminuria (1%)

Respiratory: Cough (2%)

Miscellaneous: Flu-like syndrome (2%)

Mechanism of Action Aldosterone increases blood pressure primarily by inducing sodium reabsorption. Eplerenone reduces blood pressure by blocking aldosterone binding at mineralocorticoid receptors found in the kidney, heart, blood vessels and brain.

Drug Interactions

Cytochrome P450 Effect: Substrate of CYP3A4 (major)

Increased Effect/Toxicity: ACE inhibitors, angiotensin II receptor antagonists, NSAIDs, potassium supplements, and potassium-sparing diuretics increase the risk of hyperkalemia; concomitant use with potassium supplements and potassium-sparing diuretics is contraindicated; monitor potassium levels with ACE inhibitors and angiotensin II receptor antagonists. Potent CYP3A4 inhibitors (eg, itraconazole, ketoconazole) lead to fivefold increase in eplerenone; concurrent use is contraindicated. Less potent CYP3A4 inhibitors (eg, erythromycin, fluconazole, saquinavir, verapamil) lead to approximately twofold increase in eplerenone; starting dose should be decreased to 25 mg/day. Although interaction studies have not been conducted, monitoring of lithium levels is recommended.

Decreased Effect: NSAIDs may decrease the antihypertensive effects of eplerenone. CYP3A4 inducers may decrease the levels/effects of eplerenone; example inducers include aminoglutethimide, carbamazepine, nafcillin, nevirapine, phenobarbital, phenytoin, and rifamycins.

Pharmacodynamics/Kinetics

Distribution: V_d: 43-90 L

Protein binding: ~50%; primarily to alpha$_1$-acid glycoproteins

Metabolism: Primarily hepatic via CYP3A4; metabolites inactive

Half-life elimination: 4-6 hours

Time to peak, plasma: 1.5 hours; may take up to 4 weeks for full therapeutic effect

Excretion: Urine (67%; <5% as unchanged drug), feces (32%)

Pregnancy Risk Factor B

EPO *see* Epoetin Alfa *on page 499*

Epoetin Alfa (e POE e tin AL fa)

U.S. Brand Names Epogen®; Procrit®

Canadian Brand Names Eprex®

Mexican Brand Names Epomax®; Eprex®

Generic Available No

Synonyms EPO; Erythropoietin; *r*HuEPO-α

Pharmacologic Category Colony Stimulating Factor

Use

Treatment of anemia related to zidovudine therapy in HIV-infected patients; in patients when the endogenous erythropoietin level is ≤500 mU/mL and the dose of zidovudine is ≤4200 mg/week

Treatment of anemia associated with chronic renal failure (CRF) including dialysis (end-stage renal disease, ESRD) and nondialysis patients. Prior to therapy, serum ferritin should be >100 ng/dL and transferrin saturation (serum iron/iron binding capacity x 100) of 20% to 30%; nondialysis patients should have a hematocrit <30%

Treatment of anemia in cancer patients on chemotherapy; in patients with nonmyeloid malignancies where anemia is caused by the effect of the

(Continued)

Epoetin Alfa *(Continued)*

concomitantly administered chemotherapy; to decrease the need for transfusions in patients who will be receiving chemotherapy for a minimum of 2 months

Reduction of allogeneic blood transfusion in surgery patients (with hemoglobin >10 g/dL up to 13 g/dL) scheduled to undergo elective, noncardiac, nonvascular surgery

Unlabeled/Investigational Use Anemia associated with rheumatic disease; hypogenerative anemia of Rh hemolytic disease; sickle cell anemia; acute renal failure; Gaucher's disease; Castleman's disease; paroxysmal nocturnal hemoglobinuria; anemia of critical illness (limited documentation); anemia of prematurity

Local Anesthetic/Vasoconstrictor Precautions No information available to require special precautions

Effects on Dental Treatment No significant effects or complications reported

Common Adverse Effects

>10%:

- Cardiovascular: Hypertension
- Central nervous system: Headache, fever
- Gastrointestinal: Nausea
- Neuromuscular & skeletal: Arthralgias

1% to 10%:

- Cardiovascular: Edema, chest pain
- Central nervous system: Fatigue, seizures
- Gastrointestinal: Vomiting, diarrhea
- Hematologic: Clotted access
- Neuromuscular & skeletal: Asthenia

Mechanism of Action Induces erythropoiesis by stimulating the division and differentiation of committed erythroid progenitor cells; induces the release of reticulocytes from the bone marrow into the bloodstream, where they mature to erythrocytes. There is a dose response relationship with this effect. This results in an increase in reticulocyte counts followed by a rise in hematocrit and hemoglobin levels.

Pharmacodynamics/Kinetics

Onset of action: Several days

Peak effect: 2-3 weeks

Distribution: V_d: 9 L; rapid in the plasma compartment; concentrated in liver, kidneys, and bone marrow

Metabolism: Some degradation does occur

Bioavailability: SubQ: ~21% to 31%; intraperitoneal epoetin: 3% (a few patients)

Half-life elimination: Circulating: Chronic renal failure: 4-13 hours; Healthy volunteers: 20% shorter

Time to peak, serum: SubQ: Chronic renal failure: 5-24 hours

Excretion: Feces (majority); urine (small amounts, 10% unchanged in normal volunteers)

Pregnancy Risk Factor C

Epogen® *see* Epoetin Alfa *on page 499*

Epoprostenol (e poe PROST en ole)

U.S. Brand Names Flolan®

Canadian Brand Names Flolan®

Generic Available No

Synonyms Epoprostenol Sodium; PGI_2; PGX; Prostacyclin

Pharmacologic Category Prostaglandin

Use Orphan drug: Treatment of primary pulmonary hypertension; treatment of secondary pulmonary hypertension due to intrinsic precapillary pulmonary vascular disease

Unlabeled/Investigational Use Other potential uses include pulmonary hypertension associated with ARDS, SLE, or CHF; neonatal pulmonary hypertension; cardiopulmonary bypass surgery; hemodialysis; atherosclerosis; peripheral vascular disorders; and neonatal purpura fulminans

Local Anesthetic/Vasoconstrictor Precautions No information available to require special precautions

Effects on Dental Treatment No significant effects or complications reported

Common Adverse Effects

>10%:

- Cardiovascular: Flushing, tachycardia, shock, syncope, heart failure
- Central nervous system: Fever, chills, anxiety, nervousness, dizziness, headache, hyperesthesia, pain

Gastrointestinal: Diarrhea, nausea, vomiting
Neuromuscular & skeletal: Jaw pain, myalgia, tremor, paresthesia
Respiratory: Hypoxia
Miscellaneous: Sepsis, flu-like symptoms

1% to 10%:

Cardiovascular: Bradycardia, hypotension, angina pectoris, edema, arrhythmias, pallor, cyanosis, palpitations, cerebrovascular accident, myocardial ischemia, chest pain
Central nervous system: Seizures, confusion, depression, insomnia
Dermatologic: Pruritus, rash
Endocrine & metabolic: Hypokalemia
Gastrointestinal: Abdominal pain, anorexia, constipation, weight change
Hematologic: Hemorrhage, disseminated intravascular coagulation
Hepatic: Ascites
Neuromuscular & skeletal: Arthralgias, bone pain, weakness
Ocular: Amblyopia
Respiratory: Cough increase, dyspnea, epistaxis, pleural effusion
Miscellaneous: Diaphoresis

Restrictions Orders for epoprostenol are distributed by two sources in the United States. Information on orders or reimbursement assistance may be obtained from either Accredo Health, Inc (1-800-935-6526) or TheraCom, Inc (1-877-356-5264).

Mechanism of Action Epoprostenol is also known as prostacyclin and PGI_2. It is a strong vasodilator of all vascular beds. In addition, it is a potent endogenous inhibitor of platelet aggregation. The reduction in platelet aggregation results from epoprostenol's activation of intracellular adenylate cyclase and the resultant increase in cyclic adenosine monophosphate concentrations within the platelets. Additionally, it is capable of decreasing thrombogenesis and platelet clumping in the lungs by inhibiting platelet aggregation.

Drug Interactions

Increased Effect/Toxicity: The hypotensive effects of epoprostenol may be exacerbated by other vasodilators, diuretics, or by using acetate in dialysis fluids. Patients treated with anticoagulants (heparins, warfarin, thrombin inhibitors) or antiplatelet agents (ticlopidine, clopidogrel, IIb/IIIa antagonists, aspirin) and epoprostenol should be monitored for increased bleeding risk.

Pharmacodynamics/Kinetics

Metabolism: Rapidly hydrolyzed at neutral pH in blood and subject to some enzymatic degradation to one active metabolite and 13 inactive metabolites
Half-life elimination: 2.7-6 minutes; Continuous infusion: ~15 minutes
Excretion: Urine (12% as unchanged drug)

Pregnancy Risk Factor B

Epoprostenol Sodium *see* Epoprostenol *on page 500*

Eprosartan (ep roe SAR tan)

Related Information

Cardiovascular Diseases *on page 1458*

U.S. Brand Names Teveten®

Canadian Brand Names Teveten®

Generic Available No

Pharmacologic Category Angiotensin II Receptor Blocker

Use Treatment of hypertension; may be used alone or in combination with other antihypertensives

Local Anesthetic/Vasoconstrictor Precautions No information available to require special precautions

Effects on Dental Treatment No significant effects or complications reported

Common Adverse Effects 1% to 10%:

Central nervous system: Fatigue (2%), depression (1%)
Endocrine & metabolic: Hypertriglyceridemia (1%)
Gastrointestinal: Abdominal pain (2%)
Genitourinary: Urinary tract infection (1%)
Respiratory: Upper respiratory tract infection (8%), rhinitis (4%), pharyngitis (4%), cough (4%)
Miscellaneous: Viral infection (2%), injury (2%)

Mechanism of Action Angiotensin II is formed from angiotensin I in a reaction catalyzed by angiotensin-converting enzyme (ACE, kininase II). Angiotensin II is the principal pressor agent of the renin-angiotensin system, with effects that include vasoconstriction, stimulation of synthesis and release of aldosterone, cardiac stimulation, and renal reabsorption of sodium. Eprosartan blocks the vasoconstrictor and aldosterone-secreting effects of angiotensin II by selectively blocking the binding of angiotensin II to the AT1 receptor in many (Continued)

Eprosartan *(Continued)*

tissues, such as vascular smooth muscle and the adrenal gland. Its action is therefore independent of the pathways for angiotensin II synthesis. Blockade of the renin-angiotensin system with ACE inhibitors, which inhibit the biosynthesis of angiotensin II from angiotensin I, is widely used in the treatment of hypertension. ACE inhibitors also inhibit the degradation of bradykinin, a reaction also catalyzed by ACE. Because eprosartan does not inhibit ACE (kininase II), it does not affect the response to bradykinin. Whether this difference has clinical relevance is not yet known. Eprosartan does not bind to or block other hormone receptors or ion channels known to be important in cardiovascular regulation.

Drug Interactions

Cytochrome P450 Effect: Inhibits CYP2C8/9 (weak)

Increased Effect/Toxicity: Eprosartan may increase risk of lithium toxicity. May increase risk of hyperkalemia with potassium-sparing diuretics (eg, amiloride, potassium, spironolactone, triamterene), potassium supplements, or high doses of trimethoprim.

Pharmacodynamics/Kinetics

Protein binding: 98%

Metabolism: Minimally hepatic

Bioavailability: 300 mg dose: 13%

Half-life elimination: Terminal: 5-9 hours

Time to peak, serum: Fasting: 1-2 hours

Excretion: Feces (90%); urine (7%, mostly as unchanged drug)

Clearance: 7.9 L/hour

Pregnancy Risk Factor C (1st trimester); D (2nd and 3rd trimesters)

Eprosartan and HCTZ *see* Eprosartan and Hydrochlorothiazide *on page 502*

Eprosartan and Hydrochlorothiazide

(ep roe SAR tan & hye droe klor oh THYE a zide)

U.S. Brand Names Teveten® HCT

Canadian Brand Names Teveten® HCT

Generic Available No

Synonyms Eprosartan and HCTZ; Eprosartan Mesylate and Hydrochlorothiazide; Hydrochlorothiazide and Eprosartan

Pharmacologic Category Angiotensin II Receptor Blocker Combination; Antihypertensive Agent, Combination; Diuretic, Thiazide

Use Treatment of hypertension (not indicated for initial treatment)

Local Anesthetic/Vasoconstrictor Precautions No information available to require special precautions

Effects on Dental Treatment No significant effects or complications reported

Common Adverse Effects Percentages reported with combination product; other reactions have been reported (see individual agents for additional information)

1% to 10%:

Central nervous system: Dizziness (4%), headache (3%), fatigue (2%)

Hematologic: Neutrophil count decreased (1%)

Neuromuscular & skeletal: Back pain (3%)

Renal: BUN elevated (1%)

Mechanism of Action Hydrochlorothiazide inhibits sodium reabsorption in the distal tubules causing increased excretion of sodium and water as well as potassium and hydrogen ions. **Eprosartan** blocks the vasoconstrictor and aldosterone-secreting effects of angiotensin II by selectively blocking the binding of angiotensin II to the AT1 receptor in many tissues, such as vascular smooth muscle and the adrenal gland.

Drug Interactions

Increased Effect/Toxicity: See individual agents.

Decreased Effect: See individual agents.

Pharmacodynamics/Kinetics See individual agents.

Pregnancy Risk Factor C/D (2nd and 3rd trimesters)

Eprosartan Mesylate and Hydrochlorothiazide *see* Eprosartan and Hydrochlorothiazide *on page 502*

Epsilon Aminocaproic Acid *see* Aminocaproic Acid *on page 97*

Epsom Salts *see* Magnesium Sulfate *on page 854*

EPT *see* Teniposide *on page 1269*

Eptacog Alfa (Activated) *see* Factor VIIa (Recombinant) *on page 571*

Eptifibatide (ep TIF i ba tide)

Related Information

Cardiovascular Diseases *on page 1458*

U.S. Brand Names Integrilin®

Canadian Brand Names Integrilin®

Generic Available No

Synonyms Intrifiban

Pharmacologic Category Antiplatelet Agent, Glycoprotein IIb/IIIa Inhibitor

Use Treatment of patients with acute coronary syndrome (UA/NQMI), including patients who are to be managed medically and those undergoing percutaneous coronary intervention (PCI including PTCA; intracoronary stenting)

Local Anesthetic/Vasoconstrictor Precautions No information available to require special precautions

Effects on Dental Treatment Key adverse event(s) related to dental treatment: Bleeding; patients weighing <70 kg may have an increased risk of major bleeding.

Common Adverse Effects Bleeding is the major drug-related adverse effect. Major bleeding was reported in 4.4% to 10.8%; minor bleeding was reported in 10.5% to 14.2%; requirement for transfusion was reported in 5.5% to 12.8%. Incidence of bleeding is also related to heparin intensity (aPTT goal 50-70 seconds). Patients weighing <70 kg may have an increased risk of major bleeding.

Cardiovascular: Hypotension

Local: Injection site reaction

Neuromuscular & skeletal: Back pain

1% to 10%: Hematologic: Thrombocytopenia (1.2% to 3.2%)

Mechanism of Action Eptifibatide is a cyclic heptapeptide which blocks the platelet glycoprotein IIb/IIIa receptor, the binding site for fibrinogen, von Willebrand factor, and other ligands. Inhibition of binding at this final common receptor reversibly blocks platelet aggregation and prevents thrombosis.

Drug Interactions

Increased Effect/Toxicity: Eptifibatide effect may be increased by other drugs which affect hemostasis include thrombolytics, oral anticoagulants, NSAIDs, dipyridamole, heparin, low molecular weight heparins, ticlopidine, and clopidogrel. Avoid concomitant use of other IIb/IIIa inhibitors. Cephalosporins which contain the MTT side chain may theoretically increase the risk of hemorrhage. Use with aspirin and heparin may increase bleeding over aspirin and heparin alone. However, aspirin and heparin were used concurrently in the majority of patients in the major clinical studies of eptifibatide.

Pharmacodynamics/Kinetics

Onset of action: Within 1 hour

Duration: Platelet function restored ~4 hours following discontinuation

Protein binding: ~25%

Half-life elimination: 2.5 hours

Excretion: Primarily urine (as eptifibatide and metabolites); significant renal impairment may alter disposition of this compound

Clearance: Total body: 55-58 mL/kg/hour; Renal: ~50% of total in healthy subjects

Pregnancy Risk Factor B

Equagesic® *see* Aspirin and Meprobamate *on page 156*

Equalactin® [OTC] *see* Polycarbophil *on page 1100*

Equanil *see* Meprobamate *on page 878*

Erbitux™ *see* Cetuximab *on page 300*

Ergamisol® *see* Levamisole *on page 806*

Ergocalciferol (er goe kal SIF e role)

U.S. Brand Names Calciferol™; Drisdol®

Canadian Brand Names Drisdol®; Ostoforte®

Generic Available Yes: Capsule

Synonyms Activated Ergosterol; Viosterol; Vitamin D_2

Pharmacologic Category Vitamin D Analog

Use Treatment of refractory rickets, hypophosphatemia, hypoparathyroidism; dietary supplement

Local Anesthetic/Vasoconstrictor Precautions No information available to require special precautions

(Continued)

Ergocalciferol *(Continued)*

Effects on Dental Treatment Key adverse event(s) related to dental treatment: Metallic taste and xerostomia (normal salivary flow resumes upon discontinuation).

Common Adverse Effects Generally well tolerated

Frequency not defined: Cardiac arrhythmias, hypertension (late), irritability, headache, psychosis (rare), somnolence, hyperthermia (late), pruritus, decreased libido (late), hypercholesterolemia, mild acidosis (late), polydipsia (late), nausea, vomiting, anorexia, pancreatitis, metallic taste, weight loss (rare), xerostomia, constipation, polyuria (late), increased BUN (late), increased LFTs (late), bone pain, myalgia, weakness, conjunctivitis, photophobia (late), vascular/nephrocalcinosis (rare)

Mechanism of Action Stimulates calcium and phosphate absorption from the small intestine, promotes secretion of calcium from bone to blood; promotes renal tubule phosphate resorption

Drug Interactions

Increased Effect/Toxicity: Thiazide diuretics may increase vitamin D effects. Cardiac glycosides may increase toxicity.

Decreased Effect: Cholestyramine, colestipol, mineral oil may decrease oral absorption.

Pharmacodynamics/Kinetics

Onset of action: Peak effect: ~1 month following daily doses

Absorption: Readily; requires bile

Metabolism: Inactive until hydroxylated hepatically and renally to calcifediol and then to calcitriol (most active form)

Pregnancy Risk Factor A/C (dose exceeding RDA recommendation)

Ergoloid Mesylates (ER goe loid MES i lates)

Canadian Brand Names Hydergine®

Generic Available Yes

Synonyms Dihydroergotoxine; Dihydrogenated Ergot Alkaloids; Hydergine [DSC]

Pharmacologic Category Ergot Derivative

Use Treatment of cerebrovascular insufficiency in primary progressive dementia, Alzheimer's dementia, and senile onset

Local Anesthetic/Vasoconstrictor Precautions No information available to require special precautions

Effects on Dental Treatment Key adverse event(s) related to dental treatment: Orthostatic hypotension.

Common Adverse Effects Adverse effects are minimal; most common include transient nausea, gastrointestinal disturbances and sublingual irritation with SL tablets; other common side effects include:

Cardiovascular: Orthostatic hypotension, bradycardia

Dermatologic: Skin rash, flushing

Ocular: Blurred vision

Respiratory: Nasal congestion

Mechanism of Action Ergoloid mesylates do not have the vasoconstrictor effects of the natural ergot alkaloids; exact mechanism in dementia is unknown; originally classed as peripheral and cerebral vasodilator, now considered a "metabolic enhancer"; there is no specific evidence which clearly establishes the mechanism by which ergoloid mesylate preparations produce mental effects, nor is there conclusive evidence that the drug particularly affects cerebral arteriosclerosis or cerebrovascular insufficiency

Drug Interactions

Cytochrome P450 Effect: Substrate of CYP3A4 (major)

Increased Effect/Toxicity: CYP3A4 inhibitors may increase the levels/effects of ergoloid mesylates; example inhibitors include azole antifungals, ciprofloxacin, clarithromycin, diclofenac, doxycycline, erythromycin, imatinib, isoniazid, nefazodone, nicardipine, propofol, protease inhibitors, quinidine, and verapamil. Ergot alkaloids are contraindicated with potent CYP3A4 inhibitors. Ergoloid mesylates may increase the effects of 5-HT_1 agonists (eg, sumatriptan), MAO inhibitors, sibutramine, and other serotonin agonists (serotonin syndrome). Severe vasoconstriction may occur when peripheral vasoconstrictors or beta-blockers are used in patients receiving ergot alkaloids; concurrent use is contraindicated.

Decreased Effect: Effects of ergoloid mesylates may be diminished by antipsychotics, metoclopramide. Antianginal effects of nitrates may be reduced by ergot alkaloids.

Pharmacodynamics/Kinetics
Absorption: Rapid yet incomplete
Half-life elimination, serum: 3.5 hours
Time to peak, serum: ~1 hour
Pregnancy Risk Factor C

Ergomar® *see* Ergotamine *on page 505*
Ergometrine Maleate *see* Ergonovine *on page 505*

Ergonovine (er goe NOE veen)

Generic Available No
Synonyms Ergometrine Maleate; Ergonovine Maleate
Pharmacologic Category Ergot Derivative
Use Prevention and treatment of postpartum and postabortion hemorrhage caused by uterine atony or subinvolution
Unlabeled/Investigational Use Migraine headaches, diagnostically to identify Prinzmetal's angina
Local Anesthetic/Vasoconstrictor Precautions No information available to require special precautions
Effects on Dental Treatment No significant effects or complications reported
Common Adverse Effects 1% to 10%: Gastrointestinal: Nausea, vomiting
Mechanism of Action Ergot alkaloid alpha-adrenergic agonist directly stimulates vascular smooth muscle to vasoconstrict peripheral and cerebral vessels; may also have antagonist effects on serotonin
Drug Interactions
Cytochrome P450 Effect: Substrate of CYP3A4 (major)
Increased Effect/Toxicity: CYP3A4 inhibitors may increase the levels/effects of ergonovine; example inhibitors include azole antifungals, ciprofloxacin, clarithromycin, diclofenac, doxycycline, erythromycin, imatinib, isoniazid, nefazodone, nicardipine, propofol, protease inhibitors, quinidine, and verapamil. Ergot alkaloids are contraindicated with potent CYP3A4 inhibitors. Ergonovine may increase the effects of 5-HT_1 agonists (eg, sumatriptan), MAO inhibitors, sibutramine, and other serotonin agonists (serotonin syndrome). Severe vasoconstriction may occur when peripheral vasoconstrictors or beta-blockers are used in patients receiving ergot alkaloids; concurrent use is contraindicated.
Decreased Effect: Effects of ergonovine may be diminished by antipsychotics, metoclopramide. Antianginal effects of nitrates may be reduced by ergot alkaloids.
Pharmacodynamics/Kinetics
Onset of action: I.M.: ~2-5 minutes
Duration: I.M.: Uterine effect: 3 hours; I.V.: ~45 minutes
Metabolism: Hepatic
Excretion: Primarily feces; urine
Pregnancy Risk Factor X

Ergonovine Maleate *see* Ergonovine *on page 505*

Ergotamine (er GOT a meen)

U.S. Brand Names Ergomar®
Generic Available No
Synonyms Ergotamine Tartrate
Pharmacologic Category Ergot Derivative
Use Abort or prevent vascular headaches, such as migraine, migraine variants, or so-called "histaminic cephalalgia"
Local Anesthetic/Vasoconstrictor Precautions No information available to require special precautions
Effects on Dental Treatment Key adverse event(s) related to dental treatment: Xerostomia and changes in salivation (normal salivary flow resumes upon discontinuation).
Common Adverse Effects Frequency not defined.
Cardiovascular: Absence of pulse, bradycardia, cardiac valvular fibrosis, cyanosis, edema, ECG changes, gangrene, hypertension, ischemia, precordial distress and pain, tachycardia, vasospasm
Central nervous system: Vertigo
Dermatologic: Itching
Gastrointestinal: Nausea, vomiting
Genitourinary: Retroperitoneal fibrosis
Neuromuscular & skeletal: Muscle pain, numbness, paresthesias, weakness
Respiratory: Pleuropulmonary fibrosis
Miscellaneous: Cold extremities
(Continued)

Ergotamine *(Continued)*

Mechanism of Action Has partial agonist and/or antagonist activity against tryptaminergic, dopaminergic and alpha-adrenergic receptors depending upon their site; is a highly active uterine stimulant; it causes constriction of peripheral and cranial blood vessels and produces depression of central vasomotor centers

Drug Interactions

Cytochrome P450 Effect: Substrate of CYP3A4 (major); Inhibits CYP3A4 (weak)

Increased Effect/Toxicity: CYP3A4 inhibitors may increase the levels/effects of ergotamine; example inhibitors include azole antifungals, ciprofloxacin, clarithromycin, diclofenac, doxycycline, erythromycin, imatinib, isoniazid, nefazodone, nicardipine, propofol, protease inhibitors, quinidine, and verapamil. Ergot alkaloids are contraindicated with strong CYP3A4 inhibitors. Ergotamine may increase the effects of 5-HT_1 agonists (eg, sumatriptan), MAO inhibitors, sibutramine, and other serotonin agonists (serotonin syndrome). Severe vasoconstriction may occur when peripheral vasoconstrictors or beta-blockers are used in patients receiving ergot alkaloids; concurrent use is contraindicated.

Decreased Effect: Effects of ergotamine may be diminished by antipsychotics, metoclopramide. Antianginal effects of nitrates may be reduced by ergot alkaloids.

Pharmacodynamics/Kinetics

Absorption: Oral: Erratic; enhanced by caffeine coadministration
Metabolism: Extensively hepatic
Time to peak, serum: 0.5-3 hours
Half-life elimination: 2 hours
Excretion: Feces (90% as metabolites)

Pregnancy Risk Factor X

Ergotamine and Caffeine (er GOT a meen & KAF een)

U.S. Brand Names Cafergot®; Wigraine®

Canadian Brand Names Cafergor®

Generic Available No

Synonyms Caffeine and Ergotamine; Ergotamine Tartrate and Caffeine

Pharmacologic Category Ergot Derivative; Stimulant

Use Abort or prevent vascular headaches, such as migraine, migraine variants, or so-called "histaminic cephalalgia"

Local Anesthetic/Vasoconstrictor Precautions No information available to require special precautions

Effects on Dental Treatment No significant effects or complications reported

Common Adverse Effects Frequency not defined.

Cardiovascular: Absence of pulse, bradycardia, cardiac valvular fibrosis, cyanosis, edema, ECG changes, gangrene, hypertension, ischemia, precordial distress and pain, tachycardia, vasospasm
Central nervous system: Vertigo
Dermatologic: Itching
Gastrointestinal: Anal or rectal ulcer (with overuse of suppository), nausea, vomiting
Genitourinary: Retroperitoneal fibrosis
Neuromuscular & skeletal: Muscle pain, numbness, paresthesias, weakness
Respiratory: Pleuropulmonary fibrosis
Miscellaneous: Cold extremities

Mechanism of Action Has partial agonist and/or antagonist activity against tryptaminergic, dopaminergic and alpha-adrenergic receptors depending upon their site; is a highly active uterine stimulant; it causes constriction of peripheral and cranial blood vessels and produces depression of central vasomotor centers

Drug Interactions

Cytochrome P450 Effect:

Ergotamine: **Substrate** of CYP3A4 (major); **Inhibits** CYP3A4 (weak)
Caffeine: **Substrate** of CYP1A2 (major), 2C8/9 (minor), 2D6 (minor), 2E1 (minor), 3A4 (minor); **Inhibits** CYP1A2 (weak), 3A4 (moderate)

Increased Effect/Toxicity: See Ergotamine monograph for related interactions. CYP1A2 inhibitors may increase the levels/effects of caffeine; example inhibitors include amiodarone, fluvoxamine, ketoconazole, quinolone antibiotics, and rofecoxib. CYP3A4 inhibitors may increase the levels/effects of ergotamine; example inhibitors include azole antifungals, ciprofloxacin, clarithromycin, diclofenac, doxycycline, erythromycin, imatinib, isoniazid, nefazodone, nicardipine, propofol, protease inhibitors, quinidine, and verapamil. Caffeine may increase the levels/effects of CYP3A4 substrates; example substrates include benzodiazepines, calcium channel blockers, ergot derivatives, mirtazapine, nateglinide, nefazodone, tacrolimus, and venlafaxine. Caffeine levels may be increased by quinolone antibiotics.

Decreased Effect: See Ergotamine monograph for related interactions.

Pharmacodynamics/Kinetics

Absorption: Ergotamine: Oral, rectal: Erratic; enhanced by caffeine coadministration

Metabolism: Extensively hepatic

Time to peak, serum: Ergotamine: 0.5-3 hours

Half-life elimination: 2 hours

Excretion: Feces (90% as metabolites)

Pregnancy Risk Factor X

Ergotamine Tartrate *see* Ergotamine *on page 505*

Ergotamine Tartrate and Caffeine *see* Ergotamine and Caffeine *on page 506*

Ergotamine Tartrate, Belladonna, and Phenobarbital *see* Belladonna, Phenobarbital, and Ergotamine *on page 186*

E•R•O [OTC] *see* Carbamide Peroxide *on page 259*

Errin™ *see* Norethindrone *on page 996*

Ertaczo™ *see* Sertaconazole *on page 1214*

Ertapenem (er ta PEN em)

U.S. Brand Names Invanz®

Canadian Brand Names Invanz®

Mexican Brand Names Invanz®

Generic Available No

Synonyms Ertapenem Sodium; L-749,345; MK0826

Pharmacologic Category Antibiotic, Carbapenem

Use Treatment of moderate-severe, complicated intra-abdominal infections, skin and skin structure infections, pyelonephritis, acute pelvic infections, and community-acquired pneumonia. Antibacterial coverage includes aerobic gram-positive organisms, aerobic gram-negative organisms, anaerobic organisms.

Note: Methicillin-resistant *Staphylococcus*, *Enterococcus* spp, penicillin-resistant strains of *Streptococcus pneumoniae,* beta-lactamase-positive strains of *Haemophilus influenzae* are **resistant** to ertapenem, as are most *Pseudomonas aeruginosa.*

Local Anesthetic/Vasoconstrictor Precautions No information available to require special precautions

Effects on Dental Treatment Key adverse event(s) related to dental treatment: Oral candidiasis.

Common Adverse Effects

1% to 10%:

Cardiovascular: Swelling/edema (3%), chest pain (1%), hypertension (0.7% to 2%), hypotension (1% to 2%), tachycardia (1% to 2%)

Central nervous system: Headache (6% to 7%), altered mental status (ie, agitation, confusion, disorientation, decreased mental acuity, changed mental status, somnolence, stupor) (3% to 5%), fever (2% to 5%), insomnia (3%), dizziness (2%), fatigue (1%), anxiety (0.8% to 1%)

Dermatologic: Rash (2% to 3%), pruritus (1% to 2%), erythema (1% to 2%)

Gastrointestinal: Diarrhea (9% to 10%), nausea (6% to 9%), abdominal pain (4%), vomiting (4%), constipation (3% to 4%), acid regurgitation (1% to 2%), dyspepsia (1%), oral candidiasis (0.1% to 1%)

Genitourinary: Vaginitis (1% to 3%)

Hematologic: Platelet count increased (4% to 7%), eosinophils increased (1% to 2%)

Hepatic: Hepatic enzyme elevations (7% to 9%), alkaline phosphatase increase (4% to 7%)

Local: Infused vein complications (5% to 7%), phlebitis/thrombophlebitis (1.5% to 2%), extravasation (0.7% to 2%)

Neuromuscular & skeletal: Leg pain (0.4% to 1%)

Respiratory: Dyspnea (1% to 3%), cough (1% to 2%), pharyngitis (0.7% to 1%), rales/rhonchi (0.5% to 1%), respiratory distress (0.2% to 1%)

Mechanism of Action Inhibits bacterial cell wall synthesis by binding to one or more of the penicillin binding proteins; which in turn inhibits the final transpeptidation step of peptidoglycan synthesis in bacterial cell walls, thus inhibiting cell wall biosynthesis. Bacteria eventually lyse due to ongoing activity of cell wall

(Continued)

Ertapenem *(Continued)*

autolytic enzymes (autolysins and murein hydrolases) while cell wall assembly is arrested.

Drug Interactions

Increased Effect/Toxicity: Probenecid decreases the renal clearance of ertapenem.

Pharmacodynamics/Kinetics

Absorption: I.M.: Almost complete

Distribution: V_{dss}: 8.2 L

Protein binding (concentration dependent): 85% at 300 mcg/mL, 95% at <100 mcg/mL

Metabolism: Hydrolysis to inactive metabolite

Bioavailability: I.M.: 90%

Half-life elimination: 4 hours

Time to peak: I.M.: 2.3 hours

Excretion: Urine (80% as unchanged drug and metabolite); feces (10%)

Pregnancy Risk Factor B

Ertapenem Sodium *see* Ertapenem *on page 507*

***Erwinia* Asparaginase** *see* Asparaginase *on page 150*

Eryc® *see* Erythromycin *on page 508*

Erycette® *see* Erythromycin *on page 508*

Eryderm® *see* Erythromycin *on page 508*

Erygel® *see* Erythromycin *on page 508*

EryPed® *see* Erythromycin *on page 508*

Ery-Tab® *see* Erythromycin *on page 508*

Erythra-Derm™ *see* Erythromycin *on page 508*

Erythrocin® *see* Erythromycin *on page 508*

Erythromycin (er ith roe MYE sin)

Related Information

Cardiovascular Diseases *on page 1458*

Oral Bacterial Infections *on page 1533*

Oral Viral Infections *on page 1547*

Respiratory Diseases *on page 1478*

Sexually-Transmitted Diseases *on page 1504*

U.S. Brand Names Akne-Mycin®; A/T/S®; E.E.S.®; Emgel®; Eryc®; Erycette®; Eryderm®; Erygel®; EryPed®; Ery-Tab®; Erythra-Derm™; Erythrocin®; PCE®; Romycin®; Staticin®; Theramycin Z®; T-Stat®

Canadian Brand Names Apo-Erythro Base®; Apo-Erythro E-C®; Apo-Erythro-ES®; Apo-Erythro-S®; Diomycin®; EES®; Erybid™; Eryc®; Erythromid®; Nu-Erythromycin-S; PCE®; PMS-Erythromycin; Sans Acne®

Mexican Brand Names Eryacnen®; Eryderm®; Ilosone®; Latotryd®; Lauricin®; Lauritran®; Optomicin®; Pantomicina®; Procephal®; Sans-Acne®; Stiemycin®

Generic Available Yes

Synonyms Erythromycin Base; Erythromycin Estolate; Erythromycin Ethylsuccinate; Erythromycin Gluceptate; Erythromycin Lactobionate; Erythromycin Stearate

Pharmacologic Category Antibiotic, Macrolide; Antibiotic, Ophthalmic; Antibiotic, Topical; Topical Skin Product; Topical Skin Product, Acne

Dental Use Systemic: Alternative to penicillin VK for treatment of orofacial infections

Use

Systemic: Treatment of susceptible bacterial infections including *S. pyogenes*, some *S. pneumoniae*, some *S. aureus, M. pneumoniae, Legionella pneumophila*, diphtheria, pertussis, chancroid, *Chlamydia*, erythrasma, *N. gonorrhoeae*, *E. histolytica*, syphilis and nongonococcal urethritis, and *Campylobacter* gastroenteritis; used in conjunction with neomycin for decontaminating the bowel

Ophthalmic: Treatment of superficial eye infections involving the conjunctiva or cornea; neonatal ophthalmia

Topical: Treatment of acne vulgaris

Unlabeled/Investigational Use Systemic: Treatment of gastroparesis

Local Anesthetic/Vasoconstrictor Precautions No information available to require special precautions

Effects on Dental Treatment Key adverse event(s) related to dental treatment: Oral candidiasis.

Significant Adverse Effects

Systemic:

Cardiovascular: Ventricular arrhythmias, QT_c prolongation, torsade de pointes (rare), ventricular tachycardia (rare)

Central nervous system: Headache (8%), pain (2%), fever, seizures

Dermatitis: Rash (3%), pruritus (1%)

Gastrointestinal: Abdominal pain (8%), cramping, nausea (8%), oral candidiasis, vomiting (3%), diarrhea (7%), dyspepsia (2%), flatulence (2%), anorexia, pseudomembranous colitis, hypertrophic pyloric stenosis (including cases in infants or IHPS), pancreatitis

Hematologic: Eosinophilia (1%)

Hepatic: Cholestatic jaundice (most common with estolate), increased liver function tests (2%)

Local: Phlebitis at the injection site, thrombophlebitis

Neuromuscular & skeletal: Weakness (2%)

Respiratory: Dyspnea (1%), cough (3%)

Miscellaneous: Hypersensitivity reactions, allergic reactions

Topical: 1% to 10%: Dermatologic: Erythema, desquamation, dryness, pruritus

Dosage

Neonates: Ophthalmic: Prophylaxis of neonatal gonococcal or chlamydial conjunctivitis: 0.5-1 cm ribbon of ointment should be instilled into each conjunctival sac

Infants and Children (**Note:** 400 mg ethylsuccinate = 250 mg base, stearate, or estolate salts):

Oral: 30-50 mg/kg/day divided every 6-8 hours; may double doses in severe infections

Preop bowel preparation: 20 mg/kg erythromycin base at 1, 2, and 11 PM on the day before surgery combined with mechanical cleansing of the large intestine and oral neomycin

I.V.: Lactobionate: 20-40 mg/kg/day divided every 6 hours

Adults:

Oral:

Base: 250-500 mg every 6-12 hours

Ethylsuccinate: 400-800 mg every 6-12 hours

Preop bowel preparation: Oral: 1 g erythromycin base at 1, 2, and 11 PM on the day before surgery combined with mechanical cleansing of the large intestine and oral neomycin

I.V.: Lactobionate: 15-20 mg/kg/day divided every 6 hours or 500 mg to 1 g every 6 hours, or given as a continuous infusion over 24 hours (maximum: 4 g/24 hours)

Children and Adults:

Ophthalmic: Instill ½" (1.25 cm) 2-6 times/day depending on the severity of the infection

Topical: Apply over the affected area twice daily after the skin has been thoroughly washed and patted dry

Dialysis: Slightly dialyzable (5% to 20%); no supplemental dosage necessary in hemo or peritoneal dialysis or in continuous arteriovenous or venovenous hemofiltration

Gastrointestinal prokinetic (unlabeled use): Adults: I.V., Oral: Erythromycin has been used as a prokinetic agent to improve gastric emptying time and intestinal motility. In adults, 200 mg was infused I.V. initially followed by 250 mg orally 3 times/day 30 minutes before meals. Lower dosages have been used in some trials.

Mechanism of Action Inhibits RNA-dependent protein synthesis at the chain elongation step; binds to the 50S ribosomal subunit resulting in blockage of transpeptidation

Contraindications Hypersensitivity to erythromycin or any component of the formulation

Systemic: Pre-existing liver disease (erythromycin estolate); concomitant use with ergot derivatives, pimozide, or cisapride; hepatic impairment

Warnings/Precautions Systemic: Hepatic impairment with or without jaundice has occurred, it may be accompanied by malaise, nausea, vomiting, abdominal colic, and fever; discontinue use if these occur; avoid using erythromycin lactobionate in neonates since formulations may contain benzyl alcohol which is associated with toxicity in neonates; observe for superinfections. Use in infants has been associated with infantile hypertrophic pyloric stenosis (IHPS). Macrolides have been associated with rare QT prolongation and ventricular arrhythmias, including torsade de pointes. Elderly may be at increased risk of adverse events, including hearing loss and/or torsade de pointes when dosage ≥4 g/day, particularly if concurrent renal/hepatic impairment.

(Continued)

Erythromycin *(Continued)*

Drug Interactions Substrate of CYP2B6 (minor), 3A4 (major); **Inhibits** CYP1A2 (weak), 3A4 (moderate)

Alfentanil (and possibly other narcotic analgesics): Serum levels may be increased by erythromycin; monitor for increased effect.

Antipsychotic agents (particularly mesoridazine and thioridazine): Risk of QT_c prolongation and malignant arrhythmias may be increased.

Benzodiazepines (those metabolized by CYP3A4, including alprazolam and triazolam): Serum levels may be increased by erythromycin; somnolence and confusion have been reported.

Bromocriptine: Serum levels may be increased by erythromycin; monitor for increased effect.

Buspirone: Serum levels may be increased by erythromycin; monitor.

Calcium channel blockers (felodipine, verapamil, and potentially others metabolized by CYP3A4): Serum levels may be increased by erythromycin; monitor.

Carbamazepine: Serum levels may be increased by erythromycin; monitor.

Cilostazol: Serum levels may be increased by erythromycin.

Cisapride: Serum levels may be increased by erythromycin; serious arrhythmias have occurred; concurrent use contraindicated.

Clindamycin (and lincomycin): Use with erythromycin may result in pharmacologic antagonism; manufacturer recommends avoiding this combination.

Clozapine: Serum levels may be increased by erythromycin; monitor.

Colchicine: serum levels/toxicity may be increased by erythromycin; monitor.

Cyclosporine: Serum levels may be increased by erythromycin; monitor serum levels.

CYP3A4 inducers: CYP3A4 inducers may decrease the levels/effects of erythromycin. Example inducers include aminoglutethimide, carbamazepine, nafcillin, nevirapine, phenobarbital, phenytoin, and rifamycins.

CYP3A4 inhibitors: May increase the levels/effects of erythromycin. Example inhibitors include azole antifungals, ciprofloxacin, clarithromycin, diclofenac, doxycycline, imatinib, isoniazid, nefazodone, nicardipine, propofol, protease inhibitors, quinidine, and verapamil.

CYP3A4 substrates: Erythromycin may increase the levels/effects of CYP3A4 substrates. Example substrates include benzodiazepines, calcium channel blockers, cyclosporine, mirtazapine, nateglinide, nefazodone, sildenafil (and other PDE-5 inhibitors), tacrolimus, and venlafaxine. Selected benzodiazepines (midazolam and triazolam), cisapride, ergot alkaloids, selected HMG-CoA reductase inhibitors (lovastatin and simvastatin), and pimozide are generally contraindicated with strong CYP3A4 inhibitors.

Delavirdine: Serum levels of erythromycin may be increased; also, serum levels of delavirdine may increased by erythromycin (low risk); monitor.

Digoxin: Serum levels may be increased by erythromycin; monitor digoxin levels.

Disopyramide: Serum levels may be increased by erythromycin; in addition, QT_c prolongation and risk of malignant arrhythmia may be increased; avoid combination.

Ergot alkaloids: Concurrent use may lead to acute ergot toxicity (severe peripheral vasospasm and dysesthesia).

HMG-CoA reductase inhibitors (atorvastatin, lovastatin, and simvastatin); Erythromycin may increase serum levels of "statins" metabolized by CYP3A4, increasing the risk of myopathy/rhabdomyolysis (does not include fluvastatin and pravastatin). Switch to pravastatin/fluvastatin or suspend treatment during course of erythromycin therapy.

Loratadine: Serum levels may be increased by erythromycin; monitor.

Methylprednisolone: Serum levels may be increased by erythromycin; monitor.

Neuromuscular-blocking agents: May be potentiated by erythromycin (case reports).

Phenytoin: Serum levels may be increased by erythromycin; other evidence suggested phenytoin levels may be decreased in some patients; monitor.

Pimozide: Serum levels may be increased, leading to malignant arrhythmias; concomitant use is contraindicated.

Protease inhibitors (amprenavir, nelfinavir, and ritonavir): May increase serum levels of erythromycin.

QT_c-prolonging agents: Concomitant use may increase the risk of malignant arrhythmias.

Quinidine: Serum levels may be increased by erythromycin; in addition, the risk of QT_c prolongation and malignant arrhythmias may be increased during concurrent use.

Quinolone antibiotics (sparfloxacin, gatifloxacin, and moxifloxacin): Concurrent use may increase the risk of malignant arrhythmias.

Rifabutin: Serum levels may be increased by erythromycin; monitor.

Sildenafil, tadalafil, vardenafil: Serum concentration may be substantially increased by erythromycin. Do not exceed single sildenafil doses of 25 mg in 48 hours, a single tadalafil dose of 10 mg in 72 hours, or a single vardenafil dose of 2.5 mg in 24 hours.

Tacrolimus: Serum levels may be increased by erythromycin; monitor serum concentration.

Theophylline: Serum levels may be increased by erythromycin; monitor.

Valproic acid (and derivatives): Serum levels may be increased by erythromycin; monitor.

Vinblastine (and vincristine): Serum levels may be increased by erythromycin.

Warfarin: Effects may be potentiated; monitor INR closely and adjust warfarin dose as needed or choose another antibiotic.

Zafirlukast: Serum levels may be decreased by erythromycin; monitor.

Zopiclone: Serum levels may be increased by erythromycin; monitor.

Ethanol/Nutrition/Herb Interactions

Ethanol: Avoid ethanol (may decrease absorption of erythromycin or enhance ethanol effects).

Food: Increased drug absorption with meals; erythromycin serum levels may be altered if taken with food.

Herb/Nutraceutical: St John's wort may decrease erythromycin levels.

Dietary Considerations Systemic: Drug may cause GI upset; may take with food.

Sodium content of oral suspension (ethylsuccinate) 200 mg/5 mL: 29 mg (1.3 mEq)

Sodium content of base Filmtab® 250 mg: 70 mg (3 mEq)

Pharmacodynamics/Kinetics

Absorption: Oral: Variable but better with salt forms than with base form; 18% to 45%; ethylsuccinate may be better absorbed with food

Distribution: Crosses placenta; enters breast milk

Relative diffusion from blood into CSF: Minimal even with inflammation

CSF:blood level ratio: Normal meninges: 1% to 12%; Inflamed meninges: 7% to 25%

Protein binding: 75% to 90%

Metabolism: Hepatic via demethylation

Half-life elimination: Peak: 1.5-2 hours; End-stage renal disease: 5-6 hours

Time to peak, serum: Base: 4 hours; Ethylsuccinate: 0.5-2.5 hours; delayed with food due to differences in absorption

Excretion: Primarily feces; urine (2% to 15% as unchanged drug)

Pregnancy Risk Factor B

Lactation Enters breast milk/compatible

Dosage Forms

Capsule, delayed release, enteric-coated pellets, as base (Eryc®): 250 mg

Gel, topical: 2% (30 g, 60 g)

A/T/S®: 2% (30 g)

Emgel®: 2% (27 g, 50 g)

Erygel®: 2% (30 g, 60 g)

Granules for oral suspension, as ethylsuccinate (E.E.S.®): 200 mg/5 mL (100 mL, 200 mL) [cherry flavor]

Injection, powder for reconstitution, as lactobionate (Erythrocin®): 500 mg, 1 g

Ointment, ophthalmic: 0.5% [5 mg/g] (1 g, 3.5 g)

Romycin®: 0.5% [5 mg/g] (3.5 g)

Ointment, topical (Akne-Mycin®): 2% (25 g)

Powder for oral suspension, as ethylsuccinate (EryPed®): 200 mg/5 mL (5 mL, 100 mL, 200 mL) [fruit flavor]; 400 mg/5 mL (5 mL, 60 mL, 100 mL, 200 mL) [banana flavor]

Powder for oral suspension, as ethylsuccinate [drops] (EryPed®): 100 mg/2.5 mL (50 mL) [fruit flavor]

Solution, topical: 1.5% (60 mL); 2% (60 mL)

A/T/S/®, Eryderm®, Erythra-Derm™, T-Stat®, Theramycin™ Z: 2% (60 mL)

Sans Acne®: 2% (60 mL) [contains ethyl alcohol 44%; available in Canada; not available in U.S.]

Staticin®: 1.5% (60 mL)

Suspension, oral, as estolate: 125 mg/5 mL (480 mL); 250 mg/5 mL (480 mL) [orange flavor]

Suspension, oral, as ethylsuccinate: 200 mg/5 mL (480 mL); 400 mg/5 mL (480 mL)

E.E.S.®: 200 mg/5 mL (100 mL, 480 mL) [fruit flavor]; 400 mg/5 mL (100 mL, 480 mL) [orange flavor]

Swab (Erycette®, T-Stat®): 2% (60s)

Tablet, chewable, as ethylsuccinate (EryPed®): 200 mg [fruit flavor]

(Continued)

Erythromycin *(Continued)*

Tablet, delayed release, enteric coated, as base (Ery-Tab®): 250 mg, 333 mg, 500 mg
Tablet [film coated], as base: 250 mg, 500 mg
Tablet [film coated], as ethylsuccinate (E.E.S.®): 400 mg
Tablet [film coated], as stearate (Erythrocin®): 250 mg, 500 mg
Tablet [polymer-coated particles], as base (PCE®): 333 mg, 500 mg

Comments Many patients cannot tolerate erythromycin because of abdominal pain and nausea; the mechanism of this adverse effect appears to be the motilin agonistic properties of erythromycin in the GI tract. For these patients, clindamycin is indicated as the alternative antibiotic for treatment of orofacial infections.

HMG-CoA reductase inhibitors, also known as the statins, effectively decrease the hepatic cholesterol biosynthesis resulting in the reduction of blood LDL-cholesterol concentrations. The AUC of atorvastatin (Lipitor®) was increased 33% by erythromycin administration. Combination of erythromycin and lovastatin (Mevacor®) has been associated with rhabdomyolysis (Ayanian, et al). The administration of erythromycin with cerivastatin (Baycol®) produced a 50% increase in area under the concentration curve for cerivastatin. The mechanism of erythromycin is inhibiting the CYP3A4 metabolism of atorvastatin, lovastatin, and cerivastatin. Simvastatin (Zocor®) would likely be affected in a similar manner by the coadministration of erythromycin. Clarithromycin (Biaxin®) may exert a similar effect as erythromycin on atorvastatin, lovastatin, cerivastatin, and simvastatin. Erythromycin 3 times/day had no effect on pravastatin (Pravachol®) plasma concentrations (Bottorff, et al).

Selected Readings

American Dental Association Council on Scientific Affairs, "Combating Antibiotic Resistance," *J Am Dent Assoc*, 2004, 135(4):484-7.

Ayanian JZ, Fuchs CS, and Stone RM, "Lovastatin and Rhabdomyolysis," *Ann Intern Med*, 1988, 109(8):682-3.

"Pimozide (Orap) Contraindicated With Clarithromycin (Biaxin®) and Other Macrolide Antibiotics," *FDA Medical Bulletin*, October 1996, 26(3).

Wynn RL and Bergman SA, "Antibiotics and Their Use in the Treatment of Orofacial Infections, Part I," *Gen Dent*, 1994, 42(5):398, 400, 402.

Wynn RL and Bergman SA, "Antibiotics and Their Use in the Treatment of Orofacial Infections, Part II," *Gen Dent*, 1994, 42(6):498-502.

Wynn RL, "Current Concepts of the Erythromycins," *Gen Dent*, 1991, 39(6):408,10-1.

Erythromycin and Benzoyl Peroxide

(er ith roe MYE sin & BEN zoe il per OKS ide)

Related Information

Benzoyl Peroxide *on page 194*
Erythromycin *on page 508*

U.S. Brand Names Benzamycin®; Benzamycin® Pak

Generic Available No

Synonyms Benzoyl Peroxide and Erythromycin

Pharmacologic Category Topical Skin Product; Topical Skin Product, Acne

Use Topical control of acne vulgaris

Local Anesthetic/Vasoconstrictor Precautions No information available to require special precautions

Effects on Dental Treatment No significant effects or complications reported

Drug Interactions

Cytochrome P450 Effect: Erythromycin: **Substrate** of CYP2B6 (minor), 3A4 (major); **Inhibits** CYP1A2 (weak), 3A4 (moderate)

Pharmacodynamics/Kinetics See individual agents.

Pregnancy Risk Factor C

Erythromycin and Sulfisoxazole

(er ith roe MYE sin & sul fi SOKS a zole)

Related Information

Erythromycin *on page 508*

U.S. Brand Names Eryzole®; Pediazole®

Canadian Brand Names Pediazole®

Generic Available Yes

Synonyms Sulfisoxazole and Erythromycin

Pharmacologic Category Antibiotic, Macrolide; Antibiotic, Macrolide Combination; Antibiotic, Sulfonamide Derivative

Use Treatment of susceptible bacterial infections of the upper and lower respiratory tract, otitis media in children caused by susceptible strains of *Haemophilus influenzae*, and many other infections in patients allergic to penicillin

Local Anesthetic/Vasoconstrictor Precautions No information available to require special precautions

Effects on Dental Treatment No significant effects or complications reported

Common Adverse Effects Frequency not defined.

Cardiovascular: Ventricular arrhythmias,
Central nervous system: Headache, fever
Dermatologic: Rash, Stevens-Johnson syndrome, toxic epidermal necrolysis
Gastrointestinal: Abdominal pain, cramping, nausea, vomiting, oral candidiasis, hypertrophic pyloric stenosis, diarrhea, pseudomembranous colitis
Hematologic: Agranulocytosis, aplastic anemia, eosinophilia
Hepatic: Hepatic necrosis, cholestatic jaundice
Local: Phlebitis at the injection site, thrombophlebitis
Renal: Toxic nephrosis, crystalluria
Miscellaneous: Hypersensitivity reactions

Mechanism of Action Erythromycin inhibits bacterial protein synthesis; sulfisoxazole competitively inhibits bacterial synthesis of folic acid from para-aminobenzoic acid

Drug Interactions

Cytochrome P450 Effect:

Erythromycin: **Substrate** of CYP2B6 (minor), 3A4 (major); **Inhibits** CYP1A2 (weak), 3A4 (moderate)
Sulfisoxazole: **Substrate** of CYP2C8/9 (major); **Inhibits** CYP2C8/9 (strong)

Increased Effect/Toxicity: See individual agents.

Decreased Effect: See individual agents.

Pharmacodynamics/Kinetics See individual agents (Erythromycin Systemic).

Pregnancy Risk Factor C

Erythromycin Base *see* Erythromycin *on page 508*
Erythromycin Estolate *see* Erythromycin *on page 508*
Erythromycin Ethylsuccinate *see* Erythromycin *on page 508*
Erythromycin Gluceptate *see* Erythromycin *on page 508*
Erythromycin Lactobionate *see* Erythromycin *on page 508*
Erythromycin Stearate *see* Erythromycin *on page 508*
Erythropoiesis Stimulating Protein *see* Darbepoetin Alfa *on page 399*
Erythropoietin *see* Epoetin Alfa *on page 499*
Eryzole® *see* Erythromycin and Sulfisoxazole *on page 512*

Escitalopram (es sye TAL oh pram)

Related Information

Citalopram *on page 339*

U.S. Brand Names Lexapro™

Generic Available No

Synonyms Escitalopram Oxalate; Lu-26-054; S-Citalopram

Pharmacologic Category Antidepressant, Selective Serotonin Reuptake Inhibitor

Use Treatment of major depressive disorder; generalized anxiety disorders (GAD)

Local Anesthetic/Vasoconstrictor Precautions Although caution should be used in patients taking tricyclic antidepressants, no interactions have been reported with vasoconstrictors and escitalopram, a nontricyclic antidepressant which acts to increase serotonin.

Effects on Dental Treatment Key adverse event(s) related to dental treatment: Xerostomia (normal salivary flow resumes upon discontinuation) and toothache.

Common Adverse Effects

>10%:

Central nervous system: Headache (24%), somnolence (6% to 13%), insomnia (9% to 12%)
Gastrointestinal: Nausea (15%)
Genitourinary: Ejaculation disorder (9% to 14%)

1% to 10%:

Cardiovascular: Chest pain, hypertension, palpitation
Central nervous system: Dizziness (5%), fatigue (5% to 8%), dreaming abnormal, concentration impaired, fever, irritability, lethargy, lightheadedness, migraine, vertigo, yawning
Dermatologic: Rash
Endocrine & metabolic: Libido decreased (3% to 7%), anorgasmia (2% to 6%), hot flashes, menstrual cramps, menstrual disorder

(Continued)

Escitalopram *(Continued)*

Gastrointestinal: Diarrhea (8%), xerostomia (6% to 9%), appetite decreased (3%), constipation (3% to 5%), indigestion (3%), abdominal pain (2%), abdominal cramps, appetite increased, flatulence, gastroenteritis, gastroesophageal reflux, heartburn, toothache, vomiting, weight gain/loss

Genitourinary: Impotence (3%), urinary tract infection, urinary frequency

Neuromuscular & skeletal: Arthralgia, limb pain, muscle cramp, myalgia, neck/shoulder pain, paresthesia, tremor

Ocular: Blurred vision

Otic: Earache, tinnitus

Respiratory: Rhinitis (5%), sinusitis (3%), bronchitis, coughing, nasal or sinus congestion, sinus headache

Miscellaneous: Diaphoresis (4% to 5%), flu-like syndrome (5%), allergy

Dosage Oral:

Adults: Depression, GAD: Initial: 10 mg/day; dose may be increased to 20 mg/day after at least 1 week

Elderly: 10 mg/day; bioavailability and half-life are increased by 50% in the elderly

Dosage adjustment in renal impairment:

Mild to moderate impairment: No dosage adjustment needed

Severe impairment: Cl_{cr} <20 mL/minute: Use caution

Dosage adjustment in hepatic impairment: 10 mg/day

Mechanism of Action Escitalopram is the S-enantiomer of the racemic derivative citalopram, which selectively inhibits the reuptake of serotonin with little to no effect on norepinephrine or dopamine reuptake. It has no or very low affinity for 5-HT_{1-7}, alpha- and beta-andrenergic, D_{1-5}, H_{1-3}, M_{1-5}, and benzodiazepine receptors. Escitalopram does not bind or has low affinity for Na^+, K^+, Cl^-, and Ca^{++} ion channels.

Contraindications Hypersensitivity to escitalopram, citalopram, or any component of the formulation; concomitant use or within 2 weeks of MAO inhibitors

Warnings/Precautions Potential for severe reaction when used with MAO inhibitors; serotonin syndrome (hyperthermia, muscular rigidity, mental status changes/agitation, autonomic instability) may occur. May precipitate a shift to mania or hypomania in patients with bipolar disorder. Monotherapy in patients with bipolar disorder should be avoided. Patients should be screened for bipolar disorder, since using antidepressants alone may induce manic episodes with this condition. Has a low potential to impair cognitive or motor performance; caution operating hazardous machinery or driving. The possibility of a suicide attempt is inherent in major depression and may persist until remission occurs. Monitor for worsening of depression or suicidality, especially during initiation of therapy or with dose increases or decreases. Worsening depression and severe abrupt suicidality that are not part of the presenting symptoms may require discontinuation or modification of drug therapy. Use caution in high-risk patients during initiation of therapy. Prescriptions should be written for the smallest quantity consistent with good patient care. Use caution with a previous seizure disorder or condition predisposing to seizures such as brain damage, alcoholism, or concurrent therapy with other drugs which lower the seizure threshold.

May cause hyponatremia/SIADH. May cause or exacerbate sexual dysfunction. Use caution with renal or liver impairment; concomitant CNS depressants; pregnancy (high doses of citalopram has been associated with teratogenicity in animals). Use caution with concomitant use of NSAIDs, ASA, or other drugs that affect coagulation; the risk of bleeding is potentiated. Safety and efficacy in pediatric patients have not been established.

Upon discontinuation of escitalopram therapy, gradually taper dose. If intolerable symptoms occur following a decrease in dosage or upon discontinuation of therapy, then resuming the previous dose with a more gradual taper should be considered. The patient's family or caregiver should be alerted to monitor patients for the emergence of suicidality and associated behaviors such as anxiety, agitation, panic attacks, insomnia, irritability, hostility, impulsivity, akathisia, hypomania, and mania; patients should be instructed not to abruptly discontinue this medication, but notify their healthcare provider if any of these symptoms or worsening depression occur.

Drug Interactions

Cytochrome P450 Effect: Substrate (major) of CYP2C19, 3A4; **Inhibits** CYP2D6 (weak)

Increased Effect/Toxicity: Escitalopram should not be used with nonselective MAO inhibitors (phenelzine, isocarboxazid) or other drugs with MAO inhibition (linezolid); fatal reactions have been reported. Wait 5 weeks after stopping escitalopram before starting a nonselective MAO inhibitor and 2

weeks after stopping an MAO inhibitor before starting escitalopram. Concurrent selegiline has been associated with mania, hypertension, or serotonin syndrome (risk may be reduced relative to nonselective MAO inhibitors).

CYP2C19 inhibitors may increase the levels/effects of imipramine; example inhibitors include delavirdine, fluconazole, fluvoxamine, gemfibrozil, isoniazid, omeprazole, and ticlopidine. CYP3A4 inhibitors may increase the levels/effects of escitalopram; example inhibitors include azole antifungals, ciprofloxacin, clarithromycin, diclofenac, doxycycline, erythromycin, imatinib, isoniazid, nefazodone, nicardipine, propofol, protease inhibitors, quinidine, and verapamil.

Combined use of SSRIs and buspirone, meperidine, moclobemide, nefazodone, other SSRIs, tramadol, trazodone, and venlafaxine may increase the risk of serotonin syndrome. Escitalopram increases serum levels/effects of CYP2D6 substrates (tricyclic antidepressants). Escitalopram may increase desipramine levels.

Combined use of sumatriptan (and other serotonin agonists) may result in toxicity; weakness, hyper-reflexia, and incoordination have been observed with sumatriptan and SSRIs. In addition, concurrent use may theoretically increase the risk of serotonin syndrome; includes sumatriptan, naratriptan, rizatriptan, and zolmitriptan.

Concomitant use of escitalopram and NSAIDs, aspirin, or other drugs affecting coagulation has been associated with an increased risk of bleeding; monitor.

Decreased Effect: CYP2C19 inducers may decrease the levels/effects of imipramine; example inducers include aminoglutethimide, carbamazepine, phenytoin, and rifampin. CYP3A4 inducers may decrease the levels/effects of escitalopram; example inducers include aminoglutethimide, carbamazepine, nafcillin, nevirapine, phenobarbital, phenytoin, and rifamycins.

Ethanol/Nutrition/Herb Interactions

Ethanol: Avoid ethanol (may increase CNS depression).

Herb/Nutraceutical: Avoid valerian, St John's wort, SAMe, kava kava, and gotu kola (may increase CNS depression).

Dietary Considerations May be taken with or without food.

Pharmacodynamics/Kinetics

Protein binding: 56% to plasma proteins

Metabolism: Hepatic via CYP2C19 and 3A4 to an active metabolite, S-desmethylcitalopram (S-DCT; 1/7 the activity); S-DCT is metabolized to S-didesmethylcitalopram (S-DDCT; active; 1/27 the activity) via CYP2D6

Half-life elimination: Escitalopram: 27-32 hours; S-desmethylcitalopram: 59 hours

Time to peak: Escitalopram: 5 ± 1.5 hours; S-desmethylcitalopram: 14 hours

Excretion: Urine (Escitalopram: 8%; S-DCT: 10%)

Clearance: Total body: 37-40 L/hour; Renal: Escitalopram: 2.7 L/hour; S-desmethylcitalopram: 6.9 L/hour

Pregnancy Risk Factor C

Dosage Forms SOLN, oral: 1 mg/mL (240 mL). **TAB:** 5 mg, 10 mg, 20 mg

Escitalopram Oxalate *see* Escitalopram *on page 513*

Esclim® *see* Estradiol *on page 518*

Eserine Salicylate *see* Physostigmine *on page 1084*

Esgic® *see* Butalbital, Acetaminophen, and Caffeine *on page 236*

Esgic-Plus™ *see* Butalbital, Acetaminophen, and Caffeine *on page 236*

Eskalith® *see* Lithium *on page 835*

Eskalith CR® *see* Lithium *on page 835*

Esmolol (ES moe lol)

U.S. Brand Names Brevibloc®

Canadian Brand Names Brevibloc®

Mexican Brand Names Brevibloc®

Generic Available No

Synonyms Esmolol Hydrochloride

Pharmacologic Category Antiarrhythmic Agent, Class II; Beta Blocker, Beta$_1$ Selective

Use Treatment of supraventricular tachycardia and atrial fibrillation/flutter (primarily to control ventricular rate); treatment of tachycardia and/or hypertension (especially intraoperative or postoperative)

Local Anesthetic/Vasoconstrictor Precautions No information available to require special precautions

(Continued)

Esmolol *(Continued)*

Effects on Dental Treatment Esmolol is a cardioselective beta-blocker. Local anesthetic with vasoconstrictor can be safely used in patients medicated with esmolol. Nonselective beta-blockers (ie, propranolol, nadolol) enhance the pressor response to epinephrine, resulting in hypertension and bradycardia; this has not been reported for esmolol. Many nonsteroidal anti-inflammatory drugs, such as ibuprofen and indomethacin, can reduce the hypotensive effect of beta-blockers after 3 or more weeks of therapy with the NSAID. Short-term NSAID use (ie, 3 days) requires no special precautions in patients taking beta-blockers.

Common Adverse Effects

>10%:

Cardiovascular: Asymptomatic hypotension (25%), symptomatic hypotension (12%)

Miscellaneous: Diaphoresis (10%)

1% to 10%:

Cardiovascular: Peripheral ischemia (1%)

Central nervous system: Dizziness (3%), somnolence (3%), confusion (2%), headache (2%), agitation (2%), fatigue (1%)

Gastrointestinal: Nausea (7%), vomiting (1%)

Local: Pain on injection (8%)

Mechanism of Action Class II antiarrhythmic: Competitively blocks response to $beta_1$-adrenergic stimulation with little or no effect of $beta_2$-receptors except at high doses, no intrinsic sympathomimetic activity, no membrane stabilizing activity

Drug Interactions

Increased Effect/Toxicity: Esmolol may increase the effect/toxicity of verapamil, and may increase potential for hypertensive crisis after or during withdrawal of either agent when combined with clonidine. Esmolol may extend the effect of neuromuscular blocking agents (succinylcholine). Esmolol may increase digoxin serum levels by 10% to 20% and may increase theophylline concentrations. Morphine may increase esmolol blood concentrations.

Decreased Effect: Decreased effect of beta-blockers with aluminum salts, barbiturates, calcium salts, cholestyramine, colestipol, NSAIDs, penicillins (ampicillin), rifampin, salicylates, and sulfinpyrazone due to decreased bioavailability and plasma levels. Beta-blockers may decrease the effect of sulfonylureas. Xanthines (eg, theophylline, caffeine) may decrease effects of esmolol.

Pharmacodynamics/Kinetics

Onset of action: Beta-blockade: I.V.: 2-10 minutes (quickest when loading doses are administered)

Duration: 10-30 minutes; prolonged following higher cumulative doses, extended duration of use

Protein binding: 55%

Metabolism: In blood by esterases

Half-life elimination: Adults: 9 minutes

Excretion: Urine (~69% as metabolites, 2% unchanged drug)

Pregnancy Risk Factor C (manufacturer); D (2nd and 3rd trimesters - expert analysis)

Esmolol Hydrochloride *see* Esmolol *on page 515*

Esomeprazole (es oh ME pray zol)

Related Information

Omeprazole *on page 1012*

U.S. Brand Names Nexium®

Canadian Brand Names Nexium®

Generic Available No

Synonyms Esomeprazole Magnesium

Pharmacologic Category Proton Pump Inhibitor; Substituted Benzimidazole

Use Short-term (4-8 weeks) treatment of erosive esophagitis; maintaining symptom resolution and healing of erosive esophagitis; treatment of symptomatic gastroesophageal reflux disease; as part of a multidrug regimen for *Helicobacter pylori* eradication in patients with duodenal ulcer disease (active or history of within the past 5 years)

Local Anesthetic/Vasoconstrictor Precautions No information available to require special precautions

Effects on Dental Treatment Key adverse event(s) related to dental treatment: Xerostomia (normal salivary flow resumes upon discontinuation).

Common Adverse Effects 1% to 10%:

Central nervous system: Headache (4% to 6%)

Gastrointestinal: Diarrhea (4%), nausea, flatulence, abdominal pain (4%), constipation, xerostomia

Dosage Note: Delayed-release capsules should be swallowed whole and taken at least 1 hour before eating

Children: Safety and efficacy have not been established in pediatric patients

Adults: Oral:

Erosive esophagitis (healing): 20-40 mg once daily for 4-8 weeks; maintenance: 20 mg once daily

Symptomatic GERD: 20 mg once daily for 4 weeks

Helicobacter pylori eradication: 40 mg once daily; requires combination therapy

Elderly: No dosage adjustment needed

Dosage adjustment in renal impairment: No dosage adjustment needed

Dosage adjustment in hepatic impairment:

Mild to moderate liver impairment (Child-Pugh Class A or B): No dosage adjustment needed

Severe liver impairment (Child-Pugh Class C): Dose should not exceed 20 mg/day

Mechanism of Action Proton pump inhibitor suppresses gastric acid secretion by inhibition of the H^+/K^+-ATPase in the gastric parietal cell

Contraindications Hypersensitivity to esomeprazole, substituted benzimidazoles (ie, lansoprazole, omeprazole, pantoprazole, rabeprazole), or any component of the formulation

Warnings/Precautions Relief of symptoms does not preclude the presence of a gastric malignancy. Atrophic gastritis (by biopsy) has been noted with long-term omeprazole therapy; this may also occur with esomeprazole. No reports of enterochromaffin-like (ECL) cell carcinoids, dysplasia, or neoplasia has occurred. Safety and efficacy in pediatric patients have not been established.

Drug Interactions

Cytochrome P450 Effect: Substrate of CYP2C19 (major), 3A4 (minor)

Increased Effect/Toxicity: Esomeprazole and omeprazole may increase the levels of benzodiazepines metabolized by oxidation (eg, diazepam, midazolam, triazolam) and carbamazepine.

Decreased Effect: CYP2C19 inducers may decrease the levels/effects of esomeprazole; example inducers include aminoglutethimide, carbamazepine, phenytoin, and rifampin. Proton pump inhibitors may decrease the absorption of atazanavir, indinavir, iron salts, itraconazole, and ketoconazole.

Ethanol/Nutrition/Herb Interactions Food: Absorption is decreased by 43% to 53% when taken with food.

Dietary Considerations Take at least 1 hour before meals; best if taken before breakfast.

Pharmacodynamics/Kinetics

Distribution: V_{dss}: 16 L

Protein binding: 97%

Metabolism: Hepatic via CYP2C19 and 3A4 enzymes to hydroxy, desmethyl, and sulfone metabolites (all inactive)

Bioavailability: 90% with repeat dosing

Half-life elimination: 1-1.5 hours

Time to peak: 1.5 hours

Excretion: Urine (80%); feces (20%)

Pregnancy Risk Factor B

Dosage Forms CAP, delayed release: 20 mg, 40 mg

Esomeprazole Magnesium *see* Esomeprazole *on page 516*

Esoterica® Regular [OTC] *see* Hydroquinone *on page 719*

Especol® [OTC] *see* Fructose, Dextrose, and Phosphoric Acid *on page 638*

Estar® [OTC] *see* Coal Tar *on page 367*

Estazolam (es TA zoe lam)

U.S. Brand Names ProSom®

Mexican Brand Names Tasedan®

Generic Available Yes

Pharmacologic Category Benzodiazepine

Use Short-term management of insomnia

Local Anesthetic/Vasoconstrictor Precautions No information available to require special precautions

(Continued)

Estazolam *(Continued)*

Effects on Dental Treatment Key adverse event(s) related to dental treatment: Significant xerostomia (normal salivary flow resumes upon discontinuation).

Common Adverse Effects

>10%:

Central nervous system: Somnolence

Neuromuscular & skeletal: Weakness

1% to 10%:

Cardiovascular: Flushing, palpitations

Central nervous system: Anxiety, confusion, dizziness, hypokinesia, abnormal coordination, hangover effect, agitation, amnesia, apathy, emotional lability, euphoria, hostility, seizure, sleep disorder, stupor, twitch

Dermatologic: Dermatitis, pruritus, rash, urticaria

Gastrointestinal: Xerostomia, constipation, decreased appetite, flatulence, gastritis, increased appetite, perverse taste

Genitourinary: Frequent urination, menstrual cramps, urinary hesitancy, urinary frequency, vaginal discharge/itching

Neuromuscular & skeletal: Paresthesia

Ocular: Photophobia, eye pain, eye swelling

Respiratory: Cough, dyspnea, asthma, rhinitis, sinusitis

Miscellaneous: Diaphoresis

Restrictions C-IV

Mechanism of Action Binds to stereospecific benzodiazepine receptors on the postsynaptic GABA neuron at several sites within the central nervous system, including the limbic system, reticular formation. Enhancement of the inhibitory effect of GABA on neuronal excitability results by increased neuronal membrane permeability to chloride ions. This shift in chloride ions results in hyperpolarization (a less excitable state) and stabilization.

Drug Interactions

Cytochrome P450 Effect: Substrate of CYP3A4 (minor)

Increased Effect/Toxicity: Sedative effects and/or respiratory depression may be additive with CNS depressants; includes ethanol, barbiturates, narcotic analgesics, and other sedative agents; monitor for increased effect. Levodopa therapeutic effects may be diminished in some patients following the addition of a benzodiazepine; limited/inconsistent data. Oral contraceptives may decrease the clearance of some benzodiazepines (those which undergo oxidative metabolism); monitor for increased benzodiazepine effect. Theophylline may partially antagonize some of the effects of benzodiazepines; monitor for decreased response; may require higher doses for sedation.

Pharmacodynamics/Kinetics

Onset of action: ~1 hour

Duration: Variable

Metabolism: Extensively hepatic

Half-life elimination: 10-24 hours (no significant changes in elderly)

Time to peak, serum: 0.5-1.6 hours

Excretion: Urine (<5% as unchanged drug)

Pregnancy Risk Factor X

Esterified Estrogen and Methyltestosterone *see* Estrogens (Esterified) and Methyltestosterone *on page 530*

Esterified Estrogens *see* Estrogens (Esterified) *on page 529*

Estrace® *see* Estradiol *on page 518*

Estraderm® *see* Estradiol *on page 518*

Estradiol (es tra DYE ole)

Related Information

Endocrine Disorders and Pregnancy *on page 1481*

Rheumatoid Arthritis, Osteoarthritis, and Osteoporosis *on page 1490*

U.S. Brand Names Alora®; Climara®; Delestrogen®; Depo®-Estradiol; Esclim®; Estrace®; Estraderm®; Estrasorb™; Estring®; EstroGel®; Femring™; Gynodiol®; Menostar™; Vagifem®; Vivelle®; Vivelle-Dot®

Canadian Brand Names Climara®; Delestrogen®; Depo®-Estradiol; Estrace®; Estraderm®; Estradot®; Estring®; EstroGel®; Oesclim®; Vagifem®; Vivelle®

Mexican Brand Names Climaderm®; Estraderm TTS®; Ginedisc®; Systen®

Generic Available Yes: Oral tablet, patch

Synonyms Estradiol Acetate; Estradiol Cypionate; Estradiol Hemihydrate; Estradiol Transdermal; Estradiol Valerate

Pharmacologic Category Estrogen Derivative

Use Treatment of moderate-to-severe vasomotor symptoms associated with menopause; treatment of vulvar and vaginal atrophy; hypoestrogenism (due to hypogonadism, castration, or primary ovarian failure); prostatic cancer (palliation), breast cancer (palliation), osteoporosis (prophylaxis); abnormal uterine bleeding due to hormonal imbalance; postmenopausal urogenital symptoms of the lower urinary tract (urinary urgency, dysuria)

Local Anesthetic/Vasoconstrictor Precautions No information available to require special precautions

Effects on Dental Treatment No significant effects or complications reported

Common Adverse Effects Frequency not defined.

Cardiovascular: Edema, hypertension, MI, venous thromboembolism

Central nervous system: Anxiety, dizziness, epilepsy exacerbation, headache, irritability, mental depression, migraine, mood disturbances, nervousness

Dermatologic: Chloasma, erythema multiforme, erythema nodosum, hemorrhagic eruption, hirsutism, loss of scalp hair, melasma, rash, pruritus

Endocrine & metabolic: Breast enlargement, breast tenderness, changes in libido, increased thyroid-binding globulin, increased total thyroid hormone (T_4), increased serum triglycerides/phospholipids, increased HDL-cholesterol, decreased LDL-cholesterol, impaired glucose tolerance, hypercalcemia

Gastrointestinal: Abdominal cramps, abdominal pain, bloating, cholecystitis, cholelithiasis, diarrhea, flatulence, gallbladder disease, nausea, pancreatitis, vomiting, weight gain/loss

Genitourinary: Alterations in frequency and flow of menses, changes in cervical secretions, endometrial cancer, increased size of uterine leiomyomata, Pap smear suspicious, vaginal candidiasis

Vaginal: Trauma from applicator insertion may occur in women with severely atrophic vaginal mucosa

Hematologic: Aggravation of porphyria, antithrombin III and antifactor Xa decreased, levels of fibrinogen increased, platelet aggregability increased and platelet count; increased prothrombin and factors VII, VIII, IX, X

Hepatic: Cholestatic jaundice

Local: Transdermal patches: Burning, erythema, irritation, thrombophlebitis

Neuromuscular & skeletal: Chorea, back pain

Ocular: Intolerance to contact lenses, steeping of corneal curvature

Respiratory: Pulmonary thromboembolism

Miscellaneous: Anaphylactoid/anaphylactic reactions, carbohydrate intolerance

Mechanism of Action Estrogens are responsible for the development and maintenance of the female reproductive system and secondary sexual characteristics. Estradiol is the principle intracellular human estrogen and is more potent than estrone and estriol at the receptor level; it is the primary estrogen secreted prior to menopause. Following menopause, estrone and estrone sulfate are more highly produced. Estrogens modulate the pituitary secretion of gonadotropins, luteinizing hormone, and follicle-stimulating hormone through a negative feedback system; estrogen replacement reduces elevated levels of these hormones in postmenopausal women.

Drug Interactions

Cytochrome P450 Effect: Substrate of CYP1A2 (major), 2A6 (minor), 2B6 (minor), 2C8/9 (minor), 2C19 (minor), 2D6 (minor), 2E1 (minor), 3A4 (major); **Inhibits** CYP1A2 (weak); **Induces** CYP3A4 (weak)

Increased Effect/Toxicity: Estradiol with hydrocortisone increases corticosteroid toxic potential. Anticoagulants and estradiol increase the potential for thromboembolic events.

Decreased Effect: CYP1A2 inducers may decrease the levels/effects of estradiol; example inducers include aminoglutethimide, carbamazepine, phenobarbital, and rifampin. CYP3A4 inducers may decrease the levels/effects of estradiol; example inducers include aminoglutethimide, carbamazepine, nafcillin, nevirapine, phenobarbital, phenytoin, and rifamycins.

Pharmacodynamics/Kinetics

Absorption: Oral, topical: Well absorbed

Distribution: Crosses placenta; enters breast milk

Protein binding: 37% to sex hormone-binding globulin; 61% to albumin

Metabolism: Hepatic via oxidation and conjugation in GI tract; hydroxylated via CYP3A4 to metabolites; first-pass effect; enterohepatic recirculation; reversibly converted to estrone and estriol

Excretion: Primarily urine (as metabolites estrone and estriol); feces (small amounts)

Pregnancy Risk Factor X

Estradiol Acetate *see* Estradiol *on page 518*

Estradiol and Medroxyprogesterone

(es tra DYE ole & me DROKS ee proe JES te rone)

Related Information

Endocrine Disorders and Pregnancy *on page 1481*
Estradiol *on page 518*

U.S. Brand Names Lunelle™

Synonyms E_2C and MPA; Medroxyprogesterone Acetate and Estradiol Cypionate

Pharmacologic Category Contraceptive; Estrogen and Progestin Combination

Use Prevention of pregnancy

Local Anesthetic/Vasoconstrictor Precautions No information available to require special precautions

Effects on Dental Treatment Since this is a combination estrogen-progesterone product, when prescribing antibiotics, patient must be warned to use additional methods of birth control if on hormonal contraceptives.

Common Adverse Effects Frequency not defined.

Cardiovascular: Arterial thromboembolism, cerebral hemorrhage, cerebral thrombosis, edema, hypertension, mesenteric thrombosis, myocardial infarction

Central nervous system: Dizziness, emotional lability, headache, mental depression, migraine, nervousness, premenstrual syndrome

Dermatologic: Acne, alopecia, erythema multiforme, erythema nodosum, hirsutism, melasma, rash (allergic)

Endocrine & metabolic: Amenorrhea, breast enlargement, breast secretion, breast tenderness/pain, decreased lactation (immediately postpartum), decreased libido/libido changes, dysmenorrhea, menorrhagia, metrorrhagia, temporary infertility following discontinuation

Gastrointestinal: Abdominal pain, appetite changes, enlarged abdomen, colitis, gallbladder disease, nausea, weight gain/loss (weight gain was the most common reason for discontinuing medication)

Genitourinary: Cervical changes, cystitis-like syndrome, vaginal moniliasis, vaginitis, vulvovaginal disorder

Hematologic: Hemolytic uremic syndrome, hemorrhagic eruption, porphyria

Hepatic: Budd-Chiari syndrome, hepatic adenoma, benign hepatic tumor

Local: Thrombophlebitis

Neuromuscular & skeletal: Weakness

Ocular: Cataracts, intolerance to contact lenses, retinal thrombosis

Renal: Impaired renal function

Respiratory: Pulmonary thromboembolism

Miscellaneous: Anaphylaxis, carbohydrate intolerance

Mechanism of Action Inhibits secretion of gonadotropins, leading to prevention of follicular maturation and ovulation. Also leads to thickening and reduction in volume of cervical mucus (decreases sperm penetration) and thinning of endometrium (reduces possibility of implantation).

Drug Interactions

Cytochrome P450 Effect:

Estradiol: **Substrate** of CYP1A2 (major), 2A6 (minor), 2B6 (minor), 2C8/9 (minor), 2C19 (minor), 2D6 (minor), 2E1 (minor), 3A4 (major); **Inhibits** CYP1A2 (weak); **Induces** CYP3A4 (weak)

Medroxyprogesterone: **Substrate** of CYP3A4 (major); **Induces** CYP3A4 (weak)

Increased Effect/Toxicity: Estradiol may inhibit metabolism of cyclosporine, prednisolone, and theophylline, leading to increased plasma levels.

Decreased Effect: Estradiol may decrease plasma levels of acetaminophen, clofibrate, morphine, salicylic acid, and temazepam. CYP3A4 inducers may decrease the levels/effects of medroxyprogesterone; example inducers include aminoglutethimide, carbamazepine, nafcillin, nevirapine, phenobarbital, phenytoin, and rifamycins. Griseofulvin, penicillins, and tetracyclines have been shown to alter pharmacokinetics of oral contraceptives leading to pregnancy; effects are not consistent with synthetic steroids. Aminoglutethimide and phenylbutazone may decrease contraceptive effectiveness and increase menstrual irregularities. St John's wort may induce hepatic enzymes resulting in decreased effect of contraceptive and breakthrough bleeding.

Pharmacodynamics/Kinetics

Absorption: Prolonged

Protein binding: 17-β-estradiol: 97% to sex hormone-binding globulin and albumin; MPA: 86% to albumin

Metabolism: Hepatic; estradiol via CYP1A2, 3A4, and 3A5-7 to estrone and estriol
Half-life elimination: Mean: 17 β-estradiol: 8.4 days; MPA: 14.7 days
Time to peak: 17 β-estradiol: 1-7 days; MPA: 1-10 days
Excretion: Urine
Pregnancy Risk Factor X

Estradiol and NGM *see* Estradiol and Norgestimate *on page 521*

Estradiol and Norethindrone (es tra DYE ole & nor eth IN drone)

Related Information
Estradiol *on page 518*
Norethindrone *on page* [illegible]96

U.S. Brand Names Activella™; CombiPatch®
Canadian Brand Names Estalis®; Estalis-Sequi®
Generic Available No
Synonyms Norethindrone and Estradiol
Pharmacologic Category Estrogen and Progestin Combination
Use Women with an intact uterus:
Tablet: Treatment of moderate-to-severe vasomotor symptoms associated with menopause; treatment of vulvar and vaginal atrophy; prophylaxis for postmenopausal osteoporosis
Transdermal patch: Treatment of moderate-to-severe vasomotor symptoms; treatment of vulvar and vaginal atrophy; treatment of hypoestrogenism due to hypogonadism, castration, or primary ovarian failure

Local Anesthetic/Vasoconstrictor Precautions No information available to require special precautions
Effects on Dental Treatment No significant effects or complications reported
Common Adverse Effects Frequency not defined.
Cardiovascular: Altered blood pressure, cardiovascular accident, edema, venous thromboembolism
Central nervous system: Dizziness, fatigue, headache, insomnia, mental depression, migraine, nervousness
Dermatologic: Chloasma, erythema multiforme, erythema nodosum, hemorrhagic eruption, hirsutism, itching, loss of scalp hair, melasma, pruritus, skin rash
Endocrine & metabolic: Breast enlargement, breast tenderness, breast pain, changes in libido
Gastrointestinal: Abdominal pain, bloating, changes in appetite, flatulence, gallbladder disease, nausea, pancreatitis, vomiting, weight gain/loss
Genitourinary: Alterations in frequency and flow of menses, changes in cervical secretions, cystitis-like syndrome, increased size of uterine leiomyomata, premenstrual-like syndrome, vaginal candidiasis, vaginitis
Hematologic: Aggravation of porphyria
Hepatic: Cholestatic jaundice
Local: Application site reaction (transdermal patch)
Neuromuscular & skeletal: Arthralgia, back pain, chorea, myalgia, weakness
Ocular: Intolerance to contact lenses, steeping of corneal curvature
Respiratory: Pharyngitis, pulmonary thromboembolism, rhinitis
Miscellaneous: Allergic reactions, carbohydrate intolerance, flu-like syndrome

Drug Interactions
Cytochrome P450 Effect:
Estradiol: **Substrate** of CYP1A2 (major), 2A6 (minor), 2B6 (minor), 2C8/9 (minor), 2C19 (minor), 2D6 (minor), 2E1 (minor), 3A4 (major); **Inhibits** CYP1A2 (weak); **Induces** CYP3A4 (weak)
Norethindrone: **Substrate** of CYP3A4 (major); **Induces** CYP2C19 (weak)

Pharmacodynamics/Kinetics
Activella™:
Bioavailability: Estradiol: 50%; Norethindrone: 100%
Half-life elimination: Estradiol: 12-14 hours; Norethindrone: 8-11 hours
Time to peak: Estradiol: 5-8 hours
See individual agents.
Pregnancy Risk Factor X

Estradiol and Norgestimate (es tra DYE ole & nor JES ti mate)

Related Information
Estradiol *on page 518*
U.S. Brand Names Prefest™
Generic Available No
Synonyms Estradiol and NGM; Norgestimate and Estradiol; Ortho Prefest
(Continued)

Estradiol and Norgestimate *(Continued)*

Pharmacologic Category Estrogen and Progestin Combination

Use Women with an intact uterus: Treatment of moderate to severe vasomotor symptoms associated with menopause; treatment of atrophic vaginitis; prevention of osteoporosis

Local Anesthetic/Vasoconstrictor Precautions No information available to require special precautions

Effects on Dental Treatment No significant effects or complications reported

Common Adverse Effects

>10%:

Central nervous system: Headache (23%)
Endocrine & metabolic: Breast pain (16%)
Gastrointestinal: Abdominal pain (12%)
Neuromuscular & skeletal: Back pain (12%)
Respiratory: Upper respiratory tract infection [illegible]
Miscellaneous: Flu-like symptoms (11%)

1% to 10%:

Central nervous system: Fatigue (6%), pain [illegible] depression [illegible] ness (5%)
Endocrine & metabolic: Vaginal bleeding (9%) [illegible] (7%)
Gastrointestinal: Nausea (6%), flatulence [illegible]
Neuromuscular & skeletal: Arthralgia [illegible] (5%)
Respiratory: Sinusitis (8%), pha[illegible]
Miscellaneous: Viral infe[illegible]

Additional adverse effects associated with e[illegible]s and progestins; frequency not defined:

Cardiovascular: Edema, hypertension, MI, stro[illegible]ous thrombosis
Central nervous system: Anxiety, epilepsy exace[illegible], insomnia, irritability, migraine, mood disturbances, nervousness, p[illegible], somnolence
Dermatologic: Acne, chloasma, erythema multif[illegible], erythema nodosum, hemorrhagic eruptions, hirsutism, itching, mela[illegible], pruritus, rash, scalp hair loss, urticaria
Endocrine & metabolic: Amenorrhea, breast canc[illegible]east discharge, breast enlargement, breast tenderness, carbohydrate t[illegible]ance decreased, endometrial cancer, endometrial hyperplasia, fibrocy[illegible] breast changes, galactorrhea, hypocalcemia, libido changes, ovar[illegible] cancer, triglycerides increased
Gastrointestinal: Abdominal cramps, appetite chan[illegible]s, bloating, gallbladder disease, pancreatitis, vomiting, weight gain/loss
Genitourinary: Abnormal withdrawal bleeding/flow, breakthrough bleeding, cervical secretion changes, cystitis syndrome, uterine leiomyomata size increased, vaginal candidiasis, vaginal bleeding/spotting
Hematologic: Anemia, porphyria
Hepatic: Cholestatic jaundice
Local: Thrombophlebitis
Neuromuscular & skeletal: Chorea
Ocular: Contact lens intolerance, corneal curvature steepening, neuro-ocular lesions
Respiratory: Asthma exacerbation, pulmonary embolism
Miscellaneous: Anaphylaxis

Mechanism of Action Estrogens are responsible for the development and maintenance of the female reproductive system and secondary sexual characteristics. Estradiol is the principle intracellular human estrogen and is more potent than estrone and estriol at the receptor level; it is the primary estrogen secreted prior to menopause. Following menopause, estrone and estrone sulfate are more highly produced. Estrogens modulate the pituitary secretion of gonadotropins, luteinizing hormone, and follicle-stimulating hormone through a negative feedback system; estrogen replacement reduces elevated levels of these hormones in postmenopausal women.

Progestins inhibit gonadotropin production which then prevents follicular maturation and ovulation. In women with adequate estrogen, progestins transform a proliferative endometrium into a secretory endometrium; when administered with estradiol, reduces the incidence of endometrial hyperplasia and risk of adenocarcinoma.

Drug Interactions

Cytochrome P450 Effect:

Estradiol: **Substrate** of CYP1A2 (major), 2A6 (minor), 2B6 (minor), 2C8/9 (minor), 2C19 (minor), 2D6 (minor), 2E1 (minor), 3A4 (major); **Inhibits** CYP1A2 (weak); **Induces** CYP3A4 (weak)

Increased Effect/Toxicity: Acetaminophen and ascorbic acid plasma levels of estrogen component. Atorvastatin and indina plasma levels of estrogen/progestin combinations. Estrogen/ combinations increase the plasma levels of alprazolam, chlordiaz cyclosporine, diazepam, prednisolone, selegiline, theophylline, tricycl depressants. Estrogen/progestin combinations may increase (or decre the effects of coumarin derivatives.

Decreased Effect: Estrogen/progestin combinations may decrease plasma levels of acetaminophen, clofibric acid, lorazepam, morphine, oxazepam, salicylic acid, temazepam. Estrogen/progestin levels decreased by aminoglutethimide, amprenavir, anticonvulsants, griseofulvin, lopinavir, nelfinavir, nevirapine, rifampin, and ritonavir. Estrogen/progestin combinations may decrease (or increase) the effects of coumarin derivatives.

Pharmacodynamics/Kinetics

Estradiol: See Estradiol monograph.

Norgestimate:

Protein binding: 17-deacetylnorgestimate: 99%

Metabolism: Forms 17-deacetylnorgestimate (major active metabolite) and other metabolites; first-pass effect

Half-life elimination: 17-deacetylnorgestimate: 37 hours

Excretion: Norgestimate metabolites: Urine and feces

Pregnancy Risk Factor X

Estradiol Cypionate *see* Estradiol *on page 518*

Estradiol Hemihydrate *see* Estradiol *on page 518*

Estradiol Transdermal *see* Estradiol *on page 518*

Estradiol Valerate *see* Estradiol *on page 518*

Estramustine (es tra MUS teen)

U.S. Brand Names Emcyt®

Canadian Brand Names Emcyt®

Generic Available No

Synonyms Estramustine Phosphate Sodium; NSC-89199

Pharmacologic Category Antineoplastic Agent, Alkylating Agent; Antineoplastic Agent, Hormone; Antineoplastic Agent, Hormone (Estrogen/Nitrogen Mustard)

Use Palliative treatment of prostatic carcinoma (progressive or metastatic)

Local Anesthetic/Vasoconstrictor Precautions No information available to require special precautions

Effects on Dental Treatment No significant effects or complications reported

Common Adverse Effects

>10%:

Cardiovascular: Impaired arterial circulation; ischemic heart disease; venous thromboembolism; cardiac decompensation (58%), about 50% of complications occur within the first 2 months of therapy, 85% occur within the first year; edema

Endocrine & metabolic: Sodium and water retention, gynecomastia, breast tenderness, libido decreased

Gastrointestinal: Nausea, vomiting, may be dose-limiting

Hematologic: Thrombocytopenia

Local: Thrombophlebitis (nearly 100% with I.V. administration)

Respiratory: Dyspnea

1% to 10%:

Cardiovascular: Myocardial infarction

Central nervous system: Insomnia, lethargy

Gastrointestinal: Diarrhea, anorexia, flatulence

Hematologic: Leukopenia

Hepatic: Serum transaminases increased, jaundice

Neuromuscular & skeletal: Leg cramps

Respiratory: Pulmonary embolism

Mechanism of Action Mechanism is not completely clear. It appears to bind to microtubule proteins, preventing normal tubulin function. The antitumor effect may be due solely to an estrogenic effect. Estramustine causes a marked decrease in plasma testosterone and an increase in estrogen levels.

Drug Interactions

Decreased Effect: Milk products and calcium-rich foods/drugs may impair the oral absorption of estramustine phosphate sodium.

Pharmacodynamics/Kinetics

Absorption: Oral: 75%

Metabolism:

GI tract: Initial dephosphorylation

(Continued)

stine *(Continued)*

tic: Oxidation and hydrolysis; metabolites include estramustine, strone, estradiol, nitrogen mustard
-life elimination: Terminal: 20-24 hours
me to peak, serum: 2-3 hours
Excretion: Feces (2.9% to 4.8% as unchanged drug)

Pregnancy Risk Factor C

Estramustine Phosphate Sodium *see* Estramustine *on page 523*

Estrasorb™ *see* Estradiol *on page 518*

Estratest® *see* Estrogens (Esterified) and Methyltestosterone *on page 530*

Estratest® H.S. *see* Estrogens (Esterified) and Methyltestosterone *on page 530*

Estring® *see* Estradiol *on page 518*

EstroGel® *see* Estradiol *on page 518*

Estrogenic Substances, Conjugated *see* Estrogens (Conjugated/Equine) *on page 525*

Estrogens (Conjugated A/Synthetic)

(ES troe jenz, KON joo gate ed, aye, sin THET ik)

Related Information
Endocrine Disorders and Pregnancy *on page 1481*

U.S. Brand Names Cenestin®

Generic Available No

Pharmacologic Category Estrogen Derivative

Use Treatment of moderate to severe vasomotor symptoms of menopause; treatment of vulvar and vaginal atrophy

Local Anesthetic/Vasoconstrictor Precautions No information available to require special precautions

Effects on Dental Treatment No significant effects or complications reported

Common Adverse Effects Adverse effects associated with estrogen therapy; frequency not defined

Cardiovascular: Edema, hypertension, venous thromboembolism
Central nervous system: Dizziness, headache, mental depression, migraine
Dermatologic: Chloasma, erythema multiforme, erythema nodosum, hemorrhagic eruption, hirsutism, loss of scalp hair, melasma
Endocrine & metabolic: Breast enlargement, breast tenderness, changes in libido, thyroid-binding globulin increased, total thyroid hormone (T_4) increased, serum triglycerides/phospholipids increased, HDL-cholesterol increased, LDL-cholesterol decreased, impaired glucose tolerance, hypercalcemia
Gastrointestinal: Abdominal cramps, bloating, cholecystitis, cholelithiasis, gallbladder disease, nausea, pancreatitis, vomiting, weight gain/loss
Genitourinary: Alterations in frequency and flow of menses, changes in cervical secretions, endometrial cancer, increased size of uterine leiomyomata, vaginal candidiasis
Hematologic: Aggravation of porphyria, antithrombin III and antifactor Xa decreased, levels of fibrinogen decreased, platelet aggregability and platelet count increased; prothrombin and factors VII, VIII, IX, X increased
Hepatic: Cholestatic jaundice
Neuromuscular & skeletal: Chorea
Ocular: Intolerance to contact lenses, steeping of corneal curvature
Respiratory: Pulmonary thromboembolism
Miscellaneous: Carbohydrate intolerance

Mechanism of Action Conjugated A/synthetic estrogens contain a mixture of 9 synthetic estrogen substances, including sodium estrone sulfate, sodium equilin sulfate, sodium 17 alpha-dihydroequilin, sodium 17 alpha-estradiol and sodium 17 beta-dihydroequilin. Estrogens are responsible for the development and maintenance of the female reproductive system and secondary sexual characteristics. Estradiol is the principle intracellular human estrogen and is more potent than estrone and estriol at the receptor level; it is the primary estrogen secreted prior to menopause. Following menopause, estrone and estrone sulfate are more highly produced. Estrogens modulate the pituitary secretion of gonadotropins, luteinizing hormone, and follicle-stimulating hormone through a negative feedback system; estrogen replacement reduces elevated levels of these hormones in postmenopausal women.

Drug Interactions

Cytochrome P450 Effect:
Based on estradiol and estrone: **Substrate** of CYP1A2 (major), 2A6 (minor), 2B6 (minor), 2C8/9 (minor), 2C19 (minor), 2D6 (minor), 2E1 (minor), 3A4 (major); **Inhibits** CYP1A2 (weak); **Induces** CYP3A4 (weak)

Increased Effect/Toxicity: CYP3A4 enzyme inhibitors may increase estrogen plasma concentrations leading to increased incidence of adverse effects; examples of CYP3A4 enzyme inhibitors include clarithromycin, erythromycin, itraconazole, ketoconazole, and ritonavir. Anticoagulants increase the potential for thromboembolic events Estrogens may enhance the effects of hydrocortisone and prednisone

Decreased Effect: CYP1A2 inducers may decrease the levels/effects of estrogens; example inducers include aminoglutethimide, carbamazepine, phenobarbital, and rifampin. CYP3A4 inducers may decrease the levels/effects of estrogen; example inducers include aminoglutethimide, carbamazepine, nafcillin, nevirapine, phenobarbital, phenytoin, and rifamycins.

Pharmacodynamics/Kinetics

Absorption: Readily absorbed

Protein-binding: Sex hormone-binding globulin (SHBG) and albumin

Metabolism: Hepatic to metabolites

Time to peak: 4-16 hours

Excretion: Urine

Pregnancy Risk Factor X

Estrogens (Conjugated/Equine)

(ES troe jenz KON joo gate ed, EE kwine)

Related Information

Endocrine Disorders and Pregnancy *on page 1481*

U.S. Brand Names Premarin®

Canadian Brand Names Cenestin; C.E.S.®; Congest; Premarin®

Generic Available No

Synonyms CEE; C.E.S.; Estrogenic Substances, Conjugated

Pharmacologic Category Estrogen Derivative

Use Treatment of moderate to severe vasomotor symptoms associated with menopause; treatment of vulvar and vaginal atrophy; hypoestrogenism (due to hypogonadism, castration, or primary ovarian failure); prostatic cancer (palliation); breast cancer (palliation); osteoporosis (prophylaxis, postmenopausal women at significant risk only); abnormal uterine bleeding

Unlabeled/Investigational Use Uremic bleeding

Local Anesthetic/Vasoconstrictor Precautions No information available to require special precautions

Effects on Dental Treatment No significant effects or complications reported

Common Adverse Effects

Note: Percentages reported in postmenopausal women.

>10%:

Central nervous system: Headache (26% to 32%; placebo 28%)
Endocrine & metabolic: Breast pain (7% to 12%; placebo 9%)
Gastrointestinal: Abdominal pain (15% to 17%)
Genitourinary: Vaginal hemorrhage (2% to 14%)
Neuromuscular & skeletal: Back pain (13% to 14%)

1% to 10%:

Central nervous system: Nervousness (2% to 5%)
Endocrine & metabolic: Leukorrhea (4% to 7%)
Gastrointestinal: Flatulence (6% to 7%)
Genitourinary: Vaginitis (5% to 7%), vaginal moniliasis (5% to 6%)
Neuromuscular & skeletal: Weakness (7% to 8%), leg cramps (3% to 7%)

In addition, the following have been reported with estrogen and/or progestin therapy:

Cardiovascular: Edema, hypertension, myocardial infarction, stroke, venous thromboembolism

Central nervous system: Dizziness, epilepsy exacerbation, headache, irritability, mental depression, migraine, mood disturbances, nervousness

Dermatologic: Angioedema, chloasma, erythema multiforme, erythema nodosum, hemorrhagic eruption, hirsutism, loss of scalp hair, melasma, pruritus, rash, urticaria

Endocrine & metabolic: Breast cancer, breast enlargement, breast tenderness, changes in libido, increased thyroid-binding globulin, increased total thyroid hormone (T_4), increased serum triglycerides/phospholipids, increased HDL-cholesterol, decreased LDL-cholesterol, impaired glucose tolerance, hypercalcemia, hypocalcemia

Gastrointestinal: Abdominal cramps, bloating, cholecystitis, cholelithiasis, gallbladder disease, nausea, pancreatitis, vomiting, weight gain/loss

Genitourinary: Alterations in frequency and flow of menses, changes in cervical secretions, endometrial cancer, endometrial hyperplasia, increased size of uterine leiomyomata, vaginal candidiasis

(Continued)

Estrogens (Conjugated/Equine) *(Continued)*

Hematologic: Aggravation of porphyria, decreased antithrombin III and antifactor Xa, increased levels of fibrinogen, increased platelet aggregability and platelet count; increased prothrombin and factors VII, VIII, IX, X
Hepatic: Cholestatic jaundice, hepatic hemangiomas enlarged
Neuromuscular & skeletal: Arthralgias, chorea, leg cramps
Local: Thrombophlebitis
Ocular: Intolerance to contact lenses, retinal vascular thrombosis, steeping of corneal curvature
Respiratory: Asthma exacerbation, pulmonary thromboembolism
Miscellaneous: Anaphylactoid/anaphylactic reactions, carbohydrate intolerance

Dosage Adults:

Male: Androgen-dependent prostate cancer: Oral: 1.25-2.5 mg 3 times/day

Female:

Prevention of osteoporosis in postmenopausal women: Oral: Initial: 0.3 mg/day cyclically* or daily, depending on medical assessment of patient. Dose may be adjusted based on bone mineral density and clinical response. The lowest effective dose should be used.

Moderate to severe vasomotor symptoms associated with menopause: Oral: Initial: 0.3 mg/day, cyclically* or daily, depending on medical assessment of patient. The lowest dose that will control symptoms should be used. Medication should be discontinued as soon as possible.

Vulvar and vaginal atrophy:

Oral: Initial: 0.3 mg/day; the lowest dose that will control symptoms should be used. May be given cyclically* or daily, depending on medical assessment of patient. Medication should be discontinued as soon as possible.

Vaginal cream: Intravaginal: ½ to 2 g/day given cyclically*

Abnormal uterine bleeding:

Acute/heavy bleeding:

Oral (unlabeled route): 1.25 mg, may repeat every 4 hours for 24 hours, followed by 1.25 mg once daily for 7-10 days

I.M., I.V.: 25 mg, may repeat in 6-12 hours if needed

Note: Treatment should be followed by a low-dose oral contraceptive; medroxyprogesterone acetate along with or following estrogen therapy can also be given

Nonacute/lesser bleeding: Oral (unlabeled route): 1.25 mg once daily for 7-10 days

Female hypogonadism: Oral: 0.3-0.625 mg/day given cyclically*; dose may be titrated in 6- to 12-month intervals; progestin treatment should be added to maintain bone mineral density once skeletal maturity is achieved.

Female castration, primary ovarian failure: Oral: 1.25 mg/day given cyclically*; adjust according to severity of symptoms and patient response. For maintenance, adjust to the lowest effective dose.

***Cyclic administration:** Either 3 weeks on, 1 week off **or** 25 days on, 5 days off

Male and Female:

Breast cancer palliation, metastatic disease in selected patients: Oral: 10 mg 3 times/day for at least 3 months

Uremic bleeding (unlabeled use): I.V.: 0.6 mg/kg/day for 5 days

Elderly: Refer to Adults dosing; a higher incidence of stroke and invasive breast cancer was observed in women >75 years in a WHI substudy.

Mechanism of Action Conjugated estrogens contain a mixture of estrone sulfate, equilin sulfate, 17 alpha-dihydroequilin, 17 alpha-estradiol and 17 beta-dihydroequilin. Estrogens are responsible for the development and maintenance of the female reproductive system and secondary sexual characteristics. Estradiol is the principle intracellular human estrogen and is more potent than estrone and estriol at the receptor level; it is the primary estrogen secreted prior to menopause. Following menopause, estrone and estrone sulfate are more highly produced. Estrogens modulate the pituitary secretion of gonadotropins, luteinizing hormone, and follicle-stimulating hormone through a negative feedback system; estrogen replacement reduces elevated levels of these hormones in postmenopausal women.

Contraindications Hypersensitivity to estrogens or any component of the formulation; undiagnosed abnormal vaginal bleeding; history of or current thrombophlebitis or venous thromboembolic disorders (including DVT, PE); active or recent (within 1 year) arterial thromboembolic disease (eg, stroke, MI); carcinoma of the breast (except in appropriately selected patients being treated for metastatic disease); estrogen-dependent tumor; hepatic dysfunction or disease; pregnancy

Warnings/Precautions

Cardiovascular-related considerations: Estrogens with or without progestin should not be used to prevent coronary heart disease. Use caution with cardiovascular disease or dysfunction. May increase the risks of hypertension, myocardial infarction (MI), stroke, pulmonary emboli (PE), and deep vein thrombosis; incidence of these effects was shown to be significantly increased in postmenopausal women using conjugated equine estrogens (CEE) in combination with medroxyprogesterone acetate (MPA). Nonfatal MI, PE, and thrombophlebitis have also been reported in males taking high doses of CEE (eg, for prostate cancer). Estrogen compounds are generally associated with lipid effects such as increased HDL-cholesterol and decreased LDL-cholesterol. Triglycerides may also be increased; use with caution in patients with familial defects of lipoprotein metabolism. Whenever possible, estrogens should be discontinued at least 4-6 weeks prior to surgeries associated with an increased risk of thromboembolism or during periods of prolonged immobilization.

Neurological considerations: The risk of dementia may be increased in postmenopausal women; increased incidence was observed in women ≥65 years of age taking CEE in combination with MPA.

Cancer-related considerations: Unopposed estrogens may increase the risk of endometrial carcinoma in postmenopausal women. Estrogens may increase the risk of breast cancer. An increased risk of invasive breast cancer was observed in postmenopausal women using CEE in combination with MPA; a smaller increase in risk was seen with estrogen therapy alone in observational studies. An increase in abnormal mammograms has also been reported with estrogen and progestin therapy. Estrogen use may lead to severe hypercalcemia in patients with breast cancer and bone metastases; discontinue estrogen if hypercalcemia occurs.

Estrogens may cause retinal vascular thrombosis; discontinue permanently if papilledema or retinal vascular lesions are observed on examination. Use with caution in patients with diseases which may be exacerbated by fluid retention, including asthma, epilepsy, migraine, diabetes or renal dysfunction. Use with caution in patients with a history of severe hypocalcemia, SLE, hepatic hemangiomas, porphyria, endometriosis, and gallbladder disease. Use caution with history of cholestatic jaundice associated with past estrogen use or pregnancy. Safety and efficacy in pediatric patients have not been established. Prior to puberty, estrogens may cause premature closure of the epiphyses, premature breast development in girls or gynecomastia in boys. Vaginal bleeding and vaginal cornification may also be induced in girls.

Before prescribing estrogen therapy to postmenopausal women, the risks and benefits must be weighed for each patient. Women should be informed of these risks and benefits, as well as possible effects of progestin when added to estrogen therapy. Estrogens with or without progestin should be used for shortest duration possible consistent with treatment goals. Conduct periodic risk:benefit assessments.

When used solely for prevention of osteoporosis in women at significant risk, nonestrogen treatment options should be considered. When used solely for the treatment of vulvar and vaginal atrophy, topical vaginal products should be considered. Use caution applying topical products to severely atrophic vaginal mucosa.

Drug Interactions

Cytochrome P450 Effect:

Based on estradiol and estrone: **Substrate** of CYP1A2 (major), 2A6 (minor), 2B6 (minor), 2C8/9 (minor), 2C19 (minor), 2D6 (minor), 2E1 (minor), 3A4 (major); Inhibits CYP1A2 (weak); Induces CYP3A4 (weak)

Increased Effect/Toxicity: Hydrocortisone taken with estrogen may cause corticosteroid-induced toxicity. Increased potential for thromboembolic events with anticoagulants.

Decreased Effect: CYP1A2 inducers may decrease the levels/effects of estrogens; example inducers include aminoglutethimide, carbamazepine, phenobarbital, and rifampin. CYP3A4 inducers may decrease the levels/effects of estrogens; example inducers include aminoglutethimide, carbamazepine, nafcillin, nevirapine, phenobarbital, phenytoin, and rifamycins.

Ethanol/Nutrition/Herb Interactions

Ethanol: Avoid ethanol (routine use increases estrogen level and risk of breast cancer). Ethanol may also increase the risk of osteoporosis.

Food: Folic acid absorption may be decreased.

(Continued)

Estrogens (Conjugated/Equine) *(Continued)*

Herb/Nutraceutical: St John's wort may decrease levels. Avoid black cohosh, dong quai (has estrogenic activity). Avoid red clover, saw palmetto, ginseng (due to potential hormonal effects).

Dietary Considerations Ensure adequate calcium and vitamin D intake when used for the prevention of osteoporosis.

Pharmacodynamics/Kinetics

Absorption: Well absorbed

Metabolism: Hepatic via CYP3A4; estradiol is converted to estrone and estriol; also undergoes enterohepatic recirculation; estrone sulfite is the main metabolite in postmenopausal women

Excretion: Urine (primarily estrone, also as estradiol, estriol and conjugates)

Pregnancy Risk Factor X

Dosage Forms CRM, vaginal: 0.625 mg/g (42.5 g). **INJ, powder for reconstitution:** 25 mg. **TAB:** 0.3 mg, 0.45 mg, 0.625 mg, 0.9 mg, 1.25 mg

Estrogens (Conjugated/Equine) and Medroxyprogesterone

(ES troe jenz KON joo gate ed/EE kwine & me DROKS ee proe JES te rone)

Related Information

Endocrine Disorders and Pregnancy *on page 1481*

U.S. Brand Names Premphase®; Prempro™

Canadian Brand Names Premphase®; Premplus®; Prempro™

Generic Available No

Synonyms Medroxyprogesterone and Estrogens (Conjugated); MPA and Estrogens (Conjugated)

Pharmacologic Category Estrogen and Progestin Combination

Use Women with an intact uterus: Treatment of moderate to severe vasomotor symptoms associated with menopause; treatment of atrophic vaginitis; osteoporosis (prophylaxis)

Local Anesthetic/Vasoconstrictor Precautions No information available to require special precautions

Effects on Dental Treatment No significant effects or complications reported

Common Adverse Effects

>10%:

- Central nervous system: Headache (28% to 37%), pain (11% to 13%), depression (6% to 11%)
- Endocrine & metabolic: Breast pain (32% to 38%), dysmenorrhea (8% to 13%)
- Gastrointestinal: Abdominal pain (16% to 23%), nausea (9% to 11%)
- Neuromuscular & skeletal: Back pain (13% to 16%)
- Respiratory: Pharyngitis (11% to 13%)
- Miscellaneous: Infection (16% to 18%), flu-like syndrome (10% to 13%)

1% to 10%:

- Cardiovascular: Peripheral edema (3% to 4%)
- Central nervous system: Dizziness (3% to 5%)
- Dermatologic: Pruritus (5% to 10%), rash (4% to 6%)
- Endocrine & metabolic: Leukorrhea (5% to 9%)
- Gastrointestinal: Flatulence (8% to 9%), diarrhea (5% to 6%), dyspepsia (5% to 6%)
- Genitourinary: Vaginitis (5% to 7%), cervical changes (4% to 5%), vaginal hemorrhage (1% to 3%)
- Neuromuscular & skeletal: Weakness (6% to 10%), arthralgia (7% to 9%), leg cramps (3% to 5%), hypertonia (3% to 4%)
- Respiratory: Sinusitis (7% to 8%), rhinitis (6% to 8%)

Additional adverse effects reported with conjugated estrogens and/or progestins: Abdominal cramps, acne, abnormal uterine bleeding, aggravation of porphyria, amenorrhea, anaphylactoid reactions, anaphylaxis, antifactor Xa decreased, antithrombin III decreased, appetite changes, bloating, breast enlargement, breast tenderness, cerebral embolism, cerebral thrombosis, chloasma, cholestatic jaundice, cholecystitis, cholelithiasis, chorea, contact lens intolerance, cystitis-like syndrome, decreased carbohydrate tolerance, dizziness; factors VII, VIII, IX, X, XII, VII-X complex, and II-VII-X complex increased; endometrial hyperplasia, erythema multiforme, erythema nodosum, galactorrhea, hemorrhagic eruption, fatigue, fibrinogen increased, impaired glucose tolerance, HDL-cholesterol increased, hirsutism, hypertension, increase in size of uterine leiomyomata, gallbladder disease, insomnia, LDL-cholesterol decreased, libido changes, loss of scalp hair, melasma, migraine, nervousness, optic neuritis, pancreatitis, platelet aggregability and platelet count increased, premenstrual like syndrome, PT and PTT accelerated, pulmonary embolism, pyrexia, retinal thrombosis, somnolence, steepening of corneal curvature, thrombophlebitis, thyroid-binding globulin increased, total thyroid hormone (T_4) increased, triglycerides increased, urticaria, vaginal candidiasis, vomiting, weight gain/loss

Mechanism of Action

Conjugated estrogens contain a mixture of estrone sulfate, equilin sulfate, 17 alpha-dihydroequilin, 17 alpha-estradiol, and 17 beta-dihydroequilin. Estrogens are responsible for the development and maintenance of the female reproductive system and secondary sexual characteristics. Estradiol is the principle intracellular human estrogen and is more potent than estrone and estriol at the receptor level; it is the primary estrogen secreted prior to menopause. Following menopause, estrone and estrone sulfate are more highly produced. Estrogens modulate the pituitary secretion of gonadotropins, luteinizing hormone, and follicle-stimulating hormone through a negative feedback system; estrogen replacement reduces elevated levels of these hormones in postmenopausal women.

MPA inhibits gonadotropin production which then prevents follicular maturation and ovulation. In women with adequate estrogen, MPA transforms a proliferative endometrium into a secretory endometrium; when administered with conjugated estrogens, reduces the incidence of endometrial hyperplasia and risk of adenocarcinoma.

Drug Interactions

Cytochrome P450 Effect:

Based on estradiol and estrone: **Substrate** of CYP1A2 (major), 2A6 (minor), 2B6 (minor), 2C8/9 (minor), 2C19 (minor), 2D6 (minor), 2E1 (minor), 3A4 (major); **Inhibits** CYP1A2 (weak); **Induces** CYP3A4 (weak)

Medroxyprogesterone: **Substrate** of CYP3A4 (major); **Induces** CYP3A4 (weak)

Increased Effect/Toxicity: Hydrocortisone taken with estrogen may cause corticosteroid-induced toxicity. Increased potential for thromboembolic events with anticoagulants.

Decreased Effect:

Conjugated estrogens:

Anticonvulsants which are enzyme inducers (barbiturates, carbamazepine, phenobarbital, phenytoin, primidone) may potentially decrease estrogen levels.

Rifampin, nelfinavir, and ritonavir decrease estradiol serum concentrations

MPA: Aminoglutethimide: May decrease effects by increasing hepatic metabolism

Pharmacodynamics/Kinetics See individual agents.

Pregnancy Risk Factor X

Estrogens (Esterified) (ES troe jenz, es TER i fied)

Related Information

Endocrine Disorders and Pregnancy *on page 1481*

U.S. Brand Names Menest®

Canadian Brand Names Estratab®; Menest®

Generic Available No

Synonyms Esterified Estrogens

Pharmacologic Category Estrogen Derivative

Use Treatment of moderate to severe vasomotor symptoms associated with menopause; treatment of vulvar and vaginal atrophy; hypoestrogenism (due to hypogonadism, castration, or primary ovarian failure); prostatic cancer (palliation); breast cancer (palliation); osteoporosis (prophylaxis, in women at significant risk only)

Local Anesthetic/Vasoconstrictor Precautions No information available to require special precautions

Effects on Dental Treatment No significant effects or complications reported

Common Adverse Effects Frequency not defined.

Cardiovascular: Edema, hypertension, venous thromboembolism

Central nervous system: Dizziness, headache, mental depression, migraine

Dermatologic: Chloasma, erythema multiforme, erythema nodosum, hemorrhagic eruption, hirsutism, loss of scalp hair, melasma

Endocrine & metabolic: Breast enlargement, breast tenderness, changes in libido, increased thyroid-binding globulin, increased total thyroid hormone (T_4), increased serum triglycerides/phospholipids, increased HDL-cholesterol, decreased LDL-cholesterol, impaired glucose tolerance, hypercalcemia

Gastrointestinal: Abdominal cramps, bloating, cholecystitis, cholelithiasis, gallbladder disease, nausea, pancreatitis, vomiting, weight gain/loss

(Continued)

Estrogens (Esterified) *(Continued)*

Genitourinary: Alterations in frequency and flow of menses, changes in cervical secretions, endometrial cancer, increased size of uterine leiomyomata, vaginal candidiasis

Hematologic: Aggravation of porphyria, decreased antithrombin III and antifactor Xa, increased levels of fibrinogen, increased platelet aggregability and platelet count; increased prothrombin and factors VII, VIII, IX, X

Hepatic: Cholestatic jaundice

Neuromuscular & skeletal: Chorea

Ocular: Intolerance to contact lenses, steeping of corneal curvature

Respiratory: Pulmonary thromboembolism

Miscellaneous: Carbohydrate intolerance

Mechanism of Action Esterified estrogens contain a mixture of estrogenic substances; the principle component is estrone. Preparations contain 75% to 85% sodium estrone sulfate and 6% to 15% sodium equilin sulfate such that the total is not <90%. Estrogens are responsible for the development and maintenance of the female reproductive system and secondary sexual characteristics. Estradiol is the principle intracellular human estrogen and is more potent than estrone and estriol at the receptor level; it is the primary estrogen secreted prior to menopause. In males and following menopause in females, estrone and estrone sulfate are more highly produced. Estrogens modulate the pituitary secretion of gonadotropins, luteinizing hormone, and follicle-stimulating hormone through a negative feedback system; estrogen replacement reduces elevated levels of these hormones.

Drug Interactions

Cytochrome P450 Effect: Based on estrone: **Substrate** of CYP1A2 (major), 2B6 (minor), 2C8/9 (minor), 2E1 (minor), 3A4 (major)

Increased Effect/Toxicity: Hydrocortisone taken with estrogen may cause corticosteroid-induced toxicity. Increased potential for thromboembolic events with anticoagulants.

Decreased Effect: CYP1A2 inducers may decrease the levels/effects of estrogens; example inducers include aminoglutethimide, carbamazepine, phenobarbital, and rifampin. CYP3A4 inducers may decrease the levels/ effects of estrogens; example inducers include aminoglutethimide, carbamazepine, nafcillin, nevirapine, phenobarbital, phenytoin, and rifamycins.

Pharmacodynamics/Kinetics

Absorption: Readily

Metabolism: Rapidly hepatic to estrone sulfate, conjugated and unconjugated metabolites; first-pass effect

Excretion: Urine (as unchanged drug and as glucuronide and sulfate conjugates)

Pregnancy Risk Factor X

Estrogens (Esterified) and Methyltestosterone

(ES troe jenz es TER i fied & meth il tes TOS te rone)

Related Information

Endocrine Disorders and Pregnancy *on page 1481*

U.S. Brand Names Estratest®; Estratest® H.S.

Canadian Brand Names Estratest®

Generic Available No

Synonyms Conjugated Estrogen and Methyltestosterone; Esterified Estrogen and Methyltestosterone

Pharmacologic Category Estrogen and Progestin Combination

Use Vasomotor symptoms of menopause

Local Anesthetic/Vasoconstrictor Precautions No information available to require special precautions

Effects on Dental Treatment No significant effects or complications reported

Common Adverse Effects 1% to 10%:

Cardiovascular: Increase in blood pressure, edema, thromboembolic disorder

Central nervous system: Depression, headache

Dermatologic: Chloasma, melasma

Endocrine & metabolic: Breast tenderness, change in menstrual flow, hypercalcemia

Gastrointestinal: Nausea, vomiting

Hepatic: Cholestatic jaundice

Mechanism of Action

Conjugated estrogens: Activate estrogen receptors (DNA protein complex) located in estrogen-responsive tissues. Once activated, regulate transcription of certain genes leading to observed effects.

Testosterone: Increases synthesis of DNA, RNA, and various proteins in target tissues

Drug Interactions

Cytochrome P450 Effect: Based on estrone: **Substrate** of CYP1A2 (major), 2B6 (minor), 2C8/9 (minor), 2E1 (minor), 3A4 (major)

Pharmacodynamics/Kinetics See individual agents.

Pregnancy Risk Factor X

Estropipate (ES troe pih pate)

Related Information

Endocrine Disorders and Pregnancy *on page 1481*

U.S. Brand Names Ogen®; Ortho-Est®

Canadian Brand Names Ogen®

Mexican Brand Names Ogen®

Generic Available Yes

Synonyms Ortho Est; Piperazine Estrone Sulfate

Pharmacologic Category Estrogen Derivative

Use Treatment of moderate to severe vasomotor symptoms associated with menopause; treatment of vulvar and vaginal atrophy; hypoestrogenism (due to hypogonadism, castration, or primary ovarian failure); osteoporosis (prophylaxis, in women at significant risk only)

Local Anesthetic/Vasoconstrictor Precautions No information available to require special precautions

Effects on Dental Treatment No significant effects or complications reported

Common Adverse Effects Frequency not defined.

Cardiovascular: Edema, hypertension, venous thromboembolism

Central nervous system: Dizziness, headache, mental depression, migraine

Dermatologic: Chloasma, erythema multiforme, erythema nodosum, hemorrhagic eruption, hirsutism, loss of scalp hair, melasma

Endocrine & metabolic: Breast enlargement, breast tenderness, changes in libido, increased thyroid-binding globulin, increased total thyroid hormone (T_4), increased serum triglycerides/phospholipids, increased HDL-cholesterol, decreased LDL-cholesterol, impaired glucose tolerance, hypercalcemia

Gastrointestinal: Abdominal cramps, bloating, cholecystitis, cholelithiasis, gallbladder disease, nausea, pancreatitis, vomiting, weight gain/loss

Genitourinary: Alterations in frequency and flow of menses, changes in cervical secretions, endometrial cancer, increased size of uterine leiomyomata, vaginal candidiasis

Hematologic: Aggravation of porphyria, decreased antithrombin III and antifactor Xa, increased levels of fibrinogen, increased platelet aggregability and platelet count; increased prothrombin and factors VII, VIII, IX, X

Hepatic: Cholestatic jaundice

Neuromuscular & skeletal: Chorea

Ocular: Intolerance to contact lenses, steeping of corneal curvature

Respiratory: Pulmonary thromboembolism

Miscellaneous: Carbohydrate intolerance

Mechanism of Action Estrogens are responsible for the development and maintenance of the female reproductive system and secondary sexual characteristics. Estradiol is the principle intracellular human estrogen and is more potent than estrone and estriol at the receptor level; it is the primary estrogen secreted prior to menopause. In males and following menopause in females, estrone and estrone sulfate are more highly produced. Estrogens modulate the pituitary secretion of gonadotropins, luteinizing hormone, and follicle-stimulating hormone through a negative feedback system; estrogen replacement reduces elevated levels of these hormones. Estropipate is prepared from purified crystalline estrone that has been solubilized as the sulfate and stabilized with piperazine.

Drug Interactions

Cytochrome P450 Effect: Based on estrone: **Substrate** of CYP1A2 (major), 2B6 (minor), 2C8/9 (minor), 2E1 (minor), 3A4 (major)

Increased Effect/Toxicity: Hydrocortisone taken with estrogen may cause corticosteroid-induced toxicity. Increased potential for thromboembolic events with anticoagulants.

Decreased Effect: CYP1A2 inducers may decrease the levels/effects of estrogens; example inducers include aminoglutethimide, carbamazepine, phenobarbital, and rifampin. CYP3A4 inducers may decrease the levels/effects of estrogens; example inducers include aminoglutethimide, carbamazepine, nafcillin, nevirapine, phenobarbital, phenytoin, and rifamycins.

Pharmacodynamics/Kinetics

Absorption: Well absorbed

(Continued)

Estropipate *(Continued)*

Metabolism: Hepatic and in target tissues; first-pass effect

Pregnancy Risk Factor X

Estrostep® Fe *see* Ethinyl Estradiol and Norethindrone *on page 550*

ETAF *see* Aldesleukin *on page 74*

Etanercept (et a NER sept)

Related Information

Rheumatoid Arthritis, Osteoarthritis, and Osteoporosis *on page 1490*

U.S. Brand Names Enbrel®

Canadian Brand Names Enbrel®

Generic Available No

Pharmacologic Category Antirheumatic, Disease Modifying

Use Reduction in signs and symptoms of moderately to severely active rheumatoid arthritis, moderately to severely active polyarticular juvenile arthritis, or psoriatic arthritis in patients who have had an inadequate response to one or more disease-modifying antirheumatic drugs (DMARDs); reduction in signs and symptoms of active ankylosing spondylitis (AS); treatment of chronic plaque psoriasis (moderate-to-severe)

Unlabeled/Investigational Use Crohn's disease

Local Anesthetic/Vasoconstrictor Precautions No information available to require special precautions

Effects on Dental Treatment No significant effects or complications reported

Common Adverse Effects Events reported include those >3% with incidence higher than placebo.

>10%:

- Central nervous system: Headache (17%)
- Local: Injection site reaction (37%)
- Respiratory: Respiratory tract infection (upper, 29%; other than upper, 38%), rhinitis (12%)
- Miscellaneous: Infection (35%), positive ANA (11%), positive antidouble-stranded DNA antibodies (15% by RIA, 3% by *Crithidia luciliae* assay)

≥3% to 10%:

- Central nervous system: Dizziness (7%)
- Dermatologic: Rash (5%)
- Gastrointestinal: Abdominal pain (5%), dyspepsia (4%), nausea (9%), vomiting (3%)
- Neuromuscular & skeletal: Weakness (5%)
- Respiratory: Pharyngitis (7%), respiratory disorder (5%), sinusitis (3%), cough (6%)

Pediatric patients (JRA): The percentages of patients reporting abdominal pain (17%) and vomiting (13%) were higher than in adult RA. Two patients developed varicella infection associated with aseptic meningitis which resolved without complications (see Warnings/Precautions).

Dosage SubQ:

Children 4-17 years: Juvenile rheumatoid arthritis:

- Once-weekly dosing: 0.8 mg/kg (maximum: 50 mg/dose) once weekly; maximum amount in any single injection site should be no more than 25 mg
- Twice-weekly dosing: 0.4 mg/kg (maximum: 25 mg/dose) twice weekly (individual doses should be separated by 72-96 hours)

Adults:

- Rheumatoid arthritis, psoriatic arthritis, ankylosing spondylitis:
  - Once-weekly dosing: 50 mg once weekly; the maximum amount in any single injection site should be no more than 25 mg
  - Twice weekly dosing: 25 mg given twice weekly (individual doses should be separated by 72-96 hours)
  - **Note:** If the physician determines that it is appropriate, patients may self-inject after proper training in injection technique.
- Plaque psoriasis:
  - Initial: 50 mg twice weekly, 3-4 days apart (starting doses of 25 or 50 mg once weekly have also been used successfully); maintain initial dose for 3 months
  - Maintenance dose: 50 mg weekly

Elderly: Although greater sensitivity of some elderly patients cannot be ruled out, no overall differences in safety or effectiveness were observed.

Mechanism of Action Etanercept is a recombinant DNA-derived protein composed of tumor necrosis factor receptor (TNFR) linked to the Fc portion of human IgG1. Etanercept binds tumor necrosis factor (TNF) and blocks its interaction with cell surface receptors. TNF plays an important role in the inflammatory processes of rheumatoid arthritis (RA) and the resulting joint pathology.

Contraindications Hypersensitivity to etanercept or any component of the formulation; patients with sepsis (mortality may be increased); active infections (including chronic or local infection)

Warnings/Precautions Etanercept may affect defenses against infections and malignancies. Safety and efficacy in patients with immunosuppression or chronic infections have not been evaluated. Discontinue administration if patient develops a serious infection. Do not start drug administration in patients with an active infection. Use caution in patients predisposed to infection, such as poorly-controlled diabetes.

Use caution in patients with pre-existing or recent-onset demyelinating CNS disorders. Use caution in patients with CHF. Use caution in patients with a history of significant hematologic abnormalities; has been associated with pancytopenia and aplastic anemia (rare). Discontinue if significant hematologic abnormalities are confirmed.

Treatment may result in the formation of autoimmune antibodies; cases of autoimmune disease have not been described. More cases of lymphoma were reported in patients receiving anti-TNF therapy (relative to controls).

Patients should be brought up to date with all immunizations before initiating therapy. Live vaccines should not be given concurrently. Patients with a significant exposure to varicella virus should temporarily discontinue etanercept. Treatment with varicella zoster immune globulin should be considered.

Drug Interactions

Increased Effect/Toxicity: Specific drug interaction studies have not been conducted with etanercept. An increased rate of serious infections has been noted with concurrent anakinra therapy, without additional improvement in American College of Rheumatology (ACR) response criteria.

Decreased Effect: Specific drug interaction studies have not been conducted with etanercept. Live vaccines should not be given during therapy.

Pharmacodynamics/Kinetics

Onset of action: ~2-3 weeks

Half-life elimination: 115 hours (range: 98-300 hours)

Time to peak: 72 hours (range: 48-96 hours)

Excretion: Clearance: Children: 45.9 mL/hour/m^2; Adults: 89 mL/hour (52 mL/hour/m^2)

Pregnancy Risk Factor B

Dosage Forms INJ, powder for reconstitution: 25 mg

Ethacrynate Sodium *see* Ethacrynic Acid *on page 533*

Ethacrynic Acid (eth a KRIN ik AS id)

Related Information

Cardiovascular Diseases *on page 1458*

U.S. Brand Names Edecrin®

Canadian Brand Names Edecrin®

Generic Available No

Synonyms Ethacrynate Sodium

Pharmacologic Category Diuretic, Loop

Use Management of edema associated with congestive heart failure; hepatic cirrhosis or renal disease; short-term management of ascites due to malignancy, idiopathic edema, and lymphedema

Local Anesthetic/Vasoconstrictor Precautions No information available to require special precautions

Effects on Dental Treatment No significant effects or complications reported

Common Adverse Effects Frequency not defined.

Central nervous system: Headache, fatigue, apprehension, confusion, fever, chills, encephalopathy (patients with pre-existing liver disease); vertigo

Dermatologic: Skin rash, Henoch-Schönlein purpura (in patient with rheumatic heart disease)

Endocrine & metabolic: Hyponatremia, hyperglycemia, variations in phosphorus, CO_2 content, bicarbonate, and calcium; reversible hyperuricemia, gout, hyperglycemia, hypoglycemia (occurred in two uremic patients who received doses above those recommended)

Gastrointestinal: Anorexia, malaise, abdominal discomfort or pain, dysphagia, nausea, vomiting, diarrhea, gastrointestinal bleeding, acute pancreatitis (rare)

(Continued)

Ethacrynic Acid *(Continued)*

Genitourinary: Hematuria
Hepatic: Jaundice, abnormal liver function tests
Hematology: Agranulocytosis, severe neutropenia, thrombocytopenia
Local: Thrombophlebitis (with intravenous use), local irritation and pain,
Ocular: Blurred vision
Otic: Tinnitus, temporary or permanent deafness
Renal: Serum creatinine increased

Mechanism of Action Inhibits reabsorption of sodium and chloride in the ascending loop of Henle and distal renal tubule, interfering with the chloride-binding cotransport system, thus causing increased excretion of water, sodium, chloride, magnesium, and calcium

Drug Interactions

Increased Effect/Toxicity: Ethacrynic acid-induced hypokalemia may predispose to digoxin toxicity and may increase the risk of arrhythmia with drugs which may prolong QT interval, including type Ia and type III antiarrhythmic agents, cisapride, and some quinolones (sparfloxacin, gatifloxacin, and moxifloxacin). The risk of toxicity from lithium and salicylates (high dose) may be increased by loop diuretics. Hypotensive effects and/or adverse renal effects of ACE inhibitors and NSAIDs are potentiated by ethacrynic acid-induced hypovolemia. The effects of peripheral adrenergic-blocking drugs or ganglionic blockers may be increased by ethacrynic acid.

Ethacrynic acid may increase the risk of ototoxicity with other ototoxic agents (aminoglycosides, cis-platinum), especially in patients with renal dysfunction. Synergistic diuretic effects occur with thiazide-type diuretics. Diuretics tend to be synergistic with other antihypertensive agents, and hypotension may occur. Nephrotoxicity has been associated with concomitant use of cephaloridine or cephalexin.

Decreased Effect: Probenecid decreases diuretic effects of ethacrynic acid. Glucose tolerance may be decreased by loop diuretics, requiring adjustment of hypoglycemic agents. Cholestyramine or colestipol may reduce bioavailability of ethacrynic acid. Indomethacin (and other NSAIDs) may reduce natriuretic and hypotensive effects of diuretics.

Pharmacodynamics/Kinetics

Onset of action: Diuresis: Oral: ~30 minutes; I.V.: 5 minutes
Peak effect: Oral: 2 hours; I.V.: 30 minutes
Duration: Oral: 12 hours; I.V.: 2 hours
Absorption: Oral: Rapid
Protein binding: >90%
Metabolism: Hepatic (35% to 40%) to active cysteine conjugate
Half-life elimination: Normal renal function: 2-4 hours
Excretion: Feces and urine (30% to 60% as unchanged drug)

Pregnancy Risk Factor B

Ethambutol (e THAM byoo tole)

Related Information

Tuberculosis *on page 1495*

U.S. Brand Names Myambutol®

Canadian Brand Names Etibi®

Generic Available Yes

Synonyms Ethambutol Hydrochloride

Pharmacologic Category Antitubercular Agent

Use Treatment of tuberculosis and other mycobacterial diseases in conjunction with other antituberculosis agents

Local Anesthetic/Vasoconstrictor Precautions No information available to require special precautions

Effects on Dental Treatment No significant effects or complications reported

Common Adverse Effects Frequency not defined.

Cardiovascular: Myocarditis, pericarditis
Central nervous system: Headache, confusion, disorientation, malaise, mental confusion, fever, dizziness, hallucinations
Dermatologic: Rash, pruritus, dermatitis, exfoliative dermatitis
Endocrine & metabolic: Acute gout or hyperuricemia
Gastrointestinal: Abdominal pain, anorexia, nausea, vomiting
Hematologic: Leukopenia, thrombocytopenia, eosinophilia, neutropenia, lymphadenopathy
Hepatic: Abnormal LFTs, hepatotoxicity (possibly related to concurrent therapy), hepatitis
Neuromuscular & skeletal: Peripheral neuritis, arthralgia

Ocular: Optic neuritis; symptoms may include decreased acuity, scotoma, color blindness, or visual defects (usually reversible with discontinuation, irreversible blindness has been described)

Renal: Nephritis

Respiratory: Infiltrates (with or without eosinophilia), pneumonitis

Miscellaneous: Anaphylaxis, anaphylactoid reaction; hypersensitivity syndrome (rash, eosinophilia, and organ-specific inflammation)

Mechanism of Action Suppresses mycobacteria multiplication by interfering with RNA synthesis

Drug Interactions

Decreased Effect: Decreased absorption with aluminum hydroxide. Avoid concurrent administration of aluminum-containing antacids for at least 4 hours following ethambutol.

Pharmacodynamics/Kinetics

Absorption: ~80%

Distribution: Widely throughout body; concentrated in kidneys, lungs, saliva, and red blood cells

Relative diffusion from blood into CSF: Adequate with or without inflammation (exceeds usual MICs)

CSF:blood level ratio: Normal meninges: 0%; Inflamed meninges: 25%

Protein binding: 20% to 30%

Metabolism: Hepatic (20%) to inactive metabolite

Half-life elimination: 2.5-3.6 hours; End-stage renal disease: 7-15 hours

Time to peak, serum: 2-4 hours

Excretion: Urine (~50%) and feces (20%) as unchanged drug

Pregnancy Risk Factor C

Ethambutol Hydrochloride *see* Ethambutol *on page 534*

Ethamolin® *see* Ethanolamine Oleate *on page 535*

ETH and C *see* Terpin Hydrate and Codeine *on page 1275*

Ethanolamine Oleate (ETH a nol a meen OH lee ate)

U.S. Brand Names Ethamolin®

Generic Available No

Synonyms Monoethanolamine

Pharmacologic Category Sclerosing Agent

Use Orphan drug: Sclerosing agent used for bleeding esophageal varices

Local Anesthetic/Vasoconstrictor Precautions No information available to require special precautions

Effects on Dental Treatment No significant effects or complications reported

Common Adverse Effects 1% to 10%:

Central nervous system: Pyrexia (1.8%)

Gastrointestinal: Esophageal ulcer (2%), esophageal stricture (1.3%)

Respiratory: Pleural effusion (2%), pneumonia (1.2%)

Miscellaneous: Retrosternal pain (1.6%)

Mechanism of Action Derived from oleic acid and similar in physical properties to sodium morrhuate; however, the exact mechanism of the hemostatic effect used in endoscopic injection sclerotherapy is not known. Intravenously injected ethanolamine oleate produces a sterile inflammatory response resulting in fibrosis and occlusion of the vein; a dose-related extravascular inflammatory reaction occurs when the drug diffuses through the venous wall. Autopsy results indicate that variceal obliteration occurs secondary to mural necrosis and fibrosis. Thrombosis appears to be a transient reaction.

Pregnancy Risk Factor C

Ethaverine (eth AV er een)

Synonyms Ethaverine Hydrochloride

Pharmacologic Category Vasodilator

Use Peripheral and cerebral vascular insufficiency associated with arterial spasm

Local Anesthetic/Vasoconstrictor Precautions No information available to require special precautions

Effects on Dental Treatment No significant effects or complications reported

Common Adverse Effects Frequency not defined.

Cardiovascular: Tachycardia, hypotension

Central nervous system: Depression, dizziness, vertigo, drowsiness, sedation, lethargy, headache, xerostomia

Dermatologic: Pruritus, flushing of the face

Gastrointestinal: Nausea, constipation

Hepatic: Hepatic hypersensitivity

Miscellaneous: Diaphoresis

Ethaverine Hydrochloride *see* Ethaverine *on page 535*

Ethinyl Estradiol and Desogestrel

(ETH in il es tra DYE ole & des oh JES trel)

U.S. Brand Names Apri®; Cyclessa®; Desogen®; Kariva™; Mircette®; Ortho-Cept®; Velivet™

Canadian Brand Names Marvelon®; Ortho-Cept®

Generic Available Yes

Synonyms Desogestrel and Ethinyl Estradiol; Ortho Cept

Pharmacologic Category Contraceptive; Estrogen and Progestin Combination

Use Prevention of pregnancy

Local Anesthetic/Vasoconstrictor Precautions No information available to require special precautions

Effects on Dental Treatment When prescribing antibiotics, patient must be warned to use additional methods of birth control if on oral contraceptives.

Common Adverse Effects Frequency not defined.

Cardiovascular: Arterial thromboembolism, cerebral hemorrhage, cerebral thrombosis, edema, hypertension, mesenteric thrombosis, myocardial infarction

Central nervous system: Depression, dizziness, headache, migraine, nervousness, premenstrual syndrome, stroke

Dermatologic: Acne, erythema multiforme, erythema nodosum, hirsutism, loss of scalp hair, melasma (may persist), rash (allergic)

Endocrine & metabolic: Amenorrhea, breakthrough bleeding, breast enlargement, breast secretion, breast tenderness, carbohydrate intolerance, lactation decreased (postpartum), glucose tolerance decreased, libido changes, menstrual flow changes, sex hormone-binding globulins (SHBG) increased, spotting, temporary infertility (following discontinuation), thyroid-binding globulin increased, triglycerides increased

Gastrointestinal: Abdominal cramps, appetite changes, bloating, cholestasis, colitis, gallbladder disease, jaundice, nausea, vomiting, weight gain/loss

Genitourinary: Cervical erosion changes, cervical secretion changes, cystitis-like syndrome, vaginal candidiasis, vaginitis

Hematologic: Antithrombin III decreased, folate levels decreased, hemolytic uremic syndrome, norepinephrine induced platelet aggregability increased, porphyria, prothrombin increased; factors VII, VIII, IX, and X

Hepatic: Benign liver tumors, Budd-Chiari syndrome, cholestatic jaundice, hepatic adenomas

Local: Thrombophlebitis

Ocular: Cataracts, change in corneal curvature (steepening), contact lens intolerance, optic neuritis, retinal thrombosis

Renal: Impaired renal function

Respiratory: Pulmonary thromboembolism

Miscellaneous: Hemorrhagic eruption

Dosage Oral: Adults: Female: Contraception:

Schedule 1 (Sunday starter): Dose begins on first Sunday after onset of menstruation; if the menstrual period starts on Sunday, take first tablet that very same day. **With a Sunday start, an additional method of contraception should be used until after the first 7 days of consecutive administration.**

For 21-tablet package: Dosage is 1 tablet daily for 21 consecutive days, followed by 7 days off of the medication; a new course begins on the 8th day after the last tablet is taken.

For 28-tablet package: Dosage is 1 tablet daily without interruption.

Schedule 2 (Day 1 starter): Dose starts on first day of menstrual cycle taking 1 tablet daily.

For 21-tablet package: Dosage is 1 tablet daily for 21 consecutive days, followed by 7 days off of the medication; a new course begins on the 8th day after the last tablet is taken.

For 28-tablet package: Dosage is 1 tablet daily without interruption.

If all doses have been taken on schedule and one menstrual period is missed, continue dosing cycle. If two consecutive menstrual periods are missed, pregnancy test is required before new dosing cycle is started.

Missed doses **monophasic formulations** (refer to package insert for complete information):

One dose missed: Take as soon as remembered or take 2 tablets next day

Two consecutive doses missed in the first 2 weeks: Take 2 tablets as soon as remembered or 2 tablets next 2 days. **An additional method of contraception should be used for 7 days after missed dose.**

Two consecutive doses missed in week 3 or three consecutive doses missed at any time:

Schedule 1 (Sunday starter): Continue to take 1 tablet daily until Sunday, then discard the rest of the pack, and a new pack is started that same day.

Schedule 2 (Day 1 starter): Current pack should be discarded, and a new pack started that same day. **An additional method of contraception should be used for 7 days after missed dose.**

Missed doses **biphasic/triphasic formulations** (refer to package insert for complete information):

One dose missed: Take as soon as remembered or take 2 tablets next day.

Two consecutive doses missed in week 1 or week 2 of the pack: Take 2 tablets as soon as remembered and 2 tablets the next day. Resume taking 1 tablet daily until the pack is empty. **An additional method of contraception should be used for 7 days after a missed dose.**

Two consecutive doses missed in week 3 of the pack; **an additional method of contraception must be used for 7 days after a missed dose**:

Schedule 1 (Sunday starter): Take 1 tablet every day until Sunday. Discard the remaining pack and start a new pack of pills on the same day.

Schedule 2 (Day 1 starter): Discard the remaining pack and start a new pack the same day.

Three or more consecutive doses missed; **an additional method of contraception must be used for 7 days after a missed dose**:

Schedule 1 (Sunday starter): Take 1 tablet every day until Sunday; on Sunday, discard the pack and start a new pack.

Schedule 2 (Day 1 starter): Discard the remaining pack and begin new pack of tablets starting on the same day.

Dosage adjustment in renal impairment: Specific guidelines not available; Use with caution

Dosage adjustment in hepatic impairment: Contraindicated in patients with hepatic impairment

Mechanism of Action Combination hormonal contraceptives inhibit ovulation via a negative feedback mechanism on the hypothalamus, which alters the normal pattern of gonadotropin secretion of a follicle-stimulating hormone (FSH) and luteinizing hormone by the anterior pituitary. The follicular phase FSH and midcycle surge of gonadotropins are inhibited. In addition, combination hormonal contraceptives produce alterations in the genital tract, including changes in the cervical mucus, rendering it unfavorable for sperm penetration even if ovulation occurs. Changes in the endometrium may also occur, producing an unfavorable environment for nidation. Combination hormonal contraceptive drugs may alter the tubal transport of the ova through the fallopian tubes. Progestational agents may also alter sperm fertility.

Contraindications Hypersensitivity to ethinyl estradiol, etonogestrel, desogestrel, or any component of the formulation; history of or current thrombophlebitis or venous thromboembolic disorders (including DVT, PE); active or recent (within 1 year) arterial thromboembolic disease (eg, stroke, MI); cerebral vascular disease, coronary artery disease, valvular heart disease with complications, severe hypertension; diabetes mellitus with vascular involvement; severe headache with focal neurological symptoms; known or suspected breast carcinoma, endometrial cancer, estrogen-dependent neoplasms, undiagnosed abnormal genital bleeding; hepatic dysfunction or tumor, cholestatic jaundice of pregnancy, jaundice with prior combination hormonal contraceptive use; major surgery with prolonged immobilization; heavy smoking (≥15 cigarettes/day) in patients >35 years of age; pregnancy

Warnings/Precautions Combination hormonal contraceptives do not protect against HIV infection or other sexually-transmitted diseases. The risk of cardiovascular side effects increases in women who smoke cigarettes, especially those who are >35 years of age; women who use combination hormonal contraceptives should be strongly advised not to smoke. Combination hormonal contraceptives may lead to increased risk of myocardial infarction, use with caution in patients with risk factors for coronary artery disease. May increase the risk of thromboembolism. Combination hormonal contraceptives may have a dose-related risk of vascular disease, hypertension, and gallbladder disease. Women with hypertension should be encouraged to use another form of contraception. The use of combination hormonal contraceptives has been associated with a slight increase in frequency of breast cancer, however, studies are not consistent. Combination hormonal contraceptives may cause glucose intolerance. Retinal thrombosis has been reported (rarely). Use with caution in patients with renal disease, conditions that may be aggravated by fluid retention, depression, or history of migraine. Not for use prior to menarche.

(Continued)

Ethinyl Estradiol and Desogestrel *(Continued)*

The minimum dosage combination of estrogen/progestin that will effectively treat the individual patient should be used. New patients should be started on products containing <50 mcg of estrogen per tablet.

Drug Interactions

Cytochrome P450 Effect:

Ethinyl estradiol: **Substrate** of CYP3A4 (major), 3A5-7 (minor); **Inhibits** CYP1A2 (weak), 2B6 (weak), 2C19 (weak), 3A4 (weak)

Desogestrel: **Substrate** of CYP2C19 (major)

Increased Effect/Toxicity: Acetaminophen, ascorbic acid, and repaglinide may increase plasma levels of estrogen component. Atorvastatin and indinavir increase plasma levels of combination hormonal contraceptives. Combination hormonal contraceptives increase the plasma levels of alprazolam, chlordiazepoxide, cyclosporine, diazepam, prednisolone, selegiline, theophylline, tricyclic antidepressants. Combination hormonal contraceptives may increase (or decrease) the effects of coumarin derivatives.

Decreased Effect: CYP2C19 inducers may decrease the levels/effects of desogestrel; example inducers include aminoglutethimide, carbamazepine, phenytoin, and rifampin. CYP3A4 inducers may decrease the levels/effects of ethinyl estradiol; example inducers include aminoglutethimide, carbamazepine, nafcillin, phenobarbital, phenytoin, and rifamycins. Combination hormonal contraceptives may decrease plasma levels of acetaminophen, clofibric acid, lorazepam, morphine, oxazepam, salicylic acid, temazepam. Contraceptive effect decreased by acitretin, amprenavir, griseofulvin, lopinavir, nelfinavir, nevirapine, penicillins (effect not consistent), ritonavir, tetracyclines (effect not consistent), troglitazone. Combination hormonal contraceptives may decrease (or increase) the effects of coumarin derivatives.

Ethanol/Nutrition/Herb Interactions

Food: CNS effects of caffeine may be enhanced if combination hormonal contraceptives are used concurrently with caffeine. Grapefruit juice increases ethinyl estradiol concentrations and would be expected to increase progesterone serum levels as well; clinical implications are unclear.

Herb/Nutraceutical: St John's wort may decrease the effectiveness of combination hormonal contraceptives by inducing hepatic enzymes. Avoid dong quai and black cohosh (have estrogen activity). Avoid saw palmetto, red clover, ginseng.

Dietary Considerations Should be taken at same time each day.

Pregnancy Risk Factor X

Dosage Forms TAB, low-dose (Kariva™, Mircette®): Day 1-21: Ethinyl estradiol 0.02 mg and desogestrel 0.15 mg, Day 22-23: Inactive, Day 24-28: Ethinyl estradiol 0.01 mg (28s). **TAB, monophasic:** (Apri® 28): Ethinyl estradiol 0.03 mg and desogestrel 0.15 mg (28s); (Desogen®): Ethinyl estradiol 0.03 mg and desogestrel 0.15 mg (28s); (Ortho-Cept® 28): Ethinyl estradiol 0.03 mg and desogestrel 0.15 mg (28s). **TAB, triphasic** (Cyclessa®): Day 1-7: Ethinyl estradiol 0.025 mg and desogestrel 0.1 mg, Day 8-14: Ethinyl estradiol 0.025 mg and desogestrel 0.125 mg, Day 14-21: Ethinyl estradiol 0.025 mg and desogestrel 0.15 mg, Day 21-28: Inactive (28s); (Velivet™): Day 1-7: Ethinyl estradiol 0.025 mg and desogestrel 0.1 mg, Day 8-14: Ethinyl estradiol 0.025 mg and desogestrel 0.125 mg, Day 14-21: Ethinyl estradiol 0.025 mg and desogestrel 0.15 mg, Day 21-28: Inactive (28s)

Ethinyl Estradiol and Drospirenone

(ETH in il es tra DYE ole & droh SPYE re none)

U.S. Brand Names Yasmin®

Generic Available No

Synonyms Drospirenone and Ethinyl Estradiol

Pharmacologic Category Contraceptive; Estrogen and Progestin Combination

Use Prevention of pregnancy

Local Anesthetic/Vasoconstrictor Precautions No information available to require special precautions

Effects on Dental Treatment When prescribing antibiotics, patient must be warned to use additional methods of birth control if on oral contraceptives.

Common Adverse Effects

>1%:

Central nervous system: Depression, dizziness, emotional lability, headache, migraine, nervousness

Dermatologic: Acne, pruritus, rash

Endocrine & metabolic: Amenorrhea, dysmenorrhea, intermenstrual bleeding, menstrual irregularities
Gastrointestinal: Abdominal pain, diarrhea, gastroenteritis, nausea, vomiting
Genitourinary: Cystitis, leukorrhea, vaginal moniliasis, vaginitis
Neuromuscular & skeletal: Back pain, weakness
Respiratory: Bronchitis, pharyngitis, sinusitis, upper respiratory infection
Miscellaneous: Allergic reaction, flu-like syndrome, infection

Adverse reactions reported with other oral contraceptives: Appetite changes, antithrombin III decreased, arterial thromboembolism, benign liver tumors, breast changes, Budd-Chiari syndrome, carbohydrate intolerance, cataracts, cerebral hemorrhage, cerebral thrombosis, cervical changes, change in corneal curvature (steepening), cholestatic jaundice, colitis, contact lens intolerance, decreased lactation (postpartum), deep vein thrombosis, diplopia, edema, erythema multiforme, erythema nodosum; factors VII, VIII, IX, X increased; folate serum concentrations decreased, gallbladder disease, glucose intolerance, hemorrhagic eruption, hemolytic uremic syndrome, hepatic adenomas, hirsutism, hypercalcemia, hypertension, hyperglycemia, libido changes, melasma, mesenteric thrombosis, myocardial infarction, papilledema, platelet aggregability increased, porphyria, premenstrual syndrome, proptosis, prothrombin increased, pulmonary thromboembolism, renal function impairment, retinal thrombosis, sex hormone-binding globulin increased, thrombophlebitis, thyroid-binding globulin increased, total thyroid hormone (T_4) increased, triglycerides/phospholipids increased, vaginal candidiasis, weight changes

Dosage Oral: Adults: Female: Contraception: Dosage is 1 tablet daily for 28 consecutive days. Dose should be taken at the same time each day, either after the evening meal or at bedtime. Dosing may be started on the first day of menstrual period (Day 1 starter) or on the first Sunday after the onset of the menstrual period (Sunday starter).

Day 1 starter: Dose starts on first day of menstrual cycle taking 1 tablet daily.
Sunday starter: Dose begins on first Sunday after onset of menstruation; if the menstrual period starts on Sunday, take first tablet that very same day. **With a Sunday start, an additional method of contraception should be used until after the first 7 days of consecutive administration.**
If all doses have been taken on schedule and one menstrual period is missed, continue dosing cycle. If two consecutive menstrual periods are missed, pregnancy test is required before new dosing cycle is started.
If doses have been missed during the first 3 weeks and the menstrual period is missed, pregnancy should be ruled out prior to continuing treatment.

Missed doses (monophasic formulations) (refer to package insert for complete information):
One dose missed: Take as soon as remembered or take 2 tablets next day
Two consecutive doses missed in the first 2 weeks: Take 2 tablets as soon as remembered or 2 tablets next 2 days. **An additional method of contraception should be used for 7 days after missed dose.**
Two consecutive doses missed in week 3 or three consecutive doses missed at any time: **An additional method of contraception must be used for 7 days after a missed dose.**
Day 1 starter: Current pack should be discarded, and a new pack should be started that same day.
Sunday starter: Continue dose of 1 tablet daily until Sunday, then discard the rest of the pack, and a new pack should be started that same day.
Any number of doses missed in week 4: Continue taking one pill each day until pack is empty; no back-up method of contraception is needed

Dosage adjustment in renal impairment: Contraindicated in patients with renal dysfunction (Cl_{cr} ≤50 mL/minute)
Dosage adjustment in hepatic impairment: Contraindicated in patients with hepatic dysfunction

Mechanism of Action Combination oral contraceptives inhibit ovulation via a negative feedback mechanism on the hypothalamus, which alters the normal pattern of gonadotropin secretion of a follicle-stimulating hormone (FSH) and luteinizing hormone by the anterior pituitary. The follicular phase FSH and midcycle surge of gonadotropins are inhibited. In addition, oral contraceptives produce alterations in the genital tract, including changes in the cervical mucus, rendering it unfavorable for sperm penetration even if ovulation occurs. Changes in the endometrium may also occur, producing an unfavorable environment for nidation. Oral contraceptive drugs may alter the tubal transport of the ova through the fallopian tubes. Progestational agents may also alter sperm fertility. Drospirenone is a spironolactone analogue with antimineralocorticoid and antiandrogenic activity.
(Continued)

Ethinyl Estradiol and Drospirenone *(Continued)*

Contraindications Hypersensitivity to ethinyl estradiol, drospirenone, or to any component of the formulation; history of or current thrombophlebitis or venous thromboembolic disorders (including DVT, PE); active or recent (within 1 year) arterial thromboembolic disease (eg, stroke, MI); cerebral vascular disease, coronary artery disease, severe hypertension; diabetes with vascular involvement; headache with focal neurological symptoms; known or suspected breast carcinoma, endometrial cancer, estrogen-dependent neoplasms, undiagnosed abnormal genital bleeding; renal insufficiency, hepatic dysfunction or tumor, adrenal insufficiency, cholestatic jaundice of pregnancy, jaundice with prior oral contraceptive use; heavy smoking (≥15 cigarettes/day) in patients >35 years of age; pregnancy

Warnings/Precautions Oral contraceptives do not protect against HIV infection or other sexually-transmitted diseases. The risk of cardiovascular side effects increases in women who smoke cigarettes, especially those who are >35 years of age; women who use oral contraceptives should be strongly advised not to smoke. Oral contraceptives may lead to increased risk of myocardial infarction, use with caution in patients with risk factors for coronary artery disease. May increase the risk of thromboembolism. Oral contraceptives may have a dose-related risk of vascular disease (decreases HDL), hypertension, and gallbladder disease; a preparation with the lowest effective estrogen/progesterone combination should be used. Women with high blood pressure should be encouraged to use another form of contraception. Oral contraceptives may cause glucose intolerance. Retinal thrombosis has been reported (rarely) with oral contraceptive use. Use with caution in patients with conditions that may be aggravated by fluid retention, depression, or patients with history of migraine. Not for use prior to menarche.

Drospirenone has antimineralocorticoid activity that may lead to hyperkalemia in patients with renal insufficiency, hepatic dysfunction, or adrenal insufficiency. Use caution with medications that may increase serum potassium.

Drug Interactions

Cytochrome P450 Effect:

Ethinyl estradiol: **Substrate** of CYP3A4 (major), 3A5-7 (minor); **Inhibits** CYP1A2 (weak), 2B6 (weak), 2C19 (weak), 3A4 (weak)

Drospirenone: **Substrate** of CYP3A4 (minor); **Inhibits** CYP1A2 (weak), 2C8/9 (weak), 2C19 (weak), 3A4 (weak)

Increased Effect/Toxicity: ACE inhibitors, aldosterone antagonists, angiotensin II receptor antagonists, heparin, NSAIDs (when taken daily, long term), and potassium-sparing diuretics increase risk of hyperkalemia with concomitant use. Acetaminophen, ascorbic acid, and atorvastatin may increase plasma concentrations of oral contraceptives. Ethinyl estradiol may increase plasma concentrations of cyclosporine, prednisolone, selegiline, and theophylline. Oral contraceptives may increase (or decrease) the effects of coumarin derivatives.

Decreased Effect: Oral contraceptives may decrease the plasma concentration of acetaminophen, clofibric acid, morphine, salicylic acid, and temazepam. Aminoglutethimide, anticonvulsants (carbamazepine, felbamate, phenobarbital, phenytoin, topiramate), phenylbutazone, rifampin, and ritonavir may increase metabolism leading to decreased effect of oral contraceptives. Oral contraceptives may decrease (or increase) the effects of coumarin derivatives.

Ethanol/Nutrition/Herb Interactions

Food: CNS effects of caffeine may be enhanced if oral contraceptives are used concurrently with caffeine. Grapefruit juice increases ethinyl estradiol concentrations; clinical implications are unclear.

Herb/Nutraceutical: St John's wort may decrease the effectiveness of oral contraceptives by inducing hepatic enzymes; may also result in breakthrough bleeding.

Pregnancy Risk Factor X

Dosage Forms TAB: Ethinyl estradiol 0.03 mg and drospirenone 3 mg (28s)

Ethinyl Estradiol and Ethynodiol Diacetate

(ETH in il es tra DYE ole & e thye noe DYE ole dye AS e tate)

U.S. Brand Names Demulen®; Zovia™

Canadian Brand Names Demulen® 30

Generic Available Yes

Synonyms Ethynodiol Diacetate and Ethinyl Estradiol

Pharmacologic Category Contraceptive; Estrogen and Progestin Combination

Use Prevention of pregnancy

Unlabeled/Investigational Use Treatment of hypermenorrhea, endometriosis, female hypogonadism

Local Anesthetic/Vasoconstrictor Precautions No information available to require special precautions

Effects on Dental Treatment When prescribing antibiotics, patient must be warned to use additional methods of birth control if on oral contraceptives.

Common Adverse Effects Frequency not defined.

Cardiovascular: Arterial thromboembolism, cerebral hemorrhage, cerebral thrombosis, edema, hypertension, mesenteric thrombosis, myocardial infarction

Central nervous system: Depression, dizziness, headache, migraine, nervousness, premenstrual syndrome, stroke

Dermatologic: Acne, erythema multiforme, erythema nodosum, hirsutism, loss of scalp hair, melasma (may persist), rash (allergic)

Endocrine & metabolic: Amenorrhea, breakthrough bleeding, breast enlargement, breast secretion, breast tenderness, carbohydrate intolerance, lactation decreased (postpartum), glucose tolerance decreased, libido changes, menstrual flow changes, sex hormone-binding globulins (SHBG) increased, spotting, temporary infertility (following discontinuation), thyroid-binding globulin increased, triglycerides increased

Gastrointestinal: Abdominal cramps, appetite changes, bloating, cholestasis, colitis, gallbladder disease, jaundice, nausea, vomiting, weight gain/loss

Genitourinary: Cervical erosion changes, cervical secretion changes, cystitis-like syndrome, vaginal candidiasis, vaginitis

Hematologic: Antithrombin III decreased, folate levels decreased, hemolytic uremic syndrome, norepinephrine induced platelet aggregability increased, porphyria, prothrombin increased; factors VII, VIII, IX, and X increased

Hepatic: Benign liver tumors, Budd-Chiari syndrome, cholestatic jaundice, hepatic adenomas

Local: Thrombophlebitis

Ocular: Cataracts, change in corneal curvature (steepening), contact lens intolerance, optic neuritis, retinal thrombosis

Renal: Impaired renal function

Respiratory: Pulmonary thromboembolism

Miscellaneous: Hemorrhagic eruption

Dosage Oral: Adults: Female: Contraception:

Schedule 1 (Sunday starter): Dose begins on first Sunday after onset of menstruation; if the menstrual period starts on Sunday, take first tablet that very same day. **With a Sunday start, an additional method of contraception should be used until after the first 7 days of consecutive administration.**

For 21-tablet package: 1 tablet/day for 21 consecutive days, followed by 7 days off of the medication; a new course begins on the 8th day after the last tablet is taken.

For 28-tablet package: 1 tablet/day without interruption.

Schedule 2 (Day 1 starter): Dose starts on first day of menstrual cycle taking 1 tablet daily.

For 21-tablet package: 1 tablet/day for 21 consecutive days, followed by 7 days off of the medication; a new course begins on the 8th day after the last tablet is taken.

For 28-tablet package: 1 tablet/day without interruption.

If all doses have been taken on schedule and one menstrual period is missed, continue dosing cycle. If two consecutive menstrual periods are missed, pregnancy test is required before new dosing cycle is started.

Missed doses **monophasic formulations** (refer to package insert for complete information):

One dose missed: Take as soon as remembered or take 2 tablets next day

Two consecutive doses missed in the first 2 weeks: Take 2 tablets as soon as remembered or 2 tablets next 2 days. **An additional method of contraception should be used for 7 days after missed dose.**

Two consecutive doses missed in week 3 or three consecutive doses missed at any time: **An additional method of contraception should be used for 7 days after missed dose:**

Schedule 1 (Sunday starter): Continue dose of 1 tablet daily until Sunday, then discard the rest of the pack, and a new pack should be started that same day.

Schedule 2 (Day 1 starter): Current package should be discarded, and a new pack should be started that same day.

Dosage adjustment in renal impairment: Specific guidelines not available; use with caution

(Continued)

Ethinyl Estradiol and Ethynodiol Diacetate *(Continued)*

Dosage adjustment in hepatic impairment: Contraindicated in patients with hepatic impairment

Mechanism of Action Combination hormonal contraceptives inhibit ovulation via a negative feedback mechanism on the hypothalamus, which alters the normal pattern of gonadotropin secretion of a follicle-stimulating hormone (FSH) and luteinizing hormone by the anterior pituitary. The follicular phase FSH and midcycle surge of gonadotropins are inhibited. In addition, combination hormonal contraceptives produce alterations in the genital tract, including changes in the cervical mucus, rendering it unfavorable for sperm penetration even if ovulation occurs. Changes in the endometrium may also occur, producing an unfavorable environment for nidation. Combination hormonal contraceptive drugs may alter the tubal transport of the ova through the fallopian tubes. Progestational agents may also alter sperm fertility.

Contraindications Hypersensitivity to ethinyl estradiol, ethynodiol diacetate, or any component of the formulation; history of or current thrombophlebitis or venous thromboembolic disorders (including DVT, PE); active or recent (within 1 year) arterial thromboembolic disease (eg, stroke, MI); cerebral vascular disease, coronary artery disease, valvular heart disease with complications, severe hypertension; diabetes mellitus with vascular involvement; severe headache with focal neurological symptoms; known or suspected breast carcinoma, endometrial cancer, estrogen-dependent neoplasms, undiagnosed abnormal genital bleeding; hepatic dysfunction or tumor, cholestatic jaundice of pregnancy, jaundice with prior combination hormonal contraceptive use; major surgery with prolonged immobilization; heavy smoking (≥15 cigarettes/day) in patients >35 years of age; pregnancy

Warnings/Precautions Combination hormonal contraceptives do not protect against HIV infection or other sexually-transmitted diseases. The risk of cardiovascular side effects increases in women who smoke cigarettes, especially those who are >35 years of age; women who use combination hormonal contraceptives should be strongly advised not to smoke. Combination hormonal contraceptives may lead to increased risk of myocardial infarction, use with caution in patients with risk factors for coronary artery disease. May increase the risk of thromboembolism. Combination hormonal contraceptives may have a dose-related risk of vascular disease, hypertension, and gallbladder disease. Women with hypertension should be encouraged to use a nonhormonal form of contraception. The use of combination hormonal contraceptives has been associated with a slight increase in frequency of breast cancer, however, studies are not consistent. Combination hormonal contraceptives may cause glucose intolerance. Retinal thrombosis has been reported (rarely). Use with caution in patients with renal disease, conditions that may be aggravated by fluid retention, depression, or history of migraine. Not for use prior to menarche.

The minimum dosage combination of estrogen/progestin that will effectively treat the individual patient should be used. New patients should be started on products containing <50 mcg of estrogen per tablet.

Drug Interactions

Cytochrome P450 Effect: Ethinyl estradiol: **Substrate** of CYP3A4 (major), 3A5-7 (minor); **Inhibits** CYP1A2 (weak), 2B6 (weak), 2C19 (weak), 3A4 (weak)

Increased Effect/Toxicity: Acetaminophen and ascorbic acid may increase plasma levels of estrogen component. Atorvastatin and indinavir increase plasma levels of combination hormonal contraceptives. Combination hormonal contraceptives increase the plasma levels of alprazolam, chlordiazepoxide, cyclosporine, diazepam, prednisolone, selegiline, theophylline, tricyclic antidepressants. Combination hormonal contraceptives may increase (or decrease) the effects of coumarin derivatives.

Decreased Effect: CYP3A4 inducers may decrease the levels/effects of ethinyl estradiol; example inducers include aminoglutethimide, carbamazepine, nafcillin, nevirapine, phenobarbital, phenytoin, and rifamycins. Combination hormonal contraceptives may decrease plasma levels of acetaminophen, clofibric acid, lorazepam, morphine, oxazepam, salicylic acid, temazepam. Contraceptive effect decreased by acitretin, aminoglutethimide, amprenavir, anticonvulsants, griseofulvin, lopinavir, nelfinavir, penicillins (effect not consistent), rifampin, ritonavir, tetracyclines (effect not consistent). Combination hormonal contraceptives may decrease (or increase) the effects of coumarin derivatives.

Ethanol/Nutrition/Herb Interactions

Food: CNS effects of caffeine may be enhanced if combination hormonal contraceptives are used concurrently with caffeine. Grapefruit juice increases ethinyl estradiol concentrations and would be expected to increase progesterone serum levels as well; clinical implications are unclear.

Herb/Nutraceutical: St John's wort may decrease the effectiveness of combination hormonal contraceptives by inducing hepatic enzymes. Avoid dong quai and black cohosh (have estrogen activity). Avoid saw palmetto, red clover, ginseng.

Dietary Considerations Should be taken with food at same time each day.

Pregnancy Risk Factor X

Dosage Forms TAB, monophasic: (Demulen® 1/35-28): Ethinyl estradiol 0.035 mg and ethynodiol 1 mg (28s); (Demulen® 1/50-21): Ethinyl estradiol 0.05 mg and ethynodiol 1 mg (21s); (Demulen® 1/50-28): Ethinyl estradiol 0.05 mg and ethynodiol 1 mg (28s); (Zovia™ 1/35-21): Ethinyl estradiol 0.035 mg and ethynodiol 1 mg (21s); (Zovia™ 1/35-28): Ethinyl estradiol 0.035 mg and ethynodiol 1 mg (28s); (Zovia™ 1/50-21): Ethinyl estradiol 0.05 mg and ethynodiol 1 mg (21s); (Zovia™ 1/50-28): Ethinyl estradiol 0.05 mg and ethynodiol 1 mg (28s)

Ethinyl Estradiol and Etonogestrel

(ETH in il es tra DYE ole & et oh noe JES trel)

U.S. Brand Names NuvaRing®

Generic Available No

Synonyms Etonogestrel and Ethinyl Estradiol

Pharmacologic Category Contraceptive; Estrogen and Progestin Combination

Use Prevention of pregnancy

Local Anesthetic/Vasoconstrictor Precautions No information available to require special precautions

Effects on Dental Treatment When prescribing antibiotics, patient must be warned to use additional methods of birth control if on oral contraceptives.

Common Adverse Effects Adverse reactions associated with oral combination hormonal contraceptive agents are also likely to appear with vaginally-administered products (frequency difficult to anticipate). Refer to oral contraceptive monographs for additional information.

5% to 14%:

Central nervous system: Headache

Gastrointestinal: Nausea, weight gain

Genitourinary: Leukorrhea, vaginitis

Respiratory: Sinusitis, upper respiratory tract infection

Frequency not defined:

Central nervous system: Emotional lability

Genitourinary: Coital problems, device expulsion, foreign body sensation, vaginal discomfort

Dosage Vaginal: Adults: Female: Contraception: One ring, inserted vaginally and left in place for 3 consecutive weeks, then removed for 1 week. A new ring is inserted 7 days after the last was removed (even if bleeding is not complete) and should be inserted at approximately the same time of day the ring was removed the previous week.

Initial treatment should begin as follows (pregnancy should always be ruled out first):

No hormonal contraceptive use in the past month: Using the first day of menstruation as "Day 1," insert the ring on or prior to "Day 5," even if bleeding is not complete. **An additional form of contraception should be used for the following 7 days.***

Switching from combination oral contraceptive: Ring should be inserted within 7 days after the last active tablet was taken and no later than the first day a new cycle of tablets would begin. Additional forms of contraception are not needed.

Switching from progestin-only contraceptive: **An additional form of contraception should be used for the following 7 days with any of the following.***

If previously using a progestin-only mini-pill, insert the ring on any day of the month; do not skip days between the last pill and insertion of the ring.

If previously using an implant, insert the ring on the same day of implant removal.

If previously using a progestin-containing IUD, insert the ring on day of IUD removal.

If previously using a progestin injection, insert the ring on the day the next injection would be given.

Following complete 1st trimester abortion: Insert ring within the first five days of abortion. If not inserted within five days, follow instructions for "No

(Continued)

Ethinyl Estradiol and Etonogestrel *(Continued)*

hormonal contraceptive use within the past month" and instruct patient to use a nonhormonal contraceptive in the interim.

Following delivery or 2nd trimester abortion: Insert ring 4 weeks postpartum (in women who are not breast-feeding) or following 2nd trimester abortion. **An additional form of contraception should be used for the following 7 days.***

If the ring is accidentally removed from the vagina at anytime during the 3-week period of use, it may be rinsed with cool or lukewarm water (not hot) and reinserted as soon as possible. If the ring is not reinserted within three hours, contraceptive effectiveness will be decreased. **An additional form of contraception should be used until the ring has been inserted for 7 continuous days.***

If the ring has been removed for longer than 1 week, pregnancy must be ruled out prior to restarting therapy. **An additional form of contraception should be used for the following 7 days.***

If the ring has been left in place for >3 weeks, a new ring should be inserted following a 1-week (ring-free) interval. Pregnancy must be ruled out prior to insertion and **an additional form of contraception should be used for the following 7 days.***

***Note:** Diaphragms may interfere with proper ring placement, and therefore, are not recommended for use as an additional form of contraception.

Dosage adjustment in renal impairment: Specific guidelines not available; use with caution.

Dosage adjustment in hepatic impairment: Contraindicated in patients with hepatic impairment

Mechanism of Action Combination hormonal contraceptives inhibit ovulation via a negative feedback mechanism on the hypothalamus, which alters the normal pattern of gonadotropin secretion of a follicle-stimulating hormone (FSH) and luteinizing hormone by the anterior pituitary. The follicular phase FSH and midcycle surge of gonadotropins are inhibited. In addition, combination hormonal contraceptives produce alterations in the genital tract, including changes in the cervical mucus, rendering it unfavorable for sperm penetration even if ovulation occurs. Changes in the endometrium may also occur, producing an unfavorable environment for nidation. Combination hormonal contraceptive drugs may alter the tubal transport of the ova through the fallopian tubes. Progestational agents may also alter sperm fertility.

Contraindications Hypersensitivity to ethinyl estradiol, etonogestrel, or any component of the formulation; history of or current thrombophlebitis or venous thromboembolic disorders (including DVT, PE); active or recent (within 1 year) arterial thromboembolic disease (eg, stroke, MI); major surgery with prolonged immobilization, cerebral vascular disease, coronary artery disease, valvular heart disease with complications, severe hypertension; diabetes mellitus with vascular involvement; severe headache with focal neurological symptoms; known or suspected breast carcinoma, endometrial cancer, estrogen-dependent neoplasms, undiagnosed abnormal genital bleeding; hepatic dysfunction or tumor, cholestatic jaundice of pregnancy, jaundice with prior combination hormonal contraceptive use; heavy smoking (≥15 cigarettes/day) in patients >35 years of age; conditions which make the vagina susceptible to irritation or ulceration; pregnancy

Warnings/Precautions Combination hormonal contraceptive agents do not protect against HIV infection or other sexually-transmitted diseases. The risk of cardiovascular side effects increases in women who smoke cigarettes, especially those who are >35 years of age; women who use combination hormonal contraceptives should be strongly advised not to smoke. May lead to increased risk of myocardial infarction, use with caution in patients with risk factors for coronary artery disease. May increase the risk of thromboembolism. May have a dose-related risk of vascular disease, hypertension, and gallbladder disease. Women with hypertension should be encouraged to use another form of contraception. May cause glucose intolerance. Retinal thrombosis has been reported (rarely). Use with caution in patients with renal disease, conditions that may be aggravated by fluid retention, depression, or history of migraine. Not for use prior to menarche.

Vaginally-administered combination hormonal contraceptive agents may have a similar adverse effects associated with oral contraceptive products. In order to reduce some of the possible risks, the minimum dosage combination of estrogen/progestin that will effectively treat the individual patient should be used.

Drug Interactions

Cytochrome P450 Effect:

Ethinyl estradiol: **Substrate** of CYP3A4 (major), 3A5-7 (minor); **Inhibits** CYP1A2 (weak), 2B6 (weak), 2C19 (weak), 3A4 (weak)

Etonogestrel: **Substrate** of CYP3A4 (minor)

Increased Effect/Toxicity: Acetaminophen and ascorbic acid may increase plasma levels of estrogen component. Atorvastatin and indinavir increase plasma levels of combination hormonal contraceptives. Combination hormonal contraceptives increase the plasma levels of alprazolam, chlordiazepoxide, cyclosporine, diazepam, prednisolone, selegiline, theophylline, tricyclic antidepressants. Combination hormonal contraceptives may increase (or decrease) the effects of coumarin derivatives.

Decreased Effect: Combination hormonal contraceptives may decrease plasma levels of acetaminophen, clofibric acid, lorazepam, morphine, oxazepam, salicylic acid, temazepam. Contraceptive effect decreased by acitretin, aminoglutethimide, amprenavir, anticonvulsants, griseofulvin, lopinavir, nelfinavir, nevirapine, penicillins (effect not consistent), rifampin, ritonavir, tetracyclines (effect not consistent). Combination hormonal contraceptives may decrease (or increase) the effects of coumarin derivatives.

Ethanol/Nutrition/Herb Interactions

Food: CNS effects of caffeine may be enhanced if combination hormonal contraceptives are used concurrently with caffeine. Grapefruit juice increases ethinyl estradiol concentrations and would be expected to increase progesterone serum levels as well; clinical implications are unclear.

Herb/Nutraceutical: St John's wort may decrease the effectiveness of combination hormonal contraceptives by inducing hepatic enzymes. Avoid dong quai and black cohosh (have estrogen activity). Avoid saw palmetto, red clover, ginseng.

Pregnancy Risk Factor X

Dosage Forms RING, intravaginal [3-week duration]: Ethinyl estradiol 0.015 mg/day and etonogestrel 0.12 mg/day (1s)

Ethinyl Estradiol and Levonorgestrel

(ETH in il es tra DYE ole & LEE voe nor jes trel)

U.S. Brand Names Alesse®; Aviane™; Enpresse™; Lessina™; Levlen®; Levlite™; Levora®; Nordette®; Portia™; PREVEN®; Seasonale®; Tri-Levlen®; Triphasil®; Trivora®

Canadian Brand Names Alesse®; Min-Ovral®; Triphasil®; Triquilar®

Generic Available Yes

Synonyms Levonorgestrel and Ethinyl Estradiol

Pharmacologic Category Contraceptive; Estrogen and Progestin Combination

Use Prevention of pregnancy; postcoital contraception

Unlabeled/Investigational Use Treatment of hypermenorrhea, endometriosis, female hypogonadism

Local Anesthetic/Vasoconstrictor Precautions No information available to require special precautions

Effects on Dental Treatment When prescribing antibiotics, patient must be warned to use additional methods of birth control if on oral contraceptives.

Common Adverse Effects Frequency not defined.

Cardiovascular: Arterial thromboembolism, cerebral hemorrhage, cerebral thrombosis, edema, hypertension, mesenteric thrombosis, myocardial infarction

Central nervous system: Depression, dizziness, headache, migraine, nervousness, premenstrual syndrome, stroke

Dermatologic: Acne, erythema multiforme, erythema nodosum, hirsutism, loss of scalp hair, melasma (may persist), rash (allergic)

Endocrine & metabolic: Amenorrhea, breakthrough bleeding, breast enlargement, breast secretion, breast tenderness, carbohydrate intolerance, lactation decreased (postpartum), glucose tolerance decreased, libido changes, menstrual flow changes, sex hormone-binding globulins (SHBG) increased, spotting, temporary infertility (following discontinuation), thyroid-binding globulin increased, triglycerides increased

Gastrointestinal: Abdominal cramps, appetite changes, bloating, cholestasis, colitis, gallbladder disease, jaundice, nausea, vomiting, weight gain/loss

Genitourinary: Cervical erosion changes, cervical secretion changes, cystitis-like syndrome, vaginal candidiasis, vaginitis

Hematologic: Antithrombin III decreased, folate levels decreased, hemolytic uremic syndrome, norepinephrine induced platelet aggregability increased, porphyria, prothrombin increased; factors VII, VIII, IX, and X increased

(Continued)

Ethinyl Estradiol and Levonorgestrel *(Continued)*

Hepatic: Benign liver tumors, Budd-Chiari syndrome, cholestatic jaundice, hepatic adenomas
Local: Thrombophlebitis
Ocular: Cataracts, change in corneal curvature (steepening), contact lens intolerance, optic neuritis, retinal thrombosis
Renal: Impaired renal function
Respiratory: Pulmonary thromboembolism
Miscellaneous: Hemorrhagic eruption

Dosage Oral: Adults: Female:

Contraception, 28-day cycle:

Schedule 1 (Sunday starter): Dose begins on first Sunday after onset of menstruation; if the menstrual period starts on Sunday, take first tablet that very same day. With a Sunday start, an additional method of contraception should be used until after the first 7 days of consecutive administration:

For 21-tablet package: 1 tablet/day for 21 consecutive days, followed by 7 days off of the medication; a new course begins on the 8th day after the last tablet is taken

For 28-tablet package: 1 tablet/day without interruption

Schedule 2 (Day 1 starter): Dose starts on first day of menstrual cycle taking 1 tablet/day:

For 21-tablet package: 1 tablet/day for 21 consecutive days, followed by 7 days off of the medication; a new course begins on the 8th day after the last tablet is taken

For 28-tablet package: 1 tablet/day without interruption

If all doses have been taken on schedule and one menstrual period is missed, continue dosing cycle. If two consecutive menstrual periods are missed, pregnancy test is required before new dosing cycle is started.

Missed doses **monophasic formulations** (refer to package insert for complete information):

One dose missed: Take as soon as remembered or take 2 tablets next day

Two consecutive doses missed in the first 2 weeks: Take 2 tablets as soon as remembered or 2 tablets next 2 days. An additional method of contraception should be used for 7 days after missed dose.

Two consecutive doses missed in week 3 or three consecutive doses missed at any time: An additional method of contraception must be used for 7 days after a missed dose:

Schedule 1 (Sunday starter): Continue dose of 1 tablet daily until Sunday, then discard the rest of the pack, and a new pack should be started that same day.

Schedule 2 (Day 1 starter): Current pack should be discarded, and a new pack should be started that same day.

Missed doses **biphasic/triphasic formulations** (refer to package insert for complete information):

One dose missed: Take as soon as remembered or take 2 tablets next day.

Two consecutive doses missed in week 1 or week 2 of the pack: Take 2 tablets as soon as remembered and 2 tablets the next day. Resume taking 1 tablet daily until the pack is empty. An additional method of contraception should be used for 7 days after a missed dose.

Two consecutive doses missed in week 3 of the pack: An additional method of contraception must be used for 7 days after a missed dose.

Schedule 1 (Sunday starter): Take 1 tablet every day until Sunday. Discard the remaining pack and start a new pack of pills on the same day.

Schedule 2 (Day 1 starter): Discard the remaining pack and start a new pack the same day.

Three or more consecutive doses missed: An additional method of contraception must be used for 7 days after a missed dose.

Schedule 1 (Sunday starter): Take 1 tablet every day until Sunday; on Sunday, discard the pack and start a new pack.

Schedule 2 (Day 1 starter): Discard the remaining pack and begin new pack of tablets starting on the same day.

Contraception, 91-day cycle (Seasonale®): One active tablet/day for 84 consecutive days, followed by 1 inactive tablet/day for 7 days; if all doses have been taken on schedule and one menstrual period is missed, pregnancy should be ruled out prior to continuing therapy.

Missed doses:

One dose missed: Take as soon as remembered or take 2 tablets the next day

Two consecutive doses missed: Take 2 tablets as soon as remembered or 2 tablets the next 2 days. An additional nonhormonal method of contraception should be used for 7 consecutive days after the missed dose.

Three or more consecutive doses missed: Do not take the missed doses; continue taking 1 tablet/day until pack is complete. Bleeding may occur during the following week. An additional nonhormonal method of contraception should be used for 7 consecutive days after the missed dose.

Emergency contraception (PREVEN®): Initial: 2 tablets as soon as possible (but within 72 hours of unprotected intercourse), followed by a second dose of 2 tablets 12 hours later. Repeat dose or use antiemetic if vomiting occurs within 1 hour of dose.

Dosage adjustment in renal impairment: Specific guidelines not available; use with caution

Dosage adjustment in hepatic impairment: Contraindicated in patients with hepatic impairment

Mechanism of Action Combination hormonal contraceptives inhibit ovulation via a negative feedback mechanism on the hypothalamus, which alters the normal pattern of gonadotropin secretion of a follicle-stimulating hormone (FSH) and luteinizing hormone by the anterior pituitary. The follicular phase FSH and midcycle surge of gonadotropins are inhibited. In addition, combination hormonal contraceptives produce alterations in the genital tract, including changes in the cervical mucus, rendering it unfavorable for sperm penetration even if ovulation occurs. Changes in the endometrium may also occur, producing an unfavorable environment for nidation. Combination hormonal contraceptive drugs may alter the tubal transport of the ova through the fallopian tubes. Progestational agents may also alter sperm fertility.

Contraindications Hypersensitivity to ethinyl estradiol, levonorgestrel, or any component of the formulation; history of or current thrombophlebitis or venous thromboembolic disorders (including DVT, PE); active or recent (within 1 year) arterial thromboembolic disease (eg, stroke, MI); cerebral vascular disease, coronary artery disease, valvular heart disease with complications, severe hypertension; diabetes mellitus with vascular involvement; severe headache with focal neurological symptoms; known or suspected breast carcinoma, endometrial cancer, estrogen-dependent neoplasms, undiagnosed abnormal genital bleeding; hepatic dysfunction or tumor, cholestatic jaundice of pregnancy, jaundice with prior combination hormonal contraceptive use; major surgery with prolonged immobilization; heavy smoking (≥15 cigarettes/day) in patients >35 years of age; pregnancy

Warnings/Precautions Combination hormonal contraceptives do not protect against HIV infection or other sexually-transmitted diseases. The risk of cardiovascular side effects increases in women who smoke cigarettes, especially those who are >35 years of age; women who use combination hormonal contraceptives should be strongly advised not to smoke. Combination hormonal contraceptives may lead to increased risk of myocardial infarction, use with caution in patients with risk factors for coronary artery disease. May increase the risk of thromboembolism. Combination hormonal contraceptives may have a dose-related risk of vascular disease, hypertension, and gallbladder disease. Women with hypertension should be encouraged to use another form of contraception. The use of combination hormonal contraceptives has been associated with a slight increase in frequency of breast cancer, however, studies are not consistent. Combination hormonal contraceptives may cause glucose intolerance. Retinal thrombosis has been reported (rarely). Use with caution in patients with renal disease, conditions that may be aggravated by fluid retention, depression, or history of migraine. Not for use prior to menarche.

The minimum dosage combination of estrogen/progestin that will effectively treat the individual patient should be used. New patients should be started on products containing <50 mcg of estrogen per tablet.

Drug Interactions

Cytochrome P450 Effect:

Ethinyl estradiol: **Substrate** of CYP3A4 (major), 3A5-7 (minor); **Inhibits** CYP1A2 (weak), 2B6 (weak), 2C19 (weak), 3A4 (weak)

Levonorgestrel: **Substrate** of CYP3A4 (major)

Increased Effect/Toxicity: Acetaminophen and ascorbic acid may increase plasma levels of estrogen component. Atorvastatin and indinavir increase plasma levels of combination hormonal contraceptives. Combination hormonal contraceptives increase the plasma levels of alprazolam, chlordiazepoxide, cyclosporine, diazepam, prednisolone, selegiline, theophylline, tricyclic antidepressants. Combination hormonal contraceptives may increase (or decrease) the effects of coumarin derivatives.

(Continued)

Ethinyl Estradiol and Levonorgestrel *(Continued)*

Decreased Effect: CYP3A4 inducers may decrease the levels/effects of ethinyl estradiol and/or levonorgestrel; example inducers include aminoglutethimide, carbamazepine, nafcillin, nevirapine, phenobarbital, phenytoin, and rifamycins. Combination hormonal contraceptives may decrease plasma levels of acetaminophen, clofibric acid, lorazepam, morphine, oxazepam, salicylic acid, temazepam. Contraceptive effect decreased by acitretin, aminoglutethimide, amprenavir, anticonvulsants, griseofulvin, lopinavir, nelfinavir, penicillins (effect not consistent), rifampin, ritonavir, tetracyclines (effect not consistent). Combination hormonal contraceptives may decrease (or increase) the effects of coumarin derivatives.

Ethanol/Nutrition/Herb Interactions

Food: CNS effects of caffeine may be enhanced if combination hormonal contraceptives are used concurrently with caffeine. Grapefruit juice increases ethinyl estradiol concentrations and would be expected to increase progesterone serum levels as well; clinical implications are unclear.

Herb/Nutraceutical: St John's wort may decrease the effectiveness of combination hormonal contraceptives by inducing hepatic enzymes. Avoid dong quai and black cohosh (have estrogen activity). Avoid saw palmetto, red clover, ginseng.

Dietary Considerations Should be taken at the same time each day.

Pharmacodynamics/Kinetics See individual agents.

Pregnancy Risk Factor X

Dosage Forms KIT [4 tablets and a pregnancy test] (PREVEN®): Ethinyl estradiol 0.05 mg and levonorgestrel 0.25 mg (4s). **TAB** (PREVEN®): Ethinyl estradiol 0.05 mg and levonorgestrel 0.25 mg (4s). **TAB, low-dose:** (Alesse®, Lessina™): Ethinyl estradiol 0.02 mg and levonorgestrel 0.1 mg (21s); (Alesse®, Lessina™, Levlite™): Ethinyl estradiol 0.02 mg and levonorgestrel 0.1 mg (28s); (Aviane™ 28): Ethinyl estradiol 0.02 mg and levonorgestrel 0.1 mg. **TAB, monophasic:** (Levlen®, Nordette®, Portia™): Ethinyl estradiol 0.03 mg and levonorgestrel 0.15 mg (21s, 28s); (Seasonale®): Ethinyl estradiol 0.03 mg and levonorgestrel 0.15 mg (91s). **TAB, triphasic:** (Enpresse™): Day 1-6: Ethinyl estradiol 0.03 mg and levonorgestrel 0.05, Day 7-11: Ethinyl estradiol 0.04 mg and levonorgestrel 0.075, Day 12-21: Ethinyl estradiol 0.03 mg and levonorgestrel 0.125; (Tri-Levlen® 21, Triphasil® 21): Day 1-6: Ethinyl estradiol 0.03 mg and levonorgestrel 0.05 mg, Day 7-11: Ethinyl estradiol 0.04 mg and levonorgestrel 0.075 mg, Day 12-21: Ethinyl estradiol 0.03 mg and levonorgestrel 0.125 mg (21s); (Tri-Levlen® 28, Triphasil® 28): Day 1-6: Ethinyl estradiol 0.03 mg and levonorgestrel 0.05 mg, Day 7-11: Ethinyl estradiol 0.04 mg and levonorgestrel 0.075 mg, Day 12-21: Ethinyl estradiol 0.03 mg and levonorgestrel 0.125 mg, Day 22-28: Inactive (28s); (Trivora® 28): Day 1-6: Ethinyl estradiol 0.03 mg and levonorgestrel 0.05 mg, Day 7-11: Ethinyl estradiol 0.04 mg and levonorgestrel 0.075 mg, Day 12-21: Ethinyl estradiol 0.03 mg and levonorgestrel 0.125 mg, Day 22-28: Inactive (28s)

Ethinyl Estradiol and NGM *see* Ethinyl Estradiol and Norgestimate *on page 554*

Ethinyl Estradiol and Norelgestromin

(ETH in il es tra DYE ole & nor el JES troe min)

U.S. Brand Names Ortho Evra™

Canadian Brand Names Evra™

Synonyms Norelgestromin and Ethinyl Estradiol; Ortho-Evra

Pharmacologic Category Contraceptive; Estrogen and Progestin Combination

Use Prevention of pregnancy

Local Anesthetic/Vasoconstrictor Precautions No information available to require special precautions

Effects on Dental Treatment When prescribing antibiotics, patient must be warned to use additional methods of birth control if on oral contraceptives.

Common Adverse Effects The following reactions have been reported with the contraceptive patch. Adverse reactions associated with oral combination hormonal contraceptive agents are also likely to appear with the topical contraceptive patch (frequency difficult to anticipate). Refer to individual **oral** contraceptive monographs for additional information.

9% to 22%: Abdominal pain, application site reaction, breast symptoms, headache, menstrual cramps, nausea, upper respiratory infection

Dosage Topical: Adults: Female:

Contraception: Apply one patch each week for 3 weeks (21 total days); followed by one week that is patch-free. Each patch should be applied on the same day each week ("patch change day") and only one patch should be worn at a time. No more than 7 days should pass during the patch-free interval.

Schedule 1 (Sunday starter): Dose begins on first Sunday after onset of menstruation; if the menstrual period starts on Sunday, apply one patch that very same day. **With a Sunday start, an additional method of contraception (nonhormonal) should be used until after the first 7 days of consecutive administration.** Each patch change will then occur on Sunday.

Schedule 2 (Day 1 starter): Dose starts on first day of menstrual cycle, applying one patch during the first 24 hours of menstrual cycle. No back-up method of contraception is needed as long as the patch is applied on the first day of cycle. Each patch change will then occur on that same day of the week.

Additional dosing considerations:

No bleeding during patch-free week/missed menstrual period: If patch has been applied as directed, continue treatment on usual "patch change day". If used correctly, no bleeding during patch-free week does not necessarily indicate pregnancy. However, if no withdrawal bleeding occurs for 2 consecutive cycles, pregnancy should be ruled out. If patch has not been applied as directed, and one menstrual period is missed, pregnancy should be ruled out prior to continuing treatment.

If a patch becomes partially or completely detached for <24 hours: Try to reapply to same place, or replace with a new patch immediately. Do not reapply if patch is no longer sticky, if it is sticking to itself or another surface, or if it has material sticking to it.

If a patch becomes partially or completely detached for >24 hours (or time period is unknown): Apply a new patch and use this day of the week as the new "patch change day" from this point on. **An additional method of contraception (nonhormonal) should be used until after the first 7 days of consecutive administration.**

Switching from oral contraceptives: Apply first patch on the first day of withdrawal bleeding. If there is no bleeding within 5 days of taking the last active tablet, pregnancy must first be ruled out. If patch is applied later than the first day of bleeding, **an additional method of contraception (nonhormonal) should be used until after the first 7 days of consecutive administration**

Use after childbirth: Therapy should not be started <4 weeks after childbirth. Pregnancy should be ruled out prior to treatment if menstrual periods have not restarted. **An additional method of contraception (nonhormonal) should be used until after the first 7 days of consecutive administration.**

Use after abortion or miscarriage: Therapy may be started immediately if abortion/miscarriage occur within the first trimester. If therapy is not started within 5 days, follow instructions for first time use. If abortion/miscarriage occur during the second trimester, therapy should not be started for at least 4 weeks. Follow directions for use after childbirth.

Dosage adjustment in renal impairment: Specific guidelines not available; use with caution

Dosage adjustment in hepatic impairment: Contraindicated in patients with hepatic impairment

Mechanism of Action Combination hormonal contraceptives inhibit ovulation via a negative feedback mechanism on the hypothalamus, which alters the normal pattern of gonadotropin secretion of a follicle-stimulating hormone (FSH) and luteinizing hormone by the anterior pituitary. The follicular phase FSH and midcycle surge of gonadotropins are inhibited. In addition, combination hormonal contraceptives produce alterations in the genital tract, including changes in the cervical mucus, rendering it unfavorable for sperm penetration even if ovulation occurs. Changes in the endometrium may also occur, producing an unfavorable environment for nidation. Combination hormonal contraceptive drugs may alter the tubal transport of the ova through the fallopian tubes. Progestational agents may also alter sperm fertility.

Contraindications Hypersensitivity to ethinyl estradiol, norelgestromin, or any component of the formulation; history of or current thrombophlebitis or venous thromboembolic disorders (including DVT, PE); active or recent (within 1 year) arterial thromboembolic disease (eg, stroke, MI); cerebral vascular disease, coronary artery disease, valvular heart disease with complications, severe hypertension; diabetes mellitus with vascular involvement; severe headache with focal neurological symptoms; known or suspected breast carcinoma, endometrial cancer, estrogen-dependent neoplasms, undiagnosed abnormal genital bleeding; hepatic dysfunction or tumor, cholestatic jaundice of pregnancy, jaundice with prior combination hormonal contraceptive use; major

(Continued)

Ethinyl Estradiol and Norelgestromin *(Continued)*

surgery with prolonged immobilization; heavy smoking (≥15 cigarettes/day) in patients >35 years of age; pregnancy

Warnings/Precautions Combination hormonal contraceptives do not protect against HIV infection or other sexually-transmitted diseases. The risk of cardiovascular side effects increases in women who smoke cigarettes, especially those who are >35 years of age; women who use combination hormonal contraceptives should be strongly advised not to smoke. Combination hormonal contraceptives may lead to increased risk of myocardial infarction, use with caution in patients with risk factors for coronary artery disease. May increase the risk of thromboembolism. Combination hormonal contraceptives may have a dose-related risk of vascular disease, hypertension, and gallbladder disease. Women with hypertension should be encouraged to use a nonhormonal form of contraception. The use of combination hormonal contraceptives has been associated with a slight increase in frequency of breast cancer, however, studies are not consistent. Combination hormonal contraceptives may cause glucose intolerance. Retinal thrombosis has been reported (rarely). Use with caution in patients with renal disease, conditions that may be aggravated by fluid retention, depression, or history of migraine. Not for use prior to menarche.

The combination hormonal contraceptive patch may have adverse effects similar to those associated with oral contraceptive products. The topical patch may be less effective in patients weighing ≥90 kg (198 lb) and an increased incidence of pregnancy has been reported in this population; consider another form of contraception.

Drug Interactions

Cytochrome P450 Effect:

Ethinyl estradiol: **Substrate** of CYP3A4 (major), 3A5-7 (minor); **Inhibits** CYP1A2 (weak), 2B6 (weak), 2C19 (weak), 3A4 (weak)

Norelgestromin: **Substrate** of CYP3A4 (minor)

Increased Effect/Toxicity: Acetaminophen and ascorbic acid may increase plasma levels of estrogen component. Atorvastatin and indinavir increase plasma levels of combination hormonal contraceptives. Combination hormonal contraceptives increase the plasma levels of alprazolam, chlordiazepoxide, cyclosporine, diazepam, prednisolone, selegiline, theophylline, tricyclic antidepressants. Combination hormonal contraceptives may increase (or decrease) the effects of coumarin derivatives.

Decreased Effect: CYP3A4 inducers may decrease the levels/effects of ethinyl estradiol; example inducers include aminoglutethimide, carbamazepine, nafcillin, nevirapine, phenobarbital, phenytoin, and rifamycins. Combination hormonal contraceptives may decrease plasma levels of acetaminophen, clofibric acid, lorazepam, morphine, oxazepam, salicylic acid, temazepam. Contraceptive effect decreased by acitretin, aminoglutethimide, amprenavir, anticonvulsants, griseofulvin, lopinavir, nelfinavir, penicillins (effect not consistent), rifampin, ritonavir, tetracyclines (effect not consistent), troglitazone. Combination hormonal contraceptives may decrease (or increase) the effects of coumarin derivatives.

Ethanol/Nutrition/Herb Interactions

Food: CNS effects of caffeine may be enhanced if combination hormonal contraceptives are used concurrently with caffeine. Grapefruit juice increases ethinyl estradiol concentrations and would be expected to increase progesterone serum levels as well; clinical implications are unclear.

Herb/Nutraceutical: St John's wort may decrease the effectiveness of combination hormonal contraceptives by inducing hepatic enzymes. Avoid dong quai and black cohosh (have estrogen activity). Avoid saw palmetto, red clover, ginseng.

Pregnancy Risk Factor X

Dosage Forms PATCH, transdermal: Ethinyl estradiol 0.75 mg and norelgestromin 6 mg (1s, 3s)

Ethinyl Estradiol and Norethindrone

(ETH in il es tra DYE ole & nor eth IN drone)

U.S. Brand Names Brevicon®; Estrostep® Fe; femhrt®; Junel™; Loestrin®; Loestrin® Fe; Microgestin™ Fe; Modicon®; Necon® 0.5/35; Necon® 1/35; Necon® 7/7/7; Necon® 10/11; Norinyl® 1+35; Nortrel™; Nortrel™ 7/7/7; Ortho-Novum®; Ovcon®; Tri-Norinyl®

Canadian Brand Names Brevicon® 0.5/35; Brevicon® 1/35; FemHRT®; Loestrin™ 1.5.30; Minestrin™ 1/20; Ortho® 0.5/35; Ortho® 1/35; Ortho® 7/7/7; Select™ 1/35; Synphasic®

Generic Available Yes

Synonyms Norethindrone Acetate and Ethinyl Estradiol; Ortho Novum

Pharmacologic Category Contraceptive; Estrogen and Progestin Combination

Use Prevention of pregnancy; treatment of acne; moderate to severe vasomotor symptoms associated with menopause; prevention of osteoporosis (in women at significant risk only)

Unlabeled/Investigational Use Treatment of hypermenorrhea, endometriosis, female hypogonadism

Local Anesthetic/Vasoconstrictor Precautions No information available to require special precautions

Effects on Dental Treatment When prescribing antibiotics, patient must be warned to use additional methods of birth control if on oral contraceptives.

Common Adverse Effects As reported with oral contraceptive agents. Frequency not defined.

Cardiovascular: Arterial thromboembolism, cerebral hemorrhage, cerebral thrombosis, edema, hypertension, mesenteric thrombosis, myocardial infarction

Central nervous system: Depression, dizziness, headache, migraine, nervousness, premenstrual syndrome, stroke

Dermatologic: Acne, erythema multiforme, erythema nodosum, hirsutism, loss of scalp hair, melasma (may persist), rash (allergic)

Endocrine & metabolic: Amenorrhea, breakthrough bleeding, breast enlargement, breast secretion, breast tenderness, carbohydrate intolerance, lactation decreased (postpartum), glucose tolerance decreased, libido changes, menstrual flow changes, sex hormone-binding globulins (SHBG) increased, spotting, temporary infertility (following discontinuation), thyroid-binding globulin increased, triglycerides increased

Gastrointestinal: Abdominal cramps, appetite changes, bloating, cholestasis, colitis, gallbladder disease, jaundice, nausea, vomiting, weight gain/loss

Genitourinary: Cervical erosion changes, cervical secretion changes, cystitis-like syndrome, vaginal candidiasis, vaginitis

Hematologic: Antithrombin III decreased, folate levels decreased, hemolytic uremic syndrome, norepinephrine induced platelet aggregability increased, porphyria, prothrombin increased; factors VII, VIII, IX, and X

Hepatic: Benign liver tumors, Budd-Chiari syndrome, cholestatic jaundice, hepatic adenomas

Local: Thrombophlebitis

Ocular: Cataracts, change in corneal curvature (steepening), contact lens intolerance, optic neuritis, retinal thrombosis

Renal: Impaired renal function

Respiratory: Pulmonary thromboembolism

Miscellaneous: Hemorrhagic eruption

Dosage Oral:

Adolescents ≥15 years and Adults: Female: Acne: Estrostep®: Refer to dosing for contraception

Adults: Female:

Moderate to severe vasomotor symptoms associated with menopause: femhrt® 1/5: 1 tablet daily; patients should be re-evaluated at 3- to 6-month intervals to determine if treatment is still necessary

Prevention of osteoporosis: femhrt® 1/5: 1 tablet daily

Contraception:

Schedule 1 (Sunday starter): Dose begins on first Sunday after onset of menstruation; if the menstrual period starts on Sunday, take first tablet that very same day. With a Sunday start, an additional method of contraception should be used until after the first 7 days of consecutive administration.

For 21-tablet package: Dosage is 1 tablet daily for 21 consecutive days, followed by 7 days off of the medication; a new course begins on the 8th day after the last tablet is taken.

For 28-tablet package: Dosage is 1 tablet daily without interruption.

Schedule 2 (Day 1 starter): Dose starts on first day of menstrual cycle taking 1 tablet daily.

For 21-tablet package: Dosage is 1 tablet daily for 21 consecutive days, followed by 7 days off of the medication; a new course begins on the 8th day after the last tablet is taken.

For 28-tablet package: Dosage is 1 tablet daily without interruption.

If all doses have been taken on schedule and one menstrual period is missed, continue dosing cycle. If two consecutive menstrual periods are missed, pregnancy test is required before new dosing cycle is started.

(Continued)

Ethinyl Estradiol and Norethindrone *(Continued)*

Missed doses **monophasic formulations** (refer to package insert for complete information):

One dose missed: Take as soon as remembered or take 2 tablets next day

Two consecutive doses missed in the first 2 weeks: Take 2 tablets as soon as remembered or 2 tablets next 2 days. An additional method of contraception should be used for 7 days after missed dose.

Two consecutive doses missed in week 3 or three consecutive doses missed at any time: An additional method of contraception must be used for 7 days after a missed dose.

Schedule 1 (Sunday starter): Continue dose of 1 tablet daily until Sunday, then discard the rest of the pack, and a new pack should be started that same day.

Schedule 2 (Day 1 starter): Current pack should be discarded, and a new pack should be started that same day.

Missed doses **biphasic/triphasic formulations** (refer to package insert for complete information):

One dose missed: Take as soon as remembered or take 2 tablets next day.

Two consecutive doses missed in week 1 or week 2 of the pack: Take 2 tablets as soon as remembered and 2 tablets the next day. Resume taking 1 tablet daily until the pack is empty. An additional method of contraception should be used for 7 days after a missed dose.

Two consecutive doses missed in week 3 of the pack: An additional method of contraception must be used for 7 days after a missed dose.

Schedule 1 (Sunday Starter): Take 1 tablet every day until Sunday. Discard the remaining pack and start a new pack of pills on the same day.

Schedule 2 (Day 1 starter): Discard the remaining pack and start a new pack the same day.

Three or more consecutive doses missed: An additional method of contraception must be used for 7 days after a missed dose.

Schedule 1 (Sunday Starter): Take 1 tablet every day until Sunday; on Sunday, discard the pack and start a new pack.

Schedule 2 (Day 1 Starter): Discard the remaining pack and begin new pack of tablets starting on the same day.

Dosage adjustment in renal impairment: Specific guidelines not available; use with caution.

Dosage adjustment in hepatic impairment: Contraindicated in patients with hepatic impairment.

Mechanism of Action Combination oral contraceptives inhibit ovulation via a negative feedback mechanism on the hypothalamus, which alters the normal pattern of gonadotropin secretion of a follicle-stimulating hormone (FSH) and luteinizing hormone by the anterior pituitary. The follicular phase FSH and midcycle surge of gonadotropins are inhibited. In addition, combination hormonal contraceptives produce alterations in the genital tract, including changes in the cervical mucus, rendering it unfavorable for sperm penetration even if ovulation occurs. Changes in the endometrium may also occur, producing an unfavorable environment for nidation. Combination hormonal contraceptive drugs may alter the tubal transport of the ova through the fallopian tubes. Progestational agents may also alter sperm fertility.

In postmenopausal women, exogenous estrogen is used to replace decreased endogenous production. The addition of progestin reduces the incidence of endometrial hyperplasia and risk of adenocarcinoma in women with an intact uterus.

Contraindications Hypersensitivity to ethinyl estradiol, norethindrone, norethindrone acetate, or any component of the formulation; history of or current thrombophlebitis or venous thromboembolic disorders (including DVT, PE); active or recent (within 1 year) arterial thromboembolic disease (eg, stroke, MI); cerebral vascular disease, coronary artery disease, severe hypertension; diabetes mellitus with vascular involvement; severe headache with focal neurological symptoms; known or suspected breast carcinoma, endometrial cancer, estrogen-dependent neoplasms, undiagnosed abnormal genital bleeding; hepatic dysfunction or tumor, cholestatic jaundice of pregnancy, jaundice with prior combination hormonal contraceptive use; major surgery with prolonged immobilization; heavy smoking (≥15 cigarettes/day) in patients >35 years of age; pregnancy

Warnings/Precautions Combination hormonal contraceptives do not protect against HIV infection or other sexually-transmitted diseases. The risk of cardiovascular side effects increases in women who smoke cigarettes, especially those who are >35 years of age; women who use combination hormonal contraceptives should be strongly advised not to smoke. Combination hormonal contraceptives may lead to increased risk of myocardial infarction, use with caution in patients with risk factors for coronary artery disease. May increase the risk of thromboembolism. Combination hormonal contraceptives may have a dose-related risk of vascular disease, hypertension, and gallbladder disease. Women with hypertension should be encouraged to use another form of contraception. The use of combination hormonal contraceptives has been associated with a slight increase in frequency of breast cancer, however, studies are not consistent. Combination hormonal contraceptives may cause glucose intolerance. Retinal thrombosis has been reported (rarely). Use with caution in patients with renal disease, conditions that may be aggravated by fluid retention, depression, or history of migraine. Not for use prior to menarche.

The minimum dosage combination of estrogen/progestin that will effectively treat the individual patient should be used. New patients should be started on products containing <50 mcg of estrogen per tablet.

Acne: For use only in females ≥15 years, who also desire combination hormonal contraceptive therapy, are unresponsive to topical treatments, and have no contraindications to combination hormonal contraceptive use; treatment must continue for at least 6 months.

Vasomotor symptoms associated with menopause and prevention of osteoporosis: For use only in postmenopausal women with an intact uterus. Use for shortest duration possible consistent with treatment goals. Conduct periodic risk:benefit assessments. When used for the prevention of osteoporosis, estrogen/progestin products should be reserved for use in women at significant risk only; nonestrogen therapies should be considered.

Drug Interactions

Cytochrome P450 Effect:

Ethinyl estradiol: **Substrate** of CYP3A4 (major), 3A5-7 (minor); **Inhibits** CYP1A2 (weak), 2B6 (weak), 2C19 (weak), 3A4 (weak)

Norethindrone: **Substrate** of CYP3A4 (major); Induces CYP2C19 (weak)

Increased Effect/Toxicity: Acetaminophen and ascorbic acid may increase plasma levels of estrogen component. Atorvastatin and indinavir increase plasma levels of combination hormonal contraceptives. Combination hormonal contraceptives increase the plasma levels of alprazolam, chlordiazepoxide, cyclosporine, diazepam, prednisolone, selegiline, theophylline, tricyclic antidepressants. Combination hormonal contraceptives may increase (or decrease) the effects of coumarin derivatives.

Decreased Effect: CYP3A4 inducers may decrease the levels/effects of ethinyl estradiol and norethindrone; example inducers include aminoglutethimide, carbamazepine, nafcillin, nevirapine, phenobarbital, phenytoin, and rifamycins. Combination hormonal contraceptives may decrease plasma levels of acetaminophen, clofibric acid, lorazepam, morphine, oxazepam, salicylic acid, temazepam. Contraceptive effect decreased by acitretin, aminoglutethimide, amprenavir, anticonvulsants, griseofulvin, lopinavir, nelfinavir, penicillins (effect not consistent), rifampin, ritonavir, tetracyclines (effect not consistent), troglitazone. Oral contraceptives may decrease (or increase) the effects of coumarin derivatives.

Ethanol/Nutrition/Herb Interactions

Ethanol: Routine use increases estrogen level and risk of breast cancer; avoid ethanol. Ethanol may also increase the risk of osteoporosis.

Food: CNS effects of caffeine may be enhanced if combination hormonal contraceptives are used concurrently with caffeine. Grapefruit juice increases ethinyl estradiol concentrations and would be expected to increase progesterone serum levels as well; clinical implications are unclear. Norethindrone absorption is increased by 27% following administration with food.

Herb/Nutraceutical: St John's wort may decrease the effectiveness of combination hormonal contraceptives by inducing hepatic enzymes. Avoid dong quai and black cohosh (have estrogen activity). Avoid saw palmetto, red clover, ginseng.

Dietary Considerations Should be taken at same time each day. May be taken with or without food.

Pharmacodynamics/Kinetics See individual agents.

Pregnancy Risk Factor X

Dosage Forms TAB (femhrt® 1/5): Ethinyl estradiol 0.005 mg and norethindrone 1 mg. **TAB, monophasic** (Brevicon®): Ethinyl estradiol 0.035 mg and norethindrone 0.5 mg (28s); (Junel™ 21 1/20, Loestrin® 21 1/20): Ethinyl estradiol 0.02 mg and norethindrone 1 mg (21s); (Junel™ 21 1.5/30, Loestrin® 21 1.5/30): Ethinyl estradiol 0.03 mg and norethindrone 1.5 mg (21s); (Junel™ Fe

(Continued)

Ethinyl Estradiol and Norethindrone *(Continued)*

1/20, Loestrin® Fe 1/20, Microgestin™ Fe 1/20): Ethinyl estradiol 0.02 mg and norethindrone 1 mg and ferrous fumarate 75 mg (28s); (Junel™ Fe 1.5/30, Loestrin® Fe 1.5/30, Microgestin™ Fe 1.5/30): Ethinyl estradiol 0.03 mg and norethindrone 1.5 mg and ferrous fumarate 75 mg (28s); (Modicon® 21): Ethinyl estradiol 0.035 mg and norethindrone 0.5 mg (21s); (Modicon® 28): Ethinyl estradiol 0.035 mg and norethindrone 0.5 mg (28s); (Necon® 0.5/35-21): Ethinyl estradiol 0.035 mg and norethindrone 0.5 mg (21s); (Necon® 0.5/35-28): Ethinyl estradiol 0.035 mg and norethindrone 0.5 mg (28s); (Necon® 1/35-21): Ethinyl estradiol 0.035 mg and norethindrone 1 mg (21s); (Necon® 1/35-28): Ethinyl estradiol 0.035 mg and norethindrone 1 mg (28s); (Norinyl® 1+35): Ethinyl estradiol 0.035 mg and norethindrone 1 mg (28s); (Nortrel™ 0.5/35 mg): Ethinyl estradiol 0.035 mg and norethindrone 0.5 mg (21s); Ethinyl estradiol 0.035 mg and norethindrone 0.5 mg (28s); (Nortrel™ 1/35 mg): Ethinyl estradiol 0.035 mg and norethindrone 1 mg (21s); Ethinyl estradiol 0.035 mg and norethindrone 1 mg (28s); (Ortho-Novum® 1/35 21): Ethinyl estradiol 0.035 mg and norethindrone 1 mg (21s); (Ortho-Novum® 1/35 28): Ethinyl estradiol 0.035 mg and norethindrone 1 mg (28s); (Ovcon® 35 21-day): Ethinyl estradiol 0.035 mg and norethindrone 0.4 mg (21s); (Ovcon® 35 28-day): Ethinyl estradiol 0.035 mg and norethindrone 0.4 mg (28s); (Ovcon® 50): Ethinyl estradiol 0.05 mg and norethindrone 1 mg (28s). **TAB, biphasic** (Necon® 10/11-21): Day 1-10: Ethinyl estradiol 0.035 mg and norethindrone 0.5 mg, Day 11-21: Ethinyl estradiol 0.035 mg and norethindrone 1 mg (21s); (Necon® 10/11-28): Day 1-10: Ethinyl estradiol 0.035 mg and norethindrone 0.5 mg, Day 11-21: Ethinyl estradiol 0.035 mg and norethindrone 1 mg, Day 22-28: Inactive (28s); (Ortho-Novum® 10/11-21): Day 1-10: Ethinyl estradiol 0.035 mg and norethindrone 0.5 mg, Day 11-21: Ethinyl estradiol 0.035 mg and norethindrone 1 mg (21s); (Ortho-Novum® 10/11-28): Day 1-10: Ethinyl estradiol 0.035 mg and norethindrone 0.5 mg, Day 11-21: Ethinyl estradiol 0.035 mg and norethindrone 1 mg, Day 22-28: Inactive (28s). **TAB, triphasic** (Estrostep® Fe): Day 1-5: Ethinyl estradiol 0.02 mg and norethindrone acetate 1 mg, Day 6-12: Ethinyl estradiol 0.03 mg and norethindrone acetate 1 mg, Day 13-21: Ethinyl estradiol 0.035 mg and norethindrone acetate 1 mg, Day 22-28: Ferrous fumarate 75 mg (28s); (Necon® 7/7/7, Ortho-Novum® 7/7/7 28): Day 1-7: Ethinyl estradiol 0.035 mg and norethindrone 0.5 mg, Day 8-14: Ethinyl estradiol 0.035 mg and norethindrone 0.75 mg, Day 15-21: Ethinyl estradiol 0.035 mg and norethindrone 1 mg, Day 22-28: Inactive (28s); (Nortrel™ 7/7/7 21): Day 1-7: Ethinyl estradiol 0.035 mg and norethindrone 0.5 mg; Day 8-14: Ethinyl estradiol 0.035 mg and norethindrone 0.75 mg; Day 15-21: Ethinyl estradiol 0.035 mg and norethindrone 1 mg (21s); (Nortrel™ 7/7/7 28): Day 1-7: Ethinyl estradiol 0.035 mg and norethindrone 0.5 mg; Day 8-14: Ethinyl estradiol 0.035 mg and norethindrone 0.75 mg; Day 15-21: Ethinyl estradiol 0.035 mg and norethindrone 1 mg; Day 22-28: Inactive (28s); (Ortho-Novum® 7/7/7 21): Day 1-7: Ethinyl estradiol 0.035 mg and norethindrone 0.5 mg, Day 8-14: Ethinyl estradiol 0.035 mg and norethindrone 0.75 mg, Day 15-21: Ethinyl estradiol 0.035 mg and norethindrone 1 mg (21s); (Tri-Norinyl® 28): Day 1-7: Ethinyl estradiol 0.035 mg and norethindrone 0.5 mg, Day 8-16: Ethinyl estradiol 0.035 mg and norethindrone 1 mg, Day 17-21: Ethinyl estradiol 0.035 mg and norethindrone 0.5 mg, Day 22-28: Inactive (28s). **TAB, chewable, monophasic** (Ovcon® 35 28-day): Ethinyl estradiol 0.035 mg and norethindrone 0.4 mg

Ethinyl Estradiol and Norgestimate

(ETH in il es tra DYE ole & nor JES ti mate)

U.S. Brand Names MonoNessa™; Ortho-Cyclen®; Ortho Tri-Cyclen®; Ortho Tri-Cyclen® Lo; Previfem™; Sprintec™; TriNessa™; Tri-Previfem™; Tri-Sprintec™

Canadian Brand Names Cyclen®; Tri-Cyclen®

Generic Available Yes

Synonyms Ethinyl Estradiol and NGM; Norgestimate and Ethinyl Estradiol; Ortho Cyclen; Ortho Tri Cyclen

Pharmacologic Category Contraceptive; Estrogen and Progestin Combination

Use Prevention of pregnancy; treatment of acne

Local Anesthetic/Vasoconstrictor Precautions No information available to require special precautions

Effects on Dental Treatment When prescribing antibiotics, patient must be warned to use additional methods of birth control if on oral contraceptives.

Common Adverse Effects Frequency not defined.

Cardiovascular: Arterial thromboembolism, cerebral hemorrhage, cerebral thrombosis, edema, hypertension, mesenteric thrombosis, myocardial infarction

Central nervous system: Depression, dizziness, headache, migraine, nervousness, premenstrual syndrome, stroke

Dermatologic: Acne, erythema multiforme, erythema nodosum, hirsutism, loss of scalp hair, melasma (may persist), rash (allergic)

Endocrine & metabolic: Amenorrhea, breakthrough bleeding, breast enlargement, breast secretion, breast tenderness, carbohydrate intolerance, lactation decreased (postpartum), glucose tolerance decreased, libido changes, menstrual flow changes, sex hormone-binding globulins (SHBG) increased, spotting, temporary infertility (following discontinuation), thyroid-binding globulin increased, triglycerides increased

Gastrointestinal: Abdominal cramps, appetite changes, bloating, cholestasis, colitis, gallbladder disease, jaundice, nausea, vomiting, weight gain/loss

Genitourinary: Cervical erosion changes, cervical secretion changes, cystitis-like syndrome, vaginal candidiasis, vaginitis

Hematologic: Antithrombin III decreased, folate levels decreased, hemolytic uremic syndrome, norepinephrine induced platelet aggregability increased, porphyria, prothrombin increased; factors VII, VIII, IX, and X increased

Hepatic: Benign liver tumors, Budd-Chiari syndrome, cholestatic jaundice, hepatic adenomas

Local: Thrombophlebitis

Ocular: Cataracts, change in corneal curvature (steepening), contact lens intolerance, optic neuritis, retinal thrombosis

Renal: Impaired renal function

Respiratory: Pulmonary thromboembolism

Miscellaneous: Hemorrhagic eruption

Dosage Oral:

Children ≥15 years and Adults: Female: Acne (Ortho Tri-Cyclen®): Refer to dosing for contraception

Adults: Female:

Contraception:

Schedule 1 (Sunday starter): Dose begins on first Sunday after onset of menstruation; if the menstrual period starts on Sunday, take first tablet that very same day. **With a Sunday start, an additional method of contraception should be used until after the first 7 days of consecutive administration.**

For 21-tablet package: Dosage is 1 tablet daily for 21 consecutive days, followed by 7 days off of the medication; a new course begins on the 8th day after the last tablet is taken.

For 28-tablet package: Dosage is 1 tablet daily without interruption.

Schedule 2 (Day 1 starter): Dose starts on first day of menstrual cycle taking 1 tablet daily.

For 21-tablet package: Dosage is 1 tablet daily for 21 consecutive days, followed by 7 days off of the medication; a new course begins on the 8th day after the last tablet is taken.

For 28-tablet package: Dosage is 1 tablet daily without interruption.

If all doses have been taken on schedule and one menstrual period is missed, continue dosing cycle. If two consecutive menstrual periods are missed, pregnancy test is required before new dosing cycle is started.

Missed doses **monophasic formulations** (refer to package insert for complete information):

One dose missed: Take as soon as remembered or take 2 tablets next day

Two consecutive doses missed in the first 2 weeks: Take 2 tablets as soon as remembered or 2 tablets next 2 days. **An additional method of contraception should be used for 7 days after missed dose.**

Two consecutive doses missed in week 3 or three consecutive doses missed at any time: **An additional method of contraception must be used for 7 days after a missed dose:**

Schedule 1 (Sunday starter): Continue dose of 1 tablet daily until Sunday, then discard the rest of the pack, and a new pack should be started that same day.

Schedule 2 (Day 1 starter): Current pack should be discarded, and a new pack should be started that same day.

Missed doses **biphasic/triphasic formulations** (refer to package insert for complete information):

One dose missed: Take as soon as remembered or take 2 tablets next day.

Two consecutive doses missed in week 1 or week 2 of the pack: Take 2 tablets as soon as remembered and 2 tablets the next day. Resume

(Continued)

Ethinyl Estradiol and Norgestimate *(Continued)*

taking 1 tablet daily until the pack is empty. **An additional method of contraception must be used for 7 days after a missed dose.**

Two consecutive doses missed in week 3 of the pack. **An additional method of contraception must be used for 7 days after a missed dose.**

Schedule 1 (Sunday starter): Take 1 tablet every day until Sunday. Discard the remaining pack and start a new pack of pills on the same day.

Schedule 2 (Day 1 starter): Discard the remaining pack and start a new pack the same day.

Three or more consecutive doses missed. **An additional method of contraception must be used for 7 days after a missed dose.**

Schedule 1 (Sunday starter): Take 1 tablet every day until Sunday; on Sunday, discard the pack and start a new pack.

Schedule 2 (Day 1 starter): Discard the remaining pack and begin new pack of tablets starting on the same day.

Dosage adjustment in renal impairment: Specific guidelines not available; use with caution.

Dosage adjustment in hepatic impairment: Contraindicated in patients with hepatic impairment.

Mechanism of Action Combination hormonal contraceptives inhibit ovulation via a negative feedback mechanism on the hypothalamus, which alters the normal pattern of gonadotropin secretion of a follicle-stimulating hormone (FSH) and luteinizing hormone by the anterior pituitary. The follicular phase FSH and midcycle surge of gonadotropins are inhibited. In addition, combination hormonal contraceptives produce alterations in the genital tract, including changes in the cervical mucus, rendering it unfavorable for sperm penetration even if ovulation occurs. Changes in the endometrium may also occur, producing an unfavorable environment for nidation. Combination hormonal contraceptive drugs may alter the tubal transport of the ova through the fallopian tubes. Progestational agents may also alter sperm fertility.

Contraindications Hypersensitivity to ethinyl estradiol, norgestimate, or any component of the formulation; history of or current thrombophlebitis or venous thromboembolic disorders (including DVT, PE); active or recent (within 1 year) arterial thromboembolic disease (eg, stroke, MI); cerebral vascular disease, coronary artery disease, valvular heart disease with complications, severe hypertension; severe headache with focal neurological symptoms; known or suspected breast carcinoma, endometrial cancer, estrogen-dependent neoplasms, undiagnosed abnormal genital bleeding; hepatic dysfunction or tumor, cholestatic jaundice of pregnancy, jaundice with prior combination hormonal contraceptive use; heavy smoking (≥15 cigarettes/day) in patients >35 years of age; pregnancy

Warnings/Precautions Combination hormonal contraceptives do not protect against HIV infection or other sexually-transmitted diseases. The risk of cardiovascular side effects increases in women who smoke cigarettes, especially those who are >35 years of age; women who use combination hormonal contraceptives should be strongly advised not to smoke. Combination hormonal contraceptives may lead to increased risk of myocardial infarction, use with caution in patients with risk factors for coronary artery disease. May increase the risk of thromboembolism. Combination hormonal contraceptives may have a dose-related risk of vascular disease, hypertension, and gallbladder disease. Women with hypertension should be encouraged to use a nonhormonal form of contraception. The use of combination hormonal contraceptives has been associated with a slight increase in frequency of breast cancer, however, studies are not consistent. Combination hormonal contraceptives may cause glucose intolerance. Retinal thrombosis has been reported (rarely). Use with caution in patients with renal disease, conditions that may be aggravated by fluid retention, depression, or history of migraine. Not for use prior to menarche.

The minimum dosage combination of estrogen/progestin that will effectively treat the individual patient should be used. New patients should be started on products containing <50 mcg of estrogen per tablet.

Acne: For use only in females ≥15 years, who also desire combination hormonal contraceptive therapy, are unresponsive to topical treatments, and have no contraindications to combination hormonal contraceptive use; treatment must continue for at least 6 months.

Drug Interactions

Cytochrome P450 Effect: Ethinyl estradiol: **Substrate** of CYP3A4 (major), 3A5-7 (minor); **Inhibits** CYP1A2 (weak), 2B6 (weak), 2C19 (weak), 3A4 (weak)

Increased Effect/Toxicity: Acetaminophen and ascorbic acid may increase plasma levels of estrogen component. Atorvastatin and indinavir increase plasma levels of combination hormonal contraceptives. Combination hormonal contraceptives increase the plasma levels of alprazolam, chlordiazepoxide, cyclosporine, diazepam, prednisolone, selegiline, theophylline, tricyclic antidepressants. Combination hormonal contraceptives may increase (or decrease) the effects of coumarin derivatives.

Decreased Effect: CYP3A4 inducers may decrease the levels/effects of ethinyl estradiol; example inducers include aminoglutethimide, carbamazepine, nafcillin, nevirapine, phenobarbital, phenytoin, and rifamycins. Combination hormonal contraceptives may decrease plasma levels of acetaminophen, clofibric acid, lorazepam, morphine, oxazepam, salicylic acid, temazepam. Contraceptive effect decreased by acitretin, aminoglutethimide, amprenavir, anticonvulsants, griseofulvin, lopinavir, nelfinavir, nevirapine, penicillins (effect not consistent), rifampin, ritonavir, tetracyclines (effect not consistent). Combination hormonal contraceptives may decrease (or increase) the effects of coumarin derivatives.

Ethanol/Nutrition/Herb Interactions

Food: CNS effects of caffeine may be enhanced if combination hormonal contraceptives are used concurrently with caffeine. Grapefruit juice increases ethinyl estradiol concentrations and would be expected to increase progesterone serum levels as well; clinical implications are unclear.

Herb/Nutraceutical: St John's wort may decrease the effectiveness of combination hormonal contraceptives by inducing hepatic enzymes. Avoid dong quai and black cohosh (have estrogen activity). Avoid saw palmetto, red clover, ginseng.

Dietary Considerations Should be taken at same time each day.

Pregnancy Risk Factor X

Dosage Forms TAB, monophasic (MonoNessa™, Ortho-Cyclen®, Previfem™, Sprintec™): Ethinyl estradiol 0.035 mg and norgestimate 0.25 mg (28s). **TAB, triphasic** (Ortho Tri-Cyclen®, Tri-Previfem™, TriNessa™, Tri-Sprintec™): Day 1-7: Ethinyl estradiol 0.035 mg and norgestimate 0.18 mg, Day 8-14: Ethinyl estradiol 0.035 mg and norgestimate 0.215 mg, Day 15-21: Ethinyl estradiol 0.035 mg and norgestimate 0.25 mg, Day 22-28: Inactive (28s); (Ortho Tri-Cyclen® Lo): Day 1-7: Ethinyl estradiol 0.025 mg and norgestimate 0.18 mg, Day 8-14: Ethinyl estradiol 0.025 mg and norgestimate 0.215 mg, Day 8-14: Ethinyl estradiol 0.025 and norgestimate 0.215 mg, Day 15-21: Ethinyl estradiol 0.025 mg and norgestimate 0.25 mg, Day 22-28: Inactive (28s)

Ethinyl Estradiol and Norgestrel

(ETH in il es tra DYE ole & nor JES trel)

U.S. Brand Names Cryselle™; Lo/Ovral®; Low-Ogestrel®; Ogestrel®; Ovral® [DSC]

Canadian Brand Names Ovral®

Generic Available Yes

Synonyms Morning After Pill; Norgestrel and Ethinyl Estradiol

Pharmacologic Category Contraceptive; Estrogen and Progestin Combination

Use Prevention of pregnancy; postcoital contraceptive or "morning after" pill

Unlabeled/Investigational Use Treatment of hypermenorrhea, endometriosis, female hypogonadism

Local Anesthetic/Vasoconstrictor Precautions No information available to require special precautions

Effects on Dental Treatment When prescribing antibiotics, patient must be warned to use additional methods of birth control if on oral contraceptives.

Common Adverse Effects Frequency not defined.

Cardiovascular: Arterial thromboembolism, cerebral hemorrhage, cerebral thrombosis, edema, hypertension, mesenteric thrombosis, myocardial infarction

Central nervous system: Depression, dizziness, headache, migraine, nervousness, premenstrual syndrome, stroke

Dermatologic: Acne, erythema multiforme, erythema nodosum, hirsutism, loss of scalp hair, melasma (may persist), rash (allergic)

Endocrine & metabolic: Amenorrhea, breakthrough bleeding, breast enlargement, breast secretion, breast tenderness, carbohydrate intolerance, lactation decreased (postpartum), glucose tolerance decreased, libido changes, menstrual flow changes, sex hormone-binding globulins (SHBG) increased,

(Continued)

Ethinyl Estradiol and Norgestrel *(Continued)*

spotting, temporary infertility (following discontinuation), thyroid-binding globulin increased, triglycerides increased

Gastrointestinal: Abdominal cramps, appetite changes, bloating, cholestasis, colitis, gallbladder disease, jaundice, nausea, vomiting, weight gain/loss

Genitourinary: Cervical erosion changes, cervical secretion changes, cystitis-like syndrome, vaginal candidiasis, vaginitis

Hematologic: Antithrombin III decreased, folate levels decreased, hemolytic uremic syndrome, norepinephrine induced platelet aggregability increased, porphyria, prothrombin increased; factors VII, VIII, IX, and X

Hepatic: Benign liver tumors, Budd-Chiari syndrome, cholestatic jaundice, hepatic adenomas

Local: Thrombophlebitis

Ocular: Cataracts, change in corneal curvature (steepening), contact lens intolerance, optic neuritis, retinal thrombosis

Renal: Impaired renal function

Respiratory: Pulmonary thromboembolism

Miscellaneous: Hemorrhagic eruption

Dosage Oral: Adults: Female:

Contraception:

Schedule 1 (Sunday starter): Dose begins on first Sunday after onset of menstruation; if the menstrual period starts on Sunday, take first tablet that very same day. **With a Sunday start, an additional method of contraception should be used until after the first 7 days of consecutive administration.**

For 21-tablet package: Dosage is 1 tablet daily for 21 consecutive days, followed by 7 days off of the medication; a new course begins on the 8th day after the last tablet is taken.

For 28-tablet package: Dosage is 1 tablet daily without interruption.

Schedule 2 (Day 1 starter): Dose starts on first day of menstrual cycle taking 1 tablet daily.

For 21-tablet package: Dosage is 1 tablet daily for 21 consecutive days, followed by 7 days off of the medication; a new course begins on the 8th day after the last tablet is taken.

For 28-tablet package: Dosage is 1 tablet daily without interruption.

If all doses have been taken on schedule and one menstrual period is missed, continue dosing cycle. If two consecutive menstrual periods are missed, pregnancy test is required before new dosing cycle is started.

Missed doses **monophasic formulations** (refer to package insert for complete information):

One dose missed: Take as soon as remembered or take 2 tablets next day

Two consecutive doses missed in the first 2 weeks: Take 2 tablets as soon as remembered or 2 tablets next 2 days. **An additional method of contraception should be used for 7 days after missed dose.**

Two consecutive doses missed in week 3 or three consecutive doses missed at any time:

Schedule 1 (Sunday starter): Continue to take 1 tablet daily until Sunday, then discard the rest of the pack, and a new pack is started that same day.

Schedule 2 (Day 1 starter): Current pack should be discarded, and a new pack started that same day. **An additional method of contraception should be used for 7 days after missed dose.**

Postcoital contraception:

Ethinyl estradiol 0.03 mg and norgestrel 0.3 mg formulation: 4 tablets within 72 hours of unprotected intercourse and 4 tablets 12 hours after first dose

Ethinyl estradiol 0.05 mg and norgestrel 0.5 mg formulation: 2 tablets within 72 hours of unprotected intercourse and 2 tablets 12 hours after first dose

Dosage adjustment in renal impairment: Specific guidelines not available; use with caution.

Dosage adjustment in hepatic impairment: Contraindicated in patients with hepatic impairment.

Mechanism of Action Combination hormonal contraceptives inhibit ovulation via a negative feedback mechanism on the hypothalamus, which alters the normal pattern of gonadotropin secretion of a follicle-stimulating hormone (FSH) and luteinizing hormone by the anterior pituitary. The follicular phase FSH and midcycle surge of gonadotropins are inhibited. In addition, combination hormonal contraceptives produce alterations in the genital tract, including changes in the cervical mucus, rendering it unfavorable for sperm penetration even if ovulation occurs. Changes in the endometrium may also occur, producing an unfavorable environment for nidation. Combination hormonal contraceptive drugs may alter the tubal transport of the ova through the fallopian tubes. Progestational agents may also alter sperm fertility.

Contraindications Hypersensitivity to ethinyl estradiol, norgestrel, or any component of the formulation; history of or current thrombophlebitis or venous thromboembolic disorders (including DVT, PE); active or recent (within 1 year) arterial thromboembolic disease (eg, stroke, MI); cerebral vascular disease, coronary artery disease, valvular heart disease with complications, severe hypertension; diabetes mellitus with vascular involvement; severe headache with focal neurological symptoms; known or suspected breast carcinoma, endometrial cancer, estrogen-dependent neoplasms, undiagnosed abnormal genital bleeding; hepatic dysfunction or tumor, cholestatic jaundice of pregnancy, jaundice with prior combination hormonal contraceptive use; major surgery with prolonged immobilization; heavy smoking (≥15 cigarettes/day) in patients >35 years of age; pregnancy

Warnings/Precautions Combination hormonal contraceptives do not protect against HIV infection or other sexually-transmitted diseases. The risk of cardiovascular side effects increases in women who smoke cigarettes, especially those who are >35 years of age; women who use combination hormonal contraceptives should be strongly advised not to smoke. Combination hormonal contraceptives may lead to increased risk of myocardial infarction, use with caution in patients with risk factors for coronary artery disease. May increase the risk of thromboembolism. Combination hormonal contraceptives may have a dose-related risk of vascular disease, hypertension, and gallbladder disease. Women with hypertension should be encouraged to use another form of contraception. The use of combination hormonal contraceptives has been associated with a slight increase in frequency of breast cancer, however, studies are not consistent. Combination hormonal contraceptives may cause glucose intolerance. Retinal thrombosis has been reported (rarely). Use with caution in patients with renal disease, conditions that may be aggravated by fluid retention, depression, or history of migraine. Not for use prior to menarche.

The minimum dosage combination of estrogen/progestin that will effectively treat the individual patient should be used. New patients should be started on products containing <50 mcg of estrogen per tablet.

Drug Interactions

Cytochrome P450 Effect:

Ethinyl estradiol: **Substrate** of CYP3A4 (major), 3A5-7 (minor); **Inhibits** CYP1A2 (weak), 2B6 (weak), 2C19 (weak), 3A4 (weak)

Norgestrel: **Substrate** of CYP3A4 (major)

Increased Effect/Toxicity: Acetaminophen and ascorbic acid may increase plasma levels of estrogen component. Atorvastatin and indinavir increase plasma levels of combination hormonal contraceptives. Combination hormonal contraceptives increase the plasma levels of alprazolam, chlordiazepoxide, cyclosporine, diazepam, prednisolone, selegiline, theophylline, tricyclic antidepressants. Combination hormonal contraceptives may increase (or decrease) the effects of coumarin derivatives.

Decreased Effect: CYP3A4 inducers may decrease the levels/effects of norgestrel; example inducers include aminoglutethimide, carbamazepine, nafcillin, nevirapine, phenobarbital, phenytoin, and rifamycins. Combination hormonal contraceptives may decrease plasma levels of acetaminophen, clofibric acid, lorazepam, morphine, oxazepam, salicylic acid, temazepam. Contraceptive effect decreased by acitretin, aminoglutethimide, amprenavir, anticonvulsants, griseofulvin, lopinavir, nelfinavir, nevirapine, penicillins (effect not consistent), rifampin, ritonavir, tetracyclines (effect not consistent). Combination hormonal contraceptives may decrease (or increase) the effects of coumarin derivatives.

Ethanol/Nutrition/Herb Interactions

Food: CNS effects of caffeine may be enhanced if combination hormonal contraceptives are used concurrently with caffeine. Grapefruit juice increases ethinyl estradiol concentrations and would be expected to increase progesterone serum levels as well; clinical implications are unclear.

Herb/Nutraceutical: St John's wort may decrease the effectiveness of combination hormonal contraceptives by inducing hepatic enzymes. Avoid dong quai and black cohosh (have estrogen activity). Avoid saw palmetto, red clover, ginseng.

Dietary Considerations Should be taken at same time each day.

Pharmacodynamics/Kinetics See individual agents.

Pregnancy Risk Factor X

Dosage Forms TAB, monophasic: (Cryselle™): Ethinyl estradiol 0.03 mg and norgestrel 0.3 mg (28s); (Low-Ogestrel® 28): Ethinyl estradiol 0.03 mg and (Continued)

Ethinyl Estradiol and Norgestrel *(Continued)*

norgestrel 0.3 mg (28s); (Lo/Ovral® 28): Ethinyl estradiol 0.03 mg and norgestrel 0.3 mg (28s); (Orgestrel® 28): Ethinyl estradiol 0.05 mg and norgestrel 0.5 mg (28s)

Ethiofos *see* Amifostine *on page 94*

Ethionamide (e thye on AM ide)

Related Information

Tuberculosis *on page 1495*

U.S. Brand Names Trecator®-SC

Canadian Brand Names Trecator®-SC

Generic Available No

Pharmacologic Category Antitubercular Agent

Use Treatment of tuberculosis and other mycobacterial diseases, in conjunction with other antituberculosis agents, when first-line agents have failed or resistance has been demonstrated

Local Anesthetic/Vasoconstrictor Precautions No information available to require special precautions

Effects on Dental Treatment Key adverse event(s) related to dental treatment: Postural hypotension, metallic taste, and stomatitis.

Common Adverse Effects Frequency not defined.

Cardiovascular: Postural hypotension

Central nervous system: Psychiatric disturbances, drowsiness, dizziness, seizures, headache

Dermatologic: Rash, alopecia

Endocrine & metabolic: Hypothyroidism or goiter, hypoglycemia, gynecomastia

Gastrointestinal: Metallic taste, diarrhea, anorexia, nausea, vomiting, stomatitis, abdominal pain

Hematologic: Thrombocytopenia

Hepatic: Hepatitis (5%), jaundice

Neuromuscular & skeletal: Peripheral neuritis, weakness (common)

Ocular: Optic neuritis, blurred vision

Respiratory: Olfactory disturbances

Mechanism of Action Inhibits peptide synthesis

Drug Interactions

Increased Effect/Toxicity: Cycloserine and isoniazid; increased hepatotoxicity with rifampin

Pharmacodynamics/Kinetics

Absorption: Rapid

Distribution: Crosses placenta

Protein binding: 10%

Metabolism: Extensively hepatic

Bioavailability: 80%

Half-life elimination: 2-3 hours

Time to peak, serum: ~3 hours

Excretion: Urine (as unchanged drug and active and inactive metabolites)

Pregnancy Risk Factor C

Ethmozine® *see* Moricizine *on page 946*

Ethosuximide (eth oh SUKS i mide)

U.S. Brand Names Zarontin®

Canadian Brand Names Zarontin®

Generic Available Yes

Pharmacologic Category Anticonvulsant, Succinimide

Use Management of absence (petit mal) seizures

Local Anesthetic/Vasoconstrictor Precautions No information available to require special precautions

Effects on Dental Treatment No significant effects or complications reported

Common Adverse Effects Frequency not defined.

Central nervous system: Ataxia, drowsiness, sedation, dizziness, lethargy, euphoria, headache, irritability, hyperactivity, fatigue, night terrors, disturbance in sleep, inability to concentrate, aggressiveness, mental depression (with cases of overt suicidal intentions), paranoid psychosis

Dermatologic: Stevens-Johnson syndrome, SLE, rash, hirsutism

Endocrine & metabolic: Increased libido

Gastrointestinal: Weight loss, gastric upset, cramps, epigastric pain, diarrhea, nausea, vomiting, anorexia, abdominal pain, gum hypertrophy, tongue swelling

Genitourinary: Vaginal bleeding, microscopic hematuria

Hematologic: Leukopenia, agranulocytosis, pancytopenia, eosinophilia
Ocular: Myopia
Miscellaneous: Hiccups

Mechanism of Action Increases the seizure threshold and suppresses paroxysmal spike-and-wave pattern in absence seizures; depresses nerve transmission in the motor cortex

Drug Interactions

Cytochrome P450 Effect: Substrate of CYP3A4 (major)

Increased Effect/Toxicity: Ethosuximide may elevate phenytoin levels. Valproate acid has been reported to both increase and decrease ethosuximide levels. CYP3A4 inhibitors may increase the levels/effects of ethosuximide; example inhibitors include azole antifungals, ciprofloxacin, clarithromycin, diclofenac, doxycycline, erythromycin, imatinib, isoniazid, nefazodone, nicardipine, propofol, protease inhibitors, quinidine, and verapamil.

Decreased Effect: CYP3A4 inducers may decrease the levels/effects of ethosuximide; example inducers include aminoglutethimide, carbamazepine, nafcillin, nevirapine, phenobarbital, phenytoin, and rifamycins.

Pharmacodynamics/Kinetics

Distribution: Adults: V_d: 0.62-0.72 L/kg
Metabolism: Hepatic (~80% to 3 inactive metabolites)
Half-life elimination, serum: Children: 30 hours; Adults: 50-60 hours
Time to peak, serum: Capsule: ~2-4 hours; Syrup: <2-4 hours
Excretion: Urine, slowly (50% as metabolites, 10% to 20% as unchanged drug); feces (small amounts)

Pregnancy Risk Factor C

Ethotoin (ETH oh toyn)

U.S. Brand Names Peganone®

Canadian Brand Names Peganone®

Generic Available No

Synonyms Ethylphenylhydantoin

Pharmacologic Category Anticonvulsant, Hydantoin

Use Generalized tonic-clonic or complex-partial seizures

Local Anesthetic/Vasoconstrictor Precautions No information available to require special precautions

Effects on Dental Treatment No significant effects or complications reported

Common Adverse Effects Frequency not defined.

Cardiovascular: Arrhythmias, ataxia, cardiovascular collapse, venous irritation and pain
Central nervous system: Psychiatric changes, slurred speech, trembling, dizziness, drowsiness, headache, insomnia
Dermatologic: Skin rash, Stevens-Johnson syndrome
Gastrointestinal: Constipation, nausea, vomiting, gingival hyperplasia, anorexia, weight loss
Hematologic: Leukopenia, blood dyscrasias
Hepatic: Hepatitis
Local: Thrombophlebitis
Neuromuscular & skeletal: Paresthesia, peripheral neuropathy
Renal: Serum creatinine increased
Ocular: Nystagmus
Miscellaneous: Lymphadenopathy, SLE-like syndrome

Drug Interactions

Cytochrome P450 Effect: Inhibits CYP2C19 (weak)

Pregnancy Risk Factor D

Ethoxynaphthamido Penicillin Sodium *see* Nafcillin *on page 958*
Ethyl Aminobenzoate *see* Benzocaine *on page 191*

Ethyl Chloride (ETH il KLOR ide)

U.S. Brand Names Gebauer's Ethyl Chloride®

Generic Available No

Synonyms Chloroethane

Pharmacologic Category Local Anesthetic

Use Local anesthetic in minor operative procedures and to relieve pain caused by insect stings and burns, and irritation caused by myofascial and visceral pain syndromes

Local Anesthetic/Vasoconstrictor Precautions No information available to require special precautions

Effects on Dental Treatment Key adverse event(s) related to dental treatment: Mucous membrane irritation.

(Continued)

Ethyl Chloride *(Continued)*

Common Adverse Effects 1% to 10%: Mucous membrane irritation, freezing may alter skin pigment

Pregnancy Risk Factor C

Comments Spray for a few seconds to the point of frost formation when the tissue becomes white; avoid prolonged spraying of skin beyond this point

Ethyl Chloride and Dichlorotetrafluoroethane

(ETH il KLOR ide & dye klor oh te tra floo or oh ETH ane)

Related Information

Ethyl Chloride *on page 561*

U.S. Brand Names Fluro-Ethyl®

Generic Available No

Synonyms Dichlorotetrafluoroethane and Ethyl Chloride

Pharmacologic Category Local Anesthetic

Use Topical refrigerant anesthetic to control pain associated with minor surgical procedures, dermabrasion, injections, contusions, and minor strains

Local Anesthetic/Vasoconstrictor Precautions No information available to require special precautions

Effects on Dental Treatment No significant effects or complications reported

Pregnancy Risk Factor C

Ethylphenylhydantoin *see* Ethotoin *on page 561*

Ethynodiol Diacetate and Ethinyl Estradiol *see* Ethinyl Estradiol and Ethynodiol Diacetate *on page 540*

Ethyol® *see* Amifostine *on page 94*

Etidocaine and Epinephrine (e TI doe kane & ep i NEF rin)

Related Information

Epinephrine *on page 496*

Oral Pain *on page 1526*

U.S. Brand Names Duranest® [DSC]

Canadian Brand Names Duranest®

Generic Available No

Synonyms Etidocaine Hydrochloride

Pharmacologic Category Local Anesthetic

Dental Use An amide-type local anesthetic for local infiltration anesthesia; injection near nerve trunks to produce nerve block

Use Infiltration anesthesia, peripheral nerve blocks, central neural blocks

Local Anesthetic/Vasoconstrictor Precautions No information available to require special precautions

Effects on Dental Treatment No significant effects or complications reported

Significant Adverse Effects Frequency not defined:

Cardiovascular: Myocardial depression

Central nervous system: Chills

Dermatologic: Urticaria

Otic: Tinnitus

Dosage The effective anesthetic dose varies with procedure, intensity of anesthesia needed, duration of anesthesia required, and physical condition of the patient. Always use the lowest effective dose along with careful aspiration.

# of Cartridges (1.8 mL)	Etidocaine HCl (1.5%) (mg)	Epinephrine 1:200,000 (mg)
1	27	0.009
2	54	0.018
3	81	0.027
4	108	0.036
5	135	0.045
6	162	0.054
7	189	0.063
8	216	0.072
9	243	0.081
10	270	0.090

Children <10 years: Dosage has not been established

Children >10 years and Adults: **Dental infiltration and nerve block:** 15-75 mg (1-5 mL) as a 1.5% solution; up to a maximum of 5.5 mg/kg of body weight but not to exceed 400 mg/injection of etidocaine hydrochloride with epinephrine 1:200,000.

The numbers of dental carpules (1.8 mL) in the table on previous page provide the indicated amounts of etidocaine hydrochloride 1.5% and epinephrine 1:200,000.

Mechanism of Action Blocks nervous conduction through the stabilization of neuronal membranes. By preventing the transient increase in membrane permeability to sodium, the ionic fluxes necessary for initiation and transmission of electrical impulses are inhibited and local anesthesia is induced.

Contraindications Hypersensitivity to etidocaine, other amide local anesthetics, or any component of the formulation; heart block, severe hemorrhage, severe hypotension

Warnings/Precautions Use with caution in patients with cardiac disease and hyperthyroidism; fetal bradycardia may occur up to 20% of the time; use with caution in areas of inflammation or sepsis, in debilitated or elderly patients, and those with severe cardiovascular disease or hepatic dysfunction; some products may contain sulfites

Drug Interactions Due to epinephrine component, use with tricyclic antidepressants or MAO inhibitors could result in increased pressor response; use with nonselective beta-blockers (ie, propranolol) could result in serious hypertension and reflex bradycardia

Pharmacodynamics/Kinetics

Onset of action: Anesthetic: 2-5 minutes

Duration: ~4-10 hours

Absorption: Rapid

Distribution: Wide V_d into neuronal tissues

Protein binding: High

Metabolism: Extensively hepatic

Excretion: Urine (small amounts)

Pregnancy Risk Factor B

Breast-Feeding Considerations Usual infiltration doses of etidocaine hydrochloride with epinephrine given to nursing mothers has not been shown to affect the health of the nursing infant.

Dosage Forms

Injection, solution, as hydrochloride: 1% [10 mg/mL] (30 mL)

Injection, solution, as hydrochloride, with epinephrine 1:200,000: 1% [10 mg/mL] (30 mL); 1.5% [15 mg/mL] (1.8 mL, 20 mL)

Selected Readings

Ayoub ST and Coleman AE, "A Review of Local Anesthetics," *Gen Dent*, 1992, 40(4):285-7, 289-90.

Budenz AW, "Local Anesthetics in Dentistry: Then and Now," *J Calif Dent Assoc*, 2003, 31(5):388-96.

Dower JS Jr, "A Review of Paresthesia in Association With Administration of Local Anesthesia," *Dent Today*, 2003, 22(2):64-9.

Finder RL and Moore PA, "Adverse Drug Reactions to Local Anesthesia," *Dent Clin North Am*, 2002, 46(4):747-57, x.

Haas DA, "An Update on Local Anesthetics in Dentistry," *J Can Dent Assoc*, 2002, 68(9):546-51.

Hawkins JM and Moore PA, "Local Anesthesia: Advances in Agents and Techniques," *Dent Clin North Am*, 2002, 46(4):719-32, ix.

"Injectable Local Anesthetics," *J Am Dent Assoc*, 2003, 134(5):628-9.

Jastak JT and Yagiela JA, "Vasoconstrictors and Local Anesthesia: A Review and Rationale for Use," *J Am Dent Assoc*, 1983, 107(4):623-30.

MacKenzie TA and Young ER, "Local Anesthetic Update," *Anesth Prog*, 1993, 40(2):29-34.

Malamed SF, "Allergy and Toxic Reactions to Local Anesthetics," *Dent Today*, 2003, 22(4):114-6, 118-21.

Wynn RL, "Epinephrine Interactions With Beta-Blockers," *Gen Dent*, 1994, 42(1):16, 18.

Wynn RL, "Recent Research on Mechanisms of Local Anesthetics," *Gen Dent*, 1995, 43(4):316-8.

Yagiela JA, "Local Anesthetics," *Anesth Prog*, 1991, 38(4-5):128-41.

Etidocaine Hydrochloride *see* Etidocaine and Epinephrine *on page 562*

Etidronate Disodium (e ti DROE nate dye SOW dee um)

Related Information

Rheumatoid Arthritis, Osteoarthritis, and Osteoporosis *on page 1490*

U.S. Brand Names Didronel®

Canadian Brand Names Didronel®; Gen-Etidronate

Generic Available No

Synonyms EHDP; Sodium Etidronate

Pharmacologic Category Bisphosphonate Derivative

Use Symptomatic treatment of Paget's disease and heterotopic ossification due to spinal cord injury or after total hip replacement, hypercalcemia associated with malignancy

Local Anesthetic/Vasoconstrictor Precautions No information available to require special precautions

(Continued)

Etidronate Disodium *(Continued)*

Effects on Dental Treatment Key adverse event(s) related to dental treatment: Abnormal taste.

Common Adverse Effects

>10%: Neuromuscular & skeletal: Bone pain (10% to 20%, Paget's)

1% to 10%:

Central nervous system: Fever (9%), convulsions (3%)

Endocrine & metabolic: Hypophosphatemia (3%), hypomagnesemia (3%), fluid overload (6%), hypercalcemia of malignancy

Gastrointestinal: Diarrhea and nausea (7% to 30%, dose-related), constipation (3%), abnormal taste (3%)

Hepatic: LFT changes (3%)

Respiratory: Dyspnea (3%)

Renal: Increased serum creatinine (10%)

Mechanism of Action Decreases bone resorption by inhibiting osteocystic osteolysis; decreases mineral release and matrix or collagen breakdown in bone

Drug Interactions

Increased Effect/Toxicity: Foscarnet and plicamycin may have additive hypocalcemic effect.

Pharmacodynamics/Kinetics

Onset of action: 1-3 months

Duration: Can persist for 12 months without continuous therapy

Absorption: Dose dependent

Metabolism: None

Excretion: Primarily urine (as unchanged drug); feces (as unabsorbed drug)

Pregnancy Risk Factor C

Etodolac (ee toe DOE lak)

Related Information

Rheumatoid Arthritis, Osteoarthritis, and Osteoporosis *on page 1490*

Temporomandibular Dysfunction (TMD) *on page 1564*

U.S. Brand Names Lodine®; Lodine® XL

Canadian Brand Names Apo-Etodolac®; Lodine®; Utradol™

Generic Available Yes

Synonyms Etodolic Acid

Pharmacologic Category Nonsteroidal Anti-inflammatory Drug (NSAID), Oral

Dental Use Management of postoperative pain

Use Acute and long-term use in the management of signs and symptoms of osteoarthritis and management of pain; rheumatoid arthritis; juvenile rheumatoid arthritis

Local Anesthetic/Vasoconstrictor Precautions No information available to require special precautions

Effects on Dental Treatment NSAID formulations are known to reversibly decrease platelet aggregation via mechanisms different than observed with aspirin. The dentist should be aware of the potential of abnormal coagulation. Caution should also be exercised in the use of NSAIDs in patients already on anticoagulant therapy with drugs such as warfarin (Coumadin®).

Significant Adverse Effects

1% to 10%:

Central nervous system: Depression (1% to 3%)

Dermatologic: Rash (1% to 3%), pruritus (1% to 3%)

Gastrointestinal: Abdominal cramps (3% to 9%), nausea (3% to 9%), vomiting (1% to 3%), dyspepsia (10%), diarrhea (3% to 9%), constipation (1% to 3%), flatulence (3% to 9%), melena (1% to 3%), gastritis (1% to 3%)

Genitourinary: Polyuria (1% to 3%)

Neuromuscular & skeletal: Weakness (3% to 9%)

Ocular: Blurred vision (1% to 3%)

Otic: Tinnitus (1% to 3%)

<1% (Limited to important or life-threatening): Acute renal failure, agranulocytosis, anemia, angioedema, arrhythmia, bone marrow suppression, CHF, dyspnea, erythema multiforme, exfoliative dermatitis, hemolytic anemia, hepatitis, hypertension, leukopenia, peripheral neuropathy, Stevens-Johnson syndrome, syncope, tachycardia, thrombocytopenia, toxic amblyopia, toxic epidermal necrolysis, urticaria

Dosage Single dose of 76-100 mg is comparable to the analgesic effect of aspirin 650 mg; in patients ≥65 years, no substantial differences in the pharmacokinetics or side-effects profile were seen compared with the general population

Children 6-16 years: Oral: Juvenile rheumatoid arthritis (Lodine® XL):
- 20-30 kg: 400 mg once daily
- 31-45 kg: 600 mg once daily
- 46-60 kg: 800 mg once daily
- >60 kg: 1000 mg once daily

Adults: Oral:

Acute pain: 200-400 mg every 6-8 hours, as needed, not to exceed total daily doses of 1200 mg; for patients weighing <60 kg, total daily dose should not exceed 20 mg/kg/day

Rheumatoid arthritis, osteoarthritis: Initial: 600-1200 mg/day given in divided doses: 400 mg 2 times/day; 300 mg 2 or 3 times/day; 500 mg 2 times/day; total daily dose should not exceed 1200 mg; for patients weighing <60 kg, total daily dose should not exceed 20 mg/kg/day

Lodine® XL: 400-1000 mg once daily

Elderly: Refer to adult dosing; in patients ≥65 years, no dosage adjustment required based on pharmacokinetics. The elderly are more sensitive to antiprostaglandin effects and may need dosage adjustments.

Mechanism of Action Inhibits prostaglandin synthesis by decreasing the activity of the enzyme, cyclooxygenase, which results in decreased formation of prostaglandin precursors

Contraindications Hypersensitivity to etodolac, aspirin, other NSAIDs, or any component of the formulation; active gastric/duodenal ulcer disease; patients with "aspirin triad" (bronchial asthma, aspirin intolerance, rhinitis); pregnancy (3rd trimester)

Warnings/Precautions Use with caution in patients with CHF, hypertension, dehydration, decreased renal or hepatic function, history of GI disease (bleeding or ulcers), or those receiving anticoagulants. Elderly are at a high risk for adverse effects from NSAIDs. As many as 60% of elderly can develop peptic ulceration and/or hemorrhage asymptomatically.

Use lowest effective dose for shortest period possible. Use of NSAIDs can compromise existing renal function especially when Cl_{cr} is <30 mL/minute. CNS adverse effects such as confusion, agitation, and hallucination are generally seen in overdose or high-dose situations; however, elderly may demonstrate these adverse effects at lower doses than younger adults. Withhold for at least 4-6 half-lives prior to surgical or dental procedures.

Drug Interactions

ACE inhibitors: Antihypertensive effects may be decreased by concurrent therapy with NSAIDs; monitor blood pressure.

Angiotensin II antagonists: Antihypertensive effects may be decreased by concurrent therapy with NSAIDs; monitor blood pressure.

Anticoagulants (warfarin, heparin, LMWHs) in combination with NSAIDs can cause increased risk of bleeding.

Antiplatelet agents (ticlopidine, clopidogrel, aspirin, abciximab, dipyridamole, eptifibatide, tirofiban) can cause an increased risk of bleeding.

Cholestyramine and colestipol reduce the bioavailability of some NSAIDs; separate administration times.

Corticosteroids may increase the risk of GI ulceration; avoid concurrent use.

Cyclosporine: NSAIDs may increase serum creatinine, potassium, blood pressure, and cyclosporine levels; monitor cyclosporine levels and renal function carefully.

Hydralazine's antihypertensive effect is decreased; avoid concurrent use.

Lithium levels can be increased; avoid concurrent use if possible or monitor lithium levels and adjust dose. Sulindac may have the least effect. When NSAID is stopped, lithium will need adjustment again.

Loop diuretics efficacy (diuretic and antihypertensive effect) is reduced. Indomethacin reduces this efficacy, however, it may be anticipated with any NSAID.

Methotrexate: Severe bone marrow suppression, aplastic anemia, and GI toxicity have been reported with concomitant NSAID therapy. Avoid use during moderate or high-dose methotrexate (increased and prolonged methotrexate levels). NSAID use during low-dose treatment of rheumatoid arthritis has not been fully evaluated; extreme caution is warranted.

Thiazides antihypertensive effects are decreased; avoid concurrent use.

Verapamil plasma concentration is decreased by some NSAIDs; avoid concurrent use.

Warfarin's INRs may be increased by piroxicam. Other NSAIDs may have the same effect depending on dose and duration. Monitor INR closely. Use the lowest dose of NSAIDs possible and for the briefest duration.

Ethanol/Nutrition/Herb Interactions

Ethanol: Avoid ethanol (may enhance gastric mucosal irritation).

Food: Etodolac peak serum levels may be decreased if taken with food.

(Continued)

Etodolac *(Continued)*

Herb/Nutraceutical: Avoid cat's claw, dong quai, evening primrose, feverfew, garlic, ginger, ginkgo, red clover, horse chestnut, green tea, ginseng (all have additional antiplatelet activity)

Dietary Considerations May be taken with food to decrease GI distress.

Pharmacodynamics/Kinetics

Onset of action: Analgesic: 2-4 hours; Maximum anti-inflammatory effect: A few days

Absorption: Well absorbed

Distribution: V_d: 0.4 L/kg

Protein binding: High

Metabolism: Hepatic

Half-life elimination: 7 hours

Time to peak, serum: 1 hour

Excretion: Urine

Pregnancy Risk Factor C/D (3rd trimester)

Lactation Excretion in breast milk unknown/contraindicated

Dosage Forms [DSC] = Discontinued product

Capsule (Lodine®): 200 mg, 300 mg

Tablet: 400 mg, 500 mg

Lodine®: 400 mg, 500 mg [DSC]

Tablet, extended release (Lodine® XL): 400 mg, 500 mg, 600 mg

Selected Readings

Brooks PM and Day RO, "Nonsteroidal Anti-inflammatory Drugs - Differences and Similarities," *N Engl J Med*, 1991, 324(24):1716-25.

Tucker PW, Smith JR, and Adams DF, "A Comparison of 2 Analgesic Regimens for the Control of Postoperative Periodontal Discomfort," *J Periodontol*, 1996, 67(2):125-9.

Etodolic Acid *see* Etodolac *on page 564*

Etomidate (e TOM i date)

U.S. Brand Names Amidate®

Canadian Brand Names Amidate®

Generic Available Yes

Pharmacologic Category General Anesthetic

Use Induction and maintenance of general anesthesia

Unlabeled/Investigational Use Sedation for diagnosis of seizure foci

Local Anesthetic/Vasoconstrictor Precautions No information available to require special precautions

Effects on Dental Treatment Key adverse event(s) related to dental treatment: Hiccups.

Common Adverse Effects

>10%:

Endocrine & metabolic: Adrenal suppression

Gastrointestinal: Nausea, vomiting on emergence from anesthesia

Local: Pain at injection site (30% to 80%)

Neuromuscular & skeletal: Myoclonus (33%), transient skeletal movements, uncontrolled eye movements

1% to 10%: Hiccups

Mechanism of Action Ultrashort-acting nonbarbiturate hypnotic (benzylimidazole) used for the induction of anesthesia; chemically, it is a carboxylated imidazole which produces a rapid induction of anesthesia with minimal cardiovascular effects; produces EEG burst suppression at high doses

Drug Interactions

Increased Effect/Toxicity: Fentanyl decreases etomidate elimination. Verapamil may increase the anesthetic and respiratory depressant effects of etomidate.

Pharmacodynamics/Kinetics

Onset of action: 30-60 seconds

Peak effect: 1 minute

Duration: 3-5 minutes; terminated by redistribution

Distribution: V_d: 2-4.5 L/kg

Protein binding: 76%;

Metabolism: Hepatic and plasma esterases

Half-life elimination: Terminal: 2.6 hours

Pregnancy Risk Factor C

Etonogestrel and Ethinyl Estradiol *see* Ethinyl Estradiol and Etonogestrel *on page 543*

Etopophos® *see* Etoposide Phosphate *on page 568*

Etoposide (e toe POE side)

U.S. Brand Names Toposar®; VePesid®

Canadian Brand Names VePesid®

Mexican Brand Names Etopos® [inj.]; Lastet®; VePesid®; Vp-Tec®

Generic Available Yes

Synonyms Epipodophyllotoxin; VP-16; VP-16-213

Pharmacologic Category Antineoplastic Agent, Podophyllotoxin Derivative

Use Treatment of lymphomas, ANLL, lung, testicular, bladder, and prostate carcinoma, hepatoma, rhabdomyosarcoma, uterine carcinoma, neuroblastoma, mycosis fungoides, Kaposi's sarcoma, histiocytosis, gestational trophoblastic disease, Ewing's sarcoma, Wilms' tumor, and brain tumors

Local Anesthetic/Vasoconstrictor Precautions No information available to require special precautions

Effects on Dental Treatment Key adverse event(s) related to dental treatment: Mucositis (especially at high doses).

Common Adverse Effects

>10%:

Cardiovascular: Hypotension if the drug is infused too fast

Dermatologic: Alopecia (22% to 93%)

Endocrine & metabolic: Ovarian failure (38%), amenorrhea

Gastrointestinal: Mild to moderate nausea and vomiting; mucositis, especially at high doses; anorexia (10% to 13%)

Hematologic: Myelosuppression, leukopenia (91%), thrombocytopenia (41%), anemia

Onset: 5-7 days

Nadir: 7-14 days

Recovery: 21-28 days

1% to 10%:

Gastrointestinal: Stomatitis (1% to 6%), diarrhea (1% to 13%), abdominal pain

Neuromuscular & skeletal: Peripheral neuropathies (0.7% to 2%)

Mechanism of Action Etoposide does not inhibit microtubular assembly. It has been shown to delay transit of cells through the S phase and arrest cells in late S or early G_2 phase. The drug may inhibit mitochondrial transport at the NADH dehydrogenase level or inhibit uptake of nucleosides into HeLa cells. Etoposide is a topoisomerase II inhibitor and appears to cause DNA strand breaks.

Drug Interactions

Cytochrome P450 Effect: Substrate of CYP1A2 (minor), 2E1 (minor), 3A4 (major); **Inhibits** CYP2C8/9 (weak), 3A4 (weak)

Increased Effect/Toxicity: The effects of etoposide may be increased by calcium antagonists (increased effects noted *in vitro*). Cyclosporine may increase the levels of etoposide. Etoposide may increase the effects/toxicity of methotrexate and warfarin. There have been reports of frequent hepatic dysfunction with hyperbilirubinemia, ascites, and thrombocytopenia when etoposide is combined with carmustine. CYP3A4 inhibitors may increase the levels/effects of etoposide; example inhibitors include azole antifungals, ciprofloxacin, clarithromycin, diclofenac, doxycycline, erythromycin, imatinib, isoniazid, nefazodone, nicardipine, propofol, protease inhibitors, quinidine, and verapamil.

Decreased Effect: CYP3A4 inducers may decrease the levels/effects of etoposide; example inducers include aminoglutethimide, carbamazepine, nafcillin, nevirapine, phenobarbital, phenytoin, and rifamycins.

Pharmacodynamics/Kinetics

Absorption: Oral: 25% to 75%; significant inter- and intrapatient variation

Distribution: Average V_d: 3-36 L/m^2; poor penetration across the blood-brain barrier; CSF concentrations <10% of plasma concentrations

Protein binding: 94% to 97%

Metabolism: Hepatic to hydroxy acid and cislactone metabolites

Half-life elimination: Terminal: 4-15 hours; Children: Normal renal/hepatic function: 6-8 hours

Time to peak, serum: Oral: 1-1.5 hours

Excretion:

Children: Urine (≤55% as unchanged drug)

Adults: Urine (42% to 67%; 8% to 35% as unchanged drug) within 24 hours; feces (up to 16%)

Pregnancy Risk Factor D

Etoposide Phosphate (e toe POE side FOS fate)

Related Information

Etoposide *on page 567*

U.S. Brand Names Etopophos®

Generic Available No

Pharmacologic Category Antineoplastic Agent, Podophyllotoxin Derivative

Use Treatment of refractory testicular tumors and small cell lung cancer

Local Anesthetic/Vasoconstrictor Precautions No information available to require special precautions

Effects on Dental Treatment Key adverse event(s) related to dental treatment: Mucositis (especially at high doses) and stomatitis.

Common Adverse Effects Based on **etoposide**:

>10%:

- Cardiovascular: Hypotension if the drug is infused too fast
- Dermatologic: Alopecia (22% to 93%)
- Endocrine & metabolic: Ovarian failure (38%), amenorrhea
- Gastrointestinal: Mild to moderate nausea and vomiting; mucositis, especially at high doses; anorexia (10% to 13%)
- Hematologic: Myelosuppression, leukopenia (91%), thrombocytopenia (41%), anemia
  - Onset: 5-7 days
  - Nadir: 7-14 days
  - Recovery: 21-28 days

1% to 10%:

- Gastrointestinal: Stomatitis (1% to 6%), diarrhea (1% to 13%), abdominal pain
- Neuromuscular & skeletal: Peripheral neuropathies (0.7% to 2%)

Mechanism of Action Etoposide phosphate is converted *in vivo* to the active moiety, etoposide, by dephosphorylation. Etoposide inhibits mitotic activity; inhibits cells from entering prophase; inhibits DNA synthesis. Initially thought to be mitotic inhibitors similar to podophyllotoxin, but actually have no effect on microtubule assembly. However, later shown to induce DNA strand breakage and inhibition of topoisomerase II (an enzyme which breaks and repairs DNA); etoposide acts in late S or early G2 phases.

Drug Interactions

Cytochrome P450 Effect: Substrate of CYP1A2 (minor), 2E1 (minor), 3A4 (major); **Inhibits** CYP2C8/9 (weak), 3A4 (weak)

Increased Effect/Toxicity: Etoposide taken with warfarin may result in prolongation of bleeding times. Alteration of methotrexate transport has been found as a slow efflux of methotrexate and its polyglutamated form out of the cell, leading to intercellular accumulation of methotrexate. Calcium antagonists increase the rate of VP-16-induced DNA damage and cytotoxicity *in vitro*. Use with carmustine has shown reports of frequent hepatic dysfunction with hyperbilirubinemia, ascites, and thrombocytopenia. Cyclosporine may cause additive cytotoxic effects on tumor cells. CYP3A4 inhibitors may increase the levels/effects of etoposide; example inhibitors include azole antifungals, ciprofloxacin, clarithromycin, diclofenac, doxycycline, erythromycin, imatinib, isoniazid, nefazodone, nicardipine, propofol, protease inhibitors, quinidine, and verapamil.

Decreased Effect: CYP3A4 inducers may decrease the levels/effects of etoposide; example inducers include aminoglutethimide, carbamazepine, nafcillin, nevirapine, phenobarbital, phenytoin, and rifamycins.

Pharmacodynamics/Kinetics

Distribution: Average V_d: 3-36 L/m^2; poor penetration across blood-brain barrier; concentrations in CSF being <10% that of plasma

Protein binding: 94% to 97%

Metabolism: Hepatic (with a biphasic decay)

Half-life elimination: Terminal: 4-15 hours; Children: Normal renal/hepatic function: 6-8 hours

Excretion: Urine (as unchanged drug and metabolites), feces (2% to 16%); Children: I.V.: Urine (≤55% as unchanged drug)

Pregnancy Risk Factor D

Eudal®-SR *see* Guaifenesin and Pseudoephedrine *on page 675*

Eulexin® *see* Flutamide *on page 615*

Eurax® *see* Crotamiton *on page 380*

Evac-U-Gen [OTC] *see* Senna *on page 1213*

Evista® *see* Raloxifene *on page 1166*

Evoxac® *see* Cevimeline *on page 302*

Exact® Acne Medication [OTC] *see* Benzoyl Peroxide *on page 194*

Excedrin® Extra Strength [OTC] *see* Acetaminophen, Aspirin, and Caffeine *on page 56*

Excedrin® Migraine [OTC] *see* Acetaminophen, Aspirin, and Caffeine *on page 56*

Excedrin® P.M. [OTC] *see* Acetaminophen and Diphenhydramine *on page 53*

Exelderm® *see* Sulconazole *on page 1243*

Exelon® *see* Rivastigmine *on page 1192*

Exemestane (ex e MES tane)

U.S. Brand Names Aromasin®

Canadian Brand Names Aromasin®

Generic Available No

Pharmacologic Category Antineoplastic Agent, Aromatase Inactivator

Use Treatment of advanced breast cancer in postmenopausal women whose disease has progressed following tamoxifen therapy

Local Anesthetic/Vasoconstrictor Precautions No information available to require special precautions

Effects on Dental Treatment No significant effects or complications reported

Common Adverse Effects

>10%:

Central nervous system: Fatigue (22%), pain (13%), depression (13%), insomnia (11%), anxiety (10%)

Endocrine & metabolic: Hot flashes (13%)

Gastrointestinal: Nausea (18%)

1% to 10%:

Cardiovascular: Edema (7%), hypertension (5%), chest pain

Central nervous system: Dizziness (8%), headache (8%), fever (5%), hypoesthesia, confusion

Dermatologic: Rash, itching, alopecia

Gastrointestinal: Vomiting (7%), abdominal pain (6%), anorexia (6%), constipation (5%), diarrhea (4%), increased appetite (3%), dyspepsia

Genitourinary: Urinary tract infection

Neuromuscular & skeletal: Weakness, paresthesia, pathological fracture, arthralgia

Respiratory: Dyspnea (10%), cough (6%), bronchitis, sinusitis, pharyngitis, rhinitis

Miscellaneous: Influenza-like symptoms (6%), diaphoresis (6%), lymphedema, infection

A dose-dependent decrease in sex hormone-binding globulin has been observed with daily doses of 25 mg or more. Serum luteinizing hormone and follicle-stimulating hormone levels have increased with this medicine.

Mechanism of Action Exemestane is an irreversible, steroidal aromatase inactivator. It prevents conversion of androgens to estrogens by tying up the enzyme aromatase. In breast cancers where growth is estrogen-dependent, this medicine will lower circulating estrogens.

Drug Interactions

Cytochrome P450 Effect: Substrate of CYP3A4 (minor)

Increased Effect/Toxicity: Although exemestane is a CYP3A4 substrate, ketoconazole, a CYP3A4 inhibitor, did not change the pharmacokinetics of exemestane. No other potential drug interactions have been evaluated.

Pharmacodynamics/Kinetics

Absorption: Rapid and moderate (~42%) following oral administration; absorption increases ~40% following high-fat meal

Distribution: Extensive

Protein binding: 90%, primarily to albumin and α_1-acid glycoprotein

Metabolism: Extensively hepatic; oxidation (CYP3A4) of methylene group, reduction of 17-keto group with formation of many secondary metabolites; metabolites are inactive

Half-life elimination: 24 hours

Time to peak: Women with breast cancer: 1.2 hours

Excretion: Urine (<1% as unchanged drug, 39% to 45% as metabolites); feces (36% to 48%)

Pregnancy Risk Factor D

ex-lax® [OTC] *see* Senna *on page 1213*

ex-lax® Maximum Strength [OTC] *see* Senna *on page 1213*

ex-lax® Stool Softener [OTC] *see* Docusate *on page 459*

Exorex® *see* Coal Tar *on page 367*

Extendryl *see* Chlorpheniramine, Phenylephrine, and Methscopolamine *on page 317*

Extendryl JR *see* Chlorpheniramine, Phenylephrine, and Methscopolamine *on page 317*

Extendryl SR *see* Chlorpheniramine, Phenylephrine, and Methscopolamine *on page 317*

Eye-Sine™ [OTC] *see* Tetrahydrozoline *on page 1282*

EZ-Char™ [OTC] *see* Charcoal *on page 303*

Ezetimibe (ez ET i mibe)

U.S. Brand Names Zetia™

Canadian Brand Names Ezetrol®

Generic Available No

Pharmacologic Category Antilipemic Agent, 2-Azetidinone

Use Use in combination with dietary therapy for the treatment of primary hypercholesterolemia (as monotherapy or in combination with HMG-CoA reductase inhibitors); homozygous sitosterolemia; homozygous familial hypercholesterolemia (in combination with atorvastatin or simvastatin)

Local Anesthetic/Vasoconstrictor Precautions No information available to require special precautions

Effects on Dental Treatment No significant effects or complications reported

Common Adverse Effects 1% to 10%:

Cardiovascular: Chest pain (3%), dizziness (3%), fatigue (2%)

Central nervous system: Headache (8%)

Gastrointestinal: Diarrhea (3% to 4%), abdominal pain (3%)

Neuromuscular & skeletal: Arthralgia (4%)

Respiratory: Sinusitis (4% to 5%), pharyngitis (2% to 3%, placebo 2%)

Dosage Oral:

Hyperlipidemias: Children ≥10 years and Adults: 10 mg/day

Sitosterolemia: Adults: 10 mg/day

Elderly: Refer to Adults dosing

Dosage adjustment in renal impairment: Bioavailability increased with severe impairment; no dosing adjustment recommended

Dosage adjustment in hepatic impairment: Bioavailability increased with hepatic impairment

Mild impairment (Child-Pugh score 5-6): No dosing adjustment necessary

Moderate to severe impairment (Child-Pugh score 7-15): Use of ezetimibe not recommended

Mechanism of Action Inhibits absorption of cholesterol at the brush border of the small intestine, leading to a decreased delivery of cholesterol to the liver, reduction of hepatic cholesterol stores and an increased clearance of cholesterol from the blood; decreases total C, LDL-cholesterol (LDL-C), ApoB, and triglycerides (TG) while increasing HDL-cholesterol (HDL-C).

Contraindications Hypersensitivity to ezetimibe or any component of the formulation

Warnings/Precautions Secondary causes of hyperlipidemia should be ruled out prior to therapy. Use caution with renal or mild hepatic impairment; not recommended for use with moderate or severe hepatic impairment. Safety and efficacy have not been established in patients <10 years of age.

Drug Interactions

Increased Effect/Toxicity: Cyclosporine may increase plasma levels of ezetimibe. Fibric acid derivatives may increase bioavailability of ezetimibe (safety and efficacy of concomitant use not established).

Decreased Effect: Bile acid sequestrants may decrease ezetimibe bioavailability; administer ezetimibe ≥2 hours before or ≥4 hours after bile acid sequestrants.

Dietary Considerations May be taken without regard to meals. Before initiation of therapy, patients should be placed on a standard cholesterol-lowering diet for 6 weeks and the diet should be continued during drug therapy.

Pharmacodynamics/Kinetics

Protein binding: >90% to plasma proteins

Metabolism: Undergoes conjugation in the small intestine and liver; forms metabolite (active); may undergo enterohepatic recycling

Bioavailability: Variable

Half-life: 22 hours (ezetimibe and metabolite)

Time to peak, plasma: 4-12 hours

Excretion: Feces (78%, 69% as ezetimibe); urine (11%, 9% as metabolite)

Pregnancy Risk Factor C

Dosage Forms TAB: 10 mg

F_3T *see* Trifluridine *on page 1339*

Fabrazyme® *see* Agalsidase Beta *on page 69*

Factive® *see* Gemifloxacin *on page 653*

Factor VIIa (Recombinant) (FAK ter SEV en ree KOM be nant)

U.S. Brand Names Novo-Seven®

Canadian Brand Names Niastase®

Generic Available No

Synonyms Coagulation Factor VIIa; Eptacog Alfa (Activated); rFVIIa

Pharmacologic Category Antihemophilic Agent; Blood Product Derivative

Use Treatment of bleeding episodes in patients with hemophilia A or B when inhibitors to factor VIII or factor IX are present

Local Anesthetic/Vasoconstrictor Precautions No information available to require special precautions

Effects on Dental Treatment No significant effects or complications reported

Common Adverse Effects 1% to 10%:

Cardiovascular: Hypertension

Hematologic: Hemorrhage, decreased plasma fibrinogen

Musculoskeletal: Hemarthrosis

Mechanism of Action Recombinant factor VIIa, a vitamin K-dependent glycoprotein, promotes hemostasis by activating the extrinsic pathway of the coagulation cascade. It replaces deficient activated coagulation factor VII, which complexes with tissue factor and may activate coagulation factor X to Xa and factor IX to IXa. When complexed with other factors, coagulation factor Xa converts prothrombin to thrombin, a key step in the formation of a fibrin-platelet hemostatic plug.

Pharmacodynamics/Kinetics

Distribution: V_d: 103 mL/kg (78-139)

Half-life elimination: 2.3 hours (1.7-2.7)

Excretion: Clearance: 33 mL/kg/hour (27-49)

Pregnancy Risk Factor C

Factor VIII (Human) *see* Antihemophilic Factor (Human) *on page 134*
Factor VIII (Porcine) *see* Antihemophilic Factor (Porcine) *on page 134*
Factor VIII (Recombinant) *see* Antihemophilic Factor (Recombinant) *on page 135*

Factor IX (FAK ter nyne)

U.S. Brand Names AlphaNine® SD; BeneFix®; Mononine®

Canadian Brand Names BeneFix®; Immunine® VH; Mononine®

Generic Available No

Pharmacologic Category Antihemophilic Agent; Blood Product Derivative

Use Control bleeding in patients with factor IX deficiency (hemophilia B or Christmas disease)

Local Anesthetic/Vasoconstrictor Precautions No information available to require special precautions

Effects on Dental Treatment No significant effects or complications reported

Common Adverse Effects Frequency not defined.

Cardiovascular: Angioedema, cyanosis, flushing, hypotension, tightness in chest, tightness in neck, (thrombosis following high dosages because of presence of activated clotting factors)

Central nervous system: Fever, headache, chills, somnolence, dizziness, drowsiness, lightheadedness

Dermatologic: Urticaria, rash

Gastrointestinal: Nausea, vomiting, abnormal taste

Hematologic: Disseminated intravascular coagulation (DIC)

Local: Injection site discomfort

Neuromuscular & skeletal: Tingling

Respiratory: Dyspnea, laryngeal edema, allergic rhinitis

Miscellaneous: Transient fever (following rapid administration), anaphylaxis, burning sensation in jaw/skull

Mechanism of Action Replaces deficient clotting factor IX; concentrate of factor IX; hemophilia B, or Christmas disease, is an X-linked inherited disorder of blood coagulation characterized by insufficient or abnormal synthesis of the clotting protein factor IX. Factor IX is a vitamin K-dependent coagulation factor which is synthesized in the liver. Factor IX is activated by factor XIa in the intrinsic coagulation pathway. Activated factor IX (IXa), in combination with factor VII:C activates factor X to Xa, resulting ultimately in the conversion of prothrombin to thrombin and the formation of a fibrin clot. The infusion of exogenous factor IX to replace the deficiency present in hemophilia B temporarily restores hemostasis. Depending upon the patient's level of biologically active factor IX, clinical symptoms range from moderate skin bruising or excessive hemorrhage after trauma or surgery to spontaneous hemorrhage into joints, muscles, or internal organs including the brain. Severe or recurring hemorrhages can produce death, organ dysfunction, or orthopedic deformity.

(Continued)

Factor IX *(Continued)*

Drug Interactions

Increased Effect/Toxicity: Do not coadminister with aminocaproic acid; may increase risk for thrombosis.

Pharmacodynamics/Kinetics Half-life elimination: IX component: 23-31 hours

Pregnancy Risk Factor C

Factor IX Complex (Human) (FAK ter nyne KOM pleks HYU man)

U.S. Brand Names Bebulin® VH; Profilnine® SD; Proplex® T

Generic Available No

Synonyms Prothrombin Complex Concentrate

Pharmacologic Category Antihemophilic Agent; Blood Product Derivative

Use

Control bleeding in patients with factor IX deficiency (hemophilia B or Christmas disease) **Note:** Factor IX concentrate containing **only** factor IX is also available and preferable for this indication.

Prevention/control of bleeding in hemophilia A patients with inhibitors to factor VIII

Prevention/control of bleeding in patients with factor VII deficiency

Emergency correction of the coagulopathy of warfarin excess in critical situations.

Local Anesthetic/Vasoconstrictor Precautions No information available to require special precautions

Effects on Dental Treatment No significant effects or complications reported

Common Adverse Effects 1% to 10%:

Central nervous system: Fever, headache, chills

Neuromuscular & skeletal: Tingling

Miscellaneous: Following rapid administration: Transient fever

Mechanism of Action Replaces deficient clotting factor including factor X; hemophilia B, or Christmas disease, is an X-linked recessively inherited disorder of blood coagulation characterized by insufficient or abnormal synthesis of the clotting protein factor IX. Factor IX is a vitamin K-dependent coagulation factor which is synthesized in the liver. Factor IX is activated by factor XIa in the intrinsic coagulation pathway. Activated factor IX (IXa), in combination with factor VII:C activates factor X to Xa, resulting ultimately in the conversion of prothrombin to thrombin and the formation of a fibrin clot. The infusion of exogenous factor IX to replace the deficiency present in hemophilia B temporarily restores hemostasis.

Drug Interactions

Increased Effect/Toxicity: Do not coadminister with aminocaproic acid; may increase risk for thrombosis.

Pharmacodynamics/Kinetics

Half-life elimination:

VII component: Initial: 4-6 hours; Terminal: 22.5 hours

IX component: 24 hours

Pregnancy Risk Factor C

Factrel® *see* Gonadorelin *on page 669*

Famciclovir (fam SYE kloe veer)

Related Information

Sexually-Transmitted Diseases *on page 1504*

Systemic Viral Diseases *on page 1519*

U.S. Brand Names Famvir®

Canadian Brand Names Famvir®

Generic Available No

Pharmacologic Category Antiviral Agent

Use Management of acute herpes zoster (shingles) and recurrent episodes of genital herpes; treatment of recurrent herpes simplex in immunocompetent patients

Local Anesthetic/Vasoconstrictor Precautions No information available to require special precautions

Effects on Dental Treatment No significant effects or complications reported

Common Adverse Effects 1% to 10%:

Central nervous system: Fatigue (4% to 6%), fever (1% to 3%), dizziness (3% to 5%), somnolence (1% to 2%), headache

Dermatologic: Pruritus (1% to 4%)

Gastrointestinal: Diarrhea (4% to 8%), vomiting (1% to 5%), constipation (1% to 5%), anorexia (1% to 3%), abdominal pain (1% to 4%), nausea
Neuromuscular & skeletal: Paresthesia (1% to 3%)
Respiratory: Sinusitis/pharyngitis (2%)

Mechanism of Action After undergoing rapid biotransformation to the active compound, penciclovir, famciclovir is phosphorylated by viral thymidine kinase in HSV-1, HSV-2, and VZV-infected cells to a monophosphate form; this is then converted to penciclovir triphosphate and competes with deoxyguanosine triphosphate to inhibit HSV-2 polymerase (ie, herpes viral DNA synthesis/replication is selectively inhibited)

Drug Interactions

Increased Effect/Toxicity:

Cimetidine: Penciclovir AUC may increase due to impaired metabolism.
Digoxin: C_{max} of digoxin increases by ~19%.
Probenecid: Penciclovir serum levels significantly increase.
Theophylline: Penciclovir AUC/C_{max} may increase and renal clearance decrease, although not clinically significant.

Pharmacodynamics/Kinetics

Absorption: Food decreases maximum peak concentration and delays time to peak; AUC remains the same
Distribution: V_{dss}: 0.98-1.08 L/kg
Protein binding: 20%
Metabolism: Rapidly deacetylated and oxidized to penciclovir; not via CYP
Bioavailability: 77%
Half-life elimination: Penciclovir: 2-3 hours (10, 20, and 7 hours in HSV-1, HSV-2, and VZV-infected cells, respectively); prolonged with renal impairment
Time to peak: 0.9 hours; C_{max} and T_{max} are decreased and prolonged with noncompensated hepatic impairment
Excretion: Urine (>90% as unchanged drug)

Pregnancy Risk Factor B

Famotidine (fa MOE ti deen)

Related Information

Gastrointestinal Disorders *on page 1476*

U.S. Brand Names Pepcid®; Pepcid® AC [OTC]

Canadian Brand Names Apo-Famotidine®; Gen-Famotidine; Novo-Famotidine; Nu-Famotidine; Pepcid®; Pepcid® AC; Pepcid® I.V.; ratio-Famotidine; Rhoxal-famotidine; Riva-Famotidine

Mexican Brand Names Durater®; Famoxal®; Farmotex®; Pepcidine®; Sigafam®

Generic Available Yes: Injection, tablet

Pharmacologic Category Histamine H_2 Antagonist

Use Therapy and treatment of duodenal ulcer, gastric ulcer, control gastric pH in critically-ill patients, symptomatic relief in gastritis, gastroesophageal reflux, active benign ulcer, and pathological hypersecretory conditions

OTC labeling: Relief of heartburn, acid indigestion, and sour stomach

Unlabeled/Investigational Use Part of a multidrug regimen for *H. pylori* eradication to reduce the risk of duodenal ulcer recurrence

Local Anesthetic/Vasoconstrictor Precautions No information available to require special precautions

Effects on Dental Treatment No significant effects or complications reported

Common Adverse Effects

Note: Agitation and vomiting have been reported in up to 14% of pediatric patients <1 year of age.

1% to 10%:

Central nervous system: Dizziness (1%), headache (5%)
Gastrointestinal: Constipation (1%), diarrhea (2%)

Dosage

Children: Treatment duration and dose should be individualized

Peptic ulcer: 1-16 years:

Oral: 0.5 mg/kg/day at bedtime or divided twice daily (maximum dose: 40 mg/day); doses of up to 1 mg/kg/day have been used in clinical studies
I.V.: 0.25 mg/kg every 12 hours (maximum dose: 40 mg/day); doses of up to 0.5 mg/kg have been used in clinical studies

GERD: Oral:

<3 months: 0.5 mg/kg once daily
3-12 months: 0.5 mg/kg twice daily
1-16 years: 1 mg/kg/day divided twice daily (maximum dose: 40 mg twice daily); doses of up to 2 mg/kg/day have been used in clinical studies

(Continued)

Famotidine *(Continued)*

Children ≥12 years and Adults: Heartburn, indigestion, sour stomach: OTC labeling: Oral: 10-20 mg every 12 hours; dose may be taken 15-60 minutes before eating foods known to cause heartburn

Adults:

Duodenal ulcer: Oral: Acute therapy: 40 mg/day at bedtime for 4-8 weeks; maintenance therapy: 20 mg/day at bedtime

Helicobacter pylori eradication (unlabeled use): 40 mg once daily; requires combination therapy with antibiotics

Gastric ulcer: Oral: Acute therapy: 40 mg/day at bedtime

Hypersecretory conditions: Oral: Initial: 20 mg every 6 hours, may increase in increments up to 160 mg every 6 hours

GERD: Oral: 20 mg twice daily for 6 weeks

Esophagitis and accompanying symptoms due to GERD: Oral: 20 mg or 40 mg twice daily for up to 12 weeks

Patients unable to take oral medication: I.V.: 20 mg every 12 hours

Dosing adjustment in renal impairment: Cl_{cr} <50 mL/minute: Manufacturer recommendation: Administer 50% of dose **or** increase the dosing interval to every 36-48 hours (to limit potential CNS adverse effects).

Mechanism of Action Competitive inhibition of histamine at H_2 receptors of the gastric parietal cells, which inhibits gastric acid secretion

Contraindications Hypersensitivity to famotidine, other H_2 antagonists, or any component of the formulation

Warnings/Precautions Modify dose in patients with renal impairment; chewable tablets contain phenylalanine; multidose vials contain benzyl alcohol

Drug Interactions

Decreased Effect: Decreased serum levels of ketoconazole and itraconazole (reduced absorption).

Ethanol/Nutrition/Herb Interactions

Ethanol: Avoid ethanol (may cause gastric mucosal irritation).

Food: Famotidine bioavailability may be increased if taken with food.

Dietary Considerations Phenylalanine content: Pepcid® AC chewable: Each 10 mg tablet contains phenylalanine 1.4 mg

Pharmacodynamics/Kinetics

Onset of action: GI: Oral: Within 1-3 hour

Duration: 10-12 hours

Protein binding: 15% to 20%

Bioavailability: Oral: 40% to 50%

Half-life elimination: 2.5-3.5 hours; prolonged with renal impairment; Oliguria: 20 hours

Time to peak, serum: Oral: ~1-3 hours

Excretion: Urine (as unchanged drug)

Pregnancy Risk Factor B

Dosage Forms GELCAP (Pepcid® AC): 10 mg. **INF** [premixed in NS] (Pepcid®): 20 mg (50 mL). **INJ, solution** 10 mg/mL (4 mL, 20 mL, 50 mL); (Pepcid®): 10 mg/mL (4 mL, 20 mL). **INJ, solution** [preservative free] (Pepcid®): 10 mg/mL (2 mL). **POWDER, oral suspension** (Pepcid®): 40 mg/5 mL (50 mL). **TAB, chewable** (Pepcid® AC): 10 mg. **TAB:** 10 mg [OTC], 20 mg, 40 mg; (Pepcid®): 20 mg, 40 mg; (Pepcid® AC): 10 mg, 20 mg

Famotidine, Calcium Carbonate, and Magnesium Hydroxide

(fa MOE ti deen, KAL see um KAR bun ate, & mag NEE zhum hye DROKS ide)

Related Information

Calcium Carbonate *on page 245*

Famotidine *on page 573*

U.S. Brand Names Pepcid® Complete [OTC]

Canadian Brand Names Pepcid® Complete [OTC]

Generic Available No

Synonyms Calcium Carbonate, Magnesium Hydroxide, and Famotidine; Magnesium Hydroxide, Famotidine, and Calcium Carbonate

Pharmacologic Category Antacid; Histamine H_2 Antagonist

Use Relief of heartburn due to acid indigestion

Local Anesthetic/Vasoconstrictor Precautions No information available to require special precautions

Effects on Dental Treatment No significant effects or complications reported

Common Adverse Effects See individual agents.

Mechanism of Action
Famotidine: H_2 antagonist
Calcium carbonate: Antacid
Magnesium hydroxide: Antacid

Drug Interactions
Increased Effect/Toxicity: See individual agents.
Decreased Effect: See individual agents.

Pharmacodynamics/Kinetics See individual agents.

Famvir® *see* Famciclovir *on page 572*
Fansidar® *see* Sulfadoxine and Pyrimethamine *on page 1245*
Fareston® *see* Toremifene *on page 1317*
Faslodex® *see* Fulvestrant *on page 639*

Fat Emulsion (fat e MUL shun)

U.S. Brand Names Intralipid®; Liposyn® III
Canadian Brand Names Intralipid®
Generic Available No
Synonyms Intravenous Fat Emulsion
Pharmacologic Category Caloric Agent
Use Source of calories and essential fatty acids for patients requiring parenteral nutrition of extended duration
Local Anesthetic/Vasoconstrictor Precautions No information available to require special precautions
Effects on Dental Treatment No significant effects or complications reported
Common Adverse Effects Frequency not defined.
Cardiovascular: Cyanosis, flushing, chest pain
Central nervous system: Headache, dizziness
Endocrine & metabolic: Hyperlipemia, hypertriglyceridemia
Gastrointestinal: Nausea, vomiting, diarrhea
Hematologic: Hypercoagulability, thrombocytopenia in neonates (rare)
Hepatic: Hepatomegaly, pancreatitis
Local: Thrombophlebitis
Respiratory: Dyspnea
Miscellaneous: Sepsis, diaphoresis, brown pigment deposition in the reticuloendothelial system (significance unknown)
Mechanism of Action Essential for normal structure and function of cell membranes
Pharmacodynamics/Kinetics
Metabolism: Undergoes lipolysis to free fatty acids which are utilized by reticuloendothelial cells
Half-life elimination: 0.5-1 hour
Pregnancy Risk Factor C

Fazaclo™ *see* Clozapine *on page 366*
5-FC *see* Flucytosine *on page 596*
FC1157a *see* Toremifene *on page 1317*
Feiba VH® *see* Anti-inhibitor Coagulant Complex *on page 135*

Felbamate (FEL ba mate)

U.S. Brand Names Felbatol®
Generic Available No
Pharmacologic Category Anticonvulsant, Miscellaneous
Use Not as a first-line antiepileptic treatment; only in those patients who respond inadequately to alternative treatments and whose epilepsy is so severe that a substantial risk of aplastic anemia and/or liver failure is deemed acceptable in light of the benefits conferred by its use. Patient must be fully advised of risk and provide signed written informed consent. Felbamate can be used as either monotherapy or adjunctive therapy in the treatment of partial seizures (with and without generalization) and in adults with epilepsy.
Orphan drug: Adjunctive therapy in the treatment of partial and generalized seizures associated with Lennox-Gastaut syndrome in children
Local Anesthetic/Vasoconstrictor Precautions No information available to require special precautions
Effects on Dental Treatment Key adverse event(s) related to dental treatment: Xerostomia (normal salivary flow resumes upon discontinuation) and abnormal taste.
Common Adverse Effects
>10%:
Central nervous system: Somnolence, headache, fatigue, dizziness
Gastrointestinal: Nausea, anorexia, vomiting, constipation
(Continued)

Felbamate *(Continued)*

1% to 10%:

Cardiovascular: Chest pain, palpitations, tachycardia

Central nervous system: Depression or behavior changes, nervousness, anxiety, ataxia, stupor, malaise, agitation, psychological disturbances, aggressive reaction

Dermatologic: Skin rash, acne, pruritus

Gastrointestinal: Xerostomia, diarrhea, abdominal pain, weight gain, taste perversion

Neuromuscular & skeletal: Tremor, abnormal gait, paresthesia, myalgia

Ocular: Diplopia, abnormal vision

Respiratory: Sinusitis, pharyngitis

Miscellaneous: ALT increase

Restrictions A patient "informed consent" form should be completed and signed by the patient and physician. Copies are available from Wallace Pharmaceuticals by calling 609-655-6147.

Mechanism of Action Mechanism of action is unknown but has properties in common with other marketed anticonvulsants; has weak inhibitory effects on GABA-receptor binding, benzodiazepine receptor binding, and is devoid of activity at the MK-801 receptor binding site of the NMDA receptor-ionophore complex.

Drug Interactions

Cytochrome P450 Effect: Substrate of CYP2E1 (minor), 3A4 (major); **Inhibits** CYP2C19 (weak); **Induces** CYP3A4 (weak)

Increased Effect/Toxicity: Felbamate increases serum phenytoin, phenobarbital, and valproic acid concentrations which may result in toxicity; consider decreasing phenytoin or phenobarbital dosage by 25%. A decrease in valproic acid dosage may also be necessary. CYP3A4 inhibitors may increase the levels/effects of felbamate; example inhibitors include azole antifungals, ciprofloxacin, clarithromycin, diclofenac, doxycycline, erythromycin, imatinib, isoniazid, nefazodone, nicardipine, propofol, protease inhibitors, quinidine, and verapamil.

Decreased Effect: Felbamate may decrease carbamazepine levels and increase levels of the active metabolite of carbamazepine (10,11-epoxide) resulting in carbamazepine toxicity; monitor for signs of carbamazepine toxicity (dizziness, ataxia, nystagmus, drowsiness). CYP3A4 inducers may decrease the levels/effects of felbamate; example inducers include aminoglutethimide, carbamazepine, nafcillin, nevirapine, phenobarbital, phenytoin, and rifamycins.

Pharmacodynamics/Kinetics

Absorption: Rapid and almost complete; food has no effect upon the tablet's absorption

Distribution: V_d: 0.7-1 L/kg

Protein binding: 22% to 25%, primarily to albumin

Half-life elimination: 20-23 hours (average); prolonged in renal dysfunction

Time to peak, serum: ~3 hours

Excretion: Urine (40% to 50% as unchanged drug, 40% as inactive metabolites)

Pregnancy Risk Factor C

Felbatol® *see* Felbamate *on page 575*

Feldene® *see* Piroxicam *on page 1097*

Felodipine (fe LOE di peen)

Related Information

Calcium Channel Blockers and Gingival Hyperplasia *on page 1600*

Calcium Channel Blockers, Comparative Pharmacokinetics *on page 1602*

Cardiovascular Diseases *on page 1458*

Enalapril and Felodipine *on page 491*

U.S. Brand Names Plendil®

Canadian Brand Names Plendil®; Renedil®

Mexican Brand Names Munobal®; Plendil®

Generic Available No

Pharmacologic Category Calcium Channel Blocker

Use Treatment of hypertension

Local Anesthetic/Vasoconstrictor Precautions No information available to require special precautions

Effects on Dental Treatment Key adverse event(s) related to dental treatment: Gingival hyperplasia (fewer reports than other CCBs, resolves upon discontinuation, consultation with physician is suggested).

Common Adverse Effects

>10%: Central nervous system: Headache (11% to 15%)

2% to 10%: Cardiovascular: Peripheral edema (2% to 17%), tachycardia (0.4% to 2.5%), flushing (4% to 7%)

Mechanism of Action Inhibits calcium ions from entering the "slow channels" or select voltage-sensitive areas of vascular smooth muscle and myocardium during depolarization, producing a relaxation of coronary vascular smooth muscle and coronary vasodilation; increases myocardial oxygen delivery in patients with vasospastic angina

Drug Interactions

Cytochrome P450 Effect: Substrate of CYP3A4 (major); **Inhibits** CYP2C8/9 (weak), 2D6 (weak), 3A4 (weak)

Increased Effect/Toxicity: CYP3A4 inhibitors may increase the levels/effects of felodipine; example inhibitors include azole antifungals, ciprofloxacin, clarithromycin, diclofenac, doxycycline, erythromycin, imatinib, isoniazid, nefazodone, nicardipine, propofol, protease inhibitors, quinidine, and verapamil. Beta-blockers may have increased pharmacokinetic or pharmacodynamic interactions with felodipine. Cyclosporine increases felodipine's serum concentration. Blood pressure-lowering effects may be additive with sildenafil, tadalafil, and vardenafil (use caution). Felodipine may increase tacrolimus serum levels (monitor).

Decreased Effect: Felodipine may decrease pharmacologic actions of theophylline. Calcium may reduce the calcium channel blocker's effects, particularly hypotension. Felodipine may decrease pharmacologic actions of theophylline. CYP3A4 inducers may decrease the levels/effects of felodipine; example inducers include aminoglutethimide, carbamazepine, nafcillin, nevirapine, phenobarbital, phenytoin, and rifamycins.

Pharmacodynamics/Kinetics

Onset of action: 2-5 hours

Duration: 16-24 hours

Absorption: 100%; Absolute: 20% due to first-pass effect

Protein binding: >99%

Metabolism: Hepatic; extensive first-pass effect

Half-life elimination: 11-16 hours

Excretion: Urine (as metabolites)

Pregnancy Risk Factor C

Felodipine and Enalapril *see* Enalapril and Felodipine *on page 491*

Femara® *see* Letrozole *on page 803*

femhrt® *see* Ethinyl Estradiol and Norethindrone *on page 550*

Femilax™ [OTC] *see* Bisacodyl *on page 208*

Femiron® [OTC] *see* Ferrous Fumarate *on page 586*

Femizol-M™ [OTC] *see* Miconazole *on page 922*

Fem-Prin® [OTC] *see* Acetaminophen, Aspirin, and Caffeine *on page 56*

Femring™ *see* Estradiol *on page 518*

Fenesin™ DM *see* Guaifenesin and Dextromethorphan *on page 673*

Fenofibrate (fen oh FYE brate)

Related Information

Cardiovascular Diseases *on page 1458*

U.S. Brand Names Lofibra™; TriCor®

Canadian Brand Names Apo-Fenofibrate®; Apo-Feno-Micro®; Gen-Fenofibrate Micro; Lipidil Micro®; Lipidil Supra®; Novo-Fenofibrate; Nu-Fenofibrate; PMS-Fenofibrate Micro; TriCor®

Mexican Brand Names Controlip®; Lipidil®

Generic Available No

Synonyms Procetofene; Proctofene

Pharmacologic Category Antilipemic Agent, Fibric Acid

Use Adjunct to dietary therapy for the treatment of adults with very high elevations of serum triglyceride levels (types IV and V hyperlipidemia) who are at risk of pancreatitis and who do not respond adequately to a determined dietary effort; adjunct to dietary therapy for the reduction of low density lipoprotein cholesterol (LDL-C), total cholesterol (total-C), triglycerides, and apolipoprotein B (apo B) in adult patients with primary hypercholesterolemia or mixed dyslipidemia (Fredrickson types IIa and IIb)

Local Anesthetic/Vasoconstrictor Precautions No information available to require special precautions

Effects on Dental Treatment No significant effects or complications reported

(Continued)

Fenofibrate *(Continued)*

Common Adverse Effects

1% to 10%:

Gastrointestinal: Abdominal pain (5%), constipation (2%)

Hepatic: Abnormal liver function test (7%), creatine phosphokinase increased (3%), ALT increased (3%), AST increased (3%)

Neuromuscular & skeletal: Back pain (3%)

Respiratory: Respiratory disorder (6%), rhinitis (2%)

Frequency not defined:

Cardiovascular: Angina pectoris, arrhythmias, atrial fibrillation, cardiovascular disorder, chest pain, coronary artery disorder, edema, electrocardiogram abnormality, extrasystoles, hypertension, hypotension, migraine, myocardial infarction, palpitations, peripheral edema, peripheral vascular disorder, phlebitis, tachycardia, varicose veins, vasodilatation

Central nervous system: Anxiety, depression, dizziness, fever, insomnia, malaise, nervousness, neuralgia, pain, somnolence, vertigo

Dermatologic: Acne, alopecia, bruising, contact dermatitis, eczema, fungal dermatitis, maculopapular rash, nail disorder, photosensitivity reaction, pruritus, skin disorder, skin ulcer, urticaria

Endocrine & metabolic: Diabetes mellitus, gout, gynecomastia, hypoglycemia, hyperuricemia

Gastrointestinal: Anorexia, appetite increased, colitis, diarrhea, dry mouth, duodenal ulcer, dyspepsia, eructation, esophagitis, flatulence, gastroenteritis, gastritis, gastrointestinal disorder, nausea, peptic ulcer, rectal disorder, rectal hemorrhage, tooth disorder, vomiting, weight gain/loss

Genitourinary: Cystitis, dysuria, prostatic disorder, libido decreased, pregnancy (unintended), urinary frequency, urolithiasis, vaginal moniliasis

Hematologic: Anemia, eosinophilia, leukopenia, lymphadenopathy, thrombocytopenia

Hepatic: Cholelithiasis, cholecystitis, fatty liver deposits

Neuromuscular & skeletal: Arthralgia, arthritis, arthrosis, bursitis, hypertonia, joint disorder, leg cramps, myalgia, myasthenia, myositis, paresthesia, tenosynovitis

Ocular: Abnormal vision, amblyopia, cataract, conjunctivitis, eye disorder, refraction disorder

Otic: Ear pain, otitis media

Renal: Creatinine increased, kidney function abnormality

Respiratory: Asthma, bronchitis, cough increased, dyspnea, laryngitis, pharyngitis, pneumonia, sinusitis

Miscellaneous: Accidental injury, allergic reaction, cyst, diaphoresis, herpes simplex, herpes zoster, infection

Dosage Oral:

Adults:

Hypertriglyceridemia: Initial:

Capsule: 67 mg/day with meals, up to 200 mg/day

Tablet: 54 mg/day with meals, up to 160 mg/day

Hypercholesterolemia or mixed hyperlipidemia: Initial:

Capsule: 200 mg/day with meals

Tablet: 160 mg/day with meals

Elderly: Initial: 67 mg/day (capsule) or 54 mg/day (tablet)

Dosage adjustment in renal impairment: Decrease dose or increase dosing interval for patients with renal failure: Initial: 67 mg/day (capsule) or 54 mg/day (tablet)

Hemodialysis has no effect on removal of fenofibric acid from the plasma.

Mechanism of Action Fenofibric acid is believed to increase VLDL catabolism by enhancing the synthesis of lipoprotein lipase; as a result of a decrease in VLDL levels, total plasma triglycerides are reduced by 30% to 60%; modest increase in HDL occurs in some hypertriglyceridemic patients

Contraindications Hypersensitivity to fenofibrate or any component of the formulation; hepatic or severe renal dysfunction including primary biliary cirrhosis and unexplained persistent liver function abnormalities; pre-existing gallbladder disease

Warnings/Precautions The hypoprothrombinemic effect of anticoagulants is significantly increased with concomitant fenofibrate administration. Use with caution in patients with severe renal dysfunction. Hepatic transaminases can significantly elevate (dose-related). Regular monitoring of liver function tests is required. May cause cholelithiasis. Adjustments in warfarin therapy may be required with concurrent use. Use caution when combining fenofibrate with HMG-CoA reductase inhibitors (may lead to myopathy, rhabdomyolysis). The effect of CAD morbidity and mortality has not been established. Therapy should be withdrawn if an adequate response is not obtained after 2 months of therapy at the maximal daily dose (201 mg). Rare hypersensitivity reactions may occur. Dose adjustment is required for renal impairment and elderly patients. Safety and efficacy in children have not been established.

Drug Interactions

Cytochrome P450 Effect: Substrate of CYP3A4 (minor)

Increased Effect/Toxicity: The hypolipidemic effect of fenofibrate is increased when used with cholestyramine or colestipol. Fenofibrate may increase the effect of chlorpropamide and warfarin. Concurrent use of fenofibrate with HMG-CoA reductase inhibitors (atorvastatin, cerivastatin, fluvastatin, lovastatin, pravastatin, simvastatin) may increase the risk of myopathy and rhabdomyolysis. The manufacturer warns against concomitant use. However, combination therapy with statins has been used in some patients with resistant hyperlipidemias (with great caution).

Decreased Effect: Rifampin (and potentially other enzyme inducers) may decrease levels of fenofibrate.

Dietary Considerations Take with food.

Pharmacodynamics/Kinetics

Absorption: Increased when taken with meals

Distribution: Widely to most tissues

Protein binding: >99%

Metabolism: Tissue and plasma via esterases to active form, fenofibric acid; undergoes inactivation by glucuronidation hepatically or renally

Half-life elimination: 20 hours

Time to peak: 6-8 hours

Excretion: Urine (60% as metabolites); feces (25%); hemodialysis has no effect on removal of fenofibric acid from plasma

Pregnancy Risk Factor C

Dosage Forms CAP [micronized] (Lofibra™): 67 mg, 134 mg, 200 mg. **TAB** (TriCor®): 54 mg, 160 mg

Fenoldopam (fe NOL doe pam)

U.S. Brand Names Corlopam®

Canadian Brand Names Corlopam®

Generic Available Yes

Synonyms Fenoldopam Mesylate

Pharmacologic Category Dopamine Agonist

Use Treatment of severe hypertension (up to 48 hours in adults), including in patients with renal compromise; short-term (up to 4 hours) blood pressure reduction in pediatric patients

Local Anesthetic/Vasoconstrictor Precautions No information available to require special precautions

Effects on Dental Treatment Key adverse event(s) related to dental treatment: Xerostomia and changes in salivation (normal salivary flow resumes upon discontinuation).

Common Adverse Effects Frequency not always defined.

Cardiovascular: Angina, asymptomatic T wave flattening on ECG, chest pain, edema, facial flushing (>5%), fibrillation (atrial), flutter (atrial), hypotension (>5%), tachycardia

Central nervous system: Dizziness, headache (>5%)

Endocrine & metabolic: Hypokalemia

Gastrointestinal: Abdominal pain/fullness, diarrhea, nausea (>5%), vomiting, xerostomia

Local: Injection site reactions

Ocular: Intraocular pressure (increased), blurred vision

Hepatic: Increases in portal pressure in cirrhotic patients

Mechanism of Action A selective postsynaptic dopamine agonist (D_1-receptors) which exerts hypotensive effects by decreasing peripheral vasculature resistance with increased renal blood flow, diuresis, and natriuresis; 6 times as potent as dopamine in producing renal vasodilitation; has minimal adrenergic effects

Drug Interactions

Increased Effect/Toxicity: Concurrent acetaminophen may increase fenoldopam levels (30% to 70%). Beta-blockers increase the risk of hypotension; avoid concurrent use. If used concurrently with beta-blockers, close monitoring is recommended.

Pharmacodynamics/Kinetics

Onset of action: I.V.: 10 minutes

Duration: I.V.: 1 hour

Distribution: V_d: 0.6 L/kg

Half-life elimination: I.V.: Children: 3-5 minutes; Adults: ~5 minutes

(Continued)

Fenoldopam *(Continued)*

Metabolism: Hepatic via methylation, glucuronidation, and sulfation; the 8-sulfate metabolite may have some activity; extensive first-pass effect
Excretion: Urine (90%); feces (10%)

Pregnancy Risk Factor B

Fenoldopam Mesylate *see* Fenoldopam *on page 579*

Fenoprofen (fen oh PROE fen)

Related Information

Rheumatoid Arthritis, Osteoarthritis, and Osteoporosis *on page 1490*
Temporomandibular Dysfunction (TMD) *on page 1564*

U.S. Brand Names Nalfon®

Canadian Brand Names Nalfon®

Generic Available Yes: Tablet

Synonyms Fenoprofen Calcium

Pharmacologic Category Nonsteroidal Anti-inflammatory Drug (NSAID), Oral

Use Symptomatic treatment of acute and chronic rheumatoid arthritis and osteoarthritis; relief of mild to moderate pain

Local Anesthetic/Vasoconstrictor Precautions No information available to require special precautions

Effects on Dental Treatment NSAID formulations are known to reversibly decrease platelet aggregation via mechanisms different than observed with aspirin. The dentist should be aware of the potential of abnormal coagulation. Caution should also be exercised in the use of NSAIDs in patients already on anticoagulant therapy with drugs such as warfarin (Coumadin®).

Common Adverse Effects

>10%:

Central nervous system: Dizziness (7% to 15%), somnolence (9% to 15%)
Gastrointestinal: Abdominal cramps (2% to 4%), heartburn, indigestion, nausea (8% to 14%), dyspepsia (10% to 14%), flatulence (14%), anorexia (14%), constipation (7% to 14%), occult blood in stool (14%), vomiting (3% to 14%), diarrhea (2% to 14%)

1% to 10%:

Central nervous system: Headache (9%)
Dermatologic: Itching
Endocrine & metabolic: Fluid retention

Mechanism of Action Inhibits prostaglandin synthesis by decreasing the activity of the enzyme, cyclooxygenase, which results in decreased formation of prostaglandin precursors

Drug Interactions

Increased Effect/Toxicity: Increased effect/toxicity of phenytoin, sulfonamides, sulfonylureas, salicylates, and oral anticoagulants. Serum concentration/toxicity of methotrexate may be increased.

Decreased Effect: Decreased effect with phenobarbital.

Pharmacodynamics/Kinetics

Onset of action: A few days
Absorption: Rapid, 80%
Distribution: Does not cross the placenta
Protein binding: 99%
Metabolism: Extensively hepatic
Half-life elimination: 2.5-3 hours
Time to peak, serum: ~2 hours
Excretion: Urine (2% to 5% as unchanged drug); feces (small amounts)

Pregnancy Risk Factor B/D (3rd trimester)

Fenoprofen Calcium *see* Fenoprofen *on page 580*

Fenoterol (fen oh TER ole)

Canadian Brand Names Berotec®

Mexican Brand Names Partusisten®

Synonyms Fenoterol Hydrobromide

Pharmacologic Category $Beta_2$-Adrenergic Agonist

Use Treatment and prevention of symptoms of reversible obstructive pulmonary disease (including asthma and acute bronchospasm), chronic bronchitis, emphysema

Local Anesthetic/Vasoconstrictor Precautions No information available to require special precautions

Effects on Dental Treatment No significant effects or complications reported

Common Adverse Effects Note: Frequency of most effects may be dose-related, approximate frequencies noted below. In the treatment of acute bronchospasm (high-dose nebulization), symptoms of headache (up to 12%), tremor (32%), and tachycardia (up to 21%) are frequently noted.

>10%: Endocrine & metabolic: Serum glucose increased, serum potassium decreased

1% to 10%:

Cardiovascular: Palpitations, tachycardia

Central nervous system: Headache, dizziness, nervousness

Neuromuscular & skeletal: Tremor, muscle cramps

Respiratory: Pharyngeal irritation, cough

Restrictions Not available in U.S.

Mechanism of Action Relaxes bronchial smooth muscle by action on $beta_2$ receptors with little effect on heart rate.

Drug Interactions

Increased Effect/Toxicity: When used with inhaled ipratropium, an increased duration of bronchodilation may occur. Cardiovascular effects are potentiated in patients also receiving MAO inhibitors, tricyclic antidepressants, and sympathomimetic agents (eg, amphetamine, dopamine, dobutamine). Fenoterol may increase the risk of malignant arrhythmias with inhaled anesthetics (eg, enflurane, halothane). Concurrent use with diuretics may increase the risk of hypokalemia.

Decreased Effect: When used with nonselective beta-adrenergic blockers (eg, propranolol), the effect of fenoterol is decreased.

Pharmacodynamics/Kinetics

Onset of action: 5 minutes

Peak effect: 30-60 minutes

Duration: 3-4 hours (up to 6-8 hours)

Pregnancy Risk Factor Not available; similar agents rated C

Fenoterol Hydrobromide *see* Fenoterol *on page 580*

Fentanyl (FEN ta nil)

U.S. Brand Names Actiq®; Duragesic®; Sublimaze®

Canadian Brand Names Actiq®; Duragesic®

Mexican Brand Names Durogesic®; Fentanest®

Generic Available Yes: Injection only

Synonyms Fentanyl Citrate

Pharmacologic Category Analgesic, Narcotic; General Anesthetic

Dental Use Adjunct in preoperative intravenous conscious sedation in patients undergoing dental surgery

Use Sedation, relief of pain, preoperative medication, adjunct to general or regional anesthesia, management of chronic pain (transdermal product)

Actiq® is indicated only for management of breakthrough cancer pain in patients who are tolerant to and currently receiving opioid therapy for persistent cancer pain.

Local Anesthetic/Vasoconstrictor Precautions No information available to require special precautions

Effects on Dental Treatment Key adverse event(s) related to dental treatment: Xerostomia, changes in salivation (normal salivary flow resumes upon discontinuation), and orthostatic hypotension. Actiq® may contribute to dental carries due to sugar content of oral lozenge; advise patients to maintain good oral hygiene.

Significant Adverse Effects

>10%:

Cardiovascular: Bradycardia, hypotension, peripheral vasodilation

Central nervous system: Drowsiness, sedation, increased intracranial pressure

Gastrointestinal: Nausea, vomiting

Endocrine & metabolic: Antidiuretic hormone release

Neuromuscular & skeletal: Chest wall rigidity (high dose I.V.)

Ocular: Miosis

1% to 10%:

Cardiovascular: Cardiac arrhythmias, orthostatic hypotension

Central nervous system: Confusion, CNS depression

Gastrointestinal: Constipation

Ocular: Blurred vision

Respiratory: Apnea, postoperative respiratory depression

<1% (Limited to important or life-threatening): Bronchospasm, convulsions, hypercarbia, laryngospasm, respiratory depression

Restrictions C-II

(Continued)

Fentanyl *(Continued)*

Dosage Note: These are guidelines and do not represent the maximum doses that may be required in all patients. Doses should be titrated to pain relief/prevention. Monitor vital signs routinely. Single I.M. doses have a duration of 1-2 hours, single I.V. doses last 0.5-1 hour.

Children 1-12 years:

Sedation for minor procedures/analgesia: I.M., I.V.: 1-2 mcg/kg/dose; may repeat at 30- to 60-minute intervals. **Note:** Children 18-36 months of age may require 2-3 mcg/kg/dose

Continuous sedation/analgesia: Initial I.V. bolus: 1-2 mcg/kg then 1 mcg/kg/hour; titrate upward; usual: 1-3 mcg/kg/hour

Pain control: Transdermal (limited to children >2 years who are opioid tolerant): Initial dose: 25 mcg/hour system (higher doses have been used based on equianalgesic conversion); change patch every 72 hours

Children >12 years and Adults:

Sedation for minor procedures/analgesia: I.M., I.V.: 0.5-1 mcg/kg/dose; higher doses are used for major procedures

Pain control: Transdermal: Initial: 25 mcg/hour system; if currently receiving opiates, convert to fentanyl equivalent and administer equianalgesic dosage titrated to minimize the adverse effects and provide analgesia. Change patch every 72 hours. To convert patients from oral or parenteral opioids to Duragesic®, the previous 24-hour analgesic requirement should be calculated. This analgesic requirement should be converted to the equianalgesic oral morphine dose.

Adults:

Premedication: I.M., slow I.V.: 50-100 mcg/dose 30-60 minutes prior to surgery

Adjunct to regional anesthesia: I.M., slow I.V.: 50-100 mcg/dose; if I.V. used, give over 1-2 minutes

Severe pain: I.M.: 50-100 mcg/dose every 1-2 hours as needed; patients with prior opiate exposure may tolerate higher initial doses

Adjunct to general anesthesia: Slow I.V.:

Low dose: Initial: 2 mcg/kg/dose; Maintenance: Additional doses infrequently needed

Moderate dose: Initial: 2-20 mcg/kg/dose; Maintenance: 25-100 mcg/dose may be given slow I.V. or I.M. as needed

High dose: Initial: 20-50 mcg/kg/dose; Maintenance: 25 mcg to one-half the initial loading dose may be given as needed

General anesthesia without additional anesthetic agents: Slow I.V.: 50-100 mcg/kg with O_2 and skeletal muscle relaxant

Mechanically-ventilated patients (based on 70 kg patient): Slow I.V.: 0.35-1.5 mcg/kg every 30-60 minutes as needed; infusion: 0.7-10 mcg/kg/hour

Patient-controlled analgesia (PCA): I.V.: Usual concentration: 50 mcg/mL

Demand dose: Usual: 10 mcg; range: 10-50 mcg

Lockout interval: 5-8 minutes

Equianalgesic Doses of Opioid Agonists

Drug	Equianalgesic Dose (mg)	
	I.M.	P.O.
Codeine	75	130
Hydromorphone	1.5	7.5
Levorphanol	2 (acute)	4 (acute)
Meperidine	75	300
Methadone	10 (acute)	20 (acute)
Morphine	10	30
Oxycodone	—	20
Oxymorphone	1	10 (PR)

From "Principles of Analgesic Use," *Am Pain Soc*, 1999.

Breakthrough cancer pain: Adults: Transmucosal: Actiq® dosing should be individually titrated to provide adequate analgesia with minimal side effects. It is indicated only for management of breakthrough cancer pain in patients who are tolerant to and currently receiving opioid therapy for persistent cancer pain. An initial starting dose of 200 mcg should be used for the treatment of breakthrough cancer pain. Patients should be monitored closely in order to determine the proper dose. If redosing for the same episode is necessary, the second dose may be started 15 minutes after completion of the first dose. Dosing should be titrated so that the patient's pain can be treated with one single dose. Generally, 1-2 days is required to determine the proper dose of analgesia with limited side effects. Once the dose has been determined, consumption should be limited to 4 units/day or less. Patients needing more than 4 units/day should have the dose of their long-term opioid re-evaluated. If signs of excessive opioid effects occur before a dose is complete, the unit should be removed from the patient's mouth immediately, and subsequent doses decreased.

See tables below and on previous page.

Corresponding Doses of Oral/Intramuscular Morphine and Duragesic™

P.O. 24-Hour Morphine (mg/d)	I.M. 24-Hour Morphine (mg/d)	Duragesic™ Dose (mcg/h)
45-134	8-22	25
135-224	28-37	50
225-314	38-52	75
315-404	53-67	100
405-494	68-82	125
495-584	83-97	150
585-674	98-112	175
675-764	113-127	200
765-854	128-142	225
855-944	143-157	250
945-1034	158-172	275
1035-1124	173-187	300

Product information, Duragesic™ — Janssen Pharmaceutica, January, 1991.

The dosage should not be titrated more frequently than every 3 days after the initial dose or every 6 days thereafter. The majority of patients are controlled on every 72-hour administration, however, a small number of patients require every 48-hour administration.

Elderly >65 years: Transmucosal: Actiq®: Dose should be reduced to 2.5-5 mcg/kg; elderly have been found to be twice as sensitive as younger patients to the effects of fentanyl. Patients in this age group generally require smaller doses of Actiq® than younger patients

Dosing adjustment in hepatic impairment: Actiq®: Although fentanyl kinetics may be altered in hepatic disease, Actiq® can be used successfully in the management of breakthrough cancer pain. Doses should be titrated to reach clinical effect with careful monitoring of patients with severe hepatic disease.

Mechanism of Action Binds with stereospecific receptors at many sites within the CNS, increases pain threshold, alters pain reception, inhibits ascending pain pathways

Contraindications Hypersensitivity to fentanyl or any component of the formulation; increased intracranial pressure; severe respiratory depression; severe liver or renal insufficiency; pregnancy (prolonged use or high doses near term)

Actiq® must not be used in patients who are intolerant to opioids. Patients are considered opioid-tolerant if they are taking at least 60 mg morphine/day, 50 mcg transdermal fentanyl/hour, or an equivalent dose of another opioid for ≥1 week.

Warnings/Precautions An opioid-containing analgesic regimen should be tailored to each patient's needs and based upon the type of pain being treated (acute versus chronic), the route of administration, degree of tolerance for opioids (naive versus chronic user), age, weight, and medical condition. The optimal analgesic dose varies widely among patients. Doses should be titrated to pain relief/prevention. Fentanyl shares the toxic potentials of opiate agonists, and precautions of opiate agonist therapy should be observed; use with caution in patients with bradycardia; rapid I.V. infusion may result in skeletal muscle and chest wall rigidity leading to respiratory distress and/or apnea, bronchoconstriction, laryngospasm; inject slowly over 3-5 minutes; nondepolarizing skeletal muscle relaxant may be required. Tolerance of drug dependence may result from extended use. The elderly may be particularly susceptible to the CNS depressant and constipating effects of narcotics.

Actiq® should be used only for the care of cancer patients and is intended for use by specialists who are knowledgeable in treating cancer pain. For patients who have received transmucosal product within 6-12 hours, it is recommended that if other narcotics are required, they should be used at starting doses ¼ to

(Continued)

Fentanyl *(Continued)*

1/3 those usually recommended. Actiq® preparations contain an amount of medication that can be fatal to children. Keep all units out of the reach of children and discard any open units properly. Patients and caregivers should be counseled on the dangers to children including the risk of exposure to partially-consumed units. Safety and efficacy have not been established in children <16 years of age.

Topical patches: Serum fentanyl concentrations may increase approximately one-third for patients with a body temperature of 40°C secondary to a temperature-dependent increase in fentanyl release from the system and increased skin permeability. Patients who experience adverse reactions should be monitored for at least 12 hours after removal of the patch. Safety and efficacy of transdermal system have been limited to children >2 years of age who are opioid tolerant.

Drug Interactions Substrate of CYP3A4 (major); **Inhibits** CYP3A4 (weak)

CNS depressants: Increased sedation with CNS depressants, phenothiazines

CYP3A4 inhibitors: May increase the levels/effects of fentanyl. Example inhibitors include azole antifungals, ciprofloxacin, clarithromycin, diclofenac, doxycycline, erythromycin, imatinib, isoniazid, nefazodone, nicardipine, propofol, protease inhibitors, quinidine, and verapamil.

MAO inhibitors: Not recommended to use Actiq® within 14 days. Severe and unpredictable potentiation by MAO inhibitors has been reported with opioid analgesics.

Ethanol/Nutrition/Herb Interactions

Ethanol: Avoid ethanol (may increase CNS depression).

Food: Glucose may cause hyperglycemia.

Herb/Nutraceutical: St John's wort may decrease fentanyl levels. Avoid valerian, St John's wort, kava kava, gotu kola (may increase CNS depression).

Dietary Considerations Glucose may cause hyperglycemia; monitor blood glucose concentrations. Actiq® contains 2 g sugar per unit.

Pharmacodynamics/Kinetics

Onset of action: Analgesic: I.M.: 7-15 minutes; I.V.: Almost immediate; Transmucosal: 5-15 minutes

Peak effect: Transmucosal: Analgesic: 20-30 minutes

Duration: I.M.: 1-2 hours; I.V.: 0.5-1 hour; Transmucosal: Related to blood level; respiratory depressant effect may last longer than analgesic effect

Absorption: Transmucosal: Rapid, ~25% from the buccal mucosa; 75% swallowed with saliva and slowly absorbed from GI tract

Distribution: Highly lipophilic, redistributes into muscle and fat

Metabolism: Hepatic

Bioavailability: Transmucosal: ~50% (range: 36% to 71%)

Half-life elimination: 2-4 hours; Transmucosal: 6.6 hours (range: 5-15 hours)

Excretion: Urine (primarily as metabolites, 10% as unchanged drug)

Pregnancy Risk Factor C/D (prolonged use or high doses at term)

Lactation Enters breast milk/not recommended (AAP rates "compatible")

Breast-Feeding Considerations Fentanyl is excreted in low concentrations into breast milk. Breast-feeding is considered acceptable following single doses to the mother; however, no information is available when used long-term.

Dosage Forms

Injection, solution, as citrate [preservative free]: 0.05 mg/mL (2 mL, 5 mL, 10 mL, 20 mL, 30 mL, 50 mL)

Sublimaze®: 0.05 mg/mL (2 mL, 5 mL, 10 mL, 20 mL)

Lozenge, oral transmucosal, as citrate [mounted on a plastic radiopaque handle] (Actiq®): 200 mcg, 400 mcg, 600 mcg, 800 mcg, 1200 mcg, 1600 mcg [raspberry flavor]

Transdermal system (Duragesic®): 25 mcg/hour [10 cm^2] (5s); 50 mcg/hour [20 cm^2] (5s); 75 mcg/hour [30 cm^2]; 100 mcg/hour [40 cm^2] (5s)

Comments Transdermal fentanyl should not be used as a pain reliever in dentistry due to danger of hypoventilation

Selected Readings

Dionne RA, Yagiela JA, Moore PA, et al, "Comparing Efficacy and Safety of Four Intravenous Sedation Regimens in Dental Outpatients," *Am Dent Assoc*, 2001, 132(6):740-51.

Fentanyl Citrate *see* Fentanyl *on page 581*

Feostat® [OTC] *see* Ferrous Fumarate *on page 586*

Feratab® [OTC] *see* Ferrous Sulfate *on page 586*

Fer-Gen-Sol [OTC] *see* Ferrous Sulfate *on page 586*

Fergon® [OTC] *see* Ferrous Gluconate *on page 586*

Feridex I.V.® *see* Ferumoxides *on page 587*

Fer-In-Sol® [OTC] *see* Ferrous Sulfate *on page 586*
Fer-Iron® [OTC] *see* Ferrous Sulfate *on page 586*
Fero-Grad 500® [OTC] *see* Ferrous Sulfate and Ascorbic Acid *on page 587*
Ferretts [OTC] *see* Ferrous Fumarate *on page 586*

Ferric Gluconate (FER ik GLOO koe nate)

U.S. Brand Names Ferrlecit®

Generic Available No

Synonyms Sodium Ferric Gluconate

Pharmacologic Category Iron Salt

Use Repletion of total body iron content in patients with iron-deficiency anemia who are undergoing hemodialysis in conjunction with erythropoietin therapy

Local Anesthetic/Vasoconstrictor Precautions No information available to require special precautions

Effects on Dental Treatment Key adverse event(s) related to dental treatment: Xerostomia (normal salivary flow resumes upon discontinuation). Do not prescribe tetracyclines simultaneously with iron since GI tract absorption of both tetracycline and iron may be inhibited.

Common Adverse Effects Major adverse reactions include hypotension and hypersensitivity reactions. Hypersensitivity reactions have included pruritus, chest pain, hypotension, nausea, abdominal pain, flank pain, fatigue and rash.

Cardiovascular: Hypotension (serious hypotension in 1%), chest pain, hypertension, syncope, tachycardia, angina, myocardial infarction, pulmonary edema, hypovolemia, peripheral edema

Central nervous system: Headache, fatigue, fever, malaise, dizziness, paresthesia, insomnia, agitation, somnolence, pain

Dermatologic: Pruritus, rash

Endocrine & metabolic: Hyperkalemia, hypoglycemia, hypokalemia

Gastrointestinal: Abdominal pain, nausea, vomiting, diarrhea, rectal disorder, dyspepsia, flatulence, melena, epigastric pain

Genitourinary: Urinary tract infection

Hematologic: Anemia, abnormal erythrocytes, lymphadenopathy

Local: Injection site reactions, pain

Neuromuscular & skeletal: Weakness, back pain, leg cramps, myalgia, arthralgia, paresthesia, groin pain

Ocular: Blurred vision, conjunctivitis

Respiratory: Dyspnea, cough, rhinitis, upper respiratory infection, pneumonia

Miscellaneous: Hypersensitivity reactions, infection, rigors, chills, flu-like syndrome, sepsis, carcinoma, increased diaphoresis

Mechanism of Action Supplies a source to elemental iron necessary to the function of hemoglobin, myoglobin and specific enzyme systems; allows transport of oxygen via hemoglobin

Drug Interactions

Decreased Effect: Chloramphenicol may decrease effect of ferric gluconate injection; ferric gluconate injection may decrease the absorption of oral iron

Pharmacodynamics/Kinetics Half-life elimination: Bound: 1 hour

Pregnancy Risk Factor B

Ferric Hexacyanoferrate (FER ik hex a SYE an oh fer ate)

U.S. Brand Names Radiogardase™

Generic Available No

Synonyms Ferric (III) Hexacyanoferrate (II); Insoluble Prussian Blue; Prussian Blue

Pharmacologic Category Antidote

Use Treatment of known or suspected internal contamination with radioactive cesium and/or radioactive or nonradioactive thallium

Local Anesthetic/Vasoconstrictor Precautions No information available to require special precautions

Effects on Dental Treatment No significant effects or complications reported

Common Adverse Effects

>10%: Gastrointestinal: Constipation (24%)

1% to 10%: Endocrine & metabolic: Hypokalemia (7%)

Frequency not defined: Gastrointestinal: Gastric distress, fecal discoloration (blue)

Mechanism of Action Binds to cesium and thallium isotopes in the gastrointestinal tract following their ingestion or excretion in the bile; reduces their gastrointestinal reabsorption (enterohepatic circulation)

Pharmacodynamics/Kinetics

Absorption: Ferric hexacyanoferrate: Oral: None

(Continued)

Ferric Hexacyanoferrate *(Continued)*

Half-life elimination:

Cesium-137: Effective: Adults: 80 days, decreased by 69% with ferric hexacyanoferrate; adolescents: 62 days, decreased by 46% with ferric hexacyanoferrate; children: 42 days, decreased by 43% with ferric hexacyanoferrate

Nonradioactive thallium: Biological: 8-10 days; with ferric hexacyanoferrate: 3 days

Excretion:

Cesium-137: Without ferric hexacyanoferrate: Urine (~80%); feces (~20%)

Thallium: Without ferric hexacyanoferrate: Fecal to urine excretion ration: 2:1

Ferric hexacyanoferrate: Feces (99%, unchanged)

Pregnancy Risk Factor C

Ferric (III) Hexacyanoferrate (II) *see* Ferric Hexacyanoferrate *on page 585*

Ferrlecit® *see* Ferric Gluconate *on page 585*

Ferro-Sequels® [OTC] *see* Ferrous Fumarate *on page 586*

Ferrous Fumarate (FER us FYOO ma rate)

U.S. Brand Names Femiron® [OTC]; Feostat® [OTC]; Ferretts [OTC]; Ferro-Sequels® [OTC]; Hemocyte® [OTC]; Ircon® [OTC]; Nephro-Fer® [OTC]

Canadian Brand Names Palafer®

Mexican Brand Names Ferval®

Generic Available No

Synonyms Iron Fumarate

Pharmacologic Category Iron Salt

Use Prevention and treatment of iron-deficiency anemias

Local Anesthetic/Vasoconstrictor Precautions No information available to require special precautions

Effects on Dental Treatment Key adverse event(s) related to dental treatment: Staining of teeth. Do not prescribe tetracyclines simultaneously with iron since GI tract absorption of both tetracycline and iron may be inhibited.

Mechanism of Action Replaces iron found in hemoglobin, myoglobin, and enzymes; allows the transportation of oxygen via hemoglobin

Pregnancy Risk Factor A

Ferrous Gluconate (FER us GLOO koe nate)

U.S. Brand Names Fergon® [OTC]

Canadian Brand Names Apo-Ferrous Gluconate®; Novo-Ferrogluc

Generic Available Yes

Synonyms Iron Gluconate

Pharmacologic Category Iron Salt

Use Prevention and treatment of iron-deficiency anemias

Local Anesthetic/Vasoconstrictor Precautions No information available to require special precautions

Effects on Dental Treatment Key adverse event(s) related to dental treatment: Staining of teeth. Do not prescribe tetracyclines simultaneously with iron since GI tract absorption of both tetracycline and iron may be inhibited.

Mechanism of Action Replaces iron found in hemoglobin, myoglobin, and enzymes; allows the transportation of oxygen via hemoglobin

Pregnancy Risk Factor A

Ferrous Sulfate (FER us SUL fate)

U.S. Brand Names Feratab® [OTC]; Fer-Gen-Sol [OTC]; Fer-In-Sol® [OTC]; Fer-Iron® [OTC]; Slow FE® [OTC]

Canadian Brand Names Apo-Ferrous Sulfate®; Fer-In-Sol®; Ferodan™

Mexican Brand Names Hemobion®

Generic Available Yes

Synonyms $FeSO_4$; Iron Sulfate

Pharmacologic Category Iron Salt

Use Prevention and treatment of iron-deficiency anemias

Local Anesthetic/Vasoconstrictor Precautions No information available to require special precautions

Effects on Dental Treatment Do not prescribe tetracyclines simultaneously with iron since GI tract absorption of both tetracycline and iron may be inhibited. Liquid preparations may temporarily stain the teeth.

Mechanism of Action Replaces iron, found in hemoglobin, myoglobin, and other enzymes; allows the transportation of oxygen via hemoglobin

Pregnancy Risk Factor A

Ferrous Sulfate and Ascorbic Acid

(FER us SUL fate & a SKOR bik AS id)

Related Information

Ascorbic Acid *on page 148*

U.S. Brand Names Fero-Grad 500® [OTC]; Vitelle™ Irospan® [OTC] [DSC]

Generic Available No

Synonyms Ascorbic Acid and Ferrous Sulfate; Iron Sulfate and Vitamin C

Pharmacologic Category Iron Salt; Vitamin

Use Treatment of iron deficiency in nonpregnant adults; treatment and prevention of iron deficiency in pregnant adults

Local Anesthetic/Vasoconstrictor Precautions No information available to require special precautions

Effects on Dental Treatment Do not prescribe tetracyclines simultaneously with iron since GI tract absorption of both tetracycline and iron may be inhibited. Liquid preparations may temporarily stain the teeth.

Common Adverse Effects Based on **ferrous sulfate** component:

>10%: Gastrointestinal: GI irritation, epigastric pain, nausea, dark stool, vomiting, stomach cramping, constipation

1% to 10%:

Gastrointestinal: Heartburn, diarrhea

Genitourinary: Discoloration of urine

Miscellaneous: Liquid preparations may temporarily stain the teeth

Drug Interactions

Increased Effect/Toxicity: Concurrent administration of ≥200 mg vitamin C per 30 mg elemental iron increases absorption of oral iron.

Decreased Effect: Absorption of oral preparation of iron and tetracyclines are decreased when both of these drugs are given together. Absorption of quinolones may be decreased due to formation of a ferric ion-quinolone complex when given concurrently. Concurrent administration of antacids and H_2 blockers (cimetidine) may decrease iron absorption. Iron may decrease absorption of levodopa, methyldopa, penicillamine when given at the same time. Response to iron therapy may be delayed by chloramphenicol.

Ferumoxides (fer yoo MOX ides)

U.S. Brand Names Feridex I.V.®

Generic Available No

Pharmacologic Category Radiopaque Agents

Use For I.V. administration as an adjunct to MRI (in adult patients) to enhance the T2 weighted images used in the detection and evaluation of lesions of the liver

Local Anesthetic/Vasoconstrictor Precautions No information available to require special precautions

Effects on Dental Treatment No significant effects or complications reported

Pregnancy Risk Factor C

$FeSO_4$ *see* Ferrous Sulfate *on page 586*

Fe-Tinic™ 150 [OTC] *see* Polysaccharide-Iron Complex *on page 1101*

Feverall® [OTC] *see* Acetaminophen *on page 47*

Fexofenadine (feks oh FEN a deen)

U.S. Brand Names Allegra®

Canadian Brand Names Allegra®

Mexican Brand Names Allegra®

Generic Available No

Synonyms Fexofenadine Hydrochloride

Pharmacologic Category Antihistamine, Nonsedating

Use Relief of symptoms associated with seasonal allergic rhinitis; treatment of chronic idiopathic urticaria

Local Anesthetic/Vasoconstrictor Precautions No information available to require special precautions

Effects on Dental Treatment No significant effects or complications reported

Common Adverse Effects

>10%: Central nervous system: Headache (7% to 11%)

1% to 10%:

Central nervous system: Fever (2%), dizziness (2%), pain (2%), drowsiness (1% to 2%), fatigue (1%)

Endocrine & metabolic: Dysmenorrhea (2%)

Gastrointestinal: Nausea (2%), dyspepsia (1%)

Neuromuscular & skeletal: Back pain (2% to 3%)

Otic: Otitis media (2%)

(Continued)

Fexofenadine *(Continued)*

Respiratory: Cough (4%), upper respiratory tract infection (3% to 4%), sinusitis (2%)

Miscellaneous: Viral infection (3%)

Dosage Oral:

Children 6-11 years: 30 mg twice daily

Children ≥12 years and Adults:

Seasonal allergic rhinitis: 60 mg twice daily **or** 180 mg once daily

Chronic idiopathic urticaria: 60 mg twice daily

Dosing adjustment in renal impairment: Cl_{cr} <80 mL/minute:

Children 6-11 years: Initial: 30 mg once daily

Children ≥12 years and Adults: Initial: 60 mg once daily

Mechanism of Action Fexofenadine is an active metabolite of terfenadine and like terfenadine it competes with histamine for H_1-receptor sites on effector cells in the gastrointestinal tract, blood vessels and respiratory tract; it appears that fexofenadine does not cross the blood brain barrier to any appreciable degree, resulting in a reduced potential for sedation

Contraindications Hypersensitivity to fexofenadine or any component of the formulation

Warnings/Precautions Safety and efficacy in children <6 years of age have not been established.

Drug Interactions

Cytochrome P450 Effect: Substrate of CYP3A4 (minor); **Inhibits** CYP2D6 (weak)

Increased Effect/Toxicity: Erythromycin and ketoconazole increased the levels of fexofenadine; however, no increase in adverse events or QT_c intervals was noted. The effect of other macrolide agents or azoles has not been investigated.

Decreased Effect: Aluminum- and magnesium-containing antacids decrease plasma levels of fexofenadine; separate administration is recommended.

Ethanol/Nutrition/Herb Interactions

Ethanol: Avoid ethanol (although limited with fexofenadine, may increase risk of sedation).

Herb/Nutraceutical: St John's wort may decrease fexofenadine levels.

Pharmacodynamics/Kinetics

Onset of action: 60 minutes

Duration: Antihistaminic effect: ≥12 hours

Protein binding: 60% to 70%, primarily albumin and $alpha_1$-acid glycoprotein

Metabolism: ~5% mostly by gut flora; 0.5% to 1.5% by CYP

Half-life elimination: 14.4 hours

Time to peak, serum: ~2.6 hours

Excretion: Feces (~80%) and urine (~11%) as unchanged drug

Pregnancy Risk Factor C

Dosage Forms TAB: 30 mg, 60 mg, 180 mg

Fexofenadine and Pseudoephedrine

(feks oh FEN a deen & soo doe e FED rin)

Related Information

Fexofenadine *on page 587*

Pseudoephedrine *on page 1147*

U.S. Brand Names Allegra-D®

Canadian Brand Names Allegra-D®

Generic Available No

Synonyms Pseudoephedrine and Fexofenadine

Pharmacologic Category Antihistamine/Decongestant Combination

Use Relief of symptoms associated with seasonal allergic rhinitis in adults and children ≥12 years of age

Local Anesthetic/Vasoconstrictor Precautions Use with caution since pseudoephedrine is a sympathomimetic amine which could interact with epinephrine to cause a pressor response

Effects on Dental Treatment Key adverse event(s) related to dental treatment: Pseudoephedrine: Xerostomia (normal salivary flow resumes upon discontinuation).

Common Adverse Effects See individual agents.

Drug Interactions

Cytochrome P450 Effect: Fexofenadine: **Substrate** of CYP3A4 (minor); **Inhibits** CYP2D6 (weak)

Pharmacodynamics/Kinetics See individual agents.

Pregnancy Risk Factor C

Fexofenadine Hydrochloride *see* Fexofenadine *on page 587*

Fiberall® *see* Psyllium *on page 1151*

FiberCon® [OTC] *see* Polycarbophil *on page 1100*

FiberEase™ [OTC] *see* Methylcellulose *on page 905*

Fiber-Lax® [OTC] *see* Polycarbophil *on page 1100*

FiberNorm™ [OTC] *see* Polycarbophil *on page 1100*

Fibrin Sealant Kit (FI brin SEEL ent kit)

U.S. Brand Names Crosseal™; Tisseel® VH

Canadian Brand Names Tisseel® VH

Generic Available No

Synonyms FS

Pharmacologic Category Hemostatic Agent

Use

Crosseal™: Adjunct to hemostasis in liver surgery

Tisseel® VH: Adjunct to hemostasis in cardiopulmonary bypass surgery and splenic injury (due to blunt or penetrating trauma to the abdomen) when the control of bleeding by conventional surgical techniques is ineffective or impractical; adjunctive sealant for closure of colostomies; hemostatic agent in heparinized patients undergoing cardiopulmonary bypass

Local Anesthetic/Vasoconstrictor Precautions No information available to require special precautions

Effects on Dental Treatment No significant effects or complications reported

Common Adverse Effects No adverse events were reported in clinical trials. Anaphylactoid or anaphylactic reactions have occurred with other plasma-derived products.

Mechanism of Action Formation of a biodegradable adhesive is done by duplicating the last step of the coagulation cascade, the formation of fibrin from fibrinogen. Fibrinogen is the main component of the sealant solution. The solution also contains thrombin, which transforms fibrinogen from the sealer protein solution into fibrin, and fibrinolysis inhibitor (aprotinin), which prevents the premature degradation of fibrin. When mixed as directed, a viscous solution forms that sets into an elastic coagulum.

Drug Interactions

Decreased Effect: Decreased effect (Tisseel® VH): Local concentrations/applications of alcohol, heavy-metal ions, iodine; oxycellulose preparations

Pharmacodynamics/Kinetics Onset of action:

Crosseal™: Time to hemostasis: 5.3 minutes

Tisseal® VH: Time to hemostasis: 5 minutes (65% of patients); Final prepared sealant: 70% strength: ~10 minutes; Full strength: ~2 hours

Pregnancy Risk Factor C

Filgrastim (fil GRA stim)

U.S. Brand Names Neupogen®

Canadian Brand Names Neupogen®

Mexican Brand Names Neupogen®

Generic Available No

Synonyms G-CSF; Granulocyte Colony Stimulating Factor

Pharmacologic Category Colony Stimulating Factor

Use Stimulation of granulocyte production in patients with malignancies, including myeloid malignancies; receiving myelosuppressive therapy associated with a significant risk of neutropenia; severe chronic neutropenia (SCN); receiving bone marrow transplantation (BMT); undergoing peripheral blood progenitor cell (PBPC) collection

Local Anesthetic/Vasoconstrictor Precautions No information available to require special precautions

Effects on Dental Treatment Key adverse event(s) related to dental treatment: Mucositis.

Common Adverse Effects

>10%:

Cardiovascular: Chest pain

Central nervous system: Fever

Dermatologic: Alopecia

Endocrine & metabolic: Fluid retention

Gastrointestinal: Nausea, vomiting, diarrhea, mucositis; splenomegaly - up to 33% of patients with cyclic neutropenia/congenital agranulocytosis receiving filgrastim for ≥14 days; rare in other patients

Neuromuscular & skeletal: Bone pain (24%), commonly in the lower back, posterior iliac crest, and sternum

(Continued)

Filgrastim *(Continued)*

1% to 10%:

Cardiovascular: S-T segment depression (3%)
Central nervous system: Headache
Dermatologic: Rash
Gastrointestinal: Anorexia, constipation, sore throat
Hematologic: Leukocytosis
Local: Pain at injection site
Neuromuscular & skeletal: Weakness
Respiratory: Dyspnea, cough

Mechanism of Action Stimulates the production, maturation, and activation of neutrophils, G-CSF activates neutrophils to increase both their migration and cytotoxicity. See table.

Comparative Effects — G-CSF vs GM-CSF

Proliferation/Differentiation	G-CSF (Filgrastim)	GM-CSF (Sargramostim)
Neutrophils	Yes	Yes
Eosinophils	No	Yes
Macrophages	No	Yes
Neutrophil migration	Enhanced	Inhibited

Drug Interactions

Increased Effect/Toxicity: Drugs which may potentiate the release of neutrophils (eg, lithium) should be used with caution.

Pharmacodynamics/Kinetics

Onset of action: ~24 hours; plateaus in 3-5 days
Duration: ANC decreases by 50% within 2 days after discontinuing G-CSF; white counts return to the normal range in 4-7 days; peak plasma levels can be maintained for up to 12 hours
Absorption: SubQ: 100%
Distribution: V_d: 150 mL/kg; no evidence of drug accumulation over a 11- to 20-day period
Metabolism: Systemically degraded
Half-life elimination: 1.8-3.5 hours
Time to peak, serum: SubQ: 2-6 hours

Pregnancy Risk Factor C

Finacea™ *see* Azelaic Acid *on page 173*

Finasteride (fi NAS teer ide)

U.S. Brand Names Propecia®; Proscar®
Canadian Brand Names Propecia®; Proscar®
Mexican Brand Names Propeshia®; Proscar®
Generic Available No
Pharmacologic Category 5 Alpha-Reductase Inhibitor
Use

Propecia®: Treatment of male pattern hair loss in **men only**. Safety and efficacy were demonstrated in men between 18-41 years of age.
Proscar®: Treatment of symptomatic benign prostatic hyperplasia (BPH); can be used in combination with an alpha blocker, doxazosin

Unlabeled/Investigational Use Adjuvant monotherapy after radical prostatectomy in the treatment of prostatic cancer; female hirsutism

Local Anesthetic/Vasoconstrictor Precautions No information available to require special precautions

Effects on Dental Treatment No significant effects or complications reported

Common Adverse Effects Note: "Combination therapy" refers to finasteride and doxazosin.

>10%:

Endocrine & metabolic: Impotence (19%; combination therapy 23%), libido decreased (10%; combination therapy 12%)
Genitourinary: Neuromuscular & skeletal: Weakness (5%; combination therapy 17%)

1% to 10%:

Cardiovascular: Postural hypotension (9%; combination therapy 18%), edema (1%, combination therapy 3%)
Central nervous system: Dizziness (7%; combination therapy 23%), somnolence (2%; combination therapy 3%)
Genitourinary: Ejaculation disturbances (7%; combination therapy 14%), decreased volume of ejaculate

Endocrine & metabolic: Gynecomastia (2%)
Respiratory: Dyspnea (1%; combination therapy 2%), rhinitis (1%; combination therapy 2%)

Mechanism of Action Finasteride is a competitive inhibitor of both tissue and hepatic 5-alpha reductase. This results in inhibition of the conversion of testosterone to dihydrotestosterone and markedly suppresses serum dihydrotestosterone levels

Drug Interactions

Cytochrome P450 Effect: Substrate of CYP3A4 (minor)

Pharmacodynamics/Kinetics

Onset of action: 3-6 months of ongoing therapy
Duration:
After a single oral dose as small as 0.5 mg: 65% depression of plasma dihydrotestosterone levels persists 5-7 days
After 6 months of treatment with 5 mg/day: Circulating dihydrotestosterone levels are reduced to castrate levels without significant effects on circulating testosterone; levels return to normal within 14 days of discontinuation of treatment
Distribution: V_{dss}: 76 L
Protein binding: 90%
Metabolism: Hepatic via CYP3A4; two active metabolites (<20% activity of finasteride)
Bioavailability: Mean: 63%
Half-life elimination, serum: Elderly: 8 hours; Adults: 6 hours (3-16)
Time to peak, serum: 2-6 hours
Excretion: Feces (57%) and urine (39%) as metabolites

Pregnancy Risk Factor X

Fioricet® *see* Butalbital, Acetaminophen, and Caffeine *on page 236*

Fioricet® with Codeine *see* Butalbital, Acetaminophen, Caffeine, and Codeine *on page 236*

Fiorinal® *see* Butalbital, Aspirin, and Caffeine *on page 238*

Fiorinal® With Codeine *see* Butalbital, Aspirin, Caffeine, and Codeine *on page 238*

Fisalamine *see* Mesalamine *on page 882*

FK506 *see* Tacrolimus *on page 1255*

Flagyl® *see* Metronidazole *on page 917*

Flagyl ER® *see* Metronidazole *on page 917*

Flarex® *see* Fluorometholone *on page 605*

Flatulex® [OTC] *see* Simethicone *on page 1222*

Flavoxate (fla VOKS ate)

U.S. Brand Names Urispas®

Canadian Brand Names Apo-Flavoxate®; Urispas®

Mexican Brand Names Bladuril®

Generic Available Yes

Synonyms Flavoxate Hydrochloride

Pharmacologic Category Antispasmodic Agent, Urinary

Use Antispasmodic to provide symptomatic relief of dysuria, nocturia, suprapubic pain, urgency, and incontinence due to detrusor instability and hyper-reflexia in elderly with cystitis, urethritis, urethrocystitis, urethrotrigonitis, and prostatitis

Local Anesthetic/Vasoconstrictor Precautions No information available to require special precautions

Effects on Dental Treatment Key adverse event(s) related to dental treatment: Xerostomia and changes in salivation (normal salivary flow resumes upon discontinuation), and dry throat.

Common Adverse Effects Frequency not defined.

Cardiovascular: Tachycardia, palpitations
Central nervous system: Drowsiness, confusion (especially in the elderly), nervousness, fatigue, vertigo, headache, hyperpyrexia
Dermatologic: Rash. urticaria
Gastrointestinal: Constipation, nausea, vomiting, xerostomia, dry throat
Genitourinary: Dysuria
Hematologic: Leukopenia
Ocular: Increased intraocular pressure, blurred vision

Mechanism of Action Synthetic antispasmodic with similar actions to that of propantheline; it exerts a direct relaxant effect on smooth muscles via phosphodiesterase inhibition, providing relief to a variety of smooth muscle spasms; it is especially useful for the treatment of bladder spasticity, whereby it produces an increase in urinary capacity

(Continued)

Flavoxate *(Continued)*

Pharmacodynamics/Kinetics

Onset of action: 55-60 minutes
Metabolism: To methyl; flavone carboxylic acid active
Excretion: Urine (10% to 30%) within 6 hours

Pregnancy Risk Factor B

Flavoxate Hydrochloride *see* Flavoxate *on page 591*

Flebogamma® *see* Immune Globulin (Intravenous) *on page 740*

Flecainide (fle KAY nide)

Related Information

Cardiovascular Diseases *on page 1458*

U.S. Brand Names Tambocor™

Canadian Brand Names Tambocor™

Mexican Brand Names Tambocor®

Generic Available Yes

Synonyms Flecainide Acetate

Pharmacologic Category Antiarrhythmic Agent, Class Ic

Use Prevention and suppression of documented life-threatening ventricular arrhythmias (eg, sustained ventricular tachycardia); controlling symptomatic, disabling supraventricular tachycardias in patients without structural heart disease in whom other agents fail

Local Anesthetic/Vasoconstrictor Precautions No information available to require special precautions

Effects on Dental Treatment No significant effects or complications reported

Common Adverse Effects

>10%:
- Central nervous system: Dizziness (19% to 30%)
- Ocular: Visual disturbances (16%)
- Respiratory: Dyspnea (~10%)

1% to 10%:
- Cardiovascular: Palpitations (6%), chest pain (5%), edema (3.5%), tachycardia (1% to 3%), proarrhythmic (4% to 12%), sinus node dysfunction (1.2%)
- Central nervous system: Headache (4% to 10%), fatigue (8%), nervousness (5%) additional symptoms occurring at a frequency between 1% and 3%: fever, malaise, hypoesthesia, paresis, ataxia, vertigo, syncope, somnolence, tinnitus, anxiety, insomnia, depression
- Dermatologic: Rash (1% to 3%)
- Gastrointestinal: Nausea (9%), constipation (1%), abdominal pain (3%), anorexia (1% to 3%), diarrhea (0.7% to 3%)
- Neuromuscular & skeletal: Tremor (5%), weakness (5%), paresthesias (1%)
- Ocular: Diplopia (1% to 3%), blurred vision

Mechanism of Action Class Ic antiarrhythmic; slows conduction in cardiac tissue by altering transport of ions across cell membranes; causes slight prolongation of refractory periods; decreases the rate of rise of the action potential without affecting its duration; increases electrical stimulation threshold of ventricle, His-Purkinje system; possesses local anesthetic and moderate negative inotropic effects

Drug Interactions

Cytochrome P450 Effect: Substrate of CYP1A2 (minor), 2D6 (major); **Inhibits** CYP2D6 (weak)

Increased Effect/Toxicity: CYP2D6 inhibitors may increase the levels/effects of flecainide; example inhibitors include chlorpromazine, delavirdine, fluoxetine, miconazole, paroxetine, pergolide, quinidine, quinine, ritonavir, and ropinirole. Flecainide concentrations may be increased by amiodarone (reduce flecainide 25% to 33%), and propranolol. Beta-adrenergic blockers, disopyramide, verapamil may enhance flecainide's negative inotropic effects. Alkalinizing agents (ie, high-dose antacids, cimetidine, carbonic anhydrase inhibitors, sodium bicarbonate) may decrease flecainide clearance, potentially increasing toxicity. Propranolol blood levels are increased by flecainide.

Decreased Effect: Smoking and acid urine increase flecainide clearance.

Pharmacodynamics/Kinetics

Absorption: Oral: Rapid
Distribution: Adults: V_d: 5-13.4 L/kg
Protein binding: $Alpha_1$ glycoprotein: 40% to 50%
Metabolism: Hepatic
Bioavailability: 85% to 90%

Half-life elimination: Infants: 11-12 hours; Children: 8 hours; Adults: 7-22 hours, increased with congestive heart failure or renal dysfunction; End-stage renal disease: 19-26 hours

Time to peak, serum: ~1.5-3 hours

Excretion: Urine (80% to 90%, 10% to 50% as unchanged drug and metabolites)

Pregnancy Risk Factor C

Flecainide Acetate *see* Flecainide *on page 592*

Fleet® Babylax® [OTC] *see* Glycerin *on page 667*

Fleet® Bisacodyl Enema [OTC] *see* Bisacodyl *on page 208*

Fleet® Enema [OTC] *see* Sodium Phosphates *on page 1230*

Fleet® Glycerin Suppositories [OTC] *see* Glycerin *on page 667*

Fleet® Glycerin Suppositories Maximum Strength [OTC] *see* Glycerin *on page 667*

Fleet® Liquid Glycerin Suppositories [OTC] *see* Glycerin *on page 667*

Fleet® Phospho®-Soda [OTC] *see* Sodium Phosphates *on page 1230*

Fleet® Phospho-Soda® Accu-Prep™ [OTC] *see* Sodium Phosphates *on page 1230*

Fleet® Sof-Lax® [OTC] *see* Docusate *on page 459*

Fleet® Sof-Lax® Overnight [DSC] [OTC] *see* Docusate and Casanthranol *on page 460*

Fleet® Stimulant Laxative [OTC] *see* Bisacodyl *on page 208*

Fletcher's® Castoria® [OTC] *see* Senna *on page 1213*

Flexeril® *see* Cyclobenzaprine *on page 382*

Flolan® *see* Epoprostenol *on page 500*

Flomax® *see* Tamsulosin *on page 1260*

Flonase® *see* Fluticasone *on page 616*

Florical® [OTC] *see* Calcium Carbonate *on page 245*

Florinef® *see* Fludrocortisone *on page 598*

Florone® *see* Diflorasone *on page 435*

Flovent® *see* Fluticasone *on page 616*

Flovent® Rotadisk® *see* Fluticasone *on page 616*

Floxin® *see* Ofloxacin *on page 1005*

Floxin Otic Singles *see* Ofloxacin *on page 1005*

Floxuridine (floks YOOR i deen)

U.S. Brand Names FUDR®

Canadian Brand Names FUDR®

Generic Available Yes

Synonyms Fluorodeoxyuridine; FUDR; 5-FUDR; NSC-27640

Pharmacologic Category Antineoplastic Agent, Antimetabolite (Pyrimidine Antagonist)

Use Management of hepatic metastases of colorectal and gastric cancers

Local Anesthetic/Vasoconstrictor Precautions No information available to require special precautions

Effects on Dental Treatment Key adverse event(s) related to dental treatment: Stomatitis.

Common Adverse Effects

>10%:

Gastrointestinal: Stomatitis, diarrhea; may be dose-limiting

Hematologic: Myelosuppression, may be dose-limiting; leukopenia, thrombocytopenia, anemia

Onset: 4-7 days

Nadir: 5-9 days

Recovery: 21 days

1% to 10%:

Dermatologic: Alopecia, photosensitivity, hyperpigmentation of the skin, localized erythema, dermatitis

Gastrointestinal: Anorexia

Hepatic: Biliary sclerosis, cholecystitis, jaundice

Mechanism of Action Mechanism of action and pharmacokinetics are very similar to fluorouracil; floxuridine is the deoxyribonucleotide of fluorouracil. Floxuridine is a fluorinated pyrimidine antagonist which inhibits DNA and RNA synthesis and methylation of deoxyuridylic acid to thymidylic acid.

Drug Interactions

Increased Effect/Toxicity: Any form of therapy which adds to the stress of the patient, interferes with nutrition, or depresses bone marrow function will

(Continued)

Floxuridine *(Continued)*

increase the toxicity of floxuridine. Pentostatin and floxuridine administered together has resulted in fatal pulmonary toxicity.

Decreased Effect: Patients may experience impaired immune response to vaccines; possible infection after administration of live vaccines in patients receiving immunosuppressants.

Pharmacodynamics/Kinetics

Metabolism: Hepatic; Active metabolites: Floxuridine monophosphate (FUDR-MP) and fluorouracil; Inactive metabolites: Urea, CO_2, α-fluoro-β-alanine, α-fluoro-β-guanidopropionic acid, α-fluoro-β-ureidopropionic acid, and dihydrofluorouracil

Excretion: Urine: Fluorouracil, urea, α-fluoro-β-alanine, α-fluoro-β-guanidopropionic acid, α-fluoro-β-ureidopropionic acid, and dihydrofluorouracil; exhaled gases (CO_2)

Pregnancy Risk Factor D

Flubenisolone *see* Betamethasone *on page 199*

Flucaine® *see* Proparacaine and Fluorescein *on page 1135*

Fluconazole (floo KOE na zole)

Related Information

Oral Fungal Infections *on page 1544*

Sexually-Transmitted Diseases *on page 1504*

U.S. Brand Names Diflucan®

Canadian Brand Names Apo-Fluconazole®; Diflucan®; Gen-Fluconazole; Novo-Fluconazole

Mexican Brand Names Afungil®; Diflucan®; Neofomiral®; Oxifungol®; Zonal®

Generic Available No

Pharmacologic Category Antifungal Agent, Oral; Antifungal Agent, Parenteral

Dental Use Treatment of susceptible fungal infections in the oral cavity including candidiasis, oral thrush, and chronic mucocutaneous candidiasis treatment of esophageal and oropharyngeal candidiasis caused by *Candida* species; treatment of severe, chronic mucocutaneous candidiasis caused by *Candida* species

Use Treatment of oral or vaginal candidiasis unresponsive to nystatin or clotrimazole; nonlife-threatening *Candida* infections (eg, cystitis, esophagitis); treatment of hepatosplenic candidiasis; treatment of other *Candida* infections in persons unable to tolerate amphotericin B; treatment of cryptococcal infections; secondary prophylaxis for cryptococcal meningitis in persons with AIDS; antifungal prophylaxis in allogeneic bone marrow transplant recipients

Oral fluconazole should be used in persons able to tolerate oral medications; parenteral fluconazole should be reserved for patients who are both unable to take oral medications and are unable to tolerate amphotericin B (eg, due to hypersensitivity or renal insufficiency)

Local Anesthetic/Vasoconstrictor Precautions No information available to require special precautions

Effects on Dental Treatment Key adverse event(s) related to dental treatment: Abnormal taste.

Significant Adverse Effects Frequency not always defined.

Cardiovascular: Pallor, angioedema

Central nervous system: Headache (2% to 13%), seizures, dizziness

Dermatologic: Rash (2%), alopecia, toxic epidermal necrolysis, Stevens-Johnson syndrome

Endocrine & metabolic: Hypertriglyceridemia, hypokalemia

Gastrointestinal: Nausea (4% to 7%), vomiting (2%), abdominal pain (2% to 6%), diarrhea (2% to 3%), taste perversion

Hematologic: Leukopenia, thrombocytopenia

Hepatic: Hepatic failure (rare), hepatitis, cholestasis, jaundice, increased ALT/AST, increased alkaline phosphatase

Respiratory: Dyspnea

Miscellaneous: Anaphylactic reactions (rare)

Dosage The daily dose of fluconazole is the same for oral and I.V. administration

Neonates: First 2 weeks of life, especially premature neonates: Same dose as older children every 72 hours

Children: Once-daily dosing by indication: See table on next page.

Adults: Oral, I.V.: Once-daily dosing by indication: See table on next page.

Fluconazole Once-Daily Dosing – Children

Indication	Day 1	Daily Therapy	Minimum Duration of Therapy
Oropharyngeal candidiasis	6 mg/kg	3 mg/kg	14 d
Esophageal candidiasis	6 mg/kg	3-12 mg/kg	21 d and for at least 2 wk following resolution of symptoms
Systemic candidiasis	—	6-12 mg/kg	28 d
Cryptococcal meningitis acute	12 mg/kg	6-12 mg/kg	10-12 wk after CSF culture becomes negative
relapse suppression	6 mg/kg	6 mg/kg	N/A

N/A = Not applicable.

Fluconazole Once-Daily Dosing – Adults

Indication	Day 1	Daily Therapy	Minimum Duration of Therapy
Oropharyngeal candidiasis (OPC) (long-term suppression)	200 mg	200 mg	Chronic therapy in AIDS patients with history of OPC
Esophageal candidiasis	200 mg	100-200 mg	14-21 d after clinical improvement
Prevention of candidiasis in bone marrow transplant	400 mg	400 mg	3 d before neutropenia, 7 d after neutrophils >1000 cells/mm^3
Urinary candidiasis	--	200 mg with AmB	7-14 d
Candidemia, primary, non-neutropenic	--	400-800 mg	14 d after last positive blood culture and resolution of signs/ symptoms
Candidemia, secondary, non-neutropenic	--	800 mg with AmB for 4-7 d, followed by 800 mg/day	14 d after last positive blood culture and resolution of signs/ symptoms
Candidemia, secondary, neutropenic	--	6-12 mg/ kg/day	14 d after last positive blood culture and resolution of signs/ symptoms
Cryptococcal meningitis acute	400 mg	200 mg	10-12 wk after CSF culture becomes negative
relapse suppression	200 mg	200 mg	N/A
Vaginal candidiasis	150 mg	Single dose	N/A

N/A = Not applicable. AmB = Conventional deoxycholate amphotericin B

Dosing adjustment/interval in renal impairment:
No adjustment for vaginal candidiasis single-dose therapy
For multiple dosing, administer usual load then adjust daily doses
Cl_{cr} 11-50 mL/minute: Administer 50% of recommended dose or administer every 48 hours
Hemodialysis: One dose after each dialysis
Continuous arteriovenous or venovenous hemodiafiltration effects: Dose as for Cl_{cr} 10-50 mL/minute

Mechanism of Action Interferes with cytochrome P450 activity, decreasing ergosterol synthesis (principal sterol in fungal cell membrane) and inhibiting cell membrane formation

Contraindications Hypersensitivity to fluconazole, other azoles, or any component of the formulation; concomitant administration with cisapride

Warnings/Precautions Should be used with caution in patients with renal and hepatic dysfunction or previous hepatotoxicity from other azole derivatives. Patients who develop abnormal liver function tests during fluconazole therapy should be monitored closely and discontinued if symptoms consistent with liver disease develop.

Drug Interactions **Inhibits** CYP1A2 (weak), 2C8/9 (strong), 2C19 (strong), 3A4 (moderate)

(Continued)

Fluconazole *(Continued)*

Alprazolam, triazolam, midazolam, and diazepam serum concentrations are increased; consider a benzodiazepine not metabolized by CYP3A4 or another antifungal that is metabolized by CYP3A4.

Caffeine's metabolism is decreased; monitor for tachycardia, nervousness, and anxiety.

Calcium channel blockers may have increased serum concentrations; consider another agent instead of a calcium channel blocker, another antifungal, or reduce the dose of the calcium channel blocker. Monitor blood pressure.

Cisapride's serum concentration is increased which may lead to malignant arrhythmias; concurrent use is contraindicated.

Cyclosporine's serum concentration is increased; monitor cyclosporine's serum concentration and renal function.

CYP2C8/9 substrates: Fluconazole may increase the levels/effects of CYP2C8/9 substrates. Example substrates include amiodarone, fluoxetine, glimepiride, glipizide, nateglinide, phenytoin, pioglitazone, rosiglitazone, sertraline, and warfarin.

CYP2C19 substrates: Fluconazole may increase the levels/effects of CYP2C19 substrates. Example substrates include citalopram, diazepam, methsuximide, phenytoin, propranolol, and sertraline.

CYP3A4 substrates: Fluconazole may increase the levels/effects of CYP3A4 substrates. Example substrates include benzodiazepines, calcium channel blockers, cyclosporine, mirtazapine, nateglinide, nefazodone, sildenafil (and other PDE-5 inhibitors), tacrolimus, and venlafaxine. Selected benzodiazepines (midazolam and triazolam), cisapride, ergot alkaloids, selected HMG-CoA reductase inhibitors (lovastatin and simvastatin), and pimozide are generally contraindicated with strong CYP3A4 inhibitors.

HMG-CoA reductase inhibitors (except pravastatin and fluvastatin) have increased serum concentrations; switch to pravastatin/fluvastatin or monitor for development of myopathy.

Losartan's active metabolite is reduced in concentration; consider another antihypertensive agent unaffected by the azole antifungals, another antifungal, or monitor blood pressure closely.

Phenytoin's serum concentration is increased; monitor phenytoin levels and adjust dose as needed.

Rifampin decreases fluconazole's serum concentration; monitor infection status.

Tacrolimus's serum concentration is increased; monitor tacrolimus's serum concentration and renal function.

Warfarin's effects are increased; monitor INR and adjust warfarin's dose as needed.

Dietary Considerations Take with or without regard to food.

Pharmacodynamics/Kinetics

Distribution: Widely throughout body with good penetration into CSF, eye, peritoneal fluid, sputum, skin, and urine

Relative diffusion blood into CSF: Adequate with or without inflammation (exceeds usual MICs)

CSF:blood level ratio: Normal meninges: 70% to 80%; Inflamed meninges: >70% to 80%

Protein binding, plasma: 11% to 12%

Bioavailability: Oral: >90%

Half-life elimination: Normal renal function: 25-30 hours

Time to peak, serum: Oral: ~2-4 hours

Excretion: Urine (80% as unchanged drug)

Pregnancy Risk Factor C

Lactation Excretion in breast milk unknown/use caution (AAP rates "compatible")

Dosage Forms

Infusion [premixed in sodium chloride or dextrose]: 2 mg/mL (100 mL, 200 mL)

Powder for oral suspension: 10 mg/mL (35 mL); 40 mg/mL (35 mL) [contains sodium benzoate; orange flavor]

Tablet: 50 mg, 100 mg, 150 mg, 200 mg

Flucytosine (floo SYE toe seen)

U.S. Brand Names Ancobon®

Canadian Brand Names Ancobon®

Generic Available No

Synonyms 5-FC; 5-Flurocytosine

Pharmacologic Category Antifungal Agent, Oral

Use Adjunctive treatment of susceptible fungal infections (usually *Candida* or *Cryptococcus*); synergy with amphotericin B for certain fungal infections (*Cryptococcus* spp., *Candida* spp.)

Local Anesthetic/Vasoconstrictor Precautions No information available to require special precautions

Effects on Dental Treatment No significant effects or complications reported

Common Adverse Effects Frequency not defined.

Cardiovascular: Cardiac arrest, myocardial toxicity, ventricular dysfunction, chest pain

Central nervous system: Confusion, headache, hallucinations, dizziness, drowsiness, psychosis, parkinsonism, ataxia, sedation, pyrexia, seizures, fatigue

Dermatologic: Rash, photosensitivity, pruritus, urticaria, Lyell's syndrome

Endocrine & metabolic: Temporary growth failure, hypoglycemia, hypokalemia

Gastrointestinal: Nausea, vomiting, diarrhea, abdominal pain, loss of appetite, dry mouth, hemorrhage, ulcerative colitis

Hematologic: Bone marrow suppression, anemia, leukopenia, thrombocytopenia, agranulocytosis, aplastic anemia, eosinophilia, pancytopenia

Hepatic: Liver enzymes increased, hepatitis, jaundice, azotemia, bilirubin increased

Neuromuscular & skeletal: Peripheral neuropathy, paresthesia, weakness

Otic: Hearing loss

Renal: BUN and serum creatinine increased, renal failure, azotemia, crystalluria

Respiratory: Respiratory arrest, dyspnea

Miscellaneous: Anaphylaxis, allergic reaction

Mechanism of Action Penetrates fungal cells and is converted to fluorouracil which competes with uracil interfering with fungal RNA and protein synthesis

Drug Interactions

Increased Effect/Toxicity: Increased effect with amphotericin B. Amphotericin B-induced renal dysfunction may predispose patient to flucytosine accumulation and myelosuppression.

Decreased Effect: Cytarabine may inactivate flucytosine activity.

Pharmacodynamics/Kinetics

Absorption: 75% to 90%

Distribution: Into CSF, aqueous humor, joints, peritoneal fluid, and bronchial secretions; V_d: 0.6 L/kg

Protein binding: 2% to 4%

Metabolism: Minimally hepatic; deaminated, possibly via gut bacteria, to 5-fluorouracil

Half-life elimination:

- Normal renal function: 2-5 hours
- Anuria: 85 hours (range: 30-250)
- End stage renal disease: 75-200 hours

Time to peak, serum: ~2-6 hours

Excretion: Urine (>90% as unchanged drug)

Pregnancy Risk Factor C

Fludara® *see* Fludarabine *on page 597*

Fludarabine (floo DARE a been)

U.S. Brand Names Fludara®

Canadian Brand Names Fludara®

Mexican Brand Names Fludara®

Generic Available Yes

Synonyms Fludarabine Phosphate

Pharmacologic Category Antineoplastic Agent, Antimetabolite (Purine Antagonist)

Use Treatment of chronic lymphocytic leukemia (CLL) (including refractory CLL); non-Hodgkin's lymphoma in adults

Unlabeled/Investigational Use Treatment of non-Hodgkin's lymphoma and acute leukemias in pediatric patients

Local Anesthetic/Vasoconstrictor Precautions No information available to require special precautions

Effects on Dental Treatment Key adverse event(s) related to dental treatment: Stomatitis.

Common Adverse Effects

>10%:

- Cardiovascular: Edema
- Central nervous system: Fatigue, somnolence (30%), chills, pain
- Dermatologic: Rash

(Continued)

Fludarabine *(Continued)*

Hematologic: Myelosuppression, common, dose-limiting toxicity, primarily leukopenia and thrombocytopenia
Nadir: 10-14 days
Recovery: 5-7 weeks
Neuromuscular & skeletal: Paresthesia, myalgia, weakness

1% to 10%:
Cardiovascular: Congestive heart failure
Central nervous system: Malaise, headache
Dermatologic: Alopecia
Endocrine & metabolic: Hyperglycemia
Gastrointestinal: Anorexia, stomatitis (1.5%), diarrhea (1.8%), mild nausea/vomiting (3% to 10%)
Hematologic: Eosinophilia, hemolytic anemia, may be dose-limiting, possibly fatal in some patients

Mechanism of Action Fludarabine inhibits DNA synthesis by inhibition of DNA polymerase and ribonucleotide reductase.

Drug Interactions

Increased Effect/Toxicity: Combined use with pentostatin may lead to severe, even fatal, pulmonary toxicity.

Pharmacodynamics/Kinetics

Distribution: V_d: 38-96 L/m^2; widely with extensive tissue binding
Metabolism: I.V.: Fludarabine phosphate is rapidly dephosphorylated to 2-fluoro-vidarabine, which subsequently enters tumor cells and is phosphorylated to the active triphosphate derivative; rapidly dephosphorylated in the serum
Bioavailability: 75%
Half-life elimination: 2-fluoro-vidarabine: 9 hours
Excretion: Urine (60%, 23% as 2-fluoro-vidarabine) within 24 hours

Pregnancy Risk Factor D

Fludarabine Phosphate *see* Fludarabine *on page 597*

Fludrocortisone (floo droe KOR ti sone)

U.S. Brand Names Florinef®

Canadian Brand Names Florinef®

Generic Available Yes

Synonyms Fludrocortisone Acetate; Fluohydrisone Acetate; Fluohydrocortisone Acetate; 9α-Fluorohydrocortisone Acetate

Pharmacologic Category Corticosteroid, Systemic

Use Partial replacement therapy for primary and secondary adrenocortical insufficiency in Addison's disease; treatment of salt-losing adrenogenital syndrome

Local Anesthetic/Vasoconstrictor Precautions No information available to require special precautions

Effects on Dental Treatment No significant effects or complications reported

Common Adverse Effects Frequency not defined.

Cardiovascular: Hypertension, edema, CHF
Central nervous system: Convulsions, headache, dizziness
Dermatologic: Acne, rash, bruising
Endocrine & metabolic: Hypokalemic alkalosis, suppression of growth, hyperglycemia, HPA suppression
Gastrointestinal: Peptic ulcer
Neuromuscular & skeletal: Muscle weakness
Ocular: Cataracts
Miscellaneous: Diaphoresis, anaphylaxis (generalized)

Mechanism of Action Promotes increased reabsorption of sodium and loss of potassium from renal distal tubules

Drug Interactions

Decreased Effect: Anticholinesterases effects are antagonized. Decreased corticosteroid effects by rifampin, barbiturates, and hydantoins. May decrease salicylate levels.

Pharmacodynamics/Kinetics

Absorption: Rapid and complete
Protein binding: 42%
Metabolism: Hepatic
Half-life elimination, plasma: 30-35 minutes; Biological: 18-36 hours
Time to peak, serum: ~1.7 hours

Pregnancy Risk Factor C

Fludrocortisone Acetate *see* Fludrocortisone *on page 598*
Flumadine® *see* Rimantadine *on page 1184*

Flumazenil (FLOO may ze nil)

Related Information

Dental Office Emergencies *on page 1584*

U.S. Brand Names Romazicon®

Canadian Brand Names Anexate®; Romazicon™

Mexican Brand Names Lanexat®

Generic Available No

Pharmacologic Category Antidote

Use Benzodiazepine antagonist; reverses sedative effects of benzodiazepines used in conscious sedation and general anesthesia; treatment of benzodiazepine overdose

Local Anesthetic/Vasoconstrictor Precautions No information available to require special precautions

Effects on Dental Treatment Key adverse event(s) related to dental treatment: Xerostomia (normal salivary flow resumes upon discontinuation).

Common Adverse Effects

>10%: Gastrointestinal: Vomiting, nausea

1% to 10%:

Cardiovascular: Palpitations

Central nervous system: Headache, anxiety, nervousness, insomnia, abnormal crying, euphoria, depression, agitation, dizziness, emotional lability, ataxia, depersonalization, increased tears, dysphoria, paranoia, fatigue, vertigo

Endocrine & metabolic: Hot flashes

Gastrointestinal: Xerostomia

Local: Pain at injection site

Neuromuscular & skeletal: Tremor, weakness, paresthesia

Ocular: Abnormal vision, blurred vision

Respiratory: Dyspnea, hyperventilation

Miscellaneous: Diaphoresis

Mechanism of Action Competitively inhibits the activity at the benzodiazepine recognition site on the GABA/benzodiazepine receptor complex. Flumazenil does not antagonize the CNS effect of drugs affecting GABA-ergic neurons by means other than the benzodiazepine receptor (ethanol, barbiturates, general anesthetics) and does not reverse the effects of opioids

Drug Interactions

Increased Effect/Toxicity: Flumazenil reverses the effects of these nonbenzodiazepine hypnotics (zaleplon, zolpidem, zopiclone).

Pharmacodynamics/Kinetics

Onset of action: 1-3 minutes; 80% response within 3 minutes

Peak effect: 6-10 minutes

Duration: Resedation: ~1 hour; duration related to dose given and benzodiazepine plasma concentrations; reversal effects of flumazenil may wear off before effects of benzodiazepine

Distribution: Initial V_d: 0.5 L/kg; V_{dss} 0.77-1.6 L/kg

Protein binding: 40% to 50%

Metabolism: Hepatic; dependent upon hepatic blood flow

Half-life elimination: Adults: Alpha: 7-15 minutes; Terminal: 41-79 minutes

Excretion: Feces; urine (0.2% as unchanged drug)

Pregnancy Risk Factor C

FluMist™ *see* Influenza Virus Vaccine *on page 748*

Flunisolide (floo NISS oh lide)

Related Information

Respiratory Diseases *on page 1478*

U.S. Brand Names AeroBid®; AeroBid®-M; Nasalide®; Nasarel®

Canadian Brand Names Alti-Flunisolide; Apo-Flunisolide®; Nasalide®; Rhinalar®

Generic Available No

Pharmacologic Category Corticosteroid, Inhalant (Oral); Corticosteroid, Nasal

Use Steroid-dependent asthma; nasal solution is used for seasonal or perennial rhinitis

Local Anesthetic/Vasoconstrictor Precautions No information available to require special precautions

Effects on Dental Treatment Key adverse event(s) related to dental treatment: *Candida* infections of the nose or pharynx, atrophic rhinitis, sore throat, bitter taste, palpitations, dizziness, headache, nervousness, GI irritation,

(Continued)

Flunisolide *(Continued)*

sneezing, coughing, upper respiratory tract infection, bronchitis, nasal congestion, nasal dryness and burning, increased susceptibility to infections, xerostomia (normal salivary flow resumes upon discontinuation), dry throat, loss of taste, epistaxis, and diaphoresis.

Common Adverse Effects

>10%:

- Cardiovascular: Pounding heartbeat
- Central nervous system: Dizziness, headache, nervousness
- Dermatologic: Itching, rash
- Endocrine & metabolic: Adrenal suppression, menstrual problems
- Gastrointestinal: GI irritation, anorexia, sore throat, bitter taste
- Local: Nasal burning, *Candida* infections of the nose or pharynx, atrophic rhinitis
- Respiratory: Sneezing, coughing, upper respiratory tract infection, bronchitis, nasal congestion, nasal dryness
- Miscellaneous: Increased susceptibility to infections

1% to 10%:

- Central nervous system: Insomnia, psychic changes
- Dermatologic: Acne, urticaria
- Gastrointestinal: Increase in appetite, xerostomia, dry throat, loss of taste perception
- Ocular: Cataracts
- Respiratory: Epistaxis
- Miscellaneous: Diaphoresis, loss of smell

Mechanism of Action Decreases inflammation by suppression of migration of polymorphonuclear leukocytes and reversal of increased capillary permeability; does not depress hypothalamus

Drug Interactions

Increased Effect/Toxicity: Expected interactions similar to other corticosteroids

Salmeterol: The addition of salmeterol has been demonstrated to improve response to inhaled corticosteroids (as compared to increasing steroid dosage).

Pharmacodynamics/Kinetics

- Absorption: Nasal inhalation: ~50%
- Metabolism: Rapidly hepatic to active metabolites
- Bioavailability: 40% to 50%
- Half-life elimination: 1.8 hours
- Excretion: Urine and feces (equal amounts)

Pregnancy Risk Factor C

Flunitrazepam (floo nye TRAZ e pam)

Synonyms RO5-420; Rohypnol

Pharmacologic Category Benzodiazepine

Use Europe: Treatment of insomnia and sedation (short-term therapy) and anesthesia induction or supplementation

Local Anesthetic/Vasoconstrictor Precautions No information available to require special precautions

Effects on Dental Treatment No significant effects or complications reported

Significant Adverse Effects Frequency not defined:

- Cardiovascular: Tachycardia, myocardial depression, shock, CHF, sinus tachycardia, night terrors, amnesia (anterograde), drowsiness, confusion, decreased blood pressure
- Central nervous system: Slurred speech, disorientation, anxiety, panic attacks, incoordination
- Gastrointestinal: Nausea, diarrhea
- Hematologic: Porphyria
- Neuromuscular & skeletal: Tremor
- Ophthalmic: Visual disturbances
- Renal: Urinary retention
- Respiratory: Cough, apnea
- Miscellaneous: Hiccups

Dosage

- Anesthesia induction: I.V.: 0.015-0.03 mg/kg slowly over 30-60 seconds
- Premedication for anesthesia: I.M.: 0.015-0.03 mg/kg slowly over 30-60 seconds
- Anesthesia maintenance: I.V.: 0.2-0.5 mg (0.005-0.01 mg/kg) 2-3 hours after anesthesia induction
- Insomnia: Oral: 0.5-2 mg nightly

Elderly: Dosage reduction required; 0.5 mg initial dose recommended for insomnia.

Mechanism of Action Intermediate to long-acting benzodiazepine; facilitates the gamma-aminobutyric acid-mediated neuroreceptors, producing sedative and muscle-relaxing effects which slow the response time of the central nervous system

Contraindications Hypersensitivity to flunitrazepam, nitrazepam, clonazepam, or any component of the formulation

Ethanol/Nutrition/Herb Interactions

Ethanol: Avoid use; aggravates sedative and toxic effects of flunitrazepam

Food can reduce absorption by 50%; insoluble in water.

Fluocinolone (floo oh SIN oh lone)

U.S. Brand Names Capex™; Derma-Smoothe/FS®; Synalar®

Canadian Brand Names Capex™; Derma-Smoothe/FS®; Fluoderm; Synalar®

Mexican Brand Names Synalar®

Generic Available Yes; Excludes oil, shampoo

Synonyms Fluocinolone Acetonide

Pharmacologic Category Corticosteroid, Topical

Use Relief of susceptible inflammatory dermatosis [low, medium, high potency topical corticosteroid]; psoriasis of the scalp; atopic dermatitis in children ≥2 years of age

Local Anesthetic/Vasoconstrictor Precautions No information available to require special precautions

Effects on Dental Treatment No significant effects or complications reported

Common Adverse Effects Frequency not defined.

Dermatologic: Acneiform eruptions, allergic contact dermatitis, burning, dryness, folliculitis, irritation, itching, hypertrichosis, hypopigmentation, miliaria, perioral dermatitis, skin atrophy, striae

Endocrine & metabolic: Cushing's syndrome, HPA axis suppression

Miscellaneous: Secondary infection

Mechanism of Action A synthetic corticosteroid which differs structurally from triamcinolone acetonide in the presence of an additional fluorine atom in the 6-alpha position on the steroid nucleus. The mechanism of action for all topical corticosteroids is not well defined, however, is believed to be a combination of anti-inflammatory, antipruritic, and vasoconstrictive properties.

Pharmacodynamics/Kinetics

Absorption: Dependent on strength of preparation, amount applied, nature of skin at application site, vehicle, and use of occlusive dressing; increased in areas of skin damage, inflammation, or occlusion

Distribution: Throughout local skin; absorbed drug is distributed rapidly into muscle, liver, skin, intestines, and kidneys

Metabolism: Primarily in skin; small amount absorbed into systemic circulation is primarily hepatic to inactive compounds

Excretion: Urine (primarily as glucuronide and sulfate, also as unconjugated products); feces (small amounts)

Pregnancy Risk Factor C

Fluocinolone Acetonide *see* Fluocinolone *on page 601*

Fluocinolone, Hydroquinone, and Tretinoin

(floo oh SIN oh lone, HYE droe kwin one, & TRET i noyn)

Related Information

Fluocinolone *on page 601*

U.S. Brand Names Tri-Luma™

Generic Available No

Synonyms Hydroquinone, Fluocinolone Acetonide, and Tretinoin; Tretinoin, Fluocinolone Acetonide, and Hydroquinone

Pharmacologic Category Corticosteroid, Topical; Depigmenting Agent; Retinoic Acid Derivative

Use Short-term treatment of moderate to severe melasma of the face

Local Anesthetic/Vasoconstrictor Precautions No information available to require special precautions

Effects on Dental Treatment Key adverse event(s) related to dental treatment: Xerostomia (normal salivary flow resumes upon discontinuation).

Common Adverse Effects

>10%:

Dermatologic: Erythema (41%), desquamation (38%), burning (18%), dry skin (14%), pruritus (11%)

1% to 10%:

Cardiovascular: Telangiectasia (3%)

(Continued)

Fluocinolone, Hydroquinone, and Tretinoin *(Continued)*

Central nervous system: Paresthesia (3%), hyperesthesia (2%)

Dermatologic: Acne (5%), pigmentation change (2%), irritation (2%), papules (1%), rash (1%), rosacea (1%), vesicles (1%)

Gastrointestinal: Xerostomia (1%)

Mechanism of Action Not clearly defined. Hydroquinone may interrupt melanin synthesis (tyrosine-tyrosinase pathway); reduces hyperpigmentation.

Drug Interactions

Cytochrome P450 Effect: Tretinoin: **Substrate** (minor) of CYP2A6, 2B6, 2C8/9; **Inhibits** CYP2C8/9 (weak); **Induces** CYP2E1 (weak)

Increased Effect/Toxicity: Avoid soaps/cosmetic preparations which are medicated, abrasive, irritating, or any product with strong drying effects (including alcohol, astringent, benzoyl peroxide, resorcinol, salicylic acid, sulfur). Drugs with photosensitizing effects should also be avoided (includes tetracyclines, thiazides, fluoroquinolones, phenothiazines, sulfonamides).

Pharmacodynamics/Kinetics

Absorption: Minimal

Metabolism: Hepatic for the small amount absorbed

Excretion: Urine and feces

Pregnancy Risk Factor C

Fluocinonide (floo oh SIN oh nide)

Related Information

Oral Nonviral Soft Tissue Ulcerations or Erosions *on page 1551*

U.S. Brand Names Lidex®; Lidex-E®

Canadian Brand Names Lidemol®; Lidex®; Lyderm®; Lydonide; Tiamol®; Topsyn®

Mexican Brand Names Topsyn®

Generic Available Yes

Pharmacologic Category Corticosteroid, Topical

Use Anti-inflammatory, antipruritic, relief of inflammatory and pruritic manifestations [high potency topical corticosteroid]

Local Anesthetic/Vasoconstrictor Precautions No information available to require special precautions

Effects on Dental Treatment No significant effects or complications reported

Common Adverse Effects Frequency not defined.

Cardiovascular: Intracranial hypertension

Dermatologic: Acne, hypopigmentation, allergic dermatitis, maceration of the skin, skin atrophy, striae, miliaria, telangiectasia, folliculitis, hypertrichosis

Endocrine & metabolic: HPA suppression, Cushing's syndrome, growth retardation

Local: Burning, itching, irritation, dryness,

Miscellaneous: Secondary infection

Mechanism of Action Fluorinated topical corticosteroid considered to be of high potency. The mechanism of action for all topical corticosteroids is not well defined, however, is felt to be a combination of three important properties: anti-inflammatory activity, immunosuppressive properties, and antiproliferative actions.

Pharmacodynamics/Kinetics

Absorption: Dependent on strength of product, amount applied, and nature of skin at application site; ranges from ~1% in areas of thick stratum corneum (palms, soles, elbows, etc) to 36% in areas of thin stratum corneum (face, eyelids, etc); increased in areas of skin damage, inflammation, or occlusion

Distribution: Throughout local skin; absorbed drug into muscle, liver, skin, intestines, and kidneys

Metabolism: Primarily in skin; small amount absorbed into systemic circulation is primarily hepatic to inactive compounds

Excretion: Urine (primarily as glucuronide and sulfate, also as unconjugated products); feces (small amounts as metabolites)

Pregnancy Risk Factor C

Fluohydrisone Acetate *see* Fludrocortisone *on page 598*

Fluohydrocortisone Acetate *see* Fludrocortisone *on page 598*

Fluoracaine® *see* Proparacaine and Fluorescein *on page 1135*

Fluor-A-Day [OTC] *see* Fluoride *on page 603*

Fluorescein and Proparacaine *see* Proparacaine and Fluorescein *on page 1135*

Fluoride (FLOR ide)

Related Information

Dentin Hypersensitivity, High Caries Index, and Xerostomia *on page 1555*

Management of Patients Undergoing Cancer Therapy *on page 1569*

U.S. Brand Names ACT® [OTC]; Fluor-A-Day [OTC]; Fluorigard® [OTC]; Fluorinse®; Flura-Drops®; Flura-Loz®; Gel-Kam® [OTC]; Gel-Kam® Rinse; Lozi-Flur™; Luride®; Luride® Lozi-Tab®; NeutraCare®; NeutraGard® [OTC]; Pediaflor®; Pharmaflur®; Pharmaflur® 1.1; Phos-Flur®; Phos-Flur® Rinse [OTC]; PreviDent®; PreviDent® 5000 Plus™; Stan-gard®; Stop®; Thera-Flur-N®

Canadian Brand Names Fluor-A-Day®; Fluotic®

Mexican Brand Names Audifluor®

Generic Available Yes

Synonyms Acidulated Phosphate Fluoride; Sodium Fluoride; Stannous Fluoride

Pharmacologic Category Nutritional Supplement

Use Prevention of dental caries

Local Anesthetic/Vasoconstrictor Precautions No information available to require special precautions

Effects on Dental Treatment Key adverse event(s) related to dental treatment: Products containing stannous fluoride may stain teeth.

Significant Adverse Effects <1% (Limited to important or life-threatening): Discoloration of teeth, rash, nausea, vomiting

Dosage Oral:

The recommended daily dose of oral fluoride supplement (mg), based on fluoride ion content (ppm) in drinking water (2.2 mg of sodium fluoride is equivalent to 1 mg of fluoride ion): See table.

Fluoride Ion

Fluoride Content of Drinking Water	Daily Dose, Oral (mg)
<0.3 ppm	
Birth - 6 mo	None
6 mo - 3 y	0.25
3-6 y	0.5
6-16 y	1
0.3-0.6 ppm	
Birth - 6 mo	None
6 mo - 3 y	None
3-6 y	0.25
6-16 y	0.5

Table from: Recommended dosage schedule of The American Dental Association, The American Academy of Pediatric Dentistry, and The American Academy of Pediatrics

Dental rinse or gel:

Children 6-12 years: 5-10 mL rinse or apply to teeth and spit daily after brushing

Adults: 10 mL rinse or apply to teeth and spit daily after brushing

PreviDent® rinse: Children >6 years and Adults: Once weekly, rinse 10 mL vigorously around and between teeth for 1 minute, then spit; this should be done preferably at bedtime, after thoroughly brushing teeth; for maximum benefit, do not eat, drink, or rinse mouth for at least 30 minutes after treatment; do not swallow

Fluorinse®: Children >6 years and Adults: Once weekly, vigorously swish 5-10 mL in mouth for 1 minute, then spit

Mechanism of Action Promotes remineralization of decalcified enamel; inhibits the cariogenic microbial process in dental plaque; increases tooth resistance to acid dissolution

Contraindications Hypersensitivity to fluoride, tartrazine, or any component of the formulation; when fluoride content of drinking water exceeds 0.7 ppm; low sodium or sodium-free diets; do not use 1 mg tablets in children <3 years of age or when drinking water fluoride content is ≥0.3 ppm; do not use 1 mg/5 mL rinse (as supplement) in children <6 years of age

Warnings/Precautions Prolonged ingestion with excessive doses may result in dental fluorosis and osseous changes; do **not** exceed recommended dosage; some products contain tartrazine

(Continued)

Fluoride *(Continued)*

Drug Interactions Decreased effect/absorption with magnesium-, aluminum-, and calcium-containing products

Dietary Considerations Do not administer with milk; do **not** allow eating or drinking for 30 minutes after use.

Pharmacodynamics/Kinetics

Absorption: Oral: Rapid and complete; sodium fluoride; other soluble fluoride salts; calcium, iron, or magnesium may delay absorption

Distribution: 50% of fluoride is deposited in teeth and bone after ingestion; topical application works superficially on enamel and plaque; crosses placenta; enters breast milk

Excretion: Urine and feces

Pregnancy Risk Factor C

Dosage Forms

Cream, topical, as sodium (PreviDent® 5000 Plus™): 1.1% (51 g) [fluoride 2.5 mg/dose; fruit and spearmint flavors]

Gel-drops, as sodium fluoride (Thera-Flur-N®): 1.1% (24 mL) [fluoride 0.5%; neutral pH; no artificial color or flavor]

Gel, topical, as acidulated phosphate fluoride (Phos-Flur®): 1.1% (60 g) [fluoride 0.5%; cherry and mint flavors]

Gel, topical, as sodium fluoride:
- NeutraCare®: 1.1% (60 g) [neutral pH; grape and mint flavors]
- PreviDent®: 1.1% (60 g) [fluoride 2 mg/dose; berry, cherry, and mint flavors]

Gel, topical, as stannous fluoride:
- Gel-Kam®: 0.4% (129 g) [bubblegum, cinnamon, fruit/berry, and mint flavors]
- Stan-Gard®: 0.4% (122 g) [bubblegum, cherry, cinnamon, grape, mint, and raspberry flavors]
- Stop®: 0.4% (120 g) [bubblegum, cinnamon, grape, and mint flavors]

Lozenge, as sodium:
- Flura-Loz®: 2.2 mg [fluoride 1 mg; sugar free; raspberry flavor]
- Fluor-A-Day: 2.2 mg [fluoride 1 mg; mint flavor]
- Lozi-Flur™: 2.21 mg [fluoride 1 mg; cherry flavor]

Solution, oral drops, as sodium:
- Flura-Drops®: 0.55 mg/drop (24 mL) [fluoride 0.25 mg/drop]
- Luride®: 1.1 mg/mL (50 mL) [fluoride 0.5 mg/mL; sugar free]
- Pediaflor®: 1.1 mg/mL (50 mL) [fluoride 0.5 mg/mL; contains alcohol <0.5%; sugar free; cherry flavor]

Solution, oral rinse, as sodium:
- ACT®: 0.05% (530 mL) [fluoride 0.0226%; bubblegum flavor, cinnamon flavor (contains tartrazine)]
- Fluorigard®: 0.05% (480 mL) [contains alcohol, sodium benzoate, and tartrazine; mint flavor]
- Fluorinse®: 0.2% (480 mL) [alcohol free; cinnamon and mint flavors]
- NeutraGard®: 0.05% (480 mL) [neutral pH; mint and tropical blast flavors]
- Phos-Flur®: 0.44% (500 mL) [bubblegum, cherry, grape, and mint flavors]
- PreviDent®: 0.2% (250 mL) [contains alcohol; mint flavor]

Solution, oral rinse concentrate, as stannous fluoride (Gel-Kam®): 0.63% (300 mL) [fluoride 7.1 mg/dose; cinnamon and mint flavors]

Tablet, chewable, as sodium:
- Fluor-A-Day:
  - 0.56 mg [fluoride 0.25 mg; raspberry flavor]
  - 1.1 mg [fluoride 0.5 mg; raspberry flavor]
  - 2.21 mg [fluoride 1 mg; raspberry flavor]
- Luride® Lozi-Tabs®:
  - 0.55 mg [fluoride 0.25 mg; sugar free; vanilla flavor]
  - 1.1 mg [fluoride 0.5 mg; sugar free; grape flavor]
  - 2.2 mg [fluoride 1 mg; sugar free; cherry flavor]
- Pharmaflur®: 2.2 mg [fluoride 1 mg; dye free, sugar free; cherry flavor]
- Pharmaflur® 1.1: 1.1 mg [fluoride 0.5 mg; dye free, sugar free; grape flavor]

Comments Neutral pH fluoride preparations are preferred in patients with oral mucositis to reduce tissue irritation; long-term use of acidulated fluorides has been associated with enamel demineralization and damage to porcelain crowns

Selected Readings

Wynn RC, "Fluoride: After 50 Years, a Clearer Picture of Its Mechanism," *Gen Dent*, 2002, 50(2):118-22, 124, 126.

Fluoride and Triclosan (Dental) *see* Triclosan and Fluoride *on page 1337*

Fluorides *see page 1555*

Fluorigard® [OTC] *see* Fluoride *on page 603*

Fluori-Methane® *see* Dichlorodifluoromethane and Trichloromonofluoromethane *on page 427*
Fluorinse® *see* Fluoride *on page 603*
Fluorodeoxyuridine *see* Floxuridine *on page 593*
9α-Fluorohydrocortisone Acetate *see* Fludrocortisone *on page 598*

Fluorometholone (flure oh METH oh lone)

U.S. Brand Names Eflone®; Flarex®; Fluor-Op®; FML®; FML® Forte
Canadian Brand Names Flarex®; FML®; FML Forte®; PMS-Fluorometholone
Generic Available Yes: Suspension (as base)
Pharmacologic Category Corticosteroid, Ophthalmic
Use Treatment of steroid-responsive inflammatory conditions of the eye
Local Anesthetic/Vasoconstrictor Precautions No information available to require special precautions
Effects on Dental Treatment No significant effects or complications reported
Mechanism of Action Decreases inflammation by suppression of migration of polymorphonuclear leukocytes and reversal of increased capillary permeability
Pregnancy Risk Factor C

Fluorometholone and Sulfacetamide *see* Sulfacetamide and Fluorometholone *on page 1244*
Fluor-Op® *see* Fluorometholone *on page 605*
Fluoroplex® *see* Fluorouracil *on page 605*

Fluorouracil (flure oh YOOR a sil)

Related Information
Capecitabine *on page 250*
U.S. Brand Names Adrucil®; Carac™; Efudex®; Fluoroplex®
Canadian Brand Names Adrucil®; Efudex®
Generic Available Yes: Injection
Synonyms 5-Fluorouracil; FU; 5-FU
Pharmacologic Category Antineoplastic Agent, Antimetabolite
Use Treatment of carcinomas of the breast, colon, head and neck, pancreas, rectum, or stomach; topically for the management of actinic or solar keratoses and superficial basal cell carcinomas
Local Anesthetic/Vasoconstrictor Precautions No information available to require special precautions
Effects on Dental Treatment Key adverse event(s) related to dental treatment: Stomatitis.
Common Adverse Effects Toxicity depends on route and duration of treatment

I.V.:

Cardiovascular: Angina, myocardial ischemia, nail changes
Central nervous system: Acute cerebellar syndrome, confusion, disorientation, euphoria, headache, nystagmus
Dermatologic: Alopecia, dermatitis, dry skin, fissuring, palmar-plantar erythrodysesthesia syndrome, pruritic maculopapular rash, photosensitivity, vein pigmentations
Gastrointestinal: Anorexia, bleeding, diarrhea, esophagopharyngitis, nausea, sloughing, stomatitis, ulceration, vomiting
Hematologic: Agranulocytosis, anemia, leukopenia, pancytopenia, thrombocytopenia
- Myelosuppression:
  - Onset: 7-10 days
  - Nadir: 9-14 days
  - Recovery: 21-28 days

Local: Thrombophlebitis
Ocular: Lacrimation, lacrimal duct stenosis, photophobia, visual changes
Respiratory: Epistaxis
Miscellaneous: Anaphylaxis, generalized allergic reactions, loss of nails

Topical: Note: Systemic toxicity normally associated with parenteral administration (including neutropenia, neurotoxicity, and gastrointestinal toxicity) has been associated with topical use particularly in patients with a genetic deficiency of dihydropyrimidine dehydrogenase (DPD).

Central nervous system: Headache, telangiectasia
Dermatologic: Photosensitivity, pruritus, rash, scarring
Hematologic: Leukocytosis
Local: Allergic contact dermatitis, burning, crusting, dryness, edema, erosion, erythema, hyperpigmentation, irritation, pain, soreness, ulceration
Ocular: Eye irritation (burning, watering, sensitivity, stinging, itching)
Miscellaneous: Birth defects, miscarriage

(Continued)

Fluorouracil *(Continued)*

Mechanism of Action A pyrimidine antimetabolite that interferes with DNA synthesis by blocking the methylation of deoxyuridylic acid; fluorouracil inhibits thymidylate synthetase (TS), or is incorporated into RNA. The reduced folate cofactor is required for tight binding to occur between the 5-FdUMP and TS.

Drug Interactions

Increased Effect/Toxicity: Fluorouracil may increase effects of warfarin.

Pharmacodynamics/Kinetics

Duration: ~3 weeks

Distribution: V_d: ~22% of total body water; penetrates extracellular fluid, CSF, and third space fluids (eg, pleural effusions and ascitic fluid)

Metabolism: Hepatic (90%); via a dehydrogenase enzyme; FU must be metabolized to be active

Bioavailability: <75%, erratic and undependable

Half-life elimination: Biphasic: Initial: 6-20 minutes; two metabolites, FdUMP and FUTP, have prolonged half-lives depending on the type of tissue

Excretion: Lung (large amounts as CO_2); urine (5% as unchanged drug) in 6 hours

Pregnancy Risk Factor D (injection); X (topical)

5-Fluorouracil *see* Fluorouracil *on page 605*

Fluoxetine (floo OKS e teen)

U.S. Brand Names Prozac®; Prozac® Weekly™; Sarafem™

Canadian Brand Names Alti-Fluoxetine; Apo-Fluoxetine®; CO Fluoxetine; FXT; Gen-Fluoxetine; Novo-Fluoxetine; Nu-Fluoxetine; PMS-Fluoxetine; Prozac®; Rhoxal-fluoxetine

Mexican Brand Names Fluoxac® [tabs]; Prozac®; Siquial® [caps]

Generic Available Yes; Excludes delayed release capsule

Synonyms Fluoxetine Hydrochloride

Pharmacologic Category Antidepressant, Selective Serotonin Reuptake Inhibitor

Use Treatment of major depressive disorder; treatment of binge-eating and vomiting in patients with moderate-to-severe bulimia nervosa; obsessive-compulsive disorder (OCD); premenstrual dysphoric disorder (PMDD); panic disorder with or without agoraphobia

Unlabeled/Investigational Use Selective mutism

Local Anesthetic/Vasoconstrictor Precautions Although caution should be used in patients taking tricyclic antidepressants, no interactions have been reported with vasoconstrictors and fluoxetine, a nontricyclic antidepressant which acts to increase serotonin

Effects on Dental Treatment Key adverse event(s) related to dental treatment: Xerostomia (normal salivary flow resumes upon discontinuation) and taste perversion. Problems with SSRI-induced bruxism have been reported and may preclude their use; clinicians attempting to evaluate any patient with bruxism or involuntary muscle movement, who is simultaneously being treated with an SSRI drug, should be aware of this potential association.

Common Adverse Effects Percentages listed for adverse effects as reported in placebo-controlled trials and were generally similar in adults and children; actual frequency may be dependent upon diagnosis and in some cases the range presented may be lower than or equal to placebo for a particular disorder.

>10%:

Central nervous system: Insomnia (10% to 33%), headache (21%), anxiety (6% to 15%), nervousness (8% to 14%), somnolence (5% to 17%)

Endocrine & metabolic: Libido decreased (1% to 11%)

Gastrointestinal: Nausea (12% to 29%), diarrhea (8% to 18%), anorexia (4% to 11%), xerostomia (4% to 12%)

Neuromuscular & skeletal: Weakness (7% to 21%), tremor (3% to 13%)

Respiratory: Pharyngitis (3% to 11%), yawn (<1% to 11%)

1% to 10%:

Cardiovascular: Vasodilation (1% to 5%), fever (2%), chest pain, hemorrhage, hypertension, palpitation

Central nervous system: Dizziness (9%), dream abnormality (1% to 5%), thinking abnormality (2%), agitation, amnesia, chills, confusion, emotional lability, sleep disorder

Dermatologic: Rash (2% to 6%), pruritus (4%)

Endocrine & metabolic: Ejaculation abnormal (<1% to 7%), impotence (<1% to 7%)

Gastrointestinal: Dyspepsia (6% to 10%), constipation (5%), flatulence (3%), vomiting (3%), weight loss (2%), appetite increased, taste perversion, weight gain

Genitourinary: Urinary frequency

Ocular: Vision abnormal (2%)

Otic: Ear pain, tinnitus

Respiratory: Sinusitis (1% to 6%)

Miscellaneous: Flu-like syndrome (3% to 10%), diaphoresis (2% to 8%)

Dosage Oral:

Children:

Depression: 8-18 years: 10-20 mg/day; lower-weight children can be started at 10 mg/day, may increase to 20 mg/day after 1 week if needed

OCD: 7-18 years: Initial: 10 mg/day; in adolescents and higher-weight children, dose may be increased to 20 mg/day after 2 weeks. Range: 10-60 mg/day

Selective mutism (unlabeled use):

<5 years: No dosing information available

5-18 years: Initial: 5-10 mg/day; titrate upwards as needed (usual maximum dose: 60 mg/day)

Adults: 20 mg/day in the morning; may increase after several weeks by 20 mg/day increments; maximum: 80 mg/day; doses >20 mg may be given once daily or divided twice daily. **Note:** Lower doses of 5-10 mg/day have been used for initial treatment.

Usual dosage range:

Bulimia nervosa: 60-80 mg/day

Depression: 20-40 mg/day; patients maintained on Prozac® 20 mg/day may be changed to Prozac® Weekly™ 90 mg/week, starting dose 7 days after the last 20 mg/day dose

OCD: 40-80 mg/day

Panic disorder: Initial: 10 mg/day; after 1 week, increase to 20 mg/day; may increase after several weeks; doses >60 mg/day have not been evaluated

PMDD (Sarafem™): 20 mg/day continuously, **or** 20 mg/day starting 14 days prior to menstruation and through first full day of menses (repeat with each cycle)

Elderly: Depression: Some patients may require an initial dose of 10 mg/day with dosage increases of 10 and 20 mg every several weeks as tolerated; should not be taken at night unless patient experiences sedation

Dosing adjustment in renal impairment:

Single dose studies: Pharmacokinetics of fluoxetine and norfluoxetine were similar among subjects with all levels of impaired renal function, including anephric patients on chronic hemodialysis

Chronic administration: Additional accumulation of fluoxetine or norfluoxetine may occur in patients with severely impaired renal function

Hemodialysis: Not removed by hemodialysis; use of lower dose or less frequent dosing is not usually necessary.

Dosing adjustment in hepatic impairment: Elimination half-life of fluoxetine is prolonged in patients with hepatic impairment; a lower or less frequent dose of fluoxetine should be used in these patients

Cirrhosis patients: Administer a lower dose or less frequent dosing interval

Compensated cirrhosis without ascites: Administer 50% of normal dose

Mechanism of Action Inhibits CNS neuron serotonin reuptake; minimal or no effect on reuptake of norepinephrine or dopamine; does not significantly bind to alpha-adrenergic, histamine, or cholinergic receptors

Contraindications Hypersensitivity to fluoxetine or any component of the formulation; patients currently receiving MAO inhibitors, thioridazine, or mesoridazine

Note: MAO inhibitor therapy must be stopped for 14 days before fluoxetine is initiated. Treatment with MAO inhibitors, thioridazine, or mesoridazine should not be initiated until 5 weeks after the discontinuation of fluoxetine.

Warnings/Precautions Potential for severe reaction when used with MAO inhibitors - serotonin syndrome (hyperthermia, muscular rigidity, mental status changes/agitation, autonomic instability) may occur. Fluoxetine may elevate plasma levels of thioridazine and increase the risk of QT_c interval prolongation. This may lead to serious ventricular arrhythmias such as torsade de pointes-type arrhythmias and sudden death.

Fluoxetine use has been associated with occurrences of significant rash and allergic events, including vasculitis, lupus-like syndrome, laryngospasm, anaphylactoid reactions, and pulmonary inflammatory disease.

May precipitate a shift to mania or hypomania in patients with bipolar disorder. Monotherapy in patients with bipolar disorder should be avoided. May cause

(Continued)

Fluoxetine *(Continued)*

insomnia, anxiety, nervousness, or anorexia. Use with caution in patients where weight loss is undesirable. May impair cognitive or motor performance; caution operating hazardous machinery or driving. The possibility of a suicide attempt is inherent in major depression and may persist until remission occurs. Monitor for worsening of depression or suicidality, especially during initiation of therapy or with dose increases or decreases. Worsening depression and severe abrupt suicidality that are not part of the presenting symptoms may require discontinuation or modification of drug therapy. Use caution in high-risk patients during initiation of therapy. Prescriptions should be written for the smallest quantity consistent with good patient care. Use caution in patients with a previous seizure disorder or condition predisposing to seizures such as brain damage, alcoholism, or concurrent therapy with other drugs which lower the seizure threshold. Use caution in patients with suicidal risk.

Use with caution in patients with hepatic or renal dysfunction and in elderly patients. May cause hyponatremia/SIADH. May increase the risks associated with electroconvulsive treatment. Use with caution in patients at risk of bleeding or receiving concurrent anticoagulant therapy; may cause impairment in platelet function. May alter glycemic control in patients with diabetes. Due to the long half-life of fluoxetine and its metabolites, the effects and interactions noted may persist for prolonged periods following discontinuation. May cause or exacerbate sexual dysfunction.

Drug Interactions

Cytochrome P450 Effect: Substrate of CYP1A2 (minor), 2B6 (minor), 2C8/9 (major), 2C19 (minor), 2D6 (major), 2E1 (minor), 3A4 (minor); **Inhibits** CYP1A2 (moderate), 2B6 (weak), 2C8/9 (weak), 2C19 (moderate), 2D6 (strong), 3A4 (weak)

Increased Effect/Toxicity: Fluoxetine should not be used with nonselective MAO inhibitors (phenelzine, isocarboxazid) or other drugs with MAO inhibition (linezolid); fatal reactions have been reported. Wait 5 weeks after stopping fluoxetine before starting a nonselective MAO inhibitor and 2 weeks after stopping an MAO inhibitor before starting fluoxetine. Concurrent selegiline has been associated with mania, hypertension, or serotonin syndrome (risk may be reduced relative to nonselective MAO inhibitors).

Fluoxetine may inhibit the metabolism of thioridazine or mesoridazine, resulting in increased plasma levels and increasing the risk of QT_c interval prolongation. This may lead to serious ventricular arrhythmias, such as torsade de pointes-type arrhythmias and sudden death. Do not use together. Wait at least 5 weeks after discontinuing fluoxetine prior to starting thioridazine.

Fluoxetine may increase the levels/effects of aminophylline, amphetamines, selected beta-blockers, citalopram, dextromethorphan, diazepam, fluvoxamine, lidocaine, mexiletine, methsuximide, mirtazapine, nefazodone, paroxetine, phenytoin, propranolol, risperidone, ritonavir, ropinirole, sertraline, theophylline, thioridazine, tricyclic antidepressants, trifluoperazine, venlafaxine, and other substrates of CYP1A2, 2C19, or 2D6.

Combined use of SSRIs and amphetamines, buspirone, meperidine, nefazodone, serotonin agonists (such as sumatriptan), sibutramine, other SSRIs, sympathomimetics, ritonavir, tramadol, and venlafaxine may increase the risk of serotonin syndrome. Combined use of sumatriptan (and other serotonin agonists) may result in toxicity; weakness, hyper-reflexia, and incoordination have been observed with sumatriptan and SSRIs. In addition, concurrent use may theoretically increase the risk of serotonin syndrome.

Concurrent lithium may increase risk of neurotoxicity, and lithium levels may be increased. Risk of hyponatremia may increase with concurrent use of loop diuretics (bumetanide, furosemide, torsemide). Fluoxetine may increase the hypoprothrombinemic response to warfarin. Concomitant use of fluoxetine and NSAIDs, aspirin, or other drugs affecting coagulation has been associated with an increased risk of bleeding; monitor.

The levels/effects of fluoxetine may be increased by chlorpromazine, delavirdine, fluconazole, gemfibrozil, ketoconazole, miconazole, nicardipine, NSAIDs, paroxetine, pergolide, pioglitazone, quinidine, quinine, ritonavir, ropinirole, sulfonamides, and other CYP2C8/9 or 2D6 inhibitors.

Decreased Effect: The levels/effects of fluoxetine may be decreased by carbamazepine, phenobarbital, phenytoin, rifampin, rifapentine, secobarbital and other CYP2C8/9 inducers. Fluoxetine may decrease the levels/effects of CYP2D6 prodrug substrates (eg, codeine, hydrocodone, oxycodone, tramadol). Cyproheptadine may inhibit the effects of serotonin reuptake inhibitors.

Lithium levels may be decreased by fluoxetine (in addition to reports of increased lithium levels).

Ethanol/Nutrition/Herb Interactions

Ethanol: Avoid ethanol (may increase CNS depression). Depressed patients should avoid/limit intake.

Herb/Nutraceutical: Avoid valerian, St John's wort, kava kava, gotu kola (may increase CNS depression).

Dietary Considerations May be taken with or without food.

Pharmacodynamics/Kinetics

Absorption: Well absorbed; delayed 1-2 hours with weekly formulation

Protein binding: 95%

Metabolism: Hepatic to norfluoxetine (active; equal to fluoxetine)

Half-life elimination: Adults:

Parent drug: 1-3 days (acute), 4-6 days (chronic), 7.6 days (cirrhosis)

Metabolite (norfluoxetine): 9.3 days (range: 4-16 days), 12 days (cirrhosis)

Due to long half-life, resolution of adverse reactions after discontinuation may be slow

Time to peak: 6-8 hours

Excretion: Urine (10% as norfluoxetine, 2.5% to 5% as fluoxetine)

Note: Weekly formulation results in greater fluctuations between peak and trough concentrations of fluoxetine and norfluoxetine compared to once-daily dosing (24% daily/164% weekly; 17% daily/43% weekly, respectively). Trough concentrations are 76% lower for fluoxetine and 47% lower for norfluoxetine than the concentrations maintained by 20 mg once-daily dosing. Steady-state fluoxetine concentrations are ~50% lower following the once-weekly regimen compared to 20 mg once daily. Average steady-state concentrations of once-daily dosing were highest in children ages 6 to <13 (fluoxetine 171 ng/mL; norfluoxetine 195 ng/mL), followed by adolescents ages 13 to <18 (fluoxetine 86 ng/mL; norfluoxetine 113 ng/mL); concentrations were considered to be within the ranges reported in adults (fluoxetine 91-302 ng/mL; norfluoxetine 72-258 ng/mL).

Pregnancy Risk Factor C

Dosage Forms CAP: 10 mg, 20 mg, 40 mg; (Prozac®): 10 mg, 20 mg, 40 mg; (Sarafem™): 10 mg, 20 mg. **CAP, delayed release** (Prozac® Weekly™): 90 mg. **SOLN, oral** (Prozac®): 20 mg/5 mL (120 mL). **TAB**: 10 mg, 20 mg; (Prozac®) [scored]: 10 mg

Selected Readings

Friedlander AH and Mahler ME, "Major Depressive Disorder. Psychopathology, Medical Management, and Dental Implications," *J Am Dent Assoc*, 2001, 132(5):629-38.

Gerber PE and Lynd LD, "Selective Serotonin Reuptake Inhibitor-induced Movement Disorders," *Ann Pharmacother*, 1998, 32(6):692-8.

Wynn RL, "New Antidepressant Medications," *Gen Dent*, 1997, 45(1):24-8.

Fluoxetine and Olanzapine *see* Olanzapine and Fluoxetine *on page 1009*

Fluoxetine Hydrochloride *see* Fluoxetine *on page 606*

Fluoxymesterone (floo oks i MES te rone)

U.S. Brand Names Halotestin®

Canadian Brand Names Halotestin®

Mexican Brand Names Stenox®

Generic Available Yes

Pharmacologic Category Androgen

Use Replacement of endogenous testicular hormone; in females, used as palliative treatment of breast cancer

Unlabeled/Investigational Use Stimulation of erythropoiesis, angioneurotic edema

Local Anesthetic/Vasoconstrictor Precautions No information available to require special precautions

Effects on Dental Treatment No significant effects or complications reported

Common Adverse Effects

>10%:

Male: Priapism

Female: Menstrual problems (amenorrhea), virilism, breast soreness

Cardiovascular: Edema

Dermatologic: Acne

1% to 10%:

Male: Prostatic carcinoma, hirsutism (increase in pubic hair growth), impotence, testicular atrophy

Cardiovascular: Edema

Gastrointestinal: GI irritation, nausea, vomiting

Genitourinary: Prostatic hyperplasia

Hepatic: Hepatic dysfunction

(Continued)

Fluoxymesterone *(Continued)*

Restrictions C-III

Mechanism of Action Synthetic androgenic anabolic hormone responsible for the normal growth and development of male sex hormones and development of male sex organs and maintenance of secondary sex characteristics; synthetic testosterone derivative with significant androgen activity; stimulates RNA polymerase activity resulting in an increase in protein production; increases bone development; halogenated derivative of testosterone with up to 5 times the activity of methyltestosterone

Drug Interactions

Increased Effect/Toxicity: Fluoxymesterone may suppress clotting factors II, V, VII, and X; therefore, bleeding may occur in patients on anticoagulant therapy May elevate cyclosporine serum levels. May enhance hypoglycemic effect of insulin therapy; may decrease blood glucose concentrations and insulin requirements in patients with diabetes. Lithium may potentiate EPS and other CNS effect. May potentiate the effects of narcotics including respiratory depression

Decreased Effect: May decrease barbiturate levels and fluphenazine effectiveness.

Pharmacodynamics/Kinetics

Absorption: Rapid
Protein binding: 98%
Metabolism: Hepatic; enterohepatic recirculation
Half-life elimination: 10-100 minutes
Excretion: Urine (90%)

Pregnancy Risk Factor X

Fluphenazine (floo FEN a zeen)

U.S. Brand Names Prolixin® [DSC]; Prolixin Decanoate®

Canadian Brand Names Apo-Fluphenazine®; Apo-Fluphenazine Decanoate®; Modecate®; Moditen® Enanthate; Moditen® HCl; PMS-Fluphenazine Decanoate

Generic Available Yes: Injection, tablet

Synonyms Fluphenazine Decanoate

Pharmacologic Category Antipsychotic Agent, Phenothiazine, Piperazine

Use Management of manifestations of psychotic disorders and schizophrenia; depot formulation may offer improved outcome in individuals with psychosis who are nonadherent with oral antipsychotics

Unlabeled/Investigational Use Pervasive developmental disorder

Local Anesthetic/Vasoconstrictor Precautions Most pharmacology textbooks state that in presence of phenothiazines, systemic doses of epinephrine paradoxically decrease the blood pressure. This is the so called "epinephrine reversal" phenomenon. This has never been observed when epinephrine is given by infiltration as part of the anesthesia procedure.

Effects on Dental Treatment Key adverse event(s) related to dental treatment: Xerostomia and increased salivation (normal salivary flow resumes upon discontinuation). Orthostatic hypotension and nasal congestion are possible and since the drug is a dopamine antagonist, extrapyramidal symptoms of the TMJ are a possibility.

Common Adverse Effects Frequency not defined.

Cardiovascular: Hypotension, tachycardia, fluctuations in blood pressure, hypertension, arrhythmias, edema

Central nervous system: Parkinsonian symptoms, akathisia, dystonias, tardive dyskinesia, dizziness, hyper-reflexia, headache, cerebral edema, drowsiness, lethargy, restlessness, excitement, bizarre dreams, EEG changes, depression, seizures, NMS, altered central temperature regulation

Dermatologic: Increased sensitivity to sun, rash, skin pigmentation, itching, erythema, urticaria, seborrhea, eczema, dermatitis

Endocrine & metabolic: Changes in menstrual cycle, breast pain, amenorrhea, galactorrhea, gynecomastia, changes in libido, elevated prolactin, SIADH

Gastrointestinal: Weight gain, loss of appetite, salivation, xerostomia, constipation, paralytic ileus, laryngeal edema

Genitourinary: Ejaculatory disturbances, impotence, polyuria, bladder paralysis, enuresis

Hematologic: Agranulocytosis, leukopenia, thrombocytopenia, nonthrombocytopenic purpura, eosinophilia, pancytopenia

Hepatic: Cholestatic jaundice, hepatotoxicity

Neuromuscular & skeletal: Trembling of fingers, SLE, facial hemispasm

Ocular: Pigmentary retinopathy, cornea and lens changes, blurred vision, glaucoma

Respiratory: Nasal congestion, asthma

Mechanism of Action Blocks postsynaptic mesolimbic dopaminergic D_1 and D_2 receptors in the brain; depresses the release of hypothalamic and hypophyseal hormones; believed to depress the reticular activating system thus affecting basal metabolism, body temperature, wakefulness, vasomotor tone, and emesis

Drug Interactions

Cytochrome P450 Effect: Substrate of CYP2D6 (major); **Inhibits** CYP1A2 (weak), 2C8/9 (weak), 2D6 (weak), 2E1 (weak)

Increased Effect/Toxicity: CYP2D6 inhibitors may increase the levels/effects of fluphenazine; example inhibitors include chlorpromazine, delavirdine, fluoxetine, miconazole, paroxetine, pergolide, quinidine, quinine, ritonavir, and ropinirole. Effects on CNS depression may be additive when fluphenazine is combined with CNS depressants (narcotic analgesics, ethanol, barbiturates, cyclic antidepressants, antihistamines, sedative-hypnotics). Fluphenazine may increase the effects/toxicity of anticholinergics, antihypertensives, lithium (rare neurotoxicity), trazodone, or valproic acid. Concurrent use with TCA may produce increased toxicity or altered therapeutic response. Chloroquine and propranolol may increase chlorpromazine concentrations. Hypotension may occur when fluphenazine is combined with epinephrine. May increase the risk of arrhythmia when combined with antiarrhythmics, cisapride, pimozide, sparfloxacin, or other drugs which prolong QT interval. Metoclopramide may increase risk of extrapyramidal symptoms (EPS).

Decreased Effect: Phenothiazines inhibit the activity of guanethidine, guanadrel, levodopa, and bromocriptine. Barbiturates and cigarette smoking may enhance the hepatic metabolism of fluphenazine. Fluphenazine and possibly other low potency antipsychotics may reverse the pressor effects of epinephrine.

Pharmacodynamics/Kinetics

Onset of action: I.M., SubQ (derivative dependent): Hydrochloride salt: ~1 hour

Peak effect: Neuroleptic: Decanoate: 48-96 hours

Duration: Hydrochloride salt: 6-8 hours; Decanoate: 24-72 hours

Absorption: Oral: Erratic and variable

Distribution: Crosses placenta; enters breast milk

Protein binding: 91% and 99%

Metabolism: Hepatic

Half-life elimination (derivative dependent): Hydrochloride: 33 hours; Decanoate: 163-232 hours

Excretion: Urine (as metabolites)

Pregnancy Risk Factor C

Fluphenazine Decanoate *see* Fluphenazine *on page 610*

Flura-Drops® *see* Fluoride *on page 603*

Flura-Loz® *see* Fluoride *on page 603*

Flurandrenolide (flure an DREN oh lide)

U.S. Brand Names Cordran®; Cordran® SP

Canadian Brand Names Cordran®

Generic Available No

Synonyms Flurandrenolone

Pharmacologic Category Corticosteroid, Topical

Use Inflammation of corticosteroid-responsive dermatoses [medium potency topical corticosteroid]

Local Anesthetic/Vasoconstrictor Precautions No information available to require special precautions

Effects on Dental Treatment No significant effects or complications reported

Common Adverse Effects Frequency not defined.

Cardiovascular: Intracranial hypertension

Dermatologic: Itching, dry skin, folliculitis, hypertrichosis, acneiform eruptions, hyperpigmentation, perioral dermatitis, allergic contact dermatitis, skin atrophy, striae, miliaria, acne, maceration of the skin

Endocrine & metabolic: Cushing's syndrome, growth retardation, HPA suppression

Local: Burning, irritation

Miscellaneous: Secondary infection

Mechanism of Action Decreases inflammation by suppression of migration of polymorphonuclear leukocytes and reversal of increased capillary permeability

(Continued)

Flurandrenolide *(Continued)*

Pharmacodynamics/Kinetics

Absorption: Adequate with intact skin; repeated applications lead to depot effects on skin, potentially resulting in enhanced percutaneous absorption

Metabolism: Hepatic

Excretion: Urine; feces (small amounts)

Pregnancy Risk Factor C

Flurandrenolone *see* Flurandrenolide *on page 611*

Flurazepam (flure AZ e pam)

U.S. Brand Names Dalmane®

Canadian Brand Names Apo-Flurazepam®; Dalmane®

Generic Available Yes

Synonyms Flurazepam Hydrochloride

Pharmacologic Category Benzodiazepine

Use Short-term treatment of insomnia

Local Anesthetic/Vasoconstrictor Precautions No information available to require special precautions

Effects on Dental Treatment Key adverse event(s) related to dental treatment: Xerostomia and changes in salivation (normal salivary flow resumes upon discontinuation), and bitter taste.

Common Adverse Effects Frequency not defined.

Cardiovascular: Palpitations, chest pain

Central nervous system: Drowsiness, ataxia, lightheadedness, memory impairment, depression, headache, hangover effect, confusion, nervousness, dizziness, falling, apprehension, irritability, euphoria, slurred speech, restlessness, hallucinations, paradoxical reactions, talkativeness

Dermatologic: Rash, pruritus

Gastrointestinal: Xerostomia, constipation, increased/excessive salivation, heartburn, upset stomach, nausea, vomiting, diarrhea, increased or decreased appetite, bitter taste, weight gain/loss

Hematologic: Granulocytopenia

Hepatic: Elevated AST/ALT, total bilirubin, alkaline phosphatase, cholestatic jaundice

Neuromuscular & skeletal: Dysarthria, body/joint pain, reflex slowing, weakness

Ocular: Blurred vision, burning eyes, difficulty focusing

Otic: Tinnitus

Respiratory: Apnea, dyspnea

Miscellaneous: Diaphoresis, drug dependence

Restrictions C-IV

Mechanism of Action Binds to stereospecific benzodiazepine receptors on the postsynaptic GABA neuron at several sites within the central nervous system, including the limbic system, reticular formation. Enhancement of the inhibitory effect of GABA on neuronal excitability results by increased neuronal membrane permeability to chloride ions. This shift in chloride ions results in hyperpolarization (a less excitable state) and stabilization.

Drug Interactions

Cytochrome P450 Effect: Substrate of CYP3A4 (major); **Inhibits** CYP2E1 (weak)

Increased Effect/Toxicity: CYP3A4 inhibitors may increase the levels/effects of flurazepam; example inhibitors include azole antifungals, ciprofloxacin, clarithromycin, diclofenac, doxycycline, erythromycin, imatinib, isoniazid, nefazodone, nicardipine, propofol, protease inhibitors, quinidine, and verapamil. Serum levels and response to flurazepam may be increased by cimetidine, clozapine, CNS depressants, diltiazem, disulfiram, digoxin, ethanol, fluconazole, fluoxetine, fluvoxamine, grapefruit juice, labetalol, levodopa, loxapine, metoprolol, metronidazole, nelfinavir, omeprazole, and valproic acid.

Decreased Effect: CYP3A4 inducers may decrease the levels/effects of flurazepam; example inducers include aminoglutethimide, carbamazepine, nafcillin, nevirapine, phenobarbital, phenytoin, and rifamycins.

Pharmacodynamics/Kinetics

Onset of action: Hypnotic: 15-20 minutes

Peak effect: 3-6 hours

Duration: 7-8 hours

Metabolism: Hepatic to N-desalkylflurazepam (active)

Half-life elimination: Desalkylflurazepam:

Adults: Single dose: 74-90 hours; Multiple doses: 111-113 hours

Elderly (61-85 years): Single dose: 120-160 hours; Multiple doses: 126-158 hours

Pregnancy Risk Factor X

Flurazepam Hydrochloride *see* Flurazepam *on page 612*

Flurbiprofen (flure BI proe fen)

Related Information

Rheumatoid Arthritis, Osteoarthritis, and Osteoporosis *on page 1490*

Temporomandibular Dysfunction (TMD) *on page 1564*

U.S. Brand Names Ansaid®; Ocufen®

Canadian Brand Names Alti-Flurbiprofen; Ansaid®; Apo-Flurbiprofen®; Froben®; Froben-SR®; Novo-Flurprofen; Nu-Flurprofen; Ocufen™

Mexican Brand Names Ansaid®

Generic Available Yes

Synonyms Flurbiprofen Sodium

Pharmacologic Category Nonsteroidal Anti-inflammatory Drug (NSAID), Ophthalmic; Nonsteroidal Anti-inflammatory Drug (NSAID), Oral

Dental Use Oral: Management of postoperative pain

Use

Oral: Treatment of rheumatoid arthritis and osteoarthritis

Ophthalmic: Inhibition of intraoperative miosis

Local Anesthetic/Vasoconstrictor Precautions No information available to require special precautions

Effects on Dental Treatment NSAID formulations are known to reversibly decrease platelet aggregation via mechanisms different than observed with aspirin. The dentist should be aware of the potential of abnormal coagulation. Caution should also be exercised in the use of NSAIDs in patients already on anticoagulant therapy with drugs such as warfarin (Coumadin®).

Significant Adverse Effects

Ophthalmic: Frequency not defined: Ocular: Slowing of corneal wound healing, mild ocular stinging, itching and burning, ocular irritation, fibrosis, miosis, mydriasis, bleeding tendency increased

Oral:

>1%:

Cardiovascular: Edema

Central nervous system: Amnesia, anxiety, depression, dizziness, headache, insomnia, malaise, nervousness, somnolence

Dermatologic: Rash

Gastrointestinal: Abdominal pain, constipation, diarrhea, dyspepsia, flatulence, GI bleeding, nausea, vomiting, weight changes

Hepatic: Liver enzymes elevated

Neuromuscular & skeletal: Reflexes increased, tremor, vertigo, weakness

Ocular: Vision changes

Otic: Tinnitus

Respiratory: Rhinitis

<1% (Limited to important or life-threatening): Anaphylactic reaction, anemia, angioedema, asthma, bruising, cerebrovascular ischemia, CHF, confusion, eczema, eosinophilia, epistaxis, exfoliative dermatitis, fever, gastric/peptic ulcer, hematocrit decreased, hematuria, hemoglobin decreased, hepatitis, hypertension, hyperuricemia, interstitial nephritis, jaundice, leukopenia, paresthesia, parosmia, photosensitivity, pruritus, purpura, renal failure, stomatitis, thrombocytopenia, toxic epidermal necrolysis, urticaria, vasodilation

Dosage

Oral:

Rheumatoid arthritis and osteoarthritis: 200-300 mg/day in 2-, 3-, or 4 divided doses; do not administer more than 100 mg for any single dose; maximum: 300 mg/day

Dental: Management of postoperative pain: 100 mg every 12 hours

Ophthalmic: Instill 1 drop every 30 minutes, beginning 2 hours prior to surgery (total of 4 drops in each affected eye)

Mechanism of Action Inhibits prostaglandin synthesis by decreasing the activity of the enzyme, cyclooxygenase, which results in decreased formation of prostaglandin precursors

Contraindications Hypersensitivity to flurbiprofen or any component of the formulation; dendritic keratitis; pregnancy (3rd trimester); patients with "aspirin triad" (bronchial asthma, aspirin intolerance, rhinitis)

Warnings/Precautions Use with caution in patients with CHF, dehydration, hypertension, decreased renal or hepatic function, history of GI disease (bleeding or ulcers), or those receiving anticoagulants. Elderly are at a high

(Continued)

Flurbiprofen *(Continued)*

risk for adverse effects from NSAIDs. As many as 60% of elderly can develop peptic ulceration and/or hemorrhage asymptomatically.

Use lowest effective dose for shortest period possible. Use of NSAIDs can compromise existing renal function especially when Cl_{cr} is <30 mL/minute. CNS adverse effects such as confusion, agitation, and hallucination are generally seen in overdose or high-dose situations; however, elderly may demonstrate these adverse effects at lower doses than younger adults. Withhold for at least 4-6 half-lives prior to surgical or dental procedures. Use of ophthalmic solution may increase bleeding of ocular tissue during ocular surgery.

Drug Interactions **Substrate** of CYP2C8/9 (minor); **Inhibits** CYP2C8/9 (strong)

ACE inhibitors: Antihypertensive effects may be decreased by concurrent therapy with NSAIDs; monitor blood pressure.

Angiotensin II antagonists: Antihypertensive effects may be decreased by concurrent therapy with NSAIDs; monitor blood pressure.

Anticoagulants (warfarin, heparin, LMWHs) in combination with NSAIDs can cause increased risk of bleeding.

Antiplatelet drugs (ticlopidine, clopidogrel, aspirin, abciximab, dipyridamole, eptifibatide, tirofiban) can cause an increased risk of bleeding.

Cholestyramine and colestipol reduce the bioavailability of some NSAIDs; separate administration times.

Corticosteroids may increase the risk of GI ulceration; avoid concurrent use.

Cyclosporine: NSAIDs may increase serum creatinine, potassium, blood pressure, and cyclosporine levels; monitor cyclosporine levels and renal function carefully.

CYP2C8/9 substrates: Flurbiprofen may increase the levels/effects of CYP2C8/9 substrates. Example substrates include amiodarone, fluoxetine, glimepiride, glipizide, nateglinide, phenytoin, pioglitazone, rosiglitazone, sertraline, and warfarin.

Gentamicin and amikacin serum concentrations are increased by indomethacin in premature infants. Results may apply to other aminoglycosides and NSAIDs.

Hydralazine's antihypertensive effect is decreased; avoid concurrent use.

Lithium levels can be increased; avoid concurrent use if possible or monitor lithium levels and adjust dose. Sulindac may have the least effect. When NSAID is stopped, lithium will need adjustment again.

Loop diuretics efficacy (diuretic and antihypertensive effect) is reduced. Indomethacin reduces this efficacy, however, it may be anticipated with any NSAID.

Methotrexate: Severe bone marrow suppression, aplastic anemia, and GI toxicity have been reported with concomitant NSAID therapy. Avoid use during moderate or high-dose methotrexate (increased and prolonged methotrexate levels). NSAID use during low-dose treatment of rheumatoid arthritis has not been fully evaluated; extreme caution is warranted.

Thiazides antihypertensive effects are decreased; avoid concurrent use.

Warfarin's INRs may be increased by piroxicam. Other NSAIDs may have the same effect depending on dose and duration. Monitor INR closely. Use the lowest dose of NSAIDs possible and for the briefest duration.

Verapamil plasma concentration is decreased by some NSAIDs; avoid concurrent use.

Ethanol/Nutrition/Herb Interactions

Ethanol: Avoid ethanol (may enhance gastric mucosal irritation).

Food: Food may decrease the rate but not the extent of absorption.

Herb/Nutraceutical: Avoid cat's claw, dong quai, evening primrose, feverfew, garlic, ginger, ginkgo, red clover, horse chestnut, green tea, ginseng (all have additional antiplatelet activity).

Dietary Considerations Tablet may be taken with food, milk, or antacid to decrease GI effects.

Pharmacodynamics/Kinetics

Onset of action: ~1-2 hours

Distribution: V_d: 0.12 L/kg

Protein binding: 99%, primarily albumin

Metabolism: Hepatic via CYP2C9; forms metabolites

Half-life elimination: 5.7 hours

Time to peak: 1.5 hours

Excretion: Urine

Pregnancy Risk Factor C/D (3rd trimester)

Lactation Enters breast milk/not recommended

Dosage Forms

Solution, ophthalmic, as sodium (Ocufen®): 0.03% (2.5 mL) [contains thimerosal]

Tablet (Ansaid®): 50 mg, 100 mg

Selected Readings

Ahmad N, Grad HA, Haas DA, et al, "The Efficacy of Nonopioid Analgesics for Postoperative Dental Pain: A Meta-Analysis," *Anesth Prog*, 1997, 44(4):119-26.

Bragger U, Muhle T, Fourmousis I, et al, "Effect of the NSAID Flurbiprofen on Remodeling After Periodontal Surgery," *J Periodontal Res*, 1997, 32(7):575-82.

Cooper SA and Kupperman A, "The Analgesic Efficacy of Flurbiprofen Compared to Acetaminophen With Codeine," *J Clin Dent*, 1991, 2(3):70-4.

Dionne R, "Additive Analgesia Without Opioid Side Effects," *Compend Contin Educ Dent*, 2000, 21(7):572-4, 576-7.

Dionne RA, "Suppression of Dental Pain by the Preoperative Administration of Flurbiprofen," *Am J Med*, 1986, 80(3A):41-9.

Dionne RA and Berthold CW, "Therapeutic Uses of Nonsteroidal Anti-inflammatory Drugs in Dentistry," *Crit Rev Oral Biol Med*, 2001, 12(4):315-30.

Dionne RA, Snyder J, and Hargreaves KM, "Analgesic Efficacy of Flurbiprofen in Comparison With Acetaminophen, Acetaminophen Plus Codeine, and Placebo After Impacted Third Molar Removal," *J Oral Maxillofac Surg*, 1994, 52(9):919-24.

Doroschak AM, Bowles WR, and Hargreaves KM, "Evaluation of the Combination of Flurbiprofen and Tramadol for Management of Endodontic Pain," *J Endod*, 1999, 25(10):660-3.

Forbes JA, Yorio CC, Selinger LR, et al, "An Evaluation of Flurbiprofen, Aspirin, and Placebo in Postoperative Oral Surgery Pain," *Pharmacotherapy*, 1989, 9(2):66-73.

Gallardo F and Rossi E, "Analgesic Efficacy of Flurbiprofen as Compared to Acetaminophen and Placebo After Periodontal Surgery," *J Periodontol*, 1990, 61(4):224-7.

Jeffcoat MK, Reddy MS, Haigh S, et al, "A Comparison of Topical Ketorolac, Systemic Flurbiprofen, and Placebo for the Inhibition of Bone Loss in Adult Periodontitis," *J Periodontol*, 1995, 66(5):329-38.

Jeffcoat MK, Reddy MS, Wang IC, et al, "The Effect of Systemic Flurbiprofen on Bone Supporting Dental Implants," *J Am Dent Assoc*, 1995, 126(3):305-11.

Malmberg AB and Yaksh TL, "Antinociception Produced by Spinal Delivery of the S and R Enantiomers of Flurbiprofen in the Formalin Test," *Eur J Pharmacol*, 1994, 256(2):205-9.

Nguyen AM, Graham DY, Gage T, et al, "Nonsteroidal Anti-inflammatory Drug Use in Dentistry: Gastrointestinal Implications," *Gen Dent*, 1999, 47(6):590-6.

Flurbiprofen Sodium *see* Flurbiprofen *on page 613*

5-Flurocytosine *see* Flucytosine *on page 596*

Fluro-Ethyl® *see* Ethyl Chloride and Dichlorotetrafluoroethane *on page 562*

Flutamide (FLOO ta mide)

U.S. Brand Names Eulexin®

Canadian Brand Names Apo-Flutamide®; Euflex®; Eulexin®; Novo-Flutamide; PMS-Flutamide

Mexican Brand Names Eulexin®; Fluken®; Flulem®

Generic Available Yes

Synonyms Niftolid; 4′-Nitro-3′-Trifluoromethylisobutyrantide; NSC-147834; SCH 13521

Pharmacologic Category Antineoplastic Agent, Antiandrogen

Use Treatment of metastatic prostatic carcinoma in combination therapy with LHRH agonist analogues

Unlabeled/Investigational Use Female hirsutism

Local Anesthetic/Vasoconstrictor Precautions No information available to require special precautions

Effects on Dental Treatment No significant effects or complications reported

Common Adverse Effects

>10%:

- Endocrine & metabolic: Gynecomastia, hot flashes, breast tenderness, galactorrhea (9% to 42%); impotence; decreased libido; tumor flare
- Gastrointestinal: Nausea, vomiting (11% to 12%)
- Hepatic: Increased AST (SGOT) and LDH levels, transient, mild

1% to 10%:

- Cardiovascular: Hypertension (1%), edema
- Central nervous system: Drowsiness, confusion, depression, anxiety, nervousness, headache, dizziness, insomnia
- Dermatologic: Pruritus, ecchymosis, photosensitivity, herpes zoster
- Gastrointestinal: Anorexia, increased appetite, constipation, indigestion, upset stomach (4% to 6%); diarrhea
- Hematologic: Anemia (6%), leukopenia (3%), thrombocytopenia (1%)
- Neuromuscular & skeletal: Weakness (1%)

Mechanism of Action Nonsteroidal antiandrogen that inhibits androgen uptake or inhibits binding of androgen in target tissues

Drug Interactions

Cytochrome P450 Effect: Substrate (major) of CYP1A2, 3A4; **Inhibits** CYP1A2 (weak)

(Continued)

Flutamide *(Continued)*

Increased Effect/Toxicity: CYP1A2 inhibitors may increase the levels/effects of flutamide; example inhibitors include amiodarone, ciprofloxacin, fluvoxamine, ketoconazole, lomefloxacin, ofloxacin, and rofecoxib. CYP3A4 inhibitors may increase the levels/effects of flutamide; example inhibitors include azole antifungals, ciprofloxacin, clarithromycin, diclofenac, doxycycline, erythromycin, imatinib, isoniazid, nefazodone, nicardipine, propofol, protease inhibitors, quinidine, and verapamil. Warfarin effects may be increased.

Decreased Effect: CYP1A2 inducers may decrease the levels/effects of flutamide; example inducers include aminoglutethimide, carbamazepine, phenobarbital, and rifampin. CYP3A4 inducers may decrease the levels/effects of flutamide; example inducers include aminoglutethimide, carbamazepine, nafcillin, nevirapine, phenobarbital, phenytoin, and rifamycins.

Pharmacodynamics/Kinetics

Absorption: Oral: Rapid and complete

Protein binding: Parent drug: 94% to 96%; 2-hydroxyflutamide: 92% to 94%

Metabolism: Extensively hepatic to more than 10 metabolites, primarily 2-hydroxyflutamide (active)

Half-life elimination: 5-6 hours (2-hydroxyflutamide)

Excretion: Primarily urine (as metabolites)

Pregnancy Risk Factor D

Fluticasone (floo TIK a sone)

Related Information

Fluticasone and Salmeterol *on page 619*

Respiratory Diseases *on page 1478*

U.S. Brand Names Cutivate®; Flonase®; Flovent®; Flovent® Rotadisk®

Canadian Brand Names Cutivate™; Flonase®; Flovent®; Flovent® HFA

Mexican Brand Names Cutivate®; Flixonase®; Flixotide®

Generic Available Yes: Cream, ointment

Synonyms Fluticasone Propionate

Pharmacologic Category Corticosteroid, Inhalant (Oral); Corticosteroid, Nasal; Corticosteroid, Topical; Corticosteroid, Topical (Medium Potency)

Use

Inhalation: Maintenance treatment of asthma as prophylactic therapy. It is also indicated for patients requiring oral corticosteroid therapy for asthma to assist in total discontinuation or reduction of total oral dose. NOT indicated for the relief of acute bronchospasm.

Intranasal: Management of seasonal and perennial allergic rhinitis and nonallergic rhinitis in patients ≥4 years of age

Topical: Relief of inflammation and pruritus associated with corticosteroid-responsive dermatoses in patients ≥3 months of age

Local Anesthetic/Vasoconstrictor Precautions No information available to require special precautions

Effects on Dental Treatment Localized infections with *Candida albicans* or *Aspergillus niger* have occurred frequently in the mouth and pharynx with repetitive use of oral inhaler of corticosteroids. These infections may require treatment with appropriate antifungal therapy or discontinuance of treatment with corticosteroid inhaler.

Common Adverse Effects

Oral inhalation: Frequency depends upon population studied and dosing used. Reactions reported are representative of multiple oral formulations.

>3%:

Central nervous system: Headache (2% to 22%), fever (1% to 7%)

Gastrointestinal: Nausea/vomiting (1% to 8%), viral GI infection (3% to 5%), diarrhea (1% to 4%), GI discomfort/pain (1% to 4%)

Neuromuscular & skeletal: Muscle injury (1% to 5%), musculoskeletal pain (1% to 5%), back problems (<1% to 4%)

Respiratory: Upper respiratory tract infection (14% to 22%), throat irritation (3% to 22%), nasal congestion (4% to 16%), pharyngitis (6% to 14%), oral candidiasis (<1% to 11%), sinusitis/sinus infection (3% to 10%), rhinitis (1% to 9%), influenza (3% to 8%), bronchitis (1% to 8%), dysphonia (<1% to 8%), upper respiratory inflammation (5%), allergic rhinitis (3% to 5%), cough (1% to 5%), nasal discharge (1% to 5%), viral respiratory infection (1% to 5%)

Miscellaneous: Viral infection (2% to 5%)

1% to 3%:

Cardiovascular: Chest symptoms, edema, palpitations, swelling

Central nervous system: Dizziness, fatigue, malaise, migraine, mood disorders, nervousness, paralysis of cranial nerves, pain, sleep disorders, giddiness

Dermatologic: Acne, dermatitis/dermatosis, eczema, folliculitis, fungal skin infection, photodermatitis, pruritus, skin rash, urticaria, viral skin infection

Endocrine & metabolic: Dysmenorrhea, fluid disturbances, goiter, uric acid metabolism disorder

Gastrointestinal: Abdominal discomfort/pain, appetite disturbances, colitis, dyspepsia, gastroenteritis, gastrointestinal infections, mouth/tongue disorder, oral erythema, oral rash, oral ulcerations, stomach disorder, viral gastroenteritis, weight gain

Genitourinary: Urinary tract infection

Hematologic: Hematoma

Hepatic: Cholecystitis

Local: Irritation from inhalant

Neuromuscular & skeletal: Arthralgia/articular rheumatism, limb pain, muscle cramps/spasms, musculoskeletal inflammation

Ocular: Blepharoconjunctivitis, conjunctivitis, irritation, keratitis

Otic: Earache, ear polyps, otitis

Respiratory: Chest congestion, dyspnea, epistaxis, laryngitis, lower respiratory infections, mouth irritation, nasal pain, nasopharyngitis, nose/throat polyps, oropharyngeal plaques, sneezing, throat constriction

Miscellaneous: Bacterial infections, burns, contusion, cysts, dental discomfort/pain, dental problems, fungal infections, lumps, masses, pressure-induced disorders, postoperative complications, soft tissue injury, tonsillitis, tooth decay, wounds/lacerations

Nasal inhalation:

>10%: Headache (7% to 16%), pharyngitis (6% to 8%)

1% to 10%:

Central nervous system: Dizziness (1% to 3%), fever (1% to 3%)

Gastrointestinal: Nausea/vomiting (3% to 5%), abdominal pain (1% to 3%), diarrhea (1% to 3%)

Respiratory: Epistaxis (6% to 7%), asthma symptoms (3% to 7%), cough (4%), blood in nasal mucous (1% to 3%), runny nose (1% to 3%), bronchitis (1% to 3%)

Miscellaneous: Aches and pains (1% to 3%), flu-like symptoms (1% to 3%)

Topical: Pruritus (3%), skin irritation (3%), exacerbation of eczema (2%), dryness (1%), numbness of fingers (1%)

Reported with other topical corticosteroids (in decreasing order of occurrence): Irritation, folliculitis, acneiform eruptions, hypopigmentation, perioral dermatitis, allergic contact dermatitis, secondary infection, skin atrophy, striae, miliaria, pustular psoriasis from chronic plaque psoriasis

Dosage

Children:

Asthma: Inhalation, oral:

Flovent®: Children ≥12 years: Refer to adult dosing.

Flovent® Diskus® and Rotadisk®: **Note:** Titrate to the lowest effective dose once asthma stability is achieved; children previously maintained on Flovent® Rotadisk® may require dosage adjustments when transferred to Flovent® Diskus®

Children ≥4-11 years: Dosing based on previous therapy

Bronchodilator alone: Recommended starting dose: 50 mcg twice daily; highest recommended dose: 100 mcg twice daily

Inhaled corticosteroids: Recommended starting dose: 50 mcg twice daily; highest recommended dose: 100 mcg twice daily; a higher starting dose may be considered in patients previously requiring higher doses of inhaled corticosteroids

Children ≥11 years: Refer to adult dosing.

Inflammation/pruritus associated with corticosteroid-responsive dermatoses: Topical: Children ≥3 months: Apply sparingly in a thin film twice daily; therapy should be discontinued when control is achieved. If no improvement is seen within 2 weeks, reassessment of diagnosis may be necessary. Safety and efficacy for use in pediatric patients <3 months have not been established.

Rhinitis: Intranasal: Children ≥4 years and Adolescents: Initial: 1 spray (50 mcg/spray) per nostril once daily; patients not adequately responding or patients with more severe symptoms may use 2 sprays (100 mcg) per nostril. Depending on response, dosage may be reduced to 100 mcg daily. Total daily dosage should not exceed 2 sprays in each nostril (200 mcg)/day. Dosing should be at regular intervals.

(Continued)

Fluticasone *(Continued)*

Adults:

Asthma: Inhalation, oral: Note: Titrate to the lowest effective dose once asthma stability is achieved

Flovent®: Dosing based on previous therapy

Bronchodilator alone: Recommended starting dose: 88 mcg twice daily; highest recommended dose: 440 mcg twice daily

Inhaled corticosteroids: Recommended starting dose: 88-220 mcg twice daily; highest recommended dose: 440 mcg twice daily; a higher starting dose may be considered in patients previously requiring higher doses of inhaled corticosteroids

Oral corticosteroids: Recommended starting dose: 880 mcg twice daily; highest recommended dose: 880 mcg twice daily; starting dose is patient dependent. In patients on chronic oral corticosteroids therapy, reduce prednisone dose no faster than 2.5 mg/day on a weekly basis; begin taper after ≥1 week of fluticasone therapy

Flovent® Diskus® and Rotadisk®: Dosing based on previous therapy

Bronchodilator alone: Recommended starting dose 100 mcg twice daily; highest recommended dose: 500 mcg twice daily

Inhaled corticosteroids: 100-250 mcg twice daily; highest recommended dose: 500 mcg twice daily; a higher starting dose may be considered in patients previously requiring higher doses of inhaled corticosteroids

Oral corticosteroids: 500-1000 mcg twice daily; highest recommended dose: 1000 mcg twice daily; starting dose is patient dependent. In patients on chronic oral corticosteroids therapy, reduce prednisone dose no faster than 2.5 mg/day on a weekly basis; begin taper after ≥1 week of fluticasone therapy

Inflammation/pruritus associated with corticosteroid-responsive dermatoses: Topical: Apply sparingly in a thin film twice daily; therapy should be discontinued when control is achieved. If no improvement is seen within 2 weeks, reassessment of diagnosis may be necessary.

Rhinitis: Intranasal: Initial: 2 sprays (50 mcg/spray) per nostril once daily; may also be divided into 100 mcg twice a day. After the first few days, dosage may be reduced to 1 spray per nostril once daily for maintenance therapy. Dosing should be at regular intervals.

Dosage adjustment in hepatic impairment: Fluticasone is primarily cleared in the liver. Fluticasone plasma levels may be increased in patients with hepatic impairment, use with caution; monitor.

Elderly: No differences in safety have been observed in the elderly when compared to younger patients. Based on current data, no dosage adjustment is needed based on age.

Mechanism of Action Fluticasone belongs to a new group of corticosteroids which utilizes a fluorocarbothioate ester linkage at the 17 carbon position; extremely potent vasoconstrictive and anti-inflammatory activity; has a weak HPA inhibitory potency when applied topically, which gives the drug a high therapeutic index. The effectiveness of inhaled fluticasone is due to its direct local effect. The mechanism of action for all topical corticosteroids is believed to be a combination of three important properties: anti-inflammatory activity, immunosuppressive properties, and antiproliferative actions.

Contraindications Hypersensitivity to fluticasone or any component of the formulation; primary treatment of status asthmaticus

Topical: Do not use if infection is present at treatment site, in the presence of skin atrophy, or for the treatment of rosacea or perioral dermatitis

Warnings/Precautions May cause hypercorticism or suppression of hypothalamic-pituitary-adrenal (HPA) axis, particularly in younger children or in patients receiving high doses for prolonged periods. HPA axis suppression may lead to adrenal crisis. Fluticasone may cause less HPA axis suppression than therapeutically equivalent oral doses of prednisone. Particular care is required when patients are transferred from systemic corticosteroids to inhaled products due to possible adrenal insufficiency or withdrawal from steroids, including an increase in allergic symptoms. Patients receiving 20 mg per day of prednisone (or equivalent) may be most susceptible. Concurrent use of ritonavir (and potentially other strong inhibitors of CYP3A4) may increase fluticasone levels and effects on HPA suppression.

Controlled clinical studies have shown that orally-inhaled and intranasal corticosteroids may cause a reduction in growth velocity in pediatric patients. (In studies of orally-inhaled corticosteroids, the mean reduction in growth velocity was approximately 1 centimeter per year [range 0.3-1.8 cm per year] and appears to be related to dose and duration of exposure.) To minimize the systemic effects of orally-inhaled and intranasal corticosteroids, each patient should be titrated to the lowest effective dose.

May suppress the immune system, patients may be more susceptible to infection. Use with caution, if at all, in patients with systemic infections, active or quiescent tuberculosis infection, or ocular herpes simplex. Avoid exposure to chickenpox and measles.

Supplemental steroids (oral or parenteral) may be needed during stress or severe asthma attacks. Rare cases of vasculitis (Churg-Strauss syndrome) or other eosinophilic conditions can occur. Flovent® aerosol contains chlorofluorocarbons (CFCs).

Inhalation: Not to be used in status asthmaticus or for the relief of acute bronchospasm. Flovent® Rotadisk® contains lactose; very rare anaphylactic reactions have been reported in patients with severe milk protein allergy.

Topical: May also cause suppression of HPA axis, especially when used on large areas of the body, denuded areas, for prolonged periods of time or with an occlusive dressing. Pediatric patients may be more susceptible to systemic toxicity. Safety and efficacy in pediatric patients <3 months of age have not been established.

Drug Interactions

Cytochrome P450 Effect: Substrate of CYP3A4 (major)

Increased Effect/Toxicity:

CYP3A4 inhibitors: Serum level and/or toxicity of fluticasone may be increased; this effect was shown with ketoconazole, but not erythromycin. Other potential inhibitors include amiodarone, cimetidine, clarithromycin, delavirdine, diltiazem, dirithromycin, disulfiram, fluoxetine, fluvoxamine, grapefruit juice, indinavir, itraconazole, ketoconazole, nefazodone, nevirapine, propoxyphene, quinupristin-dalfopristin, ritonavir, saquinavir, verapamil, zafirlukast, zileuton. Ritonavir may increase serum levels (due to CYP3A4 inhibition) and the potential for steroid-related adverse effects (eg, Cushing syndrome, adrenal suppression).

Salmeterol: The addition of salmeterol has been demonstrated to improve response to inhaled corticosteroids (as compared to increasing steroid dosage).

Ethanol/Nutrition/Herb Interactions Herb/Nutraceutical: In theory, St John's wort may decrease serum levels of fluticasone by inducing CYP3A4 isoenzymes.

Dietary Considerations Flovent® Rotadisk® contains lactose; very rare anaphylactic reactions have been reported in patients with severe milk protein allergy.

Pharmacodynamics/Kinetics

Absorption:

Cream: 5% (increased with inflammation)

Oral inhalation: Primarily via lungs, minimal GI absorption due to presystemic metabolism

Distribution: 4.2 L/kg

Protein binding: 91%

Metabolism: Hepatic via CYP3A4 to 17β-carboxylic acid (negligible activity)

Bioavailability: Oral inhalation: 14% to 30%

Excretion: Feces (as parent drug and metabolites); urine (<5% as metabolites)

Pregnancy Risk Factor C

Dosage Forms AERO, oral inhalation (Flovent®): 44 mcg/inhalation (7.9 g, 13 g); 110 mcg/inhalation (7.9 g, 13 g); 220 mcg/inhalation (7.9 g, 13 g). **CRM** (Cutivate®): 0.05% (15 g, 30 g, 60 g). **OINT** (Cutivate®): 0.005% (15 g, 30 g, 60 g). **POWDER, oral inhalation** (Flovent® Rotadisk®): 50 mcg: 44 mcg/inhalation (60s); 100 mcg: 88 mcg/inhalation (60s); 250 mcg: 220 mcg/inhalation (60s). **SUSP, intranasal spray** (Flonase®): 50 mcg/inhalation (16 g)

Fluticasone and Salmeterol (floo TIK a sone & sal ME te role)

Related Information

Fluticasone *on page 616*

Salmeterol *on page 1206*

U.S. Brand Names Advair Diskus®

Canadian Brand Names Advair Diskus®

Generic Available No

Synonyms Salmeterol and Fluticasone

Pharmacologic Category Beta$_2$-Adrenergic Agonist; Corticosteroid, Inhalant (Oral)

(Continued)

Fluticasone and Salmeterol *(Continued)*

Use Maintenance treatment of asthma in adults and children ≥4 years; **not** for use for relief of acute bronchospasm; maintenance treatment of COPD associated with chronic bronchitis

Local Anesthetic/Vasoconstrictor Precautions No information available to require special precautions

Effects on Dental Treatment Localized infections with *Candida albicans* or *Aspergillus niger* have occurred frequently in the mouth and pharynx with repetitive use of oral inhaler of corticosteroids. These infections may require treatment with appropriate antifungal therapy or discontinuance of treatment with corticosteroid inhaler.

Common Adverse Effects Percentages reported in patients with asthma

>10%:

Central nervous system: Headache (12% to 13%)

Endocrine & metabolic: Serum glucose increased, serum potassium decreased

Respiratory: Upper respiratory tract infection (21% to 27%), pharyngitis (10% to 13%)

>3% to 10%:

Gastrointestinal: Nausea/vomiting (4% to 6%), diarrhea (2% to 4%), GI pain/ discomfort (1% to 4%), oral candidiasis (1% to 4%)

Neuromuscular & skeletal: Musculoskeletal pain (2% to 4%)

Respiratory: Bronchitis (2% to 8%), upper respiratory tract inflammation (6% to 7%), cough (3% to 6%), sinusitis (4% to 5%), hoarseness/dysphonia (2% to 5%), viral respiratory tract infections (4%)

1% to 3%:

Cardiovascular: Chest symptoms, fluid retention, palpitations

Central nervous system: Compressed nerve syndromes, hypnagogic effects, pain, sleep disorders, tremors

Dermatologic: Hives, skin flakiness/ichthyosis, urticaria, viral skin infections

Gastrointestinal: Appendicitis, constipation, dental discomfort/pain, gastrointestinal disorder, gastrointestinal infections, gastrointestinal signs and symptoms (nonspecified), oral discomfort/pain, oral erythema/rash, oral ulcerations, unusual taste, viral GI infections (0% to 3%)

Hematologic: Contusions/hematomas, lymphatic signs and symptoms (nonspecified)

Hepatic: Abnormal liver function tests

Neuromuscular & skeletal: Arthralgia, articular rheumatism, bone/cartilage disorders, fractures, muscle injuries, muscle stiffness, tightness/rigidity

Ocular: Conjunctivitis, eye redness, keratitis

Otic: Ear signs and symptoms (nonspecified)

Respiratory: Blood in nasal mucosa, congestion, ear/nose/throat infections, lower respiratory tract infections, lower respiratory signs and symptoms (nonspecified), nasal irritation, nasal signs and symptoms (nonspecified), nasal sinus disorders, pneumonia, rhinitis, rhinorrhea/post nasal drip, sneezing, wheezing

Miscellaneous: Allergies/allergic reactions, bacterial infections, burns, candidiasis (0% to 3%), sweat/sebum disorders, diaphoresis, viral infections, wounds and lacerations

Dosage Oral inhalation: **Note:** Do not use to transfer patients from systemic corticosteroid therapy.

COPD: Adults: Fluticasone 250 mcg/salmeterol 50 mcg twice daily, 12 hours apart

Asthma:

Children 4-11 years: Fluticasone 100 mg/salmeterol 50 mg twice daily, 12 hours apart

Children ≥12 and Adults: One inhalation twice daily, morning and evening, 12 hours apart

Note: Advair™ Diskus® is available in 3 strengths, initial dose prescribed should be based upon previous asthma therapy. Dose should be increased after 2 weeks if adequate response is not achieved. Patients should be titrated to lowest effective dose once stable. (Because each strength contains salmeterol 50 mcg/inhalation, dose adjustments should be made by changing inhaler strength. No more than 1 inhalation of any strength should be taken more than twice a day). Maximum dose: Fluticasone 500 mcg/salmeterol 50 mcg, one inhalation twice daily.

Patients not currently on inhaled corticosteroids: Fluticasone 100 mcg/ salmeterol 50 mcg

Patients currently using inhaled beclomethasone dipropionate:

≤420 mcg/day: Fluticasone 100 mcg/salmeterol 50 mcg

462-840 mcg/day: Fluticasone 250 mcg/salmeterol 50 mcg

Patients currently using inhaled budesonide:

≤400 mcg/day: Fluticasone 100 mcg/salmeterol 50 mcg

800-1200 mcg/day: Fluticasone 250 mcg/salmeterol 50 mcg

1600 mcg/day: Fluticasone 500 mcg/salmeterol 50 mcg

Patients currently using inhaled flunisolide:

≤1000 mcg/day: Fluticasone 100 mcg/salmeterol 50 mcg

1250-2000 mcg/day: Fluticasone 250 mcg/salmeterol 50 mcg

Patients currently using inhaled fluticasone propionate aerosol:

≤176 mcg/day: Fluticasone 100 mcg/salmeterol 50 mcg

440 mcg/day: Fluticasone 250 mcg/salmeterol 50 mcg

660-880 mcg/day: Fluticasone 500 mcg/salmeterol 50 mcg

Patients currently using inhaled fluticasone propionate powder:

≤200 mcg/day: Fluticasone 100 mcg/salmeterol 50 mcg

500 mcg/day: Fluticasone 250 mcg/salmeterol 50 mcg

1000 mcg/day: Fluticasone 500 mcg/salmeterol 50 mcg

Patients currently using inhaled triamcinolone acetonide:

≤1000 mcg/day: Fluticasone 100 mcg/salmeterol 50 mcg

1100-1600 mcg/day: Fluticasone 250 mcg/salmeterol 50 mcg

Elderly: No differences in safety or effectiveness have been seen in studies of patients ≥65 years of age. However, increased sensitivity may be seen in the elderly. Use with caution in patients with concomitant cardiovascular disease.

Dosage adjustment in renal impairment: Specific guidelines are not available

Dosage adjustment in hepatic impairment: Fluticasone is cleared by hepatic metabolism. No dosing adjustment suggested. Use with caution in patients with impaired liver function.

Mechanism of Action Combination of fluticasone (corticosteroid) and salmeterol (long-acting beta$_2$ agonist) designed to improve pulmonary function and control over what is produced by either agent when used alone. Because fluticasone and salmeterol act locally in the lung, plasma levels do not predict therapeutic effect.

Fluticasone: The mechanism of action for all topical corticosteroids is believed to be a combination of three important properties: Anti-inflammatory activity, immunosuppressive properties, and antiproliferative actions. Fluticasone has extremely potent vasoconstrictive and anti-inflammatory activity.

Salmeterol: Relaxes bronchial smooth muscle by selective action on beta$_2$-receptors with little effect on heart rate

Contraindications Hypersensitivity to fluticasone, salmeterol, or any component of the formulation; status asthmaticus; acute episodes of asthma

Warnings/Precautions Not indicated for treatment of acute symptoms of asthma. Not for use in patients with rapidly deteriorating or life-threatening episodes of asthma. Fatalities have been reported. Do not use in conjunction with other long-acting beta$_2$ agonist inhalers. Do not exceed recommended dosage; short-acting beta$_2$ agonist should be used for acute symptoms and symptoms occurring between treatments. Do not use to transfer patients from oral corticosteroid therapy. Immediate hypersensitivity reactions (urticaria, angioedema, rash, bronchospasm) have been reported. Rare cases of vasculitis (Churg-Strauss syndrome) have been reported with fluticasone use.

May cause hypercorticism or suppression of hypothalamic-pituitary-adrenal (HPA) axis, particularly in younger children or in patients receiving high doses for prolonged periods. HPA axis suppression may lead to adrenal crisis. Withdrawal and discontinuation of a corticosteroid should be done slowly and carefully. Particular care is required when patients are transferred from systemic corticosteroids to inhaled products due to possible adrenal insufficiency or withdrawal from steroids, including an increase in allergic symptoms. Patients receiving 20 mg per day of prednisone (or equivalent) may be most susceptible. Concurrent use of ritonavir (and potentially other strong inhibitors of CYP3A4) may increase fluticasone levels and effects on HPA suppression. Fatalities have occurred due to adrenal insufficiency in asthmatic patients during and after transfer from systemic corticosteroids to aerosol steroids; aerosol steroids do **not** provide the systemic steroid needed to treat patients having trauma, surgery, or infections. May suppress the immune system; use with caution in patients with systemic infections or ocular herpes simplex. Avoid exposure to chickenpox and measles.

Controlled clinical studies have shown that orally-inhaled and intranasal corticosteroids may cause a reduction in growth velocity in pediatric patients. (In studies of orally-inhaled corticosteroids, the mean reduction in growth velocity was ~1 cm per year [range 0.3-1.8 cm per year] and appears to be related to

(Continued)

Fluticasone and Salmeterol *(Continued)*

dose and duration of exposure.) Long-term use may affect bone mineral density in adults. To minimize the systemic effects of orally-inhaled and intranasal corticosteroids, each patient should be titrated to the lowest effective dose.

Beta agonists may cause elevation in blood pressure, heart rate, and result in CNS excitement. Use caution in patients with cardiovascular disease (arrhythmia or hypertension or CHF), convulsive disorders, diabetes, glaucoma, hyperthyroidism, or hypokalemia. May increase risk of arrhythmia and may increase serum glucose or decrease serum potassium concentrations. In a large, randomized clinical trial (SMART), salmeterol was associated with a small, but statistically significant increase in asthma-related deaths (when added to usual asthma therapy); risk may be greater in African-American patients versus Caucasians. The elderly may be at greater risk of cardiovascular side effects. Safety and efficacy have not been established in children <4 years of age.

Powder for oral inhalation contains lactose; very rare anaphylactic reactions have been reported in patients with severe milk protein allergy.

Drug Interactions

Cytochrome P450 Effect: Fluticasone: **Substrate** of CYP3A4 (major)

Increased Effect/Toxicity: Diuretics (loop, thiazide): Hypokalemia from diuretics may be worsened by beta-agonists (dose related); use with caution. CYP3A4 inhibitors may increase levels and/or effects of fluticasone; example inhibitors include azole antifungals, ciprofloxacin, clarithromycin, diclofenac, doxycycline, erythromycin, imatinib, isoniazid, nefazodone, nicardipine, propofol, protease inhibitors, quinidine, and verapamil. Ritonavir may increase serum levels (due to CYP3A4 inhibition) and the potential for steroid-related adverse effects (eg, Cushing syndrome, adrenal suppression); avoid concurrent use. May cause increased cardiovascular toxicity with MAO inhibitors or tricyclic antidepressants; wait at least 2 weeks after discontinuing these agents to start fluticasone/salmeterol. Beta$_2$-agonists (long-acting) should not be coadministered with fluticasone/salmeterol combination.

Decreased Effect: Beta-adrenergic blockers (eg, propranolol) may decreased the effect of salmeterol component and may cause bronchospasm in asthmatics; use with caution.

Dietary Considerations Powder for oral inhalation contains lactose; very rare anaphylactic reactions have been reported in patients with severe milk protein allergy.

Pharmacodynamics/Kinetics

Advair™ Diskus®:

Onset of action: 30-60 minutes

Peak effect: ≥1 week for full effect

Duration: 12 hours

See individual agents.

Pregnancy Risk Factor C

Dosage Forms POWDER, oral inhalation: 100/50: Fluticasone 100 mcg and salmeterol 50 mcg (28s, 60s); 250/50: Fluticasone 250 mcg and salmeterol 50 mcg (28s, 60s); 500/50: Fluticasone 500 mcg and salmeterol 50 mcg (28s, 60s)

Fluticasone Propionate *see* Fluticasone *on page 616*

Fluvastatin (FLOO va sta tin)

Related Information

Cardiovascular Diseases *on page 1458*

U.S. Brand Names Lescol®; Lescol® XL

Canadian Brand Names Lescol®

Mexican Brand Names Canef®; Lescol®

Generic Available No

Pharmacologic Category Antilipemic Agent, HMG-CoA Reductase Inhibitor

Use To be used as a component of multiple risk factor intervention in patients at risk for atherosclerosis vascular disease due to hypercholesterolemia

Adjunct to dietary therapy to reduce elevated total cholesterol (total-C), LDL-C, triglyceride, and apolipoprotein B (apo-B) levels and to increase HDL-C in primary hypercholesterolemia and mixed dyslipidemia (Fredrickson types IIa and IIb); to slow the progression of coronary atherosclerosis in patients with coronary heart disease; reduce risk of coronary revascularization procedures in patients with coronary heart disease

Local Anesthetic/Vasoconstrictor Precautions No information available to require special precautions

Effects on Dental Treatment No significant effects or complications reported

Common Adverse Effects As reported with fluvastatin capsules; in general, adverse reactions reported with fluvastatin extended release tablet were similar, but the incidence was less.

1% to 10%:

- Central nervous system: Headache (9%), fatigue (3%), insomnia (3%)
- Gastrointestinal: Dyspepsia (8%), diarrhea (5%), abdominal pain (5%), nausea (3%)
- Genitourinary: Urinary tract infection (2%)
- Neuromuscular & skeletal: Myalgia (5%)
- Respiratory: Sinusitis (3%), bronchitis (2%)

Mechanism of Action Acts by competitively inhibiting 3-hydroxyl-3-methylglutaryl-coenzyme A (HMG-CoA) reductase, the enzyme that catalyzes the reduction of HMG-CoA to mevalonate; this is an early rate-limiting step in cholesterol biosynthesis. HDL is increased while total, LDL and VLDL cholesterols, apolipoprotein B, and plasma triglycerides are decreased.

Drug Interactions

Cytochrome P450 Effect: Substrate (minor) of CYP2C8/9, 2D6, 3A4; **Inhibits** CYP1A2 (weak), 2C8/9 (moderate), 2D6 (weak), 3A4 (weak)

Increased Effect/Toxicity: Cimetidine, omeprazole, ranitidine, and ritonavir may increase fluvastatin blood levels. Clofibrate, erythromycin, gemfibrozil, fenofibrate, and niacin may increase the risk of myopathy and rhabdomyolysis. Anticoagulant effect of warfarin may be increased by fluvastatin. Cholestyramine effect will be additive with fluvastatin if administration times are separated. Fluvastatin may increase C_{max} and decrease clearance of digoxin. Fluvastatin may increase the levels/effects of amiodarone, fluoxetine, glimepiride, glipizide, nateglinide, phenytoin, pioglitazone, rosiglitazone, sertraline, warfarin, and other CYP2C8/9 substrates.

Decreased Effect: Administration of cholestyramine at the same time with fluvastatin reduces absorption and clinical effect of fluvastatin. Separate administration times by at least 4 hours. Rifampin and rifabutin may decrease fluvastatin blood levels.

Pharmacodynamics/Kinetics

Distribution: V_d: 0.35 L/kg

Protein binding: >98%

Metabolism: To inactive and active metabolites [oxidative metabolism via CYP2C9 (75%), 2C8 (~5%), and 3A4 (~20%) isoenzymes]; active forms do not circulate systemically; extensive first-pass hepatic extraction

Bioavailability: Absolute: Capsule: 24%; Extended release tablet: 29%

Half-life elimination: Capsule: <3 hours; Extended release tablet: 9 hours

Excretion: Feces (90%): urine (5%)

Pregnancy Risk Factor X

Fluvirin® *see* Influenza Virus Vaccine *on page 748*

Fluvoxamine (floo VOKS a meen)

Canadian Brand Names Alti-Fluvoxamine; Apo-Fluvoxamine®; Luvox®; Novo-Fluvoxamine; Nu-Fluvoxamine; PMS-Fluvoxamine; Rhoxal-fluvoxamine

Mexican Brand Names Luvox®

Generic Available Yes

Synonyms Luvox

Pharmacologic Category Antidepressant, Selective Serotonin Reuptake Inhibitor

Use Treatment of obsessive-compulsive disorder (OCD) in children ≥8 years of age and adults

Unlabeled/Investigational Use Treatment of major depression; panic disorder; anxiety disorders in children

Local Anesthetic/Vasoconstrictor Precautions Although caution should be used in patients taking tricyclic antidepressants, no interactions have been reported with vasoconstrictors and fluvoxamine, a nontricyclic antidepressant which acts to increase serotonin

Effects on Dental Treatment Key adverse event(s) related to dental treatment: Xerostomia (normal salivary flow resumes upon discontinuation) and abnormal taste. Problems with SSRI-induced bruxism have been reported and may preclude their use; clinicians attempting to evaluate any patient with bruxism or involuntary muscle movement, who is simultaneously being treated with an SSRI drug, should be aware of the potential association.

(Continued)

Fluvoxamine *(Continued)*

Common Adverse Effects

>10%:

Central nervous system: Headache (22%), somnolence (22%), insomnia (21%), nervousness (12%), dizziness (11%)

Gastrointestinal: Nausea (40%), diarrhea (11%), xerostomia (14%)

Neuromuscular & skeletal: Weakness (14%)

1% to 10%:

Cardiovascular: Palpitations

Central nervous system: Somnolence, mania, hypomania, vertigo, abnormal thinking, agitation, anxiety, malaise, amnesia, yawning, hypertonia, CNS stimulation, depression

Endocrine & metabolic: Decreased libido

Gastrointestinal: Abdominal pain, vomiting, dyspepsia, constipation, abnormal taste, anorexia, flatulence, weight gain

Genitourinary: Delayed ejaculation, impotence, anorgasmia, urinary frequency, urinary retention

Neuromuscular & skeletal: Tremors

Ocular: Blurred vision

Respiratory: Dyspnea

Miscellaneous: Diaphoresis

Mechanism of Action Inhibits CNS neuron serotonin uptake; minimal or no effect on reuptake of norepinephrine or dopamine; does not significantly bind to alpha-adrenergic, histamine or cholinergic receptors

Drug Interactions

Cytochrome P450 Effect: Substrate (major) of CYP1A2, 2D6; **Inhibits** CYP1A2 (strong), 2B6 (weak), 2C8/9 (weak), 2C19 (strong), 2D6 (weak), 3A4 (weak)

Increased Effect/Toxicity: Fluvoxamine should not be used with nonselective MAO inhibitors (phenelzine, isocarboxazid) and drugs with MAO inhibitor properties (linezolid); fatal reactions have been reported. Wait 5 weeks after stopping fluvoxamine before starting a nonselective MAO inhibitor and 2 weeks after stopping an MAO inhibitor before starting fluvoxamine. Concurrent selegiline has been associated with mania, hypertension, or serotonin syndrome (risk may be reduced relative to nonselective MAO inhibitors).

Fluvoxamine may inhibit the metabolism of thioridazine or mesoridazine, resulting in increased plasma levels and increasing the risk of QT_c interval prolongation. This may lead to serious ventricular arrhythmias, such as torsade de pointes-type arrhythmias and sudden death. Do not use together. Wait at least 5 weeks after discontinuing fluvoxamine prior to starting thioridazine. Fluvoxamine may increase the levels/effects of aminophylline, citalopram, diazepam, mexiletine, mirtazapine, methsuximide, phenytoin, propranolol, ropinirole, sertraline, theophylline, trifluoperazine and other substrates of CYP1A2 or 2C19.

The levels/effects of fluvoxamine may be increased by amiodarone, amphetamines, selected beta-blockers, chlorpromazine, ciprofloxacin, delavirdine, fluoxetine, ketoconazole, miconazole, lomefloxacin, ofloxacin, paroxetine, pergolide, quinidine, quinine, ritonavir, rofecoxib, ropinirole, and other CYP1A2 or 2D6 inhibitors.

Combined use of SSRIs and amphetamines, buspirone, meperidine, nefazodone, serotonin agonists (such as sumatriptan), sibutramine, other SSRIs, sympathomimetics, ritonavir, tramadol, and venlafaxine may increase the risk of serotonin syndrome. Combined use of sumatriptan (and other serotonin agonists) may result in toxicity; weakness, hyper-reflexia, and incoordination have been observed with sumatriptan and SSRIs. In addition, concurrent use may theoretically increase the risk of serotonin syndrome; includes sumatriptan, naratriptan, rizatriptan, and zolmitriptan.

Concurrent lithium may increase risk of nephrotoxicity. Risk of hyponatremia may increase with concurrent use of loop diuretics (bumetanide, furosemide, torsemide). Fluvoxamine may increase the hypoprothrombinemic response to warfarin. Concomitant use of fluvoxamine and NSAIDs, aspirin, or other drugs affecting coagulation has been associated with an increased risk of bleeding; monitor.

Decreased Effect: The levels/effects of fluvoxamine may be decreased by aminoglutethimide, carbamazepine, phenobarbital, rifampin, and other CYP1A2 inducers. Cyproheptadine, a serotonin antagonist, may inhibit the effects of serotonin reuptake inhibitors (fluvoxamine); monitor for altered antidepressant response.

Pharmacodynamics/Kinetics

Absorption: Steady-state plasma concentrations have been noted to be 2-3 times higher in children than those in adolescents; female children demonstrated a significantly higher AUC than males

Distribution: V_d: ~25 L/kg

Protein binding: ~80%, primarily to albumin

Metabolism: Hepatic

Bioavailability: 53%; not significantly affected by food

Half-life elimination: ~15 hours

Time to peak, plasma: 3-8 hours

Excretion: Urine

Pregnancy Risk Factor C

Comments Problems with SSRI-induced bruxism have been reported and may preclude their use; clinicians attempting to evaluate any patient with bruxism or involuntary muscle movement, who is simultaneously being treated with an SSRI drug, should be aware of the potential association.

Fluzone® *see* Influenza Virus Vaccine *on page 748*

FML® *see* Fluorometholone *on page 605*

FML® Forte *see* Fluorometholone *on page 605*

FML-S® *see* Sulfacetamide and Fluorometholone *on page 1244*

Focalin™ *see* Dexmethylphenidate *on page 416*

Foille® [OTC] *see* Benzocaine *on page 191*

Foille® Medicated First Aid [OTC] *see* Benzocaine *on page 191*

Foille® Plus [OTC] *see* Benzocaine *on page 191*

Folacin *see* Folic Acid *on page 625*

Folacin, Vitamin B_{12}, and Vitamin B_6 *see* Folic Acid, Cyanocobalamin, and Pyridoxine *on page 626*

Folate *see* Folic Acid *on page 625*

Folbee *see* Folic Acid, Cyanocobalamin, and Pyridoxine *on page 626*

Folgard® [OTC] *see* Folic Acid, Cyanocobalamin, and Pyridoxine *on page 626*

Folgard RX 2.2® *see* Folic Acid, Cyanocobalamin, and Pyridoxine *on page 626*

Folic Acid (FOE lik AS id)

Canadian Brand Names Apo-Folic®

Mexican Brand Names A.f. Valdecasas®

Generic Available Yes

Synonyms Folacin; Folate; Pteroylglutamic Acid

Pharmacologic Category Vitamin, Water Soluble

Use Treatment of megaloblastic and macrocytic anemias due to folate deficiency; dietary supplement to prevent neural tube defects

Local Anesthetic/Vasoconstrictor Precautions No information available to require special precautions

Effects on Dental Treatment No significant effects or complications reported

Significant Adverse Effects <1% (Limited to important or life-threatening): Bronchospasm

Dosage

Infants: 0.1 mg/day

Children <4 years: Up to 0.3 mg/day

Children >4 years and Adults: 0.4 mg/day

Pregnant and lactating women: 0.8 mg/day

RDA:

Adult male: 0.15-0.2 mg/day

Adult female: 0.15-0.18 mg/day

Mechanism of Action Folic acid is necessary for formation of a number of coenzymes in many metabolic systems, particularly for purine and pyrimidine synthesis; required for nucleoprotein synthesis and maintenance in erythropoiesis; stimulates WBC and platelet production in folate deficiency anemia

Contraindications Pernicious, aplastic, or normocytic anemias

Warnings/Precautions Doses >0.1 mg/day may obscure pernicious anemia with continuing irreversible nerve damage progression; the dose that masks anemia is controversial, but doses of 400 mcg daily (or even less) have been reported. Resistance to treatment may occur with depressed hematopoiesis, alcoholism, deficiencies of other vitamins. Injection contains benzyl alcohol (1.5%) as preservative (use care in administration to neonates).

Drug Interactions Decreased effect: In folate-deficient patients, folic acid therapy (>15 mg/day) may increase phenytoin metabolism. Phenytoin, primidone, para-aminosalicylic acid, and sulfasalazine may decrease serum folate concentrations and cause deficiency. Oral contraceptives may also impair folate metabolism producing depletion, but the effect is unlikely to cause

(Continued)

Folic Acid *(Continued)*

anemia or megaloblastic changes. Concurrent administration of chloramphenicol and folic acid may result in antagonism of the hematopoietic response to folic acid; dihydrofolate reductase inhibitors (eg, methotrexate, trimethoprim) may interfere with folic acid utilization.

Pharmacodynamics/Kinetics

Onset of effect: Peak effect: Oral: 0.5-1 hour

Absorption: Proximal part of small intestine

Pregnancy Risk Factor A/C (dose exceeding RDA recommendation)

Lactation Enters breast milk/compatible

Dosage Forms

Injection, solution, as sodium folate: 5 mg/mL (10 mL) [contains benzyl alcohol]

Tablet: 0.4 mg, 0.8 mg, 1 mg

Folic Acid, Cyanocobalamin, and Pyridoxine

(FOE lik AS id, sye an oh koe BAL a min, & peer i DOKS een)

Related Information

Folic Acid *on page 625*

U.S. Brand Names Folbee; Folgard® [OTC]; Folgard RX 2.2®; Foltx®; Tricardio B

Generic Available Yes

Synonyms Cyanocobalamin, Folic Acid, and Pyridoxine; Folacin, Vitamin B_{12}, and Vitamin B_6; Pyridoxine, Folic Acid, and Cyanocobalamin

Pharmacologic Category Vitamin

Use Nutritional supplement in end-stage renal failure, dialysis, hyperhomocysteinemia, homocystinuria, malabsorption syndromes, dietary deficiencies

Local Anesthetic/Vasoconstrictor Precautions No information available to require special precautions

Effects on Dental Treatment No significant effects or complications reported

Common Adverse Effects See individual agents.

Folinic Acid *see* Leucovorin *on page 804*

Follistim® [DSC] *see* Follitropins *on page 626*

Follistim® AQ *see* Follitropins *on page 626*

Follitropin Alfa *see* Follitropins *on page 626*

Follitropin Alpha *see* Follitropins *on page 626*

Follitropin Beta *see* Follitropins *on page 626*

Follitropins (foe li TRO pins)

U.S. Brand Names Bravelle™; Follistim® [DSC]; Follistim® AQ; Gonal-F®

Canadian Brand Names Gonal-F®; Puregon™

Mexican Brand Names Follitrin®; Gonal-F®; Puregon® [biosyn.]

Generic Available No

Synonyms Follitropin Alfa; Follitropin Alpha; Follitropin Beta; Recombinant Human Follicle Stimulating Hormone; rFSH-alpha; rFSH-beta; rhFSH-alpha; rhFSH-beta; Urofollitropin

Pharmacologic Category Gonadotropin; Ovulation Stimulator

Use

Urofollitropin (Bravelle™): Ovulation induction in patients who previously received pituitary suppression; Assisted Reproductive Technologies (ART) ART

Follitropin alfa (Gonal-F®), Follitropin beta (Follistim®): Ovulation induction in patients in whom the cause of infertility is functional and not caused by primary ovarian failure; ART; spermatogenesis induction

Follitropin beta (Follistim® AQ): Ovulation induction in patients in whom the cause of infertility is functional and not caused by primary ovarian failure; ART

Local Anesthetic/Vasoconstrictor Precautions No information available to require special precautions

Effects on Dental Treatment No significant effects or complications reported

Common Adverse Effects Frequency varies by specific product and route of administration.

2% to 10%:

Central nervous system: Headache, dizziness, fever

Dermatologic: Acne (male), dermoid cyst (male), dry skin, body rash, hair loss, hives

Endocrine & metabolic: Ovarian hyperstimulation syndrome, adnexal torsion, mild to moderate ovarian enlargement, abdominal pain, ovarian cysts, breast tenderness, gynecomastia (male)

Gastrointestinal: Nausea, vomiting, diarrhea, abdominal cramps, bloating, flatulence, dyspepsia
Genitourinary: Urinary tract infection, menstrual disorder, intermenstrual bleeding, dysmenorrhea, cervical lesion
Local: Pain, rash, swelling, or irritation at the site of injection
Neuromuscular & skeletal: Back pain, varicose veins (male)
Respiratory: Exacerbation of asthma, sinusitis, pharyngitis
Miscellaneous: Febrile reactions accompanied by chills, musculoskeletal, joint pains, malaise, headache, and fatigue; flu-like symptoms

Mechanism of Action Urofollitropin is a preparation of highly purified follicle-stimulating hormone (FSH) extracted from the urine of postmenopausal women. Follitropin alfa and follitropin beta are human FSH preparations of recombinant DNA origin. Follitropins stimulate ovarian follicular growth in women who do not have primary ovarian failure, and stimulate spermatogenesis in men with hypogonadotrophic hypogonadism. FSH is required for normal follicular growth, maturation, gonadal steroid production, and spermatogenesis.

Pharmacodynamics/Kinetics
Onset of action: Peak effect: Spermatogenesis, median: 165 days (range: 25-327 days); Follicle development: Within cycle
Absorption: Rate limited: I.M., SubQ: Slower than elimination rate
Distribution: Mean V_d: Follitropin alfa: 10 L; Follitropin beta: 8 L
Metabolism: Total clearance of follitropin alfa was 0.6 L/hour following I.V. administration
Bioavailability: Ranges from ~66% to 82% depending on agent
Half-life elimination:
Mean: SubQ: Follitropin alfa: 24-32 hours; Follitropin beta: ~30 hours; Urofollitropin: 32-37 hours
Mean terminal: Multiple doses: I.M. follitropin alfa, SubQ follitropin beta: ~30 hours; I.M. urofollitropin: 15 hours, SubQ urofollitropin: 21 hours
Time to peak:
Follitropin alfa: SubQ: 16 hours; I.M.: 25 hours
Follitropin beta: I.M.: 27 hours
Urofollitropin: Single dose: SubQ: 15-20 hours, I.M.: 10-17 hours; Multiple doses: I.M., SubQ: 10 hours
Excretion: Clearance: Follitropin alfa: I.V.: 0.6 L/hour

Pregnancy Risk Factor X

Foltx® *see* Folic Acid, Cyanocobalamin, and Pyridoxine *on page 626*

Fomepizole (foe ME pi zole)

U.S. Brand Names Antizol®
Generic Available No
Synonyms 4-Methylpyrazole; 4-MP
Pharmacologic Category Antidote
Use Orphan drug: Treatment of methanol or ethylene glycol poisoning alone or in combination with hemodialysis
Unlabeled/Investigational Use Known or suspected propylene glycol toxicity
Local Anesthetic/Vasoconstrictor Precautions No information available to require special precautions
Effects on Dental Treatment Key adverse event(s) related to dental treatment: Bad/metallic taste.

Common Adverse Effects
>10%:
Central nervous system: Headache (14%)
Gastrointestinal: Nausea (11%)
1% to 10% (≤3% unless otherwise noted):
Cardiovascular: Bradycardia, facial flush, hypotension, phlebosclerosis, shock, tachycardia
Central nervous system: Dizziness (6%), increased drowsiness (6%), agitation, anxiety, lightheadedness, seizure, vertigo
Dermatologic: Rash
Gastrointestinal: Bad/metallic taste (6%), abdominal pain, decreased appetite, diarrhea, heartburn, vomiting
Hematologic: Anemia, disseminated intravascular coagulation, eosinophilia, lymphangitis
Hepatic: Increased liver function tests
Local: Application site reaction, inflammation at the injection site, pain during injection, phlebitis
Neuromuscular & skeletal: Backache
Ocular: Nystagmus, transient blurred vision, visual disturbances
Renal: Anuria
(Continued)

Fomepizole *(Continued)*

Respiratory: Abnormal smell, hiccups, pharyngitis
Miscellaneous: Multiorgan failure, speech disturbances

Mechanism of Action Fomepizole competitively inhibits alcohol dehydrogenase, an enzyme which catalyzes the metabolism of ethanol, ethylene glycol, and methanol to their toxic metabolites. Ethylene glycol is metabolized to glycoaldehyde, then oxidized to glycolate, glyoxylate, and oxalate. Glycolate and oxalate are responsible for metabolic acidosis and renal damage. Methanol is metabolized to formaldehyde, then oxidized to formic acid. Formic acid is responsible for metabolic acidosis and visual disturbances.

Pharmacodynamics/Kinetics

Onset of effect: Peak effect: Maximum: 1.5-2 hours
Absorption: Oral: Readily absorbed
Distribution: V_d: 0.6-1.02 L/kg; rapidly into total body water
Protein binding: Negligible
Metabolism: Hepatic to 4-carboxypyrazole (80% to 85% of dose), 4-hydroxymethylpyrazole, and their N-glucuronide conjugates; following multiple doses, induces its own metabolism via CYP oxidases after 30-40 hours
Half-life elimination: Has not been calculated; varies with dose
Excretion: Urine (1% to 3.5% as unchanged drug and metabolites)

Pregnancy Risk Factor C

Fomivirsen (foe MI vir sen)

Related Information

Systemic Viral Diseases *on page 1519*

U.S. Brand Names Vitravene™ [DSC]

Canadian Brand Names Vitravene™

Generic Available No

Synonyms Fomivirsen Sodium

Pharmacologic Category Antiviral Agent, Ophthalmic

Use Local treatment of cytomegalovirus (CMV) retinitis in patients with acquired immunodeficiency syndrome who are intolerant or insufficiently responsive to other treatments for CMV retinitis or when other treatments for CMV retinitis are contraindicated

Local Anesthetic/Vasoconstrictor Precautions No information available to require special precautions

Effects on Dental Treatment No significant effects or complications reported

Mechanism of Action Inhibits synthesis of viral protein by binding to mRNA which blocks replication of cytomegalovirus through an antisense mechanism

Fomivirsen Sodium *see* Fomivirsen *on page 628*

Fondaparinux (fon da PARE i nuks)

U.S. Brand Names Arixtra®

Canadian Brand Names Arixtra®

Generic Available No

Synonyms Fondaparinux Sodium

Pharmacologic Category Factor Xa Inhibitor

Use Prophylaxis of deep vein thrombosis (DVT) in patients undergoing surgery for hip replacement, knee replacement, or hip fracture surgery (including extended prophylaxis following hip fracture surgery); treatment of acute pulmonary embolism (PE); treatment of acute DVT without PE

Local Anesthetic/Vasoconstrictor Precautions No information available to require special precautions

Effects on Dental Treatment Key adverse event(s) related to dental treatment: Hemorrhage may occur at any site; risk increased in renal dysfunction, patients >75 years and/or <50 kg; major bleeding increased as high as 5% in patients receiving initial dose <6 hours postsurgery.

Common Adverse Effects As with all anticoagulants, bleeding is the major adverse effect. Hemorrhage may occur at any site. Risk appears increased by a number of factors including renal dysfunction, age (>75 years), and weight (<50 kg).

>10%:

Central nervous system: Fever (4% to 14%)
Gastrointestinal: Nausea (11%)
Hematologic: Anemia (20%)

1% to 10%:

Cardiovascular: Edema (9%), hypotension (4%), confusion (3%)
Central nervous system: Insomnia (5%), dizziness (4%), headache (2% to 5%), pain (2%)
Dermatologic: Rash (8%), purpura (4%), bullous eruption (3%)

Endocrine & metabolic: Hypokalemia (1% to 4%)
Gastrointestinal: Constipation (5% to 9%), nausea (3%), vomiting (6%), diarrhea (3%), dyspepsia (2%)
Genitourinary: Urinary tract infection (4%), urinary retention (3%)
Hematologic: Moderate thrombocytopenia (50,000-100,000/mm^3: 3%), major bleeding (1% to 3%), minor bleeding (3% to 4%), hematoma (3%); risk of major bleeding increased as high as 5% in patients receiving initial dose <6 hours following surgery
Hepatic: SGOT increased (2%), SGPT increased (3%)
Local: Injection site reaction (bleeding, rash, pruritus)
Miscellaneous: Wound drainage increased (5%)

Mechanism of Action Fondaparinux is a synthetic pentasaccharide that causes an antithrombin III-mediated selective inhibition of factor Xa. Neutralization of factor Xa interrupts the blood coagulation cascade and inhibits thrombin formation and thrombus development.

Drug Interactions

Increased Effect/Toxicity: Anticoagulants, antiplatelet agents, drotrecogin alfa, NSAIDs, salicylates, and thrombolytic agents may enhance the anticoagulant effect and/or increase the risk of bleeding.

Pharmacodynamics/Kinetics

Absorption: Rapid and complete
Distribution: V_d: 7-11 L; mainly in blood
Protein binding: ≥94% to antithrombin III
Bioavailability: 100%
Half-life elimination: 17-21 hours; prolonged with worsening renal impairment
Time to peak: 2-3 hours
Excretion: Urine (as unchanged drug)

Pregnancy Risk Factor B

Fondaparinux Sodium *see* Fondaparinux *on page 628*
Foradil® Aerolizer™ *see* Formoterol *on page 629*

Formoterol (for MOH te rol)

U.S. Brand Names Foradil® Aerolizer™

Canadian Brand Names Foradil®; Oxeze® Turbuhaler®

Generic Available No

Synonyms Formoterol Fumarate

Pharmacologic Category Beta$_2$-Adrenergic Agonist

Use Maintenance treatment of asthma and prevention of bronchospasm in patients ≥5 years of age with reversible obstructive airway disease, including patients with symptoms of nocturnal asthma, who require regular treatment with inhaled, short-acting beta$_2$ agonists; maintenance treatment of bronchoconstriction in patients with COPD; prevention of exercise-induced bronchospasm in patients ≥5 years of age

Local Anesthetic/Vasoconstrictor Precautions No information available to require special precautions

Effects on Dental Treatment Key adverse event(s) related to dental treatment: Xerostomia (normal salivary flow resumes upon discontinuation).

Common Adverse Effects Children are more likely to have infection, inflammation, abdominal pain, nausea, and dyspepsia.

>10%:
Endocrine & metabolic: Serum glucose increased, serum potassium decreased
Miscellaneous: Viral infection (17%)

1% to 10%:
Cardiovascular: Chest pain (2%)
Central nervous system: Tremor (2%), dizziness (2%), insomnia (2%), dysphonia (1%)
Dermatologic: Rash (1%)
Respiratory: Bronchitis (5%), infection (3%), dyspnea (2%), tonsillitis (1%)

Mechanism of Action Relaxes bronchial smooth muscle by selective action on beta$_2$ receptors with little effect on heart rate. Formoterol has a long-acting effect.

Drug Interactions

Cytochrome P450 Effect: Substrate (minor) of CYP2A6, 2C8/9, 2C19, 2D6

Increased Effect/Toxicity: Adrenergic agonists, antidepressants (tricyclic), beta-blockers, corticosteroids, diuretics, drugs that prolong QT_c interval, MAO inhibitors, theophylline derivatives

Pharmacodynamics/Kinetics

Duration: Improvement in FEV_1 observed for 12 hours in most patients
Absorption: Rapidly into plasma

(Continued)

Formoterol *(Continued)*

Protein binding: 61% to 64% *in vitro* at higher concentrations than achieved with usual dosing

Metabolism: Hepatic via direct glucuronidation and O-demethylation; CYP2D6, CYP2C8/9, CYP2C19, CYP2A6 involved in O-demethylation

Half-life elimination: ~10-14 hours

Time to peak: Maximum improvement in FEV_1 in 1-3 hours

Excretion:

Children 5-12 years: Urine (7% to 9% as direct glucuronide metabolites, 6% as unchanged drug)

Adults: Urine (15% to 18% as direct glucuronide metabolites, 10% as unchanged drug)

Pregnancy Risk Factor C

Formoterol Fumarate *see* Formoterol *on page 629*

Formula EM [OTC] *see* Fructose, Dextrose, and Phosphoric Acid *on page 638*

Formulation R™ [OTC] *see* Phenylephrine *on page 1078*

5-Formyl Tetrahydrofolate *see* Leucovorin *on page 804*

Fortamet™ *see* Metformin *on page 887*

Fortaz® *see* Ceftazidime *on page 286*

Forteo™ *see* Teriparatide *on page 1274*

Fortovase® *see* Saquinavir *on page 1207*

Fosamax® *see* Alendronate *on page 77*

Fosamprenavir (FOS am pren a veer)

Related Information

HIV Infection and AIDS *on page 1484*

U.S. Brand Names Lexiva™

Generic Available No

Synonyms Fosamprenavir Calcium; GW433908G

Pharmacologic Category Antiretroviral Agent, Protease Inhibitor

Use Treatment of HIV infections in combination with at least two other antiretroviral agents

Local Anesthetic/Vasoconstrictor Precautions No information available to require special precautions

Effects on Dental Treatment No significant effects or complications reported

Common Adverse Effects

>10%:

Central nervous system: Headache (19% to 21%), fatigue (10% to 18%)

Dermatologic: Rash (17% to 35%; moderate to severe reactions 3% to 8%)

Gastrointestinal: Nausea (37% to 39%), diarrhea (34% to 52%), vomiting (16% to 20%), abdominal pain (5% to 11%)

1% to 10%:

Central nervous system: Depression (8%), fatigue, headache, paresthesia

Dermatologic: Pruritus (3% to 8%)

Endocrine & metabolic: Hypertriglyceridemia (0% to 11%), serum lipase increased (6% to 8%), hyperglycemia (<1% to 2%)

Hematologic: Neutropenia (3%)

Hepatic: Increased transaminases (4% to 8%)

Miscellaneous: Perioral tingling/numbness (2% to 10%)

Mechanism of Action Fosamprenavir is rapidly and almost completely converted to amprenavir *in vivo*. Amprenavir binds to the protease activity site and inhibits the activity of the enzyme. HIV protease is required for the cleavage of viral polyprotein precursors into individual functional proteins found in infectious HIV. Inhibition prevents cleavage of these polyproteins, resulting in the formation of immature, noninfectious viral particles.

Drug Interactions

Cytochrome P450 Effect: As amprenavir: **Substrate** of CYP2C8/9 (minor), 3A4 (major); **Inhibits** CYP2C19 (weak), 3A4 (strong)

Increased Effect/Toxicity: Concurrent use of cisapride, midazolam, pimozide, quinidine, or triazolam is contraindicated. Concurrent use of ergot alkaloids (dihydroergotamine, ergotamine, ergonovine, methylergonovine) with amprenavir is also contraindicated (may cause vasospasm and peripheral ischemia). Concurrent use of oral solution with disulfiram or metronidazole is contraindicated, due to the risk of propylene glycol toxicity.

Serum concentrations of amiodarone, bepridil, lidocaine, quinidine and other antiarrhythmics may be increased, potentially leading to toxicity; when amprenavir is coadministered with ritonavir, flecainide and propafenone are contraindicated. HMG-CoA reductase inhibitors serum concentrations may be increased by amprenavir, increasing the risk of myopathy/rhabdomyolysis; lovastatin and simvastatin are not recommended; fluvastatin and pravastatin may be safer alternatives.

Amprenavir may increase the levels/effects of selected benzodiazepines (midazolam and triazolam are contraindicated), calcium channel blockers, cyclosporine, mirtazapine, nateglinide, nefazodone, quinidine, sildenafil (and other PDE-5 inhibitors), tacrolimus, venlafaxine, and other CYP3A4 substrates. When used with strong CYP3A4 inhibitors, dosage adjustment/limits are recommended for sildenafil and other PDE-5 inhibitors; refer to individual monographs.

Concurrent therapy with ritonavir may result in increased serum concentrations: dosage adjustment is recommended. Clarithromycin, indinavir, nelfinavir may increase serum concentrations of amprenavir.

Decreased Effect: CYP3A4 inducers may decrease the levels/effects of amprenavir; example inducers include aminoglutethimide, carbamazepine, nafcillin, nevirapine, phenobarbital, phenytoin, and rifamycins. The administration of didanosine (buffered formulation) should be separated from amprenavir by 1 hour to limit interaction between formulations. Serum concentrations of estrogen (oral contraceptives) may be decreased, use alternative (nonhormonal) forms of contraception. Dexamethasone may decrease the therapeutic effect of amprenavir. Serum concentrations of delavirdine may be decreased; may lead to loss of virologic response and possible resistance to delavirdine; concomitant use is not recommended. Efavirenz and nevirapine may decrease serum concentrations of amprenavir (dosing for combinations not established). Avoid St John's wort (may lead to subtherapeutic concentrations of amprenavir). Effect of amprenavir may be diminished when administered with methadone (consider alternative antiretroviral); in addition, effect of methadone may be reduced (dosage increase may be required).

Pharmacodynamics/Kinetics

Absorption: 63%

Bioavailability: Not established; food does not have a significant effect on absorption

Protein-binding: 90%

Half-Life elimination: 7.7 hours

Time to peak, plasma: 1.5-4 hours

Metabolism: Fosamprenavir is rapidly and almost completely converted to amprenavir by cellular phosphatases; amprenavir is hepatically metabolized via CYP isoenzymes (primarily CYP3A4)

Excretion: Feces (75%); urine (14% as metabolites; <1% as unchanged drug)

Pregnancy Risk Factor C

Fosamprenavir Calcium *see* Fosamprenavir *on page 630*

Foscarnet (fos KAR net)

Related Information

Systemic Viral Diseases *on page 1519*

U.S. Brand Names Foscavir®

Canadian Brand Names Foscavir®

Generic Available No

Synonyms PFA; Phosphonoformate; Phosphonoformic Acid

Pharmacologic Category Antiviral Agent

Use

Treatment of herpes virus infections suspected to be caused by acyclovir-resistant (HSV, VZV) or ganciclovir-resistant (CMV) strains; this occurs almost exclusively in immunocompromised persons (eg, with advanced AIDS) who have received prolonged treatment for a herpes virus infection

Treatment of CMV retinitis in persons with AIDS

Unlabeled/Investigational Use Other CMV infections in persons unable to tolerate ganciclovir; may be given in combination with ganciclovir in patients who relapse after monotherapy with either drug

Local Anesthetic/Vasoconstrictor Precautions No information available to require special precautions

Effects on Dental Treatment No significant effects or complications reported

Common Adverse Effects

>10%:

Central nervous system: Fever (65%), headache (26%), seizures (10%)

Gastrointestinal: Nausea (47%), diarrhea (30%), vomiting

Hematologic: Anemia (33%)

Renal: Abnormal renal function/decreased creatinine clearance (27%)

(Continued)

Foscarnet *(Continued)*

1% to 10%:

Central nervous system: Fatigue, malaise, dizziness, hypoesthesia, depression/confusion/anxiety (≥5%)

Dermatologic: Rash

Endocrine & metabolic: Electrolyte imbalance (especially potassium, calcium, magnesium, and phosphorus)

Gastrointestinal: Anorexia

Hematologic: Granulocytopenia, leukopenia (≥5%), thrombocytopenia, thrombosis

Local: Injection site pain

Neuromuscular & skeletal: Paresthesia, involuntary muscle contractions, rigors, neuropathy (peripheral), weakness

Ocular: Vision abnormalities

Respiratory: Coughing, dyspnea (≥5%)

Miscellaneous: Sepsis, diaphoresis (increased)

Mechanism of Action Pyrophosphate analogue which acts as a noncompetitive inhibitor of many viral RNA and DNA polymerases as well as HIV reverse transcriptase. Similar to ganciclovir, foscarnet is a virostatic agent. Foscarnet does not require activation by thymidine kinase.

Drug Interactions

Increased Effect/Toxicity: Concurrent use with ciprofloxacin (or other fluoroquinolone) increases seizure potential. Acute renal failure (reversible) has been reported with cyclosporine due most likely to a synergistic toxic effect. Nephrotoxic drugs (amphotericin B, I.V. pentamidine, aminoglycosides, etc) should be avoided, if possible, to minimize additive renal risk with foscarnet. Concurrent use of pentamidine also increases the potential for hypocalcemia. Protease inhibitors (ritonavir, saquinavir) have been associated with an increased risk of renal impairment during concurrent use of foscarnet

Pharmacodynamics/Kinetics

Distribution: Up to 28% of cumulative I.V. dose may be deposited in bone

Metabolism: Biotransformation does not occur

Half-life elimination: ~3 hours

Excretion: Urine (≤28% as unchanged drug)

Pregnancy Risk Factor C

Foscavir® *see* Foscarnet *on page 631*

Fosfomycin (fos foe MYE sin)

U.S. Brand Names Monurol™

Canadian Brand Names Monurol™

Mexican Brand Names Fosfocil®; Fosfocil® [inj.]; Monurol®

Generic Available No

Synonyms Fosfomycin Tromethamine

Pharmacologic Category Antibiotic, Miscellaneous

Use A single oral dose in the treatment of uncomplicated urinary tract infections in women due to susceptible strains of *E. coli* and *Enterococcus*; multiple doses have been investigated for complicated urinary tract infections in men; may have an advantage over other agents since it maintains high concentration in the urine for up to 48 hours

Local Anesthetic/Vasoconstrictor Precautions No information available to require special precautions

Effects on Dental Treatment No significant effects or complications reported

Common Adverse Effects >1%:

Central nervous system: Headache

Dermatologic: Rash

Gastrointestinal: Diarrhea (2% to 8%), nausea, vomiting, epigastric discomfort, anorexia

Mechanism of Action As a phosphonic acid derivative, fosfomycin inhibits bacterial wall synthesis (bactericidal) by inactivating the enzyme, pyruvyl transferase, which is critical in the synthesis of cell walls by bacteria; the tromethamine salt is preferable to the calcium salt due to its superior absorption

Drug Interactions

Decreased Effect: Antacids or calcium salts may cause precipitate formation and decrease fosfomycin absorption. Increased gastrointestinal motility due to metoclopramide may lower fosfomycin tromethamine serum concentrations and urinary excretion. This drug interaction possibly could be extrapolated to other medications which increase gastrointestinal motility.

Pharmacodynamics/Kinetics

Absorption: Well absorbed

Distribution: V_d: 2 L/kg; high concentrations in urine; well into other tissues; crosses maximally into CSF with inflamed meninges

Protein binding: <3%

Bioavailability: 34% to 58%

Half-life elimination: 4-8 hours; Cl_{cr} <10 mL/minute: 50 hours

Time to peak, serum: 2 hours

Excretion: Urine (as unchanged drug); high urinary levels (100 mcg/mL) persist for >48 hours

Pregnancy Risk Factor B

Fosfomycin Tromethamine *see* Fosfomycin *on page 632*

Fosinopril (foe SIN oh pril)

Related Information

Cardiovascular Diseases *on page 1458*

U.S. Brand Names Monopril®

Canadian Brand Names Monopril®

Generic Available Yes

Pharmacologic Category Angiotensin-Converting Enzyme (ACE) Inhibitor

Use Treatment of hypertension, either alone or in combination with other antihypertensive agents; treatment of congestive heart failure, left ventricular dysfunction after myocardial infarction

Local Anesthetic/Vasoconstrictor Precautions No information available to require special precautions

Effects on Dental Treatment Key adverse event(s) related to dental treatment: Orthostatic hypotension.

Common Adverse Effects Note: Frequency ranges include data from hypertension and heart failure trials. Higher rates of adverse reactions have generally been noted in patients with CHF. However, the frequency of adverse effects associated with placebo is also increased in this population.

>10%: Central nervous system: Dizziness (2% to 12%)

1% to 10%:

- Cardiovascular: Orthostatic hypotension (1% to 2%), palpitation (1%)
- Central nervous system: Dizziness (1% to 2%; up to 12% in CHF patients), headache (3%), weakness (1%), fatigue (1% to 2%)
- Endocrine & metabolic: Hyperkalemia (2.6%)
- Gastrointestinal: Diarrhea (2%), nausea/vomiting (1.2% to 2.2%)
- Hepatic: Increased transaminases
- Neuromuscular & skeletal: Musculoskeletal pain (<1% to 3%), noncardiac chest pain (<1% to 2%)
- Renal: Increased serum creatinine, worsening of renal function (in patients with bilateral renal artery stenosis or hypovolemia)
- Respiratory: Cough (2% to 10%)
- Miscellaneous: Upper respiratory infection (2%)

>1% but ≤ frequency in patients receiving placebo: Sexual dysfunction, fever, flu-like syndrome, dyspnea, rash, headache, insomnia

Other events reported with ACE inhibitors: Neutropenia, agranulocytosis, eosinophilic pneumonitis, cardiac arrest, pancytopenia, hemolytic anemia, anemia, aplastic anemia, thrombocytopenia, acute renal failure, hepatic failure, jaundice, symptomatic hyponatremia, bullous pemphigus, exfoliative dermatitis, Stevens-Johnson syndrome. In addition, a syndrome which may include fever, myalgia, arthralgia, interstitial nephritis, vasculitis, rash, eosinophilia and positive ANA, and elevated ESR has been reported for other ACE inhibitors.

Dosage Oral:

Children >50 kg: Hypertension: Initial: 5-10 mg once daily

Adults:

- Hypertension: Initial: 10 mg/day; most patients are maintained on 20-40 mg/day. May need to divide the dose into two if trough effect is inadequate; discontinue the diuretic, if possible 2-3 days before initiation of therapy; resume diuretic therapy carefully, if needed.
- Heart failure: Initial: 10 mg/day (5 mg if renal dysfunction present) and increase, as needed, to a maximum of 40 mg once daily over several weeks; usual dose: 20-40 mg/day. If hypotension, orthostasis, or azotemia occur during titration, consider decreasing concomitant diuretic dose, if any.

Dosing adjustment/comments in renal impairment: None needed since hepatobiliary elimination compensates adequately diminished renal elimination.

Hemodialysis: Moderately dialyzable (20% to 50%)

(Continued)

Fosinopril *(Continued)*

Mechanism of Action Competitive inhibitor of angiotensin-converting enzyme (ACE); prevents conversion of angiotensin I to angiotensin II, a potent vasoconstrictor; results in lower levels of angiotensin II which causes an increase in plasma renin activity and a reduction in aldosterone secretion; a CNS mechanism may also be involved in hypotensive effect as angiotensin II increases adrenergic outflow from CNS; vasoactive kallikreins may be decreased in conversion to active hormones by ACE inhibitors, thus reducing blood pressure

Contraindications Hypersensitivity to fosinopril or any component of the formulation; angioedema related to previous treatment with an ACE inhibitor; idiopathic or hereditary angioedema; bilateral renal artery stenosis; pregnancy (2nd and 3rd trimesters)

Warnings/Precautions Anaphylactic reactions can occur. Angioedema can occur at any time during treatment (especially following first dose). Angioedema may involve head and neck (potentially affecting the airway) or the intestine (presenting with abdominal pain). Careful blood pressure monitoring (hypotension can occur especially in volume depleted patients). Dosage adjustment needed in severe renal impairment (Cl_{cr} <10 mL/minute). Use with caution in hypovolemia; collagen vascular diseases; valvular stenosis (particularly aortic stenosis); hyperkalemia; or before, during, or immediately after anesthesia. Avoid rapid dosage escalation which may lead to renal insufficiency. Hypersensitivity reactions may be seen during hemodialysis with high-flux dialysis membranes (eg, AN69). Hyperkalemia may rarely occur. Neutropenia/agranulocytosis with myeloid hyperplasia can rarely occur. If patient has renal impairment, then a baseline WBC with differential and serum creatinine should be evaluated and monitored closely during initial therapy. Use with caution in unilateral renal artery stenosis and pre-existing renal insufficiency.

Drug Interactions

Increased Effect/Toxicity: Potassium supplements, co-trimoxazole (high dose), angiotensin II receptor antagonists (eg, candesartan, losartan, irbesartan), or potassium-sparing diuretics (amiloride, spironolactone, triamterene) may result in elevated serum potassium levels when combined with fosinopril. ACE inhibitor effects may be increased by phenothiazines or probenecid (increases levels of captopril). ACE inhibitors may increase serum concentrations/effects of digoxin, lithium, and sulfonlyureas.

Diuretics have additive hypotensive effects with ACE inhibitors, and hypovolemia increases the potential for adverse renal effects of ACE inhibitors. In patients with compromised renal function, coadministration with NSAIDs may result in further deterioration of renal function. Allopurinol and ACE inhibitors may cause a higher risk of hypersensitivity reaction when taken concurrently.

Decreased Effect: Aspirin (high dose) may reduce the therapeutic effects of ACE inhibitors; at low dosages this does not appear to be significant. Rifampin may decrease the effect of ACE inhibitors. Antacids may decrease the bioavailability of ACE inhibitors (may be more likely to occur with captopril); separate administration times by 1-2 hours. NSAIDs, specifically indomethacin, may reduce the hypotensive effects of ACE inhibitors. More likely to occur in low renin or volume dependent hypertensive patients.

Ethanol/Nutrition/Herb Interactions Herb/Nutraceutical: Avoid dong quai if using for hypertension (has estrogenic activity). Avoid ephedra, garlic, yohimbe, ginseng (may worsen hypertension).

Dietary Considerations Should not take a potassium salt supplement without the advice of healthcare provider.

Pharmacodynamics/Kinetics

Onset of action: 1 hour

Duration: 24 hours

Absorption: 36%

Protein binding: 95%

Metabolism: Prodrug, hydrolyzed to its active metabolite fosinoprilat by intestinal wall and hepatic esterases

Bioavailability: 36%

Half-life elimination, serum (fosinoprilat): 12 hours

Time to peak, serum: ~3 hours

Excretion: Urine and feces (as fosinoprilat and other metabolites in roughly equal proportions, 45% to 50%)

Pregnancy Risk Factor C/D (2nd and 3rd trimesters)

Dosage Forms TAB: 10 mg, 20 mg, 40 mg

Fosinopril and Hydrochlorothiazide

(foe SIN oh pril & hye droe klor oh THYE a zide)

Related Information

Fosinopril *on page 633*

Hydrochlorothiazide *on page 699*

U.S. Brand Names Monopril-HCT®

Canadian Brand Names Monopril-HCT®

Generic Available No

Synonyms Hydrochlorothiazide and Fosinopril

Pharmacologic Category Antihypertensive Agent, Combination

Use Treatment of hypertension; not indicated for first-line treatment

Local Anesthetic/Vasoconstrictor Precautions No information available to require special precautions

Effects on Dental Treatment No significant effects or complications reported

Common Adverse Effects

2% to 10%:

Central nervous system: Headache (7%, less than placebo), fatigue (4%), dizziness (3%), orthostatic hypotension (2%)

Neuromuscular & skeletal: Musculoskeletal pain (2%)

Respiratory: Cough (6%), upper respiratory infection (2%, less than placebo)

<2%: Abdominal pain, angioedema, breast mass, BUN elevation (similar to placebo), chest pain, creatinine elevation (similar to placebo), depression, diarrhea, dyspepsia, dysuria, edema, eosinophilia, esophagitis, fever, flushing, gastritis, gout, heartburn, hepatic necrosis, leukopenia, libido change, liver function test elevations (transaminases, LDH, alkaline phosphatase, serum bilirubin), muscle cramps, myalgia, nausea, neutropenia, numbness, paresthesia, pharyngitis, pruritus, rash, rhinitis, sexual dysfunction, sinus congestion, somnolence, syncope, tinnitus, urinary frequency, urinary tract infection, viral infection, vomiting, weakness

Other adverse events reported with **ACE inhibitors**: Aplastic anemia, bullous pemphigus, cardiac arrest, cholestatic jaundice, exfoliative dermatitis, hemolytic anemia, hyperkalemia, pancreatitis, pancytopenia, photosensitivity; syndrome that may include one or more of arthralgia/arthritis, vasculitis, serositis, myalgia, fever, rash or other dermopathy, positive ANA titer, leukocytosis, eosinophilia, and elevated ESR; thrombocytopenia

Other adverse events reported with **hydrochlorothiazide**: Agranulocytosis, anaphylactic reactions, anorexia, blurred vision (transient), constipation, cramping, glucosuria, hemolytic anemia, hypercalcemia, hyperglycemia, hyperuricemia, hypokalemia, jaundice (intrahepatic cholestatic), lightheadedness, muscle spasm, necrotizing angiitis, pancreatitis, photosensitivity, pneumonitis, pulmonary edema, purpura, respiratory distress, restlessness, sialadenitis, SLE, Stevens-Johnson syndrome, urticaria, vertigo, xanthopsia

Mechanism of Action Fosinopril is a competitive inhibitor of angiotensin-converting enzyme (ACE); prevents conversion of angiotensin I to angiotensin II, a potent vasoconstrictor; results in lower levels of angiotensin II which causes an increase in plasma renin activity and a reduction in aldosterone secretion; a CNS mechanism may also be involved in hypotensive effect as angiotensin II increases adrenergic outflow from CNS; vasoactive kallikreins may be decreased in conversion to active hormones by ACE inhibitors, thus reducing blood pressure. Hydrochlorothiazide inhibits sodium reabsorption in the distal tubules causing increased excretion of sodium and water as well as potassium and hydrogen ions.

Drug Interactions

Increased Effect/Toxicity: Alpha$_1$ blockers, diuretics increase hypotension. Beta blockers may increase hyperglycemic effect. Cyclosporine may increase risk of gout or renal toxicity. Risk of lithium toxicity may be increased. Mercaptopurine may increase risk of neutropenia. Digoxin and neuromuscular-blocking agents: Effects may be increased with hypokalemia. Potassium-sparing diuretics, potassium supplements, trimethoprim may increase risk of hyperkalemia.

Decreased Effect: Aspirin, NSAIDs may decrease antihypertensive effect. Antacids, cholestyramine, colestipol may decrease absorption.

Pharmacodynamics/Kinetics See individual agents.

Pregnancy Risk Factor C (1st trimester); D (2nd and 3rd trimester)

Fosphenytoin (FOS fen i toyn)

Related Information

Phenytoin *on page 1080*

U.S. Brand Names Cerebyx®

(Continued)

Fosphenytoin *(Continued)*

Canadian Brand Names Cerebyx®

Generic Available No

Synonyms Fosphenytoin Sodium

Pharmacologic Category Anticonvulsant, Hydantoin

Use Used for the control of generalized convulsive status epilepticus and prevention and treatment of seizures occurring during neurosurgery; indicated for short-term parenteral administration when other means of phenytoin administration are unavailable, inappropriate or deemed less advantageous (the safety and effectiveness of fosphenytoin in this use has not been systematically evaluated for more than 5 days)

Local Anesthetic/Vasoconstrictor Precautions No information available to require special precautions

Effects on Dental Treatment No significant effects or complications reported

Common Adverse Effects The more important adverse clinical events caused by the I.V. use of fosphenytoin or phenytoin are cardiovascular collapse and/or central nervous system depression. Hypotension can occur when either drug is administered rapidly by the I.V. route. Do not exceed a rate of 150 mg phenytoin equivalent/minute when administering fosphenytoin.

The adverse clinical events most commonly observed with the use of fosphenytoin in clinical trials were nystagmus, dizziness, pruritus, paresthesia, headache, somnolence, and ataxia. Paresthesia and pruritus were seen more often following fosphenytoin (versus phenytoin) administration and occurred more often with I.V. fosphenytoin than with I.M. administration. These events were dose- and rate-related (doses ≥15 mg/kg at a rate of 150 mg/minute). These sensations, generally described as itching, burning, or tingling are usually not at the infusion site. The location of the discomfort varied with the groin mentioned most frequently. The paresthesia and pruritus were transient events that occurred within several minutes of the start of infusion and generally resolved within 10 minutes after completion of infusion.

Transient pruritus, tinnitus, nystagmus, somnolence, and ataxia occurred 2-3 times more often at doses ≥15 mg/kg and rates ≥150 mg/minute.

I.V. administration (maximum dose/rate):

>10%:

Central nervous system: Nystagmus, dizziness, somnolence, ataxia
Dermatologic: Pruritus

1% to 10%:

Cardiovascular: Hypotension, vasodilation, tachycardia
Central nervous system: Stupor, incoordination, paresthesia, extrapyramidal syndrome, tremor, agitation, hypesthesia, dysarthria, vertigo, brain edema, headache
Gastrointestinal: Nausea, tongue disorder, dry mouth, vomiting
Neuromuscular & skeletal: Pelvic pain, muscle weakness, back pain
Ocular: Diplopia, amblyopia
Otic: Tinnitus, deafness
Miscellaneous: Taste perversion

I.M. administration (substitute for oral phenytoin):

1% to 10%:

Central nervous system: Nystagmus, tremor, ataxia, headache, incoordination, somnolence, dizziness, paresthesia, reflexes decreased
Dermatologic: Pruritus
Gastrointestinal: Nausea, vomiting
Hematologic/lymphatic: Ecchymosis
Neuromuscular & skeletal: Muscle weakness

Mechanism of Action Diphosphate ester salt of phenytoin which acts as a water soluble prodrug of phenytoin; after administration, plasma esterases convert fosphenytoin to phosphate, formaldehyde and phenytoin as the active moiety; phenytoin works by stabilizing neuronal membranes and decreasing seizure activity by increasing efflux or decreasing influx of sodium ions across cell membranes in the motor cortex during generation of nerve impulses

Drug Interactions

Cytochrome P450 Effect: As phenytoin: **Substrate** of CYP2C8/9 (major), 2C19 (major), 3A4 (minor); **Induces** CYP2B6 (strong), 2C8/9 (strong), 2C19 (strong), 3A4 (strong)

Increased Effect/Toxicity: The sedative effects of phenytoin may be additive with other CNS depressants including ethanol, barbiturates, sedatives, antidepressants, narcotic analgesics, and benzodiazepines. Selected anticonvulsants (felbamate, gabapentin, and topiramate) have been reported to increase phenytoin levels/effects. In addition, serum phenytoin concentrations may be increased by allopurinol, amiodarone, calcium channel blockers (including diltiazem and nifedipine), cimetidine, disulfiram, methylphenidate, metronidazole, omeprazole, selective serotonin reuptake inhibitors (SSRIs), ticlopidine, tricyclic antidepressants, trazodone, and trimethoprim. Case reports indicate ciprofloxacin may increase or decrease serum phenytoin concentrations.

The levels/effects of phenytoin may be increased by delavirdine, fluconazole, fluvoxamine, gemfibrozil, isoniazid, ketoconazole, nicardipine, NSAIDs, omeprazole, pioglitazone, sulfonamides, ticlopidine, and other CYP2C8/9 or 2C19 inhibitors.

Phenytoin enhances the conversion of primidone to phenobarbital resulting in elevated phenobarbital serum concentrations. Concurrent use of acetazolamide with phenytoin may result in an increased risk of osteomalacia. Concurrent use of phenytoin and lithium has resulted in lithium intoxication. Valproic acid (and sulfisoxazole) may displace phenytoin from binding sites; valproic acid may increase, decrease, or have no effect on phenytoin serum concentrations. Phenytoin transiently increased the response to warfarin initially; this is followed by an inhibition of the hypoprothrombinemic response. Phenytoin may enhance the hepatotoxic potential of acetaminophen overdoses. Concurrent use of dopamine and intravenous phenytoin may lead to an increased risk of hypotension.

Decreased Effect: Phenytoin may enhance the metabolism of estrogen and/or oral contraceptives, decreasing their clinical effect; an alternative method of contraception should be considered. Phenytoin may increase the metabolism of anticonvulsants including barbiturates, carbamazepine, ethosuximide, felbamate, lamotrigine, tiagabine, topiramate, and zonisamide. Valproic acid may increase, decrease, or have no effect on phenytoin serum concentrations. Phenytoin may also decrease the serum concentrations/effects of some antiarrhythmics (disopyramide, propafenone, quinidine, quetiapine) and tricyclic antidepressants may be reduced by phenytoin. Phenytoin may enhance the metabolism of doxycycline, decreasing its clinical effect; higher dosages may be required. Phenytoin may increase the metabolism of chloramphenicol or itraconazole.

Phenytoin may decrease the levels/effects of amiodarone, benzodiazepines, bupropion, calcium channel blockers, carbamazepine, citalopram, clarithromycin, cyclosporine, efavirenz, erythromycin, estrogens, fluoxetine, glimepiride, glipizide, losartan, methsuximide, mirtazapine, nateglinide, nefazodone, nevirapine, phenytoin, pioglitazone, promethazine, propranolol, protease inhibitors, proton pump inhibitors, rosiglitazone, selegiline, sertraline, sulfonamides, tacrolimus, venlafaxine. voriconazole, warfarin, zafirlukast, and other CYP2B6, 2C8/9, 2C19, or 3A4 substrates.

The levels/effects of phenytoin may be decreased by aminoglutethimide, carbamazepine, phenobarbital, rifampin, rifapentine, secobarbital, and other CYP2C8/9 or 2C19 inducers. Clozapine and vigabatrin may reduce phenytoin serum concentrations. Case reports indicate ciprofloxacin may increase or decrease serum phenytoin concentrations. Dexamethasone may decrease serum phenytoin concentrations. Replacement of folic acid has been reported to increase the metabolism of phenytoin, decreasing its serum concentrations and/or increasing seizures.

Initially, phenytoin increases the response to warfarin; this is followed by a decrease in response to warfarin. Phenytoin may inhibit the anti-Parkinson effect of levodopa. The duration of neuromuscular blockade from neuromuscular-blocking agents may be decreased by phenytoin. Phenytoin may enhance the metabolism of methadone resulting in methadone withdrawal. Phenytoin may decrease serum levels/effects of digitalis glycosides, theophylline, and thyroid hormones.

Several chemotherapeutic agents have been associated with a decrease in serum phenytoin levels; includes cisplatin, bleomycin, carmustine, methotrexate, and vinblastine. Enzyme-inducing anticonvulsant therapy may reduce the effectiveness of some chemotherapy regimens (specifically in ALL). Teniposide and methotrexate may be cleared more rapidly in these patients.

Pharmacodynamics/Kinetics Also refer to Phenytoin monograph for additional information.

Protein binding: Fosphenytoin: 95% to 99% to albumin; can displace phenytoin and increase free fraction (up to 30% unbound) during the period required for conversion of fosphenytoin to phenytoin

(Continued)

Fosphenytoin *(Continued)*

Metabolism: Fosphenytoin is rapidly converted via hydrolysis to phenytoin; phenytoin is metabolized in the liver and forms metabolites
Bioavailability: I.M.: Fosphenytoin: 100%
Half-life elimination:
Fosphenytoin: 15 minutes
Phenytoin: Variable (mean: 12-29 hours); kinetics of phenytoin are saturable
Time to peak: Conversion to phenytoin: Following I.V. administration (maximum rate of administration): 15 minutes; following I.M. administration, peak phenytoin levels are reached in 3 hours
Excretion: Phenytoin: Urine (as inactive metabolites)

Pregnancy Risk Factor D

Fosphenytoin Sodium *see* Fosphenytoin *on page 635*

Fostex® 10% BPO [OTC] *see* Benzoyl Peroxide *on page 194*

Fragmin® *see* Dalteparin *on page 395*

Freezone® [OTC] *see* Salicylic Acid *on page 1205*

Frova® *see* Frovatriptan *on page 638*

Frovatriptan (froe va TRIP tan)

U.S. Brand Names Frova®

Generic Available No

Synonyms Frovatriptan Succinate

Pharmacologic Category Antimigraine Agent; Serotonin 5-$HT_{1B, 1D}$ Receptor Agonist

Use Acute treatment of migraine with or without aura in adults

Local Anesthetic/Vasoconstrictor Precautions No information available to require special precautions

Effects on Dental Treatment Key adverse event(s) related to dental treatment: Xerostomia (normal salivary flow resumes upon discontinuation).

Common Adverse Effects 1% to 10%:
Cardiovascular: Chest pain (2%), flushing (4%), palpitation (1%)
Central nervous system: Dizziness (8%), fatigue (5%), headache (4%), hot or cold sensation (3%), anxiety (1%), dysesthesia (1%), hypoesthesia (1%), insomnia (1%), pain (1%)
Gastrointestinal: Hyposalivation (3%), dyspepsia (2%), abdominal pain (1%), diarrhea (1%), vomiting (1%)
Neuromuscular & skeletal: Paresthesia (4%), skeletal pain (3%)
Ocular: Visual abnormalities (1%)
Otic: Tinnitus (1%)
Respiratory: Rhinitis (1%), sinusitis (1%)
Miscellaneous: Diaphoresis (1%)

Mechanism of Action Selective agonist for serotonin (5-HT_{1B} and 5-HT_{1D} receptor) in cranial arteries to cause vasoconstriction and reduces sterile inflammation associated with antidromic neuronal transmission correlating with relief of migraine.

Drug Interactions

Cytochrome P450 Effect: Substrate of CYP1A2 (minor)

Increased Effect/Toxicity: The effects of frovatriptan may be increased by estrogen derivatives and propranolol. Ergot derivatives may increase the effects of frovatriptan (do not use within 24 hours of each other). SSRIs may exhibit additive toxicity with frovatriptan or other serotonin agonists (eg, antidepressants, dextromethorphan, tramadol) leading to serotonin syndrome.

Pharmacodynamics/Kinetics
Distribution: Male: 4.2 L/kg; Female: 3.0 L/kg
Protein binding: 15%
Metabolism: Primarily hepatic via CYP1A2
Bioavailability: 20% to 30%
Half-life elimination: 26 hours
Time to peak: 2-4 hours
Excretion: Feces (62%); urine (32%)

Pregnancy Risk Factor C

Frovatriptan Succinate *see* Frovatriptan *on page 638*

Fructose, Dextrose, and Phosphoric Acid

(FRUK tose, DEKS trose, & foss FOR ik AS id)

U.S. Brand Names Emetrol® [OTC]; Especol® [OTC]; Formula EM [OTC]; Kalmz [OTC]; Nausea Relief [OTC]; Nausetrol® [OTC]

Generic Available Yes

Synonyms Dextrose, Levulose and Phosphoric Acid; Levulose, Dextrose and Phosphoric Acid; Phosphorated Carbohydrate Solution; Phosphoric Acid, Levulose and Dextrose

Pharmacologic Category Antiemetic

Use Relief of nausea associated with upset stomach that occurs with intestinal flu, food indiscretions, and emotional upsets

Unlabeled/Investigational Use Relief of nausea associated with pregnancy

Local Anesthetic/Vasoconstrictor Precautions No information available to require special precautions

Effects on Dental Treatment No significant effects or complications reported

Common Adverse Effects 1% to 10%: Gastrointestinal: Abdominal pain, diarrhea

Frusemide *see* Furosemide *on page 640*
FS *see* Fibrin Sealant Kit *on page 589*
FTC *see* Emtricitabine *on page 487*
FU *see* Fluorouracil *on page 605*
5-FU *see* Fluorouracil *on page 605*
FUDR® *see* Floxuridine *on page 593*
5-FUDR *see* Floxuridine *on page 593*

Fulvestrant (fool VES trant)

U.S. Brand Names Faslodex®

Generic Available No

Synonyms ICI 182,780; Zeneca 182,780; ZM-182,780

Pharmacologic Category Antineoplastic Agent, Estrogen Receptor Antagonist

Use Treatment of hormone receptor positive metastatic breast cancer in postmenopausal women with disease progression following antiestrogen therapy.

Unlabeled/Investigational Use Endometriosis; uterine bleeding

Local Anesthetic/Vasoconstrictor Precautions No information available to require special precautions

Effects on Dental Treatment No significant effects or complications reported

Common Adverse Effects

>10%:
- Cardiovascular: Vasodilation (18%)
- Central nervous system: Pain (19%), headache (15%)
- Endocrine & metabolic: Hot flushes (19% to 24%)
- Gastrointestinal: Nausea (26%), vomiting (13%), constipation (13%), diarrhea (12%), abdominal pain (12%)
- Local: Injection site reaction (11%)
- Neuromuscular & skeletal: Weakness (23%), bone pain (16%), back pain (14%)
- Respiratory: Pharyngitis (16%), dyspnea (15%)

1% to 10%:
- Cardiovascular: Edema (9%), chest pain (7%)
- Central nervous system: Dizziness (7%), insomnia (7%), paresthesia (6%), fever (6%), depression (6%), anxiety (5%)
- Dermatologic: Rash (7%)
- Gastrointestinal: Anorexia (9%), weight gain (1% to 2%)
- Genitourinary: Pelvic pain (10%), urinary tract infection (6%), vaginitis (2% to 3%)
- Hematologic: Anemia (5%)
- Neuromuscular and skeletal: Arthritis (3%)
- Respiratory: Cough (10%)
- Miscellaneous: Diaphoresis increased (5%)

Mechanism of Action Steroidal compound which competitively binds to estrogen receptors on tumors and other tissue targets, producing a nuclear complex that decreases DNA synthesis and inhibits estrogen effects. Fulvestrant has no estrogen-receptor agonist activity. Causes down-regulation of estrogen receptors and inhibits tumor growth.

Drug Interactions

Cytochrome P450 Effect: Substrate of CYP3A4 (minor)

Pharmacodynamics/Kinetics

Duration: I.M.: Plasma levels maintained for at least 1 month
Distribution: V_d: 3-5 L/kg
Protein binding: 99%
Metabolism: Hepatic via multiple pathways (CYP3A4 substrate, relative contribution to metabolism unknown)
Bioavailability: Oral: Poor
Half-life elimination: ~40 days
(Continued)

Fulvestrant *(Continued)*

Time to peak, plasma: I.M.: 7-9 days
Excretion: Feces (>90%); urine (<1%)

Pregnancy Risk Factor D

Fulvicin® P/G *see* Griseofulvin *on page 671*
Fulvicin-U/F® *see* Griseofulvin *on page 671*
Fungi-Guard [OTC] *see* Tolnaftate *on page 1312*
Fungi-Nail® [OTC] *see* Undecylenic Acid and Derivatives *on page 1352*
Fungizone® *see* Amphotericin B (Conventional) *on page 120*
Fung-O® [OTC] *see* Salicylic Acid *on page 1205*
Fungoid® Tincture [OTC] *see* Miconazole *on page 922*
Furadantin® *see* Nitrofurantoin *on page 990*

Furazolidone (fyoor a ZOE li done)

Canadian Brand Names Furoxone®

Mexican Brand Names Furoxona®; Fuxol®; Salmocide®

Generic Available No

Synonyms Furoxone

Pharmacologic Category Antiprotozoal

Use Treatment of bacterial or protozoal diarrhea and enteritis caused by susceptible organisms *Giardia lamblia* and *Vibrio cholerae*

Local Anesthetic/Vasoconstrictor Precautions No information available to require special precautions

Effects on Dental Treatment No significant effects or complications reported

Common Adverse Effects

>10%: Genitourinary: Discoloration of urine (dark yellow to brown)
1% to 10%:
Central nervous system: Headache
Gastrointestinal: Abdominal pain, diarrhea, nausea, vomiting

Restrictions Not available in U.S.

Mechanism of Action Inhibits several vital enzymatic reactions causing antibacterial and antiprotozoal action

Drug Interactions

Increased Effect/Toxicity: Increased effect with sympathomimetic amines, tricyclic antidepressants, tyramine-containing foods, MAO inhibitors, meperidine, anorexiants, dextromethorphan, fluoxetine, paroxetine, sertraline, and trazodone. Increased effect/toxicity of levodopa. Disulfiram-like reaction with alcohol.

Pharmacodynamics/Kinetics

Absorption: Poor
Excretion: Urine (33% as active drug and metabolites)

Pregnancy Risk Factor C

Furazosin *see* Prazosin *on page 1111*

Furosemide (fyoor OH se mide)

Related Information

Cardiovascular Diseases *on page 1458*

U.S. Brand Names Lasix®

Canadian Brand Names Apo-Furosemide®; Lasix®; Lasix® Special

Mexican Brand Names Edenol®; Lasix®; Selectofur® [tabs]; Zafimida®

Generic Available Yes

Synonyms Frusemide

Pharmacologic Category Diuretic, Loop

Use Management of edema associated with congestive heart failure and hepatic or renal disease; alone or in combination with antihypertensives in treatment of hypertension

Local Anesthetic/Vasoconstrictor Precautions No information available to require special precautions

Effects on Dental Treatment No significant effects or complications reported

Common Adverse Effects Frequency not defined.

Cardiovascular: Orthostatic hypotension, necrotizing angiitis, thrombophlebitis, chronic aortitis, acute hypotension, sudden death from cardiac arrest (with I.V. or I.M. administration)

Central nervous system: Paresthesias, vertigo, dizziness, lightheadedness, headache, blurred vision, xanthopsia , fever, restlessness

Dermatologic: Exfoliative dermatitis, erythema multiforme, purpura, photosensitivity, urticaria, rash, pruritus, cutaneous vasculitis

Endocrine & metabolic: Hyperglycemia, hyperuricemia, hypokalemia, hypochloremia, metabolic alkalosis, hypocalcemia, hypomagnesemia, gout, hypernatremia

Gastrointestinal: Nausea, vomiting, anorexia, oral and gastric irritation, cramping, diarrhea, constipation, pancreatitis, intrahepatic cholestatic jaundice, ischemia hepatitis

Genitourinary: Urinary bladder spasm, urinary frequency

Hematological: Aplastic anemia (rare), thrombocytopenia, agranulocytosis (rare), hemolytic anemia, leukopenia, anemia, purpura

Neuromuscular & skeletal: Muscle spasm, weakness

Otic: Hearing impairment (reversible or permanent with rapid I.V. or I.M. administration), tinnitus, reversible deafness (with rapid I.V. or I.M. administration)

Renal: Vasculitis, allergic interstitial nephritis, glycosuria, fall in glomerular filtration rate and renal blood flow (due to overdiuresis), transient rise in BUN

Miscellaneous: Anaphylaxis (rare), exacerbate or activate systemic lupus erythematosus

Dosage

Infants and Children:

Oral: 1-2 mg/kg/dose increased in increments of 1 mg/kg/dose with each succeeding dose until a satisfactory effect is achieved to a maximum of 6 mg/kg/dose no more frequently than 6 hours.

I.M., I.V.: 1 mg/kg/dose, increasing by each succeeding dose at 1 mg/kg/dose at intervals of 6-12 hours until a satisfactory response up to 6 mg/kg/dose.

Adults:

Oral: 20-80 mg/dose initially increased in increments of 20-40 mg/dose at intervals of 6-8 hours; usual maintenance dose interval is twice daily or every day; may be titrated up to 600 mg/day with severe edematous states. Hypertension (JNC 7): 20-80 mg/day in 2 divided doses

I.M., I.V.: 20-40 mg/dose, may be repeated in 1-2 hours as needed and increased by 20 mg/dose until the desired effect has been obtained. Usual dosing interval: 6-12 hours; for acute pulmonary edema, the usual dose is 40 mg I.V. over 1-2 minutes. If not adequate, may increase dose to 80 mg.

Continuous I.V. infusion: Initial I.V. bolus dose of 0.1 mg/kg followed by continuous I.V. infusion doses of 0.1 mg/kg/hour doubled every 2 hours to a maximum of 0.4 mg/kg/hour if urine output is <1 mL/kg/hour have been found to be effective and result in a lower daily requirement of furosemide than with intermittent dosing. Other studies have used a rate of ≤4 mg/minute as a continuous I.V. infusion.

Elderly: Oral, I.M., I.V.: Initial: 20 mg/day; increase slowly to desired response.

Adults and Elderly: Refractory heart failure: Oral, I.V.: Doses up to 8 g/day have been used.

Dosing adjustment/comments in renal impairment: Acute renal failure: High doses (up to 1-3 g/day - oral/I.V.) have been used to initiate desired response; avoid use in oliguric states.

Dialysis: Not removed by hemo- or peritoneal dialysis; supplemental dose is not necessary.

Dosing adjustment/comments in hepatic disease: Diminished natriuretic effect with increased sensitivity to hypokalemia and volume depletion in cirrhosis; monitor effects, particularly with high doses.

Mechanism of Action Inhibits reabsorption of sodium and chloride in the ascending loop of Henle and distal renal tubule, interfering with the chloride-binding cotransport system, thus causing increased excretion of water, sodium, chloride, magnesium, and calcium

Contraindications Hypersensitivity to furosemide, any component, or sulfonylureas; anuria; patients with hepatic coma or in states of severe electrolyte depletion until the condition improves or is corrected

Warnings/Precautions Loop diuretics are potent diuretics; close medical supervision and dose evaluation is required to prevent fluid and electrolyte imbalance; use caution with other nephrotoxic or ototoxic drugs; use caution in patients with known hypersensitivity to sulfonamides or thiazides (due to possible cross-sensitivity; avoid in history of severe reactions).

Chemical similarities are present among sulfonamides, sulfonylureas, carbonic anhydrase inhibitors, thiazides, and loop diuretics (except ethacrynic acid). Use in patients with sulfonylurea allergy is specifically contraindicated in product labeling, however, a risk of cross-reaction exists in patients with allergy to any of these compounds; avoid use when previous reaction has been severe.

Drug Interactions

Increased Effect/Toxicity: Furosemide-induced hypokalemia may predispose to digoxin toxicity and may increase the risk of arrhythmia with drugs

(Continued)

Furosemide *(Continued)*

which may prolong QT interval, including type Ia and type III antiarrhythmic agents, cisapride, and some quinolones (sparfloxacin, gatifloxacin, and moxifloxacin). The risk of toxicity from lithium and salicylates (high dose) may be increased by loop diuretics. Hypotensive effects and/or adverse renal effects of ACE inhibitors and NSAIDs are potentiated by furosemide-induced hypovolemia. The effects of peripheral adrenergic-blocking drugs or ganglionic blockers may be increased by furosemide.

Furosemide may increase the risk of ototoxicity with other ototoxic agents (aminoglycosides, cis-platinum), especially in patients with renal dysfunction. Synergistic diuretic effects occur with thiazide-type diuretics. Diuretics tend to be synergistic with other antihypertensive agents, and hypotension may occur.

Decreased Effect: Indomethacin, aspirin, phenobarbital, phenytoin, and NSAIDs may reduce natriuretic and hypotensive effects of furosemide. Colestipol, cholestyramine, and sucralfate may reduce the effect of furosemide; separate administration by 2 hours. Furosemide may antagonize the effect of skeletal muscle relaxants (tubocurarine). Glucose tolerance may be decreased by furosemide, requiring an adjustment in the dose of hypoglycemic agents. Metformin may decrease furosemide concentrations.

Ethanol/Nutrition/Herb Interactions

Food: Furosemide serum levels may be decreased if taken with food.

Herb/Nutraceutical: Avoid dong quai if using for hypertension (has estrogenic activity). Avoid ephedra, yohimbe, ginseng (may worsen hypertension). Limit intake of natural licorice. Avoid garlic (may have increased antihypertensive effect).

Dietary Considerations This product may cause a potassium loss; your healthcare provider may prescribe a potassium supplement, another medication to help prevent the potassium loss, or recommend that you eat foods high in potassium, especially citrus fruits; do not change your diet on your own while taking this medication, especially if you are taking potassium supplements or medications to reduce potassium loss; too much potassium can be as harmful as too little; ideally, should be administered on an empty stomach; however, may be administered with food or milk if GI distress; do not mix with acidic solutions. Sodium content of 1 mL (injection): 0.162 mEq

Pharmacodynamics/Kinetics

Onset of action: Diuresis: Oral: 30-60 minutes; I.M.: 30 minutes; I.V.: ~5 minutes

Peak effect: Oral: 1-2 hours

Duration: Oral: 6-8 hours; I.V.: 2 hours

Absorption: Oral: 60% to 67%

Protein binding: >98%

Metabolism: Minimally hepatic

Half-life elimination: Normal renal function: 0.5-1.1 hours; End-stage renal disease: 9 hours

Excretion: Urine (Oral: 50%, I.V.: 80%) within 24 hours; feces (as unchanged drug); nonrenal clearance prolonged in renal impairment

Pregnancy Risk Factor C

Dosage Forms INJ, solution: 10 mg/mL (2 mL, 4 mL, 8 mL, 10 mL). **SOLN, oral:** 10 mg/mL (60 mL, 120 mL); 40 mg/5 mL (5 mL, 500 mL). **TAB** (Lasix®): 20 mg, 40 mg, 80 mg

Furoxone *see* Furazolidone *on page 640*

Fuzeon™ *see* Enfuvirtide *on page 492*

Gabapentin (GA ba pen tin)

U.S. Brand Names Neurontin®

Canadian Brand Names Apo-Gabapentin®; Neurontin®; Novo-Gabapentin; Nu-Gabapentin; PMS-Gabapentin

Mexican Brand Names Neurontin®

Generic Available No

Pharmacologic Category Anticonvulsant, Miscellaneous

Use Adjunct for treatment of partial seizures with and without secondary generalized seizures in patients >12 years of age with epilepsy; adjunct for treatment of partial seizures in pediatric patients 3-12 years of age; management of post-herpetic neuralgia (PHN) in adults

Unlabeled/Investigational Use Bipolar disorder, social phobia; chronic pain

Local Anesthetic/Vasoconstrictor Precautions No information available to require special precautions

Effects on Dental Treatment Key adverse event(s) related to dental treatment: Xerostomia (normal salivary flow resumes upon discontinuation), dry throat, and dental abnormalities.

Significant Adverse Effects As reported in patients >12 years of age, unless otherwise noted

>10%:

Central nervous system: Somnolence (20%), dizziness (17%), ataxia (12%), fatigue (11% in adults)

Miscellaneous: Viral infection (11% in children 3-12 years)

1% to 10%:

Cardiovascular: Peripheral edema (2%)

Central nervous system: Fever (10% in children 3-12 years), hostility (8% in children 3-12 years), somnolence (8% in children 3-12 years), emotional lability (4% to 6% in children 3-12 years), fatigue (3% in children 3-12 years), abnormal thinking (2% in children and adults), amnesia (2%), depression (2%), dizziness (2% in children 3-12 years), dysarthria (2%), nervousness (2%), abnormal coordination (1%), twitching (1%)

Dermatologic: Pruritus (1%)

Gastrointestinal: Nausea/vomiting (8% in children 3-12 years), weight gain (3% in adults and children), dyspepsia (2%), dry throat (2%), xerostomia (2%), appetite stimulation (1%), constipation (1%), dental abnormalities (1%)

Genitourinary: Impotence (1%)

Hematologic: Leukopenia (1%), decreased WBC (1%)

Neuromuscular & skeletal: Tremor (7%), hyperkinesia (3% to 5% in children 3-12 years), back pain (2%), myalgia (2%)

Ocular: Nystagmus (8%), diplopia (6%), blurred vision (4%)

Respiratory: Rhinitis (4%), bronchitis (3% in children 3-12 years), pharyngitis (3%), coughing (2%), respiratory infection (2% in children 3-12 years)

<1% (Limited to important or life-threatening): Allergy, alopecia, angina pectoris, angioedema, erythema multiforme, ethanol intolerance, hepatitis, hyperlipidemia, hypertension, hyponatremia, intracranial hemorrhage, jaundice, new tumor formation/worsening of existing tumors, pancreatitis, peripheral vascular disorder, pneumonia, purpura, Stevens-Johnson syndrome, subdural hematoma, vertigo

Dosage Oral:

Children: Anticonvulsant:

3-12 years: Initial: 10-15 mg/kg/day in 3 divided doses; titrate to effective dose over ~3 days; dosages of up to 50 mg/kg/day have been tolerated in clinical studies

3-4 years: Effective dose: 40 mg/kg/day in 3 divided doses

≥5-12 years: Effective dose: 25-35 mg/kg/day in 3 divided doses

Note: If gabapentin is discontinued or if another anticonvulsant is added to therapy, it should be done slowly over a minimum of 1 week

Children >12 years and Adults:

Anticonvulsant: Initial: 300 mg 3 times/day; if necessary the dose may be increased using 300 mg or 400 mg capsules 3 times/day up to 1800 mg/day

Dosage range: 900-1800 mg administered in 3 divided doses at 8-hour intervals

Pain (unlabeled use): 300-1800 mg/day given in 3 divided doses has been the most common dosage range

Bipolar disorder (unlabeled use): 300-3000 mg/day given in 3 divided doses; **Note:** Does not appear to be effective as an adjunctive treatment for bipolar disorder (Pande AC, 2000)

Neurontin® Dosing Adjustments in Renal Impairment

Creatinine Clearance (mL/min)	Total Daily Dose Range (mg/day)	Dosage Regimens Based on Renal Function (mg)				
≥60	900-3600	300 tid	400 tid	600 tid	800 tid	1200 tid
>30-59	400-1400	200 bid	300 bid	400 bid	500 bid	700 bid
>15-29	200-700	200 qd	300 qd	400 qd	500 qd	700 qd
15[1]	100-300	100 qd	125 qd	150 qd	200 qd	300 qd
Hemodialysis[2]		Posthemodialysis Supplemental Dose				
		125 mg	150 mg	200 mg	250 mg	350 mg

[1]Cl_{cr}<15 mL/minute: Reduce daily dose in proportion to creatinine clearance.

[2]Supplemental dose administered after each 4 hours of hemodialysis (maintenance doses based on renal function).

Adults: Post-herpetic neuralgia: Day 1: 300 mg, Day 2: 300 mg twice daily, Day 3: 300 mg 3 times/day; dose may be titrated as needed for pain relief

(Continued)

Gabapentin *(Continued)*

(range: 1800-3600 mg/day, daily doses >1800 mg do not generally show greater benefit)

Elderly: Studies in elderly patients have shown a decrease in clearance as age increases. This is most likely due to age-related decreases in renal function; dose reductions may be needed.

Dosing adjustment in renal impairment: Children ≥12 years and Adults: See table on previous page.

Mechanism of Action Exact mechanism of action is not known, but does have properties in common with other anticonvulsants; although structurally related to GABA, it does not interact with GABA receptors

Contraindications Hypersensitivity to gabapentin or any component of the formulation

Warnings/Precautions Avoid abrupt withdrawal, may precipitate seizures; may be associated with a slight incidence (0.6%) of status epilepticus and sudden deaths (0.0038 deaths/patient year); use cautiously in patients with severe renal dysfunction; rat studies demonstrated an association with pancreatic adenocarcinoma in male rats; clinical implication unknown. May cause CNS depression, which may impair physical or mental abilities. Patients must be cautioned about performing tasks which require mental alertness (eg, operating machinery or driving). Effects with other sedative drugs or ethanol may be potentiated. Pediatric patients (3-12 years of age) have shown increased incidence of CNS-related adverse effects, including emotional lability, hostility, thought disorder, and hyperkinesia. Safety and efficacy in children <3 years of age have not been established.

Drug Interactions

Antacids: Antacids may reduce the bioavailability of gabapentin by ~20%; gabapentin should be taken at least 2 hours following antacid administration

Cimetidine: Cimetidine may increase gabapentin serum concentrations; clearance of gabapentin is decreased by 14%

Felbamate: Serum concentrations may be increased by gabapentin; monitor for increased felbamate effect/toxicity

Morphine: Serum concentrations of gabapentin may be increased during concurrent use.

Norethindrone: Gabapentin may increase C_{max} of norethindrone by 13%

Phenytoin: Phenytoin serum concentrations may be increased by gabapentin; limited documentation; monitor. **Note:** Valproic acid, carbamazepine, and phenobarbital do not seem to be affected by gabapentin.

Ethanol/Nutrition/Herb Interactions

Ethanol: Avoid ethanol (may increase CNS depression).

Food: Does not change rate or extent of absorption.

Herb/Nutraceutical: Avoid evening primrose (seizure threshold decreased). Avoid valerian, St John's wort, kava kava, gotu kola (may increase CNS depression).

Dietary Considerations May be taken without regard to meals.

Pharmacodynamics/Kinetics

Absorption: 50% to 60%

Distribution: V_d: 0.6-0.8 L/kg

Protein binding: 0%

Bioavailability: As gabapentin dose increases, bioavailability decreases; it is absorbed from proximal small bowel into blood by L-amino transport system (which becomes saturated, therefore is a major contributor to lack of proportionality in plasma levels). Interpatient variability exists; standard gabapentin doses may result in different plasma concentrations in individual patients.

900 mg divided 3 times/day: 60%
1200 mg divided 3 times/day: 47%
2400 mg divided 3 times/day: 34%
3600 mg divided 3 times/day: 33%
4800 mg divided 3 times/day: 27%

Half-life elimination: 5-6 hours

Excretion: Urine (56% to 80%)

Pregnancy Risk Factor C

Lactation Excretion in breast milk unknown/not recommended

Breast-Feeding Considerations Gabapentin is excreted in human breast milk. A nursed infant could be exposed to ~1 mg/kg/day of gabapentin; the effect on the child is not known. Use in breast-feeding women only if the benefits to the mother outweigh the potential risk to the infant.

Dosage Forms

Capsule: 100 mg, 300 mg, 400 mg

Solution, oral: 250 mg/5 mL (480 mL) [cool strawberry anise flavor]

Tablet: 600 mg, 800 mg

Selected Readings

Laird MA and Gidal BE, "Use of Gabapentin in the Treatment of Neuropathic Pain," *Ann Pharmacother*, 2000, 34(6):802-7.

Rose MA and Kam PCA, "Gabapentin: Pharmacology and Its Use in Pain Management," *Anaesthesia*, 2002, 57:451-62.

Rosenberg JM, Harrell C, Ristic H, et al, "The Effect of Gabapentin on Neuropathic Pain," *Clin J Pain*, 1997, 13(3):251-5.

Rowbotham M, Harden N, Stacey B, et al, "Gabapentin for the Treatment of Postherpetic Neuralgia: A Randomized Controlled Trial," *JAMA*, 1998, 280(21):1837-42.

Gabitril® *see* Tiagabine *on page 1294*

Gadoteridol *see* Radiological/Contrast Media (Nonionic) *on page 1166*

Galantamine (ga LAN ta meen)

U.S. Brand Names Reminyl®

Canadian Brand Names Reminyl®

Generic Available No

Synonyms Galantamine Hydrobromide

Pharmacologic Category Acetylcholinesterase Inhibitor (Central)

Use Treatment of mild to moderate dementia of Alzheimer's disease

Local Anesthetic/Vasoconstrictor Precautions No information available to require special precautions

Effects on Dental Treatment No significant effects or complications reported

Common Adverse Effects

>10%: Gastrointestinal: Nausea (6% to 24%), vomiting (4% to 13%), diarrhea (6% to 12%)

1% to 10%:

- Cardiovascular: Bradycardia (2% to 3%), syncope (0.4% to 2.2%: dose-related), chest pain (≥1%)
- Central nervous system: Dizziness (9%), headache (8%), depression (7%), fatigue (5%), insomnia (5%), somnolence (4%), tremor (3%)
- Gastrointestinal: Anorexia (7% to 9%), weight loss (5% to 7%), abdominal pain (5%), dyspepsia (5%), flatulence (≥1%)
- Genitourinary: Urinary tract infection (8%), hematuria (<1% to 3%), incontinence (≥1%)
- Hematologic: Anemia (3%)
- Respiratory: Rhinitis (4%)

Mechanism of Action Centrally-acting cholinesterase inhibitor (competitive and reversible). It elevates acetylcholine in cerebral cortex by slowing the degradation of acetylcholine. Modulates nicotinic acetylcholine receptor to increase acetylcholine from surviving presynaptic nerve terminals. May increase glutamate and serotonin levels.

Drug Interactions

Cytochrome P450 Effect: Substrate (minor) of CYP2D6, 3A4

Increased Effect/Toxicity: Succinylcholine: increased neuromuscular blockade. Amiodarone, beta-blockers without ISA activity, diltiazem, verapamil may increase bradycardia. NSAIDs increase risk of peptic ulcer. Cimetidine, ketoconazole, paroxetine, other CYP3A4 inhibitors, other CYP2D6 inhibitors increase levels of galantamine. Concurrent cholinergic agents may have synergistic effects. Digoxin may lead to AV block.

Decreased Effect: Anticholinergic agents are antagonized by galantamine. CYP inducers may decrease galantamine levels.

Pharmacodynamics/Kinetics

Duration: 3 hours; maximum inhibition of erythrocyte acetylcholinesterase ~40% at 1 hour post 10 mg oral dose; levels return to baseline at 30 hours

Absorption: Rapid and complete

Distribution: 1.8-2.6 L/kg; levels in the brain are 2-3 times higher than in plasma

Protein binding: 18%

Metabolism: Hepatic; linear, CYP2D6 and 3A4; metabolized to epigalanthaminone and galanthaminone both of which have acetylcholinesterase inhibitory activity 130 times less than galantamine

Bioavailability: 80% to 100%

Half-life elimination: 6-8 hours

Time to peak: 1 hour

Excretion: Urine (25%)

Pregnancy Risk Factor B

Galantamine Hydrobromide *see* Galantamine *on page 645*

Gallium Nitrate (GAL ee um NYE trate)

U.S. Brand Names Ganite™

Generic Available No

Synonyms NSC-15200

Pharmacologic Category Calcium-Lowering Agent

Use Treatment of hypercalcemia

Local Anesthetic/Vasoconstrictor Precautions No information available to require special precautions

Effects on Dental Treatment No significant effects or complications reported

Mechanism of Action Inhibits bone resorption by inhibiting osteoclast function

Pregnancy Risk Factor C

Gamimune® N *see* Immune Globulin (Intravenous) *on page 740*

Gamma Benzene Hexachloride *see* Lindane *on page 829*

Gammagard® S/D *see* Immune Globulin (Intravenous) *on page 740*

Gamma Globulin *see* Immune Globulin (Intramuscular) *on page 739*

Gamma Hydroxybutyric Acid *see* Sodium Oxybate *on page 1229*

Gammaphos *see* Amifostine *on page 94*

Gammar®-P I.V. *see* Immune Globulin (Intravenous) *on page 740*

Gamunex® *see* Immune Globulin (Intravenous) *on page 740*

Ganciclovir (gan SYE kloe veer)

Related Information

Systemic Viral Diseases *on page 1519*

Valganciclovir *on page 1358*

U.S. Brand Names Cytovene®; Vitrasert®

Canadian Brand Names Cytovene®; Vitrasert®

Mexican Brand Names Cymevene®

Generic Available Yes: Capsule

Synonyms DHPG Sodium; GCV Sodium; Nordeoxyguanosine

Pharmacologic Category Antiviral Agent

Use

Parenteral: Treatment of CMV retinitis in immunocompromised individuals, including patients with acquired immunodeficiency syndrome; prophylaxis of CMV infection in transplant patients

Oral: Alternative to the I.V. formulation for maintenance treatment of CMV retinitis in immunocompromised patients, including patients with AIDS, in whom retinitis is stable following appropriate induction therapy and for whom the risk of more rapid progression is balanced by the benefit associated with avoiding daily I.V. infusions.

Implant: Treatment of CMV retinitis

Unlabeled/Investigational Use May be given in combination with foscarnet in patients who relapse after monotherapy with either drug

Local Anesthetic/Vasoconstrictor Precautions No information available to require special precautions

Effects on Dental Treatment Key adverse event(s) related to dental treatment: Xerostomia (normal salivary flow resumes upon discontinuation).

Common Adverse Effects

>10%:

Central nervous system: Fever (38% to 48%)

Dermatologic: Rash (15% oral, 10% I.V.)

Gastrointestinal: Abdominal pain (17% to 19%), diarrhea (40%), nausea (25%), anorexia (15%), vomiting (13%)

Hematologic: Anemia (20% to 25%), leukopenia (30% to 40%)

1% to 10%:

Central nervous system: Confusion, neuropathy (8% to 9%), headache (4%)

Dermatologic: Pruritus (5%)

Hematologic: Thrombocytopenia (6%), neutropenia with ANC <500/mm^3 (5% oral, 14% I.V.)

Neuromuscular & skeletal: Paresthesia (6% to 10%), weakness (6%)

Ocular: Retinal detachment (8% oral, 11% I.V.; relationship to ganciclovir not established)

Miscellaneous: Sepsis (4% oral, 15% I.V.)

Mechanism of Action Ganciclovir is phosphorylated to a substrate which competitively inhibits the binding of deoxyguanosine triphosphate to DNA polymerase resulting in inhibition of viral DNA synthesis

Drug Interactions

Increased Effect/Toxicity: Immunosuppressive agents may increase hematologic toxicity of ganciclovir. Imipenem/cilastatin may increase seizure potential. Oral ganciclovir increases blood levels of zidovudine, although zidovudine decreases steady-state levels of ganciclovir. Since both drugs have the potential to cause neutropenia and anemia, some patients may not tolerate concomitant therapy with these drugs at full dosage. Didanosine levels are increased with concurrent ganciclovir. Other nephrotoxic drugs (eg, amphotericin and cyclosporine) may have additive nephrotoxicity with ganciclovir.

Decreased Effect: A decrease in blood levels of ganciclovir AUC may occur when used with didanosine.

Pharmacodynamics/Kinetics

Distribution: V_d: 15.26 L/1.73 m^2; widely to all tissues including CSF and ocular tissue

Protein binding: 1% to 2%

Bioavailability: Oral: Fasting: 5%; Following food: 6% to 9%; Following fatty meal: 28% to 31%

Half-life elimination: 1.7-5.8 hours; prolonged with renal impairment; End-stage renal disease: 5-28 hours

Excretion: Urine (80% to 99% as unchanged drug)

Pregnancy Risk Factor C

Ganidin NR *see* Guaifenesin *on page 672*

Ganirelix (ga ni REL ix)

U.S. Brand Names Antagon®

Canadian Brand Names Antagon®; Orgalutran®

Generic Available No

Synonyms Ganirelix Acetate

Pharmacologic Category Gonadotropin Releasing Hormone Antagonist

Use Inhibits premature luteinizing hormone (LH) surges in women undergoing controlled ovarian hyperstimulation in fertility clinics.

Local Anesthetic/Vasoconstrictor Precautions No information available to require special precautions

Effects on Dental Treatment No significant effects or complications reported

Common Adverse Effects 1% to 10%:

Central nervous system: Headache (3%)

Endocrine & metabolic: Ovarian hyperstimulation syndrome (2%)

Gastrointestinal: Abdominal pain (5%), nausea (1%), and abdominal pain (1%)

Genitourinary: Vaginal bleeding (2%)

Local: Injection site reaction (1%)

Mechanism of Action Competitively blocks the gonadotropin-release hormone receptors on the pituitary gonadotroph and transduction pathway. This suppresses gonadotropin secretion and luteinizing hormone secretion preventing ovulation until the follicles are of adequate size.

Drug Interactions

Increased Effect/Toxicity: No formal studies have been performed.

Decreased Effect: No formal studies have been performed.

Pharmacodynamics/Kinetics

Absorption: SubQ: Rapid

Distribution: Mean V_d: 43.7 L

Protein binding: 81.9%

Metabolism: Hepatic to two primary metabolites (1-4 and 1-6 peptide)

Bioavailability: 91.1%

Half-life elimination: 16.2 hours

Time to peak: 1.1 hours

Excretion: Feces (75%) within 288 hours; urine (22%) within 24 hours

Pregnancy Risk Factor X

Ganirelix Acetate *see* Ganirelix *on page 647*
Ganite™ *see* Gallium Nitrate *on page 646*
Gani-Tuss® NR *see* Guaifenesin and Codeine *on page 673*
Gantrisin® *see* SulfiSOXAZOLE *on page 1250*
Garamycin® [DSC] *see* Gentamicin *on page 655*
Gastrocrom® *see* Cromolyn *on page 378*
Gastrointestinal Disorders *see page 1476*
Gas-X® [OTC] *see* Simethicone *on page 1222*
Gas-X® Extra Strength [OTC] *see* Simethicone *on page 1222*

Gatifloxacin (gat i FLOKS a sin)

Related Information

Oral Bacterial Infections *on page 1533*
Respiratory Diseases *on page 1478*
Sexually-Transmitted Diseases *on page 1504*

(Continued)

Gatifloxacin *(Continued)*

U.S. Brand Names Tequin®; Zymar™

Canadian Brand Names Tequin®

Generic Available No

Pharmacologic Category Antibiotic, Ophthalmic; Antibiotic, Quinolone

Use Treatment of the following infections when caused by susceptible bacteria: Acute bacterial exacerbation of chronic bronchitis; acute sinusitis; community-acquired pneumonia including pneumonia caused by multidrug-resistant *S. pneumoniae* (MDRSP); uncomplicated skin and skin structure infection; uncomplicated urinary tract infections (cystitis); complicated urinary tract infections; pyelonephritis; uncomplicated urethral and cervical gonorrhea; acute, uncomplicated rectal infections in women; bacterial conjunctivitis

Local Anesthetic/Vasoconstrictor Precautions No information available to require special precautions

Effects on Dental Treatment Key adverse event(s) related to dental treatment: Taste disturbance.

Common Adverse Effects

Systemic therapy:

3% to 10%:

Central nervous system: Headache (3%), dizziness (3%)

Gastrointestinal: Nausea (8%), diarrhea (4%)

Genitourinary: Vaginitis (6%)

Local: Injection site reactions (5%)

0.1% to 3%: Abdominal pain, abnormal dreams, abnormal vision, agitation, alkaline phosphatase increased, allergic reaction, anorexia, anxiety, arthralgia, back pain, chest pain, chills, confusion, constipation, diaphoresis, dry skin, dyspepsia, dyspnea, dysuria, facial edema, fever, flatulence, gastritis, glossitis, hematuria, hyperglycemia, hypertension, insomnia, leg cramps, mouth ulceration, nervousness, oral candidiasis, palpitation, paresthesia, peripheral edema, pharyngitis, pruritus, rash, serum amylase increased, serum bilirubin increased, serum transaminases increased, somnolence, stomatitis, taste perversion, thirst, tinnitus, tremor, weakness, vasodilation, vertigo, vomiting

Ophthalmic therapy:

5% to 10%: Ocular: Conjunctival irritation, keratitis, lacrimation increased, papillary conjunctivitis

1% to 4%:

Central nervous system: Headache

Gastrointestinal: Taste disturbance

Ocular: Chemosis, conjunctival hemorrhage, discharge, dry eye, edema, irritation, pain, visual acuity decreased

Mechanism of Action Gatifloxacin is a DNA gyrase inhibitor, and also inhibits topoisomerase IV. DNA gyrase (topoisomerase II) is an essential bacterial enzyme that maintains the superhelical structure of DNA. DNA gyrase is required for DNA replication and transcription, DNA repair, recombination, and transposition; inhibition is bactericidal.

Drug Interactions

Increased Effect/Toxicity: Use caution with drugs which prolong QT interval (including Class Ia and Class III antiarrhythmics, erythromycin, cisapride, antipsychotics, and cyclic antidepressants). Drugs which may induce bradycardia (eg, beta-blockers, amiodarone) should be avoided. Gatifloxacin may alter glucose control in patients receiving hypoglycemic agents with or without insulin. Cases of severe disturbances (including symptomatic hypoglycemia) have been reported, typically within 1-3 days of gatifloxacin initiation. Probenecid, loop diuretics, and cimetidine (possibly other H_2 antagonists) may increase the serum concentrations of gatifloxacin (based on experience with other quinolones). Digoxin levels may be increased in some patients by gatifloxacin. NSAIDs and foscarnet have been associated with an increased risk of seizures with some quinolones (not reported with gatifloxacin). The hypoprothrombinemic effect of warfarin is enhanced by some quinolone antibiotics. Monitoring of the INR during concurrent therapy is recommended by the manufacturer. Concurrent use of corticosteroids may increase risk of tendon rupture.

Decreased Effect: Metal cations (magnesium, aluminum, iron, and zinc) inhibit intestinal absorption of gatifloxacin (by up to 98%). Antacids, electrolyte supplements, sucralfate, quinapril, and some didanosine formulations (buffered tablets and pediatric powder for oral solution) should be avoided. Gatifloxacin should be administered 4 hours before these agents. Calcium carbonate was not found to alter the absorption of gatifloxacin. Antineoplastic agents, H_2 antagonists, and proton pump inhibitors may also decrease absorption of some quinolones. Gatifloxacin may alter glucose control in patients receiving hypoglycemic agents with or without insulin.

Pharmacodynamics/Kinetics

Absorption: Oral: Well absorbed; Ophthalmic: Not measurable

Distribution: V_d: 1.5-2.0 L/kg; concentrates in alveolar macrophages and lung parenchyma

Protein binding: 20%

Metabolism: Only 1%; no interaction with CYP

Bioavailability: 96%

Half-life elimination: 7.1-13.9 hours; ESRD/CAPD: 30-40 hours

Time to peak: Oral: 1 hour

Excretion: Urine (70% as unchanged drug, <1% as metabolites); feces (5%)

Pregnancy Risk Factor C

Gaviscon® Extra Strength [OTC] *see* Aluminum Hydroxide and Magnesium Carbonate *on page 90*

Gaviscon® Liquid [OTC] *see* Aluminum Hydroxide and Magnesium Carbonate *on page 90*

Gaviscon® Tablet [OTC] *see* Aluminum Hydroxide and Magnesium Trisilicate *on page 91*

G-CSF *see* Filgrastim *on page 589*

G-CSF (PEG Conjugate) *see* Pegfilgrastim *on page 1052*

GCV Sodium *see* Ganciclovir *on page 646*

Gebauer's Ethyl Chloride® *see* Ethyl Chloride *on page 561*

Gefitinib (ge FI tye nib)

U.S. Brand Names Iressa™

Generic Available No

Synonyms NSC-715055; ZD1839

Pharmacologic Category Antineoplastic Agent, Tyrosine Kinase Inhibitor

Use Second-line treatment of nonsmall cell lung cancer

Unlabeled/Investigational Use Brain cancer, breast cancer, colon cancer, head and neck cancer, ovarian cancer

Local Anesthetic/Vasoconstrictor Precautions No information available to require special precautions

Effects on Dental Treatment Key adverse event(s) related to dental treatment: Mouth ulceration.

Common Adverse Effects Based on 250 mg/day:

>10%:

Dermatologic: Rash (43%), acne (25%), dry skin (13%)

Gastrointestinal: Diarrhea (48%), nausea (13%), vomiting (12%)

1% to 10%:

Cardiovascular: Peripheral edema (2%)

Dermatologic: Pruritus (8%)

Gastrointestinal: Anorexia (7%), weight loss (3%), mouth ulceration (1%)

Neuromuscular & skeletal: Weakness (6%)

Ocular: Amblyopia (2%), conjunctivitis (1%)

Respiratory: Dyspnea (2%), interstitial lung disease (1%)

Mechanism of Action The mechanism of antineoplastic action is not fully understood. Gefitinib inhibits tyrosine kinases (TK) associated with transmembrane cell surface receptors found on both normal and cancer cells. One such receptor is epidermal growth factor receptor. TK activity appears to be vitally important to cell proliferation and survival.

Drug Interactions

Cytochrome P450 Effect: Substrate of CYP3A4 (major); **Inhibits** CYP2C19 (weak), 2D6 (weak)

Increased Effect/Toxicity: Gefitinib may increase the effects of warfarin. CYP3A4 inhibitors may increase the levels/effects of gefitinib; example inhibitors include azole antifungals, ciprofloxacin, clarithromycin, diclofenac, doxycycline, erythromycin, imatinib, isoniazid, nefazodone, nicardipine, propofol, protease inhibitors, quinidine, and verapamil.

Decreased Effect: Gefitinib effects may be decreased by H_2-receptor blockers and sodium bicarbonate. CYP3A4 inducers may decrease the levels/effects of gefitinib; example inducers include aminoglutethimide, carbamazepine, nafcillin, nevirapine, phenobarbital, phenytoin, and rifamycins.

Pharmacodynamics/Kinetics

Absorption: Oral: slow

Distribution: I.V.: 1400 L

Protein binding: 90%, albumin and $alpha_1$-acid glycoprotein

Metabolism: Hepatic, primarily via CYP3A4; forms metabolites

(Continued)

Gefitinib *(Continued)*

Bioavailability: 60%
Half-life elimination: I.V.: 48 hours
Time to peak, plasma: Oral: 3-7 hours
Excretion: Feces (86%); urine (<4%)

Pregnancy Risk Factor D

Gelatin (Absorbable) (JEL a tin, ab SORB a ble)

U.S. Brand Names Gelfilm®; Gelfoam®

Generic Available No

Synonyms Absorbable Gelatin Sponge

Pharmacologic Category Hemostatic Agent

Dental Use Adjunct to provide hemostasis in oral and dental surgery

Use Adjunct to provide hemostasis in surgery; open prostatic surgery

Local Anesthetic/Vasoconstrictor Precautions No information available to require special precautions

Effects on Dental Treatment Key adverse event(s) related to dental treatment: Local infection and abscess formation.

Significant Adverse Effects 1% to 10%: Local: Infection and abscess formation

Dosage Hemostasis: Apply packs or sponges dry or saturated with sodium chloride. When applied dry, hold in place with moderate pressure. When applied wet, squeeze to remove air bubbles. The powder is applied as a paste prepared by adding approximately 4 mL of sterile saline solution to the powder.

Contraindications Should not be used in closure of skin incisions since they may interfere with the healing of skin edges

Warnings/Precautions Do not sterilize by heat; do not use in the presence of infection

Drug Interactions No data reported

Pregnancy Risk Factor No data reported

Dosage Forms

Film, ophthalmic (Gelfilm®): 25 mm x 50 mm (6s)
Film, topical (Gelfilm®): 100 mm x 125 mm (1s)
Powder, topical (Gelfoam®): 1 g
Sponge, dental (Gelfoam®): Size 4 (12s)
Sponge, topical (Gelfoam®):
  Size 50 (4s)
  Size 100 (6s)
  Size 200 (6s)
  Size 2 cm (1s)
  Size 6 cm (6s)
  Size 12-7 mm (12s)

Gelclair™ *see* Maltodextrin *on page 855*
Gelfilm® *see* Gelatin (Absorbable) *on page 650*
Gelfoam® *see* Gelatin (Absorbable) *on page 650*
Gel-Kam® [OTC] *see* Fluoride *on page 603*
Gel-Kam® Rinse *see* Fluoride *on page 603*
Gelucast® *see* Zinc Gelatin *on page 1400*

Gemcitabine (jem SITE a been)

U.S. Brand Names Gemzar®

Canadian Brand Names Gemzar®

Mexican Brand Names Gemzar®

Generic Available No

Synonyms Gemcitabine Hydrochloride

Pharmacologic Category Antineoplastic Agent, Antimetabolite (Pyrimidine Antagonist)

Use

Adenocarcinoma of the pancreas; first-line therapy in locally-advanced (nonresectable stage II or stage III) or metastatic (stage IV) adenocarcinoma of the pancreas (indicated for patients previously treated with fluorouracil)

Breast cancer: First-line therapy in metastatic breast cancer after failure of an anthracycline-containing adjuvant therapy (unless contraindicated); used in combination with paclitaxel

Nonsmall-cell lung cancer: First-line therapy in locally-advanced (stage IIIA or IIIB) or metastatic (stage IV) nonsmall-cell lung cancer; used in combination with cisplatin

Local Anesthetic/Vasoconstrictor Precautions No information available to require special precautions

Effects on Dental Treatment Key adverse event(s) related to dental treatment: Stomatitis.

Common Adverse Effects Percentages reported with single-agent therapy for pancreatic cancer and other malignancies.

>10%:

Central nervous system: Pain (42% to 48%; grades 3 and 4: <1% to 9%), fever (38% to 41%; grades 3 and 4: ≤2%), somnolence (11%; grades 3 and 4: <1%). Fever was reported to occur in the absence of infection in pancreatic cancer treatment.

Dermatologic: Rash (28% to 30%; grades 3 and 4: <1%), alopecia (15% to 16%; grades 3 and 4: <1%). Rash in pancreatic cancer treatment was typically a macular or finely-granular maculopapular pruritic eruption of mild-to-moderate severity involving the trunk and extremities.

Gastrointestinal: Nausea and vomiting (69% to 71%; grades 3 and 4: 1% to 13%), constipation (23% to 31%; grades 3 and 4: <1% to 3%), diarrhea (19% to 30%; grades 3 and 4: ≤3%), stomatitis (10% to 11%; grades 3 and 4: <1%)

Hematologic: Anemia (73% to 68%; grades 3 and 4: 1% to 8%), leukopenia (62% to 64%; grades 3 and 4: <1% to 9%), neutropenia (61% to 63%; grades 3 and 4: 6% to 19%), thrombocytopenia (24% to 36%; grades 3 and 4: <1% to 7%), hemorrhage (4% to 17%; grades 3 or 4: <1%). Myelosuppression may be the dose-limiting toxicity with pancreatic cancer

Hepatic: Transaminases increased (68% to 78%; grades 3 and 4: 1% to 12%), alkaline phosphatase increased (55% to 77%; grades 3 and 4: 2% to 16%), bilirubin increased (13% to 26%; grades 3 or 4: <1% to 6%). Serious hepatotoxicity was reported rarely in pancreatic cancer treatment.

Renal: Proteinuria (32% to 45%; grades 3 and 4: <1%), hematuria (23% to 35%; grades 3 and 4: <1%), BUN increased (15% to 16%; grades 3 and 4: 0%)

Respiratory: Dyspnea (10% to 23%; grades 3 and 4: <1% to 3%)

Miscellaneous: Infection (10% to 16%; grades 3 or 4: <1% to 2%)

1% to 10%:

Local: Injection site reactions (4%)

Neuromuscular & skeletal: Paresthesias (10%)

Renal: Creatinine increased (6% to 8%)

Respiratory: Bronchospasm (<2%)

Mechanism of Action A pyrimidine antimetabolite that inhibits DNA synthesis by inhibition of DNA polymerase and ribonucleotide reductase, specific for the S-phase of the cycle.

Drug Interactions

Decreased Effect: No confirmed interactions have been reported. No specific drug interaction studies have been conducted.

Pharmacodynamics/Kinetics

Distribution: V_d: Male: 15.6 mL mL/m^2; Female: 11.3 L/m^2

Protein binding: Low

Metabolism: Hepatic, metabolites: di- and triphosphates (active); uridine derivative (inactive)

Half-life elimination: Infusion time: ≤1 hour: 32-94 minutes; Infusion time: 3-4 hours: 4-10.5 hours

Time to peak: 30 minutes

Excretion: Urine (99%, 92% to 98% as intact drug or inactive uridine metabolite); feces (<1%)

Pregnancy Risk Factor D

Gemcitabine Hydrochloride *see* Gemcitabine *on page 650*

Gemfibrozil (jem FI broe zil)

Related Information

Cardiovascular Diseases *on page 1458*

U.S. Brand Names Lopid®

Canadian Brand Names Apo-Gemfibrozil®; Gen-Gemfibrozil; Lopid®; Novo-Gemfibrozil; Nu-Gemfibrozil; PMS-Gemfibrozil

Mexican Brand Names Lopid®

Generic Available Yes

Synonyms CI-719

Pharmacologic Category Antilipemic Agent, Fibric Acid

Use Treatment of hypertriglyceridemia in types IV and V hyperlipidemia for patients who are at greater risk for pancreatitis and who have not responded to dietary intervention

Local Anesthetic/Vasoconstrictor Precautions No information available to require special precautions

(Continued)

Gemfibrozil *(Continued)*

Effects on Dental Treatment No significant effects or complications reported

Common Adverse Effects

>10% Gastrointestinal: Dyspepsia (20%)

1% to 10%:

Central nervous system: Fatigue (4%), vertigo (2%), headache (1%)

Dermatologic: Eczema (2%), rash (2%)

Gastrointestinal: Abdominal pain (10%), diarrhea (7%), nausea/vomiting (3%), constipation (1%)

Reports where causal relationship has not been established: Weight loss, extrasystoles, pancreatitis, hepatoma, colitis, confusion, seizures, syncope, retinal edema, decreased fertility (male), renal dysfunction, positive ANA, drug-induced lupus-like syndrome, thrombocytopenia, anaphylaxis, vasculitis, alopecia, photosensitivity

Dosage Adults: Oral: 1200 mg/day in 2 divided doses, 30 minutes before breakfast and dinner

Hemodialysis: Not removed by hemodialysis; supplemental dose is not necessary

Mechanism of Action The exact mechanism of action of gemfibrozil is unknown, however, several theories exist regarding the VLDL effect; it can inhibit lipolysis and decrease subsequent hepatic fatty acid uptake as well as inhibit hepatic secretion of VLDL; together these actions decrease serum VLDL levels; increases HDL-cholesterol; the mechanism behind HDL elevation is currently unknown

Contraindications Hypersensitivity to gemfibrozil or any component of the formulation; significant hepatic or renal dysfunction; primary biliary cirrhosis; pre-existing gallbladder disease

Warnings/Precautions Abnormal elevation of AST, ALT, LDH, bilirubin, and alkaline phosphatase has occurred; if no appreciable triglyceride or cholesterol lowering effect occurs after 3 months, the drug should be discontinued; not useful for type I hyperlipidemia; myositis may be more common in patients with poor renal function

Drug Interactions

Cytochrome P450 Effect: Substrate of CYP3A4 (minor); **Inhibits** CYP1A2 (moderate), 2C8/9 (strong), 2C19 (strong)

Increased Effect/Toxicity: Gemfibrozil may potentiate the effects of bexarotene (avoid concurrent use), sulfonylureas (including glyburide, chlorpropamide), and warfarin. HMG-CoA reductase inhibitors (atorvastatin, fluvastatin, lovastatin, pravastatin, simvastatin) may increase the risk of myopathy and rhabdomyolysis. The manufacturer warns against the concurrent use of lovastatin (if unavoidable, limit lovastatin to <20 mg/day). Combination therapy with statins has been used in some patients with resistant hyperlipidemias (with great caution). Gemfibrozil may increase the serum concentration of repaglinide (resulting in severe, prolonged hypoglycemia); the addition of itraconazole may augment the effects of gemfibrozil on repaglinide (consider alternative therapy). Gemfibrozil may increase the levels/effects of aminophylline, amiodarone, citalopram, diazepam, fluoxetine, fluvoxamine, glimepiride, glipizide, methsuximide, mexiletine, mirtazapine, nateglinide, phenytoin, pioglitazone, propranolol, ropinirole, rosiglitazone, sertraline, theophylline, trifluoperazine, warfarin, and other substrates of CYP1A2, 2C8/9, or 2C19.

Decreased Effect: Cyclosporine's blood levels may be reduced during concurrent therapy. Rifampin may decrease gemfibrozil blood levels.

Ethanol/Nutrition/Herb Interactions Ethanol: Avoid ethanol to decrease triglycerides.

Dietary Considerations Before initiation of therapy, patients should be placed on a standard cholesterol-lowering diet for 3-6 months and the diet should be continued during drug therapy.

Pharmacodynamics/Kinetics

Onset of action: May require several days

Absorption: Well absorbed

Protein binding: 99%

Metabolism: Hepatic via oxidation to two inactive metabolites; undergoes enterohepatic recycling

Half-life elimination: 1.4 hours

Time to peak, serum: 1-2 hours

Excretion: Urine (70% primarily as unchanged drug)

Pregnancy Risk Factor C

Dosage Forms TAB, film coated: 600 mg

Gemifloxacin (je mi FLOKS a sin)

Related Information

Oral Bacterial Infections *on page 1533*

U.S. Brand Names Factive®

Generic Available No

Synonyms DW286; Gemifloxacin Mesylate; LA 20304a; SB-265805

Pharmacologic Category Antibiotic, Quinolone

Use Treatment of acute exacerbation of chronic bronchitis; treatment of community-acquired pneumonia, including pneumonia caused by multidrug-resistant strains of *S. pneumoniae* (MDRSP)

Unlabeled/Investigational Use Acute sinusitis, uncomplicated urinary tract infection

Local Anesthetic/Vasoconstrictor Precautions No information available to require special precautions

Effects on Dental Treatment No significant effects or complications reported

Common Adverse Effects

1% to 10%:

Central nervous system: Headache (1%), dizziness (1%)

Dermatologic: Rash (3%)

Gastrointestinal: Diarrhea (4%), nausea (3%), abdominal pain (1%), vomiting (1%)

Hepatic: Transaminases increased (1% to 2%)

Important adverse effects reported with other agents in this drug class include (not reported for gemifloxacin): Allergic reactions, CNS stimulation, hepatitis, jaundice, seizures, severe dermatologic reactions (toxic epidermal necrolysis, Stevens-Johnson syndrome), pneumonitis (eosinophilic), tendon rupture, torsade de pointes, vasculitis

Mechanism of Action Gemifloxacin is a DNA gyrase inhibitor and also inhibits topoisomerase IV. DNA gyrase (topoisomerase IV) is an essential bacterial enzyme that maintains the superhelical structure of DNA. DNA gyrase is required for DNA replication and transcription, DNA repair, recombination, and transposition; bactericidal

Drug Interactions

Increased Effect/Toxicity: Gemifloxacin may prolong QT interval; avoid use with drugs which prolong QT interval (including class Ia and class III antiarrhythmics, erythromycin, cisapride, antipsychotics, and cyclic antidepressants). Concurrent use of corticosteroids may increase the risk of tendon rupture with quinolones, particularly in elderly patients (overall incidence rare). Probenecid may increase systemic exposure to gemifloxacin (blocks renal secretion). Loop diuretics and cimetidine have been shown to increase serum concentrations of some quinolones (due to decreased renal secretion). Foscarnet and NSAIDs have been associated with an increased risk of CNS effects with some quinolones. The effect of warfarin may be enhanced by some quinolone antibiotics.

Decreased Effect: Metal cations (magnesium, aluminum, iron, and zinc) bind quinolones in the gastrointestinal tract and inhibit absorption (by up to 98%). Antacids, electrolyte supplements, sucralfate, quinapril, and some didanosine formulations should be avoided. Gemifloxacin should be administered 3 hours before or 2 hours after these agents. Calcium carbonate did not result in significant changes in the absorption of gemifloxacin. Antineoplastic agents may also decrease the absorption of quinolones.

Pharmacodynamics/Kinetics

Absorption: Well absorbed from the GI tract

Bioavailability: 71%

Metabolism: Hepatic (minor); forms metabolites (CYP isoenzymes are not involved)

Time to peak, plasma: 1-2 hours

Protein binding: 60% to 70%

Half-life elimination: 7 hours (range 4-12 hours)

Excretion: Urine (30% to 40%); feces (60%)

Pregnancy Risk Factor C

Gemifloxacin Mesylate *see* Gemifloxacin *on page 653*

Gemtuzumab Ozogamicin (gem TOO zoo mab oh zog a MY sin)

U.S. Brand Names Mylotarg®

Canadian Brand Names Mylotarg™

Generic Available No

Pharmacologic Category Antineoplastic Agent, Monoclonal Antibody

(Continued)

Gemtuzumab Ozogamicin *(Continued)*

Use Treatment of acute myeloid leukemia (CD33 positive) in first relapse in patients who are ≥60 years of age and who are not considered candidates for cytotoxic chemotherapy.

Local Anesthetic/Vasoconstrictor Precautions No information available to require special precautions

Effects on Dental Treatment Key adverse event(s) related to dental treatment: Stomatitis and mucositis.

Common Adverse Effects Percentages established in adults >60 years of age. **Note:** A postinfusion symptom complex (fever, chills, less commonly hypertension, and/or dyspnea) may occur within 24 hours of administration.

>10%:

- Cardiovascular: Peripheral edema (21%), hypertension (16%), hypotension (20%)
- Central nervous system: Chills (66%), fever (82%), headache (37%), pain (25%), dizziness (11%), insomnia (18%)
- Dermatologic: Rash (23%), petechiae (21%), ecchymosis (15%), cutaneous herpes simplex (21%)
- Endocrine & metabolic: Hypokalemia (30%)
- Gastrointestinal: Nausea (68%), vomiting (58%), diarrhea (38%), anorexia (31%), abdominal pain (29%), constipation (28%), stomatitis/mucositis (25%), abdominal distention (11%), dyspepsia (11%)
- Hematologic: Neutropenia (98%; median recovery 40.5 days), thrombocytopenia (99%; median recovery 39 days); anemia (52%), bleeding (15%), lymphopenia
- Hepatic: Hyperbilirubinemia (29%), LDH increased (18%), transaminases increased (9% to 18%)
- Local: Local reaction (25%)
- Neuromuscular & skeletal: Weakness (45%), back pain (18%)
- Respiratory: Dyspnea (26%), epistaxis (29%; severe 3%), cough (19%), pharyngitis (14%)
- Miscellaneous: Infection (30%), sepsis (24%), neutropenic fever (20%)

1% to 10%:

- Cardiovascular: Tachycardia (10%)
- Central nervous system: Depression (10%), cerebral hemorrhage (2%), intracranial hemorrhage (2%)
- Dermatologic: Pruritus (6%)
- Endocrine & metabolic: Hypomagnesemia (4%), hyperglycemia (10%)
- Genitourinary: Hematuria (10%; severe 1%), vaginal hemorrhage (7%)
- Hematologic: Hemorrhage (8%), disseminated intravascular coagulation (DIC) (2%)
- Hepatic: PT increased, veno-occlusive disease (range: 1% to 20% in relapsed patients; higher frequency in patients with prior history of subsequent hematopoetic stem cell transplant)
- Neuromuscular & skeletal: Arthralgia (10%)
- Respiratory: Rhinitis (10%), hypoxia (6%), pneumonia (10%)

Mechanism of Action Antibody to CD33 antigen, which is expressed on leukemic blasts in >80% of patients with acute myeloid leukemia (AML), as well as normal myeloid cells. Binding results in internalization of the antibody-antigen complex. Following internalization, the calicheamicin derivative is released inside the myeloid cell. The calicheamicin derivative binds to DNA resulting in double strand breaks and cell death. Pluripotent stem cells and nonhematopoietic cells are not affected.

Drug Interactions

Increased Effect/Toxicity: No formal drug interaction studies have been conducted.

Decreased Effect: No formal drug interaction studies have been conducted.

Pharmacodynamics/Kinetics Half-life elimination: Calicheamicin: Total: Initial: 45 hours, Repeat dose: 60 hours; Unconjugated: 100 hours (no change noted in repeat dosing)

Pregnancy Risk Factor D

Gemzar® *see* Gemcitabine *on page 650*

Genac® [OTC] *see* Triprolidine and Pseudoephedrine *on page 1345*

Genaced™ [OTC] *see* Acetaminophen, Aspirin, and Caffeine *on page 56*

Genahist® [OTC] *see* DiphenhydrAMINE *on page 448*

Genapap® [OTC] *see* Acetaminophen *on page 47*

Genapap® Children [OTC] *see* Acetaminophen *on page 47*

Genapap® Extra Strength [OTC] *see* Acetaminophen *on page 47*

Genapap® Infant [OTC] *see* Acetaminophen *on page 47*

Genapap® Sinus Maximum Strength [OTC] *see* Acetaminophen and Pseudoephedrine *on page 53*
Genaphed® [OTC] *see* Pseudoephedrine *on page 1147*
Genaphed Plus [OTC] *see* Chlorpheniramine and Pseudoephedrine *on page 315*
Genasal [OTC] *see* Oxymetazoline *on page 1034*
Genasoft® [OTC] *see* Docusate *on page 459*
Genasoft® Plus [DSC] [OTC] *see* Docusate and Casanthranol *on page 460*
Genasyme® [OTC] *see* Simethicone *on page 1222*
Genaton Tablet [OTC] *see* Aluminum Hydroxide and Magnesium Trisilicate *on page 91*
Genatuss DM® [OTC] *see* Guaifenesin and Dextromethorphan *on page 673*
Genebs® [OTC] *see* Acetaminophen *on page 47*
Genebs® Extra Strength [OTC] *see* Acetaminophen *on page 47*
Generlac *see* Lactulose *on page 794*
Genesec® [OTC] *see* Acetaminophen and Phenyltoloxamine *on page 53*
Geneye® [OTC] *see* Tetrahydrozoline *on page 1282*
Genfiber® [OTC] *see* Psyllium *on page 1151*
Gengraf® *see* CycloSPORINE *on page 386*
Genoptic® *see* Gentamicin *on page 655*
Genotropin® *see* Human Growth Hormone *on page 694*
Genotropin Miniquick® *see* Human Growth Hormone *on page 694*
Genpril® [OTC] *see* Ibuprofen *on page 728*
Gentacidin® *see* Gentamicin *on page 655*
Gentak® *see* Gentamicin *on page 655*

Gentamicin (jen ta MYE sin)

Related Information

Cardiovascular Diseases *on page 1458*
Sexually-Transmitted Diseases *on page 1504*

U.S. Brand Names Garamycin® [DSC]; Genoptic®; Gentacidin®; Gentak®

Canadian Brand Names Alcomicin®; Diogent®; Garamycin®; Minim's Gentamicin 0.3%; SAB-Gentamicin

Mexican Brand Names Garamicina® [cream]; Garamicina® [inj.]; Genemicin® [inj.]; Genkova® [inj.]; Genrex®; Gentabac®; Gentacin® [inj.]; Genta Grin®; Gentarim®; Gentazaf®; G.I.®; Ikatin®; Servigenta®; Tondex® [inj.]; Yectamicina®

Generic Available Yes

Synonyms Gentamicin Sulfate

Pharmacologic Category Antibiotic, Aminoglycoside; Antibiotic, Ophthalmic; Antibiotic, Topical

Dental Use Prevention of bacterial endocarditis prior to dental or surgical procedures

Use Treatment of susceptible bacterial infections, normally gram-negative organisms including *Pseudomonas*, *Proteus*, *Serratia*, and gram-positive *Staphylococcus*; treatment of bone infections, respiratory tract infections, skin and soft tissue infections, as well as abdominal and urinary tract infections, endocarditis, and septicemia; used topically to treat superficial infections of the skin or ophthalmic infections caused by susceptible bacteria; prevention of bacterial endocarditis prior to dental or surgical procedures

Local Anesthetic/Vasoconstrictor Precautions No information available to require special precautions

Effects on Dental Treatment No significant effects or complications reported

Significant Adverse Effects

>10%:
- Central nervous system: Neurotoxicity (vertigo, ataxia)
- Neuromuscular & skeletal: Gait instability
- Otic: Ototoxicity (auditory), ototoxicity (vestibular)
- Renal: Nephrotoxicity, decreased creatinine clearance

1% to 10%:
- Cardiovascular: Edema
- Dermatologic: Skin itching, reddening of skin, rash

<1% (Limited to important or life-threatening): Agranulocytosis, allergic reaction, dyspnea, granulocytopenia, photosensitivity, pseudomotor cerebri, thrombocytopenia

Dosage Individualization is critical because of the low therapeutic index

Use of ideal body weight (IBW) for determining the mg/kg/dose appears to be more accurate than dosing on the basis of total body weight (TBW).

(Continued)

Gentamicin *(Continued)*

In morbid obesity, dosage requirement may best be estimated using a dosing weight of IBW + 0.4 (TBW - IBW)

Initial and periodic peak and trough plasma drug levels should be determined, particularly in critically-ill patients with serious infections or in disease states known to significantly alter aminoglycoside pharmacokinetics (eg, cystic fibrosis, burns, or major surgery)

Newborns: Intrathecal: 1 mg every day

Infants >3 months: Intrathecal: 1-2 mg/day

Infants and Children <5 years: I.M., I.V.: 2.5 mg/kg/dose every 8 hours*

Cystic fibrosis: 2.5 mg/kg/dose every 6 hours

Children >5 years: I.M., I.V.: 1.5-2.5 mg/kg/dose every 8 hours*

Prevention of bacterial endocarditis: Dental, oral, upper respiratory procedures, GI/GU procedures: 2 mg/kg with ampicillin (50 mg/kg) 30 minutes prior to procedure

*Some patients may require larger or more frequent doses (eg, every 6 hours) if serum levels document the need (ie, cystic fibrosis or febrile granulocytopenic patients)

Adults: I.M., I.V.:

Severe life-threatening infections: 2-2.5 mg/kg/dose

Urinary tract infections: 1.5 mg/kg/dose

Synergy (for gram-positive infections): 1 mg/kg/dose

Prevention of bacterial endocarditis:

Dental, oral, or upper respiratory procedures: 1.5 mg/kg not to exceed 80 mg with ampicillin (1-2 g) 30 minutes prior to procedure

GI/GU surgery: 1.5 mg/kg not to exceed 80 mg with ampicillin (2 g) 30 minutes prior to procedure

Some clinicians suggest a daily dose of 4-7 mg/kg for all patients with normal renal function. This dose is at least as efficacious with similar, if not less, toxicity than conventional dosing.

Children and Adults:

Intrathecal: 4-8 mg/day

Ophthalmic:

Ointment: Instill ½" (1.25 cm) 2-3 times/day to every 3-4 hours

Solution: Instill 1-2 drops every 2-4 hours, up to 2 drops every hour for severe infections

Topical: Apply 3-4 times/day to affected area

Dosing interval in renal impairment:

Cl_{cr} ≥60 mL/minute: Administer every 8 hours

Cl_{cr} 40-60 mL/minute: Administer every 12 hours

Cl_{cr} 20-40 mL/minute: Administer every 24 hours

Cl_{cr} <20 mL/minute: Loading dose, then monitor levels

Hemodialysis: Dialyzable; removal by hemodialysis: 30% removal of aminoglycosides occurs during 4 hours of HD; administer dose after dialysis and follow levels

Removal by continuous ambulatory peritoneal dialysis (CAPD):

Administration via CAPD fluid:

Gram-negative infection: 4-8 mg/L (4-8 mcg/mL) of CAPD fluid

Gram-positive infection (ie, synergy): 3-4 mg/L (3-4 mcg/mL) of CAPD fluid

Administration via I.V., I.M. route during CAPD: Dose as for Cl_{cr}<10 mL/minute and follow levels

Removal via continuous arteriovenous or venovenous hemofiltration: Dose as for Cl_{cr} 10-40 mL/minute and follow levels

Dosing adjustment/comments in hepatic disease: Monitor plasma concentrations

Mechanism of Action Interferes with bacterial protein synthesis by binding to 30S and 50S ribosomal subunits resulting in a defective bacterial cell membrane

Contraindications Hypersensitivity to gentamicin or other aminoglycosides

Warnings/Precautions Not intended for long-term therapy due to toxic hazards associated with extended administration; pre-existing renal insufficiency, vestibular or cochlear impairment, myasthenia gravis, hypocalcemia, conditions which depress neuromuscular transmission

Parenteral aminoglycosides have been associated with significant nephrotoxicity or ototoxicity; the ototoxicity may be directly proportional to the amount of drug given and the duration of treatment; tinnitus or vertigo are indications of vestibular injury and impending hearing loss; renal damage is usually reversible

Drug Interactions

Increased toxicity:

Aminoglycosides may potentiate the effects of neuromuscular-blocking agents.

Penicillins, cephalosporins, amphotericin B, loop diuretics may increase nephrotoxic potential

Decreased effect: Gentamicin's efficacy reduced when given concurrently with carbenicillin, ticarcillin, or piperacillin to patients with severe renal impairment (inactivation). Separate administration.

Dietary Considerations Calcium, magnesium, potassium: Renal wasting may cause hypocalcemia, hypomagnesemia, and/or hypokalemia.

Pharmacodynamics/Kinetics

Absorption: Oral: None

Distribution: Crosses placenta

V_d: Increased by edema, ascites, fluid overload; decreased with dehydration

Neonates: 0.4-0.6 L/kg

Children: 0.3-0.35 L/kg

Adults: 0.2-0.3 L/kg

Relative diffusion from blood into CSF: Minimal even with inflammation

CSF:blood level ratio: Normal meninges: Nil; Inflamed meninges: 10% to 30%

Protein binding: <30%

Half-life elimination:

Infants: <1 week old: 3-11.5 hours; 1 week to 6 months old: 3-3.5 hours

Adults: 1.5-3 hours; End-stage renal disease: 36-70 hours

Time to peak, serum: I.M.: 30-90 minutes; I.V.: 30 minutes after 30-minute infusion

Excretion: Urine (as unchanged drug)

Clearance: Directly related to renal function

Pregnancy Risk Factor C

Lactation Enters breast milk (small amounts)/use caution (AAP rates "compatible")

Breast-Feeding Considerations No data reported; however, gentamicin is not absorbed orally and other aminoglycosides may be taken while breast-feeding.

Dosage Forms [DSC] = Discontinued product

Cream, topical, as sulfate: 0.1% (15 g, 30 g)

Garamycin®: 0.1% (15 g) [DSC]

Infusion, as sulfate [premixed in NS]: 40 mg (50 mL); 60 mg (50 mL, 100 mL); 70 mg (50 mL); 80 mg (50 mL, 100 mL); 90 mg (100 mL); 100 mg (50 mL, 100 mL); 120 mg (100 mL)

Injection, solution, as sulfate [ADD-Vantage® vial]: 10 mg/mL (6 mL, 8 mL, 10 mL)

Injection, solution, as sulfate: 40 mg/mL (2 mL, 20 mL) [may contain sodium metabisulfite]

Garamycin®: 40 mg/mL (2 mL) [contains sodium bisulfite] [DSC]

Injection, solution, pediatric, as sulfate: 10 mg/mL (2 mL) [may contain sodium metabisulfite]

Injection, solution, pediatric, as sulfate [preservative free]: 10 mg/mL (2 mL)

Ointment, ophthalmic, as sulfate (Gentak®): 0.3% [3 mg/g] (3.5 g)

Ointment, topical, as sulfate: 0.1% (15 g, 30 g)

Solution, ophthalmic, as sulfate: 0.3% (5 mL, 15 mL) [contains benzalkonium chloride]

Genoptic®: 0.3% (1 mL, 5 mL) [contains benzalkonium chloride]

Gentacidin®: 0.3% (5 mL) [contains benzalkonium chloride]

Gentak®: 0.3% (5 mL, 15 mL) [contains benzalkonium chloride]

Gentamicin and Prednisolone *see* Prednisolone and Gentamicin *on page 1115*

Gentamicin Sulfate *see* Gentamicin *on page 655*

GenTeal® [OTC] *see* Hydroxypropyl Methylcellulose *on page 721*

GenTeal® Mild [OTC] *see* Hydroxypropyl Methylcellulose *on page 721*

Gentian Violet (JEN shun VYE oh let)

Generic Available Yes

Synonyms Crystal Violet; Methylrosaniline Chloride

Pharmacologic Category Antibiotic, Topical; Antifungal Agent, Topical

Use Treatment of cutaneous or mucocutaneous infections caused by *Candida albicans* and other superficial skin infections

Local Anesthetic/Vasoconstrictor Precautions No information available to require special precautions

(Continued)

Gentian Violet *(Continued)*

Effects on Dental Treatment No significant effects or complications reported

Common Adverse Effects Frequency not defined.

Dermatologic: Vesicle formation
Gastrointestinal: Esophagitis, ulceration of mucous membranes
Local: Burning, irritation
Respiratory: Laryngitis, laryngeal obstruction, tracheitis
Miscellaneous: Sensitivity reactions

Mechanism of Action Topical antiseptic/germicide effective against some vegetative gram-positive bacteria, particularly *Staphylococcus* sp, and some yeast; it is much less effective against gram-negative bacteria and is ineffective against acid-fast bacteria

Pregnancy Risk Factor C

Gentlax® [OTC] *see* Bisacodyl *on page 208*

Gentran® *see* Dextran *on page 417*

Geocillin® *see* Carbenicillin *on page 260*

Geodon® *see* Ziprasidone *on page 1401*

Geref® [DSC] *see* Sermorelin Acetate *on page 1214*

Geref® Diagnostic *see* Sermorelin Acetate *on page 1214*

Geri-Hydrolac™ [OTC] *see* Lactic Acid and Ammonium Hydroxide *on page 793*

Geri-Hydrolac™-12 [OTC] *see* Lactic Acid and Ammonium Hydroxide *on page 793*

Geritol® Tonic [OTC] *see* Vitamins (Multiple/Oral) *on page 1384*

German Measles Vaccine *see* Rubella Virus Vaccine (Live) *on page 1203*

Gevrabon® [OTC] *see* Vitamin B Complex Combinations *on page 1382*

GF196960 *see* Tadalafil *on page 1257*

GG *see* Guaifenesin *on page 672*

GHB *see* Sodium Oxybate *on page 1229*

GI87084B *see* Remifentanil *on page 1172*

Gingi-Aid® Gingival Retraction Cord *see* Aluminum Chloride *on page 90*

Gingi-Aid® Solution *see* Aluminum Chloride *on page 90*

Glargine, Insulin *see* Insulin Preparations *on page 749*

Glatiramer Acetate (gla TIR a mer AS e tate)

U.S. Brand Names Copaxone®

Canadian Brand Names Copaxone®

Generic Available No

Synonyms Copolymer-1

Pharmacologic Category Biological, Miscellaneous

Use Treatment of relapsing-remitting type multiple sclerosis; studies indicate that it reduces the frequency of attacks and the severity of disability; appears to be most effective for patients with minimal disability

Local Anesthetic/Vasoconstrictor Precautions No information available to require special precautions

Effects on Dental Treatment Key adverse event(s) related to dental treatment: Ulcerative stomatitis and salivary gland enlargement.

Common Adverse Effects Reported in >2% of patients in placebo-controlled trials:

>10%:

Cardiovascular: Chest pain (21%), vasodilation (27%), palpitations (17%)
Central nervous system: Pain (28%), anxiety (23%)
Dermatologic: Pruritus (18%), rash (18%), diaphoresis (15%)
Gastrointestinal: Nausea (22%), diarrhea (12%)
Local: Injection site reactions: Pain (73%), erythema (66%), inflammation (49%), pruritus (40%), mass (27%), induration (13%), welt (11%)
Neuromuscular & skeletal: Weakness (41%), arthralgia (24%), hypertonia (22%), back pain (16%)
Respiratory: Dyspnea (19%), rhinitis (14%)
Miscellaneous: Infection (50%), flu-like syndrome (19%), lymphadenopathy (12%)

1% to 10%:

Cardiovascular: Peripheral edema (7%), facial edema (6%), edema (3%), tachycardia (5%)
Central nervous system: Fever (8%), vertigo (6%), migraine (5%), syncope (5%), agitation (4%), chills (4%), confusion (2%), nervousness (2%), speech disorder (2%)

Dermatologic: Bruising (8%), erythema (4%), urticaria (4%), skin nodule (2%)
Endocrine & metabolic: Dysmenorrhea (6%)
Gastrointestinal: Anorexia (8%), vomiting (6%), gastrointestinal disorder (5%), gastroenteritis (3%), weight gain (3%)
Genitourinary: Urinary urgency (10%), vaginal moniliasis (8%)
Local: Injection site reactions: Hemorrhage (5%), urticaria (5%)
Neuromuscular & skeletal: Tremor (7%), foot drop (3%)
Ocular: Eye disorder (4%), nystagmus (2%)
Otic: Ear pain (7%)
Respiratory: Bronchitis (9%), laryngismus (5%)
Miscellaneous: Neck pain (8%), bacterial infection (5%), herpes simplex (4%), cyst (2%)

Mechanism of Action Glatiramer is a mixture of random polymers of four amino acids; L-alanine, L-glutamic acid, L-lysine and L-tyrosine, the resulting mixture is antigenically similar to myelin basic protein, which is an important component of the myelin sheath of nerves; glatiramer is thought to suppress T-lymphocytes specific for a myelin antigen, it is also proposed that glatiramer interferes with the antigen-presenting function of certain immune cells opposing pathogenic T-cell function

Pharmacodynamics/Kinetics
Distribution: Small amounts of intact and partial hydrolyzed drug enter lymphatic circulation
Metabolism: SubQ: Large percentage hydrolyzed locally

Pregnancy Risk Factor B

Gleevec™ *see* Imatinib *on page 734*

Gliadel® *see* Carmustine *on page 268*

Glibenclamide *see* GlyBURIDE *on page 664*

Glimepiride (GLYE me pye ride)

Related Information
Endocrine Disorders and Pregnancy *on page 1481*

U.S. Brand Names Amaryl®

Canadian Brand Names Amaryl®

Mexican Brand Names Amaryl®

Generic Available No

Pharmacologic Category Antidiabetic Agent, Sulfonylurea

Use Management of type 2 diabetes mellitus (noninsulin dependent, NIDDM) as an adjunct to diet and exercise to lower blood glucose or in combination with metformin; use in combination with insulin to lower blood glucose in patients whose hyperglycemia cannot be controlled by diet and exercise in conjunction with an oral hypoglycemic agent

Local Anesthetic/Vasoconstrictor Precautions No information available to require special precautions

Effects on Dental Treatment Glimepiride-dependent diabetics (noninsulin dependent, type 2) should be appointed for dental treatment in morning in order to minimize chance of stress-induced hypoglycemia.

Common Adverse Effects 1% to 10%: Central nervous system: Headache

Dosage Oral (allow several days between dose titrations):
Adults: Initial: 1-2 mg once daily, administered with breakfast or the first main meal; usual maintenance dose: 1-4 mg once daily; after a dose of 2 mg once daily, increase in increments of 2 mg at 1- to 2-week intervals based upon the patient's blood glucose response to a maximum of 8 mg once daily
Combination with insulin therapy (fasting glucose level for instituting combination therapy is in the range of >150 mg/dL in plasma or serum depending on the patient): initial recommended dose: 8 mg once daily with the first main meal
After starting with low-dose insulin, upward adjustments of insulin can be done approximately weekly as guided by frequent measurements of fasting blood glucose. Once stable, combination-therapy patients should monitor their capillary blood glucose on an ongoing basis, preferably daily.

Dosing adjustment/comments in renal impairment: Cl_{cr} <22 mL/minute: Initial starting dose should be 1 mg and dosage increments should be based on fasting blood glucose levels

Dosing adjustment in hepatic impairment: No data available

Elderly: Initial: 1 mg/day; dose titration and maintenance dosing should be conservative to avoid hypoglycemia

Mechanism of Action Stimulates insulin release from the pancreatic beta cells; reduces glucose output from the liver; insulin sensitivity is increased at peripheral target sites
(Continued)

Glimepiride *(Continued)*

Contraindications Hypersensitivity to glimepiride, any component of the formulation, or sulfonamides; diabetic ketoacidosis (with or without coma)

Warnings/Precautions All sulfonylurea drugs are capable of producing severe hypoglycemia. Hypoglycemia is more likely to occur when caloric intake is deficient, after severe or prolonged exercise, when ethanol is ingested, or when more than one glucose-lowering drug is used.

Chemical similarities are present among sulfonamides, sulfonylureas, carbonic anhydrase inhibitors, thiazides, and loop diuretics (except ethacrynic acid). Use in patients with sulfonamide allergy is specifically contraindicated in product labeling, however, a risk of cross-reaction exists in patients with allergy to any of these compounds; avoid use when previous reaction has been severe.

Product labeling states oral hypoglycemic drugs may be associated with an increased cardiovascular mortality as compared to treatment with diet alone or diet plus insulin. Data to support this association are limited, and several studies, including a large prospective trial (UKPDS) have not supported an association.

Drug Interactions

Cytochrome P450 Effect: Substrate of CYP2C8/9 (major)

Increased Effect/Toxicity: CYP2C8/9 inhibitors may increase the levels/effects of glimepiride; example inhibitors include delavirdine, ketoconazole, nicardipine, NSAIDs, and pioglitazone. Beta-blockers, chloramphenicol, cimetidine, clofibrate, fluconazole, gemfibrozil, pegvisomant, salicylates, sulfonamides, and tricyclic antidepressants may increase the hypoglycemic effects of glimepiride. Glimepiride may increase effects of coumarins and cyclosporine.

Decreased Effect: CYP2C8/9 inducers may decrease the levels/effects of glimepiride; example inducers include carbamazepine, phenobarbital, phenytoin, rifampin, rifapentine, and secobarbital. There may be a decreased effect of glimepiride with corticosteroids, estrogens, oral contraceptives, thiazide and other diuretics, phenothiazines, NSAIDs, thyroid products, nicotinic acid, isoniazid, sympathomimetics, urinary alkalinizers, and charcoal. **Note:** However, pooled data did **not** demonstrate drug interactions with calcium channel blockers, estrogens, NSAIDs, HMG-CoA reductase inhibitors, sulfonamides, or thyroid hormone.

Ethanol/Nutrition/Herb Interactions

Ethanol: Caution with ethanol (may cause hypoglycemia).

Herb/Nutraceutical: Caution with chromium, garlic, gymnema (may cause hypoglycemia).

Dietary Considerations Administer with breakfast or the first main meal of the day. Dietary modification based on ADA recommendations is a part of therapy. Decreases blood glucose concentration. Hypoglycemia may occur. Must be able to recognize symptoms of hypoglycemia (palpitations, sweaty palms, lightheadedness).

Pharmacodynamics/Kinetics

Onset of action: Peak effect: Blood glucose reductions: 2-3 hours

Duration: 24 hours

Absorption: 100%; delayed when given with food

Protein binding: >99.5%

Metabolism: Completely hepatic

Half-life elimination: 5-9 hours

Excretion: Urine and feces (as metabolites)

Pregnancy Risk Factor C

Dosage Forms TAB: 1 mg, 2 mg, 4 mg

GlipIZIDE (GLIP i zide)

Related Information

Endocrine Disorders and Pregnancy *on page 1481*

Glipizide and Metformin *on page 662*

U.S. Brand Names Glucotrol®; Glucotrol® XL

Mexican Brand Names Glupitel®; Minodiab®

Generic Available Yes: Not extended release formulation

Synonyms Glydiazinamide

Pharmacologic Category Antidiabetic Agent, Sulfonylurea

Use Management of type 2 diabetes mellitus (noninsulin dependent, NIDDM)

Local Anesthetic/Vasoconstrictor Precautions No information available to require special precautions

Effects on Dental Treatment Glipizide-dependent diabetics (noninsulin dependent, type 2) should be appointed for dental treatment in morning in order to minimize chance of stress-induced hypoglycemia.

Common Adverse Effects Frequency not defined.

Cardiovascular: Edema, syncope

Central nervous system: Anxiety, depression, dizziness, headache, insomnia, nervousness

Dermatologic: Rash, urticaria, photosensitivity, pruritus

Endocrine & metabolic: Hypoglycemia, hyponatremia, SIADH (rare)

Gastrointestinal: Anorexia, nausea, vomiting, diarrhea, epigastric fullness, constipation, heartburn, flatulence

Hematologic: Blood dyscrasias, aplastic anemia, hemolytic anemia, bone marrow suppression, thrombocytopenia, agranulocytosis

Hepatic: Cholestatic jaundice, hepatic porphyria

Neuromuscular & skeletal: Arthralgia, leg cramps, myalgia, tremor

Ocular: Blurred vision

Renal: Diuretic effect (minor)

Miscellaneous: Diaphoresis, disulfiram-like reaction

Dosage Oral (allow several days between dose titrations): Adults: Initial: 5 mg/day; adjust dosage at 2.5-5 mg daily increments as determined by blood glucose response at intervals of several days.

Immediate release tablet: Maximum recommended once-daily dose: 15 mg; maximum recommended total daily dose: 40 mg

Extended release tablet (Glucotrol® XL): Maximum recommended dose: 20 mg

When transferring from insulin to glipizide:

Current insulin requirement ≤20 units: Discontinue insulin and initiate glipizide at usual dose

Current insulin requirement >20 units: Decrease insulin by 50% and initiate glipizide at usual dose; gradually decrease insulin dose based on patient response. Several days should elapse between dosage changes.

Elderly: Initial: 2.5 mg/day; increase by 2.5-5 mg/day at 1- to 2-week intervals

Dosing adjustment/comments in renal impairment: Cl_{cr} <10 mL/minute: Some investigators recommend not using

Dosing adjustment in hepatic impairment: Initial dosage should be 2.5 mg/day

Mechanism of Action Stimulates insulin release from the pancreatic beta cells; reduces glucose output from the liver; insulin sensitivity is increased at peripheral target sites

Contraindications Hypersensitivity to glipizide or any component of the formulation, other sulfonamides; type 1 diabetes mellitus (insulin dependent, IDDM)

Warnings/Precautions Use with caution in patients with severe hepatic disease.

Chemical similarities are present among sulfonamides, sulfonylureas, carbonic anhydrase inhibitors, thiazides, and loop diuretics (except ethacrynic acid). Use in patients with sulfonamide allergy is specifically contraindicated in product labeling, however, a risk of cross-reaction exists in patients with allergy to any of these compounds; avoid use when previous reaction has been severe.

Product labeling states oral hypoglycemic drugs may be associated with an increased cardiovascular mortality as compared to treatment with diet alone or diet plus insulin. Data to support this association are limited, and several studies, including a large prospective trial (UKPDS) have not supported an association.

At higher dosages, sulfonylureas may block the ATP-sensitive potassium channels, which have been suggested to increase the risk of cardiovascular events. In May, 2000, the National Diabetes Center (a patient advocacy group, not a government agency) issued a warning to avoid the use of sulfonylureas at higher dosages. The clinical data supporting an association is inconsistent, and there is no consensus within the medical community to support this assertion.

Drug Interactions

Cytochrome P450 Effect: Substrate of 2C8/9 (major)

Increased Effect/Toxicity: CYP2C8/9 inhibitors may increase the levels/effects of glipizide; example inhibitors include delavirdine, fluconazole, gemfibrozil, ketoconazole, nicardipine, NSAIDs, pioglitazone, and sulfonamides. Increased effects/hypoglycemic effects of glipizide with H_2 antagonists, anticoagulants, androgens, cimetidine, salicylates, tricyclic antidepressants, probenecid, MAO inhibitors, methyldopa, digitalis glycosides, and urinary acidifiers.

(Continued)

GlipiZIDE *(Continued)*

Decreased Effect: CYP2C8/9 inducers may decrease the levels/effects of glipizide; example inducers include carbamazepine, phenobarbital, phenytoin, rifampin, rifapentine, and secobarbital. Decreased effect of glipizide with beta-blockers, cholestyramine, hydantoins, thiazide diuretics, urinary alkalinizers, and charcoal.

Ethanol/Nutrition/Herb Interactions

Ethanol: Caution with ethanol (may cause hypoglycemia or rare disulfiram reaction).

Food: A delayed release of insulin may occur if glipizide is taken with food. Immediate release tablets should be administered 30 minutes before meals to avoid erratic absorption.

Herb/Nutraceutical: Caution with chromium, garlic, gymnema (may cause hypoglycemia).

Dietary Considerations Take immediate release tablets 30 minutes before meals; extended release tablets should be taken with breakfast. Dietary modification based on ADA recommendations is a part of therapy. Decreases blood glucose concentration. Hypoglycemia may occur. Must be able to recognize symptoms of hypoglycemia (palpitations, sweaty palms, lightheadedness).

Pharmacodynamics/Kinetics

Onset of action: Peak effect: Blood glucose reductions: 1.5-2 hours
Duration: 12-24 hours
Absorption: Delayed with food
Protein binding: 92% to 99%
Metabolism: Hepatic with metabolites
Half-life elimination: 2-4 hours
Excretion: Urine (60% to 80%, 91% to 97% as metabolites); feces (11%)

Pregnancy Risk Factor C

Dosage Forms TAB (Glucotrol®): 5 mg, 10 mg. **TAB, extended release** (Glucotrol® XL): 2.5 mg, 5 mg, 10 mg

Glipizide and Metformin (GLIP i zide & met FOR min)

Related Information

GlipiZIDE *on page 660*
Metformin *on page 887*

U.S. Brand Names Metaglip™

Generic Available No

Synonyms Glipizide and Metformin Hydrochloride; Metformin and Glipizide

Pharmacologic Category Antidiabetic Agent, Biguanide; Antidiabetic Agent, Sulfonylurea

Use Initial therapy for management of type 2 diabetes mellitus (noninsulin dependent, NIDDM) when hyperglycemia cannot be managed with diet and exercise alone. Second-line therapy for management of type 2 diabetes (NIDDM) when hyperglycemia cannot be managed with a sulfonylurea or metformin along with diet and exercise.

Local Anesthetic/Vasoconstrictor Precautions No information available to require special precautions

Effects on Dental Treatment Key adverse event(s) related to dental treatment: Upper respiratory tract infection (8% to 10%). Dependent diabetics (noninsulin dependent, type 2) should be appointed for dental treatment in the morning in order to minimize chance of stress-induced hypoglycemia.

Common Adverse Effects Also see individual agents.

>10%:
- Central nervous system: Headache (12%)
- Endocrine & metabolic: Hypoglycemia (8% to 13%)
- Gastrointestinal: Diarrhea (2% to 18%)

1% to 10%:
- Cardiovascular: Hypertension (3%)
- Central nervous system: Dizziness (2% to 5%)
- Gastrointestinal: Nausea/vomiting (<1% to 8%), abdominal pain (6%)
- Neuromuscular & skeletal: Musculoskeletal pain (8%)
- Renal: Urinary tract infection (1%)
- Respiratory: Upper respiratory tract infection (8% to 10%)

Mechanism of Action The combination of glipizide and metformin is used to improve glycemic control in patients with type 2 diabetes mellitus (noninsulin dependent, NIDDM) by using two different, but complementary, mechanisms of action:

Glipizide: Stimulates insulin release from the pancreatic beta cells; reduces glucose output from the liver; insulin sensitivity is increased at peripheral target sites

Metformin: Decreases hepatic glucose production, decreasing intestinal absorption of glucose and improves insulin sensitivity (increases peripheral glucose uptake and utilization)

Drug Interactions

Cytochrome P450 Effect: Glipizide: **Substrate** of 2C8/9 (major)

Increased Effect/Toxicity: See individual agents.

Decreased Effect: See individual agents.

Pharmacodynamics/Kinetics See individual agents.

Pregnancy Risk Factor C

Glipizide and Metformin Hydrochloride *see* Glipizide and Metformin *on page 662*

Glivec *see* Imatinib *on page 734*

GlucaGen® *see* Glucagon *on page 663*

GlucaGen® Diagnostic Kit *see* Glucagon *on page 663*

Glucagon (GLOO ka gon)

U.S. Brand Names GlucaGen®; GlucaGen® Diagnostic Kit; Glucagon Diagnostic Kit; Glucagon Emergency Kit

Generic Available No

Synonyms Glucagon Hydrochloride

Pharmacologic Category Antidote; Diagnostic Agent

Use Management of hypoglycemia; diagnostic aid in radiologic examinations to temporarily inhibit GI tract movement

Unlabeled/Investigational Use Used with some success as a cardiac stimulant in management of severe cases of beta-adrenergic blocking agent overdosage; treatment of myocardial depression due to calcium channel blocker overdose

Local Anesthetic/Vasoconstrictor Precautions No information available to require special precautions

Effects on Dental Treatment No significant effects or complications reported

Common Adverse Effects Frequency not defined.

Cardiovascular: Hypotension (up to 2 hours after GI procedures), hypertension, tachycardia

Gastrointestinal: Nausea, vomiting (high incidence with rapid administration of high doses)

Miscellaneous: Hypersensitivity reactions, anaphylaxis

Mechanism of Action Stimulates adenylate cyclase to produce increased cyclic AMP, which promotes hepatic glycogenolysis and gluconeogenesis, causing a raise in blood glucose levels

Drug Interactions

Increased Effect/Toxicity: Oral anticoagulant: Hypoprothrombinemic effects may be increased possibly with bleeding; effect seen with glucagon doses of 50 mg administered over 1-2 days

Pharmacodynamics/Kinetics

Onset of action: Peak effect: Blood glucose levels: Parenteral:

I.V.: 5-20 minutes

I.M.: 30 minutes

SubQ: 30-45 minutes

Duration: Hyperglycemia: 60-90 minutes

Metabolism: Primarily hepatic; some inactivation occurring renally and in plasma

Half-life elimination, plasma: 3-10 minutes

Pregnancy Risk Factor B

Glucagon Diagnostic Kit *see* Glucagon *on page 663*

Glucagon Emergency Kit *see* Glucagon *on page 663*

Glucagon Hydrochloride *see* Glucagon *on page 663*

Glucocerebrosidase *see* Alglucerase *on page 80*

Glucophage® *see* Metformin *on page 887*

Glucophage® XR *see* Metformin *on page 887*

Glucose (Instant) (GLOO kose, IN stant)

Related Information

Dental Office Emergencies *on page 1584*

U.S. Brand Names B-D™ Glucose [OTC]; Dex4 Glucose [OTC]; Glutol™ [OTC]; Glutose™ [OTC]; Insta-Glucose® [OTC]

Generic Available Yes

Pharmacologic Category Antihypoglycemic Agent

Use Management of hypoglycemia

(Continued)

Glucose (Instant) *(Continued)*

Local Anesthetic/Vasoconstrictor Precautions No information available to require special precautions

Effects on Dental Treatment No significant effects or complications reported

Common Adverse Effects Frequency not defined: Gastrointestinal: Nausea, diarrhea

Pregnancy Risk Factor A

Glucose Polymers (GLOO kose POL i merz)

U.S. Brand Names Moducal® [OTC]; Polycose® [OTC]

Generic Available No

Pharmacologic Category Nutritional Supplement

Use Supplies calories for those persons not able to meet the caloric requirement with usual food intake

Local Anesthetic/Vasoconstrictor Precautions No information available to require special precautions

Effects on Dental Treatment No significant effects or complications reported

Glucotrol® *see* GlipiZIDE *on page 660*
Glucotrol® XL *see* GlipiZIDE *on page 660*
Glucovance® *see* Glyburide and Metformin *on page 665*
Glu-K® [OTC] *see* Potassium Gluconate *on page 1106*
Glulisine, Insulin *see* Insulin Preparations *on page 749*

Glutamic Acid (gloo TAM ik AS id)

Generic Available Yes

Synonyms Glutamic Acid Hydrochloride

Pharmacologic Category Gastrointestinal Agent, Miscellaneous

Use Treatment of hypochlorhydria and achlorhydria

Local Anesthetic/Vasoconstrictor Precautions No information available to require special precautions

Effects on Dental Treatment No significant effects or complications reported

Pregnancy Risk Factor C

Glutamic Acid Hydrochloride *see* Glutamic Acid *on page 664*
Glutol™ [OTC] *see* Glucose (Instant) *on page 663*
Glutose™ [OTC] *see* Glucose (Instant) *on page 663*
Glybenclamide *see* GlyBURIDE *on page 664*
Glybenzcyclamide *see* GlyBURIDE *on page 664*

GlyBURIDE (GLYE byoor ide)

Related Information

Endocrine Disorders and Pregnancy *on page 1481*

U.S. Brand Names Diaβeta®; Glynase® PresTab®; Micronase®

Canadian Brand Names Albert® Glyburide; Apo-Glyburide®; Diaβeta®; Euglucon®; Gen-Glybe; Novo-Glyburide; Nu-Glyburide; PMS-Glyburide; ratio-Glyburide

Mexican Brand Names Daonil®; Euglucon®; Glibenil®; Glucal®; Glucoven®; Nadib®; Norboral®

Generic Available Yes

Synonyms Diabeta; Glibenclamide; Glybenclamide; Glybenzcyclamide

Pharmacologic Category Antidiabetic Agent, Sulfonylurea

Use Management of type 2 diabetes mellitus (noninsulin dependent, NIDDM)

Unlabeled/Investigational Use Alternative to insulin in women for the treatment of gestational diabetes (11-33 weeks gestation)

Local Anesthetic/Vasoconstrictor Precautions No information available to require special precautions

Effects on Dental Treatment Glyburide-dependent diabetics (noninsulin dependent, type 2) should be appointed for dental treatment in morning in order to minimize chance of stress-induced hypoglycemia.

Common Adverse Effects Frequency not defined.

Central nervous system: Headache, dizziness

Dermatologic: Pruritus, rash, urticaria, photosensitivity reaction

Endocrine & metabolic: Hypoglycemia, hyponatremia (SIADH reported with other sulfonylureas)

Gastrointestinal: Nausea, epigastric fullness, heartburn, constipation, diarrhea, anorexia

Genitourinary: Nocturia

Hematologic: Leukopenia, thrombocytopenia, hemolytic anemia, aplastic anemia, bone marrow suppression, agranulocytosis

Hepatic: Cholestatic jaundice, hepatitis
Neuromuscular & skeletal: Arthralgia, paresthesia
Ocular: Blurred vision
Renal: Diuretic effect (minor)

Mechanism of Action Stimulates insulin release from the pancreatic beta cells; reduces glucose output from the liver; insulin sensitivity is increased at peripheral target sites

Drug Interactions

Cytochrome P450 Effect: Inhibits CYP3A4 (weak)

Increased Effect/Toxicity: Increased hypoglycemic effects of glyburide may occur with oral anticoagulants (warfarin), phenytoin, other hydantoins, salicylates, NSAIDs, sulfonamides, and beta-blockers. Ethanol ingestion may cause disulfiram reactions.

Decreased Effect: Thiazides and other diuretics, corticosteroids may decrease effectiveness of glyburide.

Pharmacodynamics/Kinetics

Onset of action: Serum insulin levels begin to increase 15-60 minutes after a single dose
Duration: ≤24 hours
Protein binding, plasma: >99%
Metabolism: To one moderately active and several inactive metabolites
Half-life elimination: 5-16 hours; may be prolonged with renal or hepatic impairment
Time to peak, serum: Adults: 2-4 hours
Excretion: Feces (50%) and urine (50%) as metabolites

Pregnancy Risk Factor C

Glyburide and Metformin (GLYE byoor ide & met FOR min)

Related Information

Endocrine Disorders and Pregnancy *on page 1481*
GlyBURIDE *on page 664*
Metformin *on page 887*

U.S. Brand Names Glucovance®

Generic Available Yes

Synonyms Glyburide and Metformin Hydrochloride; Metformin and Glyburide

Pharmacologic Category Antidiabetic Agent, Biguanide; Antidiabetic Agent, Sulfonylurea

Use Initial therapy for management of type 2 diabetes mellitus (noninsulin dependent, NIDDM). Second-line therapy for management of type 2 diabetes (NIDDM) when hyperglycemia cannot be managed with a sulfonylurea or metformin; combination therapy with a thiazolidinedione may be required to achieve additional control.

Local Anesthetic/Vasoconstrictor Precautions No information available to require special precautions

Effects on Dental Treatment Glyburide-dependent diabetics (noninsulin dependent, type 2) should be appointed for dental treatment in morning in order to minimize chance of stress-induced hypoglycemia. Metformin-dependent diabetics (noninsulin dependent, type 2) should be appointed for dental treatment in morning in order to minimize chance of stress-induced hypoglycemia.

Common Adverse Effects (Also refer to individual agents)

>10%:
Endocrine & metabolic: Hypoglycemia (11% to 38%, effects higher when increased doses were used as initial therapy)
Gastrointestinal: Diarrhea (17%)
Respiratory: Upper respiratory infection (17%)

1% to 10%:
Central nervous system: Headache (9%), dizziness (6%)
Gastrointestinal: Nausea (8%), vomiting (8%), abdominal pain (7%) (combined GI effects increased to 38% in patients taking high doses as initial therapy)

Dosage Note: Dose must be individualized. Dosages expressed as glyburide/metformin components.

Adults: Oral:

Initial therapy (no prior treatment with sulfonylurea or metformin): 1.25 mg/250 mg once daily with a meal; patients with Hb A_{1c} >9% or fasting plasma glucose (FPG) >200 mg/dL may start with 1.25 mg/250 mg twice daily

Dosage may be increased in increments of 1.25 mg/250 mg, at intervals of not less than 2 weeks; maximum daily dose: 10 mg/2000 mg (limited experience with higher doses)

(Continued)

Glyburide and Metformin *(Continued)*

Previously treated with a sulfonylurea or metformin alone: Initial: 2.5 mg/500 mg or 5 mg/500 mg twice daily; increase in increments no greater than 5 mg/500 mg; maximum daily dose: 20 mg/2000 mg

When switching patients previously on a sulfonylurea and metformin together, do not exceed the daily dose of glyburide (or glyburide equivalent) or metformin.

Note: May combine with a thiazolidinedione in patients with an inadequate response to glyburide/metformin therapy (risk of hypoglycemia may be increased).

Elderly: Oral: Conservative doses are recommended in the elderly due to potentially decreased renal function; **do not titrate to maximum dose**; should not be used in patients ≥80 years of age unless renal function is verified as normal

Dosage adjustment in renal impairment: Risk of lactic acidosis increases with degree of renal impairment; contraindicated in renal disease or renal dysfunction (see Contraindications)

Dosage adjustment in hepatic impairment: Use conservative initial and maintenance doses and avoid use in severe hepatic disease

Mechanism of Action The combination of glyburide and metformin is used to improve glycemic control in patients with type 2 diabetes mellitus by using two different, but complementary, mechanisms of action:

Glyburide: Stimulates insulin release from the pancreatic beta cells; reduces glucose output from the liver; insulin sensitivity is increased at peripheral target sites

Metformin: Decreases hepatic glucose production, decreasing intestinal absorption of glucose and improves insulin sensitivity (increases peripheral glucose uptake and utilization)

Contraindications Hypersensitivity to glyburide or other sulfonamides, metformin, or any component of the formulation; renal disease or renal dysfunction (serum creatinine ≥1.5 mg/dL in males or ≥1.4 mg/dL in females, or abnormal creatinine clearance which may also result from conditions such as cardiovascular collapse, acute myocardial infarction, and septicemia); acute or chronic metabolic acidosis with or without coma (including diabetic ketoacidosis); congestive heart failure requiring pharmacologic treatment

Note: Temporarily discontinue in patients undergoing radiologic studies in which intravascular iodinated contrast materials are utilized.

Warnings/Precautions Age, hepatic and renal impairment are independent risk factors for hypoglycemia. Use with caution in patients with hepatic impairment, malnourished or debilitated conditions, or adrenal or pituitary insufficiency. Use caution in patients with renal impairment. Lactic acidosis is a rare, but potentially severe consequence of therapy with metformin. Withhold therapy in hypoxemia, dehydration, or sepsis. The risk of lactic acidosis is increased in any patient with CHF requiring pharmacologic management. This risk is particularly high during acute or unstable CHF because of the risk of hypoperfusion and hypoxemia.

Metformin is substantially excreted by the kidney. The risk of accumulation and lactic acidosis increases with the degree of impairment of renal function. Patients with renal function below the limit of normal for their age should not receive metformin. In elderly patients, renal function should be monitored regularly; should not be used in any patient ≥80 years of age unless measurement of creatinine clearance verifies normal renal function. Use of concomitant medications that may affect renal function (ie, affect tubular secretion) may also affect metformin disposition. Metformin should be suspended in patients with dehydration and/or prerenal azotemia. Therapy should be suspended for any surgical procedures (resume only after normal intake resumed and normal renal function is verified).Intravascular iodinated contrast materials used for radiologic studies are associated with alteration of renal function and may increase risk of lactic acidosis. Discontinue Glucovance® at the time of or prior to the procedure and withhold for 48 hours subsequent to the procedure; reinstitute only after renal function has been re-evaluated and found to be normal.

Chemical similarities are present among sulfonamides, sulfonylureas, carbonic anhydrase inhibitors, thiazides, and loop diuretics (except ethacrynic acid). Use in patients with sulfonamide allergy is specifically contraindicated in product labeling, however a risk of cross-reaction exists in patients with allergy to any of these compounds; avoid use when previous reaction has been severe.

Product labeling states oral hypoglycemic drugs may be associated with an increased cardiovascular mortality as compared to treatment with diet alone or diet plus insulin. Data to support this association are limited, and several studies, including a large prospective trial (UKPDS), have not supported an association.

Drug Interactions

Increased Effect/Toxicity: See individual agents.

Decreased Effect: See individual agents.

Ethanol/Nutrition/Herb Interactions

Ethanol: May cause hypoglycemia; incidence of lactic acidosis may be increased; a disulfiram-like reaction characterized by flushing, headache, nausea, vomiting, sweating, or tachycardia has been reported with sulfonylureas; avoid or limit use.

Food: Metformin decreases absorption of vitamin B_{12}. Metformin decreases absorption of folic acid.

Dietary Considerations May cause GI upset; take with food to decrease GI upset. Dietary modification based on ADA recommendations is a part of therapy. Decreases blood glucose concentration. Hypoglycemia may occur. Must be able to recognize symptoms of hypoglycemia (palpitations, sweaty palms, lightheadedness). Monitor for signs and symptoms of vitamin B_{12} deficiency. Monitor for signs and symptoms of folic acid deficiency.

Pharmacodynamics/Kinetics

Glucovance®:

Bioavailability: 18% with 2.5 mg glyburide/500 mg metformin dose; 7% with 5 mg glyburide/500 mg metformin dose; bioavailability is greater than that of Micronase® brand of glyburide and therefore not bioequivalent

Time to peak: 2.75 hours when taken with food

Glyburide: See Glyburide monograph.

Metformin: This component of Glucovance® is bioequivalent to metformin coadministration with glyburide.

Pregnancy Risk Factor B (manufacturer); C (expert analysis)

Dosage Forms TAB, film coated: 1.25 mg/250 mg: Glyburide 1.25 mg and metformin 250 mg; 2.5 mg/500 mg: Glyburide 2.5 mg and metformin 500 mg; 5 mg/500 mg: Glyburide 5 mg and metformin 500 mg

Glyburide and Metformin Hydrochloride *see* Glyburide and Metformin *on page 665*

Glycerin (GLIS er in)

U.S. Brand Names Bausch & Lomb® Computer Eye Drops [OTC]; Fleet® Babylax® [OTC]; Fleet® Glycerin Suppositories [OTC]; Fleet® Glycerin Suppositories Maximum Strength [OTC]; Fleet® Liquid Glycerin Suppositories [OTC]; Osmoglyn®; Sani-Supp® [OTC]

Mexican Brand Names Supositorios Senosiain®

Generic Available Yes

Synonyms Glycerol

Pharmacologic Category Laxative; Ophthalmic Agent, Miscellaneous

Use Constipation; reduction of intraocular pressure; reduction of corneal edema; glycerin has been administered orally to reduce intracranial pressure

Local Anesthetic/Vasoconstrictor Precautions No information available to require special precautions

Effects on Dental Treatment No significant effects or complications reported

Common Adverse Effects Frequency not defined.

Cardiovascular: Arrhythmias

Central nervous system: Headache, confusion, dizziness, hyperosmolar nonketotic coma

Endocrine: Polydipsia, hyperglycemia, dehydration

Gastrointestinal: Nausea, vomiting, tenesmus, rectal irritation, cramping pain, diarrhea, dry mouth

Mechanism of Action Osmotic dehydrating agent which increases osmotic pressure; draws fluid into colon and thus stimulates evacuation

Pharmacodynamics/Kinetics

Onset of action:

- Decrease in intraocular pressure: Oral: 10-30 minutes
- Reduction of intracranial pressure: Oral: 10-60 minutes
- Constipation: Suppository: 15-30 minutes
- Peak effect:
  - Decrease in intraocular pressure: Oral: 60-90 minutes
  - Reduction of intracranial pressure: Oral: 60-90 minutes

Duration:

- Decrease in intraocular pressure: Oral: 4-8 hours

(Continued)

Glycerin *(Continued)*

Reduction of intracranial pressure: Oral: ~2-3 hours
Absorption: Oral: Well absorbed; Rectal: Poorly absorbed
Half-life elimination, serum: 30-45 minutes

Pregnancy Risk Factor C

Glycerol *see* Glycerin *on page 667*
Glycerol Guaiacolate *see* Guaifenesin *on page 672*
Glycerol Triacetate *see* Triacetin *on page 1329*
Glyceryl Trinitrate *see* Nitroglycerin *on page 991*

Glycopyrrolate (glye koe PYE roe late)

U.S. Brand Names Robinul®; Robinul® Forte

Generic Available Yes: Injection

Synonyms Glycopyrronium Bromide

Pharmacologic Category Anticholinergic Agent

Use Inhibit salivation and excessive secretions of the respiratory tract preoperatively; reversal of neuromuscular blockade; control of upper airway secretions; adjunct in treatment of peptic ulcer

Local Anesthetic/Vasoconstrictor Precautions No information available to require special precautions

Effects on Dental Treatment Key adverse event(s) related to dental treatment: Dysphagia, significant xerostomia (normal salivary flow resumes upon discontinuation), and dry throat.

Common Adverse Effects

>10%:
- Dermatologic: Dry skin
- Gastrointestinal: Constipation, dry throat, xerostomia
- Local: Irritation at injection site
- Respiratory: Dry nose
- Miscellaneous: Diaphoresis (decreased)

1% to 10%:
- Dermatologic: Increased sensitivity to light
- Endocrine & metabolic: Decreased flow of breast milk
- Gastrointestinal: Dysphagia

Mechanism of Action Blocks the action of acetylcholine at parasympathetic sites in smooth muscle, secretory glands, and the CNS

Drug Interactions

Increased Effect/Toxicity: Increased toxicity with amantadine and cyclopropane. Effects of other anticholinergic agents may be increased by glycopyrrolate.

Decreased Effect: Decreased effect of levodopa.

Pharmacodynamics/Kinetics

Onset of action: Oral: 50 minutes; I.M.: 20-40 minutes; I.V.: ~1 minute
Peak effect: Oral: ~1 hour
Duration: Vagal effect: 2-3 hours; Inhibition of salivation: Up to 7 hours; Anticholinergic: Oral: 8-12 hours
Absorption: Oral: Poor and erratic
Metabolism: Hepatic (minimal)
Bioavailability: ~10%
Half-life elimination: 20-40 minutes

Pregnancy Risk Factor B

Glycopyrronium Bromide *see* Glycopyrrolate *on page 668*
Glydiazinamide *see* GlipiZIDE *on page 660*
Glynase® PresTab® *see* GlyBURIDE *on page 664*
Gly-Oxide® [OTC] *see* Carbamide Peroxide *on page 259*
Glyquin® *see* Hydroquinone *on page 719*
Glyset® *see* Miglitol *on page 929*
GM-CSF *see* Sargramostim *on page 1209*
GnRH *see* Gonadorelin *on page 669*
Gold Bond® Antifungal [OTC] *see* Tolnaftate *on page 1312*

Gold Sodium Thiomalate (gold SOW dee um thye oh MAL ate)

Related Information

Rheumatoid Arthritis, Osteoarthritis, and Osteoporosis *on page 1490*

U.S. Brand Names Aurolate®

Canadian Brand Names Myochrysine®

Generic Available No

Pharmacologic Category Gold Compound

Use Treatment of progressive rheumatoid arthritis

Local Anesthetic/Vasoconstrictor Precautions No information available to require special precautions

Effects on Dental Treatment Key adverse event(s) related to dental treatment: Stomatitis, gingivitis, and glossitis.

Common Adverse Effects

>10%:

Dermatologic: Itching, rash

Gastrointestinal: Stomatitis, gingivitis, glossitis

Ocular: Conjunctivitis

1% to 10%:

Dermatologic: Urticaria, alopecia

Hematologic: Eosinophilia, leukopenia, thrombocytopenia

Renal: Proteinuria, hematuria

Mechanism of Action Unknown, may decrease prostaglandin synthesis or may alter cellular mechanisms by inhibiting sulfhydryl systems

Drug Interactions

Decreased Effect: Penicillamine and acetylcysteine may decrease effect of gold sodium thiomalate.

Pharmacodynamics/Kinetics

Onset of action: Delayed; may require up to 3 months

Half-life elimination: 5 days; may be prolonged with multiple doses

Time to peak, serum: 4-6 hours

Excretion: Urine (60% to 90%); feces (10% to 40%)

Pregnancy Risk Factor C

GoLYTELY® *see* Polyethylene Glycol-Electrolyte Solution *on page 1100*

Gonadorelin (goe nad oh RELL in)

U.S. Brand Names Factrel®

Canadian Brand Names Lutrepulse™

Mexican Brand Names Relisorm L®

Generic Available No

Synonyms GnRH; Gonadorelin Acetate; Gonadorelin Hydrochloride; Gonadotropin Releasing Hormone; LHRH; LRH; Luteinizing Hormone Releasing Hormone

Pharmacologic Category Diagnostic Agent; Gonadotropin

Use Evaluation of functional capacity and response of gonadotrophic hormones; evaluate abnormal gonadotropin regulation as in precocious puberty and delayed puberty.

Orphan drug: Lutrepulse®: Induction of ovulation in females with hypothalamic amenorrhea

Local Anesthetic/Vasoconstrictor Precautions No information available to require special precautions

Effects on Dental Treatment No significant effects or complications reported

Common Adverse Effects 1% to 10%: Local: Pain at injection site

Mechanism of Action Stimulates the release of luteinizing hormone (LH) from the anterior pituitary gland

Drug Interactions

Increased Effect/Toxicity: Increased levels/effect with androgens, estrogens, progestins, glucocorticoids, spironolactone, and levodopa.

Decreased Effect: Decreased levels/effect with oral contraceptives, digoxin, phenothiazines, and dopamine antagonists.

Pharmacodynamics/Kinetics

Onset of action: Peak effect: Maximal LH release: ~20 minutes

Duration: 3-5 hours

Half-life elimination: 4 minutes

Pregnancy Risk Factor B

Gonadorelin Acetate *see* Gonadorelin *on page 669*

Gonadorelin Hydrochloride *see* Gonadorelin *on page 669*

Gonadotropin Releasing Hormone *see* Gonadorelin *on page 669*

Gonak™ [OTC] *see* Hydroxypropyl Methylcellulose *on page 721*

Gonal-F® *see* Follitropins *on page 626*

Gonioscopic Ophthalmic Solution *see* Hydroxypropyl Methylcellulose *on page 721*

Goniosol® [OTC] *see* Hydroxypropyl Methylcellulose *on page 721*

Goody's® Extra Strength Headache Powder [OTC] *see* Acetaminophen, Aspirin, and Caffeine *on page 56*

Goody's® Extra Strength Pain Relief [OTC] *see* Acetaminophen, Aspirin, and Caffeine *on page 56*

Goody's PM® Powder *see* Acetaminophen and Diphenhydramine *on page 53*
Gordofilm® [OTC] *see* Salicylic Acid *on page 1205*
Gormel® [OTC] *see* Urea *on page 1353*

Goserelin (GOE se rel in)

U.S. Brand Names Zoladex®

Canadian Brand Names Zoladex®; Zoladex® LA

Mexican Brand Names Zoladex®

Generic Available No

Synonyms D-Ser(Bu^t)^6,Azgly^{10}-LHRH; Goserelin Acetate; ICI-118630; NSC-606864

Pharmacologic Category Gonadotropin Releasing Hormone Agonist

Use Palliative treatment of advanced breast cancer and carcinoma of the prostate; treatment of endometriosis, including pain relief and reduction of endometriotic lesions; endometrial thinning agent as part of treatment for dysfunctional uterine bleeding

Local Anesthetic/Vasoconstrictor Precautions No information available to require special precautions

Effects on Dental Treatment Key adverse event(s) related to dental treatment: Taste disturbances.

Common Adverse Effects Percentages reported in males with prostatic carcinoma and females with endometriosis using the 1-month implant:

>10%:

Central nervous system: Headache (female 75%, male 1% to 5%), emotional lability (female 60%), depression (female 54%, male 1% to 5%), pain (female 17%, male 8%), insomnia (female 11%, male 5%)

Dermatologic: Diaphoresis (female 45%, male 6%)

Endocrine & metabolic: Hot flashes (female 96%, male 62%), sexual dysfunction (21%), erections decreased (18%), libido decreased (female 61%), breast enlargement (female 18%)

Genitourinary: Lower urinary symptoms (male 13%), vaginitis (75%), dyspareunia (female 14%)

Miscellaneous: Infection (female 13%)

1% to 10%:

Cardiovascular: CHF (male 5%), arrhythmia, cerebrovascular accident, hypertension, myocardial infarction, peripheral vascular disorder, chest pain, palpitations, tachycardia, edema

Central nervous system: Lethargy (male 8%), dizziness (female 6%, male 5%), abnormal thinking, anxiety, chills, fever, malaise, migraine, somnolence

Dermatologic: Rash (female >1%, male 6%), alopecia, bruising, dry skin, skin discoloration

Endocrine & metabolic: Breast pain (female 7%), breast swelling/tenderness (male 1% to 5%), dysmenorrhea, gout, hyperglycemia

Gastrointestinal: Anorexia (female >1%, male 5%), nausea (male 5%), constipation, diarrhea, flatulence, dyspepsia, ulcer, vomiting, weight increased, xerostomia

Genitourinary: Renal insufficiency, urinary frequency, urinary obstruction, urinary tract infection, vaginal hemorrhage

Hematologic: Anemia, hemorrhage

Neuromuscular & skeletal: Arthralgia, bone mineral density decreased (female; ~4% decrease in 6 months), joint disorder, paresthesia

Ocular: Amblyopia, dry eyes

Respiratory: Upper respiratory tract infection (male 7%), COPD (male 5%), pharyngitis (female 5%), bronchitis, cough, epistaxis, rhinitis, sinusitis

Miscellaneous: Allergic reaction

Mechanism of Action Goserelin is a synthetic analog of luteinizing-hormone-releasing hormone (LHRH). Following an initial increase in luteinizing hormone (LH) and follicle stimulating hormone (FSH), chronic administration of goserelin results in a sustained suppression of pituitary gonadotropins. Serum testosterone falls to levels comparable to surgical castration. The exact mechanism of this effect is unknown, but may be related to changes in the control of LH or down-regulation of LH receptors.

Pharmacodynamics/Kinetics Note: Data reported using the 1-month implant.

Absorption: SubQ: Rapid and can be detected in serum in 10 minutes

Distribution: V_d: Male: 44.1 L; Female: 20.3 L

Time to peak, serum: SubQ: Male: 12-15 days, Female: 8-22 days

Half-life elimination: SubQ: Male: ~4 hours, Female: ~2 hours; Renal impairment: Male: 12 hours

Excretion: Urine (90%)

Pregnancy Risk Factor X (endometriosis, endometrial thinning); D (advanced breast cancer)

Goserelin Acetate *see* Goserelin *on page 670*

GP 47680 *see* Oxcarbazepine *on page 1023*

G-Phed *see* Guaifenesin and Pseudoephedrine *on page 675*

G-Phed-PD *see* Guaifenesin and Pseudoephedrine *on page 675*

GR38032R *see* Ondansetron *on page 1014*

Gramicidin, Neomycin, and Polymyxin B *see* Neomycin, Polymyxin B, and Gramicidin *on page 974*

Granisetron (gra NI se tron)

U.S. Brand Names Kytril®

Canadian Brand Names Kytril®

Mexican Brand Names Kytril®

Generic Available No

Synonyms BRL 43694

Pharmacologic Category Antiemetic; Selective 5-HT_3 Receptor Antagonist

Use Prophylaxis of chemotherapy-related emesis; prophylaxis of nausea and vomiting associated with radiation therapy, including total body irradiation and fractionated abdominal radiation; prophylaxis of postoperative nausea and vomiting (PONV)

Generally **not** recommended for treatment of existing chemotherapy-induced emesis (CIE) or for prophylaxis of nausea from agents with a low emetogenic potential.

Local Anesthetic/Vasoconstrictor Precautions No information available to require special precautions

Effects on Dental Treatment No significant effects or complications reported

Common Adverse Effects

>10%:

Central nervous system: Headache (8% to 21%)

Gastrointestinal: Constipation (3% to 18%)

1% to 10%:

Cardiovascular: Hypertension (1% to 2%)

Central nervous system: Dizziness, insomnia, anxiety, somnolence, fever (3% to 8%), pain (10%)

Gastrointestinal: Abdominal pain, diarrhea (1% to 9%), dyspepsia

Hepatic: Elevated liver enzymes (5% to 6%)

Neuromuscular & skeletal: Weakness (5% to 18%)

Mechanism of Action Selective 5-HT_3-receptor antagonist, blocking serotonin, both peripherally on vagal nerve terminals and centrally in the chemoreceptor trigger zone

Drug Interactions

Cytochrome P450 Effect: Substrate of CYP3A4 (minor)

Pharmacodynamics/Kinetics

Duration: Generally up to 24 hours

Distribution: V_d: 2-4 L/kg; widely throughout body

Protein binding: 65%

Metabolism: Hepatic via N-demethylation, oxidation, and conjugation; some metabolites may have 5-HT_3 antagonist activity

Half-life elimination: Cancer patients: 10-12 hours; Healthy volunteers: 4-5 hours; PONV: 9 hours

Excretion: Urine (12% as unchanged drug, 49% as metabolites); feces (34% as metabolites)

Pregnancy Risk Factor B

Granulex® *see* Trypsin, Balsam Peru, and Castor Oil *on page 1349*

Granulocyte Colony Stimulating Factor *see* Filgrastim *on page 589*

Granulocyte Colony Stimulating Factor (PEG Conjugate) *see* Pegfilgrastim *on page 1052*

Granulocyte-Macrophage Colony Stimulating Factor *see* Sargramostim *on page 1209*

Grifulvin® V *see* Griseofulvin *on page 671*

Griseofulvin (gri see oh FUL vin)

U.S. Brand Names Fulvicin® P/G; Fulvicin-U/F®; Grifulvin® V; Gris-PEG®

Canadian Brand Names Fulvicin® U/F

Mexican Brand Names Grisovin®

Generic Available Yes: Ultramicrosized product

Synonyms Griseofulvin Microsize; Griseofulvin Ultramicrosize

Pharmacologic Category Antifungal Agent, Oral

(Continued)

Griseofulvin *(Continued)*

Use Treatment of susceptible tinea infections of the skin, hair, and nails

Local Anesthetic/Vasoconstrictor Precautions No information available to require special precautions

Effects on Dental Treatment Key adverse event(s) related to dental treatment: May cause soreness or irritation of mouth or tongue.

Common Adverse Effects Frequency not defined.

Central nervous system: Headache, fatigue, dizziness, insomnia, mental confusion

Dermatologic: Rash (most common), urticaria (most common), photosensitivity, erythema multiforme, angioneurotic edema (rare)

Gastrointestinal: Nausea, vomiting, epigastric distress, diarrhea, GI bleeding

Genitourinary: Menstrual irregularities (rare)

Hematologic: Leukopenia, granulocytopenia

Neuromuscular & skeletal: Paresthesia (rare)

Renal: Hepatotoxicity, proteinuria, nephrosis

Miscellaneous: Oral thrush, drug-induced lupus-like syndrome (rare)

Mechanism of Action Inhibits fungal cell mitosis at metaphase; binds to human keratin making it resistant to fungal invasion

Drug Interactions

Cytochrome P450 Effect: Induces CYP1A2 (weak), 2C8/9 (weak), 3A4 (weak)

Increased Effect/Toxicity: Increased toxicity with ethanol, may cause tachycardia and flushing.

Decreased Effect: Barbiturates may decrease levels. Decreased warfarin activity. Decreased oral contraceptive effectiveness.

Pharmacodynamics/Kinetics

Absorption: Ultramicrosize griseofulvin absorption is almost complete; absorption of microsize griseofulvin is variable (25% to 70% of an oral dose); enhanced by ingestion of a fatty meal (GI absorption of ultramicrosize is ~1.5 times that of microsize)

Distribution: Crosses placenta

Metabolism: Extensively hepatic

Half-life elimination: 9-22 hours

Excretion: Urine (<1% as unchanged drug); feces; perspiration

Pregnancy Risk Factor C

Griseofulvin Microsize *see* Griseofulvin *on page 671*

Griseofulvin Ultramicrosize *see* Griseofulvin *on page 671*

Gris-PEG® *see* Griseofulvin *on page 671*

Growth Hormone *see* Human Growth Hormone *on page 694*

Guaifed® [OTC] *see* Guaifenesin and Pseudoephedrine *on page 675*

Guaifed-PD® *see* Guaifenesin and Pseudoephedrine *on page 675*

Guaifenesin (gwye FEN e sin)

Related Information

Guaifenesin and Phenylephrine *on page 674*

Guaifenesin, Pseudoephedrine, and Dextromethorphan *on page 676*

U.S. Brand Names Allfen Jr; Amibid LA [DSC]; Diabetic Tussin® EX [OTC]; Ganidin NR; Guiatuss™ [OTC]; Humibid® LA [DSC]; Humibid® Pediatric [DSC]; Iophen NR; Liquibid® [DSC]; Liquibid® 1200 [DSC]; Mucinex® [OTC]; Naldecon Senior EX® [OTC]; Organ-1 NR; Organidin® NR; Phanasin [OTC]; Phanasin® Diabetic Choice [OTC]; Q-Tussin [OTC]; Respa-GF® [DSC]; Robitussin® [OTC]; Scot-Tussin® Expectorant [OTC]; Siltussin DAS [OTC]; Siltussin SA [OTC]; Touro Ex® [DSC]; Tussin [OTC]

Canadian Brand Names Balminil Expectorant; Benylin® E Extra Strength; Koffex Expectorant; Robitussin®

Mexican Brand Names Tukol®

Generic Available Yes

Synonyms GG; Glycerol Guaiacolate

Pharmacologic Category Expectorant

Use Help loosen phlegm and thin bronchial secretions to make coughs more productive

Local Anesthetic/Vasoconstrictor Precautions No information available to require special precautions

Effects on Dental Treatment No significant effects or complications reported

Common Adverse Effects Frequency not defined.

Central nervous system: Dizziness, drowsiness, headache

Dermatologic: Rash

Endocrine & metabolic: Uric acid levels decreased

Gastrointestinal: Nausea, vomiting, stomach pain

Postmarketing and/or case reports: Kidney stone formation (with consumption of large quantities)

Mechanism of Action Thought to act as an expectorant by irritating the gastric mucosa and stimulating respiratory tract secretions, thereby increasing respiratory fluid volumes and decreasing mucus viscosity

Pharmacodynamics/Kinetics

Absorption: Well absorbed

Half-life elimination: ~1 hour

Excretion: Urine (as unchanged drug and metabolites)

Pregnancy Risk Factor C

Guaifenesin and Codeine (gwye FEN e sin & KOE deen)

Related Information

Codeine *on page 369*

Guaifenesin *on page 672*

U.S. Brand Names Brontex®; Cheracol®; Diabetic Tussin C®; Gani-Tuss® NR; Guaituss AC®; Halotussin AC; Mytussin® AC; Robafen® AC; Romilar® AC; Tussi-Organidin® NR; Tussi-Organidin® S-NR

Generic Available Yes

Synonyms Codeine and Guaifenesin

Pharmacologic Category Antitussive; Cough Preparation; Expectorant

Use Temporary control of cough due to minor throat and bronchial irritation

Local Anesthetic/Vasoconstrictor Precautions No information available to require special precautions

Effects on Dental Treatment Key adverse event(s) related to dental treatment: Xerostomia (normal salivary flow resumes upon discontinuation).

Common Adverse Effects

Based on **guaifenesin** component:

Central nervous system: Drowsiness, headache

Dermatologic: Rash

Gastrointestinal: Nausea, vomiting, stomach pain

Based on **codeine** component:

>10%:

- Central nervous system: Drowsiness
- Gastrointestinal: Constipation

1% to 10%:

- Cardiovascular: Tachycardia or bradycardia, hypotension
- Central nervous system: Dizziness, lightheadedness, false feeling of well being, malaise, headache, restlessness, paradoxical CNS stimulation, confusion
- Dermatologic: Rash, urticaria
- Gastrointestinal: Xerostomia, anorexia, nausea, vomiting,
- Genitourinary: Decreased urination, ureteral spasm
- Hepatic: Increased LFTs
- Local: Burning at injection site
- Neuromuscular & skeletal: Weakness
- Ocular: Blurred vision
- Respiratory: Dyspnea
- Miscellaneous: Histamine release

Percentage unknown: Increased AST, ALT

Restrictions C-V

Mechanism of Action

Guaifenesin is thought to act as an expectorant by irritating the gastric mucosa and stimulating respiratory tract secretions, thereby increasing respiratory fluid volumes and decreasing phlegm viscosity

Codeine is an antitussive that controls cough by depressing the medullary cough center

Drug Interactions

Increased Effect/Toxicity: See individual agents.

Decreased Effect: See individual agents.

Pharmacodynamics/Kinetics See individual agents.

Pregnancy Risk Factor C

Guaifenesin and Dextromethorphan

(gwye FEN e sin & deks troe meth OR fan)

Related Information

Dextromethorphan *on page 421*

Guaifenesin *on page 672*

(Continued)

Guaifenesin and Dextromethorphan *(Continued)*

U.S. Brand Names Aquatab® DM; Benylin® Expectorant [OTC]; Cheracol® D [OTC]; Cheracol® Plus [OTC]; Diabetic Tussin® DM [OTC]; Diabetic Tussin® DM Maximum Strength [OTC]; Duratuss® DM; Fenesin™ DM; Genatuss DM® [OTC]; Guaifenex® DM; Guiatuss-DM® [OTC]; Humibid® DM; Hydro-Tussin™ DM; Kolephrin® GG/DM [OTC]; Mytussin® DM [OTC]; Respa-DM®; Robitussin® DM [OTC]; Robitussin® Sugar Free Cough [OTC]; Safe Tussin® 30 [OTC]; Silexin® [OTC]; Tolu-Sed® DM [OTC]; Touro® DM; Tussi-Organidin® DM NR; Vicks® 44E [OTC]; Vicks® Pediatric Formula 44E [OTC]; Z-Cof LA

Canadian Brand Names Balminil DM E; Benylin® DM-E; Koffex DM-Expectorant; Robitussin® DM

Generic Available Yes

Synonyms Dextromethorphan and Guaifenesin

Pharmacologic Category Antitussive; Cough Preparation; Expectorant

Use Temporary control of cough due to minor throat and bronchial irritation

Local Anesthetic/Vasoconstrictor Precautions No information available to require special precautions

Effects on Dental Treatment No significant effects or complications reported

Common Adverse Effects Frequency not defined.

Central nervous system: Drowsiness, headache

Dermatologic: Rash

Gastrointestinal: Nausea, vomiting

Mechanism of Action

Guaifenesin is thought to act as an expectorant by irritating the gastric mucosa and stimulating respiratory tract secretions, thereby increasing respiratory fluid volumes and decreasing phlegm viscosity

Dextromethorphan is a chemical relative of morphine lacking narcotic properties except in overdose; controls cough by depressing the medullary cough center

Drug Interactions

Cytochrome P450 Effect: Dextromethorphan: **Substrate** of CYP2B6 (minor), 2C8/9 (minor), 2C19 (minor), 2D6 (major), 2E1 (minor), 3A4 (minor); **Inhibits** CYP2D6 (weak)

Increased Effect/Toxicity: See individual agents.

Decreased Effect: See individual agents.

Pharmacodynamics/Kinetics

Onset of action: Oral: Antitussive: 15-30 minutes

See individual agents.

Pregnancy Risk Factor C

Guaifenesin and Hydrocodone *see* Hydrocodone and Guaifenesin *on page 708*

Guaifenesin and Phenylephrine (gwye FEN e sin & fen il EF rin)

Related Information

Guaifenesin *on page 672*

Phenylephrine *on page 1078*

U.S. Brand Names Endal®; Entex® LA; Liquibid-D; Prolex-D

Generic Available Yes

Synonyms Phenylephrine and Guaifenesin

Pharmacologic Category Decongestant; Expectorant

Use Symptomatic relief of those respiratory conditions where tenacious mucous plugs and congestion complicate the problem such as sinusitis, pharyngitis, bronchitis, asthma, and as an adjunctive therapy in serous otitis media

Local Anesthetic/Vasoconstrictor Precautions Use with caution since phenylephrine is a sympathomimetic amine which could interact with epinephrine to cause a pressor response

Effects on Dental Treatment Key adverse event(s) related to dental treatment:

Guaifenesin: No significant effects or complications reported

Phenylephrine: Up to 10% of patients could experience tachycardia, palpitations, and xerostomia (normal salivary flow resumes upon discontinuation); use vasoconstrictor with caution

Common Adverse Effects See individual agents.

Mechanism of Action See individual agents.

Drug Interactions

Increased Effect/Toxicity: See individual agents.

Decreased Effect: See individual agents.

Pharmacodynamics/Kinetics See individual agents.

Guaifenesin and Potassium Guaiacolsulfonate

(gwye FEN e sin & poe TASS ee um gwye a kole SUL foe nate)

U.S. Brand Names Allfen *(reformulation)*; Humibid® LA *(reformulation)*

Generic Available No

Synonyms Potassium Guaiacolsulfonate and Guaifenesin

Pharmacologic Category Expectorant

Use Temporary control of cough associated with respiratory tract infections and related conditions which are complicated by tenacious mucus and/or mucus plugs and congestion

Local Anesthetic/Vasoconstrictor Precautions No information available to require special precautions

Effects on Dental Treatment No significant effects or complications reported

Mechanism of Action Guaifenesin and potassium guaiacolsulfonate are both expectorants. Guaifenesin is thought to act as an expectorant by irritating the gastric mucosa and stimulating respiratory tract secretions, thereby increasing respiratory fluid volumes and decreasing mucus viscosity.

Pregnancy Risk Factor C

Guaifenesin and Pseudoephedrine

(gwye FEN e sin & soo doe e FED rin)

Related Information

Guaifenesin *on page 672*

Pseudoephedrine *on page 1147*

U.S. Brand Names Ami-Tex PSE; Anatuss LA; Aquatab®; Aquatab® D Dose Pack; Congestac®; Deconsal® II; Defen-LA®; Duratuss™; Duratuss™ GP; Entex® PSE; Eudal®-SR; G-Phed; G-Phed-PD; Guaifed® [OTC]; Guaifed-PD®; Guaifenex® GP; Guaifenex® PSE; Guaifen PSE; Guai-Vent™/PSE; Maxifed®; Maxifed-G®; Miraphen PSE; Mucinex® D; PanMist® Jr.; PanMist® LA; PanMist® S; Pseudo GG TR; Pseudovent™; Pseudovent™-Ped; Respa-1st®; Respaire®-60 SR; Respaire®-120 SR; Robitussin-PE® [OTC]; Robitussin® Severe Congestion [OTC]; Touro LA®; V-Dec-M®; Versacaps®; Zephrex®; Zephrex LA®

Canadian Brand Names Novahistex® Expectorant with Decongestant

Generic Available Yes

Synonyms Pseudoephedrine and Guaifenesin

Pharmacologic Category Decongestant; Expectorant

Use Enhance the output of respiratory tract fluid and reduce mucosal congestion and edema in the nasal passage

Local Anesthetic/Vasoconstrictor Precautions Use with caution since pseudoephedrine is a sympathomimetic amine which could interact with epinephrine to cause a pressor response

Effects on Dental Treatment Key adverse event(s) related to dental treatment:

Guaifenesin: No significant effects or complications reported

Pseudoephedrine: Xerostomia (normal salivary flow resumes upon discontinuation).

Common Adverse Effects See individual agents.

Drug Interactions

Increased Effect/Toxicity: See individual agents.

Decreased Effect: See individual agents.

Pharmacodynamics/Kinetics See individual agents.

Pregnancy Risk Factor C

Guaifenesin and Theophylline *see* Theophylline and Guaifenesin *on page 1286*

Guaifenesin, Hydrocodone, and Pseudoephedrine *see* Hydrocodone, Pseudoephedrine, and Guaifenesin *on page 713*

Guaifenesin, Potassium Guaiacolsulfonate, and Dextromethorphan

(gwye FEN e sin, poe TASS ee um gwye a kole SUL foe nate, & deks troe meth OR fan)

U.S. Brand Names Humibid® DM *(reformulation)*

Generic Available No

Synonyms Dextromethorphan, Guaifenesin, and Potassium Guaiacolsulfonate; Potassium Guaiacolsulfonate, Dextromethorphan, and Guaifenesin

Pharmacologic Category Antitussive; Cough Preparation; Expectorant

(Continued)

Guaifenesin, Potassium Guaiacolsulfonate, and Dextromethorphan *(Continued)*

Use Temporary control of cough associated with respiratory tract infections and related conditions which are complicated by tenacious mucus and/or mucus plugs and congestion

Local Anesthetic/Vasoconstrictor Precautions No information available to require special precautions

Effects on Dental Treatment No significant effects or complications reported

Mechanism of Action Guaifenesin and potassium guaiacolsulfonate are both expectorants. Guaifenesin is thought to act as an expectorant by irritating the gastric mucosa and stimulating respiratory tract secretions, thereby increasing respiratory fluid volumes and decreasing mucus viscosity. Dextromethorphan is a chemical relative of morphine, lacking narcotic properties except in overdose; controls cough by depressing the medullary cough center.

Pregnancy Risk Factor C

Guaifenesin, Pseudoephedrine, and Codeine

(gwye FEN e sin, soo doe e FED rin, & KOE deen)

Related Information

Codeine *on page 369*

Guaifenesin *on page 672*

Pseudoephedrine *on page 1147*

U.S. Brand Names Cheratussin DAC; Codafed® Expectorant; Codafed® Pediatric Expectorant; Dihistine® Expectorant; Guiatuss™ DAC®; Halotussin® DAC; Mytussin® DAC; Nucofed® Expectorant; Nucofed® Pediatric Expectorant; Nucotuss®; Robitussin®-DAC [DSC]

Canadian Brand Names Benylin® 3.3 mg-D-E; Calmylin with Codeine

Generic Available Yes

Synonyms Codeine, Guaifenesin, and Pseudoephedrine; Pseudoephedrine, Guaifenesin, and Codeine

Pharmacologic Category Antitussive/Decongestant/Expectorant

Use Temporarily relieves nasal congestion and controls cough due to minor throat and bronchial irritation; helps loosen phlegm and thin bronchial secretions to make coughs more productive

Local Anesthetic/Vasoconstrictor Precautions Use with caution since pseudoephedrine is a sympathomimetic amine which could interact with epinephrine to cause a pressor response

Effects on Dental Treatment Key adverse event(s) related to dental treatment:

Codeine: Xerostomia (normal salivary flow resumes upon discontinuation).

Guaifenesin: No significant effects or complications reported

Pseudoephedrine: Xerostomia (normal salivary flow resumes upon discontinuation).

Common Adverse Effects See individual agents.

Restrictions C-III; C-V

Drug Interactions

Increased Effect/Toxicity: See individual agents.

Decreased Effect: See individual agents.

Pharmacodynamics/Kinetics See individual agents.

Pregnancy Risk Factor C

Guaifenesin, Pseudoephedrine, and Dextromethorphan

(gwye FEN e sin, soo doe e FED rin, & deks troe meth OR fan)

Related Information

Dextromethorphan *on page 421*

Guaifenesin *on page 672*

Pseudoephedrine *on page 1147*

U.S. Brand Names Ambifed-G DM; Aquatab® C; Dimetapp® Cold and Congestion [OTC]; Guaifenex™-Rx DM; Maxifed® DM; PanMist®-DM; Profen Forte™ DM; Profen II DM®; Protuss®-DM [DSC]; Pseudovent™ DM; Relacon-DM; Robitussin® CF [OTC]; Robitussin® Cold and Congestion [OTC]; Robitussin® Cough and Cold Infant [OTC]; Touro™ CC; Tri-Vent™ DM; Z-Cof DM

Canadian Brand Names Balminil DM + Decongestant + Expectorant; Benylin® DM-D-E; Koffex DM + Decongestant + Expectorant; Novahistex® DM Decongestant Expectorant; Novahistine® DM Decongestant Expectorant; Robitussin® Cough & Cold®

Generic Available Yes

Synonyms Dextromethorphan, Guaifenesin, and Pseudoephedrine; Pseudoephedrine, Dextromethorphan, and Guaifenesin

Pharmacologic Category Antitussive/Decongestant/Expectorant

Use Temporarily relieves nasal congestion and controls cough due to minor throat and bronchial irritation; helps loosen phlegm and thin bronchial secretions to make coughs more productive

Local Anesthetic/Vasoconstrictor Precautions Use with caution since pseudoephedrine is a sympathomimetic amine which could interact with epinephrine to cause a pressor response

Effects on Dental Treatment Key adverse event(s) related to dental treatment:

Dextromethorphan: No significant effects or complications reported

Guaifenesin: No significant effects or complications reported

Pseudoephedrine: Xerostomia (normal salivary flow resumes upon discontinuation).

Common Adverse Effects See individual agents.

Mechanism of Action See individual agents.

Drug Interactions

Cytochrome P450 Effect: Dextromethorphan: **Substrate** of CYP2B6 (minor), 2C8/9 (minor), 2C19 (minor), 2D6 (major), 2E1 (minor), 3A4 (minor); **Inhibits** CYP2D6 (weak)

Increased Effect/Toxicity: See individual agents.

Decreased Effect: See individual agents.

Pharmacodynamics/Kinetics See individual agents.

Pregnancy Risk Factor C

Guaifenex® DM *see* Guaifenesin and Dextromethorphan *on page 673*

Guaifenex® GP *see* Guaifenesin and Pseudoephedrine *on page 675*

Guaifenex® PSE *see* Guaifenesin and Pseudoephedrine *on page 675*

Guaifenex™-Rx DM *see* Guaifenesin, Pseudoephedrine, and Dextromethorphan *on page 676*

Guaifen PSE *see* Guaifenesin and Pseudoephedrine *on page 675*

Guaituss AC® *see* Guaifenesin and Codeine *on page 673*

Guai-Vent™/PSE *see* Guaifenesin and Pseudoephedrine *on page 675*

Guanabenz (GWAHN a benz)

Related Information

Cardiovascular Diseases *on page 1458*

U.S. Brand Names Wytensin® [DSC]

Canadian Brand Names Wytensin®

Generic Available Yes

Synonyms Guanabenz Acetate

Pharmacologic Category Alpha$_2$-Adrenergic Agonist

Use Management of hypertension

Local Anesthetic/Vasoconstrictor Precautions No information available to require special precautions

Effects on Dental Treatment Key adverse event(s) related to dental treatment: Taste disorder, nasal congestion, dyspnea, significant xerostomia (normal salivary flow resumes upon discontinuation).

Common Adverse Effects Higher rates with larger doses

>5% (at doses of 16 mg/day):

- Cardiovascular: Orthostasis
- Central nervous system: Drowsiness or sedation (39%), dizziness (12% to 17%), headache (5%)
- Gastrointestinal: Xerostomia (28% to 38%)
- Neuromuscular & skeletal: Weakness (~10%)

≤3% (may be similar to placebo):

- Cardiovascular: Arrhythmias, palpitations, chest pain, edema
- Central nervous system: Anxiety, ataxia, depression, sleep disturbances
- Dermatologic: Rash, pruritus
- Endocrine & metabolic: Disturbances of sexual function, gynecomastia, decreased sexual function
- Gastrointestinal: Diarrhea, vomiting, constipation, nausea
- Genitourinary: Polyuria
- Neuromuscular & skeletal: Myalgia
- Ocular: Blurring of vision
- Respiratory: Nasal congestion, dyspnea
- Miscellaneous: Taste disorders

(Continued)

Guanabenz *(Continued)*

Mechanism of Action Stimulates alpha$_2$-adrenoreceptors in the brain stem, thus activating an inhibitory neuron, resulting in reduced sympathetic outflow, producing a decrease in vasomotor tone and heart rate

Drug Interactions

Cytochrome P450 Effect: Substrate of CYP1A2 (major)

Increased Effect/Toxicity: CYP1A2 inhibitors may increase the levels/effects of guanabenz; example inhibitors include amiodarone, ciprofloxacin, fluvoxamine, ketoconazole, lomefloxacin, ofloxacin, and rofecoxib. Nitroprusside and guanabenz have additive hypotensive effects. Noncardioselective beta-blockers (nadolol, propranolol, timolol) may exacerbate rebound hypertension when guanabenz is withdrawn. The beta-blocker should be withdrawn first. The gradual withdrawal of guanabenz or a cardioselective beta-blocker could be substituted.

Hypoglycemic agents: Hypoglycemic symptoms may be reduced. Educate patient about decreased signs and symptoms of hypoglycemia or avoid use in patients with frequent episodes of hypoglycemia.

Decreased Effect: CYP1A2 inducers may decrease the levels/effects of guanabenz; example inducers include aminoglutethimide, carbamazepine, phenobarbital, and rifampin. TCAs decrease the hypotensive effect of guanabenz.

Pharmacodynamics/Kinetics

Onset of action: Antihypertensive: ~1 hour

Absorption: ~75%

Half-life elimination, serum: 7-10 hours

Pregnancy Risk Factor C

Guanabenz Acetate *see* Guanabenz *on page 677*

Guanadrel (GWAHN a drel)

Related Information

Cardiovascular Diseases *on page 1458*

U.S. Brand Names Hylorel®

Canadian Brand Names Hylorel®

Generic Available No

Synonyms Guanadrel Sulfate

Pharmacologic Category False Neurotransmitter

Use Considered a second line agent in the treatment of hypertension, usually with a diuretic

Local Anesthetic/Vasoconstrictor Precautions Manufacturer's information states that guanadrel may block vasopressor activity of epinephrine. This has not been observed during use of epinephrine as a vasoconstrictor in local anesthesia.

Effects on Dental Treatment Key adverse event(s) related to dental treatment: Coughing, xerostomia (normal salivary flow resumes upon discontinuation), glossitis, orthostatic hypotension.

Common Adverse Effects

>10%:

Cardiovascular: Palpitations (30%), chest pain (28%), peripheral edema (29%)

Central nervous system: Fatigue (64%), headache (58%), faintness (47% to 49%), drowsiness (45%), confusion (15%)

Gastrointestinal: Increased bowel movements (31%), gas pain (24% to 32%), constipation (21%), anorexia (19%), weight gain/loss (42% to 44%)

Genitourinary: Nocturia (48%), polyuria (34%), ejaculation disturbances (18%)

Neuromuscular & skeletal: Paresthesia (25%), aching limbs (43%), leg cramps (20% to 26%)

Ocular: Visual disturbances (29%)

Respiratory: Dyspnea at rest (18%), coughing (27%)

1% to 10%:

Cardiovascular: Orthostatic hypotension

Central nervous system: Psychological problems (4%), depression (2%), sleep disorders (2%)

Gastrointestinal: Glossitis (8%), nausea/vomiting (4%), xerostomia (2%)

Genitourinary: Impotence (5%)

Renal: Hematuria (2%)

Mechanism of Action Acts as a false neurotransmitter that blocks the adrenergic actions of norepinephrine; it displaces norepinephrine from its presynaptic storage granules and thus exposes it to degradation; it thereby produces a reduction in total peripheral resistance and, therefore, blood pressure

Drug Interactions

Increased Effect/Toxicity: Increased toxicity of direct-acting amines (epinephrine, norepinephrine) by guanadrel; the hypotensive effect of guanadrel may be potentiated. Increased effect of beta-blockers, vasodilators. Norepinephrine/phenylephrine have exaggerated pressor response; monitor blood pressure closely. MAO inhibitors may cause severe hypertension; give at least 1 week apart.

Decreased Effect: TCAs decrease hypotensive effect of guanadrel. Phenothiazines may inhibit the antihypertensive response to guanadrel; consider an alternative antihypertensive with different mechanism of action. Amphetamines, related sympathomimetics, and methylphenidate decrease the antihypertensive response to guanadrel; consider an alternative antihypertensive with different mechanism of action. Reassess the need for amphetamine, related sympathomimetic, or methylphenidate; consider alternatives. Ephedrine may inhibit the antihypertensive response to guanadrel; consider an alternative antihypertensive with different mechanism of action. Reassess the need for ephedrine.

Pharmacodynamics/Kinetics

Onset of action: Peak effect: 4-6 hours
Duration: 4-14 hours
Absorption: Rapid
Half-life elimination, serum: Biphasic: Initial: 1-4 hours; Terminal: 5-45 hours
Time to peak, serum: 1.5-2 hours

Pregnancy Risk Factor B

Guanadrel Sulfate *see* Guanadrel *on page 678*

Guanfacine (GWAHN fa seen)

Related Information

Cardiovascular Diseases *on page 1458*

U.S. Brand Names Tenex®

Canadian Brand Names Tenex®

Generic Available No

Synonyms Guanfacine Hydrochloride

Pharmacologic Category Alpha$_2$-Adrenergic Agonist

Use Management of hypertension

Local Anesthetic/Vasoconstrictor Precautions No information available to require special precautions

Effects on Dental Treatment Key adverse event(s) related to dental treatment: Xerostomia and changes in salivation (normal salivary flow resumes upon discontinuation).

Common Adverse Effects

>10%:

Central nervous system: Somnolence (5% to 40%), headache (3% to 13%), dizziness (2% to 15%)
Gastrointestinal: Xerostomia (10% to 54%), constipation (2% to 15%)

1% to 10%:

Central nervous system: Fatigue (2% to 10%)
Endocrine & metabolic: Impotence (up to 7%)

Mechanism of Action Stimulates alpha$_2$-adrenoreceptors in the brain stem, thus activating an inhibitory neuron, resulting in reduced sympathetic outflow, producing a decrease in vasomotor tone and heart rate

Drug Interactions

Increased Effect/Toxicity: Nitroprusside and guanfacine have additive hypotensive effects. Noncardioselective beta-blockers (nadolol, propranolol, timolol) may exacerbate rebound hypertension when guanfacine is withdrawn. The beta-blocker should be withdrawn first. The gradual withdrawal of guanfacine or a cardioselective beta-blocker could be substituted.

Decreased Effect: TCAs decrease the hypotensive effect of guanfacine.

Pharmacodynamics/Kinetics

Onset of action: Peak effect: 8-11 hours
Duration: 24 hours following single dose
Half-life elimination, serum: 17 hours
Time to peak, serum: 1-4 hours

Pregnancy Risk Factor B

Guanfacine Hydrochloride *see* Guanfacine *on page 679*

Guanidine (GWAHN i deen)

Generic Available No

Synonyms Guanidine Hydrochloride

Pharmacologic Category Cholinergic Agonist

(Continued)

Guanidine *(Continued)*

Use Reduction of the symptoms of muscle weakness associated with the myasthenic syndrome of Eaton-Lambert, not for myasthenia gravis

Local Anesthetic/Vasoconstrictor Precautions No information available to require special precautions

Effects on Dental Treatment No significant effects or complications reported

Guanidine Hydrochloride *see* Guanidine *on page 679*

Guiatuss™ [OTC] *see* Guaifenesin *on page 672*

Guiatuss™ DAC® *see* Guaifenesin, Pseudoephedrine, and Codeine *on page 676*

Guiatuss-DM® [OTC] *see* Guaifenesin and Dextromethorphan *on page 673*

Gum Benjamin *see* Benzoin *on page 193*

GW433908G *see* Fosamprenavir *on page 630*

Gynazole-1® *see* Butoconazole *on page 239*

Gyne-Lotrimin® 3 [OTC] *see* Clotrimazole *on page 363*

Gynodiol® *see* Estradiol *on page 518*

Gynol II® [OTC] *see* Nonoxynol 9 *on page 995*

Habitrol® *see* Nicotine *on page 981*

Haemophilus b Conjugate Vaccine

(he MOF fi lus bee KON joo gate vak SEEN)

Related Information

Immunizations (Vaccines) *on page 1614*

U.S. Brand Names ActHIB®; HibTITER®; PedvaxHIB®

Canadian Brand Names ActHIB®; PedvaxHIB®

Generic Available No

Synonyms Diphtheria CRM_{197} Protein Conjugate; Diphtheria Toxoid Conjugate; *Haemophilus* b Oligosaccharide Conjugate Vaccine; *Haemophilus* b Polysaccharide Vaccine; HbCV; Hib Polysaccharide Conjugate; PRP-D

Pharmacologic Category Vaccine

Use Routine immunization of children 2 months to 5 years of age against invasive disease caused by *H. influenzae*

Unimmunized children ≥5 years of age with a chronic illness known to be associated with increased risk of *Haemophilus influenzae* type b disease, specifically, persons with anatomic or functional asplenia or sickle cell anemia or those who have undergone splenectomy, should receive Hib vaccine.

Haemophilus b conjugate vaccines are not indicated for prevention of bronchitis or other infections due to *H. influenzae* in adults; adults with specific dysfunction or certain complement deficiencies who are at especially high risk of *H. influenzae* type b infection (HIV-infected adults); patients with Hodgkin's disease (vaccinated at least 2 weeks before the initiation of chemotherapy or 3 months after the end of chemotherapy)

Local Anesthetic/Vasoconstrictor Precautions No information available to require special precautions

Effects on Dental Treatment No significant effects or complications reported

Common Adverse Effects When administered during the same visit that DTP vaccine is given, the rates of systemic reactions do not differ from those observed only when DTP vaccine is administered. **All serious adverse reactions must be reported to the U.S. Department of Health and Human Services (DHHS) Vaccine Adverse Event Reporting System (VAERS) 1-800-822-7967.**

25%:
- Cardiovascular: Edema
- Dermatologic: Local erythema
- Local: Increased risk of *Haemophilus* b infections in the week after vaccination
- Miscellaneous: Warmth

>10%: Acute febrile reactions

1% to 10%:
- Central nervous system: Fever (up to 102.2°F), irritability, lethargy
- Gastrointestinal: Anorexia, diarrhea
- Local: Irritation at injection site

Mechanism of Action Stimulates production of anticapsular antibodies and provides active immunity to *Haemophilus influenzae*

Drug Interactions

Decreased Effect: Decreased effect with immunosuppressive agents, immunoglobulins within 1 month may decrease antibody production.

Pharmacodynamics/Kinetics Seroconversion following one dose of Hib vaccine for children 18 months or 24 months of age or older is 75% to 90% respectively.

Onset of action: Serum antibody response: 1-2 weeks
Duration: Immunity: 1.5 years

Pregnancy Risk Factor C

***Haemophilus* b Oligosaccharide Conjugate Vaccine** *see Haemophilus* b Conjugate Vaccine *on page 680*

***Haemophilus* b Polysaccharide Vaccine** *see Haemophilus* b Conjugate Vaccine *on page 680*

Halcinonide (hal SIN oh nide)

U.S. Brand Names Halog®; Halog®-E [DSC]
Canadian Brand Names Halog®
Mexican Brand Names Dermalog®
Generic Available No
Pharmacologic Category Corticosteroid, Topical
Use Inflammation of corticosteroid-responsive dermatoses [high potency topical corticosteroid]
Local Anesthetic/Vasoconstrictor Precautions No information available to require special precautions
Effects on Dental Treatment No significant effects or complications reported
Common Adverse Effects Frequency not defined: Itching; dry skin; folliculitis; hypertrichosis; acneiform eruptions; hypopigmentation; perioral dermatitis; allergic contact dermatitis; skin maceration; skin atrophy; striae; local burning, irritation, miliaria; secondary infection
Mechanism of Action Decreases inflammation by suppression of migration of polymorphonuclear leukocytes and reversal of increased capillary permeability
Pharmacodynamics/Kinetics

Absorption: Percutaneous absorption varies by location of topical application and use of occlusive dressings
Metabolism: Primarily hepatic
Excretion: Urine

Pregnancy Risk Factor C

Halcion® *see* Triazolam *on page 1335*
Haldol® *see* Haloperidol *on page 682*
Haldol® Decanoate *see* Haloperidol *on page 682*
Haley's M-O *see* Magnesium Hydroxide and Mineral Oil *on page 853*
Halfprin® [OTC] *see* Aspirin *on page 151*

Halobetasol (hal oh BAY ta sol)

U.S. Brand Names Ultravate®
Canadian Brand Names Ultravate®
Generic Available No
Synonyms Halobetasol Propionate
Pharmacologic Category Corticosteroid, Topical
Use Relief of inflammatory and pruritic manifestations of corticosteroid-response dermatoses [super high potency topical corticosteroid]
Local Anesthetic/Vasoconstrictor Precautions No information available to require special precautions
Effects on Dental Treatment No significant effects or complications reported
Common Adverse Effects 1% to 4%: Dermatologic: Burning, itching, stinging
Mechanism of Action Corticosteroids inhibit the initial manifestations of the inflammatory process (ie, capillary dilation and edema, fibrin deposition, and migration and diapedesis of leukocytes into the inflamed site) as well as later sequelae (angiogenesis, fibroblast proliferation)
Pharmacodynamics/Kinetics

Absorption: Percutaneous absorption varies by location of topical application; ~6% of a topically applied dose of ointment enters circulation within 96 hours
Metabolism: Primarily hepatic
Excretion: Urine

Pregnancy Risk Factor C

Halobetasol Propionate *see* Halobetasol *on page 681*

Halofantrine (ha loe FAN trin)

Generic Available No
Synonyms Halofantrine Hydrochloride
Pharmacologic Category Antimalarial Agent

(Continued)

Halofantrine *(Continued)*

Use Treatment of mild to moderate acute malaria caused by susceptible strains of *Plasmodium falciparum* and *Plasmodium vivax*

Local Anesthetic/Vasoconstrictor Precautions No information available to require special precautions

Effects on Dental Treatment No significant effects or complications reported

Common Adverse Effects

1% to 10%:

Cardiovascular: Edema

Central nervous system: Malaise, headache (3%), dizziness (5%)

Dermatologic: Pruritus (3%)

Gastrointestinal: Nausea (3%), vomiting (4%), abdominal pain (9%), diarrhea (6%), anorexia (5%)

Hematologic: Leukocytosis

Hepatic: Elevated LFTs

Local: Tenderness

Neuromuscular & skeletal: Myalgia (1%), rigors (2%)

Respiratory: Cough

Miscellaneous: Lymphadenopathy

Restrictions Not available in U.S.

Mechanism of Action Exact mechanism unknown; destruction of asexual blood forms, possible inhibition of proton pump

Drug Interactions

Cytochrome P450 Effect: Substrate of CYP2C8/9 (minor), 2D6 (minor), 3A4 (major); **Inhibits** CYP2D6 (weak)

Increased Effect/Toxicity: CYP3A4 inhibitors may increase the levels/effects of halofantrine; example inhibitors include azole antifungals, ciprofloxacin, clarithromycin, diclofenac, doxycycline, erythromycin, imatinib, isoniazid, nefazodone, nicardipine, propofol, protease inhibitors, quinidine, and verapamil. Increased toxicity (QT_c interval prolongation) with other agents that cause QT_c interval prolongation, especially mefloquine.

Decreased Effect: CYP3A4 inducers may decrease the levels/effects of halofantrine; example inducers include aminoglutethimide, carbamazepine, nafcillin, nevirapine, phenobarbital, phenytoin, and rifamycins.

Pharmacodynamics/Kinetics

Absorption: Erratic and variable; serum levels are proportional to dose up to 1000 mg; smaller doses should be divided; may be increased 60% with high fat meals

Distribution: V_d: 570 L/kg; widely to most tissues

Metabolism: Hepatic to active metabolite

Half-life elimination: 6-10 days; Metabolite: 3-4 days; may be prolonged in active disease

Excretion: Primarily in feces (hepatobiliary)

Clearance: Parasite: Mean: 40-84 hours

Pregnancy Risk Factor C

Halofantrine Hydrochloride *see* Halofantrine *on page 681*

Halog® *see* Halcinonide *on page 681*

Halog®-E [DSC] *see* Halcinonide *on page 681*

Haloperidol (ha loe PER i dole)

U.S. Brand Names Haldol®; Haldol® Decanoate

Canadian Brand Names Apo-Haloperidol®; Apo-Haloperidol LA®; Haloperidol-LA Omega; Haloperidol Long Acting; Novo-Peridol; Peridol; PMS-Haloperidol LA

Mexican Brand Names Haldol®; Haldol decanoas®; Haloperil®

Generic Available Yes

Synonyms Haloperidol Decanoate; Haloperidol Lactate

Pharmacologic Category Antipsychotic Agent, Butyrophenone

Use Management of schizophrenia; control of tics and vocal utterances of Tourette's disorder in children and adults; severe behavioral problems in children

Unlabeled/Investigational Use Treatment of psychosis; may be used for the emergency sedation of severely-agitated or delirious patients; adjunctive treatment of ethanol dependence; antiemetic

Local Anesthetic/Vasoconstrictor Precautions Manufacturer's information states that haloperidol may block vasopressor activity of epinephrine. This has not been observed during use of epinephrine as a vasoconstrictor in local anesthesia.

Effects on Dental Treatment Key adverse event(s) related to dental treatment: Orthostatic hypotension, and nasal congestion are possible; since the drug is a dopamine antagonist, extrapyramidal symptoms of the TMJ are a possibility.

Common Adverse Effects Frequency not defined.

Cardiovascular: Hypotension, hypertension, tachycardia, arrhythmias, abnormal T waves with prolonged ventricular repolarization, torsade de pointes (case-control study ~4%)

Central nervous system: Restlessness, anxiety, extrapyramidal symptoms, dystonic reactions, pseudoparkinsonian signs and symptoms, tardive dyskinesia, neuroleptic malignant syndrome (NMS), altered central temperature regulation, akathisia, tardive dystonia, insomnia, euphoria, agitation, drowsiness, depression, lethargy, headache, confusion, vertigo, seizures

Dermatologic: Hyperpigmentation, pruritus, rash, contact dermatitis, alopecia, photosensitivity (rare)

Endocrine & metabolic: Amenorrhea, galactorrhea, gynecomastia, sexual dysfunction, lactation, breast engorgement, mastalgia, menstrual irregularities, hyperglycemia, hypoglycemia, hyponatremia

Gastrointestinal: Nausea, vomiting, anorexia, constipation, diarrhea, hypersalivation, dyspepsia, xerostomia

Genitourinary: Urinary retention, priapism

Hematologic: Cholestatic jaundice, obstructive jaundice

Ocular: Blurred vision

Respiratory: Laryngospasm, bronchospasm

Miscellaneous: Heat stroke, diaphoresis

Mechanism of Action Blocks postsynaptic mesolimbic dopaminergic D_1 and D_2 receptors in the brain; depresses the release of hypothalamic and hypophyseal hormones; believed to depress the reticular activating system thus affecting basal metabolism, body temperature, wakefulness, vasomotor tone, and emesis

Drug Interactions

Cytochrome P450 Effect: Substrate of CYP1A2 (minor), 2D6 (major), 3A4 (major); **Inhibits** CYP2D6 (moderate), 3A4 (moderate)

Increased Effect/Toxicity: Haloperidol concentrations/effects may be increased by chloroquine, propranolol, and sulfadoxine-pyridoxine. The levels/effects of haloperidol may be increased by azole antifungals, chlorpromazine, ciprofloxacin, clarithromycin, delavirdine, diclofenac, doxycycline, erythromycin, fluoxetine, imatinib, isoniazid, miconazole, nefazodone, nicardipine, paroxetine, pergolide, propofol, protease inhibitors, quinidine, quinine, ritonavir, ropinirole, telithromycin, verapamil, and other CYP2D6 or 3A4 inhibitors.

Haloperidol may increase the levels/effects of amphetamines, selected beta-blockers, selected benzodiazepines, calcium channel blockers, cisapride, cyclosporine, dextromethorphan, ergot alkaloids, fluoxetine, selected HMG-CoA reductase inhibitors, lidocaine, mesoridazine, mirtazapine, nateglinide, nefazodone, paroxetine, risperidone, ritonavir, sildenafil (and other PDE-5 inhibitors), tacrolimus, thioridazine, tricyclic antidepressants, venlafaxine, and other substrates of CYP2D6 or 3A4.

Haloperidol may increase the effects of antihypertensives, CNS depressants (ethanol, narcotics, sedative-hypnotics), lithium, trazodone, and TCAs. Haloperidol in combination with indomethacin may result in drowsiness, tiredness, and confusion. Metoclopramide may increase risk of extrapyramidal symptoms (EPS).

Decreased Effect: Haloperidol may inhibit the ability of bromocriptine to lower serum prolactin concentrations. Benztropine (and other anticholinergics) may inhibit the therapeutic response to haloperidol and excess anticholinergic effects may occur. Barbiturates, carbamazepine, and cigarette smoking may enhance the hepatic metabolism of haloperidol. Haloperidol may inhibit the antiparkinsonian effect of levodopa; avoid this combination. The levels/effects of haloperidol may be decreased by aminoglutethimide, carbamazepine, nafcillin, nevirapine, phenobarbital, phenytoin, rifamycins, and other CYP3A4 inducers. Haloperidol may decrease the levels/effects of CYP2D6 prodrug substrates (eg, codeine, hydrocodone, oxycodone, tramadol).

Pharmacodynamics/Kinetics

Onset of action: Sedation: I.V.: ~1 hour

Duration: Decanoate: ~3 weeks

Distribution: Crosses placenta; enters breast milk

Protein binding: 90%

Metabolism: Hepatic to inactive compounds

Bioavailability: Oral: 60%

(Continued)

Haloperidol *(Continued)*

Half-life elimination: 20 hours
Time to peak, serum: 20 minutes
Excretion: Urine (33% to 40% as metabolites) within 5 days; feces (15%)

Pregnancy Risk Factor C

Haloperidol Decanoate *see* Haloperidol *on page 682*
Haloperidol Lactate *see* Haloperidol *on page 682*
Halotestin® *see* Fluoxymesterone *on page 609*
Halotussin AC *see* Guaifenesin and Codeine *on page 673*
Halotussin® DAC *see* Guaifenesin, Pseudoephedrine, and Codeine *on page 676*
Haltran® [OTC] [DSC] *see* Ibuprofen *on page 728*
HandClens® [OTC] *see* Benzalkonium Chloride *on page 190*
Havrix® *see* Hepatitis A Vaccine *on page 687*
Havrix® and Engerix-B® *see* Hepatitis A (Inactivated) and Hepatitis B (Recombinant) Vaccine *on page 686*
Hayfebrol® [OTC] *see* Chlorpheniramine and Pseudoephedrine *on page 315*
HbCV *see Haemophilus* b Conjugate Vaccine *on page 680*
HBIG *see* Hepatitis B Immune Globulin *on page 688*
hBNP *see* Nesiritide *on page 976*
25-HCC *see* Calcifediol *on page 242*
hCG *see* Chorionic Gonadotropin (Human) *on page 326*
HCTZ *see* Hydrochlorothiazide *on page 699*
HCTZ and Telmisartan *see* Telmisartan and Hydrochlorothiazide *on page 1265*
HDA® Toothache [OTC] *see* Benzocaine *on page 191*
HDCV *see* Rabies Virus Vaccine *on page 1165*
Head & Shoulders® Classic Clean [OTC] *see* Pyrithione Zinc *on page 1155*
Head & Shoulders® Classic Clean 2-In-1 [OTC] *see* Pyrithione Zinc *on page 1155*
Head & Shoulders® Dry Scalp Care [OTC] *see* Pyrithione Zinc *on page 1155*
Head & Shoulders® Extra Fullness [OTC] *see* Pyrithione Zinc *on page 1155*
Head & Shoulders® Refresh [OTC] *see* Pyrithione Zinc *on page 1155*
Head & Shoulders® Smooth & Silky 2-In-1 [OTC] *see* Pyrithione Zinc *on page 1155*
Healon® *see* Hyaluronate and Derivatives *on page 696*
Healon®5 *see* Hyaluronate and Derivatives *on page 696*
Healon GV® *see* Hyaluronate and Derivatives *on page 696*
Hectorol® *see* Doxercalciferol *on page 468*
Helidac® *see* Bismuth Subsalicylate, Metronidazole, and Tetracycline *on page 209*
Helistat® *see* Microfibrillar Collagen Hemostat *on page 923*
Helixate® FS *see* Antihemophilic Factor (Recombinant) *on page 135*
Hemabate® *see* Carboprost Tromethamine *on page 265*
Hemiacidrin *see* Citric Acid, Magnesium Carbonate, and Glucono-Delta-Lactone *on page 341*

Hemin (HEE min)

U.S. Brand Names Panhematin®

Generic Available No

Pharmacologic Category Blood Modifiers

Use Orphan drug: Treatment of recurrent attacks of acute intermittent porphyria (AIP) only after an appropriate period of alternate therapy has been tried

Local Anesthetic/Vasoconstrictor Precautions No information available to require special precautions

Effects on Dental Treatment No significant effects or complications reported

Common Adverse Effects Frequency not defined.

Central nervous system: Mild pyrexia
Hematologic: Leukocytosis
Local: Phlebitis
Case report: Coagulopathy

Hemocyte® [OTC] *see* Ferrous Fumarate *on page 586*
Hemodent® Gingival Retraction Cord *see* Aluminum Chloride *on page 90*
Hemofil® M *see* Antihemophilic Factor (Human) *on page 134*
Hemril-HC® *see* Hydrocortisone *on page 714*

Heparin (HEP a rin)

U.S. Brand Names Hep-Lock®

Canadian Brand Names Hepalean®; Hepalean® Leo; Hepalean®-LOK

Mexican Brand Names Proparin® [inj.]

Generic Available Yes

Synonyms Heparin Calcium; Heparin Lock Flush; Heparin Sodium

Pharmacologic Category Anticoagulant

Use Prophylaxis and treatment of thromboembolic disorders

Local Anesthetic/Vasoconstrictor Precautions No information available to require special precautions

Effects on Dental Treatment Key adverse event(s) related to dental treatment: Bleeding from the gums.

Common Adverse Effects Frequency not defined.

Cardiovascular: Chest pain, vasospasm (possibly related to thrombosis), hemorrhagic shock

Central nervous system: Fever, headache, chills

Dermatologic: Unexplained bruising, urticaria, alopecia, dysesthesia pedis, purpura, eczema, cutaneous necrosis (following deep SubQ injection), erythematous plaques (case reports)

Endocrine & metabolic: Hyperkalemia (supression of aldosterone), rebound hyperlipidemia on discontinuation

Gastrointestinal: Nausea, vomiting, constipation, hematemesis

Genitourinary: Frequent or persistent erection

Hematologic: Hemorrhage, blood in urine, bleeding from gums, epistaxis, adrenal hemorrhage, ovarian hemorrhage, retroperitoneal hemorrhage, thrombocytopenia (see note)

Hepatic: Elevated liver enzymes (AST/ALT)

Local: Irritation, ulceration, cutaneous necrosis have been rarely reported with deep SubQ injections, I.M. injection (not recommended) is associated with a high incidence of these effects

Neuromuscular & skeletal: Peripheral neuropathy, osteoporosis (chronic therapy effect)

Ocular: Conjunctivitis (allergic reaction)

Respiratory: Hemoptysis, pulmonary hemorrhage, asthma, rhinitis, bronchospasm (case reports)

Miscellaneous: Allergic reactions, anaphylactoid reactions

Note: Thrombocytopenia has been reported to occur at an incidence between 0% and 30%. It is often of no clinical significance. However, immunologically mediated heparin-induced thrombocytopenia has been estimated to occur in 1% to 2% of patients, and is marked by a progressive fall in platelet counts and, in some cases, thromboembolic complications (skin necrosis, pulmonary embolism, gangrene of the extremities, stroke or myocardial infarction); daily platelet counts for 5-7 days at initiation of therapy may help detect the onset of this complication.

Mechanism of Action Potentiates the action of antithrombin III and thereby inactivates thrombin (as well as activated coagulation factors IX, X, XI, XII, and plasmin) and prevents the conversion of fibrinogen to fibrin; heparin also stimulates release of lipoprotein lipase (lipoprotein lipase hydrolyzes triglycerides to glycerol and free fatty acids)

Drug Interactions

Increased Effect/Toxicity: The risk of hemorrhage associated with heparin may be increased by oral anticoagulants (warfarin), thrombolytics, dextran, and drugs which affect platelet function (eg, aspirin, NSAIDs, dipyridamole, ticlopidine, clopidogrel, IIb/IIIa antagonists). However, heparin is often used in conjunction with thrombolytic therapy or during the initiation of warfarin therapy to assure anticoagulation and to protect against possible transient hypercoagulability. Cephalosporins which contain the MTT side chain and parenteral penicillins (may inhibit platelet aggregation) may increase the risk of hemorrhage. Other drugs reported to increase heparin's anticoagulant effect include antihistamines, tetracycline, quinine, nicotine, and cardiac glycosides (digoxin).

Decreased Effect: Nitroglycerin (I.V.) may decrease heparin's anticoagulant effect. This interaction has not been validated in some studies, and may only occur at high nitroglycerin dosages.

Pharmacodynamics/Kinetics

Onset of action: Anticoagulation: I.V.: Immediate; SubQ: ~20-30 minutes

Absorption: Oral, rectal, I.M.: Erratic at best from all these routes of administration; SubQ absorption is also erratic, but considered acceptable for prophylactic use

Distribution: Does not cross placenta; does not enter breast milk

(Continued)

Heparin *(Continued)*

Metabolism: Hepatic; may be partially metabolized in the reticuloendothelial system

Half-life elimination: Mean: 1.5 hours; Range: 1-2 hours; affected by obesity, renal function, hepatic function, malignancy, presence of pulmonary embolism, and infections

Excretion: Urine (small amounts as unchanged drug)

Pregnancy Risk Factor C

Heparin Calcium *see* Heparin *on page 685*

Heparin Cofactor I *see* Antithrombin III *on page 136*

Heparin Lock Flush *see* Heparin *on page 685*

Heparin Sodium *see* Heparin *on page 685*

Hepatitis A (Inactivated) and Hepatitis B (Recombinant) Vaccine

(hep a TYE tis aye in ak ti VAY ted & hep a TYE tis bee ree KOM be nant vak SEEN)

Related Information

Immunizations (Vaccines) *on page 1614*

Systemic Viral Diseases *on page 1519*

U.S. Brand Names Twinrix®

Canadian Brand Names Twinrix™

Generic Available No

Synonyms Engerix-B® and Havrix®; Havrix® and Engerix-B®; Hepatitis B (Recombinant) and Hepatitis A Inactivated Vaccine

Pharmacologic Category Vaccine

Use Active immunization against disease caused by hepatitis A virus and hepatitis B virus (all known subtypes) in populations desiring protection against or at high risk of exposure to these viruses.

Populations include travelers to areas of intermediate/high endemicity for **both** HAV and HBV; those at increased risk of HBV infection due to behavioral or occupational factors; patients with chronic liver disease; laboratory workers who handle live HAV and HBV; healthcare workers, police, and other personnel who render first-aid or medical assistance; workers who come in contact with sewage; employees of day care centers and correctional facilities; patients/staff of hemodialysis units; male homosexuals; patients frequently receiving blood products; military personnel; users of injectable illicit drugs; close household contacts of patients with hepatitis A and hepatitis B infection.

Local Anesthetic/Vasoconstrictor Precautions No information available to require special precautions

Effects on Dental Treatment Key adverse event(s) related to dental treatment: Flu-like syndrome and upper respiratory tract infection.

Significant Adverse Effects **All serious adverse reactions must be reported to the U.S. Department of Health and Human Services (DHHS) Vaccine Adverse Event Reporting System (VAERS) 1-800-822-7967.**

Incidence of adverse effects of the combination product were similar to those occurring after administration of hepatitis A vaccine and hepatitis B vaccine alone. (Incidence reported is not versus placebo.)

>10%:

- Central nervous system: Headache (13% to 22%), fatigue (11% to 14%)
- Local: Injection site reaction: Soreness (37% to 41%), redness (9% to 11%)

1% to 10%:

- Central nervous system: Fever (2% to 3%)
- Gastrointestinal: Diarrhea (4% to 6%), nausea (2% to 4%), vomiting (≤1%)
- Local: Injection site reaction: Swelling (4% to 6%), induration
- Respiratory: Upper respiratory tract infection
- Miscellaneous: Flu-like syndrome

<1% (Limited to important or life-threatening): Also see individual agents: Allergic reactions, anaphylaxis, anaphylactoid reactions, arthralgia, Bell's palsy, bronchospasm, bruising at injection site, diaphoresis, dizziness, dyspnea, encephalopathy, erythema, erythema multiforme, flushing, Guillain-Barré syndrome, liver function test abnormalities, pruritus at injection site, rash, somnolence, Stevens-Johnson syndrome, syncope, urticaria, vertigo, vomiting, weakness

Dosage I.M.: Adults: Primary immunization: Three doses (1 mL each) given on a 0-, 1-, and 6-month schedule

Mechanism of Action

Hepatitis A vaccine (Havrix®), an inactivated virus vaccine, offers active immunization against hepatitis A virus infection at an effective immune response rate in up to 99% of subjects.

Recombinant hepatitis B vaccine (Engerix-B®) is a noninfectious subunit viral vaccine. The vaccine is derived from hepatitis B surface antigen (HB_sAg) produced through recombinant DNA techniques from yeast cells. The portion of the hepatitis B gene which codes for HB_sAg is cloned into yeast which is then cultured to produce hepatitis B vaccine.

In immunocompetent people, Twinrix® provides active immunization against hepatitis A virus infection (at an effective immune response rate >99% of subjects) and against hepatitis B virus infection (at an effective immune response rate of 93% to 97%) 30 days after completion of the 3-dose series. This is comparable to using hepatitis A vaccine (Havrix®) and hepatitis B vaccine (Engerix-B®) concomitantly.

Contraindications Hypersensitivity to hepatitis A vaccine or hepatitis B vaccine, or any component of the formulation

Warnings/Precautions Use caution in patients on anticoagulants, with thrombocytopenia, or bleeding disorders (bleeding may occur following intramuscular injection). Treatment for anaphylactic reactions should be immediately available. Postpone vaccination in moderate to severe acute illness (minor illness is not a contraindication). May not prevent infection if adequate antibody titers are not achieved (including immunosuppressed patients, patients on immunosuppressant therapy). Safety and efficacy in patients <18 years of age have not been established.

See individual agents.

Drug Interactions Immunosuppressant agents: May decrease immune response to vaccine

Pharmacodynamics/Kinetics

Onset of action: Seroconversion for antibodies against HAV and HBV were detected 1 month after completion of the 3-dose series.

Duration: Patients remained seropositive for at least 4 years during clinical studies.

Pregnancy Risk Factor C

Lactation Excretion in breast milk unknown/use caution

Dosage Forms Injection, suspension: Inactivated hepatitis A virus 720 ELISA units and hepatitis B surface antigen 20 mcg per mL (1 mL) [prefilled syringe; single-dose vial]

Hepatitis A Vaccine (hep a TYE tis aye vak SEEN)

Related Information

Immunizations (Vaccines) *on page 1614*

Systemic Viral Diseases *on page 1519*

U.S. Brand Names Havrix®; VAQTA®

Canadian Brand Names Avaxim®; Avaxim®-Pediatric; Epaxal Berna®; Havrix™; VAQTA®

Generic Available No

Pharmacologic Category Vaccine

Use For populations desiring protection against hepatitis A or for populations at high risk of exposure to hepatitis A virus (travelers to developing countries, household and sexual contacts of persons infected with hepatitis A), child day care employees, patients with chronic liver disease, illicit drug users, male homosexuals, institutional workers (eg, institutions for the mentally and physically handicapped persons, prisons), and healthcare workers who may be exposed to hepatitis A virus (eg, laboratory employees); protection lasts for approximately 15 years

Local Anesthetic/Vasoconstrictor Precautions No information available to require special precautions

Effects on Dental Treatment No significant effects or complications reported

Significant Adverse Effects **All serious adverse reactions must be reported to the U.S. Department of Health and Human Services (DHHS) Vaccine Adverse Event Reporting System (VAERS) 1-800-822-7967.**

Percentage unknown: Fatigue, fever (rare), transient LFT abnormalities

>10%:

- Central nervous system: Headache
- Local: Pain, tenderness, and warmth

1% to 10%:

- Endocrine & metabolic: Pharyngitis (1%)
- Gastrointestinal: Abdominal pain (1%)

(Continued)

Hepatitis A Vaccine *(Continued)*

Local: Cutaneous reactions at the injection site (soreness, edema, and redness)

Dosage I.M.:

Havrix®:

Children 2-18 years: 720 ELISA units (administered as 2 injections of 360 ELISA units [0.5 mL]) 15-30 days prior to travel with a booster 6-12 months following primary immunization; the deltoid muscle should be used for I.M. injection

Adults: 1440 ELISA units (1 mL) 15-30 days prior to travel with a booster 6-12 months following primary immunization; injection should be in the deltoid

VAQTA®:

Children 2-17 years: 25 units (0.5 mL) with 25 units (0.5 mL) booster to be given 6-18 months after primary immunization

Adults: 50 units (1 mL) with 50 units (1 mL) booster to be given 6 months after primary immunization

Mechanism of Action As an inactivated virus vaccine, hepatitis A vaccine offers active immunization against hepatitis A virus infection at an effective immune response rate in up to 99% of subjects

Contraindications Hypersensitivity to hepatitis A vaccine or any component of the formulation

Warnings/Precautions Use caution in patients with serious active infection, cardiovascular disease, or pulmonary disorders; treatment for anaphylactic reactions should be immediately available

Drug Interactions No interference of immunogenicity was reported when mixed with hepatitis B vaccine

Pharmacodynamics/Kinetics

Onset of action (protection): 3 weeks after a single dose

Duration: Neutralizing antibodies have persisted for >3 years; unconfirmed evidence indicates that antibody levels may persist for 5-10 years

Pregnancy Risk Factor C

Dosage Forms

Injection, suspension, adult [prefilled syringe; single-dose vial]:

Havrix®: Viral antigen 1440 ELISA units/mL (1 mL)

VAQTA®: HAV protein 50 units/mL (1 mL)

Injection, suspension, pediatric [prefilled syringe; single-dose vial] (Havrix®): Viral antigen 720 ELISA units/0.5 mL (0.5 mL)

Injection, suspension, pediatric/adolescent [prefilled syringe; single-dose vial] (VAQTA®): HAV protein 25 units/0.5 mL (0.5 mL)

Selected Readings

Centers for Disease Control, "Recommendations of the Advisory Committee on Immunization Practices (ACIP): General Recommendations on Immunization," *MMWR*, 1994, 43(RR-1):23.

Hepatitis B Immune Globulin

(hep a TYE tis bee i MYUN GLOB yoo lin)

Related Information

Immunizations (Vaccines) *on page 1614*

Occupational Exposure to Bloodborne Pathogens (Standard/Universal Precautions) *on page 1603*

Systemic Viral Diseases *on page 1519*

U.S. Brand Names BayHep B™; Nabi-HB®

Canadian Brand Names BayHep B™

Generic Available No

Synonyms HBIG

Pharmacologic Category Immune Globulin

Use Provide prophylactic passive immunity to hepatitis B infection to those individuals exposed; newborns of mothers known to be hepatitis B surface antigen positive; hepatitis B immune globulin is not indicated for treatment of active hepatitis B infections and is ineffective in the treatment of chronic active hepatitis B infection

Local Anesthetic/Vasoconstrictor Precautions No information available to require special precautions

Effects on Dental Treatment No significant effects or complications reported

Significant Adverse Effects Frequency not defined.

Central nervous system: Dizziness, malaise, fever, lethargy, chills

Dermatologic: Urticaria, angioedema, rash, erythema

Gastrointestinal: Vomiting, nausea

Genitourinary: Nephrotic syndrome

Local: Pain, tenderness, and muscular stiffness at injection site

Neuromuscular & skeletal: Arthralgia, myalgia

Miscellaneous: Anaphylaxis

Dosage I.M.:

Newborns: Hepatitis B: 0.5 mL as soon after birth as possible (within 12 hours); may repeat at 3 months in order for a higher rate of prevention of the carrier state to be achieved; at this time an active vaccination program with the vaccine may begin

Adults: Postexposure prophylaxis: 0.06 mL/kg as soon as possible after exposure (ie, within 24 hours of needlestick, ocular, or mucosal exposure or within 14 days of sexual exposure); usual dose: 3-5 mL; repeat at 28-30 days after exposure

Note: HBIG may be administered at the same time (but at a different site) or up to 1 month preceding hepatitis B vaccination without impairing the active immune response

Mechanism of Action Hepatitis B immune globulin (HBIG) is a nonpyrogenic sterile solution containing 10% to 18% protein of which at least 80% is monomeric immunoglobulin G (IgG). HBIG differs from immune globulin in the amount of anti-HB_s. Immune globulin is prepared from plasma that is not preselected for anti-HB_s content. HBIG is prepared from plasma preselected for high titer anti-HB_s. In the U.S., HBIG has an anti-HB_s high titer >1:100,000 by IRA. There is no evidence that the causative agent of AIDS (HTLV-III/LAV) is transmitted by HBIG.

Contraindications Hypersensitivity to hepatitis B immune globulin or any component of the formulation; allergies to gamma globulin or anti-immunoglobulin antibodies; allergies to thimerosal; IgA deficiency

Warnings/Precautions Have epinephrine 1:1000 available for anaphylactic reactions. As a product of human plasma, this product may potentially transmit disease; screening of donors, as well as testing and/or inactivation of certain viruses reduces this risk. Use caution in patients with thrombocytopenia or coagulation disorders (I.M. injections may be contraindicated), in patients with isolated IgA deficiency, or in patients with previous systemic hypersensitivity to human immunoglobulins. Not for intravenous administration.

Drug Interactions Interferes with immune response of live virus vaccines

Pharmacodynamics/Kinetics

Absorption: Slow

Time to peak, serum: 1-6 days

Pregnancy Risk Factor C

Dosage Forms

Injection, solution, neonatal [preservative free; single-dose syringe] (BayHep B™): 0.5 mL

Injection, solution [preservative free; single-dose vial] (BayHep B™, Nabi-HB®): 1 mL, 5 mL

Hepatitis B Inactivated Virus Vaccine (plasma derived) *see* Hepatitis B Vaccine *on page 689*

Hepatitis B Inactivated Virus Vaccine (recombinant DNA) *see* Hepatitis B Vaccine *on page 689*

Hepatitis B (Recombinant) and Hepatitis A Inactivated Vaccine *see* Hepatitis A (Inactivated) and Hepatitis B (Recombinant) Vaccine *on page 686*

Hepatitis B Vaccine (hep a TYE tis bee vak SEEN)

Related Information

Diphtheria, Tetanus Toxoids, Acellular Pertussis, Hepatitis B (Recombinant), and Poliovirus (Inactivated) Vaccine *on page 452*

Immunizations (Vaccines) *on page 1614*

Systemic Viral Diseases *on page 1519*

U.S. Brand Names Engerix-B®; Recombivax HB®

Canadian Brand Names Engerix-B®; Recombivax HB®

Generic Available No

Synonyms Hepatitis B Inactivated Virus Vaccine (plasma derived); Hepatitis B Inactivated Virus Vaccine (recombinant DNA)

Pharmacologic Category Vaccine

Dental Use Immunization is recommended for dentists, oral surgeons, dental hygienists, dental nurses, and dental students

Use Immunization against infection caused by all known subtypes of hepatitis B virus, in individuals considered at high risk of potential exposure to hepatitis B virus or HB_sAg-positive materials: See table on next page.

(Continued)

Pre-exposure Prophylaxis for Hepatitis B

Healthcare workers[1]

Special patient groups (eg, adolescents, infants born to HB_sAg-positive mothers, children born after 11/21/91, military personnel, etc)

- Hemodialysis patients[2](see dosing recommendations)
- Recipients of certain blood products[3]

Lifestyle factors

- Homosexual and bisexual men
- Intravenous drug abusers
- Heterosexually-active persons with multiple sexual partners or recently acquired sexually-transmitted diseases

Environmental factors

- Household and sexual contacts of HBV carriers
- Prison inmates
- Clients and staff of institutions for the mentally handicapped
- Residents, immigrants, and refugees from areas with endemic HBV infection
- International travelers at increased risk of acquiring HBV infection

[1]The risk of hepatitis B virus (HBV) infection for healthcare workers varies both between hospitals and within hospitals. Hepatitis B vaccination is recommended for all healthcare workers with blood exposure.

[2]Hemodialysis patients often respond poorly to hepatitis B vaccination; higher vaccine doses or increased number of doses are required. A special formulation of one vaccine is now available for such persons (Recombivax HB®, 40 mcg/mL). The anti-Hb_s(antibody to hepatitis B surface antigen) response of such persons should be tested after they are vaccinated, and those who have not responded should be revaccinated with 1-3 additional doses.

Patients with chronic renal disease should be vaccinated as early as possible, ideally before they require hemodialysis. In addition, their anti-HB_s levels should be monitored at 6- to 12-month intervals to assess the need for revaccination.

[3]Patients with hemophilia should be immunized subcutaneously, not intramuscularly.

Local Anesthetic/Vasoconstrictor Precautions No information available to require special precautions

Effects on Dental Treatment No significant effects or complications reported

Routine Immunization Regimen of Three I.M. Hepatitis B Vaccine Doses

Age	Initial		1 mo		6 mo	
	Recombivax HB® (mL)	Engerix-B® (mL)	Recombivax HB® (mL)	Engerix-B® (mL)	Recombivax HB® (mL)	Engerix-B® (mL)
Birth[1] to 19 y	0.5[2]	0.5[3]	0.5[2]	0.5[3]	0.5[2]	0.5[3]
≥20 y	1[4]	1[5]	1[4]	1[5]	1[4]	1[5]
Dialysis or immunocompromised patients[6]	1[7]	2[8]	1[7]	2[8]	1[7]	2[8]

[1]Infants born of HB_sAg **negative** mothers.

[2]5 mcg/0.5 mL pediatric/adolescent formulation

[3]10 mcg/0.5 mL formulation

[4]10 mcg/mL adult formulation

[5]20 mcg/mL formulation

[6]Revaccinate if anti-HB_s <10 mIU/mL ≥1-2 months after third dose.

[7]40 mcg/mL dialysis formulation

[8]Two 1 mL doses given at different sites using the 40 mcg/2 mL dialysis formulation

Significant Adverse Effects All serious adverse reactions must be reported to the U.S. Department of Health and Human Services (DHHS) Vaccine Adverse Event Reporting System (VAERS) 1-800-822-7967.

Frequency not defined. The most common adverse effects reported with both products included injection site reactions (>10%).

Cardiovascular: Hypotension

Central nervous system: Agitation, chills, dizziness, fatigue, fever (≥37.5°C / 100°F), flushing, headache, insomnia, irritability, lightheadedness, malaise, vertigo

Dermatologic: Angioedema, petechiae, pruritus, rash, urticaria

Gastrointestinal: Abdominal pain, appetite decreased, cramps, diarrhea, dyspepsia, nausea, vomiting

Genitourinary: Dysuria

Local: Injection site reactions: Ecchymosis, erythema, induration, pain, nodule formation, soreness, swelling, tenderness, warmth

Neuromuscular & skeletal: Achiness, arthralgia, back pain, myalgia, neck pain, neck stiffness, paresthesia, shoulder pain, weakness

Otic: Earache
Respiratory: Cough, pharyngitis, rhinitis, upper respiratory tract infection
Miscellaneous: Lymphadenopathy, diaphoresis

Postmarketing and/or case reports: Alopecia, anaphylaxis, arthritis, Bell's palsy, bronchospasm, conjunctivitis, constipation, eczema, encephalitis, erythema nodosum, erythema multiforme, erythrocyte sedimentation rate increased, Guillain-Barré syndrome, herpes zoster, hypoesthesia, keratitis, liver enzyme elevation, migraine, multiple sclerosis, optic neuritis, palpitations, paresis, paresthesia, purpura, seizures, serum-sickness like syndrome (may be delayed days to weeks), Stevens-Johnson syndrome, syncope, tachycardia, thrombocytopenia, transverse myelitis, visual disturbances, vertigo

Dosage I.M.:

Immunization regimen: Regimen consists of 3 doses (0, 1, and 6 months): First dose given on the elected date, second dose given 1 month later, third dose given 6 months after the first dose; see table on previous page.

Alternative dosing schedule for **Recombivax HB®:** Children 11-15 years (10 mcg/mL adult formulation): First dose of 1 mL given on the elected date, second dose given 4-6 months later

Alternative dosing schedules for **Engerix-B®:**

Children ≤10 years (10 mcg/0.5 mL formulation): High-risk children: 0.5 mL at 0, 1, 2, and 12 months; lower-risk children ages 5-10 who are candidates for an extended administration schedule may receive an alternative regimen of 0.5 mL at 0, 12, and 24 months. If booster dose is needed, revaccinate with 0.5 mL.

Adolescents 11-19 years (20 mcg/mL formulation): 1 mL at 0, 1, and 6 months. High-risk adolescents: 1 mL at 0, 1, 2, and 12 months; lower-risk adolescents 11-16 years who are candidates for an extended administration schedule may receive an alternative regimen of 0.5 mL (using the 10 mcg/0.5 mL) formulation at 0, 12, and 24 months. If booster dose is needed, revaccinate with 20 mcg.

Adults ≥20 years: High-risk adults (20 mcg/mL formulation): 1 mL at 0, 1, 2, and 12 months. If booster dose is needed, revaccinate with 1 mL.

Postexposure prophylaxis: See table.

Postexposure Prophylaxis
Recommended Dosage for Infants Born to HB_sAg-Positive Mothers

Treatment	Birth	Within 7 d	1 mo	6 mo
Engerix-B® (pediatric formulation 10 mcg/0.5 mL)[1]	Note[2]	0.5 mL[2]	0.5 mL	0.5 mL
Recombivax HB® (pediatric/adolescent formulation 5 mcg/0.5 mL)	Note[2]	0.5 mL[2]	0.5 mL	0.5 mL
Hepatitis B immune globulin	0.5 mL	—	—	—

[1]An alternate regimen is administration of the vaccine at birth, within 7 days of birth, and 1, 2, and 12 months later.

[2]The first dose may be given at birth at the same time as HBIG, but give in the opposite anterolateral thigh. This may better ensure vaccine absorption.

Mechanism of Action Recombinant hepatitis B vaccine is a noninfectious subunit viral vaccine. The vaccine is derived from hepatitis B surface antigen (HB_sAg) produced through recombinant DNA techniques from yeast cells. The portion of the hepatitis B gene which codes for HB_sAg is cloned into yeast which is then cultured to produce hepatitis B vaccine.

Contraindications Hypersensitivity to yeast, hepatitis B vaccine, or any component of the formulation

Warnings/Precautions Immediate treatment for anaphylactic/anaphylactoid reaction should be available during vaccine use; consider delaying vaccination during acute febrile illness; use caution with decreased cardiopulmonary function; unrecognized hepatitis B infection may be present, immunization may not prevent infection in these patients; patients >65 years may have lower response rates

Drug Interactions

DTaP: Vaccines may be administered together (using separate sites and syringes).

Haemophilus b conjugate vaccine (PedvaxHIB®): Vaccines may be administered together (using separate sites and syringes).

Immunosuppressant medications: The effect of the vaccine may be decreased; consider deferring vaccination for 3 months after immunosuppressant therapy is discontinued.

(Continued)

Hepatitis B Vaccine *(Continued)*

MMR: Vaccines may be administered together (using separate sites and syringes).

OPV: Vaccines may be administered together.

Pharmacodynamics/Kinetics Duration of action: Following a 3-dose series, immunity lasts ~5-7 years

Pregnancy Risk Factor C

Lactation Excretion in breast milk unknown/use caution

Dosage Forms

Injection, suspension [recombinant DNA]:

Engerix-B®:

Adult: Hepatitis B surface antigen 20 mcg/mL (1 mL) [contains trace amounts of thimerosal]

Pediatric/adolescent: Hepatitis B surface antigen 10 mcg/0.5 mL (0.5 mL) [contains trace amounts of thimerosal]

Recombivax HB®:

Adult [preservative free]: Hepatitis B surface antigen 10 mcg/mL (1 mL, 3 mL)

Dialysis [preservative free]: Hepatitis B surface antigen 40 mcg/mL (1 mL)

Pediatric/adolescent [preservative free]: Hepatitis B surface antigen 5 mcg/0.5 mL (0.5 mL)

Selected Readings

Centers for Disease Control, "Recommendations of the Advisory Committee on Immunization Practices (ACIP): General Recommendations on Immunization," *MMWR*, 1994, 43(RR-1):23.

Gardner P and Schaffner W, "Immunization of Adults," *N Engl J Med*, 1993, 328(17):1252-8.

Hep-Lock® *see* Heparin *on page 685*

Hepsera™ *see* Adefovir *on page 68*

Herceptin® *see* Trastuzumab *on page 1324*

HES *see* Hetastarch *on page 692*

Hespan® *see* Hetastarch *on page 692*

Hetastarch (HET a starch)

U.S. Brand Names Hespan®; Hextend®

Canadian Brand Names Hextend®

Mexican Brand Names HAES-steril®

Generic Available Yes: Sodium chloride infusion

Synonyms HES; Hydroxyethyl Starch

Pharmacologic Category Plasma Volume Expander, Colloid

Use Blood volume expander used in treatment of hypovolemia

Hespan®: Adjunct in leukapheresis to improve harvesting and increasing the yield of granulocytes by centrifugal means

Unlabeled/Investigational Use Hextand®: Priming fluid in pump oxygenators during cardiopulmonary bypass, and as a plasma volume expander during cardiopulmonary bypass

Local Anesthetic/Vasoconstrictor Precautions No information available to require special precautions

Effects on Dental Treatment No significant effects or complications reported

Common Adverse Effects Frequency not defined.

Cardiovascular: Circulatory overload, heart failure, peripheral edema

Central nervous system: Chills, fever, headache, intracranial bleeding

Dermatologic: Itching, pruritus, rash

Endocrine & metabolic: Amylase levels increased, parotid gland enlargement, indirect bilirubin increased, metabolic acidosis

Gastrointestinal: Vomiting

Hematologic: Bleeding, factor VIII:C plasma levels decreased, decreased plasma aggregation decreased, von Willebrand factor decreased, dilutional coagulopathy; prolongation of PT, PTT, clotting time, and bleeding time; thrombocytopenia, anemia, disseminated intravascular coagulopathy (rare), hemolysis (rare)

Neuromuscular & skeletal: Myalgia

Miscellaneous: Anaphylactoid reactions, hypersensitivity, flu-like symptoms (mild)

Mechanism of Action Produces plasma volume expansion by virtue of its highly colloidal starch structure, similar to albumin

Pharmacodynamics/Kinetics

Onset of action: Volume expansion: I.V.: ~30 minutes

Duration: 24-36 hours

Metabolism: Molecules >50,000 daltons require enzymatic degradation by the reticuloendothelial system or amylases in the blood

Excretion: Urine (~40%) within 24 hours; smaller molecular weight molecules readily excreted

Pregnancy Risk Factor C

Hexachlorocyclohexane *see* Lindane *on page 829*

Hexachlorophene (heks a KLOR oh feen)

U.S. Brand Names pHisoHex®

Canadian Brand Names pHisoHex®

Generic Available No

Pharmacologic Category Antibiotic, Topical

Use Surgical scrub and as a bacteriostatic skin cleanser; control an outbreak of gram-positive infection when other procedures have been unsuccessful

Local Anesthetic/Vasoconstrictor Precautions No information available to require special precautions

Effects on Dental Treatment No significant effects or complications reported

Mechanism of Action Bacteriostatic polychlorinated biphenyl which inhibits membrane-bound enzymes and disrupts the cell membrane

Pharmacodynamics/Kinetics

Absorption: Percutaneously through inflamed, excoriated, and intact skin

Distribution: Crosses placenta

Half-life elimination: Infants: 6.1-44.2 hours

Pregnancy Risk Factor C

Hexalen® *see* Altretamine *on page 89*

Hexamethylenetetramine *see* Methenamine *on page 892*

Hexamethylmelamine *see* Altretamine *on page 89*

HEXM *see* Altretamine *on page 89*

Hextend® *see* Hetastarch *on page 692*

Hexylresorcinol (heks il re ZOR si nole)

U.S. Brand Names Sucrets® Original [OTC]

Generic Available Yes

Pharmacologic Category Local Anesthetic

Use Minor antiseptic and local anesthetic for sore throat

Local Anesthetic/Vasoconstrictor Precautions No information available to require special precautions

Effects on Dental Treatment No significant effects or complications reported

Hibiclens® [OTC] *see* Chlorhexidine Gluconate *on page 308*

Hibistat® [OTC] *see* Chlorhexidine Gluconate *on page 308*

Hib Polysaccharide Conjugate *see Haemophilus* b Conjugate Vaccine *on page 680*

HibTITER® *see Haemophilus* b Conjugate Vaccine *on page 680*

Hiprex® *see* Methenamine *on page 892*

Hirulog *see* Bivalirudin *on page 212*

Histatab® Plus [OTC] *see* Chlorpheniramine and Phenylephrine *on page 314*

Hista-Vent® DA *see* Chlorpheniramine, Phenylephrine, and Methscopolamine *on page 317*

Histex™ *see* Chlorpheniramine and Pseudoephedrine *on page 315*

Histex™ CT *see* Carbinoxamine *on page 262*

Histex™ HC *see* Hydrocodone, Carbinoxamine, and Pseudoephedrine *on page 712*

Histex™ I/E *see* Carbinoxamine *on page 262*

Histex™ PD *see* Carbinoxamine *on page 262*

Histex™ SR *see* Brompheniramine and Pseudoephedrine *on page 220*

Histussin D® *see* Hydrocodone and Pseudoephedrine *on page 711*

Hi-Vegi-Lip® [OTC] *see* Pancreatin *on page 1042*

Hivid® *see* Zalcitabine *on page 1395*

HIV Infection and AIDS *see page 1484*

HMM *see* Altretamine *on page 89*

HMR 3647 *see* Telithromycin *on page 1263*

HMS Liquifilm® *see* Medrysone *on page 863*

Hold® DM [OTC] *see* Dextromethorphan *on page 421*

Homatropine (hoe MA troe peen)

U.S. Brand Names Isopto® Homatropine

Generic Available No

Synonyms Homatropine Hydrobromide

(Continued)

Homatropine *(Continued)*

Pharmacologic Category Anticholinergic Agent, Ophthalmic; Ophthalmic Agent, Mydriatic

Use Producing cycloplegia and mydriasis for refraction; treatment of acute inflammatory conditions of the uveal tract

Local Anesthetic/Vasoconstrictor Precautions No information available to require special precautions

Effects on Dental Treatment Key adverse event(s) related to dental treatment: Nasal congestion.

Mechanism of Action Blocks response of iris sphincter muscle and the accommodative muscle of the ciliary body to cholinergic stimulation resulting in dilation and loss of accommodation

Pregnancy Risk Factor C

Homatropine and Hydrocodone *see* Hydrocodone and Homatropine *on page 709*

Homatropine Hydrobromide *see* Homatropine *on page 693*

Horse Antihuman Thymocyte Gamma Globulin *see* Antithymocyte Globulin (Equine) *on page 136*

H.P. Acthar® Gel *see* Corticotropin *on page 376*

HTF919 *see* Tegaserod *on page 1263*

hu1124 *see* Efalizumab *on page 483*

Humalog® *see* Insulin Preparations *on page 749*

Humalog® Mix 75/25™ *see* Insulin Preparations *on page 749*

Human Antitumor Necrosis Factor-alpha *see* Adalimumab *on page 67*

Human Diploid Cell Cultures Rabies Vaccine *see* Rabies Virus Vaccine *on page 1165*

Human Growth Hormone (HYU man grothe HOR mone)

U.S. Brand Names Genotropin®; Genotropin Miniquick®; Humatrope®; Norditropin®; Norditropin® Cartridges; Nutropin®; Nutropin AQ®; Nutropin Depot® [DSC]; Protropin®; Saizen®; Serostim®; Zorbtive™

Canadian Brand Names Humatrope®; Nutropin® AQ; Nutropine®; Protropine®; Saizen®; Serostim®

Generic Available No

Synonyms Growth Hormone; Somatrem; Somatropin

Pharmacologic Category Growth Hormone

Use

Children:

- Long-term treatment of growth failure due to lack of adequate endogenous growth hormone secretion (Genotropin®, Humatrope®, Norditropin®, Nutropin®, Nutropin AQ®, Nutropin Depot®, Protropin®, Saizen®)
- Long-term treatment of short stature associated with Turner syndrome (Humatrope®, Nutropin®, Nutropin AQ®)
- Treatment of Prader-Willi syndrome (Genotropin®)
- Treatment of growth failure associated with chronic renal insufficiency (CRI) up until the time of renal transplantation (Nutropin®, Nutropin AQ®)
- Long-term treatment of growth failure in children born small for gestational age who fail to manifest catch-up growth by 2 years of age (Genotropin®)
- Long-term treatment of idiopathic short stature (nongrowth hormone-deficient short stature) defined by height standard deviation score (SDS) less than or equal to -2.25 and growth rate not likely to attain normal adult height (Humatrope®)

Adults:

- AIDS-wasting or cachexia with concomitant antiviral therapy (Serostim®)
- Replacement of endogenous growth hormone in patients with adult growth hormone deficiency who meet both of the following criteria (Genotropin®, Humatrope®, Nutropin®, Nutropin AQ®):
  - Biochemical diagnosis of adult growth hormone deficiency by means of a subnormal response to a standard growth hormone stimulation test (peak growth hormone ≤5 mcg/L)

    and
  - Adult-onset: Patients who have adult growth hormone deficiency whether alone or with multiple hormone deficiencies (hypopituitarism) as a result of pituitary disease, hypothalamic disease, surgery, radiation therapy, or trauma

    or
  - Childhood-onset: Patients who were growth hormone deficient during childhood, confirmed as an adult before replacement therapy is initiated
- Treatment of short-bowel syndrome (Zorbtive™)

Unlabeled/Investigational Use Investigational: Congestive heart failure; AIDS-wasting/cachexia in children (Serostim®)

Local Anesthetic/Vasoconstrictor Precautions No information available to require special precautions

Effects on Dental Treatment No significant effects or complications reported

Common Adverse Effects

Growth hormone deficiency: Antigrowth hormone antibodies, carpal tunnel syndrome (rare), fluid balance disturbances, glucosuria, gynocomastia (rare), headache, hematuria, hyperglycemia (mild), hypoglycemia, hypothyroidism, leukemia, lipoatrophy, muscle pain, increased growth of pre-existing nevi (rare), pain/ local reactions at the injection site, pancreatitis (rare), peripheral edema, exacerbation of psoriasis, seizures

Idiopathic short stature: Myalgia (24%), scoliosis (19%), otitis media (16%), arthralgia (11%), arthrosis (11%), hyperlipidemia (8%), gynecomastia (5%), hip pain (3%), hypertension (3%)

Prader-Willi syndrome: Aggressiveness, arthralgia, edema, hair loss, headache, benign intracranial hypertension, myalgia; fatalities associated with use in this population have been reported

Turner syndrome: Humatrope®: Surgical procedures (45%), otitis media (43%), ear disorders (18%), hypothyroidism (13%), increased nevi (11%), peripheral edema (7%)

Adult growth hormone replacement: Increased ALT, increased AST, arthralgia, back pain, carpal tunnel syndrome, diabetes mellitus, fatigue, flu-like syndrome, generalized edema, gastritis, gynocomastia (rare), headache, hypoesthesia, joint disorder, myalgia, increased growth of pre-existing nevi, pain, pancreatitis (rare), paresthesia, peripheral edema, pharyngitis, rhinitis, stiffness in extremities, weakness

AIDS wasting or cachexia (limited): Serostim®: Musculoskeletal discomfort (54%), increased tissue turgor (27%), diarrhea (26%), neuropathy (26%), nausea (26%), fatigue (17%), albuminuria (15%), increased diaphoresis (14%), anorexia (12%), anemia (12%), increased AST (12%), insomnia (11%), tachycardia (11%), hyperglycemia (10%), increased ALT (10%)

Short-bowel syndrome: Peripheral edema (69% to 81%), edema (facial 44% to 50%; peripheral 13%), arthralgia (13% to 44%), injection site reaction (19% to 31%), flatulence (25%), abdominal pain (20% to 25%), vomiting (19%), malaise (13%), nausea (13%), diaphoresis increased (13%), rhinitis (7%), dizziness (6%)

Postmarketing and/or case reports: Carpal tunnel syndrome

Small for gestational age: Mild, transient hyperglycemia; benign intracranial hypertension (rare); central precocious puberty; jaw prominence (rare); aggravation of pre-existing scoliosis (rare); injection site reactions; progression of pigmented nevi

Mechanism of Action Somatropin and somatrem are purified polypeptide hormones of recombinant DNA origin; somatropin contains the identical sequence of amino acids found in human growth hormone while somatrem's amino acid sequence is identical plus an additional amino acid, methionine; human growth hormone stimulates growth of linear bone, skeletal muscle, and organs; stimulates erythropoietin which increases red blood cell mass; exerts both insulin-like and diabetogenic effects; enhances the transmucosal transport of water, electrolytes, and nutrients across the gut

Drug Interactions

Decreased Effect: Glucocorticoid therapy may inhibit growth-promoting effects. Growth hormone may induce insulin resistance in patients with diabetes mellitus; monitor glucose and adjust insulin dose as necessary.

Pharmacodynamics/Kinetics Somatrem and somatropin have equivalent pharmacokinetic properties

Duration: Maintains supraphysiologic levels for 18-20 hours

Absorption: I.M., SubQ: Well absorbed

Metabolism: Hepatic and renal (~90%)

Half-life elimination: Preparation and route of administration dependent

Excretion: Urine

Pregnancy Risk Factor B/C (depending upon manufacturer)

Humanized IgG1 Anti-CD52 Monoclonal Antibody *see* Alemtuzumab *on page 76*

Human LFA-3/IgG(1) Fusion Protein *see* Alefacept *on page 76*

Human Thyroid Stimulating Hormone *see* Thyrotropin Alpha *on page 1294*

Humate-P® *see* Antihemophilic Factor (Human) *on page 134*

Humatin® *see* Paromomycin *on page 1046*

Humatrope® *see* Human Growth Hormone *on page 694*

Humibid® DM *see* Guaifenesin and Dextromethorphan *on page 673*

Humibid® DM *(reformulation)* *see* Guaifenesin, Potassium Guaiacolsulfonate, and Dextromethorphan *on page 675*
Humibid® LA [DSC] *see* Guaifenesin *on page 672*
Humibid® LA *(reformulation)* *see* Guaifenesin and Potassium Guaiacolsulfonate *on page 675*
Humibid® Pediatric [DSC] *see* Guaifenesin *on page 672*
Humira™ *see* Adalimumab *on page 67*
Humulin® 50/50 *see* Insulin Preparations *on page 749*
Humulin® 70/30 *see* Insulin Preparations *on page 749*
Humulin® L *see* Insulin Preparations *on page 749*
Humulin® N *see* Insulin Preparations *on page 749*
Humulin® R *see* Insulin Preparations *on page 749*
Humulin® R (Concentrated) U-500 *see* Insulin Preparations *on page 749*
Humulin® U *see* Insulin Preparations *on page 749*
Hurricaine® *see* Benzocaine *on page 191*
HXM *see* Altretamine *on page 89*
Hyalgan® *see* Hyaluronate and Derivatives *on page 696*
Hyaluronan *see* Hyaluronate and Derivatives *on page 696*

Hyaluronate and Derivatives

(hye al yoor ON ate & dah RIV ah tives)

U.S. Brand Names Biolon™; Healon®; Healon®5; Healon GV®; Hyalgan®; Hylaform®; IPM Wound Gel™ [OTC]; Orthovisc®; Provisc®; Restylane®; Supartz™; Synvisc®; Vitrax®

Canadian Brand Names Biolon™; Cystistat®; Eyestil; Healon®; Healon GV®; OrthoVisc®; Suplasyn®

Mexican Brand Names Biolon®; Healon®

Generic Available No

Synonyms Hyaluronan; Hyaluronic Acid; Hylan Polymers; Sodium Hyaluronate

Pharmacologic Category Antirheumatic Miscellaneous; Ophthalmic Agent, Viscoelastic; Skin and Mucous Membrane Agent, Miscellaneous

Use

Intra-articular injection: Treatment of pain in osteoarthritis in knee in patients who have failed nonpharmacologic treatment and simple analgesics

Intradermal: Correction of moderate-to-severe facial wrinkles or folds

Ophthalmic: Surgical aid in cataract extraction, intraocular implantation, corneal transplant, glaucoma filtration, and retinal attachment surgery

Topical: Management of skin ulcers and wounds

Local Anesthetic/Vasoconstrictor Precautions No information available to require special precautions

Effects on Dental Treatment No significant effects or complications reported

Common Adverse Effects Frequency not defined. Frequencies and/or type of local reaction may vary by formulation and site of application/injection.

Cardiovascular: Edema, flushing, hypotension, tachycardia

Central nervous system: Dizziness, headache

Dermatologic: Itching, rash

Local: Injection site: Arthralgia, bruising, desquamation, erythema, pain, rash, swelling

Ocular: Postoperative inflammatory reactions (iritis, hypopyon), corneal edema, corneal decompensation, transient postoperative increase in IOP

Miscellaneous: Abscess formation, anaphylaxis, allergic reactions, respiratory difficulties

Mechanism of Action Sodium hyaluronate is a polysaccharide which is distributed widely in the extracellular matrix of connective tissue in man (vitreous and aqueous humor of the eye, synovial fluid, skin, and umbilical cord). Sodium hyaluronate and its derivatives form a viscoelastic solution in water (at physiological pH and ionic strength) which makes it suitable for aqueous and vitreous humor in ophthalmic surgery, and functions as a tissue and/or joint lubricant which plays an important role in modulating the interactions between adjacent tissues. Intradermal injection may decrease the depth of facial wrinkles.

Drug Interactions

Increased Effect/Toxicity: Anticoagulants or antiplatelet agents may increase the risk of injection site bleeding or hematoma.

Pharmacodynamics/Kinetics

Distribution: Intravitreous injection: Diffusion occurs slowly

Excretion: Ophthalmic: Via Canal of Schlemm

Pregnancy Risk Factor C

Hyaluronic Acid *see* Hyaluronate and Derivatives *on page 696*

Hyaluronidase (hye al yoor ON i dase)

U.S. Brand Names Vitrase®

Generic Available No

Pharmacologic Category Enzyme

Use Increase the dispersion and absorption of other drugs; increase rate of absorption of parenteral fluids given by hypodermoclysis; adjunct in subcutaneous urography for improving resorption of radiopaque agents

Unlabeled/Investigational Use Management of drug extravasations

Local Anesthetic/Vasoconstrictor Precautions No information available to require special precautions

Effects on Dental Treatment No significant effects or complications reported

Common Adverse Effects Frequency not defined: Local: Injection site reactions

Mechanism of Action Modifies the permeability of connective tissue through hydrolysis of hyaluronic acid, one of the chief ingredients of tissue cement which offers resistance to diffusion of liquids through tissues; hyaluronidase increases both the distribution and absorption of locally injected substances.

Drug Interactions

Increased Effect/Toxicity: Absorption and toxicity of local anesthetics may be increased.

Pharmacodynamics/Kinetics

Onset of action: SubQ: Immediate

Duration: 24-48 hours

Pregnancy Risk Factor C

Hyate:C® *see* Antihemophilic Factor (Porcine) *on page 134*

Hycamptamine *see* Topotecan *on page 1316*

Hycamtin® *see* Topotecan *on page 1316*

hycet™ *see* Hydrocodone and Acetaminophen *on page 702*

Hycoclear Tuss *see* Hydrocodone and Guaifenesin *on page 708*

Hycodan® *see* Hydrocodone and Homatropine *on page 709*

Hycomine® Compound *see* Hydrocodone, Chlorpheniramine, Phenylephrine, Acetaminophen, and Caffeine *on page 712*

Hycosin *see* Hydrocodone and Guaifenesin *on page 708*

Hycotuss® *see* Hydrocodone and Guaifenesin *on page 708*

Hydergine [DSC] *see* Ergoloid Mesylates *on page 504*

HydrALAZINE (hye DRAL a zeen)

Related Information

Cardiovascular Diseases *on page 1458*

Canadian Brand Names Apo-Hydralazine®; Apresoline®; Novo-Hylazin; Nu-Hydral

Generic Available Yes

Synonyms Apresoline [DSC]; Hydralazine Hydrochloride

Pharmacologic Category Vasodilator

Use Management of moderate to severe hypertension, congestive heart failure, hypertension secondary to pre-eclampsia/eclampsia; treatment of primary pulmonary hypertension

Local Anesthetic/Vasoconstrictor Precautions No information available to require special precautions

Effects on Dental Treatment No significant effects or complications reported

Common Adverse Effects Frequency not defined.

Cardiovascular: Tachycardia, angina pectoris, orthostatic hypotension (rare), dizziness (rare), paradoxical hypertension, peripheral edema, vascular collapse (rare), flushing

Central nervous system: Increased intracranial pressure (I.V., in patient with pre-existing increased intracranial pressure), fever (rare), chills (rare), anxiety*, disorientation*, depression*, coma*

Dermatologic: Rash (rare), urticaria (rash), pruritus (rash)

Gastrointestinal: Anorexia, nausea, vomiting, diarrhea, constipation, adynamic ileus

Genitourinary: Difficulty in micturition, impotence

Hematologic: Hemolytic anemia (rare), eosinophilia (rare), decreased hemoglobin concentration (rare), reduced erythrocyte count (rare), leukopenia (rare), agranulocytosis (rare), thrombocytopenia (rare)

Neuromuscular & skeletal: Rheumatoid arthritis, muscle cramps, weakness, tremors, peripheral neuritis (rare)

Ocular: Lacrimation, conjunctivitis

Respiratory: Nasal congestion, dyspnea

(Continued)

HydrALAZINE *(Continued)*

Miscellaneous: Drug-induced lupus-like syndrome (dose-related; fever, arthralgia, splenomegaly, lymphadenopathy, asthenia, myalgia, malaise, pleuritic chest pain, edema, positive ANA, positive LE cells, maculopapular facial rash, positive direct Coombs' test, pericarditis, pericardial tamponade), diaphoresis

*Seen in uremic patients and severe hypertension where rapidly escalating doses may have caused hypotension leading to these effects.

Mechanism of Action Direct vasodilation of arterioles (with little effect on veins) with decreased systemic resistance

Drug Interactions

Cytochrome P450 Effect: Inhibits CYP3A4 (weak)

Increased Effect/Toxicity: Hydralazine may increase levels of beta-blockers (metoprolol, propranolol). Some beta-blockers (acebutolol, atenolol, and nadolol) are unlikely to be affected due to limited hepatic metabolism. Concurrent use of hydralazine with MAO inhibitors may cause a significant decrease in blood pressure. Propranolol may increase hydralazine serum concentrations.

Decreased Effect: NSAIDs (eg, indomethacin) may decrease the hemodynamic effects of hydralazine.

Pharmacodynamics/Kinetics

Onset of action: Oral: 20-30 minutes; I.V.: 5-20 minutes

Duration: Oral: 2-4 hours; I.V.: 2-6 hours

Distribution: Crosses placenta; enters breast milk

Protein binding: 85% to 90%

Metabolism: Hepatically acetylated; extensive first-pass effect (oral)

Bioavailability: 30% to 50%; increased with food

Half-life elimination: Normal renal function: 2-8 hours; End-stage renal disease: 7-16 hours

Excretion: Urine (14% as unchanged drug)

Pregnancy Risk Factor C

Hydralazine and Hydrochlorothiazide

(hye DRAL a zeen & hye droe klor oh THYE a zide)

Related Information

HydrALAZINE *on page 697*

Hydrochlorothiazide *on page 699*

Generic Available Yes

Synonyms Apresazide [DSC]; Hydrochlorothiazide and Hydralazine

Pharmacologic Category Antihypertensive Agent, Combination

Use Management of moderate to severe hypertension and treatment of congestive heart failure

Local Anesthetic/Vasoconstrictor Precautions No information available to require special precautions

Effects on Dental Treatment No significant effects or complications reported

Common Adverse Effects See individual agents.

Drug Interactions

Cytochrome P450 Effect: Hydralazine: **Inhibits** CYP3A4 (weak)

Increased Effect/Toxicity: See individual agents.

Pharmacodynamics/Kinetics See individual agents.

Pregnancy Risk Factor C

Hydralazine Hydrochloride *see* HydrALAZINE *on page 697*

Hydralazine, Hydrochlorothiazide, and Reserpine

(hye DRAL a zeen, hye droe klor oh THYE a zide, & re SER peen)

Related Information

HydrALAZINE *on page 697*

Hydrochlorothiazide *on page 699*

Generic Available Yes

Synonyms Hydrochlorothiazide, Hydralazine, and Reserpine; Reserpine, Hydralazine, and Hydrochlorothiazide; Ser-Ap-Es [DSC]

Pharmacologic Category Antihypertensive Agent, Combination

Use Treatment of hypertensive disorders

Local Anesthetic/Vasoconstrictor Precautions No information available to require special precautions

Effects on Dental Treatment No significant effects or complications reported

Common Adverse Effects See individual agents.

Drug Interactions

Cytochrome P450 Effect: Hydralazine: **Inhibits** CYP3A4 (weak)

Increased Effect/Toxicity: See individual agents.

Pharmacodynamics/Kinetics See individual agents.

Pregnancy Risk Factor C

Hydramine® [OTC] *see* DiphenhydrAMINE *on page 448*

Hydramine® Cough [OTC] *see* DiphenhydrAMINE *on page 448*

Hydrate® [DSC] *see* DimenhyDRINATE *on page 446*

Hydrated Chloral *see* Chloral Hydrate *on page 304*

Hydrea® *see* Hydroxyurea *on page 722*

Hydrisalic™ [OTC] *see* Salicylic Acid *on page 1205*

Hydrochlorothiazide (hye droe klor oh THYE a zide)

Related Information

Cardiovascular Diseases *on page 1458*

Moexipril and Hydrochlorothiazide *on page 941*

U.S. Brand Names Aquazide® H; Microzide™; Oretic®

Canadian Brand Names Apo-Hydro®; Novo-Hydrazide

Mexican Brand Names Diclotride®

Generic Available Yes

Synonyms HCTZ

Pharmacologic Category Diuretic, Thiazide

Use Management of mild to moderate hypertension; treatment of edema in congestive heart failure and nephrotic syndrome

Unlabeled/Investigational Use Treatment of lithium-induced diabetes insipidus

Local Anesthetic/Vasoconstrictor Precautions No information available to require special precautions

Effects on Dental Treatment Key adverse event(s) related to dental treatment: Orthostatic hypotension and hypotension.

Common Adverse Effects

1% to 10%:

- Cardiovascular: Orthostatic hypotension, hypotension
- Dermatologic: Photosensitivity
- Endocrine & metabolic: Hypokalemia
- Gastrointestinal: Anorexia, epigastric distress

Dosage Oral (effect of drug may be decreased when used every day):

Children (in pediatric patients, chlorothiazide may be preferred over hydrochlorothiazide as there are more dosage formulations [eg, suspension] available):

- <6 months: 2-3 mg/kg/day in 2 divided doses
- >6 months: 2 mg/kg/day in 2 divided doses

Adults:

- Edema: 25-100 mg/day in 1-2 doses; maximum: 200 mg/day
- Hypertension: 12.5-50 mg/day; minimal increase in response and more electrolyte disturbances are seen with doses >50 mg/day

Elderly: 12.5-25 mg once daily

Dosing adjustment/comments in renal impairment: Cl_{cr} 25-50 mL/minute: Not effective

Mechanism of Action Inhibits sodium reabsorption in the distal tubules causing increased excretion of sodium and water as well as potassium and hydrogen ions

Contraindications Hypersensitivity to hydrochlorothiazide or any component of the formulation, thiazides, or sulfonamide-derived drugs; anuria; renal decompensation; pregnancy

Warnings/Precautions Avoid in severe renal disease (ineffective). Electrolyte disturbances (hypokalemia, hypochloremic alkalosis, hyponatremia) can occur. Use with caution in severe hepatic dysfunction; hepatic encephalopathy can be caused by electrolyte disturbances. Gout can be precipitate in certain patients with a history of gout, a familial predisposition to gout, or chronic renal failure. Cautious use in diabetics; may see a change in glucose control. Hypersensitivity reactions can occur. Can cause SLE exacerbation or activation. Use with caution in patients with moderate or high cholesterol concentrations. Photosensitization may occur. Correct hypokalemia before initiating therapy.

Chemical similarities are present among sulfonamides, sulfonylureas, carbonic anhydrase inhibitors, thiazides, and loop diuretics (except ethacrynic acid). Use in patients with sulfonamide allergy is specifically contraindicated in product labeling, however, a risk of cross-reaction exists in patients with allergy

(Continued)

Hydrochlorothiazide *(Continued)*

to any of these compounds; avoid use when previous reaction has been severe.

Drug Interactions

Increased Effect/Toxicity: Increased effect of hydrochlorothiazide with furosemide and other loop diuretics. Increased hypotension and/or renal adverse effects of ACE inhibitors may result in aggressively diuresed patients. Beta-blockers increase hyperglycemic effects of thiazides in type 2 diabetes mellitus. Cyclosporine and thiazides can increase the risk of gout or renal toxicity. Digoxin toxicity can be exacerbated if a thiazide induces hypokalemia or hypomagnesemia. Lithium toxicity can occur with thiazides due to reduced renal excretion of lithium. Thiazides may prolong the duration of action with neuromuscular blocking agents.

Decreased Effect: Effects of oral hypoglycemics may be decreased. Decreased absorption of hydrochlorothiazide with cholestyramine and colestipol. NSAIDs can decrease the efficacy of thiazides, reducing the diuretic and antihypertensive effects.

Ethanol/Nutrition/Herb Interactions

Food: Hydrochlorothiazide peak serum levels may be decreased if taken with food. This product may deplete potassium, sodium, and magnesium.

Herb/Nutraceutical: Avoid dong quai if using for hypertension (has estrogenic activity). Dong quai may also cause photosensitization. Avoid ephedra, ginseng, yohimbe (may worsen hypertension). Avoid garlic (may have increased antihypertensive effect).

Pharmacodynamics/Kinetics

Onset of action: Diuresis: ~2 hours
Peak effect: 4-6 hours

Duration: 6-12 hours

Absorption: ~50% to 80%

Distribution: 3.6-7.8 L/kg

Protein binding: 68%

Metabolism: Not metabolized

Bioavailability: 50% to 80%

Half-life elimination: 5.6-14.8 hours

Time to peak: 1-2.5 hours

Excretion: Urine (as unchanged drug)

Pregnancy Risk Factor B (manufacturer); D (expert analysis)

Dosage Forms CAP (Microzide™): 12.5 mg. **TAB:** 25 mg, 50 mg; (Aquazide® H, Oretic®): 50 mg

Hydrochlorothiazide and Amiloride *see* Amiloride and Hydrochlorothiazide *on page 96*

Hydrochlorothiazide and Benazepril *see* Benazepril and Hydrochlorothiazide *on page 189*

Hydrochlorothiazide and Bisoprolol *see* Bisoprolol and Hydrochlorothiazide *on page 211*

Hydrochlorothiazide and Captopril *see* Captopril and Hydrochlorothiazide *on page 255*

Hydrochlorothiazide and Enalapril *see* Enalapril and Hydrochlorothiazide *on page 491*

Hydrochlorothiazide and Eprosartan *see* Eprosartan and Hydrochlorothiazide *on page 502*

Hydrochlorothiazide and Fosinopril *see* Fosinopril and Hydrochlorothiazide *on page 635*

Hydrochlorothiazide and Hydralazine *see* Hydralazine and Hydrochlorothiazide *on page 698*

Hydrochlorothiazide and Irbesartan *see* Irbesartan and Hydrochlorothiazide *on page 764*

Hydrochlorothiazide and Lisinopril *see* Lisinopril and Hydrochlorothiazide *on page 834*

Hydrochlorothiazide and Losartan *see* Losartan and Hydrochlorothiazide *on page 847*

Hydrochlorothiazide and Methyldopa *see* Methyldopa and Hydrochlorothiazide *on page 906*

Hydrochlorothiazide and Moexipril *see* Moexipril and Hydrochlorothiazide *on page 941*

Hydrochlorothiazide and Olmesartan Medoxomil *see* Olmesartan and Hydrochlorothiazide *on page 1010*

Hydrochlorothiazide and Propranolol *see* Propranolol and Hydrochlorothiazide *on page 1143*

Hydrochlorothiazide and Quinapril *see* Quinapril and Hydrochlorothiazide *on page 1160*

Hydrochlorothiazide and Spironolactone

(hye droe klor oh THYE a zide & speer on oh LAK tone)

Related Information

Cardiovascular Diseases *on page 1458*
Hydrochlorothiazide *on page 699*

U.S. Brand Names Aldactazide®

Canadian Brand Names Aldactazide 25®; Aldactazide 50®; Novo-Spirozine

Generic Available Yes

Synonyms Spironolactone and Hydrochlorothiazide

Pharmacologic Category Antihypertensive Agent, Combination

Use Management of mild to moderate hypertension; treatment of edema in congestive heart failure and nephrotic syndrome, and cirrhosis of the liver accompanied by edema and/or ascites

Local Anesthetic/Vasoconstrictor Precautions No information available to require special precautions

Effects on Dental Treatment No significant effects or complications reported

Common Adverse Effects See individual agents.

Drug Interactions

Increased Effect/Toxicity: See individual agents.

Pharmacodynamics/Kinetics See individual agents.

Pregnancy Risk Factor C

Hydrochlorothiazide and Telmisartan *see* Telmisartan and Hydrochlorothiazide *on page 1265*

Hydrochlorothiazide and Triamterene

(hye droe klor oh THYE a zide & trye AM ter een)

Related Information

Cardiovascular Diseases *on page 1458*
Hydrochlorothiazide *on page 699*

U.S. Brand Names Dyazide®; Maxzide®; Maxzide®-25

Canadian Brand Names Apo-Triazide®; Novo-Triamzide; Nu-Triazide; Penta-Triamterene HCTZ; Riva-Zide

Generic Available Yes

Synonyms Triamterene and Hydrochlorothiazide

Pharmacologic Category Antihypertensive Agent, Combination; Diuretic, Potassium-Sparing; Diuretic, Thiazide

Use Management of mild to moderate hypertension; treatment of edema in congestive heart failure and nephrotic syndrome

Local Anesthetic/Vasoconstrictor Precautions No information available to require special precautions

Effects on Dental Treatment No significant effects or complications reported

Common Adverse Effects Also see individual agents. Frequency not defined.

Central nervous system: Dizziness, fatigue
Dermatologic: Purpura, cracked corners of mouth
Endocrine & metabolic: Electrolyte disturbances
Gastrointestinal: Bright orange tongue, burning of tongue, loss of appetite, nausea, vomiting, stomach cramps, diarrhea, upset stomach
Hematologic: Aplastic anemia, agranulocytosis, hemolytic anemia, leukopenia, thrombocytopenia, megaloblastic anemia
Neuromuscular & skeletal: Muscle cramps
Ocular: Xanthopsia, transient blurred vision
Respiratory: Allergic pneumonitis, pulmonary edema, respiratory distress

Dosage Adults: Oral:

Hydrochlorothiazide 25 mg and triamterene 37.5 mg: 1-2 tablets/capsules once daily
Hydrochlorothiazide 50 mg and triamterene 75 mg: $^1/_2$-1 tablet daily

Mechanism of Action

Based on **triamterene** component: Competes with aldosterone for receptor sites in the distal renal tubules, increasing sodium, chloride, and water excretion while conserving potassium and hydrogen ions; may block the effect of aldosterone on arteriolar smooth muscle as well

Based on **hydrochlorothiazide** component: Inhibits sodium reabsorption in the distal tubules causing increased excretion of sodium and water as well as potassium and hydrogen ions

(Continued)

Hydrochlorothiazide and Triamterene *(Continued)*

Contraindications

Based on **hydrochlorothiazide** component: Hypersensitivity to hydrochlorothiazide or any component of the formulation, thiazides, or sulfonamide-derived drugs; anuria; renal decompensation; pregnancy

Based on **triamterene** component: Hypersensitivity to triamterene or any component of the formulation; patients receiving other potassium-sparing diuretics; anuria; severe hepatic disease; hyperkalemia or history of hyperkalemia; severe or progressive renal disease

Drug Interactions

Increased Effect/Toxicity: See individual agents.

Ethanol/Nutrition/Herb Interactions Food: Avoid food with high potassium content and potassium-containing salt substitutes.

Dietary Considerations Should be taken after meals.

Pharmacodynamics/Kinetics See individual agents.

Pregnancy Risk Factor C (per manufacturer)

Dosage Forms CAP: (Dyazide®): Hydrochlorothiazide 25 mg and triamterene 37.5 mg. **TAB:** (Maxzide®): Hydrochlorothiazide 50 mg and triamterene 75 mg; (Maxzide®-25): Hydrochlorothiazide 25 mg and triamterene 37.5 mg

Hydrochlorothiazide and Valsartan *see* Valsartan and Hydrochlorothiazide *on page 1364*

Hydrochlorothiazide, Hydralazine, and Reserpine *see* Hydralazine, Hydrochlorothiazide, and Reserpine *on page 698*

Hydrocil® [OTC] *see* Psyllium *on page 1151*

Hydrocodone and Acetaminophen

(hye droe KOE done & a seet a MIN oh fen)

Related Information

Acetaminophen *on page 47*

Oral Pain *on page 1526*

U.S. Brand Names Anexsia®; Bancap HC®; Ceta-Plus®; Co-Gesic®; hycet™; Lorcet® 10/650; Lorcet®-HD; Lorcet® Plus; Lortab®; Margesic® H; Maxidone™; Norco®; Stagesic®; Vicodin®; Vicodin® ES; Vicodin® HP; Zydone®

Generic Available Yes

Synonyms Acetaminophen and Hydrocodone

Pharmacologic Category Analgesic Combination (Narcotic)

Dental Use Treatment of postoperative pain

Use Relief of moderate to severe pain

Local Anesthetic/Vasoconstrictor Precautions No information available to require special precautions

Effects on Dental Treatment Key adverse event(s) related to dental treatment: Xerostomia (normal salivary flow resumes upon discontinuation).

Significant Adverse Effects Frequency not defined.

Cardiovascular: Bradycardia, cardiac arrest, circulatory collapse, coma, hypotension

Central nervous system: anxiety, dizziness, drowsiness, dysphoria, euphoria, fear, lethargy, lightheadedness, malaise, mental clouding, mental impairment, mood changes, physiological dependence, sedation, somnolence, stupor

Dermatologic: Pruritus, rash

Endocrine & metabolic: Hypoglycemic coma

Gastrointestinal: Abdominal pain, constipation, gastric distress, heartburn, nausea, peptic ulcer, vomiting

Genitourinary: Ureteral spasm, urinary retention, vesical sphincter spasm

Hematologic: Agranulocytosis, bleeding time prolonged, hemolytic anemia, iron deficiency anemia, occult blood loss, thrombocytopenia

Hepatic: Hepatic necrosis, hepatitis

Neuromuscular & skeletal: Skeletal muscle rigidity

Otic: Hearing impairment or loss (chronic overdose)

Renal: Renal toxicity, renal tubular necrosis

Respiratory: Acute airway obstruction, apnea, dyspnea, respiratory depression (dose related)

Miscellaneous: Allergic reactions, clamminess, diaphoresis

Restrictions C-III

Dosage Oral (doses should be titrated to appropriate analgesic effect): Analgesic:

Children 2-13 years or <50 kg: Hydrocodone 0.135 mg/kg/dose every 4-6 hours; do not exceed 6 doses/day or the maximum recommended dose of acetaminophen

Children and Adults ≥50 kg: Average starting dose in opioid naive patients: Hydrocodone 5-10 mg 4 times/day; the dosage of acetaminophen should be limited to ≤4 g/day (and possibly less in patients with hopatic impairment or ethanol use).

Dosage ranges (based on specific product labeling): Hydrocodone 2.5-10 mg every 4-6 hours; maximum: 60 mg hydrocodone/day (maximum dose of hydrocodone may be limited by the acetaminophen content of specific product)

Elderly: Doses should be titrated to appropriate analgesic effect; 2.5-5 mg of the hydrocodone component every 4-6 hours. Do not exceed 4 g/day of acetaminophen.

Dosage adjustment in hepatic impairment: Use with caution. Limited, low-dose therapy usually well tolerated in hepatic disease/cirrhosis; however, cases of hepatotoxicity at daily acetaminophen dosages <4 g/day have been reported. Avoid chronic use in hepatic impairment.

Contraindications Hypersensitivity to hydrocodone, acetaminophen, or any component of the formulation; CNS depression; severe respiratory depression

Warnings/Precautions Use with caution in patients with hypersensitivity reactions to other phenanthrene derivative opioid agonists (morphine, hydromorphone, levorphanol, oxycodone, oxymorphone); tolerance or drug dependence may result from extended use.

Respiratory depressant effects may be increased with head injuries. Use caution with acute abdominal conditions; clinical course may be obscured. Use caution with thyroid dysfunction, prostatic hyperplasia, hepatic or renal disease, and in the elderly. Causes sedation; caution must be used in performing tasks which require alertness (eg, operating machinery or driving).

Limit acetaminophen to <4 g/day. May cause severe hepatic toxicity in acute overdose; in addition, chronic daily dosing in adults has resulted in liver damage in some patients. Use with caution in patients with alcoholic liver disease; consuming ≥3 alcoholic drinks/day may increase the risk of liver damage. Use caution in patients with known G6PD deficiency.

Drug Interactions

Hydrocodone: **Substrate** of CYP2D6 (major)

Acetaminophen: **Substrate** (minor) of CYP1A2, 2A6, 2C8/9, 2D6, 2E1, 3A4; **Inhibits** CYP3A4 (weak)

Acetaminophen component: Refer to Acetaminophen monograph.

Hydrocodone component:

CYP2D6 inhibitors may decrease the effects of hydrocodone. Example inhibitors include chlorpromazine, delavirdine, fluoxetine, miconazole, paroxetine, pergolide, quinidine, quinine, ritonavir, and ropinirole.

CNS depressants (including antianxiety agents, antihistamines, antipsychotics, narcotics): CNS depression is additive; dose adjustment may be needed

MAO inhibitors: May see increased effects of MAO inhibitor and hydrocodone.

Tricyclic antidepressants (TCAs): May see increased effects of TCA and hydrocodone.

Ethanol/Nutrition/Herb Interactions

Ethanol: Avoid ethanol (may increase CNS depression); consuming ≥ 3 alcoholic drinks/day may increase the risk of liver damage

Herb/Nutraceutical: Avoid valerian, St John's wort, SAMe, kava kava (may increase risk of excessive sedation).

Pharmacodynamics/Kinetics

Acetaminophen: See Acetaminophen monograph.

Hydrocodone:

Onset of action: Narcotic analgesic: 10-20 minutes

Duration: 4-8 hours

Distribution: Crosses placenta

Metabolism: Hepatic; O-demethylation; N-demethylation and 6-ketosteroid reduction

Half-life elimination: 3.3-4.4 hours

Excretion: Urine

Pregnancy Risk Factor C/D (prolonged use or high doses near term)

Lactation Excretion in breast milk unknown/contraindicated

Breast-Feeding Considerations Acetaminophen is excreted in breast milk. The AAP considers it to be "compatible" with breast-feeding. Information is not available for hydrocodone; codeine and other opioids are excreted in breast milk and the AAP considers codeine to be "compatible" with breast-feeding. The manufacturers recommend discontinuing the medication or to discontinue nursing during therapy.

(Continued)

Hydrocodone and Acetaminophen *(Continued)*

Dosage Forms

Capsule (Bancap HC®, Ceta-Plus®, Lorcet®-HD, Margesic® H, Stagesic®): Hydrocodone bitartrate 5 mg and acetaminophen 500 mg

Elixir: Hydrocodone bitartrate 7.5 mg and acetaminophen 500 mg per 15 mL (480 mL)

Lortab®: Hydrocodone bitartrate 7.5 mg and acetaminophen 500 mg per 15 mL (480 mL) [contains alcohol 7%; tropical fruit punch flavor]

Solution, oral (hycet™): Hydrocodone bitartrate 7.5 mg and acetaminophen 325 mg per 15 mL (480 mL) [contains alcohol 7%; tropical fruit punch flavor]

Tablet:

Hydrocodone bitartrate 2.5 mg and acetaminophen 500 mg
Hydrocodone bitartrate 5 mg and acetaminophen 325 mg
Hydrocodone bitartrate 5 mg and acetaminophen 500 mg
Hydrocodone bitartrate 7.5 mg and acetaminophen 325 mg
Hydrocodone bitartrate 7.5 mg and acetaminophen 500 mg
Hydrocodone bitartrate 7.5 mg and acetaminophen 650 mg
Hydrocodone bitartrate 7.5 mg and acetaminophen 750 mg
Hydrocodone bitartrate 10 mg and acetaminophen 325 mg
Hydrocodone bitartrate 10 mg and acetaminophen 500 mg
Hydrocodone bitartrate 10 mg and acetaminophen 650 mg
Hydrocodone bitartrate 10 mg and acetaminophen 660 mg

Anexsia®:
5/500: Hydrocodone bitartrate 5 mg and acetaminophen 500 mg
7.5/650: Hydrocodone bitartrate 7.5 mg and acetaminophen 650 mg

Co-Gesic® 5/500: Hydrocodone bitartrate 5 mg and acetaminophen 500 mg

Lorcet® 10/650: Hydrocodone bitartrate 10 mg and acetaminophen 650 mg

Lorcet® Plus: Hydrocodone bitartrate 7.5 mg and acetaminophen 650 mg

Lortab®:
2.5/500: Hydrocodone bitartrate 2.5 mg and acetaminophen 500 mg
5/500: Hydrocodone bitartrate 5 mg and acetaminophen 500 mg
7.5/500: Hydrocodone bitartrate 7.5 mg and acetaminophen 500 mg
10/500: Hydrocodone bitartrate 10 mg and acetaminophen 500 mg

Maxidone™: Hydrocodone bitartrate 10 mg and acetaminophen 750 mg

Norco®:
Hydrocodone bitartrate 5 mg and acetaminophen 325 mg
Hydrocodone bitartrate 7.5 mg and acetaminophen 325 mg
Hydrocodone bitartrate 10 mg and acetaminophen 325 mg

Vicodin®: Hydrocodone bitartrate 5 mg and acetaminophen 500 mg

Vicodin® ES: Hydrocodone bitartrate 7.5 mg and acetaminophen 750 mg

Vicodin® HP: Hydrocodone bitartrate 10 mg and acetaminophen 660 mg

Zydone®:
Hydrocodone bitartrate 5 mg and acetaminophen 400 mg
Hydrocodone bitartrate 7.5 mg and acetaminophen 400 mg
Hydrocodone bitartrate 10 mg and acetaminophen 400 mg

Comments Neither hydrocodone nor acetaminophen elicit anti-inflammatory effects. Because of addiction liability of opiate analgesics, the use of hydrocodone should be limited to 2-3 days postoperatively for treatment of dental pain. Nausea is the most common adverse effect seen after use in dental patients; sedation and constipation are second. Nausea elicited by narcotic analgesics is centrally mediated and the presence or absence of food will not affect the degree nor incidence of nausea.

Acetaminophen:

A study by Hylek, et al, suggested that the combination of acetaminophen with warfarin (Coumadin®) may cause enhanced anticoagulation. The following recommendations have been made by Hylek, et al, and supported by an editorial in *JAMA* by Bell.

Dose and duration of acetaminophen should be as low as possible, individualized and monitored

The study by Hylek reported the following:

For patients who reported taking the equivalent of at least 4 regular strength (325 mg) tablets for longer than a week, the odds of having an INR >6.0 were increased 10-fold above those not taking acetaminophen. Risk decreased with lower intakes of acetaminophen reaching a background level of risk at a dose of 6 or fewer 325 mg tablets per week.

Selected Readings

Bell WR, "Acetaminophen and Warfarin: Undesirable Synergy," *JAMA*, 1998, 279(9):702-3.

Botting RM, "Mechanism of Action of Acetaminophen: Is There a Cyclooxygenase 3?" *Clin Infect Dis*, 2000, Suppl 5:S202-10.

Dart RC, Kuffner EK, and Rumack BH, "Treatment of Pain or Fever With Paracetamol (Acetaminophen) in the Alcoholic Patient: A Systematic Review," *Am J Ther*, 2000, 7(2):123-34.

Dionne RA, "New Approaches to Preventing and Treating Postoperative Pain," *J Am Dent Assoc*, 1992, 123(6):26-34.
Gobetti JP, "Controlling Dental Pain," *J Am Dent Assoc*, 1992, 123(6):47-52.
Grant JA and Weiler JM, "A Report of a Rare Immediate Reaction After Ingestion of Acetaminophen," *Ann Allergy Asthma Immunol*, 2001, 87(3):227-9.
Hylek EM, Heiman H, Skates SJ, et al, "Acetaminophen and Other Risk factors for excessive warfarin anticoagulation," *JAMA*, 1998, 279(9):657-62.
Kwan D, Bartle WR, and Walker SE, "The Effects of Acetaminophen on Pharmacokinetics and Pharmacodynamics of Warfarin," *J Clin Pharmacol*, 1999, 39(1):68-75.
McClain CJ, Price S, Barve S, et al, "Acetaminophen Hepatotoxicity: An Update," *Curr Gastroenterol Rep*, 1999, 1(1):42-9.
Shek KL, Chan LN, and Nutescu E, "Warfarin-Acetaminophen Drug Interaction Revisited," *Pharmacotherapy*, 1999, 19(10):1153-8.
Tanaka E, Yamazaki K, and Misawa S, "Update: The Clinical Importance of Acetaminophen Hepatotoxicity in Nonalcoholic and Alcoholic Subjects," *J Clin Pharm Ther*, 2000, 25(5):325-32.
Wynn RL, "Narcotic Analgesics for Dental Pain: Available Products, Strengths, and Formulations," *Gen Dent*, 2001, 49(2):126-8, 130, 132 passim.

Hydrocodone and Aspirin (hye droe KOE done & AS pir in)

Related Information
Aspirin *on page 151*

U.S. Brand Names Damason-P®

Generic Available No

Synonyms Aspirin and Hydrocodone

Pharmacologic Category Analgesic Combination (Narcotic)

Dental Use Treatment of postoperative pain

Use Relief of moderate to moderately severe pain

Local Anesthetic/Vasoconstrictor Precautions No information available to require special precautions

Effects on Dental Treatment Key adverse event(s) related to dental treatment: Nausea is the most common adverse effect seen after use in dental patients. Sedation and constipation are second. Aspirin component affects bleeding times and could influence wound-healing time. Elderly are a high-risk population for adverse effects from NSAIDs. As many as 60% of elderly patients with GI complications from NSAIDs can develop peptic ulceration and/or hemorrhage asymptomatically. Concomitant disease and drug use contribute to the risk of GI adverse effects.

Significant Adverse Effects

>10%:
- Cardiovascular: Hypotension
- Central nervous system: Lightheadedness, dizziness, sedation, drowsiness, fatigue
- Gastrointestinal: Nausea, heartburn, stomach pains, heartburn, epigastric discomfort
- Neuromuscular & skeletal: Weakness

1% to 10%:
- Cardiovascular: Bradycardia
- Central nervous system: Confusion
- Dermatologic: Rash
- Gastrointestinal: Vomiting, gastrointestinal ulceration
- Genitourinary: Decreased urination
- Hematologic: Hemolytic anemia
- Respiratory: Dyspnea
- Miscellaneous: Anaphylactic shock

<1% (Limited to important or life-threatening): Biliary tract spasm, bronchospasm, hallucinations, hepatotoxicity, histamine release, leukopenia, occult bleeding, physical and psychological dependence with prolonged use, prolongated bleeding time, thrombocytopenia, urinary tract spasm

Restrictions C-III

Dosage Adults: Oral: 1-2 tablets every 4-6 hours as needed for pain

Mechanism of Action

Based on **hydrocodone** component: Binds to opiate receptors in the CNS, altering the perception of and response to pain; suppresses cough in medullary center; produces generalized CNS depression

Based on **aspirin** component: Inhibits prostaglandin synthesis, acts on the hypothalamus heat-regulating center to reduce fever, blocks prostaglandin synthetase action which prevents formation of the platelet-aggregating substance thromboxane A_2

Contraindications

Based on **hydrocodone** component: Hypersensitivity to hydrocodone or any component of the formulation

Based on **aspirin** component: Hypersensitivity to salicylates, other NSAIDs, or any component of the formulation; asthma; rhinitis; nasal polyps; inherited or acquired bleeding disorders (including factor VII and factor IX deficiency);

(Continued)

Hydrocodone and Aspirin *(Continued)*

pregnancy (in 3rd trimester especially); do not use in children (<16 years) for viral infections (chickenpox or flu symptoms), with or without fever, due to a potential association with Reye's syndrome

Warnings/Precautions Use with caution in patients with impaired renal function, erosive gastritis, or peptic ulcer disease; children and teenagers should not use for chickenpox or flu symptoms before a physician is consulted about Reye's syndrome; tolerance or drug dependence may result from extended use

Based on **hydrocodone** component: Use with caution in patients with hypersensitivity reactions to other phenanthrene-derivative opioid agonists (morphine, codeine, hydromorphone, levorphanol, oxycodone, oxymorphone); should be used with caution in elderly or debilitated patients, and those with severe impairment of hepatic or renal function, prostatic hyperplasia, or urethral stricture. Also use caution in patients with head injury, increased intracranial pressure, acute abdomen, or impaired thyroid function. Hydrocodone suppresses the cough reflex; caution should be exercised when this agent is used postoperatively and in patients with pulmonary diseases (including asthma, emphysema, COPD)

Based on **aspirin** component: Use with caution in patients with platelet and bleeding disorders, renal dysfunction, dehydration, erosive gastritis, or peptic ulcer disease. Heavy ethanol use (>3 drinks/day) can increase bleeding risks. Avoid use in severe renal failure or in severe hepatic failure. Discontinue use if tinnitus or impaired hearing occurs. Caution in mild-moderate renal failure (only at high dosages). Patients with sensitivity to tartrazine dyes, nasal polyps and asthma may have an increased risk of salicylate sensitivity. Surgical patients should avoid ASA if possible, for 1-2 weeks prior to surgery, to reduce the risk of excessive bleeding.

Drug Interactions

Based on **hydrocodone** component: **Substrate** of CYP2D6 (major)

CNS depressants, MAO inhibitors, general anesthetics, and tricyclic antidepressants: May potentiate the effects of opiate agonists; dextroamphetamine may enhance the analgesic effect of opiate agonists.

CYP2D6 inhibitors: May decrease the effects of hydrocodone. Example inhibitors include chlorpromazine, delavirdine, fluoxetine, miconazole, paroxetine, pergolide, quinidine, quinine, ritonavir, and ropinirole.

Based on **aspirin** component: **Substrate** of CYP2C8/9 (minor)

ACE inhibitors: The effects of ACE inhibitors may be blunted by aspirin administration, particularly at higher dosages.

Buspirone increases aspirin's free % *in vitro*.

Carbonic anhydrase inhibitors and corticosteroids have been associated with alteration in salicylate serum concentrations.

Heparin and low molecular weight heparins: Concurrent use may increase the risk of bleeding

Methotrexate serum levels may be increased; consider discontinuing aspirin 2-3 days before high-dose methotrexate treatment or avoid concurrent use.

NSAIDs may increase the risk of gastrointestinal adverse effects and bleeding. Serum concentrations of some NSAIDs may be decreased by aspirin.

Platelet inhibitors (IIb/IIIa antagonists): Risk of bleeding may be increased.

Probenecid effects may be antagonized by aspirin.

Sulfonylureas: The effects of older sulfonylurea agents (tolazamide, tolbutamide) may be potentiated due to displacement from plasma proteins. This effect does not appear to be clinically significant for newer sulfonylurea agents (glyburide, glipizide, glimepiride).

Valproic acid may be displaced from its binding sites which can result in toxicity.

Verapamil may potentiate the prolongation of bleeding time associated with aspirin.

Warfarin and oral anticoagulants may increase the risk of bleeding.

Ethanol/Nutrition/Herb Interactions

Based on **hydrocodone** component: Ethanol: Avoid or limit ethanol (may increase CNS depression). Watch for sedation.

Based on **aspirin** component:

Ethanol: Avoid ethanol (may enhance gastric mucosal damage).

Food: Food may decrease the rate but not the extent of oral absorption. Take with food or or large volume of water or milk to minimize GI upset.

Herb/Nutraceutical: Avoid cat's claw, dong quai, evening primrose, feverfew, garlic, ginger, ginkgo, red clover, horse chestnut, green tea, ginseng (all have additional antiplatelet activity).

Pharmacodynamics/Kinetics

Aspirin: See Aspirin monograph.

Hydrocodone:

Onset of action: Narcotic analgesic: 10-20 minutes

Duration: 4-8 hours

Distribution: Crosses placenta

Metabolism: Hepatic; O-demethylation; N-demethylation and 6-ketosteroid reduction

Half-life elimination: 3.3-4.4 hours

Excretion: Urine

Pregnancy Risk Factor D

Lactation Enters breast milk/contraindicated

Breast-Feeding Considerations

Hydrocodone: No data reported.

Aspirin: Cautious use due to potential adverse effects in nursing infants.

Dosage Forms Tablet: Hydrocodone bitartrate 5 mg and aspirin 500 mg

Comments Because of addiction liability of opiate analgesics, the use of hydrocodone should be limited to 2-3 days postoperatively for treatment of dental pain; nausea is the most common adverse effect seen after use in dental patients; sedation and constipation are second; aspirin component affects bleeding times and could influence time of wound healing

Selected Readings

Dionne RA, "New Approaches to Preventing and Treating Postoperative Pain," *J Am Dent Assoc*, 1992, 123(6):26-34.

Gobetti JP, "Controlling Dental Pain," *J Am Dent Assoc*, 1992, 123(6):47-52.

Wynn RL, "Narcotic Analgesics for Dental Pain: Available Products, Strengths, and Formulations," *Gen Dent*, 2001, 49(2):126-8, 130, 132 passim.

Hydrocodone and Chlorpheniramine

(hye droe KOE done & klor fen IR a meen)

Related Information

Chlorpheniramine *on page 313*

U.S. Brand Names Tussionex®

Generic Available No

Synonyms Chlorpheniramine and Hydrocodone

Pharmacologic Category Antihistamine/Antitussive

Use Symptomatic relief of cough and allergy

Local Anesthetic/Vasoconstrictor Precautions No information available to require special precautions

Effects on Dental Treatment Key adverse event(s) related to dental treatment: Prolonged use will cause significant xerostomia (normal salivary flow resumes upon discontinuation).

Common Adverse Effects (Limited to important or life-threatening symptoms): Drowsiness, sedation, lethargy, anxiety, facial pruritus, constipation, nausea, ureteral spasm, respiratory depression, dryness of pharynx

Restrictions C-III

Mechanism of Action

Based on **hydrocodone** component: Binds to opiate receptors in the CNS, altering the perception of and response to pain; suppresses cough in medullary center; produces generalized CNS depression

Based on **chlorpheniramine** component: Competes with histamine for H_1-receptor sites on effector cells in the gastrointestinal tract, blood vessels, and respiratory tract

Drug Interactions

Cytochrome P450 Effect:

Hydrocodone: **Substrate** of CYP2D6 (major)

Chlorpheniramine: **Substrate** of CYP2D6 (minor), 3A4 (major); **Inhibits** CYP2D6 (weak)

Increased Effect/Toxicity:

Based on **hydrocodone** component: Increased toxicity: CNS depressants, MAO inhibitors, general anesthetics, and tricyclic antidepressants may potentiate the effects of opiate agonists; dextroamphetamine may enhance the analgesic effect of opiate agonists

Based on **chlorpheniramine** component: CYP2D6 enzyme substrate; Increased toxicity (CNS depression): CNS depressants, MAO inhibitors, tricyclic antidepressants, phenothiazines

Pharmacodynamics/Kinetics

Chlorpheniramine: See Chlorpheniramine monograph.

(Continued)

Hydrocodone and Chlorpheniramine *(Continued)*

Hydrocodone:

Onset of action: Narcotic analgesic: 10-20 minutes

Duration: 4-8 hours

Distribution: Crosses placenta

Metabolism: Hepatic; O-demethylation; N-demethylation and 6-ketosteroid reduction

Half-life elimination: 3.3-4.4 hours

Excretion: Urine

Pregnancy Risk Factor C

Hydrocodone and Guaifenesin

(hye droe KOE done & gwye FEN e sin)

Related Information

Guaifenesin *on page 672*

U.S. Brand Names Codiclear® DH; Hycosin; Hycotuss®; Kwelcof®; Pneumotussin®; Vicodin Tuss®; Vitussin

Generic Available Yes: Liquid

Synonyms Guaifenesin and Hydrocodone; Hycoclear Tuss

Pharmacologic Category Antitussive/Expectorant

Use Symptomatic relief of nonproductive coughs associated with upper and lower respiratory tract congestion

Local Anesthetic/Vasoconstrictor Precautions No information available to require special precautions

Effects on Dental Treatment Key adverse event(s) related to dental treatment: Xerostomia (normal salivary flow resumes upon discontinuation).

Common Adverse Effects Frequency not defined.

Cardiovascular: Hypertension, postural hypotension, palpitations

Central nervous system: Drowsiness, sedation, mental clouding, mental and physical impairment, anxiety, fear, dysphoria, dizziness, psychotic dependence, mood changes

Gastrointestinal: Nausea, vomiting, constipation with prolonged use

Genitourinary: Ureteral spasm, urinary retention

Ocular: Blurred vision

Respiratory: Respiratory depression (dose related)

Restrictions C-III

Mechanism of Action

Based on **hydrocodone** component: Binds to opiate receptors in the CNS, altering the perception of and response to pain; suppresses cough in medullary center; produces generalized CNS depression

Based on **guaifenesin** component: Thought to act as an expectorant by irritating the gastric mucosa and stimulating respiratory tract secretions, thereby increasing respiratory fluid volumes and decreasing phlegm viscosity

Drug Interactions

Cytochrome P450 Effect: Hydrocodone: **Substrate** of CYP2D6 (major)

Increased Effect/Toxicity:

Based on **hydrocodone** component: CNS depressants, MAO inhibitors, general anesthetics, and tricyclic antidepressants may potentiate the effects of opiate agonists; dextroamphetamine may enhance the analgesic effect of opiate agonists

Based on **guaifenesin** component: Disulfiram, MAO inhibitors, metronidazole, procarbazine

Decreased Effect:

Based on **guaifenesin** component: Disulfiram, MAO inhibitors, metronidazole, procarbazine

Pharmacodynamics/Kinetics

Guaifenesin: See Guaifenesin monograph.

Hydrocodone:

Onset of action: Narcotic analgesic: 10-20 minutes

Duration: 4-8 hours

Distribution: Crosses placenta

Metabolism: Hepatic; O-demethylation; N-demethylation and 6-ketosteroid reduction

Half-life elimination: 3.3-4.4 hours

Excretion: Urine

Pregnancy Risk Factor C

Hydrocodone and Homatropine

(hye droe KOE done & hoe MA troe peen)

Related Information

Homatropine *on page 693*

U.S. Brand Names Hycodan®; Hydromet®; Hydropane®; Tussigon®

Generic Available Yes: Syrup

Synonyms Homatropine and Hydrocodone

Pharmacologic Category Antitussive

Use Symptomatic relief of cough

Local Anesthetic/Vasoconstrictor Precautions No information available to require special precautions

Effects on Dental Treatment Key adverse event(s) related to dental treatment: Xerostomia (normal salivary flow resumes upon discontinuation).

Common Adverse Effects Frequency not defined.

Cardiovascular: Bradycardia, tachycardia, hypotension, hypertension

Central nervous system: Lightheadedness, dizziness, sedation, drowsiness, fatigue, confusion, hallucinations

Gastrointestinal: Nausea, vomiting, xerostomia, anorexia, impaired GI motility

Genitourinary: Decreased urination, urinary tract spasm

Hepatic: Biliary tract spasm

Neuromuscular & skeletal: Weakness

Ocular: Diplopia, miosis, mydriasis, blurred vision

Respiratory: Dyspnea

Miscellaneous: Histamine release, physical and psychological dependence with prolonged use

Restrictions C-III

Mechanism of Action

Based on **hydrocodone** component: Binds to opiate receptors in the CNS, altering the perception of and response to pain; suppresses cough in medullary center; produces generalized CNS depression

Based on **homatropine** component: Blocks response of iris sphincter muscle and the accommodative muscle of the ciliary body to cholinergic stimulation resulting in dilation and loss of accommodation

Drug Interactions

Cytochrome P450 Effect: Hydrocodone: **Substrate** of CYP2D6 (major)

Increased Effect/Toxicity:

Based on **hydrocodone** component: Increased toxicity: CNS depressants, MAO inhibitors, general anesthetics, and tricyclic antidepressants may potentiate the effects of opiate agonists; dextroamphetamine may enhance the analgesic effect of opiate agonists

Based on **homatropine** component:

Phenothiazine and TCAs may increase anticholinergic effects when used concurrently.

Sympathomimetic amines may cause tachyarrhythmias; avoid concurrent use

Pharmacodynamics/Kinetics Duration: Hydrocodone: 4-6 hours

Pregnancy Risk Factor C

Hydrocodone and Ibuprofen

(hye droe KOE done & eye byoo PROE fen)

Related Information

Ibuprofen *on page 728*

Oral Pain *on page 1526*

U.S. Brand Names Vicoprofen®

Canadian Brand Names Vicoprofen®

Generic Available Yes

Synonyms Ibuprofen and Hydrocodone

Pharmacologic Category Analgesic, Narcotic

Use Short-term (generally <10 days) management of moderate to severe acute pain; is not indicated for treatment of such conditions as osteoarthritis or rheumatoid arthritis

Local Anesthetic/Vasoconstrictor Precautions No information available to require special precautions

Effects on Dental Treatment Key adverse event(s) related to dental treatment: Xerostomia (normal salivary flow resumes upon discontinuation).

Significant Adverse Effects

>10%:

Central nervous system: Headache (27%), dizziness (14%), sedation (22%)

Dermatologic: Rash, urticaria

Gastrointestinal: Constipation (22%), nausea (21%), dyspepsia (12%)

(Continued)

Hydrocodone and Ibuprofen *(Continued)*

1% to 10%:

- Cardiovascular: Bradycardia, palpitations (<3%), vasodilation (<3%), edema (3% to 9%)
- Central nervous system: Headache, nervousness, confusion, fever (<3%), pain (3% to 9%), anxiety (3% to 9%), thought abnormalities
- Dermatologic: Itching (3% to 9%)
- Endocrine & metabolic: Fluid retention
- Gastrointestinal: Vomiting (3% to 9%), anorexia, diarrhea (3% to 9%), xerostomia (3% to 9%), flatulence (3% to 9%), gastritis (<3%), melena (<3%), mouth ulcers (<3%)
- Genitourinary: Polyuria (<3%)
- Neuromuscular & skeletal: Weakness (3% to 9%)
- Otic: Tinnitus
- Respiratory: Dyspnea, hiccups, pharyngitis, rhinitis
- Miscellaneous: Flu syndrome (<3%), infection (3% to 9%)

<1% (Limited to important or life-threatening): Acute renal failure, agranulocytosis, anemia, arrhythmias, aseptic meningitis, biliary tract spasm, bone marrow suppression, CHF, depression, diplopia, erythema multiforme, hallucinations, hemolytic anemia, hepatitis, histamine release, inhibition of platelet aggregation, leukopenia, neutropenia, peripheral neuropathy, physical and psychological dependence with prolonged use, Stevens-Johnson syndrome, thrombocytopenia, toxic amblyopia, toxic epidermal necrolysis, urinary tract spasm, urticaria

Restrictions C-III

Dosage Adults: Oral: 1-2 tablets every 4-6 hours as needed for pain; maximum: 5 tablets/day

Mechanism of Action

Based on **hydrocodone** component: Binds to opiate receptors in the CNS, altering the perception of and response to pain; suppresses cough in medullary center; produces generalized CNS depression

Based on **ibuprofen** component: Inhibits prostaglandin synthesis by decreasing the activity of the enzyme, cyclooxygenase, which results in decreased formation of prostaglandin precursors

Contraindications Hypersensitivity to hydrocodone, ibuprofen, aspirin, other NSAIDs, or any component of the formulation; pregnancy (3rd trimester)

Warnings/Precautions As with any opioid analgesic agent, this agent should be used with caution in elderly or debilitated patients, and those with severe impairment of hepatic or renal function, hypothyroidism, Addison's disease, prostatic hyperplasia, or urethral stricture. The usual precautions should be observed and the possibility of respiratory depression should be kept in mind. Patients with head injury, increased intracranial pressure, acute abdomen, active peptic ulcer disease, history of upper GI disease, impaired thyroid function, asthma, hypertension, edema, heart failure, and any bleeding disorder should use this agent cautiously. Hydrocodone suppresses the cough reflex; as with opioids, caution should be exercised when this agent is used postoperatively and in patients with pulmonary disease.

Drug Interactions

Hydrocodone: **Substrate** of CYP2D6 (major)

Ibuprofen: **Substrate** (minor) of CYP2C8/9, 2C19; **Inhibits** CYP2C8/9 (strong)

Also see individual agents.

Ethanol/Nutrition/Herb Interactions

Based on **hydrocodone** component: Ethanol: Avoid or limit ethanol (may increase CNS depression). Watch for sedation.

Based on **ibuprofen** component:

- Ethanol: Avoid ethanol (may enhance gastric mucosal irritation).
- Food: Ibuprofen peak serum levels may be decreased if taken with food.
- Herb/Nutraceutical: Avoid cat's claw, dong quai, evening primrose, feverfew, garlic, ginger, ginkgo, red clover, horse chestnut, green tea, ginseng (all have additional antiplatelet activity).

Pharmacodynamics/Kinetics

Ibuprofen: See Ibuprofen monograph.

Hydrocodone:

- Onset of action: Narcotic analgesic: 10-20 minutes
- Duration: 4-8 hours
- Distribution: Crosses placenta
- Protein binding: 19% to 45%
- Metabolism: Hepatic; O-demethylation; N-demethylation and 6-ketosteroid reduction
- Half-life elimination: 3.3-4.4 hours

Time to peak: 1.7 hours
Excretion: Urine

Pregnancy Risk Factor C/D (3rd trimester)

Lactation Excretion in breast milk unknown/contraindicated

Dosage Forms

Tablet: Hydrocodone bitartrate 5 mg and ibuprofen 200 mg; hydrocodone bitartrate 7.5 mg and ibuprofen 200 mg

Vicoprofen®: Hydrocodone bitartrate 7.5 mg and ibuprofen 200 mg

Selected Readings

Dionne R, "To Tame the Pain?" *Compend Contin Educ Dent*, 1998, 19(4):426-8, 430-1.

Hargreaves KM, "Management of Pain in Endodontic Patients," *Tex Dent J*, 1997, 114(10):27-31.

Sunshine A, Olson NZ, O'Neill E, et al, "Analgesic Efficacy of a Hydrocodone With Ibuprofen Combination Compared With Ibuprofen Alone for the Treatment of Acute Postoperative Pain," *J Clin Pharmacol*, 1997, 37(10):908-15.

Wynn RL, "Narcotic Analgesics for Dental Pain: Available Products, Strengths, and Formulations," *Gen Dent*, 2001, 49(2):126-8, 130, 132 passim.

Hydrocodone and Pseudoephedrine

(hye droe KOE done & soo doe e FED rin)

U.S. Brand Names Detussin®; Histussin D®; P-V Tussin Tablet

Generic Available Yes

Synonyms Pseudoephedrine and Hydrocodone

Pharmacologic Category Antitussive/Decongestant

Use Symptomatic relief of cough due to colds, nasal congestion, and cough

Local Anesthetic/Vasoconstrictor Precautions Use with caution since pseudoephedrine is a sympathomimetic amine which could interact with epinephrine to cause a pressor response

Effects on Dental Treatment Key adverse event(s) related to dental treatment: Pseudoephedrine: Xerostomia (normal salivary flow resumes upon discontinuation).

Common Adverse Effects See individual agents.

Restrictions C-III

Mechanism of Action

Based on **hydrocodone** component: Binds to opiate receptors in the CNS, altering the perception of and response to pain; suppresses cough in medullary center; produces generalized CNS depression

Based on **pseudoephedrine** component: Directly stimulates alpha-adrenergic receptors of respiratory mucosa causing vasoconstriction; directly stimulates beta-adrenergic receptors causing bronchial relaxation, increased heart rate and contractility

Drug Interactions

Cytochrome P450 Effect: Hydrocodone: **Substrate** of CYP2D6 (major)

Increased Effect/Toxicity:

Based on **hydrocodone** component: Increased toxicity: CNS depressants, MAO inhibitors, general anesthetics, and tricyclic antidepressants may potentiate the effects of opiate agonists; dextroamphetamine may enhance the analgesic effect of opiate agonists

Based on **pseudoephedrine** component: Increased toxicity: MAO inhibitors may increase blood pressure effects of pseudoephedrine; propranolol, sympathomimetic agents may increase toxicity

Decreased Effect: Based on **pseudoephedrine** component: Decreased effect of methyldopa, reserpine

Pharmacodynamics/Kinetics

Pseudoephedrine: See Pseudoephedrine monograph.

Hydrocodone:

Onset of action: Narcotic analgesic: 10-20 minutes
Duration: 4-8 hours
Distribution: Crosses placenta
Metabolism: Hepatic; O-demethylation; N-demethylation and 6-ketosteroid reduction
Half-life elimination: 3.3-4.4 hours
Excretion: Urine

Hydrocodone Bitartrate, Carbinoxamine Maleate, and Pseudoephedrine Hydrochloride *see* Hydrocodone, Carbinoxamine, and Pseudoephedrine *on page 712*

Hydrocodone Bitartrate, Phenylephrine Hydrochloride, and Diphenhydramine Hydrochloride *see* Hydrocodone, Phenylephrine, and Diphenhydramine *on page 713*

Hydrocodone, Carbinoxamine, and Pseudoephedrine

(hye droe KOE done, kar bi NOKS a meen, & soo doe e FED rin)

Related Information

Carbinoxamine and Pseudoephedrine *on page 262*
Pseudoephedrine *on page 1147*

U.S. Brand Names Histex™ HC; Tri-Vent™ HC

Generic Available Yes

Synonyms Carbinoxamine, Pseudoephedrine, and Hydrocodone; Hydrocodone Bitartrate, Carbinoxamine Maleate, and Pseudoephedrine Hydrochloride; Pseudoephedrine, Hydrocodone, and Carbinoxamine

Pharmacologic Category Antihistamine/Decongestant/Antitussive

Use Symptomatic relief of cough, congestion, and rhinorrhea associated with the common cold, influenza, bronchitis, or sinusitis

Local Anesthetic/Vasoconstrictor Precautions Use with caution since pseudoephedrine is a sympathomimetic amine which could interact with epinephrine to cause a pressor response

Effects on Dental Treatment Key adverse event(s) related to dental treatment: Pseudoephedrine: Xerostomia (normal salivary flow resumes upon discontinuation).

Common Adverse Effects See individual agents.

Restrictions C-III

Mechanism of Action

Hydrocodone binds to opiate receptors in the CNS, altering the perception of and response to pain; suppresses cough in medullary center; produces generalized CNS depression.

Carbinoxamine competes with histamine for H_1-receptor sites on effector cells in the gastrointestinal tract, blood vessels, and respiratory tract.

Pseudoephedrine is a sympathomimetic amine and isomer of ephedrine; acts as a decongestant in respiratory tract mucous membranes with less vasoconstrictor action than ephedrine in normotensive individuals.

Pharmacodynamics/Kinetics See individual agents.

Pregnancy Risk Factor C

Hydrocodone, Chlorpheniramine, Phenylephrine, Acetaminophen, and Caffeine

(hye droe KOE done, klor fen IR a meen, fen il EF rin, a seet a MIN oh fen, & KAF een)

Related Information

Acetaminophen *on page 47*
Chlorpheniramine *on page 313*
Phenylephrine *on page 1078*

U.S. Brand Names Hycomine® Compound

Generic Available No

Synonyms Acetaminophen, Caffeine, Hydrocodone, Chlorpheniramine, and Phenylephrine; Caffeine, Hydrocodone, Chlorpheniramine, Phenylephrine, and Acetaminophen; Chlorpheniramine, Hydrocodone, Phenylephrine, Acetaminophen, and Caffeine; Phenylephrine, Hydrocodone, Chlorpheniramine, Acetaminophen, and Caffeine

Pharmacologic Category Antitussive/Decongestant

Use Symptomatic relief of cough and symptoms of upper respiratory infection

Local Anesthetic/Vasoconstrictor Precautions Use with caution since phenylephrine is a sympathomimetic amine which could interact with epinephrine to cause a pressor response

Effects on Dental Treatment Key adverse event(s) related to dental treatment:

Acetaminophen: No significant effects or complications reported.

Chlorpheniramine: Prolonged use will cause significant xerostomia (normal salivary flow resumes upon discontinuation).

Phenylephrine: Up to 10% of patients could experience tachycardia, palpitations, and xerostomia; use vasoconstrictor with caution.

Common Adverse Effects Frequency not defined.

Cardiovascular: Hypertension, postural hypotension, tachycardia, palpitations

Central nervous system: Sedation, drowsiness, mental clouding, lethargy, impairment of mental and physical performance, anxiety, fear, dysphoria, dizziness, psychic dependence, mood changes

Dermatologic: Rash, pruritus

Gastrointestinal: Nausea, vomiting, constipation with prolonged use

Genitourinary: Ureteral spasms, spasm of vesical sphincters and urinary retention

Ocular: Blurred vision
Respiratory: Respiratory depression

Restrictions C-III

Drug Interactions

Cytochrome P450 Effect:

Hydrocodone: **Substrate** of CYP2D6 (major)
Chlorpheniramine: **Substrate** of CYP2D6 (minor), 3A4 (major); **Inhibits** CYP2D6 (weak)
Acetaminophen: **Substrate** (minor) of CYP1A2, 2A6, 2C8/9, 2D6, 2E1, 3A4;
Caffeine: **Substrate** of CYP1A2 (major), 2C8/9 (minor), 2D6 (minor), 2E1 (minor), 3A4 (minor); **Inhibits** CYP1A2 (weak), 3A4 (moderate)

Increased Effect/Toxicity: See individual agents.

Pharmacodynamics/Kinetics

See Chlorpheniramine, Phenylephrine, and Acetaminophen monographs.

Hydrocodone:

Onset of action: Narcotic analgesic: 10-20 minutes
Duration: 4-8 hours
Distribution: Crosses placenta
Metabolism: Hepatic; O-demethylation; N-demethylation and 6-ketosteroid reduction
Half-life elimination: 3.3-4.4 hours
Excretion: Urine

Pregnancy Risk Factor C

Hydrocodone, Phenylephrine, and Diphenhydramine

(hye droe KOE done, fen il EF rin, & dye fen HYE dra meen)

U.S. Brand Names Endal® HD

Generic Available No

Synonyms Diphenhydramine, Hydrocodone, and Phenylephrine; Hydrocodone Bitartrate, Phenylephrine Hydrochloride, and Diphenhydramine Hydrochloride; Phenylephrine, Diphenhydramine, and Hydrocodone

Pharmacologic Category Antihistamine/Decongestant/Antitussive; Antitussive; Decongestant; Histamine H_1 Antagonist

Use Symptomatic relief of cough and congestion associated with the common cold, sinusitis, or acute upper respiratory tract infections

Local Anesthetic/Vasoconstrictor Precautions Use with caution since phenylephrine is a sympathomimetic amine which could interact with epinephrine to cause a pressor response

Effects on Dental Treatment Key adverse event(s) related to dental treatment: Xerostomia (normal salivary flow resumes upon discontinuation).

Common Adverse Effects See individual agents.

Restrictions C-III

Mechanism of Action

Hydrocodone binds to opiate receptors in the CNS; suppresses cough in medullary center.

Phenylephrine is a potent, direct-acting alpha-adrenergic stimulator.

Diphenhydramine is an H_1-receptor antagonist.

Pharmacodynamics/Kinetics See individual agents.

Pregnancy Risk Factor C

Hydrocodone, Pseudoephedrine, and Guaifenesin

(hye droe KOE done, soo doe e FED rin & gwye FEN e sin)

Related Information

Guaifenesin *on page 672*
Pseudoephedrine *on page 1147*

U.S. Brand Names Duratuss® HD; Hydro-Tussin™ HD; Hydro-Tussin™ XP; Pancof®-XP; Su-Tuss®-HD; Tussend® Expectorant

Generic Available Yes

Synonyms Guaifenesin, Hydrocodone, and Pseudoephedrine; Pseudoephedrine, Hydrocodone, and Guaifenesin

Pharmacologic Category Antitussive/Decongestant/Expectorant

Use Symptomatic relief of irritating, nonproductive cough associated with respiratory conditions such as bronchitis, bronchial asthma, tracheobronchitis, and the common cold

Local Anesthetic/Vasoconstrictor Precautions Use with caution since pseudoephedrine is a sympathomimetic amine which could interact with epinephrine to cause a pressor response

Effects on Dental Treatment Key adverse event(s) related to dental treatment:

Guaifenesin: No significant effects or complications reported

(Continued)

Hydrocodone, Pseudoephedrine, and Guaifenesin *(Continued)*

Pseudoephedrine: Xerostomia (normal salivary flow resumes upon discontinuation).

Common Adverse Effects Frequency not defined.

Cardiovascular: Arrhythmias, tachycardia, hypertension

Central nervous system: Drowsiness, fear, anxiety, tenseness, restlessness, pallor, insomnia, hallucinations, CNS depression

Gastrointestinal: GI upset, nausea, constipation with prolonged use

Genitourinary: Dysuria

Hepatic: Slight elevation in serum transaminase levels

Neuromuscular & skeletal: Weakness, tremor

Respiratory: Respiratory difficulty

Patients hyper-reactive to pseudoephedrine may display ephedrine-like reactions such as tachycardia, palpitations, headache, dizziness, or nausea; patient idiosyncrasy to adrenergic agents may be manifested by insomnia, dizziness, weakness, tremor, or arrhythmias.

Restrictions C-III

Drug Interactions

Cytochrome P450 Effect: Hydrocodone: **Substrate** of CYP2D6 (major)

Pharmacodynamics/Kinetics

See Guaifenesin and Pseudoephedrine monographs.

Hydrocodone:

Onset of action: Narcotic analgesic: 10-20 minutes

Duration: 4-8 hours

Distribution: Crosses placenta

Metabolism: Hepatic; O-demethylation; N-demethylation and 6-ketosteroid reduction

Half-life elimination: 3.3-4.4 hours

Excretion: Urine

Pregnancy Risk Factor C

Hydrocortisone (hye droe KOR ti sone)

Related Information

Dental Office Emergencies *on page 1584*

U.S. Brand Names A-hydroCort®; Anucort-HC®; Anusol-HC®; Anusol® HC-1 [OTC]; Aquanil™ HC [OTC]; CaldeCORT® [OTC]; Cetacort®; Colocort™; CortaGel® Maximum Strength [OTC]; Cortaid® Intensive Therapy [OTC]; Cortaid® Maximum Strength [OTC]; Cortaid® Sensitive Skin With Aloe [OTC]; Cortef®; Corticool® [OTC]; Cortifoam®; Cortizone®-5 [OTC]; Cortizone®-10 Maximum Strength [OTC]; Cortizone®-10 Plus Maximum Strength [OTC]; Cortizone® 10 Quick Shot [OTC]; Cortizone® for Kids [OTC]; Dermarest Dricort® [OTC]; Dermtex® HC [OTC]; EarSol® HC; Hemril-HC®; Hydrocortone® [DSC]; Hydrocortone® Phosphate; Hytone®; LactiCare-HC®; Locoid®; Locoid Lipocream®; Nupercainal® Hydrocortisone Cream [OTC]; Nutracort®; Pandel®; Post Peel Healing Balm [OTC]; Preparation H® Hydrocortisone [OTC]; Proctocort®; ProctoCream® HC; Proctosol-HC®; Sarnol®-HC [OTC]; Solu-Cortef®; Summer's Eve® SpecialCare™ Medicated Anti-Itch Cream [OTC]; Texacort®; Theracort® [OTC]; Westcort®

Canadian Brand Names Aquacort®; Cortamed®; Cortate®; Cortef®; Cortenema®; Cortifoam™; Cortoderm; Emo-Cort®; Hycort™; Hyderm; HydroVal®; Locoid®; Prevex® HC; Sarna® HC; Solu-Cortef®; Westcort®

Mexican Brand Names Aquanil HC®; LactiCare-HC®; Nutracort®

Generic Available Yes

Synonyms Compound F; Cortisol; Hydrocortisone Acetate; Hydrocortisone Buteprate; Hydrocortisone Butyrate; Hydrocortisone Cypionate; Hydrocortisone Sodium Phosphate; Hydrocortisone Sodium Succinate; Hydrocortisone Valerate

Pharmacologic Category Corticosteroid, Rectal; Corticosteroid, Systemic; Corticosteroid, Topical

Dental Use Treatment of a variety of oral diseases of allergic, inflammatory, or autoimmune origin

Use Management of adrenocortical insufficiency; relief of inflammation of corticosteroid-responsive dermatoses (low and medium potency topical corticosteroid); adjunctive treatment of ulcerative colitis

Local Anesthetic/Vasoconstrictor Precautions No information available to require special precautions

Effects on Dental Treatment No significant effects or complications reported

Significant Adverse Effects

Systemic:

>10%:

Central nervous system: Insomnia, nervousness

Gastrointestinal: Increased appetite, indigestion

1% to 10%:

Dermatologic: Hirsutism

Endocrine & metabolic: Diabetes mellitus

Neuromuscular & skeletal: Arthralgia

Ocular: Cataracts

Respiratory: Epistaxis

<1% (Limited to important or life-threatening): Hypertension, edema, euphoria, headache, delirium, hallucinations, seizures, mood swings, acne, dermatitis, skin atrophy, bruising, hyperpigmentation, hypokalemia, hyperglycemia, Cushing's syndrome, sodium and water retention, bone growth suppression, amenorrhea, peptic ulcer, abdominal distention, ulcerative esophagitis, pancreatitis, muscle wasting, hypersensitivity reactions, immunosuppression

Topical:

>10%: Dermatologic: Eczema (12.5%)

1% to 10%: Dermatologic: Pruritus (6%), stinging (2%), dry skin (2%)

<1% (Limited to important or life-threatening): Allergic contact dermatitis, burning, dermal atrophy, folliculitis, HPA axis suppression, hypopigmentation; metabolic effects (hyperglycemia, hypokalemia); striae

Dosage Dose should be based on severity of disease and patient response

Acute adrenal insufficiency: I.M., I.V.:

Infants and young Children: Succinate: 1-2 mg/kg/dose bolus, then 25-150 mg/day in divided doses every 6-8 hours

Older Children: Succinate: 1-2 mg/kg bolus then 150-250 mg/day in divided doses every 6-8 hours

Adults: Succinate: 100 mg I.V. bolus, then 300 mg/day in divided doses every 8 hours or as a continuous infusion for 48 hours; once patient is stable change to oral, 50 mg every 8 hours for 6 doses, then taper to 30-50 mg/day in divided doses

Chronic adrenal corticoid insufficiency: Adults: Oral: 20-30 mg/day

Anti-inflammatory or immunosuppressive:

Infants and Children:

Oral: 2.5-10 mg/kg/day **or** 75-300 mg/m^2/day every 6-8 hours

I.M., I.V.: Succinate: 1-5 mg/kg/day **or** 30-150 mg/m^2/day divided every 12-24 hours

Adolescents and Adults: Oral, I.M., I.V.: Succinate: 15-240 mg every 12 hours

Congenital adrenal hyperplasia: Oral: Initial: 10-20 mg/m^2/day in 3 divided doses; a variety of dosing schedules have been used. **Note:** Inconsistencies have occurred with liquid formulations; tablets may provide more reliable levels. Doses must be individualized by monitoring growth, bone age, and hormonal levels. Mineralocorticoid and sodium supplementation may be required based upon electrolyte regulation and plasma renin activity.

Physiologic replacement: Children:

Oral: 0.5-0.75 mg/kg/day **or** 20-25 mg/m^2/day every 8 hours

I.M.: Succinate: 0.25-0.35 mg/kg/day **or** 12-15 mg/m^2/day once daily

Shock: I.M., I.V.: Succinate:

Children: Initial: 50 mg/kg, then repeated in 4 hours and/or every 24 hours as needed

Adolescents and Adults: 500 mg to 2 g every 2-6 hours

Status asthmaticus: Children and Adults: I.V.: Succinate: 1-2 mg/kg/dose every 6 hours for 24 hours, then maintenance of 0.5-1 mg/kg every 6 hours

Adults:

Rheumatic diseases:

Intralesional, intra-articular, soft tissue injection: Acetate:

Large joints: 25 mg (up to 37.5 mg)

Small joints: 10-25 mg

Tendon sheaths: 5-12.5 mg

Soft tissue infiltration: 25-50 mg (up to 75 mg)

Bursae: 25-37.5 mg

Ganglia: 12.5-25 mg

Stress dosing (surgery) in patients known to be adrenally-suppressed or on chronic systemic steroids: I.V.:

Minor stress (ie, inguinal herniorrhaphy): 25 mg/day for 1 day

Moderate stress (ie, joint replacement, cholecystectomy): 50-75 mg/day (25 mg every 8-12 hours) for 1-2 days

(Continued)

Hydrocortisone *(Continued)*

Major stress (pancreatoduodenectomy, esophagogastrectomy, cardiac surgery): 100-150 mg/day (50 mg every 8-12 hours) for 2-3 days

Dermatosis: Children >2 years and Adults: Topical: Apply to affected area 2-4 times/day (Buteprate: Apply once or twice daily). Therapy should be discontinued when control is achieved; if no improvement is seen, reassessment of diagnosis may be necessary.

Ulcerative colitis: Adults: Rectal: 10-100 mg 1-2 times/day for 2-3 weeks

Mechanism of Action Decreases inflammation by suppression of migration of polymorphonuclear leukocytes and reversal of increased capillary permeability

Contraindications Hypersensitivity to hydrocortisone or any component of the formulation; serious infections, except septic shock or tuberculous meningitis; viral, fungal, or tubercular skin lesions

Warnings/Precautions

Use with caution in patients with hyperthyroidism, cirrhosis, nonspecific ulcerative colitis, hypertension, osteoporosis, thromboembolic tendencies, CHF, convulsive disorders, myasthenia gravis, thrombophlebitis, peptic ulcer, diabetes, glaucoma, cataracts, or tuberculosis. Use caution in hepatic impairment.

May cause HPA axis suppression. Acute adrenal insufficiency may occur with abrupt withdrawal after long-term therapy or with stress; young pediatric patients may be more susceptible to adrenal axis suppression from topical therapy. Avoid use of topical preparations with occlusive dressings or on weeping or exudative lesions.

Because of the risk of adverse effects, systemic corticosteroids should be used cautiously in the elderly, in the smallest possible dose, and for the shortest possible time

Drug Interactions Substrate of CYP3A4 (minor); **Induces** CYP3A4 (weak)

Decreased effect:

- Insulin decreases hypoglycemic effect
- Phenytoin, phenobarbital, ephedrine, and rifampin increase metabolism of hydrocortisone and decrease steroid blood level

Increased toxicity:

- Oral anticoagulants change prothrombin time
- Potassium-depleting diuretics increase risk of hypokalemia
- Cardiac glucosides increase risk of arrhythmias or digitalis toxicity secondary to hypokalemia

Ethanol/Nutrition/Herb Interactions

Ethanol: Avoid ethanol (may enhance gastric mucosal irritation).

Food: Hydrocortisone interferes with calcium absorption.

Herb/Nutraceutical: St John's wort may decrease hydrocortisone levels. Avoid cat's claw, echinacea (have immunostimulant properties).

Dietary Considerations Systemic use of corticosteroids may require a diet with increased potassium, vitamins A, B_6, C, D, folate, calcium, zinc, phosphorus, and decreased sodium. Sodium content of 1 g (sodium succinate injection): 47.5 mg (2.07 mEq)

Pharmacodynamics/Kinetics

Onset of action:

- Hydrocortisone acetate: Slow
- Hydrocortisone sodium phosphate (water soluble): Rapid
- Hydrocortisone sodium succinate (water soluble): Rapid

Duration:

- Hydrocortisone acetate: Long
- Hydrocortisone sodium phosphate (water soluble): Short

Absorption: Rapid by all routes, except rectally

Metabolism: Hepatic

Half-life elimination: Biologic: 8-12 hours

Excretion: Urine (primarily as 17-hydroxysteroids and 17-ketosteroids)

Pregnancy Risk Factor C

Lactation Excretion in breast milk unknown/use caution

Breast-Feeding Considerations It is not known if hydrocortisone is excreted in breast milk, however, other corticosteroids are excreted. Prednisone and prednisolone are excreted in breast milk; the AAP considers them to be "usually compatible" with breast-feeding. Hypertension was reported in a nursing infant when a topical corticosteroid was applied to the nipples of the mother.

Dosage Forms [DSC] = Discontinued product

Aerosol, rectal, as acetate (Cortifoam®): 10% (15 g) [90 mg/applicator]

Aerosol, topical spray, as base

Cortizone® 10 Quick Shot: 1% (44 mL) [contains benzyl alcohol]

Dermtex® HC: 1% (52 mL) [contains menthol 1%]
Cream, rectal, as acetate (Nupercainal® Hydrocortisone Cream): 1% (30 g)
Cream, rectal, as base:
Cortizone®-10: 1% (30g) [contains aloe]
Preparation H® Hydrocortisone: 1% (27 g)
Cream, topical, as acetate: 0.5% (30 g) [available with aloe]; 1% (30 g) [available with aloe]
Cortaid® Maximum Strength: 1% (15 g, 30 g, 40 g)
Cortaid® Sensitive Skin With Aloe: 0.5% (15 g) [contains aloe vera gel]
Cream, topical, as base: 0.5% (30 g); 1% (1.5 g, 30 g, 454 g); 2.5% (20 g, 30 g, 454 g)
Anusol-HC®: 2.5% (30 g) [contains benzyl alcohol]
CaldeCORT®: 1% (15 g, 30 g)[contains aloe vera gel and benzyl alcohol]
Cortaid® Intensive Therapy: 1% (60 g)
Cortaid® Maximum Strength: 1% (15 g, 30 g, 40 g, 60 g) [contains aloe vera gel and benzyl alcohol]
Cortizone®-5: 0.5% (30 g, 60 g) [contains aloe]
Cortizone®-10 Maximum Strength: 1% (15 g, 30 g, 60 g) [contains aloe]
Cortizone®-10 Plus Maximum Strength: 1% (30 g, 60 g) [contains vitamins A, D, E and aloe]
Cortizone® for Kids: 0.5% (30 g) [contains aloe]
Dermarest® Dri-Cort: 1% (15 g, 30 g)
Hytone®: 2.5% (30 g, 60 g)
Post Peel Healing Balm: 1% (23 g)
ProctoCream® HC: 2.5% (30 g) [contains benzyl alcohol]
Proctocort®: 1% (30 g)
Proctosol-HC®: 2.5% (30 g)
Summer's Eve® SpecialCare™ Medicated Anti-Itch Cream: 1% (30 g)
Cream, topical, as butyrate (Locoid®, Locoid Lipocream®): 0.1% (15 g, 45 g)
Cream, topical, as probutate (Pandel®): 0.1% (15 g, 45 g, 80 g)
Cream, topical, as valerate (Westcort®): 0.2% (15 g, 45 g, 60 g)
Gel, topical, as base:
Corticool®: 1% (45 g)
Cortagel® Maximum Strength: 1% (15 g, 30 g) [contains aloe vera gel]
Injection, powder for reconstitution, as sodium succinate:
A-Hydrocort®: 100 mg, 250 mg [diluent contains benzyl alcohol]
Solu-Cortef®: 100 mg, 250 mg, 500 mg, 1 g [diluent contains benzyl alcohol]
Injection, solution, as sodium phosphate (Hydrocortone® Phosphate): 50 mg/mL (2 mL) [contains sodium bisulfite]
Lotion, topical, as base: 1% (120 mL); 2.5% (60 mL)
Aquanil™ HC: 1% (120 mL)
Cetacort®, Sarnol®-HC: 1% (60 mL)
Hytone®: 1% (30 mL, 120 mL); 2.5% (60 mL)
LactiCare-HC®: 1% (120 mL); 2.5% (60 mL, 120 mL)
Nutracort®: 1% (60 mL, 120 mL); 2.5% (60 mL, 120 mL)
Theracort®: 1% (120 mL)
Ointment, topical, as acetate: 1% (30 g) [available with aloe]
Anusol® HC-1: 1% (21 g)
Cortaid® Maximum Strength: 1% (15 g, 30 g)
Ointment, topical, as base: 0.5% (30 g); 1% (30 g, 454 g); 2.5% (20 g, 30 g, 454 g)
Cortizone®-5: 0.5% (30 g) [contains aloe]
Cortizone®-10 Maximum Strength: 1% (30 g, 60 g)
Hytone®: 2.5% (30 g)
Ointment, topical, as base [in Orabase®]: 1% (25 g, 110 g, 454 g)
Ointment, topical, as butyrate (Locoid®): 0.1% (15 g, 45 g)
Ointment, topical, as valerate (Westcort®): 0.2% (15 g, 45 g, 60 g)
Solution, otic, as base (EarSol® HC): 1% (30 mL) [contains alcohol 44%, benzyl benzoate, yerba santa]
Solution, rectal, as base (Colocort™): 100 mg/60 mL (7s) [packaged as single-dose enemas]
Solution, topical, as base (Texacort®): 1% (30 mL) [DSC]; 2.5% (30 mL) [contains alcohol]
Solution, topical, as butyrate (Locoid®): 0.1% (20 mL, 60 mL) [contains alcohol 50%]
Suppository, rectal, as acetate: 25 mg (12s, 24s)
Anucort™ HC: 25 mg (12s, 24s, 100s)
Anusol-HC®: 25 mg (12s, 24s)
Hemril® HC: 25 mg (12s)
Proctocort®: 30 mg (12s, 24s)
Proctosol-HC®: 25 mg (12s, 24s)
(Continued)

Hydrocortisone *(Continued)*

Suspension, oral, as cypionate (Cortef®): 10 mg/5 mL (120 mL) [contains benzoic acid] [DSC]
Tablet, as base: 20 mg
Cortef®: 5 mg, 10 mg, 20 mg
Hydrocortone®: 10 mg [DSC]

Hydrocortisone Acetate *see* Hydrocortisone *on page 714*
Hydrocortisone, Acetic Acid, and Propylene Glycol Diacetate *see* Acetic Acid, Propylene Glycol Diacetate, and Hydrocortisone *on page 60*
Hydrocortisone and Benzoyl Peroxide *see* Benzoyl Peroxide and Hydrocortisone *on page 194*
Hydrocortisone and Ciprofloxacin *see* Ciprofloxacin and Hydrocortisone *on page 336*
Hydrocortisone and Iodoquinol *see* Iodoquinol and Hydrocortisone *on page 759*
Hydrocortisone and Lidocaine *see* Lidocaine and Hydrocortisone *on page 826*
Hydrocortisone and Oxytetracycline *see* Oxytetracycline and Hydrocortisone *on page 1037*
Hydrocortisone and Pramoxine *see* Pramoxine and Hydrocortisone *on page 1109*
Hydrocortisone and Urea *see* Urea and Hydrocortisone *on page 1353*
Hydrocortisone, Bacitracin, Neomycin, and Polymyxin B *see* Bacitracin, Neomycin, Polymyxin B, and Hydrocortisone *on page 179*
Hydrocortisone Buteprate *see* Hydrocortisone *on page 714*
Hydrocortisone Butyrate *see* Hydrocortisone *on page 714*
Hydrocortisone Cypionate *see* Hydrocortisone *on page 714*
Hydrocortisone, Neomycin, and Polymyxin B *see* Neomycin, Polymyxin B, and Hydrocortisone *on page 975*
Hydrocortisone, Propylene Glycol Diacetate, and Acetic Acid *see* Acetic Acid, Propylene Glycol Diacetate, and Hydrocortisone *on page 60*
Hydrocortisone Sodium Phosphate *see* Hydrocortisone *on page 714*
Hydrocortisone Sodium Succinate *see* Hydrocortisone *on page 714*
Hydrocortisone Valerate *see* Hydrocortisone *on page 714*
Hydrocortone® [DSC] *see* Hydrocortisone *on page 714*
Hydrocortone® Phosphate *see* Hydrocortisone *on page 714*
Hydromet® *see* Hydrocodone and Homatropine *on page 709*

Hydromorphone (hye droe MOR fone)

Related Information

Oxymorphone *on page 1036*

U.S. Brand Names Dilaudid®; Dilaudid-HP®

Canadian Brand Names Dilaudid®; Dilaudid-HP®; Dilaudid-HP-Plus®; Dilaudid® Sterile Powder; Dilaudid-XP®; Hydromorph Contin®; Hydromorphone HP; PMS-Hydromorphone

Generic Available Yes

Synonyms Dihydromorphinone; Hydromorphone Hydrochloride

Pharmacologic Category Analgesic, Narcotic

Use Management of moderate to severe pain; antitussive at lower doses

Local Anesthetic/Vasoconstrictor Precautions No information available to require special precautions

Effects on Dental Treatment Key adverse event(s) related to dental treatment: Xerostomia (normal salivary flow resumes upon discontinuation).

Common Adverse Effects Frequency not defined.

Cardiovascular: Palpitations, hypotension, peripheral vasodilation, tachycardia, bradycardia, flushing of face
Central nervous system: CNS depression, increased intracranial pressure, fatigue, headache, nervousness, restlessness, dizziness, lightheadedness, drowsiness, hallucinations, mental depression, seizures
Dermatologic: Pruritus, rash, urticaria
Endocrine & metabolic: Antidiuretic hormone release
Gastrointestinal: Nausea, vomiting, constipation, stomach cramps, xerostomia, anorexia, biliary tract spasm, paralytic ileus
Genitourinary: Decreased urination, ureteral spasm, urinary tract spasm
Hepatic: LFTs increased, AST increased, ALT increased
Local: Pain at injection site (I.M.)
Neuromuscular & skeletal: Trembling, weakness, myoclonus
Ocular: Miosis

Respiratory: Respiratory depression, dyspnea

Miscellaneous: Histamine release, physical and psychological dependence

Restrictions C-II

Mechanism of Action Binds to opiate receptors in the CNS, causing inhibition of ascending pain pathways, altering the perception of and response to pain; causes cough supression by direct central action in the medulla; produces generalized CNS depression

Drug Interactions

Increased Effect/Toxicity: CNS depressants, phenothiazines, and tricyclic antidepressants may potentiate the adverse effects of hydromorphone.

Pharmacodynamics/Kinetics

Onset of action: Analgesic: Oral: 15-30 minutes

Peak effect: Oral: 30-60 minutes

Duration: 4-5 hours

Absorption: I.M.: Variable and delayed

Metabolism: Hepatic; no active metabolites

Bioavailability: 62%

Half-life elimination: 1-3 hours

Excretion: Urine (primarily as glucuronide conjugates)

Pregnancy Risk Factor B/D (prolonged use or high doses at term)

Hydromorphone Hydrochloride *see* Hydromorphone *on page 718*

Hydropane® *see* Hydrocodone and Homatropine *on page 709*

Hydroquinol *see* Hydroquinone *on page 719*

Hydroquinone (HYE droe kwin one)

U.S. Brand Names Alphaquin HP; Alustra™; Claripel™; Eldopaque® [OTC]; Eldopaque Forte®; Eldoquin® [OTC]; Eldoquin Forte®; EpiQuin™ Micro; Esoterica® Regular [OTC]; Glyquin®; Lustra®; Lustra-AF™; Melanex®; Melpaque HP®; Melquin-3®; Melquin HP®; NeoStrata AHA [OTC]; Nuquin HP®; Palmer's® Skin Success Fade Cream™ [OTC]; Solaquin® [OTC]; Solaquin Forte®

Canadian Brand Names Eldopaque™; Eldoquin™; Glyquin® XM; Lustra®; NeoStrata® HQ; Solaquin™; Solaquin Forte™; Ultraquin™

Mexican Brand Names Crema Blanca®; Eldopaque®; Eldoquin®; Hidroquin®

Generic Available Yes: 4% cream

Synonyms Hydroquinol; Quinol

Pharmacologic Category Depigmenting Agent

Use Gradual bleaching of hyperpigmented skin conditions

Local Anesthetic/Vasoconstrictor Precautions No information available to require special precautions

Effects on Dental Treatment No significant effects or complications reported

Common Adverse Effects Frequency not defined.

Dermatologic: Dermatitis, dryness, erythema, stinging, inflammatory reaction, sensitization

Local: Irritation

Mechanism of Action Produces reversible depigmentation of the skin by suppression of melanocyte metabolic processes, in particular the inhibition of the enzymatic oxidation of tyrosine to DOPA (3,4-dihydroxyphenylalanine); sun exposure reverses this effect and will cause repigmentation.

Pharmacodynamics/Kinetics Onset and duration of depigmentation produced by hydroquinone varies among individuals

Pregnancy Risk Factor C

Hydroquinone, Fluocinolone Acetonide, and Tretinoin *see* Fluocinolone, Hydroquinone, and Tretinoin *on page 601*

Hydro-Tussin™-CBX *see* Carbinoxamine and Pseudoephedrine *on page 262*

Hydro-Tussin™ DHC *see* Pseudoephedrine, Dihydrocodeine, and Chlorpheniramine *on page 1150*

Hydro-Tussin™ DM *see* Guaifenesin and Dextromethorphan *on page 673*

Hydro-Tussin™ HD *see* Hydrocodone, Pseudoephedrine, and Guaifenesin *on page 713*

Hydro-Tussin™ XP *see* Hydrocodone, Pseudoephedrine, and Guaifenesin *on page 713*

Hydroxocobalamin (hye droks oh koe BAL a min)

Mexican Brand Names Axofor®; Duradoce®

Generic Available Yes

Synonyms Vitamin B_{12}

Pharmacologic Category Vitamin, Water Soluble

(Continued)

Hydroxocobalamin *(Continued)*

Use Treatment of pernicious anemia, vitamin B_{12} deficiency, increased B_{12} requirements due to pregnancy, thyrotoxicosis, hemorrhage, malignancy, liver or kidney disease

Unlabeled/Investigational Use Neuropathies, multiple sclerosis

Local Anesthetic/Vasoconstrictor Precautions No information available to require special precautions

Effects on Dental Treatment No significant effects or complications reported

Common Adverse Effects Frequency not defined.

Cardiovascular: Peripheral vascular thrombosis
Dermatologic: Itching, urticaria
Gastrointestinal: Diarrhea
Miscellaneous: Hypersensitivity reactions

Mechanism of Action Coenzyme for various metabolic functions, including fat and carbohydrate metabolism and protein synthesis, used in cell replication and hematopoiesis

Pregnancy Risk Factor A/C (dose exceeding RDA recommendation)

Hydroxyamphetamine and Tropicamide

(hye droks ee am FET a meen & troe PIK a mide)

U.S. Brand Names Paremyd®

Generic Available No

Synonyms Hydroxyamphetamine Hydrobromide and Tropicamide; Tropicamide and Hydroxyamphetamine

Pharmacologic Category Adrenergic Agonist Agent, Ophthalmic

Use Short-term pupil dilation for diagnostic procedures and exams

Local Anesthetic/Vasoconstrictor Precautions No information available to require special precautions

Effects on Dental Treatment No significant effects or complications reported

Mechanism of Action Hydroxyamphetamine hydrobromide is an indirect acting sympathomimetic agent which causes the release of norepinephrine from adrenergic nerve terminals, resulting in mydriasis. Tropicamide is a parasympatholytic agent which produces mydriasis and paralysis by blocking the sphincter muscle in the iris and the ciliary muscle.

Pregnancy Risk Factor C

Hydroxyamphetamine Hydrobromide and Tropicamide *see* Hydroxyamphetamine and Tropicamide *on page 720*

4-Hydroxybutyrate *see* Sodium Oxybate *on page 1229*

Hydroxycarbamide *see* Hydroxyurea *on page 722*

Hydroxychloroquine (hye droks ee KLOR oh kwin)

Related Information

Rheumatoid Arthritis, Osteoarthritis, and Osteoporosis *on page 1490*

U.S. Brand Names Plaquenil®

Canadian Brand Names Apo-Hydroxyquine®; Plaquenil®

Generic Available Yes

Synonyms Hydroxychloroquine Sulfate

Pharmacologic Category Aminoquinoline (Antimalarial)

Use Suppression and treatment of acute attacks of malaria; treatment of systemic lupus erythematosus and rheumatoid arthritis

Unlabeled/Investigational Use Porphyria cutanea tarda, polymorphous light eruptions

Local Anesthetic/Vasoconstrictor Precautions No information available to require special precautions

Effects on Dental Treatment No significant effects or complications reported

Common Adverse Effects Frequency not defined.

Cardiovascular: Cardiomyopathy (rare, relationship to hydroxychloroquine unclear)
Central nervous system: Irritability, nervousness, emotional changes, nightmares, psychosis, headache, dizziness, vertigo, seizures, ataxia, lassitude
Dermatologic: Bleaching of hair, alopecia, pigmentation changes (skin and mucosal; black-blue color), rash (urticarial, morbilliform, lichenoid, maculopapular, purpuric, erythema annulare centrifugum, Stevens-Johnson syndrome, acute generalized exanthematous pustulosis, and exfoliative dermatitis)
Endocrine & metabolic: Weight loss
Gastrointestinal: Anorexia, nausea, vomiting, diarrhea, abdominal cramping
Hematologic: Aplastic anemia, agranulocytosis, leukopenia, thrombocytopenia, hemolysis (in patients with glucose-6-phosphate deficiency)

Hepatic: Abnormal liver function/hepatic failure (isolated cases)

Neuromuscular & skeletal: Myopathy, palsy, or neuromyopathy leading to progressive weakness and atrophy of proximal muscle groups (may be associated with mild sensory changes, loss of deep tendon reflexes, and abnormal nerve conduction)

Ocular: Disturbance in accommodation, keratopathy, corneal changes/deposits (visual disturbances, blurred vision, photophobia - reversible on discontinuation), macular edema, atrophy, abnormal pigmentation, retinopathy (early changes reversible - may progress despite discontinuation if advanced), optic disc pallor/atrophy, attenuation of retinal arterioles, pigmentary retinopathy, scotoma, decreased visual acuity, nystagmus

Otic: Tinnitus, deafness

Miscellaneous: Exacerbation of porphyria and nonlight sensitive psoriasis

Mechanism of Action Interferes with digestive vacuole function within sensitive malarial parasites by increasing the pH and interfering with lysosomal degradation of hemoglobin; inhibits locomotion of neutrophils and chemotaxis of eosinophils; impairs complement-dependent antigen-antibody reactions

Drug Interactions

Increased Effect/Toxicity: Cimetidine increases levels of chloroquine and probably other 4-aminoquinolones.

Decreased Effect: Chloroquine and other 4-aminoquinolones absorption may be decreased due to GI binding with kaolin or magnesium trisilicate.

Pharmacodynamics/Kinetics

Onset of action: Rheumatic disease: May require 4-6 weeks to respond

Absorption: Complete

Protein binding: 55%

Metabolism: Hepatic

Half-life elimination: 32-50 days

Time to peak: Rheumatic disease: Several months

Excretion: Urine (as metabolites and unchanged drug); may be enhanced by urinary acidification

Pregnancy Risk Factor C

Hydroxychloroquine Sulfate *see* Hydroxychloroquine *on page 720*

25-Hydroxycholecalciferol *see* Calcifediol *on page 242*

Hydroxydaunomycin Hydrochloride *see* DOXOrubicin *on page 469*

1α-Hydroxyergocalciferol *see* Doxercalciferol *on page 468*

Hydroxyethylcellulose *see* Artificial Tears *on page 148*

Hydroxyethyl Starch *see* Hetastarch *on page 692*

Hydroxyldaunorubicin Hydrochloride *see* DOXOrubicin *on page 469*

Hydroxypropyl Cellulose (hye droks ee PROE pil SEL yoo lose)

Related Information

Hydroxypropyl Methylcellulose *on page 721*

U.S. Brand Names Lacrisert®

Canadian Brand Names Lacrisert®

Generic Available No

Pharmacologic Category Ophthalmic Agent, Miscellaneous

Use Dry eyes (moderate to severe)

Local Anesthetic/Vasoconstrictor Precautions No information available to require special precautions

Effects on Dental Treatment No significant effects or complications reported

Hydroxypropyl Methylcellulose

(hye droks ee PROE pil meth il SEL yoo lose)

Related Information

Hydroxypropyl Cellulose *on page 721*

U.S. Brand Names GenTeal® [OTC]; GenTeal® Mild [OTC]; Gonak™ [OTC]; Goniosol® [OTC]; Isopto® Tears [OTC]; Tearisol® [OTC]

Canadian Brand Names Genteal®; Isopto® Tears

Mexican Brand Names Celulose Grin®; Meticel Ofteno®

Generic Available No

Synonyms Gonioscopic Ophthalmic Solution; Hypromellose

Pharmacologic Category Diagnostic Agent, Ophthalmic; Lubricant, Ocular

Use Relief of burning and minor irritation due to dry eyes; diagnostic agent in gonioscopic examination

Local Anesthetic/Vasoconstrictor Precautions No information available to require special precautions

Effects on Dental Treatment No significant effects or complications reported

Pregnancy Risk Factor C

Hydroxyurea (hye droks ee yoor EE a)

U.S. Brand Names Droxia™; Hydrea®; Mylocel™

Canadian Brand Names Gen-Hydroxyurea; Hydrea®

Mexican Brand Names Hydrea®

Generic Available Yes: Capsule

Synonyms Hydroxycarbamide

Pharmacologic Category Antineoplastic Agent, Antimetabolite

Use CML in chronic phase; radiosensitizing agent in the treatment of primary brain tumors, head and neck tumors, uterine cervix and nonsmall cell lung cancer, and psoriasis; treatment of hematologic conditions such as essential thrombocythemia, polycythemia vera, hypereosinophilia, and hyperleukocytosis due to acute leukemia. Has shown activity against renal cell cancer, melanoma, ovarian cancer, head and neck cancer (excluding lip cancer), and prostate cancer.

Orphan drug: Droxia™: Sickle cell anemia: Specifically for patients >18 years of age who have had at least three "painful crises" in the previous year - to reduce frequency of these crises and the need for blood transfusions

Unlabeled/Investigational Use Treatment of HIV; treatment of psoriasis

Local Anesthetic/Vasoconstrictor Precautions No information available to require special precautions

Effects on Dental Treatment No significant effects or complications reported

Common Adverse Effects Frequency not defined.

Cardiovascular: Edema

Central nervous system: Drowsiness (with high doses), hallucinations, headache, dizziness, disorientation, seizures, fever, chills

Dermatologic: Erythema of the hands and face, maculopapular rash, pruritus, dry skin, dermatomyositis-like skin changes, hyperpigmentation, atrophy of skin and nails, scaling and violet papules (long-term use), nail banding, skin cancer

Endocrine & metabolic: Hyperuricemia

Gastrointestinal: Nausea, vomiting, stomatitis, anorexia, diarrhea, constipation, mucositis (potentiated in patients receiving radiation), pancreatitis, ulceration of buccal mucosa and GI epithelium (severe intoxication)

Emetic potential: Low (10% to 30%)

Genitourinary: Dysuria

Hematologic: Myelosuppression (primarily leukopenia); Dose-limiting toxicity, causes a rapid drop in leukocyte count (seen in 4-5 days in nonhematologic malignancy and more rapidly in leukemia); thrombocytopenia and anemia occur less often

Onset: 24-48 hours

Nadir: 10 days

Recovery: 7 days after stopping drug (reversal of WBC count occurs rapidly but the platelet count may take 7-10 days to recover)

Other hematologic effects include megaloblastic erythropoiesis, macrocytosis, hemolysis, decreased serum iron, persistent cytopenias, secondary leukemias (long-term use)

Hepatic: Elevation of hepatic enzymes, hepatotoxicity, hyperbilirubinemia (polycythemia vera)

Neuromuscular & skeletal: Weakness, peripheral neuropathy

Renal: Increased creatinine and BUN due to impairment of renal tubular function

Respiratory: Acute diffuse pulmonary infiltrates (rare), dyspnea, pulmonary fibrosis

Mechanism of Action Thought to interfere (unsubstantiated hypothesis) with synthesis of DNA, during the S phase of cell division, without interfering with RNA synthesis; inhibits ribonucleoside diphosphate reductase, preventing conversion of ribonucleotides to deoxyribonucleotides; cell-cycle specific for the S phase and may hold other cells in the G_1 phase of the cell cycle.

Drug Interactions

Increased Effect/Toxicity: Zidovudine, zalcitabine, didanosine may increase synergy. The potential for neurotoxicity may increase with concomitant administration with fluorouracil. Hydroxyurea modulates the metabolism and cytotoxicity of cytarabine; dose reduction is recommended. Hydroxyurea may precipitate didanosine- or stavudine-induced pancreatitis, hepatotoxicity, or neuropathy; concomitant use is not recommended.

Pharmacodynamics/Kinetics

Absorption: Readily (≥80%)

Distribution: Readily crosses blood-brain barrier; well into intestine, brain, lung, kidney tissues, effusions and ascites; enters breast milk

Metabolism: Hepatic and via GI tract; 50% degradation by enzymes of intestinal bacteria
Half-life elimination: 3-4 hours
Time to peak: ~2 hours
Excretion: Urine (80%, 50% as unchanged drug, 30% as urea); exhaled gases (as CO_2)

Pregnancy Risk Factor D

25-Hydroxyvitamin D₃ *see* Calcifediol *on page 242*

HydrOXYzine (hye DROKS i zeen)

Related Information

Patients Requiring Sedation *on page 1567*

U.S. Brand Names Atarax®; Vistaril®

Canadian Brand Names Apo-Hydroxyzine®; Atarax™; Novo-Hydroxyzin; PMS-Hydroxyzine; Vistaril®

Generic Available Yes

Synonyms Hydroxyzine Hydrochloride; Hydroxyzine Pamoate

Pharmacologic Category Antiemetic; Antihistamine

Dental Use Treatment of anxiety, as a preoperative sedative in pediatric dentistry

Use Treatment of anxiety; preoperative sedative; antipruritic

Unlabeled/Investigational Use Antiemetic; ethanol withdrawal symptoms

Local Anesthetic/Vasoconstrictor Precautions No information available to require special precautions

Effects on Dental Treatment Key adverse event(s) related to dental treatment: Xerostomia (normal salivary flow resumes upon discontinuation).

Significant Adverse Effects Frequency not defined.

Central nervous system: Drowsiness, headache, fatigue, nervousness, dizziness
Gastrointestinal: Xerostomia
Neuromuscular & skeletal: Tremor, paresthesia, seizure
Ocular: Blurred vision
Respiratory: Thickening of bronchial secretions

Dosage

Children:
- Oral: 0.6 mg/kg/dose every 6 hours
- I.M.: 0.5-1.1 mg/kg/dose every 4-6 hours as needed

Adults:
- Antiemetic: I.M.: 25-100 mg/dose every 4-6 hours as needed
- Anxiety: Oral: 25-100 mg 4 times/day; maximum dose: 600 mg/day
- Preoperative sedation:
  - Oral: 50-100 mg
  - I.M.: 25-100 mg
- Management of pruritus: Oral: 25 mg 3-4 times/day

Dosing interval in hepatic impairment: Change dosing interval to every 24 hours in patients with primary biliary cirrhosis

Mechanism of Action Competes with histamine for H_1-receptor sites on effector cells in the gastrointestinal tract, blood vessels, and respiratory tract. Possesses skeletal muscle relaxing, bronchodilator, antihistamine, antiemetic, and analgesic properties.

Contraindications Hypersensitivity to hydroxyzine or any component of the formulation

Warnings/Precautions Causes sedation, caution must be used in performing tasks which require alertness (eg, operating machinery or driving). Sedative effects of CNS depressants or ethanol are potentiated. SubQ, intra-arterial, and I.V. administration are not recommended since thrombosis and digital gangrene can occur; extravasation can result in sterile abscess and marked tissue induration; should be used with caution in patients with narrow-angle glaucoma, prostatic hyperplasia, and bladder neck obstruction; should also be used with caution in patients with asthma or COPD.

Anticholinergic effects are not well tolerated in the elderly. Hydroxyzine may be useful as a short-term antipruritic, but it is not recommended for use as a sedative or anxiolytic in the elderly.

Drug Interactions Inhibits CYP2D6 (weak)

Amantadine, rimantadine: Central and/or peripheral anticholinergic syndrome can occur when administered with amantadine or rimantadine

Anticholinergic agents: Central and/or peripheral anticholinergic syndrome can occur when administered with narcotic analgesics, phenothiazines and other antipsychotics (especially with high anticholinergic activity), tricyclic antidepressants, quinidine and some other antiarrhythmics, and antihistamines

(Continued)

HydrOXYzine *(Continued)*

Antipsychotics: Hydroxyzine may antagonize the therapeutic effects of antipsychotics

CNS depressants: Sedative effects of hydroxyzine may be additive with CNS depressants; includes ethanol, benzodiazepines, barbiturates, narcotic analgesics, and other sedative agents; monitor for increased effect

Ethanol/Nutrition/Herb Interactions

Ethanol: Avoid ethanol (may increase CNS depression).

Herb/Nutraceutical: Avoid valerian, St John's wort, kava kava, gotu kola (may increase CNS depression).

Pharmacodynamics/Kinetics

Onset of action: 15-30 minutes

Duration: 4-6 hours

Absorption: Oral: Rapid

Metabolism: Exact fate unknown

Half-life elimination: 3-7 hours

Time to peak: ~2 hours

Pregnancy Risk Factor C

Lactation Enters breast milk/contraindicated

Dosage Forms [DSC] = Discontinued product

Capsule, as pamoate (Vistaril®): 25 mg, 50 mg, 100 mg

Injection, solution, as hydrochloride: 25 mg/mL (1 mL); 50 mg/mL (1 mL, 2 mL, 10 mL)

Vistaril® [DSC]: 50 mg/mL (10 mL) [contains benzyl alcohol]

Suspension, oral, as pamoate (Vistaril®): 25 mg/5 mL (120 mL, 480 mL) [lemon flavor]

Syrup, as hydrochloride: 10 mg/5 mL (120 mL, 480 mL)

Atarax®: 10 mg/5 mL (480 mL) [contains alcohol, sodium benzoate; mint flavor]

Tablet, as hydrochloride: 10 mg, 25 mg, 50 mg

Atarax®: 10 mg, 25 mg, 50 mg, 100 mg

Hydroxyzine Hydrochloride *see* HydrOXYzine *on page 723*

Hydroxyzine Pamoate *see* HydrOXYzine *on page 723*

Hygroton *see* Chlorthalidone *on page 321*

Hylaform® *see* Hyaluronate and Derivatives *on page 696*

Hylan Polymers *see* Hyaluronate and Derivatives *on page 696*

Hylorel® *see* Guanadrel *on page 678*

Hyoscine *see* Scopolamine *on page 1210*

Hyoscyamine (hye oh SYE a meen)

U.S. Brand Names Anaspaz®; Cystospaz®; Cystospaz-M®; Hyosine; Levbid®; Levsin®; Levsinex®; Levsin/SL®; NuLev™; Spacol; Spacol T/S; Symax SL; Symax SR

Canadian Brand Names Cystospaz®; Levsin®

Generic Available Yes

Synonyms Hyoscyamine Sulfate; *l*-Hyoscyamine Sulfate

Pharmacologic Category Anticholinergic Agent

Use

Oral: Adjunctive therapy for peptic ulcers, irritable bowel, neurogenic bladder/bowel; treatment of infant colic, GI tract disorders caused by spasm; to reduce rigidity, tremors, sialorrhea, and hyperhidrosis associated with parkinsonism; as a drying agent in acute rhinitis

Injection: Preoperative antimuscarinic to reduce secretions and block cardiac vagal inhibitory reflexes; to improve radiologic visibility of the kidneys; symptomatic relief of biliary and renal colic; reduce GI motility to facilitate diagnostic procedures (ie, endoscopy, hypotonic duodenography); reduce pain and hypersecretion in pancreatitis, certain cases of partial heart block associated with vagal activity; reversal of neuromuscular blockade

Local Anesthetic/Vasoconstrictor Precautions No information available to require special precautions

Effects on Dental Treatment Key adverse event(s) related to dental treatment: Xerostomia (normal salivary flow resumes upon discontinuation).

Mechanism of Action Blocks the action of acetylcholine at parasympathetic sites in smooth muscle, secretory glands and the CNS; increases cardiac output, dries secretions, antagonizes histamine and serotonin

Pregnancy Risk Factor C

Hyoscyamine, Atropine, Scopolamine, and Phenobarbital

(hye oh SYE a meen, A troe peen, skoe POL a meen, & fee noe BAR bi tal)

Related Information

Atropine *on page 166*
Hyoscyamine *on page 724*
Phenobarbital *on page 1073*
Scopolamine *on page 1210*

U.S. Brand Names Donnatal®; Donnatal Extentabs®

Canadian Brand Names Donnatal®

Generic Available No

Synonyms Atropine, Hyoscyamine, Scopolamine, and Phenobarbital; Phenobarbital, Hyoscyamine, Atropine, and Scopolamine; Scopolamine, Hyoscyamine, Atropine, and Phenobarbital

Pharmacologic Category Anticholinergic Agent; Antispasmodic Agent, Gastrointestinal

Use Adjunct in treatment of irritable bowel syndrome, acute enterocolitis, duodenal ulcer

Local Anesthetic/Vasoconstrictor Precautions No information available to require special precautions

Effects on Dental Treatment Key adverse event(s) related to dental treatment: Xerostomia, dry throat (normal salivary flow resumes upon discontinuation).

Common Adverse Effects Frequency not defined.

Cardiovascular: Palpitation, tachycardia

Central nervous system: Dizziness, drowsiness, headache, insomnia, nervousness

Dermatologic: Urticaria

Gastrointestinal: Bloating, constipation, nausea, taste loss, vomiting, xerostomia

Genitourinary: Impotence, urinary hesitancy, urinary retention

Neuromuscular & skeletal: Musculoskeletal pain, weakness

Ocular: Blurred vision, cycloplegia, mydriasis, ocular tension increased

Miscellaneous: Allergic reaction (may be severe), anaphylaxis, lactation suppressed, diaphoresis decreased

Mechanism of Action A fixed combination of belladonna alkaloids and phenobarbital which provides anticholinergic/antispasmodic action and mild sedation.

Drug Interactions

Cytochrome P450 Effect: Phenobarbital: **Substrate** (minor) of CYP2C8/9, 2C19, 2E1; **Induces** CYP1A2 (strong), 2A6 (strong), 2B6 (strong), 2C8/9 (strong), 3A4 (strong)

Increased Effect/Toxicity: Anticholinergic effects may be additive with other anticholinergic agents, or drugs with significant anticholinergic activity (antihistamine, tricyclic antidepressants, phenothiazines). When combined with other CNS depressants, ethanol, narcotic analgesics, antidepressants, or benzodiazepines, additive respiratory and CNS depression may occur. Barbiturates may enhance the hepatotoxic potential of acetaminophen overdoses. Chloramphenicol, MAO inhibitors, valproic acid, and felbamate may inhibit barbiturate metabolism. Barbiturates may impair the absorption of griseofulvin, and may enhance the nephrotoxic effects of methoxyflurane. Concurrent use of phenobarbital with meperidine may result in increased CNS depression. Concurrent use of phenobarbital with primidone may result in elevated phenobarbital serum concentrations. The levels/effects of phenobarbital may be increased by delavirdine, fluconazole, fluvoxamine, gemfibrozil, isoniazid, omeprazole, ticlopidine, and other CYP2C19 inhibitors.

Decreased Effect: Barbiturates may increase the metabolism of estrogens and reduce the efficacy of oral contraceptives; an alternative method of contraception should be considered. Barbiturates inhibit the hypoprothrombinemic effects of oral anticoagulants via increased metabolism. Barbiturates may enhance the metabolism of methadone resulting in methadone withdrawal. The levels/effects of phenobarbital may be decreased by aminoglutethimide, carbamazepine, phenytoin, rifampin, and other CYP2C19 inducers.

Phenobarbital may decrease the levels/effects of aminophylline, amiodarone, benzodiazepines, bupropion, calcium channel blockers, carbamazepine, citalopram, clarithromycin, cyclosporine diazepam, efavirenz, erythromycin, estrogens, fluoxetine, fluvoxamine, glimepiride, glipizide, ifosfamide, losartan, methsuximide, mirtazapine, nateglinide, nefazodone, nevirapine, phenytoin, pioglitazone, promethazine, propranolol, protease

(Continued)

Hyoscyamine, Atropine, Scopolamine, and Phenobarbital *(Continued)*

inhibitors, proton pump inhibitors, rifampin, ropinirole, rosiglitazone, selegiline, sertraline, sulfonamides, tacrolimus, theophylline, venlafaxine. voriconazole warfarin, zafirlukast, and other CYP1A2, 2A6, 2B6, 2C8/9, or 3A4 substrates.

Pregnancy Risk Factor C

Hyoscyamine, Atropine, Scopolamine, Kaolin, and Pectin

(hye oh SYE a meen, A troe peen, skoe POL a meen, KAY oh lin, & PEK tin)

Related Information

Atropine *on page 166*
Hyoscyamine *on page 724*
Kaolin and Pectin *on page 781*
Scopolamine *on page 1210*

Generic Available Yes

Synonyms Atropine, Hyoscyamine, Scopolamine, Kaolin, and Pectin; Kaolin, Hyoscyamine, Atropine, Scopolamine, and Pectin; Pectin, Hyoscyamine, Atropine, Scopolamine, and Kaolin; Scopolamine, Hyoscyamine, Atropine, Kaolin, and Pectin

Pharmacologic Category Anticholinergic Agent; Antidiarrheal

Use Antidiarrheal; also used in gastritis, enteritis, colitis, and acute gastrointestinal upsets, and nausea which may accompany any of these conditions

Local Anesthetic/Vasoconstrictor Precautions No information available to require special precautions

Effects on Dental Treatment Key adverse event(s) related to dental treatment: Xerostomia (normal salivary flow resumes upon discontinuation).

Pregnancy Risk Factor C

Hyoscyamine, Atropine, Scopolamine, Kaolin, Pectin, and Opium

(hye oh SYE a meen, A troe peen, skoe POL a meen, KAY oh lin, PEK tin, & OH pee um)

Related Information

Atropine *on page 166*
Hyoscyamine *on page 724*
Kaolin and Pectin *on page 781*
Opium Tincture *on page 1015*
Scopolamine *on page 1210*

U.S. Brand Names Donnapectolin-PG®; Kapectolin PG®

Generic Available Yes

Synonyms Atropine, Hyoscyamine, Scopolamine, Kaolin, Pectin, and Opium; Kaolin, Hyoscyamine, Atropine, Scopolamine, Pectin, and Opium; Opium, Hyoscyamine, Atropine, Scopolamine, Kaolin, and Pectin; Pectin, Hyoscyamine, Atropine, Scopolamine, Kaolin, and Opium; Scopolamine, Hyoscyamine, Atropine, Kaolin, Pectin, and Opium

Pharmacologic Category Anticholinergic Agent; Antidiarrheal

Use Treatment of diarrhea

Local Anesthetic/Vasoconstrictor Precautions No information available to require special precautions

Effects on Dental Treatment Key adverse event(s) related to dental treatment: Xerostomia (normal salivary flow resumes upon discontinuation).

Common Adverse Effects Frequency not defined.

Cardiovascular: Tachycardia, palpitations, hypotension

Central nervous system: Fatigue, delirium, restlessness, drowsiness, headache, ataxia, confusion, impairment of judgment and coordination

Dermatologic: Dry hot skin, skin rash

Gastrointestinal: Impaired GI motility, xerostomia, constipation

Genitourinary: Urinary hesitancy/retention

Neuromuscular & skeletal: Tremors

Ocular: Mydriasis, blurred vision, dry eyes

Respiratory: Respiratory depression (rare)

Restrictions C-V

Pregnancy Risk Factor C

Hyoscyamine, Methenamine, Sodium Biphosphate, Phenyl Salicylate, and Methylene Blue *see* Methenamine, Sodium Biphosphate, Phenyl Salicylate, Methylene Blue, and Hyoscyamine *on page 893*
Hyoscyamine Sulfate *see* Hyoscyamine *on page 724*
Hyosine *see* Hyoscyamine *on page 724*
Hyperstat® *see* Diazoxide *on page 425*
HypoTears [OTC] *see* Artificial Tears *on page 148*
HypoTears PF [OTC] *see* Artificial Tears *on page 148*
Hypromellose *see* Hydroxypropyl Methylcellulose *on page 721*
Hyrexin-50® *see* DiphenhydrAMINE *on page 448*
Hytakerol® *see* Dihydrotachysterol *on page 443*
Hytinic® [OTC] *see* Polysaccharide-Iron Complex *on page 1101*
Hytone® *see* Hydrocortisone *on page 714*
Hytrin® *see* Terazosin *on page 1271*
Hyzaar® *see* Losartan and Hydrochlorothiazide *on page 847*
Iberet® [OTC] *see* Vitamins (Multiple/Oral) *on page 1384*
Iberet®-500 [OTC] *see* Vitamins (Multiple/Oral) *on page 1384*
Iberet-Folic-500® *see* Vitamins (Multiple/Oral) *on page 1384*
Ibidomide Hydrochloride *see* Labetalol *on page 791*

Ibritumomab (ib ri TYOO mo mab)

U.S. Brand Names Zevalin™

Generic Available No

Synonyms Ibritumomab Tiuxetan; In-111 Zevalin; Y-90 Zevalin

Pharmacologic Category Antineoplastic Agent, Monoclonal Antibody; Radiopharmaceutical

Use Treatment of relapsed or refractory low-grade, follicular, or transformed B-cell non-Hodgkin's lymphoma (including rituximab-refractory follicular non-Hodgkin's lymphoma) as part of a therapeutic regimen with rituximab (Zevalin™ therapeutic regimen); **not to be used as single-agent therapy**; must be radiolabeled prior to use

Local Anesthetic/Vasoconstrictor Precautions No information available to require special precautions

Effects on Dental Treatment Key adverse event(s) related to dental treatment: Hypotension, cough, throat irritation, rhinitis.

Common Adverse Effects Severe, potentially life-threatening allergic reactions have occurred in association with infusions. Also refer to Rituximab monograph.

>10%:
- Central nervous system: Chills (24%), fever (17%), pain (13%), headache (12%)
- Gastrointestinal: Nausea (31%), abdominal pain (16%), vomiting (12%)
- Hematologic: Thrombocytopenia (95%), neutropenia (77%), anemia (61%)
  - Myelosuppressive:
    - WBC: Severe
    - Platelets: Severe
    - Nadir: 7-9 weeks
    - Recovery: 22-35 days
- Neuromuscular & skeletal: Weakness (43%)
- Respiratory: Dyspnea (14%)
- Miscellaneous: Infection (29%)

1% to 10%:
- Cardiovascular: Peripheral edema (8%), hypotension (6%), flushing (6%), angioedema (5%)
- Central nervous system: Dizziness (10%), insomnia (5%), anxiety (4%)
- Dermatologic: Pruritus (9%), rash (8%), urticaria (4%), petechia (3%)
- Gastrointestinal: Diarrhea (9%), anorexia (8%), abdominal distension (5%), constipation (5%), dyspepsia (4%), melena (2%; life threatening in 1%), gastrointestinal hemorrhage (1%)
- Hematologic: Bruising (7%), pancytopenia (2%), secondary malignancies (2%)
- Neuromuscular & skeletal: Back pain (8%), arthralgia (7%), myalgia (7%)
- Respiratory: Cough (10%), throat irritation (10%), rhinitis (6%), bronchospasm (5%), epistaxis (3%), apnea (1%)
- Miscellaneous: Diaphoresis (4%), allergic reaction (2%; life-threatening in 1%)

Mechanism of Action Ibritumomab is a monoclonal antibody directed against the CD20 antigen found on B lymphocytes (normal and malignant). Ibritumomab binding induces apoptosis in B lymphocytes *in vitro*. It is

(Continued)

Ibritumomab *(Continued)*

combined with the chelator tiuxetan, which acts as a specific chelation site for either Indium-111 (In-111) or Yttrium-90 (Y-90). The monoclonal antibody acts as a delivery system to direct the radioactive isotope to the targeted cells, however, binding has been observed in lymphoid cells throughout the body and in lymphoid nodules in organs such as the large and small intestines. Indium-111 is a gamma-emitter used to assess biodistribution of ibritumomab, while Y-90 emits beta particles. Beta-emission induces cellular damage through the formation of free radicals (in both target cells and surrounding cells).

Drug Interactions

Increased Effect/Toxicity: Due to the high incidence of thrombocytopenia associated with ibritumomab, the use of agents which decrease platelet function may be associated with a higher risk of bleeding (includes aspirin, NSAIDs, glycoprotein IIb/IIIa antagonists, clopidogrel and ticlopidine). In addition, the risk of bleeding may be increased with anticoagulant agents, including heparin, low molecular weight heparins, thrombolytics, and warfarin. The safety of live viral vaccines has not been established.

Decreased Effect: Response to vaccination may be impaired.

Pharmacodynamics/Kinetics

Duration: Beta cell recovery begins in ~12 weeks; generally in normal range within 9 months

Distribution: To lymphoid cells throughout the body and in lymphoid nodules in organs such as the large and small intestines, spleen, testes, and liver

Metabolism: Has not been characterized; the product of yttrium-90 radioactive decay is zirconium-90 (nonradioactive); Indium-111 decays to cadmium-111 (nonradioactive)

Half-life elimination: Y-90 ibritumomab: 30 hours; Indium-111 decays with a physical half-life of 67 hours; Yttrium-90 decays with a physical half-life of 64 hours

Excretion: A median of 7.2% of the radiolabeled activity was excreted in urine over 7 days

Pregnancy Risk Factor D

Ibritumomab Tiuxetan *see* Ibritumomab *on page 727*

Ibu-200 [OTC] *see* Ibuprofen *on page 728*

Ibuprofen (eye byoo PROE fen)

Related Information

Oral Pain *on page 1526*

Rheumatoid Arthritis, Osteoarthritis, and Osteoporosis *on page 1490*

Temporomandibular Dysfunction (TMD) *on page 1564*

U.S. Brand Names Advil® [OTC]; Advil® Children's [OTC]; Advil® Infants' [OTC]; Advil® Junior [OTC]; Advil® Migraine [OTC]; Genpril® [OTC]; Haltran® [OTC] [DSC]; Ibu-200 [OTC]; I-Prin [OTC]; Menadol® [OTC]; Midol® Maximum Strength Cramp Formula [OTC]; Motrin®; Motrin® Children's [OTC]; Motrin® IB [OTC]; Motrin® Infants' [OTC]; Motrin® Junior Strength [OTC]; Motrin® Migraine Pain [OTC]; Proprinal [OTC]; Ultraprin [OTC]

Canadian Brand Names Advil®; Apo-Ibuprofen®; Motrin®; Motrin® (Children's); Motrin® IB; Novo-Profen®; Nu-Ibuprofen

Mexican Brand Names Advil®; Algidol®; Citalgan®; Days® [tabs]; Dibufen®; Diprodol®; Flexafen®; Motrin®; Proartinal®; Quadrax®; Tabalon®

Generic Available Yes: Caplet, suspension, tablet

Synonyms *p*-Isobutylhydratropic Acid

Pharmacologic Category Nonsteroidal Anti-inflammatory Drug (NSAID), Oral

Dental Use Management of pain and swelling

Use Inflammatory diseases and rheumatoid disorders including juvenile rheumatoid arthritis, mild to moderate pain, fever, dysmenorrhea

Unlabeled/Investigational Use Cystic fibrosis, gout, ankylosing spondylitis, acute migraine headache

Local Anesthetic/Vasoconstrictor Precautions No information available to require special precautions

Effects on Dental Treatment NSAID formulations are known to reversibly decrease platelet aggregation via mechanisms different than observed with aspirin. The dentist should be aware of the potential of abnormal coagulation. Caution should also be exercised in the use of NSAIDs in patients already on anticoagulant therapy with drugs such as warfarin (Coumadin®).

Significant Adverse Effects

1% to 10%:

Cardiovascular: Edema (1% to 3%)

Central nervous system: Dizziness (3% to 9%), headache (1% to 3%), nervousness (1% to 3%)
Dermatologic: Itching (1% to 3%), rash (3% to 9%)
Endocrine & metabolic: Fluid retention (1% to 3%)
Gastrointestinal: Dyspepsia (1% to 3%), vomiting (1% to 3%), abdominal pain/cramps/distress (1% to 3%), heartburn (3% to 9%), nausea (3% to 9%), diarrhea (1% to 3%), constipation (1% to 3%), flatulence (1% to 3%), epigastric pain (3% to 9%), appetite decreased (1% to 3%)
Otic: Tinnitus (3% to 9%)

<1% (Limited to important or life-threatening): Acute renal failure, agranulocytosis, anaphylaxis, aplastic anemia, azotemia, blurred vision, bone marrow suppression, confusion, creatinine clearance decreased, duodenal ulcer, edema, eosinophilia, epistaxis, erythema multiforme, gastric ulcer, GI bleed, GI hemorrhage, GI ulceration, hallucinations, hearing decreased, hematuria, hematocrit decreased, hemoglobin decreased, hemolytic anemia, hepatitis, hypertension, inhibition of platelet aggregation, jaundice, liver function tests abnormal, leukopenia, melena, neutropenia, pancreatitis, Stevens-Johnson syndrome, thrombocytopenia, toxic amblyopia, toxic epidermal necrolysis, urticaria, vesiculobullous eruptions, vision changes

Dosage Oral:

Children:

Antipyretic: 6 months to 12 years: Temperature <102.5°F (39°C): 5 mg/kg/dose; temperature >102.5°F: 10 mg/kg/dose given every 6-8 hours (maximum daily dose: 40 mg/kg/day)

Juvenile rheumatoid arthritis: 30-50 mg/kg/24 hours divided every 8 hours; start at lower end of dosing range and titrate upward (maximum: 2.4 g/day)

Analgesic: 4-10 mg/kg/dose every 6-8 hours

Cystic fibrosis (unlabeled use): Chronic (>4 years) twice daily dosing adjusted to maintain serum levels of 50-100 mcg/mL has been associated with slowing of disease progression in younger patients with mild lung disease

OTC labeling (analgesic, antipyretic):

Children 6 months to 11 years: See table; use of weight to select dose is preferred; doses may be repeated every 6-8 hours (maximum: 4 doses/day)

Children ≥12 years: 200 mg every 4-6 hours as needed (maximum: 1200 mg/24 hours)

Ibuprofen Dosing

Weight (lbs)	Age	Dosage (mg)
12-17	6-11 mo	50
18-23	12-23 mo	75
24-35	2-3 y	100
35-47	4-5 y	150
48-59	6-8 y	200
60-71	9-10 y	250
72-95	11 y	300

Adults:

Inflammatory disease: 400-800 mg/dose 3-4 times/day (maximum dose: 3.2 g/day)

Analgesia/pain/fever/dysmenorrhea: 200-400 mg/dose every 4-6 hours (maximum daily dose: 1.2 g, unless directed by physician)

OTC labeling (analgesic, antipyretic): 200 mg every 4-6 hours as needed (maximum: 1200 mg/24 hours)

Dosing adjustment/comments in severe hepatic impairment: Avoid use

Mechanism of Action Inhibits prostaglandin synthesis by decreasing the activity of the enzyme, cyclooxygenase, which results in decreased formation of prostaglandin precursors

Contraindications Hypersensitivity to ibuprofen, any component of the formulation, aspirin, or other NSAIDs; patients with "aspirin triad" (bronchial asthma, aspirin intolerance, rhinitis); pregnancy (3rd trimester)

Warnings/Precautions Use with caution in patients with CHF, hypertension, dehydration, decreased renal or hepatic function, history of GI disease (bleeding or ulcers), or those receiving anticoagulants. Consuming ≥3 alcoholic beverages/day may increase the risk of GI bleeding. Elderly are at a high risk for adverse effects from NSAIDs. As many as 60% of elderly can develop peptic ulceration and/or hemorrhage asymptomatically. Fatal asthmatic and anaphylactoid reactions have occurred in patients with "aspirin triad" (see Contraindications).

(Continued)

Ibuprofen *(Continued)*

Use lowest effective dose for shortest period possible. Use of NSAIDs can compromise existing renal function especially when Cl_{cr} is <30 mL/minute. CNS adverse effects such as confusion, agitation, and hallucination are generally seen in overdose or high-dose situations; however, elderly may demonstrate these adverse effects at lower doses than younger adults. Do not exceed 3200 mg/day. Withhold for at least 4-6 half-lives prior to surgical or dental procedures.

OTC labeling: When used for self-medication, patients should be instructed to contact healthcare provider if used for fever lasting >3 days or for pain lasting >10 days in adults or >3 days in children.

Drug Interactions Substrate (minor) of CYP2C8/9, 2C19; **Inhibits** CYP2C8/9 (strong)

ACE inhibitors: Antihypertensive effects may be decreased by concurrent therapy with NSAIDs; monitor blood pressure.

Angiotensin II antagonists: Antihypertensive effects may be decreased by concurrent therapy with NSAIDs; monitor blood pressure.

Anticoagulants (warfarin, heparin, LMWHs) in combination with NSAIDs can cause increased risk of bleeding.

Antiplatelet drugs (ticlopidine, clopidogrel, aspirin, abciximab, dipyridamole, eptifibatide, tirofiban) can cause an increased risk of bleeding.

Corticosteroids: May increase the risk of GI ulceration; avoid concurrent use

Cyclosporine: NSAIDs may increase serum creatinine, potassium, blood pressure, and cyclosporine levels; monitor cyclosporine levels and renal function carefully.

CYP2C8/9 substrates: Ibuprofen may increase the levels/effects of CYP2C8/9 substrates. Example substrates include amiodarone, fluoxetine, glimepiride, glipizide, nateglinide, phenytoin, pioglitazone, rosiglitazone, sertraline, and warfarin.

Hydralazine's antihypertensive effect is decreased; avoid concurrent use

Lithium levels can be increased; avoid concurrent use if possible or monitor lithium levels and adjust dose. Sulindac may have the least effect. When NSAID is stopped, lithium will need adjustment again.

Loop diuretics efficacy (diuretic and antihypertensive effect) is reduced. Indomethacin reduces this efficacy, however, it may be anticipated with any NSAID.

Methotrexate: Severe bone marrow suppression, aplastic anemia, and GI toxicity have been reported with concomitant NSAID therapy. Avoid use during moderate or high-dose methotrexate (increased and prolonged methotrexate levels). NSAID use during low-dose treatment of rheumatoid arthritis has not been fully evaluated; extreme caution is warranted.

Warfarin's INRs may be increased by piroxicam. Other NSAIDs may have the same effect depending on dose and duration. Monitor INR closely. Use the lowest dose of NSAIDs possible and for the briefest duration. May alter the anticoagulant effects of warfarin; concurrent use with other antiplatelet agents or anticoagulants may increase risk of bleeding.

Ethanol/Nutrition/Herb Interactions

Ethanol: Avoid ethanol (may enhance gastric mucosal irritation).

Food: Ibuprofen peak serum levels may be decreased if taken with food.

Herb/Nutraceutical: Avoid cat's claw, dong quai, evening primrose, feverfew, garlic, ginger, ginkgo, red clover, horse chestnut, green tea, ginseng (all have additional antiplatelet activity).

Dietary Considerations Should be taken with food. Chewable tablets may contain phenylalanine; amount varies by product, consult manufacturers labeling.

Pharmacodynamics/Kinetics

Onset of action: Analgesic: 30-60 minutes; Anti-inflammatory: ≤7 days
Peak effect: 1-2 weeks

Duration: 4-6 hours

Absorption: Oral: Rapid (85%)

Protein binding: 90% to 99%

Metabolism: Hepatic via oxidation

Half-life elimination: 2-4 hours; End-stage renal disease: Unchanged

Time to peak: ~1-2 hours

Excretion: Urine (1% as free drug); some feces

Pregnancy Risk Factor B/D (3rd trimester)

Lactation Enters breast milk/use caution (AAP rates "compatible")

Breast-Feeding Considerations Limited data suggests minimal excretion in breast milk.

Dosage Forms [DSC] = Discontinued product

Caplet: 200 mg [OTC]
  Advil®: 200 mg [contains sodium benzoate]
  Ibu-200, Menadol®, Motrin® IB, Motrin® Migraine Pain: 200 mg
  Motrin® Junior Strength: 100 mg [contains tartrazine]
Capsule, liqui-gel:
  Advil®: 200 mg
  Advil® Migraine: 200 mg [solubilized ibuprofen]
Gelcap:
  Advil®: 200 mg
  Motrin® IB: 200 mg [contains benzyl alcohol]
Suspension, oral: 100 mg/5 mL (5 mL, 120 mL, 480 mL)
  Advil® Children's: 100 mg/5 mL (60 mL, 120 mL) [contains sodium benzoate; blue raspberry, fruit, and grape flavors]
  Motrin® Children's: 100 mg/5 mL (60 mL, 120 mL) [contains sodium benzoate; berry, dye-free berry, bubble gum, and grape flavors]
Suspension, oral drops: 40 mg/mL (15 mL)
  Advil® Infants': 40 mg/mL (15 mL) [contains sodium benzoate; fruit and grape flavors]
  Motrin® Infants': 40 mg/mL (15 mL, 30 mL) [contains sodium benzoate; berry and dye-free berry flavors]
Tablet: 200 mg [OTC], 400 mg, 600 mg, 800 mg
  Advil®: 200 mg [contains sodium benzoate]
  Advil® Junior: 100 mg [contains sodium benzoate; coated tablets]
  Genpril®, Haltran® [DSC], I-Prin, Midol® Maximum Strength Cramp Formula, Motrin® IB, Proprinal, Ultraprin: 200 mg
  Motrin®: 400 mg, 600 mg, 800 mg
Tablet, chewable:
  Advil® Children's: 50 mg [contains phenylalanine 2.1 mg; fruit and grape flavors]
  Advil® Junior: 100 mg [contains phenylalanine 2.1 mg; fruit and grape flavors]
  Motrin® Children's: 50 mg [contains phenylalanine 1.4 mg; orange flavor]
  Motrin® Junior Strength: 100 mg [contains phenylalanine 2.1 mg; grape and orange flavors]

Comments Preoperative use of ibuprofen at a dose of 400-600 mg every 6 hours 24 hours before the appointment decreases postoperative edema and hastens healing time.

Selected Readings

Ahmad N, Grad HA, Haas DA, et al, "The Efficacy of Nonopioid Analgesics for Postoperative Dental Pain: A Meta-Analysis," *Anesth Prog*, 1997, 44(4):119-26.

Beaver WT, "Review of the Analgesic Efficacy of Ibuprofen," *Int J Clin Pract*, 2003, (Suppl 135):13-7.

Dionne R, "Additive Analgesia Without Opioid Side Effects," *Compend Contin Educ Dent*, 2000, 21(7):572-4, 576-7.

Dionne R, "Relative Efficacy of Selective COX-2 Inhibitors Compared With Over-The-Counter Ibuprofen," *Int J Clin Pract Suppl*, 2003, (135):18-22.

Dionne RA and Berthold CW, "Therapeutic Uses of Nonsteroidal Anti-inflammatory Drugs in Dentistry," *Crit Rev Oral Biol Med*, 2001, 12(4):315-30.

Doyle G, Jayawardena S, Ashraf E, et al, "Efficacy and Tolerability of Nonprescription Ibuprofen Versus Celecoxib for Dental Pain," *J Clin Pharmacol*, 2002, 42(8):912-9.

Gobetti JP, "Controlling Dental Pain," *J Am Dent Assoc*, 1992, 123(6):47-52.

Hersh EV, Levin LM, Cooper SA, et al, "Ibuprofen Liquigel for Oral Surgery Pain," *Clin Ther*, 2000, 22(11):1306-18.

Olson NZ, Otero AM, Marrero I, et al, "Onset of Analgesia for Liquigel Ibuprofen 400 mg, Acetaminophen 1000 mg, Ketoprofen 25 mg, and Placebo in the Treatment of Postoperative Dental Pain," *J Clin Pharmacol*, 2001, 41(11):1238-47.

Pearlman B, Boyatzis S, Daly C, et al, "The Analgesic Efficacy of Ibuprofen in Periodontal Surgery: A Multicentre Study," *Aust Dent J*, 1997, 42(5):328-34.

Nguyen AM, Graham DY, Gage T, et al, "Nonsteroidal Anti-inflammatory Drug Use in Dentistry: Gastrointestinal Implications," *Gen Dent*, 1999, 47(6):590-6.

Wynn RL, "Update on Nonprescription Pain Relievers for Dental Pain," *Gen Dent*, 2004, 52(2):94-8.

Ibuprofen and Hydrocodone *see* Hydrocodone and Ibuprofen *on page 709*

Ibuprofen and Pseudoephedrine *see* Pseudoephedrine and Ibuprofen *on page 1149*

Ibutilide (i BYOO ti lide)

Related Information

Cardiovascular Diseases *on page 1458*

U.S. Brand Names Corvert®

Generic Available No

Synonyms Ibutilide Fumarate

Pharmacologic Category Antiarrhythmic Agent, Class III

(Continued)

Ibutilide *(Continued)*

Use Acute termination of atrial fibrillation or flutter of recent onset; the effectiveness of ibutilide has not been determined in patients with arrhythmias >90 days in duration

Local Anesthetic/Vasoconstrictor Precautions No information available to require special precautions

Effects on Dental Treatment No significant effects or complications reported

Common Adverse Effects 1% to 10%:

Cardiovascular: Sustained polymorphic ventricular tachycardia (ie, torsade de pointes) (1.7%, often requiring cardioversion), nonsustained polymorphic ventricular tachycardia (2.7%), nonsustained monomorphic ventricular tachycardia (4.9%), ventricular extrasystoles (5.1%), nonsustained monomorphic VT (4.9%), tachycardia/supraventricular tachycardia (2.7%), hypotension (2%), bundle branch block (1.9%), AV block (1.5%), bradycardia (1.2%), QT segment prolongation, hypertension (1.2%), palpitations (1%)

Central nervous system: Headache (3.6%)

Gastrointestinal: Nausea (>1%)

Mechanism of Action Exact mechanism of action is unknown; prolongs the action potential in cardiac tissue

Drug Interactions

Increased Effect/Toxicity: Class Ia antiarrhythmic drugs (disopyramide, quinidine, and procainamide) and other class III drugs such as amiodarone and sotalol should not be given concomitantly with ibutilide due to their potential to prolong refractoriness. Signs of digoxin toxicity may be masked when coadministered with ibutilide. Toxicity of ibutilide is potentiated by concurrent administration of other drugs which may prolong QT interval: phenothiazines, tricyclic and tetracyclic antidepressants, cisapride, sparfloxacin, gatifloxacin, moxifloxacin, and erythromycin.

Pharmacodynamics/Kinetics

Onset of action: ~90 minutes after start of infusion (1/2 of conversions to sinus rhythm occur during infusion)

Distribution: V_d: 11 L/kg

Protein binding: 40%

Metabolism: Extensively hepatic; oxidation

Half-life elimination: 2-12 hours (average: 6 hours)

Excretion: Urine (82%, 7% as unchanged drug and metabolites); feces (19%)

Pregnancy Risk Factor C

Ibutilide Fumarate *see* Ibutilide *on page 731*

IC-Green® *see* Indocyanine Green *on page 745*

ICI 182,780 *see* Fulvestrant *on page 639*

ICI 204, 219 *see* Zafirlukast *on page 1394*

ICI-46474 *see* Tamoxifen *on page 1258*

ICI-118630 *see* Goserelin *on page 670*

ICI-176334 *see* Bicalutamide *on page 206*

ICI-D1033 *see* Anastrozole *on page 132*

ICRF-187 *see* Dexrazoxane *on page 417*

I.D.A. *see* Acetaminophen, Isometheptene, and Dichloralphenazone *on page 59*

Idamycin PFS® *see* Idarubicin *on page 732*

Idarubicin (eye da ROO bi sin)

U.S. Brand Names Idamycin PFS®

Canadian Brand Names Idamycin®

Mexican Brand Names Idamycin®

Generic Available Yes

Synonyms 4-Demethoxydaunorubicin; 4-DMDR; Idarubicin Hydrochloride; IDR; IMI 30; NSC-256439; SC 33428

Pharmacologic Category Antineoplastic Agent, Anthracycline; Antineoplastic Agent, Antibiotic

Use Treatment of acute leukemias (AML, ANLL, ALL), accelerated phase or blast crisis of chronic myelogenous leukemia (CML), breast cancer

Local Anesthetic/Vasoconstrictor Precautions No information available to require special precautions

Effects on Dental Treatment Key adverse event(s) related to dental treatment: Stomatitis.

Common Adverse Effects

>10%:

Cardiovascular: Transient ECG abnormalities (supraventricular tachycardia, S-T wave changes, atrial or ventricular extrasystoles); generally asymptomatic and self-limiting. Congestive heart failure, dose-related. The relative cardiotoxicity of idarubicin compared to doxorubicin is unclear. Some investigators report no increase in cardiac toxicity at cumulative oral idarubicin doses up to 540 mg/m^2; other reports suggest a maximum cumulative intravenous dose of 150 mg/m^2.

Central nervous system: Headache

Dermatologic: Alopecia (25% to 30%), radiation recall, skin rash (11%), urticaria

Gastrointestinal: Nausea, vomiting (30% to 60%); diarrhea (9% to 22%); stomatitis (11%); GI hemorrhage (30%)

Genitourinary: Discoloration of urine (darker yellow)

Hematologic: Myelosuppression, primarily leukopenia; thrombocytopenia and anemia. Effects are generally less severe with oral dosing.

Nadir: 10-15 days

Recovery: 21-28 days

Hepatic: Elevations of bilirubin and transaminases (44%)

1% to 10%:

Central nervous system: Seizures

Neuromuscular & skeletal: Peripheral neuropathy

Mechanism of Action Similar to doxorubicin and daunorubicin; inhibition of DNA and RNA synthesis by intercalation between DNA base pairs

Drug Interactions

Decreased Effect: Patients may experience impaired immune response to vaccines; possible infection after administration of live vaccines in patients receiving immunosuppressants.

Pharmacodynamics/Kinetics

Absorption: Oral: Variable (4% to 77%; mean: ~30%)

Distribution: V_d: 64 L/kg (some reports indicate 2250 L); extensive tissue binding; CSF

Protein binding: 94% to 97%

Metabolism: Hepatic to idarubicinol (pharmacologically active)

Half-life elimination: Oral: 14-35 hours; I.V.: 12-27 hours

Time to peak, serum: 1-5 hours

Excretion:

Oral: Urine (~5% of dose; 0.5% to 0.7% as unchanged drug, 4% as idarubicinol); hepatic (8%)

I.V.: Urine (13% as idarubicinol, 3% as unchanged drug); hepatic (17%)

Pregnancy Risk Factor D

Idarubicin Hydrochloride *see* Idarubicin *on page 732*

IDEC-C2B8 *see* Rituximab *on page 1191*

IDR *see* Idarubicin *on page 732*

Ifex® *see* Ifosfamide *on page 733*

IFLrA *see* Interferon Alfa-2a *on page 751*

Ifosfamide (eye FOSS fa mide)

U.S. Brand Names Ifex®

Canadian Brand Names Ifex®

Mexican Brand Names Ifolem®; Ifoxan®

Generic Available Yes

Synonyms Isophosphamide; NSC-109724; Z4942

Pharmacologic Category Antineoplastic Agent, Alkylating Agent; Antineoplastic Agent, Alkylating Agent (Nitrogen Mustard)

Use Treatment of lung cancer, Hodgkin's and non-Hodgkin's lymphoma, breast cancer, acute and chronic lymphocytic leukemias, ovarian cancer, sarcomas, pancreatic and gastric carcinomas

Orphan drug: Treatment of testicular cancer

Local Anesthetic/Vasoconstrictor Precautions No information available to require special precautions

Effects on Dental Treatment No significant effects or complications reported

Common Adverse Effects

>10%:

Central nervous system: Somnolence, confusion, hallucinations (12%)

Dermatologic: Alopecia (75% to 100%)

Endocrine & metabolic: Metabolic acidosis (31%)

Gastrointestinal: Nausea and vomiting (58%), may be more common with higher doses or bolus infusions; constipation

(Continued)

Ifosfamide *(Continued)*

Genitourinary: Hemorrhagic cystitis (40% to 50%), patients should be vigorously hydrated (at least 2 L/day) and receive mesna
Hematologic: Myelosuppression, leukopenia (65% to 100%), thrombocytopenia (10%) - dose-related
Onset: 7-14 days
Nadir: 21-28 days
Recovery: 21-28 days
Renal: Hematuria (6% to 92%)

1% to 10%:
Central nervous system: Hallucinations, depressive psychoses, polyneuropathy
Dermatologic: Dermatitis, nail banding/ridging, hyperpigmentation
Endocrine & metabolic: SIADH, sterility, elevated transaminases (3%)
Hematologic: Anemia
Local: Phlebitis
Renal: Increased creatinine/BUN (6%)
Respiratory: Nasal stuffiness

Mechanism of Action Causes cross-linking of strands of DNA by binding with nucleic acids and other intracellular structures; inhibits protein synthesis and DNA synthesis

Drug Interactions

Cytochrome P450 Effect: Substrate of CYP2A6 (minor), 2B6 (minor), 2C8/9 (minor), 2C19 (minor), 3A4 (major); **Inhibits** CYP3A4 (weak); **Induces** CYP2C8/9 (weak)

Increased Effect/Toxicity: CYP3A4 inducers may increase the levels/effects of acrolein (the active metabolite of ifosfamide); example inducers include aminoglutethimide, carbamazepine, nafcillin, nevirapine, phenobarbital, phenytoin, and rifamycins.

Decreased Effect: CYP3A4 inhibitors may decrease the levels/effects of acrolein (the active metabolite of ifosfamide); example inhibitors include azole antifungals, ciprofloxacin, clarithromycin, diclofenac, doxycycline, erythromycin, imatinib, isoniazid, nefazodone, nicardipine, propofol, protease inhibitors, quinidine, and verapamil.

Pharmacodynamics/Kinetics Pharmacokinetics are dose dependent
Distribution: V_d: 5.7-49 L; does penetrate CNS, but not in therapeutic levels
Protein binding: Negligible
Metabolism: Hepatic to active metabolites phosphoramide mustard, acrolein, and inactive dichloroethylated and carboxy metabolites; acrolein is the agent implicated in development of hemorrhagic cystitis
Bioavailability: Estimated at 100%
Half-life elimination: Beta: High dose: 11-15 hours (3800-5000 mg/m^2); Lower dose: 4-7 hours (1800 mg/m^2)
Time to peak, plasma: Oral: Within 1 hour
Excretion: Urine (15% to 50% as unchanged drug, 41% as metabolites)

Pregnancy Risk Factor D

IG *see* Immune Globulin (Intramuscular) *on page 739*
IGIM *see* Immune Globulin (Intramuscular) *on page 739*
IL-1Ra *see* Anakinra *on page 131*
IL-2 *see* Aldesleukin *on page 74*
IL-11 *see* Oprelvekin *on page 1015*

Imatinib (eye MAT eh nib)

U.S. Brand Names Gleevec™
Canadian Brand Names Gleevec™
Mexican Brand Names Gleevec®
Generic Available No
Synonyms CGP 57148B; Glivec; Imatinib Mesylate; STI571
Pharmacologic Category Antineoplastic Agent, Tyrosine Kinase Inhibitor
Use Treatment of adult patients with Philadelphia chromosome-positive (Ph+) chronic myeloid leukemia (CML), including newly-diagnosed patients as well as patients in blast crisis, accelerated phase, or in chronic phase after failure of interferon-alpha therapy; treatment of pediatric patients with Ph+ CML (chronic phase) recurring following stem cell transplant or who are resistant to interferon-alpha therapy; treatment of Kit-positive (CD117) unresectable and/or (metastatic) malignant gastrointestinal stromal tumors (GIST)
Local Anesthetic/Vasoconstrictor Precautions No information available to require special precautions

Effects on Dental Treatment Key adverse event(s) related to dental treatment: Taste disturbance.

Common Adverse Effects Adverse reactions listed were established in patients with a wide variation in level of illness or specific diagnosis. In many cases, other medications were used concurrently (relationship to imatinib not specific). Effects reported in children were similar to adults, except that musculoskeletal pain was less frequent and peripheral edema was not reported.

>10%:

Central nervous system: Fatigue (29% to 41%), pyrexia (5% to 41%), headache (25% to 35%), dizziness (11% to 13%), insomnia (10% to 13%)

Dermatologic: Rash (26% to 44%), pruritus (8% to 13%), bruising (2% to 11%)

Endocrine & metabolic: Fluid retention (3% to 22% includes aggravated edema, anasarca, ascites, pericardial effusion, pleural effusion, pulmonary edema, excludes GIST); hypokalemia (5% to 13%)

Gastrointestinal: Nausea (42% to 71%), diarrhea (30% to 60%), vomiting (15% to 56%), abdominal pain (23% to 37%), weight increased (3% to 30%), dyspepsia (11% to 24), flatulence (16% to 23%), anorexia (6% to 17%), constipation (6% to 15%), taste disturbance (1% to 14%)

Hematologic: Hemorrhage (18% to 52%), neutropenia (grade 3 or 4: 2% to 48%), thrombocytopenia (grade 3 or 4: <1% to 31%)

Neuromuscular & skeletal: Muscle cramps (27% to 55%), musculoskeletal pain (11% to 46%), arthralgia (25% to 36%), joint pain (27%), myalgia (8% to 25%), weakness (5% to 12%), back pain (10% to 11%), rigors (8% to 11%)

Ocular: Lacrimation (6% to 11%)

Respiratory: Cough (12% to 26%), dyspnea (9% to 20%), nasopharyngitis (8% to 19%), upper respiratory tract infection (3% to 15%), pharyngolaryngeal pain (14%), epistaxis (5% to 13%), pneumonia (3% to 12%), sore throat (8% to 11%)

Miscellaneous: Superficial edema (53% to 76%), night sweats (10% to 14%)

1% to 10%:

Central nervous system: Paresthesia (1% to 10%)

Hematologic: Anemia (grade 3 or 4: <1% to 4%)

Hepatic: Ascites or pleural effusion (GIST: 4% to 6%), alkaline phosphatase increased (grade 3 or 4: <1% to 5%), ALT increased (grade 3 or 4: <1% to 4%), bilirubin increased (grade 3 or 4: <1% to 4%), AST increased (grade 3 or 4: <1% to 3%)

Renal: Albumin decreased (grade 3 or 4: 3% to 4%), creatine increased (grade 3 or 4: <1% to 3%)

Miscellaneous: Flu-like syndrome (<1% to 10%)

Mechanism of Action Inhibits Bcr-Abl tyrosine kinase, the constitutive abnormal gene product of the Philadelphia chromosome in chronic myeloid leukemia (CML). Inhibition of this enzyme blocks proliferation and induces apoptosis in Bcr-Abl positive cell lines as well as in fresh leukemic cells in Philadelphia chromosome positive CML. Also inhibits tyrosine kinase for platelet-derived growth factor (PDGF), stem cell factor (SCF), c-kit, and events mediated by PDGF and SCF.

Drug Interactions

Cytochrome P450 Effect: Substrate of CYP1A2 (minor), 2D6 (minor), 2C8/9 (minor), 2C19 (minor), 3A4 (major), **Inhibits** CYP2C8/9 (weak), 2D6 (weak), 3A4 (strong)

Increased Effect/Toxicity: Note: Drug interaction data are limited. Few clinical studies have been conducted. Many interactions listed here are derived by extrapolation from *in vitro* inhibition of cytochrome P450 isoenzymes. Chronic use of acetaminophen may increase potential for hepatotoxic reaction with imatinib (case report of hepatic failure with concurrent therapy).

Imatinib may increase the levels/effects of amiodarone, selected benzodiazepines, calcium channel blockers, cisapride, cyclosporine, ergot derivatives, fluoxetine, glimepiride, glipizide, HMG-CoA reductase inhibitors, nateglinide, phenytoin, phenytoin, propranolol, sertraline, mirtazapine, nateglinide, nefazodone, pioglitazone, rosiglitazone, sertraline, sildenafil (and other PDE-5 inhibitors), tacrolimus, venlafaxine, warfarin, and other substrates of CYP2C8/9 or 3A4. Selected benzodiazepines (midazolam and triazolam), cisapride, ergot alkaloids, selected HMG-CoA reductase inhibitors (lovastatin and simvastatin), mesoridazine, pimozide, and thioridazine are generally contraindicated with strong CYP3A4 inhibitors. When used with strong CYP3A4 inhibitors, dosage adjustment/limits are recommended for sildenafil and other PDE-5 inhibitors; consult individual monographs.

(Continued)

Imatinib *(Continued)*

The levels/effects of imatinib may be increased by azole antifungals, ciprofloxacin, clarithromycin, diclofenac, doxycycline, erythromycin, isoniazid, nefazodone, nicardipine, propofol, protease inhibitors, quinidine, telithromycin, verapamil, and other CYP3A4 inhibitors.

Decreased Effect: The levels/effects of imatinib may be decreased by aminoglutethimide, carbamazepine, nafcillin, nevirapine, phenobarbital, phenytoin, rifamycins, and other CYP3A4 inducers. Dosage of imatinib should be increased by at least 50% (with careful monitoring) when used concurrently with a strong inducer.

Pharmacodynamics/Kinetics

Protein binding: 95% to albumin and $alpha_1$-acid glycoprotein

Metabolism: Hepatic via CYP3A4 (minor metabolism via CYP1A2, CYP2D6, CYP2C9, CYP2C19); primary metabolite (active): N-demethylated piperazine derivative

Bioavailability: 98%

Half-life elimination: Parent drug: 18 hours; N-demethyl metabolite: 40 hours

Time to peak: 2-4 hours

Excretion: Feces (68% primarily as metabolites, 20% as unchanged drug); urine (13% primarily as metabolites, 5% as unchanged drug)

Clearance: Highly variable; Mean: 8-14 L/hour (for 50 kg and 100 kg male, respectively)

Pregnancy Risk Factor D

Imatinib Mesylate *see* Imatinib *on page 734*

IMC-C225 *see* Cetuximab *on page 300*

Imdur® *see* Isosorbide Mononitrate *on page 771*

IMI 30 *see* Idarubicin *on page 732*

Imidazol Carboxamide Dimethyltriazene *see* Dacarbazine *on page 392*

Imidazole Carboxamide *see* Dacarbazine *on page 392*

Imiglucerase (i mi GLOO ser ace)

U.S. Brand Names Cerezyme®

Canadian Brand Names Cerezyme®

Generic Available No

Pharmacologic Category Enzyme

Use Long-term enzyme replacement therapy for patients with Type 1 Gaucher's disease

Local Anesthetic/Vasoconstrictor Precautions No information available to require special precautions

Effects on Dental Treatment No significant effects or complications reported

Common Adverse Effects

1% to 10%: Miscellaneous: Hypersensitivity reaction (7%; symptoms may include pruritus, flushing, urticaria, angioedema, bronchospasm)

Individual frequency not defined, but <1.5%:

Cardiovascular: Tachycardia

Central nervous system: Headache, dizziness, fatigue, fever

Dermatologic: Rash, pruritus

Gastrointestinal: Nausea, abdominal discomfort, vomiting, diarrhea

Local: Injection site burning, swelling, or sterile abscess (<1%)

Neuromuscular & skeletal: Backache

Miscellaneous: Anaphylactoid reactions (<1%)

Mechanism of Action Imiglucerase is an analogue of glucocerebrosidase; it is produced by recombinant DNA technology using mammalian cell culture. Glucocerebrosidase is an enzyme deficient in Gaucher's disease. It is needed to catalyze the hydrolysis of glucocerebroside to glucose and ceramide.

Pharmacodynamics/Kinetics

Distribution: V_d: 0.09-0.15 L/kg

Half-life elimination: 3.6-10.4 minutes

Pregnancy Risk Factor C

Imipemide *see* Imipenem and Cilastatin *on page 736*

Imipenem and Cilastatin (i mi PEN em & sye la STAT in)

Related Information

Animal and Human Bites Guidelines *on page 1582*

U.S. Brand Names Primaxin®

Canadian Brand Names Primaxin®

Generic Available No

Synonyms Imipemide

Pharmacologic Category Antibiotic, Carbapenem

Use Treatment of respiratory tract, urinary tract, intra-abdominal, gynecologic, bone and joint, skin structure, and polymicrobic infections as well as bacterial septicemia and endocarditis. Antibacterial activity includes resistant gram-negative bacilli (*Pseudomonas aeruginosa* and *Enterobacter* sp), gram-positive bacteria (methicillin-sensitive *Staphylococcus aureus* and *Streptococcus* sp) and anaerobes.

Note: I.M. administration is not intended for severe or life-threatening infections (eg, septicemia, endocarditis, shock)

Local Anesthetic/Vasoconstrictor Precautions No information available to require special precautions

Effects on Dental Treatment No significant effects or complications reported

Common Adverse Effects 1% to 10%:

Gastrointestinal: Nausea/diarrhea/vomiting (1% to 2%)

Local: Phlebitis (3%), pain at I.M. injection site (1.2%)

Mechanism of Action Inhibits bacterial cell wall synthesis by binding to one or more of the penicillin binding proteins (PBPs); which in turn inhibits the final transpeptidation step of peptidoglycan synthesis in bacterial cell walls, thus inhibiting cell wall biosynthesis. Bacteria eventually lyse due to ongoing activity of cell wall autolytic enzymes (autolysins and murein hydrolases) while cell wall assembly is arrested. Cilastatin prevents renal metabolism of imipenem by competitive inhibition of dehydropeptidase along the brush border of the renal tubules.

Drug Interactions

Increased Effect/Toxicity: Beta-lactam antibiotics and probenecid may increase potential for toxicity.

Pharmacodynamics/Kinetics

Absorption: I.M.: Imipenem: 60% to 75%; cilastatin: 95% to 100%

Distribution: Rapidly and widely to most tissues and fluids including sputum, pleural fluid, peritoneal fluid, interstitial fluid, bile, aqueous humor, reproductive organs, and bone; highest concentrations in pleural fluid, interstitial fluid, peritoneal fluid, and reproductive organs; low concentrations in CSF; crosses placenta; enters breast milk

Metabolism: Renally by dehydropeptidase; activity is blocked by cilastatin; cilastatin is partially metabolized renally

Half-life elimination: Both drugs: 60 minutes; prolonged with renal impairment

Excretion: Both drugs: Urine (~70% as unchanged drug)

Pregnancy Risk Factor C

Imipramine (im IP ra meen)

U.S. Brand Names Tofranil®; Tofranil-PM®

Canadian Brand Names Apo-Imipramine®; Tofranil®

Mexican Brand Names Talpramin®; Tofranil®; Tofranil-PM®

Generic Available Yes: Tablet

Synonyms Imipramine Hydrochloride; Imipramine Pamoate

Pharmacologic Category Antidepressant, Tricyclic (Tertiary Amine)

Use Treatment of depression

Unlabeled/Investigational Use Enuresis in children; analgesic for certain chronic and neuropathic pain; panic disorder; attention-deficit/hyperactivity disorder (ADHD)

Local Anesthetic/Vasoconstrictor Precautions Use with caution; epinephrine, norepinephrine and levonordefrin have been shown to have an increased pressor response in combination with TCAs

Effects on Dental Treatment Key adverse event(s) related to dental treatment: Xerostomia and changes in salivation (normal salivary flow resumes upon discontinuation). Long-term treatment with TCAs, such as imipramine, increases the risk of caries by reducing salivation and salivary buffer capacity. In a study by Rundergren, et al, pathological alterations were observed in the oral mucosa of 72% of 58 patients; 55% had new carious lesions after taking TCAs for a median of 5½ years. Current research is investigating the use of the salivary stimulant pilocarpine to overcome the xerostomia from imipramine.

Common Adverse Effects Frequency not defined.

Cardiovascular: Orthostatic hypotension, arrhythmias, tachycardia, hypertension, palpitations, myocardial infarction, heart block, ECG changes, CHF, stroke

Central nervous system: Dizziness, drowsiness, headache, agitation, insomnia, nightmares, hypomania, psychosis, fatigue, confusion, hallucinations, disorientation, delusions, anxiety, restlessness, seizures

Endocrine & metabolic: Gynecomastia, breast enlargement, galactorrhea, increase or decrease in libido, increase or decrease in blood sugar, SIADH

(Continued)

Imipramine *(Continued)*

Gastrointestinal: Nausea, unpleasant taste, weight gain, xerostomia, constipation, ileus, stomatitis, abdominal cramps, vomiting, anorexia, epigastric disorders, diarrhea, black tongue, weight loss

Genitourinary: Urinary retention, impotence

Neuromuscular & skeletal: Weakness, numbness, tingling, paresthesias, incoordination, ataxia, tremor, peripheral neuropathy, extrapyramidal symptoms

Ocular: Blurred vision, disturbances of accommodation, mydriasis

Otic: Tinnitus

Miscellaneous: Diaphoresis

Mechanism of Action Traditionally believed to increase the synaptic concentration of serotonin and/or norepinephrine in the central nervous system by inhibition of their reuptake by the presynaptic neuronal membrane. However, additional receptor effects have been found including desensitization of adenyl cyclase, down regulation of beta-adrenergic receptors, and down regulation of serotonin receptors.

Drug Interactions

Cytochrome P450 Effect: Substrate of CYP1A2 (minor), 2B6 (minor), 2C19 (major), 2D6 (major), 3A4 (minor); **Inhibits** CYP1A2 (weak), 2C19 (weak), 2D6 (moderate), 2E1 (weak)

Increased Effect/Toxicity: When used with MAO inhibitors, hyperpyrexia, hypertension, tachycardia, confusion, seizures, and **deaths have been reported** (serotonin syndrome). Serotonin syndrome has also been reported with ritonavir (rare). Use of lithium with a TCA may increase the risk for neurotoxicity.

CYP2C19 inhibitors may increase the levels/effects of imipramine; example inhibitors include delavirdine, fluconazole, fluvoxamine, gemfibrozil, isoniazid, omeprazole, and ticlopidine. Imipramine increases the effects of amphetamines, anticholinergics, other CNS depressants (sedatives, hypnotics, or ethanol), chlorpropamide, tolazamide, and warfarin. CYP2D6 inhibitors may increase the levels/effects of imipramine; example inhibitors include chlorpromazine, delavirdine, fluoxetine, miconazole, paroxetine, pergolide, quinidine, quinine, ritonavir, and ropinirole.

Phenothiazines may increase concentration of some TCAs and TCAs may increase concentration of phenothiazines. Pressor response to I.V. epinephrine, norepinephrine, and phenylephrine may be enhanced in patients receiving TCAs (**Note:** Effect is unlikely with epinephrine or levonordefrin dosages typically administered as infiltration in combination with local anesthetics).

Combined use of beta-agonists or drugs which prolong QT_c (including quinidine, procainamide, disopyramide, cisapride, sparfloxacin, gatifloxacin, moxifloxacin) with TCAs may predispose patients to cardiac arrhythmias.

Decreased Effect: CYP2C19 inducers may decrease the levels/effects of imipramine; example inducers include aminoglutethimide, carbamazepine, phenytoin, and rifampin. Imipramine inhibits the antihypertensive response to bethanidine, clonidine, debrisoquin, guanadrel, guanethidine, guanabenz, and guanfacine. Cholestyramine and colestipol may bind TCAs and reduce their absorption; monitor for altered response.

Pharmacodynamics/Kinetics

Onset of action: Peak antidepressant effect: Usually after ≥2 weeks

Absorption: Well absorbed

Distribution: Crosses placenta

Metabolism: Hepatic via CYP to desipramine (active) and other metabolites; significant first-pass effect

Half-life elimination: 6-18 hours

Excretion: Urine (as metabolites)

Pregnancy Risk Factor D

Imipramine Hydrochloride *see* Imipramine *on page 737*

Imipramine Pamoate *see* Imipramine *on page 737*

Imiquimod (i mi KWI mod)

Related Information

Oral Viral Infections *on page 1547*

Systemic Viral Diseases *on page 1519*

U.S. Brand Names Aldara™

Canadian Brand Names Aldara™

Generic Available No

Pharmacologic Category Skin and Mucous Membrane Agent; Topical Skin Product

Use Treatment of external genital and perianal warts/condyloma acuminata in children ≥12 years of age and adults; nonhyperkeratotic, nonhypertrophic actinic keratosis

Unlabeled/Investigational Use Treatment of common warts, basal cell carcinoma

Local Anesthetic/Vasoconstrictor Precautions No information available to require special precautions

Effects on Dental Treatment No significant effects or complications reported

Common Adverse Effects

>10%:

- Local, mild/moderate: Erythema (54% to 61%), itching (22% to 32%), erosion (21% to 32%), burning (9% to 26%), excoriation/flaking (18% to 25%), edema (12% to 17%), scabbing (9% to 13%), fungal infections (2% to 11%)
- Respiratory: Upper respiratory infection (15%)

1% to 10%:

- Cardiovascular: Atrial fibrillation (1%)
- Central nervous system: Pain (2% to 8%), headache (4% to 5%), fatigue (actinic keratosis 1%), fever (actinic keratosis 1%), dizziness (1%)
- Endocrine & metabolic: Hypercholesterolemia (2%)
- Gastrointestinal: Diarrhea (3%), dyspepsia (3%)
- Local:
  - Severe: Hyperkeratosis (actinic keratosis 9%), erythema (4%), eczema (2%), erosion (1%), edema (1%), alopecia (actinic keratosis 1%)
  - Mild/moderate: Pain, induration, ulceration (5% to 7%), vesicles (2% to 3%), soreness (<1% to 3%)
- Neuromuscular & skeletal: Myalgia (1%), back pain (actinic keratosis 1%)
- Miscellaneous: Influenza-like symptoms (1% to 3%), squamous cell carcinoma (4%)
- Respiratory: Sinusitis (7%), pharyngitis (2%)

Mechanism of Action Mechanism of action is unknown; however, induces cytokines, including interferon-alpha and others

Drug Interactions

Cytochrome P450 Effect: Substrate (minor) of CYP1A2, 3A4

Pharmacodynamics/Kinetics

Absorption: Minimal

Excretion: Urine and feces (<0.9%)

Pregnancy Risk Factor C

Imitrex® *see* Sumatriptan *on page 1252*

Immune Globulin (Intramuscular)

(i MYUN GLOB yoo lin, IN tra MUS kyoo ler)

Related Information

Immunizations (Vaccines) *on page 1614*
Systemic Viral Diseases *on page 1519*

U.S. Brand Names BayGam®

Canadian Brand Names BayGam®

Generic Available No

Synonyms Gamma Globulin; IG; IGIM; Immune Serum Globulin; ISG

Pharmacologic Category Immune Globulin

Use Household and sexual contacts of persons with hepatitis A, measles, varicella, and possibly rubella; travelers to high-risk areas outside tourist routes; staff, attendees, and parents of diapered attendees in day-care center outbreaks

For travelers, IG is not an alternative to careful selection of foods and water; immune globulin can interfere with the antibody response to parenterally administered live virus vaccines. Frequent travelers should be tested for hepatitis A antibody, immune hemolytic anemia, and neutropenia (with ITP, I.V. route is usually used).

Local Anesthetic/Vasoconstrictor Precautions No information available to require special precautions

Effects on Dental Treatment No significant effects or complications reported

Significant Adverse Effects Frequency not defined.

- Cardiovascular: Flushing, angioedema
- Central nervous system: Chills, lethargy, fever
- Dermatologic: Urticaria, erythema
- Gastrointestinal: Nausea, vomiting
- Local: Pain, tenderness, muscle stiffness at I.M. site
- Neuromuscular & skeletal: Myalgia
- Miscellaneous: Hypersensitivity reactions

(Continued)

Immune Globulin (Intramuscular) *(Continued)*

Dosage I.M.:

Hepatitis A:

Pre-exposure prophylaxis upon travel into endemic areas (hepatitis A vaccine preferred):

0.02 mL/kg for anticipated risk 1-3 months

0.06 mL/kg for anticipated risk >3 months

Repeat approximate dose every 4-6 months if exposure continues

Postexposure prophylaxis: 0.02 mL/kg given within 7 days of exposure

Measles:

Prophylaxis: 0.25 mL/kg/dose (maximum dose: 15 mL) given within 6 days of exposure followed by live attenuated measles vaccine in 3 months or at 15 months of age (whichever is later)

For patients with leukemia, lymphoma, immunodeficiency disorders, generalized malignancy, or receiving immunosuppressive therapy: 0.5 mL/kg (maximum dose: 15 mL)

Poliomyelitis: Prophylaxis: 0.3 mL/kg/dose as a single dose

Rubella: Prophylaxis: 0.55 mL/kg/dose within 72 hours of exposure

Varicella: Prophylaxis: 0.6-1.2 mL/kg (varicella zoster immune globulin preferred) within 72 hours of exposure

IgG deficiency: 1.3 mL/kg, then 0.66 mL/kg in 3-4 weeks

Hepatitis B: Prophylaxis: 0.06 mL/kg/dose (HBIG preferred)

Mechanism of Action Provides passive immunity by increasing the antibody titer and antigen-antibody reaction potential

Contraindications Hypersensitivity to immune globulin, thimerosal, or any component of the formulation; IgA deficiency; I.M. injections in patients with thrombocytopenia or coagulation disorders

Warnings/Precautions Skin testing should not be performed as local irritation can occur and be misinterpreted as a positive reaction; IG should **not** be used to control outbreaks of measles. As a product of human plasma, this product may potentially transmit disease; screening of donors, as well as testing and/or inactivation of certain viruses reduces this risk. Epidemiologic and laboratory data indicate current IMIG products do not have a discernible risk of transmitting HIV. Use caution in patients with thrombocytopenia or coagulation disorders (I.M. injections may be contraindicated). Not for I.V. administration.

Drug Interactions Increased toxicity: Live virus, vaccines (measles, mumps, rubella); do not administer within 3 months after administration of these vaccines

Pharmacodynamics/Kinetics

Duration: Immune effect: Usually 3-4 weeks

Half-life elimination: 23 days

Time to peak, serum: I.M.: ~24-48 hours

Pregnancy Risk Factor C

Dosage Forms Injection, solution [preservative free]: 15% to 18% (2 mL, 10 mL)

Immune Globulin (Intravenous)

(i MYUN GLOB yoo lin, IN tra VEE nus)

Related Information

Systemic Viral Diseases *on page 1519*

U.S. Brand Names Carimune™; Flebogamma®; Gamimune® N; Gammagard® S/D; Gammar®-P I.V.; Gamunex®; Iveegam EN; Octagam®; Panglobulin®; Polygam® S/D; Venoglobulin®-S

Canadian Brand Names Gamimune® N; Gammagard® S/D; Gamunex®; Iveegam Immuno®

Generic Available No

Synonyms IVIG

Pharmacologic Category Immune Globulin

Use

Treatment of primary immunodeficiency syndromes (congenital agammaglobulinemia, severe combined immunodeficiency syndromes [SCIDS], common variable immunodeficiency, X-linked immunodeficiency, Wiskott-Aldrich syndrome); idiopathic thrombocytopenic purpura (ITP); Kawasaki disease (in combination with aspirin)

Prevention of bacterial infection in B-cell chronic lymphocytic leukemia (CLL); pediatric HIV infection; bone marrow transplant (BMT)

Unlabeled/Investigational Use Autoimmune diseases (myasthenia gravis, SLE, bullous pemphigoid, severe rheumatoid arthritis), Guillain-Barré syndrome; used in conjunction with appropriate anti-infective therapy to prevent or modify acute bacterial or viral infections in patients with iatrogenically-induced or disease-associated immunodepression; autoimmune hemolytic anemia or neutropenia, refractory dermatomyositis/polymyositis

Local Anesthetic/Vasoconstrictor Precautions No information available to require special precautions

Effects on Dental Treatment No significant effects or complications reported

Significant Adverse Effects Frequency not defined.

Cardiovascular: Flushing of the face, tachycardia, hypertension, hypotension, chest tightness, angioedema, lightheadedness, chest pain, myocardial infarction, CHF, pulmonary embolism

Central nervous system: Anxiety, chills, dizziness, drowsiness, fatigue, fever, headache, irritability, lethargy, malaise, aseptic meningitis syndrome

Dermatologic: Pruritus, rash, urticaria

Gastrointestinal: Abdominal cramps, diarrhea, nausea, sore throat, vomiting

Hematologic: Autoimmune hemolytic anemia, mild hemolysis

Hepatic: Liver function test increased

Local: Pain or irritation at the infusion site

Neuromuscular & skeletal: Arthralgia, back or hip pain, myalgia, nuchal rigidity

Ocular: Photophobia, painful eye movements

Renal: Acute renal failure, acute tubular necrosis, anuria, BUN increased, creatinine increased, nephrotic syndrome, oliguria, proximal tubular nephropathy, osmotic nephrosis

Respiratory: Cough, dyspnea, wheezing, nasal congestion, rhinorrhea, sinusitis

Miscellaneous: Diaphoresis, hypersensitivity reactions, anaphylaxis

Postmarketing and/or case reports: Abdominal pain, apnea, ARDS, bronchospasm, bullous dermatitis, cardiac arrest, Coombs' test positive, cyanosis, epidermolysis, erythema multiforme, hepatic dysfunction, hypoxemia, leukopenia, loss of consciousness, pancytopenia, pulmonary edema, rigors, seizure, Stevens-Johnson syndrome, thromboembolism, transfusion-related acute lung injury (TRALI), tremor, vascular collapse

Dosage Approved doses and regimens may vary between brands; check manufacturer guidelines. **Note:** Some clinicians dose IVIG on ideal body weight or an adjusted ideal body weight in morbidly obese patients. The volume of distribution of IVIG preparations in healthy subjects is similar to that observed with endogenous IgG. IVIG remains primarily in the intravascular space. Patients with congenital humoral immunodeficiencies appear to have about 70% of the IVIG available in the intravascular space.

Infants and Children: Prevention of gastroenteritis (unlabeled use): Oral: 50 mg/kg/day divided every 6 hours

Children: I.V.:

- Pediatric HIV: 400 mg/kg every 28 days
- Severe systemic viral and bacterial infections (unlabeled use): 500-1000 mg/kg/week

Children and Adults: I.V.:

- Primary immunodeficiency disorders: 200-400 mg/kg every 4 weeks or as per monitored serum IgG concentrations
  - Flebogamma®, Gamunex®, Octagam®: 300-600 mg/kg every 3-4 weeks; adjusted based on dosage and interval in conjunction with monitored serum IgG concentrations.
- B-cell chronic lymphocytic leukemia (CLL): 400 mg/kg/dose every 3 weeks
- Idiopathic thrombocytopenic purpura (ITP):
  - Acute: 400 mg/kg/day for 5 days or 1000 mg/kg/day for 1-2 days
  - Chronic: 400 mg/kg as needed to maintain platelet count >30,000/mm^3; may increase dose to 800 mg/kg (1000 mg/kg if needed)
- Kawasaki disease: Initiate therapy within 10 days of disease onset: 2 g/kg as a single dose administered over 10 hours, or 400 mg/kg/day for 4 days. **Note:** Must be used in combination with aspirin: 80-100 mg/kg/day in 4 divided doses for 14 days; when fever subsides, dose aspirin at 3-5 mg/kg once daily for ≥6-8 weeks
- Acquired immunodeficiency syndrome (patients must be symptomatic) (unlabeled use): Various regimens have been used, including:
  200-250 mg/kg/dose every 2 weeks
  or
  400-500 mg/kg/dose every month or every 4 weeks
- Autoimmune hemolytic anemia and neutropenia (unlabeled use): 1000 mg/kg/dose for 2-3 days
- Autoimmune diseases (unlabeled use): 400 mg/kg/day for 4 days
- Bone marrow transplant: 500 mg/kg beginning on days 7 and 2 pretransplant, then 500 mg/kg/week for 90 days post-transplant

(Continued)

Immune Globulin (Intravenous) *(Continued)*

Adjuvant to severe cytomegalovirus infections (unlabeled use): 500 mg/kg/dose every other day for 7 doses

Guillain-Barré syndrome (unlabeled use): Various regimens have been used, including:

400 mg/kg/day for 4 days

or

1000 mg/kg/day for 2 days

or

2000 mg/kg/day for one day

Refractory dermatomyositis (unlabeled use): 2 g/kg/dose every month x 3-4 doses

Refractory polymyositis (unlabeled use): 1 g/kg/day x 2 days every month x 4 doses

Chronic inflammatory demyelinating polyneuropathy (unlabeled use): Various regimens have been used, including:

400 mg/kg/day for 5 doses once each month

or

800 mg/kg/day for 3 doses once each month

or

1000 mg/kg/day for 2 days once each month

Dosing adjustment/comments in renal impairment: Cl_{cr} <10 mL/minute: Avoid use; in patients at risk of renal dysfunction, consider infusion at a rate less than maximum.

Mechanism of Action Replacement therapy for primary and secondary immunodeficiencies; interference with F_c receptors on the cells of the reticuloendothelial system for autoimmune cytopenias and ITP; possible role of contained antiviral-type antibodies

Contraindications Hypersensitivity to immune globulin or any component of the formulation; selective IgA deficiency

Warnings/Precautions Anaphylactic hypersensitivity reactions can occur, especially in IgA-deficient patients; studies indicate that the currently available products have no discernible risk of transmitting HIV or hepatitis B; aseptic meningitis may occur with high doses (≥2 g/kg). Use with caution in the elderly, patients with renal disease, diabetes mellitus, volume depletion, sepsis, paraproteinemia, and nephrotoxic medications due to risk of renal dysfunction. Patients should be adequately hydrated prior to therapy. Acute renal dysfunction (increased serum creatinine, oliguria, acute renal failure) can rarely occur; usually within 7 days of use (more likely with products stabilized with sucrose). Use caution in patients with a history of thrombotic events or cardiovascular disease; there is clinical evidence of a possible association between thrombotic events and administration of intravenous immune globulin. For intravenous administration only.

Drug Interactions Live virus, vaccines (eg, measles, mumps, rubella): May have impaired response to vaccines; separate administration by at least 3 months.

Dietary Considerations Octagam® contains sodium 30 mmol/L

Pharmacodynamics/Kinetics

Onset of action: I.V.: Provides immediate antibody levels

Duration: Immune effect: 3-4 weeks (variable)

Distribution: V_d: 0.09-0.13 L/kg

Intravascular portion: Healthy subjects: 41% to 57%; Patients with congenital humoral immunodeficiencies: ~70%

Half-life elimination: IgG (variable among patients): Healthy subjects: 14-24 days; Patients with congenital humoral immunodeficiencies: 26-40 days; hypermetabolism associated with fever and infection have coincided with a shortened half-life

Pregnancy Risk Factor C

Lactation Excretion in breast milk unknown

Dosage Forms

Injection, powder for reconstitution [preservative free]:

Carimune™, Panglobulin®: 1 g, 3 g, 6 g, 12 g

Gammar®-P I.V.: 1 g, 2.5 g, 5 g, 10 g [stabilized with human albumin and sucrose]

Iveegam EN: 0.5 g, 1 g, 2.5 g, 5 g [stabilized with glucose]

Injection, powder for reconstitution [preservative free, solvent detergent treated] (Gammagard® S/D): 2.5 g, 5 g, 10 g [stabilized with human albumin, glycine, glucose, and polyethylene glycol]

Injection, solution [preservative free; solvent detergent-treated]:

Gamimune® N: 10% [100 mg/mL] (10 mL, 50 mL, 100 mL, 200 mL)

Octagam®: 5% [50 mg/mL] (20 mL, 50 mL, 100 mL, 200 mL) [sucrose free; contains sodium 30 mmol/L and maltose]

Venoglobulin®-S: 5% [50 mg/mL] (50 mL, 100 mL, 200 mL); 10% [100 mg/mL] (50 mL, 100 mL, 200 mL) [stabilized with human albumin]

Injection, solution [preservative free]:

Flebogamma®: 5% (10 mL, 50 mL, 100 mL, 200 mL) [PEG precipitated/chromatography purified]

Gamunex®: 10% (10 mL, 25 mL, 50 mL, 100 mL, 200 mL) [caprylate/chromatography purified]

Immune Serum Globulin *see* Immune Globulin (Intramuscular) *on page 739*
Immunizations (Vaccines) *see page 1614*
Imodium® A-D [OTC] *see* Loperamide *on page 838*
Imogam® *see* Rabies Immune Globulin (Human) *on page 1165*
Imovax® Rabies *see* Rabies Virus Vaccine *on page 1165*
Imuran® *see* Azathioprine *on page 172*
In-111 Zevalin *see* Ibritumomab *on page 727*

Inamrinone (eye NAM ri none)

Related Information

Cardiovascular Diseases *on page 1458*

Generic Available Yes

Synonyms Amrinone Lactate

Pharmacologic Category Phosphodiesterase Enzyme Inhibitor

Use Infrequently used as a last resort, short-term therapy in patients with intractable heart failure

Local Anesthetic/Vasoconstrictor Precautions No information available to require special precautions

Effects on Dental Treatment No significant effects or complications reported

Common Adverse Effects

1% to 10%:

Cardiovascular: Arrhythmias (3%, especially in high-risk patients), hypotension (1% to 2%), (may be infusion rate-related)

Gastrointestinal: Nausea (1% to 2%)

Hematologic: Thrombocytopenia (may be dose-related)

Mechanism of Action Inhibits myocardial cyclic adenosine monophosphate (cAMP) phosphodiesterase activity and increases cellular levels of cAMP resulting in a positive inotropic effect and increased cardiac output; also possesses systemic and pulmonary vasodilator effects resulting in pre- and afterload reduction; slightly increases atrioventricular conduction

Drug Interactions

Increased Effect/Toxicity: Diuretics may cause significant hypovolemia and decrease filling pressure. Inotropic effects with digitalis are additive.

Pharmacodynamics/Kinetics

Onset of action: I.V.: 2-5 minutes

Peak effect: ~10 minutes

Duration (dose dependent): Low dose: ~30 minutes; Higher doses: ~2 hours

Half-life elimination, serum: Adults: Healthy volunteers: 3.6 hours, Congestive heart failure: 5.8 hours

Pregnancy Risk Factor C

Inapsine® *see* Droperidol *on page 477*

Indapamide (in DAP a mide)

Related Information

Cardiovascular Diseases *on page 1458*

U.S. Brand Names Lozol®

Canadian Brand Names Apo-Indapamide®; Gen-Indapamide; Lozide®; Lozol®; Novo-Indapamide; Nu-Indapamide; PMS-Indapamide

Generic Available Yes

Pharmacologic Category Diuretic, Thiazide-Related

Use Management of mild to moderate hypertension; treatment of edema in congestive heart failure and nephrotic syndrome

Local Anesthetic/Vasoconstrictor Precautions No information available to require special precautions

Effects on Dental Treatment Key adverse event(s) related to dental treatment: Orthostatic hypotension, palpitations, flushing, xerostomia (normal salivary flow resumes upon discontinuation), and rhinorrhea.

Common Adverse Effects 1% to 10%:

Cardiovascular: Orthostatic hypotension, palpitations (<5%), flushing

(Continued)

Indapamide *(Continued)*

Central nervous system: Dizziness (<5%), lightheadedness (<5%), vertigo (<5%), headache (≥5%), restlessness (<5%), drowsiness (<5%), fatigue, lethargy, malaise, lassitude, anxiety, agitation, depression, nervousness (≥5%)
Dermatologic: Rash (<5%), pruritus (<5%), hives (<5%)
Endocrine & metabolic: Hyperglycemia (<5%), hyperuricemia (<5%)
Gastrointestinal: Anorexia, gastric irritation, nausea, vomiting, abdominal pain, cramping, bloating, diarrhea, constipation, dry mouth, weight loss
Genitourinary: Nocturia, frequent urination, polyuria, impotence (<5%), reduced libido (<5%), glycosuria (<5%)
Neuromuscular & skeletal: Muscle cramps, spasm, weakness (≥5%)
Ocular: Blurred vision (<5%)
Renal: Necrotizing angiitis, vasculitis, cutaneous vasculitis (<5%)
Respiratory: Rhinorrhea (<5%)

Mechanism of Action Diuretic effect is localized at the proximal segment of the distal tubule of the nephron; it does not appear to have significant effect on glomerular filtration rate nor renal blood flow; like other diuretics, it enhances sodium, chloride, and water excretion by interfering with the transport of sodium ions across the renal tubular epithelium

Drug Interactions

Increased Effect/Toxicity: The diuretic effect of indapamide is synergistic with furosemide and other loop diuretics. Increased hypotension and/or renal adverse effects of ACE inhibitors may result in aggressively diuresed patients. Cyclosporine and thiazide-type diuretics can increase the risk of gout or renal toxicity. Digoxin toxicity can be exacerbated if a diuretic induces hypokalemia or hypomagnesemia. Lithium toxicity can occur with thiazide-type diuretics due to reduced renal excretion of lithium. Thiazide-type diuretics may prolong the duration of action of neuromuscular blocking agents.

Decreased Effect: Effects of oral hypoglycemics may be decreased. Decreased absorption of indapamide with cholestyramine and colestipol. NSAIDs can decrease the efficacy of thiazide-type diuretics, reducing the diuretic and antihypertensive effects.

Pharmacodynamics/Kinetics

Onset of action: 1-2 hours
Duration: ≤36 hours
Absorption: Complete
Protein binding, plasma: 71% to 79%
Metabolism: Extensively hepatic
Half-life elimination: 14-18 hours
Time to peak: 2-2.5 hours
Excretion: Urine (~60%) within 48 hours; feces (~16% to 23%)

Pregnancy Risk Factor B (manufacturer); D (expert analysis)

Inderal® *see* Propranolol *on page 1140*
Inderal® LA *see* Propranolol *on page 1140*
Inderide® *see* Propranolol and Hydrochlorothiazide *on page 1143*

Indinavir (in DIN a veer)

Related Information

HIV Infection and AIDS *on page 1484*
Tuberculosis *on page 1495*

U.S. Brand Names Crixivan®

Canadian Brand Names Crixivan®

Mexican Brand Names Crixivan®

Generic Available No

Synonyms Indinavir Sulfate

Pharmacologic Category Antiretroviral Agent, Protease Inhibitor

Use Treatment of HIV infection; should always be used as part of a multidrug regimen (at least three antiretroviral agents)

Local Anesthetic/Vasoconstrictor Precautions No information available to require special precautions

Effects on Dental Treatment Key adverse event(s) related to dental treatment: Abnormal taste.

Common Adverse Effects Protease inhibitors cause dyslipidemia which includes elevated cholesterol and triglycerides and a redistribution of body fat centrally to cause increased abdominal girth, buffalo hump, facial atrophy, and breast enlargement. These agents also cause hyperglycemia (exacerbation or new-onset diabetes).

10%:

Gastrointestinal: Nausea (12%)

Hepatic: Hyperbilirubinemia (14%)

Renal: Nephrolithiasis/urolithiasis (29%, pediatric patients; 12% adult patients)

1% to 10%:

Central nervous system: Headache (6%), insomnia (3%)

Gastrointestinal: Abdominal pain (9%), diarrhea/vomiting (4% to 5%), taste perversion (3%)

Neuromuscular & skeletal: Weakness (4%), flank pain (3%)

Renal: Hematuria

Mechanism of Action Indinavir is a human immunodeficiency virus protease inhibitor, binding to the protease activity site and inhibiting the activity of this enzyme. HIV protease is an enzyme required for the cleavage of viral polyprotein precursors into individual functional proteins found in infectious HIV. Inhibition prevents cleavage of these polyproteins resulting in the formation of immature noninfectious viral particles.

Drug Interactions

Cytochrome P450 Effect: Substrate of CYP2D6 (minor), 3A4 (major); **Inhibits** CYP2C8/9 (weak), 2C19 (weak), 2D6 (weak), 3A4 (strong)

Increased Effect/Toxicity: Indinavir may increase the levels/effects of selected benzodiazepines, calcium channel blockers, cyclosporine, mirtazapine, nateglinide, nefazodone, quinidine, sildenafil (and other PDE-5 inhibitors), tacrolimus, venlafaxine, and other CYP3A4 substrates. Selected benzodiazepines (midazolam, triazolam), cisapride, ergot alkaloids, selected HMG-CoA reductase inhibitors (lovastatin and simvastatin), mesoridazine, pimozide, and thioridazine are generally contraindicated with strong CYP3A4 inhibitors. When used with strong CYP3A4 inhibitors, dosage adjustment/limits are recommended for sildenafil and other PDE-5 inhibitors; refer to individual monographs.

Itraconazole or ketoconazole may increase the serum concentrations of indinavir; dosage adjustment is recommended. The levels/effects of indinavir may be increased by azole antifungals, ciprofloxacin, clarithromycin, diclofenac, doxycycline, erythromycin, imatinib, isoniazid, nefazodone, nicardipine, propofol, protease inhibitors, quinidine, verapamil, and other CYP3A4 inhibitors.

When used with delavirdine, serum levels of indinavir are increased; dosage adjustment of indinavir may be required for this combination. Serum levels of both nelfinavir and indinavir are increased with concurrent use. Serum concentrations of indinavir may be increased by ritonavir; serum levels of ritonavir and saquinavir may be increased; dosage adjustments of indinavir are required during concurrent therapy. Rifabutin serum concentrations has been increased when coadministered with indinavir; dosage adjustments of both agents required. Concurrent use or atazanavir with indinavir may increase the risk of hyperbilirubinemia.

Decreased Effect: The levels/effects of indinavir may be decreased by aminoglutethimide, carbamazepine, nafcillin, nevirapine, phenobarbital, phenytoin, rifamycins, and other CYP3A4 inducers; dosage adjustment may be recommended. Rifampin and/or St John's wort *(Hypericum perforatum)*; should not be used with indinavir.

Pharmacodynamics/Kinetics

Absorption: Administration with a high fat, high calorie diet resulted in a reduction in AUC and in maximum serum concentration (77% and 84% respectively); lighter meal resulted in little or no change in these parameters.

Protein binding, plasma: 60%

Metabolism: Hepatic via CYP3A4; seven metabolites of indinavir identified

Bioavailability: Good

Half-life elimination: 1.8 ± 0.4 hour

Time to peak: 0.8 ± 0.3 hour

Excretion: Urine and feces

Pregnancy Risk Factor C

Indinavir Sulfate *see* Indinavir *on page 744*

Indocin® *see* Indomethacin *on page 746*

Indocin® I.V. *see* Indomethacin *on page 746*

Indocin® SR *see* Indomethacin *on page 746*

Indocyanine Green (in doe SYE a neen green)

U.S. Brand Names IC-Green®

Generic Available No

Pharmacologic Category Diagnostic Agent

(Continued)

Indocyanine Green *(Continued)*

Use Determining hepatic function, cardiac output and liver blood flow and for ophthalmic angiography

Local Anesthetic/Vasoconstrictor Precautions No information available to require special precautions

Effects on Dental Treatment No significant effects or complications reported

Common Adverse Effects 1% to 10%:

Central nervous system: Headache

Dermatologic: Pruritus, skin discoloration

Miscellaneous: Diaphoresis, anaphylactoid reactions

Pregnancy Risk Factor C

Indometacin *see* Indomethacin *on page 746*

Indomethacin (in doe METH a sin)

Related Information

Rheumatoid Arthritis, Osteoarthritis, and Osteoporosis *on page 1490*

Temporomandibular Dysfunction (TMD) *on page 1564*

U.S. Brand Names Indocin®; Indocin® I.V.; Indocin® SR

Canadian Brand Names Apo-Indomethacin®; Indocid®; Indocid® P.D.A.; Indocin®; Indo-Lemmon; Indotec; Novo-Methacin; Nu-Indo; Rhodacine®

Mexican Brand Names Antalgin®; Indocid®; Malival®

Generic Available Yes: Capsule, suspension

Synonyms Indometacin; Indomethacin Sodium Trihydrate

Pharmacologic Category Nonsteroidal Anti-inflammatory Drug (NSAID), Oral; Nonsteroidal Anti-inflammatory Drug (NSAID), Parenteral

Use Management of inflammatory diseases and rheumatoid disorders; moderate pain; acute gouty arthritis, acute bursitis/tendonitis, moderate to severe osteoarthritis, rheumatoid arthritis, ankylosing spondylitis; I.V. form used as alternative to surgery for closure of patent ductus arteriosus in neonates

Local Anesthetic/Vasoconstrictor Precautions No information available to require special precautions

Effects on Dental Treatment NSAID formulations are known to reversibly decrease platelet aggregation via mechanisms different than observed with aspirin. The dentist should be aware of the potential of abnormal coagulation. Caution should also be exercised in the use of NSAIDs in patients already on anticoagulant therapy with drugs such as warfarin (Coumadin®).

Common Adverse Effects

>10%: Central nervous system: Headache (12%)

1% to 10%:

Central nervous system: Dizziness (3% to 9%), drowsiness (<1%), fatigue (<3%), vertigo (<3%), depression (<3%), malaise (<3%), somnolence (<3%)

Gastrointestinal: Nausea (3% to 9%), epigastric pain (3% to 9%), abdominal pain/cramps/distress (<3%), anorexia (<1%), GI bleeding (<1%), ulcers (<1%), perforation (<1%), heartburn (3% to 9%), indigestion (3% to 9%), constipation (<3%), diarrhea (<3%), dyspepsia (3% to 9%)

Hematologic: Inhibition of platelet aggregation (3% to 9%)

Otic: Tinnitus (<3%)

Mechanism of Action Inhibits prostaglandin synthesis by decreasing the activity of the enzyme, cyclooxygenase, which results in decreased formation of prostaglandin precursors

Drug Interactions

Cytochrome P450 Effect: Substrate (minor) of CYP2C8/9, 2C19; **Inhibits** CYP2C8/9 (strong), 2C19 (weak)

Increased Effect/Toxicity: Indomethacin may increase serum potassium with potassium-sparing diuretics. Probenecid may increase indomethacin serum concentrations. Other NSAIDs may increase GI adverse effects. May increase nephrotoxicity of cyclosporine and increase renal adverse effects of ACE inhibitors. Indomethacin may increase serum concentrations of digoxin, methotrexate, lithium, and aminoglycosides (reported with I.V. use in neonates). Indomethacin may increase the levels/effects of amiodarone, fluoxetine, glimepiride, glipizide, nateglinide, phenytoin, pioglitazone, rosiglitazone, sertraline, warfarin, and other CYP2C8/9 substrates.

Decreased Effect: May decrease antihypertensive effects of beta-blockers, hydralazine, ACE inhibitors, and angiotensin II antagonists. Indomethacin may decrease the antihypertensive and diuretic effect of thiazides (eg, hydrochlorothiazide) and loop diuretics (furosemide, bumetanide).

Pharmacodynamics/Kinetics

Onset of action: ~30 minutes

Duration: 4-6 hours

Absorption: Prompt and extensive

Distribution: V_d: 0.34-1.57 L/kg; crosses placenta; enters breast milk

Protein binding: 90%

Metabolism: Hepatic; significant enterohepatic recirculation

Half-life elimination: 4.5 hours; prolonged in neonates

Time to peak: Oral: ~3-4 hours

Excretion: Urine (primarily as glucuronide conjugates)

Pregnancy Risk Factor B/D (3rd trimester)

Indomethacin Sodium Trihydrate *see* Indomethacin *on page 746*

INF-alpha 2 *see* Interferon Alfa-2b *on page 752*

Infants' Tylenol® Cold Plus Cough Concentrated Drops [OTC] *see* Acetaminophen, Dextromethorphan, and Pseudoephedrine *on page 59*

Infasurf® *see* Calfactant *on page 247*

INFeD® *see* Iron Dextran Complex *on page 766*

Inflamase® Forte *see* PrednisoLONE *on page 1113*

Inflamase® Mild *see* PrednisoLONE *on page 1113*

Infliximab (in FLIKS e mab)

U.S. Brand Names Remicade®

Canadian Brand Names Remicade®

Generic Available No

Synonyms Infliximab, Recombinant

Pharmacologic Category Antirheumatic, Disease Modifying; Gastrointestinal Agent, Miscellaneous; Monoclonal Antibody

Use

Crohn's disease: Induction and maintenance of remission in patients with moderate to severe disease who have an inadequate response to conventional therapy; to reduce the number of draining enterocutaneous and rectovaginal fistulas and to maintain fistula closure

Rheumatoid arthritis: Inhibits the progression of structural damage and improves physical function in patients with moderate to severe disease; used with methotrexate in patients who have had an inadequate response to methotrexate alone

Local Anesthetic/Vasoconstrictor Precautions No information available to require special precautions

Effects on Dental Treatment No significant effects or complications reported

Common Adverse Effects Note: Although profile is similar, frequency of effects may be different in specific populations (Crohn's disease vs rheumatoid arthritis). Percentages reported with rheumatoid arthritis:

>10%:

Central nervous system: Headache (29%), fatigue (13%), fever (13%)

Dermatologic: Rash (18%)

Gastrointestinal: Nausea (24%), diarrhea (19%), abdominal pain (17%)

Genitourinary: Urinary tract infection (14%)

Local: Infusion reactions (20%)

Neuromuscular & skeletal: Arthralgia (13%), back pain (13%)

Respiratory: Upper respiratory tract infection (40%), cough (18%), sinusitis (20%), pharyngitis (17%)

Miscellaneous: Development of antinuclear antibodies (52%), infections (35%), development of antibodies to double-stranded DNA (17%); Crohn's patients with fistulizing disease: Development of new abscess (15%)

2% to 10%:

Cardiovascular: Chest pain (7%), hypertension (10%)

Central nervous system: Depression (8%), insomnia (6%)

Dermatologic: Pruritus (9%)

Gastrointestinal: Dyspepsia (10%)

Respiratory: Bronchitis, dyspnea (6%)

Miscellaneous: Moniliasis (8%), abscess (6%)

Mechanism of Action Infliximab is a chimeric monoclonal antibody that binds to human tumor necrosis factor alpha (TNFα), thereby interfering with endogenous TNFα activity. Biological activities of TNFα include the induction of pro-inflammatory cytokines (interleukins), enhancement of leukocyte migration, activation of neutrophils and eosinophils, and the induction of acute phase reactants and tissue degrading enzymes. Animal models have shown TNFα expression causes polyarthritis, and infliximab can prevent disease as well as allow diseased joints to heal.

(Continued)

Infliximab *(Continued)*

Drug Interactions

Increased Effect/Toxicity: Specific drug interaction studies have not been conducted.

Decreased Effect: Specific drug interaction studies have not been conducted.

Decreased toxicity: Immunosuppressants: When used with infliximab, may decrease the risk of infusion related reactions, and may decrease development of anti-double-stranded DNA antibodies

Pharmacodynamics/Kinetics

Onset of action: Crohn's disease: ~2 weeks

Half-life elimination: 8-9.5 days

Pregnancy Risk Factor B (manufacturer)

Infliximab, Recombinant *see* Infliximab *on page 747*

Influenza Virus Vaccine (in floo EN za VYE rus vak SEEN)

Related Information

Immunizations (Vaccines) *on page 1614*

U.S. Brand Names FluMist™; Fluvirin®; Fluzone®

Canadian Brand Names Fluviral S/F®; Fluzone®; Vaxigrip®

Generic Available No

Synonyms Influenza Virus Vaccine (Purified Surface Antigen); Influenza Virus Vaccine (Split-Virus); Influenza Virus Vaccine (Trivalent, Live)

Pharmacologic Category Vaccine

Use Provide active immunity to influenza virus strains contained in the vaccine

Groups at Increased Risk for Influenza-Related Complications:

- Persons ≥65 years of age
- Residents of nursing homes and other chronic-care facilities that house persons of any age with chronic medical conditions
- Adults and children with chronic disorders of the pulmonary or cardiovascular systems, including children with asthma
- Adults and children who have required regular medical follow-up or hospitalization during the preceding year because of chronic metabolic diseases (including diabetes mellitus), renal dysfunction, hemoglobinopathies, or immunosuppression (including immunosuppression caused by medications)
- Children and adolescents (6 months to 18 years of age) who are receiving long-term aspirin therapy and therefore, may be at risk for developing Reye's syndrome after influenza
- Women who will be pregnant during the influenza season
- Children 6-23 months of age

Vaccination is also recommended for persons 50-64 years of age, close contacts of children 0-23 months of age, and healthy persons who may transmit influenza to those at risk.

Local Anesthetic/Vasoconstrictor Precautions No information available to require special precautions

Effects on Dental Treatment No significant effects or complications reported

Common Adverse Effects All serious adverse reactions must be reported to the U.S. Department of Health and Human Services (DHHS) Vaccine Adverse Event Reporting System (VAERS) 1-800-822-7967.

Injection: Frequency not defined:

Central nervous system: Fever and malaise (may start within 6-12 hours and last 1-2 days; incidence equal to placebo in adults; occurs more frequently than placebo in children); GBS (previously reported with older vaccine formulations; relationship to current formulations not known, however, patients with history of GBS have a greater likelihood of developing GBS than those without)

Dermatologic: Angioedema, urticaria

Local: Tenderness, redness, or induration at the site of injection (10% to 64%; may last up to 2 days)

Neuromuscular & skeletal: Myalgia (may start within 6-12 hours and last 1-2 days; incidence equal to placebo in adults; occurs more frequently than placebo in children)

Miscellaneous: Allergic or anaphylactoid reactions (most likely to residual egg protein; includes allergic asthma, angioedema, hives, systemic anaphylaxis)

Nasal spray: **Note:** Frequency of events reported within 10 days

>10%:

Central nervous system: Headache (children 18% after first dose, < placebo after second dose; adults 40%) irritability (children 10% to 19%)

Neuromuscular & skeletal: Tiredness/weakness (adults 26%), muscle aches (children 5% to 6%; adults 17%)

Respiratory: Cough, nasal congestion/ runny nose (children 46% to 48%; adults 9% to 45%), sore throat (children < placebo; adults 28%)

Miscellaneous: Activity decreased (children 14% after first dose, < placebo after second dose)

1% to 10%:

Central nervous system: Chills,

Gastrointestinal: Abdominal pain, diarrhea, vomiting

Otic: Otitis media

Mechanism of Action Promotes immunity to influenza virus by inducing specific antibody production. Each year the formulation is standardized according to the U.S. Public Health Service. Preparations from previous seasons must not be used.

Drug Interactions

Increased Effect/Toxicity: Concomitant use of aspirin and the nasal spray formulation may increase the risk of Reye syndrome in patients 5-17 years; concomitant use in this age group is contraindicated.

Decreased Effect: Decreased effect with immunosuppressive agents; some manufacturers and clinicians recommend that the flu vaccine not be administered concomitantly with DTP due to the potential for increased febrile reactions (specifically whole-cell pertussis) and that one should wait at least 3 days. However, ACIP recommends that children at high risk for influenza may get the vaccine concomitantly with DTP. Safety and efficacy of nasal spray with other vaccines have not been established; do not give within 1 month of other live virus vaccines or within 2 weeks of inactivated or subunit vaccines.

Pharmacodynamics/Kinetics

Onset: Protective antibody levels achieved ~2 weeks after vaccination

Duration: Protective antibody levels persist approximately ≥6 months

Pregnancy Risk Factor C

Influenza Virus Vaccine (Purified Surface Antigen) *see* Influenza Virus Vaccine *on page 748*

Influenza Virus Vaccine (Split-Virus) *see* Influenza Virus Vaccine *on page 748*

Influenza Virus Vaccine (Trivalent, Live) *see* Influenza Virus Vaccine *on page 748*

Infumorph® *see* Morphine Sulfate *on page 947*

INH *see* Isoniazid *on page 769*

Innohep® *see* Tinzaparin *on page 1301*

InnoPran XL™ *see* Propranolol *on page 1140*

INOmax® *see* Nitric Oxide *on page 990*

Insect Sting Kit *see* Epinephrine and Chlorpheniramine *on page 497*

Insoluble Prussian Blue *see* Ferric Hexacyanoferrate *on page 585*

Inspra™ *see* Eplerenone *on page 498*

Insta-Glucose® [OTC] *see* Glucose (Instant) *on page 663*

Insulin Preparations (IN su lin prep a RAY shuns)

Related Information

Endocrine Disorders and Pregnancy *on page 1481*

U.S. Brand Names Apidra™; Humalog®; Humalog® Mix 75/25™; Humulin® 50/50; Humulin® 70/30; Humulin® L; Humulin® N; Humulin® R; Humulin® R (Concentrated) U-500; Humulin® U; Lantus®; Lente® Iletin® II [DSC]; Novolin® 70/30; Novolin® L [DSC]; Novolin® N; Novolin® R; NovoLog®; NovoLog® Mix 70/30; NPH Iletin® II; Regular Iletin® II; Velosulin® BR (Buffered) [DSC]

Canadian Brand Names Humalog®; Humalog® Mix 25™; Humulin®; Iletin® II Pork; Novolin® ge; NovoRapid®

Mexican Brand Names Humulin 20/80® [biosyn./ 20% sol./80% isoph.]; Humulin 30/70® [biosyn./ 30% sol./70% isoph.]; Humulin L® [biosyn.]; Humulin N® [biosyn.]; Insulin Novolin 30/70® [biosyn./ 30% sol./70% isoph.]; Insulin Novolin L® [biosyn.]; Insulin Novolin N® [biosyn.]

Generic Available No

Synonyms Aspart, Insulin; Glargine, Insulin; Glulisine, Insulin; Lente, Insulin; Lispro, Insulin; NPH, Insulin; Regular, Insulin

Pharmacologic Category Antidiabetic Agent, Insulin; Antidote

(Continued)

Insulin Preparations *(Continued)*

Use Treatment of type 1 diabetes mellitus (insulin dependent, IDDM); type 2 diabetes mellitus (noninsulin dependent, NIDDM) unresponsive to treatment with diet and/or oral hypoglycemics; adjunct to parenteral nutrition

Unlabeled/Investigational Use Hyperkalemia (regular insulin only; use with glucose to shift potassium into cells to lower serum potassium levels)

Local Anesthetic/Vasoconstrictor Precautions No information available to require special precautions

Effects on Dental Treatment Type 1 diabetics (insulin-dependent) should be appointed for dental treatment in the morning in order to minimize chance of stress-induced hypoglycemia.

Common Adverse Effects Frequency not defined.

Cardiovascular: Palpitation, tachycardia, pallor

Central nervous system: Fatigue, mental confusion, loss of consciousness, headache, hypothermia

Dermatologic: Urticaria, redness

Endocrine & metabolic: Hypoglycemia

Gastrointestinal: Hunger, nausea, numbness of mouth

Local: Itching, edema, stinging, pain or warmth at injection site; atrophy or hypertrophy of SubQ fat tissue

Neuromuscular & skeletal: Muscle weakness, paresthesia, tremors

Ocular: Transient presbyopia or blurred vision

Miscellaneous: Diaphoresis, anaphylaxis, local allergy, systemic allergic symptoms

Mechanism of Action The principal hormone required for proper glucose utilization in normal metabolic processes; it is obtained from beef or pork pancreas or a biosynthetic process converting pork insulin to human insulin; insulins are categorized into 3 groups related to promptness, duration, and intensity of action

Drug Interactions

Cytochrome P450 Effect: Induces CYP1A2 (weak)

Increased Effect/Toxicity: Increased hypoglycemic effect of insulin with alcohol, alpha-blockers, anabolic steroids, beta-blockers (nonselective beta-blockers may delay recovery from hypoglycemic episodes and mask signs/symptoms of hypoglycemia; cardioselective beta-blocker agents may be alternatives), clofibrate, guanethidine, MAO inhibitors, pentamidine, phenylbutazone, salicylates, sulfinpyrazone, and tetracyclines.

Insulin increases the risk of hypoglycemia associated with oral hypoglycemic agents (including sulfonylureas, metformin, pioglitazone, rosiglitazone, and troglitazone).

Decreased Effect: Decreased hypoglycemic effect of insulin with corticosteroids, dextrothyroxine, diltiazem, dobutamine, epinephrine, niacin, oral contraceptives, thiazide diuretics, thyroid hormone, and smoking.

Pharmacodynamics/Kinetics

Onset of action and duration: Biosynthetic NPH human insulin shows a more rapid onset and shorter duration of action than corresponding porcine insulins; human insulin and purified porcine regular insulin are similarly efficacious following SubQ administration. The duration of action of highly purified porcine insulins is shorter than that of conventional insulin equivalents. Duration depends on type of preparation and route of administration as well as patient-related variables. In general, the larger the dose of insulin, the longer the duration of activity.

Absorption: Biosynthetic regular human insulin is absorbed from the SubQ injection site more rapidly than insulins of animal origin (60-90 minutes peak vs 120-150 minutes peak respectively) and lowers the initial blood glucose much faster. Human Ultralente® insulin is absorbed about twice as quickly as its bovine equivalent, and bioavailability is also improved. Human Lente® insulin preparations are also absorbed more quickly than their animal equivalents. Insulin glargine (Lantus®) is designed to form microprecipitates when injected subcutaneously. Small amounts of insulin glargine are then released over a 24-hour period, with no pronounced peak. Insulin glargine (Lantus®) for the treatment of type 1 diabetes (insulin dependent, IDDM) and type 2 diabetes mellitus (noninsulin dependent, NIDDM) in patients who require basal (long-acting) insulin.

Bioavailability: Medium-acting SubQ Lente®-type human insulins did not differ from the corresponding porcine insulins

Insulin aspart (NovoLog®):

Onset: 0.17-0.33 hours; Peak effect: 1-3 hours; Duration: 3-5 hours

Insulin lispro (Humalog®), insulin glulisine (Apidra™):
Onset: 0.25 hours; Peak effect: 0.5-1.5 hours; Duration: 6-8 hours
Insulin, regular (Novolin® R):
Onset: 0.5-1 hours; Peak effect: 2-3 hours; Duration: 8-12 hours
Isophane insulin suspension (NPH) (Novolin® N):
Onset: 1-1.5 hours; Peak effect: 4-12 hours; Duration: 24 hours
Insulin zinc suspension (Lente®):
Onset: 1-2.5 hours; Peak effect: 8-12 hours; Duration: 18-24 hours
Isophane insulin suspension and regular insulin injection (Novolin® 70/30):
Onset: 0.5 hours; Peak effect: 2-12 hours; Duration: 24 hours
Extended insulin zinc suspension (Ultralente®):
Onset: 4-8 hours; Peak effect: 16-18 hours; Duration: >36 hours
Insulin glargine (Lantus®):
Duration: 24 hours

Pregnancy Risk Factor B; C (insulin glargine [Lantus®]; insulin aspart [NovoLog®])

Intal® *see* Cromolyn *on page 378*
Integrilin® *see* Eptifibatide *on page 503*
α-2-interferon *see* Interferon Alfa-2b *on page 752*

Interferon Alfa-2a (in ter FEER on AL fa too aye)

Related Information
Systemic Viral Diseases *on page 1519*

U.S. Brand Names Roferon-A®

Canadian Brand Names Roferon-A®

Generic Available No

Synonyms IFLrA; rIFN-A

Pharmacologic Category Interferon

Use
Patients >18 years of age: Hairy cell leukemia, AIDS-related Kaposi's sarcoma, chronic hepatitis C
Children and Adults: Chronic myelogenous leukemia (CML), Philadelphia chromosome positive, within 1 year of diagnosis (limited experience in children)

Unlabeled/Investigational Use Adjuvant therapy for malignant melanoma, AIDS-related thrombocytopenia, cutaneous ulcerations of Behçet's disease, brain tumors, metastatic ileal carcinoid tumors, cervical and colorectal cancers, genital warts, idiopathic mixed cryoglobulinemia, hemangioma, hepatitis D, hepatocellular carcinoma, idiopathic hypereosinophilic syndrome, mycosis fungoides, Sézary syndrome, low-grade non-Hodgkin's lymphoma, macular degeneration, multiple myeloma, renal cell carcinoma, basal and squamous cell skin cancer, essential thrombocythemia, cutaneous T-cell lymphoma

Local Anesthetic/Vasoconstrictor Precautions No information available to require special precautions

Effects on Dental Treatment Key adverse event(s) related to dental treatment: Significant xerostomia (normal salivary flow resumes upon discontinuation), metallic taste, taste change, loss of taste, cough, irritation of oropharynx.

Common Adverse Effects Note: A flu-like syndrome (fever, chills, tachycardia, malaise, myalgia, arthralgia, headache) occurs within 1-2 hours of administration; may last up to 24 hours and may be dose-limiting (symptoms in up to 92% of patients). For the listing below, the percentage of incidence noted generally corresponds to highest reported ranges. Incidence depends upon dosage and indication.

>10%:
Cardiovascular: Chest pain (4% to 11%), edema (11%), hypertension (11%)
Central nervous system: Psychiatric disturbances (including depression and suicidal behavior/ideation; reported incidence highly variable, generally >15%), fatigue (90%), headache (52%), dizziness (21%), irritability (15%), insomnia (14%), somnolence, lethargy, confusion, mental impairment, and motor weakness (most frequently seen at high doses [>100 million units], usually reverses within a few days); vertigo (19%); mental status changes (12%)
Dermatologic: Rash (usually maculopapular) on the trunk and extremities (7% to 18%), alopecia (19% to 22%), pruritus (13%), dry skin
Endocrine & metabolic: Hypocalcemia (10% to 51%), hyperglycemia (33% to 39%), elevation of transaminase levels (25% to 30%), elevation of alkaline phosphatase (48%)
Gastrointestinal: Loss of taste, anorexia (30% to 70%), nausea (28% to 53%), vomiting (10% to 30%, usually mild), diarrhea (22% to 34%, may be

(Continued)

Interferon Alfa-2a *(Continued)*

severe), taste change (13%), dry throat, xerostomia, abdominal cramps, abdominal pain

Hematologic (often due to underlying disease): Myelosuppression; neutropenia (32% to 70%); thrombocytopenia (22% to 70%); anemia (24% to 65%, may be dose-limiting, usually seen only during the first 6 months of therapy)

Onset: 7-10 days

Nadir: 14 days, may be delayed 20-40 days in hairy cell leukemia

Recovery: 21 days

Hepatic: Elevation of AST (SGOT) (77% to 80%), LDH (47%), bilirubin (31%)

Local: Injection site reaction (29%)

Neuromuscular & skeletal: Weakness (may be severe at doses >20,000,000 units/day); arthralgia and myalgia (5% to 73%, usually during the first 72 hours of treatment); rigors

Renal: Proteinuria (15% to 25%)

Respiratory: Cough (27%), irritation of oropharynx (14%)

Miscellaneous: Flu-like syndrome (up to 92% of patients), diaphoresis (15%)

1% to 10%:

Cardiovascular: Hypotension (6%), supraventricular tachyarrhythmias, palpitations (<3%), acute myocardial infarction (<1% to 1%)

Central nervous system: Confusion (10%), delirium

Dermatologic: Erythema (diffuse), urticaria

Endocrine & metabolic: Hyperphosphatemia (2%)

Gastrointestinal: Stomatitis, pancreatitis (<5%), flatulence, liver pain

Genitourinary: Impotence (6%), menstrual irregularities

Neuromuscular & skeletal: Leg cramps; peripheral neuropathy, paresthesias (7%), and numbness (4%) are more common in patients previously treated with vinca alkaloids or receiving concurrent vinblastine

Ocular: Conjunctivitis (4%)

Respiratory: Dyspnea (7.5%), epistaxis (4%), rhinitis (3%)

Miscellaneous: Antibody production to interferon (10%)

Mechanism of Action Following activation, multiple effects can be detected including induction of gene transcription. Inhibits cellular growth, alters the state of cellular differentiation, interferes with oncogene expression, alters cell surface antigen expression, increases phagocytic activity of macrophages, and augments cytotoxicity of lymphocytes for target cells

Drug Interactions

Cytochrome P450 Effect: Inhibits CYP1A2 (weak)

Increased Effect/Toxicity: Theophylline clearance has been reported to be decreased in hepatitis patients receiving interferon. Interferons may increase the adverse/toxic effects of ACE inhibitors, specifically the development of granulocytopenia. Agranulocytosis has been reported with concurrent use of clozapine (case report). Interferons may increase the anticoagulant effects of warfarin, and interferons may increase serum levels of zidovudine.

Decreased Effect: Prednisone may decrease the therapeutic effects of interferon alpha. A decreased response to erythropoietin has been reported (case reports) in patients receiving interferons. Interferon alpha may decrease the serum concentrations of melphalan (may or may not decrease toxicity of melphalan).

Pharmacodynamics/Kinetics

Absorption: Filtered and absorbed at the renal tubule

Distribution: V_d: 0.223-0.748 L/kg

Metabolism: Primarily renal; filtered through glomeruli and undergoes rapid proteolytic degradation during tubular reabsorption

Bioavailability: I.M.: 83%; SubQ: 90%

Half-life elimination: I.V.: 3.7-8.5 hours (mean ~5 hours)

Time to peak, serum: I.M., SubQ: ~6-8 hours

Pregnancy Risk Factor C

Interferon Alfa-2a (PEG Conjugate) *see* Peginterferon Alfa-2a *on page 1052*

Interferon Alfa-2b (in ter FEER on AL fa too bee)

Related Information

Systemic Viral Diseases *on page 1519*

U.S. Brand Names Intron® A

Canadian Brand Names Intron® A

Generic Available No

Synonyms INF-alpha 2; α-2-interferon; rLFN-α2

Pharmacologic Category Interferon

Use

Patients ≥1 year of age: Chronic hepatitis B

Patients ≥18 years of age: Condyloma acuminata, chronic hepatitis C, hairy cell leukemia, malignant melanoma, AIDS-related Kaposi's sarcoma, follicular non-Hodgkin's lymphoma

Unlabeled/Investigational Use AIDS-related thrombocytopenia, cutaneous ulcerations of Behçet's disease, carcinoid syndrome, cervical cancer, lymphomatoid granulomatosis, genital herpes, hepatitis D, chronic myelogenous leukemia (CML), non-Hodgkin's lymphomas (other than follicular lymphoma, see approved use), polycythemia vera, medullary thyroid carcinoma, multiple myeloma, renal cell carcinoma, basal and squamous cell skin cancers, essential thrombocytopenia, thrombocytopenic purpura

Investigational: West Nile virus

Local Anesthetic/Vasoconstrictor Precautions No information available to require special precautions

Effects on Dental Treatment Key adverse event(s) related to dental treatment: Xerostomia (normal salivary flow resumes upon discontinuation) and metallic taste.

Common Adverse Effects Note: In a majority of patients, a flu-like syndrome (fever, chills, tachycardia, malaise, myalgia, headache), occurs within 1-2 hours of administration; may last up to 24 hours and may be dose-limiting.

>10%:

Cardiovascular: Chest pain (2% to 28%)

Central nervous system: Fatigue (8% to 96%), headache (21% to 62%), fever (34% to 94%), depression (4% to 40%), somnolence (1% to 33%), irritability (1% to 22%), paresthesia (1% to 21%, more common in patients previously treated with vinca alkaloids or receiving concurrent vinblastine), dizziness (7% to 23%), confusion (1% to 12%), malaise (3% to 14%), pain (3% to 15%), insomnia (1% to 12%), impaired concentration (1% to 14%, usually reverses within a few days), amnesia (1% to 14%), chills (45% to 54%),

Dermatologic: Alopecia (8% to 38%), rash (usually maculopapular) on the trunk and extremities (1% to 25%), pruritus (3% to 11%), dry skin (1% to 10%)

Endocrine & metabolic: Hypocalcemia (10% to 51%), hyperglycemia (33% to 39%), amenorrhea (up to 12% in lymphoma)

Gastrointestinal: Anorexia (1% to 69%), nausea (19% to 66%), vomiting (2% to 32%, usually mild), diarrhea (2% to 45%, may be severe), taste change (2% to 24%), xerostomia (1% to 28%), abdominal pain (2% to 23%), gingivitis (2% to 14%), constipation (1% to 14%)

Hematologic: Myelosuppression; neutropenia (30% to 66%); thrombocytopenia (5% to 15%); anemia (15% to 32%, may be dose-limiting, usually seen only during the first 6 months of therapy)

Onset: 7-10 days

Nadir: 14 days, may be delayed 20-40 days in hairy cell leukemia

Recovery: 21 days

Hepatic: Increased transaminases (increased SGOT in up to 63%), elevation of alkaline phosphatase (48%), right upper quadrant pain (15% in hepatitis C)

Local: Injection site reaction (1% to 20%)

Neuromuscular & skeletal: Weakness (5% to 63%) may be severe at doses >20,000,000 units/day; mild arthralgia and myalgia (5% to 75% - usually during the first 72 hours of treatment), rigors (2% to 42%), back pain (1% to 19%), musculoskeletal pain (1% to 21%), paresthesia (1% to 21%)

Renal: Urinary tract infection (up to 5% in hepatitis C)

Respiratory: Dyspnea (1% to 34%), cough (1% to 31%), pharyngitis (1% to 31%),

Miscellaneous: Loss of smell, flu-like symptoms (5% to 79%), diaphoresis (2% to 21%)

5% to 10%:

Cardiovascular: Hypertension (9% in hepatitis C)

Central nervous system: Anxiety (1% to 9%), nervousness (1% to 3%), vertigo (up to 8% in lymphoma)

Dermatologic: Dermatitis (1% to 8%)

Endocrine & metabolic: Decreased libido (1% to 5%)

Gastrointestinal: Loose stools (1% to 21%), dyspepsia (2% to 8%)

Neuromuscular & skeletal: Hypoesthesia (1% to 10%)

Respiratory: Nasal congestion (1% to 10%)

Mechanism of Action Following activation, multiple effects can be detected including induction of gene transcription. Inhibits cellular growth, alters the state of cellular differentiation, interferes with oncogene expression, alters cell

(Continued)

Interferon Alfa-2b *(Continued)*

surface antigen expression, increases phagocytic activity of macrophages, and augments cytotoxicity of lymphocytes for target cells

Drug Interactions

Cytochrome P450 Effect: Inhibits CYP1A2 (weak)

Increased Effect/Toxicity: Theophylline clearance has been reported to be decreased in hepatitis patients receiving interferon. Interferons may increase the adverse/toxic effects of ACE inhibitors, specifically the development of granulocytopenia. Agranulocytosis has been reported with concurrent use of clozapine (case report). Interferons may increase the anticoagulant effects of warfarin, and interferons may increase serum levels of zidovudine.

Pharmacodynamics/Kinetics

Distribution: V_d: 31 L; but has been noted to be much greater (370-720 L) in leukemia patients receiving continuous infusion IFN; IFN does not penetrate the CSF

Metabolism: Primarily renal

Bioavailability: I.M.: 83%; SubQ: 90%

Half-life elimination: I.M., I.V.: 2 hours; SubQ: 3 hours

Time to peak, serum: I.M., SubQ: ~3-12 hours

Pregnancy Risk Factor C

Interferon Alfa-2b and Ribavirin

(in ter FEER on AL fa too bee & rye ba VYE rin)

Related Information

Interferon Alfa-2b *on page 752*

Ribavirin *on page 1177*

U.S. Brand Names Rebetron®

Canadian Brand Names Rebetron®

Generic Available No

Synonyms Interferon Alfa-2b and Ribavirin Combination Pack; Ribavirin and Interferon Alfa-2b Combination Pack

Pharmacologic Category Antiviral Agent; Interferon

Use Combination therapy for the treatment of chronic hepatitis C in patients with compensated liver disease previously untreated with alpha interferon or who have relapsed after alpha interferon therapy

Local Anesthetic/Vasoconstrictor Precautions No information available to require special precautions

Effects on Dental Treatment Key adverse event(s) related to dental treatment: Xerostomia (normal salivary flow resumes upon discontinuation), metallic taste, and taste perversion.

Common Adverse Effects Note: Adverse reactions listed are specific to combination regimen in previously untreated hepatitis patients. See individual agents for additional adverse reactions reported with each agent during therapy for other diseases.

>10%:

- Central nervous system: Fatigue (children 61%; adults 68%), headache (63%), insomnia (children 14%; adults 39%), fever (children 61%; adults 37%), depression (children 13%; adults 32% to 36%), irritability (children 10%; adults 23% to 32%), dizziness (17% to 23%), emotional lability (children 16%; adults 7% to 11%), impaired concentration (5% to 14%)
- Dermatologic: Alopecia (23% to 32%), pruritus (children 12%; adults 19% to 21%), rash (17% to 28%)
- Gastrointestinal: Nausea (33% to 46%), anorexia (children 51%; adults 25% to 27%), dyspepsia (children <1%; adults 14% to 16%), vomiting (children 42%; adults 9% to 11%)
- Hematologic: Leukopenia, neutropenia (usually recovers within 4 weeks of treatment discontinuation), anemia
- Hepatic: Hyperbilirubinemia (27%; only 0.9% to 2% >3.0-6 mg/dL)
- Local: Injection site inflammation (13%)
- Neuromuscular & skeletal: Myalgia (children 32%; adults 61% to 64%), rigors (40%), arthralgia (children 15%; adults 30% to 33%), musculoskeletal pain (20% to 28%)
- Respiratory: Dyspnea (children 5%; adults 18% to 19%)
- Miscellaneous: Flu-like syndrome (children 31%; adults 14% to 18%)

1% to 10%:

- Cardiovascular: Chest pain (5% to 9%)
- Central nervous system: Nervousness (3% to 4%)
- Endocrine & metabolic: Thyroid abnormalities (hyper- or hypothyroidism), serum uric acid increased, hyperglycemia
- Gastrointestinal: Taste perversion (children <1%; adults 7% to 8%)

Hematologic: Hemolytic anemia (10%), thrombocytopenia, anemia
Local: Injection site reaction (7%)
Neuromuscular & skeletal: Weakness (5% to 9%)
Respiratory: Sinusitis (children <1%; adults 9% to 10%)

Mechanism of Action

Interferon Alfa-2b: Alpha interferons are a family of proteins, produced by nucleated cells, that have antiviral, antiproliferative, and immune-regulating activity. There are 16 known subtypes of alpha interferons. Interferons interact with cells through high affinity cell surface receptors. Following activation, multiple effects can be detected including induction of gene transcription. Inhibits cellular growth, alters the state of cellular differentiation, interferes with oncogene expression, alters cell surface antigen expression, increases phagocytic activity of macrophages, and augments cytotoxicity of lymphocytes for target cells

Ribavirin: Inhibits replication of RNA and DNA viruses; inhibits influenza virus RNA polymerase activity and inhibits the initiation and elongation of RNA fragments resulting in inhibition of viral protein synthesis

Drug Interactions

Cytochrome P450 Effect: Interferon Alfa-2b: **Inhibits** CYP1A2 (weak)

Increased Effect/Toxicity: Interferon alpha: Cimetidine may augment the antitumor effects of interferon in melanoma. Theophylline clearance has been reported to be decreased in hepatitis patients receiving interferon. Vinblastine enhances interferon toxicity in several patients; increased incidence of paresthesia has also been noted. Interferons may increase the adverse/toxic effects of ACE inhibitors, specifically the development of granulocytopenia. Agranulocytosis has been reported with concurrent use of clozapine (case report). Interferons may increase the anticoagulant effects of warfarin, and interferons may increase serum levels of zidovudine. Concomitant use of ribavirin and nucleoside analogues may increase the risk of developing lactic acidosis.

Decreased Effect:

Interferon alpha: Prednisone may decrease the therapeutic effects of interferon alpha. A decreased response to erythropoietin has been reported (case reports) in patients receiving interferons. Interferon alpha may decrease the serum concentrations of melphalan (may or may not decrease toxicity of melphalan). Thyroid dysfunction has been reported during treatment; monitor response to thyroid hormones.

Ribavirin: Decreased effect of stavudine and zidovudine.

Pharmacodynamics/Kinetics See individual agents.

Pregnancy Risk Factor X

Interferon Alfa-2b and Ribavirin Combination Pack *see* Interferon Alfa-2b and Ribavirin *on page 754*

Interferon Alfa-2b (PEG Conjugate) *see* Peginterferon Alfa-2b *on page 1053*

Interferon Alfa-n3 (in ter FEER on AL fa en three)

Related Information

Systemic Viral Diseases *on page 1519*

U.S. Brand Names Alferon® N

Canadian Brand Names Alferon® N

Generic Available No

Pharmacologic Category Interferon

Use Patients ≥18 years of age: Intralesional treatment of refractory or recurring genital or venereal warts (condylomata acuminata)

Local Anesthetic/Vasoconstrictor Precautions No information available to require special precautions

Effects on Dental Treatment Key adverse event(s) related to dental treatment: Xerostomia (normal salivary flow resumes upon discontinuation), metallic taste, tongue hyperesthesia, abnormal taste, thirst, rhinitis, pharyngitis, nosebleed, and increased diaphoresis.

Common Adverse Effects Note: Adverse reaction incidence noted below is specific to intralesional administration in patients with condylomata acuminata. Flu-like reactions, consisting of headache, fever, and/or myalgia, was reported in 30% of patients, and abated with repeated dosing.

>10%:

Central nervous system: Fever (40%), headache (31%), chills (14%), fatigue (14%)
Hematologic: Decreased WBC (11%)
Neuromuscular & skeletal: Myalgia (45%)
Miscellaneous: Flu-like syndrome (30%)

(Continued)

Interferon Alfa-n3 *(Continued)*

1% to 10%:

Central nervous system: Malaise (9%), dizziness (9%), depression (2%), insomnia (2%), thirst (1%)

Dermatologic: Pruritus (2%)

Gastrointestinal: Nausea (45), vomiting (3%), dyspepsia (3%), diarrhea (2%), tongue hyperesthesia (1%), taste disturbance (1%)

Genitourinary: Groin lymph node swelling (1%)

Neuromuscular & skeletal: Arthralgia (5%), back pain (4%), cramps (1%), paresthesia (1%)

Ocular: Visual disturbance (1%)

Respiratory: Rhinitis (2%), pharyngitis (1%), nosebleed (1%)

Miscellaneous: Increased diaphoresis (2%), vasovagal reaction (2%)

Mechanism of Action Interferons interact with cells through high affinity cell surface receptors. Following activation, multiple effects can be detected including induction of gene transcription. Inhibits cellular growth, alters the state of cellular differentiation, interferes with oncogene expression, alters cell surface antigen expression, increases phagocytic activity of macrophages, and augments cytotoxicity of lymphocytes for target cells

Drug Interactions

Increased Effect/Toxicity: Interferons may increase the adverse/toxic effects of ACE inhibitors, specifically the development of granulocytopenia. Risk: Monitor A case report of agranulocytosis has been reported with concurrent use of clozapine. Case reports of decreased hematopoietic effect with erythropoietin. Interferon alpha may decrease the P450 isoenzyme metabolism of theophylline. Interferons may increase the anticoagulant effects of warfarin. Interferons may decrease the metabolism of zidovudine.

Decreased Effect: Interferon alpha may decrease the serum concentrations of melphalan; this may or may not decrease the potential toxicity of melphalan. Prednisone may decrease the therapeutic effects of Interferon alpha.

Pregnancy Risk Factor C

Interferon Beta-1a (in ter FEER on BAY ta won aye)

U.S. Brand Names Avonex®; Rebif®

Canadian Brand Names Avonex®; Rebif®

Generic Available No

Synonyms rIFN beta-1a

Pharmacologic Category Interferon

Use Treatment of relapsing forms of multiple sclerosis (MS)

Local Anesthetic/Vasoconstrictor Precautions No information available to require special precautions

Effects on Dental Treatment No significant effects or complications reported

Common Adverse Effects

>10%:

Central nervous system: Headache (Avonex® 58%; Rebif® 65% to 70%), fatigue (Rebif® 33% to 41%), fever (Avonex® 20%; Rebif® 25% to 28%), pain (Avonex® 23%), chills (Avonex® 19%), depression (Avonex® 18%), dizziness (Avonex® 14%)

Gastrointestinal: Nausea (Avonex® 23%), abdominal pain (Avonex® 8%; Rebif® 20% to 22%)

Genitourinary: Urinary tract infection (Avonex® 17%)

Hematologic: Leukopenia (Rebif® 28% to 36%)

Hepatic: ALT increased (Rebif® 20% to 27%), AST increased (Rebif® 10% to 17%)

Local: Injection site reaction (Avonex® 3%; Rebif® 89% to 92%)

Neuromuscular & skeletal: Myalgia (Avonex® 29%; Rebif® 25%), back pain (Rebif® 23% to 25%), weakness (Avonex® 24%), skeletal pain (Rebif® 10% to 15%), rigors (Rebif® 6% to 13%)

Ocular: Vision abnormal (Rebif® 7% to 13%)

Respiratory: Sinusitis (Avonex® 14%), upper respiratory tract infection (Avonex® 14%)

Miscellaneous: Flu-like symptoms (Avonex® 49%; Rebif® 56% to 59%), neutralizing antibodies (significance not known; Avonex® 5%; Rebif® 24%), lymphadenopathy (Rebif® 11% to 12%)

1% to 10% (reported with one or both products):

Cardiovascular: Chest pain, vasodilation

Central nervous system: Convulsions, malaise, migraine, somnolence

Dermatologic: Alopecia, rash

Endocrine & metabolic: Thyroid disorder

Gastrointestinal: Toothache, xerostomia
Genitourinary: Micturition frequency, urinary incontinence
Hematologic: Anemia, thrombocytopenia
Hepatic: Bilirubinemia, hepatic function abnormal
Local: Injection site bruising, injection site inflammation, injection site necrosis, injection site pain
Neuromuscular & skeletal: Arthralgia, coordination abnormal, hypertonia
Ocular: Eye disorder, xerophthalmia
Respiratory: Bronchitis
Miscellaneous: Infection

Mechanism of Action Interferon beta differs from naturally occurring human protein by a single amino acid substitution and the lack of carbohydrate side chains; alters the expression and response to surface antigens and can enhance immune cell activities. Properties of interferon beta that modify biologic responses are mediated by cell surface receptor interactions; mechanism in the treatment of MS is unknown.

Drug Interactions

Increased Effect/Toxicity: Interferons may increase the adverse/toxic effects of ACE inhibitors, specifically the development of granulocytopenia. Agranulocytosis has been reported with concurrent use of clozapine (case report). Interferons may increase the anticoagulant effects of warfarin, and interferons may increase serum levels of zidovudine.

Pharmacodynamics/Kinetics Limited data due to small doses used
Half-life elimination: Avonex®: 10 hours; Rebif®: 69 hours
Time to peak, serum: Avonex® (I.M.): 3-15 hours; Rebif® (SubQ): 16 hours

Pregnancy Risk Factor C

Interferon Beta-1b (in ter FEER on BAY ta won bee)

U.S. Brand Names Betaseron®

Canadian Brand Names Betaseron®

Generic Available No

Synonyms rIFN beta-1b

Pharmacologic Category Interferon

Use Treatment of relapsing forms of multiple sclerosis (MS)

Local Anesthetic/Vasoconstrictor Precautions No information available to require special precautions

Effects on Dental Treatment No significant effects or complications reported

Common Adverse Effects Note: Flu-like symptoms (including at least two of the following - headache, fever, chills, malaise, diaphoresis, and myalgias) are reported in the majority of patients (60%) and decrease over time (average duration ~1 week).

>10%:
Cardiovascular: Peripheral edema (15%), chest pain (11%)
Central nervous system: Headache (57%), fever (36%), pain (51%), chills (25%), dizziness (24%), insomnia (24%)
Dermatologic: Rash (24%), skin disorder (12%)
Endocrine & metabolic: Metrorrhagia (11%)
Gastrointestinal: Nausea (27%), diarrhea (19%), abdominal pain (19%), constipation (20%), dyspepsia (14%)
Genitourinary: Urinary urgency (13%)
Hematologic: Lymphopenia (88%), neutropenia (14%), leukopenia (14%)
Local: Injection site reaction (85%), inflammation (53%), pain (18%)
Neuromuscular & skeletal: Weakness (61%), myalgia (27%), hypertonia (50%), myasthenia (46%), arthralgia (31%), incoordination (21%)
Miscellaneous: Flu-like symptoms (60%)

1% to 10%:
Cardiovascular: Palpitation (4%), vasodilation (8%), hypertension (7%), tachycardia (4%), peripheral vascular disorder (6%)
Central nervous system: Anxiety (10%), malaise (8%), nervousness (7%)
Dermatologic: Alopecia (4%)
Endocrine & metabolic: Menorrhagia (8%), dysmenorrhea (7%)
Genitourinary: Impotence (9%), pelvic pain (6%), cystitis (8%), urinary frequency (7%), weight gain (7%), prostatic disorder (3%)
Hematologic: Lymphadenopathy (8%)
Hepatic: SGPT increased >5x baseline (10%), SGOT increased >5x baseline (3%)
Local: Injection site necrosis (5%), edema (3%), mass (2%)
Neuromuscular & skeletal: Leg cramps (4%)
Respiratory: Dyspnea (7%)
Miscellaneous: Diaphoresis (4%), hypersensitivity (3%)

(Continued)

Interferon Beta-1b *(Continued)*

Mechanism of Action Interferon beta-1b differs from naturally occurring human protein by a single amino acid substitution and the lack of carbohydrate side chains; alters the expression and response to surface antigens and can enhance immune cell activities. Properties of interferon beta-1b that modify biologic responses are mediated by cell surface receptor interactions; mechanism in the treatment of MS is unknown.

Drug Interactions

Increased Effect/Toxicity: Interferons may increase the adverse/toxic effects of ACE inhibitors, specifically the development of granulocytopenia. Risk: Monitor A case report of agranulocytosis has been reported with concurrent use of clozapine. Case reports of decreased hematopoietic effect with erythropoietin. Interferon alpha may decrease the P450 isoenzyme metabolism of theophylline. Interferons may increase the anticoagulant effects of warfarin. Interferons may decrease the metabolism of zidovudine.

Pharmacodynamics/Kinetics Limited data due to small doses used

Half-life elimination: 8 minutes to 4.3 hours

Time to peak, serum: 1-8 hours

Pregnancy Risk Factor C

Interferon Gamma-1b (in ter FEER on GAM ah won bee)

U.S. Brand Names Actimmune®

Canadian Brand Names Actimmune®

Generic Available No

Pharmacologic Category Interferon

Use Reduce frequency and severity of serious infections associated with chronic granulomatous disease; delay time to disease progression in patients with severe, malignant osteopetrosis

Local Anesthetic/Vasoconstrictor Precautions No information available to require special precautions

Effects on Dental Treatment No significant effects or complications reported

Common Adverse Effects Based on 50 mcg/m^2 dose administered 3 times weekly for chronic granulomatous disease

>10%:

- Central nervous system: Fever (52%), headache (33%), chills (14%), fatigue (14%)
- Dermatologic: Rash (17%)
- Gastrointestinal: Diarrhea (14%), vomiting (13%)
- Local: Injection site erythema or tenderness (14%)

1% to 10%:

- Central nervous system: Depression (3%)
- Gastrointestinal: Nausea (10%), abdominal pain (8%)
- Neuromuscular & skeletal: Myalgia (6%), arthralgia (2%), back pain (2%)

Drug Interactions

Cytochrome P450 Effect: Inhibits CYP1A2 (weak), 2E1 (weak)

Increased Effect/Toxicity: Interferon gamma-1b may increase hepatic enzymes or enhance myelosuppression when taken with other myelosuppressive agents. May decrease cytochrome P450 concentrations leading to increased serum concentrations of drugs metabolized by this pathway.

Pharmacodynamics/Kinetics

Absorption: I.M., SubQ: Slowly

Half-life elimination: I.V.: 38 minutes; I.M., SubQ: 3-6 hours

Time to peak, plasma: I.M.: 4 hours (1.5 ng/mL); SubQ: 7 hours (0.6 ng/mL)

Pregnancy Risk Factor C

Interleukin-1 Receptor antagonist *see* Anakinra *on page 131*

Interleukin-2 *see* Aldesleukin *on page 74*

Interleukin-11 *see* Oprelvekin *on page 1015*

Intralipid® *see* Fat Emulsion *on page 575*

Intravenous Fat Emulsion *see* Fat Emulsion *on page 575*

Intrifiban *see* Eptifibatide *on page 503*

Intron® A *see* Interferon Alfa-2b *on page 752*

Invanz® *see* Ertapenem *on page 507*

Inversine® *see* Mecamylamine *on page 859*

Invirase® *see* Saquinavir *on page 1207*

Iodex [OTC] *see* Iodine *on page 758*

Iodine (EYE oh dyne)

Related Information

Trace Metals *on page 1319*

U.S. Brand Names Iodex [OTC]; Iodoflex™; Iodosorb®

Generic Available Yes

Pharmacologic Category Topical Skin Product

Use Used topically as an antiseptic in the management of minor, superficial skin wounds and has been used to disinfect the skin preoperatively

Local Anesthetic/Vasoconstrictor Precautions No information available to require special precautions

Effects on Dental Treatment No significant effects or complications reported

Common Adverse Effects Frequency not defined.

Central nervous system: Fever, headache
Dermatologic: Skin rash, angioedema, urticaria, acne
Endocrine & metabolic: Hypothyroidism
Gastrointestinal: Metallic taste, diarrhea
Hematologic: Eosinophilia, hemorrhage (mucosal)
Neuromuscular & skeletal: Arthralgia
Ocular: Swelling of eyelids
Respiratory: Pulmonary edema
Miscellaneous: Lymph node enlargement

Pregnancy Risk Factor D

Iodine *see* Trace Metals *on page 1319*

Iodoflex™ *see* Iodine *on page 758*

Iodopen® *see* Trace Metals *on page 1319*

Iodoquinol (eye oh doe KWIN ole)

U.S. Brand Names Yodoxin®

Canadian Brand Names Diodoquin®

Generic Available No

Synonyms Diiodohydroxyquin

Pharmacologic Category Amebicide

Use Treatment of acute and chronic intestinal amebiasis; asymptomatic cyst passers; *Blastocystis hominis* infections; ineffective for amebic hepatitis or hepatic abscess

Local Anesthetic/Vasoconstrictor Precautions No information available to require special precautions

Effects on Dental Treatment No significant effects or complications reported

Common Adverse Effects Frequency not defined.

Central nervous system: Fever, chills, agitation, retrograde amnesia, headache
Dermatologic: Rash, urticaria, pruritus
Endocrine & metabolic: Thyroid gland enlargement
Gastrointestinal: Diarrhea, nausea, vomiting, stomach pain, abdominal cramps
Neuromuscular & skeletal: Peripheral neuropathy, weakness
Ocular: Optic neuritis, optic atrophy, visual impairment
Miscellaneous: Itching of rectal area

Mechanism of Action Contact amebicide that works in the lumen of the intestine by an unknown mechanism

Pharmacodynamics/Kinetics

Absorption: Poor and erratic
Metabolism: Hepatic
Excretion: Feces (high percentage)

Pregnancy Risk Factor C

Iodoquinol and Hydrocortisone

(eye oh doe KWIN ole & hye droe KOR ti sone)

Related Information

Hydrocortisone *on page 714*
Iodoquinol *on page 759*

U.S. Brand Names Dermazene®; Vytone®

Generic Available Yes

Synonyms Hydrocortisone and Iodoquinol

Pharmacologic Category Antifungal Agent, Topical; Corticosteroid, Topical

Dental Use Reported to be useful in the treatment of angular cheilitis

Use Treatment of eczema; infectious dermatitis; chronic eczematoid otitis externa; mycotic dermatoses

Local Anesthetic/Vasoconstrictor Precautions No information available to require special precautions

Effects on Dental Treatment No significant effects or complications reported

(Continued)

Iodoquinol and Hydrocortisone *(Continued)*

Common Adverse Effects

Based on **iodoquinol** component:

Central nervous system: Fever, chills, agitation, retrograde amnesia, headache

Dermatologic: Rash, urticaria, pruritus

Endocrine & metabolic: Thyroid gland enlargement

Gastrointestinal: Diarrhea, nausea, vomiting, stomach pain, abdominal cramps

Neuromuscular & skeletal: Peripheral neuropathy, weakness

Ocular: Optic neuritis, optic atrophy, visual impairment

Miscellaneous: Itching of rectal area

Based on **hydrocortisone** component:

>10%:

Central nervous system: Insomnia, nervousness

Gastrointestinal: Increased appetite, indigestion

1% to 10%:

Dermatologic: Hirsutism

Endocrine & metabolic: Diabetes mellitus

Neuromuscular & skeletal: Arthralgia

Ocular: Cataracts

Respiratory: Epistaxis

Drug Interactions

Cytochrome P450 Effect: Hydrocortisone: **Substrate** of CYP3A4 (minor); **Induces** CYP3A4 (weak)

Pharmacodynamics/Kinetics See individual agents.

Pregnancy Risk Factor C

Iodosorb® *see* Iodine *on page 758*

Iohexol *see* Radiological/Contrast Media (Nonionic) *on page 1166*

Ionamin® *see* Phentermine *on page 1076*

Ionil® [OTC] *see* Salicylic Acid *on page 1205*

Ionil® Plus [OTC] *see* Salicylic Acid *on page 1205*

Ionil T® [OTC] *see* Coal Tar *on page 367*

Ionil T® Plus [OTC] *see* Coal Tar *on page 367*

Iopamidol *see* Radiological/Contrast Media (Nonionic) *on page 1166*

Iophen NR *see* Guaifenesin *on page 672*

Iopidine® *see* Apraclonidine *on page 138*

Iopromide (eye oh PROE mide)

U.S. Brand Names Ultravist®

Generic Available No

Pharmacologic Category Contrast Agent, Nonionic

Use Enhance imaging in cerebral arteriography and peripheral arteriography; coronary arteriography and left ventriculography, visceral angiography and aortography; contrast-enhanced computed tomographic imaging of the head and body, excretory urography, intra-arterial digital subtraction angiography, peripheral venography

Local Anesthetic/Vasoconstrictor Precautions No information available to require special precautions

Effects on Dental Treatment No significant effects or complications reported

Mechanism of Action Iopromide opacifies vessels in its path of flow, permitting radiographic visualization of internal structures.

Pregnancy Risk Factor B

Iosat™ [OTC] *see* Potassium Iodide *on page 1106*

Ioversol *see* Radiological/Contrast Media (Nonionic) *on page 1166*

Ipecac Syrup (IP e kak SIR up)

Generic Available Yes

Synonyms Syrup of Ipecac

Pharmacologic Category Antidote

Use Treatment of acute oral drug overdosage and in certain poisonings

Local Anesthetic/Vasoconstrictor Precautions No information available to require special precautions

Effects on Dental Treatment No significant effects or complications reported

Common Adverse Effects Frequency not defined.

Cardiovascular: Cardiotoxicity

Central nervous system: Lethargy

Gastrointestinal: Protracted vomiting, diarrhea

Neuromuscular & skeletal: Myopathy

Mechanism of Action Irritates the gastric mucosa and stimulates the medullary chemoreceptor trigger zone to induce vomiting

Drug Interactions

Increased Effect/Toxicity: Phenothiazines (chlorpromazine has been associated with serious dystonic reactions).

Decreased Effect: Activated charcoal, milk, carbonated beverages decrease the effect of ipecac syrup.

Pharmacodynamics/Kinetics

Onset of action: 15-30 minutes

Duration: 20-25 minutes; 60 minutes in some cases

Absorption: Significant amounts, mainly when it does not produce emesis

Excretion: Urine; emetine (alkaloid component) may be detected in urine 60 days after excess dose or chronic use

Pregnancy Risk Factor C

IPM Wound Gel™ [OTC] *see* Hyaluronate and Derivatives *on page 696*

IPOL® *see* Poliovirus Vaccine (Inactivated) *on page 1099*

Ipratropium (i pra TROE pee um)

Related Information

Ipratropium and Albuterol *on page 761*

Respiratory Diseases *on page 1478*

U.S. Brand Names Atrovent®

Canadian Brand Names Alti-Ipratropium; Apo-Ipravent®; Atrovent®; Gen-Ipratropium; Novo-Ipramide; Nu-Ipratropium; PMS-Ipratropium

Mexican Brand Names Atrovent®

Generic Available Yes: Excludes solution for oral inhalation

Synonyms Ipratropium Bromide

Pharmacologic Category Anticholinergic Agent

Use Anticholinergic bronchodilator used in bronchospasm associated with COPD, bronchitis, and emphysema; symptomatic relief of rhinorrhea associated with the common cold and allergic and nonallergic rhinitis

Local Anesthetic/Vasoconstrictor Precautions No information available to require special precautions

Effects on Dental Treatment Key adverse event(s) related to dental treatment: Xerostomia and changes in salivation (normal salivary flow resumes upon discontinuation), and dry mucous membranes.

Common Adverse Effects Note: Ipratropium is poorly absorbed from the lung, so systemic effects are rare.

Inhalation aerosol and inhalation solution:

<10%: Respiratory: Upper respiratory infection (13%), bronchitis (15%)

1% to 10%:

Cardiovascular: Palpitations (2%)

Central nervous system: Nervousness (3%), dizziness (2%), fatigue, headache (6%), pain (4%)

Dermatologic: Rash (1%)

Gastrointestinal: Nausea, xerostomia, stomach upset, dry mucous membranes

Respiratory: Nasal congestion, dyspnea (10%), increased sputum (1%), bronchospasm (2%), pharyngitis (3%), rhinitis (2%), sinusitis (5%)

Miscellaneous: Influenza-like symptoms

Nasal spray: Epistaxis (8%), nasal dryness (5%), nausea (2%)

Mechanism of Action Blocks the action of acetylcholine at parasympathetic sites in bronchial smooth muscle causing bronchodilation

Drug Interactions

Increased Effect/Toxicity: Increased therapeutic effect with albuterol. Increased toxicity with anticholinergics or drugs with anticholinergic properties and dronabinol.

Pharmacodynamics/Kinetics

Onset of action: Bronchodilation: 1-3 minutes

Peak effect: 1.5-2 hours

Duration: ≤4-6 hours

Absorption: Negligible

Distribution: Inhalation: 15% of dose reaches lower airways

Pregnancy Risk Factor B

Ipratropium and Albuterol (i pra TROE pee um & al BYOO ter ole)

Related Information

Albuterol *on page 71*

Ipratropium *on page 761*

(Continued)

Ipratropium and Albuterol *(Continued)*

U.S. Brand Names Combivent®; DuoNeb™

Canadian Brand Names Combivent®

Generic Available No

Synonyms Albuterol and Ipratropium

Pharmacologic Category Bronchodilator

Use Treatment of COPD in those patients that are currently on a regular bronchodilator who continue to have bronchospasms and require a second bronchodilator

Local Anesthetic/Vasoconstrictor Precautions No information available to require special precautions

Effects on Dental Treatment Key adverse event(s) related to dental treatment: Xerostomia (normal salivary flow resumes upon discontinuation) and dry mucous membrane.

Common Adverse Effects

Based on **ipratropium** component: **Note:** Ipratropium is poorly absorbed from the lung, so systemic effects are rare.

Inhalation aerosol and inhalation solution:

<10%: Respiratory: Upper respiratory infection (13%), bronchitis (15%)

1% to 10%:

- Cardiovascular: Palpitations (2%)
- Central nervous system: Nervousness (3%), dizziness (2%), fatigue, headache (6%), pain (4%)
- Dermatologic: Rash (1%)
- Gastrointestinal: Nausea, xerostomia, stomach upset, dry mucous membranes
- Respiratory: Nasal congestion, dyspnea (10%), increased sputum (1%), bronchospasm (2%), pharyngitis (3%), rhinitis (2%), sinusitis (5%)
- Miscellaneous: Influenza-like symptoms

Based on **albuterol** component:

>10%:

- Cardiovascular: Tachycardia, palpitations, pounding heartbeat
- Gastrointestinal: GI upset, nausea

1% to 10%:

- Cardiovascular: Flushing of face, hypertension or hypotension
- Central nervous system: Nervousness, CNS stimulation, hyperactivity, insomnia, dizziness, lightheadedness, drowsiness, headache
- Gastrointestinal: Xerostomia, heartburn, vomiting, unusual taste
- Genitourinary: Dysuria
- Neuromuscular & skeletal: Muscle cramping, tremor, weakness
- Respiratory: Coughing
- Miscellaneous: Diaphoresis (increased)

Dosage Adults:

Inhalation: 2 inhalations 4 times/day (maximum: 12 inhalations/24 hours)

Inhalation via nebulization: Initial: 3 mL every 6 hours (maximum: 3 mL every 4 hours)

Mechanism of Action See individual agents.

Contraindications

Based on **ipratropium** component: Hypersensitivity to atropine, its derivatives, or any component of the formulation

In addition, Combivent® inhalation aerosol is contraindicated in patients with hypersensitivity to soya lecithin or related food products (eg, soybean and peanut). **Note:** Other formulations may include these components; refer to product-specific labeling.

Based on **albuterol** component: Hypersensitivity to albuterol, adrenergic amines, or any component of the formulation

Drug Interactions

Cytochrome P450 Effect: Albuterol: **Substrate** of CYP3A4 (major)

Increased Effect/Toxicity: See individual agents.

Decreased Effect: See individual agents.

Dietary Considerations Some dosage forms may contain soya lecithin. Do not use in patients allergic to soya lecithin or related food products such as soybean and peanut.

Pharmacodynamics/Kinetics See individual agents.

Pregnancy Risk Factor C

Dosage Forms AERO, oral inhalation (Combivent®): Ipratropium 18 mcg and albuterol 103 mcg per actuation (14.7 g). **SOLN, oral inhalation** (DuoNeb™): Ipratropium 0.5 mg [0.017%] and albuterol base 2.5 mg [0.083%] per 3 mL vial (30s, 60s)

Ipratropium Bromide *see* Ipratropium *on page 761*

I-Prin [OTC] *see* Ibuprofen *on page 728*

Iproveratril Hydrochloride *see* Verapamil *on page 1373*

IPV *see* Poliovirus Vaccine (Inactivated) *on page 1099*

Iquix® *see* Levofloxacin *on page 812*

Irbesartan (ir be SAR tan)

Related Information

Cardiovascular Diseases *on page 1458*

U.S. Brand Names Avapro®

Canadian Brand Names Avapro®

Mexican Brand Names Aprovel®; Avapro®

Generic Available No

Pharmacologic Category Angiotensin II Receptor Blocker

Use Treatment of hypertension alone or in combination with other antihypertensives; treatment of diabetic nephropathy in patients with type 2 diabetes mellitus (noninsulin dependent, NIDDM) and hypertension

Local Anesthetic/Vasoconstrictor Precautions No information available to require special precautions

Effects on Dental Treatment Key adverse event(s) related to dental treatment: Orthostatic hypotension.

Common Adverse Effects Unless otherwise indicated, percentage of incidence is reported for patients with hypertension.

>10%: Endocrine & metabolic: Hyperkalemia (19%, diabetic nephropathy)

1% to 10%:

- Cardiovascular: Orthostatic hypotension (5%, diabetic nephropathy)
- Central nervous system: Fatigue (4%), dizziness (10%, diabetic nephropathy)
- Gastrointestinal: Diarrhea (3%), dyspepsia (2%)
- Respiratory: Upper respiratory infection (9%), cough (2.8% versus 2.7% in placebo)

>1% but frequency ≤ placebo: Abdominal pain, anxiety, chest pain, edema, headache, influenza, musculoskeletal pain, nausea, nervousness, pharyngitis, rash, rhinitis, sinus abnormality, syncope, tachycardia, urinary tract infection, vertigo, vomiting

Dosage Oral:

Hypertension:

Children:

<6 years: Safety and efficacy have not been established.

≥6-12 years: Initial: 75 mg once daily; may be titrated to a maximum of 150 mg once daily

Children ≥13 years and Adults: 150 mg once daily; patients may be titrated to 300 mg once daily

Note: Starting dose in volume-depleted patients should be 75 mg

Nephropathy in patients with type 2 diabetes and hypertension: Adults: Target dose: 300 mg once daily

Dosage adjustment in renal impairment: No dosage adjustment necessary with mild to severe impairment unless the patient is also volume depleted.

Mechanism of Action Irbesartan is an angiotensin receptor antagonist. Angiotensin II acts as a vasoconstrictor. In addition to causing direct vasoconstriction, angiotensin II also stimulates the release of aldosterone. Once aldosterone is released, sodium as well as water are reabsorbed. The end result is an elevation in blood pressure. Irbesartan binds to the AT1 angiotensin II receptor. This binding prevents angiotensin II from binding to the receptor thereby blocking the vasoconstriction and the aldosterone secreting effects of angiotensin II.

Contraindications Hypersensitivity to irbesartan or any component of the formulation; hypersensitivity to other A-II receptor antagonists; bilateral renal artery stenosis; pregnancy (2nd and 3rd trimesters)

Warnings/Precautions Safety and efficacy have not been established in pediatric patients <6 years of age. Avoid use or use a much smaller dose in patients who are intravascularly volume-depleted; use caution in patients with unilateral or bilateral renal artery stenosis to avoid a decrease in renal function; AUCs of irbesartan (not the active metabolite) are about 50% greater in patients with Cl_{cr} <30 mL/minute and are doubled in hemodialysis patients

Drug Interactions

Cytochrome P450 Effect: Substrate of CYP2C8/9 (minor); **Inhibits** CYP2C8/9 (moderate), 2D6 (weak), 3A4 (weak)

(Continued)

Irbesartan *(Continued)*

Increased Effect/Toxicity: Potassium salts/supplements, co-trimoxazole (high dose), ACE inhibitors, and potassium-sparing diuretics (amiloride, spironolactone, triamterene) may increase the risk of hyperkalemia. Irbesartan may increase the levels/effects of amiodarone, fluoxetine, glimepiride, glipizide, nateglinide, phenytoin, pioglitazone, rosiglitazone, sertraline, warfarin, and other CYP2C8/9 substrates.

Ethanol/Nutrition/Herb Interactions Herb/Nutraceutical: Avoid dong quai if using for hypertension (has estrogenic activity). Avoid ephedra, yohimbe, ginseng (may worsen hypertension). Avoid garlic (may have increased antihypertensive effect).

Dietary Considerations May be taken with or without food.

Pharmacodynamics/Kinetics

Onset of action: Peak effect: 1-2 hours
Duration: >24 hours
Distribution: V_d: 53-93 L
Protein binding, plasma: 90%
Metabolism: Hepatic, primarily CYP2C9
Bioavailability: 60% to 80%
Half-life elimination: Terminal: 11-15 hours
Time to peak, serum: 1.5-2 hours
Excretion: Feces (80%); urine (20%)

Pregnancy Risk Factor C/D (2nd and 3rd trimesters)

Dosage Forms TAB: 75 mg, 150 mg, 300 mg

Irbesartan and Hydrochlorothiazide

(ir be SAR tan & hye droe klor oh THYE a zide)

Related Information

Cardiovascular Diseases *on page 1458*
Hydrochlorothiazide *on page 699*
Irbesartan *on page 763*

U.S. Brand Names Avalide®

Canadian Brand Names Avalide®

Generic Available No

Synonyms Avapro® HCT; Hydrochlorothiazide and Irbesartan

Pharmacologic Category Antihypertensive Agent, Combination

Use Combination therapy for the management of hypertension

Local Anesthetic/Vasoconstrictor Precautions No information available to require special precautions

Effects on Dental Treatment No significant effects or complications reported

Common Adverse Effects See individual agents.

Mechanism of Action

Irbesartan: Irbesartan is an angiotensin receptor antagonist. Angiotensin II acts as a vasoconstrictor. In addition to causing direct vasoconstriction, angiotensin II also stimulates the release of aldosterone. Once aldosterone is released, sodium as well as water are reabsorbed. The end result is an elevation in blood pressure. Irbesartan binds to the AT1 angiotensin II receptor. This binding prevents angiotensin II from binding to the receptor thereby blocking the vasoconstriction and the aldosterone secreting effects of angiotensin II.

Hydrochlorothiazide: Inhibits sodium reabsorption in the distal tubules causing increased excretion of sodium and water as well as potassium and hydrogen ions

Drug Interactions

Cytochrome P450 Effect: Irbesartan: **Substrate** of CYP2C8/9 (minor); **Inhibits** CYP2C8/9 (moderate), 2D6 (weak), 3A4 (weak)

Increased Effect/Toxicity: See individual agents.

Decreased Effect: See individual agents.

Pregnancy Risk Factor C/D (2nd and 3rd trimesters)

Ircon® [OTC] *see* Ferrous Fumarate *on page 586*

Iressa™ *see* Gefitinib *on page 649*

Irinotecan (eye rye no TEE kan)

U.S. Brand Names Camptosar®

Canadian Brand Names Camptosar®

Mexican Brand Names Camptosar®

Generic Available No

Synonyms Camptothecin-11; CPT-11; NSC-616348

Pharmacologic Category Antineoplastic Agent, Natural Source (Plant) Derivative

Use Treatment of metastatic carcinoma of the colon or rectum

Unlabeled/Investigational Use Lung cancer (small cell and nonsmall cell), cervical cancer, gastric cancer, pancreatic cancer, leukemia, lymphoma, breast cancer

Local Anesthetic/Vasoconstrictor Precautions No information available to require special precautions

Effects on Dental Treatment No significant effects or complications reported

Common Adverse Effects

>10%:

Cardiovascular: Vasodilation

Central nervous system: Insomnia, dizziness, fever (45.4%)

Dermatologic: Alopecia (60.5%), rash

Gastrointestinal: Irinotecan therapy may induce two different forms of diarrhea. Onset, symptoms, proposed mechanisms and treatment are different. Overall, 56.9% of patients treated experience abdominal pain and/or cramping during therapy. Anorexia, constipation, flatulence, stomatitis, and dyspepsia have also been reported.

Diarrhea: Dose-limiting toxicity with weekly dosing regimen

Early diarrhea (50.7% incidence, grade 3/4 8%) usually occurs during or within 24 hours of administration. May be accompanied by symptoms of cramping, vomiting, flushing, and diaphoresis. It is thought to be mediated by cholinergic effects which can be successfully managed with atropine.

Late diarrhea (87.8% incidence) usually occurs >24 hours after treatment. National Cancer Institute (NCI) grade 3 or 4 diarrhea (31%) occurs in 30.6% of patients. Late diarrhea generally occurs with a median of 11 days after therapy and lasts approximately 3 days. Patients experiencing grade 3 or 4 diarrhea were noted to have symptoms a total of 7 days. Correlated with irinotecan or SN-38 levels in plasma and bile. Due to the duration, dehydration and electrolyte imbalances are significant clinical concerns. Loperamide therapy is recommended. The incidence of grade 3 or 4 late diarrhea is significantly higher in patients ≥65 years of age; close monitoring and prompt initiation of high-dose loperamide therapy is prudent.

Emetic potential: Moderately high (86.2% incidence, however, only 12.5% grade 3 or 4 vomiting)

Hematologic: Myelosuppressive: Dose-limiting toxicity with 3 week dosing regimen

Grade 1-4 neutropenia occurred in 53.9% of patients. Patients who had previously received pelvic or abdominal radiation therapy were noted to have a significantly increased incidence of grade 3 or 4 neutropenia. White blood cell count nadir is 15 days after administration and is more frequent than thrombocytopenia. Recovery is usually within 24-28 days and cumulative toxicity has not been observed.

WBC: Mild to severe

Platelets: Mild

Onset (days): 10

Nadir (days): 14-16

Recovery (days): 21-28

Neuromuscular & skeletal: Weakness (75.7%)

Respiratory: Dyspnea (22%), coughing, rhinitis, decreased DLCO (in a few patients)

Miscellaneous: Diaphoresis

1% to 10%: **Irritant chemotherapy**; thrombophlebitis has been reported

Note: In limited pediatric experience, dehydration (often associated with severe hypokalemia and hyponatremia) was among the most significant grade 3/4 adverse events, with a frequency up to 29%. In addition, grade 3/4 infection was reported in 24%.

Mechanism of Action Irinotecan and its active metabolite (SN-38) bind reversibly to topoisomerase I and stabilize the cleavable complex so that religation of the cleaved DNA strand cannot occur. This results in the accumulation of cleavable complexes and single-strand DNA breaks. This interaction results in single-stranded DNA breaks and cell death consistent with S-phase cell cycle specificity.

Drug Interactions

Cytochrome P450 Effect: Substrate (major) of CYP2B6, 3A4

Increased Effect/Toxicity: CYP2B6 inhibitors may increase the levels/effects of irinotecan; example inhibitors include desipramine, paroxetine, and sertraline. CYP3A4 inhibitors may increase the levels/effects of irinotecan;

(Continued)

Irinotecan *(Continued)*

example inhibitors include azole antifungals, ciprofloxacin, clarithromycin, diclofenac, doxycycline, erythromycin, imatinib, isoniazid, nefazodone, nicardipine, propofol, protease inhibitors, quinidine, and verapamil.

Decreased Effect: CYP2B6 inducers may decrease the levels/effects of irinotecan; example inducers include carbamazepine, nevirapine, phenobarbital, phenytoin, and rifampin. CYP3A4 inducers may decrease the levels/effects of irinotecan; example inducers include aminoglutethimide, carbamazepine, nafcillin, nevirapine, phenobarbital, phenytoin, and rifamycins.

Pharmacodynamics/Kinetics

Distribution: V_d: 33-150 L/m^2

Protein binding, plasma: Parent drug: 30% to 68%; SN-38 (active drug): 95%

Metabolism: Via intestinal mucosa, plasma, hepatic, and perhaps in some tumors; converted to SN-38 by carboxylesterase enzymes; undergoes glucuronidation, the metabolite having much less activity than SN-38. Enterohepatic recirculation results in a second peak in the concentration of SN-38. The lactones of both irinotecan and SN-38 undergo hydrolysis to inactive hydroxy acid forms.

Half-life elimination: Parent drug: Alpha: 0.2 hours, Beta: 2.5 hours, Gamma: 14.2 hours; SN-38: 3-23.9 hours.

Time to peak: SN-38: 30-minute infusion: ~1 hour

Excretion: Urine (~20% of dose) within 24 hours; SN-38 excretion in 24 hours accounted for 0.25% of administered dose

Pregnancy Risk Factor D

Iron Dextran Complex (EYE ern DEKS tran KOM pleks)

U.S. Brand Names Dexferrum®; INFeD®

Canadian Brand Names Dexiron™; Infufer®

Generic Available No

Pharmacologic Category Iron Salt

Use Treatment of microcytic hypochromic anemia resulting from iron deficiency in patients in whom oral administration is infeasible or ineffective

Local Anesthetic/Vasoconstrictor Precautions No information available to require special precautions

Effects on Dental Treatment Key adverse event(s) related to dental treatment: Metallic taste.

Common Adverse Effects

>10%:

Cardiovascular: Flushing

Central nervous system: Dizziness, fever, headache, pain

Gastrointestinal: Nausea, vomiting, metallic taste

Local: Staining of skin at the site of I.M. injection

Miscellaneous: Diaphoresis

1% to 10%:

Cardiovascular: Hypotension (1% to 2%)

Dermatologic: Urticaria (1% to 2%), phlebitis (1% to 2%)

Gastrointestinal: Diarrhea

Genitourinary: Discoloration of urine

Note: Diaphoresis, urticaria, arthralgia, fever, chills, dizziness, headache, and nausea may be delayed 24-48 hours after I.V. administration or 3-4 days after I.M. administration.

Anaphylactoid reactions: Respiratory difficulties and cardiovascular collapse have been reported and occur most frequently within the first several minutes of administration.

Mechanism of Action The released iron, from the plasma, eventually replenishes the depleted iron stores in the bone marrow where it is incorporated into hemoglobin

Drug Interactions

Decreased Effect: Decreased effect with chloramphenicol.

Pharmacodynamics/Kinetics

Absorption:

I.M.: 50% to 90% is promptly absorbed, balance is slowly absorbed over month

I.V.: Uptake of iron by the reticuloendothelial system appears to be constant at about 10-20 mg/hour

Excretion: Urine and feces via reticuloendothelial system

Pregnancy Risk Factor C

Iron Fumarate *see* Ferrous Fumarate *on page 586*

Iron Gluconate *see* Ferrous Gluconate *on page 586*

Iron-Polysaccharide Complex *see* Polysaccharide-Iron Complex *on page 1101*

Iron Sucrose (EYE ern SOO krose)

U.S. Brand Names Venofer®

Canadian Brand Names Venofer®

Generic Available No

Pharmacologic Category Iron Salt

Use Treatment of iron-deficiency anemia in patients undergoing chronic hemodialysis who are receiving supplemental erythropoietin therapy

Local Anesthetic/Vasoconstrictor Precautions No information available to require special precautions

Effects on Dental Treatment No significant effects or complications reported

Common Adverse Effects Fatal and life-threatening anaphylactoid reactions (characterized by anaphylactic shock, loss of consciousness, collapse, hypotension, dyspnea, or convulsion) have been reported; hypotension may be related to total dose or rate of administration.

>5%:

Cardiovascular: Hypotension (36%)
Central nervous system: Headache
Gastrointestinal: Nausea, vomiting, diarrhea
Neuromuscular & skeletal: Leg cramps (23%)

1% to 5%:

Cardiovascular: Chest pain, congestive heart failure, hypertension, hypervolemia
Central nervous system: Fever, malaise, dizziness
Dermatologic: Pruritus
Gastrointestinal: Abdominal pain, taste perversion
Hepatic: Elevated enzymes
Local: Application site reaction
Neuromuscular & skeletal: Musculoskeletal pain, weakness
Respiratory: Dyspnea, pneumonia, cough
Miscellaneous: Sepsis

Mechanism of Action Iron sucrose is dissociated by the reticuloendothelial system into iron and sucrose. The released iron increases serum iron concentrations and is incorporated into hemoglobin.

Drug Interactions

Decreased Effect: Chloramphenicol may diminish the therapeutic effects of iron sucrose injection. Iron sucrose injection may reduce the absorption of oral iron preparations.

Pharmacodynamics/Kinetics

Distribution: V_{dss}: Healthy adults: 7.9 L
Metabolism: Dissociated into iron and sucrose by the reticuloendothelial system
Half-life elimination: Healthy adults: 6 hours
Excretion: Healthy adults: Urine (5%) within 24 hours

Pregnancy Risk Factor B

Iron Sulfate *see* Ferrous Sulfate *on page 586*

Iron Sulfate and Vitamin C *see* Ferrous Sulfate and Ascorbic Acid *on page 587*

ISD *see* Isosorbide Dinitrate *on page 770*

ISDN *see* Isosorbide Dinitrate *on page 770*

ISG *see* Immune Globulin (Intramuscular) *on page 739*

ISMN *see* Isosorbide Mononitrate *on page 771*

Ismo® *see* Isosorbide Mononitrate *on page 771*

Isoamyl Nitrite *see* Amyl Nitrite *on page 130*

Isobamate *see* Carisoprodol *on page 266*

Isocarboxazid (eye soe kar BOKS a zid)

U.S. Brand Names Marplan®

Generic Available No

Pharmacologic Category Antidepressant, Monoamine Oxidase Inhibitor

Use Symptomatic treatment of atypical, nonendogenous or neurotic depression

Local Anesthetic/Vasoconstrictor Precautions Attempts should be made to avoid use of vasoconstrictor due to possibility of hypertensive episodes with monoamine oxidase inhibitors

Effects on Dental Treatment Key adverse event(s) related to dental treatment: Orthostatic hypotension, xerostomia (normal salivary flow resumes upon discontinuation).

(Continued)

Isocarboxazid *(Continued)*

Common Adverse Effects

>10%:

Cardiovascular: Orthostatic hypotension
Central nervous system: Drowsiness
Endocrine & metabolic: Decreased sexual ability
Neuromuscular & skeletal: Weakness, trembling
Ocular: Blurred vision

1% to 10%:

Cardiovascular: Tachycardia, peripheral edema
Central nervous system: Nervousness, chills
Dermatologic: Xerostomia
Gastrointestinal: Diarrhea, anorexia, constipation, xerostomia

Mechanism of Action Thought to act by increasing endogenous concentrations of epinephrine, norepinephrine, dopamine, and serotonin through inhibition of the enzyme (monoamine oxidase) responsible for the breakdown of these neurotransmitters

Drug Interactions

Increased Effect/Toxicity: In general, the combined use with TCAs, venlafaxine, trazodone, dexfenfluramine, sibutramine, lithium, meperidine, fenfluramine, dextromethorphan, and SSRIs should be avoided due to the potential for severe adverse reactions (serotonin syndrome, death). MAO inhibitors (including isocarboxazid) may inhibit the metabolism of barbiturates and prolong their effect. Isocarboxazid in combination with amphetamines, other stimulants (methylphenidate), levodopa, metaraminol, reserpine, and decongestants (pseudoephedrine) may result in severe hypertensive reactions. Foods (eg, cheese) and beverages (eg, ethanol) containing tyramine should be avoided; hypertensive crisis may result. Isocarboxazid may increase the pressor response of norepinephrine and may prolong neuromuscular blockade produced by succinylcholine. Tramadol may increase the risk of seizures and serotonin syndrome in patients receiving an MAO inhibitor. Isocarboxazid may produce additive hypoglycemic effect in patients receiving hypoglycemic agents and may produce delirium in patients receiving disulfiram.

Decreased Effect: MAO inhibitors may inhibit the antihypertensive response to guanadrel or guanethidine.

Pregnancy Risk Factor C

Isoetharine (eye soe ETH a reen)

Related Information

Respiratory Diseases *on page 1478*

Canadian Brand Names Beta-2®; Bronkometer®; Bronkosol®

Generic Available Yes

Synonyms Isoetharine Hydrochloride; Isoetharine Mesylate

Pharmacologic Category Adrenergic Agonist Agent; Sympathomimetic

Use Bronchodilator in bronchial asthma and for reversible bronchospasm occurring with bronchitis and emphysema

Local Anesthetic/Vasoconstrictor Precautions Isoetharine is selective for beta-adrenergic receptors and not alpha receptors; therefore, there is no precaution in the use of vasoconstrictor such as epinephrine

Effects on Dental Treatment Key adverse event(s) related to dental treatment: Xerostomia (normal salivary flow resumes upon discontinuation).

Common Adverse Effects Frequency not defined.

Cardiovascular: Tachycardia, hypertension, pounding heartbeat
Central nervous system: Dizziness, lightheadedness, headache, nervousness, insomnia
Gastrointestinal: Xerostomia, nausea, vomiting
Neuromuscular & skeletal: Trembling, weakness
Respiratory: Paradoxical bronchospasm

Mechanism of Action Relaxes bronchial smooth muscle by action on beta$_2$-receptors with very little effect on heart rate

Drug Interactions

Increased Effect/Toxicity: Increased toxicity with other sympathomimetics (eg, epinephrine).

Decreased Effect: Decreased effect with beta-blockers.

Pharmacodynamics/Kinetics

Onset of action: Peak effect: Inhalation: 5-15 minutes
Duration: 1-4 hours
Metabolism: Hepatic, pulmonary, and other tissues
Excretion: Urine (90% primarily as metabolites)

Pregnancy Risk Factor C

Isoetharine Hydrochloride *see* Isoetharine *on page 768*

Isoetharine Mesylate *see* Isoetharine *on page 768*

Isometheptene, Acetaminophen, and Dichloralphenazone *see* Acetaminophen, Isometheptene, and Dichloralphenazone *on page 59*

Isometheptene, Dichloralphenazone, and Acetaminophen *see* Acetaminophen, Isometheptene, and Dichloralphenazone *on page 59*

Isoniazid (eye soe NYE a zid)

Related Information

Tuberculosis *on page 1495*

U.S. Brand Names Nydrazid®

Canadian Brand Names Isotamine®; PMS-Isoniazid

Generic Available Yes

Synonyms INH; Isonicotinic Acid Hydrazide

Pharmacologic Category Antitubercular Agent

Use Treatment of susceptible tuberculosis infections; prophylactically in those individuals exposed to tuberculosis

Local Anesthetic/Vasoconstrictor Precautions No information available to require special precautions

Effects on Dental Treatment Key adverse event(s) related to dental treatment: Xerostomia (normal salivary flow resumes upon discontinuation).

Common Adverse Effects

>10%:

- Gastrointestinal: Loss of appetite, nausea, vomiting, stomach pain
- Hepatic: Mild increased LFTs (10% to 20%)
- Neuromuscular & skeletal: Weakness, peripheral neuropathy (dose-related incidence, 10% to 20% incidence with 10 mg/kg/day)

1% to 10%:

- Central nervous system: Dizziness, slurred speech, lethargy
- Hepatic: Progressive liver damage (increases with age; 2.3% in patients >50 years of age)
- Neuromuscular & skeletal: Hyper-reflexia

Mechanism of Action Unknown, but may include the inhibition of myocolic acid synthesis resulting in disruption of the bacterial cell wall

Drug Interactions

Cytochrome P450 Effect: Substrate of CYP2E1 (major); **Inhibits** CYP1A2 (weak), 2A6 (moderate), 2C8/9 (moderate), 2C19 (strong), 2D6 (moderate), 2E1 (moderate), 3A4 (strong); **Induces** CYP2E1 (after discontinuation) (weak)

Increased Effect/Toxicity: Concurrent use of disulfiram may result in acute intolerance reactions. Isoniazid may increase the levels/effects of amiodarone, amphetamines, benzodiazepines, beta-blockers, calcium channel blockers, citalopram, dexmedetomidine, dextromethorphan, diazepam, fluoxetine, glimepiride, glipizide, ifosfamide, inhalational anesthetics, lidocaine, mesoridazine, methsuximide, mirtazapine, nateglinide, nefazodone, paroxetine, phenytoin, pioglitazone, propranolol, risperidone, ritonavir, rosiglitazone, sertraline, sildenafil (and other PDE-5 inhibitors) tacrolimus, theophylline, thioridazine, tricyclic antidepressants, trimethadione, venlafaxine. warfarin, and other substrates of CYP2A6, 2C8/9, 2C19, 2D6, 2E1, or 3A4. Selected benzodiazepines (midazolam and triazolam), cisapride, ergot alkaloids, selected HMG-CoA reductase inhibitors (lovastatin and simvastatin), and pimozide are generally contraindicated with strong CYP3A4 inhibitors. Mesoridazine and thioridazine are generally contraindicated with strong CYP2D6 inhibitors. When used with strong CYP3A4 inhibitors, dosage adjustment/limits are recommended for sildenafil and other PDE-5 inhibitors; consult individual monographs.

Decreased Effect: Decreased effect/levels of isoniazid with aluminum salts or antacids. Isoniazid may decrease the levels/effects of CYP2D6 prodrug substrates (eg, codeine, hydrocodone, oxycodone, tramadol).

Pharmacodynamics/Kinetics

Absorption: Rapid and complete; rate can be slowed with food

Distribution: All body tissues and fluids including CSF; crosses placenta; enters breast milk

Protein binding: 10% to 15%

Metabolism: Hepatic with decay rate determined genetically by acetylation phenotype

Half-life elimination: Fast acetylators: 30-100 minutes; Slow acetylators: 2-5 hours; may be prolonged with hepatic or severe renal impairment

Time to peak, serum: 1-2 hours

(Continued)

Isoniazid *(Continued)*

Excretion: Urine (75% to 95%); feces; saliva

Pregnancy Risk Factor C

Isoniazid and Rifampin *see* Rifampin and Isoniazid *on page 1181*

Isoniazid, Rifampin, and Pyrazinamide *see* Rifampin, Isoniazid, and Pyrazinamide *on page 1181*

Isonicotinic Acid Hydrazide *see* Isoniazid *on page 769*

Isonipecaine Hydrochloride *see* Meperidine *on page 870*

Isophosphamide *see* Ifosfamide *on page 733*

Isopropyl Alcohol Tincture of Benzylkonium Chloride *see* Benzalkonium Chloride and Isopropyl Alcohol *on page 190*

Isoproterenol (eye soe proe TER e nole)

Related Information

Cardiovascular Diseases *on page 1458*

U.S. Brand Names Isuprel®

Generic Available Yes

Synonyms Isoproterenol Hydrochloride

Pharmacologic Category $Beta_1$- & $Beta_2$-Adrenergic Agonist Agent

Use Ventricular arrhythmias due to AV nodal block; hemodynamically compromised bradyarrhythmias or atropine- and dopamine-resistant bradyarrhythmias (when transcutaneous/venous pacing is not available); temporary use in third-degree AV block until pacemaker insertion

Unlabeled/Investigational Use Temporizing measure before transvenous pacing for torsade de pointes; diagnostic aid (vasovagal syncope)

Local Anesthetic/Vasoconstrictor Precautions Isoproterenol is selective for beta-adrenergic receptors and not alpha receptors; therefore, there is no precaution in the use of vasoconstrictor such as epinephrine

Effects on Dental Treatment Key adverse event(s) related to dental treatment: Xerostomia and changes in salivation (normal salivary flow resumes upon discontinuation).

Common Adverse Effects Frequency not defined.

Cardiovascular: Premature ventricular beats, bradycardia, hypertension, hypotension, chest pain, palpitations, tachycardia, ventricular arrhythmias, myocardial infarction size increased

Central nervous system: Headache, nervousness or restlessness

Endocrine & metabolic: Serum glucose increased, serum potassium decreased, hypokalemia

Gastrointestinal: Nausea, vomiting

Respiratory: Dyspnea

Mechanism of Action Stimulates $beta_1$- and $beta_2$-receptors resulting in relaxation of bronchial, GI, and uterine smooth muscle, increased heart rate and contractility, vasodilation of peripheral vasculature

Drug Interactions

Increased Effect/Toxicity: Sympathomimetic agents may cause headaches and elevate blood pressure. General anesthetics may cause arrhythmias.

Pharmacodynamics/Kinetics

Onset of action: Bronchodilation: I.V.: Immediate

Duration: I.V.: 10-15 minutes

Metabolism: Via conjugation in many tissues including hepatic and pulmonary

Half-life elimination: 2.5-5 minutes

Excretion: Urine (primarily as sulfate conjugates)

Pregnancy Risk Factor C

Isoproterenol Hydrochloride *see* Isoproterenol *on page 770*

Isoptin® SR *see* Verapamil *on page 1373*

Isopto® Atropine *see* Atropine *on page 166*

Isopto® Carbachol *see* Carbachol *on page 255*

Isopto® Carpine *see* Pilocarpine *on page 1085*

Isopto® Homatropine *see* Homatropine *on page 693*

Isopto® Hyoscine *see* Scopolamine *on page 1210*

Isopto® Tears [OTC] *see* Artificial Tears *on page 148*

Isopto® Tears [OTC] *see* Hydroxypropyl Methylcellulose *on page 721*

Isordil® *see* Isosorbide Dinitrate *on page 770*

Isosorbide Dinitrate (eye soe SOR bide dye NYE trate)

Related Information

Cardiovascular Diseases *on page 1458*

Isosorbide Mononitrate *on page 771*

U.S. Brand Names Dilatrate®-SR; Isordil®

Canadian Brand Names Apo-ISDN®; Cedocard®-SR; Coronex®; Novo-Sorbide; PMS-Isosorbide

Mexican Brand Names Isoket®; Isorbid®

Generic Available Yes: Tablet

Synonyms ISD; ISDN

Pharmacologic Category Vasodilator

Use Prevention and treatment of angina pectoris; for congestive heart failure; to relieve pain, dysphagia, and spasm in esophageal spasm with GE reflux

Local Anesthetic/Vasoconstrictor Precautions No information available to require special precautions

Effects on Dental Treatment No significant effects or complications reported

Common Adverse Effects Frequency not defined.

Cardiovascular: Hypotension (infrequent), postural hypotension, crescendo angina (uncommon), rebound hypertension (uncommon), pallor, cardiovascular collapse, tachycardia, shock, flushing, peripheral edema

Central nervous system: Headache (most common), lightheadedness (related to blood pressure changes), syncope (uncommon), dizziness, restlessness

Gastrointestinal: Nausea, vomiting, bowel incontinence, xerostomia

Genitourinary: Urinary incontinence

Hematologic: Methemoglobinemia (rare, overdose)

Neuromuscular & skeletal: Weakness

Ocular: Blurred vision

Miscellaneous: Cold sweat

The incidence of hypotension and adverse cardiovascular events may be increased when used in combination with sildenafil (Viagra®).

Mechanism of Action Stimulation of intracellular cyclic-GMP results in vascular smooth muscle relaxation of both arterial and venous vasculature. Increased venous pooling decreases left ventricular pressure (preload) and arterial dilatation decreases arterial resistance (afterload). Therefore, this reduces cardiac oxygen demand by decreasing left ventricular pressure and systemic vascular resistance by dilating arteries. Additionally, coronary artery dilation improves collateral flow to ischemic regions; esophageal smooth muscle is relaxed via the same mechanism.

Drug Interactions

Cytochrome P450 Effect: Substrate of CYP3A4 (major)

Increased Effect/Toxicity: CYP3A4 inhibitors may increase the levels/effects of isosorbide dinitrate; example inhibitors include azole antifungals, ciprofloxacin, clarithromycin, diclofenac, doxycycline, erythromycin, imatinib, isoniazid, nefazodone, nicardipine, propofol, protease inhibitors, quinidine, and verapamil. Significant reduction of systolic and diastolic blood pressure with concurrent use of sildenafil, tadalafil, or vardenafil (contraindicated). Do not administer sildenafil, tadalafil, or vardenafil within 24 hours of a nitrate preparation.

Decreased Effect: CYP3A4 inducers may decrease the levels/effects of isosorbide dinitrate; example inducers include aminoglutethimide, carbamazepine, nafcillin, nevirapine, phenobarbital, phenytoin, and rifamycins.

Pharmacodynamics/Kinetics

Onset of action: Sublingual tablet: 2-10 minutes; Chewable tablet: 3 minutes; Oral tablet: 45-60 minutes

Duration: Sublingual tablet: 1-2 hours; Chewable tablet: 0.5-2 hours; Oral tablet: 4-6 hours

Metabolism: Extensively hepatic to conjugated metabolites, including isosorbide 5-mononitrate (active) and 2-mononitrate (active)

Half-life elimination: Parent drug: 1-4 hours; Metabolite (5-mononitrate): 4 hours

Excretion: Urine and feces

Pregnancy Risk Factor C

Isosorbide Mononitrate (eye soe SOR bide mon oh NYE trate)

Related Information

Cardiovascular Diseases *on page 1458*

Isosorbide Dinitrate *on page 770*

U.S. Brand Names Imdur®; Ismo®; Monoket®

Canadian Brand Names Imdur®

Mexican Brand Names Elantan®; Imdur®; Mono Mack®

Generic Available Yes

Synonyms ISMN

Pharmacologic Category Vasodilator

(Continued)

Isosorbide Mononitrate *(Continued)*

Use Long-acting metabolite of the vasodilator isosorbide dinitrate used for the prophylactic treatment of angina pectoris

Local Anesthetic/Vasoconstrictor Precautions No information available to require special precautions

Effects on Dental Treatment No significant effects or complications reported

Common Adverse Effects

>10%: Central nervous system: Headache (19% to 38%)

1% to 10%:

Central nervous system: Dizziness (3% to 5%)

Gastrointestinal: Nausea/vomiting (2% to 4%)

The incidence of hypotension and adverse cardiovascular events may be increased when used in combination with sildenafil (Viagra®).

Dosage Adults and Geriatrics (start with lowest recommended dose): Oral:

Regular tablet: 5-10 mg twice daily with the two doses given 7 hours apart (eg, 8 AM and 3 PM) to decrease tolerance development; then titrate to 10 mg twice daily in first 2-3 days.

Extended release tablet: Initial: 30-60 mg given in morning as a single dose; titrate upward as needed, giving at least 3 days between increases; maximum daily single dose: 240 mg

Dosing adjustment in renal impairment: Not necessary for elderly or patients with altered renal or hepatic function.

Tolerance to nitrate effects develops with chronic exposure. Dose escalation does not overcome this effect. Tolerance can only be overcome by short periods of nitrate absence from the body. Short periods (10-12 hours) of nitrate withdrawal help minimize tolerance. Recommended dosage regimens incorporate this interval. General recommendations are to take the last dose of short-acting agents no later than 7 PM; administer 2 times/day rather than 4 times/day. Administer sustained release tablet once daily in the morning.

Mechanism of Action Prevailing mechanism of action for nitroglycerin (and other nitrates) is systemic venodilation, decreasing preload as measured by pulmonary capillary wedge pressure and left ventricular end diastolic volume and pressure; the average reduction in left ventricular end diastolic volume is 25% at rest, with a corresponding increase in ejection fractions of 50% to 60%. This effect improves congestive symptoms in heart failure and improves the myocardial perfusion gradient in patients with coronary artery disease.

Contraindications Hypersensitivity to isosorbide or any component of the formulation; hypersensitivity to organic nitrates; concurrent use with phosphodiesterase-5 (PDE-5) inhibitors (sildenafil, tadalafil, or vardenafil); angle-closure glaucoma (intraocular pressure may be increased); head trauma or cerebral hemorrhage (increase intracranial pressure); severe anemia

Warnings/Precautions Postural hypotension, transient episodes of weakness, dizziness, or syncope may occur even with small doses; ethanol accentuates these effects; tolerance and cross-tolerance to nitrate antianginal and hemodynamic effects may occur during prolonged isosorbide mononitrate therapy; (minimized by using the smallest effective dose, by alternating coronary vasodilators or offering drug-free intervals of as little as 12 hours). Excessive doses may result in severe headache, blurred vision, or xerostomia; increased anginal symptoms may be a result of dosage increases. Avoid use with sildenafil.

Drug Interactions

Cytochrome P450 Effect: Substrate of CYP3A4 (major)

Increased Effect/Toxicity: CYP3A4 inhibitors may increase the levels/effects of isosorbide dinitrate; example inhibitors include azole antifungals, ciprofloxacin, clarithromycin, diclofenac, doxycycline, erythromycin, imatinib, isoniazid, nefazodone, nicardipine, propofol, protease inhibitors, quinidine, and verapamil. Significant reduction of systolic and diastolic blood pressure with concurrent use of sildenafil, tadalafil, or vardenafil (contraindicated). Do not administer sildenafil, tadalafil, or vardenafil within 24 hours of a nitrate preparation.

Ethanol/Nutrition/Herb Interactions Ethanol: Caution with ethanol (may increase risk of hypotension).

Pharmacodynamics/Kinetics

Onset of action: 30-60 minutes

Absorption: Nearly complete and low intersubject variability in its pharmacokinetic parameters and plasma concentrations

Metabolism: Hepatic

Half-life elimination: Mononitrate: ~4 hours

Excretion: Urine and feces

Pregnancy Risk Factor C

Dosage Forms TAB: 10 mg, 20 mg; (Ismo®): 20 mg; (Monoket®): 10 mg, 20 mg. **TAB, extended release** (Imdur®): 30 mg, 60 mg, 120 mg

Isotretinoin (eye soe TRET i noyn)

U.S. Brand Names Accutane®; Amnesteem™; Claravis™; Sotret®

Canadian Brand Names Accutane®; Isotrex®

Mexican Brand Names Isotrex®; Roaccutan®

Generic Available Yes

Synonyms 13-*cis*-Retinoic Acid

Pharmacologic Category Retinoic Acid Derivative

Use Treatment of severe recalcitrant nodular acne unresponsive to conventional therapy

Unlabeled/Investigational Use Investigational: Treatment of children with metastatic neuroblastoma or leukemia that does not respond to conventional therapy

Local Anesthetic/Vasoconstrictor Precautions No information available to require special precautions

Effects on Dental Treatment Key adverse event(s) related to dental treatment: Xerostomia and changes in salivation (normal salivary flow resumes upon discontinuation).

Common Adverse Effects Frequency not defined.

Cardiovascular: Palpitation, tachycardia, vascular thrombotic disease, stroke, chest pain, syncope, flushing

Central nervous system: Edema, fatigue, pseudotumor cerebri, dizziness, drowsiness, headache, insomnia, lethargy, malaise, nervousness, paresthesias, seizures, stroke, suicidal ideation, suicide attempts, suicide, depression, psychosis, aggressive or violent behavior, emotional instability

Dermatologic: Cutaneous allergic reactions, purpura, acne fulminans, alopecia, bruising, cheilitis, dry mouth, dry nose, dry skin, epistaxis, eruptive xanthomas, fragility of skin, hair abnormalities, hirsutism, hyperpigmentation, hypopigmentation, peeling of palms, peeling of soles, photoallergic reactions, photosensitizing reactions, pruritus, rash, dystrophy, paronychia, facial erythema, seborrhea, eczema, increased sunburn susceptibility, diaphoresis, urticaria, abnormal wound healing

Endocrine & metabolic: Increased triglycerides (25%), elevated blood glucose, increased HDL, increased cholesterol, abnormal menses

Gastrointestinal: Weight loss, inflammatory bowel disease, regional ileitis, pancreatitis, bleeding and inflammation of the gums, colitis, nausea, nonspecific gastrointestinal symptoms

Genitourinary: Nonspecific urogenital findings

Hematologic: Anemia, thrombocytopenia, neutropenia, agranulocytosis, pyogenic granuloma

Hepatic: Hepatitis

Neuromuscular & skeletal: Skeletal hyperostosis, calcification of tendons and ligaments, premature epiphyseal closure, arthralgia, CPK elevations, arthritis, tendonitis, bone abnormalities, weakness, back pain (29% in pediatric patients), rhabdomyolysis (rare), bone mineral density decreased

Ocular: Corneal opacities, decreased night vision, cataracts, color vision disorder, conjunctivitis, dry eyes, eyelid inflammation, keratitis, optic neuritis, photophobia, visual disturbances

Otic: Hearing impairment, tinnitus

Renal: Vasculitis, glomerulonephritis,

Respiratory: Bronchospasms, respiratory infection, voice alteration, Wegener's granulomatosis

Miscellaneous: Allergic reactions, anaphylactic reactions, lymphadenopathy, infection, disseminated herpes simplex, diaphoresis

Restrictions Prescriptions for isotretinoin may not be dispensed unless they are affixed with a yellow, self-adhesive qualification sticker filled out by the prescriber. Telephone, fax, or computer-generated prescriptions are no longer valid. Prescriptions may not be written for more than a 1-month supply and must be dispensed with a patient education guide every month. In addition, prescriptions for females must be filled within 7 days of the qualification date noted on the yellow sticker; prescriptions filled after 7 days of the noted date are considered to be expired and cannot be honored. Pharmacists may call the manufacturer to confirm the prescriber's authority to write for this medication, however, this is not mandatory.

Prescribers will be provided with qualification stickers after they have read the details of the program and have signed and mailed to the manufacturer their agreement to participate. Audits of pharmacies will be conducted to monitor program compliance.

(Continued)

Isotretinoin *(Continued)*

Mechanism of Action Reduces sebaceous gland size and reduces sebum production; regulates cell proliferation and differentiation

Drug Interactions

Increased Effect/Toxicity: Increased toxicity: Corticosteroids may cause osteoporosis; interactive effect with isotretinoin unknown; use with caution. Phenytoin may cause osteomalacia; interactive effect with isotretinoin unknown; use with caution. Cases of pseudotumor cerebri have been reported in concurrent use with tetracycline; avoid combination.

Decreased Effect: Isotretinoin may increase clearance of carbamazepine resulting in reduced carbamazepine levels. Microdosed progesterone preparations ("mini-pills") may not be an adequate form of contraception.

Pharmacodynamics/Kinetics

Distribution: Crosses placenta

Protein binding: 99% to 100%; primarily albumin

Metabolism: Hepatic via CYP2B6, 2C8, 2C9, 2D6, 3A4; forms metabolites; major metabolite: 4-oxo-isotretinoin (active)

Half-life elimination: Terminal: Parent drug: 21 hours; Metabolite: 21-24 hours

Time to peak, serum: 3-5 hours

Excretion: Urine and feces (equal amounts)

Pregnancy Risk Factor X

Isovue® *see* Radiological/Contrast Media (Nonionic) *on page 1166*

Isoxsuprine (eye SOKS syoo preen)

U.S. Brand Names Vasodilan® [DSC]

Generic Available Yes

Synonyms Isoxsuprine Hydrochloride

Pharmacologic Category Vasodilator

Use Treatment of peripheral vascular diseases, such as arteriosclerosis obliterans and Raynaud's disease

Local Anesthetic/Vasoconstrictor Precautions No information available to require special precautions

Effects on Dental Treatment May enhance effects of other vasodilators.

Common Adverse Effects Frequency not defined.

Cardiovascular: Hypotension, tachycardia, chest pain

Central nervous system: Dizziness

Dermatologic: Rash

Gastrointestinal: Nausea, vomiting

Neuromuscular & skeletal: Weakness

Mechanism of Action In studies on normal human subjects, isoxsuprine increases muscle blood flow, but skin blood flow is usually unaffected. Rather than increasing muscle blood flow by beta-receptor stimulation, isoxsuprine probably has a direct action on vascular smooth muscle. The generally accepted mechanism of action of isoxsuprine on the uterus is beta-adrenergic stimulation. Isoxsuprine was shown to inhibit prostaglandin synthetase at high serum concentrations, with low concentrations there was an increase in the P-G synthesis.

Drug Interactions

Increased Effect/Toxicity: May enhance effects of other vasodilators/hypotensive agents.

Pharmacodynamics/Kinetics

Absorption: Nearly complete

Half-life elimination, serum: Mean: 1.25 hours

Time to peak, serum: ~1 hour

Pregnancy Risk Factor C

Isoxsuprine Hydrochloride *see* Isoxsuprine *on page 774*

Isradipine (iz RA di peen)

Related Information

Calcium Channel Blockers and Gingival Hyperplasia *on page 1600*

Calcium Channel Blockers, Comparative Pharmacokinetics *on page 1602*

Cardiovascular Diseases *on page 1458*

U.S. Brand Names DynaCirc®; DynaCirc® CR

Canadian Brand Names DynaCirc®

Mexican Brand Names DynaCirc®

Generic Available No

Pharmacologic Category Calcium Channel Blocker

Use Treatment of hypertension

Local Anesthetic/Vasoconstrictor Precautions No information available to require special precautions

Effects on Dental Treatment No significant effects or complications reported

Common Adverse Effects

>10%: Central nervous system: Headache (dose-related 2% to 22%)

1% to 10%:

Cardiovascular: Edema (dose-related 1% to 9%), palpitations (dose-related 1% to 5%), flushing (dose-related 1% to 5%), tachycardia (1% to 3%), chest pain (2% to 3%)

Central nervous system: Dizziness (2% to 8%), fatigue (dose-related 1% to 9%), flushing (9%)

Dermatologic: Rash (1.5% to 2%)

Gastrointestinal: Nausea (1% to 5%), abdominal discomfort (≤3%), vomiting (≤1%), diarrhea (≤3%)

Renal: Urinary frequency (1% to 3%)

Respiratory: Dyspnea (1% to 3%)

Mechanism of Action Inhibits calcium ion from entering the "slow channels" or select voltage-sensitive areas of vascular smooth muscle and myocardium during depolarization, producing a relaxation of coronary vascular smooth muscle and coronary vasodilation; increases myocardial oxygen delivery in patients with vasospastic angina

Drug Interactions

Cytochrome P450 Effect: Substrate of CYP3A4 (major); **Inhibits** CYP3A4 (weak)

Increased Effect/Toxicity: Isradipine may increase cardiovascular adverse effects of beta-blockers. Isradipine may minimally increase cyclosporine levels. CYP3A4 inhibitors may increase the levels/effects of isradipine; example inhibitors include azole antifungals, ciprofloxacin, clarithromycin, diclofenac, doxycycline, erythromycin, imatinib, isoniazid, nefazodone, nicardipine, propofol, protease inhibitors, quinidine, and verapamil. Blood pressure-lowering effects may be additive with sildenafil, tadalafil, and vardenafil (use caution).

Decreased Effect: NSAIDs (diclofenac) may decrease the antihypertensive response of isradipine. Isradipine may cause a decrease in lovastatin effect. CYP3A4 inducers may decrease the levels/effects of isradipine; example inducers include aminoglutethimide, carbamazepine, nafcillin, nevirapine, phenobarbital, phenytoin, and rifamycins.

Pharmacodynamics/Kinetics

Duration: 8-16 hours

Absorption: 90% to 95%

Protein binding: 95%

Metabolism: Hepatic; extensive first-pass effect

Bioavailability: 15% to 24%

Half-life elimination: 8 hours

Time to peak, serum: 1-1.5 hours

Excretion: Urine (as metabolites)

Pregnancy Risk Factor C

Istalol™ *see* Timolol *on page 1299*

Isuprel® *see* Isoproterenol *on page 770*

Itch-X® [OTC] *see* Pramoxine *on page 1109*

Itraconazole (i tra KOE na zole)

Related Information

Oral Fungal Infections *on page 1544*

U.S. Brand Names Sporanox®

Canadian Brand Names Sporanox®

Mexican Brand Names Carexan®; Isox®; Itranax®; Sporanox®

Generic Available No

Pharmacologic Category Antifungal Agent, Oral

Use Treatment of susceptible fungal infections in immunocompromised and immunocompetent patients including blastomycosis and histoplasmosis; indicated for aspergillosis, and onychomycosis of the toenail; treatment of onychomycosis of the fingernail without concomitant toenail infection via a pulse-type dosing regimen; has activity against *Aspergillus, Candida, Coccidioides, Cryptococcus, Sporothrix*, tinea unguium

Oral: Useful in superficial mycoses including dermatophytoses (eg, tinea capitis), pityriasis versicolor, sebopsoriasis, vaginal and chronic mucocutaneous candidiases; systemic mycoses including candidiasis, meningeal and

(Continued)

Itraconazole *(Continued)*

disseminated cryptococcal infections, paracoccidioidomycosis, coccidioidomycoses; miscellaneous mycoses such as sporotrichosis, chromomycosis, leishmaniasis, fungal keratitis, alternariosis, zygomycosis

Oral solution: Treatment of oral and esophageal candidiasis

Intravenous solution: Indicated in the treatment of blastomycosis, histoplasmosis (nonmeningeal), and aspergillosis (in patients intolerant or refractory to amphotericin B therapy); empiric therapy of febrile neutropenic fever

Local Anesthetic/Vasoconstrictor Precautions No information available to require special precautions

Effects on Dental Treatment No significant effects or complications reported

Significant Adverse Effects Listed incidences are for higher doses appropriate for systemic fungal infections.

>10%: Gastrointestinal: Nausea (11%)

1% to 10%:

Cardiovascular: Edema (4%), hypertension (3%)

Central nervous system: Headache (4%), fatigue (2% to 3%), malaise (1%), fever (3%), dizziness (2%)

Dermatologic: Rash (9%), pruritus (3%)

Endocrine & metabolic: Decreased libido (1%), hypertriglyceridemia, hypokalemia (2%)

Gastrointestinal: Abdominal pain (2%), anorexia (1%), vomiting (5%), diarrhea (3%)

Hepatic: Abnormal LFTs (3%), hepatitis

Renal: Albuminuria (1%)

<1% (Limited to important or life-threatening): Adrenal suppression; allergic reactions (urticaria, angioedema); alopecia, anaphylactoid reactions, anaphylaxis, arrhythmia, CHF, constipation, gastritis, gynecomastia, hepatic failure, impotence, neutropenia, peripheral neuropathy, photosensitivity, pulmonary edema, somnolence, Stevens-Johnson syndrome, tinnitus

Dosage Note: Capsule: Absorption is best if taken with food, therefore, it is best to administer itraconazole after meals; Solution: Should be taken on an empty stomach.

Children: Efficacy and safety have not been established; a small number of patients 3-16 years of age have been treated with 100 mg/day for systemic fungal infections with no serious adverse effects reported. A dose of 5 mg/kg once daily was used in a pharmacokinetic study using the oral solution in patients 6 months-12 years; duration of study was 2 weeks.

Adults:

Oral:

Blastomycosis/histoplasmosis: 200 mg once daily, if no obvious improvement or there is evidence of progressive fungal disease, increase the dose in 100 mg increments to a maximum of 400 mg/day; doses >200 mg/day are given in 2 divided doses; length of therapy varies from 1 day to >6 months depending on the condition and mycological response

Aspergillosis: 200-400 mg/day

Onychomycosis: 200 mg once daily for 12 consecutive weeks

Life-threatening infections: Loading dose: 200 mg 3 times/day (600 mg/day) should be given for the first 3 days of therapy

Oropharyngeal candidiasis: Oral solution: 200 mg once daily for 1-2 weeks; in patients unresponsive or refractory to fluconazole: 100 mg twice daily (clinical response expected in 1-2 weeks)

Esophageal candidiasis: Oral solution: 100-200 mg once daily for a minimum of 3 weeks; continue dosing for 2 weeks after resolution of symptoms

I.V.: 200 mg twice daily for 4 doses, followed by 200 mg daily

Dosing adjustment in renal impairment: Not necessary; itraconazole injection is not recommended in patients with Cl_{cr} <30 mL/minute

Hemodialysis: Not dialyzable

Dosing adjustment in hepatic impairment: May be necessary, but specific guidelines are not available. Risk-to-benefit evaluation should be undertaken in patients who develop liver function abnormalities during treatment.

Mechanism of Action Interferes with cytochrome P450 activity, decreasing ergosterol synthesis (principal sterol in fungal cell membrane) and inhibiting cell membrane formation

Contraindications Hypersensitivity to itraconazole, any component of the formulation, or to other azoles; concurrent administration with cisapride, dofetilide, ergot derivatives, lovastatin, midazolam, pimozide, quinidine, simvastatin, or triazolam; treatment of onychomycosis in patients with evidence of left ventricular dysfunction, CHF, or a history of CHF

Warnings/Precautions Discontinue if signs or symptoms of CHF or neuropathy occur during treatment. Rare cases of serious cardiovascular adverse events (including death), ventricular tachycardia, and torsade de pointes have been observed due to increased cisapride concentrations induced by itraconazole. Use with caution in patients with left ventricular dysfunction or a history of CHF. Not recommended for use in patients with active liver disease, elevated liver enzymes, or prior hepatotoxic reactions to other drugs. Itraconazole has been associated with rare cases of serious hepatotoxicity (including fatal cases and cases within the first week of treatment); treatment should be discontinued in patients who develop clinical symptoms of liver dysfunction or abnormal liver function tests during itraconazole therapy except in cases where expected benefit exceeds risk. Large differences in itraconazole pharmacokinetic parameters have been observed in cystic fibrosis patients receiving the solution; if a patient with cystic fibrosis does not respond to therapy, alternate therapies should be considered. Due to differences in bioavailability, oral capsules and oral solution **cannot** be used interchangeably. Intravenous formulation should be used with caution in renal impairment; consider conversion to oral therapy if renal dysfunction/toxicity is noted. Initiation of treatment with oral solution is not recommended in patients at immediate risk for systemic candidiasis (eg, patients with severe neutropenia).

Drug Interactions Substrate of CYP3A4 (major); **Inhibits** CYP3A4 (strong)

Antacids: May decrease serum concentration of itraconazole. Administer antacids 1 hour before or 2 hours after itraconazole capsules.

Alfentanil: Serum concentrations may be increased; monitor.

Anticonvulsants: Itraconazole may increase the serum concentration of carbamazepine; carbamazepine, phenobarbital, and phenytoin may decrease the serum concentration of itraconazole.

Benzodiazepines: Alprazolam, diazepam, temazepam, triazolam, and midazolam serum concentrations may be increased; consider a benzodiazepine not metabolized by CYP3A4 (such as lorazepam) or another antifungal that is metabolized by CYP3A4

Buspirone: Serum concentrations may be increased; monitor for sedation

Busulfan: Serum concentrations may be increased; avoid concurrent use

Calcium channel blockers: Serum concentrations may be increased (applies to those agents metabolized by CYP3A4, including felodipine, nifedipine, and verapamil); consider another agent instead of a calcium channel blocker, another antifungal, or reduce the dose of the calcium channel blocker; monitor blood pressure

Cisapride; Serum concentration is increased which may lead to malignant arrhythmias; concurrent use is contraindicated

Corticosteroids: Serum levels/effects of the corticosteroid may be increased; use caution.

CYP3A4 inducers: CYP3A4 inducers may decrease the levels/effects of itraconazole. Example inducers include aminoglutethimide, carbamazepine, nafcillin, nevirapine, phenobarbital, phenytoin, and rifamycins.

CYP3A4 substrates: Itraconazole may increase the levels/effects of CYP3A4 substrates. Example substrates include benzodiazepines, calcium channel blockers, mirtazapine, nateglinide, nefazodone, tacrolimus, and venlafaxine. Selected benzodiazepines (midazolam and triazolam), cisapride, ergot alkaloids, selected HMG-CoA reductase inhibitors (lovastatin and simvastatin), and pimozide are generally contraindicated with strong CYP3A4 inhibitors.

Didanosine: May decrease absorption of itraconazole (due to buffering capacity of oral solution); applies only to oral solution formulation of didanosine

Digoxin: Serum concentrations may be increased; monitor.

Disopyramide: Serum levels/effects (including QT_c prolongation) may be increased; use caution.

Docetaxel: Serum concentrations may be increased; avoid concurrent use

Dofetilide: Serum levels/toxicity may be increased; concurrent use is contraindicated.

Ergot alkaloids: Toxicity (vasospasm, ischemia) may be significantly increased by itraconazole; concurrent use is contraindicated.

Erythromycin (and clarithromycin): May increase serum concentrations of itraconazole.

H_2 blockers: May decrease itraconazole absorption. Itraconazole depends on gastric acidity for absorption. Avoid concurrent use.

Halofantrine: Serum levels/effects (including QT_c prolongation) may be increased; use caution.

HMG-CoA reductase inhibitors (except pravastatin and fluvastatin): Serum concentrations may be increased. The risk of myopathy/rhabdomyolysis may

(Continued)

Itraconazole *(Continued)*

be increased. Switch to pravastatin/fluvastatin or suspend treatment during course of itraconazole therapy.

Hypoglycemic agents, oral: Serum concentrations may be increased; monitor.

Immunosuppressants: Cyclosporine, sirolimus, and tacrolimus: Serum concentrations may be increased; monitor serum concentrations and renal function.

Levomethadyl: Serum levels/effects may be increased by itraconazole, potentially resulting in malignant arrhythmia; concurrent use is contraindicated.

Methylprednisolone: Serum levels/effects (including QT_c prolongation) may be increased; concurrent use is contraindicated.

Nevirapine: May decrease serum concentrations of itraconazole; monitor

Oral contraceptives: Efficacy may be reduced by itraconazole (limited data); use barrier birth control method during concurrent use

Pimozide: Serum levels/toxicity may be increased; concurrent use is contraindicated.

Protease inhibitors: May increase serum concentrations of itraconazole. Includes amprenavir, indinavir, nelfinavir, ritonavir, and saquinavir; monitor. Serum concentrations of indinavir, ritonavir, or saquinavir may be increased by itraconazole.

Proton pump inhibitors: May decrease itraconazole absorption. Itraconazole depends on gastric acidity for absorption. Avoid concurrent use (includes omeprazole, lansoprazole).

Quinidine: Serum levels may be increased. Concurrent use is contraindicated.

Rifabutin: Serum concentrations may be increased; monitor.

Sildenafil: Serum concentrations may be increased by itraconazole; consider dosage reduction. A maximum sildenafil dose of 25 mg in 48 hours is recommended with other strong CYP3A4 inhibitors.

Tadalafil: Serum concentrations may be increased by itraconazole. A maximum tadalafil dose of 10 mg in 72 hours is recommended with strong CYP3A4 inhibitors.

Trimetrexate: Serum concentrations may be increased; monitor

Vardenafil: Serum concentrations may be increased by itraconazole. If itraconazole dose is 200 mg/day, limit vardenafil dose to a maximum of 5 mg/24 hours. If itraconazole dose is 400 mg/day, limit vardenafil dose to a maximum of 2.5 mg/24 hours.

Warfarin: Anticoagulant effects may be increased; monitor INR and adjust warfarin's dose as needed

Vinca alkaloids: Serum concentrations may be increased; avoid concurrent use

Zolpidem: Serum levels may be increased; monitor

Ethanol/Nutrition/Herb Interactions

Food:

Capsules: Enhanced by food and possibly by gastric acidity. cola drinks have been shown to increase the absorption of the capsules in patients with achlorhydria or those taking H_2-receptor antagonists or other gastric acid suppressors. Avoid grapefruit juice.

Solution: Decreased by food, time to peak concentration prolonged by food.

Herb/Nutraceutical: St John's wort may decrease itraconazole levels.

Dietary Considerations

Capsule: Administer with food.

Solution: Take without food, if possible.

Pharmacodynamics/Kinetics

Absorption: Requires gastric acidity; capsule better absorbed with food, solution better absorbed on empty stomach; hypochlorhydria has been reported in HIV-infected patients; therefore, oral absorption in these patients may be decreased

Distribution: V_d (average): 796 ± 185 L or 10 L/kg; highly lipophilic and tissue concentrations are higher than plasma concentrations. The highest concentrations: adipose, omentum, endometrium, cervical and vaginal mucus, and skin/nails. Aqueous fluids (eg, CSF and urine) contain negligible amounts.

Protein binding, plasma: 99.9%; metabolite hydroxy-itraconazole: 99.5%

Metabolism: Extensively hepatic via CYP3A4 into >30 metabolites including hydroxy-itraconazole (major metabolite); appears to have *in vitro* antifungal activity. Main metabolic pathway is oxidation; may undergo saturation metabolism with multiple dosing.

Bioavailability: Variable, ~ 55% (oral solution) in 1 small study; **Note:** Oral solution has a higher degree of bioavailability (149% ± 68%) relative to oral capsules; should not be interchanged

Half-life elimination: Oral: After single 200 mg dose: 21 ± 5 hours; 64 hours at steady-state; I.V.: steady-state: 35 hours; steady-state concentrations are achieved in 13 days with multiple administration of itraconazole 100-400 mg/day.

Excretion: Feces (~3% to 18%); urine (~0.03% as parent drug, 40% as metabolites)

Pregnancy Risk Factor C

Lactation Enters breast milk/not recommended

Dosage Forms

Capsule: 100 mg

Injection, solution: 10 mg/mL (25 mL) [packaged in a kit containing sodium chloride 0.9% (50 mL); filtered infusion set (1)]

Solution, oral: 100 mg/10 mL (150 mL) [cherry flavor]

Iveegam EN *see* Immune Globulin (Intravenous) *on page 740*

Ivermectin (eye ver MEK tin)

U.S. Brand Names Stromectol®

Generic Available No

Pharmacologic Category Anthelmintic

Use Treatment of the following infections: Strongyloidiasis of the intestinal tract due to the nematode parasite *Strongyloides stercoralis.* Onchocerciasis due to the nematode parasite *Onchocerca volvulus.* Ivermectin is only active against the immature form of *Onchocerca volvulus*, and the intestinal forms of *Strongyloides stercoralis.*

Unlabeled/Investigational Use Has been used for other parasitic infections including *Ascaris lumbricoides*, Bancroftian filariasis, *Brugia malayi*, scabies, *Enterobius vermicularis, Mansonella ozzardi, Trichuris trichiura.*

Local Anesthetic/Vasoconstrictor Precautions No information available to require special precautions

Effects on Dental Treatment No significant effects or complications reported

Common Adverse Effects Frequency not defined.

Cardiovascular: Hypotension, mild ECG changes, orthostasis, peripheral and facial edema, transient tachycardia

Central nervous system: Dizziness, headache, hyperthermia, insomnia, somnolence, vertigo

Dermatologic: Pruritus, rash, urticaria, toxic epidermal necrolysis

Gastrointestinal: Abdominal pain, anorexia, constipation, diarrhea, nausea, vomiting

Hematologic: Anemia, eosinophilia, leukopenia

Hepatic: ALT/AST increased

Neuromuscular & skeletal: Limbitis, myalgia, tremor, weakness

Ocular: Blurred vision, mild conjunctivitis, punctate opacity

Respiratory: Asthma exacerbation

Mazzotti reaction (with onchocerciasis): Arthralgia, edema, fever, lymphadenopathy, ocular damage, pruritus, rash, synovitis

Mechanism of Action Ivermectin is a semisynthetic antihelminthic agent; it binds selectively and with strong affinity to glutamate-gated chloride ion channels which occur in invertebrate nerve and muscle cells. This leads to increased permeability of cell membranes to chloride ions then hyperpolarization of the nerve or muscle cell, and death of the parasite.

Drug Interactions

Cytochrome P450 Effect: Substrate of CYP3A4 (minor)

Pharmacodynamics/Kinetics

Onset of action: Peak effect: 3-6 months

Absorption: Well absorbed

Distribution: Does not cross blood-brain barrier

Half-life elimination: 16-35 hours

Metabolism: Hepatic (>97%)

Excretion: Urine (<1%); feces

Pregnancy Risk Factor C

IVIG *see* Immune Globulin (Intravenous) *on page 740*

IvyBlock® [OTC] *see* Bentoquatam *on page 189*

Jantoven™ *see* Warfarin *on page 1389*

Japanese Encephalitis Virus Vaccine (Inactivated)

(jap a NEESE en sef a LYE tis VYE rus vak SEEN, in ak ti VAY ted)

Related Information

Immunizations (Vaccines) *on page 1614*

U.S. Brand Names JE-VAX®

Canadian Brand Names JE-VAX®

Generic Available No

(Continued)

Japanese Encephalitis Virus Vaccine (Inactivated) *(Continued)*

Pharmacologic Category Vaccine

Use Active immunization against Japanese encephalitis for persons 1 year of age and older who plan to spend 1 month or more in endemic areas in Asia, especially persons traveling during the transmission season or visiting rural areas; consider vaccination for shorter trips to epidemic areas or extensive outdoor activities in rural endemic areas; elderly (>55 years of age) individuals should be considered for vaccination, since they have increased risk of developing symptomatic illness after infection; those planning travel to or residence in endemic areas should consult the Travel Advisory Service (Central Campus) for specific advice

Local Anesthetic/Vasoconstrictor Precautions No information available to require special precautions

Effects on Dental Treatment No significant effects or complications reported

Common Adverse Effects Report allergic or unusual adverse reactions to the Vaccine Adverse Event Reporting System (VAERS) 1-800-822-7967.

Frequency not defined, common:

- Cardiovascular: Hypotension
- Central nervous system: Fever, headache, malaise, chills, dizziness
- Dermatologic: Rash, urticaria, itching with or without accompanying rash
- Gastrointestinal: Nausea, vomiting, abdominal pain
- Local: Tenderness, redness, and swelling at injection site
- Neuromuscular & skeletal: Myalgia

Frequency not defined, rare:

- Cardiovascular: Angioedema
- Central nervous system: Seizure, encephalitis, encephalopathy
- Dermatologic: Erythema multiforme, erythema nodosum
- Neuromuscular & skeletal: Peripheral neuropathy, joint swelling
- Respiratory: Dyspnea
- Miscellaneous: Anaphylactic reaction

Pregnancy Risk Factor C

JE-VAX® *see* Japanese Encephalitis Virus Vaccine (Inactivated) *on page 779*

Jolivette™ *see* Norethindrone *on page 996*

Junel™ *see* Ethinyl Estradiol and Norethindrone *on page 550*

K+8 *see* Potassium Chloride *on page 1105*

K+10 *see* Potassium Chloride *on page 1105*

Kadian® *see* Morphine Sulfate *on page 947*

Kala® [OTC] *see Lactobacillus on page 793*

Kaletra™ *see* Lopinavir and Ritonavir *on page 839*

Kalmz [OTC] *see* Fructose, Dextrose, and Phosphoric Acid *on page 638*

Kanamycin (kan a MYE sin)

Related Information

Tuberculosis *on page 1495*

U.S. Brand Names Kantrex®

Canadian Brand Names Kantrex®

Mexican Brand Names Koptin®

Generic Available No

Synonyms Kanamycin Sulfate

Pharmacologic Category Antibiotic, Aminoglycoside

Use Treatment of serious infections caused by susceptible strains of *E. coli, Proteus species, Enterobacter aerogenes, Klebsiella pneumoniae, Serratia marcescens,* and *Acinetobacter* species; second-line treatment of *Mycobacterium tuberculosis*

Local Anesthetic/Vasoconstrictor Precautions No information available to require special precautions

Effects on Dental Treatment No significant effects or complications reported

Common Adverse Effects Frequency not defined.

- Cardiovascular: Edema
- Central nervous system: Neurotoxicity, drowsiness, headache, pseudomotor cerebri
- Dermatologic: Skin itching, redness, rash, photosensitivity, erythema
- Gastrointestinal: Nausea, vomiting, diarrhea, malabsorption syndrome (with prolonged and high-dose therapy of hepatic coma), anorexia, weight loss, salivation increased, enterocolitis
- Hematologic: Granulocytopenia, agranulocytosis, thrombocytopenia
- Local: Burning, stinging

Neuromuscular & skeletal: Weakness, tremors, muscle cramps
Otic: Ototoxicity (auditory), ototoxicity (vestibular)
Renal: Nephrotoxicity
Respiratory: Dyspnea

Mechanism of Action Interferes with protein synthesis in bacterial cell by binding to ribosomal subunit

Drug Interactions

Increased Effect/Toxicity: Increased toxicity may occur with amphotericin B, cisplatin, loop diuretics, neuromuscular-blocking agents. Use with bisphosphonate derivatives may lead to hypocalcemia.

Pharmacodynamics/Kinetics

Distribution:
Relative diffusion from blood into CSF: Good only with inflammation (exceeds usual MICs)
CSF:blood level ratio: Normal meninges: Nil; Inflamed meninges: 43%
Half-life elimination: 2-4 hours; Anuria: 80 hours; End-stage renal disease: 40-96 hours
Time to peak, serum: I.M.: 1-2 hours (decreased in burn patients)
Excretion: Urine (entire amount)

Pregnancy Risk Factor D

Kanamycin Sulfate *see* Kanamycin *on page 780*
Kantrex® *see* Kanamycin *on page 780*
Kaodene® NN [OTC] *see* Kaolin and Pectin *on page 781*

Kaolin and Pectin (KAY oh lin & PEK tin)

U.S. Brand Names Kaodene® NN [OTC]; Kao-Spen® [OTC]; Kapectolin® [OTC]

Generic Available Yes

Synonyms Pectin and Kaolin

Pharmacologic Category Antidiarrheal

Use Treatment of uncomplicated diarrhea

Local Anesthetic/Vasoconstrictor Precautions No information available to require special precautions

Effects on Dental Treatment No significant effects or complications reported

Common Adverse Effects Gastrointestinal: Constipation, fecal impaction

Drug Interactions

Decreased Effect: May decrease absorption of many drugs, including chloroquine, atenolol, metoprolol, propranolol, diflunisal, isoniazid, penicillamine, clindamycin, digoxin (give kaolin/pectin 2 hours before or 4 hours after medication).

Pregnancy Risk Factor C

Kaolin, Hyoscyamine, Atropine, Scopolamine, and Pectin *see* Hyoscyamine, Atropine, Scopolamine, Kaolin, and Pectin *on page 726*
Kaolin, Hyoscyamine, Atropine, Scopolamine, Pectin, and Opium *see* Hyoscyamine, Atropine, Scopolamine, Kaolin, Pectin, and Opium *on page 726*
Kaon-Cl-10® *see* Potassium Chloride *on page 1105*
Kaon-Cl® 20 *see* Potassium Chloride *on page 1105*
Kaopectate® [OTC] *see* Bismuth *on page 209*
Kaopectate® Advanced Formula [DSC] [OTC] *see* Attapulgite *on page 170*
Kaopectate® Extra Strength [OTC] *see* Bismuth *on page 209*
Kaopectate® Maximum Strength Caplets [DSC] [OTC] *see* Attapulgite *on page 170*
Kao-Spen® [OTC] *see* Kaolin and Pectin *on page 781*
Kapectolin® [OTC] *see* Kaolin and Pectin *on page 781*
Kapectolin PG® *see* Hyoscyamine, Atropine, Scopolamine, Kaolin, Pectin, and Opium *on page 726*
Kariva™ *see* Ethinyl Estradiol and Desogestrel *on page 536*
Kay Ciel® *see* Potassium Chloride *on page 1105*
K+ Care® *see* Potassium Chloride *on page 1105*
K+ Care® ET *see* Potassium Bicarbonate *on page 1104*
KCl *see* Potassium Chloride *on page 1105*
K-Dur® 10 *see* Potassium Chloride *on page 1105*
K-Dur® 20 *see* Potassium Chloride *on page 1105*
Keflex® *see* Cephalexin *on page 294*
Kemadrin® *see* Procyclidine *on page 1127*
Kenalog® *see* Triamcinolone *on page 1330*
Kenalog-10® *see* Triamcinolone *on page 1330*

Kenalog-40® *see* Triamcinolone *on page 1330*
Kenalog® in Orabase® *see* Triamcinolone *on page 1330*
Kenalog® in Orabase® *see* Triamcinolone Acetonide (Dental Paste) *on page 1333*
Keoxifene Hydrochloride *see* Raloxifene *on page 1166*
Keppra® *see* Levetiracetam *on page 807*
Keralyt® [OTC] *see* Salicylic Acid *on page 1205*
Kerlone® *see* Betaxolol *on page 202*
Kerr Insta-Char® [OTC] *see* Charcoal *on page 303*
Ketalar® *see* Ketamine *on page 782*

Ketamine (KEET a meen)

U.S. Brand Names Ketalar®
Canadian Brand Names Ketalar®
Mexican Brand Names Ketalin®
Generic Available Yes
Synonyms Ketamine Hydrochloride
Pharmacologic Category General Anesthetic
Use Induction and maintenance of general anesthesia, especially when cardiovascular depression must be avoided (ie, hypotension, hypovolemia, cardiomyopathy, constrictive pericarditis); sedation; analgesia
Local Anesthetic/Vasoconstrictor Precautions No information available to require special precautions
Effects on Dental Treatment Key adverse event(s) related to dental treatment: Increased salivation.
Common Adverse Effects
>10%:
Cardiovascular: Hypertension, increased cardiac output, paradoxical direct myocardial depression, tachycardia
Central nervous system: Increased intracranial pressure, visual hallucinations, vivid dreams
Neuromuscular & skeletal: Tonic-clonic movements, tremors
Miscellaneous: Emergence reactions, vocalization
1% to 10%:
Cardiovascular: Bradycardia, hypotension
Dermatologic: Pain at injection site, skin rash
Gastrointestinal: Anorexia, nausea, vomiting
Ocular: Diplopia, nystagmus
Respiratory: Respiratory depression
Restrictions C-III
Mechanism of Action Produces a cataleptic-like state in which the patient is dissociated from the surrounding environment by direct action on the cortex and limbic system. Releases endogenous catecholamines (epinephrine, norepinephrine) which maintain blood pressure and heart rate. Reduces polysynaptic spinal reflexes.
Drug Interactions
Cytochrome P450 Effect: Substrate (major) of CYP2B6, 2C8/9, 3A4
Increased Effect/Toxicity: CYP2B6 inhibitors may increase the levels/effects of ketamine; example inhibitors include desipramine, paroxetine, and sertraline. CYP2C8/9 inhibitors may increase the levels/effects of ketamine; example inhibitors include delavirdine, fluconazole, gemfibrozil, ketoconazole, nicardipine, NSAIDs, pioglitazone, and sulfonamides. CYP3A4 inhibitors may increase the levels/effects of ketamine; example inhibitors include azole antifungals, ciprofloxacin, clarithromycin, diclofenac, doxycycline, erythromycin, imatinib, isoniazid, nefazodone, nicardipine, propofol, protease inhibitors, quinidine, and verapamil. Barbiturates, narcotics, hydroxyzine increase prolonged recovery; nondepolarizing neuromuscular blockers may increase effects. Muscle relaxants, thyroid hormones may increase blood pressure and heart rate. Halothane may decrease BP.
Pharmacodynamics/Kinetics
Onset of action:
I.V.: General anesthesia: 1-2 minutes; Sedation: 1-2 minutes
I.M.: General anesthesia: 3-8 minutes
Duration: I.V.: 5-15 minutes; I.M.: 12-25 minutes
Metabolism: Hepatic via hydroxylation and N-demethylation; the metabolite norketamine is 25% as potent as parent compound
Half-life elimination: 11-17 minutes; Elimination: 2.5-3.1 hours
Excretion: Clearance: 18 mL/kg/minute
Pregnancy Risk Factor D

Ketamine Hydrochloride *see* Ketamine *on page 782*

Ketek™ *see* Telithromycin *on page 1263*

Ketoconazole (kee toe KOE na zole)

Related Information

Oral Fungal Infections *on page 1544*

Respiratory Diseases *on page 1478*

U.S. Brand Names Nizoral®; Nizoral® A-D [OTC]

Canadian Brand Names Apo-Ketoconazole®; Ketoderm®; Nizoral®; Novo-Ketoconazole

Mexican Brand Names Akorazol®; Conazol®; Cremosan®; Fungoral®; Konaderm®; Mi-Ke-Son's®; Mycodib®; Nizoral®; Onofin-K®; Termizol®; Tiniazol®

Generic Available Yes

Pharmacologic Category Antifungal Agent, Oral; Antifungal Agent, Topical

Dental Use Treatment of susceptible fungal infections in the oral cavity including candidiasis, oral thrush, and chronic mucocutaneous candidiasis

Use Treatment of susceptible fungal infections, including candidiasis, oral thrush, blastomycosis, histoplasmosis, paracoccidioidomycosis, coccidioidomycosis, chromomycosis, candiduria, chronic mucocutaneous candidiasis, as well as certain recalcitrant cutaneous dermatophytoses; used topically for treatment of tinea corporis, tinea cruris, tinea versicolor, and cutaneous candidiasis, seborrheic dermatitis

Unlabeled/Investigational Use Treatment of prostate cancer (androgen synthesis inhibitor)

Local Anesthetic/Vasoconstrictor Precautions No information available to require special precautions

Effects on Dental Treatment No significant effects or complications reported

Significant Adverse Effects

Oral:

1% to 10%:

Dermatologic: Pruritus (2%)

Gastrointestinal: Nausea/vomiting (3% to 10%), abdominal pain (1%)

<1% (Limited to important or life-threatening): Bulging fontanelles, chills, depression, diarrhea, dizziness, fever, gynecomastia, headache, hemolytic anemia, hepatotoxicity, impotence, leukopenia, photophobia, somnolence, thrombocytopenia

Cream: Severe irritation, pruritus, stinging (~5%)

Shampoo: Increases in normal hair loss, irritation (<1%), abnormal hair texture, scalp pustules, mild dryness of skin, itching, oiliness/dryness of hair

Dosage

Fungal infections:

Oral:

Children ≥2 years: 3.3-6.6 mg/kg/day as a single dose for 1-2 weeks for candidiasis, for at least 4 weeks in recalcitrant dermatophyte infections, and for up to 6 months for other systemic mycoses

Adults: 200-400 mg/day as a single daily dose for durations as stated above

Shampoo: Apply twice weekly for 4 weeks with at least 3 days between each shampoo

Topical: Rub gently into the affected area once daily to twice daily

Prostate cancer (unlabeled use): Oral: Adults: 400 mg 3 times/day

Dosing adjustment in hepatic impairment: Dose reductions should be considered in patients with severe liver disease

Hemodialysis: Not dialyzable (0% to 5%)

Mechanism of Action Alters the permeability of the cell wall by blocking fungal cytochrome P450; inhibits biosynthesis of triglycerides and phospholipids by fungi; inhibits several fungal enzymes that results in a build-up of toxic concentrations of hydrogen peroxide; also inhibits androgen synthesis

Contraindications Hypersensitivity to ketoconazole or any component of the formulation; CNS fungal infections (due to poor CNS penetration); coadministration with ergot derivatives or cisapride is contraindicated due to risk of potentially fatal cardiac arrhythmias

Warnings/Precautions Use with caution in patients with impaired hepatic function; has been associated with hepatotoxicity, including some fatalities; perform periodic liver function tests; high doses of ketoconazole may depress adrenocortical function.

Drug Interactions Substrate of CYP3A4 (major); **Inhibits** CYP1A2 (strong), 2A6 (moderate), 2B6 (weak), 2C8/9 (strong), 2C19 (moderate), 2D6 (moderate), 3A4 (strong)

Benzodiazepines: Alprazolam, diazepam, temazepam, triazolam, and midazolam serum concentrations may be increased; consider a benzodiazepine

(Continued)

Ketoconazole *(Continued)*

not metabolized by CYP3A4 (such as lorazepam) or another antifungal that is metabolized by CYP3A4. Concurrent use is contraindicated.

Buspirone: Serum concentrations may be increased; monitor for sedation

Busulfan: Serum concentrations may be increased; avoid concurrent use

Calcium channel blockers: Serum concentrations may be increased (applies to those agents metabolized by CYP3A4, including felodipine, nifedipine, and verapamil); consider another agent instead of a calcium channel blocker, another antifungal, or reduce the dose of the calcium channel blocker; monitor blood pressure

Cisapride: Serum concentration is increased which may lead to malignant arrhythmias; concurrent use is contraindicated

CYP1A2 substrates: Ketoconazole may increase the levels/effects of CYP1A2 substrates. Example substrates include aminophylline, fluvoxamine, mexiletine, mirtazapine, ropinirole, theophylline, and trifluoperazine.

CYP2A6 substrates: Ketoconazole may increase the levels/effects of CYP2A6 substrates. Example substrates include dexmedetomidine and ifosfamide.

CYP2C8/9 substrates: Ketoconazole may increase the levels/effects of CYP2C8/9 substrates. Example substrates include amiodarone, fluoxetine, glimepiride, glipizide, nateglinide, phenytoin, pioglitazone, rosiglitazone, sertraline, and warfarin.

CYP2C19 substrates: Ketoconazole may increase the levels/effects of CYP2C19 substrates. Example substrates include citalopram, diazepam, methsuximide, phenytoin, propranolol, and sertraline.

CYP2D6 substrates: Ketoconazole may increase the levels/effects of CYP2D6 substrates. Example substrates include amphetamines, selected beta-blockers, dextromethorphan, fluoxetine, lidocaine, mirtazapine, nefazodone, paroxetine, risperidone, ritonavir, thioridazine, tricyclic antidepressants, and venlafaxine.

CYP2D6 prodrug substrates: Ketoconazole may decrease the levels/effects of CYP2D6 prodrug substrates. Example prodrug substrates include codeine, hydrocodone, oxycodone, and tramadol.

CYP3A4 inducers: CYP3A4 inducers may decrease the levels/effects of ketoconazole. Example inducers include aminoglutethimide, carbamazepine, nafcillin, nevirapine, phenobarbital, phenytoin, and rifamycins.

CYP3A4 substrates: Ketoconazole may increase the levels/effects of CYP3A4 substrates. Example substrates include benzodiazepines, calcium channel blockers, mirtazapine, nateglinide, nefazodone, tacrolimus, and venlafaxine. Selected benzodiazepines (midazolam and triazolam), cisapride, ergot alkaloids, selected HMG-CoA reductase inhibitors (lovastatin and simvastatin), and pimozide are generally contraindicated with strong CYP3A4 inhibitors.

Didanosine: May decrease absorption of ketoconazole (due to buffering capacity of oral solution); applies only to oral solution formulation of didanosine

Docetaxel: Serum concentrations may be increased; avoid concurrent use

Erythromycin (and clarithromycin): May increase serum concentrations of ketoconazole.

H_2 blockers: May decrease ketoconazole absorption. Ketoconazole depends on gastric acidity for absorption. Avoid concurrent use.

HMG-CoA reductase inhibitors (except pravastatin and fluvastatin): Serum concentrations may be increased. The risk of myopathy/rhabdomyolysis may be increased. Switch to pravastatin/fluvastatin or suspend treatment during course of ketoconazole therapy.

Immunosuppressants: Cyclosporine, sirolimus, and tacrolimus: Serum concentrations may be increased; monitor serum concentrations and renal function

Methylprednisolone: Serum concentrations may be increased; monitor

Nevirapine: May decrease serum concentrations of ketoconazole; monitor

Oral contraceptives: Efficacy may be reduced by ketoconazole (limited data); use barrier birth control method during concurrent use

Phenytoin: Serum concentrations may be increased; monitor phenytoin levels and adjust dose as needed

Protease inhibitors: May increase serum concentrations of ketoconazole. Includes amprenavir, indinavir, nelfinavir, ritonavir, and saquinavir; monitor

Proton pump inhibitors: May decrease ketoconazole absorption. Ketoconazole depends on gastric acidity for absorption. Avoid concurrent use (includes omeprazole, lansoprazole).

Quinidine: Serum levels may be increased; monitor

Rifampin: Rifampin decreases ketoconazole's serum concentration to levels which are no longer effective; avoid concurrent use.

Sildenafil: Serum concentrations may be increased by ketoconazole; consider dosage reduction. A maximum sildenafil dose of 25 mg in 48 hours is recommended with other strong CYP3A4 inhibitors.

Tadalafil: Serum concentrations may be increased by ketoconazole. A maximum tadalafil dose of 10 mg in 72 hours is recommended with strong CYP3A4 inhibitors.

Trimetrexate: Serum concentrations may be increased; monitor

Vardenafil: Serum concentrations may be increased by ketoconazole. If ketoconazole dose is 200 mg/day, limit vardenafil to a maximum of 5 mg/24 hours. If ketoconazole dose is 400 mg/day, limit vardenafil dose to a maximum of 2.5 mg/24 hours.

Warfarin: Anticoagulant effects may be increased; monitor INR and adjust warfarin's dose as needed

Vinca alkaloids: Serum concentrations may be increased; avoid concurrent use

Zolpidem: Serum levels may be increased; monitor

Ethanol/Nutrition/Herb Interactions

Food: Ketoconazole peak serum levels may be prolonged if taken with food.

Herb/Nutraceutical: St John's wort may decrease ketoconazole levels.

Dietary Considerations May be taken with food or milk to decrease GI adverse effects.

Pharmacodynamics/Kinetics

Absorption: Oral: Rapid (~75%); Shampoo: None

Distribution: Well into inflamed joint fluid, saliva, bile, urine, breast milk, sebum, cerumen, feces, tendons, skin and soft tissues, and testes; crosses blood-brain barrier poorly; only negligible amounts reach CSF

Protein binding: 93% to 96%

Metabolism: Partially hepatic via CYP3A4 to inactive compounds

Bioavailability: Decreases as gastric pH increases

Half-life elimination: Biphasic: Initial: 2 hours; Terminal: 8 hours

Time to peak, serum: 1-2 hours

Excretion: Feces (57%); urine (13%)

Pregnancy Risk Factor C

Lactation Enters breast milk/not recommended

Dosage Forms

Cream, topical: 2% (15 g, 30 g, 60 g)

Shampoo, topical (Nizoral® A-D): 1% (6 mL, 120 mL, 210 mL)

Tablet (Nizoral®): 200 mg

Ketoprofen (kee toe PROE fen)

Related Information

Oral Pain *on page 1526*

Rheumatoid Arthritis, Osteoarthritis, and Osteoporosis *on page 1490*

Temporomandibular Dysfunction (TMD) *on page 1564*

U.S. Brand Names Orudis® KT [OTC]; Oruvail®

Canadian Brand Names Apo-Keto®; Apo-Keto-E®; Apo-Keto SR®; Novo-Keto; Novo-Keto-EC; Nu-Ketoprofen; Nu-Ketoprofen-E; Orudis® SR; Oruvail®; Rhodis™; Rhodis-EC™; Rhodis SR™

Mexican Brand Names Keduril®; K-Profen®; Orudis®; Profenid®

Generic Available Yes: Capsule

Pharmacologic Category Nonsteroidal Anti-inflammatory Drug (NSAID), Oral

Dental Use Management of pain and swelling

Use Acute and long-term treatment of rheumatoid arthritis and osteoarthritis; primary dysmenorrhea; mild to moderate pain

Local Anesthetic/Vasoconstrictor Precautions No information available to require special precautions

Effects on Dental Treatment Key adverse event(s) related to dental treatment: Stomatitis.

NSAID formulations are known to reversibly decrease platelet aggregation via mechanisms different than observed with aspirin. The dentist should be aware of the potential of abnormal coagulation. Caution should also be exercised in the use of NSAIDs in patients already on anticoagulant therapy with drugs such as warfarin (Coumadin®).

Significant Adverse Effects

>10%: Gastrointestinal: Dyspepsia (11%)

1% to 10%:

Central nervous system: Headache (3% to 9%), nervousness, dizziness, somnolence, insomnia, malaise, depression

Dermatologic: Rash, itching

Endocrine & metabolic: Fluid retention

(Continued)

Ketoprofen *(Continued)*

Gastrointestinal: Vomiting (>1%), diarrhea (3% to 9%), nausea (3% to 9%), constipation (3% to 9%), abdominal distress/cramping/pain (3% to 9%), flatulence (3% to 9%), anorexia (>1%), stomatitis (>1%)

Genitourinary: Urinary tract infection (>1%)

Ocular: Visual disturbances

Otic: Tinnitus

Renal: Renal function impairment

<1% (Limited to important or life-threatening): Acute renal failure, agranulocytosis, allergic reaction, allergic rhinitis, anaphylaxis, anemia, angioedema, arrhythmias, aseptic meningitis, blurred vision, bone marrow suppression, confusion, congestive heart failure, conjunctivitis, cystitis, drowsiness, dry eyes, dyspnea, epistaxis, erythema multiforme, gastritis, GI ulceration, hallucinations, hearing decreased, hemolytic anemia, hepatitis, hot flashes, hypertension, leukopenia, peripheral neuropathy, photosensitivity, polydipsia, polyuria, Stevens-Johnson syndrome, tachycardia, thrombocytopenia, toxic amblyopia, toxic epidermal necrolysis, urticaria

Dosage Oral:

Children ≥16 years and Adults:

Rheumatoid arthritis or osteoarthritis:

Capsule: 50-75 mg 3-4 times/day up to a maximum of 300 mg/day

Capsule, extended release: 200 mg once daily

Mild to moderate pain: Capsule: 25-50 mg every 6-8 hours up to a maximum of 300 mg/day

OTC labeling: 12.5 mg every 4-6 hours, up to a maximum of 6 tablets/24 hours

Elderly: Initial dose should be decreased in patients >75 years; use caution when dosage changes are made

Dosage adjustment in renal impairment:

Mild impairment: Maximum dose: 150 mg/day

Severe impairment: Maximum dose: 100 mg/day

Dosage adjustment in hepatic impairment and serum albumin <3.5 g/dL:

Maximum dose: 100 mg/day

Mechanism of Action Inhibits prostaglandin synthesis by decreasing the activity of the enzyme, cyclooxygenase, which results in decreased formation of prostaglandin precursors

Contraindications Hypersensitivity to ketoprofen, any component of the formulation, or other NSAIDs/aspirin; pregnancy (3rd trimester)

Warnings/Precautions Use with caution in patients with CHF, hypertension, dehydration, decreased renal or hepatic function, history of GI disease (bleeding or ulcers), or those receiving anticoagulants. Elderly are at a high risk for adverse effects from NSAIDs. As many as 60% of elderly can develop peptic ulceration and/or hemorrhage asymptomatically.

Use lowest effective dose for shortest period possible. Use of NSAIDs can compromise existing renal function especially when Cl_{cr} is <30 mL/minute. CNS adverse effects such as confusion, agitation, and hallucination are generally seen in overdose or high-dose situations; however, elderly may demonstrate these adverse effects at lower doses than younger adults. Withhold for at least 4-6 half-lives prior to surgical or dental procedures. Safety and efficacy in pediatric patients have not been established.

Drug Interactions Inhibits CYP2C8/9 (weak)

ACE inhibitors: Antihypertensive effects may be decreased by concurrent therapy with NSAIDs; monitor blood pressure

Angiotensin II antagonists: Antihypertensive effects may be decreased by concurrent therapy with NSAIDs; monitor blood pressure

Anticoagulants (warfarin, heparin, LMWHs) in combination with NSAIDs can cause increased risk of bleeding.

Other antiplatelet drugs (ticlopidine, clopidogrel, aspirin, abciximab, dipyridamole, eptifibatide, tirofiban) can cause an increased risk of bleeding.

Corticosteroids may increase the risk of GI ulceration; avoid concurrent use.

Cyclosporine: NSAIDs may increase serum creatinine, potassium, blood pressure, and cyclosporine levels; monitor cyclosporine levels and renal function carefully

Gentamicin and amikacin serum concentrations are increased by indomethacin in premature infants. Results may apply to other aminoglycosides and NSAIDs.

Hydralazine's antihypertensive effect is decreased; avoid concurrent use

Lithium: Levels can be increased by NSAIDs; avoid concurrent use if possible or monitor lithium levels and adjust dose. Sulindac may have the least effect.

Loop diuretics: Efficacy (diuretic and antihypertensive effect) is reduced.

Methotrexate: NSAIDs may decrease the excretion of methotrexate; monitor.
Probenecid: Clearance of ketoprofen may be decreased.
Thiazides antihypertensive effects are decreased; avoid concurrent use
Verapamil plasma concentration is decreased by diclofenac; avoid concurrent use
Warfarin's INRs may be increased by piroxicam. Other NSAIDs may have the same effect depending on dose and duration. Monitor INR closely. Use the lowest dose of NSAIDs possible and for the briefest duration.

Ethanol/Nutrition/Herb Interactions

Ethanol: Avoid ethanol (due to GI irritation).
Food: Although food affects the bioavailability of ketoprofen, analgesic efficacy is not significantly diminished; food slows rate of absorption resulting in delayed and reduced peak serum concentrations.

Dietary Considerations In order to minimize gastrointestinal effects, ketoprofen can be prescribed to be taken with food or milk.

Pharmacodynamics/Kinetics

Absorption: Almost complete
Protein binding: >99%, primarily albumin
Metabolism: Hepatic
Half-life elimination: Capsule: 2.5 hours; Capsule, extended release: 5.4 hours
Time to peak, serum: Capsule: 0.5-2 hours; Capsule, extended release: 6-7 hours
Excretion: Urine (~80%, primarily as glucuronide conjugates)

Pregnancy Risk Factor B/D (3rd trimester)

Lactation Excretion in breast milk unknown/not recommended

Dosage Forms

Capsule: 50 mg, 75 mg
Capsule, extended release (Oruvail®): 100 mg, 150 mg, 200 mg
Tablet (Orudis® KT): 12.5 mg [contains tartrazine and sodium benzoate]

Selected Readings

Brooks PM and Day RO, "Nonsteroidal Anti-inflammatory Drugs - Differences and Similarities," *N Engl J Med*, 1991, 324(24):1716-25.
Cooper SA, "Ketoprofen in Oral Surgery Pain: A Review," *J Clin Pharmacol*, 1988, 28(12 Suppl):S40-6.
Hersh EV, "The Efficacy and Safety of Ketoprofen in Postsurgical Dental Pain," *Compendium*, 1991, 12(4):234.

Ketorolac (KEE toe role ak)

Related Information

Rheumatoid Arthritis, Osteoarthritis, and Osteoporosis *on page 1490*
Temporomandibular Dysfunction (TMD) *on page 1564*

U.S. Brand Names Acular®; Acular LS™; Acular® PF; Toradol®

Canadian Brand Names Acular®; Apo-Ketorolac®; Apo-Ketorolac Injectable®; Novo-Ketorolac; ratio-Ketorolac; Toradol®; Toradol® IM

Mexican Brand Names Acularen®; Alidol®; Dolac®; Dolotor®; Findol®; Supradol®

Generic Available Yes: Injection, tablet

Synonyms Ketorolac Tromethamine

Pharmacologic Category Nonsteroidal Anti-inflammatory Drug (NSAID), Ophthalmic; Nonsteroidal Anti-inflammatory Drug (NSAID), Oral; Nonsteroidal Anti-inflammatory Drug (NSAID), Parenteral

Use

Oral, injection: Short-term (≤5 days) management of moderately-severe acute pain requiring analgesia at the opioid level
Ophthalmic: Temporary relief of ocular itching due to seasonal allergic conjunctivitis; postoperative inflammation following cataract extraction; reduction of ocular pain and photophobia following incisional refractive surgery, reduction of ocular pain, burning and stinging following corneal refractive surgery

Local Anesthetic/Vasoconstrictor Precautions No information available to require special precautions

Effects on Dental Treatment Key adverse event(s) related to dental treatment: Xerostomia (normal salivary flow resumes upon discontinuation).
NSAID formulations are known to reversibly decrease platelet aggregation via mechanisms different than observed with aspirin. The dentist should be aware of the potential of abnormal coagulation. Caution should also be exercised in the use of NSAIDs in patients already on anticoagulant therapy with drugs such as warfarin (Coumadin®).

Significant Adverse Effects

Systemic:

>10%:
Central nervous system: Headache (17%)

(Continued)

Ketorolac *(Continued)*

Gastrointestinal: Gastrointestinal pain (13%), dyspepsia (12%), nausea (12%)

>1% to 10%:

Cardiovascular: Edema (4%), hypertension

Central nervous system: Dizziness (7%), drowsiness (6%)

Dermatologic: Pruritus, purpura, rash

Gastrointestinal: Diarrhea (7%), constipation, flatulence, gastrointestinal fullness, vomiting, stomatitis

Local: Injection site pain (2%)

Miscellaneous: Diaphoresis

≤1% (Limited to important or life-threatening): Abnormal vision, acute renal failure, anaphylactoid reaction, anaphylaxis, asthma, azotemia, bronchospasm, cholestatic jaundice, convulsions, eosinophilia, epistaxis, esophagitis, extrapyramidal symptoms, GI hemorrhage, GI perforation, hallucinations, hearing loss, hematemesis, hematuria, hepatitis, hypersensitivity reactions, liver failure, Lyell's syndrome, maculopapular rash, nephritis, peptic ulceration, Stevens-Johnson syndrome, tinnitus, toxic epidermal necrolysis, urticaria, vertigo, wound hemorrhage (postoperative)

Ophthalmic solution:

>10%: Ocular: Transient burning/stinging (Acular®: 40%; Acular® PF: 20%)

>1% to 10%:

Central nervous system: Headache

Ocular: Conjunctival hyperemia, corneal infiltrates, iritis, ocular edema, ocular inflammation, ocular irritation, ocular pain, superficial keratitis, superficial ocular infection

Miscellaneous: Allergic reactions

≤1% (Limited to important or life-threatening): Blurred vision corneal ulcer, corneal erosion, corneal perforation, corneal thinning, dry eyes, epithelial breakdown

Dosage

Children 2-16 years: **Do not exceed adult doses**

Single-dose treatment:

I.M.: 1 mg/kg (maximum: 30 mg)

I.V.: 0.5 mg/kg (maximum: 15 mg)

Oral (unlabeled): 1 mg/kg as a single dose reported in one study

Multiple-dose treatment (unlabeled): Limited pediatric studies. The maximum combined duration of treatment (for parenteral and oral) is 5 days.

I.V.: Initial dose: 0.5 mg/kg, followed by 0.25-1 mg/kg every 6 hours for up to 48 hours (maximum daily dose: 90 mg)

Oral: 0.25 mg/kg every 6 hours

Adults (pain relief usually begins within 10 minutes with parenteral forms): **Note:** The maximum combined duration of treatment (for parenteral and oral) is 5 days; do not increase dose or frequency; supplement with low-dose opioids if needed for breakthrough pain. For patients <50 kg and/or ≥65 years, see Elderly dosing.

I.M.: 60 mg as a single dose or 30 mg every 6 hours (maximum daily dose: 120 mg)

I.V.: 30 mg as a single dose or 30 mg every 6 hours (maximum daily dose: 120 mg)

Oral: 20 mg, followed by 10 mg every 4-6 hours; do not exceed 40 mg/day; oral dosing is intended to be a continuation of I.M. or I.V. therapy only

Ophthalmic: Children ≥3 years and Adults:

Allergic conjunctivitis (relief of ocular itching) (Acular®): Instill 1 drop (0.25 mg) 4 times/day for seasonal allergic conjunctivitis

Inflammation following cataract extraction (Acular®): Instill 1 drop (0.25 mg) to affected eye(s) 4 times/day beginning 24 hours after surgery; continue for 2 weeks

Pain and photophobia following incisional refractive surgery (Acular® PF): Instill 1 drop (0.25 mg) 4 times/day to affected eye for up to 3 days

Pain following corneal refractive surgery (Acular LS™): Instill 1 drop 4 times/day as needed to affected eye for up to 4 days

Elderly >65 years: Renal insufficiency or weight <50 kg: **Note:** Ketorolac has decreased clearance and increased half-life in the elderly. In addition, the elderly have reported increased incidence of GI bleeding, ulceration, and perforation. The maximum combined duration of treatment (for parenteral and oral) is 5 days.

I.M.: 30 mg as a single dose or 15 mg every 6 hours (maximum daily dose: 60 mg)

I.V.: 15 mg as a single dose or 15 mg every 6 hours (maximum daily dose: 60 mg)

Oral: 10 mg every 4-6 hours; do not exceed 40 mg/day; oral dosing is intended to be a continuation of I.M. or I.V. therapy only

Dosage adjustment in renal impairment: Do not use in patients with advanced renal impairment. Patients with moderately-elevated serum creatinine should use half the recommended dose, not to exceed 60 mg/day I.M./I.V.

Dosage adjustment in hepatic impairment: Use with caution, may cause elevation of liver enzymes

Mechanism of Action Inhibits prostaglandin synthesis by decreasing the activity of the enzyme, cyclooxygenase, which results in decreased formation of prostaglandin precursors

Contraindications Hypersensitivity to ketorolac, aspirin, other NSAIDs, or any component of the formulation; patients who have developed nasal polyps, angioedema, or bronchospastic reactions to other NSAIDs; active or history of peptic ulcer disease; recent or history of GI bleeding or perforation; patients with advanced renal disease or risk of renal failure; labor and delivery; nursing mothers; prophylaxis before major surgery; suspected or confirmed cerebrovascular bleeding; hemorrhagic diathesis; concurrent ASA or other NSAIDs; epidural or intrathecal administration; concomitant probenecid; pregnancy (3rd trimester)

Warnings/Precautions

Systemic: Treatment should be started with I.V./I.M. administration then changed to oral only as a continuation of treatment. Total therapy is not to exceed 5 days. Should not be used for minor or chronic pain. Hypersensitivity reactions have occurred flowing the first dose of ketorolac injection, including patients without prior exposure to ketorolac, aspirin, or other NSAIDs. Use extra caution and reduce dosages in the elderly because it is cleared renally somewhat slower, and the elderly are also more sensitive to the renal effects of NSAIDs and have a greater risk of GI perforation and bleeding; use with caution in patients with CHF, hypertension, dehydration, decreased renal or hepatic function, or those receiving anticoagulants. May prolong bleeding time; do not use when hemostasis is critical. Patients should be euvolemic prior to treatment. Low doses of narcotics may be needed for breakthrough pain. Withhold for at least 4-6 half-lives prior to surgical or dental procedures.

Ophthalmic: May increase bleeding time associated with ocular surgery. Use with caution in patients with known bleeding tendencies or those receiving anticoagulants. Healing time may be slowed or delayed. Corneal thinning, erosion, or ulceration have been reported with topical NSAIDs; discontinue if corneal epithelial breakdown occurs. Use caution with complicated ocular surgery, corneal denervation, corneal epithelial defects, diabetes, rheumatoid arthritis, ocular surface disease, or ocular surgeries repeated within short periods of time; risk of corneal epithelial breakdown may be increased. Use for >24 hours prior to or for >14 days following surgery also increases risk of corneal adverse effects. Do not administer while wearing soft contact lenses. Safety and efficacy in pediatric patients <3 years of age have not been established.

Drug Interactions

ACE inhibitors: Antihypertensive effects may be decreased by concurrent therapy with NSAIDs; monitor blood pressure.

Angiotensin II antagonists: Antihypertensive effects may be decreased by concurrent therapy with NSAIDs; monitor blood pressure.

Anticoagulants: Increased risk of bleeding complications with concomitant use; monitor closely.

Antiepileptic drugs (carbamazepine, phenytoin): Sporadic cases of seizures have been reported with concomitant use.

Diuretics: May see decreased effect of diuretics.

Lithium: May increase lithium levels; monitor.

Methotrexate: Severe bone marrow suppression, aplastic anemia, and GI toxicity have been reported with concomitant NSAID therapy. Avoid use during moderate or high-dose methotrexate (increased and prolonged methotrexate levels). NSAID use during low-dose treatment of rheumatoid arthritis has not been fully evaluated; extreme caution is warranted.

Nondepolarizing muscle relaxants: Concomitant use has resulted in apnea.

NSAIDs, salicylates: Concomitant use increases NSAID-induced adverse effects; contraindicated.

Probenecid: Probenecid significantly decreases ketorolac clearance, increases ketorolac plasma levels, and doubles the half-life of ketorolac; concomitant use is contraindicated.

(Continued)

Ketorolac *(Continued)*

Psychoactive drugs (alprazolam, fluoxetine, thiothixene): Hallucinations have been reported with concomitant use.

Ethanol/Nutrition/Herb Interactions

Ethanol: Avoid ethanol (may enhance gastric mucosal irritation).

Food: Oral: High-fat meals may delay time to peak (by ~1 hour) and decrease peak concentrations.

Herb/Nutraceutical: Avoid cat's claw, dong quai, evening primrose, feverfew, garlic, ginger, ginkgo, red clover, horse chestnut, green tea, ginseng (all have additional antiplatelet activity).

Dietary Considerations Administer tablet with food or milk to decrease gastrointestinal distress.

Pharmacodynamics/Kinetics

Onset of action: Analgesic: I.M.: ~10 minutes

Peak effect: Analgesic: 2-3 hours

Duration: Analgesic: 6-8 hours

Absorption: Oral: Well absorbed

Distribution: Poor penetration into CSF; crosses placenta; enters breast milk

Protein binding: 99%

Metabolism: Hepatic

Half-life elimination: 2-8 hours; prolonged 30% to 50% in elderly

Time to peak, serum: I.M.: 30-60 minutes

Excretion: Urine (61% as unchanged drug)

Pregnancy Risk Factor C/D (3rd trimester); ophthalmic: C

Lactation Enters breast milk/contraindicated (AAP rates "compatible")

Dosage Forms

Injection, solution, as tromethamine (Toradol®): 15 mg/mL (1 mL); 30 mg/mL (1 mL, 2 mL) [contains alcohol]

Solution, ophthalmic, as tromethamine:

Acular®: 0.5% (3 mL, 5 mL, 10 mL) [contains benzalkonium chloride]

Acular LS™: 0.4% (5 mL) [contains benzalkonium chloride]

Acular® P.F. [preservative free]: 0.5% (0.4 mL)

Tablet, as tromethamine (Toradol®): 10 mg

Comments According to the manufacturer, ketorolac has been used inappropriately by physicians in the past. The drug had been prescribed to NSAID-sensitive patients, patients with GI bleeding, and for long-term use; a warning has been issued regarding increased incidence and severity of GI complications with increasing doses and duration of use. Labeling now includes the statement that ketorolac inhibits platelet function and is indicated for up to 5 days use only.

Selected Readings

Ahmad N, Grad HA, Haas DA, et al, "The Efficacy of Nonopioid Analgesics for Postoperative Dental Pain: A Meta-Analysis," *Anesth Prog*, 1997, 44(4):119-26.

Balevi B, "Ketorolac Versus Ibuprofen: A Simple Cost-Efficacy Comparison for Dental Use," *J Can Dent Assoc*, 1994, 60(1):31-2.

Forbes JA, Butterworth GA, Burchfield WH, et al, "Evaluation of Ketorolac, Aspirin, and an Acetaminophen-Codeine Combination in Postoperative Oral Surgery Pain," *Pharmacotherapy*, 1990, 10(6 Pt 2): 77S-93S.

Forbes JA, Kehm CJ, Grodin CD, et al, "Evaluation of Ketorolac, Ibuprofen, Acetaminophen, and an Acetaminophen-Codeine Combination in Postoperative Oral Surgery Pain," *Pharmacotherapy*, 1990, 10(6 Pt 2):94S-105S.

Fricke JR Jr, Angelocci D, Fox K, et al, "Comparison of the Efficacy and Safety of Ketorolac and Meperidine in the Relief of Dental Pain," *J Clin Pharmacol*, 1992, 32(4):376-84.

Fricke J, Halladay SC, Bynum L, et al, "Pain Relief After Dental Impaction Surgery Using Ketorolac, Hydrocodone Plus Acetaminophen, or Placebo," *Clin Ther*, 1993, 15(3):500-9.

Pendeville PE, Van Boven MJ, Contreras V, et al, "Ketorolac Tromethamine for Postoperative Analgesia in Oral Surgery," *Acta Anaesthesiol Belg*, 1995, 46(1):25-30.

Swift JQ, Roszkowski MT, Alton T, "Effect of Intra-articular Versus Systemic Anti-inflammatory Drugs in a Rabbit Model of Temporomandibular Joint Inflammation," *J Oral Maxillofac Surg*, 1998, 56(11):1288-95; discussion 1295-6.

Walton GM, Rood JP, Snowdon AT, et al, "Ketorolac and Diclofenac for Postoperative Pain Relief Following Oral Surgery," *Br J Oral Maxillofac Surg*, 1993, 31(3):158-60.

Wynn RL, "Ketorolac (Toradol®) for Dental Pain," *Gen Dent*, 1992, 40(6):476-9.

Ketorolac Tromethamine *see* Ketorolac *on page 787*

Ketotifen (kee toe TYE fen)

U.S. Brand Names Zaditor™

Canadian Brand Names Apo-Ketotifen®; Novo-Ketotifen; Zaditen®; Zaditor™

Mexican Brand Names Kasmal®; Ventisol®; Zaditen®

Generic Available No

Synonyms Ketotifen Fumarate

Pharmacologic Category Antihistamine, H_1 Blocker, Ophthalmic

Use Temporary prevention of eye itching due to allergic conjunctivitis

Local Anesthetic/Vasoconstrictor Precautions No information available to require special precautions

Effects on Dental Treatment Key adverse event(s) related to dental treatment: Pharyngitis.

Mechanism of Action Relatively selective, noncompetitive H_1-receptor antagonist and mast cell stabilizer, inhibiting the release of mediators from cells involved in hypersensitivity reactions

Pregnancy Risk Factor C

Ketotifen Fumarate *see* Ketotifen *on page 790*
Key-E® [OTC] *see* Vitamin E *on page 1383*
Key-E® Kaps [OTC] *see* Vitamin E *on page 1383*
KI *see* Potassium Iodide *on page 1106*
Kidkare Decongestant [OTC] *see* Pseudoephedrine *on page 1147*
Kineret® *see* Anakinra *on page 131*
Kinevac® *see* Sincalide *on page 1224*
Klaron® *see* Sulfacetamide *on page 1244*
Klonopin® *see* Clonazepam *on page 356*
K-Lor™ *see* Potassium Chloride *on page 1105*
Klor-Con® *see* Potassium Chloride *on page 1105*
Klor-Con® 8 *see* Potassium Chloride *on page 1105*
Klor-Con® 10 *see* Potassium Chloride *on page 1105*
Klor-Con®/25 *see* Potassium Chloride *on page 1105*
Klor-Con®/EF *see* Potassium Bicarbonate and Potassium Citrate *on page 1105*
Klor-Con® M *see* Potassium Chloride *on page 1105*
Klotrix® *see* Potassium Chloride *on page 1105*
K-Lyte® *see* Potassium Bicarbonate and Potassium Citrate *on page 1105*
K-Lyte/Cl® *see* Potassium Bicarbonate and Potassium Chloride *on page 1104*
K-Lyte/Cl® 50 *see* Potassium Bicarbonate and Potassium Chloride *on page 1104*
K-Lyte® DS *see* Potassium Bicarbonate and Potassium Citrate *on page 1105*
Koāte®-DVI *see* Antihemophilic Factor (Human) *on page 134*
Kodet SE [OTC] *see* Pseudoephedrine *on page 1147*
Kogenate® FS *see* Antihemophilic Factor (Recombinant) *on page 135*
Kolephrin® GG/DM [OTC] *see* Guaifenesin and Dextromethorphan *on page 673*
Konsyl® [OTC] *see* Psyllium *on page 1151*
Konsyl-D® [OTC] *see* Psyllium *on page 1151*
Konsyl® Easy Mix [OTC] *see* Psyllium *on page 1151*
Konsyl® Orange [OTC] *see* Psyllium *on page 1151*
Konsyl® Tablets [OTC] *see* Polycarbophil *on page 1100*
K-Phos® MF *see* Potassium Phosphate and Sodium Phosphate *on page 1107*
K-Phos® Neutral *see* Potassium Phosphate and Sodium Phosphate *on page 1107*
K-Phos® No. 2 *see* Potassium Phosphate and Sodium Phosphate *on page 1107*
K-Phos® Original *see* Potassium Acid Phosphate *on page 1104*
Kristalose™ *see* Lactulose *on page 794*
Kronofed-A® *see* Chlorpheniramine and Pseudoephedrine *on page 315*
Kronofed-A®-Jr *see* Chlorpheniramine and Pseudoephedrine *on page 315*
K-Tab® *see* Potassium Chloride *on page 1105*
Kutrase® *see* Pancreatin *on page 1042*
Ku-Zyme® *see* Pancreatin *on page 1042*
Ku-Zyme® HP *see* Pancrelipase *on page 1042*
Kwelcof® *see* Hydrocodone and Guaifenesin *on page 708*
Kytril® *see* Granisetron *on page 671*
L-749,345 *see* Ertapenem *on page 507*
L 754030 *see* Aprepitant *on page 138*
LA 20304a *see* Gemifloxacin *on page 653*

Labetalol (la BET a lole)

Related Information

Cardiovascular Diseases *on page 1458*

U.S. Brand Names Normodyne®; Trandate®

Canadian Brand Names Apo-Labetalol®; Normodyne®; Trandate®

Generic Available Yes

Synonyms Ibidomide Hydrochloride; Labetalol Hydrochloride

Pharmacologic Category Beta Blocker With Alpha-Blocking Activity

(Continued)

Labetalol *(Continued)*

Use Treatment of mild to severe hypertension; I.V. for hypertensive emergencies

Local Anesthetic/Vasoconstrictor Precautions Use with caution; epinephrine has interacted with nonselective beta-blockers to result in initial hypertensive episode followed by bradycardia

Effects on Dental Treatment Key adverse event(s) related to dental treatment: Taste disorder.

Noncardioselective beta-blockers enhance the pressor response to epinephrine, resulting in hypertension and bradycardia. Many nonsteroidal anti-inflammatory drugs, such as ibuprofen and indomethacin, can reduce the hypotensive effect of beta-blockers after 3 or more weeks of therapy with the NSAID. Short-term NSAID use (ie, 3 days) requires no special precautions in patients taking beta-blockers.

Common Adverse Effects

>10%:

Central nervous system: Dizziness (1% to 16%)

Gastrointestinal: Nausea (0% to 19%)

1% to 10%:

Cardiovascular: Edema (0% to 2%), hypotension (1% to 5%); with IV use, hypotension may occur in up to 58%

Central nervous system: Fatigue (1% to 10%), paresthesia (1% to 5%), headache (2%), vertigo (2%), weakness (1%)

Dermatologic: Rash (1%), scalp tingling (1% to 5%)

Gastrointestinal: Vomiting (<1% to 3%), dyspepsia (1% to 4%)

Genitourinary: Ejaculatory failure (0% to 5%), impotence (1% to 4%)

Hepatic: Increased transaminases (4%)

Respiratory: Nasal congestion (1% to 6%), dyspnea (2%)

Miscellaneous: Taste disorder (1%), abnormal vision (1%)

Other adverse reactions noted with beta-adrenergic blocking agents include mental depression, catatonia, disorientation, short-term memory loss, emotional lability, clouded sensorium, intensification of pre-existing AV block, laryngospasm, respiratory distress, agranulocytosis, thrombocytopenic purpura, nonthrombocytopenic purpura, mesenteric artery thrombosis, and ischemic colitis.

Mechanism of Action Blocks alpha-, beta$_1$-, and beta$_2$-adrenergic receptor sites; elevated renins are reduced

Drug Interactions

Cytochrome P450 Effect: Substrate of CYP2D6 (major); **Inhibits** CYP2D6 (weak)

Increased Effect/Toxicity: CYP2D6 inhibitors may increase the levels/effects of labetalol; example inhibitors include chlorpromazine, delavirdine, fluoxetine, miconazole, paroxetine, pergolide, quinidine, quinine, ritonavir, and ropinirole. Cimetidine increases the bioavailability of labetalol. Labetalol has additive hypotensive effects with other antihypertensive agents. Concurrent use with alpha-blockers (prazosin, terazosin) and beta-blockers increases the risk of orthostasis. Concurrent use with diltiazem, verapamil, or digoxin may increase the risk of bradycardia with beta-blocking agents. Halothane, enflurane, isoflurane, and potentially other inhalation anesthetics may cause synergistic hypotension. Beta-blockers may affect the action or levels of ethanol, disopyramide, nondepolarizing muscle relaxants, and theophylline although the effects are difficult to predict.

Decreased Effect: Decreased effect of beta-blockers with aluminum salts, barbiturates, calcium salts, cholestyramine, colestipol, NSAIDs, penicillins (ampicillin), rifampin, salicylates, and sulfinpyrazone due to decreased bioavailability and plasma levels. Beta-blockers may decrease the effect of sulfonylureas.

Pharmacodynamics/Kinetics

Onset of action: Oral: 20 minutes to 2 hours; I.V.: 2-5 minutes

Peak effect: Oral: 1-4 hours; I.V.: 5-15 minutes

Duration: Oral: 8-24 hours (dose dependent); I.V.: 2-4 hours

Distribution: V_d: Adults: 3-16 L/kg; mean: <9.4 L/kg; moderately lipid soluble, therefore, can enter CNS; crosses placenta; small amounts enter breast milk

Protein binding: 50%

Metabolism: Hepatic, primarily via glucuronide conjugation; extensive first-pass effect

Bioavailability: Oral: 25%; increased with liver disease, elderly, and concurrent cimetidine

Half-life elimination: Normal renal function: 2.5-8 hours

Excretion: Urine (<5% as unchanged drug)

Clearance: Possibly decreased in neonates/infants

Pregnancy Risk Factor C (manufacturer); D (2nd and 3rd trimesters - expert analysis)

Labetalol Hydrochloride *see* Labetalol *on page 791*
Lac-Hydrin® *see* Lactic Acid and Ammonium Hydroxide *on page 793*
Lac-Hydrin® Five [OTC] *see* Lactic Acid and Ammonium Hydroxide *on page 793*
LAClotion™ *see* Lactic Acid and Ammonium Hydroxide *on page 793*
Lacrisert® *see* Hydroxypropyl Cellulose *on page 721*
Lactaid® [OTC] *see* Lactase *on page 793*
Lactaid® Extra Strength [OTC] *see* Lactase *on page 793*
Lactaid® Ultra [OTC] *see* Lactase *on page 793*

Lactase (LAK tase)

U.S. Brand Names Lactaid® [OTC]; Lactaid® Extra Strength [OTC]; Lactaid® Ultra [OTC]; Lactrase® [OTC]
Canadian Brand Names Dairyaid®
Generic Available No
Pharmacologic Category Enzyme
Use Help digest lactose in milk for patients with lactose intolerance
Local Anesthetic/Vasoconstrictor Precautions No information available to require special precautions
Effects on Dental Treatment No significant effects or complications reported

Lactic Acid and Ammonium Hydroxide

(LAK tik AS id with a MOE nee um hye DROKS ide)
U.S. Brand Names AmLactin® [OTC]; Geri-Hydrolac™ [OTC]; Geri-Hydrolac™-12 [OTC]; Lac-Hydrin®; Lac-Hydrin® Five [OTC]; LAClotion™
Generic Available Yes
Synonyms Ammonium Lactate
Pharmacologic Category Topical Skin Product
Use Treatment of moderate to severe xerosis and ichthyosis vulgaris
Local Anesthetic/Vasoconstrictor Precautions No information available to require special precautions
Effects on Dental Treatment No significant effects or complications reported
Common Adverse Effects
>10%: Dermatologic: Rash, including erythema and irritation (2% to 15%); burning/stinging (2% to 15%)
1% to 10%: Dermatologic: Itching (5%), dry skin (2%)
Mechanism of Action Exact mechanism of action unknown; lactic acid is a normal component in blood and tissues. When applied topically to the skin, acts as a humectant.
Pharmacodynamics/Kinetics Absorption: 6%
Pregnancy Risk Factor B

Lactic Acid and Sodium-PCA

(LAK tik AS id & SOW dee um-pee see aye)
U.S. Brand Names LactiCare® [OTC]; Lactinol®; Lactinol-E®
Generic Available No
Synonyms Sodium-PCA and Lactic Acid
Pharmacologic Category Topical Skin Product
Use Lubricate and moisturize the skin counteracting dryness and itching
Local Anesthetic/Vasoconstrictor Precautions No information available to require special precautions
Effects on Dental Treatment No significant effects or complications reported

LactiCare® [OTC] *see* Lactic Acid and Sodium-PCA *on page 793*
LactiCare-HC® *see* Hydrocortisone *on page 714*
Lactinex® [OTC] *see Lactobacillus on page 793*
Lactinol® *see* Lactic Acid and Sodium-PCA *on page 793*
Lactinol-E® *see* Lactic Acid and Sodium-PCA *on page 793*

Lactobacillus (lak toe ba SIL us)

Related Information
Bifidobacterium bifidum / Lactobacillus acidophilus on page 1415
Oral Nonviral Soft Tissue Ulcerations or Erosions *on page 1551*
U.S. Brand Names Bacid® [OTC]; Kala® [OTC]; Lactinex® [OTC]; Megadophilus® [OTC]; MoreDophilus® [OTC]; Probiotica® [OTC]; Superdophilus® [OTC]
Canadian Brand Names Bacid®; Fermalac
(Continued)

Lactobacillus (Continued)

Generic Available Yes

Synonyms *Lactobacillus acidophilus*; *Lactobacillus acidophilus* and *Lactobacillus bulgaricus*; *Lactobacillus reuteri*

Pharmacologic Category Antidiarrheal

Use Treatment of uncomplicated diarrhea particularly that caused by antibiotic therapy; re-establish normal physiologic and bacterial flora of the intestinal tract

Local Anesthetic/Vasoconstrictor Precautions No information available to require special precautions

Effects on Dental Treatment No significant effects or complications reported

Common Adverse Effects No data reported

Mechanism of Action Creates an environment unfavorable to potentially pathogenic fungi or bacteria through the production of lactic acid, and favors establishment of an aciduric flora, thereby suppressing the growth of pathogenic microorganisms; helps re-establish normal intestinal flora

Pharmacodynamics/Kinetics

Absorption: Oral: None

Distribution: Local, primarily colon

Excretion: Feces

Pregnancy Risk Factor Not available

Lactobacillus acidophilus *see* *Lactobacillus on page 793*

Lactobacillus acidophilus and Lactobacillus bulgaricus *see Lactobacillus on page 793*

Lactobacillus reuteri *see Lactobacillus on page 793*

Lactoflavin *see* Riboflavin *on page 1178*

Lactrase® [OTC] *see* Lactase *on page 793*

Lactulose (LAK tyoo lose)

U.S. Brand Names Cholac®; Constilac®; Constulose®; Enulose®; Generlac; Kristalose™

Canadian Brand Names Acilac; Apo-Lactulose®; Laxilose; PMS-Lactulose

Mexican Brand Names Lactulax®; Regulact®

Generic Available Yes

Pharmacologic Category Ammonium Detoxicant; Laxative, Miscellaneous

Use Adjunct in the prevention and treatment of portal-systemic encephalopathy; treatment of chronic constipation

Local Anesthetic/Vasoconstrictor Precautions No information available to require special precautions

Effects on Dental Treatment No significant effects or complications reported

Common Adverse Effects Frequency not defined: Gastrointestinal: Flatulence, diarrhea (excessive dose), abdominal discomfort, nausea, vomiting, cramping

Mechanism of Action The bacterial degradation of lactulose resulting in an acidic pH inhibits the diffusion of NH_3 into the blood by causing the conversion of NH_3 to NH_4+; also enhances the diffusion of NH_3 from the blood into the gut where conversion to NH_4+ occurs; produces an osmotic effect in the colon with resultant distention promoting peristalsis

Drug Interactions

Decreased Effect: Oral neomycin, laxatives, antacids

Pharmacodynamics/Kinetics

Absorption: Not appreciable

Metabolism: Via colonic flora to lactic acid and acetic acid; requires colonic flora for drug activation

Excretion: Primarily feces and urine (~3%)

Pregnancy Risk Factor B

Ladakamycin *see* Azacitidine *on page 171*

L-AmB *see* Amphotericin B (Liposomal) *on page 122*

Lamictal® *see* Lamotrigine *on page 795*

Lamisil® *see* Terbinafine *on page 1272*

Lamisil® AT™ [OTC] *see* Terbinafine *on page 1272*

Lamivudine (la MI vyoo deen)

Related Information

HIV Infection and AIDS *on page 1484*

Zidovudine and Lamivudine *on page 1399*

U.S. Brand Names Epivir®; Epivir-HBV®

Canadian Brand Names Heptovir®; 3TC®

Mexican Brand Names 3TC®
Generic Available No
Synonyms 3TC
Pharmacologic Category Antiretroviral Agent, Reverse Transcriptase Inhibitor (Nucleoside)
Use
Epivir®: Treatment of HIV infection when antiretroviral therapy is warranted; should always be used as part of a multidrug regimen (at least three antiretroviral agents)
Epivir-HBV®: Treatment of chronic hepatitis B associated with evidence of hepatitis B viral replication and active liver inflammation
Unlabeled/Investigational Use Prevention of HIV following needlesticks (with or without protease inhibitor)
Local Anesthetic/Vasoconstrictor Precautions No information available to require special precautions
Effects on Dental Treatment No significant effects or complications reported
Common Adverse Effects (As reported in adults treated for HIV infection)
>10%:
Central nervous system: Headache, fatigue
Gastrointestinal: Nausea, diarrhea, vomiting, pancreatitis (range: 0.5% to 18%; higher percentage in pediatric patients)
Neuromuscular & skeletal: Peripheral neuropathy, paresthesia, musculoskeletal pain
1% to 10%:
Central nervous system: Dizziness, depression, fever, chills, insomnia
Dermatologic: Rash
Gastrointestinal: Anorexia, abdominal pain, heartburn, elevated amylase
Hematologic: Neutropenia
Hepatic: Elevated AST, ALT
Neuromuscular & skeletal: Myalgia, arthralgia
Respiratory: Nasal signs and symptoms, cough
Mechanism of Action Lamivudine is a cytosine analog. After lamivudine is triphosphorylated, the principle mode of action is inhibition of HIV reverse transcription via viral DNA chain termination; inhibits RNA- and DNA-dependent DNA polymerase activities of reverse transcriptase. The monophosphate form of lamivudine is incorporated into the viral DNA by hepatitis B virus polymerase, resulting in DNA chain termination.
Drug Interactions
Increased Effect/Toxicity: Zidovudine concentrations increase significantly (~39%) with lamivudine coadministration. sulfamethoxazole/trimethoprim increases lamivudine's blood levels. Concomitant use of ribavirin and nucleoside analogues may increase the risk of developing lactic acidosis (includes adefovir, didanosine, lamivudine, stavudine, zalcitabine, zidovudine). Trimethoprim (and other drugs excreted by organic cation transport) may increase serum levels/effects of lamivudine.
Decreased Effect: Zalcitabine and lamivudine may inhibit the intracellular phosphorylation of each other; concomitant use should be avoided.
Pharmacodynamics/Kinetics
Absorption: Rapid
Distribution: V_d: 1.3 L/kg
Protein binding, plasma: <36%
Metabolism: 5.6% to trans-sulfoxide metabolite
Bioavailability: Absolute; Cp_{max} decreased with food although AUC not significantly affected
Children: 66%
Adults: 87%
Half-life elimination: Children: 2 hours; Adults: 5-7 hours
Excretion: Primarily urine (as unchanged drug)
Pregnancy Risk Factor C

Lamivudine, Abacavir, and Zidovudine *see* Abacavir, Lamivudine, and Zidovudine *on page 43*
Lamivudine and Zidovudine *see* Zidovudine and Lamivudine *on page 1399*

Lamotrigine (la MOE tri jeen)

U.S. Brand Names Lamictal®
Canadian Brand Names Apo-Lamotrigine®; Lamictal®; PMS-Lamotrigine; ratio-Lamotrigine
Mexican Brand Names Lamictal®
Generic Available No
Synonyms BW-430C; LTG
(Continued)

Lamotrigine *(Continued)*

Pharmacologic Category Anticonvulsant, Miscellaneous

Use Adjunctive therapy in the treatment of generalized seizures of Lennox-Gastaut syndrome and partial seizures in adults and children ≥2 years of age; conversion to monotherapy in adults with partial seizures who are receiving treatment with valproate or a single enzyme-inducing antiepileptic drug; maintenance treatment of bipolar disorder

Local Anesthetic/Vasoconstrictor Precautions No information available to require special precautions

Effects on Dental Treatment No significant effects or complications reported

Common Adverse Effects Percentages reported in adults receiving adjunctive therapy:

>10%:

Central nervous system: Headache (29%), dizziness (38%), ataxia (22%), somnolence (14%)

Gastrointestinal: Nausea (19%)

Ocular: Diplopia (28%), blurred vision (16%)

Respiratory: Rhinitis (14%)

1% to 10%:

Cardiovascular: Peripheral edema

Central nervous system: Depression (4%), anxiety (4%), irritability (3%), confusion, speech disorder (3%), difficulty concentrating (2%), malaise, seizures (includes exacerbations) (2% to 3%), incoordination (6%), insomnia (6%), pain, amnesia, hostility, memory decreased, nervousness, vertigo

Dermatologic: Hypersensitivity rash (10%; serious rash requiring hospitalization - adults 0.3%, children 0.8%), pruritus (3%)

Gastrointestinal: Abdominal pain (5%), vomiting (9%), diarrhea (6%), dyspepsia (5%), xerostomia, constipation (4%), anorexia (2%), tooth disorder (3%)

Genitourinary: Vaginitis (4%), dysmenorrhea (7%), amenorrhea (2%)

Neuromuscular & skeletal: Tremor (4%), arthralgia (2%), neck pain (2%)

Ocular: Nystagmus (2%), visual abnormality

Respiratory: Epistaxis, bronchitis, dyspnea

Miscellaneous: Flu syndrome (7%), fever (6%)

Mechanism of Action A triazine derivative which inhibits release of glutamate (an excitatory amino acid) and inhibits voltage-sensitive sodium channels, which stabilizes neuronal membranes. Lamotrigine has weak inhibitory effect on the 5-HT_3 receptor; *in vitro* inhibits dihydrofolate reductase.

Drug Interactions

Increased Effect/Toxicity: Lamotrigine may increase the epoxide metabolite of carbamazepine resulting in toxicity. Valproic acid increases blood levels of lamotrigine. Valproic acid inhibits the clearance of lamotrigine, dosage adjustment required when adding or withdrawing valproic acid; inhibition appears maximal at valproic acid 250-500 mg/day; the incidence of serious rash may be increased by valproic acid. Toxicity has been reported following addition of sertraline (limited documentation).

Decreased Effect: Acetaminophen (chronic administration), carbamazepine, oral contraceptives (estrogens), phenytoin, phenobarbital may decrease concentrations of lamotrigine; dosage adjustments may be needed when adding or withdrawing agent; monitor

Pharmacodynamics/Kinetics

Distribution: V_d: 1.1 L/kg

Protein binding: 55%

Metabolism: Hepatic and renal; metabolized by glucuronic acid conjugation to inactive metabolites

Bioavailability: 98%

Half-life elimination: Adults: 25-33 hours; Concomitant valproic acid therapy: 59-70 hours; Concomitant phenytoin or carbamazepine therapy: 13-14 hours

Time to peak, plasma: 1-4 hours

Excretion: Urine (94%, ~90% as glucuronide conjugates and ~10% unchanged); feces (2%)

Pregnancy Risk Factor C

Lamprene® *see* Clofazimine *on page 352*

Lanacane® [OTC] *see* Benzocaine *on page 191*

Lanaphilic® [OTC] *see* Urea *on page 1353*

Lanolin, Cetyl Alcohol, Glycerin, Petrolatum, and Mineral Oil

(LAN oh lin, SEE til AL koe hol, GLIS er in, pe troe LAY tum, & MIN er al oyl)

U.S. Brand Names Lubriderm® [OTC]; Lubriderm® Fragrance Free [OTC]

Generic Available Yes

Synonyms Mineral Oil, Petrolatum, Lanolin, Cetyl Alcohol, and Glycerin

Pharmacologic Category Topical Skin Product

Use Treatment of dry skin

Local Anesthetic/Vasoconstrictor Precautions No information available to require special precautions

Effects on Dental Treatment No significant effects or complications reported

Common Adverse Effects 1% to 10%: Local irritation

Pregnancy Risk Factor C

Lanoxicaps® *see* Digoxin *on page 437*

Lanoxin® *see* Digoxin *on page 437*

Lansoprazole (lan SOE pra zole)

Related Information

Gastrointestinal Disorders *on page 1476*

U.S. Brand Names Prevacid®; Prevacid® SoluTab™

Canadian Brand Names Prevacid®

Mexican Brand Names Ilsatec®; Ogastro®; Ulpax®

Generic Available No

Pharmacologic Category Proton Pump Inhibitor; Substituted Benzimidazole

Use

Oral: Short-term treatment of active duodenal ulcers; maintenance treatment of healed duodenal ulcers; as part of a multidrug regimen for *H. pylori* eradication to reduce the risk of duodenal ulcer recurrence; short-term treatment of active benign gastric ulcer; treatment of NSAID-associated gastric ulcer; to reduce the risk of NSAID-associated gastric ulcer in patients with a history of gastric ulcer who require an NSAID; short-term treatment of symptomatic GERD; short-term treatment for all grades of erosive esophagitis; to maintain healing of erosive esophagitis; long-term treatment of pathological hypersecretory conditions, including Zollinger-Ellison syndrome

I.V.: Short-term treatment (≤7 days) of erosive esophagitis in adults unable to take oral medications

Local Anesthetic/Vasoconstrictor Precautions No information available to require special precautions

Effects on Dental Treatment No significant effects or complications reported

Common Adverse Effects 1% to 10%:

Central nervous system: Headache (children 1-11 years 3%, 12-17 years 7%)

Gastrointestinal: Abdominal pain (children 12-17 years 5%; adults 2%), constipation (children 1-11 years 5%; adults 1%), diarrhea (4%; 4% to 7% at doses of 30-60 mg/day), nausea (children 12-17 years 3%; adults 1%)

Dosage

Children 1-11 years: GERD, erosive esophagitis: Oral:

≤30 kg: 15 mg once daily

>30 kg: 30 mg once daily

Note: Doses were increased in some pediatric patients if still symptomatic after 2 or more weeks of treatment (maximum dose: 30 mg twice daily)

Children 12-17 years: Oral:

Nonerosive GERD: 15 mg once daily for up to 8 weeks

Erosive esophagitis: 30 mg once daily for up to 8 weeks

Adults:

Duodenal ulcer: Oral: Short-term treatment: 15 mg once daily for 4 weeks; maintenance therapy: 15 mg once daily

Gastric ulcer: Oral: Short-term treatment: 30 mg once daily for up to 8 weeks

NSAID-associated gastric ulcer (healing): Oral: 30 mg once daily for 8 weeks; controlled studies did not extend past 8 weeks of therapy

NSAID-associated gastric ulcer (to reduce risk): Oral: 15 mg once daily for up to 12 weeks; controlled studies did not extend past 12 weeks of therapy

Symptomatic GERD: Oral: Short-term treatment: 15 mg once daily for up to 8 weeks

Erosive esophagitis:

Oral: Short-term treatment: 30 mg once daily for up to 8 weeks; continued treatment for an additional 8 weeks may be considered for recurrence or for patients that do not heal after the first 8 weeks of therapy; maintenance therapy: 15 mg once daily

(Continued)

Lansoprazole *(Continued)*

I.V.: 30 mg once daily for up to 7 days; patients should be switched to an oral formulation as soon as they can take oral medications

Hypersecretory conditions: Oral: Initial: 60 mg once daily; adjust dose based upon patient response and to reduce acid secretion to <10 mEq/hour (5 mEq/hour in patients with prior gastric surgery); doses of 90 mg twice daily have been used; administer doses >120 mg/day in divided doses

Helicobacter pylori eradication: Oral: Currently accepted recommendations (may differ from product labeling): Dose varies with regimen: 30 mg once daily or 60 mg/day in 2 divided doses; requires combination therapy with antibiotics

Elderly: No dosage adjustment is needed in elderly patients with normal hepatic function

Dosage adjustment in renal impairment: No dosage adjustment is needed

Dosing adjustment in hepatic impairment: Dose reduction is necessary for severe hepatic impairment

Mechanism of Action A proton pump inhibitor which decreases acid secretion in gastric parietal cells

Contraindications Hypersensitivity to lansoprazole, substituted benzimidazoles (ie, esomeprazole, omeprazole, pantoprazole, rabeprazole), or any component of the formulation

Warnings/Precautions Severe liver dysfunction may require dosage reductions. Symptomatic response does not exclude malignancy. Safety and efficacy have not been established in children <1 year of age.

Drug Interactions

Cytochrome P450 Effect: Substrate of CYP2C8/9 (minor), 2C19 (major), 3A4 (major); **Inhibits** CYP2C8/9 (weak), 2C19 (moderate), 2D6 (weak), 3A4 (weak); **Induces** CYP1A2 (weak)

Increased Effect/Toxicity: Lansoprazole may increase the levels/effects of citalopram, diazepam, methsuximide, phenytoin, propranolol, sertraline, and other CYP2C19 substrates.

Decreased Effect: Proton pump inhibitors may decrease the absorption of atazanavir, indinavir, itraconazole, and ketoconazole. The levels/effects of lansoprazole may be decreased by aminoglutethimide, carbamazepine, nafcillin, nevirapine, phenobarbital, phenytoin, rifamycins, and other CYP2C19 or 3A4 inducers.

Ethanol/Nutrition/Herb Interactions

Ethanol: Avoid ethanol (may cause gastric mucosal irritation).

Food: Lansoprazole serum concentrations may be decreased if taken with food.

Dietary Considerations Should be taken before eating; best if taken before breakfast. Prevacid® SoluTab™ contains phenylalanine 2.5 mg per 15 mg tablet; phenylalanine 5.1 mg per 30 mg tablet.

Pharmacodynamics/Kinetics

Duration: >1 day

Absorption: Rapid

Protein binding: 97%

Metabolism: Hepatic via CYP2C19 and 3A4, and in parietal cells to two inactive metabolites

Bioavailability: 80%; decreased 50% to 70% if given 30 minutes after food

Half-life elimination: 2 hours; Elderly: 2-3 hours; Hepatic impairment: ≤7 hours

Time to peak, plasma: 1.7 hours

Excretion: Feces (67%); urine (33%)

Pregnancy Risk Factor B

Dosage Forms CAP, delayed release (Prevacid®): 15 mg, 30 mg. **GRAN, for oral suspension, delayed release** (Prevacid®): 15 mg/packet (30s), 30 mg/packet (30s). **INJ, powder for reconstitution** (Prevacid®): 30 mg. **TAB, orally-disintegrating** (Prevacid® SoluTab™): 15 mg, 30 mg

Lansoprazole, Amoxicillin, and Clarithromycin

(lan SOE pra zole, a moks i SIL in, & kla RITH roe mye sin)

Related Information

Gastrointestinal Disorders *on page 1476*

Lansoprazole *on page 797*

U.S. Brand Names Prevpac®

Canadian Brand Names Hp-PAC®; Prevpac™

Generic Available No

Synonyms Amoxicillin, Lansoprazole, and Clarithromycin; Clarithromycin, Lansoprazole, and Amoxicillin

Pharmacologic Category Antibiotic, Macrolide Combination; Antibiotic, Penicillin; Gastrointestinal Agent, Miscellaneous

Use Eradication of *H. pylori* to reduce the risk of recurrent duodenal ulcer

Local Anesthetic/Vasoconstrictor Precautions No information available to require special precautions

Effects on Dental Treatment No significant effects or complications reported

Common Adverse Effects

Based on **lansoprazole** component: 1% to 10%: Gastrointestinal: Abdominal pain (2%), diarrhea (4%, more likely at doses of 60 mg/day), constipation (1%), nausea (1%)

Based on **amoxicillin** component: Frequency not defined:

Central nervous system: Hyperactivity, agitation, anxiety, insomnia, confusion, convulsions, behavioral changes, dizziness

Dermatologic: Erythematous maculopapular rashes, erythema multiforme, Stevens-Johnson syndrome, exfoliative dermatitis, toxic epidermal necrolysis, hypersensitivity vasculitis, urticaria

Gastrointestinal: Nausea, vomiting, diarrhea, hemorrhagic colitis, pseudomembranous colitis

Hematologic: Anemia, hemolytic anemia, thrombocytopenia, thrombocytopenia purpura, eosinophilia, leukopenia, agranulocytosis

Hepatic: Elevated AST (SGOT) and ALT (SGPT), cholestatic jaundice, hepatic cholestasis, acute cytolytic hepatitis

Based on **clarithromycin** component:

1% to 10%:

Central nervous system: Headache (adults and children 2%)

Dermatologic: Rash (children 3%)

Gastrointestinal: Diarrhea (adults 6%, children 6%); vomiting (children 6%); nausea (adults 3%); abnormal taste (adults 7%); heartburn (adults 2%); abdominal pain (adults 2%, children 3%)

Hepatic: Elevated prothrombin time (1%)

Renal: Elevated BUN (4%)

Drug Interactions

Cytochrome P450 Effect:

Lansoprazole: **Substrate** of CYP2C8/9 (minor), 2C19 (major), 3A4 (major); **Inhibits** CYP2C8/9 (weak), 2C19 (moderate), 2D6 (weak), 3A4 (weak); **Induces** CYP1A2 (weak)

Clarithromycin: **Substrate** of CYP3A4 (major); **Inhibits** CYP1A2 (weak), 3A4 (strong)

Increased Effect/Toxicity: See individual agents.

Decreased Effect: See individual agents.

Pharmacodynamics/Kinetics See individual agents.

Pregnancy Risk Factor C (clarithromycin)

Lansoprazole and Naproxen (lan SOE pra zole & na PROKS en)

Related Information

Gastrointestinal Disorders *on page 1476*
Lansoprazole *on page 797*
Naproxen *on page 965*
Oral Pain *on page 1526*

U.S. Brand Names Prevacid® NapraPAC™

Generic Available No

Synonyms NapraPAC™; Naproxen and Lansoprazole

Pharmacologic Category Nonsteroidal Anti-inflammatory Drug (NSAID), Oral; Proton Pump Inhibitor

Use Reduction of the risk of NSAID-associated gastric ulcers in patients with history of gastric ulcer who require an NSAID for the treatment of rheumatoid arthritis, osteoarthritis, and ankylosing spondylitis

Local Anesthetic/Vasoconstrictor Precautions No information available to require special precautions

Effects on Dental Treatment No significant effects or complications reported

Common Adverse Effects See individual agents.

Mechanism of Action Lansoprazole is a proton pump inhibitor which decreases acid secretion in gastric parietal cells; naproxen inhibits prostaglandin synthesis by decreasing the activity of the enzyme (cyclooxygenase) which results in decreased formation of prostaglandin precursors.

Drug Interactions

Cytochrome P450 Effect:

Lansoprazole: **Substrate** of CYP2C8/9 (minor), 2C19 (major), 3A4 (major); **Inhibits** CYP2C8/9 (weak), 2C19 (moderate), 2D6 (weak), 3A4 (weak); **Induces** CYP1A2 (weak)

(Continued)

Lansoprazole and Naproxen *(Continued)*

Naproxen: **Substrate** (minor) of CYP1A2, 2C8/9

Increased Effect/Toxicity: See individual agents.

Decreased Effect: See individual agents.

Pharmacodynamics/Kinetics See individual agents.

Pregnancy Risk Factor B (naproxen: D/third trimester)

Lantus® *see* Insulin Preparations *on page 749*

Lariam® *see* Mefloquine *on page 864*

Laronidase (lair OH ni days)

U.S. Brand Names Aldurazyme®

Generic Available No

Synonyms Recombinant α-L-Iduronidase (Glycosaminoglycan α-L-Iduronohydrolase)

Pharmacologic Category Enzyme

Use Treatment of Hurler and Hurler-Scheie forms of mucopolysaccharidosis I (MPS I); treatment of Scheie form of MPS I in patients with moderate to severe symptoms

Local Anesthetic/Vasoconstrictor Precautions No information available to require special precautions

Effects on Dental Treatment No significant effects or complications reported

Common Adverse Effects

>10%:

Cardiovascular: Vein disorder (14%)

Dermatologic: Rash (36%)

Local: Infusion reactions [31%; may be severe; includes flushing (23%), fever, and headache; frequency decreased over time during open-label extension period], injection site reaction (18%)

Neuromuscular & skeletal: Hyper-reflexia (14%), paresthesia (14%)

Respiratory: Upper respiratory tract infection (32%)

Miscellaneous: Antibody development to laronidase (91%; significance unknown)

1% to 10%:

Cardiovascular: Chest pain (9%), edema (9%), facial edema (9%), hypotension (9%)

Hematologic: Thrombocytopenia (9%)

Hepatic: Bilirubinemia

Local: Abscess (9%), injection site pain (9%)

Ocular: Corneal opacity (9%)

Mechanism of Action Laronidase is a recombinant (replacement) form of α-L-iduronidase derived from Chinese hamster cells. α-L-iduronidase is an enzyme needed to break down endogenous glycosaminoglycans (GAGs) within lysosomes. A deficiency of α-L-iduronidase leads to an accumulation of GAGs, causing cellular, tissue, and organ dysfunction as seen in MPS I. Improved pulmonary function and walking capacity have been demonstrated with the administration of laronidase to patients with Hurler, Hurler-Scheie, or Scheie (with moderate to severe symptoms) forms of MPS.

Pharmacodynamics/Kinetics

Distribution: V_d: 0.24-0.6 L/kg

Half-life elimination: 1.5-3.6 hours

Excretion: Clearance: 1.7 to 2.7 mL/minute/kg; during the first 12 weeks of therapy the clearance of laronidase increases proportionally to the amount of antibodies a given patient develops against the enzyme. However, with long-term use (≥26 weeks) antibody titers have no effect on laronidase clearance.

Pregnancy Risk Factor B

Lasix® *see* Furosemide *on page 640*

L-asparaginase *see* Asparaginase *on page 150*

Lassar's Zinc Paste *see* Zinc Oxide *on page 1400*

Latanoprost (la TA noe prost)

U.S. Brand Names Xalatan®

Canadian Brand Names Xalatan®

Mexican Brand Names Xalatan®

Generic Available No

Pharmacologic Category Ophthalmic Agent, Antiglaucoma; Prostaglandin, Ophthalmic

Use Reduction of elevated intraocular pressure in patients with open-angle glaucoma or ocular hypertension

Local Anesthetic/Vasoconstrictor Precautions No information available to require special precautions

Effects on Dental Treatment No significant effects or complications reported

Common Adverse Effects

>10%: Ocular: Blurred vision, burning and stinging, conjunctival hyperemia, foreign body sensation, itching, increased pigmentation of the iris, and punctate epithelial keratopathy

1% to 10%:

Cardiovascular: Chest pain, angina pectoris

Dermatologic: Rash, allergic skin reaction

Neuromuscular & skeletal: Myalgia, arthralgia, back pain

Ocular: Dry eye, excessive tearing, eye pain, lid crusting, lid edema, lid erythema, lid discomfort/pain, photophobia

Respiratory: Upper respiratory tract infection, cold, flu

Dosage Adults: Ophthalmic: 1 drop (1.5 mcg) in the affected eye(s) once daily in the evening; do not exceed the once daily dosage because it has been shown that more frequent administration may decrease the IOP lowering effect

Note: A medication delivery device (Xal-Ease™) is available for use with Xalatan®.

Mechanism of Action Latanoprost is a prostaglandin F_2-alpha analog believed to reduce intraocular pressure by increasing the outflow of the aqueous humor

Contraindications Hypersensitivity to latanoprost or any component of the formulation

Warnings/Precautions Latanoprost may gradually change eye color, increasing the amount of brown pigment in the iris by increasing the number of melanosome in melanocytes. The long-term effects on the melanocytes and the consequences of potential injury to the melanocytes or deposition of pigment granules to other areas of the eye is currently unknown. Patients should be examined regularly, and depending on the clinical situation, treatment may be stopped if increased pigmentation ensues.

There have been reports of bacterial keratitis associated with the use of multiple-dose containers of topical ophthalmic products. Do not administer while wearing contact lenses.

Drug Interactions

Decreased Effect: *In vitro* studies have shown that precipitation occurs when eye drops containing thimerosal are mixed with latanoprost. If such drugs are used, administer with an interval of at least 5 minutes between applications. May be used concomitantly with other topical ophthalmic drugs if administration is separated by at least 5 minutes.

Pharmacodynamics/Kinetics

Onset of action: 3-4 hours

Peak effect: Maximum: 8-12 hours

Absorption: Through the cornea where the isopropyl ester prodrug is hydrolyzed by esterases to the biologically active acid. Peak concentration is reached in 2 hours after topical administration in the aqueous humor.

Distribution: V_d: 0.16 L/kg

Metabolism: Primarily hepatic via fatty acid beta-oxidation

Half-life elimination: 17 minutes

Excretion: Urine (as metabolites)

Pregnancy Risk Factor C

Dosage Forms SOLN, ophthalmic: 0.005% (2.5 mL)

l-Bunolol Hydrochloride *see* Levobunolol *on page 808*

L-Carnitine *see* Levocarnitine *on page 810*

LCD *see* Coal Tar *on page 367*

LCR *see* VinCRIStine *on page 1378*

L-Deprenyl *see* Selegiline *on page 1212*

LDP-341 *see* Bortezomib *on page 214*

Leflunomide (le FLOO noh mide)

Related Information

Rheumatoid Arthritis, Osteoarthritis, and Osteoporosis *on page 1490*

U.S. Brand Names Arava®

Canadian Brand Names Arava®

Generic Available No

Pharmacologic Category Antirheumatic, Disease Modifying

Use Treatment of active rheumatoid arthritis; indicated to reduce signs and symptoms, and to retard structural damage and improve physical function

(Continued)

Leflunomide *(Continued)*

Local Anesthetic/Vasoconstrictor Precautions No information available to require special precautions

Effects on Dental Treatment Key adverse event(s) related to dental treatment: Stomatitis, oral candidiasis, and abnormal taste.

Common Adverse Effects

>10%:

Gastrointestinal: Diarrhea (17%)

Respiratory: Respiratory tract infection (15%)

1% to 10%:

Cardiovascular: Hypertension (10%), chest pain (2%), palpitation, tachycardia, vasculitis, vasodilation, varicose vein, edema (peripheral)

Central nervous system: Headache (7%), dizziness (4%), pain (2%), fever, malaise, migraine, anxiety, depression, insomnia, sleep disorder

Dermatologic: Alopecia (10%), rash (10%), pruritus (4%), dry skin (2%), eczema (2%), acne, dermatitis, hair discoloration, hematoma, herpes infection, nail disorder, subcutaneous nodule, skin disorder/discoloration, skin ulcer, bruising

Endocrine & metabolic: Hypokalemia (1%), diabetes mellitus, hyperglycemia, hyperlipidemia, hyperthyroidism, menstrual disorder

Gastrointestinal: Nausea (9%), abdominal pain (5%), dyspepsia (5%), weight loss (4%), anorexia (3%), gastroenteritis (3%), stomatitis (3%), vomiting (3%), cholelithiasis, colitis, constipation, esophagitis, flatulence, gastritis, gingivitis, melena, candidiasis (oral), enlarged salivary gland, tooth disorder, xerostomia, taste disturbance

Genitourinary: Urinary tract infection (5%), albuminuria, cystitis, dysuria, hematuria, vaginal candidiasis, prostate disorder, urinary frequency

Hematologic: Anemia

Hepatic: Abnormal LFTs (5%)

Neuromuscular & skeletal: Back pain (5%), joint disorder (4%), weakness (3%), tenosynovitis (3%), synovitis (2%), arthralgia (1%), paresthesia (2%), muscle cramps (1%), neck pain, pelvic pain, increased CPK, arthrosis, bursitis, myalgia, bone necrosis, bone pain, tendon rupture, neuralgia, neuritis

Ocular: Blurred vision, cataract, conjunctivitis, eye disorder

Respiratory: Bronchitis (7%), cough (3%), pharyngitis (3%), pneumonia (2%), rhinitis (2%), sinusitis (2%), asthma, dyspnea, epistaxis

Miscellaneous: Infection (4%), accidental injury (5%), allergic reactions (2%), diaphoresis

Mechanism of Action Inhibits pyrimidine synthesis, resulting in antiproliferative and anti-inflammatory effects

Drug Interactions

Cytochrome P450 Effect: Inhibits CYP2C8/9 (weak)

Increased Effect/Toxicity: Theoretically, concomitant use of drugs metabolized by this enzyme, including many NSAIDs, may result in increased serum concentrations and possible toxic effects. Coadministration with methotrexate increases the risk of hepatotoxicity. Leflunomide may also enhance the hepatotoxicity of other drugs. Tolbutamide free fraction may be increased. Rifampin may increase serum concentrations of leflunomide. Leflunomide has uricosuric activity and may enhance activity of other uricosuric agents.

Decreased Effect: Administration of cholestyramine and activated charcoal enhance the elimination of leflunomide's active metabolite.

Pharmacodynamics/Kinetics

Distribution: V_d: 0.13 L/kg

Metabolism: Hepatic to A77 1726 (MI) which accounts for nearly all pharmacologic activity; further metabolism to multiple inactive metabolites; undergoes enterohepatic recirculation

Bioavailability: 80%

Half-life elimination: Mean: 14-15 days; enterohepatic recycling appears to contribute to the long half-life of this agent, since activated charcoal and cholestyramine substantially reduce plasma half-life

Time to peak: 6-12 hours

Excretion: Feces (48%); urine (43%)

Pregnancy Risk Factor X

Legatrin PM® [OTC] *see* Acetaminophen and Diphenhydramine *on page 53*

Lente® Iletin® II [DSC] *see* Insulin Preparations *on page 749*

Lente, Insulin *see* Insulin Preparations *on page 749*

Lepirudin (leh puh ROO din)

Related Information
Cardiovascular Diseases *on page 1458*

U.S. Brand Names Refludan®

Canadian Brand Names Refludan®

Generic Available No

Synonyms Lepirudin (rDNA); Recombinant Hirudin

Pharmacologic Category Anticoagulant, Thrombin Inhibitor

Use Indicated for anticoagulation in patients with heparin-induced thrombocytopenia (HIT) and associated thromboembolic disease in order to prevent further thromboembolic complications

Unlabeled/Investigational Use Investigational: Prevention or reduction of ischemic complications associated with unstable angina

Local Anesthetic/Vasoconstrictor Precautions No information available to require special precautions

Effects on Dental Treatment No significant effects or complications reported

Common Adverse Effects As with all anticoagulants, bleeding is the most common adverse event associated with lepirudin. Hemorrhage may occur at virtually any site. Risk is dependent on multiple variables.

HIT patients:

>10%: Hematologic: Anemia (12%), bleeding from puncture sites (11%), hematoma (11%)

1% to 10%:

Cardiovascular: Heart failure (3%), pericardial effusion (1%), ventricular fibrillation (1%)
Central nervous system: Fever (7%)
Dermatologic: Eczema (3%), maculopapular rash (4%)
Gastrointestinal: GI bleeding/rectal bleeding (5%)
Genitourinary: Vaginal bleeding (2%)
Hepatic: Increased transaminases (6%)
Renal: Hematuria (4%)
Respiratory: Epistaxis (4%)

Non-HIT populations (including those receiving thrombolytics and/or contrast media):

1% to 10%: Respiratory: Bronchospasm/stridor/dyspnea/cough

Mechanism of Action Lepirudin is a highly specific direct inhibitor of thrombin; lepirudin is a recombinant hirudin derived from yeast cells

Drug Interactions

Increased Effect/Toxicity: Thrombolytics may enhance anticoagulant properties of lepirudin on aPTT and can increase the risk of bleeding complications. Bleeding risk may also be increased by oral anticoagulants (warfarin) and platelet function inhibitors (NSAIDs, dipyridamole, ticlopidine, clopidogrel, IIb/IIIa antagonists, and aspirin).

Pharmacodynamics/Kinetics

Distribution: Two-compartment model; confined to extracellular fluids.

Metabolism: Via release of amino acids via catabolic hydrolysis of parent drug

Half-life elimination: Initial: ~10 minutes: Terminal: Healthy volunteers: 1.3 hours; Marked renal impairment (Cl_{cr} <15 mL/minute and on hemodialysis): ≤2 days

Excretion: Urine (~48%, 35% as unchanged drug and unchanged drug fragments of parent drug); systemic clearance is proportional to glomerular filtration rate or creatinine clearance

Pregnancy Risk Factor B

Lepirudin (rDNA) *see* Lepirudin *on page 803*

Lescol® *see* Fluvastatin *on page 622*

Lescol® XL *see* Fluvastatin *on page 622*

Lessina™ *see* Ethinyl Estradiol and Levonorgestrel *on page 545*

Letrozole (LET roe zole)

U.S. Brand Names Femara®

Canadian Brand Names Femara®

Generic Available No

Pharmacologic Category Antineoplastic Agent, Aromatase Inhibitor

Use First-line treatment of hormone receptor positive or hormone receptor unknown, locally advanced, or metastatic breast cancer in postmenopausal women; treatment of advanced breast cancer in postmenopausal women with disease progression following antiestrogen therapy

Local Anesthetic/Vasoconstrictor Precautions No information available to require special precautions

(Continued)

Letrozole *(Continued)*

Effects on Dental Treatment No significant effects or complications reported

Common Adverse Effects

>10%:

Cardiovascular: Hot flushes (5% to 19%)

Central nervous system: Headache (8% to 12%), fatigue (6% to 13%)

Gastrointestinal: Nausea (13% to 17%)

Neuromuscular & skeletal: Musculoskeletal pain, bone pain (22%), back pain (18%), arthralgia (8% to 16%)

Respiratory: Dyspnea (7% to 18%), cough (5% to 13%)

2% to 10%:

Cardiovascular: Chest pain (3% to 8%), peripheral edema (5%), hypertension (5% to 8%)

Central nervous system: Pain (5%), insomnia (7%), dizziness (3% to 5%), somnolence (2% to 3%), depression (<5%), anxiety (<5%), vertigo (<5%)

Dermatologic: Rash (4% to 5%), alopecia (<5%), pruritus (1% to 2%)

Endocrine & metabolic: Breast pain (7%), hypercholesterolemia (3%), hypercalcemia (<5%)

Gastrointestinal: Vomiting (7%), constipation (6% to 10%), diarrhea (5% to 8%), abdominal pain (5% to 6%), anorexia (3% to 5%), dyspepsia (3% to 4%), weight loss (7%), weight gain (2%)

Neuromuscular & skeletal: Weakness (4% to 6%)

Miscellaneous: Flu (6%)

<2%: Angina, cardiac ischemia, coronary artery disease, hemiparesis, hemorrhagic stroke, bilirubin increased, transaminases increased, lymphopenia, MI, portal vein thrombosis, pulmonary embolism, thrombocytopenia, thrombophlebitis, thrombotic stroke, transient ischemic attack, vaginal bleeding, venous thrombosis

Mechanism of Action Competitive inhibitor of the aromatase enzyme system which binds to the heme group of aromatase, a cytochrome P450 enzyme which catalyzes conversion of androgens to estrogens (specifically, androstenedione to estrone and testosterone to estradiol). This leads to inhibition of the enzyme and a significant reduction in plasma estrogen levels. Does not affect synthesis of adrenal or thyroid hormones, aldosterone, or androgens.

Drug Interactions

Cytochrome P450 Effect: Substrate (minor) of CYP2A6, 3A4; **Inhibits** CYP2A6 (weak), 2C19 (weak)

Pharmacodynamics/Kinetics

Absorption: Well absorbed; not affected by food

Distribution: V_d: ~1.9 L/kg

Protein binding, plasma: Weak

Metabolism: Hepatic via CYP3A4 and CYP2A6 to an inactive carbinol metabolite

Half-life elimination: Terminal: ~2 days

Time to steady state, plasma: 2-6 weeks

Excretion: Urine (6% as unchanged drug, 75% as glucuronide carbinol metabolite)

Pregnancy Risk Factor D

Leucovorin (loo koe VOR in)

Mexican Brand Names Dalisol®; Flynoken®

Generic Available Yes

Synonyms Calcium Leucovorin; Citrovorum Factor; Folinic Acid; 5-Formyl Tetrahydrofolate; Leucovorin Calcium

Pharmacologic Category Antidote; Vitamin, Water Soluble

Use Antidote for folic acid antagonists (methotrexate, trimethoprim, pyrimethamine); treatment of megaloblastic anemias when folate is deficient as in infancy, sprue, pregnancy, and nutritional deficiency when oral folate therapy is not possible; in combination with fluorouracil in the treatment of colon cancer

Local Anesthetic/Vasoconstrictor Precautions No information available to require special precautions

Effects on Dental Treatment No significant effects or complications reported

Common Adverse Effects Frequency not defined.

Dermatologic: Rash, pruritus, erythema, urticaria

Hematologic: Thrombocytosis

Respiratory: Wheezing

Miscellaneous: Anaphylactoid reactions

Mechanism of Action A reduced form of folic acid, leucovorin supplies the necessary cofactor blocked by methotrexate, enters the cells via the same active transport system as methotrexate. Stabilizes the binding of 5-dUMP and thrymidylate synthetase, enhancing the activity of fluorouracil.

Drug Interactions

Decreased Effect: May decrease efficacy of co-trimoxazole against *Pneumocystis carinii* pneumonitis

Pharmacodynamics/Kinetics

Onset of action: Oral: ~30 minutes; I.V.: ~5 minutes

Absorption: Oral, I.M.: Rapid and well absorbed

Metabolism: Intestinal mucosa and hepatically to 5-methyl-tetrahydrofolate (5MTHF; active)

Bioavailability: 31% following 200 mg dose; 98% following doses ≤25 mg

Half-life elimination: Leucovorin: 15 minutes; 5MTHF: 33-35 minutes

Excretion: Urine (80% to 90%); feces (5% to 8%)

Pregnancy Risk Factor C

Leucovorin Calcium *see* Leucovorin *on page 804*

Leukeran® *see* Chlorambucil *on page 305*

Leukine® *see* Sargramostim *on page 1209*

Leuprolide (loo PROE lide)

U.S. Brand Names Eligard™; Lupron®; Lupron Depot®; Lupron Depot-Ped®; Viadur®

Canadian Brand Names Lupron®; Lupron® Depot®; Viadur®

Generic Available Yes: Injection (solution)

Synonyms Abbott-43818; Leuprolide Acetate; Leuprorelin Acetate; NSC-377526; TAP-144

Pharmacologic Category Gonadotropin Releasing Hormone Agonist

Use Palliative treatment of advanced prostate carcinoma; management of endometriosis as initial treatment and/or treatment of recurrent symptoms; preoperative treatment of anemia caused by uterine leiomyomata (fibroids); central precocious puberty

Unlabeled/Investigational Use Treatment of breast, ovarian, and endometrial cancer; infertility; prostatic hyperplasia

Local Anesthetic/Vasoconstrictor Precautions No information available to require special precautions

Effects on Dental Treatment No significant effects or complications reported

Common Adverse Effects

Children: 1% to 10%

Central nervous system: Pain (2%)

Dermatologic: Acne (2%), rash (2%), seborrhea (2%)

Genitourinary: Vaginitis (2%), vaginal bleeding (2%), vaginal discharge (2%)

Local: Injection site reaction (5%)

Adults (frequency dependent upon formulation and indication):

Cardiovascular: Angina, atrial fibrillation, CHF, deep vein thrombosis, edema, hot flashes, hypertension, MI, tachycardia

Central nervous system: Abnormal thinking, agitation, amnesia, confusion, convulsion, dementia, depression, dizziness, fever, headache, insomnia, pain, vertigo

Dermatologic: Alopecia, bruising, cellulitis

Endocrine & metabolic: Breast enlargement, breast tenderness, dehydration, hyperglycemia, hyperlipidemia, hyperphosphatemia, libido decreased, menstrual disorders, potassium decreased

Gastrointestinal: Anorexia, appetite increased, diarrhea, dysphagia, eructation, GI hemorrhage, gingivitis, gum hemorrhage, intestinal obstruction, nausea, peptic ulcer

Genitourinary: Balanitis, impotence, testicular atrophy, urinary disorder, vaginitis

Hematologic: Platelets decreased, PT prolonged, WBC increased

Hepatic: Hepatomegaly, liver function tests abnormal

Local: Abscess, injection site reaction

Neuromuscular & skeletal: Leg cramps, myalgia, paresthesia, weakness

Renal: BUN increased

Respiratory: Allergic reaction, emphysema, hemoptysis, hypoxia, lung edema, pulmonary embolism

Miscellaneous: Body odor, flu-like syndrome, neoplasm, voice alteration

Mechanism of Action Potent inhibitor of gonadotropin secretion; continuous daily administration results in suppression of ovarian and testicular steroidogenesis due to decreased levels of LH and FSH with subsequent decrease in testosterone (male) and estrogen (female) levels. Leuprolide may also have a direct inhibitory effect on the testes, and act by a different mechanism not directly related to reduction in serum testosterone.

(Continued)

Leuprolide *(Continued)*

Pharmacodynamics/Kinetics

Onset of action: Following transient increase, testosterone suppression occurs in ~2-4 weeks of continued therapy

Distribution: Males: V_d: 27 L

Protein binding: 43% to 49%

Metabolism: Not well defined; forms smaller, inactive peptides and metabolites

Bioavailability: Oral: None; SubQ: 94%

Half-life elimination: 3 hours

Excretion: Urine (<5% as parent and major metabolite)

Pregnancy Risk Factor X

Leuprolide Acetate *see* Leuprolide *on page 805*

Leuprorelin Acetate *see* Leuprolide *on page 805*

Leurocristine Sulfate *see* VinCRIStine *on page 1378*

Leustatin® *see* Cladribine *on page 342*

Levalbuterol (leve al BYOO ter ole)

U.S. Brand Names Xopenex®

Canadian Brand Names Xopenex®

Generic Available No

Synonyms R-albuterol

Pharmacologic Category $Beta_2$-Adrenergic Agonist

Use Treatment or prevention of bronchospasm in adults and adolescents ≥6 years of age with reversible obstructive airway disease

Local Anesthetic/Vasoconstrictor Precautions No information available to require special precautions

Effects on Dental Treatment No significant effects or complications reported

Common Adverse Effects Events reported include those ≥2% with incidence higher than placebo in patients ≥12 years of age.

>10%:

- Endocrine & metabolic: Serum glucose increased, serum potassium decreased
- Respiratory: Viral infection (7% to 12%), rhinitis (3% to 11%)

>2% to 10%:

- Central nervous system: Nervousness (3% to 10%), tremor (≤7%), anxiety (≤3%), dizziness (1% to 3%), migraine (≤3%), pain (1% to 3%)
- Cardiovascular: Tachycardia (~3%)
- Gastrointestinal: Dyspepsia (1% to 3%)
- Neuromuscular & skeletal: Leg cramps (≤3%)
- Respiratory: Cough (1% to 4%), nasal edema (1% to 3%), sinusitis (1% to 4%)
- Miscellaneous: Flu-like syndrome (1% to 4%), accidental injury (≤3%)

Mechanism of Action Relaxes bronchial smooth muscle by action on beta-2 receptors with little effect on heart rate

Drug Interactions

Increased Effect/Toxicity: May add to effects of medications which deplete potassium (eg, loop or thiazide diuretics). Cardiac effects of levalbuterol may be potentiated in patients receiving MAO inhibitors, tricyclic antidepressants, sympathomimetics (eg, amphetamine, dobutamine), or inhaled anesthetics (eg, enflurane).

Decreased Effect: Beta-blockers (particularly nonselective agents) block the effect of levalbuterol. Digoxin levels may be decreased.

Pharmacodynamics/Kinetics

Onset of action: 10-17 minutes (measured as a 15% increase in FEV_1)

Peak effect: 1.5 hours

Duration: 5-6 hours (up to 8 hours in some patients)

Absorption: A portion of inhaled dose is absorbed to systemic circulation

Half-life elimination: 3.3-4 hours

Time to peak, serum: 0.2 hours

Pregnancy Risk Factor C

Levamisole (lee VAM i sole)

U.S. Brand Names Ergamisol®

Canadian Brand Names Ergamisol®

Mexican Brand Names Decaris®

Generic Available No

Synonyms Levamisole Hydrochloride

Pharmacologic Category Immune Modulator

Use Adjuvant treatment with fluorouracil in Dukes stage C colon cancer

Local Anesthetic/Vasoconstrictor Precautions No information available to require special precautions

Effects on Dental Treatment No significant effects or complications reported

Common Adverse Effects

>10%: Gastrointestinal: Nausea, diarrhea

1% to 10%:

Cardiovascular: Edema

Central nervous system: Fatigue, fever, dizziness, headache, somnolence, depression, nervousness, insomnia

Dermatologic: Dermatitis, alopecia

Gastrointestinal: Stomatitis, vomiting, anorexia, abdominal pain, constipation, taste perversion

Hematologic: Leukopenia

Neuromuscular & skeletal: Rigors, arthralgia, myalgia, paresthesia

Miscellaneous: Infection

Mechanism of Action Clinically, combined therapy with levamisole and 5-fluorouracil has been effective in treating colon cancer patients, whereas demonstrable activity has been demonstrated. Due to the broad range of pharmacologic activities of levamisole, it has been suggested that the drug may act as a biochemical modulator (of fluorouracil, for example, in colon cancer), an effect entirely independent of immune modulation. Further studies are needed to evaluate the mechanisms of action of the drug in cancer patients.

Drug Interactions

Increased Effect/Toxicity: Increased toxicity/serum levels of phenytoin. Disulfiram-like reaction with alcohol.

Pharmacodynamics/Kinetics

Absorption: Well absorbed

Metabolism: Hepatic (>70%)

Half-life elimination: 2-6 hours

Time to peak, serum: 1-2 hours

Excretion: Urine and feces within 48 hours

Pregnancy Risk Factor C

Levamisole Hydrochloride *see* Levamisole *on page 806*

Levaquin® *see* Levofloxacin *on page 812*

Levarterenol Bitartrate *see* Norepinephrine *on page 996*

Levatol® *see* Penbutolol *on page 1055*

Levbid® *see* Hyoscyamine *on page 724*

Levetiracetam (lee va tye RA se tam)

U.S. Brand Names Keppra®

Canadian Brand Names Keppra®

Generic Available No

Pharmacologic Category Anticonvulsant, Miscellaneous

Use Indicated as adjunctive therapy in the treatment of partial onset seizures in adults with epilepsy

Unlabeled/Investigational Use Bipolar disorder; partial onset seizures in children with epilepsy

Local Anesthetic/Vasoconstrictor Precautions No information available to require special precautions

Effects on Dental Treatment No significant effects or complications reported

Common Adverse Effects

>10%:

Central nervous system: Somnolence (15%), headache (14%)

Neuromuscular & skeletal: Weakness (15%)

Miscellaneous: Infection (13%)

<10%:

Cardiovascular: Chest pain

Central nervous system: Pain (7%), psychotic symptoms (1%), amnesia (2%), ataxia (3%), depression (4%), dizziness (9%), emotional lability (2%), nervousness (4%), vertigo (3%), agitation, anger, aggression, irritability, hostility (2%), anxiety (2%), apathy, depersonalization, confusion, convulsion, fever, insomnia, thinking abnormal

Dermatologic: Bruising, rash

Gastrointestinal: Anorexia (3%), abdominal pain, constipation, diarrhea, dyspepsia, gastroenteritis, gingivitis, nausea, vomiting, weight gain

Hematologic: Decreased erythrocyte counts (3%), decreased leukocytes (2% to 3%)

Neuromuscular & skeletal: Ataxia and other coordination difficulties (3%), paresthesia (2%), arthralgia, back pain, tremor

(Continued)

Levetiracetam *(Continued)*

Ocular: Diplopia (2%), amblyopia, otitis media

Respiratory: Pharyngitis (6%), rhinitis (4%), cough (2%), sinusitis (2%), bronchitis

Miscellaneous: Flu-like symptoms

Mechanism of Action The precise mechanism by which levetiracetam exerts its antiepileptic effect is unknown and does not appear to derive from any interaction with known mechanisms involved in inhibitory and excitatory neurotransmission

Drug Interactions

Increased Effect/Toxicity: No interaction was observed in pharmacokinetic trials with other anticonvulsants, including phenytoin, carbamazepine, valproic acid, phenobarbital, lamotrigine, gabapentin, and primidone.

Pharmacodynamics/Kinetics

Onset of action: Peak effect: 1 hour

Absorption: Rapid and complete

Protein binding: <10%

Metabolism: Not extensive; primarily by enzymatic hydrolysis; forms metabolites (inactive)

Bioavailability: 100%

Half-life elimination: 6-8 hours

Excretion: Urine (66%)

Dialyzable: ~50% of pooled levetiracetam removed during standard 4-hour hemodialysis

Pregnancy Risk Factor C

Levitra® *see* Vardenafil *on page 1367*

Levlen® *see* Ethinyl Estradiol and Levonorgestrel *on page 545*

Levlite™ *see* Ethinyl Estradiol and Levonorgestrel *on page 545*

Levobetaxolol (lee voe be TAX oh lol)

U.S. Brand Names Betaxon®

Canadian Brand Names Betaxon®

Generic Available No

Pharmacologic Category Beta Blocker, $Beta_1$ Selective; Ophthalmic Agent, Antiglaucoma

Use Lowering of intraocular pressure in patients with chronic open-angle glaucoma or ocular hypertension

Local Anesthetic/Vasoconstrictor Precautions No information available to require special precautions

Effects on Dental Treatment Key adverse event(s) related to dental treatment: Tachycardia, bradycardia, hypertension, hypotension, headache, anxiety, abnormal taste, infection, bronchitis, dyspnea, pharyngitis, pneumonia, rhinitis, sinusitis, otitis media, dizziness. Levobetaxolol is a cardioselective beta-blocker. Local anesthetic with vasoconstrictor can be safely used in patients medicated with levobetaxolol. Nonselective beta-blockers (ie, propranolol, nadolol) enhance the pressor response to epinephrine, resulting in hypertension and bradycardia; this has not been reported for levobetaxolol. Many nonsteroidal anti-inflammatory drugs, such as ibuprofen and indomethacin, can reduce the hypotensive effect of beta-blockers after 3 or more weeks of therapy with the NSAID. Short-term NSAID use (ie, 3 days) requires no special precautions in patients taking beta-blockers.

Mechanism of Action Levobetaxolol is a cardioselective, $beta_1$-adrenergic receptor antagonist. It is the more active enantiomer of betaxolol. Reduces intraocular pressure by reducing the production of aqueous humor.

Pregnancy Risk Factor C

Levobunolol (lee voe BYOO noe lole)

U.S. Brand Names Betagan®

Canadian Brand Names Apo-Levobunolol®; Betagan®; Novo-Levobunolol; Optho-Bunolol®; PMS-Levobunolol

Mexican Brand Names Betagan®

Generic Available Yes

Synonyms *l*-Bunolol Hydrochloride; Levobunolol Hydrochloride

Pharmacologic Category Beta-Adrenergic Blocker, Nonselective; Ophthalmic Agent, Antiglaucoma

Use To lower intraocular pressure in chronic open-angle glaucoma or ocular hypertension

Local Anesthetic/Vasoconstrictor Precautions No information available to require special precautions

Effects on Dental Treatment Key adverse event(s) related to dental treatment: Levobunolol is a nonselective beta-blocker and may enhance the pressor response to epinephrine, resulting in hypertension and bradycardia. Many nonsteroidal anti-inflammatory drugs, such as ibuprofen and indomethacin, can reduce the hypotensive effect of beta-blockers after 3 or more weeks of therapy with the NSAID. Short-term NSAID use (ie, 3 days) requires no special precautions in patients taking beta-blockers.

Mechanism of Action A nonselective beta-adrenergic blocking agent that lowers intraocular pressure by reducing aqueous humor production and possibly increases the outflow of aqueous humor

Pregnancy Risk Factor C

Levobunolol Hydrochloride *see* Levobunolol *on page 808*

Levobupivacaine (LEE voe byoo PIV a kane)

Related Information

Oral Pain *on page 1526*

U.S. Brand Names Chirocaine®

Canadian Brand Names Chirocaine®

Generic Available No

Pharmacologic Category Local Anesthetic

Use Production of local or regional anesthesia for surgery and obstetrics, and for postoperative pain management

Local Anesthetic/Vasoconstrictor Precautions No information available to require special precautions

Effects on Dental Treatment No significant effects or complications reported

Common Adverse Effects

>10%:

Cardiovascular: Hypotension (20% to 31%)

Central nervous system: Pain (postoperative) (7% to 18%), fever (7% to 17%)

Gastrointestinal: Nausea (12% to 21%), vomiting (8% to 14%)

Hematologic: Anemia (10% to 12%)

1% to 10%:

Cardiovascular: Abnormal ECG (3%), bradycardia (2%), tachycardia (2%), hypertension (1%)

Central nervous system: Pain (4% to 8%), headache (5% to 7%), dizziness (5% to 6%), hypoesthesia (3%), somnolence (1%), anxiety (1%), hypothermia (2%)

Dermatologic: Pruritus (4% to 9%), purpura (1%)

Endocrine & metabolic: Breast pain - female (1%)

Gastrointestinal: Constipation (3% to 7%), enlarged abdomen (3%), flatulence (2%), abdominal pain (2%), dyspepsia (2%), diarrhea (1%)

Genitourinary: Urinary incontinence (1%), urine flow decreased (1%), urinary tract infection (1%)

Hematologic: Leukocytosis (1%)

Local: Anesthesia (1%)

Neuromuscular & skeletal: Back pain (6%), rigors (3%), paresthesia (2%)

Ocular: Diplopia (3%)

Renal: Albuminuria (3%), hematuria (2%)

Respiratory: Cough (1%)

Miscellaneous: Fetal distress (5% to 10%), delayed delivery (6%), hemorrhage in pregnancy (2%), uterine abnormality (2%), increased wound drainage (1%)

Mechanism of Action Levobupivacaine is the S-enantiomer of bupivacaine. It blocks both the initiation and transmission of nerve impulses by decreasing the neuronal membrane's permeability to sodium ions, which results in inhibition of depolarization with resultant blockade of conduction. Local anesthetics reversibly prevent generation and conduction of electrical impulses in neurons by decreasing the transient increase in permeability to sodium. The differential sensitivity generally depends on the size of the fiber; small fibers are more sensitive than larger fibers and require a longer period for recovery. Sensory pain fibers are usually blocked first, followed by fibers that transmit sensations of temperature, touch, and deep pressure. High concentrations block sympathetic somatic sensory and somatic motor fibers. The spread of anesthesia depends upon the distribution of the solution. This is primarily dependent on the site of administration and volume of drug injected.

Drug Interactions

Cytochrome P450 Effect: Substrate (minor) of CYP1A2, 3A4

Pharmacodynamics/Kinetics

Onset of action: Epidural: 10-14 minutes

Duration (dose dependent): 1-8 hours

(Continued)

Levobupivacaine *(Continued)*

Absorption: Dependent on route of administration and dose
Distribution: 67 L
Protein binding, plasma: >97%
Metabolism: Extensively hepatic via CYP3A4 and CYP1A2
Half-life elimination: 1.3 hours
Time to peak: Epidural: 30 minutes
Excretion: Urine (71%) and feces (24%) as metabolites

Pregnancy Risk Factor B

Levocabastine (LEE voe kab as teen)

U.S. Brand Names Livostin®

Canadian Brand Names Livostin®

Mexican Brand Names Livostin®

Generic Available No

Synonyms Levocabastine Hydrochloride

Pharmacologic Category Antihistamine, H_1 Blocker, Ophthalmic

Use Treatment of allergic conjunctivitis

Local Anesthetic/Vasoconstrictor Precautions No information available to require special precautions

Effects on Dental Treatment Key adverse event(s) related to dental treatment: Xerostomia (normal salivary flow resumes upon discontinuation).

Mechanism of Action Potent, selective histamine H_1-receptor antagonist for topical ophthalmic use

Pregnancy Risk Factor C

Levocabastine Hydrochloride *see* Levocabastine *on page 810*

Levocarnitine (lee voe KAR ni teen)

U.S. Brand Names Carnitor®

Canadian Brand Names Carnitor®

Mexican Brand Names Cardispan®

Generic Available Yes

Synonyms L-Carnitine

Pharmacologic Category Dietary Supplement

Use Orphan drug:

Oral: Primary systemic carnitine deficiency; acute and chronic treatment of patients with an inborn error of metabolism which results in secondary carnitine deficiency

I.V.: Acute and chronic treatment of patients with an inborn error of metabolism which results in secondary carnitine deficiency; prevention and treatment of carnitine deficiency in patients with end-stage renal disease (ESRD) who are undergoing hemodialysis.

Local Anesthetic/Vasoconstrictor Precautions No information available to require special precautions

Effects on Dental Treatment No significant effects or complications reported

Common Adverse Effects Frequencies noted with I.V. therapy (hemodialysis patients):

Cardiovascular: Hypertension (18% to 21%), peripheral edema (3% to 6%)
Central nervous system: Dizziness (10% to 18%), fever (5% to 12%), paresthesia (3% to 12%), depression (5% to 6%)
Endocrine & metabolic: Hypercalcemia (6% to 15%)
Gastrointestinal: Diarrhea (9% to 35%), abdominal pain (5% to 21%), vomiting (9% to 21%), nausea (5% to 12%)
Neuromuscular & skeletal: Weakness (9% to 12%)
Miscellaneous: Allergic reaction (2% to 6%)

Mechanism of Action Carnitine is a naturally occurring metabolic compound which functions as a carrier molecule for long-chain fatty acids within the mitochondria, facilitating energy production. Carnitine deficiency is associated with accumulation of excess acyl CoA esters and disruption of intermediary metabolism. Carnitine supplementation increases carnitine plasma concentrations. The effects on specific metabolic alterations have not been evaluated. ESRD patients on maintenance HD may have low plasma carnitine levels because of reduced intake of meat and dairy products, reduced renal synthesis, and dialytic losses. Certain clinical conditions (malaise, muscle weakness, cardiomyopathy and arrhythmias) in HD patients may be related to carnitine deficiency.

Pharmacodynamics/Kinetics

Metabolism: Hepatic (limited with moderate renal impairment), to trimethylamine (TMA) and trimethylamine N-oxide (TMAO)

Bioavailability: Tablet/solution: 15% to 16%
Half-life elimination: 17.4 hours
Time to peak: Tablet/solution: 3.3 hours
Excretion: Urine (4% to 9% as unchanged drug); metabolites also eliminated in urine

Pregnancy Risk Factor B

Levodopa and Carbidopa (lee voe DOE pa & kar bi DOE pa)

Related Information

Carbidopa *on page 261*

U.S. Brand Names Sinemet®; Sinemet® CR

Canadian Brand Names Apo-Levocarb®; Endo®-Levodopa/Carbidopa; Novo-Levocarbidopa; Nu-Levocarb; Sinemet®; Sinemet® CR

Generic Available Yes

Synonyms Carbidopa and Levodopa

Pharmacologic Category Anti-Parkinson's Agent, Dopamine Agonist

Use Idiopathic Parkinson's disease; postencephalitic parkinsonism; symptomatic parkinsonism

Unlabeled/Investigational Use Restless leg syndrome

Local Anesthetic/Vasoconstrictor Precautions No information available to require special precautions

Effects on Dental Treatment Key adverse event(s) related to dental treatment: Xerostomia (normal salivary flow resumes upon discontinuation). Dopaminergic therapy in Parkinson's disease (ie, treatment with levodopa and carbidopa combination) is associated with orthostatic hypotension. Patients medicated with this drug combination should be carefully assisted from the chair and observed for signs of orthostatic hypotension.

Common Adverse Effects Frequency not defined.

Cardiovascular: Orthostatic hypotension, arrhythmias, chest pain, hypertension, syncope, palpitations, phlebitis

Central nervous system: Dizziness, anxiety, confusion, nightmares, headache, hallucinations, on-off phenomenon, decreased mental acuity, memory impairment, disorientation, delusions, euphoria, agitation, somnolence, insomnia, gait abnormalities, nervousness, ataxia, EPS, falling, psychosis, peripheral neuropathy, seizures (causal relationship not established)

Dermatologic: Rash, alopecia, malignant melanoma, hypersensitivity (angioedema, urticaria, pruritus, bullous lesions, Henoch-Schönlein purpura)

Endocrine & metabolic: Increased libido

Gastrointestinal: Anorexia, nausea, vomiting, constipation, GI bleeding, duodenal ulcer, diarrhea, dyspepsia, taste alterations, sialorrhea, heartburn

Genitourinary: Discoloration of urine, urinary frequency

Hematologic: Hemolytic anemia, agranulocytosis, thrombocytopenia, leukopenia; decreased hemoglobin and hematocrit; abnormalities in AST and ALT, LDH, bilirubin, BUN, Coombs' test

Neuromuscular & skeletal: Choreiform and involuntary movements, paresthesia, bone pain, shoulder pain, muscle cramps, weakness

Ocular: Blepharospasm, oculogyric crises (may be associated with acute dystonic reactions)

Renal: Difficult urination

Respiratory: Dyspnea, cough

Miscellaneous: Hiccups, discoloration of sweat, diaphoresis (increased)

Mechanism of Action Parkinson's symptoms are due to a lack of striatal dopamine; levodopa circulates in the plasma to the blood-brain-barrier (BBB), where it crosses, to be converted by striatal enzymes to dopamine; carbidopa inhibits the peripheral plasma breakdown of levodopa by inhibiting its decarboxylation, and thereby increases available levodopa at the BBB

Drug Interactions

Increased Effect/Toxicity: Concurrent use of levodopa with nonselective MAO inhibitors may result in hypertensive reactions via an increased storage and release of dopamine, norepinephrine, or both. Use with carbidopa to minimize reactions if combination is necessary; otherwise avoid combination.

Decreased Effect: Antipsychotics, benzodiazepines, L-methionine, phenytoin, pyridoxine, spiramycin, and tacrine may inhibit the antiparkinsonian effects of levodopa; monitor for reduced effect. Antipsychotics may inhibit the antiparkinsonian effects of levodopa via dopamine receptor blockade. Use antipsychotics with low dopamine blockade (clozapine, olanzapine, quetiapine). High-protein diets may inhibit levodopa's efficacy; avoid high protein foods. Iron binds levodopa and reduces its bioavailability; separate doses of iron and levodopa.

(Continued)

Levodopa and Carbidopa *(Continued)*

Pharmacodynamics/Kinetics

Duration: Variable, 6-12 hours; longer with sustained release forms

See Carbidopa.

Pregnancy Risk Factor C

Levodopa, Carbidopa, and Entacapone

(lee voe DOE pa, kar bi DOE pa, & en TA ka pone)

Related Information

Carbidopa *on page 261*

Entacapone *on page 494*

Levodopa and Carbidopa *on page 811*

U.S. Brand Names Stalevo™

Generic Available No

Synonyms Carbidopa, Levodopa, and Entacapone; Entacapone, Carbidopa, and Levodopa

Pharmacologic Category Anti-Parkinson's Agent, COMT Inhibitor; Anti-Parkinson's Agent, Dopamine Agonist

Use Treatment of idiopathic Parkinson's disease

Local Anesthetic/Vasoconstrictor Precautions No information available to require special precautions

Effects on Dental Treatment No significant effects or complications reported

Common Adverse Effects See individual agents.

Mechanism of Action

Levodopa: The metabolic precursor of dopamine, a chemical depleted in Parkinson's disease. Levodopa is able to circulate in the plasma and cross the blood-brain-barrier (BBB), where it is converted by striatal enzymes to dopamine.

Carbidopa: Inhibits the peripheral plasma breakdown of levodopa by inhibiting its decarboxylation; increases available levodopa at the BBB

Entacapone: A reversible and selective inhibitor of catechol-O-methyltransferase (COMT). Alters the pharmacokinetics of levodopa, resulting in more sustained levodopa serum levels and increased concentrations available for absorption across the BBB.

Pharmacodynamics/Kinetics See individual agents.

Pregnancy Risk Factor C

Levo-Dromoran® *see* Levorphanol *on page 816*

Levofloxacin (lee voe FLOKS a sin)

Related Information

Sexually-Transmitted Diseases *on page 1504*

Tuberculosis *on page 1495*

U.S. Brand Names Iquix®; Levaquin®; Quixin™

Canadian Brand Names Levaquin®

Mexican Brand Names Elequine®; Tavanic®

Generic Available No

Pharmacologic Category Antibiotic, Quinolone

Use

Systemic: Treatment of mild, moderate, or severe infections caused by susceptible organisms. Includes the treatment of community-acquired pneumonia (including penicillin-resistant strains of *S. pneumoniae*); nosocomial pneumonia; chronic bronchitis (acute bacterial exacerbation); acute maxillary sinusitis; urinary tract infection (uncomplicated or complicated), including acute pyelonephritis caused by *E. coli*; prostatitis (chronic bacterial); skin or skin structure infections (uncomplicated or complicated)

Ophthalmic: Treatment of bacterial conjunctivitis caused by susceptible organisms (Quixin™ 0.5% ophthalmic solution); treatment of corneal ulcer caused by susceptible organisms (Iquix® 1.5% ophthalmic solution)

Local Anesthetic/Vasoconstrictor Precautions No information available to require special precautions

Effects on Dental Treatment No significant effects or complications reported

Common Adverse Effects 1% to 10%:

Central nervous system: Dizziness, fever, headache, insomnia

Gastrointestinal: Nausea, vomiting, diarrhea, constipation

Ocular (with ophthalmic solution use): Decreased vision (transient), foreign body sensation, transient ocular burning, ocular pain or discomfort, photophobia

Respiratory: Pharyngitis

Dosage

Oral, I.V. (infuse I.V. solution over 60 minutes): Adults:

Chronic bronchitis (acute bacterial exacerbation): 500 mg every 24 hours for at least 7 days

Maxillary sinusitis (acute): 500 mg every 24 hours for 10-14 days

Pneumonia:

Community-acquired: 500 mg every 24 hours for 7-14 days or 750 mg every 24 hours for 5 days

Nosocomial: 750 mg every 24 hours for 7-14 days

Prostatitis (chronic bacterial): 500 mg every 24 hours for 28 days

Skin infections:

Uncomplicated: 500 mg every 24 hours for 7-10 days

Complicated: 750 mg every 24 hours for 7-14 days

Urinary tract infections:

Uncomplicated: 250 mg once daily for 3 days

Complicated, including acute pyelonephritis: 250 mg every 24 hours for 10 days

Ophthalmic:

Conjunctivitis (0.5% ophthalmic solution): Children ≥1 year and Adults:

Treatment day 1 and day 2: Instill 1-2 drops into affected eye(s) every 2 hours while awake, up to 8 times/day

Treatment day 3 through day 7: Instill 1-2 drops into affected eye(s) every 4 hours while awake, up to 4 times/day

Corneal ulceration (1.5% ophthalmic solution): Children ≥6 years and Adults:

Treatment day 1 through day 3: Instill 1-2 drops into affected eye(s) every 30 minutes to 2 hours while awake and ~4-6 hours after retiring.

Treatment day 4 to treatment completion: Instill 1-2 drops into affected eye(s) every 1-4 hours while awake.

Dosing adjustment in renal impairment:

Chronic bronchitis, acute maxillary sinusitis, uncomplicated skin infection, community-acquired pneumonia, chronic bacterial prostatitis, complicated UTI, or acute pyelonephritis: First dose as indicated in patients with normal renal function (250 mg or 500 mg), followed by:

Cl_{cr} 20-49 mL/minute: 250 mg every 24 hours

Cl_{cr} 10-19 mL/minute: 250 mg every 48 hours

Uncomplicated UTI: No dosage adjustment required

Complicated skin infection, community-acquired pneumonia, or nosocomial pneumonia:

Cl_{cr} 20-49 mL/minute: Administer 750 mg every 48 hours

Cl_{cr} 10-19 mL/minute: Administer 500 mg every 48 hours (initial: 750 mg)

Hemodialysis/CAPD: 250 mg every 48 hours (initial: 500 mg for most infections; initial: 750 mg for complicated skin/soft tissue infections followed by 500 mg every 48 hours)

Mechanism of Action As the S (-) enantiomer of the fluoroquinolone, ofloxacin, levofloxacin, inhibits DNA-gyrase in susceptible organisms thereby inhibits relaxation of supercoiled DNA and promotes breakage of DNA strands. DNA gyrase (topoisomerase II), is an essential bacterial enzyme that maintains the superhelical structure of DNA and is required for DNA replication and transcription, DNA repair, recombination, and transposition.

Contraindications Hypersensitivity to levofloxacin, any component of the formulation, or other quinolones

Warnings/Precautions

Systemic: Not recommended in children <18 years of age; CNS stimulation may occur (tremor, restlessness, confusion, and very rarely hallucinations or seizures); use with caution in patients with known or suspected CNS disorders or renal dysfunction; use caution to avoid possible photosensitivity reactions during and for several days following fluoroquinolone therapy

Rare cases of torsade de pointes have been reported in patients receiving levofloxacin. Use caution in patients with bradycardia, hypokalemia, hypomagnesemia, or in those receiving concurrent therapy with Class Ia or Class III antiarrhythmics.

Severe hypersensitivity reactions, including anaphylaxis, have occurred with quinolone therapy. If an allergic reaction occurs (itching, urticaria, dyspnea or facial edema, loss of consciousness, tingling, cardiovascular collapse), discontinue drug immediately. Prolonged use may result in superinfection; pseudomembranous colitis may occur and should be considered in all patients who present with diarrhea. Tendon inflammation and/or rupture has been reported; discontinue at first sign of tendon inflammation or pain. Quinolones may exacerbate myasthenia gravis.

Ophthalmic solution: For topical use only. Do not inject subconjunctivally or introduce into anterior chamber of the eye. Contact lenses should not be

(Continued)

Levofloxacin *(Continued)*

worn during treatment for bacterial conjunctivitis. Safety and efficacy in children <1 year of age (Quixin™) or <6 years of age (Iquix®) have not been established. **Note:** Indications for ophthalmic solutions are product concentration-specific and should not be used interchangeably.

Drug Interactions

Increased Effect/Toxicity: Quinolones may cause increased levels of azlocillin and cyclosporine. Azlocillin, cimetidine, loop diuretics (furosemide, torsemide), and probenecid increase quinolone levels (decreased renal secretion). An increased incidence of seizures may occur with foscarnet or NSAIDs. The hypoprothrombinemic effect of warfarin is enhanced by some quinolone antibiotics. QT_c-prolonging agents (including Class Ia and Class III antiarrhythmics, erythromycin, cisapride, antipsychotics, and cyclic antidepressants) should be avoided with levofloxacin. Levofloxacin does not alter warfarin levels, but may alter the gastrointestinal flora. Monitor INR closely during therapy. Concurrent use of corticosteroids may increase risk of tendon rupture.

Decreased Effect: Metal cations (magnesium, aluminum, iron, and zinc) bind quinolones in the gastrointestinal tract and inhibit absorption (by up to 98%). Due to electrolyte content, antacids, electrolyte supplements, sucralfate, quinapril, and some didanosine formulations should be avoided. Levofloxacin should be administered 2 hours before or 2 hours after these agents. Antineoplastic agents may decrease the absorption of quinolones.

Dietary Considerations May be taken without regard to meals.

Pharmacodynamics/Kinetics

Absorption: Rapid and complete

Distribution: V_d: 1.25 L/kg; CSF concentrations ~15% of serum levels; high concentrations are achieved in prostate and gynecological tissues, sinus, breast milk, and saliva

Protein binding: 50%

Metabolism: Minimally hepatic

Bioavailability: 100%

Half-life elimination: 6 hours

Time to peak, serum: 1 hour

Excretion: Primarily urine (as unchanged drug)

Pregnancy Risk Factor C

Dosage Forms INF [premixed in D_5W] (Levaquin®): 5 mg/mL (50 mL, 100 mL, 150 mL). **INJ, solution** [preservative free] (Levaquin®): 25 mg/mL (20 mL, 30 mL). **SOLN, ophthalmic:** (Iquix®): 1.5% (5 mL); (Quixin™): 0.5% (5 mL). **TAB** (Levaquin®): 250 mg, 500 mg, 750 mg

Levomepromazine *see* Methotrimeprazine *on page 901*

Levomethadyl Acetate Hydrochloride

(lee voe METH a dil AS e tate hye droe KLOR ide)

U.S. Brand Names ORLAAM® [DSC]

Generic Available No

Pharmacologic Category Analgesic, Narcotic

Use Management of opiate dependence; should be reserved for use in treatment of opiate-addicted patients who fail to show an acceptable response to other adequate treatments for addiction

Local Anesthetic/Vasoconstrictor Precautions No information available to require special precautions

Effects on Dental Treatment Key adverse event(s) related to dental treatment: Xerostomia (normal salivary flow resumes upon discontinuation).

Common Adverse Effects

>10%:

Central nervous system: Malaise

Miscellaneous: Flu syndrome

1% to 10%:

Central nervous system: CNS depression, sedation, chills, abnormal dreams, anxiety, euphoria, headache, insomnia, nervousness, hypesthesia

Endocrine & metabolic: Hot flashes (males 2:1)

Gastrointestinal: Abdominal pain, constipation, diarrhea, xerostomia, nausea, vomiting

Genitourinary: Urinary tract spasm, difficult ejaculation, impotence, decreased sex drive

Neuromuscular & skeletal: Arthralgia, back pain, weakness

Ocular: Miosis, blurred vision

Restrictions C-II; must be dispensed in a designated clinic setting only

Mechanism of Action A synthetic opioid agonist with actions similar to morphine; principal actions are analgesia and sedation. Its clinical effects in the treatment of opiate abuse occur through two mechanisms: 1) cross-sensitivity for opiates of the morphine type, suppressing symptoms of withdrawal in opiate-dependent persons; 2) with chronic oral administration, can produce sufficient tolerance to block the subjective high of usual doses of parenterally administered opiates

Drug Interactions

Cytochrome P450 Effect: Substrate of CYP2B6 (minor), 3A4 (major)

Increased Effect/Toxicity: CNS depressants, including sedatives, tranquilizers, propoxyphene, antidepressants, benzodiazepines, and ethanol may result in serious overdose when used with levomethadyl. CYP3A4 inhibitors may increase the levels/effects of levomethadyl; example inhibitors include azole antifungals, ciprofloxacin, clarithromycin, diclofenac, doxycycline, erythromycin, imatinib, isoniazid, nefazodone, nicardipine, propofol, protease inhibitors, quinidine, and verapamil. Concurrent use of QT_c-prolonging agents is contraindicated (includes class I and III antiarrhythmics, cisapride, erythromycin, select quinolones, mesoridazine, thioridazine, zonisamide). Concurrent use of MAO inhibitors is contraindicated (per manufacturer), or drugs with MAO-blocking activity (linezolid). Safety of selegiline (selective MAO type B inhibitor) not established.

Decreased Effect: Levomethadyl used in combination with naloxone, naltrexone, pentazocine, nalbuphine, butorphanol, and buprenorphine may result in withdrawal symptoms. The effect of meperidine may be decreased by levomethadyl. CYP3A4 inducers may decrease the levels/effects of levomethadyl; example inducers include aminoglutethimide, carbamazepine, nafcillin, nevirapine, phenobarbital, phenytoin, and rifamycins.

Pharmacodynamics/Kinetics

Protein binding: 80%

Metabolism: Hepatic to L-alpha-noracetylmethadol and L-alpha-dinoracetylmethadol (active metabolites)

Half-life elimination: 35-60 hours

Time to peak, serum: 1.5-6 hours

Excretion: Urine (as methadol and normethadol)

Pregnancy Risk Factor C

Levonordefrin and Mepivacaine (Dental) *see* Mepivacaine and Levonordefrin *(WITHDRAWN FROM MARKET) on page 875*

Levonorgestrel (LEE voe nor jes trel)

Related Information

Endocrine Disorders and Pregnancy *on page 1481*

U.S. Brand Names Mirena®; Plan B®

Canadian Brand Names Mirena®; Norplant® Implant; Plan B™

Mexican Brand Names Microlut®

Generic Available No

Synonyms LNg 20

Pharmacologic Category Contraceptive; Progestin

Use Prevention of pregnancy

Local Anesthetic/Vasoconstrictor Precautions No information available to require special precautions

Effects on Dental Treatment No significant effects or complications reported

Common Adverse Effects

Intrauterine system:

>5%:

Cardiovascular: Hypertension

Central nervous system: Headache, depression, nervousness

Dermatologic: Acne

Endocrine & metabolic: Breast pain, dysmenorrhea, decreased libido, abnormal Pap smear, amenorrhea (20% at 1 year), enlarged follicles (12%)

Gastrointestinal: Abdominal pain, nausea, weight gain

Genitourinary: Leukorrhea, vaginitis

Neuromuscular & skeletal: Back pain

Respiratory: Upper respiratory tract infection, sinusitis

<3% and postmarketing reports: Alopecia, anemia, cervicitis, dyspareunia, eczema, failed insertion, migraine, sepsis, vomiting

Oral tablets:

>10%:

Central nervous system: Fatigue (17%), headache (17%), dizziness (11%)

(Continued)

Levonorgestrel *(Continued)*

Endocrine & metabolic: Heavier menstrual bleeding (14%), lighter menstrual bleeding (12%), breast tenderness (11%)
Gastrointestinal: Nausea (23%), abdominal pain (18%)
1% to 10%: Gastrointestinal: Vomiting (6%), diarrhea (5%)

Mechanism of Action Pregnancy may be prevented through several mechanisms: Thickening of cervical mucus, which inhibits sperm passage through the uterus and sperm survival; inhibition of ovulation, from a negative feedback mechanism on the hypothalamus, leading to reduced secretion of follicle stimulating hormone (FSH) and luteinizing hormone (LH); inhibition of implantation. Levonorgestrel is not effective once the implantation process has begun.

Drug Interactions

Cytochrome P450 Effect: Substrate of CYP3A4 (major)

Decreased Effect: CYP3A4 inducers may decrease the levels/effects of levonorgestrel; example inducers include aminoglutethimide, carbamazepine, nafcillin, nevirapine, phenobarbital, phenytoin, and rifamycins.

Pharmacodynamics/Kinetics

Duration: Intrauterine system: Up to 5 years
Absorption: Rapid and complete
Protein binding: Highly bound to albumin and sex hormone-binding globulin
Metabolism: To inactive metabolites
Bioavailability: 100%
Half-life elimination: Oral tablet: ~24 hours
Excretion: Primarily urine

Pregnancy Risk Factor X

Levonorgestrel and Ethinyl Estradiol *see* Ethinyl Estradiol and Levonorgestrel *on page 545*

Levophed® *see* Norepinephrine *on page 996*

Levora® *see* Ethinyl Estradiol and Levonorgestrel *on page 545*

Levorphanol (lee VOR fa nole)

U.S. Brand Names Levo-Dromoran®

Generic Available Yes: Tablet

Synonyms Levorphanol Tartrate; Levorphan Tartrate

Pharmacologic Category Analgesic, Narcotic

Use Relief of moderate to severe pain; also used parenterally for preoperative sedation and an adjunct to nitrous oxide/oxygen anesthesia; 2 mg levorphanol produces analgesia comparable to that produced by 10 mg of morphine

Local Anesthetic/Vasoconstrictor Precautions No information available to require special precautions

Effects on Dental Treatment Key adverse event(s) related to dental treatment: Xerostomia (normal salivary flow resumes upon discontinuation).

Common Adverse Effects Frequency not defined.

Cardiovascular: Palpitations, hypotension, bradycardia, peripheral vasodilation, cardiac arrest, shock, tachycardia
Central nervous system: CNS depression, fatigue, drowsiness, dizziness, nervousness, headache, restlessness, anorexia, malaise, confusion, coma, convulsion, insomnia, amnesia, mental depression, hallucinations, paradoxical CNS stimulation, intracranial pressure (increased)
Dermatologic: Pruritus, urticaria, rash
Endocrine & metabolic: Antidiuretic hormone release
Gastrointestinal: Nausea, vomiting, dyspepsia, stomach cramps, xerostomia, constipation, abdominal pain, dry mouth, biliary tract spasm, paralytic ileus
Genitourinary: Decreased urination, urinary tract spasm, urinary retention
Local: Pain at injection site
Neuromuscular & skeletal: Weakness
Ocular: Miosis, diplopia
Respiratory: Respiratory depression, apnea, hypoventilation, cyanosis
Miscellaneous: Histamine release, physical and psychological dependence

Restrictions C-II

Mechanism of Action Levorphanol tartrate is a synthetic opioid agonist that is classified as a morphinan derivative. Opioids interact with stereospecific opioid receptors in various parts of the central nervous system and other tissues. Analgesic potency parallels the affinity for these binding sites. These drugs do not alter the threshold or responsiveness to pain, but the perception of pain.

Drug Interactions

Increased Effect/Toxicity: CNS depression is enhanced with coadministration of other CNS depressants.

Pharmacodynamics/Kinetics
Onset of action: Oral: 10-60 minutes
Duration: 4-8 hours
Metabolism: Hepatic
Half-life elimination: 11-16 hours
Excretion: Urine (as inactive metabolite)

Pregnancy Risk Factor B/D (prolonged use or high doses at term)

Levorphanol Tartrate *see* Levorphanol *on page 816*

Levorphan Tartrate *see* Levorphanol *on page 816*

Levothroid® *see* Levothyroxine *on page 817*

Levothyroxine (lee voe thye ROKS een)

Related Information
Endocrine Disorders and Pregnancy *on page 1481*

U.S. Brand Names Levothroid®; Levoxyl®; Novothyrox; Synthroid®; Unithroid®

Canadian Brand Names Eltroxin®; Synthroid®

Mexican Brand Names Eutirox®; Tiroidine® [tabs]

Generic Available Yes: Injection

Synonyms Levothyroxine Sodium; *L*-Thyroxine Sodium; T_4

Pharmacologic Category Thyroid Product

Use Replacement or supplemental therapy in hypothyroidism; pituitary TSH suppression

Local Anesthetic/Vasoconstrictor Precautions No precautions with vasoconstrictor are necessary if patient is well controlled with levothyroxine

Effects on Dental Treatment No significant effects or complications reported

Common Adverse Effects Frequency not defined.
- Cardiovascular: Angina, arrhythmias, blood pressure increased, cardiac arrest, flushing, heart failure, MI, palpitations, pulse increased, tachycardia
- Central nervous system: Anxiety, emotional lability, fatigue, fever, headache, hyperactivity, insomnia, irritability, nervousness, pseudotumor cerebri (children), seizures (rare)
- Dermatologic: Alopecia
- Endocrine & metabolic: Fertility impaired, menstrual irregularities
- Gastrointestinal: Abdominal cramps, appetite increased, diarrhea, vomiting, weight loss
- Hepatic: Liver function tests increased
- Neuromuscular & skeletal: Bone mineral density decreased, muscle weakness, tremors, slipped capital femoral epiphysis (children)
- Respiratory: Dyspnea
- Miscellaneous: Diaphoresis, heat intolerance, hypersensitivity (to inactive ingredients, symptoms include urticaria, pruritus, rash, flushing, angioedema, GI symptoms, fever, arthralgia, serum sickness, wheezing)

Dosage Doses should be adjusted based on clinical response and laboratory parameters.

Oral:

Children: Hypothyroidism:

Newborns: Initial: 10-15 mcg/kg/day. Lower doses of 25 mcg/day should be considered in newborns at risk for cardiac failure. Newborns with T_4 levels <5 mcg/dL should be started at 50 mcg/day. Adjust dose at 4- to 6-week intervals.

Infants and Children: Dose based on body weight and age as listed below. Children with severe or chronic hypothyroidism should be started at 25 mcg/day; adjust dose by 25 mcg every 2-4 weeks. In older children, hyperactivity may be decreased by starting with 1/4 of the recommended dose and increasing by 1/4 dose each week until the full replacement dose is reached. Refer to adult dosing once growth and puberty are complete.
- 0-3 months: 10-15 mcg/kg/day
- 3-6 months: 8-10 mcg/kg/day
- 6-12 months: 6-8 mcg/kg/day
- 1-5 years: 5-6 mcg/kg/day
- 6-12 years: 4-5 mcg/kg/day
- >12 years: 2-3 mcg/kg/day

Adults:

Hypothyroidism: 1.7 mcg/kg/day in otherwise healthy adults <50 years old, children in whom growth and puberty are complete, and older adults who have been recently treated for hyperthyroidism or who have been hypothyroid for only a few months. Titrate dose every 6 weeks. Average starting dose ~100 mcg; usual doses are ≤200 mcg/day; doses ≥300 mcg/day are rare (consider poor compliance, malabsorption, and/or drug

(Continued)

Levothyroxine *(Continued)*

interactions). **Note:** For patients >50 years or patients with cardiac disease, refer to Elderly dosing.

Severe hypothyroidism: Initial: 12.5-25 mcg/day; adjust dose by 25 mcg/day every 2-4 weeks as appropriate; **Note:** Oral agents are not recommended for myxedema (see I.V. dosing).

Subclinical hypothyroidism (if treated): 1 mcg/kg/day

TSH suppression:

Well-differentiated thyroid cancer: Highly individualized; Doses >2 mcg/kg/day may be needed to suppress TSH to <0.1 mU/L.

Benign nodules and nontoxic multinodular goiter: Goal TSH suppression: 0.1-0.3 mU/L

Elderly: Hypothyroidism:

>50 years without cardiac disease **or** <50 years with cardiac disease: Initial: 25-50 mcg/day; adjust dose at 6- to 8-week intervals as needed

>50 years with cardiac disease: Initial: 12.5-25 mcg/day; adjust dose by 12.5-25 mcg increments at 4- to 6-week intervals

Note: Elderly patients may require <1 mcg/kg/day

I.M., I.V.: Children, Adults, Elderly: Hypothyroidism: 50% of the oral dose

I.V.:

Adults: Myxedema coma or stupor: 200-500 mcg, then 100-300 mcg the next day if necessary; smaller doses should be considered in patients with cardiovascular disease

Elderly: Myxedema coma: Refer to Adults dosing; lower doses may be needed

Mechanism of Action Exact mechanism of action is unknown; however, it is believed the thyroid hormone exerts its many metabolic effects through control of DNA transcription and protein synthesis; involved in normal metabolism, growth, and development; promotes gluconeogenesis, increases utilization and mobilization of glycogen stores, and stimulates protein synthesis, increases basal metabolic rate

Contraindications Hypersensitivity to levothyroxine sodium or any component of the formulation; recent MI or thyrotoxicosis; uncorrected adrenal insufficiency

Warnings/Precautions Ineffective and potentially toxic for weight reduction; high doses may produce serious or even life-threatening toxic effects particularly when used with some anorectic drugs. Use with caution and reduce dosage in patients with angina pectoris or other cardiovascular disease; use cautiously in elderly since they may be more likely to have compromised cardiovascular functions. Patients with adrenal insufficiency, myxedema, diabetes mellitus and insipidus may have symptoms exaggerated or aggravated; thyroid replacement requires periodic assessment of thyroid status. Chronic hypothyroidism predisposes patients to coronary artery disease.

Drug Interactions

Increased Effect/Toxicity: Levothyroxine may potentiate the hypoprothrombinemic effect of warfarin (and other oral anticoagulants). Tricyclic antidepressants (TCAs) coadministered with levothyroxine may increase potential for toxicity of both drugs. Coadministration with ketamine may lead to hypertension and tachycardia.

Decreased Effect: Some medications may decrease absorption of levothyroxine: Cholestyramine, colestipol (separate administration by at least 2 hours); aluminum- and magnesium-containing antacids, iron preparations, sucralfate, Kayexalate® (separate administration by at least 4 hours). Enzyme inducers (phenytoin, phenobarbital, carbamazepine, and rifampin/rifabutin) may decrease levothyroxine levels. Levothyroxine may decrease effect of oral sulfonylureas. Serum levels of digoxin and theophylline may be altered by thyroid function. Estrogens may decrease serum free-thyroxine concentrations.

Ethanol/Nutrition/Herb Interactions Food: Taking levothyroxine with enteral nutrition may cause reduced bioavailability and may lower serum thyroxine levels leading to signs or symptoms of hypothyroidism. Limit intake of goitrogenic foods (eg, asparagus, cabbage, peas, turnip greens, broccoli, spinach, Brussels sprouts, lettuce, soybeans). Soybean flour (infant formula), cottonseed meal, walnuts, and dietary fiber may decrease absorption of levothyroxine from the GI tract.

Dietary Considerations Should be taken on an empty stomach, at least 30 minutes before food.

Pharmacodynamics/Kinetics

Onset of action: Therapeutic: Oral: 3-5 days; I.V. 6-8 hours

Peak effect: I.V.: ~24 hours

Absorption: Oral: Erratic (40% to 80%); decreases with age

Protein binding: >99%
Metabolism: Hepatic to triiodothyronine (active)
Time to peak, serum: 2-4 hours
Half-life elimination: Euthyroid: 6-7 days; Hypothyroid: 9-10 days; Hyperthyroid: 3-4 days
Excretion: Urine and feces; decreases with age

Pregnancy Risk Factor A

Dosage Forms INJ, powder for reconstitution (Synthroid®): 0.2 mg, 0.5 mg. **TAB**: (Levothroid®, Levoxyl®, Novothyrox, Synthroid®): 25 mcg, 50 mcg, 75 mcg, 88 mcg, 100 mcg, 112 mcg, 125 mcg, 137 mcg, 150 mcg, 175 mcg, 200 mcg, 300 mcg; (Unithroid®): 25 mcg, 50 mcg, 75 mcg, 88 mcg, 100 mcg, 112 mcg, 125 mcg, 150 mcg, 175 mcg, 200 mcg, 300 mcg

Levothyroxine Sodium *see* Levothyroxine *on page 817*
Levoxyl® *see* Levothyroxine *on page 817*
Levsin® *see* Hyoscyamine *on page 724*
Levsinex® *see* Hyoscyamine *on page 724*
Levsin/SL® *see* Hyoscyamine *on page 724*
Levulan® Kerastick® *see* Aminolevulinic Acid *on page 99*
Levulose, Dextrose and Phosphoric Acid *see* Fructose, Dextrose, and Phosphoric Acid *on page 638*
Lexapro™ *see* Escitalopram *on page 513*
Lexiva™ *see* Fosamprenavir *on page 630*
Lexxel® *see* Enalapril and Felodipine *on page 491*
LFA-3/IgG(1) Fusion Protein, Human *see* Alefacept *on page 76*
LHRH *see* Gonadorelin *on page 669*
***l*-Hyoscyamine Sulfate** *see* Hyoscyamine *on page 724*
Librax® *see* Clidinium and Chlordiazepoxide *on page 347*
Librium® *see* Chlordiazepoxide *on page 307*
LidaMantle® *see* Lidocaine *on page 819*
Lida-Mantle® HC *see* Lidocaine and Hydrocortisone *on page 826*
Lidex® *see* Fluocinonide *on page 602*
Lidex-E® *see* Fluocinonide *on page 602*

Lidocaine (LYE doe kane)

Related Information

Cardiovascular Diseases *on page 1458*
Management of Patients Undergoing Cancer Therapy *on page 1569*
Oral Pain *on page 1526*
Oral Viral Infections *on page 1547*

U.S. Brand Names Anestacon®; Band-Aid® Hurt-Free™ Antiseptic Wash [OTC]; Burnamycin [OTC]; Burn Jel [OTC]; Burn-O-Jel [OTC]; LidaMantle®; Lidoderm®; L-M-X™ 4 [OTC]; L-M-X™ 5 [OTC]; Premjact® [OTC]; Solarcaine® Aloe Extra Burn Relief [OTC]; Topicaine® [OTC]; Xylocaine®; Xylocaine® MPF; Xylocaine® Viscous; Zilactin-L® [OTC]

Canadian Brand Names Betacaine®; Lidodan™; Lidoderm®; Xylocaine®; Xylocard®; Zilactin®

Mexican Brand Names Xylocaina®

Generic Available Yes: Gel, injection, ointment, solution

Synonyms Lidocaine Hydrochloride; Lignocaine Hydrochloride

Pharmacologic Category Analgesic, Topical; Antiarrhythmic Agent, Class Ib; Local Anesthetic

Dental Use Amide-type injectable local anesthetic and topical local anesthetic; Patch: Production of mild topical anesthesia of accessible mucous membranes of the mouth prior to superficial dental procedures

Use Local anesthetic and acute treatment of ventricular arrhythmias from myocardial infarction, cardiac manipulation, digitalis intoxication; drug of choice for ventricular ectopy, ventricular tachycardia (VT), ventricular fibrillation (VF); for pulseless VT or VF preferably administer **after** defibrillation and epinephrine; control of premature ventricular contractions, wide-complex paroxysmal supraventricular tachycardia (PSVT); control of hemodynamically compromising PVCs; hemodynamically stable VT

Rectal: Temporary relief of pain and itching due to anorectal disorders
Topical: Local anesthetic for use in laser, cosmetic, and outpatient surgeries; minor burns, cuts, and abrasions of the skin

Orphan drug: Lidoderm® Patch: Relief of allodynia (painful hypersensitivity) and chronic pain in postherpetic neuralgia

Local Anesthetic/Vasoconstrictor Precautions No information available to require special precautions

(Continued)

Lidocaine *(Continued)*

Effects on Dental Treatment No significant effects or complications reported

Significant Adverse Effects Effects vary with route of administration. Many effects are dose-related.

Frequency not defined:

Cardiovascular: Bradycardia, hypotension, heart block, arrhythmias, cardiovascular collapse, sinus node supression, increase defibrillator threshold, vascular insufficiency (periarticular injections), arterial spasms

Central nervous system: Drowsiness after administration is usually a sign of a high blood level. Other effects may include lightheadedness, dizziness, tinnitus, blurred vision, vomiting, twitching, tremors, lethargy, coma, agitation, slurred speech, seizures, anxiety, euphoria, hallucinations, paresthesia, psychosis

Dermatologic: Itching, rash, edema of the skin, contact dermatitis

Gastrointestinal: Nausea, vomiting, taste disorder

Local:Thrombophlebitis

Neuromuscular & skeletal: Transient radicular pain (subarachnoid administration; up to 1.9%)

Ocular: Blurred vision, diplopia

Respiratory: Dyspnea, respiratory depression or arrest, bronchospasm

Miscellaneous: Allergic reactions, urticaria, edema, anaphylactoid reaction

Following spinal anesthesia positional headache (3%), shivering (2%) nausea, peripheral nerve symptoms, respiratory inadequacy and double vision (<1%), hypotension, cauda equina syndrome

Postmarketing and/or case reports: ARDS (inhalation), asystole, methemoglobinemia, severe back pain

Dosage

Topical: Apply to affected area as needed; maximum: 3 mg/kg/dose; do not repeat within 2 hours.

L-M-X™ 4 cream: Apply 1/4 inch thick layer to intact skin. Leave on until adequate anesthetic effect is obtained. Remove cream and cleanse area before beginning procedure.

Rectal: Relief of pain and itching (L-M-X™ 5): Children ≥12 years and Adults: Apply topically to clean, dry area **or** using applicator insert rectally, up to 6 times/day

Injectable local anesthetic: Varies with procedure, degree of anesthesia needed, vascularity of tissue, duration of anesthesia required, and physical condition of patient; maximum: 4.5 mg/kg/dose; do not repeat within 2 hours.

Patch: Postherpetic neuralgia: Apply patch to most painful area. Up to 3 patches may be applied in a single application. Patch may remain in place for up to 12 hours in any 24-hour period.

Antiarrhythmic:

I.V.: 1-1.5 mg/kg bolus over 2-3 minutes; may repeat doses of 0.5-0.75 mg/kg in 5-10 minutes up to a total of 3 mg/kg; continuous infusion: 1-4 mg/minute

I.V. (2 g/250 mL D_5W) infusion rates (infusion pump should be used for I.V. infusion administration):

1 mg/minute: 7.5 mL/hour
2 mg/minute: 15 mL/hour
3 mg/minute: 22.5 mL/hour
4 mg/minute: 30 mL/hour

Ventricular fibrillation (after defibrillation and epinephrine): Initial: 1-1.5 mg/kg. Repeat 0.5-0.75 mg/kg bolus may be given 3-5 minutes after initial dose. Total dose should not exceed 200-300 mg during a 1-hour period or 3 mg/kg total dose. Follow with continuous infusion after return of perfusion.

Endotracheal: 2-2.5 times the I.V. dose (2-4 mg/kg diluted with NS to a total volume of 10 mL)

Decrease dose in patients with CHF, shock, or hepatic disease.

Dosage adjustment in renal impairment: Not dialyzable (0% to 5%) by hemo- or peritoneal dialysis; supplemental dose is not necessary.

Dosage adjustment in hepatic impairment: Reduce dose in acute hepatitis and decompensated cirrhosis by 50%.

Mechanism of Action Class Ib antiarrhythmic; suppresses automaticity of conduction tissue, by increasing electrical stimulation threshold of ventricle, His-Purkinje system, and spontaneous depolarization of the ventricles during diastole by a direct action on the tissues; blocks both the initiation and conduction of nerve impulses by decreasing the neuronal membrane's permeability to sodium ions, which results in inhibition of depolarization with resultant blockade of conduction

Contraindications Hypersensitivity to lidocaine or any component of the formulation; hypersensitivity to another local anesthetic of the amide type; Adam-Stokes syndrome; severe degrees of SA, AV, or intraventricular heart block (except in patients with a functioning artificial pacemaker); premixed injection may contain corn-derived dextrose and its use is contraindicated in patients with allergy to corn-related products

Warnings/Precautions

Intravenous: Constant ECG monitoring is necessary during I.V. administration. Use cautiously in hepatic impairment, any degree of heart block, Wolff-Parkinson-White syndrome, CHF, marked hypoxia, severe respiratory depression, hypovolemia, history of malignant hyperthermia, or shock. Increased ventricular rate may be seen when administered to a patient with atrial fibrillation. Correct any underlying causes of ventricular arrhythmias. Monitor closely for signs and symptoms of CNS toxicity. The elderly may be prone to increased CNS and cardiovascular side effects. Reduce dose in hepatic dysfunction and CHF.

Injectable anesthetic: Follow appropriate administration techniques so as not to administer any intravascularly. Solutions containing antimicrobial preservatives should not be used for epidural or spinal anesthesia. Some solutions contain a bisulfite; avoid in patients who are allergic to bisulfite. Resuscitative equipment, medicine and oxygen should be available in case of emergency. Use products containing epinephrine cautiously in patients with significant vascular disease, compromised blood flow, or during or following general anesthesia (increased risk of arrhythmias). Adjust the dose for the elderly, pediatric, acutely ill, and debilitated patients.

Topical: L-M-X™ 4 cream: Do not leave on large body areas for >2 hours. Observe young children closely to prevent accidental ingestion. Not for use ophthalmic use or for use on mucous membranes.

Drug Interactions Substrate of CYP1A2 (minor), 2A6 (minor), 2B6 (minor), 2C8/9 (minor), 2D6 (major), 3A4 (major); **Inhibits** CYP1A2 (strong), 2D6 (moderate), 3A4 (moderate)

Cimetidine increases lidocaine blood levels; monitor levels or use an alternative H_2 antagonist.

CYP1A2 substrates: Lidocaine may increase the levels/effects of CYP1A2 substrates. Example substrates include aminophylline, fluvoxamine, mexiletine, mirtazapine, ropinirole, theophylline, and trifluoperazine.

CYP2D6 inhibitors: May increase the levels/effects of lidocaine. Example inhibitors include chlorpromazine, delavirdine, fluoxetine, miconazole, paroxetine, pergolide, quinidine, quinine, ritonavir, and ropinirole.

CYP2D6 substrates: Lidocaine may increase the levels/effects of CYP2D6 substrates. Example substrates include amphetamines, selected beta-blockers, dextromethorphan, fluoxetine, mirtazapine, nefazodone, paroxetine, risperidone, ritonavir, thioridazine, tricyclic antidepressants, and venlafaxine.

CYP2D6 prodrug substrates: Lidocaine may decrease the levels/effects of CYP2D6 prodrug substrates. Example prodrug substrates include codeine, hydrocodone, oxycodone, and tramadol.

CYP3A4 inducers: CYP3A4 inducers may decrease the levels/effects of lidocaine. Example inducers include aminoglutethimide, carbamazepine, nafcillin, nevirapine, phenobarbital, phenytoin, and rifamycins.

CYP3A4 inhibitors: May increase the levels/effects of lidocaine. Example inhibitors include azole antifungals, ciprofloxacin, clarithromycin, diclofenac, doxycycline, erythromycin, imatinib, isoniazid, nefazodone, nicardipine, propofol, protease inhibitors, quinidine, and verapamil.

CYP3A4 substrates: Lidocaine may increase the levels/effects of CYP3A4 substrates. Example substrates include benzodiazepines, calcium channel blockers, cyclosporine, mirtazapine, nateglinide, nefazodone, sildenafil (and other PDE-5 inhibitors), tacrolimus, and venlafaxine. Selected benzodiazepines (midazolam and triazolam), cisapride, ergot alkaloids, selected HMG-CoA reductase inhibitors (lovastatin and simvastatin), and pimozide are generally contraindicated with strong CYP3A4 inhibitors.

Propranolol: Increases lidocaine blood levels.

Protease inhibitors (eg, amprenavir, ritonavir): May increase lidocaine blood levels.

Ethanol/Nutrition/Herb Interactions Herb/Nutraceutical: St John's wort may decrease lidocaine levels; avoid concurrent use.

Dietary Considerations Premixed injection may contain corn-derived dextrose and its use is contraindicated in patients with allergy to corn-related products.

(Continued)

Lidocaine *(Continued)*

Pharmacodynamics/Kinetics

Onset of action: Single bolus dose: 45-90 seconds

Duration: 10-20 minutes

Distribution: V_d: 1.1-2.1 L/kg; alterable by many patient factors; decreased in CHF and liver disease; crosses blood-brain barrier

Protein binding: 60% to 80% to $alpha_1$ acid glycoprotein

Metabolism: 90% hepatic; active metabolites monoethylglycinexylidide (MEGX) and glycinexylidide (GX) can accumulate and may cause CNS toxicity

Half-life elimination: Biphasic: Prolonged with congestive heart failure, liver disease, shock, severe renal disease; Initial: 7-30 minutes; Terminal: Infants, premature: 3.2 hours, Adults: 1.5-2 hours

Pregnancy Risk Factor B (manufacturer); C (expert analysis)

Lactation Enters breast milk (small amounts)/compatible

Dosage Forms

Cream, rectal (L-M-X™ 5): 5% (30 g) [contains benzyl alcohol; previously named ELA-Max® 5]

Cream, topical (L-M-X™ 4): 4% (5 g, 30 g) [contains benzyl alcohol; previously named ELA-Max®]

Cream, topical, as hydrochloride (LidaMantle®): 3% (30 g, 85 g)

Gel, topical:
- Burn-O-Jel: 0.5% (90 g)
- Topicaine®: 4% (1 g, 10 g, 30 g, 113 g) [contains benzyl alcohol, aloe vera, and jojoba]

Gel, topical, as hydrochloride: 2% (30 g)
- Burn Jel: 2% (3.5 g, 120 g)
- Solarcaine® Aloe Extra Burn Relief: 0.5% (226 g) [contains aloe vera gel and tartrazine]

Infusion, as hydrochloride [premixed in D_5W]: 0.4% [4 mg/mL] (250 mL, 500 mL); 0.8% [8 mg/mL] (250 mL, 500 mL)

Injection, solution, as hydrochloride: 0.5% [5 mg/mL] (50 mL); 1% [10 mg/mL] (5 mL, 20 mL, 30 mL, 50 mL); 1.5% [15 mg/mL] (20 mL); 2% [20 mg/mL] (2 mL, 5 mL, 20 mL, 30 mL, 50 mL)
- Xylocaine®: 0.5% [5 mg/mL] (50 mL); 1% [10 mg/mL] (10 mL, 20 mL, 50 mL); 2% [20 mg/mL] (1.8 mL, 10 mL, 20 mL, 50 mL); 4% [40 mg/mL] (5 mL)

Injection, solution, as hydrochloride [preservative free]: 0.5% [5 mg/mL] (50 mL); 1% [10 mg/mL] (2 mL, 5 mL, 30 mL); 1.5% [15 mg/mL] (20 mL); 2% [20 mg/mL] (5 mL, 10 mL); 4% [40 mg/mL] (5 mL); 10% [100 mg/mL] (10 mL); 20% [200 mg/mL] (10 mL)
- Xylocaine® MPF: 0.5% [5 mg/mL] (50 mL); 1% [10 mg/mL] (2 mL, 5 mL, 10 mL, 20 mL, 30 mL); 1.5% [15 mg/mL] (10 mL, 20 mL); 2% [2 mg/mL] (2 mL, 5 mL, 10 mL); 4% [40 mg/mL] (5 mL)

Injection, solution, as hydrochloride [premixed in $D_{7.5}W$, preservative free]: 5% (2 mL)
- Xylocaine®-MPF: 1.5% (2 mL)

Jelly, topical, as hydrochloride:
- Anestacon®: 2% (15 mL, 240 mL) [contains benzalkonium chloride]
- Xylocaine®: 2% (5 mL, 10 mL, 20 mL, 30 mL)

Liquid, topical (Zilactin®-L): 2.5% (7.5 mL)

Ointment, topical: 5% (37 g)
- Xylocaine®: 2.5% (35 g) [OTC]; 5% (3.5 g, 35 g) [mint or unflavored]

Patch, transdermal (Lidoderm®): 5% (30s)

Solution, topical, as hydrochloride: 2% [20 mg/mL] (15 mL, 240 mL); 4% [40 mg/mL] (50 mL)
- Band-Aid® Hurt-Free™ Antiseptic Wash: 2% (180 mL)
- Xylocaine®: 4% [40 mg/mL] (50 mL)

Solution, viscous, as hydrochloride: 2% [20 mg/mL] (20 mL, 100 mL)
- Xylocaine® Viscous: 2% [20 mg/mL] (20 mL, 100 mL, 450 mL)

Spray, topical:
- Burnamycin: 0.5% (60 mL) [contains aloe vera gel]
- Premjact®: 9.6% (13 mL)
- Solarcaine® Aloe Extra Burn Relief: 0.5% (127 g) [contains aloe vera]

Lidocaine and Bupivacaine (LYE doe kane & byoo PIV a kane)

Related Information

Bupivacaine *on page 225*
Lidocaine *on page 819*

U.S. Brand Names Duocaine™

Generic Available No

Synonyms Bupivacaine and Lidocaine; Lidocaine Hydrochloride and Bupivacaine Hydrochloride

Pharmacologic Category Local Anesthetic

Use Local or regional anesthesia in ophthalmologic surgery by peripheral nerve block techniques such as peribulbar, retrobulbar, and facial blocks; may be used with or without epinephrine

Local Anesthetic/Vasoconstrictor Precautions No information available to require special precautions

Effects on Dental Treatment No significant effects or complications reported

Common Adverse Effects Frequency not defined; reactions may be dose related or due to unintentional intravascular injection.

Cardiovascular: Bradycardia, cardiac arrest, cardiac output decreased, heart block, hypotension, myocardium depression, ventricular arrhythmia

Central nervous system: Anxiety, chills, convulsions, depression, dizziness, drowsiness, excitation, restlessness

Gastrointestinal: Nausea, vomiting

Neuromuscular & skeletal: Tremors

Ocular: Blurred vision, pupil constriction, permanent injury to extraocular muscle

Otic: Tinnitus

Respiratory: Respiratory arrest

Miscellaneous: Allergic reaction

Following unintentional subarachnoid injection: Backache, cranial nerve palsies, headache, incontinence (fecal or urinary), meningismus, paralysis, paresthesia, perineal sensation loss, persistent anesthesia, septic meningitis, sexual function loss, spinal block, urinary retention, weakness

Mechanism of Action Blocks both the initiation and conduction of nerve impulses by decreasing the neuronal membrane's permeability to sodium ions, which results in inhibition of depolarization with resultant blockade of conduction.

Drug Interactions

Cytochrome P450 Effect: Lidocaine: **Substrate** of CYP1A2 (minor), 2A6 (minor), 2B6 (minor), 2C8/9 (minor), 2D6 (major), 3A4 (major); **Inhibits** CYP1A2 (strong), 2D6 (moderate), 3A4 (moderate)

Decreased Effect: Epinephrine may be used to decrease systemic absorption of lidocaine/bupivacaine; if used, see Epinephrine monograph for Drug Interactions.

Pharmacodynamics/Kinetics Also see individual agents.

Protein binding: Lidocaine: Fraction bound decreases with increased concentration; also dependent upon plasma concentration of alpha$_1$-acid glycoprotein

Metabolism: Lidocaine: Hepatic, forms metabolites; Bupivacaine: hepatic, forms metabolites

Half-life elimination: Lidocaine: I.V.: 1.5-2 hours; Bupivacaine: I.V.: 2.7 hours

Time to peak, plasma: Following peribulbar block: Lidocaine: 20 minutes; Bupivacaine: 21 minutes

Excretion: Urine

Pregnancy Risk Factor C

Lidocaine and Epinephrine (LYE doe kane & ep i NEF rin)

Related Information

Epinephrine *on page 496*

Lidocaine *on page 819*

Oral Pain *on page 1526*

U.S. Brand Names Xylocaine® MPF With Epinephrine; Xylocaine® With Epinephrine

Canadian Brand Names Xylocaine® With Epinephrine

Generic Available Yes

Synonyms Epinephrine and Lidocaine

Pharmacologic Category Local Anesthetic

Dental Use Amide-type anesthetic used for local infiltration anesthesia injection near nerve trunks to produce nerve block

Use Local infiltration anesthesia; AVS for nerve block

Local Anesthetic/Vasoconstrictor Precautions No information available to require special precautions

Effects on Dental Treatment It is common to misinterpret psychogenic responses to local anesthetic injection as an allergic reaction. Intraoral injections are perceived by many patients as a stressful procedure in dentistry.

(Continued)

Lidocaine and Epinephrine *(Continued)*

Common symptoms to this stress are diaphoresis, palpitations, hyperventilation. Patients may exhibit hypersensitivity to bisulfites contained in local anesthetic solution to prevent oxidation of epinephrine. In general, patients reacting to bisulfites have a history of asthma and their airways are hyper-reactive to asthmatic syndrome.

Degree of adverse effects in the CNS and cardiovascular system is directly related to the blood levels of bupivacaine. Bradycardia, hypersensitivity reactions (rare; may be manifest as dermatologic reactions and edema at injection site), asthmatic syndromes

High blood levels: Anxiety, restlessness, disorientation, confusion, dizziness, tremors, seizures, CNS depression (resulting in somnolence, unconsciousness and possible respiratory arrest), nausea, and vomiting.

Significant Adverse Effects Degree of adverse effects in the central nervous system and cardiovascular system are directly related to the blood levels of lidocaine. The effects below are more likely to occur after systemic administration rather than infiltration.

Cardiovascular: Myocardial effects include a decrease in contraction force as well as a decrease in electrical excitability and myocardial conduction rate resulting in bradycardia and reduction in cardiac output.

Central nervous system: High blood levels result in anxiety, restlessness, disorientation, confusion, dizziness, tremors and seizures. This is followed by depression of CNS resulting in somnolence, unconsciousness and possible respiratory arrest. In some cases, symptoms of CNS stimulation may be absent and the primary CNS effects are somnolence and unconsciousness.

Gastrointestinal: Nausea and vomiting may occur

Hypersensitivity reactions: Extremely rare, but may be manifest as dermatologic reactions and edema at injection site. Asthmatic syndromes have occurred. Patients may exhibit hypersensitivity to bisulfites contained in local anesthetic solution to prevent oxidation of epinephrine. In general, patients reacting to bisulfites have a history of asthma and their airways are hyper-reactive to asthmatic syndrome.

Psychogenic reactions: It is common to misinterpret psychogenic responses to local anesthetic injection as an allergic reaction. Intraoral injections are perceived by many patients as a stressful procedure in dentistry. Common symptoms to this stress are diaphoresis, palpitations, hyperventilation, generalized pallor and a fainting feeling

Dosage Dosage varies with the anesthetic procedure, degree of anesthesia needed, vascularity of tissue, duration of anesthesia required, and physical condition of patient.

Dental anesthesia, infiltration, or conduction block:

Children <10 years: 20-30 mg (1-1.5 mL) of lidocaine hydrochloride as a 2% solution with epinephrine 1:100,000; maximum: 4-5 mg of lidocaine hydrochloride/kg of body weight or 100-150 mg as a single dose

Children >10 years and Adults: Do not exceed 6.6 mg/kg body weight or 300 mg of lidocaine hydrochloride and 3 mcg (0.003 mg) of epinephrine/kg of body weight or 0.2 mg epinephrine per dental appointment. The effective anesthetic dose varies with procedure, intensity of anesthesia needed, duration of anesthesia required, and physical condition of the patient. Always use the lowest effective dose along with careful aspiration.

The numbers of dental carpules (1.8 mL) provide the indicated amounts of lidocaine hydrochloride 2% and epinephrine 1:100,000 (see table on next page).

For most routine dental procedures, lidocaine hydrochloride 2% with epinephrine 1:100,000 is preferred. When a more pronounced hemostasis is required, a 1:50,000 epinephrine concentration should be used. The following numbers of dental carpules (1.8 mL) provide the indicated amounts of lidocaine hydrochloride 2% and epinephrine 1:50,000 (see table on next page).

Mechanism of Action Lidocaine blocks both the initiation and conduction of nerve impulses via decreased permeability of sodium ions; epinephrine increases the duration of action of lidocaine by causing vasoconstriction (via alpha effects) which slows the vascular absorption of lidocaine

Contraindications Hypersensitivity to local anesthetics of the amide type or any component of the formulation; myasthenia gravis; shock; cardiac conduction disease; also see individual agents

Warnings/Precautions Should be avoided in patients with uncontrolled hyperthyroidism. Should be used in minimal amounts in patients with significant cardiovascular problems (because of epinephrine component). Aspirate the syringe after tissue penetration and before injection to minimize chance of direct vascular injection.

# of Cartridges (1.8 mL)	Lidocaine HCl (2%) (mg)	Epinephrine 1:100,000 (mg)
1	36	0.018
2	72	0.036
3	108	0.054
4	144	0.072
5	180	0.090
6	216	0.108
7	252	0.126
8	288	0.144
9	324	0.162
10	360	0.180

# of Cartridges (1.8 mL)	Lidocaine HCl (2%) (mg)	Epinephrine 1:50,000 (mg)
1	36	0.036
2	72	0.072
3	108	0.108
4	144	0.144
5	180	0.180
6	216	0.216

Drug Interactions Lidocaine: **Substrate** of CYP1A2 (minor), 2A6 (minor), 2B6 (minor), 2C8/9 (minor), 2D6 (major), 3A4 (major); **Inhibits** CYP1A2 (strong), 2D6 (strong), 3A4 (moderate)

Also see individual agents.

Epinephrine (and other direct alpha-agonists): Pressor response to I.V. epinephrine, norepinephrine, and phenylephrine may be enhanced in patients receiving TCAs (**Note:** Effect is unlikely with epinephrine or levonordefrin dosages typically administered as infiltration in combination with local anesthetics)

Pharmacodynamics/Kinetics

Onset of action: Peak effect: ~5 minutes

Duration: ~2 hours; dose and anesthetic procedure dependent

See individual agents.

Pregnancy Risk Factor B

Lactation Enters breast milk/compatible

Breast-Feeding Considerations Usual infiltration doses of lidocaine with epinephrine given to nursing mothers has not been shown to affect the health of the nursing infant.

Dosage Forms

Injection, solution, as hydrochloride, with epinephrine 1:50,000 (Xylocaine® with Epinephrine): Lidocaine 2% [20 mg/mL] (1.8 mL) [contains sodium metabisulfite]

Injection, solution, as hydrochloride, with epinephrine 1:100,000: Lidocaine 1% [10 mg/mL] (20 mL, 30 mL, 50 mL); Lidocaine 2% (20 mL, 30 mL, 50 mL)

Xylocaine® with Epinephrine: Lidocaine 1% [10 mg/mL] (10 mL 20 mL, 50 mL); Lidocaine 2% (1.8 mL, 10 mL, 20 mL, 50 mL) [contains sodium metabisulfite]

Injection, solution, as hydrochloride, with epinephrine 1:200,000: Lidocaine 0.5% [5 mg/mL] (50 mL)

Xylocaine® with Epinephrine: Lidocaine 0.5% [5 mg/mL] (50 mL) [contains sodium metabisulfite]

Injection, solution, as hydrochloride, with epinephrine 1:200,000 [methylparaben free]: Lidocaine 1% [10 mg/mL] (30 mL); Lidocaine 1.5% (5 mL, 30 mL); Lidocaine 2% (20 mL) [contains sodium metabisulfite]

Xylocaine® MPF with Epinephrine: Lidocaine 1% [10 mg/mL] (5 mL, 10 mL, 30 mL); 1.5% [15 mg/mL] (5 mL, 10 mL, 30 mL); Lidocaine 2% [20 mg/mL] (5 mL, 10 mL, 20 mL) [contains sodium metabisulfite]

Selected Readings

Ayoub ST and Coleman AE, "A Review of Local Anesthetics," *Gen Dent*, 1992, 40(4):285-7, 289-90.

(Continued)

Lidocaine and Epinephrine *(Continued)*

Budenz AW, "Local Anesthetics in Dentistry: Then and Now," *J Calif Dent Assoc*, 2003, 31(5):388-96.
Dower JS Jr, "A Review of Paresthesia in Association With Administration of Local Anesthesia," *Dent Today*, 2003, 22(2):64-9.
Finder RL and Moore PA, "Adverse Drug Reactions to Local Anesthesia," *Dent Clin North Am*, 2002, 46(4):747-57, x.
Haas DA, "An Update on Local Anesthetics in Dentistry," *J Can Dent Assoc*, 2002, 68(9):546-51.
Hawkins JM and Moore PA, "Local Anesthesia: Advances in Agents and Techniques," *Dent Clin North Am*, 2002, 46(4):719-32, ix.
"Injectable Local Anesthetics," *J Am Dent Assoc*, 2003, 134(5):628-9.
Jastak JT and Yagiela JA, "Vasoconstrictors and Local Anesthesia: A Review and Rationale for Use," *J Am Dent Assoc*, 1983, 107(4):623-30.
MacKenzie TA and Young ER, "Local Anesthetic Update," *Anesth Prog*, 1993, 40(2):29-34.
Malamed SF, "Allergy and Toxic Reactions to Local Anesthetics," *Dent Today*, 2003, 22(4):114-6, 118-21.
Nusstein J, Reader A, and Beck FM, "Anesthetic Efficacy of Different Volumes of Lidocaine With Epinephrine for Inferior Alveolar Nerve Blocks," *Gen Dent*, 2002, 50(4):372-5.
Wynn RL, "Epinephrine Interactions With Beta-Blockers," *Gen Dent*, 1994, 42(1):16, 18.
Wynn RL, "Recent Research on Mechanisms of Local Anesthetics," *Gen Dent*, 1995, 43(4):316-8.
Yagiela JA, "Local Anesthetics," *Anesth Prog*, 1991, 38(4-5):128-41.

Lidocaine and Hydrocortisone

(LYE doe kane & hye droe KOR ti sone)

Related Information

Hydrocortisone *on page 714*
Lidocaine *on page 819*

U.S. Brand Names AnaMantle® HC; Lida-Mantle® HC

Generic Available No

Synonyms Hydrocortisone and Lidocaine

Pharmacologic Category Anesthetic/Corticosteroid

Use Topical anti-inflammatory and anesthetic for skin disorders; rectal for the treatment of hemorrhoids, anal fissures, pruritus ani, or similar conditions

Local Anesthetic/Vasoconstrictor Precautions No information available to require special precautions

Effects on Dental Treatment No significant effects or complications reported

Drug Interactions

Cytochrome P450 Effect:

Lidocaine: **Substrate** of CYP1A2 (minor), 2A6 (minor), 2B6 (minor), 2C8/9 (minor), 2D6 (major), 3A4 (major); **Inhibits** CYP1A2 (strong), 2D6 (strong), 3A4 (moderate)

Hydrocortisone: **Substrate** of CYP3A4 (minor); **Induces** CYP3A4 (weak)

Increased Effect/Toxicity: See individual agents.

Decreased Effect: See individual agents.

Pharmacodynamics/Kinetics See individual agents.

Pregnancy Risk Factor B

Lidocaine and Prilocaine (LYE doe kane & PRIL oh kane)

Related Information

Lidocaine *on page 819*
Prilocaine *on page 1118*

U.S. Brand Names EMLA®

Canadian Brand Names EMLA®

Generic Available Yes: Cream

Synonyms Prilocaine and Lidocaine

Pharmacologic Category Local Anesthetic

Dental Use Amide-type topical anesthetic for use on normal intact skin to provide local analgesia for minor procedures such as I.V. cannulation or venipuncture

Use Topical anesthetic for use on normal intact skin to provide local analgesia for minor procedures such as I.V. cannulation or venipuncture; has also been used for painful procedures such as lumbar puncture and skin graft harvesting; for superficial minor surgery of genital mucous membranes and as an adjunct for local infiltration anesthesia in genital mucous membranes.

Local Anesthetic/Vasoconstrictor Precautions No information available to require special precautions

Effects on Dental Treatment No significant effects or complications reported

Significant Adverse Effects Frequency not defined.

Cardiovascular: Hypotension, angioedema
Central nervous system: Shock
Dermatologic: Hyperpigmentation, erythema, itching, rash, burning, urticaria
Genitourinary: Blistering of foreskin (rare)
Local: Burning, stinging, edema

Respiratory: Bronchospasm

Miscellaneous: Alteration in temperature sensation, hypersensitivity reactions

Dosage Although the incidence of systemic adverse effects with EMLA® is very low, caution should be exercised, particularly when applying over large areas and leaving on for >2 hours

Children (intact skin): EMLA® should **not** be used in neonates with a gestation age <37 weeks nor in infants <12 months of age who are receiving treatment with methemoglobin-inducing agents

Dosing is based on child's age and weight:

Age 0-3 months or <5 kg: Apply a maximum of 1 g over no more than 10 cm^2 of skin; leave on for no longer than 1 hour

Age 3 months to 12 months and >5 kg: Apply no more than a maximum 2 g total over no more than 20 cm^2 of skin; leave on for no longer than 4 hours

Age 1-6 years and >10 kg: Apply no more than a maximum of 10 g total over no more than 100 cm^2 of skin; leave on for no longer than 4 hours.

Age 7-12 years and >20 kg: Apply no more than a maximum 20 g total over no more than 200 cm^2 of skin; leave on for no longer than 4 hours.

Note: If a patient greater than 3 months old does not meet the minimum weight requirement, the maximum total dose should be restricted to the corresponding maximum based on patient weight.

Adults (intact skin):

EMLA® cream and EMLA® anesthetic disc: A thick layer of EMLA® cream is applied to intact skin and covered with an occlusive dressing, or alternatively, an EMLA® anesthetic disc is applied to intact skin

Minor dermal procedures (eg, I.V. cannulation or venipuncture): Apply 2.5 g of cream (1/2 of the 5 g tube) over 20-25 cm of skin surface area, or 1 anesthetic disc (1 g over 10 cm^2) for at least 1 hour. **Note:** In clinical trials, 2 sites were usually prepared in case there was a technical problem with cannulation or venipuncture at the first site.

Major dermal procedures (eg, more painful dermatological procedures involving a larger skin area such as split thickness skin graft harvesting): Apply 2 g of cream per 10 cm^2 of skin and allow to remain in contact with the skin for at least 2 hours.

Adult male genital skin (eg, pretreatment prior to local anesthetic infiltration): Apply a thick layer of cream (1 g/10 cm^2) to the skin surface for 15 minutes. Local anesthetic infiltration should be performed immediately after removal of EMLA® cream.

Note: Dermal analgesia can be expected to increase for up to 3 hours under occlusive dressing and persist for 1-2 hours after removal of the cream

Adult females: Genital mucous membranes: Minor procedures (eg, removal of condylomata acuminata, pretreatment for local anesthetic infiltration): Apply 5-10 g (thick layer) of cream for 5-10 minutes

Mechanism of Action Local anesthetic action occurs by stabilization of neuronal membranes and inhibiting the ionic fluxes required for the initiation and conduction of impulses

Contraindications

Hypersensitivity to amide type anesthetic agents [ie, lidocaine, prilocaine, dibucaine, mepivacaine, bupivacaine, etidocaine]; hypersensitivity to any component of the formulation selected; application on mucous membranes or broken or inflamed skin; infants <1 month of age if gestational age is <37 weeks; infants <12 months of age receiving therapy with methemoglobin-inducing agents; children with congenital or idiopathic methemoglobinemia, or in children who are receiving medications associated with drug-induced methemoglobinemia [ie, acetaminophen (overdosage), benzocaine, chloroquine, dapsone, nitrofurantoin, nitroglycerin, nitroprusside, phenazopyridine, phenelzine, phenobarbital, phenytoin, quinine, sulfonamides]

Warnings/Precautions Use with caution in patients receiving class I antiarrhythmic drugs, since systemic absorption occurs and synergistic toxicity is possible. Although the incidence of systemic adverse reactions with EMLA® is very low, caution should be exercised, particularly when applying over large areas and leaving on for longer than 2 hours.

Drug Interactions Lidocaine: **Substrate** of CYP1A2 (minor), 2A6 (minor), 2B6 (minor), 2C8/9 (minor), 2D6 (major), 3A4 (major); **Inhibits** CYP1A2 (strong), 2D6 (strong), 3A4 (moderate)

Also see individual agents.

Increased toxicity:

Class I antiarrhythmic drugs (tocainide, mexiletine): Effects are additive and potentially synergistic

Drugs known to induce methemoglobinemia

(Continued)

Lidocaine and Prilocaine *(Continued)*

Pharmacodynamics/Kinetics

EMLA®:

Onset of action: 1 hour

Peak effect: 2-3 hours

Duration: 1-2 hours after removal

Absorption: Related to duration of application and area where applied

3-hour application: 3.6% lidocaine and 6.1% prilocaine

24-hour application: 16.2% lidocaine and 33.5% prilocaine

See individual agents.

Pregnancy Risk Factor B

Lactation Enters breast milk/compatible

Breast-Feeding Considerations Usual infiltration doses of lidocaine and prilocaine given to nursing mothers has not been shown to affect the health of the nursing infant.

Dosage Forms

Cream, topical: Lidocaine 2.5% and prilocaine 2.5% (30 g)

EMLA®: Lidocaine 2.5% and prilocaine 2.5% (5 g, 30 g) [each 5 g tube is packaged with two Tegaderm® dressings]

Disc, topical: 1 g (2s, 10s) [contains lidocaine 2.5% and prilocaine 2.5% per 10 cm^2 disc]

Selected Readings

Broadman LM, Soliman IE, Hannallah RS, et al, "Analgesic Efficacy of Eutectic Mixture of Local Anesthetics (EMLA®) vs Intradermal Infiltration Prior to Venous Cannulation in Children," *Am J Anaesth*, 1987, 34:S56.

Friskopp J and Huledal G, "Plasma Levels of Lidocaine and Prilocaine After Application of Oraqix, a New Intrapocket Anesthetic, in Patients With Advanced Periodontitis," *J Clin Periodontol*, 2001, 28(5):425-9.

Friskopp J, Nilsson M, and Isacsson G, "The Anesthetic Onset and Duration of a New Lidocaine/Prilocaine Gel Intra-Pocket Anesthetic (Oraqix) for Periodontal Scaling/Root Planing," *J Clin Periodontol*, 2001, 28(5):453-8.

Halperin DL, Koren G, Attias D, et al, "Topical Skin Anesthesia for Venous Subcutaneous Drug Reservoir and Lumbar Puncture in Children," *Pediatrics*, 1989, 84(2):281-4.

Robieux I, Kumar R, Radhakrishnan S, et al, "Assessing Pain and Analgesia With a Lidocaine-Prilocaine Emulsion in Infants and Toddlers During Venipuncture," *J Pediatr*, 1991, 118(6):971-3.

Taddio A, Shennan AT, Stevens B, et al, "Safety of Lidocaine-Prilocaine Cream in the Treatment of Preterm Neonates," *J Pediatr*, 1995, 127(6):1002-5.

Vickers ER, Mazbani N, Gerzina TM, et al, "Pharmacokinetics of EMLA Cream 5% Application to Oral Mucosa," *Anesth Prog*, 1997, 44:32-7.

Lidocaine Hydrochloride *see* Lidocaine *on page 819*

Lidocaine Hydrochloride and Bupivacaine Hydrochloride *see* Lidocaine and Bupivacaine *on page 822*

Lidocaine (Transoral) (LYE doe kane trans OR al)

Related Information

Lidocaine *on page 819*

Oral Pain *on page 1526*

U.S. Brand Names DentiPatch®

Generic Available No

Pharmacologic Category Local Anesthetic, Transoral

Use Local anesthesia of the oral mucosa prior to oral injections and soft-tissue dental procedures

Local Anesthetic/Vasoconstrictor Precautions No information available to require special precautions

Effects on Dental Treatment No significant effects or complications reported

Significant Adverse Effects No data reported

Dosage One patch on selected area of oral mucosa

Mechanism of Action Blocks both the initiation and conduction of nerve impulses by decreasing the neuronal membrane's permeability to sodium ions, which results in inhibition of depolarization with resultant blockade of conduction

Contraindications Hypersensitivity to lidocaine or any of component of the formulation

Pharmacodynamics/Kinetics

Onset of action: 2 minutes

Duration: Anesthesia: 40 minutes after 15-minute wear period

Dosage Forms Patch: 23 mg/2 cm^2; 46.1 mg/2 cm^2 (50s, 100s)

Comments Peak plasma levels were 10% of those seen following local infiltration anesthesia with 1.8 mL lidocaine and 1:100,000 epinephrine.

The manufacturer claims DentiPatch® is safe, with "negligible systemic absorption" of lidocaine. The agent is "clinically proven to prevent injection pain from

25-gauge needles that are inserted to the level of the bone." Data from controlled studies (235 patients) have shown no serious adverse effects with the application of lidocaine patch to the oral mucosa for 15 minutes.

Selected Readings

Hersh EV, Houpt MI, Cooper SA, et al, "Analgesic Efficacy and Safety of an Intraoral Lidocaine Patch," *J Am Dent Assoc*, 1996, 127(11):1626-34.

Houpt MI, Heins P, Lamster I, et al, "An Evaluation of Intraoral Lidocaine Patches in Reducing Needle-Insertion Pain," *Compend Contin Educ Dent*, 1997, 18(4):309-10, 312-4, 316.

"The Lidocaine Patch: A New Delivery System," *Biolog Ther Dent*, 1997, 13:17-22.

Lidoderm® *see* Lidocaine *on page 819*

Lignocaine Hydrochloride *see* Lidocaine *on page 819*

Lilly CT-3231 *see* Vindesine *on page 1379*

Limbitrol® *see* Amitriptyline and Chlordiazepoxide *on page 105*

Limbitrol® DS *see* Amitriptyline and Chlordiazepoxide *on page 105*

Lincocin® *see* Lincomycin *on page 829*

Lincomycin (lin koe MYE sin)

U.S. Brand Names Lincocin®

Canadian Brand Names Lincocin®

Mexican Brand Names Lincocin®; Princol®; Rimsalin®

Generic Available No

Synonyms Lincomycin Hydrochloride

Pharmacologic Category Antibiotic, Macrolide

Use Treatment of susceptible bacterial infections, mainly those caused by streptococci and staphylococci resistant to other agents

Local Anesthetic/Vasoconstrictor Precautions No information available to require special precautions

Effects on Dental Treatment No significant effects or complications reported

Common Adverse Effects Frequency not defined.

Central nervous system: Vertigo
Dermatologic: Vesiculobullous dermatitis (rare)
Gastrointestinal: Nausea, vomiting, diarrhea
Hematologic: Pancytopenia (rare)
Miscellaneous: Serum sickness (rare)

Mechanism of Action Lincosamide antibiotic which was isolated from a strain of *Streptomyces lincolnensis*; lincomycin, like clindamycin, inhibits bacterial protein synthesis by specifically binding on the 50S subunit and affecting the process of peptide chain initiation. Other macrolide antibiotics (erythromycin) also bind to the 50S subunit. Since only one molecule of antibiotic can bind to a single ribosome, the concomitant use of erythromycin and lincomycin is not recommended.

Drug Interactions

Increased Effect/Toxicity: Increased activity/toxicity of neuromuscular blocking agents.

Decreased Effect: Decreased effect with erythromycin.

Pharmacodynamics/Kinetics

Absorption: Oral: ~20% to 30%
Half-life elimination, serum: 2-11.5 hours
Time to peak, serum: Oral: 2-4 hours; I.M.: 1 hour

Pregnancy Risk Factor B

Lincomycin Hydrochloride *see* Lincomycin *on page 829*

Lindane (LIN dane)

Canadian Brand Names Hexit™; PMS-Lindane

Mexican Brand Names Herklin Shampoo®; Scabisan®

Generic Available Yes

Synonyms Benzene Hexachloride; Gamma Benzene Hexachloride; Hexachlorocyclohexane

Pharmacologic Category Antiparasitic Agent, Topical; Pediculocide; Scabicidal Agent

Use Treatment of *Sarcoptes scabiei* (scabies), *Pediculus capitis* (head lice), and *Pthirus pubis* (crab lice); FDA recommends reserving lindane as a second-line agent or with inadequate response to other therapies

Local Anesthetic/Vasoconstrictor Precautions No information available to require special precautions

Effects on Dental Treatment No significant effects or complications reported

Common Adverse Effects Frequency not defined (includes postmarketing and/or case reports).

Cardiovascular: Cardiac arrhythmia
(Continued)

Lindane *(Continued)*

Central nervous system: Ataxia, dizziness, headache, restlessness, seizures, pain
Dermatologic: Alopecia, contact dermatitis, skin and adipose tissue may act as repositories, eczematous eruptions, pruritus, urticaria
Gastrointestinal: Nausea, vomiting
Hematologic: Aplastic anemia
Hepatic: Hepatitis
Local: Burning and stinging
Neuromuscular & skeletal: Paresthesias
Renal: Hematuria
Respiratory: Pulmonary edema

Mechanism of Action Directly absorbed by parasites and ova through the exoskeleton; stimulates the nervous system resulting in seizures and death of parasitic arthropods

Drug Interactions

Increased Effect/Toxicity: Increased toxicity: Drugs which lower seizure threshold

Pharmacodynamics/Kinetics

Absorption: ≤13% systemically
Distribution: Stored in body fat; accumulates in brain; skin and adipose tissue may act as repositories
Metabolism: Hepatic
Half-life elimination: Children: 17-22 hours
Time to peak, serum: Children: 6 hours
Excretion: Urine and feces

Pregnancy Risk Factor C

Linezolid (li NE zoh lid)

U.S. Brand Names Zyvox™

Canadian Brand Names Zyvoxam®

Generic Available No

Pharmacologic Category Antibiotic, Oxazolidinone

Use Treatment of vancomycin-resistant *Enterococcus faecium* (VRE) infections, nosocomial pneumonia caused by *Staphylococcus aureus* including MRSA or *Streptococcus pneumoniae* (including multidrug-resistant strains [MDRSP]), complicated and uncomplicated skin and skin structure infections (including diabetic foot infections without concomitant osteomyelitis), and community-acquired pneumonia caused by susceptible gram-positive organisms

Local Anesthetic/Vasoconstrictor Precautions Linezolid has mild monoamine oxidase inhibitor properties. The clinician is reminded that vasoconstrictors have the potential to interact with MAOIs to result in elevation of blood pressure. Caution is suggested.

Effects on Dental Treatment Key adverse event(s) related to dental treatment: Oral moniliasis, taste alteration, and tongue discoloration.

Common Adverse Effects Percentages as reported in adults; frequency similar in pediatric patients

1% to 10%:

Cardiovascular: Hypertension (1% to 3%)
Central nervous system: Headache (0.5% to 11%), insomnia (3%), dizziness (0.4% to 2%), fever (2%)
Dermatologic: Rash (2%)
Gastrointestinal: Nausea (3% to 10%), diarrhea (3% to 11%), vomiting (1% to 4%), constipation (2%), taste alteration (1% to 2%), tongue discoloration (0.2% to 1%), oral moniliasis (0.4% to 1%), pancreatitis
Genitourinary: Vaginal moniliasis (1% to 2%)
Hematologic: Thrombocytopenia (0.3% to 10%), anemia, leukopenia, neutropenia; **Note:** Myelosuppression (including anemia, leukopenia, pancytopenia, and thrombocytopenia; may be more common in patients receiving linezolid for >2 weeks)
Hepatic: Abnormal LFTs (0.4% to 1%)
Miscellaneous: Fungal infections (0.1% to 2%)

Mechanism of Action Inhibits bacterial protein synthesis by binding to bacterial 23S ribosomal RNA of the 50S subunit. This prevents the formation of a functional 70S initiation complex that is essential for the bacterial translation process. Linezolid is bacteriostatic against enterococci and staphylococci and bactericidal against most strains of streptococci.

Drug Interactions

Increased Effect/Toxicity: Linezolid is a reversible, nonselective inhibitor of MAO. Serotonergic agents (eg, TCAs, venlafaxine, trazodone, sibutramine, meperidine, dextromethorphan, and SSRIs) may cause a serotonin syndrome (eg, hyperpyrexia, cognitive dysfunction) when used concomitantly. Adrenergic agents (eg, phenylpropanolamine, pseudoephedrine, sympathomimetic agents, vasopressor or dopaminergic agents) may cause hypertension. Tramadol may increase the risk of seizures when used concurrently with linezolid. Myelosuppressive medications may increase risk of myelosuppression when used concurrently with linezolid.

Pharmacodynamics/Kinetics

Absorption: Rapid and extensive

Distribution: V_{dss}: Adults: 40-50 L

Protein binding: Adults: 31%

Metabolism: Hepatic via oxidation of the morpholine ring, resulting in two inactive metabolites (aminoethoxyacetic acid, hydroxyethyl glycine); does not involve CYP

Bioavailability: 100%

Half-life elimination: Children ≥1 week (full-term) to 11 years: 1.5-3 hours; Adults: 4-5 hours

Time to peak: Adults: Oral: 1-2 hours

Excretion: Urine (30% as parent drug, 50% as metabolites); feces (9% as metabolites)

Nonrenal clearance: 65%; increased in children ≥1 week to 11 years

Pregnancy Risk Factor C

Lioresal® *see* Baclofen *on page 180*

Liothyronine (lye oh THYE roe neen)

Related Information

Endocrine Disorders and Pregnancy *on page 1481*

U.S. Brand Names Cytomel®; Triostat®

Canadian Brand Names Cytomel®

Mexican Brand Names Triyotex®

Generic Available No

Synonyms Liothyronine Sodium; Sodium *L*-Triiodothyronine; T_3 Sodium

Pharmacologic Category Thyroid Product

Use

Oral: Replacement or supplemental therapy in hypothyroidism; management of nontoxic goiter; a diagnostic aid

I.V.: Treatment of myxedema coma/precoma

Local Anesthetic/Vasoconstrictor Precautions No precautions with vasoconstrictor are necessary if patient is well controlled with liothyronine

Effects on Dental Treatment No significant effects or complications reported

Common Adverse Effects 1% to 10%: Cardiovascular: Arrhythmia (6%), tachycardia (3%), cardiopulmonary arrest (2%), hypotension (2%), MI (2%)

Mechanism of Action Exact mechanism of action is unknown; however, it is believed the thyroid hormone exerts its many metabolic effects through control of DNA transcription and protein synthesis; involved in normal metabolism, growth, and development; promotes gluconeogenesis, increases utilization and mobilization of glycogen stores, and stimulates protein synthesis, increases basal metabolic rate

Drug Interactions

Increased Effect/Toxicity: Thyroid products may potentiate the hypoprothrombinemic effect of warfarin (and other oral anticoagulants). Tricyclic antidepressants (TCAs) may increase potential for toxicity of both drugs. Coadministration with ketamine may lead to hypertension and tachycardia.

Decreased Effect: Some medications may decrease absorption of liothyronine: Cholestyramine, colestipol (separate administration by at least 2 hours); aluminum- and magnesium-containing antacids, iron preparations, sucralfate, Kayexalate® (separate administration by at least 4 hours). Enzyme inducers (phenytoin, phenobarbital, carbamazepine, and rifampin/rifabutin) may decrease thyroid hormone levels. Thyroid hormone may decrease effect of oral sulfonylureas. Serum levels of digoxin and theophylline may be altered by thyroid function. Estrogens may decrease serum free-thyroxine concentrations.

Pharmacodynamics/Kinetics

Onset of action: 2-4 hours

Peak response: 2-3 days

Absorption: Oral: Well absorbed (95% in 4 hours)

Half-life elimination: 2.5 days

Excretion: Urine

Pregnancy Risk Factor A

Liothyronine Sodium *see* Liothyronine *on page 831*

Liotrix (LYE oh triks)

Related Information

Endocrine Disorders and Pregnancy *on page 1481*

U.S. Brand Names Thyrolar®

Canadian Brand Names Thyrolar®

Generic Available No

Synonyms T_3/T_4 Liotrix

Pharmacologic Category Thyroid Product

Use Replacement or supplemental therapy in hypothyroidism (uniform mixture of T_4:T_3 in 4:1 ratio by weight); little advantage to this product exists and cost is not justified

Local Anesthetic/Vasoconstrictor Precautions No precautions with vasoconstrictor are necessary if patient is well controlled with liotrix

Effects on Dental Treatment No significant effects or complications reported

Common Adverse Effects Frequency not defined.

Cardiovascular: Palpitations, cardiac arrhythmias, tachycardia, chest pain
Central nervous system: Nervousness, headache, insomnia, fever, ataxia
Dermatologic: Alopecia
Endocrine & metabolic: Changes in menstrual cycle, weight loss, increased appetite
Gastrointestinal: Diarrhea, abdominal cramps, constipation, vomiting
Neuromuscular & skeletal: Myalgia, hand tremors, tremor
Respiratory: Dyspnea
Miscellaneous: Diaphoresis, allergic skin reactions (rare)

Mechanism of Action The primary active compound is T_3 (triiodothyronine), which may be converted from T_4 (thyroxine) and then circulates throughout the body to influence growth and maturation of various tissues. Liotrix is uniform mixture of synthetic T_4 and T_3 in 4:1 ratio; exact mechanism of action is unknown; however, it is believed the thyroid hormone exerts its many metabolic effects through control of DNA transcription and protein synthesis; involved in normal metabolism, growth, and development; promotes gluconeogenesis, increases utilization and mobilization of glycogen stores and stimulates protein synthesis, increases basal metabolic rate

Drug Interactions

Increased Effect/Toxicity: Thyroid products may potentiate the hypoprothrombinemic effect of warfarin (and other oral anticoagulants). Effect of warfarin may be dramatically increased when thyroid is added. However, the addition of warfarin in a patient previously receiving a stable dose of thyroid hormone does not require a significantly different dosing strategy. Tricyclic antidepressants (TCAs) may increase potential for toxicity of both drugs. Excessive thyroid replacement in patients receiving growth hormone may lead to accelerated epiphyseal closure; inadequate replacement interferes with growth response. Coadministration with ketamine may lead to hypertension and tachycardia.

Decreased Effect: Aluminum- and magnesium-containing antacids, iron preparations, sucralfate, cholestyramine, colestipol, and Kayexalate® may decrease absorption (separate administration by 8 hours). Thyroid hormone may decrease effect of oral sulfonylureas. Dosage of thyroid hormone may need to be increased when SSRIs are added. Serum levels of digoxin and theophylline may be altered by thyroid function.

Pharmacodynamics/Kinetics

Absorption: 50% to 95%
Metabolism: Partially hepatic, renal, and in intestines
Half-life elimination: 6-7 days
Time to peak, serum: 12-48 hours
Excretion: Partially feces (as conjugated metabolites)

Pregnancy Risk Factor A

Lipancreatin *see* Pancrelipase *on page 1042*

Lipitor® *see* Atorvastatin *on page 162*

Liposyn® III *see* Fat Emulsion *on page 575*

Lipram 4500 *see* Pancrelipase *on page 1042*

Lipram-CR *see* Pancrelipase *on page 1042*

Lipram-PN *see* Pancrelipase *on page 1042*

Lipram-UL *see* Pancrelipase *on page 1042*

Liquibid® [DSC] *see* Guaifenesin *on page 672*

Liquibid® 1200 [DSC] *see* Guaifenesin *on page 672*

Liquibid-D *see* Guaifenesin and Phenylephrine *on page 674*

Liqui-Char® [OTC] [DSC] *see* Charcoal *on page 303*

Liquid Antidote *see* Charcoal *on page 303*

Liquifilm® Tears [OTC] *see* Artificial Tears *on page 148*

Lisinopril (lyse IN oh pril)

Related Information

Cardiovascular Diseases *on page 1458*

U.S. Brand Names Prinivil®; Zestril®

Canadian Brand Names Apo-Lisinopril®; Prinivil®; Zestril®

Mexican Brand Names Prinivil®; Zestril®

Generic Available Yes

Pharmacologic Category Angiotensin-Converting Enzyme (ACE) Inhibitor

Use Treatment of hypertension, either alone or in combination with other antihypertensive agents; adjunctive therapy in treatment of CHF (afterload reduction); treatment of acute myocardial infarction within 24 hours in hemodynamically-stable patients to improve survival; treatment of left ventricular dysfunction after myocardial infarction

Local Anesthetic/Vasoconstrictor Precautions No information available to require special precautions

Effects on Dental Treatment Key adverse event(s) related to dental treatment: Orthostatic effects.

Common Adverse Effects Note: Frequency ranges include data from hypertension and heart failure trials. Higher rates of adverse reactions have generally been noted in patients with CHF. However, the frequency of adverse effects associated with placebo is also increased in this population.

1% to 10%:

Cardiovascular: Orthostatic effects (1%), hypotension (1% to 4%)

Central nervous system: Headache (4% to 6%), dizziness (5% to 12%), fatigue (3%), weakness (1%)

Dermatologic: Rash (1% to 2%)

Endocrine & metabolic: Hyperkalemia (2% to 5%)

Gastrointestinal: Diarrhea (3% to 4%), nausea (2%), vomiting (1%), abdominal pain (2%)

Genitourinary: Impotence (1%)

Hematologic: Decreased hemoglobin (small)

Neuromuscular & skeletal: Chest pain (3%)

Renal: Increased serum creatinine (often transient), increased BUN (2%); deterioration in renal function (in patients with bilateral renal artery stenosis or hypovolemia)

Respiratory: Cough (4% to 9%), upper respiratory infection (2% to 2%)

Dosage Oral:

Hypertension:

Children ≥6 years: Initial: 0.07 mg/kg once daily (up to 5 mg); increase dose at 1- to 2-week intervals; doses >0.61 mg/kg or >40 mg have not been evaluated.

Adults: Initial: 10 mg/day; increase doses 5-10 mg/day at 1- to 2-week intervals; maximum daily dose: 40 mg

Elderly: Initial: 2.5-5 mg/day; increase doses 2.5-5 mg/day at 1- to 2-week intervals; maximum daily dose: 40 mg

Patients taking diuretics should have them discontinued 2-3 days prior to initiating lisinopril if possible. Restart diuretic after blood pressure is stable if needed. If diuretic cannot be discontinued prior to therapy, begin with 5 mg with close supervision until stable blood pressure. In patients with hyponatremia (<130 mEq/L), start dose at 2.5 mg/day,

Congestive heart failure: Adults: Initial: 5 mg; then increase by no more than 10 mg increments at intervals no less than 2 weeks to a maximum daily dose of 40 mg. Usual maintenance: 5-40 mg/day as a single dose. Patients should start/continue standard therapy, including diuretics, beta-blockers, and digoxin, as indicated.

Acute myocardial infarction (within 24 hours in hemodynamically stable patients): Oral: 5 mg immediately, then 5 mg at 24 hours, 10 mg at 48 hours, and 10 mg every day thereafter for 6 weeks. Patients should continue to receive standard treatments such as thrombolytics, aspirin, and beta-blockers.

Dosing adjustment in renal impairment:

Adults: Initial doses should be modified and upward titration should be cautious, based on response (maximum: 40 mg/day)

Cl_{cr} >30 mL/minute: Initial: 10 mg/day

Cl_{cr} 10-30 mL/minute: Initial: 5 mg/day

Hemodialysis: Initial: 2.5 mg/day; dialyzable (50%)

Children: Use in not recommended in pediatric patients with GFR <30 mL/minute/1.73 m^2

(Continued)

Lisinopril *(Continued)*

Mechanism of Action Competitive inhibitor of angiotensin-converting enzyme (ACE); prevents conversion of angiotensin I to angiotensin II, a potent vasoconstrictor; results in lower levels of angiotensin II which causes an increase in plasma renin activity and a reduction in aldosterone secretion; a CNS mechanism may also be involved in hypotensive effect as angiotensin II increases adrenergic outflow from CNS; vasoactive kallikreins may be decreased in conversion to active hormones by ACE inhibitors, thus reducing blood pressure

Contraindications Hypersensitivity to lisinopril or any component of the formulation; angioedema related to previous treatment with an ACE inhibitor; bilateral renal artery stenosis; pregnancy (2nd and 3rd trimesters)

Warnings/Precautions Anaphylactic reactions can occur. Angioedema can occur at any time during treatment (especially following first dose). Angioedema may involve head and neck (potentially affecting the airway) or the intestine (presenting with abdominal pain). Careful blood pressure monitoring with first dose (hypotension can occur especially in volume depleted patients). Dosage adjustment needed in renal impairment. Use with caution in hypovolemia; collagen vascular diseases; valvular stenosis (particularly aortic stenosis); hyperkalemia; or before, during, or immediately after anesthesia. Avoid rapid dosage escalation, which may lead to renal insufficiency. Neutropenia/agranulocytosis with myeloid hyperplasia can rarely occur. If patient has renal impairment then a baseline WBC with differential and serum creatinine should be evaluated and monitored closely during the first 3 months of therapy. Hypersensitivity reactions may be seen during hemodialysis with high-flux dialysis membranes (eg, AN69). Deterioration in renal function can occur with initiation. Use with caution in unilateral renal artery stenosis and pre-existing renal insufficiency. Safety and efficacy have not been established in children <6 years of age.

Drug Interactions

Increased Effect/Toxicity: Potassium supplements, co-trimoxazole (high dose), angiotensin II receptor antagonists (eg, candesartan, losartan, irbesartan), or potassium-sparing diuretics (amiloride, spironolactone, triamterene) may result in elevated serum potassium levels when combined with lisinopril. ACE inhibitor effects may be increased by phenothiazines or probenecid (increases levels of captopril). ACE inhibitors may increase serum concentrations/effects of digoxin, lithium, and sulfonlyureas.

Diuretics have additive hypotensive effects with ACE inhibitors, and hypovolemia increases the potential for adverse renal effects of ACE inhibitors. In patients with compromised renal function, coadministration with NSAIDs may result in further deterioration of renal function. Allopurinol and ACE inhibitors may cause a higher risk of hypersensitivity reaction when taken concurrently.

Decreased Effect: Aspirin (high dose) may reduce the therapeutic effects of ACE inhibitors; at low dosages this does not appear to be significant. Rifampin may decrease the effect of ACE inhibitors. Antacids may decrease the bioavailability of ACE inhibitors (may be more likely to occur with captopril); separate administration times by 1-2 hours. NSAIDs, specifically indomethacin, may reduce the hypotensive effects of ACE inhibitors. More likely to occur in low renin or volume dependent hypertensive patients.

Ethanol/Nutrition/Herb Interactions Herb/Nutraceutical: Avoid dong quai if using for hypertension (has estrogenic activity). Avoid ephedra, yohimbe, ginseng (may worsen hypertension). Avoid garlic (may have increased antihypertensive effect).

Pharmacodynamics/Kinetics

Onset of action: 1 hour

Peak effect: Hypotensive: Oral: ~6 hours

Duration: 24 hours

Absorption: Well absorbed; unaffected by food

Protein binding: 25%

Half-life elimination: 11-12 hours

Excretion: Primarily urine (as unchanged drug)

Pregnancy Risk Factor C/D (2nd and 3rd trimesters)

Dosage Forms TAB: 2.5 mg, 5 mg, 10 mg, 20 mg, 30 mg, 40 mg

Lisinopril and Hydrochlorothiazide

(lyse IN oh pril & hye droe klor oh THYE a zide)

Related Information

Cardiovascular Diseases *on page 1458*
Hydrochlorothiazide *on page 699*
Lisinopril *on page 833*

U.S. Brand Names Prinzide®; Zestoretic®

Canadian Brand Names Prinzide®; Zestoretic®

Generic Available Yes

Synonyms Hydrochlorothiazide and Lisinopril

Pharmacologic Category Antihypertensive Agent, Combination

Use Treatment of hypertension

Local Anesthetic/Vasoconstrictor Precautions No information available to require special precautions

Effects on Dental Treatment No significant effects or complications reported

Common Adverse Effects See individual agents.

Drug Interactions

Increased Effect/Toxicity: See individual agents.

Decreased Effect: See individual agents.

Pharmacodynamics/Kinetics See individual agents.

Pregnancy Risk Factor C/D (2nd and 3rd trimesters)

Lispro, Insulin *see* Insulin Preparations *on page 749*

Lithium (LITH ee um)

U.S. Brand Names Eskalith®; Eskalith CR®; Lithobid®

Canadian Brand Names Apo-Lithium®; Carbolith™; Duralith®; Lithane™; PMS-Lithium Carbonate; PMS-Lithium Citrate

Mexican Brand Names Carbolit®; Litheum®

Generic Available Yes

Synonyms Lithium Carbonate; Lithium Citrate

Pharmacologic Category Lithium

Use Management of bipolar disorders; treatment of mania in individuals with bipolar disorder (maintenance treatment prevents or diminishes intensity of subsequent episodes)

Unlabeled/Investigational Use Potential augmenting agent for antidepressants; aggression, post-traumatic stress disorder, conduct disorder in children

Local Anesthetic/Vasoconstrictor Precautions No information available to require special precautions

Effects on Dental Treatment Avoid NSAIDs if analgesics are required since lithium toxicity has been reported with concomitant administration; acetaminophen products (ie, singly or with narcotics) are recommended.

Common Adverse Effects Frequency not defined.

Cardiovascular: Cardiac arrhythmias, hypotension, sinus node dysfunction, flattened or inverted T waves (reversible), edema, bradycardia, syncope

Central nervous system: Dizziness, vertigo, slurred speech, blackout spells, seizures, sedation, restlessness, confusion, psychomotor retardation, stupor, coma, dystonia, fatigue, lethargy, headache, pseudotumor cerebri, slowed intellectual functioning, tics

Dermatologic: Dry or thinning of hair, folliculitis, alopecia, exacerbation of psoriasis, rash

Endocrine & metabolic: Euthyroid goiter and/or hypothyroidism, hyperthyroidism, hyperglycemia, diabetes insipidus

Gastrointestinal: Polydipsia, anorexia, nausea, vomiting, diarrhea, xerostomia, metallic taste, weight gain, salivary gland swelling, excessive salivation

Genitourinary: Incontinence, polyuria, glycosuria, oliguria, albuminuria

Hematologic: Leukocytosis

Neuromuscular & skeletal: Tremor, muscle hyperirritability, ataxia, choreoathetoid movements, hyperactive deep tendon reflexes, myasthenia gravis (rare)

Ocular: Nystagmus, blurred vision, transient scotoma

Miscellaneous: Coldness and painful discoloration of fingers and toes

Mechanism of Action Alters cation transport across cell membrane in nerve and muscle cells and influences reuptake of serotonin and/or norepinephrine; second messenger systems involving the phosphatidylinositol cycle are inhibited; postsynaptic D2 receptor supersensitivity is inhibited

Drug Interactions

Increased Effect/Toxicity: Concurrent use of lithium with carbamazepine, diltiazem, SSRIs (fluoxetine, fluvoxamine), haloperidol, methyldopa, metronidazole (rare), phenothiazines, phenytoin, TCAs, and verapamil may increase the risk for neurotoxicity. A rare encephalopathic syndrome has been reported in association with haloperidol (causal relationship not established). Lithium concentrations/toxicity may be increased by diuretics, NSAIDs (sulindac and aspirin may be exceptions), ACE inhibitors, angiotensin receptor antagonists (losartan), tetracyclines, or COX-2 inhibitors (celecoxib).

(Continued)

Lithium *(Continued)*

Lithium and MAO inhibitors should generally be avoided due to use reports of fatal malignant hyperpyrexia; risk with selective MAO type B inhibitors (selegiline) appears to be lower. Potassium iodide may enhance the hypothyroid effects of lithium. Combined use of lithium with tricyclic antidepressants or sibutramine may increase the risk of serotonin syndrome; this combination is best avoided. Lithium may potentiate effect of neuromuscular blockers.

Decreased Effect: Combined use of lithium and chlorpromazine may lower serum concentrations of both drugs. Lithium may blunt the pressor response to sympathomimetics (epinephrine, norepinephrine). Caffeine (xanthine derivatives) may lower lithium serum concentrations by increasing urinary lithium excretion (monitor).

Pharmacodynamics/Kinetics

Absorption: Rapid and complete

Distribution: V_d: Initial: 0.3-0.4 L/kg; V_{dss}: 0.7-1 L/kg; crosses placenta; enters breast milk at 35% to 50% the concentrations in serum; distribution is complete in 6-10 hours

CSF, liver concentrations: $\frac{1}{3}$ to $\frac{1}{2}$ of serum concentration

Erythrocyte concentration: ~$\frac{1}{2}$ of serum concentration

Heart, lung, kidney, muscle concentrations: Equivalent to serum concentration

Saliva concentration: 2-3 times serum concentration

Thyroid, bone, brain tissue concentrations: Increase 50% over serum concentrations

Protein binding: Not protein bound

Metabolism: Not metabolized

Bioavailability: Not affected by food; Capsule, immediate release tablet: 95% to 100%; Extended release tablet: 60% to 90%; Syrup: 100%

Half-life elimination: 18-24 hours; can increase to more than 36 hours in elderly or with renal impairment

Time to peak, serum: Nonsustained release: ~0.5-2 hours; slow release: 4-12 hours; syrup: 15-60 minutes

Excretion: Urine (90% to 98% as unchanged drug); sweat (4% to 5%); feces (1%)

Clearance: 80% of filtered lithium is reabsorbed in the proximal convoluted tubules; therefore, clearance approximates 20% of GFR or 20-40 mL/minute

Pregnancy Risk Factor D

Lithium Carbonate *see* Lithium *on page 835*
Lithium Citrate *see* Lithium *on page 835*
Lithobid® *see* Lithium *on page 835*
Lithostat® *see* Acetohydroxamic Acid *on page 61*
Livostin® *see* Levocabastine *on page 810*
L-Lysine Hydrochloride *see* Lysine *on page 851*
LMD® *see* Dextran *on page 417*
L-M-X™ 4 [OTC] *see* Lidocaine *on page 819*
L-M-X™ 5 [OTC] *see* Lidocaine *on page 819*
LNg 20 *see* Levonorgestrel *on page 815*
Locoid® *see* Hydrocortisone *on page 714*
Locoid Lipocream® *see* Hydrocortisone *on page 714*
Lodine® *see* Etodolac *on page 564*
Lodine® XL *see* Etodolac *on page 564*
Lodosyn® *see* Carbidopa *on page 261*

Lodoxamide (loe DOKS a mide)

U.S. Brand Names Alomide®

Canadian Brand Names Alomide®

Generic Available No

Synonyms Lodoxamide Tromethamine

Pharmacologic Category Mast Cell Stabilizer

Use Treatment of vernal keratoconjunctivitis, vernal conjunctivitis, and vernal keratitis

Local Anesthetic/Vasoconstrictor Precautions No information available to require special precautions

Effects on Dental Treatment No significant effects or complications reported

Common Adverse Effects

>10%: Local: Transient burning, stinging, discomfort

1% to 10%:
Central nervous system: Headache
Ocular: Blurred vision, corneal erosion/ulcer, eye pain, corneal abrasion, blepharitis

Mechanism of Action Mast cell stabilizer that inhibits the *in vivo* type I immediate hypersensitivity reaction to increase cutaneous vascular permeability associated with IgE and antigen-mediated reactions

Pharmacodynamics/Kinetics Absorption: Topical: Negligible

Pregnancy Risk Factor B

Lodoxamide Tromethamine *see* Lodoxamide *on page 836*
Lodrane® *see* Brompheniramine and Pseudoephedrine *on page 220*
Lodrane® 12D *see* Brompheniramine and Pseudoephedrine *on page 220*
Lodrane® LD *see* Brompheniramine and Pseudoephedrine *on page 220*
Loestrin® *see* Ethinyl Estradiol and Norethindrone *on page 550*
Loestrin® Fe *see* Ethinyl Estradiol and Norethindrone *on page 550*
Lofibra™ *see* Fenofibrate *on page 577*
L-OHP *see* Oxaliplatin *on page 1020*
LoKara™ *see* Desonide *on page 410*

Lomefloxacin (loe me FLOKS a sin)

Related Information
Sexually-Transmitted Diseases *on page 1504*

U.S. Brand Names Maxaquin®

Mexican Brand Names Lomacin®; Maxaquin®

Generic Available No

Synonyms Lomefloxacin Hydrochloride

Pharmacologic Category Antibiotic, Quinolone

Use Lower respiratory infections, acute bacterial exacerbation of chronic bronchitis, and urinary tract infections caused by *E. coli*, *K. pneumoniae*, *P. mirabilis*, *P. aeruginosa*; also has gram-positive activity including *S. pneumoniae* and some staphylococci; surgical prophylaxis (transrectal prostate biopsy or transurethral procedures)

Local Anesthetic/Vasoconstrictor Precautions No information available to require special precautions

Effects on Dental Treatment No significant effects or complications reported

Common Adverse Effects 1% to 10%:
Central nervous system: Headache (3%), dizziness (2%)
Dermatologic: Photosensitivity (2%)
Gastrointestinal: Nausea (4%)

Mechanism of Action Inhibits DNA-gyrase in susceptible organisms thereby inhibits relaxation of supercoiled DNA and promotes breakage of DNA strands. DNA gyrase (topoisomerase II), is an essential bacterial enzyme that maintains the superhelical structure of DNA and is required for DNA replication and transcription, DNA repair, recombination, and transposition.

Drug Interactions

Cytochrome P450 Effect: Inhibits CYP1A2 (strong)

Increased Effect/Toxicity: Azlocillin, imipenem, cimetidine, loop diuretics, and probenecid may increase lomefloxacin serum levels. Increased CNS stimulation may occur with caffeine, theophylline, NSAIDs. Foscarnet has been associated with seizures in patients receiving quinolones. Concurrent use of corticosteroids may increase risk of tendon rupture. Lomefloxacin may increase the levels/effects of aminophylline, fluvoxamine, mexiletine, mirtazapine, ropinirole, theophylline, trifluoperazine, and other CYP1A2 substrates. Quinolones can cause elevated levels/effects of warfarin, and cyclosporine.

Decreased Effect: Decreased absorption with antacids containing aluminum, magnesium, and/or calcium (by up to 98% if given at the same time). Antineoplastic agents may decrease quinolone absorption.

Pharmacodynamics/Kinetics
Absorption: Well absorbed
Distribution: V_d: 2.4-3.5 L/kg; into bronchus, prostatic tissue, and urine
Protein binding: 20%
Half-life elimination: 5-7.5 hours
Excretion: Primarily urine (as unchanged drug)

Pregnancy Risk Factor C

Lomefloxacin Hydrochloride *see* Lomefloxacin *on page 837*
Lomotil® *see* Diphenoxylate and Atropine *on page 451*

Lomustine (loe MUS teen)

U.S. Brand Names CeeNU®

Canadian Brand Names CeeNU®

Mexican Brand Names CeeNU®

Generic Available No

Synonyms CCNU

Pharmacologic Category Antineoplastic Agent, Alkylating Agent

Use Treatment of brain tumors and Hodgkin's disease, non-Hodgkin's lymphoma, melanoma, renal carcinoma, lung cancer, colon cancer

Local Anesthetic/Vasoconstrictor Precautions No information available to require special precautions

Effects on Dental Treatment No significant effects or complications reported

Common Adverse Effects

>10%:

Gastrointestinal: Nausea and vomiting, usually within 3-6 hours after oral administration. Administration of the dose at bedtime, with an antiemetic, significantly reduces both the incidence and severity of nausea.

Hematologic: Myelosuppression, common, dose-limiting, may be cumulative and irreversible

Onset: 10-14 days

Nadir: Leukopenia: 6 weeks

Thrombocytopenia: 4 weeks

Recovery: 6-8 weeks

1% to 10%:

Dermatologic: Rash

Gastrointestinal: Anorexia, stomatitis, diarrhea

Genitourinary: Progressive azotemia, renal failure, decrease in kidney size

Hematologic: Anemia

Hepatic: Elevated liver enzymes, transient, reversible

Mechanism of Action Inhibits DNA and RNA synthesis via carbamylation of DNA polymerase, alkylation of DNA, and alteration of RNA, proteins, and enzymes

Drug Interactions

Cytochrome P450 Effect: Substrate of CYP2D6 (major); **Inhibits** CYP2D6 (weak), 3A4 (weak)

Increased Effect/Toxicity: CYP2D6 inhibitors may increase the levels/effects of lomustine; example inhibitors include chlorpromazine, delavirdine, fluoxetine, miconazole, paroxetine, pergolide, quinidine, quinine, ritonavir, and ropinirole. Increased toxicity with cimetidine, reported to cause bone marrow depression or to potentiate the myelosuppressive effects of lomustine.

Decreased Effect: Decreased effect with phenobarbital, resulting in reduced efficacy of both drugs.

Pharmacodynamics/Kinetics

Duration: Marrow recovery: ≤6 weeks

Absorption: Complete; appears in plasma within 3 minutes after administration

Distribution: Crosses blood-brain barrier to a greater degree than BCNU; CNS concentrations are equal to that of plasma

Protein binding: 50%

Metabolism: Rapidly hepatic via hydroxylation producing at least two active metabolites; enterohepatically recycled

Half-life elimination: Parent drug: 16-72 hours; Active metabolite: Terminal: 1.3-2 days

Time to peak, serum: Active metabolite: ~3 hours

Excretion: Urine; feces (<5%); expired air (<10%)

Pregnancy Risk Factor D

Loniten® *see* Minoxidil *on page 934*

Lonox® *see* Diphenoxylate and Atropine *on page 451*

Lo/Ovral® *see* Ethinyl Estradiol and Norgestrel *on page 557*

Loperamide (loe PER a mide)

U.S. Brand Names Imodium® A-D [OTC]

Canadian Brand Names Apo-Loperamide®; Diarr-Eze; Imodium®; Loperacap; Novo-Loperamide; PMS-Loperamine; Rho®-Loperamine; Riva-Loperamine

Mexican Brand Names Cryoperacid®; Pramidal®; Top-Dal® [tabs]

Generic Available Yes

Synonyms Loperamide Hydrochloride

Pharmacologic Category Antidiarrheal

Use Treatment of acute diarrhea and chronic diarrhea associated with inflammatory bowel disease; chronic functional diarrhea (idiopathic), chronic diarrhea caused by bowel resection or organic lesions; to decrease the volume of ileostomy discharge

Unlabeled/Investigational Use Treatment of traveler's diarrhea in combination with trimethoprim-sulfamethoxazole (co-trimoxazole) (3-day therapy)

Local Anesthetic/Vasoconstrictor Precautions No information available to require special precautions

Effects on Dental Treatment No significant effects or complications reported

Common Adverse Effects Frequency not defined.

Cardiovascular: Shock

Central nervous system: Dizziness, drowsiness, fatigue, sedation

Dermatologic: Rash, toxic epidermal necrolysis

Gastrointestinal: Abdominal cramping, abdominal distention, constipation, dry mouth, nausea, paralytic ileus, vomiting

Miscellaneous: Anaphylaxis

Mechanism of Action Acts directly on intestinal muscles to inhibit peristalsis and prolongs transit time enhancing fluid and electrolyte movement through intestinal mucosa; reduces fecal volume, increases viscosity, and diminishes fluid and electrolyte loss; demonstrates antisecretory activity; exhibits peripheral action

Drug Interactions

Increased Effect/Toxicity: Loperamide may potentiate the adverse effects of CNS depressants, phenothiazines, tricyclic antidepressants.

Pharmacodynamics/Kinetics

Onset of action: 0.5-1 hour

Absorption: <40%

Distribution: Low amounts enter breast milk

Protein binding: 97%

Metabolism: Hepatic (>50%) to inactive compounds

Half-life elimination: 7-14 hours

Excretion: Urine and feces (1% as metabolites, 30% to 40% as unchanged drug)

Pregnancy Risk Factor B

Loperamide Hydrochloride *see* Loperamide *on page 838*

Lopid® *see* Gemfibrozil *on page 651*

Lopinavir and Ritonavir (loe PIN a veer & rit ON uh veer)

Related Information

HIV Infection and AIDS *on page 1484*

U.S. Brand Names Kaletra™

Canadian Brand Names Kaletra™

Generic Available No

Synonyms Ritonavir and Lopinavir

Pharmacologic Category Antiretroviral Agent, Protease Inhibitor

Use Treatment of HIV infection in combination with other antiretroviral agents

Local Anesthetic/Vasoconstrictor Precautions No information available to require special precautions

Effects on Dental Treatment No significant effects or complications reported

Common Adverse Effects Protease inhibitors cause dyslipidemia which includes elevated cholesterol and triglycerides and a redistribution of body fat centrally to cause increased abdominal girth, buffalo hump, facial atrophy, and breast enlargement. These agents also cause hyperglycemia.

>10%:

Endocrine & metabolic: Hypercholesterolemia (9% to 28%), triglycerides increased (9% to 28%)

Gastrointestinal: Diarrhea (16% to 24%), nausea (3% to 15%)

Hepatic: GGT increased (4% to 25%)

2% to 10%:

Central nervous system: Headache (2% to 7%), pain (0% to 2%), insomnia (1% to 2%)

Dermatologic: Rash (1% to 4%)

Endocrine & metabolic: Hyperglycemia (1% to 4%), hyperuricemia (up to 4%), sodium decreased (3% children), organic phosphorus decreased (up to 2%), amylase increased (2% to 10%)

Gastrointestinal: Abnormal stools (up to 6%), abdominal pain (2% to 4%), vomiting (2% to 5%), dyspepsia (0.5% to 2%)

Hematologic: Platelets decreased (4% children), neutrophils decreased (1% to 3%)

(Continued)

Lopinavir and Ritonavir *(Continued)*

Hepatic: AST increased (2% to 9%), ALT increased (4% to 8%), bilirubin increased (children 3%)

Neuromuscular & skeletal: Weakness (4% to 7%)

Mechanism of Action A coformulation of lopinavir and ritonavir. The lopinavir component is the active inhibitor of HIV protease. Lopinavir inhibits HIV protease and renders the enzyme incapable of processing polyprotein precursor which leads to production of noninfectious immature HIV particles. The ritonavir component inhibits the CYP3A metabolism of lopinavir, allowing increased plasma levels of lopinavir.

Drug Interactions

Cytochrome P450 Effect:

Lopinavir: **Substrate** of 3A4 (minor)

Ritonavir: **Substrate** of CYP1A2 (minor), 2B6 (minor), 2D6 (major), 3A4 (major); **Inhibits** CYP2C8/9 (weak), 2C19 (weak), 2D6 (strong), 2E1 (weak), 3A4 (strong); **Induces** CYP1A2 (weak), 2C8/9 (weak), 3A4 (weak)

Increased Effect/Toxicity: Concurrent use of cisapride, ergot alkaloids, (dihydroergotamine, ergonovine, methylergonovine), lovastatin, midazolam, pimozide, simvastatin, and triazolam is contraindicated. Antiarrhythmic agents (including amiodarone, bepridil, flecainide, propafenone, lidocaine (systemic), and quinidine) should be used with caution; life-threatening arrhythmias may result from concurrent use.

Ritonavir may increase the levels/effects of amphetamines, selected beta-blockers, selected benzodiazepines (midazolam and triazolam contraindicated), calcium channel blockers, dextromethorphan, fluoxetine, lidocaine, HMG-CoA reductase inhibitors (lovastatin and simvastatin are not recommended), mesoridazine, mirtazapine, nateglinide, nefazodone, paroxetine, risperidone, sildenafil (and other PDE-5 inhibitors), thioridazine, tricyclic antidepressants, venlafaxine, and other substrates of CYP2D6 or 3A4. Mesoridazine and thioridazine are generally contraindicated with strong CYP2D6 inhibitors. When used with strong CYP3A4 inhibitors, dosage adjustment/limits are recommended for sildenafil and other PDE-5 inhibitors; refer to individual monographs. Warfarin levels/effects may also be increased. High dosages of itraconazole or ketoconazole (>200 mg/day) are not recommended.

Serum levels of protease inhibitors may be altered during concurrent therapy. Ritonavir may increase serum concentrations of amprenavir, indinavir, or saquinavir. Delavirdine increases levels of lopinavir; dosing recommendations are not yet established.

Lopinavir/ritonavir solution contains alcohol, concurrent use with disulfiram or metronidazole should be avoided. May cause disulfiram-like reaction. Serum concentrations of meperidine's neuroexcitatory metabolite (normeperidine) are increased by ritonavir, which may increase the risk of CNS toxicity/seizures. Rifabutin and rifabutin metabolite serum concentrations may be increased by ritonavir; reduce rifabutin dose to 150 mg every other day.

Decreased Effect: The levels/effects of ritonavir may be decreased by aminoglutethimide, carbamazepine, nafcillin, nevirapine, phenobarbital, phenytoin, rifamycins, and other CYP3A4 inducers. Concurrent use of rifampin is not recommended. Ritonavir may decrease the levels/effects of CYP2D6 prodrug substrates (eg, codeine, hydrocodone, oxycodone, tramadol). Non-nucleoside reverse transcriptase inhibitors (efavirenz, nevirapine) may decrease levels of lopinavir. To avoid incompatibility with didanosine, administer didanosine 1 hour before or 2 hours after lopinavir/ritonavir. Decreased levels of ethinyl estradiol may result from concurrent use (alternative contraception is recommended). Lopinavir/ritonavir may decrease levels of abacavir, atovaquone, or zidovudine. Voriconazole serum levels are reduced by ritonavir (concurrent use is contraindicated).

Pharmacodynamics/Kinetics

Ritonavir: See Ritonavir monograph.

Lopinavir:

Protein binding: 98% to 99%

Metabolism: Hepatic via CYP3A; 13 metabolites identified

Half-life elimination: 5-6 hours

Excretion: Feces (83%, 20% as unchanged drug); urine (2%)

Pregnancy Risk Factor C

Lopremone *see* Protirelin *on page 1145*

Lopressor® *see* Metoprolol *on page 915*

Loprox® *see* Ciclopirox *on page 327*

Lorabid® *see* Loracarbef *on page 841*

Loracarbef (lor a KAR bef)

U.S. Brand Names Lorabid®

Canadian Brand Names Lorabid™

Mexican Brand Names Carbac®; Lorabid®

Generic Available No

Pharmacologic Category Antibiotic, Carbacephem

Use Infections caused by susceptible organisms involving the respiratory tract, acute otitis media, sinusitis, skin and skin structure, bone and joint, and urinary tract and gynecologic

Local Anesthetic/Vasoconstrictor Precautions No information available to require special precautions

Effects on Dental Treatment No significant effects or complications reported

Common Adverse Effects ≥1%:

Central nervous system: Headache (1% to 3%), somnolence (<2%)

Dermatologic: Rash (1% to 3%)

Gastrointestinal: Diarrhea (4% to 6%), nausea (2%), vomiting (1% to 3%), anorexia (<2%), abdominal pain (1%)

Genitourinary: Vaginitis (1%)

Respiratory: Rhinitis (2% to 6%)

Mechanism of Action Inhibits bacterial cell wall synthesis by binding to one or more of the penicillin binding proteins (PBPs); inhibits the final transpeptidation step of peptidoglycan synthesis in bacterial cell walls, thus inhibiting cell wall biosynthesis. It is thought that beta-lactam antibiotics inactivate transpeptidase via acylation of the enzyme with cleavage of the CO-N bond of the beta-lactam ring. Upon exposure to beta-lactam antibiotics, bacteria eventually lyse due to ongoing activity of cell wall autolytic enzymes (autolysins and murein hydrolases) while cell wall assembly is arrested.

Drug Interactions

Increased Effect/Toxicity: Loracarbef serum levels are increased with coadministered probenecid.

Pharmacodynamics/Kinetics

Absorption: Rapid

Half-life elimination: ~1 hour

Time to peak, serum: ~1 hour

Excretion: Clearance: Plasma: ~200-300 mL/minute

Pregnancy Risk Factor B

Loratadine (lor AT a deen)

U.S. Brand Names Alavert™ [OTC]; Claritin® [OTC]; Claritin® Hives Relief [OTC]; Dimetapp® Children's ND [OTC]; Tavist® ND [OTC]

Canadian Brand Names Apo-Loratadine®; Claritin®; Claritin® Kids

Mexican Brand Names Clarityne®; Lertamine®; Sensibit®

Generic Available Yes: Excludes syrup

Pharmacologic Category Antihistamine, Nonsedating

Use Relief of nasal and non-nasal symptoms of seasonal allergic rhinitis; treatment of chronic idiopathic urticaria

Local Anesthetic/Vasoconstrictor Precautions No information available to require special precautions

Effects on Dental Treatment Key adverse event(s) related to dental treatment: Xerostomia (normal salivary flow resumes upon discontinuation).

Common Adverse Effects

Adults:

Central nervous system: Headache (12%), somnolence (8%), fatigue (4%)

Gastrointestinal: Xerostomia (3%)

Children:

Central nervous system: Nervousness (4% ages 6-12 years), fatigue (3% ages 6-12 years, 2% to 3% ages 2-5 years), malaise (2% ages 6-12 years)

Dermatologic: Rash (2% to 3% ages 2-5 years)

Gastrointestinal: Abdominal pain (2% ages 6-12 years), stomatitis (2% to 3% ages 2-5 years)

Neuromuscular & skeletal: Hyperkinesia (3% ages 6-12 years)

Ocular: Conjunctivitis (2% ages 6-12 years)

Respiratory: Wheezing (4% ages 6-12 years), dysphonia (2% ages 6-12 years), upper respiratory infection (2% ages 6-12 years), epistaxis (2% to 3% ages 2-5 years), pharyngitis (2% to 3% ages 2-5 years), flu-like symptoms (2% to 3% ages 2-5 years)

Miscellaneous: Viral infection (2% to 3% ages 2-5 years)

Mechanism of Action Long-acting tricyclic antihistamine with selective peripheral histamine H_1-receptor antagonistic properties

(Continued)

Loratadine *(Continued)*

Drug Interactions

Cytochrome P450 Effect: Substrate (minor) of CYP2D6, 3A4; **Inhibits** CYP2C19 (moderate), 2D6 (weak)

Increased Effect/Toxicity: Increased toxicity with procarbazine, other antihistamines. Protease inhibitors (amprenavir, ritonavir, nelfinavir) may increase the serum levels of loratadine. Loratadine may increase the levels/effects of citalopram, diazepam, methsuximide, phenytoin, propranolol, sertraline, and other CYP2C19 substrates.

Pharmacodynamics/Kinetics

Onset of action: 1-3 hours

Peak effect: 8-12 hours

Duration: >24 hours

Absorption: Rapid

Distribution: Significant amounts enter breast milk

Metabolism: Extensively hepatic via CYP2D6 and 3A4 to active metabolite

Half-life elimination: 12-15 hours

Excretion: Urine (40%) and feces (40%) as metabolites

Pregnancy Risk Factor B

Loratadine and Pseudoephedrine

(lor AT a deen & soo doe e FED rin)

Related Information

Loratadine *on page 841*

Oral Bacterial Infections *on page 1533*

Pseudoephedrine *on page 1147*

U.S. Brand Names Alavert™ Allergy and Sinus [OTC]; Claritin-D® 12-Hour [OTC]; Claritin-D® 24-Hour [OTC]

Canadian Brand Names Chlor-Tripolon ND®; Claritin® Extra; Claritin® Liberator

Generic Available Yes

Synonyms Pseudoephedrine and Loratadine

Pharmacologic Category Antihistamine/Decongestant Combination

Use Temporary relief of symptoms of seasonal allergic rhinitis and nasal congestion

Local Anesthetic/Vasoconstrictor Precautions Use with caution since pseudoephedrine is a sympathomimetic amine which could interact with epinephrine to cause a pressor response

Effects on Dental Treatment Key adverse event(s) related to dental treatment: Pseudoephedrine: Xerostomia (normal salivary flow resumes upon discontinuation).

Common Adverse Effects 1% to 10%:

Central nervous system: Headache, fatigue (3%), dizziness (4%), slight to moderate drowsiness (6%), nervousness (3%), insomnia (5%)

Gastrointestinal: Weight gain, nausea (3%), diarrhea, abdominal pain, dry mouth, xerostomia (8%), anorexia (2%)

Genitourinary: Dysuria, dysmenorrhea (2%)

Neuromuscular & skeletal: Arthralgia, weakness

Respiratory: Pharyngitis (5%), thickening of bronchial secretions, cough

Miscellaneous: Diaphoresis

Drug Interactions

Cytochrome P450 Effect: Loratadine: **Substrate** (minor) of CYP2D6, 3A4; **Inhibits** CYP2C19, 2D6

Increased Effect/Toxicity: See individual agents.

Pharmacodynamics/Kinetics See individual agents.

Pregnancy Risk Factor B

Lorazepam (lor A ze pam)

Related Information

Patients Requiring Sedation *on page 1567*

Temporomandibular Dysfunction (TMD) *on page 1564*

U.S. Brand Names Ativan®; Lorazepam Intensol®

Canadian Brand Names Apo-Lorazepam®; Ativan®; Novo-Lorazepam; Nu-Loraz; PMS-Lorazepam; Riva-Lorazepam

Mexican Brand Names Ativan®; Sinestron®

Generic Available Yes

Pharmacologic Category Benzodiazepine

Use

Oral: Management of anxiety disorders or short-term relief of the symptoms of anxiety or anxiety associated with depressive symptoms

I.V.: Status epilepticus, preanesthesia for desired amnesia, antiemetic adjunct

Unlabeled/Investigational Use Ethanol detoxification; insomnia; psychogenic catatonia; partial complex seizures; agitation (I.V.)

Local Anesthetic/Vasoconstrictor Precautions No information available to require special precautions

Effects on Dental Treatment Key adverse event(s) related to dental treatment: Xerostomia (normal salivary flow resumes upon discontinuation).

Significant Adverse Effects

>10%:

Central nervous system: Sedation

Respiratory: Respiratory depression

1% to 10%:

Cardiovascular: Hypotension

Central nervous system: Confusion, dizziness, akathisia, unsteadiness, headache, depression, disorientation, amnesia

Dermatologic: Dermatitis, rash

Gastrointestinal: Weight gain/loss, nausea, changes in appetite

Neuromuscular & skeletal: Weakness

Respiratory: Nasal congestion, hyperventilation, apnea

<1% (Limited to important or life-threatening): Menstrual irregularities, increased salivation, blood dyscrasias, reflex slowing, physical and psychological dependence with prolonged use, polyethylene glycol or propylene glycol poisoning (prolonged I.V. infusion)

Restrictions C-IV

Dosage

Antiemetic:

Children 2-15 years: I.V.: 0.05 mg/kg (up to 2 mg/dose) prior to chemotherapy

Adults: Oral, I.V. (**Note:** May be administered sublingually; not a labeled route): 0.5-2 mg every 4-6 hours as needed

Anxiety and sedation:

Infants and Children: Oral, I.M., I.V.: Usual: 0.05 mg/kg/dose (range: 0.02-0.09 mg/kg) every 4-8 hours

I.V.: May use smaller doses (eg, 0.01-0.03 mg/kg) and repeat every 20 minutes, as needed to titrate to effect

Adults: Oral: 1-10 mg/day in 2-3 divided doses; usual dose: 2-6 mg/day in divided doses

Elderly: 0.5-4 mg/day; initial dose not to exceed 2 mg

Insomnia: Adults: Oral: 2-4 mg at bedtime

Preoperative: Adults:

I.M.: 0.05 mg/kg administered 2 hours before surgery (maximum: 4 mg/dose)

I.V.: 0.044 mg/kg 15-20 minutes before surgery (usual maximum: 2 mg/dose)

Operative amnesia: Adults: I.V.: Up to 0.05 mg/kg (maximum: 4 mg/dose)

Sedation (preprocedure): Infants and Children:

Oral, I.M., I.V.: Usual: 0.05 mg/kg (range: 0.02-0.09 mg/kg);

I.V.: May use smaller doses (eg, 0.01-0.03 mg/kg) and repeat every 20 minutes, as needed to titrate to effect

Status epilepticus: I.V.:

Infants and Children: 0.1 mg/kg slow I.V. over 2-5 minutes; do not exceed 4 mg/single dose; may repeat second dose of 0.05 mg/kg slow I.V. in 10-15 minutes if needed

Adolescents: 0.07 mg/kg slow I.V. over 2-5 minutes; maximum: 4 mg/dose; may repeat in 10-15 minutes

Adults: 4 mg/dose slow I.V. over 2-5 minutes; may repeat in 10-15 minutes; usual maximum dose: 8 mg

Rapid tranquilization of agitated patient (administer every 30-60 minutes):

Oral: 1-2 mg

I.M.: 0.5-1 mg

Average total dose for tranquilization: Oral, I.M.: 4-8 mg

Agitation in the ICU patient (unlabeled):

I.V.: 0.02-0.06 mg/kg every 2-6 hours

I.V. infusion: 0.01-0.1 mg/kg/hour

Mechanism of Action Binds to stereospecific benzodiazepine receptors on the postsynaptic GABA neuron at several sites within the central nervous system, including the limbic system, reticular formation. Enhancement of the inhibitory effect of GABA on neuronal excitability results by increased neuronal membrane permeability to chloride ions. This shift in chloride ions results in hyperpolarization (a less excitable state) and stabilization.

Contraindications Hypersensitivity to lorazepam or any component of the formulation (cross-sensitivity with other benzodiazepines may exist); acute narrow-angle glaucoma; sleep apnea (parenteral); intra-arterial injection of

(Continued)

Lorazepam *(Continued)*

parenteral formulation; severe respiratory insufficiency (except during mechanical ventilation); pregnancy

Warnings/Precautions Use with caution in elderly or debilitated patients, patients with hepatic disease (including alcoholics) or renal impairment. Use with caution in patients with respiratory disease or impaired gag reflex. Initial doses in elderly or debilitated patients should not exceed 2 mg. Prolonged lorazepam use may have a possible relationship to GI disease, including esophageal dilation.

The parenteral formulation of lorazepam contains polyethylene glycol and propylene glycol. Each agent has been associated with specific toxicities when administered in prolonged infusions at high dosages. Also contains benzyl alcohol - avoid rapid injection in neonates or prolonged infusions. Intra-arterial injection or extravasation should be avoided. Concurrent administration with scopolamine results in an increased risk of hallucinations, sedation, and irrational behavior.

Causes CNS depression (dose-related) resulting in sedation, dizziness, confusion, or ataxia which may impair physical and mental capabilities. Patients must be cautioned about performing tasks which require mental alertness (eg, operating machinery or driving). Use with caution in patients receiving other CNS depressants or psychoactive agents. Effects with other sedative drugs or ethanol may be potentiated. Benzodiazepines have been associated with falls and traumatic injury and should be used with extreme caution in patients who are at risk of these events (especially the elderly).

Lorazepam may cause anterograde amnesia. Paradoxical reactions, including hyperactive or aggressive behavior have been reported with benzodiazepines, particularly in adolescent/pediatric or psychiatric patients. Does not have analgesic, antidepressant, or antipsychotic properties.

Use caution in patients with depression, particularly if suicidal risk may be present. Use with caution in patients with a history of drug dependence. Benzodiazepines have been associated with dependence and acute withdrawal symptoms on discontinuation or reduction in dose. Acute withdrawal, including seizures, may be precipitated after administration of flumazenil to patients receiving long-term benzodiazepine therapy.

As a hypnotic agent, should be used only after evaluation of potential causes of sleep disturbance. Failure of sleep disturbance to resolve after 7-10 days may indicate psychiatric or medical illness. A worsening of insomnia or the emergence of new abnormalities of thought or behavior may represent unrecognized psychiatric or medical illness and requires immediate and careful evaluation.

Drug Interactions

CNS depressants: Sedative effects and/or respiratory depression may be additive with CNS depressants; includes ethanol, barbiturates, narcotic analgesics, and other sedative agents; monitor for increased effect

Levodopa: Lorazepam may decrease the antiparkinsonian efficacy of levodopa (limited documentation); monitor

Loxapine: There are rare reports of significant respiratory depression, stupor, and/or hypotension with concomitant use of loxapine and lorazepam; use caution if concomitant administration of loxapine and CNS drugs is required

Scopolamine: May increase the incidence of sedation, hallucinations, and irrational behavior; reported only with parenteral lorazepam

Theophylline: May partially antagonize some of the effects of benzodiazepines; monitor for decreased response; may require higher doses for sedation

Ethanol/Nutrition/Herb Interactions

Ethanol: Avoid or limit ethanol (may increase CNS depression).

Herb/Nutraceutical: Avoid valerian, St John's wort, kava kava, gotu kola (may increase CNS depression).

Pharmacodynamics/Kinetics

Onset of action:
- Hypnosis: I.M.: 20-30 minutes
- Sedation: I.V.: 5-20 minutes
- Anticonvulsant: I.V.: 5 minutes, oral: 30-60 minutes

Duration: 6-8 hours

Absorption: Oral, I.M.: Prompt

Distribution:
- V_d: Neonates: 0.76 L/kg, Adults: 1.3 L/kg; crosses placenta; enters breast milk

Protein binding: 85%; free fraction may be significantly higher in elderly

Metabolism: Hepatic to inactive compounds

Half-life elimination: Neonates: 40.2 hours; Older children: 10.5 hours; Adults: 12.9 hours; Elderly: 15.9 hours; End-stage renal disease: 32-70 hours

Excretion: Urine; feces (minimal)

Pregnancy Risk Factor D

Lactation Enters breast milk/contraindicated (AAP rates "of concern")

Breast-Feeding Considerations Crosses into breast milk and no data on clinical effects on the infant. AAP states MAY BE OF CONCERN.

Dosage Forms

Injection, solution (Ativan®): 2 mg/mL (1 mL, 10 mL); 4 mg/mL (1 mL, 10 mL) [contains benzyl alcohol]

Solution, oral concentrate (Lorazepam Intensol®): 2 mg/mL (30 mL) [alcohol free, dye free]

Tablet (Ativan®): 0.5 mg, 1 mg, 2 mg

Lorazepam Intensol® *see* Lorazepam *on page 842*

Lorcet® 10/650 *see* Hydrocodone and Acetaminophen *on page 702*

Lorcet®-HD *see* Hydrocodone and Acetaminophen *on page 702*

Lorcet® Plus *see* Hydrocodone and Acetaminophen *on page 702*

Loroxide® [OTC] *see* Benzoyl Peroxide *on page 194*

Lortab® *see* Hydrocodone and Acetaminophen *on page 702*

Losartan (loe SAR tan)

Related Information

Cardiovascular Diseases *on page 1458*

U.S. Brand Names Cozaar®

Canadian Brand Names Cozaar®

Mexican Brand Names Cozaar®

Generic Available No

Synonyms DuP 753; Losartan Potassium; MK594

Pharmacologic Category Angiotensin II Receptor Blocker

Use Treatment of hypertension (HTN); treatment of diabetic nephropathy in patients with type 2 diabetes mellitus (noninsulin dependent, NIDDM) and a history of hypertension; stroke risk reduction in patients with HTN and left ventricular hypertrophy (LVH)

Local Anesthetic/Vasoconstrictor Precautions No information available to require special precautions

Effects on Dental Treatment No significant effects or complications reported

Common Adverse Effects

>10%:

Cardiovascular: Chest pain (12% diabetic nephropathy)

Central nervous system: Fatigue (14% diabetic nephropathy)

Endocrine: Hypoglycemia (14% diabetic nephropathy)

Gastrointestinal: Diarrhea (2% hypertension to 15% diabetic nephropathy)

Genitourinary: Urinary tract infection (13% diabetic nephropathy)

Hematologic: Anemia (14% diabetic nephropathy)

Neuromuscular & skeletal: Weakness (14% diabetic nephropathy), back pain (2% hypertension to 12% diabetic nephropathy)

Respiratory: Cough (11% diabetic nephropathy; 17% to 29% hypertension but similar to that associated with hydrochlorothiazide or placebo therapy)

1% to 10%:

Cardiovascular: Hypotension (7% diabetic nephropathy), orthostatic hypotension (4% hypertension to 4% diabetic nephropathy), first-dose hypotension (dose-related: <1% with 50 mg, 2% with 100 mg)

Central nervous system: Dizziness (4%), hypoesthesia (5% diabetic nephropathy), fever (4% diabetic nephropathy), insomnia (1%)

Dermatology: Cellulitis (7% diabetic nephropathy)

Endocrine: Hyperkalemia (<1% hypertension to 7% diabetic nephropathy)

Gastrointestinal: Gastritis (5% diabetic nephropathy), weight gain (4% diabetic nephropathy), dyspepsia (1% to 4%), abdominal pain (2%), nausea (2%)

Neuromuscular & skeletal: Muscular weakness (7% diabetic nephropathy), knee pain (5% diabetic nephropathy), leg pain (1% to 5%), muscle cramps (1%), myalgia (1%)

Respiratory: Bronchitis (10% diabetic nephropathy), upper respiratory infection (8%), nasal congestion (2%), sinusitis (1% hypertension to 6% diabetic nephropathy)

Miscellaneous: Infection (5% diabetic nephropathy), flu-like syndrome (10% diabetic nephropathy)

(Continued)

Losartan *(Continued)*

Dosage Oral:

Hypertension:

Children 6-16 years: 0.7 mg/kg once daily (maximum: 50 mg/day); adjust dose based on response; doses >1.4 mg/kg (maximum: 100 mg) have not been studied

Adults: Usual starting dose: 50 mg once daily; can be administered once or twice daily with total daily doses ranging from 25-100 mg

Patients receiving diuretics or with intravascular volume depletion: Usual initial dose: 25 mg

Nephropathy in patients with type 2 diabetes and hypertension: Adults: Initial: 50 mg once daily; can be increased to 100 mg once daily based on blood pressure response

Stroke reduction (HTN with LVH): Adults: 50 mg once daily (maximum daily dose: 100 mg); may be used in combination with a thiazide diuretic

Dosing adjustment in renal impairment:

Children: Use is not recommended if Cl_{cr} <30 mL/minute.

Adults: No adjustment necessary.

Dosing adjustment in hepatic impairment: Reduce the initial dose to 25 mg/day; divide dosage intervals into two.

Mechanism of Action As a selective and competitive, nonpeptide angiotensin II receptor antagonist, losartan blocks the vasoconstrictor and aldosterone-secreting effects of angiotensin II; losartan interacts reversibly at the AT1 and AT2 receptors of many tissues and has slow dissociation kinetics; its affinity for the AT1 receptor is 1000 times greater than the AT2 receptor. Angiotensin II receptor antagonists may induce a more complete inhibition of the renin-angiotensin system than ACE inhibitors, they do not affect the response to bradykinin, and are less likely to be associated with nonrenin-angiotensin effects (eg, cough and angioedema). Losartan increases urinary flow rate and in addition to being natriuretic and kaliuretic, increases excretion of chloride, magnesium, uric acid, calcium, and phosphate.

Contraindications Hypersensitivity to losartan or any component of the formulation; hypersensitivity to other A-II receptor antagonists; bilateral renal artery stenosis; pregnancy (2nd and 3rd trimesters)

Warnings/Precautions Avoid use or use a much smaller dose in patients who are volume-depleted; correct depletion first. Use with caution in patients with pre-existing renal insufficiency or significant aortic/mitral stenosis. Use caution in patients with unilateral or bilateral renal artery stenosis to avoid a decrease in renal function. AUCs of losartan (not the active metabolite) are about 50% greater in patients with Cl_{cr} <30 mL/minute and are doubled in hemodialysis patients. When used to reduce the risk of stroke in patients with HTN and LVH, may not be effective in African-American population. Use caution with hepatic dysfunction, dose adjustment may be needed.

Drug Interactions

Cytochrome P450 Effect: Substrate (major) of CYP2C8/9, 3A4; **Inhibits** CYP1A2 (weak), 2C8/9 (moderate), 2C19 (weak), 3A4 (weak)

Increased Effect/Toxicity: Cimetidine may increase the absorption of losartan by 18% (clinical effect is unknown). Potassium salts/supplements, co-trimoxazole (high dose), ACE inhibitors, and potassium-sparing diuretics (amiloride, spironolactone, triamterene) may increase the risk of hyperkalemia. Risk of lithium toxicity may be increased by losartan. Losartan may increase the levels/effects of amiodarone, fluoxetine, glimepiride, glipizide, nateglinide, phenytoin, pioglitazone, rosiglitazone, sertraline, warfarin, and other CYP2C8/9 substrates. Fluconazole may increase the levels/effects of losartan.

Decreased Effect: The levels/effects of losartan may be decreased by aminoglutethimide, carbamazepine, nafcillin, nevirapine, phenobarbital, phenytoin, rifampin, rifapentine, secobarbital, and other CYP2C8/9 or 3A4 inducers. NSAIDs may decrease the efficacy of losartan.

Ethanol/Nutrition/Herb Interactions Herb/Nutraceutical: St John's wort may decrease levels. Avoid dong quai if using for hypertension (has estrogenic activity). Avoid ephedra, yohimbe, ginseng (may worsen hypertension). Avoid garlic (may have increased antihypertensive effect).

Dietary Considerations May be taken with or without food.

Pharmacodynamics/Kinetics

Onset of action: 6 hours

Distribution: V_d: Losartan: 34 L; E-3174: 12 L; does not cross blood brain barrier

Protein binding, plasma: High

Metabolism: Hepatic (14%) via CYP2C9 and 3A4 to active metabolite, E-3174 (40 times more potent than losartan); extensive first-pass effect

Bioavailability: 25% to 33%; AUC of E-3174 is four times greater than that of losartan

Half-life elimination: Losartan: 1.5-2 hours; E-3174: 6-9 hours

Time to peak, serum: Losartan: 1 hour; E-3174: 3-4 hours

Excretion: Urine (4% as unchanged drug, 6% as active metabolite)

Clearance: Plasma: Losartan: 600 mL/minute; Active metabolite: 50 mL/minute

Pregnancy Risk Factor C/D (2nd and 3rd trimesters)

Dosage Forms TAB, film coated: 25 mg, 50 mg, 100 mg

Losartan and Hydrochlorothiazide

(loe SAR tan & hye droe klor oh THYE a zide)

Related Information

Hydrochlorothiazide *on page 699*

Losartan *on page 845*

U.S. Brand Names Hyzaar®

Canadian Brand Names Hyzaar®; Hyzaar® DS

Generic Available No

Synonyms Hydrochlorothiazide and Losartan

Pharmacologic Category Angiotensin II Receptor Blocker Combination; Antihypertensive Agent, Combination; Diuretic, Thiazide

Use Treatment of hypertension

Local Anesthetic/Vasoconstrictor Precautions No information available to require special precautions

Effects on Dental Treatment No significant effects or complications reported

Common Adverse Effects See individual agents.

Dosage Oral (dosage must be individualized): Adults: 1 tablet daily

Contraindications

Based on **losartan** component: Hypersensitivity to losartan or any component of the formulation; hypersensitivity to other A-II receptor antagonists; bilateral renal artery stenosis; pregnancy (2nd and 3rd trimesters)

Based on **hydrochlorothiazide** component: Hypersensitivity to hydrochlorothiazide, thiazides, sulfonamide-derived drugs, or any component of the formulation; anuria; renal decompensation; pregnancy (2nd and 3rd trimesters)

Drug Interactions

Cytochrome P450 Effect: Losartan: **Substrate** (major) of CYP2C8/9, 3A4; **Inhibits** CYP1A2 (weak), 2C8/9 (moderate), 2C19 (weak), 3A4 (weak)

Increased Effect/Toxicity: See individual agents.

Pharmacodynamics/Kinetics See individual agents.

Pregnancy Risk Factor C/D (2nd and 3rd trimesters)

Dosage Forms TAB, film coated: 50-12.5: Losartan potassium 50 mg and hydrochlorothiazide 12.5 mg; 100-25: Losartan potassium 100 mg and hydrochlorothiazide 25 mg

Losartan Potassium *see* Losartan *on page 845*

Lotemax® *see* Loteprednol *on page 847*

Lotensin® *see* Benazepril *on page 187*

Lotensin® HCT *see* Benazepril and Hydrochlorothiazide *on page 189*

Loteprednol (loe te PRED nol)

U.S. Brand Names Alrex®; Lotemax®

Canadian Brand Names Alrex®; Lotemax®

Generic Available No

Synonyms Loteprednol Etabonate

Pharmacologic Category Corticosteroid, Ophthalmic

Use

Suspension, 0.2% (Alrex™): Temporary relief of signs and symptoms of seasonal allergic conjunctivitis

Suspension, 0.5% (Lotemax™): Inflammatory conditions (treatment of steroid-responsive inflammatory conditions of the palpebral and bulbar conjunctiva, cornea, and anterior segment of the globe such as allergic conjunctivitis, acne rosacea, superficial punctate keratitis, herpes zoster keratitis, iritis, cyclitis, selected infective conjunctivitis, when the inherent hazard of steroid use is accepted to obtain an advisable diminution in edema and inflammation) and treatment of postoperative inflammation following ocular surgery

(Continued)

Loteprednol *(Continued)*

Local Anesthetic/Vasoconstrictor Precautions No information available to require special precautions

Effects on Dental Treatment No significant effects or complications reported

Mechanism of Action Corticosteroids inhibit the inflammatory response including edema, capillary dilation, leukocyte migration, and scar formation. Loteprednol is highly lipid soluble and penetrates cells readily to induce the production of lipocortins. These proteins modulate the activity of prostaglandins and leukotrienes.

Pregnancy Risk Factor C

Loteprednol Etabonate *see* Loteprednol *on page 847*

Lotrel® *see* Amlodipine and Benazepril *on page 110*

Lotrimin® AF Athlete's Foot Cream [OTC] *see* Clotrimazole *on page 363*

Lotrimin® AF Athlete's Foot Solution [OTC] *see* Clotrimazole *on page 363*

Lotrimin® AF Jock Itch Cream [OTC] *see* Clotrimazole *on page 363*

Lotrimin® AF Powder/Spray [OTC] *see* Miconazole *on page 922*

Lotrimin® Ultra™ [OTC] *see* Butenafine *on page 239*

Lotrisone® *see* Betamethasone and Clotrimazole *on page 201*

Lotronex® *see* Alosetron *on page 83*

Lovastatin (LOE va sta tin)

Related Information

Cardiovascular Diseases *on page 1458*

U.S. Brand Names Altocor™ [DSC]; Altoprev™; Mevacor®

Canadian Brand Names Apo-Lovastatin®; Gen-Lovastatin; Mevacor®; Novo-Lovastatin; Nu-Lovastatin; PMS-Lovastatin; ratio-Lovastatin

Mexican Brand Names Mevacor®

Generic Available Yes: Immediate release tablet

Synonyms Mevinolin; Monacolin K

Pharmacologic Category Antilipemic Agent, HMG-CoA Reductase Inhibitor

Use

Adjunct to dietary therapy to decrease elevated serum total and LDL-cholesterol concentrations in primary hypercholesterolemia

Primary prevention of coronary artery disease (patients without symptomatic disease with average to moderately elevated total and LDL-cholesterol and below average HDL-cholesterol); slow progression of coronary atherosclerosis in patients with coronary heart disease

Adjunct to dietary therapy in adolescent patients (10-17 years of age, females >1 year postmenarche) with heterozygous familial hypercholesterolemia having LDL >189 mg/dL, **or** LDL >160 mg/dL with positive family history of premature cardiovascular disease (CVD), **or** LDL >160 mg/dL with the presence of at least two other CVD risk factors

Local Anesthetic/Vasoconstrictor Precautions No information available to require special precautions

Effects on Dental Treatment No significant effects or complications reported

Common Adverse Effects Percentages as reported with immediate release tablets; similar adverse reactions seen with extended release tablets.

>10%: Neuromuscular & skeletal: Increased CPK (>2x normal) (11%)

1% to 10%:

- Central nervous system: Headache (2% to 3%), dizziness (0.5% to 1%)
- Dermatologic: Rash (0.8% to 1%)
- Gastrointestinal: Abdominal pain (2% to 3%), constipation (2% to 4%), diarrhea (2% to 3%), dyspepsia (1% to 2%), flatulence (4% to 5%), nausea (2% to 3%)
- Neuromuscular & skeletal: Myalgia (2% to 3%), weakness (1% to 2%), muscle cramps (0.6% to 1%)
- Ocular: Blurred vision (0.8% to 1%)

Dosage Oral:

Adolescents 10-17 years: Immediate release tablet:

- LDL reduction <20%: Initial: 10 mg/day with evening meal
- LDL reduction ≥20%: Initial: 20 mg/day with evening meal
- Usual range: 10-40 mg with evening meal, then adjust dose at 4-week intervals

Adults: Initial: 20 mg with evening meal, then adjust at 4-week intervals; maximum dose: 80 mg/day immediate release tablet **or** 60 mg/day extended release tablet; before initiation of therapy, patients should be placed on a standard cholesterol-lowering diet for 3-6 months and the diet should be continued during drug therapy. Patients receiving immunosuppressant drugs should start at 10 mg/day and not exceed 20 mg/day. Patients receiving concurrent therapy with fibrates should not exceed 20 mg lovastatin. Patients receiving amiodarone, niacin, or verapamil should not exceed 40 mg lovastatin daily.

Mechanism of Action Lovastatin acts by competitively inhibiting 3-hydroxyl-3-methylglutaryl-coenzyme A (HMG-CoA) reductase, the enzyme that catalyzes the rate-limiting step in cholesterol biosynthesis

Contraindications Hypersensitivity to lovastatin or any component of the formulation; active liver disease; unexplained persistent elevations of serum transaminases; pregnancy; breast-feeding

Warnings/Precautions May elevate aminotransferases; LFTs should be performed before and every 4- 6 weeks during the first 12-15 months of therapy and periodically thereafter. Can also cause myalgia and rhabdomyolysis. Rhabdomyolysis with acute renal failure has occurred. Risk is increased with concurrent use of clarithromycin, danazol, diltiazem, fluvoxamine, indinavir, nefazodone, nelfinavir, ritonavir, verapamil, troleandomycin, cyclosporine, fibric acid derivatives, erythromycin, niacin, azole antifungals, or large quantities of grapefruit juice. Weigh the risk versus benefit when combining any of these drugs with lovastatin. Temporarily discontinue in any patient experiencing an acute or serious condition predisposing to renal failure secondary to rhabdomyolysis. Use with caution in patients who consume large amounts of alcohol or have a history of liver disease. Safety and efficacy of the immediate release tablet have not been evaluated in prepubertal patients, patients <10 years of age, or doses >40 mg/day in appropriately-selected adolescents; extended release tablets have not been studied in patients <20 years of age.

Drug Interactions

Cytochrome P450 Effect: Substrate of CYP3A4 (major); **Inhibits** CYP2C8/9 (weak), 2D6 (weak), 3A4 (weak)

Increased Effect/Toxicity: CYP3A4 inhibitors may increase the levels/effects of lovastatin; example inhibitors include azole antifungals, ciprofloxacin, clarithromycin, diclofenac, doxycycline, erythromycin, imatinib, isoniazid, nefazodone, nicardipine, propofol, protease inhibitors, quinidine, and verapamil. Limit dose to ≤40 mg with amiodarone or verapamil. Suspend lovastatin therapy during concurrent clarithromycin, erythromycin, itraconazole, or ketoconazole therapy. Cyclosporine, clofibrate, fenofibrate, gemfibrozil, and niacin also may increase the risk of myopathy and rhabdomyolysis. Limit dose to ≤20 mg with concurrent gemfibrozil. The effect/toxicity of warfarin (elevated PT) and levothyroxine may be increased by lovastatin. Digoxin, norethindrone, and ethinyl estradiol levels may be increased. Effects are additive with other lipid-lowering therapies.

Decreased Effect: Cholestyramine taken with lovastatin reduces lovastatin absorption and effect.

Ethanol/Nutrition/Herb Interactions

Ethanol: Avoid excessive ethanol consumption (due to potential hepatic effects).

Food: The therapeutic effect of lovastatin may be decreased if taken with food. Lovastatin serum concentrations may be increased if taken with grapefruit juice; avoid concurrent intake of large quantities (>1 quart/day).

Herb/Nutraceutical: St John's wort may decrease lovastatin levels.

Dietary Considerations Before initiation of therapy, patients should be placed on a standard cholesterol-lowering diet for 6 weeks and the diet should be continued during drug therapy. Avoid intake of large quantities of grapefruit juice (≥1 quart/day); may increase toxicity.

Pharmacodynamics/Kinetics

Onset of action: LDL-cholesterol reductions: 3 days

Absorption: 30%; increased with extended release tablets

Protein binding: 95%

Metabolism: Hepatic; extensive first-pass effect; hydrolyzed to B-hydroxy acid (active)

Bioavailability: Increased with extended release tablets

Half-life elimination: 1.1-1.7 hours

Time to peak, serum: 2-4 hours

Excretion: Feces (~80% to 85%); urine (10%)

Pregnancy Risk Factor X

Dosage Forms TAB: (Mevacor®): 20 mg, 40 mg. **TAB, extended release:** (Altoprev™) 10 mg, 20 mg, 40 mg, 60 mg

Lovastatin and Niacin *see* Niacin and Lovastatin *on page 979*

Lovenox® *see* Enoxaparin *on page 493*

Low-Ogestrel® *see* Ethinyl Estradiol and Norgestrel *on page 557*

Loxapine (LOKS a peen)

U.S. Brand Names Loxitane®; Loxitane® C

Canadian Brand Names Apo-Loxapine®; Nu-Loxapine; PMS-Loxapine

Generic Available Yes

Synonyms Loxapine Hydrochloride; Loxapine Succinate; Oxilapine Succinate

Pharmacologic Category Antipsychotic Agent, Dibenzoxazepine

Use Management of psychotic disorders

Local Anesthetic/Vasoconstrictor Precautions Most pharmacology textbooks state that in presence of phenothiazines, systemic doses of epinephrine paradoxically decrease the blood pressure. This is the so called "epinephrine reversal" phenomenon. This has never been observed when epinephrine is given by infiltration as part of the anesthesia procedure.

Effects on Dental Treatment Key adverse event(s) related to dental treatment:

Xerostomia and changes in salivation (normal salivary flow resumes upon discontinuation).

Significant hypotension may occur, especially when the drug is administered parenterally; orthostatic hypotension is due to alpha-receptor blockade, the elderly are at greater risk for orthostatic hypotension.

Tardive dyskinesia: Prevalence rate may be 40% in elderly; development of the syndrome and the irreversible nature are proportional to duration and total cumulative dose over time. Extrapyramidal reactions are more common in elderly with up to 50% developing these reactions after 60 years of age. Drug-induced Parkinson's syndrome occurs often; akathisia is the most common extrapyramidal reaction in elderly.

Increased confusion, memory loss, psychotic behavior, and agitation frequently occur as a consequence of anticholinergic effects. Antipsychotic associated sedation in nonpsychotic patients is extremely unpleasant due to feelings of depersonalization, derealization, and dysphoria.

Common Adverse Effects Frequency not defined.

Cardiovascular: Orthostatic hypotension, tachycardia, arrhythmias, abnormal T-waves with prolonged ventricular repolarization, hypertension, hypotension, lightheadedness, syncope

Central nervous system: Drowsiness, extrapyramidal symptoms (dystonia, akathisia, pseudoparkinsonism, tardive dyskinesia, akinesia), dizziness, faintness, ataxia, insomnia, agitation, tension, seizures, slurred speech, confusion, headache, neuroleptic malignant syndrome (NMS), altered central temperature regulation

Dermatologic: Rash, pruritus, photosensitivity, dermatitis, alopecia, seborrhea

Endocrine & metabolic: Enlargement of breasts, galactorrhea, amenorrhea, gynecomastia, menstrual irregularity

Gastrointestinal: Xerostomia, constipation, nausea, vomiting, weight gain/loss, adynamic ileus, polydipsia

Genitourinary: Urinary retention, sexual dysfunction

Hematologic: Agranulocytosis, leukopenia, thrombocytopenia

Neuromuscular & skeletal: Weakness

Ocular: Blurred vision

Respiratory: Nasal congestion

Mechanism of Action Blocks postsynaptic mesolimbic D_1 and D_2 receptors in the brain, and also possesses serotonin 5-HT_2 blocking activity

Drug Interactions

Increased Effect/Toxicity: Loxapine concentrations may be increased by chloroquine, propranolol, sulfadoxine-pyrimethamine. Loxapine may increased the effect and/or toxicity of antihypertensives, lithium, TCAs, CNS depressants (ethanol, narcotics), and trazodone. There are rare reports of significant respiratory depression, stupor, and/or hypotension with the concomitant use of loxapine and lorazepam. Use caution if the concomitant administration of loxapine and CNS drugs is required. Metoclopramide may increase risk of extrapyramidal symptoms (EPS). Effects on QT_c interval may be additive with antipsychotics, increasing the risk of malignant arrhythmias; other QT_c-prolonging agents include type Ia antiarrhythmics, TCAs, and some quinolone antibiotics (sparfloxacin, moxifloxacin and gatifloxacin). Concomitant use with thioridazine is contraindicated.

Decreased Effect: Antipsychotics inhibit the activity of bromocriptine and levodopa. Benztropine (and other anticholinergics) may inhibit the therapeutic response to loxapine and excess anticholinergic effects may occur. Loxapine and possibly other low potency antipsychotic may reverse the pressor effects of epinephrine.

Pharmacodynamics/Kinetics

Onset of action: Neuroleptic: Oral: 20-30 minutes

Peak effect: 1.5-3 hours
Duration: ~12 hours
Metabolism: Hepatic to glucuronide conjugates
Half-life elimination: Biphasic: Initial: 5 hours; Terminal: 12-19 hours
Excretion: Urine; feces (small amounts)

Pregnancy Risk Factor C

Loxapine Hydrochloride *see* Loxapine *on page 850*
Loxapine Succinate *see* Loxapine *on page 850*
Loxitane® *see* Loxapine *on page 850*
Loxitane® C *see* Loxapine *on page 850*
Lozi-Flur™ *see* Fluoride *on page 603*
Lozol® *see* Indapamide *on page 743*
L-PAM *see* Melphalan *on page 866*
LRH *see* Gonadorelin *on page 669*
L-Sarcolysin *see* Melphalan *on page 866*
LTG *see* Lamotrigine *on page 795*
***L*-Thyroxine Sodium** *see* Levothyroxine *on page 817*
Lu-26-054 *see* Escitalopram *on page 513*
Lubriderm® [OTC] *see* Lanolin, Cetyl Alcohol, Glycerin, Petrolatum, and Mineral Oil *on page 797*
Lubriderm® Fragrance Free [OTC] *see* Lanolin, Cetyl Alcohol, Glycerin, Petrolatum, and Mineral Oil *on page 797*
Ludiomil *see* Maprotiline *on page 856*
Lufyllin® *see* Dyphylline *on page 480*
Lugol's Solution *see* Potassium Iodide *on page 1106*
Lumigan® *see* Bimatoprost *on page 207*
Luminal® Sodium *see* Phenobarbital *on page 1073*
Lumitene™ *see* Beta-Carotene *on page 198*
Lunelle™ *see* Estradiol and Medroxyprogesterone *on page 520*
LupiCare™ Dandruff [OTC] *see* Salicylic Acid *on page 1205*
LupiCare™ II Psoriasis [OTC] *see* Salicylic Acid *on page 1205*
LupiCare™ Psoriasis [OTC] *see* Salicylic Acid *on page 1205*
Lupron® *see* Leuprolide *on page 805*
Lupron Depot® *see* Leuprolide *on page 805*
Lupron Depot-Ped® *see* Leuprolide *on page 805*
Luride® *see* Fluoride *on page 603*
Luride® Lozi-Tab® *see* Fluoride *on page 603*
Lustra® *see* Hydroquinone *on page 719*
Lustra-AF™ *see* Hydroquinone *on page 719*
Luteinizing Hormone Releasing Hormone *see* Gonadorelin *on page 669*
Luvox *see* Fluvoxamine *on page 623*
Luxiq® *see* Betamethasone *on page 199*
LY139603 *see* Atomoxetine *on page 161*
LY146032 *see* Daptomycin *on page 399*
LY170053 *see* Olanzapine *on page 1007*
LY231514 *see* Pemetrexed *on page 1054*
Lymphocyte Immune Globulin *see* Antithymocyte Globulin (Equine) *on page 136*
Lymphocyte Mitogenic Factor *see* Aldesleukin *on page 74*

Lysine (el LYE seen)

U.S. Brand Names Lysinyl [OTC]
Generic Available Yes
Synonyms L-Lysine Hydrochloride
Pharmacologic Category Nutritional Supplement
Use Improves utilization of vegetable proteins
Local Anesthetic/Vasoconstrictor Precautions No information available to require special precautions
Effects on Dental Treatment No significant effects or complications reported
Pregnancy Risk Factor C

Lysinyl [OTC] *see* Lysine *on page 851*
Lysodren® *see* Mitotane *on page 937*
Maalox® [OTC] *see* Aluminum Hydroxide, Magnesium Hydroxide, and Simethicone *on page 92*
Maalox® Max [OTC] *see* Aluminum Hydroxide, Magnesium Hydroxide, and Simethicone *on page 92*

Maalox® TC (Therapeutic Concentrate) [OTC] [DSC] *see* Aluminum Hydroxide and Magnesium Hydroxide *on page 91*

Macrobid® *see* Nitrofurantoin *on page 990*

Macrodantin® *see* Nitrofurantoin *on page 990*

Mafenide (MA fe nide)

U.S. Brand Names Sulfamylon®

Generic Available No

Synonyms Mafenide Acetate

Pharmacologic Category Antibiotic, Topical

Use Adjunct in the treatment of second- and third-degree burns to prevent septicemia caused by susceptible organisms such as *Pseudomonas aeruginosa*

Orphan drug: Prevention of graft loss of meshed autografts on excised burn wounds

Local Anesthetic/Vasoconstrictor Precautions No information available to require special precautions

Effects on Dental Treatment No significant effects or complications reported

Mechanism of Action Interferes with bacterial folic acid synthesis through competitive inhibition of para-aminobenzoic acid

Pregnancy Risk Factor C

Mafenide Acetate *see* Mafenide *on page 852*

Magaldrate and Simethicone (MAG al drate & sye METH i kone)

Related Information

Simethicone *on page 1222*

U.S. Brand Names Riopan Plus® [OTC]; Riopan Plus® Double Strength [OTC]

Generic Available Yes

Synonyms Simethicone and Magaldrate

Pharmacologic Category Antacid; Antiflatulent

Use Relief of hyperacidity associated with peptic ulcer, gastritis, peptic esophagitis and hiatal hernia which are accompanied by symptoms of gas

Local Anesthetic/Vasoconstrictor Precautions No information available to require special precautions

Effects on Dental Treatment No significant effects or complications reported

Common Adverse Effects Frequency not defined.

Based on **magaldrate** component:

Central nervous system: Encephalopathy

Gastrointestinal: Constipation, chalky taste, stomach cramps, fecal impaction, diarrhea, nausea, vomiting, discoloration of feces (white speckles), rebound hyperacidity

Endocrine & metabolic: Hypophosphatemia, hypermagnesemia, milk-alkali syndrome

Neuromuscular & metabolic: Osteomalacia

Miscellaneous: Aluminum intoxication

Based on **simethicone** component: No data reported

Drug Interactions

Increased Effect/Toxicity: See individual agents.

Pregnancy Risk Factor C

Mag Delay® [OTC] *see* Magnesium Chloride *on page 852*

Mag G® [OTC] *see* Magnesium Gluconate *on page 853*

Maginex™ [OTC] *see* Magnesium L-aspartate Hydrochloride *on page 854*

Maginex™ DS [OTC] *see* Magnesium L-aspartate Hydrochloride *on page 854*

Magnesia Magma *see* Magnesium Hydroxide *on page 853*

Magnesium Carbonate and Aluminum Hydroxide *see* Aluminum Hydroxide and Magnesium Carbonate *on page 90*

Magnesium Chloride (mag NEE zhum KLOR ide)

U.S. Brand Names Chloromag®; Mag Delay® [OTC]; Mag-SR® [OTC]; Slow-Mag® [OTC]

Generic Available Yes: Injection

Pharmacologic Category Magnesium Salt

Use Correction or prevention of hypomagnesemia

Local Anesthetic/Vasoconstrictor Precautions No information available to require special precautions

Effects on Dental Treatment Key adverse event(s) related to dental treatment: Magnesium products may prevent GI absorption of tetracyclines by forming a large ionized chelated molecule with the tetracyclines in the stomach. Tetracyclines should be given at least 1 hour before magnesium.

Pregnancy Risk Factor D

Magnesium Citrate (mag NEE zhum SIT rate)

Canadian Brand Names Citro-Mag®

Generic Available Yes

Synonyms Citrate of Magnesia

Pharmacologic Category Laxative, Saline; Magnesium Salt

Use Evacuation of bowel prior to certain surgical and diagnostic procedures or overdose situations

Local Anesthetic/Vasoconstrictor Precautions No information available to require special precautions

Effects on Dental Treatment Key adverse event(s) related to dental treatment: Magnesium products may prevent GI absorption of tetracyclines by forming a large ionized chelated molecule with the tetracyclines in the stomach. Tetracyclines should be given at least 1 hour before magnesium.

Mechanism of Action Promotes bowel evacuation by causing osmotic retention of fluid which distends the colon with increased peristaltic activity

Pregnancy Risk Factor B

Magnesium Gluconate (mag NEE zhum GLOO koe nate)

U.S. Brand Names Almora® [OTC]; Mag G® [OTC]; Magonate® [OTC]; Magonate® Sport [OTC]; Magtrate® [OTC]

Generic Available Yes: Tablet

Pharmacologic Category Magnesium Salt

Use Dietary supplement for treatment of magnesium deficiencies

Local Anesthetic/Vasoconstrictor Precautions No information available to require special precautions

Effects on Dental Treatment Key adverse event(s) related to dental treatment: Magnesium products may prevent GI absorption of tetracyclines by forming a large ionized chelated molecule with the tetracyclines in the stomach. Tetracyclines should be given at least 1 hour before magnesium.

Mechanism of Action Magnesium is important as a cofactor in many enzymatic reactions in the body involving protein synthesis and carbohydrate metabolism (at least 300 enzymatic reactions require magnesium). Actions on lipoprotein lipase have been found to be important in reducing serum cholesterol and on sodium/potassium ATPase in promoting polarization (ie, neuromuscular functioning).

Magnesium Hydroxide (mag NEE zhum hye DROKS ide)

U.S. Brand Names Dulcolax® Milk of Magnesia [OTC]; Phillips'® Milk of Magnesia [OTC]

Generic Available Yes: Liquid

Synonyms Magnesia Magma; Milk of Magnesia; MOM

Pharmacologic Category Antacid; Magnesium Salt

Use Short-term treatment of occasional constipation and symptoms of hyperacidity, magnesium replacement therapy

Local Anesthetic/Vasoconstrictor Precautions No information available to require special precautions

Effects on Dental Treatment Key adverse event(s) related to dental treatment: Magnesium products may prevent GI absorption of tetracyclines by forming a large ionized chelated molecule with the tetracyclines in the stomach. Tetracyclines should be given at least 1 hour before magnesium.

Mechanism of Action Promotes bowel evacuation by causing osmotic retention of fluid which distends the colon with increased peristaltic activity; reacts with hydrochloric acid in stomach to form magnesium chloride

Pregnancy Risk Factor B

Magnesium Hydroxide, Aluminum Hydroxide, and Simethicone *see* Aluminum Hydroxide, Magnesium Hydroxide, and Simethicone *on page 92*

Magnesium Hydroxide and Aluminum Hydroxide *see* Aluminum Hydroxide and Magnesium Hydroxide *on page 91*

Magnesium Hydroxide and Calcium Carbonate *see* Calcium Carbonate and Magnesium Hydroxide *on page 245*

Magnesium Hydroxide and Mineral Oil

(mag NEE zhum hye DROKS ide & MIN er al oyl)

Related Information

Magnesium Hydroxide *on page 853*

U.S. Brand Names Phillips' M-O® [OTC]

Generic Available No

Synonyms Haley's M-O; MOM/Mineral Oil Emulsion

(Continued)

Magnesium Hydroxide and Mineral Oil *(Continued)*

Pharmacologic Category Laxative

Use Short-term treatment of occasional constipation

Local Anesthetic/Vasoconstrictor Precautions No information available to require special precautions

Effects on Dental Treatment Key adverse event(s) related to dental treatment: Magnesium products may prevent GI absorption of tetracyclines by forming a large ionized chelated molecule with the tetracyclines in the stomach. Tetracyclines should be given at least 1 hour before magnesium.

Pregnancy Risk Factor B

Magnesium Hydroxide, Famotidine, and Calcium Carbonate *see* Famotidine, Calcium Carbonate, and Magnesium Hydroxide *on page 574*

Magnesium L-aspartate Hydrochloride

(mag NEE zhum el as PAR tate hye droe KLOR ide)

U.S. Brand Names Maginex™ [OTC]; Maginex™ DS [OTC]

Synonyms MAH™

Pharmacologic Category Electrolyte Supplement, Oral

Use Dietary supplement

Local Anesthetic/Vasoconstrictor Precautions No information available to require special precautions

Effects on Dental Treatment Key adverse event(s) related to dental treatment: Magnesium ions prevent GI absorption of tetracycline by forming a large, ionized, chelated molecule with the magnesium ion and tetracyclines in the stomach. Magnesium supplement should not be taken within 2-4 hours of oral tetracycline or other members of the tetracycline family.

Common Adverse Effects Frequency not defined: Gastrointestinal: Diarrhea, loose stools

Magnesium Oxide (mag NEE zhum OKS ide)

U.S. Brand Names Mag-Ox® 400 [OTC]; Uro-Mag® [OTC]

Generic Available Yes: Tablet

Pharmacologic Category Electrolyte Supplement, Oral

Use Electrolyte replacement

Local Anesthetic/Vasoconstrictor Precautions No information available to require special precautions

Effects on Dental Treatment Key adverse event(s) related to dental treatment: Magnesium products may prevent GI absorption of tetracyclines by forming a large ionized chelated molecule with the tetracyclines in the stomach. Tetracyclines should be given at least 1 hour before magnesium.

Pregnancy Risk Factor B

Magnesium Salicylate (mag NEE zhum sa LIS i late)

Related Information

Rheumatoid Arthritis, Osteoarthritis, and Osteoporosis *on page 1490*

Temporomandibular Dysfunction (TMD) *on page 1564*

U.S. Brand Names Doan's® [OTC]; Doan's® Extra Strength [OTC]; Mobidin® [DSC]; Momentum® [OTC]

Mexican Brand Names Myoflex®

Generic Available Yes

Pharmacologic Category Salicylate

Use Mild to moderate pain, fever, various inflammatory conditions

Local Anesthetic/Vasoconstrictor Precautions No information available to require special precautions

Effects on Dental Treatment NSAID formulations are known to reversibly decrease platelet aggregation via mechanisms different than observed with aspirin. The dentist should be aware of the potential of abnormal coagulation. Caution should also be exercised in the use of NSAIDs in patients already on anticoagulant therapy with drugs such as warfarin (Coumadin®).

Drug Interactions

Decreased Effect: Decreased absorption of aminoquinolones, digoxin, nitrofurantoin, penicillamine, and tetracyclines may occur with magnesium salts.

Magnesium Sulfate (mag NEE zhum SUL fate)

Generic Available Yes

Synonyms Epsom Salts

Pharmacologic Category Antacid; Anticonvulsant, Miscellaneous; Electrolyte Supplement, Parenteral; Laxative, Saline; Magnesium Salt

Use Treatment and prevention of hypomagnesemia; seizure prevention in severe pre-eclampsia or eclampsia, pediatric acute nephritis; short-term treatment torsade de pointes; treatment of cardiac arrhythmias (VT/VF) caused by hypomagnesemia; short-term treatment of constipation or soaking aid

Local Anesthetic/Vasoconstrictor Precautions No information available to require special precautions

Effects on Dental Treatment Key adverse event(s) related to dental treatment: Magnesium products may prevent GI absorption of tetracyclines by forming a large ionized chelated molecule with the tetracyclines in the stomach. Tetracyclines should be given at least 1 hour before magnesium.

Mechanism of Action Promotes bowel evacuation by causing osmotic retention of fluid which distends the colon with increased peristaltic activity when taken orally; parenterally, decreases acetylcholine in motor nerve terminals and acts on myocardium by slowing rate of S-A node impulse formation and prolonging conduction time

Pregnancy Risk Factor B

Magnesium Trisilicate and Aluminum Hydroxide *see* Aluminum Hydroxide and Magnesium Trisilicate *on page 91*

Magonate® [OTC] *see* Magnesium Gluconate *on page 853*

Magonate® Sport [OTC] *see* Magnesium Gluconate *on page 853*

Mag-Ox® 400 [OTC] *see* Magnesium Oxide *on page 854*

Mag-SR® [OTC] *see* Magnesium Chloride *on page 852*

Magtrate® [OTC] *see* Magnesium Gluconate *on page 853*

MAH™ *see* Magnesium L-aspartate Hydrochloride *on page 854*

Malarone™ *see* Atovaquone and Proguanil *on page 165*

Maltodextrin (mal toe DEK strin)

U.S. Brand Names Gelclair™; Multidex® [OTC]; OraRinse™ [OTC]

Generic Available No

Pharmacologic Category Anti-inflammatory, Locally Applied

Dental Use Oral: Management and relief of pain due to oral lesions (including mucositis/stomatitis), oral ulcers, or irritation; treatment of aphthous ulcers

Use Topical: Treatment of infected or noninfected wounds

Local Anesthetic/Vasoconstrictor Precautions No information available to require special precautions

Effects on Dental Treatment No significant effects or complications reported

Dosage Adults:

Oral: Management of pain due to oral lesions:

Gelclair™: Using contents of 1 reconstituted packet, rinse around mouth for ~1 minute, 3 times/day or more if needed; gargle and expectorate. May be used undiluted or with less dilution if adequate pain relief is not achieved.

OraRinse™: 1 tablespoonful, swish or gargle for ~1 minute, 4 times/day or more if needed

Topical: Wound dressing: Multidex®: After debridement and irrigation of wound, apply and cover with a nonadherent, nonocclusive dressing. May be applied to moist or dry, infected or noninfected wounds.

Mechanism of Action Forms a protective barrier over wound providing an environment which promotes tissue growth.

Contraindications Hypersensitivity to maltodextrin or any component of the formulation

Warnings/Precautions Oral: Avoid eating or drinking for 1 hour; products are not harmful if accidentally swallowed; notify healthcare provider if improvement is not seen within 7 days

Dosage Forms

Gel, oral [concentrate] (Gelclair™): 15 mL/packet (21s) [contains benzalkonium chloride and sodium benzoate]

Gel, topical dressing (Multidex®): (4 mL, 7 mL, 14 mL, 85 mL)

Powder, for oral suspension (OraRinse™): (19 g) [contains phenylalanine; also contains aloe vera, fructose, and sodium benzoate; vanilla flavor]

Powder, topical dressing (Multidex®): (6 g, 12 g, 25 g, 45 g)

Comments

Gelclair™: Store at room temperature away from direct sunlight. Do not refrigerate. Gel may become darker or thicker over time; efficacy and safety are not affected if used prior to labeled expiration date. Mix contents of one packet with 40 mL of water. Stir and use at once. Product may be used undiluted if water is unavailable.

OraRinse™: Fill bottle with water to first arrow; shake vigorously until suspended; continue to fill to second arrow; shake well

Malt Soup Extract (malt soop EKS trakt)

U.S. Brand Names Maltsupex® [OTC]

Generic Available No

Pharmacologic Category Laxative

Use Short-term treatment of constipation

Local Anesthetic/Vasoconstrictor Precautions No information available to require special precautions

Effects on Dental Treatment No significant effects or complications reported

Common Adverse Effects Frequency not defined: Gastrointestinal: Abdominal cramps, diarrhea, rectal obstruction

Maltsupex® [OTC] *see* Malt Soup Extract *on page 856*
m-AMSA *see* Amsacrine *on page 129*
Management of Patients Undergoing Cancer Therapy *see page 1569*
Management of Sialorrhea *see page 1557*
Mandelamine® *see* Methenamine *on page 892*
Mandol® [DSC] *see* Cefamandole *on page 277*
Mandrake *see* Podophyllum Resin *on page 1099*
Manganese *see* Trace Metals *on page 1319*
Mantoux *see* Tuberculin Tests *on page 1349*
Mapap® [OTC] *see* Acetaminophen *on page 47*
Mapap® Arthritis [OTC] *see* Acetaminophen *on page 47*
Mapap® Children's [OTC] *see* Acetaminophen *on page 47*
Mapap® Extra Strength [OTC] *see* Acetaminophen *on page 47*
Mapap® Infants [OTC] *see* Acetaminophen *on page 47*
Mapap Sinus Maximum Strength [OTC] *see* Acetaminophen and Pseudoephedrine *on page 53*

Maprotiline (ma PROE ti leen)

Canadian Brand Names Novo-Maprotiline

Mexican Brand Names Ludiomil®

Generic Available Yes

Synonyms Ludiomil; Maprotiline Hydrochloride

Pharmacologic Category Antidepressant, Tetracyclic

Use Treatment of depression and anxiety associated with depression

Unlabeled/Investigational Use Bulimia; duodenal ulcers; enuresis; urinary symptoms of multiple sclerosis; pain; panic attacks; tension headache; cocaine withdrawal

Local Anesthetic/Vasoconstrictor Precautions Although maprotiline is not a tricyclic antidepressant, it does block norepinephrine reuptake within CNS synapses as part of its mechanisms. It has been suggested that vasoconstrictor be administered with caution and to monitor vital signs in dental patients taking antidepressants that affect norepinephrine in this way, including maprotiline. Epinephrine, norepinephrine and levonordefrin have been shown to have an increased pressor response in combination with TCAs.

Effects on Dental Treatment Key adverse event(s) related to dental treatment: Xerostomia and changes in salivation (normal salivary flow resumes upon discontinuation).

Common Adverse Effects

>10%:

Central nervous system: Drowsiness

Gastrointestinal: Xerostomia

1% to 10%:

Central nervous system: Insomnia, nervousness, anxiety, agitation, dizziness, fatigue, headache

Gastrointestinal: Constipation, nausea

Neuromuscular & skeletal: Tremor, weakness

Ocular: Blurred vision

Mechanism of Action Traditionally believed to increase the synaptic concentration of norepinephrine in the central nervous system by inhibition of their reuptake by the presynaptic neuronal membrane. However, additional receptor effects have been found including desensitization of adenyl cyclase, down regulation of beta-adrenergic receptors, and down regulation of serotonin receptors.

Drug Interactions

Cytochrome P450 Effect: Substrate of CYP2D6 (major)

Increased Effect/Toxicity: Maprotiline may increase the effects of amphetamines, anticholinergics, other CNS depressants (sedatives, hypnotics, or ethanol), carbamazepine, tolazamide, chlorpropamide, and warfarin. When used with MAO inhibitors, hyperpyrexia, hypertension, tachycardia, confusion, seizures, and **deaths have been reported** (serotonin syndrome). CYP2D6 inhibitors may increase the levels/effects of maprotiline; example inhibitors include chlorpromazine, delavirdine, fluoxetine, miconazole, paroxetine, pergolide, quinidine, quinine, ritonavir, and ropinirole. Cimetidine, fenfluramine, grapefruit juice, indinavir, methylphenidate, diltiazem, valproate, and verapamil may increase the serum concentrations of cyclic antidepressants. Use of lithium with a cyclic antidepressant may increase the risk for neurotoxicity. Phenothiazines may increase concentration of some cyclic antidepressants and cyclic antidepressants may increase the concentration of phenothiazines. Pressor response to I.V. epinephrine, norepinephrine, and phenylephrine may be enhanced in patients receiving cyclic antidepressants (**Note:** Effect is unlikely with epinephrine or levonordefrin dosages typically administered as infiltration in combination with local anesthetics). Combined use of beta-agonists or drugs which prolong QT_c (including quinidine, procainamide, disopyramide, cisapride, sparfloxacin, gatifloxacin, moxifloxacin) with cyclic antidepressants may predispose patients to cardiac arrhythmias.

Decreased Effect: Maprotiline inhibits the antihypertensive response to bethanidine, clonidine, debrisoquin, guanadrel, guanethidine, guanabenz, or guanfacine. Cholestyramine and colestipol may bind cyclic antidepressants and reduce their absorption.

Pharmacodynamics/Kinetics

Absorption: Slow

Protein binding: 88%

Metabolism: Hepatic to active and inactive compounds

Half-life elimination, serum: 27-58 hours (mean: 43 hours)

Time to peak, serum: Within 12 hours

Excretion: Urine (70%); feces (30%)

Pregnancy Risk Factor B

Maprotiline Hydrochloride *see* Maprotiline *on page 856*

Marcaine® *see* Bupivacaine *on page 225*

Marcaine® Spinal *see* Bupivacaine *on page 225*

Marcaine® with Epinephrine *see* Bupivacaine and Epinephrine *on page 227*

Marezine® [OTC] *see* Cyclizine *on page 381*

Margesic® H *see* Hydrocodone and Acetaminophen *on page 702*

Marinol® *see* Dronabinol *on page 477*

Marplan® *see* Isocarboxazid *on page 767*

Matulane® *see* Procarbazine *on page 1125*

3M™ Avagard™ [OTC] *see* Chlorhexidine Gluconate *on page 308*

Mavik® *see* Trandolapril *on page 1321*

Maxair™ Autohaler™ *see* Pirbuterol *on page 1096*

Maxalt® *see* Rizatriptan *on page 1193*

Maxalt-MLT® *see* Rizatriptan *on page 1193*

Maxaquin® *see* Lomefloxacin *on page 837*

Maxidex® *see* Dexamethasone *on page 411*

Maxidone™ *see* Hydrocodone and Acetaminophen *on page 702*

Maxifed® *see* Guaifenesin and Pseudoephedrine *on page 675*

Maxifed® DM *see* Guaifenesin, Pseudoephedrine, and Dextromethorphan *on page 676*

Maxifed-G® *see* Guaifenesin and Pseudoephedrine *on page 675*

Maxiflor® [DSC] *see* Diflorasone *on page 435*

Maxipime® *see* Cefepime *on page 281*

Maxitrol® *see* Neomycin, Polymyxin B, and Dexamethasone *on page 974*

Maxivate® *see* Betamethasone *on page 199*

Maxzide® *see* Hydrochlorothiazide and Triamterene *on page 701*

Maxzide®-25 *see* Hydrochlorothiazide and Triamterene *on page 701*

May Apple *see* Podophyllum Resin *on page 1099*

3M™ Cavilon™ Skin Cleanser [OTC] *see* Benzalkonium Chloride *on page 190*

MCH *see* Microfibrillar Collagen Hemostat *on page 923*

m-Cresyl Acetate (em-KREE sil AS e tate)

U.S. Brand Names Cresylate®

Generic Available No

Pharmacologic Category Otic Agent, Anti-infective

Use Provides an acid medium; for external otitis infections caused by susceptible bacteria or fungus

(Continued)

m-Cresyl Acetate *(Continued)*

Local Anesthetic/Vasoconstrictor Precautions No information available to require special precautions

Effects on Dental Treatment No significant effects or complications reported

MCT Oil® [OTC] *see* Medium Chain Triglycerides *on page 861*

MDL 73,147EF *see* Dolasetron *on page 461*

ME-500® *see* Methionine *on page 894*

Measles, Mumps, and Rubella Vaccines (Combined)

(MEE zels, mumpz & roo BEL a vak SEENS, kom BINED)

Related Information

Immunizations (Vaccines) *on page 1614*

U.S. Brand Names M-M-R® II

Canadian Brand Names M-M-R® II; Priorix™

Generic Available No

Synonyms MMR; Mumps, Measles and Rubella Vaccines, Combined; Rubella, Measles and Mumps Vaccines, Combined

Pharmacologic Category Vaccine, Live Virus

Use Measles, mumps, and rubella prophylaxis

Local Anesthetic/Vasoconstrictor Precautions No information available to require special precautions

Effects on Dental Treatment No significant effects or complications reported

Common Adverse Effects All serious adverse reactions must be reported to the U.S. Department of Health and Human Services (DHHS) Vaccine Adverse Event Reporting System (VAERS) 1-800-822-7967.

Frequency not defined:

- Cardiovascular: Syncope, vasculitis
- Central nervous system: Ataxia, dizziness, febrile convulsions, fever, encephalitis, encephalopathy, Guillain-Barré syndrome, headache, irritability, malaise, measles inclusion body encephalitis, polyneuritis, polyneuropathy, seizures, subacute sclerosing panencephalitis,
- Dermatologic: Angioneurotic edema, erythema multiforme, purpura, rash, Stevens-Johnson syndrome, urticaria
- Endocrine & metabolic: Diabetes mellitus, parotitis
- Gastrointestinal: Diarrhea, nausea, pancreatitis, sore throat, vomiting
- Genitourinary: Orchitis
- Hematologic: Leukocytosis, thrombocytopenia
- Local: Injection site reactions which include burning, induration, redness, stinging, swelling, tenderness, wheal and flare, vesiculation
- Neuromuscular & skeletal: Arthralgia/arthritis (variable; highest rates in women, 12% to 26% versus children, up to 3%), myalgia, paresthesia
- Ocular: Ocular palsies
- Otic: Otitis media
- Renal: Conjunctivitis, retinitis, optic neuritis, papillitis, retrobulbar neuritis
- Respiratory: Bronchospasm, cough, pneumonitis, rhinitis
- Miscellaneous: Anaphylactoid reactions, anaphylaxis, atypical measles, panniculitis, regional lymphadenopathy

Mechanism of Action As a live, attenuated vaccine, MMR vaccine offers active immunity to disease caused by the measles, mumps, and rubella viruses.

Drug Interactions

Decreased Effect: The effect of the vaccine may be decreased in individuals who are receiving immunosuppressant drugs (including high dose systemic corticosteroids). Effect of vaccine may be decreased when given with immune globulin; do not administer with vaccine. Effectiveness of MMR may be decreased if given within 30 days of varicella vaccine (effectiveness not decreased when administered simultaneously).

Pregnancy Risk Factor C

Measles Virus Vaccine (Live) (MEE zels VYE rus vak SEEN, live)

Related Information

Immunizations (Vaccines) *on page 1614*

U.S. Brand Names Attenuvax®

Generic Available No

Synonyms More Attenuated Enders Strain; Rubeola Vaccine

Pharmacologic Category Vaccine, Live Virus

Use Adults born before 1957 are generally considered to be immune. All those born in or after 1957 without documentation of live vaccine on or after first birthday, physician-diagnosed measles, or laboratory evidence of immunity should be vaccinated, ideally with two doses of vaccine separated by no less than 1 month. For those previously vaccinated with one dose of measles vaccine, revaccination is recommended for students entering colleges and other institutions of higher education, for healthcare workers at the time of employment, and for international travelers who visit endemic areas.

MMR is the vaccine of choice if recipients are likely to be susceptible to rubella and/or mumps as well as to measles. Persons vaccinated between 1963 and 1967 with a killed measles vaccine, followed by live vaccine within 3 months, or with a vaccine of unknown type should be revaccinated with live measles virus vaccine.

Local Anesthetic/Vasoconstrictor Precautions No information available to require special precautions

Effects on Dental Treatment No significant effects or complications reported

Common Adverse Effects All serious adverse reactions must be reported to the U.S. Department of Health and Human Services (DHHS) Vaccine Adverse Event Reporting System (VAERS) 1-800-822-7967.

>10%:
- Cardiovascular: Edema
- Central nervous system: Fever (<100°F)
- Local: Burning or stinging, induration

1% to 10%:
- Central nervous system: Fever between 100°F and 103°F usually between 5th and 12th days postvaccination
- Dermatologic: Rash (rarely generalized)

Mechanism of Action Promotes active immunity to measles virus by inducing specific measles IgG and IgM antibodies.

Pregnancy Risk Factor X

Mebaral® *see* Mephobarbital *on page 873*

Mebendazole (me BEN da zole)

U.S. Brand Names Vermox®

Canadian Brand Names Vermox®

Mexican Brand Names Revapol®; Vermicol®; Vermidil®; Vermin®

Generic Available Yes

Pharmacologic Category Anthelmintic

Use Treatment of pinworms (*Enterobius vermicularis*), whipworms (*Trichuris trichiura*), roundworms (*Ascaris lumbricoides*), and hookworms (*Ancylostoma duodenale*)

Local Anesthetic/Vasoconstrictor Precautions No information available to require special precautions

Effects on Dental Treatment No significant effects or complications reported

Mechanism of Action Selectively and irreversibly blocks glucose uptake and other nutrients in susceptible adult intestine-dwelling helminths

Pregnancy Risk Factor C

Mecamylamine (mek a MIL a meen)

U.S. Brand Names Inversine®

Canadian Brand Names Inversine®

Generic Available No

Synonyms Mecamylamine Hydrochloride

Pharmacologic Category Ganglionic Blocking Agent

Use Treatment of moderately severe to severe hypertension and in uncomplicated malignant hypertension

Unlabeled/Investigational Use Tourette's syndrome

Local Anesthetic/Vasoconstrictor Precautions No information available to require special precautions

Effects on Dental Treatment Key adverse event(s) related to dental treatment: Xerostomia (normal salivary flow resumes upon discontinuation).

Mechanism of Action Mecamylamine is a ganglionic blocker. This agent inhibits acetylcholine at the autonomic ganglia, causing a decrease in blood pressure. Mecamylamine also blocks central nicotinic cholinergic receptors, which inhibits the effects of nicotine and may suppress the desire to smoke.

Pregnancy Risk Factor C

Mecamylamine Hydrochloride *see* Mecamylamine *on page 859*

Meclizine (MEK li zeen)

U.S. Brand Names Antivert®; Bonine® [OTC]; Dramamine® Less Drowsy Formula [OTC]

Canadian Brand Names Antivert®; Bonamine™; Bonine®

(Continued)

Meclizine *(Continued)*

Generic Available Yes

Synonyms Meclizine Hydrochloride; Meclozine Hydrochloride

Pharmacologic Category Antiemetic; Antihistamine

Use Prevention and treatment of symptoms of motion sickness; management of vertigo with diseases affecting the vestibular system

Local Anesthetic/Vasoconstrictor Precautions No information available to require special precautions

Effects on Dental Treatment Key adverse event(s) related to dental treatment: Slight to moderate drowsiness, thickening of bronchial secretions, significant xerostomia (normal salivary flow resumes upon discontinuation).

Common Adverse Effects

>10%:

Central nervous system: Slight to moderate drowsiness

Respiratory: Thickening of bronchial secretions

1% to 10%:

Central nervous system: Headache, fatigue, nervousness, dizziness

Gastrointestinal: Appetite increase, weight gain, nausea, diarrhea, abdominal pain, xerostomia

Neuromuscular & skeletal: Arthralgia

Respiratory: Pharyngitis

Mechanism of Action Has central anticholinergic action by blocking chemoreceptor trigger zone; decreases excitability of the middle ear labyrinth and blocks conduction in the middle ear vestibular-cerebellar pathways

Drug Interactions

Increased Effect/Toxicity: Increased toxicity with CNS depressants, neuroleptics, and anticholinergics.

Pharmacodynamics/Kinetics

Onset of action: ~1 hour

Duration: 8-24 hours

Metabolism: Hepatic

Half-life elimination: 6 hours

Excretion: Urine (as metabolites); feces (as unchanged drug)

Pregnancy Risk Factor B

Meclizine Hydrochloride *see* Meclizine *on page 859*

Meclofenamate (me kloe fen AM ate)

Related Information

Rheumatoid Arthritis, Osteoarthritis, and Osteoporosis *on page 1490*

Temporomandibular Dysfunction (TMD) *on page 1564*

Canadian Brand Names Meclomen®

Generic Available Yes

Synonyms Meclofenamate Sodium

Pharmacologic Category Nonsteroidal Anti-inflammatory Drug (NSAID), Oral

Use Treatment of inflammatory disorders, arthritis, mild to moderate pain, dysmenorrhea

Local Anesthetic/Vasoconstrictor Precautions No information available to require special precautions

Effects on Dental Treatment NSAID formulations are known to reversibly decrease platelet aggregation via mechanisms different than observed with aspirin. The dentist should be aware of the potential of abnormal coagulation. Caution should also be exercised in the use of NSAIDs in patients already on anticoagulant therapy with drugs such as warfarin (Coumadin®). Recovery of platelet function usually occurs 1-2 days after discontinuation of NSAIDs.

Common Adverse Effects

>10%:

Central nervous system: Dizziness

Dermatologic: Rash

Gastrointestinal: Abdominal cramps, heartburn, indigestion, nausea

1% to 10%:

Central nervous system: Headache, nervousness

Dermatologic: Itching

Endocrine & metabolic: Fluid retention

Gastrointestinal: Vomiting

Otic: Tinnitus

Mechanism of Action Inhibits prostaglandin synthesis by decreasing the activity of the enzyme, cyclooxygenase, which results in decreased formation of prostaglandin precursors

Drug Interactions

Increased Effect/Toxicity: Anticoagulants (warfarin, heparin, LMWHs) in combination with NSAIDs can cause increased risk of bleeding. Other antiplatelet drugs (ticlopidine, clopidogrel, aspirin, abciximab, dipyridamole, eptifibatide, tirofiban) can cause an increased risk of bleeding. NSAIDs may increase serum creatinine, potassium, blood pressure, and cyclosporine levels during concurrent therapy; monitor cyclosporine levels and renal function carefully. Lithium levels can be increased; avoid concurrent use if possible or monitor lithium levels and adjust dose. Sulindac may have the least effect. When NSAID is stopped, lithium will need adjustment again. Corticosteroids may increase the risk of GI ulceration; avoid concurrent use. Serum concentration/toxicity of methotrexate may be increased.

Decreased Effect: Antihypertensive effects of ACE inhibitors, angiotensin antagonists, diuretics, and hydralazine may be decreased by concurrent therapy with NSAIDs; monitor blood pressure. Cholestyramine and colestipol reduce the bioavailability of diclofenac; separate administration times.

Pharmacodynamics/Kinetics

Duration: 2-4 hours

Distribution: Crosses placenta

Protein binding: 99%

Half-life elimination: 2-3.3 hours

Time to peak, serum: 0.5-1.5 hours

Excretion: Primarily urine and feces (as metabolites)

Pregnancy Risk Factor B/D (3rd trimester)

Meclofenamate Sodium *see* Meclofenamate *on page 860*

Meclozine Hydrochloride *see* Meclizine *on page 859*

Medicinal Carbon *see* Charcoal *on page 303*

Medicinal Charcoal *see* Charcoal *on page 303*

Medicone® [OTC] *see* Phenylephrine *on page 1078*

Mediplast® [OTC] *see* Salicylic Acid *on page 1205*

Medi-Synal [OTC] *see* Acetaminophen and Pseudoephedrine *on page 53*

Medium Chain Triglycerides

(mee DEE um chane trye GLIS er ides)

U.S. Brand Names MCT Oil® [OTC]

Canadian Brand Names MCT Oil®

Generic Available No

Synonyms Triglycerides, Medium Chain

Pharmacologic Category Nutritional Supplement

Use Dietary supplement for those who cannot digest long chain fats; malabsorption associated with disorders such as pancreatic insufficiency, bile salt deficiency, and bacterial overgrowth of the small bowel; induce ketosis as a prevention for seizures (akinetic, clonic, and petit mal)

Local Anesthetic/Vasoconstrictor Precautions No information available to require special precautions

Effects on Dental Treatment No significant effects or complications reported

Common Adverse Effects Frequency not defined.

Central nervous system: May result in **narcosis** and **coma** in cirrhotic patients due to high levels of medium chain fatty acids in the serum which then enter the cerebral spinal fluid; electroencephalogram effects include slowing of the alpha wave (can occur during infusion of fatty acids of 2-6 carbon lengths)

Endocrine & metabolic:

MCT therapy does not produce recognized metabolic side effects of any clinical importance, nor do they interfere with the metabolism of other food stuffs or with the absorption of drugs; when administered in the form of a mixed diet with carbohydrates and protein, there is no clinical evidence of **hyperketonemia**; hyperketonemia may occur in normal or diabetic subjects in the absence of carbohydrates; has been reported that MCT may increase hepatic free fatty acid synthesis and reduce ketone clearance

Fecal water, sodium and potassium excretion are decreased in patients with steatorrhea who are treated with MCT; enhanced calcium absorption has been demonstrated in patients with steatorrhea who are given MCT

Gastrointestinal: Nausea, occasional vomiting, gastritis and distention, diarrhea, and borborygmi are common adverse reactions occurring in about 10% of the patients receiving supplements or diets containing MCT; these symptoms may be related to rapid hydrolysis of MCT, high concentrations of free fatty acids in the stomach and small intestine, hyperosmolarity causing influx of large amounts of fluid, and lactose intolerance; abdominal cramps, nausea

(Continued)

Medium Chain Triglycerides *(Continued)*

and vomiting occurred despite cautionary administration of MCT in small sips throughout meals, but subsided with continued administration

Pregnancy Risk Factor C

Medrol® *see* MethylPREDNISolone *on page 910*

MedroxyPROGESTERone (me DROKS ee proe JES te rone)

Related Information

Endocrine Disorders and Pregnancy *on page 1481*

U.S. Brand Names Depo-Provera®; Depo-Provera® Contraceptive; Provera®

Canadian Brand Names Alti-MPA; Apo-Medroxy®; Depo-Prevera®; Gen-Medroxy; Novo-Medrone; Provera®

Generic Available Yes: Tablet

Synonyms Acetoxymethylprogesterone; Medroxyprogesterone Acetate; Methylacetoxyprogesterone

Pharmacologic Category Contraceptive; Progestin

Use Endometrial carcinoma or renal carcinoma as well as secondary amenorrhea or abnormal uterine bleeding due to hormonal imbalance; reduction of endometrial hyperplasia in postmenopausal women receiving 0.625 mg conjugated estrogens for 12-14 consecutive days per month; Depo-Provera® injection is used for the prevention of pregnancy

Unlabeled/Investigational Use Hypoventilation disorders, advanced breast cancer

Local Anesthetic/Vasoconstrictor Precautions No information available to require special precautions

Effects on Dental Treatment Progestins may predispose the patient to gingival bleeding.

Common Adverse Effects Frequency not defined.

Cardiovascular: Edema, embolism, central thrombosis

Central nervous system: Mental depression, fever, insomnia, somnolence, headache (rare), dizziness

Dermatologic: Melasma or chloasma, allergic rash with or without pruritus, acne, hirsutism, angioneurotic edema

Endocrine & metabolic: Breakthrough bleeding, spotting, changes in menstrual flow, amenorrhea, increased breast tenderness, changes in cervical erosion and secretions

Gastrointestinal: Weight gain/loss, anorexia, nausea

Hepatic: Cholestatic jaundice

Local: Pain at injection site, sterile abscess, thrombophlebitis

Neuromuscular & skeletal: Weakness

Respiratory: Pulmonary embolism

Miscellaneous: Anaphylaxis

Mechanism of Action Inhibits secretion of pituitary gonadotropins, which prevents follicular maturation and ovulation, stimulates growth of mammary tissue

Drug Interactions

Cytochrome P450 Effect: Substrate of CYP3A4 (major); **Induces** CYP3A4 (weak)

Decreased Effect: Aminoglutethimide may decrease effects by increasing hepatic metabolism. CYP3A4 inducers may decrease the levels/effects of medroxyprogesterone; example inducers include aminoglutethimide, carbamazepine, nafcillin, nevirapine, phenobarbital, phenytoin, and rifamycins.

Pharmacodynamics/Kinetics

Absorption: Oral: Well absorbed; I.M.: Slow

Protein binding: 90% primarily to albumin; not to sex hormone-binding globulin

Metabolism: Oral: Hepatic via hydroxylated and conjugated

Bioavailability: 0.6% to 10%

Time to peak: Oral: 2-4 hours

Half-life elimination: Oral: 38-46 hours; I.M.: Acetate: 50 days

Excretion: Oral: Urine and feces

Pregnancy Risk Factor X

Medroxyprogesterone Acetate *see* MedroxyPROGESTERone *on page 862*

Medroxyprogesterone Acetate and Estradiol Cypionate *see* Estradiol and Medroxyprogesterone *on page 520*

Medroxyprogesterone and Estrogens (Conjugated) *see* Estrogens (Conjugated/Equine) and Medroxyprogesterone *on page 528*

Medrysone (ME dri sone)

U.S. Brand Names HMS Liquifilm®

Generic Available No

Pharmacologic Category Corticosteroid, Ophthalmic

Use Treatment of allergic conjunctivitis, vernal conjunctivitis, episcleritis, ophthalmic epinephrine sensitivity reaction

Local Anesthetic/Vasoconstrictor Precautions No information available to require special precautions

Effects on Dental Treatment No significant effects or complications reported

Mechanism of Action Decreases inflammation by suppression of migration of polymorphonuclear leukocytes and reversal of increased capillary permeability

Pregnancy Risk Factor C

Mefenamic Acid (me fe NAM ik AS id)

Related Information

Rheumatoid Arthritis, Osteoarthritis, and Osteoporosis *on page 1490*
Temporomandibular Dysfunction (TMD) *on page 1564*

U.S. Brand Names Ponstel®

Canadian Brand Names Apo-Mefenamic®; Nu-Mefenamic; PMS-Mefenamic Acid; Ponstan®; Ponstel®

Mexican Brand Names Ponstan®

Generic Available No

Pharmacologic Category Nonsteroidal Anti-inflammatory Drug (NSAID), Oral

Use Short-term relief of mild to moderate pain including primary dysmenorrhea

Local Anesthetic/Vasoconstrictor Precautions No information available to require special precautions

Effects on Dental Treatment NSAID formulations are known to reversibly decrease platelet aggregation via mechanisms different than observed with aspirin. The dentist should be aware of the potential of abnormal coagulation. Caution should also be exercised in the use of NSAIDs in patients already on anticoagulant therapy with drugs such as warfarin (Coumadin®). Recovery of platelet function usually occurs 1-2 days after discontinuation of NSAIDs.

Common Adverse Effects 1% to 10%:

Central nervous system: Headache, nervousness, dizziness (3% to 9%)
Dermatologic: Itching, rash
Endocrine & metabolic: Fluid retention
Gastrointestinal: Abdominal cramps, heartburn, indigestion, nausea (1% to 10%), vomiting (1% to 10%), diarrhea (1% to 10%), constipation (1% to 10%), abdominal distress/cramping/pain (1% to 10%), dyspepsia (1% to 10%), flatulence (1% to 10%), gastric or duodenal ulcer with bleeding or perforation (1% to 10%), gastritis (1% to 10%)
Hematologic: Bleeding (1% to 10%)
Hepatic: Elevated LFTs (1% to 10%)
Otic: Tinnitus (1% to 10%)

Mechanism of Action Inhibits prostaglandin synthesis by decreasing the activity of the enzyme, cyclooxygenase, which results in decreased formation of prostaglandin precursors

Drug Interactions

Cytochrome P450 Effect: Substrate of CYP2C8/9 (minor); **Inhibits** CYP2C8/9 (strong)

Increased Effect/Toxicity: Anticoagulants (warfarin, heparin, LMWHs) in combination with NSAIDs can cause increased risk of bleeding. Other antiplatelet drugs (ticlopidine, clopidogrel, aspirin, abciximab, dipyridamole, eptifibatide, tirofiban) can cause an increased risk of bleeding. Mefenamic acid may increase the levels/effects of CYP2C8/9 substrates (eg, amiodarone, fluoxetine, glimepiride, glipizide, nateglinide, phenytoin, pioglitazone, rosiglitazone, sertraline, warfarin). NSAIDs may increase serum creatinine, potassium, blood pressure, and cyclosporine levels during concurrent therapy; monitor cyclosporine levels and renal function carefully. Lithium levels can be increased; avoid concurrent use if possible or monitor lithium levels and adjust dose. Sulindac may have the least effect. When NSAID is stopped, lithium will need adjustment again. Corticosteroids may increase the risk of GI ulceration; avoid concurrent use. Serum concentration/toxicity of methotrexate may be increased.

Decreased Effect: Antihypertensive effects of ACE inhibitors, angiotensin antagonists, diuretics, and hydralazine may be decreased by concurrent therapy with NSAIDs; monitor blood pressure. Cholestyramine and colestipol reduce the bioavailability of diclofenac; separate administration times.

(Continued)

Mefenamic Acid *(Continued)*

Pharmacodynamics/Kinetics

Onset of action: Peak effect: 2-4 hours

Duration: ≤6 hours

Protein binding: High

Metabolism: Conjugated hepatically

Half-life elimination: 3.5 hours

Excretion: Urine (50%) and feces as unchanged drug and metabolites

Pregnancy Risk Factor C/D (3rd trimester)

Mefloquine (ME floe kwin)

U.S. Brand Names Lariam®

Canadian Brand Names Apo-Mefloquine®; Lariam®

Generic Available Yes

Synonyms Mefloquine Hydrochloride

Pharmacologic Category Antimalarial Agent

Use Treatment of acute malarial infections and prevention of malaria

Local Anesthetic/Vasoconstrictor Precautions No information available to require special precautions

Effects on Dental Treatment No significant effects or complications reported

Common Adverse Effects

Frequency not defined: Neuropsychiatric events

1% to 10%:

- Central nervous system: Headache, fever, chills, fatigue
- Dermatologic: Rash
- Gastrointestinal: Vomiting (3%), diarrhea, stomach pain, nausea, appetite decreased
- Neuromuscular & skeletal: Myalgia
- Otic: Tinnitus

Restrictions A medication guide must be provided to all patients when mefloquine is dispensed.

Mechanism of Action Mefloquine is a quinoline-methanol compound structurally similar to quinine; mefloquine's effectiveness in the treatment and prophylaxis of malaria is due to the destruction of the asexual blood forms of the malarial pathogens that affect humans, *Plasmodium falciparum*, *P. vivax*, *P. malariae*, *P. ovale*

Drug Interactions

Cytochrome P450 Effect: Substrate of CYP3A4 (major); **Inhibits** CYP2D6 (weak), 3A4 (weak)

Increased Effect/Toxicity: Use caution with drugs that alter cardiac conduction; increased toxicity with chloroquine, quinine, and quinidine (hold treatment until at least 12 hours after these later drugs); increased toxicity with halofantrine (concurrent use is contraindicated). CYP3A4 inhibitors may increase the levels/effects of mefloquine; example inhibitors include azole antifungals, ciprofloxacin, clarithromycin, diclofenac, doxycycline, erythromycin, imatinib, isoniazid, nefazodone, nicardipine, propofol, protease inhibitors, quinidine, and verapamil.

Decreased Effect: Mefloquine may decrease the effect of valproic acid, carbamazepine, phenobarbital, and phenytoin. CYP3A4 inducers may decrease the levels/effects of mefloquine; example inducers include aminoglutethimide, carbamazepine, nafcillin, nevirapine, phenobarbital, phenytoin, and rifamycins.

Pharmacodynamics/Kinetics

Absorption: Well absorbed

Distribution: V_d: 19 L/kg; blood, urine, CSF, tissues; enters breast milk

Protein binding: 98%

Metabolism: Extensively hepatic; main metabolite is inactive

Bioavailability: Increased by food

Half-life elimination: 21-22 days

Time to peak, plasma: 6-24 hours (median: ~17 hours)

Excretion: Primarily bile and feces; urine (9% as unchanged drug, 4% as primary metabolite)

Pregnancy Risk Factor C

Mefloquine Hydrochloride *see* Mefloquine *on page 864*

Mefoxin® *see* Cefoxitin *on page 284*

Megace® *see* Megestrol *on page 865*

Megadophilus® [OTC] *see Lactobacillus on page 793*

Megestrol (me JES trole)

U.S. Brand Names Megace®

Canadian Brand Names Apo-Megestrol®; Lin-Megestrol; Megace®; Megace® OS; Nu-Megestrol

Generic Available Yes

Synonyms 5071-1DL(6); Megestrol Acetate; NSC-10363

Pharmacologic Category Antineoplastic Agent, Hormone; Appetite Stimulant; Progestin

Use Palliative treatment of breast and endometrial carcinoma

Orphan drug: Treatment of anorexia, cachexia, or significant weight loss (≥10% baseline body weight) and confirmed diagnosis of AIDS

Unlabeled/Investigational Use Uterine bleeding

Local Anesthetic/Vasoconstrictor Precautions No information available to require special precautions

Effects on Dental Treatment No significant effects or complications reported

Common Adverse Effects

Cardiovascular: Edema, hypertension (≤8%), cardiomyopathy, palpitations

Central nervous system: Insomnia, fever (2% to 6%), headache (≤10%), pain (≤6%, similar to placebo), confusion (1% to 3%), convulsions (1% to 3%), depression (1% to 3%)

Dermatologic: Allergic rash (2% to 12%) with or without pruritus, alopecia

Endocrine & metabolic: Breakthrough bleeding and amenorrhea, spotting, changes in menstrual flow, changes in cervical erosion and secretions, increased breast tenderness, changes in vaginal bleeding pattern, edema, fluid retention, hyperglycemia (≤6%), diabetes, HPA axis suppression, adrenal insufficiency, Cushing's syndrome

Gastrointestinal: Weight gain (not attributed to edema or fluid retention), nausea, vomiting (7%), diarrhea (8% to 15%, similar to placebo), flatulence (≤10%), constipation (1% to 3%)

Genitourinary: Impotence (4% to 14%), decreased libido (≤5%)

Hepatic: Cholestatic jaundice, hepatotoxicity, hepatomegaly (1% to 3%)

Local: Thrombophlebitis

Neuromuscular & skeletal: Carpal tunnel syndrome, weakness, paresthesia (1% to 3%)

Respiratory: Hyperpnea, dyspnea (1% to 3%), cough (1% to 3%)

Miscellaneous: Diaphoresis

Mechanism of Action A synthetic progestin with antiestrogenic properties which disrupt the estrogen receptor cycle. Megestrol interferes with the normal estrogen cycle and results in a lower LH titer. May also have a direct effect on the endometrium. Megestrol is an antineoplastic progestin thought to act through an antileutenizing effect mediated via the pituitary.

Pharmacodynamics/Kinetics

Absorption: Well absorbed orally

Metabolism: Completely hepatic to free steroids and glucuronide conjugates

Time to peak, serum: 1-3 hours

Half-life elimination: 15-100 hours

Excretion: Urine (57% to 78% as steroid metabolites and inactive compound); feces (8% to 30%)

Pregnancy Risk Factor X

Megestrol Acetate *see* Megestrol *on page 865*

Melanex® *see* Hydroquinone *on page 719*

Melfiat® *see* Phendimetrazine *on page 1072*

Mellaril® [DSC] *see* Thioridazine *on page 1289*

Meloxicam (mel OKS i kam)

U.S. Brand Names MOBIC®

Canadian Brand Names MOBIC®; Mobicox®

Mexican Brand Names Masflex®; Mobicox®

Generic Available No

Pharmacologic Category Nonsteroidal Anti-inflammatory Drug (NSAID), Oral

Use Relief of signs and symptoms of osteoarthritis

Local Anesthetic/Vasoconstrictor Precautions No information available to require special precautions

Effects on Dental Treatment Key adverse event(s) related to dental treatment: Taste perversion, ulcerative stomatitis, and xerostomia (normal salivary flow resumes upon discontinuation).

Common Adverse Effects 2% to 10%:

Cardiovascular: Edema (2% to 5%)

(Continued)

Meloxicam *(Continued)*

Central nervous system: Headache and dizziness occurred in 2% to 8% of patients, but occurred less frequently than placebo in controlled trials
Dermatologic: Rash (1% to 3%)
Gastrointestinal: Diarrhea (3% to 8%), dyspepsia (5%), nausea (4%), flatulence (3%), abdominal pain (2% to 3%)
Respiratory: Upper respiratory infection (2% to 3%), pharyngitis (1% to 3%)
Miscellaneous: Flu-like symptoms (5% to 6%), falls (3%)

Mechanism of Action Inhibits prostaglandin synthesis by decreasing the activity of the enzyme, cyclooxygenase, which results in decreased formation of prostaglandin precursors

Drug Interactions

Cytochrome P450 Effect: Substrate (minor) of CYP2C8/9, 3A4; **Inhibits** CYP2C8/9 (weak)

Increased Effect/Toxicity: Anticoagulants (warfarin, heparin, LMWHs) in combination with NSAIDs can cause increased risk of bleeding. Antiplatelet drugs (ticlopidine, clopidogrel, aspirin, abciximab, dipyridamole, eptifibatide, tirofiban) can cause an increased risk of bleeding. Aspirin increases serum concentrations (AUC) of meloxicam (in addition to potential for additive adverse effects); concurrent use is not recommended. Corticosteroids may increase the risk of GI ulceration; avoid concurrent use. NSAIDs may increase serum creatinine, potassium, blood pressure, and cyclosporine levels; monitor cyclosporine levels and renal function carefully. Lithium levels can be increased; avoid concurrent use if possible or monitor lithium levels and adjust dose. When NSAID is stopped, lithium will need adjustment again. Serum concentration/toxicity of methotrexate may be increased. Warfarin INRs may be increased by meloxicam. Monitor INR closely, particularly during initiation or change in dose. May increase risk of bleeding. Use lowest possible dose for shortest duration possible.

Decreased Effect: Cholestyramine (and possibly colestipol) increases the clearance of meloxicam. Hydralazine's antihypertensive effect is decreased; avoid concurrent use. Loop diuretic efficacy (diuretic and antihypertensive effect) may be reduced by NSAIDs. Antihypertensive effects of thiazide diuretics are decreased; avoid concurrent use.

Pharmacodynamics/Kinetics

Distribution: 10 L
Protein binding: 99.4%
Metabolism: Hepatic via CYP2C9 and CYP3A4 (minor)
Bioavailability: 89%
Half-life elimination: 15-20 hours
Time to peak: 5-10 hours
Excretion: Urine and feces (as inactive metabolites)

Pregnancy Risk Factor C/D (3rd trimester)

Melpaque HP® *see* Hydroquinone *on page 719*

Melphalan (MEL fa lan)

U.S. Brand Names Alkeran®
Canadian Brand Names Alkeran®
Mexican Brand Names Alkeran®
Generic Available No
Synonyms L-PAM; L-Sarcolysin; Phenylalanine Mustard
Pharmacologic Category Antineoplastic Agent, Alkylating Agent
Use Palliative treatment of multiple myeloma and nonresectable epithelial ovarian carcinoma; neuroblastoma, rhabdomyosarcoma, breast cancer
Local Anesthetic/Vasoconstrictor Precautions No information available to require special precautions
Effects on Dental Treatment Key adverse event(s) related to dental treatment: Stomatitis.

Common Adverse Effects

>10%: Hematologic: Myelosuppressive: Leukopenia and thrombocytopenia are the most common effects of melphalan; irreversible bone marrow failure has been reported
WBC: Moderate
Platelets: Moderate
Onset: 7 days
Nadir: 8-10 days and 27-32 days
Recovery: 42-50 days

1% to 10%:
Cardiovascular: Vasculitis
Dermatologic: Vesiculation of skin, alopecia, pruritus, rash

Endocrine & metabolic: SIADH, sterility, amenorrhea

Gastrointestinal: Nausea and vomiting are mild; stomatitis and diarrhea are infrequent

Genitourinary: Hemorrhagic cystitis, bladder irritation

Hematologic: Anemia, agranulocytosis, hemolytic anemia

Hepatic: Transaminases increased (hepatitis, jaundice have been reported)

Respiratory: Pulmonary fibrosis, interstitial pneumonitis

Miscellaneous: Hypersensitivity, secondary malignancy

Mechanism of Action Alkylating agent which is a derivative of mechlorethamine that inhibits DNA and RNA synthesis via formation of carbonium ions; cross-links strands of DNA

Drug Interactions

Increased Effect/Toxicity: Cyclosporine: Risk of nephrotoxicity is increased by melphalan.

Decreased Effect: Cimetidine and other H_2 antagonists: The reduction in gastric pH has been reported to decrease bioavailability of melphalan by 30%.

Pharmacodynamics/Kinetics

Absorption: Oral: Variable and incomplete

Distribution: V_d: 0.5-0.6 L/kg throughout total body water

Bioavailability: Unpredictable, decreasing from 85% to 58% with repeated doses

Half-life elimination: Terminal: 1.5 hours

Time to peak, serum: ~2 hours

Excretion: Oral: Feces (20% to 50%); urine (10% to 30% as unchanged drug)

Pregnancy Risk Factor D

Melquin-3® *see* Hydroquinone *on page 719*

Melquin HP® *see* Hydroquinone *on page 719*

Memantine (me MAN teen)

U.S. Brand Names Namenda™

Generic Available No

Synonyms Memantine Hydrochloride

Pharmacologic Category N-Methyl-D-Aspartate Receptor Antagonist

Use Treatment of moderate-to-severe dementia of the Alzheimer's type

Local Anesthetic/Vasoconstrictor Precautions No information available to require special precautions

Effects on Dental Treatment No significant effects or complications reported

Common Adverse Effects

1% to 10%:

Cardiovascular: Hypertension (4%), cardiac failure, syncope, cerebrovascular accident, transient ischemic attack

Central nervous system: Dizziness (7%), confusion (6%), headache (6%), hallucinations (3%), pain (3%), somnolence (3%), fatigue (2%), aggressive reaction, ataxia, vertigo

Dermatologic: Rash

Gastrointestinal: Constipation (5%), vomiting (3%), weight loss

Genitourinary: Micturition

Hematologic: Anemia

Hepatic: Alkaline phosphatase increased

Neuromuscular & skeletal: Back pain (3%), hypokinesia

Ocular: Cataract, conjunctivitis

Respiratory: Cough (4%), dyspnea (2%), pneumonia

Mechanism of Action Memantine reduces the decline in function in Alzheimer's disease by binding to N-methyl-D-aspartate (NMDA) receptors and blocking the actions of glutamate. Glutamate is an amino acid which may contribute to the pathogenesis of Alzheimer's disease by over-stimulating the NMDA receptor. Memantine does not prevent or slow neurodegeneration associated with Alzheimer's disease.

Drug Interactions

Increased Effect/Toxicity: Clearance of memantine is decreased 80% at urinary pH 8; use caution with medications (carbonic anhydrase inhibitors, sodium bicarbonate) which may increase urinary pH.

Pharmacodynamics/Kinetics

Distribution: 9-11 L/kg

Protein binding: 45%

Metabolism: Forms three metabolites (minimal activity)

Half-life elimination: Terminal: 60-80 hours

Time to peak, serum: 3-7 hours

Excretion: Urine (57% to 82% unchanged); excretion affected by urine pH

Pregnancy Risk Factor B

Memantine Hydrochloride *see* Memantine *on page 867*

Menadol® [OTC] *see* Ibuprofen *on page 728*

Menest® *see* Estrogens (Esterified) *on page 529*

Meningococcal Polysaccharide Vaccine (Groups A, C, Y, and W-135)

(me NIN joe kok al pol i SAK a ride vak SEEN groops aye, see, why & dubl yoo won thur tee fyve)

Related Information

Immunizations (Vaccines) *on page 1614*

U.S. Brand Names Menomune®-A/C/Y/W-135

Generic Available No

Pharmacologic Category Vaccine

Use Provide active immunity to meningococcal serogroups contained in the vaccine; prevention and control of outbreaks of serogroup C meningococcal disease; recommended for use in:

Immunization of persons ≥2 years of age in epidemic or endemic areas as might be determined in a population delineated by neighborhood, school, dormitory, or other reasonable boundary. The prevalent serogroup in such a situation should match a serogroup in the vaccine. Individuals at particular high-risk include persons with terminal component complement deficiencies and those with anatomic or functional asplenia.

Travelers visiting areas of a country that are recognized as having hyperendemic or epidemic meningococcal disease

Vaccinations should be considered for household or institutional contacts of persons with meningococcal disease as an adjunct to appropriate antibiotic chemoprophylaxis as well as medical and laboratory personnel at risk of exposure to meningococcal disease

Local Anesthetic/Vasoconstrictor Precautions No information available to require special precautions

Effects on Dental Treatment No significant effects or complications reported

Common Adverse Effects All serious adverse reactions must be reported to the U.S. Department of Health and Human Services (DHHS) Vaccine Adverse Event Reporting System (VAERS) 1-800-822-7967. Incidence of erythema, swelling, or tenderness may be higher in children

>10%: Local: Tenderness (9% to 36% as reported in adults)

1% to 10%:

Central nervous system: Headache (2% to 5%), malaise (2%), fever (100°F to 106°F: 3%), chills (2%)

Local: Pain at injection site (2% to 3%), erythema (1% to 4%), induration (1% to 4%)

Mechanism of Action Induces the formation of bactericidal antibodies to meningococcal antigens; the presence of these antibodies is strongly correlated with immunity to meningococcal disease caused by *Neisseria meningitidis* groups A, C, Y and W-135.

Drug Interactions

Increased Effect/Toxicity: Should not be administered with whole-cell pertussis or whole-cell typhoid vaccines due to combined endotoxin content.

Decreased Effect: Decreased effect with administration of immunoglobulin within 1 month.

Pharmacodynamics/Kinetics

Onset of action: Antibody levels: 7-10 days

Duration: Antibodies against group A and C polysaccharides decline markedly (to prevaccination levels) over the first 3 years following a single dose of vaccine, especially in children <4 years of age

Pregnancy Risk Factor C

Menomune®-A/C/Y/W-135 *see* Meningococcal Polysaccharide Vaccine (Groups A, C, Y, and W-135) *on page 868*

Menostar™ *see* Estradiol *on page 518*

Menotropins (men oh TROE pins)

U.S. Brand Names Pergonal®; Repronex®

Canadian Brand Names Pergonal®; Repronex®

Mexican Brand Names HMG Massone® [inj.]; Humegon®

Generic Available No

Pharmacologic Category Gonadotropin; Ovulation Stimulator

Use Sequentially with hCG to induce ovulation and pregnancy in the infertile woman with functional anovulation or in patients who have previously received pituitary suppression; stimulation of multiple follicle development in ovulatory patients as part of an *in vitro* fertilization program; used with hCG in men to stimulate spermatogenesis in those with primary hypogonadotropic hypogonadism

Local Anesthetic/Vasoconstrictor Precautions No information available to require special precautions

Effects on Dental Treatment No significant effects or complications reported

Common Adverse Effects

Male:

>10%: Endocrine & metabolic: Gynecomastia

1% to 10%: Erythrocytosis (dyspnea, dizziness, anorexia, syncope, epistaxis)

Female:

1% to 10%:

Central nervous system: Headache

Endocrine & metabolic: Breast tenderness

Gastrointestinal: Abdominal cramping, abdominal pain, diarrhea, enlarged abdomen, nausea, vomiting

Genitourinary: Ectopic pregnancy, OHSS (% is dose related), ovarian disease, vaginal hemorrhage

Local: Injection site edema/reaction

Miscellaneous: Infection, pelvic pain

Percentage not reported:

Cardiovascular: Stroke, tachycardia, thrombosis (venous or arterial)

Central nervous system: Dizziness

Dermatologic: Angioedema, urticaria

Genitourinary: Adnexal torsion, hemoperitoneum, ovarian enlargement

Neuromuscular & skeletal: Limb necrosis

Respiratory: Acute respiratory distress syndrome, atelectasis, dyspnea, embolism, laryngeal edema pulmonary infarction tachypnea

Miscellaneous: Allergic reactions, anaphylaxis, rash

Mechanism of Action Actions occur as a result of both follicle stimulating hormone (FSH) effects and luteinizing hormone (LH) effects; menotropins stimulate the development and maturation of the ovarian follicle (FSH), cause ovulation (LH), and stimulate the development of the corpus luteum (LH); in males it stimulates spermatogenesis (LH)

Drug Interactions

Increased Effect/Toxicity: Clomiphene may decrease the amount of human menopausal gonadotropin (HMG) needed to induce ovulation (Gonadorelin, Factrel®); should not be used with drugs that stimulate ovulation.

Pharmacodynamics/Kinetics Excretion: Urine (~10% as unchanged drug)

Pregnancy Risk Factor X

Mentax® *see* Butenafine *on page 239*

Mepenzolate (me PEN zoe late)

U.S. Brand Names Cantil®

Canadian Brand Names Cantil®

Generic Available No

Synonyms Mepenzolate Bromide

Pharmacologic Category Anticholinergic Agent; Antispasmodic Agent, Gastrointestinal

Use Adjunctive treatment of peptic ulcer disease

Local Anesthetic/Vasoconstrictor Precautions No information available to require special precautions

Effects on Dental Treatment Key adverse event(s) related to dental treatment: Xerostomia (normal salivary flow resumes upon discontinuation) and dry throat.

Common Adverse Effects Frequency not defined.

Cardiovascular: Palpitations, tachycardia

Central nervous system: Headache, nervousness, drowsiness, dizziness, CNS stimulation may be produced with large doses, confusion, insomnia

Dermatologic: Dry skin, urticaria

Gastrointestinal: Constipation, xerostomia, dysphagia, nausea, vomiting, delayed gastric emptying, loss of taste

Genitourinary: Impotence, urinary hesitation, urinary retention

Neuromuscular & skeletal: Weakness

Ophthalmic: Cycloplegia, blurred vision, ocular tension increased, pupil dilation

(Continued)

Mepenzolate *(Continued)*

Miscellaneous: Diaphoresis decreased, hypersensitivity reactions, anaphylaxis, lactation suppressed

Mechanism of Action Mepenzolate is a post-ganglionic parasympathetic inhibitor. It decreases gastric acid and pepsin secretion and suppresses spontaneous contractions of the colon.

Pharmacodynamics/Kinetics

Absorption: Oral: Low

Excretion: Urine (3% to 33%); feces

Pregnancy Risk Factor B

Mepenzolate Bromide *see* Mepenzolate *on page 869*

Mepergan *see* Meperidine and Promethazine *on page 872*

Meperidine (me PER i deen)

Related Information

Oral Pain *on page 1526*

U.S. Brand Names Demerol®; Meperitab®

Canadian Brand Names Demerol®

Generic Available Yes

Synonyms Isonipecaine Hydrochloride; Meperidine Hydrochloride; Pethidine Hydrochloride

Pharmacologic Category Analgesic, Narcotic

Dental Use Adjunct in preoperative intravenous conscious sedation in patients undergoing dental surgery; alternate oral narcotic in patients allergic to codeine to treat moderate to moderate-severe pain

Use Management of moderate to severe pain; adjunct to anesthesia and preoperative sedation

Local Anesthetic/Vasoconstrictor Precautions No information available to require special precautions

Effects on Dental Treatment Key adverse event(s) related to dental treatment: Xerostomia (normal salivary flow resumes upon discontinuation).

Significant Adverse Effects Frequency not defined.

Cardiovascular: Hypotension

Central nervous system: Fatigue, drowsiness, dizziness, nervousness, headache, restlessness, malaise, confusion, mental depression, hallucinations, paradoxical CNS stimulation, increased intracranial pressure, seizures (associated with metabolite accumulation)

Dermatologic: Rash, urticaria

Gastrointestinal: Nausea, vomiting, constipation, anorexia, stomach cramps, xerostomia, biliary spasm, paralytic ileus

Genitourinary: Ureteral spasms, decreased urination

Local: Pain at injection site

Neuromuscular & skeletal: Weakness

Respiratory: Dyspnea

Miscellaneous: Histamine release, physical and psychological dependence

Restrictions C-II

Dosage Note: Doses should be titrated to necessary analgesic effect. When changing route of administration, note that oral doses are about half as effective as parenteral dose. Oral route not recommended for chronic pain. These are guidelines and do not represent the maximum doses that may be required in all patients.

Children: Pain: Oral, I.M., I.V., SubQ: 1-1.5 mg/kg/dose every 3-4 hours as needed; 1-2 mg/kg as a single dose preoperative medication may be used; maximum 100 mg/dose

Adults: Pain:

- Oral: Initial: Opiate-naive: 50 mg every 3-4 hours as needed; usual dosage range: 50-150 mg every 2-4 hours as needed
- I.M., SubQ: Initial: Opiate-naive: 50-75 mg every 3-4 hours as needed; patients with prior opiate exposure may require higher initial doses; usual dosage range: 50-150 mg every 2-4 hours as needed
  - Preoperatively: 50-100 mg given 30-90 minutes before the beginning of anesthesia
- Slow I.V.: Initial: 5-10 mg every 5 minutes as needed
- Patient-controlled analgesia (PCA): Usual concentration: 10 mg/mL
  - Initial dose: 10 mg
  - Demand dose: 1-5 mg (manufacturer recommendations); range 5-25 mg (American Pain Society, 1999).
  - Lockout interval: 5-10 minutes

Elderly:

Oral: 50 mg every 4 hours

I.M.: 25 mg every 4 hours

Dosing adjustment in renal impairment: Avoid repeated administration of meperidine in renal dysfunction:

Cl_{cr} 10-50 mL/minute: Administer at 75% of normal dose

Cl_{cr} <10 mL/minute: Administer at 50% of normal dose

Dosing adjustment/comments in hepatic disease: Increased narcotic effect in cirrhosis; reduction in dose more important for oral than I.V. route

Mechanism of Action Binds to opiate receptors in the CNS, causing inhibition of ascending pain pathways, altering the perception of and response to pain; produces generalized CNS depression

Contraindications Hypersensitivity to meperidine or any component of the formulation; patients receiving MAO inhibitors presently or in the past 14 days; pregnancy (prolonged use or high doses near term)

Warnings/Precautions An opioid-containing analgesic regimen should be tailored to each patient's needs and based upon the type of pain being treated (acute versus chronic), the route of administration, degree of tolerance for opioids (naive versus chronic user), age, weight, and medical condition. The optimal analgesic dose varies widely among patients. Doses should be titrated to pain relief/prevention. Use for chronic pain management not recommended. Oral meperidine not recommended for acute pain management.

Use with caution in patients with pulmonary, hepatic, renal disorders, or increased intracranial pressure; use with caution in patients with renal failure or seizure disorders or those receiving high-dose meperidine; normeperidine (an active metabolite and CNS stimulant) may accumulate and precipitate twitches, tremors, or seizures; some preparations contain sulfites which may cause allergic reaction; not recommended as a drug of first choice for the treatment of chronic pain in the elderly due to the accumulation of normeperidine; for acute pain, its use should be limited to 1-2 doses; tolerance or drug dependence may result from extended use. Use only with extreme caution **(if at all)** in patients with head injury or increased intracranial pressure (ICP); potential to elevate ICP may be greatly exaggerated in these patients.

Drug Interactions

Acyclovir: May increase meperidine metabolite concentrations. Use caution.

Barbiturates: May decrease analgesic efficacy and increase sedative and/or respiratory depressive effects of meperidine.

Cimetidine: May increase meperidine metabolite concentrations; use caution.

CNS depressants (including benzodiazepines): May potentiate the sedative and/or respiratory depressive effects of meperidine.

MAO inhibitors: Greatly potentiate the effects of meperidine; acute opioid overdosage symptoms can be seen, including severe toxic reactions. Concurrent use within 14 days of an MAO inhibitor is contraindicated.

Phenothiazines: May potentiate the sedative and/or respiratory depressive effects of meperidine; may increase the incidence of hypotension.

Phenytoin: May decrease the analgesic effects of meperidine

Ritonavir: May increase meperidine metabolite concentrations; use caution.

Serotonin agonists: Serotonin agonists may enhance the adverse/toxic effect of meperidine. Serotonin syndrome may occur.

Serotonin reuptake inhibitors: May potentiate the effects of meperidine; including severe toxic reactions

Tricyclic antidepressants: May potentiate the sedative and/or respiratory depressive effects of meperidine. In addition, potentially may increase the risk of serotonin syndrome.

Ethanol/Nutrition/Herb Interactions

Ethanol: Avoid or limit ethanol (may increase CNS depression). Watch for sedation.

Food: Glucose may cause hyperglycemia; monitor blood glucose concentrations.

Herb/Nutraceutical: Avoid valerian, St John's wort, kava kava, gotu kola (may increase CNS depression).

Pharmacodynamics/Kinetics

Onset of action: Analgesic: Oral, SubQ, I.M.: 10-15 minutes; I.V.: ~5 minutes

Peak effect: Oral, SubQ, I.M.: ~1 hour

Duration: Oral, SubQ, I.M.: 2-4 hours

Distribution: Crosses placenta; enters breast milk

Protein binding: 65% to 75%

Metabolism: Hepatic; active metabolite (normeperidine)

Bioavailability: ~50% to 60%; increased with liver disease

(Continued)

Meperidine *(Continued)*

Half-life elimination:

Parent drug: Terminal phase: Neonates: 23 hours (range: 12-39 hours); Adults: 2.5-4 hours, Liver disease: 7-11 hours

Normeperidine (active metabolite): 15-30 hours; can accumulate with high doses or with decreased renal function

Pregnancy Risk Factor C/D (prolonged use or high doses at term)

Lactation Enters breast milk/contraindicated (AAP rates "compatible")

Breast-Feeding Considerations Meperidine is excreted in breast milk and may cause CNS and/or respiratory depression in the nursing infant.

Dosage Forms

Injection, solution, as hydrochloride [ampul]: 50 mg/mL (1.5 mL, 2 mL)

Injection, solution, as hydrochloride [prefilled syringe]: 25 mg/mL (1 mL); 50 mg/mL (1 mL); 75 mg/mL (1 mL); 100 mg/mL (1 mL)

Injection, solution, as hydrochloride [prefilled syringe for PCA pump]: 10 mg/mL (50 mL)

Injection, solution, as hydrochloride [vial]: 50 mg/mL (1 mL, 30 mL); 100 mg/mL (20 mL) [may contain sodium metabisulfite]

Syrup, as hydrochloride: 50 mg/5 mL (5 mL, 500 mL) [contains sodium benzoate]

Demerol®: 50 mg/5 mL (480 mL) [contains benzoic acid; banana flavor]

Tablet, as hydrochloride (Demerol®, Meperitab®): 50 mg, 100 mg

Comments Meperidine is not to be used as the narcotic drug of first choice. It is recommended only to be used in codeine-allergic patients when a narcotic analgesic is indicated. Meperidine is not an anti-inflammatory agent. Meperidine, as with other narcotic analgesics, is recommended only for limited acute dosing (ie, 3 days or less); common adverse effects in the dental patient are nausea, sedation, and constipation. Meperidine has a significant addiction liability, especially when given long-term.

Meperidine and Promethazine

(me PER i deen & proe METH a zeen)

Related Information

Meperidine *on page 870*

Promethazine *on page 1130*

Generic Available Yes

Synonyms Mepergan; Promethazine and Meperidine

Pharmacologic Category Analgesic Combination (Narcotic)

Use Management of moderate to severe pain

Local Anesthetic/Vasoconstrictor Precautions No information available to require special precautions

Effects on Dental Treatment Key adverse event(s) related to dental treatment: Xerostomia (normal salivary flow resumes upon discontinuation).

Common Adverse Effects Frequency not defined.

Based on **meperidine** component:

Cardiovascular: Hypotension

Central nervous system: Fatigue, drowsiness, dizziness, nervousness, headache, restlessness, malaise, confusion, mental depression, hallucinations, paradoxical CNS stimulation, increased intracranial pressure

Dermatologic: Rash, urticaria

Gastrointestinal: Nausea, vomiting, constipation, anorexia, stomach cramps, xerostomia, biliary spasm

Genitourinary: Ureteral spasms, decreased urination, paralytic ileus

Local: Pain at injection site

Neuromuscular & skeletal: Weakness

Respiratory: Dyspnea

Miscellaneous: Histamine release, physical and psychological dependence

Based on **promethazine** component:

Cardiovascular: Postural hypotension, tachycardia, dizziness, nonspecific QT changes

Central nervous system: Drowsiness, dystonias, akathisia, pseudoparkinsonism, tardive dyskinesia, neuroleptic malignant syndrome, seizures

Dermatologic: Photosensitivity, dermatitis, skin pigmentation (slate gray)

Endocrine & metabolic: Lactation, breast engorgement, false-positive pregnancy test, amenorrhea, gynecomastia, hyper- or hypoglycemia

Gastrointestinal: Xerostomia, constipation, nausea

Genitourinary: Urinary retention, ejaculatory disorder, impotence

Hematologic: Agranulocytosis, eosinophilia, leukopenia, hemolytic anemia, aplastic anemia, thrombocytopenic purpura

Hepatic: Jaundice

Ocular: Blurred vision, corneal and lenticular changes, epithelial keratopathy, pigmentary retinopathy

Restrictions C-II

Drug Interactions

Cytochrome P450 Effect: Promethazine: **Substrate** (major) of CYP2B6, 2D6; **Inhibits** CYP2D6 (weak)

Pharmacodynamics/Kinetics See individual agents.

Pregnancy Risk Factor B/D (prolonged use or high doses at term)

Meperidine Hydrochloride *see* Meperidine *on page 870*

Meperitab® *see* Meperidine *on page 870*

Mephobarbital (me foe BAR bi tal)

U.S. Brand Names Mebaral®

Canadian Brand Names Mebaral®

Generic Available No

Synonyms Methylphenobarbital

Pharmacologic Category Barbiturate

Use Sedative; treatment of grand mal and petit mal epilepsy

Local Anesthetic/Vasoconstrictor Precautions No information available to require special precautions

Effects on Dental Treatment No significant effects or complications reported

Common Adverse Effects

>10%: Central nervous system: Dizziness, lightheadedness, drowsiness, "hangover" effect

1% to 10%:

Central nervous system: Confusion, mental depression, unusual excitement, nervousness, faint feeling, headache, insomnia, nightmares

Gastrointestinal: Constipation, nausea, vomiting

Restrictions C-IV

Mechanism of Action Increases seizure threshold in the motor cortex; depresses monosynaptic and polysynaptic transmission in the CNS

Drug Interactions

Cytochrome P450 Effect: Substrate of CYP2B6 (minor), 2C8/9 (minor), 2C19 (major); **Inhibits** CYP2C19 (weak); **Induces** CYP2A6 (weak)

Increased Effect/Toxicity: When combined with other CNS depressants, ethanol, narcotic analgesics, antidepressants, or benzodiazepines, additive respiratory and CNS depression may occur. Barbiturates may enhance the hepatotoxic potential of acetaminophen overdoses. Chloramphenicol, MAO inhibitors, valproic acid, and felbamate may inhibit barbiturate metabolism. Barbiturates may impair the absorption of griseofulvin, and may enhance the nephrotoxic effects of methoxyflurane. Concurrent use of phenobarbital with meperidine may result in increased CNS depression. CYP2C19 inhibitors may increase the levels/effects of mephobarbital; example inhibitors include delavirdine, fluconazole, fluvoxamine, gemfibrozil, isoniazid, omeprazole, and ticlopidine.

Decreased Effect: Barbiturates are hepatic enzyme inducers, and may increase the metabolism of antipsychotics, some beta-blockers (unlikely with atenolol and nadolol), calcium channel blockers, chloramphenicol, cimetidine, corticosteroids, cyclosporine, disopyramide, doxycycline, ethosuximide, felbamate, furosemide, griseofulvin, lamotrigine, phenytoin, propafenone, quinidine, tacrolimus, TCAs, and theophylline. Barbiturates may increase the metabolism of estrogens and reduce the efficacy of oral contraceptives; an alternative method of contraception should be considered. Barbiturates inhibit the hypoprothrombinemic effects of oral anticoagulants via increased metabolism. Barbiturates may enhance the metabolism of methadone resulting in methadone withdrawal. CYP2C19 inducers may decrease the levels/effects of mephobarbital; example inducers include aminoglutethimide, carbamazepine, phenytoin, and rifampin.

Pharmacodynamics/Kinetics

Onset of action: 20-60 minutes

Duration: 6-8 hours

Absorption: ~50%

Half-life elimination, serum: 34 hours

Pregnancy Risk Factor D

Mephyton® *see* Phytonadione *on page 1084*

Mepivacaine (me PIV a kane)

U.S. Brand Names Carbocaine® [DSC]; Polocaine®; Polocaine® MPF

Canadian Brand Names Carbocaine®; Polocaine®

(Continued)

Mepivacaine *(Continued)*

Generic Available No

Synonyms Mepivacaine Hydrochloride

Pharmacologic Category Local Anesthetic

Dental Use Local anesthesia by nerve block, infiltration in dental procedures

Use Not for use in spinal anesthesia

Local Anesthetic/Vasoconstrictor Precautions No information available to require special precautions

Effects on Dental Treatment Key adverse event(s) related to dental treatment: Degree of adverse effects in the CNS and cardiovascular system is directly related to blood levels of mepivacaine (frequency not defined; more likely to occur after systemic administration rather than infiltration): Bradycardia, cardiovascular collapse, hypotension, myocardial depression, ventricular arrhythmias, nausea, vomiting, respiratory arrest, anaphylactoid reactions, blurred vision, heart block, transient stinging or burning at injection site

High blood levels: Anxiety, restlessness, disorientation, confusion, dizziness, and seizures, followed by CNS depression resulting in somnolence, unconsciousness, and possible respiratory arrest.

In some cases, symptoms of CNS stimulation may be absent and the primary CNS effects are somnolence and unconsciousness.

Significant Adverse Effects Degree of adverse effects in the CNS and cardiovascular system are directly related to the blood levels of mepivacaine. The effects below are more likely to occur after systemic administration rather than infiltration.

Cardiovascular: Bradycardia, cardiovascular collapse, edema, heart block, hypotension, myocardial depression, ventricular arrhythmias, angioneurotic edema

Central nervous system: High blood levels result in anxiety, restlessness, disorientation, confusion, dizziness, and seizures. This is followed by depression of CNS resulting in somnolence, unconsciousness, and possible respiratory arrest. In some cases, symptoms of CNS stimulation may be absent and the primary CNS effects are somnolence and unconsciousness.

Dermatologic: Cutaneous lesions, urticaria

Gastrointestinal: Nausea, vomiting

Local: Transient stinging or burning at injection site

Ophthalmic: Blurred vision

Otic: Tinnitus

Respiratory: Respiratory arrest

Miscellaneous: Anaphylactoid reactions

Dosage Children and Adults: Injectable local anesthetic: Varies with procedure, degree of anesthesia needed, vascularity of tissue, duration of anesthesia required, and physical condition of patient

Mechanism of Action Mepivacaine is an amino amide local anesthetic similar to lidocaine; like all local anesthetics, mepivacaine acts by preventing the generation and conduction of nerve impulses

Contraindications Hypersensitivity to mepivacaine, any component of the formulation, or other amide anesthetics; allergy to sodium bisulfate

Warnings/Precautions Use with caution in patients with cardiac disease, renal disease, and hyperthyroidism; convulsions due to systemic toxicity leading to cardiac arrest have been reported presumably due to intravascular injection

Pharmacodynamics/Kinetics

Onset of action: Epidural: 7-15 minutes

Duration: 2-2.5 hours; similar onset and duration following infiltration

Protein binding: 70% to 85%

Metabolism: Primarily hepatic via N-demethylation, hydroxylation, and glucuronidation

Half-life elimination: 1.9 hours

Excretion: Urine (95% as metabolites)

Pregnancy Risk Factor C

Lactation Excretion in breast milk unknown/compatible

Dosage Forms [DSC] = Discontinued product

Injection, solution, as hydrochloride:

Carbocaine® [DSC]: 1% (30 mL, 50 mL); 2% (20 mL, 50 mL)

Polocaine®: 1% (50 mL); 2% (50 mL)

Polocaine® MPF: 1% (30 mL); 1.5% (30 mL); 3% (20 mL)

Mepivacaine and Levonordefrin *(WITHDRAWN FROM MARKET)* (me PIV a kane & lee voe nor DEF rin)

Related Information

Mepivacaine *on page 873*

Oral Pain *on page 1526*

U.S. Brand Names Carbocaine® 2% with Neo-Cobefrin® [DSC]

Canadian Brand Names Polocaine® 2% and Levonordefrin 1:20,000

Generic Available No

Synonyms Levonordefrin and Mepivacaine (Dental)

Pharmacologic Category Local Anesthetic

Dental Use Amide-type anesthetic used for local infiltration anesthesia; injection near nerve trunks to produce nerve block

Local Anesthetic/Vasoconstrictor Precautions No information available to require special precautions

Effects on Dental Treatment It is common to misinterpret psychogenic responses to local anesthetic injection as an allergic reaction. Intraoral injections are perceived by many patients as a stressful procedure in dentistry. Common symptoms to this stress are diaphoresis, palpitations, hyperventilation, generalized pallor and a fainting feeling. Patients may exhibit hypersensitivity to bisulfites contained in local anesthetic solution to prevent oxidation of levonordefrin. In general, patients reacting to bisulfites have a history of asthma and their airways are hyper-reactive to asthmatic syndrome.

Degree of adverse effects in the CNS and cardiovascular system is directly related to the blood levels of mepivacaine (frequency not defined; more likely to occur after systemic administration rather than infiltration): Bradycardia and reduction in cardiac output, nausea, vomiting, tremors, hypersensitivity reactions (extremely rare; may be manifest as dermatologic reactions and edema at injection site), asthmatic syndromes

High blood levels: Anxiety, restlessness, disorientation, confusion, dizziness, and seizures, followed by CNS depression resulting in somnolence, unconsciousness and possible respiratory arrest.

In some cases, symptoms of CNS stimulation may be absent and the primary CNS effects are somnolence and unconsciousness.

Significant Adverse Effects Degree of adverse effects in the CNS and cardiovascular system are directly related to the blood levels of mepivacaine. The effects below are more likely to occur after systemic administration rather than infiltration.

Cardiovascular: Myocardial effects include a decrease in contraction force as well as a decrease in electrical excitability and myocardial conduction rate resulting in bradycardia and reduction in cardiac output.

Central nervous system: High blood levels result in anxiety, restlessness, disorientation, confusion, dizziness, and seizures. This is followed by depression of CNS resulting in somnolence, unconsciousness and possible respiratory arrest. In some cases, symptoms of CNS stimulation may be absent and the primary CNS effects are somnolence and unconsciousness.

Gastrointestinal: Nausea and vomiting may occur

Hypersensitivity reactions: Extremely rare, but may be manifest as dermatologic reactions and edema at injection site. Asthmatic syndromes have occurred. Patients may exhibit hypersensitivity to bisulfites contained in local anesthetic solution to prevent oxidation of levonordefrin. In general, patients reacting to bisulfites have a history of asthma and their airways are hyper-reactive to asthmatic syndrome.

Neuromuscular & skeletal: Tremors

Psychogenic reactions: It is common to misinterpret psychogenic responses to local anesthetic injection as an allergic reaction. Intraoral injections are perceived by many patients as a stressful procedure in dentistry. Common symptoms to this stress are diaphoresis, palpitations, hyperventilation, generalized pallor and a fainting feeling.

Dosage

Children <10 years: Maximum pediatric dosage must be carefully calculated on the basis of patient's weight but should not exceed 6.6 mg/kg of body weight or 180 mg of mepivacaine hydrochloride as a 2% solution with levonordefrin 1:20,000

Children >10 years and Adults:

Dental infiltration and nerve block, single site: 36 mg (1.8 mL) of mepivacaine hydrochloride as a 2% solution with levonordefrin 1:20,000

Entire oral cavity: 180 mg (9 mL) of mepivacaine hydrochloride as a 2% solution with levonordefrin 1:20,000; up to a maximum of 6.6 mg/kg of body weight but not to exceed 400 mg of mepivacaine hydrochloride per

(Continued)

Mepivacaine and Levonordefrin *(WITHDRAWN FROM MARKET)* *(Continued)*

appointment. The effective anesthetic dose varies with procedure, intensity of anesthesia needed, duration of anesthesia required, and physical condition of the patient. Always use the lowest effective dose along with careful aspiration.

The following numbers of dental carpules (1.8 mL) provide the indicated amounts of mepivacaine hydrochloride 2% and levonordefrin 1:20,000. See table.

# of Cartridges (1.8 mL)	Mg Mepivacaine (2%)	Mg Vasoconstrictor (Levonordefrin 1:20,000)
1	36	0.090
2	72	0.180
3	108	0.270
4	144	0.360
5	180	0.450
6	216	0.540
7	252	0.630
8	288	0.720
9	324	0.810
10	360	0.900

Note: Adult and children doses of mepivacaine hydrochloride with levonordefrin cited from USP Dispensing Information (USP DI), 17th ed, The United States Pharmacopeial Convention, Inc, Rockville, MD, 1997, 139.

Mechanism of Action Local anesthetics bind selectively to the intracellular surface of sodium channels to block influx of sodium into the axon. As a result, depolarization necessary for action potential propagation and subsequent nerve function is prevented. The block at the sodium channel is reversible. When drug diffuses away from the axon, sodium channel function is restored and nerve propagation returns.

Levonordefrin prolongs the duration of the anesthetic actions of mepivacaine by causing vasoconstriction (alpha adrenergic receptor agonist) of the vasculature surrounding the nerve axons. This prevents the diffusion of mepivacaine away from the nerves resulting in a longer retention in the axon.

Contraindications Hypersensitivity to local anesthetics of the amide-type or any component of the formulation

Warnings/Precautions Should be avoided in patients with uncontrolled hyperthyroidism. Should be used in minimal amounts in patients with significant cardiovascular problems (because of levonordefrin component). Aspirate the syringe after tissue penetration and before injection to minimize chance of direct vascular injection.

Drug Interactions Due to levonordefrin component, use with tricyclic antidepressants or MAO inhibitors could result in increased pressor response; use with nonselective beta-blockers (ie, propranolol) could result in serious hypertension and reflex bradycardia

Pharmacodynamics/Kinetics

Duration: Upper jaw: 1-2.5 hours; Lower jaw: 2.5-5.5 hours

Infiltration: 50 minutes

Inferior alveolar block: 60-75 minutes

Pregnancy Risk Factor C

Breast-Feeding Considerations Usual infiltration doses of mepivacaine with levonordefrin given to nursing mothers has not been shown to affect the health of the nursing infant.

Dosage Forms Injection: Mepivacaine hydrochloride 2% with levonordefrin 1:20,000 (1.8 mL dental cartridges) [DSC]

Selected Readings

Ayoub ST and Coleman AE, "A Review of Local Anesthetics," *Gen Dent*, 1992, 40(4):285-7, 289-90.

Jastak JT and Yagiela JA, "Vasoconstrictors and Local Anesthesia: A Review and Rationale for Use," *J Am Dent Assoc*, 1983, 107(4):623-30.

MacKenzie TA and Young ER, "Local Anesthetic Update," *Anesth Prog*, 1993, 40(2):29-34.

Wynn RL, "Epinephrine Interactions With Beta-Blockers," *Gen Dent*, 1994, 42(1):16, 18.

Wynn RL, "Recent Research on Mechanisms of Local Anesthetics," *Gen Dent*, 1995, 43(4):316-8.

Yagiela JA, "Local Anesthetics," *Anesth Prog*, 1991, 38(4-5):128-41.

Mepivacaine (Dental Anesthetic) (me PIV a kane)

Related Information

Mepivacaine *on page 873*

Oral Pain *on page 1526*

U.S. Brand Names Carbocaine® 3%

Canadian Brand Names Polocaine®

Generic Available Yes

Pharmacologic Category Local Anesthetic

Dental Use Amide-type anesthetic used for local infiltration anesthesia; injection near nerve trunks to produce nerve block

Local Anesthetic/Vasoconstrictor Precautions No information available to require special precautions

Effects on Dental Treatment It is common to misinterpret psychogenic responses to local anesthetic injection as an allergic reaction. Intraoral injections are perceived by many patients as a stressful procedure in dentistry. Common symptoms to this stress are diaphoresis, palpitations, hyperventilation, generalized pallor, and a fainting feeling.

Degree of adverse effects in the CNS and cardiovascular system is directly related to the blood levels of mepivacaine.

Frequency not defined: Bradycardia and reduction in cardiac output, nausea, vomiting, tremors, asthmatic syndromes, hypersensitivity reactions (may manifest as dermatologic reactions and edema at injection site)

High blood levels: Anxiety, restlessness, disorientation, confusion, dizziness, tremors and seizures, followed by CNS depression resulting in somnolence, unconsciousness and possible respiratory arrest. In some cases, symptoms of CNS stimulation may be absent and the primary CNS effects are somnolence and unconsciousness.

Significant Adverse Effects Degree of adverse effects in the CNS and cardiovascular system are directly related to the blood levels of local anesthetic.

Cardiovascular: Myocardial effects include a decrease in contraction force as well as a decrease in electrical excitability and myocardial conduction rate resulting in bradycardia and reduction in cardiac output

Central nervous system: High blood levels result in anxiety, restlessness, disorientation, confusion, dizziness, and seizures. This is followed by depression of CNS resulting in somnolence, unconsciousness and possible respiratory arrest. In some cases, symptoms of CNS stimulation may be absent and the primary CNS effects are somnolence and unconsciousness.

Gastrointestinal: Nausea and vomiting may occur

Hypersensitivity reactions: May manifest as dermatologic reactions and edema at injection site. Asthmatic syndromes have occurred.

Neuromuscular & skeletal: Tremors

Psychogenic reactions: It is common to misinterpret psychogenic responses to local anesthetic injection as an allergic reaction. Intraoral injection is perceived by many patients as a stressful procedure in dentistry. Common symptoms to this stress are diaphoresis, palpitations, hyperventilation, generalized pallor and a fainting feeling.

Dosage

Children <10 years: Up to 5-6 mg/kg of body weight; maximum pediatric dosage must be carefully calculated on the basis of patient's weight but must not exceed 270 mg (9 mL) of the 3% solution

Children >10 years and Adults:

Dental anesthesia, single site in upper or lower jaw: 54 mg (1.8 mL) as a 3% solution

# of Cartridges (1.8 mL)	Mg Mepivacaine (3%)
1	54
2	108
3	162
4	216
5	270
6	324
7	378
8	432

Infiltration and nerve block of entire oral cavity: 270 mg (9 mL) as a 3% solution; up to a maximum of 6.6 mg/kg of body weight but not to exceed

(Continued)

Mepivacaine (Dental Anesthetic) *(Continued)*

300 mg per appointment. Manufacturer's maximum recommended dose is not more than 400 mg to normal healthy adults. The effective anesthetic dose varies with procedure, intensity of anesthesia needed, duration of anesthesia required, and physical condition of the patient. Always use the lowest effective dose along with careful aspiration.

The number of dental carpules (1.8 mL) provide the indicated amounts of mepivacaine dental anesthetic 3%. See table on previous page.

Note: Adult and children doses of mepivacaine dental anesthetic cited from USP Dispensing Information (USP DI), 17th ed, The United States Pharmacopeial Convention, Inc, Rockville, MD, 1997, 138-9.

Mechanism of Action Local anesthetics bind selectively to the intracellular surface of sodium channels to block influx of sodium into the axon. As a result, depolarization necessary for action potential propagation and subsequent nerve function is prevented. The block at the sodium channel is reversible. When drug diffuses away from the axon, sodium channel function is restored and nerve propagation returns.

Contraindications Hypersensitivity to local anesthetics of the amide type or any component of the formulation

Warnings/Precautions Aspirate the syringe after tissue penetration and before injection to minimize chance of direct vascular injection

Drug Interactions No data reported

Pharmacodynamics/Kinetics

Onset of action: Upper jaw: 30-120 seconds; Lower jaw: 1-4 minutes

Duration: Upper jaw: 20 minutes; Lower jaw: 40 minutes

Half-life elimination, serum: 1.9 hours

Pregnancy Risk Factor C

Breast-Feeding Considerations Usual infiltration doses of mepivacaine dental anesthetic given to nursing mothers has not been shown to affect the health of the nursing infant.

Dosage Forms Injection: Mepivacaine hydrochloride 3% (1.8 mL dental cartridges)

Selected Readings

Ayoub ST and Coleman AE, "A Review of Local Anesthetics," *Gen Dent*, 1992, 40(4):285-7, 289-90.

Budenz AW, "Local Anesthetics in Dentistry: Then and Now," *J Calif Dent Assoc*, 2003, 31(5):388-96.

Dower JS Jr, "A Review of Paresthesia in Association With Administration of Local Anesthesia," *Dent Today*, 2003, 22(2):64-9.

Finder RL and Moore PA, "Adverse Drug Reactions to Local Anesthesia," *Dent Clin North Am*, 2002, 46(4):747-57, x.

Haas DA, "An Update on Local Anesthetics in Dentistry," *J Can Dent Assoc*, 2002, 68(9):546-51.

Hawkins JM and Moore PA, "Local Anesthesia: Advances in Agents and Techniques," *Dent Clin North Am*, 2002, 46(4):719-32, ix.

"Injectable Local Anesthetics," *J Am Dent Assoc*, 2003, 134(5):628-9.

Malamed SF, "Allergy and Toxic Reactions to Local Anesthetics," *Dent Today*, 2003, 22(4):114-6, 118-21.

Wynn RL, "Recent Research on Mechanisms of Local Anesthetics," *Gen Dent*, 1995, 43(4):316-8.

Mepivacaine Hydrochloride *see* Mepivacaine *on page 873*

Meprobamate (me proe BA mate)

U.S. Brand Names Miltown®

Canadian Brand Names Novo-Mepro

Generic Available Yes

Synonyms Equanil

Pharmacologic Category Antianxiety Agent, Miscellaneous

Dental Use Treatment of muscle spasm associated with acute temporomandibular joint pain; management of dental anxiety disorders

Use Management of anxiety disorders

Unlabeled/Investigational Use Demonstrated value for muscle contraction, headache, premenstrual tension, external sphincter spasticity, muscle rigidity, opisthotonos-associated with tetanus

Local Anesthetic/Vasoconstrictor Precautions No information available to require special precautions

Effects on Dental Treatment No significant effects or complications reported

Significant Adverse Effects Frequency not defined.

Cardiovascular: Syncope, peripheral edema, palpitations, tachycardia, arrhythmia

Central nervous system: Drowsiness, ataxia, dizziness, paradoxical excitement, confusion, slurred speech, headache, euphoria, chills, vertigo, paresthesia, overstimulation

Dermatologic: Rashes, purpura, dermatitis, Stevens-Johnson syndrome, petechiae, ecchymosis
Gastrointestinal: Diarrhea, vomiting, nausea
Hematologic: Leukopenia, eosinophilia, agranulocytosis, aplastic anemia
Neuromuscular & skeletal: Weakness
Ocular: Blurred vision, impairment of accommodation
Renal: Renal failure
Respiratory: Wheezing, dyspnea, bronchospasm, angioneurotic edema

Restrictions C-IV

Dosage Oral:
Children 6-12 years: Anxiety: 100-200 mg 2-3 times/day
Adults: Anxiety: 400 mg 3-4 times/day, up to 2400 mg/day

Dosing interval in renal impairment:
Cl_{cr} 10-50 mL/minute: Administer every 9-12 hours
Cl_{cr} <10 mL/minute: Administer every 12-18 hours
Hemodialysis: Moderately dialyzable (20% to 50%)

Dosing adjustment in hepatic impairment: Probably necessary in patients with liver disease

Mechanism of Action Affects the thalamus and limbic system; also appears to inhibit multineuronal spinal reflexes

Contraindications Hypersensitivity to meprobamate, related compounds (including carisoprodol), or any component of the formulation; acute intermittent porphyria; pre-existing CNS depression; narrow-angle glaucoma; severe uncontrolled pain; pregnancy

Warnings/Precautions Physical and psychological dependence and abuse may occur; abrupt cessation may precipitate withdrawal. Use with caution in patients with depression or suicidal tendencies, or in patients with a history of drug abuse. May cause CNS depression, which may impair physical or mental abilities. Patients must be cautioned about performing tasks which require mental alertness (eg, operating machinery or driving). Effects with other sedative drugs or ethanol may be potentiated. Not recommended in children <6 years of age; allergic reaction may occur in patients with history of dermatological condition (usually by fourth dose). Use with caution in patients with renal or hepatic impairment, or with a history of seizures. Use caution in the elderly as it may cause confusion, cognitive impairment, or excessive sedation.

Drug Interactions CNS depressants: Sedative effects may be additive with other CNS depressants; monitor for increased effect; includes barbiturates, benzodiazepines, narcotic analgesics, ethanol, and other sedative agents

Ethanol/Nutrition/Herb Interactions
Ethanol: Avoid ethanol (may increase CNS depression).
Herb/Nutraceutical: Avoid valerian, St John's wort, kava kava, gotu kola (may increase CNS depression).

Pharmacodynamics/Kinetics
Onset of action: Sedation: ~1 hour
Distribution: Crosses placenta; enters breast milk
Metabolism: Hepatic
Half-life elimination: 10 hours
Excretion: Urine (8% to 20% as unchanged drug); feces (10% as metabolites)

Pregnancy Risk Factor D

Lactation Enters breast milk/not recommended

Breast-Feeding Considerations Breast milk concentrations are higher than plasma; effects are unknown.

Dosage Forms Tablet: 200 mg, 400 mg

Meprobamate and Aspirin *see* Aspirin and Meprobamate *on page 156*
Mepron® *see* Atovaquone *on page 164*

Mequinol and Tretinoin (ME kwi nole & TRET i noyn)

U.S. Brand Names Solagé™

Canadian Brand Names Solagé™

Generic Available No

Synonyms Tretinoin and Mequinol

Pharmacologic Category Retinoic Acid Derivative; Vitamin A Derivative; Vitamin, Topical

Use Treatment of solar lentigines; the efficacy of using Solagé™ daily for >24 weeks has not been established. The local cutaneous safety of Solagé™ in non-Caucasians has not been adequately established.

Local Anesthetic/Vasoconstrictor Precautions No information available to require special precautions

Effects on Dental Treatment No significant effects or complications reported

(Continued)

Mequinol and Tretinoin *(Continued)*

Common Adverse Effects

>10%: Dermatologic: Erythema (49%), burning, stinging or tingling (26%), desquamation (14%), pruritus (12%),

1% to 10%: Dermatologic: Skin irritation (5%), hypopigmentation (5%), halo hypopigmentation (7%), rash (3%), dry skin (3%), crusting (3%), vesicular bullae rash (2%), contact allergic reaction (1%)

Mechanism of Action Solar lentigines are localized, pigmented, macular lesions of the skin on areas of the body chronically exposed to the sun. Mequinol is a substrate for the enzyme tyrosinase and acts as a competitive inhibitor of the formation of melanin precursors. The mechanisms of depigmentation for both drugs is unknown.

Drug Interactions

Cytochrome P450 Effect: Tretinoin: **Substrate** (minor) of CYP2A6, 2B6, 2C8/9; **Inhibits** CYP2C8/9 (weak); **Induces** CYP2E1 (weak)

Increased Effect/Toxicity:

Topical products with skin drying effects (eg, those containing alcohol, astringents, spices, or lime; medicated soaps or shampoos; permanent wave solutions; hair depilatories or waxes; and others) may increase skin irritation. Avoid concurrent use.

Photosensitizing drugs (eg, thiazides, tetracyclines, fluoroquinolones, phenothiazines, sulfonamides) can further increase sun sensitivity. Avoid concurrent use.

Pharmacodynamics/Kinetics

Absorption: Percutaneous absorption was 4.4% of tretinoin when applied as 0.8 mL of Solagé™ to a 400 cm^2 area of the back

Time to peak: Mequinol: 2 hours

Pregnancy Risk Factor X

Merbromin (mer BROE min)

U.S. Brand Names Mercurochrome®

Generic Available Yes

Pharmacologic Category Topical Skin Product

Use Topical antiseptic

Local Anesthetic/Vasoconstrictor Precautions No information available to require special precautions

Effects on Dental Treatment No significant effects or complications reported

Mercaptopurine (mer kap toe PYOOR een)

U.S. Brand Names Purinethol®

Canadian Brand Names Purinethol®

Mexican Brand Names Purinethol®

Generic Available Yes

Synonyms 6-Mercaptopurine; 6-MP; NSC-755

Pharmacologic Category Antineoplastic Agent, Antimetabolite

Use Maintenance therapy in acute lymphoblastic leukemia (ALL); other (less common) uses include chronic granulocytic leukemia, induction therapy in ALL, and treatment of non-Hodgkin's lymphomas

Local Anesthetic/Vasoconstrictor Precautions No information available to require special precautions

Effects on Dental Treatment Key adverse event(s) related to dental treatment: Stomatitis and mucositis.

Common Adverse Effects

>10%:

Hematologic: Myelosuppression; leukopenia, thrombocytopenia, anemia

Onset: 7-10 days

Nadir: 14-16 days

Recovery: 21-28 days

Hepatic: Intrahepatic cholestasis and focal centralobular necrosis (40%), characterized by hyperbilirubinemia, increased alkaline phosphatase and AST, jaundice, ascites, encephalopathy; more common at doses >2.5 mg/kg/day. Usually occurs within 2 months of therapy but may occur within 1 week, or be delayed up to 8 years.

1% to 10%:

Central nervous system: Drug fever

Dermatologic: Hyperpigmentation, rash

Endocrine & metabolic: Hyperuricemia

Gastrointestinal: Nausea, vomiting, diarrhea, stomatitis, anorexia, stomach pain, mucositis

Renal: Renal toxicity

Restrictions Note: I.V. formulation is not commercially available in the U.S.

Mechanism of Action Purine antagonist which inhibits DNA and RNA synthesis; acts as false metabolite and is incorporated into DNA and RNA, eventually inhibiting their synthesis; specific for the S phase of the cell cycle

Drug Interactions

Increased Effect/Toxicity:

Allopurinol can cause increased levels of mercaptopurine by inhibition of xanthine oxidase. Decrease dose of mercaptopurine by 75% when both drugs are used concomitantly. Seen only with oral mercaptopurine usage, not with I.V. May potentiate effect of bone marrow suppression (reduce mercaptopurine to 25% of dose).

Doxorubicin: Synergistic liver toxicity with mercaptopurine in >50% of patients, which resolved with discontinuation of the mercaptopurine.

Hepatotoxic drugs: Any agent which could potentially alter the metabolic function of the liver could produce higher drug levels and greater toxicities from either mercaptopurine or thioguanine (6-TG).

Aminosalicylates (olsalazine, mesalamine, sulfasalazine): May inhibit TPMT, increasing toxicity/myelosuppression of mercaptopurine.

Decreased Effect: mercaptopurine inhibits the anticoagulation effect of warfarin by an unknown mechanism.

Pharmacodynamics/Kinetics

Absorption: Variable and incomplete (16% to 50%)

Distribution: V_d = total body water; CNS penetration is poor

Protein binding: 30%

Metabolism: Hepatic and in GI mucosa; hepatically via xanthine oxidase and methylation to sulfate conjugates, 6-thiouric acid, and other inactive compounds; first-pass effect

Half-life elimination (age dependent): Children: 21 minutes; Adults: 47 minutes

Time to peak, serum: ~2 hours

Excretion: Urine; following high (1 g/m^2) I.V. doses, 20% to 40% excreted unchanged; at lower doses renal elimination minor

Pregnancy Risk Factor D

6-Mercaptopurine *see* Mercaptopurine *on page 880*

Mercapturic Acid *see* Acetylcysteine *on page 61*

Mercuric Oxide (mer KYOOR ik OKS ide)

Generic Available Yes

Synonyms Yellow Mercuric Oxide

Pharmacologic Category Antibiotic, Ophthalmic

Use Treatment of irritation and minor infections of the eyelids

Local Anesthetic/Vasoconstrictor Precautions No information available to require special precautions

Effects on Dental Treatment No significant effects or complications reported

Mercurochrome® *see* Merbromin *on page 880*

Meridia® *see* Sibutramine *on page 1218*

Meropenem (mer oh PEN em)

U.S. Brand Names Merrem® I.V.

Canadian Brand Names Merrem®

Mexican Brand Names Merrem®

Generic Available No

Pharmacologic Category Antibiotic, Carbapenem

Use Intra-abdominal infections (complicated appendicitis and peritonitis) caused by viridans group streptococci, *E. coli*, *K. pneumoniae*, *P. aeruginosa*, *B. fragilis*, *B. thetaiotaomicron*, and *Peptostreptococcus* sp; also indicated for bacterial meningitis in pediatric patients >3 months of age caused by *S. pneumoniae*, *H. influenzae*, and *N. meningitidis*; meropenem has also been used to treat soft tissue infections, febrile neutropenia, and urinary tract infections

Local Anesthetic/Vasoconstrictor Precautions No information available to require special precautions

Effects on Dental Treatment Key adverse event(s) related to dental treatment: Oral moniliasis (pediatric patients) and glossitis.

Common Adverse Effects 1% to 10%:

Central nervous system: Headache (2%)

Dermatologic: Rash (2% to 3%, includes diaper-area moniliasis in pediatrics), pruritus (1%)

Gastrointestinal: Diarrhea (4% to 5%), nausea/vomiting (1% to 4%), constipation (1%), oral moniliasis (up to 2% in pediatric patients), glossitis

Local: Inflammation at the injection site (2%), phlebitis/thrombophlebitis (1%), injection site reaction (1%)

(Continued)

Meropenem *(Continued)*

Respiratory: Apnea (1%)
Miscellaneous: Sepsis (2%), septic shock (1%)

Mechanism of Action Inhibits bacterial cell wall synthesis by binding to several of the penicillin-binding proteins, which in turn inhibit the final transpeptidation step of peptidoglycan synthesis in bacterial cell walls, thus inhibiting cell wall biosynthesis; bacteria eventually lyse due to ongoing activity of cell wall autolytic enzymes (autolysins and murein hydrolases) while cell wall assembly is arrested

Drug Interactions

Increased Effect/Toxicity: Probenecid interferes with renal excretion of meropenem.

Decreased Effect: Serum concentrations of valproic acid may be reduced during meropenem therapy (potentially to subtherapeutic levels).

Pharmacodynamics/Kinetics

Distribution: V_d: Adults: ~0.3 L/kg, Children: 0.4-0.5 L/kg; penetrates well into most body fluids and tissues; CSF concentrations approximate those of the plasma
Protein binding: 2%
Metabolism: Hepatic; metabolized to open beta-lactam form (inactive)
Half-life elimination:
Normal renal function: 1-1.5 hours
Cl_{cr} 30-80 mL/minute: 1.9-3.3 hours
Cl_{cr} 2-30 mL/minute: 3.82-5.7 hours
Time to peak, tissue: 1 hour following infusion
Excretion: Urine (~25% as inactive metabolites)

Pregnancy Risk Factor B

Merrem® I.V. *see* Meropenem *on page 881*
Mersol® [OTC] *see* Thimerosal *on page 1288*
Merthiolate® [OTC] *see* Thimerosal *on page 1288*
Meruvax® II *see* Rubella Virus Vaccine (Live) *on page 1203*

Mesalamine (me SAL a meen)

U.S. Brand Names Asacol®; Canasa™; Pentasa®; Rowasa®

Canadian Brand Names Asacol®; Mesasal®; Novo-5 ASA; Pentasa®; Quintasa®; Rowasa®; Salofalk®

Mexican Brand Names Salofalk®

Generic Available No

Synonyms 5-Aminosalicylic Acid; 5-ASA; Fisalamine; Mesalazine

Pharmacologic Category 5-Aminosalicylic Acid Derivative

Use

Oral: Treatment and maintenance of remission of mildly to moderately active ulcerative colitis
Rectal: Treatment of active mild to moderate distal ulcerative colitis, proctosigmoiditis, or proctitis

Local Anesthetic/Vasoconstrictor Precautions No information available to require special precautions

Effects on Dental Treatment Key adverse event(s) related to dental treatment: Pharyngitis.

Common Adverse Effects Adverse effects vary depending upon dosage form. Effects as reported with tablets, unless otherwise noted:

>10%:
Central nervous system: Pain (14%)
Gastrointestinal: Abdominal pain (18%; enema: 8%)
Genitourinary: Eructation (16%)
Respiratory: Pharyngitis (11%)

1% to 10%:
Cardiovascular: Chest pain (3%), peripheral edema (3%)
Central nervous system: Chills (3%), dizziness (suppository: 3%), fever (enema: 3%; suppository: 1%), insomnia (2%), malaise (2%)
Dermatologic: Rash (6%; suppository: 1%), pruritus (3%; enema: 1%), acne (2%; suppository: 1%)
Gastrointestinal: Dyspepsia (6%), constipation (5%), vomiting (5%), colitis exacerbation (3%; suppository: 1%), nausea (capsule: 3%), flatulence (enema: 6%), hemorrhoids (enema: 1%), nausea and vomiting (capsule: 1%), rectal pain (enema: 1%; suppository: 2%)
Local: Pain on insertion of enema tip (enema: 1%)
Neuromuscular & skeletal: Back pain (7%; enema: 1%), arthralgia (5%), hypertonia (5%), myalgia (3%), arthritis (2%), leg/joint pain (enema: 2%)

Ocular: Conjunctivitis (2%)

Respiratory: Flu-like syndrome (3%; enema: 5%), diaphoresis (3%), cough increased (2%)

Mechanism of Action Mesalamine (5-aminosalicylic acid) is the active component of sulfasalazine; the specific mechanism of action of mesalamine is unknown; however, it is thought that it modulates local chemical mediators of the inflammatory response, especially leukotrienes; action appears topical rather than systemic

Drug Interactions

Increased Effect/Toxicity: Mesalamine may increase the risk of myelosuppression from azathioprine, mercaptopurine, and thioguanine.

Decreased Effect: Decreased digoxin bioavailability.

Pharmacodynamics/Kinetics

Absorption: Rectal: Variable and dependent upon retention time, underlying GI disease, and colonic pH; Oral: Tablet: ~28%, Capsule: ~20% to 30%

Metabolism: Hepatic and via GI tract to acetyl-5-aminosalicylic acid

Half-life elimination: 5-ASA: 0.5-1.5 hours; acetyl-5-ASA: 5-10 hours

Time to peak, serum: 4-7 hours

Excretion: Urine (as metabolites); feces (<2%)

Pregnancy Risk Factor B

Mesalazine *see* Mesalamine *on page 882*

Mesoridazine (mez oh RID a zeen)

U.S. Brand Names Serentil® [DSC]

Canadian Brand Names Serentil®

Generic Available No

Synonyms Mesoridazine Besylate

Pharmacologic Category Antipsychotic Agent, Phenothiazine, Piperidine

Use Management of schizophrenic patients who fail to respond adequately to treatment with other antipsychotic drugs, either because of insufficient effectiveness or the inability to achieve an effective dose due to intolerable adverse effects from these drugs

Unlabeled/Investigational Use Psychosis

Local Anesthetic/Vasoconstrictor Precautions No information available to require special precautions

Effects on Dental Treatment Key adverse event(s) related to dental treatment: Orthostatic hypotension.

Common Adverse Effects Frequency not defined.

Cardiovascular: Hypotension, orthostatic hypotension, tachycardia, QT prolongation (dose dependent, up to 100% of patients at higher dosages), syncope, edema

Central nervous system: Pseudoparkinsonism, akathisia, dystonias, tardive dyskinesia, dizziness, drowsiness, restlessness, ataxia, slurred speech, neuroleptic malignant syndrome (NMS), impairment of temperature regulation, lowering of seizure threshold

Dermatologic: Increased sensitivity to sun, rash, itching, angioneurotic edema, dermatitis, discoloration of skin (blue-gray)

Endocrine & metabolic: Changes in menstrual cycle, changes in libido, gynecomastia, lactation, galactorrhea

Gastrointestinal: Constipation, xerostomia, weight gain, nausea, vomiting, stomach pain

Genitourinary: Difficulty in urination, ejaculatory disturbances, impotence, enuresis, incontinence, priapism, urinary retention

Hematologic: Agranulocytosis, leukopenia, eosinophilia, thrombocytopenia, anemia, aplastic anemia

Hepatic: Cholestatic jaundice, hepatotoxicity

Neuromuscular & skeletal: Weakness, tremor, rigidity

Ocular: Pigmentary retinopathy, photophobia, blurred vision, cornea and lens changes

Respiratory: Nasal congestion

Miscellaneous: Diaphoresis (decreased), lupus-like syndrome

Mechanism of Action Blockade of postsynaptic CNS dopamine$_2$ receptors in the mesolimbic and mesocortical areas

Drug Interactions

Increased Effect/Toxicity: Use of mesoridazine with other agents known to prolong QT_c may increase the risk of malignant arrhythmias; concurrent use is contraindicated - includes type I and type III antiarrhythmics, TCAs, and some quinolone antibiotics (sparfloxacin, moxifloxacin, gatifloxacin). Mesoridazine may increase the effect and/or toxicity of antihypertensives, (Continued)

Mesoridazine *(Continued)*

anticholinergics, lithium, CNS depressants (ethanol, narcotics), and trazodone. Metoclopramide may increase risk of extrapyramidal symptoms (EPS).

Decreased Effect: Mesoridazine may inhibit the activity of bromocriptine and levodopa. Benztropine (and other anticholinergics) may inhibit the therapeutic response to mesoridazine and excess anticholinergic effects may occur. Mesoridazine and possibly other low potency antipsychotic may reverse the pressor effects of epinephrine.

Pharmacodynamics/Kinetics

Duration: 4-6 hours
Absorption: Tablet: Erratic; Liquid: More dependable
Protein binding: 91% to 99%
Half-life elimination: 24-48 hours
Time to peak, serum: 2-4 hours; Steady-state serum: 4-7 days
Excretion: Urine

Pregnancy Risk Factor C

Mesoridazine Besylate *see* Mesoridazine *on page 883*
Mestinon® *see* Pyridostigmine *on page 1153*
Mestinon® Timespan® *see* Pyridostigmine *on page 1153*

Mestranol and Norethindrone (MES tra nole & nor eth IN drone)

Related Information

Endocrine Disorders and Pregnancy *on page 1481*
Norethindrone *on page 996*

U.S. Brand Names Necon® 1/50; Norinyl® 1+50; Ortho-Novum® 1/50

Canadian Brand Names Ortho-Novum® 1/50

Generic Available Yes

Synonyms Norethindrone and Mestranol; Ortho Novum 1/50

Pharmacologic Category Contraceptive; Estrogen and Progestin Combination

Use Prevention of pregnancy

Unlabeled/Investigational Use Treatment of hypermenorrhea, endometriosis, female hypogonadism

Local Anesthetic/Vasoconstrictor Precautions No information available to require special precautions

Effects on Dental Treatment When prescribing antibiotics, patient must be advised to use additional methods of birth control if on hormonal contraceptives.

Common Adverse Effects Frequency not defined.

Cardiovascular: Arterial thromboembolism, cerebral hemorrhage, cerebral thrombosis, edema, hypertension, mesenteric thrombosis, myocardial infarction

Central nervous system: Depression, dizziness, headache, migraine, nervousness, premenstrual syndrome, stroke

Dermatologic: Acne, erythema multiforme, erythema nodosum, hirsutism, loss of scalp hair, melasma (may persist), rash (allergic)

Endocrine & metabolic: Amenorrhea, breakthrough bleeding, breast enlargement, breast secretion, breast tenderness, carbohydrate intolerance, lactation decreased (postpartum), glucose tolerance decreased, libido changes, menstrual flow changes, sex hormone-binding globulins (SHBG) increased, spotting, temporary infertility (following discontinuation), thyroid-binding globulin increased, triglycerides increased

Gastrointestinal: Abdominal cramps, appetite changes, bloating, cholestasis, colitis, gallbladder disease, jaundice, nausea, vomiting, weight gain/loss

Genitourinary: Cervical erosion changes, cervical secretion changes, cystitis-like syndrome, vaginal candidiasis, vaginitis

Hematologic: Antithrombin III decreased, folate levels decreased, hemolytic uremic syndrome, norepinephrine induced platelet aggregability increased, porphyria, prothrombin increased; factors VII, VIII, IX, and X increased

Hepatic: Benign liver tumors, Budd-Chiari syndrome, cholestatic jaundice, hepatic adenomas

Local: Thrombophlebitis

Ocular: Cataracts, change in corneal curvature (steepening), contact lens intolerance, optic neuritis, retinal thrombosis

Renal: Impaired renal function

Respiratory: Pulmonary thromboembolism

Miscellaneous: Hemorrhagic eruption

Mechanism of Action Combination oral contraceptives inhibit ovulation via a negative feedback mechanism on the hypothalamus, which alters the normal pattern of gonadotropin secretion of a follicle-stimulating hormone (FSH) and luteinizing hormone by the anterior pituitary. The follicular phase FSH and midcycle surge of gonadotropins are inhibited. In addition, combination hormonal contraceptives produce alterations in the genital tract, including changes in the cervical mucus, rendering it unfavorable for sperm penetration even if ovulation occurs. Changes in the endometrium may also occur, producing an unfavorable environment for nidation. Combination hormonal contraceptive drugs may alter the tubal transport of the ova through the fallopian tubes. Progestational agents may also alter sperm fertility.

Drug Interactions

Cytochrome P450 Effect:

Mestranol: **Substrate** of CYP2C19 (major); Based on active metabolite ethinyl estradiol: **Substrate** of CYP3A4 (major), 3A5-7 (minor); **Inhibits** CYP1A2 (weak), 2B6 (weak), 2C19 (weak), 3A4 (weak)

Norethindrone: **Substrate** of CYP3A4 (major); **Induces** CYP2C19 (weak)

Increased Effect/Toxicity: Acetaminophen and ascorbic acid may increase plasma levels of estrogen component. Atorvastatin and indinavir increase plasma levels of combination hormonal contraceptives. Combination hormonal contraceptives increase the plasma levels of alprazolam, chlordiazepoxide, cyclosporine, diazepam, prednisolone, selegiline, theophylline, tricyclic antidepressants. Combination hormonal contraceptives may increase (or decrease) the effects of coumarin derivatives.

Decreased Effect: CYP2C8/9 inhibitors may decrease the levels of ethinyl estradiol (active metabolite of mestranol); example inhibitors include delavirdine, fluconazole, gemfibrozil, ketoconazole, nicardipine, NSAIDs, pioglitazone, and sulfonamides. CYP3A4 inducers may decrease the levels of ethinyl estradiol (active metabolite of mestranol); example inducers include aminoglutethimide, carbamazepine, nafcillin, nevirapine, phenobarbital, phenytoin, and rifamycins. Combination hormonal contraceptives may decrease plasma levels of acetaminophen, clofibric acid, lorazepam, morphine, oxazepam, salicylic acid, temazepam. Contraceptive effect decreased by acitretin, aminoglutethimide, amprenavir, griseofulvin, lopinavir, nelfinavir, nevirapine, penicillins (effect not consistent), ritonavir, tetracyclines (effect not consistent) troglitazone. Combination hormonal contraceptives may decrease (or increase) the effects of coumarin derivatives.

Pharmacodynamics/Kinetics

Mestranol: Metabolism: Hepatic via demethylation to ethinyl estradiol

Norethindrone: See Norethindrone monograph for additional information.

Pregnancy Risk Factor X

Metacortandralone *see* PrednisoLONE *on page 1113*

Metadate® CD *see* Methylphenidate *on page 908*

Metadate™ ER *see* Methylphenidate *on page 908*

Metaglip™ *see* Glipizide and Metformin *on page 662*

Metamucil® [OTC] *see* Psyllium *on page 1151*

Metamucil® Smooth Texture [OTC] *see* Psyllium *on page 1151*

Metaproterenol (met a proe TER e nol)

Related Information

Respiratory Diseases *on page 1478*

U.S. Brand Names Alupent®

Generic Available Yes; Excludes inhaler

Synonyms Metaproterenol Sulfate; Orciprenaline Sulfate

Pharmacologic Category $Beta_2$-Adrenergic Agonist

Use Bronchodilator in reversible airway obstruction due to asthma or COPD; because of its delayed onset of action (1 hour) and prolonged effect (4 or more hours), this may not be the drug of choice for assessing response to a bronchodilator

Local Anesthetic/Vasoconstrictor Precautions No information available to require special precautions

Effects on Dental Treatment Key adverse event(s) related to dental treatment: Bad taste and xerostomia (normal salivary flow resumes upon discontinuation).

Common Adverse Effects

>10%:

Cardiovascular: Tachycardia (<17%)

Central nervous system: Nervousness (3% to 14%)

Endocrine & metabolic: Serum glucose increased, serum potassium decreased

Neuromuscular & skeletal: Tremor (1% to 33%)

(Continued)

Metaproterenol *(Continued)*

1% to 10%:

Cardiovascular: Palpitations (<4%)

Central nervous system: Headache (<4%), dizziness (1% to 4%), insomnia (2%)

Gastrointestinal: Nausea, vomiting, bad taste, heartburn (≥4%), xerostomia

Neuromuscular & skeletal: Trembling, muscle cramps, weakness (1%)

Respiratory: Coughing, pharyngitis (≤4%)

Miscellaneous: Diaphoresis (increased) (≤4%)

Mechanism of Action Relaxes bronchial smooth muscle by action on $beta_2$-receptors with very little effect on heart rate

Drug Interactions

Increased Effect/Toxicity: Sympathomimetics, TCAs, MAO inhibitors taken with metaproterenol may result in toxicity. Inhaled ipratropium may increase duration of bronchodilation. Halothane may increase risk of malignant arrhythmias; avoid concurrent use.

Decreased Effect: Decreased effect of beta-blockers.

Pharmacodynamics/Kinetics

Onset of action: Bronchodilation: Oral: ~15 minutes; Inhalation: ~60 seconds

Peak effect: Oral: ~1 hour

Duration: ~1-5 hours

Pregnancy Risk Factor C

Metaproterenol Sulfate *see* Metaproterenol *on page 885*

Metaxalone (me TAKS a lone)

U.S. Brand Names Skelaxin®

Canadian Brand Names Skelaxin®

Generic Available No

Pharmacologic Category Skeletal Muscle Relaxant

Use Relief of discomfort associated with acute, painful musculoskeletal conditions

Local Anesthetic/Vasoconstrictor Precautions No information available to require special precautions

Effects on Dental Treatment No significant effects or complications reported

Common Adverse Effects Frequency not defined.

Central nervous system: Paradoxical stimulation, headache, drowsiness, dizziness, irritability

Dermatologic: Allergic dermatitis

Gastrointestinal: Nausea, vomiting, stomach cramps

Hematologic: Leukopenia, hemolytic anemia

Hepatic: Hepatotoxicity

Miscellaneous: Anaphylaxis

Dosage Children >12 years and Adults: Oral: 800 mg 3-4 times/day

Mechanism of Action Does not have a direct effect on skeletal muscle; most of its therapeutic effect comes from actions on the central nervous system

Contraindications Hypersensitivity to metaxalone or any component of the formulation; impaired hepatic or renal function, history of drug-induced hemolytic anemias or other anemias

Warnings/Precautions Use with caution in patients with impaired hepatic function

Drug Interactions

Increased Effect/Toxicity: Additive effects with ethanol or CNS depressants

Ethanol/Nutrition/Herb Interactions Ethanol: Avoid ethanol (may increase CNS depression).

Dietary Considerations Administration with food may increase serum concentrations.

Pharmacodynamics/Kinetics

Onset of action: ~1 hour

Duration: ~4-6 hours

Metabolism: Hepatic

Bioavailability: Not established; food may increase

Half-life elimination: 9 hours

Time to peak: T_{max}: 3 hours

Excretion: Urine (as metabolites)

Pregnancy Risk Factor C

Dosage Forms TAB: 400 mg, 800 mg

Metformin (met FOR min)

Related Information

Endocrine Disorders and Pregnancy *on page 1481*
Glipizide and Metformin *on page 662*
Rosiglitazone and Metformin *on page 1201*

U.S. Brand Names Fortamet™; Glucophage®; Glucophage® XR; Riomet™

Canadian Brand Names Alti-Metformin; Apo-Metformin®; Gen-Metformin; Glucophage®; Glycon; Novo-Metformin; Nu-Metformin; PMS-Metformin; Rho®-Metformin; Rhoxal-metformin FC

Mexican Brand Names Dabex® [tabs]; Dimefor®; Glucophage®

Generic Available Yes: Excludes solution

Synonyms Metformin Hydrochloride

Pharmacologic Category Antidiabetic Agent, Biguanide

Use Management of type 2 diabetes mellitus (noninsulin dependent, NIDDM) as monotherapy when hyperglycemia cannot be managed on diet alone. May be used concomitantly with a sulfonylurea or insulin to improve glycemic control.

Unlabeled/Investigational Use Treatment of HIV lipodystrophy syndrome

Local Anesthetic/Vasoconstrictor Precautions No information available to require special precautions

Effects on Dental Treatment No significant effects or complications reported

Common Adverse Effects

>10%:

Gastrointestinal: Nausea/vomiting (6% to 25%), diarrhea (10% to 53%), flatulence (12%)

Neuromuscular & skeletal: Weakness (9%)

1% to 10%:

Cardiovascular: Chest discomfort, flushing, palpitation

Central nervous system: Headache (6%), chills, dizziness, lightheadedness

Dermatologic: Rash

Endocrine & metabolic: Hypoglycemia

Gastrointestinal: Indigestion (7%), abdominal discomfort (6%), abdominal distention, abnormal stools, constipation, dyspepsia/ heartburn, taste disorder

Neuromuscular & skeletal: Myalgia

Respiratory: Dyspnea, upper respiratory tract infection

Miscellaneous: Decreased vitamin B_{12} levels (7%), increased diaphoresis, flu-like syndrome, nail disorder

Dosage Note: Allow 1-2 weeks between dose titrations: Generally, clinically significant responses are not seen at doses <1500 mg daily; however, a lower recommended starting dose and gradual increased dosage is recommended to minimize gastrointestinal symptoms

Children 10-16 years: Management of type 2 diabetes mellitus: Oral (500 mg tablet or oral solution): Initial: 500 mg twice daily (given with the morning and evening meals); increases in daily dosage should be made in increments of 500 mg at weekly intervals, given in divided doses, up to a maximum of 2000 mg/day

Adults ≥17 years: Management of type 2 diabetes mellitus: Oral:

Immediate release tablet or oral solution: Initial: 500 mg twice daily (give with the morning and evening meals) **or** 850 mg once daily; increase dosage incrementally.

Incremental dosing recommendations based on dosage form:

500 mg tablet: One tablet/day at weekly intervals
850 mg tablet: One tablet/day every other week
Oral solution: 500 mg twice daily every other week

Doses of up to 2000 mg/day may be given twice daily. If a dose > 2000 mg/day is required, it may be better tolerated in three divided doses. Maximum recommended dose 2550 mg/day.

Extended release tablet: Initial: 500 mg once daily (with the evening meal); dosage may be increased by 500 mg weekly; maximum dose: 2000 mg once daily. If glycemic control is not achieved at maximum dose, may divide dose to 1000 mg twice daily. If doses >2000 mg/day are needed, switch to regular release tablets and titrate to maximum dose of 2550 mg/day.

Elderly: The initial and maintenance dosing should be conservative, due to the potential for decreased renal function. Generally, elderly patients should not be titrated to the maximum dose of metformin. Do not use in patients ≥80 years of age unless normal renal function has been established.

Transfer from other antidiabetic agents: No transition period is generally necessary except when transferring from chlorpropamide. When transferring

(Continued)

Metformin *(Continued)*

from chlorpropamide, care should be exercised during the first 2 weeks because of the prolonged retention of chlorpropamide in the body, leading to overlapping drug effects and possible hypoglycemia.

Concomitant metformin and oral sulfonylurea therapy: If patients have not responded to 4 weeks of the maximum dose of metformin monotherapy, consider a gradual addition of an oral sulfonylurea, even if prior primary or secondary failure to a sulfonylurea has occurred. Continue metformin at the maximum dose.

Failed sulfonylurea therapy: Patients with prior failure on glyburide may be treated by gradual addition of metformin. Initiate with glyburide 20 mg and metformin 500 mg daily. Metformin dosage may be increased by 500 mg/day at weekly intervals, up to a maximum of 2500 mg/day (dosage of glyburide maintained at 20 mg/day).

Concomitant metformin and insulin therapy: Initial: 500 mg metformin once daily, continue current insulin dose; increase by 500 mg metformin weekly until adequate glycemic control is achieved

Maximum dose: 2500 mg metformin; 2000 mg metformin extended release

Decrease insulin dose 10% to 25% when FPG <120 mg/dL; monitor and make further adjustments as needed

Dosing adjustment/comments in renal impairment: The plasma and blood half-life of metformin is prolonged and the renal clearance is decreased in proportion to the decrease in creatinine clearance. Per the manufacturer, metformin is contraindicated in the presence of renal dysfunction defined as a serum creatinine >1.5 mg/dL in males, or >1.4 mg/dL in females and in patients with abnormal clearance. Clinically, it has been recommended that metformin be avoided in patients with Cl_{cr} <60-70 mL/minute (DeFronzo, 1999).

Dosing adjustment in hepatic impairment: Avoid metformin; liver disease is a risk factor for the development of lactic acidosis during metformin therapy.

Mechanism of Action Decreases hepatic glucose production, decreasing intestinal absorption of glucose and improves insulin sensitivity (increases peripheral glucose uptake and utilization)

Contraindications Hypersensitivity to metformin or any component of the formulation; renal disease or renal dysfunction (serum creatinine ≥1.5 mg/dL in males or ≥1.4 mg/dL in females or abnormal creatinine clearance from any cause, including shock, acute myocardial infarction, or septicemia); congestive heart failure requiring pharmacological management; acute or chronic metabolic acidosis with or without coma (including diabetic ketoacidosis)

Note: Temporarily discontinue in patients undergoing radiologic studies in which intravascular iodinated contrast materials are utilized.

Warnings/Precautions Lactic acidosis is a rare, but potentially severe consequence of therapy with metformin. Lactic acidosis should be suspected in any diabetic patient receiving metformin who has evidence of acidosis when evidence of ketoacidosis is lacking. Discontinue metformin in clinical situations predisposing to hypoxemia, including conditions such as cardiovascular collapse, respiratory failure, acute myocardial infarction, acute congestive heart failure, and septicemia.

Metformin is substantially excreted by the kidney. The risk of accumulation and lactic acidosis increases with the degree of impairment of renal function. Patients with renal function below the limit of normal for their age should not receive metformin. In elderly patients, renal function should be monitored regularly; should not be used in any patient ≥80 years of age unless measurement of creatinine clearance verifies normal renal function. Use of concomitant medications that may affect renal function (ie, affect tubular secretion) may also affect metformin disposition. Metformin should be suspended in patients with dehydration and/or prerenal azotemia. Therapy should be suspended for any surgical procedures (resume only after normal intake resumed and normal renal function is verified). Metformin should also be temporarily discontinued for 48 hours in patients undergoing radiologic studies involving the intravascular administration of iodinated contrast materials (potential for acute alteration in renal function).

Avoid use in patients with impaired liver function. Patient must be instructed to avoid excessive acute or chronic ethanol use. Administration of oral antidiabetic drugs has been reported to be associated with increased cardiovascular mortality; metformin does not appear to share this risk. Safety and efficacy of metformin have been established for use in children ≥10 years of age; the extended release preparation is for use in patients ≥17 years of age.

Drug Interactions

Increased Effect/Toxicity: Furosemide and cimetidine may increase metformin blood levels. Cationic drugs (eg, amiloride, digoxin, morphine, procainamide, quinidine, quinine, ranitidine, triamterene, trimethoprim, and vancomycin) which are eliminated by renal tubular secretion have the potential to increase metformin levels by competing for common renal tubular transport systems. Contrast agents may increase the risk of metformin-induced lactic acidosis; discontinue metformin prior to exposure and withhold for 48 hours.

Decreased Effect: Drugs which tend to produce hyperglycemia (eg, diuretics, corticosteroids, phenothiazines, thyroid products, estrogens, oral contraceptives, phenytoin, nicotinic acid, sympathomimetics, calcium channel blocking drugs, isoniazid) may lead to a loss of glucose control.

Ethanol/Nutrition/Herb Interactions

Ethanol: Avoid or limit ethanol (incidence of lactic acidosis may be increased; may cause hypoglycemia).

Food: Food decreases the extent and slightly delays the absorption. May decrease absorption of vitamin B_{12} and/or folic acid.

Herb/Nutraceutical: Caution with chromium, garlic, gymnema (may cause hypoglycemia).

Dietary Considerations Drug may cause GI upset; take with food (to decrease GI upset). Take at the same time each day. Dietary modification based on ADA recommendations is a part of therapy. Monitor for signs and symptoms of vitamin B_{12} and/or folic acid deficiency; supplementation may be required.

Pharmacodynamics/Kinetics

Onset of action: Within days; maximum effects up to 2 weeks

Distribution: V_d: 654 ± 358 L

Protein binding: Negligible

Bioavailability: Absolute: Fasting: 50% to 60%

Half-life elimination, plasma: 6.2 hours

Excretion: Urine (90% as unchanged drug)

Pregnancy Risk Factor B

Dosage Forms SOLN, oral (Riomet™): 100 mg/mL (118 mL, 473 mL). **TAB** (Glucophage®): 500 mg, 850 mg, 1000 mg. **TAB, extended release:** 500 mg; (Fortamet™): 500 mg, 1000 mg; (Glucophage® XR): 500 mg, 750 mg

Metformin and Glipizide *see* Glipizide and Metformin *on page 662*

Metformin and Glyburide *see* Glyburide and Metformin *on page 665*

Metformin and Rosiglitazone *see* Rosiglitazone and Metformin *on page 1201*

Metformin Hydrochloride *see* Metformin *on page 887*

Metformin Hydrochloride and Rosiglitazone Maleate *see* Rosiglitazone and Metformin *on page 1201*

Methadone (METH a done)

U.S. Brand Names Dolophine®; Methadone Intensol™; Methadose®

Canadian Brand Names Dolophine®; Metadol™; Methadose®

Generic Available Yes

Synonyms Methadone Hydrochloride

Pharmacologic Category Analgesic, Narcotic

Use Management of severe pain; detoxification and maintenance treatment of narcotic addiction (if used for detoxification and maintenance treatment of narcotic addiction, it must be part of an FDA-approved program)

Local Anesthetic/Vasoconstrictor Precautions No information available to require special precautions

Effects on Dental Treatment Key adverse event(s) related to dental treatment: Significant xerostomia (normal salivary flow resumes upon discontinuation).

Common Adverse Effects Frequency not defined. During prolonged administration, adverse effects may decrease over several weeks; however, constipation and sweating may persist.

Cardiovascular: Bradycardia, peripheral vasodilation, cardiac arrest, syncope, faintness, shock, hypotension, edema, arrhythmias, bigeminal rhythms, extrasystoles, tachycardia, torsade de pointes, ventricular fibrillation, ventricular tachycardia, EKG changes, QT interval prolonged, T-wave inversion, cardiomyopathy, flushing, heart failure, palpitations, phlebitis, orthostatic hypotension,

Central nervous system: Euphoria, dysphoria, headache, insomnia, agitation, disorientation, drowsiness, dizziness, lightheadedness, sedation, confusion, seizures

Dermatologic: Pruritus, urticaria, rash, hemorrhagic urticaria

(Continued)

Methadone *(Continued)*

Endocrine & metabolic: Libido decreased, hypokalemia, hypomagnesemia, antidiuretic effect, amenorrhea
Gastrointestinal: Nausea, vomiting, constipation, anorexia, stomach cramps, xerostomia, biliary tract spasm, abdominal pain, glossitis, weight gain
Genitourinary: Urinary retention or hesitancy, impotence
Hematologic: Thrombocytopenia (reversible, reported in patients with chronic hepatitis)
Neuromuscular & skeletal: Weakness
Local: I.M./SubQ injection: Pain, erythema, swelling; I.V. injection: pruritus, urticaria, rash, hemorrhagic urticaria (rare)
Ocular: Miosis, visual disturbances
Respiratory: Respiratory depression, respiratory arrest, pulmonary edema
Miscellaneous: Physical and psychological dependence, death, diaphoresis

Restrictions C-II

Treatment of narcotic addiction: May only be dispensed by pharmacies or maintenance programs approved by the FDA and designated state authority. Prior approval must be obtained for doses >120 mg administered at a clinic or >100 mg to be taken at home.

Mechanism of Action Binds to opiate receptors in the CNS, causing inhibition of ascending pain pathways, altering the perception of and response to pain; produces generalized CNS depression

Drug Interactions

Cytochrome P450 Effect: Substrate of CYP2C8/9 (minor), 2C19 (minor), 2D6 (minor), 3A4 (major); **Inhibits** CYP2D6 (moderate), 3A4 (weak)

Increased Effect/Toxicity: CYP3A4 inhibitors may increase the levels/effects of methadone (eg, azole antifungals, ciprofloxacin, clarithromycin, diclofenac, doxycycline, erythromycin, imatinib, isoniazid, nefazodone, nicardipine, propofol, protease inhibitors, quinidine, verapamil). Methadone may increase the levels/effects of CYP2D6 substrates (eg, amphetamines, selected beta-blockers, dextromethorphan, fluoxetine, lidocaine, mirtazapine, nefazodone, paroxetine, risperidone, ritonavir, thioridazine, tricyclic antidepressants, venlafaxine). Methadone may increase bioavailability and toxic effects of zidovudine. CNS depressants (including but not limited to opioid analgesics, general anesthetics, sedatives, hypnotics, ethanol) may cause respiratory depression, hypotension, profound sedation, or coma. Levels of desipramine may be increased by methadone. Effects/toxicity of QT_c interval-prolonging agents may be increased; use with caution (including but may not be limited to amitriptyline, astemizole, bepridil, disopyramide, erythromycin, haloperidol, imipramine, quinidine, pimozide, procainamide, sotalol, thioridazine).

Decreased Effect: Agonist/antagonist analgesics (buprenorphine, butorphanol, nalbuphine, pentazocine) may decrease analgesic effect of methadone and precipitate withdrawal symptoms; use is not recommended. Efavirenz and nevirapine may decrease levels of methadone (opioid withdrawal syndrome has been reported). Methadone may decrease bioavailability of didanosine and stavudine. Ritonavir (and combinations) may decrease levels of methadone; withdrawal symptoms have inconsistently been observed, monitor. CYP3A4 inducers may decrease the levels/effects of methadone (eg, aminoglutethimide, carbamazepine, nafcillin, nevirapine, phenobarbital, phenytoin, rifamycins). Monitor for methadone withdrawal. Larger doses of methadone may be required. Methadone may decrease the levels/effects of CYP2D6 prodrug substrates (eg, codeine, hydrocodone, oxycodone, tramadol).

Pharmacodynamics/Kinetics

Onset of action: Oral: Analgesic: 0.5-1 hour; Parenteral: 10-20 minutes
Peak effect: Parenteral: 1-2 hours
Duration: Oral: 6-8 hours, increases to 22-48 hours with repeated doses
Distribution: V_d: 2-6 L/kg; crosses placenta; enters breast milk
Protein binding: 85% to 90%
Metabolism: Hepatic; N-demethylation via CYP3A4 and 2D6 to inactive metabolites
Half-life elimination: 8-59 hours; may be prolonged with alkaline pH, decreased during pregnancy
Excretion: Urine (<10% as unchanged drug); increased with urine pH <6

Pregnancy Risk Factor C/D (prolonged use or high doses at term)

Methadone Hydrochloride *see* Methadone *on page 889*
Methadone Intensol™ *see* Methadone *on page 889*
Methadose® *see* Methadone *on page 889*

Methaminodiazepoxide Hydrochloride *see* Chlordiazepoxide *on page 307*

Methamphetamine (meth am FET a meen)

U.S. Brand Names Desoxyn®

Canadian Brand Names Desoxyn®

Generic Available No

Synonyms Desoxyephedrine Hydrochloride; Methamphetamine Hydrochloride

Pharmacologic Category Stimulant

Use Treatment of attention-deficit/hyperactivity disorder (ADHD); exogenous obesity (short-term adjunct)

Unlabeled/Investigational Use Narcolepsy

Local Anesthetic/Vasoconstrictor Precautions Use vasoconstrictor with caution in patients taking methamphetamine. Amphetamines enhance the sympathomimetic response of epinephrine and norepinephrine leading to potential hypertension and cardiotoxicity.

Effects on Dental Treatment Key adverse event(s) related to dental treatment: Xerostomia (normal salivary flow resumes upon discontinuation). Up to 10% of patients taking dextroamphetamines may present with hypertension. The use of local anesthetic without vasoconstrictor is recommended in these patients.

Common Adverse Effects Frequency not defined.

Cardiovascular: Hypertension, tachycardia, palpitations

Central nervous system: Restlessness, headache, exacerbation of motor and phonic tics and Tourette's syndrome, dizziness, psychosis, dysphoria, overstimulation, euphoria, insomnia

Dermatologic: Rash, urticaria

Endocrine & metabolic: Change in libido

Gastrointestinal: Diarrhea, nausea, vomiting, stomach cramps, constipation, anorexia, weight loss, xerostomia, unpleasant taste

Genitourinary: Impotence

Neuromuscular & skeletal: Tremor

Miscellaneous: Suppression of growth in children, tolerance and withdrawal with prolonged use

Restrictions C-II

Mechanism of Action A sympathomimetic amine related to ephedrine and amphetamine with CNS stimulant activity; peripheral actions include elevation of systolic and diastolic blood pressure and weak bronchodilator and respiratory stimulant action

Drug Interactions

Cytochrome P450 Effect: Substrate of CYP2D6 (major)

Increased Effect/Toxicity: Amphetamines may precipitate hypertensive crisis or serotonin syndrome in patients receiving MAO inhibitors (selegiline >10 mg/day, isocarboxazid, phenelzine, tranylcypromine, furazolidone). Serotonin syndrome has also been associated with combinations of amphetamines and SSRIs; these combinations should be avoided. TCAs may enhance the effects of amphetamines, potentially leading to hypertensive crisis. CYP2D6 inhibitors may increase the levels/effects of methamphetamine; example inhibitors include chlorpromazine, delavirdine, fluoxetine, miconazole, paroxetine, pergolide, quinidine, quinine, ritonavir, and ropinirole. Large doses of antacids or urinary alkalinizers increase the half-life and duration of action of amphetamines. May precipitate arrhythmias in patients receiving general anesthetics. Inhibitors of CYP2D6 may increase the effects of amphetamines (includes amiodarone, cimetidine, delavirdine, fluoxetine, paroxetine, propafenone, quinidine, and ritonavir).

Decreased Effect: Amphetamines inhibit the antihypertensive response to guanethidine and guanadrel. Urinary acidifiers decrease the half-life and duration of action of amphetamines. Enzyme inducers (barbiturates, carbamazepine, phenytoin, and rifampin) may decrease serum concentrations of amphetamines.

Pharmacodynamics/Kinetics

Absorption: Rapid from GI tract

Metabolism: Hepatic

Half-Life elimination: 4-5 hours

Excretion: Urine primarily (dependent on urine pH)

Pregnancy Risk Factor C

Methamphetamine Hydrochloride *see* Methamphetamine *on page 891*

Methazolamide (meth a ZOE la mide)

U.S. Brand Names Neptazane® [DSC]

Canadian Brand Names Apo-Methazolamide®

(Continued)

Methazolamide *(Continued)*

Generic Available Yes

Pharmacologic Category Carbonic Anhydrase Inhibitor; Diuretic, Carbonic Anhydrase Inhibitor; Ophthalmic Agent, Antiglaucoma

Use Adjunctive treatment of open-angle or secondary glaucoma; short-term therapy of narrow-angle glaucoma when delay of surgery is desired

Local Anesthetic/Vasoconstrictor Precautions No information available to require special precautions

Effects on Dental Treatment No significant effects or complications reported

Common Adverse Effects Frequency not defined.

Central nervous system: Malaise, fever, mental depression, drowsiness, dizziness, nervousness, headache, confusion, seizures, fatigue, trembling, unsteadiness

Dermatologic: Urticaria, pruritus, photosensitivity, rash, Stevens-Johnson syndrome

Endocrine & metabolic: Hyperchloremic metabolic acidosis, hypokalemia, hyperglycemia

Gastrointestinal: Metallic taste, anorexia, nausea, vomiting, diarrhea, constipation, weight loss, GI irritation, xerostomia, black tarry stools

Genitourinary: Polyuria, crystalluria, hematuria, polyuria, renal calculi, impotence

Hematologic: Bone marrow depression, thrombocytopenia, thrombocytopenic purpura, hemolytic anemia, leukopenia, pancytopenia, agranulocytosis

Hepatic: Hepatic insufficiency

Neuromuscular & skeletal: Weakness, ataxia, paresthesias

Miscellaneous: Hypersensitivity

Mechanism of Action Noncompetitive inhibition of the enzyme carbonic anhydrase; thought that carbonic anhydrase is located at the luminal border of cells of the proximal tubule. When the enzyme is inhibited, there is an increase in urine volume and a change to an alkaline pH with a subsequent decrease in the excretion of titratable acid and ammonia.

Drug Interactions

Increased Effect/Toxicity: Methazolamide may induce hypokalemia which would sensitize a patient to digitalis toxicity. Hypokalemia may be compounded with concurrent diuretic use or steroids. Methazolamide may increase the potential for salicylate toxicity. Primidone absorption may be delayed.

Decreased Effect: Increased lithium excretion and altered excretion of other drugs by alkalinization of the urine, such as amphetamines, quinidine, procainamide, methenamine, phenobarbital, and salicylates.

Pharmacodynamics/Kinetics

Onset of action: Slow in comparison with acetazolamide (2-4 hours)

Peak effect: 6-8 hours

Duration: 10-18 hours

Absorption: Slow

Distribution: Well into tissue

Protein binding: ~55%

Metabolism: Slowly from GI tract

Half-life elimination: ~14 hours

Excretion: Urine (~25% as unchanged drug)

Pregnancy Risk Factor C

Methenamine (meth EN a meen)

U.S. Brand Names Hiprex®; Mandelamine®; Urex®

Canadian Brand Names Dehydral®; Hiprex®; Mandelamine®; Urasal®; Urex®

Generic Available Yes

Synonyms Hexamethylenetetramine; Methenamine Hippurate; Methenamine Mandelate

Pharmacologic Category Antibiotic, Miscellaneous

Use Prophylaxis or suppression of recurrent urinary tract infections; urinary tract discomfort secondary to hypermotility

Local Anesthetic/Vasoconstrictor Precautions No information available to require special precautions

Effects on Dental Treatment No significant effects or complications reported

Common Adverse Effects 1% to 10%:

Dermatologic: Rash (4%)

Gastrointestinal: Nausea, dyspepsia (4%)

Genitourinary: Dysuria (4%)

Mechanism of Action Methenamine is hydrolyzed to formaldehyde and ammonia in acidic urine; formaldehyde has nonspecific bactericidal action

Drug Interactions

Increased Effect/Toxicity: Sulfonamides may precipitate in the urine.

Decreased Effect: Sodium bicarbonate and acetazolamide will decrease effect secondary to alkalinization of urine.

Pharmacodynamics/Kinetics

Absorption: Readily

Metabolism: Gastric juices: Hydrolyze 10% to 30% unless protected via enteric coating; Hepatic: ~10% to 25%

Half-life elimination: 3-6 hours

Excretion: Urine (~70% to 90% as unchanged drug) within 24 hours

Pregnancy Risk Factor C

Methenamine Hippurate *see* Methenamine *on page 892*

Methenamine Mandelate *see* Methenamine *on page 892*

Methenamine, Sodium Biphosphate, Phenyl Salicylate, Methylene Blue, and Hyoscyamine

(meth EN a meen, SOW dee um bye FOS fate, fen nil sa LIS i late, METH i leen bloo, & hye oh SYE a meen)

Related Information

Hyoscyamine *on page 724*

Methenamine *on page 892*

U.S. Brand Names Urimar-T; Urimax®

Generic Available No

Synonyms Hyoscyamine, Methenamine, Sodium Biphosphate, Phenyl Salicylate, and Methylene Blue; Methylene Blue, Methenamine, Sodium Biphosphate, Phenyl Salicylate, and Hyoscyamine; Phenyl Salicylate, Methenamine, Methylene Blue, Sodium Biphosphate, and Hyoscyamine; Sodium Biphosphate, Methenamine, Methylene Blue, Phenyl Salicylate, and Hyoscyamine

Pharmacologic Category Antibiotic, Miscellaneous

Use Treatment of symptoms of irritative voiding; relief of local symptoms associated with urinary tract infections; relief of urinary tract symptoms caused by diagnostic procedures

Local Anesthetic/Vasoconstrictor Precautions No information available to require special precautions

Effects on Dental Treatment No significant effects or complications reported

Common Adverse Effects Frequency not defined.

Cardiovascular: Tachycardia, flushing

Central nervous system: Dizziness

Gastrointestinal: Xerostomia, nausea, vomiting

Genitourinary: Urinary retention (acute), micturition difficulty, discoloration of urine (blue)

Ocular: Blurred vision

Respiratory: Dyspnea, shortness of breath

Drug Interactions

Increased Effect/Toxicity: Refer to individual monographs for Hyoscyamine and Methenamine.

Decreased Effect: Refer to individual monographs for Hyoscyamine and Methenamine.

Pregnancy Risk Factor C

Methergine® *see* Methylergonovine *on page 907*

Methimazole (meth IM a zole)

Related Information

Endocrine Disorders and Pregnancy *on page 1481*

U.S. Brand Names Tapazole®

Canadian Brand Names Tapazole®

Generic Available Yes

Synonyms Thiamazole

Pharmacologic Category Antithyroid Agent

Use Palliative treatment of hyperthyroidism, return the hyperthyroid patient to a normal metabolic state prior to thyroidectomy, and to control thyrotoxic crisis that may accompany thyroidectomy. The use of antithyroid thioamides is as effective in elderly as they are in younger adults; however, the expense, potential adverse effects, and inconvenience (compliance, monitoring) make them undesirable. The use of radioiodine due to ease of administration and less concern for long-term side effects and reproduction problems (some older males) makes it a more appropriate therapy.

(Continued)

Methimazole *(Continued)*

Local Anesthetic/Vasoconstrictor Precautions No information available to require special precautions

Effects on Dental Treatment No significant effects or complications reported

Common Adverse Effects Frequency not defined.

Cardiovascular: Edema

Central nervous system: Headache, vertigo, drowsiness, CNS stimulation, depression

Dermatologic: Skin rash, urticaria, pruritus, erythema nodosum, skin pigmentation, exfoliative dermatitis, alopecia

Endocrine & metabolic: Goiter

Gastrointestinal: Nausea, vomiting, stomach pain, abnormal taste, constipation, weight gain, salivary gland swelling

Hematologic: Leukopenia, agranulocytosis, granulocytopenia, thrombocytopenia, aplastic anemia, hypoprothrombinemia

Hepatic: Cholestatic jaundice, jaundice, hepatitis

Neuromuscular & skeletal: Arthralgia, paresthesia

Renal: Nephrotic syndrome

Miscellaneous: SLE-like syndrome

Mechanism of Action Inhibits the synthesis of thyroid hormones by blocking the oxidation of iodine in the thyroid gland, blocking iodine's ability to combine with tyrosine to form thyroxine and triiodothyronine (T_3), does not inactivate circulating T_4 and T_3

Drug Interactions

Cytochrome P450 Effect: Inhibits CYP1A2 (weak), 2A6 (weak), 2B6 (weak), 2C8/9 (weak), 2C19 (weak), 2D6 (moderate), 2E1 (weak), 3A4 (weak)

Increased Effect/Toxicity: Dosage of some drugs (including beta-blockers, digoxin, and theophylline) require adjustment during treatment of hyperthyroidism. Methimazole may increase the levels/effects of CYP2D6 substrates (eg, amphetamines, selected beta-blockers, dextromethorphan, fluoxetine, lidocaine, mirtazapine, nefazodone, paroxetine, risperidone, ritonavir, thioridazine, tricyclic antidepressants, venlafaxine).

Decreased Effect: Anticoagulant effect of warfarin may be decreased. Methimazole may decrease the levels/effects of CYP2D6 prodrug substrates (eg, codeine, hydrocodone, oxycodone, tramadol).

Pharmacodynamics/Kinetics

Onset of action: Antithyroid: Oral: 12-18 hours

Duration: 36-72 hours

Distribution: Concentrated in thyroid gland; crosses placenta; enters breast milk (1:1)

Protein binding, plasma: None

Metabolism: Hepatic

Bioavailability: 80% to 95%

Half-life elimination: 4-13 hours

Excretion: Urine (80%)

Pregnancy Risk Factor D

Methionine (me THYE oh neen)

U.S. Brand Names ME-500®; Pedameth®

Generic Available Yes

Pharmacologic Category Nutritional Supplement

Use Treatment of diaper rash and control of odor, dermatitis and ulceration caused by ammoniacal urine

Local Anesthetic/Vasoconstrictor Precautions No information available to require special precautions

Effects on Dental Treatment No significant effects or complications reported

Methitest® *see* MethylTESTOSTERone *on page 912*

Methocarbamol (meth oh KAR ba mole)

Related Information

Temporomandibular Dysfunction (TMD) *on page 1564*

U.S. Brand Names Robaxin®

Canadian Brand Names Robaxin®

Generic Available Yes: Tablet

Pharmacologic Category Skeletal Muscle Relaxant

Dental Use Treatment of muscle spasm associated with acute temporomandibular joint pain

Use Treatment of muscle spasm associated with acute painful musculoskeletal conditions; supportive therapy in tetanus

Local Anesthetic/Vasoconstrictor Precautions No information available to require special precautions

Effects on Dental Treatment Key adverse event(s) related to dental treatment: Metallic taste.

Significant Adverse Effects Frequency not defined.

Cardiovascular: Flushing of face, bradycardia, hypotension, syncope

Central nervous system: Drowsiness, dizziness, lightheadedness, convulsion, vertigo, headache, fever, amnesia, confusion, insomnia, sedation, coordination impaired (mild)

Dermatologic: Allergic dermatitis, urticaria, pruritus, rash, angioneurotic edema

Gastrointestinal: Nausea, vomiting, metallic taste, dyspepsia

Hematologic: Leukopenia

Hepatic: Jaundice

Local: Pain at injection site, thrombophlebitis

Ocular: Nystagmus, blurred vision, diplopia, conjunctivitis

Renal: Renal impairment

Respiratory: Nasal congestion

Miscellaneous: Allergic manifestations, anaphylactic reaction

Dosage

Tetanus: I.V.:

Children: Recommended **only** for use in tetanus: 15 mg/kg/dose or 500 mg/m^2/dose, may repeat every 6 hours if needed; maximum dose: 1.8 g/m^2/day for 3 days only

Adults: Initial dose: 1-3 g; may repeat dose every 6 hours until oral dosing is possible; injection should not be used for more than 3 consecutive days

Muscle spasm: Children ≥16 years and Adults:

Oral: 1.5 g 4 times/day for 2-3 days (up to 8 g/day may be given in severe conditions), then decrease to 4-4.5 g/day in 3-6 divided doses

I.M., I.V.: 1 g every 8 hours if oral not possible; injection should not be used for more than 3 consecutive days. If condition persists, may repeat course of therapy after a drug-free interval of 48 hours.

Elderly: Muscle spasm: Oral: Initial: 500 mg 4 times/day; titrate to response

Dosing adjustment/comments in renal impairment: Do not administer parenteral formulation to patients with renal dysfunction.

Dosing adjustment in hepatic impairment: Specific dosing guidelines are not available; plasma protein binding and clearance are decreased; half-life is increased

Mechanism of Action Causes skeletal muscle relaxation by general CNS depression

Contraindications Hypersensitivity to methocarbamol or any component of the formulation; renal impairment (injection formulation)

Warnings/Precautions

Oral: Use caution with renal or hepatic impairment.

Injection: Rate of injection should not exceed 3 mL/minute; solution is hypertonic; avoid extravasation. Use with caution in patients with a history of seizures. Use caution with hepatic impairment.

Drug Interactions Increased effect/toxicity with CNS depressants; pyridostigmine (a single case of worsening myasthenia has been reported following methocarbamol administration)

Ethanol/Nutrition/Herb Interactions

Ethanol: Avoid ethanol (may increase CNS depression).

Herb/Nutraceutical: Avoid valerian, St John's wort, kava kava, gotu kola (may increase CNS depression).

Pharmacodynamics/Kinetics

Onset of action: Muscle relaxation: Oral: ~30 minutes

Protein binding: 46% to 50%

Metabolism: Hepatic via dealkylation and hydroxylation

Half-life elimination: 1-2 hours

Time to peak, serum: ~2 hours

Excretion: Urine (as metabolites)

Pregnancy Risk Factor C

Lactation Excretion in breast milk unknown/use caution

Dosage Forms

Injection, solution: 100 mg/mL (10 mL) [in polyethylene glycol; vial stopper contains latex]

Tablet: 500 mg, 750 mg

Methohexital (meth oh HEKS i tal)

U.S. Brand Names Brevital® Sodium

Canadian Brand Names Brevital®

Generic Available No

(Continued)

Methohexital *(Continued)*

Synonyms Methohexital Sodium

Pharmacologic Category Barbiturate

Use Induction and maintenance of general anesthesia for short procedures

Can be used in pediatric patients ≥1 month of age as follows: For rectal or intramuscular induction of anesthesia prior to the use of other general anesthetic agents, as an adjunct to subpotent inhalational anesthetic agents for short surgical procedures, or for short surgical, diagnostic, or therapeutic procedures associated with minimal painful stimuli

Unlabeled/Investigational Use Wada test

Local Anesthetic/Vasoconstrictor Precautions No information available to require special precautions

Effects on Dental Treatment No significant effects or complications reported

Significant Adverse Effects Frequency not defined.

Cardiovascular: Hypotension, peripheral vascular collapse

Central nervous system: Seizures, headache

Gastrointestinal: Cramping, diarrhea, rectal bleeding, nausea, vomiting, abdominal pain

Hematologic: Hemolytic anemia, thrombophlebitis

Hepatic: Elevated transaminases

Local: Pain on I.M. injection

Neuromuscular & skeletal: Tremor, twitching, rigidity, involuntary muscle movement, radial nerve palsy

Respiratory: Apnea, respiratory depression, laryngospasm, coughing, hiccups

Restrictions C-IV

Dosage Doses must be titrated to effect

Manufacturer's recommendations:

Infants <1 month: Safety and efficacy not established

Infants ≥1 month and Children:

I.M.: Induction: 6.6-10 mg/kg of a 5% solution

Rectal: Induction: Usual: 25 mg/kg of a 1% solution

Alternative pediatric dosing:

Children 3-12 years:

I.M.: Preoperative: 5-10 mg/kg/dose

I.V.: Induction: 1-2 mg/kg/dose

Rectal: Preoperative/induction: 20-35 mg/kg/dose; usual: 25 mg/kg/dose; maximum dose: 500 mg/dose; give as 10% aqueous solution

Adults: I.V.:

Induction: 50-120 mg to start; 20-40 mg every 4-7 minutes

Wada test (unlabeled): 3-4 mg over 3 second; following signs of recovery, administer a second dose of 2 mg over 2 seconds

Dosing adjustment/comments in hepatic impairment: Lower dosage and monitor closely

Mechanism of Action Ultra short-acting I.V. barbiturate anesthetic

Contraindications Hypersensitivity to methohexital or any component of the formulation; porphyria

Warnings/Precautions Use with extreme caution in patients with liver impairment, asthma, cardiovascular instability

Drug Interactions

Acetaminophen: Barbiturates may enhance the hepatotoxic potential of acetaminophen overdoses

Antiarrhythmics: Barbiturates may increase the metabolism of antiarrhythmics, decreasing their clinical effect; includes disopyramide, propafenone, and quinidine

Anticonvulsants: Barbiturates may increase the metabolism of anticonvulsants; includes ethosuximide, felbamate (possibly), lamotrigine, phenytoin, tiagabine, topiramate, and zonisamide; does not appear to affect gabapentin or levetiracetam

Antineoplastics: Limited evidence suggests that enzyme-inducing anticonvulsant therapy may reduce the effectiveness of some chemotherapy regimens (specifically in ALL); teniposide and methotrexate may be cleared more rapidly in these patients

Antipsychotics: Barbiturates may enhance the metabolism (decrease the efficacy) of antipsychotics; monitor for altered response; dose adjustment may be needed

Beta-blockers: Metabolism of beta-blockers may be increased and clinical effect decreased; atenolol and nadolol are unlikely to interact given their renal elimination

Calcium channel blockers: Barbiturates may enhance the metabolism of calcium channel blockers, decreasing their clinical effect

Chloramphenicol: Barbiturates may increase the metabolism of chloramphenicol and chloramphenicol may inhibit barbiturate metabolism; monitor for altered response

Cimetidine: Barbiturates may enhance the metabolism of cimetidine, decreasing its clinical effect

CNS depressants: Sedative effects and/or respiratory depression with barbiturates may be additive with other CNS depressants; monitor for increased effect; includes ethanol, sedatives, antidepressants, narcotic analgesics, and benzodiazepines

Corticosteroids: Barbiturates may enhance the metabolism of corticosteroids, decreasing their clinical effect

Cyclosporine: Levels may be decreased by barbiturates; monitor

Doxycycline: Barbiturates may enhance the metabolism of doxycycline, decreasing its clinical effect; higher dosages may be required

Estrogens: Barbiturates may increase the metabolism of estrogens and reduce their efficacy

Felbamate may inhibit the metabolism of barbiturates and barbiturates may increase the metabolism of felbamate

Griseofulvin: Barbiturates may impair the absorption of griseofulvin, and griseofulvin metabolism may be increased by barbiturates, decreasing clinical effect

Guanfacine: Effect may be decreased by barbiturates

Immunosuppressants: Barbiturates may enhance the metabolism of immunosuppressants, decreasing its clinical effect; includes both cyclosporine and tacrolimus

Loop diuretics: Metabolism may be increased and clinical effects decreased; established for furosemide, effect with other loop diuretics not established

MAO inhibitors: Metabolism of barbiturates may be inhibited, increasing clinical effect or toxicity of the barbiturates

Methadone: Barbiturates may enhance the metabolism of methadone resulting in methadone withdrawal

Methoxyflurane: Barbiturates may enhance the nephrotoxic effects of methoxyflurane

Oral contraceptives: Barbiturates may enhance the metabolism of oral contraceptives, decreasing their clinical effect; an alternative method of contraception should be considered

Theophylline: Barbiturates may increase metabolism of theophylline derivatives and decrease their clinical effect

Tricyclic antidepressants: Barbiturates may increase metabolism of tricyclic antidepressants and decrease their clinical effect; sedative effects may be additive

Valproic acid: Metabolism of barbiturates may be inhibited by valproic acid; monitor for excessive sedation; a dose reduction may be needed

Warfarin: Barbiturates inhibit the hypoprothrombinemic effects of oral anticoagulants via increased metabolism; this combination should generally be avoided

Dietary Considerations Should not be given to patients with food in stomach because of danger of vomiting during anesthesia.

Pharmacodynamics/Kinetics

Onset of action: I.V.: Immediately

Duration: Single dose: 10-20 minutes

Pregnancy Risk Factor C

Dosage Forms Injection, powder for reconstitution, as sodium: 500 mg, 2.5 g, 5 g

Selected Readings

Buchtel HA, Passaro EA, Selwa LM, et al, "Sodium Methohexital (Brevital) as an Anesthetic in the Wada Test," *Epilepsia*, 2002, 43(9):1056-61.

Cote' CJ, "Sedation for the Pediatric Patient," *Pediatr Clin North Am*, 1994, 41(1):31-58.

Dionne RA, Yagiela JA, Moore PA, et al, "Comparing Efficacy and Safety of Four Intravenous Sedation Regimens in Dental Outpatients," *Am Dent Assoc*, 2001, 132(6):740-51.

Methohexital Sodium *see* Methohexital *on page 895*

Methotrexate (meth oh TREKS ate)

Related Information

Rheumatoid Arthritis, Osteoarthritis, and Osteoporosis *on page 1490*

U.S. Brand Names Rheumatrex®; Trexall™

Canadian Brand Names Apo-Methotrexate®; ratio-Methotrexate

Mexican Brand Names Ledertrexate®; Texate®; Trixilem®

Generic Available Yes

Synonyms Amethopterin; Methotrexate Sodium; MTX; NSC-740

Pharmacologic Category Antineoplastic Agent, Antimetabolite

(Continued)

Methotrexate *(Continued)*

Use Treatment of trophoblastic neoplasms; leukemias; psoriasis; rheumatoid arthritis (RA), including polyarticular-course juvenile rheumatoid arthritis (JRA); breast, head and neck, and lung carcinomas; osteosarcoma; soft-tissue sarcomas; carcinoma of gastrointestinal tract, esophagus, testes; lymphomas

Local Anesthetic/Vasoconstrictor Precautions No information available to require special precautions

Effects on Dental Treatment Key adverse event(s) related to dental treatment: Ulcerative stomatitis, gingivitis, glossitis, and mucositis (dose dependent; appears 3-7 days post-therapy and resolves within 2 weeks).

Common Adverse Effects **Note:** Adverse reactions vary by route and dosage. Hematologic and/or gastrointestinal toxicities may be common at dosages used in chemotherapy; these reactions are much less frequent when used at typical dosages for rheumatic diseases.

>10%:

Central nervous system (with I.T. administration or very high-dose therapy):
- Arachnoiditis: Acute reaction manifested as severe headache, nuchal rigidity, vomiting, and fever; may be alleviated by reducing the dose
- Subacute toxicity: 10% of patients treated with 12-15 mg/m^2 of I.T. methotrexate may develop this in the second or third week of therapy; consists of motor paralysis of extremities, cranial nerve palsy, seizures, or coma. This has also been seen in pediatric cases receiving very high-dose I.V. methotrexate (when enough methotrexate can get across into the CSF).
- Demyelinating encephalopathy: Seen months or years after receiving methotrexate; usually in association with cranial irradiation or other systemic chemotherapy

Dermatologic: Reddening of skin

Endocrine & metabolic: Hyperuricemia, defective oogenesis or spermatogenesis

Gastrointestinal: Ulcerative stomatitis, glossitis, gingivitis, nausea, vomiting, diarrhea, anorexia, intestinal perforation, mucositis (dose dependent; appears in 3-7 days after therapy, resolving within 2 weeks)
- Emetic potential:
  - <100 mg: Moderately low (10% to 30%)
  - ≥100 mg or <250 mg: Moderate (30% to 60%)
  - ≥250 mg: Moderately high (60% to 90%)

Hematologic: Leukopenia, thrombocytopenia

Renal: Renal failure, azotemia, nephropathy

Respiratory: Pharyngitis

1% to 10%:

Cardiovascular: Vasculitis

Central nervous system: Dizziness, malaise, encephalopathy, seizures, fever, chills

Dermatologic: Alopecia, rash, photosensitivity, depigmentation or hyperpigmentation of skin

Endocrine & metabolic: Diabetes

Genitourinary: Cystitis

Hematologic: Hemorrhage

Myelosuppressive: This is the primary dose-limiting factor (along with mucositis) of methotrexate; occurs about 5-7 days after methotrexate therapy, and should resolve within 2 weeks
- WBC: Mild
- Platelets: Moderate
- Onset: 7 days
- Nadir: 10 days
- Recovery: 21 days

Hepatic: Cirrhosis and portal fibrosis have been associated with chronic methotrexate therapy; acute elevation of liver enzymes are common after high-dose methotrexate, and usually resolve within 10 days.

Neuromuscular & skeletal: Arthralgia

Ocular: Blurred vision

Renal: Renal dysfunction: Manifested by an abrupt rise in serum creatinine and BUN and a fall in urine output; more common with high-dose methotrexate, and may be due to precipitation of the drug. The best treatment is prevention: Aggressively hydrate with 3 L/m^2/day starting 12 hours before therapy and continue for 24-36 hours; alkalinize the urine by adding 50 mEq of bicarbonate to each liter of fluid; keep urine flow over 100 mL/hour and urine pH >7.

Respiratory: Pneumonitis: Associated with fever, cough, and interstitial pulmonary infiltrates; treatment is to withhold methotrexate during the acute reaction; interstitial pneumonitis has been reported to occur with an incidence of 1% in patients with RA (dose 7.5-15 mg/week)

Dosage Refer to individual protocols.

Note: Doses between 100-500 mg/m^2 **may require** leucovorin rescue. Doses >500 mg/m^2 **require** leucovorin rescue.

Children:

Dermatomyositis: Oral: 15-20 mg/m^2/week as a single dose once weekly **or** 0.3-1 mg/kg/dose once weekly

Juvenile rheumatoid arthritis: Oral, I.M.: 10 mg/m^2 once weekly, then 5-15 mg/m^2/week as a single dose **or** as 3 divided doses given 12 hours apart

Antineoplastic dosage range:

Oral, I.M.: 7.5-30 mg/m^2/week **or** every 2 weeks

I.V.: 10-18,000 mg/m^2 bolus dosing **or** continuous infusion over 6-42 hours

For dosing schedules, see table:

Methotrexate Dosing Schedules

Dose	Route	Frequency
Conventional		
15-20 mg/m^2	P.O.	Twice weekly
30-50 mg/m^2	P.O., I.V.	Weekly
15 mg/day for 5 days	P.O., I.M.	Every 2-3 weeks
Intermediate		
50-150 mg/m^2*	I.V. push	Every 2-3 weeks
240 mg/m^2*	I.V. infusion	Every 4-7 days
0.5-1 g/m^2**	I.V. infusion	Every 2-3 weeks
High		
1-25 g/m^2*	I.V. infusion	Every 1-3 weeks

*Doses between 100-500 mg/m^2 may require leucovorin rescue in some patients.

**Followed with leucovorin rescue - refer to Leucovorin monograph for details.

Pediatric solid tumors (high-dose): I.V.:

<12 years: 12-25 g/m^2

≥12 years: 8 g/m^2

Acute lymphocytic leukemia (intermediate-dose): I.V.: Loading: 100 mg/m^2 bolus dose, followed by 900 mg/m^2/day infusion over 23-41 hours.

Meningeal leukemia: I.T.: 10-15 mg/m^2 (maximum dose: 15 mg) **or** an age-based dosing regimen; one possible system is:

≤3 months: 3 mg/dose

4-11 months: 6 mg/dose

1 year: 8 mg/dose

2 years: 10 mg/dose

≥3 years: 12 mg/dose

Adults: I.V.: Range is wide from 30-40 mg/m^2/week to 100-12,000 mg/m^2 with leucovorin rescue

Trophoblastic neoplasms:

Oral, I.M.: 15-30 mg/day for 5 days; repeat in 7 days for 3-5 courses

I.V.: 11 mg/m^2 days 1 through 5 every 3 weeks

Head and neck cancer: Oral, I.M., I.V.: 25-50 mg/m^2 once weekly

Mycosis fungoides (cutaneous T-cell lymphoma): Oral, I.M.: Initial (early stages):

5-50 mg once weekly **or**

15-37.5 mg twice weekly

Bladder cancer: I.V.:

30 mg/m^2 day 1 and 8 every 3 weeks **or**

30 mg/m^2 day 1, 15, and 22 every 4 weeks

Breast cancer: I.V.: 30-60 mg/m^2 days 1 and 8 every 3-4 weeks

Gastric cancer: I.V.:1500 mg/m^2 every 4 weeks

Lymphoma, non-Hodgkin's: I.V.:

30 mg/m^2 days 3 and 10 every 3 weeks **or**

120 mg/m^2 day 8 and 15 every 3-4 weeks **or**

200 mg/m^2 day 8 and 15 every 3 weeks **or**

400 mg/m^2 every 4 weeks for 3 cycles **or**

1 g/m^2 every 3 weeks **or**

1.5 g/m^2 every 4 weeks

Sarcoma: I.V.: 8-12 g/m^2 weekly for 2-4 weeks

Rheumatoid arthritis: Oral: 7.5 mg once weekly **or** 2.5 mg every 12 hours for 3 doses/week, not to exceed 20 mg/week

(Continued)

Methotrexate *(Continued)*

Psoriasis:

Oral: 2.5-5 mg/dose every 12 hours for 3 doses given weekly **or**
Oral, I.M.: 10-25 mg/dose given once weekly

Ectopic pregnancy: I.M., I.V.: 50 mg/m^2 as a single dose

Elderly: Rheumatoid arthritis/psoriasis: Oral: Initial: 5-7.5 mg/week, not to exceed 20 mg/week

Dosing adjustment in renal impairment:

Cl_{cr} 61-80 mL/minute: Reduce dose to 75% of usual dose
Cl_{cr} 51-60 mL/minute: Reduce dose to 70% of usual dose
Cl_{cr} 10-50 mL/minute: Reduce dose to 30% to 50% of usual dose
Cl_{cr} <10 mL/minute: Avoid use

Hemodialysis: Not dialyzable (0% to 5%); supplemental dose is not necessary
Peritoneal dialysis: Supplemental dose is not necessary

Dosage adjustment in hepatic impairment:

Bilirubin 3.1-5 mg/dL **or** AST >180 units: Administer 75% of usual dose
Bilirubin >5 mg/dL: Do not use

Mechanism of Action Methotrexate is a folate antimetabolite that inhibits DNA synthesis. Methotrexate irreversibly binds to dihydrofolate reductase, inhibiting the formation of reduced folates, and thymidylate synthetase, resulting in inhibition of purine and thymidylic acid synthesis. Methotrexate is cell cycle specific for the S phase of the cycle.

The MOA in the treatment of rheumatoid arthritis is unknown, but may affect immune function. In psoriasis, methotrexate is thought to target rapidly proliferating epithelial cells in the skin.

Contraindications Hypersensitivity to methotrexate or any component of the formulation; severe renal or hepatic impairment; pre-existing profound bone marrow suppression in patients with psoriasis or rheumatoid arthritis, alcoholic liver disease, AIDS, pre-existing blood dyscrasias; pregnancy (in patients with psoriasis or rheumatoid arthritis); breast-feeding

Warnings/Precautions The U.S. Food and Drug Administration (FDA) currently recommends that procedures for proper handling and disposal of antineoplastic agents be considered.

May cause potentially life-threatening pneumonitis (may occur at any time during therapy and at any dosage); monitor closely for pulmonary symptoms, particularly dry, nonproductive cough. Methotrexate may cause photosensitivity and/or severe dermatologic reactions which are not dose-related. Methotrexate has been associated with acute and chronic hepatotoxicity, fibrosis, and cirrhosis. Risk is related to cumulative dose and prolonged exposure. Ethanol abuse, obesity, advanced age, and diabetes may increase the risk of hepatotoxic reactions.

Methotrexate may cause renal failure, gastrointestinal toxicity, or bone marrow depression. Use with caution in patients with renal impairment, peptic ulcer disease, ulcerative colitis, or pre-existing bone marrow suppression. Gastrointestinal toxicity may be severe: diarrhea and ulcerative stomatitis may require interruption of therapy; death from hemorrhagic enteritis or intestinal perforation has been reported. Methotrexate penetrates slowly into 3rd space fluids, such as pleural effusions or ascites, and exits slowly from these compartments (slower than from plasma). The potential for toxicity may be increased under these conditions. Dosage reduction may be necessary in patients with renal or hepatic impairment, ascites, and pleural effusion. Toxicity from methotrexate or any immunosuppressive is increased in the elderly.

Severe bone marrow suppression, aplastic anemia, and GI toxicity have occurred during concomitant administration with NSAIDs. Use caution when used with other hepatotoxic agents (azathioprine, retinoids, sulfasalazine). Methotrexate given concomitantly with radiotherapy may increase the risk of soft tissue necrosis and osteonecrosis. Immune suppression may lead to opportunistic infections.

For rheumatoid arthritis and psoriasis, immunosuppressive therapy should only be used when disease is active and less toxic; traditional therapy is ineffective. Discontinue therapy in RA or psoriasis if a significant decrease in hematologic components is noted. Methotrexate formulations and/or diluents containing preservatives should not be used for intrathecal or high-dose therapy. Methotrexate injection may contain benzyl alcohol and should not be used in neonates.

Drug Interactions

Increased Effect/Toxicity: Concurrent therapy with NSAIDs has resulted in severe bone marrow suppression, aplastic anemia, and GI toxicity. NSAIDs should not be used during moderate or high-dose methotrexate due to increased and prolonged methotrexate levels (may increase toxicity); NSAID use during treatment of rheumatoid arthritis has not been fully explored, but continuation of prior regimen has been allowed in some circumstances, with cautious monitoring. Salicylates may increase methotrexate levels, however salicylate doses used for prophylaxis of cardiovascular events are not likely to be of concern.

Penicillins, probenecid, sulfonamides, tetracyclines may increase methotrexate concentrations due to a reduction in renal tubular secretion; primarily a concern with high doses of methotrexate. Hepatotoxic agents (acitretin, azathioprine, retinoids, sulfasalazine) may increase the risk of hepatotoxic reactions with methotrexate.

Concomitant administration of cyclosporine with methotrexate may increase levels and toxicity of each. Methotrexate may increase mercaptopurine or theophylline levels. Methotrexate, when administered prior to cytarabine, may enhance the efficacy and toxicity of cytarabine; some combination treatment regimens (eg, hyper-CVAD) have been designed to take advantage of this interaction.

Concurrent use of live virus vaccines may result in infections.

Decreased Effect: Cholestyramine may decrease levels of methotrexate. Corticosteroids may decrease uptake of methotrexate into leukemia cells. Administration of these drugs should be separated by 12 hours. Dexamethasone has been reported to not affect methotrexate influx into cells.

Ethanol/Nutrition/Herb Interactions

Ethanol: Avoid ethanol (may be associated with increased liver injury).

Food: Methotrexate peak serum levels may be decreased if taken with food. Milk-rich foods may decrease methotrexate absorption. Folate may decrease drug response.

Herb/Nutraceutical: Avoid echinacea (has immunostimulant properties).

Dietary Considerations

Sodium content of 100 mg injection: 20 mg (0.86 mEq)

Sodium content of 100 mg (low sodium) injection: 15 mg (0.65 mEq)

Pharmacodynamics/Kinetics

Onset of action: Antirheumatic: 3-6 weeks; additional improvement may continue longer than 12 weeks

Absorption: Oral: Rapid; well absorbed at low doses (<30 mg/m^2), incomplete after large doses; I.M.: Complete

Distribution: Penetrates slowly into 3rd space fluids (eg, pleural effusions, ascites), exits slowly from these compartments (slower than from plasma); crosses placenta; small amounts enter breast milk; sustained concentrations retained in kidney and liver

Protein binding: 50%

Metabolism: <10%; degraded by intestinal flora to DAMPA by carboxypeptidase; hepatic aldehyde oxidase converts methotrexate to 7-OH methotrexate; polyglutamates are produced intracellularly and are just as potent as methotrexate; their production is dose- and duration-dependent and they are slowly eliminated by the cell once formed

Half-life elimination: Low dose: 3-10 hours; High dose: 8-12 hours

Time to peak, serum: Oral: 1-2 hours; I.M.: 30-60 minutes

Excretion: Urine (44% to 100%); feces (small amounts)

Pregnancy Risk Factor X (psoriasis, rheumatoid arthritis)

Dosage Forms INJ, powder for reconstitution [preservative free]: 20 mg, 1 g. **INJ, solution:** 25 mg/mL (2 mL, 10 mL). **INJ, solution** [preservative free]: 25 mg/mL (2 mL, 4 mL, 8 mL, 10 mL). **TAB:** 2.5 mg; (Rheumatrex®): 2.5 mg; (Trexall™): 5 mg, 7.5 mg, 10 mg, 15 mg. **TAB** [dose pack] (Rheumatrex® Dose Pack): 2.5 mg (4 cards with 2, 3, 4, 5, or 6 tablets each)

Methotrexate Sodium *see* Methotrexate *on page 897*

Methotrimeprazine (meth oh trye MEP ra zeen)

Canadian Brand Names Apo-Methoprazine®; Novo-Meprazine; Nozinan®

Mexican Brand Names Levocina® [tabs]; Sinogan® [tabs]; Sinogan® [inj.]

Generic Available No

Synonyms Levomepromazine; Methotrimeprazine Hydrochloride

Pharmacologic Category Analgesic, Non-narcotic

Use Treatment of schizophrenia or psychosis; management of pain, including pain caused by neuralgia or cancer; adjunct to general anesthesia; management of nausea and vomiting; sedation

Unlabeled/Investigational Use Bipolar disorder, agitation

Local Anesthetic/Vasoconstrictor Precautions No information available to require special precautions

(Continued)

Methotrimeprazine *(Continued)*

Effects on Dental Treatment Key adverse event(s) related to dental treatment: Anticholinergic side effects can cause a reduction of saliva production or secretion, contributing to discomfort and dental disease (ie, caries, oral candidiasis, and periodontal disease). Phenothiazines can cause extrapyramidal reactions which may appear as muscle twitching or increased motor activity of the face, neck, or head.

Common Adverse Effects Note: Frequencies not defined; some reactions listed are based on reports for other agents in this same pharmacologic class, and may not be specifically reported for methotrimeprazine.

Cardiovascular: Hypotension, orthostatic hypotension, tachycardia, QT_c prolongation (rare)

Central nervous system: Extrapyramidal symptoms (pseudoparkinsonism, akathisia, dystonias, tardive dyskinesia), dizziness, seizures, headache, drowsiness, neuroleptic malignant syndrome (NMS), impairment of temperature regulation

Dermatologic: Photosensitivity (rare), rash

Endocrine & metabolic: Gynecomastia, weight gain, menstrual irregularity, changes in libido

Gastrointestinal: Constipation, vomiting, nausea, xerostomia, ileus

Genitourinary: Difficulty in urination, ejaculatory disturbances, incontinence, polyuria, ejaculating dysfunction, priapism

Hematologic: Agranulocytosis (rare), leukopenia, eosinophilia, hemolytic anemia, thrombocytopenic purpura, pancytopenia

Hepatic: Cholestatic jaundice, hepatotoxicity

Miscellaneous: Diaphoresis

Restrictions Not available in U.S.

Mechanism of Action Dopamine antagonist; also binds alpha-1, alpha-2, and serotonin receptors

Drug Interactions

Cytochrome P450 Effect: Inhibits CYP2D6

Increased Effect/Toxicity: Concurrent use of MAO inhibitors may result in toxicity; these combinations are best avoided. Methotrimeprazine may produce additive CNS depressant effects with CNS depressants (ethanol, narcotics). If a patient is receiving methotrimeprazine, the dose of a barbiturate or narcotic should be reduced by 50%. Chloroquine, propranolol, and sulfadoxine-pyrimethamine may increase methotrimeprazine concentrations. Concurrent use with TCA may produce increased toxicity or altered therapeutic response. A phenothiazine plus lithium may rarely produce neurotoxicity. Metoclopramide may increase risk of extrapyramidal symptoms (EPS).

Methotrimeprazine may increase the levels/effects of amphetamines, selected beta blockers, dextromethorphan, fluoxetine, lidocaine, mesoridazine, mirtazapine, nefazodone, paroxetine, risperidone, ritonavir, thioridazine, tricyclic antidepressants, venlafaxine, and other CYP2D6 substrates.

Decreased Effect: Benztropine (and other anticholinergics) may inhibit the therapeutic response to phenothiazines. Antipsychotics such as methotrimeprazine inhibit the ability of bromocriptine to lower serum prolactin concentrations. The antihypertensive effects of guanethidine and guanadrel may be inhibited by phenothiazines. Methotrimeprazine may inhibit the antiparkinsonian effect of levodopa. Low potency antipsychotics may reverse the pressor effects of epinephrine. Methotrimeprazine may decrease the levels/effects of CYP2D6 prodrug substrates (eg, codeine, hydrocodone, oxycodone, tramadol).

Pharmacodynamics/Kinetics

Onset of action: Injection: 1 hour

Duration of action: 2-4 hours

Bioavailability: 50%

Time to peak, serum: I.M.: 0.5-1.5 hours; Oral: 1-3 hours

Half-life elimination: 30 hours

Pregnancy Risk Factor C

Methotrimeprazine Hydrochloride *see* Methotrimeprazine *on page 901*

Methoxsalen (meth OKS a len)

U.S. Brand Names 8-MOP®; Oxsoralen®; Oxsoralen-Ultra®; Uvadex®

Canadian Brand Names 8-MOP®; Oxsoralen™; Oxsoralen-Ultra™; Ultramop™; Uvadex®

Mexican Brand Names Dermox®; Meladinina®; Oxsoralen®

Generic Available No

Synonyms Methoxypsoralen; 8-Methoxypsoralen; 8-MOP

Pharmacologic Category Psoralen

Use

Oral: Symptomatic control of severe, recalcitrant disabling psoriasis; repigmentation of idiopathic vitiligo; palliative treatment of skin manifestations of cutaneous T-cell lymphoma (CTCL)

Topical: Repigmentation of idiopathic vitiligo

Extracorporeal: Palliative treatment of skin manifestations of CTCL

Local Anesthetic/Vasoconstrictor Precautions No information available to require special precautions

Effects on Dental Treatment No significant effects or complications reported

Common Adverse Effects Frequency not always defined.

Cardiovascular: Severe edema, hypotension

Central nervous system: Nervousness, vertigo, depression, dizziness, headache, malaise

Dermatologic: Painful blistering, burning, and peeling of skin; pruritus (10%), freckling, hypopigmentation, rash, cheilitis, erythema, itching, urticaria

Gastrointestinal: Nausea (10%)

Neuromuscular & skeletal: Loss of muscle coordination, leg cramps

Miscellaneous: Miliaria

Mechanism of Action Bonds covalently to pyrimidine bases in DNA, inhibits the synthesis of DNA, and suppresses cell division. The augmented sunburn reaction involves excitation of the methoxsalen molecule by radiation in the long-wave ultraviolet light (UVA), resulting in transference of energy to the methoxsalen molecule producing an excited state ("triplet electronic state"). The molecule, in this "triplet state", then reacts with cutaneous DNA.

Drug Interactions

Cytochrome P450 Effect: Substrate of CYP2A6 (minor); **Inhibits** CYP1A2 (strong), 2A6 (strong), 2C8/9 (weak), 2C19 (weak), 2D6 (weak), 2E1 (weak), 3A4 (weak)

Increased Effect/Toxicity: Methoxsalen may increase the levels/effects of CYP1A2 substrates (eg, aminophylline, fluvoxamine, mexiletine, mirtazapine, ropinirole, theophylline, trifluoperazine) and CYP2A6 substrates (eg, dexmedetomidine, ifosfamide).

Pharmacodynamics/Kinetics

Protein binding: Reversibly bound to albumin

Metabolism: Hepatic; forms metabolites

Bioavailability: Bioavailability increased with soft-gelatin capsules compared to hard-gelatin capsules; exposure using UVAR® system is ~200 times less than with oral administration

Time to peak, serum:

Hard-gelatin capsules: 1.5-6 hours (peak photosensitivity: ~4 hours)

Soft-gelatin capsules: 0.5-4 hours (peak photosensitivity: 1.5-2 hours)

Half-life elimination: ~2 hours

Excretion: Urine (~95% as metabolites)

Pregnancy Risk Factor C/D (Uvadex®)

Methoxypsoralen *see* Methoxsalen *on page 902*

8-Methoxypsoralen *see* Methoxsalen *on page 902*

Methscopolamine (meth skoe POL a meen)

U.S. Brand Names Pamine®; Pamine® Forte

Canadian Brand Names Pamine®

Generic Available No

Synonyms Methscopolamine Bromide

Pharmacologic Category Anticholinergic Agent

Use Adjunctive therapy in the treatment of peptic ulcer

Local Anesthetic/Vasoconstrictor Precautions No information available to require special precautions

Effects on Dental Treatment Key adverse event(s) related to dental treatment: Xerostomia and changes in salivation (normal salivary flow resumes upon discontinuation), and dry throat and nose. Anticholinergic side effects can cause a reduction of saliva production or secretion, contributing to discomfort and dental disease (ie, caries, oral candidiasis and periodontal disease).

Common Adverse Effects Frequency not defined.

Cardiovascular: Palpitations, tachycardia

Central nervous system: Headache, insomnia, flushing, nervousness, drowsiness, dizziness, confusion, fever, CNS stimulation may be produced with large doses

Dermatologic: Dry skin, urticaria

Endocrine & metabolic: Lactation suppressed

(Continued)

Methscopolamine *(Continued)*

Gastrointestinal: Constipation, xerostomia, dry throat, dysphagia, nausea, vomiting, loss of taste

Genitourinary: Impotence, urinary hesitancy, urinary retention

Neuromuscular & skeletal: Weakness

Ocular: Blurred vision, cycloplegia, ocular tension increased, pupil dilation

Respiratory: Dry nose

Miscellaneous: Allergic reaction, diaphoresis decreased, hypersensitivity reactions, anaphylaxis

Mechanism of Action Methscopolamine is a peripheral anticholinergic agent with limited ability to cross the blood-brain barrier and provides a peripheral blockade of muscarinic receptors. This agent reduces the volume and the total acid content of gastric secretions, inhibits salivation, and reduces gastrointestinal motility.

Drug Interactions

Increased Effect/Toxicity: Antipsychotic agents and TCAs may produce additive anticholinergic effects.

Decreased Effect: Antacids may decrease the absorption of methscopolamine.

Pharmacodynamics/Kinetics

Onset: 1 hour

Duration: 4-6 hours

Excretion: Bile, urine

Pregnancy Risk Factor C

Methscopolamine Bromide *see* Methscopolamine *on page 903*

Methscopolamine, Chlorpheniramine, and Phenylephrine *see* Chlorpheniramine, Phenylephrine, and Methscopolamine *on page 317*

Methsuximide (meth SUKS i mide)

U.S. Brand Names Celontin®

Canadian Brand Names Celontin®

Generic Available No

Pharmacologic Category Anticonvulsant, Succinimide

Use Control of absence (petit mal) seizures that are refractory to other drugs

Unlabeled/Investigational Use Partial complex (psychomotor) seizures

Local Anesthetic/Vasoconstrictor Precautions No information available to require special precautions

Effects on Dental Treatment No significant effects or complications reported

Common Adverse Effects Frequency not defined.

Cardiovascular: Hyperemia

Central nervous system: Ataxia, dizziness, drowsiness, headache, aggressiveness, mental depression, irritability, nervousness, insomnia, confusion, psychosis, suicidal behavior, auditory hallucinations

Dermatologic: Stevens-Johnson syndrome, rash, urticaria, pruritus

Gastrointestinal: Anorexia, nausea, vomiting, weight loss, diarrhea, epigastric and abdominal pain, constipation

Genitourinary: Proteinuria, hematuria (microscopic); cases of blood dyscrasias have been reported with succinimides

Hematologic: Leukopenia, pancytopenia, eosinophilia, monocytosis

Neuromuscular & skeletal: Cases of systemic lupus erythematosus have been reported

Ocular: Blurred vision, photophobia, peripheral edema

Mechanism of Action Increases the seizure threshold and suppresses paroxysmal spike-and-wave pattern in absence seizures; depresses nerve transmission in the motor cortex

Drug Interactions

Cytochrome P450 Effect: Substrate of CYP2C19 (major); **Inhibits** CYP2C19 (weak)

Increased Effect/Toxicity: CYP2C19 inhibitors may increase the levels/effects of methsuximide; example inhibitors include delavirdine, fluconazole, fluvoxamine, gemfibrozil, isoniazid, omeprazole, and ticlopidine. Sedative effects and/or respiratory depression may be additive with CNS depressants; includes ethanol, benzodiazepines, barbiturates, narcotic analgesics, and other sedative agents. Methsuximide may increase phenobarbital and/or phenytoin concentration.

Decreased Effect: CYP2C19 inducers may decrease the levels/effects of methsuximide; example inducers include aminoglutethimide, carbamazepine, phenytoin, and rifampin.

Pharmacodynamics/Kinetics
Metabolism: Hepatic; rapidly demethylated to N-desmethylmethsuximide (active metabolite)
Half-life elimination: 2-4 hours
Time to peak, serum: Within 1-3 hours
Excretion: Urine (<1% as unchanged drug)
Pregnancy Risk Factor C

Methyclothiazide (meth i kloe THYE a zide)

Related Information
Cardiovascular Diseases *on page 1458*
U.S. Brand Names Aquatensen®; Enduron®
Canadian Brand Names Aquatensen®; Enduron®
Generic Available Yes
Pharmacologic Category Diuretic, Thiazide
Use Management of mild to moderate hypertension; treatment of edema in congestive heart failure and nephrotic syndrome
Local Anesthetic/Vasoconstrictor Precautions No information available to require special precautions
Effects on Dental Treatment No significant effects or complications reported
Common Adverse Effects 1% to 10%:
Cardiovascular: Orthostatic hypotension
Dermatologic: Photosensitivity
Endocrine & metabolic: Hypokalemia
Gastrointestinal: Anorexia, epigastric distress
Mechanism of Action Inhibits sodium reabsorption in the distal tubules causing increased excretion of sodium and water, as well as, potassium and hydrogen ions
Drug Interactions
Increased Effect/Toxicity: Increased effect of methyclothiazide with furosemide and other loop diuretics. Increased hypotension and/or renal adverse effects of ACE inhibitors may result in aggressively diuresed patients. Beta-blockers increase hyperglycemic effects of thiazides in Type 2 diabetes mellitus. Cyclosporine and thiazides can increase the risk of gout or renal toxicity. Digoxin toxicity can be exacerbated if a thiazide induces hypokalemia or hypomagnesemia. Lithium toxicity can occur with thiazides due to reduced renal excretion of lithium. Thiazides may prolong the duration of action with neuromuscular blocking agents.
Decreased Effect: Effects of oral hypoglycemics may be decreased. Decreased absorption of thiazides with cholestyramine and colestipol. NSAIDs can decrease the efficacy of thiazides, reducing the diuretic and antihypertensive effects.
Pharmacodynamics/Kinetics
Onset of action: Diuresis: 2 hours
Peak effect: 6 hours
Duration: ~1 day
Distribution: Crosses placenta; enters breast milk
Excretion: Urine (as unchanged drug)
Pregnancy Risk Factor B

Methyclothiazide and Deserpidine

(meth i kloe THYE a zide & de SER pi deen)
Related Information
Methyclothiazide *on page 905*
U.S. Brand Names Enduronyl®; Enduronyl® Forte
Canadian Brand Names Enduronyl®; Enduronyl® Forte
Generic Available No
Synonyms Deserpidine and Methyclothiazide
Pharmacologic Category Antihypertensive Agent, Combination
Use Management of mild to moderately severe hypertension
Local Anesthetic/Vasoconstrictor Precautions No information available to require special precautions
Effects on Dental Treatment No significant effects or complications reported
Common Adverse Effects See individual agents.
Pregnancy Risk Factor C

Methylacetoxyprogesterone *see* MedroxyPROGESTERone *on page 862*

Methylcellulose (meth il SEL yoo lose)

U.S. Brand Names Citrucel® [OTC]; FiberEase™ [OTC]
Generic Available No
(Continued)

Methylcellulose *(Continued)*

Pharmacologic Category Laxative

Use Adjunct in treatment of constipation

Local Anesthetic/Vasoconstrictor Precautions No information available to require special precautions

Effects on Dental Treatment No significant effects or complications reported

Pregnancy Risk Factor C

Methyldopa (meth il DOE pa)

Related Information

Cardiovascular Diseases *on page 1458*

Canadian Brand Names Apo-Methyldopa®; Nu-Medopa

Mexican Brand Names Aldomet®

Generic Available Yes

Synonyms Aldomet; Methyldopate Hydrochloride

Pharmacologic Category Alpha-Adrenergic Inhibitor

Use Management of moderate to severe hypertension

Local Anesthetic/Vasoconstrictor Precautions No information available to require special precautions

Effects on Dental Treatment Key adverse event(s) related to dental treatment: Xerostomia (normal salivary flow resumes upon discontinuation). Anticholinergic side effects can cause a reduction of saliva production or secretion, contributing to discomfort and dental disease (ie, caries, oral candidiasis, and periodontal disease).

Common Adverse Effects

>10%: Cardiovascular: Peripheral edema

1% to 10%:

- Central nervous system: Drug fever, mental depression, anxiety, nightmares, drowsiness, headache
- Gastrointestinal: Dry mouth

Mechanism of Action Stimulation of central alpha-adrenergic receptors by a false transmitter that results in a decreased sympathetic outflow to the heart, kidneys, and peripheral vasculature

Drug Interactions

Increased Effect/Toxicity: Beta-blockers, MAO inhibitors, phenothiazines, and sympathomimetics (including epinephrine) may result in hypertension (sometimes severe) when combined with methyldopa. Methyldopa may increase lithium serum levels resulting in lithium toxicity. Levodopa may cause enhanced blood pressure lowering; methyldopa may also potentiate the effect of levodopa. Tolbutamide, haloperidol, and anesthetics effects/toxicity are increased with methyldopa.

Decreased Effect: Iron supplements can interact and cause a significant **increase** in blood pressure. Ferrous sulfate and ferrous gluconate decrease bioavailability. Barbiturates and TCAs may reduce response to methyldopa.

Pharmacodynamics/Kinetics

Onset of action: Peak effect: Hypotensive: Oral/parenteral: 3-6 hours

Duration: 12-24 hours

Distribution: Crosses placenta; enters breast milk

Protein binding: <15%

Metabolism: Intestinal and hepatic

Half-life elimination: 75-80 minutes; End-stage renal disease: 6-16 hours

Excretion: Urine (85% as metabolites) within 24 hours

Pregnancy Risk Factor B

Methyldopa and Hydrochlorothiazide

(meth il DOE pa & hye droe klor oh THYE a zide)

Related Information

Hydrochlorothiazide *on page 699*

U.S. Brand Names Aldoril®; Aldoril® D

Canadian Brand Names Apo-Methazide®

Generic Available Yes

Synonyms Hydrochlorothiazide and Methyldopa

Pharmacologic Category Antihypertensive Agent, Combination

Use Management of moderate to severe hypertension

Local Anesthetic/Vasoconstrictor Precautions No information available to require special precautions

Effects on Dental Treatment Key adverse event(s) related to dental treatment: Anticholinergic side effects can cause a reduction of saliva production or secretion, contributing to discomfort and dental disease (ie, caries, oral candidiasis, and periodontal disease).

Common Adverse Effects See individual agents.

Drug Interactions

Increased Effect/Toxicity: See individual agents.

Decreased Effect: See individual agents.

Pharmacodynamics/Kinetics See individual agents.

Pregnancy Risk Factor C

Methyldopate Hydrochloride *see* Methyldopa *on page 906*

Methylene Blue, Methenamine, Sodium Biphosphate, Phenyl Salicylate, and Hyoscyamine *see* Methenamine, Sodium Biphosphate, Phenyl Salicylate, Methylene Blue, and Hyoscyamine *on page 893*

Methylergometrine Maleate *see* Methylergonovine *on page 907*

Methylergonovine (meth il er goe NOE veen)

U.S. Brand Names Methergine®

Canadian Brand Names Methergine®

Generic Available No

Synonyms Methylergometrine Maleate; Methylergonovine Maleate

Pharmacologic Category Ergot Derivative

Use Prevention and treatment of postpartum and postabortion hemorrhage caused by uterine atony or subinvolution

Local Anesthetic/Vasoconstrictor Precautions No information available to require special precautions

Effects on Dental Treatment No significant effects or complications reported

Common Adverse Effects Frequency not defined.

Cardiovascular: Hypertension, temporary chest pain, palpitations
Central nervous system: Hallucinations, dizziness, seizures, headache
Endocrine & metabolic: Water intoxication
Gastrointestinal: Nausea, vomiting, diarrhea, foul taste
Local: Thrombophlebitis
Neuromuscular & skeletal: Leg cramps
Otic: Tinnitus
Renal: Hematuria
Respiratory: Dyspnea, nasal congestion
Miscellaneous: Diaphoresis

Mechanism of Action Similar smooth muscle actions as seen with ergotamine; however, it affects primarily uterine smooth muscles producing sustained contractions and thereby shortens the third stage of labor

Drug Interactions

Cytochrome P450 Effect: Substrate of CYP3A4 (major)

Increased Effect/Toxicity: CYP3A4 inhibitors may increase the levels/effects of methylergonovine; example inhibitors include azole antifungals, ciprofloxacin, clarithromycin, diclofenac, doxycycline, erythromycin, imatinib, isoniazid, nefazodone, nicardipine, propofol, protease inhibitors, quinidine, and verapamil. Ergot alkaloids are contraindicated with potent CYP3A4 inhibitors. Methylergonovine may increase the effects of 5-HT_1 agonists (eg, sumatriptan), MAO inhibitors, sibutramine, and other serotonin agonists (serotonin syndrome). Severe vasoconstriction may occur when peripheral vasoconstrictors or beta-blockers are used in patients receiving ergot alkaloids; concurrent use is contraindicated.

Decreased Effect: Effects of methylergonovine may be diminished by antipsychotics, metoclopramide/

Pharmacodynamics/Kinetics

Onset of action: Oxytocic: Oral: 5-10 minutes; I.M.: 2-5 minutes; I.V.: Immediately
Duration: Oral: ~3 hours; I.M.: ~3 hours; I.V.: 45 minutes
Absorption: Rapid
Distribution: Rapid; primarily to plasma and extracellular fluid following I.V. administration; tissues
Metabolism: Hepatic
Half-life elimination: Biphasic: Initial: 1-5 minutes; Terminal: 0.5-2 hours
Time to peak, serum: 0.5-3 hours
Excretion: Urine and feces

Pregnancy Risk Factor C

Methylergonovine Maleate *see* Methylergonovine *on page 907*

Methylin™ *see* Methylphenidate *on page 908*

Methylin™ ER *see* Methylphenidate *on page 908*

Methylmorphine *see* Codeine *on page 369*

Methylphenidate (meth il FEN i date)

U.S. Brand Names Concerta®; Metadate® CD; Metadate™ ER; Methylin™; Methylin™ ER; Ritalin®; Ritalin® LA; Ritalin-SR®

Canadian Brand Names Concerta®; PMS-Methylphenidate; Riphenidate; Ritalin®; Ritalin® SR

Mexican Brand Names Ritalin®

Generic Available Yes: Tablet

Synonyms Methylphenidate Hydrochloride

Pharmacologic Category Central Nervous System Stimulant

Use Treatment of attention-deficit/hyperactivity disorder (ADHD); symptomatic management of narcolepsy

Unlabeled/Investigational Use Depression (especially elderly or medically ill)

Local Anesthetic/Vasoconstrictor Precautions No information available to require special precautions

Effects on Dental Treatment Key adverse event(s) related to dental treatment: Up to 10% of patients taking dextroamphetamines or amphetamine-like drugs may present with hypertension. The use of local anesthetic without vasoconstrictor is recommended in these patients.

Common Adverse Effects Frequency not defined.

Cardiovascular: Angina, cardiac arrhythmias, cerebral arteritis, cerebral occlusion, hypertension, hypotension, palpitations, pulse increase/decrease, tachycardia

Central nervous system: Depression, dizziness, drowsiness, fever, headache, insomnia, nervousness, neuroleptic malignant syndrome (NMS), Tourette's syndrome, toxic psychosis

Dermatologic: Erythema multiforme, exfoliative dermatitis, hair loss, rash, urticaria

Endocrine & metabolic: Growth retardation

Gastrointestinal: Abdominal pain, anorexia, nausea, vomiting, weight loss

Hematologic: Anemia, leukopenia, thrombocytopenic purpura

Hepatic: Abnormal liver function tests, hepatic coma, transaminase elevation

Neuromuscular & skeletal: Arthralgia, dyskinesia

Ocular: Blurred vision

Renal: Necrotizing vasculitis

Respiratory: Cough increased, pharyngitis, sinusitis, upper respiratory tract infection

Miscellaneous: Hypersensitivity reactions

Restrictions C-II

Dosage Oral (discontinue periodically to re-evaluate or if no improvement occurs within 1 month):

Children ≥6 years: ADHD: Initial: 0.3 mg/kg/dose or 2.5-5 mg/dose given before breakfast and lunch; increase by 0.1 mg/kg/dose or by 5-10 mg/day at weekly intervals; usual dose: 0.5-1 mg/kg/day; maximum dose: 2 mg/kg/day or 90 mg/day

Extended release products:

Metadate™ ER, Methylin™ ER, Ritalin® SR: Duration of action is 8 hours. May be given in place of regular tablets, once the daily dose is titrated using the regular tablets and the titrated 8-hour dosage corresponds to sustained release tablet size.

Metadate® CD, Ritalin® LA: Initial: 20 mg once daily; may be adjusted in 10-20 mg increments at weekly intervals; maximum: 60 mg/day

Concerta®: Duration of action is 12 hours:

Children not currently taking methylphenidate:

Initial: 18 mg once daily in the morning

Adjustment: May increase to maximum of 54 mg/day in increments of 18 mg/day; dose may be adjusted at weekly intervals

Children currently taking methylphenidate: **Note:** Dosing based on current regimen and clinical judgment; suggested dosing listed below:

Patients taking methylphenidate 5 mg 2-3 times/day or 20 mg/day sustained release formulation: Initial dose: 18 mg once every morning (maximum: 54 mg/day)

Patients taking methylphenidate 10 mg 2-3 times/day or 40 mg/day sustained release formulation: Initial dose: 36 mg once every morning (maximum: 54 mg/day)

Patients taking methylphenidate 15 mg 2-3 times/day or 60 mg/day sustained release formulation: Initial dose: 54 mg once every morning (maximum: 54 mg/day)

Note: A 27 mg dosage strength is available for situations in which a dosage between 18 mg and 36 mg is desired.

Adults:

Narcolepsy: 10 mg 2-3 times/day, up to 60 mg/day

Depression (unlabeled use): Initial: 2.5 mg every morning before 9 AM; dosage may be increased by 2.5-5 mg every 2-3 days as tolerated to a maximum of 20 mg/day; may be divided (ie, 7 AM and 12 noon), but should not be given after noon; do not use sustained release product

Mechanism of Action Mild CNS stimulant; blocks the reuptake mechanism of dopaminergic neurons; appears to stimulate the cerebral cortex and subcortical structures similar to amphetamines

Contraindications Hypersensitivity to methylphenidate, any component of the formulation, or idiosyncrasy to sympathomimetic amines; marked anxiety, tension, and agitation; glaucoma; use during or within 14 days following MAO inhibitor therapy; Tourette's syndrome or tics

Warnings/Precautions Methylphenidate has a high potential for abuse; avoid abrupt discontinuation in patients who have received for prolonged periods. Has demonstrated value as part of a comprehensive treatment program for ADHD. May have value in selected patients as an antidepressant.

Safety and efficacy in children <6 years of age not established. Use with caution in patients with bipolar disorder, diabetes mellitus, cardiovascular disease, seizure disorders, insomnia, porphyria, or mild hypertension (stage I). May exacerbate symptoms of behavior and thought disorder in psychotic patients. Do not use to treat severe depression or fatigue states. Stimulant use has been associated with growth suppression. Concerta® should not be used in patients with pre-existing severe gastrointestinal narrowing (small bowel disease, short gut syndrome, history of peritonitis, cystic fibrosis, chronic intestinal pseudo-obstruction, Meckel's diverticulum)

Drug Interactions

Cytochrome P450 Effect: Substrate of CYP2D6 (major); **Inhibits** CYP2D6 (weak)

Increased Effect/Toxicity: Methylphenidate may cause hypertensive effects when used in combination with MAO inhibitors or drugs with MAO-inhibiting activity (linezolid). Risk may be less with selegiline (MAO type B selective at low doses); it is best to avoid this combination. CYP2D6 inhibitors may increase the levels/effects of methylphenidate; example inhibitors include chlorpromazine, delavirdine, fluoxetine, miconazole, paroxetine, pergolide, quinidine, quinine, ritonavir, and ropinirole. NMS has been reported in a patient receiving methylphenidate and venlafaxine. Methylphenidate may increase levels of phenytoin, phenobarbital, TCAs, and warfarin. Increased toxicity with clonidine and sibutramine.

Decreased Effect: Effectiveness of antihypertensive agents may be decreased. Carbamazepine may decrease the effect of methylphenidate.

Ethanol/Nutrition/Herb Interactions

Ethanol: Avoid ethanol (may cause CNS depression).

Food: Food may increase oral absorption; Concerta® formulation is not affected. Food delays early peak and high-fat meals increase C_{max} and AUC of Metadate® CD formulation.

Herb/Nutraceutical: Avoid ephedra (may cause hypertension or arrhythmias) and yohimbe (also has CNS stimulatory activity).

Dietary Considerations Should be taken 30-45 minutes before meals. Concerta® is not affected by food and should be taken with water, milk, or juice. Metadate® CD should be taken before breakfast. Metadate™ ER should be taken before breakfast and lunch.

Pharmacodynamics/Kinetics

Onset of action: Peak effect:

Immediate release tablet: Cerebral stimulation: ~2 hours

Extended release capsule (Metadate® CD): Biphasic; initial peak similar to immediate release product, followed by second rising portion (corresponding to extended release portion)

Sustained release tablet: 4-7 hours

Osmotic release tablet (Concerta®): Initial: 1-2 hours

Duration: Immediate release tablet: 3-6 hours; Sustained release tablet: 8 hours

Absorption: Readily

Metabolism: Hepatic via de-esterification to active metabolite

Half-life elimination: 2-4 hours

Time to peak: C_{max}: 6-8 hours

Excretion: Urine (90% as metabolites and unchanged drug)

Pregnancy Risk Factor C

Dosage Forms CAP, extended release (Metadate® CD): 10 mg, 20 mg, 30 mg; (Ritalin® LA): 10 mg, 20 mg, 30 mg, 40 mg. **TAB** (Methylin™, Ritalin®): 5 mg, 10 mg, 20 mg. **TAB, extended release:** 20 mg; (Concerta®): 18 mg, 27

(Continued)

Methylphenidate *(Continued)*

mg, 36 mg, 54 mg; (Metadate™ ER, Methylin™ ER): 10 mg, 20 mg. **TAB, sustained release** (Ritalin-SR®): 20 mg

Methylphenidate Hydrochloride *see* Methylphenidate *on page 908*

Methylphenobarbital *see* Mephobarbital *on page 873*

Methylphenoxy-Benzene Propanamine *see* Atomoxetine *on page 161*

Methylphenyl Isoxazolyl Penicillin *see* Oxacillin *on page 1020*

Methylphytyl Napthoquinone *see* Phytonadione *on page 1084*

MethylPREDNISolone (meth il pred NIS oh lone)

Related Information

Respiratory Diseases *on page 1478*

U.S. Brand Names A-Methapred®; Depo-Medrol®; Medrol®; Solu-Medrol®

Canadian Brand Names Depo-Medrol®; Medrol®; Solu-Medrol®

Generic Available Yes

Synonyms 6-α-Methylprednisolone; Methylprednisolone Acetate; Methylprednisolone Sodium Succinate

Pharmacologic Category Corticosteroid, Systemic

Dental Use Treatment of a variety of oral diseases of allergic, inflammatory, or autoimmune origin

Use Primarily as an anti-inflammatory or immunosuppressant agent in the treatment of a variety of diseases including those of hematologic, allergic, inflammatory, neoplastic, and autoimmune origin. Prevention and treatment of graft-versus-host disease following allogeneic bone marrow transplantation.

Unlabeled/Investigational Use Treatment of fibrosing-alveolitis phase of adult respiratory distress syndrome (ARDS)

Local Anesthetic/Vasoconstrictor Precautions No information available to require special precautions

Effects on Dental Treatment No significant effects or complications reported

Significant Adverse Effects Frequency not defined.

Cardiovascular: Edema, hypertension, arrhythmias

Central nervous system: Insomnia, nervousness, vertigo, seizures, psychoses, pseudotumor cerebri, headache, mood swings, delirium, hallucinations, euphoria

Dermatologic: Hirsutism, acne, skin atrophy, bruising, hyperpigmentation

Endocrine & metabolic: Diabetes mellitus, adrenal suppression, hyperlipidemia, Cushing's syndrome, pituitary-adrenal axis suppression, growth suppression, glucose intolerance, hypokalemia, alkalosis, amenorrhea, sodium and water retention, hyperglycemia

Gastrointestinal: Increased appetite, indigestion, peptic ulcer, nausea, vomiting, abdominal distention, ulcerative esophagitis, pancreatitis

Hematologic: Transient leukocytosis

Neuromuscular & skeletal: Arthralgia, muscle weakness, osteoporosis, fractures

Ocular: Cataracts, glaucoma

Miscellaneous: Infections, hypersensitivity reactions, avascular necrosis, secondary malignancy, intractable hiccups

Dosage Dosing should be based on the lesser of ideal body weight or actual body weight

Only sodium succinate may be given I.V.; methylprednisolone sodium succinate is highly soluble and has a rapid effect by I.M. and I.V. routes. Methylprednisolone acetate has a low solubility and has a sustained I.M. effect.

Children:

Anti-inflammatory or immunosuppressive: Oral, I.M., I.V. (sodium succinate): 0.5-1.7 mg/kg/day **or** 5-25 mg/m^2/day in divided doses every 6-12 hours; "Pulse" therapy: 15-30 mg/kg/dose over ≥30 minutes given once daily for 3 days

Status asthmaticus: I.V. (sodium succinate): Loading dose: 2 mg/kg/dose, then 0.5-1 mg/kg/dose every 6 hours for up to 5 days

Acute spinal cord injury: I.V. (sodium succinate): 30 mg/kg over 15 minutes, followed in 45 minutes by a continuous infusion of 5.4 mg/kg/hour for 23 hours

Lupus nephritis: I.V. (sodium succinate): 30 mg/kg over ≥30 minutes every other day for 6 doses

Adults: **Only sodium succinate may be given I.V.;** methylprednisolone sodium succinate is highly soluble and has a rapid effect by I.M. and I.V. routes. Methylprednisolone acetate has a low solubility and has a sustained I.M. effect.

Acute spinal cord injury: I.V. (sodium succinate): 30 mg/kg over 15 minutes, followed in 45 minutes by a continuous infusion of 5.4 mg/kg/hour for 23 hours

Anti-inflammatory or immunosuppressive:

Oral: 2-60 mg/day in 1-4 divided doses to start, followed by gradual reduction in dosage to the lowest possible level consistent with maintaining an adequate clinical response.

I.M. (sodium succinate): 10-80 mg/day once daily

I.M. (acetate): 10-80 mg every 1-2 weeks

I.V. (sodium succinate): 10-40 mg over a period of several minutes and repeated I.V. or I.M. at intervals depending on clinical response; when high dosages are needed, give 30 mg/kg over a period ≥30 minutes and may be repeated every 4-6 hours for 48 hours.

Status asthmaticus: I.V. (sodium succinate): Loading dose: 2 mg/kg/dose, then 0.5-1 mg/kg/dose every 6 hours for up to 5 days

High-dose therapy for acute spinal cord injury: I.V. bolus: 30 mg/kg over 15 minutes, followed 45 minutes later by an infusion of 5.4 mg/kg/hour for 23 hours

Lupus nephritis: High-dose "pulse" therapy: I.V. (sodium succinate): 1 g/day for 3 days

Aplastic anemia: I.V. (sodium succinate): 1 mg/kg/day or 40 mg/day (whichever dose is higher), for 4 days. After 4 days, change to oral and continue until day 10 or until symptoms of serum sickness resolve, then rapidly reduce over approximately 2 weeks.

Pneumocystis pneumonia in AIDs patients: I.V.: 40-60 mg every 6 hours for 7-10 days

Intra-articular (acetate): Administer every 1-5 weeks.

Large joints: 20-80 mg

Small joints: 4-10 mg

Intralesional (acetate): 20-60 mg every 1-5 weeks

Mechanism of Action In a tissue-specific manner, corticosteroids regulate gene expression subsequent to binding specific intracellular receptors and translocation into the nucleus. Corticosteroids exert a wide array of physiologic effects including modulation of carbohydrate, protein, and lipid metabolism and maintenance of fluid and electrolyte homeostasis. Moreover cardiovascular, immunologic, musculoskeletal, endocrine, and neurologic physiology are influenced by corticosteroids. Decreases inflammation by suppression of migration of polymorphonuclear leukocytes and reversal of increased capillary permeability.

Contraindications Hypersensitivity to methylprednisolone or any component of the formulation; viral, fungal, or tubercular skin lesions; administration of live virus vaccines; serious infections, except septic shock or tuberculous meningitis. Methylprednisolone formulations containing benzyl alcohol preservative are contraindicated in infants.

Warnings/Precautions Use with caution in patients with hyperthyroidism, cirrhosis, nonspecific ulcerative colitis, hypertension, osteoporosis, thromboembolic tendencies, CHF, convulsive disorders, myasthenia gravis, thrombophlebitis, peptic ulcer, diabetes, glaucoma, cataracts, or tuberculosis. Use caution in hepatic impairment. Because of the risk of adverse effects, systemic corticosteroids should be used cautiously in the elderly, in the smallest possible dose, and for the shortest possible time

Acute adrenal insufficiency may occur with abrupt withdrawal after long-term therapy or with stress; young pediatric patients may be more susceptible to adrenal axis suppression from topical therapy

Drug Interactions Substrate of CYP3A4 (minor); **Inhibits** CYP3A4 (weak)

Decreased effect:

Phenytoin, phenobarbital, rifampin increase clearance of methylprednisolone

Potassium depleting diuretics enhance potassium depletion

Increased toxicity:

Skin test antigens, immunizations decrease response and increase potential infections

Methylprednisolone may increase circulating glucose levels and may need adjustments of insulin or oral hypoglycemics

Ethanol/Nutrition/Herb Interactions

Ethanol: Avoid ethanol (may increase gastric mucosal irritation).

Food: Methylprednisolone interferes with calcium absorption. Limit caffeine.

Herb/Nutraceutical: St John's wort may decrease methylprednisolone levels. Avoid cat's claw, echinacea (have immunostimulant properties).

Dietary Considerations Should be taken after meals or with food or milk; need diet rich in pyridoxine, vitamin C, vitamin D, folate, calcium, phosphorus, and protein.

(Continued)

MethylPREDNISolone *(Continued)*

Sodium content of 1 g sodium succinate injection: 2.01 mEq; 53 mg of sodium succinate salt is equivalent to 40 mg of methylprednisolone base

Methylprednisolone acetate: Depo-Medrol®

Methylprednisolone sodium succinate: Solu-Medrol®

Pharmacodynamics/Kinetics

Onset of action: Peak effect (route dependent): Oral: 1-2 hours; I.M.: 4-8 days; Intra-articular: 1 week; methylprednisolone sodium succinate is highly soluble and has a rapid effect by I.M. and I.V. routes

Duration (route dependent): Oral: 30-36 hours; I.M.: 1-4 weeks; Intra-articular: 1-5 weeks; methylprednisolone acetate has a low solubility and has a sustained I.M. effect

Distribution: V_d: 0.7-1.5 L/kg

Half-life elimination: 3-3.5 hours; reduced in obese

Excretion: Clearance: Reduced in obese

Pregnancy Risk Factor C

Lactation Excretion in breast milk unknown

Dosage Forms

Injection, powder for reconstitution, as sodium succinate: 40 mg, 125 mg, 500 mg

A-Methapred®: 40 mg, 125 mg, 500 mg, 1000 mg [diluent contains benzyl alcohol]

Solu-Medrol®: 40 mg, 125 mg, 500 mg, 1 g, 2 g [packaged with diluent; diluent contains benzyl alcohol]

Solu-Medrol®: 500 mg, 1 g

Injection, suspension, as acetate (Depo-Medrol®): 20 mg/mL (5 mL); 40 mg/mL (5 mL); 80 mg/mL (5 mL) [contains benzyl alcohol]

Injection, suspension, as acetate [single-dose vial] (Depo-Medrol®): 40 mg/mL (1 mL); 80 mg/mL (1 mL)

Tablet: 4 mg

Medrol®: 2 mg, 4 mg, 8 mg, 16 mg, 32 mg

Tablet, dose-pack: 4 mg (21s)

6-α-Methylprednisolone *see* MethylPREDNISolone *on page 910*

Methylprednisolone Acetate *see* MethylPREDNISolone *on page 910*

Methylprednisolone Sodium Succinate *see* MethylPREDNISolone *on page 910*

4-Methylpyrazole *see* Fomepizole *on page 627*

Methylrosaniline Chloride *see* Gentian Violet *on page 657*

MethylTESTOSTERone (meth il tes TOS te rone)

U.S. Brand Names Android®; Methitest®; Testred®; Virilon®

Generic Available No

Pharmacologic Category Androgen

Use

Male: Hypogonadism; delayed puberty; impotence and climacteric symptoms

Female: Palliative treatment of metastatic breast cancer

Local Anesthetic/Vasoconstrictor Precautions No information available to require special precautions

Effects on Dental Treatment No significant effects or complications reported

Common Adverse Effects Frequency not defined.

Male: Virilism, priapism, prostatic hyperplasia, prostatic carcinoma, impotence, testicular atrophy, gynecomastia

Female: Virilism, menstrual problems (amenorrhea), breast soreness, hirsutism (increase in pubic hair growth) atrophy

Cardiovascular: Edema

Central nervous system: Headache, anxiety, depression

Dermatologic: Acne, "male pattern" baldness, seborrhea

Endocrine & metabolic: Hypercalcemia, hypercholesterolemia

Gastrointestinal: GI irritation, nausea, vomiting

Hematologic: Leukopenia, polycythemia

Hepatic: Hepatic dysfunction, hepatic necrosis, cholestatic hepatitis

Miscellaneous: Hypersensitivity reactions

Restrictions C-III

Mechanism of Action Stimulates receptors in organs and tissues to promote growth and development of male sex organs and maintains secondary sex characteristics in androgen-deficient males

Drug Interactions

Increased Effect/Toxicity: Effects of oral anticoagulants and hypoglycemic agents may be increased. Toxicity may occur with cyclosporine; avoid concurrent use.

Decreased Effect: Decreased oral anticoagulant effect

Pharmacodynamics/Kinetics

Metabolism: Hepatic

Excretion: Urine

Pregnancy Risk Factor X

Methysergide (meth i SER jide)

U.S. Brand Names Sansert® [DSC]

Canadian Brand Names Sansert®

Generic Available No

Synonyms Methysergide Maleate

Pharmacologic Category Ergot Derivative

Use Prophylaxis of vascular headache

Local Anesthetic/Vasoconstrictor Precautions No information available to require special precautions

Effects on Dental Treatment No significant effects or complications reported

Common Adverse Effects Frequency not defined.

Cardiovascular: Postural hypotension, peripheral ischemia, peripheral edema, tachycardia, bradycardia, edema

Central nervous system: Insomnia, drowsiness, euphoria, dizziness, seizures, fever

Dermatologic: Rash, telangiectasia, flushing

Endocrine & metabolic: Weight gain

Gastrointestinal: Nausea, vomiting, abdominal pain, diarrhea, heartburn

Hematologic: Neutropenia, eosinophilia, thrombocytopenia

Neuromuscular & skeletal: Weakness, myalgia, arthralgia

Note: Fibrotic complications: Retroperitoneal, pleuropulmonary, cardiac (aortic root, aortic valve, mitral valve) fibrosis, and Peyronie's disease have been reported.

Mechanism of Action Ergotamine congener, however, actions appear to differ; methysergide has minimal ergotamine-like oxytocic or vasoconstrictive properties, and has significantly greater serotonin-like properties

Drug Interactions

Cytochrome P450 Effect: Substrate of CYP3A4 (major)

Increased Effect/Toxicity: Effects of methysergide may be increased by MAO inhibitors and sumatriptan (vasospasm). Methysergide may increase the effects of sibutramine and other serotonin agonists (serotonin syndrome). CYP3A4 inhibitors may increase the levels/effects of methysergide; example inhibitors include azole antifungals, ciprofloxacin, clarithromycin, diclofenac, doxycycline, erythromycin, imatinib, isoniazid, nefazodone, nicardipine, propofol, protease inhibitors, quinidine, and verapamil.

Pharmacodynamics/Kinetics

Metabolism: Hepatic to methylergonovine and glucuronide metabolite

Half-life elimination: ~10 hours

Pregnancy Risk Factor X

Methysergide Maleate *see* Methysergide *on page 913*

Metipranolol (met i PRAN oh lol)

U.S. Brand Names OptiPranolol®

Canadian Brand Names OptiPranolol®

Generic Available Yes

Synonyms Metipranolol Hydrochloride

Pharmacologic Category Beta-Adrenergic Blocker, Nonselective; Ophthalmic Agent, Antiglaucoma

Use Agent for lowering intraocular pressure in patients with chronic open-angle glaucoma

Local Anesthetic/Vasoconstrictor Precautions No information available to require special precautions

Effects on Dental Treatment Metipranolol is a nonselective beta-blocker and may enhance the pressor response to epinephrine, resulting in hypertension and bradycardia. Many nonsteroidal anti-inflammatory drugs, such as ibuprofen and indomethacin, can reduce the hypotensive effect of beta-blockers after 3 or more weeks of therapy with the NSAID. Short-term NSAID use (ie, 3 days) requires no special precautions in patients taking beta-blockers.

(Continued)

Metipranolol *(Continued)*

Mechanism of Action Beta-adrenoceptor-blocking agent; lacks intrinsic sympathomimetic activity and membrane-stabilizing effects and possesses only slight local anesthetic activity; mechanism of action of metipranolol in reducing intraocular pressure appears to be via reduced production of aqueous humor. This effect may be related to a reduction in blood flow to the iris root-ciliary body. It remains unclear if the reduction in intraocular pressure observed with beta-blockers is actually secondary to beta-adrenoceptor blockade.

Pregnancy Risk Factor C

Metipranolol Hydrochloride *see* Metipranolol *on page 913*

Metoclopramide (met oh kloe PRA mide)

Related Information

Endocrine Disorders and Pregnancy *on page 1481*

U.S. Brand Names Reglan®

Canadian Brand Names Apo-Metoclop®; Nu-Metoclopramide

Mexican Brand Names Plasil®

Generic Available Yes

Pharmacologic Category Antiemetic; Gastrointestinal Agent, Prokinetic

Use Prevention and/or treatment of nausea and vomiting associated with chemotherapy, radiation therapy, or postsurgery; symptomatic treatment of diabetic gastric stasis; gastroesophageal reflux; facilitation of intubation of the small intestine

Local Anesthetic/Vasoconstrictor Precautions No information available to require special precautions

Effects on Dental Treatment Key adverse event(s) related to dental treatment: Xerostomia (normal salivary flow resumes upon discontinuation).

Common Adverse Effects Adverse reactions are more common/severe at dosages used for prophylaxis of chemotherapy-induced emesis.

>10%:

- Central nervous system: Restlessness, drowsiness, extrapyramidal symptoms (high-dose, up to 34%)
- Gastrointestinal: Diarrhea (may be dose-limiting)
- Neuromuscular & skeletal: Weakness

1% to 10%:

- Central nervous system: Insomnia, depression
- Dermatologic: Rash
- Endocrine & metabolic: Breast tenderness, prolactin stimulation
- Gastrointestinal: Nausea, xerostomia

Mechanism of Action Blocks dopamine receptors and (when given in higher doses) also blocks serotonin receptors in chemoreceptor trigger zone of the CNS; enhances the response to acetylcholine of tissue in upper GI tract causing enhanced motility and accelerated gastric emptying without stimulating gastric, biliary, or pancreatic secretions

Drug Interactions

Cytochrome P450 Effect: Substrate (minor) of CYP1A2, 2D6; **Inhibits** CYP2D6 (weak)

Increased Effect/Toxicity: Opiate analgesics may increase CNS depression. Metoclopramide may increase extrapyramidal symptoms (EPS) or risk when used concurrently with antipsychotic agents.

Decreased Effect: Anticholinergic agents antagonize metoclopramide's actions.

Pharmacodynamics/Kinetics

Onset of action: Oral: 0.5-1 hour; I.V.: 1-3 minutes

Duration: Therapeutic: 1-2 hours, regardless of route

Distribution: V_d: 2-4 L/kg; Crosses placenta; enters breast milk

Protein binding: 30% to 40%, primarily to α_1-acid glycoprotein

Half-life elimination: Normal renal function: 4-7 hours (may be dose dependent)

Time to peak, serum: Oral: 1-3 hours; I.M.: 2-3 hours; I.V.: Within 5 minutes; Rectal: 1-8 hours

Excretion: Urine (70% to 85%, ~19% as unchanged drug); feces (2% to 3%)

Pregnancy Risk Factor B

Metolazone (me TOLE a zone)

Related Information

Cardiovascular Diseases *on page 1458*

U.S. Brand Names Mykrox® [DSC]; Zaroxolyn®

Canadian Brand Names Mykrox®; Zaroxolyn®

Generic Available Yes

Pharmacologic Category Diuretic, Thiazide-Related

Use Management of mild to moderate hypertension; treatment of edema in congestive heart failure and nephrotic syndrome, impaired renal function

Local Anesthetic/Vasoconstrictor Precautions No information available to require special precautions

Effects on Dental Treatment No significant effects or complications reported

Mechanism of Action Inhibits sodium reabsorption in the distal tubules causing increased excretion of sodium and water, as well as, potassium and hydrogen ions

Pregnancy Risk Factor B (manufacturer); D (expert analysis)

Metoprolol (me toe PROE lole)

Related Information

Cardiovascular Diseases *on page 1458*

U.S. Brand Names Lopressor®; Toprol-XL®

Canadian Brand Names Apo-Metoprolol®; Betaloc®; Betaloc® Durules®; Lopressor®; Novo-Metoprolol; Nu-Metop; PMS-Metoprolol; Toprol-XL®

Mexican Brand Names Lopresor®; Proken M®; Prolaken®; Ritmolol® [tabs]; Selectadril® [tabs]; Seloken®

Generic Available Yes: Injection, tablet (nonextended release)

Synonyms Metoprolol Succinate; Metoprolol Tartrate

Pharmacologic Category Beta Blocker, Beta$_1$ Selective

Use Treatment of hypertension and angina pectoris; prevention of myocardial infarction, atrial fibrillation, flutter, symptomatic treatment of hypertrophic subaortic stenosis; to reduce mortality/hospitalization in patients with congestive heart failure (stable NYHA Class II or III) in patients already receiving ACE inhibitors, diuretics, and/or digoxin (sustained-release only)

Unlabeled/Investigational Use Treatment of ventricular arrhythmias, atrial ectopy, migraine prophylaxis, essential tremor, aggressive behavior

Local Anesthetic/Vasoconstrictor Precautions No information available to require special precautions

Effects on Dental Treatment Metoprolol is a cardioselective beta-blocker. Local anesthetic with vasoconstrictor can be safely used in patients medicated with metoprolol. Nonselective beta-blockers (ie, propranolol, nadolol) enhance the pressor response to epinephrine, resulting in hypertension and bradycardia; this has not been reported for metoprolol. Many nonsteroidal anti-inflammatory drugs, such as ibuprofen and indomethacin, can reduce the hypotensive effect of beta-blockers after 3 or more weeks of therapy with the NSAID. Short-term NSAID use (ie, 3 days) requires no special precautions in patients taking beta-blockers.

Common Adverse Effects

>10%:

- Central nervous system: Drowsiness, insomnia
- Endocrine & metabolic: Decreased sexual ability

1% to 10%:

- Cardiovascular: Bradycardia, palpitations, edema, CHF, reduced peripheral circulation
- Central nervous system: Mental depression
- Gastrointestinal: Diarrhea or constipation, nausea, stomach discomfort
- Respiratory: Bronchospasm
- Miscellaneous: Cold extremities

Dosage

Children: Oral: 1-5 mg/kg/24 hours divided twice daily; allow 3 days between dose adjustments

Adults:

Hypertension: Oral: 100-450 mg/day in 2-3 divided doses, begin with 50 mg twice daily and increase doses at weekly intervals to desired effect; usual dosage range (JNC 7): 50-100 mg/day

Extended release: Same daily dose administered as a single dose

Angina, SVT, MI prophylaxis: Oral: 100-450 mg/day in 2-3 divided doses, begin with 50 mg twice daily and increase doses at weekly intervals to desired effect

Extended release: Same daily dose administered as a single dose

Hypertension/ventricular rate control: I.V. (in patients having nonfunctioning GI tract): Initial: 1.25-5 mg every 6-12 hours; titrate initial dose to response. Initially, low doses may be appropriate to establish response; however, up to 15 mg every 3-6 hours has been employed.

Congestive heart failure: Oral (extended release): Initial: 25 mg once daily (reduce to 12.5 mg once daily in NYHA class higher than class II); may double dosage every 2 weeks as tolerated, up to 200 mg/day

(Continued)

Metoprolol *(Continued)*

Myocardial infarction (acute): I.V.: 5 mg every 2 minutes for 3 doses in early treatment of myocardial infarction; thereafter give 50 mg orally every 6 hours 15 minutes after last I.V. dose and continue for 48 hours; then administer a maintenance dose of 100 mg twice daily.

Elderly: Oral: Initial: 25 mg/day; usual range: 25-300 mg/day

Extended release: 25-50 mg/day initially as a single dose; increase at 1- to 2-week intervals.

Hemodialysis: Administer dose posthemodialysis or administer 50 mg supplemental dose; supplemental dose is not necessary following peritoneal dialysis

Dosing adjustment/comments in hepatic disease: Reduced dose probably necessary

Mechanism of Action Selective inhibitor of beta$_1$-adrenergic receptors; competitively blocks beta$_1$-receptors, with little or no effect on beta$_2$-receptors at doses <100 mg; does not exhibit any membrane stabilizing or intrinsic sympathomimetic activity

Contraindications Hypersensitivity to metoprolol or any component of the formulation; sinus bradycardia; heart block greater than first degree (except in patients with a functioning artificial pacemaker); cardiogenic shock; uncompensated cardiac failure; pregnancy (2nd and 3rd trimesters)

Warnings/Precautions Abrupt withdrawal of the drug should be avoided (may result in an exaggerated cardiac beta-adrenergic response, tachycardia, hypertension, ischemia, angina, myocardial infarction, and sudden death), drug should be discontinued over 1-2 weeks. Must use care in compensated heart failure and monitor closely for a worsening of the condition (efficacy has not been established for metoprolol). Avoid abrupt discontinuation in patients with a history of CAD; slowly wean while monitoring for signs and symptoms of ischemia. Use caution in patients with PVD (can aggravate arterial insufficiency). Use caution with concurrent use of beta-blockers and either verapamil or diltiazem; bradycardia or heart block can occur. Avoid concurrent I.V. use of both agents. In general, beta-blockers should be avoided in patients with bronchospastic disease. Metoprolol, with B1 selectivity, should be used cautiously in bronchospastic disease with close monitoring, since selectivity can be lost with higher doses. Beta-blockers may increase the risk of anaphylaxis (in predisposed patients) and blunt response to epinephrine. Use cautiously in diabetics because it can mask prominent hypoglycemic symptoms. Can mask signs of thyrotoxicosis. Can cause fetal harm when administered in pregnancy. Use cautiously in the hepatically impaired. Use care with anesthetic agents which decrease myocardial function.

Drug Interactions

Cytochrome P450 Effect: Substrate of CYP2C19 (minor), 2D6 (major); **Inhibits** CYP2D6 (weak)

Increased Effect/Toxicity: CYP2D6 inhibitors may increase the levels/effects of metoprolol; example inhibitors include chlorpromazine, delavirdine, fluoxetine, miconazole, paroxetine, pergolide, quinidine, quinine, ritonavir, and ropinirole. Metoprolol may increase the effects of other drugs which slow AV conduction (digoxin, verapamil, diltiazem), alpha-blockers (prazosin, terazosin), and alpha-adrenergic stimulants (epinephrine, phenylephrine). Metoprolol may mask the tachycardia from hypoglycemia caused by insulin and oral hypoglycemics. In patients receiving concurrent therapy, the risk of hypertensive crisis is increased when either clonidine or the beta-blocker is withdrawn. Reserpine has been shown to enhance the effect of beta-blockers. Beta-blockers may increase the action or levels of ethanol, disopyramide, nondepolarizing muscle relaxants, and theophylline although the effects are difficult to predict.

Decreased Effect: Decreased effect of beta-blockers with aluminum salts, barbiturates, calcium salts, cholestyramine, colestipol, NSAIDs, penicillins (ampicillin), rifampin, salicylates, and sulfinpyrazone due to decreased bioavailability and plasma levels. Beta-blockers may decrease the effect of sulfonylureas.

Ethanol/Nutrition/Herb Interactions

Food: Food increases absorption. Metoprolol serum levels may be increased if taken with food.

Herb/Nutraceutical: Avoid dong quai if using for hypertension (has estrogenic activity). Avoid ephedra, yohimbe, ginseng (may worsen hypertension). Avoid garlic (may have increased antihypertensive effect).

Dietary Considerations Regular tablets should be taken with food. Extended release tablets may be taken without regard to meals.

Pharmacodynamics/Kinetics
Onset of action: Peak effect: Antihypertensive: Oral: 1.5-4 hours
Duration: 10-20 hours
Absorption: 95%
Protein binding: 8%
Metabolism: Extensively hepatic; significant first-pass effect
Bioavailability: Oral: 40% to 50%
Half-life elimination: 3-4 hours; End-stage renal disease: 2.5-4.5 hours
Excretion: Urine (3% to 10% as unchanged drug)

Pregnancy Risk Factor C (manufacturer); D (2nd and 3rd trimesters - expert analysis)

Dosage Forms INJ, solution, as tartrate (Lopressor®): 1 mg/mL (5 mL). **TAB, as tartrate:** 25 mg, 50 mg, 100 mg; (Lopressor®): 50 mg, 100 mg. **TAB, extended release, as succinate** (Toprol XL®): 25 mg, 50 mg, 100 mg, 200 mg

Selected Readings

Foster CA and Aston SJ, "Propranolol-Epinephrine Interaction: A Potential Disaster," *Plast Reconstr Surg*, 1983, 72(1):74-8.

Wong DG, Spence JD, Lamki L, et al, "Effect of Nonsteroidal Anti-inflammatory Drugs on Control of Hypertension of Beta-Blockers and Diuretics," *Lancet*, 1986, 1(8488):997-1001.

Wynn RL, "Dental Nonsteroidal Anti-inflammatory Drugs and Prostaglandin-Based Drug Interactions, Part Two," *Gen Dent*, 1992, 40(2):104, 106, 108.

Wynn RL, "Epinephrine Interactions With Beta-Blockers," *Gen Dent*, 1994, 42(1):16, 18.

Metoprolol Succinate *see* Metoprolol *on page 915*

Metoprolol Tartrate *see* Metoprolol *on page 915*

Metrizamide *see* Radiological/Contrast Media (Nonionic) *on page 1166*

MetroCream® *see* Metronidazole *on page 917*

MetroGel® *see* Metronidazole *on page 917*

MetroGel-Vaginal® *see* Metronidazole *on page 917*

MetroLotion® *see* Metronidazole *on page 917*

Metronidazole (me troe NI da zole)

Related Information

Gastrointestinal Disorders *on page 1476*
Oral Bacterial Infections *on page 1533*
Oral Nonviral Soft Tissue Ulcerations or Erosions *on page 1551*
Periodontal Diseases *on page 1542*
Sexually-Transmitted Diseases *on page 1504*

U.S. Brand Names Flagyl®; Flagyl ER®; MetroCream®; MetroGel®; MetroGel-Vaginal®; MetroLotion®; Noritate®; Rozex™

Canadian Brand Names Apo-Metronidazole®; Flagyl®; Florazole® ER; MetroCream™; Metrogel®; Nidagel™; Noritate®; Novo-Nidazol; Trikacide

Mexican Brand Names Ameblin®; Flagenase® [syrup]; Flagenase® [tabs]; Flagyl®; Fresenizol® [inj.]; MetroGel®; Nidrozol® [syrup]; Nidrozol® [tabs]; Selegil® [syrup]; Selegil® [tabs]; Servizol®; Servizol® [liqu. oral]; Vertisal®

Generic Available Yes: Cream, infusion, tablet

Synonyms Metronidazole Hydrochloride

Pharmacologic Category Amebicide; Antibiotic, Topical; Antibiotic, Miscellaneous; Antiprotozoal, Nitroimidazole

Dental Use Treatment of oral soft tissue infections due to anaerobic bacteria including all anaerobic cocci, anaerobic gram-negative bacilli (*Bacteroides*), and gram-positive spore-forming bacilli (*Clostridium*). Useful as single agent or in combination with amoxicillin, Augmentin®, or ciprofloxacin in the treatment of periodontitis associated with the presence of *Actinobacillus actinomycetemcomitans* (AA).

Use Treatment of susceptible anaerobic bacterial and protozoal infections in the following conditions: Amebiasis, symptomatic and asymptomatic trichomoniasis; skin and skin structure infections; CNS infections; intra-abdominal infections (as part of combination regimen); systemic anaerobic infections; treatment of antibiotic-associated pseudomembranous colitis (AAPC), bacterial vaginosis; as part of a multidrug regimen for *H. pylori* eradication to reduce the risk of duodenal ulcer recurrence
Topical: Treatment of inflammatory lesions and erythema of rosacea

Unlabeled/Investigational Use Crohn's disease

Local Anesthetic/Vasoconstrictor Precautions No information available to require special precautions

Effects on Dental Treatment Key adverse event(s) related to dental treatment: Unusual/metallic taste, glossitis, stomatitis, and xerostomia (normal salivary flow resumes upon discontinuation).

Significant Adverse Effects
Systemic: Frequency not defined:
Cardiovascular: Flattening of the T-wave, flushing

(Continued)

Metronidazole *(Continued)*

Central nervous system: Ataxia, confusion, coordination impaired, dizziness, fever, headache, insomnia, irritability, seizures, vertigo

Dermatologic: Erythematous rash, urticaria

Endocrine & metabolic: Disulfiram-like reaction, dysmenorrhea, libido decreased

Gastrointestinal: Nausea (~12%), anorexia, abdominal cramping, constipation, diarrhea, furry tongue, glossitis, proctitis, stomatitis, unusual/metallic taste, vomiting, xerostomia

Genitourinary: Cystitis, darkened urine (rare), dysuria, incontinence, polyuria, vaginitis

Hematologic: Neutropenia (reversible), thrombocytopenia (reversible, rare)

Neuromuscular & skeletal: Peripheral neuropathy, weakness

Respiratory: Nasal congestion, rhinitis, sinusitis, pharyngitis

Miscellaneous: Flu-like syndrome, moniliasis

Topical: Frequency not defined:

Central nervous system: Headache

Dermatologic: Burning, contact dermatitis, dryness, erythema, irritation, pruritus, rash

Gastrointestinal: Unusual/metallic taste, nausea, constipation

Local: Local allergic reaction

Neuromuscular & skeletal: Tingling/numbness of extremities

Ocular: Eye irritation

Dosage

Infants and Children:

Amebiasis: Oral: 35-50 mg/kg/day in divided doses every 8 hours for 10 days

Trichomoniasis: Oral: 15-30 mg/kg/day in divided doses every 8 hours for 7 days

Anaerobic infections:

Oral: 15-35 mg/kg/day in divided doses every 8 hours

I.V.: 30 mg/kg/day in divided doses every 6 hours

Clostridium difficile (antibiotic-associated colitis): Oral: 20 mg/kg/day divided every 6 hours

Maximum dose: 2 g/day

Adults:

Treatment of periodontitis associated with AA: Oral:

Single agent: 200-400 mg 3 times/day for 7-10 days

In combination: Metronidazole plus Augmentin® 250 mg 3 times/day each for 7 days; metronidazole 250 mg plus amoxicillin 250 mg each 3 times/day for 7 days; metronidazole plus ciprofloxacin 500 mg each twice daily for 8 days

Amebiasis: Oral: 500-750 mg every 8 hours for 5-10 days

Trichomoniasis: Oral: 250 mg every 8 hours for 7 days **or** 375 mg twice daily for 7 days **or** 2 g as a single dose

Anaerobic infections: Oral, I.V.: 500 mg every 6-8 hours, not to exceed 4 g/day

Antibiotic-associated pseudomembranous colitis: Oral: 250-500 mg 3-4 times/day for 10-14 days

Helicobacter pylori eradication: Oral: 250-500 mg with meals and at bedtime for 14 days; requires combination therapy with at least one other antibiotic and an acid-suppressing agent (proton pump inhibitor or H_2 blocker)

Bacterial vaginosis:

Oral: 750 mg (extended release tablet) once daily for 7 days

Vaginal: 1 applicatorful (~37.5 mg metronidazole) intravaginally once or twice daily for 5 days; apply once in morning and evening if using twice daily, if daily, use at bedtime

Acne rosacea: Topical:

0.75%: Apply and rub a thin film twice daily, morning and evening, to entire affected areas after washing. Significant therapeutic results should be noticed within 3 weeks. Clinical studies have demonstrated continuing improvement through 9 weeks of therapy.

1%: Apply thin film to affected area once daily

Elderly: Use lower end of dosing recommendations for adults, do not administer as a single dose

Dosing adjustment in renal impairment: Cl_{cr} <10 mL/minute: Administer 50% of dose or every 12 hours

Hemodialysis: Extensively removed by hemodialysis and peritoneal dialysis (50% to 100%); administer dose posthemodialysis

Peritoneal dialysis: Dose as for Cl_{cr} <10 mL/minute

Continuous arteriovenous or venovenous hemofiltration: Administer usual dose

Dosing adjustment/comments in hepatic disease: Unchanged in mild liver disease; reduce dosage in severe liver disease

Mechanism of Action After diffusing into the organism, interacts with DNA to cause a loss of helical DNA structure and strand breakage resulting in inhibition of protein synthesis and cell death in susceptible organisms

Contraindications Hypersensitivity to metronidazole, nitroimidazole derivatives, or any component of the formulation; pregnancy (1st trimester - found to be carcinogenic in rats)

Warnings/Precautions Use with caution in patients with liver impairment due to potential accumulation, blood dyscrasias; history of seizures, CHF, or other sodium retaining states; reduce dosage in patients with severe liver impairment, CNS disease, and severe renal failure (Cl_{cr} <10 mL/minute); if *H. pylori* is not eradicated in patients being treated with metronidazole in a regimen, it should be assumed that metronidazole-resistance has occurred and it should not again be used; seizures and neuropathies have been reported especially with increased doses and chronic treatment; if this occurs, discontinue therapy

Drug Interactions Inhibits CYP2C8/9 (weak), 3A4 (moderate)

Cimetidine may increase metronidazole levels.

Cisapride: May inhibit metabolism of cisapride, causing potential arrhythmias; avoid concurrent use

CYP3A4 substrates: Metronidazole may increase the levels/effects of CYP3A4 substrates. Example substrates include benzodiazepines, calcium channel blockers, cyclosporine, mirtazapine, nateglinide, nefazodone, sildenafil (and other PDE-5 inhibitors), tacrolimus, and venlafaxine. Selected benzodiazepines (midazolam and triazolam), cisapride, ergot alkaloids, selected HMG-CoA reductase inhibitors (lovastatin and simvastatin), and pimozide are generally contraindicated with strong CYP3A4 inhibitors.

Ethanol: Ethanol results in disulfiram-like reactions.

Lithium: Metronidazole may increase lithium levels/toxicity; monitor lithium levels.

Phenytoin, phenobarbital may increase metabolism of metronidazole, potentially decreasing its effect.

Warfarin: Metronidazole increases P-T prolongation with warfarin.

Ethanol/Nutrition/Herb Interactions

Ethanol: The manufacturer recommends to avoid all ethanol or any ethanol-containing drugs (may cause disulfiram-like reaction characterized by flushing, headache, nausea, vomiting, sweating or tachycardia).

Food: Peak antibiotic serum concentration lowered and delayed, but total drug absorbed not affected.

Dietary Considerations Take on an empty stomach. Drug may cause GI upset; if GI upset occurs, take with food. Extended release tablets should be taken on an empty stomach (1 hour before or 2 hours after meals). Sodium content of 500 mg (I.V.): 322 mg (14 mEq). The manufacturer recommends that ethanol be avoided during treatment and for 3 days after therapy is complete.

Pharmacodynamics/Kinetics

Absorption: Oral: Well absorbed; Topical: Concentrations achieved systemically after application of 1 g topically are 10 times less than those obtained after a 250 mg oral dose

Distribution: To saliva, bile, seminal fluid, breast milk, bone, liver, and liver abscesses, lung and vaginal secretions; crosses placenta and blood-brain barrier

CSF:blood level ratio: Normal meninges: 16% to 43%; Inflamed meninges: 100%

Protein binding: <20%

Metabolism: Hepatic (30% to 60%)

Half-life elimination: Neonates: 25-75 hours; Others: 6-8 hours, prolonged with hepatic impairment; End-stage renal disease: 21 hours

Time to peak, serum: Oral: Immediate release: 1-2 hours

Excretion: Urine (20% to 40% as unchanged drug); feces (6% to 15%)

Pregnancy Risk Factor B (may be contraindicated in 1st trimester)

Lactation Enters breast milk/not recommended (AAP rates "of concern")

Breast-Feeding Considerations It is suggested to stop breast-feeding for 12-24 hours following single dose therapy to allow excretion of dose.

(Continued)

Metronidazole *(Continued)*

Dosage Forms [DSC] = Discontinued product

Capsule (Flagyl®): 375 mg

Cream, topical: 0.75% (45 g)

MetroCream®: 0.75% (45 g) [contains benzyl alcohol]

Noritate®: 1% (60 g)

Emulsion, topical (Rozex™): 0.75% (60 g) [contains benzyl alcohol]

Gel, topical (MetroGel®): 0.75% [7.5 mg/mL] (45 g)

Gel, vaginal (MetroGel-Vaginal®): 0.75% (70 g)

Infusion [premixed iso-osmotic sodium chloride solution]: 500 mg (100 mL)

Injection, powder for reconstitution, as hydrochloride (Flagyl®): 500 mg [DSC]

Lotion, topical (MetroLotion®): 0.75% (60 mL) [contains benzyl alcohol]

Tablet (Flagyl®): 250 mg, 500 mg

Tablet, extended release (Flagyl® ER): 750 mg

Selected Readings

Eisenberg L, Suchow R, Coles RS, et al, "The Effects of Metronidazole Administration on Clinical and Microbiologic Parameters of Periodontal Disease," *Clin Prev Dent*, 1991, 13(1):28-34.

Herrera D, Sanz M, Jepsen S, et al, "A Systematic Review on the Effect of Systemic Antimicrobials as an Adjunct to Scaling and Root Planing in Periodontitis Patients," *J Clin Periodontol*, 2002, 29(Suppl 3):136-59, discussion 160-2.

Jansson H, Bratthall G, and Soderholm G, "Clinical Outcome Observed in Subjects With Recurrent Periodontal Disease Following Local Treatment With 25% Metronidazole Gel," *J Periodontol*, 2003, 74(3):372-7.

Jenkins WM, MacFarlane TW, Gilmour WH, et al, "Systemic Metronidazole in the Treatment of Periodontitis," *J Clin Periodontol*, 1989, 16(7):433-50.

Loesche WJ, Giordano JR, Hujoel P, et al, "Metronidazole in Periodontitis: Reduced Need for Surgery," *J Clin Periodontol*, 1992, 19(2):103-12.

Loesche WJ, Schmidt E, Smith BA, et al, "Effects of Metronidazole on Periodontal Treatment Needs," *J Periodontol*, 1991, 62(4):247-57.

Noiri Y, Okami Y, Narimatsu M, et al, "Effects of Chlorhexidine, Minocycline, and Metronidazole on Porphyromonas Gingivalis Strain 381 in Biofilms," *J Periodontol*, 2003, 74(11):1647-51.

Soder PO, Frithiof L, Wikner S, et al, "The Effect of Systemic Metronidazole After Nonsurgical Treatment in Moderate and Advanced Periodontitis in Young Adults," *J Periodontol*, 1990, 61(5):281-8.

Wynn RL, Bergman SA, Meiller TF, et al, "Antibiotics in Treating Oral-Facial Infections of Odontogenic Origin: An Update," *Gen Dent*, 2001, 49(3):238-40, 242, 244 passim.

Metronidazole, Bismuth Subsalicylate, and Tetracycline *see* Bismuth Subsalicylate, Metronidazole, and Tetracycline *on page 209*

Metronidazole Hydrochloride *see* Metronidazole *on page 917*

Metronidazole, Tetracycline, and Bismuth Subsalicylate *see* Bismuth Subsalicylate, Metronidazole, and Tetracycline *on page 209*

Metyrosine (me TYE roe seen)

U.S. Brand Names Demser®

Canadian Brand Names Demser®

Generic Available No

Synonyms AMPT; OGMT

Pharmacologic Category Tyrosine Hydroxylase Inhibitor

Use Short-term management of pheochromocytoma before surgery, long-term management when surgery is contraindicated or when chronic malignant pheochromocytoma exists

Local Anesthetic/Vasoconstrictor Precautions No information available to require special precautions

Effects on Dental Treatment Key adverse event(s) related to dental treatment: Xerostomia (normal salivary flow resumes upon discontinuation).

Common Adverse Effects

>10%:

Central nervous system: Drowsiness, extrapyramidal symptoms

Gastrointestinal: Diarrhea

1% to 10%:

Endocrine & metabolic: Galactorrhea, edema of the breasts

Gastrointestinal: Nausea, vomiting, xerostomia

Genitourinary: Impotence

Respiratory: Nasal congestion

Mechanism of Action Blocks the rate-limiting step in the biosynthetic pathway of catecholamines. It is a tyrosine hydroxylase inhibitor, blocking the conversion of tyrosine to dihydroxyphenylalanine. This inhibition results in decreased levels of endogenous catecholamines. Catecholamine biosynthesis is reduced by 35% to 80% in patients treated with metyrosine 1-4 g/day.

Drug Interactions

Increased Effect/Toxicity: Phenothiazines, haloperidol may potentiate EPS

Pharmacodynamics/Kinetics

Half-life elimination: 7.2 hours

Excretion: Primarily urine (as unchanged drug)

Pregnancy Risk Factor C

Mevacor® *see* Lovastatin *on page 848*

Mevinolin *see* Lovastatin *on page 848*

Mexiletine (MEKS i le teen)

Related Information

Cardiovascular Diseases *on page 1458*

U.S. Brand Names Mexitil®

Canadian Brand Names Novo-Mexiletine

Generic Available Yes

Pharmacologic Category Antiarrhythmic Agent, Class Ib

Use Management of serious ventricular arrhythmias; suppression of PVCs

Unlabeled/Investigational Use Diabetic neuropathy

Local Anesthetic/Vasoconstrictor Precautions No information available to require special precautions

Effects on Dental Treatment Key adverse event(s) related to dental treatment: Xerostomia (normal salivary flow resumes upon discontinuation).

Common Adverse Effects

>10%:

Central nervous system: Lightheadedness (11% to 25%), dizziness (20% to 25%), nervousness (5% to 10%), incoordination (10%)

Gastrointestinal: GI distress (41%), nausea/vomiting (40%)

Neuromuscular & skeletal: Trembling, unsteady gait, tremor (13%), ataxia (10% to 20%)

1% to 10%:

Cardiovascular: Chest pain (3% to 8%), premature ventricular contractions (1% to 2%), palpitations (4% to 8%), angina (2%), proarrhythmic (10% to 15% in patients with malignant arrhythmias)

Central nervous system: Confusion, headache, insomnia (5% to 7%), depression (2%)

Dermatologic: Rash (4%)

Gastrointestinal: Constipation or diarrhea (4% to 5%), xerostomia (3%), abdominal pain (1%)

Neuromuscular & skeletal: Weakness (5%), numbness of fingers or toes (2% to 4%), paresthesias (2%), arthralgias (1%)

Ocular: Blurred vision (5% to 7%), nystagmus (6%)

Otic: Tinnitus (2% to 3%)

Respiratory: Dyspnea (3%)

Mechanism of Action Class IB antiarrhythmic, structurally related to lidocaine, which inhibits inward sodium current, decreases rate of rise of phase 0, increases effective refractory period/action potential duration ratio

Drug Interactions

Cytochrome P450 Effect: Substrate (major) of CYP1A2, 2D6; **Inhibits** CYP1A2 (strong)

Increased Effect/Toxicity: Mexiletine may increase the levels/effects of aminophylline, fluvoxamine, mirtazapine, ropinirole, trifluoperazine, or other CYP1A2 substrates. The levels/effects of mexiletine; example inhibitors include amiodarone, chlorpromazine, ciprofloxacin, delavirdine, fluoxetine, fluvoxamine, ketoconazole, lomefloxacin, miconazole, ofloxacin, paroxetine, pergolide, quinidine, quinine, ritonavir, rofecoxib, ropinirole, and other CYP1A2 or 2D6 inhibitors. Mexiletine and caffeine or theophylline may result in elevated levels of theophylline and caffeine. Quinidine and urinary alkalinizers (antacids, sodium bicarbonate, acetazolamide) may increase mexiletine blood levels.

Decreased Effect: The levels/effects of mexiletine may be decreased by aminoglutethimide, carbamazepine, phenobarbital, rifampin, and other CYP1A2 inducers. Urinary acidifying agents may decrease mexiletine levels.

Pharmacodynamics/Kinetics

Absorption: Elderly have a slightly slower rate, but extent of absorption is the same as young adults

Distribution: V_d: 5-7 L/kg

Protein binding: 50% to 70%

Metabolism: Hepatic; low first-pass effect

Half-life elimination: Adults: 10-14 hours (average: elderly: 14.4 hours, younger adults: 12 hours); prolonged with hepatic impairment or heart failure

Time to peak: 2-3 hours

Excretion: Urine (10% to 15% as unchanged drug); urinary acidification increases excretion, alkalinization decreases excretion

Pregnancy Risk Factor C

Mexitil® *see* Mexiletine *on page 921*
M-FA-142 *see* Amonafide *on page 112*
MG 217® [OTC] *see* Coal Tar *on page 367*
MG 217® Medicated Tar [OTC] *see* Coal Tar *on page 367*
MG217 Sal-Acid® [OTC] *see* Salicylic Acid *on page 1205*
Miacalcin® *see* Calcitonin *on page 243*
Micaderm® [OTC] *see* Miconazole *on page 922*
Micardis® *see* Telmisartan *on page 1265*
Micardis® HCT *see* Telmisartan and Hydrochlorothiazide *on page 1265*
Micatin® [OTC] *see* Miconazole *on page 922*

Miconazole (mi KON a zole)

Related Information

Sexually-Transmitted Diseases *on page 1504*

U.S. Brand Names Aloe Vesta® 2-n-1 Antifungal [OTC]; Baza® Antifungal [OTC]; Carrington Antifungal [OTC]; Femizol-M™ [OTC]; Fungoid® Tincture [OTC]; Lotrimin® AF Powder/Spray [OTC]; Micaderm® [OTC]; Micatin® [OTC]; Micro-Guard® [OTC]; Mitrazol™ [OTC]; Monistat® 1 Combination Pack [OTC]; Monistat® 3 [OTC]; Monistat® 7 [OTC]; Monistat-Derm®; Triple Care® Antifungal [OTC]; Zeasorb®-AF [OTC]

Canadian Brand Names Dermazole; Micatin®; Micozole; Monistat®; Monistat®-3

Mexican Brand Names Aloid®; Daktarin®; Dermifun®; Lotrimin AF®; Neomicol®

Generic Available Yes

Synonyms Miconazole Nitrate

Pharmacologic Category Antifungal Agent, Topical; Antifungal Agent, Vaginal

Use Treatment of vulvovaginal candidiasis and a variety of skin and mucous membrane fungal infections

Local Anesthetic/Vasoconstrictor Precautions No information available to require special precautions

Effects on Dental Treatment No significant effects or complications reported

Common Adverse Effects Frequency not defined.

Topical: Allergic contact dermatitis, burning, maceration

Vaginal: Abdominal cramps, burning, irritation, itching

Mechanism of Action Inhibits biosynthesis of ergosterol, damaging the fungal cell wall membrane, which increases permeability causing leaking of nutrients

Drug Interactions

Cytochrome P450 Effect: Substrate of CYP3A4 (major); **Inhibits** CYP1A2 (moderate), 2A6 (strong), 2B6 (weak), 2C8/9 (strong), 2C19 (strong), 2D6 (strong), 2E1 (moderate), 3A4 (strong)

Increased Effect/Toxicity: Note: The majority of reported drug interactions were observed following intravenous miconazole administration. Although systemic absorption following topical and/or vaginal administration is low, potential interactions due to CYP isoenzyme inhibition may occur (rarely). This may be particularly true in situations where topical absorption may be increased (ie, inflamed tissue).

Miconazole coadministered with warfarin has increased the anticoagulant effect of warfarin (including reports associated with vaginal miconazole therapy of as little as 3 days). Concurrent administration of cisapride is contraindicated due to an increased risk of cardiotoxicity. Miconazole may increase the serum levels/effects of amiodarone, amphetamines, benzodiazepines, beta-blockers, buspirone, busulfan, calcium channel blockers, citalopram, dexmedetomidine, dextromethorphan, diazepam, digoxin, docetaxel, fluoxetine, fluvoxamine, glimepiride, glipizide, ifosfamide, inhalational anesthetics, lidocaine, mesoridazine, methsuximide, mexiletine, mirtazapine, nateglinide, nefazodone, paroxetine, phenytoin, pioglitazone, propranolol, risperidone, ritonavir, ropinirole, rosiglitazone, sertraline, sirolimus, tacrolimus, theophylline, thioridazine, tricyclic antidepressants, trifluoperazine, trimetrexate, venlafaxine, vincristine, vinblastine, warfarin, zolpidem, and other substrates of CYP1A2, 2A6, 2C8/9, 2C19, 2D6, or 3A4. Selected benzodiazepines (midazolam and triazolam), cisapride, ergot alkaloids, selected HMG-CoA reductase inhibitors (lovastatin and simvastatin), and pimozide are generally contraindicated with strong CYP3A4 inhibitors. Mesoridazine and thioridazine are generally contraindicated with strong CYP2D6 inhibitors. When used with strong CYP3A4 inhibitors, dosage adjustment/limits are recommended for sildenafil and other PDE-5 inhibitors; consult individual monographs.

Decreased Effect: Amphotericin B may decrease antifungal effect of both agents. The levels/effects of miconazole may be decreased by aminoglutethimide, carbamazepine, nafcillin, nevirapine, phenobarbital, phenytoin, rifamycins or other CYP3A4 inducers. Miconazole may decrease the levels/effects of CYP2D6 prodrug substrates (eg, codeine, hydrocodone, oxycodone, tramadol).

Pharmacodynamics/Kinetics

Absorption: Topical: Negligible

Distribution: Widely to body tissues; penetrates well into inflamed joints, vitreous humor of eye, and peritoneal cavity, but poorly into saliva and sputum; crosses blood-brain barrier but only to a small extent

Protein binding: 91% to 93%

Metabolism: Hepatic

Half-life elimination: Multiphasic: Initial: 40 minutes; Secondary: 126 minutes; Terminal: 24 hours

Excretion: Feces (~50%); urine (<1% as unchanged drug)

Pregnancy Risk Factor C

Miconazole Nitrate *see* Miconazole *on page 922*

MICRhoGAM® *see* Rh_0(D) Immune Globulin *on page 1176*

Microfibrillar Collagen Hemostat

(mye kro FI bri lar KOL la jen HEE moe stat)

U.S. Brand Names Avitene®; Helistat®

Generic Available No

Synonyms Collagen; MCH

Pharmacologic Category Hemostatic Agent

Use Adjunct to hemostasis when control of bleeding by ligature is ineffective or impractical

Local Anesthetic/Vasoconstrictor Precautions No information available to require special precautions

Effects on Dental Treatment No significant effects or complications reported

Significant Adverse Effects Potentiation of infection, allergic reaction, adhesion formation, foreign body reaction

Dosage Apply dry directly to source of bleeding

Mechanism of Action Microfibrillar collagen hemostat is an absorbable topical hemostatic agent prepared from purified bovine corium collagen and shredded into fibrils. Physically, microfibrillar collagen hemostat yields a large surface area. Chemically, it is collagen with hydrochloric acid noncovalently bound to some of the available amino groups in the collagen molecules. When in contact with a bleeding surface, microfibrillar collagen hemostat attracts platelets which adhere to its fibrils and undergo the release phenomenon. This triggers aggregation of the platelets into thrombi in the interstices of the fibrous mass, initiating the formation of a physiologic platelet plug.

Contraindications Hypersensitivity to any component of the formulation; closure of skin incisions, contaminated wounds

Warnings/Precautions Fragments of MCH may pass through filters of blood scavenging systems, avoid reintroduction of blood from operative sites treated with MCH; after several minutes remove excess material

Drug Interactions No data reported

Pharmacodynamics/Kinetics Absorption: By animal tissue in 3 months

Pregnancy Risk Factor C

Dosage Forms Sponge:

Avitene® [bovine collagen]: 2 cm x 6.25 cm x 7 mm (12s); 8 cm x 6.25 cm x 1 cm (6s); 8 cm x 12.5 cm x 1 cm (6s); 8 cm x 12.5 cm x 3 mm (6s); 8 cm x 25 cm x 1 cm (6s)

Helisat® [bovine collagen]: 0.5 inch x 1 inch x 7 mm (18s) [packaged as 3 strips of 6 sponges]

Microgestin™ Fe *see* Ethinyl Estradiol and Norethindrone *on page 550*

Micro-Guard® [OTC] *see* Miconazole *on page 922*

microK® *see* Potassium Chloride *on page 1105*

microK® 10 *see* Potassium Chloride *on page 1105*

Micronase® *see* GlyBURIDE *on page 664*

microNefrin® *see* Epinephrine (Racemic) *on page 497*

Micronor® *see* Norethindrone *on page 996*

Microzide™ *see* Hydrochlorothiazide *on page 699*

Midamor® [DSC] *see* Amiloride *on page 95*

Midazolam (MID aye zoe lam)

U.S. Brand Names Versed® [DSC]

Canadian Brand Names Apo-Midazolam®

Mexican Brand Names Dormicum®

Generic Available Yes: Injection

Synonyms Midazolam Hydrochloride

Pharmacologic Category Benzodiazepine

Dental Use Sedation component in I.V. conscious sedation in oral surgery patients; syrup formulation is used for children to help alleviate anxiety before a dental procedure

Use Preoperative sedation and provides conscious sedation prior to diagnostic or radiographic procedures; ICU sedation (continuous infusion); intravenous anesthesia (induction); intravenous anesthesia (maintenance)

Unlabeled/Investigational Use Anxiety, status epilepticus

Local Anesthetic/Vasoconstrictor Precautions No information available to require special precautions

Effects on Dental Treatment No significant effects or complications reported

Significant Adverse Effects As reported in adults unless otherwise noted:

>10%: Respiratory: Decreased tidal volume and/or respiratory rate decrease, apnea (3% children)

1% to 10%:

Cardiovascular: Hypotension (3% children)

Central nervous system: Drowsiness (1%), oversedation, headache (1%), seizure-like activity (1% children)

Gastrointestinal: Nausea (3%), vomiting (3%)

Local: Pain and local reactions at injection site (4% I.M., 5% I.V.; severity less than diazepam)

Ocular: Nystagmus (1% children)

Respiratory: Cough (1%)

Miscellaneous: Physical and psychological dependence with prolonged use, hiccups (4%, 1% children), paradoxical reaction (2% children)

<1% (Limited to important or life-threatening): Agitation, amnesia, bigeminy, bronchospasm, emergence delirium, euphoria, hallucinations, laryngospasm, rash

Restrictions C-IV

Dosage The dose of midazolam needs to be individualized based on the patient's age, underlying diseases, and concurrent medications. Decrease dose (by ~30%) if narcotics or other CNS depressants are administered concomitantly. **Personnel and equipment needed for standard respiratory resuscitation should be immediately available during midazolam administration.**

Children <6 years may require higher doses and closer monitoring than older children; calculate dose on ideal body weight

Conscious sedation for procedures or preoperative sedation:

Oral: 0.25-0.5 mg/kg as a single dose preprocedure, up to a maximum of 20 mg; administer 30-45 minutes prior to procedure. Children <6 years or less cooperative patients may require as much as 1 mg/kg as a single dose; 0.25 mg/kg may suffice for children 6-16 years of age.

Intranasal (not an approved route): 0.2 mg/kg (up to 0.4 mg/kg in some studies), to a maximum of 15 mg; may be administered 30-45 minutes prior to procedure

I.M.: 0.1-0.15 mg/kg 30-60 minutes before surgery or procedure; range 0.05-0.15 mg/kg; doses up to 0.5 mg/kg have been used in more anxious patients; maximum total dose: 10 mg

I.V.:

Infants <6 months: Limited information is available in nonintubated infants; dosing recommendations not clear; infants <6 months are at higher risk for airway obstruction and hypoventilation; titrate dose in small increments to desired effect; monitor carefully

Infants 6 months to Children 5 years: Initial: 0.05-0.1 mg/kg; titrate dose carefully; total dose of 0.6 mg/kg may be required; usual maximum total dose: 6 mg

Children 6-12 years: Initial: 0.025-0.05 mg/kg; titrate dose carefully; total doses of 0.4 mg/kg may be required; usual maximum total dose: 10 mg

Children 12-16 years: Dose as adults; usual maximum total dose: 10 mg

Conscious sedation during mechanical ventilation: Children: Loading dose: 0.05-0.2 mg/kg, followed by initial continuous infusion: 0.06-0.12 mg/kg/hour (1-2 mcg/kg/minute); titrate to the desired effect; usual range: 0.4-6 mcg/kg/minute

Status epilepticus refractory to standard therapy (unlabeled use): Infants >2 months and Children: Loading dose: 0.15 mg/kg followed by a continuous infusion of 1 mcg/kg/minute; titrate dose upward every 5 minutes until clinical seizure activity is controlled; mean infusion rate required in 24 children was 2.3 mcg/kg/minute with a range of 1-18 mcg/kg/minute

Adults:

Preoperative sedation:

I.M.: 0.07-0.08 mg/kg 30-60 minutes prior to surgery/procedure; usual dose: 5 mg; **Note:** Reduce dose in patients with COPD, high-risk patients, patients ≥60 years of age, and patients receiving other narcotics or CNS depressants

I.V.: 0.02-0.04 mg/kg; repeat every 5 minutes as needed to desired effect or up to 0.1-0.2 mg/kg

Intranasal (not an approved route): 0.2 mg/kg (up to 0.4 mg/kg in some studies); administer 30-45 minutes prior to surgery/procedure

Conscious sedation: I.V.: Initial: 0.5-2 mg slow I.V. over at least 2 minutes; slowly titrate to effect by repeating doses every 2-3 minutes if needed; usual total dose: 2.5-5 mg; use decreased doses in elderly

Healthy Adults <60 years: Some patients respond to doses as low as 1 mg; no more than 2.5 mg should be administered over a period of 2 minutes. Additional doses of midazolam may be administered after a 2-minute waiting period and evaluation of sedation after each dose increment. A total dose >5 mg is generally not needed. If narcotics or other CNS depressants are administered concomitantly, the midazolam dose should be reduced by 30%.

Anesthesia: I.V.:

Induction:

Unpremedicated patients: 0.3-0.35 mg/kg (up to 0.6 mg/kg in resistant cases)

Premedicated patients: 0.15-0.35 mg/kg

Maintenance: 0.05-0.3 mg/kg as needed, or continuous infusion 0.25-1.5 mcg/kg/minute

Sedation in mechanically-ventilated patients: I.V. continuous infusion: 100 mg in 250 mL D_5W or NS (if patient is fluid-restricted, may concentrate up to a maximum of 0.5 mg/mL); initial dose: 0.02-0.08 mg/kg (~1 mg to 5 mg in 70 kg adult) initially and either repeated at 5-15 minute intervals until adequate sedation is achieved or continuous infusion rates of 0.04-0.2 mg/kg/hour and titrate to reach desired level of sedation

Elderly: I.V.: Conscious sedation: Initial: 0.5 mg slow I.V.; give no more than 1.5 mg in a 2-minute period; if additional titration is needed, give no more than 1 mg over 2 minutes, waiting another 2 or more minutes to evaluate sedative effect; a total dose of >3.5 mg is rarely necessary

Dosage adjustment in renal impairment:

Hemodialysis: Supplemental dose is not necessary

Peritoneal dialysis: Significant drug removal is unlikely based on physiochemical characteristics

Mechanism of Action Binds to stereospecific benzodiazepine receptors on the postsynaptic GABA neuron at several sites within the central nervous system, including the limbic system, reticular formation. Enhancement of the inhibitory effect of GABA on neuronal excitability results by increased neuronal membrane permeability to chloride ions. This shift in chloride ions results in hyperpolarization (a less excitable state) and stabilization.

Contraindications Hypersensitivity to midazolam or any component of the formulation, including benzyl alcohol (cross-sensitivity with other benzodiazepines may exist); parenteral form is not for intrathecal or epidural injection; narrow-angle glaucoma; concurrent use of potent inhibitors of CYP3A4 (amprenavir, atazanavir, or ritonavir); pregnancy

Warnings/Precautions May cause severe respiratory depression, respiratory arrest, or apnea. Use with extreme caution, particularly in noncritical care settings. Appropriate resuscitative equipment and qualified personnel must be available for administration and monitoring. Initial dosing must be cautiously titrated and individualized, particularly in elderly or debilitated patients, patients with hepatic impairment (including alcoholics), or in renal impairment, particularly if other CNS depressants (including opiates) are used concurrently. Initial doses in elderly or debilitated patients should not exceed 2.5 mg. Use with caution in patients with respiratory disease or impaired gag reflex. Use during upper airway procedures may increase risk of hypoventilation. Prolonged responses have been noted following extended administration by continuous infusion (possibly due to metabolite accumulation) or in the presence of drugs which inhibit midazolam metabolism.

(Continued)

Midazolam *(Continued)*

May cause hypotension - hemodynamic events are more common in pediatric patients or patients with hemodynamic instability. Hypotension and/or respiratory depression may occur more frequently in patients who have received narcotic analgesics. Use with caution in obese patients, chronic renal failure, and CHF. Parenteral form contains benzyl alcohol - avoid rapid injection in neonates or prolonged infusions. Does not protect against increases in heart rate or blood pressure during intubation. Should not be used in shock, coma, or acute alcohol intoxication. Avoid intra-arterial administration or extravasation of parenteral formulation.

Causes CNS depression (dose-related) resulting in sedation, dizziness, confusion, or ataxia which may impair physical and mental capabilities. Patients must be cautioned about performing tasks which require mental alertness (eg, operating machinery or driving). A minimum of 1 day should elapse after midazolam administration before attempting these tasks. Use with caution in patients receiving other CNS depressants or psychoactive agents. Effects with other sedative drugs or ethanol may be potentiated. Benzodiazepines have been associated with falls and traumatic injury and should be used with extreme caution in patients who are at risk of these events (especially the elderly).

Midazolam causes anterograde amnesia. Paradoxical reactions, including hyperactive or aggressive behavior have been reported with benzodiazepines, particularly in adolescent/pediatric or psychiatric patients. Does not have analgesic, antidepressant, or antipsychotic properties.

Benzodiazepines have been associated with dependence and acute withdrawal symptoms on discontinuation or reduction in dose. Acute withdrawal, including seizures, may be precipitated after administration of flumazenil to patients receiving long-term benzodiazepine therapy.

Drug Interactions Substrate of CYP2B6 (minor), 3A4 (major); **Inhibits** CYP2C8/9 (weak), 3A4 (weak)

CNS depressants: Sedative effects and/or respiratory depression may be additive with CNS depressants; includes ethanol, barbiturates, narcotic analgesics, and other sedative agents; monitor for increased effect. **If narcotics or other CNS depressants are administered concomitantly, the midazolam dose should be reduced by 30% if <65 years of age, or by at least 50% if >65 years of age.**

CYP3A4 inducers: CYP3A4 inducers may decrease the levels/effects of midazolam. Example inducers include aminoglutethimide, carbamazepine, nafcillin, nevirapine, phenobarbital, phenytoin, and rifamycins.

CYP3A4 inhibitors: May increase the levels/effects of midazolam. Example inhibitors include azole antifungals, ciprofloxacin, clarithromycin, diclofenac, doxycycline, erythromycin, imatinib, isoniazid, nefazodone, nicardipine, propofol, protease inhibitors, quinidine, and verapamil.

Levodopa: Therapeutic effects may be diminished in some patients following the addition of a benzodiazepine; limited/inconsistent data

Oral contraceptives: May decrease the clearance of some benzodiazepines (those which undergo oxidative metabolism); monitor for increased benzodiazepine effect

Saquinavir: A 56% reduction in clearance and a doubling of midazolam's half-life were seen with concurrent administration with saquinavir.

Theophylline: May partially antagonize some of the effects of benzodiazepines; monitor for decreased response; may require higher doses for sedation

Ethanol/Nutrition/Herb Interactions

Ethanol: Avoid ethanol (may increase CNS depression).

Food: Grapefruit juice may increase serum concentrations of midazolam; avoid concurrent use with oral form.

Herb/Nutraceutical: Avoid concurrent use with St John's wort (may decrease midazolam levels, may increase CNS depression). Avoid concurrent use with valerian, kava kava, gotu kola (may increase CNS depression).

Dietary Considerations Injection: Sodium content of 1 mL: 0.14 mEq

Pharmacodynamics/Kinetics

Onset of action: I.M.: Sedation: ~15 minutes; I.V.: 1-5 minutes

Peak effect: I.M.: 0.5-1 hour

Duration: I.M.: Up to 6 hours; Mean: 2 hours

Absorption: Oral: Rapid

Distribution: V_d: 0.8-2.5 L/kg; increased with congestive heart failure (CHF) and chronic renal failure

Protein binding: 95%

Metabolism: Extensively hepatic via CYP3A4

Bioavailability: Mean: 45%

Half-life elimination: 1-4 hours; prolonged with cirrhosis, congestive heart failure, obesity, and elderly

Excretion: Urine (as glucuronide conjugated metabolites); feces (~2% to 10%)

Pregnancy Risk Factor D

Lactation Enters breast milk/not recommended (AAP rates "of concern")

Dosage Forms [DSC] = Discontinued product

Injection, solution, as hydrochloride (Versed® [DSC]): 1 mg/mL (2 mL, 5 mL, 10 mL); 5 mg/mL (1 mL, 2 mL, 5 mL, 10 mL) [contains benzyl alcohol 1%]

Injection, solution, as hydrochloride [preservative free]: 1 mg/mL (2 mL, 5 mL); 5 mg/mL (1 mL, 2 mL)

Syrup, as hydrochloride (Versed® [DSC]): 2 mg/mL (118 mL) [contains sodium benzoate; cherry flavor]

Selected Readings

Dionne RA, Yagiela JA, Moore PA, et al, "Comparing Efficacy and Safety of Four Intravenous Sedation Regimens in Dental Outpatients," *Am Dent Assoc*, 2001, 132(6):740-51.

Midazolam Hydrochloride *see* Midazolam *on page 924*

Midodrine (MI doe dreen)

U.S. Brand Names ProAmatine®

Canadian Brand Names Amatine®

Generic Available Yes

Synonyms Midodrine Hydrochloride

Pharmacologic Category Alpha$_1$ Agonist

Use Orphan drug: Treatment of symptomatic orthostatic hypotension

Unlabeled/Investigational Use Investigational: Management of urinary incontinence

Local Anesthetic/Vasoconstrictor Precautions No information available to require special precautions

Effects on Dental Treatment Key adverse event(s) related to dental treatment: Xerostomia (normal salivary flow resumes upon discontinuation).

Common Adverse Effects

>10%:

- Dermatologic: Piloerection (13%), pruritus (12%)
- Genitourinary: Urinary urgency, retention, or polyuria, dysuria (up to 13%)
- Neuromuscular & skeletal: Paresthesia (18.3%)

1% to 10%:

- Cardiovascular: Supine hypertension (7%), facial flushing
- Central nervous system: Confusion, anxiety, dizziness, chills (5%)
- Dermatologic: Rash, dry skin (2%)
- Gastrointestinal: Xerostomia, nausea, abdominal pain
- Neuromuscular & skeletal: Pain (5%)

Causes of Orthostatic Hypotension

Primary Autonomic Causes
Pure autonomic failure (Bradbury-Eggleston syndrome, idiopathic orthostatic hypotension)
Autonomic failure with multiple system atrophy (Shy-Drager syndrome)
Familial dysautonomia (Riley-Day syndrome)
Dopamine beta-hydroxylase deficiency
Secondary Autonomic Causes
Chronic alcoholism
Parkinson's disease
Diabetes mellitus
Porphyria
Amyloidosis
Various carcinomas
Vitamin B_1 or B_{12} deficiency
Nonautonomic Causes
Hypovolemia (such as associated with hemorrhage, burns, or hemodialysis) and dehydration
Diminished homeostatic regulation (such as associated with aging, pregnancy, fever, or prolonged bedrest)
Medications (eg, antihypertensives, insulin, tricyclic antidepressants)

Mechanism of Action Midodrine forms an active metabolite, desglymidodrine, that is an alpha$_1$-agonist. This agent increases arteriolar and venous tone

(Continued)

Midodrine *(Continued)*

resulting in a rise in standing, sitting, and supine systolic and diastolic blood pressure in patients with orthostatic hypotension. See table on previous page.

Drug Interactions

Increased Effect/Toxicity: Concomitant fludrocortisone results in hypernatremia or an increase in intraocular pressure and glaucoma. Bradycardia may be accentuated with concomitant administration of cardiac glycosides, psychotherapeutics, and beta-blockers. Alpha agonists may increase the pressure effects and alpha antagonists may negate the effects of midodrine.

Pharmacodynamics/Kinetics

Onset of action: ~1 hour

Duration: 2-3 hours

Absorption: Rapid

Distribution: V_d (desglymidodrine): <1.6 L/kg; poorly across membrane (eg, blood brain barrier)

Protein binding: Minimal

Metabolism: Hepatic; rapid deglycination to desglymidodrine occurs in many tissues and plasma

Bioavailability: Absolute: 93%

Half-life elimination: Active drug: ~3-4 hours; Prodrug: 25 minutes

Time to peak, serum: Active drug: 1-2 hours; Prodrug: 30 minutes

Excretion: Urine (2% to 4%)

Clearance: Desglymidodrine: 385 mL/minute (predominantly by renal secretion)

Pregnancy Risk Factor C

Midodrine Hydrochloride *see* Midodrine *on page 927*

Midol® Maximum Strength Cramp Formula [OTC] *see* Ibuprofen *on page 728*

Midrin® *see* Acetaminophen, Isometheptene, and Dichloralphenazone *on page 59*

Mifeprex® *see* Mifepristone *on page 928*

Mifepristone (mi FE pris tone)

Related Information

Endocrine Disorders and Pregnancy *on page 1481*

U.S. Brand Names Mifeprex®

Generic Available No

Synonyms RU-486; RU-38486

Pharmacologic Category Abortifacient; Antineoplastic Agent, Hormone Antagonist; Antiprogestin

Use Medical termination of intrauterine pregnancy, through day 49 of pregnancy. Patients may need treatment with misoprostol and possibly surgery to complete therapy

Unlabeled/Investigational Use Treatment of unresectable meningioma; has been studied in the treatment of breast cancer, ovarian cancer, and adrenal cortical carcinoma

Local Anesthetic/Vasoconstrictor Precautions No information available to require special precautions

Effects on Dental Treatment No significant effects or complications reported

Common Adverse Effects Vaginal bleeding and uterine cramping are expected to occur when this medication is used to terminate a pregnancy; 90% of women using this medication for this purpose also report adverse reactions

>10%:

Central nervous system: Headache (2% to 31%), dizziness (1% to 12%)

Gastrointestinal: Abdominal pain (cramping) (96%), nausea (43% to 61%), vomiting (18% to 26%), diarrhea (12% to 20%)

Genitourinary: Uterine cramping (83%)

1% to 10%:

Cardiovascular: Syncope (1%)

Central nervous system: Fatigue (10%), fever (4%), insomnia (3%), anxiety (2%), fainting (2%)

Gastrointestinal: Dyspepsia (3%)

Genitourinary: Uterine hemorrhage (5%), vaginitis (3%), pelvic pain (2%)

Hematologic: Decreased hemoglobin >2 g/dL (6%), anemia (2%), leukorrhea (2%)

Neuromuscular & skeletal: Back pain (9%), rigors (3%), leg pain (2%), weakness (2%)

Respiratory: Sinusitis (2%)

Miscellaneous: Viral infection (4%)

Restrictions There are currently no clinical trials with mifepristone in oncology open in the U.S.; investigators wishing to obtain the agent for use in oncology patients must apply for a patient-specific IND from the FDA. Mifepristone will be supplied only to licensed physicians who sign and return a "Prescriber's Agreement." Distribution of mifepristone will be subject to specific requirements imposed by the distributor. Mifepristone will **not** be available to the public through licensed pharmacies.

Mechanism of Action Mifepristone, a synthetic steroid, competitively binds to the intracellular progesterone receptor, blocking the effects of progesterone. When used for the termination of pregnancy, this leads to contraction-inducing activity in the myometrium. In the absence of progesterone, mifepristone acts as a partial progesterone agonist. Mifepristone also has weak antiglucocorticoid and antiandrogenic properties; it blocks the feedback effect of cortisol on corticotropin secretion.

Drug Interactions

Cytochrome P450 Effect: Substrate of CYP3A4 (minor); **Inhibits** CYP2D6 (weak), 3A4 (weak)

Increased Effect/Toxicity: There are no reported interactions. It might be anticipated that the effects of one or both agents would be minimized if mifepristone were administered concurrently with a progestin (exogenous).

Pharmacodynamics/Kinetics

Protein binding: 98% to albumin and α_1-acid glycoprotein

Metabolism: Hepatic via CYP3A4 to three metabolites (may possess some antiprogestin and antiglucocorticoid activity)

Bioavailability: 69%

Half-life elimination: Terminal: 18 hours following a slower phase where 50% eliminated between 12-72 hours

Time to peak: 90 minutes

Excretion: Feces (83%); urine (9%)

Pregnancy Risk Factor X

Miglitol (MIG li tol)

Related Information

Endocrine Disorders and Pregnancy *on page 1481*

U.S. Brand Names Glyset®

Canadian Brand Names Glyset®

Generic Available No

Pharmacologic Category Antidiabetic Agent, Alpha-Glucosidase Inhibitor

Use Type 2 diabetes mellitus (noninsulin-dependent, NIDDM):

Monotherapy adjunct to diet to improve glycemic control in patients with type 2 diabetes mellitus (noninsulin-dependent, NIDDM) whose hyperglycemia cannot be managed with diet alone

Combination therapy with a sulfonylurea when diet plus either miglitol or a sulfonylurea alone do not result in adequate glycemic control. The effect of miglitol to enhance glycemic control is additive to that of sulfonylureas when used in combination.

Local Anesthetic/Vasoconstrictor Precautions No information available to require special precautions

Effects on Dental Treatment No significant effects or complications reported

Common Adverse Effects

>10%: Gastrointestinal: Flatulence (42%), diarrhea (29%), abdominal pain (12%)

1% to 10%: Dermatologic: Rash

Mechanism of Action In contrast to sulfonylureas, miglitol does not enhance insulin secretion; the antihyperglycemic action of miglitol results from a reversible inhibition of membrane-bound intestinal alpha-glucosidases which hydrolyze oligosaccharides and disaccharides to glucose and other monosaccharides in the brush border of the small intestine; in diabetic patients, this enzyme inhibition results in delayed glucose absorption and lowering of postprandial hyperglycemia

Drug Interactions

Decreased Effect: Miglitol may decrease the absorption and bioavailability of digoxin, propranolol, and ranitidine. Digestive enzymes (amylase, pancreatin, charcoal) may reduce the effect of miglitol and should **not** be taken concomitantly.

Pharmacodynamics/Kinetics

Absorption: Saturable at high doses: 25 mg dose: Completely absorbed; 100 mg dose: 50% to 70% absorbed

Distribution: V_d: 0.18 L/kg

Protein binding: <4%

Metabolism: None

(Continued)

Miglitol *(Continued)*

Half-life elimination: ~2 hours
Time to peak: 2-3 hours
Excretion: Urine (as unchanged drug)

Pregnancy Risk Factor B

Miglustat (MIG loo stat)

U.S. Brand Names Zavesca®
Generic Available No
Synonyms OGT-918
Pharmacologic Category Enzyme Inhibitor
Use Treatment of mild-to-moderate type 1 Gaucher disease when enzyme replacement therapy is not a therapeutic option
Local Anesthetic/Vasoconstrictor Precautions No information available to require special precautions
Effects on Dental Treatment No significant effects or complications reported
Common Adverse Effects Percentages reported from open-label, uncontrolled monotherapy trials.

>10%:

Central nervous system: Headache (21% to 22%), dizziness (up to 11%)
Gastrointestinal: Diarrhea (89%; up to 100% in other studies), weight loss (39% to 67%), abdominal pain (18% to 50%), flatulence (29% to 44%), nausea (14% to 22%), vomiting (4% to 11%), cramps (up to 11%)
Neuromuscular & skeletal: Tremor (11%; up to 30% in other studies), leg cramps (4% to 11%),
Ocular: visual disturbances (up to 17%)

1% to 10%:

Central nervous system: headache (up to 6%)
Endocrine & metabolic: Menstrual disorder (up to 6%)
Gastrointestinal: Anorexia (up to 7%), dyspepsia (up to 7%), epigastric pain (up to 6%)
Hematologic: Thrombocytopenia (6% to 7%)
Neuromuscular & skeletal: Paresthesia (up to 7%)

Mechanism of Action Miglustat inhibits the enzyme needed to produce glycosphingolipids and decreases the rate of glycosphingolipid glucosylceramide formation. Glucosylceramide accumulates in type 1 Gaucher disease, causing complications specific to this disease.

Drug Interactions

Decreased Effect: Miglustat increases the clearance of imiglucerase; combination therapy is not indicated.

Pharmacodynamics/Kinetics

Distribution: V_d: 83-105 L
Protein binding: No binding to plasma proteins
Bioavailability: 97%
Half-life elimination: 6-7 hours
Time to peak, plasma: 2-2.5 hours
Excretion: Urine (as unchanged drug)

Pregnancy Risk Factor X

Migranal® *see* Dihydroergotamine *on page 442*

Migrin-A *see* Acetaminophen, Isometheptene, and Dichloralphenazone *on page 59*

Milk of Magnesia *see* Magnesium Hydroxide *on page 853*

Milrinone (MIL ri none)

Related Information

Cardiovascular Diseases *on page 1458*

U.S. Brand Names Primacor®
Canadian Brand Names Primacor®
Generic Available Yes: Injection
Synonyms Milrinone Lactate
Pharmacologic Category Phosphodiesterase Enzyme Inhibitor
Use Short-term I.V. therapy of congestive heart failure; calcium antagonist intoxication
Local Anesthetic/Vasoconstrictor Precautions No information available to require special precautions
Effects on Dental Treatment No significant effects or complications reported
Common Adverse Effects

>10%: Cardiovascular: Ventricular arrhythmia (ectopy 9%, NSVT 3%, sustained ventricular tachycardia 1%, ventricular fibrillation <1%);

life-threatening arrhythmias are infrequent, often associated with underlying factors (eg, pre-existing arrhythmia, electrolyte disturbances, catheter insertion)

1% to 10%:

Cardiovascular: Supraventricular arrhythmia (4%), hypotension

Central nervous system: Headache

Mechanism of Action Phosphodiesterase inhibitor resulting in vasodilation

Pharmacodynamics/Kinetics

Onset of action: I.V.: 5-15 minutes

Serum level: I.V.: Following a 125 mcg/kg dose, peak plasma concentrations ~1000 ng/mL were observed at 2 minutes postinjection, decreasing to <100 ng/mL in 2 hours

Drug concentration levels:

Therapeutic:

Serum levels of 166 ng/mL, achieved during I.V. infusions of 0.25-1 mcg/kg/minute, were associated with sustained hemodynamic benefit in severe congestive heart failure patients over a 24-hour period

Maximum beneficial effects on cardiac output and pulmonary capillary wedge pressure following I.V. infusion have been associated with plasma milrinone concentrations of 150-250 ng/mL

Toxic: Serum concentrations >250-300 ng/mL have been associated with marked reductions in mean arterial pressure and tachycardia; however, more studies are required to determine the toxic serum levels for milrinone

Distribution: V_{dss}: 0.32 L/kg; Severe congestive heart failure (CHF): V_d: 0.33-0.47 L/kg; not significantly bound to tissues; excretion in breast milk unknown

Protein binding, plasma: ~70%

Metabolism: Hepatic (12%)

Half-life elimination: I.V.: 136 minutes in patients with CHF; patients with severe CHF have a more prolonged half-life, with values ranging from 1.7-2.7 hours. Patients with CHF have a reduction in the systemic clearance of milrinone, resulting in a prolonged elimination half-life. Alternatively, one study reported that 1 month of therapy with milrinone did not change the pharmacokinetic parameters for patients with CHF despite improvement in cardiac function.

Excretion: I.V.: Urine (85% as unchanged drug) within 24 hours; active tubular secretion is a major elimination pathway for milrinone

Clearance: I.V. bolus: 25.9 ± 5.7 L/hour (0.37 L/hour/kg); Severe congestive heart failure: 0.11-0.13 L/hour/kg. The reduction in clearance may be a result of reduced renal function. Creatinine clearance values were 1/2 those reported for healthy adults in patients with severe congestive heart failure (52 vs 119 mL/minute).

Pregnancy Risk Factor C

Milrinone Lactate *see* Milrinone *on page 930*

Miltown® *see* Meprobamate *on page 878*

Mineral Oil, Petrolatum, Lanolin, Cetyl Alcohol, and Glycerin *see* Lanolin, Cetyl Alcohol, Glycerin, Petrolatum, and Mineral Oil *on page 797*

Minidyne® [OTC] *see* Povidone-Iodine *on page 1107*

Minipress® *see* Prazosin *on page 1111*

Minitran™ *see* Nitroglycerin *on page 991*

Minizide® *see* Prazosin and Polythiazide *on page 1112*

Minocin® *see* Minocycline *on page 931*

Minocycline (mi noe SYE kleen)

Related Information

Sexually-Transmitted Diseases *on page 1504*

U.S. Brand Names Dynacin®; Minocin®

Canadian Brand Names Alti-Minocycline; Apo-Minocycline®; Gen-Minocycline; Minocin®; Novo-Minocycline; PMS-Minocycline; Rhoxal-minocycline

Mexican Brand Names Minocin®

Generic Available Yes: Capsule

Synonyms Minocycline Hydrochloride

Pharmacologic Category Antibiotic, Tetracycline Derivative

Dental Use Treatment of periodontitis associated with presence of *Actinobacillus actinomycetemcomitans* (AA); as adjunctive therapy in recurrent aphthous ulcers

Use Treatment of susceptible bacterial infections of both gram-negative and gram-positive organisms; treatment of anthrax (inhalational, cutaneous, and gastrointestinal); acne; meningococcal carrier state; Rickettsial diseases

(Continued)

Minocycline *(Continued)*

(including Rocky Mountain spotted fever, Q fever); nongonococcal urethritis, gonorrhea; acute intestinal amebiasis

Local Anesthetic/Vasoconstrictor Precautions No information available to require special precautions

Effects on Dental Treatment Key adverse event(s) related to dental treatment: Discoloration of teeth (children). Opportunistic "superinfection" with *Candida albicans*; tetracyclines are not recommended for use during pregnancy or in children ≤8 years of age since they have been reported to cause enamel hypoplasia and permanent teeth discoloration. The use of tetracycline's should only be used in these patients if other agents are contraindicated or alternative antimicrobials will not eradicate the organism. Long-term use associated with oral candidiasis.

Significant Adverse Effects

>10%: Miscellaneous: Discoloration of teeth (in children)

1% to 10%:

Central nervous system: Lightheadedness, vertigo

Dermatologic: Photosensitivity

Gastrointestinal: Nausea, diarrhea

<1%: Acute renal failure, anaphylaxis, angioedema, diabetes insipidus, eosinophilia, erythema multiforme, esophagitis, exfoliative dermatitis, hemolytic anemia, hepatitis, hepatic failure, neutropenia, paresthesia, pericarditis, pigmentation of nails, pseudotumor cerebri, rash, Stevens-Johnson syndrome, superinfections, thrombocytopenia, thyroid dysfunction (extremely rare), tinnitus, vomiting

Dosage

Children >8 years: Oral, I.V.: Initial: 4 mg/kg followed by 2 mg/kg/dose every 12 hours

Adults:

Infection: Oral, I.V.: 200 mg stat, 100 mg every 12 hours not to exceed 400 mg/24 hours

Acne: Oral: 50 mg 1-3 times/day

Dosage adjustment in renal impairment: Consider decreasing dose or increasing dosing interval with renal impairment.

Mechanism of Action Inhibits bacterial protein synthesis by binding with the 30S and possibly the 50S ribosomal subunit(s) of susceptible bacteria; cell wall synthesis is not affected

Contraindications Hypersensitivity to minocycline, other tetracyclines, or any component of the formulation; pregnancy

Warnings/Precautions Avoid use during tooth development (children ≤8 years of age) unless other drugs are not likely to be effective or are contraindicated. May be associated with increases in BUN secondary to anti-anabolic effects. Avoid in renal insufficiency (associated with hepatotoxicity). CNS effects (lightheadedness, vertigo) may occur, potentially affecting a patient's ability to drive or operate heavy machinery. Has been associated (rarely) with pseudotumor cerebri. May cause photosensitivity.

Drug Interactions

Calcium-, magnesium-, or aluminum-containing antacids, oral contraceptives, iron, zinc, sodium bicarbonate, penicillins, cimetidine: May decrease absorption of tetracyclines

Although no clinical evidence exists, tetracyclines may bind with bismuth or calcium carbonate, an excipient in bismuth subsalicylate, during treatment for *H. pylori*.

Digoxin: Tetracyclines may rarely increase digoxin serum levels.

Methoxyflurane anesthesia when concurrent with tetracyclines may cause fatal nephrotoxicity.

Oral contraceptives: Anecdotal reports suggesting decreased contraceptive efficacy with tetracyclines have been refuted by more rigorous scientific and clinical data.

Warfarin: Hypoprothrombinemic response may be increased with tetracyclines; monitor INR closely during initiation or discontinuation.

Ethanol/Nutrition/Herb Interactions

Food: Minocycline serum concentrations are not altered if taken with dairy products.

Herb/Nutraceutical: Avoid dong quai, St John's wort (may also cause photosensitization).

Dietary Considerations May be taken with food or milk.

Pharmacodynamics/Kinetics

Absorption: Well absorbed

Distribution: Majority deposits for extended periods in fat; crosses placenta; enters breast milk

Protein binding: 70% to 75%

Half-life elimination: 15 hours

Excretion: Urine

Pregnancy Risk Factor D

Lactation Enters breast milk/not recommended (AAP rates "compatible")

Breast-Feeding Considerations Although tetracyclines are excreted in limited amounts, the potential for staining of unerupted teeth has led some experts to recommend against breast-feeding. The AAP identified tetracyclines as "compatible" with breast-feeding.

Dosage Forms

Capsule, as hydrochloride: 50 mg, 75 mg, 100 mg

Dynacin®: 50 mg, 75 mg, 100 mg

Capsule, pellet-filled, as hydrochloride (Minocin®): 50 mg, 100 mg

Injection, powder for reconstitution, as hydrochloride (Minocin®): 100 mg

Tablet, as hydrochloride (Dynacin®): 50 mg, 75 mg, 100 mg

Minocycline Hydrochloride *see* Minocycline *on page 931*

Minocycline Hydrochloride (Periodontal)

Related Information

Minocycline *on page 931*

U.S. Brand Names Arestin™

Generic Available No

Pharmacologic Category Antibiotic, Tetracycline Derivative

Dental Use Adjunct to scaling and root planing procedures for reduction of pocket depth in patients with adult periodontitis. May be used as part of a periodontal maintenance program which includes good oral hygiene, scaling, and root planing.

Local Anesthetic/Vasoconstrictor Precautions No information available to require special precautions

Effects on Dental Treatment Key adverse event(s) related to dental treatment: Patients should avoid the following postadministration: Eating hard, crunchy, or sticky foods for 1 week; brushing for a 12-hour period; touching treated areas; use of interproximal cleaning devices for 10 days.

Significant Adverse Effects Frequency not defined.

Central nervous system: Headache, pain

Gastrointestinal: Periodontitis, tooth disorder, dental caries, dental pain, gingivitis, stomatitis, mouth ulceration, dyspepsia, dental infection, mucous membrane disorder

Respiratory: Pharyngitis

Miscellaneous: Infection, flu syndrome

Dosage Arestin™ is a variable dose product; dependent upon the size, shape, and number of pockets being treated.

Administration of Arestin™ does not require local anesthesia. Professional subgingival administration is accomplished by inserting the unit-dose cartridge to the base of the periodontal pocket and then pressing the thumb ring in the handle mechanism to expel the powder while gradually withdrawing the tip from the base of the pocket. The handle mechanism should be sterilized between patients. Arestin™ does not have to be removed (it is bioresorbable) nor is an adhesive dressing required.

Mechanism of Action Minocycline, a member of the tetracycline class of antibiotics, has a broad spectrum of activity. It is bacteriostatic and exerts its antimicrobial activity by inhibiting protein synthesis.

Contraindications Known hypersensitivity to minocycline, tetracyclines, or any component of the formulation; pregnancy

Warnings/Precautions The use of the tetracycline class during tooth development (last half of pregnancy, infancy, and childhood to 8 years of age) may cause permanent discoloration of the teeth (yellow-gray brown). This adverse reaction is more common during long-term use of the drugs, but has been observed following repeated short-term courses. Enamel hypoplasia has also been reported. Tetracycline drugs, therefore, should not be used in this age group, or in pregnant or nursing women, unless the potential benefits are considered to outweigh the potential risks. Results of animal studies indicate that tetracyclines cross the placenta, are found in fetal tissues, and can have toxic effects on the developing fetus (often related to retardation of skeletal development). Evidence of embryotoxicity has also been noted in animals treated early in pregnancy. If any tetracyclines are used during pregnancy, or if the patient becomes pregnant while taking this drug, the patient should be apprised of the potential hazard to the fetus. Photosensitivity manifested by an

(Continued)

Minocycline Hydrochloride (Periodontal) *(Continued)*

exaggerated sunburn reaction has been observed in some individuals taking tetracyclines. Patients apt to be exposed to direct sunlight or ultraviolet light should be advised that this reaction can occur with tetracycline drugs, and treatment should be discontinued at the first evidence of skin erythema.

The use of Arestin™ in an acutely abscessed periodontal pocket has not been studied and is not recommended. While no overgrowth by opportunistic microorganisms, such as yeast, were noted during clinical studies, as with other antimicrobials, the use of Arestin™ may result in overgrowth of nonsusceptible microorganisms including fungi. The effects of treatment for >6 months have not been studied. Arestin™ should be used with caution in patients having a history of predisposition to oral candidiasis. The safety and effectiveness of Arestin™ have not been established for the treatment of periodontitis in patients with coexistent oral candidiasis. Arestin™ has not been clinically tested in immunocompromised patients (such as those immunocompromised by diabetes, chemotherapy, radiation therapy, or infection with HIV). If superinfection is suspected, appropriate measures should be taken. Arestin™ has not been clinically tested for use in the regeneration of alveolar bone, either in preparation for or in conjunction with the placement of endosseous (dental) implants or in the treatment of failing implants.

Pregnancy Risk Factor D

Dosage Forms Injection, powder, sustained release [microspheres for subgingival application] (Arestin™): 1 mg (12s) [each unit-dose cartridge delivers minocycline hydrochloride equivalent to minocycline free base 1 mg]

Minoxidil (mi NOKS i dil)

Related Information

Cardiovascular Diseases *on page 1458*

U.S. Brand Names Loniten®; Rogaine® Extra Strength for Men [OTC]; Rogaine® for Men [OTC]; Rogaine® for Women [OTC]

Canadian Brand Names Apo-Gain®; Minox; Rogaine®

Mexican Brand Names Regaine®

Generic Available Yes

Pharmacologic Category Topical Skin Product; Vasodilator

Use Management of severe hypertension (usually in combination with a diuretic and beta-blocker); treatment (topical formulation) of alopecia androgenetica in males and females

Local Anesthetic/Vasoconstrictor Precautions No information available to require special precautions

Effects on Dental Treatment No significant effects or complications reported

Common Adverse Effects

Oral: Incidence of reactions not always reported.

Cardiovascular: Peripheral edema (7%), sodium and water retention, CHF, tachycardia, angina pectoris, pericardial effusion with or without tamponade, pericarditis, ECG changes (T-wave changes, 60%), rebound hypertension (in children after a gradual withdrawal)

Central nervous system: Headache (rare), fatigue

Dermatologic: Hypertrichosis (common, 80%), transient pruritus, changes in pigmentation (rare), serosanguineous bullae (rare), rash (rare), Stevens-Johnson syndrome

Hepatic: Increased alkaline phosphatase

Renal: Transient increase in serum BUN and creatinine

Respiratory: Pulmonary edema

Topical: Incidence of adverse events is not always reported.

Cardiovascular: Increased left ventricular end-diastolic volume, increased cardiac output, increased left ventricular mass, dizziness, tachycardia, edema, transient chest pain, palpitation, increase or decrease in blood pressure, increase or decrease in pulse rate (1.5%, placebo 1.6%)

Central nervous system: Headache, dizziness, weakness, taste alterations, faintness, lightheadedness (3.4%, placebo 3.5%), vertigo (1.2%, placebo 1.2%), anxiety (rare), mental depression (rare), fatigue (rare 0.4%, placebo 1%)

Dermatologic: Local irritation, dryness, erythema, allergic contact dermatitis (7.4%, placebo 5.4%), pruritus, scaling/flaking, eczema, seborrhea, papular rash, folliculitis, local erythema, flushing, exacerbation of hair loss, alopecia, hypertrichosis, increased hair growth outside the area of application (face, beard, eyebrows, ear, arm)

Gastrointestinal: Diarrhea, nausea, vomiting (4.3%, placebo 6.6%), weight gain (1.2%, placebo 1.3%)

Neuromuscular & skeletal: Fractures, back pain, retrosternal chest pain of muscular origin, tendonitis (2.6%, placebo 2.2%)
Ocular: Conjunctivitis, visual disturbances, decreased visual acuity
Respiratory: Bronchitis, upper respiratory infections, sinusitis (7.2%, placebo 8.6%)

Mechanism of Action Produces vasodilation by directly relaxing arteriolar smooth muscle, with little effect on veins; effects may be mediated by cyclic AMP; stimulation of hair growth is secondary to vasodilation, increased cutaneous blood flow and stimulation of resting hair follicles

Drug Interactions

Increased Effect/Toxicity: Concurrent use of guanethidine can cause severe orthostasis; avoid concurrent use - discontinue 1-3 weeks prior to initiating minoxidil. Effects of other antihypertensives may be additive with minoxidil.

Pharmacodynamics/Kinetics

Onset of action: Hypotensive: Oral: ~30 minutes
Peak effect: 2-8 hours
Duration: 2-5 days
Protein binding: None
Metabolism: 88%, primarily via glucuronidation
Bioavailability: Oral: 90%
Half-life elimination: Adults: 3.5-4.2 hours
Excretion: Urine (12% as unchanged drug)

Pregnancy Risk Factor C

Mintezol® *see* Thiabendazole *on page 1286*
Miochol-E® *see* Acetylcholine *on page 61*
Miostat® *see* Carbachol *on page 255*
MiraLax™ *see* Polyethylene Glycol-Electrolyte Solution *on page 1100*
Mirapex® *see* Pramipexole *on page 1108*
Miraphen PSE *see* Guaifenesin and Pseudoephedrine *on page 675*
Mircette® *see* Ethinyl Estradiol and Desogestrel *on page 536*
Mirena® *see* Levonorgestrel *on page 815*

Mirtazapine (mir TAZ a peen)

U.S. Brand Names Remeron®; Remeron SolTab®
Canadian Brand Names Remeron®
Mexican Brand Names Remeron®
Generic Available Yes
Pharmacologic Category Antidepressant, Alpha-2 Antagonist
Use Treatment of depression

Local Anesthetic/Vasoconstrictor Precautions Although mirtazapine is not a tricyclic antidepressant, it does block norepinephrine reuptake within CNS synapses as part of its mechanisms. It has been suggested that vasoconstrictor be administered with caution and to monitor vital signs in dental patients taking antidepressants that affect norepinephrine in this way, including mirtazapine.

Effects on Dental Treatment Key adverse event(s) related to dental treatment: Significant xerostomia (normal salivary flow resumes upon discontinuation).

Common Adverse Effects

>10%:
Central nervous system: Somnolence (54%)
Endocrine & metabolic: Increased cholesterol
Gastrointestinal: Constipation (13%), xerostomia (25%), increased appetite (17%), weight gain (12%; weight gain of >7% reported in 8% of adults, ≤49% of pediatric patients)

1% to 10%:
Cardiovascular: Hypertension, vasodilatation, peripheral edema (2%), edema (1%)
Central nervous system: Dizziness (7%), abnormal dreams (4%), abnormal thoughts (3%), confusion (2%), malaise
Endocrine & metabolic: Increased triglycerides
Gastrointestinal: Vomiting, anorexia, abdominal pain
Genitourinary: Urinary frequency (2%)
Neuromuscular & skeletal: Myalgia (2%), back pain (2%), arthralgias, tremor (2%), weakness (8%)
Respiratory: Dyspnea (1%)
Miscellaneous: Flu-like symptoms (5%), thirst

Mechanism of Action Mirtazapine is a tetracyclic antidepressant that works by its central presynaptic $alpha_2$-adrenergic antagonist effects, which results in

(Continued)

Mirtazapine *(Continued)*

increased release of norepinephrine and serotonin. It is also a potent antagonist of 5-HT_2 and 5-HT_3 serotonin receptors and H1 histamine receptors and a moderate peripheral $alpha_1$-adrenergic and muscarinic antagonist; it does not inhibit the reuptake of norepinephrine or serotonin.

Drug Interactions

Cytochrome P450 Effect: Substrate of CYP1A2 (major), 2C8/9 (minor), 2D6 (major), 3A4 (major); **Inhibits** CYP1A2 (weak), 3A4 (weak)

Increased Effect/Toxicity: Contraindicated with drugs which inhibit MAO (including linezolid, selegiline, sibutramine, and MAOIs); severe/fatal reactions may occur. CYP1A2 inhibitors may increase the levels/effects of mirtazapine; example inhibitors include amiodarone, ciprofloxacin, fluvoxamine, ketoconazole, lomefloxacin, ofloxacin, and rofecoxib. CYP2D6 inhibitors may increase the levels/effects of mirtazapine; example inhibitors include chlorpromazine, delavirdine, fluoxetine, miconazole, paroxetine, pergolide, quinidine, quinine, ritonavir, and ropinirole. CYP3A4 inhibitors may increase the levels/effects of mirtazapine; example inhibitors include azole antifungals, ciprofloxacin, clarithromycin, diclofenac, doxycycline, erythromycin, imatinib, isoniazid, nefazodone, nicardipine, propofol, protease inhibitors, quinidine, and verapamil. Increased sedative effect seen with CNS depressants.

Decreased Effect: CYP1A2 inducers may decrease the levels/effects of mirtazapine; example inducers include aminoglutethimide, carbamazepine, phenobarbital, and rifampin. Decreased effect seen with clonidine. CYP3A4 inducers may decrease the levels/effects of mirtazapine; example inducers include aminoglutethimide, carbamazepine, nafcillin, nevirapine, phenobarbital, phenytoin, and rifamycins.

Pharmacodynamics/Kinetics

Protein binding: 85%

Metabolism: Extensively hepatic via CYP1A2, 2C9, 2D6, 3A4 and via demethylation and hydroxylation

Bioavailability: 50%

Half-life elimination: 20-40 hours; hampered with renal or hepatic impairment

Time to peak, serum: 2 hours

Excretion: Urine (75%) and feces (15%) as metabolites

Pregnancy Risk Factor C

Misoprostol (mye soe PROST ole)

U.S. Brand Names Cytotec®

Canadian Brand Names Apo-Misoprostol®; Cytotec®; Novo-Misoprostol

Mexican Brand Names Cytotec®

Generic Available Yes

Pharmacologic Category Prostaglandin

Use Prevention of NSAID-induced gastric ulcers; medical termination of pregnancy of ≤49 days (in conjunction with mifepristone)

Unlabeled/Investigational Use Cervical ripening and labor induction; NSAID-induced nephropathy; fat malabsorption in cystic fibrosis

Local Anesthetic/Vasoconstrictor Precautions No information available to require special precautions

Effects on Dental Treatment No significant effects or complications reported

Common Adverse Effects

>10%: Gastrointestinal: Diarrhea, abdominal pain

1% to 10%:

Central nervous system: Headache

Gastrointestinal: Constipation, flatulence, nausea, dyspepsia, vomiting

Mechanism of Action Misoprostol is a synthetic prostaglandin E_1 analog that replaces the protective prostaglandins consumed with prostaglandin-inhibiting therapies (eg, NSAIDs); has been shown to induce uterine contractions

Drug Interactions

Decreased Effect: Antacids may diminish absorption (not clinically significant)

Pharmacodynamics/Kinetics

Absorption: Rapid

Metabolism: Hepatic; rapidly de-esterified to misoprostol acid (active)

Half-life elimination: Metabolite: 20-40 minutes

Time to peak, serum: Active metabolite: Fasting: 15-30 minutes

Excretion: Urine (64% to 73%) and feces (15%) within 24 hours

Pregnancy Risk Factor X

Misoprostol and Diclofenac *see* Diclofenac and Misoprostol *on page 430*

Mitomycin (mye toe MYE sin)

U.S. Brand Names Mutamycin®

Canadian Brand Names Mutamycin®

Mexican Brand Names Mitocin®

Generic Available Yes

Synonyms Mitomycin-C; Mitomycin-X; MTC; NSC-26980

Pharmacologic Category Antineoplastic Agent, Antibiotic

Use Treatment of adenocarcinoma of stomach or pancreas, bladder cancer, breast cancer, or colorectal cancer

Unlabeled/Investigational Use Prevention of excess scarring in glaucoma filtration procedures in patients at high risk of bleb failure

Local Anesthetic/Vasoconstrictor Precautions No information available to require special precautions

Effects on Dental Treatment Key adverse event(s) related to dental treatment: Stomatitis.

Common Adverse Effects

>10%:

- Cardiovascular: Congestive heart failure (3% to 15%) (doses >30 mg/m^2)
- Central nervous system: Fever (14%)
- Dermatologic: Alopecia, nail banding/discoloration
- Gastrointestinal: Nausea, vomiting and anorexia (14%)
- Hematologic: Anemia (19% to 24%); myelosuppression, common, dose-limiting, delayed
  - Onset: 3 weeks
  - Nadir: 4-6 weeks
  - Recovery: 6-8 weeks

1% to 10%:

- Dermatologic: Rash
- Gastrointestinal: Stomatitis
- Neuromuscular: Paresthesias
- Renal: Creatinine increase (2%)
- Respiratory: Interstitial pneumonitis, infiltrates, dyspnea, cough (7%)

Mechanism of Action Acts like an alkylating agent and produces DNA cross-linking (primarily with guanine and cytosine pairs); cell-cycle nonspecific; inhibits DNA and RNA synthesis; degrades preformed DNA, causes nuclear lysis and formation of giant cells. While not phase-specific *per se*, mitomycin has its maximum effect against cells in late G and early S phases.

Drug Interactions

Increased Effect/Toxicity: *Vinca* alkaloids or doxorubicin may enhance cardiac toxicity when coadministered with mitomycin.

Pharmacodynamics/Kinetics

Distribution: V_d: 22 L/m^2; high drug concentrations found in kidney, tongue, muscle, heart, and lung tissue; probably not distributed into the CNS

Metabolism: Hepatic

Half-life elimination: 23-78 minutes; Terminal: 50 minutes

Excretion: Urine (<10% as unchanged drug), with elevated serum concentrations

Pregnancy Risk Factor D

Mitomycin-C *see* Mitomycin *on page 937*

Mitomycin-X *see* Mitomycin *on page 937*

Mitotane (MYE toe tane)

U.S. Brand Names Lysodren®

Canadian Brand Names Lysodren®

Generic Available No

Synonyms NSC-38721; o,p′-DDD

Pharmacologic Category Antineoplastic Agent, Miscellaneous

Use Treatment of adrenocortical carcinoma

Unlabeled/Investigational Use Treatment of Cushing's syndrome

Local Anesthetic/Vasoconstrictor Precautions No information available to require special precautions

Effects on Dental Treatment No significant effects or complications reported

Common Adverse Effects

>10%:

- Central nervous system: CNS depression (32%), dizziness (15%)
- Dermatologic: Skin rash (12%)
- Gastrointestinal: Anorexia (24%), nausea (39%), vomiting (37%), diarrhea (13%)
- Neuromuscular & skeletal: Weakness (12%)

(Continued)

Mitotane *(Continued)*

1% to 10%:

Central nervous system: Headache (5%), confusion (3%)

Neuromuscular & skeletal: Muscle tremor (3%)

Mechanism of Action Causes adrenal cortical atrophy; drug affects mitochondria in adrenal cortical cells and decreases production of cortisol; also alters the peripheral metabolism of steroids

Drug Interactions

Increased Effect/Toxicity: CNS depressants taken with mitotane may enhance CNS depression.

Decreased Effect: Mitotane may enhance the clearance of barbiturates and warfarin by induction of the hepatic microsomal enzyme system resulting in a decreased effect. Coadministration of spironolactone has resulted in negation of mitotane's effect. Mitotane may increase clearance of phenytoin by microsomal enzyme stimulation.

Pharmacodynamics/Kinetics

Absorption: Oral: ~35% to 40%

Distribution: Stored mainly in fat tissue but is found in all body tissues

Metabolism: Hepatic and other tissues

Half-life elimination: 18-159 days

Time to peak, serum: 3-5 hours

Excretion: Urine and feces (as metabolites)

Pregnancy Risk Factor C

Mitoxantrone (mye toe ZAN trone)

U.S. Brand Names Novantrone®

Canadian Brand Names Novantrone®

Mexican Brand Names Mitroxone® [inj.]; Novantrone®

Generic Available No

Synonyms DAD; DHAD; DHAQ; Dihydroxyanthracenedione Dihydrochloride; Mitoxantrone Hydrochloride CL-232315; Mitozantrone; NSC-301739

Pharmacologic Category Antineoplastic Agent, Anthracenedione

Use Treatment of acute leukemias, lymphoma, breast cancer, pediatric sarcoma, progressive or relapsing-remitting multiple sclerosis, prostate cancer

Local Anesthetic/Vasoconstrictor Precautions No information available to require special precautions

Effects on Dental Treatment Key adverse event(s) related to dental treatment: Mucositis and stomatitis.

Common Adverse Effects Reported with any indication; incidence varies based on treatment/dose

>10%:

Cardiovascular: Abnormal ECG, arrhythmia (3% to 18%), edema, nail bed changes

Central nervous system: Fatigue, fever, headache (6% to 13%)

Dermatologic: Alopecia (20% to 61%)

Endocrine & metabolic: Amenorrhea, menstrual disorder

Gastrointestinal: Abdominal pain, anorexia, nausea (29% to 76%), constipation, diarrhea (16% to 47%), GI bleeding, mucositis (10% to 29%), stomatitis, vomiting, weight gain/loss

Genitourinary: Abnormal urine, urinary tract infection

Hematologic: Decreased hemoglobin, leukopenia, lymphopenia, petechiae/bruising; myelosuppressive effects of chemotherapy:

WBC: Mild

Platelets: Mild

Onset: 7-10 days

Nadir: 14 days

Recovery: 21 days

Hepatic: Increased GGT

Neuromuscular & skeletal: Weakness (24%)

Respiratory: Cough, dyspnea, upper respiratory tract infection

Miscellaneous: Fungal infections, infection, sepsis

1% to 10%:

Cardiovascular: CHF (2% to 3%; risk is much lower with anthracyclines, some reports suggest cumulative doses >160 mg/mL cause CHF in ~10% of patients), ECG changes, hypotension, ischemia, LVEF decreased (≤5%)

Central nervous system: Chills, anxiety, depression, seizures

Dermatologic: Skin infection

Endocrine & metabolic: Hypocalcemia, hypokalemia, hyponatremia, hyperglycemia

Gastrointestinal: Dyspepsia, aphthosis

Genitourinary: Impotence, proteinuria, renal failure, sterility
Hematologic: Anemia, granulocytopenia, hemorrhage
Hepatic: Jaundice, increased SGOT, increased SGPT
Neuromuscular & skeletal: Back pain, myalgia, arthralgia
Ocular: Blurred vision, conjunctivitis
Renal: Hematuria
Respiratory: Pneumonia, rhinitis, sinusitis
Miscellaneous: Systemic infection, sweats, development of secondary leukemia

Mechanism of Action Analogue of the anthracyclines, mitoxantrone intercalates DNA; binds to nucleic acids and inhibits DNA and RNA synthesis by template disordering and steric obstruction; replication is decreased by binding to DNA topoisomerase II and seems to inhibit the incorporation of uridine into RNA and thymidine into DNA; active throughout entire cell cycle

Drug Interactions

Cytochrome P450 Effect: Inhibits CYP3A4 (weak)

Decreased Effect: Patients may experience impaired immune response to vaccines; possible infection after administration of live vaccines in patients receiving immunosuppressants.

Pharmacodynamics/Kinetics

Absorption: Oral: Poor
Distribution: V_d: 14 L/kg; distributes into pleural fluid, kidney, thyroid, liver, heart, and red blood cells
Protein binding: >95%, 76% to albumin
Metabolism: Hepatic; pathway not determined
Half-life elimination: Terminal: 23-215 hours; may be prolonged with hepatic impairment
Excretion: Urine (6% to 11%) and feces as unchanged drug and metabolites

Pregnancy Risk Factor D

Mitoxantrone Hydrochloride CL-232315 *see* Mitoxantrone *on page 938*
Mitozantrone *see* Mitoxantrone *on page 938*
Mitrazol™ [OTC] *see* Miconazole *on page 922*
MK383 *see* Tirofiban *on page 1304*
MK462 *see* Rizatriptan *on page 1193*
MK594 *see* Losartan *on page 845*
MK0826 *see* Ertapenem *on page 507*
MK 869 *see* Aprepitant *on page 138*
MLN341 *see* Bortezomib *on page 214*
MMF *see* Mycophenolate *on page 952*
MMR *see* Measles, Mumps, and Rubella Vaccines (Combined) *on page 858*
M-M-R® II *see* Measles, Mumps, and Rubella Vaccines (Combined) *on page 858*
Moban® *see* Molindone *on page 942*
MOBIC® *see* Meloxicam *on page 865*
Mobidin® [DSC] *see* Magnesium Salicylate *on page 854*
Mobisyl® [OTC] *see* Triethanolamine Salicylate *on page 1338*

Modafinil (moe DAF i nil)

U.S. Brand Names Provigil®

Canadian Brand Names Alertec®; Provigil®

Generic Available No

Pharmacologic Category Stimulant

Use Improve wakefulness in patients with excessive daytime sleepiness associated with narcolepsy and shift work sleep disorder (SWSD); adjunctive therapy for obstructive sleep apnea/hypopnea syndrome (OSAHS)

Unlabeled/Investigational Use Attention-deficit/hyperactivity disorder (ADHD); treatment of fatigue in MS and other disorders

Local Anesthetic/Vasoconstrictor Precautions No information available to require special precautions

Effects on Dental Treatment Key adverse event(s) related to dental treatment: Xerostomia (normal salivary flow resumes upon discontinuation), oral ulceration, and gingivitis.

Common Adverse Effects

>10%:

Central nervous system: Headache (34%, dose related)
Gastrointestinal: Nausea (11%)

1% to 10%:

Cardiovascular: Chest pain (3%), hypertension (3%), palpitation (2%), tachycardia (2%), vasodilation (2%), edema (1%)

(Continued)

Modafinil *(Continued)*

Central nervous system: Nervousness (7%), dizziness (5%), depression (2%), anxiety (5%, dose related), insomnia (5%), somnolence (2%), chills (1%), agitation (1%), confusion (1%), emotional lability (1%), vertigo (1%)
Gastrointestinal: Diarrhea (6%), dyspepsia (5%), xerostomia (4%), anorexia (4%), constipation (2%), flatulence (1%), mouth ulceration (1%), taste perversion (1%)
Genitourinary: Abnormal urine (1%), hematuria (1%), pyuria (1%)
Hematologic: Eosinophilia (1%)
Hepatic: Abnormal LFTs (2%)
Neuromuscular & skeletal: Back pain (6%), paresthesias (2%), dyskinesia (1%), hyperkinesia (1%), hypertonia (1%), neck rigidity (1%), tremor (1%)
Ocular: Amblyopia (1%), abnormal vision (1%), eye pain (1%)
Respiratory: Pharyngitis (4%), rhinitis (7%), lung disorder (2%), asthma (1%), epistaxis (1%)
Miscellaneous: Diaphoresis

Postmarketing and/or case reports: Agranulocytosis, mania, psychosis

Restrictions C-IV

Mechanism of Action The exact mechanism of action is unclear, it does not appear to alter the release of dopamine or norepinephrine, it may exert its stimulant effects by decreasing GABA-mediated neurotransmission, although this theory has not yet been fully evaluated; several studies also suggest that an intact central alpha-adrenergic system is required for modafinil's activity; the drug increases high-frequency alpha waves while decreasing both delta and theta wave activity, and these effects are consistent with generalized increases in mental alertness

Drug Interactions

Cytochrome P450 Effect: Substrate of CYP3A4 (major); **Inhibits** CYP1A2 (weak), 2A6 (weak), 2C8/9 (weak), 2C19 (strong), 2E1 (weak), 3A4 (weak); **Induces** CYP1A2 (weak), 2B6 (weak), 3A4 (weak)

Increased Effect/Toxicity: Modafinil may increase the levels/effects of citalopram, diazepam, methsuximide, phenytoin, propranolol, sertraline, or other CYP2C19 substrates. Modafinil may increase levels of warfarin. In populations deficient in the CYP2D6 isoenzyme, where CYP2C19 acts as a secondary metabolic pathway, concentrations of tricyclic antidepressants and selective serotonin reuptake inhibitors may be increased during coadministration. The levels/effects of modafinil may be increased by azole antifungals, ciprofloxacin, clarithromycin, diclofenac, doxycycline, erythromycin, imatinib, isoniazid, nefazodone, nicardipine, propofol, protease inhibitors, quinidine, telithromycin, verapamil, or other CYP3A4 inhibitors.

Decreased Effect: Modafinil may decrease serum concentrations of oral contraceptives, cyclosporine, and to a lesser degree, theophylline. The levels/effects of modafinil may be decreased by aminoglutethimide, carbamazepine, nafcillin, nevirapine, phenobarbital, phenytoin, rifamycins, and other CYP3A4 inducers. There is also evidence to suggest that modafinil may induce its own metabolism.

Pharmacodynamics/Kinetics Modafinil is a racemic compound (10% *d*-isomer and 90% *l*-isomer at steady state) whose enantiomers have different pharmacokinetics

Distribution: V_d: 0.9 L/kg
Protein binding: 60%, primarily to albumin
Metabolism: Hepatic; multiple pathways including CYP3A4
Half-life elimination: Effective half-life: 15 hours; Steady-state: 2-4 days
Time to peak, serum: 2-4 hours
Excretion: Urine (as metabolites, <10% as unchanged drug)

Pregnancy Risk Factor C

Modane® Bulk [OTC] *see* Psyllium *on page 1151*
Modane Tablets® [OTC] *see* Bisacodyl *on page 208*
Modicon® *see* Ethinyl Estradiol and Norethindrone *on page 550*
Modified Dakin's Solution *see* Sodium Hypochlorite Solution *on page 1228*
Modified Shohl's Solution *see* Sodium Citrate and Citric Acid *on page 1228*
Moducal® [OTC] *see* Glucose Polymers *on page 664*
Moduretic® [DSC] *see* Amiloride and Hydrochlorothiazide *on page 96*

Moexipril (mo EKS i pril)

Related Information

Cardiovascular Diseases *on page 1458*
Moexipril and Hydrochlorothiazide *on page 941*

U.S. Brand Names Univasc®

Generic Available No

Synonyms Moexipril Hydrochloride

Pharmacologic Category Angiotensin-Converting Enzyme (ACE) Inhibitor

Use Treatment of hypertension, alone or in combination with thiazide diuretics; treatment of left ventricular dysfunction after myocardial infarction

Local Anesthetic/Vasoconstrictor Precautions No information available to require special precautions

Effects on Dental Treatment No significant effects or complications reported

Common Adverse Effects 1% to 10%:

Cardiovascular: Hypotension, peripheral edema

Central nervous system: Headache, dizziness, fatigue

Dermatologic: Rash, alopecia, flushing, rash

Endocrine & metabolic: Hyperkalemia, hyponatremia

Gastrointestinal: Diarrhea, nausea, heartburn

Genitourinary: Polyuria

Neuromuscular & skeletal: Myalgia

Renal: Reversible increases in creatinine or BUN

Respiratory: Cough, pharyngitis, upper respiratory infection, sinusitis

Mechanism of Action Competitive inhibitor of angiotensin-converting enzyme (ACE); prevents conversion of angiotensin I to angiotensin II, a potent vasoconstrictor; results in lower levels of angiotensin II which causes an increase in plasma renin activity and a reduction in aldosterone secretion

Drug Interactions

Increased Effect/Toxicity: Potassium supplements, co-trimoxazole (high dose), angiotensin II receptor antagonists (eg, candesartan, losartan, irbesartan), or potassium-sparing diuretics (amiloride, spironolactone, triamterene) may result in elevated serum potassium levels when combined with moexipril. ACE inhibitor effects may be increased by probenecid (increases levels of captopril). ACE inhibitors may increase serum concentrations/effects of digoxin, lithium, and sulfonlyureas.

Diuretics have additive hypotensive effects with ACE inhibitors, and hypovolemia increases the potential for adverse renal effects of ACE inhibitors. In patients with compromised renal function, coadministration with NSAIDs may result in further deterioration of renal function. Allopurinol and ACE inhibitors may cause a higher risk of hypersensitivity reaction when taken concurrently.

Decreased Effect: Aspirin (high dose) may reduce the therapeutic effects of ACE inhibitors; at low dosages this does not appear to be significant. Rifampin may decrease the effect of ACE inhibitors. Antacids may decrease the bioavailability of ACE inhibitors (may be more likely to occur with captopril); separate administration times by 1-2 hours. NSAIDs, specifically indomethacin, may reduce the hypotensive effects of ACE inhibitors. More likely to occur in low renin or volume dependent hypertensive patients.

Pharmacodynamics/Kinetics

Onset of action: Peak effect: 1-2 hours

Duration: >24 hours

Distribution: V_d (moexiprilat): 180 L

Protein binding, plasma: Moexipril: 90%; Moexiprilat: 50% to 70%

Metabolism: Parent drug: Hepatic and via GI tract to moexiprilat, 1000 times more potent than parent

Bioavailability: Moexiprilat: 13%; reduced with food (AUC decreased by ~40%)

Half-life elimination: Moexipril: 1 hour; Moexiprilat: 2-9 hours

Time to peak: 1.5 hours

Excretion: Feces (50%)

Pregnancy Risk Factor C/D (2nd and 3rd trimesters)

Moexipril and Hydrochlorothiazide

(mo EKS i pril & hye droe klor oh THYE a zide)

Related Information

Hydrochlorothiazide *on page 699*

Moexipril *on page 940*

U.S. Brand Names Uniretic®

Canadian Brand Names Uniretic™

Generic Available No

Synonyms Hydrochlorothiazide and Moexipril

Pharmacologic Category Antihypertensive Agent, Combination

Use Combination therapy for hypertension, however, not indicated for initial treatment of hypertension; replacement therapy in patients receiving separate dosage forms (for patient convenience); when monotherapy with one component fails to achieve desired antihypertensive effect, or when dose-limiting adverse effects limit upward titration of monotherapy

(Continued)

Moexipril and Hydrochlorothiazide *(Continued)*

Local Anesthetic/Vasoconstrictor Precautions No information available to require special precautions

Effects on Dental Treatment No significant effects or complications reported

Common Adverse Effects See individual agents.

Mechanism of Action See individual agents.

Drug Interactions

Increased Effect/Toxicity: See individual agents.

Decreased Effect: See individual agents.

Pharmacodynamics/Kinetics See individual agents.

Pregnancy Risk Factor C/D (2nd and 3rd trimesters)

Moexipril Hydrochloride *see* Moexipril *on page 940*
Moi-Stir® [OTC] *see* Saliva Substitute *on page 1205*
Moisture® Eyes [OTC] *see* Artificial Tears *on page 148*
Moisture® Eyes PM [OTC] *see* Artificial Tears *on page 148*

Molindone (moe LIN done)

U.S. Brand Names Moban®

Canadian Brand Names Moban®

Generic Available No

Synonyms Molindone Hydrochloride

Pharmacologic Category Antipsychotic Agent, Dihydroindoline

Use Management of schizophrenia

Unlabeled/Investigational Use Management of psychotic disorders

Local Anesthetic/Vasoconstrictor Precautions No information available to require special precautions

Effects on Dental Treatment Key adverse event(s) related to dental treatment: Xerostomia and changes in salivation (normal salivary flow resumes upon discontinuation). Anticholinergic side effects can cause a reduction of saliva production or secretion, contributing to discomfort and dental disease (ie, caries, oral candidiasis, and periodontal disease). Molindone can cause extrapyramidal reactions which may appear as muscle twitching or increased motor activity of the face, neck, or head.

Common Adverse Effects Frequency not defined.

Cardiovascular: Orthostatic hypotension, tachycardia, arrhythmias

Central nervous system: Extrapyramidal reactions (akathisia, pseudoparkinsonism, dystonia, tardive dyskinesia), mental depression, altered central temperature regulation, sedation, drowsiness, restlessness, anxiety, hyperactivity, euphoria, seizures, neuroleptic malignant syndrome (NMS)

Dermatologic: Pruritus, rash, photosensitivity

Endocrine & metabolic: Change in menstrual periods, edema of breasts, amenorrhea, galactorrhea, gynecomastia

Gastrointestinal: Constipation, xerostomia, nausea, salivation, weight gain (minimal compared to other antipsychotics), weight loss

Genitourinary: Urinary retention, priapism

Hematologic: Leukopenia, leukocytosis

Ocular: Blurred vision, retinal pigmentation

Miscellaneous: Diaphoresis (decreased)

Mechanism of Action Mechanism of action mimics that of chlorpromazine; however, it produces more extrapyramidal symptoms and less sedation than chlorpromazine

Drug Interactions

Increased Effect/Toxicity: Molindone concentrations may be increased by chloroquine, propranolol, sulfadoxine-pyrimethamine. Molindone may increase the effect and/or toxicity of antihypertensives, lithium, TCAs, CNS depressants (ethanol, narcotics), and trazodone. Metoclopramide may increase risk of extrapyramidal symptoms (EPS).

Decreased Effect: Antipsychotics inhibit the activity of bromocriptine and levodopa. Benztropine (and other anticholinergics) may inhibit the therapeutic response to molindone and excess anticholinergic effects may occur. Barbiturates and cigarette smoking may enhance the hepatic metabolism of molindone. Molindone and possibly other low potency antipsychotic may reverse the pressor effects of epinephrine.

Pharmacodynamics/Kinetics

Metabolism: Hepatic

Half-life elimination: 1.5 hours

Time to peak, serum: ~1.5 hours

Excretion: Urine and feces (90%) within 24 hours

Pregnancy Risk Factor C

Molindone Hydrochloride *see* Molindone *on page 942*
Molybdenum *see* Trace Metals *on page 1319*
Molypen® *see* Trace Metals *on page 1319*
MOM *see* Magnesium Hydroxide *on page 853*
Momentum® [OTC] *see* Magnesium Salicylate *on page 854*

Mometasone Furoate (moe MET a sone FYOOR oh ate)

Related Information

Respiratory Diseases *on page 1478*

U.S. Brand Names Elocon®; Nasonex®

Canadian Brand Names Elocom®; Nasonex®

Generic Available Yes: Ointment

Pharmacologic Category Corticosteroid, Nasal; Corticosteroid, Topical

Use Relief of the inflammatory and pruritic manifestations of corticosteroid-responsive dermatoses (medium potency topical corticosteroid); treatment of nasal symptoms of seasonal and perennial allergic rhinitis in adults and children ≥2 years of age; prevention of nasal symptoms associated with seasonal allergic rhinitis in children ≥12 years of age and adults

Local Anesthetic/Vasoconstrictor Precautions No information available to require special precautions

Effects on Dental Treatment No significant effects or complications reported

Common Adverse Effects

Nasal:

>10%:

Central nervous system: Headache (17% to 26%)

Respiratory: Pharyngitis (10% to 12%), cough (7% to 13%), epistaxis (8% to 11%)

Miscellaneous: Viral infection (8% to 14%)

1% to 10%:

Cardiovascular: Chest pain

Endocrine & metabolic: Dysmenorrhea (1% to 5%)

Gastrointestinal: Vomiting (1% to 5%), diarrhea, dyspepsia, nausea

Neuromuscular & skeletal: Musculoskeletal pain (1% to 5%), arthralgia, myalgia

Ocular: Conjunctivitis

Otic: Earache, otitis media

Respiratory: Upper respiratory tract infection (5% to 6%), sinusitis (4% to 5%), asthma, bronchitis, nasal irritation, rhinitis, wheezing

Miscellaneous: Flu-like symptoms

Topical:

1% to 10%: Dermatologic: Bacterial skin infection, burning, furunculosis, pruritus, skin atrophy, tingling/stinging

Cataract formation, reduction in growth velocity, and HPA axis suppression have been reported with other corticosteroids

Dosage

Nasal spray:

Children 2-11 years: 1 spray (50 mcg) in each nostril daily

Children ≥12 years and Adults: 2 sprays (100 mcg) in each nostril daily; when used for the prevention of allergic rhinitis, treatment should begin 2-4 weeks prior to pollen season

Topical: Apply sparingly, do not use occlusive dressings. Therapy should be discontinued when control is achieved; if no improvement is seen in 2 weeks, reassessment of diagnosis may be necessary.

Cream, ointment: Children ≥2 years and Adults: Apply a thin film to affected area once daily; do not use in pediatric patients for longer than 3 weeks

Lotion: Children ≥12 years and Adults: Apply a few drops to affected area once daily

Mechanism of Action May depress the formation, release, and activity of endogenous chemical mediators of inflammation (kinins, histamine, liposomal enzymes, prostaglandins). Leukocytes and macrophages may have to be present for the initiation of responses mediated by the above substances. Inhibits the margination and subsequent cell migration to the area of injury, and also reverses the dilatation and increased vessel permeability in the area resulting in decreased access of cells to the sites of injury.

Contraindications Hypersensitivity to mometasone or any component of the formulation; fungal, viral, or tubercular skin lesions, herpes simplex or zoster

Warnings/Precautions

Nasal: Use caution if replacing systemic corticosteroid with nasal; may cause symptoms of withdrawal or acute adrenal insufficiency May cause suppression of hypothalamic-pituitary-adrenal (HPA) axis, particularly in younger

(Continued)

Mometasone Furoate *(Continued)*

children or in patients receiving high doses for prolonged periods. Controlled clinical studies have shown that intranasal corticosteroids may cause a reduction in growth velocity in pediatric patients; titrate to the lowest effective dose. May suppress the immune system, patients may be more susceptible to infection. Use with caution, if at all, in patients with systemic infections, active or quiescent tuberculosis infection, or ocular herpes simplex. Avoid exposure to chickenpox and measles.

Topical: May cause suppression of HPA axis, especially when used on large areas of the body, denuded areas, for prolonged periods of time or with an occlusive dressing. Pediatric patients may be more susceptible to systemic toxicity.

Drug Interactions

Cytochrome P450 Effect: Substrate of CYP3A4 (minor)

Pharmacodynamics/Kinetics

Absorption:

Nasal: Mometasone furoate monohydrate: Undetectable in plasma

Ointment: 0.7%; increased by occlusive dressings

Protein binding: Mometasone furoate: 98% to 99%

Metabolism: Mometasone furoate: Hepatic via CYP3A4; forms metabolite

Half-life elimination: I.V.: 5.8 hours

Excretion: Bile, urine

Pregnancy Risk Factor C

Dosage Forms CRM, topical (Elocon®): 0.1% (15 g, 45 g). **LOTION, topical** (Elocon®): 0.1% (30 mL, 60 mL). **OINT, topical** (Elocon®): 0.1% (15 g, 45 g). **SUSP, intranasal spray** (Nasonex®): 50 mcg/spray (17 g)

MOM/Mineral Oil Emulsion *see* Magnesium Hydroxide and Mineral Oil *on page 853*

Monacolin K *see* Lovastatin *on page 848*

Monarc® M *see* Antihemophilic Factor (Human) *on page 134*

Monistat® 1 Combination Pack [OTC] *see* Miconazole *on page 922*

Monistat® 3 [OTC] *see* Miconazole *on page 922*

Monistat® 7 [OTC] *see* Miconazole *on page 922*

Monistat-Derm® *see* Miconazole *on page 922*

Monobenzone (mon oh BEN zone)

U.S. Brand Names Benoquin®

Generic Available No

Pharmacologic Category Topical Skin Product

Use Final depigmentation in extensive vitiligo

Local Anesthetic/Vasoconstrictor Precautions No information available to require special precautions

Effects on Dental Treatment No significant effects or complications reported

Common Adverse Effects 1% to 10%: Irritation, burning sensation, dermatitis

Pregnancy Risk Factor C

Monoclate-P® *see* Antihemophilic Factor (Human) *on page 134*

Monoclonal Antibody *see* Muromonab-CD3 *on page 952*

Monodox® *see* Doxycycline *on page 471*

Monoethanolamine *see* Ethanolamine Oleate *on page 535*

Mono-Gesic® *see* Salsalate *on page 1207*

Monoket® *see* Isosorbide Mononitrate *on page 771*

MonoNessa™ *see* Ethinyl Estradiol and Norgestimate *on page 554*

Mononine® *see* Factor IX *on page 571*

Monopril® *see* Fosinopril *on page 633*

Monopril-HCT® *see* Fosinopril and Hydrochlorothiazide *on page 635*

Montelukast (mon te LOO kast)

Related Information

Respiratory Diseases *on page 1478*

U.S. Brand Names Singulair®

Canadian Brand Names Singulair®

Mexican Brand Names Singulair®

Generic Available No

Synonyms Montelukast Sodium

Pharmacologic Category Leukotriene-Receptor Antagonist

Use Prophylaxis and chronic treatment of asthma in adults and children ≥1 year of age; relief of symptoms of seasonal allergic rhinitis in adults and children ≥2 years of age

Local Anesthetic/Vasoconstrictor Precautions No information available to require special precautions

Effects on Dental Treatment No significant effects or complications reported

Common Adverse Effects (As reported in adults with asthma)

>10%: Central nervous system: Headache (18%)

1% to 10%:

Central nervous system: Dizziness (2%), fatigue (2%), fever (2%)

Dermatologic: Rash (2%)

Gastrointestinal: Dyspepsia (2%), dental pain (2%), gastroenteritis (2%), abdominal pain (3%)

Neuromuscular & skeletal: Weakness (2%)

Respiratory: Cough (3%), nasal congestion (2%)

Miscellaneous: Flu-like symptoms (4%), trauma (1%)

Dosage Oral:

Children:

<1 year: Safety and efficacy have not been established

12-23 months: Asthma: 4 mg (oral granules) once daily, taken in the evening

2-5 years: Asthma or seasonal allergic rhinitis: 4 mg (chewable tablet or oral granules) once daily, taken in the evening

6-14 years: Asthma or seasonal allergic rhinitis: Chew one 5 mg chewable tablet/day, taken in the evening

Children ≥15 years and Adults: Asthma or seasonal allergic rhinitis: 10 mg/day, taken in the evening

Dosing adjustment in hepatic impairment: Mild to moderate: No adjustment necessary

Mechanism of Action Selective leukotriene receptor antagonist that inhibits the cysteinyl leukotriene receptor. Cysteinyl leukotrienes and leukotriene receptor occupation have been correlated with the pathophysiology of asthma, including airway edema, smooth muscle contraction, and altered cellular activity associated with the inflammatory process, which contribute to the signs and symptoms of asthma.

Contraindications Hypersensitivity to montelukast or any component of the formulation

Warnings/Precautions Montelukast is not indicated for use in the reversal of bronchospasm in acute asthma attacks, including status asthmaticus. Should not be used as monotherapy for the treatment and management of exercise-induced bronchospasm. Advise patients to have appropriate rescue medication available. Appropriate clinical monitoring and caution are recommended when systemic corticosteroid reduction is considered in patients receiving montelukast. Inform phenylketonuric patients that the chewable tablet contains phenylalanine. Safety and efficacy in children <1 year of age have not been established.

In rare cases, patients on therapy with montelukast may present with systemic eosinophilia, sometimes presenting with clinical features of vasculitis consistent with Churg-Strauss syndrome, a condition which is often treated with systemic corticosteroid therapy. Healthcare providers should be alert to eosinophilia, vasculitic rash, worsening pulmonary symptoms, cardiac complications, and/or neuropathy presenting in their patients. A causal association between montelukast and these underlying conditions has not been established.

Drug Interactions

Cytochrome P450 Effect: Substrate (major) of CYP2C8/9, 3A4; **Inhibits** CYP2C8/9 (weak)

Decreased Effect: CYP2C8/9 inducers may decrease the levels/effects of montelukast; example inducers include carbamazepine, phenobarbital, phenytoin, rifampin, rifapentine, and secobarbital. CYP3A4 inducers may decrease the levels/effects of montelukast; example inducers include aminoglutethimide, carbamazepine, nafcillin, nevirapine, phenobarbital, phenytoin, and rifamycins.

Ethanol/Nutrition/Herb Interactions Herb/Nutraceutical: St John's wort may decrease montelukast levels.

Dietary Considerations Tablet, chewable: 4 mg strength contains phenylalanine 0.674 mg; 5 mg strength contains phenylalanine 0.842 mg

Pharmacodynamics/Kinetics

Duration: >24 hours

Absorption: Rapid

Distribution: V_d: 8-11 L

Protein binding, plasma: >99%

(Continued)

Montelukast *(Continued)*

Metabolism: Extensively hepatic via CYP3A4 and 2C8/9
Bioavailability: Tablet: 10 mg: Mean: 64%; 5 mg: 63% to 73%
Half-life elimination, plasma: Mean: 2.7-5.5 hours
Time to peak, serum: Tablet: 10 mg: 3-4 hours; 5 mg: 2-2.5 hours; 4 mg: 2 hours
Excretion: Feces (86%); urine (<0.2%)

Pregnancy Risk Factor B

Dosage Forms GRAN: 4 mg/packet. **TAB:** 10 mg. **TAB, chewable:** 4 mg, 5 mg

Montelukast Sodium *see* Montelukast *on page 944*
Monurol™ *see* Fosfomycin *on page 632*
8-MOP® *see* Methoxsalen *on page 902*
More Attenuated Enders Strain *see* Measles Virus Vaccine (Live) *on page 858*
MoreDophilus® [OTC] *see Lactobacillus on page 793*

Moricizine (mor I siz een)

Related Information
Cardiovascular Diseases *on page 1458*

U.S. Brand Names Ethmozine®

Canadian Brand Names Ethmozine®

Generic Available No

Synonyms Moricizine Hydrochloride

Pharmacologic Category Antiarrhythmic Agent, Class I

Use Treatment of ventricular tachycardia and life-threatening ventricular arrhythmias

Unlabeled/Investigational Use PVCs, complete and nonsustained ventricular tachycardia, atrial arrhythmias

Local Anesthetic/Vasoconstrictor Precautions No information available to require special precautions

Effects on Dental Treatment No significant effects or complications reported

Common Adverse Effects
>10%: Central nervous system: Dizziness
1% to 10%:
Cardiovascular: Proarrhythmia, palpitations, cardiac death, ECG abnormalities, CHF
Central nervous system: Headache, fatigue, insomnia
Endocrine & metabolic: Decreased libido
Gastrointestinal: Nausea, diarrhea, ileus
Ocular: Blurred vision, periorbital edema
Respiratory: Dyspnea

Mechanism of Action Class I antiarrhythmic agent; reduces the fast inward current carried by sodium ions, shortens Phase I and Phase II repolarization, resulting in decreased action potential duration and effective refractory period

Drug Interactions

Cytochrome P450 Effect: Substrate of CYP3A4 (major); **Induces** CYP1A2 (weak), 3A4 (weak)

Increased Effect/Toxicity: CYP3A4 inhibitors may increase the levels/effects of moricizine; example inhibitors include azole antifungals, ciprofloxacin, clarithromycin, diclofenac, doxycycline, erythromycin, imatinib, isoniazid, nefazodone, nicardipine, propofol, protease inhibitors, quinidine, and verapamil. Moricizine levels may be increased by cimetidine and diltiazem. Digoxin may result in additive prolongation of the PR interval when combined with moricizine (but not rate of second- and third-degree AV block). Drugs which may prolong QT interval (including cisapride, erythromycin, phenothiazines, cyclic antidepressants, and some quinolones) are contraindicated with type Ia antiarrhythmics. Moricizine has some type Ia activity, and caution should be used.

Decreased Effect: Moricizine may decrease levels of theophylline (50%) and diltiazem. CYP3A4 inducers may decrease the levels/effects of moricizine; example inducers include aminoglutethimide, carbamazepine, nafcillin, nevirapine, phenobarbital, phenytoin, and rifamycins.

Pharmacodynamics/Kinetics
Protein binding, plasma: 95%
Metabolism: Significant first-pass effect; some enterohepatic recycling
Bioavailability: 38%
Half-life elimination: Healthy volunteers: 3-4 hours; Cardiac disease: 6-13 hours
Excretion: Feces (56%); urine (39%)

Pregnancy Risk Factor B

Moricizine Hydrochloride *see* Moricizine *on page 946*

Morning After Pill *see* Ethinyl Estradiol and Norgestrel *on page 557*

Morphine Sulfate (MOR feen SUL fate)

Related Information

Dental Office Emergencies *on page 1584*

Oxymorphone *on page 1036*

U.S. Brand Names Astramorph/PF™; Avinza™; DepoDur™; Duramorph®; Infumorph®; Kadian®; MS Contin®; MSIR®; Oramorph SR®; RMS®; Roxanol®; Roxanol 100®; Roxanol®-T

Canadian Brand Names Kadian®; M-Eslon®; Morphine HP®; Morphine LP® Epidural; M.O.S.-Sulfate®; MS Contin®; MS-IR®; PMS-Morphine Sulfate SR; ratio-Morphine SR; Statex®

Mexican Brand Names Analfin®; Duralmor L.P.®; Graten® [inj.]; Kapanol®; MST Continus®

Generic Available Yes: Excludes capsule, controlled release tablet, sustained release tablet, extended release liposomal suspension for injection

Pharmacologic Category Analgesic, Narcotic

Use Relief of moderate to severe acute and chronic pain; relief of pain of myocardial infarction; relief of dyspnea of acute left ventricular failure and pulmonary edema; preanesthetic medication

DepoDur™: Epidural (lumbar) single-dose management of surgical pain

Orphan drug: Infumorph™: Used in microinfusion devices for intraspinal administration in treatment of intractable chronic pain

Local Anesthetic/Vasoconstrictor Precautions No information available to require special precautions

Effects on Dental Treatment Key adverse event(s) related to dental treatment: Xerostomia (normal salivary flow resumes upon discontinuation). Anticholinergic side effects can cause a reduction of saliva production or secretion, contributing to discomfort and dental disease (ie, caries, oral candidiasis, and periodontal disease).

Common Adverse Effects Note: Percentages are based on a study in 19 chronic cancer pain patients (*J Pain Symptom Manage*, 1995, 10:416-22). Chronic use of various opioids in cancer pain is accompanied by similar adverse reactions; individual patient differences are unpredictable, and percentage may differ in acute pain (surgical) treatment.

Frequency not defined: Flushing, CNS depression, sedation, antidiuretic hormone release, physical and psychological dependence, diaphoresis

>10%:

- Cardiovascular: Palpitations, hypotension, bradycardia
- Central nervous system: Drowsiness (48%, tolerance usually develops to drowsiness with regular dosing for 1-2 weeks); dizziness (20%); confusion
- Dermatologic: Pruritus (may be secondary to histamine release)
- Gastrointestinal: Nausea (28%, tolerance usually develops to nausea and vomiting with chronic use); vomiting (9%); constipation (40%, tolerance develops very slowly if at all); xerostomia (78%)
- Genitourinary: Urinary retention (16%)
- Local: Pain at injection site
- Neuromuscular & skeletal: Weakness
- Miscellaneous: Histamine release

1% to 10%:

- Central nervous system: Restlessness, headache, false feeling of well being
- Gastrointestinal: Anorexia, GI irritation, paralytic ileus
- Genitourinary: Decreased urination
- Neuromuscular & skeletal: Trembling
- Ocular: Vision problems
- Respiratory: Respiratory depression, dyspnea

Restrictions C-II

Mechanism of Action Binds to opiate receptors in the CNS, causing inhibition of ascending pain pathways, altering the perception of and response to pain; produces generalized CNS depression

Drug Interactions

Cytochrome P450 Effect: Substrate of CYP2D6 (minor)

Increased Effect/Toxicity: CNS depressants (phenothiazines, tranquilizers, anxiolytics, sedatives, hypnotics, or alcohol), tricyclic antidepressants may potentiate the effects of morphine and other opiate agonists. Dextroamphetamine may enhance the analgesic effect of morphine and other opiate agonists. Concurrent use of MAO inhibitors and meperidine has been associated

(Continued)

Morphine Sulfate *(Continued)*

with significant adverse effects. Use caution with morphine. Some manufacturers recommend avoiding use within 14 days of MAO inhibitors.

Decreased Effect: Diuretic effects may be decreased (due to antidiuretic hormone release).

Pharmacodynamics/Kinetics

Onset of action: Oral: 1 hour; I.V.: 5-10 minutes

Duration: Pain relief (immediate release forms): 4 hours

Absorption: Variable

Distribution: Binds to opioid receptors in the CNS and periphery (eg, GI tract)

Metabolism: Hepatic via conjugation with glucuronic acid to morphine-3-glucuronide (inactive), morphine-6-glucuronide (active), and in lesser amounts, morphine-3-6-diglucuronide; other minor metabolites include normorphine (active) and the 3-ethereal sulfate

Bioavailability: Oral: 17% to 33% (first-pass effect limits oral bioavailability; oral:parenteral effectiveness reportedly varies from 1:6 in opioid naive patients to 1:3 with chronic use)

Half-life elimination: Adults: 2-4 hours (immediate release forms)

Excretion: Urine (primarily as morphine-3-glucuronide, ~2% to 12% excreted unchanged); feces (~7% to 10%). It has been suggested that accumulation of morphine-6-glucuronide might cause toxicity with renal insufficiency. All of the metabolites (ie, morphine-3-glucuronide, morphine-6-glucuronide, and normorphine) have been suggested as possible causes of neurotoxicity (eg, myoclonus).

Pregnancy Risk Factor C/D (prolonged use or high doses at term)

Morrhuate Sodium (MOR yoo ate SOW dee um)

U.S. Brand Names Scleromate™

Generic Available No

Pharmacologic Category Sclerosing Agent

Use Treatment of small, uncomplicated varicose veins of the lower extremities

Local Anesthetic/Vasoconstrictor Precautions No information available to require special precautions

Effects on Dental Treatment No significant effects or complications reported

Mechanism of Action Both varicose veins and esophageal varices are treated by the thrombotic action of morrhuate sodium. By causing inflammation of the vein's intima, a thrombus is formed. Occlusion secondary to the fibrous tissue and the thrombus results in the obliteration of the vein.

Pregnancy Risk Factor C

Mosco® Corn and Callus Remover [OTC] *see* Salicylic Acid *on page 1205*

Motofen® *see* Difenoxin and Atropine *on page 434*

Motrin® *see* Ibuprofen *on page 728*

Motrin® Children's [OTC] *see* Ibuprofen *on page 728*

Motrin® Cold and Sinus [OTC] *see* Pseudoephedrine and Ibuprofen *on page 1149*

Motrin® Cold, Children's [OTC] *see* Pseudoephedrine and Ibuprofen *on page 1149*

Motrin® IB [OTC] *see* Ibuprofen *on page 728*

Motrin® Infants' [OTC] *see* Ibuprofen *on page 728*

Motrin® Junior Strength [OTC] *see* Ibuprofen *on page 728*

Motrin® Migraine Pain [OTC] *see* Ibuprofen *on page 728*

Mouthkote® [OTC] *see* Saliva Substitute *on page 1205*

Mouth Pain, Cold Sore, and Canker Sore Products *see page 1633*

Mouthwash (Antiseptic) (MOUTH wosh)

Related Information

Antiplaque Agents *on page 1556*

Dentin Hypersensitivity, High Caries Index, and Xerostomia *on page 1555*

Oral Bacterial Infections *on page 1533*

Oral Nonviral Soft Tissue Ulcerations or Erosions *on page 1551*

Oral Rinse Products *on page 1638*

Periodontal Diseases *on page 1542*

Synonyms Antiseptic Mouthwash

Pharmacologic Category Antimicrobial Mouth Rinse; Antiplaque Agent; Mouthwash

Dental Use Aid in prevention and reduction of plaque and gingivitis; halitosis

Local Anesthetic/Vasoconstrictor Precautions No information available to require special precautions

Effects on Dental Treatment No significant effects or complications reported

Significant Adverse Effects No data reported

Dosage Rinse full strength for 30 seconds with 20 mL (2/3 fluid ounce or 4 teaspoonfuls) morning and night

Contraindications Hypersensitivity to any component of the formulation

Dosage Forms Rinse: 250 mL, 500 mL, 1000 mL

Comments Active ingredients:

Listerine® Antiseptic: Thymol 0.064%, eucalyptus 0.092%, methyl salicylate 0.060%, menthol 0.042%, alcohol 26.9%, water, benzoic acid, poloxamer 407, sodium benzoate, caramel

Fresh Burst Listerine® Antiseptic: Thymol 0.064%, eucalyptus 0.092%, methyl salicylate 0.060%, menthol 0.042%, alcohol 26.9%, water, benzoic acid, poloxamer 407, sodium benzoate, flavoring, sodium, saccharin, sodium citrate, citric acid, D&C yellow #10, FD&C green #3

Cool Mint Listerine® Antiseptic: Thymol 0.064%, eucalyptus 0.092%, methyl salicylate 0.060%, menthol 0.042%, alcohol 26.9%, water, benzoic acid, poloxamer 407, sodium benzoate, flavoring, sodium, saccharin, sodium citrate, citric acid, FD&C green #3

The following information is endorsed on the label of the Listerine® products by the Council on Scientific Affairs, American Dental Association: "Listerine® Antiseptic has been shown to help prevent and reduce supragingival plaque accumulation and gingivitis when used in a conscientiously applied program of oral hygiene and regular professional care. Its effect on periodontitis has not been determined."

Moxifloxacin (moxs i FLOKS a sin)

Related Information

Oral Bacterial Infections *on page 1533*

Respiratory Diseases *on page 1478*

U.S. Brand Names Avelox®; Avelox® I.V.; Vigamox™

Canadian Brand Names Avelox®

Generic Available No

Synonyms Moxifloxacin Hydrochloride

Pharmacologic Category Antibiotic, Ophthalmic; Antibiotic, Quinolone

Use Treatment of mild-to-moderate community-acquired pneumonia, including multidrug-resistant *Streptococcus pneumoniae* (MDRSP); acute bacterial exacerbation of chronic bronchitis; acute bacterial sinusitis; uncomplicated skin infections; bacterial conjunctivitis (ophthalmic formulation)

Local Anesthetic/Vasoconstrictor Precautions No information available to require special precautions

Effects on Dental Treatment No significant effects or complications reported

Common Adverse Effects

Systemic:

3% to 10%:

Central nervous system: Dizziness (3%)

Gastrointestinal: Nausea (7%), diarrhea (6%)

0.1% to 3%:

Cardiovascular: Chest pain, hypertension, palpitation, peripheral edema, QT prolongation, tachycardia

Central nervous system: Anxiety, chills, confusion, headache, insomnia, nervousness, pain, somnolence, tremor, vertigo

Dermatologic: Dry skin, pruritus, rash (maculopapular, purpuric, pustular)

Endocrine & metabolic: Serum chloride increased (≥2%), serum ionized calcium increased (≥2%), serum glucose decreased (≥2%)

Gastrointestinal: Abdominal pain, amylase increased, amylase decreased (≥2%), anorexia, constipation, dry mouth, dyspepsia, flatulence, glossitis, lactic dehydrogenase increased, stomatitis, taste perversion, vomiting

Hematologic: Eosinophilia, leukopenia, prothrombin time prolonged, increased INR, thrombocythemia, thrombocytopenia

Increased serum levels of the following (≥2%): MCH, neutrophils, WBC

Decreased serum levels of the following (≥2%): Basophils, eosinophils, hemoglobin, RBC, neutrophils

Hepatic: Bilirubin decreased (≥2%), cholestatic jaundice, GGTP increased, liver function test abnormal

Local: Injection site reaction

Neuromuscular & skeletal: Arthralgia, back pain, leg pain, myalgia, paresthesia, malaise, weakness

Renal: Serum albumin increased (≥2%)

Respiratory: Dyspnea, pharyngitis, pneumonia, rhinitis, sinusitis, PO_2 increased (≥2%)

Miscellaneous: Allergic reaction, infection, moniliasis, diaphoresis

(Continued)

Moxifloxacin *(Continued)*

Additional reactions with **ophthalmic** preparation: 1% to 6%: Conjunctivitis, dry eye, ocular discomfort, ocular hyperemia, ocular pain, ocular pruritus, subconjunctival hemorrhage, tearing, visual acuity decreased

Mechanism of Action Moxifloxacin is a DNA gyrase inhibitor, and also inhibits topoisomerase IV. DNA gyrase (topoisomerase II) is an essential bacterial enzyme that maintains the superhelical structure of DNA. DNA gyrase is required for DNA replication and transcription, DNA repair, recombination, and transposition; inhibition is bactericidal.

Drug Interactions

Increased Effect/Toxicity: Drugs which prolong QT interval (including Class Ia and Class III antiarrhythmics, erythromycin, cisapride, antipsychotics, and cyclic antidepressants) are contraindicated with moxifloxacin. Cimetidine and probenecid increase quinolone levels. An increased incidence of seizures may occur with foscarnet or NSAIDs. Serum levels of some quinolones are increased by loop diuretic administration. Digoxin levels may be increased in some patients by quinolones. The hypoprothrombinemic effect of warfarin is enhanced by some quinolone antibiotics. Although moxifloxacin has not been shown to alter warfarin disposition, monitoring of the INR during concurrent therapy is recommended by the manufacturer. Concurrent use of corticosteroids may increase risk of tendon rupture.

Decreased Effect: Metal cations (magnesium, aluminum, iron, and zinc) bind quinolones in the gastrointestinal tract and inhibit absorption (by up to 98%). Antacids, multivitamins with minerals, sucralfate, and some didanosine formulations should be avoided. Moxifloxacin should be administered 4 hours before or 8 hours (a minimum of 2 hours before and 2 hours after) after these agents. Antineoplastic agents may decrease the absorption of quinolones.

Pharmacodynamics/Kinetics

Absorption: Well absorbed; not affected by high fat meal or yogurt

Distribution: V_d: 1.7 to 2.7 L/kg; tissue concentrations often exceed plasma concentrations in respiratory tissues, alveolar macrophages, and sinus tissues

Protein binding: 50%

Metabolism: Hepatic (52% of dose) via glucuronide (14%) and sulfate (38%) conjugation

Bioavailability: 90%

Half-life elimination: Oral: 12 hours; I.V.: 15 hours

Excretion: Approximately 45% of a dose is excreted in feces (25%) and urine (20%) as unchanged drug

Metabolites: Sulfate conjugates in feces, glucuronide conjugates in urine

Pregnancy Risk Factor C

Moxifloxacin Hydrochloride *see* Moxifloxacin *on page 949*

Moxilin® *see* Amoxicillin *on page 114*

4-MP *see* Fomepizole *on page 627*

6-MP *see* Mercaptopurine *on page 880*

MPA *see* Mycophenolate *on page 952*

MPA and Estrogens (Conjugated) *see* Estrogens (Conjugated/Equine) and Medroxyprogesterone *on page 528*

MS Contin® *see* Morphine Sulfate *on page 947*

MSIR® *see* Morphine Sulfate *on page 947*

MTA *see* Pemetrexed *on page 1054*

MTC *see* Mitomycin *on page 937*

M.T.E.-4® *see* Trace Metals *on page 1319*

M.T.E.-5® *see* Trace Metals *on page 1319*

M.T.E.-6® *see* Trace Metals *on page 1319*

M.T.E.-7® *see* Trace Metals *on page 1319*

MTX *see* Methotrexate *on page 897*

Mucinex® [OTC] *see* Guaifenesin *on page 672*

Mucinex® D *see* Guaifenesin and Pseudoephedrine *on page 675*

Mucomyst® *see* Acetylcysteine *on page 61*

Multidex® [OTC] *see* Maltodextrin *on page 855*

Multiple Vitamins *see* Vitamins (Multiple/Oral) *on page 1384*

Multitargeted Antifolate *see* Pemetrexed *on page 1054*

Multitest CMI® *see* Skin Test Antigens (Multiple) *on page 1226*

Multitrace™-4 *see* Trace Metals *on page 1319*

Multitrace™-4 Neonatal *see* Trace Metals *on page 1319*

Multitrace™-4 Pediatric *see* Trace Metals *on page 1319*
Multitrace™-5 *see* Trace Metals *on page 1319*
Multivitamin Products *see page 1644*
Mumps, Measles and Rubella Vaccines, Combined *see* Measles, Mumps, and Rubella Vaccines (Combined) *on page 858*
Mumpsvax® *see* Mumps Virus Vaccine (Live/Attenuated) *on page 951*

Mumps Virus Vaccine (Live/Attenuated)

(mumpz VYE rus vak SEEN, live, a ten YOO ate ed)

Related Information

Immunizations (Vaccines) *on page 1614*

U.S. Brand Names Mumpsvax®

Canadian Brand Names Mumpsvax®

Generic Available No

Pharmacologic Category Vaccine

Use Mumps prophylaxis by promoting active immunity

Note: Trivalent measles-mumps-rubella (MMR) vaccine is the preferred agent for most children and many adults; persons born prior to 1957 are generally considered immune and need not be vaccinated

Local Anesthetic/Vasoconstrictor Precautions No information available to require special precautions

Effects on Dental Treatment No significant effects or complications reported

Common Adverse Effects All serious adverse reactions must be reported to the U.S. Department of Health and Human Services (DHHS) Vaccine Adverse Event Reporting System (VAERS) 1-800-822-7967.

>10%: Local: Burning or stinging at injection site

1% to 10%:

Central nervous system: Fever (≤100°F)

Dermatologic: Rash

Endocrine & metabolic: Parotitis

Mechanism of Action Promotes active immunity to mumps virus by inducing specific antibodies.

Pregnancy Risk Factor X

Mupirocin

(myoo PEER oh sin)

U.S. Brand Names Bactroban®; Bactroban® Nasal

Canadian Brand Names Bactroban®

Mexican Brand Names Bactroban®

Generic Available Yes: Topical ointment

Synonyms Mupirocin Calcium; Pseudomonic Acid A

Pharmacologic Category Antibiotic, Topical

Use

Intranasal: Eradication of nasal colonization with MRSA in adult patients and healthcare workers

Topical treatment of impetigo due to *Staphylococcus aureus*, beta-hemolytic *Streptococcus*, and *S. pyogenes*

Unlabeled/Investigational Use Intranasal: Surgical prophylaxis to prevent wound infections

Local Anesthetic/Vasoconstrictor Precautions No information available to require special precautions

Effects on Dental Treatment No significant effects or complications reported

Common Adverse Effects Frequency not defined.

Central nervous system: Dizziness, headache

Dermatologic: Pruritus, rash, erythema, dry skin, cellulitis, dermatitis

Gastrointestinal: Nausea, taste perversion

Local: Burning, stinging, tenderness, edema, pain

Respiratory: Rhinitis, upper respiratory tract infection, pharyngitis, cough

Mechanism of Action Binds to bacterial isoleucyl transfer-RNA synthetase resulting in the inhibition of protein and RNA synthesis

Pharmacodynamics/Kinetics

Absorption: Topical: Penetrates outer layers of skin; systemic absorption minimal through intact skin

Protein binding: 95%

Metabolism: Skin: 3% to monic acid

Half-life elimination: 17-36 minutes

Excretion: Urine

Pregnancy Risk Factor B

Mupirocin Calcium *see* Mupirocin *on page 951*
Murine® Ear [OTC] *see* Carbamide Peroxide *on page 259*

Murine® Tears [OTC] *see* Artificial Tears *on page 148*
Murine® Tears Plus [OTC] *see* Tetrahydrozoline *on page 1282*
Muro 128® [OTC] *see* Sodium Chloride *on page 1227*
Murocel® [OTC] *see* Artificial Tears *on page 148*
Murocoll-2® *see* Phenylephrine and Scopolamine *on page 1079*

Muromonab-CD3 (myoo roe MOE nab see dee three)

U.S. Brand Names Orthoclone OKT® 3
Canadian Brand Names Orthoclone OKT® 3
Mexican Brand Names Orthoclone OKT3®
Generic Available No
Synonyms Monoclonal Antibody; OKT3
Pharmacologic Category Immunosuppressant Agent
Use Treatment of acute allograft rejection in renal transplant patients; treatment of acute hepatic, kidney, and pancreas rejection episodes resistant to conventional treatment. Acute graft-versus-host disease following bone marrow transplantation resistant to conventional treatment.
Local Anesthetic/Vasoconstrictor Precautions No information available to require special precautions
Effects on Dental Treatment No significant effects or complications reported
Common Adverse Effects

>10%:

"First-dose" (cytokine release) effects: Onset: 1-3 hours after the dose; duration: 12-16 hours. Severity is mild to life-threatening. Signs and symptoms include fever, chilling, dyspnea, wheezing, chest pain, chest tightness, nausea, vomiting, and diarrhea. Hypervolemic pulmonary edema, nephrotoxicity, meningitis, and encephalopathy are possible. Reactions tend to decrease with repeated doses.

Cardiovascular: Tachycardia (including ventricular)
Central nervous system: Dizziness, faintness
Gastrointestinal: Diarrhea, nausea, vomiting
Hematologic: Transient lymphopenia
Neuromuscular & skeletal: Trembling
Respiratory: Dyspnea

1% to 10%:

Central nervous system: Headache
Neuromuscular & skeletal: Stiff neck
Ocular: Photophobia
Respiratory: Pulmonary edema

Mechanism of Action Reverses graft rejection by binding to T cells and interfering with their function by binding T-cell receptor-associated CD3 glycoprotein
Drug Interactions

Increased Effect/Toxicity: Recommend decreasing dose of prednisone to 0.5 mg/kg, azathioprine to 0.5 mg/kg (approximate 50% decrease in dose), and discontinuing cyclosporine while patient is receiving OKT3.

Decreased Effect: Decreased effect with immunosuppressive drugs.

Pharmacodynamics/Kinetics

Duration: 7 days after discontinuation
Time to peak: Steady-state: Trough: 3-14 days

Pregnancy Risk Factor C

Muse® *see* Alprostadil *on page 87*
Mutamycin® *see* Mitomycin *on page 937*
Myambutol® *see* Ethambutol *on page 534*
Mycelex® *see* Clotrimazole *on page 363*
Mycelex®-3 [OTC] *see* Butoconazole *on page 239*
Mycelex®-7 [OTC] *see* Clotrimazole *on page 363*
Mycelex® Twin Pack [OTC] *see* Clotrimazole *on page 363*
Myciguent [OTC] *see* Neomycin *on page 973*
Mycinettes® [OTC] *see* Benzocaine *on page 191*
Mycobutin® *see* Rifabutin *on page 1179*
Mycolog®-II [DSC] *see* Nystatin and Triamcinolone *on page 1004*
Myco-Nail [OTC] *see* Triacetin *on page 1329*

Mycophenolate (mye koe FEN oh late)

U.S. Brand Names CellCept®; Myfortic®
Canadian Brand Names CellCept®
Generic Available No

Synonyms MMF; MPA; Mycophenolate Mofetil; Mycophenolate Sodium; Mycophenolic Acid

Pharmacologic Category Immunosuppressant Agent

Use Prophylaxis of organ rejection concomitantly with cyclosporine and corticosteroids in patients receiving allogenic renal (CellCept®, Myfortic®), cardiac (CellCept®), or hepatic (CellCept®) transplants

Unlabeled/Investigational Use Treatment of rejection in liver transplant patients unable to tolerate tacrolimus or cyclosporine due to neurotoxicity; mild rejection in heart transplant patients; treatment of moderate-severe psoriasis; treatment of proliferative lupus nephritis

Local Anesthetic/Vasoconstrictor Precautions No information available to require special precautions

Effects on Dental Treatment No significant effects or complications reported

Common Adverse Effects As reported in adults following oral dosing of CellCept® alone in renal, cardiac, and hepatic allograft rejection studies. In general, lower doses used in renal rejection patients had less adverse effects than higher doses. Rates of adverse effects were similar for each indication, except for those unique to the specific organ involved. The type of adverse effects observed in pediatric patients was similar to those seen in adults; abdominal pain, anemia, diarrhea, fever, hypertension, infection, pharyngitis, respiratory tract infection, sepsis, and vomiting were seen in higher proportion; lymphoproliferative disorder was the only type of malignancy observed. Percentages of adverse reactions were similar in studies comparing CellCept® to Myfortic® in patients following renal transplant.

>20%:

- Cardiovascular: Hypertension (28% to 77%), peripheral edema (27% to 64%), edema (27% to 28%), tachycardia (20% to 22%)
- Central nervous system: Pain (31% to 76%), headache (16% to 54%), insomnia (41% to 52%), fever (21% to 52%), anxiety (28%)
- Dermatologic: Rash (22%)
- Endocrine & metabolic: Hypercholesterolemia (41%), hypokalemia (32% to 37%)
- Gastrointestinal: Abdominal pain (25% to 62%), nausea (20% to 54%), diarrhea (31% to 52%), constipation (18% to 41%), vomiting (33% to 34%), anorexia (25%), dyspepsia (22%)
- Genitourinary: Urinary tract infection (37%)
- Hematologic: Leukopenia (23% to 46%), leukocytosis (22% to 40%), hypochromic anemia (25%)
- Hepatic: Liver function tests abnormal (25%), ascites (24%)
- Neuromuscular & skeletal: Back pain (35% to 47%), weakness (35% to 43%), tremor (24% to 34%), paresthesia (21%)
- Respiratory: Dyspnea (31% to 37%), respiratory tract infection (22% to 37%), cough (31%), lung disorder (22% to 30%)
- Miscellaneous: Infection (18% to 27%), *Candida* (11% to 22%), herpes simplex (10% to 21%)

3% to <20%:

- Cardiovascular: Angina, arrhythmia, arterial thrombosis, atrial fibrillation, atrial flutter, bradycardia, cardiac arrest, cardiac failure, CHF, extrasystole, facial edema, hypervolemia, hypotension, pallor, palpitation, pericardial effusion, peripheral vascular disorder, postural hypotension, supraventricular extrasystoles, supraventricular tachycardia, syncope, thrombosis, vasodilation, vasospasm, venous pressure increased, ventricular extrasystole, ventricular tachycardia
- Central nervous system: Agitation, chills with fever, confusion, convulsion, delirium, depression, emotional lability, hallucinations, hypesthesia, malaise, nervousness, psychosis, somnolence, thinking abnormal, vertigo
- Dermatologic: Acne, alopecia, bruising, cellulitis, hirsutism, pruritus, skin carcinoma, skin hypertrophy
- Endocrine & metabolic: Acidosis, Cushing's syndrome, dehydration, diabetes mellitus, gout, hypercalcemia, hyperlipemia, hyperphosphatemia, hyperuricemia, hypothyroidism, parathyroid disorder
- Gastrointestinal: Abdomen enlarged, dry mouth, dysphagia, esophagitis, flatulence, gastritis, gastroenteritis, gastrointestinal hemorrhage, gastrointestinal moniliasis, gingivitis, gum hyperplasia, melena, mouth ulceration, oral moniliasis, stomach disorder, stomatitis
- Genitourinary: Impotence, pelvic pain, prostatic disorder, urinary frequency, urinary incontinence, urinary retention, urinary tract disorder
- Hematologic: Coagulation disorder, hemorrhage, pancytopenia, polycythemia, prothrombin time increased, thromboplastin increased

(Continued)

Mycophenolate *(Continued)*

Hepatic: Alkaline phosphatase increased, alkalosis, bilirubinemia, cholangitis, cholestatic jaundice, GGT increased, hepatitis, jaundice, liver damage

Local: Abscess, ALT increased, AST increased

Neuromuscular & skeletal: Arthralgia, hypertonia, joint disorder, leg cramps, myalgia, myasthenia, neck pain, neuropathy, osteoporosis

Ocular: Amblyopia, cataract, conjunctivitis, eye hemorrhage, lacrimation disorder, vision abnormal

Otic: Deafness, ear disorder, ear pain, tinnitus

Renal: Albuminuria, creatinine increased, dysuria, hematuria, hydronephrosis, kidney failure, kidney tubular necrosis, oliguria

Respiratory: Apnea, asthma, atelectasis, bronchitis, epistaxis, hemoptysis, hiccup, hyperventilation, hypoxia, respiratory acidosis, lung edema, pharyngitis, pleural effusion, pneumonia, pneumothorax, pulmonary hypertension, respiratory moniliasis, rhinitis, sinusitis, sputum increased, voice alteration

Miscellaneous: CMV viremia/syndrome (12% to 14%), CMV tissue invasive disease (6% to 11%), herpes zoster cutaneous disease (4% to 10%), cyst, diaphoresis, flu-like syndrome, fungal dermatitis, healing abnormal, hernia, ileus infection, lactic dehydrogenase increased, peritonitis, pyelonephritis, scrotal edema, thirst

Mechanism of Action MPA exhibits a cytostatic effect on T and B lymphocytes. It is an inhibitor of inosine monophosphate dehydrogenase (IMPDH) which inhibits *de novo* guanosine nucleotide synthesis. T and B lymphocytes are dependent on this pathway for proliferation.

Drug Interactions

Increased Effect/Toxicity: Acyclovir and ganciclovir levels may increase due to competition for tubular secretion of these drugs. Probenecid may increase mycophenolate levels due to inhibition of tubular secretion. High doses of salicylates may increase free fraction of mycophenolic acid. Azathioprine's bone marrow suppression may be potentiated; do not administer together.

Decreased Effect: Antacids decrease serum levels (C_{max} and AUC); **do not administer together**. Cholestyramine resin decreases serum levels; **do not administer together**. Avoid use of live vaccines; vaccinations may be less effective. Influenza vaccine may be of value. During concurrent use of oral contraceptives, progesterone levels are not significantly affected, however, effect on estrogen component varies; an additional form of contraception should be used.

Pharmacodynamics/Kinetics

Onset of action: Peak effect: Correlation of toxicity or efficacy is still being developed, however, one study indicated that 12-hour AUCs >40 mcg/mL/hour were correlated with efficacy and decreased episodes of rejection

T_{max}: Oral: MPA:

CellCept®: 1-1.5 hours

Myfortic®: 1.5-2.5 hours

Absorption: AUC values for MPA are lower in the early post-transplant period versus later (>3 months) post-transplant period. The extent of absorption in pediatrics is similar to that seen in adults, although there was wide variability reported.

Oral: Myfortic®: 93%

Distribution:

CellCept®: MPA: Oral: 4 L/kg; I.V.: 3.6 L/kg

Myfortic®: MPA: Oral: 54 L (at steady state); 112 L (elimination phase)

Protein binding: MPA: 97%, MPAG 82%

Metabolism: Hepatic and via GI tract; CellCept® is completely hydrolyzed in the liver to mycophenolic acid (MPA; active metabolite); enterohepatic recirculation of MPA may occur; MPA is glucuronidated to MPAG (inactive metabolite)

Bioavailability: Oral: CellCept®: 94%; Myfortic®: 72%

Half-life elimination:

CellCept®: MPA: Oral: 18 hours; I.V.: 17 hours

Myfortic®: MPA: Oral: 8-16 hours; MPAG: 13-17 hours

Excretion:

CellCept®: MPA: Urine (<1%), feces (6%); MPAG: Urine (87%)

Myfortic®: MPA: Urine (3%), feces; MPAG: Urine (>60%)

Pregnancy Risk Factor C (manufacturer)

Mycophenolate Mofetil *see* Mycophenolate *on page 952*

Mycophenolate Sodium *see* Mycophenolate *on page 952*

Mycophenolic Acid *see* Mycophenolate *on page 952*
Mycostatin® *see* Nystatin *on page 1003*
Mydfrin® *see* Phenylephrine *on page 1078*
Mydriacyl® *see* Tropicamide *on page 1348*
Myfortic® *see* Mycophenolate *on page 952*
Mykrox® [DSC] *see* Metolazone *on page 914*
Mylanta® Children's [OTC] *see* Calcium Carbonate *on page 245*
Mylanta® Gas [OTC] *see* Simethicone *on page 1222*
Mylanta® Gas Maximum Strength [OTC] *see* Simethicone *on page 1222*
Mylanta® Gelcaps® [OTC] *see* Calcium Carbonate and Magnesium Hydroxide *on page 245*
Mylanta® Liquid [OTC] *see* Aluminum Hydroxide, Magnesium Hydroxide, and Simethicone *on page 92*
Mylanta® Maximum Strength Liquid [OTC] *see* Aluminum Hydroxide, Magnesium Hydroxide, and Simethicone *on page 92*
Mylanta® Supreme [OTC] *see* Calcium Carbonate and Magnesium Hydroxide *on page 245*
Mylanta® Ultra [OTC] *see* Calcium Carbonate and Magnesium Hydroxide *on page 245*
Myleran® *see* Busulfan *on page 234*
Mylicon® Infants [OTC] *see* Simethicone *on page 1222*
Mylocel™ *see* Hydroxyurea *on page 722*
Mylotarg® *see* Gemtuzumab Ozogamicin *on page 653*
Myobloc® *see* Botulinum Toxin Type B *on page 217*
Myoflex® [OTC] *see* Triethanolamine Salicylate *on page 1338*
Mysoline® *see* Primidone *on page 1122*
Mytelase® *see* Ambenonium *on page 93*
Mytussin® AC *see* Guaifenesin and Codeine *on page 673*
Mytussin® DAC *see* Guaifenesin, Pseudoephedrine, and Codeine *on page 676*
Mytussin® DM [OTC] *see* Guaifenesin and Dextromethorphan *on page 673*
Nabi-HB® *see* Hepatitis B Immune Globulin *on page 688*

Nabumetone (na BYOO me tone)

Related Information

Rheumatoid Arthritis, Osteoarthritis, and Osteoporosis *on page 1490*
Temporomandibular Dysfunction (TMD) *on page 1564*

U.S. Brand Names Relafen®

Canadian Brand Names Apo-Nabumetone®; Gen-Nabumetone; Relafen™; Rhoxal-nabumetone

Mexican Brand Names Relifex®

Generic Available Yes

Pharmacologic Category Nonsteroidal Anti-inflammatory Drug (NSAID), Oral

Use Management of osteoarthritis and rheumatoid arthritis

Unlabeled/Investigational Use Sunburn, mild to moderate pain

Local Anesthetic/Vasoconstrictor Precautions No information available to require special precautions

Effects on Dental Treatment Key adverse event(s) related to dental treatment: Xerostomia (normal salivary flow resumes upon discontinuation). NSAID formulations are known to reversibly decrease platelet aggregation via mechanisms different than observed with aspirin. The dentist should be aware of the potential of abnormal coagulation. Caution should also be exercised in the use of NSAIDs in patients already on anticoagulant therapy with drugs such as warfarin (Coumadin®).

Common Adverse Effects

>10%:
- Central nervous system: Dizziness
- Dermatologic: Rash
- Gastrointestinal: Abdominal cramps, abdominal pain (12%), diarrhea (14%), dyspepsia (13%), heartburn, indigestion, nausea

1% to 10%:
- Central nervous system: Headache, nervousness
- Dermatologic: Itching
- Endocrine & metabolic: Fluid retention
- Gastrointestinal: Vomiting
- Otic: Tinnitus

Mechanism of Action Nabumetone is a nonacidic NSAID that is rapidly metabolized after absorption to a major active metabolite,

(Continued)

Nabumetone *(Continued)*

6-methoxy-2-naphthylacetic acid. As found with previous NSAIDs, nabumetone's active metabolite inhibits the cyclooxygenase enzyme which is indirectly responsible for the production of inflammation and pain during arthritis by way of enhancing the production of endoperoxides and prostaglandins E_2 and I_2 (prostacyclin). The active metabolite of nabumetone is felt to be the compound primarily responsible for therapeutic effect. Comparatively, the parent drug is a poor inhibitor of prostaglandin synthesis.

Drug Interactions

Increased Effect/Toxicity: NSAIDs may increase digoxin, methotrexate, and lithium serum concentrations. The renal adverse effects of ACE inhibitors may be potentiated by NSAIDs. Potential for bleeding may be increased with anticoagulants or antiplatelet agents. Concurrent use of corticosteroids may increase the risk of GI ulceration.

Decreased Effect: NSAIDs may decrease the effect of some antihypertensive agents, including ACE inhibitors, angiotensin receptor antagonists, and hydralazine. The efficacy of diuretics (loop and/or thiazide) may be decreased.

Pharmacodynamics/Kinetics

Onset of action: Several days

Distribution: Diffusion occurs readily into synovial fluid

Protein binding: >99%

Metabolism: Prodrug, rapidly metabolized to an active metabolite (6-methoxy-2-naphthylacetic acid); extensive first-pass effect

Half-life elimination: Major metabolite: 24 hours

Time to peak, serum: Metabolite: Oral: 3-6 hours; Synovial fluid: 4-12 hours

Excretion: Urine (80%) and feces (10%) with little as unchanged drug

Pregnancy Risk Factor C/D (3rd trimester)

NAC *see* Acetylcysteine *on page 61*

***N*-Acetylcysteine** *see* Acetylcysteine *on page 61*

***N*-Acetyl-L-cysteine** *see* Acetylcysteine *on page 61*

N-Acetyl-P-Aminophenol *see* Acetaminophen *on page 47*

NaCl *see* Sodium Chloride *on page 1227*

Nadolol (nay DOE lole)

Related Information

Cardiovascular Diseases *on page 1458*

U.S. Brand Names Corgard®

Canadian Brand Names Alti-Nadolol; Apo-Nadol®; Corgard®; Novo-Nadolol

Generic Available Yes

Pharmacologic Category Beta-Adrenergic Blocker, Nonselective

Use Treatment of hypertension and angina pectoris; prophylaxis of migraine headaches

Local Anesthetic/Vasoconstrictor Precautions Use with caution; epinephrine has interacted with nonselective beta-blockers to result in initial hypertensive episode followed by bradycardia

Effects on Dental Treatment Nadolol is a nonselective beta-blocker and may enhance the pressor response to epinephrine, resulting in hypertension and bradycardia. Many nonsteroidal anti-inflammatory drugs, such as ibuprofen and indomethacin, can reduce the hypotensive effect of beta-blockers after 3 or more weeks of therapy with the NSAID. Short-term NSAID use (ie, 3 days) requires no special precautions in patients taking beta-blockers.

Common Adverse Effects

>10%:

- Central nervous system: Drowsiness, insomnia
- Endocrine & metabolic: Decreased sexual ability

1% to 10%:

- Cardiovascular: Bradycardia, palpitations, edema, CHF, reduced peripheral circulation
- Central nervous system: Mental depression
- Gastrointestinal: Diarrhea or constipation, nausea, vomiting, stomach discomfort
- Respiratory: Bronchospasm
- Miscellaneous: Cold extremities

Mechanism of Action Competitively blocks response to $beta_1$- and $beta_2$-adrenergic stimulation; does not exhibit any membrane stabilizing or intrinsic sympathomimetic activity

Drug Interactions

Increased Effect/Toxicity: The heart rate lowering effects of nadolol are additive with other drugs which slow AV conduction (digoxin, verapamil, diltiazem). Concurrent use of alpha-blockers (prazosin, terazosin) with beta-blockers may increase risk of orthostasis. Nadolol may mask the tachycardia from hypoglycemia caused by insulin and oral hypoglycemics. In patients receiving concurrent therapy, the risk of hypertensive crisis is increased when either clonidine or the beta-blocker is withdrawn. Reserpine has been shown to enhance the effect of beta-blockers. Avoid using with alpha-adrenergic stimulants (phenylephrine, epinephrine, etc) which may have exaggerated hypertensive responses. Beta-blockers may affect the action or levels of ethanol, disopyramide, nondepolarizing muscle relaxants, and theophylline although the effects are difficult to predict. The vasoconstrictive effects of ergot alkaloids may be enhanced.

Decreased Effect: Decreased effect of beta-blockers with aluminum salts, barbiturates, calcium salts, cholestyramine, colestipol, NSAIDs, penicillins (ampicillin), rifampin, salicylates, and sulfinpyrazone due to decreased bioavailability and plasma levels. Beta-blockers may decrease the effect of sulfonylureas (possibly hyperglycemia). Nonselective beta-blockers blunt the effect of beta-2 adrenergic agonists (albuterol).

Pharmacodynamics/Kinetics

Duration: 17-24 hours

Absorption: 30% to 40%

Distribution: Concentration in human breast milk is 4.6 times higher than serum

Protein binding: 28%

Half-life elimination: Adults: 10-24 hours; prolonged with renal impairment; End-stage renal disease: 45 hours

Time to peak, serum: 2-4 hours

Excretion: Urine (as unchanged drug)

Pregnancy Risk Factor C

Nadolol and Bendroflumethiazide

(nay DOE lole & ben droe floo meth EYE a zide)

U.S. Brand Names Corzide®

Generic Available No

Synonyms Bendroflumethiazide and Nadolol

Pharmacologic Category Antihypertensive Agent, Combination; Beta-Adrenergic Blocker, Nonselective; Diuretic, Thiazide

Use Treatment of hypertension; combination product should not be used for initial therapy

Local Anesthetic/Vasoconstrictor Precautions Use with caution; epinephrine has interacted with nonselective beta-blockers to result in initial hypertensive episode followed by bradycardia

Effects on Dental Treatment Nadolol is a nonselective beta-blocker and may enhance the pressor response to epinephrine, resulting in hypertension and bradycardia. Many nonsteroidal anti-inflammatory drugs, such as ibuprofen and indomethacin, can reduce the hypotensive effect of beta-blockers after 3 or more weeks of therapy with the NSAID. Short-term NSAID use (ie, 3 days) requires no special precautions in patients taking beta-blockers.

Common Adverse Effects See individual agents.

Mechanism of Action See individual agents.

Drug Interactions

Increased Effect/Toxicity: See individual agents.

Decreased Effect: See individual agents.

Pharmacodynamics/Kinetics Also see individual agents.

Bioavailability: Bendroflumethiazide: When used in this combination, bioavailability is increased 30% compared to single agent administration.

Pregnancy Risk Factor C

Nafarelin (NAF a re lin)

U.S. Brand Names Synarel®

Canadian Brand Names Synarel®

Mexican Brand Names Synarel®

Generic Available No

Synonyms Nafarelin Acetate

Pharmacologic Category Gonadotropin Releasing Hormone Agonist

Use Treatment of endometriosis, including pain and reduction of lesions; treatment of central precocious puberty (gonadotropin-dependent precocious puberty) in children of both sexes

(Continued)

Nafarelin *(Continued)*

Local Anesthetic/Vasoconstrictor Precautions No information available to require special precautions

Effects on Dental Treatment No significant effects or complications reported

Common Adverse Effects

>10%:

Central nervous system: Headache, emotional lability
Dermatologic: Acne
Endocrine & metabolic: Hot flashes, decreased libido, decreased breast size
Genitourinary: Vaginal dryness
Neuromuscular & skeletal: Myalgia
Respiratory: Nasal irritation

1% to 10%:

Cardiovascular: Edema, chest pain
Central nervous system: Insomnia
Dermatologic: Urticaria, rash, pruritus, seborrhea
Respiratory: Dyspnea

Mechanism of Action Potent synthetic decapeptide analogue of gonadotropin-releasing hormone (GnRH; LHRH) which is approximately 200 times more potent than GnRH in terms of pituitary release of luteinizing hormone (LH) and follicle-stimulating hormone (FSH). Effects on the pituitary gland and sex hormones are dependent upon its length of administration. After acute administration, an initial stimulation of the release of LH and FSH from the pituitary is observed; an increase in androgens and estrogens subsequently follows. Continued administration of nafarelin, however, suppresses gonadotrope responsiveness to endogenous GnRH resulting in reduced secretion of LH and FSH and, secondarily, decreased ovarian and testicular steroid production.

Pharmacodynamics/Kinetics

Protein binding, plasma: 80%
Time to peak, serum: 10-45 minutes

Pregnancy Risk Factor X

Nafarelin Acetate *see* Nafarelin *on page 957*

Nafcillin (naf SIL in)

Canadian Brand Names Nallpen®; Unipen®

Generic Available Yes

Synonyms Ethoxynaphthamido Penicillin Sodium; Nafcillin Sodium; Nallpen; Sodium Nafcillin

Pharmacologic Category Antibiotic, Penicillin

Use Treatment of infections such as osteomyelitis, septicemia, endocarditis, and CNS infections caused by susceptible strains of staphylococci species

Local Anesthetic/Vasoconstrictor Precautions No information available to require special precautions

Effects on Dental Treatment Key adverse event(s) related to dental treatment: Prolonged use of penicillins may lead to the development of oral candidiasis.

Common Adverse Effects Frequency not defined.

Central nervous system: Pain, fever
Dermatologic: Rash
Gastrointestinal: Nausea, diarrhea
Hematologic: Agranulocytosis, bone marrow depression, neutropenia
Local: Pain, swelling, inflammation, phlebitis, skin sloughing, and thrombophlebitis at the injection site; oxacillin (less likely to cause phlebitis) is often preferred in pediatric patients
Renal: Interstitial nephritis (acute)
Miscellaneous: Hypersensitivity reactions

Mechanism of Action Interferes with bacterial cell wall synthesis during active multiplication, causing cell wall death and resultant bactericidal activity against susceptible bacteria

Drug Interactions

Cytochrome P450 Effect: Induces CYP3A4 (strong)

Increased Effect/Toxicity: Probenecid may cause an increase in nafcillin levels. Penicillins may increase the exposure to methotrexate during concurrent therapy; monitor.

Decreased Effect: Chloramphenicol may decrease nafcillin efficacy. If taken concomitantly with warfarin, nafcillin may inhibit the anticoagulant response to warfarin. This effect may persist for up to 30 days after nafcillin has been discontinued. Subtherapeutic cyclosporine levels may result when taken concomitantly with nafcillin. Although anecdotal reports suggest oral contraceptive efficacy could be reduced by penicillins, this has been refuted by more rigorous scientific and clinical data. Nafcillin may decrease the levels/effects of benzodiazepines, calcium channel blockers, clarithromycin, cyclosporine, erythromycin, estrogens, mirtazapine, nateglinide, nefazodone, nevirapine, protease inhibitors, tacrolimus, venlafaxine, and other CYP3A4 substrates.

Pharmacodynamics/Kinetics

Distribution: Widely distributed; CSF penetration is poor but enhanced by meningeal inflammation; crosses placenta

Protein binding: 70% to 90%

Metabolism: Primarily hepatic; undergoes enterohepatic recirculation

Half-life elimination:

- Neonates: <3 weeks: 2.2-5.5 hours; 4-9 weeks: 1.2-2.3 hours
- Children 3 months to 14 years: 0.75-1.9 hours
- Adults: 30 minutes to 1.5 hours with normal renal and hepatic function

Time to peak, serum: I.M.: 30-60 minutes

Excretion: Primarily feces; urine (10% to 30% as unchanged drug)

Pregnancy Risk Factor B

Nafcillin Sodium *see* Nafcillin *on page 958*

Nafidimide *see* Amonafide *on page 112*

Naftifine (NAF ti feen)

Related Information

Oral Fungal Infections *on page 1544*

U.S. Brand Names Naftin®

Generic Available No

Synonyms Naftifine Hydrochloride

Pharmacologic Category Antifungal Agent, Topical

Use Topical treatment of tinea cruris (jock itch), tinea corporis (ringworm), and tinea pedis (athlete's foot)

Local Anesthetic/Vasoconstrictor Precautions No information available to require special precautions

Effects on Dental Treatment No significant effects or complications reported

Common Adverse Effects

>10%: Local: Burning, stinging

1% to 10%:

- Dermatologic: Erythema, itching
- Local: Dryness, irritation

Mechanism of Action Synthetic, broad-spectrum antifungal agent in the allylamine class; appears to have both fungistatic and fungicidal activity. Exhibits antifungal activity by selectively inhibiting the enzyme squalene epoxidase in a dose-dependent manner which results in the primary sterol, ergosterol, within the fungal membrane not being synthesized.

Pharmacodynamics/Kinetics

Absorption: Systemic: Cream: 6%; Gel: ≤4%

Half-life elimination: 2-3 days

Excretion: Urine and feces (as metabolites)

Pregnancy Risk Factor B

Naftifine Hydrochloride *see* Naftifine *on page 959*

Naftin® *see* Naftifine *on page 959*

$NaHCO_3$ *see* Sodium Bicarbonate *on page 1226*

Nalbuphine (NAL byoo feen)

U.S. Brand Names Nubain®

Canadian Brand Names Nubain®

Mexican Brand Names Bufigen®; Nalcryn® [inj.]; Nubain®

Generic Available Yes

Synonyms Nalbuphine Hydrochloride

Pharmacologic Category Analgesic, Narcotic

Use Relief of moderate to severe pain; preoperative analgesia, postoperative and surgical anesthesia, and obstetrical analgesia during labor and delivery

Local Anesthetic/Vasoconstrictor Precautions No information available to require special precautions

Effects on Dental Treatment Key adverse event(s) related to dental treatment: Anticholinergic side effects can cause a reduction of saliva production or secretion, contributing to discomfort and dental disease (ie, caries, oral candidiasis, and periodontal disease).

(Continued)

Nalbuphine *(Continued)*

Common Adverse Effects

>10%:

Central nervous system: Fatigue, drowsiness

Miscellaneous: Histamine release

1% to 10%:

Cardiovascular: Hypotension

Central nervous system: Headache, nightmares, dizziness

Gastrointestinal: Anorexia, nausea, vomiting, dry mouth

Local: Pain at injection site

Neuromuscular & skeletal: Weakness

Mechanism of Action Binds to opiate receptors in the CNS, causing inhibition of ascending pain pathways, altering the perception of and response to pain; produces generalized CNS depression

Drug Interactions

Increased Effect/Toxicity: Barbiturate anesthetics may increase CNS depression.

Pharmacodynamics/Kinetics

Onset of action: Peak effect: I.M.: 30 minutes; I.V.: 1-3 minutes

Metabolism: Hepatic

Half-life elimination: 3.5-5 hours

Excretion: Feces; urine (~7% as metabolites)

Pregnancy Risk Factor B/D (prolonged use or high doses at term)

Nalbuphine Hydrochloride *see* Nalbuphine *on page 959*

Naldecon Senior EX® [OTC] *see* Guaifenesin *on page 672*

Nalex®-A *see* Chlorpheniramine, Phenylephrine, and Phenyltoloxamine *on page 317*

Nalfon® *see* Fenoprofen *on page 580*

Nalidixic Acid (nal i DIKS ik AS id)

U.S. Brand Names NegGram®

Canadian Brand Names NegGram®

Generic Available No

Synonyms Nalidixinic Acid

Pharmacologic Category Antibiotic, Quinolone

Use Treatment of urinary tract infections

Local Anesthetic/Vasoconstrictor Precautions No information available to require special precautions

Effects on Dental Treatment No significant effects or complications reported

Mechanism of Action Inhibits DNA polymerization in late stages of chromosomal replication

Pregnancy Risk Factor B

Nalidixinic Acid *see* Nalidixic Acid *on page 960*

Nallpen *see* Nafcillin *on page 958*

***N*-allylnoroxymorphine Hydrochloride** *see* Naloxone *on page 961*

Nalmefene (NAL me feen)

U.S. Brand Names Revex®

Generic Available No

Synonyms Nalmefene Hydrochloride

Pharmacologic Category Antidote

Use Complete or partial reversal of opioid drug effects, including respiratory depression induced by natural or synthetic opioids; reversal of postoperative opioid depression; management of known or suspected opioid overdose

Local Anesthetic/Vasoconstrictor Precautions No information available to require special precautions

Effects on Dental Treatment No significant effects or complications reported

Common Adverse Effects

>10%: Gastrointestinal: Nausea

1% to 10%:

Cardiovascular: Tachycardia, hypertension, hypotension, vasodilation

Central nervous system: Fever, dizziness, headache, chills

Gastrointestinal: Vomiting

Miscellaneous: Postoperative pain

Mechanism of Action As a 6-methylene analog of naltrexone, nalmefene acts as a competitive antagonist at opioid receptor sites, preventing or reversing the respiratory depression, sedation, and hypotension induced by opiates; no pharmacologic activity of its own (eg, opioid agonist activity) has been demonstrated

Drug Interactions

Increased Effect/Toxicity: Potential increased risk of seizures may exist with use of flumazenil and nalmefene coadministration.

Pharmacodynamics/Kinetics

Onset of action: I.M., SubQ: 5-15 minutes

Distribution: V_d: 8.6 L/kg; rapid

Protein binding: 45%

Metabolism: Hepatic via glucuronide conjugation to metabolites with little or no activity

Bioavailability: I.M., I.V., SubQ: 100%

Half-life elimination: 10.8 hours

Time to peak, serum: I.M.: 2.3 hours; I.V.: <2 minutes; SubQ: 1.5 hours

Excretion: Feces (17%); urine (<5% as unchanged drug)

Clearance: 0.8 L/hour/kg

Pregnancy Risk Factor B

Nalmefene Hydrochloride *see* Nalmefene *on page 960*

Naloxone (nal OKS one)

Related Information

Dental Office Emergencies *on page 1584*

U.S. Brand Names Narcan®

Canadian Brand Names Narcan®

Mexican Brand Names Narcanti®

Generic Available Yes

Synonyms *N*-allylnoroxymorphine Hydrochloride; Naloxone Hydrochloride

Pharmacologic Category Antidote

Dental Use Reverse overdose effects of the two narcotic agents, fentanyl and meperidine, used in the technique of I.V. conscious sedation

Use

Complete or partial reversal of opioid depression, including respiratory depression, induced by natural and synthetic opioids, including propoxyphene, methadone, and certain mixed agonist-antagonist analgesics: nalbuphine, pentazocine, and butorphanol

Diagnosis of suspected opioid tolerance or acute opioid overdose

Adjunctive agent to increase blood pressure in the management of septic shock

Unlabeled/Investigational Use PCP and ethanol ingestion

Local Anesthetic/Vasoconstrictor Precautions No information available to require special precautions

Effects on Dental Treatment No significant effects or complications reported

Significant Adverse Effects Frequency not defined.

Cardiovascular: Hypertension, hypotension, tachycardia, ventricular arrhythmias, cardiac arrest

Central nervous system: Irritability, anxiety, narcotic withdrawal, restlessness, seizures

Gastrointestinal: Nausea, vomiting, diarrhea

Neuromuscular & skeletal: Tremulousness

Respiratory: Dyspnea, pulmonary edema, runny nose, sneezing

Miscellaneous: Diaphoresis

Dosage I.M., I.V. (preferred), intratracheal, SubQ:

Postanesthesia narcotic reversal: Infants and Children: 0.01 mg/kg; may repeat every 2-3 minutes, as needed based on response

Opiate intoxication:

Children:

Birth (including premature infants) to 5 years or <20 kg: 0.1 mg/kg; repeat every 2-3 minutes if needed; may need to repeat doses every 20-60 minutes

>5 years or ≥20 kg: 2 mg/dose; if no response, repeat every 2-3 minutes; may need to repeat doses every 20-60 minutes

Children and Adults: Continuous infusion: I.V.: If continuous infusion is required, calculate dosage/hour based on effective intermittent dose used and duration of adequate response seen, titrate dose 0.04-0.16 mg/kg/hour for 2-5 days in children, adult dose typically 0.25-6.25 mg/hour (short-term infusions as high as 2.4 mg/kg/hour have been tolerated in adults during treatment for septic shock); alternatively, continuous infusion utilizes $^2/_3$ of the initial naloxone bolus on an hourly basis; add 10 times this dose to each liter of D_5W and infuse at a rate of 100 mL/hour; $^1/_2$ of the initial bolus dose should be readministered 15 minutes after initiation of the

(Continued)

Naloxone *(Continued)*

continuous infusion to prevent a drop in naloxone levels; increase infusion rate as needed to assure adequate ventilation

Narcotic overdose: Adults: I.V.: 0.4-2 mg every 2-3 minutes as needed; may need to repeat doses every 20-60 minutes, if no response is observed after 10 mg, question the diagnosis. **Note:** Use 0.1-0.2 mg increments in patients who are opioid dependent and in postoperative patients to avoid large cardiovascular changes.

Mechanism of Action Pure opioid antagonist that competes and displaces narcotics at opioid receptor sites

Contraindications Hypersensitivity to naloxone or any component of the formulation

Warnings/Precautions Due to an association between naloxone and acute pulmonary edema, use with caution in patients with cardiovascular disease or in patients receiving medications with potential adverse cardiovascular effects (eg, hypotension, pulmonary edema or arrhythmias). Excessive dosages should be avoided after use of opiates in surgery. Abrupt postoperative reversal may result in nausea, vomiting, sweating, tachycardia, hypertension, seizures, and other cardiovascular events (including pulmonary edema and arrhythmias). May precipitate withdrawal symptoms in patients addicted to opiates, including pain, hypertension, sweating, agitation, irritability; in neonates: shrill cry, failure to feed. Recurrence of respiratory depression is possible if the opioid involved is long-acting; observe patients until there is no reasonable risk of recurrent respiratory depression.

Drug Interactions Narcotic analgesics: Decreased effect of narcotic analgesics; may precipitate acute withdrawal reaction in physically dependent patients

Pharmacodynamics/Kinetics

Onset of action: Endotracheal, I.M., SubQ: 2-5 minutes; I.V.: ~2 minutes

Duration: 20-60 minutes; since shorter than that of most opioids, repeated doses are usually needed

Distribution: Crosses placenta

Metabolism: Primarily hepatic via glucuronidation

Half-life elimination: Neonates: 1.2-3 hours; Adults: 1-1.5 hours

Excretion: Urine (as metabolites)

Pregnancy Risk Factor C

Lactation Excretion in breast milk unknown/not recommended

Breast-Feeding Considerations No data reported. Since naloxone is used for opiate reversal the concern should be on opiate drug levels in a breast-feeding mother and transfer to the infant rather than naloxone exposure. The safest approach would be **not** to breast-feed.

Dosage Forms

Injection, neonatal solution, as hydrochloride: 0.02 mg/mL (2 mL)

Injection, solution, as hydrochloride: 0.4 mg/mL (1 mL, 10 mL); 1 mg/mL (2 mL, 10 mL)

Naloxone and Buprenorphine *see* Buprenorphine and Naloxone *on page 230*

Naloxone Hydrochloride *see* Naloxone *on page 961*

Naloxone Hydrochloride and Pentazocine Hydrochloride *see* Pentazocine *on page 1063*

Naloxone Hydrochloride Dihydrate and Buprenorphine Hydrochloride *see* Buprenorphine and Naloxone *on page 230*

Naltrexone (nal TREKS one)

U.S. Brand Names ReVia®

Canadian Brand Names ReVia®

Generic Available Yes

Synonyms Naltrexone Hydrochloride

Pharmacologic Category Antidote

Use Treatment of ethanol dependence; blockade of the effects of exogenously administered opioids

Local Anesthetic/Vasoconstrictor Precautions No information available to require special precautions

Effects on Dental Treatment No significant effects or complications reported

Common Adverse Effects

>10%:

Central nervous system: Insomnia, nervousness, headache, low energy

Gastrointestinal: Abdominal cramping, nausea, vomiting

Neuromuscular & skeletal: Arthralgia

1% to 10%:
- Central nervous system: Increased energy, feeling down, irritability, dizziness, anxiety, somnolence
- Dermatologic: Rash
- Endocrine & metabolic: Polydipsia
- Gastrointestinal: Diarrhea, constipation
- Genitourinary: Delayed ejaculation, impotency

Mechanism of Action Naltrexone (a pure opioid antagonist) is a cyclopropyl derivative of oxymorphone similar in structure to naloxone and nalorphine (a morphine derivative); it acts as a competitive antagonist at opioid receptor sites

Drug Interactions

Increased Effect/Toxicity: Lethargy and somnolence have been reported with the combination of naltrexone and thioridazine.

Decreased Effect: Naltrexone decreases effects of opioid-containing products.

Pharmacodynamics/Kinetics

Duration: 50 mg: 24 hours; 100 mg: 48 hours; 150 mg: 72 hours

Absorption: Almost complete

Distribution: V_d: 19 L/kg; widely throughout the body but considerable interindividual variation exists

Protein binding: 21%

Metabolism: Extensive first-pass effect to 6-β-naltrexol

Half-life elimination: 4 hours; 6-β-naltrexol: 13 hours

Time to peak, serum: ~60 minutes

Excretion: Primarily urine (as metabolites and unchanged drug)

Pregnancy Risk Factor C

Naltrexone Hydrochloride *see* Naltrexone *on page 962*
Namenda™ *see* Memantine *on page 867*

Nandrolone (NAN droe lone)

U.S. Brand Names Deca-Durabolin® [DSC]

Canadian Brand Names Deca-Durabolin®; Durabolin®

Generic Available Yes

Synonyms Nandrolone Decanoate; Nandrolone Phenpropionate

Pharmacologic Category Androgen

Use Control of metastatic breast cancer; management of anemia of renal insufficiency

Local Anesthetic/Vasoconstrictor Precautions No information available to require special precautions

Effects on Dental Treatment No significant effects or complications reported

Common Adverse Effects

Male:

Postpubertal:

>10%:
- Dermatologic: Acne
- Endocrine & metabolic: Gynecomastia
- Genitourinary: Bladder irritability, priapism

1% to 10%:
- Central nervous system: Insomnia, chills
- Endocrine & metabolic: Decreased libido, hepatic dysfunction
- Gastrointestinal: Nausea, diarrhea
- Genitourinary: Prostatic hyperplasia (elderly)
- Hematologic: Iron deficiency anemia, suppression of clotting factors

Prepubertal:

>10%:
- Dermatologic: Acne
- Endocrine & metabolic: Virilism

1% to 10%:
- Central nervous system: Chills, insomnia
- Dermatologic: Hyperpigmentation
- Gastrointestinal: Diarrhea, nausea
- Hematologic: Iron deficiency anemia, suppression of clotting

Female:

>10%: Endocrine & metabolic: Virilism

1% to 10%:
- Central nervous system: Chills, insomnia
- Endocrine & metabolic: Hypercalcemia
- Gastrointestinal: Nausea, diarrhea
- Hematologic: Iron deficiency anemia, suppression of clotting factors
- Hepatic: Hepatic dysfunction

(Continued)

Nandrolone *(Continued)*

Restrictions C-III

Mechanism of Action Promotes tissue-building processes, increases production of erythropoietin, causes protein anabolism; increases hemoglobin and red blood cell volume

Drug Interactions

Increased Effect/Toxicity: Nandrolone may increase the effect of oral anticoagulants, insulin, oral hypoglycemic agents, adrenal steroids, or ACTH when taken together.

Pharmacodynamics/Kinetics

Onset of action: 3-6 months
Duration: Up to 30 days
Absorption: I.M.: 77%
Metabolism: Hepatic
Excretion: Urine

Pregnancy Risk Factor X

Nandrolone Decanoate *see* Nandrolone *on page 963*

Nandrolone Phenpropionate *see* Nandrolone *on page 963*

Naphazoline (naf AZ oh leen)

U.S. Brand Names AK-Con™; Albalon®; Allersol®; Clear Eyes® [OTC]; Clear Eyes® ACR [OTC]; Naphcon® [OTC]; Privine® [OTC]; VasoClear® [OTC]

Canadian Brand Names Naphcon Forte®; Vasocon®

Mexican Brand Names Afazol Grin®

Generic Available Yes: Ophthalmic solution

Synonyms Naphazoline Hydrochloride

Pharmacologic Category Alpha$_1$ Agonist; Ophthalmic Agent, Vasoconstrictor

Use Topical ocular vasoconstrictor; will temporarily relieve congestion, itching, and minor irritation, and to control hyperemia in patients with superficial corneal vascularity; treatment of nasal congestion; adjunct for sinusitis

Local Anesthetic/Vasoconstrictor Precautions No information available to require special precautions

Effects on Dental Treatment No significant effects or complications reported

Common Adverse Effects Frequency not defined.

Cardiovascular: Systemic cardiovascular stimulation
Central nervous system: Dizziness, headache, nervousness
Gastrointestinal: Nausea
Local: Transient stinging, nasal mucosa irritation, dryness, rebound congestion
Ocular: Mydriasis, increased intraocular pressure, blurring of vision
Respiratory: Sneezing

Mechanism of Action Stimulates alpha-adrenergic receptors in the arterioles of the conjunctiva and the nasal mucosa to produce vasoconstriction

Pharmacodynamics/Kinetics

Onset of action: Decongestant: Topical: ~10 minutes
Duration: 2-6 hours

Pregnancy Risk Factor C

Naphazoline and Antazoline (naf AZ oh leen & an TAZ oh leen)

Related Information

Naphazoline *on page 964*

U.S. Brand Names Vasocon-A® [OTC]

Canadian Brand Names Albalon®-A Liquifilm; Vasocon-A®

Generic Available No

Synonyms Antazoline and Naphazoline

Pharmacologic Category Ophthalmic Agent, Vasoconstrictor

Use Topical ocular congestion, irritation and itching

Local Anesthetic/Vasoconstrictor Precautions No information available to require special precautions

Effects on Dental Treatment No significant effects or complications reported

Pregnancy Risk Factor C

Naphazoline and Pheniramine

(naf AZ oh leen & fen NIR a meen)

Related Information

Naphazoline *on page 964*

U.S. Brand Names Naphcon-A® [OTC]; Opcon-A® [OTC]; Visine-A™ [OTC]

Canadian Brand Names Naphcon-A®

Generic Available Yes

Synonyms Pheniramine and Naphazoline

Pharmacologic Category Ophthalmic Agent, Vasoconstrictor

Use Treatment of ocular congestion, irritation, and itching

Local Anesthetic/Vasoconstrictor Precautions No information available to require special precautions

Effects on Dental Treatment No significant effects or complications reported

Pregnancy Risk Factor C

Naphazoline Hydrochloride *see* Naphazoline *on page 964*

Naphcon® [OTC] *see* Naphazoline *on page 964*

Naphcon-A® [OTC] *see* Naphazoline and Pheniramine *on page 964*

NapraPAC™ *see* Lansoprazole and Naproxen *on page 799*

Naprelan® *see* Naproxen *on page 965*

Naprosyn® *see* Naproxen *on page 965*

Naproxen (na PROKS en)

Related Information

Oral Pain *on page 1526*

Rheumatoid Arthritis, Osteoarthritis, and Osteoporosis *on page 1490*

Temporomandibular Dysfunction (TMD) *on page 1564*

U.S. Brand Names Aleve® [OTC]; Anaprox®; Anaprox® DS; EC-Naprosyn®; Naprelan®; Naprosyn®; Pamprin® Maximum Strength All Day Relief [OTC]

Canadian Brand Names Anaprox®; Anaprox® DS; Apo-Napro-Na®; Apo-Napro-Na DS®; Apo-Naproxen®; Apo-Naproxen SR®; Gen-Naproxen EC; Naprosyn®; Naxen®; Novo-Naproc EC; Novo-Naprox; Novo-Naprox Sodium; Novo-Naprox Sodium DS; Novo-Naprox SR; Nu-Naprox; Riva-Naproxen

Mexican Brand Names Artron®; Dafloxen® [syrup]; Dafloxen® [caps, tabs]; Flanax®; Flogen® [caps]; Fuxen®; Naprodil® [syrup]; Naprodil® [tabs]; Naxen®; Neonaxil®; Nixal®; Novaxen®; Pactens®; Pronaxil®; Tandax®

Generic Available Yes

Synonyms Naproxen Sodium

Pharmacologic Category Nonsteroidal Anti-inflammatory Drug (NSAID), Oral

Dental Use Management of pain and swelling

Use Management of inflammatory disease and rheumatoid disorders (including juvenile rheumatoid arthritis); acute gout; mild to moderate pain; dysmenorrhea; fever, migraine headache

Local Anesthetic/Vasoconstrictor Precautions No information available to require special precautions

Effects on Dental Treatment Key adverse event(s) related to dental treatment: Stomatitis. NSAID formulations are known to reversibly decrease platelet aggregation via mechanisms different than observed with aspirin. The dentist should be aware of the potential of abnormal coagulation. Caution should also be exercised in the use of NSAIDs in patients already on anticoagulant therapy with drugs such as warfarin (Coumadin®).

Significant Adverse Effects

1% to 10%:

- Central nervous system: Headache (11%), nervousness, malaise (<3%), somnolence (3% to 9%)
- Dermatologic: Itching, pruritus, rash, ecchymosis (3% to 9%)
- Endocrine & metabolic: Fluid retention (3% to 9%)
- Gastrointestinal: Abdominal discomfort, nausea (3% to 9%), heartburn, constipation (3% to 9%), GI bleeding, ulcers, perforation, indigestion, diarrhea (<3%), abdominal distress/cramps/pain (3% to 9%), dyspepsia (<3%), stomatitis (<3%), heartburn (<3%)
- Hematologic: Hemolysis (3% to 9%), ecchymosis (3% to 9%)
- Otic: Tinnitus (3% to 9%)
- Respiratory: Dyspnea (3% to 9%)

<1% (Limited to important or life-threatening): Acute renal failure, agranulocytosis, allergic rhinitis, anemia, angioedema, arrhythmias, aseptic meningitis, bone marrow suppression, bronchospasm, CHF, erythema multiforme, GI ulceration, hallucinations, hemolytic anemia, hepatitis, hypertension, leukopenia, mental depression, peripheral neuropathy, renal dysfunction, Stevens-Johnson syndrome, thrombocytopenia, toxic amblyopia, toxic epidermal necrolysis, urticaria, vomiting

Dosage Oral:

Children >2 years:

- Fever: 2.5-10 mg/kg/dose; maximum: 10 mg/kg/day
- Juvenile arthritis: 10 mg/kg/day in 2 divided doses

(Continued)

Naproxen *(Continued)*

Adults:

Rheumatoid arthritis, osteoarthritis, and ankylosing spondylitis: 500-1000 mg/day in 2 divided doses; may increase to 1.5 g/day of naproxen base for limited time period

Mild to moderate pain or dysmenorrhea: Initial: 500 mg, then 250 mg every 6-8 hours; maximum: 1250 mg/day naproxen base

OTC labeling: Pain/fever:

Children ≥12 years and Adults ≤65 years: 200 mg naproxen base every 8-12 hours; if needed, may take 400 mg naproxen base for the initial dose; maximum: 600 mg naproxen base/24 hours

Adults >65 years: 200 mg naproxen base every 12 hours

Dosing adjustment in hepatic impairment: Reduce dose to 50%

Mechanism of Action Inhibits prostaglandin synthesis by decreasing the activity of the enzyme, cyclooxygenase, which results in decreased formation of prostaglandin precursors

Contraindications Hypersensitivity to naproxen, aspirin, other NSAIDs, or any component of the formulation; patients with "aspirin triad" (bronchial asthma, aspirin intolerance, rhinitis); pregnancy (3rd trimester)

Warnings/Precautions Use with caution in patients with GI disease (bleeding or ulcers), cardiovascular disease (CHF, hypertension), dehydration, renal or hepatic impairment, and patients receiving anticoagulants; perform ophthalmologic evaluation for those who develop eye complaints during therapy (blurred vision, diminished vision, changes in color vision, retinal changes); NSAIDs may mask signs/symptoms of infections; photosensitivity reported. Consuming ≥3 alcoholic beverages per day may increase risk of GI bleeding. Elderly are at a high risk for adverse effects (including gastrointestinal and CNS adverse effects) from NSAIDs. As many as 60% of elderly can develop peptic ulceration and/or hemorrhage asymptomatically. Use lowest effective dose for shortest period possible. Use of NSAIDs can compromise existing renal function especially when Cl_{cr} is <30 mL/minute. Withhold for at least 4-6 half-lives prior to surgical or dental procedures.

OTC labeling: When used for self-medication, patients should be instructed to contact healthcare provider if used for fever lasting >3 days or pain lasting >10 days.

Drug Interactions Substrate (minor) of CYP1A2, 2C8/9

ACE inhibitors: Antihypertensive effects may be decreased by concurrent therapy with NSAIDs; monitor blood pressure.

Angiotensin II antagonists: Antihypertensive effects may be decreased by concurrent therapy with NSAIDs; monitor blood pressure.

Anticoagulants (warfarin, heparin, LMWHs) in combination with NSAIDs can cause increased risk of bleeding.

Antiplatelet drugs (ticlopidine, clopidogrel, aspirin, abciximab, dipyridamole, eptifibatide, tirofiban) can cause an increased risk of bleeding.

Corticosteroids may increase the risk of GI ulceration; avoid concurrent use.

Cyclosporine: NSAIDs may increase serum creatinine, potassium, blood pressure, and cyclosporine levels; monitor cyclosporine levels and renal function carefully.

Hydralazine's antihypertensive effect is decreased; avoid concurrent use.

Lithium levels can be increased; avoid concurrent use if possible or monitor lithium levels and adjust dose. Sulindac may have the least effect. When NSAID is stopped, lithium will need adjustment again.

Loop diuretics efficacy (diuretic and antihypertensive effect) is reduced. Indomethacin reduces this efficacy, however, it may be anticipated with any NSAID.

Methotrexate: Severe bone marrow suppression, aplastic anemia, and GI toxicity have been reported with concomitant NSAID therapy. Avoid use during moderate or high-dose methotrexate (increased and prolonged methotrexate levels). NSAID use during low-dose treatment of rheumatoid arthritis has not been fully evaluated; extreme caution is warranted.

Thiazides antihypertensive effects are decreased; avoid concurrent use.

Warfarin's INRs may be increased by naproxen. Other NSAIDs may have the same effect depending on dose and duration. Monitor INR closely. Use the lowest dose of NSAIDs possible and for the briefest duration.

Ethanol/Nutrition/Herb Interactions

Ethanol: Avoid or limit ethanol (may enhance gastric mucosal irritation).

Food: Naproxen absorption rate may be decreased if taken with food.

Herb/Nutraceutical: Avoid cat's claw, dong quai, evening primrose, feverfew, garlic, ginger, ginkgo, red clover, horse chestnut, green tea, ginseng (all have additional antiplatelet activity).

Dietary Considerations Drug may cause GI upset, bleeding, ulceration, perforation; take with food or milk to minimize GI upset.

Pharmacodynamics/Kinetics

Onset of action: Analgesic: 1 hour; Anti-inflammatory: ~2 weeks

Peak effect: Anti-inflammatory: 2-4 weeks

Duration: Analgesic: ≤7 hours; Anti-inflammatory: ≤12 hours

Absorption: Almost 100%

Protein binding: >90%; increased free fraction in elderly

Half-life elimination: Normal renal function: 12-15 hours; End-stage renal disease: Unchanged

Time to peak, serum: 1-2 hours

Excretion: Urine (95%)

Pregnancy Risk Factor B/D (3rd trimester)

Lactation Enters breast milk/compatible

Dosage Forms

Caplet, as sodium (Aleve®, Pamprin® Maximum Strength All Day Relief): 220 mg [equivalent to naproxen 200 mg and sodium 20 mg]

Gelcap, as sodium (Aleve®): 220 mg [equivalent to naproxen 200 mg and sodium 20 mg]

Suspension, oral (Naprosyn®): 125 mg/5 mL (480 mL) [contains sodium 0.3 mEq/mL; orange-pineapple flavor]

Tablet (Naprosyn®): 250 mg, 375 mg, 500 mg

Tablet, as sodium: 220 mg [equivalent to naproxen 200 mg and sodium 20 mg]; 275 mg [equivalent to naproxen 250 mg and sodium 25 mg]; 550 mg [equivalent to naproxen 500 mg and sodium 50 mg]

Aleve®: 220 mg [equivalent to naproxen 200 mg and sodium 20 mg]

Anaprox®: 275 mg [equivalent to naproxen 250 mg and sodium 25 mg]

Anaprox® DS: 550 mg [equivalent to naproxen 500 mg and sodium 50 mg]

Tablet, controlled release, as sodium: 550 mg [equivalent to naproxen 500 mg and sodium 50 mg]

Naprelan®: 421.5 mg [equivalent to naproxen 375 mg and sodium 37.5 mg]; 550 mg [equivalent to naproxen 500 mg and sodium 50 mg]

Tablet, delayed release (EC-Naprosyn®): 375 mg, 500 mg

Selected Readings

Ahmad N, Grad HA, Haas DA, et al, "The Efficacy of Nonopioid Analgesics for Postoperative Dental Pain: A Meta-Analysis," *Anesth Prog*, 1997, 44(4):119-26.

Brooks PM and Day RO, "Nonsteroidal Anti-inflammatory Drugs - Differences and Similarities," *N Engl J Med*, 1991, 324(24):1716-25.

Dionne R, "Additive Analgesia Without Opioid Side Effects," *Compend Contin Educ Dent*, 2000, 21(7):572-4, 576-7.

Dionne RA and Berthold CW, "Therapeutic Uses of Nonsteroidal Anti-inflammatory Drugs in Dentistry," *Crit Rev Oral Biol Med*, 2001, 12(4):315-30.

Forbes JA, Keller CK, Smith JW, et al, "Analgesic Effect of Naproxen Sodium, Codeine, a Naproxen-Codeine Combination and Aspirin on the Postoperative Pain of Oral Surgery," *Pharmacotherapy*, 1986, 6(5):211-8.

Nguyen AM, Graham DY, Gage T, et al, "Nonsteroidal Anti-inflammatory Drug Use in Dentistry: Gastrointestinal Implications," *Gen Dent*, 1999, 47(6):590-6.

Naproxen and Lansoprazole *see* Lansoprazole and Naproxen *on page 799*

Naproxen Sodium *see* Naproxen *on page 965*

Naqua® *see* Trichlormethiazide *on page 1337*

Naratriptan (NAR a trip tan)

U.S. Brand Names Amerge®

Canadian Brand Names Amerge®

Mexican Brand Names Naramig®

Generic Available No

Synonyms Naratriptan Hydrochloride

Pharmacologic Category Serotonin $5\text{-}HT_{1D}$ Receptor Agonist

Use Treatment of acute migraine headache with or without aura

Local Anesthetic/Vasoconstrictor Precautions No information available to require special precautions

Effects on Dental Treatment No significant effects or complications reported

Common Adverse Effects 1% to 10%:

Central nervous system: Dizziness, drowsiness, malaise/fatigue

Gastrointestinal: Nausea, vomiting

Neuromuscular & skeletal: Paresthesias

Miscellaneous: Pain or pressure in throat or neck

Mechanism of Action The therapeutic effect for migraine is due to serotonin agonist activity

(Continued)

Naratriptan *(Continued)*

Drug Interactions

Increased Effect/Toxicity: Ergot-containing drugs (dihydroergotamine or methysergide) may cause vasospastic reactions when taken with naratriptan. Avoid concomitant use with ergots; separate dose of naratriptan and ergots by at least 24 hours. Oral contraceptives taken with naratriptan reduced the clearance of naratriptan ~30% which may contribute to adverse effects. Selective serotonin reuptake inhibitors (SSRIs) (eg, fluoxetine, fluvoxamine, paroxetine, sertraline) may cause lack of coordination, hyper-reflexia, or weakness and should be avoided when taking naratriptan.

Decreased Effect: Smoking increases the clearance of naratriptan.

Pharmacodynamics/Kinetics

Onset of action: 30 minutes
Absorption: Well absorbed
Protein binding, plasma: 28% to 31%
Metabolism: Hepatic via CYP
Bioavailability: 70%
Time to peak: 2-3 hours
Excretion: Urine

Pregnancy Risk Factor C

Naratriptan Hydrochloride *see* Naratriptan *on page 967*
Narcan® *see* Naloxone *on page 961*
Nardil® *see* Phenelzine *on page 1072*
Naropin® *see* Ropivacaine *on page 1199*
Nasacort® [DSC] *see* Triamcinolone *on page 1330*
Nasacort® AQ *see* Triamcinolone *on page 1330*
NaSal™ [OTC] *see* Sodium Chloride *on page 1227*
Nasalcrom® [OTC] *see* Cromolyn *on page 378*
Nasalide® *see* Flunisolide *on page 599*
Nasal Moist® [OTC] *see* Sodium Chloride *on page 1227*
Nasarel® *see* Flunisolide *on page 599*
Nascobal® *see* Cyanocobalamin *on page 380*
Nasonex® *see* Mometasone Furoate *on page 943*
Natacyn® *see* Natamycin *on page 968*

Natamycin (na ta MYE sin)

U.S. Brand Names Natacyn®
Canadian Brand Names Natacyn®
Generic Available No
Synonyms Pimaricin
Pharmacologic Category Antifungal Agent, Ophthalmic
Use Treatment of blepharitis, conjunctivitis, and keratitis caused by susceptible fungi (*Aspergillus, Candida*), *Cephalosporium, Curvularia, Fusarium, Penicillium, Microsporum, Epidermophyton, Blastomyces dermatitidis, Coccidioides immitis, Cryptococcus neoformans, Histoplasma capsulatum, Sporothrix schenckii*, and *Trichomonas vaginalis*
Local Anesthetic/Vasoconstrictor Precautions No information available to require special precautions
Effects on Dental Treatment No significant effects or complications reported
Mechanism of Action Increases cell membrane permeability in susceptible fungi
Pregnancy Risk Factor C

Nateglinide (na te GLYE nide)

Related Information

Endocrine Disorders and Pregnancy *on page 1481*

U.S. Brand Names Starlix®
Canadian Brand Names Starlix®
Generic Available No
Pharmacologic Category Antidiabetic Agent, Miscellaneous
Use Management of type 2 diabetes mellitus (noninsulin dependent, NIDDM) as monotherapy when hyperglycemia cannot be managed by diet and exercise alone; in combination with metformin or a thiazolidinedione to lower blood glucose in patients whose hyperglycemia cannot be controlled by exercise, diet, or a single agent alone
Local Anesthetic/Vasoconstrictor Precautions No information available to require special precautions
Effects on Dental Treatment No significant effects or complications reported

Common Adverse Effects As reported with nateglinide monotherapy:
1% to 10%:
Central nervous system: Dizziness (4%)
Endocrine & metabolic: Hypoglycemia (2%), increased uric acid
Gastrointestinal: Weight gain
Neuromuscular & skeletal: Arthropathy (3%)
Respiratory: Upper respiratory infection (10%)
Miscellaneous: Flu-like symptoms (4%)

Mechanism of Action A phenylalanine derivative, nonsulfonylurea hypoglycemic agent used in the management of type 2 diabetes mellitus (noninsulin dependent, NIDDM); stimulates insulin release from the pancreatic beta cells to reduce postprandial hyperglycemia; amount of insulin release is dependent upon existing glucose levels

Drug Interactions

Cytochrome P450 Effect: Substrate (major) of CYP2C8/9, 3A4; **Inhibits** CYP2C8/9 (weak)

Increased Effect/Toxicity: CYP2C8/9 inhibitors may increase the levels/effects of nateglinide; example inhibitors include delavirdine, fluconazole, gemfibrozil, ketoconazole, nicardipine, NSAIDs, pioglitazone, and sulfonamides. CYP3A4 inhibitors may increase the levels/effects of nateglinide; example inhibitors include azole antifungals, ciprofloxacin, clarithromycin, diclofenac, doxycycline, erythromycin, imatinib, isoniazid, nefazodone, nicardipine, propofol, protease inhibitors, quinidine, and verapamil. Possible increased hypoglycemic effect may be seen with salicylates, MAO inhibitors, and nonselective beta-adrenergic blocking agents; monitor glucose closely when agents are initiated, modified, or discontinued.

Decreased Effect: CYP2C8/9 inducers may decrease the levels/effects of nateglinide; example inducers include carbamazepine, phenobarbital, phenytoin, rifampin, rifapentine, and secobarbital. CYP3A4 inducers may decrease the levels/effects of nateglinide; example inducers include aminoglutethimide, carbamazepine, nafcillin, nevirapine, phenobarbital, phenytoin, and rifamycins. Possible decreased hypoglycemic effect may be seen with thiazides, corticosteroids, thyroid products, and sympathomimetic drugs; monitor glucose closely when agents are initiated, modified, or discontinued.

Pharmacodynamics/Kinetics
Onset of action: Insulin secretion: ~20 minutes
Peak effect: 1 hour
Duration: 4 hours
Absorption: Rapid
Distribution: 10 L
Protein binding: 98%, primarily to albumin
Metabolism: Hepatic via hydroxylation followed by glucuronide conjugation via CYP2C9 (70%) and CYP3A4 (30%) to metabolites
Bioavailability: 73%
Half-life elimination: 1.5 hours
Time to peak: ≤1 hour
Excretion: Urine (83%, 16% as unchanged drug); feces (10%)

Pregnancy Risk Factor C

Natrecor® *see* Nesiritide *on page 976*
Natriuretic Peptide *see* Nesiritide *on page 976*
Natural Lung Surfactant *see* Beractant *on page 198*
Natural Products: Herbal and Dietary Supplements *see page 1409*
Nature's Tears® [OTC] *see* Artificial Tears *on page 148*
Nature-Throid® NT *see* Thyroid *on page 1293*
Naturetin® [DSC] *see* Bendroflumethiazide *on page 189*
Nausea Relief [OTC] *see* Fructose, Dextrose, and Phosphoric Acid *on page 638*
Nausetrol® [OTC] *see* Fructose, Dextrose, and Phosphoric Acid *on page 638*
Navane® *see* Thiothixene *on page 1291*
Navelbine® *see* Vinorelbine *on page 1380*
Na-Zone® [OTC] *see* Sodium Chloride *on page 1227*
***n*-Docosanol** *see* Docosanol *on page 459*
Nebcin® *see* Tobramycin *on page 1306*
NebuPent® *see* Pentamidine *on page 1062*
Necon® 0.5/35 *see* Ethinyl Estradiol and Norethindrone *on page 550*
Necon® 1/35 *see* Ethinyl Estradiol and Norethindrone *on page 550*
Necon® 1/50 *see* Mestranol and Norethindrone *on page 884*
Necon® 7/7/7 *see* Ethinyl Estradiol and Norethindrone *on page 550*
Necon® 10/11 *see* Ethinyl Estradiol and Norethindrone *on page 550*

Nedocromil (ne doe KROE mil)

Related Information

Respiratory Diseases *on page 1478*

U.S. Brand Names Alocril™; Tilade®

Canadian Brand Names Alocril™; Tilade®

Generic Available No

Synonyms Nedocromil Sodium

Pharmacologic Category Mast Cell Stabilizer

Use

Aerosol: Maintenance therapy in patients with mild to moderate bronchial asthma

Ophthalmic: Treatment of itching associated with allergic conjunctivitis

Local Anesthetic/Vasoconstrictor Precautions No information available to require special precautions

Effects on Dental Treatment No significant effects or complications reported

Common Adverse Effects

Inhalation aerosol:

>10%: Gastrointestinal: Unpleasant taste

1% to 10%:

Cardiovascular: Chest pain

Central nervous system: Dizziness, dysphonia, headache, fatigue

Dermatologic: Rash

Gastrointestinal: Nausea, vomiting, dyspepsia, diarrhea, abdominal pain, xerostomia, unpleasant taste

Hepatic: Increased ALT

Neuromuscular & skeletal: Arthritis, tremor

Respiratory: Cough, pharyngitis, rhinitis, bronchitis, upper respiratory infection, bronchospasm, increased sputum production

Ophthalmic solution:

>10%:

Central nervous system: Headache (40%)

Gastrointestinal: Unpleasant taste

Ocular: Burning, irritation, stinging

Respiratory: Nasal congestion

1% to 10%:

Ocular: Conjunctivitis, eye redness, photophobia

Respiratory: Asthma, rhinitis

Mechanism of Action Inhibits the activation of and mediator release from a variety of inflammatory cell types associated with asthma including eosinophils, neutrophils, macrophages, mast cells, monocytes, and platelets; it inhibits the release of histamine, leukotrienes, and slow-reacting substance of anaphylaxis; it inhibits the development of early and late bronchoconstriction responses to inhaled antigen

Pharmacodynamics/Kinetics

Duration: Therapeutic effect: 2 hours

Protein binding, plasma: 89%

Bioavailability: 7% to 9%

Half-life elimination: 1.5-2 hours

Excretion: Urine (as unchanged drug)

Pregnancy Risk Factor B

Nedocromil Sodium *see* Nedocromil *on page 970*

Nefazodone (nef AY zoe done)

U.S. Brand Names Serzone® [DSC]

Canadian Brand Names Apo-Nefazodone®; Lin-Nefazodone [DSC]; Serzone-5HT$_2$® [DSC]

Generic Available Yes

Synonyms Nefazodone Hydrochloride

Pharmacologic Category Antidepressant, Serotonin Reuptake Inhibitor/Antagonist

Use Treatment of depression

Unlabeled/Investigational Use Post-traumatic stress disorder

Local Anesthetic/Vasoconstrictor Precautions Although nefazodone is not a tricyclic antidepressant, it does block norepinephrine reuptake within CNS synapses as part of its mechanisms. It has been suggested that vasoconstrictor be administered with caution and to monitor vital signs in dental patients taking antidepressants that affect norepinephrine in this way, including nefazodone.

Effects on Dental Treatment Key adverse event(s) related to dental treatment: Significant xerostomia (normal salivary flow resumes upon discontinuation).

Common Adverse Effects

>10%:

Central nervous system: Headache, drowsiness, insomnia, agitation, dizziness

Gastrointestinal: Xerostomia, nausea, constipation

Neuromuscular & skeletal: Weakness

1% to 10%:

Cardiovascular: Bradycardia, hypotension, peripheral edema, postural hypotension, vasodilation

Central nervous system: Chills, fever, incoordination, lightheadedness, confusion, memory impairment, abnormal dreams, decreased concentration, ataxia, psychomotor retardation, tremor

Dermatologic: Pruritus, rash

Endocrine & metabolic: Breast pain, impotence, libido decreased

Gastrointestinal: Gastroenteritis, vomiting, dyspepsia, diarrhea, increased appetite, thirst, taste perversion

Genitourinary: Urinary frequency, urinary retention

Hematologic: Hematocrit decreased

Neuromuscular & skeletal: Arthralgia, hypertonia, paresthesia, neck rigidity, tremor

Ocular: Blurred vision (9%), abnormal vision (7%), eye pain, visual field defect

Otic: Tinnitus

Respiratory: Bronchitis, cough, dyspnea, pharyngitis

Miscellaneous: Flu syndrome, infection

Mechanism of Action Inhibits neuronal reuptake of serotonin and norepinephrine; also blocks 5-HT_2 and $alpha_1$ receptors; has no significant affinity for $alpha_2$, beta-adrenergic, 5-HT_{1A}, cholinergic, dopaminergic, or benzodiazepine receptors

Drug Interactions

Cytochrome P450 Effect: Substrate (major) of CYP2D6, 3A4; **Inhibits** CYP1A2 (weak), 2B6 (weak), 2D6 (weak), 3A4 (strong)

Increased Effect/Toxicity: Concurrent use of carbamazepine, cisapride, or pimozide is contraindicated. Concurrent therapy with triazolam or alprazolam is generally contraindicated (dosage must be reduced by 75% for triazolam and 50% for alprazolam; such reductions may not be possible with available dosage forms). Concurrent use of ergot alkaloids and/or selected HMG-CoA reductase inhibitors (lovastatin and simvastatin) is generally contraindicated with strong CYP3A4 inhibitors.

Concurrent use of MAO inhibitors may lead to serotonin syndrome; avoid concurrent use or use within 14 days (includes phenelzine, isocarboxazid, and linezolid). Selegiline may increase the risk of serotonin syndrome, particularly at higher doses (>10 mg/day, where selectivity for MAO type B is decreased). Theoretically, concurrent use of buspirone, meperidine, serotonin agonists (sumatriptan and rizatriptan), SSRIs, and venlafaxine may result in serotonin syndrome.

Nefazodone may increase the serum levels/effects of antiarrhythmics (amiodarone, lidocaine, propafenone, quinidine), some antipsychotics (clozapine, haloperidol, mesoridazine, quetiapine, and risperidone), some benzodiazepines (triazolam is contraindicated; decrease alprazolam dose by 50%), buspirone (limit buspirone dose to <2.5 mg/day), Nefazodone may increase the levels/effects of calcium channel blockers, cyclosporine, mirtazapine, nateglinide, nefazodone, quinidine, sildenafil (and other PDE-5 inhibitors), tacrolimus, venlafaxine, and other CYP3A4 substrates. When used with strong CYP3A4 inhibitors, dosage adjustment/limits are recommended for sildenafil and other PDE-5 inhibitors; refer to individual monographs.

CYP3A4 inhibitors may increase The levels/effects of nefazodone may be increased by azole antifungals, chlorpromazine, ciprofloxacin, clarithromycin, delavirdine, diclofenac, doxycycline, erythromycin, fluoxetine, imatinib, isoniazid, miconazole, nicardipine, paroxetine, pergolide, propofol, protease inhibitors, quinidine, quinine, ritonavir, ropinirole, verapamil, and other CYP2D6 or 3A4 inhibitors.

Decreased Effect: Carbamazepine may reduce serum concentrations of nefazodone; concurrent administration should be avoided. The levels/effects of nefazodone may be decreased by aminoglutethimide, nafcillin, nevirapine, phenobarbital, phenytoin, and rifamycins and other CYP3A4 inducers.

(Continued)

Nefazodone *(Continued)*

Pharmacodynamics/Kinetics

Onset of action: Therapeutic: Up to 6 weeks

Metabolism: Hepatic to three active metabolites: Triazoledione, hydroxynefazodone, and m-chlorophenylpiperazine (mCPP)

Bioavailability: 20% (variable)

Half-life elimination: Parent drug: 2-4 hours; active metabolites persist longer

Time to peak, serum: 1 hour, prolonged in presence of food

Excretion: Primarily urine (as metabolites); feces

Pregnancy Risk Factor C

Nefazodone Hydrochloride *see* Nefazodone *on page 970*

NegGram® *see* Nalidixic Acid *on page 960*

Nelfinavir (nel FIN a veer)

Related Information

HIV Infection and AIDS *on page 1484*

Oral Viral Infections *on page 1547*

Tuberculosis *on page 1495*

U.S. Brand Names Viracept®

Canadian Brand Names Viracept®

Generic Available No

Synonyms NFV

Pharmacologic Category Antiretroviral Agent, Protease Inhibitor

Use In combination with other antiretroviral therapy in the treatment of HIV infection

Local Anesthetic/Vasoconstrictor Precautions No information available to require special precautions

Effects on Dental Treatment Key adverse event(s) related to dental treatment: Mouth ulcers.

Common Adverse Effects

>10%: Gastrointestinal: Diarrhea

2% to 10%:

- Dermatologic: Rash
- Gastrointestinal: Nausea, flatulence
- Hematologic: Abnormal creatine kinase, hemoglobin, lymphocytes, neutrophils
- Hepatic: Abnormal ALT, AST

Mechanism of Action Inhibits the HIV-1 protease; inhibition of the viral protease prevents cleavage of the gag-pol polyprotein resulting in the production of immature, noninfectious virus

Drug Interactions

Cytochrome P450 Effect: Substrate of CYP2C8/9 (minor), 2C19 (major), 2D6 (minor), 3A4 (major); **Inhibits** CYP1A2 (weak), 2B6 (weak), 2C8/9 (weak), 2C19 (weak), 2D6 (weak), 3A4 (strong)

Increased Effect/Toxicity: Nelfinavir effects may be increased by azithromycin, delavirdine, and protease inhibitors. Nelfinavir may increase the levels/effects of selected benzodiazepines, calcium channel blockers, cyclosporine, mirtazapine, nateglinide, nefazodone, quinidine, sildenafil (and other PDE-5 inhibitors), tacrolimus, venlafaxine, and other CYP3A4 substrates. Selected benzodiazepines (midazolam, triazolam), cisapride, ergot alkaloids, selected HMG-CoA reductase inhibitors (lovastatin and simvastatin), and pimozide are generally contraindicated with strong CYP3A4 inhibitors. When used with strong CYP3A4 inhibitors, dosage adjustment/limits are recommended for sildenafil and other PDE-5 inhibitors; refer to individual monographs.

Decreased Effect: The levels/effects of nelfinavir may be decreased by aminoglutethimide, carbamazepine, nafcillin, nevirapine, phenobarbital, phenytoin, rifamycins, or other inducers of CYP2C19 or 3A4. Nelfinavir effects may be decreased by St John's wort. Nelfinavir may decrease the effects of delavirdine, methadone, and oral contraceptives

Pharmacodynamics/Kinetics

Absorption: Food increases plasma concentration-time curve (AUC) by two- to threefold

Distribution: V_d: 2-7 L/kg

Protein binding: 98%

Metabolism: Hepatic via CYP2C19 and 3A4; major metabolite has activity comparable to parent drug

Half-life elimination: 3.5-5 hours

Time to peak, serum: 2-4 hours

Excretion: Feces (98% to 99%, 78% as metabolites, 22% as unchanged drug); urine (1% to 2%)

Pregnancy Risk Factor B

Nembutal® *see* Pentobarbital *on page 1065*

NeoCeuticals™ Acne Spot Treatment [OTC] *see* Salicylic Acid *on page 1205*

NeoDecadron® *see* Neomycin and Dexamethasone *on page 973*

Neo-Fradin™ *see* Neomycin *on page 973*

Neomycin (nee oh MYE sin)

Related Information

Neomycin and Polymyxin B *on page 973*
Neomycin, Polymyxin B, and Dexamethasone *on page 974*
Neomycin, Polymyxin B, and Prednisolone *on page 975*

U.S. Brand Names Myciguent [OTC]; Neo-Fradin™; Neo-Rx

Generic Available Yes

Synonyms Neomycin Sulfate

Pharmacologic Category Ammonium Detoxicant; Antibiotic, Aminoglycoside; Antibiotic, Topical

Use Orally to prepare GI tract for surgery; topically to treat minor skin infections; treatment of diarrhea caused by *E. coli*; adjunct in the treatment of hepatic encephalopathy; bladder irrigation; ocular infections

Local Anesthetic/Vasoconstrictor Precautions No information available to require special precautions

Effects on Dental Treatment No significant effects or complications reported

Common Adverse Effects

Oral: >10%: Gastrointestinal: Nausea, diarrhea, vomiting, irritation or soreness of the mouth or rectal area

Topical: >10%: Dermatologic: Contact dermatitis

Mechanism of Action Interferes with bacterial protein synthesis by binding to 30S ribosomal subunits

Drug Interactions

Increased Effect/Toxicity: Oral neomycin may potentiate the effects of oral anticoagulants. Neomycin may increase the adverse effects with other neurotoxic, ototoxic, or nephrotoxic drugs.

Decreased Effect: May decrease GI absorption of digoxin and methotrexate.

Pharmacodynamics/Kinetics

Absorption: Oral, percutaneous: Poor (3%)
Distribution: V_d: 0.36 L/kg
Metabolism: Slightly hepatic
Half-life elimination (age and renal function dependent): 3 hours
Time to peak, serum: Oral: 1-4 hours; I.M.: ~2 hours
Excretion: Feces (97% of oral dose as unchanged drug); urine (30% to 50% of absorbed drug as unchanged drug)

Pregnancy Risk Factor C

Neomycin and Dexamethasone

(nee oh MYE sin & deks a METH a sone)

Related Information

Dexamethasone *on page 411*

U.S. Brand Names NeoDecadron®

Generic Available No

Synonyms Dexamethasone and Neomycin

Pharmacologic Category Antibiotic/Corticosteroid, Ophthalmic

Use Treatment of steroid responsive inflammatory conditions of the palpebral and bulbar conjunctiva, lid, cornea, and anterior segment of the globe

Local Anesthetic/Vasoconstrictor Precautions No information available to require special precautions

Effects on Dental Treatment No significant effects or complications reported

Pregnancy Risk Factor C

Neomycin and Polymyxin B (nee oh MYE sin & pol i MIKS in bee)

Related Information

Neomycin *on page 973*
Polymyxin B *on page 1100*

U.S. Brand Names Neosporin® G.U. Irrigant

Canadian Brand Names Neosporin® Irrigating Solution

Generic Available No

Synonyms Polymyxin B and Neomycin

(Continued)

Neomycin and Polymyxin B *(Continued)*

Pharmacologic Category Antibiotic, Topical

Use Short-term as a continuous irrigant or rinse in the urinary bladder to prevent bacteriuria and gram-negative rod septicemia associated with the use of indwelling catheters; to help prevent infection in minor cuts, scrapes, and burns

Local Anesthetic/Vasoconstrictor Precautions No information available to require special precautions

Effects on Dental Treatment No significant effects or complications reported

Common Adverse Effects Frequency not defined.

Dermatologic: Contact dermatitis, erythema, rash, urticaria
Genitourinary: Bladder irritation
Local: Burning
Neuromuscular & skeletal: Neuromuscular blockade
Otic: Ototoxicity
Renal: Nephrotoxicity

Mechanism of Action See individual agents.

Pharmacodynamics/Kinetics

Absorption: Topical: Not absorbed following application to intact skin; absorbed through denuded or abraded skin, peritoneum, wounds, or ulcers
See individual agents.

Pregnancy Risk Factor C/D (for G.U. irrigant)

Neomycin, Bacitracin, and Polymyxin B *see* Bacitracin, Neomycin, and Polymyxin B *on page 179*

Neomycin, Bacitracin, Polymyxin B, and Hydrocortisone *see* Bacitracin, Neomycin, Polymyxin B, and Hydrocortisone *on page 179*

Neomycin, Bacitracin, Polymyxin B, and Pramoxine *see* Bacitracin, Neomycin, Polymyxin B, and Pramoxine *on page 180*

Neomycin, Polymyxin B, and Dexamethasone

(nee oh MYE sin, pol i MIKS in bee, & deks a METH a sone)

Related Information

Dexamethasone *on page 411*
Neomycin *on page 973*
Polymyxin B *on page 1100*

U.S. Brand Names AK-Trol®; Dexacidin®; Dexacine™; Maxitrol®

Canadian Brand Names Dioptrol®; Maxitrol®

Generic Available Yes

Synonyms Dexamethasone, Neomycin, and Polymyxin B; Polymyxin B, Neomycin, and Dexamethasone

Pharmacologic Category Antibiotic/Corticosteroid, Ophthalmic

Use Steroid-responsive inflammatory ocular conditions in which a corticosteroid is indicated and where bacterial infection or a risk of bacterial infection exists

Local Anesthetic/Vasoconstrictor Precautions No information available to require special precautions

Effects on Dental Treatment No significant effects or complications reported

Mechanism of Action See individual agents.

Pregnancy Risk Factor C

Neomycin, Polymyxin B, and Gramicidin

(nee oh MYE sin, pol i MIKS in bee, & gram i SYE din)

Related Information

Neomycin *on page 973*

U.S. Brand Names Neosporin® Ophthalmic Solution

Canadian Brand Names Neosporin®; Optimyxin Plus®

Generic Available Yes

Synonyms Gramicidin, Neomycin, and Polymyxin B; Polymyxin B, Neomycin, and Gramicidin

Pharmacologic Category Antibiotic, Ophthalmic

Use Treatment of superficial ocular infection

Local Anesthetic/Vasoconstrictor Precautions No information available to require special precautions

Effects on Dental Treatment No significant effects or complications reported

Mechanism of Action Interferes with bacterial protein synthesis by binding to 30S ribosomal subunits; binds to phospholipids, alters permeability, and damages the bacterial cytoplasmic membrane permitting leakage of intracellular constituents

Pregnancy Risk Factor C

Neomycin, Polymyxin B, and Hydrocortisone

(nee oh MYE sin, pol i MIKS in bee, & hye droe KOR ti sone)

Related Information

Hydrocortisone *on page 714*
Neomycin *on page 973*

U.S. Brand Names AntibiOtic® Ear; Cortisporin® Cream; Cortisporin® Ophthalmic; Cortisporin® Otic; PediOtic®

Canadian Brand Names Cortimyxin®; Cortisporin® Otic

Generic Available Yes

Synonyms Hydrocortisone, Neomycin, and Polymyxin B; Polymyxin B, Neomycin, and Hydrocortisone

Pharmacologic Category Antibiotic/Corticosteroid, Ophthalmic; Antibiotic/Corticosteroid, Otic; Topical Skin Product

Use Steroid-responsive inflammatory condition for which a corticosteroid is indicated and where bacterial infection or a risk of bacterial infection exists

Local Anesthetic/Vasoconstrictor Precautions No information available to require special precautions

Effects on Dental Treatment No significant effects or complications reported

Common Adverse Effects Frequency not defined.

Dermatologic: Contact dermatitis, erythema, rash, urticaria
Local: Burning, itching, swelling, pain, stinging
Ocular: Intraocular pressure increased, glaucoma, cataracts, conjunctival erythema, transient irritation, burning, stinging, itching, inflammation, angioneurotic edema, urticaria, vesicular and maculopapular dermatitis
Otic: Ototoxicity
Miscellaneous: Hypersensitivity, sensitization to neomycin, secondary infections

Mechanism of Action See individual agents.

Drug Interactions

Cytochrome P450 Effect: Hydrocortisone: **Substrate** of CYP3A4 (minor); **Induces** CYP3A4 (weak)

Pharmacodynamics/Kinetics See individual agents.

Pregnancy Risk Factor C

Neomycin, Polymyxin B, and Prednisolone

(nee oh MYE sin, pol i MIKS in bee, & pred NIS oh lone)

Related Information

Neomycin *on page 973*
Polymyxin B *on page 1100*
PrednisoLONE *on page 1113*

U.S. Brand Names Poly-Pred®

Generic Available No

Synonyms Polymyxin B, Neomycin, and Prednisolone; Prednisolone, Neomycin, and Polymyxin B

Pharmacologic Category Antibiotic/Corticosteroid, Ophthalmic

Use Steroid-responsive inflammatory ocular condition in which bacterial infection or a risk of bacterial ocular infection exists

Local Anesthetic/Vasoconstrictor Precautions No information available to require special precautions

Effects on Dental Treatment No significant effects or complications reported

Mechanism of Action See individual agents.

Pregnancy Risk Factor C

Neomycin Sulfate *see* Neomycin *on page 973*
Neonatal Trace Metals *see* Trace Metals *on page 1319*
Neoral® *see* CycloSPORINE *on page 386*
Neo-Rx *see* Neomycin *on page 973*
Neosporin® G.U. Irrigant *see* Neomycin and Polymyxin B *on page 973*
Neosporin® Neo To Go® [OTC] *see* Bacitracin, Neomycin, and Polymyxin B *on page 179*
Neosporin® Ophthalmic Ointment *see* Bacitracin, Neomycin, and Polymyxin B *on page 179*
Neosporin® Ophthalmic Solution *see* Neomycin, Polymyxin B, and Gramicidin *on page 974*
Neosporin® + Pain Ointment [OTC] *see* Bacitracin, Neomycin, Polymyxin B, and Pramoxine *on page 180*
Neosporin® Topical [OTC] *see* Bacitracin, Neomycin, and Polymyxin B *on page 179*
NeoStrata AHA [OTC] *see* Hydroquinone *on page 719*
Neo-Synephrine® 12 Hour [OTC] *see* Oxymetazoline *on page 1034*

Neo-Synephrine® 12 Hour Extra Moisturizing [OTC] *see* Oxymetazoline *on page 1034*
Neo-Synephrine® Extra Strength [OTC] *see* Phenylephrine *on page 1078*
Neo-Synephrine® Mild [OTC] *see* Phenylephrine *on page 1078*
Neo-Synephrine® Ophthalmic *see* Phenylephrine *on page 1078*
Neo-Synephrine® Regular Strength [OTC] *see* Phenylephrine *on page 1078*
Neotrace-4® *see* Trace Metals *on page 1319*
NephPlex® Rx *see* Vitamin B Complex Combinations *on page 1382*
Nephro-Calci® [OTC] *see* Calcium Carbonate *on page 245*
Nephrocaps® *see* Vitamin B Complex Combinations *on page 1382*
Nephro-Fer® [OTC] *see* Ferrous Fumarate *on page 586*
Nephron FA® *see* Vitamin B Complex Combinations *on page 1382*
Nephro-Vite® *see* Vitamin B Complex Combinations *on page 1382*
Nephro-Vite® Rx *see* Vitamin B Complex Combinations *on page 1382*
Neptazane® [DSC] *see* Methazolamide *on page 891*
Nesacaine® *see* Chloroprocaine *on page 310*
Nesacaine®-MPF *see* Chloroprocaine *on page 310*

Nesiritide (ni SIR i tide)

U.S. Brand Names Natrecor®

Generic Available No

Synonyms B-type Natriuretic Peptide (Human); hBNP; Natriuretic Peptide

Pharmacologic Category Natriuretic Peptide, B-Type, Human; Vasodilator

Use Treatment of acutely decompensated congestive heart failure (CHF) in patients with dyspnea at rest or with minimal activity

Local Anesthetic/Vasoconstrictor Precautions No information available to require special precautions

Effects on Dental Treatment No significant effects or complications reported

Common Adverse Effects Note: Frequencies cited below were recorded in VMAC trial at dosages similar to approved labeling. Higher frequencies have been observed in trials using higher dosages of nesiritide.

>10%:

Cardiovascular: Hypotension (total: 11%; symptomatic: 4% at recommended dose, up to 17% at higher doses)

Renal: Increased serum creatinine (28% with >0.5 mg/dL increase over baseline)

1% to 10%:

Cardiovascular: Ventricular tachycardia (3%)*, ventricular extrasystoles (3%)*, angina (2%)*, bradycardia (1%), tachycardia, atrial fibrillation, AV node conduction abnormalities

Central nervous system: Headache (8%)*, dizziness (3%)*, insomnia (2%), anxiety (3%), fever, confusion, paresthesia, somnolence, tremor

Dermatologic: Pruritus, rash

Gastrointestinal: Nausea (4%)*, abdominal pain (1%)*, vomiting (1%)*

Hematologic: Anemia

Local: Injection site reaction

Neuromuscular & skeletal: Back pain (4%), leg cramps

Ocular: Amblyopia

Respiratory: Cough (increased), hemoptysis, apnea

Miscellaneous: Increased diaphoresis

*Frequency less than or equal to placebo or other standard therapy

Mechanism of Action Binds to guanylate cyclase receptor on vascular smooth muscle and endothelial cells, increasing intracellular cyclic GMP, resulting in smooth muscle cell relaxation. Has been shown to produce dose-dependent reductions in pulmonary capillary wedge pressure (PCWP) and systemic arterial pressure.

Drug Interactions

Increased Effect/Toxicity: An increased frequency of symptomatic hypotension was observed with concurrent administration of ACE inhibitors. Other hypotensive agents are likely to have additive effects on hypotension. In patients receiving diuretic therapy leading to depletion of intravascular volume, the risk of hypotension and/or renal impairment may be increased. Nesiritide should be avoided in patients with low filling pressures.

Pharmacodynamics/Kinetics

Onset of action: 15 minutes (60% of 3-hour effect achieved)

Duration: >60 minutes (up to several hours) for systolic blood pressure; hemodynamic effects persist longer than serum half-life would predict

Distribution: V_{ss}: 0.19 L/kg

Metabolism: Proteolytic cleavage by vascular endopeptidases and proteolysis following receptor binding and cellular internalization

Half-life elimination: Initial (distribution) 2 minutes; Terminal: 18 minutes

Time to peak: 1 hour

Excretion: Urine

Pregnancy Risk Factor C

Neulasta™ *see* Pegfilgrastim *on page 1052*

Neumega® *see* Oprelvekin *on page 1015*

Neupogen® *see* Filgrastim *on page 589*

Neurontin® *see* Gabapentin *on page 642*

Neut® *see* Sodium Bicarbonate *on page 1226*

NeutraCare® *see* Fluoride *on page 603*

NeutraGard® [OTC] *see* Fluoride *on page 603*

Neutra-Phos® [OTC] *see* Potassium Phosphate and Sodium Phosphate *on page 1107*

Neutra-Phos®-K [OTC] *see* Potassium Phosphate *on page 1107*

Neutrexin® *see* Trimetrexate Glucuronate *on page 1342*

Neutrogena® Acne Mask [OTC] *see* Benzoyl Peroxide *on page 194*

Neutrogena® Acne Wash [OTC] *see* Salicylic Acid *on page 1205*

Neutrogena® Body Clear™ [OTC] *see* Salicylic Acid *on page 1205*

Neutrogena® Clear Pore [OTC] *see* Salicylic Acid *on page 1205*

Neutrogena® Clear Pore Shine Control [OTC] *see* Salicylic Acid *on page 1205*

Neutrogena® Healthy Scalp [OTC] *see* Salicylic Acid *on page 1205*

Neutrogena® Maximum Strength T/Sal® [OTC] *see* Salicylic Acid *on page 1205*

Neutrogena® On The Spot® Acne Patch [OTC] *see* Salicylic Acid *on page 1205*

Neutrogena® On The Spot® Acne Treatment [OTC] *see* Benzoyl Peroxide *on page 194*

Neutrogena® T/Gel [OTC] *see* Coal Tar *on page 367*

Neutrogena® T/Gel Extra Strength [OTC] *see* Coal Tar *on page 367*

Nevirapine (ne VYE ra peen)

Related Information

HIV Infection and AIDS *on page 1484*

Tuberculosis *on page 1495*

U.S. Brand Names Viramune®

Canadian Brand Names Viramune®

Mexican Brand Names Viramune®

Generic Available No

Synonyms NVP

Pharmacologic Category Antiretroviral Agent, Reverse Transcriptase Inhibitor (Non-nucleoside)

Use In combination therapy with other antiretroviral agents for the treatment of HIV-1

Local Anesthetic/Vasoconstrictor Precautions No information available to require special precautions

Effects on Dental Treatment Key adverse event(s) related to dental treatment: Ulcerative stomatitis and oral lesions.

Common Adverse Effects

>10%:

Central nervous system: Headache (11%), fever (8% to 11%)

Dermatologic: Rash (15% to 20%)

Gastrointestinal: Diarrhea (15% to 20%)

Hematologic: Neutropenia (10% to 11%)

1% to 10%:

Gastrointestinal: Ulcerative stomatitis (4%), nausea, abdominal pain (2%)

Hematologic: Anemia

Hepatic: Hepatitis, increased LFTs (2% to 4%)

Neuromuscular & skeletal: Peripheral neuropathy, paresthesia (2%), myalgia

Hypersensitivity (frequency not defined): Symptoms of severe hypersensitivity/dermatologic reactions may include: Severe rash (or rash with fever), blisters, oral lesions, conjunctivitis, facial edema, muscle or joint aches, general malaise, hepatitis, eosinophilia, granulocytopenia, lymphadenopathy, or renal dysfunction. Nevirapine should be permanently discontinued.

Mechanism of Action As a non-nucleoside reverse transcriptase inhibitor, nevirapine has activity against HIV-1 by binding to reverse transcriptase. It

(Continued)

Nevirapine *(Continued)*

consequently blocks the RNA-dependent and DNA-dependent DNA polymerase activities including HIV-1 replication. It does not require intracellular phosphorylation for antiviral activity.

Drug Interactions

Cytochrome P450 Effect: Substrate of CYP2B6 (minor), 2D6 (minor), 3A4 (major); **Inhibits** CYP1A2 (weak), 2D6 (weak), 3A4 (weak); **Induces** CYP2B6 (strong), 3A4 (strong)

Increased Effect/Toxicity: Cimetidine, itraconazole, ketoconazole, and some macrolide antibiotics may increase nevirapine plasma concentrations. Concurrent administration of prednisone for the initial 14 days of nevirapine therapy was associated with an increased incidence and severity of rash. Rifabutin concentrations are increased by nevirapine.

Decreased Effect: The levels/effects of nevirapine may be decreased by aminoglutethimide, carbamazepine, nafcillin, nevirapine, phenobarbital, phenytoin, and rifamycins, and other CYP3A4 inducers; avoid concurrent use. Nevirapine may decrease the levels/effects of benzodiazepines, bupropion, calcium channel blockers, clarithromycin, cyclosporine, efavirenz, erythromycin, estrogens, mirtazapine, nateglinide, nefazodone, promethazine, selegiline, sertraline, tacrolimus, venlafaxine, and other CYP2B6 or 3A4 substrates. Nevirapine may decrease serum concentrations of some protease inhibitors (AUC of indinavir, lopinavir, nelfinavir, and saquinavir may be decreased, however, no effect noted with ritonavir); specific dosage adjustments have not been recommended; no adjustment recommended for ritonavir, unless combined with lopinavir (Kaletra™). Nevirapine may decrease the effectiveness of oral contraceptives; suggest alternate method or additional form of birth control. Nevirapine also decreases the effect of ketoconazole and methadone.

Pharmacodynamics/Kinetics

Absorption: >90%

Distribution: Widely; V_d: 1.2-1.4 L/kg; crosses placenta; enters breast milk; CSF penetration approximates 50% of plasma

Protein binding, plasma: 50% to 60%

Metabolism: Extensively hepatic via CYP3A4 (hydroxylation to inactive compounds); may undergo enterohepatic recycling

Half-life elimination: Decreases over 2- to 4-week time with chronic dosing due to autoinduction (ie, half-life = 45 hours initially and decreases to 23 hours)

Time to peak, serum: 2-4 hours

Excretion: Urine (as metabolites, <3% as unchanged drug)

Pregnancy Risk Factor C

Nexium® *see* Esomeprazole *on page 516*

NFV *see* Nelfinavir *on page 972*

Niacin (NYE a sin)

Related Information

Cardiovascular Diseases *on page 1458*

U.S. Brand Names Niacor®; Niaspan®; Nicotinex [OTC]; Slo-Niacin® [OTC]

Canadian Brand Names Niaspan®

Mexican Brand Names Hipocol®; Pepevit®

Generic Available Yes

Synonyms Nicotinic Acid; Vitamin B_3

Pharmacologic Category Antilipemic Agent, Miscellaneous; Vitamin, Water Soluble

Use Adjunctive treatment of dyslipidemias (alone or with lovastatin or bile acid sequestrant); peripheral vascular disease and circulatory disorders; treatment of pellagra; dietary supplement

Local Anesthetic/Vasoconstrictor Precautions No information available to require special precautions

Effects on Dental Treatment No significant effects or complications reported

Common Adverse Effects Frequency not defined.

Cardiovascular: Arrhythmias, atrial fibrillation, edema, flushing, hypotension, orthostasis, palpitations, syncope (rare), tachycardia

Central nervous system: Chills, dizziness, insomnia, migraine

Dermatologic: Acanthosis nigricans, dry skin, hyperpigmentation, maculopapular rash, pruritus, rash, urticaria

Endocrine & metabolic: Glucose tolerance decreased, gout, phosphorous levels decreased, uric acid level increased

Gastrointestinal: Abdominal pain, nausea, peptic ulcers, vomiting

Hepatic: Hepatic necrosis (rare), jaundice, liver enzymes elevated

Neuromuscular & skeletal: Myalgia, myopathy (with concurrent HMG-CoA reductase inhibitor), rhabdomyolysis (with concurrent HMG-CoA reductase inhibitor; rare), weakness
Ocular: Cystoid macular edema, toxic amblyopia
Respiratory: Dyspnea
Miscellaneous: Diaphoresis

Mechanism of Action Component of two coenzymes which is necessary for tissue respiration, lipid metabolism, and glycogenolysis; inhibits the synthesis of very low density lipoproteins

Drug Interactions

Increased Effect/Toxicity: Use with adrenergic blocking agents may result in additive vasodilating effect and postural hypotension.

Decreased Effect: The effect of oral hypoglycemics may be decreased by niacin. Niacin may inhibit uricosuric effects of sulfinpyrazone and probenecid. Aspirin (or other NSAIDs) decreases niacin-induced flushing. Bile acid sequestrants decrease the absorption of niacin.

Pharmacodynamics/Kinetics

Absorption: Rapid and extensive
Distribution: Mainly to hepatic, renal, and adipose tissue
Metabolism: Extensive first-pass effects; converted to nicotinamide (dose dependent); niacinamide (30%) hepatically metabolized
Half-life elimination: 45 minutes
Time to peak, serum: Immediate release formulation: ~45 minutes; extended release formulation: 4-5 hours
Excretion: Urine (unchanged drug and metabolites); with larger doses, greater percentage as unchanged drug

Pregnancy Risk Factor A/C (dose exceeding RDA recommendation)

Niacinamide (nye a SIN a mide)

Generic Available Yes

Synonyms Nicotinamide; Vitamin B_3

Pharmacologic Category Vitamin, Water Soluble

Use Prophylaxis and treatment of pellagra

Local Anesthetic/Vasoconstrictor Precautions No information available to require special precautions

Effects on Dental Treatment No significant effects or complications reported

Common Adverse Effects Frequency not defined.

Cardiovascular: Tachycardia
Dermatologic: Increased sebaceous gland activity, rash
Gastrointestinal: Bloating, flatulence, nausea
Neuromuscular & skeletal: Paresthesia in extremities
Ocular: Blurred vision
Respiratory: Wheezing

Mechanism of Action Used by the body as a source of niacin; is a component of two coenzymes which is necessary for tissue respiration, lipid metabolism, and glycogenolysis; inhibits the synthesis of very low density lipoproteins; does not have hypolipidemia or vasodilating effects

Pharmacodynamics/Kinetics

Absorption: Rapid
Metabolism: Hepatic
Half-life elimination: 45 minutes
Time to peak, serum: 20-70 minutes
Excretion: Urine

Pregnancy Risk Factor A/C (dose exceeding RDA recommendation)

Niacin and Lovastatin (NYE a sin & LOE va sta tin)

Related Information

Lovastatin *on page 848*
Niacin *on page 978*

U.S. Brand Names Advicor™

Generic Available No

Synonyms Lovastatin and Niacin

Pharmacologic Category Antilipemic Agent, HMG-CoA Reductase Inhibitor; Antilipemic Agent, Miscellaneous

Use Treatment of primary hypercholesterolemia (heterozygous familial and nonfamilial) and mixed dyslipidemia (Fredrickson types IIa and IIb) in patients previously treated with either agent alone (patients who require further lowering of triglycerides (TG) or increase in HDL-cholesterol (HDL-C) from addition of niacin or further lowering of LDL-cholesterol (LDL-C) from addition of lovastatin). Combination product; not intended for initial treatment.

(Continued)

Niacin and Lovastatin *(Continued)*

Local Anesthetic/Vasoconstrictor Precautions No information available to require special precautions

Effects on Dental Treatment No significant effects or complications reported

Common Adverse Effects

>10%: Cardiovascular: Flushing

1% to 10%:

Central nervous system: Headache (9%), pain (8%)

Dermatologic: Pruritus (7%), rash (5%)

Endocrine & metabolic: Hyperglycemia (4%)

Gastrointestinal: Nausea (7%), diarrhea (6%), abdominal pain (4%), dyspepsia (3%), vomiting (3%)

Neuromuscular & skeletal: Back pain (5%), weakness (5%), myalgia (3%)

Miscellaneous: Flu-like syndrome (6%)

Mechanism of Action Lovastatin acts by competitively inhibiting 3-hydroxyl-3-methylglutaryl-coenzyme A (HMG-CoA) reductase, the enzyme that catalyzes the rate-limiting step in cholesterol biosynthesis. Niacin is a component of two coenzymes which is necessary for tissue respiration, lipid metabolism, and glycogenolysis; inhibits the synthesis of very low density lipoproteins.

Drug Interactions

Cytochrome P450 Effect: Lovastatin: **Substrate** of CYP3A4 (major); **Inhibits** CYP2C8/9 (weak), 2D6 (weak), 3A4 (weak)

Increased Effect/Toxicity: See individual agents.

Decreased Effect: See individual agents.

Pharmacodynamics/Kinetics See individual agents.

Pregnancy Risk Factor X

Niacor® *see* Niacin *on page 978*

Niaspan® *see* Niacin *on page 978*

NiCARdipine (nye KAR de peen)

Related Information

Calcium Channel Blockers and Gingival Hyperplasia *on page 1600*

Calcium Channel Blockers, Comparative Pharmacokinetics *on page 1602*

Cardiovascular Diseases *on page 1458*

U.S. Brand Names Cardene®; Cardene® I.V.; Cardene® SR

Mexican Brand Names Ridene® [caps]

Generic Available Yes: Capsule

Synonyms Nicardipine Hydrochloride

Pharmacologic Category Calcium Channel Blocker

Use Chronic stable angina (immediate-release product only); management of essential hypertension (immediate and sustained release; parenteral only for short time that oral treatment is not feasible)

Unlabeled/Investigational Use Congestive heart failure

Local Anesthetic/Vasoconstrictor Precautions No information available to require special precautions

Effects on Dental Treatment Key adverse event(s) related to dental treatment: Xerostomia (normal salivary flow resumes upon discontinuation). Other drugs of this class can cause gingival hyperplasia (ie, nifedipine). The first case of nicardipine-induced gingival hyperplasia has been reported in a child taking 40-50 mg daily for 20 months.

Common Adverse Effects

1% to 10%:

Cardiovascular: Flushing (6% to 10%), palpitations (3% to 4%), tachycardia (1% to 4%), peripheral edema (dose-related 7% to 8%), increased angina (dose-related 6%), hypotension (I.V. 6%), orthostasis (I.V. 1%)

Central nervous system: Headache (6% to 15%), dizziness (4% to 7%), somnolence (4% to 6%), paresthesia (1%)

Dermatologic: Rash (1%)

Gastrointestinal: Nausea (2% to 5%), dry mouth (1%)

Genitourinary: Polyuria (1%)

Local: Injection site reaction (I.V. 1%)

Neuromuscular & skeletal: Weakness (4% to 6%), myalgia (1%)

Miscellaneous: Diaphoresis

Mechanism of Action Inhibits calcium ion from entering the "slow channels" or select voltage-sensitive areas of vascular smooth muscle and myocardium during depolarization, producing a relaxation of coronary vascular smooth muscle and coronary vasodilation; increases myocardial oxygen delivery in patients with vasospastic angina

Drug Interactions

Cytochrome P450 Effect: Substrate of CYP1A2 (minor), 2C8/9 (minor), 2D6 (minor), 2E1 (minor), 3A4 (major); **Inhibits** CYP2C8/9 (strong), 2C19 (moderate), 2D6 (moderate), 3A4 (strong)

Increased Effect/Toxicity: H_2 blockers (cimetidine) may increase the bioavailability of nicardipine. The levels/effects of nicardipine may be increased by azole antifungals, ciprofloxacin, clarithromycin, diclofenac, doxycycline, erythromycin, imatinib, isoniazid, nefazodone, propofol, protease inhibitors, quinidine, verapamil and other CYP3A4 inhibitors.

Nicardipine may increase the effect of vecuronium (reduce dose 25%). Nicardipine increase the levels/effects of amiodarone, amphetamines, selected benzodiazepines, selected beta-blockers, calcium channel blockers, cisapride, citalopram, cyclosporine, dextromethorphan, diazepam, ergot derivatives, fluoxetine, glimepiride, glipizide, HMG-CoA reductase inhibitors, lidocaine, methsuximide, mirtazapine, nateglinide, nefazodone, paroxetine, phenytoin, pioglitazone, propranolol, risperidone, ritonavir, rosiglitazone, sertraline, sildenafil (and other PDE-5 inhibitors), tacrolimus, thioridazine, tricyclic antidepressants, venlafaxine, warfarin, and other substrates of CYP2C8/9, 2C19, 2D6, or 3A4.

Decreased Effect: The levels/effects of nicardipine may be decreased by aminoglutethimide, carbamazepine, nafcillin, nevirapine, phenobarbital, phenytoin, rifamycins, and other CYP3A4 inducers. Nicardipine may decrease the levels/effects of CYP2D6 prodrug substrates (eg, codeine, hydrocodone, oxycodone, tramadol). Calcium may reduce the calcium channel blocker's effects, particularly hypotension.

Pharmacodynamics/Kinetics

Onset of action: Oral: 1-2 hours; I.V.: 10 minutes; Hypotension: ~20 minutes
Duration: 2-6 hours
Absorption: Oral: ~100%
Protein binding: 95%
Metabolism: Hepatic; extensive first-pass effect
Bioavailability: 35%
Half-life elimination: 2-4 hours
Time to peak, serum: 20-120 minutes
Excretion: Urine (as metabolites)

Pregnancy Risk Factor C

Nicardipine Hydrochloride *see* NiCARdipine *on page 980*
NicoDerm® CQ® [OTC] *see* Nicotine *on page 981*
Nicorette® [OTC] *see* Nicotine *on page 981*
Nicotinamide *see* Niacinamide *on page 979*

Nicotine (nik oh TEEN)

Related Information

Chemical Dependency and Smoking Cessation *on page 1576*

U.S. Brand Names Commit™ [OTC]; NicoDerm® CQ® [OTC]; Nicorette® [OTC]; Nicotrol® Inhaler; Nicotrol® NS; Nicotrol® Patch [OTC]

Canadian Brand Names Habitrol®; Nicoderm®; Nicorette®; Nicorette® Plus; Nicotrol®

Mexican Brand Names Nicotinell TTS®

Generic Available Yes: Transdermal patch and gum

Synonyms Habitrol®

Pharmacologic Category Smoking Cessation Aid

Use Treatment to aid smoking cessation for the relief of nicotine withdrawal symptoms (including nicotine craving)

Unlabeled/Investigational Use Management of ulcerative colitis (transdermal)

Local Anesthetic/Vasoconstrictor Precautions No information available to require special precautions

Effects on Dental Treatment Key adverse event(s) related to dental treatment: Chewing gum: Excessive salivation, mouth/throat soreness, jaw muscle ache, hiccups, tachycardia, headache (mild), vomiting, belching, nausea, xerostomia (normal salivary flow resumes upon discontinuation), dizziness, nervousness, GI distress, hoarseness, hiccups, and muscle pain.

Significant Adverse Effects

Chewing gum/lozenge:

>10%:

Cardiovascular: Tachycardia
Central nervous system: Headache (mild)
Gastrointestinal: Nausea, vomiting, indigestion, excessive salivation, belching, increased appetite

(Continued)

Nicotine *(Continued)*

Miscellaneous: Mouth or throat soreness, jaw muscle ache, hiccups

1% to 10%:

Central nervous system: Insomnia, dizziness, nervousness
Endocrine & metabolic: Dysmenorrhea
Gastrointestinal: GI distress, eructation
Neuromuscular & skeletal: Muscle pain
Respiratory: Hoarseness
Miscellaneous: Hiccups

<1% (Limited to important or life-threatening): Atrial fibrillation, erythema, hypersensitivity reactions, itching

Transdermal systems:

>10%:

Central nervous system: Insomnia, abnormal dreams
Dermatologic: Pruritus, erythema
Local: Application site reaction
Respiratory: Rhinitis, cough, pharyngitis, sinusitis

1% to 10%:

Cardiovascular: Chest pain
Central nervous system: Dysphoria, anxiety, difficulty concentrating, dizziness, somnolence
Dermatologic: Rash
Gastrointestinal: Diarrhea, dyspepsia, nausea, xerostomia, constipation, anorexia, abdominal pain
Neuromuscular & skeletal: Arthralgia, myalgia

<1% (Limited to important or life-threatening): Atrial fibrillation, hypersensitivity reactions, itching, nervousness, taste perversion, thirst, tremor

Dosage

Smoking deterrent: Patients should be advised to completely stop smoking upon initiation of therapy.

Gum: Chew 1 piece of gum when urge to smoke, up to 30 pieces/day; most patients require 10-12 pieces of gum/day

Inhaler: Usually 6 to 16 cartridges per day; best effect was achieved by frequent continuous puffing (20 minutes); recommended duration of treatment is 3 months, after which patients may be weaned from the inhaler by gradual reduction of the daily dose over 6-12 weeks

Lozenge: Patients who smoke their first cigarette within 30 minutes of waking should use the 4 mg strength; otherwise the 2 mg strength is recommended.

Weeks 1-6: One lozenge every 1-2 hours
Weeks 7-9: One lozenge every 2-4 hours
Weeks 10-12: One lozenge every 4-8 hours

Note: Use at least 9 lozenges/day during first 6 weeks to improve chances of quitting; do not use more than one lozenge at a time (maximum: 5 lozenges every 6 hours, 20 lozenges/day)

Transdermal patch: Apply new patch every 24 hours to nonhairy, clean, dry skin on the upper body or upper outer arm; each patch should be applied to a different site. **Note:** Adjustment may be required during initial treatment (move to higher dose if experiencing withdrawal symptoms; lower dose if side effects are experienced).

Habitrol®, NicoDerm CQ®:

Patients smoking ≥10 cigarettes/day: Begin with **step 1** (21 mg/day) for 4-6 weeks, followed by **step 2** (14 mg/day) for 2 weeks; finish with **step 3** (7 mg/day) for 2 weeks

Patients smoking <10 cigarettes/day: Begin with **step 2** (14 mg/day) for 6 weeks, followed by **step 3** (7 mg/day) for 2 weeks

Note: Initial starting dose for patients <100 pounds, history of cardiovascular disease: 14 mg/day for 4-6 weeks, followed by 7 mg/day for 2-4 weeks

Note: Patients receiving >600 mg/day of cimetidine: Decrease to the next lower patch size

Nicotrol®: One patch daily for 6 weeks

Note: Benefits of use of nicotine transdermal patches beyond 3 months have not been demonstrated.

Spray: 1-2 sprays/hour; do not exceed more than 5 doses (10 sprays) per hour; each dose (2 sprays) contains 1 mg of nicotine. **Warning:** A dose of 40 mg can cause fatalities.

Ulcerative colitis (unlabeled use): Transdermal: Titrated to 22-25 mg/day

Mechanism of Action Nicotine is one of two naturally-occurring alkaloids which exhibit their primary effects via autonomic ganglia stimulation. The other alkaloid is lobeline which has many actions similar to those of nicotine but is less potent. Nicotine is a potent ganglionic and central nervous system stimulant, the actions of which are mediated via nicotine-specific receptors. Biphasic actions are observed depending upon the dose administered. The main effect of nicotine in small doses is stimulation of all autonomic ganglia; with larger doses, initial stimulation is followed by blockade of transmission. Biphasic effects are also evident in the adrenal medulla; discharge of catecholamines occurs with small doses, whereas prevention of catecholamines release is seen with higher doses as a response to splanchnic nerve stimulation. Stimulation of the central nervous system (CNS) is characterized by tremors and respiratory excitation. However, convulsions may occur with higher doses, along with respiratory failure secondary to both central paralysis and peripheral blockade to respiratory muscles.

Contraindications Hypersensitivity to nicotine or any component of the formulation; patients who are smoking during the postmyocardial infarction period; patients with life-threatening arrhythmias, or severe or worsening angina pectoris; active temporomandibular joint disease (gum); pregnancy; not for use in nonsmokers

Warnings/Precautions The risk versus the benefits must be weighed for each of these groups: patients with CAD, serious cardiac arrhythmias, vasospastic disease. Use caution in patients with hyperthyroidism, pheochromocytoma, or insulin-dependent diabetes. Use with caution in oropharyngeal inflammation and in patients with history of esophagitis, peptic ulcer, coronary artery disease, vasospastic disease, angina, hypertension, hyperthyroidism, pheochromocytoma, diabetes, severe renal dysfunction, and hepatic dysfunction. The inhaler should be used with caution in patients with bronchospastic disease (other forms of nicotine replacement may be preferred). Safety and efficacy have not been established in pediatric patients. Cautious use of topical nicotine in patients with certain skin diseases. Hypersensitivity to the topical products can occur. Dental problems may be worsened by chewing the gum. Urge patients to stop smoking completely when initiating therapy.

Drug Interactions **Substrate** (minor) of CYP1A2, 2A6, 2B6, 2C8/9, 2C19, 2D6, 2E1, 3A4; **Inhibits** CYP2A6 (weak), 2E1 (weak)

Adenosine: Nicotine increases the hemodynamic and AV blocking effects of adenosine; monitor

Bupropion: Monitor for treatment-emergent hypertension in patients treated with the combination of nicotine patch and bupropion

Cimetidine; May increases nicotine concentrations; therefore, may decrease amount of gum or patches needed

Ethanol/Nutrition/Herb Interactions Food: Lozenge: Acidic foods/beverages decrease absorption of nicotine.

Dietary Considerations Each lozenge contains phenylalanine 3.4 mg.

Pharmacodynamics/Kinetics

Onset of action: Intranasal: More closely approximate the time course of plasma nicotine levels observed after cigarette smoking than other dosage forms

Duration: Transdermal: 24 hours

Absorption: Transdermal: Slow

Metabolism: Hepatic, primarily to cotinine ($^1/_5$ as active)

Half-life elimination: 4 hours

Time to peak, serum: Transdermal: 8-9 hours

Excretion: Urine

Clearance: Renal: pH dependent

Pregnancy Risk Factor D (transdermal); X (chewing gum)

Lactation Excretion in breast milk unknown/contraindicated

Dosage Forms

Gum, chewing, as polacrilex (Nicorette®): 2 mg/square (48s, 108s, 168s); 4 mg/square (48s, 108s, 168s) [mint, orange, and original flavors]

Lozenge, as polacrilex (Commit™): 2 mg, 4 mg [contains phenylalanine 3.4 mg/lozenge; mint flavor]

Oral inhalation system (Nicotrol® Inhaler): 10 mg cartridge [delivering 4 mg nicotine] (42s) [each unit consists of 1 mouthpiece, 7 storage trays each containing 6 cartridges, and 1 storage case]

Patch, transdermal: 7 mg/24 (7s, 30s); 14 mg/24 hours (7s, 14s, 30s); 21 mg/24 hours (7s, 14s, 30s)

Kit: Step 1: 21 mg/24 hours (28s); Step 2: 14 mg/24 hours (14s); Step 3: 7 mg/24 hours (14s) [kit also contains support material]

NicoDerm® CQ® [clear patch]: 7 mg/24 hours (14s); 14 mg/24 hours (14s); 21 mg/24 hours (14s)

NicoDerm® CQ® [tan patch]: 7 mg/24 hours (14s); 14 mg/24 hours (14s); 21 mg/24 hours (7s, 14s)

Nicotrol®: 15 mg/16 hours (7s)

(Continued)

Nicotine *(Continued)*

Solution, intranasal spray (Nicotrol® NS): 10 mg/mL (10 mL) [delivers 0.5 mg/spray; 200 sprays]

Selected Readings

Christen AG and Christen JA, "The Prescription of Transdermal Nicotine Patches for Tobacco-Using Dental Patients: Current Status in Indiana," *J Indiana Dent Assoc*, 1992, 71(6):12-8.

Davies GM, Willner P, James DL, et al, "Influence of Nicotine Gum on Acute Cravings for Cigarettes," *J Psychopharmacol*, 2004, 18(1):83-7.

Li Wan Po A, "Transdermal Nicotine in Smoking Cessation. A Meta-Analysis," *Eur J Clin Pharmacol*, 1993, 45(6):519-28.

Stafne EE, "The Nicotine Transdermal Patch: Use in the Dental Office Tobacco Cessation Program," *Northwest Dent*, 1994, 73(3):19-22.

Tonstad S and Johnston JA, "Does Bupropion Have Advantages Over Other Medical Therapies in the Cessation of Smoking?" *Expert Opin Pharmacother*, 2004, 5(4):727-34.

Transdermal Nicotine Study Group, "Transdermal Nicotine for Smoking Cessation. Six-Month Results From Two Multicenter Controlled Clinical Trials," *JAMA*, 1991, 266(22):3133-8.

Westman EC, Levin ED, and Rose JE, "The Nicotine Patch in Smoking Cessation," *Arch Intern Med*, 1993, 153(16):1917-23.

Wynn RL, "Nicotine Patches in Smoking Cessation," *AGD Impact*, 1994, 22:14.

Nicotinex [OTC] *see* Niacin *on page 978*

Nicotinic Acid *see* Niacin *on page 978*

Nicotrol® Inhaler *see* Nicotine *on page 981*

Nicotrol® NS *see* Nicotine *on page 981*

Nicotrol® Patch [OTC] *see* Nicotine *on page 981*

Nifedical™ XL *see* NIFEdipine *on page 984*

NIFEdipine (nye FED i peen)

Related Information

Calcium Channel Blockers and Gingival Hyperplasia *on page 1600*
Calcium Channel Blockers, Comparative Pharmacokinetics *on page 1602*
Cardiovascular Diseases *on page 1458*

U.S. Brand Names Adalat® CC; Nifedical™ XL; Procardia®; Procardia XL®

Canadian Brand Names Adalat® XL®; Apo-Nifed®; Apo-Nifed PA®; Novo-Nifedin; Nu Nifed; Procardia®

Mexican Brand Names Adalat®; Corotrend®; Nifedipres®

Generic Available Yes

Pharmacologic Category Calcium Channel Blocker

Use Angina and hypertension (sustained release only), pulmonary hypertension

Local Anesthetic/Vasoconstrictor Precautions No information available to require special precautions

Effects on Dental Treatment Nifedipine has been reported to cause 10% incidence of gingival hyperplasia; effects from 30-100 mg/day have appeared after 1-9 months. Discontinuance results in complete disappearance or marked regression of symptoms; symptoms will reappear upon remedication. Marked regression occurs after 1 week and complete disappearance of symptoms has occurred within 15 days. If a gingivectomy is performed and use of the drug is continued or resumed, hyperplasia usually will recur. The success of the gingivectomy usually requires that the medication be discontinued or that a switch to a noncalcium channel blocker be made. If for some reason nifedipine cannot be discontinued, hyperplasia has not recurred after gingivectomy when extensive plaque control was performed. If nifedipine is changed to another class of cardiovascular agent, the gingival hyperplasia will probably regress and resolve. Switching to another calcium channel blocker may result in continued hyperplasia.

Common Adverse Effects

>10%:

Cardiovascular: Flushing (10% to 25%), peripheral edema (dose-related 7% to 10%; up to 50%)

Central nervous system: Dizziness/lightheadedness/giddiness (10% to 27%), headache (10% to 23%)

Gastrointestinal: Nausea/heartburn (10% to 11%)

Neuromuscular & skeletal: Weakness (10% to 12%)

≥1% to 10%:

Cardiovascular: Palpitations (≤2% to 7%), transient hypotension (dose-related 5%), CHF (2%)

Central nervous system: Nervousness/mood changes (≤2% to 7%), shakiness (≤2%), jitteriness (≤2%), sleep disturbances (≤2%), difficulties in balance (≤2%), fever (≤2%), chills (≤2%)

Dermatologic: Dermatitis (≤2%), pruritus (≤2%), urticaria (≤2%)

Endocrine & metabolic: Sexual difficulties (≤2%)

Gastrointestinal: Diarrhea (≤2%), constipation (≤2%), cramps (≤2%), flatulence (≤2%), gingival hyperplasia (≤10%)

Neuromuscular & skeletal: Muscle cramps/tremor (≤2% to 8%), weakness (10%), inflammation (≤2%), joint stiffness (≤2%)

Ocular: Blurred vision (≤2%)

Respiratory: Dyspnea/cough/wheezing (6%), nasal congestion/sore throat (≤2% to 6%), chest congestion (≤2%), dyspnea (≤2%)

Miscellaneous: Diaphoresis (≤2%)

Dosage Oral:

Children: Hypertrophic cardiomyopathy: 0.6-0.9 mg/kg/24 hours in 3-4 divided doses

Adolescents and Adults: (**Note:** When switching from immediate release to sustained release formulations, total daily dose will start the same)

Initial: 30 mg once daily as sustained release formulation, or if indicated, 10 mg 3 times/day as capsules

Usual dose: 10-30 mg 3 times/day as capsules or 30-60 mg once daily as sustained release

Maximum dose: 120-180 mg/day

Increase sustained release at 7- to 14-day intervals

Hemodialysis: Supplemental dose is not necessary.

Peritoneal dialysis effects: Supplemental dose is not necessary.

Dosing adjustment in hepatic impairment: Reduce oral dose by 50% to 60% in patients with cirrhosis.

Mechanism of Action Inhibits calcium ion from entering the "slow channels" or select voltage-sensitive areas of vascular smooth muscle and myocardium during depolarization, producing a relaxation of coronary vascular smooth muscle and coronary vasodilation; increases myocardial oxygen delivery in patients with vasospastic angina

Contraindications Hypersensitivity to nifedipine or any component of the formulation; immediate release preparation for treatment of urgent or emergent hypertension; acute MI

Warnings/Precautions The routine use of short-acting nifedipine capsules in hypertensive emergencies and pseudoemergencies is not recommended. **The use of sublingual short-acting nifedipine in hypertensive emergencies is neither safe or effective and SHOULD BE ABANDONED!** Serious adverse events (cerebrovascular ischemia, syncope, heart block, stroke, sinus arrest, severe hypotension, acute myocardial infarction, ECG changes, and fetal distress) have been reported in relation to the administration of short-acting nifedipine in hypertensive emergencies.

Increased angina may be seen upon starting or increasing doses; may increase frequency, duration, and severity of angina during initiation of therapy; use with caution in patients with CHF or aortic stenosis (especially with concomitant beta-adrenergic blocker); severe left ventricular dysfunction, hepatic or renal impairment, hypertrophic cardiomyopathy (especially obstructive), concomitant therapy with beta-blockers or digoxin, edema

Mild and transient elevations in liver function enzymes may be apparent within 8 weeks of therapy initiation.

Therapeutic potential of sustained-release formulation (elementary osmotic pump, gastrointestinal therapeutic system [GITS]) may be decreased in patients with certain GI disorders that accelerate intestinal transit time (eg, short bowel syndrome, inflammatory bowel disease, severe diarrhea).

Note: Elderly patients may experience a greater hypotensive response and the use of the immediate release formulation in patients >71 years of age has been associated with a nearly fourfold increased risk for all-cause mortality when compared to beta-blockers, ACE inhibitors, or other classes of calcium channel blockers

Drug Interactions

Cytochrome P450 Effect: Substrate of CYP2D6 (minor), 3A4 (major); **Inhibits** CYP1A2 (moderate), 2C8/9 (weak), 2D6 (weak), 3A4 (weak)

Increased Effect/Toxicity: The levels/effects of nifedipine may be increased by azole antifungals, ciprofloxacin, clarithromycin, diclofenac, doxycycline, erythromycin, imatinib, isoniazid, nefazodone, nicardipine, propofol, protease inhibitors, quinidine, telithromycin, verapamil, and other CYP3A4 inhibitors. Cimetidine may also increase nifedipine levels. Nifedipine may increase the levels/effects of aminophylline, digoxin, fluvoxamine, mexiletine, mirtazapine, ropinirole, trifluoperazine, vincristine, and other CYP1A2 substrates. Digoxin, phenytoin, and vincristine levels may also be increased by nifedipine. Blood pressure-lowering effects may be additive with sildenafil, tadalafil, and vardenafil (use caution).

(Continued)

NIFEdipine *(Continued)*

Decreased Effect: Nifedipine may decrease quinidine serum levels. Calcium may reduce the hypotension from of calcium channel blockers. The levels/effects of nifedipine may be decreased by aminoglutethimide, carbamazepine, nafcillin, nevirapine, phenobarbital, phenytoin, rifamycins, and other CYP3A4 inducers.

Ethanol/Nutrition/Herb Interactions

Ethanol: Avoid ethanol (may increase CNS depression).

Food: Nifedipine serum levels may be decreased if taken with food. Food may decrease the rate but not the extent of absorption of Procardia XL®. Increased therapeutic and vasodilator side effects, including severe hypotension and myocardial ischemia, may occur if nifedipine is taken by patients ingesting grapefruit.

Herb/Nutraceutical: St John's wort may decrease nifedipine levels. Avoid dong quai if using for hypertension (has estrogenic activity). Avoid ephedra, yohimbe, ginseng (may worsen hypertension). Avoid garlic (may have increased antihypertensive effect).

Dietary Considerations Capsule is rapidly absorbed orally if it is administered without food, but may result in vasodilator side effects; administration with low-fat meals may decrease flushing. Avoid grapefruit juice.

Pharmacodynamics/Kinetics

Onset of action: ~20 minutes

Protein binding (concentration dependent): 92% to 98%

Metabolism: Hepatic to inactive metabolites

Bioavailability: Capsules: 45% to 75%; Sustained release: 65% to 86%

Half-life elimination: Adults: Healthy: 2-5 hours, Cirrhosis: 7 hours; Elderly: 6.7 hours

Excretion: Urine

Pregnancy Risk Factor C

Dosage Forms CAP, liquid-filled (Procardia®): 10 mg, 20 mg. **TAB, extended release:** 30 mg, 60 mg, 90 mg; (Adalat® CC, Procardia XL®): 30 mg, 60 mg, 90 mg; (Nifedical™ XL): 30 mg, 60 mg

Selected Readings

Deen-Duggins L, Fry HR, Clay JR, et al, "Nifedipine-Associated Gingival Overgrowth: A Survey of the Literature and Report of Four Cases," *Quintessence Int*, 1996, 27(3):163-70.

Desai P and Silver JG, "Drug-Induced Gingival Enlargements," *J Can Dent Assoc*, 1998, 64(4):263-8.

Harel-Raviv M, Eckler M, Lalani K, et al, "Nifedipine-Induced Gingival Hyperplasia. A Comprehensive Review and Analysis," *Oral Surg Oral Med Oral Pathol Oral Radiol Endod*, 1995, 79(6):715-22.

Lederman D, Lumerman H, Reuben S, et al, "Gingival Hyperplasia Associated With Nifedipine Therapy," *Oral Surg Oral Med Oral Pathol*, 1984, 57(6):620-2.

Lucas RM, Howell LP, and Wall BA, "Nifedipine-Induced Gingival Hyperplasia: A Histochemical and Ultrastructural Study," *J Periodontol*, 1985, 56(4):211-5.

Nery EB, Edson RG, Lee KK, et al, "Prevalence of Nifedipine-Induced Gingival Hyperplasia," *J Periodontol*, 1995, 66(7):572-8.

Nishikawa SJ, Tada H, Hamasaki A, et al, "Nifedipine-Induced Gingival Hyperplasia: A Clinical and In Vitro Study," *J Periodontol*, 1991, 62(1):30-5.

Pilloni A, Camargo PM, Carere M, et al, "Surgical Treatment of Cyclosporine A- and Nifedipine-Induced Gingival Enlargement: Gingivectomy Versus Periodontal Flap," *J Periodontol*, 1998, 69(7):791-7.

Saito K, Mori S, Iwakura M, et al, "Immunohistochemical Localization of Transforming Growth Factor Beta, Basic Fibroblast Growth Factor and Heparin Sulphate Glycosaminoglycan in Gingival Hyperplasia Induced by Nifedipine and Phenytoin," *J Periodontal Res*, 1996, 31(8):545-5.

Silverstein LH, Koch JP, Lefkove MD, et al, "Nifedipine-Induced Gingival Enlargement Around Dental Implants: A Clinical Report," *J Oral Implantol*, 1995, 21(2):116-20.

Westbrook P, Bednarczyk EM, Carlson M, et al, "Regression of Nifedipine-Induced Gingival Hyperplasia Following Switch to a Same Class Calcium Channel Blocker, Isradipine," *J Periodontol*, 1997, 68(7):645-50.

Wynn RL, "Calcium Channel Blockers and Gingival Hyperplasia," *Gen Dent*, 1991, 39(4):240-3.

Wynn RL, "Update on Calcium Channel Blocker-Induced Gingival Hyperplasia," *Gen Dent*, 1995, 43(3):218-22.

Niferex® [OTC] *see* Polysaccharide-Iron Complex *on page 1101*

Niferex® 150 [OTC] *see* Polysaccharide-Iron Complex *on page 1101*

Niftolid *see* Flutamide *on page 615*

Nilandron® *see* Nilutamide *on page 986*

Nilutamide (ni LOO ta mide)

U.S. Brand Names Nilandron®

Canadian Brand Names Anandron®

Generic Available No

Synonyms RU-23908

Pharmacologic Category Antiandrogen; Antineoplastic Agent, Antiandrogen

Use Treatment of metastatic prostate cancer

Local Anesthetic/Vasoconstrictor Precautions No information available to require special precautions

Effects on Dental Treatment Key adverse event(s) related to dental treatment: Xerostomia (normal salivary flow resumes upon discontinuation).

Common Adverse Effects

>10%:

Central nervous system: Headache, insomnia

Endocrine & metabolic: Hot flashes (30% to 67%), gynecomastia (10%)

Gastrointestinal: Nausea (mild - 10% to 32%), abdominal pain (10%), constipation, anorexia

Genitourinary: Testicular atrophy (16%), libido decreased

Hepatic: Transient elevation in serum transaminases (8% to 13%)

Ocular: Impaired dark adaptation (13% to 57%), usually reversible with dose reduction, may require discontinuation of the drug in 1% to 2% of patients

Respiratory: Dyspnea (11%)

1% to 10%:

Cardiovascular: Chest pain, edema, heart failure, hypertension, syncope

Central nervous system: Dizziness, drowsiness, malaise, hypesthesia, depression

Dermatologic: Pruritus, alopecia, dry skin, rash

Endocrine & metabolic: Disulfiram-like reaction (hot flashes, rashes) (5%); Flu-like syndrome, fever

Gastrointestinal: Vomiting, diarrhea, dyspepsia, GI hemorrhage, melena, weight loss, xerostomia

Genitourinary: Hematuria, nocturia

Hematologic: Anemia

Hepatic: Hepatitis (1%)

Neuromuscular & skeletal: Arthritis, paresthesia

Ocular: Chromatopsia (9%), abnormal vision (6% to 7%), cataracts, photophobia

Respiratory: Interstitial pneumonitis (2% - typically exertional dyspnea, cough, chest pain, and fever; most often occurring within the first 3 months of treatment); rhinitis

Miscellaneous: Diaphoresis

Mechanism of Action Nonsteroidal antiandrogen that inhibits androgen uptake or inhibits binding of androgen in target tissues. It specifically blocks the action of androgens by interacting with cytosolic androgen receptor F sites in target tissue

Drug Interactions

Cytochrome P450 Effect: Substrate of CYP2C19 (major); **Inhibits** CYP2C19 (weak)

Increased Effect/Toxicity: CYP2C19 inhibitors may increase the levels/effects of nilutamide; example inhibitors include delavirdine, fluconazole, fluvoxamine, gemfibrozil, isoniazid, omeprazole, and ticlopidine.

Decreased Effect: CYP2C19 inducers may decrease the levels/effects of nilutamide; example inducers include aminoglutethimide, carbamazepine, phenytoin, and rifampin.

Pharmacodynamics/Kinetics

Absorption: Rapid and complete

Protein binding: 72% to 85%

Metabolism: Hepatic, forms active metabolites

Half-life elimination: Terminal: 23-87 hours; Metabolites: 35-137 hours

Excretion: Urine (up to 78% at 120 hours; <1% as unchanged drug); feces (1% to 7%)

Pregnancy Risk Factor C

Nimodipine (nye MOE di peen)

Related Information

Calcium Channel Blockers and Gingival Hyperplasia *on page 1600*

Calcium Channel Blockers, Comparative Pharmacokinetics *on page 1602*

Cardiovascular Diseases *on page 1458*

U.S. Brand Names Nimotop®

Canadian Brand Names Nimotop®

Mexican Brand Names Nimotop®

Generic Available No

Pharmacologic Category Calcium Channel Blocker

Use Spasm following subarachnoid hemorrhage from ruptured intracranial aneurysms regardless of the patients neurological condition postictus (Hunt and Hess grades I-V)

Local Anesthetic/Vasoconstrictor Precautions No information available to require special precautions

(Continued)

Nimodipine *(Continued)*

Effects on Dental Treatment Other drugs of this class can cause gingival hyperplasia (ie, nifedipine) but there have been no reports for nimodipine.

Common Adverse Effects 1% to 10%:

Cardiovascular: Reductions in systemic blood pressure (1% to 8%)
Central nervous system: Headache (1% to 4%)
Dermatologic: Rash (1% to 2%)
Gastrointestinal: Diarrhea (2% to 4%), abdominal discomfort (2%)

Mechanism of Action Nimodipine shares the pharmacology of other calcium channel blockers; animal studies indicate that nimodipine has a greater effect on cerebral arterials than other arterials; this increased specificity may be due to the drug's increased lipophilicity and cerebral distribution as compared to nifedipine; inhibits calcium ion from entering the "slow channels" or select voltage sensitive areas of vascular smooth muscle and myocardium during depolarization

Drug Interactions

Cytochrome P450 Effect: Substrate of CYP3A4 (major)

Increased Effect/Toxicity: Calcium channel blockers and nimodipine may result in enhanced cardiovascular effects of other calcium channel blockers. Cimetidine, omeprazole, and valproic acid may increase serum nimodipine levels. The effects of antihypertensive agents may be increased by nimodipine. Blood pressure-lowering effects may be additive with sildenafil, tadalafil, and vardenafil (use caution). CYP3A4 inhibitors may increase the levels/effects of nimodipine; example inhibitors include azole antifungals, ciprofloxacin, clarithromycin, diclofenac, doxycycline, erythromycin, imatinib, isoniazid, nefazodone, nicardipine, propofol, protease inhibitors, quinidine, and verapamil.

Decreased Effect: CYP3A4 inducers may decrease the levels/effects of nimodipine; example inducers include aminoglutethimide, carbamazepine, nafcillin, nevirapine, phenobarbital, phenytoin, and rifamycins.

Pharmacodynamics/Kinetics

Protein binding: >95%
Metabolism: Extensively hepatic
Bioavailability: 13%
Half-life elimination: 3 hours; prolonged with renal impairment
Time to peak, serum: ~1 hour
Excretion: Urine (50%) and feces (32%) within 4 days

Pregnancy Risk Factor C

Nimotop® *see* Nimodipine *on page 987*
Nipent® *see* Pentostatin *on page 1065*

Nisoldipine (NYE sole di peen)

Related Information

Calcium Channel Blockers, Comparative Pharmacokinetics *on page 1602*
Cardiovascular Diseases *on page 1458*

U.S. Brand Names Sular®

Mexican Brand Names Sular®; Syscor®

Generic Available No

Pharmacologic Category Calcium Channel Blocker

Use Management of hypertension, alone or in combination with other antihypertensive agents

Local Anesthetic/Vasoconstrictor Precautions No information available to require special precautions

Effects on Dental Treatment Key adverse event(s) related to dental treatment: Xerostomia (normal salivary flow resumes upon discontinuation).

Common Adverse Effects

>10%:

Cardiovascular: Peripheral edema (dose-related 7% to 29%)
Central nervous system: Headache (22%)

1% to 10%:

Cardiovascular: Chest pain (2%), palpitations (3%), vasodilation (4%)
Central nervous system: Dizziness (3% to 10%)
Dermatologic: Rash (2%)
Gastrointestinal: Nausea (2%)
Respiratory: Pharyngitis (5%), sinusitis (3%), dyspnea (3%), cough (5%)

Mechanism of Action As a dihydropyridine calcium channel blocker, structurally similar to nifedipine, nisoldipine impedes the movement of calcium ions into vascular smooth muscle and cardiac muscle. Dihydropyridines are potent vasodilators and are not as likely to suppress cardiac contractility and slow cardiac conduction as other calcium antagonists such as verapamil and diltiazem; nisoldipine is 5-10 times as potent a vasodilator as nifedipine.

Drug Interactions

Cytochrome P450 Effect: Substrate of CYP3A4 (major); **Inhibits** CYP1A2 (weak), 3A4 (weak)

Increased Effect/Toxicity: CYP3A4 inhibitors may increase the levels/effects of nisoldipine; example inhibitors include azole antifungals, ciprofloxacin, clarithromycin, diclofenac, doxycycline, erythromycin, imatinib, isoniazid, nefazodone, nicardipine, propofol, protease inhibitors, quinidine, and verapamil. Calcium may reduce the calcium channel blocker's effects, particularly hypotension. Blood pressure-lowering effects may be additive with sildenafil, tadalafil, and vardenafil (use caution). Digoxin and nisoldipine may increase digoxin effect.

Decreased Effect: CYP3A4 inducers may decrease the levels/effects of nisoldipine; example inducers include aminoglutethimide, carbamazepine, nafcillin, nevirapine, phenobarbital, phenytoin, and rifamycins. Calcium may decrease the hypotension from calcium channel blockers.

Pharmacodynamics/Kinetics

Duration: >24 hours

Absorption: Well absorbed

Metabolism: Extensively hepatic to inactive metabolites; first-pass effect

Bioavailability: 5%

Half-life elimination: 7-12 hours

Time to peak: 6-12 hours

Excretion: Urine

Pregnancy Risk Factor C

Nitalapram *see* Citalopram *on page 339*

Nitazoxanide (nye ta ZOX a nide)

U.S. Brand Names Alinia™

Mexican Brand Names Colufase®; NTZ®

Generic Available No

Synonyms NTZ

Pharmacologic Category Antiprotozoal

Use Treatment of diarrhea caused by *Cryptosporidium parvum* and *Giardia lamblia* in pediatric patients 1-11 years of age

Local Anesthetic/Vasoconstrictor Precautions No information available to require special precautions

Effects on Dental Treatment No significant effects or complications reported

Common Adverse Effects Rates of adverse effects were similar to those reported with placebo.

1% to 10%:

Central nervous system: Headache (1%)

Gastrointestinal: Abdominal pain (8%), diarrhea (2%), vomiting (1%)

Mechanism of Action Nitazoxanide is rapidly metabolized to the active metabolite tizoxanide *in vivo*. Activity may be due to interference with the pyruvate:ferredoxin oxidoreductase (PFOR) enzyme-dependent electron transfer reaction which is essential to anaerobic metabolism. *In vitro*, nitazoxanide and tizoxanide inhibit the growth of sporozoites and oocysts of *Cryptosporidium parvum* and trophozoites of *Giardia lamblia*.

Pharmacodynamics/Kinetics

Protein binding: Tizoxanide: >99%

Metabolism: Hepatic, to an active metabolite, tizoxanide. Tizoxanide undergoes conjugation to form tizoxanide glucuronide. Nitazoxanide is not detectable in the serum following oral administration.

Time to peak, plasma: Tizoxanide and tizoxanide glucuronide: 1-4 hours

Excretion: Tizoxanide: Urine, bile, and feces; Tizoxanide glucuronide: Urine and bile

Pregnancy Risk Factor B

Nitisinone (ni TIS i known)

U.S. Brand Names Orfadin®

Generic Available No

Pharmacologic Category 4-Hydroxyphenylpyruvate Dioxygenase Inhibitor

Use Treatment of hereditary tyrosinemia type 1 (HT-1); to be used with dietary restriction of tyrosine and phenylalanine

Local Anesthetic/Vasoconstrictor Precautions No information available to require special precautions

Effects on Dental Treatment No significant effects or complications reported

(Continued)

Nitisinone *(Continued)*

Mechanism of Action In patients with HT-1, tyrosine metabolism is interrupted due to a lack of the enzyme (fumarylacetoacetate hydrolase) needed in the last step of tyrosine degradation. Toxic metabolites of tyrosine accumulate and cause liver and kidney toxicity. Nitisinone competitively inhibits 4-hydroxyphenyl-pyruvate dioxygenase, an enzyme needed earlier in the tyrosine degradation pathway, and therefore prevents the build-up of the damaging metabolites.

Pregnancy Risk Factor C

Nitrek® *see* Nitroglycerin *on page 991*

Nitric Oxide (NYE trik OKS ide)

U.S. Brand Names INOmax®

Canadian Brand Names INOmax®

Generic Available No

Pharmacologic Category Vasodilator, Pulmonary

Use Treatment of term and near-term (>34 weeks) neonates with hypoxic respiratory failure associated with pulmonary hypertension; used concurrently with ventilatory support and other agents

Unlabeled/Investigational Use Treatment of adult respiratory distress syndrome (ARDS)

Local Anesthetic/Vasoconstrictor Precautions No information available to require special precautions

Effects on Dental Treatment No significant effects or complications reported

Common Adverse Effects

>10%:

Cardiovascular: Hypotension (13%)

Miscellaneous: Withdrawal syndrome (12%)

1% to 10%:

Dermatologic: Cellulitis (5%)

Endocrine & metabolic: Hyperglycemia (8%)

Genitourinary: Hematuria (8%)

Respiratory: Atelectasis (9% - same as placebo), stridor (5%)

Miscellaneous: Sepsis (7%), infection (6%)

Mechanism of Action In neonates with persistent pulmonary hypertension, nitric oxide improves oxygenation. Nitric oxide relaxes vascular smooth muscle by binding to the heme moiety of cytosolic guanylate cyclase, activating guanylate cyclase and increasing intracellular levels of cyclic guanosine 3',5'-monophosphate, which leads to vasodilation. When inhaled, pulmonary vasodilation occurs and an increase in the partial pressure of arterial oxygen results. Dilation of pulmonary vessels in well ventilated lung areas redistributes blood flow away from lung areas where ventilation/perfusion ratios are poor.

Drug Interactions

Increased Effect/Toxicity: Concurrent use of sodium nitroprusside, nitroglycerin, or prilocaine may result in an increased risk of developing methemoglobinemia.

Pharmacodynamics/Kinetics

Absorption: Systemic after inhalation

Metabolism: Nitric oxide combines with hemoglobin that is 60% to 100% oxygenated. Nitric oxide combines with oxyhemoglobin to produce methemoglobin and nitrate. Within the pulmonary system, nitric oxide can combine with oxygen and water to produce nitrogen dioxide and nitrite respectively, which interact with oxyhemoglobin to then produce methemoglobin and nitrate. At 80 ppm the methemoglobin percent is ~5% after 8 hours of administration. Methemoglobin levels >7% were attained only in patients receiving 80 ppm.

Excretion: Urine (as nitrate)

Clearance: Nitrate: At a rate approaching the glomerular filtration rate

Pregnancy Risk Factor C

4'-Nitro-3'-Trifluoromethylisobutyrantide *see* Flutamide *on page 615*

Nitro-Bid® *see* Nitroglycerin *on page 991*

Nitro-Dur® *see* Nitroglycerin *on page 991*

Nitrofurantoin (nye troe fyoor AN toyn)

U.S. Brand Names Furadantin®; Macrobid®; Macrodantin®

Canadian Brand Names Apo-Nitrofurantoin®; MacroBID®; Macrodantin®; Novo-Furantoin

Mexican Brand Names Macrodantina®

Generic Available Yes: Excludes suspension

Pharmacologic Category Antibiotic, Miscellaneous

Use Prevention and treatment of urinary tract infections caused by susceptible gram-negative and some gram-positive organisms; *Pseudomonas*, *Serratia*, and most species of *Proteus* are generally resistant to nitrofurantoin

Local Anesthetic/Vasoconstrictor Precautions No information available to require special precautions

Effects on Dental Treatment No significant effects or complications reported

Common Adverse Effects Frequency not defined.

Cardiovascular: Chest pain, cyanosis, ECG changes (associated with pulmonary toxicity)

Central nervous system: Chills, depression, dizziness, drowsiness, fatigue, fever, headache, pseudotumor cerebri, psychotic reaction

Dermatologic: Alopecia, erythema multiforme, exfoliative dermatitis, pruritus, rash, Stevens-Johnson syndrome

Gastrointestinal: Abdominal pain, *C. difficile*-colitis, constipation, diarrhea, dyspepsia, loss of appetite, nausea (most common), pancreatitis, sore throat, vomiting

Hematologic: Agranulocytosis, aplastic anemia, eosinophilia, hemolytic anemia, methemoglobinemia, thrombocytopenia

Hepatic: Cholestasis, hepatitis, hepatic necrosis, serum transaminases increased, jaundice (cholestatic)

Neuromuscular & skeletal: Arthralgia, numbness, paresthesia, peripheral neuropathy, weakness

Ocular: Amblyopia, nystagmus, optic neuritis (rare)

Respiratory: Cough, dyspnea, pneumonitis, pulmonary fibrosis

Miscellaneous: Hypersensitivity (including acute pulmonary hypersensitivity), lupus-like syndrome

Mechanism of Action Inhibits several bacterial enzyme systems including acetyl coenzyme A interfering with metabolism and possibly cell wall synthesis

Drug Interactions

Increased Effect/Toxicity: Probenecid decreases renal excretion of nitrofurantoin.

Decreased Effect: Antacids decrease absorption of nitrofurantoin.

Pharmacodynamics/Kinetics

Absorption: Well absorbed; macrocrystalline form absorbed more slowly due to slower dissolution (causes less GI distress)

Distribution: V_d: 0.8 L/kg; crosses placenta; enters breast milk

Protein binding: 60% to 90%

Metabolism: Body tissues (except plasma) metabolize 60% of drug to inactive metabolites

Bioavailability: Increased with food

Half-life elimination: 20-60 minutes; prolonged with renal impairment

Excretion:

Suspension: Urine (40%) and feces (small amounts) as metabolites and unchanged drug

Macrocrystals: Urine (20% to 25% as unchanged drug)

Pregnancy Risk Factor B (contraindicated at term)

Nitrogard® *see* Nitroglycerin *on page 991*

Nitroglycerin (nye troe GLI ser in)

Related Information

Cardiovascular Diseases *on page 1458*
Dental Office Emergencies *on page 1584*

U.S. Brand Names Minitran™; Nitrek®; Nitro-Bid®; Nitro-Dur®; Nitrogard®; Nitrol® [DSC]; Nitrolingual®; NitroQuick®; Nitrostat®; Nitro-Tab®; NitroTime®

Canadian Brand Names Gen-Nitro; Minitran™; Nitro-Dur®; Nitrol®; Nitrostat™; Rho-Nitro; Transderm-Nitro®

Mexican Brand Names Anglix®; Cardinit®; Minitran®; Nitradisc®; Nitroderm TTS®; Nitro-DUR®; Nitro-Dur®

Generic Available Yes: Capsule, injection, patch, tablet

Synonyms Glyceryl Trinitrate; Nitroglycerol; NTG

Pharmacologic Category Vasodilator

Use Treatment of angina pectoris; I.V. for congestive heart failure (especially when associated with acute myocardial infarction); pulmonary hypertension; hypertensive emergencies occurring perioperatively (especially during cardiovascular surgery)

Local Anesthetic/Vasoconstrictor Precautions No information available to require special precautions

Effects on Dental Treatment No significant effects or complications reported

(Continued)

Nitroglycerin *(Continued)*

Common Adverse Effects

Spray or patch:

>10%: Central nervous system: Headache (patch 63%, spray 50%)

1% to 10%:

Cardiovascular: Hypotension (patch 4%), increased angina (patch 2%)

Central nervous system: Lightheadedness (patch 6%), syncope (patch 4%)

Topical, sublingual, intravenous: Frequency not defined:

Cardiovascular: Hypotension (infrequent), postural hypotension, crescendo angina (uncommon), rebound hypertension (uncommon), pallor, cardiovascular collapse, tachycardia, shock, flushing, peripheral edema

Central nervous system: Headache (most common), lightheadedness (related to blood pressure changes), syncope (uncommon), dizziness, restlessness

Gastrointestinal: Nausea, vomiting, bowel incontinence, xerostomia

Genitourinary: Urinary incontinence

Hematologic: Methemoglobinemia (rare, overdose)

Neuromuscular & skeletal: Weakness

Ocular: Blurred vision

Miscellaneous: Cold sweat

The incidence of hypotension and adverse cardiovascular events may be increased when used in combination with sildenafil (Viagra®).

Dosage Note: Hemodynamic and antianginal tolerance often develop within 24-48 hours of continuous nitrate administration

Children: Pulmonary hypertension: Continuous infusion: Start 0.25-0.5 mcg/kg/minute and titrate by 1 mcg/kg/minute at 20- to 60-minute intervals to desired effect; usual dose: 1-3 mcg/kg/minute; maximum: 5 mcg/kg/minute

Adults:

Buccal: Initial: 1 mg every 3-5 hours while awake (3 times/day); titrate dosage upward if angina occurs with tablet in place

Oral: 2.5-9 mg 2-4 times/day (up to 26 mg 4 times/day)

I.V.: 5 mcg/minute, increase by 5 mcg/minute every 3-5 minutes to 20 mcg/minute; if no response at 20 mcg/minute increase by 10 mcg/minute every 3-5 minutes, up to 200 mcg/minute

Ointment: $1/2$" upon rising and $1/2$" 6 hours later; the dose may be doubled and even doubled again as needed

Patch, transdermal: Initial: 0.2-0.4 mg/hour, titrate to doses of 0.4-0.8 mg/hour; tolerance is minimized by using a patch-on period of 12-14 hours and patch-off period of 10-12 hours

Sublingual: 0.2-0.6 mg every 5 minutes for maximum of 3 doses in 15 minutes; may also use prophylactically 5-10 minutes prior to activities which may provoke an attack

Translingual: 1-2 sprays into mouth under tongue every 3-5 minutes for maximum of 3 doses in 15 minutes, may also be used 5-10 minutes prior to activities which may provoke an attack prophylactically

Hemodialysis: Supplemental dose is not necessary

Peritoneal dialysis: Supplemental dose is not necessary

May need to use nitrate-free interval (10-12 hours/day) to avoid tolerance development; gradually decrease dose in patients receiving NTG for prolonged period to avoid withdrawal reaction

Elderly: In general, dose selection should be cautious, usually starting at the low end of the dosing range

Mechanism of Action Reduces cardiac oxygen demand by decreasing left ventricular pressure and systemic vascular resistance; dilates coronary arteries and improves collateral flow to ischemic regions

Contraindications Hypersensitivity to organic nitrates; hypersensitivity to isosorbide, nitroglycerin, or any component of the formulation; concurrent use with phosphodiesterase-5 (PDE-5) inhibitors (sildenafil, tadalafil, or vardenafil); angle-closure glaucoma (intraocular pressure may be increased); head trauma or cerebral hemorrhage (increase intracranial pressure); severe anemia; allergy to adhesive (transdermal product)

I.V. product: Hypotension; uncorrected hypovolemia; inadequate cerebral circulation; increased intracranial pressure; constrictive pericarditis; pericardial tamponade

Warnings/Precautions Do not use extended release preparations in patients with GI hypermotility or malabsorptive syndrome; use with caution in patients with hepatic impairment, CHF, or acute myocardial infarction; available preparations of I.V. nitroglycerin differ in concentration or volume; pay attention to dilution and dosage; I.V. preparations contain alcohol and/or propylene glycol;

avoid loss of nitroglycerin in standard PVC tubing; dosing instructions must be followed with care when the appropriate infusion sets are used

Hypotension may occur, use with caution in patients who are volume-depleted, are hypotensive, have inadequate circulation; nitrate therapy may aggravate angina caused by hypertrophic cardiomyopathy

Drug Interactions

Increased Effect/Toxicity: Significant reduction of systolic and diastolic blood pressure with concurrent use of sildenafil, tadalafil, or vardenafil (contraindicated); do not administer sildenafil, tadalafil, or vardenafil within 24 hours of a nitrate preparation. Ethanol can cause hypotension when nitrates are taken 1 hour or more after ethanol ingestion.

Decreased Effect: I.V. nitroglycerin may antagonize the anticoagulant effect of heparin (possibly only at high nitroglycerin dosages); monitor closely. May need to decrease heparin dosage when nitroglycerin is discontinued. Alteplase (tissue plasminogen activator) has a lesser effect when used with I.V. nitroglycerin; avoid concurrent use. Ergot alkaloids may cause an increase in blood pressure and decrease in antianginal effects; avoid concurrent use.

Pharmacodynamics/Kinetics

Onset of action: Sublingual tablet: 1-3 minutes; Translingual spray: 2 minutes; Buccal tablet: 2-5 minutes; Sustained release: 20-45 minutes; Topical: 15-60 minutes; Transdermal: 40-60 minutes; I.V. drip: Immediate

Peak effect: Sublingual tablet: 4-8 minutes; Translingual spray: 4-10 minutes; Buccal tablet: 4-10 minutes; Sustained release: 45-120 minutes; Topical: 30-120 minutes; Transdermal: 60-180 minutes; I.V. drip: Immediate

Duration: Sublingual tablet: 30-60 minutes; Translingual spray: 30-60 minutes; Buccal tablet: 2 hours; Sustained release: 4-8 hours; Topical: 2-12 hours; Transdermal: 18-24 hours; I.V. drip: 3-5 minutes

Protein binding: 60%

Metabolism: Extensive first-pass effect

Half-life elimination: 1-4 minutes

Excretion: Urine (as inactive metabolites)

Pregnancy Risk Factor C

Dosage Forms AERO, translingual (Nitrolingual® Pumpspray): 0.4 mg/metered spray (12 g). **CAP, extended release** (Nitro-Time®): 2.5 mg, 6.5 mg, 9 mg. **INF** [premixed in D_5W]: 0.1 mg/mL (250 mL, 500 mL); 0.2 mg/mL (250 mL); 0.4 mg/mL (250 mL, 500 mL). **INJ, solution**: 5 mg/mL (5 mL, 10 mL). **OINT, topical** (Nitro-Bid®): 2% [20 mg/g] (30 g, 60 g). **PATCH, transdermal:** Systems deliver 0.1 mg/hour (30s), 0.2 mg/hour (30s), 0.4 mg/hour (30s), 0.6 mg/hour (30s); (Minitran™): 0.1 mg/hour (30s), 0.2 mg/hour (30s), 0.4 mg/hour (30s), 0.6 mg/hour (30s); (Nitrek®): 0.2 mg/hour (30s), 0.4 mg/hour (30s), 0.6 mg/hour (30s); (Nitro-Dur®): 0.1 mg/hour (30s), 0.2 mg/hour (30s), 0.3 mg/hour (30s), 0.4 mg/hour (30s), 0.6 mg/hour (30s), 0.8 mg/hour (30s). **TAB, buccal, extended release** (Nitrogard®): 2 mg, 3 mg. **TAB, sublingual** (NitroQuick®, Nitrostat®, NitroTab®): 0.3 mg, 0.4 mg, 0.6 mg.

Nitroglycerol *see* Nitroglycerin *on page 991*

Nitrol® [DSC] *see* Nitroglycerin *on page 991*

Nitrolingual® *see* Nitroglycerin *on page 991*

Nitropress® *see* Nitroprusside *on page 993*

Nitroprusside (nye troe PRUS ide)

Related Information

Cardiovascular Diseases *on page 1458*

U.S. Brand Names Nitropress®

Canadian Brand Names Nipride®

Generic Available Yes: Solution

Synonyms Nitroprusside Sodium; Sodium Nitroferricyanide; Sodium Nitroprusside

Pharmacologic Category Vasodilator

Use Management of hypertensive crises; congestive heart failure; used for controlled hypotension to reduce bleeding during surgery

Local Anesthetic/Vasoconstrictor Precautions No information available to require special precautions

Effects on Dental Treatment No significant effects or complications reported

Common Adverse Effects 1% to 10%:

Cardiovascular: Excessive hypotensive response, palpitations, substernal distress

Central nervous system: Disorientation, psychosis, headache, restlessness

Endocrine & metabolic: Thyroid suppression

(Continued)

Nitroprusside *(Continued)*

Gastrointestinal: Nausea, vomiting
Neuromuscular & skeletal: Weakness, muscle spasm
Otic: Tinnitus
Respiratory: Hypoxia
Miscellaneous: Diaphoresis, thiocyanate toxicity

Mechanism of Action Causes peripheral vasodilation by direct action on venous and arteriolar smooth muscle, thus reducing peripheral resistance; will increase cardiac output by decreasing afterload; reduces aortal and left ventricular impedance

Pharmacodynamics/Kinetics

Onset of action: BP reduction <2 minutes
Duration: 1-10 minutes
Metabolism: Nitroprusside is converted to cyanide ions in the bloodstream; decomposes to prussic acid which in the presence of sulfur donor is converted to thiocyanate (hepatic and renal rhodanase systems)
Half-life elimination: Parent drug: <10 minutes; Thiocyanate: 2.7-7 days
Excretion: Urine (as thiocyanate)

Pregnancy Risk Factor C

Nitroprusside Sodium *see* Nitroprusside *on page 993*

NitroQuick® *see* Nitroglycerin *on page 991*

Nitrostat® *see* Nitroglycerin *on page 991*

Nitro-Tab® *see* Nitroglycerin *on page 991*

NitroTime® *see* Nitroglycerin *on page 991*

Nitrous Oxide (NYE trus OKS ide)

Related Information

Patients Requiring Sedation *on page 1567*

Generic Available Yes

Pharmacologic Category Dental Gases; General Anesthetic

Dental Use Induction of sedation and analgesia in anxious dental patients

Use Produces sedation and analgesia; principal adjunct to inhalation and intravenous general anesthesia

Local Anesthetic/Vasoconstrictor Precautions No information available to require special precautions

Effects on Dental Treatment No significant effects or complications reported

Significant Adverse Effects Personnel exposed to unscavenged nitrous oxide have an increased risk of renal and hepatic diseases and peripheral neuropathy similar to that of vitamin B_{12} deficiency. Female dental personnel who were exposed to unscavenged nitrous oxide for more than 5 hours/week were significantly less fertile than women who were not exposed, or who were exposed to lower levels of scavenged or unscavenged nitrous oxide.

Dosage Children and Adults:

Surgical: For sedation and analgesia: Concentrations of 25% to 50% nitrous oxide with oxygen. For general anesthesia, concentrations of 40% to 70% via mask or endotracheal tube. Minimal alveolar concentration (MAC), which can be considered the ED_{50} of inhalational anesthetics, is 105%; therefore delivery in a hyperbaric chamber is necessary to use as a complete anesthetic. When administered at 70%, reduces the MAC of other anesthetics by half.

Dental: For sedation and analgesia: Concentrations of 25% to 50% nitrous oxide with oxygen

Mechanism of Action General CNS depressant action; may act similarly as inhalant general anesthetics by stabilizing axonal membranes to partially inhibit action potentials leading to sedation; may partially act on opiate receptor systems to cause mild analgesia

Contraindications Hypersensitivity to nitrous oxide or any component of the formulation; nitrous oxide should not be administered without oxygen; should not be given to patients after a full meal

Warnings/Precautions Nausea and vomiting occurs postoperatively in ~15% of patients. Prolonged use may produce bone marrow suppression and/or neurologic dysfunction. Oxygen should be briefly administered during emergence from prolonged anesthesia with nitrous oxide to prevent diffusion hypoxia. Patients with vitamin B_{12} deficiency (pernicious anemia) and those with other nutritional deficiencies (alcoholics) are at increased risk of developing neurologic disease and bone marrow suppression with exposure to nitrous oxide. May be addictive.

Drug Interactions No data reported

Pharmacodynamics/Kinetics
Onset of action: Inhalation: 2-5 minutes
Absorption: Rapid via lungs; blood/gas partition coefficient is 0.47
Metabolism: Body: <0.004%
Excretion: Primarily exhaled gases; skin (minimal amounts)
Pregnancy Risk Factor No data reported
Dosage Forms Supplied in blue cylinders

Nix® [OTC] *see* Permethrin *on page 1070*

Nizatidine (ni ZA ti deen)

Related Information
Gastrointestinal Disorders *on page 1476*
U.S. Brand Names Axid®; Axid® AR [OTC]
Canadian Brand Names Apo-Nizatidine®; Axid®; Gen-Nizatidine; Novo-Nizatidine; Nu-Nizatidine; PMS-Nizatidine
Mexican Brand Names Axid®
Generic Available Yes: Capsule
Pharmacologic Category Histamine H_2 Antagonist
Use Treatment and maintenance of duodenal ulcer; treatment of benign gastric ulcer; treatment of gastroesophageal reflux disease (GERD); OTC tablet used for the prevention of meal-induced heartburn, acid indigestion, and sour stomach
Unlabeled/Investigational Use Part of a multidrug regimen for *H. pylori* eradication to reduce the risk of duodenal ulcer recurrence
Local Anesthetic/Vasoconstrictor Precautions No information available to require special precautions
Effects on Dental Treatment Key adverse event(s) related to dental treatment: Xerostomia (normal salivary flow resumes upon discontinuation).
Common Adverse Effects
>10%: Central nervous system: Headache (16%)
1% to 10%:
Central nervous system: Anxiety, dizziness, fever (reported in children), insomnia, irritability (reported in children), somnolence, nervousness
Dermatologic: Pruritus, rash
Gastrointestinal: Abdominal pain, anorexia, constipation, diarrhea, dry mouth, flatulence, heartburn, nausea, vomiting
Respiratory: Reported in children: Cough, nasal congestion, nasopharyngitis
Mechanism of Action Competitive inhibition of histamine at H2-receptors of the gastric parietal cells resulting in reduced gastric acid secretion, gastric volume and hydrogen ion concentration reduced. In healthy volunteers, nizatidine suppresses gastric acid secretion induced by pentagastrin infusion or food.
Drug Interactions
Cytochrome P450 Effect: Inhibits 3A4 (weak)
Decreased Effect: May decrease the absorption of itraconazole or ketoconazole.
Pharmacodynamics/Kinetics
Distribution: V_d: 0.8-1.5 L/kg
Protein binding: 35% to α_1-acid glycoprotein
Metabolism: Partially hepatic; forms metabolites
Bioavailability: >70%
Half-life elimination: 1-2 hours; prolonged with renal impairment
Time to peak, plasma: 0.5-3.0 hours
Excretion: Urine (90%; ~60% as unchanged drug); feces (<6%)
Pregnancy Risk Factor B

Nizoral® *see* Ketoconazole *on page 783*
Nizoral® A-D [OTC] *see* Ketoconazole *on page 783*
N-Methylhydrazine *see* Procarbazine *on page 1125*
Nolahist® [OTC] *see* Phenindamine *on page 1073*
Nolvadex® *see* Tamoxifen *on page 1258*

Nonoxynol 9 (non OKS i nole nine)

U.S. Brand Names Advantage-S™ [OTC]; Aqua Lube Plus [OTC]; Conceptrol® [OTC]; Delfen® [OTC]; Emko® [OTC]; Encare® [OTC]; Gynol II® [OTC]; Semicid® [OTC]; Shur-Seal® [OTC]; VCF™ [OTC]
Canadian Brand Names Advantage 24™
Generic Available No
Pharmacologic Category Spermicide
Use Spermatocide in contraception
(Continued)

Nonoxynol 9 *(Continued)*

Local Anesthetic/Vasoconstrictor Precautions No information available to require special precautions

Effects on Dental Treatment No significant effects or complications reported

Common Adverse Effects Frequency not defined: Genitourinary: Irritation of mucous membranes (including vaginal/urethral)

Pregnancy Risk Factor C

Nonviral Infectious Diseases *see page 1495*

Nora-BE™ *see* Norethindrone *on page 996*

Noradrenaline *see* Norepinephrine *on page 996*

Noradrenaline Acid Tartrate *see* Norepinephrine *on page 996*

Norco® *see* Hydrocodone and Acetaminophen *on page 702*

Nordeoxyguanosine *see* Ganciclovir *on page 646*

Nordette® *see* Ethinyl Estradiol and Levonorgestrel *on page 545*

Norditropin® *see* Human Growth Hormone *on page 694*

Norditropin® Cartridges *see* Human Growth Hormone *on page 694*

Norelgestromin and Ethinyl Estradiol *see* Ethinyl Estradiol and Norelgestromin *on page 548*

Norepinephrine (nor ep i NEF rin)

U.S. Brand Names Levophed®

Canadian Brand Names Levophed®

Generic Available No

Synonyms Levarterenol Bitartrate; Noradrenaline; Noradrenaline Acid Tartrate; Norepinephrine Bitartrate

Pharmacologic Category Alpha/Beta Agonist

Use Treatment of shock which persists after adequate fluid volume replacement

Local Anesthetic/Vasoconstrictor Precautions No information available to require special precautions

Effects on Dental Treatment No significant effects or complications reported

Mechanism of Action Stimulates $beta_1$-adrenergic receptors and alpha-adrenergic receptors causing increased contractility and heart rate as well as vasoconstriction, thereby increasing systemic blood pressure and coronary blood flow; clinically alpha effects (vasoconstriction) are greater than beta effects (inotropic and chronotropic effects)

Pregnancy Risk Factor C

Norepinephrine Bitartrate *see* Norepinephrine *on page 996*

Norethindrone (nor eth IN drone)

Related Information

Endocrine Disorders and Pregnancy *on page 1481*

U.S. Brand Names Aygestin®; Camila™; Errin™; Jolivette™; Micronor®; Nora-BE™; Nor-QD®

Canadian Brand Names Micronor®; Norlutate®

Generic Available Yes

Synonyms Norethindrone Acetate; Norethisterone

Pharmacologic Category Contraceptive; Progestin

Use Treatment of amenorrhea; abnormal uterine bleeding; endometriosis, oral contraceptive; **higher rate of failure with progestin only contraceptives**

Local Anesthetic/Vasoconstrictor Precautions No information available to require special precautions

Effects on Dental Treatment Until we know more about the mechanism of interaction, caution is required in prescribing antibiotics to female dental patients taking progestin-only hormonal contraceptives.

Common Adverse Effects

>10%:

- Cardiovascular: Edema
- Endocrine & metabolic: Breakthrough bleeding, spotting, changes in menstrual flow, amenorrhea
- Gastrointestinal: Anorexia
- Local: Pain at injection site
- Neuromuscular & skeletal: Weakness

1% to 10%:

- Cardiovascular: Edema
- Central nervous system: Mental depression, fever, insomnia
- Dermatologic: Melasma or chloasma, allergic rash with or without pruritus
- Endocrine & metabolic: Increased breast tenderness
- Gastrointestinal: Weight gain/loss

Genitourinary: Changes in cervical erosion and secretions
Hepatic: Cholestatic jaundice

Mechanism of Action Inhibits secretion of pituitary gonadotropin (LH) which prevents follicular maturation and ovulation

Drug Interactions

Cytochrome P450 Effect: Substrate of CYP3A4 (major); **Induces** CYP2C19 (weak)

Decreased Effect: Nelfinavir decreases the pharmacologic effect of norethindrone. CYP3A4 inducers may decrease the levels/effects of norethindrone; example inducers include aminoglutethimide, carbamazepine, nafcillin, nevirapine, phenobarbital, phenytoin, and rifamycins.

Pharmacodynamics/Kinetics

Absorption: Oral, transdermal: Rapidly absorbed
Distribution: V_d: 2-4 L/kg
Protein binding: 61% to albumin; 36% to sex hormone-binding globulin (SHBG); SHBG capacity affected by plasma ethinyl estradiol levels
Metabolism: Oral: Hepatic via reduction and conjugation; first-pass effect
Bioavailability: 64%
Half-life elimination: 5-14 hours
Time to peak: 1-2 hours
Excretion: Primarily urine (as metabolites)

Pregnancy Risk Factor X

Norethindrone Acetate *see* Norethindrone *on page 996*

Norethindrone Acetate and Ethinyl Estradiol *see* Ethinyl Estradiol and Norethindrone *on page 550*

Norethindrone and Estradiol *see* Estradiol and Norethindrone *on page 521*

Norethindrone and Mestranol *see* Mestranol and Norethindrone *on page 884*

Norethisterone *see* Norethindrone *on page 996*

Norflex™ *see* Orphenadrine *on page 1017*

Norfloxacin (nor FLOKS a sin)

Related Information

Sexually-Transmitted Diseases *on page 1504*

U.S. Brand Names Noroxin®

Canadian Brand Names Apo-Norflox®; Norfloxacine®; Novo-Norfloxacin; PMS-Norfloxacin; Riva-Norfloxacin

Mexican Brand Names Difoxacil®; Floxacin®; Noroxin®; Oranor®

Generic Available No

Pharmacologic Category Antibiotic, Quinolone

Use Uncomplicated urinary tract infections and cystitis caused by susceptible gram-negative and gram-positive bacteria; sexually-transmitted disease (eg, uncomplicated urethral and cervical gonorrhea) caused by *N. gonorrhoeae*; prostatitis due to *E. coli*

Local Anesthetic/Vasoconstrictor Precautions No information available to require special precautions

Effects on Dental Treatment No significant effects or complications reported

Common Adverse Effects 1% to 10%:

Central nervous system: Headache (3%), dizziness (3%)
Gastrointestinal: Nausea (4%)
Neuromuscular & skeletal: Weakness (1%)

Mechanism of Action Norfloxacin is a DNA gyrase inhibitor. DNA gyrase is an essential bacterial enzyme that maintains the superhelical structure of DNA. DNA gyrase is required for DNA replication and transcription, DNA repair, recombination, and transposition; bactericidal

Drug Interactions

Cytochrome P450 Effect: Inhibits CYP1A2 (strong), 3A4 (moderate)

Increased Effect/Toxicity: Quinolones cause increased levels of caffeine, warfarin, cyclosporine, and theophylline. Cimetidine and probenecid may increase norfloxacin serum levels. Concurrent use of corticosteroids may increase risk of tendon rupture. Norfloxacin may increase the levels/effects of CYP3A4 substrates (eg, benzodiazepines, calcium channel blockers, cyclosporine, mirtazapine, nateglinide, nefazodone, sildenafil and other PDE-5 inhibitors, tacrolimus, and venlafaxine. Selected benzodiazepines (midazolam and triazolam), cisapride, ergot alkaloids, selected HMG-CoA reductase inhibitors (lovastatin and simvastatin), and pimozide are generally contraindicated with strong CYP3A4 inhibitors.

Decreased Effect: Decreased absorption with antacids containing aluminum, magnesium, and/or calcium (by up to 98% if given at the same time); decreased serum levels of fluoroquinolones by antineoplastics; nitrofurantoin may antagonize effects of norfloxacin; phenytoin serum levels may

(Continued)

Norfloxacin *(Continued)*

be decreased by fluoroquinolones; didanosine (chewable/buffered or pediatric powder) may decrease quinolone absorption

Pharmacodynamics/Kinetics

Absorption: Oral: Rapid, up to 40%

Distribution: Crosses placenta; small amounts enter breast milk

Protein binding: 15%

Metabolism: Hepatic

Half-life elimination: 3-4 hours; Renal impairment (Cl_{cr} ≤30 mL/minute): 6.5 hours; Elderly: 4 hours

Time to peak, serum: 1-2 hours

Excretion: Urine (26% to 36%); feces (30%)

Pregnancy Risk Factor C

Norgesic™ *see* Orphenadrine, Aspirin, and Caffeine *on page 1018*

Norgesic™ Forte *see* Orphenadrine, Aspirin, and Caffeine *on page 1018*

Norgestimate and Estradiol *see* Estradiol and Norgestimate *on page 521*

Norgestimate and Ethinyl Estradiol *see* Ethinyl Estradiol and Norgestimate *on page 554*

Norgestrel (nor JES trel)

Related Information

Endocrine Disorders and Pregnancy *on page 1481*

U.S. Brand Names Ovrette®

Canadian Brand Names Ovrette®

Generic Available No

Pharmacologic Category Contraceptive; Progestin

Use Prevention of pregnancy; **progestin only products have higher risk of failure in contraceptive use**

Local Anesthetic/Vasoconstrictor Precautions No information available to require special precautions

Effects on Dental Treatment Until we know more about the mechanism of interaction, caution is required in prescribing antibiotics to female dental patients taking progestin-only hormonal contraceptives.

Common Adverse Effects Frequency not defined.

Cardiovascular: Embolism, cerebral thrombosis, edema

Central nervous system: Mental depression, fever, insomnia

Dermatologic: Melasma or chloasma, allergic rash with or without pruritus

Endocrine & metabolic: Breakthrough bleeding, spotting, changes in menstrual flow, amenorrhea, changes in cervical erosion and secretions, increased breast tenderness

Gastrointestinal: Weight gain/loss, anorexia

Hepatic: Cholestatic jaundice

Local: Thrombophlebitis

Neuromuscular & skeletal: Weakness

Mechanism of Action Inhibits secretion of pituitary gonadotropin (LH) which prevents follicular maturation and ovulation

Drug Interactions

Cytochrome P450 Effect: Substrate of CYP3A4 (major)

Increased Effect/Toxicity: Oral contraceptives may increase toxicity of acetaminophen, anticoagulants, benzodiazepines, caffeine, corticosteroids, metoprolol, theophylline, and tricyclic antidepressants.

Decreased Effect: CYP3A4 inducers may decrease the levels/effects of norgestrel; example inducers include aminoglutethimide, carbamazepine, nafcillin, nevirapine, phenobarbital, phenytoin, and rifamycins. Antibiotics (penicillins, tetracyclines, griseofulvin) were reported to decrease efficacy of oral contraceptives, but this has not been validated in more rigorous investigations.

Pharmacodynamics/Kinetics

Absorption: Oral: Well absorbed

Protein binding: >97% to sex hormone-binding globulin

Metabolism: Primarily hepatic via reduction and conjugation

Half-life elimination: ~20 hours

Excretion: Urine (as metabolites)

Pregnancy Risk Factor X

Norgestrel and Ethinyl Estradiol *see* Ethinyl Estradiol and Norgestrel *on page 557*

Norinyl® 1+35 *see* Ethinyl Estradiol and Norethindrone *on page 550*

Norinyl® 1+50 *see* Mestranol and Norethindrone *on page 884*

Noritate® *see* Metronidazole *on page 917*

Normal Blood Values *see page 1620*
Normal Saline *see* Sodium Chloride *on page 1227*
Normodyne® *see* Labetalol *on page 791*
Noroxin® *see* Norfloxacin *on page 997*
Norpace® *see* Disopyramide *on page 455*
Norpace® CR *see* Disopyramide *on page 455*
Norpramin® *see* Desipramine *on page 407*
Nor-QD® *see* Norethindrone *on page 996*
Nortrel™ *see* Ethinyl Estradiol and Norethindrone *on page 550*
Nortrel™ 7/7/7 *see* Ethinyl Estradiol and Norethindrone *on page 550*

Nortriptyline (nor TRIP ti leen)

U.S. Brand Names Aventyl® HCl; Pamelor®

Canadian Brand Names Alti-Nortriptyline; Apo-Nortriptyline®; Aventyl®; Gen-Nortriptyline; Norventyl; Novo-Nortriptyline; Nu-Nortriptyline; PMS-Nortriptyline

Generic Available Yes

Synonyms Nortriptyline Hydrochloride

Pharmacologic Category Antidepressant, Tricyclic (Secondary Amine)

Use Treatment of symptoms of depression

Unlabeled/Investigational Use Chronic pain, anxiety disorders, enuresis, attention-deficit/hyperactivity disorder (ADHD)

Local Anesthetic/Vasoconstrictor Precautions Use with caution; epinephrine, norepinephrine and levonordefrin have been shown to have an increased pressor response in combination with TCAs

Effects on Dental Treatment Key adverse event(s) related to dental treatment: Xerostomia (normal salivary flow resumes upon discontinuation). Long-term treatment with TCAs, such as nortriptyline, increases the risk of caries by reducing salivation and salivary buffer capacity.

Common Adverse Effects Frequency not defined.

Cardiovascular: Postural hypotension, arrhythmias, hypertension, heart block, tachycardia, palpitations, myocardial infarction

Central nervous system: Confusion, delirium, hallucinations, restlessness, insomnia, disorientation, delusions, anxiety, agitation, panic, nightmares, hypomania, exacerbation of psychosis, incoordination, ataxia, extrapyramidal symptoms, seizures

Dermatologic: Alopecia, photosensitivity, rash, petechiae, urticaria, itching

Endocrine & metabolic: Sexual dysfunction, gynecomastia, breast enlargement, galactorrhea, increase or decrease in libido, increase in blood sugar, SIADH

Gastrointestinal: Xerostomia, constipation, vomiting, anorexia, diarrhea, abdominal cramps, black tongue, nausea, unpleasant taste, weight gain/loss

Genitourinary: Urinary retention, delayed micturition, impotence, testicular edema

Hematologic: Rarely agranulocytosis, eosinophilia, purpura, thrombocytopenia

Hepatic: Increased liver enzymes, cholestatic jaundice

Neuromuscular & skeletal: Tremor, numbness, tingling, paresthesias, peripheral neuropathy

Ocular: Blurred vision, eye pain, disturbances in accommodation, mydriasis

Otic: Tinnitus

Miscellaneous: Diaphoresis (excessive), allergic reactions

Dosage Oral:

- Nocturnal enuresis:
  - Children:
    - 6-7 years (20-25 kg): 10 mg/day
    - 8-11 years (25-35 kg): 10-20 mg/day
    - >11 years (35-54 kg): 25-35 mg/day
- Depression or ADHD (unlabeled use):
  - Children 6-12 years: 1-3 mg/kg/day or 10-20 mg/day in 3-4 divided doses
  - Adolescents: 30-100 mg/day in divided doses
- Depression:
  - Adults: 25 mg 3-4 times/day up to 150 mg/day
  - Elderly (**Note:** Nortriptyline is one of the best tolerated TCAs in the elderly)
    - Initial: 10-25 mg at bedtime
    - Dosage can be increased by 25 mg every 3 days for inpatients and weekly for outpatients if tolerated
    - Usual maintenance dose: 75 mg as a single bedtime dose or 2 divided doses; however, lower or higher doses may be required to stay within the therapeutic window

(Continued)

Nortriptyline *(Continued)*

Dosing adjustment in hepatic impairment: Lower doses and slower titration dependent on individualization of dosage is recommended

Mechanism of Action Traditionally believed to increase the synaptic concentration of serotonin and/or norepinephrine in the central nervous system by inhibition of their reuptake by the presynaptic neuronal membrane. However, additional receptor effects have been found including desensitization of adenyl cyclase, down regulation of beta-adrenergic receptors, and down regulation of serotonin receptors.

Contraindications Hypersensitivity to nortriptyline and similar chemical class, or any component of the formulation; use of MAO inhibitors within 14 days; use in a patient during the acute recovery phase of MI; pregnancy

Warnings/Precautions May cause sedation, resulting in impaired performance of tasks requiring alertness (eg, operating machinery or driving). Sedative effects may be additive with other CNS depressants and/or ethanol. The degree of sedation is low-moderate relative to other antidepressants. May worsen psychosis in some patients or precipitate a shift to mania or hypomania in patients with bipolar disease. May increase the risks associated with electroconvulsive therapy. This agent should be discontinued, when possible, prior to elective surgery. Therapy should not be abruptly discontinued in patients receiving high doses for prolonged periods. May alter glucose regulation - use caution in patients with diabetes.

May cause orthostatic hypotension (risk is low relative to other antidepressants) - use with caution in patients at risk of hypotension or in patients where transient hypotensive episodes would be poorly tolerated (cardiovascular disease or cerebrovascular disease). The degree of anticholinergic blockade produced by this agent is moderate relative to other cyclic antidepressants, however, caution should still be used in patients with urinary retention, benign prostatic hypertrophy, narrow-angle glaucoma, xerostomia, visual problems, constipation, or history of bowel obstruction.

The possibility of a suicide attempt is inherent in major depression and may persist until remission occurs. Use caution in high-risk patients during initiation of therapy. Prescriptions should be written for the smallest quantity consistent with good patient care. Use with caution in patients with a history of cardiovascular disease (including previous MI, stroke, tachycardia, or conduction abnormalities). The risk conduction abnormalities with this agent is moderate relative to other antidepressants. Use caution in patients with a previous seizure disorder or condition predisposing to seizures such as brain damage, alcoholism, or concurrent therapy with other drugs which lower the seizure threshold. Use with caution in hyperthyroid patients or those receiving thyroid supplementation. Use with caution in patients with hepatic or renal dysfunction and in elderly patients.

Drug Interactions

Cytochrome P450 Effect: Substrate of CYP1A2 (minor), 2C19 (minor), 2D6 (major), 3A4 (minor); **Inhibits** CYP2D6 (weak), 2E1 (weak)

Increased Effect/Toxicity: Nortriptyline increases the effects of amphetamines, anticholinergics, other CNS depressants (sedatives, hypnotics, ethanol), chlorpropamide, tolazamide, and warfarin. When used with MAO inhibitors, hyperpyrexia, hypertension, tachycardia, confusion, seizures, and **deaths have been reported** (serotonin syndrome). Serotonin syndrome has also been reported with ritonavir (rare). CYP2D6 inhibitors may increase the levels/effects of nortriptyline; example inhibitors include chlorpromazine, delavirdine, fluoxetine, miconazole, paroxetine, pergolide, quinidine, quinine, ritonavir, and ropinirole. Cimetidine, grapefruit juice, indinavir, methylphenidate, diltiazem, and verapamil may increase the serum concentrations of TCAs. Use of lithium with a TCA may increase the risk for neurotoxicity. Phenothiazines may increase concentration of some TCAs and TCAs may increase concentration of phenothiazines. Pressor response to I.V. epinephrine, norepinephrine, and phenylephrine may be enhanced in patients receiving TCAs (**Note:** Effect is unlikely with epinephrine or levonordefrin dosages typically administered as infiltration in combination with local anesthetics). Combined use of beta-agonists or drugs which prolong QT_c (including quinidine, procainamide, disopyramide, cisapride, sparfloxacin, gatifloxacin, moxifloxacin) with TCAs may predispose patients to cardiac arrhythmias. Use with altretamine may cause orthostatic hypotension.

Decreased Effect: Carbamazepine, phenobarbital, and rifampin may increase the metabolism of nortriptyline resulting in decreased effect of nortriptyline. Nortriptyline inhibits the antihypertensive response to bethanidine, clonidine, debrisoquin, guanadrel, guanethidine, guanabenz, or guanfacine. Cholestyramine and colestipol may bind TCAs and reduce their absorption; monitor for altered response.

Ethanol/Nutrition/Herb Interactions

Ethanol: Avoid ethanol (may increase CNS depression).

Food: Grapefruit juice may inhibit the metabolism of some TCAs and clinical toxicity may result.

Herb/Nutraceutical: Avoid valerian, St John's wort, SAMe, kava kava (may increase risk of serotonin syndrome and/or excessive sedation).

Pharmacodynamics/Kinetics

Onset of action: Therapeutic: 1-3 weeks

Distribution: V_d: 21 L/kg

Protein binding: 93% to 95%

Metabolism: Primarily hepatic; extensive first-pass effect

Half-life elimination: 28-31 hours

Time to peak, serum: 7-8.5 hours

Excretion: Urine (as metabolites and small amounts of unchanged drug); feces (small amounts)

Pregnancy Risk Factor D

Dosage Forms CAP: 10 mg, 25 mg, 50 mg, 75 mg; (Aventyl® HCl): 10 mg, 25 mg; (Pamelor®): 10 mg, 25 mg, 50 mg, 75 mg. **SOLN** (Aventyl® HCl, Pamelor®): 10 mg/5 mL (473 mL)

Selected Readings

Friedlander AH and Mahler ME, "Major Depressive Disorder. Psychopathology, Medical Management, and Dental Implications," *J Am Dent Assoc*, 2001, 132(5):629-38.

Ganzberg S, "Psychoactive Drugs," *ADA Guide to Dental Therapeutics*, 2nd ed, Chicago, IL: ADA Publishing, a Division of ADA Business Enterprises, Inc, 2000, 376-405.

Jastak JT and Yagiela JA, "Vasoconstrictors and Local Anesthesia: A Review and Rationale for Use," *J Am Dent Assoc*, 1983, 107(4):623-30.

Rundegren J, van Dijken J, Mörnstad H, et al, "Oral Conditions in Patients Receiving Long-Term Treatment With Cyclic Antidepressant Drugs," *Swed Dent J*, 1985, 9(2):55-64.

Yagiela JA, "Adverse Drug Interactions in Dental Practice: Interactions Associated With Vasoconstrictors. Part V of a Series," *J Am Dent Assoc*, 1999, 130(5):701-9.

Nortriptyline Hydrochloride *see* Nortriptyline *on page 999*

Norvasc® *see* Amlodipine *on page 108*

Norvir® *see* Ritonavir *on page 1189*

Nostril® [OTC] *see* Phenylephrine *on page 1078*

Nōstrilla® [OTC] *see* Oxymetazoline *on page 1034*

Novantrone® *see* Mitoxantrone *on page 938*

Novarel™ *see* Chorionic Gonadotropin (Human) *on page 326*

Novocain® *see* Procaine *on page 1125*

Novolin® 70/30 *see* Insulin Preparations *on page 749*

Novolin® L [DSC] *see* Insulin Preparations *on page 749*

Novolin® N *see* Insulin Preparations *on page 749*

Novolin® R *see* Insulin Preparations *on page 749*

NovoLog® *see* Insulin Preparations *on page 749*

NovoLog® Mix 70/30 *see* Insulin Preparations *on page 749*

Novo-Seven® *see* Factor VIIa (Recombinant) *on page 571*

Novothyrox *see* Levothyroxine *on page 817*

NPH Iletin® II *see* Insulin Preparations *on page 749*

NPH, Insulin *see* Insulin Preparations *on page 749*

NSC-740 *see* Methotrexate *on page 897*

NSC-752 *see* Thioguanine *on page 1288*

NSC-755 *see* Mercaptopurine *on page 880*

NSC-3053 *see* Dactinomycin *on page 394*

NSC-3088 *see* Chlorambucil *on page 305*

NSC-10363 *see* Megestrol *on page 865*

NSC-13875 *see* Altretamine *on page 89*

NSC-15200 *see* Gallium Nitrate *on page 646*

NSC-26271 *see* Cyclophosphamide *on page 384*

NSC-26980 *see* Mitomycin *on page 937*

NSC-27640 *see* Floxuridine *on page 593*

NSC-38721 *see* Mitotane *on page 937*

NSC-49842 *see* VinBLAStine *on page 1377*

NSC-63878 *see* Cytarabine *on page 390*

NSC-67574 *see* VinCRIStine *on page 1378*

NSC-77213 *see* Procarbazine *on page 1125*

NSC-82151 *see* DAUNOrubicin Hydrochloride *on page 401*

NSC-85998 *see* Streptozocin *on page 1240*
NSC-89199 *see* Estramustine *on page 523*
NSC-102816 *see* Azacitidine *on page 171*
NSC-106977 (*Erwinia*) *see* Asparaginase *on page 150*
NSC-109229 (*E. coli*) *see* Asparaginase *on page 150*
NSC-109724 *see* Ifosfamide *on page 733*
NSC-122758 *see* Tretinoin (Oral) *on page 1328*
NSC-123127 *see* DOXOrubicin *on page 469*
NSC-125066 *see* Bleomycin *on page 213*
NSC-125973 *see* Paclitaxel *on page 1038*
NSC-147834 *see* Flutamide *on page 615*
NSC-180973 *see* Tamoxifen *on page 1258*
NSC-218321 *see* Pentostatin *on page 1065*
NSC-245467 *see* Vindesine *on page 1379*
NSC-249992 *see* Amsacrine *on page 129*
NSC-256439 *see* Idarubicin *on page 732*
NSC-266046 *see* Oxaliplatin *on page 1020*
NSC-301739 *see* Mitoxantrone *on page 938*
NSC-308847 *see* Amonafide *on page 112*
NSC-352122 *see* Trimetrexate Glucuronate *on page 1342*
NSC-362856 *see* Temozolomide *on page 1268*
NSC-373364 *see* Aldesleukin *on page 74*
NSC-377526 *see* Leuprolide *on page 805*
NSC-409962 *see* Carmustine *on page 268*
NSC-603071 *see* Aminocamptothecin *on page 96*
NSC-606864 *see* Goserelin *on page 670*
NSC-609699 *see* Topotecan *on page 1316*
NSC-616348 *see* Irinotecan *on page 764*
NSC-628503 *see* Docetaxel *on page 458*
NSC-644954 *see* Pegaspargase *on page 1051*
NSC-698037 *see* Pemetrexed *on page 1054*
NSC-715055 *see* Gefitinib *on page 649*
NTG *see* Nitroglycerin *on page 991*
***N*-trifluoroacetyladriamycin-14-valerate** *see* Valrubicin *on page 1362*
NTZ *see* Nitazoxanide *on page 989*
Nubain® *see* Nalbuphine *on page 959*
Nucofed® Expectorant *see* Guaifenesin, Pseudoephedrine, and Codeine *on page 676*
Nucofed® Pediatric Expectorant *see* Guaifenesin, Pseudoephedrine, and Codeine *on page 676*
Nucotuss® *see* Guaifenesin, Pseudoephedrine, and Codeine *on page 676*
Nu-Iron® 150 [OTC] *see* Polysaccharide-Iron Complex *on page 1101*
NuLev™ *see* Hyoscyamine *on page 724*
Nullo® [OTC] *see* Chlorophyll *on page 310*
NuLytely® *see* Polyethylene Glycol-Electrolyte Solution *on page 1100*
Numorphan® *see* Oxymorphone *on page 1036*
Nupercainal® [OTC] *see* Dibucaine *on page 426*
Nupercainal® Hydrocortisone Cream [OTC] *see* Hydrocortisone *on page 714*
Nuquin HP® *see* Hydroquinone *on page 719*
Nu-Tears® [OTC] *see* Artificial Tears *on page 148*
Nu-Tears® II [OTC] *see* Artificial Tears *on page 148*
Nutracort® *see* Hydrocortisone *on page 714*
Nutraplus® [OTC] *see* Urea *on page 1353*
Nutropin® *see* Human Growth Hormone *on page 694*
Nutropin AQ® *see* Human Growth Hormone *on page 694*
Nutropin Depot® [DSC] *see* Human Growth Hormone *on page 694*
NuvaRing® *see* Ethinyl Estradiol and Etonogestrel *on page 543*
NVB *see* Vinorelbine *on page 1380*
NVP *see* Nevirapine *on page 977*
Nydrazid® *see* Isoniazid *on page 769*

Nylidrin (NYE li drin)

U.S. Brand Names Arlidin®

Canadian Brand Names Arlidin®

Pharmacologic Category Vasodilator, Peripheral

Use Considered "possibly effective" for increasing blood supply to treat peripheral disease (arteriosclerosis obliterans, diabetic vascular disease, nocturnal leg cramps, Raynaud's disease, frost bite, ischemic ulcer, thrombophlebitis) and circulatory disturbances of the inner ear (cochlear ischemia, macular or ampullar ischemia, etc)

Local Anesthetic/Vasoconstrictor Precautions No information available to require special precautions

Effects on Dental Treatment No significant effects or complications reported

Common Adverse Effects

1% to 10%:

Central nervous system: Nervousness

Neuromuscular & skeletal: Trembling

Mechanism of Action Nylidrin is a peripheral vasodilator; this results from direct relaxation of vascular smooth muscle and beta agonist action. Nylidrin does not appear to affect cutaneous blood flow; it reportedly increases heart rate and cardiac output; cutaneous blood flow is not enhanced to any appreciable extent.

Pregnancy Risk Factor C

Nystatin (nye STAT in)

Related Information

Management of Patients Undergoing Cancer Therapy *on page 1569*

Oral Fungal Infections *on page 1544*

Sexually-Transmitted Diseases *on page 1504*

U.S. Brand Names Bio-Statin®; Mycostatin®; Nystat-Rx®; Nystop®; Pedi-Dri®

Canadian Brand Names Candistatin®; Mycostatin®; Nilstat; Nyaderm; PMS-Nystatin

Mexican Brand Names Micostatin®

Generic Available Yes: Cream, ointment, powder, suspension, tablet

Pharmacologic Category Antifungal Agent, Oral Nonabsorbed; Antifungal Agent, Topical; Antifungal Agent, Vaginal

Use Treatment of susceptible cutaneous, mucocutaneous, and oral cavity fungal infections normally caused by the *Candida* species

Local Anesthetic/Vasoconstrictor Precautions No information available to require special precautions

Effects on Dental Treatment No significant effects or complications reported

Significant Adverse Effects

Frequency not defined: Dermatologic: Contact dermatitis, Stevens-Johnson syndrome

1% to 10%: Gastrointestinal: Nausea, vomiting, diarrhea, stomach pain

<1% (Limited to important or life-threatening): Hypersensitivity reactions

Dosage

Oral candidiasis:

Suspension (swish and swallow orally):

Premature infants: 100,000 units 4 times/day

Infants: 200,000 units 4 times/day or 100,000 units to each side of mouth 4 times/day

Children and Adults: 400,000-600,000 units 4 times/day

Troche: Children and Adults: 200,000-400,000 units 4-5 times/day

Powder for compounding: Children and Adults: $^1/_8$ teaspoon (500,000 units) to equal approximately $^1/_2$ cup of water; give 4 times/day

Mucocutaneous infections: Children and Adults: Topical: Apply 2-3 times/day to affected areas; very moist topical lesions are treated best with powder

Intestinal infections: Adults: Oral: 500,000-1,000,000 units every 8 hours

Vaginal infections: Adults: Vaginal tablets: Insert 1 tablet/day at bedtime for 2 weeks

Mechanism of Action Binds to sterols in fungal cell membrane, changing the cell wall permeability allowing for leakage of cellular contents

Contraindications Hypersensitivity to nystatin or any component of the formulation

Drug Interactions No data reported

Pharmacodynamics/Kinetics

Onset of action: Symptomatic relief from candidiasis: 24-72 hours

Absorption: Topical: None through mucous membranes or intact skin; Oral: Poorly absorbed

Excretion: Feces (as unchanged drug)

Pregnancy Risk Factor B/C (oral)

Lactation Does not enter breast milk/compatible (not absorbed orally)

(Continued)

Nystatin *(Continued)*

Dosage Forms [DSC] = Discontinued product

Capsule (Bio-Statin®): 500,000 units, 1 million units
Cream: 100,000 units/g (15 g, 30 g)
Mycostatin®: 100,000 units/g (30 g)
Lozenge (Mycostatin®): 200,000 units [DSC]
Ointment, topical: 100,000 units/g (15 g, 30 g)
Powder, for prescription compounding: 50 million units (10 g); 150 million units (30 g); 500 million units (100 g); 2 billion units (400 g)
Nystat-Rx®: 50 million units (10 g); 150 million units (30 g); 500 million units (100 g); 1 billion units (190 g); 2 billion units (350 g)
Powder, topical:
Mycostatin®: 100,000 units/g (15 g)
Nystop®: 100,000 units/g (15 g, 30 g, 60 g)
Pedi-Dri®: 100,000 units/g (56.7 g)
Suspension, oral: 100,000 units/mL (5 mL, 60 mL, 480 mL)
Mycostatin® [DSC]: 100,000 units/mL (60 mL, 480 mL) [contains alcohol ≤1%; cherry-mint flavor]
Tablet: 500,000 units
Tablet, vaginal: 100,000 units (15s) [packaged with applicator]

Nystatin and Triamcinolone (nye STAT in & trye am SIN oh lone)

Related Information

Nystatin *on page 1003*
Oral Fungal Infections *on page 1544*
Triamcinolone *on page 1330*

U.S. Brand Names Mycolog®-II [DSC]

Generic Available Yes

Synonyms Triamcinolone and Nystatin

Pharmacologic Category Antifungal Agent, Topical; Corticosteroid, Topical

Use Treatment of cutaneous candidiasis

Local Anesthetic/Vasoconstrictor Precautions No information available to require special precautions

Effects on Dental Treatment No significant effects or complications reported

Common Adverse Effects 1% to 10%:

Dermatologic: Dryness, folliculitis, hypertrichosis, acne, hypopigmentation, allergic dermatitis, maceration of the skin, skin atrophy
Local: Burning, itching, irritation
Miscellaneous: Increased incidence of secondary infection

Mechanism of Action Nystatin is an antifungal agent that binds to sterols in fungal cell membrane, changing the cell wall permeability allowing for leakage of cellular contents. Triamcinolone is a synthetic corticosteroid; it decreases inflammation by suppression of migration of polymorphonuclear leukocytes and reversal of increased capillary permeability. It suppresses the immune system reducing activity and volume of the lymphatic system. It suppresses adrenal function at high doses.

Pharmacodynamics/Kinetics See individual agents.

Pregnancy Risk Factor C

Nystat-Rx® *see* Nystatin *on page 1003*
Nystop® *see* Nystatin *on page 1003*
Nytol® [OTC] *see* DiphenhydrAMINE *on page 448*
Nytol® Maximum Strength [OTC] *see* DiphenhydrAMINE *on page 448*
Obezine® *see* Phendimetrazine *on page 1072*
OCBZ *see* Oxcarbazepine *on page 1023*
Occlusal®-HP [OTC] *see* Salicylic Acid *on page 1205*
Occupational Exposure to Bloodborne Pathogens (Standard/Universal Precautions) *see page 1603*
Ocean® [OTC] *see* Sodium Chloride *on page 1227*
Octagam® *see* Immune Globulin (Intravenous) *on page 740*

Octreotide (ok TREE oh tide)

U.S. Brand Names Sandostatin®; Sandostatin LAR®

Canadian Brand Names Sandostatin®; Sandostatin LAR®

Mexican Brand Names Sandostatina®

Generic Available No

Synonyms Octreotide Acetate

Pharmacologic Category Antidiarrheal; Somatostatin Analog

Use Control of symptoms in patients with metastatic carcinoid and vasoactive intestinal peptide-secreting tumors (VIPomas); pancreatic tumors, gastrinoma, secretory diarrhea, acromegaly

Unlabeled/Investigational Use AIDS-associated secretory diarrhea, control of bleeding of esophageal varices, breast cancer, cryptosporidiosis, Cushing's syndrome, insulinomas, small bowel fistulas, postgastrectomy dumping syndrome, chemotherapy-induced diarrhea, graft-versus-host disease (GVHD) induced diarrhea, Zollinger-Ellison syndrome, congenital hyperinsulinism

Local Anesthetic/Vasoconstrictor Precautions No information available to require special precautions

Effects on Dental Treatment No significant effects or complications reported

Common Adverse Effects

>10%:

Cardiovascular: Sinus bradycardia (19% to 25%)

Endocrine & metabolic: Hyperglycemia (15% acromegaly, 27% carcinoid)

Gastrointestinal: Diarrhea (36% to 58% acromegaly), abdominal pain (30% to 44% acromegaly), flatulence (13% to 26% acromegaly), constipation (9% to 19% acromegaly), nausea (10% to 30%)

1% to 10%:

Cardiovascular: Flushing, edema, conduction abnormalities (9% to 10%), arrhythmias (3% to 9%)

Central nervous system: Fatigue, headache, dizziness, vertigo, anorexia, depression

Endocrine & metabolic: Hypoglycemia (2% acromegaly, 4% carcinoid), hyperglycemia (1%), hypothyroidism, galactorrhea

Gastrointestinal: Nausea, vomiting, diarrhea, constipation, abdominal pain, cramping, discomfort, fat malabsorption, loose stools, flatulence, tenesmus

Hepatic: Jaundice, hepatitis, increase LFTs, cholelithiasis has occurred, presumably by altering fat absorption and decreasing the motility of the gallbladder

Local: Pain at injection site (dose-related)

Neuromuscular & skeletal: Weakness

Mechanism of Action Mimics natural somatostatin by inhibiting serotonin release, and the secretion of gastrin, VIP, insulin, glucagon, secretin, motilin, and pancreatic polypeptide. Decreases growth hormone and IGF-1 in acromegaly.

Drug Interactions

Increased Effect/Toxicity: Octreotide may increase the effect of insulin or sulfonylurea agents which may result in hypoglycemia. Octreotide may increase serum levels of bromocriptine.

Decreased Effect: Octreotide may lower cyclosporine serum levels (case report of a transplant rejection due to reduction of serum cyclosporine levels). Codeine effect may be reduced.

Pharmacodynamics/Kinetics

Duration: SubQ: 6-12 hours

Absorption: SubQ: Rapid

Distribution: V_d: 14 L

Protein binding: 65% to lipoproteins

Metabolism: Extensively hepatic

Bioavailability: SubQ: 100%

Half-life elimination: 60-110 minutes

Excretion: Urine (32%)

Pregnancy Risk Factor B

Octreotide Acetate *see* Octreotide *on page 1004*

OcuClear® [OTC] [DSC] *see* Oxymetazoline *on page 1034*

OcuCoat® [OTC] *see* Artificial Tears *on page 148*

OcuCoat® PF [OTC] *see* Artificial Tears *on page 148*

Ocufen® *see* Flurbiprofen *on page 613*

Ocuflox® *see* Ofloxacin *on page 1005*

Ocupress® [DSC] *see* Carteolol *on page 269*

Ocusulf-10 *see* Sulfacetamide *on page 1244*

Ofloxacin (oh FLOKS a sin)

Related Information

Sexually-Transmitted Diseases *on page 1504*

Tuberculosis *on page 1495*

U.S. Brand Names Floxin®; Ocuflox®

Canadian Brand Names Apo-Oflox®; Floxin®; Ocuflox®

Mexican Brand Names Bactocin®; Floxil®; Floxstat®; Ocuflox®

Generic Available Yes: Tablet, ophthalmic solution

Synonyms Floxin Otic Singles

Pharmacologic Category Antibiotic, Quinolone

(Continued)

Ofloxacin *(Continued)*

Use Quinolone antibiotic for the treatment of acute exacerbations of chronic bronchitis, community-acquired pneumonia, skin and skin structure infections (uncomplicated), urethral and cervical gonorrhea (acute, uncomplicated), urethritis and cervicitis (nongonococcal), mixed infections of the urethra and cervix, pelvic inflammatory disease (acute), cystitis (uncomplicated), urinary tract infections (complicated), prostatitis

Ophthalmic: Treatment of superficial ocular infections involving the conjunctiva or cornea due to strains of susceptible organisms

Otic: Otitis externa, chronic suppurative otitis media, acute otitis media

Unlabeled/Investigational Use Epididymitis (gonorrhea)

Local Anesthetic/Vasoconstrictor Precautions No information available to require special precautions

Effects on Dental Treatment No significant effects or complications reported

Common Adverse Effects

Systemic:

1% to 10%:

Cardiovascular: Chest pain (1% to 3%)

Central nervous system: Headache (1% to 9%), insomnia (3% to 7%), dizziness (1% to 5%), fatigue (1% to 3%), somnolence (1% to 3%), sleep disorders (1% to 3%), nervousness (1% to 3%), pyrexia (1% to 3%)

Dermatologic: Rash/pruritus (1% to 3%)

Gastrointestinal: Diarrhea (1% to 4%), vomiting (1% to 4%), GI distress (1% to 3%), abdominal cramps (1% to 3%), flatulence (1% to 3%), abnormal taste (1% to 3%), xerostomia (1% to 3%), decreased appetite (1% to 3%), nausea (3% to 10%), constipation (1% to 3%)

Genitourinary: Vaginitis (1% to 5%), external genital pruritus in women (1% to 3%)

Ocular: Visual disturbances (1% to 3%)

Respiratory: Pharyngitis (1% to 3%)

Miscellaneous: Trunk pain

Ophthalmic: Frequency not defined:

Central nervous system: Dizziness

Gastrointestinal: Nausea

Ocular: Blurred vision, burning, chemical conjunctivitis/keratitis, discomfort, dryness, edema, eye pain, foreign body sensation, itching, photophobia, redness, stinging, tearing

Otic:

>10%: Local: Application site reaction (<1% to 17%)

1% to 10%:

Central nervous system: Dizziness (≤1%), vertigo (≤1%)

Dermatologic: Pruritus (1% to 4%), rash (1%)

Gastrointestinal: Taste perversion (7%)

Neuromuscular & skeletal: Paresthesia (1%)

Mechanism of Action Ofloxacin is a DNA gyrase inhibitor. DNA gyrase is an essential bacterial enzyme that maintains the superhelical structure of DNA. DNA gyrase is required for DNA replication and transcription, DNA repair, recombination, and transposition; bactericidal

Drug Interactions

Cytochrome P450 Effect: Inhibits CYP1A2 (strong)

Increased Effect/Toxicity: Ofloxacin may increase the levels/effects of aminophylline, fluvoxamine, mexiletine, mirtazapine, ropinirole, theophylline, trifluoperazine, and other CYP1A2 substrates. Quinolones can cause increased levels/effects of caffeine, warfarin, and cyclosporine. Azlocillin, cimetidine, and probenecid may increase ofloxacin serum levels. Foscarnet and NSAIDs have been associated with an increased risk of seizures with some quinolones. Serum levels of some quinolones are increased by loop diuretic administration. The hypoprothrombinemic effect of warfarin is enhanced by some quinolone antibiotics. Ofloxacin does not alter warfarin levels, but may alter the gastrointestinal flora which may increase warfarin's effect. Concurrent use of corticosteroids may increase risk of tendon rupture.

Decreased Effect: Metal cations (magnesium, aluminum, iron, and zinc) bind quinolones in the gastrointestinal tract and inhibit absorption (as much as 98%). Antacids, electrolyte supplements, sucralfate, quinapril, and some didanosine formulations should be avoided. Ofloxacin should be administered 2 hours before or 2 hours after these agents. Antineoplastic agents may decrease the absorption of quinolones.

Pharmacodynamics/Kinetics

Absorption: Well absorbed; food causes only minor alterations

Distribution: V_d: 2.4-3.5 L/kg

Protein binding: 20%
Bioavailability: Oral: 98%
Half-life elimination: Biphasic: 5-7.5 hours and 20-25 hours (accounts for <5%); prolonged with renal impairment
Excretion: Primarily urine (as unchanged drug)

Pregnancy Risk Factor C

Ogen® *see* Estropipate *on page 531*

Ogestrel® *see* Ethinyl Estradiol and Norgestrel *on page 557*

OGMT *see* Metyrosine *on page 920*

OGT-918 *see* Miglustat *on page 930*

OKT3 *see* Muromonab-CD3 *on page 952*

Olanzapine (oh LAN za peen)

U.S. Brand Names Zyprexa®; Zyprexa® Zydis®

Canadian Brand Names Zyprexa®; Zyprexa® Zydis®

Mexican Brand Names Zyprexa®

Generic Available No

Synonyms LY170053; Zyprexa Zydis

Pharmacologic Category Antipsychotic Agent, Thienobenzodiazepine

Use Treatment of the manifestations of schizophrenia; treatment of acute mania episodes associated with bipolar disorder (as monotherapy or in combination with lithium or valproate); maintenance treatment of bipolar disorder; acute agitation (patients with schizophrenia or bipolar mania)

Unlabeled/Investigational Use Treatment of psychotic symptoms; chronic pain

Local Anesthetic/Vasoconstrictor Precautions No information available to require special precautions

Effects on Dental Treatment No significant effects or complications reported

Common Adverse Effects

>10%:
- Central nervous system: Headache, somnolence, insomnia, agitation, nervousness, hostility, dizziness
- Gastrointestinal: Dyspepsia, constipation, weight gain (clinically and long term)
- Neuromuscular & skeletal: Weakness

1% to 10%:
- Cardiovascular: Postural hypotension, tachycardia, hypotension, peripheral edema, chest pain, hypertension
- Central nervous system: Dystonic reactions, parkinsonian events, amnesia, euphoria, stuttering, akathisia, anxiety, personality changes, fever, abnormal dreams, speech disorder
- Dermatologic: Rash, bruising
- Endocrine & metabolic: Prolactin increased, amenorrhea
- Gastrointestinal: Xerostomia, abdominal pain, appetite increased, vomiting, salivation increased
- Genitourinary: Premenstrual syndrome, incontinence
- Hematologic: Leukopenia
- Neuromuscular & skeletal: Arthralgia, neck rigidity, twitching, hypertonia, tremor, back pain, abnormal gait, akathisia, falling (particularly in older patients)
- Ocular: Amblyopia
- Respiratory: Rhinitis, cough, pharyngitis, dyspnea
- Miscellaneous: Diaphoresis

Additional significant effects reported with I.M. administration: Articulation impairment, AV block, injection site pain, syncope

Dosage

Children: Schizophrenia/bipolar disorder: Oral: Initial: 2.5 mg/day; titrate as necessary to 20 mg/day (0.12-0.29 mg/kg/day)

Adults:
- Schizophrenia: Oral: Usual starting dose: 5-10 mg once daily; increase to 10 mg once daily within 5-7 days, thereafter adjust by 5-10 mg/day at 1-week intervals, up to a maximum of 20 mg/day; doses of 30-50 mg/day have been used; typical dosage range: 10-30 mg/day
- Bipolar mania: Oral:
  - Monotherapy: Usual starting dose: 10-15 mg once daily; increase by 5 mg/day at intervals of not less than 24 hours; maintenance: 5-20 mg/day; maximum dose: 20 mg/day
  - Combination therapy (olanzapine in combination with lithium or valproate): Initial: 10 mg once daily; dosing range: 5-20 mg/day

(Continued)

Olanzapine *(Continued)*

Agitation (acute, associated with bipolar disorder or schizophrenia): I.M.: Initial dose: 5-10 mg (a lower dose of 2.5 mg may be considered when clinical factors warrant); additional doses (2.5-10 mg) may be considered; however, 2-4 hours should be allowed between doses to evaluate response (maximum total daily dose: 30 mg, per manufacturer's recommendation)

Elderly: Schizophrenia: Oral: Usual starting dose: 2.5 mg/day, increase as clinically indicated and monitor blood pressure; typical dosage range: 2.5-10 mg/day

Dosage comment in renal impairment: Not removed by dialysis

Mechanism of Action Olanzapine is a thienobenzodiazepine neuroleptic; thought to work by antagonizing dopamine and serotonin activities. It is a selective monoaminergic antagonist with high affinity binding to serotonin 5-HT_{2A} and 5-HT_{2C}, dopamine D_{1-4}, muscarinic M_{1-5}, histamine H_1- and alpha$_1$-adrenergic receptor sites. Olanzapine binds weakly to GABA-A, BZD, and beta-adrenergic receptors.

Contraindications Hypersensitivity to olanzapine or any component of the formulation

Warnings/Precautions Moderate to highly sedating, use with caution in disorders where CNS depression is a feature. Use with caution in Parkinson's disease and Alzheimer's disease. Caution in patients with hemodynamic instability; bone marrow suppression; predisposition to seizures; subcortical brain damage; severe cardiac, hepatic, renal, or respiratory disease. Esophageal dysmotility and aspiration have been associated with antipsychotic use - use with caution in patients at risk of pneumonia (ie, Alzheimer's disease). Caution in breast cancer or other prolactin-dependent tumors (may elevate prolactin levels). May alter temperature regulation or mask toxicity of other drugs due to antiemetic effects. Life-threatening arrhythmias have occurred with therapeutic doses of some neuroleptics. An increased incidence of cerebrovascular adverse events (including fatalities) has been reported in elderly patients with dementia-related psychosis. Significant weight gain may occur.

May cause anticholinergic effects (constipation, xerostomia, blurred vision, urinary retention); therefore, they should be used with caution in patients with decreased gastrointestinal motility, urinary retention, BPH, xerostomia, or visual problems. Conditions which also may be exacerbated by cholinergic blockade include narrow-angle glaucoma (screening is recommended) and worsening of myasthenia gravis. Relative to other neuroleptics, olanzapine has a moderate potency of cholinergic blockade.

May cause extrapyramidal reactions, including pseudoparkinsonism, acute dystonic reactions, akathisia, and tardive dyskinesia (risk of these reactions is very low relative to other neuroleptics). May be associated with neuroleptic malignant syndrome (NMS). May cause hyperglycemia; in some cases may be extreme and associated with ketoacidosis, hyperosmolar coma, or death. Use with caution in patients with diabetes or other disorders of glucose regulation; monitor for worsening of glucose control.

Drug Interactions

Cytochrome P450 Effect: Substrate (minor) of CYP1A2, 2D6; **Inhibits** CYP1A2 (weak), 2C8/9 (weak), 2C19 (weak), 2D6 (weak), 3A4 (weak)

Increased Effect/Toxicity: Olanzapine levels may be increased by CYP1A2 inhibitors such as cimetidine and fluvoxamine. Sedations from olanzapine is increased with ethanol or other CNS depressants. The risk of hypotension and orthostatic hypotension from olanzapine is increased by concurrent antihypertensives. Metoclopramide may increase risk of extrapyramidal symptoms (EPS).

Decreased Effect: Olanzapine levels may be decreased by cytochrome P450 enzyme inducers such as rifampin, omeprazole, and carbamazepine (also cigarette smoking). Olanzapine may antagonize the effects of levodopa and dopamine agonists.

Ethanol/Nutrition/Herb Interactions

Ethanol: Avoid ethanol (may increase CNS depression).

Herb/Nutraceutical: Avoid dong quai, St John's wort (may also cause photosensitization). Avoid kava kava, gotu kola, valerian, St John's wort (may increase CNS depression).

Dietary Considerations Tablets may be taken with or without food/meals. Zyprexa® Zydis®: 5 mg tablet contains phenylalanine 0.34 mg; 10 mg tablet contains phenylalanine 0.45 mg; 15 mg tablet contains phenylalanine 0.67 mg; 20 mg tablet contains phenylalanine 0.9 mg

Pharmacodynamics/Kinetics

Absorption:

I.M.: Rapidly absorbed

Oral: Well absorbed; not affected by food; tablets and orally-disintegrating tablets are bioequivalent

Distribution: V_d: Extensive, 1000 L

Protein binding, plasma: 93% bound to albumin and alpha$_1$-glycoprotein

Metabolism: Highly metabolized via direct glucuronidation and cytochrome P450 mediated oxidation (CYP1A2, CYP2D6)

Bioavailability: >57%

Half-life elimination: 21-54 hours; ~1.5 times greater in elderly

Time to peak, plasma: Maximum plasma concentrations after I.M. administration are 5 times higher than maximum plasma concentrations produced by an oral dose.

I.M.: 15-45 minutes

Oral: ~6 hours

Excretion: 40% removed via first pass metabolism; urine (57%, 7% as unchanged drug); feces (30%)

Clearance: 40% increase in olanzapine clearance in smokers

Pregnancy Risk Factor C

Dosage Forms INJ, powder for reconstitution (Zyprexa® IntraMuscular): 10 mg. **TAB** (Zyprexa®): 2.5 mg, 5 mg, 7.5 mg, 10 mg, 15 mg, 20 mg. **TAB, orally-disintegrating** (Zyprexa® Zydis®): 5 mg, 10 mg, 15 mg, 20 mg

Olanzapine and Fluoxetine (oh LAN za peen & floo OKS e teen)

Related Information

Fluoxetine *on page 606*

Olanzapine *on page 1007*

U.S. Brand Names Symbyax™

Generic Available No

Synonyms Fluoxetine and Olanzapine; Olanzapine and Fluoxetine Hydrochloride

Pharmacologic Category Antidepressant, Selective Serotonin Reuptake Inhibitor; Antipsychotic Agent, Thienobenzodiazepine

Use Treatment of depressive episodes associated with bipolar disorder

Local Anesthetic/Vasoconstrictor Precautions No information available to require special precautions

Effects on Dental Treatment Key adverse event(s) related to dental treatment: Xerostomia or salivation increased (normal salivary flow resumes upon discontinuation), tooth disorder, and taste perversion.

Common Adverse Effects As reported with combination product (also see individual agents):

>10%:

Central nervous system: Somnolence (21% to 22%)

Gastrointestinal: Weight gain (17% to 21%), diarrhea (8% to 19%), appetite increased (13% to 16%), xerostomia (11% to 16%)

Neuromuscular & skeletal: Weakness (13% to 15%)

1% to 10%:

Cardiovascular: Peripheral edema (4% to 8%), edema (up to 5%), hypertension (2%), tachycardia (2%), vasodilation

Central nervous system: Thinking abnormal (6%), fever (3% to 4%), amnesia (1% to 3%), personality disorder (1% to 2%), sleep disorder (1% to 2%), speech disorder (up to 2%), chills, migraine

Dermatologic: Photosensitivity

Endocrine & metabolic: Ejaculation abnormal (2% to 7%), impotence (2% to 4%), libido decreased (2% to 4%), anorgasmia (1% to 3%), breast pain, menorrhagia

Gastrointestinal: Tooth disorder (1% to 2%), salivation increased, taste perversion, thirst, weight loss

Genitourinary: Urinary frequency, urinary incontinence, urinary tract infection

Neuromuscular & skeletal: Tremor (8% to 9%), twitching (2% to 6%), arthralgia (3% to 5%), hyperkinesias (1% to 2%), joint disorder (1% to 2%), bruising, neck pain/rigidity

Ocular: Amblyopia (4% to 5%), vision abnormal

Otic: Ear pain (1% to 2%), otitis media (up to 2%), tinnitus

Respiratory: Pharyngitis (4% to 6%), dyspnea (1% to 2%), bronchitis, lung disorder

Frequency not defined: Alkaline phosphate increased, cholesterol increased, GGT increased, hemoglobin decreased, prolactin increased, uric acid increased

(Continued)

Olanzapine and Fluoxetine *(Continued)*

Mechanism of Action Olanzapine is a thienobenzodiazepine neuroleptic; thought to work by antagonizing dopamine and serotonin activities. It is a selective monoaminergic antagonist with high affinity binding to serotonin 5-HT_{2A} and 5-HT_{2C}, dopamine D_{1-4}, muscarinic M_{1-5}, histamine H_1- and alpha$_1$-adrenergic receptor sites. Olanzapine binds weakly to GABA-A, BZD, and beta-adrenergic receptors. Fluoxetine inhibits CNS neuron serotonin reuptake; minimal or no effect on reuptake of norepinephrine or dopamine; does not significantly bind to alpha-adrenergic, histamine, or cholinergic receptors. The enhanced antidepressant effect of the combination may be due to synergistic increases in serotonin, norepinephrine and dopamine.

Pharmacodynamics/Kinetics See individual agents.

Pregnancy Risk Factor C

Olanzapine and Fluoxetine Hydrochloride *see* Olanzapine and Fluoxetine *on page 1009*

Oleovitamin A *see* Vitamin A *on page 1382*

Oleum Ricini *see* Castor Oil *on page 273*

Olmesartan (ole me SAR tan)

U.S. Brand Names Benicar™

Generic Available No

Synonyms Olmesartan Medoxomil

Pharmacologic Category Angiotensin II Receptor Blocker

Use Treatment of hypertension with or without concurrent use of other antihypertensive agents

Local Anesthetic/Vasoconstrictor Precautions No information available to require special precautions

Effects on Dental Treatment No significant effects or complications reported

Common Adverse Effects 1% to 10%:

Central nervous system: Dizziness (3%), headache
Endocrine & metabolic: Hyperglycemia, hypertriglyceridemia
Gastrointestinal: Diarrhea
Neuromuscular & skeletal: Back pain, CPK increased
Renal: Hematuria
Respiratory: Bronchitis, pharyngitis, rhinitis, sinusitis
Miscellaneous: Flu-like syndrome

Mechanism of Action As a selective and competitive, nonpeptide angiotensin II receptor antagonist, olmesartan blocks the vasoconstrictor and aldosterone-secreting effects of angiotensin II; olmesartan interacts reversibly at the AT1 and AT2 receptors of many tissues and has slow dissociation kinetics; its affinity for the AT1 receptor is 12,500 times greater than the AT2 receptor. Angiotensin II receptor antagonists may induce a more complete inhibition of the renin-angiotensin system than ACE inhibitors, they do not affect the response to bradykinin, and are less likely to be associated with nonrenin-angiotensin effects (eg, cough and angioedema). Olmesartan increases urinary flow rate and, in addition to being natriuretic and kaliuretic, increases excretion of chloride, magnesium, uric acid, calcium, and phosphate.

Drug Interactions

Increased Effect/Toxicity: The risk of hyperkalemia may be increased during concomitant use with potassium-sparing diuretics, potassium supplements, and trimethoprim; may increase risk of lithium toxicity.

Decreased Effect: NSAIDs may decrease the efficacy of olmesartan.

Pharmacodynamics/Kinetics

Distribution: 17 L; does not cross the blood-brain barrier (animal studies)
Protein binding: 99%
Metabolism: Olmesartan medoxomil is hydrolyzed in the GI tract to active olmesartan. No further metabolism occurs.
Bioavailability: 26%
Half-life elimination: Terminal: 13 hours
Time to peak: 1-2 hours
Excretion: All as unchanged drug: Feces (50% to 65%); urine (35% to 50%)

Pregnancy Risk Factor C/D (2nd and 3rd trimesters)

Olmesartan and Hydrochlorothiazide

(ole me SAR tan & hye droe klor oh THYE a zide)

Related Information

Olmesartan *on page 1010*

U.S. Brand Names Benicar HCT™

Generic Available No

Synonyms Hydrochlorothiazide and Olmesartan Medoxomil; Olmesartan Medoxomil and Hydrochlorothiazide

Pharmacologic Category Angiotensin II Receptor Blocker; Diuretic, Thiazide

Use Treatment of hypertension (not recommended for initial treatment)

Local Anesthetic/Vasoconstrictor Precautions No information available to require special precautions

Effects on Dental Treatment No significant effects or complications reported

Common Adverse Effects Frequencies reported with combination product. See individual monographs for additional adverse effects reported with each agent.

Cardiovascular: Chest pain, peripheral edema
Central nervous system: Dizziness (9%), vertigo
Dermatologic: Rash
Endocrine & metabolic: Hyperuricemia (4%), hyperglycemia
Gastrointestinal: Nausea (3%), abdominal pain, dyspepsia, gastroenteritis, diarrhea
Genitourinary: Hematuria
Hepatic: Transaminases increased
Neuromuscular & skeletal: Back pain, arthritis, arthralgia, myalgia
Respiratory: Upper respiratory infection (7%), cough
Miscellaneous: CPK increased

Angioedema and rhabdomyolysis have been reported with angiotensin-receptor blockers. Severe dermatologic reactions, hypokalemia, and pancreatitis have been reported with hydrochlorothiazide.

Mechanism of Action Olmesartan blocks the vasoconstrictor and aldosterone-secreting effects of angiotensin II. Hydrochlorothiazide inhibits sodium reabsorption in the distal tubules causing increased excretion of sodium and water as well as potassium and hydrogen ions.

Pharmacodynamics/Kinetics See individual agents.

Pregnancy Risk Factor C/D (2nd and 3rd trimesters)

Olmesartan Medoxomil *see* Olmesartan *on page 1010*

Olmesartan Medoxomil and Hydrochlorothiazide *see* Olmesartan and Hydrochlorothiazide *on page 1010*

Olopatadine (oh loe pa TA deen)

U.S. Brand Names Patanol®

Canadian Brand Names Patanol®

Generic Available No

Pharmacologic Category Antihistamine; Ophthalmic Agent, Miscellaneous

Use Treatment of the signs and symptoms of allergic conjunctivitis

Local Anesthetic/Vasoconstrictor Precautions No information available to require special precautions

Effects on Dental Treatment No significant effects or complications reported

Pregnancy Risk Factor C

Olsalazine (ole SAL a zeen)

U.S. Brand Names Dipentum®

Canadian Brand Names Dipentum®

Generic Available No

Synonyms Olsalazine Sodium

Pharmacologic Category 5-Aminosalicylic Acid Derivative

Use Maintenance of remission of ulcerative colitis in patients intolerant to sulfasalazine

Local Anesthetic/Vasoconstrictor Precautions No information available to require special precautions

Effects on Dental Treatment No significant effects or complications reported

Common Adverse Effects

>10%: Gastrointestinal: Diarrhea, cramps, abdominal pain

1% to 10%:
- Central nervous system: Headache, fatigue, depression
- Dermatologic: Rash, itching
- Gastrointestinal: Nausea, heartburn, bloating, anorexia
- Neuromuscular & skeletal: Arthralgia

Mechanism of Action The mechanism of action appears to be topical rather than systemic

Drug Interactions

Increased Effect/Toxicity: Olsalazine has been reported to increase the prothrombin time in patients taking warfarin. Olsalazine may increase the risk of myelosuppression with azathioprine, mesalamine, or sulfasalazine.

(Continued)

Olsalazine *(Continued)*

Pharmacodynamics/Kinetics

Absorption: <3%; very little intact olsalazine is systemically absorbed
Protein binding, plasma: >99%
Metabolism: Primarily via colonic bacteria to active drug, 5-aminosalicylic acid
Half-life elimination: 56 minutes
Time to peak: ~1 hour
Excretion: Primarily feces

Pregnancy Risk Factor C

Olsalazine Sodium *see* Olsalazine *on page 1011*

Olux® *see* Clobetasol *on page 351*

Omalizumab (oh mah lye ZOO mab)

U.S. Brand Names Xolair®

Generic Available No

Synonyms rhuMAb-E25

Pharmacologic Category Monoclonal Antibody, Anti-Asthmatic

Use Treatment of moderate-to-severe, persistent allergic asthma not adequately controlled with inhaled corticosteroids

Local Anesthetic/Vasoconstrictor Precautions No information available to require special precautions

Effects on Dental Treatment No significant effects or complications reported

Common Adverse Effects

>10%:

Central nervous system: Headache (15%)
Local: Injection site reaction (45%; placebo 43%), severe injection site reactions (12%; placebo 9%). Most reactions occurred within 1 hour, lasted <8 days, and decreased in frequency with additional dosing.
Respiratory: Upper respiratory tract infection (23%), sinusitis (16%), pharyngitis (11%)
Miscellaneous: Viral infection (23%)

1% to 10%:

Central nervous system: Pain (7%), fatigue (3%), dizziness (3%)
Dermatologic: Dermatitis (2%), pruritus (2%)
Neuromuscular & skeletal: Arthralgia (8%), leg pain (4%), arm pain (2%), fracture (2%)
Otic: Earache (2%)

Mechanism of Action Omalizumab is an IgG monoclonal antibody (recombinant DNA-derived) which inhibits IgE binding to the high-affinity IgE receptor on mast cells and basophils. By decreasing bound IgE, the activation and release of mediators in the allergic response (early and late phase) is limited. Serum free IgE levels and the number of high-affinity IgE receptors are decreased. Long-term treatment in patients with allergic asthma showed a decrease in asthma exacerbations and corticosteroid usage.

Pharmacodynamics/Kinetics

Absorption: Slow following SubQ injection
Distribution: V_d: 78 ± 32 mL/kg
Metabolism: Hepatic; IgG degradation by reticuloendothelial system and endothelial cells
Bioavailability: 62%
Half-life elimination: 26 days
Time to peak: 7-8 days
Excretion: Primarily via hepatic degradation; intact IgG may be secreted in bile

Pregnancy Risk Factor B

Omeprazole (oh ME pray zol)

Related Information

Esomeprazole *on page 516*
Gastrointestinal Disorders *on page 1476*

U.S. Brand Names Prilosec®; Prilosec OTC™ [OTC]; Zegerid™

Canadian Brand Names Losec®

Mexican Brand Names Inhibitron®; Losec®; Losec® [inj.]; Olexin®; Osiren®; Prazidec®; Prazolit®; Ulsen®

Generic Available Yes

Pharmacologic Category Proton Pump Inhibitor; Substituted Benzimidazole

Use Short-term (4-8 weeks) treatment of active duodenal ulcer disease or active benign gastric ulcer; treatment of heartburn and other symptoms associated with gastroesophageal reflux disease (GERD); short-term (4-8 weeks) treatment of endoscopically-diagnosed erosive esophagitis; maintenance healing of erosive esophagitis; long-term treatment of pathological hypersecretory conditions; as part of a multidrug regimen for *H. pylori* eradication to reduce the risk of duodenal ulcer recurrence

OTC labeling: Short-term treatment of frequent, uncomplicated heartburn occurring ≥2 days/week

Unlabeled/Investigational Use Healing NSAID-induced ulcers; prevention of NSAID-induced ulcers

Local Anesthetic/Vasoconstrictor Precautions No information available to require special precautions

Effects on Dental Treatment Key adverse event(s) related to dental treatment: Taste perversion, dry mouth, esophageal candidiasis, and mucosal atrophy (tongue).

Common Adverse Effects 1% to 10%:

Central nervous system: Headache (7%), dizziness (2%)

Dermatologic: Rash (2%)

Gastrointestinal: Diarrhea (3%), abdominal pain (2%), nausea (2%), vomiting (2%), constipation (1%), taste perversion (<1% to 15%)

Neuromuscular & skeletal: Weakness (1%), back pain (1%)

Respiratory: Upper respiratory infection (2%), cough (1%)

Dosage Oral:

Children ≥2 years: GERD or other acid-related disorders:

<20 kg: 10 mg once daily

≥20 kg: 20 mg once daily

Adults:

Active duodenal ulcer: 20 mg/day for 4-8 weeks

Gastric ulcers: 40 mg/day for 4-8 weeks

Symptomatic GERD: 20 mg/day for up to 4 weeks

Erosive esophagitis: 20 mg/day for 4-8 weeks

Helicobacter pylori eradication: Dose varies with regimen: 20 mg once daily **or** 40 mg/day as single dose or in 2 divided doses; requires combination therapy with antibiotics

Pathological hypersecretory conditions: Initial: 60 mg once daily; doses up to 120 mg 3 times/day have been administered; administer daily doses >80 mg in divided doses

Frequent heartburn (OTC labeling): 20 mg/day for 14 days; treatment may be repeated after 4 months if needed

Dosage adjustment in hepatic impairment: Specific guidelines are not available; bioavailability is increased with chronic liver disease

Mechanism of Action Suppresses gastric acid secretion by inhibiting the parietal cell H+/K+ ATP pump

Contraindications Hypersensitivity to omeprazole, substituted benzimidazoles (ie, esomeprazole, lansoprazole, pantoprazole, rabeprazole), or any component of the formulation

Warnings/Precautions In long-term (2-year) studies in rats, omeprazole produced a dose-related increase in gastric carcinoid tumors. While available endoscopic evaluations and histologic examinations of biopsy specimens from human stomachs have not detected a risk from short-term exposure to omeprazole, further human data on the effect of sustained hypochlorhydria and hypergastrinemia are needed to rule out the possibility of an increased risk for the development of tumors in humans receiving long-term therapy. Bioavailability may be increased in the elderly, Asian population, and with hepatic dysfunction. Use Zegerid™ with caution in patients with Bartter's syndrome, hypokalemia, and respiratory alkalosis. Safety and efficacy have not been established in children <2 years of age. When used for self-medication (OTC), do not use for >14 days; treatment should not be repeated more often than every 4 months; not approved for OTC use in children <18 years of age.

Drug Interactions

Cytochrome P450 Effect: Substrate of CYP2A6 (minor), 2C8/9 (minor), 2C19 (major), 2D6 (minor), 3A4 (minor); **Inhibits** CYP1A2 (weak), 2C8/9 (moderate), 2C19 (strong), 2D6 (weak), 3A4 (weak); **Induces** CYP1A2 (weak)

Increased Effect/Toxicity: Esomeprazole and omeprazole may increase the levels of benzodiazepines metabolized by oxidation (eg, diazepam, midazolam, triazolam) and carbamazepine. Elimination of phenytoin or warfarin may be prolonged when used concomitantly with omeprazole. Omeprazole may increase the levels/effects of amiodarone, citalopram, diazepam, fluoxetine, glimepiride, glipizide, methsuximide, nateglinide, phenytoin, pioglitazone, propranolol, rosiglitazone, sertraline, warfarin, and other CYP2C8/9 or 2C19 substrates.

Decreased Effect: Proton pump inhibitors may decrease the absorption of atazanavir, indinavir, itraconazole, and ketoconazole. The levels/effects of

(Continued)

Omeprazole *(Continued)*

omeprazole may be decreased by aminoglutethimide, carbamazepine, phenytoin, rifampin, and other CYP2C19 inducers.

Ethanol/Nutrition/Herb Interactions

Ethanol: Avoid ethanol (may cause gastric mucosal irritation).

Food: Food delays absorption. When Zegerid™ is given 1 hour after a meal, absorption is reduced.

Herb/Nutraceutical: St John's wort may decrease omeprazole levels.

Dietary Considerations

Should be taken on an empty stomach; best if taken before breakfast.

Zegerid™: Take 1 hour before a meal; contains sodium bicarbonate 1680 mg (20 mEq), equivalent to sodium 460 mg (20 mEq) per dose

Pharmacodynamics/Kinetics

Onset of action: Antisecretory: ~1 hour

Peak effect: 2 hours

Duration: 72 hours

Protein binding: 95%

Metabolism: Extensively hepatic to inactive metabolites

Bioavailability: Oral: 30% to 40%; increased in Asian patients and with hepatic dysfunction

Half-life elimination: 0.5-1 hour

Excretion: Urine (77% as metabolites, very small amount as unchanged drug); feces

Pregnancy Risk Factor C

Dosage Forms CAP, delayed release: 10 mg, 20 mg; (Prilosec®): 10 mg, 20 mg, 40 mg; (Prilosec OTC™): 20 mg. **POWDER for oral suspension** (Zegerid™): 20 mEq/packet (30s)

Omnicef® *see* Cefdinir *on page 279*

Omnipaque® *see* Radiological/Contrast Media (Nonionic) *on page 1166*

Oncaspar® *see* Pegaspargase *on page 1051*

Oncovin® [DSC] *see* VinCRIStine *on page 1378*

Ondansetron (on DAN se tron)

U.S. Brand Names Zofran®; Zofran® ODT

Canadian Brand Names Zofran®; Zofran® ODT

Mexican Brand Names Zofran®

Generic Available No

Synonyms GR38032R; Ondansetron Hydrochloride

Pharmacologic Category Antiemetic; Selective 5-HT_3 Receptor Antagonist

Use Prevention of nausea and vomiting associated with moderately- to highly-emetogenic cancer chemotherapy; radiotherapy in patients receiving total body irradiation or fractions to the abdomen; prevention and treatment of postoperative nausea and vomiting

Generally **not** recommended for treatment of existing chemotherapy-induced emesis (CIE) or for prophylaxis of nausea from agents with a low emetogenic potential.

Unlabeled/Investigational Use Treatment of early-onset alcoholism

Local Anesthetic/Vasoconstrictor Precautions No information available to require special precautions

Effects on Dental Treatment Key adverse event(s) related to dental treatment: Xerostomia (normal salivary flow resumes upon discontinuation).

Common Adverse Effects

>10%:

Cardiovascular: Malaise/fatigue (9% to 13%)

Central nervous system: Headache (9% to 27%)

1% to 10%:

Central nervous system: Drowsiness (8%), fever (2% to 8%), dizziness (4% to 7%), anxiety (6%), cold sensation (2%)

Dermatologic: Pruritus (2% to 5%), rash (1%)

Gastrointestinal: Constipation (6% to 9%), diarrhea (3% to 7%)

Genitourinary: Gynecological disorder (7%), urinary retention (5%)

Hepatic: Increased ALT/AST (1% to 2%)

Local: Injection site reaction (4%)

Neuromuscular & skeletal: Paresthesia (2%)

Respiratory: Hypoxia (9%)

Mechanism of Action Selective 5-HT_3-receptor antagonist, blocking serotonin, both peripherally on vagal nerve terminals and centrally in the chemoreceptor trigger zone

Drug Interactions

Cytochrome P450 Effect: Substrate of CYP1A2 (minor), 2C8/9 (minor), 2D6 (minor), 2E1 (minor), 3A4 (major); **Inhibits** CYP1A2 (weak), 2C8/9 (weak), 2D6 (weak)

Decreased Effect: CYP3A4 inducers may decrease the levels/effects of ondansetron; example inducers include aminoglutethimide, carbamazepine, nafcillin, nevirapine, phenobarbital, phenytoin, and rifamycins.

Pharmacodynamics/Kinetics

Onset of action: ~30 minutes

Distribution: V_d: 2.2-2.5 L/kg

Protein binding, plasma: 70% to 76%

Metabolism: Extensively hepatic via hydroxylation, followed by glucuronide or sulfate conjugation; CYP1A2, CYP2D6, and CYP3A4 substrate; some demethylation occurs

Bioavailability: Oral: 56% to 71%; Rectal: 58% to 74%

Half-life elimination: Children <15 years: 2-3 hours; Adults: 3-6 hours

Time to peak: Oral: ~2 hours

Excretion: Urine (44% to 60% as metabolites, 5% to 10% as unchanged drug); feces (~25%)

Pregnancy Risk Factor B

Ondansetron Hydrochloride *see* Ondansetron *on page 1014*

One-A-Day® 50 Plus Formula [OTC] *see* Vitamins (Multiple/Oral) *on page 1384*

One-A-Day® Active Formula [OTC] *see* Vitamins (Multiple/Oral) *on page 1384*

One-A -Day® Essential Formula [OTC] *see* Vitamins (Multiple/Oral) *on page 1384*

One-A-Day® Maximum Formula [OTC] *see* Vitamins (Multiple/Oral) *on page 1384*

One-A- Day® Men's Formula [OTC] *see* Vitamins (Multiple/Oral) *on page 1384*

One-A-Day® Today [OTC] *see* Vitamins (Multiple/Oral) *on page 1384*

One-A-Day® Women's Formula [OTC] *see* Vitamins (Multiple/Oral) *on page 1384*

ONTAK® *see* Denileukin Diftitox *on page 405*

Onxol™ *see* Paclitaxel *on page 1038*

Ony-Clear [OTC] [DSC] *see* Benzalkonium Chloride *on page 190*

OPC-13013 *see* Cilostazol *on page 329*

OPC-14597 *see* Aripiprazole *on page 142*

OP-CCK *see* Sincalide *on page 1224*

Opcon-A® [OTC] *see* Naphazoline and Pheniramine *on page 964*

o,p'-DDD *see* Mitotane *on page 937*

Operand® [OTC] *see* Povidone-Iodine *on page 1107*

Operand® Chlorhexidine Gluconate [OTC] *see* Chlorhexidine Gluconate *on page 308*

Ophthetic® *see* Proparacaine *on page 1134*

Opium and Belladonna *see* Belladonna and Opium *on page 186*

Opium, Hyoscyamine, Atropine, Scopolamine, Kaolin, and Pectin *see* Hyoscyamine, Atropine, Scopolamine, Kaolin, Pectin, and Opium *on page 726*

Opium Tincture (OH pee um TING chur)

Generic Available Yes

Synonyms DTO; Opium Tincture, Deodorized

Pharmacologic Category Analgesic, Narcotic; Antidiarrheal

Use Treatment of diarrhea or relief of pain

Local Anesthetic/Vasoconstrictor Precautions No information available to require special precautions

Effects on Dental Treatment No significant effects or complications reported

Mechanism of Action Contains many narcotic alkaloids including morphine; its mechanism for gastric motility inhibition is primarily due to this morphine content; it results in a decrease in digestive secretions, an increase in GI muscle tone, and therefore a reduction in GI propulsion

Pregnancy Risk Factor B/D (prolonged use or high doses at term)

Opium Tincture, Deodorized *see* Opium Tincture *on page 1015*

Oprelvekin (oh PREL ve kin)

U.S. Brand Names Neumega®

Generic Available No

Synonyms IL-11; Interleukin-11; Recombinant Human Interleukin-11; Recombinant Interleukin-11; rhIL-11; rIL-11

(Continued)

Oprelvekin *(Continued)*

Pharmacologic Category Biological Response Modulator; Human Growth Factor

Use Prevention of severe thrombocytopenia and the reduction of the need for platelet transfusions following myelosuppressive chemotherapy

Local Anesthetic/Vasoconstrictor Precautions No information available to require special precautions

Effects on Dental Treatment No significant effects or complications reported

Common Adverse Effects

>10%:

- Cardiovascular: Tachycardia (19% to 30%), palpitations (14% to 24%), atrial arrhythmias (12%), peripheral edema (60% to 75%), syncope (6% to 13%)
- Central nervous system: Headache (41%), dizziness (38%), insomnia (33%), fatigue (30%), fever (36%)
- Dermatologic: Rash (25%)
- Endocrine & metabolic: Fluid retention
- Gastrointestinal: Nausea (50% to 77%), vomiting, anorexia
- Hematologic: Anemia (100%), probably a dilutional phenomena; appears within 3 days of initiation of therapy, resolves in about 2 weeks after cessation of oprelvekin
- Neuromuscular & skeletal: Arthralgia, myalgias
- Respiratory: Dyspnea (48%), pleural effusions (10%)

1% to 10%: Gastrointestinal: Weight gain (5%)

Mechanism of Action Oprelvekin stimulates multiple stages of megakaryocytopoiesis and thrombopoiesis, resulting in proliferation of megakaryocyte progenitors and megakaryocyte maturation

Pharmacodynamics/Kinetics

Metabolism: Uncertain
Half-life elimination: Terminal: 5-8 hours
Time to peak, serum: 1-6 hours
Excretion: Urine (primarily as metabolites)

Pregnancy Risk Factor C

Opticaine® *see* Tetracaine *on page 1278*

Opticrom® *see* Cromolyn *on page 378*

Opticyl® *see* Tropicamide *on page 1348*

Optigene® 3 [OTC] *see* Tetrahydrozoline *on page 1282*

OptiPranolol® *see* Metipranolol *on page 913*

Optiray® *see* Radiological/Contrast Media (Nonionic) *on page 1166*

Optivar® *see* Azelastine *on page 173*

Orabase®-B [OTC] *see* Benzocaine *on page 191*

Oracit® *see* Sodium Citrate and Citric Acid *on page 1228*

Orajel® [OTC] *see* Benzocaine *on page 191*

Orajel® Baby [OTC] *see* Benzocaine *on page 191*

Orajel® Baby Nighttime [OTC] *see* Benzocaine *on page 191*

Orajel® Maximum Strength [OTC] *see* Benzocaine *on page 191*

Orajel® Perioseptic® Spot Treatment [OTC] *see* Carbamide Peroxide *on page 259*

Oral Bacterial Infections *see page 1533*

Oral Fungal Infections *see page 1544*

Oral Nonviral Soft Tissue Ulcerations or Erosions *see page 1551*

Oral Pain *see page 1526*

Oral Rinse Products *see page 1638*

Oral Viral Infections *see page 1547*

Oramorph SR® *see* Morphine Sulfate *on page 947*

Oranyl [OTC] *see* Pseudoephedrine *on page 1147*

Orap® *see* Pimozide *on page 1088*

Orapred® *see* PrednisoLONE *on page 1113*

OraRinse™ [OTC] *see* Maltodextrin *on page 855*

Orasol® [OTC] *see* Benzocaine *on page 191*

Orazinc® [OTC] *see* Zinc Sulfate *on page 1401*

Orciprenaline Sulfate *see* Metaproterenol *on page 885*

Oretic® *see* Hydrochlorothiazide *on page 699*

Orfadin® *see* Nitisinone *on page 989*

Organ-1 NR *see* Guaifenesin *on page 672*

Organidin® NR *see* Guaifenesin *on page 672*

Orgaran® [DSC] *see* Danaparoid *on page 395*

Orinase Diagnostic® [DSC] *see* TOLBUTamide *on page 1309*

ORLAAM® [DSC] *see* Levomethadyl Acetate Hydrochloride *on page 814*

Orlistat (OR li stat)

U.S. Brand Names Xenical®

Canadian Brand Names Xenical®

Mexican Brand Names Xenical®

Generic Available No

Pharmacologic Category Lipase Inhibitor

Use Management of obesity, including weight loss and weight management when used in conjunction with a reduced-calorie diet; reduce the risk of weight regain after prior weight loss; indicated for obese patients with an initial body mass index (BMI) ≥30 kg/m^2 or ≥27 kg/m^2 in the presence of other risk factors

Local Anesthetic/Vasoconstrictor Precautions No information available to require special precautions

Effects on Dental Treatment No significant effects or complications reported

Common Adverse Effects

>10%:

Central nervous system: Headache (31%)

Gastrointestinal: Oily spotting (27%), abdominal pain/discomfort (26%), flatus with discharge (24%), fatty/oily stool (20%), fecal urgency (22%), oily evacuation (12%), increased defecation (11%)

Neuromuscular & skeletal: Back pain (14%)

Respiratory: Upper respiratory infection (38%)

1% to 10%:

Central nervous system: Fatigue (7%), anxiety (5%), sleep disorder (4%)

Dermatologic: Dry skin (2%)

Endocrine & metabolic: Menstrual irregularities (10%)

Gastrointestinal: Fecal incontinence (8%), nausea (8%), infectious diarrhea (5%), rectal pain/discomfort (5%), vomiting (4%)

Neuromuscular & skeletal: Arthritis (5%), myalgia (4%)

Otic: Otitis (4%)

Mechanism of Action A reversible inhibitor of gastric and pancreatic lipases thus inhibiting absorption of dietary fats by 30% (at doses of 120 mg 3 times/day).

Drug Interactions

Decreased Effect: Orlistat may decrease amiodarone absorption (monitor). Coadministration with cyclosporine may decrease plasma levels of cyclosporine (administer cyclosporine 2 hours before or after orlistat and monitor). Orlistat does not alter the pharmacokinetics of warfarin, however, vitamin K absorption may be decreased during orlistat therapy (patients stabilized on warfarin should be monitored for changes in warfarin effects).

Pharmacodynamics/Kinetics

Absorption: Minimal

Metabolism: Metabolized within the gastrointestinal wall; forms inactive metabolites

Excretion: Feces (83% as unchanged drug)

Pregnancy Risk Factor B

Ornex® [OTC] *see* Acetaminophen and Pseudoephedrine *on page 53*

Ornex® Maximum Strength [OTC] *see* Acetaminophen and Pseudoephedrine *on page 53*

Orphenadrine (or FEN a dreen)

Related Information

Temporomandibular Dysfunction (TMD) *on page 1564*

U.S. Brand Names Norflex™

Canadian Brand Names Norflex™; Orphenace®; Rhoxal-orphendrine

Generic Available Yes

Synonyms Orphenadrine Citrate

Pharmacologic Category Anti-Parkinson's Agent, Anticholinergic; Skeletal Muscle Relaxant

Use Treatment of muscle spasm associated with acute painful musculoskeletal conditions; supportive therapy in tetanus

Local Anesthetic/Vasoconstrictor Precautions No information available to require special precautions

Effects on Dental Treatment The peripheral anticholinergic effects of orphenadrine may decrease or inhibit salivary flow; normal salivation will return with cessation of drug therapy.

(Continued)

Orphenadrine *(Continued)*

Common Adverse Effects

>10%:

Central nervous system: Drowsiness, dizziness
Ocular: Blurred vision

1% to 10%:

Cardiovascular: Flushing of face, tachycardia, syncope
Dermatologic: Rash
Gastrointestinal: Nausea, vomiting, constipation
Genitourinary: Decreased urination
Neuromuscular & skeletal: Weakness
Ocular: Nystagmus, increased intraocular pressure
Respiratory: Nasal congestion

Mechanism of Action Indirect skeletal muscle relaxant thought to work by central atropine-like effects; has some euphorigenic and analgesic properties

Drug Interactions

Cytochrome P450 Effect: Substrate (minor) of CYP1A2, 2B6, 2D6, 3A4; **Inhibits** CYP1A2 (weak), 2A6 (weak), 2B6 (weak), 2C8/9 (weak), 2C19 (weak), 2D6 (weak), 2E1 (weak), 3A4 (weak)

Increased Effect/Toxicity: Orphenadrine may increase potential for anticholinergic adverse effects of anticholinergic agents; includes drugs with high anticholinergic activity (diphenhydramine, TCAs, phenothiazines). Sedative effects of may be additive in concurrent use of orphenadrine and CNS depressants (monitor). Effects of levodopa may be decreased by orphenadrine. Monitor.

Pharmacodynamics/Kinetics

Onset of effect: Peak effect: Oral: 2-4 hours
Duration: 4-6 hours
Protein binding: 20%
Metabolism: Extensively hepatic
Half-life elimination: 14-16 hours
Excretion: Primarily urine (8% as unchanged drug)

Pregnancy Risk Factor C

Orphenadrine, Aspirin, and Caffeine

(or FEN a dreen, AS pir in, & KAF een)

Related Information

Aspirin *on page 151*
Orphenadrine *on page 1017*

U.S. Brand Names Norgesic™; Norgesic™ Forte; Orphengesic; Orphengesic Forte

Canadian Brand Names Norgesic™; Norgesic™ Forte

Generic Available Yes

Synonyms Aspirin, Orphenadrine, and Caffeine; Caffeine, Orphenadrine, and Aspirin

Pharmacologic Category Skeletal Muscle Relaxant

Use Relief of discomfort associated with skeletal muscular conditions

Local Anesthetic/Vasoconstrictor Precautions No information available to require special precautions

Effects on Dental Treatment The peripheral anticholinergic effects of orphenadrine may decrease or inhibit salivary flow; normal salivation will return with cessation of drug therapy.

Drug Interactions

Cytochrome P450 Effect:

Orphenadrine: **Substrate** (minor) of CYP1A2, 2B6, 2D6, 3A4; **Inhibits** CYP1A2 (weak), 2A6 (weak), 2B6 (weak), 2C8/9 (weak), 2C19 (weak), 2D6 (weak), 2E1 (weak), 3A4 (weak)

Aspirin: **Substrate** of CYP2C8/9 (minor)

Caffeine: **Substrate** of CYP1A2 (major), 2C8/9 (minor), 2D6 (minor), 2E1 (minor), 3A4 (minor); **Inhibits** CYP1A2 (weak), 3A4 (moderate)

Pharmacodynamics/Kinetics See individual agents.

Pregnancy Risk Factor D

Orphenadrine Citrate *see* Orphenadrine *on page 1017*
Orphengesic *see* Orphenadrine, Aspirin, and Caffeine *on page 1018*
Orphengesic Forte *see* Orphenadrine, Aspirin, and Caffeine *on page 1018*
Ortho-Cept® *see* Ethinyl Estradiol and Desogestrel *on page 536*
Orthoclone OKT® 3 *see* Muromonab-CD3 *on page 952*
Ortho-Cyclen® *see* Ethinyl Estradiol and Norgestimate *on page 554*
Ortho-Est® *see* Estropipate *on page 531*

Ortho Evra™ *see* Ethinyl Estradiol and Norelgestromin *on page 548*
Ortho-Novum® *see* Ethinyl Estradiol and Norethindrone *on page 550*
Ortho-Novum® 1/50 *see* Mestranol and Norethindrone *on page 884*
Ortho Prefest *see* Estradiol and Norgestimate *on page 521*
Ortho Tri-Cyclen® *see* Ethinyl Estradiol and Norgestimate *on page 554*
Ortho Tri-Cyclen® Lo *see* Ethinyl Estradiol and Norgestimate *on page 554*
Orthovisc® *see* Hyaluronate and Derivatives *on page 696*
Orudis® KT [OTC] *see* Ketoprofen *on page 785*
Oruvail® *see* Ketoprofen *on page 785*
Os-Cal® 500 [OTC] *see* Calcium Carbonate *on page 245*

Oseltamivir (oh sel TAM i vir)

Related Information

Systemic Viral Diseases *on page 1519*

U.S. Brand Names Tamiflu®

Canadian Brand Names Tamiflu®

Generic Available No

Pharmacologic Category Antiviral Agent; Neuraminidase Inhibitor

Use Treatment of uncomplicated acute illness due to influenza (A or B) infection in adults and children >1 year of age who have been symptomatic for no more than 2 days; prophylaxis against influenza (A or B) infection in adults and adolescents ≥13 years of age

Local Anesthetic/Vasoconstrictor Precautions No information available to require special precautions

Effects on Dental Treatment No significant effects or complications reported

Common Adverse Effects

As seen with **treatment** doses: 1% to 10%:

- Central nervous system: Insomnia (adults 1%), vertigo (adults 1%)
- Gastrointestinal: Nausea (adults 10%), vomiting (adults 9%, children 15%), abdominal pain (children 5%)
- Ocular: Conjunctivitis (children 1%)
- Otic: Ear disorder (children 2%)
- Respiratory: Epistaxis (children 3%)

Similar adverse effects were seen in **prophylactic** use, however, the incidence was generally less. The following reactions were seen more commonly with prophylactic use: Headache (20%), fatigue (8%), diarrhea (3%)

Mechanism of Action Oseltamivir, a prodrug, is hydrolyzed to the active form, oseltamivir carboxylate. It is thought to inhibit influenza virus neuraminidase, with the possibility of alteration of virus particle aggregation and release. In clinical studies of the influenza virus, 1.3% of post-treatment isolates had decreased neuraminidase susceptibility to oseltamivir carboxylate.

Drug Interactions

Increased Effect/Toxicity: Cimetidine and amoxicillin have no effect on plasma concentrations. Probenecid increases oseltamivir carboxylate serum concentration by twofold. Dosage adjustments are not required.

Pharmacodynamics/Kinetics

Absorption: Well absorbed

Distribution: V_d: 23-26 L (oseltamivir carboxylate)

Protein binding, plasma: Oseltamivir carboxylate: 3%; Oseltamivir: 42%

Metabolism: Hepatic (90%) to oseltamivir carboxylate; neither the parent drug nor active metabolite has any effect on CYP

Bioavailability: 75% reaches systemic circulation in active form

Half-life elimination: Oseltamivir carboxylate: 6-10 hours; similar in geriatrics (68-78 years)

Time to peak: C_{max}: Oseltamivir: 65 ng/mL; Oseltamivir carboxylate: 348 ng/mL

Excretion: Urine (as carboxylate metabolite)

Pregnancy Risk Factor C

Osmoglyn® *see* Glycerin *on page 667*
Otrivin® [OTC] [DSC] *see* Xylometazoline *on page 1393*
Otrivin® Pediatric [OTC] [DSC] *see* Xylometazoline *on page 1393*
Ovace™ *see* Sulfacetamide *on page 1244*
Ovcon® *see* Ethinyl Estradiol and Norethindrone *on page 550*
Ovidrel® *see* Chorionic Gonadotropin (Recombinant) *on page 326*
Ovral® [DSC] *see* Ethinyl Estradiol and Norgestrel *on page 557*
Ovrette® *see* Norgestrel *on page 998*

Oxacillin (oks a SIL in)

Generic Available Yes

Synonyms Methylphenyl Isoxazolyl Penicillin; Oxacillin Sodium

Pharmacologic Category Antibiotic, Penicillin

Use Treatment of infections such as osteomyelitis, septicemia, endocarditis, and CNS infections caused by susceptible strains of *Staphylococcus*

Local Anesthetic/Vasoconstrictor Precautions No information available to require special precautions

Effects on Dental Treatment Key adverse event(s) related to dental treatment: Prolonged use of penicillins may lead to development of oral candidiasis.

Common Adverse Effects Frequency not defined.

Central nervous system: Fever

Dermatologic: Rash

Gastrointestinal: Nausea, diarrhea, vomiting

Hematologic: Eosinophilia, leukopenia, neutropenia, thrombocytopenia, agranulocytosis

Hepatic: Hepatotoxicity, AST increased

Renal: Acute interstitial nephritis, hematuria

Miscellaneous: Serum sickness-like reactions

Mechanism of Action Inhibits bacterial cell wall synthesis by binding to one or more of the penicillin binding proteins (PBPs); which in turn inhibits the final transpeptidation step of peptidoglycan synthesis in bacterial cell walls, thus inhibiting cell wall biosynthesis. Bacteria eventually lyse due to ongoing activity of cell wall autolytic enzymes (autolysins and murein hydrolases) while cell wall assembly is arrested.

Drug Interactions

Increased Effect/Toxicity: Probenecid increases penicillin levels. Penicillins and anticoagulants may increase the effect of anticoagulants. Penicillins may increase the exposure to methotrexate during concurrent therapy; monitor.

Decreased Effect: Although anecdotal reports suggest oral contraceptive efficacy could be reduced by penicillins, this has been refuted by more rigorous scientific and clinical data.

Pharmacodynamics/Kinetics

Distribution: Into bile, synovial and pleural fluids, bronchial secretions, peritoneal, and pericardial fluids; crosses placenta; enters breast milk; penetrates the blood-brain barrier only when meninges are inflamed

Protein binding: ~94%

Metabolism: Hepatic to active metabolites

Half-life elimination: Children 1 week to 2 years: 0.9-1.8 hours; Adults: 23-60 minutes; prolonged in neonates and with renal impairment

Time to peak, serum: I.M.: 30-60 minutes

Excretion: Urine and feces (small amounts as unchanged drug and metabolites)

Pregnancy Risk Factor B

Oxacillin Sodium *see* Oxacillin *on page 1020*

Oxaliplatin (ox AL i pla tin)

U.S. Brand Names Eloxatin™

Generic Available No

Synonyms Diaminocyclohexane Oxalatoplatinum; L-OHP; NSC-266046

Pharmacologic Category Antineoplastic Agent, Alkylating Agent

Use Treatment of advanced colon or rectal carcinoma

Unlabeled/Investigational Use Head and neck cancer, nonsmall cell lung cancer, non-Hodgkin's lymphoma, ovarian cancer

Local Anesthetic/Vasoconstrictor Precautions No information available to require special precautions

Effects on Dental Treatment No significant effects or complications reported

Common Adverse Effects Based on clinical trial data using oxaliplatin alone. Some adverse effects (eg, thrombocytopenia, hemorrhagic events, neutropenia) may be increased when therapy is combined with fluorouracil/leucovorin.

>10%:

Central nervous system: Fatigue (61%), fever (25%), pain (14%), headache (13%), insomnia (11%)

Gastrointestinal: Nausea (64%), diarrhea (46%), vomiting (37%), abdominal pain (31%), constipation (31%), anorexia (20%), stomatitis (14%)

Hematologic: Anemia (64%), thrombocytopenia (30%), leukopenia (13%)

Hepatic: SGOT increased (54%), SGPT increased (36%); total bilirubin increased (13%)
Neuromuscular & skeletal: Neuropathy (may be dose-limiting), peripheral (acute 56%, persistent 48%), back pain (11%)
Respiratory: Dyspnea (13%), coughing (11%)

1% to 10%:
Cardiovascular: Edema (10%), chest pain (5%), flushing (3%), thrombosis (2% to 6%), thromboembolism (6% to 9%)
Central nervous system: Rigors (9%), dizziness (7%), hand-foot syndrome (1%)
Dermatologic: Rash (5%), alopecia (3%)
Endocrine & metabolic: Dehydration (5%), hypokalemia (3%)
Gastrointestinal: Dyspepsia (7%), taste perversion (5%), flatulence (3%), mucositis (2%), gastroesophageal reflux (1%), dysphagia (acute 1% to 2%)
Genitourinary: Dysuria (1%)
Hematologic: Neutropenia (7%)
Local: Injection site reaction (9%)
Neuromuscular & skeletal: Arthralgia (7%)
Ocular: Abnormal lacrimation (1%)
Renal: Serum creatinine increased (10%)
Respiratory: URI (7%), rhinitis (6%), epistaxis (2%), pharyngitis (2%), pharyngolaryngeal dysesthesia (1% to 2%)
Miscellaneous: Allergic reactions (3%), hiccup (2%)

Mechanism of Action Oxaliplatin is an alkylating agent. Following intracellular hydrolysis, the platinum compound binds to DNA, RNA, or proteins. Cytotoxicity is cell-cycle nonspecific.

Drug Interactions

Increased Effect/Toxicity: Taxane derivatives may increase oxaliplatin toxicity if administered before the platin as a sequential infusion; nephrotoxic agents (aminoglycosides) may increase oxaliplatin toxicity

Pharmacodynamics/Kinetics
Distribution: 400 L
Protein binding: >90% primarily albumin and gamma globulin (irreversible binding to platinum)
Metabolism: Nonenzymatic (rapid and extensive), forms active and inactive derivatives
Half-life elimination: 391 hours; Distribution: 0.4-16.8 hours
Excretion: Primarily urine

Pregnancy Risk Factor D

Oxandrin® *see* Oxandrolone *on page 1021*

Oxandrolone (oks AN droe lone)

U.S. Brand Names Oxandrin®

Generic Available No

Pharmacologic Category Androgen

Use Adjunctive therapy to promote weight gain after weight loss following extensive surgery, chronic infections, or severe trauma, and in some patients who, without definite pathophysiologic reasons, fail to gain or to maintain normal weight; to offset protein catabolism with prolonged corticosteroid administration; relief of bone pain associated with osteoporosis

Local Anesthetic/Vasoconstrictor Precautions No information available to require special precautions

Effects on Dental Treatment No significant effects or complications reported

Common Adverse Effects Frequency not defined.
Cardiovascular: Edema
Central nervous system: Depression, excitation, insomnia
Dermatologic: Acne (females and prepubertal males)
Also reported in females: Hirsutism, male-pattern baldness
Endocrine & metabolic: Electrolyte imbalances, glucose intolerance, gonadotropin secretion inhibited, gynecomastia
Also reported in females: Clitoral enlargement, menstrual irregularities
Genitourinary:
Prepubertal males: Increased or persistent erections, penile enlargement
Postpubertal males: Bladder irritation, epididymitis, impotence, oligospermia, priapism (chronic), testicular atrophy, testicular function
Hepatic: Alkaline phosphatase increased, AST increased, bilirubin increased, cholestatic jaundice, hepatic necrosis (rare), hepatocellular neoplasms, peliosis hepatitis (with long-term therapy)
Neuromuscular & skeletal: CPK increased, premature closure of epiphyses (in children)

(Continued)

Oxandrolone *(Continued)*

Renal: Creatinine excretion increased

Miscellaneous: Bromsulfophthalein retention, habituation, voice alteration (deepening, in females)

Restrictions C-III

Mechanism of Action Synthetic testosterone derivative with similar androgenic and anabolic actions

Drug Interactions

Increased Effect/Toxicity: ACTH, adrenal steroids may increase risk of edema and acne. Oxandrolone enhances the hypoprothrombinemic effects of oral anticoagulants, and enhances the hypoglycemic effects of insulin and sulfonylureas (oral hypoglycemics).

Pregnancy Risk Factor X

Oxaprozin (oks a PROE zin)

Related Information

Rheumatoid Arthritis, Osteoarthritis, and Osteoporosis *on page 1490*

Temporomandibular Dysfunction (TMD) *on page 1564*

U.S. Brand Names Daypro®

Canadian Brand Names Apo-Oxaprozin®; Daypro®; Rhoxal-oxaprozin

Generic Available Yes

Pharmacologic Category Nonsteroidal Anti-inflammatory Drug (NSAID), Oral

Use Acute and long-term use in the management of signs and symptoms of osteoarthritis and rheumatoid arthritis; juvenile rheumatoid arthritis

Local Anesthetic/Vasoconstrictor Precautions No information available to require special precautions

Effects on Dental Treatment NSAID formulations are known to reversibly decrease platelet aggregation via mechanisms different than observed with aspirin. The dentist should be aware of the potential of abnormal coagulation. Caution should also be exercised in the use of NSAIDs in patients already on anticoagulant therapy with drugs such as warfarin (Coumadin®).

Common Adverse Effects

1% to 10%:

Cardiovascular: Edema

Central nervous system: Confusion, depression, dizziness, headache, sedation, sleep disturbance, somnolence

Dermatologic: Pruritus, rash

Gastrointestinal: Abdominal distress, abdominal pain, anorexia, constipation, diarrhea, flatulence, gastrointestinal ulcer, gross bleeding with perforation, heartburn, nausea, vomiting

Hematologic: Anemia, bleeding time increased

Hepatic: Liver enzyme elevation

Otic: Tinnitus

Renal: Dysuria, renal function abnormal, urinary frequency

Mechanism of Action Inhibits prostaglandin synthesis by decreasing the activity of the enzyme, cyclooxygenase, which results in decreased formation of prostaglandin precursors

Drug Interactions

Increased Effect/Toxicity: Oxaprozin may increase cyclosporine, digoxin, lithium, and methotrexate serum concentrations. The renal adverse effects of ACE inhibitors may be potentiated by NSAIDs. Corticosteroids may increase the risk of GI ulceration. The risk of bleeding with anticoagulants (warfarin, antiplatelet agents, low molecular weight heparins) may be increased.

Decreased Effect: Oxaprozin may decrease the effect of some antihypertensive agents (including ACE inhibitors and angiotensin antagonists) and diuretics.

Pharmacodynamics/Kinetics

Absorption: Almost complete

Protein binding: >99%

Metabolism: Hepatic via oxidation and glucuronidation; no active metabolites

Half-life elimination: 40-50 hours

Time to peak: 2-4 hours

Excretion: Urine (5% unchanged, 65% as metabolites); feces (35% as metabolites)

Pregnancy Risk Factor C/D (3rd trimester)

Oxazepam (oks A ze pam)

Related Information

Patients Requiring Sedation *on page 1567*

U.S. Brand Names Serax®

Canadian Brand Names Apo-Oxazepam®; Novoxapram®; Oxpram®; PMS-Oxazepam

Generic Available Yes: Capsule

Pharmacologic Category Benzodiazepine

Use Treatment of anxiety; management of ethanol withdrawal

Unlabeled/Investigational Use Anticonvulsant in management of simple partial seizures; hypnotic

Local Anesthetic/Vasoconstrictor Precautions No information available to require special precautions

Effects on Dental Treatment Key adverse event(s) related to dental treatment: Xerostomia (normal salivary flow resumes upon discontinuation).

Common Adverse Effects Frequency not defined.

Cardiovascular: Syncope (rare), edema

Central nervous system: Drowsiness, ataxia, dizziness, vertigo, memory impairment, headache, paradoxical reactions (excitement, stimulation of effect), lethargy, amnesia, euphoria

Dermatologic: Rash

Endocrine & metabolic: Decreased libido, menstrual irregularities

Genitourinary: Incontinence

Hematologic: Leukopenia, blood dyscrasias

Hepatic: Jaundice

Neuromuscular & skeletal: Dysarthria, tremor, reflex slowing

Ocular: Blurred vision, diplopia

Miscellaneous: Drug dependence

Restrictions C-IV

Mechanism of Action Binds to stereospecific benzodiazepine receptors on the postsynaptic GABA neuron at several sites within the central nervous system, including the limbic system, reticular formation. Enhancement of the inhibitory effect of GABA on neuronal excitability results by increased neuronal membrane permeability to chloride ions. This shift in chloride ions results in hyperpolarization (a less excitable state) and stabilization.

Drug Interactions

Increased Effect/Toxicity: Ethanol and other CNS depressants may increase the CNS effects of oxazepam. Oxazepam may decrease the antiparkinsonian efficacy of levodopa. Flumazenil may cause seizures if administered following long-term benzodiazepine treatment.

Decreased Effect: Oral contraceptives may increase the clearance of oxazepam. Theophylline and other CNS stimulants may antagonize the sedative effects of oxazepam. Phenytoin may increase the clearance of oxazepam.

Pharmacodynamics/Kinetics

Absorption: Almost complete

Protein binding: 86% to 99%

Metabolism: Hepatic to inactive compounds (primarily as glucuronides)

Half-life elimination: 2.8-5.7 hours

Time to peak, serum: 2-4 hours

Excretion: Urine (as unchanged drug (50%) and metabolites)

Pregnancy Risk Factor D

Oxcarbazepine (ox car BAZ e peen)

U.S. Brand Names Trileptal®

Canadian Brand Names Trileptal®

Mexican Brand Names Trileptal®

Generic Available No

Synonyms GP 47680; OCBZ

Pharmacologic Category Anticonvulsant, Miscellaneous

Use Monotherapy or adjunctive therapy in the treatment of partial seizures in adults and children (4-16 years of age) with epilepsy

Unlabeled/Investigational Use Bipolar disorder

Local Anesthetic/Vasoconstrictor Precautions No information available to require special precautions

Effects on Dental Treatment No significant effects or complications reported

Common Adverse Effects As reported in adults with doses of up to 2400 mg/day (includes patients on monotherapy, adjunctive therapy, and those not previously on AEDs); incidence in children was similar.

>10%:

Central nervous system: Dizziness (22% to 49%), somnolence (20% to 36%), headache (13% to 32%, placebo 23%), ataxia (5% to 31%), fatigue (12% to 15%), vertigo (6% to 15%)

(Continued)

Oxcarbazepine *(Continued)*

Gastrointestinal: Vomiting (7% to 36%), nausea (15% to 29%), abdominal pain (10% to 13%)
Neuromuscular & skeletal: Abnormal gait (5% to 17%), tremor (3% to 16%)
Ocular: Diplopia (14% to 40%), nystagmus (7% to 26%), abnormal vision (4% to 14%)

1% to 10%:

Cardiovascular: Hypotension (1% to 2%), leg edema (1% to 2%, placebo 1%)
Central nervous system: Nervousness (2% to 5%, placebo 1% to 2%), amnesia (4%), abnormal thinking (2% to 4%), insomnia (2% to 4%), speech disorder (1% to 3%), EEG abnormalities (2%), abnormal feelings (1% to 2%), agitation (1% to 2%, placebo 1%), confusion (1% to 2%, placebo 1%)
Dermatologic: Rash (4%), acne (1% to 2%)
Endocrine & metabolic: Hyponatremia (1% to 3%, placebo 1%)
Gastrointestinal: Diarrhea (5% to 7%), dyspepsia (5% to 6%), constipation (2% to 6%, placebo 0% to 4%), gastritis (1% to 2%, placebo 1%), weight gain (1% to 2%, placebo 1%)
Neuromuscular & skeletal: Weakness (3% to 6%, placebo 5%), back pain (4%), falling down (4%), abnormal coordination (1% to 4%, placebo 1% to 2%), dysmetria (1% to 3%), sprains/strains (2%), muscle weakness (1% to 2%)
Ocular: Abnormal accommodation (2%)
Respiratory: Upper respiratory tract infection (7%), rhinitis (2% to 5%, placebo 4%), chest infection (4%), epistaxis (4%), sinusitis (4%)

Mechanism of Action Pharmacological activity results from both oxcarbazepine and its monohydroxy metabolite (MHD). Precise mechanism of anticonvulsant effect has not been defined. Oxcarbazepine and MHD block voltage sensitive sodium channels, stabilizing hyperexcited neuronal membranes, inhibiting repetitive firing, and decreasing the propagation of synaptic impulses. These actions are believed to prevent the spread of seizures. Oxcarbazepine and MHD also increase potassium conductance and modulate the activity of high-voltage activated calcium channels.

Drug Interactions

Cytochrome P450 Effect: Inhibits CYP2C19 (weak); **Induces** CYP3A4 (strong)

Increased Effect/Toxicity: Serum concentrations of phenytoin and phenobarbital are increased by oxcarbazepine.

Decreased Effect: Oxcarbazepine serum concentrations may be reduced by carbamazepine, phenytoin, phenobarbital, valproic acid and verapamil (decreases levels of active oxcarbazepine metabolite). Oxcarbazepine reduces the serum concentrations oral contraceptives; use alternative contraceptive measures. Oxcarbazepine may decrease the levels/effects of benzodiazepines, calcium channel blockers, clarithromycin, cyclosporine, erythromycin, estrogens, mirtazapine, nateglinide, nefazodone, nevirapine, protease inhibitors, tacrolimus, venlafaxine, and other CYP3A4 substrates.

Pharmacodynamics/Kinetics

Absorption: Complete; food has no affect on rate or extent
Distribution: MHD: V_d: 49 L
Protein binding, serum: MHD: 40%
Metabolism: Hepatic to 10-monohydroxy metabolite (MHC; active); MHD is further conjugated to DHD (inactive)
Bioavailability: Decreased in children <8 years; increased in elderly >60 years
Half-life elimination: Parent drug: 2 hours; MHD: 9 hours; renal impairment (Cl_{cr} 30 mL/minute): 19 hours
Time to peak, serum: 4.5 hours (3-13 hours)
Excretion: Urine (95%, <1% as unchanged oxcarbazepine, 27% as unchanged MHD, 49% as MHD glucuronides); feces (<4%)

Pregnancy Risk Factor C

Oxiconazole (oks i KON a zole)

Related Information

Oral Fungal Infections *on page 1544*

U.S. Brand Names Oxistat®

Canadian Brand Names Oxistat®; Oxizole®

Mexican Brand Names Gyno-Myfungar®; Myfungar®; Oxistat®

Generic Available No

Synonyms Oxiconazole Nitrate

Pharmacologic Category Antifungal Agent, Topical

Use Treatment of tinea pedis (athlete's foot), tinea cruris (jock itch), and tinea corporis (ringworm)

Local Anesthetic/Vasoconstrictor Precautions No information available to require special precautions

Effects on Dental Treatment No significant effects or complications reported

Common Adverse Effects 1% to 10%:

Dermatologic: Itching, erythema

Local: Transient burning, local irritation, stinging, dryness

Mechanism of Action The cytoplasmic membrane integrity of fungi is destroyed by oxiconazole which exerts a fungicidal activity through inhibition of ergosterol synthesis. Effective for treatment of tinea pedis, tinea cruris, tinea corporis, and tinea versicolor. Active against *Trichophyton rubrum*, *Trichophyton mentagrophytes*, *Trichophyton violaceum*, *Microsporum canis*, *Microsporum audouini*, *Microsporum gypseum*, *Epidermophyton floccosum*, *Candida albicans*, and *Malassezia furfur*.

Pharmacodynamics/Kinetics

Absorption: In each layer of the dermis; very little systemically after one topical dose

Distribution: To each layer of the dermis; enters breast milk

Excretion: Urine (<0.3%)

Pregnancy Risk Factor B

Oxiconazole Nitrate *see* Oxiconazole *on page 1024*

Oxidized Regenerated Cellulose *see* Cellulose (Oxidized/Regenerated) *on page 293*

Oxilapine Succinate *see* Loxapine *on page 850*

Oxipor® VHC [OTC] *see* Coal Tar *on page 367*

Oxistat® *see* Oxiconazole *on page 1024*

Oxpentifylline *see* Pentoxifylline *on page 1066*

Oxprenolol (ox PREN oh lole)

Canadian Brand Names Slow-Trasicor®; Trasicor®

Generic Available No

Synonyms Oxprenolol Hydrochloride

Pharmacologic Category Antihypertensive; Beta-Adrenergic Blocker, Noncardioselective

Use Treatment of mild or moderate hypertension

Unlabeled/Investigational Use Treatment of nonsevere hypertension in pregnancy (second-line agent)

Local Anesthetic/Vasoconstrictor Precautions No information available to require special precautions

Effects on Dental Treatment Nonselective beta-blockers may enhance the pressor response to epinephrine, resulting in hypertension and bradycardia. Many nonsteroidal anti-inflammatory drugs, such as ibuprofen and indomethacin, can reduce the hypotensive effect of beta-blockers after 3 or more weeks of therapy with the NSAID. Short-term NSAID use (ie, 3 days) requires no special precautions in patients taking beta-blockers.

Common Adverse Effects Frequency not defined

Cardiovascular: Congestive heart failure, pulmonary edema, cardiac enlargement, postural hypotension, severe bradycardia, lengthening of PR interval, second- and third-degree AV block, sinus arrest, palpitations, chest pain; peripheral vascular disorders, Raynaud's phenomenon, claudication, hot flashes

Central nervous system: Vertigo, syncope, lightheadedness, headache, dizziness, anxiety, mental depression, nervousness, irritability, hallucinations, sleep disturbances, nightmares, insomnia, weakness, sedation, vivid dreams, slurred speech

Dermatological: Dry skin, rash, pruritus

Endocrine & metabolic: Decreased libido, impotence, weight gain; elevated transaminases, alkaline phosphatase, and bilirubin; hypoglycemia

Gastrointestinal: Diarrhea, constipation, flatulence, heartburn, anorexia, nausea, vomiting, abdominal pain, dry mouth

Hematological: Thrombocytopenia, leukopenia

Neuromuscular & skeletal: Paresthesia

Ocular: Keratoconjunctivitis, dry eyes, itching eyes, blurred vision

Otic: Tinnitus

Renal: Elevated BUN

Respiratory: Dyspnea, wheezing, bronchospasm, status asthmaticus

Miscellaneous: Diaphoresis, nasal stuffiness, exertional tiredness

Restrictions Not available in U.S.

(Continued)

Oxprenolol *(Continued)*

Mechanism of Action Oxprenolol has a competitive ability to antagonize catecholamine-induced tachycardia at the beta-receptor sites in the heart, thus decreasing cardiac output, inhibits of renin release by the kidneys, and inhibits the vasomotor centers.

Drug Interactions

Cytochrome P450 Effect: Inhibits CYP2D6 (weak)

Increased Effect/Toxicity: Antiarrhythmic agents (eg, quinidine, amiodarone) may potentiate the negative inotropic and dromotropic effect of antiarrhythmic agents (quinidine, amiodarone) may be potentiated by oxprenolol. Concomitant use of I.V. calcium channel blockers with AV-blocking potential (eg, diltiazem and verapamil) may lead to severe hypotension, cardiac arrhythmias and cardiac arrest may occur. Catecholamine-depleting drugs (reserpine, guanethidine) may produce any excessive reduction of sympathetic activity, leading to severe bradycardia and hypotension.

Ergot alkaloids may cause deterioration in peripheral blood flow, leading to peripheral ischemia. Inhalational anesthetics may cause cardiodepressant effects in patients receiving oxprenolol. Oxprenolol may potentiate hypoglycemic effects of insulin and hypoglycemic agents. Concomitant use of MAO inhibitors may produce any excessive reduction of sympathetic activity. CNS depressants (opiate analgesics, antihistamines, ethanol, and psycho-active drugs) may potentiate CNS depressant effects of oxprenolol.

Decreased Effect: Concomitant use of NSAIDs (indomethacin) may decrease antihypertensive effect of oxprenolol. Concomitant use of sympathomimetic agents (eg, epinephrine) may cause hypertensive reactions.

Pharmacodynamics/Kinetics

Duration of beta-blocking effects: Immediate-release tablet: 8-12 hours; Slow-release tablet: Up to 24 hours

Absorption: 20% to 70%

Distribution: 1.3 L/kg

Protein binding: 80%

Metabolism: Hepatic first-pass effect

Half-life elimination: 1.3-1.5 hours

Time to peak, serum: Immediate-release tablet: 0.5-1.5 hours; Slow-release tablet: 2-4 hours

Excretion: Urine (as inactive metabolites, <5% as unchanged drug); major metabolite is glucuronide

Pregnancy Risk Factor Not assigned (similar agents rated C/D)

Oxprenolol Hydrochloride *see* Oxprenolol *on page 1025*

Oxsoralen® *see* Methoxsalen *on page 902*

Oxsoralen-Ultra® *see* Methoxsalen *on page 902*

Oxy 10® Balanced Medicated Face Wash [OTC] *see* Benzoyl Peroxide *on page 194*

Oxy 10® Balance Spot Treatment [OTC] *see* Benzoyl Peroxide *on page 194*

Oxy Balance® [OTC] *see* Salicylic Acid *on page 1205*

Oxy® Balance Deep Pore [OTC] *see* Salicylic Acid *on page 1205*

Oxybutynin (oks i BYOO ti nin)

U.S. Brand Names Ditropan®; Ditropan® XL; Oxytrol™

Canadian Brand Names Ditropan®; Ditropan® XL; Gen-Oxybutynin; Novo-Oxybutynin; Nu-Oxybutyn; PMS-Oxybutynin

Mexican Brand Names Tavor®

Generic Available Yes: Excludes extended release formulation or transdermal patch

Synonyms Oxybutynin Chloride

Pharmacologic Category Antispasmodic Agent, Urinary

Use Antispasmodic for neurogenic bladder (urgency, frequency, urge incontinence) and uninhibited bladder

Local Anesthetic/Vasoconstrictor Precautions No information available to require special precautions

Effects on Dental Treatment Key adverse event(s) related to dental treatment: Xerostomia and changes in salivation (normal salivary flow resumes upon discontinuation), and taste perversion.

Common Adverse Effects

Oral:

>10%:

Central nervous system: Dizziness (6% to 16%), somnolence (12% to 13%)

Gastrointestinal: Xerostomia (61% to 71%), constipation (13%)

Genitourinary: Urination impaired (11%)

1% to 10%:

Cardiovascular: Palpitation (2% to <5%), peripheral edema (2% to <5%), hypertension (2% to <5%), vasodilation (2% to <5%)

Central nervous system: Headache (6% to 10%), pain (7%), confusion (2% to <5%), insomnia (2% to <5%), nervousness (2% to <5%)

Dermatologic: Dry skin (2% to <5%), skin rash (2% to <5%)

Gastrointestinal: Nausea (9% to 10%), dyspepsia (7%), abdominal pain (2% to 6%), diarrhea (5% to 9%), flatulence (2% to <5%), gastrointestinal reflux (2% to <5%), taste perversion (2% to <5%)

Genitourinary: Post-void residuals increased (2% to 9%), urinary tract infection (5%)

Neuromuscular & skeletal: Weakness (2% to 7%)

Ocular: Blurred vision (8% to 9%), dry eyes (2% to 6%)

Respiratory: Rhinitis (6%), dry nasal and sinus membranes (2% to <5%)

Transdermal:

>10%: Local: Application site reaction (17%), pruritus (14%)

1% to 10%:

Gastrointestinal: Xerostomia (4% to 10%), diarrhea (3%), constipation (3%)

Genitourinary: Dysuria (2%)

Local: Erythema (6% to 8%), vesicles (3%), rash (3%)

Ocular: Vision changes (3%)

Mechanism of Action Direct antispasmodic effect on smooth muscle, also inhibits the action of acetylcholine on smooth muscle (exhibits $^1/_5$ the anticholinergic activity of atropine, but is 4-10 times the antispasmodic activity); does not block effects at skeletal muscle or at autonomic ganglia; increases bladder capacity, decreases uninhibited contractions, and delays desire to void; therefore, decreases urgency and frequency

Drug Interactions

Cytochrome P450 Effect: Substrate of CYP3A4 (minor); **Inhibits** CYP2D6 (weak), 3A4 (weak)

Increased Effect/Toxicity: Additive sedation with CNS depressants and ethanol. Additive anticholinergic effects with antihistamines and anticholinergic agents.

Pharmacodynamics/Kinetics

Onset of action: Oral: 30-60 minutes

Peak effect: 3-6 hours

Duration: 6-10 hours

Absorption: Oral: Rapid and well absorbed; Transdermal: High

Distribution: V_d: 193 L

Metabolism: Hepatic via CYP3A4; Oral: High first-pass metabolism; I.V.: Forms active and inactive metabolites

Half-life elimination: I.V.: ~2 hours (parent drug), 7-8 hours (metabolites)

Time to peak, serum: Oral: ~60 minutes; Transdermal: 24-48 hours

Excretion: Urine (<0.1%)

Pregnancy Risk Factor B

Oxybutynin Chloride *see* Oxybutynin *on page 1026*

Oxychlorosene (oks i KLOR oh seen)

U.S. Brand Names Clorpactin® WCS-90 [OTC]

Generic Available No

Synonyms Oxychlorosene Sodium

Pharmacologic Category Antibiotic, Topical

Use Treatment of localized infections

Local Anesthetic/Vasoconstrictor Precautions No information available to require special precautions

Effects on Dental Treatment No significant effects or complications reported

Oxychlorosene Sodium *see* Oxychlorosene *on page 1027*

Oxycodone (oks i KOE done)

Related Information

Oral Pain *on page 1526*

Oxycodone and Aspirin *on page 1032*

U.S. Brand Names OxyContin®; Oxydose™; OxyFast®; OxyIR®; Roxicodone™; Roxicodone™ Intensol™

Canadian Brand Names OxyContin®; Oxy.IR®; Supeudol®

Mexican Brand Names OxyContin®

Generic Available Yes

Synonyms Dihydrohydroxycodeinone; Oxycodone Hydrochloride

Pharmacologic Category Analgesic, Narcotic

Dental Use Treatment of postoperative pain

(Continued)

Oxycodone *(Continued)*

Use Management of moderate to severe pain, normally used in combination with non-narcotic analgesics

OxyContin® is indicated for around-the-clock management of moderate to severe pain when an analgesic is needed for an extended period of time. **Note:** OxyContin® is not intended for use as an "as needed" analgesic or for immediately-postoperative pain management (should be used postoperatively only if the patient has received it prior to surgery or if severe, persistent pain is anticipated).

Local Anesthetic/Vasoconstrictor Precautions No information available to require special precautions

Effects on Dental Treatment Key adverse event(s) related to dental treatment: Xerostomia (normal salivary flow resumes upon discontinuation).

Significant Adverse Effects

>10%:

Central nervous system: Fatigue, drowsiness, dizziness, somnolence
Dermatologic: Pruritus
Gastrointestinal: Nausea, vomiting, constipation
Neuromuscular & skeletal: Weakness

1% to 10%:

Cardiovascular: Postural hypotension
Central nervous system: Nervousness, headache, restlessness, malaise, confusion, anxiety, abnormal dreams, euphoria, thought abnormalities
Dermatologic: Rash
Gastrointestinal: Anorexia, stomach cramps, xerostomia, biliary spasm, abdominal pain, dyspepsia, gastritis
Genitourinary: Ureteral spasms, decreased urination
Local: Pain at injection site
Respiratory: Dyspnea, hiccoughs
Miscellaneous: Diaphoresis

<1% (Limited to important or life-threatening): Anaphylaxis, anaphylactoid reaction, dysphagia, exfoliative dermatitis, hallucinations, histamine release, hyponatremia, ileus, intracranial pressure increased, mental depression, paradoxical CNS stimulation, paralytic ileus, physical and psychological dependence, SIADH, syncope, urinary retention, urticaria, vasodilation, withdrawal syndrome (may include seizures)

Note: Deaths due to overdose have been reported due to misuse/abuse after crushing the sustained release tablets.

Restrictions C-II

Dosage Oral:

Immediate release:

Children:

6-12 years: 1.25 mg every 6 hours as needed
>12 years: 2.5 mg every 6 hours as needed

Adults: 5 mg every 6 hours as needed

Controlled release: Adults:

Opioid naive (not currently on opioid): 10 mg every 12 hours

Currently on opioid/ASA or acetaminophen or NSAID combination:

1-5 tablets: 10-20 mg every 12 hours
6-9 tablets: 20-30 mg every 12 hours
10-12 tablets: 30-40 mg every 12 hours
May continue the nonopioid as a separate drug.

Currently on opioids: Use standard conversion chart to convert daily dose to oxycodone equivalent. Divide daily dose in 2 (for every 12-hour dosing) and round down to nearest dosage form.

Note: 80 mg or 160 mg tablets are for use **only** in opioid-tolerant patients. Special safety considerations must be addressed when converting to OxyContin® doses ≥160 mg every 12 hours. Dietary caution must be taken when patients are initially titrated to 160 mg tablets.

Dosing adjustment in hepatic impairment: Reduce dosage in patients with severe liver disease

Mechanism of Action Binds to opiate receptors in the CNS, causing inhibition of ascending pain pathways, altering the perception of and response to pain; produces generalized CNS depression

Contraindications Hypersensitivity to oxycodone or any component of the formulation; significant respiratory depression; hypercarbia; acute or severe bronchial asthma; OxyContin® is also contraindicated in paralytic ileus (known or suspected); pregnancy (prolonged use or high doses at term)

Warnings/Precautions Use with caution in patients with hypersensitivity reactions to other phenanthrene derivative opioid agonists (morphine, hydrocodone, hydromorphone, levorphanol, oxycodone, oxymorphone), respiratory diseases including asthma, emphysema, or COPD. Use with caution in pancreatitis or biliary tract disease, acute alcoholism (including delirium tremens), adrenocortical insufficiency, CNS depression/coma, kyphoscoliosis (or other skeletal disorder which may alter respiratory function), hypothyroidism (including myxedema), prostatic hyperplasia, urethral stricture, and toxic psychosis.

Use with caution in the elderly, debilitated, severe hepatic or renal function. Hemodynamic effects (hypotension, orthostasis) may be exaggerated in patients with hypovolemia, concurrent vasodilating drugs, or in patients with head injury. Respiratory depressant effects and capacity to elevate CSF pressure may be exaggerated in presence of head injury, other intracranial lesion, or pre-existing intracranial pressure. Tolerance or drug dependence may result from extended use. Healthcare provider should be alert to problems of abuse, misuse, and diversion. Do **not** crush controlled-release tablets. Some preparations contain sulfites which may cause allergic reactions. OxyContin® 80 mg and 160 mg strengths are for use only in opioid-tolerant patients requiring high daily dosages >160 mg (80 mg formulation) or >320 mg (160 mg formulation).

Drug Interactions Substrate of CYP2D6 (major)

CNS depressants, MAO inhibitors, general anesthetics, and tricyclic antidepressants: May potentiate the effects of opiate agonists; dextroamphetamine may enhance the analgesic effect of opiate agonists

CYP2D6 inhibitors: May decrease the effects of oxycodone. Example inhibitors include chlorpromazine, delavirdine, fluoxetine, miconazole, paroxetine, pergolide, quinidine, quinine, ritonavir, and ropinirole.

Ethanol/Nutrition/Herb Interactions

Ethanol: Avoid ethanol (may increase CNS depression).

Food: When taken with a high-fat meal, peak concentration is 25% greater following a single OxyContin® 160 mg tablet as compared to two 80 mg tablets.

Herb/Nutraceutical: Avoid valerian, St John's wort, kava kava, gotu kola (may increase CNS depression).

Dietary Considerations Instruct patient to avoid high-fat meals when taking OxyContin® 160 mg tablets.

Pharmacodynamics/Kinetics

Onset of action: Pain relief: 10-15 minutes

Peak effect: 0.5-1 hour

Duration: 3-6 hours; Controlled release: ≤12 hours

Metabolism: Hepatic

Half-life elimination: 2-3 hours

Excretion: Urine

Pregnancy Risk Factor B/D (prolonged use or high doses at term)

Lactation Enters breast milk/use caution

Dosage Forms

Capsule, immediate release, as hydrochloride (OxyIR®): 5 mg

Solution, oral, as hydrochloride: 5 mg/5 mL (500 mL)

Roxicodone™: 5 mg/5 mL (5 mL, 500 mL) [contains alcohol]

Solution, oral concentrate, as hydrochloride: 20 mg/mL (30 mL)

Oxydose™: 20 mg/mL (30 mL) [contains sodium benzoate; berry flavor]

OxyFast®, Roxicodone™ Intensol™: 20 mg/mL (30 mL) [contains sodium benzoate]

Tablet, as hydrochloride: 5 mg

Roxicodone™: 5 mg, 15 mg, 30 mg

Tablet, controlled release, as hydrochloride (OxyContin®): 10 mg, 20 mg, 40 mg, 80 mg, 160 mg

Tablet, extended release, as hydrochloride: 80 mg

Selected Readings

Wynn RL, "Narcotic Analgesics for Dental Pain: Available Products, Strengths, and Formulations," *Gen Dent*, 2001, 49(2)126-36.

Oxycodone and Acetaminophen

(oks i KOE done & a seet a MIN oh fen)

Related Information

Acetaminophen *on page 47*

Oral Pain *on page 1526*

Oxycodone *on page 1027*

U.S. Brand Names Endocet®; Percocet®; Roxicet™; Roxicet™ 5/500; Tylox®

Canadian Brand Names Endocet®; Oxycocet®; Percocet®; Percocet®-Demi; PMS-Oxycodone-Acetaminophen

(Continued)

Oxycodone and Acetaminophen *(Continued)*

Generic Available Yes

Synonyms Acetaminophen and Oxycodone

Pharmacologic Category Analgesic, Narcotic

Dental Use Treatment of postoperative pain

Use Management of moderate to severe pain

Local Anesthetic/Vasoconstrictor Precautions No information available to require special precautions

Effects on Dental Treatment Key adverse event(s) related to dental treatment: Nausea, sedation, constipation, and xerostomia (normal salivary flow resumes upon discontinuation).

Significant Adverse Effects Frequency not defined (also see individual agents): Allergic reaction, constipation, dizziness, dysphoria, euphoria, lightheadedness, nausea, pruritus, respiratory depression, sedation, skin rash, vomiting

Restrictions C-II

Dosage Oral: Doses should be given every 4-6 hours as needed and titrated to appropriate analgesic effects. **Note:** Initial dose is based on the **oxycodone** content; however, the maximum daily dose is based on the **acetaminophen** content.

Children: Maximum acetaminophen dose: Children <45 kg: 90 mg/kg/day; children >45 kg: 4 g/day

Mild to moderate pain: Initial dose, **based on oxycodone content:** 0.05-0.1 mg/kg/dose

Severe pain: Initial dose, **based on oxycodone content:** 0.3 mg/kg/dose

Adults:

Mild to moderate pain: Initial dose, **based on oxycodone content:** 5 mg

Severe pain: Initial dose, **based on oxycodone content:** 15-30 mg. Do not exceed acetaminophen 4 g/day.

Elderly: Doses should be titrated to appropriate analgesic effects: Initial dose, **based on oxycodone content:** 2.5-5 mg every 6 hours. Do not exceed acetaminophen 4 g/day.

Dosage adjustment in hepatic impairment: Dose should be reduced in patients with severe liver disease.

Mechanism of Action

Oxycodone, as with other narcotic (opiate) analgesics, blocks pain perception in the cerebral cortex by binding to specific receptor molecules (opiate receptors) within the neuronal membranes of synapses. This binding results in a decreased synaptic chemical transmission throughout the CNS thus inhibiting the flow of pain sensations into the higher centers. Mu and kappa are the two subtypes of the opiate receptor which oxycodone binds to to cause analgesia.

Acetaminophen inhibits the synthesis of prostaglandins in the CNS and peripherally blocks pain impulse generation; produces antipyresis from inhibition of hypothalamic heat-regulating center

Contraindications Hypersensitivity to oxycodone, acetaminophen, or any component of the formulation; severe respiratory depression (in absence of resuscitative equipment or ventilatory support); pregnancy (prolonged periods or high doses at term)

Warnings/Precautions Use with caution in patients with hypersensitivity reactions to other phenanthrene-derivative opioid agonists (morphine, codeine, hydrocodone, hydromorphone, levorphanol, oxymorphone); respiratory diseases including asthma, emphysema, COPD, or severe liver or renal insufficiency, hypothyroidism, Addison's disease, prostatic hypertrophy, or urethral stricture; some preparations contain sulfites which may cause allergic reactions; may be habit-forming

Use with caution in patients with head injury and increased intracranial pressure (respiratory depressant effects increased and may also elevate CSF pressure). May mask diagnosis or clinical course in patients with acute abdominal conditions.

Enhanced analgesia has been seen in elderly patients on therapeutic doses of narcotics; duration of action may be increased in the elderly; the elderly may be particularly susceptible to the CNS depressant and constipating effects of narcotics

Drug Interactions Also see individual agents.

Oxycodone: **Substrate** of CYP2D6 (major)

Acetaminophen: **Substrate** (minor) of CYP1A2, 2A6, 2C8/9, 2D6, 2E1, 3A4

Anesthetics, general: May have additive CNS depression; consider lowering dose of one or both agents

Anticholinergics: Concomitant use may lead to paralytic ileus
CNS depressants: May have additive CNS depression; consider lowering dose of one or both agents
CYP2D6 inhibitors: May decrease the effects of oxycodone. Example inhibitors include chlorpromazine, delavirdine, fluoxetine, miconazole, paroxetine, pergolide, quinidine, quinine, ritonavir, and ropinirole.
Phenothiazines: May have additive CNS depression with phenothiazine and other tranquilizers; consider lowering dose of one or both agents
Sedative hypnotics: May have additive CNS depression; consider lowering dose of one or both agents

Ethanol/Nutrition/Herb Interactions Ethanol: May have additive CNS depression. In addition, excessive intake of ethanol may increase the risk of acetaminophen-induced hepatotoxicity. Avoid ethanol or limit to <3 drinks/day.

Pharmacodynamics/Kinetics See individual agents.

Pregnancy Risk Factor C/D (prolonged periods or high doses at term)

Lactation Enters breast milk/use caution

Breast-Feeding Considerations

Oxycodone: Excreted in breast milk. If occasional doses are used during breast-feeding, monitor infant for sedation, GI effects and changes in feeding pattern.
Acetaminophen: May be taken while breast-feeding

Dosage Forms

Caplet (Roxicet™ 5/500): Oxycodone hydrochloride 5 mg and acetaminophen 500 mg
Capsule: Oxycodone hydrochloride 5 mg and acetaminophen 500 mg
  Tylox®: Oxycodone hydrochloride 5 mg and acetaminophen 500 mg [contains sodium benzoate and sodium metabisulfite]
Solution, oral (Roxicet™): Oxycodone hydrochloride 5 mg and acetaminophen 325 mg per 5 mL (5 mL, 500 mL) [contains alcohol <0.5%]
Tablet: Oxycodone hydrochloride 5 mg and acetaminophen 325 mg; oxycodone hydrochloride 7.5 mg and acetaminophen 325 mg; oxycodone hydrochloride 7.5 mg and acetaminophen 500 mg; oxycodone hydrochloride 10 mg and acetaminophen 325 mg; oxycodone hydrochloride 10 mg and acetaminophen 650 mg
  Endocet® 5/325 [scored]: Oxycodone hydrochloride 5 mg and acetaminophen 325 mg
  Endocet® 7.5/325: Oxycodone hydrochloride 7.5 mg and acetaminophen 325 mg
  Endocet® 7.5/500: Oxycodone hydrochloride 7.5 mg and acetaminophen 500 mg
  Endocet® 10/325: Oxycodone hydrochloride 10 mg and acetaminophen 325 mg
  Endocet® 10/650: Oxycodone hydrochloride 10 mg and acetaminophen 650 mg
  Percocet® 2.5/325: Oxycodone hydrochloride 2.5 mg and acetaminophen 325 mg
  Percocet® 5/325 [scored]: Oxycodone hydrochloride 5 mg and acetaminophen 325 mg
  Percocet® 7.5/325: Oxycodone hydrochloride 7.5 mg and acetaminophen 325 mg
  Percocet® 7.5/500: Oxycodone hydrochloride 7.5 mg and acetaminophen 500 mg
  Percocet® 10/325: Oxycodone hydrochloride 10 mg and acetaminophen 325 mg
  Percocet® 10/650: Oxycodone hydrochloride 10 mg and acetaminophen 650 mg
  Roxicet™ [scored]: Oxycodone hydrochloride 5 mg and acetaminophen 325 mg

Comments Oxycodone, as with other narcotic analgesics, is recommended only for limited acute dosing (ie, 3 days or less). Oxycodone has an addictive liability, especially when given long-term. The acetaminophen component requires use with caution in patients with alcoholic liver disease.

Acetaminophen: A study by Hylek, et al, suggested that the combination of acetaminophen with warfarin (Coumadin®) may cause enhanced anticoagulation. The following recommendations have been made by Hylek, et al, and supported by an editorial in *JAMA* by Bell.
Dose and duration of acetaminophen should be as low as possible, individualized and monitored
For patients who reported taking the equivalent of at least 4 regular strength (325 mg) tablets for longer than a week, the odds of having an INR >6.0 were increased 10-fold above those not taking acetaminophen. Risk decreased
(Continued)

Oxycodone and Acetaminophen *(Continued)*

with lower intakes of acetaminophen reaching a background level of risk at a dose of 6 or fewer 325 mg tablets per week.

Selected Readings

Bell WR, "Acetaminophen and Warfarin: Undesirable Synergy," *JAMA*, 1998, 279(9):702-3.

Botting RM, "Mechanism of Action of Acetaminophen: Is There a Cyclooxygenase 3?" *Clin Infect Dis*, 2000, Suppl 5:S202-10.

Cooper SA, Precheur H, Rauch D, et al, "Evaluation of Oxycodone and Acetaminophen in Treatment of Postoperative Pain," *Oral Surg Oral Med Oral Pathol*, 1980, 50(6):496-501.

Dart RC, Kuffner EK, and Rumack BH, "Treatment of Pain or Fever With Paracetamol (Acetaminophen) in the Alcoholic Patient: A Systematic Review," *Am J Ther*, 2000, 7(2):123-34.

Dionne RA, "New Approaches to Preventing and Treating Postoperative Pain," *J Am Dent Assoc*, 1992, 123(6):26-34.

Gobetti JP, "Controlling Dental Pain," *J Am Dent Assoc*, 1992, 123(6):47-52.

Grant JA and Weiler JM, "A Report of a Rare Immediate Reaction After Ingestion of Acetaminophen," *Ann Allergy Asthma Immunol*, 2001, 87(3):227-9.

Hylek EM, Heiman H, Skates SJ, et al, "Acetaminophen and Other Risk Factors for Excessive Warfarin Anticoagulation 1998," *JAMA*, 1998, 279(9):702-3.

Kwan D, Bartle WR, and Walker SE, "The Effects of Acetaminophen on Pharmacokinetics and Pharmacodynamics of Warfarin," *J Clin Pharmacol*, 1999, 39(1):68-75.

McClain CJ, Price S, Barve S, et al, "Acetaminophen Hepatotoxicity: An Update," *Curr Gastroenterol Rep*, 1999, 1(1):42-9.

Shek KL, Chan LN, and Nutescu E, "Warfarin-Acetaminophen Drug Interaction Revisited," *Pharmacotherapy*, 1999, 19(10):1153-8.

Tanaka E, Yamazaki K, and Misawa S, "Update: The Clinical Importance of Acetaminophen Hepatotoxicity in Nonalcoholic and Alcoholic Subjects," *J Clin Pharm Ther*, 2000, 25(5):325-32.

Wynn RL, "Narcotic Analgesics for Dental Pain: Available Products, Strengths, and Formulations," *Gen Dent*, 2001, 49(2):126-8, 130, 132 passim.

Oxycodone and Aspirin (oks i KOE done & AS pir in)

Related Information

Aspirin *on page 151*

Oral Pain *on page 1526*

Oxycodone *on page 1027*

U.S. Brand Names Endodan®; Percodan®; Percodan®-Demi [DSC]

Canadian Brand Names Endodan®; Oxycodan®; Percodan®; Percodan®-Demi

Generic Available Yes

Synonyms Aspirin and Oxycodone

Pharmacologic Category Analgesic, Narcotic

Dental Use Treatment of postoperative pain

Use Management of moderate to severe pain

Local Anesthetic/Vasoconstrictor Precautions No information available to require special precautions

Effects on Dental Treatment Key adverse event(s) related to dental treatment: Nausea, sedation, constipation, and xerostomia (normal salivary flow resumes upon discontinuation). May have anticoagulant effects which may affect bleeding time. The elderly are a high-risk population for adverse effects from NSAIDs. As many as 60% of elderly patients with GI complications from NSAIDs can develop peptic ulceration and/or hemorrhage asymptomatically. Concomitant disease and drug use contribute to the risk of GI adverse effects. Enhanced analgesia has been seen with therapeutic doses of narcotics; duration of action may be increased. Elderly may also be particularly susceptible to the CNS depressant effects of narcotics.

Significant Adverse Effects

>10%:

- Cardiovascular: Hypotension
- Central nervous system: Dizziness, sedation, somnolence
- Gastrointestinal: Nausea, vomiting

1% to 10%:

- Central nervous system: Headache, nervousness
- Neuromuscular & skeletal: Weakness
- Gastrointestinal: Biliary spasm, constipation, stomach cramps, xerostomia
- Genitourinary: Ureteral spasms
- Respiratory: Dyspnea

Restrictions C-II

Dosage Oral (based on oxycodone combined salts):

Children: 0.05-0.15 mg/kg/dose every 4-6 hours as needed; maximum: 5 mg/dose (1 tablet Percodan® or 2 tablets Percodan®-Demi/dose)

Adults: Percodan®: 1 tablet every 6 hours as needed for pain or Percodan®-Demi: 1-2 tablets every 6 hours as needed for pain

Dosing adjustment in hepatic impairment: Dose should be reduced in patients with severe liver disease

Mechanism of Action

Oxycodone, as with other narcotic (opiate) analgesics, blocks pain perception in the cerebral cortex by binding to specific receptor molecules (opiate receptors) within the neuronal membranes of synapses. This binding results in a decreased synaptic chemical transmission throughout the CNS thus inhibiting the flow of pain sensations into the higher centers. Mu and kappa are the two subtypes of the opiate receptor which oxycodone binds to to cause analgesia.

Aspirin inhibits prostaglandin synthesis by decreasing the activity of the enzyme, cyclooxygenase, which results in decreased formation of prostaglandin precursors, acts on the hypothalamic heat-regulating center to reduce fever, blocks thromboxane synthetase action which prevents formation of the platelet-aggregating substance thromboxane A_2

Contraindications Hypersensitivity to oxycodone, aspirin, or any component of the formulation; severe respiratory depression; pregnancy

Warnings/Precautions Use with caution in patients with hypersensitivity to other phenanthrene derivative opioid agonists (morphine, codeine, hydrocodone, hydromorphone, oxymorphone, levorphanol); children and teenagers should not be given aspirin products if chickenpox or flu symptoms are present; aspirin use has been associated with Reye's syndrome; severe liver or renal insufficiency, pre-existing CNS and depression

Enhanced analgesia has been seen in elderly patients on therapeutic doses of narcotics; duration of action may be increased in the elderly; the elderly may be particularly susceptible to the CNS depressant and constipating effects of narcotics

Drug Interactions

Oxycodone: **Substrate** of CYP2D6 (major)

Aspirin: **Substrate** of CYP2C8/9 (minor)

Also see individual agents.

CYP2D6 inhibitors: May decrease the effects of oxycodone. Example inhibitors include chlorpromazine, delavirdine, fluoxetine, miconazole, paroxetine, pergolide, quinidine, quinine, ritonavir, and ropinirole.

Increased effect/toxicity with CNS depressants, TCAs, dextroamphetamine

Dietary Considerations May be taken with food or water.

Pharmacodynamics/Kinetics See individual agents.

Pregnancy Risk Factor D

Lactation Enters breast milk/use caution due to aspirin content

Breast-Feeding Considerations

Aspirin: Caution is suggested due to potential adverse effects in nursing infants.

Oxycodone: No data reported.

Dosage Forms [DSC] = Discontinued product

Tablet: Oxycodone hydrochloride 4.5 mg, oxycodone terephthalate 0.38 mg, and aspirin 325 mg

Endodan®, Percodan®: Oxycodone hydrochloride 4.5 mg, oxycodone terephthalate 0.38 mg, and aspirin 325 mg

Percodan®-Demi [DSC]: Oxycodone hydrochloride 2.25 mg, oxycodone terephthalate 0.19 mg, and aspirin 325 mg

Comments Oxycodone, as with other narcotic analgesics, is recommended only for limited acute dosing (ie, 3 days or less). Oxycodone has an addictive liability, especially when given long-term. The oxycodone with aspirin could have anticoagulant effects and could possibly affect bleeding times.

Selected Readings

Dionne RA, "New Approaches to Preventing and Treating Postoperative Pain," *J Am Dent Assoc*, 1992, 123(6):26-34.

Gobetti JP, "Controlling Dental Pain," *J Am Dent Assoc*, 1992, 123(6):47-52.

Wynn RL, "Narcotic Analgesics for Dental Pain: Available Products, Strengths, and Formulations," *Gen Dent*, 2001, 49(2):126-8, 130, 132 passim.

Oxycodone Hydrochloride *see* Oxycodone *on page 1027*

OxyContin® *see* Oxycodone *on page 1027*

Oxydose™ *see* Oxycodone *on page 1027*

OxyFast® *see* Oxycodone *on page 1027*

Oxygen (OKS i jen)

Related Information

Dental Office Emergencies *on page 1584*

Generic Available Yes

Pharmacologic Category Dental Gases

Dental Use Administered as a supplement with nitrous oxide to ensure adequate ventilation during sedation; a resuscitative agent for medical emergencies in dental office

(Continued)

Oxygen *(Continued)*

Use Treatment of various clinical disorders, both respiratory and nonrespiratory; relief of arterial hypoxia and secondary complications; treatment of pulmonary hypertension, polycythemia secondary to hypoxemia, chronic disease states complicated by anemia, cancer, migraine headaches, coronary artery disease, seizure disorders, sickle-cell crisis, and sleep apnea

Local Anesthetic/Vasoconstrictor Precautions No information available to require special precautions

Effects on Dental Treatment No significant effects or complications reported

Significant Adverse Effects No data reported

Dosage Children and Adults: Average rate of 2 L/minute

Mechanism of Action Increased oxygen in tidal volume and oxygenation of tissues at molecular level

Contraindications No data reported

Warnings/Precautions Oxygen-induced hypoventilation is the greatest potential hazard of oxygen therapy. In patients with severe COPD, the respiratory drive results from hypoxic stimulation of the carotid chemoreceptors. If this hypoxic drive is diminished by excessive oxygen therapy, hypoventilation may occur and further carbon dioxide retention with possible cessation of ventilation.

Drug Interactions No data reported

Pregnancy Risk Factor No data reported

Dosage Forms Liquid system with large reservoir holding 75-100 lb of liquid oxygen; compressed gas system consisting of high-pressure tank; tank sizes are "H" (6900 L of oxygen), "E" (622 L of oxygen) and "D" (356 L of oxygen)

OxyIR® *see* Oxycodone *on page 1027*

Oxymetazoline (oks i met AZ oh leen)

Related Information

Oral Bacterial Infections *on page 1533*

U.S. Brand Names Afrin® [OTC]; Afrin® Extra Moisturizing [OTC]; Afrin® Original [OTC]; Afrin® Severe Congestion [OTC]; Afrin® Sinus [OTC]; Duramist® Plus [OTC]; Duration® [OTC]; Genasal [OTC]; Neo-Synephrine® 12 Hour [OTC]; Neo-Synephrine® 12 Hour Extra Moisturizing [OTC]; Nōstrilla® [OTC]; OcuClear® [OTC] [DSC]; Twice-A-Day® [OTC]; Vicks Sinex® 12 Hour Ultrafine Mist [OTC]; Visine® L.R. [OTC]; 4-Way® Long Acting [OTC]

Canadian Brand Names Claritin® Allergic Decongestant; Dristan® Long Lasting Nasal; Drixoral® Nasal

Mexican Brand Names Afrin®; Iliadin®; Ocuclear®; Oxylin®; Visine A.D.®

Generic Available Yes

Synonyms Oxymetazoline Hydrochloride

Pharmacologic Category Adrenergic Agonist Agent; Vasoconstrictor

Dental Use Symptomatic relief of nasal mucosal congestion

Use Adjunctive therapy of middle ear infections, associated with acute or chronic rhinitis, the common cold, sinusitis, hay fever, or other allergies

Ophthalmic: Relief of redness of eye due to minor eye irritations

Local Anesthetic/Vasoconstrictor Precautions No information available to require special precautions

Effects on Dental Treatment No significant effects or complications reported

Significant Adverse Effects

>10%:

- Local: Transient burning, stinging
- Respiratory: Dryness of the nasal mucosa, sneezing

1% to 10%:

- Cardiovascular: Hypertension, palpitations
- Respiratory: Rebound congestion with prolonged use

Dosage

Intranasal (therapy should not exceed 3-5 days):

- Children 2-5 years: 0.025% solution: Instill 2-3 drops in each nostril twice daily
- Children ≥6 years and Adults: 0.05% solution: Instill 2-3 drops or 2-3 sprays into each nostril twice daily

Ophthalmic: Children >6 years and Adults: 0.025% solution: Instill 1-2 drops in affected eye(s) every 6 hours as needed or as directed by healthcare provider

Mechanism of Action Stimulates alpha-adrenergic receptors in the arterioles of the nasal mucosa to produce vasoconstriction

Contraindications Hypersensitivity to oxymetazoline or any component of the formulation

Warnings/Precautions Rebound congestion may occur with extended use (>3 days); use with caution in the presence of hypertension, diabetes, hyperthyroidism, heart disease, coronary artery disease, cerebral arteriosclerosis, or long-standing bronchial asthma

Drug Interactions Increased toxicity with MAO inhibitors

Pharmacodynamics/Kinetics

Onset of action: Intranasal: 5-10 minutes

Duration: 5-6 hours

Pregnancy Risk Factor C

Dosage Forms [DSC] = Discontinued product

Solution, intranasal spray, as hydrochloride: 0.05% (15 mL, 30 mL)

Afrin®, Afrin® Extra Moisturizing, Afrin® Sinus: 0.05% (15 mL) [contains benzyl alcohol; no drip formula]

Afrin® Original: 0.05% (15 mL, 30 mL, 45 mL)

Afrin® Severe Congestion: 0.05% (15 mL) [contains benzyl alcohol and menthol; no drip formula]

Duramist® Plus, Neo-Synephrine® 12 Hour, Nōstrilla®, Vicks Sinex® 12 Hour Ultrafine Mist, 4-Way® Long Acting Nasal: 0.05% (15 mL)

Duration®: 0.05% (30 mL)

Genasal: 0.05% (15 mL, 30 mL)

Neo-Synephrine® 12 Hour Extra Moisturizing: 0.05% (15 mL) [contains glycerin]

Solution, ophthalmic, as hydrochloride (OcuClear® [DSC], Visine® L.R.): 0.025% (15 mL, 30 mL) [contains benzalkonium chloride]

Oxymetazoline Hydrochloride *see* Oxymetazoline *on page 1034*

Oxymetholone (oks i METH oh lone)

U.S. Brand Names Anadrol®

Generic Available No

Pharmacologic Category Anabolic Steroid

Use Anemias caused by the administration of myelotoxic drugs

Local Anesthetic/Vasoconstrictor Precautions No information available to require special precautions

Effects on Dental Treatment No significant effects or complications reported

Common Adverse Effects

Male:

Postpubertal:

>10%:

- Dermatologic: Acne
- Endocrine & metabolic: Gynecomastia
- Genitourinary: Bladder irritability, priapism

1% to 10%:

- Central nervous system: Insomnia, chills
- Endocrine & metabolic: Decreased libido
- Gastrointestinal: Nausea, diarrhea
- Genitourinary: Prostatic hyperplasia (elderly)
- Hematologic: Iron-deficiency anemia, suppression of clotting factors
- Hepatic: Hepatic dysfunction

Prepubertal:

>10%:

- Dermatologic: Acne
- Endocrine & metabolic: Virilism

1% to 10%:

- Central nervous system: Chills, insomnia
- Dermatologic: Hyperpigmentation
- Gastrointestinal: Diarrhea, nausea
- Hematologic: Iron-deficiency anemia, suppression of clotting factors

Female:

>10%: Endocrine & metabolic: Virilism

1% to 10%:

- Central nervous system: Chills, insomnia
- Endocrine & metabolic: Hypercalcemia
- Gastrointestinal: Nausea, diarrhea
- Hematologic: Iron deficiency anemia, suppression of clotting factors
- Hepatic: Hepatic dysfunction

Restrictions C-III

Mechanism of Action Stimulates receptors in organs and tissues to promote growth and development of male sex organs and maintains secondary sex characteristics in androgen-deficient males

(Continued)

Oxymetholone *(Continued)*

Drug Interactions

Increased Effect/Toxicity: Oxymetholone may increase prothrombin times with patients receiving warfarin leading to toxicity. Insulin effects may be enhanced leading to hypoglycemia.

Pharmacodynamics/Kinetics

Onset of action: 2-6 months

Half-life elimination: 9 hours

Excretion: Urine (20% to 25%)

Pregnancy Risk Factor X

Oxymorphone (oks i MOR fone)

U.S. Brand Names Numorphan®

Canadian Brand Names Numorphan®

Generic Available No

Synonyms Oxymorphone Hydrochloride

Pharmacologic Category Analgesic, Narcotic

Use Management of moderate to severe pain and preoperatively as a sedative and a supplement to anesthesia

Local Anesthetic/Vasoconstrictor Precautions No information available to require special precautions

Effects on Dental Treatment Key adverse event(s) related to dental treatment: Anticholinergic side effects can cause a reduction of saliva production or secretion, contributing to discomfort and dental disease (ie, caries, oral candidiasis, and periodontal disease).

Common Adverse Effects

>10%:

Cardiovascular: Hypotension

Central nervous system: Fatigue, drowsiness, dizziness

Gastrointestinal: Nausea, vomiting, constipation

Neuromuscular & skeletal: Weakness

Miscellaneous: Histamine release

1% to 10%:

Central nervous system: Nervousness, headache, restlessness, malaise, confusion

Gastrointestinal: Anorexia, stomach cramps, xerostomia, biliary spasm

Genitourinary: Decreased urination, ureteral spasms

Local: Pain at injection site

Respiratory: Dyspnea

Restrictions C-II

Mechanism of Action Oxymorphone hydrochloride (Numorphan®) is a potent narcotic analgesic with uses similar to those of morphine. The drug is a semisynthetic derivative of morphine (phenanthrene derivative) and is closely related to hydromorphone chemically (Dilaudid®).

Drug Interactions

Increased Effect/Toxicity: Increased effect/toxicity with CNS depressants (phenothiazines, tranquilizers, anxiolytics, sedatives, hypnotics, alcohol), tricyclic antidepressants, and dextroamphetamine.

Decreased Effect: Decreased effect with phenothiazines.

Pharmacodynamics/Kinetics

Onset of action: Analgesic: I.V., I.M., SubQ: 5-10 minutes; Rectal: 15-30 minutes

Duration: Analgesic: Parenteral, rectal: 3-4 hours

Metabolism: Hepatic via glucuronidation

Excretion: Urine

Pregnancy Risk Factor B/D (prolonged use or high doses at term)

Oxymorphone Hydrochloride *see* Oxymorphone *on page 1036*

Oxytetracycline (oks i tet ra SYE kleen)

U.S. Brand Names Terramycin® I.M.

Canadian Brand Names Terramycin®

Mexican Brand Names Oxitraklin®; Terramicina®

Generic Available No

Synonyms Oxytetracycline Hydrochloride

Pharmacologic Category Antibiotic, Tetracycline Derivative

Use Treatment of susceptible bacterial infections; both gram-positive and gram-negative, as well as, *Rickettsia* and *Mycoplasma* organisms

Local Anesthetic/Vasoconstrictor Precautions No information available to require special precautions

Effects on Dental Treatment Tetracyclines are not recommended for use during pregnancy or in children ≤8 years of age since they have been reported to cause enamel hypoplasia and permanent teeth discoloration. Tetracyclines should only be used in these patients if other agents are contraindicated or alternative antimicrobials will not eradicate the organism. Long-term use associated with oral candidiasis.

Common Adverse Effects Frequency not defined; also refer to Tetracycline monograph

Cardiovascular: Pericarditis

Central nervous system: Bulging fontanels (infants), intracranial hypertension (adults)

Dermatologic: Angioneurotic edema, erythematous rash, exfoliative dermatitis (uncommon), maculopapular rash, photosensitivity, urticaria

Gastrointestinal: Anogenital inflammatory lesions, diarrhea, dysphagia, enamel hypoplasia, enterocolitis, glossitis, nausea, tooth discoloration, vomiting

Hematologic: Anemia, eosinophilia, neutropenia, thrombocytopenia

Local: Irritation

Renal: BUN increased

Miscellaneous: Anaphylactoid purpura, anaphylaxis, hypersensitivity reaction, SLE exacerbation

Mechanism of Action Inhibits bacterial protein synthesis by binding with the 30S and possibly the 50S ribosomal subunit(s) of susceptible bacteria, cell wall synthesis is not affected

Drug Interactions

Increased Effect/Toxicity: Oral anticoagulant (warfarin) effects may be increased.

Decreased Effect: Barbiturates, phenytoin, and carbamazepine decrease serum levels of tetracyclines. Although anecdotal reports suggest oral contraceptive efficacy could be reduced by tetracyclines, this has been refuted by more rigorous scientific and clinical data.

Pharmacodynamics/Kinetics

Absorption: Poor

Distribution: Crosses placenta

Metabolism: Hepatic (small amounts)

Half-life elimination: 8.5-9.6 hours; prolonged with renal impairment

Excretion: Urine; feces

Pregnancy Risk Factor D

Oxytetracycline and Hydrocortisone

(oks i tet ra SYE kleen & hye droe KOR ti sone)

Related Information

Hydrocortisone *on page 714*

Oxytetracycline *on page 1036*

U.S. Brand Names Terra-Cortril® [DSC]

Generic Available No

Synonyms Hydrocortisone and Oxytetracycline

Pharmacologic Category Antibiotic/Corticosteroid, Ophthalmic

Use Treatment of susceptible ophthalmic bacterial infections with associated swelling

Local Anesthetic/Vasoconstrictor Precautions No information available to require special precautions

Effects on Dental Treatment No significant effects or complications reported

Pregnancy Risk Factor C

Oxytetracycline and Polymyxin B

(oks i tet ra SYE kleen & pol i MIKS in bee)

Related Information

Oxytetracycline *on page 1036*

Polymyxin B *on page 1100*

U.S. Brand Names Terramycin® w/Polymyxin B Ophthalmic

Generic Available No

Synonyms Polymyxin B and Oxytetracycline

Pharmacologic Category Antibiotic, Ophthalmic

Use Treatment of superficial ocular infections involving the conjunctiva and/or cornea

Local Anesthetic/Vasoconstrictor Precautions No information available to require special precautions

Effects on Dental Treatment No significant effects or complications reported

Pregnancy Risk Factor D

Oxytetracycline Hydrochloride *see* Oxytetracycline *on page 1036*

Oxytocin (oks i TOE sin)

U.S. Brand Names Pitocin®
Canadian Brand Names Pitocin®; Syntocinon®
Mexican Brand Names Syntocinon®; Xitocin®
Generic Available Yes
Synonyms Pit
Pharmacologic Category Oxytocic Agent
Use Induction of labor at term; control of postpartum bleeding; adjunctive therapy in management of abortion
Local Anesthetic/Vasoconstrictor Precautions No information available to require special precautions
Effects on Dental Treatment No significant effects or complications reported
Common Adverse Effects Frequency not defined.
Fetus or neonate:
Cardiovascular: Arrhythmias (including premature ventricular contractions), bradycardia
Central nervous system: Brain or CNS damage (permanent), neonatal seizures
Hepatic: Neonatal jaundice
Ocular: Neonatal retinal hemorrhage
Miscellaneous: Fetal death, low Apgar score (5 minute)
Mother:
Cardiovascular: Arrhythmias, hypertensive episodes, premature ventricular contractions
Gastrointestinal: Nausea, vomiting
Genitourinary: Pelvic hematoma, postpartum hemorrhage, uterine hypertonicity, tetanic contraction of the uterus, uterine rupture, uterine spasm
Hematologic: Afibrinogenemia (fatal)
Miscellaneous: Anaphylactic reaction, subarachnoid hemorrhage
Mechanism of Action Produces the rhythmic uterine contractions characteristic to delivery
Pharmacodynamics/Kinetics
Onset of action: Uterine contractions: I.M.: 3-5 minutes; I.V.: ~1 minute
Duration: I.M.: 2-3 hour; I.V.: 1 hour
Metabolism: Rapidly hepatic and via plasma (by oxytocinase) and to a smaller degree the mammary gland
Half-life elimination: 1-5 minutes
Excretion: Urine
Pregnancy Risk Factor X

Oxytrol™ *see* Oxybutynin *on page 1026*
Oysco 500 [OTC] *see* Calcium Carbonate *on page 245*
Oyst-Cal 500 [OTC] *see* Calcium Carbonate *on page 245*
P-071 *see* Cetirizine *on page 298*
Pacerone® *see* Amiodarone *on page 101*

Paclitaxel (PAK li taks el)

U.S. Brand Names Onxol™; Taxol®
Canadian Brand Names Taxol®
Mexican Brand Names Bris Taxol®; Praxel®
Generic Available Yes
Synonyms NSC-125973
Pharmacologic Category Antineoplastic Agent, Antimicrotubular; Antineoplastic Agent, Natural Source (Plant) Derivative
Use Treatment of breast, lung (small cell and nonsmall cell), and ovarian cancers
Local Anesthetic/Vasoconstrictor Precautions No information available to require special precautions
Effects on Dental Treatment No significant effects or complications reported
Common Adverse Effects
>10%:
Allergic: Appear to be primarily nonimmunologically mediated release of histamine and other vasoactive substances; almost always seen within the first hour of an infusion (~75% occur within 10 minutes of starting the infusion); incidence is significantly reduced by premedication
Cardiovascular: Bradycardia (transient, 25%)
Dermatologic: Alopecia (87%), venous erythema, tenderness, discomfort
Hematologic: Myelosuppression, leukopenia, neutropenia (6% to 21%), thrombocytopenia
Hepatic: Mild increases in liver enzymes

Onset: 8-11 days
Nadir: 15-21 days
Recovery: 21 days

Neurotoxicity: Sensory and/or autonomic neuropathy (numbness, tingling, burning pain), myopathy or myopathic effects (25% to 55%), and central nervous system toxicity. May be cumulative and dose-limiting. **Note:** Motor neuropathy is uncommon at doses <250 mg/m^2; sensory neuropathy is almost universal at doses >250 mg/m^2; myopathic effects are common with doses >250 mg/m^2, generally occurring within 2-3 days of treatment, resolving over 5-6 days; pre-existing neuropathy may increase the risk of neuropathy.

Gastrointestinal: Severe, potentially dose-limiting mucositis, stomatitis (15%), most common at doses >390 mg/m^2

Neuromuscular & skeletal: Arthralgia, myalgia

1% to 10%:

Cardiovascular: Myocardial infarction

Dermatologic: Phlebitis (2%)

Gastrointestinal: Mild nausea and vomiting (5% to 6%), diarrhea (5% to 6%)

Hematologic: Anemia

Mechanism of Action Paclitaxel promotes microtubule assembly by enhancing the action of tubulin dimers, stabilizing existing microtubules, and inhibiting their disassembly, interfering with the late G_2 mitotic phase, and inhibiting cell replication. In addition, the drug can distort mitotic spindles, resulting in the breakage of chromosomes. Paclitaxel may also suppress cell proliferation and modulate immune response.

Drug Interactions

Cytochrome P450 Effect: Substrate (major) of CYP2C8/9, 3A4; **Induces** CYP3A4 (weak)

Increased Effect/Toxicity: CYP2C8/9 inhibitors may increase the levels/effects of paclitaxel; example inhibitors include delavirdine, fluconazole, gemfibrozil, ketoconazole, nicardipine, NSAIDs, pioglitazone, and sulfonamides. CYP3A4 inhibitors may increase the levels/effects of paclitaxel; example inhibitors include azole antifungals, ciprofloxacin, clarithromycin, diclofenac, doxycycline, erythromycin, imatinib, isoniazid, nefazodone, nicardipine, propofol, protease inhibitors, quinidine, and verapamil. In Phase I trials, myelosuppression was more profound when given after cisplatin than with alternative sequence. administered as sequential infusions, studies indicate a potential for increased toxicity when platinum derivatives (carboplatin, cisplatin) are administered before taxane derivatives (docetaxel, paclitaxel). Paclitaxel may increase doxorubicin levels/toxicity.

Decreased Effect: CYP2C8/9 inducers may decrease the levels/effects of paclitaxel; example inducers include carbamazepine, phenobarbital, phenytoin, rifampin, rifapentine, and secobarbital. CYP3A4 inducers may decrease the levels/effects of paclitaxel; example inducers include aminoglutethimide, carbamazepine, nafcillin, nevirapine, phenobarbital, phenytoin, and rifamycins.

Pharmacodynamics/Kinetics

Distribution:

V_d: Widely distributed into body fluids and tissues; affected by dose and duration of infusion

V_{dss}:

1- to 6-hour infusion: 67.1 L/m^2
24-hour infusion: 227-688 L/m^2

Protein binding: 89% to 98%

Metabolism: Hepatic via CYP2C8/9 and 3A4; forms metabolites

Half-life elimination:

1- to 6-hour infusion: Mean (beta): 6.4 hours
3-hour infusion: Mean (terminal): 13.1-20.2 hours
24-hour infusion: Mean (terminal): 15.7-52.7 hours

Excretion: Feces (~70%, 5% as unchanged drug); urine (14%)

Clearance: Mean: Total body: After 1- and 6-hour infusions: 5.8-16.3 L/hour/m^2; After 24-hour infusions: 14.2-17.2 L/hour/m^2

Pregnancy Risk Factor D

Pain-A-Lay® [OTC] *see* Phenol *on page 1075*

Pain-Off [OTC] *see* Acetaminophen, Aspirin, and Caffeine *on page 56*

Palgic *see* Carbinoxamine *on page 262*

Palgic®-D *see* Carbinoxamine and Pseudoephedrine *on page 262*

Palgic®-DS *see* Carbinoxamine and Pseudoephedrine *on page 262*

Palivizumab (pah li VIZ u mab)

U.S. Brand Names Synagis®

Canadian Brand Names Synagis®

Generic Available No

Pharmacologic Category Monoclonal Antibody

Use Prevention of serious lower respiratory tract disease caused by respiratory syncytial virus (RSV) in infants and children <2 years of age at high risk of RSV disease

Local Anesthetic/Vasoconstrictor Precautions No information available to require special precautions

Effects on Dental Treatment No significant effects or complications reported

Common Adverse Effects The incidence of adverse events was similar between the palivizumab and placebo groups.

>1%:

Central nervous system: Nervousness, fever
Dermatologic: Fungal dermatitis, eczema, seborrhea, rash
Gastrointestinal: Diarrhea, vomiting, gastroenteritis
Hematologic: Anemia
Hepatic: ALT increase, abnormal LFTs
Local: Injection site reaction, erythema, induration
Ocular: Conjunctivitis
Otic: Otitis media
Respiratory: Cough, wheezing, bronchiolitis, pneumonia, bronchitis, asthma, croup, dyspnea, sinusitis, apnea, upper respiratory infection, rhinitis
Miscellaneous: Oral moniliasis, failure to thrive, viral infection, flu syndrome

Postmarketing and/or case reports: Hypersensitivity reactions, anaphylaxis (very rare)

Mechanism of Action Exhibits neutralizing and fusion-inhibitory activity against RSV; these activities inhibit RSV replication in laboratory and clinical studies

Pharmacodynamics/Kinetics

Half-life elimination: Children <24 months: 20 days; Adults: 18 days
Time to peak, serum: 48 hours

Pregnancy Risk Factor C

Palmer's® Skin Success Acne [OTC] *see* Benzoyl Peroxide *on page 194*

Palmer's® Skin Success Acne Cleanser [OTC] *see* Salicylic Acid *on page 1205*

Palmer's® Skin Success Fade Cream™ [OTC] *see* Hydroquinone *on page 719*

Palmitate-A® [OTC] *see* Vitamin A *on page 1382*

Palonosetron (pal oh NOE se tron)

U.S. Brand Names Aloxi™

Generic Available No

Synonyms Palonosetron Hydrochloride; RS-25259; RS-25259-197

Pharmacologic Category Antiemetic; Selective 5-HT_3 Receptor Antagonist

Use Prevention of acute (within 24 hours) and delayed (2-5 days) chemotherapy-induced nausea and vomiting

Unlabeled/Investigational Use Prevention of postoperative vomiting

Local Anesthetic/Vasoconstrictor Precautions No information available to require special precautions

Effects on Dental Treatment No significant effects or complications reported

Common Adverse Effects

>10%: Dermatologic: Pruritus (8% to 22%)

1% to 10%:

Cardiovascular: Bradycardia (1%), hypotension (1%), tachycardia (nonsustained) (1%)
Central nervous system: Headache (6% to 9%), anxiety (1% to 5%), dizziness (1%)
Endocrine & metabolic: Hyperkalemia (1%)
Gastrointestinal: Constipation (5% to 10%), diarrhea (1%)
Neuromuscular & skeletal: Weakness (1%)

Mechanism of Action Selective 5-HT_3 receptor antagonist, blocking serotonin, both peripherally on vagal nerve terminals and centrally in the chemoreceptor trigger zone

Drug Interactions

Cytochrome P450 Effect: Substrate (minor) of CYP1A2, 2D6, 3A4

Increased Effect/Toxicity: No drug interactions of concern have been identified.

Pharmacodynamics/Kinetics

Distribution: V_d: 8.3 ± 2.5 L/kg

Protein binding: 62%

Metabolism: ~50% metabolized via CYP enzymes (and likely other pathways) to relatively inactive metabolites; CYP1A2, 2D6, and 3A4 contribute to its metabolism

Half-life elimination: Terminal: 40 hours

Excretion: Urine (80%, 40% as unchanged drug)

Pregnancy Risk Factor B

Palonosetron Hydrochloride *see* Palonosetron *on page 1040*

Pamelor® *see* Nortriptyline *on page 999*

Pamidronate (pa mi DROE nate)

U.S. Brand Names Aredia®

Canadian Brand Names Aredia®

Generic Available Yes

Synonyms Pamidronate Disodium

Pharmacologic Category Antidote; Bisphosphonate Derivative

Use Treatment of hypercalcemia associated with malignancy; treatment of osteolytic bone lesions associated with multiple myeloma or metastatic breast cancer; moderate to severe Paget's disease of bone

Local Anesthetic/Vasoconstrictor Precautions No information available to require special precautions

Effects on Dental Treatment No significant effects or complications reported

Common Adverse Effects As reported with hypercalcemia of malignancy; percentage of adverse effect varies upon dose and duration of infusion.

>10%:

Central nervous system: Fever (18% to 26%), fatigue (12%)

Endocrine & metabolic: Hypophosphatemia (9% to 18%), hypokalemia (4% to 18%), hypomagnesemia (4% to 12%), hypocalcemia (1% to 12%)

Gastrointestinal: Nausea (up to 18%), anorexia (1% to 12%)

Local: Infusion site reaction (up to 18%)

1% to 10%:

Cardiovascular: Atrial fibrillation (up to 6%), hypertension (up to 6%), syncope (up to 6%), tachycardia (up to 6%), atrial flutter (up to 1%), cardiac failure (up to 1%)

Central nervous system: Somnolence (1% to 6%), psychosis (up to 4%), insomnia (up to 1%)

Endocrine & metabolic: Hypothyroidism (6%)

Gastrointestinal: Constipation (4% to 6%), stomatitis (up to 1%)

Hematologic: Leukopenia (up to 4%), neutropenia (up to 1%), thrombocytopenia (up to 1%)

Neuromuscular & skeletal: Myalgia (up to 1%)

Renal: Uremia (up to 4%)

Respiratory: Rales (up to 6%), rhinitis (up to 6%), upper respiratory tract infection (up to 3%)

Mechanism of Action A biphosphonate which inhibits bone resorption via actions on osteoclasts or on osteoclast precursors. Does not appear to produce any significant effects on renal tubular calcium handling and is poorly absorbed following oral administration (high oral doses have been reported effective); therefore, I.V. therapy is preferred.

Pharmacodynamics/Kinetics

Onset of action: 24-48 hours

Peak effect: Maximum: 5-7 days

Absorption: Poor; pharmacokinetic studies lacking

Metabolism: Not metabolized

Half-life elimination: 21-35 hours

Excretion: Biphasic; urine (~50% as unchanged drug) within 120 hours

Pregnancy Risk Factor D

Pamidronate Disodium *see* Pamidronate *on page 1041*

Pamine® *see* Methscopolamine *on page 903*

Pamine® Forte *see* Methscopolamine *on page 903*

p-Aminoclonidine *see* Apraclonidine *on page 138*

Pamprin® Maximum Strength All Day Relief [OTC] *see* Naproxen *on page 965*

Pan-2400™ [OTC] *see* Pancreatin *on page 1042*

Pan-B Antibody *see* Rituximab *on page 1191*

Pancof® *see* Pseudoephedrine, Dihydrocodeine, and Chlorpheniramine *on page 1150*

Pancof®-XP *see* Hydrocodone, Pseudoephedrine, and Guaifenesin *on page 713*

Pancrease® *see* Pancrelipase *on page 1042*

Pancrease® MT *see* Pancrelipase *on page 1042*

Pancreatin (PAN kree a tin)

U.S. Brand Names Hi-Vegi-Lip® [OTC]; Kutrase®; Ku-Zyme®; Pan-2400™ [OTC]; Pancreatin 4X [OTC]; Pancreatin 8X [OTC]; Veg-Pancreatin 4X [OTC]

Mexican Brand Names Creon®; Optifree®; Pancrease®; Selecto®

Generic Available Yes

Pharmacologic Category Enzyme

Use Relief of functional indigestion due to enzyme deficiency or imbalance

Local Anesthetic/Vasoconstrictor Precautions No information available to require special precautions

Effects on Dental Treatment No significant effects or complications reported

Common Adverse Effects Frequency not defined.

Gastrointestinal: Loose stools (decrease dose)

Respiratory: Mucous membrane irritation or precipitation of asthma attack (due to inhalation of airborne powder)

Mechanism of Action An enzyme supplement, not a replacement, which contains a combination of lipase, amylase and protease. Enhances the digestion of proteins, starch and fat in the stomach and intestines.

Pregnancy Risk Factor C

Pancreatin 4X [OTC] *see* Pancreatin *on page 1042*

Pancreatin 8X [OTC] *see* Pancreatin *on page 1042*

Pancrecarb MS® *see* Pancrelipase *on page 1042*

Pancrelipase (pan kre LI pase)

U.S. Brand Names Creon®; Ku-Zyme® HP; Lipram 4500; Lipram-CR; Lipram-PN; Lipram-UL; Pancrease®; Pancrease® MT; Pancrecarb MS®; Pangestyme™ CN; Pangestyme™ EC; Pangestyme™ MT; Pangestyme™ UL; Ultrase®; Ultrase® MT; Viokase®

Canadian Brand Names Cotazym®; Creon® 5; Creon® 10; Creon® 20; Creon® 25; Pancrease®; Pancrease® MT; Ultrase®; Ultrase® MT; Viokase®

Generic Available Yes

Synonyms Lipancreatin

Pharmacologic Category Enzyme

Use Replacement therapy in symptomatic treatment of malabsorption syndrome caused by pancreatic insufficiency

Unlabeled/Investigational Use Treatment of occluded feeding tubes

Local Anesthetic/Vasoconstrictor Precautions No information available to require special precautions

Effects on Dental Treatment No significant effects or complications reported

Common Adverse Effects Frequency not defined; occurrence of events may be dose related.

Central nervous system: Pain

Dermatologic: Rash

Endocrine & metabolic: Hyperuricemia

Gastrointestinal: Nausea, cramps, constipation, diarrhea, perianal irritation/inflammation (large doses), irritation of the mouth, abdominal pain, intestinal obstruction, vomiting, flatulence, melena, weight loss, fibrotic strictures, greasy stools

Ocular: Lacrimation

Renal: Hyperuricosuria

Respiratory: Sneezing, dyspnea, bronchospasm

Miscellaneous: Allergic reactions

Mechanism of Action Pancrelipase is a natural product harvested from the hog pancreas. It contains a combination of lipase, amylase, and protease. Products are formulated to dissolve in the more basic pH of the duodenum so that they may act locally to break down fats, protein, and starch.

Pharmacodynamics/Kinetics

Absorption: None; acts locally in GI tract

Excretion: Feces

Pregnancy Risk Factor B/C (product specific)

Pandel® *see* Hydrocortisone *on page 714*

Pangestyme™ CN *see* Pancrelipase *on page 1042*

Pangestyme™ EC *see* Pancrelipase *on page 1042*

Pangestyme™ MT *see* Pancrelipase *on page 1042*

Pangestyme™ UL *see* Pancrelipase *on page 1042*

Panglobulin® *see* Immune Globulin (Intravenous) *on page 740*
Panhematin® *see* Hemin *on page 684*
Panixine DisperDose™ *see* Cephalexin *on page 294*
Panlor® DC *see* Acetaminophen, Caffeine, and Dihydrocodeine *on page 57*
Panlor® SS *see* Acetaminophen, Caffeine, and Dihydrocodeine *on page 57*
PanMist®-DM *see* Guaifenesin, Pseudoephedrine, and Dextromethorphan *on page 676*
PanMist® Jr. *see* Guaifenesin and Pseudoephedrine *on page 675*
PanMist® LA *see* Guaifenesin and Pseudoephedrine *on page 675*
PanMist® S *see* Guaifenesin and Pseudoephedrine *on page 675*
PanOxyl® *see* Benzoyl Peroxide *on page 194*
PanOxyl®-AQ *see* Benzoyl Peroxide *on page 194*
PanOxyl® Aqua Gel *see* Benzoyl Peroxide *on page 194*
PanOxyl® Bar [OTC] *see* Benzoyl Peroxide *on page 194*
Panretin® *see* Alitretinoin *on page 81*
Panthoderm® [OTC] *see* Dexpanthenol *on page 416*

Pantoprazole (pan TOE pra zole)

Related Information

Gastrointestinal Disorders *on page 1476*

U.S. Brand Names Protonix®

Canadian Brand Names Panto™ IV; Pantoloc™; Protonix®

Mexican Brand Names Pantozol®; Zurcal®

Generic Available No

Pharmacologic Category Proton Pump Inhibitor; Substituted Benzimidazole

Use

Oral: Treatment and maintenance of healing of erosive esophagitis associated with GERD; reduction in relapse rates of daytime and nighttime heartburn symptoms in GERD; hypersecretory disorders associated with Zollinger-Ellison syndrome or other neoplastic disorders

I.V.: As an alternative to oral therapy in patients unable to continue oral pantoprazole; hypersecretory disorders associated with Zollinger-Ellison syndrome or other neoplastic disorders

Unlabeled/Investigational Use Peptic ulcer disease, active ulcer bleeding (parenteral formulation); adjunct treatment with antibiotics for *Helicobacter pylori* eradication

Local Anesthetic/Vasoconstrictor Precautions No information available to require special precautions

Effects on Dental Treatment No significant effects or complications reported

Common Adverse Effects

1% to 10%:

Cardiovascular: Chest pain

Central nervous system: Pain, migraine, anxiety, dizziness

Endocrine & metabolic: Hyperglycemia (1%), hyperlipidemia

Gastrointestinal: Diarrhea (4%), constipation, dyspepsia, gastroenteritis, nausea, rectal disorder, vomiting

Genitourinary: Urinary frequency, urinary tract infection

Hepatic: Liver function test abnormality increased SGPT

Neuromuscular & skeletal: Weakness, back pain, neck pain, arthralgia, hypertonia

Respiratory: Bronchitis, increased cough, dyspnea, pharyngitis, rhinitis, sinusitis, upper respiratory tract infection

Miscellaneous: Flu syndrome, infection

Dosage Adults:

Oral:

Erosive esophagitis associated with GERD:

Treatment: 40 mg once daily for up to 8 weeks; an additional 8 weeks may be used in patients who have not healed after an 8-week course

Maintenance of healing: 40 mg once daily

Note: Lower doses (20 mg once daily) have been used successfully in mild GERD treatment and maintenance of healing

Hypersecretory disorders (including Zollinger-Ellison): Initial: 40 mg twice daily; adjust dose based on patient needs; doses up to 240 mg/day have been administered

Helicobacter pylori eradication (unlabeled use): Doses up to 40 mg twice daily have been used as part of combination therapy

I.V.:

Erosive esophagitis associated with GERD: 40 mg once daily for 7-10 days

(Continued)

Pantoprazole *(Continued)*

Hypersecretory disorders: 80 mg twice daily; adjust dose based on acid output measurements; 160-240 mg/day in divided doses has been used for a limited period (up to 7 days)

Prevention of rebleeding in peptic ulcer bleed (unlabeled use): 80 mg, followed by 8 mg/hour infusion for 72 hours

Elderly: Dosage adjustment not required

Dosage adjustment in renal impairment: Not required; pantoprazole is not removed by hemodialysis

Dosage adjustment in hepatic impairment: Not required

Mechanism of Action Suppresses gastric acid secretin by inhibiting the parietal cell H^+/K^+ ATP pump

Contraindications Hypersensitivity to pantoprazole, substituted benzamidazoles (ie, esomeprazole, lansoprazole, omeprazole, rabeprazole), or any component of the formulation

Warnings/Precautions Symptomatic response does not preclude gastric malignancy. Not indicated for maintenance therapy; safety and efficacy for use beyond 16 weeks have not been established. Prolonged treatment (typically >3 years) may lead to vitamin B_{12} malabsorption. Intravenous preparation contains edetate sodium (EDTA); use caution in patients who are risk for zinc deficiency if other EDTA-containing solutions are coadministered. Safety and efficacy in pediatric patients have not been established.

Drug Interactions

Cytochrome P450 Effect: Substrate of CYP2C19 (major), 3A4 (minor); **Inhibits** 2C8/9 (moderate); **Induces** CYP1A2 (weak), 3A4 (weak)

Increased Effect/Toxicity: Pantoprazole may increase the levels/effects of amiodarone, fluoxetine, glimepiride, glipizide, nateglinide, phenytoin, pioglitazone, rosiglitazone, sertraline, warfarin, and other CYP2C8/9 substrates.

Decreased Effect: Proton pump inhibitors may decrease the absorption of ampicillin esters, atazanavir, indinavir, iron salts, itraconazole, and ketoconazole. The levels/effects of pantoprazole may be decreased by aminoglutethimide, carbamazepine, phenytoin, rifampin, and other CYP2C19 inducers.

Ethanol/Nutrition/Herb Interactions Ethanol: Avoid ethanol (may cause gastric mucosal irritation).

Dietary Considerations

Oral: May be taken with or without food; best if taken before breakfast.

I.V.: Due to EDTA in preparation, zinc supplementation may be needed in patients prone to zinc deficiency.

Pharmacodynamics/Kinetics

Absorption: Well absorbed

Distribution: V_d: 11-24 L

Protein binding: 98%, primarily to albumin

Metabolism: Extensively hepatic; CYP2C19 (demethylation), CYP3A4; no evidence that metabolites have pharmacologic activity

Bioavailability: 77%

Half-life elimination: 1 hour

Time to peak: Oral: 2.5 hours

Excretion: Urine (71%); feces (18%)

Pregnancy Risk Factor B

Dosage Forms INJ, powder for reconstitution: 40 mg. **TAB, delayed release:** 20 mg, 40 mg

Pantothenic Acid (pan toe THEN ik AS id)

Generic Available Yes

Synonyms Calcium Pantothenate; Vitamin B_5

Pharmacologic Category Vitamin, Water Soluble

Use Pantothenic acid deficiency

Local Anesthetic/Vasoconstrictor Precautions No information available to require special precautions

Effects on Dental Treatment No significant effects or complications reported

Pregnancy Risk Factor A/C (dose exceeding RDA recommendation)

Pantothenyl Alcohol *see* Dexpanthenol *on page 416*

Papaverine (pa PAV er een)

U.S. Brand Names Para-Time S.R.®

Generic Available Yes

Synonyms Papaverine Hydrochloride; Pavabid [DSC]

Pharmacologic Category Vasodilator

Use Oral: Relief of peripheral and cerebral ischemia associated with arterial spasm and myocardial ischemia complicated by arrhythmias

Unlabeled/Investigational Use Investigational: Parenteral: Various vascular spasms associated with muscle spasms as in myocardial infarction, angina, peripheral and pulmonary embolism, peripheral vascular disease, angiospastic states, and visceral spasm (ureteral, biliary, and GI colic); testing for impotence

Local Anesthetic/Vasoconstrictor Precautions No information available to require special precautions

Effects on Dental Treatment No significant effects or complications reported

Common Adverse Effects Frequency not defined.

Cardiovascular: Arrhythmias (with rapid I.V. use), flushing of the face, mild hypertension, tachycardias

Central nervous system: Drowsiness, headache, lethargy, sedation, vertigo

Gastrointestinal: Abdominal distress, anorexia, constipation, diarrhea, nausea

Hepatic: Chronic hepatitis, hepatic hypersensitivity

Respiratory: Apnea (with rapid I.V. use)

Mechanism of Action Smooth muscle spasmolytic producing a generalized smooth muscle relaxation including: vasodilatation, gastrointestinal sphincter relaxation, bronchiolar muscle relaxation, and potentially a depressed myocardium (with large doses); muscle relaxation may occur due to inhibition or cyclic nucleotide phosphodiesterase, increasing cyclic AMP; muscle relaxation is unrelated to nerve innervation; papaverine increases cerebral blood flow in normal subjects; oxygen uptake is unaltered

Drug Interactions

Decreased Effect: Papaverine decreases the effects of levodopa.

Pharmacodynamics/Kinetics

Onset of action: Oral: Rapid

Protein binding: 90%

Metabolism: Rapidly hepatic

Half-life elimination: 0.5-1.5 hours

Excretion: Primarily urine (as metabolites)

Pregnancy Risk Factor C

Papaverine Hydrochloride *see* Papaverine *on page 1044*

Para-Aminosalicylate Sodium *see* Aminosalicylic Acid *on page 100*

Paracetamol *see* Acetaminophen *on page 47*

Parafon Forte® DSC *see* Chlorzoxazone *on page 322*

Paraplatin® *see* Carboplatin *on page 264*

Parathyroid Hormone (1-34) *see* Teriparatide *on page 1274*

Para-Time S.R.® *see* Papaverine *on page 1044*

Paregoric (par e GOR ik)

Generic Available Yes

Synonyms Camphorated Tincture of Opium

Pharmacologic Category Analgesic, Narcotic

Use Treatment of diarrhea or relief of pain; neonatal opiate withdrawal

Local Anesthetic/Vasoconstrictor Precautions No information available to require special precautions

Effects on Dental Treatment No significant effects or complications reported

Mechanism of Action Increases smooth muscle tone in GI tract, decreases motility and peristalsis, diminishes digestive secretions

Pregnancy Risk Factor B/D (prolonged use or high doses)

Paremyd® *see* Hydroxyamphetamine and Tropicamide *on page 720*

Paricalcitol (pah ri KAL si tole)

U.S. Brand Names Zemplar™

Canadian Brand Names Zemplar™

Generic Available No

Pharmacologic Category Vitamin D Analog

Use Prevention and treatment of secondary hyperparathyroidism associated with chronic renal failure. Has been evaluated only in hemodialysis patients.

Local Anesthetic/Vasoconstrictor Precautions No information available to require special precautions

Effects on Dental Treatment No significant effects or complications reported

Common Adverse Effects The three most frequently reported events in clinical studies were nausea, vomiting, and edema, which are commonly seen in hemodialysis patients.

>10%: Gastrointestinal: Nausea (13%)

(Continued)

Paricalcitol *(Continued)*

1% to 10%:

Cardiovascular: Palpitations, peripheral edema (7%)
Central nervous system: Chills, malaise, fever, lightheadedness (5%)
Gastrointestinal: Vomiting (8%), GI bleeding (5%), xerostomia (3%)
Respiratory: Pneumonia (5%)
Miscellaneous: Flu-like symptoms, sepsis

Mechanism of Action Synthetic vitamin D analog which has been shown to reduce PTH serum concentrations

Drug Interactions

Increased Effect/Toxicity: Phosphate or vitamin D-related compounds should not be taken concurrently. Digitalis toxicity is potentiated by hypercalcemia.

Pharmacodynamics/Kinetics

Protein binding: >99%

Excretion: Feces (74%) in healthy subjects; urine (16%); 51% to 59% as metabolites

Pregnancy Risk Factor C

Pariprazole *see* Rabeprazole *on page 1164*
Parlodel® *see* Bromocriptine *on page 219*
Parnate® *see* Tranylcypromine *on page 1323*

Paromomycin (par oh moe MYE sin)

U.S. Brand Names Humatin®

Canadian Brand Names Humatin®

Generic Available Yes

Synonyms Paromomycin Sulfate

Pharmacologic Category Amebicide

Use Treatment of acute and chronic intestinal amebiasis; hepatic coma

Unlabeled/Investigational Use Treatment of cryptosporidiosis

Local Anesthetic/Vasoconstrictor Precautions No information available to require special precautions

Effects on Dental Treatment No significant effects or complications reported

Common Adverse Effects

1% to 10%: Gastrointestinal: Diarrhea, abdominal cramps, nausea, vomiting, heartburn

Mechanism of Action Acts directly on ameba; has antibacterial activity against normal and pathogenic organisms in the GI tract; interferes with bacterial protein synthesis by binding to 30S ribosomal subunits

Pharmacodynamics/Kinetics

Absorption: None

Excretion: Feces (100% as unchanged drug)

Pregnancy Risk Factor C

Paromomycin Sulfate *see* Paromomycin *on page 1046*

Paroxetine (pa ROKS e teen)

U.S. Brand Names Paxil®; Paxil CR™; Pexeva™

Canadian Brand Names Paxil®; Paxil CR™

Mexican Brand Names Aropax®; Paxil®

Generic Available Yes: Tablet, as hydrochloride

Synonyms Paroxetine Hydrochloride; Paroxetine Mesylate

Pharmacologic Category Antidepressant, Selective Serotonin Reuptake Inhibitor

Use Treatment of depression in adults; treatment of panic disorder with or without agoraphobia; obsessive-compulsive disorder (OCD) in adults; social anxiety disorder (social phobia); generalized anxiety disorder (GAD); post-traumatic stress disorder (PTSD)

Paxil CR™: Treatment of depression; panic disorder; premenstrual dysphoric disorder (PMDD); social anxiety disorder (social phobia)

Unlabeled/Investigational Use May be useful in eating disorders, impulse control disorders, self-injurious behavior; premenstrual disorders, vasomotor symptoms of menopause; treatment of depression and obsessive-compulsive disorder (OCD) in children

Local Anesthetic/Vasoconstrictor Precautions Although caution should be used in patients taking tricyclic antidepressants, no interactions have been reported with vasoconstrictor and paroxetine, a nontricyclic antidepressant which acts to increase serotonin

Effects on Dental Treatment Key adverse event(s) related to dental treatment: Xerostomia and changes in salivation (normal salivary flow resumes upon discontinuation), postural hypotension, and abnormal taste. Problems with SSRI-induced bruxism have been reported and may preclude their use; clinicians attempting to evaluate any patient with bruxism or involuntary muscle movement, who is simultaneously being treated with an SSRI drug, should be aware of the potential association. Prolonged use may decrease or inhibit salivary flow; normal salivation resumes upon discontinuation.

Common Adverse Effects

>10%:

- Central nervous system: Headache, somnolence, dizziness, insomnia
- Gastrointestinal: Nausea, xerostomia, constipation, diarrhea
- Genitourinary: Ejaculatory disturbances
- Neuromuscular & skeletal: Weakness
- Miscellaneous: Diaphoresis

1% to 10%:

- Cardiovascular: Palpitations, vasodilation, postural hypotension
- Central nervous system: Nervousness, anxiety, yawning, abnormal dreams, agitation
- Dermatologic: Rash
- Endocrine & metabolic: Libido decreased, delayed ejaculation
- Gastrointestinal: Anorexia, flatulence, vomiting, dyspepsia, taste perversion, weight gain
- Genitourinary: Urinary frequency, impotence
- Neuromuscular & skeletal: Tremor, paresthesia, myopathy, myalgia
- Ocular: Blurred vision
- Respiratory: Rhinitis

Dosage Oral:

Children:

- Depression (unlabeled use; not recommended by FDA): Initial: 10 mg/day and adjusted upward on an individual basis to 20 mg/day
- OCD (unlabeled use): Initial: 10 mg/day and titrate up as necessary to 60 mg/day
- Self-injurious behavior (unlabeled use): 20 mg/day
- Social phobia (unlabeled use): 2.5-15 mg/day

Adults:

- Depression:
  - Paxil®, Pexeva™: Initial: 20 mg once daily, preferably in the morning; increase if needed by 10 mg/day increments at intervals of at least 1 week; maximum dose: 50 mg/day
  - Paxil CR™: Initial: 25 mg once daily; increase if needed by 12.5 mg/day increments at intervals of at least 1 week; maximum dose: 62.5 mg/day
- GAD (Paxil®): Initial: 20 mg once daily, preferably in the morning; doses of 20-50 mg/day were used in clinical trials, however, no greater benefit was seen with doses >20 mg. If dose is increased, adjust in increments of 10 mg/day at 1-week intervals.
- OCD (Paxil®, Pexeva™): Initial: 20 mg once daily, preferably in the morning; increase if needed by 10 mg/day increments at intervals of at least 1 week; recommended dose: 40 mg/day; range: 20-60 mg/day; maximum dose: 60 mg/day
- Panic disorder:
  - Paxil®, Pexeva™: Initial: 10 mg once daily, preferably in the morning; increase if needed by 10 mg/day increments at intervals of at least 1 week; recommended dose: 40 mg/day; range: 10-60 mg/day; maximum dose: 60 mg/day
  - Paxil CR™: Initial: 12.5 mg once daily; increase if needed by 12.5 mg/day at intervals of at least 1 week; maximum dose: 75 mg/day
- PMDD (Paxil CR™): Initial: 12.5 mg once daily in the morning; may be increased to 25 mg/day; dosing changes should occur at intervals of at least 1 week. May be given daily throughout the menstrual cycle or limited to the luteal phase.
- PTSD (Paxil®): Initial: 20 mg once daily, preferably in the morning; increase if needed by 10 mg/day increments at intervals of at least 1 week; range: 20-50 mg
- Social anxiety disorder:
  - Paxil®: Initial: 20 mg once daily, preferably in the morning; recommended dose: 20 mg/day; range: 20-60 mg/day; doses >20 mg may not have additional benefit
  - Paxil CR™: Initial: 12.5 mg once daily, preferably in the morning; may be increased by 12.5 mg/day at intervals of at least 1 week; maximum dose: 37.5 mg/day

(Continued)

Paroxetine *(Continued)*

Vasomotor symptoms of menopause (unlabeled use, Paxil CR™): 12.5-25 mg/day

Elderly: C_{min} concentrations 70% to 80% greater in the elderly compared to nonelderly patients; clearance is also decreased.

Paxil®, Pexeva™: Initial: 10 mg/day; increase if needed by 10 mg/day increments at intervals of at least 1 week; maximum dose: 40 mg/day

Paxil CR™; Initial: 12.5 mg/day; increase if needed by 12.5 mg/day increments at intervals of at least 1 week; maximum dose: 50 mg/day

Note: Upon discontinuation of paroxetine therapy, gradually taper dose:

Paxil®: Taper-phase regimen used in PTSD/GAD clinical trials involved an incremental decrease in the daily dose by 10 mg/day at weekly intervals; when 20 mg/day dose was reached, this dose was continued for 1 week before treatment was discontinued.

Paxil CR™: Patients receiving 37.5 mg/day in clinical trials had their dose decreased by 12.5 mg/day to a dose of 25 mg/day and remained at a dose of 25 mg/day for 1 week before treatment was discontinued.

Dosage adjustment in severe renal/hepatic impairment: Adults:

Cl_{cr} <30 mL/minute: Mean plasma concentration is ~4 times that seen in normal function.

Cl_{cr} 30-60 mL/minute and hepatic dysfunction: Plasma concentration is 2 times that seen in normal function.

Paxil®, Pexeva™: Initial: 10 mg/day; increase if needed by 10 mg/day increments at intervals of at least 1 week; maximum dose: 40 mg/day

Paxil CR™: Initial: 12.5 mg/day; increase if needed by 12.5 mg/day increments at intervals of at least 1 week; maximum dose: 50 mg/day

Mechanism of Action Paroxetine is a selective serotonin reuptake inhibitor, chemically unrelated to tricyclic, tetracyclic, or other antidepressants; presumably, the inhibition of serotonin reuptake from brain synapse stimulated serotonin activity in the brain

Contraindications Hypersensitivity to paroxetine or any component of the formulation; use of MAO inhibitors or within 14 days; concurrent use with thioridazine or mesoridazine

Warnings/Precautions Use cautiously in children or during breast-feeding in lactating women. Upon discontinuation of paroxetine therapy, gradually taper dose and monitor for discontinuation symptoms (eg, dizziness, dysphoric mood, irritability, agitation, confusion, paresthesias). If intolerable symptoms occur following a decrease in dosage or upon discontinuation of therapy, then resuming the previous dose with a more gradual taper should be considered. Potential for severe reaction when used with MAO inhibitors - serotonin syndrome (hyperthermia, muscular rigidity, mental status changes/agitation, autonomic instability) may occur. May precipitate a shift to mania or hypomania in patients with bipolar disorder. Monotherapy in patients with bipolar disorder should be avoided. The possibility of a suicide attempt is inherent in major depression and may persist until remission occurs. Monitor for worsening of depression or suicidality, especially during initiation of therapy or with dose increases or decreases. Worsening depression and severe abrupt suicidality that are not part of the presenting symptoms may require discontinuation or modification of drug therapy. Use caution in high-risk patients during initiation of therapy. Prescriptions should be written for the smallest quantity consistent with good patient care. The patient's family or caregiver should be alerted to monitor patients for the emergence of suicidality and associated behaviors such as anxiety, agitation, panic attacks, insomnia, irritability, hostility, impulsivity, akathisia, hypomania, and mania; patients should be instructed to notify their healthcare provider if any of these symptoms or worsening depression occur. Has a low potential to impair cognitive or motor performance; caution operating hazardous machinery or driving. Low potential for sedation or anticholinergic effects relative to cyclic antidepressants. Use caution in patients with a previous seizure disorder or condition predisposing to seizures such as brain damage, alcoholism, or concurrent therapy with other drugs which lower the seizure threshold. Use with caution in patients with hepatic or dysfunction and in elderly patients. May cause hyponatremia/SIADH. Use with caution in patients at risk of bleeding or receiving anticoagulant therapy - may cause impairment in platelet aggregation. Use with caution in patients with renal insufficiency or other concurrent illness (due to limited experience). May cause or exacerbate sexual dysfunction.

Drug Interactions

Cytochrome P450 Effect: Substrate of CYP2D6 (major); **Inhibits** CYP1A2 (weak), 2B6 (moderate), 2C8/9 (weak), 2C19 (weak), 2D6 (strong), 3A4 (weak)

Increased Effect/Toxicity: Paroxetine should not be used with nonselective MAO inhibitors (phenelzine, isocarboxazid) or other drugs with MAO inhibition (linezolid); fatal reactions have been reported. Wait 5 weeks after stopping fluoxetine before starting a nonselective MAO inhibitor and 2 weeks after stopping an MAO inhibitor before starting paroxetine. Concurrent selegiline has been associated with mania, hypertension, or serotonin syndrome (risk may be reduced relative to nonselective MAO inhibitors).

Paroxetine may inhibit the metabolism of thioridazine or mesoridazine, resulting in increased plasma levels and increasing the risk of QT_c interval prolongation. This may lead to serious ventricular arrhythmias, such as torsade de pointes-type arrhythmias and sudden death. Do not use together. Wait at least 5 weeks after discontinuing paroxetine prior to starting thioridazine.

The levels/effects of paroxetine may be increased by chlorpromazine, delavirdine, fluoxetine, miconazole, pergolide, quinidine, quinine, ritonavir, ropinirole, and other CYP2D6 inhibitors. Paroxetine may increase the levels/effects of amphetamines, selected beta-blockers, bupropion, dextromethorphan, fluoxetine, lidocaine, mirtazapine, nefazodone, promethazine, propofol, risperidone, ritonavir, sertraline, tricyclic antidepressants, venlafaxine, and other CYP2B6 or 2D6 substrates.

Concomitant use of paroxetine and NSAIDs, aspirin, or other drugs affecting coagulation has been associated with an increased risk of bleeding. Paroxetine may increase the hypoprothrombinemic response to warfarin. Paroxetine increases levels of procyclidine; this may result in increased anticholinergic effects; procyclidine dose reduction may be necessary.

Combined use of SSRIs and amphetamines, buspirone, meperidine, nefazodone, serotonin agonists (such as sumatriptan), sibutramine, other SSRIs, sympathomimetics, ritonavir, tramadol, and venlafaxine may increase the risk of serotonin syndrome. Combined use of sumatriptan (and other serotonin agonists) may result in toxicity; weakness, hyper-reflexia, and incoordination have been observed with sumatriptan and SSRIs. In addition, concurrent use may theoretically increase the risk of serotonin syndrome; includes sumatriptan, naratriptan, rizatriptan, and zolmitriptan. Combination with tryptophan, a may cause agitation, restlessness, headache, nausea, sweating, and dizziness; this combination is best avoided. Concurrent lithium may increase risk of nephrotoxicity. Risk of hyponatremia may increase with concurrent use of loop diuretics (bumetanide, furosemide, torsemide).

Decreased Effect: Cyproheptadine, a serotonin antagonist, may inhibit the effects of serotonin reuptake inhibitors (paroxetine). Paroxetine may decrease the levels/effects of CYP2D6 prodrug substrates (eg, codeine, hydrocodone, oxycodone, tramadol).

Ethanol/Nutrition/Herb Interactions

Ethanol: Avoid ethanol.

Food: Peak concentration is increased, but bioavailability is not significantly altered by food.

Herb/Nutraceutical: Avoid valerian, St John's wort, SAMe, kava kava.

Dietary Considerations May be taken with or without food.

Pharmacodynamics/Kinetics

Absorption: Completely absorbed following oral administration

Distribution: V_d: 8.7 L/kg (3-28 L/kg)

Protein binding: 93% to 95%

Metabolism: Extensively hepatic via CYP enzymes via oxidation and methylation; nonlinear pharmacokinetics may be seen with higher doses and longer duration of therapy. Saturation of CYP2D6 appears to account for the nonlinearity.

Half-life elimination: 21 hours (3-65 hours)

Time to peak, serum: Immediate release: 5.2 hours; controlled release: 6-10 hours

Excretion: As metabolites in urine and bile; 2% as unchanged drug in urine

Pregnancy Risk Factor C

Dosage Forms SUSP, oral, as hydrochloride (Paxil®): 10 mg/5 mL (250 mL). **TAB, as hydrochloride** (Paxil®): 10 mg, 20 mg, 30 mg, 40 mg. **TAB, as mesylate** (Pexeva™): 10 mg, 20 mg, 30 mg, 40 mg. **TAB, controlled release, as hydrochloride** (Paxil CR™): 12.5 mg, 25 mg, 37.5 mg

Paroxetine Hydrochloride *see* Paroxetine *on page 1046*

Paroxetine Mesylate *see* Paroxetine *on page 1046*

PAS *see* Aminosalicylic Acid *on page 100*

Paser® *see* Aminosalicylic Acid *on page 100*

Patanol® *see* Olopatadine *on page 1011*
Patients Requiring Sedation *see page 1567*
Pavabid [DSC] *see* Papaverine *on page 1044*
Paxil® *see* Paroxetine *on page 1046*
Paxil CR™ *see* Paroxetine *on page 1046*
PBZ® *see* Tripelennamine *on page 1344*
PBZ-SR® *see* Tripelennamine *on page 1344*
PCA *see* Procainamide *on page 1124*
PCE® *see* Erythromycin *on page 508*
PCEC *see* Rabies Virus Vaccine *on page 1165*
PCV7 *see* Pneumococcal Conjugate Vaccine (7-Valent) *on page 1098*
Pectin and Kaolin *see* Kaolin and Pectin *on page 781*
Pectin, Hyoscyamine, Atropine, Scopolamine, and Kaolin *see* Hyoscyamine, Atropine, Scopolamine, Kaolin, and Pectin *on page 726*
Pectin, Hyoscyamine, Atropine, Scopolamine, Kaolin, and Opium *see* Hyoscyamine, Atropine, Scopolamine, Kaolin, Pectin, and Opium *on page 726*
Pedameth® *see* Methionine *on page 894*
PediaCare® Cold and Allergy [OTC] *see* Chlorpheniramine and Pseudoephedrine *on page 315*
PediaCare® Decongestant Infants [OTC] *see* Pseudoephedrine *on page 1147*
Pediacare® Decongestant Plus Cough [OTC] *see* Pseudoephedrine and Dextromethorphan *on page 1148*
PediaCare® Infants' Long-Acting Cough [OTC] *see* Dextromethorphan *on page 421*
Pediacare® Long Acting Cough Plus Cold [OTC] *see* Pseudoephedrine and Dextromethorphan *on page 1148*
Pediacof® *see* Chlorpheniramine, Phenylephrine, Codeine, and Potassium Iodide *on page 318*
Pediaflor® *see* Fluoride *on page 603*
Pediamist® [OTC] *see* Sodium Chloride *on page 1227*
Pediapred® *see* PrednisoLONE *on page 1113*
Pediarix™ *see* Diphtheria, Tetanus Toxoids, Acellular Pertussis, Hepatitis B (Recombinant), and Poliovirus (Inactivated) Vaccine *on page 452*
Pediatex™ *see* Carbinoxamine *on page 262*
Pediatex™-D *see* Carbinoxamine and Pseudoephedrine *on page 262*
Pediatex™-DM *see* Carbinoxamine, Pseudoephedrine, and Dextromethorphan *on page 263*
Pediazole® *see* Erythromycin and Sulfisoxazole *on page 512*
Pedi-Boro® [OTC] *see* Aluminum Sulfate and Calcium Acetate *on page 92*
Pedi-Dri® *see* Nystatin *on page 1003*
PediOtic® *see* Neomycin, Polymyxin B, and Hydrocortisone *on page 975*
Pedisilk® [OTC] *see* Salicylic Acid *on page 1205*
Pedtrace-4® *see* Trace Metals *on page 1319*
PedvaxHIB® *see Haemophilus* b Conjugate Vaccine *on page 680*

Pegademase Bovine (peg A de mase BOE vine)

U.S. Brand Names Adagen®
Canadian Brand Names Adagen®
Generic Available No
Pharmacologic Category Enzyme
Use Orphan drug: Enzyme replacement therapy for adenosine deaminase (ADA) deficiency in patients with severe combined immunodeficiency disease (SCID) who can not benefit from bone marrow transplant; not a cure for SCID, unlike bone marrow transplants, injections must be used the rest of the child's life, therefore is not really an alternative
Local Anesthetic/Vasoconstrictor Precautions No information available to require special precautions
Effects on Dental Treatment No significant effects or complications reported
Mechanism of Action Adenosine deaminase is an enzyme that catalyzes the deamination of both adenosine and deoxyadenosine. Hereditary lack of adenosine deaminase activity results in severe combined immunodeficiency disease, a fatal disorder of infancy characterized by profound defects of both cellular and humoral immunity. It is estimated that 25% of patients with the autosomal recessive form of severe combined immunodeficiency lack adenosine deaminase.
Pharmacodynamics/Kinetics
Absorption: Rapid

Half-life elimination: 48-72 hours

Time to peak: Plasma adenosine deaminase activity: 2-3 weeks

Pregnancy Risk Factor C

Peganone® *see* Ethotoin *on page 561*

Pegaspargase (peg AS par jase)

Related Information

Asparaginase *on page 150*

U.S. Brand Names Oncaspar®

Generic Available No

Synonyms NSC-644954; PEG-L-asparaginase

Pharmacologic Category Antineoplastic Agent, Miscellaneous

Use Treatment of acute lymphocytic leukemia, blast crisis of chronic lymphocytic leukemia (CLL), salvage therapy of non-Hodgkin's lymphoma; may be used in some patients who have had hypersensitivity reactions to *E. coli* asparaginase

Local Anesthetic/Vasoconstrictor Precautions No information available to require special precautions

Effects on Dental Treatment No significant effects or complications reported

Common Adverse Effects In general, pegaspargase toxicities tend to be less frequent and appear somewhat later than comparable toxicities of asparaginase. Intramuscular rather than intravenous injection may decrease the incidence of coagulopathy; GI, hepatic, and renal toxicity.

>10%:

- Cardiovascular: Edema
- Central nervous system: Fatigue, disorientation (10%)
- Gastrointestinal: Nausea, vomiting (50% to 60%), generally mild to moderate, but may be severe and protracted in some patients; anorexia (33%); abdominal pain (38%); diarrhea (28%); increased serum lipase and amylase
- Hematologic: Hypofibrinogenemia and depression of clotting factors V and VII, variable decreases in factors VII and IX, severe protein C deficiency and decrease in antithrombin III - overt bleeding is uncommon, but may be dose-limiting, or fatal in some patients
- Hypersensitivity: Acute allergic reactions, including fever, rash, urticaria, arthralgia, hypotension, angioedema, bronchospasm, anaphylaxis (10% to 30%) - dose-limiting in some patients
- Neuromuscular & skeletal: Weakness (33%)

1% to 10%:

- Cardiovascular: Hypotension, tachycardia, thrombosis
- Dermatologic: Urticaria, erythema, lip edema
- Endocrine & metabolic: Hyperglycemia (3%)
- Gastrointestinal: Acute pancreatitis (1%)

Mechanism of Action Pegaspargase is a modified version of asparaginase. Leukemic cells, especially lymphoblasts, require exogenous asparagine; normal cells can synthesize asparagine. Asparaginase contains L-asparaginase amidohydrolase type EC-2 which inhibits protein synthesis by deaminating asparagine to aspartic acid and ammonia in the plasma and extracellular fluid and therefore deprives tumor cells of the amino acid for protein synthesis. Asparaginase is cycle-specific for the G_1 phase of the cell cycle.

Drug Interactions

Increased Effect/Toxicity:

- Aspirin, dipyridamole, heparin, warfarin, NSAIDs: Imbalances in coagulation factors have been noted with the use of pegaspargase - use with caution.
- Vincristine and prednisone: An increased toxicity has been noticed when asparaginase is administered with VCR and prednisone.
- Cyclophosphamide (decreased metabolism)
- Mercaptopurine (increased hepatotoxicity)
- Vincristine (increased neuropathy)
- Prednisone (hyperglycemia)

Decreased Effect: Asparaginase terminates methotrexate action by inhibition of protein synthesis and prevention of cell entry into the S Phase.

Pharmacodynamics/Kinetics

Duration: Asparaginase was measurable for at least 15 days following initial treatment with pegaspargase

Distribution: V_d: 4-5 L/kg; 70% to 80% of plasma volume; does not penetrate the CSF

Metabolism: Systemically degraded

Half-life elimination: 5.73 days; unaffected by age, renal or hepatic function

Excretion: Urine (trace amounts)

Pregnancy Risk Factor C

Pegasys® *see* Peginterferon Alfa-2a *on page 1052*

Pegfilgrastim (peg fil GRA stim)

U.S. Brand Names Neulasta™

Generic Available No

Synonyms G-CSF (PEG Conjugate); Granulocyte Colony Stimulating Factor (PEG Conjugate)

Pharmacologic Category Colony Stimulating Factor

Use Decrease the incidence of infection, by stimulation of granulocyte production, in patients with nonmyeloid malignancies receiving myelosuppressive therapy associated with a significant risk of febrile neutropenia

Local Anesthetic/Vasoconstrictor Precautions No information available to require special precautions

Effects on Dental Treatment No significant effects or complications reported

Common Adverse Effects

>10%

- Neuromuscular & skeletal: Bone pain (medullary, 26%)
- Hepatic: Increased LDH (19%)

1% to 10%

- Endocrine & metabolic: Uric acid increased (8%)
- Hepatic: Alkaline phosphatase increased (9%)

Mechanism of Action Stimulates the production, maturation, and activation of neutrophils, pegfilgrastim activates neutrophils to increase both their migration and cytotoxicity. Pegfilgrastim has a prolonged duration of effect relative to filgrastim and a reduced renal clearance.

Drug Interactions

Increased Effect/Toxicity: No formal drug interactions studies have been conducted. Lithium may potentiate release of neutrophils.

Pharmacodynamics/Kinetics Half-life elimination: SubQ: 15-80 hours

Pregnancy Risk Factor C

Peginterferon Alfa-2a (peg in ter FEER on AL fa too aye)

U.S. Brand Names Pegasys®

Canadian Brand Names Pegasys®

Generic Available No

Synonyms Interferon Alfa-2a (PEG Conjugate); Pegylated Interferon Alfa-2a

Pharmacologic Category Interferon

Use Treatment of chronic hepatitis C, alone or in combination with ribavirin, in patients with compensated liver disease

Local Anesthetic/Vasoconstrictor Precautions No information available to require special precautions

Effects on Dental Treatment No significant effects or complications reported

Common Adverse Effects Note: Percentages indicated as "with ribavirin" are those which have been seen with peginterferon alfa-2b/ribavirin combination therapy.

>10%:

- Central nervous system: Headache (54%), fatigue (50%), pyrexia (36%), insomnia (19%; 30% with ribavirin), depression (1% to 18%), dizziness (16%), irritability (13%), irritability/anxiety/nervousness (33% with ribavirin), pain (11%)
- Dermatologic: Alopecia (23%), pruritus (12%; 19% with ribavirin), dermatitis (16% with ribavirin)
- Gastrointestinal: Nausea (5% to 23%), anorexia (17%; 24% with ribavirin), diarrhea (16%), abdominal pain (15%)
- Hematologic: Neutropenia (21%), lymphopenia (14% with ribavirin), anemia (11% with ribavirin)
- Local: Injection site reaction (22%)
- Neuromuscular & skeletal: Myalgia (37%), rigors (32%), arthralgia (28%)
- Respiratory: Dyspnea (13% with ribavirin)

1% to 10%:

- Central nervous system: Concentration impaired (8%), anxiety (6%), memory impaired (5%)
- Dermatologic: Dermatitis (8%), rash (5%), eczema (5% with ribavirin)
- Endocrine & metabolic: Hypothyroidism (4%), hyperthyroidism (1%)
- Gastrointestinal: Xerostomia (6%), vomiting (5%)
- Hematologic: Thrombocytopenia (5%), platelets decreased <50,000/mm^3 (5%)
- Neuromuscular & skeletal: Back pain (9%), weakness (5%)

Miscellaneous: Diaphoresis (6%)

Mechanism of Action Alpha interferons are a family of proteins, produced by nucleated cells, that have antiviral, antiproliferative, and immune-regulating activity. There are 16 known subtypes of alpha interferons. Interferons interact with cells through high affinity cell surface receptors. Following activation, multiple effects can be detected including induction of gene transcription. Inhibits cellular growth, alters the state of cellular differentiation, interferes with oncogene expression, alters cell surface antigen expression, increases phagocytic activity of macrophages, and augments cytotoxicity of lymphocytes for target cells.

Drug Interactions

Cytochrome P450 Effect: Inhibits CYP1A2 (weak)

Increased Effect/Toxicity: Interferons may increase the risk of neutropenia when used with ACE inhibitors; fluorouracil concentrations doubled with interferon alpha-2b; interferon alpha may decrease the metabolism of theophylline and zidovudine; interferons may increase the anticoagulant effects of warfarin

Decreased Effect: Prednisone may decrease the therapeutic effects of interferon alpha; interferon alpha may decrease the serum concentrations of melphalan

Pharmacodynamics/Kinetics

Half-life elimination: Terminal: 80 hours; increased with renal dysfunction

Time to peak, serum: 72-96 hours

Pregnancy Risk Factor C

Peginterferon Alfa-2b (peg in ter FEER on AL fa too bee)

Related Information

Systemic Viral Diseases *on page 1519*

U.S. Brand Names PEG-Intron®

Canadian Brand Names PEG-Intron®

Generic Available No

Synonyms Interferon Alfa-2b (PEG Conjugate); Pegylated Interferon Alfa-2b

Pharmacologic Category Interferon

Use Treatment of chronic hepatitis C (as monotherapy or in combination with ribavirin) in adult patients who have never received interferon alpha and have compensated liver disease

Local Anesthetic/Vasoconstrictor Precautions No information available to require special precautions

Effects on Dental Treatment No significant effects or complications reported

Common Adverse Effects

>10%:

Central nervous system: Headache (56%), fatigue (52%), depression (16% to 29%), anxiety/emotional liability/irritability (28%), insomnia (23%), fever (22%), dizziness (12%), impaired concentration (5% to 12%), pain (12%)

Dermatologic: Alopecia (22%), pruritus (12%), dry skin (11%)

Gastrointestinal: Nausea (26%), anorexia (20%), diarrhea (18%), abdominal pain (15%), weight loss (11%)

Local: Injection site inflammation/reaction (47%),

Neuromuscular & skeletal: Musculoskeletal pain (56%), myalgia (38% to 42%), rigors (23% to 45%)

Respiratory: Epistaxis (14%), nasopharyngitis (11%)

Miscellaneous: Flu-like syndrome (46%), viral infection (11%)

>1% to 10%:

Cardiovascular: Flushing (6%)

Central nervous system: Malaise (8%)

Dermatologic: Rash (6%), dermatitis (7%)

Endocrine & metabolic: Hypothyroidism (5%)

Gastrointestinal: Vomiting (7%), dyspepsia (6%), taste perversion

Hematologic: Neutropenia, thrombocytopenia

Hepatic: Transient increase in transaminases (10%), hepatomegaly (6%)

Local: Injection site pain (2%)

Neuromuscular & skeletal: Hypertonia (5%)

Respiratory: Pharyngitis (10%), sinusitis (7%), cough (6%)

Miscellaneous: Diaphoresis (6%)

Mechanism of Action Alpha interferons are a family of proteins, produced by nucleated cells, that have antiviral, antiproliferative, and immune-regulating activity. There are 16 known subtypes of alpha interferons. Interferons interact with cells through high affinity cell surface receptors. Following activation, multiple effects can be detected including induction of gene transcription. Inhibits cellular growth, alters the state of cellular differentiation, interferes with

(Continued)

Peginterferon Alfa-2b *(Continued)*

oncogene expression, alters cell surface antigen expression, increases phagocytic activity of macrophages, and augments cytotoxicity of lymphocytes for target cells.

Drug Interactions

Cytochrome P450 Effect: Inhibits CYP1A2 (weak)

Increased Effect/Toxicity: ACE inhibitors, clozapine, erythropoietin may increase risk of bone marrow suppression. Fluorouracil, theophylline, zidovudine concentrations may increase. Warfarin's anticoagulant effect may increase.

Decreased Effect: Melphalan concentrations may decrease. Prednisone may decrease effects of interferon alpha.

Pharmacodynamics/Kinetics

Bioavailability: Increases with chronic dosing
Half-life elimination: 40 hours
Time to peak: 15-44 hours
Excretion: Urine (30%)

Pregnancy Risk Factor C (manufacturer) as monotherapy; X in combination with ribavirin

PEG-Intron® *see* Peginterferon Alfa-2b *on page 1053*
PEG-L-asparaginase *see* Pegaspargase *on page 1051*
Pegylated Interferon Alfa-2a *see* Peginterferon Alfa-2a *on page 1052*
Pegylated Interferon Alfa-2b *see* Peginterferon Alfa-2b *on page 1053*
PemADD® *see* Pemoline *on page 1055*
PemADD® CT *see* Pemoline *on page 1055*

Pemetrexed (pem e TREKS ed)

U.S. Brand Names Alimta®

Synonyms LY231514; MTA; Multitargeted Antifolate; NSC-698037

Pharmacologic Category Antineoplastic Agent, Antimetabolite; Antineoplastic Agent, Antimetabolite (Antifolate)

Use Treatment of malignant pleural mesothelioma in combination with cisplatin

Unlabeled/Investigational Use Bladder, breast, cervical, colorectal, esophageal, gastric, head and neck, nonsmall cell lung, ovarian, pancreatic, and renal cell cancers

Local Anesthetic/Vasoconstrictor Precautions No information available to require special precautions

Effects on Dental Treatment No significant effects or complications reported

Common Adverse Effects

>10%:
- Cardiovascular: Chest pain (40%)
- Central nervous system: Fatigue (80%), fever (17%), depression (14%)
- Dermatologic: Rash (22%)
- Gastrointestinal: Nausea (84%; grade 3 or 4 in 12%), vomiting (58%; grade 3 or 4 in 11%), constipation (44%), anorexia (35%), stomatitis/pharyngitis (28%), diarrhea (26%)
- Hematologic: Neutropenia (58%), leukopenia (55%), anemia (33%), thrombocytopenia (27%)
  - Nadir: 8-10 days
  - Recovery: 12-17 days
- Neuromuscular & skeletal: Neuropathy (17%)
- Renal: Creatinine increased (16%)
- Respiratory: Dyspnea (66%)
- Miscellaneous: Infection (17%)

1% to 10%:
- Cardiovascular: Thrombosis/embolism (7%)
- Endocrine & metabolic: Dehydration (7%)
- Gastrointestinal: Dysphagia/esophagitis/odynophagia (6%)
- Renal: Renal failure (2%)
- Miscellaneous: Allergic reaction (2%)

Mechanism of Action Inhibits thymidylate synthase (TS), dihydrofolate reductase (DHFR), glycinamide ribonucleotide formyltransferase (GARFT), and aminoimidazole carboxamide ribonucleotide formyltransferase (AICARFT), the enzymes involved in folate metabolism and DNA synthesis, resulting in inhibition of purine and thymidine nucleotide and protein synthesis.

Drug Interactions

Increased Effect/Toxicity: NSAIDs may increase the toxicity of pemetrexed.

Pharmacodynamics/Kinetics
Duration: V_{dss}: 16.1 L
Protein binding: ~81%
Metabolism: Minimal
Half-life elimination: Normal renal function: 3.5 hours
Excretion: Urine (70% to 90% as unchanged drug)
Pregnancy Risk Factor D

Pemirolast (pe MIR oh last)

U.S. Brand Names Alamast™
Canadian Brand Names Alamast™
Generic Available No
Pharmacologic Category Mast Cell Stabilizer; Ophthalmic Agent, Miscellaneous
Use Prevention of itching of the eye due to allergic conjunctivitis
Local Anesthetic/Vasoconstrictor Precautions No information available to require special precautions
Effects on Dental Treatment No significant effects or complications reported
Mechanism of Action Mast cell stabilizer that inhibits the *in vivo* type I immediate hypersensitivity reaction; in addition, inhibits chemotaxis of eosinophils into the ocular tissue and blocks their release of mediators; also reported to prevent calcium influx into mast cells following antigen stimulation
Pregnancy Risk Factor C

Pemoline (PEM oh leen)

U.S. Brand Names Cylert®; PemADD®; PemADD® CT
Generic Available Yes
Synonyms Phenylisohydantoin; PIO
Pharmacologic Category Stimulant
Use Treatment of attention-deficit/hyperactivity disorder (ADHD) (not first-line)
Unlabeled/Investigational Use Narcolepsy
Local Anesthetic/Vasoconstrictor Precautions Pemoline has minimal sympathomimetic effects; there are no precautions in using vasoconstrictors
Effects on Dental Treatment No significant effects or complications reported
Common Adverse Effects Frequency not defined.
Central nervous system: Insomnia, dizziness, drowsiness, mental depression, increased irritability, seizures, precipitation of Tourette's syndrome, hallucinations, headache, movement disorders
Dermatologic: Rash
Endocrine & metabolic: Suppression of growth in children
Gastrointestinal: Anorexia, weight loss, stomach pain, nausea
Hematologic: Aplastic anemia
Hepatic: Increased liver enzyme (usually reversible upon discontinuation), hepatitis, jaundice, hepatic failure
Restrictions C-IV
Mechanism of Action Blocks the reuptake mechanism of dopaminergic neurons, appears to act at the cerebral cortex and subcortical structures; CNS and respiratory stimulant with weak sympathomimetic effects; actions may be mediated via increase in CNS dopamine
Drug Interactions
Increased Effect/Toxicity: Use caution when pemoline is used with other CNS-acting medications.
Decreased Effect: Pemoline in combination with antiepileptic medications may decrease seizure threshold.
Pharmacodynamics/Kinetics
Onset of action: Peak effect: 4 hours
Duration: 8 hours
Protein binding: 50%
Metabolism: Partially hepatic
Half-life elimination: Children: 7-8.6 hours; Adults: 12 hours
Time to peak, serum: 2-4 hours
Excretion: Urine; feces (negligible amounts)
Pregnancy Risk Factor B

Penbutolol (pen BYOO toe lole)

Related Information
Cardiovascular Diseases *on page 1458*
U.S. Brand Names Levatol®
Canadian Brand Names Levatol®
Generic Available No
(Continued)

Penbutolol *(Continued)*

Synonyms Penbutolol Sulfate

Pharmacologic Category Beta Blocker With Intrinsic Sympathomimetic Activity

Use Treatment of mild to moderate arterial hypertension

Local Anesthetic/Vasoconstrictor Precautions No information available to require special precautions

Effects on Dental Treatment Key adverse event(s) related to dental treatment: Xerostomia (normal salivary flow resumes upon discontinuation). Penbutolol is a nonselective beta-blocker and may enhance the pressor response to epinephrine, resulting in hypertension and bradycardia. Many nonsteroidal anti-inflammatory drugs, such as ibuprofen and indomethacin, can reduce the hypotensive effect of beta-blockers after 3 or more weeks of therapy with the NSAID. Short-term NSAID use (ie, 3 days) requires no special precautions in patients taking beta-blockers.

Common Adverse Effects 1% to 10%:

Cardiovascular: Congestive heart failure, arrhythmia

Central nervous system: Mental depression, headache, dizziness, fatigue

Gastrointestinal: Nausea, diarrhea, dyspepsia

Neuromuscular & skeletal: Arthralgia

Mechanism of Action Blocks both beta$_1$- and beta$_2$-receptors and has mild intrinsic sympathomimetic activity; has negative inotropic and chronotropic effects and can significantly slow AV nodal conduction

Drug Interactions

Increased Effect/Toxicity: The heart rate lowering effects of propranolol are beta-blockers are additive with other drugs which slow AV conduction (digoxin, verapamil, diltiazem). Concurrent use of beta-blockers may increase the effects of alpha-blockers (prazosin, terazosin), alpha-adrenergic stimulants (epinephrine, phenylephrine), and the vasoconstrictive effects of ergot alkaloids. Beta-blockers may mask the tachycardia from hypoglycemia caused by insulin and oral hypoglycemics. In patients receiving concurrent therapy, the risk of hypertensive crisis is increased when either clonidine or the beta blocker is withdrawn. Beta-blockers may increase the action or levels of ethanol, disopyramide, nondepolarizing muscle relaxants, and theophylline although the effects are difficult to predict.

Beta-blocker effects may be enhanced by oral contraceptives, flecainide, haloperidol (hypotensive effects), H$_2$-antagonists (cimetidine, possibly ranitidine), hydralazine, loop diuretics, possibly MAO inhibitors, phenothiazines, propafenone, quinidine (in extensive metabolizers), ciprofloxacin, thyroid hormones (when hypothyroid patient is converted to euthyroid state). Beta-blockers may increase the effect/toxicity of flecainide, haloperidol (hypotensive effects), hydralazine, phenothiazines, acetaminophen, anticoagulants (warfarin), and benzodiazepines.

Decreased Effect: Aluminum salts, barbiturates, calcium salts, cholestyramine, colestipol, NSAIDs, penicillins (ampicillin), rifampin, salicylates, and sulfinpyrazone decrease effect of beta-blockers due to decreased bioavailability and plasma levels. Beta-blockers may decrease the effect of sulfonylureas. Nonselective beta-blockers blunt the response to beta-2 adrenergic agonists (albuterol).

Pharmacodynamics/Kinetics

Absorption: ~100%

Protein binding: 80% to 98%

Metabolism: Extensively hepatic (oxidation and conjugation)

Bioavailability: ~100%

Half-life elimination: 5 hours

Excretion: Urine

Pregnancy Risk Factor C (manufacturer); D (2nd and 3rd trimester - expert analysis)

Penbutolol Sulfate *see* Penbutolol *on page 1055*

Penciclovir (pen SYE kloe veer)

Related Information

Oral Viral Infections *on page 1547*

Systemic Viral Diseases *on page 1519*

U.S. Brand Names Denavir®

Generic Available No

Pharmacologic Category Antiviral Agent

Use Topical treatment of herpes simplex labialis (cold sores)

Local Anesthetic/Vasoconstrictor Precautions No information available to require special precautions

Effects on Dental Treatment No significant effects or complications reported

Significant Adverse Effects

>10%: Dermatologic: Mild erythema (50%)

1% to 10%: Central nervous system: Headache (5.3%)

<1%: Local anesthesia (0.9%)

Postmarketing and/or case reports: Application site reaction, local edema, urticaria, pain, pruritus, paresthesia, skin discoloration, erythematous rash, oropharyngeal edema, parosmia

Dosage Children ≥12 years and Adults: Topical: Apply cream at the first sign or symptom of cold sore (eg, tingling, swelling); apply every 2 hours during waking hours for 4 days

Mechanism of Action In cells infected with HSV-1 or HSV-2, viral thymidine kinase phosphorylates penciclovir to a monophosphate form which, in turn, is converted to penciclovir triphosphate by cellular kinases. Penciclovir triphosphate inhibits HSV polymerase competitively with deoxyguanosine triphosphate. Consequently, herpes viral DNA synthesis and, therefore, replication are selectively inhibited

Contraindications Hypersensitivity to the penciclovir or any component of the formulation; previous and significant adverse reactions to famciclovir

Warnings/Precautions Penciclovir should only be used on herpes labialis on the lips and face; because no data are available, application to mucous membranes is not recommended. Avoid application in or near eyes since it may cause irritation. The effect of penciclovir has not been established in immunocompromised patients.

Drug Interactions No data reported

Pharmacodynamics/Kinetics Absorption: Topical: None

Pregnancy Risk Factor B

Lactation Excretion in breast milk unknown

Dosage Forms Cream: 1% (1.5 g)

Penicillamine (pen i SIL a meen)

U.S. Brand Names Cuprimine®; Depen®

Canadian Brand Names Cuprimine®; Depen®

Mexican Brand Names Adalken®; Sufortan®; Sufortanon®

Generic Available No

Synonyms D-3-Mercaptovaline; β,β-Dimethylcysteine; D-Penicillamine

Pharmacologic Category Chelating Agent

Use Treatment of Wilson's disease, cystinuria, adjunct in the treatment of rheumatoid arthritis

Unlabeled/Investigational Use Lead, mercury, copper, and possibly gold poisoning (**Note:** Oral succimer [DMSA] is preferable for lead or mercury poisoning)

Local Anesthetic/Vasoconstrictor Precautions No information available to require special precautions

Effects on Dental Treatment No significant effects or complications reported

Common Adverse Effects

>10%:

- Dermatologic: Rash, urticaria, itching (44% to 50%)
- Gastrointestinal: Hypogeusia (25% to 33%), diarrhea (17%), altered taste perception (12%)
- Neuromuscular & skeletal: Arthralgia

1% to 10%:

- Cardiovascular: Edema of the face, feet, or lower legs
- Central nervous system: Fever, chills
- Gastrointestinal: Weight gain, sore throat, anorexia, epigastric pain
- Genitourinary: Bloody or cloudy urine
- Hematologic: Aplastic or hemolytic anemia, leukopenia (2%), thrombocytopenia (4%)
- Renal: Proteinuria (6%)
- Miscellaneous: White spots on lips or mouth, positive ANA

Mechanism of Action Chelates with lead, copper, mercury and other heavy metals to form stable, soluble complexes that are excreted in urine; depresses circulating IgM rheumatoid factor, depresses T-cell but not B-cell activity; combines with cystine to form a compound which is more soluble, thus cystine calculi are prevented

Drug Interactions

Increased Effect/Toxicity: Increased effect or toxicity of gold, antimalarials, immunosuppressants, and phenylbutazone (hematologic, renal toxicity).

(Continued)

Penicillamine *(Continued)*

Decreased Effect: Decreased effect of penicillamine when taken with iron and zinc salts, antacids (magnesium, calcium, aluminum), and food. Digoxin levels may be decreased when taken with penicillamine.

Pharmacodynamics/Kinetics

Absorption: 40% to 70%
Protein binding: 80% to albumin
Metabolism: Hepatic (small amounts)
Half-life elimination: 1.7-3.2 hours
Time to peak, serum: ~2 hours
Excretion: Urine (30% to 60% as unchanged drug)

Pregnancy Risk Factor D

Penicillin G Benzathine (pen i SIL in jee BENZ a theen)

Related Information

Sexually-Transmitted Diseases *on page 1504*

U.S. Brand Names Bicillin® L-A; Permapen® Isoject®

Mexican Brand Names Bencelin®; Benzanil®; Benzetacil®

Generic Available No

Synonyms Benzathine Benzylpenicillin; Benzathine Penicillin G; Benzylpenicillin Benzathine

Pharmacologic Category Antibiotic, Penicillin

Use Active against some gram-positive organisms, few gram-negative organisms such as *Neisseria gonorrhoeae*, and some anaerobes and spirochetes; used in the treatment of syphilis; used only for the treatment of mild to moderately severe infections caused by organisms susceptible to low concentrations of penicillin G or for prophylaxis of infections caused by these organisms

Local Anesthetic/Vasoconstrictor Precautions No information available to require special precautions

Effects on Dental Treatment No significant effects or complications reported

Common Adverse Effects Frequency not defined.

Central nervous system: Convulsions, confusion, drowsiness, myoclonus, fever
Dermatologic: Rash
Endocrine & metabolic: Electrolyte imbalance
Hematologic: Positive Coombs' reaction, hemolytic anemia
Local: Pain, thrombophlebitis
Renal: Acute interstitial nephritis
Miscellaneous: Anaphylaxis, hypersensitivity reactions, Jarisch-Herxheimer reaction

Mechanism of Action Interferes with bacterial cell wall synthesis during active multiplication, causing cell wall death and resultant bactericidal activity against susceptible bacteria

Drug Interactions

Increased Effect/Toxicity: Probenecid increases penicillin levels. Aminoglycosides may lead to synergistic efficacy. Penicillins may increase the exposure to methotrexate during concurrent therapy; monitor.

Decreased Effect: Tetracyclines may decrease penicillin effectiveness. Although anecdotal reports suggest oral contraceptive efficacy could be reduced by penicillins, this has been refuted by more rigorous scientific and clinical data.

Pharmacodynamics/Kinetics

Duration: 1-4 weeks (dose dependent); larger doses result in more sustained levels
Absorption: I.M.: Slow
Time to peak, serum: 12-24 hours

Pregnancy Risk Factor B

Penicillin G Benzathine and Penicillin G Procaine

(pen i SIL in jee BENZ a theen & pen i SIL in jee PROE kane)

U.S. Brand Names Bicillin® C-R; Bicillin® C-R 900/300

Generic Available No

Synonyms Penicillin G Procaine and Benzathine Combined

Pharmacologic Category Antibiotic, Penicillin

Use May be used in specific situations in the treatment of streptococcal infections

Local Anesthetic/Vasoconstrictor Precautions No information available to require special precautions

Effects on Dental Treatment No significant effects or complications reported

Common Adverse Effects Frequency not defined.

Central nervous system: CNS toxicity (convulsions, confusion, drowsiness, myoclonus)
Hematologic: Positive Coombs' reaction, hemolytic anemia
Renal: Interstitial nephritis
Miscellaneous: Hypersensitivity reactions, Jarisch-Herxheimer reaction

Mechanism of Action Inhibits bacterial cell wall synthesis by binding to one or more of the penicillin binding proteins (PBPs); which in turn inhibits the final transpeptidation step of peptidoglycan synthesis in bacterial cell walls, thus inhibiting cell wall biosynthesis. Bacteria eventually lyse due to ongoing activity of cell wall autolytic enzymes (autolysins and murein hydrolases) while cell wall assembly is arrested.

Drug Interactions

Increased Effect/Toxicity: Probenecid increases penicillin levels. Aminoglycosides may lead to synergistic efficacy. Warfarin effects may be increased. Penicillins may increase the exposure to methotrexate during concurrent therapy; monitor.

Decreased Effect: Tetracyclines may decrease penicillin effectiveness. Although anecdotal reports suggest oral contraceptive efficacy could be reduced by penicillins, this has been refuted by more rigorous scientific and clinical data.

Pregnancy Risk Factor B

Penicillin G (Parenteral/Aqueous)

(pen i SIL in jee, pa REN ter al, AYE kwee us)

Related Information

Sexually-Transmitted Diseases *on page 1504*

U.S. Brand Names Pfizerpen®

Canadian Brand Names Pfizerpen®

Generic Available Yes

Synonyms Benzylpenicillin Potassium; Benzylpenicillin Sodium; Crystalline Penicillin; Penicillin G Potassium; Penicillin G Sodium

Pharmacologic Category Antibiotic, Penicillin

Use Active against some gram-positive organisms, generally not *Staphylococcus aureus*; some gram-negative organisms such as *Neisseria gonorrhoeae*, and some anaerobes and spirochetes

Local Anesthetic/Vasoconstrictor Precautions No information available to require special precautions

Effects on Dental Treatment No significant effects or complications reported

Common Adverse Effects Frequency not defined.

Central nervous system: Convulsions, confusion, drowsiness, myoclonus, fever
Dermatologic: Rash
Endocrine & metabolic: Electrolyte imbalance
Hematologic: Positive Coombs' reaction, hemolytic anemia
Local: Thrombophlebitis
Renal: Acute interstitial nephritis
Miscellaneous: Anaphylaxis, hypersensitivity reactions, Jarisch-Herxheimer reaction

Mechanism of Action Interferes with bacterial cell wall synthesis during active multiplication, causing cell wall death and resultant bactericidal activity against susceptible bacteria

Drug Interactions

Increased Effect/Toxicity: Probenecid increases penicillin levels. Aminoglycosides may lead to synergistic efficacy. Penicillins may increase the exposure to methotrexate during concurrent therapy; monitor.

Decreased Effect: Tetracyclines may decrease penicillin effectiveness. Although anecdotal reports suggest oral contraceptive efficacy could be reduced by penicillins, this has been refuted by more rigorous scientific and clinical data.

Pharmacodynamics/Kinetics

Distribution: Poor penetration across blood-brain barrier, despite inflamed meninges; crosses placenta; enters breast milk

Relative diffusion from blood into CSF: Good only with inflammation (exceeds usual MICs)

CSF:blood level ratio: Normal meninges: <1%; Inflamed meninges: 3% to 5%

Protein binding: 65%

Metabolism: Hepatic (30%) to penicilloic acid

Half-life elimination:

Neonates: <6 days old: 3.2-3.4 hours; 7-13 days old: 1.2-2.2 hours; >14 days old: 0.9-1.9 hours

(Continued)

Penicillin G (Parenteral/Aqueous) *(Continued)*

Children and Adults: Normal renal function: 20-50 minutes
End-stage renal disease: 3.3-5.1 hours
Time to peak, serum: I.M.: ~30 minutes; I.V. ~1 hour
Excretion: Urine

Pregnancy Risk Factor B

Penicillin G Potassium *see* Penicillin G (Parenteral/Aqueous) *on page 1059*

Penicillin G Procaine (pen i SIL in jee PROE kane)

Related Information

Sexually-Transmitted Diseases *on page 1504*

Canadian Brand Names Pfizerpen-AS®; Wycillin®

Generic Available Yes

Synonyms APPG; Aqueous Procaine Penicillin G; Procaine Benzylpenicillin; Procaine Penicillin G; Wycillin [DSC]

Pharmacologic Category Antibiotic, Penicillin

Use Moderately severe infections due to *Treponema pallidum* and other penicillin G-sensitive microorganisms that are susceptible to low, but prolonged serum penicillin concentrations; anthrax due to *Bacillus anthracis* (postexposure) to reduce the incidence or progression of disease following exposure to aerolized *Bacillus anthracis*

Local Anesthetic/Vasoconstrictor Precautions No information available to require special precautions

Effects on Dental Treatment No significant effects or complications reported

Common Adverse Effects Frequency not defined.

Cardiovascular: Myocardial depression, vasodilation, conduction disturbances
Central nervous system: Confusion, drowsiness, myoclonus, CNS stimulation, seizures
Hematologic: Positive Coombs' reaction, hemolytic anemia, neutropenia
Local: Pain at injection site, thrombophlebitis, sterile abscess at injection site
Renal: Interstitial nephritis
Miscellaneous: Pseudoanaphylactic reactions, hypersensitivity reactions, Jarisch-Herxheimer reaction, serum sickness

Mechanism of Action Inhibits bacterial cell wall synthesis by binding to one or more of the penicillin binding proteins (PBPs); which in turn inhibits the final transpeptidation step of peptidoglycan synthesis in bacterial cell walls, thus inhibiting cell wall biosynthesis. Bacteria eventually lyse due to ongoing activity of cell wall autolytic enzymes (autolysins and murein hydrolases) while cell wall assembly is arrested.

Drug Interactions

Increased Effect/Toxicity: Probenecid increases penicillin levels. Aminoglycosides may lead to synergistic efficacy. Penicillins may increase the exposure to methotrexate during concurrent therapy; monitor.

Decreased Effect: Tetracyclines may decrease penicillin effectiveness. Although anecdotal reports suggest oral contraceptive efficacy could be reduced by penicillins, this has been refuted by more rigorous scientific and clinical data.

Pharmacodynamics/Kinetics

Duration: Therapeutic: 15-24 hours
Absorption: I.M.: Slow
Distribution: Penetration across the blood-brain barrier is poor, despite inflamed meninges; enters breast milk
Protein binding: 65%
Metabolism: ~30% hepatically inactivated
Time to peak, serum: 1-4 hours
Excretion: Urine (60% to 90% as unchanged drug)
Clearance: Renal: Delayed in neonates, young infants, and with impaired renal function

Pregnancy Risk Factor B

Penicillin G Procaine and Benzathine Combined *see* Penicillin G Benzathine and Penicillin G Procaine *on page 1058*

Penicillin G Sodium *see* Penicillin G (Parenteral/Aqueous) *on page 1059*

Penicillin V Potassium (pen i SIL in vee poe TASS ee um)

Related Information

Antibiotic Prophylaxis, Preprocedural Guidelines for Dental Patients *on page 1509*
Oral Bacterial Infections *on page 1533*
Oral Viral Infections *on page 1547*

U.S. Brand Names Veetids®

Canadian Brand Names Apo-Pen VK®; Nadopen-V®; Novo-Pen-VK; Nu-Pen-VK; PVF® K

Generic Available Yes

Synonyms Pen VK; Phenoxymethyl Penicillin

Pharmacologic Category Antibiotic, Penicillin

Dental Use Antibiotic of first choice in treatment of common orofacial infections caused by aerobic gram-positive cocci and anaerobes. These orofacial infections include cellulitis, periapical abscess, periodontal abscess, acute suppurative pulpitis, oronasal fistula, pericoronitis, osteitis, osteomyelitis, postsurgical and post-traumatic infection. **This agent is no longer recommended for dental procedure prophylaxis.**

Use Treatment of infections caused by susceptible organisms involving the respiratory tract, otitis media, sinusitis, skin, and urinary tract; prophylaxis in rheumatic fever

Local Anesthetic/Vasoconstrictor Precautions No information available to require special precautions

Effects on Dental Treatment Key adverse event(s) related to dental treatment: Oral candidiasis (prolonged use).

Significant Adverse Effects

>10%: Gastrointestinal: Mild diarrhea, vomiting, nausea, oral candidiasis

<1% (Limited to important or life-threatening): Acute interstitial nephritis, convulsions, hemolytic anemia, positive Coombs' reaction

Dosage Oral:

Systemic infections:

- Children <12 years: 25-50 mg/kg/day in divided doses every 6-8 hours; maximum dose: 3 g/day
- Children ≥12 years and Adults: 125-500 mg every 6-8 hours

Prophylaxis of pneumococcal infections:

- Children <5 years: 125 mg twice daily
- Children ≥5 years and Adults: 250 mg twice daily

Prophylaxis of recurrent rheumatic fever:

- Children <5 years: 125 mg twice daily
- Children ≥5 years and Adults: 250 mg twice daily

Dosing interval in renal impairment: Cl_{cr} <10 mL/minute: Administer 250 mg every 6 hours

Mechanism of Action Inhibits bacterial cell wall synthesis by binding to one or more of the penicillin binding proteins (PBPs); which in turn inhibits the final transpeptidation step of peptidoglycan synthesis in bacterial cell walls, thus inhibiting cell wall biosynthesis. Bacteria eventually lyse due to ongoing activity of cell wall autolytic enzymes (autolysins and murein hydrolases) while cell wall assembly is arrested.

Contraindications Hypersensitivity to penicillin or any component of the formulation

Warnings/Precautions Use with caution in patients with severe renal impairment (modify dosage), history of seizures, or hypersensitivity to cephalosporins

Drug Interactions

Aminoglycosides: May be synergistic against selected organisms

Methotrexate: Penicillins may increase the exposure to methotrexate during concurrent therapy; monitor.

Oral contraceptives: Anecdotal reports suggesting decreased contraceptive efficacy with penicillins have been refuted by more rigorous scientific and clinical data.

Probenecid, disulfiram: May increase penicillin levels

Tetracyclines: May decrease penicillin effectiveness

Warfarin: Effects of warfarin may be increased

Ethanol/Nutrition/Herb Interactions Food: Decreases drug absorption rate; decreases drug serum concentration.

Dietary Considerations Take on an empty stomach 1 hour before or 2 hours after meals.

Pharmacodynamics/Kinetics

Absorption: 60% to 73%

Distribution: Enters breast milk

Protein binding, plasma: 80%

Half-life elimination: 30 minutes; prolonged with renal impairment

Time to peak, serum: 0.5-1 hour

Excretion: Urine (as unchanged drug and metabolites)

Pregnancy Risk Factor B

Lactation Enters breast milk (other penicillins are compatible with breast-feeding)

(Continued)

Penicillin V Potassium *(Continued)*

Breast-Feeding Considerations No data reported; however, other penicillins may be taken while breast-feeding.

Dosage Forms Note: 250 mg = 400,000 units

Powder for oral solution: 125 mg/5 mL (100 mL, 200 mL); 250 mg/5 mL (100 mL, 200 mL)

Tablet: 250 mg, 500 mg

Selected Readings

Wynn RL and Bergman SA, "Antibiotics and Their Use in the Treatment of Orofacial Infections, Part I," *Gen Dent*, 1994, 42(5):398, 400, 402.

Wynn RL and Bergman SA, "Antibiotics and Their Use in the Treatment of Orofacial Infections, Part II," *Gen Dent*, 1994, 42(6):498-502.

Wynn RL, Bergman SA, Meiller TF, et al, "Antibiotics in Treating Oral-Facial Infections of Odontogenic Origin: An Update," *Gen Dent*, 2001, 49(3):238-40, 242, 244 passim.

Penicilloyl-polylysine *see* Benzylpenicilloyl-polylysine *on page 196*

Penlac™ *see* Ciclopirox *on page 327*

Pentahydrate *see* Sodium Thiosulfate *on page 1230*

Pentam-300® *see* Pentamidine *on page 1062*

Pentamidine (pen TAM i deen)

U.S. Brand Names NebuPent®; Pentam-300®

Canadian Brand Names Pentacarinat®

Generic Available Yes: Injection

Synonyms Pentamidine Isethionate

Pharmacologic Category Antibiotic, Miscellaneous

Use Treatment and prevention of pneumonia caused by *Pneumocystis carinii* (PCP)

Unlabeled/Investigational Use Treatment of trypanosomiasis and visceral leishmaniasis

Local Anesthetic/Vasoconstrictor Precautions No information available to require special precautions

Effects on Dental Treatment No significant effects or complications reported

Common Adverse Effects Injection (I); Aerosol (A)

>10%:

- Cardiovascular: Chest pain (A - 10% to 23%)
- Central nervous system: Fatigue (A - 50% to 70%); dizziness (A - 31% to 47%)
- Dermatologic: Rash (31% to 47%)
- Endocrine & metabolic: Hyperkalemia
- Gastrointestinal: Anorexia (A - 50% to 70%), nausea (A - 10% to 23%)
- Local: Local reactions at injection site
- Renal: Increased creatinine (I - 23%)
- Respiratory: Wheezing (A - 10% to 23%), dyspnea (A - 50% to 70%), coughing (A - 31% to 47%), pharyngitis (10% to 23%)

1% to 10%:

- Cardiovascular: Hypotension (I - 4%)
- Central nervous system: Confusion/hallucinations (1% to 2%), headache (A - 1% to 5%)
- Dermatologic: Rash (I - 3.3%)
- Endocrine & metabolic: Hypoglycemia <25 mg/dL (I - 2.4%)
- Gastrointestinal: Nausea/anorexia (I - 6%), diarrhea (A - 1% to 5%), vomiting
- Hematologic: Severe leukopenia (I - 2.8%), thrombocytopenia <20,000/mm^3 (I - 1.7%), anemia (A - 1% to 5%)
- Hepatic: Increased LFTs (I - 8.7%)

Mechanism of Action Interferes with RNA/DNA, phospholipids and protein synthesis, through inhibition of oxidative phosphorylation and/or interference with incorporation of nucleotides and nucleic acids into RNA and DNA, in protozoa

Drug Interactions

Cytochrome P450 Effect: Substrate of CYP2C19 (major); **Inhibits** CYP2C8/9 (weak), 2C19 (weak), 2D6 (weak), 3A4 (weak)

Increased Effect/Toxicity: CYP2C19 inhibitors may increase the levels/effects of pentamidine; example inhibitors include delavirdine, fluconazole, fluvoxamine, gemfibrozil, isoniazid, omeprazole, and ticlopidine. Pentamidine may potentiate the effect of other drugs which prolong QT interval (cisapride, sparfloxacin, gatifloxacin, moxifloxacin, pimozide, and type Ia and type III antiarrhythmics).

Decreased Effect: CYP2C19 inducers may decrease the levels/effects of pentamidine; example inducers include aminoglutethimide, carbamazepine, phenytoin, and rifampin.

Pharmacodynamics/Kinetics

Absorption: I.M.: Well absorbed; Inhalation: Limited systemic absorption

Half-life elimination: Terminal: 6.4-9.4 hours; may be prolonged with severe renal impairment

Excretion: Urine (33% to 66% as unchanged drug)

Pregnancy Risk Factor C

Pentamidine Isethionate *see* Pentamidine *on page 1062*

Pentasa® *see* Mesalamine *on page 882*

Pentaspan® *see* Pentastarch *on page 1063*

Pentastarch (PEN ta starch)

U.S. Brand Names Pentaspan®

Canadian Brand Names Pentaspan®

Mexican Brand Names Pentaspan®

Generic Available No

Pharmacologic Category Blood Modifiers

Use Orphan drug: Adjunct in leukapheresis to improve harvesting and increase yield of leukocytes by centrifugal means

Local Anesthetic/Vasoconstrictor Precautions No information available to require special precautions

Effects on Dental Treatment No significant effects or complications reported

Pentazocine (pen TAZ oh seen)

U.S. Brand Names Talwin®; Talwin® NX

Canadian Brand Names Talwin®

Generic Available Yes: Tablet

Synonyms Naloxone Hydrochloride and Pentazocine Hydrochloride; Pentazocine Hydrochloride; Pentazocine Hydrochloride and Naloxone Hydrochloride; Pentazocine Lactate

Pharmacologic Category Analgesic, Narcotic

Use Relief of moderate to severe pain; has also been used as a sedative prior to surgery and as a supplement to surgical anesthesia

Local Anesthetic/Vasoconstrictor Precautions No information available to require special precautions

Effects on Dental Treatment No significant effects or complications reported

Common Adverse Effects Frequency not defined.

Cardiovascular: Hypotension, circulatory depression, shock, tachycardia, syncope, flushing

Central nervous system: Malaise, headache, nightmares, insomnia, CNS depression, sedation, hallucinations, confusion, disorientation, dizziness, euphoria, drowsiness, lightheadedness, irritability, chills, excitement

Dermatologic: Rash, pruritus, dermatitis, urticaria, Stevens-Johnson syndrome, toxic epidermal necrolysis, erythema multiforme

Gastrointestinal: Nausea, vomiting, xerostomia, constipation, anorexia, diarrhea, abdominal distress

Genitourinary: Urinary retention

Hematologic: WBCs decreased, eosinophilia

Local: Tissue damage and irritation with I.M./SubQ use

Neuromuscular & skeletal: Weakness, tremor, paresthesia

Ocular: Blurred vision, miosis

Otic: Tinnitus

Respiratory: Dyspnea, respiratory depression (rare)

Miscellaneous: Physical and psychological dependence, facial edema, diaphoresis, anaphylaxis

Restrictions C-IV

Mechanism of Action Binds to opiate receptors in the CNS, causing inhibition of ascending pain pathways, altering the perception of and response to pain; produces generalized CNS depression; partial agonist-antagonist

Drug Interactions

Increased Effect/Toxicity: Increased effect/toxicity with tripelennamine (can be lethal), CNS depressants (eg, phenothiazines, tranquilizers, anxiolytics, sedatives, hypnotics, alcohol).

Decreased Effect: May potentiate or reduce analgesic effect of opiate agonist (eg, morphine) depending on patients tolerance to opiates; can precipitate withdrawal in narcotic addicts.

Pharmacodynamics/Kinetics

Onset of action: Oral, I.M., SubQ: 15-30 minutes; I.V.: 2-3 minutes

Duration: Oral: 4-5 hours; Parenteral: 2-3 hours

Protein binding: 60%

(Continued)

Pentazocine *(Continued)*

Metabolism: Hepatic via oxidative and glucuronide conjugation pathways; extensive first-pass effect

Bioavailability: Oral: ~20%; increased to 60% to 70% with cirrhosis

Half-life elimination: 2-3 hours; prolonged with hepatic impairment

Excretion: Urine (small amounts as unchanged drug)

Pregnancy Risk Factor C/D (prolonged use or high doses at term)

Pentazocine and Acetaminophen

(pen TAZ oh seen & a seet a MIN oh fen)

Related Information

Acetaminophen *on page 47*

Pentazocine *on page 1063*

U.S. Brand Names Talacen®

Generic Available Yes

Synonyms Acetaminophen and Pentazocine; Pentazocine Hydrochloride and Acetaminophen

Pharmacologic Category Analgesic Combination (Narcotic)

Use Relief of mild to moderate pain

Local Anesthetic/Vasoconstrictor Precautions No information available to require special precautions

Effects on Dental Treatment No significant effects or complications reported

Significant Adverse Effects Frequency not defined.

Cardiovascular: Tachycardia, hypotension, syncope, flushing

Central nervous system: Headache, dizziness, drowsiness, lightheadedness, sedation, insomnia, hallucinations, euphoria, depression, confusion, disorientation, chills, irritability, excitement

Dermatologic: Rash, urticaria, erythema multiforme, Stevens-Johnson syndrome, toxic epidermal necrolysis

Gastrointestinal: Nausea, vomiting, biliary spasm, constipation, anorexia, diarrhea, abdominal distress

Genitourinary: Urinary retention

Hematologic: WBCs decreased, eosinophilia, thrombocytopenic purpura, hemolytic anemia, agranulocytosis

Neuromuscular & skeletal: Weakness, tremor, paresthesia

Ocular: Blurred vision

Otic: Tinnitus

Respiratory: Respiratory depression

Miscellaneous: Diaphoresis, facial edema, anaphylaxis

Restrictions C-IV

Dosage Oral: Adults: Analgesic: 1 caplet every 4 hours, up to a maximum of 6 caplets

Mechanism of Action

Pentazocine: Binds to opiate receptors in the CNS, causing inhibition of ascending pain pathways, altering the perception of and response to pain; produces generalized CNS depression; partial agonist-antagonist

Acetaminophen: Inhibits the synthesis of prostaglandins in the central nervous system and peripherally blocks pain impulse generation

Contraindications Hypersensitivity to pentazocine, acetaminophen, or any component of the formulation; pregnancy (prolonged use or high doses at term)

Warnings/Precautions Contains sodium metasulfite; may cause allergic-type reactions; potential for elevating CSF pressure due to respiratory effects which may be exaggerated in presence of head injury, intracranial lesions, or pre-existing increase in intracranial lesions. May experience hallucinations, disorientation, and confusion. May cause psychological and physical dependence. Use with caution in patients with myocardial infarction who have nausea or vomiting, patients with respiratory depression, severely limited respiratory reserve, severe bronchial asthma, other obstructive respiratory conditions or cyanosis, impaired renal or hepatic function, patients prone to seizures. Abrupt discontinuation may result in withdrawal symptoms. Pentazocine may precipitate opiate withdrawal symptoms in patients who have been receiving opiates regularly.

Ethanol/Nutrition/Herb Interactions

Ethanol: Avoid ethanol (may increase CNS depression).

Herb/Nutraceutical: Avoid valerian, St John's wort, kava kava, gotu kola (may increase CNS depression).

Pharmacodynamics/Kinetics See individual agents.

Pregnancy Risk Factor C/D (prolonged use or high doses at term)

Lactation Excretion in breast milk unknown/use caution

Breast-Feeding Considerations Excretion of pentazocine in breast milk is unknown; acetaminophen is excreted in breast milk

Dosage Forms Caplet (Talacen®): Pentazocine hydrochloride 25 mg and acetaminophen 650 mg [contains sodium metabisulfite]

Pentazocine Hydrochloride *see* Pentazocine *on page 1063*

Pentazocine Hydrochloride and Acetaminophen *see* Pentazocine and Acetaminophen *on page 1064*

Pentazocine Hydrochloride and Naloxone Hydrochloride *see* Pentazocine *on page 1063*

Pentazocine Lactate *see* Pentazocine *on page 1063*

Pentobarbital (pen toe BAR bi tal)

U.S. Brand Names Nembutal®

Canadian Brand Names Nembutal® Sodium

Generic Available No

Synonyms Pentobarbital Sodium

Pharmacologic Category Anticonvulsant, Barbiturate; Barbiturate

Use Sedative/hypnotic; preanesthetic; high-dose barbiturate coma for treatment of increased intracranial pressure or status epilepticus unresponsive to other therapy

Local Anesthetic/Vasoconstrictor Precautions No information available to require special precautions

Effects on Dental Treatment No significant effects or complications reported

Mechanism of Action Short-acting barbiturate with sedative, hypnotic, and anticonvulsant properties. Barbiturates depress the sensory cortex, decrease motor activity, alter cerebellar function, and produce drowsiness, sedation, and hypnosis. In high doses, barbiturates exhibit anticonvulsant activity; barbiturates produce dose-dependent respiratory depression.

Pregnancy Risk Factor D

Pentobarbital Sodium *see* Pentobarbital *on page 1065*

Pentosan Polysulfate Sodium

(PEN toe san pol i SUL fate SOW dee um)

U.S. Brand Names Elmiron®

Canadian Brand Names Elmiron™

Generic Available No

Synonyms PPS

Pharmacologic Category Analgesic, Urinary

Use Orphan drug: Relief of bladder pain or discomfort due to interstitial cystitis

Local Anesthetic/Vasoconstrictor Precautions No information available to require special precautions

Effects on Dental Treatment No significant effects or complications reported

Common Adverse Effects 1% to 10%:

Central nervous system: Headache (3%), dizziness (1%), depression (2%)
Dermatologic: Alopecia, rash, pruritus
Gastrointestinal: Diarrhea, nausea, dyspepsia, abdominal pain
Hepatic: Liver function test abnormalities (1%)

Mechanism of Action Although pentosan polysulfate sodium is a low-molecular weight heparinoid, it is not known whether these properties play a role in its mechanism of action in treating interstitial cystitis; the drug appears to adhere to the bladder wall mucosa where it may act as a buffer to protect the tissues from irritating substances in the urine.

Drug Interactions

Increased Effect/Toxicity: Although there is no information about potential drug interactions, it is expected that pentosan polysulfate sodium would have at least additive anticoagulant effects when administered with anticoagulant drugs such as warfarin or heparin, and possible similar effects when administered with aspirin or thrombolytics.

Pharmacodynamics/Kinetics

Absorption: ~3%
Metabolism: Hepatic and via spleen
Half-life elimination: 4.8 hours
Excretion: Urine (3% as unchanged drug)

Pregnancy Risk Factor B

Pentostatin (PEN toe stat in)

U.S. Brand Names Nipent®

Canadian Brand Names Nipent®

Generic Available No

(Continued)

Pentostatin *(Continued)*

Synonyms CL-825; Co-Vidarabine; dCF; Deoxycoformycin; 2′-Deoxycoformycin; NSC-218321

Pharmacologic Category Antineoplastic Agent, Antibiotic; Antineoplastic Agent, Antimetabolite

Use Treatment of hairy cell leukemia; non-Hodgkin's lymphoma, cutaneous T-cell lymphoma

Local Anesthetic/Vasoconstrictor Precautions No information available to require special precautions

Effects on Dental Treatment Key adverse event(s) related to dental treatment: Stomatitis.

Common Adverse Effects

>10%:

Central nervous system: Fever, chills, headache

Dermatologic: Skin rashes (25% to 30%), alopecia (10%)

Gastrointestinal: Mild to moderate nausea, vomiting (60%), stomatitis, diarrhea (13%), anorexia

Genitourinary: Acute renal failure (35%)

Hematologic: Thrombocytopenia (50%), dose-limiting in 25% of patients; anemia (40% to 45%), neutropenia, mild to moderate, not dose-limiting (11%)

Nadir: 7 days

Recovery: 10-14 days

Hepatic: Mild to moderate increases in transaminase levels (30%), usually transient; hepatitis (19%), usually reversible

Respiratory: Pulmonary edema (15%), may be exacerbated by fludarabine

Miscellaneous: Infection (57%; 35% severe, life-threatening)

1% to 10%:

Cardiovascular: Chest pain, arrhythmia, peripheral edema

Central nervous system: Opportunistic infections (8%); anxiety, confusion, depression, dizziness, insomnia, nervousness, somnolence, myalgias, malaise

Dermatologic: Dry skin, eczema, pruritus

Gastrointestinal: Constipation, flatulence, weight loss

Neuromuscular & skeletal: Paresthesia, weakness

Ocular: Moderate to severe keratoconjunctivitis, abnormal vision, eye pain

Otic: Ear pain

Respiratory: Dyspnea, pneumonia, bronchitis, pharyngitis, rhinitis, epistaxis, sinusitis (3% to 7%)

Mechanism of Action Pentostatin is a purine antimetabolite that inhibits adenosine deaminase, preventing the deamination of adenosine to inosine. Accumulation of deoxyadenosine (dAdo) and deoxyadenosine 5′-triphosphate (dATP) results in a reduction of purine metabolism and DNA synthesis and cell death.

Drug Interactions

Increased Effect/Toxicity: Increased toxicity with vidarabine and allopurinol; combined use with fludarabine may lead to severe, even fatal, pulmonary toxicity

Pharmacodynamics/Kinetics

Distribution: I.V.: V_d: 36.1 L (20.1 L/m^2); rapidly to body tissues

Half-life elimination: Distribution half-life: 30-85 minutes; Terminal: 5-15 hours

Excretion: Urine (~50% to 96%) within 24 hours (30% to 90% as unchanged drug)

Pregnancy Risk Factor D

Pentothal® *see* Thiopental *on page 1289*

Pentoxifylline (pen toks I fi leen)

U.S. Brand Names Pentoxil®; Trental®

Canadian Brand Names Albert® Pentoxifylline; Apo-Pentoxifylline SR®; Nu-Pentoxifylline SR; ratio-Pentoxifylline; Trental®

Mexican Brand Names Fixoten®; Kentadin®; Peridane®; Sufisal®; Trental®; Vasofyl®

Generic Available Yes

Synonyms Oxpentifylline

Pharmacologic Category Blood Viscosity Reducer Agent

Use Treatment of intermittent claudication on the basis of chronic occlusive arterial disease of the limbs; may improve function and symptoms, but not intended to replace more definitive therapy

Unlabeled/Investigational Use AIDS patients with increased TNF, CVA, cerebrovascular diseases, diabetic atherosclerosis, diabetic neuropathy, gangrene, hemodialysis shunt thrombosis, vascular impotence, cerebral malaria, septic shock, sickle cell syndromes, and vasculitis

Local Anesthetic/Vasoconstrictor Precautions No information available to require special precautions

Effects on Dental Treatment No significant effects or complications reported

Common Adverse Effects 1% to 10%:

Central nervous system: Dizziness, headache

Gastrointestinal: Dyspepsia, nausea, vomiting

Mechanism of Action Mechanism of action remains unclear; is thought to reduce blood viscosity and improve blood flow by altering the rheology of red blood cells

Drug Interactions

Cytochrome P450 Effect: Inhibits CYP1A2 (weak)

Increased Effect/Toxicity: Pentoxifylline levels may be increased with cimetidine and other H_2 antagonists. May increase anticoagulation with warfarin. Pentoxifylline may increase the serum levels of theophylline.

Decreased Effect: Blood pressure changes (decreases) have been observed with the addition of pentoxifylline therapy in patients receiving antihypertensives.

Pharmacodynamics/Kinetics

Absorption: Well absorbed

Metabolism: Hepatic and via erythrocytes; extensive first-pass effect

Half-life elimination: Parent drug: 24-48 minutes; Metabolites: 60-96 minutes

Time to peak, serum: 2-4 hours

Excretion: Primarily urine

Pregnancy Risk Factor C

Pentoxil® *see* Pentoxifylline *on page 1066*

Pentrax® [OTC] *see* Coal Tar *on page 367*

Pen VK *see* Penicillin V Potassium *on page 1060*

Pepcid® *see* Famotidine *on page 573*

Pepcid® AC [OTC] *see* Famotidine *on page 573*

Pepcid® Complete [OTC] *see* Famotidine, Calcium Carbonate, and Magnesium Hydroxide *on page 574*

Pepto-Bismol® [OTC] *see* Bismuth *on page 209*

Pepto-Bismol® Maximum Strength [OTC] *see* Bismuth *on page 209*

Percocet® *see* Oxycodone and Acetaminophen *on page 1029*

Percodan® *see* Oxycodone and Aspirin *on page 1032*

Percodan®-Demi [DSC] *see* Oxycodone and Aspirin *on page 1032*

Percogesic® [OTC] *see* Acetaminophen and Phenyltoloxamine *on page 53*

Percogesic® Extra Strength [OTC] *see* Acetaminophen and Diphenhydramine *on page 53*

Perdiem® Fiber Therapy [OTC] *see* Psyllium *on page 1151*

Pergolide (PER go lide)

U.S. Brand Names Permax®

Canadian Brand Names Permax®

Mexican Brand Names Permax®

Generic Available Yes

Synonyms Pergolide Mesylate

Pharmacologic Category Anti-Parkinson's Agent, Dopamine Agonist; Ergot Derivative

Use Adjunctive treatment to levodopa/carbidopa in the management of Parkinson's disease

Unlabeled/Investigational Use Tourette's disorder, chronic motor or vocal tic disorder

Local Anesthetic/Vasoconstrictor Precautions No information available to require special precautions

Effects on Dental Treatment Key adverse event(s) related to dental treatment: Xerostomia (normal salivary flow resumes upon discontinuation). Prolonged use may decrease or inhibit salivary flow, contributing to discomfort and dental disease (ie, oral candidiasis and periodontal disease).

Common Adverse Effects

>10%:

Central nervous system: Dizziness (19%), hallucinations (14%), dystonia (12%), somnolence (10%), confusion (10%)

Gastrointestinal: Nausea (24%), constipation (11%)

Neuromuscular & skeletal: Dyskinesia (62%)

Respiratory: Rhinitis (12%)

(Continued)

Pergolide *(Continued)*

1% to 10%:

Cardiovascular: Hypotension or postural hypotension (10%), peripheral edema (7%), chest pain (4%), vasodilation (3%), palpitation (2%), syncope (2%), arrhythmias (1%), hypertension (2%), MI (1%)

Central nervous system: Insomnia (8%), pain (7%), anxiety (6%), psychosis (2%), EPS (2%), incoordination (2%), chills (1%)

Dermatologic: Rash (3%)

Gastrointestinal: Diarrhea (6%), dyspepsia (6%), abdominal pain (6%), anorexia (5%), xerostomia (4%), vomiting (3%), dysphagia (1%), nausea (1%)

Hematologic: Anemia (1%)

Neuromuscular & skeletal: Myalgia (1%), neuralgia (1%)

Ocular: Abnormal vision (6%), diplopia (2%)

Respiratory: Dyspnea (5%), epistaxis (2%)

Miscellaneous: Flu syndrome (3%), hiccups (1%)

Mechanism of Action Pergolide is a semisynthetic ergot alkaloid similar to bromocriptine but stated to be more potent (10-1000 times) and longer-acting; it is a centrally-active dopamine agonist stimulating both D_1 and D_2 receptors. Pergolide is believed to exert its therapeutic effect by directly stimulating post-synaptic dopamine receptors in the nigrostriatal system.

Drug Interactions

Cytochrome P450 Effect: Substrate of CYP3A4 (major); **Inhibits** CYP2D6 (strong), 3A4 (weak)

Increased Effect/Toxicity: Effects of pergolide may be increased by levodopa (hallucinations) and MAO inhibitors. Pergolide may increase the levels/effects of amphetamines, selected beta-blockers, dextromethorphan, fluoxetine, lidocaine, mirtazapine, nefazodone, paroxetine, risperidone, ritonavir, thioridazine, tricyclic antidepressants, venlafaxine, and other CYP2D6 substrates. Pergolide may increase the levels/effects of sibutramine and other serotonin agonists (serotonin syndrome). The levels/effects of pergolide may be increased by azole antifungals, ciprofloxacin, clarithromycin, diclofenac, doxycycline, erythromycin, imatinib, isoniazid, nefazodone, nicardipine, propofol, protease inhibitors, quinidine, telithromycin, verapamil, and other CYP3A4 inhibitors.

Decreased Effect: Effects of pergolide may be diminished by antipsychotics, metoclopramide. Pergolide may decrease the levels/effects of CYP2D6 prodrug substrates (eg, codeine, hydrocodone, oxycodone, tramadol).

Pharmacodynamics/Kinetics

Absorption: Well absorbed

Protein binding, plasma: 90%

Metabolism: Extensively hepatic

Half-life elimination: 27 hours

Excretion: Urine (~50%); feces (50%)

Pregnancy Risk Factor B

Pergolide Mesylate *see* Pergolide *on page 1067*

Pergonal® *see* Menotropins *on page 868*

Periactin *see* Cyproheptadine *on page 389*

Peri-Colace® [DSC] [OTC] *see* Docusate and Casanthranol *on page 460*

Peridex® *see* Chlorhexidine Gluconate *on page 308*

Perindopril Erbumine (per IN doe pril er BYOO meen)

Related Information

Cardiovascular Diseases *on page 1458*

U.S. Brand Names Aceon®

Canadian Brand Names Coversyl®

Mexican Brand Names Coversyl®

Generic Available No

Pharmacologic Category Angiotensin-Converting Enzyme (ACE) Inhibitor

Use Treatment of stage I or II hypertension and congestive heart failure; treatment of left ventricular dysfunction after myocardial infarction

Local Anesthetic/Vasoconstrictor Precautions No information available to require special precautions

Effects on Dental Treatment No significant effects or complications reported

Common Adverse Effects

>10%: Central nervous system: Headache (23%)

1% to 10%:

Cardiovascular: edema (4%), chest pain (2%)

Central nervous system: Dizziness (8%), sleep disorders (3%), depression (2%), fever (2%), weakness (8%), nervousness (1%)

Dermatologic: Rash (2%)

Endocrine & metabolic: Hyperkalemia (1%), increased triglycerides (1%)

Gastrointestinal: Nausea (2%), diarrhea (4%), vomiting (2%), dyspepsia (2%), abdominal pain (3%), flatulence (1%)

Genitourinary: Sexual dysfunction (male: 1%)

Hepatic: Increased ALT (2%)

Neuromuscular & skeletal: Back pain (6%), upper extremity pain (3%), lower extremity pain (5%), paresthesia (2%), joint pain (1%), myalgia (1%), arthritis (1%)

Renal: Proteinuria (2%)

Respiratory: Cough (incidence is higher in women, 3:1) (12%), sinusitis (5%), rhinitis (5%), pharyngitis (3%)

Otic: Tinnitus (2%)

Miscellaneous: Viral infection (3%)

Note: Some reactions occurred at an incidence >1% but ≤ placebo.

Additional adverse effects associated with with **ACE inhibitors** include agranulocytosis (especially in patients with renal impairment or collagen vascular disease), neutropenia, decreases in creatinine clearance in some elderly hypertensive patients or those with chronic renal failure, and worsening of renal function in patients with bilateral renal artery stenosis or hypovolemic patients (diuretic therapy). In addition, a syndrome which may include fever, myalgia, arthralgia, interstitial nephritis, vasculitis, rash, eosinophilia and positive ANA, and elevated ESR has been reported with ACE inhibitors.

Mechanism of Action Competitive inhibitor of angiotensin-converting enzyme (ACE); prevents conversion of angiotensin I to angiotensin II, a potent vasoconstrictor; results in lower levels of angiotensin II which, in turn, causes an increase in plasma renin activity and a reduction in aldosterone secretion

Drug Interactions

Increased Effect/Toxicity: Potassium supplements, co-trimoxazole (high dose), angiotensin II receptor antagonists (eg, candesartan, losartan, irbesartan), or potassium-sparing diuretics (amiloride, spironolactone, triamterene) may result in elevated serum potassium levels when combined with perindopril. ACE inhibitor effects may be increased by phenothiazines or probenecid (increases levels of captopril). ACE inhibitors may increase serum concentrations/effects of digoxin, lithium, and sulfonlyureas.

Diuretics have additive hypotensive effects with ACE inhibitors, and hypovolemia increases the potential for adverse renal effects of ACE inhibitors. In patients with compromised renal function, coadministration with NSAIDs may result in further deterioration of renal function. Allopurinol and ACE inhibitors may cause a higher risk of hypersensitivity reaction when taken concurrently.

Decreased Effect: Aspirin (high dose) may reduce the therapeutic effects of ACE inhibitors; at low dosages this does not appear to be significant. Rifampin may decrease the effect of ACE inhibitors. Antacids may decrease the bioavailability of ACE inhibitors (may be more likely to occur with captopril); separate administration times by 1-2 hours. NSAIDs, specifically indomethacin, may reduce the hypotensive effects of ACE inhibitors. More likely to occur in low renin or volume dependent hypertensive patients.

Pharmacodynamics/Kinetics

Onset of action: Peak effect: 1-2 hours

Distribution: Small amounts enter breast milk

Protein binding: Perindopril: 60%; Perindoprilat: 10% to 20%

Metabolism: Hepatically hydrolyzed to active metabolite, perindoprilat (~17% to 20% of a dose) and other inactive metabolites

Bioavailability: Perindopril: 65% to 95%

Half-life elimination: Parent drug: 1.5-3 hours; Metabolite: Effective: 3-10 hours, Terminal: 30-120 hours

Time to peak: Chronic therapy: Perindopril: 1 hour; Perindoprilat: 3-4 hours (maximum perindoprilat serum levels are 2-3 times higher and T_{max} is shorter following chronic therapy); CHF: Perindoprilat: 6 hours

Excretion: Urine (75%, 10% as unchanged drug)

Pregnancy Risk Factor D (especially 2nd and 3rd trimesters)

PerioChip® *see* Chlorhexidine Gluconate *on page 308*

Periodontal Diseases *see page 1542*

PerioGard® *see* Chlorhexidine Gluconate *on page 308*

Periostat® *see* Doxycycline (Subantimicrobial) *on page 476*

Permapen® Isoject® *see* Penicillin G Benzathine *on page 1058*

Permax® *see* Pergolide *on page 1067*

Permethrin (per METH rin)

U.S. Brand Names A200® Lice [OTC]; Acticin®; Elimite®; Nix® [OTC]; Rid® Spray [OTC]

Canadian Brand Names Kwellada-P™; Nix®

Mexican Brand Names Novo-Herklin 2000®

Generic Available Yes: Excludes spray

Pharmacologic Category Antiparasitic Agent, Topical; Scabicidal Agent

Use Single-application treatment of infestation with *Pediculus humanus capitis* (head louse) and its nits or *Sarcoptes scabiei* (scabies); indicated for prophylactic use during epidemics of lice

Local Anesthetic/Vasoconstrictor Precautions No information available to require special precautions

Effects on Dental Treatment No significant effects or complications reported

Common Adverse Effects 1% to 10%:

Dermatologic: Pruritus, erythema, rash of the scalp

Local: Burning, stinging, tingling, numbness or scalp discomfort, edema

Mechanism of Action Inhibits sodium ion influx through nerve cell membrane channels in parasites resulting in delayed repolarization and thus paralysis and death of the pest

Pharmacodynamics/Kinetics

Absorption: <2%

Metabolism: Hepatic via ester hydrolysis to inactive metabolites

Excretion: Urine

Pregnancy Risk Factor B

Perphenazine (per FEN a zeen)

U.S. Brand Names Trilafon® [DSC]

Canadian Brand Names Apo-Perphenazine®; Trilafon®

Mexican Brand Names Leptopsique®

Generic Available Yes

Pharmacologic Category Antipsychotic Agent, Phenothiazine, Piperazine

Use Treatment of schizophrenia; nausea and vomiting

Unlabeled/Investigational Use Ethanol withdrawal; dementia in elderly; Tourette's syndrome; Huntington's chorea; spasmodic torticollis; Reye's syndrome; psychosis

Local Anesthetic/Vasoconstrictor Precautions Most pharmacology textbooks state that in presence of phenothiazines, systemic doses of epinephrine paradoxically decrease the blood pressure. This is the so called "epinephrine reversal" phenomenon. This has never been observed when epinephrine is given by infiltration as part of the anesthesia procedure.

Effects on Dental Treatment Key adverse event(s) related to dental treatment:

Significant hypotension may occur, especially when the drug is administered parenterally; orthostatic hypotension is due to alpha-receptor blockade, the elderly are at greater risk for orthostatic hypotension.

Tardive dyskinesia: Prevalence rate may be 40% in elderly; development of the syndrome and the irreversible nature are proportional to duration and total cumulative dose over time. Extrapyramidal reactions are more common in elderly with up to 50% developing these reactions after 60 years of age. Drug-induced Parkinson's syndrome occurs often; akathisia is the most common extrapyramidal reaction in elderly.

Common Adverse Effects Frequency not defined.

Cardiovascular: Hypotension, orthostatic hypotension, hypertension, tachycardia, bradycardia, dizziness, cardiac arrest

Central nervous system: Extrapyramidal symptoms (pseudoparkinsonism, akathisia, dystonias, tardive dyskinesia), dizziness, cerebral edema, seizures, headache, drowsiness, paradoxical excitement, restlessness, hyperactivity, insomnia, neuroleptic malignant syndrome (NMS), impairment of temperature regulation

Dermatologic: Increased sensitivity to sun, rash, discoloration of skin (blue-gray)

Endocrine & metabolic: Hypoglycemia, hyperglycemia, galactorrhea, lactation, breast enlargement, gynecomastia, menstrual irregularity, amenorrhea, SIADH, changes in libido

Gastrointestinal: Constipation, weight gain, vomiting, stomach pain, nausea, xerostomia, salivation, diarrhea, anorexia, ileus

Genitourinary: Difficulty in urination, ejaculatory disturbances, incontinence, polyuria, ejaculating dysfunction, priapism

Hematologic: Agranulocytosis, leukopenia, eosinophilia, hemolytic anemia, thrombocytopenic purpura, pancytopenia

Hepatic: Cholestatic jaundice, hepatotoxicity
Neuromuscular & skeletal: Tremor
Ocular: Pigmentary retinopathy, blurred vision, cornea and lens changes
Respiratory: Nasal congestion
Miscellaneous: Diaphoresis

Mechanism of Action Blocks postsynaptic mesolimbic dopaminergic receptors in the brain; exhibits alpha-adrenergic blocking effect and depresses the release of hypothalamic and hypophyseal hormones

Drug Interactions

Cytochrome P450 Effect: Substrate of CYP1A2 (minor), 2C8/9 (minor), 2C19 (minor), 2D6 (major), 3A4 (minor); **Inhibits** CYP1A2 (weak), 2D6 (weak)

Increased Effect/Toxicity: CYP2D6 inhibitors may increase the levels/effects of perphenazine; example inhibitors include chlorpromazine, delavirdine, fluoxetine, miconazole, paroxetine, pergolide, quinidine, quinine, ritonavir, and ropinirole. Effects on CNS depression may be additive when perphenazine is combined with CNS depressants (narcotic analgesics, ethanol, barbiturates, cyclic antidepressants, antihistamines, or sedative-hypnotics). Perphenazine may increase the effects/toxicity of anticholinergics, antihypertensives, lithium (rare neurotoxicity), trazodone, or valproic acid. Concurrent use with TCA may produce increased toxicity or altered therapeutic response. Chloroquine and propranolol may increase perphenazine concentrations. Hypotension may occur when perphenazine is combined with epinephrine. May increase the risk of arrhythmia when combined with antiarrhythmics, cisapride, pimozide, sparfloxacin, or other drugs which prolong QT interval. Metoclopramide may increase risk of extrapyramidal symptoms (EPS).

Decreased Effect: Phenothiazines inhibit the ability of bromocriptine to lower serum prolactin concentrations. Benztropine (and other anticholinergics) may inhibit the therapeutic response to perphenazine and excess anticholinergic effects may occur. Cigarette smoking and barbiturates may enhance the hepatic metabolism of chlorpromazine. Antihypertensive effects of guanethidine and guanadrel may be inhibited by perphenazine. Perphenazine may inhibit the antiparkinsonian effect of levodopa. Perphenazine and possibly other low potency antipsychotics may reverse the pressor effects of epinephrine.

Pharmacodynamics/Kinetics

Absorption: Oral: Well absorbed
Distribution: Crosses placenta
Metabolism: Extensively hepatic to metabolites via sulfoxidation, hydroxylation, dealkylation, and glucuronidation
Half-life elimination: Perphenazine: 9-12 hours; 7-hydroxyperphenazine: 11.3 hours
Time to peak, serum: Perphenazine: 1-3 hours; 7-hydroxyperphenazine: 2-4 hours
Excretion: Urine and feces

Pregnancy Risk Factor C

Perphenazine and Amitriptyline *see* Amitriptyline and Perphenazine *on page 106*
Persantine® *see* Dipyridamole *on page 453*
Pertussin® DM [OTC] *see* Dextromethorphan *on page 421*
Pethidine Hydrochloride *see* Meperidine *on page 870*
Pexeva™ *see* Paroxetine *on page 1046*
PFA *see* Foscarnet *on page 631*
Pfizerpen® *see* Penicillin G (Parenteral/Aqueous) *on page 1059*
PGE_1 *see* Alprostadil *on page 87*
PGE_2 *see* Dinoprostone *on page 447*
PGI_2 *see* Epoprostenol *on page 500*
PGX *see* Epoprostenol *on page 500*
Phanasin [OTC] *see* Guaifenesin *on page 672*
Phanasin® Diabetic Choice [OTC] *see* Guaifenesin *on page 672*
Pharmacology of Drug Metabolism and Interactions *see page 24*
Pharmaflur® *see* Fluoride *on page 603*
Pharmaflur® 1.1 *see* Fluoride *on page 603*
Phazyme® Quick Dissolve [OTC] *see* Simethicone *on page 1222*
Phazyme® Ultra Strength [OTC] *see* Simethicone *on page 1222*
Phenadoz™ *see* Promethazine *on page 1130*

Phenazopyridine (fen az oh PEER i deen)

U.S. Brand Names Azo-Gesic® [OTC]; Azo-Standard® [OTC]; Prodium® [OTC]; Pyridium®; ReAzo [OTC]; Uristat® [OTC]; UTI Relief® [OTC]

Canadian Brand Names Phenazo™; Pyridium®

Generic Available Yes

Synonyms Phenazopyridine Hydrochloride; Phenylazo Diamino Pyridine Hydrochloride

Pharmacologic Category Analgesic, Urinary

Use Symptomatic relief of urinary burning, itching, frequency and urgency in association with urinary tract infection or following urologic procedures

Local Anesthetic/Vasoconstrictor Precautions No information available to require special precautions

Effects on Dental Treatment No significant effects or complications reported

Common Adverse Effects 1% to 10%:

Central nervous system: Headache, dizziness
Gastrointestinal: Stomach cramps

Mechanism of Action An azo dye which exerts local anesthetic or analgesic action on urinary tract mucosa through an unknown mechanism

Pharmacodynamics/Kinetics

Metabolism: Hepatic and via other tissues
Excretion: Urine (65% as unchanged drug)

Pregnancy Risk Factor B

Phenazopyridine Hydrochloride *see* Phenazopyridine *on page 1072*

Phendimetrazine (fen dye ME tra zeen)

U.S. Brand Names Bontril PDM®; Bontril® Slow-Release; Melfiat®; Obezine®; Prelu-2®

Canadian Brand Names Bontril®; Plegine®; Statobex®

Generic Available Yes

Synonyms Phendimetrazine Tartrate

Pharmacologic Category Anorexiant

Use Appetite suppressant during the first few weeks of dieting to help establish new eating habits; its effectiveness lasts only for short periods (3-12 weeks)

Local Anesthetic/Vasoconstrictor Precautions Use vasoconstrictor with caution in patients taking phendimetrazine. Phendimetrazine can enhance the sympathomimetic response to epinephrine leading to potential hypertension and cardiotoxicity.

Effects on Dental Treatment No significant effects or complications reported

Common Adverse Effects Frequency not defined.

Cardiovascular: Hypertension, tachycardia, arrhythmias
Central nervous system: Euphoria, nervousness, insomnia, confusion, mental depression, restlessness, headache
Dermatologic: Alopecia
Endocrine & metabolic: Changes in libido
Gastrointestinal: Nausea, vomiting, constipation, diarrhea, abdominal cramps
Genitourinary: Dysuria
Hematologic: Blood dyscrasias
Neuromuscular & skeletal: Tremor, myalgia
Ocular: Blurred vision
Renal: Polyuria
Respiratory: Dyspnea
Miscellaneous: Diaphoresis (increased)

Restrictions C-III

Pregnancy Risk Factor C

Phendimetrazine Tartrate *see* Phendimetrazine *on page 1072*

Phenelzine (FEN el zeen)

U.S. Brand Names Nardil®

Canadian Brand Names Nardil®

Generic Available No

Synonyms Phenelzine Sulfate

Pharmacologic Category Antidepressant, Monoamine Oxidase Inhibitor

Use Symptomatic treatment of atypical, nonendogenous, or neurotic depression

Unlabeled/Investigational Use Selective mutism

Local Anesthetic/Vasoconstrictor Precautions Attempts should be made to avoid use of vasoconstrictor due to possibility of hypertensive episodes with monoamine oxidase inhibitors

Effects on Dental Treatment Key adverse event(s) related to dental treatment: Orthostatic hypotension, xerostomia and changes in salivation (normal salivary flow resumes upon discontinuation). Avoid use as an analgesic due to toxic reactions with MAO inhibitors.

Mechanism of Action Thought to act by increasing endogenous concentrations of norepinephrine, dopamine, and serotonin through inhibition of the enzyme (monoamine oxidase) responsible for the breakdown of these neurotransmitters

Pregnancy Risk Factor C

Phenelzine Sulfate *see* Phenelzine *on page 1072*

Phenergan® *see* Promethazine *on page 1130*

Phenergan® With Codeine *see* Promethazine and Codeine *on page 1131*

Phenindamine (fen IN dah meen)

U.S. Brand Names Nolahist® [OTC]

Canadian Brand Names Nolahist®

Generic Available No

Synonyms Phenindamine Tartrate

Pharmacologic Category Antihistamine

Use Treatment of perennial and seasonal allergic rhinitis and chronic urticaria

Local Anesthetic/Vasoconstrictor Precautions No information available to require special precautions

Effects on Dental Treatment No significant effects or complications reported

Phenindamine Tartrate *see* Phenindamine *on page 1073*

Pheniramine and Naphazoline *see* Naphazoline and Pheniramine *on page 964*

Phenobarbital (fee noe BAR bi tal)

U.S. Brand Names Luminal® Sodium

Canadian Brand Names PMS-Phenobarbital

Generic Available Yes

Synonyms Phenobarbital Sodium; Phenobarbitone; Phenylethylmalonylurea

Pharmacologic Category Anticonvulsant, Barbiturate; Barbiturate

Use Management of generalized tonic-clonic (grand mal) and partial seizures; sedative

Unlabeled/Investigational Use Febrile seizures in children; may also be used for prevention and treatment of neonatal hyperbilirubinemia and lowering of bilirubin in chronic cholestasis; neonatal seizures; management of sedative/hypnotic withdrawal

Local Anesthetic/Vasoconstrictor Precautions No information available to require special precautions

Effects on Dental Treatment No significant effects or complications reported

Common Adverse Effects Frequency not defined.

- Cardiovascular: Bradycardia, hypotension, syncope
- Central nervous system: Drowsiness, lethargy, CNS excitation or depression, impaired judgment, "hangover" effect, confusion, somnolence, agitation, hyperkinesia, ataxia, nervousness, headache, insomnia, nightmares, hallucinations, anxiety, dizziness
- Dermatologic: Rash, exfoliative dermatitis, Stevens-Johnson syndrome
- Gastrointestinal: Nausea, vomiting, constipation
- Hematologic: Agranulocytosis, thrombocytopenia, megaloblastic anemia
- Local: Pain at injection site, thrombophlebitis with I.V. use
- Renal: Oliguria
- Respiratory: Laryngospasm, respiratory depression, apnea (especially with rapid I.V. use), hypoventilation
- Miscellaneous: Gangrene with inadvertent intra-arterial injection

Restrictions C-IV

Dosage

Children:
- Sedation: Oral: 2 mg/kg 3 times/day
- Hypnotic: I.M., I.V., SubQ: 3-5 mg/kg at bedtime
- Preoperative sedation: Oral, I.M., I.V.: 1-3 mg/kg 1-1.5 hours before procedure

Adults:
- Sedation: Oral, I.M.: 30-120 mg/day in 2-3 divided doses
- Hypnotic: Oral, I.M., I.V., SubQ: 100-320 mg at bedtime
- Preoperative sedation: I.M.: 100-200 mg 1-1.5 hours before procedure

Anticonvulsant: Status epilepticus: **Loading dose:** I.V.:
- Infants and Children: 10-20 mg/kg in a single or divided dose; in select patients may administer additional 5 mg/kg/dose every 15-30 minutes until seizure is controlled or a total dose of 40 mg/kg is reached

(Continued)

Phenobarbital *(Continued)*

Adults: 300-800 mg initially followed by 120-240 mg/dose at 20-minute intervals until seizures are controlled or a total dose of 1-2 g

Anticonvulsant maintenance dose: Oral, I.V.:

Infants: 5-8 mg/kg/day in 1-2 divided doses

Children:

1-5 years: 6-8 mg/kg/day in 1-2 divided doses

5-12 years: 4-6 mg/kg/day in 1-2 divided doses

Children >12 years and Adults: 1-3 mg/kg/day in divided doses or 50-100 mg 2-3 times/day

Sedative/hypnotic withdrawal (unlabeled use): Initial daily requirement is determined by substituting phenobarbital 30 mg for every 100 mg pentobarbital used during tolerance testing; then daily requirement is decreased by 10% of initial dose

Dosing interval in renal impairment: Cl_{cr} <10 mL/minute: Administer every 12-16 hours

Hemodialysis: Moderately dialyzable (20% to 50%)

Dosing adjustment/comments in hepatic disease: Increased side effects may occur in severe liver disease; monitor plasma levels and adjust dose accordingly

Mechanism of Action Short-acting barbiturate with sedative, hypnotic, and anticonvulsant properties. Barbiturates depress the sensory cortex, decrease motor activity, alter cerebellar function, and produce drowsiness, sedation, and hypnosis. In high doses, barbiturates exhibit anticonvulsant activity; barbiturates produce dose-dependent respiratory depression.

Contraindications Hypersensitivity to barbiturates or any component of the formulation; marked hepatic impairment; dyspnea or airway obstruction; porphyria; pregnancy

Warnings/Precautions Use with caution in patients with hypovolemic shock, CHF, hepatic impairment, respiratory dysfunction or depression, previous addiction to the sedative/hypnotic group, chronic or acute pain, renal dysfunction, and the elderly, due to its long half-life and risk of dependence, phenobarbital is not recommended as a sedative in the elderly; tolerance or psychological and physical dependence may occur with prolonged use. Use with caution in patients with depression or suicidal tendencies, or in patients with a history of drug abuse. **Abrupt withdrawal in patients with epilepsy may precipitate status epilepticus.**

Drug Interactions

Cytochrome P450 Effect: Substrate of CYP2C8/9 (minor), 2C19 (major), 2E1 (minor); **Induces** CYP1A2 (strong), 2A6 (strong), 2B6 (strong), 2C8/9 (strong), 3A4 (strong)

Increased Effect/Toxicity: When combined with other CNS depressants, ethanol, narcotic analgesics, antidepressants, or benzodiazepines, additive respiratory and CNS depression may occur. Barbiturates may enhance the hepatotoxic potential of acetaminophen overdoses. Chloramphenicol, MAO inhibitors, valproic acid, and felbamate may inhibit barbiturate metabolism. Barbiturates may impair the absorption of griseofulvin, and may enhance the nephrotoxic effects of methoxyflurane. Concurrent use of phenobarbital with meperidine may result in increased CNS depression. Concurrent use of phenobarbital with primidone may result in elevated phenobarbital serum concentrations. The levels/effects of phenobarbital may be increased by delavirdine, fluconazole, fluvoxamine, gemfibrozil, isoniazid, omeprazole, ticlopidine, and other CYP2C19 inhibitors.

Decreased Effect: Barbiturates may increase the metabolism of estrogens and reduce the efficacy of oral contraceptives; an alternative method of contraception should be considered. Barbiturates inhibit the hypoprothrombinemic effects of oral anticoagulants via increased metabolism. Barbiturates may enhance the metabolism of methadone resulting in methadone withdrawal. The levels/effects of phenobarbital may be decreased by aminoglutethimide, carbamazepine, phenytoin, rifampin, and other CYP2C19 inducers.

Phenobarbital may decrease the levels/effects of aminophylline, amiodarone, benzodiazepines, bupropion, calcium channel blockers, carbamazepine, citalopram, clarithromycin, cyclosporine, diazepam, efavirenz, erythromycin, estrogens, fluoxetine, fluvoxamine, glimepiride, glipizide, ifosfamide, losartan, methsuximide, mirtazapine, nateglinide, nefazodone, nevirapine, phenytoin, pioglitazone, promethazine, propranolol, protease inhibitors, proton pump inhibitors, rifampin, ropinirole, rosiglitazone, selegiline, sertraline, sulfonamides, tacrolimus, theophylline, venlafaxine, voriconazole, warfarin, zafirlukast, and other CYP1A2, 2A6, 2B6, 2C8/9, or 3A4 substrates.

Ethanol/Nutrition/Herb Interactions

Ethanol: Avoid ethanol (may increase CNS depression).

Food: May cause decrease in vitamin D and calcium.

Herb/Nutraceutical: Avoid evening primrose (seizure threshold decreased). Avoid valerian, St John's wort, kava kava, gotu kola (may increase CNS depression).

Dietary Considerations Vitamin D: Loss in vitamin D due to malabsorption; increase intake of foods rich in vitamin D. Supplementation of vitamin D and/or calcium may be necessary. Sodium content of injection (65 mg, 1 mL): 6 mg (0.3 mEq).

Pharmacodynamics/Kinetics

Onset of action: Oral: Hypnosis: 20-60 minutes; I.V.: ~5 minutes

Peak effect: I.V.: ~30 minutes

Duration: Oral: 6-10 hours; I.V.: 4-10 hours

Absorption: Oral: 70% to 90%

Protein binding: 20% to 45%; decreased in neonates

Metabolism: Hepatic via hydroxylation and glucuronide conjugation

Half-life elimination: Neonates: 45-500 hours; Infants: 20-133 hours; Children: 37-73 hours; Adults: 53-140 hours

Time to peak, serum: Oral: 1-6 hours

Excretion: Urine (20% to 50% as unchanged drug)

Pregnancy Risk Factor D

Dosage Forms ELIX: 20 mg/5 mL (5 mL, 7.5 mL, 15 mL, 473 mL, 946 mL, 4000 mL). **INJ, solution, as sodium:** 60 mg/mL (1 mL); 130 mg/mL (1 mL); (Luminal® Sodium): 60 mg/mL (1 mL); 130 mg/mL (1 mL). **TAB:** 15 mg, 30 mg, 32 mg, 60 mg, 65 mg, 100 mg

Phenobarbital, Belladonna, and Ergotamine Tartrate *see* Belladonna, Phenobarbital, and Ergotamine *on page 186*

Phenobarbital, Hyoscyamine, Atropine, and Scopolamine *see* Hyoscyamine, Atropine, Scopolamine, and Phenobarbital *on page 725*

Phenobarbital Sodium *see* Phenobarbital *on page 1073*

Phenobarbitone *see* Phenobarbital *on page 1073*

Phenol (FEE nol)

Related Information

Mouth Pain, Cold Sore, and Canker Sore Products *on page 1633*

U.S. Brand Names Cēpastat® [OTC]; Cēpastat® Extra Strength [OTC]; Chloraseptic® Gargle [OTC]; Chloraseptic® Mouth Pain Spray [OTC]; Chloraseptic® Rinse [OTC]; Chloraseptic® Spray [OTC]; Chloraseptic® Spray for Kids [OTC]; Pain-A-Lay® [OTC]; Ulcerease® [OTC]

Canadian Brand Names P & S™ Liquid Phenol

Generic Available Yes: Oral spray

Synonyms Carbolic Acid

Pharmacologic Category Pharmaceutical Aid

Use Relief of sore throat pain, mouth, gum, and throat irritations; neurologic pain, rectal prolapse, hemorrhoids, hydrocele

Local Anesthetic/Vasoconstrictor Precautions No information available to require special precautions

Effects on Dental Treatment No significant effects or complications reported

Pregnancy Risk Factor C

Phenol and Camphor *see* Camphor and Phenol *on page 248*

Phenoptic® *see* Phenylephrine *on page 1078*

Phenoxybenzamine (fen oks ee BEN za meen)

U.S. Brand Names Dibenzyline®

Canadian Brand Names Dibenzyline®

Generic Available No

Synonyms Phenoxybenzamine Hydrochloride

Pharmacologic Category Alpha$_1$ Blocker

Use Symptomatic management of pheochromocytoma; treatment of hypertensive crisis caused by sympathomimetic amines

Unlabeled/Investigational Use Micturition problems associated with neurogenic bladder, functional outlet obstruction, and partial prostate obstruction

Local Anesthetic/Vasoconstrictor Precautions No information available to require special precautions

Effects on Dental Treatment No significant effects or complications reported

Common Adverse Effects Frequency not defined.

(Continued)

Phenoxybenzamine *(Continued)*

Cardiovascular: Postural hypotension, tachycardia, syncope, shock
Central nervous system: Lethargy, headache, confusion, fatigue
Gastrointestinal: Vomiting, nausea, diarrhea, xerostomia
Genitourinary: Inhibition of ejaculation
Neuromuscular & skeletal: Weakness
Ocular: Miosis
Respiratory: Nasal congestion

Mechanism of Action Produces long-lasting noncompetitive alpha-adrenergic blockade of postganglionic synapses in exocrine glands and smooth muscle; relaxes urethra and increases opening of the bladder

Drug Interactions

Increased Effect/Toxicity: Beta-blockers may result in increased toxicity (hypotension, tachycardia). Blood pressure-lowering effects are additive with sildenafil (use with extreme caution at a dose ≤25 mg), tadalafil (use is contraindicated by the manufacturer), and vardenafil (use is contraindicated by the manufacturer).

Decreased Effect: Alpha adrenergic agonists decrease the effect of phenoxybenzamine.

Pharmacodynamics/Kinetics

Onset of action: ~2 hours
Peak effect: 4-6 hours
Duration: ≥4 days
Half-life elimination: 24 hours
Excretion: Primarily urine and feces

Pregnancy Risk Factor C

Phenoxybenzamine Hydrochloride *see* Phenoxybenzamine *on page 1075*
Phenoxymethyl Penicillin *see* Penicillin V Potassium *on page 1060*

Phentermine (FEN ter meen)

U.S. Brand Names Adipex-P®; Ionamin®

Canadian Brand Names Ionamin®

Mexican Brand Names Ifa Reduccing "S"®

Generic Available Yes

Synonyms Phentermine Hydrochloride

Pharmacologic Category Anorexiant

Use Short-term adjunct in a regimen of weight reduction based on exercise, behavioral modification, and caloric reduction in the management of exogenous obesity for patients with an initial body mass index ≥30 kg/m^2 or ≥27 kg/m^2 in the presence of other risk factors (diabetes, hypertension)

Local Anesthetic/Vasoconstrictor Precautions Use vasoconstrictor with caution in patients taking phentermine. Amphetamines enhance the sympathomimetic response of epinephrine and norepinephrine leading to potential hypertension and cardiotoxicity.

Effects on Dental Treatment Key adverse event(s) related ot dental treatment: Up to 10% of patients may present with hypertension. The use of local anesthetic without vasoconstrictor is recommended in these patients.

Common Adverse Effects Frequency not defined.

Cardiovascular: Hypertension, palpitations, tachycardia, primary pulmonary hypertension and/or regurgitant cardiac valvular disease
Central nervous system: Euphoria, insomnia, overstimulation, dizziness, dysphoria, headache, restlessness, psychosis
Dermatologic: Urticaria
Endocrine & metabolic: Changes in libido, impotence
Gastrointestinal: Nausea, constipation, xerostomia, unpleasant taste, diarrhea
Hematologic: Blood dyscrasias
Neuromuscular & skeletal: Tremor
Ocular: Blurred vision

Restrictions C-IV

Mechanism of Action Phentermine is structurally similar to dextroamphetamine and is comparable to dextroamphetamine as an appetite suppressant, but is generally associated with a lower incidence and severity of CNS side effects. Phentermine, like other anorexiants, stimulates the hypothalamus to result in decreased appetite; anorexiant effects are most likely mediated via norepinephrine and dopamine metabolism. However, other CNS effects or metabolic effects may be involved.

Drug Interactions

Increased Effect/Toxicity: Dosage of hypoglycemic agents may need to be adjusted when phentermine is used in a diabetic receiving a special diet.

Concurrent use of MAO inhibitors and drugs with MAO activity (furazolidone, linezolid) may be associated with hypertensive episodes. Concurrent use of SSRIs may be associated with a risk of serotonin syndrome.

Decreased Effect: Phentermine may decrease the effect of antihypertensive medications The efficacy of anorexiants may be decreased by antipsychotics; in addition, amphetamines or related compounds may induce an increase in psychotic symptoms in some patients. Amphetamines (and related compounds) inhibit the antihypertensive response to guanethidine; probably also may occur with guànadrel.

Pharmacodynamics/Kinetics

Duration: Resin produces more prolonged clinical effects

Absorption: Well absorbed; resin absorbed slower

Half-life elimination: 20 hours

Excretion: Primarily urine (as unchanged drug)

Pregnancy Risk Factor C

Comments Many diet physicians have prescribed fenfluramine ("fen") and phentermine ("phen"). When taken together the combination is known as "fen-phen". The diet drug dexfenfluramine (Redux®) is chemically similar to fenfluramine (Pondimin®) and was also used in combination with phentermine called "Redux-phen". While each of the three drugs alone had approval from the FDA for sale in the treatment of obesity, neither combination had an official approval. The use of the combinations in the treatment of obesity was considered an "off-label" use. Reports in medical literature have been accumulating for some years about significant side effects associated with fenfluramine and dexfenfluramine. In 1997, the manufacturers, at the urging of the FDA, agreed to voluntarily withdraw the drugs from the market. The action was based on findings from physicians who evaluated patients taking fenfluramine and dexfenfluramine with echocardiograms. The findings indicated that approximately 30% of patients had abnormal echocardiograms, even though they had no symptoms. This was a much higher than expected percentage of abnormal test results. This conclusion was based on a sample of 291 patients examined by five different physicians. Under normal conditions, fewer than 1% of patients would be expected to show signs of heart valve disease. The findings suggested that fenfluramine and dexfenfluramine were the likely cause of heart valve problems of the type that promoted FDA's earlier warnings concerning "fen-phen". The earlier warning included the following: The mitral valve and other valves in the heart are damaged by a strange white coating and allow blood to flow back, causing heart muscle damage. In several cases, valve replacement surgery has been done. As a rule, the person must, thereafter for life, be on a blood thinner to prevent clots from the mechanical valve. This type of valve damage had only been seen before in persons who were exposed to large amounts of serotonin. The fenfluramine increases the availability of serotonin.

Phentermine Hydrochloride *see* Phentermine *on page 1076*

Phentolamine (fen TOLE a meen)

Canadian Brand Names Regitine®; Rogitine®

Mexican Brand Names Z-Max®

Generic Available Yes

Synonyms Phentolamine Mesylate; Regitine [DSC]

Pharmacologic Category Alpha$_1$ Blocker

Use Diagnosis of pheochromocytoma and treatment of hypertension associated with pheochromocytoma or other forms of hypertension caused by excess sympathomimetic amines; as treatment of dermal necrosis after extravasation of drugs with alpha-adrenergic effects (norepinephrine, dopamine, epinephrine)

Unlabeled/Investigational Use Treatment of pralidoxime-induced hypertension

Local Anesthetic/Vasoconstrictor Precautions Although the alpha-adrenergic blocking effects could antagonize epinephrine, there is no information available to require special precautions

Effects on Dental Treatment No significant effects or complications reported

Common Adverse Effects Frequency not defined.

Cardiovascular: Hypotension, tachycardia, arrhythmia, flushing, orthostatic hypotension

Central nervous system: Weakness, dizziness

Gastrointestinal: Nausea, vomiting, diarrhea

Respiratory: Nasal congestion

Case report: Pulmonary hypertension

Mechanism of Action Competitively blocks alpha-adrenergic receptors to produce brief antagonism of circulating epinephrine and norepinephrine to

(Continued)

Phentolamine *(Continued)*

reduce hypertension caused by alpha effects of these catecholamines; also has a positive inotropic and chronotropic effect on the heart

Drug Interactions

Increased Effect/Toxicity: Phentolamine's toxicity is increased with ethanol (disulfiram reaction). Blood pressure-lowering effects are additive with sildenafil (use with extreme caution at a dose ≤25 mg), tadalafil (use is contraindicated by the manufacturer), and vardenafil (use is contraindicated by the manufacturer).

Decreased Effect: Decreased effect of phentolamine with epinephrine and ephedrine.

Pharmacodynamics/Kinetics

Onset of action: I.M.: 15-20 minutes; I.V.: Immediate
Duration: I.M.: 30-45 minutes; I.V.: 15-30 minutes
Metabolism: Hepatic
Half-life elimination: 19 minutes
Excretion: Urine (10% as unchanged drug)

Pregnancy Risk Factor C

Phentolamine Mesylate *see* Phentolamine *on page 1077*

Phenylalanine Mustard *see* Melphalan *on page 866*

Phenylazo Diamino Pyridine Hydrochloride *see* Phenazopyridine *on page 1072*

Phenylephrine (fen il EF rin)

Related Information

Guaifenesin and Phenylephrine *on page 674*

U.S. Brand Names AK-Dilate®; AK-Nefrin®; Formulation R™ [OTC]; Medicone® [OTC]; Mydfrin®; Neo-Synephrine® Extra Strength [OTC]; Neo-Synephrine® Mild [OTC]; Neo-Synephrine® Ophthalmic; Neo-Synephrine® Regular Strength [OTC]; Nostril® [OTC]; Phenoptic®; Prefrin™ [DSC]; Relief® [OTC]; Vicks® Sinex® Nasal Spray [OTC]; Vicks® Sinex® UltraFine Mist [OTC]

Canadian Brand Names Dionephrine®; Mydfrin®; Neo-Synephrine®

Generic Available Yes: Excludes nasal drops and spray

Synonyms Phenylephrine Hydrochloride

Pharmacologic Category Alpha/Beta Agonist; Ophthalmic Agent, Antiglaucoma; Ophthalmic Agent, Mydriatic

Use Treatment of hypotension, vascular failure in shock; as a vasoconstrictor in regional analgesia; as a mydriatic in ophthalmic procedures and treatment of wide-angle glaucoma; supraventricular tachycardia

For OTC use as symptomatic relief of nasal and nasopharyngeal mucosal congestion, treatment of hemorrhoids, relief of redness of the eye due to irritation

Local Anesthetic/Vasoconstrictor Precautions Use with caution since phenylephrine is a sympathomimetic amine which could interact with epinephrine to cause a pressor response

Effects on Dental Treatment Key adverse event(s) related to dental treatment: Tachycardia, palpitations (use vasoconstrictor with caution), and xerostomia (normal salivary flow resumes upon discontinuation).

Common Adverse Effects Frequency not defined.

Cardiovascular: Reflex bradycardia, excitability, restlessness, arrhythmias (rare), precordial pain or discomfort, pallor, hypertension, severe peripheral and visceral vasoconstriction, decreased cardiac output
Central nervous system: Headache, anxiety, weakness, dizziness, tremor, paresthesia, restlessness
Endocrine & metabolic: Metabolic acidosis
Local: I.V.: Extravasation which may lead to necrosis and sloughing of surrounding tissue, blanching of skin
Neuromuscular & skeletal: Pilomotor response, weakness
Renal: Decreased renal perfusion, reduced urine output, reduced urine output
Respiratory: Respiratory distress

Mechanism of Action Potent, direct-acting alpha-adrenergic stimulator with weak beta-adrenergic activity; causes vasoconstriction of the arterioles of the nasal mucosa and conjunctiva; activates the dilator muscle of the pupil to cause contraction; produces vasoconstriction of arterioles in the body; produces systemic arterial vasoconstriction

Drug Interactions

Increased Effect/Toxicity: Phenylephrine, taken with sympathomimetics, may induce tachycardia or arrhythmias. If taken with MAO inhibitors or oxytocic agents, actions may be potentiated.

Decreased Effect: Alpha- and beta-adrenergic blocking agents may have a decreased effect if taken with phenylephrine.

Pharmacodynamics/Kinetics

Onset of action: I.M., SubQ: 10-15 minutes; I.V.: Immediate

Duration: I.M.: 0.5-2 hours; I.V.: 15-30 minutes; SubQ: 1 hour

Metabolism: Hepatic, via intestinal monoamine oxidase to phenolic conjugates

Half-life elimination: 2.5 hours; prolonged after long-term infusion

Excretion: Urine (90%)

Pregnancy Risk Factor C

Phenylephrine and Chlorpheniramine *see* Chlorpheniramine and Phenylephrine *on page 314*

Phenylephrine and Cyclopentolate *see* Cyclopentolate and Phenylephrine *on page 384*

Phenylephrine and Guaifenesin *see* Guaifenesin and Phenylephrine *on page 674*

Phenylephrine and Promethazine *see* Promethazine and Phenylephrine *on page 1132*

Phenylephrine and Scopolamine

(fen il EF rin & skoe POL a meen)

Related Information

Phenylephrine *on page 1078*

Scopolamine *on page 1210*

U.S. Brand Names Murocoll-2®

Generic Available No

Synonyms Scopolamine and Phenylephrine

Pharmacologic Category Anticholinergic/Adrenergic Agonist

Use Mydriasis, cycloplegia, and to break posterior synechiae in iritis

Local Anesthetic/Vasoconstrictor Precautions Use with caution since phenylephrine is a sympathomimetic amine which could interact with epinephrine to cause a pressor response

Effects on Dental Treatment This form of phenylephrine will have no effect on dental treatment when given as eye drops.

Pharmacodynamics/Kinetics See individual agents.

Pregnancy Risk Factor C

Phenylephrine and Zinc Sulfate (fen il EF rin & zingk SUL fate)

Related Information

Phenylephrine *on page 1078*

U.S. Brand Names Zincfrin® [OTC]

Canadian Brand Names Zincfrin®

Generic Available No

Synonyms Zinc Sulfate and Phenylephrine

Pharmacologic Category Adrenergic Agonist Agent

Use Soothe, moisturize, and remove redness due to minor eye irritation

Local Anesthetic/Vasoconstrictor Precautions No information available to require special precautions

Effects on Dental Treatment No significant effects or complications reported

Pharmacodynamics/Kinetics See individual agents.

Phenylephrine, Chlorpheniramine, and Dextromethorphan *see* Chlorpheniramine, Phenylephrine, and Dextromethorphan *on page 316*

Phenylephrine, Chlorpheniramine, and Methscopolamine *see* Chlorpheniramine, Phenylephrine, and Methscopolamine *on page 317*

Phenylephrine, Chlorpheniramine, and Phenyltoloxamine *see* Chlorpheniramine, Phenylephrine, and Phenyltoloxamine *on page 317*

Phenylephrine, Chlorpheniramine, Codeine, and Potassium Iodide *see* Chlorpheniramine, Phenylephrine, Codeine, and Potassium Iodide *on page 318*

Phenylephrine, Diphenhydramine, and Hydrocodone *see* Hydrocodone, Phenylephrine, and Diphenhydramine *on page 713*

Phenylephrine, Ephedrine, Chlorpheniramine, and Carbetapentane *see* Chlorpheniramine, Ephedrine, Phenylephrine, and Carbetapentane *on page 316*

Phenylephrine Hydrochloride *see* Phenylephrine *on page 1078*

Phenylephrine, Hydrocodone, Chlorpheniramine, Acetaminophen, and Caffeine *see* Hydrocodone, Chlorpheniramine, Phenylephrine, Acetaminophen, and Caffeine *on page 712*

Phenylephrine, Promethazine, and Codeine *see* Promethazine, Phenylephrine, and Codeine *on page 1132*

Phenylephrine Tannate, Carbetapentane Tannate, and Pyrilamine Tannate *see* Carbetapentane, Phenylephrine, and Pyrilamine *on page 261*

Phenylethylmalonylurea *see* Phenobarbital *on page 1073*

Phenylgesic® [OTC] *see* Acetaminophen and Phenyltoloxamine *on page 53*

Phenylisohydantoin *see* Pemoline *on page 1055*

Phenyl Salicylate, Methenamine, Methylene Blue, Sodium Biphosphate, and Hyoscyamine *see* Methenamine, Sodium Biphosphate, Phenyl Salicylate, Methylene Blue, and Hyoscyamine *on page 893*

Phenyltoloxamine and Acetaminophen *see* Acetaminophen and Phenyltoloxamine *on page 53*

Phenyltoloxamine, Chlorpheniramine, and Phenylephrine *see* Chlorpheniramine, Phenylephrine, and Phenyltoloxamine *on page 317*

Phenytek™ *see* Phenytoin *on page 1080*

Phenytoin (FEN i toyn)

Related Information

Cardiovascular Diseases *on page 1458*
Fosphenytoin *on page 635*

U.S. Brand Names Dilantin®; Phenytek™

Canadian Brand Names Dilantin®

Mexican Brand Names Epamin®; Fenidantoin® [tabs]; Fenitron® [tabs]; Hidantoina®

Generic Available Yes: Excludes chewable tablet, extended release capsule

Synonyms Diphenylhydantoin; DPH; Phenytoin Sodium; Phenytoin Sodium, Extended; Phenytoin Sodium, Prompt

Pharmacologic Category Antiarrhythmic Agent, Class Ib; Anticonvulsant, Hydantoin

Use Management of generalized tonic-clonic (grand mal), complex partial seizures; prevention of seizures following head trauma/neurosurgery

Unlabeled/Investigational Use Ventricular arrhythmias, including those associated with digitalis intoxication, prolonged QT interval and surgical repair of congenital heart diseases in children; epidermolysis bullosa

Local Anesthetic/Vasoconstrictor Precautions No information available to require special precautions

Effects on Dental Treatment Gingival hyperplasia is a common problem observed during the first 6 months of phenytoin therapy appearing as gingivitis or gum inflammation. To minimize severity and growth rate of gingival tissue begin a program of professional cleaning and patient plaque control within 10 days of starting anticonvulsant therapy.

Common Adverse Effects I.V. effects: Hypotension, bradycardia, cardiac arrhythmias, cardiovascular collapse (especially with rapid I.V. use), venous irritation and pain, thrombophlebitis

Effects not related to plasma phenytoin concentrations: Hypertrichosis, gingival hypertrophy, thickening of facial features, carbohydrate intolerance, folic acid deficiency, peripheral neuropathy, vitamin D deficiency, osteomalacia, systemic lupus erythematosus

Concentration-related effects: Nystagmus, blurred vision, diplopia, ataxia, slurred speech, dizziness, drowsiness, lethargy, coma, rash, fever, nausea, vomiting, gum tenderness, confusion, mood changes, folic acid depletion, osteomalacia, hyperglycemia

Related to elevated concentrations:

>20 mcg/mL: Far lateral nystagmus
>30 mcg/mL: 45° lateral gaze nystagmus and ataxia
>40 mcg/mL: Decreased mentation
>100 mcg/mL: Death

Cardiovascular: Hypotension, bradycardia, cardiac arrhythmias, cardiovascular collapse

Central nervous system: Psychiatric changes, slurred speech, dizziness, drowsiness, headache, insomnia

Dermatologic: Rash

Gastrointestinal: Constipation, nausea, vomiting, gingival hyperplasia, enlargement of lips

Hematologic: Leukopenia, thrombocytopenia, agranulocytosis

Hepatic: Hepatitis

Local: Thrombophlebitis

Neuromuscular & skeletal: Tremor, peripheral neuropathy, paresthesia

Ocular: Diplopia, nystagmus, blurred vision

Rarely seen effects: SLE-like syndrome, lymphadenopathy, hepatitis, Stevens-Johnson syndrome, blood dyscrasias, dyskinesias, pseudolymphoma, lymphoma, venous irritation and pain, coarsening of the facial features, hypertrichosis

Dosage

Status epilepticus: I.V.:

Infants and Children: Loading dose: 15-20 mg/kg in a single or divided dose; maintenance dose: Initial: 5 mg/kg/day in 2 divided doses; usual doses:

6 months to 3 years: 8-10 mg/kg/day

4-6 years: 7.5-9 mg/kg/day

7-9 years: 7-8 mg/kg/day

10-16 years: 6-7 mg/kg/day, some patients may require every 8 hours dosing

Adults: Loading dose: Manufacturer recommends 10-15 mg/kg, however, 15-25 mg/kg has been used clinically; maintenance dose: 300 mg/day or 5-6 mg/kg/day in 3 divided doses or 1-2 divided doses using extended release

Anticonvulsant: Children and Adults: Oral:

Loading dose: 15-20 mg/kg; based on phenytoin serum concentrations and recent dosing history; administer oral loading dose in 3 divided doses given every 2-4 hours to decrease GI adverse effects and to ensure complete oral absorption; maintenance dose: same as I.V.

Neurosurgery (prophylactic): 100-200 mg at approximately 4-hour intervals during surgery and during the immediate postoperative period

Dosing adjustment/comments in renal impairment or hepatic disease: Safe in usual doses in mild liver disease; clearance may be substantially reduced in cirrhosis and plasma level monitoring with dose adjustment advisable. Free phenytoin levels should be monitored closely.

Mechanism of Action Stabilizes neuronal membranes and decreases seizure activity by increasing efflux or decreasing influx of sodium ions across cell membranes in the motor cortex during generation of nerve impulses; prolongs effective refractory period and suppresses ventricular pacemaker automaticity, shortens action potential in the heart

Contraindications Hypersensitivity to phenytoin, other hydantoins, or any component of the formulation; pregnancy

Warnings/Precautions May increase frequency of petit mal seizures; I.V. form may cause hypotension, skin necrosis at I.V. site; avoid I.V. administration in small veins; use with caution in patients with porphyria; discontinue if rash or lymphadenopathy occurs; use with caution in patients with hepatic dysfunction, sinus bradycardia, S-A block, or AV block; use with caution in elderly or debilitated patients, or in any condition associated with low serum albumin levels, which will increase the free fraction of phenytoin in the serum and, therefore, the pharmacologic response. Sedation, confusional states, or cerebellar dysfunction (loss of motor coordination) may occur at higher total serum concentrations, or at lower total serum concentrations when the free fraction of phenytoin is increased. Abrupt withdrawal may precipitate status epilepticus.

Drug Interactions

Cytochrome P450 Effect: Substrate of CYP2C8/9 (major), 2C19 (major), 3A4 (minor); **Induces** CYP2B6 (strong), 2C8/9 (strong), 2C19 (strong), 3A4 (strong)

Increased Effect/Toxicity: The sedative effects of phenytoin may be additive with other CNS depressants including ethanol, barbiturates, sedatives, antidepressants, narcotic analgesics, and benzodiazepines. Selected anticonvulsants (felbamate, gabapentin, and topiramate) have been reported to increase phenytoin levels/effects. In addition, serum phenytoin concentrations may be increased by allopurinol, amiodarone, calcium channel blockers (including diltiazem and nifedipine), cimetidine, disulfiram, methylphenidate, metronidazole, omeprazole, selective serotonin reuptake inhibitors (SSRIs), ticlopidine, tricyclic antidepressants, trazodone, and trimethoprim. Case reports indicate ciprofloxacin may increase or decrease serum phenytoin concentrations.

The levels/effects of phenytoin may be increased by delavirdine, fluconazole, fluvoxamine, gemfibrozil, isoniazid, ketoconazole, nicardipine, NSAIDs, omeprazole, pioglitazone, sulfonamides, ticlopidine, and other CYP2C8/9 or 2C19 inhibitors.

Phenytoin enhances the conversion of primidone to phenobarbital resulting in elevated phenobarbital serum concentrations. Concurrent use of acetazolamide with phenytoin may result in an increased risk of osteomalacia. Concurrent use of phenytoin and lithium has resulted in lithium intoxication. Valproic acid (and sulfisoxazole) may displace phenytoin from binding sites;

(Continued)

Phenytoin *(Continued)*

valproic acid may increase, decrease, or have no effect on phenytoin serum concentrations. Phenytoin transiently increased the response to warfarin initially; this is followed by an inhibition of the hypoprothrombinemic response. Phenytoin may enhance the hepatotoxic potential of acetaminophen overdoses. Concurrent use of dopamine and intravenous phenytoin may lead to an increased risk of hypotension.

Decreased Effect: Phenytoin may enhance the metabolism of estrogen and/ or oral contraceptives, decreasing their clinical effect; an alternative method of contraception should be considered. Phenytoin may increase the metabolism of anticonvulsants including barbiturates, carbamazepine, ethosuximide, felbamate, lamotrigine, tiagabine, topiramate, and zonisamide. Valproic acid may increase, decrease, or have no effect on phenytoin serum concentrations. Phenytoin may also decrease the serum concentrations/effects of some antiarrhythmics (disopyramide, propafenone, quinidine, quetiapine) and tricyclic antidepressants may be reduced by phenytoin. Phenytoin may enhance the metabolism of doxycycline, decreasing its clinical effect; higher dosages may be required. Phenytoin may increase the metabolism of chloramphenicol or itraconazole.

Phenytoin may decrease the levels/effects of amiodarone, benzodiazepines, bupropion, calcium channel blockers, carbamazepine, citalopram, clarithromycin, cyclosporine, efavirenz, erythromycin, estrogens, fluoxetine, glimepiride, glipizide, losartan, methsuximide, mirtazapine, nateglinide, nefazodone, nevirapine, phenytoin, pioglitazone, promethazine, propranolol, protease inhibitors, proton pump inhibitors, rosiglitazone, selegiline, sertraline, sulfonamides, tacrolimus, venlafaxine. voriconazole, warfarin, zafirlukast, and other CYP2B6, 2C8/9, 2C19, or 3A4 substrates.

The levels/effects of phenytoin may be decreased by aminoglutethimide, carbamazepine, phenobarbital, rifampin, rifapentine, secobarbital, and other CYP2C8/9 or 2C19 inducers. Clozapine and vigabatrin may reduce phenytoin serum concentrations. Case reports indicate ciprofloxacin may increase or decrease serum phenytoin concentrations. Dexamethasone may decrease serum phenytoin concentrations. Replacement of folic acid has been reported to increase the metabolism of phenytoin, decreasing its serum concentrations and/or increasing seizures.

Initially, phenytoin increases the response to warfarin; this is followed by a decrease in response to warfarin. Phenytoin may inhibit the anti-Parkinson effect of levodopa. The duration of neuromuscular blockade from neuromuscular-blocking agents may be decreased by phenytoin. Phenytoin may enhance the metabolism of methadone resulting in methadone withdrawal. Phenytoin may decrease serum levels/effects of digitalis glycosides, theophylline, and thyroid hormones.

Several chemotherapeutic agents have been associated with a decrease in serum phenytoin levels; includes cisplatin, bleomycin, carmustine, methotrexate, and vinblastine. Enzyme-inducing anticonvulsant therapy may reduce the effectiveness of some chemotherapy regimens (specifically in ALL). Teniposide and methotrexate may be cleared more rapidly in these patients.

Ethanol/Nutrition/Herb Interactions

Ethanol:

Acute use: Avoid or limit ethanol (inhibits metabolism of phenytoin). Watch for sedation.

Chronic use: Avoid or limit ethanol (stimulates metabolism of phenytoin).

Food: Phenytoin serum concentrations may be altered if taken with food. If taken with enteral nutrition, phenytoin serum concentrations may be decreased. Tube feedings decrease bioavailability; hold tube feedings 2 hours before and 2 hours after phenytoin administration. May decrease calcium, folic acid, and vitamin D levels.

Herb/Nutraceutical: Avoid evening primrose (seizure threshold decreased). Avoid valerian, St John's wort, kava kava, gotu kola (may increase CNS depression).

Dietary Considerations

Folic acid: Phenytoin may decrease mucosal uptake of folic acid; to avoid folic acid deficiency and megaloblastic anemia, some clinicians recommend giving patients on anticonvulsants prophylactic doses of folic acid and cyanocobalamin. However, folate supplementation may increase seizures in some patients (dose dependent). Discuss with healthcare provider prior to using any supplements.

Calcium: Hypocalcemia has been reported in patients taking prolonged high-dose therapy with an anticonvulsant. Some clinicians have given an additional 4000 units/week of vitamin D (especially in those receiving poor nutrition and getting no sun exposure) to prevent hypocalcemia.

Vitamin D: Phenytoin interferes with vitamin D metabolism and osteomalacia may result; may need to supplement with vitamin D

Tube feedings: Tube feedings decrease phenytoin absorption. To avoid decreased serum levels with continuous NG feeds, hold feedings for 2 hours prior to and 2 hours after phenytoin administration, if possible. There is a variety of opinions on how to administer phenytoin with enteral feedings. Be **consistent** throughout therapy.

Sodium content of 1 g injection: 88 mg (3.8 mEq)

Pharmacodynamics/Kinetics

Onset of action: I.V.: ~0.5-1 hour

Absorption: Oral: Slow

Distribution: V_d:

Neonates: Premature: 1-1.2 L/kg; Full-term: 0.8-0.9 L/kg

Infants: 0.7-0.8 L/kg

Children: 0.7 L/kg

Adults: 0.6-0.7 L/kg

Protein binding:

Neonates: ≥80% (≤20% free)

Infants: ≥85% (≤15% free)

Adults: 90% to 95%

Others: Decreased protein binding

Disease states resulting in a decrease in serum albumin concentration: Burns, hepatic cirrhosis, nephrotic syndrome, pregnancy, cystic fibrosis

Disease states resulting in an apparent decrease in affinity of phenytoin for serum albumin: Renal failure, jaundice (severe), other drugs (displacers), hyperbilirubinemia (total bilirubin >15 mg/dL), Cl_{cr} <25 mL/minute (unbound fraction is increased two- to threefold in uremia)

Metabolism: Follows dose-dependent capacity-limited (Michaelis-Menten) pharmacokinetics with increased V_{max} in infants >6 months of age and children versus adults; major metabolite (via oxidation), HPPA, undergoes enterohepatic recirculation

Bioavailability: Form dependent

Half-life elimination: Oral: 22 hours (range: 7-42 hours)

Time to peak, serum (form dependent): Oral: Extended-release capsule: 4-12 hours; Immediate release preparation: 2-3 hours

Excretion: Urine (<5% as unchanged drug); as glucuronides

Clearance: Highly variable, dependent upon intrinsic hepatic function and dose administered; increased clearance and decreased serum concentrations with febrile illness

Pregnancy Risk Factor D

Dosage Forms CAP, extended release: (Dilantin®): 30 mg, 100 mg; (Phenytek™): 200 mg, 300 mg. **CAP, prompt release:** 100 mg. **INJ, solution:** 50 mg/mL (2 mL, 5 mL). **SUSP, oral** (Dilantin®): 125 mg/5 mL (240 mL). **TAB, chewable** (Dilantin®): 50 mg

Selected Readings

Dooley G and Vasan N, "Dilantin® Hyperplasia: A Review of the Literature," *J N Z Soc Periodontol*, 1989, 68:19-22.

Iacopino AM, Doxey D, Cutler CW, et al, "Phenytoin and Cyclosporine A Specifically Regulate Macrophage Phenotype and Expression of Platelet-Derived Growth Factor and Interleukin-1 *In Vitro* and *In Vivo*: Possible Molecular Mechanism of Drug-Induced Gingival Hyperplasia," *J Periodontol*, 1997, 68(1):73-83.

Pihlstrom BL, "Prevention and Treatment of Dilantin®-Associated Gingival Enlargement," *Compendium*, 1990, 14:S506-10.

Saito K, Mori S, Iwakura M, et al, "Immunohistochemical Localization of Transforming Growth Factor Beta, Basic Fibroblast Growth Factor and Heparin Sulphate Glycosaminoglycan in Gingival Hyperplasia Induced by Nifedipine and Phenytoin," *J Periodontal Res*, 1996, 31(8):545-5.

Zhou LX, Pihlstrom B, Hardwick JP, et al, "Metabolism of Phenytoin by the Gingiva of Normal Humans: The Possible Role of Reactive Metabolites of Phenytoin in the Initiation of Gingival Hyperplasia," *Clin Pharmacol Ther*, 1996, 60(2):191-8.

Phenytoin Sodium *see* Phenytoin *on page 1080*

Phenytoin Sodium, Extended *see* Phenytoin *on page 1080*

Phenytoin Sodium, Prompt *see* Phenytoin *on page 1080*

Phillips'® Fibercaps [OTC] *see* Polycarbophil *on page 1100*

Phillips'® Milk of Magnesia [OTC] *see* Magnesium Hydroxide *on page 853*

Phillips' M-O® [OTC] *see* Magnesium Hydroxide and Mineral Oil *on page 853*

Phillips'® Stool Softener Laxative [OTC] *see* Docusate *on page 459*

pHisoHex® *see* Hexachlorophene *on page 693*

Phos-Flur® *see* Fluoride *on page 603*
Phos-Flur® Rinse [OTC] *see* Fluoride *on page 603*
PhosLo® *see* Calcium Acetate *on page 245*
Phosphate, Potassium *see* Potassium Phosphate *on page 1107*
Phospholine Iodide® *see* Echothiophate Iodide *on page 481*
Phosphonoformate *see* Foscarnet *on page 631*
Phosphonoformic Acid *see* Foscarnet *on page 631*
Phosphorated Carbohydrate Solution *see* Fructose, Dextrose, and Phosphoric Acid *on page 638*
Phosphoric Acid, Levulose and Dextrose *see* Fructose, Dextrose, and Phosphoric Acid *on page 638*
Photofrin® *see* Porfimer *on page 1103*
Phrenilin® with Caffeine and Codeine *see* Butalbital, Aspirin, Caffeine, and Codeine *on page 238*
***p*-Hydroxyampicillin** *see* Amoxicillin *on page 114*
Phylloquinone *see* Phytonadione *on page 1084*

Physostigmine (fye zoe STIG meen)

Canadian Brand Names Eserine®; Isopto® Eserine

Generic Available Yes

Synonyms Eserine Salicylate; Physostigmine Salicylate; Physostigmine Sulfate

Pharmacologic Category Acetylcholinesterase Inhibitor

Use Reverse toxic CNS effects caused by anticholinergic drugs

Local Anesthetic/Vasoconstrictor Precautions No information available to require special precautions

Effects on Dental Treatment Key adverse event(s) related to dental treatment: Salivation.

Common Adverse Effects Frequency not defined.
- Cardiovascular: Palpitations, bradycardia
- Central nervous system: Restlessness, nervousness, hallucinations, seizures
- Gastrointestinal: Nausea, salivation, diarrhea, stomach pains
- Genitourinary: Frequent urge to urinate
- Neuromuscular & skeletal: Muscle twitching
- Ocular: Lacrimation, miosis
- Respiratory: Dyspnea, bronchospasm, respiratory paralysis, pulmonary edema
- Miscellaneous: Diaphoresis

Mechanism of Action Inhibits destruction of acetylcholine by acetylcholinesterase which facilitates transmission of impulses across myoneural junction and prolongs the central and peripheral effects of acetylcholine

Drug Interactions

Increased Effect/Toxicity: Increased toxicity with bethanechol, methacholine. Succinylcholine may increase neuromuscular blockade with systemic administration.

Pharmacodynamics/Kinetics
- Onset of action: ~5 minutes
- Duration: 0.5-5 hours
- Absorption: I.M., SubQ: Readily absorbed
- Distribution: Crosses blood-brain barrier readily and reverses both central and peripheral anticholinergic effects
- Metabolism: Hepatic and via hydrolysis by cholinesterases
- Half-life elimination: 15-40 minutes

Pregnancy Risk Factor C

Physostigmine Salicylate *see* Physostigmine *on page 1084*
Physostigmine Sulfate *see* Physostigmine *on page 1084*
Phytomenadione *see* Phytonadione *on page 1084*

Phytonadione (fye toe na DYE one)

U.S. Brand Names AquaMEPHYTON® [DSC]; Mephyton®

Canadian Brand Names AquaMEPHYTON®; Konakion; Mephyton®

Mexican Brand Names Konakion®

Generic Available Yes: Injection

Synonyms Methylphytyl Napthoquinone; Phylloquinone; Phytomenadione; Vitamin K_1

Pharmacologic Category Vitamin, Fat Soluble

Use Prevention and treatment of hypoprothrombinemia caused by drug-induced or anticoagulant-induced vitamin K deficiency, hemorrhagic disease of the newborn; phytonadione is more effective and is preferred to other vitamin K preparations in the presence of impending hemorrhage; oral absorption depends on the presence of bile salts

Local Anesthetic/Vasoconstrictor Precautions No information available to require special precautions

Effects on Dental Treatment No significant effects or complications reported

Mechanism of Action Promotes liver synthesis of clotting factors (II, VII, IX, X); however, the exact mechanism as to this stimulation is unknown. Menadiol is a water soluble form of vitamin K; phytonadione has a more rapid and prolonged effect than menadione; menadiol sodium diphosphate (K_4) is half as potent as menadione (K_3).

Drug Interactions

Decreased Effect: The anticoagulant effects of warfarin, dicumarol, anisindione are reversed by phytonadione.

Pharmacodynamics/Kinetics

Onset of action: Increased coagulation factors: Oral: 6-12 hours; Parenteral: 1-2 hours; prothrombin may become normal after 12-14 hours

Absorption: Oral: From intestines in presence of bile

Metabolism: Rapidly hepatic

Excretion: Urine and feces

Pregnancy Risk Factor C

α_1-PI *see* Alpha₁-Proteinase Inhibitor *on page 84*

Pidorubicin *see* Epirubicin *on page 498*

Pidorubicin Hydrochloride *see* Epirubicin *on page 498*

Pilocar® *see* Pilocarpine *on page 1085*

Pilocarpine (pye loe KAR peen)

Related Information

Management of Patients Undergoing Cancer Therapy *on page 1569*

U.S. Brand Names Isopto® Carpine; Pilocar®; Pilopine HS®; Piloptic®

Canadian Brand Names Diocarpine; Isopto® Carpine; Pilopine HS®

Generic Available Yes: Hydrochloride solution

Synonyms Pilocarpine Hydrochloride; Pilocarpine Nitrate

Pharmacologic Category Cholinergic Agonist; Ophthalmic Agent, Antiglaucoma; Ophthalmic Agent, Miotic

Use Ophthalmic: Management of chronic simple glaucoma, chronic and acute angle-closure glaucoma

Unlabeled/Investigational Use Counter effects of cycloplegics

Local Anesthetic/Vasoconstrictor Precautions No information available to require special precautions

Effects on Dental Treatment No significant effects or complications reported

Significant Adverse Effects Ophthalmic (frequency not defined):

Gastrointestinal: Diarrhea

Ocular: Burning, ciliary spasm, conjunctival vascular congestion, corneal granularity (gel 10%), lacrimation, lens opacity, myopia, retinal detachment,

Respiratory: Pulmonary edema

Dosage Adults:

Ophthalmic:

Glaucoma:

Solution: Instill 1-2 drops up to 6 times/day; adjust the concentration and frequency as required to control elevated intraocular pressure

Gel: Instill 0.5" ribbon into lower conjunctival sac once daily at bedtime.

Ocular systems: Systems are labeled in terms of mean rate of release of pilocarpine over 7 days; begin with 20 mcg/hour at night and adjust based on response.

To counteract the mydriatic effects of sympathomimetic agents (unlabeled use): Solution: Instill 1 drop of a 1% solution into the affected eye(s).

Mechanism of Action Directly stimulates cholinergic receptors in the eye causing miosis (by contraction of the iris sphincter), loss of accommodation (by constriction of ciliary muscle), and lowering of intraocular pressure (with decreased resistance to aqueous humor outflow)

Contraindications Hypersensitivity to pilocarpine or any component of the formulation; acute inflammatory disease of the anterior chamber of the eye

Warnings/Precautions Ophthalmic products may cause decreased visual acuity, especially at night or with reduced lighting. Use caution with cardiovascular disease; patients may have difficulty compensating for transient changes in hemodynamics or rhythm induced by pilocarpine.

Drug Interactions Inhibits CYP2A6 (weak), 2E1 (weak), 3A4 (weak)

Concurrent use with beta-blockers may cause conduction disturbances. Pilocarpine may antagonize the effects of anticholinergic drugs.

(Continued)

Pilocarpine *(Continued)*

Ethanol/Nutrition/Herb Interactions Food: Avoid administering oral formulation with high-fat meal; fat decreases the rate of absorption, maximum concentration and increases the time it takes to reach maximum concentration.

Pharmacodynamics/Kinetics Ophthalmic:

Onset of action:
- Miosis: 10-30 minutes
- Intraocular pressure reduction: 1 hour

Duration:
- Miosis: 4-8 hours
- Intraocular pressure reduction: 4-12 hours

Pregnancy Risk Factor C

Lactation Excretion in breast milk unknown/not recommended

Breast-Feeding Considerations The excretion in breast milk is unknown; however, breast-feeding in women receiving this medication is not recommended.

Dosage Forms

Gel, ophthalmic, as hydrochloride (Pilopine HS®): 4% (3.5 g) [contains benzalkonium chloride]

Solution, ophthalmic, as hydrochloride: 1% (15 mL); 2% (15 mL); 4% (15 mL); 6% (15 mL) [may contain benzalkonium chloride]
- Isopto® Carpine: 1% (15 mL); 2% (15 mL, 30 mL); 4% (15 mL, 30 mL); 6% (15 mL); 8% (15 mL) [contains benzalkonium chloride]
- Pilocar®: 0.5% (15 mL); 1% (1 mL, 15 mL); 2% (1 mL, 15 mL); 3% (15 mL); 4% (1 mL, 15 mL); 6% (15 mL) [contains benzalkonium chloride]
- Piloptic®: 0.5% (15 mL); 1% (15 mL); 2% (15 mL); 3% (15 mL); 4% (15 mL); 6% (15 mL) [contains benzalkonium chloride]

Pilocarpine (Dental) (pye loe KAR peen DEN tal)

Related Information

Dentin Hypersensitivity, High Caries Index, and Xerostomia *on page 1555*
Pilocarpine *on page 1085*

U.S. Brand Names Salagen®

Canadian Brand Names Salagen®

Generic Available No

Pharmacologic Category Cholinergic Agonist

Dental Use Treatment of xerostomia caused by radiation therapy in patients with head and neck cancer and from Sjögren's syndrome

Local Anesthetic/Vasoconstrictor Precautions No information available to require special precautions

Effects on Dental Treatment Key adverse event(s) related to dental treatment: Increased salivation (therapeutic effect).

Significant Adverse Effects Oral (frequency varies by indication and dose):

>10%: Genitourinary: Urinary frequency (9% to 12%)

1% to 10%:
- Cardiovascular: Edema (<1% to 5%)
- Dermatologic: Pruritus, rash
- Gastrointestinal: Diarrhea (4% to 7%), constipation, flatulence
- Genitourinary: Vaginitis, urinary incontinence
- Neuromuscular & skeletal: Myalgias
- Ocular: Lacrimation (6%), amblyopia (4%), conjunctivitis
- Otic: Tinnitus
- Miscellaneous: Allergic reaction, voice alteration

<1%: Abnormal dreams, abnormal thinking, alopecia, angina pectoris, anorexia, anxiety, aphasia, appetite increased, arrhythmia, arthralgia, arthritis, bilirubinemia, body odor, bone disorder, bradycardia, breast pain, bronchitis, cataract, cholelithiasis, colitis, confusion, contact dermatitis, cyst, deafness, depression, dry eyes, dry mouth, dry skin, dyspnea, dysuria, ear pain, ECG abnormality, eczema, emotional lability, eructation, erythema nodosum, esophagitis, exfoliative dermatitis, eye hemorrhage, eye pain, gastritis, gastroenteritis, gastrointestinal disorder, gingivitis, glaucoma, hematuria, hepatitis, herpes simplex, hiccup, hyperkinesias, hypesthesia, hypoglycemia, hypotension, hypothermia, insomnia, intracranial hemorrhage, laryngismus, laryngitis, leg cramps, leukopenia, liver function test abnormal, lymphadenopathy, mastitis, melena, menorrhagia, metrorrhagia, migraine, moniliasis, myasthenia, MI, neck pain, photosensitivity reaction, nervousness, ovarian disorder, pancreatitis, paresthesias, parotid gland enlargement, peripheral edema, platelet abnormality, pneumonia, pyuria, salivary gland enlargement, salpingitis, seborrhea, skin ulcer, speech disorder, sputum increased, stridor, syncope, taste loss, tendon disorder,

tenosynovitis, thrombocythemia, thrombocytopenia, thrombosis, tongue disorder, twitching, urethral pain, urinary impairment, urinary urgency, vaginal hemorrhage, vaginal moniliasis, vesiculobullous rash, WBC abnormality, yawning

Dosage Oral: Adults: 1-2 tablets 3-4 times/day not to exceed 30 mg/day (minimum 90-day therapy required for optimum effects)

Mechanism of Action Stimulates the muscarinic-type acetylcholine receptors in the salivary glands within the parasympathetic division of the autonomic nervous system to cause an increase in serous-type saliva

Contraindications Hypersensitivity to pilocarpine or any component of the formulation; uncontrolled asthma, angle-closure glaucoma, severe hepatic impairment

Warnings/Precautions Use caution with cardiovascular disease (patients may have difficulty compensating for transient changes in hemodynamics or rhythm induced by pilocarpine); controlled asthma, chronic bronchitis, or COPD (may increase airway resistance, bronchial smooth muscle tone, bronchial secretions); cholelithiasis, biliary tract disease, and nephrolithiasis. Adjust dose with moderate hepatic impairment.

Drug Interactions Increased Effect/Toxicity: Concurrent use with anticholinergics may cause antagonism of pilocarpine's cholinergic effect; medications with cholinergic actions may result in additive cholinergic effects. Beta-adrenergic receptor blocking drugs when used with pilocarpine may increase the possibility of myocardial conduction disturbances.

Pharmacodynamics/Kinetics

Onset of action: 20 minutes after single dose

Duration: 3-5 hours

Halflife, elimination: 0.76 hours

Time to peak: 1.25 hours

Breast-Feeding Considerations The excretion in breast milk is unknown; however, breast-feeding in women receiving this medication is not recommended.

Dosage Forms Tablet, as hydrochloride (Salagen®): 5 mg

Comments Pilocarpine may have potential as a salivary stimulant in individuals suffering from xerostomia induced by antidepressants and other medications. At the present time however, the FDA has not approved pilocarpine for use in drug-induced xerostomia (clinical studies required). In an attempt to discern the efficacy of pilocarpine as a salivary stimulant in patients suffering from Sjögren's syndrome (SS), Rhodus and Schuh studied 9 patients with SS given daily doses of pilocarpine over a 6-week period. A dose of 5 mg daily produced a significant overall increase in both whole unstimulated salivary flow and parotid stimulated salivary flow. These results support the use of pilocarpine to increase salivary flow in patients with SS.

Selected Readings

Davies AN and Singer J, "A Comparison of Artificial Saliva and Pilocarpine in Radiation-Induced Xerostomia," *J Laryngol Otol*, 1994, 108(8):663-5.

Fox PC, "Management of Dry Mouth," *Dent Clin North Am*, 1997, 41(4):863-75.

Fox PC, Atkinson JC, Macynski AA, et al, "Pilocarpine Treatment of Salivary Gland Hypofunction and Dry Mouth (Xerostomia)," *Arch Intern Med*, 1991, 151(6):1149-52.

Fox PC, "Salivary Enhancement Therapies," *Caries Res*, 2004, 38(3):241-6.

Garg AK and Malo M, "Manifestations and Treatment of Xerostomia and Associated Oral Effects Secondary to Head and Neck Radiation Therapy," *J Am Dent Assoc*, 1997, 128(8):1128-33.

Gotrick B, Akerman S, Ericson D, et al, "Oral Pilocarpine for Treatment of Opioid-Induced Oral Dryness in Healthy Adults," *J Dent Res*, 2004, 83(5):393-7.

Hendrickson RG, Morocco AP, and Greenberg MI, "Pilocarpine Toxicity and the Treatment of Xerostomia," *J Emerg Med*, 2004, 26(4):429-32.

Johnson JT, Ferretti GA, Nethery WJ, et al, "Oral Pilocarpine for Postirradiation Xerostomia in Patients With Head and Neck Cancer," *N Engl J Med*, 1993, 329(6):390-5.

Mosqueda-Taylor A, Luna-Ortiz K, Irigoyen-Camacho ME, et al, "Effect of Pilocarpine Hydrochloride on Salivary Production in Previously Irradiated Head and Neck Cancer Patients," *Med Oral*, 2004, 9(3):204-11.

Nagler RM and Laufer D, "Protection Against Irradiation-Induced Damage to Salivary Glands by Adrenergic Agonist Administration," *Int J Radiat Oncol Biol Phys*, 1998, 40(2):477-81.

Nelson JD, Friedlaender M, Yeatts RP, et al, "Oral Pilocarpine for Symptomatic Relief of Keratoconjunctivitis Sicca in Patients With Sjögren's Syndrome. The MGI PHARMA Sjögren's Syndrome Study Group," *Adv Exp Med Biol*, 1998, 438:979-83.

Rhodus NL and Schuh MJ, "Effects of Pilocarpine on Salivary Flow in Patients With Sjögren's Syndrome," *Oral Surg Oral Med Oral Pathol*, 1991, 72(5):545-9.

Rieke JW, Hafermann MD, Johnson JT, et al, "Oral Pilocarpine for Radiation-Induced Xerostomia: Integrated Efficacy and Safety Results From Two Prospective Randomized Clinical Trials," *Int J Radiat Oncol Biol Phys*, 1995, 31(3):661-9.

Rousseau P, "Pilocarpine in Radiation-Induced Xerostomia," *Am J Hosp Palliat Care*, 1995, 12(2):38-9.

Schuller DE, Stevens P, Clausen KP, et al, "Treatment of Radiation Side Effects With Pilocarpine," *J Surg Oncol*, 1989, 42(4):272-6.

Singhal S, Mehta J, Rattenbury H, et al, "Oral Pilocarpine Hydrochloride for the Treatment of Refractory Xerostomia Associated With Chronic Graft-Versus-Host Disease," *Blood*, 1995, 85(4):1147-8.

(Continued)

Pilocarpine (Dental) *(Continued)*

Valdez IH, Wolff A, Atkinson JC, et al, "Use of Pilocarpine During Head and Neck Radiation Therapy to Reduce Xerostomia Salivary Dysfunction," *Cancer*, 1993, 71(5):1848-51.

Wiseman LR and Faulds D, "Oral Pilocarpine: A Review of Its Pharmacological Properties and Clinical Potential in Xerostomia," *Drugs*, 1995, 49(1):143-55.

Wynn RL, "Oral Pilocarpine (Salagen®) - A Recently Approved Salivary Stimulant," *Gen Dent*, 1996, 44(1):26,29-30.

Zimmerman RP, Mark RJ, Tran LM, et al, "Concomitant Pilocarpine During Head and Neck Irradiation Is Associated With Decreased Post-Treatment Xerostomia," *Int J Radiat Oncol Biol Phys*, 1997, 37(3):571-5.

Pilocarpine Hydrochloride *see* Pilocarpine *on page 1085*

Pilocarpine Nitrate *see* Pilocarpine *on page 1085*

Pilopine HS® *see* Pilocarpine *on page 1085*

Piloptic® *see* Pilocarpine *on page 1085*

Pima® *see* Potassium Iodide *on page 1106*

Pimaricin *see* Natamycin *on page 968*

Pimecrolimus (pim e KROE li mus)

U.S. Brand Names Elidel®

Canadian Brand Names Elidel®

Generic Available No

Pharmacologic Category Immunosuppressant Agent; Topical Skin Product

Use Short-term and intermittent long-term treatment of mild to moderate atopic dermatitis in patients not responsive to conventional therapy or when conventional therapy is not appropriate

Local Anesthetic/Vasoconstrictor Precautions No information available to require special precautions

Effects on Dental Treatment No significant effects or complications reported

Common Adverse Effects

>10%:

Central nervous system: Headache (7% to 25%), pyrexia (1% to 13%)

Local: Burning at application site (2% to 26%)

Respiratory: Nasopharyngitis (8% to 27%), cough (2% to 16%), upper respiratory tract infection (4% to 19%), bronchitis (0.4% to 11%)

Miscellaneous: Influenza (3% to 13%)

1% to 10%:

Dermatologic: Skin papilloma (warts) (up to 3%), molluscum contagiosum (0.7% to 2%), herpes simplex dermatitis (up to 2%)

Gastrointestinal: Diarrhea (0.6% to 8%), constipation (up to 4%)

Local: Irritation at application site (0.4% to 6%), erythema at application site (0.4% to 2%), pruritus at application site (0.6% to 6%)

Ocular: Eye infection (up to 1%)

Otic: Ear infection (0.6% to 6%)

Respiratory: Pharyngitis (0.7% to 8%), sinusitis (0.6% to 3%), nasal congestion (0.6% to 3%)

Miscellaneous: Viral infection (up to 7%), herpes simplex infections (0.4% to 4%), tonsillitis (0.4% to 6%)

Adverse events ≤ placebo: Abdominal pain, acne, arthralgias, asthma exacerbation, back pain, bacterial infection, conjunctivitis, dyspnea, dysmenorrhea, earache, epistaxis, folliculitis, hypersensitivity, impetigo, nausea, otitis media, pharyngitis (streptococcal), pneumonia, rhinorrhea, rhinitis, sinus congestion, skin infection, sore throat, Staphylococcal infection, toothache, urticaria, vomiting, wheezing

Mechanism of Action Penetrates inflamed epidermis to inhibit T cell activation by blocking transcription of proinflammatory cytokine genes such as interleukin-2, interferon gamma (Th1-type), interleukin-4, and interleukin-10 (Th2-type). Blocks catalytic function of calcineurin. Prevents release of inflammatory cytokines and mediators from mast cells *in vitro* after stimulation by antigen/IgE.

Drug Interactions

Cytochrome P450 Effect: Substrate of CYP3A4 (minor)

Increased Effect/Toxicity: CYP3A inhibitors may increase pimecrolimus levels in patients where increased absorption expected.

Pharmacodynamics/Kinetics Absorption: Poor when applied to 13% to 62% body surface area for up to a year

Pregnancy Risk Factor C

Pimozide (PI moe zide)

U.S. Brand Names Orap®

Canadian Brand Names Orap®

Generic Available No

Pharmacologic Category Antipsychotic Agent, Diphenylbutylperidine

Use Suppression of severe motor and phonic tics in patients with Tourette's disorder who have failed to respond satisfactorily to standard treatment

Unlabeled/Investigational Use Psychosis; reported use in individuals with delusions focused on physical symptoms (ie, preoccupation with parasitic infestation); Huntington's chorea

Local Anesthetic/Vasoconstrictor Precautions No information available to require special precautions

Effects on Dental Treatment Key adverse event(s) related to dental treatment: Tourette's disorder: Xerostomia and increased salivation (normal salivary flow resumes upon discontinuation), and taste disturbance.

Common Adverse Effects

Frequencies >1% reported in adults (limited data) and/or children with Tourette's disorder:

Cardiovascular: Abnormal ECG (3%)

Central nervous system: Somnolence (up to 28% in children), sedation (14%), akathisia (8%), drowsiness (7%), hyperkinesias (6%), insomnia (2%), depression (2%), headache (1%), nervousness (1% to 8%)

Dermatologic: Rash (8%)

Gastrointestinal: Xerostomia (25%), constipation (20%), increased salivation (14%), diarrhea (5%), thirst (5%), appetite increased (5%), taste disturbance (5%), dysphagia (3%)

Genitourinary: Impotence (15%)

Neuromuscular & skeletal: Weakness (22%), muscle tightness (15%), rigidity (10%), myalgia (3%), torticollis (3%), tremor (3%)

Ocular: Visual disturbance (6% to 20%), accommodation decreased (20%)

Miscellaneous: Speech disorder (10%)

Frequency not established (reported in disorders other than Tourette's disorder): Blood dyscrasias, breast edema, chest pain, dizziness, extrapyramidal symptoms (akathisia, akinesia, dystonia, pseudoparkinsonism, tardive dyskinesia); facial edema, gingival hyperplasia (case report), hypertension, hyponatremia, hypotension, jaundice, libido decreased, neuroleptic malignant syndrome, orthostatic hypotension, palpitations, periorbital edema, postural hypotension, QT_c prolongation, seizure, tachycardia, ventricular arrhythmias, vomiting, weight gain/loss

Mechanism of Action A potent centrally-acting dopamine-receptor antagonist resulting in its characteristic neuroleptic effects

Drug Interactions

Cytochrome P450 Effect: Substrate (major) of CYP1A2, 3A4; **Inhibits** CYP2C19 (weak), 2D6 (weak), 2E1 (weak), 3A4 (weak)

Increased Effect/Toxicity: Concurrent use with QT_c-prolonging agents is contraindicated including Class Ia and Class III antiarrhythmics, arsenic trioxide, chlorpromazine, dolasetron, droperidol, halofantrine, levomethadyl, mefloquine, pentamidine, probucol, tacrolimus, ziprasidone, mesoridazine, thioridazine, tricyclic antidepressants, and some quinolone antibiotics (sparfloxacin, moxifloxacin, and gatifloxacin).

CYP1A2 inhibitors may increase the levels/effects of pimozide; example inhibitors include amiodarone, ciprofloxacin, fluvoxamine, ketoconazole, lomefloxacin, ofloxacin, and rofecoxib. Chloroquine, propranolol, and sulfadoxine-pyrimethamine also may increase pimozide concentrations. Concurrent use with TCA may produce increased toxicity or altered therapeutic response. Pimozide plus lithium may (rarely) produce neurotoxicity. Pimozide and CNS depressants (ethanol, narcotics) may produce additive CNS depressant effects. Pimozide with fluoxetine has been associated with the development of bradycardia (case report). Metoclopramide may increase risk of extrapyramidal symptoms (EPS).

CYP3A4 inhibitors may increase the levels/effects of pimozide; example inhibitors include azole antifungals, ciprofloxacin, clarithromycin, diclofenac, doxycycline, erythromycin, imatinib, isoniazid, nefazodone, nicardipine, propofol, protease inhibitors, quinidine, and verapamil. Concurrent use of strong CYP3A4 inhibitors with pimozide is contraindicated.

Decreased Effect: CYP1A2 inducers may decrease the levels/effects of pimozide; example inducers include aminoglutethimide, carbamazepine, phenobarbital, and rifampin. CYP3A4 inducers may decrease the levels/effects of pimozide; example inducers include aminoglutethimide, carbamazepine, nafcillin, nevirapine, phenobarbital, phenytoin, and rifamycins. Benztropine (and other anticholinergics) may inhibit the therapeutic response to pimozide. Antipsychotics such as pimozide inhibit the ability of bromocriptine to lower serum prolactin concentrations. The antihypertensive effects of guanethidine and guanadrel may be inhibited by pimozide. Pimozide may

(Continued)

Pimozide *(Continued)*

inhibit the antiparkinsonian effect of levodopa. Pimozide (and possibly other low potency antipsychotics) may reverse the pressor effects of epinephrine.

Pharmacodynamics/Kinetics

Absorption: 50%

Protein binding: 99%

Metabolism: Hepatic; significant first-pass effect

Half-life elimination: 50 hours

Time to peak, serum: 6-8 hours

Excretion: Urine

Pregnancy Risk Factor C

Pindolol (PIN doe lole)

Related Information

Cardiovascular Diseases *on page 1458*

Canadian Brand Names Apo-Pindol®; Gen-Pindolol; Novo-Pindol; Nu-Pindol; PMS-Pindolol; Visken®

Generic Available Yes

Pharmacologic Category Beta Blocker With Intrinsic Sympathomimetic Activity

Use Management of hypertension

Unlabeled/Investigational Use Potential augmenting agent for antidepressants; ventricular arrhythmias/tachycardia, antipsychotic-induced akathisia, situational anxiety; aggressive behavior associated with dementia

Local Anesthetic/Vasoconstrictor Precautions Use with caution; epinephrine has interacted with nonselective beta-blockers to result in initial hypertensive episode followed by bradycardia

Effects on Dental Treatment Pindolol is a nonselective beta-blocker and may enhance the pressor response to epinephrine, resulting in hypertension and bradycardia. Many nonsteroidal anti-inflammatory drugs, such as ibuprofen and indomethacin, can reduce the hypotensive effect of beta-blockers after 3 or more weeks of therapy with the NSAID. Short-term NSAID use (ie, 3 days) requires no special precautions in patients taking beta-blockers.

Common Adverse Effects 1% to 10%:

Cardiovascular: Chest pain (3%), edema (6%)

Central nervous system: Nightmares/vivid dreams (5%), dizziness (9%), insomnia (10%), fatigue (8%), nervousness (7%), anxiety (<2%)

Dermatologic: Rash, itching (4%)

Gastrointestinal: Nausea (5%), abdominal discomfort (4%)

Neuromuscular & skeletal: Weakness (4%), paresthesia (3%), arthralgia (7%), muscle pain (10%)

Respiratory: Dyspnea (5%)

Mechanism of Action Blocks both beta$_1$- and beta$_2$-receptors and has mild intrinsic sympathomimetic activity; pindolol has negative inotropic and chronotropic effects and can significantly slow AV nodal conduction. Augmentive action of antidepressants thought to be mediated via a serotonin 1A autoreceptor antagonism.

Drug Interactions

Cytochrome P450 Effect: Substrate of CYP2D6 (major); **Inhibits** CYP2D6 (weak)

Increased Effect/Toxicity: CYP2D6 inhibitors may increase the levels/effects of pindolol; example inhibitors include chlorpromazine, delavirdine, fluoxetine, miconazole, paroxetine, pergolide, quinidine, quinine, ritonavir, and ropinirole. Pindolol may increase the effects of other drugs which slow AV conduction (digoxin, verapamil, diltiazem), alpha-blockers (prazosin, terazosin), and alpha-adrenergic stimulants (epinephrine, phenylephrine). Pindolol may mask the tachycardia from hypoglycemia caused by insulin and oral hypoglycemics. In patients receiving concurrent therapy, the risk of hypertensive crisis is increased when either clonidine or the beta-blocker is withdrawn. Reserpine has been shown to enhance the effect of beta-blockers. Beta-blockers may increase the action or levels of ethanol, disopyramide, nondepolarizing muscle relaxants, and theophylline although the effects are difficult to predict.

Decreased Effect: Decreased levels/effect of pindolol with aluminum salts, barbiturates, calcium salts, cholestyramine, colestipol, NSAIDs, penicillins (ampicillin), rifampin, salicylates, and sulfinpyrazone due to decreased bioavailability and plasma levels. Beta-blockers may decrease the effect of sulfonylureas (possibly hyperglycemia). Nonselective beta-blockers blunt the effect of beta-2 adrenergic agonists (albuterol).

Pharmacodynamics/Kinetics

Absorption: Rapid, 50% to 95%

Protein binding: 50%

Metabolism: Hepatic (60% to 65%) to conjugates

Half-life elimination: 2.5-4 hours; prolonged with renal impairment, age, and cirrhosis

Time to peak, serum: 1-2 hours

Excretion: Urine (35% to 50% as unchanged drug)

Pregnancy Risk Factor B

Pink Bismuth *see* Bismuth *on page 209*

Pin-X® [OTC] *see* Pyrantel Pamoate *on page 1151*

PIO *see* Pemoline *on page 1055*

Pioglitazone (pye oh GLI ta zone)

U.S. Brand Names Actos®

Canadian Brand Names Actos®

Generic Available No

Pharmacologic Category Antidiabetic Agent, Thiazolidinedione

Use

Type 2 diabetes mellitus (noninsulin dependent, NIDDM), monotherapy: Adjunct to diet and exercise, to improve glycemic control

Type 2 diabetes mellitus (noninsulin dependent, NIDDM), combination therapy with sulfonylurea, metformin, or insulin: When diet, exercise, and a single agent alone does not result in adequate glycemic control

Local Anesthetic/Vasoconstrictor Precautions No information available to require special precautions

Effects on Dental Treatment Pioglitazone-dependent diabetics should be appointed for dental treatment in morning in order to minimize chance of stress-induced hypoglycemia.

Common Adverse Effects

>10%:

Endocrine & metabolic: Serum triglycerides decreased, HDL-cholesterol increased

Gastrointestinal: Weight gain

Respiratory: Upper respiratory tract infection (13%)

1% to 10%:

Cardiovascular: Edema (5%) (in combination trials with sulfonylureas or insulin, the incidence of edema was as high as 15%)

Central nervous system: Headache (9%), fatigue (4%)

Endocrine & metabolic: Aggravation of diabetes mellitus (5%), hypoglycemia (range 2% to 15% when used in combination with sulfonylureas or insulin)

Hematologic: Anemia (1%)

Neuromuscular & skeletal: Myalgia (5%)

Respiratory: Sinusitis (6%), pharyngitis (5%)

Dosage Adults: Oral:

Monotherapy: Initial: 15-30 mg once daily; if response is inadequate, the dosage may be increased in increments up to 45 mg once daily; maximum recommended dose: 45 mg once daily

Combination therapy (doses >30 mg/day have not been evaluated in combination regimens):

With sulfonylureas: Initial: 15-30 mg once daily; dose of sulfonylurea should be reduced if the patient reports hypoglycemia

With metformin: Initial: 15-30 mg once daily; it is unlikely that the dose of metformin will need to be reduced due to hypoglycemia

With insulin: Initial: 15-30 mg once daily; dose of insulin should be reduced by 10% to 25% if the patient reports hypoglycemia or if the plasma glucose falls to <100 mg/dL.

Elderly: No dosage adjustment is recommended in elderly patients.

Dosage adjustment in renal impairment: No dosage adjustment is required.

Dosage adjustment in hepatic impairment: Clearance is significantly lower in hepatic impairment. Therapy should not be initiated if the patient exhibits active liver disease or increased transaminases (>2.5 times the upper limit of normal) at baseline.

Mechanism of Action Thiazolidinedione antidiabetic agent that lowers blood glucose by improving target cell response to insulin, without increasing pancreatic insulin secretion. It has a mechanism of action that is dependent on the presence of insulin for activity. Pioglitazone is a potent and selective agonist for peroxisome proliferator-activated receptor-gamma (PPARgamma). Activation of nuclear PPARgamma receptors influences the production of a number of gene products involved in glucose and lipid metabolism.

(Continued)

Pioglitazone *(Continued)*

Contraindications Hypersensitivity to pioglitazone or any component of the formulation; active liver disease (transaminases >2.5 times the upper limit of normal at baseline); patients who have experienced jaundice during troglitazone therapy

Warnings/Precautions Should not be used in diabetic ketoacidosis. Mechanism requires the presence of insulin, therefore use in type 1 diabetes is not recommended. May potentiate hypoglycemia when used in combination with sulfonylureas or insulin. Use with caution in premenopausal, anovulatory women - may result in a resumption of ovulation, increasing the risk of pregnancy. Use with caution in patients with anemia (may reduce hemoglobin and hematocrit). Use with caution in patients with edema; may increase plasma volume and/or increase cardiac hypertrophy. Monitor closely for signs and symptoms of heart failure (including weight gain, edema, or dyspnea). Not recommended for use in patients with NYHA Class III or IV heart failure. Discontinue if heart failure develops. Use with caution in patients with minor elevations in transaminases (AST or ALT). Idiosyncratic hepatotoxicity has been reported with another thiazolidinedione agent (troglitazone) and postmarketing case reports of hepatitis (with rare hepatic failure) have been received for pioglitazone. Monitoring should include periodic determinations of liver function. Not for use in children <18 years of age.

Drug Interactions

Cytochrome P450 Effect: Substrate (major) of CYP2C8/9, 3A4; **Inhibits** CYP2C8/9 (strong), 2C19 (weak), 2D6 (moderate); **Induces** CYP3A4 (weak)

Increased Effect/Toxicity: Concomitant use with thioridazine is contraindicated, due to a risk of arrhythmias. The levels/effects of pioglitazone may be increased by azole antifungals, ciprofloxacin, clarithromycin, delavirdine, diclofenac, doxycycline, erythromycin, fluconazole, gemfibrozil, imatinib, isoniazid, itraconazole, ketoconazole, nefazodone, nicardipine, NSAIDs, propofol, protease inhibitors, quinidine, sulfonamides, verapamil, and other CYP2C8/9 or 3A4 inhibitors.

Pioglitazone may increase the levels/effects of amiodarone, amphetamines, selected beta-blockers, dextromethorphan, fluoxetine, glimepiride, glipizide, lidocaine, mirtazapine, nateglinide, nefazodone, paroxetine, phenytoin, risperidone, ritonavir, rosiglitazone, sertraline, thioridazine, warfarin, and other CYP2D6 or 2C8/9 substrates.

Decreased Effect: The levels/effects of pioglitazone may be decreased by aminoglutethimide, carbamazepine, nafcillin, nevirapine, phenobarbital, phenytoin, rifamycins, secobarbital, and other CYP2C8/9 or CYP3A4 inducers. Pioglitazone may decrease the levels/effects of CYP2D6 prodrug substrates (eg, codeine, hydrocodone, oxycodone, tramadol). Effects of oral contraceptives (hormonal) may be decreased, based on data from a related compound. This has not been specifically evaluated for pioglitazone. Bile acid sequestrants may decrease pioglitazone levels.

Ethanol/Nutrition/Herb Interactions

Ethanol: Caution with ethanol (may cause hypoglycemia).

Food: Peak concentrations are delayed when administered with food, but the extent of absorption is not affected. Pioglitazone may be taken without regard to meals.

Herb/Nutraceutical: St John's wort may decrease levels. Caution with chromium, garlic, gymnema (may cause hypoglycemia).

Dietary Considerations Management of type 2 diabetes mellitus (noninsulin dependent, NIDDM) should include diet control. May be taken without regard to meals.

Pharmacodynamics/Kinetics

Onset of action: Delayed

Peak effect: Glucose control: Several weeks

Distribution: V_{ss} (apparent): 0.63 L/kg

Protein binding: 99.8%

Metabolism: Hepatic (99%) via CYP2C8/9 and 3A4 to both active and inactive metabolites

Half-life elimination: Parent drug: 3-7 hours; Total: 16-24 hours

Time to peak: ~2 hours

Excretion: Urine (15% to 30%) and feces as metabolites

Pregnancy Risk Factor C

Dosage Forms TAB: 15 mg, 30 mg, 45 mg

Piperacillin (pi PER a sil in)

U.S. Brand Names Pipracil® [DSC]

Canadian Brand Names Pipracil®

Generic Available No

Synonyms Piperacillin Sodium

Pharmacologic Category Antibiotic, Penicillin

Use Treatment of susceptible infections such as septicemia, acute and chronic respiratory tract infections, skin and soft tissue infections, and urinary tract infections due to susceptible strains of *Pseudomonas*, *Proteus*, and *Escherichia coli* and *Enterobacter*; active against some streptococci and some anaerobic bacteria; febrile neutropenia (as part of combination regimen)

Local Anesthetic/Vasoconstrictor Precautions No information available to require special precautions

Effects on Dental Treatment Key adverse event(s) related to dental treatment: Prolonged use of penicillins may lead to development of oral candidiasis.

Common Adverse Effects Frequency not defined.

Central nervous system: Confusion, convulsions, drowsiness, fever, Jarisch-Herxheimer reaction

Dermatologic: Rash

Endocrine & metabolic: Electrolyte imbalance

Hematologic: Abnormal platelet aggregation and prolonged PT (high doses), hemolytic anemia, Coombs' reaction (positive)

Local: Thrombophlebitis

Neuromuscular & skeletal: Myoclonus

Renal: Acute interstitial nephritis

Miscellaneous: Anaphylaxis, hypersensitivity reactions

Mechanism of Action Inhibits bacterial cell wall synthesis by binding to one or more of the penicillin binding proteins (PBPs); which in turn inhibits the final transpeptidation step of peptidoglycan synthesis in bacterial cell walls, thus inhibiting cell wall biosynthesis. Bacteria eventually lyse due to ongoing activity of cell wall autolytic enzymes (autolysins and murein hydrolases) while cell wall assembly is arrested.

Drug Interactions

Increased Effect/Toxicity: Probenecid may increase penicillin levels. Neuromuscular blockers may increase duration of blockade. Penicillins may increase the exposure to methotrexate during concurrent therapy; monitor.

Decreased Effect: Tetracyclines may decrease penicillin effectiveness. High concentrations of piperacillin may cause physical inactivation of aminoglycosides and lead to potential toxicity in patients with mild-moderate renal dysfunction. Although anecdotal reports suggest oral contraceptive efficacy could be reduced by penicillins, this has been refuted by more rigorous scientific and clinical data.

Pharmacodynamics/Kinetics

Absorption: I.M.: 70% to 80%

Distribution: Crosses placenta; low concentrations enter breast milk

Protein binding: 22%

Half-life elimination (dose dependent; prolonged with moderately severe renal or hepatic impairment):

Neonates: 1-5 days old: 3.6 hours; >6 days old: 2.1-2.7 hours

Children: 1-6 months: 0.79 hour; 6 months to 12 years: 0.39-0.5 hour

Adults: 36-80 minutes

Time to peak, serum: I.M.: 30-50 minutes

Excretion: Primarily urine; partially feces

Pregnancy Risk Factor B

Piperacillin and Tazobactam Sodium

(pi PER a sil in & ta zoe BAK tam SOW dee um)

Related Information

Piperacillin *on page 1092*

U.S. Brand Names Zosyn®

Canadian Brand Names Tazocin®

Generic Available No

Synonyms Piperacillin Sodium and Tazobactam Sodium

Pharmacologic Category Antibiotic, Penicillin

Use Treatment of infections caused by susceptible organisms, including infections of the lower respiratory tract (community-acquired pneumonia, nosocomial pneumonia); urinary tract; skin and skin structures; gynecologic (endometritis, pelvic inflammatory disease); bone and joint infections; intra-abdominal infections (appendicitis with rupture/abscess, peritonitis); and septicemia. Tazobactam expands activity of piperacillin to include beta-lactamase producing strains of *S. aureus*, *H. influenzae*, *Bacteroides*, and other gram-negative bacteria.

(Continued)

Piperacillin and Tazobactam Sodium *(Continued)*

Local Anesthetic/Vasoconstrictor Precautions No information available to require special precautions

Effects on Dental Treatment Key adverse event(s) related to dental treatment: Prolonged use of penicillins may lead to development of oral candidiasis.

Common Adverse Effects

>10%: Gastrointestinal: Diarrhea (11%)

1% to 10%:

Cardiovascular: Hypertension (2%)

Central nervous system: Insomnia (7%), headache (7% to 8%), agitation (2%), fever (2%), dizziness (1%)

Dermatologic: Rash (4%), pruritus (3%)

Gastrointestinal: Constipation (7% to 8%), nausea (7%), vomiting/dyspepsia (3%)

Hepatic: Transaminases increased

Respiratory: Rhinitis/dyspnea (~1%)

Miscellaneous: Serum sickness-like reaction

Several laboratory abnormalities have rarely been associated with piperacillin/tazobactam including reversible eosinophilia, and neutropenia (associated most often with prolonged therapy), positive direct Coombs' test, prolonged PT and aPTT, transient elevations of LFT, increases in creatinine

Mechanism of Action Inhibits bacterial cell wall synthesis by binding to one or more of the penicillin binding proteins (PBPs); which in turn inhibits the final transpeptidation step of peptidoglycan synthesis in bacterial cell walls, thus inhibiting cell wall biosynthesis. Bacteria eventually lyse due to ongoing activity of cell wall autolytic enzymes (autolysins and murein hydrolases) while cell wall assembly is arrested. Tazobactam inhibits many beta-lactamases, including staphylococcal penicillinase and Richmond and Sykes types II, III, IV, and V, including extended spectrum enzymes; it has only limited activity against class I beta-lactamases other than class Ic types.

Drug Interactions

Increased Effect/Toxicity: Probenecid may increase penicillin levels. Neuromuscular blockers may increase duration of blockade. Penicillins may increase methotrexate exposure; clinical significance has not been established.

Decreased Effect: Tetracyclines may decrease penicillin effectiveness. Aminoglycosides may cause physical inactivation of aminoglycosides in the presence of high concentrations of piperacillin and potential toxicity in patients with mild-moderate renal dysfunction. Although anecdotal reports suggest oral contraceptive efficacy could be reduced by penicillins, this has been refuted by more rigorous scientific and clinical data.

Pharmacodynamics/Kinetics Both AUC and peak concentrations are dose proportional; hepatic impairment does not affect kinetics

Distribution: Well into lungs, intestinal mucosa, skin, muscle, uterus, ovary, prostate, gallbladder, and bile; penetration into CSF is low in subject with noninflamed meninges

Protein binding: Piperacillin: ~26% to 33%; Tazobactam: 31% to 32%

Metabolism: Piperacillin: 6% to 9%; Tazobactam: ~26%

Half-life elimination: Piperacillin: 1 hour; Metabolite: 1-1.5 hours; Tazobactam: 0.7-0.9 hour

Excretion: Both piperacillin and tazobactam are directly proportional to renal function

Piperacillin: Urine (50% to 70%); feces (10% to 20%)

Tazobactam: Urine (26% as inactive metabolite) within 24 hours

Pregnancy Risk Factor B

Piperacillin Sodium *see* Piperacillin *on page 1092*

Piperacillin Sodium and Tazobactam Sodium *see* Piperacillin and Tazobactam Sodium *on page 1093*

Piperazine (PI per a zeen)

Canadian Brand Names Entacyl®

Mexican Brand Names Desparasil®

Generic Available Yes

Synonyms Piperazine Citrate

Pharmacologic Category Anthelmintic

Use Treatment of pinworm and roundworm infections (used as an alternative to first-line agents, mebendazole, or pyrantel pamoate)

Local Anesthetic/Vasoconstrictor Precautions No information available to require special precautions

Effects on Dental Treatment No significant effects or complications reported

Mechanism of Action Causes muscle paralysis of the roundworm by blocking the effects of acetylcholine at the neuromuscular junction

Drug Interactions

Decreased Effect: Pyrantel pamoate (antagonistic mode of action).

Pharmacodynamics/Kinetics

Absorption: Well absorbed

Time to peak, serum: 1 hour

Excretion: Urine (as unchanged drug and metabolites)

Pregnancy Risk Factor B

Piperazine Citrate *see* Piperazine *on page 1094*

Piperazine Estrone Sulfate *see* Estropipate *on page 531*

Piperonyl Butoxide and Pyrethrins *see* Pyrethrins and Piperonyl Butoxide *on page 1153*

Pipotiazine (pip oh TYE a zeen)

Canadian Brand Names Piportil® L_4

Generic Available No

Synonyms Pipotiazine Palmitate

Pharmacologic Category Antipsychotic Agent, Phenothiazine, Piperidine

Use Management of schizophrenia

Local Anesthetic/Vasoconstrictor Precautions No information available to require special precautions

Effects on Dental Treatment No significant effects or complications reported

Common Adverse Effects Frequency not defined.

Cardiovascular: Tachycardia, hypotension, syncope, edema, ECG changes, QT_c prolongation, cardiac arrest

Central nervous system; Extrapyramidal symptoms (tremor, akathisia, dystonia, dyskinesia, oculogyric crisis, opisthotonos, hyper-reflexia, pseudo-Parkinsonism, rigidity, sialorrhea); tardive dyskinesia, sleep disturbance, dizziness, drowsiness, fatigue, insomnia, depression, agitation, anxiety, restlessness, excitement, bizarre dreams, fever, headache, cerebral edema, EEG changes, seizures, paradoxical psychosis

Dermatologic: Pruritus, dermatitis, rash, erythema, urticaria, seborrhea, eczema, exfoliative dermatitis, photosensitivity, skin pigmentation (prolonged therapy), epithelial keratopathy

Endocrine & metabolic: Anorexia, menstrual irregularities, thirst, weight changes, appetite increased, galactorrhea, gynecomastia, changes in libido

Gastrointestinal: Nausea, constipation, xerostomia, vomiting, salivation, adynamic ileus, fecal impaction, cholestasis, jaundice

Genitourinary: Urinary retention, bladder paralysis, incontinence, polyuria, impotence

Hematologic: Agranulocytosis, anemia, eosinophilia, leukopenia, pancytopenia, thrombocytopenia

Ocular: Blurred vision, glaucoma, corneal deposits (prolonged therapy), lenticular deposits, pigmentary retinopathy (prolonged therapy)

Respiratory: Nasal congestion, pneumonia, pneumonitis

Miscellaneous: Angioedema, diaphoresis increased, Lupus-like syndrome

Restrictions Not available in U.S.

Mechanism of Action Blocks postsynaptic mesolimbic dopaminergic receptors in the brain; depresses the release of hypothalamic and hypophyseal hormones. Relative to other piperidine phenothiazines, pipotiazine appears to be less sedating, with less potential to potentiate other CNS depressants, and may possess a lower propensity to cause hypotension. However, it has a relatively high propensity for cause extrapyramidal reactions.

Drug Interactions

Cytochrome P450 Effect: No published data on CYP metabolism. Based on structural analysis, pipotiazine may be a substrate of CYP2D6 and 3A4.

Increased Effect/Toxicity: The levels/effects of pipotiazine may be increased by azole antifungals, chlorpromazine, ciprofloxacin, clarithromycin, delavirdine, diclofenac, doxycycline, erythromycin, fluoxetine, imatinib, isoniazid, miconazole, nefazodone, nicardipine, paroxetine, pergolide, propofol, protease inhibitors, quinidine, quinine, ritonavir, ropinirole, verapamil and other CYP2D6 or 3A4 inhibitors.

Drugs which alter the QT_c interval may be additive with pipotiazine, increasing the risk of malignant arrhythmias; includes type Ia antiarrhythmics, TCAs, and some quinolone antibiotics (sparfloxacin, moxifloxacin

(Continued)

Pipotiazine *(Continued)*

and gatifloxacin). **These agents are contraindicated with other piperadine phenothiazines (thioridazine)** Potassium depleting agents may increase the risk of serious arrhythmias with pipotiazine (includes many diuretics, aminoglycosides, and amphotericin).

Phenothiazines inhibit the ability of bromocriptine to lower serum prolactin concentrations. The sedative effects of CNS depressants or ethanol may be additive with phenothiazines. Phenothiazines and trazodone may produce additive hypotensive effects. Metoclopramide may increase risk of extrapyramidal symptoms (EPS). Concurrent use of antihypertensives may result in additive hypotensive effects (particularly orthostasis).

Phenothiazines may produce neurotoxicity with lithium; this is a rare effect. Rare cases of respiratory paralysis have been reported with concurrent use of phenothiazines and polypeptide antibiotics. Naltrexone in combination with pipotiazine has been reported to cause lethargy and somnolence. Phenylpropanolamine has been reported to result in cardiac arrhythmias when combined with some phenothiazines.

Decreased Effect: Aluminum salts may decrease the absorption of phenothiazines. The efficacy of amphetamines may be diminished by antipsychotics; in addition, amphetamines may increase psychotic symptoms; avoid concurrent use. Anticholinergics may inhibit the therapeutic response to phenothiazines and excess anticholinergic effects may occur (includes benztropine, trihexyphenidyl, biperiden, and drugs with significant anticholinergic activity). Low potency antipsychotics (such as pipotiazine) may diminish the pressor effects of epinephrine. The antihypertensive effects of guanethidine or guanadrel may be inhibited by phenothiazines. Phenothiazines may inhibit the antiparkinsonian effect of levodopa. Enzyme inducers may enhance the hepatic metabolism of phenothiazines; larger doses may be required; includes rifampin, rifabutin, barbiturates, phenytoin, and cigarette smoking.

Pharmacodynamics/Kinetics

Onset: I.M.: 2-3 days

Duration: 3-6 weeks

Pipotiazine Palmitate *see* Pipotiazine *on page 1095*

Pipracil® [DSC] *see* Piperacillin *on page 1092*

Pirbuterol (peer BYOO ter ole)

Related Information

Respiratory Diseases *on page 1478*

U.S. Brand Names Maxair™ Autohaler™

Generic Available No

Synonyms Pirbuterol Acetate

Pharmacologic Category Beta$_2$-Adrenergic Agonist

Use Prevention and treatment of reversible bronchospasm including asthma

Local Anesthetic/Vasoconstrictor Precautions No information available to require special precautions

Effects on Dental Treatment Key adverse event(s) related to dental treatment: Xerostomia (normal salivary flow resumes upon discontinuation).

Common Adverse Effects

>10%:

- Central nervous system: Nervousness (7%)
- Endocrine & metabolic: Serum glucose increased, serum potassium decreased
- Neuromuscular & skeletal: Trembling (6%)

1% to 10%:

- Cardiovascular: Palpitations (2%), tachycardia (1%)
- Central nervous system: Headache (2%), dizziness (1%)
- Gastrointestinal: Nausea (2%)
- Respiratory: Cough (1%)

Mechanism of Action Pirbuterol is a beta$_2$-adrenergic agonist with a similar structure to albuterol, specifically a pyridine ring has been substituted for the benzene ring in albuterol. The increased beta$_2$ selectivity of pirbuterol results from the substitution of a tertiary butyl group on the nitrogen of the side chain, which additionally imparts resistance of pirbuterol to degradation by monoamine oxidase and provides a lengthened duration of action in comparison to the less selective previous beta-agonist agents.

Drug Interactions

Increased Effect/Toxicity: Increased toxicity with other beta agonists, MAO inhibitors, tricyclic antidepressants.

Decreased Effect: Decreased effect with beta-blockers.

Pharmacodynamics/Kinetics

Onset of action: Peak effect: Therapeutic: Oral: 2-3 hours with peak serum concentration of 6.2-9.8 mcg/L; Inhalation: 0.5-1 hour

Half-life elimination: 2-3 hours

Metabolism: Hepatic

Excretion: Urine (10% as unchanged drug)

Pregnancy Risk Factor C

Pirbuterol Acetate *see* Pirbuterol *on page 1096*

Piroxicam (peer OKS i kam)

Related Information

Rheumatoid Arthritis, Osteoarthritis, and Osteoporosis *on page 1490*

Temporomandibular Dysfunction (TMD) *on page 1564*

U.S. Brand Names Feldene®

Canadian Brand Names Apo-Piroxicam®; Feldene™; Gen-Piroxicam; Novo-Pirocam; Nu-Pirox; Pexicam®

Mexican Brand Names Androxicam®; Artinor®; Brexicam®; Citoken® [caps]; Dixonal®; Dolzycam®; Facicam®; Feldene®; Osteral®; Oxicanol®; Piroxan®; Rogal®

Generic Available Yes

Pharmacologic Category Nonsteroidal Anti-inflammatory Drug (NSAID), Oral

Use Symptomatic treatment of acute and chronic rheumatoid arthritis and osteoarthritis

Unlabeled/Investigational Use Ankylosing spondylitis

Local Anesthetic/Vasoconstrictor Precautions No information available to require special precautions

Effects on Dental Treatment NSAID formulations are known to reversibly decrease platelet aggregation via mechanisms different than observed with aspirin. The dentist should be aware of the potential of abnormal coagulation. Caution should also be exercised in the use of NSAIDs in patients already on anticoagulant therapy with drugs such as warfarin (Coumadin®).

Common Adverse Effects

>10%:

- Central nervous system: Dizziness
- Dermatologic: Rash
- Gastrointestinal: Abdominal cramps, heartburn, indigestion, nausea

1% to 10%:

- Central nervous system: Headache, nervousness
- Dermatologic: Itching
- Endocrine & metabolic: Fluid retention
- Gastrointestinal: Vomiting
- Otic: Tinnitus

Mechanism of Action Inhibits prostaglandin synthesis, acts on the hypothalamus heat-regulating center to reduce fever, blocks prostaglandin synthetase action which prevents formation of the platelet-aggregating substance thromboxane A_2; decreases pain receptor sensitivity. Other proposed mechanisms of action for salicylate anti-inflammatory action are lysosomal stabilization, kinin and leukotriene production, alteration of chemotactic factors, and inhibition of neutrophil activation. This latter mechanism may be the most significant pharmacologic action to reduce inflammation.

Drug Interactions

Cytochrome P450 Effect: Substrate of CYP2C8/9 (minor); **Inhibits** CYP2C8/9 (strong)

Increased Effect/Toxicity: Increased effect/toxicity of lithium and methotrexate (controversial). Piroxicam may increase the levels/effects of amiodarone, fluoxetine, glimepiride, glipizide, nateglinide, phenytoin, pioglitazone, rosiglitazone, sertraline, warfarin, and other CYP2C8/9 substrates.

Decreased Effect: Decreased effect of diuretics, beta-blockers. Decreased effect with aspirin, antacids, and cholestyramine.

Pharmacodynamics/Kinetics

Onset of action: Analgesic: ~1 hour

Peak effect: 3-5 hours

Protein binding: 99%

Metabolism: Hepatic

Half-life elimination: 45-50 hours

Excretion: Primarily urine and feces (small amounts) as unchanged drug (5%) and metabolites

Pregnancy Risk Factor B/D (3rd trimester or near term)

p-Isobutylhydratropic Acid *see* Ibuprofen *on page 728*
Pit *see* Oxytocin *on page 1038*
Pitocin® *see* Oxytocin *on page 1038*
Pitressin® *see* Vasopressin *on page 1369*
Pix Carbonis *see* Coal Tar *on page 367*
Plague Vaccine *see page 1614*
Plan B® *see* Levonorgestrel *on page 815*
Plantago Seed *see* Psyllium *on page 1151*
Plantain Seed *see* Psyllium *on page 1151*
Plaquenil® *see* Hydroxychloroquine *on page 720*
Platinol®-AQ *see* Cisplatin *on page 337*
Plavix® *see* Clopidogrel *on page 361*
Plenaxis™ *see* Abarelix *on page 43*
Plendil® *see* Felodipine *on page 576*
Pletal® *see* Cilostazol *on page 329*
PMPA *see* Tenofovir *on page 1270*
Pneumococcal 7-Valent Conjugate Vaccine *see* Pneumococcal Conjugate Vaccine (7-Valent) *on page 1098*

Pneumococcal Conjugate Vaccine (7-Valent)

(noo moe KOK al KON ju gate vak SEEN, seven vay lent)

Related Information
Immunizations (Vaccines) *on page 1614*

U.S. Brand Names Prevnar®

Canadian Brand Names Prevnar®

Generic Available No

Synonyms Diphtheria CRM_{197} Protein; PCV7; Pneumococcal 7-Valent Conjugate Vaccine

Pharmacologic Category Vaccine

Use Immunization of infants and toddlers against *Streptococcus pneumoniae* infection caused by serotypes included in the vaccine

Advisory Committee on Immunization Practices (ACIP) guidelines also recommend PCV7 for use in:
- Children ≥2-59 months with cochlear implants
- All children ≥23 months
- Children ages 24-59 months with: Sickle cell disease (including other sickle cell hemoglobinopathies, asplenia, splenic dysfunction), HIV infection, immunocompromising conditions (congenital immunodeficiencies, renal failure, nephrotic syndrome, diseases associated with immunosuppressive or radiation therapy, solid organ transplant), chronic illnesses (cardiac disease, cerebrospinal fluid leaks, diabetes mellitus, pulmonary disease excluding asthma unless on high dose corticosteroids)
- Consider use in all children 24-59 months with priority given to:
  - Children 24-35 months
  - Children 24-59 months who are of Alaska native, American Indian, or African-American descent
  - Children 24-59 months who attend group day care centers

Local Anesthetic/Vasoconstrictor Precautions No information available to require special precautions

Effects on Dental Treatment No significant effects or complications reported

Common Adverse Effects All serious adverse reactions must be reported to the U.S. Department of Health and Human Services (DHHS) Vaccine Adverse Event Reporting System (VAERS) 1-800-822-7967.

>10%:
- Central nervous system: Fever, irritability, drowsiness, restlessness
- Dermatologic: Erythema
- Gastrointestinal: Decreased appetite, vomiting, diarrhea
- Local: Induration, tenderness, nodule

1% to 10%: Dermatologic: Rash (0.5% to 1.4%)

Mechanism of Action Contains saccharides of capsular antigens of serotypes 4, 6B, 9V, 18C, 19F, and 23F, individually conjugated to CRM197 protein

Pregnancy Risk Factor C

Pneumococcal Polysaccharide Vaccine (Polyvalent) *see page 1614*
Pneumotussin® *see* Hydrocodone and Guaifenesin *on page 708*
Podocon-25® *see* Podophyllum Resin *on page 1099*

Podofilox (po do FIL oks)

U.S. Brand Names Condylox®

Canadian Brand Names Condyline™; Wartec®

Generic Available Yes: Topical solution

Pharmacologic Category Keratolytic Agent; Topical Skin Product

Use Treatment of external genital warts

Local Anesthetic/Vasoconstrictor Precautions No information available to require special precautions

Effects on Dental Treatment No significant effects or complications reported

Pregnancy Risk Factor C

Podophyllin *see* Podophyllum Resin *on page 1099*

Podophyllum Resin (po DOF fil um REZ in)

U.S. Brand Names Podocon-25®

Canadian Brand Names Podofilm®

Generic Available No

Synonyms Mandrake; May Apple; Podophyllin

Pharmacologic Category Keratolytic Agent

Use Topical treatment of benign growths including external genital and perianal warts, papillomas, fibroids; compound benzoin tincture generally is used as the medium for topical application

Local Anesthetic/Vasoconstrictor Precautions No information available to require special precautions

Effects on Dental Treatment No significant effects or complications reported

Common Adverse Effects 1% to 10%:

Dermatologic: Pruritus

Gastrointestinal: Nausea, vomiting, abdominal pain, diarrhea

Mechanism of Action Directly affects epithelial cell metabolism by arresting mitosis through binding to a protein subunit of spindle microtubules (tubulin)

Pregnancy Risk Factor X

Poliovirus Vaccine (Inactivated)

(POE lee oh VYE rus vak SEEN, in ak ti VAY ted)

Related Information

Diphtheria, Tetanus Toxoids, Acellular Pertussis, Hepatitis B (Recombinant), and Poliovirus (Inactivated) Vaccine *on page 452*

Immunizations (Vaccines) *on page 1614*

U.S. Brand Names IPOL®

Canadian Brand Names IPOL™

Generic Available No

Synonyms Enhanced-potency Inactivated Poliovirus Vaccine; IPV; Salk Vaccine

Pharmacologic Category Vaccine

Use

As the global eradication of poliomyelitis continues, the risk for importation of wild-type poliovirus into the United States decreases dramatically. To eliminate the risk for vaccine-associated paralytic poliomyelitis (VAPP), an all-IPV schedule is recommended for routine childhood vaccination in the United States. All children should receive four doses of IPV (at age 2 months, age 4 months, between ages 6-18 months, and between ages 4-6 years). Oral poliovirus vaccine (OPV), if available, may be used only for the following special circumstances:

- Mass vaccination campaigns to control outbreaks of paralytic polio
- Unvaccinated children who will be traveling within 4 weeks to areas where polio is endemic or epidemic
- Children of parents who do not accept the recommended number of vaccine injections; these children may receive OPV only for the third or fourth dose or both. In this situation, healthcare providers should administer OPV only after discussing the risk for VAPP with parents or caregivers.

OPV supplies are expected to be very limited in the United States after inventories are depleted. ACIP reaffirms its support for the global eradication initiative and use of OPV as the vaccine of choice to eradicate polio where it is endemic.

Local Anesthetic/Vasoconstrictor Precautions No information available to require special precautions

Effects on Dental Treatment No significant effects or complications reported

(Continued)

Poliovirus Vaccine (Inactivated) *(Continued)*

Common Adverse Effects All serious adverse reactions must be reported to the U.S. Department of Health and Human Services (DHHS) Vaccine Adverse Event Reporting System (VAERS) 1-800-822-7967.

1% to 10%:

Central nervous system: Fever (>101.3°F)

Dermatologic: Rash

Local: Tenderness or pain at injection site

Pregnancy Risk Factor C

Polocaine® *see* Mepivacaine *on page 873*

Polocaine® MPF *see* Mepivacaine *on page 873*

Polycarbophil (KAL see um pol i KAR boe fil)

U.S. Brand Names Equalactin® [OTC]; FiberCon® [OTC]; Fiber-Lax® [OTC]; FiberNorm™ [OTC]; Konsyl® Tablets [OTC]; Phillips'® Fibercaps [OTC]

Mexican Brand Names Fibercon®

Generic Available Yes: Chewable tablet

Pharmacologic Category Antidiarrheal; Laxative, Bulk-Producing

Use Treatment of constipation or diarrhea

Local Anesthetic/Vasoconstrictor Precautions No information available to require special precautions

Effects on Dental Treatment Oral medication should be given at least 1 hour prior to taking the bulk-producing laxative in order to prevent decreased absorption of medication.

Mechanism of Action Restoring a more normal moisture level and providing bulk in the patient's intestinal tract

Pregnancy Risk Factor C

Polycitra® *see* Citric Acid, Sodium Citrate, and Potassium Citrate *on page 341*

Polycitra®-K *see* Potassium Citrate and Citric Acid *on page 1106*

Polycitra®-LC *see* Citric Acid, Sodium Citrate, and Potassium Citrate *on page 341*

Polycose® [OTC] *see* Glucose Polymers *on page 664*

Polyethylene Glycol-Electrolyte Solution

(pol i ETH i leen GLY kol ee LEK troe lite soe LOO shun)

U.S. Brand Names Colyte®; GoLYTELY®; MiraLax™; NuLytely®; TriLyte™

Canadian Brand Names Colyte™; Klean-Prep®; Klean-Prep®; Lyteprep™; PegLyte®; Peglyte™

Generic Available Yes

Synonyms Electrolyte Lavage Solution

Pharmacologic Category Cathartic; Laxative, Bowel Evacuant

Use Bowel cleansing prior to GI examination or following toxic ingestion (electrolyte containing solutions only); treatment of occasional constipation (MiraLax™)

Local Anesthetic/Vasoconstrictor Precautions No information available to require special precautions

Effects on Dental Treatment No significant effects or complications reported

Common Adverse Effects Frequency not defined.

Dermatologic: Dermatitis, rash, urticaria

Gastrointestinal: Nausea, abdominal fullness, bloating, abdominal cramps, vomiting, anal irritation, diarrhea, flatulence

Mechanism of Action Induces catharsis by strong electrolyte and osmotic effects

Drug Interactions

Decreased Effect: Oral medications should not be administered within 1 hour of start of therapy.

Pharmacodynamics/Kinetics Onset of effect: Oral: Bowel cleansing: ~1-2 hours; Constipation: 48-96 hours

Pregnancy Risk Factor C

Polygam® S/D *see* Immune Globulin (Intravenous) *on page 740*

Polymyxin B (pol i MIKS in bee)

Related Information

Neomycin and Polymyxin B *on page 973*

Neomycin, Polymyxin B, and Dexamethasone *on page 974*

Neomycin, Polymyxin B, and Prednisolone *on page 975*

U.S. Brand Names Poly-Rx

Generic Available Yes

Synonyms Polymyxin B Sulfate

Pharmacologic Category Antibiotic, Irrigation; Antibiotic, Miscellaneous

Use Treatment of acute infections caused by susceptible strains of *Pseudomonas aeruginosa*; used occasionally for gut decontamination; parenteral use of polymyxin B has mainly been replaced by less toxic antibiotics, reserved for life-threatening infections caused by organisms resistant to the preferred drugs (eg, pseudomonal meningitis - intrathecal administration)

Local Anesthetic/Vasoconstrictor Precautions No information available to require special precautions

Effects on Dental Treatment No significant effects or complications reported

Common Adverse Effects Frequency not defined.

Cardiovascular: Facial flushing

Central nervous system: Neurotoxicity (irritability, drowsiness, ataxia, perioral paresthesia, numbness of the extremities, and blurring of vision); dizziness, drug fever, meningeal irritation with intrathecal administration

Dermatologic: Urticarial rash

Endocrine & metabolic: Hypocalcemia, hyponatremia, hypokalemia, hypochloremia

Local: Pain at injection site

Neuromuscular & skeletal: Neuromuscular blockade, weakness

Renal: Nephrotoxicity

Respiratory: Respiratory arrest

Miscellaneous: Anaphylactoid reaction

Mechanism of Action Binds to phospholipids, alters permeability, and damages the bacterial cytoplasmic membrane permitting leakage of intracellular constituents

Drug Interactions

Increased Effect/Toxicity: Increased/prolonged effect of neuromuscular blocking agents.

Pharmacodynamics/Kinetics

Absorption: Well absorbed from peritoneum; minimal from GI tract (except in neonates) from mucous membranes or intact skin

Distribution: Minimal into CSF; does not cross placenta

Half-life elimination: 4.5-6 hours; prolonged with renal impairment

Time to peak, serum: I.M.: ~2 hours

Excretion: Urine (>60% primarily as unchanged drug)

Pregnancy Risk Factor B (per expert opinion)

Polymyxin B and Bacitracin *see* Bacitracin and Polymyxin B *on page 178*

Polymyxin B and Neomycin *see* Neomycin and Polymyxin B *on page 973*

Polymyxin B and Oxytetracycline *see* Oxytetracycline and Polymyxin B *on page 1037*

Polymyxin B and Trimethoprim *see* Trimethoprim and Polymyxin B *on page 1342*

Polymyxin B, Bacitracin, and Neomycin *see* Bacitracin, Neomycin, and Polymyxin B *on page 179*

Polymyxin B, Bacitracin, Neomycin, and Hydrocortisone *see* Bacitracin, Neomycin, Polymyxin B, and Hydrocortisone *on page 179*

Polymyxin B, Neomycin, and Dexamethasone *see* Neomycin, Polymyxin B, and Dexamethasone *on page 974*

Polymyxin B, Neomycin, and Gramicidin *see* Neomycin, Polymyxin B, and Gramicidin *on page 974*

Polymyxin B, Neomycin, and Hydrocortisone *see* Neomycin, Polymyxin B, and Hydrocortisone *on page 975*

Polymyxin B, Neomycin, and Prednisolone *see* Neomycin, Polymyxin B, and Prednisolone *on page 975*

Polymyxin B, Neomycin, Bacitracin, and Pramoxine *see* Bacitracin, Neomycin, Polymyxin B, and Pramoxine *on page 180*

Polymyxin B Sulfate *see* Polymyxin B *on page 1100*

Poly-Pred® *see* Neomycin, Polymyxin B, and Prednisolone *on page 975*

Poly-Rx *see* Polymyxin B *on page 1100*

Polysaccharide-Iron Complex

(pol i SAK a ride-EYE ern KOM pleks)

U.S. Brand Names Fe-Tinic™ 150 [OTC]; Hytinic® [OTC]; Niferex® [OTC]; Niferex® 150 [OTC]; Nu-Iron® 150 [OTC]

Generic Available Yes: Capsule

Synonyms Iron-Polysaccharide Complex

Pharmacologic Category Iron Salt

Use Prevention and treatment of iron-deficiency anemias

(Continued)

Polysaccharide-Iron Complex *(Continued)*

Local Anesthetic/Vasoconstrictor Precautions No information available to require special precautions

Effects on Dental Treatment No significant effects or complications reported

Common Adverse Effects

>10%: Gastrointestinal: Stomach cramping, constipation, nausea, vomiting, dark stools, GI irritation, epigastric pain, nausea

1% to 10%:

Gastrointestinal: Heartburn, diarrhea

Genitourinary: Discolored urine

Miscellaneous: Staining of teeth

Pregnancy Risk Factor A

Polysporin® Ophthalmic *see* Bacitracin and Polymyxin B *on page 178*

Polysporin® Topical [OTC] *see* Bacitracin and Polymyxin B *on page 178*

Polytar® [OTC] *see* Coal Tar *on page 367*

Polythiazide (pol i THYE a zide)

Related Information

Cardiovascular Diseases *on page 1458*

U.S. Brand Names Renese®

Generic Available No

Pharmacologic Category Diuretic, Thiazide

Use Adjunctive therapy in treatment of edema and hypertension

Local Anesthetic/Vasoconstrictor Precautions No information available to require special precautions

Effects on Dental Treatment No significant effects or complications reported

Mechanism of Action The diuretic mechanism of action of the thiazides is primarily inhibition of sodium, chloride, and water reabsorption in the renal distal tubules, thereby producing diuresis with a resultant reduction in plasma volume. The antihypertensive mechanism of action of the thiazides is unknown. It is known that doses of thiazides produce greater reductions in blood pressure than equivalent diuretic doses of loop diuretics (eg, furosemide). There has been speculation that the thiazides may have some influence on vascular tone mediated through sodium depletion, but this remains to be proven.

Pregnancy Risk Factor D

Polythiazide and Prazosin *see* Prazosin and Polythiazide *on page 1112*

Polytrim® *see* Trimethoprim and Polymyxin B *on page 1342*

Polyvinyl Alcohol *see* Artificial Tears *on page 148*

Ponstel® *see* Mefenamic Acid *on page 863*

Pontocaine® *see* Tetracaine *on page 1278*

Pontocaine® With Dextrose *see* Tetracaine and Dextrose *on page 1279*

Poractant Alfa (por AKT ant AL fa)

U.S. Brand Names Curosurf®

Canadian Brand Names Curosurf®

Generic Available No

Pharmacologic Category Lung Surfactant

Use Orphan drug: Treatment and prevention of respiratory distress syndrome (RDS) in premature infants

Local Anesthetic/Vasoconstrictor Precautions No information available to require special precautions

Effects on Dental Treatment No significant effects or complications reported

Common Adverse Effects Frequency not defined.

Cardiovascular: Bradycardia, hypotension

Gastrointestinal: Endotracheal tube blockage

Respiratory: Oxygen desaturation

Mechanism of Action Endogenous pulmonary surfactant reduces surface tension at the air-liquid interface of the alveoli during ventilation and stabilizes the alveoli against collapse at resting transpulmonary pressures. A deficiency of pulmonary surfactant in preterm infants results in respiratory distress syndrome characterized by poor lung expansion, inadequate gas exchange, and atelectasis. Poractant alpha compensates for the surfactant deficiency and restores surface activity to the infant's lungs. It reduces mortality and pneumothoraces associated with RDS.

Pharmacodynamics/Kinetics Information limited to animal models. No human information about pharmacokinetics exists.

Porfimer (POR fi mer)

U.S. Brand Names Photofrin®

Canadian Brand Names Photofrin®

Generic Available No

Synonyms CL-184116; Dihematoporphyrin Ether; Porfimer Sodium

Pharmacologic Category Antineoplastic Agent, Miscellaneous

Use Adjunct to laser light therapy for obstructing esophageal cancer, obstructing endobronchial nonsmall cell lung cancer (NSCLC), ablation of high-grade dysplasia in Barrett's esophagus

Unlabeled/Investigational Use Transitional cell carcinoma *in situ* of the urinary bladder; gastric and rectal cancers

Local Anesthetic/Vasoconstrictor Precautions No information available to require special precautions

Effects on Dental Treatment No significant effects or complications reported

Common Adverse Effects

>10%:

Cardiovascular: Atrial fibrillation (10%), chest pain (5% to 22%)

Central nervous system: Insomnia (14%), hyperthermia (31%)

Dermatologic: Photosensitivity reaction (10% to 80%, minor reactions may occur in up to 100%)

Gastrointestinal: Abdominal pain (20%), constipation (23%), dysphagia, nausea (24%), vomiting (17%)

Genitourinary: Urinary tract irritation including frequency, urgency, nocturia, painful urination, or bladder spasm (~100% of bladder cancer patients)

Hematologic: Anemia (26% of esophageal cancer patients)

Neuromuscular & skeletal: Back pain

Respiratory: Dyspnea (20%), pharyngitis (11%), pleural effusion (32% of esophageal cancer patients), pneumonia (18%), respiratory insufficiency

Miscellaneous: Mild-moderate allergic-type reactions (34% of lung cancer patients)

1% to 10%:

Cardiovascular: Hypertension (6% to 7%), hypotension (6% to 7%), edema, cardiac failure (6% to 7%), tachycardia (6%), chest pain (substernal)

Central nervous system: Anxiety (7%), confusion (8%)

Dermatologic: Increased hair growth, skin discoloration, skin wrinkles, skin nodules, increased skin fragility

Endocrine & metabolic: Dehydration

Gastrointestinal: Diarrhea (5%), dyspepsia (6%), eructation (5%), esophageal edema (8%), esophageal tumor bleeding, esophageal stricture, esophagitis, hematemesis, melena, weight loss, anorexia

Genitourinary: Urinary tract infection

Neuromuscular & skeletal: Weakness

Respiratory: Coughing, tracheoesophageal fistula

Miscellaneous: Moniliasis, surgical complication

Mechanism of Action Porfimer's cytotoxic activity is dependent on light and oxygen. Following administration, the drug is selectively retained in neoplastic tissues. Exposure of the drug to laser light at wavelengths >630 nm results in the production of oxygen free-radicals. Release of thromboxane A_2, leading to vascular occlusion and ischemic necrosis, may also occur.

Drug Interactions

Increased Effect/Toxicity: Concomitant administration of other photosensitizing agents (eg, tetracyclines, sulfonamides, phenothiazines, sulfonylureas, thiazide diuretics, griseofulvin) could increase the photosensitivity reaction.

Decreased Effect: Compounds that quench active oxygen species or scavenge radicals (eg, dimethyl sulfoxide, beta-carotene, ethanol, mannitol) would be expected to decrease photodynamic therapy (PDT) activity. Allopurinol, calcium channel blockers, and some prostaglandin synthesis inhibitors could interfere with porfimer. Drugs that decrease clotting, vasoconstriction, or platelet aggregation could decrease the efficacy of PDT. Glucocorticoid hormones may decrease the efficacy of the treatment.

Pharmacodynamics/Kinetics

Distribution: V_{dss}: 0.49 L/kg

Protein binding, plasma: 90%

Half-life elimination: Mean: 21.5 days (range: 11-28 days)

Time to peak, serum: ~2 hours

Excretion: Feces; Clearance: Plasma: Total: 0.051 mL/minute/kg

Pregnancy Risk Factor C

Porfimer Sodium *see* Porfimer *on page 1103*

Portia™ *see* Ethinyl Estradiol and Levonorgestrel *on page 545*

Post Peel Healing Balm [OTC] *see* Hydrocortisone *on page 714*
Posture® [OTC] *see* Calcium Phosphate (Tribasic) *on page 247*

Potassium Acetate (poe TASS ee um AS e tate)

Generic Available Yes

Pharmacologic Category Electrolyte Supplement, Parenteral

Use Potassium deficiency; to avoid chloride when high concentration of potassium is needed, source of bicarbonate

Local Anesthetic/Vasoconstrictor Precautions No information available to require special precautions

Effects on Dental Treatment No significant effects or complications reported

Mechanism of Action Potassium is the major cation of intracellular fluid and is essential for the conduction of nerve impulses in heart, brain, and skeletal muscle; contraction of cardiac, skeletal and smooth muscles; maintenance of normal renal function, acid-base balance, carbohydrate metabolism, and gastric secretion

Pregnancy Risk Factor C

Potassium Acetate, Potassium Bicarbonate, and Potassium Citrate

(poe TASS ee um AS e tate, poe TASS ee um bye KAR bun ate, & poe TASS ee um SIT rate)

U.S. Brand Names Tri-K®

Generic Available No

Synonyms Potassium Acetate, Potassium Citrate, and Potassium Bicarbonate; Potassium Bicarbonate, Potassium Acetate, and Potassium Citrate; Potassium Bicarbonate, Potassium Citrate, and Potassium Acetate; Potassium Citrate, Potassium Acetate, and Potassium Bicarbonate; Potassium Citrate, Potassium Bicarbonate, and Potassium Acetate

Pharmacologic Category Electrolyte Supplement, Oral

Use Treatment or prevention of hypokalemia

Local Anesthetic/Vasoconstrictor Precautions No information available to require special precautions

Effects on Dental Treatment No significant effects or complications reported

Pregnancy Risk Factor C

Potassium Acetate, Potassium Citrate, and Potassium Bicarbonate *see* Potassium Acetate, Potassium Bicarbonate, and Potassium Citrate *on page 1104*

Potassium Acid Phosphate (poe TASS ee um AS id FOS fate)

U.S. Brand Names K-Phos® Original

Generic Available No

Pharmacologic Category Urinary Acidifying Agent

Use Acidifies urine and lowers urinary calcium concentration; reduces odor and rash caused by ammoniacal urine; increases the antibacterial activity of methenamine

Local Anesthetic/Vasoconstrictor Precautions No information available to require special precautions

Effects on Dental Treatment No significant effects or complications reported

Mechanism of Action The principal intracellular cation; involved in transmission of nerve impulses, muscle contractions, enzyme activity, and glucose utilization

Pregnancy Risk Factor C

Potassium Bicarbonate (poe TASS ee um bye KAR bun ate)

U.S. Brand Names K+ Care® ET

Mexican Brand Names Kaliolite®; K-Dur®

Generic Available Yes

Pharmacologic Category Electrolyte Supplement, Oral

Use Potassium deficiency, hypokalemia

Local Anesthetic/Vasoconstrictor Precautions No information available to require special precautions

Effects on Dental Treatment No significant effects or complications reported

Pregnancy Risk Factor C

Potassium Bicarbonate and Potassium Chloride

(poe TASS ee um bye KAR bun ate & poe TASS ee um KLOR ide)

U.S. Brand Names K-Lyte/Cl®; K-Lyte/Cl® 50

Generic Available No

Synonyms Potassium Bicarbonate and Potassium Chloride (Effervescent)

Pharmacologic Category Electrolyte Supplement, Oral

Use Treatment or prevention of hypokalemia

Local Anesthetic/Vasoconstrictor Precautions No information available to require special precautions

Effects on Dental Treatment No significant effects or complications reported

Pregnancy Risk Factor C

Potassium Bicarbonate and Potassium Chloride (Effervescent) *see* Potassium Bicarbonate and Potassium Chloride *on page 1104*

Potassium Bicarbonate and Potassium Citrate

(poe TASS ee um bye KAR bun ate & poe TASS ee um SIT rate)

U.S. Brand Names Effer-K™; Klor-Con®/EF; K-Lyte®; K-Lyte® DS

Generic Available Yes

Synonyms Potassium Bicarbonate and Potassium Citrate (Effervescent)

Pharmacologic Category Electrolyte Supplement, Oral

Use Treatment or prevention of hypokalemia

Local Anesthetic/Vasoconstrictor Precautions No information available to require special precautions

Effects on Dental Treatment No significant effects or complications reported

Mechanism of Action Needed for the conduction of nerve impulses in heart, brain, and skeletal muscle; contraction of cardiac, skeletal and smooth muscles; maintenance of normal renal function

Pregnancy Risk Factor C

Potassium Bicarbonate and Potassium Citrate (Effervescent) *see* Potassium Bicarbonate and Potassium Citrate *on page 1105*

Potassium Bicarbonate, Potassium Acetate, and Potassium Citrate *see* Potassium Acetate, Potassium Bicarbonate, and Potassium Citrate *on page 1104*

Potassium Bicarbonate, Potassium Citrate, and Potassium Acetate *see* Potassium Acetate, Potassium Bicarbonate, and Potassium Citrate *on page 1104*

Potassium Chloride (poe TASS ee um KLOR ide)

U.S. Brand Names K+8; K+10; Kaon-Cl-10®; Kaon-Cl® 20; Kay Ciel®; K+ Care®; K-Dur® 10; K-Dur® 20; K-Lor™; Klor-Con®; Klor-Con® 8; Klor-Con® 10; Klor-Con®/25; Klor-Con® M; Klotrix®; K-Tab®; microK®; microK® 10; Rum-K®

Canadian Brand Names Apo-K®; K-10®; K-Dur®; K-Lor®; K-Lyte®/Cl; Micro-K Extencaps®; Roychlor®; Slow-K®

Generic Available Yes

Synonyms KCl

Pharmacologic Category Electrolyte Supplement, Oral; Electrolyte Supplement, Parenteral

Use Treatment or prevention of hypokalemia

Local Anesthetic/Vasoconstrictor Precautions No information available to require special precautions

Effects on Dental Treatment No significant effects or complications reported

Mechanism of Action Potassium is the major cation of intracellular fluid and is essential for the conduction of nerve impulses in heart, brain, and skeletal muscle; contraction of cardiac, skeletal and smooth muscles; maintenance of normal renal function, acid-base balance, carbohydrate metabolism, and gastric secretion

Pregnancy Risk Factor A

Potassium Citrate (poe TASS ee um SIT rate)

U.S. Brand Names Urocit®-K

Canadian Brand Names K-Citra®; K-Lyte®; Polycitra®-K

Generic Available No

Pharmacologic Category Alkalinizing Agent, Oral

Use Prevention of uric acid nephrolithiasis; prevention of calcium renal stones in patients with hypocitraturia; urinary alkalinizer when sodium citrate is contraindicated

Local Anesthetic/Vasoconstrictor Precautions No information available to require special precautions

Effects on Dental Treatment No significant effects or complications reported

Pregnancy Risk Factor Not available

Potassium Citrate and Citric Acid

(poe TASS ee um SIT rate & SI trik AS id)

U.S. Brand Names Cytra-K; Polycitra®-K

Generic Available Yes

Synonyms Citric Acid and Potassium Citrate

Pharmacologic Category Alkalinizing Agent, Oral

Use Treatment of metabolic acidosis; alkalinizing agent in conditions where long-term maintenance of an alkaline urine is desirable

Local Anesthetic/Vasoconstrictor Precautions No information available to require special precautions

Effects on Dental Treatment No significant effects or complications reported

Drug Interactions

Increased Effect/Toxicity: Concurrent administration with potassium-containing medications, potassium-sparing diuretics, ACE inhibitors, or cardiac glycosides could lead to toxicity.

Pharmacodynamics/Kinetics

Metabolism: To potassium bicarbonate; citric acid is metabolized to CO_2 and H_2O

Excretion: Urine

Pregnancy Risk Factor A

Potassium Citrate, Citric Acid, and Sodium Citrate *see* Citric Acid, Sodium Citrate, and Potassium Citrate *on page 341*

Potassium Citrate, Potassium Acetate, and Potassium Bicarbonate *see* Potassium Acetate, Potassium Bicarbonate, and Potassium Citrate *on page 1104*

Potassium Citrate, Potassium Bicarbonate, and Potassium Acetate *see* Potassium Acetate, Potassium Bicarbonate, and Potassium Citrate *on page 1104*

Potassium Gluconate (poe TASS ee um GLOO coe nate)

U.S. Brand Names Glu-K® [OTC]

Canadian Brand Names Kaon®

Generic Available Yes

Pharmacologic Category Electrolyte Supplement, Oral

Use Treatment or prevention of hypokalemia

Local Anesthetic/Vasoconstrictor Precautions No information available to require special precautions

Effects on Dental Treatment No significant effects or complications reported

Mechanism of Action Potassium is the major cation of intracellular fluid and is essential for the conduction of nerve impulses in heart, brain, and skeletal muscle; contraction of cardiac, skeletal and smooth muscles; maintenance of normal renal function, acid-base balance, carbohydrate metabolism, and gastric secretion

Pregnancy Risk Factor A

Potassium Guaiacolsulfonate and Guaifenesin *see* Guaifenesin and Potassium Guaiacolsulfonate *on page 675*

Potassium Guaiacolsulfonate, Dextromethorphan, and Guaifenesin *see* Guaifenesin, Potassium Guaiacolsulfonate, and Dextromethorphan *on page 675*

Potassium Iodide (poe TASS ee um EYE oh dide)

Related Information

Endocrine Disorders and Pregnancy *on page 1481*

U.S. Brand Names Iosat™ [OTC]; Pima®; SSKI®

Generic Available Yes

Synonyms KI; Lugol's Solution; Strong Iodine Solution

Pharmacologic Category Antithyroid Agent; Expectorant

Use Expectorant for the symptomatic treatment of chronic pulmonary diseases complicated by mucous; reduce thyroid vascularity prior to thyroidectomy and management of thyrotoxic crisis; block thyroidal uptake of radioactive isotopes of iodine in a radiation emergency or other exposure to radioactive iodine

Unlabeled/Investigational Use Lymphocutaneous and cutaneous sporotrichosis

Local Anesthetic/Vasoconstrictor Precautions No information available to require special precautions

Effects on Dental Treatment No significant effects or complications reported

Common Adverse Effects Frequency not defined.

Cardiovascular: Irregular heart beat

Central nervous system: Confusion, tiredness, fever

Dermatologic: Skin rash

Endocrine & metabolic: Goiter, salivary gland swelling/tenderness, thyroid adenoma, swelling of neck/throat, myxedema, lymph node swelling

Gastrointestinal: Diarrhea, gastrointestinal bleeding, metallic taste, nausea, stomach pain, stomach upset, vomiting

Neuromuscular & skeletal: Numbness, tingling, weakness

Miscellaneous: Chronic iodine poisoning (with prolonged treatment/high doses); iodism, hypersensitivity reactions (angioedema, cutaneous and mucosal hemorrhage, serum sickness-like symptoms)

Mechanism of Action Reduces viscosity of mucus by increasing respiratory tract secretions; inhibits secretion of thyroid hormone, fosters colloid accumulation in thyroid follicles

Drug Interactions

Increased Effect/Toxicity: Lithium may cause additive hypothyroid effects; ACE inhibitors, potassium-sparing diuretics, and potassium/potassium-containing products may lead to hyperkalemia, cardiac arrhythmias, or cardiac arrest

Pharmacodynamics/Kinetics

Onset of action: 24-48 hours

Peak effect: 10-15 days after continuous therapy

Duration: May persist for up to 6 weeks

Excretion: Clearance: Euthyroid patient: Renal: 2 times that of thyroid

Pregnancy Risk Factor D

Potassium Iodide, Chlorpheniramine, Phenylephrine, and Codeine *see* Chlorpheniramine, Phenylephrine, Codeine, and Potassium Iodide *on page 318*

Potassium Phosphate (poe TASS ee um FOS fate)

U.S. Brand Names Neutra-Phos®-K [OTC]

Generic Available Yes

Synonyms Phosphate, Potassium

Pharmacologic Category Electrolyte Supplement, Oral; Electrolyte Supplement, Parenteral

Use Treatment and prevention of hypophosphatemia or hypokalemia

Local Anesthetic/Vasoconstrictor Precautions No information available to require special precautions

Effects on Dental Treatment No significant effects or complications reported

Pregnancy Risk Factor C

Potassium Phosphate and Sodium Phosphate

(poe TASS ee um FOS fate & SOW dee um FOS fate)

U.S. Brand Names K-Phos® MF; K-Phos® Neutral; K-Phos® No. 2; Neutra-Phos® [OTC]; Uro-KP-Neutral®

Generic Available Yes

Synonyms Sodium Phosphate and Potassium Phosphate

Pharmacologic Category Electrolyte Supplement, Oral

Use Treatment of conditions associated with excessive renal phosphate loss or inadequate GI absorption of phosphate; to acidify the urine to lower calcium concentrations; to increase the antibacterial activity of methenamine; reduce odor and rash caused by ammonia in urine

Local Anesthetic/Vasoconstrictor Precautions No information available to require special precautions

Effects on Dental Treatment No significant effects or complications reported

Pregnancy Risk Factor C

Povidone-Iodine (POE vi done EYE oh dyne)

Related Information

Animal and Human Bites Guidelines *on page 1582*

Management of Patients Undergoing Cancer Therapy *on page 1569*

U.S. Brand Names ACU-dyne® [OTC]; Betadine® [OTC]; Betadine® Ophthalmic; Minidyne® [OTC]; Operand® [OTC]; Summer's Eve® Medicated Douche [OTC]; Vagi-Gard® [OTC]

Canadian Brand Names Betadine®; Proviodine

Mexican Brand Names Isodine®; Yodine®

Generic Available Yes

Pharmacologic Category Antibiotic, Ophthalmic; Antibiotic, Topical; Antibiotic, Vaginal; Topical Skin Product

Use External antiseptic with broad microbicidal spectrum against bacteria, fungi, viruses, protozoa, and yeasts

Local Anesthetic/Vasoconstrictor Precautions No information available to require special precautions

(Continued)

Povidone-Iodine *(Continued)*

Effects on Dental Treatment No significant effects or complications reported

Common Adverse Effects 1% to 10%:

Dermatologic: Rash, pruritus

Local: Local edema

Mechanism of Action Povidone-iodine is known to be a powerful broad spectrum germicidal agent effective against a wide range of bacteria, viruses, fungi, protozoa, and spores.

Pharmacodynamics/Kinetics Absorption: Topical: Healthy volunteers: Little systemic absorption; Vaginal: Rapid, serum concentrations of total iodine and inorganic iodide are increased significantly

Pregnancy Risk Factor D

PPD *see* Tuberculin Tests *on page 1349*

PPI-149 *see* Abarelix *on page 43*

PPL *see* Benzylpenicilloyl-polylysine *on page 196*

PPS *see* Pentosan Polysulfate Sodium *on page 1065*

Pramipexole (pra mi PEKS ole)

U.S. Brand Names Mirapex®

Canadian Brand Names Mirapex®

Generic Available No

Pharmacologic Category Anti-Parkinson's Agent, Dopamine Agonist

Use Treatment of the signs and symptoms of idiopathic Parkinson's disease

Unlabeled/Investigational Use Treatment of depression

Local Anesthetic/Vasoconstrictor Precautions No information available to require special precautions

Effects on Dental Treatment No significant effects or complications reported

Common Adverse Effects

>10%:

Cardiovascular: Postural hypotension

Central nervous system: Asthenia, dizziness, somnolence, insomnia, hallucinations, abnormal dreams

Gastrointestinal: Nausea, constipation

Neuromuscular & skeletal: Weakness, dyskinesia, EPS

1% to 10%:

Cardiovascular: Edema, syncope, tachycardia, chest pain

Central nervous system: Malaise, confusion, amnesia, dystonias, akathisia, thinking abnormalities, myoclonus, hyperesthesia, paranoia, fever

Endocrine & metabolic: Decreased libido

Gastrointestinal: Anorexia, weight loss, xerostomia, dysphagia

Genitourinary: Urinary frequency, impotence, urinary incontinence

Neuromuscular & skeletal: Muscle twitching, leg cramps, arthritis, bursitis, myasthenia, gait abnormalities, hypertonia

Ocular: Vision abnormalities

Respiratory: Dyspnea, rhinitis

Mechanism of Action Pramipexole is a nonergot dopamine agonist with specificity for the D_2 subfamily dopamine receptor, and has also been shown to bind to D_3 and D_4 receptors. By binding to these receptors, it is thought that pramipexole can stimulate dopamine activity on the nerves of the striatum and substantia nigra.

Drug Interactions

Increased Effect/Toxicity: Cimetidine in combination with pramipexole produced a 50% increase in AUC and a 40% increase in half-life. Drugs secreted by the cationic transport system (diltiazem, triamterene, verapamil, quinidine, quinine, ranitidine) decrease the clearance of pramipexole by ~20%.

Decreased Effect: Dopamine antagonists (antipsychotics, metoclopramide) may decrease the efficiency of pramipexole.

Pharmacodynamics/Kinetics

Protein binding: 15%

Bioavailability: 90%

Half-life elimination: ~8 hours; Elderly: 12-14 hours

Time to peak, serum: ~2 hours

Excretion: Urine (90% as unchanged drug)

Pregnancy Risk Factor C

Pramosone® *see* Pramoxine and Hydrocortisone *on page 1109*

Pramoxine (pra MOKS een)

U.S. Brand Names Anusol® Ointment [OTC]; Itch-X® [OTC]; Prax® [OTC]; ProctoFoam® NS [OTC]; Tronolane® [OTC]

Generic Available No

Synonyms Pramoxine Hydrochloride

Pharmacologic Category Local Anesthetic

Use Temporary relief of pain and itching associated with anogenital pruritus or irritation; dermatosis, minor burns, or hemorrhoids

Local Anesthetic/Vasoconstrictor Precautions No information available to require special precautions

Effects on Dental Treatment No significant effects or complications reported

Common Adverse Effects 1% to 10%:

Dermatologic: Angioedema

Local: Contact dermatitis, burning, stinging

Mechanism of Action Pramoxine, like other anesthetics, decreases the neuronal membrane's permeability to sodium ions; both initiation and conduction of nerve impulses are blocked, thus depolarization of the neuron is inhibited

Pharmacodynamics/Kinetics

Onset of action: Therapeutic: 2-5 minutes

Peak effect: 3-5 minutes

Duration: Several days

Pregnancy Risk Factor C

Pramoxine and Hydrocortisone

(pra MOKS een & hye droe KOR ti sone)

Related Information

Hydrocortisone *on page 714*

Pramoxine *on page 1109*

U.S. Brand Names Analpram-HC®; Enzone®; Epifoam®; Pramosone®; ProctoFoam®-HC; Zone-A®; Zone-A Forte®

Canadian Brand Names Pramox® HC; Proctofoam™-HC

Generic Available No

Synonyms Hydrocortisone and Pramoxine

Pharmacologic Category Anesthetic/Corticosteroid

Use Relief of inflammatory and pruritic manifestations of corticosteroid-responsive dermatoses

Local Anesthetic/Vasoconstrictor Precautions No information available to require special precautions

Effects on Dental Treatment No significant effects or complications reported

Common Adverse Effects See individual agents.

Drug Interactions

Cytochrome P450 Effect: Hydrocortisone: **Substrate** of CYP3A4 (minor); **Induces** CYP3A4 (weak)

Increased Effect/Toxicity: See individual agents.

Decreased Effect: See individual agents.

Pharmacodynamics/Kinetics See individual agents.

Pregnancy Risk Factor C

Pramoxine Hydrochloride *see* Pramoxine *on page 1109*

Pramoxine, Neomycin, Bacitracin, and Polymyxin B *see* Bacitracin, Neomycin, Polymyxin B, and Pramoxine *on page 180*

Prandin® *see* Repaglinide *on page 1173*

Pravachol® *see* Pravastatin *on page 1109*

Pravastatin (PRA va stat in)

Related Information

Cardiovascular Diseases *on page 1458*

U.S. Brand Names Pravachol®

Canadian Brand Names Apo-Pravastatin®; Lin-Pravastatin; Novo-Pravastatin; PMS-Pravastatin; Pravachol®; ratio-Pravastatin

Mexican Brand Names Pravacol®

Generic Available No

Synonyms Pravastatin Sodium

Pharmacologic Category Antilipemic Agent, HMG-CoA Reductase Inhibitor

Use Use with dietary therapy for the following:

Primary prevention of coronary events: In hypercholesterolemic patients without established coronary heart disease to reduce cardiovascular morbidity (myocardial infarction, coronary revascularization procedures) and mortality.

(Continued)

Pravastatin *(Continued)*

Secondary prevention of cardiovascular events in patients with established coronary heart disease: To slow the progression of coronary atherosclerosis; to reduce cardiovascular morbidity (myocardial infarction, coronary vascular procedures) and to reduce mortality; to reduce the risk of stroke and transient ischemic attacks

Hyperlipidemias: Reduce elevations in total cholesterol, LDL-C, apolipoprotein B, and triglycerides (elevations of 1 or more components are present in Fredrickson type IIa, IIb, III, and IV hyperlipidemias)

Heterozygous familial hypercholesterolemia (HeFH): In pediatric patients, 8-18 years of age, with HeFH having LDL-C ≥190 mg/dL **or** LDL ≥160 mg/dL with positive family history of premature cardiovascular disease (CVD) or 2 or more CVD risk factors in the pediatric patient

Local Anesthetic/Vasoconstrictor Precautions No information available to require special precautions

Effects on Dental Treatment No significant effects or complications reported

Common Adverse Effects As reported in short-term trials; safety and tolerability with long-term use were similar to placebo

1% to 10%:

Cardiovascular: Chest pain (4%)

Central nervous system: Headache (2% to 6%), fatigue (4%), dizziness (1% to 3%)

Dermatologic: Rash (4%)

Gastrointestinal: Nausea/vomiting (7%), diarrhea (6%), heartburn (3%)

Hepatic: Increased transaminases (>3x normal on two occasions - 1%)

Neuromuscular & skeletal: Myalgia (2%)

Respiratory: Cough (3%)

Miscellaneous: Influenza (2%)

Additional class-related events or case reports (not necessarily reported with pravastatin therapy): Angioedema, cataracts, depression, dyspnea, eosinophilia, erectile dysfunction, facial paresis, hypersensitivity reaction, impaired extraocular muscle movement, impotence, leukopenia, malaise, memory loss, ophthalmoplegia, paresthesia, peripheral neuropathy, photosensitivity, psychic disturbance, skin discoloration, thrombocytopenia, thyroid dysfunction, toxic epidermal necrolysis, transaminases increased, vomiting

Dosage Oral: **Note:** Doses should be individualized according to the baseline LDL-cholesterol levels, the recommended goal of therapy, and patient response; adjustments should be made at intervals of 4 weeks or more; doses may need adjusted based on concomitant medications

Children: HeFH:

8-13 years: 20 mg/day

14-18 years: 40 mg/day

Dosage adjustment for pravastatin based on concomitant immunosuppressants (ie, cyclosporine): Refer to Adults dosing section

Adults: Hyperlipidemias, primary prevention of coronary events, secondary prevention of cardiovascular events: Initial: 40 mg once daily; titrate dosage to response; usual range: 10-80 mg; (maximum dose: 80 mg once daily)

Dosage adjustment for pravastatin based on concomitant immunosuppressants (ie, cyclosporine): Initial: 10 mg/day, titrate with caution (maximum dose: 20 mg/day)

Elderly: No specific dosage recommendations. Clearance is reduced in the elderly, resulting in an increase in AUC between 25% to 50%. However, substantial accumulation is not expected.

Dosing adjustment in renal impairment: Initial: 10 mg/day

Dosing adjustment in hepatic impairment: Initial: 10 mg/day

Mechanism of Action Pravastatin is a competitive inhibitor of 3-hydroxy-3-methylglutaryl coenzyme A (HMG-CoA) reductase, which is the rate-limiting enzyme involved in *de novo* cholesterol synthesis.

Contraindications Hypersensitivity to pravastatin or any component of the formulation; active liver disease; unexplained persistent elevations of serum transaminases; pregnancy; breast-feeding

Warnings/Precautions Secondary causes of hyperlipidemia should be ruled out prior to therapy. Liver function must be monitored by periodic laboratory assessment. Rhabdomyolysis with acute renal failure has occurred. Risk may be increased with concurrent use of other drugs which may cause rhabdomyolysis (including gemfibrozil, fibric acid derivatives, or niacin at doses ≥1 g/day). Temporarily discontinue in any patient experiencing an acute or serious condition predisposing to renal failure secondary to rhabdomyolysis. Use caution in patients with previous liver disease or heavy ethanol use. Treatment in patients <8 years of age is not recommended.

Drug Interactions

Cytochrome P450 Effect: Substrate of CYP3A4 (minor); **Inhibits** CYP2C8/9 (weak), 2D6 (weak), 3A4 (weak)

Increased Effect/Toxicity: Clofibrate, cyclosporine, fenofibrate, gemfibrozil, and niacin may increase the risk of myopathy and rhabdomyolysis. Imidazole antifungals (itraconazole, ketoconazole), P-glycoprotein inhibitors may increase pravastatin concentrations.

Decreased Effect: Concurrent administration of cholestyramine or colestipol can decrease pravastatin absorption.

Ethanol/Nutrition/Herb Interactions

Ethanol: Consumption of large amounts of ethanol may increase the risk of liver damage with HMG-CoA reductase inhibitors.

Herb/Nutraceutical: St John's wort may decrease pravastatin levels.

Dietary Considerations May be taken without regard to meals. Before initiation of therapy, patients should be placed on a standard cholesterol-lowering diet for 6 weeks and the diet should be continued during drug therapy.

Pharmacodynamics/Kinetics

Onset of action: Several days

Peak effect: 4 weeks

Absorption: Rapidly absorbed; average absorption 34%

Protein binding: 50%

Metabolism: Hepatic to at least two metabolites

Bioavailability: 17%

Half-life elimination: ~2-3 hours

Time to peak, serum: 1-1.5 hours

Excretion: Feces (70%); urine (≤20%, 8% as unchanged drug)

Pregnancy Risk Factor X

Dosage Forms TAB: 10 mg, 20 mg, 40 mg, 80 mg

Pravastatin and Aspirin *see* Aspirin and Pravastatin *on page 157*

Pravastatin Sodium *see* Pravastatin *on page 1109*

Pravigard™ PAC *see* Aspirin and Pravastatin *on page 157*

Prax® [OTC] *see* Pramoxine *on page 1109*

Praziquantel (pray zi KWON tel)

U.S. Brand Names Biltricide®

Canadian Brand Names Biltricide®

Mexican Brand Names Cesol®; Cisticid®

Generic Available No

Pharmacologic Category Anthelmintic

Use All stages of schistosomiasis caused by all *Schistosoma* species pathogenic to humans; clonorchiasis and opisthorchiasis

Unlabeled/Investigational Use Cysticercosis and many intestinal tapeworms

Local Anesthetic/Vasoconstrictor Precautions No information available to require special precautions

Effects on Dental Treatment No significant effects or complications reported

Common Adverse Effects 1% to 10%:

Central nervous system: Dizziness, drowsiness, headache, malaise, CSF reaction syndrome in patients being treated for neurocysticercosis

Gastrointestinal: Abdominal pain, loss of appetite, nausea, vomiting

Miscellaneous: Diaphoresis

Mechanism of Action Increases the cell permeability to calcium in schistosomes, causing strong contractions and paralysis of worm musculature leading to detachment of suckers from the blood vessel walls and to dislodgment

Drug Interactions

Cytochrome P450 Effect: Inhibits CYP2D6 (weak)

Pharmacodynamics/Kinetics

Absorption: Oral: ~80%

Distribution: CSF concentration is 14% to 20% of plasma concentration; enters breast milk

Protein binding: ~80%

Metabolism: Extensive first-pass effect

Half-life elimination: Parent drug: 0.8-1.5 hours; Metabolites: 4.5 hours

Time to peak, serum: 1-3 hours

Excretion: Urine (99% as metabolites)

Pregnancy Risk Factor B

Prazosin (PRA zoe sin)

Related Information

Cardiovascular Diseases *on page 1458*

U.S. Brand Names Minipress®

(Continued)

Prazosin *(Continued)*

Canadian Brand Names Apo-Prazo®; Minipress™; Novo-Prazin; Nu-Prazo

Mexican Brand Names Minipres®; Sinozzard®

Generic Available Yes

Synonyms Furazosin; Prazosin Hydrochloride

Pharmacologic Category $Alpha_1$ Blocker

Use Treatment of hypertension

Unlabeled/Investigational Use Benign prostatic hyperplasia; Raynaud's syndrome

Local Anesthetic/Vasoconstrictor Precautions No information available to require special precautions

Effects on Dental Treatment Key adverse event(s) related to dental treatment: Significant xerostomia (normal salivary flow resumes upon discontinuation). Significant orthostatic hypotension is a possibility; monitor patient when getting out of dental chair.

Common Adverse Effects

>10%: Central nervous system: Dizziness (10%)

1% to 10%:

- Cardiovascular: Palpitations (5%), edema, orthostatic hypotension, syncope (1%)
- Central nervous system: Headache (8%), drowsiness (8%), weakness (7%), vertigo, depression, nervousness
- Dermatologic: Rash (1% to 4%)
- Endocrine & metabolic: Decreased energy (7%)
- Gastrointestinal: Nausea (5%), vomiting, diarrhea, constipation
- Genitourinary: Urinary frequency (1% to 5%)
- Ocular: Blurred vision, reddened sclera, xerostomia
- Respiratory: Dyspnea, epistaxis, nasal congestion

Mechanism of Action Competitively inhibits postsynaptic alpha-adrenergic receptors which results in vasodilation of veins and arterioles and a decrease in total peripheral resistance and blood pressure

Drug Interactions

Increased Effect/Toxicity: Prazosin's hypotensive effect may be increased with beta-blockers, diuretics, ACE inhibitors, calcium channel blockers, other antihypertensive medications, sildenafil (use with extreme caution at a dose ≤25 mg), tadalafil (use is contraindicated by the manufacturer), and vardenafil (use is contraindicated by the manufacturer). Concurrent use with tricyclic antidepressants (TCAs) and low-potency antipsychotics may increase risk of orthostasis.

Decreased Effect: Decreased antihypertensive effect if taken with NSAIDs.

Pharmacodynamics/Kinetics

Onset of action: BP reduction: ~2 hours

Maximum decrease: 2-4 hours

Duration: 10-24 hours

Distribution: Hypertensive adults: V_d: 0.5 L/kg

Protein binding: 92% to 97%

Metabolism: Extensively hepatic

Bioavailability: 43% to 82%

Half-life elimination: 2-4 hours; prolonged with congestive heart failure

Excretion: Urine (6% to 10% as unchanged drug)

Pregnancy Risk Factor C

Prazosin and Polythiazide (PRA zoe sin & pol i THYE a zide)

Related Information

Polythiazide *on page 1102*

Prazosin *on page 1111*

U.S. Brand Names Minizide®

Generic Available No

Synonyms Polythiazide and Prazosin

Pharmacologic Category Antihypertensive Agent, Combination

Use Management of mild to moderate hypertension

Local Anesthetic/Vasoconstrictor Precautions No information available to require special precautions

Effects on Dental Treatment Key adverse event(s) related to dental treatment: Significant xerostomia (normal salivary flow resumes upon discontinuation). Significant orthostatic hypotension is a possibility; monitor patient when getting out of dental chair.

Common Adverse Effects See individual agents.

Pharmacodynamics/Kinetics See individual agents.

Pregnancy Risk Factor C

Prazosin Hydrochloride *see* Prazosin *on page 1111*
Precedex™ *see* Dexmedetomidine *on page 415*
Precose® *see* Acarbose *on page 45*
Pred Forte® *see* PrednisoLONE *on page 1113*
Pred-G® *see* Prednisolone and Gentamicin *on page 1115*
Pred Mild® *see* PrednisoLONE *on page 1113*

Prednicarbate (PRED ni kar bate)

U.S. Brand Names Dermatop®

Canadian Brand Names Dermatop®

Generic Available No

Pharmacologic Category Corticosteroid, Topical

Use Relief of the inflammatory and pruritic manifestations of corticosteroid-responsive dermatoses (medium potency topical corticosteroid)

Local Anesthetic/Vasoconstrictor Precautions No information available to require special precautions

Effects on Dental Treatment No significant effects or complications reported

Mechanism of Action Topical corticosteroids have anti-inflammatory, antipruritic, vasoconstrictive, and antiproliferative actions

Pregnancy Risk Factor C

PrednisoLONE (pred NISS oh lone)

Related Information

Neomycin, Polymyxin B, and Prednisolone *on page 975*
PredniSONE *on page 1115*
Respiratory Diseases *on page 1478*

U.S. Brand Names AK-Pred®; Econopred®; Econopred® Plus; Inflamase® Forte; Inflamase® Mild; Orapred®; Pediapred®; Pred Forte®; Pred Mild®; Prelone®

Canadian Brand Names Diopred®; Hydeltra T.B.A.®; Inflamase® Forte; Inflamase® Mild; Novo-Prednisolone®; Ophtho-Tate®; Pediapred®; Pred Forte®; Pred Mild®; Sab-Prenase

Generic Available Yes

Synonyms Deltahydrocortisone; Metacortandralone; Prednisolone Acetate; Prednisolone Acetate, Ophthalmic; Prednisolone Sodium Phosphate; Prednisolone Sodium Phosphate, Ophthalmic

Pharmacologic Category Corticosteroid, Ophthalmic; Corticosteroid, Systemic

Dental Use Treatment of a variety of oral diseases of allergic, inflammatory, or autoimmune origin

Use Treatment of palpebral and bulbar conjunctivitis; corneal injury from chemical, radiation, thermal burns, or foreign body penetration; endocrine disorders, rheumatic disorders, collagen diseases, dermatologic diseases, allergic states, ophthalmic diseases, respiratory diseases, hematologic disorders, neoplastic diseases, edematous states, and gastrointestinal diseases; useful in patients with inability to activate prednisone (liver disease)

Local Anesthetic/Vasoconstrictor Precautions No information available to require special precautions

Effects on Dental Treatment No significant effects or complications reported

Significant Adverse Effects Systemic:

>10%:
- Central nervous system: Insomnia, nervousness
- Gastrointestinal: Increased appetite, indigestion

1% to 10%:
- Central nervous system: Dizziness or lightheadedness, headache
- Dermatologic: Hirsutism, hypopigmentation
- Endocrine & metabolic: Diabetes mellitus
- Neuromuscular & skeletal: Arthralgia
- Ocular: Cataracts, glaucoma
- Respiratory: Epistaxis
- Miscellaneous: Diaphoresis

<1% (Limited to important or life-threatening): Cushing's syndrome, edema, fractures, hallucinations, hypersensitivity reactions, hypertension, muscle wasting, osteoporosis, pancreatitis, pituitary-adrenal axis suppression, pseudotumor cerebri, seizures

Dosage Dose depends upon condition being treated and response of patient; dosage for infants and children should be based on severity of the disease and response of the patient rather than on strict adherence to dosage indicated by age, weight, or body surface area. Consider alternate day therapy for

(Continued)

PrednisoLONE *(Continued)*

long-term therapy. Discontinuation of long-term therapy requires gradual withdrawal by tapering the dose.

Children: Oral:

Acute asthma: 1-2 mg/kg/day in divided doses 1-2 times/day for 3-5 days

Anti-inflammatory or immunosuppressive dose: 0.1-2 mg/kg/day in divided doses 1-4 times/day

Nephrotic syndrome:

Initial (first 3 episodes): 2 mg/kg/day **or** 60 mg/m²/day (maximum: 80 mg/day) in divided doses 3-4 times/day until urine is protein free for 3 consecutive days (maximum: 28 days); followed by 1-1.5 mg/kg/dose **or** 40 mg/m²/dose given every other day for 4 weeks

Maintenance (long-term maintenance dose for frequent relapses): 0.5-1 mg/kg/dose given every other day for 3-6 months

Children and Adults: Ophthalmic suspension/solution: Instill 1-2 drops into conjunctival sac every hour during day, every 2 hours at night until favorable response is obtained, then use 1 drop every 4 hours

Adults: Oral:

Usual range: 5-60 mg/day

Multiple sclerosis: 200 mg/day for 1 week followed by 80 mg every other day for 1 month

Rheumatoid arthritis: Initial: 5-7.5 mg/day; adjust dose as necessary

Elderly: Use lowest effective dose

Dosing adjustment in hyperthyroidism: Prednisolone dose may need to be increased to achieve adequate therapeutic effects

Hemodialysis: Slightly dialyzable (5% to 20%); administer dose posthemodialysis

Peritoneal dialysis: Supplemental dose is not necessary

Mechanism of Action Decreases inflammation by suppression of migration of polymorphonuclear leukocytes and reversal of increased capillary permeability; suppresses the immune system by reducing activity and volume of the lymphatic system

Contraindications Hypersensitivity to prednisolone or any component of the formulation; acute superficial herpes simplex keratitis; systemic fungal infections; varicella

Warnings/Precautions Use with caution in patients with hyperthyroidism, cirrhosis, nonspecific ulcerative colitis, hypertension, osteoporosis, thromboembolic tendencies, CHF, convulsive disorders, myasthenia gravis, thrombophlebitis, peptic ulcer, diabetes; acute adrenal insufficiency may occur with abrupt withdrawal after long-term therapy or with stress; young pediatric patients may be more susceptible to adrenal axis suppression from topical therapy. Because of the risk of adverse effects, systemic corticosteroids should be used cautiously in the elderly, in the smallest possible dose, and for the shortest possible time.

Drug Interactions **Substrate** of CYP3A4 (minor); **Inhibits** CYP3A4 (weak)

Decreased effect:

Barbiturates, phenytoin, rifampin decrease corticosteroid effectiveness

Decreases salicylates

Decreases vaccines

Decreases toxoids effectiveness

Ethanol/Nutrition/Herb Interactions

Ethanol: Avoid ethanol (may increase gastric mucosal irritation).

Food: Prednisolone interferes with calcium absorption. Limit caffeine.

Herb/Nutraceutical: St John's wort may decrease prednisolone levels. Avoid cat's claw, echinacea (have immunostimulant properties).

Dietary Considerations Should be taken after meals or with food or milk to decrease GI effects; increase dietary intake of pyridoxine, vitamin C, vitamin D, folate, calcium, and phosphorus.

Pharmacodynamics/Kinetics

Duration: 18-36 hours

Protein binding (concentration dependent): 65% to 91%

Metabolism: Primarily hepatic, but also metabolized in most tissues, to inactive compounds

Half-life elimination: 3.6 hours; End-stage renal disease: 3-5 hours

Excretion: Primarily urine (as glucuronides, sulfates, and unconjugated metabolites)

Pregnancy Risk Factor C

Lactation Enters breast milk/compatible

Dosage Forms

Solution, ophthalmic, as sodium phosphate: 1% (5 mL, 10 mL, 15 mL) [contains benzalkonium chloride]

AK-Pred®: 1% (5 mL, 15 mL) [contains benzalkonium chloride]

Inflamase® Forte: 1% (5 mL, 10 mL, 15 mL) [contains benzalkonium chloride]

Inflamase® Mild: 0.125% (5 mL, 10 mL) [contains benzalkonium chloride]

Solution, oral, as sodium phosphate: Prednisolone base 5 mg/5 mL (120 mL)

Orapred®: 20 mg/5 mL (240 mL) [equivalent to prednisolone base 15 mg/5 mL; dye free; contains alcohol 2%, sodium benzoate; grape flavor]

Pediapred®: 6.7 mg/5 mL (120 mL) [equivalent to prednisolone base 5 mg/5 mL; dye free; raspberry flavor]

Suspension, ophthalmic, as acetate: 1% (5 mL, 10 mL, 15 mL) [contains benzalkonium chloride]

Econopred®: 0.125% (5 mL, 10 mL) [contains benzalkonium chloride]

Econopred® Plus: 1% (5 mL, 10 mL) [contains benzalkonium chloride]

Pred Forte®: 1% (1 mL, 5 mL, 10 mL, 15 mL) [contains benzalkonium chloride and sodium bisulfite]

Pred Mild®: 0.12% (5 mL, 10 mL) [contains benzalkonium chloride and sodium bisulfite]

Syrup, as base: 5 mg/5 mL (120 mL); 15 mg/5 mL (240 mL, 480 mL)

Prelone®: 5 mg/5 mL (120 mL) [dye free, sugar free; contains alcohol ≤0.4%, benzoic acid; wild cherry flavor]; 15 mg/5 mL (240 mL, 480 mL) [contains alcohol 5%, benzoic acid; wild cherry flavor]

Tablet, as base: 5 mg [contains sodium benzoate]

Prednisolone Acetate *see* PrednisoLONE *on page 1113*

Prednisolone Acetate, Ophthalmic *see* PrednisoLONE *on page 1113*

Prednisolone and Gentamicin

(pred NIS oh lone & jen ta MYE sin)

Related Information

PrednisoLONE *on page 1113*

U.S. Brand Names Pred-G®

Generic Available No

Synonyms Gentamicin and Prednisolone

Pharmacologic Category Antibiotic/Corticosteroid, Ophthalmic

Use Treatment of steroid responsive inflammatory conditions and superficial ocular infections due to microorganisms susceptible to gentamicin

Local Anesthetic/Vasoconstrictor Precautions No information available to require special precautions

Effects on Dental Treatment No significant effects or complications reported

Pregnancy Risk Factor C

Prednisolone and Sulfacetamide *see* Sulfacetamide and Prednisolone *on page 1245*

Prednisolone, Neomycin, and Polymyxin B *see* Neomycin, Polymyxin B, and Prednisolone *on page 975*

Prednisolone Sodium Phosphate *see* PrednisoLONE *on page 1113*

Prednisolone Sodium Phosphate, Ophthalmic *see* PrednisoLONE *on page 1113*

PredniSONE (PRED ni sone)

Related Information

Oral Nonviral Soft Tissue Ulcerations or Erosions *on page 1551*

PrednisoLONE *on page 1113*

Respiratory Diseases *on page 1478*

Rheumatoid Arthritis, Osteoarthritis, and Osteoporosis *on page 1490*

U.S. Brand Names Deltasone®; Prednisone Intensol™; Sterapred®; Sterapred® DS

Canadian Brand Names Apo-Prednisone®; Winpred™

Mexican Brand Names Meticorten®; Prednidib®

Generic Available Yes

Synonyms Deltacortisone; Deltadehydrocortisone

Pharmacologic Category Corticosteroid, Systemic

Dental Use Treatment of a variety of oral diseases of allergic, inflammatory, or autoimmune origin

Use Treatment of a variety of diseases including adrenocortical insufficiency, hypercalcemia, rheumatic, and collagen disorders; dermatologic, ocular, respiratory, gastrointestinal, and neoplastic diseases; organ transplantation and a variety of diseases including those of hematologic, allergic, inflammatory, and autoimmune in origin; not available in injectable form, prednisolone must be used

(Continued)

PredniSONE *(Continued)*

Unlabeled/Investigational Use Investigational: Prevention of postherpetic neuralgia and relief of acute pain in the early stages

Local Anesthetic/Vasoconstrictor Precautions No information available to require special precautions

Effects on Dental Treatment No significant effects or complications reported

Significant Adverse Effects

>10%:

Central nervous system: Insomnia, nervousness

Gastrointestinal: Increased appetite, indigestion

1% to 10%:

Central nervous system: Dizziness or lightheadedness, headache

Dermatologic: Hirsutism, hypopigmentation

Endocrine & metabolic: Diabetes mellitus, glucose intolerance, hyperglycemia

Neuromuscular & skeletal: Arthralgia

Ocular: Cataracts, glaucoma

Respiratory: Epistaxis

Miscellaneous: Diaphoresis

<1% (Limited to important or life-threatening): Cushing's syndrome, edema, fractures, hallucinations, hypertension, muscle-wasting, osteoporosis, pancreatitis, pituitary-adrenal axis suppression, seizures

Dosage Oral: Dose depends upon condition being treated and response of patient; dosage for infants and children should be based on severity of the disease and response of the patient rather than on strict adherence to dosage indicated by age, weight, or body surface area. Consider alternate day therapy for long-term therapy. Discontinuation of long-term therapy requires gradual withdrawal by tapering the dose.

Children:

Anti-inflammatory or immunosuppressive dose: 0.05-2 mg/kg/day divided 1-4 times/day

Acute asthma: 1-2 mg/kg/day in divided doses 1-2 times/day for 3-5 days

Alternatively (for 3- to 5-day "burst"):

<1 year: 10 mg every 12 hours

1-4 years: 20 mg every 12 hours

5-13 years: 30 mg every 12 hours

>13 years: 40 mg every 12 hours

Asthma long-term therapy (alternative dosing by age):

<1 year: 10 mg every other day

1-4 years: 20 mg every other day

5-13 years: 30 mg every other day

>13 years: 40 mg every other day

Nephrotic syndrome:

Initial (first 3 episodes): 2 mg/kg/day **or** 60 mg/m^2/day (maximum: 80 mg/day) in divided doses 3-4 times/day until urine is protein free for 3 consecutive days (maximum: 28 days); followed by 1-1.5 mg/kg/dose **or** 40 mg/m^2/dose given every other day for 4 weeks

Maintenance dose (long-term maintenance dose for frequent relapses): 0.5-1 mg/kg/dose given every other day for 3-6 months

Children and Adults: Physiologic replacement: 4-5 mg/m^2/day

Children ≥5 years and Adults: Asthma:

Moderate persistent: Inhaled corticosteroid (medium dose) or inhaled corticosteroid (low-medium dose) with a long-acting bronchodilator

Severe persistent: Inhaled corticosteroid (high dose) and corticosteroid tablets or syrup long term: 2 mg/kg/day, generally not to exceed 60 mg/day

Adults:

Immunosuppression/chemotherapy adjunct: Range: 5-60 mg/day in divided doses 1-4 times/day

Allergic reaction (contact dermatitis):

Day 1: 30 mg divided as 10 mg before breakfast, 5 mg at lunch, 5 mg at dinner, 10 mg at bedtime

Day 2: 5 mg at breakfast, 5 mg at lunch, 5 mg at dinner, 10 mg at bedtime

Day 3: 5 mg 4 times/day (with meals and at bedtime)

Day 4: 5 mg 3 times/day (breakfast, lunch, bedtime)

Day 5: 5 mg 2 times/day (breakfast, bedtime)

Day 6: 5 mg before breakfast

Pneumocystis carinii pneumonia (PCP):

40 mg twice daily for 5 days **followed by**

40 mg once daily for 5 days **followed by**

20 mg once daily for 11 days or until antimicrobial regimen is completed

Thyrotoxicosis: Oral: 60 mg/day

Chemotherapy (refer to individual protocols): Oral: Range: 20 mg/day to 100 mg/m²/day

Rheumatoid arthritis: Oral: Use lowest possible daily dose (often ≤7.5 mg/day)

Idiopathic thrombocytopenia purpura (ITP): Oral: 60 mg daily for 4-6 weeks, gradually tapered over several weeks

Systemic lupus erythematosus (SLE): Oral:

Acute: 1-2 mg/kg/day in 2-3 divided doses

Maintenance: Reduce to lowest possible dose, usually <1 mg/kg/day as single dose (morning)

Elderly: Use the lowest effective dose

Dosing adjustment in hepatic impairment: Prednisone is inactive and must be metabolized by the liver to prednisolone. This conversion may be impaired in patients with liver disease, however, prednisolone levels are observed to be higher in patients with severe liver failure than in normal patients. Therefore, compensation for the inadequate conversion of prednisone to prednisolone occurs.

Dosing adjustment in hyperthyroidism: Prednisone dose may need to be increased to achieve adequate therapeutic effects

Hemodialysis: Supplemental dose is not necessary

Peritoneal dialysis: Supplemental dose is not necessary

Mechanism of Action Decreases inflammation by suppression of migration of polymorphonuclear leukocytes and reversal of increased capillary permeability; suppresses the immune system by reducing activity and volume of the lymphatic system; suppresses adrenal function at high doses. Antitumor effects may be related to inhibition of glucose transport, phosphorylation, or induction of cell death in immature lymphocytes. Antiemetic effects are thought to occur due to blockade of cerebral innervation of the emetic center via inhibition of prostaglandin synthesis.

Contraindications Hypersensitivity to prednisone or any component of the formulation; serious infections, except tuberculous meningitis; systemic fungal infections; varicella

Warnings/Precautions Withdraw therapy with gradual tapering of dose, may retard bone growth. Use with caution in patients with hypothyroidism, cirrhosis, CHF, ulcerative colitis, thromboembolic disorders, and patients at increased risk for peptic ulcer disease. Corticosteroids should be used with caution in patients with diabetes, hypertension, osteoporosis, glaucoma, cataracts, or tuberculosis. Use caution in hepatic impairment. Because of the risk of adverse effects, systemic corticosteroids should be used cautiously in the elderly, in the smallest possible dose, and for the shortest possible time.

Drug Interactions **Substrate** of CYP3A4 (minor); **Induces** CYP2C19 (weak), 3A4 (weak)

Decreased effect:

Barbiturates, phenytoin, rifampin decrease corticosteroid effectiveness

Decreases salicylates

Decreases vaccines

Decreases toxoids effectiveness

Increased effect/toxicity: NSAIDs: Concurrent use of prednisone may increase the risk of GI ulceration

Ethanol/Nutrition/Herb Interactions

Ethanol: Avoid ethanol (may increase gastric mucosal irritation)

Food: Prednisone interferes with calcium absorption, Limit caffeine.

Herb/Nutraceutical: St John's wort may decrease prednisone levels. Avoid cat's claw, echinacea (have immunostimulant properties).

Dietary Considerations Should be taken after meals or with food or milk; increase dietary intake of pyridoxine, vitamin C, vitamin D, folate, calcium, and phosphorus.

Pharmacodynamics/Kinetics

Protein binding (concentration dependent): 65% to 91%

Metabolism: Hepatically converted from prednisone (inactive) to prednisolone (active); may be impaired with hepatic dysfunction

Half-life elimination: Normal renal function: 2.5-3.5 hours

See Prednisolone monograph for complete information.

Pregnancy Risk Factor B

Lactation Enters breast milk/compatible

Breast-Feeding Considerations Crosses into breast milk. No data on clinical effects on the infant. AAP considers **compatible** with breast-feeding.

Dosage Forms

Solution, oral: 1 mg/mL (5 mL, 120 mL, 500 mL) [contains alcohol 5%, sodium benzoate; vanilla flavor]

(Continued)

PredniSONE *(Continued)*

Solution, oral concentrate (Prednisone Intensol™): 5 mg/mL (30 mL) [contains alcohol 30%]

Tablet: 1 mg, 2.5 mg, 5 mg, 10 mg, 20 mg, 50 mg

Deltasone®: 2.5 mg, 10 mg, 20 mg, 50 mg

Sterapred®: 5 mg [supplied as 21 tablet 6-day unit-dose package or 48 tablet 12-day unit-dose package]

Sterapred® DS: 10 mg [supplied as 21 tablet 6-day unit-dose package or 48 tablet 12-day unit-dose package]

Prednisone Intensol™ *see* PredniSONE *on page 1115*

Prefest™ *see* Estradiol and Norgestimate *on page 521*

Prefrin™ [DSC] *see* Phenylephrine *on page 1078*

Pregnenedione *see* Progesterone *on page 1128*

Pregnyl® *see* Chorionic Gonadotropin (Human) *on page 326*

Prelone® *see* PrednisoLONE *on page 1113*

Prelu-2® *see* Phendimetrazine *on page 1072*

Premarin® *see* Estrogens (Conjugated/Equine) *on page 525*

Premjact® [OTC] *see* Lidocaine *on page 819*

Premphase® *see* Estrogens (Conjugated/Equine) and Medroxyprogesterone *on page 528*

Prempro™ *see* Estrogens (Conjugated/Equine) and Medroxyprogesterone *on page 528*

Preparation H® Hydrocortisone [OTC] *see* Hydrocortisone *on page 714*

Pre-Pen® *see* Benzylpenicilloyl-polylysine *on page 196*

Prepidil® *see* Dinoprostone *on page 447*

Pretz-D® [OTC] *see* Ephedrine *on page 495*

Pretz® Irrigation [OTC] *see* Sodium Chloride *on page 1227*

Prevacid® *see* Lansoprazole *on page 797*

Prevacid® NapraPAC™ *see* Lansoprazole and Naproxen *on page 799*

Prevacid® SoluTab™ *see* Lansoprazole *on page 797*

Prevalite® *see* Cholestyramine Resin *on page 323*

PREVEN® *see* Ethinyl Estradiol and Levonorgestrel *on page 545*

PreviDent® *see* Fluoride *on page 603*

PreviDent® 5000 Plus™ *see* Fluoride *on page 603*

Previfem™ *see* Ethinyl Estradiol and Norgestimate *on page 554*

Prevnar® *see* Pneumococcal Conjugate Vaccine (7-Valent) *on page 1098*

Prevpac® *see* Lansoprazole, Amoxicillin, and Clarithromycin *on page 798*

Priftin® *see* Rifapentine *on page 1182*

Prilocaine (PRIL oh kane)

Related Information

Oral Pain *on page 1526*

U.S. Brand Names Citanest® Plain

Canadian Brand Names Citanest® Plain

Generic Available No

Pharmacologic Category Local Anesthetic

Dental Use Amide-type anesthetic used for local infiltration anesthesia; injection near nerve trunks to produce nerve block

Local Anesthetic/Vasoconstrictor Precautions No information available to require special precautions

Effects on Dental Treatment It is common to misinterpret psychogenic responses to local anesthetic injection as an allergic reaction. Intraoral injections are perceived by many patients as a stressful procedure in dentistry. Common symptoms to this stress are diaphoresis, palpitations, hyperventilation, generalized pallor and a fainting feeling.

Degree of adverse effects in the CNS and cardiovascular system is directly related to blood levels of prilocaine (frequency not defined; more likely to occur after systemic administration rather than infiltration): Bradycardia and reduction in cardiac output, hypersensitivity reactions (may be manifest as dermatologic reactions and edema at injection site), asthmatic syndromes

High blood levels: Anxiety, restlessness, disorientation, confusion, dizziness, tremors, and seizures, followed by CNS depression, resulting in somnolence, unconsciousness and possible respiratory arrest; nausea and vomiting

In some cases, symptoms of CNS stimulation may be absent and the primary CNS effects are somnolence and unconsciousness.

Significant Adverse Effects

1% to 10%: Cardiovascular: Hypotension

<1% (Limited to important or life-threatening): Anaphylactoid reaction, aseptic meningitis resulting in paralysis, chills, CNS stimulation followed by CNS depression, miosis, nausea, skin discoloration, tinnitus, vomiting

Dosage

Children <10 years: Doses >40 mg (1 mL) as a 4% solution per procedure rarely needed

Children >10 years and Adults: Dental anesthesia, infiltration, or conduction block: Initial: 40-80 mg (1-2 mL) as a 4% solution; up to a maximum of 400 mg (10 mL) as a 4% solution within a 2-hour period. Manufacturer's maximum recommended dose is not more than 600 mg to normal healthy adults. The effective anesthetic dose varies with procedure, intensity of anesthesia needed, duration of anesthesia required and physical condition of the patient. Always use the lowest effective dose along with careful aspiration.

The following numbers of dental carpules (1.8 mL) provide the indicated amounts of prilocaine hydrochloride 4%. See table.

Prilocaine

# of Cartridges (1.8 mL)	Mg Prilocaine (4%)
1	72
2	144
3	216
4	288
5	360
6	432
7	504
8	576

Note: Adult and children doses of prilocaine hydrochloride cited from USP Dispensing Information (USP DI), 17th ed, The United States Pharmacopeial Convention, Inc, Rockville, MD, 1997, 139.

Mechanism of Action Local anesthetics bind selectively to the intracellular surface of sodium channels to block influx of sodium into the axon. As a result, depolarization necessary for action potential propagation and subsequent nerve function is prevented. The block at the sodium channel is reversible. When drug diffuses away from the axon, sodium channel function is restored and nerve propagation returns.

Contraindications Hypersensitivity to local anesthetics of the amide type or any component of the formulation

Warnings/Precautions Aspirate the syringe after tissue penetration and before injection to minimize chance of direct vascular injection

Drug Interactions No data reported

Pharmacodynamics/Kinetics

Onset of action: Infiltration: ~2 minutes; Inferior alveolar nerve block: ~3 minutes

Duration: Infiltration: Complete anesthesia for procedures lasting 20 minutes; Inferior alveolar nerve block: ~2.5 hours

Distribution: V_d: 0.7-4.4 L/kg; crosses blood-brain barrier

Protein binding: 55%

Metabolism: Hepatic and renal

Half-life elimination: 10-150 minutes; prolonged with hepatic or renal impairment

Pregnancy Risk Factor B

Breast-Feeding Considerations Usual infiltration doses of prilocaine given to nursing mothers has not been shown to affect the health of the nursing infant.

Dosage Forms Injection, solution: Prilocaine hydrochloride 4% (1.8 mL) [prefilled cartridge]

Selected Readings

Budenz AW, "Local Anesthetics in Dentistry: Then and Now," *J Calif Dent Assoc*, 2003, 31(5):388-96.

Dower JS Jr, "A Review of Paresthesia in Association With Administration of Local Anesthesia," *Dent Today*, 2003, 22(2):64-9.

Finder RL and Moore PA, "Adverse Drug Reactions to Local Anesthesia," *Dent Clin North Am*, 2002, 46(4):747-57, x.

Haas DA, "An Update on Local Anesthetics in Dentistry," *J Can Dent Assoc*, 2002, 68(9):546-51.

Hawkins JM and Moore PA, "Local Anesthesia: Advances in Agents and Techniques," *Dent Clin North Am*, 2002, 46(4):719-32, ix.

(Continued)

Prilocaine *(Continued)*

"Injectable Local Anesthetics," *J Am Dent Assoc*, 2003, 134(5):628-9.
Jastak JT and Yagiela JA, "Vasoconstrictors and Local Anesthesia: A Review and Rationale for Use," *J Am Dent Assoc*, 1983, 107(4):623-30.
MacKenzie TA and Young ER, "Local Anesthetic Update," *Anesth Prog*, 1993, 40(2):29-34.
Malamed SF, "Allergy and Toxic Reactions to Local Anesthetics," *Dent Today*, 2003, 22(4):114-6, 118-21.
Wahl MJ, Schmitt MM, Overton DA, et al, "Injection Pain of Bupivacaine With Epinephrine vs. Prilocaine Plain," *J Am Dent Assoc*, 2002, 133(12):1652-6.
Wynn RL, "Epinephrine Interactions With Beta-Blockers," *Gen Dent*, 1994, 42(1):16, 18.
Yagiela JA, "Local Anesthetics," *Anesth Prog*, 1991, 38(4-5):128-41.

Prilocaine and Epinephrine (PRIL oh kane with ep i NEF rin)

Related Information

Oral Pain *on page 1526*
Prilocaine *on page 1118*

U.S. Brand Names Citanest® Forte

Canadian Brand Names Citanest® Forte

Generic Available No

Synonyms Epinephrine and Prilocaine (Dental)

Pharmacologic Category Local Anesthetic

Dental Use Amide-type anesthetic used for local infiltration anesthesia; injection near nerve trunks to produce nerve block

Local Anesthetic/Vasoconstrictor Precautions No information available to require special precautions

Effects on Dental Treatment It is common to misinterpret psychogenic responses to local anesthetic injection as an allergic reaction. Intraoral injections are perceived by many patients as a stressful procedure in dentistry. Common symptoms to this stress are diaphoresis, palpitations, hyperventilation, generalized pallor and a fainting feeling. Patients may exhibit hypersensitivity to bisulfites contained in local anesthetic solution to prevent oxidation of epinephrine. In general, patients reacting to bisulfites have a history of asthma and their airways are hyper-reactive to asthmatic syndrome.

Degree of adverse effects in the CNS and cardiovascular system is directly related to blood levels of prilocaine (frequency not defined; more likely to occur after systemic administration rather than infiltration): Bradycardia and reduction in cardiac output, hypersensitivity reactions (extremely rare; may be manifest as dermatologic reactions and edema at injection site), asthmatic syndromes

High blood levels: Anxiety, restlessness, disorientation, confusion, dizziness, tremors, and seizures, followed by CNS depression, resulting in somnolence, unconsciousness and possible respiratory arrest; nausea and vomiting

In some cases, symptoms of CNS stimulation may be absent and the primary CNS effects are somnolence and unconsciousness.

Significant Adverse Effects Degree of adverse effects in the CNS and cardiovascular system are directly related to the blood levels of prilocaine. The effects below are more likely to occur after systemic administration rather than infiltration.

Cardiovascular: Myocardial effects include a decrease in contraction force as well as a decrease in electrical excitability and myocardial conduction rate resulting in bradycardia and reduction in cardiac output.

Central nervous system: High blood levels result in anxiety, restlessness, disorientation, confusion, dizziness, tremors and seizures. This is followed by depression of CNS resulting in somnolence, unconsciousness and possible respiratory arrest. Nausea and vomiting may also occur. In some cases, symptoms of CNS stimulation may be absent and the primary CNS effects are somnolence and unconsciousness.

Hypersensitivity reactions: Extremely rare, but may be manifest as dermatologic reactions and edema at injection site. Asthmatic syndromes have occurred. Patients may exhibit hypersensitivity to bisulfites contained in local anesthetic solution to prevent oxidation of epinephrine. In general, patients reacting to bisulfites have a history of asthma and their airways are hyper-reactive to asthmatic syndrome.

Psychogenic reactions: It is common to misinterpret psychogenic responses to local anesthetic injection as an allergic reaction. Intraoral injections are perceived by many patients as a stressful procedure in dentistry. Common symptoms to this stress are diaphoresis, palpitations, hyperventilation, generalized pallor, and a fainting feeling.

Dosage

Children <10 years: Doses >40 mg (1 mL) of prilocaine hydrochloride as a 4% solution with epinephrine 1:200,000 are rarely needed

Children >10 years and Adults: Dental anesthesia, infiltration, or conduction block: Initial: 40-80 mg (1-2 mL) of prilocaine hydrochloride as a 4% solution with epinephrine 1:200,000; up to a maximum of 400 mg (10 mL) of prilocaine hydrochloride within a 2-hour period. The effective anesthetic dose varies with procedure, intensity of anesthesia needed, duration of anesthesia required, and physical condition of the patient. Always use the lowest effective dose along with careful aspiration.

The following numbers of dental carpules (1.8 mL) provide the indicated amounts of prilocaine hydrochloride 4% and epinephrine 1:200,000. See table.

Prilocaine With Epinephrine

# of Cartridges (1.8 mL)	Mg Prilocaine (4%)	Mg Vasoconstrictor (Epinephrine 1:200,000)
1	72	0.009
2	144	0.018
3	216	0.027
4	288	0.036
5	360	0.045
6	432	0.054
7	504	0.063
8	576	0.072

Note: Adult and children doses of prilocaine hydrochloride with epinephrine cited from USP Dispensing Information (USP DI), 17th ed, The United States Pharmacopeial Convention, Inc, Rockville, MD, 1997, 140.

Mechanism of Action Local anesthetics bind selectively to the intracellular surface of sodium channels to block influx of sodium into the axon. As a result, depolarization necessary for action potential propagation and subsequent nerve function is prevented. The block at the sodium channel is reversible. When drug diffuses away from the axon, sodium channel function is restored and nerve propagation returns.

Epinephrine prolongs the duration of the anesthetic actions of prilocaine by causing vasoconstriction (alpha adrenergic receptor agonist) of the vasculature surrounding the nerve axons. This prevents the diffusion of prilocaine away from the nerves resulting in a longer retention in the axon.

Contraindications Hypersensitivity to local anesthetics of the amide-type or any component of the formulation

Warnings/Precautions Should be avoided in patients with uncontrolled hyperthyroidism. Should be used in minimal amounts in patients with significant cardiovascular problems (because of epinephrine component). Aspirate the syringe after tissue penetration and before injection to minimize chance of direct vascular injection

Drug Interactions

Beta-blockers, nonselective (ie, propranolol): Concurrent use could result in serious hypertension and reflex bradycardia

MAO inhibitors: Administration of local anesthetic solutions containing epinephrine may produce severe, prolonged hypertension

Tricyclic antidepressants: Pressor response to I.V. epinephrine, norepinephrine, and phenylephrine may be enhanced in patients receiving TCAs (**Note:** Effect is unlikely with epinephrine or levonordefrin dosages typically administered as infiltration in combination with local anesthetics)

Pharmacodynamics/Kinetics

Onset of action: Infiltration: <2 minutes; Inferior alveolar nerve block: <3 minutes

Duration: Infiltration: 2.25 hours; Inferior alveolar nerve block: 3 hours

Pregnancy Risk Factor C

Breast-Feeding Considerations Usual infiltration doses of prilocaine with epinephrine given to nursing mothers has not been shown to affect the health of the nursing infant.

Dosage Forms Injection: Prilocaine hydrochloride 4% with epinephrine 1:200,000 (1.8 mL cartridges, in boxes of 100)

Selected Readings

Ayoub ST and Coleman AE, "A Review of Local Anesthetics," *Gen Dent*, 1992, 40(4):285-7, 289-90.

Blanton PL and Roda RS, "The Anatomy of Local Anesthesia," *J Calif Dent Assoc*, 1995, 23(4):55-65.

Budenz AW, "Local Anesthetics in Dentistry: Then and Now," *J Calif Dent Assoc*, 2003, 31(5):388-96.

(Continued)

Prilocaine and Epinephrine *(Continued)*

Dower JS Jr, "A Review of Paresthesia in Association With Administration of Local Anesthesia," *Dent Today*, 2003, 22(2):64-9.

Finder RL and Moore PA, "Adverse Drug Reactions to Local Anesthesia," *Dent Clin North Am*, 2002, 46(4):747-57, x.

Haas DA, "An Update on Local Anesthetics in Dentistry," *J Can Dent Assoc*, 2002, 68(9):546-51.

Hawkins JM and Moore PA, "Local Anesthesia: Advances in Agents and Techniques," *Dent Clin North Am*, 2002, 46(4):719-32, ix.

"Injectable Local Anesthetics," *J Am Dent Assoc*, 2003, 134(5):628-9.

Jastak JT and Yagiela JA, "Vasoconstrictors and Local Anesthesia: A Review and Rationale for Use," *J Am Dent Assoc*, 1983, 107(4):623-30.

MacKenzie TA and Young ER, "Local Anesthetic Update," *Anesth Prog*, 1993, 40(2):29-34.

Malamed SF, "Allergy and Toxic Reactions to Local Anesthetics," *Dent Today*, 2003, 22(4):114-6, 118-21.

Wynn RL, "Epinephrine Interactions With Beta-Blockers," *Gen Dent*, 1994, 42(1):16, 18.

Yagiela JA, "Local Anesthetics," *Anesth Prog*, 1991, 38(4-5):128-41.

Yagiela JA, "Vasoconstrictor Agents for Local Anesthesia," *Anesth Prog*, 1995, 42(3-4):116-20.

Prilocaine and Lidocaine *see* Lidocaine and Prilocaine *on page 826*

Prilosec® *see* Omeprazole *on page 1012*

Prilosec OTC™ [OTC] *see* Omeprazole *on page 1012*

Primaclone *see* Primidone *on page 1122*

Primacor® *see* Milrinone *on page 930*

Primaquine (PRIM a kween)

Generic Available Yes

Synonyms Primaquine Phosphate; Prymaccone

Pharmacologic Category Aminoquinoline (Antimalarial)

Use Treatment of malaria

Unlabeled/Investigational Use Prevention of malaria; treatment *Pneumocystis carinii* pneumonia

Local Anesthetic/Vasoconstrictor Precautions No information available to require special precautions

Effects on Dental Treatment No significant effects or complications reported

Common Adverse Effects Frequency not defined.

Cardiovascular: Arrhythmias

Central nervous system: Headache

Dermatologic: Pruritus

Gastrointestinal: Abdominal pain, nausea, vomiting

Hematologic: Agranulocytosis, hemolytic anemia in G6PD deficiency, leukopenia, leukocytosis, methemoglobinemia in NADH-methemoglobin reductase-deficient individuals

Ocular: Interference with visual accommodation

Mechanism of Action Eliminates the primary tissue exoerythrocytic forms of *P. falciparum*; disrupts mitochondria and binds to DNA

Drug Interactions

Cytochrome P450 Effect: Substrate of CYP3A4 (major); **Inhibits** CYP1A2 (strong), 2D6 (weak), 3A4 (weak); **Induces** CYP1A2 (weak)

Increased Effect/Toxicity: Increased toxicity/levels with quinacrine. Primaquine may increase the levels/effects of aminophylline, fluvoxamine, mexiletine, mirtazapine, ropinirole, theophylline, trifluoperazine, and other CYP1A2 substrates.

Decreased Effect: The levels/effects of primaquine may be decreased by aminoglutethimide, carbamazepine, nafcillin, nevirapine, phenobarbital, phenytoin, rifamycins, and other CYP3A4 inducers.

Pharmacodynamics/Kinetics

Absorption: Well absorbed

Metabolism: Hepatic to carboxyprimaquine (active)

Half-life elimination: 3.7-9.6 hours

Time to peak, serum: 1-2 hours

Excretion: Urine (small amounts as unchanged drug)

Pregnancy Risk Factor C

Primaquine Phosphate *see* Primaquine *on page 1122*

Primaxin® *see* Imipenem and Cilastatin *on page 736*

Primidone (PRI mi done)

U.S. Brand Names Mysoline®

Canadian Brand Names Apo-Primidone®; Mysoline®

Mexican Brand Names Mysoline®

Generic Available Yes

Synonyms Desoxyphenobarbital; Primaclone

Pharmacologic Category Anticonvulsant, Miscellaneous; Barbiturate

Use Management of grand mal, psychomotor, and focal seizures

Unlabeled/Investigational Use Benign familial tremor (essential tremor)

Local Anesthetic/Vasoconstrictor Precautions No information available to require special precautions

Effects on Dental Treatment No significant effects or complications reported

Common Adverse Effects Frequency not defined.

Central nervous system: Drowsiness, vertigo, ataxia, lethargy, behavior change, fatigue, hyperirritability

Dermatologic: Rash

Gastrointestinal: Nausea, vomiting, anorexia

Genitourinary: Impotence

Hematologic: Agranulocytopenia, agranulocytosis, anemia

Ocular: Diplopia, nystagmus

Mechanism of Action Decreases neuron excitability, raises seizure threshold similar to phenobarbital; primidone has two active metabolites, phenobarbital and phenylethylmalonamide (PEMA); PEMA may enhance the activity of phenobarbital

Drug Interactions

Cytochrome P450 Effect: Metabolized to phenobarbital; **Induces** CYP1A2 (strong), 2B6 (strong), 2C8/9 (strong), 3A4 (strong)

Increased Effect/Toxicity: When combined with other CNS depressants, ethanol, narcotic analgesics, antidepressants, or benzodiazepines, additive respiratory and CNS depression may occur. Barbiturates may enhance the hepatotoxic potential of acetaminophen overdoses. Chloramphenicol, MAO inhibitors, valproic acid, and felbamate may inhibit barbiturate metabolism. Barbiturates may impair the absorption of griseofulvin, and may enhance the nephrotoxic effects of methoxyflurane. Concurrent use of phenobarbital with meperidine may result in increased CNS depression. Concurrent use of phenobarbital with primidone may result in elevated phenobarbital serum concentrations. CYP2C19 inhibitors may increase the levels/effects of primidone; example inhibitors include delavirdine, fluconazole, fluvoxamine, gemfibrozil, isoniazid, omeprazole, and ticlopidine.

Decreased Effect: Barbiturates may increase the metabolism of estrogens and reduce the efficacy of oral contraceptives; an alternative method of contraception should be considered. Barbiturates inhibit the hypoprothrombinemic effects of oral anticoagulants via increased metabolism. Barbiturates may enhance the metabolism of methadone resulting in methadone withdrawal. The levels/effects of primidone may be decreased by aminoglutethimide, carbamazepine, phenytoin, rifampin, and other CYP2C19 inducers.

Primidone may decrease the levels/effects of aminophylline, amiodarone, benzodiazepines, bupropion, calcium channel blockers, carbamazepine, citalopram, clarithromycin, cyclosporine, diazepam, efavirenz, erythromycin, estrogens, fluoxetine, fluvoxamine, glimepiride, glipizide, ifosfamide, losartan, methsuximide, mirtazapine, nateglinide, nefazodone, nevirapine, phenytoin, pioglitazone, promethazine, propranolol, protease inhibitors, proton pump inhibitors, rifampin, ropinirole, rosiglitazone, selegiline, sertraline, sulfonamides, tacrolimus, theophylline, venlafaxine. voriconazole, warfarin, zafirlukast, and other CYP1A2, 2A6, 2B6, 2C8/9, or 3A4 substrates.

Pharmacodynamics/Kinetics

Distribution: Adults: V_d: 2-3 L/kg

Protein binding: 99%

Metabolism: Hepatic to phenobarbital (active) and phenylethylmalonamide (PEMA)

Bioavailability: 60% to 80%

Half-life elimination (age dependent): Primidone: 10-12 hours; PEMA: 16 hours; Phenobarbital: 52-118 hours

Time to peak, serum: ~4 hours

Excretion: Urine (15% to 25% as unchanged drug and active metabolites)

Pregnancy Risk Factor D

Primsol® *see* Trimethoprim *on page 1341*

Principen® *see* Ampicillin *on page 124*

Prinivil® *see* Lisinopril *on page 833*

Prinzide® *see* Lisinopril and Hydrochlorothiazide *on page 834*

Priscoline® [DSC] *see* Tolazoline *on page 1309*

Pristinamycin *see* Quinupristin and Dalfopristin *on page 1163*

Privine® [OTC] *see* Naphazoline *on page 964*

ProAmatine® *see* Midodrine *on page 927*

Probampacin® *see* Ampicillin and Probenecid *on page 126*

Probenecid (proe BEN e sid)

Related Information

Sexually-Transmitted Diseases *on page 1504*

Canadian Brand Names Benuryl™

Mexican Brand Names Benecid®

Generic Available Yes

Synonyms Benemid [DSC]

Pharmacologic Category Uricosuric Agent

Use Prevention of gouty arthritis; hyperuricemia; prolongation of beta-lactam effect (ie, serum levels)

Local Anesthetic/Vasoconstrictor Precautions No information available to require special precautions

Effects on Dental Treatment No significant effects or complications reported

Common Adverse Effects Frequency not defined.

Cardiovascular: Flushing of face
Central nervous system: Headache, dizziness
Dermatologic: Rash, itching
Gastrointestinal: Anorexia, nausea, vomiting, sore gums
Genitourinary: Painful urination
Hematologic: Aplastic anemia, hemolytic anemia, leukopenia
Hepatic: Hepatic necrosis
Neuromuscular & skeletal: Gouty arthritis (acute)
Renal: Renal calculi, nephrotic syndrome, urate nephropathy
Miscellaneous: Anaphylaxis

Mechanism of Action Competitively inhibits the reabsorption of uric acid at the proximal convoluted tubule, thereby promoting its excretion and reducing serum uric acid levels; increases plasma levels of weak organic acids (penicillins, cephalosporins, or other beta-lactam antibiotics) by competitively inhibiting their renal tubular secretion

Drug Interactions

Cytochrome P450 Effect: Inhibits CYP2C19 (weak)

Increased Effect/Toxicity: Increases methotrexate toxic potential. Probenecid increases the serum concentrations of quinolones and beta-lactams such as penicillins and cephalosporins. Also increases levels/toxicity of acyclovir, diflunisal, ketorolac, thiopental, benzodiazepines, dapsone, fluoroquinolones, methotrexate, NSAIDs, sulfonylureas, zidovudine.

Decreased Effect: Salicylates (high-dose) may decrease uricosuria. Decreased urinary levels of nitrofurantoin may decrease efficacy.

Pharmacodynamics/Kinetics

Onset of action: Effect on penicillin levels: 2 hours
Absorption: Rapid and complete
Metabolism: Hepatic
Half-life elimination (dose dependent): Normal renal function: 6-12 hours
Time to peak, serum: 2-4 hours
Excretion: Urine

Pregnancy Risk Factor B

Probenecid and Ampicillin (Dental) *see* Ampicillin and Probenecid *on page 126*

Probenecid and Colchicine *see* Colchicine and Probenecid *on page 372*

Probiotica® [OTC] *see Lactobacillus on page 793*

Procainamide (proe kane A mide)

Related Information

Cardiovascular Diseases *on page 1458*

U.S. Brand Names Procanbid®; Pronestyl® [DSC]; Pronestyl-SR® [DSC]

Canadian Brand Names Apo-Procainamide®; Procan® SR; Pronestyl®-SR

Generic Available Yes: Excludes tablet

Synonyms PCA; Procainamide Hydrochloride; Procaine Amide Hydrochloride

Pharmacologic Category Antiarrhythmic Agent, Class Ia

Use Treatment of ventricular tachycardia (VT), premature ventricular contractions, paroxysmal atrial tachycardia (PSVT), and atrial fibrillation (AF); prevent recurrence of ventricular tachycardia, paroxysmal supraventricular tachycardia, atrial fibrillation or flutter

Unlabeled/Investigational Use ACLS guidelines:

Intermittent/recurrent VF or pulseless VT not responsive to earlier interventions
Monomorphic VT (EF >40%, no CHF)
Polymorphic VT with normal baseline QT interval
Wide complex tachycardia of unknown type (EF >40%, no CHF, patient stable)
Refractory paroxysmal SVT

Atrial fibrillation or flutter (EF >40%, no CHF) including pre-excitation syndrome

Local Anesthetic/Vasoconstrictor Precautions No information available to require special precautions

Effects on Dental Treatment No significant effects or complications reported

Mechanism of Action Decreases myocardial excitability and conduction velocity and may depress myocardial contractility, by increasing the electrical stimulation threshold of ventricle, His-Purkinje system and through direct cardiac effects

Pregnancy Risk Factor C

Procainamide Hydrochloride *see* Procainamide *on page 1124*

Procaine (PROE kane)

U.S. Brand Names Novocain®

Canadian Brand Names Novocain®

Generic Available Yes

Synonyms Procaine Hydrochloride

Pharmacologic Category Local Anesthetic

Use Produces spinal anesthesia and epidural and peripheral nerve block by injection and infiltration methods

Local Anesthetic/Vasoconstrictor Precautions No information available to require special precautions

Effects on Dental Treatment This is no longer a useful anesthetic in dentistry due to high incidence of allergic reactions.

Mechanism of Action Blocks both the initiation and conduction of nerve impulses by decreasing the neuronal membrane's permeability to sodium ions, which results in inhibition of depolarization with resultant blockade of conduction

Pregnancy Risk Factor C

Procaine Amide Hydrochloride *see* Procainamide *on page 1124*

Procaine Benzylpenicillin *see* Penicillin G Procaine *on page 1060*

Procaine Hydrochloride *see* Procaine *on page 1125*

Procaine Penicillin G *see* Penicillin G Procaine *on page 1060*

Procanbid® *see* Procainamide *on page 1124*

Procarbazine (proe KAR ba zeen)

U.S. Brand Names Matulane®

Canadian Brand Names Matulane®; Natulan®

Mexican Brand Names Natulan®

Generic Available No

Synonyms Benzmethyzin; N-Methylhydrazine; NSC-77213; Procarbazine Hydrochloride

Pharmacologic Category Antineoplastic Agent, Alkylating Agent

Use Treatment of Hodgkin's disease

Unlabeled/Investigational Use Treatment of non-Hodgkin's lymphoma, brain tumors, melanoma, lung cancer, multiple myeloma

Local Anesthetic/Vasoconstrictor Precautions No information available to require special precautions

Effects on Dental Treatment No significant effects or complications reported

Common Adverse Effects Frequency not defined.

Central nervous system: Reports of neurotoxicity with procarbazine generally originate from early usage with single agent oral (continuous) or I.V. dosing; CNS depression is commonly reported to be additive with other CNS depressants

Hematologic: Myelosuppression, hemolysis in patients with G6PD deficiency

Gastrointestinal: Nausea and vomiting (60% to 90%); increasing the dose in a stepwise fashion over several days may minimize this

Genitourinary: Reproductive dysfunction >10% (in animals, hormone treatment has prevented azoospermia)

Respiratory: Pulmonary toxicity (<1%); the most commonly reported pulmonary toxicity is a hypersensitivity pneumonitis which responds to steroids and discontinuation of the drug. At least one report of persistent pulmonary fibrosis has been reported, however, a higher incidence (18%) of pulmonary toxicity (fibrosis) was reported when procarbazine was given prior to BCNU (BCNU alone does cause pulmonary fibrosis).

Miscellaneous: Second malignancies (cumulative incidence 2% to 15% reported with MOPP combination therapy)

(Continued)

Procarbazine *(Continued)*

Mechanism of Action Mechanism of action is not clear, methylating of nucleic acids; inhibits DNA, RNA, and protein synthesis; may damage DNA directly and suppresses mitosis; metabolic activation required by host

Drug Interactions

Increased Effect/Toxicity: Procarbazine exhibits weak MAO inhibitor activity. Foods containing high amounts of tyramine should, therefore, be avoided. When an MAO inhibitor is given with food high in tyramine, hypertensive crisis, intracranial bleeding, and headache have been reported.

Sympathomimetic amines (epinephrine and amphetamines) and antidepressants (tricyclics) should be used cautiously with procarbazine. Barbiturates, narcotics, phenothiazines, and other CNS depressants can cause somnolence, ataxia, and other symptoms of CNS depression. Ethanol has caused a disulfiram-like reaction with procarbazine. May result in headache, respiratory difficulties, nausea, vomiting, sweating, thirst, hypotension, and flushing.

Pharmacodynamics/Kinetics

Absorption: Rapid and complete

Distribution: Crosses blood-brain barrier; distributes into CSF

Metabolism: Hepatic and renal

Half-life elimination: 1 hour

Excretion: Urine and respiratory tract (<5% as unchanged drug, 70% as metabolites)

Pregnancy Risk Factor D

Procarbazine Hydrochloride *see* Procarbazine *on page 1125*

Procardia® *see* NIFEdipine *on page 984*

Procardia XL® *see* NIFEdipine *on page 984*

Procetofene *see* Fenofibrate *on page 577*

Prochieve™ *see* Progesterone *on page 1128*

Prochlorperazine (proe klor PER a zeen)

U.S. Brand Names Compazine® [DSC]; Compro™

Canadian Brand Names Apo-Prochlorperazine®; Compazine®; Nu-Prochlor; Stemetil®

Generic Available Yes: Injection, tablet, suppository

Synonyms Chlormeprazine; Prochlorperazine Edisylate; Prochlorperazine Maleate

Pharmacologic Category Antiemetic; Antipsychotic Agent, Phenothiazine, Piperazine

Use Management of nausea and vomiting; psychosis; anxiety

Unlabeled/Investigational Use Behavioral syndromes in dementia

Local Anesthetic/Vasoconstrictor Precautions Most pharmacology textbooks state that in presence of phenothiazines, systemic doses of epinephrine paradoxically decrease the blood pressure. This is the so called "epinephrine reversal" phenomenon. This has never been observed when epinephrine is given by infiltration as part of the anesthesia procedure.

Effects on Dental Treatment Key adverse event(s) related to dental treatment: Xerostomia and changes in salivation (normal salivary flow resumes upon discontinuation). Significant hypotension may occur, especially when the drug is administered parenterally; orthostatic hypotension is due to alpha-receptor blockade, the elderly are at greater risk for orthostatic hypotension.

Tardive dyskinesia: Prevalence rate may be 40% in elderly; development of the syndrome and the irreversible nature are proportional to duration and total cumulative dose over time. Extrapyramidal reactions are more common in elderly with up to 50% developing these reactions after 60 years of age. Drug-induced Parkinson's syndrome occurs often; akathisia is the most common extrapyramidal reaction in elderly.

Common Adverse Effects Frequency not defined.

Cardiovascular: Hypotension, orthostatic hypotension, hypertension, tachycardia, bradycardia, dizziness, cardiac arrest

Central nervous system: Extrapyramidal signs (pseudoparkinsonism, akathisia, dystonias, tardive dyskinesia), dizziness, cerebral edema, seizures, headache, drowsiness, paradoxical excitement, restlessness, hyperactivity, insomnia, neuroleptic malignant syndrome (NMS), impairment of temperature regulation

Dermatologic: Increased sensitivity to sun, rash, discoloration of skin (blue-gray)

Endocrine & metabolic: Hypoglycemia, hyperglycemia, galactorrhea, lactation, breast enlargement, gynecomastia, menstrual irregularity, amenorrhea, SIADH, changes in libido

Gastrointestinal: Constipation, weight gain, vomiting, stomach pain, nausea, xerostomia, salivation, diarrhea, anorexia, ileus

Genitourinary: Difficulty in urination, ejaculatory disturbances, incontinence, polyuria, ejaculating dysfunction, priapism

Hematologic: Agranulocytosis, leukopenia, eosinophilia, hemolytic anemia, thrombocytopenic purpura, pancytopenia

Hepatic: Cholestatic jaundice, hepatotoxicity

Neuromuscular & skeletal: Tremor

Ocular: Pigmentary retinopathy, blurred vision, cornea and lens changes

Respiratory: Nasal congestion

Miscellaneous: Diaphoresis

Mechanism of Action Blocks postsynaptic mesolimbic dopaminergic D_1 and D_2 receptors in the brain, including the medullary chemoreceptor trigger zone; exhibits a strong alpha-adrenergic and anticholinergic blocking effect and depresses the release of hypothalamic and hypophyseal hormones; believed to depress the reticular activating system, thus affecting basal metabolism, body temperature, wakefulness, vasomotor tone and emesis

Drug Interactions

Increased Effect/Toxicity: Chloroquine, propranolol, and sulfadoxine-pyrimethamine may increase prochlorperazine concentrations. Concurrent use with TCA may produce increased toxicity or altered therapeutic response. Prochlorperazine plus lithium may rarely produce neurotoxicity. Prochlorperazine may produce additive CNS depressant effects with CNS depressants (ethanol, narcotics). Metoclopramide may increase risk of extrapyramidal symptoms (EPS).

Decreased Effect: Barbiturates and carbamazepine may increase the metabolism of prochlorperazine, lowering its serum levels. Benztropine (and other anticholinergics) may inhibit the therapeutic response to prochlorperazine. Antipsychotics such as prochlorperazine inhibit the ability of bromocriptine to lower serum prolactin concentrations. The antihypertensive effects of guanethidine and guanadrel may be inhibited by prochlorperazine. Prochlorperazine may inhibit the antiparkinsonian effect of levodopa. Prochlorperazine (and possibly other low potency antipsychotics) may reverse the pressor effects of epinephrine.

Pharmacodynamics/Kinetics

Onset of action: Oral: 30-40 minutes; I.M.: 10-20 minutes; Rectal: ~60 minutes

Duration: I.M., oral extended-release: 12 hours; Rectal, immediate release: 3-4 hours

Distribution: V_d: 1400-1548 L; crosses placenta; enters breast milk

Metabolism: Primarily hepatic; N-desmethyl prochlorperazine (major active metabolite)

Bioavailability: Oral: 12.5%

Half-life elimination: Oral: 3-5 hours; I.V.: ~7 hours

Pregnancy Risk Factor C

Prochlorperazine Edisylate *see* Prochlorperazine *on page 1126*

Prochlorperazine Maleate *see* Prochlorperazine *on page 1126*

Procrit® *see* Epoetin Alfa *on page 499*

Proctocort® *see* Hydrocortisone *on page 714*

ProctoCream® HC *see* Hydrocortisone *on page 714*

Proctofene *see* Fenofibrate *on page 577*

ProctoFoam®-HC *see* Pramoxine and Hydrocortisone *on page 1109*

ProctoFoam® NS [OTC] *see* Pramoxine *on page 1109*

Proctosol-HC® *see* Hydrocortisone *on page 714*

Procyclidine (proe SYE kli deen)

U.S. Brand Names Kemadrin®

Canadian Brand Names PMS-Procyclidine; Procyclid™

Generic Available No

Synonyms Procyclidine Hydrochloride

Pharmacologic Category Anticholinergic Agent; Anti-Parkinson's Agent, Anticholinergic

Use Relieves symptoms of parkinsonian syndrome and drug-induced extrapyramidal symptoms

Local Anesthetic/Vasoconstrictor Precautions No information available to require special precautions

Effects on Dental Treatment Key adverse event(s) related to dental treatment: Xerostomia (normal salivary flow resumes upon discontinuation) and dry

(Continued)

Procyclidine *(Continued)*

throat and nose. Prolonged use of antidyskinetics may decrease or inhibit salivary flow, contributing to discomfort and dental disease (ie, caries, oral candidiasis, and periodontal disease).

Common Adverse Effects Frequency not defined.

Cardiovascular: Tachycardia, palpitations

Central nervous system: Confusion, drowsiness, headache, loss of memory, fatigue, ataxia, giddiness, lightheadedness

Dermatologic: Dry skin, increased sensitivity to light, rash

Gastrointestinal: Constipation, xerostomia, dry throat, nausea, vomiting, epigastric distress

Genitourinary: Difficult urination

Neuromuscular & skeletal: Weakness

Ocular: Increased intraocular pain, blurred vision, mydriasis

Respiratory: Dry nose

Miscellaneous: Diaphoresis (decreased)

Mechanism of Action Thought to act by blocking excess acetylcholine at cerebral synapses; many of its effects are due to its pharmacologic similarities with atropine; it exerts an antispasmodic effect on smooth muscle, is a potent mydriatic; inhibits salivation

Drug Interactions

Increased Effect/Toxicity: Central and/or peripheral anticholinergic syndrome can occur when administered with amantadine, rimantadine, narcotic analgesics, phenothiazines and other antipsychotics (especially with high anticholinergic activity), tricyclic antidepressants, quinidine and some other antiarrhythmics, and antihistamines.

Decreased Effect: May increase gastric degradation of levodopa and decrease the amount of levodopa absorbed by delaying gastric emptying; the opposite may be true for digoxin. Therapeutic effects of cholinergic agents (tacrine, donepezil) and neuroleptics may be antagonized.

Pharmacodynamics/Kinetics

Onset of action: 30-40 minutes

Duration: 4-6 hours

Pregnancy Risk Factor C

Procyclidine Hydrochloride *see* Procyclidine *on page 1127*

Prodium® [OTC] *see* Phenazopyridine *on page 1072*

Profen Forte™ DM *see* Guaifenesin, Pseudoephedrine, and Dextromethorphan *on page 676*

Profen II DM® *see* Guaifenesin, Pseudoephedrine, and Dextromethorphan *on page 676*

Profilnine® SD *see* Factor IX Complex (Human) *on page 572*

Progestasert® *see* Progesterone *on page 1128*

Progesterone (proe JES ter one)

U.S. Brand Names Crinone®; Prochieve™; Progestasert®; Prometrium®

Canadian Brand Names Crinone®; Prometrium®

Mexican Brand Names Crinone®

Generic Available Yes: Injection

Synonyms Pregnenedione; Progestin

Pharmacologic Category Progestin

Use

Oral: Prevention of endometrial hyperplasia in nonhysterectomized, postmenopausal women who are receiving conjugated estrogen tablets; secondary amenorrhea

I.M.: Amenorrhea; abnormal uterine bleeding due to hormonal imbalance

Intrauterine device (IUD): Contraception in women who have had at least one child, are in a stable and mutually-monogamous relationship, and have no history of pelvic inflammatory disease; amenorrhea; functional uterine bleeding

Intravaginal gel: Part of assisted reproductive technology (ART) for infertile women with progesterone deficiency; secondary amenorrhea

Local Anesthetic/Vasoconstrictor Precautions No information available to require special precautions

Effects on Dental Treatment Key adverse event(s) related to dental treatment: Progestins may predispose the patient to gingival bleeding.

Common Adverse Effects

Intrauterine device:

Cardiovascular: Bradycardia and syncope (secondary to insertion)

Central nervous system: Pain

Endocrine & metabolic: Amenorrhea, delayed menses, dysmenorrhea, ectopic pregnancy, endometritis, pregnancy, septic abortion, prolonged menstrual flow, spontaneous abortion, spotting

Genitourinary: Cervical erosion, dyspareunia, leukorrhea, pelvic infection, tubal damage, tubo-ovarian abscess, vaginitis

Hematologic: Anemia

Local: Embedment or fragmentation of the IUD, perforation of uterus and cervix

Neuromuscular & skeletal: Backache

Miscellaneous: Abscess formation and erosion of adjacent area, abdominal adhesions, complete or partial IUD expulsion, congenital anomalies, cramping, cystic masses in the pelvis, death, difficult removal, fetal damage, hormonal imbalance, intestinal penetration, intestinal obstruction, local inflammatory reaction, loss of fertility, peritonitis, septicemia

Injection (I.M.):

Cardiovascular: Edema

Central nervous system: Depression, fever, insomnia, somnolence

Dermatologic: Acne, allergic rash (rare), alopecia, hirsutism, pruritus, rash, urticaria

Endocrine & metabolic: Amenorrhea, breakthrough bleeding, breast tenderness, galactorrhea, menstrual flow changes, spotting

Gastrointestinal: Nausea, weight gain, weight loss

Genitourinary: Cervical erosion changes, cervical secretion changes

Hepatic: Cholestatic jaundice

Local: Pain at the injection site

Miscellaneous: Anaphylactoid reactions

Oral capsule:

>10%:

Central nervous system: Dizziness (16%)

Endocrine & metabolic: Breast pain (11%)

5% to 10%:

Central nervous system: Headache (10%), fatigue (7%), emotional lability (6%), irritability (5%)

Gastrointestinal: Abdominal pain (10%), abdominal distention (6%)

Neuromuscular & skeletal: Musculoskeletal pain (6%)

Respiratory: Upper respiratory tract infection (5%)

Miscellaneous: Viral infection (7%)

Mechanism of Action Natural steroid hormone that induces secretory changes in the endometrium, promotes mammary gland development, relaxes uterine smooth muscle, blocks follicular maturation and ovulation, and maintains pregnancy

Drug Interactions

Cytochrome P450 Effect: Substrate of CYP1A2 (minor), 2A6 (minor), 2C8/9 (minor), 2C19 (major), 2D6 (minor), 3A4 (major); **Inhibits** CYP2C8/9 (weak), 2C19 (weak), 3A4 (weak)

Increased Effect/Toxicity: Ketoconazole may increase the bioavailability of progesterone. Progesterone may increase concentrations of estrogenic compounds during concurrent therapy with conjugated estrogens.

Decreased Effect: CYP2C19 inducers may decrease the levels/effects of progesterone; example inducers include aminoglutethimide, carbamazepine, phenytoin, and rifampin. CYP3A4 inducers may decrease the levels/effects of progesterone; example inducers include aminoglutethimide, carbamazepine, nafcillin, nevirapine, phenobarbital, phenytoin, and rifamycins.

Pharmacodynamics/Kinetics

Duration: 24 hours

Protein binding: 96% to 99%

Metabolism: Hepatic

Half-life elimination: 5 minutes

Time to peak: Oral: 1.5-2.3 hours

Excretion: Urine (50% to 60%); feces (~10%)

Pregnancy Risk Factor B (Prometrium®, per manufacturer); none established for gel (Crinone®), injection (contraindicated), or intrauterine device (contraindicated)

Progestin *see* Progesterone *on page 1128*

Proglycem® *see* Diazoxide *on page 425*

Prograf® *see* Tacrolimus *on page 1255*

Proguanil and Atovaquone *see* Atovaquone and Proguanil *on page 165*

ProHance® *see* Radiological/Contrast Media (Nonionic) *on page 1166*

Prolastin® *see* Alpha$_1$-Proteinase Inhibitor *on page 84*

Proleukin® *see* Aldesleukin *on page 74*
Prolex-D *see* Guaifenesin and Phenylephrine *on page 674*
Prolixin® [DSC] *see* Fluphenazine *on page 610*
Prolixin Decanoate® *see* Fluphenazine *on page 610*
Proloprim® *see* Trimethoprim *on page 1341*

Promethazine (proe METH a zeen)

U.S. Brand Names Phenadoz™; Phenergan®

Canadian Brand Names Phenergan®

Generic Available Yes

Synonyms Promethazine Hydrochloride

Pharmacologic Category Antiemetic; Antihistamine; Phenothiazine Derivative; Sedative

Use Symptomatic treatment of various allergic conditions; antiemetic; motion sickness; sedative; postoperative pain (adjunctive therapy); anesthetic (adjunctive therapy); anaphylactic reactions (adjunctive therapy)

Local Anesthetic/Vasoconstrictor Precautions Most pharmacology textbooks state that in presence of phenothiazines, systemic doses of epinephrine paradoxically decrease the blood pressure. This is the so called "epinephrine reversal" phenomenon. This has never been observed when epinephrine is given by infiltration as part of the anesthesia procedure.

Effects on Dental Treatment Key adverse event(s) related to dental treatment: Xerostomia (normal salivary flow resumes upon discontinuation). Significant hypotension may occur, especially when the drug is administered parenterally; orthostatic hypotension is due to alpha-receptor blockade, the elderly are at greater risk for orthostatic hypotension.

Tardive dyskinesia: Prevalence rate may be 40% in elderly; development of the syndrome and the irreversible nature are proportional to duration and total cumulative dose over time. Extrapyramidal reactions are more common in elderly with up to 50% developing these reactions after 60 years of age. Drug-induced Parkinson's syndrome occurs often; akathisia is the most common extrapyramidal reaction in elderly.

Increased confusion, memory loss, psychotic behavior, and agitation frequently occur as a consequence of anticholinergic effects. Antipsychotic associated sedation in nonpsychotic patients is extremely unpleasant due to feelings of depersonalization, derealization, and dysphoria.

Common Adverse Effects Frequency not defined.

Cardiovascular: Bradycardia, hypertension, postural hypotension, tachycardia, nonspecific QT changes

Central nervous system: Catatonic states, confusion, disorientation, dizziness, drowsiness, dystonias, euphoria, excitation, extrapyramidal symptoms, fatigue, hallucinations, hysteria, insomnia, akathisia, pseudoparkinsonism, tardive dyskinesia, nervousness, neuroleptic malignant syndrome, sedation, seizures, somnolence

Dermatologic: Angioneurotic edema, photosensitivity, dermatitis, skin pigmentation (slate gray), urticaria

Endocrine & metabolic: Lactation, breast engorgement, amenorrhea, gynecomastia, hyper- or hypoglycemia

Gastrointestinal: Xerostomia, constipation, nausea, vomiting

Genitourinary: Urinary retention, ejaculatory disorder, impotence

Hematologic: Agranulocytosis, eosinophilia, leukopenia, hemolytic anemia, aplastic anemia, thrombocytopenia, thrombocytopenic purpura

Hepatic: Jaundice

Neuromuscular & skeletal: Incoordination, tremors

Ocular: Blurred vision, corneal and lenticular changes, diplopia, epithelial keratopathy, pigmentary retinopathy

Otic: Tinnitus

Respiratory: Apnea, respiratory depression

Mechanism of Action Blocks postsynaptic mesolimbic dopaminergic receptors in the brain; exhibits a strong alpha-adrenergic blocking effect and depresses the release of hypothalamic and hypophyseal hormones; competes with histamine for the H_1-receptor; reduces stimuli to the brainstem reticular system

Drug Interactions

Cytochrome P450 Effect: Substrate (major) of CYP2B6, 2D6; **Inhibits** CYP2D6 (weak)

Increased Effect/Toxicity: CYP2B6 inhibitors may increase the levels/effects of promethazine; example inhibitors include desipramine, paroxetine, and sertraline. CYP2D6 inhibitors may increase the levels/effects of promethazine; example inhibitors include chlorpromazine, delavirdine, fluoxetine, miconazole, paroxetine, pergolide, quinidine, quinine, ritonavir, and ropinirole. Chloroquine, propranolol, and sulfadoxine-pyrimethamine also may increase promethazine concentrations. Concurrent use with TCA may produce increased toxicity or altered therapeutic response. Promethazine plus lithium may rarely produce neurotoxicity. Concurrent use of promethazine and CNS depressants (ethanol, narcotics) may produce additive depressant effects.

Decreased Effect: CYP2B6 inducers may decrease the levels/effects of promethazine; example inducers include carbamazepine, nevirapine, phenobarbital, phenytoin, and rifampin. Benztropine (and other anticholinergics) may inhibit the therapeutic response to promethazine. Promethazine may inhibit the ability of bromocriptine to lower serum prolactin concentrations. The antihypertensive effects of guanethidine and guanadrel may be inhibited by promethazine. Promethazine may inhibit the antiparkinsonian effect of levodopa. Promethazine (and possibly other low potency antipsychotics) may reverse the pressor effects of epinephrine.

Pharmacodynamics/Kinetics

Onset of action: I.M.: ~20 minutes; I.V.: 3-5 minutes

Peak effect: C_{max}: 9.04 ng/mL (suppository); 19.3 ng/mL (syrup)

Duration: 2-6 hours

Absorption:

I.M.: Bioavailability may be greater than with oral or rectal administration

Oral: Rapid and complete; large first pass effect limits systemic bioavailability

Distribution: V_d: 171 L

Protein binding: 93%

Metabolism: Hepatic; primarily oxidation; forms metabolites

Half-life elimination: 9-16 hours

Time to maximum serum concentration: 4.4 hours (syrup); 6.7-8.6 hours (suppositories)

Excretion: Primarily urine and feces (as inactive metabolites)

Pregnancy Risk Factor C

Promethazine and Codeine (proe METH a zeen & KOE deen)

Related Information

Codeine *on page 369*

Promethazine *on page 1130*

U.S. Brand Names Phenergan® With Codeine

Generic Available Yes

Synonyms Codeine and Promethazine

Pharmacologic Category Antihistamine/Antitussive

Use Temporary relief of coughs and upper respiratory symptoms associated with allergy or the common cold

Local Anesthetic/Vasoconstrictor Precautions No information available to require special precautions

Effects on Dental Treatment Although promethazine is a phenothiazine derivative, extrapyramidal reactions or tardive dyskinesias are not seen with the use of this drug.

Restrictions C-V

Drug Interactions

Cytochrome P450 Effect: Promethazine: **Substrate** (major) of CYP2B6, 2D6; **Inhibits** CYP2D6 (weak)

Pharmacodynamics/Kinetics See individual agents.

Pregnancy Risk Factor C

Promethazine and Dextromethorphan

(proe METH a zeen & deks troe meth OR fan)

Related Information

Dextromethorphan *on page 421*

Promethazine *on page 1130*

Canadian Brand Names Promatussin® DM

Generic Available Yes

Synonyms Dextromethorphan and Promethazine

Pharmacologic Category Antihistamine/Antitussive

Use Temporary relief of coughs and upper respiratory symptoms associated with allergy or the common cold

Local Anesthetic/Vasoconstrictor Precautions No information available to require special precautions

Effects on Dental Treatment Although promethazine is a phenothiazine derivative, extrapyramidal reactions or tardive dyskinesias are not seen with the use of this drug.

(Continued)

Promethazine and Dextromethorphan *(Continued)*

Drug Interactions

Cytochrome P450 Effect:

Promethazine: **Substrate** (major) of CYP2B6, 2D6; **Inhibits** CYP2D6 (weak)

Dextromethorphan: **Substrate** of CYP2B6 (minor), 2C8/9 (minor), 2C19 (minor), 2D6 (major), 2E1 (minor), 3A4 (minor); **Inhibits** CYP2D6 (weak)

Pharmacodynamics/Kinetics See individual agents.

Pregnancy Risk Factor C

Promethazine and Meperidine *see* Meperidine and Promethazine *on page 872*

Promethazine and Phenylephrine

(proe METH a zeen & fen il EF rin)

Related Information

Phenylephrine *on page 1078*

Promethazine *on page 1130*

Generic Available Yes

Synonyms Phenylephrine and Promethazine

Pharmacologic Category Antihistamine/Decongestant Combination

Use Temporary relief of upper respiratory symptoms associated with allergy or the common cold

Local Anesthetic/Vasoconstrictor Precautions

Phenylephrine: Use with caution since phenylephrine is a sympathomimetic amine which could interact with epinephrine to cause a pressor response

Promethazine: No information available to require special precautions

Effects on Dental Treatment Key adverse event(s) related to dental treatment: Phenylephrine: Tachycardia, palpitations, xerostomia (normal salivary flow resumes upon discontinuation); use vasoconstrictor with caution. Although promethazine is a phenothiazine derivative, extrapyramidal reactions or tardive dyskinesias are not seen with the use of this drug.

Drug Interactions

Cytochrome P450 Effect: Promethazine: **Substrate** (major) of CYP2B6, 2D6; **Inhibits** CYP2D6 (weak)

Pharmacodynamics/Kinetics See individual agents.

Pregnancy Risk Factor C

Promethazine Hydrochloride *see* Promethazine *on page 1130*

Promethazine, Phenylephrine, and Codeine

(proe METH a zeen, fen il EF rin, & KOE deen)

Related Information

Codeine *on page 369*

Phenylephrine *on page 1078*

Promethazine *on page 1130*

Generic Available Yes

Synonyms Codeine, Promethazine, and Phenylephrine; Phenylephrine, Promethazine, and Codeine

Pharmacologic Category Antihistamine/Decongestant/Antitussive

Use Temporary relief of coughs and upper respiratory symptoms including nasal congestion

Local Anesthetic/Vasoconstrictor Precautions

Phenylephrine: Use with caution since phenylephrine is a sympathomimetic amine which could interact with epinephrine to cause a pressor response

Promethazine: No information available to require special precautions

Effects on Dental Treatment Key adverse event(s) related to dental treatment: Phenylephrine: Tachycardia, palpitations, xerostomia (normal salivary flow resumes upon discontinuation); use vasoconstrictor with caution. Although promethazine is a phenothiazine derivative, extrapyramidal reactions or tardive dyskinesias are not seen with the use of this drug.

Restrictions C-V

Drug Interactions

Cytochrome P450 Effect:

Promethazine: **Substrate** (major) of CYP2B6, 2D6; **Inhibits** CYP2D6 (weak)

Codeine: **Substrate** of CYP2D6 (major), 3A4 (minor); **Inhibits** CYP2D6 (weak)

Pharmacodynamics/Kinetics See individual agents.

Pregnancy Risk Factor C

Prometrium® *see* Progesterone *on page 1128*

Promit® *see* Dextran 1 *on page 418*

Pronap-100® *see* Propoxyphene and Acetaminophen *on page 1137*
Pronestyl® [DSC] *see* Procainamide *on page 1124*
Pronestyl-SR® [DSC] *see* Procainamide *on page 1124*
Pronto® [OTC] *see* Pyrethrins and Piperonyl Butoxide *on page 1153*

Propafenone (proe pa FEEN one)

Related Information
Cardiovascular Diseases *on page 1458*

U.S. Brand Names Rythmol®; Rythmol® SR

Canadian Brand Names Apo-Propafenone®; Rythmol® Gen-Propafenone

Mexican Brand Names Nistaken® [tabs]; Norfenon®

Generic Available Yes

Synonyms Propafenone Hydrochloride

Pharmacologic Category Antiarrhythmic Agent, Class Ic

Use Treatment of life-threatening ventricular arrhythmias
Rythmol® SR: Maintenance of normal sinus rhythm in patients with symptomatic atrial fibrillation

Unlabeled/Investigational Use Supraventricular tachycardias, including those patients with Wolff-Parkinson-White syndrome

Local Anesthetic/Vasoconstrictor Precautions In some patients, propafenone has been reported to induce new or worsened arrhythmias (proarrhythmic effect). It is suggested that vasoconstrictors be used with caution since epinephrine has the potential to stimulate the heart rate when given in the anesthetic regimen.

Effects on Dental Treatment Key adverse event(s) related to dental treatment: Unusual taste and significant xerostomia (normal salivary flow resumes upon discontinuation).

Common Adverse Effects 1% to 10%:
Cardiovascular: New or worsened arrhythmias (proarrhythmic effect) (2% to 10%), angina (2% to 5%), CHF (1% to 4%), ventricular tachycardia (1% to 3%), palpitations (1% to 3%), AV block (first-degree) (1% to 3%), syncope (1% to 2%), increased QRS interval (1% to 2%), chest pain (1% to 2%), PVCs (1% to 2%), bradycardia (1% to 2%), edema (0% to 1%), bundle branch block (0% to 1%), atrial fibrillation (1%), hypotension (0% to 1%), intraventricular conduction delay (0% to 1%)
Central nervous system: Dizziness (4% to 15%), fatigue (2% to 6%), headache (2% to 5%), weakness (1% to 2%), ataxia (0% to 2%), insomnia (0% to 2%), anxiety (1% to 2%), drowsiness (1%)
Dermatologic: Rash (1% to 3%)
Gastrointestinal: Nausea/vomiting (2% to 11%), unusual taste (3% to 23%), constipation (2% to 7%), dyspepsia (1% to 3%), diarrhea (1% to 3%), xerostomia (1% to 2%), anorexia (1% to 2%), abdominal pain (1% to 2%), flatulence (0% to 1%)
Neuromuscular & skeletal: Tremor (0% to 1%), arthralgia (0% to 1%)
Ocular: Blurred vision (1% to 6%)
Respiratory: Dyspnea (2% to 5%)
Miscellaneous: Diaphoresis (1%)

Mechanism of Action Propafenone is a class 1c antiarrhythmic agent which possesses local anesthetic properties, blocks the fast inward sodium current, and slows the rate of increase of the action potential. Prolongs conduction and refractoriness in all areas of the myocardium, with a slightly more pronounced effect on intraventricular conduction; it prolongs effective refractory period, reduces spontaneous automaticity and exhibits some beta-blockade activity.

Drug Interactions
Cytochrome P450 Effect: Substrate of CYP1A2 (minor), 2D6 (major), 3A4 (minor); **Inhibits** CYP1A2 (weak), 2C8/9 (weak), 2D6 (weak)
Increased Effect/Toxicity: Amprenavir, cimetidine, metoprolol, propranolol, quinidine, and ritonavir may increase propafenone levels; concurrent use is contraindicated. CYP2D6 inhibitors may increase the levels/effects of propafenone; example inhibitors include chlorpromazine, delavirdine, fluoxetine, miconazole, paroxetine, pergolide, quinidine, quinine, ritonavir, and ropinirole. Digoxin (reduce dose by 25%), cyclosporine, local anesthetics, theophylline, and warfarin blood levels are increased by propafenone.
Decreased Effect: Enzyme inducers (phenobarbital, phenytoin, rifabutin, rifampin) may decrease propafenone blood levels.

Pharmacodynamics/Kinetics
Absorption: Well absorbed
Metabolism: Hepatic; two genetically determined metabolism groups exist: fast or slow metabolizers; 10% of Caucasians are slow metabolizers; exhibits nonlinear pharmacokinetics; when dose is increased from 300-900 mg/day,
(Continued)

Propafenone *(Continued)*

serum concentrations increase tenfold; this nonlinearity is thought to be due to saturable first-pass effect

Bioavailability: 150 mg: 3.4%; 300 mg: 10.6%

Half-life elimination: Single dose (100-300 mg): 2-8 hours; Chronic dosing: 10-32 hours

Time to peak: 150 mg dose: 2 hours, 300 mg dose: 3 hours

Pregnancy Risk Factor C

Propafenone Hydrochloride *see* Propafenone *on page 1133*

Propantheline (proe PAN the leen)

Canadian Brand Names Propanthel™

Generic Available Yes

Synonyms Propantheline Bromide

Pharmacologic Category Anticholinergic Agent

Dental Use Induce dry field (xerostomia) in oral cavity

Use Adjunctive treatment of peptic ulcer, irritable bowel syndrome, pancreatitis, ureteral and urinary bladder spasm; reduce duodenal motility during diagnostic radiologic procedures

Local Anesthetic/Vasoconstrictor Precautions No information available to require special precautions

Effects on Dental Treatment Key adverse event(s) related to dental treatment: Significant xerostomia (therapeutic effect; normal salivary flow resumes upon discontinuation), dry throat, nasal dryness, and dysphagia.

Significant Adverse Effects Frequency not defined.

Dermatologic: Dry skin

Gastrointestinal: Constipation, dry mouth and throat, dysphagia

Respiratory: Dry nose

Miscellaneous: Diaphoresis (decreased)

Dosage Oral:

Antisecretory:

Children: 1-2 mg/kg/day in 3-4 divided doses

Adults: 15 mg 3 times/day before meals or food and 30 mg at bedtime

Elderly: 7.5 mg 3 times/day before meals and at bedtime

Antispasmodic:

Children: 2-3 mg/kg/day in divided doses every 4-6 hours and at bedtime

Adults: 15 mg 3 times/day before meals or food and 30 mg at bedtime

Mechanism of Action Competitively blocks the action of acetylcholine at postganglionic parasympathetic receptor sites

Contraindications Hypersensitivity to propantheline or any component of the formulation; ulcerative colitis, toxic megacolon, obstructive disease of the GI or urinary tract; narrow-angle glaucoma; myasthenia gravis

Warnings/Precautions Use with caution in patients with hyperthyroidism, hepatic, cardiac, or renal disease, hypertension, GI infections, or other endocrine diseases.

Drug Interactions

Decreased effect with antacids (decreased absorption); decreased effect of sustained release dosage forms (decreased absorption)

Increased effect/toxicity with anticholinergics, disopyramide, narcotic analgesics, bretylium, type I antiarrhythmics, antihistamines, phenothiazines, TCAs, corticosteroids (increased IOP), CNS depressants (sedation), adenosine, amiodarone, beta-blockers, amoxapine

Dietary Considerations Should be taken 30 minutes before meals so that the drug's peak effect occurs at the proper time.

Pharmacodynamics/Kinetics

Onset of action: 30-45 minutes

Duration: 4-6 hours

Half-life elimination, serum: Average: 1.6 hours

Pregnancy Risk Factor C

Lactation Excretion in breast milk unknown

Breast-Feeding Considerations No data reported; however, atropine may be taken while breast-feeding.

Dosage Forms Tablet, as bromide: 15 mg

Propantheline Bromide *see* Propantheline *on page 1134*

Propa pH [OTC] *see* Salicylic Acid *on page 1205*

Proparacaine (proe PAR a kane)

U.S. Brand Names Alcaine®; Ophthetic®

Canadian Brand Names Alcaine®; Diocaine®

Generic Available Yes

Synonyms Proparacaine Hydrochloride; Proxymetacaine

Pharmacologic Category Local Anesthetic, Ophthalmic

Use Anesthesia for tonometry, gonioscopy; suture removal from cornea; removal of corneal foreign body; cataract extraction, glaucoma surgery; short operative procedure involving the cornea and conjunctiva

Local Anesthetic/Vasoconstrictor Precautions No information available to require special precautions

Effects on Dental Treatment No significant effects or complications reported

Mechanism of Action Prevents initiation and transmission of impulse at the nerve cell membrane by decreasing ion permeability through stabilizing

Pregnancy Risk Factor C

Proparacaine and Fluorescein

(proe PAR a kane & FLURE e seen)

Related Information

Proparacaine *on page 1134*

U.S. Brand Names Flucaine®; Fluoracaine®

Generic Available Yes

Synonyms Fluorescein and Proparacaine

Pharmacologic Category Diagnostic Agent; Local Anesthetic

Use Anesthesia for tonometry, gonioscopy; suture removal from cornea; removal of corneal foreign body; cataract extraction, glaucoma surgery

Local Anesthetic/Vasoconstrictor Precautions No information available to require special precautions

Effects on Dental Treatment No significant effects or complications reported

Common Adverse Effects 1% to 10%: Local: Burning, stinging of eye

Mechanism of Action Prevents initiation and transmission of impulse at the nerve cell membrane by decreasing ion permeability through stabilizing

Pharmacodynamics/Kinetics

Onset of action: ~20 seconds

Duration: 15-20 minutes

Pregnancy Risk Factor C

Proparacaine Hydrochloride *see* Proparacaine *on page 1134*

Propecia® *see* Finasteride *on page 590*

Propine® *see* Dipivefrin *on page 453*

Proplex® T *see* Factor IX Complex (Human) *on page 572*

Propofol (PROE po fole)

U.S. Brand Names Diprivan®

Canadian Brand Names Diprivan®

Mexican Brand Names Diprivan®; Fresofol®; Recofol®

Generic Available Yes

Pharmacologic Category General Anesthetic

Use Induction of anesthesia for inpatient or outpatient surgery in patients ≥3 years of age; maintenance of anesthesia for inpatient or outpatient surgery in patients >2 months of age; in adults, for the induction and maintenance of monitored anesthesia care sedation during diagnostic procedures; treatment of agitation in intubated, mechanically-ventilated ICU patients

Unlabeled/Investigational Use Postoperative antiemetic; refractory delirium tremens (case reports); conscious sedation

Local Anesthetic/Vasoconstrictor Precautions No information available to require special precautions

Effects on Dental Treatment No significant effects or complications reported

Common Adverse Effects

>10%:

- Cardiovascular: Hypotension (children 17%, adults 3% to 26%)
- Central nervous system: Dystonic or choreoform movement (children 17%)
- Local: Injection site burning, stinging, or pain (children 10%, adults 18%)
- Respiratory: Apnea lasting 30-60 seconds (children 10%, adults 24%); apnea lasting >60 seconds (children 5%, adults 12%)

1% to 10%:

- Cardiovascular: Hypertension (children 8%), arrhythmia, bradycardia, cardiac output decreased, tachycardia
- Central nervous system: Movement (adults)
- Dermatologic: Pruritus (children 2%), rash (children 5%)
- Endocrine & metabolic: Hyperlipidemia, hypertriglyceridemia
- Respiratory: Respiratory acidosis during weaning

(Continued)

Propofol *(Continued)*

Mechanism of Action Propofol is a hindered phenolic compound with intravenous general anesthetic properties. The drug is unrelated to any of the currently used barbiturate, opioid, benzodiazepine, arylcyclohexylamine, or imidazole intravenous anesthetic agents.

Drug Interactions

Cytochrome P450 Effect: Substrate of CYP1A2 (minor), 2A6 (minor), 2B6 (major), 2C8/9 (major), 2C19 (minor), 2D6 (minor), 2E1 (minor), 3A4 (minor); **Inhibits** CYP1A2 (moderate), 2C8/9 (weak), 2C19 (moderate), 2D6 (weak), 2E1 (weak), 3A4 (strong)

Increased Effect/Toxicity: Additive CNS depression and respiratory depression may necessitate dosage reduction when used with anesthetics, benzodiazepines, opiates, ethanol, narcotics, phenothiazines. The levels/effects of propofol may be increased by delavirdine, desipramine, fluconazole, gemfibrozil, ketoconazole, nicardipine, NSAIDs, paroxetine, sertraline, sulfonamides, and other inhibitors of CYP2B6 or 2C8/9.

Propofol may potentiate the neuromuscular blockade of vecuronium (and possibly other neuromuscular-blocking agents). Propofol may increase the levels/effects of aminophylline, benzodiazepines, calcium channel blockers, cyclosporine, fluvoxamine, selected HMG-CoA reductase inhibitors, mexiletine, mirtazapine, nateglinide, nefazodone, ropinirole, sildenafil (and other PDE-5 inhibitors) tacrolimus, theophylline, trifluoperazine, venlafaxine, and other CYP1A2 or 3A4 substrates. Selected benzodiazepines (midazolam and triazolam), cisapride, ergot alkaloids, selected HMG-CoA reductase inhibitors (lovastatin and simvastatin), and pimozide are generally contraindicated with strong CYP3A4 inhibitors.

Pharmacodynamics/Kinetics

Onset of action: Anesthetic: Bolus infusion (dose dependent): 9-51 seconds (average 30 seconds)

Duration (dose and rate dependent): 3-10 minutes

Distribution: V_d: 2-10 L/kg; highly lipophilic

Protein binding: 97% to 99%

Metabolism: Hepatic to water-soluble sulfate and glucuronide conjugates

Half-life elimination: Biphasic: Initial: 40 minutes; Terminal: 4-7 hours (up to 1-3 days)

Excretion: Urine (~88% as metabolites, 40% as glucuronide metabolite); feces (<2%)

Clearance: 20-30 mL/kg/minute; total body clearance exceeds liver blood flow

Pregnancy Risk Factor B

Propoxyphene (proe POKS i feen)

U.S. Brand Names Darvon®; Darvon-N®

Canadian Brand Names Darvon-N®; 642® Tablet

Generic Available Yes: Capsule

Synonyms Dextropropoxyphene; Propoxyphene Hydrochloride; Propoxyphene Napsylate

Pharmacologic Category Analgesic, Narcotic

Use Management of mild to moderate pain

Local Anesthetic/Vasoconstrictor Precautions No information available to require special precautions

Effects on Dental Treatment Key adverse event(s) related to dental treatment: Xerostomia (normal salivary flow resumes upon discontinuation).

Common Adverse Effects Frequency not defined.

Cardiovascular: Hypotension, bundle branch block

Central nervous system: Dizziness, lightheadedness, sedation, paradoxical excitement and insomnia, fatigue, drowsiness, mental depression, hallucinations, paradoxical CNS stimulation, increased intracranial pressure, nervousness, headache, restlessness, malaise, confusion, dysphoria, vertigo

Dermatologic: Rash, urticaria

Endocrine & metabolic: Hypoglycemia, urinary 17-OHCS decreased

Gastrointestinal: Anorexia, stomach cramps, xerostomia, biliary spasm, nausea, vomiting, constipation, paralytic ileus, abdominal pain

Genitourinary: Urination decreased, ureteral spasms

Neuromuscular & skeletal: Weakness

Hepatic: LFTs increased, jaundice

Ocular: Visual disturbances

Respiratory: Dyspnea

Miscellaneous: Psychologic and physical dependence with prolonged use, histamine release, hypersensitivity reaction

Restrictions C-IV

Mechanism of Action Propoxyphene is a weak narcotic analgesic which acts through binding to opiate receptors to inhibit ascending pain pathways. Propoxyphene, as with other narcotic (opiate) analgesics, blocks pain perception in the cerebral cortex by binding to specific receptor molecules (opiate receptors) within the neuronal membranes of synapses. This binding results in a decreased synaptic chemical transmission throughout the CNS thus inhibiting the flow of pain sensations into the higher centers. Mu and kappa are the two subtypes of the opiate receptor which propoxyphene binds to to cause analgesia.

Drug Interactions

Cytochrome P450 Effect: Inhibits CYP2C8/9 (weak), 2D6 (weak), 3A4 (weak)

Increased Effect/Toxicity: CNS depressants (phenothiazines, tranquilizers, anxiolytics, sedatives, hypnotics, or alcohol) may potentiate pharmacologic effects. Propoxyphene may inhibit the metabolism and increase the serum concentrations of carbamazepine, phenobarbital, MAO inhibitors, tricyclic antidepressants, and warfarin.

Decreased Effect: Decreased effect with cigarette smoking.

Pharmacodynamics/Kinetics

Onset of action: 0.5-1 hour

Duration: 4-6 hours

Metabolism: Hepatic to active metabolite (norpropoxyphene) and inactive metabolites; first-pass effect

Half-life elimination: Adults: Parent drug: 6-12 hours; Norpropoxyphene: 30-36 hours

Excretion: Urine (primarily as metabolites)

Pregnancy Risk Factor C/D (prolonged use)

Propoxyphene and Acetaminophen

(proe POKS i feen & a seet a MIN oh fen)

Related Information

Acetaminophen *on page 47*

Propoxyphene *on page 1136*

U.S. Brand Names Darvocet A500™; Darvocet-N® 50; Darvocet-N® 100; Pronap-100®

Canadian Brand Names Darvocet-N® 50; Darvocet-N® 100

Generic Available Yes

Synonyms Propoxyphene Hydrochloride and Acetaminophen; Propoxyphene Napsylate and Acetaminophen

Pharmacologic Category Analgesic Combination (Narcotic)

Dental Use Management of postoperative pain

Use Management of mild to moderate pain

Local Anesthetic/Vasoconstrictor Precautions No information available to require special precautions

Effects on Dental Treatment Key adverse event(s) related to dental treatment: Xerostomia (normal salivary flow resumes upon discontinuation).

Significant Adverse Effects See individual agents.

Restrictions C-IV

Dosage Oral: Adults:

Darvocet A500™, Darvocet-N® 100: 1 tablet every 4 hours as needed; maximum: 600 mg propoxyphene napsylate/day

Darvocet-N® 50: 1-2 tablets every 4 hours as needed; maximum: 600 mg propoxyphene napsylate/day

Note: Dosage of acetaminophen should not exceed 4 g/day (6 tablets of Darvocet-N® 100); possibly less in patients with ethanol

Elderly: Refer to Adults dosing

Dosing adjustment in renal/hepatic impairment: Serum concentrations of propoxyphene may be increased or elimination may be delayed; specific dosing recommendations not available.

Mechanism of Action

Propoxyphene is a weak narcotic analgesic which acts through binding to opiate receptors to inhibit ascending pain pathways

Propoxyphene, as with other narcotic (opiate) analgesics, blocks pain perception in the cerebral cortex by binding to specific receptor molecules (opiate receptors) within the neuronal membranes of synapses. This binding results in a decreased synaptic chemical transmission throughout the CNS thus inhibiting the flow of pain sensations into the higher centers. Mu and kappa are the two subtypes of the opiate receptor which propoxyphene binds to to cause analgesia.

(Continued)

Propoxyphene and Acetaminophen *(Continued)*

Acetaminophen inhibits the synthesis of prostaglandins in the CNS and peripherally blocks pain impulse generation; produces antipyresis from inhibition of hypothalamic heat-regulating center

Contraindications Hypersensitivity to propoxyphene, acetaminophen, or any component of the formulation

Warnings/Precautions When given in excessive doses, either alone or in combination with other CNS depressants, propoxyphene is a major cause of drug-related deaths; do not exceed recommended dosage; give with caution in patients dependent on opiates, substitution may result in acute opiate withdrawal symptoms. Avoid use in severely-depressed or suicidal patients. Tolerance or drug dependence may result from extended use.

Propoxyphene should be used with caution in patients with renal or hepatic dysfunction or in the elderly; consider dosing adjustment. Acetaminophen should be used with caution in patients with liver disease; consuming ≥3 alcoholic drinks/day may increase risk of liver damage. Use caution in patients with known G6PD deficiency. Safety and efficacy of this combination have not been established in pediatric patients.

Drug Interactions

Propoxyphene: **Inhibits** CYP2C8/9 (weak), 2D6 (weak), 3A4 (weak)

Acetaminophen: **Substrate** (minor) of CYP1A2, 2A6, 2C8/9, 2D6, 2E1, 3A4; **Inhibits** CYP3A4 (weak)

Also see individual agents.

Ethanol/Nutrition/Herb Interactions

Based on **propoxyphene** component:

Ethanol: Avoid or limit ethanol (may increase CNS depression). Watch for sedation.

Food: May decrease rate of absorption, but may slightly increase bioavailability.

Based on **acetaminophen** component:

Ethanol: Excessive intake of ethanol may increase the risk of acetaminophen-induced hepatotoxicity. Avoid ethanol or limit to <3 drinks/day.

Food: Rate of absorption may be decreased when given with food.

Herb/Nutraceutical: St John's wort may decrease acetaminophen levels.

Dietary Considerations May be taken with food if gastrointestinal distress occurs.

Pharmacodynamics/Kinetics See individual agents.

Pregnancy Risk Factor C

Lactation Enters breast milk/compatible

Breast-Feeding Considerations Propoxyphene, norpropoxyphene and acetaminophen are excreted in breast milk. The AAP considers propoxyphene and acetaminophen to be "compatible" with breast-feeding.

Dosage Forms Tablet: Propoxyphene hydrochloride 65 mg and acetaminophen 650 mg, propoxyphene napsylate 100 mg, and acetaminophen 650 mg

Darvocet A500™: Propoxyphene napsylate 100 mg and acetaminophen 500 mg [contains lactose]

Darvocet-N® 50: Propoxyphene napsylate 50 mg and acetaminophen 325 mg

Darvocet-N® 100, Pronap-100®: Propoxyphene napsylate 100 mg and acetaminophen 650 mg

Comments Propoxyphene is a narcotic analgesic and shares many properties including addiction liability. The acetaminophen component requires use with caution in patients with alcoholic liver disease.

Selected Readings

Botting RM, "Mechanism of Action of Acetaminophen: Is There a Cyclooxygenase 3?" *Clin Infect Dis*, 2000, Suppl 5:S202-10.

Dart RC, Kuffner EK, and Rumack BH, "Treatment of Pain or Fever with Paracetamol (Acetaminophen) in the Alcoholic Patient: A Systematic Review," *Am J Ther*, 2000, 7(2):123-34.

Grant JA and Weiler JM, "A Report of a Rare Immediate Reaction After Ingestion of Acetaminophen," *Ann Allergy Asthma Immunol*, 2001, 87(3):227-9.

Kwan D, Bartle WR, and Walker SE, "The Effects of Acetaminophen on Pharmacokinetics and Pharmacodynamics of Warfarin," *J Clin Pharmacol*, 1999, 39(1):68-75.

McClain CJ, Price S, Barve S, et al, "Acetaminophen Hepatotoxicity: An Update," *Curr Gastroenterol Rep*, 1999, 1(1):42-9.

Shek KL, Chan LN, and Nutescu E, "Warfarin-Acetaminophen Drug Interaction Revisited," *Pharmacotherapy*, 1999, 19(10):1153-8.

Tanaka E, Yamazaki K, and Misawa S, "Update: The Clinical Importance of Acetaminophen Hepatotoxicity in Nonalcoholic and Alcoholic Subjects," *J Clin Pharm Ther*, 2000, 25(5):325-32.

Propoxyphene, Aspirin, and Caffeine

(proe POKS i feen, AS pir in, & KAF een)

Related Information

Aspirin *on page 151*

Propoxyphene *on page 1136*

U.S. Brand Names Darvon® Compound

Generic Available No

Synonyms Aspirin, Caffeine, and Propoxyphene; Caffeine, Propoxyphene, and Aspirin; Propoxyphene Hydrochloride, Aspirin, and Caffeine

Pharmacologic Category Analgesic Combination (Narcotic)

Use Treatment of mild-to-moderate pain

Local Anesthetic/Vasoconstrictor Precautions No information available to require special precautions

Effects on Dental Treatment Key adverse event(s) related to dental treatment: As with all drugs which may affect hemostasis, bleeding is associated with aspirin. Hemorrhage may occur at virtually any site; risk is dependent on multiple variables including dosage, concurrent use of multiple agents which alter hemostasis, and patient susceptibility. Many adverse effects of aspirin are dose-related, and are rare at low dosages. Other serious reactions are idiosyncratic, related to allergy or individual sensitivity.

Elderly are a high-risk population for adverse effects from nonsteroidal anti-inflammatory agents. As many as 60% of elderly patients with GI complications from NSAIDs can develop peptic ulceration and/or hemorrhage asymptomatically. Concomitant disease and drug use contribute to the risk of GI adverse effects. Use lowest effective dose for shortest period possible. Consider renal function decline with age.

Significant Adverse Effects See individual agents.

Restrictions C-IV

Dosage Oral: Adults: Pain: One capsule (providing propoxyphene 32 mg or 65 mg) every 4 hours as needed; maximum propoxyphene 390 mg/day. This will also provide aspirin 389 mg and caffeine 32.4 mg per capsule.

Elderly: Refer to Adults dosing; consider increasing dosing interval

Dosage adjustment in renal impairment: Serum concentrations of propoxyphene may be increased or elimination may be delayed; specific dosing recommendations not available. Avoid use with Cl_{cr} <10 mL/minute.

Dosage adjustment in hepatic impairment: Serum concentrations or propoxyphene may be increased or elimination may be delayed; specific dosing recommendations not available.

Mechanism of Action Propoxyphene is a weak narcotic analgesic which acts through binding to opiate receptors to inhibit ascending pain pathways. Propoxyphene, as with other narcotic (opiate) analgesics, blocks pain perception in the cerebral cortex by binding to specific receptor molecules (opiate receptors) within the neuronal membranes of synapses. This binding results in a decreased synaptic chemical transmission throughout the CNS thus inhibiting the flow of pain sensations into the higher centers. Mu and kappa are the two subtypes of the opiate receptor which propoxyphene binds to to cause analgesia.

Aspirin inhibits prostaglandin synthesis, acts on the hypothalamus heat-regulating center to reduce fever, blocks prostaglandin synthetase action which prevents formation of the platelet-aggregating substance thromboxane A_2.

Caffeine is a CNS stimulant; use with propoxyphene and aspirin increases the level of analgesia provided by each agent.

Contraindications Hypersensitivity to propoxyphene, aspirin, caffeine, or any component of the formulation

Warnings/Precautions When given in excessive doses, either alone or in combination with other CNS depressants, propoxyphene is a major cause of drug-related deaths; do not exceed recommended dosage; give with caution in patients dependent on opiates, substitution may result in acute opiate withdrawal symptoms. Avoid use in severely-depressed or suicidal patients. Tolerance or drug dependence may result from extended use. Propoxyphene should be used with caution in patients with renal or hepatic dysfunction or in the elderly; consider dosing adjustment

Aspirin should be used with caution in patients with ulcers or coagulation abnormalities. Patients with sensitivity to tartrazine dyes, nasal polyps and asthma may have an increased risk of salicylate sensitivity. Surgical patients should avoid ASA if possible, for 1-2 weeks prior to surgery, to reduce the risk of excessive bleeding. Heavy ethanol use (≥3 drinks/day) can increase bleeding risks. Aspirin should be avoided in children (<16 years of age) with viral infections (chickenpox or flu symptoms), with or without fever, due to a potential association with Reye's syndrome. Safety and efficacy of this combination product in children have not been established.

Drug Interactions See individual agents for Propoxyphene and Aspirin.

(Continued)

Propoxyphene, Aspirin, and Caffeine *(Continued)*

Ethanol/Nutrition/Herb Interactions Based on **propoxyphene** component:

Ethanol: Avoid or limit ethanol (may increase CNS depression). Watch for sedation.

Food: May decrease rate of absorption, but may slightly increase bioavailability.

Pharmacodynamics/Kinetics See individual agents.

Pregnancy Risk Factor C

Lactation Enters breast milk/use caution

Breast-Feeding Considerations Propoxyphene, norpropoxyphene, aspirin, and caffeine are excreted in breast milk. The AAP recommends that aspirin be used "with caution" during breast-feeding; propoxyphene and caffeine (moderate intake) are considered "compatible."

Dosage Forms Capsule:

Darvon® Compound 32: Propoxyphene hydrochloride 32 mg, aspirin 389 mg, and caffeine 32.4 mg

Darvon® Compound 65: Propoxyphene hydrochloride 65 mg, aspirin 389 mg, and caffeine 32.4 mg

Comments Propoxyphene is a narcotic analgesic and shares many properties including addiction liability. The aspirin component could have anticoagulant effects and could possibly affect bleeding times.

Propoxyphene Hydrochloride *see* Propoxyphene *on page 1136*

Propoxyphene Hydrochloride and Acetaminophen *see* Propoxyphene and Acetaminophen *on page 1137*

Propoxyphene Hydrochloride, Aspirin, and Caffeine *see* Propoxyphene, Aspirin, and Caffeine *on page 1138*

Propoxyphene Napsylate *see* Propoxyphene *on page 1136*

Propoxyphene Napsylate and Acetaminophen *see* Propoxyphene and Acetaminophen *on page 1137*

Propranolol (proe PRAN oh lole)

Related Information

Cardiovascular Diseases *on page 1458*

Endocrine Disorders and Pregnancy *on page 1481*

U.S. Brand Names Inderal®; Inderal® LA; InnoPran XL™; Propranolol Intensol™

Canadian Brand Names Apo-Propranolol®; Inderal®; Inderal®-LA; Nu-Propranolol

Generic Available Yes: Excludes capsule

Synonyms Propranolol Hydrochloride

Pharmacologic Category Antiarrhythmic Agent, Class II; Beta-Adrenergic Blocker, Nonselective

Use Management of hypertension; angina pectoris; pheochromocytoma; essential tremor; tetralogy of Fallot cyanotic spells; arrhythmias (such as atrial fibrillation and flutter, AV nodal re-entrant tachycardias, and catecholamine-induced arrhythmias); prevention of myocardial infarction; migraine headache; symptomatic treatment of hypertrophic subaortic stenosis

Unlabeled/Investigational Use Tremor due to Parkinson's disease; ethanol withdrawal; aggressive behavior; antipsychotic-induced akathisia; prevention of bleeding esophageal varices; anxiety; schizophrenia; acute panic; gastric bleeding in portal hypertension; thyrotoxicosis

Local Anesthetic/Vasoconstrictor Precautions Use with caution; epinephrine has interacted with nonselective beta-blockers to result in initial hypertensive episode followed by bradycardia

Effects on Dental Treatment Propranolol is a nonselective beta-blocker and may enhance the pressor response to epinephrine, resulting in hypertension and bradycardia. Many nonsteroidal anti-inflammatory drugs, such as ibuprofen and indomethacin, can reduce the hypotensive effect of beta-blockers after 3 or more weeks of therapy with the NSAID. Short-term NSAID use (ie, 3 days) requires no special precautions in patients taking beta-blockers.

Common Adverse Effects Frequency not defined.

Cardiovascular: Bradycardia, CHF, reduced peripheral circulation, chest pain, hypotension, impaired myocardial contractility, worsening of AV conduction disturbance, cardiogenic shock, Raynaud's syndrome, mesenteric thrombosis (rare)

Central nervous system: Mental depression, lightheadedness, amnesia, emotional lability, confusion, hallucinations, dizziness, insomnia, fatigue, vivid dreams, lethargy, cold extremities, vertigo, syncope, cognitive dysfunction, psychosis, hypersomnolence

Dermatologic: Rash, alopecia, exfoliative dermatitis, psoriasiform eruptions, eczematous eruptions, hyperkeratosis, nail changes, pruritus, urticaria, ulcerative lichenoid, contact dermatitis

Endocrine & metabolic: Hypoglycemia, hyperglycemia, hyperlipidemia, hyperkalemia

Gastrointestinal: Diarrhea, nausea, vomiting, stomach discomfort, constipation, anorexia

Genitourinary: Impotence, proteinuria (rare), oliguria (rare), interstitial nephritis (rare), Peyronie's disease

Hematologic: Agranulocytosis, thrombocytopenia, thrombocytopenic purpura

Neuromuscular & skeletal: Weakness, carpal tunnel syndrome (rare), paresthesias, myotonus, polyarthritis, arthropathy

Respiratory: Wheezing, pharyngitis, bronchospasm, pulmonary edema

Ocular: Hyperemia of the conjunctiva, decreased tear production, decreased visual acuity, mydriasis

Miscellaneous: Lupus-like syndrome (rare)

Dosage

Akathisia: Oral: Adults: 30-120 mg/day in 2-3 divided doses

Angina: Oral: Adults: 80-320 mg/day in doses divided 2-4 times/day

Long-acting formulation: Initial: 80 mg once daily; maximum dose: 320 mg once daily

Essential tremor: Oral: Adults: 20-40 mg twice daily initially; maintenance doses: usually 120-320 mg/day

Hypertension:

Oral:

Children: Initial: 0.5-1 mg/kg/day in divided doses every 6-12 hours; increase gradually every 5-7 days; maximum: 16 mg/kg/24 hours

Adults: Initial: 40 mg twice daily; increase dosage every 3-7 days; usual dose: ≤320 mg divided in 2-3 doses/day; maximum daily dose: 640 mg; usual dosage range (JNC 7): 40-160 mg/day in 2 divided doses

Long-acting formulation: Initial: 80 mg once daily; usual maintenance: 120-160 mg once daily; maximum daily dose: 640 mg; usual dosage range (JNC 7): 60-180 mg/day once daily

I.V.: Children: 0.01-0.05 mg/kg over 1 hour; maximum dose: 10 mg

Hypertrophic subaortic stenosis: Oral: Adults: 20-40 mg 3-4 times/day

Long-acting formulation: 80-160 mg once daily

Migraine headache prophylaxis: Oral:

Children: Initial: 2-4 mg/kg/day **or**

≤35 kg: 10-20 mg 3 times/day

>35 kg: 20-40 mg 3 times/day

Adults: Initial: 80 mg/day divided every 6-8 hours; increase by 20-40 mg/dose every 3-4 weeks to a maximum of 160-240 mg/day given in divided doses every 6-8 hours; if satisfactory response not achieved within 6 weeks of starting therapy, drug should be withdrawn gradually over several weeks

Long-acting formulation: Initial: 80 mg once daily; effective dose range: 160-240 mg once daily

Myocardial infarction prophylaxis: Oral: Adults: 180-240 mg/day in 3-4 divided doses

Pheochromocytoma: Oral: Adults: 30-60 mg/day in divided doses

Tachyarrhythmias:

Oral:

Children: Initial: 0.5-1 mg/kg/day in divided doses every 6-8 hours; titrate dosage upward every 3-7 days; usual dose: 2-6 mg/kg/day; higher doses may be needed; do not exceed 16 mg/kg/day or 60 mg/day

Adults: 10-30 mg/dose every 6-8 hours

Elderly: Initial: 10 mg twice daily; increase dosage every 3-7 days; usual dosage range: 10-320 mg given in 2 divided doses

I.V.:

Children: 0.01-0.1 mg/kg/dose slow IVP over 10 minutes; maximum dose: 1 mg for infants; 3 mg for children

Adults (in patients having nonfunctional GI tract): 1 mg/dose slow IVP; repeat every 5 minutes up to a total of 5 mg; titrate initial dose to desired response

Tetralogy spells: Children:

Oral: Palliation: Initial: 1 mg/kg/day every 6 hours; if ineffective, may increase dose after 1 week by 1 mg/kg/day to a maximum of 5 mg/kg/day; if patient becomes refractory, may increase slowly to a maximum of 10-15 mg/kg/day. Allow 24 hours between dosing changes.

(Continued)

Propranolol *(Continued)*

I.V.: 0.01-0.2 mg/kg/dose infused over 10 minutes; maximum initial dose: 1 mg

Thyrotoxicosis:

Oral:

Children: 2 mg/kg/day, divided every 6-8 hours, titrate to effective dose

Adolescents and Adults: Oral: 10-40 mg/dose every 6 hours

I.V.: Adults: 1-3 mg/dose slow IVP as a single dose

Dosing adjustment/comments in renal impairment: Not dialyzable (0% to 5%); supplemental dose is not necessary. Peritoneal dialysis effects: Supplemental dose is not necessary.

Dosing adjustment/comments in hepatic disease: Marked slowing of heart rate may occur in cirrhosis with conventional doses; low initial dose and regular heart rate monitoring

Mechanism of Action Nonselective beta-adrenergic blocker (class II antiarrhythmic); competitively blocks response to $beta_1$- and $beta_2$-adrenergic stimulation which results in decreases in heart rate, myocardial contractility, blood pressure, and myocardial oxygen demand

Contraindications Hypersensitivity to propranolol, beta-blockers, or any component of the formulation; uncompensated congestive heart failure (unless the failure is due to tachyarrhythmias being treated with propranolol), cardiogenic shock, bradycardia or heart block (2nd or 3rd degree), pulmonary edema, severe hyperactive airway disease (asthma or COPD), Raynaud's disease; pregnancy (2nd and 3rd trimesters)

Warnings/Precautions Administer cautiously in compensated heart failure and monitor for a worsening of the condition (efficacy of propranolol in CHF has not been demonstrated). Beta-blocker therapy should not be withdrawn abruptly (particularly in patients with CAD), but gradually tapered (over 2 weeks) to avoid acute tachycardia, hypertension, and/or ischemia. Use caution in patient with PVD. Use caution with concurrent use of beta-blockers and either verapamil or diltiazem; bradycardia or heart block can occur. Avoid concurrent I.V. use of both agents. Use cautiously in diabetics because it can mask prominent hypoglycemic symptoms. Can mask signs of thyrotoxicosis. Can cause fetal harm when administered in pregnancy. Use cautiously in hepatic dysfunction (dosage adjustment required). Use care with anesthetic agents which decrease myocardial function. Not indicated for hypertensive emergencies.

Drug Interactions

Cytochrome P450 Effect: Substrate of CYP1A2 (major), 2C19 (minor), 2D6 (major), 3A4 (minor); **Inhibits** CYP1A2 (weak), 2D6 (weak)

Increased Effect/Toxicity: CYP1A2 inhibitors may increase the levels/effects of propranolol; example inhibitors include amiodarone, ciprofloxacin, fluvoxamine, ketoconazole, lomefloxacin, ofloxacin, and rofecoxib. CYP2D6 inhibitors may increase the levels/effects of propranolol; example inhibitors include chlorpromazine, delavirdine, fluoxetine, miconazole, paroxetine, pergolide, quinidine, quinine, ritonavir, and ropinirole. The heart rate-lowering effects of propranolol are additive with other drugs which slow AV conduction (digoxin, verapamil, diltiazem). Reserpine increases the effects of propranolol. Concurrent use of propranolol may increase the effects of alpha-blockers (prazosin, terazosin), alpha-adrenergic stimulants (epinephrine, phenylephrine), and the vasoconstrictive effects of ergot alkaloids. Propranolol may mask the tachycardia from hypoglycemia caused by insulin and oral hypoglycemics. In patients receiving concurrent therapy, the risk of hypertensive crisis is increased when either clonidine or the beta-blocker is withdrawn. Beta-blockers may increase the action or levels of ethanol, disopyramide, nondepolarizing muscle relaxants, and theophylline although the effects are difficult to predict. Propranolol may increase the bioavailability of serotonin 5-HT_{1D} receptor agonists. Propranolol may decrease the metabolism of lidocaine.

Beta-blocker effects may be enhanced by oral contraceptives, flecainide, haloperidol (hypotensive effects), cimetidine, hydralazine, phenothiazines, propafenone, thyroid hormones (when hypothyroid patient is converted to euthyroid state). Beta-blockers may increase the effect/toxicity of flecainide, haloperidol (hypotensive effects), hydralazine, phenothiazines, acetaminophen, anticoagulants (warfarin), and benzodiazepines.

Decreased Effect: CYP1A2 inducers may decrease the levels/effects of propranolol; example inducers include aminoglutethimide, carbamazepine, phenobarbital, and rifampin. Aluminum salts, calcium salts, cholestyramine, colestipol, NSAIDs, penicillins (ampicillin), salicylates, and sulfinpyrazone decrease effect of beta-blockers due to decreased bioavailability and plasma levels. Beta-blockers may decrease the effect of sulfonylureas. Ascorbic acid decreases propranolol Cp_{max} and AUC and increases the T_{max} significantly resulting in a greater decrease in the reduction of heart rate, possibly due to decreased absorption and first pass metabolism (n=5). Nefazodone decreased peak plasma levels and AUC of propranolol and increases time to reach steady-state; monitoring of clinical response is recommended. Nonselective beta-blockers blunt the response to beta-2 adrenergic agonists (albuterol).

Ethanol/Nutrition/Herb Interactions

Ethanol: Ethanol may decrease plasma levels of propranolol by increasing metabolism.

Food: Propranolol serum levels may be increased if taken with food. Protein-rich foods may increase bioavailability; a change in diet from high carbohydrate/low protein to low carbohydrate/high protein may result in increased oral clearance.

Cigarette: Smoking may decrease plasma levels of propranolol by increasing metabolism.

Herb/Nutraceutical: Avoid dong quai if using for hypertension (has estrogenic activity). Avoid ephedra, yohimbe, ginseng (may worsen hypertension or arrhythmia). Avoid natural licorice (causes sodium and water retention and increases potassium loss). Avoid garlic (may have increased antihypertensive effect).

Dietary Considerations Tablets should be taken on an empty stomach; capsules may be taken with or without food, but should always be taken consistently (with food or on an empty stomach)

Pharmacodynamics/Kinetics

Onset of action: Beta-blockade: Oral: 1-2 hours

Duration: ~6 hours

Distribution: V_d: 3.9 L/kg in adults; crosses placenta; small amounts enter breast milk

Protein binding: Newborns: 68%; Adults: 93%

Metabolism: Hepatic to active and inactive compounds; extensive first-pass effect

Bioavailability: 30% to 40%; may be increased in Down syndrome

Half-life elimination: Neonates and Infants: Possible increased half-life; Children: 3.9-6.4 hours; Adults: 4-6 hours

Excretion: Urine (96% to 99%)

Pregnancy Risk Factor C (manufacturer); D (2nd and 3rd trimesters - expert analysis)

Dosage Forms CAP, extended release (InnPran™): 80 mg, 120 mg. **CAP, sustained release** (Inderal® LA): 60 mg, 80 mg, 120 mg, 160 mg. **INJ, solution** (Inderal®): 1 mg/mL (1 mL). **SOLN, oral:** 4 mg/mL (5 mL, 500 mL); 8 mg/mL (500 mL). **SOLN, oral concentrate** (Propranolol Intensol™): 80 mg/mL (30 mL). **TAB** (Inderal®): 10 mg, 20 mg, 40 mg, 60 mg, 80 mg

Selected Readings

Foster CA and Aston SJ, "Propranolol-Epinephrine Interaction: A Potential Disaster," *Plast Reconstr Surg*, 1983, 72(1):74-8.

Wong DG, Spence JD, Lamki L, et al, "Effect of Nonsteroidal Anti-inflammatory Drugs on Control of Hypertension of Beta-Blockers and Diuretics," *Lancet*, 1986, 1(8488):997-1001.

Wynn RL, "Dental Nonsteroidal Anti-inflammatory Drugs and Prostaglandin-Based Drug Interactions, Part Two," *Gen Dent*, 1992, 40(2):104, 106, 108.

Wynn RL, "Epinephrine Interactions With Beta-Blockers," *Gen Dent*, 1994, 42(1):16, 18.

Propranolol and Hydrochlorothiazide

(proe PRAN oh lole & hye droe klor oh THYE a zide)

Related Information

Hydrochlorothiazide *on page 699*

Propranolol *on page 1140*

U.S. Brand Names Inderide®

Generic Available Yes

Synonyms Hydrochlorothiazide and Propranolol

Pharmacologic Category Antihypertensive Agent, Combination

Use Management of hypertension

Local Anesthetic/Vasoconstrictor Precautions Use with caution; epinephrine has interacted with nonselective beta-blockers to result in initial hypertensive episode followed by bradycardia

Effects on Dental Treatment Noncardioselective beta-blockers (ie, propranolol, nadolol) enhance the pressor response to epinephrine, resulting in hypertension and bradycardia. Many nonsteroidal anti-inflammatory drugs, such as ibuprofen and indomethacin, can reduce the hypotensive effect of beta-blockers after 3 or more weeks of therapy with the NSAID. Short-term

(Continued)

Propranolol and Hydrochlorothiazide *(Continued)*

NSAID use (ie, 3 days) requires no special precautions in patients taking beta-blockers.

Common Adverse Effects See individual agents.

Drug Interactions

Cytochrome P450 Effect: Propranolol: **Substrate** of CYP1A2 (major), 2C19 (major), 2D6 (major), 3A4 (minor); **Inhibits** CYP1A2 (weak), 2D6 (weak)

Pharmacodynamics/Kinetics See individual agents.

Pregnancy Risk Factor C

Propranolol Hydrochloride *see* Propranolol *on page 1140*

Propranolol Intensol™ *see* Propranolol *on page 1140*

Proprinal [OTC] *see* Ibuprofen *on page 728*

Propulsid® *see* Cisapride *on page 336*

Propylene Glycol Diacetate, Acetic Acid, and Hydrocortisone *see* Acetic Acid, Propylene Glycol Diacetate, and Hydrocortisone *on page 60*

Propylene Glycol Diacetate, Hydrocortisone, and Acetic Acid *see* Acetic Acid, Propylene Glycol Diacetate, and Hydrocortisone *on page 60*

Propylhexedrine (proe pil HEKS e dreen)

U.S. Brand Names Benzedrex® [OTC]

Generic Available No

Pharmacologic Category Adrenergic Agonist Agent

Use Topical nasal decongestant

Local Anesthetic/Vasoconstrictor Precautions No information available to require special precautions

Effects on Dental Treatment No significant effects or complications reported

2-Propylpentanoic Acid *see* Valproic Acid and Derivatives *on page 1359*

Propylthiouracil (proe pil thye oh YOOR a sil)

Related Information

Endocrine Disorders and Pregnancy *on page 1481*

Canadian Brand Names Propyl-Thyracil®

Generic Available Yes

Synonyms PTU

Pharmacologic Category Antithyroid Agent

Use Palliative treatment of hyperthyroidism as an adjunct to ameliorate hyperthyroidism in preparation for surgical treatment or radioactive iodine therapy; management of thyrotoxic crisis

Local Anesthetic/Vasoconstrictor Precautions No information available to require special precautions

Effects on Dental Treatment No significant effects or complications reported

Common Adverse Effects Frequency not defined.

- Cardiovascular: Edema, cutaneous vasculitis, leukocytoclastic vasculitis, ANCA-positive vasculitis
- Central nervous system: Fever, drowsiness, vertigo, headache, drug fever, dizziness, neuritis
- Dermatologic: Skin rash, urticaria, pruritus, exfoliative dermatitis, alopecia, erythema nodosum
- Endocrine & metabolic: Goiter, weight gain, swollen salivary glands
- Gastrointestinal: Nausea, vomiting, loss of taste perception, stomach pain, constipation
- Hematologic: Leukopenia, agranulocytosis, thrombocytopenia, bleeding, aplastic anemia
- Hepatic: Cholestatic jaundice, hepatitis
- Neuromuscular & skeletal: Arthralgia, paresthesia
- Renal: Nephritis, glomerulonephritis, acute renal failure
- Respiratory: Interstitial pneumonitis, alveolar hemorrhage
- Miscellaneous: SLE-like syndrome

Mechanism of Action Inhibits the synthesis of thyroid hormones by blocking the oxidation of iodine in the thyroid gland; blocks synthesis of thyroxine and triiodothyronine

Drug Interactions

Increased Effect/Toxicity: Propylthiouracil may increase the anticoagulant activity of warfarin.

Decreased Effect: Oral anticoagulant activity is increased only until metabolic effect stabilizes. Anticoagulants may be potentiated by antivitamin K effect of propylthiouracil. Correction of hyperthyroidism may alter disposition of beta-blockers, digoxin, and theophylline, necessitating a dose reduction of these agents.

Pharmacodynamics/Kinetics

Onset of action: Therapeutic: 24-36 hours

Peak effect: Remission: 4 months of continued therapy

Duration: 2-3 hours

Distribution: Concentrated in the thyroid gland

Protein binding: 75% to 80%

Metabolism: Hepatic

Bioavailability: 80% to 95%

Half-life elimination: 1.5-5 hours; End-stage renal disease: 8.5 hours

Time to peak, serum: ~1 hour

Excretion: Urine (35%)

Pregnancy Risk Factor D

2-Propylvaleric Acid *see* Valproic Acid and Derivatives *on page 1359*

Proscar® *see* Finasteride *on page 590*

ProSom® *see* Estazolam *on page 517*

Prostacyclin *see* Epoprostenol *on page 500*

Prostaglandin E_1 *see* Alprostadil *on page 87*

Prostaglandin E_2 *see* Dinoprostone *on page 447*

Prostin E_2® *see* Dinoprostone *on page 447*

Prostin VR Pediatric® *see* Alprostadil *on page 87*

Protamine Sulfate (PROE ta meen SUL fate)

Generic Available Yes

Pharmacologic Category Antidote

Use Treatment of heparin overdosage; neutralize heparin during surgery or dialysis procedures

Unlabeled/Investigational Use Treatment of low molecular weight heparin (LMWH) overdose

Local Anesthetic/Vasoconstrictor Precautions No information available to require special precautions

Effects on Dental Treatment No significant effects or complications reported

Common Adverse Effects Frequency not defined.

Cardiovascular: Sudden fall in blood pressure, bradycardia, flushing, hypotension

Central nervous system: Lassitude

Gastrointestinal: Nausea, vomiting

Hematologic: Hemorrhage

Respiratory: Dyspnea, pulmonary hypertension

Miscellaneous: Hypersensitivity reactions

Mechanism of Action Combines with strongly acidic heparin to form a stable complex (salt) neutralizing the anticoagulant activity of both drugs

Pharmacodynamics/Kinetics Onset of action: I.V.: Heparin neutralization: ~5 minutes

Pregnancy Risk Factor C

Protein C (Activated), Human, Recombinant *see* Drotrecogin Alfa *on page 478*

Prothrombin Complex Concentrate *see* Factor IX Complex (Human) *on page 572*

Protirelin (proe TYE re lin)

U.S. Brand Names Thyrel® TRH [DSC]

Canadian Brand Names Relefact® TRH

Generic Available No

Synonyms Lopremone; Thyrotropin Releasing Hormone; TRH

Pharmacologic Category Diagnostic Agent

Use Adjunct in the diagnostic assessment of thyroid function, and an adjunct to other diagnostic procedures in patients with pituitary or hypothalamic dysfunction; also causes release of prolactin from the pituitary and is used to detect defective control of prolactin secretion

Local Anesthetic/Vasoconstrictor Precautions No information available to require special precautions

Effects on Dental Treatment Key adverse event(s) related to dental treatment: Xerostomia (normal salivary flow resumes upon discontinuation).

Common Adverse Effects

>10%:

Central nervous system: Headache, lightheadedness

Dermatologic: Flushing of face

(Continued)

Protirelin *(Continued)*

Gastrointestinal: Nausea, xerostomia
Genitourinary: Urge to urinate

1% to 10%:

Central nervous system: Anxiety
Endocrine & metabolic: Breast enlargement and leaking in lactating women
Gastrointestinal: Bad taste in mouth, abdominal discomfort
Neuromuscular & skeletal: Tingling
Miscellaneous: Diaphoresis

Mechanism of Action Increase release of thyroid stimulating hormone from the anterior pituitary

Drug Interactions

Decreased Effect: Aspirin, levodopa, thyroid hormones, adrenocorticoid drugs

Pharmacodynamics/Kinetics

Onset of action: Peak effect: TSH: 20-30 minutes
Duration: TSH returns to baseline after ~3 hours
Half-life elimination, serum: Mean plasma: 5 minutes

Pregnancy Risk Factor C

Protonix® *see* Pantoprazole *on page 1043*
Protopic® *see* Tacrolimus *on page 1255*

Protriptyline (proe TRIP ti leen)

U.S. Brand Names Vivactil®

Generic Available No

Synonyms Protriptyline Hydrochloride

Pharmacologic Category Antidepressant, Tricyclic (Secondary Amine)

Use Treatment of depression

Local Anesthetic/Vasoconstrictor Precautions No information available to require special precautions

Effects on Dental Treatment Key adverse event(s) related to dental treatment: Xerostomia and changes in salivation (normal salivary flow resumes upon discontinuation). Long-term treatment with TCAs, such as protriptyline, increases the risk of caries by reducing salivation and salivary buffer capacity.

Common Adverse Effects Frequency not defined.

Cardiovascular: Arrhythmias, hypotension, myocardial infarction, stroke, heart block, hypertension, tachycardia, palpitations
Central nervous system: Dizziness, drowsiness, headache, confusion, delirium, hallucinations, restlessness, insomnia, nightmares, fatigue, delusions, anxiety, agitation, hypomania, exacerbation of psychosis, panic, seizures, incoordination, ataxia, EPS
Dermatologic: Alopecia, photosensitivity, rash, petechiae, urticaria, itching
Endocrine & metabolic: Breast enlargement, galactorrhea, SIADH, gynecomastia, increased or decreased libido
Gastrointestinal: Xerostomia, constipation, unpleasant taste, weight gain/loss, increased appetite, nausea, diarrhea, heartburn, vomiting, anorexia, trouble with gums, decreased lower esophageal sphincter tone may cause GE reflux
Genitourinary: Difficult urination, impotence, testicular edema
Hematologic: Agranulocytosis, leukopenia, eosinophilia, thrombocytopenia, purpura
Hepatic: Cholestatic jaundice, increased liver enzymes
Neuromuscular & skeletal: Fine muscle tremors, weakness, tremor, numbness, tingling
Ocular: Blurred vision, eye pain, increased intraocular pressure
Otic: Tinnitus
Miscellaneous: Diaphoresis (excessive), allergic reactions

Mechanism of Action Increases the synaptic concentration of serotonin and/or norepinephrine in the central nervous system by inhibition of their reuptake by the presynaptic neuronal membrane

Drug Interactions

Cytochrome P450 Effect: Substrate of CYP2D6 (major)

Increased Effect/Toxicity: Protriptyline increases the effects of amphetamines, anticholinergics, other CNS depressants (sedatives, hypnotics, or ethanol), chlorpropamide, tolazamide, and warfarin. When used with MAO inhibitors, hyperpyrexia, hypertension, tachycardia, confusion, seizures, and **deaths have been reported** (serotonin syndrome). The SSRIs (to varying degrees), cimetidine, grapefruit juice, indinavir, methylphenidate, ritonavir, quinidine, diltiazem, and verapamil inhibit the metabolism of TCAs. Levels/effects of protriptyline may be increased by chlorpromazine, delavirdine, fluoxetine, miconazole, paroxetine, pergolide, quinidine, quinine, ritonavir, ropinirole, and other CYP2D6 inhibitors. Use of lithium with a TCA may increase the risk for neurotoxicity. Phenothiazines may increase concentration of some TCAs and TCAs may increase concentration of phenothiazines. Pressor response to I.V. epinephrine, norepinephrine, and phenylephrine may be enhanced in patients receiving TCAs (**Note:** Effect is unlikely with epinephrine or levonordefrin dosages typically administered as infiltration in combination with local anesthetics). Combined use of beta-agonists or drugs which prolong QT_c (including quinidine, procainamide, disopyramide, cisapride, sparfloxacin, gatifloxacin, moxifloxacin) with TCAs may predispose patients to cardiac arrhythmias.

Decreased Effect: Carbamazepine, phenobarbital, and rifampin may increase the metabolism of protriptyline, decreasing its effects. Protriptyline inhibits the antihypertensive response to bethanidine, clonidine, debrisoquin, guanadrel, guanethidine, guanabenz, guanfacine. Cimetidine and methylphenidate may decrease the metabolism of protriptyline. Cholestyramine and colestipol may bind TCAs and reduce their absorption.

Pharmacodynamics/Kinetics

Distribution: Crosses placenta

Protein binding: 92%

Metabolism: Extensively hepatic via N-oxidation, hydroxylation, and glucuronidation; first-pass effect (10% to 25%)

Half-life elimination: 54-92 hours (average: 74 hours)

Time to peak, serum: 24-30 hours

Excretion: Urine

Pregnancy Risk Factor C

Protriptyline Hydrochloride *see* Protriptyline *on page 1146*

Protropin® *see* Human Growth Hormone *on page 694*

Protuss®-DM [DSC] *see* Guaifenesin, Pseudoephedrine, and Dextromethorphan *on page 676*

Proventil® *see* Albuterol *on page 71*

Proventil® HFA *see* Albuterol *on page 71*

Proventil® Repetabs® *see* Albuterol *on page 71*

Provera® *see* MedroxyPROGESTERone *on page 862*

Provigil® *see* Modafinil *on page 939*

Provisc® *see* Hyaluronate and Derivatives *on page 696*

Proxymetacaine *see* Proparacaine *on page 1134*

Prozac® *see* Fluoxetine *on page 606*

Prozac® Weekly™ *see* Fluoxetine *on page 606*

PRP-D *see Haemophilus* b Conjugate Vaccine *on page 680*

Prudoxin™ *see* Doxepin *on page 467*

Prussian Blue *see* Ferric Hexacyanoferrate *on page 585*

Prymaccone *see* Primaquine *on page 1122*

PS-341 *see* Bortezomib *on page 214*

Pseudoephedrine (soo doe e FED rin)

Related Information

Diphenhydramine and Pseudoephedrine *on page 451*

Guaifenesin, Pseudoephedrine, and Dextromethorphan *on page 676*

Oral Bacterial Infections *on page 1533*

U.S. Brand Names Biofed [OTC]; Decofed® [OTC]; Dimetapp® 12-Hour Non-Drowsy Extentabs® [OTC]; Dimetapp® Decongestant [OTC]; Genaphed® [OTC]; Kidkare Decongestant [OTC]; Kodet SE [OTC]; Oranyl [OTC]; PediaCare® Decongestant Infants [OTC]; Silfedrine Children's [OTC]; Sudafed® [OTC]; Sudafed® 12 Hour [OTC]; Sudafed® 24 Hour [OTC]; Sudafed® Children's [OTC]; Sudodrin [OTC]; Triaminic® Allergy Congestion [OTC]

Canadian Brand Names Balminil Decongestant; Contac® Cold 12 Hour Relief Non Drowsy; Drixoral® ND; Eltor®; PMS-Pseudoephedrine; Pseudofrin; Robidrine®; Sudafed® Decongestant; Triaminic® Allergy Congestion

Mexican Brand Names Lertamine-D®; Sudafed®

Generic Available Yes: Tablet, syrup

Synonyms *d*-Isoephedrine Hydrochloride; Pseudoephedrine Hydrochloride; Pseudoephedrine Sulfate

Pharmacologic Category Alpha/Beta Agonist

Use Temporary symptomatic relief of nasal congestion due to common cold, upper respiratory allergies, and sinusitis; also promotes nasal or sinus drainage

Local Anesthetic/Vasoconstrictor Precautions Use with caution since pseudoephedrine is a sympathomimetic amine which could interact with epinephrine to cause a pressor response

(Continued)

Pseudoephedrine *(Continued)*

Effects on Dental Treatment Key adverse event(s) related to dental treatment: Xerostomia (normal salivary flow resumes upon discontinuation).

Common Adverse Effects Frequency not defined.

Cardiovascular: Tachycardia, palpitations, arrhythmias

Central nervous system: Nervousness, transient stimulation, insomnia, excitability, dizziness, drowsiness, convulsions, hallucinations, headache

Gastrointestinal: Nausea, vomiting

Genitourinary: Dysuria

Neuromuscular & skeletal: Weakness, tremor

Respiratory: Dyspnea

Miscellaneous: Diaphoresis

Mechanism of Action Directly stimulates alpha-adrenergic receptors of respiratory mucosa causing vasoconstriction; directly stimulates beta-adrenergic receptors causing bronchial relaxation, increased heart rate and contractility

Drug Interactions

Increased Effect/Toxicity: MAO inhibitors may increase blood pressure effects of pseudoephedrine. Sympathomimetic agents may increase toxicity.

Decreased Effect: Decreased effect of methyldopa, reserpine.

Pharmacodynamics/Kinetics

Onset of action: Decongestant: Oral: 15-30 minutes

Duration: Immediate release tablet: 4-6 hours; Extended release: ≤12 hours

Absorption: Rapid

Metabolism: Partially hepatic

Half-life elimination: 9-16 hours

Excretion: Urine (70% to 90% as unchanged drug, 1% to 6% as active norpseudoephedrine); dependent on urine pH and flow rate; alkaline urine decreases renal elimination of pseudoephedrine

Pregnancy Risk Factor C

Pseudoephedrine, Acetaminophen, and Chlorpheniramine *see* Acetaminophen, Chlorpheniramine, and Pseudoephedrine *on page 58*

Pseudoephedrine, Acetaminophen, and Dextromethorphan *see* Acetaminophen, Dextromethorphan, and Pseudoephedrine *on page 59*

Pseudoephedrine and Acetaminophen *see* Acetaminophen and Pseudoephedrine *on page 53*

Pseudoephedrine and Acrivastine *see* Acrivastine and Pseudoephedrine *on page 62*

Pseudoephedrine and Brompheniramine *see* Brompheniramine and Pseudoephedrine *on page 220*

Pseudoephedrine and Carbinoxamine *see* Carbinoxamine and Pseudoephedrine *on page 262*

Pseudoephedrine and Chlorpheniramine *see* Chlorpheniramine and Pseudoephedrine *on page 315*

Pseudoephedrine and Dexbrompheniramine *see* Dexbrompheniramine and Pseudoephedrine *on page 414*

Pseudoephedrine and Dextromethorphan

(soo doe e FED rin & deks troe meth OR fan)

Related Information

Dextromethorphan *on page 421*

Pseudoephedrine *on page 1147*

U.S. Brand Names Children's Sudafed® Cough & Cold [OTC]; Pediacare® Decongestant Plus Cough [OTC]; Pediacare® Long Acting Cough Plus Cold [OTC]; Robitussin® Maximum Strength Cough & Cold [OTC]; Robitussin® Pediatric Cough & Cold [OTC]; Vicks® 44D Cough & Head Congestion [OTC]

Canadian Brand Names Balminil DM D; Benylin® DM-D; Koffex DM-D; Novahistex® DM Decongestant; Novahistine® DM Decongestant; Robitussin® Childrens Cough & Cold

Generic Available Yes: Liquid

Synonyms Dextromethorphan and Pseudoephedrine

Pharmacologic Category Antitussive/Decongestant

Use Temporary symptomatic relief of nasal congestion due to common cold, upper respiratory allergies, and sinusitis; also promotes nasal or sinus drainage; symptomatic relief of coughs caused by minor viral upper respiratory tract infections or inhaled irritants; most effective for a chronic nonproductive cough

Local Anesthetic/Vasoconstrictor Precautions Use with caution since pseudoephedrine is a sympathomimetic amine which could interact with epinephrine to cause a pressor response

Effects on Dental Treatment Key adverse event(s) related to dental treatment: Pseudoephedrine: Xerostomia (normal salivary flow resumes upon discontinuation).

Common Adverse Effects Frequency not defined.

Based on **pseudoephedrine** component:

Cardiovascular: Tachycardia, palpitations, arrhythmias

Central nervous system: Nervousness, transient stimulation, insomnia, excitability, dizziness, drowsiness, convulsions, hallucinations, headache

Gastrointestinal: Nausea, vomiting

Genitourinary: Dysuria

Neuromuscular & skeletal: Weakness, tremor

Respiratory: Dyspnea

Miscellaneous: Diaphoresis

Based on **dextromethorphan** component: Abdominal discomfort coma, constipation, dizziness, drowsiness, GI upset, nausea, respiratory depression

Drug Interactions

Cytochrome P450 Effect: Dextromethorphan: **Substrate** of CYP2B6 (minor), 2C8/9 (minor), 2C19 (minor), 2D6 (major), 2E1 (minor), 3A4 (minor); **Inhibits** CYP2D6 (weak)

Increased Effect/Toxicity: Based on **pseudoephedrine** component: MAO inhibitors may increase blood pressure effects of pseudoephedrine. Sympathomimetic agents may increase toxicity.

Decreased Effect: Based on **pseudoephedrine** component: Decreased effect of methyldopa, reserpine.

Pharmacodynamics/Kinetics See individual agents.

Pseudoephedrine and Diphenhydramine *see* Diphenhydramine and Pseudoephedrine *on page 451*

Pseudoephedrine and Fexofenadine *see* Fexofenadine and Pseudoephedrine *on page 588*

Pseudoephedrine and Guaifenesin *see* Guaifenesin and Pseudoephedrine *on page 675*

Pseudoephedrine and Hydrocodone *see* Hydrocodone and Pseudoephedrine *on page 711*

Pseudoephedrine and Ibuprofen

(soo doe e FED rin & eye byoo PROE fen)

Related Information

Ibuprofen *on page 728*

Pseudoephedrine *on page 1147*

U.S. Brand Names Advil® Cold, Children's [OTC]; Advil® Cold & Sinus [OTC]; Dristan® Sinus [OTC]; Motrin® Cold and Sinus [OTC]; Motrin® Cold, Children's [OTC]

Canadian Brand Names Advil® Cold & Sinus; Dristan® Sinus; Sudafed® Sinus Advance

Generic Available No

Synonyms Ibuprofen and Pseudoephedrine

Pharmacologic Category Decongestant/Analgesic

Use For temporary relief of cold, sinus and flu symptoms (including nasal congestion, headache, sore throat, minor body aches and pains, and fever)

Local Anesthetic/Vasoconstrictor Precautions Use with caution since pseudoephedrine is a sympathomimetic amine which could interact with epinephrine to cause a pressor response

Effects on Dental Treatment Key adverse event(s) related to dental treatment: Pseudoephedrine: Xerostomia (normal salivary flow resumes upon discontinuation).

Common Adverse Effects See individual agents.

Drug Interactions

Cytochrome P450 Effect: Ibuprofen: **Substrate** (minor) of CYP2C8/9, 2C19; **Inhibits** CYP2C8/9 (strong)

Increased Effect/Toxicity: See individual agents.

Decreased Effect: See individual agents.

Pharmacodynamics/Kinetics See individual agents.

Pregnancy Risk Factor Ibuprofen: B/D (3rd trimester)

Pseudoephedrine and Loratadine *see* Loratadine and Pseudoephedrine *on page 842*

Pseudoephedrine and Triprolidine *see* Triprolidine and Pseudoephedrine *on page 1345*

Pseudoephedrine, Carbinoxamine, and Dextromethorphan *see* Carbinoxamine, Pseudoephedrine, and Dextromethorphan *on page 263*

Pseudoephedrine, Chlorpheniramine, and Acetaminophen *see* Acetaminophen, Chlorpheniramine, and Pseudoephedrine *on page 58*

Pseudoephedrine, Chlorpheniramine, and Codeine *see* Chlorpheniramine, Pseudoephedrine, and Codeine *on page 319*

Pseudoephedrine, Chlorpheniramine, and Dihydrocodeine *see* Pseudoephedrine, Dihydrocodeine, and Chlorpheniramine *on page 1150*

Pseudoephedrine, Dextromethorphan, and Acetaminophen *see* Acetaminophen, Dextromethorphan, and Pseudoephedrine *on page 59*

Pseudoephedrine, Dextromethorphan, and Carbinoxamine *see* Carbinoxamine, Pseudoephedrine, and Dextromethorphan *on page 263*

Pseudoephedrine, Dextromethorphan, and Guaifenesin *see* Guaifenesin, Pseudoephedrine, and Dextromethorphan *on page 676*

Pseudoephedrine, Dihydrocodeine, and Chlorpheniramine

(soo doe e FED rin, dye hye droe KOE, & klor fen IR a meen)

U.S. Brand Names DiHydro-CP; Hydro-Tussin™ DHC; Pancof®; Uni-Cof

Generic Available Yes

Synonyms Chlorpheniramine, Pseudoephedrine, and Dihydrocodeine; Dihydrocodeine Bitartrate, Pseudoephedrine Hydrochloride, and Chlorpheniramine Maleate; Pseudoephedrine, Chlorpheniramine, and Dihydrocodeine

Pharmacologic Category Antihistamine; Antihistamine/Decongestant/Antitussive; Antitussive; Decongestant

Use Temporary relief of cough, congestion, and sneezing due to colds, respiratory infections, or hay fever

Local Anesthetic/Vasoconstrictor Precautions Use with caution since pseudoephedrine is a sympathomimetic amine which could interact with epinephrine to cause a pressor response

Effects on Dental Treatment Key adverse event(s) related to dental treatment:

Chlorpheniramine: Prolonged use will cause significant xerostomia (normal salivary flow resumes upon discontinuation).

Pseudoephedrine: Xerostomia (prolonged use worsens; normal salivary flow resumes upon discontinuation).

Common Adverse Effects See individual agents.

Restrictions C-III

Mechanism of Action

Pseudoephedrine: Directly stimulates alpha-adrenergic receptors of respiratory mucosa causing vasoconstriction; directly stimulates beta-adrenergic receptors causing bronchial relaxation

Dihydrocodeine: Binds to opiate receptors in the CNS; suppresses cough in medullary center

Chlorpheniramine: Competes with histamine for H_1-receptor sites on effector cells in the gastrointestinal tract, blood vessels, and respiratory tract

Drug Interactions

Cytochrome P450 Effect:

Dihydrocodeine: **Substrate** of CYP2D6 (major)

Chlorpheniramine: **Substrate** of CYP2D6 (minor), 3A4 (major); Inhibits CYP2D6 (weak).

Increased Effect/Toxicity: Also see individual agents. CYP3A4 inhibitors may increase the levels/effects of chlorpheniramine (example inhibitors include azole antifungals, ciprofloxacin, clarithromycin, diclofenac, doxycycline, erythromycin, imatinib, isoniazid, nefazodone, nicardipine, propofol, protease inhibitors, quinidine, and verapamil).

Decreased Effect: Also see individual agents. CYP2D6 inhibitors may decrease the effects of dihydrocodeine (example inhibitors include chlorpromazine, delavirdine, fluoxetine, miconazole, paroxetine, pergolide, quinidine, quinine, ritonavir, and ropinirole).

Pharmacodynamics/Kinetics See individual agents.

Pregnancy Risk Factor C

Pseudoephedrine, Guaifenesin, and Codeine *see* Guaifenesin, Pseudoephedrine, and Codeine *on page 676*

Pseudoephedrine Hydrochloride *see* Pseudoephedrine *on page 1147*

Pseudoephedrine Hydrochloride and Cetirizine Hydrochloride *see* Cetirizine and Pseudoephedrine *on page 299*

Pseudoephedrine, Hydrocodone, and Carbinoxamine *see* Hydrocodone, Carbinoxamine, and Pseudoephedrine *on page 712*

Pseudoephedrine, Hydrocodone, and Guaifenesin *see* Hydrocodone, Pseudoephedrine, and Guaifenesin *on page 713*

Pseudoephedrine Sulfate *see* Pseudoephedrine *on page 1147*

Pseudoephedrine, Triprolidine, and Codeine Pseudoephedrine, Codeine, and Triprolidine *see* Triprolidine, Pseudoephedrine, and Codeine *on page 1346*

Pseudo GG TR *see* Guaifenesin and Pseudoephedrine *on page 675*

Pseudomonic Acid A *see* Mupirocin *on page 951*

Pseudovent™ *see* Guaifenesin and Pseudoephedrine *on page 675*

Pseudovent™ DM *see* Guaifenesin, Pseudoephedrine, and Dextromethorphan *on page 676*

Pseudovent™-Ped *see* Guaifenesin and Pseudoephedrine *on page 675*

Psorcon® *see* Diflorasone *on page 435*

Psorcon® e™ *see* Diflorasone *on page 435*

Psoriatec™ *see* Anthralin *on page 133*

PsoriGel® [OTC] *see* Coal Tar *on page 367*

Psyllium (SIL i yum)

U.S. Brand Names Fiberall®; Genfiber® [OTC]; Hydrocil® [OTC]; Konsyl® [OTC]; Konsyl-D® [OTC]; Konsyl® Easy Mix [OTC]; Konsyl® Orange [OTC]; Metamucil® [OTC]; Metamucil® Smooth Texture [OTC]; Modane® Bulk [OTC]; Perdiem® Fiber Therapy [OTC]; Reguloid® [OTC]; Serutan® [OTC]

Canadian Brand Names Metamucil®; Novo-Mucilax

Generic Available Yes: Powder

Synonyms Plantago Seed; Plantain Seed; Psyllium Hydrophilic Mucilloid

Pharmacologic Category Antidiarrheal; Laxative, Bulk-Producing

Use Treatment of chronic atonic or spastic constipation and in constipation associated with rectal disorders; management of irritable bowel syndrome; labeled for OTC use as fiber supplement, treatment of constipation

Local Anesthetic/Vasoconstrictor Precautions No information available to require special precautions

Effects on Dental Treatment No significant effects or complications reported

Common Adverse Effects Frequency not defined.

Gastrointestinal: Esophageal or bowel obstruction, diarrhea, constipation, abdominal cramps

Respiratory: Bronchospasm

Miscellaneous: Anaphylaxis upon inhalation in susceptible individuals, rhinoconjunctivitis

Mechanism of Action Adsorbs water in the intestine to form a viscous liquid which promotes peristalsis and reduces transit time

Drug Interactions

Decreased Effect: Decreased effect of warfarin, digitalis, potassium-sparing diuretics, salicylates, tetracyclines, nitrofurantoin when taken together. Separate administration times to reduce potential for drug-drug interaction.

Pharmacodynamics/Kinetics

Onset of action: 12-24 hours

Peak effect: 2-3 days

Absorption: None; small amounts of grain extracts present in the preparation have been reportedly absorbed following colonic hydrolysis

Pregnancy Risk Factor B

Psyllium Hydrophilic Mucilloid *see* Psyllium *on page 1151*

P.T.E.-4® *see* Trace Metals *on page 1319*

P.T.E.-5® *see* Trace Metals *on page 1319*

Pteroylglutamic Acid *see* Folic Acid *on page 625*

PTU *see* Propylthiouracil *on page 1144*

Pulmicort Respules® *see* Budesonide *on page 221*

Pulmicort Turbuhaler® *see* Budesonide *on page 221*

Pulmozyme® *see* Dornase Alfa *on page 463*

Puralube® Tears [OTC] *see* Artificial Tears *on page 148*

Purge® [OTC] *see* Castor Oil *on page 273*

Purified Chick Embryo Cell *see* Rabies Virus Vaccine *on page 1165*

Purinethol® *see* Mercaptopurine *on page 880*

P-V Tussin Tablet *see* Hydrocodone and Pseudoephedrine *on page 711*

Pyrantel Pamoate (pi RAN tel PAM oh ate)

U.S. Brand Names Pin-X® [OTC]; Reese's® Pinworm Medicine [OTC]

Canadian Brand Names Combantrin™

Mexican Brand Names Combantrin®

(Continued)

Pyrantel Pamoate *(Continued)*

Generic Available No

Pharmacologic Category Anthelmintic

Use Treatment of pinworms (*Enterobius vermicularis*) and roundworms (*Ascaris lumbricoides*)

Unlabeled/Investigational Use Treatment of whipworms (*Trichuris trichiura*) and hookworms (*Ancylostoma duodenale*)

Local Anesthetic/Vasoconstrictor Precautions No information available to require special precautions

Effects on Dental Treatment No significant effects or complications reported

Common Adverse Effects Frequency not defined.

Central nervous system: Dizziness, drowsiness, insomnia, headache

Dermatologic: Rash

Gastrointestinal: Anorexia, nausea, vomiting, abdominal cramps, diarrhea, tenesmus

Hepatic: Elevated liver enzymes

Neuromuscular & skeletal: Weakness

Mechanism of Action Causes the release of acetylcholine and inhibits cholinesterase; acts as a depolarizing neuromuscular blocker, paralyzing the helminths

Drug Interactions

Decreased Effect: Decreased effect with piperazine

Pharmacodynamics/Kinetics

Absorption: Oral: Poor

Metabolism: Partially hepatic

Time to peak, serum: 1-3 hours

Excretion: Feces (50% as unchanged drug); urine (7% as unchanged drug)

Pregnancy Risk Factor C

Pyrazinamide (peer a ZIN a mide)

Related Information

Tuberculosis *on page 1495*

Canadian Brand Names Tebrazid™

Generic Available Yes

Synonyms Pyrazinoic Acid Amide

Pharmacologic Category Antitubercular Agent

Use Adjunctive treatment of tuberculosis in combination with other anti-tuberculosis agents

Local Anesthetic/Vasoconstrictor Precautions No information available to require special precautions

Effects on Dental Treatment No significant effects or complications reported

Common Adverse Effects 1% to 10%:

Central nervous system: Malaise

Gastrointestinal: Nausea, vomiting, anorexia

Neuromuscular & skeletal: Arthralgia, myalgia

Mechanism of Action Converted to pyrazinoic acid in susceptible strains of *Mycobacterium* which lowers the pH of the environment; exact mechanism of action has not been elucidated

Drug Interactions

Increased Effect/Toxicity: Combination therapy with rifampin and pyrazinamide has been associated with severe and fatal hepatotoxic reactions.

Pharmacodynamics/Kinetics Bacteriostatic or bactericidal depending on drug's concentration at infection site

Absorption: Well absorbed

Distribution: Widely into body tissues and fluids including liver, lung, and CSF

- Relative diffusion from blood into CSF: Adequate with or without inflammation (exceeds usual MICs)
- CSF:blood level ratio: Inflamed meninges: 100%

Protein binding: 50%

Metabolism: Hepatic

Half-life elimination: 9-10 hours

Time to peak, serum: Within 2 hours

Excretion: Urine (4% as unchanged drug)

Pregnancy Risk Factor C

Pyrazinamide, Rifampin, and Isoniazid *see* Rifampin, Isoniazid, and Pyrazinamide *on page 1181*

Pyrazinoic Acid Amide *see* Pyrazinamide *on page 1152*

Pyrethrins and Piperonyl Butoxide

(pye RE thrins & pi PER oh nil byo TOKS ide)

U.S. Brand Names A-200® Maximum Strength [OTC]; Pronto® [OTC]; Pyrinyl Plus® [OTC]; RID® Maximum Strength [OTC]; Tisit® [OTC]; Tisit® Blue Gel [OTC]

Canadian Brand Names Pronto® Lice Control; R & C™ II; R & C™ Shampoo/Conditioner; RID® Mousse

Generic Available Yes: Shampoo

Synonyms Piperonyl Butoxide and Pyrethrins

Pharmacologic Category Antiparasitic Agent, Topical; Pediculocide; Shampoo, Pediculocide

Use Treatment of *Pediculus humanus* infestations (head lice, body lice, pubic lice and their eggs)

Local Anesthetic/Vasoconstrictor Precautions No information available to require special precautions

Effects on Dental Treatment No significant effects or complications reported

Common Adverse Effects Frequency not defined.

Dermatologic: Pruritus

Local: Burning, stinging, irritation with repeat use

Mechanism of Action Pyrethrins are derived from flowers that belong to the chrysanthemum family. The mechanism of action on the neuronal membranes of lice is similar to that of DDT. Piperonyl butoxide is usually added to pyrethrin to enhance the product's activity by decreasing the metabolism of pyrethrins in arthropods.

Pharmacodynamics/Kinetics

Onset of action: ~30 minutes

Absorption: Minimal

Metabolism: Via ester hydrolysis and hydroxylation

Pregnancy Risk Factor C

Pyridium® *see* Phenazopyridine *on page 1072*

Pyridostigmine (peer id oh STIG meen)

U.S. Brand Names Mestinon®; Mestinon® Timespan®

Canadian Brand Names Mestinon®; Mestinon®-SR

Generic Available Yes: Tablet

Synonyms Pyridostigmine Bromide

Pharmacologic Category Acetylcholinesterase Inhibitor

Use Symptomatic treatment of myasthenia gravis; antidote for nondepolarizing neuromuscular blockers

Military use: Pretreatment for Soman nerve gas exposure

Local Anesthetic/Vasoconstrictor Precautions No information available to require special precautions

Effects on Dental Treatment No significant effects or complications reported

Common Adverse Effects Frequency not defined.

Cardiovascular: Arrhythmias (especially bradycardia), hypotension, decreased carbon monoxide, tachycardia, AV block, nodal rhythm, nonspecific ECG changes, cardiac arrest, syncope, flushing

Central nervous system: Convulsions, dysarthria, dysphonia, dizziness, loss of consciousness, drowsiness, headache

Dermatologic: Skin rash, thrombophlebitis (I.V.), urticaria

Gastrointestinal: Hyperperistalsis, nausea, vomiting, salivation, diarrhea, stomach cramps, dysphagia, flatulence, abdominal pain

Genitourinary: Urinary urgency

Neuromuscular & skeletal: Weakness, fasciculations, muscle cramps, spasms, arthralgias, myalgia

Ocular: Small pupils, lacrimation, amblyopia

Respiratory: Increased bronchial secretions, laryngospasm, bronchiolar constriction, respiratory muscle paralysis, dyspnea, respiratory depression, respiratory arrest, bronchospasm

Miscellaneous: Diaphoresis (increased), anaphylaxis, allergic reactions

Mechanism of Action Inhibits destruction of acetylcholine by acetylcholinesterase which facilitates transmission of impulses across myoneural junction

Drug Interactions

Increased Effect/Toxicity: Increased effect of depolarizing neuromuscular blockers (succinylcholine). Increased toxicity with edrophonium. Increased bradycardia/hypotension with beta-blockers.

Decreased Effect: Neuromuscular blockade reversal effect of pyridostigmine may be decreased by aminoglycosides, quinolones, tetracyclines, bacitracin,

(Continued)

Pyridostigmine *(Continued)*

colistin, polymyxin B, sodium colistimethate, quinidine, elevated serum magnesium concentrations.

Pharmacodynamics/Kinetics

Onset of action: Oral, I.M.: 15-30 minutes; I.V. injection: 2-5 minutes
Duration: Oral: Up to 6-8 hours (due to slow absorption); I.V.: 2-3 hours
Absorption: Oral: Very poor
Distribution: 19 ± 12 L
Metabolism: Hepatic
Bioavailability: 10% to 20%
Half-life elimination: 1-2 hours; Renal failure: ≤6 hours
Excretion: Urine (80% to 90% as unchanged drug)

Pregnancy Risk Factor B

Pyridostigmine Bromide *see* Pyridostigmine *on page 1153*

Pyridoxine (peer i DOKS een)

U.S. Brand Names Aminoxin® [OTC]

Generic Available Yes

Synonyms Pyridoxine Hydrochloride; Vitamin B_6

Pharmacologic Category Vitamin, Water Soluble

Use Prevention and treatment of vitamin B_6 deficiency, pyridoxine-dependent seizures in infants; adjunct to treatment of acute toxicity from isoniazid, cycloserine, or hydralazine overdose

Local Anesthetic/Vasoconstrictor Precautions No information available to require special precautions

Effects on Dental Treatment No significant effects or complications reported

Common Adverse Effects Frequency not defined.

Central nervous system: Headache, seizures (following very large I.V. doses), sensory neuropathy
Endocrine & metabolic: Decreased serum folic acid secretions
Gastrointestinal: Nausea
Hepatic: Increased AST
Neuromuscular & skeletal: Paresthesia
Miscellaneous: Allergic reactions

Mechanism of Action Precursor to pyridoxal, which functions in the metabolism of proteins, carbohydrates, and fats; pyridoxal also aids in the release of liver and muscle-stored glycogen and in the synthesis of GABA (within the central nervous system) and heme

Drug Interactions

Decreased Effect: Pyridoxine may decrease serum levels of levodopa, phenobarbital, and phenytoin (patients taking levodopa without carbidopa should avoid supplemental vitamin B_6 >5 mg per day, which includes multivitamin preparations).

Pharmacodynamics/Kinetics

Absorption: Enteral, parenteral: Well absorbed
Metabolism: Via 4-pyridoxic acid (active form) and other metabolites
Half-life elimination: 15-20 days
Excretion: Urine

Pregnancy Risk Factor A/C (dose exceeding RDA recommendation)

Pyridoxine, Folic Acid, and Cyanocobalamin *see* Folic Acid, Cyanocobalamin, and Pyridoxine *on page 626*

Pyridoxine Hydrochloride *see* Pyridoxine *on page 1154*

Pyrilamine, Phenylephrine, and Carbetapentane *see* Carbetapentane, Phenylephrine, and Pyrilamine *on page 261*

Pyrimethamine (peer i METH a meen)

U.S. Brand Names Daraprim®

Canadian Brand Names Daraprim®

Mexican Brand Names Daraprim®

Generic Available No

Pharmacologic Category Antimalarial Agent

Use Prophylaxis of malaria due to susceptible strains of plasmodia; used in conjunction with quinine and sulfadiazine for the treatment of uncomplicated attacks of chloroquine-resistant *P. falciparum* malaria; used in conjunction with fast-acting schizonticide to initiate transmission control and suppression cure; synergistic combination with sulfonamide in treatment of toxoplasmosis

Local Anesthetic/Vasoconstrictor Precautions No information available to require special precautions

Effects on Dental Treatment Key adverse event(s) related to dental treatment: Atrophic glossitis has been reported.

Common Adverse Effects Frequency not defined.

Cardiovascular: Arrhythmias (large doses)

Central nervous system: Depression, fever, insomnia, lightheadedness, malaise, seizures

Dermatologic: Abnormal skin pigmentation, dermatitis, erythema multiforme, rash, Stevens-Johnson syndrome, toxic epidermal necrolysis

Gastrointestinal: Anorexia, abdominal cramps, vomiting, diarrhea, xerostomia, atrophic glossitis

Genitourinary: Hematuria

Hematologic: Megaloblastic anemia, leukopenia, pancytopenia, thrombocytopenia, pulmonary eosinophilia

Miscellaneous: Anaphylaxis

Mechanism of Action Inhibits parasitic dihydrofolate reductase, resulting in inhibition of vital tetrahydrofolic acid synthesis

Drug Interactions

Cytochrome P450 Effect: Inhibits CYP2C8/9 (moderate), 2D6 (moderate)

Increased Effect/Toxicity: Serum levels of antipsychotic agents may be increased by pyrimethamine. Sulfonamides (synergy), methotrexate, TMP/SMZ, and zidovudine may increase the risk of bone marrow suppression. Pyrimethamine may increase the levels/effects of amiodarone, amphetamines, selected beta-blockers, dextromethorphan, fluoxetine, glimepiride, glipizide, lidocaine, mirtazapine, nateglinide, nefazodone, paroxetine, phenytoin, pioglitazone, risperidone, ritonavir, rosiglitazone, sertraline, thioridazine, tricyclic antidepressants, venlafaxine, warfarin, and other CYP2C8/9 or 2D6 substrates.

Decreased Effect: Pyrimethamine may decrease the levels/effects of CYP2D6 prodrug substrates (eg, codeine, hydrocodone, oxycodone, tramadol).

Pharmacodynamics/Kinetics

Onset of action: ~1 hour

Absorption: Well absorbed

Distribution: Widely, mainly in blood cells, kidneys, lungs, liver, and spleen; crosses into CSF; crosses placenta; enters breast milk

Protein binding: 80% to 87%

Metabolism: Hepatic

Half-life elimination: 80-95 hours

Time to peak, serum: 1.5-8 hours

Excretion: Urine (20% to 30% as unchanged drug)

Pregnancy Risk Factor C

Pyrimethamine and Sulfadoxine *see* Sulfadoxine and Pyrimethamine *on page 1245*

Pyrinyl Plus® [OTC] *see* Pyrethrins and Piperonyl Butoxide *on page 1153*

Pyrithione Zinc (peer i THYE one zingk)

U.S. Brand Names DHS™ Zinc [OTC]; Head & Shoulders® Classic Clean [OTC]; Head & Shoulders® Classic Clean 2-In-1 [OTC]; Head & Shoulders® Dry Scalp Care [OTC]; Head & Shoulders® Extra Fullness [OTC]; Head & Shoulders® Refresh [OTC]; Head & Shoulders® Smooth & Silky 2-In-1 [OTC]; Zincon® [OTC]; ZNP® Bar [OTC]

Mexican Brand Names ZNP Shampoo®

Generic Available No

Pharmacologic Category Topical Skin Product

Use Relieves the itching, irritation and scalp flaking associated with dandruff and/or seborrheal dermatitis

Local Anesthetic/Vasoconstrictor Precautions No information available to require special precautions

Effects on Dental Treatment No significant effects or complications reported

Q-Tussin [OTC] *see* Guaifenesin *on page 672*

Quaternium-18 Bentonite *see* Bentoquatam *on page 189*

Quazepam (KWAY ze pam)

U.S. Brand Names Doral®

Canadian Brand Names Doral®

Generic Available No

Pharmacologic Category Benzodiazepine

Use Treatment of insomnia

Local Anesthetic/Vasoconstrictor Precautions No information available to require special precautions

(Continued)

Quazepam *(Continued)*

Effects on Dental Treatment Key adverse event(s) related to dental treatment: Xerostomia (normal salivary flow resumes upon discontinuation).

Common Adverse Effects Frequency not defined.

Cardiovascular: Palpitations

Central nervous system: Drowsiness, fatigue, ataxia, memory impairment, anxiety, depression, headache, confusion, nervousness, dizziness, incoordination, hypo- and hyperkinesia, agitation, euphoria, paranoid reaction, nightmares, abnormal thinking

Dermatologic: Dermatitis, pruritus, rash

Endocrine & metabolic: Decreased libido, menstrual irregularities

Gastrointestinal: Xerostomia, constipation, diarrhea, dyspepsia, anorexia, abnormal taste perception, nausea, vomiting, increased or decreased appetite, abdominal pain

Genitourinary: Impotence, incontinence

Hematologic: Blood dyscrasias

Neuromuscular & skeletal: Dysarthria, rigidity, tremor, muscle cramps, reflex slowing

Ocular: Blurred vision

Miscellaneous: Drug dependence

Restrictions C-IV

Mechanism of Action Binds to stereospecific benzodiazepine receptors on the postsynaptic GABA neuron at several sites within the central nervous system, including the limbic system, reticular formation. Enhancement of the inhibitory effect of GABA on neuronal excitability results by increased neuronal membrane permeability to chloride ions. This shift in chloride ions results in hyperpolarization (a less excitable state) and stabilization.

Drug Interactions

Cytochrome P450 Effect: Substrate of CYP3A4 (minor)

Increased Effect/Toxicity: Serum levels and/or toxicity of quazepam may be increased by cimetidine, ciprofloxacin, clarithromycin, clozapine, CNS depressants, diltiazem, disulfiram, digoxin, erythromycin, ethanol, fluconazole, fluoxetine, fluvoxamine, grapefruit juice, isoniazid, itraconazole, ketoconazole, labetalol, levodopa, loxapine, metoprolol, metronidazole, miconazole, nefazodone, omeprazole, phenytoin, rifabutin, rifampin, troleandomycin, valproic acid, and verapamil.

Pharmacodynamics/Kinetics

Absorption: Rapid

Protein binding: 95%

Half-life elimination, serum: Parent drug: 25-41 hours; Active metabolite: 40-114 hours

Pregnancy Risk Factor X

Quelicin® *see* Succinylcholine *on page 1241*

Questran® *see* Cholestyramine Resin *on page 323*

Questran® Light *see* Cholestyramine Resin *on page 323*

Quetiapine (kwe TYE a peen)

U.S. Brand Names Seroquel®

Canadian Brand Names Seroquel®

Mexican Brand Names Seroquel®

Generic Available No

Synonyms Quetiapine Fumarate

Pharmacologic Category Antipsychotic Agent, Dibenzothiazepine

Use Treatment of schizophrenia; treatment of acute manic episodes associated with bipolar disorder (as monotherapy or in combination with lithium or valproate)

Unlabeled/Investigational Use Autism, psychosis (children)

Local Anesthetic/Vasoconstrictor Precautions No information available to require special precautions

Effects on Dental Treatment No significant effects or complications reported

Common Adverse Effects

>10%:

Central nervous system: Agitation, dizziness, headache, somnolence

Endocrine & metabolic: Cholesterol increased (11%), triglycerides increased (17%)

Gastrointestinal: Weight gain (≥7% body weight, dose related), xerostomia

1% to 10%:

Cardiovascular: Postural hypotension, tachycardia, palpitations, peripheral edema

Central nervous system: Anxiety, fever, pain
Dermatologic: Rash
Gastrointestinal: Abdominal pain (dose related), constipation, dyspepsia (dose related), anorexia, vomiting, gastroenteritis
Hematologic: Leukopenia
Hepatic: AST increased, ALT increased, GGT increased
Neuromuscular & skeletal: Dysarthria, back pain, weakness, tremor, hypertonia, dysarthria
Ocular: Amblyopia
Respiratory: Rhinitis, pharyngitis, cough, dyspnea
Miscellaneous: Diaphoresis, flu-like syndrome

Dosage Oral:

Children and Adolescents:

Autism (unlabeled use): 100-350 mg/day (1.6-5.2 mg/kg/day)

Psychosis and mania (unlabeled use): Initial: 25 mg twice daily; titrate as necessary to 450 mg/day

Adults:

Schizophrenia/psychoses: Initial: 25 mg twice daily; increase in increments of 25-50 mg 2-3 times/day on the second and third day, if tolerated, to a target dose of 300-400 mg in 2-3 divided doses by day 4. Make further adjustments as needed at intervals of at least 2 days in adjustments of 25-50 mg twice daily. Usual maintenance range: 300-800 mg/day

Mania: Initial: 50 mg twice daily on day 1, increase dose in increments of 100 mg/day to 200 mg twice daily on day 4; may increase to a target dose of 800 mg/day by day 6 at increments of ≤200 mg/day. Usual dosage range: 400-800 mg/day

Elderly: 40% lower mean oral clearance of quetiapine in adults >65 years of age; higher plasma levels expected and, therefore, dosage adjustment may be needed; elderly patients usually require 50-200 mg/day

Dosing comments in renal insufficiency: 25% lower mean oral clearance of quetiapine than normal subjects; however, plasma concentrations similar to normal subjects receiving the same dose; no dosage adjustment required

Dosing comments in hepatic insufficiency: 30% lower mean oral clearance of quetiapine than normal subjects; higher plasma levels expected in hepatically impaired subjects; dosage adjustment may be needed

Initial: 25 mg/day, increase dose by 25-50 mg/day to effective dose, based on clinical response and tolerability to patient

Mechanism of Action Mechanism of action of quetiapine, as with other antipsychotic drugs, is unknown. However, it has been proposed that this drug's antipsychotic activity is mediated through a combination of dopamine type 2 (D_2) and serotonin type 2 ($5\text{-}HT_2$) antagonism. It is an antagonist at multiple neurotransmitter receptors in the brain: serotonin $5\text{-}HT_{1A}$ and $5\text{-}HT_2$, dopamine D_1 and D_2, histamine H_1, and adrenergic alpha$_1$- and alpha$_2$- receptors; but appears to have no appreciable affinity at cholinergic muscarinic and benzodiazepine receptors.

Antagonism at receptors other than dopamine and $5\text{-}HT_2$ with similar receptor affinities may explain some of the other effects of quetiapine. The drug's antagonism of histamine H_1-receptors may explain the somnolence observed with it. The drug's antagonism of adrenergic alpha$_1$-receptors may explain the orthostatic hypotension observed with it.

Contraindications Hypersensitivity to quetiapine or any component of the formulation; severe CNS depression; bone marrow suppression; blood dyscrasias; severe hepatic disease, coma

Warnings/Precautions May induce orthostatic hypotension associated with dizziness, tachycardia, and, in some cases, syncope, especially during the initial dose titration period. Should be used with particular caution in patients with known cardiovascular disease (history of MI or ischemic heart disease, heart failure, or conduction abnormalities), cerebrovascular disease, or conditions that predispose to hypotension. Development of cataracts has been observed in animal studies, therefore, lens examinations should be made upon initiation of therapy and every 6 months thereafter.

Neuroleptic malignant syndrome (NMS) is a potentially fatal symptom complex that has been reported in association with administration of antipsychotic drugs. Clinical manifestations of NMS are hyperpyrexia, muscle rigidity, altered mental status, and evidence of autonomic instability (irregular pulse or blood pressure, tachycardia, diaphoresis, and cardiac dysrhythmia). Management of NMS should include immediate discontinuation of antipsychotic drugs and other drugs not essential to concurrent therapy, intensive symptomatic treatment and medication monitoring, and treatment of any concomitant medical problems for which specific treatment are available.

(Continued)

Quetiapine *(Continued)*

Tardive dyskinesia; caution in patients with a history of seizures, decreases in total free thyroxine, pre-existing hyperprolactinemia, elevations of liver enzymes, cholesterol levels and/or triglyceride increases.

May cause hyperglycemia; in some cases may be extreme and associated with ketoacidosis, hyperosmolar coma, or death. Use with caution in patients with diabetes or other disorders of glucose regulation; monitor for worsening of glucose control.

Drug Interactions

Cytochrome P450 Effect: Substrate of CYP2D6 (minor), 3A4 (major)

Increased Effect/Toxicity: Quetiapine increases levels of lorazepam. The effects of other centrally-acting drugs, sedatives, or ethanol may be potentiated by quetiapine. Quetiapine may enhance the effects of antihypertensive agents. CYP3A4 inhibitors may increase the levels/effects of quetiapine; example inhibitors include azole antifungals, ciprofloxacin, clarithromycin, diclofenac, doxycycline, erythromycin, imatinib, isoniazid, nefazodone, nicardipine, propofol, protease inhibitors, quinidine, and verapamil; ketoconazole increased serum concentrations of quetiapine by 335%. Concomitant use of quetiapine and divalproex increased the mean maximum plasma concentration of quetiapine at by 17% at steady state (the mean oral clearance of valproic acid was increased by 11%). Cimetidine increases blood levels of quetiapine (quetiapine's clearance is reduced by by 20%). Metoclopramide may increase risk of extrapyramidal symptoms (EPS).

Decreased Effect: Thioridazine increases quetiapine's clearance (by 65%), decreasing serum levels. CYP3A4 inducers may decrease the levels/effects of quetiapine. Example inducers include aminoglutethimide, carbamazepine, nafcillin, nevirapine, phenobarbital, phenytoin, and rifamycins.

Ethanol/Nutrition/Herb Interactions

Ethanol: Avoid ethanol (may cause excessive impairment in cognition/motor function).

Food: In healthy volunteers, administration of quetiapine with food resulted in an increase in the peak serum concentration and AUC (each by ~15%) compared to the fasting state.

Herb/Nutraceutical: St John's wort may decrease quetiapine levels. Avoid valerian, St John's wort, kava kava, gotu kola (may increase CNS depression).

Dietary Considerations May be taken with or without food.

Pharmacodynamics/Kinetics

Absorption: Rapidly absorbed following oral administration
Distribution: V_d: 10 ± 4 L/kg; V_{dss}: ~2 days
Protein binding, plasma: 83%
Metabolism: Primarily hepatic; via CYP3A4; forms two inactive metabolites
Bioavailability: 9% ± 4%; tablet is 100% bioavailable relative to solution
Half-life elimination: Mean: Terminal: ~6 hours
Time to peak, plasma: 1.5 hours
Excretion: Urine (73% as metabolites, <1% as unchanged drug); feces (20%)

Pregnancy Risk Factor C

Dosage Forms TAB: 25 mg, 100 mg, 200 mg, 300 mg

Quetiapine Fumarate *see* Quetiapine *on page 1156*
Quibron® *see* Theophylline and Guaifenesin *on page 1286*
Quibron®-T *see* Theophylline *on page 1285*
Quibron®-T/SR *see* Theophylline *on page 1285*
Quinaglute® Dura-Tabs® [DSC] *see* Quinidine *on page 1160*
Quinalbarbitone Sodium *see* Secobarbital *on page 1211*

Quinapril (KWIN a pril)

Related Information

Cardiovascular Diseases *on page 1458*

U.S. Brand Names Accupril®

Canadian Brand Names Accupril™

Mexican Brand Names Acupril®

Generic Available No

Synonyms Quinapril Hydrochloride

Pharmacologic Category Angiotensin-Converting Enzyme (ACE) Inhibitor

Use Management of hypertension; treatment of congestive heart failure

Unlabeled/Investigational Use Treatment of left ventricular dysfunction after myocardial infarction

Local Anesthetic/Vasoconstrictor Precautions No information available to require special precautions

Effects on Dental Treatment No significant effects or complications reported

Common Adverse Effects Note: Frequency ranges include data from hypertension and heart failure trials. Higher rates of adverse reactions have generally been noted in patients with CHF. However, the frequency of adverse effects associated with placebo is also increased in this population.

1% to 10%:

Cardiovascular: Hypotension (3%), chest pain (2%), first-dose hypotension (up to 3%)

Central nervous system: Dizziness (4% to 8%), headache (2% to 6%), fatigue (3%)

Dermatologic: Rash (1%)

Endocrine & metabolic: Hyperkalemia (2%)

Gastrointestinal: Vomiting/nausea (1% to 2%), diarrhea (2%)

Neuromuscular & skeletal: Myalgias (2% to 5%), back pain (1%)

Renal: Increased BUN/serum creatinine (2%, transient elevations may occur with a higher frequency), worsening of renal function (in patients with bilateral renal artery stenosis or hypovolemia)

Respiratory: Upper respiratory symptoms, cough (2% to 4%; up to 13% in some studies), dyspnea (2%)

Dosage

Adults: Oral:

Hypertension: Initial: 10-20 mg once daily, adjust according to blood pressure response at peak and trough blood levels; initial dose may be reduced to 5 mg in patients receiving diuretic therapy if the diuretic is continued; usual dose range (JNC 7): 10-40 mg once daily

Congestive heart failure or post-MI: Initial: 5 mg once daily, titrated at weekly intervals to 20-40 mg daily in 2 divided doses

Elderly: Initial: 2.5-5 mg/day; increase dosage at increments of 2.5-5 mg at 1- to 2-week intervals.

Dosing adjustment in renal impairment: Lower initial doses should be used; after initial dose (if tolerated), administer initial dose twice daily; may be increased at weekly intervals to optimal response:

Hypertension: Initial:

Cl_{cr} >60 mL/minute: Administer 10 mg/day

Cl_{cr} 30-60 mL/minute: Administer 5 mg/day

Cl_{cr} 10-30 mL/minute: Administer 2.5 mg/day

Congestive heart failure: Initial:

Cl_{cr} >30 mL/minute: Administer 5 mg/day

Cl_{cr} 10-30 mL/minute: Administer 2.5 mg/day

Dosing comments in hepatic impairment: In patients with alcoholic cirrhosis, hydrolysis of quinapril to quinaprilat is impaired; however, the subsequent elimination of quinaprilat is unaltered.

Mechanism of Action Competitive inhibitor of angiotensin-converting enzyme (ACE); prevents conversion of angiotensin I to angiotensin II, a potent vasoconstrictor; results in lower levels of angiotensin II which causes an increase in plasma renin activity and a reduction in aldosterone secretion; a CNS mechanism may also be involved in hypotensive effect as angiotensin II increases adrenergic outflow from CNS; vasoactive kallikreins may be decreased in conversion to active hormones by ACE inhibitors, thus reducing blood pressure

Contraindications Hypersensitivity to quinapril or any component of the formulation; angioedema related to previous treatment with an ACE inhibitor; bilateral renal artery stenosis; patients with idiopathic or hereditary angioedema; pregnancy (2nd and 3rd trimesters)

Warnings/Precautions Use with caution in patients with renal insufficiency, autoimmune disease, renal artery stenosis; excessive hypotension may be more likely in volume-depleted patients, the elderly, and following the first dose (first dose phenomenon); quinapril should be discontinued if laryngeal stridor or angioedema is observed. Angioedema can occur at any time during treatment (especially following first dose); it may involve head and neck (potentially affecting the airway) or the intestine (presenting with abdominal pain).

Drug Interactions

Increased Effect/Toxicity: Potassium supplements, co-trimoxazole (high dose), angiotensin II receptor antagonists (eg, candesartan, losartan, irbesartan), or potassium-sparing diuretics (amiloride, spironolactone, triamterene) may result in elevated serum potassium levels when combined with quinapril. ACE inhibitor effects may be increased by phenothiazines or probenecid (increases levels of captopril). ACE inhibitors may increase serum concentrations/effects of digoxin, lithium, and sulfonlyureas.

Diuretics have additive hypotensive effects with ACE inhibitors, and hypovolemia increases the potential for adverse renal effects of ACE inhibitors. In patients with compromised renal function, coadministration with NSAIDs may

(Continued)

Quinapril *(Continued)*

result in further deterioration of renal function. Allopurinol and ACE inhibitors may cause a higher risk of hypersensitivity reaction when taken concurrently.

Decreased Effect: Quinapril may reduce the absorption of quinolones and tetracycline antibiotics. Aspirin (high dose) may reduce the therapeutic effects of ACE inhibitors; at low dosages this does not appear to be significant. Rifampin may decrease the effect of ACE inhibitors. Antacids may decrease the bioavailability of ACE inhibitors (may be more likely to occur with captopril); separate administration times by 1-2 hours. NSAIDs, specifically indomethacin, may reduce the hypotensive effects of ACE inhibitors.

Ethanol/Nutrition/Herb Interactions Herb/Nutraceutical: Avoid dong quai if using for hypertension (has estrogenic activity). Avoid ephedra, yohimbe, ginseng (may worsen hypertension). Avoid garlic (may have increased antihypertensive effect).

Pharmacodynamics/Kinetics

Onset of action: 1 hour

Duration: 24 hours

Absorption: Quinapril: ≥60%

Protein binding: Quinapril: 97%; Quinaprilat: 97%

Metabolism: Rapidly hydrolyzed to quinaprilat, the active metabolite

Half-life elimination: Quinapril: 0.8 hours; Quinaprilat: 3 hours; increases as Cl_{cr} decreases

Time to peak, serum: Quinapril: 1 hour; Quinaprilat: ~2 hours

Excretion: Urine (50% to 60% primarily as quinaprilat)

Pregnancy Risk Factor C/D (2nd and 3rd trimesters)

Dosage Forms TAB: 5 mg, 10 mg, 20 mg, 40 mg

Quinapril and Hydrochlorothiazide

(KWIN a pril & hye droe klor oh THYE a zide)

Related Information

Hydrochlorothiazide *on page 699*

Quinapril *on page 1158*

U.S. Brand Names Accuretic™

Canadian Brand Names Accuretic™

Generic Available No

Synonyms Hydrochlorothiazide and Quinapril

Pharmacologic Category Angiotensin-Converting Enzyme (ACE) Inhibitor; Antihypertensive; Diuretic, Thiazide

Use Treatment of hypertension (not for initial therapy)

Local Anesthetic/Vasoconstrictor Precautions No information available to require special precautions

Effects on Dental Treatment No significant effects or complications reported

Common Adverse Effects

1% to 10%:

- Central nervous system: Dizziness (5%), somnolence (1%)
- Neuromuscular & skeletal: Weakness (1%)
- Renal: Serum creatinine increase (3%), blood urea nitrogen increase (4%)
- Respiratory: Cough (3%), bronchitis (1%)

Drug Interactions

Increased Effect/Toxicity: See individual agents.

Decreased Effect: See individual agents.

Pharmacodynamics/Kinetics See individual agents.

Pregnancy Risk Factor C (1st trimester); D (2nd and 3rd trimesters)

Quinapril Hydrochloride *see* Quinapril *on page 1158*

Quinidine (KWIN i deen)

Related Information

Cardiovascular Diseases *on page 1458*

U.S. Brand Names Quinaglute® Dura-Tabs® [DSC]

Canadian Brand Names Apo-Quin-G®; Apo-Quinidine®; BioQuin® Durules™; Novo-Quinidin; Quinate®

Generic Available Yes

Synonyms Quinidine Gluconate; Quinidine Polygalacturonate; Quinidine Sulfate

Pharmacologic Category Antiarrhythmic Agent, Class Ia

Use Prophylaxis after cardioversion of atrial fibrillation and/or flutter to maintain normal sinus rhythm; prevent recurrence of paroxysmal supraventricular tachycardia, paroxysmal AV junctional rhythm, paroxysmal ventricular tachycardia, paroxysmal atrial fibrillation, and atrial or ventricular premature contractions; has activity against *Plasmodium falciparum* malaria

Local Anesthetic/Vasoconstrictor Precautions No information available to require special precautions

Effects on Dental Treatment When taken over a long period of time, the anticholinergic side effects from quinidine can cause a reduction of saliva production or secretion contributing to discomfort and dental disease (ie, caries, oral candidiasis and periodontal disease).

Common Adverse Effects

Frequency not defined: Hypotension, syncope

>10%:

Cardiovascular: QT_c prolongation (modest prolongation is common, however, excessive prolongation is rare and indicates toxicity)

Central nervous system: Lightheadedness (15%)

Gastrointestinal: Diarrhea (35%), upper GI distress, bitter taste, diarrhea, anorexia, nausea, vomiting, stomach cramping (22%)

1% to 10%:

Cardiovascular: Angina (6%), palpitation (7%), new or worsened arrhythmias (proarrhythmic effect)

Central nervous system: Syncope (1% to 8%), headache (7%), fatigue (7%), weakness (5%), sleep disturbance (3%), tremor (2%), nervousness (2%), incoordination (1%)

Dermatologic: Rash (5%)

Ocular: Blurred vision

Otic: Tinnitus

Respiratory: Wheezing

Note: Cinchonism, a syndrome which may include tinnitus, high-frequency hearing loss, deafness, vertigo, blurred vision, diplopia, photophobia, headache, confusion, and delirium has been associated with quinidine use. Usually associated with chronic toxicity, this syndrome has also been described after brief exposure to a moderate dose in sensitive patients. Vomiting and diarrhea may also occur as isolated reactions to therapeutic quinidine levels.

Mechanism of Action Class 1a antiarrhythmic agent; depresses phase O of the action potential; decreases myocardial excitability and conduction velocity, and myocardial contractility by decreasing sodium influx during depolarization and potassium efflux in repolarization; also reduces calcium transport across cell membrane

Drug Interactions

Cytochrome P450 Effect: Substrate of CYP2C8/9 (minor), 2E1 (minor), 3A4 (major); **Inhibits** CYP2C8/9 (weak), 2D6 (strong), 3A4 (strong)

Increased Effect/Toxicity: Effects may be additive with drugs which prolong the QT interval, including amiodarone, amitriptyline, bepridil, cisapride (use is contraindicated), disopyramide, erythromycin, haloperidol, imipramine, pimozide, procainamide, sotalol, thioridazine, and some quinolones (sparfloxacin, gatifloxacin, moxifloxacin - concurrent use is contraindicated). Concurrent use of amprenavir, or ritonavir is contraindicated. Quinidine increases digoxin serum concentrations; digoxin dosage may need to be reduced (by 50%) when quinidine is initiated; new steady-state digoxin plasma concentrations occur in 5-7 days.

Quinidine may increase the levels/effects of amphetamines, selected beta-blockers, selected benzodiazepines, calcium channel blockers, cisapride, cyclosporine, dextromethorphan, ergot alkaloids, fluoxetine, selected HMG-CoA reductase inhibitors, lidocaine, mesoridazine, mirtazapine, nateglinide, nefazodone, paroxetine, risperidone, ritonavir, sildenafil (and other PDE-5 inhibitors), tacrolimus, thioridazine, tricyclic antidepressants, venlafaxine, and other substrates of CYP2D6 or 3A4. Selected benzodiazepines (midazolam and triazolam), cisapride, ergot alkaloids, selected HMG-CoA reductase inhibitors (lovastatin and simvastatin), mesoridazine, pimozide, and thioridazine are generally contraindicated with strong CYP3A4 inhibitors. When used with strong CYP3A4 inhibitors, dosage adjustment/limits are recommended for sildenafil and other PDE-5 inhibitors; refer to individual monographs.

The levels/effects of quinidine may be increased by azole antifungals, ciprofloxacin, clarithromycin, diclofenac, doxycycline, erythromycin, imatinib, isoniazid, nefazodone, nicardipine, propofol, protease inhibitors (amprenavir and ritonavir are contraindicated), verapamil, and other CYP3A4 inhibitors. Quinidine potentiates nondepolarizing and depolarizing muscle relaxants. When combined with quinidine, amiloride may cause prolonged ventricular conduction leading to arrhythmias. Urinary alkalinizers (antacids, sodium

(Continued)

Quinidine *(Continued)*

bicarbonate, acetazolamide) increase quinidine blood levels. Warfarin effects may be increased by quinidine.

Decreased Effect: The levels/effects of quinidine may be decreased by aminoglutethimide, carbamazepine, nafcillin, nevirapine, phenobarbital, phenytoin, rifamycins, and other CYP3A4 inducers. Quinidine may decrease the levels/effects of CYP2D6 prodrug substrates (eg, codeine, hydrocodone, oxycodone, tramadol).

Pharmacodynamics/Kinetics

Distribution: V_d: Adults: 2-3.5 L/kg, decreased with congestive heart failure, malaria; increased with cirrhosis; crosses placenta; enters breast milk

Protein binding:

Newborns: 60% to 70%; decreased protein binding with cyanotic congenital heart disease, cirrhosis, or acute myocardial infarction

Adults: 80% to 90%

Metabolism: Extensively hepatic (50% to 90%) to inactive compounds

Bioavailability: Sulfate: 80%; Gluconate: 70%

Half-life elimination, plasma: Children: 2.5-6.7 hours; Adults: 6-8 hours; prolonged with elderly, cirrhosis, and congestive heart failure

Excretion: Urine (15% to 25% as unchanged drug)

Pregnancy Risk Factor C

Quinidine Gluconate *see* Quinidine *on page 1160*

Quinidine Polygalacturonate *see* Quinidine *on page 1160*

Quinidine Sulfate *see* Quinidine *on page 1160*

Quinine (KWYE nine)

Canadian Brand Names Quinine-Odan™

Generic Available Yes

Synonyms Quinine Sulfate

Pharmacologic Category Antimalarial Agent

Use In conjunction with other antimalarial agents, suppression or treatment of chloroquine-resistant *P. falciparum* malaria; treatment of *Babesia microti* infection in conjunction with clindamycin

Unlabeled/Investigational Use Prevention and treatment of nocturnal recumbency leg muscle cramps

Local Anesthetic/Vasoconstrictor Precautions No information available to require special precautions

Effects on Dental Treatment No significant effects or complications reported

Common Adverse Effects Frequency not defined.

Central nervous system: Severe headache

Gastrointestinal: Nausea, vomiting, diarrhea

Ocular: Blurred vision

Otic: Tinnitus

Miscellaneous: Cinchonism (risk of cinchonism is directly related to dose and duration of therapy)

Mechanism of Action Depresses oxygen uptake and carbohydrate metabolism; intercalates into DNA, disrupting the parasite's replication and transcription; affects calcium distribution within muscle fibers and decreases the excitability of the motor end-plate region; cardiovascular effects similar to quinidine

Drug Interactions

Cytochrome P450 Effect: Substrate (minor) of CYP1A2, 2C19, 3A4; **Inhibits** CYP2C8/9 (moderate), 2D6 (strong), 3A4 (weak)

Increased Effect/Toxicity: Quinine may increase the levels/effects of CYP2D6 substrates (eg, amphetamines, selected beta-blockers, dextromethorphan, fluoxetine, lidocaine, mirtazapine, nefazodone, paroxetine, risperidone, ritonavir, thioridazine, tricyclic antidepressants, venlafaxine). Beta-blockers with quinine may increase bradycardia. Quinine may enhance warfarin anticoagulant effect. Quinine potentiates nondepolarizing and depolarizing muscle relaxants. Quinine may increase plasma concentration of digoxin. Closely monitor digoxin concentrations. Digoxin dosage may need to be reduced (by one-half) when quinine is initiated. New steady-state digoxin plasma concentrations occur in 5-7 days. Verapamil, amiodarone, alkalinizing agents, and cimetidine may increase quinine serum concentrations.

Decreased Effect: Phenobarbital, phenytoin, and rifampin may decrease quinine serum concentrations. Quinine may decrease the levels/effects of CYP2D6 prodrug substrates (eg, codeine, hydrocodone, oxycodone, tramadol).

Pharmacodynamics/Kinetics

Absorption: Readily, mainly from upper small intestine
Protein binding: 70% to 95%
Metabolism: Primarily hepatic
Half-life elimination: Children: 6-12 hours; Adults: 8-14 hours
Time to peak, serum: 1-3 hours
Excretion: Feces and saliva; urine (<5% as unchanged drug)

Pregnancy Risk Factor X

Quinine Sulfate *see* Quinine *on page 1162*

Quinol *see* Hydroquinone *on page 719*

Quinupristin and Dalfopristin

(kwi NYOO pris tin & dal FOE pris tin)

U.S. Brand Names Synercid®

Canadian Brand Names Synercid®

Generic Available No

Synonyms Pristinamycin; RP-59500

Pharmacologic Category Antibiotic, Streptogramin

Use Treatment of serious or life-threatening infections associated with vancomycin-resistant *Enterococcus faecium* bacteremia; treatment of complicated skin and skin structure infections caused by methcillin-susceptible *Staphylococcus aureus* or *Streptococcus pyogenes*

Has been studied in the treatment of a variety of infections caused by *Enterococcus faecium* (not *E. fecalis*) including vancomycin-resistant strains. May also be effective in the treatment of serious infections caused by *Staphylococcus* species including those resistant to methicillin.

Local Anesthetic/Vasoconstrictor Precautions No information available to require special precautions

Effects on Dental Treatment No significant effects or complications reported

Common Adverse Effects

>10%:

Hepatic: Hyperbilirubinemia (3% to 35%)
Local: Inflammation at infusion site (38% to 42%), local pain (40% to 44%), local edema (17% to 18%), infusion site reaction (12% to 13%)

1% to 10%:

Central nervous system: Pain (2% to 3%), headache (2%)
Dermatologic: Pruritus (2%), rash (3%)
Endocrine & metabolic: Hyperglycemia (1%)
Gastrointestinal: Nausea (3% to 5%), diarrhea (3%), vomiting (3% to 4%)
Hematologic: Anemia (3%)
Hepatic: Increased LDH (3%), increased GGT (2%)
Local: Thrombophlebitis (2%)
Neuromuscular & skeletal: Arthralgia (<1% to 8%), myalgia (<1% to 5%), Increased CPK (2%)

Mechanism of Action Quinupristin/dalfopristin inhibits bacterial protein synthesis by binding to different sites on the 50S bacterial ribosomal subunit thereby inhibiting protein synthesis

Drug Interactions

Cytochrome P450 Effect: Quinupristin: **Inhibits** CYP3A4 (weak)

Increased Effect/Toxicity: The manufacturer states that quinupristin/dalfopristin may increase cisapride concentrations and cause QT_c prolongation, and recommends to avoid concurrent use with cisapride. Quinupristin/dalfopristin may increase cyclosporine concentrations; monitor.

Pharmacodynamics/Kinetics

Distribution: Quinupristin: 0.45 L/kg; Dalfopristin: 0.24 L/kg
Protein binding: Moderate
Metabolism: To active metabolites via nonenzymatic reactions
Half-life elimination: Quinupristin: 0.85 hour; Dalfopristin: 0.7 hour (mean elimination half-lives, including metabolites: 3 and 1 hours, respectively)
Excretion: Feces (75% to 77% as unchanged drug and metabolites); urine (15% to 19%)

Pregnancy Risk Factor B

Quixin™ *see* Levofloxacin *on page 812*

QVAR® *see* Beclomethasone *on page 184*

R-3827 *see* Abarelix *on page 43*

RabAvert® *see* Rabies Virus Vaccine *on page 1165*

Rabeprazole (ra BE pray zole)

U.S. Brand Names Aciphex®

Canadian Brand Names Aciphex®; Pariet®

Mexican Brand Names Pariet®

Generic Available No

Synonyms Pariprazole

Pharmacologic Category Proton Pump Inhibitor; Substituted Benzimidazole

Use Short-term (4-8 weeks) treatment and maintenance of erosive or ulcerative gastroesophageal reflux disease (GERD); symptomatic GERD; short-term (up to 4 weeks) treatment of duodenal ulcers; long-term treatment of pathological hypersecretory conditions, including Zollinger-Ellison syndrome; *H. pylori* eradication (in combination with amoxicillin and clarithromycin)

Unlabeled/Investigational Use Maintenance of duodenal ulcer

Local Anesthetic/Vasoconstrictor Precautions No information available to require special precautions

Effects on Dental Treatment No significant effects or complications reported

Common Adverse Effects 1% to 10%: Central nervous system: Headache

Dosage Oral: Adults >18 years and Elderly:

GERD: 20 mg once daily for 4-8 weeks; maintenance: 20 mg once daily

Duodenal ulcer: 20 mg/day before breakfast for 4 weeks

H. pylori eradication: 20 mg twice daily for 7 days; to be administered with amoxicillin 1000 mg and clarithromycin 500 mg, also given twice daily for 7 days.

Hypersecretory conditions: 60 mg once daily; dose may need to be adjusted as necessary. Doses as high as 100 mg once daily and 60 mg twice daily have been used.

Dosage adjustment in renal impairment: No dosage adjustment required

Dosage adjustment in hepatic impairment:

Mild to moderate: Elimination decreased; no dosage adjustment required

Severe: Use caution

Mechanism of Action Potent proton pump inhibitor; suppresses gastric acid secretion by inhibiting the parietal cell H^+/K^+ ATP pump

Contraindications Hypersensitivity to rabeprazole, substituted benzimidazoles (ie, esomeprazole, lansoprazole, omeprazole, pantoprazole), or any component of the formulation

Warnings/Precautions Use caution in severe hepatic impairment; relief of symptoms with rabeprazole does not preclude the presence of a gastric malignancy

Drug Interactions

Cytochrome P450 Effect: Substrate (major) of CYP2C19, 3A4; **Inhibits** CYP2C19 (moderate), 2DC (weak), 3A4 (weak)

Increased Effect/Toxicity: Rabeprazole may increase the levels/effects of citalopram, diazepam, methsuximide, phenytoin, propranolol, sertraline, or other CYP2C19 substrates.

Decreased Effect: Proton pump inhibitors may decrease the absorption of atazanavir, indinavir, itraconazole, and ketoconazole. The levels/effects of rabeprazole may be decreased by aminoglutethimide, carbamazepine, nafcillin, nevirapine, phenobarbital, phenytoin, rifampin, and other CYP2C19 or 3A4 inducers.

Ethanol/Nutrition/Herb Interactions

Ethanol: Avoid ethanol (may cause gastric mucosal irritation).

Food: High-fat meals may delay absorption, but C_{max} and AUC are not altered.

Dietary Considerations May be taken with or without food; best if taken before breakfast.

Pharmacodynamics/Kinetics

Onset of action: 1 hour

Duration: 24 hours

Absorption: Oral: Well absorbed within 1 hour

Distribution: 96.3%

Protein binding, serum: 94.8% to 97.5%

Metabolism: Hepatic via CYP3A and 2C19 to inactive metabolites

Bioavailability: Oral: 52%

Half-life elimination (dose dependent): 0.85-2 hours

Time to peak, plasma: 2-5 hours

Excretion: Urine (90% primarily as thioether carboxylic acid); remainder in feces

Pregnancy Risk Factor B

Dosage Forms TAB, delayed release, enteric coated: 20 mg

Rabies Immune Globulin (Human)

(RAY beez i MYUN GLOB yoo lin, HYU man)

Related Information

Animal and Human Bites Guidelines *on page 1582*
Immunizations (Vaccines) *on page 1614*

U.S. Brand Names BayRab®; Imogam®

Canadian Brand Names BayRab™; Imogam® Rabies Pasteurized

Generic Available No

Synonyms RIG

Pharmacologic Category Immune Globulin

Use Part of postexposure prophylaxis of persons with rabies exposure who lack a history of pre-exposure or postexposure prophylaxis with rabies vaccine or a recently documented neutralizing antibody response to previous rabies vaccination; although it is preferable to administer RIG with the first dose of vaccine, it can be given up to 8 days after vaccination

Local Anesthetic/Vasoconstrictor Precautions No information available to require special precautions

Effects on Dental Treatment No significant effects or complications reported

Common Adverse Effects 1% to 10%:

Central nervous system: Fever (mild)
Local: Soreness at injection site

Mechanism of Action Rabies immune globulin is a solution of globulins dried from the plasma or serum of selected adult human donors who have been immunized with rabies vaccine and have developed high titers of rabies antibody. It generally contains 10% to 18% of protein of which not less than 80% is monomeric immunoglobulin G.

Pregnancy Risk Factor C

Rabies Virus Vaccine (RAY beez VYE rus vak SEEN)

Related Information

Animal and Human Bites Guidelines *on page 1582*
Immunizations (Vaccines) *on page 1614*

U.S. Brand Names Imovax® Rabies; RabAvert®

Canadian Brand Names Imovax® Rabies

Generic Available No

Synonyms HDCV; Human Diploid Cell Cultures Rabies Vaccine; PCEC; Purified Chick Embryo Cell

Pharmacologic Category Vaccine

Use Pre-exposure immunization: Vaccinate persons with greater than usual risk due to occupation or avocation including veterinarians, rangers, animal handlers, certain laboratory workers, and persons living in or visiting countries for longer than 1 month where rabies is a constant threat.

Postexposure prophylaxis: If a bite from a carrier animal is unprovoked, if it is not captured and rabies is present in that species and area, administer rabies immune globulin (RIG) and the vaccine as indicated

Local Anesthetic/Vasoconstrictor Precautions No information available to require special precautions

Effects on Dental Treatment No significant effects or complications reported

Common Adverse Effects All serious adverse reactions must be reported to the U.S. Department of Health and Human Services (DHHS) Vaccine Adverse Event Reporting System (VAERS) 1-800-822-7967.

Frequency not defined.

Cardiovascular: Edema
Central nervous system: Dizziness, malaise, encephalomyelitis, transverse myelitis, fever, pain, headache, neuroparalytic reactions
Gastrointestinal: Nausea, abdominal pain
Local: Local discomfort, pain at injection site, itching, erythema, swelling or pain
Neuromuscular & skeletal: Myalgia

Mechanism of Action Rabies vaccine is an inactivated virus vaccine which promotes immunity by inducing an active immune response. The production of specific antibodies requires about 7-10 days to develop. Rabies immune globulin or antirabies serum, equine (ARS) is given in conjunction with rabies vaccine to provide immune protection until an antibody response can occur.

Pharmacodynamics/Kinetics

Onset of action: I.M.: Rabies antibody: ~7-10 days
Peak effect: ~30-60 days
Duration: ≥1 year

Pregnancy Risk Factor C

Radiogardase™ *see* Ferric Hexacyanoferrate *on page 585*

Radiological/Contrast Media (Nonionic)

(ray deo LOG ik al/KON trast MEE dia non eye ON ik)

U.S. Brand Names Amipaque® [DSC]; Isovue®; Omnipaque®; Optiray®; ProHance®

Generic Available Yes

Synonyms Gadoteridol; Iohexol; Iopamidol; Ioversol; Metrizamide

Pharmacologic Category Radiopaque Agents

Use Enhance visualization of structures during radiologic procedures

Local Anesthetic/Vasoconstrictor Precautions No information available to require special precautions

Effects on Dental Treatment Key adverse event(s) related to dental treatment: Taste perversion, xerostomia (normal salivary flow resumes upon discontinuation), edematous and/or itching tongue, and gingivitis.

Drug Interactions

Increased Effect/Toxicity: Interleukins may increase the risk of hypersensitivity reactions. Risk of metformin-induced acidosis may be increased by iodinated contrast agents; discontinue metformin prior to contrast exposure and withhold for 48 hours.

rAHF *see* Antihemophilic Factor (Recombinant) *on page 135*

R-albuterol *see* Levalbuterol *on page 806*

Raloxifene (ral OKS i feen)

Related Information

Endocrine Disorders and Pregnancy *on page 1481*

Rheumatoid Arthritis, Osteoarthritis, and Osteoporosis *on page 1490*

U.S. Brand Names Evista®

Canadian Brand Names Evista®

Mexican Brand Names Evista®

Generic Available No

Synonyms Keoxifene Hydrochloride; Raloxifene Hydrochloride

Pharmacologic Category Selective Estrogen Receptor Modulator (SERM)

Use Prevention and treatment of osteoporosis in postmenopausal women

Local Anesthetic/Vasoconstrictor Precautions No information available to require special precautions

Effects on Dental Treatment No significant effects or complications reported

Common Adverse Effects Note: Has been associated with increased risk of thromboembolism (DVT, PE) and superficial thrombophlebitis; risk is similar to reported risk of HRT

≥2%:

Cardiovascular: Chest pain

Central nervous system: Migraine, depression, insomnia, fever

Dermatologic: Rash

Endocrine & metabolic: Hot flashes

Gastrointestinal: Nausea, dyspepsia, vomiting, flatulence, gastroenteritis, weight gain

Genitourinary: Vaginitis, urinary tract infection, cystitis, leukorrhea

Neuromuscular & skeletal: Leg cramps, arthralgia, myalgia, arthritis

Respiratory: Sinusitis, pharyngitis, cough, pneumonia, laryngitis

Miscellaneous: Infection, flu syndrome, diaphoresis

Dosage Adults: Female: Oral: 60 mg/day which may be administered any time of the day without regard to meals

Mechanism of Action A selective estrogen receptor modulator, meaning that it affects some of the same receptors that estrogen does, but not all, and in some instances, it antagonizes or blocks estrogen; it acts like estrogen to prevent bone loss and improve lipid profiles (decreases total and LDL-cholesterol but does not raise triglycerides), but it has the potential to block some estrogen effects such as those that lead to breast cancer and uterine cancer

Contraindications Hypersensitivity to raloxifene or any component of the formulation; active thromboembolic disorder; pregnancy (not intended for use in premenopausal women)

Warnings/Precautions History of venous thromboembolism/pulmonary embolism; patients with cardiovascular disease; history of cervical/uterine carcinoma; renal/hepatic insufficiency (however, pharmacokinetic data are lacking);

concurrent use of estrogens; women with a history of elevated triglycerides in response to treatment with oral estrogens (or estrogen/progestin)

Drug Interactions

Increased Effect/Toxicity: Raloxifene has the potential to interact with highly protein-bound drugs (increase effects of either agent). Use caution with highly protein-bound drugs, warfarin, clofibrate, indomethacin, naproxen, ibuprofen, diazepam, phenytoin, or tamoxifen.

Decreased Effect: Ampicillin and cholestyramine reduce raloxifene absorption/blood levels.

Ethanol/Nutrition/Herb Interactions Ethanol: Avoid ethanol (may increase risk of osteoporosis).

Pharmacodynamics/Kinetics

Onset of action: 8 weeks
Absorption: ~60%
Distribution: 2348 L/kg
Protein binding: >95% to albumin and α-glycoprotein
Metabolism: Extensive first-pass effect
Bioavailability: ~2%
Half-life elimination: 27.7-32.5 hours
Excretion: Primarily feces; urine (0.2%)

Pregnancy Risk Factor X

Dosage Forms TAB: 60 mg

Raloxifene Hydrochloride *see* Raloxifene *on page 1166*

Ramipril (ra MI pril)

Related Information

Cardiovascular Diseases *on page 1458*

U.S. Brand Names Altace®

Canadian Brand Names Altace®

Mexican Brand Names Ramace®; Tritace®

Generic Available No

Pharmacologic Category Angiotensin-Converting Enzyme (ACE) Inhibitor

Use Treatment of hypertension, alone or in combination with thiazide diuretics; treatment of congestive heart failure; treatment of left ventricular dysfunction after myocardial infarction; to reduce risk of heart attack, stroke, and death in patients at increased risk for these problems

Local Anesthetic/Vasoconstrictor Precautions No information available to require special precautions

Effects on Dental Treatment No significant effects or complications reported

Common Adverse Effects Note: Frequency ranges include data from hypertension and heart failure trials. Higher rates of adverse reactions have generally been noted in patients with CHF. However, the frequency of adverse effects associated with placebo is also increased in this population.

>10%: Respiratory: Cough (increased) (7% to 12%)

1% to 10%:

- Cardiovascular: Hypotension (11%), angina (3%), postural hypotension (2%), syncope (2%)
- Central nervous system: Headache (1% to 5%), dizziness (2% to 4%), fatigue (2%), vertigo (2%)
- Endocrine & metabolic: Hyperkalemia (1% to 10%)
- Gastrointestinal: Nausea/vomiting (1% to 2%)
- Neuromuscular & skeletal: Chest pain (noncardiac) (1%)
- Renal: Renal dysfunction (1%), elevation in serum creatinine (1% to 2%), increased BUN (<1% to 3%); transient elevations of creatinine and/or BUN may occur more frequently
- Respiratory: Cough (estimated 1% to 10%)

Worsening of renal function may occur in patients with bilateral renal artery stenosis or in hypovolemia. In addition, a syndrome which may include fever, myalgia, arthralgia, interstitial nephritis, vasculitis, rash, eosinophilia and positive ANA, and elevated ESR has been reported with ACE inhibitors. Risk of pancreatitis and agranulocytosis may be increased in patients with collagen vascular disease or renal impairment.

Dosage Adults: Oral:

Hypertension: 2.5-5 mg once daily, maximum: 20 mg/day

Reduction in risk of MI, stroke, and death from cardiovascular causes: Initial: 2.5 mg once daily for 1 week, then 5 mg once daily for the next 3 weeks, then increase as tolerated to 10 mg once daily (may be given as divided dose)

Heart failure postmyocardial infarction: Initial: 2.5 mg twice daily titrated upward, if possible, to 5 mg twice daily.

(Continued)

Ramipril *(Continued)*

Note: The dose of any concomitant diuretic should be reduced. If the diuretic cannot be discontinued, initiate therapy with 1.25 mg. After the initial dose, the patient should be monitored carefully until blood pressure has stabilized.

Dosing adjustment in renal impairment:

Cl_{cr} <40 mL/minute: Administer 25% of normal dose.

Renal failure and hypertension: Administer 1.25 mg once daily, titrated upward as possible.

Renal failure and heart failure: Administer 1.25 mg once daily, increasing to 1.25 mg twice daily up to 2.5 mg twice daily as tolerated.

Mechanism of Action Ramipril is an ACE inhibitor which prevents the formation of angiotensin II from angiotensin I and exhibits pharmacologic effects that are similar to captopril. Ramipril must undergo enzymatic saponification by esterases in the liver to its biologically active metabolite, ramiprilat. The pharmacodynamic effects of ramipril result from the high-affinity, competitive, reversible binding of ramiprilat to angiotensin-converting enzyme thus preventing the formation of the potent vasoconstrictor angiotensin II. This isomerized enzyme-inhibitor complex has a slow rate of dissociation, which results in high potency and a long duration of action; a CNS mechanism may also be involved in the hypotensive effect as angiotensin II increases adrenergic outflow from CNS; vasoactive kallikreins may be decreased in conversion to active hormones by ACE inhibitors, thus reducing blood pressure

Contraindications Hypersensitivity to ramipril or any component of the formulation; prior hypersensitivity (including angioedema) to ACE inhibitors; bilateral renal artery stenosis; pregnancy (2nd and 3rd trimesters)

Warnings/Precautions Anaphylactic or anaphylactoid reactions can occur. Use with caution and modify dosage in patients with renal impairment (especially renal artery stenosis), severe CHF. Severe hypotension may occur in the elderly and patients who are sodium and/or volume depleted, initiate lower doses and monitor closely when starting therapy in these patients. Should be discontinued if laryngeal stridor or angioedema of the face, tongue, or glottis is observed. Angioedema can occur at any time during treatment (especially following first dose). Angioedema may involve head and neck (potentially affecting the airway) or the intestine (presenting with abdominal pain). Careful blood pressure monitoring with first dose (hypotension can occur especially in volume depleted patients). Use with caution in hypovolemia; collagen vascular diseases; valvular stenosis (particularly aortic stenosis); hyperkalemia; or before, during, or immediately after anesthesia. Avoid rapid dosage escalation, which may lead to renal insufficiency. Neutropenia/agranulocytosis with myeloid hyperplasia can rarely occur. If patient has renal impairment then a baseline WBC with differential and serum creatinine should be evaluated and monitored closely during the first 3 months of therapy. Hypersensitivity reactions may be seen during hemodialysis with high-flux dialysis membranes (eg, AN69).

Drug Interactions

Increased Effect/Toxicity: Potassium supplements, co-trimoxazole (high dose), angiotensin II receptor antagonists (eg, candesartan, losartan, irbesartan), or potassium-sparing diuretics (amiloride, spironolactone, triamterene) may result in elevated serum potassium levels when combined with ramipril. ACE inhibitor effects may be increased by phenothiazines or probenecid (increases levels of captopril). ACE inhibitors may increase serum concentrations/effects of digoxin, lithium, and sulfonlyureas.

Diuretics have additive hypotensive effects with ACE inhibitors, and hypovolemia increases the potential for adverse renal effects of ACE inhibitors. In patients with compromised renal function, coadministration with NSAIDs may result in further deterioration of renal function. Allopurinol and ACE inhibitors may cause a higher risk of hypersensitivity reaction when taken concurrently.

Decreased Effect: Aspirin (high dose) may reduce the therapeutic effects of ACE inhibitors; at low dosages this does not appear to be significant. Rifampin may decrease the effect of ACE inhibitors. Antacids may decrease the bioavailability of ACE inhibitors (may be more likely to occur with captopril); separate administration times by 1-2 hours. NSAIDs, specifically indomethacin, may reduce the hypotensive effects of ACE inhibitors. More likely to occur in low renin or volume dependent hypertensive patients.

Ethanol/Nutrition/Herb Interactions Herb/Nutraceutical: Avoid dong quai if using for hypertension (has estrogenic activity). Avoid ephedra, yohimbe, ginseng (may worsen hypertension). Avoid garlic (may have increased antihypertensive effect).

Pharmacodynamics/Kinetics

Onset of action: 1-2 hours

Duration: 24 hours
Absorption: Well absorbed (50% to 60%)
Distribution: Plasma levels decline in a triphasic fashion; rapid decline is a distribution phase to peripheral compartment, plasma protein and tissue ACE (half-life 2-4 hours); 2nd phase is an apparent elimination phase representing the clearance of free ramiprilat (half-life: 9-18 hours); and final phase is the terminal elimination phase representing the equilibrium phase between tissue binding and dissociation
Metabolism: Hepatic to the active form, ramiprilat
Half-life elimination: Ramiprilat: Effective: 13-17 hours; Terminal: >50 hours
Time to peak, serum: ~1 hour
Excretion: Urine (60%) and feces (40%) as parent drug and metabolites

Pregnancy Risk Factor C/D (2nd and 3rd trimesters)

Dosage Forms CAP: 1.25 mg, 2.5 mg, 5 mg, 10 mg

Raniclor™ *see* Cefaclor *on page 274*

Ranitidine (ra NI ti deen)

Related Information

Gastrointestinal Disorders *on page 1476*

U.S. Brand Names Zantac®; Zantac® 75 [OTC]

Canadian Brand Names Alti-Ranitidine; Apo-Ranitidine®; Gen-Ranidine; Novo-Ranidine; Nu-Ranit; PMS-Ranitidine; Rhoxal-ranitidine; Zantac®; Zantac 75®

Mexican Brand Names Acloral®; Alter-H!2®; Alvidina®; Anistal®; Azanplus®; Azantac®; Credaxol®; Galidrin®; Neugal®; Ranifur® [tabs]; Ranifur® [inj.]; Ranisen®; Raudil®; Serviradine®; Ulcedin®; Ulsaven®; Ultran®

Generic Available Yes; Excludes effervescent granules and tablets, injection

Synonyms Ranitidine Hydrochloride

Pharmacologic Category Histamine H_2 Antagonist

Use

Zantac®: Short-term and maintenance therapy of duodenal ulcer, gastric ulcer, gastroesophageal reflux, active benign ulcer, erosive esophagitis, and pathological hypersecretory conditions; as part of a multidrug regimen for *H. pylori* eradication to reduce the risk of duodenal ulcer recurrence

Zantac® 75 [OTC]: Relief of heartburn, acid indigestion, and sour stomach

Unlabeled/Investigational Use Recurrent postoperative ulcer, upper GI bleeding, prevention of acid-aspiration pneumonitis during surgery, and prevention of stress-induced ulcers

Local Anesthetic/Vasoconstrictor Precautions No information available to require special precautions

Effects on Dental Treatment No significant effects or complications reported

Common Adverse Effects Frequency not defined.

Cardiovascular: Atrioventricular block, bradycardia, premature ventricular beats, tachycardia, vasculitis
Central nervous system: Agitation, dizziness, depression, hallucinations, headache, insomnia, malaise, mental confusion, somnolence, vertigo
Dermatologic: Alopecia, erythema multiforme, rash
Endocrine & metabolic: Gynocomastia, impotence, increased prolactin levels, loss of libido
Gastrointestinal: Abdominal discomfort/pain, constipation, diarrhea, nausea, pancreatitis, vomiting
Hematologic: Acquired hemolytic anemia, agranulocytosis, aplastic anemia, granulocytopenia, leukopenia, pancytopenia, thrombocytopenia
Hepatic: Hepatic failure, hepatitis
Local: Transient pain, burning or itching at the injection site
Neuromuscular & skeletal: Arthralgia, involuntary motor disturbance, myalgia
Ocular: Blurred vision
Renal: Increased serum creatinine
Miscellaneous: Anaphylaxis, angioneurotic edema, hypersensitivity reactions

Dosage

Children 1 month to 16 years:
- Duodenal and gastric ulcer:
  - Oral:
    - Treatment: 2-4 mg/kg/day divided twice daily; maximum treatment dose: 300 mg/day
    - Maintenance: 2-4 mg/kg once daily; maximum maintenance dose: 150 mg/day
  - I.V.: 2-4 mg/kg/day divided every 6-8 hours; maximum: 150 mg/day
- GERD and erosive esophagitis:
  - Oral: 5-10 mg/kg/day divided twice daily; maximum: GERD: 300 mg/day, erosive esophagitis: 600 mg/day

(Continued)

Ranitidine *(Continued)*

I.V.: 2-4 mg/kg/day divided every 6-8 hours; maximum: 150 mg/day **or as an alternative**

Continuous infusion: Initial: 1 mg/kg/dose for one dose followed by infusion of 0.08-0.17 mg/kg/hour or 2-4 mg/kg/day

Children ≥12 years: Prevention of heartburn: Oral: Zantac® 75 [OTC]: 75 mg 30-60 minutes before eating food or drinking beverages which cause heartburn; maximum: 150 mg/24 hours; do not use for more than 14 days

Adults:

Duodenal ulcer: Oral: Treatment: 150 mg twice daily, or 300 mg once daily after the evening meal or at bedtime; maintenance: 150 mg once daily at bedtime

Helicobacter pylori eradication: 150 mg twice daily; requires combination therapy

Pathological hypersecretory conditions:

Oral: 150 mg twice daily; adjust dose or frequency as clinically indicated; doses of up to 6 g/day have been used

I.V.: Continuous infusion for Zollinger-Ellison: 1 mg/kg/hour; measure gastric acid output at 4 hours, if >10 mEq or if patient is symptomatic, increase dose in increments of 0.5 mg/kg/hour; doses of up to 2.5 mg/kg/hour have been used

Gastric ulcer, benign: Oral: 150 mg twice daily; maintenance: 150 mg once daily at bedtime

Erosive esophagitis: Oral: Treatment: 150 mg 4 times/day; maintenance: 150 mg twice daily

Prevention of heartburn: Oral: Zantac® 75 [OTC]: 75 mg 30-60 minutes before eating food or drinking beverages which cause heartburn; maximum: 150 mg in 24 hours; do not use for more than 14 days

Patients not able to take oral medication:

I.M.: 50 mg every 6-8 hours

I.V.: Intermittent bolus or infusion: 50 mg every 6-8 hours

Continuous I.V. infusion: 6.25 mg/hour

Elderly: Ulcer healing rates and incidence of adverse effects are similar in the elderly, when compared to younger patients; dosing adjustments not necessary based on age alone

Dosing adjustment in renal impairment: Adults: Cl_{cr} <50 mL/minute:

Oral: 150 mg every 24 hours; adjust dose cautiously if needed

I.V.: 50 mg every 18-24 hours; adjust dose cautiously if needed

Hemodialysis: Adjust dosing schedule so that dose coincides with the end of hemodialysis

Dosing adjustment/comments in hepatic disease: Patients with hepatic impairment may have minor changes in ranitidine half-life, distribution, clearance, and bioavailability; dosing adjustments not necessary, monitor

Mechanism of Action Competitive inhibition of histamine at H_2-receptors of the gastric parietal cells, which inhibits gastric acid secretion, gastric volume, and hydrogen ion concentration are reduced. Does not affect pepsin secretion, pentagastrin-stimulated intrinsic factor secretion, or serum gastrin.

Contraindications Hypersensitivity to ranitidine or any component of the formulation

Warnings/Precautions Use with caution in patients with hepatic impairment; use with caution in renal impairment, dosage modification required; avoid use in patients with history of acute porphyria (may precipitate attacks); long-term therapy may be associated with vitamin B_{12} deficiency; EFFERdose® formulations contain phenylalanine; safety and efficacy have not been established for pediatric patients <1 month of age

Drug Interactions

Cytochrome P450 Effect: Substrate (minor) of CYP1A2, 2C19, 2D6; **Inhibits** CYP1A2 (weak), 2D6 (weak)

Increased Effect/Toxicity: Increased the effect/toxicity of cyclosporine (increased serum creatinine), gentamicin (neuromuscular blockade), glipizide, glyburide, midazolam (increased concentrations), metoprolol, pentoxifylline, phenytoin, quinidine, and triazolam.

Decreased Effect:

Decreased effect: Variable effects on warfarin; antacids may decrease absorption of ranitidine; ketoconazole and itraconazole absorptions are decreased; may produce altered serum levels of procainamide and ferrous sulfate; decreased effect of nondepolarizing muscle relaxants, cefpodoxime, cyanocobalamin (decreased absorption), diazepam, oxaprozin

Decreased toxicity of atropine

Ethanol/Nutrition/Herb Interactions

Ethanol: Avoid ethanol (may cause gastric mucosal irritation).

Food: Does not interfere with absorption of ranitidine.

Dietary Considerations Oral dosage forms may be taken with or without food.

Zantac® EFFERdose®:

Granules contain sodium 7.55 mEq/packet and phenylalanine 16.84 mg/packet

Effervescent tablet 25 mg contains sodium 1.33 mEq/tablet and phenylalanine 2.81 mg/tablet

Effervescent tablet 150 mg contains sodium 7.96 mEq/tablet and phenylalanine 16.84 mg/tablet

Pharmacodynamics/Kinetics

Absorption: Oral: 50%

Distribution: Normal renal function: V_d: 1.7 L/kg; Cl_{cr} 25-35 mL/minute: 1.76 L/kg minimally penetrates the blood-brain barrier; enters breast milk

Protein binding: 15%

Metabolism: Hepatic to N-oxide, S-oxide, and N-desmethyl metabolites

Bioavailability: Oral: 48%

Half-life elimination:

Oral: Normal renal function: 2.5-3 hours; Cl_{cr} 25-35 mL/minute: 4.8 hours

I.V.: Normal renal function: 2-2.5 hours

Time to peak, serum: Oral: 2-3 hours; I.M.: ≤15 minutes

Excretion: Urine: Oral: 30%, I.V.: 70% (as unchanged drug); feces (as metabolites)

Pregnancy Risk Factor B

Dosage Forms CAP: 150 mg, 300 mg. **INF** [premixed in NaCl 0.45%; preservative free] (Zantac®): 50 mg (50 mL). **INJ, solution** (Zantac®): 25 mg/mL (2 mL, 6 mL, 40 mL). **SYR:** 15 mg/mL (10 mL); (Zantac®): 15 mg/mL (473 mL). **TAB:** 75 mg [OTC], 150 mg, 300 mg; (Zantac®): 150 mg, 300 mg; (Zantac® 75): 75 mg. **TAB, effervescent** (Zantac® EFFERdose®): 25 mg, 150 mg

Ranitidine Hydrochloride *see* Ranitidine *on page 1169*

Rapamune® *see* Sirolimus *on page 1224*

Raptiva™ *see* Efalizumab *on page 483*

Rasburicase (ras BYOOR i kayse)

U.S. Brand Names Elitek™

Generic Available No

Pharmacologic Category Enzyme; Enzyme, Urate-Oxidase (Recombinant)

Use Initial management of uric acid levels in pediatric patients with leukemia, lymphoma, and solid tumor malignancies receiving anticancer therapy expected to result in tumor lysis and elevation of plasma uric acid

Local Anesthetic/Vasoconstrictor Precautions No information available to require special precautions

Effects on Dental Treatment No significant effects or complications reported

Common Adverse Effects As reported in patients receiving rasburicase with antitumor therapy versus active-control:

>10%:

Central nervous system: Fever (5% to 46%), headache (26%)

Dermatologic: Rash (13%)

Gastrointestinal: Vomiting (50%), nausea (27%), abdominal pain (20%), constipation (20%), mucositis (2% to 15%), diarrhea (≤1% to 20%)

1% to 10%:

Hematologic: Neutropenia with fever (4%), neutropenia (2%)

Respiratory: Respiratory distress (3%)

Miscellaneous: Sepsis (3%)

Mechanism of Action Rasburicase is a recombinant urate-oxidase enzyme, which converts uric acid to allantoin (an inactive and soluble metabolite of uric acid); it does not inhibit the formation of uric acid.

Pharmacodynamics/Kinetics

Distribution: Pediatric patients: 110-127 mL/kg

Half-life elimination: Pediatric patients: 18 hours

Pregnancy Risk Factor C

Rauwolfia Serpentina (rah WOOL fee a ser pen TEEN ah)

Generic Available Yes

Synonyms Whole Root Rauwolfia

Pharmacologic Category Rauwolfia Alkaloid

Use Mild essential hypertension; relief of agitated psychotic states

Local Anesthetic/Vasoconstrictor Precautions No information available to require special precautions

(Continued)

Rauwolfia Serpentina *(Continued)*

Effects on Dental Treatment No significant effects or complications reported

Pregnancy Risk Factor C

Rea-Lo® [OTC] *see* Urea *on page 1353*

ReAzo [OTC] *see* Phenazopyridine *on page 1072*

Rebetol® *see* Ribavirin *on page 1177*

Rebetron® *see* Interferon Alfa-2b and Ribavirin *on page 754*

Rebif® *see* Interferon Beta-1a *on page 756*

Recombinant α-L-Iduronidase (Glycosaminoglycan α-L-Iduronohydrolase) *see* Laronidase *on page 800*

Recombinant Hirudin *see* Lepirudin *on page 803*

Recombinant Human Deoxyribonuclease *see* Dornase Alfa *on page 463*

Recombinant Human Follicle Stimulating Hormone *see* Follitropins *on page 626*

Recombinant Human Interleukin-11 *see* Oprelvekin *on page 1015*

Recombinant Human Parathyroid Hormone (1-34) *see* Teriparatide *on page 1274*

Recombinant Human Platelet-Derived Growth Factor B *see* Becaplermin *on page 184*

Recombinant Interleukin-11 *see* Oprelvekin *on page 1015*

Recombinant Plasminogen Activator *see* Reteplase *on page 1175*

Recombinate™ *see* Antihemophilic Factor (Recombinant) *on page 135*

Recombivax HB® *see* Hepatitis B Vaccine *on page 689*

Redutemp® [OTC] *see* Acetaminophen *on page 47*

Reese's® Pinworm Medicine [OTC] *see* Pyrantel Pamoate *on page 1151*

ReFacto® *see* Antihemophilic Factor (Recombinant) *on page 135*

Refludan® *see* Lepirudin *on page 803*

Refresh® [OTC] *see* Artificial Tears *on page 148*

Refresh Liquigel™ [OTC] *see* Carboxymethylcellulose *on page 265*

Refresh® Plus [OTC] *see* Artificial Tears *on page 148*

Refresh Plus® [OTC] *see* Carboxymethylcellulose *on page 265*

Refresh® Tears [OTC] *see* Artificial Tears *on page 148*

Refresh Tears® [OTC] *see* Carboxymethylcellulose *on page 265*

Regitine [DSC] *see* Phentolamine *on page 1077*

Reglan® *see* Metoclopramide *on page 914*

Regranex® *see* Becaplermin *on page 184*

Regular Iletin® II *see* Insulin Preparations *on page 749*

Regular, Insulin *see* Insulin Preparations *on page 749*

Reguloid® [OTC] *see* Psyllium *on page 1151*

Relacon-DM *see* Guaifenesin, Pseudoephedrine, and Dextromethorphan *on page 676*

Relafen® *see* Nabumetone *on page 955*

Relenza® *see* Zanamivir *on page 1396*

Relief® [OTC] *see* Phenylephrine *on page 1078*

Relpax® *see* Eletriptan *on page 486*

Remeron® *see* Mirtazapine *on page 935*

Remeron SolTab® *see* Mirtazapine *on page 935*

Reme-t™ [OTC] *see* Coal Tar *on page 367*

Remicade® *see* Infliximab *on page 747*

Remifentanil (rem i FEN ta nil)

U.S. Brand Names Ultiva®

Canadian Brand Names Ultiva®

Mexican Brand Names Ultiva®

Generic Available No

Synonyms GI87084B

Pharmacologic Category Analgesic, Narcotic

Use Analgesic for use during the induction and maintenance of general anesthesia; for continued analgesia into the immediate postoperative period; analgesic component of monitored anesthesia

Unlabeled/Investigational Use Management of pain in mechanically-ventilated patients

Local Anesthetic/Vasoconstrictor Precautions No information available to require special precautions

Effects on Dental Treatment No significant effects or complications reported

Common Adverse Effects

>10%: Gastrointestinal: Nausea, vomiting

1% to 10%:

Cardiovascular: Hypotension (dose dependent), bradycardia (dose dependent), tachycardia, hypertension

Central nervous system: Dizziness, headache, agitation, fever

Dermatologic: Pruritus

Neuromuscular & skeletal: Muscle rigidity (dose dependent)

Ocular: Visual disturbances

Respiratory: Respiratory depression, apnea, hypoxia

Miscellaneous: Shivering, postoperative pain

Restrictions C-II

Mechanism of Action Binds with stereospecific mu-opioid receptors at many sites within the CNS, increases pain threshold, alters pain reception, inhibits ascending pain pathways

Drug Interactions

Increased Effect/Toxicity: Additive effects with other CNS depressants. Synergistic with other anesthetics, may need to decrease thiopental, propofol, isoflurane, and midazolam by up to 75%.

Pharmacodynamics/Kinetics

Onset of action: I.V.: 1-3 minutes

Distribution: V_d: 100 mL/kg; increased in children

Protein binding: ~70% (primarily $alpha_1$ acid glycoprotein)

Metabolism: Rapid via blood and tissue esterases

Half-life elimination (dose dependent): Terminal: 10-20 minutes; effective: 3-10 minutes

Excretion: Urine

Pregnancy Risk Factor C

Reminyl® *see* Galantamine *on page 645*

Remodulin™ *see* Treprostinil *on page 1327*

Renacidin® *see* Citric Acid, Magnesium Carbonate, and Glucono-Delta-Lactone *on page 341*

Renagel® *see* Sevelamer *on page 1217*

Renese® *see* Polythiazide *on page 1102*

Renova® *see* Tretinoin (Topical) *on page 1329*

ReoPro® *see* Abciximab *on page 44*

Repaglinide (re pa GLI nide)

Related Information

Endocrine Disorders and Pregnancy *on page 1481*

U.S. Brand Names Prandin®

Canadian Brand Names GlucoNorm®; Prandin®

Generic Available No

Pharmacologic Category Antidiabetic Agent, Miscellaneous

Use Management of type 2 diabetes mellitus (noninsulin dependent, NIDDM); may be used in combination with metformin or thiazolidinediones

Local Anesthetic/Vasoconstrictor Precautions No information available to require special precautions

Effects on Dental Treatment No significant effects or complications reported

Common Adverse Effects

>10%:

Central nervous system: Headache (9% to 11%)

Endocrine & metabolic: Hypoglycemia (16% to 31%)

Respiratory: Upper respiratory tract infection (10% to 16%)

1% to 10%:

Cardiovascular: Chest pain (2% to 3%)

Gastrointestinal: Nausea (3% to 5%), heartburn (2% to 4%), vomiting (2% to 3%) constipation (2% to 3%), diarrhea (4% to 5%), tooth disorder (<1% to 2%)

Genitourinary: Urinary tract infection (2% to 3%)

Neuromuscular & skeletal: Arthralgia (3% to 6%), back pain (5% to 6%), paresthesia (2% to 3%)

Respiratory: Sinusitis (3% to 6%), rhinitis (3% to 7%), bronchitis (2% to 6%)

Miscellaneous: Allergy (1% to 2%)

Mechanism of Action Nonsulfonylurea hypoglycemic agent of the meglitinide class (the nonsulfonylurea moiety of glyburide) used in the management of type 2 diabetes mellitus; stimulates insulin release from the pancreatic beta cells

(Continued)

Repaglinide *(Continued)*

Drug Interactions

Cytochrome P450 Effect: Substrate of CYP2C8/9 (minor), 3A4 (major)

Increased Effect/Toxicity: Concurrent use of other hypoglycemic agents may increase risk of hypoglycemia. Gemfibrozil may increase the serum concentration of repaglinide (resulting in severe, prolonged hypoglycemia), and the addition of itraconazole may augment the effects of gemfibrozil on repaglinide. CYP3A4 inhibitors may increase the levels/effects of repaglinide; example inhibitors include azole antifungals, ciprofloxacin, clarithromycin, diclofenac, doxycycline, erythromycin, imatinib, isoniazid, nefazodone, nicardipine, propofol, protease inhibitors, quinidine, and verapamil.

Decreased Effect: Certain drugs (thiazides, diuretics, corticosteroids, phenothiazines, thyroid products, estrogens, oral contraceptives, phenytoin, nicotinic acid, sympathomimetics, calcium channel blockers, isoniazid) tend to produce hyperglycemia and may lead to loss of glycemic control. CYP3A4 inducers may decrease the levels/effects of repaglinide; example inducers include aminoglutethimide, carbamazepine, nafcillin, nevirapine, phenobarbital, phenytoin, and rifamycins.

Pharmacodynamics/Kinetics

Onset of action: Single dose: Increased insulin levels: ~15-60 minutes

Duration: 4-6 hours

Absorption: Rapid and complete

Distribution: V_d: 31 L

Protein binding, plasma: >98%

Metabolism: Hepatic via CYP3A4 isoenzyme and glucuronidation to inactive metabolites

Bioavailability: Mean absolute: ~56%

Half-life elimination: 1 hour

Time to peak, plasma: ~1 hour

Excretion: Within 96 hours: Feces (~90%, <2% as parent drug); Urine (~8%)

Pregnancy Risk Factor C

Repan® *see* Butalbital, Acetaminophen, and Caffeine *on page 236*

Repronex® *see* Menotropins *on page 868*

Requip® *see* Ropinirole *on page 1197*

Rescriptor® *see* Delavirdine *on page 403*

Rescula® *see* Unoprostone *on page 1352*

Reserpine (re SER peen)

Related Information

Cardiovascular Diseases *on page 1458*

Generic Available Yes

Pharmacologic Category Rauwolfia Alkaloid

Use Management of mild to moderate hypertension

Unlabeled/Investigational Use Management of tardive dyskinesia, schizophrenia

Local Anesthetic/Vasoconstrictor Precautions No information available to require special precautions

Effects on Dental Treatment Key adverse event(s) related to dental treatment: Xerostomia and changes in salivation (normal salivary flow resumes upon discontinuation).

Mechanism of Action Reduces blood pressure via depletion of sympathetic biogenic amines (norepinephrine and dopamine); this also commonly results in sedative effects

Pregnancy Risk Factor C

Reserpine, Hydralazine, and Hydrochlorothiazide *see* Hydralazine, Hydrochlorothiazide, and Reserpine *on page 698*

Respa-1st® *see* Guaifenesin and Pseudoephedrine *on page 675*

Respa-DM® *see* Guaifenesin and Dextromethorphan *on page 673*

Respa-GF® [DSC] *see* Guaifenesin *on page 672*

Respaire®-60 SR *see* Guaifenesin and Pseudoephedrine *on page 675*

Respaire®-120 SR *see* Guaifenesin and Pseudoephedrine *on page 675*

Respiratory Diseases *see page 1478*

Respiratory Synctial Virus Immune Globulin *see page 1614*

Restasis™ *see* CycloSPORINE *on page 386*

Restoril® *see* Temazepam *on page 1266*

Restylane® *see* Hyaluronate and Derivatives *on page 696*

Retavase® *see* Reteplase *on page 1175*

Reteplase (RE ta plase)

Related Information

Cardiovascular Diseases *on page 1458*

U.S. Brand Names Retavase®

Canadian Brand Names Retavase®

Generic Available No

Synonyms Recombinant Plasminogen Activator; r-PA

Pharmacologic Category Thrombolytic Agent

Use Management of acute myocardial infarction (AMI); improvement of ventricular function; reduction of the incidence of CHF and the reduction of mortality following AMI

Local Anesthetic/Vasoconstrictor Precautions No information available to require special precautions

Effects on Dental Treatment No significant effects or complications reported

Common Adverse Effects Bleeding is the most frequent adverse effect associated with reteplase. Heparin and aspirin have been administered concurrently with reteplase in clinical trials. The incidence of adverse events is a reflection of these combined therapies, and are comparable with comparison thrombolytics.

>10%: Local: Injection site bleeding (4.6% to 48.6%)

1% to 10%:

Gastrointestinal: Bleeding (1.8% to 9.0%)

Genitourinary: Bleeding (0.9% to 9.5%)

Hematologic: Anemia (0.9% to 2.6%)

Other adverse effects noted are frequently associated with myocardial infarction (and therefore may or may not be attributable to Retavase®) and include arrhythmias, hypotension, cardiogenic shock, pulmonary edema, cardiac arrest, reinfarction, pericarditis, tamponade, thrombosis, and embolism.

Mechanism of Action Reteplase is a nonglycosylated form of tPA produced by recombinant DNA technology using *E. coli*; it initiates local fibrinolysis by binding to fibrin in a thrombus (clot) and converts entrapped plasminogen to plasmin

Drug Interactions

Increased Effect/Toxicity: The risk of bleeding associated with reteplase may be increased by oral anticoagulants (warfarin), heparin, low molecular weight heparins, and drugs which affect platelet function (eg, NSAIDs, dipyridamole, ticlopidine, clopidogrel, IIb/IIIa antagonists). Concurrent use with aspirin and heparin may increase the risk of bleeding; however, aspirin and heparin were used concomitantly with reteplase in the majority of patients in clinical studies.

Decreased Effect: Aminocaproic acid (antifibrinolytic agent) may decrease effectiveness of thrombolytic agents.

Pharmacodynamics/Kinetics

Onset of action: Thrombolysis: 30-90 minutes

Half-life elimination: 13-16 minutes

Excretion: Feces and urine

Clearance: Plasma: 250-450 mL/minute

Pregnancy Risk Factor C

Retin-A® *see* Tretinoin (Topical) *on page 1329*

Retin-A® Micro *see* Tretinoin (Topical) *on page 1329*

Retinoic Acid *see* Tretinoin (Topical) *on page 1329*

Retrovir® *see* Zidovudine *on page 1398*

Reversol® *see* Edrophonium *on page 483*

Revex® *see* Nalmefene *on page 960*

Rēv-Eyes™ *see* Dapiprazole *on page 398*

ReVia® *see* Naltrexone *on page 962*

Reyataz® *see* Atazanavir *on page 158*

rFSH-alpha *see* Follitropins *on page 626*

rFSH-beta *see* Follitropins *on page 626*

rFVIIa *see* Factor VIIa (Recombinant) *on page 571*

R-Gene® *see* Arginine *on page 141*

rGM-CSF *see* Sargramostim *on page 1209*

r-h α-GAL *see* Agalsidase Beta *on page 69*

r-hCG *see* Chorionic Gonadotropin (Recombinant) *on page 326*

Rheumatoid Arthritis, Osteoarthritis, and Osteoporosis *see page 1490*

Rheumatrex® *see* Methotrexate *on page 897*

rhFSH-alpha *see* Follitropins *on page 626*

rhFSH-beta *see* Follitropins *on page 626*

RhIG *see* $Rh_o(D)$ Immune Globulin *on page 1176*

rhIL-11 *see* Oprelvekin *on page 1015*

Rhinocort® Aqua® *see* Budesonide *on page 221*

Rhinosyn® [OTC] *see* Chlorpheniramine and Pseudoephedrine *on page 315*

Rhinosyn-PD® [OTC] *see* Chlorpheniramine and Pseudoephedrine *on page 315*

$Rh_o(D)$ Immune Globulin (ar aych oh (dee) i MYUN GLOB yoo lin)

Related Information

Immunizations (Vaccines) *on page 1614*

U.S. Brand Names BayRho-D® Full-Dose; BayRho-D® Mini-Dose; MICRhoGAM®; RhoGAM®; Rhophylac®; WinRho SDF®

Canadian Brand Names BayRho-D® Full-Dose

Generic Available No

Synonyms RhIG; Rho(D) Immune Globulin (Human); RhoIGIV; RhoIVIM

Pharmacologic Category Immune Globulin

Use

Suppression of Rh isoimmunization: Use in the following situations when an $Rh_o(D)$-negative individual is exposed to $Rh_o(D)$-positive blood: During delivery of an $Rh_o(D)$-positive infant; abortion; amniocentesis; chorionic villus sampling; ruptured tubal pregnancy; abdominal trauma; transplacental hemorrhage. Used when the mother is $Rh_o(D)$ negative, the father of the child is either $Rh_o(D)$ positive or $Rh_o(D)$ unknown, the baby is either either $Rh_o(D)$ positive or $Rh_o(D)$ unknown.

Transfusion: Suppression of Rh isoimmunization in $Rh_o(D)$-negative female children and female adults in their childbearing years transfused with $Rh_o(D)$ antigen-positive RBCs or blood components containing $Rh_o(D)$ antigen-positive RBCs

Treatment of idiopathic thrombocytopenic purpura (ITP): Used in the following nonsplenectomized $Rh_o(D)$ positive individuals: Children with acute or chronic ITP, adults with chronic ITP, children and adults with ITP secondary to HIV infection

Local Anesthetic/Vasoconstrictor Precautions No information available to require special precautions

Effects on Dental Treatment No significant effects or complications reported

Common Adverse Effects Frequency not defined.

Cardiovascular: Hypotension, pallor, tachycardia, vasodilation

Central nervous system: Chills, dizziness, fever, headache, malaise, somnolence

Dermatologic: Pruritus, rash

Gastrointestinal: Abdominal pain, diarrhea, nausea, vomiting

Hematologic: Hemoglobin decreased (patients with ITP), intravascular hemolysis (patients with ITP)

Hepatic: LDH increased

Local: Injection site reaction: Discomfort, induration, mild pain, redness, swelling

Neuromuscular & skeletal: Back pain, hyperkinesia, myalgia, weakness

Miscellaneous: Anaphylaxis, diaphoresis

Mechanism of Action

Rh suppression: Suppresses the immune response and antibody formation of $Rh_o(D)$ negative individuals to $Rh_o(D)$ positive red blood cells.

ITP: Coats the patients $Rh_o(D)$ positive red blood cells with antibody, so that as they are cleared by the spleen, the spleens ability to clear antibody-coated cells is saturated, sparing the platelets.

Drug Interactions

Decreased Effect: $Rh_o(D)$ immune globulin may interfere with the response of live vaccines; vaccines should not be administered within 3 months after $Rh_o(D)$

Pharmacodynamics/Kinetics

Onset of platelet increase: ITP: 1-3 days

Duration: Suppression of Rh isoimmunization: ~12 weeks; Treatment of ITP: 3-4 weeks

Distribution: V_d: I.M.: 8.59 L

Half-life elimination: 21-30 days

Time to peak, plasma: I.M.: 5-10 days

Pregnancy Risk Factor C

Rho(D) Immune Globulin (Human) *see* $Rh_o(D)$ Immune Globulin *on page 1176*

RhoGAM® *see* $Rh_o(D)$ Immune Globulin *on page 1176*

RhoIGIV *see* Rh$_0$(D) Immune Globulin *on page 1176*
RhoIVIM *see* Rh$_0$(D) Immune Globulin *on page 1176*
Rhophylac® *see* Rh$_0$(D) Immune Globulin *on page 1176*
rhPTH(1-34) *see* Teriparatide *on page 1274*
rHuEPO-α *see* Epoetin Alfa *on page 499*
rhuMAb-E25 *see* Omalizumab *on page 1012*
rhuMAb-VEGF *see* Bevacizumab *on page 204*
Ribasphere™ *see* Ribavirin *on page 1177*

Ribavirin (rye ba VYE rin)

Related Information

Systemic Viral Diseases *on page 1519*

U.S. Brand Names Copegus®; Rebetol®; Ribasphere™; Virazole®

Canadian Brand Names Virazole®

Mexican Brand Names Vilona®; Virazide®

Generic Available Yes: Capsule

Synonyms RTCA; Tribavirin

Pharmacologic Category Antiviral Agent

Use

Inhalation: Treatment of patients with respiratory syncytial virus (RSV) infections; specially indicated for treatment of severe lower respiratory tract RSV infections in patients with an underlying compromising condition (prematurity, bronchopulmonary dysplasia and other chronic lung conditions, congenital heart disease, immunodeficiency, immunosuppression), and recent transplant recipients

Oral capsule:

In combination with interferon alfa-2b (Intron® A) injection for the treatment of chronic hepatitis C in patients with compensated liver disease who have relapsed after alpha interferon therapy or were previously untreated with alpha interferons

In combination with peginterferon alfa-2b (PEG-Intron®) injection for the treatment of chronic hepatitis C in patients with compensated liver disease who were previously untreated with alpha interferons

Oral solution: In combination with interferon alfa 2b (Intron® A) injection for the treatment of chronic hepatitis C in patients ≥3 years of age with compensated liver disease who were previously untreated with alpha interferons or patients ≥18 years of age who have relapsed after alpha interferon therapy

Oral tablet: In combination with peginterferon alfa-2a (Pegasys®) injection for the treatment of chronic hepatitis C in patients with compensated liver disease who were previously untreated with alpha interferons

Unlabeled/Investigational Use Used in other viral infections including influenza A and B and adenovirus

Local Anesthetic/Vasoconstrictor Precautions No information available to require special precautions

Effects on Dental Treatment No significant effects or complications reported

Common Adverse Effects

Inhalation:

1% to 10%:

Central nervous system: Fatigue, headache, insomnia

Gastrointestinal: Nausea, anorexia

Hematologic: Anemia

Note: Incidence of adverse effects (approximate) in healthcare workers: Headache (51%); conjunctivitis (32%); rhinitis, nausea, rash, dizziness, pharyngitis, and lacrimation (10% to 20%)

Oral (all adverse reactions are documented while receiving combination therapy with interferon alpha-2b; percentages as reported in adults):

>10%:

Central nervous system: Dizziness (17% to 26%), headache (63% to 66%)*, fatigue (60% to 70%)*, fever (32% to 41%)*, insomnia (26% to 39%), irritability (23% to 32%), depression (23% to 36%)*, emotional lability (7% to 12%)*, impaired concentration (10% to 14%)*

Dermatologic: Alopecia (27% to 32%), rash (20% to 28%), pruritus (13% to 21%)

Gastrointestinal: Nausea (38% to 47%), anorexia (21% to 27%), dyspepsia (14% to 16%), vomiting (9% to 12%)*

Hematologic: Decreased hemoglobin (25% to 36%), decreased WBC, absolute neutrophil count <0.5 x 10^9/L (5% to 11%), thrombocytopenia (6% to 14%), hyperbilirubinemia (24% to 34%), hemolysis

Neuromuscular & skeletal: Myalgia (61% to 64%)*, arthralgia (29% to 33%)*, musculoskeletal pain (20% to 28%), rigors (40% to 43%)

(Continued)

Ribavirin *(Continued)*

Respiratory: Dyspnea (17% to 19%), sinusitis (9% to 12%)*, nasal congestion

Miscellaneous: Flu-like syndrome (13% to 18%)*

*Similar to interferon alone

1% to 10%:

Cardiovascular: Chest pain (5% to 9%)*

Central nervous system: Nervousness (~5%)*

Gastrointestinal: Taste perversion (6% to 8%)

Hematologic: Hemolytic anemia (~10%)

Neuromuscular & skeletal: Weakness (9% to 10%)

*Similar to interferon alone

Incidence of anorexia, headache, fever, suicidal ideation, and vomiting are higher in children.

Mechanism of Action Inhibits replication of RNA and DNA viruses; inhibits influenza virus RNA polymerase activity and inhibits the initiation and elongation of RNA fragments resulting in inhibition of viral protein synthesis

Drug Interactions

Increased Effect/Toxicity: Concomitant use of ribavirin and nucleoside analogues may increase the risk of developing lactic acidosis (includes adefovir, didanosine, lamivudine, stavudine, zalcitabine, zidovudine). Concurrent use with didanosine has been noted to increase the risk of pancreatitis and/or peripheral neuropathy in addition to lactic acidosis. Suspend therapy if signs/symptoms of toxicity are present.

Decreased Effect: Decreased effect of stavudine and zidovudine (*in vitro*).

Pharmacodynamics/Kinetics

Absorption: Inhalation: Systemic; dependent upon respiratory factors and method of drug delivery; maximal absorption occurs with the use of aerosol generator via endotracheal tube; highest concentrations in respiratory tract and erythrocytes

Distribution: Oral capsule: Single dose: V_d 2825 L; distribution significantly prolonged in the erythrocyte (16-40 days), which can be used as a marker for intracellular metabolism

Protein binding: Oral: None

Metabolism: Hepatically and intracellularly (forms active metabolites); may be necessary for drug action

Bioavailability: Oral: 64%

Half-life elimination, plasma:

Children: Inhalation: 6.5-11 hours

Adults: Oral capsule, single dose: 24 hours in healthy adults, 44 hours with chronic hepatitis C infection (increases to ~298 hours at steady state)

Time to peak, serum: Inhalation: At end of inhalation period; Oral capsule: Multiple doses: 3 hours

Excretion: Inhalation: Urine (40% as unchanged drug and metabolites); Oral capsule: Urine (61%), feces (12%)

Pregnancy Risk Factor X

Ribavirin and Interferon Alfa-2b Combination Pack *see* Interferon Alfa-2b and Ribavirin *on page 754*

Riboflavin (RYE boe flay vin)

Generic Available Yes

Synonyms Lactoflavin; Vitamin B_2; Vitamin G

Pharmacologic Category Vitamin, Water Soluble

Use Prevention of riboflavin deficiency and treatment of ariboflavinosis

Local Anesthetic/Vasoconstrictor Precautions No information available to require special precautions

Effects on Dental Treatment No significant effects or complications reported

Significant Adverse Effects Frequency not defined: Genitourinary: Discoloration of urine (yellow-orange)

Dosage Oral:

Riboflavin deficiency:

Children: 2.5-10 mg/day in divided doses

Adults: 5-30 mg/day in divided doses

Recommended daily allowance:

Children: 0.4-1.8 mg

Adults: 1.2-1.7 mg

Mechanism of Action Component of flavoprotein enzymes that work together, which are necessary for normal tissue respiration; also needed for activation of pyridoxine and conversion of tryptophan to niacin

Warnings/Precautions Riboflavin deficiency often occurs in the presence of other B vitamin deficiencies

Drug Interactions Decreased absorption with probenecid

Pharmacodynamics/Kinetics

Absorption: Readily via GI tract, however, food increases extent; decreased with hepatitis, cirrhosis, or biliary obstruction

Metabolism: None

Half-life elimination: Biologic: 66-84 minutes

Excretion: Urine (9%) as unchanged drug

Pregnancy Risk Factor A/C (dose exceeding RDA recommendation)

Lactation Enters breast milk/compatible

Dosage Forms

Capsule: 100 mg

Tablet: 25 mg, 50 mg, 100 mg

Ridaura® *see* Auranofin *on page 170*

RID® Maximum Strength [OTC] *see* Pyrethrins and Piperonyl Butoxide *on page 1153*

Rid® Spray [OTC] *see* Permethrin *on page 1070*

Rifabutin (rif a BYOO tin)

Related Information

Systemic Viral Diseases *on page 1519*

Tuberculosis *on page 1495*

U.S. Brand Names Mycobutin®

Canadian Brand Names Mycobutin®

Generic Available No

Synonyms Ansamycin

Pharmacologic Category Antibiotic, Miscellaneous; Antitubercular Agent

Use Prevention of disseminated *Mycobacterium avium* complex (MAC) in patients with advanced HIV infection

Unlabeled/Investigational Use Utilized in multidrug regimens for treatment of MAC

Local Anesthetic/Vasoconstrictor Precautions No information available to require special precautions

Effects on Dental Treatment No significant effects or complications reported

Common Adverse Effects

>10%:

Dermatologic: Rash (11%)

Genitourinary: Discoloration of urine (30%)

Hematologic: Neutropenia (25%), leukopenia (17%)

1% to 10%:

Central nervous system: Headache (3%)

Gastrointestinal: Vomiting/nausea (3%), abdominal pain (4%), diarrhea (3%), anorexia (2%), flatulence (2%), eructation (3%)

Hematologic: Anemia, thrombocytopenia (5%)

Hepatic: Increased AST/ALT (7% to 9%)

Neuromuscular & skeletal: Myalgia

Mechanism of Action Inhibits DNA-dependent RNA polymerase at the beta subunit which prevents chain initiation

Drug Interactions

Cytochrome P450 Effect: Substrate (major) of CYP1A2, 3A4; **Induces** CYP3A4 (strong)

Increased Effect/Toxicity: Rifabutin may increase the therapeutic effect of clopidogrel; concurrent use with isoniazid may increase risk of hepatotoxicity; the levels/toxicity of rifabutin may be increased by imidazole antifungals, macrolide antibiotics, and protease inhibitors

Decreased Effect: Rifabutin may decrease the levels/effects of alfentanil, amiodarone, angiotensin II receptor blockers (irbesartan, losartan), CYP3A4 substrates (eg, clarithromycin, erythromycin, mirtazapine, nefazodone, venlafaxine), 5-HT_3 antagonists, imidazole antifungals, aprepitant, barbiturates, benzodiazepines (metabolized by oxidation), beta blockers, buspirone, calcium channel blockers, chloramphenicol, corticosteroids, cyclosporine, dapsone, disopyramide, estrogen and progestin contraceptives, fluconazole, gefitinib, HMG-CoA reductase inhibitors, methadone, morphine, phenytoin, propafenone, protease inhibitors, quinidine, repaglinide, reverse transcriptase inhibitors (non-nucleoside), tacrolimus, tamoxifen, terbinafine, tocainide, tricyclic antidepressants, warfarin, zaleplon, zolpidem. The effects of rifabutin may be decreased by CYP3A4 inducers (eg, aminoglutethimide, carbamazepine, nafcillin, nevirapine, phenobarbital, phenytoin).

(Continued)

Rifabutin *(Continued)*

Pharmacodynamics/Kinetics

Absorption: Readily, 53%

Distribution: V_d: 9.32 L/kg; distributes to body tissues including the lungs, liver, spleen, eyes, and kidneys

Protein binding: 85%

Metabolism: To active and inactive metabolites

Bioavailability: Absolute: HIV: 20%

Half-life elimination: Terminal: 45 hours (range: 16-69 hours)

Time to peak, serum: 2-4 hours

Excretion: Urine (10% as unchanged drug, 53% as metabolites); feces (10% as unchanged drug, 30% as metabolites)

Pregnancy Risk Factor B

Rifadin® *see* Rifampin *on page 1180*

Rifamate® *see* Rifampin and Isoniazid *on page 1181*

Rifampicin *see* Rifampin *on page 1180*

Rifampin (RIF am pin)

Related Information

Rifapentine *on page 1182*

Tuberculosis *on page 1495*

U.S. Brand Names Rifadin®; Rimactane®

Canadian Brand Names Rifadin®; Rofact™

Mexican Brand Names Pestarin®; Rifadin®; Rimactan®

Generic Available Yes

Synonyms Rifampicin

Pharmacologic Category Antibiotic, Miscellaneous; Antitubercular Agent

Use Management of active tuberculosis in combination with other agents; eliminate meningococci from asymptomatic carriers

Unlabeled/Investigational Use Prophylaxis of *Haemophilus influenzae* type b infection; *Legionella* pneumonia; used in combination with other anti-infectives in the treatment of staphylococcal infections; treatment of *M. leprae* infections

Local Anesthetic/Vasoconstrictor Precautions No information available to require special precautions

Effects on Dental Treatment No significant effects or complications reported

Common Adverse Effects

Frequency not defined:

- Cardiovascular: Flushing, edema
- Central nervous system: Headache, drowsiness, dizziness, confusion, numbness, behavioral changes, ataxia
- Dermatologic: Pruritus, urticaria, pemphigoid reaction
- Hematologic: Eosinophilia, leukopenia, hemolysis, hemolytic anemia, thrombocytopenia (especially with high-dose therapy)
- Hepatic: Hepatitis (rare)
- Neuromuscular & skeletal: Myalgia, weakness, osteomalacia
- Ocular: Visual changes, exudative conjunctivitis

1% to 10%:

- Dermatologic: Rash (1% to 5%)
- Gastrointestinal (1% to 2%): Epigastric distress, anorexia, nausea, vomiting, diarrhea, cramps, pseudomembranous colitis, pancreatitis
- Hepatic: Increased LFTs (up to 14%)

Mechanism of Action Inhibits bacterial RNA synthesis by binding to the beta subunit of DNA-dependent RNA polymerase, blocking RNA transcription

Drug Interactions

Cytochrome P450 Effect: Substrate (major) of CYP2A6, 2C8/9, 3A4; **Induces** CYP1A2 (strong), 2A6 (strong), 2B6 (strong), 2C8/9 (strong), 2C19 (strong), 3A4 (strong)

Increased Effect/Toxicity: Rifampin may increase the therapeutic effect of clopidogrel; concurrent use with isoniazid or pyrazinamide may increase risk of hepatotoxicity; macrolide antibiotics may increase levels/toxicity of rifampin

Decreased Effect: Rifampin may decrease the levels/effects of the following drugs: acetaminophen, alfentanil, amiodarone, angiotensin II receptor blockers (irbesartan and losartan), 5-HT_3 antagonists, imidazole antifungals, aprepitant, barbiturates, benzodiazepines (metabolized by oxidation), beta blockers, buspirone, calcium channel blockers, chloramphenicol, corticosteroids, cyclosporine; CYP1A2, 2A6, 2B6, 2C8/9, 2C19, and 3A4 substrates (eg, aminophylline, amiodarone, bupropion, fluoxetine, fluvoxamine, ifosfamide, methsuximide, mirtazapine, nateglinide, pioglitazone, promethazine, proton pump inhibitors, ropinirole, rosiglitazone, selegiline, sertraline, theophylline, venlafaxine, and zafirlukast); dapsone, disopyramide, estrogen and progestin contraceptives, fexofenadine, fluconazole, fusidic acid, gefitinib, HMG-CoA reductase inhibitors, methadone, morphine, phenytoin, propafenone, protease inhibitors, quinidine, repaglinide, reverse transcriptase inhibitors (non-nucleoside), sulfonylureas, tacrolimus, tamoxifen, terbinafine, tocainide, tricyclic antidepressants, warfarin, zaleplon, zidovudine, zolpidem. The effects of rifampin may be decreased by CYP2A6, 2C8/9, and 3A4 inducers (eg, aminoglutethimide, barbiturates, carbamazepine, nafcillin, nevirapine, and phenytoin).

Pharmacodynamics/Kinetics

Duration: ≤24 hours

Absorption: Oral: Well absorbed; food may delay or slightly reduce peak

Distribution: Highly lipophilic; crosses blood-brain barrier well

Relative diffusion from blood into CSF: Adequate with or without inflammation (exceeds usual MICs)

CSF:blood level ratio: Inflamed meninges: 25%

Protein binding: 80%

Metabolism: Hepatic; undergoes enterohepatic recirculation

Half-life elimination: 3-4 hours; prolonged with hepatic impairment; End-stage renal disease: 1.8-11 hours

Time to peak, serum: Oral: 2-4 hours

Excretion: Feces (60% to 65%) and urine (~30%) as unchanged drug

Pregnancy Risk Factor C

Rifampin and Isoniazid (RIF am pin & eye soe NYE a zid)

Related Information

Isoniazid *on page 769*

Rifampin *on page 1180*

U.S. Brand Names Rifamate®

Canadian Brand Names Rifamate®

Generic Available No

Synonyms Isoniazid and Rifampin

Pharmacologic Category Antibiotic, Miscellaneous

Use Management of active tuberculosis; see individual agents for additional information

Local Anesthetic/Vasoconstrictor Precautions No information available to require special precautions

Effects on Dental Treatment No significant effects or complications reported

Drug Interactions

Cytochrome P450 Effect:

Rifampin: **Substrate** (major) of CYP2A6, 2C8/9, 3A4; **Induces** CYP1A2 (strong), 2A6 (strong), 2B6 (strong), 2C8/9 (strong), 2C19 (strong), 3A4 (strong)

Isoniazid: **Substrate** of CYP2E1 (major); **Inhibits** CYP1A2 (weak), 2A6 (moderate), 2C8/9 (moderate), 2C19 (strong), 2D6 (moderate), 2E1 (moderate), 3A4 (strong); **Induces** CYP2E1 (after discontinuation) (weak)

Pharmacodynamics/Kinetics See individual agents.

Pregnancy Risk Factor C

Rifampin, Isoniazid, and Pyrazinamide

(RIF am pin, eye soe NYE a zid, & peer a ZIN a mide)

Related Information

Isoniazid *on page 769*

Pyrazinamide *on page 1152*

Rifampin *on page 1180*

U.S. Brand Names Rifater®

Canadian Brand Names Rifater™

Generic Available No

Synonyms Isoniazid, Rifampin, and Pyrazinamide; Pyrazinamide, Rifampin, and Isoniazid

Pharmacologic Category Antibiotic, Miscellaneous

Use Management of active tuberculosis; see individual agents for additional information

Local Anesthetic/Vasoconstrictor Precautions No information available to require special precautions

Effects on Dental Treatment No significant effects or complications reported

Common Adverse Effects See individual agents.

(Continued)

Rifampin, Isoniazid, and Pyrazinamide *(Continued)*

Drug Interactions

Cytochrome P450 Effect:

Rifampin: **Substrate** (major) of CYP2A6, 2C8/9, 3A4; **Induces** CYP1A2 (strong), 2A6 (strong), 2B6 (strong), 2C8/9 (strong), 2C19 (strong), 3A4 (strong)

Isoniazid: **Substrate** of CYP2E1 (major); **Inhibits** CYP1A2 (weak), 2A6 (moderate), 2C8/9 (moderate), 2C19 (strong), 2D6 (moderate), 2E1 (moderate), 3A4 (strong); CYP2E1 (after discontinuation) (weak)

Increased Effect/Toxicity: Increased effect/toxicity: Combination therapy with rifampin and pyrazinamide has been associated with severe and fatal hepatotoxic reactions.

Based on **rifampin** component: Rifampin levels may be increased when given with co-trimoxazole, probenecid, or ritonavir. Rifampin given with halothane or isoniazid increases the potential for hepatotoxicity.

Pharmacodynamics/Kinetics See individual agents.

Pregnancy Risk Factor C

Rifapentine (RIF a pen teen)

Related Information

Rifampin *on page 1180*

U.S. Brand Names Priftin®

Canadian Brand Names Priftin®

Generic Available No

Pharmacologic Category Antitubercular Agent

Use Treatment of pulmonary tuberculosis; rifapentine must always be used in conjunction with at least one other antituberculosis drug to which the isolate is susceptible; it may also be necessary to add a third agent (either streptomycin or ethambutol) until susceptibility is known.

Local Anesthetic/Vasoconstrictor Precautions No information available to require special precautions

Effects on Dental Treatment No significant effects or complications reported

Common Adverse Effects

>10%: Endocrine & metabolic: Hyperuricemia (most likely due to pyrazinamide from initiation phase combination therapy)

1% to 10%:

Cardiovascular: Hypertension

Central nervous system: Headache, dizziness

Dermatologic: Rash, pruritus, acne

Gastrointestinal: Anorexia, nausea, vomiting, dyspepsia, diarrhea

Hematologic: Neutropenia, lymphopenia, anemia, leukopenia, thrombocytosis

Hepatic: Increased ALT/AST

Neuromuscular & skeletal: Arthralgia, pain

Renal: Pyuria, proteinuria, hematuria, urinary casts

Respiratory: Hemoptysis

Mechanism of Action Inhibits DNA-dependent RNA polymerase in susceptible strains of *Mycobacterium tuberculosis* (but not in mammalian cells). Rifapentine is bactericidal against both intracellular and extracellular MTB organisms. MTB resistant to other rifamycins including rifampin are likely to be resistant to rifapentine. Cross-resistance does not appear between rifapentine and other nonrifamycin antimycobacterial agents.

Drug Interactions

Cytochrome P450 Effect: Induces CYP2C8/9 (strong), 3A4 (strong)

Increased Effect/Toxicity: Rifapentine may increase the therapeutic effect of clopidogrel; concurrent use with isoniazid may increase risk of hepatotoxicity

Decreased Effect: Rifapentine may decrease the levels/effects of the following drugs: alfentanil, amiodarone, angiotensin II receptor blockers (irbesartan, losartan), 5-HT_3 antagonists, imidazole antifungals, aprepitant, barbiturates, benzodiazepines (metabolized by oxidation), beta blockers, buspirone, calcium channel blockers, corticosteroids, cyclosporine; CYP2C8/9 and 3A4 substrates (eg, amiodarone, clarithromycin, erythromycin, fluoxetine, mirtazapine, nateglinide, nefazodone, nevirapine, pioglitazone, rosiglitazone, sertraline, venlafaxine, and zafirlukast); dapsone, disopyramide, estrogen and progestin contraceptives, fluconazole, gefitinib, HMG-CoA reductase inhibitors, methadone, morphine, phenytoin, propafenone, protease inhibitors, quinidine, repaglinide, reverse transcriptase inhibitors (non-nucleoside), tacrolimus, tamoxifen, terbinafine, tocainide, tricyclic antidepressants, warfarin, zaleplon, zidovudine, and zolpidem.

Pharmacodynamics/Kinetics

Absorption: Food increases AUC and C_{max} by 43% and 44% respectively.

Distribution: V_d: ~70.2 L; rifapentine and metabolite accumulate in human monocyte-derived macrophages with intracellular/extracellular ratios of 24:1 and 7:1 respectively

Protein binding: Rifapentine and 25-desacetyl metabolite: 97.7% and 93.2%, primarily to albumin

Metabolism: Hepatic; hydrolyzed by an esterase and esterase enzyme to form the active metabolite 25-desacetyl rifapentine

Bioavailability: ~70%

Half-life elimination: Rifapentine: 14-17 hours; 25-desacetyl rifapentine: 13 hours

Time to peak, serum: 5-6 hours

Excretion: Urine (17% primarily as metabolites)

Pregnancy Risk Factor C

Rifater® *see* Rifampin, Isoniazid, and Pyrazinamide *on page 1181*

Rifaximin (rif AX i min)

U.S. Brand Names Xifaxan™

Generic Available No

Pharmacologic Category Antibiotic, Miscellaneous

Use Treatment of travelers' diarrhea caused by noninvasive strains of *E. coli*

Local Anesthetic/Vasoconstrictor Precautions No information available to require special precautions

Effects on Dental Treatment No significant effects or complications reported

Common Adverse Effects Incidence of adverse effects reported as ≥2% occurred more in the placebo group than the rifaximin group except for headache.

2% to 10%: Central nervous system: Headache (10%; placebo 9%)

Mechanism of Action Rifaximin inhibits bacterial RNA synthesis by binding to bacterial DNA-dependent RNA polymerase.

Drug Interactions

Cytochrome P450 Effect: Induces CYP3A4 (minor)

Pharmacodynamics/Kinetics

Absorption: Oral: <0.4%

Distribution: 80% to 90% in the gut

Half-life elimination: ~6 hours

Excretion: Feces (~97% as unchanged drug); urine (<1%)

Pregnancy Risk Factor C

rIFN-A *see* Interferon Alfa-2a *on page 751*

rIFN beta-1a *see* Interferon Beta-1a *on page 756*

rIFN beta-1b *see* Interferon Beta-1b *on page 757*

RIG *see* Rabies Immune Globulin (Human) *on page 1165*

rIL-11 *see* Oprelvekin *on page 1015*

Rilutek® *see* Riluzole *on page 1183*

Riluzole (RIL yoo zole)

U.S. Brand Names Rilutek®

Canadian Brand Names Rilutek®

Mexican Brand Names Rilutek®

Generic Available No

Synonyms 2-Amino-6-Trifluoromethoxy-benzothiazole; RP-54274

Pharmacologic Category Glutamate Inhibitor

Use Orphan drug: Treatment of amyotrophic lateral sclerosis (ALS); riluzole can extend survival or time to tracheostomy

Local Anesthetic/Vasoconstrictor Precautions No information available to require special precautions

Effects on Dental Treatment No significant effects or complications reported

Common Adverse Effects

>10%:

- Gastrointestinal: Nausea (10% to 21%)
- Neuromuscular & skeletal: Weakness (15% to 20%)
- Respiratory: Decreased lung function (10% to 16%)

1% to 10%:

- Cardiovascular: Hypertension, tachycardia, postural hypotension, edema
- Central nervous system: headache, dizziness, somnolence, insomnia, malaise, depression, vertigo, agitation, tremor, circumoral paresthesia
- Dermatologic: Pruritus, eczema, alopecia

(Continued)

Riluzole *(Continued)*

Gastrointestinal: Abdominal pain, diarrhea, anorexia, dyspepsia, vomiting, stomatitis

Neuromuscular & skeletal: Arthralgia, back pain

Respiratory: Rhinitis, increased cough

Miscellaneous: Aggravation reaction

Mechanism of Action Inhibitory effect on glutamate release, inactivation of voltage-dependent sodium channels; and ability to interfere with intracellular events that follow transmitter binding at excitatory amino acid receptors

Drug Interactions

Cytochrome P450 Effect: Substrate of CYP1A2 (major)

Increased Effect/Toxicity: CYP1A2 inhibitors may increase the levels/effects of riluzole; example inhibitors include amiodarone, ciprofloxacin, fluvoxamine, ketoconazole, lomefloxacin, ofloxacin, and rofecoxib.

Decreased Effect: CYP1A2 inducers may decrease the levels/effects of riluzole; example inducers include aminoglutethimide, carbamazepine, phenobarbital, and rifampin.

Pharmacodynamics/Kinetics

Absorption: 90%; high fat meal decreases AUC by 20%, peak blood levels by 45%

Protein binding, plasma: 96%, primarily to albumin and lipoproteins

Metabolism: Extensively hepatic to six major and a number of minor metabolites via CYP1A2 dependent hydroxylation and glucuronidation

Bioavailability: Oral: Absolute: 50%

Half-life elimination: 12 hours

Excretion: Urine (90%; 85% as metabolites, 2% as unchanged drug) and feces (5%) within 7 days

Pregnancy Risk Factor C

Rimactane® *see* Rifampin *on page 1180*

Rimantadine (ri MAN ta deen)

Related Information

Systemic Viral Diseases *on page 1519*

U.S. Brand Names Flumadine®

Canadian Brand Names Flumadine®

Generic Available Yes: Tablet

Synonyms Rimantadine Hydrochloride

Pharmacologic Category Antiviral Agent

Use Prophylaxis (adults and children >1 year of age) and treatment (adults) of influenza A viral infection

Local Anesthetic/Vasoconstrictor Precautions No information available to require special precautions

Effects on Dental Treatment Key adverse event(s) related to dental treatment: Xerostomia (normal salivary flow resumes upon discontinuation).

Common Adverse Effects 1% to 10%:

Cardiovascular: Orthostatic hypotension, edema

Central nervous system: Dizziness (2%), confusion, headache (1%), insomnia (2%), difficulty in concentrating, anxiety (1%), restlessness, irritability, hallucinations; incidence of CNS side effects may be less than that associated with amantadine

Gastrointestinal: Nausea (3%), vomiting (2%), xerostomia (2%), abdominal pain (1%), anorexia (2%)

Genitourinary: Urinary retention

Mechanism of Action Exerts its inhibitory effect on three antigenic subtypes of influenza A virus (H1N1, H2N2, H3N2) early in the viral replicative cycle, possibly inhibiting the uncoating process; it has no activity against influenza B virus and is two- to eightfold more active than amantadine

Drug Interactions

Increased Effect/Toxicity: Cimetidine increases blood levels/toxicity of rimantadine.

Decreased Effect: Acetaminophen may cause a small reduction in AUC and peak concentration of rimantadine. Peak plasma and AUC concentrations of rimantadine are slightly reduced by aspirin.

Pharmacodynamics/Kinetics

Onset of action: Antiviral activity: No data exist establishing a correlation between plasma concentration and antiviral effect

Absorption: Tablet and syrup formulations are equally absorbed

Metabolism: Extensively hepatic

Half-life elimination: 25.4 hours; prolonged in elderly

Time to peak: 6 hours
Excretion: Urine (<25% as unchanged drug)
Clearance: Hemodialysis does not contribute to clearance

Pregnancy Risk Factor C

Rimantadine Hydrochloride *see* Rimantadine *on page 1184*

Rimexolone (ri MEKS oh lone)

U.S. Brand Names Vexol®

Canadian Brand Names Vexol®

Generic Available No

Pharmacologic Category Corticosteroid, Ophthalmic

Use Treatment of inflammation after ocular surgery and the treatment of anterior uveitis

Local Anesthetic/Vasoconstrictor Precautions No information available to require special precautions

Effects on Dental Treatment No significant effects or complications reported

Mechanism of Action Decreases inflammation by suppression of migration of polymorphonuclear leukocytes and reversal of increased capillary permeability

Pregnancy Risk Factor C

Riomet™ *see* Metformin *on page 887*

Riopan Plus® [OTC] *see* Magaldrate and Simethicone *on page 852*

Riopan Plus® Double Strength [OTC] *see* Magaldrate and Simethicone *on page 852*

Risedronate (ris ED roe nate)

Related Information

Rheumatoid Arthritis, Osteoarthritis, and Osteoporosis *on page 1490*

U.S. Brand Names Actonel®

Canadian Brand Names Actonel®

Generic Available No

Synonyms Risedronate Sodium

Pharmacologic Category Bisphosphonate Derivative

Use Paget's disease of the bone; treatment and prevention of glucocorticoid-induced osteoporosis; treatment and prevention of osteoporosis in postmenopausal women

Local Anesthetic/Vasoconstrictor Precautions No information available to require special precautions

Effects on Dental Treatment No significant effects or complications reported

Common Adverse Effects

Seen in patients taking 30 mg/day for Paget's disease:

- >10%:
  - Central nervous system: Headache (18%)
  - Dermatologic: Rash (11%)
  - Gastrointestinal: Diarrhea (20%), abdominal pain (11%)
  - Neuromuscular & skeletal: Arthralgia (33%)
  - Miscellaneous: Flu-like syndrome (10%)
- 1% to 10%:
  - Cardiovascular: Peripheral edema (8%)
  - Central nervous system: Chest pain (7%), dizziness (7%)
  - Gastrointestinal: Nausea (10%), constipation (7%), belching (3%), colitis (3%, placebo 3%)
  - Neuromuscular & skeletal: Weakness (5%), bone pain (5%, placebo 5%), leg cramps (3%, placebo 3%), myasthenia (3%)
  - Ocular: Amblyopia (3%, placebo 3%), dry eye (3%)
  - Otic: Tinnitus (3%, placebo 3%)
  - Respiratory: Sinusitis (5%), bronchitis (3%, placebo 5%)
  - Miscellaneous: Neoplasm (3%)

Seen in patient taking 5 mg/day for osteoporosis (events similar to those seen with placebo)

- >10%:
  - Central nervous system: Pain (14%)
  - Gastrointestinal: Abdominal pain (12%), diarrhea (11%), nausea (11%)
  - Genitourinary: Urinary tract infection (11%)
  - Neuromuscular & skeletal: Back pain (26%), arthralgia (24%)
- 1% to 10%:
  - Cardiovascular: Hypertension (10%), chest pain (5%), cardiovascular disorder (2%), angina (2%)
  - Central nervous system: Depression (7%), dizziness (6%), insomnia (5%), anxiety (4%), vertigo (3%)

(Continued)

Risedronate *(Continued)*

Dermatologic: Rash (8%), bruising (4%), pruritus (3%), skin carcinoma (2%)
Gastrointestinal: Flatulence (5), gastritis (2%), gastrointestinal disorder (2%), rectal disorder (2%), tooth disorder (2%)
Genitourinary: Cystitis (4%)
Hematologic: Anemia (2%)
Neuromuscular & skeletal: Joint disorder (7%), myalgia (7%), neck pain (5%), asthenia (5%), bone pain (5%), bone disorder (4%), neuralgia (4%), leg cramps (4%), bursitis (3%), tendon disorder (3%), hypertonia (2%), paresthesia (2%)
Ocular: Cataract (6%), conjunctivitis (3%)
Otic: Otitis media (2%)
Respiratory: Pharyngitis (6%), rhinitis (6%), dyspnea (4%), pneumonia (3%)
Miscellaneous: Neoplasm(3%), hernia (3%)

Dosage Risedronate should be taken at least 30 minutes before the first food or drink of the day other than water. Oral:

Adults (patients should receive supplemental calcium and vitamin D if dietary intake is inadequate):

Paget's disease of bone: 30 mg once daily for 2 months

Retreatment may be considered (following post-treatment observation of at least 2 months) if relapse occurs, or if treatment fails to normalize serum alkaline phosphatase. For retreatment, the dose and duration of therapy are the same as for initial treatment. No data are available on more than one course of retreatment.

Osteoporosis (postmenopausal) prevention and treatment: 5 mg once daily; efficacy for use longer than 1 year has not been established; **alternatively,** a dose of 35 mg once weekly has been demonstrated to be effective

Osteoporosis (glucocorticoid-induced) prevention and treatment: 5 mg once daily

Elderly: Dosage adjustment is not necessary in patients with Cl_{cr} ≥30 mL/minute.

Dosage adjustment in renal impairment: Cl_{cr} <30 mL/minute: **Not** recommended for use

Mechanism of Action A bisphosphonate which inhibits bone resorption via actions on osteoclasts or on osteoclast precursors; decreases the rate of bone resorption direction, leading to an indirect decrease in bone formation

Contraindications Hypersensitivity to risedronate, bisphosphonates, or any component of the formulation; hypocalcemia; abnormalities of the esophagus which delay esophageal emptying such as stricture or achalasia; inability to stand or sit upright for at least 30 minutes; severe renal impairment (Cl_{cr} <30 mL/minute)

Warnings/Precautions Bisphosphonates may cause upper gastrointestinal disorders such as dysphagia, esophageal ulcer, and gastric ulcer. Use caution in patients with renal impairment; hypocalcemia must be corrected before therapy initiation with alendronate; ensure adequate calcium and vitamin D intake, especially for patients with Paget's disease in whom the pretreatment rate of bone turnover may be greatly elevated.

Drug Interactions

Decreased Effect: Calcium supplements and antacids interfere with absorption of risedronate (take at a different time of the day than risedronate).

Ethanol/Nutrition/Herb Interactions

Ethanol: Avoid ethanol (may increase risk of osteoporosis).
Food: Food may reduce absorption (similar to other bisphosphonates); mean oral bioavailability is decreased when given with food.

Dietary Considerations Take ≥30 minutes before the first food or drink of the day other than water.

Pharmacodynamics/Kinetics

Onset of action: May require weeks
Absorption: Rapid
Distribution: V_d: 6.3 L/kg
Protein binding: ~24%
Metabolism: None
Bioavailability: Poor, ~0.54% to 0.75%
Half-life elimination: Terminal: 480 hours
Excretion: Urine (up to 80%); feces (as unabsorbed drug)

Pregnancy Risk Factor C

Dosage Forms TAB: 5 mg, 30 mg, 35 mg

Risedronate Sodium *see* Risedronate *on page 1185*

Risperdal® *see* Risperidone *on page 1187*
Risperdal® Consta™ *see* Risperidone *on page 1187*
Risperdal M-Tab™ *see* Risperidone *on page 1187*

Risperidone (ris PER i done)

U.S. Brand Names Risperdal®; Risperdal® Consta™

Canadian Brand Names Risperdal®

Mexican Brand Names Risperdal®

Generic Available No

Synonyms Risperdal M-Tab™

Pharmacologic Category Antipsychotic Agent, Benzisoxazole

Use Treatment of schizophrenia; treatment of acute mania or mixed episodes associated with bipolar I disorder (as monotherapy or in combination with lithium or valproate)

Unlabeled/Investigational Use Behavioral symptoms associated with dementia in elderly; treatment of Tourette's disorder; treatment of pervasive developmental disorder and autism in children and adolescents

Local Anesthetic/Vasoconstrictor Precautions No information available to require special precautions

Effects on Dental Treatment Key adverse event(s) related to dental treatment: Significant xerostomia (normal salivary flow resumes upon discontinuation).

Common Adverse Effects

Frequency not defined: Gastrointestinal: Dysphagia, esophageal dysmotility

>10%:

Central nervous system: Insomnia, agitation, anxiety, headache, extrapyramidal symptoms (dose dependent), dizziness (I.M. injection)

Gastrointestinal: Weight gain

Respiratory: Rhinitis (I.M. injection)

1% to 10%:

Cardiovascular: Hypotension (especially orthostatic), tachycardia

Central nervous system: Sedation, dizziness (oral formulation), restlessness, dystonic reactions, pseudoparkinsonism, tardive dyskinesia, neuroleptic malignant syndrome, altered central temperature regulation, nervousness, fatigue, somnolence, hallucination, tremor, hypoesthesia, akathisia

Dermatologic: Photosensitivity (rare), rash, dry skin, seborrhea, acne

Endocrine & metabolic: Amenorrhea, galactorrhea, gynecomastia, sexual dysfunction

Gastrointestinal: Constipation, GI upset, xerostomia, dyspepsia, vomiting, abdominal pain, nausea, anorexia, diarrhea, weight changes

Genitourinary: Polyuria

Neuromuscular & skeletal: Myalgia

Ocular: Abnormal vision

Respiratory: Rhinitis (oral formulation), coughing, sinusitis, pharyngitis, dyspnea

Dosage

Oral:

Children and Adolescents:

Pervasive developmental disorder (unlabeled use): Initial: 0.25 mg twice daily; titrate up 0.25 mg/day every 5-7 days; optimal dose range: 0.75-3 mg/day

Autism (unlabeled use): Initial: 0.25 mg at bedtime; titrate to 1 mg/day (0.1 mg/kg/day)

Schizophrenia (unlabeled use): Initial: 0.5 mg once or twice daily; titrate as necessary up to 2-6 mg/day

Bipolar disorder (unlabeled use): Initial: 0.5 mg; titrate to 0.5-3 mg/day

Tourette's disorder (unlabeled use): Initial: 0.5 mg; titrate to 2-4 mg/day

Adults:

Schizophrenia: Recommended starting dose: 0.5-1 mg twice daily; slowly increase to the optimum range of 3-6 mg/day; may be given as a single daily dose once maintenance dose is achieved; daily dosages >10 mg does not appear to confer any additional benefit, and the incidence of extrapyramidal symptoms is higher than with lower doses

Bipolar mania: Recommended starting dose: 2-3 mg once daily; if needed, adjust dose by 1 mg/day in intervals ≥24 hours; dosing range: 1-6 mg/day

Elderly: A starting dose of 0.25-1 mg in 1-2 divided doses, and titration should progress slowly. Additional monitoring of renal function and orthostatic blood pressure may be warranted. If once-a-day dosing in the elderly or debilitated patient is considered, a twice daily regimen should be used to

(Continued)

Risperidone *(Continued)*

titrate to the target dose, and this dose should be maintained for 2-3 days prior to attempts to switch to a once-daily regimen.

I.M.: Adults: Schizophrenia (Risperdal® Consta™): 25 mg every 2 weeks; some patients may benefit from larger doses; maximum dose not to exceed 50 mg every 2 weeks. Dosage adjustments should not be made more frequently than every 4 weeks.

Note: Oral risperidone (or other antipsychotic) should be administered with the initial injection of Risperdal® Consta™ and continued for 3 weeks (then discontinued) to maintain adequate therapeutic plasma concentrations prior to main release phase of risperidone from injection site.

Dosing adjustment in renal impairment: Oral: Starting dose of 0.25-0.5 mg twice daily; clearance of the active moiety is decreased by 60% in patients with moderate to severe renal disease compared to healthy subjects.

Dosing adjustment in hepatic impairment: Oral: Starting dose of 0.25-0.5 mg twice daily; the mean free fraction of risperidone in plasma was increased by 35% compared to healthy subjects.

Mechanism of Action Risperidone is a benzisoxazole derivative, mixed serotonin-dopamine antagonist; binds to 5-HT_2-receptors in the CNS and in the periphery with a very high affinity; binds to dopamine-D_2 receptors with less affinity. The binding affinity to the dopamine-D_2 receptor is 20 times lower than the 5-HT_2 affinity. The addition of serotonin antagonism to dopamine antagonism (classic neuroleptic mechanism) is thought to improve negative symptoms of psychoses and reduce the incidence of extrapyramidal side effects. $Alpha_1$, $alpha_2$ adrenergic, and histaminergic receptors are also antagonized with high affinity. Risperidone has low to moderate affinity for 5-HT_{1C}, 5-HT_{1D}, and 5-HT_{1A} receptors, weak affinity for D_1 and no affinity for muscarinics or $beta_1$ and $beta_2$ receptors

Contraindications Hypersensitivity to risperidone or any component of the formulation

Warnings/Precautions Low to moderately sedating, use with caution in disorders where CNS depression is a feature. Use with caution in Parkinson's disease. Caution in patients with hemodynamic instability; bone marrow suppression; predisposition to seizures; subcortical brain damage; severe cardiac, hepatic, or respiratory disease. Use with caution in renal dysfunction. Esophageal dysmotility and aspiration have been associated with antipsychotic use - use with caution in patients at risk of aspiration pneumonia (ie, Alzheimer's disease). Caution in breast cancer or other prolactin-dependent tumors (may elevate prolactin levels). May alter temperature regulation or mask toxicity of other drugs due to antiemetic effects.

May cause orthostasis; an increased incidence of cerebrovascular events has been associated with risperidone use in elderly demented patients. Use with caution in patients with cardiovascular diseases (eg, heart failure, history of myocardial infarction or ischemia, cerebrovascular disease, conduction abnormalities). Use caution in patients receiving medications for hypertension (orthostatic effects may be exacerbated) or in patients with hypovolemia or dehydration. May alter cardiac conduction; life-threatening arrhythmias have occurred with therapeutic doses of neuroleptics.

May cause anticholinergic effects (confusion, agitation, constipation, xerostomia, blurred vision, urinary retention); therefore, they should be used with caution in patients with decreased gastrointestinal motility, urinary retention, BPH, xerostomia, or visual problems. Conditions which also may be exacerbated by cholinergic blockade include narrow-angle glaucoma (screening is recommended) and worsening of myasthenia gravis. Relative to other neuroleptics, risperidone has a low potency of cholinergic blockade.

May cause extrapyramidal symptoms, including pseudoparkinsonism, acute dystonic reactions, akathisia, and tardive dyskinesia (risk of these reactions is low relative to other neuroleptics, and is dose dependent). May be associated with neuroleptic malignant syndrome (NMS). May rarely cause hyperglycemia - use with caution in patients with diabetes or other disorders of glucose regulation.

Drug Interactions

Cytochrome P450 Effect: Substrate of CYP2D6 (major), 3A4 (minor); **Inhibits** CYP2D6 (weak), 3A4 (weak)

Increased Effect/Toxicity: CYP2D6 inhibitors may increase the levels/effects of risperidone; example inhibitors include chlorpromazine, delavirdine, fluoxetine, miconazole, paroxetine, pergolide, quinidine, quinine, ritonavir, and ropinirole. Risperidone may enhance the hypotensive effects of antihypertensive agents. Clozapine decreases clearance of risperidone. Metoclopramide may increase risk of extrapyramidal symptoms (EPS).

Decreased Effect: Risperidone may antagonize effects of levodopa. Carbamazepine decreases risperidone serum concentrations.

Ethanol/Nutrition/Herb Interactions

Ethanol: Avoid ethanol (may increase CNS depression).

Herb/Nutraceutical: Avoid kava kava, gotu kola, valerian, St John's wort (may increase CNS depression).

Dietary Considerations May be taken with or without food. Risperdal® M-Tabs™ contain phenylalanine.

Pharmacodynamics/Kinetics

Absorption:

Oral: Rapid and well absorbed; food does not affect rate or extent

Injection: <1% absorbed initially; main release occurs at ~3 weeks and is maintained from 4-6 weeks

Distribution: V_d: 1-2 L/kg

Protein binding, plasma: Risperidone 90%; 9-hydroxyrisperidone: 77%

Metabolism: Extensively hepatic via CYP2D6 to 9-hydroxyrisperidone (similar pharmacological activity as risperidone); *N*-dealkylation is a second minor pathway

Bioavailability: Solution: 70%; Tablet: 66%; orally-disintegrating tablets are bioequivalent to tablets

Half-life elimination: Active moiety (risperidone and its active metabolite 9-hydroxyrisperidone)

Oral: 20 hours (mean)

Extensive metabolizers: Risperidone: 3 hours; 9-hydroxyrisperidone: 21 hours

Poor metabolizers: Risperidone: 20 hours; 9-hydroxyrisperidone: 30 hours

Injection: 3-6 days; related to microsphere erosion and subsequent absorption of risperidone

Time to peak, plasma: Oral: Risperidone: Within 1 hour; 9-hydroxyrisperidone: Extensive metabolizers: 3 hours; Poor metabolizers: 17 hours

Excretion: Urine (70%); feces (15%)

Pregnancy Risk Factor C

Dosage Forms INJ, microspheres for reconstitution, extended release (Risperdal® Consta™): 25 mg, 37.5 mg, 50 mg. **SOLN, oral:** 1 mg/mL (30 mL). **TAB:** 0.25 mg, 0.5 mg, 1 mg, 2 mg, 3 mg, 4 mg. **TAB, orally disintegrating** (Risperdal® M-Tab™): 0.5 mg, 1 mg, 2 mg

Ritalin® *see* Methylphenidate *on page 908*

Ritalin® LA *see* Methylphenidate *on page 908*

Ritalin-SR® *see* Methylphenidate *on page 908*

Ritonavir (ri TOE na veer)

Related Information

HIV Infection and AIDS *on page 1484*

Tuberculosis *on page 1495*

U.S. Brand Names Norvir®

Canadian Brand Names Norvir®; Norvir® SEC

Mexican Brand Names Norvir®

Generic Available No

Pharmacologic Category Antiretroviral Agent, Protease Inhibitor

Use Treatment of HIV infection; should always be used as part of a multidrug regimen (at least three antiretroviral agents)

Local Anesthetic/Vasoconstrictor Precautions No information available to require special precautions

Effects on Dental Treatment Key adverse event(s) related to dental treatment: Xerostomia (normal salivary flow resumes upon discontinuation).

Common Adverse Effects Protease inhibitors cause dyslipidemia which includes elevated cholesterol and triglycerides and a redistribution of body fat centrally to cause increased abdominal girth, buffalo hump, facial atrophy, and breast enlargement. These agents also cause hyperglycemia.

>10%:

Endocrine & metabolic: Triglycerides increased

Gastrointestinal: Diarrhea, nausea, vomiting, taste perversion

Hematologic: Anemia, WBCs decreased

Hepatic: GGT increased

Neuromuscular & skeletal: Weakness

1% to 10%:

Cardiovascular: Vasodilation

(Continued)

Ritonavir *(Continued)*

Central nervous system: Fever, headache, malaise, dizziness, insomnia, somnolence, thinking abnormally

Dermatologic: Rash

Endocrine & metabolic: Hyperlipidemia, uric acid increased, glucose increased

Gastrointestinal: Abdominal pain, anorexia, constipation, dyspepsia, flatulence, local throat irritation

Hematologic: Neutropenia, eosinophilia, neutrophilia, prolonged PT, leukocytosis

Hepatic: LFTs increased

Neuromuscular & skeletal: CPK increased, myalgia, paresthesia

Respiratory: Pharyngitis

Miscellaneous: Diaphoresis, potassium increased, calcium increased

Mechanism of Action Ritonavir inhibits HIV protease and renders the enzyme incapable of processing of polyprotein precursor which leads to production of noninfectious immature HIV particles

Drug Interactions

Cytochrome P450 Effect: Substrate of CYP1A2 (minor), 2B6 (minor), 2D6 (minor), 3A4 (major); **Inhibits** CYP2C8/9 (weak), 2C19 (weak), 2D6 (strong), 2E1 (weak), 3A4 (strong); **Induces** CYP1A2 (weak), 2C8/9 (weak), 3A4 (weak)

Increased Effect/Toxicity: Concurrent use of amiodarone, bepridil, cisapride, ergot alkaloids (dihydroergotamine, ergonovine, methylergonovine), flecainide, lovastatin, midazolam, pimozide, propafenone, quinidine, simvastatin, and triazolam is contraindicated.

Saquinavir's serum concentrations are increased by ritonavir; the dosage of both agents should be reduced to 400 mg twice daily. Concurrent therapy with amprenavir may result in increased serum concentrations: dosage adjustment is recommended. Metronidazole or disulfiram may cause disulfiram reaction (oral solution contains 43% ethanol). Serum levels/effects of corticosteroids (eg, dexamethasone, fluticasone, prednisone) and immunosuppressants (cyclosporine, sirolimus, tacrolimus; monitor) may be increased by ritonavir. Serum concentrations of meperidine's neuroexcitatory metabolite (normeperidine) are increased by ritonavir, which may increase the risk of CNS toxicity/seizures. Rifabutin and rifabutin metabolite serum concentrations may be increased by ritonavir; reduce rifabutin dose to 150 mg every other day.

Ritonavir may increase the levels/effects of amphetamines, selected beta-blockers, selected benzodiazepines (midazolam and triazolam contraindicated), calcium channel blockers (bepridil contraindicated), cisapride (contraindicated), dextromethorphan, ergot alkaloids (contraindicated), fluoxetine, lidocaine, HMG-CoA reductase inhibitors (lovastatin and simvastatin are contraindicated), mesoridazine, mirtazapine, nateglinide, nefazodone, paroxetine, pimozide (contraindicated), propafenone (contraindicated), risperidone, sildenafil (and other PDE-5 inhibitors), thioridazine, tricyclic antidepressants, venlafaxine, and other substrates of CYP2D6 or 3A4. Mesoridazine and thioridazine are generally contraindicated with strong CYP2D6 inhibitors. When used with strong CYP3A4 inhibitors, dosage adjustment/limits are recommended for sildenafil and other PDE-5 inhibitors; refer to individual monographs.

Decreased Effect: The administration of didanosine (buffered formulation) should be separated from ritonavir by 2.5 hours to limit interaction with ritonavir. Concurrent use of rifampin, rifabutin, dexamethasone, and many anticonvulsants may lower serum concentration of ritonavir. Ritonavir may reduce the concentration of ethinyl estradiol which may result in loss of contraception (including combination products). Theophylline concentrations may be reduced in concurrent therapy. Levels of didanosine and zidovudine may be decreased by ritonavir, however, no dosage adjustment is necessary. Voriconazole serum levels are reduced by ritonavir (concurrent use is contraindicated). In addition, ritonavir may decrease the serum concentrations of the following drugs: Atovaquone, divalproex, lamotrigine, methadone, phenytoin, warfarin. The levels/effects of ritonavir may be decreased by aminoglutethimide, carbamazepine, nafcillin, nevirapine, phenobarbital, phenytoin, rifamycins, and other CYP3A4 inducers. Ritonavir may decrease the levels/effects of CYP2D6 prodrug substrates (eg, codeine, hydrocodone, oxycodone, tramadol).

Pharmacodynamics/Kinetics

Absorption: Variable, with or without food

Distribution: High concentrations in serum and lymph nodes

Protein binding: 98% to 99%
Metabolism: Hepatic; five metabolites, low concentration of an active metabolite achieved in plasma (oxidative); see Drug Interactions
Half-life elimination: 3-5 hours
Excretion: Urine (negligible amounts)

Pregnancy Risk Factor B

Ritonavir and Lopinavir *see* Lopinavir and Ritonavir *on page 839*

Rituxan® *see* Rituximab *on page 1191*

Rituximab (ri TUK si mab)

U.S. Brand Names Rituxan®

Canadian Brand Names Rituxan®

Mexican Brand Names Mabthera®

Generic Available No

Synonyms Anti-CD20 Monoclonal Antibody; C2B8; C2B8 Monoclonal Antibody; IDEC-C2B8; Pan-B Antibody

Pharmacologic Category Antineoplastic Agent, Monoclonal Antibody

Use Treatment of relapsed or refractory CD20 positive, B-cell non-Hodgkin's lymphoma

Local Anesthetic/Vasoconstrictor Precautions No information available to require special precautions

Effects on Dental Treatment No significant effects or complications reported

Common Adverse Effects Note: Abdominal pain, anemia, dyspnea, hypotension, and neutropenia are more common in patients with bulky disease.

>10%:
- Central nervous system: Fever (53%), chills (33%), headache (19%), pain (12%)
- Dermatologic: Rash (15%), pruritus (14%), angioedema (11%)
- Gastrointestinal: Nausea (23%), abdominal pain (14%)
- Hematologic: Lymphopenia (48%; Grade 3/4: 40%; mean duration 14 days), leukopenia (14%; Grade 3/4: 4%), neutropenia (14%; Grade 3/4: 6%; mean duration 13 days), thrombocytopenia (12%; Grade 3/4: 2%)
- Neuromuscular & skeletal: Weakness (26%)
- Respiratory: Cough (13%), rhinitis (12%)
- Miscellaneous: Infection (31%), night sweats (15%)
  - Infusion-related reactions: Chills, fever, rigors, dizziness, hypertension,myalgia, nausea, pruritus, rash and vomiting (first dose 77%; fourth dose 30%; eighth dose 14%)

1% to 10%:
- Cardiovascular: Dizziness (10%), hypotension (10%), peripheral edema (8%), hypertension (6%), anxiety (5%), flushing (5%)
- Central nervous system: Agitation (<5%), depression (<5%), edema (<5%), insomnia (<5%), malaise (<5%), nervousness (<5%), somnolence (<5%), vertigo (<5%)
- Dermatologic: Urticaria (8%)
- Endocrine & metabolic: Hyperglycemia (9%), hypoglycemia (<5%)
- Gastrointestinal: Diarrhea (10%), vomiting (10%), anorexia (<5%), weight loss (<5%)
- Hematologic: Anemia (8%; Grade 3/4: 3%)
- Local: Pain at the injection site (<5%)
- Neuromuscular & skeletal: Arthralgia (10%), back pain (10%), myalgia (10%), arthritis (<5%), hyperkinesia (<5%), hypertonia (<5%), hypesthesia (<5%), neuritis (<5%), neuropathy (<5%), paresthesia (<5%)
- Ocular: Conjunctivitis (<5%), lacrimation disorder (<5%)
- Respiratory: Throat irritation (9%), bronchospasm (8%), dyspnea (7%), sinusitis (6%), dyspepsia (<5%)
- Miscellaneous: LDH increased (7%)

Mechanism of Action Rituximab is a monoclonal antibody directed against the CD20 antigen on B-lymphocytes. CD20 regulates cell cycle initiation; and, possibly, functions as a calcium channel. Rituximab binds to the antigen on the cell surface, activating complement-dependent cytotoxicity; and to human Fc receptors, mediating cell killing through an antibody-dependent cellular toxicity.

Pharmacodynamics/Kinetics

Duration: Detectable in serum 3-6 months after completion of treatment; B-cell recovery begins ~6 months following completion of treatment; median B-cell levels return to normal by 12 months following completion of treatment
Absorption: I.V.: Immediate and results in a rapid and sustained depletion of circulating and tissue-based B cells
Half-life elimination:
>100 mg/m^2: 4.4 days (range 1.6-10.5 days)

(Continued)

Rituximab *(Continued)*

375 mg/m^2: 50 hours (following first dose) to 174 hours (following fourth dose)

Excretion: Uncertain; may undergo phagocytosis and catabolism in the reticuloendothelial system (RES)

Pregnancy Risk Factor C

Rivastigmine (ri va STIG meen)

U.S. Brand Names Exelon®

Canadian Brand Names Exelon®

Mexican Brand Names Exelon®

Generic Available No

Synonyms ENA 713; SDZ ENA 713

Pharmacologic Category Acetylcholinesterase Inhibitor (Central)

Use Mild to moderate dementia from Alzheimer's disease

Local Anesthetic/Vasoconstrictor Precautions No information available to require special precautions

Effects on Dental Treatment No significant effects or complications reported

Common Adverse Effects

>10%:

Central nervous system: Dizziness (21%), headache (17%)

Gastrointestinal: Nausea (47%), vomiting (31%), diarrhea (19%), anorexia (17%), abdominal pain (13%)

2% to 10%:

Cardiovascular: Syncope (3%), hypertension (3%)

Central nervous system: Fatigue (9%), insomnia (9%), confusion (8%), depression (6%), anxiety (5%), malaise (5%), somnolence (5%), hallucinations (4%), aggressiveness (3%)

Gastrointestinal: Dyspepsia (9%), constipation (5%), flatulence (4%), weight loss (3%), eructation (2%)

Genitourinary: Urinary tract infection (7%)

Neuromuscular & skeletal: Weakness (6%), tremor (4%)

Respiratory: Rhinitis (4%)

Miscellaneous: Increased diaphoresis (4%), flu-like syndrome (3%)

>2% (but frequency equal to placebo): Chest pain, peripheral edema, vertigo, back pain, arthralgia, pain, bone fracture, agitation, nervousness, delusion, paranoid reaction, upper respiratory tract infections, infection, coughing, pharyngitis, bronchitis, rash, urinary incontinence.

<2% (Limited to important or life-threatening symptoms; reactions may be at a similar frequency to placebo): Fever, edema, allergy, periorbital or facial edema, hypothermia, hypotension, postural hypotension, cardiac failure, ataxia, convulsions, apraxia, aphasia, dysphonia, hyperkinesia, hypertonia, hypokinesia, migraine, neuralgia, peripheral neuropathy, hypothyroidism, peptic ulcer, gastroesophageal reflux, GI hemorrhage, intestinal obstruction, pancreatitis, colitis, atrial fibrillation, bradycardia, AV block, bundle branch block, sick sinus syndrome, cardiac arrest, supraventricular tachycardia, tachycardia, abnormal hepatic function, cholecystitis, dehydration, arthritis, angina pectoris, myocardial infarction, epistaxis, hematoma, thrombocytopenia, purpura, delirium, emotional lability, psychosis, anemia, bronchospasm, apnea, rashes (maculopapular, eczema, bullous, exfoliative, psoriaform, erythematous), urticaria, acute renal failure, peripheral ischemia, pulmonary embolism, thrombosis, thrombophlebitis, intracranial hemorrhage, conjunctival hemorrhage, diplopia, glaucoma, lymphadenopathy, leukocytosis.

Mechanism of Action A deficiency of cortical acetylcholine is thought to account for some of the symptoms of Alzheimer's disease; rivastigmine increases acetylcholine in the central nervous system through reversible inhibition of its hydrolysis by cholinesterase

Drug Interactions

Increased Effect/Toxicity:

Beta-blockers without ISA activity may increase risk of bradycardia.

Calcium channel blockers (diltiazem or verapamil) may increase risk of bradycardia.

Cholinergic agonists effects may be increased with rivastigmine.

Cigarette use increases the clearance of rivastigmine by 23%.

Depolarizing neuromuscular blocking agents effects may be increased with rivastigmine.

Digoxin may increase risk of bradycardia.

Decreased Effect: Anticholinergic agents effects may be reduced with rivastigmine.

Pharmacodynamics/Kinetics

Absorption: Fasting: Rapid and complete within 1 hour

Distribution: V_d: 1.8-2.7 L/kg

Protein binding: 40%

Metabolism: Extensively via cholinesterase-mediated hydrolysis in the brain; metabolite undergoes N-demethylation and/or sulfate conjugation hepatically; CYP minimally involved; linear kinetics at 3 mg twice daily, but nonlinear at higher doses

Bioavailability: 40%

Half-life elimination: 1.5 hours

Time to peak: 1 hour

Excretion: Urine (97% as metabolites); feces (0.4%)

Pregnancy Risk Factor B

Rizatriptan (rye za TRIP tan)

U.S. Brand Names Maxalt®; Maxalt-MLT®

Canadian Brand Names Maxalt™; Maxalt RPD™

Mexican Brand Names Maxalt®

Generic Available No

Synonyms MK462

Pharmacologic Category Serotonin 5-HT_{1D} Receptor Agonist

Use Acute treatment of migraine with or without aura

Local Anesthetic/Vasoconstrictor Precautions No information available to require special precautions

Effects on Dental Treatment Key adverse event(s) related to dental treatment: Xerostomia (normal salivary flow resumes upon discontinuation).

Common Adverse Effects 1% to 10%:

Cardiovascular: Systolic/diastolic blood pressure increases (5-10 mm Hg), chest pain (5%), palpitation

Central nervous system: Dizziness, drowsiness, fatigue (13% to 30%, dose related)

Dermatologic: Skin flushing

Endocrine & metabolic: Mild increase in growth hormone, hot flashes

Gastrointestinal: Nausea, abdominal pain, dry mouth (<5%)

Respiratory: Dyspnea

Mechanism of Action Selective agonist for serotonin (5-HT_{1D} receptor) in cranial arteries to cause vasoconstriction and reduce sterile inflammation associated with antidromic neuronal transmission correlating with relief of migraine

Drug Interactions

Increased Effect/Toxicity: Use within 24 hours of another selective 5-HT_1 antagonist or ergot-containing drug should be avoided due to possible additive vasoconstriction. Use with propranolol increased plasma concentration of rizatriptan by 70%. Rarely, concurrent use with SSRIs results in weakness and incoordination; monitor closely. MAO inhibitors and nonselective MAO inhibitors increase concentration of rizatriptan.

Pharmacodynamics/Kinetics

Onset of action: ~30 minutes

Duration: 14-16 hours

Protein binding: 14%

Metabolism: Via monoamine oxidase-A; first-pass effect

Bioavailability: 40% to 50%

Half-life elimination: 2-3 hours

Time to peak: 1-1.5 hours

Excretion: Urine (82%, 8% to 16% as unchanged drug); feces (12%)

Pregnancy Risk Factor C

rLFN-α2 *see* Interferon Alfa-2b *on page 752*

RMS® *see* Morphine Sulfate *on page 947*

RO5-420 *see* Flunitrazepam *on page 600*

Ro 5488 *see* Tretinoin (Oral) *on page 1328*

Robafen® AC *see* Guaifenesin and Codeine *on page 673*

Robaxin® *see* Methocarbamol *on page 894*

Robinul® *see* Glycopyrrolate *on page 668*

Robinul® Forte *see* Glycopyrrolate *on page 668*

Robitussin® [OTC] *see* Guaifenesin *on page 672*

Robitussin® CF [OTC] *see* Guaifenesin, Pseudoephedrine, and Dextromethorphan *on page 676*

Robitussin® Cold and Congestion [OTC] *see* Guaifenesin, Pseudoephedrine, and Dextromethorphan *on page 676*

Robitussin® Cough and Cold Infant [OTC] *see* Guaifenesin, Pseudoephedrine, and Dextromethorphan *on page 676*
Robitussin® CoughGels™[OTC] *see* Dextromethorphan *on page 421*
Robitussin®-DAC [DSC] *see* Guaifenesin, Pseudoephedrine, and Codeine *on page 676*
Robitussin® DM [OTC] *see* Guaifenesin and Dextromethorphan *on page 673*
Robitussin® Honey Cough [OTC] *see* Dextromethorphan *on page 421*
Robitussin® Maximum Strength Cough [OTC] *see* Dextromethorphan *on page 421*
Robitussin® Maximum Strength Cough & Cold [OTC] *see* Pseudoephedrine and Dextromethorphan *on page 1148*
Robitussin-PE® [OTC] *see* Guaifenesin and Pseudoephedrine *on page 675*
Robitussin® Pediatric Cough [OTC] *see* Dextromethorphan *on page 421*
Robitussin® Pediatric Cough & Cold [OTC] *see* Pseudoephedrine and Dextromethorphan *on page 1148*
Robitussin® Severe Congestion [OTC] *see* Guaifenesin and Pseudoephedrine *on page 675*
Robitussin® Sugar Free Cough [OTC] *see* Guaifenesin and Dextromethorphan *on page 673*
Rocaltrol® *see* Calcitriol *on page 244*
Rocephin® *see* Ceftriaxone *on page 288*

Rofecoxib (roe fe COX ib)

Related Information

Oral Pain *on page 1526*
Rheumatoid Arthritis, Osteoarthritis, and Osteoporosis *on page 1490*

U.S. Brand Names Vioxx®

Canadian Brand Names Vioxx®

Generic Available No

Pharmacologic Category Nonsteroidal Anti-inflammatory Drug (NSAID), COX-2 Selective

Dental Use Management of acute pain in adults

Use Relief of the signs and symptoms of osteoarthritis and rheumatoid arthritis; management of acute pain; treatment of primary dysmenorrhea; treatment of migraine attacks

Local Anesthetic/Vasoconstrictor Precautions No information available to require special precautions

Effects on Dental Treatment In models of postoperative dental pain, rofecoxib was effective against dental pain rated as moderate to severe. The analgesic efficacy of a single 50 mg dose of rofecoxib was apparently similar to 40 mg of ibuprofen or 550 mg of naproxen sodium. The onset of analgesia for postoperative dental pain with a single 50 mg dose of rofecoxib was 45 minutes.

Platelets: Bleeding time was not altered after a single dose of 500 mg or 1000 mg of rofecoxib. In addition, according to the manufacturer, multiple doses of rofecoxib 12.5 mg, 25 mg, and up to 375 mg administered daily up to 12 days, had no effect on bleeding time relative to placebo. However, according to the manufacturer, rofecoxib may increase the INR in patients receiving warfarin (see Drug Interactions).

Significant Adverse Effects

2% to 10%:

- Cardiovascular: Peripheral edema (4%), hypertension (up to 10%)
- Central nervous system: Headache (5%), dizziness (3%), weakness (2%)
- Gastrointestinal: Diarrhea (7%), nausea (5%), heartburn (4%), epigastric discomfort (4%), dyspepsia (4%), abdominal pain (3%), dry socket (post-dental extraction alveolitis 2%)
- Genitourinary: Urinary tract infection (3%)
- Neuromuscular & skeletal: Back pain (3%)
- Respiratory: Upper respiratory infection (9%), bronchitis (2%), sinusitis (3%)
- Miscellaneous: Flu-like syndrome (3%)

<2% (Limited to important or life-threatening): Allergy, alopecia, angina, arrhythmia, asthma, atopic dermatitis, atrial fibrillation, blurred vision, decreased mental acuity, depression, dyspnea, esophageal reflux, esophagitis, fluid retention, gastritis, hematochezia, hematoma, hemorrhoids, muscle cramps, neuropathy, paresthesia, pruritus, rash, somnolence, syncope, tendonitis, tinnitus, transaminases increased (>3 times ULN), urinary retention, urticaria, venous insufficiency, vertigo

<0.1% (Limited to important or life-threatening): Breast cancer, cholecystitis, colitis, colonic neoplasm, CHF, deep vein thrombosis, duodenal ulcer, gastrointestinal bleeding, intestinal obstruction, lymphoma, myocardial

infarction, pancreatitis, prostatic cancer, stroke, transient ischemic attack, unstable angina, urolithiasis

Dosage Adults: Oral:

Osteoarthritis: 12.5 mg once daily; may be increased to a maximum of 25 mg once daily

Acute pain and management of dysmenorrhea: 50 mg once daily as needed (use for longer than 5 days has not been studied)

Migraine attack: 25 mg once daily, as needed; may be increased to a maximum of 50 mg once daily

Rheumatoid arthritis: 25 mg once daily

Elderly: No specific adjustment is recommended. However, the AUC in elderly patients may be increased by 34% as compared to younger subjects. Use the lowest recommended dose.

Dosing comment in renal impairment: Use in advanced renal disease is not recommended

Dosing adjustment in hepatic impairment: Moderate hepatic dysfunction (Child-Pugh score 7-9): Maximum dose: 12.5 mg/day

Mechanism of Action Inhibits prostaglandin synthesis by decreasing the activity of the enzyme, cyclooxygenase-2 (COX-2), which results in decreased formation of prostaglandin precursors. Rofecoxib does not inhibit cyclooxygenase-1 (COX-1) at therapeutic concentrations.

Contraindications Hypersensitivity to rofecoxib or any component of the formulation, aspirin, or other NSAIDs; patients with "aspirin triad" (bronchial asthma, aspirin intolerance, rhinitis); pregnancy (3rd trimester)

Warnings/Precautions Gastrointestinal irritation, ulceration, bleeding, and perforation may occur with NSAIDs (rofecoxib has been associated with rates of these events which are lower than naproxen, a nonselective NSAID); use the lowest effective dose for the shortest duration possible to decrease risk. Use with caution in patients with a history of GI disease (bleeding or ulcers), decreased renal function, hepatic disease, CHF, hypertension, or asthma. Edema, GI irritation, and/or hypertension occur at an increased frequency with chronic use of 50 mg/day. Use with caution in patients with ischemic heart disease; antiplatelet therapies should be considered (rofecoxib is not a substitute for antiplatelet agents). Anaphylactoid reactions may occur, even with no prior exposure to rofecoxib. Safety and efficacy in pediatric patients and use in cluster headaches have not been established.

Drug Interactions **Substrate** of CYP2C8/9 (minor); **Inhibits** CYP1A2 (weak); **Induces** CYP3A4 (weak)

ACE inhibitors: Antihypertensive effects may be reduced by rofecoxib.

Aspirin: Rofecoxib may be used with low-dose aspirin, however, rates of gastrointestinal bleeding may be increased with coadministration.

Cimetidine increases AUC of rofecoxib by 23%.

Diuretics: Thiazide diuretics, loop diuretics: Effects may be diminished by rofecoxib.

Lithium: Serum concentrations/toxicity may be increased by rofecoxib; monitor.

Methotrexate: Severe bone marrow suppression, aplastic anemia, and GI toxicity have been reported with concomitant NSAID therapy. Selective COX-2 inhibitors appear to have a lower risk of this toxicity, however, caution is warranted.

Rifampin reduces the serum concentration of rofecoxib by ~50%; consider using initial dose of 25 mg/day for osteoarthritis.

Theophylline: Serum concentrations may be increased during therapy with rofecoxib; monitor.

Warfarin: Rofecoxib may increase the INR in patients receiving warfarin and may increase the risk of bleeding complications. However, rofecoxib does not appear to inhibit platelet aggregation.

Ethanol/Nutrition/Herb Interactions

Ethanol: Avoid ethanol (may increase gastric mucosal irritation)

Food: Time to peak concentrations are delayed when taken with a high-fat meal, however, peak concentration and AUC are unchanged.

Dietary Considerations May be taken without regard to meals.

Pharmacodynamics/Kinetics

Onset of action: 45 minutes

Duration: Up to >24 hours

Distribution: V_{dss} (apparent): 86-91 L

Protein binding: 87%

Metabolism: Hepatic (99%); minor metabolism via CYP2C8/9 isoenzyme; metabolites inactive

Bioavailability: 93%

Half-life elimination: 17 hours

Time to peak: 2-3 hours

(Continued)

Rofecoxib *(Continued)*

Excretion: Urine (72% as metabolites, <1% as unchanged drug); feces (14% as unchanged drug)

Pregnancy Risk Factor C/D (3rd trimester)

Lactation Excretion in breast milk unknown/not recommended

Breast-Feeding Considerations In animal studies, rofecoxib has been found to be excreted in milk. It is not known whether rofecoxib is excreted in human milk. Because many drugs are excreted in milk, and the potential for serious adverse reactions exists, a decision should be made whether to discontinue nursing or discontinue the drug, taking into account the importance of the drug to the mother.

Dosage Forms

Suspension, oral: 12.5 mg/5 mL (150 mL); 25 mg/5 mL (150 mL) [strawberry flavor]

Tablet: 12.5 mg, 25 mg, 50 mg

Comments Recent news reports have noted an association between selective COX-2 inhibitors and increased cardiovascular risk. This was prompted by the publication of a meta-analysis entitled, "Risk of Cardiovascular Events Associated With Selective COX-2 Inhibitors" in the August 22, 2001 edition of the *Journal of the American Medical Association* (JAMA), viewable at http://jama.ama-assn.org/issues/v286n8/rfull/jsc10193.html. The researchers reanalyzed four previously published trials, assessing cardiovascular events in patients receiving either celecoxib or rofecoxib. They found an association between the use of COX-2 inhibitors and cardiovascular events (including myocardial infarction and ischemic stroke). The annualized myocardial infarction rate was found to be significantly higher in patients receiving celecoxib or rofecoxib than in the control (placebo) group from a recent meta-analysis of primary prevention trials. Although cause and effect cannot be established (these trials were originally designed to assess GI effects, not cardiovascular effects), the authors believe the available data raise a cautionary flag concerning the risk of cardiovascular events with the use of COX-2 inhibitors. The manufacturers of these agents dispute the methods and validity of the study's conclusions.

New indications, warnings added to Vioxx® labeling - April, 2002: The FDA has approved new labeling which extends its approved indications to the symptomatic management of rheumatoid arthritis in adults and emphasized differences in the adverse event profile as compared to nonselective NSAIDs. A reduction in GI adverse events relative to a nonselective NSAID (naproxen) is noted. Precautions concerning the use in cardiovascular disease (including ischemic disease) have also been added. The potential development of edema and hypertension with rofecoxib, particularly at high dosages (50 mg/day), is emphasized. Prescribers are reminded that rofecoxib does not possess antiplatelet activity, which may influence risk of ischemic events (as compared to nonselective NSAIDs). Data concerning ischemic cardiovascular events, including myocardial infarction, are presented but it is noted that prospective studies to evaluate cardiovascular risk have not been conducted.

Selected Readings

Bombardier C, Laine L, Reicin A, et al, "Comparison of Upper Gastrointestinal Toxicity of Rofecoxib and Naproxen in Patients With Rheumatoid Arthritis. VIGOR Study Group," *N Engl J Med*, 2000, 343(21):1520-8.

Chang DJ, Desjardins PJ, Chen E, et al, "Comparison of the Analgesic Efficacy of Rofecoxib and Enteric-Coated Diclofenac Sodium in the Treatment of Postoperative Dental Pain: A Randomized, Placebo-Controlled Clinical Trial," *Clin Ther*, 2002, 24(4):490-503.

Chang DJ, Fricke JR, Bird SR, et al, "Rofecoxib Versus Codeine/Acetaminophen in Postoperative Dental Pain: A Double-Blind, Randomized, Placebo- and Active Comparator-Controlled Clinical Trial," *Clin Ther*, 2001, 23(9):1446-55.

Dionne R, "COX-2 Inhibitors: Better Than Ibuprofen for Dental Pain?" *Compend Contin Educ Dent*, 1999, 20(6):518-20, 522-4.

Ehrich EW, Dallob A, De Lepeleire I, et al, "Characterization of Rofecoxib as a Cyclo-oxygenase-2 Isoform Inhibitor and Demonstration of Analgesia in the Dental Pain Model," *Clin Pharmacol Ther*, 1999, 65(3):336-47.

Fricke J, Varkalis J, Zwillich S, et al, "Valdecoxib is More Efficacious Than Rofecoxib in Relieving Pain Associated With Oral Surgery," *Am J Ther*, 2002, 9(2):89-97.

Gopikrishna V and Parameswaran A, "Effectiveness of Prophylactic Use of Rofecoxib in Comparison With Ibuprofen on Postendodontic Pain," *J Endod*, 2003, 29(1):62-4.

Graham GG, Graham RI, and Day RO, "Comparative Analgesia, Cardiovascular and Renal Effects of Celecoxib, Rofecoxib and Acetaminophen (Paracetamol)," *Curr Pharm Des*, 2002, 8(12):1063-75.

Greenberg HE, Gottesdiener K, Huntington M, et al, "A New Cyclo-oxygenase-2 Inhibitor, Rofecoxib (Vioxx®), Did Not Alter the Antiplatelet Effects of Low-Dose Aspirin in Healthy Volunteers," *J Clin Pharmacol*, 2000, 40(12 Pt 2):1509-15.

Hawkey CJ, Jackson L, Harper SE, et al, "Review Article: The Gastrointestinal Safety Profile of Rofecoxib, a Highly Selective Inhibitor of Cyclo-oxygenase-2 in Humans," *Aliment Pharmacol Ther*, 2001, 15(1):1-9.

Jeske AH, "COX-2 Inhibitors and Dental Pain Control," *J Gt Houst Dent Soc*, 1999, 71(4):39-40.

Kellstein D, Ott D, Jayawardene S, et al, "Analgesic Efficacy of a Single Dose of Lumiracoxib Compared With Rofecoxib, Celecoxib and Placebo in the Treatment of Post-Operative Dental Pain," *Int J Clin Pract*, 2004, 58(3):244-50.

Malmstrom K, Daniels S, Kotey P, et al, "Comparison of Rofecoxib and Celecoxib, two Cyclooxygenase-2 Inhibitors, in Postoperative Dental Pain: A Randomized Placebo- and Active-Comparator-Controlled Clinical Trial," *Clin Ther*, 1999, 21(10):1653-63.

Malmstrom K, Fricke JR, Kotey P, et al, "A Comparison of Rofecoxib Versus Celecoxib in Treating Pain After Dental Surgery: A Single-Center, Randomized, Double-Blind, Placebo- and Active-Comparator-Controlled, Parallel-Group, Single-Dose Study Using the Dental Impaction Pain Model," *Clin Ther*, 2002, 24(10):1549-60.

Moore PA and Hersh EV, "Celecoxib and Rofecoxib. The Role of COX-2 Inhibitors in Dental Practice," *J Am Dent Assoc*, 2001, 132(4):451-6.

Morrison BW, Christensen S, Yuan W, et al, "Analgesic Efficacy of the Cyclo-oxygenase-2-Specific Inhibitor Rofecoxib in Postdental Surgery Pain: A Randomized, Controlled Trial," *Clin Ther*, 1999, 21(6):943-53.

Morrison BW, Fricke J, Brown J, et al, "The Optimal Analgesic Dose of Rofecoxib: Overview of Six Randomized Controlled Trials," *J Am Dent Assoc*, 2000, 131(12):1729-37.

"Rofecoxib Compared to Oxycodone/Acetaminophen for Postoperative Dental Pain," *Pain Med*, 2002, 3(2):185-186.

Wynn RL, "The New COX-2 Inhibitors: Rofecoxib (Vioxx®) and Celecoxib (Celebrex™)," *Gen Dent*, 2000, 48(1):16-20.

Roferon-A® *see* Interferon Alfa-2a *on page 751*

Rogaine® Extra Strength for Men [OTC] *see* Minoxidil *on page 934*

Rogaine® for Men [OTC] *see* Minoxidil *on page 934*

Rogaine® for Women [OTC] *see* Minoxidil *on page 934*

Rohypnol *see* Flunitrazepam *on page 600*

Rolaids® [OTC] *see* Calcium Carbonate and Magnesium Hydroxide *on page 245*

Rolaids® Extra Strength [OTC] *see* Calcium Carbonate and Magnesium Hydroxide *on page 245*

Romazicon® *see* Flumazenil *on page 599*

Romilar® AC *see* Guaifenesin and Codeine *on page 673*

Romycin® *see* Erythromycin *on page 508*

Rondec®-DM Drops *see* Carbinoxamine, Pseudoephedrine, and Dextromethorphan *on page 263*

Rondec® Drops *see* Carbinoxamine and Pseudoephedrine *on page 262*

Rondec® Syrup *see* Brompheniramine and Pseudoephedrine *on page 220*

Rondec® Tablets *see* Carbinoxamine and Pseudoephedrine *on page 262*

Rondec-TR® *see* Carbinoxamine and Pseudoephedrine *on page 262*

Ropinirole (roe PIN i role)

U.S. Brand Names Requip®

Canadian Brand Names ReQuip™

Generic Available No

Synonyms Ropinirole Hydrochloride

Pharmacologic Category Anti-Parkinson's Agent, Dopamine Agonist

Use Treatment of idiopathic Parkinson's disease; in patients with early Parkinson's disease who were not receiving concomitant levodopa therapy as well as in patients with advanced disease on concomitant levodopa

Local Anesthetic/Vasoconstrictor Precautions No information available to require special precautions

Effects on Dental Treatment Key adverse event(s) related to dental treatment: Xerostomia and increased salivation (normal salivary flow resumes upon discontinuation).

Common Adverse Effects

Early Parkinson's disease (without levodopa):

>10%:

- Cardiovascular: Syncope (12%)
- Central nervous system: Dizziness (40%), somnolence (40%), fatigue (11%)
- Gastrointestinal: Nausea (60%), vomiting (12%)
- Miscellaneous: Viral infection (11%)

1% to 10%:

- Cardiovascular: Dependent/leg edema (6% to 7%), orthostasis (6%), hypertension (5%), chest pain (4%), flushing (3%), palpitations (3%), peripheral ischemia (3%), hypotension (2%), tachycardia (2%)
- Central nervous system: Pain (8%), confusion (5%), hallucinations (5%, dose related), hypoesthesia (4%), amnesia (3%), malaise (3%), vertigo (2%), yawning (3%)
- Gastrointestinal: Constipation (>5%), dyspepsia (10%), abdominal pain (6%), xerostomia (5%), anorexia (4%), flatulence (3%)
- Genitourinary: Urinary tract infection (5%), impotence (3%)
- Hepatic: Elevated alkaline phosphatase (3%)
- Neuromuscular & skeletal: Weakness (6%)

(Continued)

Ropinirole *(Continued)*

Ocular: Abnormal vision (6%), xerophthalmia (2%)
Respiratory: Pharyngitis (6%), rhinitis (4%), sinusitis (4%), dyspnea (3%)
Miscellaneous: Diaphoresis (increased) (6%)

Advanced Parkinson's disease (with levodopa):

>10%:

Central nervous system: Dizziness (26%), somnolence (20%), headache (17%)
Gastrointestinal: Nausea (30%)
Neuromuscular & skeletal: Dyskinesias (34%)

1% to 10%:

Cardiovascular: Syncope (3%), hypotension (2%)
Central nervous system: Hallucinations (10%, dose related), aggravated parkinsonism, confusion (9%), pain (5%), paresis (3%), amnesia (5%), anxiety (6%), abnormal dreaming (3%), insomnia
Gastrointestinal: Abdominal pain (9%), vomiting (7%), constipation (6%), diarrhea (5%), dysphagia (2%), flatulence (2%), increased salivation (2%), xerostomia, weight loss (2%)
Genitourinary: Urinary tract infections
Hematologic: Anemia (2%)
Neuromuscular & skeletal: Falls (10%), arthralgia (7%), tremor (6%), hypokinesia (5%), paresthesia (5%), arthritis (3%)
Respiratory: Upper respiratory tract infection (9%), dyspnea (3%)
Miscellaneous: Injury, increased diaphoresis (7%), viral infection, increased drug level (7%)

Other adverse effects (all phase 2/3 trials):

1% to 10%:

Central nervous system: Neuralgia (>1%)
Renal: Elevated BUN (>1%)

Mechanism of Action Ropinirole has a high relative *in vitro* specificity and full intrinsic activity at the D_2 and D_3 dopamine receptor subtypes, binding with higher affinity to D_3 than to D_2 or D_4 receptor subtypes; relevance of D_3 receptor binding in Parkinson's disease is unknown. Ropinirole has moderate *in vitro* affinity for opioid receptors. Ropinirole and its metabolites have negligible *in vitro* affinity for dopamine D_1, 5-HT_1, 5-HT_2, benzodiazepine, GABA, muscarinic, alpha$_1$-, alpha$_2$-, and beta-adrenoreceptors. Although precise mechanism of action of ropinirole is unknown, it is believed to be due to stimulation of postsynaptic dopamine D_2-type receptors within the caudate-putamen in the brain. Ropinirole caused decreases in systolic and diastolic blood pressure at doses >0.25 mg. The mechanism of ropinirole-induced postural hypotension is believed to be due to D_2-mediated blunting of the noradrenergic response to standing and subsequent decrease in peripheral vascular resistance.

Drug Interactions

Cytochrome P450 Effect: Substrate of CYP1A2 (major), 3A4 (minor); **Inhibits** CYP1A2 (weak), 2D6 (strong)

Increased Effect/Toxicity: The levels/effects of ropinirole may be increased by amiodarone, ciprofloxacin, fluvoxamine, ketoconazole, lomefloxacin, ofloxacin, rofecoxib, and other CYP1A2 inhibitors. Estrogens may also reduce the metabolism of ropinirole; dosage adjustments may be needed. Ropinirole may increase the levels/effects of amphetamines, selected beta-blockers, dextromethorphan, fluoxetine, lidocaine, mirtazapine, nefazodone, paroxetine, risperidone, ritonavir, thioridazine, tricyclic antidepressants, venlafaxine, and other CYP2D6 substrates.

Decreased Effect: The levels/effects of ropinirole may be decreased by aminoglutethimide, carbamazepine, phenobarbital, rifampin, and other CYP1A2 inducers. Antipsychotics, cigarette smoking, and metoclopramide may reduce the effect or serum concentrations of ropinirole. Ropinirole may decrease the levels/effects of CYP2D6 prodrug substrates (eg, codeine, hydrocodone, oxycodone, tramadol).

Pharmacodynamics/Kinetics

Absorption: Not affected by food
Distribution: V_d: 525 L
Metabolism: Extensively hepatic via CYP1A2 to inactive metabolites; first-pass effect
Bioavailability: Absolute: 55%
Half-life elimination: ~6 hours
Time to peak: ~1-2 hours; T_{max} increased by 2.5 hours when drug taken with food
Excretion: Clearance: Reduced by 30% in patients >65 years of age

Pregnancy Risk Factor C

Ropinirole Hydrochloride *see* Ropinirole *on page 1197*

Ropivacaine (roe PIV a kane)

Related Information

Oral Pain *on page 1526*

U.S. Brand Names Naropin®

Canadian Brand Names Naropin®

Mexican Brand Names Naropin®

Generic Available No

Synonyms Ropivacaine Hydrochloride

Pharmacologic Category Local Anesthetic

Use Local anesthetic (injectable) for use in surgery, postoperative pain management, and obstetrical procedures when local or regional anesthesia is needed. It can be administered via local infiltration, epidural block and epidural infusion, or intermittent bolus.

Local Anesthetic/Vasoconstrictor Precautions No information available to require special precautions

Effects on Dental Treatment No significant effects or complications reported

Common Adverse Effects

>5% (dose and route related):

- Cardiovascular: Hypotension, bradycardia
- Central nervous system: Headache
- Dermatologic: Pruritus
- Gastrointestinal: Nausea, vomiting
- Neuromuscular & skeletal: Back pain, paresthesia
- Miscellaneous: Shivering

1% to 5% (dose related):

- Cardiovascular: Hypertension, tachycardia
- Central nervous system: Dizziness, anxiety, lightheadedness
- Endocrine & metabolic: Hypokalemia
- Neuromuscular & skeletal: Hypoesthesia, rigors, circumoral paresthesia
- Otic: Tinnitus
- Respiratory: Dyspnea

Mechanism of Action Blocks both the initiation and conduction of nerve impulses by decreasing the neuronal membrane's permeability to sodium ions, which results in inhibition of depolarization with resultant blockade of conduction

Drug Interactions

Cytochrome P450 Effect: Substrate (minor) of CYP1A2, 2B6, 2D6, 3A4

Increased Effect/Toxicity: Other local anesthetics or agents structurally related to the amide-type anesthetics. Increased toxicity possible (but not yet reported) with drugs that decrease cytochrome P450 1A enzyme function. SSRIs may increase ropivacaine levels.

Pharmacodynamics/Kinetics

Onset of action: Anesthesia (route dependent): 3-15 minutes

Duration (dose and route dependent): 3-15 hours

Metabolism: Hepatic

Half-life elimination: Epidural: 5-7 hours; I.V.: 2.4 hours

Excretion: Urine (86% as metabolites)

Pregnancy Risk Factor B

Comments Not available with vasoconstrictor (epinephrine) and not available in dental (1.8 mL) carpules

Ropivacaine Hydrochloride *see* Ropivacaine *on page 1199*

Rosiglitazone (roh si GLI ta zone)

Related Information

Rosiglitazone and Metformin *on page 1201*

U.S. Brand Names Avandia®

Canadian Brand Names Avandia®

Generic Available No

Pharmacologic Category Antidiabetic Agent, Thiazolidinedione

Use Type 2 diabetes mellitus (noninsulin dependent, NIDDM):

Monotherapy: Improve glycemic control as an adjunct to diet and exercise

Combination therapy: In combination with a sulfonylurea, metformin, or insulin when diet, exercise, and a single agent do not result in adequate glycemic control

Local Anesthetic/Vasoconstrictor Precautions No information available to require special precautions

(Continued)

Rosiglitazone *(Continued)*

Effects on Dental Treatment Rosiglitazone-dependent diabetics should be appointed for dental treatment in morning in order to minimize chance of stress-induced hypoglycemia.

Common Adverse Effects Rare cases of hepatocellular injury have been reported in men in their 60s within 2-3 weeks after initiation of rosiglitazone therapy. LFTs in these patients revealed severe hepatocellular injury which responded with rapid improvement of liver function and resolution of symptoms upon discontinuation of rosiglitazone. Patients were also receiving other potentially hepatotoxic medications (*Ann Intern Med*, 2000, 132:121-4; 132:164-6).

>10%: Endocrine & metabolic: Weight gain, increase in total cholesterol, increased LDL-cholesterol, increased HDL-cholesterol

1% to 10%:

- Cardiovascular: Edema (5%)
- Central nervous system: Headache (6%), fatigue (4%)
- Endocrine & metabolic: Hyperglycemia (4%), hypoglycemia (1% to 2%)
- Gastrointestinal: Diarrhea (2%)
- Hematologic: Anemia (2%)
- Neuromuscular & skeletal: Back pain (4%)
- Respiratory: Upper respiratory tract infection (10%), sinusitis (3%)
- Miscellaneous: Injury (8%)

Dosage Oral:

Adults:

Monotherapy: Initial: 4 mg daily as a single daily dose or in divided doses twice daily. If response is inadequate after 12 weeks of treatment, the dosage may be increased to 8 mg daily as a single daily dose or in divided doses twice daily. In clinical trials, the 4 mg twice-daily regimen resulted in the greatest reduction in fasting plasma glucose and Hb A_{1c}.

Combination therapy:

With sulfonylureas: Initial: 4 mg daily as a single daily dose or in divided doses twice daily; dose of sulfonylurea should be reduced if the patient reports hypoglycemia. Doses of rosiglitazone >4 mg/day are not indicated in combination with sulfonylureas.

With metformin: Initial: 4 mg daily as a single daily dose or in divided doses twice daily. If response is inadequate after 12 weeks of treatment, the dosage may be increased to 8 mg daily as a single daily dose or in divided doses twice daily. It is unlikely that the dose of metformin will need to be reduced due to hypoglycemia

With insulin: Initial: 4 mg daily as a single daily dose or in divided doses twice daily. Dose of insulin should be reduced by 10% to 25% if the patient reports hypoglycemia or if the plasma glucose falls to <100 mg/dL. Doses of rosiglitazone >4 mg/day are not indicated in combination with insulin.

Elderly: No dosage adjustment is recommended

Dosage adjustment in renal impairment: No dosage adjustment is required

Dosage comment in hepatic impairment: Clearance is significantly lower in hepatic impairment. Therapy should not be initiated if the patient exhibits active liver disease of increased transaminases (>2.5 times the upper limit of normal) at baseline.

Mechanism of Action Thiazolidinedione antidiabetic agent that lowers blood glucose by improving target cell response to insulin, without increasing pancreatic insulin secretion. It has a mechanism of action that is dependent on the presence of insulin for activity.

Contraindications Hypersensitivity to rosiglitazone or any component of the formulation; active liver disease (transaminases >2.5 times the upper limit of normal at baseline); contraindicated in patients who previously experienced jaundice during troglitazone therapy

Warnings/Precautions Should not be used in diabetic ketoacidosis. Mechanism requires the presence of insulin, therefore use in type 1 diabetes is not recommended. Use with caution in premenopausal, anovulatory women; may result in resumption of ovulation, increasing the risk of pregnancy. May result in hormonal imbalance; development of menstrual irregularities should prompt reconsideration of therapy. Use with caution in patients with anemia or depressed leukocyte counts (may reduce hemoglobin, hematocrit, and/or WBC). Use with caution in patients with edema; may increase in plasma volume and/or increase cardiac hypertrophy. Assess for fluid accumulation in patients with unusually rapid weight gain. Not recommended for use in patients with NYHA Class III or IV heart failure. Discontinue if heart failure develops. Use with caution in patients with elevated transaminases (AST or ALT). Idiosyncratic hepatotoxicity has been reported with another thiazolidinedione agent (troglitazone). Monitoring should include periodic determinations of liver function.

Drug Interactions

Cytochrome P450 Effect: Substrate of CYP2C8/9 (major); **Inhibits** CYP2C8/9 (moderate), 2C19 (weak), 2D6 (weak)

Increased Effect/Toxicity: The levels/effects of rosiglitazone may be increased by delavirdine, fluconazole, gemfibrozil, ketoconazole, nicardipine, NSAIDs, pioglitazone, sulfonamides, and other CYP2C8/9 inhibitors. Gemfibrozil may increase rosiglitazone levels; severe hypoglycemic episodes have been reported. Rosiglitazone may increase the levels/effects of amiodarone, fluoxetine, glimepiride, glipizide, nateglinide, phenytoin, pioglitazone, sertraline, warfarin, and other CYP2C8/9 substrates.

Decreased Effect: The levels/effects of rosiglitazone may be decreased by carbamazepine, phenobarbital, phenytoin, rifampin, rifapentine, and secobarbital, and other CYP2C8/9 inducers. Bile acid sequestrants may decrease rosiglitazone levels.

Ethanol/Nutrition/Herb Interactions

Ethanol: Avoid ethanol (may cause hypoglycemia).

Food: Peak concentrations are lower by 28% and delayed when administered with food, but these effects are not believed to be clinically significant.

Herb/Nutraceutical: Avoid garlic, gymnema (may cause hypoglycemia).

Dietary Considerations Management of type 2 diabetes mellitus (noninsulin dependent, NIDDM) should include diet control. May be taken without regard to meals.

Pharmacodynamics/Kinetics

Onset of action: Delayed; Maximum effect: Up to 12 weeks

Distribution: V_{dss} (apparent): 17.6 L

Protein binding: 99.8%

Metabolism: Hepatic (99%) via CYP2C8; minor metabolism via CYP2C9

Bioavailability: 99%

Half-life elimination: 3.15-3.59 hours

Time to peak: 1 hour

Excretion: Urine (64%) and feces (23%) as metabolites

Pregnancy Risk Factor C

Dosage Forms TAB: 2 mg, 4 mg, 8 mg

Rosiglitazone and Metformin (roh si GLI ta zone & met FOR min)

Related Information

Metformin *on page 887*

Rosiglitazone *on page 1199*

U.S. Brand Names Avandamet™

Canadian Brand Names Avandamet™

Generic Available No

Synonyms Metformin and Rosiglitazone; Metformin Hydrochloride and Rosiglitazone Maleate; Rosiglitazone Maleate and Metformin Hydrochloride

Pharmacologic Category Antidiabetic Agent, Biguanide; Antidiabetic Agent, Thiazolidinedione

Use Management of type 2 diabetes mellitus (noninsulin dependent, NIDDM) in patients who are already treated with the combination of rosiglitazone and metformin, or who are not adequately controlled on metformin alone. Used as an adjunct to diet and exercise to lower the blood glucose when hyperglycemia cannot be controlled satisfactorily by diet and exercise alone

Local Anesthetic/Vasoconstrictor Precautions No information available to require special precautions

Effects on Dental Treatment Dependent diabetics (noninsulin dependent, type 2) should be appointed for dental treatment in the morning in order to minimize chance of stress-induced hypoglycemia.

Common Adverse Effects Also see individual agents. Percentages of adverse effects as reported with the combination product.

>10%:

- Gastrointestinal: Diarrhea (13%)
- Respiratory: Upper respiratory tract infection (16%)

1% to 10%:

- Cardiovascular: Edema (4%)
- Central nervous system: Headache (7%), fatigue (6%)
- Endocrine & metabolic: Hypoglycemia (3%), hyperglycemia (2%)
- Hematologic: Anemia (7%)
- Neuromuscular & skeletal: Arthralgia (5%), back pain (5%)
- Respiratory: Sinusitis (6%)
- Miscellaneous: Viral infection (5%)

(Continued)

Rosiglitazone and Metformin *(Continued)*

Mechanism of Action Rosiglitazone is a thiazolidinedione antidiabetic agent that lowers blood glucose by improving target cell response to insulin, without increasing pancreatic insulin secretion. It has a mechanism of action that is dependent on the presence of insulin for activity. Metformin decreases hepatic glucose production, decreasing intestinal absorption of glucose, and improves insulin sensitivity (increases peripheral glucose uptake and utilization).

Drug Interactions

Cytochrome P450 Effect: Rosiglitazone: **Substrate** of CYP2C8/9 (major); **Inhibits** CYP2C8/9 (moderate), 2C19 (weak), 2D6 (weak)

Increased Effect/Toxicity: See individual agents.

Decreased Effect: See individual agents.

Pharmacodynamics/Kinetics See individual agents.

Pregnancy Risk Factor C

Rosiglitazone Maleate and Metformin Hydrochloride *see* Rosiglitazone and Metformin *on page 1201*

Rosuvastatin (roe SOO va sta tin)

U.S. Brand Names Crestor®

Canadian Brand Names Crestor®

Generic Available No

Synonyms Rosuvastatin Calcium

Pharmacologic Category Antilipemic Agent, HMG-CoA Reductase Inhibitor

Use Used with dietary therapy for hyperlipidemias to reduce elevations in total cholesterol (TC), LDL-C, apolipoprotein B, and triglycerides (TG) in patients with primary hypercholesterolemia (elevations of 1 or more components are present in Fredrickson type IIa, IIb, and IV hyperlipidemias); treatment of homozygous familial hypercholesterolemia (FH)

Local Anesthetic/Vasoconstrictor Precautions No information available to require special precautions

Effects on Dental Treatment No significant effects or complications reported

Common Adverse Effects

2% to 10%:

Cardiovascular: Chest pain, hypertension, peripheral edema

Central nervous system: Headache (6%), depression, dizziness, insomnia, pain

Dermatologic: Rash

Gastrointestinal: Pharyngitis (9%), abdominal pain, constipation, gastroenteritis

Neuromuscular & skeletal: Myalgia (3%), arthritis, arthralgia, hypertonia, paresthesia

Respiratory: Bronchitis, cough

≥1% (Limited to important or life-threatening): Anemia, angina, anxiety, bruising, neuralgia, palpitation, pruritus, vertigo, vomiting

Mechanism of Action Inhibitor of 3-hydroxy-3-methylglutaryl coenzyme A (HMG-CoA) reductase, the rate-limiting enzyme in cholesterol synthesis (reduces the production of mevalonic acid from HMG-CoA); this then results in a compensatory increase in the expression of LDL receptors on hepatocyte membranes and a stimulation of LDL catabolism

Drug Interactions

Cytochrome P450 Effect: Substrate (minor) of CYP2C9, 3A4

Increased Effect/Toxicity: Cyclosporine may increase serum concentrations of rosuvastatin (up to 10-fold); limit dose to 5 mg/day. Serum concentrations of rosuvastatin may be increased (doubled) during concurrent administration of gemfibrozil; combination should be avoided; limit dose to 10 mg/day. Clofibrate, fenofibrate, or niacin may increase the risk of myopathy and rhabdomyolysis with HMG-CoA reductase inhibitors; the effects on lipids may be additive. The anticoagulant effects of warfarin may be increased by rosuvastatin (monitor). Rosuvastatin increases serum concentrations of hormonal contraceptives (ethinyl estradiol and norgestrel).

Decreased Effect: Plasma concentrations of rosuvastatin may be decreased when given with magnesium/aluminum hydroxide-containing antacids; antacids should be administered at least 2 hours after rosuvastatin. Cholestyramine and colestipol (bile acid sequestrants) may reduce absorption of several HMG-CoA reductase inhibitors; separate administration times by at least 4 hours; cholesterol-lowering effects are additive.

Pharmacodynamics/Kinetics

Onset: Within 1 week; maximal at 4 weeks

Distribution: V_d: 134 L

Protein binding: 90%

Metabolism: Hepatic (10%), via CYP2C9 (1 active metabolite identified)
Bioavailability: 20% (high first-pass extraction by liver)
Half-life elimination: 19 hours
Time to peak, plasma: 3-5 hours
Excretion: Feces (90%), primarily as unchanged drug

Pregnancy Risk Factor X

Rosuvastatin Calcium *see* Rosuvastatin *on page 1202*
Rowasa® *see* Mesalamine *on page 882*
Roxanol® *see* Morphine Sulfate *on page 947*
Roxanol 100® *see* Morphine Sulfate *on page 947*
Roxanol®-T *see* Morphine Sulfate *on page 947*
Roxicet™ *see* Oxycodone and Acetaminophen *on page 1029*
Roxicet™ 5/500 *see* Oxycodone and Acetaminophen *on page 1029*
Roxicodone™ *see* Oxycodone *on page 1027*
Roxicodone™ Intensol™ *see* Oxycodone *on page 1027*
Rozex™ *see* Metronidazole *on page 917*
RP-6976 *see* Docetaxel *on page 458*
RP-54274 *see* Riluzole *on page 1183*
RP-59500 *see* Quinupristin and Dalfopristin *on page 1163*
r-PA *see* Reteplase *on page 1175*
rPDGF-BB *see* Becaplermin *on page 184*
RS-25259 *see* Palonosetron *on page 1040*
RS-25259-197 *see* Palonosetron *on page 1040*
RTCA *see* Ribavirin *on page 1177*
RU-486 *see* Mifepristone *on page 928*
RU-23908 *see* Nilutamide *on page 986*
RU-38486 *see* Mifepristone *on page 928*
Rubella, Measles and Mumps Vaccines, Combined *see* Measles, Mumps, and Rubella Vaccines (Combined) *on page 858*

Rubella Virus Vaccine (Live) (rue BEL a VYE rus vak SEEN, live)

Related Information

Immunizations (Vaccines) *on page 1614*

U.S. Brand Names Meruvax® II

Generic Available No

Synonyms German Measles Vaccine

Pharmacologic Category Vaccine

Use Selective active immunization against rubella; vaccination is routinely recommended for persons from 12 months of age to puberty. All adults, both male and female, lacking documentation of live vaccine on or after first birthday, or laboratory evidence of immunity (particularly women of child-bearing age and young adults who work in or congregate in hospitals, colleges, and on military bases) should be vaccinated. Susceptible travelers should be vaccinated.

Note: Trivalent measles - mumps - rubella (MMR) vaccine is the preferred immunizing agent for most children and many adults.

Local Anesthetic/Vasoconstrictor Precautions No information available to require special precautions

Effects on Dental Treatment No significant effects or complications reported

Common Adverse Effects All serious adverse reactions must be reported to the U.S. Department of Health and Human Services (DHHS) Vaccine Adverse Event Reporting System (VAERS) 1-800-822-7967.

Frequency not defined.

Cardiovascular: Syncope, vasculitis

Central nervous system: Dizziness, encephalitis, fever, Guillain-Barré syndrome, headache, irritability, malaise, polyneuritis, polyneuropathy

Dermatologic: Angioneurotic edema, erythema multiforme, purpura, rash, Stevens-Johnson syndrome, urticaria

Gastrointestinal: Diarrhea, nausea, sore throat, vomiting

Hematologic: Leukocytosis, thrombocytopenia

Local: Injection site reactions which include burning, induration, pain, redness, stinging, wheal and flare

Neuromuscular & skeletal: Arthralgia/arthritis (variable; highest rates in women, 12% to 26% versus children, up to 3%), myalgia, paresthesia

Ocular: Conjunctivitis, optic neuritis, papillitis, retrobulbar neuritis

Otic: Nerve deafness, otitis media

Respiratory: Bronchial spasm, cough, rhinitis

(Continued)

Rubella Virus Vaccine (Live) *(Continued)*

Miscellaneous: Anaphylactoid reactions, anaphylaxis, regional lymphadenopathy

Mechanism of Action Rubella vaccine is a live attenuated vaccine that contains the Wistar Institute RA 27/3 strain, which is adapted to and propagated in human diploid cell culture. Promotes active immunity by inducing rubella hemagglutination-inhibiting antibodies.

Drug Interactions

Decreased Effect: The effect of the vaccine may be decreased in individuals who are receiving immunosuppressant drugs (including high-dose systemic corticosteroids). Effect of vaccine may be decreased in given with immune globulin, whole blood or plasma; do not administer with vaccine. Effectiveness may be decreased if given within 30 days of varicella vaccine (effectiveness not decreased when administered simultaneously).

Pharmacodynamics/Kinetics Onset of action: Antibodies to vaccine: 2-4 weeks

Pregnancy Risk Factor C

Rubeola Vaccine *see* Measles Virus Vaccine (Live) *on page 858*

Rubex® *see* DOXOrubicin *on page 469*

Rubidomycin Hydrochloride *see* DAUNOrubicin Hydrochloride *on page 401*

Rulox *see* Aluminum Hydroxide and Magnesium Hydroxide *on page 91*

Rulox No. 1 *see* Aluminum Hydroxide and Magnesium Hydroxide *on page 91*

Rum-K® *see* Potassium Chloride *on page 1105*

Ryna® [OTC] [DSC] *see* Chlorpheniramine and Pseudoephedrine *on page 315*

Rynatan® *see* Chlorpheniramine and Phenylephrine *on page 314*

Rynatan® Pediatric Suspension *see* Chlorpheniramine and Phenylephrine *on page 314*

Rynatuss® *see* Chlorpheniramine, Ephedrine, Phenylephrine, and Carbetapentane *on page 316*

Rynatuss® Pediatric *see* Chlorpheniramine, Ephedrine, Phenylephrine, and Carbetapentane *on page 316*

Rythmol® *see* Propafenone *on page 1133*

Rythmol® SR *see* Propafenone *on page 1133*

S-2® *see* Epinephrine (Racemic) *on page 497*

Sacrosidase (sak ROE si dase)

U.S. Brand Names Sucraid®

Canadian Brand Names Sucraid®

Generic Available No

Pharmacologic Category Enzyme, Gastrointestinal

Use Orphan drug: Oral replacement therapy in sucrase deficiency, as seen in congenital sucrase-isomaltase deficiency (CSID)

Local Anesthetic/Vasoconstrictor Precautions No information available to require special precautions

Effects on Dental Treatment No significant effects or complications reported

Common Adverse Effects 1% to 10%: Gastrointestinal: Abdominal pain, vomiting, nausea, diarrhea, constipation

Mechanism of Action Sacrosidase is a naturally-occurring gastrointestinal enzyme which breaks down the disaccharide sucrose to its monosaccharide components. Hydrolysis is necessary to allow absorption of these nutrients.

Drug Interactions

Increased Effect/Toxicity: Drug-drug interactions have not been evaluated.

Pharmacodynamics/Kinetics

Absorption: Amino acids

Metabolism: GI tract to individual amino acids

Pregnancy Risk Factor C

Safe Tussin® 30 [OTC] *see* Guaifenesin and Dextromethorphan *on page 673*

Saizen® *see* Human Growth Hormone *on page 694*

SalAc® [OTC] *see* Salicylic Acid *on page 1205*

Sal-Acid® [OTC] *see* Salicylic Acid *on page 1205*

Salactic® [OTC] *see* Salicylic Acid *on page 1205*

Salagen® *see* Pilocarpine (Dental) *on page 1086*

Salbutamol *see* Albuterol *on page 71*

Salflex® *see* Salsalate *on page 1207*

Salicylazosulfapyridine *see* Sulfasalazine *on page 1249*

Salicylic Acid (sal i SIL ik AS id)

U.S. Brand Names Compound W® [OTC]; Compound W® One Step Wart Remover [OTC]; DHS™ Sal [OTC]; Dr. Scholl's® Callus Remover [OTC]; Dr. Scholl's® Clear Away [OTC]; DuoFilm® [OTC]; DuoPlant® [DSC] [OTC]; Freezone® [OTC]; Fung-O® [OTC]; Gordofilm® [OTC]; Hydrisalic™ [OTC]; Ionil® [OTC]; Ionil® Plus [OTC]; Keralyt® [OTC]; LupiCare™ Dandruff [OTC]; LupiCare™ II Psoriasis [OTC]; LupiCare™ Psoriasis [OTC]; Mediplast® [OTC]; MG217 Sal-Acid® [OTC]; Mosco® Corn and Callus Remover [OTC]; NeoCeuticals™ Acne Spot Treatment [OTC]; Neutrogena® Acne Wash [OTC]; Neutrogena® Body Clear™ [OTC]; Neutrogena® Clear Pore [OTC]; Neutrogena® Clear Pore Shine Control [OTC]; Neutrogena® Healthy Scalp [OTC]; Neutrogena® Maximum Strength T/Sal® [OTC]; Neutrogena® On The Spot® Acne Patch [OTC]; Occlusal®-HP [OTC]; Oxy Balance® [OTC]; Oxy® Balance Deep Pore [OTC]; Palmer's Skin Success Acne Cleanser [OTC]; Pedisilk® [OTC]; Propa pH [OTC]; SalAc® [OTC]; Sal-Acid® [OTC]; Salactic® [OTC]; Sal-Plant® [OTC]; Stri-dex® [OTC]; Stri-dex® Body Focus [OTC]; Stri-dex® Facewipes To Go™ [OTC]; Stri-dex® Maximum Strength [OTC]; Tinamed® [OTC]; Tiseb® [OTC]; Trans-Ver-Sal® [OTC]; Wart-Off® Maximum Strength [OTC]; Zapzyt® Acne Wash [OTC]; Zapzyt® Pore Treatment [OTC]

Canadian Brand Names Duofilm®; Duoforte® 27; Occlusal™; Occlusal™-HP; Sebcur®; Soluver®; Soluver® Plus; Trans-Plantar®; Trans-Ver-Sal®

Mexican Brand Names DuoPlant®; Ionil®; Ionil Plus®; Trans-Ver-Sal®

Generic Available Yes: Gel, soap

Pharmacologic Category Keratolytic Agent

Use Topically for its keratolytic effect in controlling seborrheic dermatitis or psoriasis of body and scalp, dandruff, and other scaling dermatoses; also used to remove warts, corns, and calluses; acne

Local Anesthetic/Vasoconstrictor Precautions No information available to require special precautions

Effects on Dental Treatment No significant effects or complications reported

Mechanism of Action Produces desquamation of hyperkeratotic epithelium via dissolution of the intercellular cement which causes the cornified tissue to swell, soften, macerate, and desquamate. Salicylic acid is keratolytic at concentrations of 3% to 6%; it becomes destructive to tissue at concentrations >6%. Concentrations of 6% to 60% are used to remove corns and warts and in the treatment of psoriasis and other hyperkeratotic disorders.

Pregnancy Risk Factor C

Salicylic Acid and Coal Tar *see* Coal Tar and Salicylic Acid *on page 367*

Salicylsalicylic Acid *see* Salsalate *on page 1207*

SalineX® [OTC] *see* Sodium Chloride *on page 1227*

Salivart® [OTC] *see* Saliva Substitute *on page 1205*

Saliva Substitute (sa LYE vu SUB sti toot)

Related Information

Management of Patients Undergoing Cancer Therapy *on page 1569*

U.S. Brand Names Entertainer's Secret® [OTC]; Moi-Stir® [OTC]; Mouthkote® [OTC]; Salivart® [OTC]; Saliva Substitute™ [OTC]; Salix® [OTC]

Generic Available No

Pharmacologic Category Gastrointestinal Agent, Miscellaneous

Dental Use Relief of dry mouth and throat in xerostomia

Use Relief of dry mouth and throat in xerostomia

Local Anesthetic/Vasoconstrictor Precautions No information available to require special precautions

Effects on Dental Treatment No significant effects or complications reported

Dosage Use as needed

Dosage Forms

Lozenge:

Salix®: Sorbitol, malic acid, sodium citrate, citric acid, dibasic calcium phosphate, sodium carboxymethylcellulose, propylene glycol, hydrogenated cottonseed oil, silicon dioxide, magnesium stearate [fruit flavor]

Solution, oral:

Entertainer's Secret®: Sodium carboxymethylcellulose, aloe vera gel, glycerin (60 mL) [honey-apple flavor]

Saliva Substitute®: Sorbitol, sodium carboxymethylcellulose, methylparaben (5 mL, 120 mL)

Spray, oral:

Moi-Stir®: Water, sorbitol, sodium carboxymethylcellulose, methylparaben, propylparaben, potassium chloride, dibasic sodium phosphate, calcium chloride, magnesium chloride, sodium chloride (120 mL)

(Continued)

Saliva Substitute *(Continued)*

Mouthkote®: Water, xylitol, sorbitol, yerba santa, citric acid, ascorbic acid, sodium saccharin, sodium benzoate (60 mL, 240 mL) [lemon-lime flavor]
Salivart™: Water, sodium carboxymethylcellulose, sorbitol, sodium chloride, potassium chloride, calcium chloride, magnesium chloride, potassium phosphate (70 mL)
Swabsticks, oral:
Moi-Stir®: Water, sorbitol, sodium carboxymethylcellulose, methylparaben, propylparaben, potassium chloride, dibasic sodium phosphate, calcium chloride, magnesium chloride, sodium chloride (300s)

Salix® [OTC] *see* Saliva Substitute *on page 1205*

Salk Vaccine *see* Poliovirus Vaccine (Inactivated) *on page 1099*

Salmeterol (sal ME te role)

Related Information

Fluticasone and Salmeterol *on page 619*
Respiratory Diseases *on page 1478*

U.S. Brand Names Serevent® [DSC]; Serevent® Diskus®

Canadian Brand Names Serevent®

Mexican Brand Names Serevent®

Generic Available No

Synonyms Salmeterol Xinafoate

Pharmacologic Category Beta$_2$-Adrenergic Agonist

Use Maintenance treatment of asthma and in prevention of bronchospasm (inhalation aerosol in patients >12 years of age; inhalation powder in patients ≥4 years of age) with reversible obstructive airway disease, including patients with symptoms of nocturnal asthma, who require regular treatment with inhaled, short-acting beta$_2$ agonists; prevention of exercise-induced bronchospasm; maintenance treatment of bronchospasm associated with COPD

Local Anesthetic/Vasoconstrictor Precautions No information available to require special precautions

Effects on Dental Treatment No significant effects or complications reported

Common Adverse Effects

>10%:
Central nervous system: Headache
Endocrine & metabolic: Serum glucose increased, serum potassium decreased
Respiratory: Pharyngitis

1% to 10%:
Cardiovascular: Tachycardia, palpitations, elevation or depression of blood pressure, cardiac arrhythmias
Central nervous system: Nervousness, CNS stimulation, hyperactivity, insomnia, malaise, dizziness
Gastrointestinal: GI upset, diarrhea, nausea
Neuromuscular & skeletal: Tremors (may be more common in the elderly), myalgias, back pain, arthralgia
Respiratory: Upper respiratory infection, cough, bronchitis

Mechanism of Action Relaxes bronchial smooth muscle by selective action on beta$_2$-receptors with little effect on heart rate; because salmeterol acts locally in the lung, therapeutic effect is not predicted by plasma levels

Drug Interactions

Increased Effect/Toxicity:
Increased toxicity (cardiovascular): MAO inhibitors, tricyclic antidepressants
Increased effect: Inhaled corticosteroids: The addition of salmeterol has been demonstrated to improve response to inhaled corticosteroids (as compared to increasing steroid dosage).

Decreased Effect: Beta-adrenergic blockers (eg, propranolol)

Pharmacodynamics/Kinetics

Onset of action: 5-20 minutes (average 10 minutes)
Peak effect: 2-4 hours
Duration: 12 hours
Protein binding: 94% to 98%
Metabolism: Hepatically hydroxylated
Half-life elimination: 3-4 hours

Pregnancy Risk Factor C

Salmeterol and Fluticasone *see* Fluticasone and Salmeterol *on page 619*

Salmeterol Xinafoate *see* Salmeterol *on page 1206*

Sal-Plant® [OTC] *see* Salicylic Acid *on page 1205*

Salsalate (SAL sa late)

Related Information

Rheumatoid Arthritis, Osteoarthritis, and Osteoporosis *on page 1490*

Temporomandibular Dysfunction (TMD) *on page 1564*

U.S. Brand Names Amigesic®; Disalcid® [DSC]; Mono-Gesic®; Salflex®

Canadian Brand Names Amigesic®; Salflex®

Generic Available Yes

Synonyms Disalicylic Acid; Salicylsalicylic Acid

Pharmacologic Category Salicylate

Use Treatment of minor pain or fever; arthritis

Local Anesthetic/Vasoconstrictor Precautions No information available to require special precautions

Effects on Dental Treatment NSAID formulations are known to reversibly decrease platelet aggregation via mechanisms different than observed with aspirin. The dentist should be aware of the potential of abnormal coagulation. Caution should also be exercised in the use of NSAIDs in patients already on anticoagulant therapy with drugs such as warfarin (Coumadin®).

Common Adverse Effects

>10%: Gastrointestinal: Nausea, heartburn, stomach pains, dyspepsia

1% to 10%:

Central nervous system: Fatigue
Dermatologic: Rash
Gastrointestinal: Gastrointestinal ulceration
Hematologic: Hemolytic anemia
Neuromuscular & skeletal: Weakness
Respiratory: Dyspnea
Miscellaneous: Anaphylactic shock

Mechanism of Action Inhibits prostaglandin synthesis, acts on the hypothalamus heat-regulating center to reduce fever, blocks prostaglandin synthetase action which prevents formation of the platelet-aggregating substance thromboxane A_2

Drug Interactions

Increased Effect/Toxicity: Increased effect/toxicity of oral anticoagulants, hypoglycemics, and methotrexate.

Decreased Effect: Decreased effect with urinary alkalinizers, antacids, and corticosteroids. Decreased effect of uricosurics and spironolactone.

Pharmacodynamics/Kinetics

Onset of action: Therapeutic: 3-4 days of continuous dosing
Absorption: Complete from small intestine
Metabolism: Hepatically hydrolyzed to two moles of salicylic acid (active)
Half-life elimination: 7-8 hours
Excretion: Primarily urine

Pregnancy Risk Factor C/D (3rd trimester)

Salt *see* Sodium Chloride *on page 1227*
Sal-Tropine™ *see* Atropine *on page 166*
Sal-Tropine™ *see* Atropine Sulfate (Dental Tablets) *on page 169*
Sandimmune® *see* CycloSPORINE *on page 386*
Sandostatin® *see* Octreotide *on page 1004*
Sandostatin LAR® *see* Octreotide *on page 1004*
Sani-Supp® [OTC] *see* Glycerin *on page 667*
Sansert® [DSC] *see* Methysergide *on page 913*
Santyl® *see* Collagenase *on page 375*

Saquinavir (sa KWIN a veer)

Related Information

HIV Infection and AIDS *on page 1484*

Tuberculosis *on page 1495*

U.S. Brand Names Fortovase®; Invirase®

Canadian Brand Names Fortovase®; Invirase®

Mexican Brand Names Invirase®

Generic Available No

Synonyms Saquinavir Mesylate

Pharmacologic Category Antiretroviral Agent, Protease Inhibitor

Use Treatment of HIV infection; used in combination with at least two other antiretroviral agents

Local Anesthetic/Vasoconstrictor Precautions No information available to require special precautions

Effects on Dental Treatment No significant effects or complications reported

(Continued)

Saquinavir *(Continued)*

Common Adverse Effects Protease inhibitors cause dyslipidemia which includes elevated cholesterol and triglycerides and a redistribution of body fat centrally to cause increased abdominal girth, buffalo hump, facial atrophy, and breast enlargement. These agents also cause hyperglycemia.

10%: Gastrointestinal: Diarrhea, nausea

1% to 10%:

Cardiovascular: Chest pain

Central nervous system: Anxiety, depression, fatigue, headache, insomnia, pain

Dermatologic: Rash, verruca

Endocrine & metabolic: Hyperglycemia, hypoglycemia, hyperkalemia, libido disorder, serum amylase increased

Gastrointestinal: Abdominal discomfort, abdominal pain, appetite decreased, buccal mucosa ulceration, constipation, dyspepsia, flatulence, taste alteration, vomiting

Hepatic: AST increased, ALT increased, bilirubin increased

Neuromuscular & skeletal: Paresthesia, weakness, CPK increased

Renal: Creatinine kinase increased

Mechanism of Action As an inhibitor of HIV protease, saquinavir prevents the cleavage of viral polyprotein precursors which are needed to generate functional proteins in and maturation of HIV-infected cells

Drug Interactions

Cytochrome P450 Effect: Substrate of CYP2D6 (minor), 3A4 (major); **Inhibits** CYP2C8/9 (weak), 2C19 (weak), 2D6 (weak), 3A4 (moderate)

Increased Effect/Toxicity: Concurrent use of amiodarone, bepridil, cisapride, flecainide, midazolam, pimozide, propafenone, quinidine, rifampin, triazolam, or ergot derivatives is contraindicated.

Saquinavir may increase the levels/effects of selected benzodiazepines, calcium channel blockers, cisapride, cyclosporine, ergot alkaloids, selected HMG-CoA reductase inhibitors, mirtazapine, nateglinide, nefazodone, pimozide, quinidine, sildenafil (and other PDE-5 inhibitors), tacrolimus, venlafaxine, and other CYP3A4 substrates. The effects of warfarin may also be increased.

Serum concentrations of saquinavir may be increased by azole antifungals (itraconazole, ketoconazole); dose adjustment was not needed at the study dose when used for a limited time (ketoconazole 400 mg once daily and Fortovase® 1200 mg 3 times/day). Saquinavir serum concentrations may be increased by delavirdine. Indinavir and ritonavir may increase serum levels of saquinavir. Serum levels of saquinavir and nelfinavir may be increased with concurrent use. Lopinavir/ritonavir (combination product) may increase serum levels of saquinavir.

Serum concentrations of saquinavir and clarithromycin may both be increased. Dose adjustment not was not needed at the study dose when used for 7 days (clarithromycin 500 mg twice daily and Fortovase® 1200 mg 3 times/day); dosage adjustment of clarithromycin is recommended in patients with renal impairment.

Serum concentrations of saquinavir are decreased and levels of rifabutin are increased when used together. Saquinavir should not be used as the sole protease inhibitor when given with rifabutin.

Decreased Effect: The levels/effects of saquinavir may be reduced by aminoglutethimide, carbamazepine, nafcillin, nevirapine, phenobarbital, phenytoin, rifamycins, and other CYP3A4 inducers. Loss of efficacy and potential resistance may occur. Concurrent use with rifampin is contraindicated.

Serum concentrations of methadone may be decreased; an increased dose may be needed when administered with saquinavir. Serum levels of the hormones in oral contraceptives may decrease significantly with administration of saquinavir. Patients should use alternative methods of contraceptives during saquinavir therapy.

Serum levels of saquinavir and efavirenz may be decreased with concurrent use; saquinavir should not be used as the sole protease inhibitor with efavirenz or nevirapine.

Dexamethasone may decrease serum concentrations of saquinavir; use with caution. Serum concentrations of saquinavir are decreased and levels of rifabutin are increased when used together. Saquinavir should not be used as the sole protease inhibitor when given with rifabutin.

Pharmacodynamics/Kinetics

Absorption: Poor; increased with high fat meal; Fortovase® has improved absorption over Invirase®

Distribution: V_d: 700 L; does not distribute into CSF

Protein binding, plasma: ~98%

Metabolism: Extensively hepatic via CYP3A4; extensive first-pass effect

Bioavailability: Invirase®: ~4%; Fortovase®: 12% to 15%

Excretion: Feces (81% to 88%), urine (1% to 3%) within 5 days

Pregnancy Risk Factor B

Saquinavir Mesylate *see* Saquinavir *on page 1207*

Sarafem™ *see* Fluoxetine *on page 606*

Sargramostim (sar GRAM oh stim)

U.S. Brand Names Leukine®

Canadian Brand Names Leukine™

Generic Available No

Synonyms GM-CSF; Granulocyte-Macrophage Colony Stimulating Factor; rGM-CSF

Pharmacologic Category Colony Stimulating Factor

Use

Myeloid reconstitution after autologous bone marrow transplantation: Non-Hodgkin's lymphoma (NHL), acute lymphoblastic leukemia (ALL), Hodgkin's lymphoma, metastatic breast cancer

Myeloid reconstitution after allogeneic bone marrow transplantation

Peripheral stem cell transplantation: Metastatic breast cancer, non-Hodgkin's lymphoma, Hodgkin's lymphoma, multiple myeloma

Orphan drug:

Acute myelogenous leukemia (AML) following induction chemotherapy in older adults to shorten time to neutrophil recovery and to reduce the incidence of severe and life-threatening infections and infections resulting in death

Bone marrow transplant (allogeneic or autologous) failure or engraftment delay

Safety and efficacy of GM-CSF given simultaneously with cytotoxic chemotherapy have not been established. Concurrent treatment may increase myelosuppression.

Local Anesthetic/Vasoconstrictor Precautions No information available to require special precautions

Effects on Dental Treatment No significant effects or complications reported

Common Adverse Effects

>10%:

Cardiovascular: Hypotension, tachycardia, flushing, and syncope may occur with the first dose of a cycle ("first-dose effect"); peripheral edema (11%)

Central nervous system: Headache (26%)

Dermatologic: Rash, alopecia

Endocrine & metabolic: Polydypsia

Gastrointestinal: Diarrhea (52% to 89%), stomatitis, mucositis

Local: Local reactions at the injection site (~50%)

Neuromuscular & skeletal: Myalgia (18%), arthralgia (21%), bone pain

Renal: Increased serum creatinine (14%)

Respiratory: Dyspnea (28%)

1% to 10%:

Cardiovascular: Transient supraventricular arrhythmias; chest pain; capillary leak syndrome; pericardial effusion (4%)

Central nervous system: Headache

Gastrointestinal: Nausea, vomiting

Hematologic: Leukocytosis, thrombocytopenia

Neuromuscular & skeletal: Weakness

Respiratory: Cough; pleural effusion (1%)

Comparative Effects — G-CSF vs GM-CSF

Proliferation/Differentiation	G-CSF (Filgrastim)	GM-CSF (Sargramostim)
Neutrophils	Yes	Yes
Eosinophils	No	Yes
Macrophages	No	Yes
Neutrophil migration	Enhanced	Inhibited

(Continued)

Sargramostim *(Continued)*

Mechanism of Action Stimulates proliferation, differentiation and functional activity of neutrophils, eosinophils, monocytes, and macrophages, as indicated: See table on previous page.

Drug Interactions

Increased Effect/Toxicity: Lithium, corticosteroids may potentiate myeloproliferative effects.

Pharmacodynamics/Kinetics

Onset of action: Increase in WBC: 7-14 days

Duration: WBCs return to baseline within 1 week of discontinuing drug

Half-life elimination: 2 hours

Time to peak, serum: SubQ: 1-2 hours

Pregnancy Risk Factor C

Sarnol®-HC [OTC] *see* Hydrocortisone *on page 714*

SB-265805 *see* Gemifloxacin *on page 653*

SC 33428 *see* Idarubicin *on page 732*

SCH 13521 *see* Flutamide *on page 615*

S-Citalopram *see* Escitalopram *on page 513*

Scleromate™ *see* Morrhuate Sodium *on page 948*

Scopace™ *see* Scopolamine *on page 1210*

Scopolamine (skoe POL a meen)

U.S. Brand Names Isopto® Hyoscine; Scopace™; Transderm Scōp®

Canadian Brand Names Buscopan®; Transderm-V®

Generic Available Yes

Synonyms Hyoscine; Scopolamine Hydrobromide

Pharmacologic Category Anticholinergic Agent

Use Preoperative medication to produce amnesia and decrease salivary and respiratory secretions; to produce cycloplegia and mydriasis; treatment of iridocyclitis; prevention of motion sickness; prevention of nausea/vomiting associated with anesthesia or opiate analgesia (patch); symptomatic treatment of postencephalitic parkinsonism and paralysis agitans (oral); inhibits excessive motility and hypertonus of the genitourinary or gastrointestinal tract in such conditions as the irritable colon syndrome, mild dysentery, diverticulitis, pylorospasm, and cardiospasm

Local Anesthetic/Vasoconstrictor Precautions No information available to require special precautions

Effects on Dental Treatment Key adverse event(s) related to dental treatment: Significant xerostomia (normal salivary flow resumes upon discontinuation) and dry throat (transdermal).

Common Adverse Effects Frequency not defined.

Ophthalmic: Note: Systemic adverse effects have been reported following ophthalmic administration.

Cardiovascular: Vascular congestion, edema

Central nervous system: Drowsiness

Dermatologic: Eczematoid dermatitis

Ocular: Blurred vision, photophobia, local irritation, increased intraocular pressure, follicular conjunctivitis, exudate

Respiratory: Congestion

Systemic:

Cardiovascular: Orthostatic hypotension, ventricular fibrillation, tachycardia, palpitations

Central nervous system: Confusion, drowsiness, headache, loss of memory, ataxia, fatigue

Dermatologic: Dry skin, increased sensitivity to light, rash

Endocrine & metabolic: Decreased flow of breast milk

Gastrointestinal: Constipation, xerostomia, dry throat, dysphagia, bloated feeling, nausea, vomiting

Genitourinary: Dysuria

Local: Irritation at injection site

Neuromuscular & skeletal: Weakness

Ocular: Increased intraocular pain, blurred vision

Respiratory: Dry nose, diaphoresis (decreased)

Mechanism of Action Blocks the action of acetylcholine at parasympathetic sites in smooth muscle, secretory glands and the CNS; increases cardiac output, dries secretions, antagonizes histamine and serotonin

Drug Interactions

Increased Effect/Toxicity: Additive adverse effects with other anticholinergic agents.

Decreased Effect: Decreased effect of acetaminophen, levodopa, ketoconazole, digoxin, riboflavin, and potassium chloride in wax matrix preparations.

Pharmacodynamics/Kinetics

Onset of action: Oral, I.M.: 0.5-1 hour; I.V.: 10 minutes

Peak effect: 20-60 minutes; may take 3-7 days for full recovery; transdermal: 24 hours

Duration: Oral, I.M.: 4-6 hours; I.V.: 2 hours

Absorption: Well absorbed from all routes

Protein binding, plasma: Reversible

Metabolism: Hepatic

Half-life elimination: 4.8 hours

Excretion: Urine (as metabolites)

Pregnancy Risk Factor C

Scopolamine and Phenylephrine *see* Phenylephrine and Scopolamine *on page 1079*

Scopolamine Hydrobromide *see* Scopolamine *on page 1210*

Scopolamine, Hyoscyamine, Atropine, and Phenobarbital *see* Hyoscyamine, Atropine, Scopolamine, and Phenobarbital *on page 725*

Scopolamine, Hyoscyamine, Atropine, Kaolin, and Pectin *see* Hyoscyamine, Atropine, Scopolamine, Kaolin, and Pectin *on page 726*

Scopolamine, Hyoscyamine, Atropine, Kaolin, Pectin, and Opium *see* Hyoscyamine, Atropine, Scopolamine, Kaolin, Pectin, and Opium *on page 726*

Scot-Tussin DM® Cough Chasers [OTC] *see* Dextromethorphan *on page 421*

Scot-Tussin® Expectorant [OTC] *see* Guaifenesin *on page 672*

SDZ ENA 713 *see* Rivastigmine *on page 1192*

SeaMist® [OTC] *see* Sodium Chloride *on page 1227*

Seasonale® *see* Ethinyl Estradiol and Levonorgestrel *on page 545*

Seba-Gel™ *see* Benzoyl Peroxide *on page 194*

Secobarbital (see koe BAR bi tal)

U.S. Brand Names Seconal®

Generic Available No

Synonyms Quinalbarbitone Sodium; Secobarbital Sodium

Pharmacologic Category Barbiturate

Use Preanesthetic agent; short-term treatment of insomnia

Local Anesthetic/Vasoconstrictor Precautions No information available to require special precautions

Effects on Dental Treatment No significant effects or complications reported

Mechanism of Action Depresses CNS activity by binding to barbiturate site at GABA-receptor complex enhancing GABA activity, depressing reticular activity system; higher doses may be gabamimetic

Pregnancy Risk Factor D

Secobarbital and Amobarbital *see* Amobarbital and Secobarbital *on page 112*

Secobarbital Sodium *see* Secobarbital *on page 1211*

Seconal® *see* Secobarbital *on page 1211*

SecreFlo™ *see* Secretin *on page 1211*

Secretin (SEE kre tin)

U.S. Brand Names SecreFlo™

Generic Available No

Pharmacologic Category Diagnostic Agent

Use Secretin-stimulation testing to aid in diagnosis of pancreatic exocrine dysfunction; diagnosis of gastrinoma (Zollinger-Ellison syndrome); facilitation of ERCP visualization

Unlabeled/Investigational Use Diagnosis of some hepatobiliary disease such as obstructive jaundice

Local Anesthetic/Vasoconstrictor Precautions No information available to require special precautions

Effects on Dental Treatment No significant effects or complications reported

Common Adverse Effects 1% to 10%: Gastrointestinal: Abdominal discomfort (1%), nausea (1%)

Mechanism of Action SecreFlo™ is a synthetic formulation of the porcine hormone secretin. This hormone is normally secreted by duodenal mucosa and upper jejunal mucosa which increases the volume and bicarbonate content of pancreatic juice; stimulates the flow of hepatic bile with a high bicarbonate concentration; stimulates gastrin release in patients with Zollinger-Ellison syndrome.

(Continued)

Secretin *(Continued)*

Drug Interactions

Decreased Effect: The response to secretin stimulation may be blunted by drugs with high anticholinergic activity such as tricyclic antidepressants, phenothiazines, and antihistamines as well as anticholinergic agents (ie, atropine, benztropine, biperiden).

Pharmacodynamics/Kinetics

Peak output of pancreatic secretions: ~30 minutes
Duration: At least 2 hours
Half-life elimination: 27 minutes

Pregnancy Risk Factor C

Sectral® *see* Acebutolol *on page 46*

Selegiline (se LE ji leen)

U.S. Brand Names Eldepryl®

Canadian Brand Names Apo-Selegiline®; Eldepryl®; Gen-Selegiline; Novo-Selegiline; Nu-Selegiline

Mexican Brand Names Niar®

Generic Available Yes

Synonyms Deprenyl; L-Deprenyl; Selegiline Hydrochloride

Pharmacologic Category Antidepressant, Monoamine Oxidase Inhibitor; Anti-Parkinson's Agent, MAO Type B Inhibitor

Use Adjunct in the management of parkinsonian patients in which levodopa/carbidopa therapy is deteriorating

Unlabeled/Investigational Use Early Parkinson's disease; attention-deficit/hyperactivity disorder (ADHD); negative symptoms of schizophrenia; extrapyramidal symptoms; depression; Alzheimer's disease (studies have shown some improvement in behavioral and cognitive performance)

Local Anesthetic/Vasoconstrictor Precautions Selegiline in doses of 10 mg a day or less does not inhibit type-A MAO. Therefore, there are no precautions with the use of vasoconstrictors.

Effects on Dental Treatment Key adverse event(s) related to dental treatment: Xerostomia and changes in salivation (normal salivary flow resumes upon discontinuation). Anticholinergic side effects can cause a reduction of saliva production or secretion, contributing to discomfort and dental disease (ie, caries, oral candidiasis, and periodontal disease).

Common Adverse Effects Frequency not defined.

Cardiovascular: Orthostatic hypotension, hypertension, arrhythmias, palpitations, angina, tachycardia, peripheral edema, bradycardia, syncope
Central nervous system: Hallucinations, dizziness, confusion, anxiety, depression, drowsiness, behavior/mood changes, dreams/nightmares, fatigue, delusions
Dermatologic: Rash, photosensitivity
Gastrointestinal: Xerostomia, nausea, vomiting, constipation, weight loss, anorexia, diarrhea, heartburn
Genitourinary: Nocturia, prostatic hyperplasia, urinary retention, sexual dysfunction
Neuromuscular & skeletal: Tremor, chorea, loss of balance, restlessness, bradykinesia
Ocular: Blepharospasm, blurred vision
Miscellaneous: Diaphoresis (increased)

Mechanism of Action Potent monoamine oxidase (MAO) type-B inhibitor; MAO type B plays a major role in the metabolism of dopamine; selegiline may also increase dopaminergic activity by interfering with dopamine reuptake at the synapse

Drug Interactions

Cytochrome P450 Effect: Substrate of CYP1A2 (minor), 2A6 (minor), 2B6 (major), 2C8/9 (major), 2D6 (minor), 3A4 (minor); **Inhibits** CYP1A2 (weak), 2A6 (weak), 2C8/9 (weak), 2C19 (weak), 2D6 (weak), 2E1 (weak), 3A4 (weak)

Increased Effect/Toxicity: CYP2B6 inhibitors may increase the levels/effects of selegiline; example inhibitors include desipramine, paroxetine, and sertraline. CYP2C8/9 inhibitors may increase the levels/effects of selegiline; example inhibitors include delavirdine, fluconazole, gemfibrozil, ketoconazole, nicardipine, NSAIDs, and sulfonamides. Concurrent use of selegiline (high dose) in combination with amphetamines, methylphenidate, dextromethorphan, fenfluramine, meperidine, nefazodone, sibutramine, tramadol, trazodone, tricyclic antidepressants, and venlafaxine may result in serotonin syndrome; these combinations are best avoided. Concurrent use of selegiline with an SSRI may result in mania or hypertension; it is generally best to avoid these combinations. Selegiline (>10 mg/day) in combination with tyramine (cheese, ethanol) may increase the pressor response; avoid high tyramine-containing foods in patients receiving >10 mg/day of selegiline. The toxicity of levodopa (hypertension), lithium (hyperpyrexia), and reserpine may be increased by MAO inhibitors.

Decreased Effect: CYP2B6 inducers may decrease the levels/effects of selegiline; example inducers include carbamazepine, nevirapine, phenobarbital, phenytoin, and rifampin. CYP2C8/9 inducers may decrease the levels/effects of selegiline; example inducers include carbamazepine, phenobarbital, phenytoin, rifampin, rifapentine, and secobarbital.

Pharmacodynamics/Kinetics

Onset of action: Therapeutic: Within 1 hour

Duration: 24-72 hours

Half-life elimination: Steady state: 10 hours

Metabolism: Hepatic to amphetamine and methamphetamine

Pregnancy Risk Factor C

Selegiline Hydrochloride *see* Selegiline *on page 1212*

Selenium (se LEE nee um)

Related Information

Trace Metals *on page 1319*

U.S. Brand Names Selepen®

Generic Available Yes

Pharmacologic Category Trace Element, Parenteral

Use Trace metal supplement

Local Anesthetic/Vasoconstrictor Precautions No information available to require special precautions

Effects on Dental Treatment No significant effects or complications reported

Common Adverse Effects Frequency not defined.

Central nervous system: Lethargy

Dermatologic: Alopecia or hair discoloration

Gastrointestinal: Vomiting following long-term use on damaged skin; abdominal pain, garlic breath

Local: Irritation

Neuromuscular & skeletal: Tremor

Miscellaneous: Diaphoresis

Mechanism of Action Part of glutathione peroxidase which protects cell components from oxidative damage due to peroxidases produced in cellular metabolism

Pharmacodynamics/Kinetics Excretion: Urine, feces, lungs, skin

Pregnancy Risk Factor C

Selenium *see* Trace Metals *on page 1319*

Selepen® *see* Selenium *on page 1213*

Selepen® *see* Trace Metals *on page 1319*

Semicid® [OTC] *see* Nonoxynol 9 *on page 995*

Semprex®-D *see* Acrivastine and Pseudoephedrine *on page 62*

Senexon® [OTC] *see* Senna *on page 1213*

Senna (SEN na)

U.S. Brand Names Agoral® Maximum Strength Laxative [OTC]; Evac-U-Gen [OTC]; ex-lax® [OTC]; ex-lax® Maximum Strength [OTC]; Fletcher's® Castoria® [OTC]; Senexon® [OTC]; Senna-Gen® [OTC]; Sennatural™ [OTC]; Senokot® [OTC]; Senokot® Children's [OTC]; SenokotXTRA® [OTC]; X-Prep® [OTC]

Generic Available Yes: Tablet

Pharmacologic Category Laxative, Stimulant

Use Short-term treatment of constipation; evacuate the colon for bowel or rectal examinations

Local Anesthetic/Vasoconstrictor Precautions No information available to require special precautions

Effects on Dental Treatment No significant effects or complications reported

Common Adverse Effects Frequency not defined: Gastrointestinal: Nausea, vomiting, diarrhea, abdominal cramps

Senna-Gen® [OTC] *see* Senna *on page 1213*

Sennatural™ [OTC] *see* Senna *on page 1213*

Senokot® [OTC] *see* Senna *on page 1213*

Senokot® Children's [OTC] *see* Senna *on page 1213*

SenokotXTRA® [OTC] *see* Senna *on page 1213*

Sensipar™ *see* Cinacalcet *on page 331*

Sensorcaine® *see* Bupivacaine *on page 225*
Sensorcaine®-MPF *see* Bupivacaine *on page 225*
Septocaine™ *see* Articaine Hydrochloride and Epinephrine (U.S.) *on page 145*
Septra® *see* Sulfamethoxazole and Trimethoprim *on page 1246*
Septra® DS *see* Sulfamethoxazole and Trimethoprim *on page 1246*
Ser-Ap-Es [DSC] *see* Hydralazine, Hydrochlorothiazide, and Reserpine *on page 698*
Serax® *see* Oxazepam *on page 1022*
Serentil® [DSC] *see* Mesoridazine *on page 883*
Serevent® [DSC] *see* Salmeterol *on page 1206*
Serevent® Diskus® *see* Salmeterol *on page 1206*

Sermorelin Acetate (ser moe REL in AS e tate)

U.S. Brand Names Geref® [DSC]; Geref® Diagnostic
Mexican Brand Names Geref®
Generic Available No
Pharmacologic Category Diagnostic Agent; Growth Hormone
Use

Geref® Diagnostic: For evaluation of the ability of the pituitary gland to secrete growth hormone (GH)

Geref® injection: Treatment of idiopathic growth hormone deficiency in children

Orphan drug: Sermorelin has been designated an orphan product for AIDS-associated catabolism or weight loss, and as an adjunct to gonadotropin on ovulation induction.

Local Anesthetic/Vasoconstrictor Precautions No information available to require special precautions

Effects on Dental Treatment No significant effects or complications reported

Common Adverse Effects Frequency not defined.

Cardiovascular: Tightness in the chest
Central nervous system: Headache, dizziness, hyperactivity, somnolence
Dermatologic: Transient flushing of the face, urticaria
Gastrointestinal: Dysphagia, nausea, vomiting
Local: Pain, redness, and/or swelling at the injection site

Drug Interactions

Decreased Effect: The test should not be conducted in the presence of drugs that directly affect the pituitary secretion of somatotropin. These include preparations that contain or release somatostatin, insulin, glucocorticoids, or cyclooxygenase inhibitors such as ASA or indomethacin. Somatotropin levels may be transiently elevated by clonidine, levodopa, and insulin-induced hypoglycemia. Response to sermorelin may be blunted in patients who are receiving muscarinic antagonists (atropine) or who are hypothyroid or being treated with antithyroid medications such as propylthiouracil. Obesity, hyperglycemia, and elevated plasma fatty acids generally are associated with subnormal GH responses to sermorelin. Exogenous growth hormone therapy should be discontinued at least 1 week before administering the test.

Pharmacodynamics/Kinetics Onset of action: Peak response: Diagnostic: Children 30 ± 27 minutes; Adults: 35 ± 29 minutes

Pregnancy Risk Factor C

Seromycin® *see* CycloSERINE *on page 385*
Serophene® *see* ClomiPHENE *on page 354*
Seroquel® *see* Quetiapine *on page 1156*
Serostim® *see* Human Growth Hormone *on page 694*

Sertaconazole (ser ta KOE na zole)

U.S. Brand Names Ertaczo™
Generic Available No
Synonyms Sertaconazole Nitrate
Pharmacologic Category Antifungal Agent, Topical
Use Topical treatment of tinea pedis (athlete's foot)

Local Anesthetic/Vasoconstrictor Precautions No information available to require special precautions

Effects on Dental Treatment No significant effects or complications reported

Common Adverse Effects 1% to 10%: Dermatologic: Burning, contact dermatitis, dry skin, tenderness

Mechanism of Action Alters fungal cell wall membrane permeability; inhibits the CYP450-dependent synthesis of ergosterol

Pharmacodynamics/Kinetics

Absorption: Topical: Minimal

Pregnancy Risk Factor C

Sertaconazole Nitrate *see* Sertaconazole *on page 1214*

Sertraline (SER tra leen)

U.S. Brand Names Zoloft®

Canadian Brand Names Apo-Sertraline®; Gen-Sertraline; Novo-Sertraline; Nu-Sertraline; PMS-Sertraline; ratio-Sertraline; Rhoxal-sertraline; Zoloft®

Mexican Brand Names Altruline®

Generic Available No

Synonyms Sertraline Hydrochloride

Pharmacologic Category Antidepressant, Selective Serotonin Reuptake Inhibitor

Use Treatment of major depression; obsessive-compulsive disorder (OCD); panic disorder; post-traumatic stress disorder (PTSD); premenstrual dysphoric disorder (PMDD); social anxiety disorder

Unlabeled/Investigational Use Eating disorders; generalized anxiety disorder (GAD); impulse control disorders

Local Anesthetic/Vasoconstrictor Precautions Although caution should be used in patients taking tricyclic antidepressants, no interactions have been reported with vasoconstrictor and sertraline, a nontricyclic antidepressant which acts to increase serotonin

Effects on Dental Treatment No significant effects or complications reported

Common Adverse Effects

>10%:

Central nervous system: Insomnia, somnolence, dizziness, headache, fatigue

Gastrointestinal: Xerostomia, diarrhea, nausea

Genitourinary: Ejaculatory disturbances

1% to 10%:

Cardiovascular: Palpitations

Central nervous system: Agitation, anxiety, nervousness

Dermatologic: Rash

Endocrine & metabolic: Decreased libido

Gastrointestinal: Constipation, anorexia, dyspepsia, flatulence, vomiting, weight gain

Genitourinary: Micturition disorders

Neuromuscular & skeletal: Tremors, paresthesia

Ocular: Visual difficulty, abnormal vision

Otic: Tinnitus

Miscellaneous: Diaphoresis (increased)

Additional adverse reactions reported in pediatric patients (frequency >2%): Aggressiveness, epistaxis, hyperkinesia, purpura, sinusitis, urinary incontinence

Dosage Oral:

Children and Adolescents: OCD:

6-12 years: Initial: 25 mg once daily

13-17 years: Initial: 50 mg once daily

Note: May increase daily dose, at intervals of not less than 1 week, to a maximum of 200 mg/day. If somnolence is noted, give at bedtime.

Adults:

Depression/OCD: Oral: Initial: 50 mg/day (see "Note" above)

Panic disorder, PTSD, social anxiety disorder: Initial: 25 mg once daily; increase to 50 mg once daily after 1 week (see "Note" above)

PMDD: 50 mg/day either daily throughout menstrual cycle **or** limited to the luteal phase of menstrual cycle, depending on physician assessment. Patients not responding to 50 mg/day may benefit from dose increases (50 mg increments per menstrual cycle) up to 150 mg/day when dosing throughout menstrual cycle **or** up to 100 mg day when dosing during luteal phase only. If a 100 mg/day dose has been established with luteal phase dosing, a 50 mg/day titration step for 3 days should be utilized at the beginning of each luteal phase dosing period.

Elderly: Depression/OCD: Start treatment with 25 mg/day in the morning and increase by 25 mg/day increments every 2-3 days if tolerated to 50-100 mg/day; additional increases may be necessary; maximum dose: 200 mg/day

Dosage adjustment/comment in renal impairment: Multiple-dose pharmacokinetics are unaffected by renal impairment.

Hemodialysis: Not removed by hemodialysis

Dosage adjustment/comment in hepatic impairment: Sertraline is extensively metabolized by the liver; caution should be used in patients with hepatic impairment; a lower dose or less frequent dosing should be used.

(Continued)

Sertraline *(Continued)*

Mechanism of Action Antidepressant with selective inhibitory effects on presynaptic serotonin (5-HT) reuptake and only very weak effects on norepinephrine and dopamine neuronal uptake. *In vitro* studies demonstrate no significant affinity for adrenergic, cholinergic, GABA, dopaminergic, histaminergic, serotonergic, or benzodiazepine receptors.

Contraindications Hypersensitivity to sertraline or any component of the formulation; use of MAO inhibitors within 14 days; concurrent use of pimozide; concurrent use of sertraline oral concentrate with disulfiram

Warnings/Precautions Do not use in combination with MAO inhibitor or within 14 days of discontinuing treatment or initiating treatment with a MAO inhibitor due to the risk of serotonin syndrome; use with caution in patients with pre-existing seizure disorders, patients in whom weight loss is undesirable, patients with recent myocardial infarction, unstable heart disease, hepatic or renal impairment, patients taking other psychotropic medications, agitated or hyperactive patients as drug may produce or activate mania or hypomania. Monotherapy in patients with bipolar disorder should be avoided. The possibility of a suicide attempt is inherent in major depression and may persist until remission occurs. Monitor for worsening of depression or suicidality, especially during initiation of therapy or with dose increases or decreases. Worsening depression and severe abrupt suicidality that are not part of the presenting symptoms may require discontinuation or modification of drug therapy. Use caution in high-risk patients during initiation of therapy. Prescriptions should be written for the smallest quantity consistent with good patient care. Use oral concentrate formulation with caution in patients with latex sensitivity; dropper dispenser contains dry natural rubber. Monitor growth in pediatric patients. Safety and efficacy in pediatric patients ≥6 years of age have been established only in the treatment of OCD.

Drug Interactions

Cytochrome P450 Effect: Substrate of CYP2B6 (minor), 2C8/9 (minor), 2C19 (major), 2D6 (major), 3A4 (minor); **Inhibits** CYP1A2 (weak), 2B6(moderate), 2C8/9 (weak), 2C19 (moderate), 2D6 (moderate), 3A4 (moderate)

Increased Effect/Toxicity: Sertraline should not be used with nonselective MAO inhibitors (phenelzine, isocarboxazid) or other drugs with MAO inhibition (linezolid); fatal reactions have been reported. Wait 5 weeks after stopping sertraline before starting a nonselective MAO inhibitor and 2 weeks after stopping an MAO inhibitor before starting sertraline. Concurrent selegiline has been associated with mania, hypertension, or serotonin syndrome (risk may be reduced relative to nonselective MAO inhibitors). Sertraline may increase serum concentrations of pimozide; concurrent use is contraindicated. Avoid use of oral concentrate with disulfiram.

Sertraline may inhibit the metabolism of thioridazine or mesoridazine, resulting in increased plasma levels and increasing the risk of QT_c interval prolongation. This may lead to serious ventricular arrhythmias, such as torsade de pointes-type arrhythmias and sudden death. Do not use together. Wait at least 5 weeks after discontinuing sertraline prior to starting thioridazine.

Sertraline may increase the levels/effects of levels/effects of amphetamines, selected beta-blockers, bupropion, selected benzodiazepines, calcium channel blockers, cisapride, cyclosporine, dextromethorphan, ergot alkaloids, fluoxetine, selected HMG-CoA reductase inhibitors, lidocaine, mesoridazine, mirtazapine, nateglinide, nefazodone, paroxetine,promethazine, propofol, risperidone, ritonavir, selegiline, sildenafil (and other PDE-5 inhibitors), tacrolimus, thioridazine, tricyclic antidepressants, venlafaxine, and other substrates of CYP2B6, 2D6 or 3A4. Sertraline may increase the hypoprothrombinemic response to warfarin.

The levels/effects of sertraline may be increased by chlorpromazine, delavirdine, fluconazole, fluoxetine, fluvoxamine, gemfibrozil, isoniazid, miconazole, omeprazole, paroxetine, pergolide, quinidine, quinine, ritonavir, ropinirole, ticlopidine, and other CYP2C19 or 2D6 inhibitors.

Combined use of SSRIs and amphetamines, buspirone, meperidine, nefazodone, serotonin agonists (such as sumatriptan), sibutramine, other SSRIs, sympathomimetics, ritonavir, tramadol, and venlafaxine may increase the risk of serotonin syndrome. Combined use of sumatriptan (and other serotonin agonists) may result in toxicity; weakness, hyper-reflexia, and incoordination have been observed with sumatriptan and SSRIs. In addition, concurrent use may theoretically increase the risk of serotonin syndrome; includes sumatriptan, naratriptan, rizatriptan, and zolmitriptan.

Concurrent lithium may increase risk of nephrotoxicity. Risk of hyponatremia may increase with concurrent use of loop diuretics (bumetanide, furosemide, torsemide). Concomitant use of sertraline and NSAIDs, aspirin, or other drugs affecting coagulation has been associated with an increased risk of bleeding; monitor.

Decreased Effect: The levels/effects of sertraline may be decreased by aminoglutethimide, carbamazepine, phenytoin, rifampin, and other CYP2C19 inducers. Sertraline may decrease the metabolism of tolbutamide; monitor for changes in glucose control. Sertraline may decrease the levels/effects of CYP2D6 prodrug substrates (eg, codeine, hydrocodone, oxycodone, tramadol).

Ethanol/Nutrition/Herb Interactions

Ethanol: Avoid ethanol (may increase CNS depression).

Food: Sertraline average peak serum levels may be increased if taken with food.

Herb/Nutraceutical: Avoid valerian, St John's wort, kava kava, gotu kola (may increase CNS depression).

Pharmacodynamics/Kinetics

Absorption: Slow

Protein binding: High

Metabolism: Hepatic; extensive first-pass metabolism

Bioavailability: 88%

Half-life elimination: Parent drug: 26 hours; Metabolite N-desmethylsertraline: 66 hours (range: 62-104 hours)

Time to peak, plasma: 4.5-8.4 hours

Excretion: Urine and feces

Pregnancy Risk Factor C

Dosage Forms Note: Available as sertraline hydrochloride; mg strength refers to sertraline. **SOLN, oral concentrate:** 20 mg/mL (60 mL). **TAB:** 25 mg, 50 mg, 100 mg

Comments Problems with SSRI-induced bruxism have been reported and may preclude their use; clinicians attempting to evaluate any patient with bruxism or involuntary muscle movement, who is simultaneously being treated with an SSRI drug, should be aware of the potential association.

Selected Readings

Gerber PE and Lynd LD, "Selective Serotonin Reuptake Inhibitor-Induced Movement Disorders," *Ann Pharmacother*, 1998, 32(6):692-8.

Sertraline Hydrochloride *see* Sertraline *on page 1215*

Serutan® [OTC] *see* Psyllium *on page 1151*

Serzone® [DSC] *see* Nefazodone *on page 970*

Sevelamer (se VEL a mer)

U.S. Brand Names Renagel®

Canadian Brand Names Renagel®

Generic Available No

Synonyms Sevelamer Hydrochloride

Pharmacologic Category Phosphate Binder

Use Reduction of serum phosphorous in patients with end-stage renal disease

Local Anesthetic/Vasoconstrictor Precautions No information available to require special precautions

Effects on Dental Treatment No significant effects or complications reported

Common Adverse Effects

>10%:

Cardiovascular: Hypotension (11%), thrombosis (10%)

Central nervous system: Headache (10%)

Endocrine & metabolic: Decreased absorption of vitamins D, E, K and folic acid

Gastrointestinal: Diarrhea (16%), dyspepsia (5% to 11%), vomiting (12%)

Neuromuscular & skeletal: Pain (13%)

Miscellaneous: Infection (15%)

1% to 10%:

Cardiovascular: Hypertension (9%)

Gastrointestinal: Nausea (7%), flatulence (4%), diarrhea (4%), constipation (2%)

Respiratory: Cough (4%)

Mechanism of Action Sevelamer (a polymeric compound) binds phosphate within the intestinal lumen, limiting absorption and decreasing serum phosphate concentrations without altering calcium, aluminum, or bicarbonate concentrations

(Continued)

Sevelamer *(Continued)*

Drug Interactions

Decreased Effect: Sevelamer may bind to some drugs in the gastrointestinal tract and decrease their absorption. When changes in absorption of oral medications may have significant clinical consequences (such as antiarrhythmic and antiseizure medications), these medications should be taken at least 1 hour before or 3 hours after a dose of sevelamer.

Pharmacodynamics/Kinetics

Absorption: None

Excretion: Feces

Pregnancy Risk Factor C

Sevelamer Hydrochloride *see* Sevelamer *on page 1217*

Sexually-Transmitted Diseases *see page 1504*

Shur-Seal® [OTC] *see* Nonoxynol 9 *on page 995*

Sibutramine (si BYOO tra meen)

U.S. Brand Names Meridia®

Canadian Brand Names Meridia®

Mexican Brand Names Raductil®; Reductil®

Generic Available No

Synonyms Sibutramine Hydrochloride Monohydrate

Pharmacologic Category Anorexiant

Use Management of obesity, including weight loss and maintenance of weight loss, and should be used in conjunction with a reduced calorie diet

Local Anesthetic/Vasoconstrictor Precautions No information available to require special precautions

Effects on Dental Treatment No significant effects or complications reported

Common Adverse Effects

>10%

Central nervous system: Headache, insomnia

Gastrointestinal: Anorexia, xerostomia, constipation

Respiratory: Rhinitis

1% to 10%

Cardiovascular: Tachycardia, vasodilation, hypertension, palpitations, chest pain, edema

Central nervous system: Migraine, dizziness, nervousness, anxiety, depression, somnolence, CNS stimulation, emotional liability

Dermatologic: Rash

Endocrine & metabolic: Dysmenorrhea

Gastrointestinal: Increased appetite, nausea, dyspepsia, gastritis, vomiting, taste perversion, abdominal pain

Neuromuscular & skeletal: Weakness, arthralgia, back pain

Respiratory: Pharyngitis, sinusitis, cough, laryngitis

Miscellaneous: Diaphoresis, flu-like syndrome, allergic reactions, thirst

Restrictions C-IV; recommended only for obese patients with a body mass index ≥30 kg/m^2 or ≥27 kg/m^2 in the presence of other risk factors such as hypertension, diabetes, and/or dyslipidemia

Mechanism of Action Sibutramine blocks the neuronal uptake of norepinephrine and, to a lesser extent, serotonin and dopamine

Drug Interactions

Cytochrome P450 Effect: Substrate of CYP3A4 (major)

Increased Effect/Toxicity: Serotonergic agents such as buspirone, selective serotonin reuptake inhibitors (eg, citalopram, fluoxetine, fluvoxamine, paroxetine, sertraline), sumatriptan (and similar serotonin agonists), dihydroergotamine, lithium, tryptophan, some opioid/analgesics (eg, meperidine, tramadol), and venlafaxine, when combined with sibutramine may result in serotonin syndrome. Dextromethorphan, MAO inhibitors and other drugs that can raise the blood pressure (eg decongestants, centrally-acting weight loss products, amphetamines, and amphetamine-like compounds) can increase the possibility of sibutramine-associated cardiovascular complications. Sibutramine may increase serum levels of tricyclic antidepressants. CYP3A4 inhibitors may increase the levels/effects of sibutramine; example inhibitors include azole antifungals, ciprofloxacin, clarithromycin, diclofenac, doxycycline, erythromycin, imatinib, isoniazid, nefazodone, nicardipine, propofol, protease inhibitors, quinidine, and verapamil.

Decreased Effect: Inducers of CYP3A4 (including phenytoin, phenobarbital, carbamazepine, and rifampin) theoretically may reduce sibutramine serum concentrations.

Pharmacodynamics/Kinetics
Absorption: Rapid
Protein binding, plasma: 94% to 97%
Metabolism: Hepatic; undergoes first-pass metabolism via CYP3A4
Time to peak: Within 3-4 hours
Excretion: Primarily urine (77%); feces

Pregnancy Risk Factor C

Comments The mechanism of action is thought to be different from the "fen" drugs. Sibutramine works to suppress the appetite by inhibiting the reuptake of norepinephrine and serotonin. Unlike dexfenfluramine and fenfluramine, it is not a serotonin releaser. Sibutramine is closer chemically to the widely used antidepressants such as fluoxetine (Prozac®). The FDA approved sibutramine over the objections of its own advisory panel, who called the drug too risky. FDA reported that the drug causes blood pressure to increase, generally by a small amount, though in some patients the increases were higher. It is now recommended that patients taking sibutramine have their blood pressure evaluated regularly.

Sibutramine Hydrochloride Monohydrate *see* Sibutramine *on page 1218*
Siladryl® Allergy [OTC] *see* DiphenhydrAMINE *on page 448*
Silafed® [OTC] *see* Triprolidine and Pseudoephedrine *on page 1345*
Silapap® Children's [OTC] *see* Acetaminophen *on page 47*
Silapap® Infants [OTC] *see* Acetaminophen *on page 47*
Sildec *see* Carbinoxamine and Pseudoephedrine *on page 262*
Sildec-DM *see* Carbinoxamine, Pseudoephedrine, and Dextromethorphan *on page 263*

Sildenafil (sil DEN a fil)

U.S. Brand Names Viagra®
Canadian Brand Names Viagra®
Mexican Brand Names Viagra®
Generic Available No
Synonyms UK92480
Pharmacologic Category Phosphodiesterase-5 Enzyme Inhibitor
Use Treatment of erectile dysfunction
Unlabeled/Investigational Use Psychotropic-induced sexual dysfunction; primary pulmonary hypertension
Local Anesthetic/Vasoconstrictor Precautions No information available to require special precautions
Effects on Dental Treatment No significant effects or complications reported

Common Adverse Effects
>10%: Central nervous system: Headache
Note: Dyspepsia and abnormal vision (color changes, blurred or increased sensitivity to light) occurred at an incidence of >10% with doses of 100 mg.
1% to 10%:
Cardiovascular: Flushing
Central nervous system: Dizziness
Dermatologic: Rash
Genitourinary: Urinary tract infection
Ophthalmic: Abnormal vision (color changes, blurred or increased sensitivity to light)
Respiratory: Nasal congestion
<2% (Limited to important of life-threatening): Allergic reaction, angina pectoris anorgasmia, asthma, AV block, cardiac arrest, cardiomyopathy, cataract, cerebral thrombosis, colitis, dyspnea, edema, exfoliative dermatitis, eye hemorrhage, gout, heart failure, hyperglycemia, hypotension, migraine, myocardial ischemia, neuralgia, photosensitivity, postural hypotension, priapism, rectal hemorrhage, seizures, shock, syncope, vertigo

Dosage Adults: Oral:
Erectile dysfunction: For most patients, the recommended dose is 50 mg taken as needed, approximately 1 hour before sexual activity. However, sildenafil may be taken anywhere from 30 minutes to 4 hours before sexual activity. Based on effectiveness and tolerance, the dose may be increased to a maximum recommended dose of 100 mg or decreased to 25 mg. The maximum recommended dosing frequency is once daily.
Primary pulmonary hypertension (unlabeled use): 25 mg twice daily, titrated based on response. Dosages up to 100 mg 5 times/day have been used (limited data).

Dosage adjustment for patients >65 years of age, hepatic impairment (cirrhosis), severe renal impairment (creatinine clearance <30 mL/minute), or concomitant use of potent cytochrome P450 3A4 inhibitors
(Continued)

Sildenafil *(Continued)*

(erythromycin, ketoconazole, itraconazole, ritonavir, amprenavir): Higher plasma levels have been associated which may result in increase in efficacy and adverse effects and a starting dose of 25 mg should be considered

Mechanism of Action Does not directly cause penile erections, but affects the response to sexual stimulation. The physiologic mechanism of erection of the penis involves release of nitric oxide (NO) in the corpus cavernosum during sexual stimulation. NO then activates the enzyme guanylate cyclase, which results in increased levels of cyclic guanosine monophosphate (cGMP), producing smooth muscle relaxation and inflow of blood to the corpus cavernosum. Sildenafil enhances the effect of NO by inhibiting phosphodiesterase type 5 (PDE-5), which is responsible for degradation of cGMP in the corpus cavernosum; when sexual stimulation causes local release of NO, inhibition of PDE-5 by sildenafil causes increased levels of cGMP in the corpus cavernosum, resulting in smooth muscle relaxation and inflow of blood to the corpus cavernosum; at recommended doses, it has no effect in the absence of sexual stimulation.

Contraindications Hypersensitivity to sildenafil or any component of the formulation; concurrent use of organic nitrates (nitroglycerin) in any form (potentiates the hypotensive effects)

Warnings/Precautions There is a degree of cardiac risk associated with sexual activity; therefore, physicians may wish to consider the cardiovascular status of their patients prior to initiating any treatment for erectile dysfunction. Agents for the treatment of erectile dysfunction should be used with caution in patients with anatomical deformation of the penis (angulation, cavernosal fibrosis, or Peyronie's disease), or in patients who have conditions which may predispose them to priapism (sickle cell anemia, multiple myeloma, leukemia).

The safety and efficacy of sildenafil with other treatments for erectile dysfunction have not been studied and are, therefore, not recommended as combination therapy.

A minority of patients with retinitis pigmentosa have generic disorders of retinal phosphodiesterases. There is no safety information on the administration of sildenafil to these patients and sildenafil should be administered with caution.

Drug Interactions

Cytochrome P450 Effect: Substrate of CYP2C8/9 (minor), 3A4 (major); **Inhibits** CYP1A2 (weak), 2C8/9 (weak), 2C19 (weak), 2D6 (weak), 2E1 (weak), 3A4 (weak)

Increased Effect/Toxicity: Sildenafil potentiates the hypotensive effects of nitrates (amyl nitrate, isosorbide dinitrate, isosorbide mononitrate, nitroglycerin); severe reactions have occurred and concurrent use is contraindicated. Concomitant use of alpha-blockers (doxazosin) may lead to symptomatic hypotension in some patients (sildenafil in doses >25 mg should not be given within 4 hours of administering an alpha-blocker).

CYP3A4 inhibitors may increase the levels/effects of sildenafil; example inhibitors include azole antifungals, ciprofloxacin, clarithromycin, diclofenac, doxycycline, erythromycin, imatinib, isoniazid, nefazodone, nicardipine, propofol, protease inhibitors, quinidine, and verapamil. Sildenafil may potentiate the effect of other antihypertensives. Sildenafil may potentiate bleeding in patients receiving heparin. Reduce sildenafil dose to 25 mg/24 hours in patients receiving azole antifungals or protease inhibitors.

Decreased Effect: Enzyme inducers (including phenytoin, carbamazepine, phenobarbital, rifampin) may decrease the serum concentration and efficacy of sildenafil.

Ethanol/Nutrition/Herb Interactions

Food: Amount and rate of absorption of sildenafil is reduced when taken with a high-fat meal. Serum concentrations/toxicity may be increased with grapefruit juice; avoid concurrent use.

Herb/Nutraceutical: St John's wort may decrease sildenafil levels.

Pharmacodynamics/Kinetics

Onset of action: ~60 minutes
Duration: 2-4 hours
Absorption: Rapid
Protein binding, plasma: ~96%
Metabolism: Hepatic via CYP3A4 (major) and CYP2C9 (minor route)
Bioavailability: 40%
Half-life elimination: 4 hours
Time to peak: 30-120 minutes
Excretion: Feces (80%); urine (13%)

Pregnancy Risk Factor B

Dosage Forms TAB: 25 mg, 50 mg, 100 mg

Silexin® [OTC] *see* Guaifenesin and Dextromethorphan *on page 673*
Silfedrine Children's [OTC] *see* Pseudoephedrine *on page 1147*
Silphen® [OTC] *see* DiphenhydrAMINE *on page 448*
Silphen DM® [OTC] *see* Dextromethorphan *on page 421*
Siltussin DAS [OTC] *see* Guaifenesin *on page 672*
Siltussin SA [OTC] *see* Guaifenesin *on page 672*
Silvadene® *see* Silver Sulfadiazine *on page 1221*

Silver Nitrate (SIL ver NYE trate)

Generic Available Yes

Synonyms $AgNO_3$

Pharmacologic Category Antibiotic, Topical; Cauterizing Agent, Topical; Topical Skin Product, Antibacterial

Use Cauterization of wounds and sluggish ulcers, removal of granulation tissue and warts; aseptic prophylaxis of burns

Local Anesthetic/Vasoconstrictor Precautions No information available to require special precautions

Effects on Dental Treatment No significant effects or complications reported

Common Adverse Effects Frequency not defined.

Dermatologic: Burning and skin irritation, staining of the skin
Endocrine & metabolic: Hyponatremia
Hematologic: Methemoglobinemia

Mechanism of Action Free silver ions precipitate bacterial proteins by combining with chloride in tissue forming silver chloride; coagulates cellular protein to form an eschar; silver ions or salts or colloidal silver preparations can inhibit the growth of both gram-positive and gram-negative bacteria. This germicidal action is attributed to the precipitation of bacterial proteins by liberated silver ions. Silver nitrate coagulates cellular protein to form an eschar, and this mode of action is the postulated mechanism for control of benign hematuria, rhinitis, and recurrent pneumothorax.

Pharmacodynamics/Kinetics

Absorption: Because silver ions readily combine with protein, there is minimal GI and cutaneous absorption of the 0.5% and 1% preparations

Excretion: Highest amounts of silver noted on autopsy have been in kidneys, excretion in urine is minimal

Pregnancy Risk Factor C

Silver Sulfadiazine (SIL ver sul fa DYE a zeen)

U.S. Brand Names Silvadene®; SSD®; SSD® AF; Thermazene®

Canadian Brand Names Dermazin™; Flamazine®; SSD™

Generic Available Yes

Pharmacologic Category Antibiotic, Topical

Use Prevention and treatment of infection in second and third degree burns

Local Anesthetic/Vasoconstrictor Precautions No information available to require special precautions

Effects on Dental Treatment No significant effects or complications reported

Common Adverse Effects Frequency not defined.

Dermatologic: Itching, rash, erythema multiforme, discoloration of skin, photosensitivity
Hematologic: Hemolytic anemia, leukopenia, agranulocytosis, aplastic anemia
Hepatic: Hepatitis
Renal: Interstitial nephritis
Miscellaneous: Allergic reactions may be related to sulfa component

Mechanism of Action Acts upon the bacterial cell wall and cell membrane. Bactericidal for many gram-negative and gram-positive bacteria and is effective against yeast. Active against *Pseudomonas aeruginosa*, *Pseudomonas maltophilia*, *Enterobacter* species, *Klebsiella* species, *Serratia* species, *Escherichia coli*, *Proteus mirabilis*, *Morganella morganii*, *Providencia rettgeri*, *Proteus vulgaris*, *Providencia* species, *Citrobacter* species, *Acinetobacter calcoaceticus*, *Staphylococcus aureus*, *Staphylococcus epidermidis*, *Enterococcus* species, *Candida albicans*, *Corynebacterium diphtheriae*, and *Clostridium perfringens*

Drug Interactions

Decreased Effect: Topical proteolytic enzymes are inactivated by silver sulfadiazine.

Pharmacodynamics/Kinetics

Absorption: Significant percutaneous absorption of silver sulfadiazine can occur especially when applied to extensive burns

(Continued)

Silver Sulfadiazine *(Continued)*

Half-life elimination: 10 hours; prolonged with renal impairment
Time to peak, serum: 3-11 days of continuous therapy
Excretion: Urine (~50% as unchanged drug)

Pregnancy Risk Factor B

Simethicone (sye METH i kone)

U.S. Brand Names Alka-Seltzer® Gas Relief [OTC]; Baby Gasz [OTC]; Flatulex® [OTC]; Gas-X® [OTC]; Gas-X® Extra Strength [OTC]; Genasyme® [OTC]; Mylanta® Gas [OTC]; Mylanta® Gas Maximum Strength [OTC]; Mylicon® Infants [OTC]; Phazyme® Quick Dissolve [OTC]; Phazyme® Ultra Strength [OTC]

Canadian Brand Names Ovol®; Phazyme™

Generic Available Yes: Tablet, suspension

Synonyms Activated Dimethicone; Activated Methylpolysiloxane

Pharmacologic Category Antiflatulent

Use Relieves flatulence and functional gastric bloating, and postoperative gas pains

Local Anesthetic/Vasoconstrictor Precautions No information available to require special precautions

Effects on Dental Treatment No significant effects or complications reported

Common Adverse Effects No data reported

Mechanism of Action Decreases the surface tension of gas bubbles thereby disperses and prevents gas pockets in the GI system

Pregnancy Risk Factor C

Simethicone, Aluminum Hydroxide, and Magnesium Hydroxide *see* Aluminum Hydroxide, Magnesium Hydroxide, and Simethicone *on page 92*

Simethicone and Calcium Carbonate *see* Calcium Carbonate and Simethicone *on page 245*

Simethicone and Magaldrate *see* Magaldrate and Simethicone *on page 852*

Simply Cough® [OTC] *see* Dextromethorphan *on page 421*

Simply Saline™ [OTC] *see* Sodium Chloride *on page 1227*

Simulect® *see* Basiliximab *on page 182*

Simvastatin (SIM va stat in)

Related Information

Cardiovascular Diseases *on page 1458*

U.S. Brand Names Zocor®

Canadian Brand Names Apo-Simvastatin®; Gen-Simvastatin; ratio-Simvastatin; Riva-Simvastatin; Zocor®

Mexican Brand Names Zocor®

Generic Available No

Pharmacologic Category Antilipemic Agent, HMG-CoA Reductase Inhibitor

Use Used with dietary therapy for the following:

Secondary prevention of cardiovascular events in hypercholesterolemic patients with established coronary heart disease (CHD) or at high risk for CHD: To reduce cardiovascular morbidity (myocardial infarction, coronary revascularization procedures) and mortality; to reduce the risk of stroke and transient ischemic attacks

Hyperlipidemias: To reduce elevations in total cholesterol, LDL-C, apolipoprotein B, and triglycerides in patients with primary hypercholesterolemia (elevations of 1 or more components are present in Fredrickson type IIa, IIb, III, and IV hyperlipidemias); treatment of homozygous familial hypercholesterolemia

Heterozygous familial hypercholesterolemia (HeFH): In adolescent patients (10-17 years of age, females >1 year postmenarche) with HeFH having LDL-C ≥190 mg/dL **or** LDL ≥160 mg/dL with positive family history of premature cardiovascular disease (CVD), or 2 or more CVD risk factors in the adolescent patient

Local Anesthetic/Vasoconstrictor Precautions No information available to require special precautions

Effects on Dental Treatment No significant effects or complications reported

Common Adverse Effects 1% to 10%:

Gastrointestinal: Constipation (2%), dyspepsia (1%), flatulence (2%)
Neuromuscular & skeletal: CPK elevation (>3x normal on one or more occasions - 5%)
Respiratory: Upper respiratory infection (2%)

Additional class-related events or case reports (not necessarily reported with simvastatin therapy): Alopecia, alteration in taste, anaphylaxis, angioedema, anorexia, anxiety, arthritis, cataracts, chills, cholestatic jaundice, cirrhosis, decreased libido, depression, dermatomyositis, dryness of skin/mucous membranes, dyspnea, elevated transaminases, eosinophilia, erectile dysfunction/impotence, erythema multiforme, facial paresis, fatty liver, fever, flushing, fulminant hepatic necrosis, gynecomastia, hemolytic anemia, hepatitis, hepatoma, hyperbilirubinemia, hypersensitivity reaction, impaired extraocular muscle movement, increased alkaline phosphatase, increased CPK (>10x normal), increased ESR, increased GGT, leukopenia, malaise, memory loss, myopathy, nail changes, nodules, ophthalmoplegia, pancreatitis, paresthesia, peripheral nerve palsy, peripheral neuropathy, photosensitivity, polymyalgia rheumatica, positive ANA, pruritus, psychic disturbance, purpura, rash, renal failure (secondary to rhabdomyolysis), rhabdomyolysis, skin discoloration, Stevens-Johnson syndrome, systemic lupus erythematosus-like syndrome, thrombocytopenia, thyroid dysfunction, toxic epidermal necrolysis, tremor, urticaria, vasculitis, vertigo, vomiting

Dosage Oral: **Note:** Doses should be individualized according to the baseline LDL-cholesterol levels, the recommended goal of therapy, and the patient's response; adjustments should be made at intervals of 4 weeks or more; doses may need adjusted based on concomitant medications

Children 10-17 years (females >1 year postmenarche): HeFH: 10 mg once daily in the evening; range: 10-40 mg/day (maximum: 40 mg/day)

Dosage adjustment for simvastatin with concomitant cyclosporine, fibrates, niacin, amiodarone, or verapamil: Refer to drug-specific dosing in Adults dosing section

Adults:

Homozygous familial hypercholesterolemia: 40 mg once daily in the evening **or** 80 mg/day (given as 20 mg, 20 mg, and 40 mg evening dose)

Prevention of cardiovascular events, hyperlipidemias: 20-40 mg once daily in the evening; range: 5-80 mg/day

Patients requiring only moderate reduction of LDL-cholesterol may be started at 10 mg once daily

Patients requiring reduction of >45% in low-density lipoprotein (LDL) cholesterol may be started at 40 mg once daily in the evening

Patients with CHD or at high risk for CHD: Dosing should be started at 40 mg once daily in the evening; simvastatin may be started simultaneously with diet

Dosage adjustment with concomitant medications:

Cyclosporine: Initial: 5 mg simvastatin, should **not** exceed 10 mg/day

Fibrates or niacin: Simvastatin dose should **not** exceed 10 mg/day

Amiodarone or verapamil: Simvastatin dose should **not** exceed 20 mg/day

Dosing adjustment/comments in renal impairment: Because simvastatin does not undergo significant renal excretion, modification of dose should not be necessary in patients with mild to moderate renal insufficiency.

Severe renal impairment: Cl_{cr} <10 mL/minute: Initial: 5 mg/day with close monitoring.

Mechanism of Action Simvastatin is a methylated derivative of lovastatin that acts by competitively inhibiting 3-hydroxy-3-methylglutaryl-coenzyme A (HMG-CoA) reductase, the enzyme that catalyzes the rate-limiting step in cholesterol biosynthesis

Contraindications Hypersensitivity to simvastatin or any component of the formulation; acute liver disease; unexplained persistent elevations of serum transaminases; pregnancy; breast-feeding

Warnings/Precautions Secondary causes of hyperlipidemia should be ruled out prior to therapy. Liver function must be monitored by laboratory assessment. Rhabdomyolysis with acute renal failure has occurred. Risk is increased with concurrent use of clarithromycin, danazol, diltiazem, fluvoxamine, indinavir, nefazodone, nelfinavir, ritonavir, verapamil, troleandomycin, cyclosporine, fibric acid derivatives, erythromycin, niacin, or azole antifungals. Weigh the risk versus benefit when combining any of these drugs with simvastatin. Temporarily discontinue in any patient experiencing an acute or serious condition predisposing to renal failure secondary to rhabdomyolysis. Use with caution in patients who consume large amounts of ethanol or have a history of liver disease. Safety and efficacy have not been established in patients <10 years or in premenarcheal girls.

Drug Interactions

Cytochrome P450 Effect: Substrate of CYP3A4 (major); **Inhibits** CYP2C8/9 (weak), 2D6 (weak)

Increased Effect/Toxicity: Risk of myopathy/rhabdomyolysis may be increased by concurrent use of lipid-lowering agents which may cause rhabdomyolysis (gemfibrozil, fibric acid derivatives, or niacin at doses ≥1 g/day), or during concurrent use of strong CYP3A4 inhibitors.

(Continued)

Simvastatin *(Continued)*

CYP3A4 inhibitors may increase the levels/effects of simvastatin; example inhibitors include azole antifungals, ciprofloxacin, clarithromycin, diclofenac, doxycycline, erythromycin, imatinib, isoniazid, nefazodone, nicardipine, propofol, protease inhibitors, quinidine, and verapamil. In large quantities (ie, >1 quart/day), grapefruit juice may also increase simvastatin serum concentrations, increasing the risk of rhabdomyolysis. In general, concurrent use with CYP3A4 inhibitors is not recommended; manufacturer recommends limiting simvastatin dose to 20 mg/day when used with amiodarone or verapamil, and 10 mg/day when used with cyclosporine, gemfibrozil, or fibric acid derivatives.

The anticoagulant effect of warfarin may be increased by simvastatin. Cholesterol-lowering effects are additive with bile-acid sequestrants (colestipol and cholestyramine).

Decreased Effect: When taken within 1 before or up to 2 hours after cholestyramine, a decrease in absorption of simvastatin can occur.

Ethanol/Nutrition/Herb Interactions

Ethanol: Avoid excessive ethanol consumption (due to potential hepatic effects).

Food: Simvastatin serum concentration may be increased when taken with grapefruit juice; avoid concurrent intake of large quantities (>1 quart/day).

Herb/Nutraceutical: St John's wort may decrease simvastatin levels.

Pharmacodynamics/Kinetics

Onset of action: >3 days

Peak effect: 2 weeks

Absorption: 85%

Protein binding: ~95%

Metabolism: Hepatic via CYP3A4; extensive first-pass effect

Bioavailability: <5%

Half-life elimination: Unknown

Time to peak: 1.3-2.4 hours

Excretion: Feces (60%); urine (13%)

Pregnancy Risk Factor X

Dosage Forms TAB: 5 mg, 10 mg, 20 mg, 40 mg, 80 mg

Sincalide (SIN ka lide)

U.S. Brand Names Kinevac®

Generic Available No

Synonyms C8-CCK; OP-CCK

Pharmacologic Category Diagnostic Agent

Use Postevacuation cholecystography; gallbladder bile sampling; stimulate pancreatic secretion for analysis

Local Anesthetic/Vasoconstrictor Precautions No information available to require special precautions

Effects on Dental Treatment No significant effects or complications reported

Mechanism of Action Stimulates contraction of the gallbladder and simultaneous relaxation of the sphincter of Oddi, inhibits gastric emptying, and increases intestinal motility. Graded doses have been shown to produce graded decreases in small intestinal transit time, thought to be mediated by acetylcholine.

Pregnancy Risk Factor B

Sinemet® *see* Levodopa and Carbidopa *on page 811*

Sinemet® CR *see* Levodopa and Carbidopa *on page 811*

Sinequan® *see* Doxepin *on page 467*

Singulair® *see* Montelukast *on page 944*

Sinus-Relief® [OTC] *see* Acetaminophen and Pseudoephedrine *on page 53*

Sinutab® Sinus [OTC] *see* Acetaminophen and Pseudoephedrine *on page 53*

Sinutab® Sinus Allergy Maximum Strength [OTC] *see* Acetaminophen, Chlorpheniramine, and Pseudoephedrine *on page 58*

Sirdalud® *see* Tizanidine *on page 1305*

Sirolimus (sir OH li mus)

U.S. Brand Names Rapamune®

Canadian Brand Names Rapamune®

Generic Available No

Pharmacologic Category Immunosuppressant Agent

Use Prophylaxis of organ rejection in patients receiving renal transplants, in combination with corticosteroids and cyclosporine (cyclosporine may be withdrawn in low-to-moderate immunological risk patients after 2-4 months, in conjunction with an increase in sirolimus dosage)

Unlabeled/Investigational Use Investigational: Immunosuppression in other forms of solid organ transplantation

Local Anesthetic/Vasoconstrictor Precautions No information available to require special precautions

Effects on Dental Treatment No significant effects or complications reported

Common Adverse Effects Incidence of many adverse effects is dose related

>20%:

Cardiovascular: Hypertension (39% to 49%), peripheral edema (54% to 64%), edema (16% to 24%), chest pain (16% to 24%)

Central nervous system: Fever (23% to 34%), headache (23% to 34%), pain (24% to 33%), insomnia (13% to 22%)

Dermatologic: Acne (20% to 31%)

Endocrine & metabolic: Hypercholesterolemia (38% to 46%), hypophosphatemia (15% to 23%), hyperlipidemia (38% to 57%), hypokalemia (11% to 21%)

Gastrointestinal: Abdominal pain (28% to 36%), nausea (25% to 36%), vomiting (19% to 25%), diarrhea (25% to 42%), constipation (28% to 38%), dyspepsia (17% to 25%), weight gain (8% to 21%)

Genitourinary: Urinary tract infection (20% to 33%)

Hematologic: Anemia (23% to 37%), thrombocytopenia (13% to 40%)

Neuromuscular & skeletal: Arthralgia (25% to 31%), weakness (22% to 40%), back pain (16% to 26%), tremor (21% to 31%)

Renal: Increased serum creatinine (35% to 40%)

Respiratory: Dyspnea (22% to 30%), upper respiratory infection (20% to 26%), pharyngitis (16% to 21%)

3% to 20%:

Cardiovascular: Atrial fibrillation, CHF, hypervolemia, hypotension, palpitation, peripheral vascular disorder, postural hypotension, syncope, tachycardia, thrombosis, vasodilation, venous thromboembolism

Central nervous system: Chills, malaise, anxiety, confusion, depression, dizziness, emotional lability, hypesthesia, hypotonia, insomnia, neuropathy, somnolence

Dermatologic: Dermatitis (fungal), hirsutism, pruritus, skin hypertrophy, dermal ulcer, ecchymosis, cellulitis, rash (10% to 20%)

Endocrine & metabolic: Cushing's syndrome, diabetes mellitus, glycosuria, acidosis, dehydration, hypercalcemia, hyperglycemia, hyperphosphatemia, hypocalcemia, hypoglycemia, hypomagnesemia, hyponatremia, hyperkalemia (12% to 17%)

Gastrointestinal: Enlarged abdomen, anorexia, dysphagia, eructation, esophagitis, flatulence, gastritis, gastroenteritis, gingivitis, gingival hyperplasia, ileus, mouth ulceration, oral moniliasis, stomatitis, weight loss

Genitourinary: Pelvic pain, scrotal edema, testis disorder, impotence

Hematologic: Leukocytosis, polycythemia, TTP, hemolytic-uremic syndrome, hemorrhage, leukopenia (9% to 15%)

Hepatic: Abnormal liver function tests, increased alkaline phosphatase, increased LDH, increased transaminases, ascites

Local: Thrombophlebitis

Neuromuscular & skeletal: Increased CPK, arthrosis, bone necrosis, leg cramps, myalgia, osteoporosis, tetany, hypertonia, paresthesia

Ocular: Abnormal vision, cataract, conjunctivitis

Otic: Ear pain, deafness, otitis media, tinnitus

Renal: Increased BUN, albuminuria, bladder pain, dysuria, hematuria, hydronephrosis, kidney pain, tubular necrosis, nocturia, oliguria, pyuria, nephropathy (toxic), urinary frequency, urinary incontinence, urinary retention

Respiratory: Asthma, atelectasis, bronchitis, cough, epistaxis, hypoxia, lung edema, pleural effusion, pneumonia, rhinitis, sinusitis

Miscellaneous: Abscess, facial edema, flu-like syndrome, hernia, infection, lymphadenopathy, lymphocele, peritonitis, sepsis, diaphoresis

Mechanism of Action Sirolimus inhibits T-lymphocyte activation and proliferation in response to antigenic and cytokine stimulation. Its mechanism differs from other immunosuppressants. It inhibits acute rejection of allografts and prolongs graft survival.

Drug Interactions

Cytochrome P450 Effect: Substrate of CYP3A4 (major); **Inhibits** CYP3A4 (weak)

(Continued)

Sirolimus *(Continued)*

Increased Effect/Toxicity: Cyclosporine increases sirolimus concentrations during concurrent therapy, and cyclosporine levels may be increased; sirolimus should be taken 4 hours after cyclosporine oral solution (modified) and/or cyclosporine capsules (modified). CYP3A4 inhibitors may increase the levels/effects of sirolimus; example inhibitors include azole antifungals, ciprofloxacin, clarithromycin, diclofenac, doxycycline, erythromycin, imatinib, isoniazid, nefazodone, nicardipine, propofol, protease inhibitors, quinidine, and verapamil; avoid concurrent use. Vaccination may be less effective and use of live vaccines should be avoided during sirolimus therapy.

Decreased Effect: CYP3A4 inducers may decrease the levels/effects of sirolimus; example inducers include aminoglutethimide, carbamazepine, nafcillin, nevirapine, phenobarbital, phenytoin, and rifamycins.

Pharmacodynamics/Kinetics

Absorption: Rapid
Distribution: 12 L/kg (± 7.52 L/kg)
Protein binding: 92%, primarily to albumin
Metabolism: Extensively hepatic via CYP3A4 and P-glycoprotein
Bioavailability: 14%
Half-life elimination: Mean: 62 hours
Time to peak: 1-3 hours
Excretion: Feces (91%); urine (2.2%)

Pregnancy Risk Factor C

SK *see* Streptokinase *on page 1238*
SK and F 104864 *see* Topotecan *on page 1316*
Skelaxin® *see* Metaxalone *on page 886*
Skelid® *see* Tiludronate *on page 1298*
SKF 104864 *see* Topotecan *on page 1316*
SKF 104864-A *see* Topotecan *on page 1316*

Skin Test Antigens (Multiple) (skin test AN tee gens, MUL ti pul)

U.S. Brand Names Multitest CMI®

Canadian Brand Names Multitest® CMI

Generic Available No

Pharmacologic Category Diagnostic Agent

Use Detection of nonresponsiveness to antigens by means of delayed hypersensitivity skin testing

Local Anesthetic/Vasoconstrictor Precautions No information available to require special precautions

Effects on Dental Treatment No significant effects or complications reported

Common Adverse Effects 1% to 10%: Local: Irritation

Pregnancy Risk Factor C

Sleepinal® [OTC] *see* DiphenhydrAMINE *on page 448*
Slo-Niacin® [OTC] *see* Niacin *on page 978*
Slow FE® [OTC] *see* Ferrous Sulfate *on page 586*
Slow-Mag® [OTC] *see* Magnesium Chloride *on page 852*
Smallpox Vaccine *see page 1614*
Smelling Salts *see* Ammonia Spirit (Aromatic) *on page 111*
SMZ-TMP *see* Sulfamethoxazole and Trimethoprim *on page 1246*
Sodium 4-Hydroxybutyrate *see* Sodium Oxybate *on page 1229*
Sodium Acid Carbonate *see* Sodium Bicarbonate *on page 1226*
Sodium Benzoate and Caffeine *see* Caffeine and Sodium Benzoate *on page 242*

Sodium Bicarbonate (SOW dee um bye KAR bun ate)

U.S. Brand Names Brioschi® [OTC]; Neut®

Generic Available Yes

Synonyms Baking Soda; $NaHCO_3$; Sodium Acid Carbonate; Sodium Hydrogen Carbonate

Pharmacologic Category Alkalinizing Agent; Antacid; Electrolyte Supplement, Oral; Electrolyte Supplement, Parenteral

Use Management of metabolic acidosis; gastric hyperacidity; as an alkalinization agent for the urine; treatment of hyperkalemia; management of overdose of certain drugs, including tricyclic antidepressants and aspirin

Local Anesthetic/Vasoconstrictor Precautions No information available to require special precautions

Effects on Dental Treatment No significant effects or complications reported

Common Adverse Effects Frequency not defined.

Cardiovascular: Cerebral hemorrhage, CHF (aggravated), edema

Central nervous system: Tetany

Gastrointestinal: Belching, flatulence (with oral), gastric distension

Endocrine & metabolic: Hypernatremia, hyperosmolality, hypocalcemia, hypokalemia, increased affinity of hemoglobin for oxygen-reduced pH in myocardial tissue necrosis when extravasated, intracranial acidosis, metabolic alkalosis, milk-alkali syndrome (especially with renal dysfunction)

Respiratory: Pulmonary edema

Mechanism of Action Dissociates to provide bicarbonate ion which neutralizes hydrogen ion concentration and raises blood and urinary pH

Drug Interactions

Increased Effect/Toxicity: Increased toxicity/levels of amphetamines, ephedrine, pseudoephedrine, flecainide, quinidine, and quinine due to urinary alkalinization.

Decreased Effect: Decreased effect/levels of lithium, chlorpropamide, and salicylates due to urinary alkalinization.

Pharmacodynamics/Kinetics

Onset of action: Oral: Rapid; I.V.: 15 minutes

Duration: Oral: 8-10 minutes; I.V.: 1-2 hours

Absorption: Oral: Well absorbed

Excretion: Urine (<1%)

Pregnancy Risk Factor C

Sodium Biphosphate, Methenamine, Methylene Blue, Phenyl Salicylate, and Hyoscyamine *see* Methenamine, Sodium Biphosphate, Phenyl Salicylate, Methylene Blue, and Hyoscyamine *on page 893*

Sodium Cellulose Phosphate *see* Cellulose Sodium Phosphate *on page 294*

Sodium Chloride (SOW dee um KLOR ide)

U.S. Brand Names Altamist [OTC]; Ayr® Baby Saline [OTC]; Ayr® Saline [OTC]; Ayr® Saline Mist [OTC]; Breathe Right® Saline [OTC]; Broncho Saline® [OTC]; Entsol® [OTC]; Muro 128® [OTC]; NaSal™ [OTC]; Nasal Moist® [OTC]; Na-Zone® [OTC]; Ocean® [OTC]; Pediamist® [OTC]; Pretz® Irrigation [OTC]; SalineX® [OTC]; SeaMist® [OTC]; Simply Saline™ [OTC]; Wound Wash Saline™ [OTC]

Generic Available Yes

Synonyms NaCl; Normal Saline; Salt

Pharmacologic Category Electrolyte Supplement, Oral; Electrolyte Supplement, Parenteral; Lubricant, Ocular; Sodium Salt

Use

Parenteral: Restores sodium ion in patients with restricted oral intake (especially hyponatremia states or low salt syndrome). In general, parenteral saline uses:

Bacteriostatic sodium chloride: Dilution or dissolving drugs for I.M., I.V., or SubQ injections

Concentrated sodium chloride: Additive for parenteral fluid therapy

Hypertonic sodium chloride: For severe hyponatremia and hypochloremia

Hypotonic sodium chloride: Hydrating solution

Normal saline: Restores water/sodium losses

Pharmaceutical aid/diluent for infusion of compatible drug additives

Ophthalmic: Reduces corneal edema

Oral: Restores sodium losses

Inhalation: Restores moisture to pulmonary system; loosens and thins congestion caused by colds or allergies; diluent for bronchodilator solutions that require dilution before inhalation

Intranasal: Restores moisture to nasal membranes

Irrigation: Wound cleansing, irrigation, and flushing

Local Anesthetic/Vasoconstrictor Precautions No information available to require special precautions

Effects on Dental Treatment No significant effects or complications reported

Common Adverse Effects Frequency not defined.

Cardiovascular: Congestive conditions

Endocrine & metabolic: Extravasation, hypervolemia, hypernatremia, dilution of serum electrolytes, overhydration, hypokalemia

Local: Thrombosis, phlebitis, extravasation

Respiratory: Pulmonary edema

Mechanism of Action Principal extracellular cation; functions in fluid and electrolyte balance, osmotic pressure control, and water distribution

(Continued)

Sodium Chloride *(Continued)*

Drug Interactions

Decreased Effect: Lithium serum concentrations may be decreased.

Pharmacodynamics/Kinetics

Absorption: Oral, I.V.: Rapid

Distribution: Widely distributed

Excretion: Primarily urine; also sweat, tears, saliva

Pregnancy Risk Factor C

Sodium Citrate and Citric Acid

(SOW dee um SIT rate & SI trik AS id)

U.S. Brand Names Bicitra®; Cytra-2; Oracit®

Canadian Brand Names PMS-Dicitrate

Generic Available Yes

Synonyms Modified Shohl's Solution

Pharmacologic Category Alkalinizing Agent, Oral

Use Treatment of metabolic acidosis; alkalinizing agent in conditions where long-term maintenance of an alkaline urine is desirable

Local Anesthetic/Vasoconstrictor Precautions No information available to require special precautions

Effects on Dental Treatment No significant effects or complications reported

Common Adverse Effects Frequency not defined. Generally well tolerated with normal renal function.

Central nervous system: Tetany

Endocrine & metabolic: Metabolic alkalosis, hyperkalemia

Gastrointestinal: Diarrhea, nausea, vomiting

Drug Interactions

Increased Effect/Toxicity: Increased toxicity/levels of amphetamines, ephedrine, pseudoephedrine, flecainide, quinidine, and quinine due to urinary alkalinization.

Decreased Effect: Decreased effect/levels of lithium, chlorpropamide, and salicylates due to urinary alkalinization.

Pharmacodynamics/Kinetics

Metabolism: Oxidized to sodium bicarbonate

Excretion: Urine (<5% as sodium citrate)

Pregnancy Risk Factor Not established

Sodium Citrate, Citric Acid, and Potassium Citrate *see* Citric Acid, Sodium Citrate, and Potassium Citrate *on page 341*

Sodium Edetate *see* Edetate Disodium *on page 482*

Sodium Etidronate *see* Etidronate Disodium *on page 563*

Sodium Ferric Gluconate *see* Ferric Gluconate *on page 585*

Sodium Fluoride *see* Fluoride *on page 603*

Sodium Hyaluronate *see* Hyaluronate and Derivatives *on page 696*

Sodium Hyaluronate-Chrondroitin Sulfate *see* Chondroitin Sulfate and Sodium Hyaluronate *on page 325*

Sodium Hydrogen Carbonate *see* Sodium Bicarbonate *on page 1226*

Sodium Hypochlorite Solution

(SOW dee um hye poe KLOR ite soe LOO shun)

U.S. Brand Names Dakin's Solution

Generic Available No

Synonyms Modified Dakin's Solution

Pharmacologic Category Disinfectant, Antibacterial (Topical)

Use Treatment of athlete's foot (0.5%); wound irrigation (0.5%); disinfection of utensils and equipment (5%)

Local Anesthetic/Vasoconstrictor Precautions No information available to require special precautions

Effects on Dental Treatment No significant effects or complications reported

Common Adverse Effects Frequency not defined.

Dermatologic: Irritating to skin

Hematologic: Dissolves blood clots, delays clotting

Pregnancy Risk Factor C

Sodium Hyposulfate *see* Sodium Thiosulfate *on page 1230*

Sodium *L*-Triiodothyronine *see* Liothyronine *on page 831*

Sodium Nafcillin *see* Nafcillin *on page 958*

Sodium Nitroferricyanide *see* Nitroprusside *on page 993*

Sodium Nitroprusside *see* Nitroprusside *on page 993*

Sodium Oxybate (SOW dee um ox i BATE)

U.S. Brand Names Xyrem®

Generic Available No

Synonyms Gamma Hydroxybutyric Acid; GHB; 4-Hydroxybutyrate; Sodium 4-Hydroxybutyrate

Pharmacologic Category Central Nervous System Depressant

Use Orphan drug: Treatment of cataplexy in patients with narcolepsy

Local Anesthetic/Vasoconstrictor Precautions No information available to require special precautions

Effects on Dental Treatment No significant effects or complications reported

Common Adverse Effects Percentages reported in controlled clinical trials:

>10%:

Central nervous system: Dizziness (23% to 34%), headache (9% to 31%), pain (9% to 20%), somnolence (12% to 15%), confusion (9% to 14%), sleep disorder (6% to 14%)

Dermatologic: Diaphoresis (3% to 11%)

Gastrointestinal: Nausea (6% to 34%), vomiting (6% to 11%)

Genitourinary: Urinary incontinence (5% to 14%, usually nocturnal)

Respiratory: Pharyngitis (11%)

Miscellaneous: Infection (7% to 15%)

1% to 10%:

Cardiovascular: Hypertension (6%), edema

Central nervous system: Dream abnormality (3% to 9%), sleepwalking (7%), depression (6%), amnesia (3% to 6%), anxiety (3% to 6%), thinking abnormality (3% to 6%), insomnia (5%), agitation, ataxia, chills, convulsion, stupor, tremor

Dermatologic: Acne, alopecia, rash

Endocrine & metabolic: Dysmenorrhea (3% to 6%)

Gastrointestinal: Dyspepsia (6% to 9%), diarrhea (6% to 8%), abdominal pain (6%), nausea and vomiting (6%), anorexia, constipation, weight gain

Hepatic: Alkaline phosphatase increased, hypercholesteremia, hypocalcemia

Neuromuscular & skeletal: Hypesthesia (6%), weakness (6% to 8%), myasthenia (3% to 6%), arthritis, leg cramps, myalgia

Ocular: Amblyopia (6%)

Otic: Tinnitus (6%)

Renal: Albuminuria, cystitis, hematuria, metrorrhagia, urinary frequency

Respiratory: Rhinitis (8%), dyspnea

Miscellaneous: Viral infection (3% to 9%), allergic reaction

Restrictions C-I (illicit use); C-III (medical use)

Sodium oxybate oral solution will be available only to prescribers enrolled in the Xyrem® Success Program[SM] and dispensed to the patient through the designated centralized pharmacy. Prior to dispensing the first prescription, prescribers will be sent educational materials to be reviewed with the patient and enrollment forms for the postmarketing surveillance program. Patients must be seen at least every 3 months; prescriptions can be written for a maximum of 3 months (the first prescription may only be written for a 1-month supply).

Mechanism of Action The exact mechanism for the efficacy of sodium oxybate the treatment of cataplexy in patients with narcolepsy is not known.

Drug Interactions

Increased Effect/Toxicity: CNS depressants: CNS depressant effects are potentiated; concomitant use with sodium oxybate is contraindicated.

Pharmacodynamics/Kinetics

Absorption: Rapid

Distribution: 190-384 mL/kg

Protein binding: <1%

Metabolism: Primarily via the Krebs cycle to form water and carbon dioxide; secondarily via beta oxidation; significant first-pass effect; no active metabolites; metabolic pathways are saturable

Bioavailability: 25%

Half-life elimination: 30-60 minutes

Time to peak: 30-75 minutes

Excretion: Primarily pulmonary (as carbon dioxide); urine (<5% unchanged drug)

Pregnancy Risk Factor B

Comments Sodium oxybate is a known substance of abuse. When used illegally, it has been referred to as a "date-rape drug". The dentist should be aware of patients showing signs of CNS depression, as with all other drugs in this class.

Sodium PAS *see* Aminosalicylic Acid *on page 100*

Sodium-PCA and Lactic Acid *see* Lactic Acid and Sodium-PCA *on page 793*

Sodium Phenylbutyrate (SOW dee um fen il BYOO ti rate)

U.S. Brand Names Buphenyl®

Generic Available No

Synonyms Ammonapse

Pharmacologic Category Urea Cycle Disorder (UCD) Treatment Agent

Use Orphan drug: Adjunctive therapy in the chronic management of patients with urea cycle disorder involving deficiencies of carbamoylphosphate synthetase, ornithine transcarbamylase, or argininosuccinic acid synthetase

Local Anesthetic/Vasoconstrictor Precautions No information available to require special precautions

Effects on Dental Treatment No significant effects or complications reported

Common Adverse Effects

>10%: Endocrine & metabolic: Amenorrhea, menstrual dysfunction

1% to 10%:

Gastrointestinal: Anorexia, abnormal taste

Miscellaneous: Offensive body odor

Mechanism of Action Sodium phenylbutyrate is a prodrug that, when given orally, is rapidly converted to phenylacetate, which is in turn conjugated with glutamine to form the active compound phenylacetylglutamine; phenylacetylglutamine serves as a substitute for urea and is excreted in the urine whereby it carries with it 2 moles of nitrogen per mole of phenylacetylglutamine and can thereby assist in the clearance of nitrogenous waste in patients with urea cycle disorders

Pregnancy Risk Factor C

Sodium Phosphate and Potassium Phosphate *see* Potassium Phosphate and Sodium Phosphate *on page 1107*

Sodium Phosphates (SOW dee um FOS fates)

U.S. Brand Names Fleet® Enema [OTC]; Fleet® Phospho®-Soda [OTC]; Fleet® Phospho-Soda® Accu-Prep™ [OTC]; Visicol™

Canadian Brand Names Fleet Enema®; Fleet® Phospho®-Soda Oral Laxative

Generic Available Yes: Enema, injection

Pharmacologic Category Cathartic; Electrolyte Supplement, Oral; Electrolyte Supplement, Parenteral; Laxative, Bowel Evacuant

Use

Oral, rectal: Short-term treatment of constipation and to evacuate the colon for rectal and bowel exams

I.V.: Source of phosphate in large volume I.V. fluids and parenteral nutrition; treatment and prevention of hypophosphatemia

Local Anesthetic/Vasoconstrictor Precautions No information available to require special precautions

Effects on Dental Treatment No significant effects or complications reported

Mechanism of Action As a laxative, exerts osmotic effect in the small intestine by drawing water into the lumen of the gut, producing distention and promoting peristalsis and evacuation of the bowel; phosphorous participates in bone deposition, calcium metabolism, utilization of B complex vitamins, and as a buffer in acid-base equilibrium

Pregnancy Risk Factor C

Sodium Sulfacetamide *see* Sulfacetamide *on page 1244*

Sodium Thiosulfate (SOW dee um thye oh SUL fate)

U.S. Brand Names Versiclear™

Generic Available Yes: Injection

Synonyms Disodium Thiosulfate Pentahydrate; Pentahydrate; Sodium Hyposulfate; Sodium Thiosulphate; Thiosulfuric Acid Disodium Salt

Pharmacologic Category Antidote

Use

Parenteral: Used alone or with sodium nitrite or amyl nitrite in cyanide poisoning or arsenic poisoning; reduce the risk of nephrotoxicity associated with cisplatin therapy

Topical: Treatment of tinea versicolor

Unlabeled/Investigational Use Management of I.V. extravasation

Local Anesthetic/Vasoconstrictor Precautions No information available to require special precautions

Effects on Dental Treatment No significant effects or complications reported

Common Adverse Effects 1% to 10%:

Cardiovascular: Hypotension

Central nervous system: Coma, CNS depression secondary to thiocyanate intoxication, psychosis, confusion

Dermatologic: Contact dermatitis, local irritation

Neuromuscular & skeletal: Weakness

Otic: Tinnitus

Mechanism of Action

Cyanide toxicity: Increases the rate of detoxification of cyanide by the enzyme rhodanese by providing an extra sulfur

Cisplatin toxicity: Complexes with cisplatin to form a compound that is nontoxic to either normal or cancerous cells

Pharmacodynamics/Kinetics

Absorption: Oral: Poor

Distribution: Extracellular fluid

Half-life elimination: 0.65 hour

Excretion: Urine (28.5% as unchanged drug)

Pregnancy Risk Factor C

Sodium Thiosulphate *see* Sodium Thiosulfate *on page 1230*

Solagé™ *see* Mequinol and Tretinoin *on page 879*

Solaquin® [OTC] *see* Hydroquinone *on page 719*

Solaquin Forte® *see* Hydroquinone *on page 719*

Solaraze™ *see* Diclofenac *on page 427*

Solarcaine® [OTC] *see* Benzocaine *on page 191*

Solarcaine® Aloe Extra Burn Relief [OTC] *see* Lidocaine *on page 819*

Solu-Cortef® *see* Hydrocortisone *on page 714*

Solu-Medrol® *see* MethylPREDNISolone *on page 910*

Soma® *see* Carisoprodol *on page 266*

Soma® Compound *see* Carisoprodol and Aspirin *on page 266*

Soma® Compound w/Codeine *see* Carisoprodol, Aspirin, and Codeine *on page 267*

Somatrem *see* Human Growth Hormone *on page 694*

Somatropin *see* Human Growth Hormone *on page 694*

Sominex® [OTC] *see* DiphenhydrAMINE *on page 448*

Sominex® Maximum Strength [OTC] *see* DiphenhydrAMINE *on page 448*

Somnote™ *see* Chloral Hydrate *on page 304*

Sonata® *see* Zaleplon *on page 1396*

Sorbitol (SOR bi tole)

Generic Available Yes

Pharmacologic Category Genitourinary Irrigant; Laxative, Miscellaneous

Use Genitourinary irrigant in transurethral prostatic resection or other transurethral resection or other transurethral surgical procedures; diuretic; humectant; sweetening agent; hyperosmotic laxative; facilitate the passage of sodium polystyrene sulfonate through the intestinal tract

Local Anesthetic/Vasoconstrictor Precautions No information available to require special precautions

Effects on Dental Treatment No significant effects or complications reported

Common Adverse Effects Frequency not defined.

Cardiovascular: Edema

Endocrine & metabolic: Fluid and electrolyte losses, hyperglycemia, lactic acidosis

Gastrointestinal: Diarrhea, nausea, vomiting, abdominal discomfort, xerostomia

Mechanism of Action A polyalcoholic sugar with osmotic cathartic actions

Pharmacodynamics/Kinetics

Onset of action: 0.25-1 hour

Absorption: Oral, rectal: Poor

Metabolism: Primarily hepatic to fructose

Pregnancy Risk Factor C

Sorine® *see* Sotalol *on page 1231*

Sotalol (SOE ta lole)

Related Information

Cardiovascular Diseases *on page 1458*

U.S. Brand Names Betapace®; Betapace AF®; Sorine®

(Continued)

Sotalol *(Continued)*

Canadian Brand Names Alti-Sotalol; Apo-Sotalol®; Betapace AF™; Gen-Sotalol; Lin-Sotalol; Novo-Sotalol; Nu-Sotalol; PMS-Sotalol; Rho®-Sotalol; Sotacor®

Generic Available Yes

Synonyms Sotalol Hydrochloride

Pharmacologic Category Antiarrhythmic Agent, Class II; Antiarrhythmic Agent, Class III; Beta-Adrenergic Blocker, Nonselective

Use Treatment of documented ventricular arrhythmias (ie, sustained ventricular tachycardia), that in the judgment of the physician are life-threatening; maintenance of normal sinus rhythm in patients with symptomatic atrial fibrillation and atrial flutter who are currently in sinus rhythm. Manufacturer states substitutions should not be made for Betapace AF® since Betapace AF® is distributed with a patient package insert specific for atrial fibrillation/flutter.

Local Anesthetic/Vasoconstrictor Precautions Use with caution; epinephrine has interacted with nonselective beta-blockers to result in initial hypertensive episode followed by bradycardia

Effects on Dental Treatment Sotalol is a nonselective beta-blocker and may enhance the pressor response to epinephrine, resulting in hypertension and bradycardia. Many nonsteroidal anti-inflammatory drugs, such as ibuprofen and indomethacin, can reduce the hypotensive effect of beta-blockers after 3 or more weeks of therapy with the NSAID. Short-term NSAID use (ie, 3 days) requires no special precautions in patients taking beta-blockers.

Common Adverse Effects

>10%:

- Cardiovascular: Bradycardia (16%), chest pain (16%), palpitations (14%)
- Central nervous system: Fatigue (20%), dizziness (20%), lightheadedness (12%)
- Neuromuscular & skeletal: Weakness (13%)
- Respiratory: Dyspnea (21%)

1% to 10%:

- Cardiovascular: Congestive heart failure (5%), peripheral vascular disorders (3%), edema (8%), abnormal ECG (7%), hypotension (6%), proarrhythmia (5%), syncope (5%)
- Central nervous system: Mental confusion (6%), anxiety (4%), headache (8%), sleep problems (8%), depression (4%)
- Dermatologic: Itching/rash (5%)
- Endocrine & metabolic: Decreased sexual ability (3%)
- Gastrointestinal: Diarrhea (7%), nausea/vomiting (10%), stomach discomfort (3% to 6%), flatulence (2%)
- Genitourinary: Impotence (2%)
- Hematologic: Bleeding (2%)
- Neuromuscular & skeletal: Paresthesia (4%), extremity pain (7%), back pain (3%)
- Ocular: Visual problems (5%)
- Respiratory: Upper respiratory problems (5% to 8%), asthma (2%)

Mechanism of Action

Beta-blocker which contains both beta-adrenoreceptor-blocking (Vaughan Williams Class II) and cardiac action potential duration prolongation (Vaughan Williams Class III) properties

Class II effects: Increased sinus cycle length, slowed heart rate, decreased AV nodal conduction, and increased AV nodal refractoriness

Class III effects: Prolongation of the atrial and ventricular monophasic action potentials, and effective refractory prolongation of atrial muscle, ventricular muscle, and atrioventricular accessory pathways in both the antegrade and retrograde directions

Sotalol is a racemic mixture of *d*- and *l*-sotalol; both isomers have similar Class III antiarrhythmic effects while the *l*-isomer is responsible for virtually all of the beta-blocking activity

Sotalol has both $beta_1$- and $beta_2$-receptor blocking activity

The beta-blocking effect of sotalol is a noncardioselective [half maximal at about 80 mg/day and maximal at doses of 320-640 mg/day]. Significant beta-blockade occurs at oral doses as low as 25 mg/day.

The Class III effects are seen only at oral doses ≥160 mg/day

Drug Interactions

Increased Effect/Toxicity: Increased effect/toxicity of beta-blockers with calcium blockers since there may be additive effects on AV conduction or ventricular function. Other agents which prolong QT interval, including Class I antiarrhythmic agents, bepridil, cisapride, erythromycin, haloperidol, pimozide, phenothiazines, tricyclic antidepressants, and specific quinolones (including sparfloxacin, gatifloxacin, moxifloxacin) may increase the effect of sotalol on the prolongation of QT interval. Amiodarone may cause additive effects on QT_c prolongation as well as decreased heart rate, and has been associated with cardiac arrest in patients receiving some beta-blockers. When used concurrently with clonidine, sotalol may increase the risk of rebound hypertension after or during withdrawal of either agent. Beta-blocker and catecholamine depleting agents (reserpine or guanethidine) may result in additive hypotension or bradycardia. Beta-blockers may increase the action or levels of ethanol, nondepolarizing muscle relaxants, and theophylline although the effects are difficult to predict.

Decreased Effect: Decreased effect of sotalol may occur with aluminum-magnesium antacids (if taken within 2 hours), aluminum salts, barbiturates, calcium salts, cholestyramine, colestipol, NSAIDs, penicillins (ampicillin), rifampin, salicylates, and sulfinpyrazone due to decreased bioavailability and plasma levels. Beta-blockers may decrease the effect of sulfonylureas. Beta-agonists such as albuterol, terbutaline may have less of a therapeutic effect when administered concomitantly.

Pharmacodynamics/Kinetics

Onset of action: Rapid, 1-2 hours

Peak effect: 2.5-4 hours

Duration: 8-16 hours

Absorption: Decreased 20% to 30% by meals compared to fasting

Distribution: Low lipid solubility; enters milk of laboratory animals and is reported to be present in human milk

Protein binding: None

Metabolism: None

Bioavailability: 90% to 100%

Half-life elimination: 12 hours; Children: 9.5 hours; terminal half-life decreases with age <2 years (may by ≥1 week in neonates)

Excretion: Urine (as unchanged drug)

Pregnancy Risk Factor B

Sotalol Hydrochloride *see* Sotalol *on page 1231*

Sotret® *see* Isotretinoin *on page 773*

Spacol *see* Hyoscyamine *on page 724*

Spacol T/S *see* Hyoscyamine *on page 724*

Sparfloxacin (spar FLOKS a sin)

U.S. Brand Names Zagam®

Generic Available No

Pharmacologic Category Antibiotic, Quinolone

Use Treatment of adults with community-acquired pneumonia caused by *C. pneumoniae*, *H. influenzae*, *H. parainfluenzae*, *M. catarrhalis*, *M. pneumoniae* or *S. pneumoniae*; treatment of acute bacterial exacerbations of chronic bronchitis caused by *C. pneumoniae*, *E. cloacae*, *H. influenzae*, *H. parainfluenzae*, *K. pneumoniae*, *M. catarrhalis*, *S. aureus* or *S. pneumoniae*

Local Anesthetic/Vasoconstrictor Precautions No information available to require special precautions

Effects on Dental Treatment Key adverse event(s) related to dental treatment: Taste perversion.

Common Adverse Effects 1% to 10%:

Cardiovascular: QT_c interval prolongation (1%), vasodilation (1%)

Central nervous system: Insomnia (2%), dizziness (2%), headache (4%)

Dermatologic: Photosensitivity reaction (8%; severe <1%), pruritus (2%)

Gastrointestinal: Diarrhea (5%), dyspepsia (2%), nausea (4%), abdominal pain (2%), vomiting (1%), flatulence (1%), taste perversion (2%)

Hepatic: Increased LFTs

Mechanism of Action Inhibits DNA-gyrase in susceptible organisms; inhibits relaxation of supercoiled DNA and promotes breakage of double-stranded DNA

Drug Interactions

Increased Effect/Toxicity: Quinolones cause increased levels of warfarin and cyclosporine. Cimetidine, and probenecid increase quinolone levels. An increased incidence of seizures may occur with foscarnet and NSAIDs. Sparfloxacin does not appear to alter warfarin levels, but warfarin effect may be increased due possible effects on gastrointestinal flora. Concurrent use of corticosteroids may increase risk of tendon rupture.

Decreased Effect: Decreased absorption with antacids containing aluminum, magnesium, and/or calcium, sucralfate, didanosine and by products containing zinc and iron salts when administered concurrently. Take >4 hours after sparfloxacin. Phenytoin serum levels may be reduced by

(Continued)

Sparfloxacin *(Continued)*

quinolones; antineoplastic agents may also decrease serum levels of fluoroquinolones

Pharmacodynamics/Kinetics

Absorption: Unaffected by food or milk; reduced ~50% by concurrent administration of aluminum- and magnesium-containing antacids

Distribution: Widely throughout the body; V_d: 3.9 L/kg

Protein binding: 45%

Metabolism: Hepatic, primarily by phase II glucuronidation

Half-life elimination: Mean terminal: 20 hours (range: 16-30 hours)

Time to peak, serum: 3-5 hours

Excretion: Urine (50%; ~10% as unchanged drug); feces (50%)

Pregnancy Risk Factor C

Spectazole® *see* Econazole *on page 481*

Spectinomycin (spek ti noe MYE sin)

Related Information

Sexually-Transmitted Diseases *on page 1504*

U.S. Brand Names Trobicin®

Mexican Brand Names Trobicin®

Generic Available No

Synonyms Spectinomycin Hydrochloride

Pharmacologic Category Antibiotic, Miscellaneous

Use Treatment of uncomplicated gonorrhea

Local Anesthetic/Vasoconstrictor Precautions No information available to require special precautions

Effects on Dental Treatment No significant effects or complications reported

Mechanism of Action A bacteriostatic antibiotic that selectively binds to the 30s subunits of ribosomes, and thereby inhibiting bacterial protein synthesis

Pharmacodynamics/Kinetics

Duration: Up to 8 hours

Absorption: I.M.: Rapid and almost complete

Distribution: Concentrates in urine; does not distribute well into the saliva

Half-life elimination: 1.7 hours

Time to peak: ~1 hour

Excretion: Urine (70% to 100% as unchanged drug)

Pregnancy Risk Factor B

Spectinomycin Hydrochloride *see* Spectinomycin *on page 1234*

Spectracef™ *see* Cefditoren *on page 280*

Spectrocin Plus™ [OTC] *see* Bacitracin, Neomycin, Polymyxin B, and Pramoxine *on page 180*

Spiramycin (speer a MYE sin)

Canadian Brand Names Rovamycine®

Generic Available No

Pharmacologic Category Antibiotic, Macrolide

Use Treatment of infections of the respiratory tract, buccal cavity, skin and soft tissues due to susceptible organisms. *N. gonorrhoeae*: as an alternate choice of treatment for gonorrhea in patients allergic to the penicillins. Before treatment of gonorrhea, the possibility of concomitant infection due to *T. pallidum* should be excluded.

Unlabeled/Investigational Use Treatment of *Toxoplasma gondii* to prevent transmission from mother to fetus

Local Anesthetic/Vasoconstrictor Precautions No information available to require special precautions

Effects on Dental Treatment No significant effects or complications reported

Common Adverse Effects Frequency not defined.

Central nervous system: Paresthesia (rare)

Dermatologic: Rash, urticaria, pruritus, angioedema (rare)

Gastrointestinal: Nausea, vomiting, diarrhea, pseudomembranous colitis (rare)

Hepatic: Transaminases increased

Miscellaneous: Anaphylactic shock (rare)

Restrictions Not available in U.S.

Mechanism of Action Inhibits growth of susceptible organisms; mechanism not established.

Drug Interactions

Cytochrome P450 Effect: Substrate of CYP3A4 (major)

Increased Effect/Toxicity: CYP3A4 inhibitors may increase the levels/effects of spiramycin; example inhibitors include azole antifungals, ciprofloxacin, clarithromycin, diclofenac, doxycycline, erythromycin, imatinib, isoniazid, nefazodone, nicardipine, propofol, protease inhibitors, quinidine, and verapamil.

Decreased Effect: Spiramycin has been reported to decrease carbidopa absorption and decrease levodopa concentrations. CYP3A4 inducers may decrease the levels/effects of spiramycin; example inducers include aminoglutethimide, carbamazepine, nafcillin, nevirapine, phenobarbital, phenytoin, and rifamycins.

Pregnancy Risk Factor Not assigned (other macrolides rated B); C per expert analysis

Spirapril (SPYE ra pril)

Generic Available No

Pharmacologic Category Angiotensin-Converting Enzyme (ACE) Inhibitor

Use Management of mild to severe hypertension; treatment of left ventricular dysfunction after myocardial infarction

Local Anesthetic/Vasoconstrictor Precautions No information available to require special precautions

Effects on Dental Treatment Key adverse event(s) related to dental treatment: Orthostatic hypotension.

Common Adverse Effects Frequency not defined.

Cardiovascular: Hypotension (orthostatic), angioedema

Central nervous system: Headache, dizziness, migraine headache (exacerbation of), hypoesthesia

Dermatologic: Skin rash

Gastrointestinal: Nausea, diarrhea, vomiting

Neuromuscular & skeletal: Back pain

Ocular: Conjunctivitis

Respiratory: Cough

Restrictions Not available in U.S.

Mechanism of Action ACE inhibitor; inhibits renin-angiotensin system

Pharmacodynamics/Kinetics

Absorption: 53% to 60%; delayed by high fat meals

Half-life elimination, serum: 1-2 hours

Pregnancy Risk Factor C (1st trimester); D (2nd and 3rd trimesters)

Spiriva® *see* Tiotropium *on page 1303*

Spironolactone (speer on oh LAK tone)

Related Information

Cardiovascular Diseases *on page 1458*

U.S. Brand Names Aldactone®

Canadian Brand Names Aldactone®; Novo-Spiroton

Mexican Brand Names Aldactone®

Generic Available Yes

Pharmacologic Category Diuretic, Potassium-Sparing; Selective Aldosterone Blocker

Use Management of edema associated with excessive aldosterone excretion; hypertension; primary hyperaldosteronism; hypokalemia; treatment of hirsutism; cirrhosis of liver accompanied by edema or ascites. The benefits of spironolactone were additive to the benefits of ACE inhibition in patients with severe CHF (further reducing mortality by 30% over 2 years) in RALES - a large controlled clinical trial.

Local Anesthetic/Vasoconstrictor Precautions No information available to require special precautions

Effects on Dental Treatment No significant effects or complications reported

Common Adverse Effects Incidence of adverse events is not always reported. (Mean daily dose: 26 mg)

Cardiovascular: Edema (2%, placebo 2%)

Central nervous system: Disorders (23%, placebo 21%) which may include drowsiness, lethargy, headache, mental confusion, drug fever, ataxia, fatigue

Dermatologic: Maculopapular, erythematous cutaneous eruptions, urticaria, hirsutism, eosinophilia

Endocrine & metabolic: Gynecomastia (men 9%; placebo 1%), breast pain (men 2%; placebo 0.1%), serious hyperkalemia (2%, placebo 1%), hyponatremia, dehydration, hyperchloremic metabolic acidosis in decompensated

(Continued)

Spironolactone *(Continued)*

hepatic cirrhosis, inability to achieve or maintain an erection, irregular menses, amenorrhea, postmenopausal bleeding

Gastrointestinal: Disorders (29%, placebo 29%) which may include anorexia, nausea, cramping, diarrhea, gastric bleeding, ulceration, gastritis, vomiting

Genitourinary: Disorders (12%, placebo 11%)

Hematologic: Agranulocytosis

Hepatic: Cholestatic/hepatocellular toxicity

Renal: Increased BUN concentration

Respiratory: Disorders (32%, placebo 34%)

Miscellaneous: Deepening of the voice, anaphylactic reaction, breast cancer

Dosage To reduce delay in onset of effect, a loading dose of 2 or 3 times the daily dose may be administered on the first day of therapy. Oral:

Neonates: Diuretic: 1-3 mg/kg/day divided every 12-24 hours

Children:

- Diuretic, hypertension: 1.5-3.5 mg/kg/day **or** 60 mg/m^2/day in divided doses every 6-24 hours
- Diagnosis of primary aldosteronism: 125-375 mg/m^2/day in divided doses
- Vaso-occlusive disease: 7.5 mg/kg/day in divided doses twice daily (not FDA approved)

Adults:

- Edema, hypokalemia: 25-200 mg/day in 1-2 divided doses
- Hypertension (JNC 7): 25-50 mg/day in 1-2 divided doses
- Diagnosis of primary aldosteronism: 100-400 mg/day in 1-2 divided doses
- Hirsutism in women: 50-200 mg/day in 1-2 divided doses
- CHF, severe (with ACE inhibitor and a loop diuretic ± digoxin): 25 mg/day, increased or reduced depending on individual response and evidence of hyperkalemia

Elderly: Initial: 25-50 mg/day in 1-2 divided doses, increasing by 25-50 mg every 5 days as needed.

Dosing interval in renal impairment:

- Cl_{cr} 10-50 mL/minute: Administer every 12-24 hours.
- Cl_{cr} <10 mL/minute: Avoid use.

Mechanism of Action Competes with aldosterone for receptor sites in the distal renal tubules, increasing sodium chloride and water excretion while conserving potassium and hydrogen ions; may block the effect of aldosterone on arteriolar smooth muscle as well

Contraindications Hypersensitivity to spironolactone or any component of the formulation; anuria; acute renal insufficiency; significant impairment of renal excretory function; hyperkalemia; pregnancy (pregnancy-induced hypertension - per expert analysis)

Warnings/Precautions Avoid potassium supplements, potassium-containing salt substitutes, a diet rich in potassium, or other drugs that can cause hyperkalemia. Monitor for fluid and electrolyte imbalances. Gynecomastia is related to dose and duration of therapy. Diuretic therapy should be carefully used in severe hepatic dysfunction; electrolyte and fluid shifts can cause or exacerbate encephalopathy. Discontinue use prior to adrenal vein catheterization.

Drug Interactions

Increased Effect/Toxicity: Concurrent use of spironolactone with other potassium-sparing diuretics, potassium supplements, angiotensin receptor antagonists, co-trimoxazole (high dose), and ACE inhibitors can increase the risk of hyperkalemia, especially in patients with renal impairment. Cholestyramine can cause hyperchloremic acidosis in cirrhotic patients; avoid concurrent use.

Decreased Effect: The effects of digoxin (loss of positive inotropic effect) and mitotane may be reduced by spironolactone. Salicylates and NSAIDs (indomethacin) may decrease the natriuretic effect of spironolactone.

Ethanol/Nutrition/Herb Interactions

Food: Food increases absorption.

Herb/Nutraceutical: Avoid natural licorice (due to mineralocorticoid activity)

Dietary Considerations Should be taken with food to decrease gastrointestinal irritation and to increase absorption. Excessive potassium intake (eg, salt substitutes, low-salt foods, bananas, nuts) should be avoided.

Pharmacodynamics/Kinetics

Protein binding: 91% to 98%

Metabolism: Hepatic to multiple metabolites, including canrenone (active)

Half-life elimination: 78-84 minutes

Time to peak, serum: 1-3 hours (primarily as the active metabolite)

Excretion: Urine and feces

Pregnancy Risk Factor C/D in pregnancy-induced hypertension (per expert analysis)

Dosage Forms TAB: 25 mg, 50 mg, 100 mg

Spironolactone and Hydrochlorothiazide *see* Hydrochlorothiazide and Spironolactone *on page 701*
Sporanox® *see* Itraconazole *on page 775*
Sportscreme® [OTC] *see* Triethanolamine Salicylate *on page 1338*
Sprintec™ *see* Ethinyl Estradiol and Norgestimate *on page 554*
SSD® *see* Silver Sulfadiazine *on page 1221*
SSD® AF *see* Silver Sulfadiazine *on page 1221*
SSKI® *see* Potassium Iodide *on page 1106*
Stadol® *see* Butorphanol *on page 240*
Stadol® NS [DSC] *see* Butorphanol *on page 240*
Stagesic® *see* Hydrocodone and Acetaminophen *on page 702*
Stalevo™ *see* Levodopa, Carbidopa, and Entacapone *on page 812*
Standard Conversions *see page 1598*
Stan-gard® *see* Fluoride *on page 603*
Stannous Fluoride *see* Fluoride *on page 603*

Stanozolol (stan OH zoe lole)

U.S. Brand Names Winstrol®

Generic Available No

Pharmacologic Category Anabolic Steroid

Use Prophylactic use against hereditary angioedema

Local Anesthetic/Vasoconstrictor Precautions No information available to require special precautions

Effects on Dental Treatment No significant effects or complications reported

Common Adverse Effects

Male:

Postpubertal:

>10%:

Dermatologic: Acne
Endocrine & metabolic: Gynecomastia
Genitourinary: Bladder irritability, priapism

1% to 10%:

Central nervous system: Insomnia, chills
Endocrine & metabolic: Decreased libido, hepatic dysfunction
Gastrointestinal: Nausea, diarrhea
Genitourinary: Prostatic hyperplasia (elderly)
Hematologic: Iron deficiency anemia, suppression of clotting factors

Prepubertal:

>10%:

Dermatologic: Acne
Endocrine & metabolic: Virilism

1% to 10%:

Central nervous system: Chills, insomnia, factors
Dermatologic: Hyperpigmentation
Gastrointestinal: Diarrhea, nausea
Hematologic: Iron deficiency anemia, suppression of clotting

Female:

>10%: Endocrine & metabolic: Virilism

1% to 10%:

Central nervous system: Chills, insomnia
Endocrine & metabolic: Hypercalcemia
Gastrointestinal: Nausea, diarrhea
Hematologic: Iron deficiency anemia, suppression of clotting factors
Hepatic: Hepatic dysfunction

Restrictions C-III

Mechanism of Action Synthetic testosterone derivative with similar androgenic and anabolic actions

Drug Interactions

Increased Effect/Toxicity: ACTH, adrenal steroids may increase risk of edema and acne. Stanozolol enhances the hypoprothrombinemic effects of oral anticoagulants and enhances the hypoglycemic effects of insulin and sulfonylureas (oral hypoglycemics).

Pharmacodynamics/Kinetics

Metabolism: Hepatic
Excretion: Urine (90%); feces (6%)

Pregnancy Risk Factor X

Starlix® *see* Nateglinide *on page 968*

Staticin® *see* Erythromycin *on page 508*

Stavudine (STAV yoo deen)

Related Information

HIV Infection and AIDS *on page 1484*

U.S. Brand Names Zerit®

Canadian Brand Names Zerit®

Mexican Brand Names Zerit®

Generic Available No

Synonyms d4T

Pharmacologic Category Antiretroviral Agent, Reverse Transcriptase Inhibitor (Nucleoside)

Use Treatment of HIV infection in combination with other antiretroviral agents

Local Anesthetic/Vasoconstrictor Precautions No information available to require special precautions

Effects on Dental Treatment No significant effects or complications reported

Common Adverse Effects All adverse reactions reported below were similar to comparative agent, zidovudine, except for peripheral neuropathy, which was greater for stavudine. Selected adverse events reported as monotherapy or in combination therapy include:

>10%:
- Central nervous system: Headache
- Dermatologic: Rash
- Gastrointestinal: Nausea, vomiting, diarrhea
- Hepatic: Hepatic transaminases increased
- Neuromuscular & skeletal: Peripheral neuropathy
- Miscellaneous: Amylase increased

1% to 10%:
- Hepatic: Bilirubin increased

Mechanism of Action Stavudine is a thymidine analog which interferes with HIV viral DNA dependent DNA polymerase resulting in inhibition of viral replication; nucleoside reverse transcriptase inhibitor

Drug Interactions

Increased Effect/Toxicity: Risk of pancreatitis may be increased with concurrent didanosine use; cases of fatal lactic acidosis have been reported with this combination when used during pregnancy (use only if clearly needed). Risk of hepatotoxicity or pancreatitis may be increased with concurrent hydroxyurea use. Zalcitabine may increase risk of peripheral neuropathy; concurrent use not recommended.

Decreased Effect: Zidovudine inhibits intracellular phosphorylation of stavudine; concurrent use not recommended. Doxorubicin may inhibit intracellular phosphorylation of stavudine; use with caution. Ribavirin may inhibit intracellular phosphorylation of stavudine; use with caution.

Pharmacodynamics/Kinetics

Distribution: V_d: 0.5 L/kg
Bioavailability: 86.4%
Metabolism: Undergoes intracellular phosphorylation to an active metabolite
Half-life elimination: 1-1.6 hours
Time to peak, serum: 1 hour
Excretion: Urine (40% as unchanged drug)

Pregnancy Risk Factor C

Stelazine® [DSC] *see* Trifluoperazine *on page 1338*

Sterapred® *see* PredniSONE *on page 1115*

Sterapred® DS *see* PredniSONE *on page 1115*

STI571 *see* Imatinib *on page 734*

Stimate™ *see* Desmopressin *on page 409*

St. Joseph® Adult Aspirin [OTC] *see* Aspirin *on page 151*

Stop® *see* Fluoride *on page 603*

Strattera™ *see* Atomoxetine *on page 161*

Streptase® *see* Streptokinase *on page 1238*

Streptokinase (strep toe KYE nase)

Related Information

Cardiovascular Diseases *on page 1458*

U.S. Brand Names Streptase®

Canadian Brand Names Streptase®

Mexican Brand Names Streptase®

Generic Available No

Synonyms SK

Pharmacologic Category Thrombolytic Agent

Use Thrombolytic agent used in treatment of recent severe or massive deep vein thrombosis, pulmonary emboli, myocardial infarction, and occluded arteriovenous cannulas

Local Anesthetic/Vasoconstrictor Precautions No information available to require special precautions

Effects on Dental Treatment No significant effects or complications reported

Common Adverse Effects As with all drugs which may affect hemostasis, bleeding is the major adverse effect associated with streptokinase. Hemorrhage may occur at virtually any site. Risk is dependent on multiple variables, including the dosage administered, concurrent use of multiple agents which alter hemostasis, and patient predisposition (including hypertension). Rapid lysis of coronary artery thrombi by thrombolytic agents may be associated with reperfusion-related atrial and/or ventricular arrhythmias.

>10%:

- Cardiovascular: Hypotension
- Local: Injection site bleeding

1% to 10%:

- Central nervous system: Fever (1% to 4%)
- Dermatologic: Bruising, rash, pruritus
- Gastrointestinal: Gastrointestinal hemorrhage, nausea, vomiting
- Genitourinary: Genitourinary hemorrhage
- Hematologic: Anemia
- Neuromuscular & skeletal: Muscle pain
- Ocular: Eye hemorrhage, periorbital edema
- Respiratory: Bronchospasm, epistaxis
- Miscellaneous: Diaphoresis hemorrhage, gingival hemorrhage

Additional cardiovascular events associated with use in myocardial infarction: Asystole, AV block, cardiac arrest, cardiac tamponade, cardiogenic shock, electromechanical dissociation, heart failure, mitral regurgitation, myocardial rupture, pericardial effusion, pericarditis, pulmonary edema, recurrent ischemia/infarction, thromboembolism, ventricular tachycardia

Mechanism of Action Activates the conversion of plasminogen to plasmin by forming a complex, exposing plasminogen-activating site, and cleaving a peptide bond that converts plasminogen to plasmin; plasmin degrades fibrin, fibrinogen and other procoagulant proteins into soluble fragments; effective both outside and within the formed thrombus/embolus

Drug Interactions

Increased Effect/Toxicity: The risk of bleeding with streptokinase is increased by oral anticoagulants (warfarin), heparin, low molecular weight heparins, and drugs which affect platelet function (eg, NSAIDs, dipyridamole, ticlopidine, clopidogrel, IIb/IIIa antagonists). Although concurrent use with aspirin and heparin may increase the risk of bleeding. Aspirin and heparin were used concomitantly with streptokinase in the majority of patients in clinical studies of MI.

Decreased Effect: Antifibrinolytic agents (aminocaproic acid) may decrease effectiveness to thrombolytic agents.

Pharmacodynamics/Kinetics

Onset of action: Activation of plasminogen occurs almost immediately

Duration: Fibrinolytic effect: Several hours; Anticoagulant effect: 12-24 hours

Half-life elimination: 83 minutes

Excretion: By circulating antibodies and the reticuloendothelial system

Pregnancy Risk Factor C

Streptomycin (strep toe MYE sin)

Related Information

Tuberculosis *on page 1495*

Generic Available Yes

Synonyms Streptomycin Sulfate

Pharmacologic Category Antibiotic, Aminoglycoside; Antitubercular Agent

Use Part of combination therapy of active tuberculosis; used in combination with other agents for treatment of streptococcal or enterococcal endocarditis, mycobacterial infections, plague, tularemia, and brucellosis

Local Anesthetic/Vasoconstrictor Precautions No information available to require special precautions

Effects on Dental Treatment No significant effects or complications reported

Common Adverse Effects Frequency not defined.

Cardiovascular: Hypotension

(Continued)

Streptomycin *(Continued)*

Central nervous system: Neurotoxicity, drowsiness, headache, drug fever, paresthesia
Dermatologic: Skin rash
Gastrointestinal: Nausea, vomiting
Hematologic: Eosinophilia, anemia
Neuromuscular & skeletal: Arthralgia, weakness, tremor
Otic: Ototoxicity (auditory), ototoxicity (vestibular)
Renal: Nephrotoxicity
Respiratory: Difficulty in breathing

Mechanism of Action Inhibits bacterial protein synthesis by binding directly to the 30S ribosomal subunits causing faulty peptide sequence to form in the protein chain

Drug Interactions

Increased Effect/Toxicity: Increased/prolonged effect with depolarizing and nondepolarizing neuromuscular blocking agents. Concurrent use with amphotericin or loop diuretics may increase nephrotoxicity.

Pharmacodynamics/Kinetics

Absorption: I.M.: Well absorbed
Distribution: To extracellular fluid including serum, abscesses, ascitic, pericardial, pleural, synovial, lymphatic, and peritoneal fluids; crosses placenta; small amounts enter breast milk
Protein binding: 34%
Half-life elimination: Newborns: 4-10 hours; Adults: 2-4.7 hours, prolonged with renal impairment
Time to peak: Within 1 hour
Excretion: Urine (90% as unchanged drug); feces, saliva, sweat, and tears (<1%)

Pregnancy Risk Factor D

Streptomycin Sulfate *see* Streptomycin *on page 1239*

Streptozocin (strep toe ZOE sin)

U.S. Brand Names Zanosar®

Canadian Brand Names Zanosar®

Generic Available No

Synonyms NSC-85998

Pharmacologic Category Antineoplastic Agent, Alkylating Agent

Use Treatment of metastatic islet cell carcinoma of the pancreas, carcinoid tumor and syndrome, Hodgkin's disease, palliative treatment of colorectal cancer

Local Anesthetic/Vasoconstrictor Precautions No information available to require special precautions

Effects on Dental Treatment No significant effects or complications reported

Common Adverse Effects

>10%:

Gastrointestinal: Nausea and vomiting (100%)
Hepatic: Increased LFTs
Miscellaneous: Hypoalbuminemia
Renal: BUN increased, Cl_{cr} decreased, hypophosphatemia, nephrotoxicity (25% to 75%), proteinuria, renal dysfunction (65%), renal tubular acidosis

1% to 10%:

Endocrine & metabolic: Hypoglycemia (6%)
Gastrointestinal: Diarrhea (10%)
Local: Pain at injection site

Mechanism of Action Interferes with the normal function of DNA by alkylation and cross-linking the strands of DNA, and by possible protein modification

Drug Interactions

Increased Effect/Toxicity: Doxorubicin toxicity may be increased with concurrent use of streptozocin. Manufacturer recommends doxorubicin dosage adjustment be considered.

Decreased Effect: Phenytoin results in negation of streptozocin cytotoxicity.

Pharmacodynamics/Kinetics

Duration: Disappears from serum in 4 hours
Distribution: Concentrates in liver, intestine, pancreas, and kidney
Metabolism: Rapidly hepatic
Half-life elimination: 35-40 minutes
Excretion: Urine (60% to 70% as metabolites); exhaled gases (5%); feces (1%)

Pregnancy Risk Factor D

Stresstabs® B-Complex [OTC] *see* Vitamin B Complex Combinations *on page 1382*
Stresstabs® B-Complex + Iron [OTC] *see* Vitamin B Complex Combinations *on page 1382*
Stresstabs® B-Complex + Zinc [OTC] *see* Vitamin B Complex Combinations *on page 1382*
Striant™ *see* Testosterone *on page 1276*
Stri-dex® [OTC] *see* Salicylic Acid *on page 1205*
Stri-dex® Body Focus [OTC] *see* Salicylic Acid *on page 1205*
Stri-dex® Facewipes To Go™ [OTC] *see* Salicylic Acid *on page 1205*
Stri-dex® Maximum Strength [OTC] *see* Salicylic Acid *on page 1205*
Stromectol® *see* Ivermectin *on page 779*
Strong Iodine Solution *see* Potassium Iodide *on page 1106*
Sublimaze® *see* Fentanyl *on page 581*
Suboxone® *see* Buprenorphine and Naloxone *on page 230*
Subutex® *see* Buprenorphine *on page 228*

Succinylcholine (suks in il KOE leen)

U.S. Brand Names Anectine® [DSC]; Quelicin®

Canadian Brand Names Quelicin®

Mexican Brand Names Anectine®

Generic Available Yes

Synonyms Succinylcholine Chloride; Suxamethonium Chloride

Pharmacologic Category Neuromuscular Blocker Agent, Depolarizing

Use Adjunct to general anesthesia to facilitate both rapid sequence and routine endotracheal intubation and to relax skeletal muscles during surgery; to reduce the intensity of muscle contractions of pharmacologically- or electrically-induced convulsions; does not relieve pain or produce sedation

Local Anesthetic/Vasoconstrictor Precautions No information available to require special precautions

Effects on Dental Treatment No significant effects or complications reported

Common Adverse Effects

>10%:

Ocular: Increased intraocular pressure

Miscellaneous: Postoperative stiffness

1% to 10%:

Cardiovascular: Bradycardia, hypotension, cardiac arrhythmias, tachycardia

Gastrointestinal: Intragastric pressure, salivation

Causes of prolonged neuromuscular blockade: Excessive drug administration; cumulative drug effect, decreased metabolism/excretion (hepatic and/or renal impairment); accumulation of active metabolites; electrolyte imbalance (hypokalemia, hypocalcemia, hypermagnesemia, hypernatremia); hypothermia; drug interactions; increased sensitivity to muscle relaxants (eg, neuromuscular disorders such as myasthenia gravis or polymyositis)

Mechanism of Action Acts similar to acetylcholine, produces depolarization of the motor endplate at the myoneural junction which causes sustained flaccid skeletal muscle paralysis produced by state of accommodation that developes in adjacent excitable muscle membranes

Drug Interactions

Increased Effect/Toxicity:

Increased toxicity: Anticholinesterase drugs (neostigmine, physostigmine, or pyridostigmine) in combination with succinylcholine can cause cardiorespiratory collapse; cyclophosphamide, oral contraceptives, lidocaine, thiotepa, pancuronium, lithium, magnesium salts, aprotinin, chloroquine, metoclopramide, terbutaline, and procaine enhance and prolong the effects of succinylcholine

Prolonged neuromuscular blockade: Inhaled anesthetics, local anesthetics, calcium channel blockers, antiarrhythmics (eg, quinidine or procainamide), antibiotics (eg, aminoglycosides, tetracyclines, vancomycin, clindamycin), immunosuppressants (eg, cyclosporine)

Pharmacodynamics/Kinetics

Onset of action: I.M.: 2-3 minutes; I.V.: Complete muscular relaxation: 30-60 seconds

Duration: I.M.: 10-30 minutes; I.V.: 4-6 minutes with single administration

Metabolism: Rapidly hydrolyzed by plasma pseudocholinesterase

Pregnancy Risk Factor C

Succinylcholine Chloride *see* Succinylcholine *on page 1241*
Sucraid® *see* Sacrosidase *on page 1204*

Sucralfate (soo KRAL fate)

Related Information

Management of Patients Undergoing Cancer Therapy *on page 1569*

U.S. Brand Names Carafate®

Canadian Brand Names Apo-Sucralate®; Novo-Sucralate; Nu-Sucralate; PMS-Sucralate; Sulcrate®; Sulcrate® Suspension Plus

Generic Available Yes

Synonyms Aluminum Sucrose Sulfate, Basic

Pharmacologic Category Gastrointestinal Agent, Miscellaneous

Use Short-term management of duodenal ulcers; maintenance of duodenal ulcers

Unlabeled/Investigational Use Gastric ulcers; suspension may be used topically for treatment of stomatitis due to cancer chemotherapy and other causes of esophageal and gastric erosions; GERD, esophagitis; treatment of NSAID mucosal damage; prevention of stress ulcers; postsclerotherapy for esophageal variceal bleeding

Local Anesthetic/Vasoconstrictor Precautions No information available to require special precautions

Effects on Dental Treatment No significant effects or complications reported

Common Adverse Effects 1% to 10%: Gastrointestinal: Constipation

Mechanism of Action Forms a complex by binding with positively charged proteins in exudates, forming a viscous paste-like, adhesive substance. This selectively forms a protective coating that protects the lining against peptic acid, pepsin, and bile salts.

Drug Interactions

Decreased Effect: Sucralfate may alter the absorption of digoxin, phenytoin (hydantoins), warfarin, ketoconazole, quinidine, quinolones, tetracycline, theophylline. Because of the potential for sucralfate to alter the absorption of some drugs; separate administration (take other medications at least 2 hours before sucralfate). The potential for decreased absorption should be considered when alterations in bioavailability are believed to be critical.

Pharmacodynamics/Kinetics

Onset of action: Paste formation and ulcer adhesion: 1-2 hours

Duration: Up to 6 hours

Absorption: Oral: <5%

Distribution: Acts locally at ulcer sites; unbound in GI tract to aluminum and sucrose octasulfate

Metabolism: None

Excretion: Urine (small amounts as unchanged compounds)

Pregnancy Risk Factor B

Sucrets® [OTC] *see* Dyclonine *on page 480*

Sucrets® Original [OTC] *see* Hexylresorcinol *on page 693*

Sudafed® [OTC] *see* Pseudoephedrine *on page 1147*

Sudafed® 12 Hour [OTC] *see* Pseudoephedrine *on page 1147*

Sudafed® 24 Hour [OTC] *see* Pseudoephedrine *on page 1147*

Sudafed® Children's [OTC] *see* Pseudoephedrine *on page 1147*

Sudafed® Severe Cold [OTC] *see* Acetaminophen, Dextromethorphan, and Pseudoephedrine *on page 59*

Sudafed® Sinus & Allergy [OTC] *see* Chlorpheniramine and Pseudoephedrine *on page 315*

Sudafed® Sinus and Cold [OTC] *see* Acetaminophen and Pseudoephedrine *on page 53*

Sudafed® Sinus Headache [OTC] *see* Acetaminophen and Pseudoephedrine *on page 53*

Sudodrin [OTC] *see* Pseudoephedrine *on page 1147*

SudoGest Sinus [OTC] *see* Acetaminophen and Pseudoephedrine *on page 53*

Sufenta® *see* Sufentanil *on page 1242*

Sufentanil (soo FEN ta nil)

U.S. Brand Names Sufenta®

Canadian Brand Names Sufenta®

Generic Available Yes

Synonyms Sufentanil Citrate

Pharmacologic Category Analgesic, Narcotic; General Anesthetic

Use Analgesic supplement in maintenance of balanced general anesthesia

Local Anesthetic/Vasoconstrictor Precautions No information available to require special precautions

Effects on Dental Treatment No significant effects or complications reported

Common Adverse Effects
>10%:
Cardiovascular: Bradycardia, hypotension
Central nervous system: Somnolence
Gastrointestinal: Nausea, vomiting
Respiratory: Respiratory depression
1% to 10%:
Cardiovascular: Cardiac arrhythmias, orthostatic hypotension
Central nervous system: CNS depression, confusion
Gastrointestinal: Biliary spasm
Ocular: Blurred vision

Restrictions C-II

Mechanism of Action Binds to opioid receptors throughout the CNS. Once receptor binding occurs, effects are exerted by opening K+ channels and inhibiting Ca++ channels. These mechanisms increase pain threshold, alter pain perception, inhibit ascending pain pathways; short-acting narcotic

Drug Interactions
Cytochrome P450 Effect: Substrate of CYP3A4 (major)
Increased Effect/Toxicity: Additive effect/toxicity with CNS depressants or beta-blockers. May increase response to neuromuscular-blocking agents. CYP3A4 inhibitors may increase the levels/effects of sufentanil; example inhibitors include azole antifungals, ciprofloxacin, clarithromycin, diclofenac, doxycycline, erythromycin, imatinib, isoniazid, nefazodone, nicardipine, propofol, protease inhibitors, quinidine, and verapamil.

Pharmacodynamics/Kinetics
Onset of action: 1-3 minutes
Duration: Dose dependent
Metabolism: Primarily hepatic

Pregnancy Risk Factor C

Sufentanil Citrate *see* Sufentanil *on page 1242*
Sular® *see* Nisoldipine *on page 988*
Sulbactam and Ampicillin *see* Ampicillin and Sulbactam *on page 126*

Sulconazole (sul KON a zole)

U.S. Brand Names Exelderm®
Canadian Brand Names Exelderm®
Generic Available No
Synonyms Sulconazole Nitrate
Pharmacologic Category Antifungal Agent, Topical
Use Treatment of superficial fungal infections of the skin, including tinea cruris (jock itch), tinea corporis (ringworm), tinea versicolor, and possibly tinea pedis (athlete's foot, cream only)
Local Anesthetic/Vasoconstrictor Precautions No information available to require special precautions
Effects on Dental Treatment No significant effects or complications reported
Common Adverse Effects 1% to 10%:
Dermatologic: Itching
Local: Burning, stinging, redness

Mechanism of Action Substituted imidazole derivative which inhibits metabolic reactions necessary for the synthesis of ergosterol, an essential membrane component. The end result is usually fungistatic; however, sulconazole may act as a fungicide in *Candida albicans* and parapsilosis during certain growth phases.

Drug Interactions
Cytochrome P450 Effect: Inhibits CYP1A2 (weak), 2A6 (weak), 2C8/9 (weak), 2C19 (weak), 2D6 (weak), 2E1 (weak), 3A4 (weak)

Pharmacodynamics/Kinetics
Absorption: Topical: ~8.7% percutaneously
Excretion: Primarily urine

Pregnancy Risk Factor C

Sulconazole Nitrate *see* Sulconazole *on page 1243*
Sulf-10® *see* Sulfacetamide *on page 1244*

Sulfabenzamide, Sulfacetamide, and Sulfathiazole

(sul fa BENZ a mide, sul fa SEE ta mide, & sul fa THYE a zole)

Related Information
Sulfacetamide *on page 1244*

U.S. Brand Names V.V.S.®
Generic Available Yes
(Continued)

Sulfabenzamide, Sulfacetamide, and Sulfathiazole *(Continued)*

Synonyms Triple Sulfa

Pharmacologic Category Antibiotic, Vaginal

Use Treatment of *Haemophilus vaginalis* vaginitis

Local Anesthetic/Vasoconstrictor Precautions No information available to require special precautions

Effects on Dental Treatment No significant effects or complications reported

Common Adverse Effects Frequency not defined.

Dermatologic: Pruritus, urticaria, Stevens-Johnson syndrome
Local: Local irritation
Miscellaneous: Allergic reactions

Mechanism of Action Interferes with microbial folic acid synthesis and growth via inhibition of para-aminobenzoic acid metabolism

Pharmacodynamics/Kinetics

Absorption: Absorption from vagina is variable and unreliable
Metabolism: Primarily via acetylation
Excretion: Urine

Pregnancy Risk Factor C (avoid if near term)

Sulfacetamide (sul fa SEE ta mide)

U.S. Brand Names AK-Sulf®; Bleph®-10; Carmol® Scalp; Klaron®; Ocusulf-10; Ovace™; Sulf-10®

Canadian Brand Names Cetamide™; Diosulf™; Sodium Sulamyd®

Mexican Brand Names Ceta Sulfa®

Generic Available Yes: Ointment, solution

Synonyms Sodium Sulfacetamide; Sulfacetamide Sodium

Pharmacologic Category Antibiotic, Ophthalmic; Antibiotic, Sulfonamide Derivative

Use

Ophthalmic: Treatment and prophylaxis of conjunctivitis due to susceptible organisms; corneal ulcers; adjunctive treatment with systemic sulfonamides for therapy of trachoma

Dermatologic: Scaling dermatosis (seborrheic); bacterial infections of the skin; acne vulgaris

Local Anesthetic/Vasoconstrictor Precautions No information available to require special precautions

Effects on Dental Treatment No significant effects or complications reported

Common Adverse Effects Frequency not defined.

Cardiovascular: Edema
Dermatologic: Burning, erythema, irritation, itching, stinging, Stevens-Johnson syndrome
Ocular (following ophthalmic application): Burning, conjunctivitis, conjunctival hyperemia, corneal ulcers, irritation, stinging
Miscellaneous: Allergic reactions, systemic lupus erythematosus

Mechanism of Action Interferes with bacterial growth by inhibiting bacterial folic acid synthesis through competitive antagonism of PABA

Drug Interactions

Decreased Effect: Silver containing products are incompatible with sulfacetamide solutions.

Pharmacodynamics/Kinetics

Half-life elimination: 7-13 hours
Excretion: When absorbed, primarily urine (as unchanged drug)

Pregnancy Risk Factor C

Sulfacetamide and Fluorometholone

(sul fa SEE ta mide SOW dee um & flure oh METH oh lone)

Related Information

Fluorometholone *on page 605*
Sulfacetamide *on page 1244*

U.S. Brand Names FML-S®

Generic Available No

Synonyms Fluorometholone and Sulfacetamide

Pharmacologic Category Antibiotic/Corticosteroid, Ophthalmic

Use Steroid-responsive inflammatory ocular conditions where infection is present or there is a risk of infection

Local Anesthetic/Vasoconstrictor Precautions No information available to require special precautions

Effects on Dental Treatment No significant effects or complications reported

Pregnancy Risk Factor C

Sulfacetamide and Prednisolone

(sul fa SEE ta mide & pred NIS oh lone)

Related Information

PrednisoLONE *on page 1113*

Sulfacetamide *on page 1244*

U.S. Brand Names Blephamide®; Vasocidin®

Canadian Brand Names Blephamide®; Dioptimyd®; Vasocidin®

Generic Available Yes: Suspension

Synonyms Prednisolone and Sulfacetamide

Pharmacologic Category Antibiotic/Corticosteroid, Ophthalmic

Use Steroid-responsive inflammatory ocular conditions where infection is present or there is a risk of infection; ophthalmic suspension may be used as an otic preparation

Local Anesthetic/Vasoconstrictor Precautions No information available to require special precautions

Effects on Dental Treatment No significant effects or complications reported

Mechanism of Action Interferes with bacterial growth by inhibiting bacterial folic acid synthesis through competitive antagonism of PABA; decreases inflammation by suppression of migration of polymorphonuclear leukocytes and reversal of increased capillary permeability; suppresses the immune system by reducing activity and volume of the lymphatic system

Pregnancy Risk Factor C

Sulfacetamide Sodium *see* Sulfacetamide *on page 1244*

SulfaDIAZINE (sul fa DYE a zeen)

Generic Available Yes

Pharmacologic Category Antibiotic, Sulfonamide Derivative

Use Treatment of urinary tract infections and nocardiosis; adjunctive treatment in toxoplasmosis; uncomplicated attack of malaria

Unlabeled/Investigational Use Rheumatic fever prophylaxis

Local Anesthetic/Vasoconstrictor Precautions No information available to require special precautions

Effects on Dental Treatment No significant effects or complications reported

Mechanism of Action Interferes with bacterial growth by inhibiting bacterial folic acid synthesis through competitive antagonism of PABA

Pregnancy Risk Factor B/D (at term)

Sulfadoxine and Pyrimethamine

(sul fa DOKS een & peer i METH a meen)

Related Information

Pyrimethamine *on page 1154*

U.S. Brand Names Fansidar®

Generic Available No

Synonyms Pyrimethamine and Sulfadoxine

Pharmacologic Category Antimalarial Agent

Use Treatment of *Plasmodium falciparum* malaria in patients in whom chloroquine resistance is suspected; malaria prophylaxis for travelers to areas where chloroquine-resistant malaria is endemic

Local Anesthetic/Vasoconstrictor Precautions No information available to require special precautions

Effects on Dental Treatment No significant effects or complications reported

Common Adverse Effects Frequency not defined.

Cardiovascular: Myocarditis (allergic), pericarditis (allergic), periorbital edema

Central nervous system: Ataxia, hallucinations, headache, polyneuritis, seizures

Dermatologic: Photosensitization, Stevens-Johnson syndrome, erythema multiforme, toxic epidermal necrolysis, rash

Endocrine & metabolic: Thyroid function dysfunction

Gastrointestinal: Anorexia, atrophic glossitis, gastritis, pancreatitis, vomiting

Genitourinary: Crystalluria

Hematologic: Megaloblastic anemia, leukopenia, thrombocytopenia, pancytopenia

Hepatic: Hepatic necrosis, hepatitis

Neuromuscular & skeletal: Tremors

Renal: BUN increased, interstitial nephritis, renal failure, serum creatinine increased

Respiratory: Respiratory failure, alveolitis (resembling eosinophilic or allergic)

(Continued)

Sulfadoxine and Pyrimethamine *(Continued)*

Miscellaneous: Anaphylactoid reaction, drug fever, hypersensitivity, Lupus-like syndrome, periarteritis nodosum

Mechanism of Action Sulfadoxine interferes with bacterial folic acid synthesis and growth via competitive inhibition of para-aminiobenzoic acid; pyrimethamine inhibits microbial dihydrofolate reductase, resulting in inhibition of tetrahydrofolic acid synthesis

Drug Interactions

Cytochrome P450 Effect: Pyrimethamine: **Inhibits** CYP2C8/9 (moderate), 2D6 (moderate)

Increased Effect/Toxicity: Effect of oral hypoglycemics (rare, but severe) may occur. Combination with methenamine may result in crystalluria; avoid use. May increase methotrexate-induced bone marrow suppression. NSAIDs and salicylates may increase sulfonamide concentrations. Pyrimethamine may increase the levels/effects of amiodarone, amphetamines, selected beta-blockers, dextromethorphan, fluoxetine, glimepiride, glipizide, lidocaine, mirtazapine, nateglinide, nefazodone, paroxetine, phenytoin, pioglitazone, risperidone, ritonavir, rosiglitazone, sertraline, thioridazine, tricyclic antidepressants, venlafaxine, warfarin, and other CYP2C8/9 and 2D6 substrates.

Decreased Effect: Cyclosporine concentrations may be decreased; monitor levels and renal function. PABA (para-aminobenzoic acid - may be found in some vitamin supplements): interferes with the antibacterial activity of sulfonamides; avoid concurrent use. Pyrimethamine may decrease the levels/effects of CYP2D6 prodrug substrates (eg, codeine, hydrocodone, oxycodone, tramadol).

Pharmacodynamics/Kinetics

Absorption: Well absorbed

Distribution: Sulfadoxine: Well distributed like other sulfonamides; Pyrimethamine: Widely distributed, mainly in blood cells, kidneys, lungs, liver, and spleen

Metabolism: Pyrimethamine: Hepatic; Sulfadoxine: None

Half-life elimination: Pyrimethamine: 80-95 hours; Sulfadoxine: 5-8 days

Time to peak, serum: 2-8 hours

Excretion: Urine (as unchanged drug and several unidentified metabolites)

Pregnancy Risk Factor C/D (at term)

Sulfamethoxazole and Trimethoprim

(sul fa meth OKS a zole & trye METH oh prim)

Related Information

Animal and Human Bites Guidelines *on page 1582*
Sexually-Transmitted Diseases *on page 1504*
Trimethoprim *on page 1341*

U.S. Brand Names Bactrim™; Bactrim™ DS; Septra®; Septra® DS

Canadian Brand Names Apo-Sulfatrim®; Novo-Trimel; Novo-Trimel D.S.; Nu-Cotrimox; Septra®; Septra® DS; Septra® Injection

Generic Available Yes

Synonyms Co-Trimoxazole; SMZ-TMP; Sulfatrim; TMP-SMZ; Trimethoprim and Sulfamethoxazole

Pharmacologic Category Antibiotic, Sulfonamide Derivative; Antibiotic, Miscellaneous

Use

Oral treatment of urinary tract infections due to *E. coli*, *Klebsiella* and *Enterobacter* sp, *M. morganii*, *P. mirabilis* and *P. vulgaris*; acute otitis media in children and acute exacerbations of chronic bronchitis in adults due to susceptible strains of *H. influenzae* or *S. pneumoniae*; prophylaxis of *Pneumocystis carinii* pneumonitis (PCP), traveler's diarrhea due to enterotoxigenic *E. coli* or *Cyclospora*

I.V. treatment or severe or complicated infections when oral therapy is not feasible, for documented PCP, empiric treatment of PCP in immune compromised patients; treatment of documented or suspected shigellosis, typhoid fever, *Nocardia asteroides* infection, or other infections caused by susceptible bacteria

Unlabeled/Investigational Use Cholera and salmonella-type infections and nocardiosis; chronic prostatitis; as prophylaxis in neutropenic patients with *P. carinii* infections, in leukemics, and in patients following renal transplantation, to decrease incidence of PCP

Local Anesthetic/Vasoconstrictor Precautions No information available to require special precautions

Effects on Dental Treatment No significant effects or complications reported

Common Adverse Effects The most common adverse reactions include gastrointestinal upset (nausea, vomiting, anorexia) and dermatologic reactions (rash or urticaria). Rare, life-threatening reactions have been associated with co-trimoxazole, including severe dermatologic reactions and hepatotoxic reactions. Most other reactions listed are rare, however, frequency cannot be accurately estimated.

Cardiovascular: Allergic myocarditis

Central nervous system: Confusion, depression, hallucinations, seizures, aseptic meningitis, peripheral neuritis, fever, ataxia, kernicterus in neonates

Dermatologic: Rashes, pruritus, urticaria, photosensitivity; rare reactions include erythema multiforme, Stevens-Johnson syndrome, toxic epidermal necrolysis, exfoliative dermatitis, and Henoch-Schönlein purpura

Endocrine & metabolic: Hyperkalemia (generally at high dosages), hypoglycemia

Gastrointestinal: Nausea, vomiting, anorexia, stomatitis, diarrhea, pseudomembranous colitis, pancreatitis

Hematologic: Thrombocytopenia, megaloblastic anemia, granulocytopenia, eosinophilia, pancytopenia, aplastic anemia, methemoglobinemia, hemolysis (with G6PD deficiency), agranulocytosis

Hepatic: Elevated serum transaminases, hepatotoxicity (including hepatitis, cholestasis, and hepatic necrosis), hyperbilirubinemia

Neuromuscular & skeletal: Arthralgia, myalgia, rhabdomyolysis

Renal: Interstitial nephritis, crystalluria, renal failure, nephrotoxicity (in association with cyclosporine), diuresis

Respiratory: Cough, dyspnea, pulmonary infiltrates

Miscellaneous: Serum sickness, angioedema, periarteritis nodosa (rare), systemic lupus erythematosus (rare)

Dosage Dosage recommendations are based on the trimethoprim component

Children >2 months:

- Mild to moderate infections: Oral, I.V.: 8 mg TMP/kg/day in divided doses every 12 hours
- Serious infection/*Pneumocystis*: I.V.: 20 mg TMP/kg/day in divided doses every 6 hours
- Urinary tract infection prophylaxis: Oral: 2 mg TMP/kg/dose daily
- Prophylaxis of *Pneumocystis*: Oral, I.V.: 10 mg TMP/kg/day or 150 mg TMP/m^2/day in divided doses every 12 hours for 3 days/week; dose should not exceed 320 mg trimethoprim and 1600 mg sulfamethoxazole 3 days/week
- Cholera: Oral, I.V.: 5 mg TMP/kg twice daily for 3 days
- *Cyclospora:* Oral, I.V.: 5 mg TMP/kg twice daily for 7 days

Adults:

- Urinary tract infection/chronic bronchitis: Oral: 1 double strength tablet every 12 hours for 10-14 days
- Sepsis: I.V.: 20 TMP/kg/day divided every 6 hours
- *Pneumocystis carinii*:
  - Prophylaxis: Oral: 1 double strength tablet daily or 3 times/week
  - Treatment: Oral, I.V.: 15-20 mg TMP/kg/day in 3-4 divided doses
- Cholera: Oral, I.V.: 160 mg TMP twice daily for 3 days
- *Cyclospora:* Oral, I.V.: 160 mg TMP twice daily for 7 days
- *Nocardia*: Oral, I.V.: 640 mg TMP/day in divided doses for several months (duration is controversial; an average of 7 months has been reported)

Dosing adjustment in renal impairment: Adults:

I.V.:

- Cl_{cr} 15-30 mL/minute: Administer 2.5-5 mg/kg every 12 hours
- Cl_{cr} <15 mL/minute: Administer 2.5-5 mg/kg every 24 hours

Oral:

- Cl_{cr} 15-30 mL/minute: Administer 1 double strength tablet every 24 hours or 1 single strength tablet every 12 hours
- Cl_{cr} <15 mL/minute: Not recommended

Mechanism of Action Sulfamethoxazole interferes with bacterial folic acid synthesis and growth via inhibition of dihydrofolic acid formation from para-aminobenzoic acid; trimethoprim inhibits dihydrofolic acid reduction to tetrahydrofolate resulting in sequential inhibition of enzymes of the folic acid pathway

Contraindications Hypersensitivity to any sulfa drug, trimethoprim, or any component of the formulation; porphyria; megaloblastic anemia due to folate deficiency; infants <2 months of age; marked hepatic damage; severe renal disease; pregnancy (at term)

Warnings/Precautions Use with caution in patients with G6PD deficiency, impaired renal or hepatic function or potential folate deficiency (malnourished, chronic anticonvulsant therapy, or elderly); maintain adequate hydration to

(Continued)

Sulfamethoxazole and Trimethoprim *(Continued)*

prevent crystalluria; adjust dosage in patients with renal impairment. Injection vehicle contains benzyl alcohol and sodium metabisulfite.

Chemical similarities are present among sulfonamides, sulfonylureas, carbonic anhydrase inhibitors, thiazides, and loop diuretics (except ethacrynic acid). Use in patients with sulfonamide allergy is specifically contraindicated in product labeling, however, a risk of cross-reaction exists in patients with allergy to any of these compounds; avoid use when previous reaction has been severe.

Fatalities associated with severe reactions including Stevens-Johnson syndrome, toxic epidermal necrolysis, hepatic necrosis, agranulocytosis, aplastic anemia and other blood dyscrasias; discontinue use at first sign of rash. Elderly patients appear at greater risk for more severe adverse reactions. May cause hypoglycemia, particularly in malnourished, or patients with renal or hepatic impairment. Use with caution in patients with porphyria or thyroid dysfunction. Slow acetylators may be more prone to adverse reactions. Caution in patients with allergies or asthma. May cause hyperkalemia (associated with high doses of trimethoprim). Incidence of adverse effects appears to be increased in patients with AIDS.

Drug Interactions

Cytochrome P450 Effect:

Sulfamethoxazole: **Substrate** of CYP2C8/9 (major), 3A4 (minor); **Inhibits** CYP2C8/9 (moderate)

Trimethoprim: **Substrate** (major) of CYP2C8/9, 3A4; **Inhibits** CYP2C8/9 (moderate)

Increased Effect/Toxicity: Sulfamethoxazole/trimethoprim may increase toxicity of methotrexate. Sulfamethoxazole/trimethoprim may increase the serum levels of procainamide. Concurrent therapy with pyrimethamine (in doses >25 mg/week) may increase the risk of megaloblastic anemia. Sulfamethoxazole/trimethoprim may increase the levels/effects of amiodarone, fluoxetine, glimepiride, glipizide, nateglinide, phenytoin, pioglitazone, rosiglitazone, sertraline, warfarin, and other CYP2C8/9 substrates.

ACE inhibitors, angiotensin receptor antagonists, or potassium-sparing diuretics may increase the risk of hyperkalemia. Concurrent use with cyclosporine may result in an increased risk of nephrotoxicity when used with sulfamethoxazole/trimethoprim. Trimethoprim may increase the serum concentration of dapsone.

Decreased Effect: The levels/effects of sulfamethoxazole may be decreased by carbamazepine, phenobarbital, phenytoin, rifampin, rifapentine, secobarbital, and other CYP2C8/9 inducers. Although occasionally recommended to limit or reverse hematologic toxicity of high-dose sulfamethoxazole/trimethoprim, concurrent use has been associated with a decreased effectiveness in treating *Pneumocystis carinii*.

Ethanol/Nutrition/Herb Interactions Herb/Nutraceutical: Avoid dong quai, St John's wort (may also cause photosensitization).

Dietary Considerations Should be taken with 8 oz of water on empty stomach.

Pharmacodynamics/Kinetics

Absorption: Oral: Almost completely, 90% to 100%

Protein binding: SMX: 68%, TMP: 45%

Metabolism: SMX: N-acetylated and glucuronidated; TMP: Metabolized to oxide and hydroxylated metabolites

Half-life elimination: SMX: 9 hours, TMP: 6-17 hours; both are prolonged in renal failure

Time to peak, serum: Within 1-4 hours

Excretion: Both are excreted in urine as metabolites and unchanged drug

Effects of aging on the pharmacokinetics of both agents has been variable; increase in half-life and decreases in clearance have been associated with reduced creatinine clearance

Pregnancy Risk Factor C/D (at term - expert analysis)

Dosage Forms Note: The 5:1 ratio (SMX:TMP) remains constant in all dosage forms. **INJ, solution:** Sulfamethoxazole 80 mg and trimethoprim 16 mg per mL (5 mL, 10 mL, 30 mL); (Septra®): Sulfamethoxazole 80 mg and trimethoprim 16 mg per mL (10 mL, 20 mL). **SUSP, oral:** Sulfamethoxazole 200 mg and trimethoprim 40 mg per 5 mL (20 mL, 100 mL, 480 mL); (Septra®): Sulfamethoxazole 200 mg and trimethoprim 40 mg per 5 mL (100 mL, 480 mL). **TAB:** Sulfamethoxazole 400 mg and trimethoprim 80 mg; (Bactrim™, Septra®): Sulfamethoxazole 400 mg and trimethoprim 80 mg. **TAB, double strength:**

Sulfamethoxazole 800 mg and trimethoprim 160 mg; (Bactrim™ DS, Septra® DS): Sulfamethoxazole 800 mg and trimethoprim 160 mg

Sulfamylon® *see* Mafenide *on page 852*

Sulfasalazine (sul fa SAL a zeen)

U.S. Brand Names Azulfidine®; Azulfidine® EN-tabs®

Canadian Brand Names Alti-Sulfasalazine; Salazopyrin®; Salazopyrin En-Tabs®

Generic Available Yes: Tablet; excludes delayed release

Synonyms Salicylazosulfapyridine

Pharmacologic Category 5-Aminosalicylic Acid Derivative

Use Management of ulcerative colitis; enteric coated tablets are also used for rheumatoid arthritis (including juvenile rheumatoid arthritis) in patients who inadequately respond to analgesics and NSAIDs

Unlabeled/Investigational Use Ankylosing spondylitis, collagenous colitis, Crohn's disease, psoriasis, psoriatic arthritis, juvenile chronic arthritis

Local Anesthetic/Vasoconstrictor Precautions No information available to require special precautions

Effects on Dental Treatment No significant effects or complications reported

Common Adverse Effects

>10%:

Central nervous system: Headache (33%)

Dermatologic: Photosensitivity

Gastrointestinal: Anorexia, nausea, vomiting, diarrhea (33%), gastric distress

Genitourinary: Reversible oligospermia (33%)

<3%:

Dermatologic: Urticaria/pruritus (<3%)

Hematologic: Hemolytic anemia (<3%), Heinz body anemia (<3%)

Additional events reported with sulfonamides and/or 5-ASA derivatives: Cholestatic jaundice, eosinophilia pneumonitis, erythema multiforme, fibrosing alveolitis, hepatic necrosis, Kawasaki-like syndrome, SLE-like syndrome, pericarditis, seizures, transverse myelitis

Mechanism of Action Acts locally in the colon to decrease the inflammatory response and systemically interferes with secretion by inhibiting prostaglandin synthesis

Drug Interactions

Increased Effect/Toxicity: Sulfasalazine may increase hydantoin levels. Effects of thiopental, oral hypoglycemics, and oral anticoagulants may be increased. Sulfasalazine may increase the risk of myelosuppression with azathioprine, mercaptopurine, or thioguanine (due to TPMT inhibition); may also increase the toxicity of methotrexate. Risk of thrombocytopenia may be increased with thiazide diuretics. Concurrent methenamine may increase risk of crystalluria.

Decreased Effect: Decreased effect with iron, digoxin and PABA or PABA metabolites of drugs (eg, procaine, proparacaine, tetracaine).

Pharmacodynamics/Kinetics

Absorption: 10% to 15% as unchanged drug from small intestine

Distribution: Small amounts enter feces and breast milk

Metabolism: Via colonic intestinal flora to sulfapyridine and 5-aminosalicylic acid (5-ASA); following absorption, sulfapyridine undergoes N-acetylation and ring hydroxylation while 5-ASA undergoes N-acetylation

Half-life elimination: 5.7-10 hours

Excretion: Primarily urine (as unchanged drug, components, and acetylated metabolites)

Pregnancy Risk Factor B/D (at term)

Sulfatrim *see* Sulfamethoxazole and Trimethoprim *on page 1246*

Sulfinpyrazone (sul fin PEER a zone)

Canadian Brand Names Apo-Sulfinpyrazone®; Nu-Sulfinpyrazone

Generic Available Yes

Synonyms Anturane

Pharmacologic Category Uricosuric Agent

Use Treatment of chronic gouty arthritis and intermittent gouty arthritis

Unlabeled/Investigational Use To decrease the incidence of sudden death postmyocardial infarction

Local Anesthetic/Vasoconstrictor Precautions No information available to require special precautions

Effects on Dental Treatment No significant effects or complications reported

Common Adverse Effects Frequency not defined.

Cardiovascular: Flushing

(Continued)

Sulfinpyrazone *(Continued)*

Central nervous system: Dizziness, headache
Dermatologic: Dermatitis, rash
Gastrointestinal (most frequent adverse effects): Nausea, vomiting, stomach pain
Genitourinary: Polyuria
Hematologic: Anemia, leukopenia, increased bleeding time (decreased platelet aggregation)
Hepatic: Hepatic necrosis
Renal: Nephrotic syndrome, uric acid stones

Mechanism of Action Acts by increasing the urinary excretion of uric acid, thereby decreasing blood urate levels; this effect is therapeutically useful in treating patients with acute intermittent gout, chronic tophaceous gout, and acts to promote resorption of tophi; also has antithrombic and platelet inhibitory effects

Drug Interactions

Cytochrome P450 Effect: Substrate of CYP2C8/9 (major), 3A4 (minor); **Inhibits** CYP2C8/9 (moderate); **Induces** CYP3A4 (weak)

Increased Effect/Toxicity: Risk of acetaminophen hepatotoxicity is increased, while therapeutic effects may be reduced. Sulfinpyrazone may increase the levels/effects of CYP2C8/9 substrates (eg, amiodarone, fluoxetine, glimepiride, glipizide, nateglinide, phenytoin, pioglitazone, rosiglitazone, sertraline, warfarin).

Decreased Effect: CYP2C8/9 inducers may decrease the levels/effects of sulfinpyrazone; example inducers include carbamazepine, phenobarbital, phenytoin, rifampin, rifapentine, and secobarbital. Decreased effect/levels of theophylline, verapamil. Decreased uricosuric activity with salicylates, niacins.

Pharmacodynamics/Kinetics

Absorption: Rapid and complete
Metabolism: Hepatic to two active metabolites
Half-life elimination: 2.7-6 hours
Time to peak, serum: 1.6 hours
Excretion: Urine (22% to 50% as unchanged drug)

Pregnancy Risk Factor C/D (near term - expert analysis)

SulfiSOXAZOLE (sul fi SOKS a zole)

U.S. Brand Names Gantrisin®

Canadian Brand Names Novo-Soxazole®; Sulfizole®

Generic Available Yes: Tablet

Synonyms Sulfisoxazole Acetyl; Sulphafurazole

Pharmacologic Category Antibiotic, Sulfonamide Derivative

Use Treatment of urinary tract infections, otitis media, *Chlamydia*; nocardiosis

Local Anesthetic/Vasoconstrictor Precautions No information available to require special precautions

Effects on Dental Treatment No significant effects or complications reported

Mechanism of Action Interferes with bacterial growth by inhibiting bacterial folic acid synthesis through competitive antagonism of PABA

Pregnancy Risk Factor B/D (near term)

Sulfisoxazole Acetyl *see* SulfiSOXAZOLE *on page 1250*

Sulfisoxazole and Erythromycin *see* Erythromycin and Sulfisoxazole *on page 512*

Sulfonated Phenolics in Aqueous Solution

U.S. Brand Names Debacterol®

Generic Available No

Pharmacologic Category Aphthous Ulcer Treatment Agent

Dental Use Therapeutic cauterization in the treatment of oral mucosal lesions (aphthous stomatitis, gingivitis, moderate to severe periodontitis)

Local Anesthetic/Vasoconstrictor Precautions No information available to require special precautions

Effects on Dental Treatment No significant effects or complications reported

Significant Adverse Effects Frequency not defined: Local: Irritation upon administration

Mechanism of Action Semiviscous, chemical cautery agent which provides controlled, focal debridement and sterilization of necrotic tissues; relieving pain, sealing damaged tissue, and providing local antiseptic action

Contraindications For external use only

Warnings/Precautions Prolonged use of Debacterol® on normal tissue should be avoided. If ingested, do not induce vomiting; immediately dilute with milk or water and get medical help or contact a Poison Control Center. If eye exposure occurs, immediately remove contact lenses, irrigate eyes for at least 15 minutes with lukewarm water, and contact a physician. Safety and efficacy in children <12 years have not been established.

Pregnancy Risk Factor C

Breast-Feeding Considerations Unknown if excreted in breast milk; use with caution

Dosage Forms Solution, topical [for oral mucosa] (Debacterol®): Sulfonated phenolics 22% and sulfuric acid 30% (1 mL)

Comments Prior to application/treatment, the ulcerated mucosal area should be thoroughly dried with a cotton-tipped applicator or similar method. After drying, dip a cotton-tipped applicator into the solution and apply directly to the ulcerated area (most patients experience a brief stinging sensation immediately) and hold the applicator in contact with the ulcer for at least 5-10 seconds. The patient should then thoroughly rinse out the mouth with water and spit out the rinse water. The stinging sensation and ulcer pain will subside almost immediately after the rinse, larger ulcers may require 1-2 minutes for relief. One application per ulcer is usually sufficient. If the ulcer pain returns shortly after rinsing, additional applications may be applied as part of the same treatment session until the ulcer remains pain-free after rinsing. It is not recommended that more than one treatment be applied to each ulcer. If excess irritation occurs during use, a rinse with sodium bicarbonate (baking soda) solution will neutralize the reaction (use 0.5 teaspoon in 120 mL water).

Note: Currently available only by direct distribution to healthcare providers from the manufacturer. Contact Northern Research Laboratories at (888) 884-4675.

Selected Readings

Rhodus NL and Bereuter J, "An Evaluation of a Chemical Cautery Agent and an Anti-inflammatory Ointment for the Treatment of Recurrent Aphthous Stomatitis: A Pilot Study," *Quintessence Int*, 1998, 29(12):769-73.

Sulindac (sul IN dak)

Related Information

Rheumatoid Arthritis, Osteoarthritis, and Osteoporosis *on page 1490*

Temporomandibular Dysfunction (TMD) *on page 1564*

U.S. Brand Names Clinoril®

Canadian Brand Names Apo-Sulin®; Novo-Sundac; Nu-Sundac

Mexican Brand Names Clinoril®; Copal®; Kenalin®

Generic Available Yes

Pharmacologic Category Nonsteroidal Anti-inflammatory Drug (NSAID), Oral

Use Management of inflammatory disease, rheumatoid disorders, acute gouty arthritis, ankylosing spondylitis, bursitis, tendonitis

Local Anesthetic/Vasoconstrictor Precautions No information available to require special precautions

Effects on Dental Treatment NSAID formulations are known to reversibly decrease platelet aggregation via mechanisms different than observed with aspirin. The dentist should be aware of the potential of abnormal coagulation. Caution should also be exercised in the use of NSAIDs in patients already on anticoagulant therapy with drugs such as warfarin (Coumadin®).

Common Adverse Effects 1% to 10%:

Cardiovascular: Edema

Central nervous system: Dizziness, headache, nervousness

Dermatologic: Pruritus, rash

Gastrointestinal: GI pain, heartburn, nausea, vomiting, diarrhea, constipation, flatulence, anorexia, abdominal cramps

Otic: Tinnitus

Mechanism of Action Inhibits prostaglandin synthesis by decreasing the activity of the enzyme, cyclooxygenase, which results in decreased formation of prostaglandin precursors

Drug Interactions

Increased Effect/Toxicity: Increased toxicity with probenecid, NSAIDs. Increased toxicity of digoxin, anticoagulants, methotrexate, lithium, aminoglycosides antibiotics (reported in neonates), cyclosporine (increased nephrotoxicity), and potassium-sparing diuretics (hyperkalemia).

Decreased Effect: Decreased effect of diuretics, beta-blockers, hydralazine, and captopril.

Pharmacodynamics/Kinetics

Onset of action: Analgesic: ~1 hour

(Continued)

Sulindac *(Continued)*

Duration: 12-24 hours
Absorption: 90%
Metabolism: Hepatic; prodrug requiring metabolic activation to sulfide metabolite (active) for therapeutic effects and to sulfone metabolites (inactive)
Half-life elimination: Parent drug: 7 hours; Active metabolite: 18 hours
Excretion: Urine (50%); feces (25%)

Pregnancy Risk Factor B/D (3rd trimester)

Sulphafurazole *see* SulfiSOXAZOLE *on page 1250*

Sumatriptan (soo ma TRIP tan SUKS i nate)

U.S. Brand Names Imitrex®
Canadian Brand Names Imitrex®
Mexican Brand Names Imigran®
Generic Available No
Synonyms Sumatriptan Succinate
Pharmacologic Category Serotonin 5-HT_{1D} Receptor Agonist
Use Acute treatment of migraine with or without aura
Sumatriptan injection: Acute treatment of cluster headache episodes

Local Anesthetic/Vasoconstrictor Precautions No information available to require special precautions

Effects on Dental Treatment Key adverse event(s) related to dental treatment: Bad taste, hyposalivation (tablet), mouth/tongue discomfort (injection).

Common Adverse Effects

>10%:

Central nervous system: Dizziness (injection 12%), warm/hot sensation (injection 11%)
Gastrointestinal: Bad taste (nasal spray 13% to 24%), nausea (nasal spray 11% to 13%), vomiting (nasal spray 11% to 13%)
Local: Injection: Pain at the injection site (59%)
Neuromuscular & skeletal: Tingling (injection 13%)

1% to 10%:

Cardiovascular: Chest pain/tightness/heaviness/pressure (injection 2% to 3%, tablet 1% to 2%)
Central nervous system: Burning (injection 7%), dizziness (nasal spray 1% to 2%, tablet >1%), feeling of heaviness (injection 7%), flushing (injection 7%), pressure sensation (injection 7%), feeling of tightness (injection 5%), numbness (injection 5%), drowsiness (injection 3%, tablet >1%), malaise/fatigue (tablet 2% to 3%, injection 1%), feeling strange (injection 2%), headache (injection 2%, tablet >1%), tight feeling in head (injection 2%), nonspecified pain (tablet 1% to 2%, placebo 1%), vertigo (tablet <1% to 2%, nasal spray 1% to 2%), migraine (tablet >1%), sleepiness (tablet >1%), cold sensation (injection 1%), anxiety (injection 1%)
Gastrointestinal: Nausea (tablet >1%), vomiting (tablet >1%), hyposalivation (tablet >1%), abdominal discomfort (injection 1%), dysphagia (injection 1%)
Neuromuscular & skeletal: Neck, throat, and jaw pain/tightness/pressure (injection 2% to 5%, tablet 2% to 3%), mouth/tongue discomfort (injection 5%), paresthesia (tablet 3% to 5%), weakness (injection 5%), myalgia (injection 2%), muscle cramps (injection 1%)
Ocular: Vision alterations (injection 1%)
Respiratory: Nasal disorder/discomfort (nasal spray 2% to 4%, injection 2%), throat discomfort (injection 3%, nasal spray 1% to 2%)
Miscellaneous: Warm/cold sensation (tablet 2% to 3%, placebo 2%), nonspecified pressure/tightness/heaviness (tablet 1% to 3%, placebo 2%), diaphoresis (injection 2%)

Dosage Adults:

Oral: A single dose of 25 mg, 50 mg, or 100 mg (taken with fluids). If a satisfactory response has not been obtained at 2 hours, a second dose may be administered. Results from clinical trials show that initial doses of 50 mg and 100 mg are more effective than doses of 25 mg, and that 100 mg doses do not provide a greater effect than 50 mg and may have increased incidence of side effects. Although doses of up to 300 mg/day have been studied, the total daily dose should not exceed 200 mg. The safety of treating an average of >4 headaches in a 30-day period have not been established.

Intranasal: A single dose of 5 mg, 10 mg, or 20 mg administered in one nostril. A 10 mg dose may be achieved by administering a single 5 mg dose in each nostril. If headache returns, the dose may be repeated once after 2 hours, not to exceed a total daily dose of 40 mg. The safety of treating an average of >4 headaches in a 30-day period has not been established.

SubQ: 6 mg; a second injection may be administered at least 1 hour after the initial dose, but not more than 2 injections in a 24-hour period. If side effects are dose-limiting, lower doses may be used.

Dosage adjustment in renal impairment: Dosage adjustment not necessary

Dosage adjustment in hepatic impairment: Bioavailability of oral sumatriptan is increased with liver disease. If treatment is needed, do not exceed single doses of 50 mg. The nasal spray has not been studied in patients with hepatic impairment, however, because the spray does not undergo first-pass metabolism, levels would not be expected to alter. Use of all dosage forms is contraindicated with severe hepatic impairment.

Elderly: Due to increased risk of CAD, decreased hepatic function, and more pronounced blood pressure increases, use of the tablet dosage form in elderly patients is not recommended. Use of the nasal spray has not been studied in the elderly. Pharmacokinetics of injectable sumatriptan in the elderly are similar to healthy patients.

Mechanism of Action Selective agonist for serotonin (5-HT_{1D} receptor) in cranial arteries to cause vasoconstriction and reduces sterile inflammation associated with antidromic neuronal transmission correlating with relief of migraine

Contraindications Hypersensitivity to sumatriptan or any component of the formulation; patients with ischemic heart disease or signs or symptoms of ischemic heart disease (including Prinzmetal's angina, angina pectoris, myocardial infarction, silent myocardial ischemia); cerebrovascular syndromes (including strokes, transient ischemic attacks); peripheral vascular syndromes (including ischemic bowel disease); uncontrolled hypertension; use within 24 hours of ergotamine derivatives; use with in 24 hours of another 5-HT_1 agonist; concurrent administration or within 2 weeks of discontinuing an MAO inhibitor, specifically MAO type A inhibitors; management of hemiplegic or basilar migraine; prophylactic treatment of migraine; severe hepatic impairment; not for I.V. administration

Warnings/Precautions

Sumatriptan is indicated only in patients ≥18 years of age with a clear diagnosis of migraine or cluster headache

Cardiac events (coronary artery vasospasm, transient ischemia, myocardial infarction, ventricular tachycardia/fibrillation, cardiac arrest and death), cerebral/subarachnoid hemorrhage, and stroke have been reported with 5-HT_1 agonist administration

Do not give to patients with risk factors for CAD until a cardiovascular evaluation has been performed; if evaluation is satisfactory, the healthcare provider should administer the first dose and cardiovascular status should be periodically evaluated

Significant elevation in blood pressure, including hypertensive crisis, has also been reported on rare occasions in patients with and without a history of hypertension. Vasospasm-related reactions have been reported other than coronary artery vasospasm. Peripheral vascular ischemia and colonic ischemia with abdominal pain and bloody diarrhea have occurred.

Use with caution in patients with a history of seizure disorder or in patients with a lowered seizure threshold. Safety and efficacy in pediatric patients have not been established

Drug Interactions

Increased Effect/Toxicity: Increased toxicity with ergot-containing drugs, avoid use, wait 24 hours from last ergot containing drug (dihydroergotamine, or methysergide) before administering sumatriptan. MAO inhibitors decrease clearance of sumatriptan increasing the risk of systemic sumatriptan toxic effects. Sumatriptan may enhance CNS toxic effects when taken with selective serotonin reuptake inhibitors (SSRIs) like fluoxetine, fluvoxamine, paroxetine, or sertraline. **Note:** Use cautiously in patients receiving concomitant medications that can lower the seizure threshold.

Pharmacodynamics/Kinetics

Onset of action: ~30 minutes

Distribution: V_d: 2.4 L/kg

Protein binding: 14% to 21%

Bioavailability: SubQ: 97% ± 16% of that following I.V. injection

Half-life elimination: Injection, tablet: 2.5 hours; Nasal spray: 2 hours

Time to peak, serum: 5-20 minutes

Excretion:

Injection: Urine (38% as indole acetic acid metabolite, 22% as unchanged drug)

Nasal spray: Urine (42% as indole acetic acid metabolite, 3% as unchanged drug)

(Continued)

Sumatriptan *(Continued)*

Tablet: Urine (60% as indole acetic acid metabolite, 3% as unchanged drug); feces (40%)

Pregnancy Risk Factor C

Dosage Forms Note: Expressed as sumatriptan base. **INJ, solution:** 12 mg/mL (0.5 mL). **SOLN, intranasal spray:** 5 mg (100 μL unit dose spray device); 20 mg (100 μL unit dose spray device). **TAB:** 25 mg, 50 mg, 100 mg

Sumatriptan Succinate *see* Sumatriptan *on page 1252*
Summer's Eve® Medicated Douche [OTC] *see* Povidone-Iodine *on page 1107*
Summer's Eve® SpecialCare™ Medicated Anti-Itch Cream [OTC] *see* Hydrocortisone *on page 714*
Sumycin® *see* Tetracycline *on page 1280*
Supartz™ *see* Hyaluronate and Derivatives *on page 696*
Superdophilus® [OTC] *see Lactobacillus on page 793*
Suprax® *see* Cefixime *on page 282*
Surbex-T® [OTC] *see* Vitamin B Complex Combinations *on page 1382*
Sureprin 81™ [OTC] *see* Aspirin *on page 151*
Surfak® [OTC] *see* Docusate *on page 459*
Surgicel® *see* Cellulose (Oxidized/Regenerated) *on page 293*
Surmontil® *see* Trimipramine *on page 1343*
Survanta® *see* Beractant *on page 198*
Sus-Phrine® (Dental) *see* Epinephrine *on page 496*
Sustiva® *see* Efavirenz *on page 484*
Su-Tuss®-HD *see* Hydrocodone, Pseudoephedrine, and Guaifenesin *on page 713*
Suxamethonium Chloride *see* Succinylcholine *on page 1241*
Sween Cream® [OTC] *see* Vitamin A and Vitamin D *on page 1382*
Symax SL *see* Hyoscyamine *on page 724*
Symax SR *see* Hyoscyamine *on page 724*
Symbyax™ *see* Olanzapine and Fluoxetine *on page 1009*
Symmetrel® *see* Amantadine *on page 92*
Synacthen *see* Cosyntropin *on page 378*
Synagis® *see* Palivizumab *on page 1040*
Synalar® *see* Fluocinolone *on page 601*
Synalgos®-DC *see* Dihydrocodeine, Aspirin, and Caffeine *on page 441*
Synarel® *see* Nafarelin *on page 957*
Synercid® *see* Quinupristin and Dalfopristin *on page 1163*
Synthroid® *see* Levothyroxine *on page 817*
Synvisc® *see* Hyaluronate and Derivatives *on page 696*
Syrup of Ipecac *see* Ipecac Syrup *on page 760*
Systemic Viral Diseases *see page 1519*
T_3 Sodium *see* Liothyronine *on page 831*
T_3/T_4 Liotrix *see* Liotrix *on page 832*
T_4 *see* Levothyroxine *on page 817*
T-20 *see* Enfuvirtide *on page 492*

Tacrine (TAK reen)

U.S. Brand Names Cognex®

Generic Available No

Synonyms Tacrine Hydrochloride; Tetrahydroaminoacrine; THA

Pharmacologic Category Acetylcholinesterase Inhibitor (Central)

Use Treatment of mild to moderate dementia of the Alzheimer's type

Local Anesthetic/Vasoconstrictor Precautions No information available to require special precautions

Effects on Dental Treatment No significant effects or complications reported

Common Adverse Effects

>10%:

Central nervous system: Headache, dizziness
Gastrointestinal: Nausea, vomiting, diarrhea
Miscellaneous: Elevated transaminases

1% to 10%:

Cardiovascular: Flushing
Central nervous system: Confusion, ataxia, insomnia, somnolence, depression, anxiety, fatigue
Dermatologic: Rash

Gastrointestinal: Dyspepsia, anorexia, abdominal pain, flatulence, constipation, weight loss

Neuromuscular & skeletal: Myalgia, tremor

Respiratory: Rhinitis

Mechanism of Action Centrally-acting cholinesterase inhibitor. It elevates acetylcholine in cerebral cortex by slowing the degradation of acetylcholine.

Drug Interactions

Cytochrome P450 Effect: Substrate of CYP1A2 (major); **Inhibits** CYP1A2 (weak)

Increased Effect/Toxicity: CYP1A2 inhibitors may increase the levels/effects of tacrine; example inhibitors include amiodarone, ciprofloxacin, fluvoxamine, ketoconazole, lomefloxacin, ofloxacin, and rofecoxib. Tacrine in combination with other cholinergic agents (eg, ambenonium, edrophonium, neostigmine, pyridostigmine, bethanechol), will likely produce additive cholinergic effects. Tacrine in combination with beta-blockers may produce additive bradycardia. Tacrine may increase the levels/effect of succinylcholine and theophylline. in elevated plasma levels. Fluvoxamine, enoxacin, and cimetidine increase tacrine concentrations via enzyme inhibition (CYP1A2).

Decreased Effect: CYP1A2 inducers may decrease the levels/effects of tacrine; example inducers include aminoglutethimide, carbamazepine, phenobarbital, rifampin, and cigarette smoking, Tacrine may worsen Parkinson's disease and inhibit the effects of levodopa. Tacrine may antagonize the therapeutic effect of anticholinergic agents (benztropine, trihexphenidyl).

Pharmacodynamics/Kinetics

Absorption: Oral: Rapid

Distribution: V_d: Mean: 349 L; reduced by food

Protein binding, plasma: 55%

Metabolism: Extensively by CYP450 to multiple metabolites; first pass effect

Bioavailability: Absolute: 17%

Half-life elimination, serum: 2-4 hours; Steady-state: 24-36 hours

Time to peak, plasma: 1-2 hours

Pregnancy Risk Factor C

Tacrine Hydrochloride *see* Tacrine *on page 1254*

Tacrolimus (ta KROE li mus)

U.S. Brand Names Prograf®; Protopic®

Canadian Brand Names Prograf®; Protopic®

Mexican Brand Names Prograf®

Generic Available No

Synonyms FK506

Pharmacologic Category Immunosuppressant Agent; Topical Skin Product

Use

Oral/injection: Potent immunosuppressive drug used in liver or kidney transplant recipients

Topical: Moderate to severe atopic dermatitis in patients not responsive to conventional therapy or when conventional therapy is not appropriate

Unlabeled/Investigational Use Potent immunosuppressive drug used in heart, lung, small bowel transplant recipients; immunosuppressive drug for peripheral stem cell/bone marrow transplantation

Local Anesthetic/Vasoconstrictor Precautions No information available to require special precautions

Effects on Dental Treatment No significant effects or complications reported

Common Adverse Effects

Oral, I.V.:

≥15%:

Cardiovascular: Chest pain, hypertension

Central nervous system: Dizziness, headache, insomnia, tremor (headache and tremor are associated with high whole blood concentrations and may respond to decreased dosage)

Dermatologic: Pruritus, rash

Endocrine & metabolic: Diabetes mellitus, hyperglycemia, hyperkalemia, hyperlipemia, hypomagnesemia, hypophosphatemia

Gastrointestinal: Abdominal pain, constipation, diarrhea, dyspepsia, nausea, vomiting

Genitourinary: Urinary tract infection

Hematologic: Anemia, leukocytosis, thrombocytopenia

Hepatic: Ascites

Neuromuscular & skeletal: Arthralgia, back pain, weakness, paresthesia

(Continued)

Tacrolimus *(Continued)*

Renal: Abnormal kidney function, increased creatinine, oliguria, urinary tract infection, increased BUN

Respiratory: Atelectasis, dyspnea, increased cough

3% to 15% (Limited to important or life-threatening symptoms):

Cardiovascular: Abnormal ECG, angina pectoris, deep thrombophlebitis, hemorrhage, hypotension, postural hypotension, thrombosis

Central nervous system: Agitation, amnesia, anxiety, confusion, depression, encephalopathy, hallucinations, psychosis, somnolence

Dermatologic: Acne, alopecia, exfoliative dermatitis, hirsutism, photosensitivity reaction, skin discoloration

Endocrine & metabolic: Cushing's syndrome, decreased bicarbonate, decreased serum iron, diabetes mellitus, hypercalcemia, hypercholesterolemia, hyperphosphatemia

Gastrointestinal: Dysphagia, esophagitis, GI perforation/hemorrhage, ileus

Hematologic: Coagulation disorder, decreased prothrombin, leukopenia

Hepatic: Cholangitis, jaundice, hepatitis

Neuromuscular & skeletal: Incoordination, myasthenia, neuropathy, osteoporosis

Respiratory: Asthma, pneumothorax, pulmonary edema

Miscellaneous: Abscess, allergic reaction, flu-like syndrome, peritonitis, sepsis

Postmarketing and/or case reports: Acute renal failure, anaphylaxis, coma, deafness, delirium, hearing loss, hemolytic-uremic syndrome, leukoencephalopathy, lymphoproliferative disorder (related to EBV), myocardial hypertrophy (associated with ventricular dysfunction), pancreatitis, seizures, Stevens-Johnson syndrome, thrombocytopenic purpura, torsade de pointes

Topical:

>10%:

Central nervous system: Headache (5% to 20%), fever (1% to 21%)

Dermatologic: Skin burning (43% to 58%), pruritus (41% to 46%), erythema (12% to 28%)

Respiratory: Increased cough (18% children)

Miscellaneous: Flu-like syndrome (23% to 28%), allergic reaction (4% to 12%)

Mechanism of Action Suppresses cellular immunity (inhibits T-lymphocyte activation), possibly by binding to an intracellular protein, FKBP-12

Drug Interactions

Cytochrome P450 Effect: Substrate of CYP3A4 (major); **Inhibits** CYP3A4 (weak)

Increased Effect/Toxicity: Amphotericin B and other nephrotoxic antibiotics have the potential to increase tacrolimus-associated nephrotoxicity. Cisapride and metaclopramide may increase tacrolimus levels. Synergistic immunosuppression results from concurrent use of cyclosporine. Voriconazole may increase tacrolimus serum concentrations; decrease tacrolimus dosage by 66% when initiating voriconazole. CYP3A4 inhibitors may increase the levels/effects of tacrolimus; example inhibitors include azole antifungals, ciprofloxacin, clarithromycin, diclofenac, doxycycline, erythromycin, imatinib, isoniazid, nefazodone, nicardipine, propofol, protease inhibitors, quinidine, and verapamil.

Decreased Effect: Antacids impair tacrolimus absorption (separate administration by at least 2 hours). St John's wort may reduce tacrolimus serum concentrations (avoid concurrent use). CYP3A4 inducers may decrease the levels/effects of tacrolimus; example inducers include aminoglutethimide, carbamazepine, nafcillin, nevirapine, phenobarbital, phenytoin, and rifamycins.

Pharmacodynamics/Kinetics

Absorption: Better in resected patients with a closed stoma; unlike cyclosporine, clamping of the T-tube in liver transplant patients does not alter trough concentrations or AUC

Oral: Incomplete and variable; food within 15 minutes of administration decreases absorption (27%)

Topical: Serum concentrations range from undetectable to 20 ng/mL (<5 ng/mL in majority of adult patients studied)

Protein binding: 99%

Metabolism: Extensively hepatic via CYP3A4 to eight possible metabolites (major metabolite, 31-demethyl tacrolimus, shows same activity as tacrolimus *in vitro*)

Bioavailability: Oral: Adults: 7% to 28%, Children: 10% to 52%; Topical: <0.5%; Absolute: Unknown

Half-life elimination: Variable, 21-61 hours in healthy volunteers
Time to peak: 0.5-4 hours
Excretion: Feces (~92%); feces/urine (<1% as unchanged drug)

Pregnancy Risk Factor C

Tadalafil (tah DA la fil)

U.S. Brand Names Cialis®

Generic Available No

Synonyms GF196960

Pharmacologic Category Phosphodiesterase-5 Enzyme Inhibitor

Use Treatment of erectile dysfunction

Local Anesthetic/Vasoconstrictor Precautions No information available to require special precautions

Effects on Dental Treatment No significant effects or complications reported

Common Adverse Effects

>10%:
- Central nervous system: Headache (11% to 15%)
- Gastrointestinal: Dyspepsia (4% to 10%)

2% to 10%:
- Cardiovascular: Flushing (2% to 3%)
- Neuromuscular & skeletal: CPK increased (2%), back pain (3% to 6%), myalgia (1% to 3%)
- Respiratory: Nasal congestion (2% to 3%)
- Miscellaneous: Limb pain (1% to 3%)

Dosage Oral: Adults: Erectile dysfunction: 10 mg prior to anticipated sexual activity (dosing range: 5-20 mg); to be given as one single dose and not given more than once daily. **Note:** Erectile function may be improved for up to 36 hours following a single dose; adjust dose.

Elderly: Dosage is based on renal function; refer to "Dosage adjustment in renal impairment"

Dosing adjustment with concomitant medications: CYP3A4 inhibitors: Dose reduction of tadalafil is recommended with strong CYP3A4 inhibitors. The dose of tadalafil should not exceed 10 mg, and tadalafil should not be taken more frequently than once every 72 hours. Examples of such inhibitors include azole antifungals, clarithromycin, diclofenac, doxycycline, erythromycin, grapefruit juice, imatinib, isoniazid, nefazodone, nicardipine, propofol, protease inhibitors, quinidine, and verapamil.

Dosage adjustment in renal impairment:

Cl_{cr} 31-50 mL/minute: Initial dose 5 mg once daily; maximum dose 10 mg not to be given more frequently than every 48 hours.

Cl_{cr} <30 mL/minute or hemodialysis: Maximum dose 5 mg.

Dosage adjustment in hepatic impairment:

Mild-to-moderate hepatic impairment (Child-Pugh class A or B): Dose should not exceed 10 mg once daily

Severe hepatic impairment: Use is not recommended

Mechanism of Action Does not directly cause penile erections, but affects the response to sexual stimulation. The physiologic mechanism of erection of the penis involves release of nitric oxide (NO) in the corpus cavernosum during sexual stimulation. NO then activates the enzyme guanylate cyclase, which results in increased levels of cyclic guanosine monophosphate (cGMP), producing smooth muscle relaxation and inflow of blood to the corpus cavernosum. Tadalafil enhances the effect of NO by inhibiting phosphodiesterase type 5 (PDE-5), which is responsible for degradation of cGMP in the corpus cavernosum; when sexual stimulation causes local release of NO, inhibition of PDE-5 by tadalafil causes increased levels of cGMP in the corpus cavernosum, resulting in smooth muscle relaxation and inflow of blood to the corpus cavernosum. At recommended doses, it has no effect in the absence of sexual stimulation.

Contraindications Hypersensitivity to tadalafil or any component of the formulation; concurrent use of organic nitrates (nitroglycerin) in any form; concurrent use of alpha-adrenergic antagonists (except tamsulosin 0.4 mg/day)

Warnings/Precautions There is a degree of cardiac risk associated with sexual activity; therefore, physicians may wish to consider the cardiovascular status of their patients prior to initiating any treatment for erectile dysfunction. Use caution in patients with left ventricular outflow obstruction (aortic stenosis or IHSS); may be more sensitive to hypotensive actions. Use caution in patients receiving strong CYP3A4 inhibitors, the elderly, or those with hepatic impairment or renal impairment; dosage adjustment/limitation is needed. Use caution in patients with peptic ulcer disease.

Agents for the treatment of erectile dysfunction should be used with caution in patients with anatomical deformation of the penis (angulation, cavernosal

(Continued)

Tadalafil *(Continued)*

fibrosis, or Peyronie's disease), or in patients who have conditions which may predispose them to priapism (sickle cell anemia, multiple myeloma, leukemia). All patients should be instructed to seek medical attention if erection persists >4 hours. The safety and efficacy of tadalafil with other treatments for erectile dysfunction have not been studied and are, therefore, not recommended as combination therapy.

Safety and efficacy have not been studied in patients with the following conditions, therefore, use in these patients is not recommended: Arrhythmias, hypotension, uncontrolled hypertension, unstable angina or angina during intercourse, cardiac failure (NYHA Class II or greater), recent myocardial infarction, or stroke within the last 6 months. A minority of patients with retinitis pigmentosa have genetic disorders of retinal phosphodiesterases. There is no safety information on the administration of tadalafil to these patients; administer with caution.

Drug Interactions

Cytochrome P450 Effect: Substrate of CYP3A4 (major)

Ethanol/Nutrition/Herb Interactions

Ethanol: Substantial consumption of ethanol may increase the risk of hypotension and orthostasis. Lower ethanol consumption has not been associated with significant changes in blood pressure or increase in orthostatic symptoms.

Food: Rate and extent of absorption are not affected by food. Grapefruit juice may increase serum levels/toxicity of tadalafil. Do not give more than a single 10 mg dose of tadalafil more frequently than every 72 hours in patients who regularly consume grapefruit juice.

Dietary Considerations May be taken with or without food.

Pharmacodynamics/Kinetics

Onset: Within 1 hour
Duration: Up to 36 hours
Distribution: V_d: 63 L
Protein binding: 94%
Metabolism: Hepatic, via CYP3A4 to metabolites (inactive)
Half-life elimination: 17.5 hours
Time to peak, plasma: 2 hours
Excretion: Feces (61%, as metabolites); urine (36%, as metabolites)

Pregnancy Risk Factor B

Dosage Forms TAB: 5 mg, 10 mg, 20 mg

Tagamet® *see* Cimetidine *on page 330*
Tagamet® HB 200 [OTC] *see* Cimetidine *on page 330*
Talacen® *see* Pentazocine and Acetaminophen *on page 1064*
Talwin® *see* Pentazocine *on page 1063*
Talwin® NX *see* Pentazocine *on page 1063*
TAM *see* Tamoxifen *on page 1258*
Tambocor™ *see* Flecainide *on page 592*
Tamiflu® *see* Oseltamivir *on page 1019*

Tamoxifen (ta MOKS i fen)

U.S. Brand Names Nolvadex®

Canadian Brand Names Apo-Tamox®; Gen-Tamoxifen; Nolvadex®; Nolvadex®-D; Novo-Tamoxifen; PMS-Tamoxifen; Tamofen®

Mexican Brand Names Nolvadex®; Taxus® [tabs]; Tecnofen® [tabs]

Generic Available Yes

Synonyms ICI-46474; NSC-180973; TAM; Tamoxifen Citrate

Pharmacologic Category Antineoplastic Agent, Estrogen Receptor Antagonist

Use Palliative or adjunctive treatment of advanced breast cancer; reduce the incidence of breast cancer in women at high risk; reduce risk of invasive breast cancer in women with ductal carcinoma *in situ* (DCIS); metastatic male breast cancer; treatment of melanoma, desmoid tumors

Unlabeled/Investigational Use Treatment of mastalgia, gynecomastia, pancreatic carcinoma; induction of ovulation; treatment of precocious puberty in females, secondary to McCune-Albright syndrome

Local Anesthetic/Vasoconstrictor Precautions No information available to require special precautions

Effects on Dental Treatment No significant effects or complications reported

Common Adverse Effects Note: Differences in the frequency of some adverse events may be related to use for a specific indication.

Frequency not defined: Depression, dizziness, headache, hypercalcemia, lightheadedness, peripheral edema, pruritus vulvae, taste disturbance, vaginal dryness

>10%:

Cardiovascular: Fluid retention (32%)

Central nervous system: Mood changes (up to 12%; may include depression)

Dermatologic: Skin changes (19%)

Endocrine & metabolic: Hot flashes (64% to 80%), weight loss (23%)

Gastrointestinal: Nausea (26%)

Genitourinary: Vaginal bleeding (up to 23%), vaginal discharge (30% to 55%), menstrual irregularities (25%)

Neuromuscular & skeletal: Bone pain, tumor pain, and local disease flare (including increase in lesion size and erythema) during treatment of metastatic breast cancer (generally resolves with continuation)

1% to 10%:

Dermatologic: Alopecia (<1% to 5%)

Gastrointestinal: Constipation (up to 4%)

Hematologic: Thrombocytopenia (<1% to 2%)

Hepatic: SGOT increased (2%), serum bilirubin increased (2%)

Renal: Serum creatinine increased (up to 2%)

Miscellaneous: Infection/sepsis (up to 6%), allergic reaction (up to 3%)

Dosage Oral (refer to individual protocols):

Children: Female: Precocious puberty and McCune-Albright syndrome (unlabeled use): A dose of 20 mg/day has been reported in patients 2-10 years of age; safety and efficacy have not been established for treatment of longer than 1 year duration

Adults:

Breast cancer:

Metastatic (males and females) or adjuvant therapy (females): 20-40 mg/day

Prevention (high-risk females): 20 mg/day for 5 years

DCIS (females): 20 mg once daily for 5 years

Note: Higher dosages (up to 700 mg/day) have been investigated for use in modulation of multidrug resistance (MDR), but are not routinely used in clinical practice

Induction of ovulation (unlabeled use): 5-40 mg twice daily for 4 days

Mechanism of Action Competitively binds to estrogen receptors on tumors and other tissue targets, producing a nuclear complex that decreases DNA synthesis and inhibits estrogen effects; nonsteroidal agent with potent antiestrogenic properties which compete with estrogen for binding sites in breast and other tissues; cells accumulate in the G_0 and G_1 phases; therefore, tamoxifen is cytostatic rather than cytocidal.

Contraindications Hypersensitivity to tamoxifen or any component of the formulation; concurrent warfarin therapy (when used for cancer risk reduction); pregnancy

Warnings/Precautions Serious, life-threatening, or fatal events (including endometrial cancer, uterine sarcoma, stroke, pulmonary embolism) have occurred in women taking tamoxifen. Healthcare providers should discuss the potential benefits versus the potential risks of these serious events with women considering tamoxifen therapy to reduce their risk of developing breast cancer. Use with caution in patients with leukopenia, thrombocytopenia, or hyperlipidemias; ovulation may be induced; "hot flashes" may be countered by Bellergal-S® tablets or clonidine; decreased visual acuity, retinopathy and corneal changes have been reported with use for more than 1 year at doses above recommended; hypercalcemia in patients with bone metastasis; hepatocellular carcinomas have been reported in animal studies. Endometrial hyperplasia and polyps have occurred.

Drug Interactions

Cytochrome P450 Effect: Substrate of CYP2A6 (minor), 2B6 (minor), 2C8/9 (major), 2D6 (major), 2E1 (minor), 3A4 (major); **Inhibits** CYP2B6 (weak), 2C8/9 (weak), 3A4 (weak)

Increased Effect/Toxicity: Allopurinol and tamoxifen results in exacerbation of allopurinol-induced hepatotoxicity. Cyclosporine serum levels may be increased when taken with tamoxifen. Concomitant use of warfarin is contraindicated when used for risk reduction; results in significant enhancement of the anticoagulant effects of warfarin. CYP2C8/9 inhibitors may increase the levels/effects of tamoxifen; example inhibitors include delavirdine, fluconazole, gemfibrozil, ketoconazole, nicardipine, NSAIDs, pioglitazone, and sulfonamides. CYP2D6 inhibitors may increase the levels/effects of

(Continued)

Tamoxifen *(Continued)*

tamoxifen; example inhibitors include chlorpromazine, delavirdine, fluoxetine, miconazole, paroxetine, pergolide, quinidine, quinine, ritonavir, and ropinirole. CYP3A4 inhibitors may increase the levels/effects of tamoxifen; example inhibitors include azole antifungals, ciprofloxacin, clarithromycin, diclofenac, doxycycline, erythromycin, imatinib, isoniazid, nefazodone, nicardipine, propofol, protease inhibitors, quinidine, and verapamil.

Decreased Effect: CYP2C8/9 inducers may decrease the levels/effects of tamoxifen; example inducers include carbamazepine, phenobarbital, phenytoin, rifampin, rifapentine, and secobarbital. CYP3A4 inducers may decrease the levels/effects of tamoxifen; example inducers include aminoglutethimide, carbamazepine, nafcillin, nevirapine, phenobarbital, phenytoin, and rifamycins. Letrozole serum levels may be reduced by tamoxifen.

Ethanol/Nutrition/Herb Interactions Herb/Nutraceutical: Avoid black cohosh, dong quai in estrogen-dependent tumors.

Pharmacodynamics/Kinetics

Absorption: Well absorbed

Distribution: High concentrations found in uterus, endometrial and breast tissue

Protein binding: 99%

Metabolism: Hepatic (via CYP3A4) to major metabolites, desmethyltamoxifen and 4-hydroxytamoxifen; undergoes enterohepatic recirculation

Half-life elimination: Distribution: 7-14 hours; Elimination: 5-7 days; Metabolites: 14 days

Time to peak, serum: 5 hours

Excretion: Feces (26% to 51%); urine (9% to 13%)

Pregnancy Risk Factor D

Dosage Forms TAB: 10 mg, 20 mg

Tamoxifen Citrate *see* Tamoxifen *on page 1258*

Tamsulosin (tam SOO loe sin)

U.S. Brand Names Flomax®

Canadian Brand Names Flomax®

Mexican Brand Names Secotex®

Generic Available No

Synonyms Tamsulosin Hydrochloride

Pharmacologic Category Alpha$_1$ Blocker

Use Treatment of signs and symptoms of benign prostatic hyperplasia (BPH)

Local Anesthetic/Vasoconstrictor Precautions No information available to require special precautions

Effects on Dental Treatment No significant effects or complications reported

Common Adverse Effects

>10%:

Cardiovascular: Studies specific for orthostatic hypotension: Overall, at least one positive test was observed in 16% of patients receiving 0.4 mg and 19% of patients receiving the 0.8 mg dose. "First-dose" orthostatic hypotension following a 0.4 mg dose was reported as 7% at 4 hours postdose and 6% at 8 hours postdose.

Central nervous system: Headache (19% to 21%), dizziness (15% to 17%)

Genitourinary: Abnormal ejaculation (8% to 18%)

Respiratory: Rhinitis (13% to 18%)

1% to 10%:

Cardiovascular: Chest pain (~4%)

Central nervous system: Somnolence (3% to 4%), insomnia (1% to 2%), vertigo (0.6% to 1%)

Endocrine & metabolic: Libido decreased (1% to 2%)

Gastrointestinal: Diarrhea (4% to 6%), nausea (3% to 4%), stomach discomfort (2% to 3%), bitter taste (2% to 3%)

Neuromuscular & skeletal: Weakness (8% to 9%), back pain (7% to 8%)

Ocular: Amblyopia (0.2% to 2%)

Respiratory: Pharyngitis (5% to 6%), cough (3% to 5%), sinusitis (2% to 4%)

Miscellaneous: Infection (9% to 11%), tooth disorder (1% to 2%)

Dosage Oral: Adults: 0.4 mg once daily ~30 minutes after the same meal each day; dose may be increased after 2-4 weeks to 0.8 mg once daily in patients who fail to respond. If therapy is interrupted for several days, restart with 0.4 mg once daily.

Dosage adjustment in renal impairment:

Cl_{cr} ≥10 mL/minute: No adjustment needed

Cl_{cr} <10 mL/minute: Not studied

Mechanism of Action Tamsulosin is an antagonist of alpha$_{1A}$ adrenoreceptors in the prostate. Smooth muscle tone in the prostate is mediated by alpha$_{1A}$ adrenoreceptors; blocking them leads to relaxation of smooth muscle in the bladder neck and prostate causing an improvement of urine flow and decreased symptoms of BPH. Approximately 75% of the alpha$_1$ receptors in the prostate are of the alpha$_{1A}$ subtype.

Contraindications Hypersensitivity to tamsulosin or any component of the formulation; concurrent use with phosphodiesterase-5 (PDE-5) inhibitors including sildenafil (>25 mg), tadalafil (if tamsulosin dose >0.4 mg/day), or vardenafil

Warnings/Precautions Not intended for use as an antihypertensive drug. May cause orthostasis, syncope or dizziness. Patients should avoid situations where injury may occur as a result of syncope. Rule out prostatic carcinoma before beginning therapy with tamsulosin.

Drug Interactions

Cytochrome P450 Effect: Substrate (major) of CYP2D6, 3A4

Increased Effect/Toxicity: Alpha-adrenergic blockers and calcium channel blockers may increase risk of hypotension. Risk of first-dose orthostatic hypotension may increase with beta-blockers. Cimetidine may decrease tamsulosin clearance. Blood pressure-lowering effects are additive with sildenafil (use with extreme caution), tadalafil (may be used when tamsulosin dose is ≤0.4 mg/day), and vardenafil (use is contraindicated by the manufacturer).

CYP2D6 inhibitors may increase the levels/effects of tamsulosin; example inhibitors include chlorpromazine, delavirdine, fluoxetine, miconazole, paroxetine, pergolide, quinidine, quinine, ritonavir, and ropinirole. CYP3A4 inhibitors may increase the levels/effects of tamsulosin; example inhibitors include azole antifungals, ciprofloxacin, clarithromycin, diclofenac, doxycycline, erythromycin, imatinib, isoniazid, nefazodone, nicardipine, propofol, protease inhibitors, quinidine, and verapamil.

Decreased Effect: CYP3A4 inducers may decrease the levels/effects of tamsulosin; example inducers include aminoglutethimide, carbamazepine, nafcillin, nevirapine, phenobarbital, phenytoin, and rifamycins.

Ethanol/Nutrition/Herb Interactions

Food: Fasting increases bioavailability by 30% and peak concentration 40% to 70%.

Herb/Nutraceutical: Avoid saw palmetto (due to limited experience with this combination).

Dietary Considerations Take once daily, 30 minutes after the same meal each day.

Pharmacodynamics/Kinetics

Absorption: >90%

Protein binding: 94% to 99%, primarily to alpha$_1$ acid glycoprotein (AAG)

Metabolism: Hepatic via CYP; metabolites undergo extensive conjugation to glucuronide or sulfate

Bioavailability: Fasting: 30% increase

Distribution: V_d: 16 L

Steady-state: By the fifth day of once-daily dosing

Half-life elimination: Healthy volunteers: 9-13 hours; Target population: 14-15 hours

Time to peak: Fasting: 4-5 hours; With food: 6-7 hours

Excretion: Urine (76%, <10% as unchanged drug); feces (21%)

Pregnancy Risk Factor B

Dosage Forms CAP: 0.4 mg

Tamsulosin Hydrochloride *see* Tamsulosin *on page 1260*

Tanafed® *see* Chlorpheniramine and Pseudoephedrine *on page 315*

Tanafed DP™ *see* Chlorpheniramine and Pseudoephedrine *on page 315*

Tannate 12 S *see* Carbetapentane and Chlorpheniramine *on page 260*

Tannic-12 *see* Carbetapentane and Chlorpheniramine *on page 260*

Tannic-12 S *see* Carbetapentane and Chlorpheniramine *on page 260*

Tannihist-12 RF *see* Carbetapentane and Chlorpheniramine *on page 260*

Tao® *see* Troleandomycin *on page 1348*

TAP-144 *see* Leuprolide *on page 805*

Tapazole® *see* Methimazole *on page 893*

Targretin® *see* Bexarotene *on page 205*

Tarka® *see* Trandolapril and Verapamil *on page 1322*

Tarsum® [OTC] *see* Coal Tar and Salicylic Acid *on page 367*

Tasmar® *see* Tolcapone *on page 1310*

Tavist® Allergy [OTC] *see* Clemastine *on page 346*

Tavist® ND [OTC] *see* Loratadine *on page 841*
Taxol® *see* Paclitaxel *on page 1038*
Taxotere® *see* Docetaxel *on page 458*

Tazarotene (taz AR oh teen)

U.S. Brand Names Avage™; Tazorac®
Canadian Brand Names Tazorac®
Generic Available No
Pharmacologic Category Keratolytic Agent
Use Topical treatment of facial acne vulgaris; topical treatment of stable plaque psoriasis of up to 20% body surface area involvement; mitigation (palliation) of facial skin wrinkling, facial mottled hyper/hypopigmentation, and benign facial lentigines
Local Anesthetic/Vasoconstrictor Precautions No information available to require special precautions
Effects on Dental Treatment No significant effects or complications reported
Common Adverse Effects Percentage of incidence varies with formulation and/or strength:

>10%: Dermatologic: Burning/stinging, desquamation, dry skin, erythema, pruritus, skin pain, worsening of psoriasis
1% to 10%: Dermatologic: Contact dermatitis, discoloration, fissuring, hypertriglyceridemia, inflammation, irritation, localized bleeding, rash

Frequency not defined:
Dermatologic: Photosensitization
Neuromuscular & skeletal: Peripheral neuropathy

Mechanism of Action Synthetic, acetylenic retinoid which modulates differentiation and proliferation of epithelial tissue and exerts some degree of anti-inflammatory and immunological activity
Drug Interactions
Increased Effect/Toxicity: Increased toxicity may occur with sulfur, benzoyl peroxide, salicylic acid, resorcinol, or any product with strong drying effects (including alcohol-containing compounds) due to increased drying actions. May augment phototoxicity of sensitizing medications (thiazides, tetracyclines, fluoroquinolones, phenothiazines, sulfonamides).
Pharmacodynamics/Kinetics
Duration: Therapeutic: Psoriasis: Effects have been observed for up to 3 months after a 3-month course of topical treatment
Absorption: Minimal following cutaneous application (≤6% of dose)
Distribution: Retained in skin for prolonged periods after topical application.
Protein binding: >99%
Metabolism: Prodrug, rapidly metabolized via esterases to an active metabolite (tazarotenic acid) following topical application and systemic absorption; tazarotenic acid undergoes further hepatic metabolism
Half-life elimination: 18 hours
Excretion: Urine and feces (as metabolites)
Pregnancy Risk Factor X

Tazicef® *see* Ceftazidime *on page 286*
Tazorac® *see* Tazarotene *on page 1262*
Taztia XT™ *see* Diltiazem *on page 444*
3TC *see* Lamivudine *on page 794*
3TC, Abacavir, and Zidovudine *see* Abacavir, Lamivudine, and Zidovudine *on page 43*
T-Cell Growth Factor *see* Aldesleukin *on page 74*
TCGF *see* Aldesleukin *on page 74*
TCN *see* Tetracycline *on page 1280*
TDF *see* Tenofovir *on page 1270*
Teargen® [OTC] *see* Artificial Tears *on page 148*
Teargen® II [OTC] *see* Artificial Tears *on page 148*
Tearisol® [OTC] *see* Artificial Tears *on page 148*
Tearisol® [OTC] *see* Hydroxypropyl Methylcellulose *on page 721*
Tears Again® [OTC] *see* Artificial Tears *on page 148*
Tears Again® Gel Drops™ [OTC] *see* Carboxymethylcellulose *on page 265*
Tears Again® Night and Day™ [OTC] *see* Carboxymethylcellulose *on page 265*
Tears Naturale® [OTC] *see* Artificial Tears *on page 148*
Tears Naturale® Free [OTC] *see* Artificial Tears *on page 148*
Tears Naturale® II [OTC] *see* Artificial Tears *on page 148*
Tears Plus® [OTC] *see* Artificial Tears *on page 148*

Tears Renewed® [OTC] *see* Artificial Tears *on page 148*

Tegaserod (teg a SER od)

U.S. Brand Names Zelnorm®

Canadian Brand Names Zelnorm®

Mexican Brand Names Zelmac®

Generic Available No

Synonyms HTF919; Tegaserod Maleate

Pharmacologic Category Serotonin 5-HT_4 Receptor Agonist

Use Short-term treatment of constipation-predominate irritable bowel syndrome (IBS) in women

Local Anesthetic/Vasoconstrictor Precautions No information available to require special precautions

Effects on Dental Treatment No significant effects or complications reported

Common Adverse Effects

>10%:
- Central nervous system: Headache (15%)
- Gastrointestinal: Abdominal pain (12%)

1% to 10%:
- Central nervous system: Dizziness (4%), migraine (2%)
- Gastrointestinal: Diarrhea (9%; severe <1%), nausea (8%), flatulence (6%)
- Neuromuscular & skeletal: Back pain (5%), arthropathy (2%), leg pain (1%)

Mechanism of Action Tegaserod is a partial neuronal 5-HT_4 receptor agonist. Its action at the receptor site leads to stimulation of the peristaltic reflex and intestinal secretion, and moderation of visceral sensitivity.

Pharmacodynamics/Kinetics

Distribution: V_d: 368 ± 223 L

Protein binding: 98% primarily to α_1-acid glycoprotein

Metabolism: GI: Hydrolysis in the stomach; Hepatic: Oxidation, conjugation, and glucuronidation; metabolite (negligible activity); significant first-pass effect

Bioavailability: Fasting: 10%

Half-life elimination: I.V.: 11 ± 5 hours

Time to peak: 1 hour

Excretion: Feces (~66% as unchanged drug); urine (~33% as metabolites)

Pregnancy Risk Factor B

Tegaserod Maleate *see* Tegaserod *on page 1263*

Tegretol® *see* Carbamazepine *on page 255*

Tegretol®-XR *see* Carbamazepine *on page 255*

Tegrin® [OTC] *see* Coal Tar *on page 367*

Telithromycin (tel ith roe MYE sin)

U.S. Brand Names Ketek™

Canadian Brand Names Ketek™

Generic Available No

Synonyms HMR 3647

Pharmacologic Category Antibiotic, Ketolide

Use Treatment of community-acquired pneumonia (mild to moderate) caused by susceptible strains of *Streptococcus pneumoniae* (including multidrug-resistant isolates), *Haemophilus influenzae, Chlamydia pneumoniae, Moraxella catarrhalis,* and *Mycoplasma pneumoniae*; treatment of bacterial exacerbation of chronic bronchitis caused by susceptible strains of *S. pneumoniae, H. influenzae,* and *Moraxella catarrhalis*; treatment of acute bacterial sinusitis caused by *Streptococcus pneumoniae, Haemophilus influenza,* and *Moraxella catarrhalis*

Unlabeled/Investigational Use Approved in Canada for use in the treatment of tonsillitis/pharyngitis due to *S. pyogenes* (as an alternative to beta-lactam antibiotics when necessary/appropriate)

Local Anesthetic/Vasoconstrictor Precautions Telithromycin is associated with prolongation of cardiac repolarization. It produces a block of myocardial potassium currents resulting in prolonged QT_c interval which may give rise to ventricular tachycardia, ventricular fibrillation or torsade de pointes. Vasoconstrictor should be used with caution; if possible, wait until the patients complete their course of antibiotic therapy prior to using vasoconstrictor. The overall risk of ventricular arrhythmias by telithromycin is small and can be further reduced by the cautious use of vasoconstrictor.

Effects on Dental Treatment Key adverse event(s) related to dental treatment: Xerostomia (normal salivary flow resumes upon discontinuation), glossitis, stomatitis, and tooth discoloration.

(Continued)

Telithromycin *(Continued)*

Common Adverse Effects

2% to 10%:

Central nervous system: Headache (2% to 6%), dizziness (3% to 4%)

Gastrointestinal: Diarrhea (10%), nausea (7% to 8%), vomiting (2% to 3%), loose stools (2%)

≥0.2% to <2%:

Central nervous system: Vertigo, fatigue, somnolence, insomnia

Dermatologic: Rash

Gastrointestinal: Abdominal distension, abdominal pain, anorexia, constipation, dyspepsia, flatulence, gastritis, gastroenteritis, GI upset, glossitis, stomatitis, watery stools, xerostomia

Genitourinary: Vaginal candidiasis

Hematologic: Platelets increased

Hepatic: Transaminases increased, hepatitis

Ocular: Blurred vision, accommodation delayed, diplopia

Miscellaneous: Candidiasis, diaphoresis increased, exacerbation of myasthenia gravis (rare)

Additional effects also reported with telithromycin:

Cardiovascular: Bundle branch block, palpitation, QT_c prolongation, vasculitis

Central nervous system: Abnormal dreams, nervousness, tremor

Endocrine & metabolic: Appetite decreased, hypokalemia, hyperkalemia

Gastrointestinal: Esophagitis, pharyngolaryngeal pain, pseudomembranous colitis, reflux esophagitis, tooth discoloration

Genitourinary: Vaginal irritation, urine discoloration, polyuria

Hematologic: Anemia, coagulation disorder, leukopenia, neutropenia, thrombocytopenia, lymphopenia

Hepatic: Cholestasis

Neuromuscular & skeletal: Weakness

Renal: Serum creatinine increased

Miscellaneous: Hypersensitivity

Mechanism of Action Inhibits bacterial protein synthesis by binding to two sites on the 50S ribosomal subunit. Telithromycin has also been demonstrated to alter secretion of IL-1alpha and TNF-alpha; the clinical significance of this immunomodulatory effect has not been evaluated.

Drug Interactions

Cytochrome P450 Effect: Substrate of CYP1A2 (minor), 3A4 (major); **Inhibits** CYP2D6 (weak), 3A4 (strong)

Increased Effect/Toxicity: Concurrent use of cisapride or pimozide is contraindicated. Concurrent use with antiarrhythmics (eg, class Ia and class III) or other drugs which prolong QT_c (eg, gatifloxacin, mesoridazine, moxifloxacin, pimozide, sparfloxacin, thioridazine) may be additive; serious arrhythmias may occur. Neuromuscular-blocking agents may be potentiated by telithromycin.

Telithromycin may increase the levels/effects of selected benzodiazepines, calcium channel blockers, cyclosporine, ergot alkaloids, selected HMG-CoA reductase inhibitors, mirtazapine, nateglinide, nefazodone, pimozide, quinidine, sildenafil (and other PDE-5 inhibitors), tacrolimus, venlafaxine, and other CYP3A4 substrates. Selected benzodiazepines (midazolam, triazolam), and selected HMG-CoA reductase inhibitors (lovastatin and simvastatin) are generally contraindicated with strong CYP3A4 inhibitors. When used with strong CYP3A4 inhibitors, dosage adjustment/limits are recommended for sildenafil and other PDE-5 inhibitors; refer to individual monographs.

The levels/effects of telithromycin may be increased by azole antifungals, ciprofloxacin, clarithromycin, diclofenac, doxycycline, erythromycin, imatinib, isoniazid, nefazodone, nicardipine, propofol, protease inhibitors, quinidine, verapamil, and other CYP3A4 inhibitors.

Decreased Effect: The levels/effects of telithromycin may be decreased by aminoglutethimide, carbamazepine, nafcillin, nevirapine, phenobarbital, phenytoin, rifamycins, and other CYP3A4 inducers; avoid concurrent use.

Pharmacodynamics/Kinetics

Absorption: Rapid

Distribution: 2.9 L/kg

Protein binding: 60% to 70%

Metabolism: Hepatic, via CYP3A4 (50%) and non-CYP-mediated pathways

Bioavailability: 57% (significant first-pass metabolism)

Half-life elimination: 10 hours

Time to peak, plasma: 1 hour

Excretion: Urine (13% unchanged drug, remainder as metabolites); feces (7%)

Pregnancy Risk Factor C

Telmisartan (tel mi SAR tan)

Related Information

Cardiovascular Diseases *on page 1458*

U.S. Brand Names Micardis®

Canadian Brand Names Micardis®

Generic Available No

Pharmacologic Category Angiotensin II Receptor Blocker

Use Treatment of hypertension; may be used alone or in combination with other antihypertensive agents

Local Anesthetic/Vasoconstrictor Precautions No information available to require special precautions

Effects on Dental Treatment No significant effects or complications reported

Common Adverse Effects May be associated with worsening of renal function in patients dependent on renin-angiotensin-aldosterone system.

1% to 10%:

- Cardiovascular: Hypertension (1%), chest pain (1%), peripheral edema (1%)
- Central nervous system: Headache (1%), dizziness (1%), pain (1%), fatigue (1%)
- Gastrointestinal: Diarrhea (3%), dyspepsia (1%), nausea (1%), abdominal pain (1%)
- Genitourinary: Urinary tract infection (1%)
- Neuromuscular & skeletal: Back pain (3%), myalgia (1%)
- Respiratory: Upper respiratory infection (7%), sinusitis (3%), pharyngitis (1%), cough (2%)
- Miscellaneous: Flu-like syndrome (1%)

Mechanism of Action Angiotensin II acts as a vasoconstrictor. In addition to causing direct vasoconstriction, angiotensin II also stimulates the release of aldosterone. Once aldosterone is released, sodium as well as water are reabsorbed. The end result is an elevation in blood pressure. Telmisartan is a nonpeptide AT1 angiotensin II receptor antagonist. This binding prevents angiotensin II from binding to the receptor thereby blocking the vasoconstriction and the aldosterone secreting effects of angiotensin II.

Drug Interactions

Cytochrome P450 Effect: Inhibits CYP2C19 (weak)

Increased Effect/Toxicity: Telmisartan may increase serum digoxin concentrations. Potassium salts/supplements, co-trimoxazole (high dose), ACE inhibitors, and potassium-sparing diuretics (amiloride, spironolactone, triamterene) may increase the risk of hyperkalemia with telmisartan.

Decreased Effect: Telmisartan decreased the trough concentrations of warfarin during concurrent therapy, however, INR was not changed.

Pharmacodynamics/Kinetics Orally active, not a prodrug

Onset of action: 1-2 hours

Peak effect: 0.5-1 hours

Duration: Up to 24 hours

Protein binding: >99.5%

Metabolism: Hepatic via conjugation to inactive metabolites; not metabolized via CYP

Bioavailability (dose dependent): 42% to 58%

Half-life elimination: Terminal: 24 hours

Excretion: Feces (97%)

Clearance: Total body: 800 mL/minute

Pregnancy Risk Factor C (1st trimester); D (2nd and 3rd trimesters)

Telmisartan and HCTZ *see* Telmisartan and Hydrochlorothiazide *on page 1265*

Telmisartan and Hydrochlorothiazide

(tel mi SAR tan & hye droe klor oh THYE a zide)

Related Information

Hydrochlorothiazide *on page 699*

Telmisartan *on page 1265*

U.S. Brand Names Micardis® HCT

Canadian Brand Names Micardis® Plus

Generic Available No

Synonyms HCTZ and Telmisartan; Hydrochlorothiazide and Telmisartan; Telmisartan and HCTZ

Pharmacologic Category Angiotensin II Receptor Blocker Combination; Antihypertensive Agent, Combination; Diuretic, Thiazide

(Continued)

Telmisartan and Hydrochlorothiazide *(Continued)*

Use Treatment of hypertension; combination product should not be used for initial therapy

Local Anesthetic/Vasoconstrictor Precautions No information available to require special precautions

Effects on Dental Treatment No significant effects or complications reported

Common Adverse Effects The following reactions have been reported with the combination product; see individual agents for additional adverse reactions that may be expected from each agent.

2% to 10%:

Central nervous system: Dizziness (5%)
Gastrointestinal: Diarrhea (3%), nausea (2%)
Renal: BUN increased (3%)
Respiratory: Upper respiratory tract infection (8%), sinusitis (4%)
Miscellaneous: Flu-like syndrome (2%)

<2%: Abdominal pain, back pain, bilirubin increased, bronchitis, dyspepsia, hematocrit decreased, hemoglobin decreased, hypokalemia, liver enzymes increased, pharyngitis, postural hypotension, rash, serum creatinine increased, tachycardia, vomiting; rhabdomyolysis has been reported (rarely) with angiotensin-receptor antagonists

Mechanism of Action

Telmisartan: Telmisartan is an angiotensin receptor antagonist. Angiotensin II acts as a vasoconstrictor. In addition to causing direct vasoconstriction, angiotensin II also stimulates the release of aldosterone. Once aldosterone is released, sodium as well as water are reabsorbed. The end result is an elevation in blood pressure. Telmisartan binds to the AT1 angiotensin II receptor. This binding prevents angiotensin II from binding to the receptor thereby blocking the vasoconstriction and the aldosterone secreting effects of angiotensin II.

Hydrochlorothiazide: Inhibits sodium reabsorption in the distal tubules causing increased excretion of sodium and water as well as potassium and hydrogen ions

Drug Interactions

Cytochrome P450 Effect: Telmisartan: **Inhibits** CYP2C19 (weak)

Increased Effect/Toxicity: See individual agents.

Decreased Effect: See individual agents.

Pharmacodynamics/Kinetics See individual agents.

Pregnancy Risk Factor C (1st trimester); D (2nd and 3rd trimesters)

Temazepam (te MAZ e pam)

U.S. Brand Names Restoril®

Canadian Brand Names Apo-Temazepam®; CO Temazepam; Gen-Temazepam; Novo-Temazepam; Nu-Temazepam; PMS-Temazepam; ratio-Temazepam; Restoril®

Generic Available Yes

Pharmacologic Category Benzodiazepine

Use Short-term treatment of insomnia

Unlabeled/Investigational Use Treatment of anxiety; adjunct in the treatment of depression; management of panic attacks

Local Anesthetic/Vasoconstrictor Precautions No information available to require special precautions

Effects on Dental Treatment Key adverse event(s) related to dental treatment: Significant xerostomia (normal salivary flow resumes upon discontinuation).

Common Adverse Effects

1% to 10%:

Central nervous system: Confusion, dizziness, drowsiness, fatigue, anxiety, headache, lethargy, hangover, euphoria, vertigo
Dermatologic: Rash
Endocrine & metabolic: Decreased libido
Gastrointestinal: Diarrhea
Neuromuscular & skeletal: Dysarthria, weakness
Ocular: Blurred vision
Miscellaneous: Diaphoresis

Restrictions C-IV

Dosage Oral:

Adults: 15-30 mg at bedtime
Elderly or debilitated patients: 15 mg

Mechanism of Action Binds to stereospecific benzodiazepine receptors on the postsynaptic GABA neuron at several sites within the central nervous system, including the limbic system, reticular formation. Enhancement of the inhibitory effect of GABA on neuronal excitability results by increased neuronal membrane permeability to chloride ions. This shift in chloride ions results in hyperpolarization (a less excitable state) and stabilization.

Contraindications Hypersensitivity to temazepam or any component of the formulation (cross-sensitivity with other benzodiazepines may exist); narrow-angle glaucoma (not in product labeling, however, benzodiazepines are contraindicated); pregnancy

Warnings/Precautions Should be used only after evaluation of potential causes of sleep disturbance. Failure of sleep disturbance to resolve after 7-10 days may indicate psychiatric or medical illness. A worsening of insomnia or the emergence of new abnormalities of thought or behavior may represent unrecognized psychiatric or medical illness and requires immediate and careful evaluation.

Use with caution in elderly or debilitated patients, patients with hepatic disease (including alcoholics), or renal impairment. Use with caution in patients with respiratory disease, or impaired gag reflex. Avoid use inpatients with sleep apnea.

Causes CNS depression (dose-related) resulting in sedation, dizziness, confusion, or ataxia which may impair physical and mental capabilities. Patients must be cautioned about performing tasks which require mental alertness (eg, operating machinery or driving). Use with caution in patients receiving other CNS depressants or psychoactive agents. Effects with other sedative drugs or ethanol may be potentiated. Benzodiazepines have been associated with falls and traumatic injury and should be used with extreme caution in patients who are at risk of these events (especially the elderly).

Use caution in patients with suicidal risk. Use with caution in patients with a history of drug dependence. Benzodiazepines have been associated with dependence and acute withdrawal symptoms on discontinuation or reduction in dose (may occur after as little as 10 days). Acute withdrawal, including seizures, may be precipitated after administration of flumazenil to patients receiving long-term benzodiazepine therapy.

Benzodiazepines have been associated with anterograde amnesia. Paradoxical reactions, including hyperactive or aggressive behavior, have been reported with benzodiazepines, particularly in adolescent/pediatric or psychiatric patients. Does not have analgesic, antidepressant, or antipsychotic properties.

Drug Interactions

Cytochrome P450 Effect: Substrate (minor) of CYP2B6, 2C8/9, 2C19, 3A4

Increased Effect/Toxicity: Temazepam potentiates the CNS depressant effects of narcotic analgesics, barbiturates, phenothiazines, ethanol, antihistamines, MAO inhibitors, sedative-hypnotics, and cyclic antidepressants. Serum levels of temazepam may be increased by inhibitors of CYP3A4, including cimetidine, ciprofloxacin, clarithromycin, clozapine, diltiazem, disulfiram, digoxin, erythromycin, ethanol, fluconazole, fluoxetine, fluvoxamine, grapefruit juice, isoniazid, itraconazole, ketoconazole, labetalol, levodopa, loxapine, metoprolol, metronidazole, miconazole, nefazodone, omeprazole, phenytoin, rifabutin, rifampin, troleandomycin, valproic acid, and verapamil.

Decreased Effect: Oral contraceptives may increase the clearance of temazepam. Temazepam may decrease the antiparkinsonian efficacy of levodopa. Theophylline and other CNS stimulants may antagonize the sedative effects of temazepam. Carbamazepine, rifampin, rifabutin may enhance the metabolism of temazepam and decrease its therapeutic effect.

Ethanol/Nutrition/Herb Interactions

Ethanol: Avoid ethanol (may increase CNS depression).

Food: Serum levels may be increased by grapefruit juice.

Herb/Nutraceutical: St John's wort may decrease temazepam levels. Avoid valerian, St John's wort, kava kava, gotu kola (may increase CNS depression).

Pharmacodynamics/Kinetics

Distribution: V_d: 1.4 L/kg

Protein binding: 96%

Metabolism: Hepatic

Half-life elimination: 9.5-12.4 hours

Time to peak, serum: 2-3 hours

Excretion: Urine (80% to 90% as inactive metabolites)

Pregnancy Risk Factor X

Dosage Forms CAP: 15 mg, 30 mg; (Restoril®): 7.5 mg, 15 mg, 30 mg

Temodar® *see* Temozolomide *on page 1268*

Temovate® *see* Clobetasol *on page 351*
Temovate E® *see* Clobetasol *on page 351*

Temozolomide (te moe ZOE loe mide)

U.S. Brand Names Temodar®
Canadian Brand Names Temodal™; Temodar®
Generic Available No
Synonyms NSC-362856; TMZ
Pharmacologic Category Antineoplastic Agent, Alkylating Agent
Use Treatment of adult patients with refractory (first relapse) anaplastic astrocytoma who have experienced disease progression on nitrosourea and procarbazine
Unlabeled/Investigational Use Glioma, melanoma
Local Anesthetic/Vasoconstrictor Precautions No information available to require special precautions
Effects on Dental Treatment No significant effects or complications reported
Common Adverse Effects

>10%:

Cardiovascular: Peripheral edema (11%)
Central nervous system: Headache (41%), fatigue (34%), convulsions (23%), hemiparesis (29%), dizziness (19%), fever (11%), coordination abnormality (11%), amnesia (10%), insomnia (10%), somnolence. In the case of CNS malignancies, it is difficult to distinguish the relative contributions of temozolomide and progressive disease to CNS symptoms.
Gastrointestinal: Nausea (53%), vomiting (42%), constipation (33%), diarrhea (16%)
Hematologic: Neutropenia (grade 3-4, 14%), thrombocytopenia (grade 3-4 19%)
Neuromuscular & skeletal: Weakness (13%)

1% to 10%:

Central nervous system: Ataxia (8%), confusion (5%), anxiety (7%), depression (6%)
Dermatologic: Rash (8%), pruritus (8%)
Endocrine & metabolic: Hypercorticism (8%), breast pain (6%), weight gain (5%)
Gastrointestinal: Dysphagia (7%), abdominal pain (9%), anorexia (9%)
Genitourinary: Increased micturition frequency (6%)
Hematologic: Anemia (8%; grade 3-4, 4%)
Neuromuscular & skeletal: Paresthesia (9%), back pain (8%), myalgia (5%)
Ocular: Diplopia (5%), vision abnormality (5%)
Respiratory: Pharyngitis (8%), sinusitis (6%), cough (5%)

Mechanism of Action Like dacarbazine, temozolomide is converted to the active alkylating metabolite MTIC [(methyl-triazene-1-yl)-imidazole-4-carboxamide]. Unlike dacarbazine, however, this conversion is spontaneous, nonenzymatic, and occurs under physiologic conditions in all tissues to which the drug distributes.

Drug Interactions

Decreased Effect: Although valproic acid reduces the clearance of temozolomide by 5%, the clinical significance of this is unknown.

Pharmacodynamics/Kinetics

Distribution: V_d: Parent drug: 0.4 L/kg
Protein binding: 15%
Metabolism: Prodrug, hydrolyzed to the active form, MTIC; MTIC is eventually eliminated as CO_2 and 5-aminoimidazole-4-carboxamide (AIC), a natural constituent in urine
Bioavailability: 100%
Half-life elimination: Mean: Parent drug: 1.8 hours
Time to peak: Empty stomach: 1 hour
Excretion: Urine (5% to 7% of total)

Pregnancy Risk Factor D

Temporomandibular Dysfunction (TMD) *see page 1564*

Tenecteplase (ten EK te plase)

Related Information

Cardiovascular Diseases *on page 1458*

U.S. Brand Names TNKase™
Canadian Brand Names TNKase™
Generic Available No
Pharmacologic Category Thrombolytic Agent

Use Thrombolytic agent used in the management of acute myocardial infarction for the lysis of thrombi in the coronary vasculature to restore perfusion and reduce mortality.

Local Anesthetic/Vasoconstrictor Precautions No information available to require special precautions

Effects on Dental Treatment No significant effects or complications reported

Common Adverse Effects As with all drugs which may affect hemostasis, bleeding is the major adverse effect associated with tenecteplase. Hemorrhage may occur at virtually any site. Risk is dependent on multiple variables, including the dosage administered, concurrent use of multiple agents which alter hemostasis, and patient predisposition. Rapid lysis of coronary artery thrombi by thrombolytic agents may be associated with reperfusion-related arterial and/or ventricular arrhythmias. The incidence of stroke and bleeding increase in patients >65 years.

>10%:

- Hematologic: Bleeding (22% minor: ASSENT-2 trial)
- Local: Hematoma (12% minor)

1% to 10%:

- Central nervous system: Stroke (2%)
- Gastrointestinal: GI hemorrhage (1% major, 2% minor), epistaxis (2% minor)
- Genitourinary: GU bleeding (4% minor)
- Hematologic: Bleeding (5% major: ASSENT-2 trial)
- Local: Bleeding at catheter puncture site (4% minor), hematoma (2% major)
- Respiratory: Pharyngeal bleeding (3% minor)

Additional cardiovascular events associated with use in myocardial infarction: Cardiogenic shock, arrhythmias, AV block, pulmonary edema, heart failure, cardiac arrest, recurrent myocardial ischemia, myocardial reinfarction, myocardial rupture, cardiac tamponade, pericarditis, pericardial effusion, mitral regurgitation, thrombosis, embolism, electromechanical dissociation, hypotension, fever, nausea, vomiting

Mechanism of Action Initiates fibrinolysis by binding to fibrin and converting plasminogen to plasmin.

Drug Interactions

Increased Effect/Toxicity: Drugs which affect platelet function (eg, NSAIDs, dipyridamole, ticlopidine, clopidogrel, IIb/IIIa antagonists) may potentiate the risk of hemorrhage; use with caution.

Heparin and aspirin: Use with aspirin and heparin may increase bleeding. However, aspirin and heparin were used concomitantly with tenecteplase in the majority of patients in clinical studies.

Warfarin or oral anticoagulants: Risk of bleeding may be increased during concurrent therapy.

Decreased Effect: Aminocaproic acid (antifibrinolytic agent) may decrease effectiveness.

Pharmacodynamics/Kinetics

Distribution: V_d is weight related and approximates plasma volume

Metabolism: Primarily hepatic

Half-life elimination: 90-130 minutes

Excretion: Clearance: Plasma: 99-119 mL/minute

Pregnancy Risk Factor C

Tenex® *see* Guanfacine *on page 679*

Teniposide (ten i POE side)

U.S. Brand Names Vumon

Canadian Brand Names Vumon®

Mexican Brand Names Vumon®

Generic Available No

Synonyms EPT; VM-26

Pharmacologic Category Antineoplastic Agent, Miscellaneous

Use Treatment of acute lymphocytic leukemia, small cell lung cancer

Local Anesthetic/Vasoconstrictor Precautions No information available to require special precautions

Effects on Dental Treatment No significant effects or complications reported

Common Adverse Effects

>10%:

- Gastrointestinal: Mucositis (75%); diarrhea, nausea, vomiting (20% to 30%); anorexia
- Hematologic: Myelosuppression, leukopenia, neutropenia (95%), thrombocytopenia (65% to 80%), anemia
  - Onset: 5-7 days
  - Nadir: 7-10 days

(Continued)

Teniposide *(Continued)*

Recovery: 21-28 days

1% to 10%:

Cardiovascular: Hypotension (2%), associated with rapid (<30 minutes) infusions

Dermatologic: Alopecia (9%), rash (3%)

Miscellaneous: Anaphylactoid reactions (5%) (fever, rash, hypertension, hypotension, dyspnea, bronchospasm), usually seen with rapid (<30 minutes) infusions

Mechanism of Action Teniposide does not inhibit microtubular assembly; it has been shown to delay transit of cells through the S phase and arrest cells in late S or early G_2 phase. Teniposide is a topoisomerase II inhibitor, and appears to cause DNA strand breaks by inhibition of strand-passing and DNA ligase action.

Drug Interactions

Cytochrome P450 Effect: Substrate of CYP3A4 (major); **Inhibits** CYP2C8/9 (weak), 3A4 (weak)

Increased Effect/Toxicity: May increase toxicity of methotrexate. Sodium salicylate, sulfamethizole, and tolbutamide displace teniposide from protein-binding sites which could cause substantial increases in free drug levels, resulting in potentiation of toxicity. Concurrent use of vincristine may increase the incidence of peripheral neuropathy. CYP3A4 inhibitors may increase the levels/effects of teniposide; example inhibitors include azole antifungals, ciprofloxacin, clarithromycin, diclofenac, doxycycline, erythromycin, imatinib, isoniazid, nefazodone, nicardipine, propofol, protease inhibitors, quinidine, and verapamil.

Decreased Effect: CYP3A4 inducers may decrease the levels/effects of teniposide; example inducers include aminoglutethimide, carbamazepine, nafcillin, nevirapine, phenobarbital, phenytoin, and rifamycins.

Pharmacodynamics/Kinetics

Distribution: V_d: 0.28 L/kg; Adults: 8-44 L; Children: 3-11 L; mainly into liver, kidneys, small intestine, and adrenals; crosses blood-brain barrier to a limited extent

Protein binding: 99.4%

Metabolism: Extensively hepatic

Half-life elimination: 5 hours

Excretion: Urine (44%, 21% as unchanged drug); feces (≤10%)

Pregnancy Risk Factor D

Tenofovir (te NOE fo veer)

Related Information

HIV Infection and AIDS *on page 1484*

U.S. Brand Names Viread®

Generic Available No

Synonyms PMPA; TDF; Tenofovir Disoproxil Fumarate

Pharmacologic Category Antiretroviral Agent, Reverse Transcriptase Inhibitor (Nucleotide)

Use Management of HIV infections in combination with at least two other antiretroviral agents

Local Anesthetic/Vasoconstrictor Precautions No information available to require special precautions

Effects on Dental Treatment No significant effects or complications reported

Common Adverse Effects Clinical trials involved addition to prior antiretroviral therapy. Frequencies listed are treatment-emergent adverse effects noted at higher frequency than in the placebo group.

>10%: Gastrointestinal: Nausea (8% to 11%), diarrhea (11% to 16%)

1% to 10%:

Central nervous system: Headache (5% to 8%), depression (5% to 8%), dizziness (1% to 3%), insomnia (1% to 4%)

Endocrine & metabolic: Glycosuria (3%, frequency equal to placebo); other metabolic effects (hyperglycemia, hypertriglyceridemia) noted at frequencies less than placebo

Gastrointestinal: Vomiting (4% to 7%), flatulence (3% to 4%), abdominal pain (4% to 7%), anorexia (3% to 4%)

Hematologic: Neutropenia (1% to 2%)

Hepatic: Transaminases increased (2% to 4%)

Neuromuscular & skeletal: Weakness (7% to 11%), back pain (3% to 4%), myalgia (3% to 4%), neuropathy (1% to 3%)

Note: Uncommon, but significant adverse reactions reported with other reverse transcriptase inhibitors include pancreatitis, peripheral neuropathy, and myopathy.

Mechanism of Action Tenofovir disoproxil fumarate (TDF) is an analog of adenosine 5'-monophosphate; it interferes with the HIV viral RNA dependent DNA polymerase resulting in inhibition of viral replication. TDF is first converted intracellularly by hydrolysis to tenofovir and subsequently phosphorylated to the active tenofovir diphosphate; nucleotide reverse transcriptase inhibitor.

Drug Interactions

Cytochrome P450 Effect: Inhibits CYP1A2 (weak)

Increased Effect/Toxicity: Concurrent use has been noted to increase serum concentrations/exposure to didanosine and its metabolites, potentially increasing the risk of didanosine toxicity (pancreatitis, peripheral neuropathy, or lactic acidosis); use caution and monitor closely; suspend therapy if signs/symptoms of toxicity are present. Drugs which may compete for renal tubule secretion (including acyclovir, cidofovir, ganciclovir, valacyclovir, valganciclovir) may increase the serum concentrations of tenofovir. Drugs causing nephrotoxicity may reduce elimination of tenofovir. Lopinavir/ritonavir may increase serum concentrations of tenofovir.

Decreased Effect: Serum levels of lopinavir and/or ritonavir may be decreased by tenofovir. Tenofovir may decrease serum concentrations of atazanavir, resulting in a loss of virologic response (specific atazanavir dosing recommendations provided by manufacturer).

Pharmacodynamics/Kinetics

Distribution: 1.2-1.3 L/kg

Protein binding: 7% to serum proteins

Metabolism: Tenofovir disoproxil fumarate (TDF) is converted intracellularly by hydrolysis (by nonCYP enzymes) to tenofovir, then phosphorylated to the active tenofovir diphosphate

Bioavailability: 25% (fasting); increases ~40% with high-fat meal

Time to peak, serum: Fasting: 1 hour; With food: 2 hours

Excretion: Urine (70% to 80%) via filtration and active secretion, primarily as unchanged tenofovir

Pregnancy Risk Factor B

Tenofovir Disoproxil Fumarate *see* Tenofovir *on page 1270*

Tenoretic® *see* Atenolol and Chlorthalidone *on page 161*

Tenormin® *see* Atenolol *on page 159*

Tenuate® *see* Diethylpropion *on page 434*

Tenuate® Dospan® *see* Diethylpropion *on page 434*

Tequin® *see* Gatifloxacin *on page 647*

Terazol® 3 *see* Terconazole *on page 1274*

Terazol® 7 *see* Terconazole *on page 1274*

Terazosin (ter AY zoe sin)

Related Information

Cardiovascular Diseases *on page 1458*

U.S. Brand Names Hytrin®

Canadian Brand Names Alti-Terazosin; Apo-Terazosin®; Hytrin®; Novo-Terazosin; Nu-Terazosin; PMS-Terazosin

Mexican Brand Names Adecur®; Hytrin®

Generic Available Yes

Pharmacologic Category Alpha$_1$ Blocker

Use Management of mild to moderate hypertension; alone or in combination with other agents such as diuretics or beta-blockers; benign prostate hyperplasia (BPH)

Local Anesthetic/Vasoconstrictor Precautions No information available to require special precautions

Effects on Dental Treatment Key adverse event(s) related to dental treatment: Xerostomia (normal salivary flow resumes upon discontinuation).

Common Adverse Effects Asthenia, postural hypotension, dizziness, somnolence, nasal congestion/rhinitis, and impotence were the only events noted in clinical trials to occur at a frequency significantly greater than placebo ($p < 0.05$).

>10%: Central nervous system: Dizziness, headache, muscle weakness

1% to 10%:

Cardiovascular: Edema, palpitations, chest pain, peripheral edema (3%), orthostatic hypotension (2.7% to 3.9%), tachycardia

Central nervous system: Fatigue, nervousness, drowsiness

(Continued)

Terazosin *(Continued)*

Gastrointestinal: Dry mouth
Genitourinary: Urinary incontinence
Ocular: Blurred vision
Respiratory: Dyspnea, nasal congestion

Dosage Oral: Adults:

Hypertension: Initial: 1 mg at bedtime; slowly increase dose to achieve desired blood pressure, up to 20 mg/day; usual dose range (JNC 7): 1-20 mg once daily

Dosage reduction may be needed when adding a diuretic or other antihypertensive agent; if drug is discontinued for greater than several days, consider beginning with initial dose and retitrate as needed; dosage may be given on a twice daily regimen if response is diminished at 24 hours and hypotensive is observed at 2-4 hours following a dose

Benign prostatic hyperplasia: Initial: 1 mg at bedtime, increasing as needed; most patients require 10 mg day; if no response after 4-6 weeks of 10 mg/day, may increase to 20 mg/day

Mechanism of Action Alpha$_1$-specific blocking agent with minimal alpha$_2$ effects; this allows peripheral postsynaptic blockade, with the resultant decrease in arterial tone, while preserving the negative feedback loop which is mediated by the peripheral presynaptic alpha$_2$-receptors; terazosin relaxes the smooth muscle of the bladder neck, thus reducing bladder outlet obstruction

Contraindications Hypersensitivity to quinazolines (doxazosin, prazosin, terazosin) or any component of the formulation; concurrent use with phosphodiesterase-5 (PDE-5) inhibitors including sildenafil (>25 mg), tadalafil, or vardenafil

Warnings/Precautions Marked orthostatic hypotension, syncope, and loss of consciousness may occur with first dose ("first dose phenomenon"). This reaction is more likely to occur in patients receiving beta-blockers, diuretics, low sodium diets, or first doses >1 mg/dose in adults; avoid rapid increase in dose; use with caution in patients with renal impairment.

Drug Interactions

Increased Effect/Toxicity: Terazosin's hypotensive effect is increased with beta-blockers, diuretics, ACE inhibitors, calcium channel blockers, other antihypertensive medications, sildenafil (use with extreme caution at a dose ≤25 mg), tadalafil (use is contraindicated by the manufacturer), and vardenafil (use is contraindicated by the manufacturer).

Decreased Effect: Decreased antihypertensive response with NSAIDs. Alpha-blockers reduce the response to pressor agents (norepinephrine).

Ethanol/Nutrition/Herb Interactions Herb/Nutraceutical: Avoid dong quai if using for hypertension (has estrogenic activity). Avoid ephedra, yohimbe, ginseng (may worsen hypertension). Avoid saw palmetto. Avoid garlic (may have increased antihypertensive effect).

Dietary Considerations May be taken without regard to meals at the same time each day.

Pharmacodynamics/Kinetics

Onset of action: 1-2 hours
Absorption: Rapid
Protein binding: 90% to 95%
Metabolism: Extensively hepatic
Half-life elimination: 9.2-12 hours
Time to peak, serum: ~1 hour
Excretion: Feces (60%); urine (40%)

Pregnancy Risk Factor C

Dosage Forms CAP (Hytrin®): 1 mg, 2 mg, 5 mg, 10 mg. **TAB:** 1 mg, 2 mg, 5 mg, 10 mg

Terbinafine (TER bin a feen)

U.S. Brand Names Lamisil®; Lamisil® AT™ [OTC]

Canadian Brand Names Apo-Terbinafine®; Gen-Terbinafine; Lamisil®; Novo-Terbinafine; PMS-Terbinafine

Mexican Brand Names Lamisil®

Generic Available No

Synonyms Terbinafine Hydrochloride

Pharmacologic Category Antifungal Agent, Oral; Antifungal Agent, Topical

Use Active against most strains of *Trichophyton mentagrophytes, Trichophyton rubrum*; may be effective for infections of *Microsporum gypseum* and *M. nanum, Trichophyton verrucosum, Epidermophyton floccosum, Candida albicans*, and *Scopulariopsis brevicaulis*

Oral: Onychomycosis of the toenail or fingernail due to susceptible dermatophytes

Topical: Antifungal for the treatment of tinea pedis (athlete's foot), tinea cruris (jock itch), and tinea corporis (ringworm) [OTC/prescription formulations]; tinea versicolor [prescription formulations]

Local Anesthetic/Vasoconstrictor Precautions No information available to require special precautions

Effects on Dental Treatment No significant effects or complications reported

Common Adverse Effects

Oral:

1% to 10%:

Central nervous system: Headache, dizziness, vertigo

Dermatologic: Rash, pruritus, urticaria

Gastrointestinal: Diarrhea, dyspepsia, abdominal pain, appetite decrease, taste disturbance

Hematologic: Lymphocytopenia

Hepatic: Liver enzymes increased

Ocular: Visual disturbance

Topical: 1% to 10%:

Dermatologic: Pruritus, contact dermatitis, irritation, burning, dryness

Local: Irritation, stinging

Mechanism of Action Synthetic alkylamine derivative which inhibits squalene epoxidase, a key enzyme in sterol biosynthesis in fungi. This results in a deficiency in ergosterol within the fungal cell wall and results in fungal cell death.

Drug Interactions

Cytochrome P450 Effect: Substrate (minor) of 1A2, 2C8/9, 2C19, 3A4; **Inhibits** CYP2D6 (strong); **Induces** CYP3A4 (weak)

Increased Effect/Toxicity: Terbinafine may increase the levels/effects of amphetamines, beta-blockers, dextromethorphan, fluoxetine, lidocaine, mirtazapine, nefazodone, paroxetine, risperidone, ritonavir, thioridazine, tricyclic antidepressants, venlafaxine, and other CYP2D6 substrates. The effects of warfarin may be increased.

Decreased Effect: Terbinafine may decrease the levels/effects of CYP2D6 prodrug substrates (eg, codeine, hydrocodone, oxycodone, tramadol).

Pharmacodynamics/Kinetics

Absorption: Topical: Limited (<5%); Oral: >70%

Distribution: V_d: 2000 L; distributed to sebum and skin predominantly

Protein binding, plasma: >99%

Metabolism: Hepatic; no active metabolites; first-pass effect; little effect on CYP

Bioavailability: Oral: 40%

Half-life elimination:

Topical: 22-26 hours

Oral: Terminal half-life: 200-400 hours; very slow release of drug from skin and adipose tissues occurs; effective half-life: ~36 hours

Time to peak, plasma: 1-2 hours

Excretion: Urine (70% to 75%)

Pregnancy Risk Factor B

Terbinafine Hydrochloride *see* Terbinafine *on page 1272*

Terbutaline (ter BYOO ta leen)

Related Information

Respiratory Diseases *on page 1478*

U.S. Brand Names Brethine®

Canadian Brand Names Bricanyl® [DSC]

Mexican Brand Names Bricanyl®; Taziken® [tabs]

Generic Available Yes

Synonyms Brethaire [DSC]; Bricanyl [DSC]

Pharmacologic Category $Beta_2$-Adrenergic Agonist

Use Bronchodilator in reversible airway obstruction and bronchial asthma; tocolytic agent

Unlabeled/Investigational Use Tocolytic agent (management of preterm labor)

Local Anesthetic/Vasoconstrictor Precautions No information available to require special precautions

Effects on Dental Treatment Key adverse event(s) related to dental treatment: Xerostomia (normal salivary flow resumes upon discontinuation).

Common Adverse Effects

>10%:

Central nervous system: Nervousness, restlessness

(Continued)

Terbutaline *(Continued)*

Endocrine & metabolic: Serum glucose increased, serum potassium decreased
Neuromuscular & skeletal: Trembling

1% to 10%:
Cardiovascular: Tachycardia, hypertension
Central nervous system: Dizziness, drowsiness, headache, insomnia
Gastrointestinal: Xerostomia, nausea, vomiting, bad taste in mouth
Neuromuscular & skeletal: Muscle cramps, weakness
Miscellaneous: Diaphoresis

Mechanism of Action Relaxes bronchial smooth muscle by action on beta$_2$-receptors with less effect on heart rate

Drug Interactions

Increased Effect/Toxicity: Increased toxicity with MAO inhibitors, tricyclic antidepressants.

Decreased Effect: Decreased effect with beta-blockers.

Pharmacodynamics/Kinetics

Onset of action: Oral: 30-45 minutes; SubQ: 6-15 minutes
Protein binding: 25%
Metabolism: Hepatic to inactive sulfate conjugates
Bioavailability: SubQ doses are more bioavailable than oral
Half-life elimination: 11-16 hours
Excretion: Urine

Pregnancy Risk Factor B

Terconazole (ter KONE a zole)

Related Information

Sexually-Transmitted Diseases *on page 1504*

U.S. Brand Names Terazol® 3; Terazol® 7

Canadian Brand Names Terazol®

Mexican Brand Names Fungistat®

Generic Available No

Synonyms Triaconazole

Pharmacologic Category Antifungal Agent, Vaginal

Use Local treatment of vulvovaginal candidiasis

Local Anesthetic/Vasoconstrictor Precautions No information available to require special precautions

Effects on Dental Treatment No significant effects or complications reported

Common Adverse Effects 1% to 10%:

Central nervous system; Fever, chills
Gastrointestinal: Abdominal pain
Genitourinary: Vulvar/vaginal burning, dysmenorrhea

Mechanism of Action Triazole ketal antifungal agent; involves inhibition of fungal cytochrome P450. Specifically, terconazole inhibits cytochrome P450-dependent 14-alpha-demethylase which results in accumulation of membrane disturbing 14-alpha-demethylsterols and ergosterol depletion.

Pharmacodynamics/Kinetics Absorption: Extent of systemic absorption after vaginal administration may be dependent on presence of a uterus; 5% to 8% in women who had a hysterectomy versus 12% to 16% in nonhysterectomy women

Pregnancy Risk Factor C

Teriparatide (ter i PAR a tide)

U.S. Brand Names Forteo™

Generic Available No

Synonyms Parathyroid Hormone (1-34); Recombinant Human Parathyroid Hormone (1-34); rhPTH(1-34)

Pharmacologic Category Parathyroid Hormone Analog

Use Treatment of osteoporosis in postmenopausal women at high risk of fracture; treatment of primary or hypogonadal osteoporosis in men at high risk of fracture

Local Anesthetic/Vasoconstrictor Precautions No information available to require special precautions

Effects on Dental Treatment No significant effects or complications reported

Common Adverse Effects 1% to 10%:

Cardiovascular: Chest pain (3%), syncope (3%)
Central nervous system: Dizziness (8%), depression (4%), vertigo (4%)
Dermatologic: Rash (5%)
Endocrine & metabolic: Hypercalcemia (transient increases noted 4-6 hours postdose in 11% of women and 6% of men)

Gastrointestinal: Nausea (9%), dyspepsia (5%), vomiting (3%), tooth disorder (2%)
Genitourinary: Hyperuricemia (3%)
Neuromuscular & skeletal: Arthralgia (10%), weakness (9%), leg cramps (3%)
Respiratory: Rhinitis (10%), pharyngitis (6%), dyspnea (4%), pneumonia (4%)
Miscellaneous: Antibodies to teriparatide (3% of women in long-term treatment; hypersensitivity reactions or decreased efficacy were not associated in preclinical trials)

Mechanism of Action Teriparatide is a recombinant formulation of endogenous parathyroid hormone (PTH), containing a 34-amino-acid sequence which is identical to the N-terminal portion of this hormone. The pharmacologic activity of teriparatide is similar to the physiologic activity of PTH, stimulating osteoblast function, increasing gastrointestinal calcium absorption, increasing renal tubular reabsorption of calcium. Treatment with teriparatide increases bone mineral density, bone mass, and strength. In postmenopausal women, it has been shown to decrease osteoporosis-related fractures.

Drug Interactions

Increased Effect/Toxicity: Digitalis serum concentrations are not affected, however, transient hypercalcemia may increase risk of digitalis toxicity (case reports).

Pharmacodynamics/Kinetics

Distribution: V_d: 0.12 L/kg
Metabolism: Hepatic (nonspecific proteolysis)
Bioavailability: 95%
Half-life elimination: Serum: I.V.: 5 minutes; SubQ: 1 hour
Excretion: Urine (as metabolites)

Pregnancy Risk Factor C

Terpin Hydrate and Codeine (TER pin HYE drate & KOE deen)

Related Information

Codeine *on page 369*

Generic Available Yes

Synonyms ETH and C

Pharmacologic Category Expectorant

Use Symptomatic relief of cough

Local Anesthetic/Vasoconstrictor Precautions No information available to require special precautions

Effects on Dental Treatment No significant effects or complications reported

Pregnancy Risk Factor C

Terra-Cortril® [DSC] *see* Oxytetracycline and Hydrocortisone *on page 1037*

Terramycin® I.M. *see* Oxytetracycline *on page 1036*

Terramycin® w/Polymyxin B Ophthalmic *see* Oxytetracycline and Polymyxin B *on page 1037*

Teslac® *see* Testolactone *on page 1275*

TESPA *see* Thiotepa *on page 1291*

Tessalon® *see* Benzonatate *on page 193*

Testim™ *see* Testosterone *on page 1276*

Testoderm® [DSC] *see* Testosterone *on page 1276*

Testoderm® with Adhesive [DSC] *see* Testosterone *on page 1276*

Testolactone (tes toe LAK tone)

U.S. Brand Names Teslac®

Canadian Brand Names Teslac®

Generic Available No

Pharmacologic Category Androgen

Use Palliative treatment of advanced or disseminated breast carcinoma

Local Anesthetic/Vasoconstrictor Precautions No information available to require special precautions

Effects on Dental Treatment No significant effects or complications reported

Common Adverse Effects Frequency not defined.

Cardiovascular: Edema, blood pressure increased
Central nervous system: Malaise
Dermatologic: Maculopapular rash, alopecia (rare)
Endocrine & metabolic: Hypercalcemia
Gastrointestinal: Anorexia, diarrhea, nausea, edema of the tongue
Neuromuscular & skeletal: Paresthesias, peripheral neuropathies
Miscellaneous: Nail growth disturbance (rare)

Restrictions C-III

(Continued)

Testolactone *(Continued)*

Mechanism of Action Testolactone is a synthetic testosterone derivative without significant androgen activity. The drug inhibits steroid aromatase activity, thereby blocking the production of estradiol and estrone from androgen precursors such as testosterone and androstenedione. Unfortunately, the enzymatic block provided by testolactone is transient and is usually limited to a period of 3 months.

Drug Interactions

Increased Effect/Toxicity: Increased effects of oral anticoagulants.

Pharmacodynamics/Kinetics

Absorption: Well absorbed

Metabolism: Hepatic (forms metabolites)

Excretion: Urine

Pregnancy Risk Factor C

Testopel® *see* Testosterone *on page 1276*

Testosterone (tes TOS ter one)

U.S. Brand Names Androderm®; AndroGel®; Delatestryl®; Depo®-Testosterone; Striant™; Testim™; Testoderm® [DSC]; Testoderm® with Adhesive [DSC]; Testopel®

Canadian Brand Names Andriol®; Androderm®; AndroGel®; Andropository; Delatestryl®; Depotest® 100; Everone® 200; Testoderm®; Virilon® IM

Generic Available No

Synonyms Testosterone Cypionate; Testosterone Enanthate

Pharmacologic Category Androgen

Use

Injection: Androgen replacement therapy in the treatment of delayed male puberty; male hypogonadism (primary or hypogonadotropic); inoperable female breast cancer (enanthate only)

Pellet: Androgen replacement therapy in the treatment of delayed male puberty; male hypogonadism (primary or hypogonadotropic)

Buccal, topical: Male hypogonadism (primary or hypogonadotropic)

Local Anesthetic/Vasoconstrictor Precautions No information available to require special precautions

Effects on Dental Treatment No significant effects or complications reported

Common Adverse Effects Frequency not defined.

Cardiovascular: Flushing, edema

Central nervous system: Excitation, aggressive behavior, sleeplessness, anxiety, mental depression, headache

Dermatologic: Hirsutism (increase in pubic hair growth), acne

Endocrine & metabolic: Menstrual problems (amenorrhea), virilism, breast soreness, gynecomastia, hypercalcemia, hypoglycemia

Gastrointestinal: Nausea, vomiting, GI irritation

Following buccal administration: Bitter taste, gum edema, gum or mouth irritation, gum tenderness, taste perversion

Genitourinary: Prostatic hyperplasia, prostatic carcinoma, impotence, testicular atrophy, epididymitis, priapism, bladder irritability

Hepatic: Hepatic dysfunction, cholestatic hepatitis, hepatic necrosis

Hematologic: Leukopenia, polycythemia, suppression of clotting factors

Miscellaneous: Hypersensitivity reactions

Restrictions C-III

Mechanism of Action Principal endogenous androgen responsible for promoting the growth and development of the male sex organs and maintaining secondary sex characteristics in androgen-deficient males

Drug Interactions

Cytochrome P450 Effect: Substrate (minor) of CYP2B6, 2C8/9, 2C19, 3A4; **Inhibits** CYP3A4 (weak)

Increased Effect/Toxicity: Warfarin and testosterone: Effects of oral anticoagulants may be enhanced. Testosterone may increase levels of oxyphenbutazone. May enhance fluid retention from corticosteroids.

Pharmacodynamics/Kinetics

Duration (route and ester dependent): I.M.: Cypionate and enanthate esters have longest duration, ≤2-4 weeks

Absorption: Transdermal gel: ~10% of dose

Distribution: Crosses placenta; enters breast milk

Protein binding: 98% bound to sex hormone-binding globulin (40%) and albumin

Metabolism: Hepatic; forms metabolites

Half-life elimination: 10-100 minutes

Excretion: Urine (90%); feces (6%)

Pregnancy Risk Factor X

Testosterone Cypionate *see* Testosterone *on page 1276*
Testosterone Enanthate *see* Testosterone *on page 1276*
Testred® *see* MethylTESTOSTERone *on page 912*
Tetanus Antitoxin *see page 1614*
Tetanus Immune Globulin (Human) *see page 1614*

Tetanus Immune Globulin (Human)

(TET a nus i MYUN GLOB yoo lin HYU man)

Related Information

Animal and Human Bites Guidelines *on page 1582*

U.S. Brand Names BayTet™

Canadian Brand Names BayTet™

Generic Available No

Synonyms TIG

Pharmacologic Category Immune Globulin

Use Passive immunization against tetanus; tetanus immune globulin is preferred over tetanus antitoxin for treatment of active tetanus; part of the management of an unclean, wound in a person whose history of previous receipt of tetanus toxoid is unknown or who has received less than three doses of tetanus toxoid; elderly may require TIG more often than younger patients with tetanus infection due to declining antibody titers with age

Local Anesthetic/Vasoconstrictor Precautions No information available to require special precautions

Effects on Dental Treatment No significant effects or complications reported

Common Adverse Effects

>10%: Local: Pain, tenderness, erythema at injection site

1% to 10%:

- Central nervous system: Fever (mild)
- Dermatologic: Urticaria, angioedema
- Neuromuscular & skeletal: Muscle stiffness
- Miscellaneous: Anaphylaxis reaction

Mechanism of Action Passive immunity toward tetanus

Pharmacodynamics/Kinetics Absorption: Well absorbed

Pregnancy Risk Factor C

Tetanus Toxoid (Adsorbed) *see page 1614*

Tetanus Toxoid (Adsorbed)

(TET a nus TOKS oyd, ad SORBED)

Related Information

Diphtheria, Tetanus Toxoids, Acellular Pertussis, Hepatitis B (Recombinant), and Poliovirus (Inactivated) Vaccine *on page 452*

Generic Available No

Pharmacologic Category Toxoid

Use Selective induction of active immunity against tetanus in selected patients. **Note:** Tetanus and diphtheria toxoids for adult use (Td) is the preferred immunizing agent for most adults and for children after their seventh birthday. Young children should receive trivalent DTwP or DTaP (diphtheria/tetanus/pertussis - whole cell or acellular), as part of their childhood immunization program, unless pertussis is contraindicated, then TD is warranted.

Local Anesthetic/Vasoconstrictor Precautions No information available to require special precautions

Effects on Dental Treatment No significant effects or complications reported

Common Adverse Effects

>10%: Local: Induration/redness at injection site

1% to 10%:

- Central nervous system: Chills, fever
- Local: Sterile abscess at injection site
- Miscellaneous: Allergic reaction

Mechanism of Action Tetanus toxoid preparations contain the toxin produced by virulent tetanus bacilli (detoxified growth products of *Clostridium tetani*). The toxin has been modified by treatment with formaldehyde so that it has lost toxicity but still retains ability to act as antigen and produce active immunity; the aluminum salt, a mineral adjuvant, delays the rate of absorption and prolongs and enhances its properties; duration ~10 years.

Pharmacodynamics/Kinetics Duration: Primary immunization: ~10 years

Pregnancy Risk Factor C

Tetanus Toxoid (Fluid) *see page 1614*

Tetanus Toxoid (Fluid) (TET a nus TOKS oyd FLOO id)

Related Information

Diphtheria, Tetanus Toxoids, Acellular Pertussis, Hepatitis B (Recombinant), and Poliovirus (Inactivated) Vaccine *on page 452*

Generic Available No

Synonyms Tetanus Toxoid Plain

Pharmacologic Category Toxoid

Use Indicated as booster dose in the active immunization against tetanus in the rare adult or child who is allergic to the aluminum adjuvant (a product containing adsorbed tetanus toxoid is preferred); not indicated for primary immunization

Unlabeled/Investigational Use Anergy testing (no longer recommended)

Local Anesthetic/Vasoconstrictor Precautions No information available to require special precautions

Effects on Dental Treatment No significant effects or complications reported

Common Adverse Effects All serious adverse reactions must be reported to the U.S. Department of Health and Human Services (DHHS) Vaccine Adverse Event Reporting System (VAERS) 1-800-822-7967.

Frequency not defined.

Cardiovascular: Hypotension

Central nervous system: Brachial neuritis, fever, Guillain-Barré syndrome, malaise

Dermatologic: Rash, urticaria

Gastrointestinal: Nausea

Local: Edema, induration (with or without tenderness), redness, warmth

Neuromuscular & skeletal: Arthralgia

Miscellaneous: Anaphylaxis, Arthus-type hypersensitivity reactions (severe local reaction developing 2-8 hours following injection)

Mechanism of Action Tetanus toxoid preparations contain the toxin produced by virulent tetanus bacilli (detoxified growth products of *Clostridium tetani*). The toxin has been modified by treatment with formaldehyde so that is has lost toxicity but still retains ability to act as antigen and produce active immunity.

Drug Interactions

Increased Effect/Toxicity: Increased bleeding and bruising may occur from I.M. injection in patients on anticoagulants.

Decreased Effect: Decreased effect of vaccine may occur with corticosteroids (greater than physiologic doses) or immunosuppressive agents

Pregnancy Risk Factor C

Tetanus Toxoid Plain *see* Tetanus Toxoid (Fluid) *on page 1278*

Tetracaine (TET ra kane)

Related Information

Mouth Pain, Cold Sore, and Canker Sore Products *on page 1633*

Oral Nonviral Soft Tissue Ulcerations or Erosions *on page 1551*

Oral Pain *on page 1526*

U.S. Brand Names AK-T-Caine™; Cēpacol Viractin® [OTC]; Opticaine®; Pontocaine®

Canadian Brand Names Ametop™; Pontocaine®

Generic Available Yes: Ophthalmic solution

Synonyms Amethocaine Hydrochloride; Tetracaine Hydrochloride

Pharmacologic Category Local Anesthetic

Dental Use Ester-type local anesthetic; applied topically to throat for various diagnostic procedures and on cold sores and fever blisters for pain

Use Spinal anesthesia; local anesthesia in the eye for various diagnostic and examination purposes; topically applied to nose and throat for various diagnostic procedures; topical gel [OTC] for treatment of pain associated with cold sores and fever blisters

Local Anesthetic/Vasoconstrictor Precautions No information available to require special precautions

Effects on Dental Treatment No significant effects or complications reported

Significant Adverse Effects Frequency not defined.

Injection:

Cardiovascular: Cardiac arrest, hypotension

Central nervous system: Chills, convulsions, dizziness, drowsiness, nervousness, unconsciousness

Gastrointestinal: Nausea, vomiting

Neuromuscular & skeletal: Tremors

Ocular: Blurred vision, pupil constriction

Otic: Tinnitus

Respiratory: Respiratory arrest
Miscellaneous: Allergic reaction

Ophthalmic: Ocular: Chemosis, lacrimation, photophobia, transient stinging
With chronic use: Corneal erosions, corneal healing retardation, corneal opacification (permanent), corneal scarring, keratitis (severe)

Dosage

Children ≥2 years and Adults: Topical gel [OTC]: Cold sores and fever blisters: Apply to affected area up to 3-4 times/day for up to 7 days

Adults:
- Ophthalmic solution (not for prolonged use): Instill 1-2 drops
- Spinal anesthesia:
  - High, medium, low, and saddle blocks: 0.2% to 0.3% solution
  - Prolonged (2-3 hours): 1% solution
  - Subarachnoid injection: 5-20 mg
  - Saddle block: 2-5 mg; a 1% solution should be diluted with equal volume of CSF before administration
- Topical mucous membranes (2% solution): Apply as needed; dose should not exceed 20 mg

Mechanism of Action Ester local anesthetic blocks both the initiation and conduction of nerve impulses by decreasing the neuronal membrane's permeability to sodium ions, which results in inhibition of depolarization with resultant blockade of conduction

Contraindications Hypersensitivity to tetracaine or any component of the formulation; ophthalmic secondary bacterial infection; liver disease; CNS disease or meningitis (if used for epidural or spinal anesthesia); myasthenia gravis

Warnings/Precautions Ophthalmic preparations may delay wound healing; use with caution in patients with cardiac disease and hyperthyroidism

Drug Interactions Decreased effect: Aminosalicylic acid, sulfonamides effects may be antagonized

Pharmacodynamics/Kinetics

Onset of action: Anesthetic: Ophthalmic: ~60 seconds; Topical or spinal injection: 3-8 minutes after applied to mucous membranes or when saddle block administered for spinal anesthesia

Metabolism: Hepatic; detoxified by plasma esterases to aminobenzoic acid

Excretion: Urine

Pregnancy Risk Factor C

Dosage Forms

Gel, as hydrochloride (Cēpacol Viractin®): 2% (7.1 g)

Injection, solution, as hydrochloride (Pontocaine®): 1% [10 mg/mL] (2 mL) [contains sodium bisulfite]

Injection, solution, as hydrochloride [premixed in dextrose 6%] (Pontocaine®): 0.3% [3 mg/mL] (5 mL)

Injection, powder for reconstitution, as hydrochloride (Pontocaine®): 20 mg

Solution, ophthalmic, as hydrochloride: 0.5% [5 mg/mL] (15 mL)
- AK-T-Caine™, Opticaine®: 0.5% (15 mL)
- Pontocaine®: 0.5% (15 mL, 59 mL)

Solution, topical, as hydrochloride (Pontocaine®): 2% [20 mg/mL] (30 mL, 118 mL)

Tetracaine and Dextrose (TET ra kane & DEKS trose)

Related Information

Oral Pain *on page 1526*
Tetracaine *on page 1278*

U.S. Brand Names Pontocaine® With Dextrose

Generic Available Yes

Synonyms Dextrose and Tetracaine

Pharmacologic Category Local Anesthetic

Use Spinal anesthesia (saddle block)

Local Anesthetic/Vasoconstrictor Precautions No information available to require special precautions

Effects on Dental Treatment No significant effects or complications reported

Pharmacodynamics/Kinetics See Tetracaine monograph.

Pregnancy Risk Factor C

Tetracaine Hydrochloride *see* Tetracaine *on page 1278*

Tetracaine Hydrochloride, Benzocaine Butyl Aminobenzoate, and Benzalkonium Chloride *see* Benzocaine, Butyl Aminobenzoate, Tetracaine, and Benzalkonium Chloride *on page 193*

Tetracosactide *see* Cosyntropin *on page 378*

Tetracycline (tet ra SYE kleen)

Related Information

Gastrointestinal Disorders *on page 1476*
Oral Bacterial Infections *on page 1533*
Oral Nonviral Soft Tissue Ulcerations or Erosions *on page 1551*
Periodontal Diseases *on page 1542*
Sexually-Transmitted Diseases *on page 1504*

U.S. Brand Names Sumycin®; Wesmycin®

Canadian Brand Names Apo-Tetra®; Novo-Tetra; Nu-Tetra

Mexican Brand Names Tetra-Atlantis®

Generic Available Yes: Capsule

Synonyms Achromycin; TCN; Tetracycline Hydrochloride

Pharmacologic Category Antibiotic, Tetracycline Derivative

Dental Use Treatment of periodontitis associated with presence of *Actinobacillus actinomycetemcomitans* (AA); as adjunctive therapy in recurrent aphthous ulcers

Use Treatment of susceptible bacterial infections of both gram-positive and gram-negative organisms; also infections due to *Mycoplasma*, *Chlamydia*, and *Rickettsia*; indicated for acne, exacerbations of chronic bronchitis, and treatment of gonorrhea and syphilis in patients that are allergic to penicillin; as part of a multidrug regimen for *H. pylori* eradication to reduce the risk of duodenal ulcer recurrence

Local Anesthetic/Vasoconstrictor Precautions No information available to require special precautions

Effects on Dental Treatment Key adverse event(s) related to dental treatment: Esophagitis, superinfections, and candidal superinfection. Opportunistic "superinfection" with *Candida albicans*; tetracyclines are not recommended for use during pregnancy or in children ≤8 years of age since they have been reported to cause enamel hypoplasia and permanent teeth discoloration. The use of tetracyclines should only be used in these patients if other agents are contraindicated or alternative antimicrobials will not eradicate the organism. Long-term use associated with oral candidiasis.

Significant Adverse Effects Frequency not defined.

Cardiovascular: Pericarditis

Central nervous system: Intracranial pressure increased, bulging fontanels in infants, pseudotumor cerebri, paresthesia

Dermatologic: Photosensitivity, pruritus, pigmentation of nails, exfoliative dermatitis

Endocrine & metabolic: Diabetes insipidus syndrome

Gastrointestinal: Discoloration of teeth and enamel hypoplasia (young children), nausea, diarrhea, vomiting, esophagitis, anorexia, abdominal cramps, antibiotic-associated pseudomembranous colitis, staphylococcal enterocolitis, pancreatitis

Hematologic: Thrombophlebitis

Hepatic: Hepatotoxicity

Renal: Acute renal failure, azotemia, renal damage

Miscellaneous: Superinfections, anaphylaxis, hypersensitivity reactions, candidal superinfection

Dosage Oral:

Children >8 years: 25-50 mg/kg/day in divided doses every 6 hours

Adults: 250-500 mg/dose every 6 hours

Helicobacter pylori eradication: 500 mg 2-4 times/day depending on regimen; requires combination therapy with at least one other antibiotic and an acid-suppressing agent (proton pump inhibitor or H_2 blocker)

Dosing interval in renal impairment:

Cl_{cr} 50-80 mL/minute: Administer every 8-12 hours

Cl_{cr} 10-50 mL/minute: Administer every 12-24 hours

Cl_{cr} <10 mL/minute: Administer every 24 hours

Dialysis: Slightly dialyzable (5% to 20%) via hemo- and peritoneal dialysis or via continuous arteriovenous or venovenous hemofiltration; no supplemental dosage necessary

Dosing adjustment in hepatic impairment: Avoid use or maximum dose is 1 g/day

Mechanism of Action Inhibits bacterial protein synthesis by binding with the 30S and possibly the 50S ribosomal subunit(s) of susceptible bacteria; may also cause alterations in the cytoplasmic membrane

Contraindications Hypersensitivity to tetracycline or any component of the formulation; do not administer to children ≤8 years of age; pregnancy

Warnings/Precautions Use of tetracyclines during tooth development may cause permanent discoloration of the teeth and enamel, hypoplasia and retardation of skeletal development and bone growth with risk being the greatest for children <4 years and those receiving high doses; use with caution in patients with renal or hepatic impairment (eg, elderly); dosage modification required in patients with renal impairment since it may increase BUN as an antianabolic agent; pseudotumor cerebri has been reported with tetracycline use (usually resolves with discontinuation); outdated drug can cause nephropathy; superinfection possible; use protective measure to avoid photosensitivity

Drug Interactions **Substrate** of CYP3A4 (major); **Inhibits** CYP3A4 (moderate)

Antacids: May decrease tetracycline absorption; separate doses.

Calcium supplements (oral): May decrease tetracycline absorption; separate doses.

CYP3A4 inducers: CYP3A4 inducers may decrease the levels/effects of tetracycline. Example inducers include aminoglutethimide, carbamazepine, nafcillin, nevirapine, phenobarbital, phenytoin, and rifamycins.

CYP3A4 substrates: Tetracycline may increase the levels/effects of CYP3A4 substrates. Example substrates include benzodiazepines, calcium channel blockers, cyclosporine, mirtazapine, nateglinide, nefazodone, sildenafil (and other PDE-5 inhibitors), tacrolimus, and venlafaxine. Selected benzodiazepines (midazolam and triazolam), cisapride, ergot alkaloids, selected HMG-CoA reductase inhibitors (lovastatin and simvastatin), and pimozide are generally contraindicated with strong CYP3A4 inhibitors.

Didanosine: May decrease tetracycline absorption; separate doses.

Digoxin: Tetracyclines may rarely increase digoxin serum levels.

Iron: May decrease tetracycline absorption; separate doses.

Methoxyflurane anesthesia when concurrent with tetracycline may cause fatal nephrotoxicity.

Oral contraceptives: Anecdotal reports suggesting decreased contraceptive efficacy with tetracyclines have been refuted by more rigorous scientific and clinical data.

Quinapril: May decrease tetracycline absorption; separate doses.

Warfarin with tetracyclines may result in increased anticoagulation.

Ethanol/Nutrition/Herb Interactions

Food: Tetracycline serum concentrations may be decreased if taken with dairy products.

Herb/Nutraceutical: Avoid dong quai, St John's wort (may also cause photosensitization)

Pharmacodynamics/Kinetics

Absorption: Oral: 75%

Distribution: Small amount appears in bile

Relative diffusion from blood into CSF: Good only with inflammation (exceeds usual MICs)

CSF:blood level ratio: Inflamed meninges: 25%

Protein binding: ~65%

Half-life elimination: Normal renal function: 8-11 hours; End-stage renal disease: 57-108 hours

Time to peak, serum: Oral: 2-4 hours

Excretion: Urine (60% as unchanged drug); feces (as active form)

Pregnancy Risk Factor D

Lactation Enters breast milk/not recommended (AAP rates "compatible")

Breast-Feeding Considerations Negligible absorption by infant; potential to stain infants' unerupted teeth

Dosage Forms

Capsule, as hydrochloride: 250 mg, 500 mg

Wesmycin®: 250 mg

Suspension, oral, as hydrochloride (Sumycin®): 125 mg/5 mL (480 mL) [contains sodium benzoate and sodium metabisulfite; fruit flavor]

Tablet, as hydrochloride (Sumycin®): 250 mg, 500 mg

Selected Readings

Gordon JM and Walker CB, "Current Status of Systemic Antibiotic Usage in Destructive Periodontal Disease," *J Periodontol*, 1993, 64(8 Suppl): 760-71.

Rams TE and Slots J, "Antibiotics in Periodontal Therapy: An Update," *Compendium*, 1992, 13(12):1130, 1132, 1134.

Seymour RA and Heasman PA, "Tetracyclines in the Management of Periodontal Diseases. A Review," *J Clin Periodontol*, 1995, 22(1):22-35.

Seymour RA and Heasman PA, "Pharmacological Control of Periodontal Disease. II. Antimicrobial Agents," *J Dent*, 1995, 23(1):5-14

Tetracycline, Bismuth Subsalicylate, and Metronidazole *see* Bismuth Subsalicylate, Metronidazole, and Tetracycline *on page 209*

Tetracycline Hydrochloride *see* Tetracycline *on page 1280*

Tetracycline, Metronidazole, and Bismuth Subsalicylate *see* Bismuth Subsalicylate, Metronidazole, and Tetracycline *on page 209*

Tetracycline (Periodontal)

(tet ra SYE kleen per ee oh DON tal FYE bers)

Related Information

Tetracycline *on page 1280*

U.S. Brand Names Actisite®

Generic Available No

Pharmacologic Category Antibacterial, Dental

Dental Use Treatment of adult periodontitis; as an adjunct to scaling and root planing for the reduction of pocket depth and bleeding on probing in selected patients with adult periodontitis

Use Used exclusively in dental applications

Local Anesthetic/Vasoconstrictor Precautions No information available to require special precautions

Effects on Dental Treatment Key adverse event(s) related to dental treatment: Gingival inflammation, mouth pain, glossitis, candidiasis, staining of tongue, local erythema following removal, and discomfort from fiber placement.

Significant Adverse Effects 1% to 10%:

Dermatologic: Local erythema following removal

Miscellaneous: Discomfort from fiber placement

Dosage

Children: Has not been established

Adults: Insert fiber to fill the periodontal pocket; each fiber contains 12.7 mg of tetracycline in 23 cm (9 inches) and provides continuous release of drug for 10 days; fibers are to be secured in pocket with cyanoacrylate adhesive and left in place for 10 days

Mechanism of Action Tetracycline is an antibiotic which inhibits growth of susceptible microorganisms. Tetracycline binds primarily to the 30S subunits of bacterial ribosomes, and appears to prevent access of aminoacyl tRNA to the acceptor site on the mRNA-ribosome complex. The fiber releases tetracycline into the periodontal site at a rate of 2 mcg/cm/hour.

Contraindications Hypersensitivity to tetracyclines or any component of the formulation

Warnings/Precautions Use of tetracyclines is not recommended during pregnancy because of interference with fetal bone and dental development

Drug Interactions No data reported

Pharmacodynamics/Kinetics

The fiber releases tetracycline at a rate of 2 mcg/cm/hour

Tissue fluid concentrations:

Gingival fluid: ~1590 mcg/mL of tetracycline per site over 10 days

Plasma: During fiber treatment of up to 11 teeth, the tetracycline plasma concentration was below any detectable levels (<0.1 mcg/mL)

Oral: 500 mg of tetracycline produces a peak plasma level of 3-4 mcg/mL

Saliva: ~50.7 mcg/mL of tetracycline immediately after fiber treatment of 9 teeth

Pregnancy Risk Factor C

Lactation Excretion in breast milk unknown

Dosage Forms Fibers: 23 cm (9") in length [12.7 mg of tetracycline hydrochloride per fiber]

Selected Readings

Baer PN, "Actisite (Tetracycline Hydrochloride Periodontal Fiber): A Critique," *Periodontal Clin Investig*, 1994, 16(2):5-7.

Greenstein G, "Treating Periodontal Diseases With Tetracycline-Impregnated Fibers: Data and Controversies," *Compend Contin Educ Dent*, 1995, 16(5)448-55.

Kerry G, "Tetracycline-Loaded Fibers as Adjunctive Treatment in Periodontal Disease," *J Am Dent Assoc*, 1994, 125(9):1199-203.

Michalowicz BS, Pihlstrom BL, Drisko CL, et al, "Evaluation of Periodontal Treatments Using Controlled-Release Tetracycline Fibers: Maintenance Response," *J Periodontol*, 1995, 66(8):708-15.

Mombelli A, Lehmann B, Tonetti M, et al, "Clinical Response to Local Delivery of Tetracycline in Relation to Overall and Local Periodontal Conditions," *J Clin Periodontol*, 1997, 24(7):470-77.

Vandekerckhove BN, Quirynen M, and van Steenberghe D, "The Use of Tetracycline-Containing Controlled-Release Fibers in the Treatment of Refractory Periodontitis," *J Periodontol*, 1997, 68(4):353-61.

Tetrahydroaminoacrine *see* Tacrine *on page 1254*

Tetrahydrocannabinol *see* Dronabinol *on page 477*

Tetrahydrozoline (tet ra hye DROZ a leen)

U.S. Brand Names Eye-Sine™ [OTC]; Geneye® [OTC]; Murine® Tears Plus [OTC]; Optigene® 3 [OTC]; Tyzine®; Tyzine® Pediatric; Visine® Advanced Relief [OTC]; Visine® Original [OTC]

Mexican Brand Names Visine®

Generic Available Yes: Ophthalmic solution

Synonyms Tetrahydrozoline Hydrochloride; Tetryzoline

Pharmacologic Category Adrenergic Agonist Agent; Ophthalmic Agent, Vasoconstrictor

Use Symptomatic relief of nasal congestion and conjunctival congestion

Local Anesthetic/Vasoconstrictor Precautions No information available to require special precautions

Effects on Dental Treatment No significant effects or complications reported

Common Adverse Effects

>10%:

Local: Transient stinging

Respiratory: Sneezing

1% to 10%:

Cardiovascular: Tachycardia, palpitations, hypertension, heart rate

Central nervous system: Headache

Neuromuscular & skeletal: Tremor

Ocular: Blurred vision

Mechanism of Action Stimulates alpha-adrenergic receptors in the arterioles of the conjunctiva and the nasal mucosa to produce vasoconstriction

Pharmacodynamics/Kinetics

Onset of action: Decongestant: Intranasal: 4-8 hours

Duration: Ophthalmic vasoconstriction: 2-3 hours

Pregnancy Risk Factor C

Tetrahydrozoline Hydrochloride *see* Tetrahydrozoline *on page 1282*

Tetra Tannate Pediatric *see* Chlorpheniramine, Ephedrine, Phenylephrine, and Carbetapentane *on page 316*

Tetryzoline *see* Tetrahydrozoline *on page 1282*

Teveten® *see* Eprosartan *on page 501*

Teveten® HCT *see* Eprosartan and Hydrochlorothiazide *on page 502*

Texacort® *see* Hydrocortisone *on page 714*

TG *see* Thioguanine *on page 1288*

6-TG *see* Thioguanine *on page 1288*

THA *see* Tacrine *on page 1254*

Thalidomide (tha LI doe mide)

Related Information

HIV Infection and AIDS *on page 1484*

Oral Nonviral Soft Tissue Ulcerations or Erosions *on page 1551*

U.S. Brand Names Thalomid®

Canadian Brand Names Thalomid®

Generic Available No

Pharmacologic Category Immunosuppressant Agent

Use Treatment and maintenance of cutaneous manifestations of erythema nodosum leprosum

Unlabeled/Investigational Use Treatment of Crohn's disease; treatment or prevention of graft-versus-host reactions after bone marrow transplantation; AIDS-related aphthous stomatitis; Behçet's syndrome; Waldenström's macroglobulinemia; Langerhans cell histiocytosis; may be effective in rheumatoid arthritis, discoid lupus erythematosus, and erythema multiforme

Local Anesthetic/Vasoconstrictor Precautions No information available to require special precautions

Effects on Dental Treatment Key adverse event(s) related to dental treatment: Oral moniliasis (HIV-seropositive patients), toothache, xerostomia (normal salivary flow resumes upon discontinuation), and aphthous stomatitis.

Common Adverse Effects

Controlled clinical trials: ENL:

>10%:

Central nervous system: Somnolence (37.5%), headache (12.5%)

Dermatologic: Rash (20.8%)

1% to 10%:

Cardiovascular: Peripheral edema

Central nervous system: Dizziness (4.2%), vertigo (8.3%), chills, malaise (8.3%),

Dermatologic: Dermatitis (fungal) (4.2%), nail disorder (4.2%), pruritus (8.3%), rash (maculopapular) (4.2%)

Gastrointestinal (4.2%): Constipation, diarrhea, nausea, moniliasis, tooth pain, abdominal pain

Genitourinary: Impotence (8.2%)

(Continued)

Thalidomide *(Continued)*

Neuromuscular & skeletal: Asthenia (8.3%), pain (8.3%), back pain (4.2%), neck pain (4.2%), neck rigidity (4.2%), tremor (4.2%)
Respiratory (4.2%): Pharyngitis, rhinitis, sinusitis

HIV-seropositive:

General: An increased viral load has been noted in patients treated with thalidomide. This is of uncertain clinical significance

>10%:

Central nervous system: Somnolence (36% to 37%), dizziness (18.7% to 19.4%), fever (19.4% to 21.9%), headache (16.7% to 18.7%)
Dermatologic: Rash (25%), maculopapular rash (16.7% to 18.7%), acne (3.1% to 11.1%)
Gastrointestinal: AST increase (2.8% to 12.5%), diarrhea (11.1% to 18.7%), nausea (≤12.5%), oral moniliasis (6.3% to 11.1%)
Hematologic: Leukopenia (16.7% to 25%), anemia (5.6% to 12.5%)
Neuromuscular & skeletal: Paresthesia (5.6% to 15.6%), weakness (5.6% to 21.9%)
Miscellaneous: Diaphoresis (≤12.5%), lymphadenopathy (5.6% to 12.5%)

1% to 10%:

Cardiovascular: Peripheral edema (3.1% to 8.3%)
Central nervous system: Nervousness (2.8% to 9.4%), insomnia (≤9.4%), agitation (≤9.4%), chills (≤9.4%), neuropathy (up to 8% in HIV-seropositive patients)
Dermatologic: Dermatitis (fungal) (5.6% to 9.4%), nail disorder (≤3.1%), pruritus (2.8% to 6.3%)
Gastrointestinal: Anorexia (2.8% to 9.4%), constipation (2.8% to 9.4%), dry mouth (8.3% to 9.4%), flatulence (8.3% to 9.4%), multiple abnormalities LFTs (≤9.4%), abdominal pain (2.8% to 3.1%)
Neuromuscular & skeletal: Back pain (≤5%), pain (≤3.1%)
Respiratory: Pharyngitis (6.3% to 8.3%), sinusitis (3.1% to 8.3%)
Miscellaneous: Accidental injury (≤5.6%), infection (6.3% to 8.3%)

Restrictions Thalidomide is approved for marketing only under a special distribution program. This program, called the "System for Thalidomide Education and Prescribing Safety" (STEPS™), has been approved by the FDA. Prescribing and dispensing of thalidomide is restricted to prescribers and pharmacists registered with the program. Prior to dispensing, an authorization number must be obtained (1-888-423-5436) from Celgene (write authorization number on prescription). No more than a 4-week supply should be dispensed. Blister packs should be dispensed intact (do not repackage capsules). Prescriptions must be filled within 7 days.

Mechanism of Action A derivative of glutethimide; mode of action for immunosuppression is unclear; inhibition of neutrophil chemotaxis and decreased monocyte phagocytosis may occur; may cause 50% to 80% reduction of tumor necrosis factor - alpha

Drug Interactions

Increased Effect/Toxicity: Thalidomide may enhance the sedative activity of other drugs such as ethanol, barbiturates, reserpine, and chlorpromazine. Drugs which may cause peripheral neuropathy should be used with caution in patients receiving thalidomide. Women using any drug which may decrease the serum concentrations and/or efficacy of hormonal contraceptives must use 2 other methods of contraception or abstain from heterosexual contact.

Pharmacodynamics/Kinetics

Distribution: V_d: 120 L
Protein binding: 55% to 66%
Metabolism: Nonenzymatic hydrolysis in plasma; forms multiple metabolites
Half-life elimination: 5-7 hours
Time to peak, plasma: 2-6 hours
Excretion: Urine (<1%)

Pregnancy Risk Factor X

Thalitone® *see* Chlorthalidone *on page 321*
Thalomid® *see* Thalidomide *on page 1283*
THAM® *see* Tromethamine *on page 1348*
THC *see* Dronabinol *on page 477*
Theo-24® *see* Theophylline *on page 1285*
Theochron® *see* Theophylline *on page 1285*
Theolair™ *see* Theophylline *on page 1285*
Theolair-SR® [DSC] *see* Theophylline *on page 1285*
Theolate *see* Theophylline and Guaifenesin *on page 1286*

Theophylline (thee OFF i lin)

Related Information

Aminophylline *on page 99*

Respiratory Diseases *on page 1478*

U.S. Brand Names Elixophyllin®; Quibron®-T; Quibron®-T/SR; Theo-24®; Theochron®; Theolair™; Theolair-SR® [DSC]; T-Phyl®; Uniphyl®

Canadian Brand Names Apo-Theo LA®; Novo-Theophyl SR; PMS-Theophylline; Pulmophylline; Quibron®-T/SR; ratio-Theo-Bronc; Theochron® SR; Theo-Dur®; Theolair™; Uniphyl® SRT

Mexican Brand Names Slo-Bid®; Teolong®; Uni-Dur®

Generic Available Yes: Elixir, extended release tablet, infusion, oral solution

Synonyms Theophylline Anhydrous

Pharmacologic Category Theophylline Derivative

Use Treatment of symptoms and reversible airway obstruction due to chronic asthma, chronic bronchitis, or COPD

Local Anesthetic/Vasoconstrictor Precautions No information available to require special precautions

Effects on Dental Treatment Prescribe erythromycin products with caution to patients taking theophylline products. Erythromycin will delay the normal metabolic inactivation of theophyllines leading to increased blood levels; this has resulted in nausea, vomiting, and CNS restlessness. Azithromycin does not cause these effects in combination with theophylline products.

Common Adverse Effects

Adverse reactions/theophylline serum level: (Adverse effects do not necessarily occur according to serum levels. Arrhythmia and seizure can occur without seeing the other adverse effects).

15-25 mcg/mL: GI upset, diarrhea, nausea/vomiting, abdominal pain, nervousness, headache, insomnia, agitation, dizziness, muscle cramp, tremor

25-35 mcg/mL: Tachycardia, occasional PVC

>35 mcg/mL: Ventricular tachycardia, frequent PVC, seizure

Uncommon at serum theophylline concentrations ≤20 mcg/mL

1% to 10%:

Cardiovascular: Tachycardia

Central nervous system: Nervousness, restlessness

Gastrointestinal: Nausea, vomiting

Mechanism of Action Causes bronchodilatation, diuresis, CNS and cardiac stimulation, and gastric acid secretion by blocking phosphodiesterase which increases tissue concentrations of cyclic adenine monophosphate (cAMP) which in turn promotes catecholamine stimulation of lipolysis, glycogenolysis, and gluconeogenesis and induces release of epinephrine from adrenal medulla cells

Drug Interactions

Cytochrome P450 Effect: Substrate of CYP1A2 (major), 2C8/9 (minor), 2D6 (minor), 2E1 (major), 3A4 (major); **Inhibits** CYP1A2 (weak)

Increased Effect/Toxicity: CYP1A2 inhibitors may increase the levels/effects of theophylline; example inhibitors include amiodarone, ciprofloxacin, fluvoxamine, ketoconazole, lomefloxacin, ofloxacin, and rofecoxib. CYP2E1 inhibitors may increase the levels/effects of theophylline; example inhibitors include disulfiram, isoniazid, and miconazole. Changes in diet may affect the elimination of theophylline. CYP3A4 inhibitors may increase the levels/effects of theophylline; example inhibitors include azole antifungals, ciprofloxacin, clarithromycin, diclofenac, doxycycline, erythromycin, imatinib, isoniazid, nefazodone, nicardipine, propofol, protease inhibitors, quinidine, and verapamil.

Decreased Effect: CYP1A2 inducers may decrease the levels/effects of theophylline; example inducers include aminoglutethimide, carbamazepine, phenobarbital, and rifampin. CYP3A4 inducers may decrease the levels/effects of theophylline; example inducers include aminoglutethimide, carbamazepine, nafcillin, nevirapine, phenobarbital, phenytoin, and rifamycins.

Pharmacodynamics/Kinetics

Absorption: Oral: Dosage form dependent

Distribution: 0.45 L/kg based on ideal body weight

Metabolism: Children >1 year and Adults: Hepatic; involves CYP1A2, 2E1 and 3A4; forms active metabolites (caffeine and 3-methylxanthine)

Half-life elimination: Highly variable and dependent upon age, liver function, cardiac function, lung disease, and smoking history

(Continued)

Theophylline *(Continued)*

Time to peak, serum:

Oral: Liquid: 1 hour; Tablet, enteric-coated: 5 hours; Tablet, uncoated: 2 hours

I.V.: Within 30 minutes

Excretion: Urine

Neonates: 50% unchanged

Children >3 months and Adults: 10% unchanged

Pregnancy Risk Factor C

Theophylline and Guaifenesin (thee OFF i lin & gwye FEN e sin)

Related Information

Guaifenesin *on page 672*

Theophylline *on page 1285*

U.S. Brand Names Elixophyllin-GG®; Quibron®; Theolate

Generic Available No

Synonyms Guaifenesin and Theophylline

Pharmacologic Category Theophylline Derivative

Use Symptomatic treatment of bronchospasm associated with bronchial asthma, chronic bronchitis, and pulmonary emphysema

Local Anesthetic/Vasoconstrictor Precautions No information available to require special precautions

Effects on Dental Treatment Prescribe erythromycin products with caution to patients taking theophylline products. Erythromycin will delay the normal metabolic inactivation of theophyllines leading to increased blood levels; this has resulted in nausea, vomiting, and CNS restlessness.

Drug Interactions

Cytochrome P450 Effect: Theophylline: **Substrate** of CYP1A2 (major), 2C8/9 (minor), 2D6 (minor), 2E1 (major), 3A4 (major); **Inhibits** CYP1A2 (weak)

Pharmacodynamics/Kinetics See individual agents.

Pregnancy Risk Factor C

Theophylline Anhydrous *see* Theophylline *on page 1285*

Theophylline Ethylenediamine *see* Aminophylline *on page 99*

Theracort® [OTC] *see* Hydrocortisone *on page 714*

TheraCys® *see* BCG Vaccine *on page 183*

Thera-Flu® Cold and Sore Throat Night Time [OTC] *see* Acetaminophen, Chlorpheniramine, and Pseudoephedrine *on page 58*

Thera-Flur-N® *see* Fluoride *on page 603*

Thera-Flu® Severe Cold Non-Drowsy [OTC] [DSC] *see* Acetaminophen, Dextromethorphan, and Pseudoephedrine *on page 59*

Theragran® Heart Right™ [OTC] *see* Vitamins (Multiple/Oral) *on page 1384*

Theragran-M® Advanced Formula [OTC] *see* Vitamins (Multiple/Oral) *on page 1384*

Theramycin Z® *see* Erythromycin *on page 508*

TheraPatch® Warm [OTC] *see* Capsaicin *on page 252*

Therapeutic Multivitamins *see* Vitamins (Multiple/Oral) *on page 1384*

Theratears® *see* Carboxymethylcellulose *on page 265*

Thermazene® *see* Silver Sulfadiazine *on page 1221*

Thiabendazole (thye a BEN da zole)

U.S. Brand Names Mintezol®

Generic Available No

Synonyms Tiabendazole

Pharmacologic Category Anthelmintic

Use Treatment of strongyloidiasis, cutaneous larva migrans, visceral larva migrans, dracunculiasis, trichinosis, and mixed helminthic infections

Unlabeled/Investigational Use Cutaneous larva migrans (topical application)

Local Anesthetic/Vasoconstrictor Precautions No information available to require special precautions

Effects on Dental Treatment No significant effects or complications reported

Common Adverse Effects Frequency not defined.

Central nervous system: Seizures, hallucinations, delirium, dizziness, drowsiness, headache, chills

Dermatologic: Rash, Stevens-Johnson syndrome, pruritus, angioedema

Endocrine & metabolic: Hyperglycemia

Gastrointestinal: Anorexia, diarrhea, nausea, vomiting, drying of mucous membranes, abdominal pain

Genitourinary: Malodor of urine, hematuria, crystalluria, enuresis
Hematologic: Leukopenia
Hepatic: Jaundice, cholestasis, hepatic failure, hepatotoxicity
Neuromuscular & skeletal: Numbness, incoordination
Ocular: Abnormal sensation in eyes, blurred vision, dry eyes, Sicca syndrome, vision decreased, xanthopsia
Otic: Tinnitus
Renal: Nephrotoxicity
Miscellaneous: Anaphylaxis, hypersensitivity reactions, lymphadenopathy

Mechanism of Action Inhibits helminth-specific mitochondrial fumarate reductase

Drug Interactions

Cytochrome P450 Effect: Substrate of CYP1A2 (minor); **Inhibits** CYP1A2 (strong)

Increased Effect/Toxicity: Thiabendazole may increase the levels/effects of aminophylline, fluvoxamine, mexiletine, mirtazapine, ropinirole, theophylline, trifluoperazine, and other CYP1A2 substrates.

Pharmacodynamics/Kinetics

Absorption: Rapid and well absorbed
Metabolism: Rapidly hepatic; metabolized to 5-hydroxy form
Half-life elimination: 1.2 hours
Time to peak, plasma: Oral suspension: Within 1-2 hours
Excretion: Urine (90%) and feces (5%) primarily as conjugated metabolites

Pregnancy Risk Factor C

Thiamazole *see* Methimazole *on page 893*
Thiamilate® [OTC] *see* Thiamine *on page 1287*

Thiamine (THYE a min)

U.S. Brand Names Thiamilate® [OTC]

Canadian Brand Names Betaxin®

Mexican Brand Names Beneva®

Generic Available Yes

Synonyms Aneurine Hydrochloride; Thiamine Hydrochloride; Thiaminium Chloride Hydrochloride; Vitamin B_1

Pharmacologic Category Vitamin, Water Soluble

Use Treatment of thiamine deficiency including beriberi, Wernicke's encephalopathy syndrome, and peripheral neuritis associated with pellagra, alcoholic patients with altered sensorium; various genetic metabolic disorders

Local Anesthetic/Vasoconstrictor Precautions No information available to require special precautions

Effects on Dental Treatment No significant effects or complications reported

Mechanism of Action An essential coenzyme in carbohydrate metabolism by combining with adenosine triphosphate to form thiamine pyrophosphate

Pharmacodynamics/Kinetics

Absorption: Oral: Adequate; I.M.: Rapid and complete
Excretion: Urine (as unchanged drug and as pyrimidine after body storage sites become saturated)

Pregnancy Risk Factor A/C (dose exceeding RDA recommendation)

Thiamine Hydrochloride *see* Thiamine *on page 1287*
Thiaminium Chloride Hydrochloride *see* Thiamine *on page 1287*

Thiethylperazine (thye eth il PER a zeen)

U.S. Brand Names Torecan® [DSC]

Canadian Brand Names Torecan®

Mexican Brand Names Torecan®

Generic Available No

Synonyms Thiethylperazine Maleate

Pharmacologic Category Antiemetic; Phenothiazine Derivative

Use Relief of nausea and vomiting

Unlabeled/Investigational Use Treatment of vertigo

Local Anesthetic/Vasoconstrictor Precautions No information available to require special precautions

Effects on Dental Treatment Key adverse event(s) related to dental treatment: Orthostatic hypotension.

Common Adverse Effects

>10%:

Central nervous system: Drowsiness, dizziness
Gastrointestinal: Xerostomia
Respiratory: Dry nose

(Continued)

Thiethylperazine *(Continued)*

1% to 10%:
- Cardiovascular: Tachycardia, orthostatic hypotension
- Central nervous system: Confusion, convulsions, extrapyramidal symptoms, tardive dyskinesia, fever, headache
- Hematologic: Agranulocytosis
- Hepatic: Cholestatic jaundice
- Otic: Tinnitus

Mechanism of Action Blocks postsynaptic mesolimbic dopaminergic receptors in the brain; exhibits a strong alpha-adrenergic blocking effect and depresses the release of hypothalamic and hypophyseal hormones; acts directly on chemoreceptor trigger zone and vomiting center; may also inhibit impulses from peripheral autonomic afferents to the vomiting center

Drug Interactions

Increased Effect/Toxicity: Increased effect with CNS depressants (eg, anesthetics, opiates, tranquilizers, alcohol), lithium, atropine, epinephrine, MAO inhibitors, TCAs

Pharmacodynamics/Kinetics

Onset of action: Antiemetic: ~30 minutes

Duration: ~4 hours

Pregnancy Risk Factor X

Thiethylperazine Maleate *see* Thiethylperazine *on page 1287*

Thimerosal (thye MER oh sal)

U.S. Brand Names Mersol® [OTC]; Merthiolate® [OTC]

Generic Available Yes

Pharmacologic Category Antibiotic, Topical

Use Organomercurial antiseptic with sustained bacteriostatic and fungistatic activity

Local Anesthetic/Vasoconstrictor Precautions No information available to require special precautions

Effects on Dental Treatment No significant effects or complications reported

Thioguanine (thye oh GWAH neen)

Canadian Brand Names Lanvis®

Generic Available Yes

Synonyms 2-Amino-6-Mercaptopurine; NSC-752; TG; 6-TG; 6-Thioguanine; Tioguanine

Pharmacologic Category Antineoplastic Agent, Antimetabolite (Purine Antagonist)

Use Treatment of acute myelogenous (nonlymphocytic) leukemia; treatment of chronic myelogenous leukemia and granulocytic leukemia

Local Anesthetic/Vasoconstrictor Precautions No information available to require special precautions

Effects on Dental Treatment Key adverse event(s) related to dental treatment: Stomatitis.

Common Adverse Effects

>10%:
- Hematologic: Myelosuppressive:
  - WBC: Moderate
  - Platelets: Moderate
  - Onset (days): 7-10
  - Nadir (days): 14
  - Recovery (days): 21

1% to 10%:
- Dermatologic: Skin rash
- Endocrine & metabolic: Hyperuricemia
- Gastrointestinal: Mild nausea or vomiting, anorexia, stomatitis, diarrhea
- Neuromuscular & skeletal: Unsteady gait

Mechanism of Action Purine analog that is incorporated into DNA and RNA resulting in the blockage of synthesis and metabolism of purine nucleotides

Drug Interactions

Increased Effect/Toxicity: Allopurinol can be used in full doses with thioguanine unlike mercaptopurine. Use with busulfan may cause hepatotoxicity and esophageal varices. Aminosalicylates (olsalazine, mesalamine, sulfasalazine) may inhibit TPMT, increasing toxicity/myelosuppression of thioguanine.

Pharmacodynamics/Kinetics

Absorption: 30% (highly variable)

Distribution: Crosses placenta

Metabolism: Rapidly and extensively hepatic to 2-amino-6-methylthioguanine (active) and inactive compounds

Half-life elimination: Terminal: 11 hours

Time to peak, serum: Within 8 hours

Excretion: Urine

Pregnancy Risk Factor D

6-Thioguanine *see* Thioguanine *on page 1288*

Thiola® *see* Tiopronin *on page 1303*

Thiopental (thye oh PEN tal)

U.S. Brand Names Pentothal®

Canadian Brand Names Pentothal®

Mexican Brand Names Pentothal Sodico®; Sodipental® [inj.]

Generic Available Yes

Synonyms Thiopental Sodium

Pharmacologic Category Anticonvulsant, Barbiturate; Barbiturate; General Anesthetic

Use Induction of anesthesia; adjunct for intubation in head injury patients; control of convulsive states; treatment of elevated intracranial pressure

Local Anesthetic/Vasoconstrictor Precautions No information available to require special precautions

Effects on Dental Treatment No significant effects or complications reported

Mechanism of Action Short-acting barbiturate with sedative, hypnotic, and anticonvulsant properties. Barbiturates depress the sensory cortex, decrease motor activity, alter cerebellar function, and produce drowsiness, sedation, and hypnosis. In high doses, barbiturates exhibit anticonvulsant activity; barbiturates produce dose-dependent respiratory depression.

Pregnancy Risk Factor C

Thiopental Sodium *see* Thiopental *on page 1289*

Thiophosphoramide *see* Thiotepa *on page 1291*

Thioplex® [DSC] *see* Thiotepa *on page 1291*

Thioridazine (thye oh RID a zeen)

U.S. Brand Names Mellaril® [DSC]; Thioridazine Intensol™

Canadian Brand Names Apo-Thioridazine®; Mellaril®

Mexican Brand Names Melleril®

Generic Available Yes

Synonyms Thioridazine Hydrochloride

Pharmacologic Category Antipsychotic Agent, Phenothiazine, Piperidine

Use Management of schizophrenic patients who fail to respond adequately to treatment with other antipsychotic drugs, either because of insufficient effectiveness or the inability to achieve an effective dose due to intolerable adverse effects from those medications

Unlabeled/Investigational Use Psychosis

Local Anesthetic/Vasoconstrictor Precautions Most pharmacology textbooks state that in presence of phenothiazines, systemic doses of epinephrine paradoxically decrease the blood pressure. This is the so called "epinephrine reversal" phenomenon. This has never been observed when epinephrine is given by infiltration as part of the anesthesia procedure.

Effects on Dental Treatment Key adverse event(s) related to dental treatment: Xerostomia and changes in salivation (normal salivary flow resumes upon discontinuation). Significant hypotension may occur, especially when the drug is administered parenterally; orthostatic hypotension is due to alpha-receptor blockade, the elderly are at greater risk for orthostatic hypotension.

Tardive dyskinesia; Prevalence rate may be 40% in elderly; development of the syndrome and the irreversible nature are proportional to duration and total cumulative dose over time. Extrapyramidal reactions are more common in elderly with up to 50% developing these reactions after 60 years of age. Drug-induced Parkinson's syndrome occurs often; akathisia is the most common extrapyramidal reaction in elderly.

Common Adverse Effects Frequency not defined.

Cardiovascular: Hypotension, orthostatic hypotension, peripheral edema, ECG changes

Central nervous system: EPS (pseudoparkinsonism, akathisia, dystonias, tardive dyskinesia), dizziness, drowsiness, neuroleptic malignant syndrome (NMS), impairment of temperature regulation, lowering of seizures threshold, seizure

(Continued)

Thioridazine *(Continued)*

Dermatologic: Increased sensitivity to sun, rash, discoloration of skin (blue-gray)
Endocrine & metabolic: Changes in menstrual cycle, changes in libido, breast pain, galactorrhea, amenorrhea
Gastrointestinal: Constipation, weight gain, nausea, vomiting, stomach pain, xerostomia, nausea, vomiting, diarrhea
Genitourinary: Difficulty in urination, ejaculatory disturbances, urinary retention, priapism
Hematologic: Agranulocytosis, leukopenia
Hepatic: Cholestatic jaundice, hepatotoxicity
Neuromuscular & skeletal: Tremor
Ocular: Pigmentary retinopathy, blurred vision, cornea and lens changes
Respiratory: Nasal congestion

Mechanism of Action Blocks postsynaptic mesolimbic dopaminergic receptors in the brain; exhibits a strong alpha-adrenergic blocking effect and depresses the release of hypothalamic and hypophyseal hormones

Drug Interactions

Cytochrome P450 Effect: Substrate of CYP2C19 (minor), 2D6 (major); **Inhibits** CYP1A2 (weak), 2C8/9 (weak), 2D6 (moderate), 2E1 (weak)

Increased Effect/Toxicity: Concurrent use fluvoxamine, propranolol, and pindolol. The levels/effects of thioridazine may be increased by chlorpromazine, delavirdine, fluoxetine, miconazole, paroxetine, pergolide, quinidine, quinine, ritonavir, ropinirole, and other CYP2D6 inhibitors. **Thioridazine is contraindicated with strong inhibitors of this enzyme.**

Drugs which alter the QT_c interval may be additive with thioridazine, increasing the risk of malignant arrhythmias; includes type Ia antiarrhythmics, TCAs, and some quinolone antibiotics (sparfloxacin, moxifloxacin and gatifloxacin). **These agents are contraindicated with thioridazine.** Potassium depleting agents may increase the risk of serious arrhythmias with thioridazine (includes many diuretics, aminoglycosides, and amphotericin).

Phenothiazines inhibit the ability of bromocriptine to lower serum prolactin concentrations. The sedative effects of CNS depressants or ethanol may be additive with phenothiazines. Phenothiazines and trazodone may produce additive hypotensive effects. Metoclopramide may increase risk of extrapyramidal symptoms (EPS). Concurrent use of antihypertensives may result in additive hypotensive effects (particularly orthostasis).

Thioridazine may increase the levels/effects of amphetamines, beta-blockers, dextromethorphan, fluoxetine, lidocaine, mirtazapine, nefazodone, paroxetine, risperidone, ritonavir, tricyclic antidepressants, venlafaxine, and other CYP2D6 substrates. **Concurrent use with fluvoxamine is contraindicated.**

Phenothiazines may produce neurotoxicity with lithium; this is a rare effect. Rare cases of respiratory paralysis have been reported with concurrent use of phenothiazines and polypeptide antibiotics. Naltrexone in combination with thioridazine has been reported to cause lethargy and somnolence. Phenylpropanolamine has been reported to result in cardiac arrhythmias when combined with thioridazine.

Decreased Effect: Aluminum salts may decrease the absorption of phenothiazines. The efficacy of amphetamines may be diminished by antipsychotics; in addition, amphetamines may increase psychotic symptoms; avoid concurrent use. Anticholinergics may inhibit the therapeutic response to phenothiazines and excess anticholinergic effects may occur (includes benztropine, trihexyphenidyl, biperiden, and drugs with significant anticholinergic activity). Chlorpromazine (and possibly other low potency antipsychotics) may diminish the pressor effects of epinephrine. The antihypertensive effects of guanethidine or guanadrel may be inhibited by phenothiazines. Phenothiazines may inhibit the antiparkinsonian effect of levodopa. Enzyme inducers may enhance the hepatic metabolism of phenothiazines; larger doses may be required; includes rifampin, rifabutin, barbiturates, phenytoin, and cigarette smoking. Thioridazine may decrease the levels/effects of CYP2D6 prodrug substrates (eg, codeine, hydrocodone, oxycodone, tramadol).

Pharmacodynamics/Kinetics

Duration: 4-5 days
Half-life elimination: 21-25 hours
Time to peak, serum: ~1 hour

Pregnancy Risk Factor C

Thioridazine Hydrochloride *see* Thioridazine *on page 1289*

Thioridazine Intensol™ *see* Thioridazine *on page 1289*
Thiosulfuric Acid Disodium Salt *see* Sodium Thiosulfate *on page 1230*

Thiotepa (thye oh TEP a)

U.S. Brand Names Thioplex® [DSC]
Generic Available Yes
Synonyms TESPA; Thiophosphoramide; Triethylenethiophosphoramide; TSPA
Pharmacologic Category Antineoplastic Agent, Alkylating Agent
Use Treatment of superficial tumors of the bladder; palliative treatment of adenocarcinoma of breast or ovary; lymphomas and sarcomas; controlling intracavitary effusions caused by metastatic tumors; I.T. use: CNS leukemia/lymphoma, CNS metastases
Local Anesthetic/Vasoconstrictor Precautions No information available to require special precautions
Effects on Dental Treatment No significant effects or complications reported
Common Adverse Effects
>10%:
Hematopoietic: Dose-limiting toxicity which is dose-related and cumulative; moderate to severe leukopenia and severe thrombocytopenia have occurred. Anemia and pancytopenia may become fatal, so careful hematologic monitoring is required; intravesical administration may cause bone marrow suppression as well.
Hematologic: Myelosuppressive:
WBC: Moderate
Platelets: Severe
Onset: 7-10 days
Nadir: 14 days
Recovery: 28 days
Local: Pain at injection site
1% to 10%:
Central nervous system: Dizziness, fever, headache
Dermatologic: Alopecia, rash, pruritus, hyperpigmentation with high-dose therapy
Endocrine & metabolic: Hyperuricemia
Gastrointestinal: Anorexia, nausea and vomiting rarely occur
Emetic potential: Low (<10%)
Genitourinary: Hemorrhagic cystitis
Renal: Hematuria
Miscellaneous: Tightness of the throat, allergic reactions
Mechanism of Action Alkylating agent that reacts with DNA phosphate groups to produce cross-linking of DNA strands leading to inhibition of DNA, RNA, and protein synthesis; mechanism of action has not been explored as thoroughly as the other alkylating agents, it is presumed that the aziridine rings open and react as nitrogen mustard; reactivity is enhanced at a lower pH
Drug Interactions
Cytochrome P450 Effect: Inhibits CYP2B6 (weak)
Increased Effect/Toxicity: Other alkylating agents or irradiation used concomitantly with thiotepa intensifies toxicity rather than enhancing therapeutic response. Prolonged muscular paralysis and respiratory depression may occur when neuromuscular blocking agents are administered. Succinylcholine and other neuromuscular blocking agents' action can be prolonged due to thiotepa inhibiting plasma pseudocholinesterase.
Pharmacodynamics/Kinetics
Absorption: Intracavitary instillation: Unreliable (10% to 100%) through bladder mucosa; I.M.: variable
Metabolism: Extensively hepatic
Half-life elimination: Terminal (dose-dependent clearance): 109 minutes
Excretion: Urine (as metabolites and unchanged drug)
Pregnancy Risk Factor D

Thiothixene (thye oh THIKS een)

U.S. Brand Names Navane®
Canadian Brand Names Navane®
Generic Available Yes
Synonyms Tiotixene
Pharmacologic Category Antipsychotic Agent, Thioxanthene Derivative
Use Management of schizophrenia
Unlabeled/Investigational Use Psychotic disorders
Local Anesthetic/Vasoconstrictor Precautions Most pharmacology textbooks state that in presence of phenothiazines, systemic doses of epinephrine
(Continued)

Thiothixene *(Continued)*

paradoxically decrease the blood pressure. This is the so called "epinephrine reversal" phenomenon. This has never been observed when epinephrine is given by infiltration as part of the anesthesia procedure.

Effects on Dental Treatment Key adverse event(s) related to dental treatment: Significant hypotension may occur, especially when the drug is administered parenterally; orthostatic hypotension is due to alpha-receptor blockade, the elderly are at greater risk for orthostatic hypotension.

Tardive dyskinesia: Prevalence rate may be 40% in elderly; development of the syndrome and the irreversible nature are proportional to duration and total cumulative dose over time. Extrapyramidal reactions are more common in elderly with up to 50% developing these reactions after 60 years of age. Drug-induced Parkinson's syndrome occurs often; akathisia is the most common extrapyramidal reaction in elderly.

Common Adverse Effects Frequency not defined.

Cardiovascular: Hypotension, tachycardia, syncope, nonspecific ECG changes

Central nervous system: Extrapyramidal signs (pseudoparkinsonism, akathisia, dystonias, lightheadedness, tardive dyskinesia), dizziness, drowsiness, restlessness, agitation, insomnia

Dermatologic: Discoloration of skin (blue-gray), rash, pruritus, urticaria, photosensitivity

Endocrine & metabolic: Changes in menstrual cycle, changes in libido, breast pain, galactorrhea, lactation, amenorrhea, gynecomastia, hyperglycemia, hypoglycemia

Gastrointestinal: Weight gain, nausea, vomiting, stomach pain, constipation, xerostomia, increased salivation

Genitourinary: Difficulty in urination, ejaculatory disturbances, impotence

Hematologic: Leukopenia, leukocytes

Neuromuscular & skeletal: Tremors

Ocular: Pigmentary retinopathy, blurred vision

Respiratory: Nasal congestion

Miscellaneous: Diaphoresis

Mechanism of Action Elicits antipsychotic activity by postsynaptic blockade of CNS dopamine receptors resulting in inhibition of dopamine-mediated effects; also has alpha-adrenergic blocking activity

Drug Interactions

Cytochrome P450 Effect: Substrate of CYP1A2 (major); **Inhibits** CYP2D6 (weak)

Increased Effect/Toxicity: CYP1A2 inhibitors may increase the levels/effects of thiothixene; example inhibitors include amiodarone, ciprofloxacin, fluvoxamine, ketoconazole, lomefloxacin, ofloxacin, and rofecoxib. Thiothixene and CNS depressants (ethanol, narcotics) may produce additive CNS depressant effects. Thiothixene may increase the effect/toxicity of antihypertensives, benztropine (and other anticholinergic agents), lithium, trazodone, and TCAs. Thiothixene's concentrations may be increased by chloroquine, sulfadoxine-pyrimethamine, and propranolol. Metoclopramide may increase risk of extrapyramidal symptoms (EPS).

Decreased Effect: CYP1A2 inducers may decrease the levels/effects of thiothixene; example inducers include aminoglutethimide, carbamazepine, phenobarbital, and rifampin. Thiothixene inhibits the activity of guanadrel, guanethidine, levodopa, and bromocriptine. Benztropine (and other anticholinergics) may inhibit the therapeutic response to thiothixene. Thiothixene and low potency antipsychotics may reverse the pressor effects of epinephrine.

Pharmacodynamics/Kinetics

Metabolism: Extensively hepatic

Half-life elimination: >24 hours with chronic use

Pregnancy Risk Factor C

Thorazine® [DSC] *see* ChlorproMAZINE *on page 319*

Thrombate III® *see* Antithrombin III *on page 136*

Thrombin-JMI® *see* Thrombin (Topical) *on page 1292*

Thrombin (Topical) (THROM bin, TOP i kal)

U.S. Brand Names Thrombin-JMI®; Thrombogen®

Canadian Brand Names Thrombostat™

Generic Available No

Pharmacologic Category Hemostatic Agent

Use Hemostasis whenever minor bleeding from capillaries and small venules is accessible

Local Anesthetic/Vasoconstrictor Precautions No information available to require special precautions

Effects on Dental Treatment No significant effects or complications reported

Significant Adverse Effects 1% to 10%:

Central nervous system: Fever

Miscellaneous: Allergic type reaction

Dosage Use 1000-2000 units/mL of solution where bleeding is profuse; apply powder directly to the site of bleeding or on oozing surfaces; use 100 units/mL for bleeding from skin or mucosal surfaces

Mechanism of Action Catalyzes the conversion of fibrinogen to fibrin

Contraindications Hypersensitivity to thrombin or any component of the formulation

Warnings/Precautions Do not inject, for topical use only

Drug Interactions No data reported

Pregnancy Risk Factor C

Dosage Forms Powder for reconstitution, topical

Thrombin-JMI®: 1000 units, 5000 units, 10,000 units, 20,000 units, 50,000 units

Thrombin-JMI® Spray Kit: 5000 unit, 10,000 units, 20,000 units

Thrombin-JMI® Syringe Spray Kit: 10,000 units, 20,000 units

Thrombogen®: 5000 units, 20,000 units

Thrombogen® Spray Kit: 10,000 units, 20,000 units

Thrombogen® *see* Thrombin (Topical) *on page 1292*

Thymocyte Stimulating Factor *see* Aldesleukin *on page 74*

Thyrel® TRH [DSC] *see* Protirelin *on page 1145*

Thyrogen® *see* Thyrotropin Alpha *on page 1294*

Thyroid (THYE roid)

Related Information

Endocrine Disorders and Pregnancy *on page 1481*

U.S. Brand Names Armour® Thyroid; Nature-Throid® NT; Westhroid®

Generic Available Yes

Synonyms Desiccated Thyroid; Thyroid Extract; Thyroid USP

Pharmacologic Category Thyroid Product

Use Replacement or supplemental therapy in hypothyroidism; pituitary TSH suppressants (thyroid nodules, thyroiditis, multinodular goiter, thyroid cancer), thyrotoxicosis, diagnostic suppression tests

Local Anesthetic/Vasoconstrictor Precautions No precautions with vasoconstrictor are necessary if patient is well controlled with thyroid preparations

Effects on Dental Treatment No significant effects or complications reported

Mechanism of Action The primary active compound is T_3 (triiodothyronine), which may be converted from T_4 (thyroxine) and then circulates throughout the body to influence growth and maturation of various tissues; exact mechanism of action is unknown; however, it is believed the thyroid hormone exerts its many metabolic effects through control of DNA transcription and protein synthesis; involved in normal metabolism, growth, and development; promotes gluconeogenesis, increases utilization and mobilization of glycogen stores and stimulates protein synthesis, increases basal metabolic rate

Drug Interactions

Increased Effect/Toxicity: Thyroid may potentiate the hypoprothrombinemic effect of oral anticoagulants. Tricyclic antidepressants (TAD) coadministered with thyroid hormone may increase potential for toxicity of both drugs.

Decreased Effect: Thyroid hormones increase the therapeutic need for oral hypoglycemics or insulin. Cholestyramine can bind thyroid and reduce its absorption. Phenytoin may decrease thyroxine serum levels. Thyroid hormone may decrease effect of oral sulfonylureas.

Pharmacodynamics/Kinetics

Absorption: T_4: 48% to 79%; T_3: 95%; desiccated thyroid contains thyroxine, liothyronine, and iodine (primarily bound)

Metabolism: Thyroxine: Largely converted to liothyronine

Half-life elimination, serum: Liothyronine: 1-2 days; Thyroxine: 6-7 days

Pregnancy Risk Factor A

Thyroid Extract *see* Thyroid *on page 1293*

Thyroid USP *see* Thyroid *on page 1293*

Thyrolar® *see* Liotrix *on page 832*

Thyrotropin Alpha (thye roe TROH pin AL fa)

U.S. Brand Names Thyrogen®

Canadian Brand Names Thyrogen®

Generic Available No

Synonyms Human Thyroid Stimulating Hormone; TSH

Pharmacologic Category Diagnostic Agent

Use As an adjunctive diagnostic tool for serum thyroglobulin (Tg) testing with or without radioiodine imaging in the follow-up of patients with well-differentiated thyroid cancer

Potential clinical use:

1. Patients with an undetectable Tg on thyroid hormone suppressive therapy to exclude the diagnosis of residual or recurrent thyroid cancer
2. Patients requiring serum Tg testing and radioiodine imaging who are unwilling to undergo thyroid hormone withdrawal testing and whose treating physician believes that use of a less sensitive test is justified
3. Patients who are either unable to mount an adequate endogenous TSH response to thyroid hormone withdrawal or in whom withdrawal is medically contraindicated

Local Anesthetic/Vasoconstrictor Precautions No information available to require special precautions

Effects on Dental Treatment No significant effects or complications reported

Common Adverse Effects

1% to 10%:

Central nervous system: Headache, chills, fever, dizziness
Gastrointestinal: Nausea, vomiting
Neuromuscular & skeletal: Weakness, paresthesia
Miscellaneous: Flu-like syndrome

Adverse reactions which may be related to local edema or hemorrhage at metastatic sites:

Ocular: Acute visual loss
Respiratory: Laryngeal edema with respiratory distress, stridor
Miscellaneous: Enlargement of locally-recurring papillary carcinoma

Mechanism of Action An exogenous source of human TSH that offers an additional diagnostic tool in the follow-up of patients with a history of well-differentiated thyroid cancer. Binding of thyrotropin alpha to TSH receptors on normal thyroid epithelial cells or on well-differentiated thyroid cancer tissue stimulates iodine uptake and organification and synthesis and secretion of thyroglobulin, triiodothyronine, and thyroxine.

Pharmacodynamics/Kinetics

Half-life elimination: 25 ± 10 hours
Time to peak: Mean: 3-24 hours after injection

Pregnancy Risk Factor C

Thyrotropin Releasing Hormone *see* Protirelin *on page 1145*
Tiabendazole *see* Thiabendazole *on page 1286*

Tiagabine (tye AG a been)

U.S. Brand Names Gabitril®

Canadian Brand Names Gabitril®

Generic Available No

Synonyms Tiagabine Hydrochloride

Pharmacologic Category Anticonvulsant, Miscellaneous

Use Adjunctive therapy in adults and children ≥12 years of age in the treatment of partial seizures

Unlabeled/Investigational Use Bipolar disorder

Local Anesthetic/Vasoconstrictor Precautions No information available to require special precautions

Effects on Dental Treatment No significant effects or complications reported

Common Adverse Effects

>10%:

Central nervous system: Dizziness, somnolence
Gastrointestinal: Nausea
Neuromuscular & skeletal: Weakness

1% to 10%:

Central nervous system: Nervousness, difficulty with concentration, insomnia, ataxia, confusion, speech disorder, depression, emotional lability, abnormal gait, hostility
Dermatologic: Rash, pruritus
Gastrointestinal: Diarrhea, vomiting, increased appetite
Neuromuscular & skeletal: Tremor, paresthesia
Ocular: Nystagmus

Otic: Hearing impairment

Respiratory: Pharyngitis, cough

Mechanism of Action The exact mechanism by which tiagabine exerts antiseizure activity is not definitively known; however, *in vitro* experiments demonstrate that it enhances the activity of gamma aminobutyric acid (GABA), the major neuroinhibitory transmitter in the nervous system; it is thought that binding to the GABA uptake carrier inhibits the uptake of GABA into presynaptic neurons, allowing an increased amount of GABA to be available to postsynaptic neurons; based on *in vitro* studies, tiagabine does not inhibit the uptake of dopamine, norepinephrine, serotonin, glutamate, or choline

Drug Interactions

Cytochrome P450 Effect: Substrate of 3A4 (major)

Increased Effect/Toxicity: CYP3A4 inhibitors may increase the levels/effects of tiagabine; example inhibitors include azole antifungals, ciprofloxacin, clarithromycin, diclofenac, doxycycline, erythromycin, imatinib, isoniazid, nefazodone, nicardipine, propofol, protease inhibitors, quinidine, and verapamil. Valproate increased free tiagabine concentrations by 40%.

Decreased Effect: CYP3A4 inducers may decrease the levels/effects of tiagabine; example inducers include aminoglutethimide, carbamazepine, nafcillin, nevirapine, phenobarbital, phenytoin, and rifamycins.

Pharmacodynamics/Kinetics

Absorption: Rapid (within 1 hour); prolonged with food

Protein binding: 96%, primarily to albumin and α_1-acid glycoprotein

Metabolism: Hepatic via CYP (primarily 3A4)

Bioavailability: Oral: Absolute: 90%

Half-life elimination: 6.7 hours

Time to peak, plasma: 45 minutes

Excretion: Feces (63%) and urine (25%, 2% as unchanged drug); primarily as metabolites

Pregnancy Risk Factor C

Tiagabine Hydrochloride *see* Tiagabine *on page 1294*

Tiazac® *see* Diltiazem *on page 444*

Ticar® *see* Ticarcillin *on page 1295*

Ticarcillin (tye kar SIL in)

U.S. Brand Names Ticar®

Generic Available No

Synonyms Ticarcillin Disodium

Pharmacologic Category Antibiotic, Penicillin

Use Treatment of susceptible infections such as septicemia, acute and chronic respiratory tract infections, skin and soft tissue infections, and urinary tract infections due to susceptible strains of *Pseudomonas*, and other gram-negative bacteria

Local Anesthetic/Vasoconstrictor Precautions No information available to require special precautions

Effects on Dental Treatment Key adverse event(s) related to dental treatment: Prolonged use of penicillins may lead to development of oral candidiasis.

Common Adverse Effects Frequency not defined.

Central nervous system: Confusion, convulsions, drowsiness, fever, Jarisch-Herxheimer reaction

Dermatologic: Rash

Endocrine & metabolic: Electrolyte imbalance

Gastrointestinal: *Clostridium difficile* colitis

Hematologic: Bleeding, eosinophilia, hemolytic anemia, leukopenia, neutropenia, positive Coombs' reaction, thrombocytopenia

Hepatic: Hepatotoxicity, jaundice

Local: Thrombophlebitis

Neuromuscular & skeletal: Myoclonus

Renal: Interstitial nephritis (acute)

Miscellaneous: Anaphylaxis, hypersensitivity reactions

Mechanism of Action Inhibits bacterial cell wall synthesis by binding to one or more of the penicillin binding proteins (PBPs); which in turn inhibits the final transpeptidation step of peptidoglycan synthesis in bacterial cell walls, thus inhibiting cell wall biosynthesis. Bacteria eventually lyse due to ongoing activity of cell wall autolytic enzymes (autolysins and murein hydrolases) while cell wall assembly is arrested.

(Continued)

Ticarcillin *(Continued)*

Drug Interactions

Increased Effect/Toxicity: Probenecid may increase penicillin levels. Neuromuscular blockers may have an increased duration of action (neuromuscular blockade). Penicillins may increase the exposure to methotrexate during concurrent therapy; monitor.

Decreased Effect: Tetracyclines may decrease penicillin effectiveness. Aminoglycosides may cause physical inactivation of aminoglycosides in the presence of high concentrations of ticarcillin and potential toxicity in patients with mild-moderate renal dysfunction. Although anecdotal reports suggest oral contraceptive efficacy could be reduced by penicillins, this has been refuted by more rigorous scientific and clinical data.

Pharmacodynamics/Kinetics

Absorption: I.M.: 86%

Distribution: Blister fluid, lymph tissue, and gallbladder; low concentrations into CSF increasing with inflamed meninges, otherwise widely distributed; crosses placenta; enters breast milk (low concentrations)

Protein binding: 45% to 65%

Half-life elimination:

Neonates: <1 week old: 3.5-5.6 hours; 1-8 weeks old: 1.3-2.2 hours

Children 5-13 years: 0.9 hour

Adults: 66-72 minutes; prolonged with renal and/or hepatic impairment

Time to peak, serum: I.M.: 30-75 minutes

Excretion: Almost entirely urine (as unchanged drug and metabolites); feces (3.5%)

Pregnancy Risk Factor B

Ticarcillin and Clavulanate Potassium

(tye kar SIL in & klav yoo LAN ate poe TASS ee um)

Related Information

Ticarcillin *on page 1295*

U.S. Brand Names Timentin®

Canadian Brand Names Timentin®

Generic Available No

Synonyms Ticarcillin and Clavulanic Acid

Pharmacologic Category Antibiotic, Penicillin

Use Treatment of infections of lower respiratory tract, urinary tract, skin and skin structures, bone and joint, and septicemia caused by susceptible organisms. Clavulanate expands activity of ticarcillin to include beta-lactamase producing strains of *S. aureus*, *H. influenzae*, *Bacteroides* species, and some other gram-negative bacilli

Local Anesthetic/Vasoconstrictor Precautions No information available to require special precautions

Effects on Dental Treatment Key adverse event(s) related to dental treatment: Prolonged use of penicillins may lead to development of oral candidiasis.

Common Adverse Effects Frequency not defined.

Central nervous system: Confusion, convulsions, drowsiness, fever, Jarisch-Herxheimer reaction

Dermatologic: Rash, erythema multiforme, toxic epidermal necrolysis, Stevens-Johnson syndrome

Endocrine & metabolic: Electrolyte imbalance

Gastrointestinal: *Clostridium difficile* colitis

Hematologic: Bleeding, hemolytic anemia, leukopenia, neutropenia, positive Coombs' reaction, thrombocytopenia

Hepatic: Hepatotoxicity, jaundice

Local: Thrombophlebitis

Neuromuscular & skeletal: Myoclonus

Renal: Interstitial nephritis (acute)

Miscellaneous: Anaphylaxis, hypersensitivity reactions

Mechanism of Action Inhibits bacterial cell wall synthesis by binding to one or more of the penicillin binding proteins (PBPs); which in turn inhibits the final transpeptidation step of peptidoglycan synthesis in bacterial cell walls, thus inhibiting cell wall biosynthesis. Bacteria eventually lyse due to ongoing activity of cell wall autolytic enzymes (autolysins and murein hydrolases) while cell wall assembly is arrested.

Drug Interactions

Increased Effect/Toxicity: Probenecid may increase penicillin levels. Neuromuscular blockers may have an increased duration of action (neuromuscular blockade). Penicillins may increase the exposure to methotrexate during concurrent therapy; monitor.

Decreased Effect: Tetracyclines may decrease penicillin effectiveness. Aminoglycosides may cause physical inactivation of aminoglycosides in the presence of high concentrations of ticarcillin and potential toxicity in patients with mild-moderate renal dysfunction. Although anecdotal reports suggest oral contraceptive efficacy could be reduced by penicillins, this has been refuted by more rigorous scientific and clinical data.

Pharmacodynamics/Kinetics

Ticarcillin: See Ticarcillin monograph.

Clavulanic acid:

Protein binding: 9% to 30%

Metabolism: Hepatic

Half-life elimination: 66-90 minutes

Excretion: Urine (45% as unchanged drug)

Clearance: Does not affect clearance of ticarcillin

Pregnancy Risk Factor B

Ticarcillin and Clavulanic Acid *see* Ticarcillin and Clavulanate Potassium *on page 1296*

Ticarcillin Disodium *see* Ticarcillin *on page 1295*

TICE® BCG *see* BCG Vaccine *on page 183*

Ticlid® *see* Ticlopidine *on page 1297*

Ticlopidine (tye KLOE pi deen)

Related Information

Cardiovascular Diseases *on page 1458*

U.S. Brand Names Ticlid®

Canadian Brand Names Alti-Ticlopidine; Apo-Ticlopidine®; Gen-Ticlopidine; Novo-Ticlopidine; Nu-Ticlopidine; PMS-Ticlopidine; Rhoxal-ticlopidine; Ticlid®

Mexican Brand Names Ticlid®

Generic Available Yes

Synonyms Ticlopidine Hydrochloride

Pharmacologic Category Antiplatelet Agent

Use Platelet aggregation inhibitor that reduces the risk of thrombotic stroke in patients who have had a stroke or stroke precursors. **Note:** Due to its association with life-threatening hematologic disorders, ticlopidine should be reserved for patients who are intolerant to aspirin, or who have failed aspirin therapy. Adjunctive therapy (with aspirin) following successful coronary stent implantation to reduce the incidence of subacute stent thrombosis.

Unlabeled/Investigational Use Protection of aortocoronary bypass grafts, diabetic microangiopathy, ischemic heart disease, prevention of postoperative DVT, reduction of graft loss following renal transplant

Local Anesthetic/Vasoconstrictor Precautions No information available to require special precautions

Effects on Dental Treatment No significant effects or complications reported; if a patient is to undergo elective surgery and an antiplatelet effect is not desired, ticlopidine should be discontinued at least 7 days prior to surgery.

Common Adverse Effects As with all drugs which may affect hemostasis, bleeding is associated with ticlopidine. Hemorrhage may occur at virtually any site. Risk is dependent on multiple variables, including the use of multiple agents which alter hemostasis and patient susceptibility.

>10%:

Endocrine & metabolic: Increased total cholesterol (increases of ~8% to 10% within 1 month of therapy)

Gastrointestinal: Diarrhea (13%)

1% to 10%:

Central nervous system: Dizziness (1%)

Dermatologic: Rash (5%), purpura (2%), pruritus (1%)

Gastrointestinal: Nausea (7%), dyspepsia (7%), gastrointestinal pain (4%), vomiting (2%), flatulence (2%), anorexia (1%)

Hematologic: Neutropenia (2%)

Hepatic: Abnormal liver function test (1%)

Mechanism of Action Ticlopidine is an inhibitor of platelet function with a mechanism which is different from other antiplatelet drugs. The drug significantly increases bleeding time. This effect may not be solely related to ticlopidine's effect on platelets. The prolongation of the bleeding time caused

(Continued)

Ticlopidine *(Continued)*

by ticlopidine is further increased by the addition of aspirin in *ex vivo* experiments. Although many metabolites of ticlopidine have been found, none have been shown to account for *in vivo* activity.

Drug Interactions

Cytochrome P450 Effect: Substrate of CYP3A4 (major); **Inhibits** CYP1A2 (weak), 2C8/9 (weak), 2C19 (strong), 2D6 (moderate), 2E1 (weak), 3A4 (weak)

Increased Effect/Toxicity: Ticlopidine may increase effect/toxicity of aspirin, anticoagulants, theophylline, and NSAIDs. Cimetidine may increase ticlopidine blood levels. Ticlopidine may increase the levels/effects of amphetamines, selected beta-blockers, citalopram, dextromethorphan, diazepam, fluoxetine, lidocaine, methsuximide, mirtazapine, nefazodone, paroxetine, phenytoin, sertraline, risperidone, ritonavir, thioridazine, tricyclic antidepressants, venlafaxine, and other CYP2C19 or 2D6 substrates.

Decreased Effect: Decreased effect of ticlopidine with antacids (decreased absorption). Ticlopidine may decrease the effect of digoxin or cyclosporine. The levels/effects of ticlopidine may be decreased by aminoglutethimide, carbamazepine, nafcillin, nevirapine, phenobarbital, phenytoin, rifamycins, and other CYP3A4 inducers. Ticlopidine may decrease the levels/effects of CYP2D6 prodrug substrates (eg, codeine, hydrocodone, oxycodone, tramadol).

Pharmacodynamics/Kinetics

Onset of action: ~6 hours

Peak effect: 3-5 days; serum levels do not correlate with clinical antiplatelet activity

Metabolism: Extensively hepatic; has at least one active metabolite

Half-life elimination: 24 hours

Pregnancy Risk Factor B

Ticlopidine Hydrochloride *see* Ticlopidine *on page 1297*

TIG *see* Tetanus Immune Globulin (Human) *on page 1277*

Tigan® *see* Trimethobenzamide *on page 1341*

Tikosyn™ *see* Dofetilide *on page 460*

Tilade® *see* Nedocromil *on page 970*

Tiludronate (tye LOO droe nate)

U.S. Brand Names Skelid®

Generic Available No

Synonyms Tiludronate Disodium

Pharmacologic Category Bisphosphonate Derivative

Use Treatment of Paget's disease of the bone in patients who have a level of serum alkaline phosphatase (SAP) at least twice the upper limit of normal, or who are symptomatic, or who are at risk for future complications of their disease

Local Anesthetic/Vasoconstrictor Precautions No information available to require special precautions

Effects on Dental Treatment No significant effects or complications reported

Common Adverse Effects The following events occurred >2% and at a frequency greater than placebo:

1% to 10%:

Cardiovascular: Chest pain (3%), edema (3%)

Central nervous system: Dizziness (4%), paresthesia (4%)

Dermatologic: Rash (3%), skin disorder (3%)

Gastrointestinal: Nausea (9%), diarrhea (9%), heartburn (5%), vomiting (4%), flatulence (3%)

Neuromuscular & skeletal: Arthrosis (3%)

Ocular: cataract (3%), conjunctivitis (3%), glaucoma (3%)

Respiratory: Rhinitis (5%), sinusitis (5%), coughing (3%), pharyngitis (3%)

Mechanism of Action Inhibition of normal and abnormal bone resorption. Inhibits osteoclasts through at least two mechanisms: disruption of the cytoskeletal ring structure, possibly by inhibition of protein-tyrosine-phosphatase, thus leading to the detachment of osteoclasts from the bone surface area and the inhibition of the osteoclast proton pump.

Drug Interactions

Increased Effect/Toxicity: Administration of indomethacin increases bioavailability of tiludronate two- to fourfold.

Decreased Effect: Concurrent administration of calcium salts, aluminum- or magnesium-containing antacids, and aspirin markedly decrease absorption/

bioavailability (by 50% to 60%) of tiludronate if given within 2 hours of a dose.

Pharmacodynamics/Kinetics

Onset of action: Delayed, may require several weeks

Absorption: Rapid

Distribution: Widely to bone and soft tissue

Protein binding: 90%, primarily to albumin

Metabolism: Little, if any

Bioavailability: 6%; reduced by food

Half-life elimination: Healthy volunteers: 50 hours; Pagetic patients: 150 hours

Time to peak, plasma: ~2 hours

Excretion: Urine (60% as unchanged drug) within 13 days

Pregnancy Risk Factor C

Tiludronate Disodium *see* Tiludronate *on page 1298*

Timentin® *see* Ticarcillin and Clavulanate Potassium *on page 1296*

Timolol (TYE moe lole)

Related Information

Cardiovascular Diseases *on page 1458*

U.S. Brand Names Betimol®; Blocadren®; Istalol™; Timoptic®; Timoptic® OcuDose®; Timoptic-XE®

Canadian Brand Names Alti-Timolol; Apo-Timol®; Apo-Timop®; Gen-Timolol; Nu-Timolol; Phoxal-timolol; PMS-Timolol; Tim-AK; Timoptic®; Timoptic-XE®

Mexican Brand Names Shemol®; Timoptol®

Generic Available Yes; Excludes hemihydrate ophthalmic solutions

Synonyms Timolol Hemihydrate; Timolol Maleate

Pharmacologic Category Beta-Adrenergic Blocker, Nonselective; Ophthalmic Agent, Antiglaucoma

Use Ophthalmic dosage form used in treatment of elevated intraocular pressure such as glaucoma or ocular hypertension; oral dosage form used for treatment of hypertension and angina, to reduce mortality following myocardial infarction, and for prophylaxis of migraine

Local Anesthetic/Vasoconstrictor Precautions Epinephrine has interacted with nonselective beta blockers such as propranolol to result in initial hypertensive episode followed by bradycardia. Timolol is also a nonselective beta blocker. Timolol is available as an eye drop and oral dose form. When administered as an eye drop, the significance of a potential systemic interaction with epinephrine is unknown. However, it is suggested that cautionary procedures be used, particularly if vasoconstrictor is used immediately following an ophthalmic dose of timolol taken by the patient. If patients are taking the oral form of timolol, then the significance of a potential systemic interaction is well known and cautionary use of epinephrine is advised.

Effects on Dental Treatment Timolol is a nonselective beta-blocker and may enhance the pressor response to epinephrine, resulting in hypertension and bradycardia. Many nonsteroidal anti-inflammatory drugs, such as ibuprofen and indomethacin, can reduce the hypotensive effect of beta-blockers after 3 or more weeks of therapy with the NSAID. Short-term NSAID use (ie, 3 days) requires no special precautions in patients taking beta-blockers.

Common Adverse Effects

Ophthalmic:

>10%: Ocular: Burning, stinging

1% to 10%:

Cardiovascular: Hypertension

Central nervous system: Headache

Ocular: Blurred vision, cataract, conjunctival injection, itching, visual acuity decreased

Miscellaneous: Infection

Systemic:

1% to 10%:

Cardiovascular: Bradycardia

Central nervous system: Fatigue, dizziness

Respiratory: Dyspnea

Frequency not defined (reported with any dosage form):

Cardiovascular: Angina pectoris, arrhythmia, bradycardia, cardiac failure, cardiac arrest, cerebral vascular accident, cerebral ischemia, edema, hypotension, heart block, palpitation, Raynaud's phenomenon

Central nervous system: Anxiety, confusion, depression, disorientation, dizziness, hallucinations, insomnia, memory loss, nervousness, nightmares, somnolence

(Continued)

Timolol *(Continued)*

Dermatologic: Alopecia, angioedema, pseudopemphigoid, psoriasiform rash, psoriasis exacerbation, rash, urticaria
Endocrine & metabolic: Hypoglycemia masked, libido decreased
Gastrointestinal: Anorexia, diarrhea, dyspepsia, nausea, xerostomia
Genitourinary: Impotence, retoperitoneal fibrosis
Hematologic: Claudication
Neuromuscular & skeletal: Myasthenia gravis exacerbation, paresthesia
Ocular: Blepharitis, conjunctivitis, corneal sensitivity decreased, cystoid macular edema, diplopia, dry eyes, foreign body sensation, keratitis, ocular discharge, ocular pain, ptosis, refractive changes, tearing, visual disturbances
Otic: Tinnitus
Respiratory: Bronchospasm, cough, dyspnea, nasal congestion, pulmonary edema, respiratory failure
Miscellaneous: Allergic reactions, cold hands/feet, Peyronie's disease, systemic lupus erythematosus

Mechanism of Action Blocks both beta$_1$- and beta$_2$-adrenergic receptors, reduces intraocular pressure by reducing aqueous humor production or possibly outflow; reduces blood pressure by blocking adrenergic receptors and decreasing sympathetic outflow, produces a negative chronotropic and inotropic activity through an unknown mechanism

Drug Interactions

Cytochrome P450 Effect: Substrate of CYP2D6 (major); **Inhibits** CYP2D6 (weak)

Increased Effect/Toxicity: CYP2D6 inhibitors may increase the levels/effects of timolol; example inhibitors include chlorpromazine, delavirdine, fluoxetine, miconazole, paroxetine, pergolide, quinidine, quinine, ritonavir, and ropinirole. The heart rate-lowering effects of timolol are additive with other drugs which slow AV conduction (digoxin, verapamil, diltiazem). Reserpine increases the effects of timolol. Concurrent use of timolol may increase the effects of alpha-blockers (prazosin, terazosin), alpha-adrenergic stimulants (epinephrine, phenylephrine), and the vasoconstrictive effects of ergot alkaloids. Timolol may mask the tachycardia from hypoglycemia caused by insulin and oral hypoglycemics. In patients receiving concurrent therapy, the risk of hypertensive crisis is increased when either clonidine or the beta-blocker is withdrawn. Beta-blockers may increase the action or levels of ethanol, disopyramide, nondepolarizing muscle relaxants, and theophylline although the effects are difficult to predict.

Decreased Effect: Decreased effect of timolol with aluminum salts, barbiturates, calcium salts, cholestyramine, colestipol, NSAIDs, penicillins (ampicillin), rifampin, salicylates, and sulfinpyrazone due to decreased bioavailability and plasma levels. Beta-blockers may decrease the effect of sulfonylureas. Beta-blockers may affect the action or levels of ethanol, disopyramide, nondepolarizing muscle relaxants, and theophylline, although the effects are difficult to predict.

Pharmacodynamics/Kinetics

Onset of action:
Hypotensive: Oral: 15-45 minutes
Peak effect: 0.5-2.5 hours
Intraocular pressure reduction: Ophthalmic: 30 minutes
Peak effect: 1-2 hours
Duration: ~4 hours; Ophthalmic: Intraocular: 24 hours
Protein binding: 60%
Metabolism: Extensively hepatic; extensive first-pass effect
Half-life elimination: 2-2.7 hours; prolonged with renal impairment
Excretion: Urine (15% to 20% as unchanged drug)

Pregnancy Risk Factor C (manufacturer); D (2nd and 3rd trimesters - expert analysis)

Timolol and Dorzolamide *see* Dorzolamide and Timolol *on page 464*
Timolol Hemihydrate *see* Timolol *on page 1299*
Timolol Maleate *see* Timolol *on page 1299*
Timoptic® *see* Timolol *on page 1299*
Timoptic® OcuDose® *see* Timolol *on page 1299*
Timoptic-XE® *see* Timolol *on page 1299*
Tinactin® Antifungal [OTC] *see* Tolnaftate *on page 1312*
Tinactin® Antifungal Jock Itch [OTC] *see* Tolnaftate *on page 1312*
Tinaderm [OTC] *see* Tolnaftate *on page 1312*
Tinamed® [OTC] *see* Salicylic Acid *on page 1205*

TinBen® [OTC] [DSC] *see* Benzoin *on page 193*

Tindamax™ *see* Tinidazole *on page 1301*

Tine Test *see* Tuberculin Tests *on page 1349*

Ting® [OTC] *see* Tolnaftate *on page 1312*

Tinidazole (tye NI da zole)

U.S. Brand Names Tindamax™

Generic Available No

Pharmacologic Category Amebicide; Antibiotic, Miscellaneous; Antiprotozoal, Nitroimidazole

Use Treatment of trichomoniasis caused by *T. vaginalis*; treatment of giardiasis caused by *G. duodenalis (G. lamblia)*; treatment of intestinal amebiasis and amebic liver abscess caused by *E. histolytica*

Local Anesthetic/Vasoconstrictor Precautions No information available to require special precautions

Effects on Dental Treatment Key adverse event(s) related to dental treatment: Xerostomia and changes in salivation (normal salivary flow resumes upon discontinuation), metallic/bitter taste, oral candidiasis, tongue discoloration, stomatitis, furry tongue.

Common Adverse Effects

1% to 10%:

- Central nervous system: Weakness/fatigue/malaise (1% to 2%), dizziness (≤1%), headache (≤1%)
- Gastrointestinal: Metallic/bitter taste (4% to 6%), nausea (3% to 5%), anorexia (2% to 3%), dyspepsia/cramps/epigastric discomfort (1% to 2%), vomiting (1% to 2%), constipation (≤1%)

Frequency not defined.

- Cardiovascular: Flushing, palpitations
- Central nervous system: Ataxia, coma, confusion, convulsions, depression, drowsiness, fever, giddiness, insomnia, vertigo
- Dermatologic: Angioedema, pruritus, rash, urticaria
- Gastrointestinal: Diarrhea, furry tongue, oral candidiasis, salivation, stomatitis, thirst, tongue discoloration, xerostomia
- Genitourinary: Urine darkened, vaginal discharge increased
- Hematologic: Leukopenia (transient), neutropenia (transient), thrombocytopenia (reversible)
- Hepatic: Transaminases increased
- Neuromuscular & skeletal: Arthralgia, arthritis, myalgia, peripheral neuropathy (transient, includes numbness and paresthesia)
- Respiratory: Bronchospasm, dyspnea, pharyngitis
- Miscellaneous: Burning sensation, *Candida* overgrowth, diaphoresis

Mechanism of Action After diffusing into the organism, it is proposed that tinidazole causes cytotoxicity by damaging DNA and preventing further DNA synthesis.

Drug Interactions

Cytochrome P450 Effect: Substrate of CYP3A4 (major)

Increased Effect/Toxicity: Specific interaction studies have not been conducted. Refer to Metronidazole monograph *on page 917*.

Decreased Effect: Specific interaction studies have not been conducted. Refer to Metronidazole monograph *on page 917*.

Pharmacodynamics/Kinetics

Absorption: Rapid and complete

Distribution: V_d: 50 L

Protein binding: 12%

Metabolism: Hepatic via CYP3A4 (primarily); undergoes oxidation, hydroxylation and conjugation; forms a metabolite

Half-life elimination: 13 hours

Excretion: Urine (20% to 25%); feces (12%)

Pregnancy Risk Factor C

Comments Although this drug is a member of the metronidazole family, there is no specific dental indication for its use. Just as with metronidazole, alcohol in any form is contraindicated while the patient is on this medication because of the danger of a disulfiram-type reaction.

Tinzaparin (tin ZA pa rin)

Related Information

Cardiovascular Diseases *on page 1458*

U.S. Brand Names Innohep®

Canadian Brand Names Innohep®

Generic Available No

(Continued)

Tinzaparin *(Continued)*

Synonyms Tinzaparin Sodium

Pharmacologic Category Low Molecular Weight Heparin

Use Treatment of acute symptomatic deep vein thrombosis, with or without pulmonary embolism, in conjunction with warfarin sodium

Local Anesthetic/Vasoconstrictor Precautions No information available to require special precautions

Effects on Dental Treatment No significant effects or complications reported

Common Adverse Effects As with all anticoagulants, bleeding is the major adverse effect of tinzaparin. Hemorrhage may occur at virtually any site. Risk is dependent on multiple variables.

>10%:

Hepatic: Increased ALT (13%)

Local: Injection site hematoma (16%)

1% to 10%:

Cardiovascular: Angina pectoris, chest pain (2%), hypertension, hypotension, tachycardia

Central nervous system: Confusion, dizziness, fever (2%), headache (2%), insomnia, pain (2%)

Dermatologic: Bullous eruption, pruritus, rash (1%), skin disorder

Gastrointestinal: Constipation (1%), dyspepsia, flatulence, nausea (2%), nonspecified gastrointestinal disorder, vomiting (1%)

Genitourinary: Dysuria, urinary retention, urinary tract infection (4%)

Hematologic: Anemia, hematoma, hemorrhage (2%), thrombocytopenia (1%)

Hepatic: Increased AST (9%)

Local: Deep vein thrombosis, injection site hematoma

Neuromuscular & skeletal: Back pain (2%)

Renal: Hematuria (1%)

Respiratory: Dyspnea (1%), epistaxis (2%), pneumonia, pulmonary embolism (2%), respiratory disorder

Miscellaneous: Impaired healing, infection, unclassified reactions

Mechanism of Action Standard heparin consists of components with molecular weights ranging from 4000-30,000 daltons with a mean of 16,000 daltons. Heparin acts as an anticoagulant by enhancing the inhibition rate of clotting proteases by antithrombin III, impairing normal hemostasis and inhibition of factor Xa. Low molecular weight heparins have a small effect on the activated partial thromboplastin time and strongly inhibit factor Xa. The primary inhibitory activity of tinzaparin is through antithrombin. Tinzaparin is derived from porcine heparin that undergoes controlled enzymatic depolymerization. The average molecular weight of tinzaparin ranges between 5500 and 7500 daltons which is distributed as (<10%) 2000 daltons (60% to 72%) 2000-8000 daltons, and (22% to 36%) >8000 daltons. The antifactor Xa activity is approximately 100 int. units/mg.

Drug Interactions

Increased Effect/Toxicity: Drugs which affect platelet function (eg, aspirin, NSAIDs, dipyridamole, ticlopidine, clopidogrel, sulfinpyrazone, dextran) may potentiate the risk of hemorrhage. Thrombolytic agents increase the risk of hemorrhage.

Warfarin: Risk of bleeding may be increased during concurrent therapy. Tinzaparin is commonly continued during the initiation of warfarin therapy to assure anticoagulation and to protect against possible transient hypercoagulability

Pharmacodynamics/Kinetics

Onset of action: 2-3 hours

Distribution: 3-5 L

Half-life elimination: 3-4 hours

Metabolism: Partially metabolized by desulphation and depolymerization

Bioavailability: 87%

Time to peak: 4-5 hours

Excretion: Urine

Pregnancy Risk Factor B

Tinzaparin Sodium *see* Tinzaparin *on page 1301*

Tioconazole (tye oh KONE a zole)

U.S. Brand Names 1-Day™ [OTC]; Vagistat®-1 [OTC]

Generic Available No

Pharmacologic Category Antifungal Agent, Vaginal

Use Local treatment of vulvovaginal candidiasis

Local Anesthetic/Vasoconstrictor Precautions No information available to require special precautions

Effects on Dental Treatment No significant effects or complications reported

Common Adverse Effects Frequency not defined.

Central nervous system: Headache

Gastrointestinal: Abdominal pain

Dermatologic: Burning, desquamation

Genitourinary: Discharge, dyspareunia, dysuria, irritation, itching, nocturia, vaginal pain, vaginitis, vulvar swelling

Mechanism of Action A 1-substituted imidazole derivative with a broad antifungal spectrum against a wide variety of dermatophytes and yeasts, including *Trichophyton mentagrophytes*, *T. rubrum*, *T. erinacei*, *T. tonsurans*, *Microsporum canis*, *Microsporum gypseum*, and *Candida albicans*. Both agents appear to be similarly effective against *Epidermophyton floccosum*.

Drug Interactions

Cytochrome P450 Effect: Inhibits CYP1A2 (weak), 2A6 (weak), 2C8/9 (weak), 2C19 (weak), 2D6 (weak), 2E1 (weak)

Pharmacodynamics/Kinetics

Onset of action: Some improvement: Within 24 hours; Complete relief: Within 7 days

Absorption: Intravaginal: Systemic (small amounts)

Distribution: Vaginal fluid: 24-72 hours

Excretion: Urine and feces

Pregnancy Risk Factor C

Tioguanine *see* Thioguanine *on page 1288*

Tiopronin (tye oh PROE nin)

U.S. Brand Names Thiola®

Canadian Brand Names Thiola™

Generic Available No

Pharmacologic Category Urinary Tract Product

Use Prevention of kidney stone (cystine) formation in patients with severe homozygous cystinuric who have urinary cystine >500 mg/day who are resistant to treatment with high fluid intake, alkali, and diet modification, or who have had adverse reactions to penicillamine

Local Anesthetic/Vasoconstrictor Precautions No information available to require special precautions

Effects on Dental Treatment No significant effects or complications reported

Pregnancy Risk Factor C

Tiotixene *see* Thiothixene *on page 1291*

Tiotropium (ty oh TRO pee um)

U.S. Brand Names Spiriva®

Canadian Brand Names Spiriva®

Synonyms Tiotropium Bromide Monohydrate

Pharmacologic Category Anticholinergic Agent

Use Maintenance treatment of bronchospasm associated with COPD (bronchitis and emphysema)

Local Anesthetic/Vasoconstrictor Precautions No information available to require special precautions

Effects on Dental Treatment Key adverse event(s) related to dental treatment: Xerostomia (normal salivary flow resumes upon discontinuation) and ulcerative stomatitis.

Common Adverse Effects

>10%:

Gastrointestinal: Xerostomia (16%)

Respiratory: Upper respiratory tract infection (41% vs 37% with placebo), sinusitis (11% vs 9% with placebo), pharyngeal irritation (frequency not specified)

1% to 10%:

Cardiovascular: Angina, edema (dependent, 5%)

Central nervous system: Paresthesia, depression

Dermatologic: Rash (4%)

Endocrine & metabolic: Hypercholesterolemia, hyperglycemia

Gastrointestinal: Dyspepsia (6%), abdominal pain (5%), constipation (4%), vomiting (4%), reflux, ulcerative stomatitis

Genitourinary: Urinary tract infection (7%)

Neuromuscular & skeletal: Myalgia (4%), leg pain, skeletal pain

Ocular: Cataract

(Continued)

Tiotropium *(Continued)*

Respiratory: Pharyngitis (9%), rhinitis (6%), epistaxis (4%), dysphonia, laryngitis

Miscellaneous: Infection (4%), moniliasis (4%), allergic reaction, herpes zoster

Mechanism of Action Blocks the action of acetylcholine at parasympathetic sites in bronchial smooth muscle causing bronchodilation

Drug Interactions

Cytochrome P450 Effect: Substrate (minor) of CYP2D6, 3A4

Increased Effect/Toxicity: Increased toxicity with anticholinergics or drugs with anticholinergic properties.

Pharmacodynamics/Kinetics

Absorption: Poorly absorbed from GI tract, systemic absorption may occur from lung

Distribution: V_d: 32 L/kg

Protein binding: 72%

Metabolism: Hepatic (minimal), via CYP2D6 and CYP3A4

Bioavailability: Following inhalation, 19.5%; oral solution: 2% to 3%

Half-life elimination: 5-6 days

Time to peak, plasma: 5 minutes (following inhalation)

Excretion: Urine (74% as unchanged drug)

Pregnancy Risk Factor C

Tiotropium Bromide Monohydrate *see* Tiotropium *on page 1303*

TipTapToe [OTC] *see* Tolnaftate *on page 1312*

Tirofiban (tye roe FYE ban)

Related Information

Cardiovascular Diseases *on page 1458*

U.S. Brand Names Aggrastat®

Canadian Brand Names Aggrastat®

Mexican Brand Names Agrastat®

Generic Available No

Synonyms MK383; Tirofiban Hydrochloride

Pharmacologic Category Antiplatelet Agent, Glycoprotein IIb/IIIa Inhibitor

Use In combination with heparin, is indicated for the treatment of acute coronary syndrome, including patients who are to be managed medically and those undergoing PTCA or atherectomy. In this setting, it has been shown to decrease the rate of a combined endpoint of death, new myocardial infarction or refractory ischemia/repeat cardiac procedure.

Local Anesthetic/Vasoconstrictor Precautions No information available to require special precautions

Effects on Dental Treatment No significant effects or complications reported

Common Adverse Effects Bleeding is the major drug-related adverse effect. Patients received background treatment with aspirin and heparin. Major bleeding was reported in 1.4% to 2.2%; minor bleeding in 10.5% to 12%; transfusion was required in 4% to 4.3%.

>1% (nonbleeding adverse events):

Cardiovascular: Bradycardia (4%), coronary artery dissection (5%), edema (2%)

Central nervous system: Dizziness (3%), fever (>1%), headache (>1%), vasovagal reaction (2%)

Gastrointestinal: Nausea (>1%)

Genitourinary: Pelvic pain (6%)

Hematologic: Thrombocytopenia: <90,000/mm^3 (1.5%), <50,000/mm^3 (0.3%)

Neuromuscular & skeletal: Leg pain (3%)

Miscellaneous: Diaphoresis (2%)

Mechanism of Action A reversible antagonist of fibrinogen binding to the GP IIb/IIIa receptor, the major platelet surface receptor involved in platelet aggregation. When administered intravenously, it inhibits *ex vivo* platelet aggregation in a dose- and concentration-dependent manner. When given according to the recommended regimen, >90% inhibition is attained by the end of the 30-minute infusion. Platelet aggregation inhibition is reversible following cessation of the infusion.

Drug Interactions

Increased Effect/Toxicity: Use of tirofiban with aspirin and heparin is associated with an increase in bleeding over aspirin and heparin alone; however, efficacy of tirofiban is improved. Risk of bleeding is increased when used with thrombolytics, oral anticoagulants, NSAIDs, dipyridamole, ticlopidine, and clopidogrel. Avoid concomitant use of other IIb/IIIa antagonists.

Cephalosporins which contain the MTT side chain may theoretically increase the risk of hemorrhage.

Decreased Effect: Levothyroxine and omeprazole decrease tirofiban levels; however, the clinical significance of this interaction remains to be demonstrated.

Pharmacodynamics/Kinetics

Distribution: 35% unbound

Metabolism: Minimally hepatic

Half-life elimination: 2 hours

Excretion: Urine (65%) and feces (25%) primarily as unchanged drug

Clearance: Elderly: Reduced by 19% to 26%

Pregnancy Risk Factor B

Tirofiban Hydrochloride *see* Tirofiban *on page 1304*

Tiseb® [OTC] *see* Salicylic Acid *on page 1205*

Tisit® [OTC] *see* Pyrethrins and Piperonyl Butoxide *on page 1153*

Tisit® Blue Gel [OTC] *see* Pyrethrins and Piperonyl Butoxide *on page 1153*

Tisseel® VH *see* Fibrin Sealant Kit *on page 589*

Titralac ™ [OTC] *see* Calcium Carbonate *on page 245*

Titralac™ Extra Strength [OTC] *see* Calcium Carbonate *on page 245*

Titralac® Plus [OTC] *see* Calcium Carbonate and Simethicone *on page 245*

Tizanidine (tye ZAN i deen)

U.S. Brand Names Zanaflex®

Canadian Brand Names Zanaflex®

Mexican Brand Names Sirdalud®

Generic Available Yes

Synonyms Sirdalud®

Pharmacologic Category Alpha$_2$-Adrenergic Agonist

Use Skeletal muscle relaxant used for treatment of muscle spasticity

Unlabeled/Investigational Use Tension headaches, low back pain, and trigeminal neuralgia

Local Anesthetic/Vasoconstrictor Precautions No information available to require special precautions

Effects on Dental Treatment Key adverse event(s) related to dental treatment: Significant xerostomia (normal salivary flow resumes upon discontinuation).

Common Adverse Effects

>10%:

Cardiovascular: Hypotension

Central nervous system: Sedation, daytime drowsiness, somnolence

Gastrointestinal: Xerostomia

1% to 10%:

Cardiovascular: Bradycardia, syncope

Central nervous system: Fatigue, dizziness, anxiety, nervousness, insomnia

Dermatologic: Pruritus, skin rash

Gastrointestinal: Nausea, vomiting, dyspepsia, constipation, diarrhea

Hepatic: Elevation of liver enzymes

Neuromuscular & skeletal: Muscle weakness, tremor

Dosage

Adults: 2-4 mg 3 times/day

Usual initial dose: 4 mg, may increase by 2-4 mg as needed for satisfactory reduction of muscle tone every 6-8 hours to a maximum of three doses in any 24 hour period

Maximum dose: 36 mg/day

Dosing adjustment in renal/hepatic impairment: May require dose reductions or less frequent dosing

Mechanism of Action An alpha$_2$-adrenergic agonist agent which decreases excitatory input to alpha motor neurons; an imidazole derivative chemically-related to clonidine, which acts as a centrally acting muscle relaxant with alpha$_2$-adrenergic agonist properties; acts on the level of the spinal cord

Contraindications Hypersensitivity to tizanidine or any component of the formulation

Warnings/Precautions Reduce dose in patients with liver or renal disease; use with caution in patients with hypotension or cardiac disease. Tizanidine clearance is reduced by more than 50% in elderly patients with renal insufficiency (Cl_{cr} <25 mL/minute) compared to healthy elderly subjects; this may lead to a longer duration of effects and, therefore, should be used with caution in renally impaired patients.

(Continued)

Tizanidine *(Continued)*

Drug Interactions

Increased Effect/Toxicity:

Increased effect: Oral contraceptives

Increased toxicity: Additive hypotensive effects may be seen with diuretics, other alpha adrenergic agonists, or antihypertensives; CNS depression with alcohol, baclofen or other CNS depressants

Ethanol/Nutrition/Herb Interactions

Ethanol: Avoid ethanol (may increase CNS depression).

Food: Increases maximum concentration of tizanidine by 33% and reduces the time to peak by 40 minutes; extent of absorption is unchanged.

Herb/Nutraceutical: Avoid valerian, St John's wort, kava kava, gotu kola (may increase CNS depression).

Pharmacodynamics/Kinetics

Duration: 3-6 hours

Bioavailability: 40%

Half-life elimination: 2.5 hours

Time to peak, serum: 1-5 hours

Pregnancy Risk Factor C

Dosage Forms TAB: 2 mg, 4 mg

TMP *see* Trimethoprim *on page 1341*

TMP-SMZ *see* Sulfamethoxazole and Trimethoprim *on page 1246*

TMZ *see* Temozolomide *on page 1268*

TNKase™ *see* Tenecteplase *on page 1268*

TOBI® *see* Tobramycin *on page 1306*

TobraDex® *see* Tobramycin and Dexamethasone *on page 1307*

Tobramycin (toe bra MYE sin)

U.S. Brand Names AKTob®; Nebcin®; TOBI®; Tobrex®

Canadian Brand Names Apo-Tobramycin®; Nebcin®; PMS-Tobramycin; TOBI®; Tobrex®; Tomycine™

Mexican Brand Names Tobrox®; Trazil®

Generic Available Yes; Excludes ophthalmic ointment, powder for injection, solution for nebulization

Synonyms Tobramycin Sulfate

Pharmacologic Category Antibiotic, Aminoglycoside; Antibiotic, Ophthalmic

Use Treatment of documented or suspected infections caused by susceptible gram-negative bacilli including *Pseudomonas aeruginosa*; topically used to treat superficial ophthalmic infections caused by susceptible bacteria. Tobramycin solution for inhalation is indicated for the management of cystic fibrosis patients (>6 years of age) with *Pseudomonas aeruginosa*.

Local Anesthetic/Vasoconstrictor Precautions No information available to require special precautions

Effects on Dental Treatment No significant effects or complications reported

Common Adverse Effects

Injection: Frequency not defined:

- Central nervous system: Confusion, disorientation, dizziness, fever, headache, lethargy, vertigo
- Dermatologic: Exfoliative dermatitis, itching, rash, urticaria
- Endocrine & metabolic: Serum calcium, magnesium, potassium, and/or sodium decreased
- Gastrointestinal: Diarrhea, nausea, vomiting
- Hematologic: Anemia, eosinophilia, granulocytopenia, leukocytosis, leukopenia, thrombocytopenia
- Hepatic: ALT, AST, bilirubin, and/or LDH increased
- Local: Pain at the injection site
- Otic: Hearing loss, tinnitus, ototoxicity (auditory), ototoxicity (vestibular), roaring in the ears
- Renal: BUN increased, cylindruria, serum creatinine increased, oliguria, proteinuria

Inhalation:

>10%:

- Gastrointestinal: Sputum discoloration (21%)
- Respiratory: Voice alteration (13%)

1% to 10%:

- Central nervous system: Malaise (6%)
- Otic: Tinnitus (3%)

Mechanism of Action Interferes with bacterial protein synthesis by binding to 30S and 50S ribosomal subunits resulting in a defective bacterial cell membrane

Drug Interactions

Increased Effect/Toxicity: Increased antimicrobial effect of tobramycin with extended spectrum penicillins (synergistic). Neuromuscular blockers may have an increased duration of action (neuromuscular blockade). Amphotericin B, cephalosporins, and loop diuretics may increase the risk of nephrotoxicity.

Pharmacodynamics/Kinetics

Absorption: I.M.: Rapid and complete

Distribution: V_d: 0.2-0.3 L/kg; Pediatrics: 0.2-0.7 L/kg; to extracellular fluid including serum, abscesses, ascitic, pericardial, pleural, synovial, lymphatic, and peritoneal fluids; crosses placenta; poor penetration into CSF, eye, bone, prostate

Protein binding: <30%

Half-life elimination:

Neonates: ≤1200 g: 11 hours; >1200 g: 2-9 hours

Adults: 2-3 hours; directly dependent upon glomerular filtration rate

Adults with impaired renal function: 5-70 hours

Time to peak, serum: I.M.: 30-60 minutes; I.V.: ~30 minutes

Excretion: Normal renal function: Urine (~90% to 95%) within 24 hours

Pregnancy Risk Factor D (injection, inhalation); B (ophthalmic)

Tobramycin and Dexamethasone

(toe bra MYE sin & deks a METH a sone)

Related Information

Dexamethasone *on page 411*

Tobramycin *on page 1306*

U.S. Brand Names TobraDex®

Canadian Brand Names Tobradex®

Generic Available No

Synonyms Dexamethasone and Tobramycin

Pharmacologic Category Antibiotic/Corticosteroid, Ophthalmic

Use Treatment of external ocular infection caused by susceptible gram-negative bacteria and steroid responsive inflammatory conditions of the palpebral and bulbar conjunctiva, lid, cornea, and anterior segment of the globe

Local Anesthetic/Vasoconstrictor Precautions No information available to require special precautions

Effects on Dental Treatment No significant effects or complications reported

Common Adverse Effects Frequency not defined.

Dermatologic: Allergic contact dermatitis, delayed wound healing

Ocular: Lacrimation, itching, edema of eyelid, keratitis, increased intraocular pressure, glaucoma, cataract formation

Mechanism of Action Refer to individual monographs for Dexamethasone and Tobramycin

Drug Interactions

Cytochrome P450 Effect: Dexamethasone: **Substrate** of CYP3A4 (minor); **Induces** CYP2A6 (weak), 2B6 (weak), 2C8/9 (weak), 3A4 (weak)

Increased Effect/Toxicity: See individual agents.

Decreased Effect: See individual agents.

Pharmacodynamics/Kinetics

Absorption: Into aqueous humor

Time to peak, serum: 1-2 hours in the cornea and aqueous humor

Pregnancy Risk Factor B

Tobramycin Sulfate *see* Tobramycin *on page 1306*

Tobrex® *see* Tobramycin *on page 1306*

Tocainide (toe KAY nide)

Related Information

Cardiovascular Diseases *on page 1458*

U.S. Brand Names Tonocard® [DSC]

Canadian Brand Names Tonocard®

Generic Available No

Synonyms Tocainide Hydrochloride

Pharmacologic Category Antiarrhythmic Agent, Class Ib

Use Suppression and prevention of symptomatic life-threatening ventricular arrhythmias

Unlabeled/Investigational Use Trigeminal neuralgia

(Continued)

Tocainide *(Continued)*

Local Anesthetic/Vasoconstrictor Precautions No information available to require special precautions

Effects on Dental Treatment No significant effects or complications reported

Common Adverse Effects

>10%:

Central nervous system: Dizziness (8% to 15%)

Gastrointestinal: Nausea (14% to 15%)

1% to 10%:

Cardiovascular: Tachycardia (3%), bradycardia/angina/palpitations (0.5% to 1.8%), hypotension (3%)

Central nervous system: Nervousness (0.5% to 1.5%), confusion (2% to 3%), headache (4.6%), anxiety, incoordination, giddiness, vertigo

Dermatologic: Rash (0.5% to 8.4%)

Gastrointestinal: Vomiting (4.5%), diarrhea (4% to 5%), anorexia (1% to 2%), loss of taste

Neuromuscular & skeletal: Paresthesia (3.5% to 9%), tremor (dose-related: 2.9% to 8.4%), ataxia (dose-related: 2.9% to 8.4%), hot and cold sensations

Ocular: Blurred vision (~1.5%), nystagmus (1%)

Note: Rare, potentially severe hematologic reactions, have occurred (generally within the first 12 weeks of therapy). These may include agranulocytosis, bone marrow depression, aplastic anemia, hypoplastic anemia, hemolytic anemia, anemia, leukopenia, neutropenia, thrombocytopenia, and eosinophilia.

Mechanism of Action Class 1B antiarrhythmic agent; suppresses automaticity of conduction tissue, by increasing electrical stimulation threshold of ventricle, His-Purkinje system, and spontaneous depolarization of the ventricles during diastole by a direct action on the tissues; blocks both the initiation and conduction of nerve impulses by decreasing the neuronal membrane's permeability to sodium ions, which results in inhibition of depolarization with resultant blockade of conduction

Drug Interactions

Cytochrome P450 Effect: Inhibits CYP1A2 (weak)

Increased Effect/Toxicity: Tocainide may increase serum levels of caffeine and theophylline.

Decreased Effect: Decreased tocainide plasma levels with cimetidine, phenobarbital, phenytoin, rifampin, and other hepatic enzyme inducers.

Pharmacodynamics/Kinetics

Absorption: Oral: 99% to 100%

Distribution: V_d: 1.62-3.2 L/kg

Protein binding: 10% to 20%

Metabolism: Hepatic to inactive metabolites; negligible first-pass effect

Half-life elimination: 11-14 hours; Renal and hepatic impairment: 23-27 hours

Time to peak, serum: 30-160 minutes

Excretion: Urine (40% to 50% as unchanged drug)

Pregnancy Risk Factor C

Tocainide Hydrochloride *see* Tocainide *on page 1307*

Tofranil® *see* Imipramine *on page 737*

Tofranil-PM® *see* Imipramine *on page 737*

TOLAZamide (tole AZ a mide)

Related Information

Endocrine Disorders and Pregnancy *on page 1481*

U.S. Brand Names Tolinase®

Canadian Brand Names Tolinase®

Generic Available Yes

Pharmacologic Category Antidiabetic Agent, Sulfonylurea

Use Adjunct to diet for the management of mild to moderately severe, stable, type 2 diabetes mellitus (noninsulin dependent, NIDDM)

Local Anesthetic/Vasoconstrictor Precautions No information available to require special precautions

Effects on Dental Treatment Use salicylates with caution in patients taking tolazamide due to potential increased hypoglycemia; NSAIDs such as ibuprofen and naproxen may be safely used. Tolazamide-dependent diabetics (noninsulin dependent, type 2) should be appointed for dental treatment in morning in order to minimize chance of stress-induced hypoglycemia.

Common Adverse Effects Frequency not defined.

Central nervous system: Headache, dizziness

Dermatologic: Rash, urticaria, photosensitivity
Endocrine & metabolic: Hypoglycemia, SIADH
Gastrointestinal: Anorexia, nausea, vomiting, diarrhea, constipation, heartburn, epigastric fullness
Hematologic: Aplastic anemia, hemolytic anemia, bone marrow suppression, thrombocytopenia, agranulocytosis
Hepatic: Cholestatic jaundice
Renal: Diuretic effect

Mechanism of Action Stimulates insulin release from the pancreatic beta cells; reduces glucose output from the liver; insulin sensitivity is increased at peripheral target sites

Drug Interactions

Increased Effect/Toxicity: Salicylates, anticoagulants, H_2 antagonists, TCAs, MAO inhibitors, beta-blockers, and thiazides may increase effect of sulfonylureas.

Decreased Effect: Many drugs, including corticosteroids, beta-blockers, and thiazides may alter response to oral hypoglycemics.

Pharmacodynamics/Kinetics

Onset of action: 4-6 hours
Duration: 10-24 hours
Protein binding: >98%
Metabolism: Extensively hepatic to one active and three inactive metabolites
Half-life elimination: 7 hours
Excretion: Urine

Pregnancy Risk Factor D

Tolazoline (tole AZ oh leen)

U.S. Brand Names Priscoline® [DSC]

Generic Available No

Synonyms Benzazoline Hydrochloride; Tolazoline Hydrochloride

Pharmacologic Category Vasodilator

Use Treatment of persistent pulmonary vasoconstriction and hypertension of the newborn (persistent fetal circulation), peripheral vasospastic disorders

Local Anesthetic/Vasoconstrictor Precautions No information available to require special precautions

Effects on Dental Treatment No significant effects or complications reported

Common Adverse Effects Frequency not defined.

Cardiovascular: Hypotension, peripheral vasodilation, tachycardia, hypertension, arrhythmias
Endocrine & metabolic: Hypochloremic alkalosis
Gastrointestinal: GI bleeding, abdominal pain, nausea, diarrhea
Hematologic: Thrombocytopenia, increased agranulocytosis, pancytopenia
Local: Burning at injection site
Neuromuscular & skeletal: Increased pilomotor activity
Ocular: Mydriasis
Renal: Acute renal failure, oliguria
Respiratory: Pulmonary hemorrhage
Miscellaneous: Increased secretions

Mechanism of Action Competitively blocks alpha-adrenergic receptors to produce brief antagonism of circulating epinephrine and norepinephrine; reduces hypertension caused by catecholamines and causes vascular smooth muscle relaxation (direct action); results in peripheral vasodilation and decreased peripheral resistance

Drug Interactions

Increased Effect/Toxicity: Disulfiram reaction may possibly be seen with concomitant ethanol use.

Decreased Effect: Decreased effect (vasopressor) of epinephrine followed by a rebound increase in blood pressure.

Pharmacodynamics/Kinetics

Half-life elimination: Neonates: 3-10 hours; prolonged with renal impairment
Time to peak, serum: Within 30 minutes
Excretion: Urine (primarily as unchanged drug)

Pregnancy Risk Factor C

Tolazoline Hydrochloride *see* Tolazoline *on page 1309*

TOLBUTamide (tole BYOO ta mide)

Related Information

Endocrine Disorders and Pregnancy *on page 1481*

U.S. Brand Names Orinase Diagnostic® [DSC]; Tol-Tab®

Canadian Brand Names Apo-Tolbutamide®

(Continued)

TOLBUTamide *(Continued)*

Mexican Brand Names Diaval®; Rastinon®

Generic Available Yes: Tablet

Synonyms Tolbutamide Sodium

Pharmacologic Category Antidiabetic Agent, Sulfonylurea

Use Adjunct to diet for the management of mild to moderately severe, stable, type 2 diabetes mellitus (noninsulin dependent, NIDDM)

Local Anesthetic/Vasoconstrictor Precautions No information available to require special precautions

Effects on Dental Treatment Use salicylates with caution in patients taking tolazamide due to potential increased hypoglycemia; NSAIDs such as ibuprofen and naproxen may be safely used. Tolbutamide-dependent diabetics (noninsulin dependent, type 2) should be appointed for dental treatment in morning in order to minimize chance of stress-induced hypoglycemia.

Common Adverse Effects Frequency not defined.

Cardiovascular: Venospasm

Central nervous system: Headache, dizziness

Dermatologic: Skin rash, urticaria, photosensitivity

Endocrine & metabolic: Hypoglycemia, SIADH

Gastrointestinal: Constipation, diarrhea, heartburn, anorexia, epigastric fullness, taste alteration

Hematologic: Aplastic anemia, hemolytic anemia, bone marrow suppression, thrombocytopenia, leukopenia, agranulocytosis

Hepatic: Cholestatic jaundice

Local: Thrombophlebitis

Otic: Tinnitus

Miscellaneous: Hypersensitivity reaction, disulfiram-like reactions

Mechanism of Action Stimulates insulin release from the pancreatic beta cells; reduces glucose output from the liver; insulin sensitivity is increased at peripheral target sites, suppression of glucagon may also contribute

Drug Interactions

Cytochrome P450 Effect: Substrate of CYP2C8/9 (major), 2C19 (minor); **Inhibits** CYP2C8/9 (strong)

Increased Effect/Toxicity: A number of drugs increase the effect of first-generation sulfonylureas (tolbutamide) including salicylates, chloramphenicol, anticoagulants, H_2 antagonists, tricyclic antidepressants, MAO inhibitors, beta-blockers, and thiazide diuretics. CYP2C8/9 inhibitors may increase the levels/effects of tolbutamide; example inhibitors include delavirdine, fluconazole, gemfibrozil, ketoconazole, nicardipine, NSAIDs, and sulfonamides.

Decreased Effect: CYP2C8/9 inducers may decrease the levels/effects of tolbutamide; example inducers include carbamazepine, phenobarbital, phenytoin, rifampin, rifapentine, and secobarbital. Drugs with increase glucose (corticosteroids, thiazides) may decrease the effect of tolbutamide.

Pharmacodynamics/Kinetics

Onset of action: Peak effect: Hypoglycemic action: Oral: 1-3 hours; I.V.: 30 minutes

Duration: Oral: 6-24 hours; I.V.: 3 hours

Absorption: Oral: Rapid

Distribution: V_d: 6-10 L; increased with decreased albumin concentrations

Protein binding: 95% to 97%, primarily to albumin

Metabolism: Hepatic to hydroxymethyltolbutamide (mildly active) and carboxytolbutamide (inactive); metabolism does not appear to be affected by age

Half-life elimination: Plasma: 4-25 hours; Elimination: 4-9 hours

Time to peak, serum: 3-5 hours

Excretion: Urine (<2% as unchanged drug, primarily as metabolites)

Pregnancy Risk Factor D

Tolbutamide Sodium *see* TOLBUTamide *on page 1309*

Tolcapone (TOLE ka pone)

U.S. Brand Names Tasmar®

Mexican Brand Names Tasmar®

Generic Available No

Pharmacologic Category Anti-Parkinson's Agent, COMT Inhibitor

Use Adjunct to levodopa and carbidopa for the treatment of signs and symptoms of idiopathic Parkinson's disease

Local Anesthetic/Vasoconstrictor Precautions No information available to require special precautions

Effects on Dental Treatment Dopaminergic therapy in Parkinson's disease (ie, treatment with levodopa) is associated with orthostatic hypotension. Tolcapone enhances levodopa bioavailability and may increase the occurrence of hypotension/syncope in the dental patient. The patient should be carefully assisted from the chair and observed for signs of orthostatic hypotension.

Common Adverse Effects

>10%:

Cardiovascular: Orthostatic hypotension

Central nervous system: Sleep disorder, excessive dreaming, somnolence, headache

Gastrointestinal: Nausea, diarrhea, anorexia

Neuromuscular & skeletal: Dyskinesia, dystonia, muscle cramps

1% to 10%:

Central nervous system: Hallucinations, fatigue, loss of balance, hyperkinesia

Gastrointestinal: Vomiting, constipation, xerostomia, abdominal pain, flatulence, dyspepsia

Genitourinary: Urine discoloration

Neuromuscular & skeletal: Paresthesia, stiffness

Miscellaneous: Diaphoresis (increased)

Mechanism of Action Tolcapone is a selective and reversible inhibitor of catechol-o-methyltransferase (COMT)

Drug Interactions

Cytochrome P450 Effect: Inhibits CYP2C8/9 (weak)

Increased Effect/Toxicity: Tolcapone may increase the effect/levels of methyldopa, dobutamine, apomorphine, and isoproterenol due to inhibition of catechol-O-methyl transferase enzymes (COMT).

Pharmacodynamics/Kinetics

Absorption: Rapid

Protein binding: >99.0%

Metabolism: Glucuronidation

Bioavailability: 65%

Half-life elimination: 2-3 hours

Time to peak: ~2 hours

Excretion: Urine and feces (40%)

Pregnancy Risk Factor C

Tolectin® *see* Tolmetin *on page 1311*

Tolectin® DS *see* Tolmetin *on page 1311*

Tolinase® *see* TOLAZamide *on page 1308*

Tolmetin (TOLE met in)

Related Information

Rheumatoid Arthritis, Osteoarthritis, and Osteoporosis *on page 1490*

Temporomandibular Dysfunction (TMD) *on page 1564*

U.S. Brand Names Tolectin®; Tolectin® DS

Canadian Brand Names Tolectin®

Mexican Brand Names Tolectin®

Generic Available Yes

Synonyms Tolmetin Sodium

Pharmacologic Category Nonsteroidal Anti-inflammatory Drug (NSAID), Oral

Use Treatment of rheumatoid arthritis and osteoarthritis, juvenile rheumatoid arthritis

Local Anesthetic/Vasoconstrictor Precautions No information available to require special precautions

Effects on Dental Treatment NSAID formulations are known to reversibly decrease platelet aggregation via mechanisms different than observed with aspirin. The dentist should be aware of the potential of abnormal coagulation. Caution should also be exercised in the use of NSAIDs in patients already on anticoagulant therapy with drugs such as warfarin (Coumadin®).

Common Adverse Effects 1% to 10%:

Cardiovascular: Chest pain, hypertension, edema

Central nervous system: Headache, dizziness, drowsiness, depression

Dermatologic: Skin irritation

Endocrine & metabolic: Weight gain/loss

Gastrointestinal: Heartburn, abdominal pain, diarrhea, flatulence, vomiting, constipation, gastritis, peptic ulcer, nausea

Genitourinary: Urinary Tract Infection

Hematologic: Elevated BUN, transient decreases in hemoglobin/hematocrit

(Continued)

Tolmetin *(Continued)*

Ocular: Visual disturbances
Otic: Tinnitus

Mechanism of Action Inhibits prostaglandin synthesis by decreasing the activity of the enzyme, cyclooxygenase, which results in decreased formation of prostaglandin precursors

Drug Interactions

Increased Effect/Toxicity: Increased toxicity of digoxin, methotrexate, cyclosporine, lithium, insulin, sulfonylureas, potassium-sparing diuretics, and aspirin.

Decreased Effect: Decreased effect with aspirin. Decreased effect of thiazides and furosemide.

Pharmacodynamics/Kinetics

Onset of action: Analgesic: 1-2 hours; Anti-inflammatory: Days to weeks
Absorption: Well absorbed
Bioavailability: Reduced 16% with food or milk
Half-life elimination: Biphasic: Rapid: 1-2 hours; Slow: 5 hours
Time to peak, serum: 30-60 minutes
Excretion: Urine (as inactive metabolites or conjugates) within 24 hours

Pregnancy Risk Factor C/D (3rd trimester or at term)

Tolmetin Sodium *see* Tolmetin *on page 1311*

Tolnaftate (tole NAF tate)

U.S. Brand Names Absorbine Jr.® Antifungal [OTC]; Aftate® Antifungal [OTC]; Blis-To-Sol® [OTC]; Dermasept Antifungal [OTC]; Fungi-Guard [OTC]; Gold Bond® Antifungal [OTC]; Tinactin® Antifungal [OTC]; Tinactin® Antifungal Jock Itch [OTC]; Tinaderm [OTC]; Ting® [OTC]; TipTapToe [OTC]

Canadian Brand Names Pitrex

Mexican Brand Names Tinaderm®

Generic Available Yes: Cream, powder, solution, swabs

Pharmacologic Category Antifungal Agent, Topical

Use Treatment of tinea pedis, tinea cruris, tinea corporis

Local Anesthetic/Vasoconstrictor Precautions No information available to require special precautions

Effects on Dental Treatment No significant effects or complications reported

Common Adverse Effects Frequency not defined.

Dermatologic: Pruritus, contact dermatitis
Local: Irritation, stinging

Mechanism of Action Distorts the hyphae and stunts mycelial growth in susceptible fungi

Pharmacodynamics/Kinetics Onset of action: 24-72 hours

Pregnancy Risk Factor C

Tol-Tab® *see* TOLBUTamide *on page 1309*

Tolterodine (tole TER oh deen)

U.S. Brand Names Detrol®; Detrol® LA

Canadian Brand Names Detrol®; Unidet®

Mexican Brand Names Detrusitol®

Generic Available No

Synonyms Tolterodine Tartrate

Pharmacologic Category Anticholinergic Agent

Use Treatment of patients with an overactive bladder with symptoms of urinary frequency, urgency, or urge incontinence

Local Anesthetic/Vasoconstrictor Precautions No information available to require special precautions

Effects on Dental Treatment The anticholinergic effects of tolterodine are selective for the urinary bladder rather than salivary glands; xerostomia should not be significant (normal salivary flow resumes upon discontinuation).

Common Adverse Effects As reported with immediate release tablet, unless otherwise specified

>10%: Gastrointestinal: Dry mouth (35%; extended release capsules 23%)

1% to 10%:

Cardiovascular: Chest pain (2%)

Central nervous system: Headache (7%; extended release capsules 6%), somnolence (3%; extended release capsules 3%), fatigue (4%; extended release capsules 2%), dizziness (5%; extended release capsules 2%), anxiety (extended release capsules 1%)

Dermatologic: Dry skin (1%)

Gastrointestinal: Abdominal pain (5%; extended release capsules 4%), constipation (7%; extended release capsules 6%), dyspepsia (4%; extended release capsules 3%), diarrhea (4%), weight gain (1%)

Genitourinary: Dysuria (2%; extended release capsules 1%)

Neuromuscular & skeletal: Arthralgia (2%)

Ocular: Abnormal vision (2%; extended release capsules 1%), dry eyes (3%; extended release capsules 3%)

Respiratory: Bronchitis (2%), sinusitis (extended release capsules 2%)

Dosage

Children: Safety and efficacy in pediatric patients have not been established

Adults: Treatment of overactive bladder: Oral:

Immediate release tablet: 2 mg twice daily; the dose may be lowered to 1 mg twice daily based on individual response and tolerability

Dosing adjustment in patients concurrently taking CYP3A4 inhibitors: 1 mg twice daily

Extended release capsule: 4 mg once a day; dose may be lowered to 2 mg daily based on individual response and tolerability

Dosing adjustment in patients concurrently taking CYP3A4 inhibitors: 2 mg daily

Elderly: Safety and efficacy in patients >64 years was found to be similar to that in younger patients; no dosage adjustment is needed based on age

Dosing adjustment in renal impairment: Use with caution (studies conducted in patients with Cl_{cr} 10-30 mL/minute):

Immediate release tablet: 1 mg twice daily

Extended release capsule: 2 mg daily

Dosing adjustment in hepatic impairment:

Immediate release tablet: 1 mg twice daily

Extended release capsule: 2 mg daily

Mechanism of Action Tolterodine is a competitive antagonist of muscarinic receptors. In animal models, tolterodine demonstrates selectivity for urinary bladder receptors over salivary receptors. Urinary bladder contraction is mediated by muscarinic receptors. Tolterodine increases residual urine volume and decreases detrusor muscle pressure.

Contraindications Hypersensitivity to tolterodine or any component of the formulation; urinary retention; gastric retention; uncontrolled narrow-angle glaucoma; myasthenia gravis

Warnings/Precautions Use with caution in patients with bladder flow obstruction, may increase the risk of urinary retention. Use with caution in patients with gastrointestinal obstructive disorders (ie, pyloric stenosis), may increase the risk of gastric retention. Use with caution in patients with controlled (treated) narrow-angle glaucoma; metabolized in the liver and excreted in the urine and feces, dosage adjustment is required for patients with renal or hepatic impairment. Patients on CYP3A4 inhibitors require lower dose. Safety and efficacy in pediatric patients have not been established.

Drug Interactions

Cytochrome P450 Effect: Substrate of CYP2C8/9 (minor), 2C19 (minor), 2D6 (major), 3A4 (major)

Increased Effect/Toxicity: CYP2D6 inhibitors may increase the levels/effects of tolterodine; example inhibitors include chlorpromazine, delavirdine, fluoxetine, miconazole, paroxetine, pergolide, quinidine, quinine, ritonavir, and ropinirole. No dosage adjustment was needed in patients coadministered tolterodine and fluoxetine. CYP3A4 inhibitors may increase the levels/effects of tolterodine; example inhibitors include azole antifungals, ciprofloxacin, clarithromycin, diclofenac, doxycycline, erythromycin, imatinib, isoniazid, nefazodone, nicardipine, propofol, protease inhibitors, quinidine, and verapamil.

Decreased Effect: CYP3A4 inducers may decrease the levels/effects of tolterodine; example inducers include aminoglutethimide, carbamazepine, nafcillin, nevirapine, phenobarbital, phenytoin, and rifamycins.

Ethanol/Nutrition/Herb Interactions

Food: Increases bioavailability (~53% increase) of tolterodine tablets, but does not affect the pharmacokinetics of tolterodine extended release capsules; adjustment of dose is not needed. As a CYP3A4 inhibitor, grapefruit juice may increase the serum level and/or toxicity of tolterodine, but unlikely secondary to high oral bioavailability.

Herb/Nutraceutical: St John's wort (*Hypericum*) appears to induce CYP3A enzymes.

Pharmacodynamics/Kinetics

Absorption: Immediate release tablet: Rapid

Distribution: I.V.: V_d: 113 ± 27 L

(Continued)

Tolterodine *(Continued)*

Protein binding: Highly bound to alpha$_1$-acid glycoprotein

Metabolism: Extensively hepatic, primarily via CYP2D6 (some metabolites share activity) and 3A4 usually (minor pathway). In patients with a genetic deficiency of CYP2D6, metabolism via 3A4 predominates. Forms three active metabolites.

Bioavailability: Immediate release tablet: 77%; increased with food

Half-life elimination:

Immediate release tablet: Extensive metabolizers: ~2 hours; Poor metabolizers: ~10 hours

Extended release capsule: Extensive metabolizers: ~7 hours; Poor metabolizers: ~18 hours

Time to peak: Immediate release tablet: 1-2 hours; Extended release tablet: 2-6 hours

Excretion: Urine (77% as unchanged drug, 5% to 14% as metabolites, <1% as metabolites in poor metabolizers); feces (17%, <1% as unchanged drug, <2.5% in poor metabolizers)

Pregnancy Risk Factor C

Dosage Forms CAP, extended release (Detrol® LA): 2 mg, 4 mg. **TAB** (Detrol®): 1 mg, 2 mg

Tolterodine Tartrate *see* Tolterodine *on page 1312*

Tolu-Sed® DM [OTC] *see* Guaifenesin and Dextromethorphan *on page 673*

Tomoxetine *see* Atomoxetine *on page 161*

Tonocard® [DSC] *see* Tocainide *on page 1307*

Top 200 Most Prescribed Drugs in 2003 *see page 1642*

Topamax® *see* Topiramate *on page 1314*

Topicaine® [OTC] *see* Lidocaine *on page 819*

Topicort® *see* Desoximetasone *on page 410*

Topicort®-LP *see* Desoximetasone *on page 410*

Topiramate (toe PYRE a mate)

U.S. Brand Names Topamax®

Canadian Brand Names Topamax®

Mexican Brand Names Topamax®

Generic Available No

Pharmacologic Category Anticonvulsant, Miscellaneous

Use In adults and pediatric patients, adjunctive therapy for partial onset seizures and adjunctive therapy of primary generalized tonic-clonic seizures; treatment of seizures associated with Lennox-Gastaut syndrome

Unlabeled/Investigational Use Bipolar disorder, infantile spasms, neuropathic pain, migraine, cluster headache

Local Anesthetic/Vasoconstrictor Precautions No information available to require special precautions

Effects on Dental Treatment Key adverse event(s) related to dental treatment: Gingivitis and xerostomia (normal salivary flow resumes upon discontinuation).

Common Adverse Effects

>10%:

Central nervous system: Dizziness, ataxia, somnolence, psychomotor slowing, nervousness, memory difficulties, speech problems, fatigue

Endocrine & metabolic: Serum bicarbonate decreased (up to 67%; marked reductions to <17 mEq/L have been reported in up to 11% of patients)

Gastrointestinal: Nausea

Neuromuscular & skeletal: Paresthesia, tremor

Ocular: Nystagmus, diplopia, abnormal vision

Respiratory: Upper respiratory infections

1% to 10%:

Cardiovascular: Chest pain, edema

Central nervous system: Language problems, abnormal coordination, confusion, depression, difficulty concentrating, hypoesthesia, hallucination, psychosis, suicide attempt

Endocrine & metabolic: Hot flashes; metabolic acidosis (hyperchloremia, nonanion gap); dehydration

Gastrointestinal: Dyspepsia, abdominal pain, anorexia, constipation, xerostomia, gingivitis, weight loss, diarrhea, vomiting

Genitourinary: Impotence, dysuria

Neuromuscular & skeletal: Myalgia, weakness, back pain, leg pain, rigors, hypertonia, arthralgia

Ocular: Conjunctivitis

Otic: Hearing decreased
Renal: Nephrolithiasis, renal calculus
Respiratory: Pharyngitis, sinusitis, epistaxis
Miscellaneous: Flu-like symptoms

Dosage Oral:

Children 2-16 years: Partial seizures (adjunctive therapy), primary generalized tonic-clonic seizures (adjunctive therapy), or seizure associated with Lennox-Gastaut syndrome: Initial dose titration should begin at 25 mg (or less, based on a range of 1-3 mg/kg/day) nightly for the first week; dosage may be increased in increments of 1-3 mg/kg/day (administered in 2 divided doses) at 1- or 2-week intervals to a total daily dose of 5-9 mg/kg/day.

Adults:

Partial onset seizures (adjunctive therapy), primary generalized tonic-clonic seizures (adjunctive therapy): Initial: 25-50 mg/day; titrate in increments of 25-50 mg per week until an effective daily dose is reached; the daily dose may be increased by 25 mg at weekly intervals for the first 4 weeks; thereafter, the daily dose may be increased by 25-50 mg weekly to an effective daily dose (usually at least 400 mg); usual maximum dose: 1600 mg/day

Note: A more rapid titration schedule has been previously recommended (ie, 50 mg/week), and may be attempted in some clinical situations; however, this may reduce the patient's ability to tolerate topiramate.

Migraine, cluster headache (unlabeled uses): Initial: 25 mg/day, titrated at weekly intervals in 25 mg increments, up to 200 mg/day

Dosing adjustment in renal impairment: Cl_{cr} <70 mL/minute: Administer 50% dose and titrate more slowly

Hemodialysis: Supplemental dose may be needed during hemodialysis

Dosing adjustment in hepatic impairment: Clearance may be reduced

Mechanism of Action Mechanism is not fully understood, it is thought to decrease seizure frequency by blocking sodium channels in neurons, enhancing GABA activity and by blocking glutamate activity

Contraindications Hypersensitivity to topiramate or any component of the formulation

Warnings/Precautions Avoid abrupt withdrawal of topiramate therapy, it should be withdrawn slowly to minimize the potential of increased seizure frequency; the risk of kidney stones is about 2-4 times that of the untreated population, the risk of this event may be reduced by increasing fluid intake. May be associated (rarely) with severe oligohydrosis and hyperthermia, most frequently in children; use caution and monitor closely during strenuous exercise, during exposure to high environmental temperature, or in patients receiving drugs with anticholinergic activity.

Topiramate may decrease serum bicarbonate concentrations, due to inhibition of carbonic anhydrase and increased renal bicarbonate loss. Decreased serum bicarbonate may occur commonly (up to 67% of patients), while treatment-emergent metabolic acidosis is less common. Risk may be increased in patients with a predisposing condition (renal, respiratory and/or hepatic impairment), ketogenic diet, or concurrent treatment with other drugs which may cause acidosis. Serum bicarbonate should be monitored, as well as potential complications of chronic acidosis (nephrolithiasis, osteomalacia, and reduced growth rates in children). Dose reduction or discontinuation (by tapering dose) should be considered in patients with persistent or severe metabolic acidosis. If treatment is continued, alkali supplementation should be considered.

Use cautiously in patients with hepatic or renal impairment and during pregnancy. Has been associated with secondary angle-closure glaucoma in adults and children, typically within 1 month of initiation. Discontinue in patients with acute onset of decreased visual acuity or ocular pain. Safety and efficacy have not been established in children <2 years of age.

Drug Interactions

Cytochrome P450 Effect: Inhibits CYP2C19 (weak); **Induces** CYP3A4 (weak)

Increased Effect/Toxicity: Concomitant administration with other CNS depressants will increase its sedative effects. Coadministration with other carbonic anhydrase inhibitors may increase the chance of nephrolithiasis and/or hyperthermia (includes acetazolamide). Topiramate may increase phenytoin concentration by 25%. Concurrent administration with anticholinergic drugs may increase the risk of oligohydrosis and/or hyperthermia (includes drugs with high anticholinergic activity such as antihistamines, cyclic antidepressants, and antipsychotics); use caution.

Decreased Effect: Phenytoin can decrease topiramate levels by as much as 48%, carbamazepine reduces it by 40%, and valproic acid reduces topiramate by 14%. Digoxin levels and ethinyl estradiol blood levels are decreased

(Continued)

Topiramate *(Continued)*

when coadministered with topiramate. Topiramate may decrease valproic acid concentration by 11%.

Ethanol/Nutrition/Herb Interactions

Ethanol: Avoid ethanol (may increase CNS depression).
Herb/Nutraceutical: Avoid evening primrose (seizure threshold decreased).

Pharmacodynamics/Kinetics

Absorption: Good; unaffected by food
Protein binding: 13% to 17%
Metabolism: Minimally hepatic via hydroxylation, hydrolysis, glucuronidation
Bioavailability: 80%
Half-life elimination: Mean: Adults: 21 hours; shorter in pediatric patients; clearance is 50% higher in pediatric patients
Time to peak, serum: ~2-4 hours
Excretion: Urine (~70% as unchanged drug)
Dialyzable: ~30%

Pregnancy Risk Factor C

Dosage Forms CAP, sprinkle: 15 mg, 25 mg. **TAB:** 25 mg, 100 mg, 200 mg

TOPO *see* Topotecan *on page 1316*
Toposar® *see* Etoposide *on page 567*

Topotecan (toe poe TEE kan)

U.S. Brand Names Hycamtin®

Canadian Brand Names Hycamtin™

Generic Available No

Synonyms Hycamptamine; NSC-609699; SK and F 104864; SKF 104864; SKF 104864-A; TOPO; Topotecan Hydrochloride; TPT

Pharmacologic Category Antineoplastic Agent, Natural Source (Plant) Derivative

Use Treatment of ovarian cancer, small cell lung cancer

Unlabeled/Investigational Use Investigational: Treatment of nonsmall cell lung cancer, sarcoma (pediatrics)

Local Anesthetic/Vasoconstrictor Precautions No information available to require special precautions

Effects on Dental Treatment No significant effects or complications reported

Common Adverse Effects

>10%:

- Central nervous system: Headache, fatigue, fever, pain
- Dermatologic: Alopecia (reversible), rash
- Gastrointestinal: Nausea, vomiting, diarrhea, constipation, abdominal pain, stomatitis, anorexia
- Hematologic: Myelosuppressive: Principle dose-limiting toxicity; white blood cell count nadir is 8-11 days and is more frequent than thrombocytopenia (at lower doses); recover is usually within 21 days and cumulative toxicity has not been noted.
- Neuromuscular & skeletal: Weakness
- Respiratory: Dyspnea (22%), cough

1% to 10%:

- Hepatic: Transient increases in liver enzymes
- Neuromuscular & skeletal: Paresthesia

Mechanism of Action Binds to topoisomerase I and stabilizes the cleavable complex so that religation of the cleaved DNA strand cannot occur. This results in the accumulation of cleavable complexes and single-strand DNA breaks. Topotecan acts in S phase.

Drug Interactions

Increased Effect/Toxicity: Concurrent administration of TPT and G-CSF in clinical trials results in severe myelosuppression. If G-CSF is to be used, manufacturer recommends that it should not be initiated until 24 hours after the completion of treatment with topotecan. Concurrent *in vitro* exposure to TPT and the topoisomerase II inhibitor etoposide results in no altered effect; sequential exposure results in potentiation. Concurrent exposure to TPT and 5-azacytidine results in potentiation both *in vitro* and *in vivo*. Myelosuppression was more severe when given in combination with cisplatin.

Pharmacodynamics/Kinetics

Absorption: Oral: ~30%
Distribution: V_{dss} of the lactone is high (mean: 87.3 L/mm^2; range: 25.6-186 L/mm^2), suggesting wide distribution and/or tissue sequestering
Protein binding: 35%
Metabolism: Undergoes a rapid, pH-dependent opening of the lactone ring to yield a relatively inactive hydroxy acid in plasma

Half-life elimination: 2-3 hours
Excretion: Urine (30%) within 24 hours

Pregnancy Risk Factor D

Topotecan Hydrochloride *see* Topotecan *on page 1316*
Toprol-XL® *see* Metoprolol *on page 915*
Toradol® *see* Ketorolac *on page 787*
Torecan® [DSC] *see* Thiethylperazine *on page 1287*

Toremifene (TORE em i feen)

U.S. Brand Names Fareston®

Canadian Brand Names Fareston®

Mexican Brand Names Fareston®

Generic Available No

Synonyms FC1157a; Toremifene Citrate

Pharmacologic Category Antineoplastic Agent, Estrogen Receptor Antagonist

Use Treatment of advanced breast cancer; management of desmoid tumors and endometrial carcinoma

Local Anesthetic/Vasoconstrictor Precautions No information available to require special precautions

Effects on Dental Treatment No significant effects or complications reported

Common Adverse Effects

>10%:
- Endocrine & metabolic: Vaginal discharge, hot flashes
- Gastrointestinal: Nausea, vomiting
- Miscellaneous: Diaphoresis

1% to 10%:
- Cardiovascular: Thromboembolism: Tamoxifen has been associated with the occurrence of venous thrombosis and pulmonary embolism; arterial thrombosis has also been described in a few case reports; cardiac failure, myocardial infarction, edema
- Central nervous system: Dizziness
- Endocrine & metabolic: Hypercalcemia may occur in patients with bone metastases; galactorrhea and vitamin deficiency, menstrual irregularities
- Genitourinary: Vaginal bleeding or discharge, endometriosis, priapism, possible endometrial cancer
- Ocular: Ophthalmologic effects (visual acuity changes, cataracts, or retinopathy), corneal opacities, dry eyes

Mechanism of Action Nonsteroidal, triphenylethylene derivative. Competitively binds to estrogen receptors on tumors and other tissue targets, producing a nuclear complex that decreases DNA synthesis and inhibits estrogen effects. Nonsteroidal agent with potent antiestrogenic properties which compete with estrogen for binding sites in breast and other tissues; cells accumulate in the G_0 and G_1 phases; therefore, toremifene is cytostatic rather than cytocidal.

Drug Interactions

Cytochrome P450 Effect: Substrate of CYP1A2 (minor), 3A4 (major)

Increased Effect/Toxicity: Concurrent therapy with warfarin results in significant enhancement of anticoagulant effects; has been speculated that a decrease in antitumor effect of tamoxifen may also occur due to alterations in the percentage of active tamoxifen metabolites.

Decreased Effect: CYP3A4 inducers may decrease the levels/effects of toremifene; example inducers include aminoglutethimide, carbamazepine, nafcillin, nevirapine, phenobarbital, phenytoin, and rifamycins.

Pharmacodynamics/Kinetics

Absorption: Well absorbed
Distribution: V_d: 580 L
Protein binding, plasma: >99.5%, primarily to albumin
Metabolism: Extensively hepatic, principally by CYP3A4 to N-demethyltoremifene, which is also antiestrogenic but with weak *in vivo* antitumor potency
Half-life elimination: ~5 days
Time to peak, serum: ~3 hours
Excretion: Primarily feces; urine (10%) during a 1-week period

Pregnancy Risk Factor D

Toremifene Citrate *see* Toremifene *on page 1317*

Torsemide (TORE se mide)

Related Information

Cardiovascular Diseases *on page 1458*

(Continued)

Torsemide *(Continued)*

U.S. Brand Names Demadex®

Generic Available Yes: Tablet

Pharmacologic Category Diuretic, Loop

Use Management of edema associated with congestive heart failure and hepatic or renal disease; used alone or in combination with antihypertensives in treatment of hypertension; I.V. form is indicated when rapid onset is desired

Local Anesthetic/Vasoconstrictor Precautions No information available to require special precautions

Effects on Dental Treatment No significant effects or complications reported

Common Adverse Effects 1% to 10%:

Cardiovascular: Edema (1.1%), EKG abnormality (2%), chest pain (1.2%)

Central nervous system: Headache (7.3%), dizziness (3.2%), insomnia (1.2%), nervousness (1%)

Endocrine & metabolic: Hyperglycemia, hyperuricemia, hypokalemia

Gastrointestinal: Diarrhea (2%), constipation (1.8%), nausea (1.8%), dyspepsia (1.6%), sore throat (1.6%)

Genitourinary: Excessive urination (6.7%)

Neuromuscular & skeletal: Weakness (2%), arthralgia (1.8%), myalgia (1.6%)

Respiratory: Rhinitis (2.8%), cough increase (2%)

Mechanism of Action Inhibits reabsorption of sodium and chloride in the ascending loop of Henle and distal renal tubule, interfering with the chloride-binding cotransport system, thus causing increased excretion of water, sodium, chloride, magnesium, and calcium; does not alter GFR, renal plasma flow, or acid-base balance

Drug Interactions

Cytochrome P450 Effect: Substrate of CYP2C8/9 (major); **Inhibits** CYP2C19 (weak)

Increased Effect/Toxicity: Torsemide-induced hypokalemia may predispose to digoxin toxicity and may increase the risk of arrhythmia with drugs which may prolong QT interval, including type Ia and type III antiarrhythmic agents, cisapride, and some quinolones (sparfloxacin, gatifloxacin, and moxifloxacin). The risk of toxicity from lithium and salicylates (high dose) may be increased by loop diuretics. Hypotensive effects and/or adverse renal effects of ACE inhibitors and NSAIDs are potentiated by bumetanide-induced hypovolemia. The effects of peripheral adrenergic-blocking drugs or ganglionic blockers may be increased by bumetanide.

Torsemide may increase the risk of ototoxicity with other ototoxic agents (aminoglycosides, cis-platinum), especially in patients with renal dysfunction. Synergistic diuretic effects occur with thiazide-type diuretics. Diuretics tend to be synergistic with other antihypertensive agents, and hypotension may occur.

Decreased Effect: Torsemide action may be reduced with probenecid. Diuretic action may be impaired in patients with cirrhosis and ascites if used with salicylates. Glucose tolerance may be decreased when used with sulfonylureas. CYP2C8/9 inducers may decrease the levels/effects of torsemide; example inducers include carbamazepine, phenobarbital, phenytoin, rifampin, rifapentine, and secobarbital. Torsemide efficacy may be decreased with NSAIDs.

Pharmacodynamics/Kinetics

Onset of action: Diuresis: 30-60 minutes

Peak effect: 1-4 hours

Duration: ~6 hours

Absorption: Oral: Rapid

Protein binding, plasma: ~97% to 99%

Metabolism: Hepatic (80%) via CYP

Bioavailability: 80% to 90%

Half-life elimination: 2-4; Cirrhosis: 7-8 hours

Excretion: Urine (20% as unchanged drug)

Pregnancy Risk Factor B

Touro™ Allergy *see* Brompheniramine and Pseudoephedrine *on page 220*

Touro™ CC *see* Guaifenesin, Pseudoephedrine, and Dextromethorphan *on page 676*

Touro® DM *see* Guaifenesin and Dextromethorphan *on page 673*

Touro Ex® [DSC] *see* Guaifenesin *on page 672*

Touro LA® *see* Guaifenesin and Pseudoephedrine *on page 675*

tPA *see* Alteplase *on page 88*

T-Phyl® *see* Theophylline *on page 1285*

TPT *see* Topotecan *on page 1316*

tRA *see* Tretinoin (Oral) *on page 1328*

Trace Metals (trase MET als)

Related Information

Chromium *on page 1420*
Iodine *on page 758*
Selenium *on page 1213*

U.S. Brand Names Iodopen®; Molypen®; M.T.E.-4®; M.T.E.-5®; M.T.E.-6®; M.T.E.-7®; Multitrace™-4; Multitrace™-4 Neonatal; Multitrace™-4 Pediatric; Multitrace™-5; Neotrace-4®; Pedtrace-4®; P.T.E.-4®; P.T.E.-5®; Selepen®

Generic Available Yes

Synonyms Chromium; Copper; Iodine; Manganese; Molybdenum; Neonatal Trace Metals; Selenium; Zinc

Pharmacologic Category Trace Element, Parenteral

Use Prevention and correction of trace metal deficiencies

Local Anesthetic/Vasoconstrictor Precautions No information available to require special precautions

Effects on Dental Treatment No significant effects or complications reported

Pregnancy Risk Factor C

Tracleer® *see* Bosentan *on page 214*

Tramadol (TRA ma dole)

U.S. Brand Names Ultram®

Canadian Brand Names Ultram®

Mexican Brand Names Nobligan®; Prontofort®; Tradol®

Generic Available Yes

Synonyms Tramadol Hydrochloride

Pharmacologic Category Analgesic, Non-narcotic

Dental Use Relief of moderate to moderately-severe dental pain

Use Relief of moderate to moderately-severe pain

Local Anesthetic/Vasoconstrictor Precautions No information available to require special precautions

Effects on Dental Treatment Key adverse event(s) related to dental treatment: Xerostomia and changes in salivation (normal salivary flow resumes upon discontinuation).

Significant Adverse Effects Incidence of some adverse effects may increase over time

>10%:
- Central nervous system: Dizziness, headache, somnolence, vertigo
- Gastrointestinal: Constipation, nausea

1% to 10%:
- Cardiovascular: Vasodilation
- Central nervous system: Agitation, anxiety, confusion, coordination impaired, emotional lability, euphoria, hallucinations, malaise, nervousness, sleep disorder, tremor
- Dermatologic: Pruritus, rash
- Endocrine & metabolic: Menopausal symptoms
- Gastrointestinal: Abdominal pain, anorexia, diarrhea, dry mouth, dyspepsia, flatulence, vomiting
- Genitourinary: Urinary frequency, urinary retention
- Neuromuscular & skeletal: Hypertonia, spasticity, weakness
- Ocular: Miosis, visual disturbance
- Miscellaneous: Diaphoresis

<1% (Limited to important or life-threatening): Allergic reaction, amnesia, anaphylaxis, angioedema, bronchospasm, cognitive dysfunction, creatinine increased, death, depression, dyspnea, gastrointestinal bleeding, liver failure, seizure, serotonin syndrome, Stevens-Johnson syndrome, suicidal tendency, syncope, toxic epidermal necrolysis, vesicles

A withdrawal syndrome may occur with abrupt discontinuation; includes anxiety, diarrhea, hallucinations (rare), nausea, pain, piloerection, rigors, sweating, and tremors. Uncommon discontinuation symptoms may include severe anxiety, panic attacks, or paresthesia.

Dosage Oral:

Adults: Moderate to severe chronic pain: 50-100 mg every 4-6 hours, not to exceed 400 mg/day

For patients not requiring rapid onset of effect, tolerability may be improved by starting dose at 25 mg/day and titrating dose by 25 mg every 3 days, until reaching 25 mg 4 times/day. Dose may then be increased by 50 mg every 3 days as tolerated, to reach dose of 50 mg 4 times/day.

(Continued)

Tramadol *(Continued)*

Elderly: >75 years: 50-100 mg every 4-6 hours (not to exceed 300 mg/day); see dosing adjustments for renal and hepatic impairment

Dosing adjustment in renal impairment: Cl_{cr} <30 mL/minute: Administer 50-100 mg dose every 12 hours (maximum: 200 mg/day)

Dosing adjustment in hepatic impairment: Cirrhosis: Recommended dose: 50 mg every 12 hours

Mechanism of Action Binds to μ-opiate receptors in the CNS causing inhibition of ascending pain pathways, altering the perception of and response to pain; also inhibits the reuptake of norepinephrine and serotonin, which also modifies the ascending pain pathway

Contraindications Hypersensitivity to tramadol, opioids, or any component of the formulation; opioid-dependent patients; acute intoxication with alcohol, hypnotics, centrally-acting analgesics, opioids, or psychotropic drugs

Warnings/Precautions Should be used only with extreme caution in patients receiving MAO inhibitors. May cause CNS depression and/or respiratory depression, particularly when combined with other CNS depressants. Use with caution and reduce dosage when administered to patients receiving other CNS depressants. An increased risk of seizures may occur in patients receiving serotonin reuptake inhibitors (SSRIs or anorectics), tricyclic antidepressants, other cyclic compounds (including cyclobenzaprine, promethazine), neuroleptics, MAO inhibitors, or drugs which may lower seizure threshold. Patients with a history of seizures, or with a risk of seizures (head trauma, metabolic disorders, CNS infection, or malignancy, or during ethanol/drug withdrawal) are also at increased risk.

Elderly patients and patients with chronic respiratory disorders may be at greater risk of adverse events. Use with caution in patients with increased intracranial pressure or head injury. Use tramadol with caution and reduce dosage in patients with liver disease or renal dysfunction and in patients with myxedema, hypothyroidism, or hypoadrenalism. Not recommended during pregnancy or in nursing mothers. Tolerance or drug dependence may result from extended use (withdrawal symptoms have been reported); abrupt discontinuation should be avoided. Tapering of dose at the time of discontinuation limits the risk of withdrawal symptoms. Safety and efficacy in pediatric patients have not been established.

Drug Interactions Substrate of CYP2D6 (major), 3A4 (minor)

Amphetamines: May increase the risk of seizures with tramadol.

Carbamazepine: Decreases half-life of tramadol by 33% to 50%.

CYP2D6 inhibitors: May decrease the effects of tramadol. Example inhibitors include chlorpromazine, delavirdine, fluoxetine, miconazole, paroxetine, pergolide, quinidine, quinine, ritonavir, and ropinirole.

Digoxin: Rare reports of digoxin toxicity with concomitant tramadol use.

Linezolid: May be associated with increased risk of seizures (due to MAO inhibition)

MAO inhibitors: May increases the risk of seizures.

Naloxone: May increase the risk of seizures (if administered in tramadol overdose)

Neuroleptic agents: May increase the risk of tramadol-associated seizures and may have additive CNS depressant effects.

Opioids: May increase the risk of seizures, and may have additive CNS depressant effects.

Quinidine: May increase the tramadol serum concentrations.

Selegiline: An increased risk of seizures has been associated with MAO inhibitors. It is not clear if drugs with selective MAO type B inhibition are safer than nonselective agents.

SSRIs: May increase the risk of seizures with tramadol. Includes citalopram, fluoxetine, paroxetine, sertraline.

Tricyclic antidepressants: May increase the risk of seizures.

Warfarin: Concomitant use may lead to an elevation of prothrombin times; monitor.

Ethanol/Nutrition/Herb Interactions

Ethanol: Avoid ethanol (may increase CNS depression).

Food: Does not affect the rate or extent of absorption.

Herb/Nutraceutical: Avoid valerian, St John's wort, kava kava, gotu kola (may increase CNS depression).

Dietary Considerations May be taken with or without food.

Pharmacodynamics/Kinetics

Onset of action: ~1 hour

Duration of action: 9 hours

Absorption: Rapid and complete

Distribution: V_d: 2.5-3 L/kg

Protein binding, plasma: 20%

Metabolism: Extensively hepatic via demethylation, glucuronidation, and sulfation; has pharmacologically active metabolite formed by CYP2D6

Bioavailability: 75%

Half-life elimination: Tramadol: ~6 hours; Active metabolite: 7 hours; prolonged in elderly, hepatic or renal impairment

Time to peak: 2 hours

Excretion: Urine (as metabolites)

Pregnancy Risk Factor C

Lactation Enters breast milk/contraindicated

Breast-Feeding Considerations Not recommended for postdelivery analgesia in nursing mothers.

Dosage Forms Tablet, as hydrochloride: 50 mg

Comments Literature reports suggest that the efficacy of tramadol in oral surgery pain is equivalent to the combination of aspirin and codeine. One study (Olson et al 1990) showed acetaminophen and dextropropoxyphene combination to be superior to tramadol and another study showed tramadol to be superior to acetaminophen and dextropropoxyphene combination. Tramadol appears to be at least equal to if not better than codeine alone. Seizures have been reported with the use of tramadol.

Selected Readings

Collins M, Young I, Sweeney P, et al, "The Effect of Tramadol on Dento-Alveolar Surgical Pain," *Br J Oral Maxillofac Surg*, 1997, 35(1):54-8.

Doroschak AM, Bowles WR, and Hargreaves KM, "Evaluation of the Combination of Flurbiprofen and Tramadol for Management of Endodontic Pain," *J Endod*, 1999, 25(10):660-3.

Kahn LH, Alderfer RJ, and Graham DJ, "Seizures Reported With Tramadol," *JAMA*, 1997, 278(20):1661.

Lewis KS and Han NH, "Tramadol: A New Centrally Acting Analgesic," *Am J Health Syst Pharm*, 1997, 54(6):643-52.

Moore PA, "Pain Management in Dental Practice: Tramadol vs. Codeine Combinations," *J Am Dent Assoc*, 1999, 130(7):1075-9.

Moore PA, Crout RJ, Jackson DL, et al, "Tramadol Hydrochloride: Analgesic Efficacy Compared With Codeine, Aspirin With Codeine, and Placebo After Dental Extraction," *J Clin Pharmacol*, 1998, 38(6):554-60.

Roelofse JA and Payne KA, "Oral Tramadol: Analgesic Efficacy in Children Following Multiple Dental Extractions," *Eur J Anaesthesiol*, 1999, 16(7):441-7.

Sunshine A, "New Clinical Experience With Tramadol," *Drugs*, 1994, 47(Suppl 1):8-18.

Sunshine A, Olson NZ, Zighelboim I, et al, "Analgesic Oral Efficacy of Tramadol Hydrochloride in Postoperative Pain," *Clin Pharmacol Ther*, 1992; 51(6):740-6.

Wynn RL, "Tramadol (Ultram) - A New Kind of Analgesic," *Gen Dent*, 1996, 44(3):216-8,220.

Tramadol Hydrochloride *see* Tramadol *on page 1319*

Tramadol Hydrochloride and Acetaminophen *see* Acetaminophen and Tramadol *on page 54*

Trandate® *see* Labetalol *on page 791*

Trandolapril (tran DOE la pril)

Related Information

Cardiovascular Diseases *on page 1458*

U.S. Brand Names Mavik®

Canadian Brand Names Mavik™

Mexican Brand Names Gopten®

Generic Available No

Pharmacologic Category Angiotensin-Converting Enzyme (ACE) Inhibitor

Use Management of hypertension alone or in combination with other antihypertensive agents; treatment of left ventricular dysfunction after myocardial infarction

Unlabeled/Investigational Use As a class, ACE inhibitors are recommended in the treatment of systolic congestive heart failure

Local Anesthetic/Vasoconstrictor Precautions No information available to require special precautions

Effects on Dental Treatment No significant effects or complications reported

Common Adverse Effects Note: Frequency ranges include data from hypertension and heart failure trials. Higher rates of adverse reactions have generally been noted in patients with CHF. However, the frequency of adverse effects associated with placebo is also increased in this population.

>1%:

Cardiovascular: Hypotension (<1% to 11%), bradycardia (<1% to 4.7%), intermittent claudication (3.8%), stroke (3.3%)

Central nervous system: Dizziness (1.3% to 23%), syncope (5.9%), asthenia (3.3%)

Endocrine & metabolic: Elevated uric acid (15%), hyperkalemia (5.3%), hypocalcemia (4.7%)

(Continued)

Trandolapril *(Continued)*

Gastrointestinal: Dyspepsia (6.4%), gastritis (4.2%)
Neuromuscular & skeletal: Myalgia (4.7%)
Renal: Elevated BUN (9%), elevated serum creatinine (1.1% to 4.7%) Respiratory: Cough (1.9% to 35%)

Mechanism of Action Trandolapril is an ACE inhibitor which prevents the formation of angiotensin II from angiotensin I. Trandolapril must undergo enzymatic hydrolysis, mainly in liver, to its biologically active metabolite, trandolaprilat. A CNS mechanism may also be involved in the hypotensive effect as angiotensin II increases adrenergic outflow from the CNS. Vasoactive kallikrein's may be decreased in conversion to active hormones by ACE inhibitors, thus, reducing blood pressure.

Drug Interactions

Increased Effect/Toxicity: Potassium supplements, co-trimoxazole (high dose), angiotensin II receptor antagonists (eg, candesartan, losartan, irbesartan), or potassium-sparing diuretics (amiloride, spironolactone, triamterene) may result in elevated serum potassium levels when combined with trandolapril. ACE inhibitor effects may be increased by phenothiazines or probenecid (increases levels of captopril). ACE inhibitors may increase serum concentrations/effects of digoxin, lithium, and sulfonlyureas.

Diuretics have additive hypotensive effects with ACE inhibitors, and hypovolemia increases the potential for adverse renal effects of ACE inhibitors. In patients with compromised renal function, coadministration with NSAIDs may result in further deterioration of renal function. Allopurinol and ACE inhibitors may cause a higher risk of hypersensitivity reaction when taken concurrently.

Decreased Effect: Aspirin (high dose) may reduce the therapeutic effects of ACE inhibitors; at low dosages this does not appear to be significant. Rifampin may decrease the effect of ACE inhibitors. Antacids may decrease the bioavailability of ACE inhibitors (may be more likely to occur with captopril); separate administration times by 1-2 hours. NSAIDs, specifically indomethacin, may reduce the hypotensive effects of ACE inhibitors. More likely to occur in low renin or volume dependent hypertensive patients.

Pharmacodynamics/Kinetics

Onset of action: 1-2 hours
Peak effect: Reduction in blood pressure: 6 hours
Duration: Prolonged; 72 hours after single dose
Absorption: Rapid
Distribution: Trandolaprilat (active metabolite) is very lipophilic in comparison to other ACE inhibitors
Protein binding: 80%
Metabolism: Hepatically hydrolyzed to active metabolite, trandolaprilat
Half-life elimination:
Trandolapril: 6 hours; Trandolaprilat: Effective: 10 hours, Terminal: 24 hours
Elimination: As metabolites in urine;
Time to peak: Parent: 1 hour; Active metabolite trandolaprilat: 4-10 hours
Excretion: Urine (as metabolites)
Clearance: Reduce dose in renal failure; creatinine clearances ≤30 mL/minute result in accumulation of active metabolite

Pregnancy Risk Factor C/D (2nd and 3rd trimesters)

Trandolapril and Verapamil (tran DOE la pril & ver AP a mil)

Related Information

Trandolapril *on page 1321*
Verapamil *on page 1373*

U.S. Brand Names Tarka®

Canadian Brand Names Tarka®

Generic Available No

Synonyms Verapamil and Trandolapril

Pharmacologic Category Antihypertensive Agent, Combination

Use Combination drug for the treatment of hypertension, however, not indicated for initial treatment of hypertension; replacement therapy in patients receiving separate dosage forms (for patient convenience); when monotherapy with one component fails to achieve desired antihypertensive effect, or when dose-limiting adverse effects limit upward titration of monotherapy

Local Anesthetic/Vasoconstrictor Precautions No information available to require special precautions

Effects on Dental Treatment No significant effects or complications reported

Common Adverse Effects See individual agents.

Drug Interactions

Cytochrome P450 Effect: Verapamil: **Substrate** of CYP1A2 (major), 2B6 (minor), 2C8/9 (minor), 2C19 (minor), 2E1 (minor), 3A4 (major); **Inhibits** CYP1A2 (weak), 2C8/9 (weak), 2D6 (weak), 3A4 (moderate)

Pharmacodynamics/Kinetics See individual agents.

Pregnancy Risk Factor C/D (2nd and 3rd trimesters)

Tranexamic Acid (tran eks AM ik AS id)

U.S. Brand Names Cyklokapron®

Canadian Brand Names Cyklokapron®

Generic Available No

Pharmacologic Category Antihemophilic Agent

Use Short-term use (2-8 days) in hemophilia patients during and following tooth extraction to reduce or prevent hemorrhage

Unlabeled/Investigational Use Has been used as an alternative to aminocaproic acid for subarachnoid hemorrhage

Local Anesthetic/Vasoconstrictor Precautions No information available to require special precautions

Effects on Dental Treatment No significant effects or complications reported

Common Adverse Effects

>10%: Gastrointestinal: Nausea, diarrhea, vomiting

1% to 10%:

Cardiovascular: Hypotension, thrombosis

Ocular: Blurred vision

Mechanism of Action Forms a reversible complex that displaces plasminogen from fibrin resulting in inhibition of fibrinolysis; it also inhibits the proteolytic activity of plasmin

Drug Interactions

Increased Effect/Toxicity: Chlorpromazine may increase cerebral vasospasm and ischemia. Coadministrations of Factor IX complex or anti-inhibitor coagulant concentrates may increase risk of thrombosis.

Pharmacodynamics/Kinetics

Half-life elimination: 2-10 hours

Excretion: Urine (>90% as unchanged drug)

Pregnancy Risk Factor B

Comments Antifibrinolytic drugs are useful for the control of bleeding after dental extractions in patients with hemophilia because the oral mucosa and saliva are rich in plasminogen activators. In a clinical trial, tranexamic acid reduced recurrent bleeding and the amount of clotting-factor-replacement therapy needed. In adults, the oral dose was 20-25 mg/kg tranexamic acid every 8 hours until the dental sockets were completely healed. Mouthwashes containing tranexamic acid are effective for preventing oral bleeding in patients with hemophilia and in patients requiring dental extraction while receiving long-term oral anticoagulant therapy.

Immediately before dental extraction in hemophilic patients, administer 10 mg/kg tranexamic acid I.V. together with replacement therapy. Following surgery, a dose of 25 mg/kg may be given orally 3-4 times/day for 2-8 days.

Transamine Sulphate *see* Tranylcypromine *on page 1323*

Transderm Scōp® *see* Scopolamine *on page 1210*

***trans*-Retinoic Acid** *see* Tretinoin (Oral) *on page 1328*

***trans*-Retinoic Acid** *see* Tretinoin (Topical) *on page 1329*

Trans-Ver-Sal® [OTC] *see* Salicylic Acid *on page 1205*

Tranxene® *see* Clorazepate *on page 362*

Tranxene® SD™ *see* Clorazepate *on page 362*

Tranxene® SD™-Half Strength *see* Clorazepate *on page 362*

Tranxene T-Tab® *see* Clorazepate *on page 362*

Tranylcypromine (tran il SIP roe meen)

U.S. Brand Names Parnate®

Canadian Brand Names Parnate®

Generic Available No

Synonyms Transamine Sulphate; Tranylcypromine Sulfate

Pharmacologic Category Antidepressant, Monoamine Oxidase Inhibitor

Use Treatment of major depressive episode without melancholia

Unlabeled/Investigational Use Post-traumatic stress disorder

Local Anesthetic/Vasoconstrictor Precautions Attempts should be made to avoid use of vasoconstrictor due to possibility of hypertensive episodes with monoamine oxidase inhibitors

(Continued)

Tranylcypromine *(Continued)*

Effects on Dental Treatment Key adverse event(s) related to dental treatment: Orthostatic hypotension. Avoid use as an analgesic due to toxic reactions with MAO inhibitors.

Common Adverse Effects Frequency not defined.

Cardiovascular: Orthostatic hypotension, edema

Central nervous system: Dizziness, headache, drowsiness, sleep disturbances, fatigue, hyper-reflexia, twitching, ataxia, mania, akinesia, confusion, disorientation, memory loss

Dermatologic: Rash, pruritus, urticaria, localized scleroderma, cystic acne (flare), alopecia

Endocrine & metabolic: Sexual dysfunction (anorgasmia, ejaculatory disturbances, impotence), hypernatremia, hypermetabolic syndrome, SIADH

Gastrointestinal: Xerostomia, constipation, weight gain

Genitourinary: Urinary retention, incontinence

Hematologic: Leukopenia, agranulocytosis

Hepatic: Hepatitis

Neuromuscular & skeletal: Weakness, tremor, myoclonus

Ocular: Blurred vision, glaucoma

Miscellaneous: Diaphoresis

Mechanism of Action Thought to act by increasing endogenous concentrations of epinephrine, norepinephrine, dopamine and serotonin through inhibition of the enzyme (monoamine oxidase) responsible for the breakdown of these neurotransmitters

Drug Interactions

Cytochrome P450 Effect: Inhibits CYP1A2 (moderate), 2A6 (strong), 2C8/9 (weak), 2C19 (moderate), 2D6 (moderate), 2E1 (weak), 3A4 (weak)

Increased Effect/Toxicity: In general, the combined use of tranylcypromine with TCAs, venlafaxine, trazodone, dexfenfluramine, sibutramine, lithium, meperidine, fenfluramine, dextromethorphan, and SSRIs should be avoided due to the potential for severe adverse reactions (serotonin syndrome, death). Tranylcypromine in combination with amphetamines, other stimulants (methylphenidate), levodopa, metaraminol, buspirone, bupropion, reserpine, and decongestants (pseudoephedrine) may result in severe hypertensive reactions. MAO inhibitors (including tranylcypromine) may inhibit the metabolism of barbiturates and prolong their effect. Foods (eg, cheese) and beverages (eg, ethanol) containing tyramine should be avoided; hypertensive crisis may result.

Tranylcypromine may increase the levels/effects of aminophylline, amphetamines, selected beta-blockers, citalopram, dexmedetomidine, dextromethorphan, diazepam, fluvoxamine, ifosfamide, lidocaine, mesoridazine, mexiletine, methsuximide, mirtazapine, nefazodone, paroxetine, phenytoin, propranolol, risperidone, ritonavir, ropinirole, sertraline, theophylline, thioridazine, tricyclic antidepressants, trifluoperazine, venlafaxine, and other substrates of CYP1A2, 2A6, 2C19, or 2D6.

Tranylcypromine may increase the pressor response of norepinephrine and may prolong neuromuscular blockade produced by succinylcholine. Tramadol may increase the risk of seizures and serotonin syndrome in patients receiving an MAO inhibitor. Tranylcypromine may produce additive hypoglycemic effect in patients receiving hypoglycemic agents and may produce delirium in patients receiving disulfiram. Tryptophan combined use with an MAO inhibitor has been reported to cause disorientation, confusion, anxiety, delirium, agitation, hypomanic signs, ataxia, and myoclonus; concurrent use is contraindicated.

Decreased Effect: Tranylcypromine inhibits the antihypertensive response to guanadrel or guanethidine. Tranylcypromine may decrease the levels/effects of CYP2D6 prodrug substrates (eg, codeine, hydrocodone, oxycodone, tramadol).

Pharmacodynamics/Kinetics

Onset of action: Therapeutic: 2-3 weeks continued dosing

Half-life elimination: 90-190 minutes

Time to peak, serum: ~2 hours

Excretion: Urine

Pregnancy Risk Factor C

Tranylcypromine Sulfate *see* Tranylcypromine *on page 1323*

Trastuzumab (tras TU zoo mab)

U.S. Brand Names Herceptin®

Canadian Brand Names Herceptin®

Generic Available No

Pharmacologic Category Monoclonal Antibody

Use

Single agent for the treatment of patients with metastatic breast cancer whose tumors overexpress the HER-2/*neu* protein and who have received one or more chemotherapy regimens for their metastatic disease

Combination therapy with paclitaxel for the treatment of patients with metastatic breast cancer whose tumors overexpress the HER-2/*neu* protein and who have not received chemotherapy for their metastatic disease

Unlabeled/Investigational Use Treatment of ovarian, gastric, colorectal, endometrial, lung, bladder, prostate, and salivary gland tumors

Local Anesthetic/Vasoconstrictor Precautions No information available to require special precautions

Effects on Dental Treatment No significant effects or complications reported

Common Adverse Effects Note: The most common adverse effects are infusion-related, occurring in up to 40% of patients, consisting of fever and chills (mild to moderate, often with other systemic symptoms). Treatment with acetaminophen, diphenhydramine, and/or meperidine is usually effective.

>10%:

- Central nervous system: Pain (47%), fever (36%), chills (32%), headache (26%)
- Dermatologic: Rash (18%)
- Gastrointestinal: Nausea (33%), diarrhea (25%), vomiting (23%), abdominal pain (22%), anorexia (14%)
- Neuromuscular & skeletal: Weakness (42%), back pain (22%)
- Respiratory: Cough (26%), dyspnea (22%), rhinitis (14%), pharyngitis (12%)
- Miscellaneous: Infection (20%); infusion reaction (40%, chills and fever most common)

1% to 10%:

- Cardiovascular: Peripheral edema (10%), CHF (7%), tachycardia (5%)
- Central nervous system: Insomnia (14%), dizziness (13%), paresthesia (9%), depression (6%), peripheral neuritis (2%), neuropathy (1%)
- Dermatologic: Herpes simplex (2%), acne (2%)
- Genitourinary: Urinary tract infection (5%)
- Hematologic: Anemia (4%), leukopenia (3%)
- Neuromuscular & skeletal: Bone pain (7%), arthralgia (6%)
- Respiratory: Sinusitis (9%)
- Miscellaneous: Flu syndrome (10%), accidental injury (6%), allergic reaction (3%)

Mechanism of Action Trastuzumab is a monoclonal antibody which binds to the extracellular domain of the human epidermal growth factor receptor 2 protein (HER2); it mediates antibody-dependent cellular cytotoxicity against cells which overproduce HER2

Drug Interactions

Increased Effect/Toxicity: Paclitaxel may result in a decrease in clearance of trastuzumab, increasing serum concentrations. Combined use with anthracyclines or cyclophosphamide may increase the incidence/severity of cardiac dysfunction. Trastuzumab may increase the incidence of neutropenia and/or febrile neutropenia when used in combination with myelosuppressive chemotherapy.

Pharmacodynamics/Kinetics

Distribution: V_d: 44 mL/kg

Half-life elimination: Mean: 5.8 days (range: 1-32 days)

Pregnancy Risk Factor B

Trasylol® *see* Aprotinin *on page 139*

Travatan® *see* Travoprost *on page 1325*

Travoprost (TRA voe prost)

U.S. Brand Names Travatan®

Canadian Brand Names Travatan®

Mexican Brand Names Travatan®

Generic Available No

Pharmacologic Category Prostaglandin, Ophthalmic

Use Reduction of elevated intraocular pressure in patients with open-angle glaucoma or ocular hypertension who are intolerant of the other IOP-lowering medications or insufficiently responsive (failed to achieve target IOP determined after multiple measurements over time) to another IOP-lowering medication

Local Anesthetic/Vasoconstrictor Precautions No information available to require special precautions

(Continued)

Travoprost *(Continued)*

Effects on Dental Treatment No significant effects or complications reported

Mechanism of Action A selective FP prostanoid receptor agonist which lowers intraocular pressure by increasing outflow

Pregnancy Risk Factor C

Trazodone (TRAZ oh done)

U.S. Brand Names Desyrel®

Canadian Brand Names Alti-Trazodone; Apo-Trazodone®; Apo-Trazodone D®; Desyrel®; Gen-Trazodone; Novo-Trazodone; Nu-Trazodone; PMS-Trazodone

Generic Available Yes

Synonyms Trazodone Hydrochloride

Pharmacologic Category Antidepressant, Serotonin Reuptake Inhibitor/Antagonist

Use Treatment of depression

Unlabeled/Investigational Use Potential augmenting agent for antidepressants, hypnotic

Local Anesthetic/Vasoconstrictor Precautions No information available to require special precautions

Effects on Dental Treatment Key adverse event(s) related to dental treatment: Xerostomia (especially in the elderly; may contribute to periodontal diseases and oral discomfort; normal salivary flow resumes upon discontinuation). Trazodone elicits anticholinergic effects; much less frequent than with tricyclic antidepressants.

Common Adverse Effects

>10%:

Central nervous system: Dizziness, headache, sedation

Gastrointestinal: Nausea, xerostomia

Ocular: Blurred vision

1% to 10%:

Cardiovascular: Syncope, hypertension, hypotension, edema

Central nervous system: Confusion, decreased concentration, fatigue, incoordination

Gastrointestinal: Diarrhea, constipation, weight gain/loss

Neuromuscular & skeletal: Tremor, myalgia

Respiratory: Nasal congestion

Dosage Oral: Therapeutic effects may take up to 6 weeks to occur; therapy is normally maintained for 6-12 months after optimum response is reached to prevent recurrence of depression

Children 6-12 years: Depression: Initial: 1.5-2 mg/kg/day in divided doses; increase gradually every 3-4 days as needed; maximum: 6 mg/kg/day in 3 divided doses

Adolescents: Depression: Initial: 25-50 mg/day; increase to 100-150 mg/day in divided doses

Adults:

Depression: Initial: 150 mg/day in 3 divided doses (may increase by 50 mg/day every 3-7 days); maximum: 600 mg/day

Sedation/hypnotic (unlabeled use): 25-50 mg at bedtime (often in combination with daytime SSRIs); may increase up to 200 mg at bedtime

Elderly: 25-50 mg at bedtime with 25-50 mg/day dose increase every 3 days for inpatients and weekly for outpatients, if tolerated; usual dose: 75-150 mg/day

Mechanism of Action Inhibits reuptake of serotonin, causes adrenoreceptor subsensitivity, and induces significant changes in 5-HT presynaptic receptor adrenoreceptors. Trazodone also significantly blocks histamine (H_1) and alpha$_1$-adrenergic receptors.

Contraindications Hypersensitivity to trazodone or any component of the formulation

Warnings/Precautions Safety and efficacy in children <18 years of age have not been established; monitor closely and use with extreme caution in patients with cardiac disease or arrhythmias. Very sedating, but little anticholinergic effects; therapeutic effects may take up to 4 weeks to occur; therapy is normally maintained for several months after optimum response is reached to prevent recurrence of depression. The possibility of a suicide attempt is inherent in major depression and may persist until remission occurs. Use caution in high-risk patients during initiation of therapy. Prescriptions should be written for the smallest quantity consistent with good patient care.

Drug Interactions

Cytochrome P450 Effect: Substrate of CYP2D6 (minor), 3A4 (major); **Inhibits** CYP2D6 (moderate), 3A4 (weak)

Increased Effect/Toxicity: Trazodone, in combination with other serotonergic agents (buspirone, MAO inhibitors), may produce additive serotonergic effects, including serotonin syndrome. Trazodone, in combination with other psychotropics (low potency antipsychotics), may result in additional hypotension. Fluoxetine may inhibit the metabolism of trazodone resulting in elevated plasma levels.

Trazodone may increase the levels/effects of amphetamines, beta-blockers, dextromethorphan, fluoxetine, lidocaine, mirtazapine, nefazodone, paroxetine, risperidone, ritonavir, thioridazine, tricyclic antidepressants, venlafaxine, and other CYP2D6 substrates. The levels/effects of trazodone may be increased by azole antifungals, ciprofloxacin, clarithromycin, diclofenac, doxycycline, erythromycin, imatinib, isoniazid, nefazodone, nicardipine, propofol, protease inhibitors, quinidine, telithromycin, verapamil, and other CYP3A4 inhibitors.

Decreased Effect: Trazodone inhibits the hypotensive response to clonidine. The levels/effects of trazodone may be decreased by aminoglutethimide, carbamazepine, nafcillin, nevirapine, phenobarbital, phenytoin, rifamycins, and other CYP3A4 inducers. Trazodone may decrease the levels/effects of CYP2D6 prodrug substrates (eg, codeine, hydrocodone, oxycodone, tramadol).

Ethanol/Nutrition/Herb Interactions

Ethanol: Avoid ethanol (may increase CNS depression).

Food: Time to peak serum levels may be increased if trazodone is taken with food.

Herb/Nutraceutical: Avoid valerian, St John's wort, SAMe, kava kava (may increase risk of serotonin syndrome and/or excessive sedation).

Pharmacodynamics/Kinetics

Onset of action: Therapeutic (antidepressant): 1-3 weeks; sleep aid: 1-3 hours

Protein binding: 85% to 95%

Metabolism: Hepatic via CYP3A4 to an active metabolite (mCPP)

Half-life elimination: 7-8 hours, two compartment kinetics

Time to peak, serum: 30-100 minutes; delayed with food (up to 2.5 hours)

Excretion: Primarily urine; secondarily feces

Pregnancy Risk Factor C

Dosage Forms TAB: 50 mg, 100 mg, 150 mg, 300 mg

Trazodone Hydrochloride *see* Trazodone *on page 1326*

Trecator®-SC *see* Ethionamide *on page 560*

Trelstar™ Depot *see* Triptorelin *on page 1346*

Trelstar™ LA *see* Triptorelin *on page 1346*

Trental® *see* Pentoxifylline *on page 1066*

Treprostinil (tre PROST in il)

U.S. Brand Names Remodulin™

Generic Available No

Synonyms Treprostinil Sodium

Pharmacologic Category Vasodilator

Use Treatment of pulmonary arterial hypertension (PAH) in patients with NYHA Class II-IV symptoms to decrease exercise-associated symptoms

Local Anesthetic/Vasoconstrictor Precautions No information available to require special precautions

Effects on Dental Treatment No significant effects or complications reported

Common Adverse Effects >10%:

Cardiovascular: Vasodilation (11%)

Central nervous system: Headache (27%)

Dermatologic: Rash (14%)

Gastrointestinal: Diarrhea (25%), nausea (22%)

Local: Infusion site pain (85%), infusion site reaction (83%)

Miscellaneous: Jaw pain (13%)

Mechanism of Action Treprostinil is a direct dilator of both pulmonary and systemic arterial vascular beds; also inhibits platelet aggregation.

Drug Interactions

Increased Effect/Toxicity: Concomitant use of treprostinil with other agents that inhibit platelet aggregation (eg, NSAIDs, ASA, antiplatelet agents) or promote anticoagulation (eg, warfarin) may increase the risk of bleeding.

Pharmacodynamics/Kinetics

Absorption: SubQ: Rapidly and completely

(Continued)

Treprostinil *(Continued)*

Distribution: 14 L/70 kg lean body weight
Protein binding: 91%
Metabolism: Hepatic (enzymes unknown); forms metabolites
Bioavailability: 100%
Half-life elimination: Terminal: 2-4 hours
Excretion: Urine (4% as unchanged drug; 64% as metabolites); feces (13%)

Pregnancy Risk Factor B

Treprostinil Sodium *see* Treprostinil *on page 1327*

Tretinoin and Mequinol *see* Mequinol and Tretinoin *on page 879*

Tretinoin, Fluocinolone Acetonide, and Hydroquinone *see* Fluocinolone, Hydroquinone, and Tretinoin *on page 601*

Tretinoin (Oral) (TRET i noyn, oral)

U.S. Brand Names Vesanoid®

Canadian Brand Names Vesanoid®

Generic Available No

Synonyms All-*trans*-Retinoic Acid; ATRA; NSC-122758; Ro 5488; tRA; *trans*-Retinoic Acid

Pharmacologic Category Antineoplastic Agent, Miscellaneous

Use Induction of remission in patients with acute promyelocytic leukemia (APL), French American British (FAB) classification M3 (including the M3 variant)

Local Anesthetic/Vasoconstrictor Precautions No information available to require special precautions

Effects on Dental Treatment Key adverse event(s) related to dental treatment: Xerostomia (normal salivary flow resumes upon discontinuation).

Common Adverse Effects Virtually all patients experience some drug-related toxicity, especially headache, fever, weakness and fatigue. These adverse effects are seldom permanent or irreversible nor do they usually require therapy interruption

>10%:

Cardiovascular: Arrhythmias, flushing, hypotension, hypertension, peripheral edema, chest discomfort, edema
Central nervous system: Dizziness, anxiety, insomnia, depression, confusion, malaise, pain
Dermatologic: Burning, redness, cheilitis, inflammation of lips, dry skin, pruritus, photosensitivity
Endocrine & metabolic: Increased serum concentration of triglycerides
Gastrointestinal: GI hemorrhage, abdominal pain, other GI disorders, diarrhea, constipation, dyspepsia, abdominal distention, weight gain/loss, xerostomia
Hematologic: Hemorrhage, disseminated intravascular coagulation
Local: Phlebitis, injection site reactions
Neuromuscular & skeletal: Bone pain, arthralgia, myalgia, paresthesia
Ocular: Itching of eye
Renal: Renal insufficiency
Respiratory: Upper respiratory tract disorders, dyspnea, respiratory insufficiency, pleural effusion, pneumonia, rales, expiratory wheezing, dry nose
Miscellaneous: Infections, shivering

1% to 10%:

Cardiovascular: Cardiac failure, cardiac arrest, myocardial infarction, enlarged heart, heart murmur, ischemia, stroke, myocarditis, pericarditis, pulmonary hypertension, secondary cardiomyopathy, cerebral hemorrhage, pallor
Central nervous system: Intracranial hypertension, agitation, hallucination, agnosia, aphasia, cerebellar edema, cerebellar disorders, convulsions, coma, CNS depression, encephalopathy, hypotaxia, no light reflex, neurologic reaction, spinal cord disorder, unconsciousness, dementia, forgetfulness, somnolence, slow speech, hypothermia
Dermatologic: Skin peeling on hands or soles of feet, rash, cellulitis
Endocrine & metabolic: Fluid imbalance, acidosis
Gastrointestinal: Hepatosplenomegaly, ulcer
Genitourinary: Dysuria, polyuria, enlarged prostate
Hepatic: Ascites, hepatitis
Neuromuscular & skeletal: Tremor, leg weakness, hyporeflexia, dysarthria, facial paralysis, hemiplegia, flank pain, asterixis, abnormal gait
Ocular: Dry eyes, photophobia
Renal: Acute renal failure, renal tubular necrosis
Respiratory: Lower respiratory tract disorders, pulmonary infiltration, bronchial asthma, pulmonary/larynx edema, unspecified pulmonary disease

Miscellaneous: Face edema, lymph disorders

Mechanism of Action Tretinoin appears to bind one or more nuclear receptors and inhibits clonal proliferation and/or granulocyte differentiation

Drug Interactions

Cytochrome P450 Effect: Substrate (minor) of CYP2A6, 2B6, 2C8/9; **Inhibits** CYP2C8/9 (weak); **Induces** CYP2E1 (weak)

Increased Effect/Toxicity: Ketoconazole increases the mean plasma AUC of tretinoin. Other drugs which inhibit CYP3A4 would be expected to increase tretinoin concentrations, potentially increasing toxicity.

Pharmacodynamics/Kinetics

Protein binding: >95%

Metabolism: Hepatic via CYP; primary metabolite: 4-oxo-all-*trans*-retinoic acid

Half-life elimination: Terminal: Parent drug: 0.5-2 hours

Time to peak, serum: 1-2 hours

Excretion: Urine (63%); feces (30%)

Pregnancy Risk Factor D

Tretinoin (Topical) (TRET i noyn, TOP i kal)

U.S. Brand Names Altinac™; Avita®; Renova®; Retin-A®; Retin-A® Micro

Canadian Brand Names Rejuva-A®; Retin-A®; Retin-A® Micro; Retinova®

Generic Available Yes: Cream, gel

Synonyms Retinoic Acid; *trans*-Retinoic Acid; Vitamin A Acid

Pharmacologic Category Retinoic Acid Derivative

Use Treatment of acne vulgaris; photodamaged skin; palliation of fine wrinkles, mottled hyperpigmentation, and tactile roughness of facial skin as part of a comprehensive skin care and sun avoidance program

Unlabeled/Investigational Use Some skin cancers

Local Anesthetic/Vasoconstrictor Precautions No information available to require special precautions

Effects on Dental Treatment No significant effects or complications reported

Common Adverse Effects

>10%: Dermatologic: Excessive dryness, erythema, scaling of the skin, pruritus

1% to 10%:

Dermatologic: Hyperpigmentation or hypopigmentation, photosensitivity, initial acne flare-up

Local: Edema, blistering, stinging

Mechanism of Action Keratinocytes in the sebaceous follicle become less adherent which allows for easy removal; inhibits microcomedone formation and eliminates lesions already present

Drug Interactions

Cytochrome P450 Effect: Substrate (minor) of CYP2A6, 2B6, 2C8/9; **Inhibits** CYP2C8/9 (weak); **Induces** CYP2E1 (weak)

Increased Effect/Toxicity: Topical application of sulfur, benzoyl peroxide, salicylic acid, resorcinol, or any product with strong drying effects potentiates adverse reactions with tretinoin.

Photosensitizing medications (thiazides, tetracyclines, fluoroquinolones, phenothiazines, sulfonamides) augment phototoxicity and should not be used when treating palliation of fine wrinkles, mottled hyperpigmentation, and tactile roughness of facial skin.

Pharmacodynamics/Kinetics

Absorption: Minimal

Metabolism: Hepatic for the small amount absorbed

Excretion: Urine and feces

Pregnancy Risk Factor C

Trexall™ *see* Methotrexate *on page 897*

TRH *see* Protirelin *on page 1145*

Triacetin (trye a SEE tin)

U.S. Brand Names Myco-Nail [OTC]

Generic Available No

Synonyms Glycerol Triacetate

Pharmacologic Category Antifungal Agent, Topical

Use Fungistat for athlete's foot and other superficial fungal infections

Local Anesthetic/Vasoconstrictor Precautions No information available to require special precautions

Effects on Dental Treatment No significant effects or complications reported

Triacetyloleandomycin *see* Troleandomycin *on page 1348*

Triacin-C® [DSC] *see* Triprolidine, Pseudoephedrine, and Codeine *on page 1346*
Triaconazole *see* Terconazole *on page 1274*

Triamcinolone (trye am SIN oh lone)

Related Information

Oral Nonviral Soft Tissue Ulcerations or Erosions *on page 1551*
Respiratory Diseases *on page 1478*
Triamcinolone Acetonide (Dental Paste) *on page 1333*

U.S. Brand Names Aristocort®; Aristocort® A; Aristocort® Forte; Aristospan®; Azmacort®; Kenalog®; Kenalog-10®; Kenalog-40®; Kenalog® in Orabase®; Nasacort® [DSC]; Nasacort® AQ; Triderm®; Tri-Nasal®

Canadian Brand Names Aristocort®; Aristospan®; Azmacort®; Kenalog®; Kenalog® in Orabase; Nasacort® AQ; Oracort; Triaderm; Trinasal®

Mexican Brand Names Triamsicort®

Generic Available Yes: Cream, lotion, ointment, paste

Synonyms Triamcinolone Acetonide, Aerosol; Triamcinolone Acetonide, Parenteral; Triamcinolone Diacetate, Oral; Triamcinolone Diacetate, Parenteral; Triamcinolone Hexacetonide; Triamcinolone, Oral

Pharmacologic Category Corticosteroid, Adrenal; Corticosteroid, Inhalant (Oral); Corticosteroid, Nasal; Corticosteroid, Systemic; Corticosteroid, Topical

Dental Use Oral, topical: Adjunctive treatment and temporary relief of symptoms associated with oral inflammatory lesions and ulcerative lesions resulting from trauma

Use

Nasal inhalation: Management of seasonal and perennial allergic rhinitis in patients ≥6 years of age

Oral inhalation: Control of bronchial asthma and related bronchospastic conditions

Oral topical: Adjunctive treatment and temporary relief of symptoms associated with oral inflammatory lesions and ulcerative lesions resulting from trauma

Systemic: Adrenocortical insufficiency, rheumatic disorders, allergic states, respiratory diseases, systemic lupus erythematosus (SLE), and other diseases requiring anti-inflammatory or immunosuppressive effects

Topical: Inflammatory dermatoses responsive to steroids

Local Anesthetic/Vasoconstrictor Precautions No information available to require special precautions

Effects on Dental Treatment Key adverse event(s) related to dental treatment: Ulcerative esophagitis, perioral dermatitis, atrophy of oral mucosa, burning, and irritation.

Significant Adverse Effects

Systemic: Frequency not defined:

Cardiovascular: CHF, hypertension

Central nervous system: Convulsions, fever, headache, intracranial pressure increased, vertigo

Dermatologic: Bruising, facial erythema, petechiae, photosensitivity, rash, thin/fragile skin, wound healing impaired

Endocrine & metabolic: Adrenocortical/pituitary unresponsiveness (particularly during stress), carbohydrate tolerance decreased, cushingoid state, diabetes mellitus (manifestations of latent disease), fluid retention, growth suppression (children), hypokalemic alkalosis, menstrual irregularities, negative nitrogen balance, potassium loss, sodium retention

Gastrointestinal: Abdominal distention, diarrhea, dyspepsia, nausea, oral *Monilia* (oral inhaler), pancreatitis, peptic ulcer, ulcerative esophagitis, weight gain

Local: Skin atrophy (at the injection site)

Neuromuscular & skeletal: Femoral/humeral head aseptic necrosis, muscle mass decreased, muscle weakness, osteoporosis, pathologic fracture of long bones, steroid myopathy, vertebral compression fractures

Ocular: Cataracts, intraocular pressure increased, exophthalmos, glaucoma

Respiratory: Cough increased (nasal spray), epistaxis (nasal inhaler/spray), pharyngitis (nasal spray/oral inhaler), sinusitis (oral inhaler), voice alteration (oral inhaler)

Miscellaneous: Anaphylaxis, diaphoresis increased, suppression to skin tests

Topical: Frequency not defined:

Dermatologic: Itching, allergic contact dermatitis, dryness, folliculitis, skin infection (secondary), itching, hypertrichosis, acneiform eruptions, hypopigmentation, skin maceration, skin atrophy, striae, miliaria, perioral dermatitis, atrophy of oral mucosa

Local: Burning, irritation

Dosage The lowest possible dose should be used to control the condition; when dose reduction is possible, the dose should be reduced gradually. Parenteral dose is usually $1/3$ to $1/2$ the oral dose given every 12 hours. In life-threatening situations, parenteral doses larger than the oral dose may be needed.

Injection:

Acetonide:

Intra-articular, intrabursal, tendon sheaths: Adults: Initial: Smaller joints: 2.5-5 mg, larger joints: 5-15 mg

Intradermal: Adults: Initial: 1 mg

I.M.: Range: 2.5-60 mg/day

Children 6-12 years: Initial: 40 mg

Children >12 years and Adults: Initial: 60 mg

Diacetate: Adults:

Intra-articular, Intrasynovial: Range: 5-40 mg; duration of effect varies from 1 week to 2 months, although more frequent dosing may be needed in acutely-inflamed joints

Average dose: Knee: 25 mg, finger: 2-5 mg

Intralesional, sublesional: Range: 5-48 mg, dependent upon size of lesion

Maximum: 12.5 mg/injection site, 25 mg/lesion, 75 mg/week

Usual treatment course: 2-3 injections at 1- to 2-week intervals

I.M.: Initial range: 3-48 mg/day; average dose: 40 mg/week

Hexacetonide: Adults:

Intralesional, sublesional: Up to 0.5 mg/square inch of affected skin

Intra-articular: Range: 2-20 mg

Triamcinolone Dosing

	Acetonide	Diacetate	Hexacetonide
Intrasynovial	2.5-40 mg	5-40 mg	
Intralesional	1-30 mg (usually 1 mg per injection site); 10 mg/mL suspension usually used	5-48 mg (not >25 mg per lesion)	Up to 0.5 mg/sq inch affected area
Sublesional	1-30 mg		
Systemic I.M.	2.5-60 mg/dose (usual adult dose: 60 mg; may repeat with 20-100 mg dose when symptoms recur)	~40 mg/wk	
Intra-articular	2.5-40 mg	2-40 mg	2-20 mg average
large joints	5-15 mg		10-20 mg
small joints	2.5-5 mg		2-6 mg
Tendon sheaths	2.5-10 mg		
Intradermal	1 mg/site		

Intranasal: Perennial allergic rhinitis, seasonal allergic rhinitis:

Nasal spray:

Children 6-11 years: 110 mcg/day as 1 spray in each nostril once daily.

Children ≥12 years and Adults: 220 mcg/day as 2 sprays in each nostril once daily

Nasal inhaler:

Children 6-11 years: Initial: 220 mcg/day as 2 sprays in each nostril once daily

Children ≥12 years and Adults: Initial: 220 mcg/day as 2 sprays in each nostril once daily; may increase dose to 440 mcg/day (given once daily or divided and given 2 or 4 times/day)

Oral: Adults:

Acute rheumatic carditis: Initial: 20-60 mg/day; reduce dose during maintenance therapy

Acute seasonal or perennial allergic rhinitis: 8-12 mg/day

Adrenocortical insufficiency: Range 4-12 mg/day

Bronchial asthma: 8-16 mg/day

Dermatological disorders, contact/atopic dermatitis: Initial: 8-16 mg/day

Ophthalmic disorders: 12-40 mg/day

Rheumatic disorders: Range: 8-16 mg/day

(Continued)

Triamcinolone *(Continued)*

SLE: Initial: 20-32 mg/day, some patients may need initial doses ≥48 mg; reduce dose during maintenance therapy

Oral inhalation: Asthma:

Children 6-12 years: 100-200 mcg 3-4 times/day **or** 200-400 mcg twice daily; maximum dose: 1200 mg/day

Children >12 years and Adults: 200 mcg 3-4 times/day **or** 400 mcg twice daily; maximum dose: 1600 mcg/day

Oral topical: Oral inflammatory lesions/ulcers: Press a small dab (about 1/4 inch) to the lesion until a thin film develops. A larger quantity may be required for coverage of some lesions. For optimal results use only enough to coat the lesion with a thin film; do not rub in.

Topical:

Cream, Ointment: Apply thin film to affected areas 2-4 times/day

Spray: Apply to affected area 3-4 times/day

Mechanism of Action Decreases inflammation by suppression of migration of polymorphonuclear leukocytes and reversal of increased capillary permeability; suppresses the immune system by reducing activity and volume of the lymphatic system; suppresses adrenal function at high doses

Contraindications Hypersensitivity to triamcinolone or any component of the formulation; systemic fungal infections; serious infections (except septic shock or tuberculous meningitis); primary treatment of status asthmaticus; fungal, viral, or bacterial infections of the mouth or throat (oral topical formulation)

Warnings/Precautions May cause suppression of hypothalamic-pituitary-adrenal (HPA) axis, particularly in younger children or in patients receiving high doses for prolonged periods. Particular care is required when patients are transferred from systemic corticosteroids to inhaled products due to possible adrenal insufficiency or withdrawal from steroids, including an increase in allergic symptoms. Patients receiving 20 mg per day of prednisone (or equivalent) may be most susceptible. Fatalities have occurred due to adrenal insufficiency in asthmatic patients during and after transfer from systemic corticosteroids to aerosol steroids; aerosol steroids do **not** provide the systemic steroid needed to treat patients having trauma, surgery, or infections. Withdrawal and discontinuation of the corticosteroid should be done slowly and carefully

Use with caution in patients with hypothyroidism, cirrhosis, nonspecific ulcerative colitis and patients at increased risk for peptic ulcer disease. Corticosteroids should be used with caution in patients with diabetes, hypertension, osteoporosis, glaucoma, cataracts, or tuberculosis. Use caution in hepatic impairment. Do not use occlusive dressings on weeping or exudative lesions and general caution with occlusive dressings should be observed; discontinue if skin irritation or contact dermatitis should occur; do not use in patients with decreased skin circulation; avoid the use of high potency steroids on the face.

Because of the risk of adverse effects, systemic corticosteroids should be used cautiously in the elderly, in the smallest possible dose, and for the shortest possible time. Azmacort® (metered dose inhaler) comes with its own spacer device attached and may be easier to use in older patients.

Controlled clinical studies have shown that orally-inhaled and intranasal corticosteroids may cause a reduction in growth velocity in pediatric patients. (In studies of orally-inhaled corticosteroids, the mean reduction in growth velocity was approximately 1 centimeter per year [range 0.3-1.8 cm per year] and appears to be related to dose and duration of exposure.) The growth of pediatric patients receiving inhaled corticosteroids, should be monitored routinely (eg, via stadiometry). To minimize the systemic effects of orally-inhaled and intranasal corticosteroids, each patient should be titrated to the lowest effective dose.

May suppress the immune system, patients may be more susceptible to infection. Use with caution in patients with systemic infections or ocular herpes simplex. Avoid exposure to chickenpox and measles.

Oral topical: Discontinue if local irritation or sensitization should develop. If significant regeneration or repair of oral tissues has not occurred in seven days, re-evaluation of the etiology of the oral lesion is advised.

Drug Interactions

Decreased effect: Barbiturates, phenytoin, rifampin increase metabolism of triamcinolone; vaccine and toxoid effects may be reduced

Increased effect: Salmeterol: The addition of salmeterol has been demonstrated to improve response to inhaled corticosteroids (as compared to increasing steroid dosage).

Increased toxicity: Salicylates may increase risk of GI ulceration

Ethanol/Nutrition/Herb Interactions

Ethanol: Avoid ethanol (may enhance gastric mucosal irritation).

Food: Triamcinolone interferes with calcium absorption.

Herb/Nutraceutical: Avoid cat's claw, echinacea (have immunostimulant properties).

Dietary Considerations May be taken with food to decrease GI distress.

Pharmacodynamics/Kinetics

Duration: Oral: 8-12 hours

Absorption: Topical: Systemic

Time to peak: I.M.: 8-10 hours

Half-life elimination: Biologic: 18-36 hours

Pregnancy Risk Factor C

Lactation Excretion in breast milk unknown/use caution

Breast-Feeding Considerations It is not known if triamcinolone is excreted in breast milk, however, other corticosteroids are excreted. Prednisone and prednisolone are excreted in breast milk; the AAP considers them to be "usually compatible" with breast-feeding. Hypertension was reported in a nursing infant when a topical corticosteroid was applied to the nipples of the mother.

Dosage Forms [DSC] = Discontinued product

Aerosol for nasal inhalation, as acetonide (Nasacort® [DSC]): 55 mcg/inhalation (10 g) [100 doses]

Aerosol for nasal inhalation, as acetonide [spray]:

Nasacort® AQ: 55 mcg/inhalation (16.5 g) [120 doses]

Tri-Nasal®: 50 mcg/inhalation (15 mL) [120 doses]

Aerosol for oral inhalation, as acetonide (Azmacort®): 100 mcg per actuation (20 g) [240 actuations]

Aerosol, topical, as acetonide (Kenalog®): 0.2 mg/2-second spray (63 g)

Cream, as acetonide: 0.025% (15 g, 80 g); 0.1% (15 g, 80 g, 454 g, 2270 g); 0.5% (15 g)

Aristocort® A: 0.025% (15 g, 60 g); 0.1% (15 g, 60 g); 0.5% (15 g) [contains benzyl alcohol]

Kenalog®: 0.1% (15 g, 60 g, 80 g); 0.5% (20 g)

Triderm®: 0.1% (30 g, 85 g)

Injection, suspension, as acetonide:

Kenalog-10®: 10 mg/mL (5 mL) [contains benzyl alcohol; not for I.V. or I.M. use]

Kenalog-40®: 40 mg/mL (1 mL, 5 mL, 10 mL) [contains benzyl alcohol; not for I.V. or intradermal use]

Injection, suspension, as diacetate:

Aristocort®: 25 mg/mL (5 mL) [contains benzyl alcohol; not for I.V. use]

Aristocort® Forte: 40 mg/mL (1 mL, 5mL) [contains benzyl alcohol; not for I.V. use]

Injection, suspension, as hexacetonide (Aristospan®): 5 mg/mL (5 mL); 20 mg/mL (1 mL, 5 mL) [contains benzyl alcohol; not for I.V. use]

Lotion, as acetonide (Kenalog®): 0.025% (60 mL); 0.1% (60 mL)

Ointment, topical, as acetonide: 0.025% (80 g); 0.1% (15 g, 80 g, 454 g)

Aristocort® A, Kenalog®: 0.1% (15 g, 60 g)

Paste, oral, topical, as acetonide (Kenalog® in Orabase®): 0.1% (5 g)

Tablet (Aristocort®): 4 mg [contains lactose and sodium benzoate]

Triamcinolone Acetonide, Aerosol *see* Triamcinolone *on page 1330*

Triamcinolone Acetonide (Dental Paste)

(trye am SIN oh lone a SEE toe nide paste)

Related Information

Triamcinolone *on page 1330*

U.S. Brand Names Kenalog® in Orabase®

Canadian Brand Names Oracort®

Generic Available Yes

Pharmacologic Category Anti-inflammatory Agent; Corticosteroid, Topical

Dental Use For adjunctive treatment and for the temporary relief of symptoms associated with oral inflammatory lesions and ulcerative lesions resulting from trauma

Local Anesthetic/Vasoconstrictor Precautions No information available to require special precautions

Effects on Dental Treatment No significant effects or complications reported

Significant Adverse Effects No data reported

Dosage Press a small dab (about 1/4 inch) to the lesion until a thin film develops. A larger quantity may be required for coverage of some lesions. For optimal results use only enough to coat the lesion with a thin film.

(Continued)

Triamcinolone Acetonide (Dental Paste) *(Continued)*

Mechanism of Action Decreases inflammation by suppression of migration of polymorphonuclear leukocytes and reversal of increased capillary permeability; suppresses the immune system by reducing activity and volume of the lymphatic system; suppresses adrenal function at high doses

Contraindications Hypersensitivity to triamcinolone or any component of the formulation; contraindicated in the presence of fungal, viral, or bacterial infections of the mouth or throat

Warnings/Precautions Patients with tuberculosis, peptic ulcer or diabetes mellitus should not be treated with any corticosteroid preparation without the advice of the patient's physician. Normal immune responses of the oral tissues are depressed in patients receiving topical corticosteroid therapy. Virulent strains of oral microorganisms may multiply without producing the usual warning symptoms of oral infections. The small amount of steroid released from the topical preparation makes systemic effects very unlikely. If local irritation or sensitization should develop, the preparation should be discontinued. If significant regeneration or repair of oral tissues has not occurred in seven days, re-evaluation of the etiology of the oral lesion is advised.

Drug Interactions No data reported

Pharmacodynamics/Kinetics

Absorption: Systemic

Half-life elimination, serum: Biological: 18-36 hours

Pregnancy Risk Factor C

Dosage Forms Tube: 5 g [each g provides 1 mg (0.1%) triamcinolone in emollient dental paste containing gelatin, pectin, and carboxymethylcellulose sodium in a polyethylene and mineral oil gel base]

Triamcinolone Acetonide, Parenteral *see* Triamcinolone *on page 1330*

Triamcinolone and Nystatin *see* Nystatin and Triamcinolone *on page 1004*

Triamcinolone Diacetate, Oral *see* Triamcinolone *on page 1330*

Triamcinolone Diacetate, Parenteral *see* Triamcinolone *on page 1330*

Triamcinolone Hexacetonide *see* Triamcinolone *on page 1330*

Triamcinolone, Oral *see* Triamcinolone *on page 1330*

Triaminic® Allergy Congestion [OTC] *see* Pseudoephedrine *on page 1147*

Triaminic® Cold and Allergy [OTC] *see* Chlorpheniramine and Pseudoephedrine *on page 315*

Triaminic® Cough and Sore Throat Formula [OTC] *see* Acetaminophen, Dextromethorphan, and Pseudoephedrine *on page 59*

Triamterene (trye AM ter een)

Related Information

Cardiovascular Diseases *on page 1458*

U.S. Brand Names Dyrenium®

Generic Available No

Pharmacologic Category Diuretic, Potassium-Sparing

Use Alone or in combination with other diuretics in treatment of edema and hypertension; decreases potassium excretion caused by kaliuretic diuretics

Local Anesthetic/Vasoconstrictor Precautions No information available to require special precautions

Effects on Dental Treatment No significant effects or complications reported

Common Adverse Effects 1% to 10%:

Cardiovascular: Hypotension, edema, CHF, bradycardia

Central nervous system: Dizziness, headache, fatigue

Gastrointestinal: Constipation, nausea

Respiratory: Dyspnea

Mechanism of Action Interferes with potassium/sodium exchange (active transport) in the distal tubule, cortical collecting tubule and collecting duct by inhibiting sodium, potassium-ATPase; decreases calcium excretion; increases magnesium loss

Drug Interactions

Increased Effect/Toxicity: ACE inhibitors or spironolactone can cause hyperkalemia, especially in patients with renal impairment, potassium-rich diets, or on other drugs causing hyperkalemia; avoid concurrent use or monitor closely. Potassium supplements may further increase potassium retention and cause hyperkalemia; avoid concurrent use.

Pharmacodynamics/Kinetics

Onset of action: Diuresis: 2-4 hours

Duration: 7-9 hours

Absorption: Unreliable

Pregnancy Risk Factor B (manufacturer); D (expert analysis)

Triamterene and Hydrochlorothiazide *see* Hydrochlorothiazide and Triamterene *on page 701*

Triavil® *see* Amitriptyline and Perphenazine *on page 106*

Triaz® *see* Benzoyl Peroxide *on page 194*

Triaz® Cleanser *see* Benzoyl Peroxide *on page 194*

Triazolam (trye AY zoe lam)

Related Information

Patients Requiring Sedation *on page 1567*

U.S. Brand Names Halcion®

Canadian Brand Names Apo-Triazo®; Gen-Triazolam; Halcion®

Mexican Brand Names Halcion®

Generic Available Yes

Pharmacologic Category Benzodiazepine

Dental Use Oral premedication before dental procedures

Use Short-term treatment of insomnia

Local Anesthetic/Vasoconstrictor Precautions No information available to require special precautions

Effects on Dental Treatment No significant effects or complications reported

Significant Adverse Effects

>10%: Central nervous system: Drowsiness, anteriograde amnesia

1% to 10%:

Central nervous system: Headache, dizziness, nervousness, lightheadedness, ataxia

Gastrointestinal: Nausea, vomiting

<1% (Limited to important or life-threatening): Confusion, depression, euphoria, memory impairment

Restrictions C-IV

Dosage Oral (onset of action is rapid, patient should be in bed when taking medication):

Children <18 years: Dosage not established

Adults:

Hypnotic: 0.125-0.25 mg at bedtime (maximum dose: 0.5 mg/day)

Preprocedure sedation (dental): 0.25 mg taken the evening before oral surgery; or 0.25 mg 1 hour before procedure

Elderly: Insomnia (short-term use): 0.0625-0.125 mg at bedtime; maximum dose: 0.25 mg/day

Dosing adjustment/comments in hepatic impairment: Reduce dose or avoid use in cirrhosis

Mechanism of Action Binds to stereospecific benzodiazepine receptors on the postsynaptic GABA neuron at several sites within the central nervous system, including the limbic system, reticular formation. Enhancement of the inhibitory effect of GABA on neuronal excitability results by increased neuronal membrane permeability to chloride ions. This shift in chloride ions results in hyperpolarization (a less excitable state) and stabilization.

Contraindications Hypersensitivity to triazolam or any component of the formulation (cross-sensitivity with other benzodiazepines may exist); concurrent therapy with atazanavir, ketoconazole, itraconazole, nefazodone, and ritonavir; pregnancy

Warnings/Precautions Should be used only after evaluation of potential causes of sleep disturbance. Failure of sleep disturbance to resolve after 7-10 days may indicate psychiatric or medical illness. A worsening of insomnia or the emergence of new abnormalities of thought or behavior may represent unrecognized psychiatric or medical illness and requires immediate and careful evaluation. Prescription should be written for a maximum of 7-10 days and should not be prescribed in quantities exceeding a 1-month supply. Abrupt discontinuation after sustained use (generally >10 days) may cause withdrawal symptoms.

An increase in daytime anxiety may occur after as few as 10 days of continuous use, which may be related to withdrawal reaction in some patients. Anterograde amnesia may occur at a higher rate with triazolam than with other benzodiazepines. Use with caution in elderly or debilitated patients, patients with hepatic disease (including alcoholics), or renal impairment. Use with caution in patients with respiratory disease or impaired gag reflex. Avoid use in patients with sleep apnea.

Causes CNS depression (dose-related) resulting in sedation, dizziness, confusion, or ataxia which may impair physical and mental capabilities. Patients must be cautioned about performing tasks which require mental alertness (eg, operating machinery or driving). Use with caution in patients receiving other CNS depressants or psychoactive agents. Effects with other sedative drugs or

(Continued)

Triazolam *(Continued)*

ethanol may be potentiated. Benzodiazepines have been associated with falls and traumatic injury and should be used with extreme caution in patients who are at risk of these events (especially the elderly).

Use caution with potent CYP3A4 inhibitors, as they may significantly decreased the clearance of triazolam. Use caution in patients with depression, particularly if suicidal risk may be present. Use with caution in patients with a history of drug dependence. Benzodiazepines have been associated with dependence and acute withdrawal symptoms on discontinuation or reduction in dose. Acute withdrawal, including seizures, may be precipitated after administration of flumazenil to patients receiving long-term benzodiazepine therapy.

Paradoxical reactions, including hyperactive or aggressive behavior have been reported with benzodiazepines, particularly in adolescent/pediatric or psychiatric patients. Does not have analgesic, antidepressant, or antipsychotic properties.

Drug Interactions Substrate of CYP3A4 (major); **Inhibits** CYP2C8/9 (weak)

CNS depressants: Sedative effects and/or respiratory depression may be additive with CNS depressants; includes ethanol, barbiturates, narcotic analgesics, and other sedative agents; monitor for increased effect

CYP3A4 inducers: CYP3A4 inducers may decrease the levels/effects of triazolam. Example inducers include aminoglutethimide, carbamazepine, nafcillin, nevirapine, phenobarbital, phenytoin, and rifamycins.

CYP3A4 inhibitors: May increase the levels/effects of triazolam. Example inhibitors include azole antifungals, ciprofloxacin, clarithromycin, diclofenac, doxycycline, erythromycin, imatinib, isoniazid, nefazodone, nicardipine, propofol, protease inhibitors, quinidine, and verapamil.

Isoniazid: Isoniazid may increase triazolam levels.

Levodopa: Therapeutic effects may be diminished in some patients following the addition of a benzodiazepine; limited/inconsistent data

Oral contraceptives: May decrease the clearance and increase the half-life of triazolam; monitor for increased triazolam effect

Ranitidine: Ranitidine may increase triazolam levels.

Theophylline: May partially antagonize some of the effects of benzodiazepines; monitor for decreased response; may require higher doses for sedation

Ethanol/Nutrition/Herb Interactions

Ethanol: Avoid ethanol (may increase CNS depression).

Food: Food may decrease the rate of absorption. Triazolam serum concentration may be increased by grapefruit juice; avoid concurrent use.

Herb/Nutraceutical: St John's wort may decrease levels. Avoid valerian, St John's wort, kava kava, gotu kola (may increase CNS depression).

Pharmacodynamics/Kinetics

Onset of action: Hypnotic: 15-30 minutes

Duration: 6-7 hours

Distribution: V_d: 0.8-1.8 L/kg

Protein binding: 89%

Metabolism: Extensively hepatic

Half-life elimination: 1.7-5 hours

Excretion: Urine as unchanged drug and metabolites

Pregnancy Risk Factor X

Lactation Excretion in breast milk unknown/not recommended

Breast-Feeding Considerations It is not known if triazolam is excreted in breast milk; however, other benzodiazepines are known to be excreted in breast milk. The AAP rates use of related agents as "of concern" and breast-feeding is not recommended.

Dosage Forms Tablet: 0.125 mg, 0.25 mg [contains sodium benzoate]

Comments Triazolam (0.25 mg) 1 hour prior to dental procedure has been used as an oral pre-op sedative

Selected Readings

Berthold CW, Dionne RA, and Corey SE, "Comparison of Sublingually and Orally Administered Triazolam for Premedication Before Oral Surgery," *Oral Surg Oral Med Oral Pathol Oral Radiol Endod*, 1997, 84(2):119-24.

Berthold CW, Schneider A, and Dionne RA, "Using Triazolam to Reduce Dental Anxiety," *J Am Dent Assoc*, 1993, 124(11):58-64.

Flanagan D, "Oral Triazolam Sedation in Implant Dentistry," *J Oral Implantol*, 2004, 30(2):93-7.

Goodchild JH, Feck AS, and Silverman MD, "Anxiolysis in General Dental Practice," *Dent Today*, 2003, 22(3):106-11.

Kaufman E, Hargreaves KM, and Dionne RA, "Comparison of Oral Triazolam and Nitrous Oxide With Placebo and Intravenous Diazepam for Outpatient Premedication," *Oral Surg Oral Med Oral Pathol*, 1993, 75(2):156-64.

Kurzrock M, "Triazolam and Dental Anxiety," *J Am Dent Assoc*, 1994, 125(4):358, 360.

Lieblich SE and Horswell B, "Attenuation of Anxiety in Ambulatory Oral Surgery Patients With Oral Triazolam," *J Oral Maxillofac Surg*, 1991, 49(8):792-7.

Milgrom P, Quarnstrom FC, Longley A, et al, "The Efficacy and Memory Effects of Oral Triazolam Premedication in Highly Anxious Dental Patients," *Anesth Prog*, 1994, 41(3):70-6.

Quarnstrom F, "Should Dentists Do Oral Sedation?" *Dent Today*, 2004, 23(3):16-8.

Tribavirin *see* Ribavirin *on page 1177*

Tricalcium Phosphate *see* Calcium Phosphate (Tribasic) *on page 247*

Tricardio B *see* Folic Acid, Cyanocobalamin, and Pyridoxine *on page 626*

Tri-Chlor® *see* Trichloroacetic Acid *on page 1337*

Trichlormethiazide (trye klor meth EYE a zide)

Related Information

Cardiovascular Diseases *on page 1458*

U.S. Brand Names Naqua®

Canadian Brand Names Metahydrin®; Metatensin®; Naqua®; Trichlorex®

Generic Available Yes

Pharmacologic Category Diuretic, Thiazide

Use Management of mild to moderate hypertension; treatment of edema in congestive heart failure and nephrotic syndrome

Local Anesthetic/Vasoconstrictor Precautions No information available to require special precautions

Effects on Dental Treatment No significant effects or complications reported

Mechanism of Action The diuretic mechanism of action of the thiazides is primarily inhibition of sodium, chloride, and water reabsorption in the renal distal tubules, thereby producing diuresis with a resultant reduction in plasma volume. The antihypertensive mechanism of action of the thiazides is unknown. It is known that doses of thiazides produce greater reduction in blood pressure than equivalent diuretic doses of loop diuretics. There has been speculation that the thiazides may have some influence on vascular tone mediated through sodium depletion, but this remains to be proven.

Pregnancy Risk Factor D

Trichloroacetaldehyde Monohydrate *see* Chloral Hydrate *on page 304*

Trichloroacetic Acid (trye klor oh a SEE tik AS id)

U.S. Brand Names Tri-Chlor®

Generic Available Yes

Pharmacologic Category Keratolytic Agent

Use Debride callous tissue

Local Anesthetic/Vasoconstrictor Precautions No information available to require special precautions

Effects on Dental Treatment No significant effects or complications reported

Trichloromonofluoromethane and Dichlorodifluoromethane *see* Dichlorodifluoromethane and Trichloromonofluoromethane *on page 427*

Triclosan and Fluoride (trye KLOE san & FLOR ide)

Related Information

Fluoride *on page 603*

Periodontal Diseases *on page 1542*

U.S. Brand Names Colgate Total® Toothpaste

Synonyms Fluoride and Triclosan (Dental)

Pharmacologic Category Antibacterial, Dental; Mineral, Oral (Topical)

Dental Use Anticavity, antigingivitis, antiplaque toothpaste

Use Used exclusively in dental applications

Local Anesthetic/Vasoconstrictor Precautions No information available to require special precautions

Effects on Dental Treatment No significant effects or complications reported

Common Adverse Effects No data reported

Mechanism of Action Triclosan is an antibacterial agent which helps to prevent gingivitis with regular use. Fluoride promotes remineralization of decalcified enamel, inhibits the cariogenic microbial process in dental plaque, and increases tooth resistance to acid dissolution

Pregnancy Risk Factor No data reported

Comments It has been shown that stannous fluoride and triclosan when formulated into a toothpaste vehicle provide plaque inhibitory effects. To provide a longer retention time of the triclosan in plaque, a polymer has been added to the toothpaste vehicle. The polymer is known as PVM/MA which stands for polyvinylmethyl ether/maleic acid copolymer, and is listed as an inactive ingredient (PVM/MA Copolymer) on the manufacturer's label. Studies have reported that the retention of triclosan in plaque (exceeding the minimal inhibitory concentration) after polymer application was 14 hours after brushing. Ongoing

(Continued)

Triclosan and Fluoride *(Continued)*

studies are evaluating the effects of triclosan/copolymer on alveolar bone loss. Rosling et al. have reported that the daily use of Colgate Total® reduced (1) the frequency of deep periodontal pockets and (2) the number of sites that exhibited additional probing attachment and bone loss.

TriCor® *see* Fenofibrate *on page 577*

Tricosal *see* Choline Magnesium Trisalicylate *on page 324*

Triderm® *see* Triamcinolone *on page 1330*

Tridesilon® *see* Desonide *on page 410*

Tridione® *see* Trimethadione *on page 1340*

Triethanolamine Polypeptide Oleate-Condensate

(trye eth a NOLE a meen pol i PEP tide OH lee ate-KON den sate)

U.S. Brand Names Cerumenex®

Canadian Brand Names Cerumenex®

Generic Available No

Pharmacologic Category Otic Agent, Cerumenolytic

Use Removal of ear wax (cerumen)

Local Anesthetic/Vasoconstrictor Precautions No information available to require special precautions

Effects on Dental Treatment No significant effects or complications reported

Mechanism of Action Emulsifies and disperses accumulated cerumen

Pregnancy Risk Factor C

Triethanolamine Salicylate (trye eth a NOLE a meen sa LIS i late)

U.S. Brand Names Mobisyl® [OTC]; Myoflex® [OTC]; Sportscreme® [OTC]

Canadian Brand Names Antiphlogistine Rub A-535 No Odour; Myoflex®

Generic Available Yes

Pharmacologic Category Analgesic, Topical; Salicylate; Topical Skin Product

Use Relief of pain of muscular aches, rheumatism, neuralgia, sprains, arthritis on intact skin

Local Anesthetic/Vasoconstrictor Precautions No information available to require special precautions

Effects on Dental Treatment No significant effects or complications reported

Common Adverse Effects 1% to 10%:

Central nervous system: Confusion, drowsiness
Gastrointestinal: Nausea, vomiting, diarrhea
Respiratory: Hyperventilation

Triethylenethiophosphoramide *see* Thiotepa *on page 1291*

Trifluoperazine (trye floo oh PER a zeen)

U.S. Brand Names Stelazine® [DSC]

Canadian Brand Names Apo-Trifluoperazine®; Novo-Trifluzine; PMS-Trifluoperazine; Terfluzine

Mexican Brand Names Flupazine® [tabs]; Stelazine®

Generic Available Yes: Tablet

Synonyms Trifluoperazine Hydrochloride

Pharmacologic Category Antipsychotic Agent, Phenothiazine, Piperazine

Use Treatment of schizophrenia

Unlabeled/Investigational Use Management of psychotic disorders

Local Anesthetic/Vasoconstrictor Precautions Most pharmacology textbooks state that in presence of phenothiazines, systemic doses of epinephrine paradoxically decrease the blood pressure. This is the so called "epinephrine reversal" phenomenon. This has never been observed when epinephrine is given by infiltration as part of the anesthesia procedure.

Effects on Dental Treatment Key adverse event(s) related to dental treatment: Significant hypotension may occur, especially when the drug is administered parenterally; orthostatic hypotension is due to alpha-receptor blockade, the elderly are at greater risk for orthostatic hypotension.

Tardive dyskinesia: Prevalence rate may be 40% in elderly; development of the syndrome and the irreversible nature are proportional to duration and total cumulative dose over time. Extrapyramidal reactions are more common in elderly with up to 50% developing these reactions after 60 years of age. Drug-induced Parkinson's syndrome occurs often; akathisia is the most common extrapyramidal reaction in elderly.

Common Adverse Effects Frequency not defined.

Cardiovascular: Hypotension, orthostatic hypotension, cardiac arrest

Central nervous system: Extrapyramidal signs (pseudoparkinsonism, akathisia, dystonias, tardive dyskinesia), dizziness, headache, neuroleptic malignant syndrome (NMS), impairment of temperature regulation, lowering of seizures threshold

Dermatologic: Increased sensitivity to sun, rash, discoloration of skin (blue-gray)

Endocrine & metabolic: Changes in menstrual cycle, changes in libido, breast pain, hyperglycemia, hypoglycemia, gynecomastia, lactation, galactorrhea

Gastrointestinal: Constipation, weight gain, nausea, vomiting, stomach pain, xerostomia

Genitourinary: Difficulty in urination, ejaculatory disturbances, urinary retention, priapism

Hematologic: Agranulocytosis, leukopenia, pancytopenia, thrombocytopenic purpura, eosinophilia, hemolytic anemia, aplastic anemia

Hepatic: Cholestatic jaundice, hepatotoxicity

Neuromuscular & skeletal: Tremor

Ocular: Pigmentary retinopathy, cornea and lens changes

Respiratory: Nasal congestion

Mechanism of Action Blocks postsynaptic mesolimbic dopaminergic receptors in the brain; exhibits alpha-adrenergic blocking effect and depresses the release of hypothalamic and hypophyseal hormones

Drug Interactions

Cytochrome P450 Effect: Substrate of CYP1A2 (major)

Increased Effect/Toxicity: CYP1A2 inhibitors may increase the levels/effects of trifluoperazine; example inhibitors include amiodarone, ciprofloxacin, fluvoxamine, ketoconazole, lomefloxacin, ofloxacin, and rofecoxib. Trifluoperazine's effects on CNS depression may be additive when trifluoperazine is combined with CNS depressants (narcotic analgesics, ethanol, barbiturates, cyclic antidepressants, antihistamines, or sedative-hypnotics). Trifluoperazine may increase the effects/toxicity of anticholinergics, antihypertensives, lithium (rare neurotoxicity), trazodone, or valproic acid. Concurrent use with TCA may produce increased toxicity or altered therapeutic response. Chloroquine and propranolol may increase trifluoperazine concentrations. Hypotension may occur when trifluoperazine is combined with epinephrine. May increase the risk of arrhythmia when combined with antiarrhythmics, cisapride, pimozide, sparfloxacin, or other drugs which prolong QT interval. Metoclopramide may increase risk of extrapyramidal symptoms (EPS).

Decreased Effect: CYP1A2 inducers may decrease the levels/effects of trifluoperazine; example inducers include aminoglutethimide, carbamazepine, phenobarbital, and rifampin. Phenothiazines inhibit the effects of levodopa, guanadrel, guanethidine, and bromocriptine. Benztropine (and other anticholinergics) may inhibit the therapeutic response to trifluoperazine and excess anticholinergic effects may occur. Cigarette smoking may enhance the hepatic metabolism of trifluoperazine. Trifluoperazine and possibly other low potency antipsychotics may reverse the pressor effects of epinephrine.

Pharmacodynamics/Kinetics

Metabolism: Extensively hepatic

Half-life elimination: >24 hours with chronic use

Pregnancy Risk Factor C

Trifluoperazine Hydrochloride *see* Trifluoperazine *on page 1338*

Trifluorothymidine *see* Trifluridine *on page 1339*

Trifluridine (trye FLURE i deen)

Related Information

Systemic Viral Diseases *on page 1519*

U.S. Brand Names Viroptic®

Canadian Brand Names Viroptic®

Generic Available Yes

Synonyms F_3T; Trifluorothymidine

Pharmacologic Category Antiviral Agent, Ophthalmic

Use Treatment of primary keratoconjunctivitis and recurrent epithelial keratitis caused by herpes simplex virus types I and II

Local Anesthetic/Vasoconstrictor Precautions No information available to require special precautions

Effects on Dental Treatment No significant effects or complications reported

Mechanism of Action Interferes with viral replication by incorporating into viral DNA in place of thymidine, inhibiting thymidylate synthetase resulting in the formation of defective proteins

Pregnancy Risk Factor C

Triglycerides, Medium Chain *see* Medium Chain Triglycerides *on page 861*

Trihexyphenidyl (trye heks ee FEN i dil)

Canadian Brand Names Apo-Trihex®

Mexican Brand Names Hipokinon®

Generic Available Yes

Synonyms Artane; Benzhexol Hydrochloride; Trihexyphenidyl Hydrochloride

Pharmacologic Category Anticholinergic Agent; Anti-Parkinson's Agent, Anticholinergic

Use Adjunctive treatment of Parkinson's disease; treatment of drug-induced extrapyramidal symptoms

Local Anesthetic/Vasoconstrictor Precautions No information available to require special precautions

Effects on Dental Treatment Key adverse event(s) related to dental treatment: Xerostomia, dry throat (normal salivary flow resumes upon discontinuation). Prolonged xerostomia may contribute to discomfort and dental disease (ie, caries, periodontal disease, and oral candidiasis).

Common Adverse Effects Frequency not defined.

Cardiovascular: Tachycardia

Central nervous system: Confusion, agitation, euphoria, drowsiness, headache, dizziness, nervousness, delusions, hallucinations, paranoia

Dermatologic: Dry skin, increased sensitivity to light, rash

Gastrointestinal: Constipation, xerostomia, dry throat, ileus, nausea, vomiting, parotitis

Genitourinary: Urinary retention

Neuromuscular & skeletal: Weakness

Ocular: Blurred vision, mydriasis, increase in intraocular pressure, glaucoma, blindness (long-term use in narrow-angle glaucoma)

Respiratory: Dry nose

Miscellaneous: Diaphoresis (decreased)

Mechanism of Action Exerts a direct inhibitory effect on the parasympathetic nervous system. It also has a relaxing effect on smooth musculature; exerted both directly on the muscle itself and indirectly through parasympathetic nervous system (inhibitory effect)

Drug Interactions

Increased Effect/Toxicity: Central and/or peripheral anticholinergic syndrome can occur when administered with amantadine, rimantadine, narcotic analgesics, phenothiazines and other antipsychotics (especially with high anticholinergic activity), tricyclic antidepressants, MAO inhibitors, quinidine and some other antiarrhythmics, and antihistamines. CNS depressants (cannabinoids, ethanol, barbiturates, and narcotic analgesics) may have additive effects with trihexyphenidyl; an abuse potential exits.

Decreased Effect: May increase gastric degradation of levodopa and decrease the amount of levodopa absorbed by delaying gastric emptying; the opposite may be true for digoxin. Therapeutic effects of cholinergic agents (tacrine, donepezil, rivastigmine, galantamine) and neuroleptics may be antagonized.

Pharmacodynamics/Kinetics

Onset of action: Peak effect: ~1 hour

Half-life elimination: 3.3-4.1 hours

Time to peak, serum: 1-1.5 hours

Excretion: Primarily urine

Pregnancy Risk Factor C

Trihexyphenidyl Hydrochloride *see* Trihexyphenidyl *on page 1340*

Tri-K® *see* Potassium Acetate, Potassium Bicarbonate, and Potassium Citrate *on page 1104*

Trilafon® [DSC] *see* Perphenazine *on page 1070*

Trileptal® *see* Oxcarbazepine *on page 1023*

Tri-Levlen® *see* Ethinyl Estradiol and Levonorgestrel *on page 545*

Trilisate® [DSC] *see* Choline Magnesium Trisalicylate *on page 324*

Tri-Luma™ *see* Fluocinolone, Hydroquinone, and Tretinoin *on page 601*

TriLyte™ *see* Polyethylene Glycol-Electrolyte Solution *on page 1100*

Trimethadione (trye meth a DYE one)

U.S. Brand Names Tridione®

Generic Available No

Synonyms Troxidone

Pharmacologic Category Anticonvulsant, Oxazolidinedione

Use Control absence (petit mal) seizures refractory to other drugs

Local Anesthetic/Vasoconstrictor Precautions No information available to require special precautions

Effects on Dental Treatment No significant effects or complications reported

Mechanism of Action An oxazolidinedione with anticonvulsant sedative properties; elevates the cortical and basal seizure thresholds, and reduces the synaptic response to low frequency impulses

Pregnancy Risk Factor D

Trimethobenzamide (trye meth oh BEN za mide)

U.S. Brand Names Tigan®

Canadian Brand Names Tigan®

Generic Available Yes: Injection

Synonyms Trimethobenzamide Hydrochloride

Pharmacologic Category Anticholinergic Agent; Antiemetic

Use Treatment of nausea and vomiting

Local Anesthetic/Vasoconstrictor Precautions No information available to require special precautions

Effects on Dental Treatment No significant effects or complications reported

Common Adverse Effects Frequency not defined.

Cardiovascular: Hypotension

Central nervous system: Coma, depression, disorientation, dizziness, drowsiness, EPS, headache, opisthotonos, Parkinson-like syndrome, seizures

Hematologic: Blood dyscrasias

Hepatic: Jaundice

Neuromuscular & skeletal: Muscle cramps

Ocular: Blurred vision

Miscellaneous: Hypersensitivity reactions

Mechanism of Action Acts centrally to inhibit the medullary chemoreceptor trigger zone

Pharmacodynamics/Kinetics

Onset of action: Antiemetic: Oral: 10-40 minutes; I.M.: 15-35 minutes

Duration: 3-4 hours

Absorption: Rectal: ~60%

Bioavailability: Oral: 100%

Half-life elimination: 7-9 hours

Time to peak: Oral: 45 minutes; I.M.: 30 minutes

Excretion: Urine (30% to 50%)

Pregnancy Risk Factor C

Trimethobenzamide Hydrochloride *see* Trimethobenzamide *on page 1341*

Trimethoprim (trye METH oh prim)

U.S. Brand Names Primsol®; Proloprim®

Canadian Brand Names Apo-Trimethoprim®; Proloprim®

Generic Available Yes: Tablet

Synonyms TMP

Pharmacologic Category Antibiotic, Miscellaneous

Use Treatment of urinary tract infections due to susceptible strains of *E. coli*, *P. mirabilis*, *K. pneumoniae*, *Enterobacter* sp and coagulase-negative *Staphylococcus* including *S. saprophyticus*; acute otitis media in children; acute exacerbations of chronic bronchitis in adults; in combination with other agents for treatment of toxoplasmosis, *Pneumocystis carinii*; treatment of superficial ocular infections involving the conjunctiva and cornea

Local Anesthetic/Vasoconstrictor Precautions No information available to require special precautions

Effects on Dental Treatment No significant effects or complications reported

Common Adverse Effects Frequency not defined.

Central nervous system: Aseptic meningitis (rare), fever

Dermatologic: Maculopapular rash (3% to 7% at 200 mg/day; incidence higher with larger daily doses), erythema multiforme (rare), exfoliative dermatitis (rare), pruritus (common), phototoxic skin eruptions, Stevens-Johnson syndrome (rare), toxic epidermal necrolysis (rare)

Endocrine & metabolic: Hyperkalemia, hyponatremia

Gastrointestinal: Epigastric distress, glossitis, nausea, vomiting

Hematologic: Leukopenia, megaloblastic anemia, methemoglobinemia, neutropenia, thrombocytopenia

Hepatic: Liver enzyme elevation, cholestatic jaundice (rare)

Renal: BUN and creatinine increased

Miscellaneous: Anaphylaxis, hypersensitivity reactions

Mechanism of Action Inhibits folic acid reduction to tetrahydrofolate, and thereby inhibits microbial growth

(Continued)

Trimethoprim *(Continued)*

Drug Interactions

Cytochrome P450 Effect: Substrate (major) of CYP2C8/9, 3A4; **Inhibits** CYP2C8/9 (moderate)

Increased Effect/Toxicity: Increased effect/toxicity/levels of phenytoin. Concurrent use with ACE inhibitors increases risk of hyperkalemia. Increased myelosuppression with methotrexate. May increase levels of digoxin. Concurrent use with dapsone may increase levels of dapsone and trimethoprim. Concurrent use with procainamide may increase levels of procainamide and trimethoprim. Trimethoprim may increase the levels/effects of amiodarone, fluoxetine, glimepiride, glipizide, nateglinide, phenytoin, pioglitazone, rosiglitazone, sertraline, warfarin, and other CYP2C8/9 substrates.

Decreased Effect: The levels/effects of trimethoprim may be decreased by aminoglutethimide, carbamazepine, nafcillin, nevirapine, phenobarbital, phenytoin, rifampin, rifapentine, secobarbital, and other CYP2C8/9 or 3A4 inducers.

Pharmacodynamics/Kinetics

Absorption: Readily and extensive

Distribution: Widely into body tissues and fluids (middle ear, prostate, bile, aqueous humor, CSF); crosses placenta; enters breast milk

Protein binding: 42% to 46%

Metabolism: Partially hepatic

Half-life elimination: 8-14 hours; prolonged with renal impairment

Time to peak, serum: 1-4 hours

Excretion: Urine (60% to 80%) as unchanged drug

Pregnancy Risk Factor C

Trimethoprim and Polymyxin B

(trye METH oh prim & pol i MIKS in bee)

Related Information

Polymyxin B *on page 1100*

U.S. Brand Names Polytrim®

Canadian Brand Names PMS-Polytrimethoprim; Polytrim™

Generic Available Yes

Synonyms Polymyxin B and Trimethoprim

Pharmacologic Category Antibiotic, Ophthalmic

Use Treatment of surface ocular bacterial conjunctivitis and blepharoconjunctivitis

Local Anesthetic/Vasoconstrictor Precautions No information available to require special precautions

Effects on Dental Treatment No significant effects or complications reported

Pregnancy Risk Factor C

Trimethoprim and Sulfamethoxazole *see* Sulfamethoxazole and Trimethoprim *on page 1246*

Trimetrexate Glucuronate (tri me TREKS ate gloo KYOOR oh nate)

U.S. Brand Names Neutrexin®

Generic Available No

Synonyms NSC-352122

Pharmacologic Category Antineoplastic Agent, Miscellaneous

Use Alternative therapy for the treatment of moderate-to-severe *Pneumocystis carinii* pneumonia (PCP) in immunocompromised patients, including patients with acquired immunodeficiency syndrome (AIDS), who are intolerant of, or are refractory to, co-trimoxazole therapy or for whom co-trimoxazole and pentamidine are contraindicated. **Concurrent folinic acid (leucovorin) must always be administered.**

Unlabeled/Investigational Use Treatment of nonsmall cell lung cancer, metastatic colorectal cancer, metastatic head and neck cancer, pancreatic adenocarcinoma

Local Anesthetic/Vasoconstrictor Precautions No information available to require special precautions

Effects on Dental Treatment Key adverse event(s) related to dental treatment: Stomatitis.

Common Adverse Effects

>10%:

Hematologic: Neutropenia

Hepatic: LFTs increased

1% to 10%:

Central nervous system: Seizures, fever

Dermatologic: Rash
Gastrointestinal: Stomatitis, nausea, vomiting
Hematologic: Thrombocytopenia, anemia
Neuromuscular & skeletal: Peripheral neuropathy
Renal: Increased serum creatinine
Miscellaneous: Flu-like illness, hypersensitivity reactions, anaphylactoid reactions

Mechanism of Action Trimetrexate is a folate antimetabolite that inhibits DNA synthesis by inhibition of dihydrofolate reductase (DHFR); DHFR inhibition reduces the formation of reduced folates and thymidylate synthetase, resulting in inhibition of purine and thymidylic acid synthesis.

Drug Interactions

Increased Effect/Toxicity: Cimetidine, clotrimazole, and ketoconazole may decrease trimetrexate metabolism, resulting in increased serum levels. Trimetrexate may increase toxicity (infections) of live virus vaccines.

Pharmacodynamics/Kinetics

Distribution: V_d: 0.62 L/kg
Metabolism: Extensively hepatic
Half-life elimination: 15-17 hours

Pregnancy Risk Factor D

Trimipramine (trye MI pra meen)

U.S. Brand Names Surmontil®

Canadian Brand Names Apo-Trimip®; Novo-Tripramine; Nu-Trimipramine; Rhotrimine®; Surmontil®

Generic Available No

Synonyms Trimipramine Maleate

Pharmacologic Category Antidepressant, Tricyclic (Tertiary Amine)

Use Treatment of depression

Local Anesthetic/Vasoconstrictor Precautions Use with caution; epinephrine, norepinephrine and levonordefrin have been shown to have an increased pressor response in combination with TCAs

Effects on Dental Treatment Key adverse event(s) related to dental treatment: Xerostomia (normal salivary flow resumes upon discontinuation). Long-term treatment with TCAs, such as trimipramine, increases the risk of caries by reducing salivation and salivary buffer capacity.

Common Adverse Effects Frequency not defined.

Cardiovascular: Arrhythmias, hypotension, hypertension, tachycardia, palpitations, heart block, stroke, myocardial infarction
Central nervous system: Headache, exacerbation of psychosis, confusion, delirium, hallucinations, nervousness, restlessness, delusions, agitation, insomnia, nightmares, anxiety, seizures, drowsiness
Dermatologic: Photosensitivity, rash, petechiae, itching
Endocrine & metabolic: Sexual dysfunction, breast enlargement, galactorrhea, SIADH
Gastrointestinal: Xerostomia, constipation, increased appetite, nausea, unpleasant taste, weight gain, diarrhea, heartburn, vomiting, anorexia, trouble with gums, decreased lower esophageal sphincter tone may cause GE reflux
Genitourinary: Difficult urination, urinary retention, testicular edema
Hematologic: Agranulocytosis, eosinophilia, purpura, thrombocytopenia
Hepatic: Cholestatic jaundice, increased liver enzymes
Neuromuscular & skeletal: Tremors, numbness, tingling, paresthesia, incoordination, ataxia, peripheral neuropathy, extrapyramidal symptoms
Ocular: Blurred vision, eye pain, disturbances in accommodation, mydriasis, increased intraocular pressure
Otic: Tinnitus
Miscellaneous: Allergic reactions

Mechanism of Action Increases the synaptic concentration of serotonin and/or norepinephrine in the central nervous system by inhibition of their reuptake by the presynaptic neuronal membrane

Drug Interactions

Cytochrome P450 Effect: Substrate (major) of CYP2C19, 2D6, 3A4

Increased Effect/Toxicity: Pressor response to I.V. epinephrine, norepinephrine, and phenylephrine may be enhanced in patients receiving TCAs (**Note:** Effect is unlikely with epinephrine or levonordefrin dosages typically administered as infiltration in combination with local anesthetics). Trimipramine increases the effects of amphetamines, anticholinergics, other CNS depressants (sedatives, hypnotics, or ethanol), chlorpropamide, tolazamide, and warfarin. When used with MAO inhibitors, hyperpyrexia, hypertension,

(Continued)

Trimipramine *(Continued)*

tachycardia, confusion, seizures, and **deaths have been reported** (serotonin syndrome). Serotonin syndrome has also been reported with ritonavir (rare).

CYP2C19 inhibitors may increase the levels/effects of trimipramine; example inhibitors include delavirdine, fluconazole, fluvoxamine, gemfibrozil, isoniazid, omeprazole, and ticlopidine. CYP2D6 inhibitors may increase the levels/effects of trimipramine; example inhibitors include chlorpromazine, delavirdine, fluoxetine, miconazole, paroxetine, pergolide, quinidine, quinine, ritonavir, and ropinirole. CYP3A4 inhibitors may increase the levels/effects of trimipramine; example inhibitors include azole antifungals, ciprofloxacin, clarithromycin, diclofenac, doxycycline, erythromycin, imatinib, isoniazid, nefazodone, nicardipine, propofol, protease inhibitors, quinidine, and verapamil. Use of lithium with a TCA may increase the risk for neurotoxicity. Phenothiazines may increase concentration of some TCAs and TCAs may increase concentration of phenothiazines. Combined use of beta-agonists or drugs which prolong QT_c (including quinidine, procainamide, disopyramide, cisapride, sparfloxacin, gatifloxacin, moxifloxacin) with TCAs may predispose patients to cardiac arrhythmias.

Decreased Effect: CYP2C19 inducers may decrease the levels/effects of trimipramine; example inducers include aminoglutethimide, carbamazepine, phenytoin, and rifampin. Trimipramine inhibits the antihypertensive response to bethanidine, clonidine, debrisoquin, guanadrel, guanethidine, guanabenz, and guanfacine. Cholestyramine and colestipol may bind TCAs and reduce their absorption; monitor for altered response. CYP3A4 inducers may decrease the levels/effects of trimipramine; example inducers include aminoglutethimide, carbamazepine, nafcillin, nevirapine, phenobarbital, phenytoin, and rifamycins.

Pharmacodynamics/Kinetics

Distribution: V_d: 17-48 L/kg
Protein binding: 95%; free drug: 3% to 7%
Metabolism: Hepatic; significant first-pass effect
Bioavailability: 18% to 63%
Half-life elimination: 16-40 hours
Excretion: Urine

Pregnancy Risk Factor C

Trimipramine Maleate *see* Trimipramine *on page 1343*
Trimox® *see* Amoxicillin *on page 114*
Tri-Nasal® *see* Triamcinolone *on page 1330*
TriNessa™ *see* Ethinyl Estradiol and Norgestimate *on page 554*
Tri-Norinyl® *see* Ethinyl Estradiol and Norethindrone *on page 550*
Trinsicon® *see* Vitamin B Complex Combinations *on page 1382*
Triostat® *see* Liothyronine *on page 831*

Tripelennamine (tri pel ENN a meen)

U.S. Brand Names PBZ®; PBZ-SR®

Generic Available Yes

Synonyms Tripelennamine Citrate; Tripelennamine Hydrochloride

Pharmacologic Category Antihistamine

Use Perennial and seasonal allergic rhinitis and other allergic symptoms including urticaria

Local Anesthetic/Vasoconstrictor Precautions No information available to require special precautions

Effects on Dental Treatment Key adverse event(s) related to dental treatment: Xerostomia and changes in salivation (normal salivary flow resumes upon discontinuation). Chronic use of antihistamines will inhibit salivary flow, particularly in elderly patients; this may contribute to periodontal disease and oral discomfort.

Common Adverse Effects

>10%:
Central nervous system: Slight to moderate drowsiness
Respiratory: Thickening of bronchial secretions

1% to 10%:
Central nervous system: Headache, fatigue, nervousness, dizziness
Gastrointestinal: Appetite increase, weight gain, nausea, diarrhea, abdominal pain, xerostomia
Neuromuscular & skeletal: Arthralgia
Respiratory: Pharyngitis

Mechanism of Action Competes with histamine for H_1-receptor sites on effector cells in the gastrointestinal tract, blood vessels, and respiratory tract

Drug Interactions

Cytochrome P450 Effect: Inhibits CYP2D6 (moderate)

Increased Effect/Toxicity: Increased effect/toxicity with alcohol, CNS depressants, and MAO inhibitors. Tripelennamine may increase the levels/effects of amphetamines, beta-blockers, dextromethorphan, fluoxetine, lidocaine, mirtazapine, nefazodone, paroxetine, risperidone, ritonavir, thioridazine, tricyclic antidepressants, venlafaxine, and other CYP2D6 substrates.

Decreased Effect: Tripelennamine may decrease the levels/effects of CYP2D6 prodrug substrates (eg, codeine, hydrocodone, oxycodone, tramadol).

Pharmacodynamics/Kinetics

Onset of action: Antihistaminic: 15-30 minutes

Duration: 4-6 hours (up to 8 hours with PBZ-SR®)

Metabolism: Almost completely hepatic

Excretion: Urine

Pregnancy Risk Factor B

Tripelennamine Citrate *see* Tripelennamine *on page 1344*

Tripelennamine Hydrochloride *see* Tripelennamine *on page 1344*

Triphasil® *see* Ethinyl Estradiol and Levonorgestrel *on page 545*

Triple Antibiotic *see* Bacitracin, Neomycin, and Polymyxin B *on page 179*

Triple Care® Antifungal [OTC] *see* Miconazole *on page 922*

Triple Sulfa *see* Sulfabenzamide, Sulfacetamide, and Sulfathiazole *on page 1243*

Tri-Previfem™ *see* Ethinyl Estradiol and Norgestimate *on page 554*

Triprolidine and Pseudoephedrine

(trye PROE li deen & soo doe e FED rin)

Related Information

Pseudoephedrine *on page 1147*

U.S. Brand Names Actifed® Cold and Allergy [OTC]; Allerfrim® [OTC]; Allerphed® [OTC]; Aphedrid™ [OTC]; Aprodine® [OTC]; Genac® [OTC]; Silafed® [OTC]; Tri-Sudo® [OTC]; Uni-Fed® [OTC]

Canadian Brand Names Actifed®

Generic Available Yes

Synonyms Pseudoephedrine and Triprolidine

Pharmacologic Category Alpha/Beta Agonist; Antihistamine

Use Temporary relief of nasal congestion, decongest sinus openings, running nose, sneezing, itching of nose or throat and itchy, watery eyes due to common cold, hay fever, or other upper respiratory allergies

Local Anesthetic/Vasoconstrictor Precautions Use with caution since pseudoephedrine is a sympathomimetic amine which could interact with epinephrine to cause a pressor response

Effects on Dental Treatment Key adverse event(s) related to dental treatment: Pseudoephedrine: Xerostomia (normal salivary flow resumes upon discontinuation). Chronic use of antihistamines will inhibit salivary flow, particularly in elderly patients; this may contribute to periodontal disease and oral discomfort.

Common Adverse Effects Frequency not defined.

Cardiovascular: Tachycardia

Central nervous system: Drowsiness, nervousness, insomnia, transient stimulation, headache, fatigue, dizziness

Respiratory: Thickening of bronchial secretions, pharyngitis

Gastrointestinal: Appetite increase, weight gain, nausea, diarrhea, abdominal pain, xerostomia

Genitourinary: Dysuria

Neuromuscular & skeletal: Arthralgia, weakness

Miscellaneous: Diaphoresis

Mechanism of Action Refer to Pseudoephedrine monograph

Triprolidine is a member of the propylamine (alkylamine) chemical class of H_1-antagonist antihistamines. As such, it is considered to be relatively less sedating than traditional antihistamines of the ethanolamine, phenothiazine, and ethylenediamine classes of antihistamines. Triprolidine has a shorter half-life and duration of action than most of the other alkylamine antihistamines. Like all H_1-antagonist antihistamines, the mechanism of action of triprolidine is believed to involve competitive blockade of H_1-receptor sites resulting in the inability of histamine to combine with its receptor sites and exert its usual effects on target cells. Antihistamines do not interrupt any effects of histamine which have already occurred. Therefore, these agents

(Continued)

Triprolidine and Pseudoephedrine *(Continued)*

are used more successfully in the prevention rather than the treatment of histamine-induced reactions.

Drug Interactions

Cytochrome P450 Effect: Triprolidine: **Inhibits** CYP2D6 (weak)

Increased Effect/Toxicity: Increased toxicity with MAO inhibitors or drugs with MAO inhibiting activity such as linezolid or furazolidone (hypertensive crisis). May increase toxicity of sympathomimetics, CNS depressants, and alcohol.

Decreased Effect: Decreased effect of guanethidine, reserpine, methyldopa.

Pharmacodynamics/Kinetics See Pseudoephedrine monograph.

Pregnancy Risk Factor C

Triprolidine, Codeine, and Pseudoephedrine *see* Triprolidine, Pseudoephedrine, and Codeine *on page 1346*

Triprolidine, Pseudoephedrine, and Codeine

(trye PROE li deen, soo doe e FED rin, & KOE deen)

Related Information

Codeine *on page 369*

Pseudoephedrine *on page 1147*

U.S. Brand Names Triacin-C® [DSC]

Canadian Brand Names CoActifed®; Covan®; ratio-Cotridin

Generic Available No

Synonyms Codeine, Pseudoephedrine, and Triprolidine; Pseudoephedrine, Triprolidine, and Codeine Pseudoephedrine, Codeine, and Triprolidine; Triprolidine, Codeine, and Pseudoephedrine; Triprolidine, Pseudoephedrine, and Codeine, Triprolidine, and Pseudoephedrine

Pharmacologic Category Antihistamine/Decongestant/Antitussive

Use Symptomatic relief of upper respiratory symptoms and cough

Local Anesthetic/Vasoconstrictor Precautions Use with caution since pseudoephedrine is a sympathomimetic amine which could interact with epinephrine to cause a pressor response

Effects on Dental Treatment Key adverse event(s) related to dental treatment: Pseudoephedrine: Xerostomia (normal salivary flow resumes upon discontinuation).

Common Adverse Effects Frequency not defined.

Cardiovascular: Hypotension

Central nervous system: Sedation, dizziness, drowsiness, increased ICP, lightheadedness, dysphoria, euphoria, headache, agitation, hallucinations, seizures, respiratory depression

Dermatologic: Pruritus, rash

Gastrointestinal: Constipation, nausea, vomiting, anorexia, xerostomia, taste disturbance, biliary tract spasm

Genitourinary: Urinary retention, urinary tract spasm

Neuromuscular & skeletal: Muscle tremor, paresthesia, muscular rigidity (rare)

Ocular: Blurred vision, nystagmus

Miscellaneous: Diaphoresis, physical or psychological dependence with continued use, withdrawal syndrome

Restrictions C-V (CDSA-I)

Drug Interactions

Cytochrome P450 Effect:

Triprolidine: **Inhibits** CYP2D6 (weak)

Codeine: **Substrate** of CYP2D6 (major), 3A4 (minor); **Inhibits** CYP2D6 (weak)

Pharmacodynamics/Kinetics See Pseudoephedrine and Codeine monographs.

Pregnancy Risk Factor C

Triprolidine, Pseudoephedrine, and Codeine, Triprolidine, and Pseudoephedrine *see* Triprolidine, Pseudoephedrine, and Codeine *on page 1346*

TripTone® [OTC] *see* DimenhyDRINATE *on page 446*

Triptoraline *see* Triptorelin *on page 1346*

Triptorelin (trip toe REL in)

U.S. Brand Names Trelstar™ Depot; Trelstar™ LA

Canadian Brand Names Trelstar™ Depot

Generic Available No

Synonyms AY-25650; CL-118,532; D-Trp(6)-LHRH; Triptoraline; Triptorelin Pamoate; Tryptoreline

Pharmacologic Category Gonadotropin Releasing Hormone Agonist

Use Palliative treatment of advanced prostate cancer as an alternative to orchiectomy or estrogen administration

Unlabeled/Investigational Use Treatment of endometriosis, growth hormone deficiency, hyperandrogenism, *in vitro* fertilization, ovarian carcinoma, pancreatic carcinoma, precocious puberty, uterine leiomyomata

Local Anesthetic/Vasoconstrictor Precautions No information available to require special precautions

Effects on Dental Treatment No significant effects or complications reported

Common Adverse Effects As reported with Trelstar™ Depot and Trelstar™ LA; frequency of effect may vary by product:

>10%:

- Central nervous system: Headache (30% to 60%)
- Endocrine & metabolic: Hot flashes (95% to 100%), glucose increased, hemoglobin decreased, RBC count decreased
- Hepatic: Alkaline phosphatase increased, ALT increased, AST increased
- Neuromuscular & skeletal: Skeletal pain (12% to 13%)
- Renal: BUN increased

1% to 10%:

- Cardiovascular: Leg edema (6%), hypertension (4%), chest pain (2%), peripheral edema (1%)
- Central nervous system: Dizziness (1% to 3%), pain (2% to 3%), emotional lability (1%), fatigue (2%), insomnia (2%)
- Dermatologic: Rash (2%), pruritus (1%)
- Endocrine & metabolic: Alkaline phosphatase increased (2%), breast pain (2%), gynocomastia (2%), libido decreased (2%), tumor flare (8%)
- Gastrointestinal: Nausea (3%), anorexia (2%), constipation (2%), dyspepsia (2%), vomiting (2%), abdominal pain (1%), diarrhea (1%)
- Genitourinary: Dysuria (5%), impotence (2% to 7%), urinary retention (1%), urinary tract infection (1%)
- Hematologic: Anemia (1%)
- Local: Injection site pain (4%)
- Neuromuscular & skeletal: Leg pain (2% to 5%), back pain (3%), arthralgia (2%), leg cramps (2%), myalgia (1%), weakness (1%)
- Ocular: Conjunctivitis (1%), eye pain (1%)
- Respiratory: Cough (2%), dyspnea (1%), pharyngitis (1%)

Postmarketing and/or case reports: Anaphylaxis, angioedema, hypersensitivity reactions, spinal cord compression, renal dysfunction

Mechanism of Action Causes suppression of ovarian and testicular steroidogenesis due to decreased levels of LH and FSH with subsequent decrease in testosterone (male) and estrogen (female) levels. After chronic and continuous administration, usually 2-4 weeks after initiation, a sustained decrease in LH and FSH secretion occurs.

Drug Interactions

Increased Effect/Toxicity: Not studied. Hyperprolactinemic drugs (dopamine antagonists such as antipsychotics, and metoclopramide) are contraindicated.

Decreased Effect: Not studied. Hyperprolactinemic drugs (dopamine antagonists such as antipsychotics, and metoclopramide) are contraindicated.

Pharmacodynamics/Kinetics

Absorption: Oral: Not active

Distribution: V_d: 30-33 L

Protein binding: None

Metabolism: Unknown; unlikely to involve CYP; no known metabolites

Half-life elimination: 2.8 ± 1.2 hours

- Moderate to severe renal impairment: 6.5-7.7 hours
- Hepatic impairment: 7.6 hours

Time to peak: 1-3 hours

Excretion: Urine (42% as intact peptide); hepatic

Pregnancy Risk Factor X

Triptorelin Pamoate *see* Triptorelin *on page 1346*

Tris Buffer *see* Tromethamine *on page 1348*

Tris(hydroxymethyl)aminomethane *see* Tromethamine *on page 1348*

Tri-Sprintec™ *see* Ethinyl Estradiol and Norgestimate *on page 554*

Tri-Sudo® [OTC] *see* Triprolidine and Pseudoephedrine *on page 1345*

Tri-Vent™ DM *see* Guaifenesin, Pseudoephedrine, and Dextromethorphan *on page 676*

Tri-Vent™ HC *see* Hydrocodone, Carbinoxamine, and Pseudoephedrine *on page 712*

Trivora® *see* Ethinyl Estradiol and Levonorgestrel *on page 545*

Trizivir® *see* Abacavir, Lamivudine, and Zidovudine *on page 43*

Trobicin® *see* Spectinomycin *on page 1234*

Trocaine® [OTC] *see* Benzocaine *on page 191*

Troleandomycin (troe lee an doe MYE sin)

U.S. Brand Names Tao®

Generic Available No

Synonyms Triacetyloleandomycin

Pharmacologic Category Antibiotic, Macrolide

Use Antibiotic with spectrum of activity similar to erythromycin

Local Anesthetic/Vasoconstrictor Precautions No information available to require special precautions

Effects on Dental Treatment No significant effects or complications reported

Mechanism of Action Decreases methylprednisolone clearance from a linear first order decline to a nonlinear decline in plasma concentration. Troleandomycin also has an undefined action independent of its effects on steroid elimination. Inhibits RNA-dependent protein synthesis at the chain elongation step; binds to the 50S ribosomal subunit resulting in blockage of transpeptidation.

Pregnancy Risk Factor C

Tromethamine (troe METH a meen)

U.S. Brand Names THAM®

Generic Available No

Synonyms Tris Buffer; Tris(hydroxymethyl)aminomethane

Pharmacologic Category Alkalinizing Agent, Parenteral

Use Correction of metabolic acidosis associated with cardiac bypass surgery or cardiac arrest; to correct excess acidity of stored blood that is preserved with acid citrate dextrose; to prime the pump-oxygenator during cardiac bypass surgery; indicated in infants needing alkalinization after receiving maximum sodium bicarbonate (8-10 mEq/kg/24 hours); (advantage of THAM® is that it alkalinizes without increasing pCO_2 and sodium)

Local Anesthetic/Vasoconstrictor Precautions No information available to require special precautions

Effects on Dental Treatment No significant effects or complications reported

Common Adverse Effects 1% to 10%:

Cardiovascular: Venospasm

Local: Tissue irritation, necrosis with extravasation

Mechanism of Action Acts as a proton acceptor, which combines with hydrogen ions to form bicarbonate buffer, to correct acidosis

Pharmacodynamics/Kinetics

Absorption: 30% of dose is not ionized

Excretion: Urine (>75%) within 3 hours

Pregnancy Risk Factor C

Tronolane® [OTC] *see* Pramoxine *on page 1109*

Tropicacyl® *see* Tropicamide *on page 1348*

Tropicamide (troe PIK a mide)

U.S. Brand Names Mydriacyl®; Opticyl®; Tropicacyl®

Canadian Brand Names Diotrope®; Mydriacyl®

Generic Available Yes

Synonyms Bistropamide

Pharmacologic Category Ophthalmic Agent, Mydriatic

Use Short-acting mydriatic used in diagnostic procedures; as well as preoperatively and postoperatively; treatment of some cases of acute iritis, iridocyclitis, and keratitis

Local Anesthetic/Vasoconstrictor Precautions No information available to require special precautions

Effects on Dental Treatment No significant effects or complications reported

Mechanism of Action Prevents the sphincter muscle of the iris and the muscle of the ciliary body from responding to cholinergic stimulation

Pregnancy Risk Factor C

Tropicamide and Hydroxyamphetamine *see* Hydroxyamphetamine and Tropicamide *on page 720*

Trovafloxacin (TROE va floks a sin)

U.S. Brand Names Trovan® [DSC]

Mexican Brand Names Trovan®

Generic Available No

Synonyms Alatrofloxacin Mesylate; CP-99,219-27

Pharmacologic Category Antibiotic, Quinolone

Use Should be used only in life- or limb-threatening infections

Treatment of nosocomial pneumonia, community-acquired pneumonia, complicated intra-abdominal infections, gynecologic/pelvic infections, complicated skin and skin structure infections

Local Anesthetic/Vasoconstrictor Precautions No information available to require special precautions

Effects on Dental Treatment No significant effects or complications reported

Common Adverse Effects Note: Fatalities have occurred in patients developing hepatic necrosis.

1% to 10% (range reported in clinical trials):

Central nervous system: Dizziness (2% to 11%), lightheadedness (<1% to 4%), headache (1% to 5%)

Dermatologic: Rash (<1% to 2%), pruritus (<1% to 2%)

Gastrointestinal: Nausea (4% to 8%), abdominal pain (<1% to 1%), vomiting, diarrhea

Genitourinary: Vaginitis (<1% to 1%)

Hepatic: Increased LFTs

Local: Injection site reaction, pain, or inflammation

Mechanism of Action Inhibits DNA-gyrase in susceptible organisms; inhibits relaxation of supercoiled DNA and promotes breakage of double-stranded DNA

Drug Interactions

Increased Effect/Toxicity: Concurrent use of corticosteroids may increase risk of tendon rupture.

Decreased Effect: Coadministration with antacids containing aluminum or magnesium, citric acid/sodium citrate, sucralfate, and iron markedly reduces absorption of trovafloxacin. Separate oral administration by at least 2 hours. Coadministration of intravenous morphine also reduces absorption. Separate I.V. morphine by 2 hours (when trovafloxacin is taken in fasting state) or 4 hours (when taken with food). Do not administer multivalent cations (eg, calcium, magnesium) through the same intravenous line.

Pharmacodynamics/Kinetics

Distribution: Concentration in most tissues greater than plasma or serum

Protein binding: 76%

Metabolism: Hepatic conjugation; glucuronidation 13%, acetylation 9%

Bioavailability: 88%

Half-life elimination: 9-12 hours

Time to peak, serum: Oral: Within 2 hours

Excretion: Feces (43% as unchanged drug); urine (6% as unchanged drug)

Pregnancy Risk Factor C

Trovan® [DSC] *see* Trovafloxacin *on page 1348*

Troxidone *see* Trimethadione *on page 1340*

Trusopt® *see* Dorzolamide *on page 464*

Trypsin, Balsam Peru, and Castor Oil

(TRIP sin, BAL sam pe RUE, & KAS tor oyl)

U.S. Brand Names Granulex®

Generic Available Yes

Synonyms Balsam Peru, Trypsin, and Castor Oil; Castor Oil, Trypsin, and Balsam Peru

Pharmacologic Category Protectant, Topical

Use Treatment of decubitus ulcers, varicose ulcers, debridement of eschar, dehiscent wounds and sunburn

Local Anesthetic/Vasoconstrictor Precautions No information available to require special precautions

Effects on Dental Treatment No significant effects or complications reported

Tryptoreline *see* Triptorelin *on page 1346*

TSH *see* Thyrotropin Alpha *on page 1294*

TSPA *see* Thiotepa *on page 1291*

TST *see* Tuberculin Tests *on page 1349*

T-Stat® *see* Erythromycin *on page 508*

T-Tab® *see* Clorazepate *on page 362*

Tuberculin Purified Protein Derivative *see* Tuberculin Tests *on page 1349*

Tuberculin Skin Test *see* Tuberculin Tests *on page 1349*

Tuberculin Tests (too BER kyoo lin tests)

U.S. Brand Names Aplisol®; Tubersol®

Generic Available No

(Continued)

Tuberculin Tests *(Continued)*

Synonyms Mantoux; PPD; Tine Test; TST; Tuberculin Purified Protein Derivative; Tuberculin Skin Test

Pharmacologic Category Diagnostic Agent

Use Skin test in diagnosis of tuberculosis, cell-mediated immunodeficiencies

Local Anesthetic/Vasoconstrictor Precautions No information available to require special precautions

Effects on Dental Treatment No significant effects or complications reported

Common Adverse Effects Frequency not defined.

Dermatologic: Ulceration, necrosis, vesiculation

Local: Pain at injection site

Mechanism of Action Tuberculosis results in individuals becoming sensitized to certain antigenic components of the *M. tuberculosis* organism. Culture extracts called tuberculins are contained in tuberculin skin test preparations. Upon intracutaneous injection of these culture extracts, a classic delayed (cellular) hypersensitivity reaction occurs. This reaction is characteristic of a delayed course (peak occurs >24 hours after injection, induration of the skin secondary to cell infiltration, and occasional vesiculation and necrosis). Delayed hypersensitivity reactions to tuberculin may indicate infection with a variety of nontuberculosis mycobacteria, or vaccination with the live attenuated mycobacterial strain of *M. bovis* vaccine, BCG, in addition to previous natural infection with *M. tuberculosis*.

Pharmacodynamics/Kinetics

Onset of action: Delayed hypersensitivity reactions: 5-6 hours

Peak effect: 48-72 hours

Duration: Reactions subside over a few days

Pregnancy Risk Factor C

Tuberculosis *see page 1495*

Tubersol® *see* Tuberculin Tests *on page 1349*

Tuinal® [DSC] *see* Amobarbital and Secobarbital *on page 112*

Tums® [OTC] *see* Calcium Carbonate *on page 245*

Tums® 500 [OTC] *see* Calcium Carbonate *on page 245*

Tums® E-X [OTC] *see* Calcium Carbonate *on page 245*

Tums® Extra Strength Sugar Free [OTC] *see* Calcium Carbonate *on page 245*

Tums® Smooth Dissolve [OTC] *see* Calcium Carbonate *on page 245*

Tums® Ultra [OTC] *see* Calcium Carbonate *on page 245*

Tussafed® *see* Carbinoxamine, Pseudoephedrine, and Dextromethorphan *on page 263*

Tussend® Expectorant *see* Hydrocodone, Pseudoephedrine, and Guaifenesin *on page 713*

Tussi-12® *see* Carbetapentane and Chlorpheniramine *on page 260*

Tussi-12® D *see* Carbetapentane, Phenylephrine, and Pyrilamine *on page 261*

Tussi-12® DS *see* Carbetapentane, Phenylephrine, and Pyrilamine *on page 261*

Tussi-12 S™ *see* Carbetapentane and Chlorpheniramine *on page 260*

Tussigon® *see* Hydrocodone and Homatropine *on page 709*

Tussin [OTC] *see* Guaifenesin *on page 672*

Tussionex® *see* Hydrocodone and Chlorpheniramine *on page 707*

Tussi-Organidin® DM NR *see* Guaifenesin and Dextromethorphan *on page 673*

Tussi-Organidin® NR *see* Guaifenesin and Codeine *on page 673*

Tussi-Organidin® S-NR *see* Guaifenesin and Codeine *on page 673*

Tussizone-12 RF™ *see* Carbetapentane and Chlorpheniramine *on page 260*

Tusstat® *see* DiphenhydrAMINE *on page 448*

Twice-A-Day® [OTC] *see* Oxymetazoline *on page 1034*

Twilite® [OTC] *see* DiphenhydrAMINE *on page 448*

Twinrix® *see* Hepatitis A (Inactivated) and Hepatitis B (Recombinant) Vaccine *on page 686*

Tylenol® [OTC] *see* Acetaminophen *on page 47*

Tylenol® 8 Hour [OTC] *see* Acetaminophen *on page 47*

Tylenol® Allergy Sinus [OTC] *see* Acetaminophen, Chlorpheniramine, and Pseudoephedrine *on page 58*

Tylenol® Arthritis Pain [OTC] *see* Acetaminophen *on page 47*

Tylenol® Children's [OTC] *see* Acetaminophen *on page 47*

Tylenol® Cold Day Non-Drowsy [OTC] *see* Acetaminophen, Dextromethorphan, and Pseudoephedrine *on page 59*

Tylenol® Cold, Infants [OTC] *see* Acetaminophen and Pseudoephedrine *on page 53*
Tylenol® Extra Strength [OTC] *see* Acetaminophen *on page 47*
Tylenol® Flu Non-Drowsy Maximum Strength [OTC] *see* Acetaminophen, Dextromethorphan, and Pseudoephedrine *on page 59*
Tylenol® Infants [OTC] *see* Acetaminophen *on page 47*
Tylenol® Junior Strength [OTC] *see* Acetaminophen *on page 47*
Tylenol® PM Extra Strength [OTC] *see* Acetaminophen and Diphenhydramine *on page 53*
Tylenol® Severe Allergy [OTC] *see* Acetaminophen and Diphenhydramine *on page 53*
Tylenol® Sinus, Children's [OTC] *see* Acetaminophen and Pseudoephedrine *on page 53*
Tylenol® Sinus Day Non-Drowsy [OTC] *see* Acetaminophen and Pseudoephedrine *on page 53*
Tylenol® Sore Throat [OTC] *see* Acetaminophen *on page 47*
Tylenol® With Codeine *see* Acetaminophen and Codeine *on page 50*
Tylox® *see* Oxycodone and Acetaminophen *on page 1029*
Typhim Vi® *see* Typhoid Vaccine *on page 1351*

Typhoid Vaccine (TYE foid vak SEEN)

Related Information

Immunizations (Vaccines) *on page 1614*

U.S. Brand Names Typhim Vi®; Vivotif Berna®

Canadian Brand Names Vivotif Berna®

Generic Available No

Synonyms Typhoid Vaccine Live Oral Ty21a

Pharmacologic Category Vaccine

Use Typhoid vaccine: Live, attenuated Ty21a typhoid vaccine should not be administered to immunocompromised persons, including those known to be infected with HIV. Parenteral inactivated vaccine is a theoretically safer alternative for this group.

Parenteral: Promotes active immunity to typhoid fever for patients intimately exposed to a typhoid carrier or foreign travel to a typhoid fever endemic area

Oral: For immunization of children >6 years of age and adults who expect intimate exposure of or household contact with typhoid fever, travelers to areas of world with risk of exposure to typhoid fever, and workers in microbiology laboratories with expected frequent contact with *S. typhi*

Local Anesthetic/Vasoconstrictor Precautions No information available to require special precautions

Effects on Dental Treatment No significant effects or complications reported

Common Adverse Effects All serious adverse reactions must be reported to the U.S. Department of Health and Human Services (DHHS) Vaccine Adverse Event Reporting System (VAERS) 1-800-822-7967.

Oral: 1% to 10%:

Central nervous system: Headache, fever

Dermatologic: Rash

Gastrointestinal: Abdominal discomfort, stomach cramps, diarrhea, nausea, vomiting

Injection:

>10%:

Central nervous system: Headache (13% to 20%), fever (3% to 11%), malaise (4% to 24%)

Dermatologic: Local tenderness (13% to 98%), induration (5% to 15%), pain at injection site (7% to 41%)

1% to 10%:

Central nervous system: Fever ≥100°F (2%)

Gastrointestinal: Nausea (2% to 8%), diarrhea (3% to 4%), vomiting (2%)

Local: Erythema at injection site (4% to 5%)

Neuromuscular & skeletal: Myalgia (3% to 7%)

Mechanism of Action Virulent strains of *Salmonella typhi* cause disease by penetrating the intestinal mucosa and entering the systemic circulation via the lymphatic vasculature. One possible mechanism of conferring immunity may be the provocation of a local immune response in the intestinal tract induced by oral ingesting of a live strain with subsequent aborted infection. The ability of *Salmonella typhi* to produce clinical disease (and to elicit an immune response) is dependent on the bacteria having a complete lipopolysaccharide. The live attenuate Ty21a strain lacks the enzyme UDP-4-galactose epimerase so that lipopolysaccharide is only synthesized under conditions that induce bacterial autolysis. Thus, the strain remains avirulent despite the production of

(Continued)

Typhoid Vaccine *(Continued)*

sufficient lipopolysaccharide to evoke a protective immune response. Despite low levels of lipopolysaccharide synthesis, cells lyse before gaining a virulent phenotype due to the intracellular accumulation of metabolic intermediates.

Pharmacodynamics/Kinetics

Onset of action: Immunity to *Salmonella typhi*: Oral: ~1 week

Duration: Immunity: Oral: ~5 years; Parenteral: ~3 years

Pregnancy Risk Factor C

Typhoid Vaccine Live Oral Ty21a *see* Typhoid Vaccine *on page 1351*
Tyzine® *see* Tetrahydrozoline *on page 1282*
Tyzine® Pediatric *see* Tetrahydrozoline *on page 1282*
U-90152S *see* Delavirdine *on page 403*
UCB-P071 *see* Cetirizine *on page 298*
UK92480 *see* Sildenafil *on page 1219*
UK109496 *see* Voriconazole *on page 1385*
Ulcerease® [OTC] *see* Phenol *on page 1075*
Ultiva® *see* Remifentanil *on page 1172*
Ultracet™ *see* Acetaminophen and Tramadol *on page 54*
Ultram® *see* Tramadol *on page 1319*
Ultra Mide® *see* Urea *on page 1353*
Ultraprin [OTC] *see* Ibuprofen *on page 728*
Ultrase® *see* Pancrelipase *on page 1042*
Ultrase® MT *see* Pancrelipase *on page 1042*
Ultra Tears® [OTC] *see* Artificial Tears *on page 148*
Ultravate® *see* Halobetasol *on page 681*
Ultravist® *see* Iopromide *on page 760*
Unasyn® *see* Ampicillin and Sulbactam *on page 126*

Undecylenic Acid and Derivatives

(un de sil EN ik AS id & dah RIV ah tivs)

U.S. Brand Names Fungi-Nail® [OTC]

Generic Available No

Synonyms Zinc Undecylenate

Pharmacologic Category Antifungal Agent, Topical

Use Treatment of athlete's foot (tinea pedis); ringworm (except nails and scalp)

Local Anesthetic/Vasoconstrictor Precautions No information available to require special precautions

Effects on Dental Treatment No significant effects or complications reported

Uni-Cof *see* Pseudoephedrine, Dihydrocodeine, and Chlorpheniramine *on page 1150*
Uni-Fed® [OTC] *see* Triprolidine and Pseudoephedrine *on page 1345*
Uniphyl® *see* Theophylline *on page 1285*
Uniretic® *see* Moexipril and Hydrochlorothiazide *on page 941*
Unisom® Maximum Strength SleepGels® [OTC] *see* DiphenhydrAMINE *on page 448*
Unithroid® *see* Levothyroxine *on page 817*
Univasc® *see* Moexipril *on page 940*
Unna's Boot *see* Zinc Gelatin *on page 1400*
Unna's Paste *see* Zinc Gelatin *on page 1400*

Unoprostone

(yoo noe PROS tone)

U.S. Brand Names Rescula®

Generic Available No

Synonyms Unoprostone Isopropyl

Pharmacologic Category Ophthalmic Agent, Miscellaneous

Use To lower intraocular pressure (IOP) in patients with open-angle glaucoma or ocular hypertension; should be used in patients who are not tolerant of, or failed treatment with other IOP-lowering medications

Local Anesthetic/Vasoconstrictor Precautions No information available to require special precautions

Effects on Dental Treatment No significant effects or complications reported

Mechanism of Action The exact mechanism of action is unknown; however, unoprostone decreases IOP by increasing the outflow of aqueous humor. Cardiovascular and pulmonary function were not affected in clinical studies. IOP was decreased by 3-4 mm Hg in patients with a mean baseline IOP of 23 mm Hg.

Pregnancy Risk Factor C

Unoprostone Isopropyl *see* Unoprostone *on page 1352*

Urea (yoor EE a)

U.S. Brand Names Amino-Cerv™; Aquacare® [OTC]; Aquaphilic® With Carbamide [OTC]; Carmol® 10 [OTC]; Carmol® 20 [OTC]; Carmol® 40; Carmol® Deep Cleaning; DPM™ [OTC]; Gormel® [OTC]; Lanaphilic® [OTC]; Nutraplus® [OTC]; Rea-Lo® [OTC]; Ultra Mide®; Ureacin® [OTC]; Vanamide™

Canadian Brand Names UltraMide 25™; Uremol®; Urisec®

Mexican Brand Names Derma Keri®; Dermoplast®

Generic Available No

Synonyms Carbamide

Pharmacologic Category Diuretic, Osmotic; Keratolytic Agent; Topical Skin Product

Use

Topical: Keratolytic agent to soften nails or skin; OTC: Moisturizer for dry, rough skin

Vaginal: Treatment of cervicitis

Local Anesthetic/Vasoconstrictor Precautions No information available to require special precautions

Effects on Dental Treatment No significant effects or complications reported

Common Adverse Effects Frequency not defined: Topical: Local: Transient stinging, local irritation

Mechanism of Action

Topical: Urea softens hyperkeratotic areas by dissolving the intracellular matrix, resulting in loosening the horny layer of the skin, or softening and debridement of the nail plate

Vaginal: Urea aids in debridement, promotes epithelialization and prevents excessive tissue formation

Pregnancy Risk Factor C

Urea and Hydrocortisone (yoor EE a & hye droe KOR ti sone)

Related Information

Hydrocortisone *on page 714*
Urea *on page 1353*

U.S. Brand Names Carmol-HC®

Canadian Brand Names Ti-U-Lac® H; Uremol® HC

Generic Available No

Synonyms Hydrocortisone and Urea

Pharmacologic Category Corticosteroid, Topical

Use Inflammation of corticosteroid-responsive dermatoses

Local Anesthetic/Vasoconstrictor Precautions No information available to require special precautions

Effects on Dental Treatment No significant effects or complications reported

Drug Interactions

Cytochrome P450 Effect: Hydrocortisone: **Substrate** of CYP3A4 (minor); **Induces** CYP3A4 (weak)

Pharmacodynamics/Kinetics See individual agents.

Pregnancy Risk Factor C

Ureacin® [OTC] *see* Urea *on page 1353*

Urea Peroxide *see* Carbamide Peroxide *on page 259*

Urecholine® *see* Bethanechol *on page 203*

Urex® *see* Methenamine *on page 892*

Urimar-T *see* Methenamine, Sodium Biphosphate, Phenyl Salicylate, Methylene Blue, and Hyoscyamine *on page 893*

Urimax® *see* Methenamine, Sodium Biphosphate, Phenyl Salicylate, Methylene Blue, and Hyoscyamine *on page 893*

Urispas® *see* Flavoxate *on page 591*

Uristat® [OTC] *see* Phenazopyridine *on page 1072*

Urocit®-K *see* Potassium Citrate *on page 1105*

Urofollitropin *see* Follitropins *on page 626*

Uro-KP-Neutral® *see* Potassium Phosphate and Sodium Phosphate *on page 1107*

Uro-Mag® [OTC] *see* Magnesium Oxide *on page 854*

Uroxatral™ *see* Alfuzosin *on page 80*

Urso® *see* Ursodiol *on page 1354*

Ursodeoxycholic Acid *see* Ursodiol *on page 1354*

Ursodiol (ER soe dye ole)

U.S. Brand Names Actigall®; Urso®

Canadian Brand Names Urso®

Mexican Brand Names Ursofalk®

Generic Available Yes: Capsule

Synonyms Ursodeoxycholic Acid

Pharmacologic Category Gallstone Dissolution Agent

Use Actigall®: Gallbladder stone dissolution; prevention of gallstones in obese patients experiencing rapid weight loss; Urso®: Primary biliary cirrhosis

Unlabeled/Investigational Use Liver transplantation

Local Anesthetic/Vasoconstrictor Precautions No information available to require special precautions

Effects on Dental Treatment No significant effects or complications reported

Common Adverse Effects

>10%:

- Central nervous system: Headache (up to 25%), dizziness (up to 17%)
- Gastrointestinal: In treatment of primary biliary cirrhosis: Constipation (up to 26%)

1% to 10%:

- Dermatologic: Rash (<1% to 3%), alopecia (<1% to 5%)
- Gastrointestinal:
  - In gallstone dissolution: Most GI events (diarrhea, nausea, vomiting) are similar to placebo and attributable to gallstone disease.
  - In treatment of primary biliary cirrhosis: Diarrhea (1%)
- Hematologic: Leukopenia (3%)
- Miscellaneous: Allergy (5%)

Mechanism of Action Decreases the cholesterol content of bile and bile stones by reducing the secretion of cholesterol from the liver and the fractional reabsorption of cholesterol by the intestines. Mechanism of action in primary biliary cirrhosis is not clearly defined.

Drug Interactions

Decreased Effect: Decreased effect with aluminum-containing antacids, cholestyramine, colestipol, clofibrate, and oral contraceptives (estrogens).

Pharmacodynamics/Kinetics

Metabolism: Undergoes extensive enterohepatic recycling; following hepatic conjugation and biliary secretion, the drug is hydrolyzed to active ursodiol, where it is recycled or transformed to lithocholic acid by colonic microbial flora

Half-life elimination: 100 hours

Excretion: Feces

Pregnancy Risk Factor B

UTI Relief® [OTC] *see* Phenazopyridine *on page 1072*

Uvadex® *see* Methoxsalen *on page 902*

Vagifem® *see* Estradiol *on page 518*

Vagi-Gard® [OTC] *see* Povidone-Iodine *on page 1107*

Vagistat®-1 [OTC] *see* Tioconazole *on page 1302*

Valacyclovir (val ay SYE kloe veer)

Related Information

Acyclovir *on page 64*

Sexually-Transmitted Diseases *on page 1504*

Systemic Viral Diseases *on page 1519*

U.S. Brand Names Valtrex®

Canadian Brand Names Valtrex®

Generic Available No

Synonyms Valacyclovir Hydrochloride

Pharmacologic Category Antiviral Agent, Oral

Use Treatment of herpes zoster (shingles) in immunocompetent patients; treatment of first-episode genital herpes; episodic treatment of recurrent genital herpes; suppression of recurrent genital herpes and reduction of heterosexual transmission of genital herpes in immunocompetent patients; suppression of genital herpes in HIV-infected individuals; treatment of herpes labialis (cold sores)

Local Anesthetic/Vasoconstrictor Precautions No information available to require special precautions

Effects on Dental Treatment No significant effects or complications reported

Significant Adverse Effects

>10%: Central nervous system: Headache (14% to 35%)

1% to 10%:

Central nervous system: Dizziness (2% to 4%), depression (0% to 7%)
Endocrine: Dysmenorrhea (≤1% to 8%)
Gastrointestinal: Abdominal pain (2% to 11%), vomiting (<1% to 6%), nausea (6% to 15%)
Hematologic: Leukopenia (≤1%), thrombocytopenia (≤1%)
Hepatic: AST increased (1% to 4%)
Neuromuscular & skeletal: Arthralgia (≤1 to 6%)

<1% (Limited to important or life-threatening): Acute hypersensitivity reactions (angioedema, anaphylaxis, dyspnea, pruritus, rash, urticaria); agitation, alopecia, aplastic anemia, coma, confusion, dysarthria, encephalopathy, erythema multiforme, hallucinations (auditory and visual), hemolytic uremic syndrome (HUS), hepatitis, leukocytoclastic vasculitis, mania, photosensitivity reaction, psychosis, rash, renal failure, thrombotic thrombocytopenic purpura/hemolytic uremic syndrome, tremors

Dosage Oral:

Adolescents and Adults: Herpes labialis (cold sores): 2 g twice daily for 1 day (separate doses by ~12 hours)

Adults:

Herpes zoster (shingles): 1 g 3 times/day for 7 days
Genital herpes:
Initial episode: 1 g twice daily for 10 days
Recurrent episode: 500 mg twice daily for 3 days
Reduction of transmission: 500 mg once daily (source partner)
Suppressive therapy:
Immunocompetent patients: 1000 mg once daily (500 mg once daily in patients with <9 recurrences per year)
HIV-infected patients (CD4 ≥100 cells/mm^3): 500 mg twice daily

Dosing interval in renal impairment:

Herpes zoster: Adults:
Cl_{cr} 30-49 mL/minute: 1 g every 12 hours
Cl_{cr} 10-29 mL/minute: 1 g every 24 hours
Cl_{cr} <10 mL/minute: 500 mg every 24 hours

Genital herpes: Adults:
Initial episode:
Cl_{cr} 10-29 mL/minute: 1 g every 24 hours
Cl_{cr} <10 mL/minute: 500 mg every 24 hours
Recurrent episode: Cl_{cr} <10-29 mL/minute: 500 mg every 24 hours
Suppressive therapy: Cl_{cr} <10-29 mL/minute:
For usual dose of 1 g every 24 hours, decrease dose to 500 mg every 24 hours
For usual dose of 500 mg every 24 hours, decrease dose to 500 mg every 48 hours
HIV-infected patients: 500 mg every 24 hours

Herpes labialis: Adolescents and Adults:
Cl_{cr} 30-49 mL/minute: 1 g every 12 hours for 2 doses
Cl_{cr} 10-29 mL/minute: 500 mg every 12 hours for 2 doses
Cl_{cr} <10 mL/minute: 500 mg as a single dose

Hemodialysis: Dialyzable (~33% removed during 4-hour session); administer dose postdialysis

Chronic ambulatory peritoneal dialysis/continuous arteriovenous hemofiltration dialysis: Pharmacokinetic parameters are similar to those in patients with ESRD; supplemental dose not needed following dialysis

Mechanism of Action Valacyclovir is rapidly and nearly completely converted to acyclovir by intestinal and hepatic metabolism. Acyclovir is converted to acyclovir monophosphate by virus-specific thymidine kinase then further converted to acyclovir triphosphate by other cellular enzymes. Acyclovir triphosphate inhibits DNA synthesis and viral replication by competing with deoxyguanosine triphosphate for viral DNA polymerase and being incorporated into viral DNA.

Contraindications Hypersensitivity to valacyclovir, acyclovir, or any component of the formulation

Warnings/Precautions Thrombotic thrombocytopenic purpura/hemolytic uremic syndrome has occurred in immunocompromised patients (at doses of 8 g/day); use caution and adjust the dose in elderly patients or those with renal insufficiency and in patients receiving concurrent nephrotoxic agents; treatment should begin as soon as possible after the first signs and symptoms (within 72 hours of onset of first diagnosis or within 24 hours of onset of recurrent episodes). Safety and efficacy in prepubertal patients have not been established.

(Continued)

Valacyclovir *(Continued)*

Drug Interactions

Cimetidine: Decreased renal clearance of acyclovir; no dosage adjustment needed in patients with normal renal function

Probenecid: Decreased renal clearance of acyclovir; no dosage adjustment needed in patients with normal renal function

Dietary Considerations May be taken with or without food.

Pharmacodynamics/Kinetics

Absorption: Rapid

Distribution: Acyclovir is widely distributed throughout the body including brain, kidney, lungs, liver, spleen, muscle, uterus, vagina, and CSF

Protein binding: 13.5% to 17.9%

Metabolism: Hepatic; valacyclovir is rapidly and nearly completely converted to acyclovir and L-valine by first-pass effect; acyclovir is hepatically metabolized to a very small extent by aldehyde oxidase and by alcohol and aldehyde dehydrogenase (inactive metabolites)

Bioavailability: ~55% once converted to acyclovir

Half-life elimination: Normal renal function: Adults: Acyclovir: 2.5-3.3 hours, Valacyclovir: ~30 minutes; End-stage renal disease: Acyclovir: 14-20 hours

Excretion: Urine, primarily as acyclovir (88%); **Note:** Following oral administration of radiolabeled valacyclovir, 46% of the label is eliminated in the feces (corresponding to nonabsorbed drug), while 47% of the radiolabel is eliminated in the urine.

Pregnancy Risk Factor B

Lactation Enters breast milk/use caution

Breast-Feeding Considerations Avoid use in breast-feeding, if possible, since the drug distributes in high concentrations in breast milk.

Dosage Forms Caplet, as hydrochloride: 500 mg, 1000 mg

Valacyclovir Hydrochloride *see* Valacyclovir *on page 1354*

Valcyte™ *see* Valganciclovir *on page 1358*

Valdecoxib (val de KOKS ib)

Related Information

Rheumatoid Arthritis, Osteoarthritis, and Osteoporosis *on page 1490*

U.S. Brand Names Bextra®

Canadian Brand Names Bextra®

Generic Available No

Pharmacologic Category Nonsteroidal Anti-inflammatory Drug (NSAID), COX-2 Selective

Dental Use Treatment of postoperative pain

Use Relief of signs and symptoms of osteoarthritis and adult rheumatoid arthritis; treatment of primary dysmenorrhea

Local Anesthetic/Vasoconstrictor Precautions No information available to require special precautions

Effects on Dental Treatment Key adverse event(s) related to dental treatment: Stomatitis, abnormal taste, and xerostomia (normal salivary flow resumes upon discontinuation).

Significant Adverse Effects

2% to 10%:

Cardiovascular: Peripheral edema (2% to 3%), hypertension (2%)

Central nervous system: Headache (5% to 9%), dizziness (3%)

Dermatologic: Rash (1% to 2%)

Gastrointestinal: Dyspepsia (8% to 9%), abdominal pain (7% to 8%), nausea (6% to 7%), diarrhea (5% to 6%), flatulence (3% to 4%), abdominal fullness (2%)

Neuromuscular & skeletal: Back pain (2% to 3%), myalgia (2%)

Otic: Earache, tinnitus

Respiratory: Upper respiratory tract infection (6% to 7%), sinusitis (2% to 3%)

Miscellaneous: Influenza-like symptoms (2%)

<2% (Limited to important or life threatening): Allergy, anaphylaxis, aneurysm, angina, angioedema, aortic stenosis, arrhythmia, atrial fibrillation, bradycardia, breast neoplasm, cardiomyopathy, carotid stenosis, colitis, CHF, convulsion, coronary thrombosis, depression exacerbation, diabetes mellitus, diverticulosis, duodenal ulcer, emphysema, erythema multiforme, esophageal perforation, exfoliative dermatitis, facial edema, gastric ulcer, gastroesophageal reflux, gastrointestinal bleeding, gout, heart block, hepatitis, hiatal hernia, hyperlipemia, hyperparathyroidism, hypertension exacerbation, hypertensive encephalopathy, hypotension, impotence, intermittent claudication, liver function tests increased, lymphadenopathy, lymphangitis,

lymphopenia, migraine, mitral insufficiency, myocardial infarction, myocardial ischemia, neuropathy, osteoporosis, ovarian cyst (malignant), pericarditis, periorbital swelling, photosensitivity, pneumonia, rash (erythematous, maculopapular, psoriaform), Stevens-Johnson syndrome, syncope, tachycardia, thrombocytopenia, thrombophlebitis, toxic epidermal necrolysis, unstable angina, urinary tract infection, vaginal hemorrhage, ventricular fibrillation, vertigo

Dosage Oral: Adults:

Osteoarthritis and rheumatoid arthritis: 10 mg once daily; **Note:** No additional benefits seen with 20 mg/day

Primary dysmenorrhea: 20 mg twice daily as needed

Dosage adjustment in renal impairment: Not recommended for use in advanced disease

Dosage adjustment in hepatic impairment: Not recommended for use in advanced liver dysfunction (Child-Pugh Class C)

Mechanism of Action Inhibits prostaglandin synthesis by decreasing the activity of the enzyme, cyclooxygenase-2 (COX-2), which results in decreased formation of prostaglandin precursors. Does not affect platelet function.

Contraindications Hypersensitivity to valdecoxib, sulfonamides, or any component of the formulation; patients who have experienced asthma, urticaria, or allergic-type reactions to aspirin or NSAIDs; pregnancy (3rd trimester)

Warnings/Precautions Gastrointestinal irritation, ulceration, bleeding, and perforation may occur with NSAIDs (it is unclear whether valdecoxib is associated with rates of these events which are similar to nonselective NSAIDs). Use with caution in patients with a history of GI disease (bleeding or ulcers) or risk factor for GI bleeding, use lowest dose for shortest time possible. Anaphylactic/anaphylactoid reactions may occur, even with no prior exposure to valdecoxib. Serious dermatologic reactions have been reported; discontinue in any patients who develop rash or any signs of hypersensitivity. Use with caution in patients with decreased renal function, hepatic disease, CHF, hypertension, fluid retention, dehydration, or asthma. Use caution in patients with known or suspected deficiency of cytochrome P450 isoenzyme 2C9. Use in patients with severe hepatic impairment (Child-Pugh Class C) is not recommended. Safety and efficacy have not been established for patients <18 years of age.

Drug Interactions Substrate (minor) of CYP2C8/9, 3A4; **Inhibits** CYP2C8/9 (weak), 2C19 (weak)

ACE inhibitors: Antihypertensive effects may be decreased by concurrent therapy with NSAIDs; monitor blood pressure.

Angiotensin II antagonists: Antihypertensive effects may be decreased by concurrent therapy with NSAIDs; monitor blood pressure.

Anticoagulants (warfarin, heparin, LMWHs): In combination with NSAIDs, can cause increased risk of bleeding.

Antiplatelet drugs (ticlopidine, clopidogrel, aspirin, abciximab, dipyridamole, eptifibatide, tirofiban): Can cause an increased risk of bleeding.

Azole antifungals: May increase valdecoxib concentrations.

Corticosteroids: May increase the risk of GI ulceration; avoid concurrent use

Cyclosporine: NSAIDs may increase serum creatinine, potassium, blood pressure, and cyclosporine levels; monitor cyclosporine levels and renal function carefully.

Hydralazine: Antihypertensive effect is decreased; avoid concurrent use

Lithium levels can be increased; avoid concurrent use if possible or monitor lithium levels and adjust dose. When NSAID is stopped, lithium will need adjustment again.

Loop diuretics: Diuretic and antihypertensive efficacy is reduced. May be anticipated with any NSAID.

Methotrexate: Severe bone marrow suppression, aplastic anemia, and GI toxicity have been reported with concomitant NSAID therapy. Selective COX-2 inhibitors appear to have a lower risk of this toxicity, however, caution is warranted.

Thiazides: Diuretic efficacy is reduced.

Warfarin: Valdecoxib (40 mg twice daily) may increase plasma warfarin exposure (12% R-warfarin, 15% S-warfarin). May increase the anticoagulant effects of warfarin. Monitor INR closely.

Ethanol/Nutrition/Herb Interactions

Ethanol: Avoid ethanol (may enhance gastric mucosal irritation).

Food: Time to peak level is delayed by 1-2 hours when taken with high-fat meal, but other parameters are unaffected.

Herb/Nutraceutical: Avoid cat's claw, dong quai, evening primrose, feverfew, garlic, ginger, ginkgo, red clover, horse chestnut, green tea, ginseng (may cause increased risk of bleeding).

(Continued)

Valdecoxib *(Continued)*

Dietary Considerations May be taken with or without food.

Pharmacodynamics/Kinetics

Onset of action: Dysmenorrhea: 60 minutes

Distribution: V_d: 86 L

Protein binding: 98%

Metabolism: Extensively hepatic via CYP3A4 and 2C9; glucuronidation; forms metabolite (active)

Bioavailability: 83%

Half-life elimination: 8-11 hours

Time to peak: 2.25-3 hours

Excretion: Primarily urine (as metabolites)

Pregnancy Risk Factor C/D (3rd trimester)

Lactation Excretion in breast milk unknown/not recommended

Dosage Forms Tablet: 10 mg, 20 mg

Valganciclovir (val gan SYE kloh veer)

Related Information

Ganciclovir *on page 646*

U.S. Brand Names Valcyte™

Canadian Brand Names Valcyte™

Generic Available No

Synonyms Valganciclovir Hydrochloride

Pharmacologic Category Antiviral Agent

Use Treatment of cytomegalovirus (CMV) retinitis in patients with acquired immunodeficiency syndrome (AIDS); prevention of CMV disease in high-risk patients (donor CMV positive/recipient CMV negative) undergoing kidney, heart, or kidney/pancreas transplantation

Local Anesthetic/Vasoconstrictor Precautions No information available to require special precautions

Effects on Dental Treatment No significant effects or complications reported

Common Adverse Effects

>10%:

Central nervous system: Fever (31%), headache (9% to 22%), insomnia (16%)

Gastrointestinal: Diarrhea (16% to 41%), nausea (8% to 30%), vomiting (21%), abdominal pain (15%)

Hematologic: Granulocytopenia (11% to 27%), anemia (8% to 26%)

Ocular: Retinal detachment (15%)

1% to 10%:

Central nervous system: Peripheral neuropathy (9%), paresthesia (8%), seizures (<5%), psychosis, hallucinations (<5%), confusion (<5%), agitation (<5%)

Hematologic: Thrombocytopenia (8%), pancytopenia (<5%), bone marrow depression (<5%), aplastic anemia (<5%), bleeding (potentially life-threatening due to thrombocytopenia <5%)

Renal: Decreased renal function (<5%)

Miscellaneous: Local and systemic infections, including sepsis (<5%); allergic reaction (<5%)

Mechanism of Action Valganciclovir is rapidly converted to ganciclovir in the body. The bioavailability of ganciclovir from valganciclovir is increased 10-fold compared to the oral ganciclovir. A dose of 900 mg achieved systemic exposure of ganciclovir comparable to that achieved with the recommended doses of intravenous ganciclovir of 5 mg/kg. Ganciclovir is phosphorylated to a substrate which competitively inhibits the binding of deoxyguanosine triphosphate to DNA polymerase resulting in inhibition of viral DNA synthesis.

Drug Interactions

Increased Effect/Toxicity: Reported for ganciclovir: Immunosuppressive agents may increase hematologic toxicity of ganciclovir. Imipenem/cilastatin may increase seizure potential. Oral ganciclovir increases blood levels of zidovudine, although zidovudine decreases steady-state levels of ganciclovir. Since both drugs have the potential to cause neutropenia and anemia, some patients may not tolerate concomitant therapy with these drugs at full dosage. Didanosine levels are increased with concurrent ganciclovir. Other nephrotoxic drugs (eg, amphotericin and cyclosporine) may have additive nephrotoxicity with ganciclovir.

Decreased Effect: Reported for ganciclovir: A decrease in blood levels of ganciclovir AUC may occur when used with didanosine.

Pharmacodynamics/Kinetics

Absorption: Well absorbed; high-fat meal increases AUC by 30%

Distribution: Ganciclovir: V_d: 15.26 L/1.73 m^2; widely to all tissues including CSF and ocular tissue
Protein binding: 1% to 2%
Metabolism: Converted to ganciclovir by intestinal mucosal cells and hepatocytes
Bioavailability: With food: 60%
Half-life elimination: Ganciclovir: 4.08 hours; prolonged with renal impairment; Severe renal impairment: Up to 68 hours
Excretion: Urine (primarily as ganciclovir)

Pregnancy Risk Factor C

Valganciclovir Hydrochloride *see* Valganciclovir *on page 1358*

Valium® *see* Diazepam *on page 423*

Valorin [OTC] *see* Acetaminophen *on page 47*

Valorin Extra [OTC] *see* Acetaminophen *on page 47*

Valproate Semisodium *see* Valproic Acid and Derivatives *on page 1359*

Valproate Sodium *see* Valproic Acid and Derivatives *on page 1359*

Valproic Acid *see* Valproic Acid and Derivatives *on page 1359*

Valproic Acid and Derivatives

(val PROE ik AS id & dah RIV ah tives)

U.S. Brand Names Depacon®; Depakene®; Depakote® Delayed Release; Depakote® ER; Depakote® Sprinkle®

Canadian Brand Names Alti-Divalproex; Apo-Divalproex®; Depakene®; Epival® ER; Epival® I.V.; Gen-Divalproex; Novo-Divalproex; Nu-Divalproex; PMS-Valproic Acid; PMS-Valproic Acid E.C.; Rhoxal-valproic

Mexican Brand Names Cryoval® [caps]; Depakene®; Epival®; Leptilan®; Valprosid®

Generic Available Yes: Valproic acid, valproate sodium

Synonyms Dipropylacetic Acid; Divalproex Sodium; DPA; 2-Propylpentanoic Acid; 2-Propylvaleric Acid; Valproate Semisodium; Valproate Sodium; Valproic Acid

Pharmacologic Category Anticonvulsant, Miscellaneous

Use Monotherapy and adjunctive therapy in the treatment of patients with complex partial seizures; monotherapy and adjunctive therapy of simple and complex absence seizures; adjunctive therapy patients with multiple seizure types that include absence seizures
Mania associated with bipolar disorder (Depakote®)
Migraine prophylaxis (Depakote®, Depakote® ER)

Unlabeled/Investigational Use Behavior disorders in Alzheimer's disease; status epilepticus

Local Anesthetic/Vasoconstrictor Precautions No information available to require special precautions

Effects on Dental Treatment No significant effects or complications reported

Common Adverse Effects

Adverse reactions reported when used as monotherapy for complex partial seizures:

>10%:
Central nervous system: Somnolence (18% to 30%), dizziness (13% to 18%), insomnia (9% to 15%), nervousness (7% to 11%)
Dermatologic: Alopecia (13% to 24%)
Gastrointestinal: Nausea (26% to 34%), diarrhea (19% to 23%), vomiting (15% to 23%), abdominal pain (9% to 12%), dyspepsia (10% to 11%), anorexia (4% to 11%)
Hematologic: Thrombocytopenia (1% to 24%)
Neuromuscular & skeletal: Tremor (19% to 57%), weakness (10% to 21%)
Respiratory: Respiratory tract infection (13% to 20%), pharyngitis (2% to 8%), dyspnea (1% to 5%)

1% to 10%
Cardiovascular: Hypertension, palpitation, peripheral edema (3% to 8%), tachycardia, chest pain
Central nervous system: Amnesia (4% to 7%), abnormal dreams, anxiety, confusion, depression (4% to 5%), malaise, personality disorder
Dermatologic: Bruising (4% to 5%), dry skin, petechia, pruritus, rash
Endocrine & metabolic: Amenorrhea, dysmenorrhea
Gastrointestinal: Eructation, flatulence, hematemesis, increased appetite, pancreatitis, periodontal abscess, taste perversion, weight gain (4% to 9%)
Genitourinary: Urinary frequency, urinary incontinence, vaginitis
Hepatic: AST and ALT increased
Neuromuscular & skeletal: Abnormal gait, arthralgia, back pain, hypertonia, incoordination, leg cramps, myalgia, myasthenia, paresthesia, twitching

(Continued)

Valproic Acid and Derivatives *(Continued)*

Ocular: Amblyopia/blurred vision (4% to 8%), abnormal vision, nystagmus (1% to 7%)

Otic: Deafness, otitis media, tinnitus (1% to 7%)

Respiratory: Epistaxis, increased cough, pneumonia, sinusitis

Additional adverse effects: Frequency not defined:

Cardiovascular: Bradycardia

Central nervous system: Aggression, ataxia, behavioral deterioration, cerebral atrophy (reversible), dementia, emotional upset, encephalopathy (rare), fever, hallucinations, headache, hostility, hyperactivity, hypesthesia, incoordination, Parkinsonism, psychosis, vertigo

Dermatologic: Cutaneous vasculitis, erythema multiforme, photosensitivity, Stevens-Johnson syndrome, toxic epidermal necrolysis (rare)

Endocrine & metabolic: Breast enlargement, galactorrhea, hyperammonemia, hyponatremia, inappropriate ADH secretion, irregular menses, parotid gland swelling, polycystic ovary disease (rare), abnormal thyroid function tests

Genitourinary: Enuresis, urinary tract infection

Hematologic: Anemia, aplastic anemia, bone marrow suppression, eosinophilia, hematoma formation, hemorrhage, hypofibrinogenemia, intermittent porphyria, leukopenia, lymphocytosis, macrocytosis, pancytopenia

Hepatic: Bilirubin increased, hyperammonemic encephalopathy (in patients with UCD)

Neuromuscular & skeletal: Asterixis, bone pain, dysarthria

Ocular: Diplopia, "spots before the eyes"

Renal: Fanconi-like syndrome (rare, in children)

Miscellaneous: Anaphylaxis, decreased carnitine, hyperglycinemia, lupus

Dosage

Seizures:

Children >10 years and Adults:

Oral: Initial: 10-15 mg/kg/day in 1-3 divided doses; increase by 5-10 mg/kg/day at weekly intervals until therapeutic levels are achieved; maintenance: 30-60 mg/kg/day. Adult usual dose: 1000-2500 mg/day. **Note:** Regular release and delayed release formulations are usually given in 2-4 divided doses/day, extended release formulation (Depakote® ER) is usually given once daily. Conversion to Depakote® ER from a stable dose of Depakote® may require an increase in the total daily dose between 8% and 20% to maintain similar serum concentrations.

Children receiving more than one anticonvulsant (ie, polytherapy) may require doses up to 100 mg/kg/day in 3-4 divided doses

I.V.: Administer as a 60-minute infusion (≤20 mg/minute) with the same frequency as oral products; switch patient to oral products as soon as possible. Alternatively, rapid infusions have been given: ≤15 mg/kg over 5-10 minutes (1.5-3 mg/kg/minute).

Rectal (unlabeled): Dilute syrup 1:1 with water for use as a retention enema; loading dose: 17-20 mg/kg one time; maintenance: 10-15 mg/kg/dose every 8 hours

Status epilepticus (unlabeled use): Adults:

Loading dose: I.V.: 15-25 mg/kg administered at 3 mg/kg/minute.

Maintenance dose: I.V. infusion: 1-4 mg/kg/hour; titrate dose as needed based upon patient response and evaluation of drug-drug interactions

Mania: Adults: Oral: 750-1500 mg/day in divided doses; dose should be adjusted as rapidly as possible to desired clinical effect; a loading dose of 20 mg/kg may be used; maximum recommended dosage: 60 mg/kg/day

Migraine prophylaxis: Adults: Oral:

Extended release tablets: 500 mg once daily for 7 days, then increase to 1000 mg once daily; adjust dose based on patient response; usual dosage range 500-1000 mg/day

Delayed release tablets: 250 mg twice daily; adjust dose based on patient response, up to 1000 mg/day

Elderly: Elimination is decreased in the elderly. Studies of elderly patients with dementia show a high incidence of somnolence. In some patients, this was associated with weight loss. Starting doses should be lower and increases should be slow, with careful monitoring of nutritional intake and dehydration. Safety and efficacy for use in patients >65 years have not been studied for migraine prophylaxis.

Dosing adjustment in renal impairment: A 27% reduction in clearance of unbound valproate is seen in patients with Cl_{cr} <10 mL/minute. Hemodialysis reduces valproate concentrations by 20%, therefore no dose adjustment is needed in patients with renal failure. Protein binding is reduced, monitoring only total valproate concentrations may be misleading.

Dosing adjustment/comments in hepatic impairment: Reduce dose. Clearance is decreased with liver impairment. Hepatic disease is also associated with decreased albumin concentrations and 2- to 2.6-fold increase in the unbound fraction. Free concentrations of valproate may be elevated while total concentrations appear normal.

Mechanism of Action Causes increased availability of gamma-aminobutyric acid (GABA), an inhibitory neurotransmitter, to brain neurons or may enhance the action of GABA or mimic its action at postsynaptic receptor sites

Contraindications Hypersensitivity to valproic acid, derivatives, or any component of the formulation; hepatic dysfunction; urea cycle disorders; pregnancy

Warnings/Precautions Hepatic failure resulting in fatalities has occurred in patients; children <2 years of age are at considerable risk; other risk factors include organic brain disease, mental retardation with severe seizure disorders, congenital metabolic disorders, and patients on multiple anticonvulsants. Hepatotoxicity has been reported after 3 days to 6 months of therapy. Monitor patients closely for appearance of malaise, weakness, facial edema, anorexia, jaundice, and vomiting; may cause severe thrombocytopenia, inhibition of platelet aggregation and bleeding; tremors may indicate overdosage; use with caution in patients receiving other anticonvulsants.

Cases of life-threatening pancreatitis, occurring at the start of therapy or following years of use, have been reported in adults and children. Some cases have been hemorrhagic with rapid progression of initial symptoms to death.

May cause teratogenic effects such as neural tube defects (eg, spina bifida). Use in women of childbearing potential requires that benefits of use in mother be weighed against the potential risk to fetus, especially when used for conditions not associated with permanent injury or risk of death (eg, migraine).

Hyperammonemic encephalopathy, sometimes fatal, has been reported following the initiation of valproate therapy in patients with known or suspected urea cycle disorders (UCD), particularly those with ornithine transcarbamylase deficiency. Although a rare genetic disorder, UCD evaluation should be considered for the following patients, prior to the start of therapy: History of unexplained encephalopathy or coma; encephalopathy associated with protein load; pregnancy or postpartum encephalopathy; unexplained mental retardation; history of elevated plasma ammonia or glutamine; history of cyclical vomiting and lethargy; episodic extreme irritability, ataxia; low BUN or protein avoidance; family history of UCD or unexplained infant deaths (particularly male); signs or symptoms of UCD (hyperammonemia, encephalopathy, respiratory alkalosis). Patients who develop symptoms of hyperammonemic encephalopathy during therapy with valproate should receive prompt evaluation for UCD and valproate should be discontinued.

Hyperammonemia may occur with therapy and may be present with normal liver function tests. Ammonia levels should be measured in patients who develop unexplained lethargy and vomiting, or changes in mental status. Discontinue therapy if ammonia levels are increased and evaluate for possible UCD.

In vitro studies have suggested valproate stimulates the replication of HIV and CMV viruses under experimental conditions. The clinical consequence of this is unknown, but should be considered when monitoring affected patients.

Anticonvulsants should not be discontinued abruptly because of the possibility of increasing seizure frequency; valproate should be withdrawn gradually to minimize this risk, unless safety concerns require a more rapid withdrawal. Concomitant use with clonazepam may induce absence status.

Hyperammonemia may occur, even in the absence of overt liver function abnormalities. Asymptomatic elevations require continued surveillance; symptomatic elevations should prompt modification or discontinuation of valproate therapy. CNS depression may occur with valproate use. Patients must be cautioned about performing tasks which require mental alertness (operating machinery or driving). Effects with other sedative drugs or ethanol may be potentiated.

Drug Interactions

Cytochrome P450 Effect: For valproic acid: **Substrate** (minor) of CYP2A6, 2B6, 2C8/9, 2C19, 2E1; **Inhibits** CYP2C8/9 (weak), 2C19 (weak), 2D6 (weak), 3A4 (weak); **Induces** CYP2A6 (weak)

Increased Effect/Toxicity: Absence seizures have been reported in patients receiving VPA and clonazepam. Valproic acid may increase, decrease, or have no effect on carbamazepine and phenytoin levels. Valproic acid may increase serum concentrations of carbamazepine-

(Continued)

Valproic Acid and Derivatives *(Continued)*

epoxide (active metabolite). Valproic acid may increase serum concentrations of diazepam, lamotrigine, nimodipine, and phenobarbital, and tricyclic antidepressants. Chlorpromazine (and possibly other phenothiazines), macrolide antibiotics (clarithromycin, erythromycin, troleandomycin), felbamate, and isoniazid may inhibit the metabolism of valproic acid. Aspirin or other salicylates may displace valproic acid from protein-binding sites, leading to acute toxicity.

Decreased Effect: Valproic acid may displace clozapine from protein binding site resulting in decreased clozapine serum concentrations. Cholestyramine (and possibly colestipol) may bind valproic acid in GI tract, decreasing absorption. Acyclovir may reduce valproic acid levels. Mefloquine may decrease serum concentration of valproic acid.

Ethanol/Nutrition/Herb Interactions

Ethanol: Avoid ethanol (may increase CNS depression).

Food: Food may delay but does not affect the extent of absorption. Valproic acid serum concentrations may be decreased if taken with food. Milk has no effect on absorption.

Herb/Nutraceutical: Avoid evening primrose (seizure threshold decreased)

Dietary Considerations Valproic acid may cause GI upset; take with large amount of water or food to decrease GI upset. May need to split doses to avoid GI upset.

Coated particles of divalproex sodium may be mixed with semisolid food (eg, applesauce or pudding) in patients having difficulty swallowing; particles should be swallowed and not chewed

Valproate sodium oral solution will generate valproic acid in carbonated beverages and may cause mouth and throat irritation; do not mix valproate sodium oral solution with carbonated beverages; sodium content of valproate sodium syrup (5 mL): 23 mg (1 mEq)

Pharmacodynamics/Kinetics

Distribution: Total valproate: 11 L/1.73 m^2; free valproate 92 L/1.73 m^2

Protein binding (dose dependent): 80% to 90%

Metabolism: Extensively hepatic via glucuronide conjugation and mitochondrial beta-oxidation. The relationship between dose and total valproate concentration is nonlinear; concentration does not increase proportionally with the dose, but increases to a lesser extent due to saturable plasma protein binding. The kinetics of unbound drug are linear.

Bioavailability: Extended release: 90% of I.V. dose and 81% to 90% of delayed release dose

Half-life elimination: (increased in neonates and with liver disease): Children: 4-14 hours; Adults: 9-16 hours

Time to peak, serum: 1-4 hours; Divalproex (enteric coated): 3-5 hours

Excretion: Urine (30% to 50% as glucuronide conjugate, 3% as unchanged drug)

Pregnancy Risk Factor D

Dosage Forms CAP, as valproic acid (Depakene®): 250 mg. **CAP, sprinkles, as divalproex sodium** (Depakote® Sprinkle®): 125 mg. **INJ, solution, as valproate sodium** (Depacon®): 100 mg/mL (5 mL). **SYR, as valproic acid:** 250 mg/5 mL (5 mL, 480 mL); (Depakene®): 250 mg/5 mL (480 mL). **TAB, delayed release, as divalproex sodium** (Depakote®): 125 mg, 250 mg, 500 mg. **TAB, extended release, as divalproex sodium** (Depakote® ER): 250 mg, 500 mg

Selected Readings

Redington K, Wells C, and Petito F, "Erythromycin and Valproic Acid Interaction," *Ann Intern Med*, 1992, 116(10):877-8.

Valrubicin (val ROO bi sin)

U.S. Brand Names Valstar® [DSC]

Canadian Brand Names Valstar®; Valtaxin®

Generic Available No

Synonyms AD3L; *N*-trifluoroacetyladriamycin-14-valerate

Pharmacologic Category Antineoplastic Agent, Anthracycline

Use Intravesical therapy of BCG-refractory carcinoma *in situ* of the urinary bladder

Local Anesthetic/Vasoconstrictor Precautions No information available to require special precautions

Effects on Dental Treatment No significant effects or complications reported

Common Adverse Effects

>10%: Genitourinary: Frequency (61%), dysuria (56%), urgency (57%), bladder spasm (31%), hematuria (29%), bladder pain (28%), urinary incontinence (22%), cystitis (15%), urinary tract infection (15%)

1% to 10%:

Cardiovascular: Chest pain (2%), vasodilation (2%), peripheral edema (1%)

Central nervous system: Headache (4%), malaise (4%), dizziness (3%), fever (2%)

Dermatologic: Rash (3%)

Endocrine & metabolic: Hyperglycemia (1%)

Gastrointestinal: Abdominal pain (5%), nausea (5%), diarrhea (3%), vomiting (2%), flatulence (1%)

Genitourinary: Nocturia (7%), burning symptoms (5%), urinary retention (4%), urethral pain (3%), pelvic pain (1%), hematuria (microscopic) (3%)

Hematologic: Anemia (2%)

Neuromuscular & skeletal: Weakness (4%), back pain (3%), myalgia (1%)

Respiratory: Pneumonia (1%)

Mechanism of Action Blocks function of DNA topoisomerase II; inhibits DNA synthesis, causes extensive chromosomal damage, and arrests cell development; unlike other anthracyclines, does not appear to intercalate DNA

Drug Interactions

Increased Effect/Toxicity: No specific drug interactions studies have been performed. Systemic exposure to valrubicin is negligible, and interactions are unlikely.

Decreased Effect: No specific drug interactions studies have been performed. Systemic exposure to valrubicin is negligible, and interactions are unlikely.

Pharmacodynamics/Kinetics

Absorption: Well absorbed into bladder tissue, negligible systemic absorption. Trauma to mucosa may increase absorption, and perforation greatly increases absorption with significant systemic myelotoxicity.

Metabolism: Negligible after intravesical instillation and 2 hour retention

Excretion: Urine when expelled from urinary bladder (98.6% as intact drug; 0.4% as *N*-trifluoroacetyladriamycin)

Pregnancy Risk Factor C

Valsartan (val SAR tan)

Related Information

Cardiovascular Diseases *on page 1458*

U.S. Brand Names Diovan®

Canadian Brand Names Diovan®

Mexican Brand Names Diovan®

Generic Available No

Pharmacologic Category Angiotensin II Receptor Blocker

Use Alone or in combination with other antihypertensive agents in treating essential hypertension; treatment of heart failure (NYHA Class II-IV) in patients intolerant to angiotensin converting enzyme (ACE) inhibitors

Local Anesthetic/Vasoconstrictor Precautions No information available to require special precautions

Effects on Dental Treatment No significant effects or complications reported

Common Adverse Effects

Hypertension: Similar incidence to placebo; independent of race, age, and gender.

>1%:

Central nervous system: Dizziness (2% to 8%), fatigue (2%)

Endocrine & metabolic: Serum potassium increased (4.4%)

Gastrointestinal: Abdominal pain (2%)

Hematologic: Neutropenia (1.9%)

Respiratory: Cough (2.6% versus 1.5% in placebo)

Miscellaneous: Viral infection (3%)

>1% but frequency ≤ placebo: Headache, upper respiratory infection, cough, diarrhea, rhinitis, sinusitis, nausea, pharyngitis, edema, arthralgia

Heart failure:

>10%: Central nervous system: Dizziness (17%)

1% to 10%:

Cardiovascular: Hypotension (7%), postural hypotension (2%)

Central nervous system: Fatigue (3%)

Endocrine & metabolic: Hyperkalemia (2%)

Gastrointestinal: Diarrhea (5%)

Neuromuscular & skeletal: Arthralgia (3%), back pain (3%)

Renal: Creatinine elevated >50% (4%)

Dosage Adults: Oral:

Hypertension: Initial: 80 mg or 160 mg once daily (in patients who are not volume depleted); majority of effect within 2 weeks, maximal effects in 4-6

(Continued)

Valsartan *(Continued)*

weeks; dose may be increased to achieve desired effect; maximum recommended dose: 320 mg/day

Heart failure: Initial: 40 mg twice daily; titrate dose to 80-160 mg twice daily, as tolerated; maximum daily dose: 320 mg. **Note:** Do not use with ACE inhibitors and beta blockers.

Dosing adjustment in renal impairment: No dosage adjustment necessary if Cl_{cr} >10 mL/minute.

Dosing adjustment in hepatic impairment (mild - moderate): ≤80 mg/day

Dialysis: Not significantly removed

Mechanism of Action As a prodrug, valsartan produces direct antagonism of the angiotensin II (AT2) receptors, unlike the ACE inhibitors. It displaces angiotensin II from the AT1 receptor and produces its blood pressure lowering effects by antagonizing AT1-induced vasoconstriction, aldosterone release, catecholamine release, arginine vasopressin release, water intake, and hypertrophic responses. This action results in more efficient blockade of the cardiovascular effects of angiotensin II and fewer side effects than the ACE inhibitors.

Contraindications Hypersensitivity to valsartan or any component of the formulation; hypersensitivity to other A-II receptor antagonists; bilateral renal artery stenosis; pregnancy (2nd and 3rd trimesters)

Warnings/Precautions Use extreme caution with concurrent administration of potassium-sparing diuretics or potassium supplements, in patients with mild to moderate hepatic dysfunction (adjust dose), in those who may be sodium/water depleted (eg, on high-dose diuretics), and in the elderly; avoid use in patients with CHF, unilateral renal artery stenosis, aortic/mitral valve stenosis, coronary artery disease, or hypertrophic cardiomyopathy, if possible

Drug Interactions

Cytochrome P450 Effect: Inhibits CYP2C8/9 (weak)

Increased Effect/Toxicity: Valsartan blood levels may be increased by cimetidine and monoxidine; clinical effect is unknown. Concurrent use of potassium salts/supplements, co-trimoxazole (high dose), ACE inhibitors, and potassium-sparing diuretics (amiloride, spironolactone, triamterene) may increase the risk of hyperkalemia.

Decreased Effect: Phenobarbital, ketoconazole, troleandomycin, sulfaphenazole

Ethanol/Nutrition/Herb Interactions

Food: Decreases rate and extent of absorption by 50% and 40%, respectively.

Herb/Nutraceutical: Avoid dong quai if using for hypertension (has estrogenic activity). Avoid ephedra, yohimbe, ginseng (may worsen hypertension). Avoid garlic (may have increased antihypertensive effect).

Dietary Considerations Avoid salt substitutes which contain potassium. May be taken with or without food.

Pharmacodynamics/Kinetics

Onset of action: Peak antihypertensive effect: 2-4 weeks

Distribution: V_d: 17 L (adults)

Protein binding: 95%, primarily albumin

Metabolism: To inactive metabolite

Bioavailability: 25% (range 10% to 35%)

Half-life elimination: 6 hours

Time to peak, serum: 2-4 hours

Excretion: Feces (83%) and urine (13%) as unchanged drug

Pregnancy Risk Factor C/D (2nd and 3rd trimesters)

Dosage Forms TAB: 40 mg, 80 mg, 160 mg, 320 mg

Valsartan and Hydrochlorothiazide

(val SAR tan & hye droe klor oh THYE a zide)

Related Information

Cardiovascular Diseases *on page 1458*

Hydrochlorothiazide *on page 699*

Valsartan *on page 1363*

U.S. Brand Names Diovan HCT®

Canadian Brand Names Diovan HCT®

Generic Available No

Synonyms Hydrochlorothiazide and Valsartan

Pharmacologic Category Angiotensin II Receptor Blocker Combination; Antihypertensive Agent, Combination; Diuretic, Thiazide

Use Treatment of hypertension (not indicated for initial therapy)

Local Anesthetic/Vasoconstrictor Precautions No information available to require special precautions

Effects on Dental Treatment No significant effects or complications reported

Common Adverse Effects Percentages reported with combination product; other reactions have been reported (see individual agents for additional information)

1% to 10%:

Central nervous system: Dizziness (9%; dose related), fatigue (5%)

Gastrointestinal: Diarrhea (3%)

Respiratory: Pharyngitis (3%), cough (3%)

Drug Interactions

Cytochrome P450 Effect: Valsartan: **Inhibits** CYP2C8/9 (weak)

Increased Effect/Toxicity: See individual agents.

Decreased Effect: See individual agents.

Pharmacodynamics/Kinetics See individual agents.

Pregnancy Risk Factor C/D (2nd and 3rd trimester)

Valstar® [DSC] *see* Valrubicin *on page 1362*

Valtrex® *see* Valacyclovir *on page 1354*

Vanamide™ *see* Urea *on page 1353*

Vancocin® *see* Vancomycin *on page 1365*

Vancomycin (van koe MYE sin)

Related Information

Cardiovascular Diseases *on page 1458*

U.S. Brand Names Vancocin®

Canadian Brand Names Vancocin®

Mexican Brand Names Vancocin®; Vanmicina®

Generic Available Yes: Injection

Synonyms Vancomycin Hydrochloride

Pharmacologic Category Antibiotic, Miscellaneous

Use Treatment of patients with infections caused by staphylococcal species and streptococcal species; used orally for staphylococcal enterocolitis or for antibiotic-associated pseudomembranous colitis produced by *C. difficile*

Local Anesthetic/Vasoconstrictor Precautions No information available to require special precautions

Effects on Dental Treatment Key adverse event(s) related to dental treatment: Bitter taste. The "red man syndrome" characterized by skin rash and hypotension is not an allergic reaction but rather is associated with too rapid infusion of the drug. To alleviate or prevent the reaction, infuse vancomycin at a rate of ≥30 minutes for each 500 mg of drug being administered (eg, 1 g over ≥60 minutes); 1.5 g over ≥90 minutes.

Significant Adverse Effects

Oral:

>10%: Gastrointestinal: Bitter taste, nausea, vomiting, stomatitis

1% to 10%:

Central nervous system: Chills, drug fever

Hematologic: Eosinophilia

<1% (Limited to important or life-threatening): Interstitial nephritis, ototoxicity, renal failure, skin rash, thrombocytopenia, vasculitis

Parenteral:

>10%:

Cardiovascular: Hypotension accompanied by flushing

Dermatologic: Erythematous rash on face and upper body (red neck or red man syndrome)

1% to 10%:

Central nervous system: Chills, drug fever

Hematologic: Eosinophilia

<1% (Limited to important or life-threatening): Ototoxicity, renal failure, thrombocytopenia, vasculitis

Dosage Initial dosage recommendation: I.V.:

Neonates:

Postnatal age ≤7 days:

<1200 g: 15 mg/kg/dose every 24 hours

1200-2000 g: 10 mg/kg/dose every 12 hours

>2000 g: 15 mg/kg/dose every 12 hours

Postnatal age >7 days:

<1200 g: 15 mg/kg/dose every 24 hours

≥1200 g: 10 mg/kg/dose divided every 8 hours

Infants >1 month and Children:

40 mg/kg/day in divided doses every 6 hours

(Continued)

Vancomycin *(Continued)*

Prophylaxis for bacterial endocarditis:

Dental, oral, or upper respiratory tract surgery: 20 mg/kg 1 hour prior to the procedure

GI/GU procedure: 20 mg/kg plus gentamicin 2 mg/kg 1 hour prior to surgery

Infants >1 month and Children with staphylococcal central nervous system infection: 60 mg/kg/day in divided doses every 6 hours

Adults:

With normal renal function: 1 g **or** 10-15 mg/kg/dose every 12 hours

Prophylaxis for bacterial endocarditis:

Dental, oral, or upper respiratory tract surgery: 1 g 1 hour before surgery

GI/GU procedure: 1 g plus 1.5 mg/kg gentamicin 1 hour prior to surgery

Dosing interval in renal impairment (vancomycin levels should be monitored in patients with any renal impairment):

Cl_{cr} >60 mL/minute: Start with 1 g or 10-15 mg/kg/dose every 12 hours

Cl_{cr} 40-60 mL/minute: Start with 1 g or 10-15 mg/kg/dose every 24 hours

Cl_{cr} <40 mL/minute: Will need longer intervals; determine by serum concentration monitoring

Hemodialysis: Not dialyzable (0% to 5%); generally not removed; exception minimal-moderate removal by some of the newer high-flux filters; dose may need to be administered more frequently; monitor serum concentrations

Continuous ambulatory peritoneal dialysis (CAPD): Not significantly removed; administration via CAPD fluid: 15-30 mg/L (15-30 mcg/mL) of CAPD fluid

Continuous arteriovenous hemofiltration: Dose as for Cl_{cr} 10-40 mL/minute

Antibiotic lock technique (for catheter infections): 2 mg/mL in SWI/NS or D_5W; instill 3-5 mL into catheter port as a flush solution instead of heparin lock (**Note:** Do not mix with any other solutions)

Intrathecal: Vancomycin is available as a powder for injection and may be diluted to 1-5 mg/mL concentration in preservative-free 0.9% sodium chloride for administration into the CSF

Neonates: 5-10 mg/day

Children: 5-20 mg/day

Adults: Up to 20 mg/day

Oral: Pseudomembranous colitis produced by *C. difficile*:

Neonates: 10 mg/kg/day in divided doses

Children: 40 mg/kg/day in divided doses, added to fluids

Adults: 125 mg 4 times/day for 10 days

Mechanism of Action Inhibits bacterial cell wall synthesis by blocking glycopeptide polymerization through binding tightly to D-alanyl-D-alanine portion of cell wall precursor

Contraindications Hypersensitivity to vancomycin or any component of the formulation; avoid in patients with previous severe hearing loss

Warnings/Precautions Use with caution in patients with renal impairment or those receiving other nephrotoxic or ototoxic drugs; dosage modification required in patients with impaired renal function (especially elderly)

Drug Interactions Increased toxicity: Anesthetic agents; other ototoxic or nephrotoxic agents

Dietary Considerations May be taken with food.

Pharmacodynamics/Kinetics

Absorption: Oral: Poor; I.M.: Erratic; Intraperitoneal: ~38%

Distribution: Widely in body tissues and fluids. except for CSF

Relative diffusion from blood into CSF: Good only with inflammation (exceeds usual MICs)

CSF:blood level ratio: Normal meninges: Nil; Inflamed meninges: 20% to 30%

Protein binding: 10% to 50%

Half-life elimination: Biphasic: Terminal:

Newborns: 6-10 hours

Infants and Children 3 months to 4 years: 4 hours

Children >3 years: 2.2-3 hours

Adults: 5-11 hours; significantly prolonged with renal impairment

End-stage renal disease: 200-250 hours

Time to peak, serum: I.V.: 45-65 minutes

Excretion: I.V.: Urine (80% to 90% as unchanged drug); Oral: Primarily feces

Pregnancy Risk Factor C

Lactation Enters breast milk/use caution

Breast-Feeding Considerations Vancomycin is excreted in breast milk but is poorly absorbed from the gastrointestinal tract. Therefore, systemic absorption would not be expected. Theoretically, vancomycin in the GI tract may affect the normal bowel flora in the infant, resulting in diarrhea.

Dosage Forms [DSC] = Discontinued product

Capsule, as hydrochloride (Vancocin®): 125 mg, 250 mg

Infusion [premixed in iso-osmotic dextrose]: 500 mg (100 mL); 1 g (200 mL)

Injection, powder for reconstitution, as hydrochloride: 500 mg, 1 g, 5 g, 10 g

Vancocin® [DSC]: 500 mg, 1 g, 10 g

Vancomycin Hydrochloride *see* Vancomycin *on page 1365*

Vanex Forte™-D *see* Chlorpheniramine, Phenylephrine, and Methscopolamine *on page 317*

Vaniqa™ *see* Eflornithine *on page 485*

Vanoxide-HC® *see* Benzoyl Peroxide and Hydrocortisone *on page 194*

Vanquish® Extra Strength Pain Reliever [OTC] *see* Acetaminophen, Aspirin, and Caffeine *on page 56*

Van R Gingibraid® *see* Epinephrine (Racemic) and Aluminum Potassium Sulfate *on page 497*

Vantin® *see* Cefpodoxime *on page 285*

Vaponefrin® *see* Epinephrine (Racemic) *on page 497*

VAQTA® *see* Hepatitis A Vaccine *on page 687*

Vardenafil (var DEN a fil)

U.S. Brand Names Levitra®

Mexican Brand Names Levitra®

Generic Available No

Synonyms Vardenafil Hydrochloride

Pharmacologic Category Phosphodiesterase-5 Enzyme Inhibitor

Use Treatment of erectile dysfunction

Local Anesthetic/Vasoconstrictor Precautions No information available to require special precautions

Effects on Dental Treatment No significant effects or complications reported

Common Adverse Effects

>10%:
- Cardiovascular: Flushing (11%)
- Central nervous system: Headache (15%)

2% to 10%:
- Central nervous system: Dizziness (2%)
- Gastrointestinal: Dyspepsia (4%), nausea (2%)
- Neuromuscular & skeletal: CPK increased (2%)
- Respiratory: Rhinitis (9%), sinusitis (3%)
- Miscellaneous: Flu-like syndrome (3%)

Dosage Oral: Adults: Erectile dysfunction: 10 mg 60 minutes prior to sexual activity; dosing range: 5-20 mg; to be given as one single dose and not given more than once daily

Dosing adjustment with concomitant medications:
- Erythromycin: Maximum vardenafil dose: 5 mg/24 hours
- Indinavir: Maximum vardenafil dose: 2.5 mg/24 hours
- Itraconazole:
  - 200 mg/day: Maximum vardenafil dose: 5 mg/24 hours
  - 400 mg/day: Maximum vardenafil dose: 2.5 mg/24 hours
- Ketoconazole:
  - 200 mg/day: Maximum vardenafil dose: 5 mg/24 hours
  - 400 mg/day: Maximum vardenafil dose: 2.5 mg/24 hours
- Ritonavir: Maximum vardenafil dose: 2.5 mg/72 hours

Elderly ≥65 years: Initial: 5 mg 60 minutes prior to sexual activity; to be given as one single dose and not given more than once daily

Dosage adjustment in renal impairment: Dose adjustment not needed for mild, moderate, or severe impairment; use has not been studied in patients on renal dialysis

Dosage adjustment in hepatic impairment: Child-Pugh class B: Initial: 5 mg 60 minutes prior to sexual activity (maximum dose: 10 mg); to be given as one single dose and not given more than once daily

Mechanism of Action Does not directly cause penile erections, but affects the response to sexual stimulation. The physiologic mechanism of erection of the penis involves release of nitric oxide (NO) in the corpus cavernosum during sexual stimulation. NO then activates the enzyme guanylate cyclase, which results in increased levels of cyclic guanosine monophosphate (cGMP), producing smooth muscle relaxation and inflow of blood to the corpus cavernosum. Vardenafil enhances the effect of NO by inhibiting phosphodiesterase type 5 (PDE-5), which is responsible for degradation of cGMP in the corpus cavernosum; when sexual stimulation causes local release of NO, inhibition of

(Continued)

Vardenafil *(Continued)*

PDE-5 by vardenafil causes increased levels of cGMP in the corpus cavernosum, resulting in smooth muscle relaxation and inflow of blood to the corpus cavernosum; at recommended doses, it has no effect in the absence of sexual stimulation.

Contraindications Hypersensitivity to vardenafil or any component of the formulation; concurrent use of organic nitrates (nitroglycerin; scheduled dosing or as needed); concomitant use of alpha blockers

Warnings/Precautions There is a degree of cardiac risk associated with sexual activity; therefore, physicians may wish to consider the patient's cardiovascular status prior to initiating any treatment for erectile dysfunction. Use caution in patients with anatomical deformation of the penis (angulation, cavernosal fibrosis, or Peyronie's disease) and in patients who have conditions which may predispose them to priapism (sickle cell anemia, multiple myeloma, leukemia). Patients should be instructed to seek medical attention if erection persists >4 hours.

Not recommended for use in patients with congenital QT prolongation or those taking Class Ia or III antiarrhythmics. Use caution with effective CYP3A4 inhibitors, the elderly, or those with hepatic impairment (Child-Pugh class B); dosage adjustment is needed.

Safety and efficacy have not been studied in patients with the following conditions, therefore, use in these patients is not recommended at this time: Hypotension, uncontrolled hypertension, unstable angina, severe cardiac failure; a life-threatening arrhythmia, myocardial infarction,or stroke within the last 6 months; severe hepatic impairment (Child-Pugh class C); end-stage renal disease requiring dialysis; retinitis pigmentosa or other degenerative retinal disorders. The safety and efficacy of vardenafil with other treatments for erectile dysfunction have not been studied and are not recommended as combination therapy.

Drug Interactions

Cytochrome P450 Effect: Substrate of CYP2C (minor), 3A5 (minor), 3A4 (major)

Increased Effect/Toxicity: CYP3A4 inhibitors may increase the levels/effects of vardenafil; example inhibitors include azole antifungals, ciprofloxacin, clarithromycin, diclofenac, doxycycline, erythromycin, imatinib, isoniazid, nefazodone, nicardipine, propofol, protease inhibitors, quinidine, and verapamil. Alpha blockers and nitroglycerin may lead to excessive hypotension; concomitant use is contraindicated.

Ethanol/Nutrition/Herb Interactions

Food: High-fat meals decrease maximum serum concentration 18% to 50%. Serum concentrations/toxicity may be increased with grapefruit juice; avoid concurrent use.

Dietary Considerations May take with or without food

Pharmacodynamics/Kinetics

Absorption: Rapid

Distribution: V_d: 208 L; <0.01% found in semen 1.5 hours after dose

Metabolism: Hepatic via CYP3A4 (major), CYP2C and 3A5 (minor); forms metabolite (active)

Bioavailability: 15%; Elderly (≥65 years): 52%; Hepatic impairment (Child-Pugh class B): 160%

Half-life elimination: Terminal: Vardenafil and metabolite: 4-5 hours

Time to peak, plasma: 0.5-2 hours

Excretion: Feces (91% to 95% as metabolites); urine (2% to 6%)

Clearance: 56 L/hour

Pregnancy Risk Factor B

Dosage Forms TAB, film-coated: 2.5 mg, 5 mg, 10 mg, 20 mg

Vardenafil Hydrochloride *see* Vardenafil *on page 1367*

Varicella Virus Vaccine *see page 1614*

Varicella-Zoster Immune Globulin (Human)

(var i SEL a- ZOS ter i MYUN GLOB yoo lin HYU man)

Related Information

Immunizations (Vaccines) *on page 1614*

Generic Available No

Synonyms VZIG

Pharmacologic Category Immune Globulin

Use Passive immunization of susceptible immunodeficient patients after exposure to varicella; most effective if begun within 96 hours of exposure; there is no evidence VZIG modifies established varicella-zoster infections.

Restrict administration to those patients meeting the following criteria:

Neoplastic disease (eg, leukemia or lymphoma)

Congenital or acquired immunodeficiency

Immunosuppressive therapy with steroids, antimetabolites or other immunosuppressive treatment regimens

Newborn of mother who had onset of chickenpox within 5 days before delivery or within 48 hours after delivery

Premature (≥28 weeks gestation) whose mother has no history of chickenpox

Premature (<28 weeks gestation or ≤1000 g VZIG) regardless of maternal history

One of the following types of exposure to chickenpox or zoster patient(s) may warrant administration:

Continuous household contact

Playmate contact (>1 hour play indoors)

Hospital contact (in same 2-4 bedroom or adjacent beds in a large ward or prolonged face-to-face contact with an infectious staff member or patient)

Susceptible to varicella-zoster

Age <15 years; administer to immunocompromised adolescents and adults and to other older patients on an individual basis

An acceptable alternative to VZIG prophylaxis is to treat varicella, if it occurs, with high-dose I.V. acyclovir

Age is the most important risk factor for reactivation of varicella zoster; persons <50 years of age have incidence of 2.5 cases per 1000, whereas those 60-79 have 6.5 cases per 1000 and those >80 years have 10 cases per 1000

Local Anesthetic/Vasoconstrictor Precautions No information available to require special precautions

Effects on Dental Treatment No significant effects or complications reported

Common Adverse Effects 1% to 10%: Local: Discomfort at the site of injection (pain, redness, edema)

Mechanism of Action The exact mechanism has not been clarified but the antibodies in varicella-zoster immune globulin most likely neutralize the varicella-zoster virus and prevent its pathological actions

Pregnancy Risk Factor C

Vascor® [DSC] *see* Bepridil *on page 197*

Vaseretic® *see* Enalapril and Hydrochlorothiazide *on page 491*

Vasocidin® *see* Sulfacetamide and Prednisolone *on page 1245*

VasoClear® [OTC] *see* Naphazoline *on page 964*

Vasocon-A® [OTC] *see* Naphazoline and Antazoline *on page 964*

Vasodilan® [DSC] *see* Isoxsuprine *on page 774*

Vasopressin (vay soe PRES in)

U.S. Brand Names Pitressin®

Canadian Brand Names Pressyn®; Pressyn® AR

Generic Available No

Synonyms ADH; Antidiuretic Hormone; 8-Arginine Vasopressin; Vasopressin Tannate

Pharmacologic Category Antidiuretic Hormone Analog; Hormone, Posterior Pituitary

Use Treatment of diabetes insipidus; prevention and treatment of postoperative abdominal distention; differential diagnosis of diabetes insipidus

Unlabeled/Investigational Use Adjunct in the treatment of GI hemorrhage and esophageal varices; pulseless ventricular tachycardia (VT)/ventricular fibrillation (VF); vasodilatory shock (septic shock); out-of-hospital asystole

Local Anesthetic/Vasoconstrictor Precautions No information available to require special precautions

Effects on Dental Treatment No significant effects or complications reported

Common Adverse Effects Frequency not defined.

Cardiovascular: Increased blood pressure, arrhythmias, venous thrombosis, vasoconstriction (with higher doses), angina, myocardial infarction

Central nervous system: Pounding in the head, fever, vertigo

Dermatologic: Urticaria, circumoral pallor

Gastrointestinal: Flatulence, abdominal cramps, nausea, vomiting

Genitourinary: Uterine contraction

Neuromuscular & skeletal: Tremor

Respiratory: Bronchial constriction

Miscellaneous: Diaphoresis

Mechanism of Action Increases cyclic adenosine monophosphate (cAMP) which increases water permeability at the renal tubule resulting in decreased

(Continued)

Vasopressin *(Continued)*

urine volume and increased osmolality; causes peristalsis by directly stimulating the smooth muscle in the GI tract

Drug Interactions

Increased Effect/Toxicity: Chlorpropamide, urea, clofibrate, carbamazepine, and fludrocortisone potentiate antidiuretic response.

Decreased Effect: Lithium, epinephrine, demeclocycline, heparin, and ethanol block antidiuretic activity to varying degrees.

Pharmacodynamics/Kinetics

Onset of action: Nasal: 1 hour

Duration: Nasal: 3-8 hours; I.M., SubQ: 2-8 hours

Metabolism: Nasal/Parenteral: Hepatic, renal

Half-life elimination: Nasal: 15 minutes; Parenteral: 10-20 minutes

Excretion: Nasal: Urine; SubQ: Urine (5% as unchanged drug) after 4 hours

Pregnancy Risk Factor C

Vasopressin Tannate *see* Vasopressin *on page 1369*

Vasotec® *see* Enalapril *on page 488*

VCF™ [OTC] *see* Nonoxynol 9 *on page 995*

VCR *see* VinCRIStine *on page 1378*

V-Dec-M® *see* Guaifenesin and Pseudoephedrine *on page 675*

Veetids® *see* Penicillin V Potassium *on page 1060*

Veg-Pancreatin 4X [OTC] *see* Pancreatin *on page 1042*

Velban® [DSC] *see* VinBLAStine *on page 1377*

Velcade™ *see* Bortezomib *on page 214*

Velivet™ *see* Ethinyl Estradiol and Desogestrel *on page 536*

Velosef® *see* Cephradine *on page 296*

Velosulin® BR (Buffered) [DSC] *see* Insulin Preparations *on page 749*

Venlafaxine (VEN la faks een)

U.S. Brand Names Effexor®; Effexor® XR

Canadian Brand Names Effexor®; Effexor® XR

Mexican Brand Names Efexor®

Generic Available No

Pharmacologic Category Antidepressant, Serotonin/Norepinephrine Reuptake Inhibitor

Use Treatment of major depressive disorder; generalized anxiety disorder (GAD), social anxiety disorder (social phobia)

Unlabeled/Investigational Use Obsessive-compulsive disorder (OCD), chronic fatigue syndrome; hot flashes; neuropathic pain; attention-deficit/hyperactivity disorder (ADHD) and autism in children

Local Anesthetic/Vasoconstrictor Precautions Although venlafaxine is not a tricyclic antidepressant, it does block norepinephrine reuptake within CNS synapses as part of its mechanisms. It has been suggested that vasoconstrictor be administered with caution and to monitor vital signs in dental patients taking antidepressants that affect norepinephrine in this way. This is particularly important in patients taking venlafaxine, which has been noted to produce a sustained increase in diastolic blood pressure and heart rate as a side effect.

Effects on Dental Treatment Key adverse event(s) related to dental treatment: Significant xerostomia (normal salivary flow resumes upon discontinuation); may contribute to oral discomfort, especially in the elderly

Common Adverse Effects

≥10%:

- Central nervous system: Headache (25%), somnolence (23%), dizziness (19%), insomnia (18%), nervousness (13%)
- Gastrointestinal: Nausea (37%), xerostomia (22%), constipation (15%), anorexia (11%)
- Genitourinary: Abnormal ejaculation/orgasm (12%)
- Neuromuscular & skeletal: Weakness (12%)
- Miscellaneous: Diaphoresis (12%)

1% to 10%:

- Cardiovascular: Vasodilation (4%), hypertension (dose-related; 3% in patients receiving <100 mg/day, up to 13% in patients receiving >300 mg/day), tachycardia (2%), chest pain (2%), postural hypotension (1%)
- Central nervous system: Anxiety (6%), abnormal dreams (4%), yawning (3%), agitation (2%), confusion (2%), abnormal thinking (2%), depersonalization (1%), depression (1%)
- Dermatologic: Rash (3%), pruritus (1%)

Endocrine & metabolic: Decreased libido
Gastrointestinal: Diarrhea (8%), vomiting (6%), dyspepsia (5%), flatulence (3%), taste perversion (2%), weight loss (1%)
Genitourinary: Impotence (6%), urinary frequency (3%), impaired urination (2%), orgasm disturbance (2%), urinary retention (1%)
Neuromuscular & skeletal: Tremor (5%), hypertonia (3%), paresthesia (3%), twitching (1%)
Ocular: Blurred vision (6%), mydriasis (2%)
Otic: Tinnitus (2%)
Miscellaneous: Infection (6%), chills (3%), trauma (2%)

Dosage Oral:

Children and Adolescents:

ADHD (unlabeled use): Initial: 12.5 mg/day

Children <40 kg: Increase by 12.5 mg/week to maximum of 50 mg/day in 2 divided doses

Children ≥40 kg: Increase by 25 mg/week to maximum of 75 mg/day in 3 divided doses.

Mean dose: 60 mg or 1.4 mg/kg administered in 2-3 divided doses

Autism (unlabeled use): Initial: 12.5 mg/day; adjust to 6.25-50 mg/day

Adults:

Depression:

Immediate-release tablets: 75 mg/day, administered in 2 or 3 divided doses, taken with food; dose may be increased in 75 mg/day increments at intervals of at least 4 days, up to 225-375 mg/day

Extended-release capsules: 75 mg once daily taken with food; for some new patients, it may be desirable to start at 37.5 mg/day for 4-7 days before increasing to 75 mg once daily; dose may be increased by up to 75 mg/day increments every 4 days as tolerated, up to a maximum of 225 mg/day

GAD, social anxiety disorder: Extended-release capsules: 75 mg once daily taken with food; for some new patients, it may be desirable to start at 37.5 mg/day for 4-7 days before increasing to 75 mg once daily; dose may be increased by up to 75 mg/day increments every 4 days as tolerated, up to a maximum of 225 mg/day

Note: When discontinuing this medication after more than 1 week of treatment, it is generally recommended that the dose be tapered. If venlafaxine is used for 6 weeks or longer, the dose should be tapered over 2 weeks when discontinuing its use.

Dosing adjustment in renal impairment: Cl_{cr} 10-70 mL/minute: Decrease dose by 25%; decrease total daily dose by 50% if dialysis patients; dialysis patients should receive dosing after completion of dialysis

Dosing adjustment in moderate hepatic impairment: Reduce total daily dosage by 50%

Mechanism of Action Venlafaxine and its active metabolite o-desmethylvenlafaxine (ODV) are potent inhibitors of neuronal serotonin and norepinephrine reuptake and weak inhibitors of dopamine reuptake. Venlafaxine and ODV have no significant activity for muscarinic cholinergic, H_1-histaminergic, or alpha$_2$-adrenergic receptors. Venlafaxine and ODV do not possess MAO-inhibitory activity.

Contraindications Hypersensitivity to venlafaxine or any component of the formulation; use of MAO inhibitors within 14 days; should not initiate MAO inhibitor within 7 days of discontinuing venlafaxine

Warnings/Precautions Potential for severe reactions when used with MAO inhibitors (myoclonus, diaphoresis, hyperthermia, NMS features, seizures, and death). May cause sustained increase in blood pressure or tachycardia, use caution in patients with recent history of MI, unstable heart disease, or hyperthyroidism; may cause increase in anxiety, nervousness, insomnia; may cause weight loss (use with caution in patients where weight loss is undesirable); may cause increases in serum cholesterol. Use caution with hepatic or renal impairment. Venlafaxine has been associated with the development of SIADH and hyponatremia.

May worsen psychosis in some patients or precipitate a shift to mania or hypomania in patients with bipolar disorder. Monotherapy in patients with bipolar disorder should be avoided. Patients should be screened for bipolar disorder, since using antidepressants alone may induce manic episodes with this condition. May increase the risks associated with electroconvulsive therapy. Use cautiously in patients with a history of seizures. The possibility of a suicide attempt is inherent in major depression and may persist until remission occurs. Monitor for worsening of depression or suicidality, especially during initiation of therapy or with dose increases or decreases. Worsening depression and severe abrupt suicidality that are not part of the presenting

(Continued)

Venlafaxine *(Continued)*

symptoms may require discontinuation or modification of drug therapy. Use caution in high-risk patients during initiation of therapy. Prescriptions should be written for the smallest quantity consistent with good patient care. The risks of cognitive or motor impairment, as well as the potential for anticholinergic effects are very low. May cause or exacerbate sexual dysfunction. May impair platelet aggregation, resulting in bleeding.

Abrupt discontinuation or dosage reduction after extended (≥6 weeks) therapy may lead to agitation, dysphoria, nervousness, anxiety, and other symptoms. When discontinuing therapy, dosage should be tapered gradually over at least a 2-week period. If intolerable symptoms occur following a decrease in dosage or upon discontinuation of therapy, then resuming the previous dose with a more gradual taper should be considered. Use caution in patients with increased intraocular pressure or at risk of acute narrow-angle glaucoma. Higher frequencies of suicidal ideation and hostility were noted in children (<18 years of age) during clinical trials evaluating treatment of major depression and/or GAD (not approved uses of venlafaxine).

The patient's family or caregiver should be alerted to monitor patients for the emergence of suicidality and associated behaviors such as anxiety, agitation, panic attacks, insomnia, irritability, hostility, impulsivity, akathisia, hypomania, and mania; patients should be instructed not to abruptly discontinue this medication, but notify their healthcare provider if any of these symptoms or worsening depression occur.

Drug Interactions

Cytochrome P450 Effect: Substrate of CYP2C8/9 (minor), 2C19 (minor), 2D6 (major), 3A4 (major); **Inhibits** CYP2B6 (weak), 2D6 (weak), 3A4 (weak)

Increased Effect/Toxicity: Concurrent use of MAO inhibitors (phenelzine, isocarboxazid), or drugs with MAO inhibitor activity (linezolid) may result in serotonin syndrome; should not be used within 2 weeks of each other. Selegiline may have a lower risk of this effect, particularly at low dosages, due to selectivity for MAO type B. In addition, concurrent use of buspirone, lithium, meperidine, nefazodone, selegiline, serotonin agonists (sumatriptan, naratriptan), sibutramine, SSRIs, trazodone, or tricyclic antidepressants may increase the risk of serotonin syndrome. Serum levels of haloperidol may be increased by venlafaxine. CYP2D6 inhibitors may increase the levels/effects of venlafaxine; example inhibitors include chlorpromazine, delavirdine, fluoxetine, miconazole, paroxetine, pergolide, quinidine, quinine, ritonavir, and ropinirole. CYP3A4 inhibitors may increase the levels/effects of venlafaxine; example inhibitors include azole antifungals, ciprofloxacin, clarithromycin, diclofenac, doxycycline, erythromycin, imatinib, isoniazid, nefazodone, nicardipine, propofol, protease inhibitors, quinidine, and verapamil.

Decreased Effect: Serum levels of indinavir may be reduced be venlafaxine (AUC reduced by 28%); clinical significance not determined. CYP3A4 inducers may decrease the levels/effects of venlafaxine; example inducers include aminoglutethimide, carbamazepine, nafcillin, nevirapine, phenobarbital, phenytoin, and rifamycins.

Ethanol/Nutrition/Herb Interactions

Ethanol: Avoid ethanol (may increase CNS effects).

Herb/Nutraceutical: Avoid valerian, St John's wort, SAMe, kava kava, tryptophan (may increase risk of serotonin syndrome and/or excessive sedation).

Dietary Considerations Should be taken with food.

Pharmacodynamics/Kinetics

Absorption: Oral: 92% to 100%; food has no significant effect on the absorption of venlafaxine or formation of the active metabolite O-desmethylvenlafaxine (ODV)

Distribution: At steady state: Venlafaxine 7.5 ± 3.7 L/kg, ODV 5.7 ± 1.8 L/Kg

Protein binding: Bound to human plasma protein: Venlafaxine 27%, ODV 30%

Metabolism: Hepatic via CYP2D6 to active metabolite, O-desmethylvenlafaxine (ODV); other metabolites include N-desmethylvenlafaxine and N,O-didesmethylvenlafaxine

Bioavailability: Absolute: ~45%

Half-life elimination: Venlafaxine: 3-7 hours; ODV: 9-13 hours; Steady-state, plasma: Venlafaxine/ODV: Within 3 days of multiple-dose therapy; prolonged with cirrhosis (Adults: Venlafaxine: ~30%, ODV: ~60%) and with dialysis (Adults: Venlafaxine: ~180%, ODV: ~142%)

Time to peak:

Immediate release: Venlafaxine: 2 hours, ODV: 3 hours

Extended release: Venlafaxine: 5.5 hours, ODV: 9 hours

Excretion: Urine (~87%, 5% as unchanged drug, 29% as unconjugated ODV, 26% as conjugated ODV, 27% as minor metabolites) within 48 hours

Clearance at steady state: Venlafaxine: 1.3 ± 0.6 L/hour/kg, ODV: 0.4 ± 0.2 L/hour/kg

Clearance decreased with:

Cirrhosis: Adults: Venlafaxine: ~50%, ODV: ~30%

Severe cirrhosis: Adults: Venlafaxine: ~90%

Renal impairment (Cl_{cr} 10-70 mL/minute): Adults: Venlafaxine: ~24%

Dialysis: Adults: Venlafaxine: ~57%, ODV: ~56%; due to large volume of distribution, a significant amount of drug is not likely to be removed.

Pregnancy Risk Factor C

Dosage Forms CAP, extended release (Effexor® XR): 37.5 mg, 75 mg, 150 mg. **TAB** (Effexor®): 25 mg, 37.5 mg, 50 mg, 75 mg, 100 mg

Selected Readings

Ganzber S, "Psychoactive Drugs," *ADA Guide to Dental Therapeutics,* 2nd edition, Chapter 21, Chicago, IL: ADA Publishing, 2000, 381.

Venofer® *see* Iron Sucrose *on page 767*

Venoglobulin®-S *see* Immune Globulin (Intravenous) *on page 740*

Ventolin® [DSC] *see* Albuterol *on page 71*

Ventolin® HFA *see* Albuterol *on page 71*

VePesid® *see* Etoposide *on page 567*

Veracolate [OTC] *see* Bisacodyl *on page 208*

Verapamil (ver AP a mil)

Related Information

Calcium Channel Blockers and Gingival Hyperplasia *on page 1600*

Calcium Channel Blockers, Comparative Pharmacokinetics *on page 1602*

Cardiovascular Diseases *on page 1458*

U.S. Brand Names Calan®; Calan® SR; Covera-HS®; Isoptin® SR; Verelan®; Verelan® PM

Canadian Brand Names Alti-Verapamil; Apo-Verap®; Calan®; Chronovera®; Covera®; Gen-Verapamil; Gen-Verapamil SR; Isoptin®; Isoptin® I.V.; Isoptin® SR; Novo-Veramil; Novo-Veramil SR; Nu-Verap

Mexican Brand Names Cronovera®; Dilacoran®

Generic Available Yes

Synonyms Iproveratril Hydrochloride; Verapamil Hydrochloride

Pharmacologic Category Antiarrhythmic Agent, Class IV; Calcium Channel Blocker

Use Orally for treatment of angina pectoris (vasospastic, chronic stable, unstable) and hypertension; I.V. for supraventricular tachyarrhythmias (PSVT, atrial fibrillation, atrial flutter)

Unlabeled/Investigational Use Migraine; hypertrophic cardiomyopathy; bipolar disorder (manic manifestations)

Local Anesthetic/Vasoconstrictor Precautions No information available to require special precautions

Effects on Dental Treatment Key adverse event(s) related to dental treatment: Gingival hyperplasia. Calcium channel blockers (CCB) have been reported to cause gingival hyperplasia (GH). Verapamil induced GH has appeared 11 months or more after subjects took daily doses of 240-360 mg. The severity of hyperplastic syndrome does not seem to be dose-dependent. Gingivectomy is only successful if CCB therapy is discontinued. GH regresses markedly 1 week after CCB discontinuance with all symptoms resolving in 2 months. If a patient must continue CCB therapy, begin a program of professional cleaning and patient plaque control to minimize severity and growth rate of gingival tissue.

Common Adverse Effects

>10%: Gastrointestinal: Gingival hyperplasia (19%)

1% to 10%:

Cardiovascular: Bradycardia (1.4% oral, 1.2% I.V.); first-, second-, or third-degree AV block (1.2% oral, unknown I.V.); CHF (1.8% oral); hypotension (2.5% oral, 3% I.V.); peripheral edema (1.9% oral), symptomatic hypotension (1.5% I.V.); severe tachycardia (1% I.V.)

Central nervous system: Dizziness (3.3% oral, 1.2% I.V.), fatigue (1.7% oral), headache (2.2% oral, 1.2% I.V.)

Dermatologic: Rash (1.2% oral)

Gastrointestinal: Constipation (12% up to 42% in clinical trials), nausea (2.7% oral, 0.9% I.V.)

Respiratory: Dyspnea (1.4% oral)

Dosage

Children: SVT:

I.V.:

<1 year: 0.1-0.2 mg/kg over 2 minutes; repeat every 30 minutes as needed

(Continued)

Verapamil *(Continued)*

1-15 years: 0.1-0.3 mg/kg over 2 minutes; maximum: 5 mg/dose, may repeat dose in 15 minutes if adequate response not achieved; maximum for second dose: 10 mg/dose

Oral (dose not well established):

1-5 years: 4-8 mg/kg/day in 3 divided doses **or** 40-80 mg every 8 hours

>5 years: 80 mg every 6-8 hours

Adults:

SVT: I.V.: 2.5-5 mg (over 2 minutes); second dose of 5-10 mg (~0.15 mg/kg) may be given 15-30 minutes after the initial dose if patient tolerates, but does not respond to initial dose; maximum total dose: 20 mg

Angina: Oral: Initial dose: 80-120 mg 3 times/day (elderly or small stature: 40 mg 3 times/day); range: 240-480 mg/day in 3-4 divided doses

Hypertension: Oral:

Immediate release: 80 mg 3 times/day; usual dose range (JNC 7): 80-320 mg/day in 2 divided doses

Sustained release: 240 mg/day; usual dose range (JNC 7): 120-360 mg/day in 1-2 divided doses; 120 mg/day in the elderly or small patients (no evidence of additional benefit in doses >360 mg/day).

Extended release:

Covera-HS®: Usual dose range (JNC 7): 120-360 mg once daily (once-daily dosing is recommended at bedtime)

Verelan® PM: Usual dose range: 200-400 mg once daily at bedtime

Dosing adjustment in renal impairment: Cl_{cr} <10 mL/minute: Administer at 50% to 75% of normal dose.

Dialysis: Not dialyzable (0% to 5%) via hemo- or peritoneal dialysis; supplemental dose is not necessary.

Dosing adjustment/comments in hepatic disease: Reduce dose in cirrhosis, reduce dose to 20% to 50% of normal and monitor ECG.

Mechanism of Action Inhibits calcium ion from entering the "slow channels" or select voltage-sensitive areas of vascular smooth muscle and myocardium during depolarization; produces a relaxation of coronary vascular smooth muscle and coronary vasodilation; increases myocardial oxygen delivery in patients with vasospastic angina; slows automaticity and conduction of AV node.

Contraindications Hypersensitivity to verapamil or any component of the formulation; severe left ventricular dysfunction; hypotension (systolic pressure <90 mm Hg) or cardiogenic shock; sick sinus syndrome (except in patients with a functioning artificial pacemaker); second- or third-degree AV block (except in patients with a functioning artificial pacemaker); atrial flutter or fibrillation and an accessory bypass tract (WPW, Lown-Ganong-Levine syndrome)

Warnings/Precautions Use with caution in sick-sinus syndrome, severe left ventricular dysfunction, hepatic or renal impairment, hypertrophic cardiomyopathy (especially obstructive), abrupt withdrawal may cause increased duration and frequency of chest pain; avoid I.V. use in neonates and young infants due to severe apnea, bradycardia, or hypotensive reactions; elderly may experience more constipation and hypotension. Monitor ECG and blood pressure closely in patients receiving I.V. therapy particularly in patients with supraventricular tachycardia. May prolong recovery from nondepolarizing neuromuscular-blocking agents.

Drug Interactions

Cytochrome P450 Effect: Substrate of CYP1A2 (minor), 2B6 (minor), 2C8/9 (minor), 2C18 (minor), 2E1 (minor), 3A4 (major); **Inhibits** CYP1A2 (weak), 2C8/9 (weak), 2D6 (weak), 3A4 (moderate)

Increased Effect/Toxicity: Use of verapamil with amiodarone, beta-blockers, or flecainide may lead to bradycardia and decreased cardiac output. Aspirin and concurrent verapamil use may increase bleeding times. Lithium neurotoxicity may result when verapamil is added. Effect of nondepolarizing neuromuscular blocker is prolonged by verapamil. Grapefruit juice may increase verapamil serum concentrations. Blood pressure-lowering effects may be additive with sildenafil, tadalafil, and vardenafil (use caution).

Cisapride levels may be increased by verapamil, potentially resulting in life-threatening arrhythmias; avoid concurrent use. Verapamil may increase the levels/effects of selected benzodiazepines, other calcium channel blockers, cyclosporine, ergot alkaloids, selected HMG-CoA reductase inhibitors, mirtazapine, nateglinide, nefazodone, pimozide, quinidine, sildenafil (and other PDE-5 inhibitors), tacrolimus, venlafaxine, and other CYP3A4 substrates. In addition, serum concentrations of the following drugs may be increased by verapamil: Alfentanil, digoxin, doxorubicin, ethanol, prazosin, and theophylline.

The levels/effects of verapamil may be increased by azole antifungals, ciprofloxacin, clarithromycin, diclofenac, doxycycline, erythromycin, imatinib, isoniazid, nefazodone, nicardipine, propofol, protease inhibitors, quinidine, and other CYP3A4 inhibitors.

Decreased Effect: The levels/effects of verapamil may be decreased by aminoglutethimide, carbamazepine, nafcillin, nevirapine, phenobarbital, phenytoin, rifamycins, and other CYP3A4 inducers. Lithium levels may be decreased by verapamil. Nafcillin decreases plasma concentration of verapamil.

Ethanol/Nutrition/Herb Interactions

Ethanol: Avoid or limit ethanol (may increase ethanol levels).

Food: Grapefruit juice may increase the serum concentration of verapamil; avoid concurrent use.

Herb/Nutraceutical: St John's wort may decrease levels. Avoid dong quai if using for hypertension (has estrogenic activity). Avoid ephedra, yohimbe, ginseng (may worsen arrhythmia or hypertension). Avoid garlic (may have increased antihypertensive effect).

Dietary Considerations Calan® SR and Isoptin® SR products may be taken with food or milk, other formulations may be administered without regard to meals; sprinkling contents of Verelan® or Verelan® PM capsule onto applesauce does not affect oral absorption.

Pharmacodynamics/Kinetics

Onset of action: Peak effect: Oral: Immediate release: 2 hours; I.V.: 1-5 minutes

Duration: Oral: Immediate release tablets: 6-8 hours; I.V.: 10-20 minutes

Protein binding: 90%

Metabolism: Hepatic via multiple CYP isoenzymes; extensive first-pass effect

Bioavailability: Oral: 20% to 30%

Half-life elimination: Infants: 4.4-6.9 hours; Adults: Single dose: 2-8 hours, Multiple doses: Up to 12 hours; prolonged with hepatic cirrhosis

Excretion: Urine (70%, 3% to 4% as unchanged drug); feces (16%)

Pregnancy Risk Factor C

Dosage Forms CAP, extended release: 120 mg, 180 mg, 240 mg; (Verelan® PM): 100 mg, 200 mg, 300 mg. **CAPLET, sustained release** (Calan® SR): 120 mg, 180 mg, 240 mg. **CAP, sustained release** (Verelan®): 120 mg, 180 mg, 240 mg, 360 mg. **INJ, solution:** 2.5 mg/mL (2 mL, 4 mL). **TAB** (Calan®): 40 mg, 80 mg, 120 mg. **TAB, extended release:** 120 mg, 180 mg, 240 mg; (Covera HS®): 180 mg, 240 mg. **TAB, sustained release** (Isoptin® SR): 120 mg, 180 mg, 240 mg

Selected Readings

Wynn RL, "Update on Calcium Channel Blocker Induced Gingival Hyperplasia," *Gen Dent*, 1995, 43(3):218-22.

Verapamil and Trandolapril *see* Trandolapril and Verapamil *on page 1322*

Verapamil Hydrochloride *see* Verapamil *on page 1373*

Verelan® *see* Verapamil *on page 1373*

Verelan® PM *see* Verapamil *on page 1373*

Vermox® *see* Mebendazole *on page 859*

Versacaps® *see* Guaifenesin and Pseudoephedrine *on page 675*

Versed® [DSC] *see* Midazolam *on page 924*

Versiclear™ *see* Sodium Thiosulfate *on page 1230*

Verteporfin (ver te POR fin)

U.S. Brand Names Visudyne®

Canadian Brand Names Visudyne®

Generic Available No

Pharmacologic Category Ophthalmic Agent

Use Treatment of predominantly classic subfoveal choroidal neovascularization due to macular degeneration, presumed ocular histoplasmosis, or pathologic myopia

Unlabeled/Investigational Use Predominantly **occult** subfoveal choroidal neovascularization

Local Anesthetic/Vasoconstrictor Precautions No information available to require special precautions

Effects on Dental Treatment No significant effects or complications reported

Mechanism of Action Following intravenous administration, verteporfin is transported by lipoproteins to the neovascular endothelium in the affected eye(s), including choroidal neovasculature and the retina. Verteporfin then needs to be activated by nonthermal red light, which results in local damage to the endothelium, leading to temporary choroidal vessel occlusion.

Pregnancy Risk Factor C

Vesanoid® *see* Tretinoin (Oral) *on page 1328*
Vexol® *see* Rimexolone *on page 1185*
VFEND® *see* Voriconazole *on page 1385*
Viadur® *see* Leuprolide *on page 805*
Viagra® *see* Sildenafil *on page 1219*
Vibramycin® *see* Doxycycline *on page 471*
Vibra-Tabs® *see* Doxycycline *on page 471*
Vicks® 44® Cough Relief [OTC] *see* Dextromethorphan *on page 421*
Vicks® 44D Cough & Head Congestion [OTC] *see* Pseudoephedrine and Dextromethorphan *on page 1148*
Vicks® 44E [OTC] *see* Guaifenesin and Dextromethorphan *on page 673*
Vicks® DayQuil® Multi-Symptom Cold and Flu [OTC] *see* Acetaminophen, Dextromethorphan, and Pseudoephedrine *on page 59*
Vicks® Pediatric Formula 44E [OTC] *see* Guaifenesin and Dextromethorphan *on page 673*
Vicks Sinex® 12 Hour Ultrafine Mist [OTC] *see* Oxymetazoline *on page 1034*
Vicks® Sinex® Nasal Spray [OTC] *see* Phenylephrine *on page 1078*
Vicks® Sinex® UltraFine Mist [OTC] *see* Phenylephrine *on page 1078*
Vicodin® *see* Hydrocodone and Acetaminophen *on page 702*
Vicodin® ES *see* Hydrocodone and Acetaminophen *on page 702*
Vicodin® HP *see* Hydrocodone and Acetaminophen *on page 702*
Vicodin Tuss® *see* Hydrocodone and Guaifenesin *on page 708*
Vicon Forte® *see* Vitamins (Multiple/Oral) *on page 1384*
Vicon Plus® [OTC] *see* Vitamins (Multiple/Oral) *on page 1384*
Vicoprofen® *see* Hydrocodone and Ibuprofen *on page 709*

Vidarabine (vye DARE a been)

Related Information
Oral Viral Infections *on page 1547*
Systemic Viral Diseases *on page 1519*

U.S. Brand Names Vira-A® [DSC]

Generic Available No

Synonyms Adenine Arabinoside; Ara-A; Arabinofuranosyladenine; Vidarabine Monohydrate

Pharmacologic Category Antiviral Agent, Ophthalmic

Use Treatment of acute keratoconjunctivitis and epithelial keratitis due to herpes simplex virus type 1 and 2; superficial keratitis caused by herpes simplex virus

Local Anesthetic/Vasoconstrictor Precautions No information available to require special precautions

Effects on Dental Treatment No significant effects or complications reported

Mechanism of Action Inhibits viral DNA synthesis by blocking DNA polymerase

Pregnancy Risk Factor C

Vidarabine Monohydrate *see* Vidarabine *on page 1376*
Vi-Daylin® + Iron Liquid [OTC] *see* Vitamins (Multiple/Oral) *on page 1384*
Vi-Daylin® Liquid [OTC] *see* Vitamins (Multiple/Oral) *on page 1384*
Videx® *see* Didanosine *on page 433*
Videx® EC *see* Didanosine *on page 433*

Vigabatrin (vye GA ba trin)

Canadian Brand Names Sabril®

Mexican Brand Names Sabril®

Generic Available No

Pharmacologic Category Anticonvulsant, Miscellaneous

Use Active management of partial or secondary generalized seizures not controlled by usual treatments; treatment of infantile spasms

Unlabeled/Investigational Use Spasticity, tardive dyskinesias

Local Anesthetic/Vasoconstrictor Precautions No information available to require special precautions

Effects on Dental Treatment No significant effects or complications reported

Common Adverse Effects

>10%

Central nervous system: Fatigue (27%), headache (26%), drowsiness (22%), dizziness (19%), depression (13%), tremor (11%), agitation (11%). **Note:** In pediatric use, hyperactivity (hyperkinesia, agitation, excitation, or restlessness) was reported in 11% of patients.

Endocrine & metabolic: Weight gain (12%)

Ophthalmic: Visual field defects, abnormal vision (11%)

1% to 10%

Cardiovascular: Edema (dependent), chest pain

Central nervous system: Amnesia, confusion, paresthesia, impaired concentration, insomnia, anxiety, emotional lability, abnormal thinking, speech disorder, vertigo, aggression, nervousness, personality disorder

Dermatologic: Rash (5%, similar to placebo), skin disorder

Endocrine & metabolic: Increased appetite, dysmenorrhea, menstrual disorder

Gastrointestinal: Nausea, diarrhea, abdominal pain, constipation, vomiting

Genitourinary: Urinary tract infection

Hematologic: Purpura

Neuromuscular & skeletal: Ataxia, arthralgia, back pain, abnormal coordination, abnormal gait, weakness, hyporeflexia, arthrosis

Ophthalmologic: Nystagmus, diplopia, eye pain

Otic: Ear pain

Respiratory: Throat irritation, nasal congestion, upper respiratory tract infection, sinusitis

Restrictions Not available in U.S.

Mechanism of Action Irreversibly inhibits gamma-aminobutyric acid transaminase (GABA-T), increasing the levels of the inhibitory compound gamma amino butyric acid (GABA) within the brain. Duration of effect is dependent upon rate of GABA-T resynthesis.

Drug Interactions

Decreased Effect: Serum concentrations of phenytoin and phenobarbital may be decreased by vigabatrin.

Pharmacodynamics/Kinetics

Duration (rate of GABA-T resynthesis dependent): Variable (not strictly correlated to serum concentrations)

Absorption: Rapid

Metabolism: Minimal

Half-life elimination: 5-8 hours; Elderly: Up to 13 hours

Time to peak: 2 hours

Excretion: Urine (70%, as unchanged drug)

Pregnancy Risk Factor Not assigned; contraindicated per manufacturer

Vigamox™ *see* Moxifloxacin *on page 949*

VinBLAStine (vin BLAS teen)

U.S. Brand Names Velban® [DSC]

Canadian Brand Names Velban®

Mexican Brand Names Lemblastine®

Generic Available Yes

Synonyms NSC-49842; Vinblastine Sulfate; VLB

Pharmacologic Category Antineoplastic Agent, Natural Source (Plant) Derivative; Antineoplastic Agent, Vinca Alkaloid

Use Treatment of Hodgkin's and non-Hodgkin's lymphoma, testicular, lung, head and neck, breast, and renal carcinomas, Mycosis fungoides, Kaposi's sarcoma, histiocytosis, choriocarcinoma, and idiopathic thrombocytopenic purpura

Local Anesthetic/Vasoconstrictor Precautions No information available to require special precautions

Effects on Dental Treatment Key adverse event(s) related to dental treatment: Stomatitis, metallic taste, and jaw pain.

Common Adverse Effects

>10%:

Dermatologic: Alopecia

Endocrine & metabolic: SIADH

Gastrointestinal: Diarrhea (less common), stomatitis, anorexia, metallic taste

Hematologic: May cause severe bone marrow suppression and is the dose-limiting toxicity of VLB (unlike vincristine); severe granulocytopenia and thrombocytopenia may occur following the administration of VLB and nadir 5-10 days after treatment

Myelosuppression (primarily leukopenia, may be dose limiting)

Onset: 4-7 days

Nadir: 5-10 days

Recovery: 4-21 days

1% to 10%:

Cardiovascular: Hypertension, Raynaud's phenomenon

Central nervous system: Depression, malaise, headache, seizures

Dermatologic: Rash, photosensitivity, dermatitis

(Continued)

VinBLAStine *(Continued)*

Endocrine & metabolic: Hyperuricemia
Gastrointestinal: Constipation, abdominal pain, nausea (mild), vomiting (mild), paralytic ileus, stomatitis
Genitourinary: Urinary retention
Neuromuscular & skeletal: Jaw pain, myalgia, paresthesia
Respiratory: Bronchospasm

Mechanism of Action Vinblastine binds to tubulin and inhibits microtubule formation, therefore, arresting the cell at metaphase by disrupting the formation of the mitotic spindle; it is specific for the M and S phases. Vinblastine may also interfere with nucleic acid and protein synthesis by blocking glutamic acid utilization.

Drug Interactions

Cytochrome P450 Effect: Substrate of CYP2D6 (minor), 3A4 (major); **Inhibits** CYP2D6 (weak), 3A4 (weak)

Increased Effect/Toxicity: CYP3A4 inhibitors may increase the levels/effects of vinblastine; example inhibitors include azole antifungals, ciprofloxacin, clarithromycin, diclofenac, doxycycline, erythromycin, imatinib, isoniazid, nefazodone, nicardipine, propofol, protease inhibitors, quinidine, and verapamil.

Previous or simultaneous use with mitomycin-C has resulted in acute shortness of breath and severe bronchospasm within minutes or several hours after *Vinca* alkaloid injection and may occur up to 2 weeks after the dose of mitomycin. Mitomycin-C in combination with administration of VLB may cause acute shortness of breath and severe bronchospasm, onset may be within minutes or several hours after VLB injection.

Decreased Effect: CYP3A4 inducers may decrease the levels/effects of vinblastine; example inducers include aminoglutethimide, carbamazepine, nafcillin, nevirapine, phenobarbital, phenytoin (may reduce vinblastine serum concentrations), and rifamycins.

Pharmacodynamics/Kinetics

Distribution: V_d: 27.3 L/kg; binds extensively to tissues; does not penetrate CNS or other fatty tissues; distributes to liver
Protein binding: 99%
Metabolism: Hepatic to active metabolite
Half-life elimination: Biphasic: Initial: 0.164 hours; Terminal: 25 hours
Excretion: Feces (95%); urine (<1% as unchanged drug)

Pregnancy Risk Factor D

Vinblastine Sulfate *see* VinBLAStine *on page 1377*
Vincasar PFS® *see* VinCRIStine *on page 1378*

VinCRIStine (vin KRIS teen)

U.S. Brand Names Oncovin® [DSC]; Vincasar PFS®

Canadian Brand Names Oncovin®; Vincasar® PFS®

Mexican Brand Names Citomid® [inj.]; Vintec®

Generic Available Yes

Synonyms LCR; Leurocristine Sulfate; NSC-67574; VCR; Vincristine Sulfate

Pharmacologic Category Antineoplastic Agent, Natural Source (Plant) Derivative; Antineoplastic Agent, Vinca Alkaloid

Use Treatment of leukemias, Hodgkin's disease, non-Hodgkin's lymphomas, Wilms' tumor, neuroblastoma, rhabdomyosarcoma

Local Anesthetic/Vasoconstrictor Precautions No information available to require special precautions

Effects on Dental Treatment No significant effects or complications reported

Common Adverse Effects

>10%:

Dermatologic: Alopecia occurs in 20% to 70% of patients
Extravasation: VCR is a vesicant and can cause tissue irritation and necrosis if infiltrated; if extravasation occurs, follow institutional policy, which may include hyaluronidase and hot compresses
Vesicant chemotherapy

1% to 10%:

Cardiovascular: Orthostatic hypotension or hypertension, hypertension, hypotension
Central nervous system: Motor difficulties, seizures, headache, CNS depression, cranial nerve paralysis, fever
Dermatologic: Rash
Endocrine & metabolic: Hyperuricemia

SIADH: Rarely occurs, but may be related to the neurologic toxicity; may cause symptomatic hyponatremia with seizures; the increase in serum ADH concentration usually subsides within 2-3 days after onset

Gastrointestinal: Constipation and possible paralytic ileus secondary to neurologic toxicity; oral ulceration, abdominal cramps, anorexia, metallic taste, bloating, nausea (mild), vomiting, weight loss, diarrhea

Local: Phlebitis

Neurologic: Alterations in mental status such as depression, confusion, or insomnia; constipation, paralytic ileus, and urinary tract disturbances may occur. All patients should be on a prophylactic bowel management regimen. Cranial nerve palsies, headaches, jaw pain, optic atrophy with blindness have been reported. Intrathecal administration of VCR has uniformly caused death; VCR should **never** be administered by this route. Neurologic effects of VCR may be additive with those of other neurotoxic agents and spinal cord irradiation.

Neuromuscular & skeletal: Jaw pain, leg pain, myalgia, cramping, numbness, weakness

Peripheral neuropathy: Frequently the dose-limiting toxicity of VCR. Most frequent in patients >40 years of age; occurs usually after an average of 3 weekly doses, but may occur after just one dose. Manifested as loss of the deep tendon reflexes in the lower extremities, numbness, tingling, pain, paresthesias of the fingers and toes (stocking glove sensation), and "foot drop" or "wrist drop"

Ocular: Photophobia

Mechanism of Action Binds to tubulin and inhibits microtubule formation; therefore arresting the cell at metaphase by disrupting the formation of the mitotic spindle; it is specific for the M and S phases. Vincristine may also interfere with nucleic acid and protein synthesis by blocking glutamic acid utilization.

Drug Interactions

Cytochrome P450 Effect: Substrate of CYP3A4 (major); **Inhibits** CYP3A4 (weak)

Increased Effect/Toxicity: Vincristine should be given 12-24 hours before asparaginase to minimize toxicity (may decrease the hepatic clearance of vincristine). Acute pulmonary reactions may occur with mitomycin-C. Previous or simultaneous use with mitomycin-C has resulted in acute shortness of breath and severe bronchospasm within minutes or several hours after *Vinca* alkaloid injection and may occur up to 2 weeks after the dose of mitomycin.

CYP3A4 inhibitors may increase the levels/effects of vincristine. Example inhibitors include azole antifungals, ciprofloxacin, clarithromycin, diclofenac, doxycycline, erythromycin, imatinib, isoniazid, nefazodone, nicardipine, propofol, protease inhibitors, quinidine, and verapamil. Digoxin plasma levels and renal excretion may decrease with combination chemotherapy including vincristine.

Decreased Effect: Digoxin levels may decrease with combination chemotherapy. CYP3A4 inducers may decrease the levels/effects of vincristine; example inducers include aminoglutethimide, carbamazepine, nafcillin, nevirapine, phenobarbital, phenytoin, and rifamycins.

Pharmacodynamics/Kinetics

Absorption: Oral: Poor

Distribution: V_d: 163-165 L/m^2; Poor penetration into CSF; rapidly removed from bloodstream and tightly bound to tissues; penetrates blood-brain barrier poorly

Protein binding: 75%

Metabolism: Extensively hepatic

Half-life elimination: Terminal: 24 hours

Excretion: Feces (~80%); urine (<1% as unchanged drug)

Pregnancy Risk Factor D

Vincristine Sulfate *see* VinCRIStine *on page 1378*

Vindesine (VIN de seen)

Generic Available No

Synonyms DAVA; Deacetyl Vinblastine Carboxamide; Desacetyl Vinblastine Amide Sulfate; DVA; Eldisine Lilly 99094; Lilly CT-3231; NSC-245467; Vindesine Sulfate

Pharmacologic Category Antineoplastic Agent, Vinca Alkaloid

Unlabeled/Investigational Use Investigational: Management of acute lymphocytic leukemia, chronic myelogenous leukemia; breast, head, neck, and lung cancers; lymphomas (Hodgkin's and non-Hodgkin's)

(Continued)

Vindesine *(Continued)*

Local Anesthetic/Vasoconstrictor Precautions No information available to require special precautions

Effects on Dental Treatment Key adverse event(s) related to dental treatment: Loss of taste and facial paralysis.

Common Adverse Effects

>10%:

Central nervous system: Pyrexia, malaise (up to 60%)

Dermatologic: Alopecia (6% to 92%)

Gastrointestinal: Mild nausea and vomiting (7% to 27%), constipation (10% to 17%) - related to the neurotoxicity

Hematologic: Leukopenia (50%) and thrombocytopenia (14% to 26%), may be dose-limiting; thrombocytosis (20% to 28%)

Nadir: 6-12 days

Recovery: Days 14-18

Neuromuscular & skeletal: Paresthesias (40% to 70%); loss of deep tendon reflexes (35% to 60%, may be dose-limiting); myalgia (up to 60%)

1% to 10%:

Dermatologic: Rashes

Gastrointestinal: Loss of taste

Hematologic: Anemia

Local: Phlebitis

Neuromuscular & skeletal: Facial paralysis

Mechanism of Action Vindesine is a semisynthetic vinca alkaloid, having a mechanism of action similar to the other vinca derivatives. It arrests cell division in metaphase through inhibition of microtubular formation of the mitotic spindle. The drug is cell-cycle specific for the S phase.

Pharmacodynamics/Kinetics

Distribution: V_d: 8 L/kg; minimal distribution to adipose tissue or CNS

Metabolism: Hepatic

Half-life elimination:

Triphasic; Alpha: 2 minutes; Beta: 1 hour

Terminal: 24 hours

Excretion: Feces; urine (~3% to 25% of dose as unchanged drug)

Vindesine Sulfate *see* Vindesine *on page 1379*

Vinorelbine (vi NOR el been)

U.S. Brand Names Navelbine®

Canadian Brand Names Navelbine®

Mexican Brand Names Navelbine®

Generic Available Yes

Synonyms Dihydroxydeoxynorvinkaleukoblastine; NVB; Vinorelbine Tartrate

Pharmacologic Category Antineoplastic Agent, Natural Source (Plant) Derivative; Antineoplastic Agent, Vinca Alkaloid

Use Treatment of nonsmall cell lung cancer

Unlabeled/Investigational Use Treatment of breast cancer, ovarian carcinoma, Hodgkin's disease, non-Hodgkin's lymphoma

Local Anesthetic/Vasoconstrictor Precautions No information available to require special precautions

Effects on Dental Treatment No significant effects or complications reported

Common Adverse Effects

>10%:

Central nervous system: Fatigue (27%)

Dermatologic: Alopecia (12%)

Gastrointestinal: Nausea (44%, severe <2%) and vomiting (20%) are most common and are easily controlled with standard antiemetics; constipation (35%), diarrhea (17%)

Emetic potential: Moderate (30% to 60%)

Hematologic: May cause severe bone marrow suppression and is the dose-limiting toxicity of vinorelbine; severe granulocytopenia (90%) may occur following the administration of vinorelbine; leukopenia (92%), anemia (83%)

Myelosuppressive:

WBC: Moderate - severe

Onset: 4-7 days

Nadir: 7-10 days

Recovery: 14-21 days

Hepatic: Elevated SGOT (67%), elevated total bilirubin (13%)

Local: Injection site reaction (28%), injection site pain (16%)

Neuromuscular & skeletal: Weakness (36%), peripheral neuropathy (20% to 25%)

1% to 10%:

Cardiovascular: Chest pain (5%)

Gastrointestinal: Paralytic ileus (1%)

Hematologic: Thrombocytopenia (5%)

Local: Extravasation: Vesicant and can cause tissue irritation and necrosis if infiltrated; if extravasation occurs, follow institutional policy, which may include hyaluronidase and hot compresses; phlebitis (7%)

Vesicant chemotherapy

Neuromuscular & skeletal: Mild to moderate peripheral neuropathy manifested by paresthesia and hyperesthesia, loss of deep tendon reflexes (<5%); myalgia (<5%), arthralgia (<5%), jaw pain (<5%)

Respiratory: Dyspnea (3% to 7%)

Mechanism of Action Semisynthetic vinca alkaloid which binds to tubulin and inhibits microtubule formation, therefore, arresting the cell at metaphase by disrupting the formation of the mitotic spindle; it is specific for the M and S phases. Vinorelbine may also interfere with nucleic acid and protein synthesis by blocking glutamic acid utilization.

Drug Interactions

Cytochrome P450 Effect: Substrate of CYP2D6 (minor), 3A4 (major); **Inhibits** CYP2D6 (weak), 3A4 (weak)

Increased Effect/Toxicity: Previous or simultaneous use with mitomycin-C has resulted in acute shortness of breath and severe bronchospasm within minutes or several hours after *Vinca* alkaloid injection and may occur up to 2 weeks after the dose of mitomycin. CYP3A4 inhibitors may increase the levels/effects of vinorelbine; example inhibitors include azole antifungals, ciprofloxacin, clarithromycin, diclofenac, doxycycline, erythromycin, imatinib, isoniazid, nefazodone, nicardipine, propofol, protease inhibitors, quinidine, and verapamil. Incidence of granulocytopenia is significantly higher in cisplatin/vinorelbine combination therapy than with single-agent vinorelbine.

Decreased Effect: CYP3A4 inducers may decrease the levels/effects of vinorelbine; example inducers include aminoglutethimide, carbamazepine, nafcillin, nevirapine, phenobarbital, phenytoin, and rifamycins.

Pharmacodynamics/Kinetics

Absorption: Unreliable; must be given I.V.

Distribution: V_d: 25.4-40.1 L/kg; binds extensively to human platelets and lymphocytes (79.6% to 91.2%)

Protein binding: 80% to 90%

Metabolism: Extensively hepatic to two metabolites, deacetylvinorelbine (active) and vinorelbine N-oxide

Bioavailability: Oral: 26% to 45%

Half-life elimination: Triphasic: Terminal: 27.7-43.6 hours

Excretion: Feces (46%); urine (18%, 10% to 12% as unchanged drug)

Clearance: Plasma: Mean: 0.97-1.26 L/hour/kg

Pregnancy Risk Factor D

Vinorelbine Tartrate *see* Vinorelbine *on page 1380*

Viokase® *see* Pancrelipase *on page 1042*

Viosterol *see* Ergocalciferol *on page 503*

Vioxx® *see* Rofecoxib *on page 1194*

Vira-A® [DSC] *see* Vidarabine *on page 1376*

Viracept® *see* Nelfinavir *on page 972*

Viramune® *see* Nevirapine *on page 977*

Virazole® *see* Ribavirin *on page 1177*

Viread® *see* Tenofovir *on page 1270*

Virilon® *see* MethylTESTOSTERone *on page 912*

Viroptic® *see* Trifluridine *on page 1339*

Viroxyn® [OTC] *see* Benzalkonium Chloride and Isopropyl Alcohol *on page 190*

Viscoat® *see* Chondroitin Sulfate and Sodium Hyaluronate *on page 325*

Visicol™ *see* Sodium Phosphates *on page 1230*

Visine-A™ [OTC] *see* Naphazoline and Pheniramine *on page 964*

Visine® Advanced Relief [OTC] *see* Tetrahydrozoline *on page 1282*

Visine® L.R. [OTC] *see* Oxymetazoline *on page 1034*

Visine® Original [OTC] *see* Tetrahydrozoline *on page 1282*

Vistaril® *see* HydrOXYzine *on page 723*

Vistide® *see* Cidofovir *on page 327*

Visudyne® *see* Verteporfin *on page 1375*

Vita-C® [OTC] *see* Ascorbic Acid *on page 148*
Vitacon Forte *see* Vitamins (Multiple/Oral) *on page 1384*

Vitamin A (VYE ta min aye)

U.S. Brand Names Aquasol A®; Palmitate-A® [OTC]
Generic Available Yes: Capsule
Synonyms Oleovitamin A
Pharmacologic Category Vitamin, Fat Soluble
Use Treatment and prevention of vitamin A deficiency; parenteral (I.M.) route is indicated when oral administration is not feasible or when absorption is insufficient (malabsorption syndrome)
Local Anesthetic/Vasoconstrictor Precautions No information available to require special precautions
Effects on Dental Treatment No significant effects or complications reported
Common Adverse Effects 1% to 10%:
Central nervous system: Irritability, vertigo, lethargy, malaise, fever, headache
Dermatologic: Drying or cracking of skin
Endocrine & metabolic: Hypercalcemia
Gastrointestinal: Weight loss
Ocular: Visual changes
Miscellaneous: Hypervitaminosis A
Mechanism of Action Needed for bone development, growth, visual adaptation to darkness, testicular and ovarian function, and as a cofactor in many biochemical processes
Drug Interactions
Increased Effect/Toxicity: Retinoids may have additive adverse effects.
Decreased Effect: Cholestyramine resin decreases absorption of vitamin A. Neomycin and mineral oil may also interfere with vitamin A absorption.
Pharmacodynamics/Kinetics
Absorption: Vitamin A in dosages **not** exceeding physiologic replacement is well absorbed after oral administration; water miscible preparations are absorbed more rapidly than oil preparations; large oral doses, conditions of fat malabsorption, low protein intake, or hepatic or pancreatic disease reduces oral absorption
Distribution: Large amounts concentrate for storage in the liver; enters breast milk
Metabolism: Conjugated with glucuronide; undergoes enterohepatic recirculation
Excretion: Feces
Pregnancy Risk Factor A/X (dose exceeding RDA recommendation)

Vitamin A Acid *see* Tretinoin (Topical) *on page 1329*

Vitamin A and Vitamin D (VYE ta min aye & VYE ta min dee)

U.S. Brand Names A and D® Ointment [OTC]; Baza® Clear [OTC]; Clocream® [OTC]; Sween Cream® [OTC]
Generic Available Yes: Capsule, ointment
Synonyms Cod Liver Oil
Pharmacologic Category Topical Skin Product
Use Temporary relief of discomfort due to chapped skin, diaper rash, minor burns, abrasions, as well as irritations associated with ostomy skin care
Local Anesthetic/Vasoconstrictor Precautions No information available to require special precautions
Effects on Dental Treatment No significant effects or complications reported
Common Adverse Effects Frequency not defined: Local: Irritation
Pregnancy Risk Factor B

Vitamin B_1 *see* Thiamine *on page 1287*
Vitamin B_2 *see* Riboflavin *on page 1178*
Vitamin B_3 *see* Niacin *on page 978*
Vitamin B_3 *see* Niacinamide *on page 979*
Vitamin B_5 *see* Pantothenic Acid *on page 1044*
Vitamin B_6 *see* Pyridoxine *on page 1154*
Vitamin B_{12} *see* Cyanocobalamin *on page 380*
Vitamin B_{12} *see* Hydroxocobalamin *on page 719*

Vitamin B Complex Combinations
(VYE ta min bee KOM pleks kom bi NAY shuns)

U.S. Brand Names Allbee® C-800 [OTC]; Allbee® C-800 + Iron [OTC]; Allbee® with C [OTC]; Apatate® [OTC]; Diatx™; DiatxFe™; Gevrabon® [OTC]; Neph-Plex® Rx; Nephrocaps®; Nephron FA®; Nephro-Vite®; Nephro-Vite® Rx;

Stresstabs® B-Complex [OTC]; Stresstabs® B-Complex + Iron [OTC]; Stresstabs® B-Complex + Zinc [OTC]; Surbex-T® [OTC]; Trinsicon®; Z-Bec® [OTC]

Generic Available Yes

Synonyms B Complex Combinations; B Vitamin Combinations

Pharmacologic Category Vitamin

Use Supplement for use in the wasting syndrome in chronic renal failure, uremia, impaired metabolic functions of the kidney, dialysis; labeled for OTC use as a dietary supplement

Local Anesthetic/Vasoconstrictor Precautions No information available to require special precautions

Effects on Dental Treatment No significant effects or complications reported

Common Adverse Effects Frequency not defined.

Central nervous system: Somnolence
Dermatologic: Itching
Gastrointestinal: Bloating, constipation, diarrhea, flatulence, nausea, vomiting
Hematologic: Peripheral vascular thrombosis, polycythemia vera
Neuromuscular & skeletal: Paresthesia
Miscellaneous: Allergic reaction

Pregnancy Risk Factor A (RDA recommended doses)

Vitamin C *see* Ascorbic Acid *on page 148*

Vitamin D_2 *see* Ergocalciferol *on page 503*

Vitamin E (VYE ta min ee)

U.S. Brand Names Aqua Gem E® [OTC]; Aquasol E® [OTC]; E-Gems® [OTC]; Key-E® [OTC]; Key-E® Kaps [OTC]

Generic Available Yes

Synonyms *d*-Alpha Tocopherol; *dl*-Alpha Tocopherol

Pharmacologic Category Vitamin, Fat Soluble

Use Prevention and treatment hemolytic anemia secondary to vitamin E deficiency, dietary supplement

Unlabeled/Investigational Use To reduce the risk of bronchopulmonary dysplasia or retrolental fibroplasia in infants exposed to high concentrations of oxygen; prevention and treatment of tardive dyskinesia and Alzheimer's disease

Local Anesthetic/Vasoconstrictor Precautions No information available to require special precautions

Effects on Dental Treatment No significant effects or complications reported

Significant Adverse Effects <1% (Limited to important or life-threatening): Blurred vision, contact dermatitis with topical preparation, gonadal dysfunction

Dosage One unit of vitamin E = 1 mg *dl*-alpha-tocopherol acetate. Oral:

Recommended daily allowance (RDA):

- Premature infants ≤3 months: 17 mg (25 units)
- Infants:
  - ≤6 months: 3 mg (4.5 units)
  - 7-12 months: 4 mg (6 units)
- Children:
  - 1-3 years: 6 mg (9 units); upper limit of intake should not exceed 200 mg/day
  - 4-8 years: 7 mg (10.5 units); upper limit of intake should not exceed 300 mg/day
  - 9-13 years: 11 mg (16.5 units); upper limit of intake should not exceed 600 mg/day
  - 14-18 years: 15 mg (22.5 units); upper limit of intake should not exceed 800 mg/day
- Adults: 15 mg (22.5 units); upper limit of intake should not exceed 1000 mg/day
- Pregnant female:
  - ≤18 years: 15 mg (22.5 units); upper level of intake should not exceed 800 mg/day
  - 19-50 years: 15 mg (22.5 units); upper level of intake should not exceed 1000 mg/day
- Lactating female:
  - ≤18 years: 19 mg (28.5 units); upper level of intake should not exceed 800 mg/day
  - 19-50 years: 19 mg (28.5 units); upper level of intake should not exceed 1000 mg/day

Vitamin E deficiency:

- Children (with malabsorption syndrome): 1 unit/kg/day of water miscible vitamin E (to raise plasma tocopherol concentrations to the normal range within 2 months and to maintain normal plasma concentrations)

(Continued)

Vitamin E *(Continued)*

Adults: 60-75 units/day

Prevention of vitamin E deficiency: Adults: 30 units/day

Prevention of retinopathy of prematurity or BPD secondary to O_2 therapy (AAP considers this use investigational and routine use is not recommended):

Retinopathy prophylaxis: 15-30 units/kg/day to maintain plasma levels between 1.5-2 mcg/mL (may need as high as 100 units/kg/day)

Cystic fibrosis, beta-thalassemia, sickle cell anemia may require higher daily maintenance doses:

Children:

Cystic fibrosis: 100-400 units/day

Beta-thalassemia: 750 units/day

Adults:

Sickle cell: 450 units/day

Alzheimer's disease: 1000 units twice daily

Tardive dyskinesia: 1600 units/day

Mechanism of Action Prevents oxidation of vitamin A and C; protects polyunsaturated fatty acids in membranes from attack by free radicals and protects red blood cells against hemolysis

Contraindications Hypersensitivity to vitamin E or any component of the formulation; I.V. route

Warnings/Precautions May induce vitamin K deficiency; necrotizing enterocolitis has been associated with oral administration of large dosages (eg, >200 units/day) of a hyperosmolar vitamin E preparation in low birth weight infants

Drug Interactions

Cholestyramine (and colestipol): May reduce absorption of vitamin E

Iron: Vitamin E may impair the hematologic response to iron in children with iron-deficiency anemia; monitor

Orlistat: May reduce absorption of vitamin E

Warfarin: Vitamin E may alter the effect of vitamin K actions on clotting factors resulting in an increase hypoprothrombinemic response to warfarin; monitor

Pharmacodynamics/Kinetics

Absorption: Oral: Depends on presence of bile; reduced in conditions of malabsorption, in low birth weight premature infants, and as dosage increases; water miscible preparations are better absorbed than oil preparations

Distribution: To all body tissues, especially adipose tissue, where it is stored

Metabolism: Hepatic to glucuronides

Excretion: Feces

Pregnancy Risk Factor A/C (dose exceeding RDA recommendation)

Lactation Excretion in breast milk unknown/compatible

Dosage Forms

Capsule: 100 units, 200 units, 400 units, 500 units, 600 units, 1000 units

Aqua Gem E®: 200 units, 400 units

E-Gems®: 30 units, 100 units, 600 units, 800 units, 1000 units, 1200 units

Key-E Kaps®: 200 units, 400 units

Cream: 100 units/g (60 g)

Key-E®: 30 units/g (60 g, 120 g, 480 g)

Oil: 100 units/0.25 mL (60 mL); 1150 units/0.25 mL (30 mL, 60 mL, 120 mL)

E-Gem®: 100 units/10 drops (15 mL, 60 mL)

Ointment, topical (Key-E®): 30 units/g (60 g, 120 g, 480 g)

Powder (Key-E®): 700 units/dose (15 g, 75 g, 1000 g)

Solution, oral drops (Aquasol E®): 15 units/0.3 mL (12 mL, 30 mL)

Spray (Key-E®): 30 units/3 seconds (105 g)

Suppository (Key-E®): 30 units (12s, 24s)

Tablet: 100 units, 200 units, 400 units, 500 units, 800 units

Key-E®: 100 units, 200 units, 400 units

Vitamin G *see* Riboflavin *on page 1178*

Vitamin K_1 *see* Phytonadione *on page 1084*

Vitamins (Multiple/Oral) (VYE ta mins, MUL ti pul/OR al)

U.S. Brand Names Centrum® [OTC]; Centrum® Performance™ [OTC]; Centrum® Silver® [OTC]; Geritol® Tonic [OTC]; Iberet® [OTC]; Iberet®-500 [OTC]; Iberet-Folic-500®; One-A-Day® 50 Plus Formula [OTC]; One-A-Day® Active Formula [OTC]; One-A -Day® Essential Formula [OTC]; One-A-Day® Maximum Formula [OTC]; One-A- Day® Men's Formula [OTC]; One-A-Day® Today [OTC]; One-A-Day® Women's Formula [OTC]; Theragran® Heart Right™ [OTC]; Theragran-M® Advanced Formula [OTC]; Vicon Forte®; Vicon Plus® [OTC]; Vi-Daylin® + Iron Liquid [OTC]; Vi-Daylin® Liquid [OTC]; Vitacon Forte

Generic Available Yes

Synonyms Multiple Vitamins; Therapeutic Multivitamins; Vitamins, Multiple (Oral); Vitamins, Multiple (Therapeutic); Vitamins, Multiple With Iron

Pharmacologic Category Vitamin

Use Prevention/treatment of vitamin and mineral deficiencies; labeled for OTC use as a dietary supplement

Local Anesthetic/Vasoconstrictor Precautions No information available to require special precautions

Effects on Dental Treatment No significant effects or complications reported

Significant Adverse Effects Refer to individual vitamin monographs.

Dosage Oral: Adults: Daily dose of adult preparations varies by product. Generally, 1 tablet or capsule or 5-15 mL of liquid per day. Consult package labeling. Prescription doses may be higher for burn or cystic fibrosis patients.

Contraindications Hypersensitivity to any component of the formulation; pre-existing hypervitaminosis

Warnings/Precautions RDA values are not requirements, but are recommended daily intakes of certain essential nutrients; use with caution in patients with severe renal or hepatic dysfunction or failure. Adult preparations may contain amounts of ethanol or iron which should not be used in children.

Ethanol/Nutrition/Herb Interactions Food: Iron absorption is inhibited by eggs and milk.

Dietary Considerations May be taken with food to decrease stomach upset.

Pregnancy Risk Factor A (at RDA recommended dose)

Lactation Enters breast milk/compatible

Dosage Forms Content varies depending on product used.

For more detailed information on ingredients in these and other multivitamins, please refer to Multivitamin Products *on page 1644*.

Vitamins, Multiple (Therapeutic) *see* Vitamins (Multiple/Oral) *on page 1384*

Vitamins, Multiple With Iron *see* Vitamins (Multiple/Oral) *on page 1384*

Vitelle™ Irospan® [OTC] [DSC] *see* Ferrous Sulfate and Ascorbic Acid *on page 587*

Vitrase® *see* Hyaluronidase *on page 697*

Vitrasert® *see* Ganciclovir *on page 646*

Vitravene™ [DSC] *see* Fomivirsen *on page 628*

Vitrax® *see* Hyaluronate and Derivatives *on page 696*

Vitussin *see* Hydrocodone and Guaifenesin *on page 708*

Vivactil® *see* Protriptyline *on page 1146*

Viva-Drops® [OTC] *see* Artificial Tears *on page 148*

Vivelle® *see* Estradiol *on page 518*

Vivelle-Dot® *see* Estradiol *on page 518*

Vivotif Berna® *see* Typhoid Vaccine *on page 1351*

VLB *see* VinBLAStine *on page 1377*

VM-26 *see* Teniposide *on page 1269*

Volmax® *see* Albuterol *on page 71*

Voltaren® *see* Diclofenac *on page 427*

Voltaren Ophthalmic® *see* Diclofenac *on page 427*

Voltaren®-XR *see* Diclofenac *on page 427*

Voriconazole (vor i KOE na zole)

U.S. Brand Names VFEND®

Generic Available No

Synonyms UK109496

Pharmacologic Category Antifungal Agent, Oral; Antifungal Agent, Parenteral

Use Treatment of invasive aspergillosis; treatment of esophageal candidiasis; treatment of serious fungal infections caused by *Scedosporium apiospermum* and *Fusarium* spp (including *Fusarium solani*) in patients intolerant of, or refractory to, other therapy

Local Anesthetic/Vasoconstrictor Precautions No information available to require special precautions

Effects on Dental Treatment Key adverse event(s) related to dental treatment: Xerostomia (normal salivary flow resumes upon discontinuation).

Significant Adverse Effects Note: Includes adverse reactions reported from all trials, including trials conducted in immunocompromised patients; cause:effect relationship not established for many reactions

>10%: Ocular: Visual changes (photophobia, color changes, increased or decreased visual acuity, or blurred vision occur in ~30%)

(Continued)

Voriconazole *(Continued)*

1% to 10%:

Cardiovascular: Tachycardia (3%), hypertension (2%), hypotension (2%), vasodilation (2%), peripheral edema (1%)

Central nervous system: Fever (6%), chills (4%), headache (3%), hallucinations (3%), dizziness (1%)

Dermatologic: Rash (6%), pruritus (1%)

Endocrine & metabolic: Hypokalemia (2%), hypomagnesemia (1%)

Gastrointestinal: Nausea (6%), vomiting (5%), abdominal pain (2%), diarrhea (1%), xerostomia (1%)

Hematologic: Thrombocytopenia (1%)

Hepatic: Alkaline phosphatase increased (4%), serum transaminases increased (2%), AST increased (2%), ALT increased (2%), cholestatic jaundice (1%)

Renal: Acute renal failure (1%)

<1% (Limited to important or life-threatening): Acute tubular necrosis, adrenal cortical insufficiency, agranulocytosis, allergic reaction, anaphylactoid reaction, anemia (aplastic), anemia (macrocytic, megaloblastic, or microcytic), angioedema, aplastic anemia, ataxia, atrial arrhythmia, atrial fibrillation, AV block, bigeminy, bone marrow depression, bone necrosis, bradycardia, brain edema, bundle branch block, cardiac arrest, cerebral hemorrhage, cholecystitis, cholelithiasis, color blindness, coma, congestive heart failure, convulsion, delirium, dementia, depersonalization, depression, DIC, discoid lupus erythematosus, duodenal ulcer perforation, dyspnea, encephalopathy, enlarged liver, enlarged spleen, eosinophilia, erythema multiforme, exfoliative dermatitis, extrapyramidal symptoms, fixed drug eruption, gastrointestinal hemorrhage, grand mal seizure, Guillain-Barré syndrome, hematemesis, hemolytic anemia, hepatic coma, hepatic failure, hepatitis, intestinal perforation, intracranial hypertension, leukopenia, lung edema, myasthenia, myocardial infarction, neuropathy, night blindness, optic atrophy, optic neuritis, pancreatitis, pancytopenia, papilledema, paresthesia, photosensitivity, psychosis, pulmonary embolus, QT interval prolongation, respiratory distress syndrome, sepsis, Stevens-Johnson syndrome, suicidal ideation, supraventricular tachycardia, syncope, thrombotic thrombocytopenic purpura, toxic epidermal necrolysis, ventricular arrhythmia, ventricular fibrillation, ventricular tachycardia, torsade de pointes, vertigo, visual field defect

Dosage

Children <12 years: No data available

Children ≥12 years and Adults:

Invasive aspergillosis and other serious fungal infections: I.V.: Initial: Loading dose: 6 mg/kg every 12 hours for 2 doses; followed by maintenance dose of 4 mg/kg every 12 hours

Conversion to oral dosing:

Patients <40 kg: 100 mg every 12 hours; increase to 150 mg every 12 hours in patients who fail to respond adequately

Patients ≥40 kg: 200 mg every 12 hours; increase to 300 mg every 12 hours in patients who fail to respond adequately

Esophageal candidiasis: Oral:

Patients <40 kg: 100 mg every 12 hours

Patients ≥40 kg: 200 mg every 12 hours

Note: Treatment should continue for a minimum of 14 days, and for at least 7 days following resolution of symptoms.

Dosage adjustment in patients unable to tolerate treatment:

I.V.: Dose may be reduced to 3 mg/kg every 12 hours

Oral: Dose may be reduced in 50 mg increments to a minimum dosage of 200 mg every 12 hours in patients weighing ≥40 kg (100 mg every 12 hours in patients <40 kg)

Dosage adjustment in patients receiving concomitant phenytoin:

I.V.: Increase maintenance dosage to 5 mg/kg every 12 hours

Oral: Increase dose from 200 mg to 400 mg every 12 hours in patients ≥40 kg (100 mg to 200 mg every 12 hours in patients <40 kg)

Dosage adjustment in renal impairment: In patients with Cl_{cr} <50 mL/minute, accumulation of the intravenous vehicle (SBECD) occurs. After initial loading dose, oral voriconazole should be administered to these patients, unless an assessment of the benefit:risk to the patient justifies the use of I.V. voriconazole. Monitor serum creatinine and change to oral voriconazole therapy when possible.

Dosage adjustment in hepatic impairment:

Mild-to-moderate hepatic dysfunction (Child-Pugh Class A and B): Following standard loading dose, reduce maintenance dosage by 50%

Severe hepatic impairment: Should only be used if benefit outweighs risk; monitor closely for toxicity

Mechanism of Action Interferes with fungal cytochrome P450 activity, decreasing ergosterol synthesis (principal sterol in fungal cell membrane) and inhibiting fungal cell membrane formation.

Contraindications Hypersensitivity to voriconazole or any component of the formulation (cross-reaction with other azole antifungal agents may occur but has not been established, use caution); coadministration of CYP3A4 substrates which may lead to QT_c prolongation (cisapride, pimozide, or quinidine); coadministration with barbiturates (long acting), carbamazepine, efavirenz, ergot alkaloids, rifampin, rifabutin, ritonavir, and sirolimus; pregnancy (unless risk:benefit justifies use)

Warnings/Precautions Visual changes are commonly associated with treatment, including blurred vision, changes in visual acuity, color changes, and photophobia. Patients should be warned to avoid tasks which depend on vision, including operating machinery or driving. Changes are reversible on discontinuation following brief exposure/treatment regimens (≤28 days); reversibility following long-term administration has not been evaluated.

Serious hepatic reactions (including hepatitis, cholestasis, and fulminant hepatic failure) have occurred during treatment, primarily in patients with serious concomitant medical conditions, including hematological malignancy. However, hepatotoxicity has occurred in patients with no identifiable risk factors. Use caution in patients with pre-existing hepatic impairment (dose adjustment required).

Voriconazole tablets contain lactose; avoid administration in hereditary galactose intolerance, Lapp lactase deficiency, or glucose-galactose malabsorption. Suspension contains sucrose; use caution with fructose intolerance, sucrose-isomaltase deficiency, or glucose-galactose malabsorption. Avoid/limit use of intravenous formulation in patients with renal impairment; intravenous formulation contains excipient sulfobutyl ether beta-cyclodextrin (SBECD), which may accumulate in renal insufficiency. Infusion-related reactions may occur with intravenous dosing. Consider discontinuation of infusion if reaction is severe.

Use caution in patients with an increased risk of arrhythmia (concurrent QT_c-prolonging drugs, hypokalemia, cardiomyopathy, or prior cardiotoxic therapy). Use caution in patients receiving concurrent non-nucleoside reverse transcriptase inhibitors (efavirenz is contraindicated).

Avoid use in pregnancy, unless an evaluation of the potential benefit justifies possible risk to the fetus. Safety and efficacy have not been established in children <12 years of age.

Drug Interactions Substrate of CYP2C8/9 (major), 2C19 (major), 3A4 (minor); **Inhibits** CYP2C8/9 (weak), 2C19 (weak), 3A4 (moderate)

Antiarrhythmics (class Ia and III): May increase risk of torsade de pointes (also see "QT_c-prolonging agents")

Barbiturates (phenobarbital, secobarbital): May decrease the serum levels/effects of voriconazole; concurrent use is contraindicated.

Benzodiazepines (metabolized by oxidation): Alprazolam, diazepam, temazepam, triazolam, and midazolam serum concentrations/toxicity may be increased.

Buspirone: Serum concentrations may be increased; monitor for sedation.

Busulfan: Serum concentrations may be increased; avoid concurrent use.

Calcium channel blockers: Serum concentrations may be increased (applies to those agents metabolized by CYP3A4, including felodipine, nifedipine, and verapamil).

Carbamazepine: May decrease the serum levels/effects of voriconazole; concurrent use is contraindicated.

Cisapride: Serum concentrations may be increased which may lead to malignant arrhythmias; concurrent use is contraindicated.

CYP2C8/9 inducers: May decrease the levels/effects of voriconazole. Example inducers include carbamazepine, phenobarbital, phenytoin, rifampin, rifapentine, and secobarbital.

CYP2C19 inducers: May decrease the levels/effects of voriconazole. Example inducers include aminoglutethimide, carbamazepine, phenytoin, and rifampin.

CYP3A4 substrates: Voriconazole may increase the levels/effects of CYP3A4 substrates. Example substrates include benzodiazepines, calcium channel blockers, cyclosporine, mirtazapine, nateglinide, nefazodone, sildenafil (and other PDE-5 inhibitors), tacrolimus, and venlafaxine. Selected benzodiazepines (midazolam and triazolam), cisapride, ergot alkaloids, selected

(Continued)

Voriconazole *(Continued)*

HMG-CoA reductase inhibitors (lovastatin and simvastatin), and pimozide are generally contraindicated with strong CYP3A4 inhibitors.

Docetaxel: Serum concentrations may be increased; avoid concurrent use.

Dofetilide: Serum levels/toxicity may be increased; avoid concurrent use.

Efavirenz: Serum concentrations of voriconazole may be reduced, and efavirenz levels increased, during concurrent therapy; concurrent use is contraindicated.

Ergot alkaloids: Serum levels may be increased by voriconazole, leading to ergot toxicity; concurrent use is contraindicated.

HMG-CoA reductase inhibitors (except pravastatin and fluvastatin): Serum concentrations may be increased. The risk of myopathy/rhabdomyolysis may be increased. Switch to pravastatin/fluvastatin or monitor for development of myopathy.

Immunosuppressants (cyclosporine, sirolimus, and tacrolimus): Serum concentrations may be increased; monitor serum concentrations and renal function. Concurrent use of sirolimus is contraindicated. Decrease cyclosporine dosage by 50% when initiating voriconazole, decreased tacrolimus dosage by 66% when initiating voriconazole.

Methylprednisolone: Serum concentrations may be increased; monitor.

Phenytoin: Serum concentrations of voriconazole may be decreased; adjust dose of voriconazole; monitor phenytoin levels and adjust dose as needed.

Pimozide: Serum levels/toxicity may be increased; concurrent use is contraindicated.

Protease inhibitors: Indinavir did not appear to alter voriconazole serum concentrations during concurrent treatment. Other protease inhibitors may result in increased voriconazole concentrations.

Proton pump inhibitors: Changes in gastric acidity do not appear to significantly affect voriconazole absorption. However, voriconazole may significantly increase serum levels of omeprazole. For omeprazole dosages >40 mg/day, reduce omeprazole dosage by 50%. Serum levels of other proton pump inhibitors may also be increased.

QT_c-prolonging agents: Risk of arrhythmia (torsade de pointes) may be increased.

Quinidine: Serum levels may be increased; concurrent use is contraindicated.

Reverse transcriptase inhibitors (non-nucleoside) (NNRTIs): Effects on serum concentrations may be difficult to predict. Serum levels of voriconazole may be increased by delavirdine. Serum levels may be decreased by efavirenz or nevirapine. Monitor closely for efficacy/toxicity. Concurrent use with efavirenz is contraindicated.

Rifabutin; Rifabutin serum levels are increased by voriconazole; concurrent use is contraindicated.

Rifampin: Rifampin decreases voriconazole's serum concentration to levels which are no longer effective; concurrent use is contraindicated.

Ritonavir: Serum levels of voriconazole are reduced; concurrent use is contraindicated.

Sulfonylureas: Serum levels may be increased by voriconazole, potentially leading to hypoglycemia; monitor.

Trimetrexate: Serum concentrations may be increased; monitor.

Warfarin: Anticoagulant effects may be increased; monitor INR.

Vinca alkaloids: Serum concentrations may be increased; consider reduced dosage of vinca alkaloid.

Zolpidem: Serum levels may be increased; monitor.

Ethanol/Nutrition/Herb Interactions

Food: May decrease voriconazole absorption. Voriconazole should be taken 1 hour before or 1 hour after a meal. Avoid grapefruit juice (may increase voriconazole serum levels).

Herb/Nutraceutical: St John's wort may decrease voriconazole levels.

Dietary Considerations Oral: Should be taken 1 hour before or 1 hour after a meal. Voriconazole tablets contain lactose; avoid administration in hereditary galactose intolerance, Lapp lactase deficiency, or glucose-galactose malabsorption. Suspension contains sucrose; use caution with fructose intolerance, sucrose-isomaltase deficiency, or glucose-galactose malabsorption.

Pharmacodynamics/Kinetics

Absorption: Well absorbed after oral administration

Distribution: V_d: 4.6 L/kg

Protein binding: 58%

Metabolism: Hepatic, via CYP2C19 (major pathway) and CYP2C9 and CYP3A4 (less significant); saturable (may demonstrate nonlinearity)

Bioavailability: 96%

Half-life elimination: Variable, dose-dependent

Time to peak: 1-2 hours

Excretion: Urine (as inactive metabolites)

Pregnancy Risk Factor D

Lactation Excretion in breast milk unknown/not recommended

Breast-Feeding Considerations Excretion in breast milk has not been investigated; avoid breast-feeding until additional data are available.

Dosage Forms

Injection, powder for reconstitution: 200 mg [contains SBECD 3200 mg]

Powder for oral suspension: 200 mg/5 mL (70 mL) [contains sodium benzoate and sucrose; orange flavor]

Tablet: 50 mg, 200 mg [contains lactose]

VōSoL® HC *see* Acetic Acid, Propylene Glycol Diacetate, and Hydrocortisone *on page 60*

VoSpire ER™ *see* Albuterol *on page 71*

VP-16 *see* Etoposide *on page 567*

VP-16-213 *see* Etoposide *on page 567*

Vumon *see* Teniposide *on page 1269*

V.V.S.® *see* Sulfabenzamide, Sulfacetamide, and Sulfathiazole *on page 1243*

Vytone® *see* Iodoquinol and Hydrocortisone *on page 759*

VZIG *see* Varicella-Zoster Immune Globulin (Human) *on page 1368*

Warfarin (WAR far in)

Related Information

Cardiovascular Diseases *on page 1458*

U.S. Brand Names Coumadin®; Jantoven™

Canadian Brand Names Apo-Warfarin®; Coumadin®; Gen-Warfarin; Taro-Warfarin

Generic Available Yes: Tablet

Synonyms Warfarin Sodium

Pharmacologic Category Anticoagulant, Coumarin Derivative

Use Prophylaxis and treatment of venous thrombosis, pulmonary embolism and thromboembolic disorders; atrial fibrillation with risk of embolism and as an adjunct in the prophylaxis of systemic embolism after myocardial infarction

Unlabeled/Investigational Use Prevention of recurrent transient ischemic attacks and to reduce risk of recurrent myocardial infarction

Local Anesthetic/Vasoconstrictor Precautions No information available to require special precautions

Effects on Dental Treatment Signs of warfarin overdose may first appear as bleeding from gingival tissue; consultation with prescribing physician is advisable prior to surgery to determine temporary dose reduction or withdrawal of medication.

Common Adverse Effects As with all anticoagulants, bleeding is the major adverse effect of warfarin. Hemorrhage may occur at virtually any site. Risk is dependent on multiple variables, including the intensity of anticoagulation and patient susceptibility.

Additional adverse effects are often related to idiosyncratic reactions, and the frequency cannot be accurately estimated.

Cardiovascular: Vasculitis, edema, hemorrhagic shock

Central nervous system: Fever, lethargy, malaise, asthenia, pain, headache, dizziness, stroke

Dermatologic: Rash, dermatitis, bullous eruptions, urticaria, pruritus, alopecia

Gastrointestinal: Anorexia, nausea, vomiting, stomach cramps, abdominal pain, diarrhea, flatulence, gastrointestinal bleeding, taste disturbance, mouth ulcers

Genitourinary: Priapism, hematuria

Hematologic: Hemorrhage, leukopenia, unrecognized bleeding sites (eg, colon cancer) may be uncovered by anticoagulation, retroperitoneal hematoma, agranulocytosis

Hepatic: Increased transaminases, hepatic injury, jaundice,

Neuromuscular & skeletal: Paresthesia, osteoporosis

Respiratory: Hemoptysis, epistaxis, pulmonary hemorrhage, tracheobronchial calcification

Miscellaneous: Hypersensitivity/allergic reactions

Skin necrosis/gangrene, due to paradoxical local thrombosis, is a known but rare risk of warfarin therapy. Its onset is usually within the first few days of therapy and is frequently localized to the limbs, breast or penis. The risk of this effect is increased in patients with protein C or S deficiency.

(Continued)

Warfarin *(Continued)*

"Purple toes syndrome," caused by cholesterol microembolization, also occurs rarely. Typically, this occurs after several weeks of therapy, and may present as a dark, purplish, mottled discoloration of the plantar and lateral surfaces. Other manifestations of cholesterol microembolization may include rash; livedo reticularis; gangrene; abrupt and intense pain in lower extremities; abdominal, flank, or back pain; hematuria, renal insufficiency; hypertension; cerebral ischemia; spinal cord infarction; or other symptom of vascular compromise.

Dosage

Oral:

Infants and Children: 0.05-0.34 mg/kg/day; infants <12 months of age may require doses at or near the high end of this range; consistent anticoagulation may be difficult to maintain in children <5 years of age

Adults: Initial dosing must be individualized. Consider the patient (hepatic function, cardiac function, age, nutritional status, concurrent therapy, risk of bleeding) in addition to prior dose response (if available) and the clinical situation. Start 5-10 mg daily for 2 days. Adjust dose according to INR results; usual maintenance dose ranges from 2-10 mg daily (individual patients may require loading and maintenance doses outside these general guidelines).

Note: Lower starting doses may be required for patients with hepatic impairment, poor nutrition, CHF, elderly, or a high risk of bleeding. Higher initial doses may be reasonable in selected patients (ie, receiving enzyme-inducing agents and with low risk of bleeding).

I.V. (administer as a slow bolus injection): 2-5 mg/day

Dosing adjustment/comments in hepatic disease: Monitor effect at usual doses; the response to oral anticoagulants may be markedly enhanced in obstructive jaundice (due to reduced vitamin K absorption) and also in hepatitis and cirrhosis (due to decreased production of vitamin K-dependent clotting factors); prothrombin index should be closely monitored

Mechanism of Action Interferes with hepatic synthesis of vitamin K-dependent coagulation factors (II, VII, IX, X)

Contraindications Hypersensitivity to warfarin or any component of the formulation; hemorrhagic tendencies; hemophilia; thrombocytopenia purpura; leukemia; recent or potential surgery of the eye or CNS; major regional lumbar block anesthesia or surgery resulting in large, open surfaces; patients bleeding from the GI, respiratory, or GU tract; threatened abortion; aneurysm; ascorbic acid deficiency; history of bleeding diathesis; prostatectomy; continuous tube drainage of the small intestine; polyarthritis; diverticulitis; emaciation; malnutrition; cerebrovascular hemorrhage; eclampsia/pre-eclampsia; blood dyscrasias; severe uncontrolled or malignant hypertension; severe hepatic disease; pericarditis or pericardial effusion; subacute bacterial endocarditis; visceral carcinoma; following spinal puncture and other diagnostic or therapeutic procedures with potential for significant bleeding; history of warfarin-induced necrosis; an unreliable, noncompliant patient; alcoholism; patient who has a history of falls or is a significant fall risk; pregnancy

Warnings/Precautions

Do not switch brands once desired therapeutic response has been achieved

Use with caution in patients with active tuberculosis or diabetes

Concomitant use with vitamin K may decrease anticoagulant effect; monitor carefully

Concomitant use with NSAIDs or aspirin may cause severe GI irritation and also increase the risk of bleeding due to impaired platelet function

Salicylates may further increase warfarin's effect by displacing it from plasma protein binding sites

Patients with protein C or S deficiency are at increased risk of skin necrosis syndrome

Before committing an elderly patient to long-term anticoagulation therapy, their risk for bleeding complications secondary to falls, drug interactions, living situation, and cognitive status should be considered. The risk for bleeding complications decreases with the duration of therapy and may increase with advancing age.

If a patient is to undergo an invasive surgical procedure (dental to actual minor/major surgery), warfarin should be stopped 3 days before the scheduled surgery date and the INR/PT should be checked prior to the procedure

Drug Interactions

Cytochrome P450 Effect: Substrate of CYP1A2 (minor), 2C8/9 (major), 2C19 (minor), 3A4 (minor); **Inhibits** CYP2C8/9 (moderate), 2C19 (weak)

Increased Effect/Toxicity: CYP2C8/9 inhibitors may increase the levels/effects of warfarin (eg, delavirdine, fluconazole, gemfibrozil, ketoconazole, nicardipine, NSAIDs, sulfonamides). Warfarin may increase the levels/

effects of CYP2C8/9 substrates (eg, amiodarone, fluoxetine, glimepiride, glipizide, nateglinide, phenytoin, pioglitazone, rosiglitazone, sertraline).

Also see tables.

Increased Bleeding Tendency

Inhibit Platelet Aggregation	Inhibit Procoagulant Factors	Ulcerogenic Drugs
Cephalosporins	Antimetabolites	Adrenal corticosteroids
Clopidogrel	Quinidine	Indomethacin
Dipyridamole	Quinine	Potassium products
Indomethacin	Salicylates	Salicylates
Penicillin, parenteral		
Salicylates		
Sulfinpyrazone		
Ticlopidine		

Use of these agents with oral anticoagulants may increase the chances of hemorrhage.

Enhanced Anticoagulant Effects

Decrease Vitamin K	Displace Anticoagulant	Inhibit Metabolism	Other
Oral antibiotics: Can ↑/↓ INR. Check INR 3 days after a patient begins antibiotics to see the INR value and adjust the warfarin dose accordingly	Chloral hydrate	Allopurinol	Acetaminophen
	Clofibrate	Amiodarone	Anabolic steroids
	Diazoxide	Azole antifungals	Capecitabine
	Ethacrynic acid	Capecitabine	Celecoxib
	Miconazole (including intravaginal use)	Chloramphenicol	Clarithromycin
	Nalidixic acid	Chlorpropamide	Clofibrate
	Salicylates	Cimetidine	Danazol
	Sulfonamides	Ciprofloxacin	Erythromycin
	Sulfonylureas	Co-trimoxazole	Fenofibrate
		Disulfiram	Gemfibrozil
		Ethanol (acute ingestion)[1]	Glucagon
		Flutamide	Influenza vaccine
		Isoniazid	Propranolol
		Metronidazole	Propylthiouracil
		Norfloxacin	Ranitidine
		Ofloxacin	Rofecoxib
		Omeprazole	SSRIs
		Phenytoin	Sulindac
		Propafenone	Tetracycline
		Propoxyphene	Thyroid drugs
		Quinidine	Vitamin E (≥400 int. units)
		"Statins"[2]	
		Sulfinpyrazone	
		Sulfonamides	
		Tamoxifen	
		Tolbutamide	
		Zafirlukast	
		Zileuton	

[1]The hypoprothrombinemic effect of oral anticoagulants has been reported to be both increased and decreased during chronic and excessive alcohol ingestion. Data are insufficient to predict the direction of this interaction in alcoholic patients.

[2]Particularly lovastatin and fluvastatin; others (atorvastatin, pravastatin) rarely associated with increased PT.

Decreased Effect: CYP2C8/9 inducers may decrease the levels/effects of warfarin; example inducers include carbamazepine, phenobarbital, phenytoin, rifampin, rifapentine, and secobarbital. Also see table.

Decreased Anticoagulant Effects

Induction of Enzymes		Increased Procoagulant Factors	Decreased Drug Absorption	Other
Antithyroid drugs	Nafcillin	Estrogens	Aluminum hydroxide	Ethchlorvynol
Barbiturates	Phenytoin	Oral contraceptives	Cholestyramine[1]	Griseofulvin
Bosentan	Rifampin	Vitamin K (including nutritional supplements)	Colestipol[1]	Spironolactone[2]
Carbamazepine				Sucralfate
Glutethimide				
Griseofulvin				

Decreased anticoagulant effect may occur when these drugs are administered with oral anticoagulants.

[1]Cholestyramine and colestipol may increase the anticoagulant effect by binding vitamin K in the gut; yet, the decreased drug absorption appears to be of more concern.

[2]Diuretic-induced hemoconcentration with subsequent concentration of clotting factors has been reported to decrease the effects of oral anticoagulants.

(Continued)

Warfarin *(Continued)*

Ethanol/Nutrition/Herb Interactions

Ethanol: Avoid ethanol. Acute ethanol ingestion (binge drinking) decreases the metabolism of warfarin and increases PT/INR. Chronic daily ethanol use increases the metabolism of warfarin and decreases PT/INR.

Food: The anticoagulant effects of warfarin may be decreased if taken with foods rich in vitamin K. Vitamin E may increase warfarin effect. Cranberry juice may increase warfarin effect.

Herb/Nutraceutical: St John's wort may decrease warfarin levels. Alfalfa contains large amounts of vitamin K as do many enteral products. Coenzyme Q_{10} may decrease response to warfarin. Avoid cat's claw, dong quai, bromelains, evening primrose, feverfew, red clover, horse chestnut, garlic, green tea, ginseng, ginkgo (all have additional antiplatelet activity).

Dietary Considerations Foods high in vitamin K (eg, beef liver, pork liver, green tea and leafy green vegetables) inhibit anticoagulant effect. Do not change dietary habits once stabilized on warfarin therapy; a balanced diet with a consistent intake of vitamin K is essential; avoid large amounts of alfalfa, asparagus, broccoli, Brussels sprouts, cabbage, cauliflower, green teas, kale, lettuce, spinach, turnip greens, watercress decrease efficacy of warfarin. It is recommended that the diet contain a CONSISTENT vitamin K content of 70-140 mcg/day. Check with healthcare provider before changing diet.

Pharmacodynamics/Kinetics

Onset of action: Anticoagulation: Oral: 36-72 hours

Peak effect: Full therapeutic effect: 5-7 days; INR may increase in 36-72 hours

Duration: 2-5 days

Absorption: Oral: Rapid

Metabolism: Hepatic

Half-life elimination: 20-60 hours; Mean: 40 hours; highly variable among individuals

Pregnancy Risk Factor X

Dosage Forms INJ, powder for reconstitution (Coumadin®): 5 mg. **TAB** (Coumadin®, Jantoven™): 1 mg, 2 mg, 2.5 mg, 3 mg, 4 mg, 5 mg, 6 mg, 7.5 mg, 10 mg

Selected Readings

Jeske AH, Suchko GD, ADA Council on Scientific Affairs and Division of Science, et al, "Lack of a Scientific Basis for Routine Discontinuation of Oral Anticoagulation Therapy Before Dental Treatment," *J Am Dent Assoc*, 2003, 134(11):1492-7.

Little JW, Miller CS, Henry RG, et al, "Antithrombotic Agents: Implications in Dentistry," *Oral Surg Oral Med Oral Pathol Oral Radiol Endod*, 2002, 93(5):544-51.

Scully C and Wolff A, "Oral Surgery in Patients on Anticoagulant Therapy," *Oral Surg Oral Med Oral Pathol Oral Radiol Endod*, 2002, 94(1):57-64.

Warfarin Sodium *see* Warfarin *on page 1389*

Wart-Off® Maximum Strength [OTC] *see* Salicylic Acid *on page 1205*

4-Way® Long Acting [OTC] *see* Oxymetazoline *on page 1034*

WelChol® *see* Colesevelam *on page 373*

Wellbutrin® *see* BuPROPion *on page 230*

Wellbutrin SR® *see* BuPROPion *on page 230*

Wellbutrin XL™ *see* BuPROPion *on page 230*

Wesmycin® *see* Tetracycline *on page 1280*

Westcort® *see* Hydrocortisone *on page 714*

Westhroid® *see* Thyroid *on page 1293*

Whole Root Rauwolfia *see* Rauwolfia Serpentina *on page 1171*

Wigraine® *see* Ergotamine and Caffeine *on page 506*

WinRho SDF® *see* Rh_0(D) Immune Globulin *on page 1176*

Winstrol® *see* Stanozolol *on page 1237*

Wound Wash Saline™ [OTC] *see* Sodium Chloride *on page 1227*

WR2721 *see* Amifostine *on page 94*

WR-139007 *see* Dacarbazine *on page 392*

WR-139013 *see* Chlorambucil *on page 305*

WR-139021 *see* Carmustine *on page 268*

Wycillin [DSC] *see* Penicillin G Procaine *on page 1060*

Wytensin® [DSC] *see* Guanabenz *on page 677*

Xalatan® *see* Latanoprost *on page 800*

Xanax® *see* Alprazolam *on page 84*

Xanax XR® *see* Alprazolam *on page 84*

Xeloda® *see* Capecitabine *on page 250*

Xenical® *see* Orlistat *on page 1017*

Xifaxan™ *see* Rifaximin *on page 1183*
Xigris® *see* Drotrecogin Alfa *on page 478*
Xolair® *see* Omalizumab *on page 1012*
Xopenex® *see* Levalbuterol *on page 806*
X-Prep® [OTC] *see* Senna *on page 1213*
X-Seb™ T [OTC] *see* Coal Tar and Salicylic Acid *on page 367*
Xylocaine® *see* Lidocaine *on page 819*
Xylocaine® MPF *see* Lidocaine *on page 819*
Xylocaine® MPF With Epinephrine *see* Lidocaine and Epinephrine *on page 823*
Xylocaine® Viscous *see* Lidocaine *on page 819*
Xylocaine® With Epinephrine *see* Lidocaine and Epinephrine *on page 823*

Xylometazoline (zye loe met AZ oh leen)

U.S. Brand Names Otrivin® [OTC] [DSC]; Otrivin® Pediatric [OTC] [DSC]

Canadian Brand Names Balminil; Decongest

Generic Available No

Synonyms Xylometazoline Hydrochloride

Pharmacologic Category Vasoconstrictor, Nasal

Use Symptomatic relief of nasal and nasopharyngeal mucosal congestion

Local Anesthetic/Vasoconstrictor Precautions No information available to require special precautions

Effects on Dental Treatment No significant effects or complications reported

Common Adverse Effects Frequency not defined.

Cardiovascular: Palpitations
Central nervous system: Drowsiness, dizziness, seizures, headache
Ocular: Blurred vision, ocular irritation, photophobia
Miscellaneous: Diaphoresis

Mechanism of Action Stimulates alpha-adrenergic receptors in the arterioles of the conjunctiva and the nasal mucosa to produce vasoconstriction

Pharmacodynamics/Kinetics

Onset of action: Intranasal: Local vasoconstriction: 5-10 minutes
Duration: 5-6 hours

Pregnancy Risk Factor C

Xylometazoline Hydrochloride *see* Xylometazoline *on page 1393*
Xyrem® *see* Sodium Oxybate *on page 1229*
Y-90 Zevalin *see* Ibritumomab *on page 727*
Yasmin® *see* Ethinyl Estradiol and Drospirenone *on page 538*
Yellow Fever Vaccine *see page 1614*
Yellow Mercuric Oxide *see* Mercuric Oxide *on page 881*
YM-08310 *see* Amifostine *on page 94*
Yocon® *see* Yohimbine *on page 1393*
Yodoxin® *see* Iodoquinol *on page 759*

Yohimbine (yo HIM bine)

Related Information

Yohimbe *on page 1451*

U.S. Brand Names Aphrodyne®; Yocon®

Canadian Brand Names PMS-Yohimbine; Yocon®

Generic Available Yes

Synonyms Yohimbine Hydrochloride

Pharmacologic Category Miscellaneous Product

Unlabeled/Investigational Use Treatment of SSRI-induced sexual dysfunction; weight loss; impotence; sympathicolytic and mydriatic; may have activity as an aphrodisiac

Local Anesthetic/Vasoconstrictor Precautions No information available to require special precautions

Effects on Dental Treatment No significant effects or complications reported

Common Adverse Effects Frequency not defined.

Cardiovascular: Tachycardia, hypertension, hypotension (orthostatic), flushing
Central nervous system: Anxiety, mania, hallucinations, irritability, dizziness, psychosis, insomnia, headache, panic attacks
Gastrointestinal: Nausea, vomiting, anorexia, salivation
Neuromuscular & skeletal: Tremors
Miscellaneous: Antidiuretic action, diaphoresis

Mechanism of Action Derived from the bark of the yohimbe tree (*Corynanthe yohimbe*), this indole alkaloid produces a presynaptic $alpha_2$-adrenergic blockade. Peripheral autonomic effect is to increase cholinergic and decrease

(Continued)

Yohimbine *(Continued)*

adrenergic activity; yohimbine exerts a stimulating effect on the mood and a mild antidiuretic effect.

Drug Interactions

Cytochrome P450 Effect: Substrate of CYP2D6 (minor); **Inhibits** CYP2D6 (weak)

Increased Effect/Toxicity: Caution with other CNS acting drugs. When used in combination with CYP3A4 inhibitors, serum level and/or toxicity of yohimbine may be increased; inhibitors include amiodarone, cimetidine, clarithromycin, erythromycin, delavirdine, diltiazem, dirithromycin, disulfiram, fluoxetine, fluvoxamine, grapefruit juice, indinavir, itraconazole, ketoconazole, metronidazole, nefazodone, nevirapine, propoxyphene, quinupristin-dalfopristin, ritonavir, saquinavir, verapamil, zafirlukast, zileuton; monitor for altered response. MAO inhibitors or drugs with MAO inhibition (linezolid, furazolidone) theoretically may increase toxicity or adverse effects

Pharmacodynamics/Kinetics

Duration of action: Usually 3-4 hours, but may last 36 hours

Absorption: 33%

Distribution: V_d: 0.3-3 L/kg

Half-life elimination: 0.6 hour

Yohimbine Hydrochloride *see* Yohimbine *on page 1393*

Z4942 *see* Ifosfamide *on page 733*

Zaditor™ *see* Ketotifen *on page 790*

Zafirlukast (za FIR loo kast)

Related Information

Respiratory Diseases *on page 1478*

U.S. Brand Names Accolate®

Canadian Brand Names Accolate®

Mexican Brand Names Accolate®

Generic Available No

Synonyms ICI 204, 219

Pharmacologic Category Leukotriene-Receptor Antagonist

Use Prophylaxis and chronic treatment of asthma in adults and children ≥5 years of age

Local Anesthetic/Vasoconstrictor Precautions No information available to require special precautions

Effects on Dental Treatment No significant effects or complications reported

Common Adverse Effects

>10%: Central nervous system: Headache (12.9%)

1% to 10%:

- Central nervous system: Dizziness, pain, fever
- Gastrointestinal: Nausea, diarrhea, abdominal pain, vomiting, dyspepsia
- Hepatic: SGPT elevation
- Neuromuscular & skeletal: Back pain, myalgia, weakness

Mechanism of Action Zafirlukast is a selectively and competitive leukotriene-receptor antagonist (LTRA) of leukotriene D4 and E4 (LTD4 and LTE4), components of slow-reacting substance of anaphylaxis (SRSA). Cysteinyl leukotriene production and receptor occupation have been correlated with the pathophysiology of asthma, including airway edema, smooth muscle constriction and altered cellular activity associated with the inflammatory process, which contribute to the signs and symptoms of asthma.

Drug Interactions

Cytochrome P450 Effect: Substrate of CYP2C8/9 (major); **Inhibits** CYP1A2 (weak), 2C8/9 (moderate), 2C19 (weak), 2D6 (weak), 3A4 (weak)

Increased Effect/Toxicity: Zafirlukast concentrations are increased by aspirin. Zafirlukast may increase theophylline levels. Zafirlukast may increase the levels/effects of amiodarone, fluoxetine, glimepiride, glipizide, nateglinide, phenytoin, pioglitazone, rosiglitazone, sertraline, warfarin, and other CYP2C8/9 substrates.

Decreased Effect: The levels/effects of zafirlukast may be decreased by carbamazepine, phenobarbital, phenytoin, rifampin, rifapentine, secobarbital, and other CYP2C8/9 inducers. Zafirlukast concentrations may be reduced by erythromycin.

Pharmacodynamics/Kinetics

Protein binding: >99%, primarily to albumin

Metabolism: Extensively hepatic via CYP2C9

Bioavailability: Reduced 40% with food

Half-life elimination: 10 hours

Time to peak, serum: 3 hours
Excretion: Urine (10%); feces

Pregnancy Risk Factor B

Zagam® *see* Sparfloxacin *on page 1233*

Zalcitabine (zal SITE a been)

Related Information

HIV Infection and AIDS *on page 1484*

U.S. Brand Names Hivid®

Canadian Brand Names Hivid®

Mexican Brand Names Hivid®

Generic Available No

Synonyms ddC; Dideoxycytidine

Pharmacologic Category Antiretroviral Agent, Reverse Transcriptase Inhibitor (Nucleoside)

Use In combination with at least two other antiretrovirals in the treatment of patients with HIV infection; it is not recommended that zalcitabine be given in combination with didanosine, stavudine, or lamivudine due to overlapping toxicities, virologic interactions, or lack of clinical data

Local Anesthetic/Vasoconstrictor Precautions No information available to require special precautions

Effects on Dental Treatment Key adverse event(s) related to dental treatment: Oral ulcerations.

Common Adverse Effects

>10%:
- Central nervous system: Fever (5% to 17%), malaise (2% to 13%)
- Neuromuscular & skeletal: Peripheral neuropathy (28%)

1% to 10%:
- Central nervous system: Headache (2%), dizziness (1%), fatigue (4%), seizures (1.3%)
- Dermatologic: Rash (2% to 11%), pruritus (3% to 5%)
- Endocrine & metabolic: Hypoglycemia (2% to 6%), hyponatremia (4%), hyperglycemia (1% to 6%)
- Gastrointestinal: Nausea (3%), dysphagia (1% to 4%), anorexia (4%), abdominal pain (3% to 8%), vomiting (1% to 3%), diarrhea (<1% to 10%), weight loss, oral ulcers (3% to 7%), increased amylase (3% to 8%)
- Hematologic: Anemia (occurs as early as 2-4 weeks), granulocytopenia (usually after 6-8 weeks)
- Hepatic: Abnormal hepatic function (9%), hyperbilirubinemia (2% to 5%)
- Neuromuscular & skeletal: Myalgia (1% to 6%), foot pain
- Respiratory: Pharyngitis (2%), cough (6%), nasal discharge (4%)

Mechanism of Action Purine nucleoside (cytosine) analog, zalcitabine or 2′,3′-dideoxycytidine (ddC) is converted to active metabolite ddCTP; lack the presence of the 3′-hydroxyl group necessary for phosphodiester linkages during DNA replication. As a result viral replication is prematurely terminated. ddCTP acts as a competitor for binding sites on the HIV-RNA dependent DNA polymerase (reverse transcriptase) to further contribute to inhibition of viral replication.

Drug Interactions

Increased Effect/Toxicity: Amphotericin, foscarnet, and aminoglycosides may potentiate the risk of developing peripheral neuropathy or other toxicities associated with zalcitabine by interfering with the renal elimination of zalcitabine. Other drugs associated with peripheral neuropathy include chloramphenicol, cisplatin, dapsone, disulfiram, ethionamide, glutethimide, gold, hydralazine, iodoquinol, isoniazid, metronidazole, nitrofurantoin, phenytoin, ribavirin, and vincristine. Concomitant use with zalcitabine may increase risk of peripheral neuropathy. Concomitant use of zalcitabine with didanosine is not recommended. Concomitant use of ribavirin and nucleoside analogues may increase the risk of developing lactic acidosis (includes adefovir, didanosine, lamivudine, stavudine, zalcitabine, zidovudine).

Decreased Effect: It is not recommended that zalcitabine be given in combination with didanosine, stavudine, or lamivudine due to overlapping toxicities, virologic interactions, or lack of clinical data. Doxorubicin and lamivudine have been shown *in vitro* to decrease zalcitabine phosphorylation. Magnesium/aluminum-containing antacids and metoclopramide may decrease the absorption of zalcitabine.

Pharmacodynamics/Kinetics

Absorption: Well, but variable; decreased 39% with food
Distribution: Minimal data available; variable CSF penetration
Protein binding: <4%
(Continued)

Zalcitabine *(Continued)*

Metabolism: Intracellularly to active triphosphorylated agent
Bioavailability: >80%
Half-life elimination: 2.9 hours; Renal impairment: ≤8.5 hours
Excretion: Urine (>70% as unchanged drug)

Pregnancy Risk Factor C

Zaleplon (ZAL e plon)

U.S. Brand Names Sonata®
Canadian Brand Names Sonata®; Starnoc®
Generic Available No
Pharmacologic Category Hypnotic, Nonbenzodiazepine
Use Short-term (7-10 days) treatment of insomnia (has been demonstrated to be effective for up to 5 weeks in controlled trial)
Local Anesthetic/Vasoconstrictor Precautions No information available to require special precautions
Effects on Dental Treatment No significant effects or complications reported
Common Adverse Effects

1% to 10%:

Cardiovascular: Peripheral edema, chest pain
Central nervous system: Amnesia, anxiety, depersonalization, dizziness, hallucinations, hypesthesia, somnolence, vertigo, malaise, depression, lightheadedness, impaired coordination, fever, migraine
Dermatologic: Photosensitivity reaction, rash, pruritus
Gastrointestinal: Abdominal pain, anorexia, colitis, dyspepsia, nausea, constipation, xerostomia
Genitourinary: Dysmenorrhea
Neuromuscular & skeletal: Paresthesia, tremor, myalgia, weakness, back pain, arthralgia
Ocular: Abnormal vision, eye pain
Otic: Hyperacusis
Miscellaneous: Parosmia

Restrictions C-IV
Mechanism of Action Zaleplon is unrelated to benzodiazepines, barbiturates, or other hypnotics. However, it interacts with the benzodiazepine GABA receptor complex. Nonclinical studies have shown that it binds selectively to the brain omega-1 receptor situated on the alpha subunit of the GABA-A receptor complex.
Drug Interactions

Cytochrome P450 Effect: Substrate of CYP3A4 (minor)

Increased Effect/Toxicity: Zaleplon potentiates the CNS effects of CNS depressants, including ethanol, anticonvulsants, antipsychotics, barbiturates, benzodiazepines, narcotic agonists, and other sedative agents. Cimetidine increases concentrations of zaleplon. Avoid concurrent use or use 5 mg zaleplon as starting dose in patient receiving cimetidine.

Pharmacodynamics/Kinetics

Onset of action: Rapid
Peak effect: ~1 hour
Duration: 6-8 hours
Absorption: Rapid and almost complete
Distribution: V_d: 1.4 L/kg
Protein binding: 60% ± 15%
Metabolism: Extensive, primarily via aldehyde oxidase to form 5-oxo-zaleplon and to a lesser extent by CYP3A4 to desethylzaleplon; all metabolites are pharmacologically inactive
Bioavailability: 30%
Half-life elimination: 1 hour
Time to peak, serum: 1 hour
Excretion: Urine (primarily metabolites, <1% as unchanged drug)
Clearance: Plasma: Oral: 3 L/hour/kg

Pregnancy Risk Factor C

Zanaflex® *see* Tizanidine *on page 1305*

Zanamivir (za NA mi veer)

Related Information

Systemic Viral Diseases *on page 1519*

U.S. Brand Names Relenza®
Canadian Brand Names Relenza®
Generic Available No
Pharmacologic Category Antiviral Agent; Neuraminidase Inhibitor

Use Treatment of uncomplicated acute illness due to influenza virus in adults and children ≥7 years of age; should not be used in patients with underlying airway disease. Treatment should only be initiated in patients who have been symptomatic for no more than 2 days.

Unlabeled/Investigational Use Investigational: Prophylaxis against influenza A/B infections

Local Anesthetic/Vasoconstrictor Precautions No information available to require special precautions

Effects on Dental Treatment No significant effects or complications reported

Common Adverse Effects Most adverse reactions occurred at a frequency which was equal to the control (lactose vehicle).

>1.5%:

Central nervous system: Headache (2%), dizziness (2%)

Gastrointestinal: Nausea (3%), diarrhea (3% adults, 2% children), vomiting (1% adults, 2% children)

Respiratory: Sinusitis (3%), bronchitis (2%), cough (2%), other nasal signs and symptoms (2%), infection (ear, nose, and throat; 2% adults, 5% children)

Mechanism of Action Zanamivir inhibits influenza virus neuraminidase enzymes, potentially altering virus particle aggregation and release.

Drug Interactions

Increased Effect/Toxicity: No clinically significant pharmacokinetic interactions are predicted.

Decreased Effect: No clinically significant pharmacokinetic interactions are predicted.

Pharmacodynamics/Kinetics

Absorption: Inhalation: 4% to 17%

Protein binding, plasma: <10%

Metabolism: None

Half-life elimination, serum: 2.5-5.1 hours

Excretion: Urine (as unchanged drug); feces (unabsorbed drug)

Pregnancy Risk Factor C

Zanosar® *see* Streptozocin *on page 1240*

Zantac® *see* Ranitidine *on page 1169*

Zantac® 75 [OTC] *see* Ranitidine *on page 1169*

Zapzyt® [OTC] *see* Benzoyl Peroxide *on page 194*

Zapzyt® Acne Wash [OTC] *see* Salicylic Acid *on page 1205*

Zapzyt® Pore Treatment [OTC] *see* Salicylic Acid *on page 1205*

Zarontin® *see* Ethosuximide *on page 560*

Zaroxolyn® *see* Metolazone *on page 914*

Zavesca® *see* Miglustat *on page 930*

Z-Bec® [OTC] *see* Vitamin B Complex Combinations *on page 1382*

Z-Cof DM *see* Guaifenesin, Pseudoephedrine, and Dextromethorphan *on page 676*

Z-Cof LA *see* Guaifenesin and Dextromethorphan *on page 673*

ZD1033 *see* Anastrozole *on page 132*

ZD1839 *see* Gefitinib *on page 649*

ZDV *see* Zidovudine *on page 1398*

ZDV, Abacavir, and Lamivudine *see* Abacavir, Lamivudine, and Zidovudine *on page 43*

Zeasorb®-AF [OTC] *see* Miconazole *on page 922*

Zebeta® *see* Bisoprolol *on page 210*

Zebutal™ *see* Butalbital, Acetaminophen, and Caffeine *on page 236*

Zegerid™ *see* Omeprazole *on page 1012*

Zeldox *see* Ziprasidone *on page 1401*

Zelnorm® *see* Tegaserod *on page 1263*

Zemaira™ *see* Alpha$_1$-Proteinase Inhibitor *on page 84*

Zemplar™ *see* Paricalcitol *on page 1045*

Zenapax® *see* Daclizumab *on page 393*

Zeneca 182,780 *see* Fulvestrant *on page 639*

Zephiran® [OTC] *see* Benzalkonium Chloride *on page 190*

Zephrex® *see* Guaifenesin and Pseudoephedrine *on page 675*

Zephrex LA® *see* Guaifenesin and Pseudoephedrine *on page 675*

Zerit® *see* Stavudine *on page 1238*

Zestoretic® *see* Lisinopril and Hydrochlorothiazide *on page 834*

Zestril® *see* Lisinopril *on page 833*

Zetar® [OTC] *see* Coal Tar *on page 367*

Zetia™ *see* Ezetimibe *on page 570*
Zevalin™ *see* Ibritumomab *on page 727*
Ziac® *see* Bisoprolol and Hydrochlorothiazide *on page 211*
Ziagen® *see* Abacavir *on page 42*

Zidovudine (zye DOE vyoo deen)

Related Information

HIV Infection and AIDS *on page 1484*
Systemic Viral Diseases *on page 1519*
Zidovudine and Lamivudine *on page 1399*

U.S. Brand Names Retrovir®

Canadian Brand Names Apo-Zidovudine®; AZT™; Novo-AZT; Retrovir®

Mexican Brand Names Isadol®; Retrovir AZT®

Generic Available No

Synonyms Azidothymidine; AZT; Compound S; ZDV

Pharmacologic Category Antiretroviral Agent, Reverse Transcriptase Inhibitor (Nucleoside)

Use Management of patients with HIV infections in combination with at least two other antiretroviral agents; for prevention of maternal/fetal HIV transmission as monotherapy

Unlabeled/Investigational Use Postexposure prophylaxis for HIV exposure as part of a multidrug regimen

Local Anesthetic/Vasoconstrictor Precautions No information available to require special precautions

Effects on Dental Treatment No significant effects or complications reported

Common Adverse Effects

>10%:

- Central nervous system: Severe headache (42%), fever (16%)
- Dermatologic: Rash (17%)
- Gastrointestinal: Nausea (46% to 61%), anorexia (11%), diarrhea (17%), pain (20%), vomiting (6% to 25%)
- Hematologic: Anemia (23% in children), leukopenia, granulocytopenia (39% in children)
- Neuromuscular & skeletal: Weakness (19%)

1% to 10%:

- Central nervous system: Malaise (8%), dizziness (6%), insomnia (5%), somnolence (8%)
- Dermatologic: Hyperpigmentation of nails (bluish-brown)
- Gastrointestinal: Dyspepsia (5%)
- Hematologic: Changes in platelet count
- Neuromuscular & skeletal: Paresthesia (6%)

Mechanism of Action Zidovudine is a thymidine analog which interferes with the HIV viral RNA dependent DNA polymerase resulting in inhibition of viral replication; nucleoside reverse transcriptase inhibitor

Drug Interactions

Cytochrome P450 Effect: Substrate (minor) of CYP2A6, 2C8/9, 2C19, 3A4

Increased Effect/Toxicity: Coadministration of zidovudine with drugs that are nephrotoxic (amphotericin B), cytotoxic (flucytosine, vincristine, vinblastine, doxorubicin, interferon), inhibit glucuronidation or excretion (acetaminophen, cimetidine, indomethacin, lorazepam, probenecid, aspirin), or interfere with RBC/WBC number or function (acyclovir, ganciclovir, pentamidine, dapsone). Clarithromycin may increase blood levels of zidovudine (although total body exposure was unaffected, peak plasma concentrations were increased). Valproic acid significantly increases zidovudine's blood levels (believed due to inhibition first pass metabolism). Concomitant use of ribavirin and nucleoside analogues may increase the risk of developing lactic acidosis (includes adefovir, didanosine, lamivudine, stavudine, zalcitabine, zidovudine).

Decreased Effect: *In vitro* evidence suggests zidovudine's antiretroviral activity may be antagonized by doxorubicin and ribavirin; avoid concurrent use. Zidovudine may decrease the antiviral activity of stavudine (based on *in vitro* data); avoid concurrent use.

Pharmacodynamics/Kinetics

Absorption: Oral: 66% to 70%

Distribution: Significant penetration into the CSF; crosses placenta

- Relative diffusion from blood into CSF: Adequate with or without inflammation (exceeds usual MICs)
- CSF:blood level ratio: Normal meninges: ~60%

Protein binding: 25% to 38%

Metabolism: Hepatic via glucuronidation to inactive metabolites; extensive first-pass effect
Half-life elimination: Terminal: 60 minutes
Time to peak, serum: 30-90 minutes
Excretion:
Oral: Urine (72% to 74% as metabolites, 14% to 18% as unchanged drug)
I.V.: Urine (45% to 60% as metabolites, 18% to 29% as unchanged drug)

Pregnancy Risk Factor C

Zidovudine, Abacavir, and Lamivudine *see* Abacavir, Lamivudine, and Zidovudine *on page 43*

Zidovudine and Lamivudine

(zye DOE vyoo deen & la MI vyoo deen)

Related Information

HIV Infection and AIDS *on page 1484*
Lamivudine *on page 794*
Zidovudine *on page 1398*

U.S. Brand Names Combivir®

Canadian Brand Names Combivir®

Generic Available No

Synonyms AZT + 3TC; Lamivudine and Zidovudine

Pharmacologic Category Antiretroviral Agent, Reverse Transcriptase Inhibitor (Nucleoside)

Use Treatment of HIV infection when therapy is warranted based on clinical and/or immunological evidence of disease progression. Combivir® given twice daily, provides an alternative regimen to lamivudine 150 mg twice daily plus zidovudine 600 mg/day in divided doses; this drug form reduces capsule/tablet intake for these two drugs to 2 per day instead of up to 8.

Local Anesthetic/Vasoconstrictor Precautions No information available to require special precautions

Effects on Dental Treatment No significant effects or complications reported

Common Adverse Effects See individual agents.

Mechanism of Action The combination of zidovudine and lamivudine are believed to act synergistically to inhibit reverse transcriptase via DNA chain termination after incorporation of the nucleoside analogue as well as to delay the emergence of mutations conferring resistance

Drug Interactions

Cytochrome P450 Effect: Zidovudine: **Substrate** (minor) of CYP2A6, 2C8/9, 2C19, 3A4

Increased Effect/Toxicity: See individual agents.

Decreased Effect: See individual agents.

Pharmacodynamics/Kinetics See individual agents.

Pregnancy Risk Factor C

Zilactin®-B [OTC] *see* Benzocaine *on page 191*
Zilactin® Baby [OTC] *see* Benzocaine *on page 191*
Zilactin-L® [OTC] *see* Lidocaine *on page 819*

Zileuton (zye LOO ton)

Related Information

Respiratory Diseases *on page 1478*

U.S. Brand Names Zyflo™ [DSC]

Generic Available No

Pharmacologic Category 5-Lipoxygenase Inhibitor

Use Prophylaxis and chronic treatment of asthma in children ≥12 years of age and adults

Local Anesthetic/Vasoconstrictor Precautions No information available to require special precautions

Effects on Dental Treatment No significant effects or complications reported

Common Adverse Effects

>10%:
Central nervous system: Headache (24.6%)
Hepatic: ALT elevation (12%)

1% to 10%:
Cardiovascular: Chest pain
Central nervous system: Pain, dizziness, fever, insomnia, malaise, nervousness, somnolence
Gastrointestinal: Dyspepsia, nausea, abdominal pain, constipation, flatulence
Hematologic: Low white blood cell count

(Continued)

Zileuton *(Continued)*

Neuromuscular & skeletal: Myalgia, arthralgia, weakness
Ocular: Conjunctivitis

Mechanism of Action Specific inhibitor of 5-lipoxygenase and thus inhibits leukotriene (LTB4, LTC4, LTD4 and LTE4) formation. Leukotrienes are substances that induce numerous biological effects including augmentation of neutrophil and eosinophil migration, neutrophil and monocyte aggregation, leukocyte adhesion, increased capillary permeability and smooth muscle contraction.

Drug Interactions

Cytochrome P450 Effect: Substrate (minor) of CYP1A2, 2C8/9, 3A4; **Inhibits** CYP1A2 (weak)

Increased Effect/Toxicity: Zileuton increases concentrations/effects of of beta-blockers (propranolol), theophylline, and warfarin. Potentially, it may increase levels of many drugs, including cisapride, due to inhibition of CYP3A4.

Pharmacodynamics/Kinetics

Absorption: Rapid
Distribution: 1.2 L/kg
Protein binding: 93%
Metabolism: Several metabolites in plasma and urine; metabolized by CYP1A2, 2C9, and 3A4
Bioavailability: Unknown
Half-life elimination: 2.5 hours
Time to peak, serum: 1.7 hours
Excretion: Urine (~95% primarily as metabolites); feces (~2%)

Pregnancy Risk Factor C

Zinacef® *see* Cefuroxime *on page 289*

Zinc *see* Trace Metals *on page 1319*

Zincate® *see* Zinc Sulfate *on page 1401*

Zinc Chloride (zink KLOR ide)

Generic Available Yes

Pharmacologic Category Trace Element

Use Cofactor for replacement therapy to different enzymes helps maintain normal growth rates, normal skin hydration and senses of taste and smell

Local Anesthetic/Vasoconstrictor Precautions No information available to require special precautions

Effects on Dental Treatment No significant effects or complications reported

Pregnancy Risk Factor C

Zincfrin® [OTC] *see* Phenylephrine and Zinc Sulfate *on page 1079*

Zinc Gelatin (zink JEL ah tin)

U.S. Brand Names Gelucast®

Generic Available Yes

Synonyms Dome Paste Bandage; Unna's Boot; Unna's Paste; Zinc Gelatin Boot

Pharmacologic Category Topical Skin Product

Use As a protectant and to support varicosities and similar lesions of the lower limbs

Local Anesthetic/Vasoconstrictor Precautions No information available to require special precautions

Effects on Dental Treatment No significant effects or complications reported

Common Adverse Effects 1% to 10%: Local: Irritation

Zinc Gelatin Boot *see* Zinc Gelatin *on page 1400*

Zincon® [OTC] *see* Pyrithione Zinc *on page 1155*

Zinc Oxide (zink OKS ide)

U.S. Brand Names Ammens® Medicated Deodorant [OTC]; Balmex® [OTC]; Boudreaux's® Butt Paste [OTC]; Critic-Aid Skin Care® [OTC]; Desitin® [OTC]; Desitin® Creamy [OTC]

Canadian Brand Names Zincofax®

Generic Available Yes: Ointment

Synonyms Base Ointment; Lassar's Zinc Paste

Pharmacologic Category Topical Skin Product

Use Protective coating for mild skin irritations and abrasions, soothing and protective ointment to promote healing of chapped skin, diaper rash

Local Anesthetic/Vasoconstrictor Precautions No information available to require special precautions

Effects on Dental Treatment No significant effects or complications reported

Common Adverse Effects 1% to 10%: Local: Skin sensitivity, irritation

Mechanism of Action Mild astringent with weak antiseptic properties

Zinc Sulfate (zink SUL fate)

U.S. Brand Names Orazinc® [OTC]; Zincate®

Canadian Brand Names Anuzinc; Rivasol

Generic Available Yes

Pharmacologic Category Trace Element

Use Zinc supplement (oral and parenteral); may improve wound healing in those who are deficient

Local Anesthetic/Vasoconstrictor Precautions No information available to require special precautions

Effects on Dental Treatment No significant effects or complications reported

Pregnancy Risk Factor C

Zinc Sulfate and Phenylephrine *see* Phenylephrine and Zinc Sulfate *on page 1079*

Zinc Undecylenate *see* Undecylenic Acid and Derivatives *on page 1352*

Zinecard® *see* Dexrazoxane *on page 417*

Ziprasidone (zi PRAY si done)

U.S. Brand Names Geodon®

Generic Available No

Synonyms Zeldox; Ziprasidone Hydrochloride; Ziprasidone Mesylate

Pharmacologic Category Antipsychotic Agent, Benzylisothiazolylpiperazine

Use Treatment of schizophrenia

Unlabeled/Investigational Use Tourette's syndrome

Local Anesthetic/Vasoconstrictor Precautions No information available to require special precautions

Effects on Dental Treatment Key adverse event(s) related to dental treatment: Xerostomia (normal salivary flow resumes upon discontinuation).

Common Adverse Effects Note: Although minor QT_c prolongation (mean 10 msec at 160 mg/day) may occur more frequently (incidence not specified), clinically relevant prolongation (>500 msec) was rare (0.06%).

>10%:

- Central nervous system: Somnolence (8% to 20%), headache (3% to 13%)
- Gastrointestinal: Nausea (4% to 12%)

1% to 10%:

- Cardiovascular: Bradycardia (2%), hypertension (2%), tachycardia (2%), postural hypotension (1% to 5%), vasodilation (1%)
- Central nervous system: Akathisia (2% to 8%), dizziness (3% to 10%), extrapyramidal symptoms (2% to 5%), dystonia (4%), hypertonia (3%), insomnia (3%), agitation (2%), anxiety (2%), speech disorder (2%), psychosis (1%)
- Dermatologic: Rash (with urticaria, 4% to 5%), fungal dermatitis (2%), furunculosis (2%)
- Endocrine & metabolic: Dysmenorrhea (2%)
- Gastrointestinal: Constipation (2% to 9%), dyspepsia (1% to 8%), diarrhea (3% to 5%), xerostomia (1% to 4%), vomiting (3%), abdominal pain (2%), anorexia (2%), weight gain (10%), rectal hemorrhage (2%)
- Genitourinary: Priapism (1%)
- Local: Pain at injection site (7% to 9%)
- Neuromuscular & skeletal: Weakness (2% to 5%), paresthesia (2%), cogwheel rigidity (1%), hypertonia (1%), myalgia (1%)
- Ocular: Abnormal vision (3%)
- Respiratory: Respiratory disorder (8%, primarily cold symptoms, upper respiratory infection), rhinitis (1% to 4%), cough increased (3%)
- Miscellaneous: Accidental injury (4%), diaphoresis (2%)

Mechanism of Action The exact mechanism of action is unknown. However, *in vitro* radioligand studies show that ziprasidone has high affinity for D_2, 5-HT_{2A}, 5-HT_{1A}, 5-HT_{2C} and 5-HT_{1D}, moderate affinity for alpha_1 adrenergic and histamine H_1 receptors, and low affinity for alpha_2 adrenergic, beta adrenergic, 5-HT_3, 5-HT_4, cholinergic, mu, sigma, or benzodiazepine receptors. Ziprasidone moderately inhibits the reuptake of serotonin and norepinephrine.

Drug Interactions

Cytochrome P450 Effect: Substrate (minor) of CYP1A2, 3A4; **Inhibits** CYP2D6 (weak), 3A4 (weak)

(Continued)

Ziprasidone *(Continued)*

Increased Effect/Toxicity:

Ketoconazole may increase serum concentrations of ziprasidone. Other CYP3A4 inhibitors may share this potential.

Concurrent use with QT_c-prolonging agents may result in additive effects on cardiac conduction, potentially resulting in malignant or lethal arrhythmias. Concurrent use is contraindicated. Includes amiodarone, arsenic trioxide, chlorpromazine, cisapride; class Ia antiarrhythmics (quinidine, procainamide); dofetilide, dolasetron, droperidol, halofantrine, levomethadyl, mefloquine, mesoridazine, pentamidine, pimozide; some quinolone antibiotics (moxifloxacin, sparfloxacin, gatifloxacin); sotalol, tacrolimus, and thioridazine. Potassium- or magnesium-depleting agents (diuretics, aminoglycosides, cyclosporine, and amphotericin B) may increase the risk of QT_c prolongation. Antihypertensive agents may increase the risk of orthostatic hypotension. CNS depressants may increase the degree of sedation caused by ziprasidone. Metoclopramide may increase risk of extrapyramidal symptoms (EPS).

Decreased Effect: Carbamazepine may decrease serum concentrations of ziprasidone. Other enzyme-inducing agents may share this potential. Amphetamines may decrease the efficacy of ziprasidone. Ziprasidone may inhibit the efficacy of levodopa.

Pharmacodynamics/Kinetics

Absorption: Well absorbed

Distribution: V_d: 1.5 L/kg

Protein binding: 99%, primarily to albumin and alpha-1-acid glycoprotein

Metabolism: Extensively hepatic, primarily via aldehyde oxidase; less than 1/3 of total metabolism via CYP3A4 and CYP1A2 (minor)

Bioavailability: Oral (with food): 60% (up to twofold increase with food); I.M.: 100%

Half-life elimination: Oral: 7 hours; I.M.: 2-5 hours

Time to peak: Oral: 6-8 hours; I.M.: ≤60 minutes

Excretion: Feces (66%) and urine (20%) as metabolites; little as unchanged drug (1% urine, 4% feces)

Pregnancy Risk Factor C

Ziprasidone Hydrochloride *see* Ziprasidone *on page 1401*

Ziprasidone Mesylate *see* Ziprasidone *on page 1401*

Zithromax® *see* Azithromycin *on page 174*

Zithromax® TRI-PAK™ *see* Azithromycin *on page 174*

Zithromax® Z-PAK® *see* Azithromycin *on page 174*

ZM-182,780 *see* Fulvestrant *on page 639*

ZNP® Bar [OTC] *see* Pyrithione Zinc *on page 1155*

Zocor® *see* Simvastatin *on page 1222*

Zofran® *see* Ondansetron *on page 1014*

Zofran® ODT *see* Ondansetron *on page 1014*

Zoladex® *see* Goserelin *on page 670*

Zoledronate *see* Zoledronic Acid *on page 1402*

Zoledronic Acid (ZOE le dron ik AS id)

U.S. Brand Names Zometa®

Canadian Brand Names Zometa®

Mexican Brand Names Zometa®

Generic Available No

Synonyms CGP-42446; Zoledronate

Pharmacologic Category Adjuvant Analgesic, Bisphosphonate

Use Treatment of hypercalcemia and bone metastases of solid tumors

Unlabeled/Investigational Use Investigational: Prevention of bone metastases from breast or prostate cancer; treatment of metabolic bone diseases

Local Anesthetic/Vasoconstrictor Precautions No information available to require special precautions

Effects on Dental Treatment Key adverse event(s) related to dental treatment: Mucositis.

Common Adverse Effects

>10%:

Cardiovascular: Leg edema (up to 19%)

Central nervous system: Fatigue (36%), fever (30% to 44%), headache (up to 18%), insomnia (15%), anxiety (9% to 14%), dizziness (14%), agitation (13%), depression (12%)

Dermatologic: Alopecia (11%)

Endocrine & metabolic: Hypophosphatemia (13%), hypokalemia (12%), dehydration (up to 12%)
Gastrointestinal: Nausea (29% to 45%), constipation (27% to 28%), vomiting (14% to 30%), diarrhea (17% to 22%), abdominal pain (12% to 16%)
Genitourinary: Urinary tract infection (11% to 14%)
Hematologic: Anemia (22% to 29%), neutropenia (11%)
Neuromuscular & skeletal: Myalgia (21%), paresthesias (18%), arthralgia (up to 18%) skeletal pain (12%)
Respiratory: Dyspnea (22% to 24%), coughing (12% to 19%)
Miscellaneous Moniliasis (12%)

1% to 10%:
Cardiovascular: Hypotension (10%), chest pain
Central nervous system: Hypoesthesia (10%)
Dermatologic: Dermatitis (10%)
Endocrine & metabolic: Hypomagnesemia (up to 10%), hypocalcemia, hypophosphatemia (9%), hypermagnesemia (Grade 3: 2%)
Gastrointestinal: Anorexia (9%), mucositis, dysphagia
Genitourinary: Urinary tract infection (14%)
Hematologic: Thrombocytopenia, pancytopenia, granulocytopenia
Neuromuscular & skeletal: Rigors (10%), weakness
Renal: Serum creatinine increased
Respiratory: Pleural effusion, upper respiratory tract infection (8%)

Symptoms of hypercalcemia include polyuria, nephrolithiasis, anorexia, nausea, vomiting, constipation, weakness, fatigue, confusion, stupor, and coma. These may not be drug-related adverse events, but related to the underlying metabolic condition.

Mechanism of Action A bisphosphonate which inhibits bone resorption via actions on osteoclasts or on osteoclast precursors; inhibits osteoclastic activity and skeletal calcium release induced by tumors. Decreases serum calcium and phosphorus, and increases their elimination.

Drug Interactions

Increased Effect/Toxicity: Aminoglycosides may also lower serum calcium levels; loop diuretics increase risk of hypocalcemia; thalidomide increases renal toxicity

Pharmacodynamics/Kinetics

Onset of action: Maximum effect may not been seen for 7 days
Distribution: Binds to bone
Protein binding: ~22%
Half-life elimination: Triphasic; Terminal: 146 hours
Excretion: Urine (39% ± 16% as unchanged drug) within 24 hours; feces (<3%)

Pregnancy Risk Factor D

Zolmitriptan (zohl mi TRIP tan)

U.S. Brand Names Zomig®; Zomig-ZMT™

Canadian Brand Names Zomig®; Zomig® Rapimelt

Mexican Brand Names Zomig®

Generic Available No

Synonyms 311C90

Pharmacologic Category Serotonin 5-HT_{1D} Receptor Agonist

Use Acute treatment of migraine with or without aura

Local Anesthetic/Vasoconstrictor Precautions No information available to require special precautions

Effects on Dental Treatment Key adverse event(s) related to dental treatment: Xerostomia (normal salivary flow resumes upon discontinuation).

Common Adverse Effects Percentages noted from oral preparations.

1% to 10%:
Cardiovascular: Chest pain (2% to 4%), palpitations (up to 2%)
Central nervous system: Dizziness (6% to 10%), somnolence (5% to 8%), pain (2% to 3%), vertigo (≤2%)
Gastrointestinal: Nausea (4% to 9%), xerostomia (3% to 5%), dyspepsia (1% to 3%), dysphagia (≤2%)
Neuromuscular & skeletal: Paresthesia (5% to 9%), weakness (3% to 9%), warm/cold sensation (5% to 7%), hypesthesia (1% to 2%), myalgia (1% to 2%), myasthenia (up to 2%)
Miscellaneous: Neck/throat/jaw pain (4% to 10%), diaphoresis (up to 3%), allergic reaction (up to 1%)

Mechanism of Action Selective agonist for serotonin (5-HT_{1B} and 5-HT_{1D} receptors) in cranial arteries to cause vasoconstriction and reduce sterile inflammation associated with antidromic neuronal transmission correlating with relief of migraine

(Continued)

Zolmitriptan *(Continued)*

Drug Interactions

Cytochrome P450 Effect: Substrate of CYP1A2 (minor)

Increased Effect/Toxicity: Ergot-containing drugs may lead to vasospasm; cimetidine, MAO inhibitors, oral contraceptives, propranolol increase levels of zolmitriptan; concurrent use with SSRIs and sibutramine may lead to serotonin syndrome.

Pharmacodynamics/Kinetics

Onset of action: 0.5-1 hour

Absorption: Well absorbed

Distribution: V_d: 7 L/kg

Protein binding: 25%

Metabolism: Converted to an active N-desmethyl metabolite (2-6 times more potent than zolmitriptan)

Half-life elimination: 2.8-3.7 hours

Bioavailability: 40%

Time to peak, serum: Tablet: 1.5 hours; Orally-disintegrating tablet and nasal spray: 3 hours

Excretion: Urine (~60% to 65% total dose); feces (30% to 40%)

Pregnancy Risk Factor C

Zoloft® *see* Sertraline *on page 1215*

Zolpidem (zole PI dem)

U.S. Brand Names Ambien®

Canadian Brand Names Ambien®

Generic Available No

Synonyms Zolpidem Tartrate

Pharmacologic Category Hypnotic, Nonbenzodiazepine

Use Short-term treatment of insomnia

Local Anesthetic/Vasoconstrictor Precautions No information available to require special precautions

Effects on Dental Treatment No significant effects or complications reported

Common Adverse Effects 1% to 10%:

Cardiovascular: Palpitations

Central nervous system: Headache, drowsiness, dizziness, lethargy, lightheadedness, depression, abnormal dreams, amnesia

Dermatologic: Rash

Gastrointestinal: Nausea, diarrhea, xerostomia, constipation

Respiratory: Sinusitis, pharyngitis

Restrictions C-IV

Dosage Duration of therapy should be limited to 7-10 days

Adults: Oral: 10 mg immediately before bedtime; maximum dose: 10 mg

Elderly: 5 mg immediately before bedtime

Hemodialysis: Not dialyzable

Dosing adjustment in hepatic impairment: Decrease dose to 5 mg

Mechanism of Action Structurally dissimilar to benzodiazepine, however, has much or all of its actions explained by its effects on benzodiazepine (BZD) receptors, especially the omega-1 receptor (with a high affinity ratio of the alpha 1/alpha 5 subunits); retains hypnotic and much of the anxiolytic properties of the BZD, but has reduced effects on skeletal muscle and seizure threshold.

Contraindications Hypersensitivity to zolpidem or any component of the formulation

Warnings/Precautions Should be used only after evaluation of potential causes of sleep disturbance. Failure of sleep disturbance to resolve after 7-10 days may indicate psychiatric or medical illness. Use with caution in patients with depression. Behavioral changes have been associated with sedative-hypnotics. Causes CNS depression, which may impair physical and mental capabilities. Effects with other sedative drugs or ethanol may be potentiated. Closely monitor elderly or debilitated patients for impaired cognitive or motor performance; not recommended for use in children <18 years of age. Avoid use in patients with sleep apnea or a history of sedative-hypnotic abuse.

Drug Interactions

Cytochrome P450 Effect: Substrate of CYP1A2 (minor), 2C8/9 (minor), 2C19 (minor), 2D6 (minor), 3A4 (major)

Increased Effect/Toxicity: Use of zolpidem in combination with other centrally-acting drugs may produce additive CNS depression. CYP3A4 inhibitors may increase the levels/effects of zolpidem; example inhibitors include azole antifungals, ciprofloxacin, clarithromycin, diclofenac, doxycycline, erythromycin, imatinib, isoniazid, nefazodone, nicardipine, propofol, protease inhibitors, quinidine, and verapamil.

Decreased Effect: CYP3A4 inducers may decrease the levels/effects of zolpidem; example inducers include aminoglutethimide, carbamazepine, nafcillin, nevirapine, phenobarbital, phenytoin, and rifamycins.

Ethanol/Nutrition/Herb Interactions

Ethanol: Avoid ethanol (may increase CNS depression).

Herb/Nutraceutical: St John's wort may decrease zolpidem levels. Avoid valerian, St John's wort, kava kava, gotu kola (may increase CNS depression).

Pharmacodynamics/Kinetics

Onset of action: 30 minutes

Duration: 6-8 hours

Absorption: Rapid

Distribution: Very low amounts enter breast milk

Protein binding: 92%

Metabolism: Hepatic to inactive metabolites

Half-life elimination: 2-2.6 hours; Cirrhosis: Up to 9.9 hours

Pregnancy Risk Factor B

Dosage Forms TAB: 5 mg, 10 mg

Zolpidem Tartrate *see* Zolpidem *on page 1404*

Zometa® *see* Zoledronic Acid *on page 1402*

Zomig® *see* Zolmitriptan *on page 1403*

Zomig-ZMT™ *see* Zolmitriptan *on page 1403*

Zonalon® *see* Doxepin *on page 467*

Zone-A® *see* Pramoxine and Hydrocortisone *on page 1109*

Zone-A Forte® *see* Pramoxine and Hydrocortisone *on page 1109*

Zonegran® *see* Zonisamide *on page 1405*

Zonisamide (zoe NIS a mide)

U.S. Brand Names Zonegran®

Canadian Brand Names Zonegran®

Generic Available No

Pharmacologic Category Anticonvulsant, Miscellaneous

Use Adjunct treatment of partial seizures in children >16 years of age and adults with epilepsy

Unlabeled/Investigational Use Bipolar disorder

Local Anesthetic/Vasoconstrictor Precautions No information available to require special precautions

Effects on Dental Treatment Key adverse event(s) related to dental treatment: Xerostomia (normal salivary flow resumes upon discontinuation) and abnormal taste.

Common Adverse Effects Adjunctive Therapy: Frequencies noted in patients receiving other anticonvulsants:

>10%:

Central nervous system: Somnolence (17%), dizziness (13%)

Gastrointestinal: Anorexia (13%)

1% to 10%:

Central nervous system: Headache (10%), agitation/irritability (9%), fatigue (8%), tiredness (7%), ataxia (6%), confusion (6%), decreased concentration (6%), memory impairment (6%), depression (6%), insomnia (6%), speech disorders (5%), mental slowing (4%), anxiety (3%), nervousness (2%), schizophrenic/schizophreniform behavior (2%), difficulty in verbal expression (2%), status epilepticus (1%), tremor (1%), convulsion (1%), hyperesthesia (1%), incoordination (1%)

Dermatologic: Rash (3%), bruising (2%), pruritus (1%)

Gastrointestinal: Nausea (9%), abdominal pain (6%), diarrhea (5%), dyspepsia (3%), weight loss (3%), constipation (2%), dry mouth (2%), taste perversion (2%), vomiting (1%)

Neuromuscular & skeletal: Paresthesia (4%), weakness (1%), abnormal gait (1%)

Ocular: Diplopia (6%), nystagmus (4%), amblyopia (1%)

Otic: Tinnitus (1%)

Respiratory: Rhinitis (2%), pharyngitis (1%), increased cough (1%)

Miscellaneous: Flu-like syndrome (4%) accidental injury (1%)

Mechanism of Action The exact mechanism of action is not known. May stabilize neuronal membranes and suppress neuronal hypersynchronization through action at sodium and calcium channels. Does not affect GABA activity.

(Continued)

Zonisamide *(Continued)*

Drug Interactions

Cytochrome P450 Effect: Substrate of CYP2C19 (minor), 3A4 (major)

Increased Effect/Toxicity: Sedative effects may be additive with other CNS depressants; monitor for increased effect (includes barbiturates, benzodiazepines, narcotic analgesics, ethanol, and other sedative agents). CYP3A4 inhibitors may increase the levels/effects of zonisamide; example inhibitors include azole antifungals, ciprofloxacin, clarithromycin, diclofenac, doxycycline, erythromycin, imatinib, isoniazid, nefazodone, nicardipine, propofol, protease inhibitors, quinidine, and verapamil.

Decreased Effect: CYP3A4 inducers may decrease the levels/effects of zonisamide; example inducers include aminoglutethimide, carbamazepine, nafcillin, nevirapine, phenobarbital, phenytoin, and rifamycins.

Pharmacodynamics/Kinetics

Distribution: V_d: 1.45 L/kg

Protein binding: 40%

Metabolism: Hepatic via CYP3A4; forms N-acetyl zonisamide and 2-sulfamoylacetyl phenol (SMAP)

Half-life elimination: 63 hours

Time to peak: 2-6 hours

Excretion: Urine (62%, 35% as unchanged drug, 65% as metabolites); feces (3%)

Pregnancy Risk Factor C

Zopiclone (ZOE pi clone)

Canadian Brand Names Alti-Zopiclone; Apo-Zopiclone®; Gen-Zopiclone; Imovane®; Nu-Zopiclone; Rhovane®

Mexican Brand Names Imovane®

Generic Available Yes

Pharmacologic Category Hypnotic, Nonbenzodiazepine

Use Symptomatic relief of transient and short-term insomnia

Local Anesthetic/Vasoconstrictor Precautions No information available to require special precautions

Effects on Dental Treatment No significant effects or complications reported

Common Adverse Effects Frequency not defined.

Cardiovascular: Palpitations

Central nervous system: Drowsiness, somnolence, dizziness, confusion, anterograde amnesia, chills, memory impairment, euphoria, nightmares, agitation, anxiety, nervousness, hostility, depression, asthenia, speech abnormalities, headache

Dermatological: Rash, spots on skin

Endocrine & metabolic: Anorexia; libido decreased; alkaline phosphatase, ALT, and AST increased; appetite increased

Gastrointestinal: Constipation, coated tongue, diarrhea, dry mouth, dyspepsia, halitosis, nausea, taste alteration (bitter taste, common), vomiting

Neuromuscular & skeletal: Hypotonia, impaired coordination, limb heaviness, muscle spasms, paresthesia, tremors

Ocular: Amblyopia

Respiratory: Dyspnea

Miscellaneous: Diaphoresis

Restrictions Not available in U.S.

Mechanism of Action Zopiclone is a cyclopyrrolone derivative and has a pharmacological profile similar to benzodiazepines. Zopiclone reduces sleep latency, increases duration of sleep, and decreases the number of nocturnal awakenings.

Drug Interactions

Cytochrome P450 Effect: Substrate (major) of CYP2C8/9, 3A4

Increased Effect/Toxicity: Zopiclone may produce additive CNS depressant effects when coadministered with ethanol, sedatives, antihistamines, anticonvulsants, or psychotropic medications. CYP2C8/9 inhibitors may increase the levels/effects of zopiclone; example inhibitors include delavirdine, fluconazole, gemfibrozil, ketoconazole, nicardipine, NSAIDs, and sulfonamides. CYP3A4 inhibitors may increase the levels/effects of zopiclone; example inhibitors include azole antifungals, ciprofloxacin, clarithromycin, diclofenac, doxycycline, erythromycin, imatinib, isoniazid, nefazodone, nicardipine, propofol, protease inhibitors, quinidine, and verapamil.

Decreased Effect: CYP2C8/9 inducers may decrease the levels/effects of zopiclone; example inducers include carbamazepine, phenobarbital, phenytoin, rifampin, rifapentine, and secobarbital. CYP3A4 inducers may decrease the levels/effects of zopiclone; example inducers include aminoglutethimide, carbamazepine, nafcillin, nevirapine, phenobarbital, phenytoin, and rifamycins.

Pharmacodynamics/Kinetics

Absorption: Elderly: 75% to 94%

Distribution: Rapidly from vascular compartment

Protein binding: ~45%

Metabolism: Extensively hepatic

Half-life elimination: 5 hours; Elderly: 7 hours; Hepatic impairment: 11.9 hours

Time to peak, serum: <2 hours; Hepatic impairment: 3.5 hours

Excretion: Urine (75%); feces (16%)

Pregnancy Risk Factor Not assigned; similar agents rated D

Zorbtive™ *see* Human Growth Hormone *on page 694*

ZORprin® *see* Aspirin *on page 151*

Zostrix® [OTC] *see* Capsaicin *on page 252*

Zostrix®-HP [OTC] *see* Capsaicin *on page 252*

Zosyn® *see* Piperacillin and Tazobactam Sodium *on page 1093*

Zovia™ *see* Ethinyl Estradiol and Ethynodiol Diacetate *on page 540*

Zovirax® *see* Acyclovir *on page 64*

Zyban® *see* BuPROPion *on page 230*

Zydone® *see* Hydrocodone and Acetaminophen *on page 702*

Zyflo™ [DSC] *see* Zileuton *on page 1399*

Zyloprim® *see* Allopurinol *on page 82*

Zymar™ *see* Gatifloxacin *on page 647*

Zyprexa® *see* Olanzapine *on page 1007*

Zyprexa® Zydis® *see* Olanzapine *on page 1007*

Zyrtec® *see* Cetirizine *on page 298*

Zyrtec-D 12 Hour™ *see* Cetirizine and Pseudoephedrine *on page 299*

Zyvox™ *see* Linezolid *on page 830*

NATURAL PRODUCTS: HERBAL AND DIETARY SUPPLEMENTS

Medical problem: " I have a toothache."
2000 BC response: "Here, eat this root."
1000 AD: "That root is heathen; here, say this prayer."
1850 AD: "That prayer is superstitious; here, drink this potion."
1940 AD: "That potion is snake oil; here, swallow this pill."
1985 AD: "That pill is ineffective; here, take this new antibiotic."
2000 AD: "That antibiotic is artificial; here, eat this root."
Adapted from an anonymous Internet communication.

INTRODUCTION

For centuries, Eastern and Western civilizations have attributed a large number of medical uses to plants and herbs. Over time, modern scientific methodologies have emerged from some of these remedies. Conversely, some of these agents have fallen into less popularity as more medical knowledge has evolved. In spite of this dichotomy, herbal and natural therapies for treatment of common medical ailments have become exceedingly popular. In America, people consistently seek out natural products that may be able to offset some perceived ailment or assist in the prevention of an ailment. One area of particular interest to those individuals using herbal or natural remedies has commonly been weight loss. There are numerous systemic considerations when some of the natural products that have been attributed weight loss powers are utilized. Many of these products are sold under the blanket of dietary supplements and, therefore, have avoided some of the more stringent Food and Drug Administration legislation. However, in 1994, that legislation was modified to include herbs, vitamins, minerals, and amino acids that may be taken as dietary supplements and the federal guidelines were further modified in 1999. This information must be made available to patients taking these types of products.

The real concern lies in the fact that health claims need not be approved by the FDA, but advertisements must include a disclaimer saying that the product has not yet been fully evaluated. Claims of medicinal use/value are often drawn from popular use, not necessarily from scientific studies. Safety is a concern when these agents are taken in combination with other prescription drugs due to the medical risk which might result. Many of these natural products may have real medicinal value but caution on the part of the dental clinician is prudent. It is impossible to cover all of the natural products, therefore, this chapter has been limited to some of the most popular dietary and herbal supplements and natural remedies used by patients you might treat and what we know about the effects of some of these agents on the body's various systems. For each of the natural products described in this section, potential/suspected drug interactions have been compiled from:

- anecdotal reports,
- scientific studies (when available), and
- any known similarities of pharmacologic effects with prescription and OTC drugs.

Most drug interactions between prescription and OTC medications and natural products have not been subject to exhaustive investigation. Readers are encouraged to consult current and comprehensive references, as well as the evolving medical literature on these interactions, for additional data. An extensive reading list is provided for further research.

ALPHABETICAL LISTING OF NATURAL PRODUCTS

Aesculus hippocastanum *see* Horse Chestnut *on page 1437*
ALA *see* Flaxseed Oil *on page 1427*
Allium savitum *see* Garlic *on page 1428*

Aloe

Synonyms Aloe Barbadensis; Aloe Capensis; Aloe vera; Cape

Use Aloe has been used as an analgesic, antibacterial, antifungal, antiviral, anti-inflammatory, emollient/moisturizer, laxative, wound-healing, and hypoglycemic agent. Topical treatment of minor burns, cuts, and skin irritations, including irritant and roentgen dermatitis. Aloe has been used as an oral rinse for gums and soft tissue. Aloe has been used to reduce discomfort following oral and periodontal surgery and in reducing pain from mouth ulcers. Aloe has been shown to reduce bleeding times after dental surgery and to accelerate the healing process after surgeries. When placed over an extraction site immediately after a tooth has been removed, the application of aloe resulted in significant reduction in postoperative pain, swelling, and bleeding. Aloe promotes wound healing and shows tremendous therapeutic value in a wide variety of soft tissue injuries including tissue insults within the oral cavity. Juice may be taken internally for digestive disorders (eg, constipation, peptic ulcers, irritable bowel syndrome) and as a blood purifier; root ingested for colic. Gel used in many cosmetic and pharmaceutical formulations.

Local Anesthetic/Vasoconstrictor Precautions No information available to require special precautions

Effects on Bleeding None reported

Adverse Reactions Frequency not defined.

Central nervous system: Catharsis
Dermatologic: Contact dermatitis (allergic)
Endocrine & metabolic: Hypokalemia, electrolyte imbalance
Gastrointestinal: Abdominal cramps, diarrhea, nausea, vomiting
Renal: Albuminuria, hematuria (may cause red discoloration of urine), proteinuria

Dosage

Oral: Drink 4-8 oz/day 100% aloe vera juice plain or mixed with juice; may be used as a rinse to gargle with and swallow
Topical: Apply gel 3-5 times/day to affected area (fresh gel from plant is best as some compounds break down quickly)
Per Commission E: Constipation: 50-200 mg aloe latex (residue left after liquid from gel evaporated) taken as liquid or capsule once daily for up to 10 days

Mechanism of Action/Effect The thin, clear, gel found inside the cactus-like leaves contains barbaloin (a glycoside of anthraquinone origin), bradykinase (a protease inhibitor), emodin, mannans, tannins, volatile oils, calcium, sodium, potassium, manganese, magnesium, iron, lecithin zinc, and aloin. Aloin is a harsh, bitter-tasting substance which acts as a local irritant in the GI tract and is responsible for aloe's laxative properties. When aloe juice is taken internally, it has a protective and healing effect on the digestive system by increasing lubrication and peristaltic action in the colon; mannans (a class of compounds) are thought to stimulate wound healing. Studies indicate that aloe may also lower blood sugar levels and act as a restorative agent in the liver by purifying the blood. Topical application is therapeutic in a wide variety of soft tissue injuries as it penetrates injured tissues and dilates capillaries, thereby increasing blood flow to the injury. It prevents progressive dermal ischemia following burns, frostbite, and electrical injuries; has antithromboxane activity, yet maintains prostaglandin ratio without causing injured blood vessels to collapse.

Contraindications Pregnancy and lactation (oral ingestion only); injection (illegal in U.S. and have caused the deaths of several people)

Warnings Use with caution in diabetics and those taking hypoglycemic agents or insulin; may lower blood sugar. Some juice products may have high sodium content. Some wound healing may be delayed when administered topically. May alter GI absorption of other herbs or drugs. Avoid other herbs with hypoglycemic or laxative properties (see below). Chronic ingestion of juice may lead to electrolyte abnormalities, especially potassium (if not using as laxative, look for juice products that do not contain the chemical anthranoids responsible for laxative properties); should not be used as a laxative for >2 weeks.

Potential/Suspected Interactions Increased effect/toxicity:

Herbs with hypoglycemic properties: Alfalfa, bilberry, bitter melon, burdock, celery, damiana, fenugreek, garcinia, garlic, ginger, ginseng (American), gymnema, marshmallow, stinging nettle
Herbs with laxative properties: Cascara, eyebright, plantain, psyllium, rhubarb, senna, yellow dock

Aloe Barbadensis *see* Aloe *on page 1412*

Aloe Capensis *see* Aloe *on page 1412*

Aloe vera *see* Aloe *on page 1412*

Alpha-linolenic Acid *see* Flaxseed Oil *on page 1427*

Alpha-lipoate *see* Alpha-Lipoic Acid *on page 1413*

Alpha-Lipoic Acid

Synonyms Alpha-lipoate; Lipoic Acid; Thioctic acid

Use Antioxidant; treatment of diabetes, diabetic neuropathy, glaucoma; prevention of cataracts and neurologic disorders including stroke

Local Anesthetic/Vasoconstrictor Precautions No information available to require special precautions

Effects on Bleeding None reported

Adverse Reactions Frequency not defined.

Dermatologic: Rash

Dosage Oral: Range: 20-600 mg/day; Common dosage: 25-50 mg twice daily

Stage II open angle glaucoma: 150 mg/day (studies showed significant improvement after 2 months)

Mechanism of Action/Effect Sulfur-containing cofactor for pyruvate dehydrogenase (PDH) and alpha-ketoglutarate dehydrogenase; one of the most potent antioxidants and is metabolized to dihydrolipoic acid (DHLA), which also has antioxidant properties. It is fat- and water-soluble and may improve recycling of other antioxidants (eg, coenzyme Q10, glutathione, vitamins C and E). This antioxidant activity may limit development of diabetic complications by increasing muscle cell glucose uptake and insulin sensitivity in (type 2 diabetics), increasing neuronal blood flow and distal nerve conduction, improving glucose utilization and regeneration of glutathione, and reducing oxidative stress. In HIV-infected individuals, it is useful in blocking activation of NF-kappa B (required for HIV virus transcription) and improving T-helper lymphocytes and T-helper/suppressor cell ratio.

Warnings Use with caution in individuals predisposed to hypoglycemia including those receiving antidiabetic agents.

Potential/Suspected Interactions Increased effect/toxicity:

Insulin and oral hypoglycemics

Herbs with hypoglycemic properties: Alfalfa, aloe, bilberry, bitter melon, burdock, celery, damiana, fenugreek, garcinia, garlic, ginger, ginseng (American), gymnema, marshmallow, stinging nettle

Herbs with estrogenic activity: Black cohosh, dong quai, evening primrose

Altamisa *see* Feverfew *on page 1426*

Amber Touch-and-Feel *see* St John's Wort *on page 1447*

American Coneflower *see Echinacea on page 1423*

Anas comosus *see* Bromelain *on page 1416*

Andro *see* Androstenedione *on page 1413*

Androstenedione

Synonyms Andro

Use Androgenic, anabolic; Athletic performance and libido enhancement; believed to facilitate faster recovery from exercise, increase strength, and promote muscle development in response to training (studies inconclusive)

Local Anesthetic/Vasoconstrictor Precautions No information available to require special precautions

Effects on Bleeding None reported

Adverse Reactions Frequency not defined.

Cardiovascular: Hypertension

Central nervous system: Aggressive behavior, cerebrovascular accident, depression, euphoria, psychosis

Dermatologic: Acne, edema, exacerbation of psoriasis, hirsutism (increase in pubic hair growth), hypertrichosis, pruritus

Endocrine & metabolic: Amenorrhea, breast enlargement, breast soreness, clitoral enlargement, gynecomastia, hirsutism, hypercalcemia, hypoprolactinemia, increased libido, infertility (males), virilism

Gastrointestinal: GI irritation, nausea, vomiting

Genitourinary: Azoospermia, benign prostatic hyperplasia (BPA), bladder irritability, clitoral enlargement, epididymitis, impotence, testicular atrophy, oligospermia, priapism, prostatic carcinoma

Hematologic: Leukopenia or neutropenia (agranulocytosis, granulocytopenia), polycythemia

Hepatic: Aminotransferase level elevation (asymptomatic), cholestatic hepatitis, cholestatic jaundice, hepatic dysfunction, hepatic necrosis (especially with water-based oral preparations), hepatocellular carcinoma, jaundice

Neuromuscular & skeletal: Piloerection

Miscellaneous: Hypersensitivity reactions

(Continued)

Androstenedione *(Continued)*

Dosage Adults: Oral: 50-100 mg/day (usually about 1 hour before exercising)

Mechanism of Action/Effect A weak androgenic steroid hormone produced through natural gonadal and adrenal synthesis; precursor to testosterone and estrone (elevates serum testosterone from 15% to 300%) with androgenic and anabolic properties

Contraindications Hypertension

Warnings Use with caution in individuals with CHF, prostate conditions, or hormone-sensitive tumors. The FDA requires specific labeling noting that it "contains steroid hormones that may cause breast enlargement, testicular shrinkage, and infertility in males, and increased facial/body hair, voice-deepening, and clitoral enlargement in females." Avoid herbs with hypertensive properties (see below).

Potential/Suspected Interactions

Increased effect/toxicity:

Androgenic drugs and estrogens

Herbs with hypertensive properties: Bayberry, blue cohosh, cayenne, ephedra, ginger, ginseng, kola nut (caffeine), licorice

Decreased Effect: Requires cobalt, calcium, and zinc for conversion to testosterone; maintain selenium required for excretion of excess

Angelica sinensis *see* Dong Quai *on page 1423*

Arctostaphylos uva-ursi *see* Uva Ursi *on page 1448*

Asian Ginseng *see* Ginseng, Panax *on page 1430*

Astragalus

Synonyms *Astragalus membranaceus*; Milk Vetch

Use Adaptogen, antibacterial, diuretic, immunostimulant/immunosupportive, radioprotective, vasodilator; treatment of cancer (adjunct to chemotherapy/radiation), hepatitis, peripheral vascular diseases, respiratory infections; disease resistance, stamina, tissue oxygenation; promotes adrenal cortical function

Unlabeled/Investigational: Treatment of HIV/AIDS; antiaging

Local Anesthetic/Vasoconstrictor Precautions No information available to require special precautions

Effects on Bleeding None reported

Dosage Oral:

Children: 1/3 of adult dose

Adults: 20-500 mg 4 times/day (standardized to 0.5% glycosides and 70% polysaccharides per dose); Typical dose: 400 mg twice daily; Acute symptoms: 500 mg every 3 hours

Tea: 9-30 g dried root steeped in boiling water for 15 minutes; drink 3 cups/day

Tincture: 30 drops 3 times/day

Mechanism of Action/Effect Contains bioflavonoids, choline, isoflavones, polysaccharides (including astragalan B) saponins, and triterpenoids (including astragalosides I-VIII); astragalan B binds to cholesterol on outer membranes of viruses, allowing the immune system to attack by destabilizing and weakening the invader. Animal studies have shown that astragalan B controls bacterial infections and protects against many toxins. Saponins and triterpenoids have structural similarity to steroid hormone precursors and appear to increase adrenal activity. Polysaccharides stimulate natural killer (NK) cells, augment T-cell function, and increase interferon production; administration has been shown to increase phagocytosis by reticuloendothelial cells, decrease T-suppressor cell function, and improve T-killer cell function; may decrease cyclophosphamide-induced immune suppression; stabilizes heart rhythms

Warnings Use with caution in individuals with acute infection, especially when fever is present.

Potential/Suspected Interactions

Increased effect/toxicity: May enhance effects of immune stimulants

Decreased effect: May limit effects of immunosuppressants

Astragalus membranaceus *see* Astragalus *on page 1414*

Awa *see* Kava *on page 1439*

Bachelor's Button *see* Feverfew *on page 1426*

Bearberry *see* Uva Ursi *on page 1448*

Bifidobacterium bifidum / Lactobacillus acidophilus

Use Antidiarrheal, digestive aid; treatment of GI complaints.

B. bifidum: Maintenance of anaerobic microflora in the colon; treatment of Crohn's disease, diarrhea, ulcerative colitis

L. acidophilus: Recolonization of the GI tract with beneficial bacteria during and after antibiotic use; treatment of constipation, infant diarrhea, lactose intolerance

Local Anesthetic/Vasoconstrictor Precautions No information available to require special precautions

Effects on Bleeding None reported

Adverse Reactions No known toxicity or serious side effect

Dosage Oral: 5-10 billion colony forming units (CFU)/day [dairy free] (refrigerate to maintain optimum potency)

Mechanism of Action/Effect Natural components of colonic flora used to facilitate recolonization with benign symbiotic organisms; promotes vitamin K synthesis and absorption

Potential/Suspected Interactions Antibiotics eliminate *B. bifidum* and *L. acidophilus*

Bilberry

Synonyms *Vaccinium myrtillus*

Use Anticoagulant, antioxidant; treatment of ophthalmic disorders (cataracts, diabetic retinopathy, day/night blindness, diminished visual acuity, macular degeneration, myopia) and vascular disorders (phlebitis, varicose veins); helps maintain capillary integrity and reduce hyperpermeability

Local Anesthetic/Vasoconstrictor Precautions No information available to require special precautions

Effects on Bleeding May see increased bleeding due to inhibition of platelet aggregation

Dosage Oral: 80 mg 2-3 times/day

Mechanism of Action/Effect Inhibits a variety of inflammatory mediators, including histamine, proteases, leukotrienes, and prostaglandins; may decrease capillary permeability and inhibit platelet aggregation

Contraindications Active bleeding (eg, intracranial bleeding, peptic ulcer)

Warnings Use with caution in diabetics (may lower blood sugar), individuals with a history of bleeding, hemostatic or drug-related hemostatic disorders, those taking anticoagulants (eg, aspirin or aspirin-containing products, NSAIDs, and warfarin) or antiplatelet agents (eg, ticlopidine, clopidogrel, and dipyridamole), hypoglycemic agents or insulin. Avoid other herbs with anticoagulant/antiplatelet and/or hypoglycemic properties (see below). May alter absorption of calcium, copper, magnesium, and zinc due to tannins. Discontinue at least 14 days prior to dental or surgical procedures.

Potential/Suspected Interactions Increased effect/toxicity:

Anticoagulant or antiplatelet agents and insulin or oral hypoglycemics

Herbs with anticoagulant/antiplatelet properties: Alfalfa, anise, bladderwrack, bromelain, cat's claw, celery, coleus, cordyceps, dong quai, evening primrose, fenugreek, feverfew, garlic, ginger, ginkgo biloba, ginseng (American/Panax/Siberian), grape seed, green tea, guggul, horse chestnut seed, horseradish, licorice, prickly ash, red clover, reishi, sweet clover, turmeric, white willow

Herbs with hypoglycemic properties: Alfalfa, aloe, bitter melon, burdock, celery, damiana, fenugreek, garcinia, garlic, ginger, ginseng (American), gymnema, marshmallow, stinging nettle

Black Cohosh

Synonyms *Cimicifuga racemosa*

Use Analgesic, anti-inflammatory, phytoestrogenic; treatment of rheumatoid arthritis, mild depression, vasomotor symptoms of menopause and premenstrual syndrome (PMS)

Local Anesthetic/Vasoconstrictor Precautions No information available to require special precautions

Effects on Bleeding None reported

Adverse Reactions Frequency not defined (high doses).

Cardiovascular: Hypotension

Central nervous system: Headache

Gastrointestinal: Nausea, vomiting

Dosage Oral: 20-40 mg twice daily (standardized to contain 1 mg triterpenes per dose)

Mechanism of Action/Effect Active components are cimicifugosides (reported to affect hypothalamus/pituitary function) and isoflavones (eg,

(Continued)

Black Cohosh *(Continued)*

formononetin); also contains triterpene glycosides (eg, acetin and 27-deoxyactein), aromatic and fatty acids, starches, sugars, resins, small amounts of salicylic acid, and tannins; phytoestrogenic compounds mimic the body's natural estrogen but have not been associated with the adverse effects of synthetic estrogen. Further clinical trials are needed to determine whether black cohosh has significant estrogenic actions in the body.

Contraindications History of endometrial cancer or estrogen-dependent tumors, lactation, pregnancy (may stimulate uterine contractions)

Warnings Use with caution in individuals taking hormonal contraceptives or receiving hormone replacement therapy (HRT), those with endometrial cancer, history of estrogen-dependent tumors, hypotension, thromboembolic disease, stroke, or salicylate allergy (unknown whether amount of salicylic acid may affect platelet aggregation or have other effects associated with salicylates). Monitor serum hormone levels after 6 months of therapy. Avoid other hypotensive or phytoestrogenic herbs (see below).

Potential/Suspected Interactions Increased effect:

Antihypertensive agents, hormonal contraceptives, hormone replacement therapy (HRT), sedatives

Herbs with hypotensive properties: Aconite, arnica, baneberry, bryony, California poppy, choke cherry, coleus, golden seal, green (false) hellebore, hawthorn, immortal, Indian tobacco, jaborandi, mistletoe, night blooming cereus, pasque flower, pleurisy root, quinine, shepherd's purse

Phytoestrogenic herbs: Alfalfa, blood root, hops, kudzu, licorice, pomegranate, red clover, soybean, thyme, yucca

Black Susans *see Echinacea on page 1423*

BN-52063 *see* Ginkgo Biloba *on page 1429*

Bromelain

Synonyms *Anas comosus*

Use Anticoagulant, anti-inflammatory, digestive aid; treatment of arthritis, dyspepsia, sinusitis

Local Anesthetic/Vasoconstrictor Precautions No information available to require special precautions

Effects on Bleeding May cause increased bleeding due to inhibition of platelet aggregation

Dosage Oral:

Digestive enzyme: 500 mg 3 times/day with meals

Inflammation: 1000 mg twice daily either 1 hour before or 2 hours after meals

Mechanism of Action/Effect Inhibits the enzyme, thromboxane synthetase, which converts prostaglandin H_2 into proinflammatory prostaglandins and thromboxanes; early reports found ingesting bromelain to be beneficial in inflammatory conditions (arthritis) but research using enteric-coated bromelain at low dosages reported no benefit (studies inconclusive)

Contraindications Active bleeding (eg, peptic ulcer, intracranial bleeding)

Warnings Use with caution in individuals with cardiovascular disease (eg, CHF, hypertension), GI ulceration, history of bleeding, hemostatic or drug-related hemostatic disorders, those taking anticoagulants (eg, aspirin or aspirin-containing products, NSAIDs, warfarin), or antiplatelet agents (eg, ticlopidine, clopidogrel, dipyridamole). Avoid other herbs with anticoagulant/antiplatelet properties (see below). Discontinue at least 14 days prior to dental or surgical procedures.

Potential/Suspected Interactions Increased effect/toxicity:

Anticoagulant or antiplatelet agents

Herbs with anticoagulant/antiplatelet properties: Alfalfa, anise, bilberry, bladderwrack, cat's claw, celery, coleus, cordyceps, dong quai, evening primrose, fenugreek, feverfew, garlic, ginger, ginkgo biloba, ginseng (American/Panax/Siberian), grape seed, green tea, guggul, horse chestnut seed, horseradish, licorice, prickly ash, red clover, reishi, sweet clover, turmeric, white willow

Calendula

Synonyms *Calendula officinalis*

Use Analgesic, anti-inflammatory, antimicrobial (antibacterial, antifungal, antiviral), antiprotozoal, antiseptic, antispasmodic, immunostimulant, wound-healing agent; treatment of minor burns, cuts, and other skin irritation

Local Anesthetic/Vasoconstrictor Precautions No information available to require special precautions

Effects on Bleeding None reported

Dosage Topical: Apply to affected area as needed

Mechanism of Action/Effect Stimulates phagocytosis and increases granulation

Warnings Use with caution in individuals with plant allergies.

Potential/Suspected Interactions Decreased effect: Depleted by valproic acid and zidovudine

Calendula officinalis *see* Calendula *on page 1416*

Camellia sinensis *see* Green Tea *on page 1436*

Cape *see* Aloe *on page 1412*

Capsicum annuum *see* Cayenne *on page 1418*

Capsicum frutescens *see* Cayenne *on page 1418*

Carnitine

Synonyms L-Carnitine

Use Treatment of CHF, hyperlipidemia, male infertility; athletic performance enhancement, weight loss

Local Anesthetic/Vasoconstrictor Precautions No information available to require special precautions

Effects on Bleeding None reported

Dosage Oral: ODA: 500-2000 mg/day in divided doses

Mechanism of Action/Effect Normally synthesized in humans from two amino acids, methionine and lysine, physiologically, participates in the transport of long-chain fatty acids across mitochondrial membranes to allow energy production; assists in the oxidation of branched-chain amino acids (a substrate for muscle during stress) and ketones when necessary; may lower serum cholesterol and triglycerides; claimed to improve efficiency of energy production in muscle tissue, including the myocardium. Improved energy generation has been proposed to improve cardiac performance and increase energy and endurance.

Potential/Suspected Interactions Decreased effect: Depleted by valproic acid and zidovudine

Cascara

Synonyms Cascara Sagrada

Use Temporary relief of constipation; sometimes used with milk of magnesia ("black and white" mixture)

Local Anesthetic/Vasoconstrictor Precautions No information available to require special precautions

Effects on Bleeding None reported

Adverse Reactions 1% to 10%:
- Endocrine & metabolic: Electrolyte and fluid imbalance
- Gastrointestinal: Abdominal cramps, diarrhea, nausea
- Genitourinary: Discoloration of urine (reddish pink or brown)

Dosage Fluid extract is 5 times more potent than aromatic fluid extract.

Oral (aromatic fluid extract):
- Infants: 1.25 mL/day (range: 0.5-1.5 mL) as needed
- Children 2-11 years: 2.5 mL/day (range: 1-3 mL) as needed
- Children ≥12 years and Adults: 5 mL/day (range: 2-6 mL) as needed at bedtime (1 tablet as needed at bedtime)

Mechanism of Action/Effect Direct chemical irritation of the intestinal mucosa resulting in an increased rate of colonic motility and change in fluid and electrolyte secretion

Cascara Sagrada *see* Cascara *on page 1417*

Cat's Claw

Synonyms *Uncaria tomentosa*

Use Anticoagulant, anti-inflammatory, antimicrobial (antibacterial, antifungal, antiviral), antiplatelet, antioxidant, immunosupportive; treatment of allergies and minor infections or inflammatory conditions

Local Anesthetic/Vasoconstrictor Precautions No information available to require special precautions

Effects on Bleeding May cause increased bleeding due to inhibition of platelet aggregation

Dosage 250-1000 mg 3 times/day (standardized to contain ≥3% pentacyclic oxindole alkaloids and ≤0.06% tetracyclic oxindole alkaloids per dose)

Mechanism of Action/Effect Unclear due to the number of potentially active components; immunomodulatory and anti-inflammatory activity may be derived from multiple components. Several glycosides are reported to stimulate phagocytosis. Isopteridine is claimed to have immunostimulatory properties. Triterpenoid alkaloids and quinovic acid glycosides may inhibit replication of some (Continued)

Cat's Claw *(Continued)*

DNA viruses. In animal studies, sterols have demonstrated anti-inflammatory activity, while glycosidic components may reduce inflammation and edema. Rhynchophylline may inhibit platelet aggregation and thrombus formation. Proanthocyanidins (PCOs) appear to be potent antioxidants, improve capillary fragility, and inhibit platelet-activating factor (PAF).

Contraindications Active bleeding (eg, intracranial bleeding, peptic ulcer), pregnancy

Warnings Use with caution in individuals taking anticoagulants (eg, aspirin or aspirin-containing products, NSAIDs, warfarin) or antiplatelet agents (eg, clopidogrel, dipyridamole, ticlopidine), therapeutic immunosuppression or I.V. immunoglobulin therapy (eg, transplant recipients), those with a history of bleeding, and hemostatic or drug-related hemostatic disorders. Avoid other herbs with anticoagulant/antiplatelet properties (see below). Discontinue at least 14 days prior to dental or surgical procedures.

Potential/Suspected Interactions Increased Effect:

Anticoagulant or antiplatelet agents, immunosuppressant therapy, and I.V. immunoglobulin therapy

Herbs with anticoagulant/antiplatelet properties: Alfalfa, anise, bilberry, bladderwrack, bromelain, celery, coleus, cordyceps, dong quai, evening primrose, fenugreek, feverfew, garlic, ginger, ginkgo biloba, ginseng (American/Panax/Siberian), grape seed, green tea, guggul, horse chestnut seed, horseradish, licorice, prickly ash, red clover, reishi, sweet clover, turmeric, white willow

Cayenne

Related Information

Capsaicin *on page 252*

Synonyms *Capsicum annuum*; *Capsicum frutescens*

Use Analgesic, anti-inflammatory, digestive stimulant, sympathomimetic; treatment of arthritis (osteo and rheumatoid), diabetic neuropathy, postmastectomy pain syndrome, postherpetic neuralgia, pruritus, psoriasis; appetite suppressant, bronchial relaxation, cardiovascular circulatory support, decongestant

Local Anesthetic/Vasoconstrictor Precautions No information available to require special precautions

Effects on Bleeding None reported

Adverse Reactions

Frequency not defined.

- Cardiovascular: Hypertension, increased heart rate, vasoconstriction
- Central nervous system: Insomnia

High doses:

- Central nervous system: Dizziness, headache, hyperactivity, irritability, tremor
- Gastrointestinal: Anorexia, xerostomia

Dosage

Oral: 400 mg 3 times/day (standardized to contain ≥0.25% capsaicin per dose)

Topical: Apply as directed by manufacturer's labeling

Mechanism of Action/Effect Contains a resinous and pungent substance known as capsaicin which increases mucosal blood flow and/or vascular permeability and may inhibit gastric motility and activate duodenal motility. Capsaicin selectively activates certain populations of unmyelinated primary afferent sensory neurons (type "C"); many positive cardiovascular effects are due to its excitation of a distinct population of these neurons in the vagus nerve. Gastric and duodenal mucosa are believed to contain capsaicin-sensitive areas that, when stimulated by capsaicin, protect against acid and drug-induced ulcers.

Contraindications Anticoagulant or antiplatelet agents, cardiovascular disease (eg, arrhythmias, hypertension), diabetes, hyperthyroidism, pregnancy, psychiatric disorders

Warnings Use with caution in individuals with GI ulceration, hypertension, and those taking MAO inhibitors. May alter GI absorption of other herbs or drugs; avoid other herbs with hypertensive or sympathomimetic properties (see below).

Potential/Suspected Interactions Increased effect/toxicity:

Anticoagulant or antiplatelet agents, and MAO inhibitors (due to increased catecholamine secretion), stimulants (eg, OTC decongestants):

Herbs with anticoagulant/antiplatelet properties: Alfalfa, anise, bilberry, bladderwrack, bromelain, cat's claw, celery, coleus, cordyceps, dong quai, evening primrose, fenugreek, feverfew, garlic, ginger, ginkgo biloba, ginseng

(American/Panax/Siberian), grape seed, green tea, guggul, horse chestnut seed, horseradish, licorice, prickly ash, red clover, reishi, sweet clover, turmeric, white willow

Herbs with hypertensive properties: Bayberry, blue cohosh, ephedra, ginger, ginseng (American), kola nut (caffeine), licorice

Herbs with sympathomimetic properties: Calamus, ephedra, Fu-tse (Fo-tzu), kola nut (caffeine), guarana, night blooming cereus, peyote (mescal buttons), scotch broom tops, Syrian rue, yellow jasmine, yohimbe

Decreased Effect: Antihypertensives and salicylates

Centella asiatica *see* Gotu Kola *on page 1434*

Chamomile

Synonyms *Matricaria chamomilla*; *Matricaria recutita*

Use Antibacterial, anti-inflammatory, antispasmodic, antiulcer agent, anxiolytic, appetite stimulant, carminative, digestive aid, sedative (mild); treatment of eczema and psoriasis, hemorrhoids, inflammatory skin conditions, indigestion and irritable bowel syndrome (IBS), insomnia, leg ulcers, mastitis, premenstrual syndrome (PMS)

Local Anesthetic/Vasoconstrictor Precautions No information available to require special precautions

Effects on Bleeding None reported

Adverse Reactions Frequency not defined.

Dermatologic: Contact dermatitis (rare)

Gastrointestinal: Emesis (dried flower buds), GI upset (high doses)

Respiratory: Nasal congestion, sneezing

Miscellaneous: Anaphylaxis, hypersensitivity (atopic individuals)

Dosage Oral: 400-1600 mg/day in divided doses (standardized to contain 1% apigenin and 0.5% essential oil per dose)

Liquid extract: 1-4 mL 3 times/day

Rinse: Gargle with liquid extract 2-3 times/day as needed

Tea: ±3 g dried flowers steeped in ±150 mL boiling water for 5-10 minutes; drink 3-4 times/day

Topical: Apply to affected area as needed

Mechanism of Action/Effect Contains many active compounds; principle components are the volatile oil, alpha bisabolol which is responsible for the antispasmotic and anti-inflammatory effect, and the flavonoid, apifenin, which provides the antianxiety effect; topical ointments containing alpha bisabolol have been reported to be more effective than hydrocortisone in the treatment of inflammatory skin conditions

Contraindications Hypersensitivity to pollen from asters, chrysanthemums, daisies, feverfew, ragweed, or sunflowers; lactation and pregnancy

Warnings Use with caution in individuals with allergies and asthma (cross sensitivity may occur in those with allergies to asters, chrysanthemums, daisies, feverfew, sunflowers, or ragweed), and those taking anticoagulants, antiplatelets, and sedatives. Avoid other herbs with allergenic, anticoagulant, or antiplatelet properties (see below).

Potential/Suspected Interactions Increased effect:

Anticoagulant/antiplatelet agents (coumarin-type anticoagulants with high doses), anxiolytics, barbiturates, benzodiazepines, CNS depressants, sedatives

Allergenic herbs: Bittersweet, devil's dung, echinacea, feverfew, flaxseed, garlic, ginseng, gotu kola, male fern, propolis, yucca

Herbs with anticoagulant/antiplatelet properties: Alfalfa, anise, bilberry, bladderwrack, bromelain, cat's claw, celery, coleus, cordyceps, dong quai, evening primrose, fenugreek, feverfew, garlic, ginger, ginkgo biloba, ginseng (American/Panax/Siberian), grape seed, green tea, guggul, horse chestnut seed, horseradish, licorice, prickly ash, red clover, reishi, sweet clover, turmeric, white willow

Chasteberry

Synonyms Chastetree; *Vitex agnus-castus*

Use Treatment of acne vulgaris, amenorrhea, corpus luteum insufficiency, endometriosis, hyperprolactinemia, lactation insufficiency, menopausal symptoms, premenstrual syndrome [PMS]

Local Anesthetic/Vasoconstrictor Precautions No information available to require special precautions

Effects on Bleeding None reported

Dosage Oral: 400 mg/day in the morning on an empty stomach (standardized to contain 0.5% agnuside and 0.6% aucubin per dose)

(Continued)

Chasteberry *(Continued)*

Mechanism of Action/Effect Reported to have a significant effect on pituitary function; demonstrates progesterone-like action; may stimulate luteinizing hormone (LH) and inhibit follicle-stimulating hormone (FSH)

Contraindications Lactation and pregnancy (based on case reports of uterine stimulation and emmenagogue effects)

Warnings Use with caution in individuals taking hormonal contraceptives or receiving hormone replacement therapy (HRT). Avoid other phytoprogestogenic herbs (see below).

Potential/Suspected Interactions Increased effect/toxicity:

Dopamine antagonists (eg, antipsychotics, levodopa, metoclopramide), hormonal contraceptives, and hormone replacement therapy (HRT)

Phytoprogestogenic herbs: Blood root, oregano, yucca

Chastetree *see* Chasteberry *on page 1419*

Chinese angelica *see* Dong Quai *on page 1423*

Chondroitin Sulfate

Use Treatment of osteoarthritis

Local Anesthetic/Vasoconstrictor Precautions No information available to require special precautions

Effects on Bleeding None reported

Dosage Oral: 300-1500 mg/day

Mechanism of Action/Effect Reported to act synergistically with glucosamine to support maintenance of strong, healthy cartilage and joint function (studies inconclusive); inhibits synovial enzymes, hyaluronidase and elastase which may contribute to cartilage destruction and loss of joint function

Warnings No known toxicity or serious side effects

Chromium

Related Information

Trace Metals *on page 1319*

Use Treatment of hyper- and hypoglycemia, hyperlipidemia, hypercholesterolemia, obesity

Local Anesthetic/Vasoconstrictor Precautions No information available to require special precautions

Effects on Bleeding None reported

Adverse Reactions Frequency not defined.

Central nervous system: Cognitive impairment

Gastrointestinal: Changes in appetite, flatulence, loose stools

Hematologic: Anemia (isolated reports)

Renal: Renal failure

Dosage Oral: 50-600 mcg/day

Mechanism of Action/Effect In its trivalent form, chromium picolinate (the only active form of chromium), appears to increase insulin sensitivity, improve glucose transport into cells, and improve lipid profile by decreasing total cholesterol and triglycerides, increasing the "good" high-density lipoprotein (HDL). The mechanism of action could include one or more of the following: Enhancing beta cell activity in the pancreas and insulin binding to target tissues, increasing the number of insulin receptors, promoting activation of insulin-receptor tyrosine dinase activity. Picolinic acid causes notable changes in brain chemicals (dopamine, norepinephrine, and serotonin).

Contraindications Behavioral disorders

Potential/Suspected Interactions Drugs that may affect blood sugar levels (eg, beta blockers, insulin, oral hypoglycemics, thiazides)

Cimicifuga racemosa *see* Black Cohosh *on page 1415*

Citrus paradisi *see* Grapefruit Seed *on page 1434*

Coenzyme 1 *see* Nicotinamide Adenine Dinucleotide *on page 1443*

Coenzyme Q_{10}

Synonyms CoQ_{10}; Ubiquinone

Use Antioxidant; treatment of angina, breast cancer, cardiovascular diseases (eg, CHF), chronic fatigue syndrome, diabetes, hypertension, muscular dystrophy, obesity, periodontal disease

Local Anesthetic/Vasoconstrictor Precautions No information available to require special precautions

Effects on Bleeding None reported

Dosage Oral: 30-200 mg/day

Breast cancer, cardiovascular disease, and diabetes: >300 mg/day (per case reports)

Mechanism of Action/Effect Involved in ATP generation, the primary source of energy in human physiology; functions as a lipid-soluble antioxidant, providing protection against free radical damage within mitochondria

Warnings Avoid other agents with hypoglycemic properties (see below).

Potential/Suspected Interactions

Increased effect: Antidiabetic agents

Herbs with hypoglycemic properties: Alfalfa, aloe, bilberry, bitter melon, burdock, celery, damiana, fenugreek, garcinia, garlic, ginger, ginseng (American), gymnema, marshmallow, stinging nettle

Decreased effect: May decrease response to warfarin; potential of decreased effect with beta blockers, biguanides, chlorpromazine, clonidine, diazoxide, haloperidol, HMG-C_0A, reductase inhibitors, hydralazine, methyldopa, sulfonylureas, thiazide diuretics, and tricyclic antidepressants

Comb Flower *see* *Echinacea on page 1423*

Comphor of the Poor *see* Garlic *on page 1428*

CoQ$_{10}$ *see* Coenzyme Q$_{10}$ *on page 1420*

Cranberry

Synonyms *Vaccinium macrocarpon*

Use Treatment of urinary tract infection and prevention of nephrolithiasis

Local Anesthetic/Vasoconstrictor Precautions No information available to require special precautions

Effects on Bleeding None reported

Dosage Oral: 100% cranberry juice 300-400 mg twice daily or 8-16 oz/day

Mechanism of Action/Effect Current research indicates that a cranberry-derived glycoprotein inhibits *E. coli* adherence to the epithelial cells of the urinary tract.

Potential/Suspected Interactions Decreased effect: Caffeine may block effects

Crataegus laevigata *see* Hawthorn *on page 1437*

Crataegus monogyna *see* Hawthorn *on page 1437*

Crataegus oxyacantha *see* Hawthorn *on page 1437*

Crataegus pinnatifida *see* Hawthorn *on page 1437*

Creatine

Use Athletic performance enhancement, energy production, and protein synthesis for muscle building

Local Anesthetic/Vasoconstrictor Precautions No information available to require special precautions

Effects on Bleeding None reported

Dosage Oral: Loading dose: 10-20 g/day in divided doses for 1 week; Maintenance: 5 g/day

Mechanism of Action/Effect A naturally occurring crystalline molecule that includes atoms of carbon, hydrogen, nitrogen, and oxygen; enhances formation of polyamines, a powerful growth promoting substance; promotes protein synthesis for quick energy; combines with phosphate to form phosphocreatine released in muscle contraction

Curcuma longa *see* Turmeric *on page 1448*

Dehydroepiandrosterone

Synonyms DHEA

Use Antiaging; treatment of depression, diabetes, fatigue, lupus

Local Anesthetic/Vasoconstrictor Precautions No information available to require special precautions

Effects on Bleeding None reported

Adverse Reactions No known toxicity or serious side effects; no long-term studies conducted

Dosage Oral: 5-50 mg/day; 100 mg/day sometimes used in elderly

Mechanism of Action/Effect Precursor for synthesis of >50 additional hormones (eg, estrogen, testosterone); secreted by adrenal glands; may increase circulating testosterone levels; stimulates production of insulin growth factor-1 (IGF-1), a hormone which enhances insulin sensitivity, energy production, anabolic metabolism, and muscle growth

Contraindications History of breast or prostate cancer

Warnings Use with caution in individuals with diabetes, hepatic dysfunction, or those predisposed to hypoglycemia (monitor blood glucose and dosage of antidiabetic agents). Avoid other agents with hypoglycemic properties (see below).

(Continued)

Dehydroepiandrosterone *(Continued)*

Potential/Suspected Interactions

Increased effect/toxicity:

Androgens, corticosteroids, hormonal contraceptives, hormone replacement therapy (HRT), insulin, oral hypoglycemic agents, and testosterone

Herbs with hypoglycemic properties: Alfalfa, aloe, bilberry, bitter melon, burdock, celery, damiana, fenugreek, garcinia, garlic, ginger, ginseng (American), gymnema, marshmallow, stinging nettle

Devil's Claw

Synonyms *Harpagophytum procumbens*

Use Anti-inflammatory, cardiotonic; treatment of back pain, gout, osteoarthritis, and other inflammatory conditions

Local Anesthetic/Vasoconstrictor Precautions No information available to require special precautions

Effects on Bleeding May see increased bleeding due to inhibition of platelet aggregation

Adverse Reactions Frequency not defined.

Cardiovascular: Cardiomegaly, cardiomyopathy, hypertension, palpitations, tachycardia, vasculitis, vasoconstriction

Central nervous system: Agitation, anxiety, auditory and visual hallucination, CNS-stimulating effects, excitation, fear, headache, insomnia, irritability, nervousness, psychosis, restlessness, sympathetic storm, tension

Endocrine & metabolic: Hypokalemia

Gastrointestinal: Anorexia, nausea

Hepatic: Aminotransferase level elevation (asymptomatic)

Neuromuscular & skeletal: Tremors, weakness

Dosage Oral: 100-200 m 1-2 times/day (standardized to contain 5% harpagosides per dose)

Mechanism of Action/Effect Reportedly improves joint mobility and reduces pain and swelling in arthritis (may be more effective for osteoarthritis and chronic symptoms compared to rheumatoid and acute symptoms). Anti-inflammatory activity has reported for constituents, harpagoside and beta sitosterol; therapeutic effect comparable to phenylbutazone (studies inconclusive); may have chronotropic and inotropic effects

Contraindications Active bleeding (eg, intracranial bleeding, peptic ulcer), GI disorders, lactation, pregnancy (may stimulate uterine contractions)

Warnings Use with caution in individuals with history of bleeding, hemostatic or drug-related hemostatic disorders, and those taking anticoagulants (eg, aspirin or aspirin-containing products, NSAIDs, warfarin) or antiplatelet agents (eg, clopidogrel, dipyridamole, ticlopidine), antiarrhythmic agents, or cardiac glycosides (eg, digoxin). Avoid herbs with anticoagulant/antiplatelet properties (see below). Discontinue at least 14 days prior to dental or surgical procedures.

Potential/Suspected Interactions Increased effect:

Antiarrhythmics or cardiac glycosides and anticoagulant or antiplatelet agents

Herbs with anticoagulant/antiplatelet properties: Alfalfa, anise, bilberry, bladderwrack, bromelain, cat's claw, celery, coleus, cordyceps, dong quai, evening primrose, fenugreek, feverfew, garlic, ginger, ginkgo biloba, ginseng (American/Panax/Siberian), grape seed, green tea, guggul, horse chestnut seed, horseradish, licorice, prickly ash, red clover, reishi, sweet clover, turmeric, white willow

DHA *see* Docosahexaenoic Acid *on page 1422*

DHEA *see* Dehydroepiandrosterone *on page 1421*

Dimethyl Sulfone *see* Methyl Sulfonyl Methane *on page 1442*

Dioscorea villosa *see* Wild Yam *on page 1450*

$DMSO_2$ *see* Methyl Sulfonyl Methane *on page 1442*

Docosahexaenoic Acid

Synonyms DHA

Use Treatment of Alzheimer's disease, attention deficit disorder (ADD) and attention deficit hyperactivity disorder (ADHD), Crohn's disease, diabetes, eczema and psoriasis, hypertension, hypertriglyceridemia, and rheumatoid arthritis; coronary heart disease risk reduction

Local Anesthetic/Vasoconstrictor Precautions No information available to require special precautions

Effects on Bleeding None reported

Dosage Oral: 125-250 mg 1-2 times/day

Mechanism of Action/Effect A long-chain, unsaturated, omega-3 fatty acid critical in the development of infants' brains and retinas; highly concentrated in synaptosomes in the brain (the region where nerve cells communicate with each other), photoreceptors (the portion of the retina that receives light stimulation), the cerebral cortex, and the mitochondria. Alpha-linolenic acid (ALA) is the precursor for the other omega-3 fatty acids, however, it is estimated that only a small percentage gets converted to DHA; the primary dietary source of DHA is from cold water or oily fish (herring, mackerel, salmon, sardines, and tuna).

Warnings Use caution with individuals taking anticoagulants (eg, aspirin or aspirin-containing products, NSAIDs, warfarin) or antiplatelet agents (eg, clopidogrel, dipyridamole, ticlopidine), insulin or oral hypoglycemics. Avoid herbs with anticoagulant/antiplatelet properties (see below); may intensify the blood-thinning effect

Potential/Suspected Interactions Increased effect:

Anticoagulant or antiplatelet agents

Herbs with anticoagulant/antiplatelet properties: Alfalfa, anise, bilberry, bladderwrack, bromelain, cat's claw, celery, coleus, cordyceps, dong quai, evening primrose, fenugreek, feverfew, garlic, ginger, ginkgo biloba, ginseng (American/Panax/Siberian), grape seed, green tea, guggul, horse chestnut seed, horseradish, licorice, prickly ash, red clover, reishi, sweet clover, turmeric, white willow

Dong Quai

Synonyms *Angelica sinensis*; Chinese angelica

Use Anabolic, anticoagulant; treatment of amenorrhea, anemia, dysmenorrhea, hypertension, menopausal symptoms, premenstrual syndrome (PMS); female vitality

Local Anesthetic/Vasoconstrictor Precautions No information available to require special precautions

Effects on Bleeding Has potential for decreasing platelet aggregation and may increase bleeding

Dosage Adults: Oral: 200 mg twice daily (standardized to contain 0.8% to 1.1% ligustilide per dose)

Mechanism of Action/Effect Reported to cause vasodilation; may have hematopoietic properties; rich in phytoestrogens, which may demonstrate similar pharmacological effects, but are less potent than pure estrogenic compounds

Contraindications Active bleeding (eg, peptic ulcer, intracranial bleeding), prolonged exposure to sunlight or other sources of ultraviolet radiation (eg, tanning booths)

Warnings May alter hemostasis, potentiate effects of warfarin, and/or cause photosensitization; use with caution in lactation, pregnancy, cardiovascular or cerebrovascular disease, endometrial cancer, estrogen-dependent tumors, hemostatic or drug-related hemostatic disorders, history of bleeding, hypotension, stroke, thromboembolic disease, and individuals taking anticoagulants (eg, aspirin or aspirin-containing products, NSAIDs, warfarin), antiplatelet agents (eg, clopidogrel, dipyridamole, ticlopidine), antihypertensive medications, hormonal contraceptives or hormone replacement therapy (HRT), or steroids. Avoid other herbs with anabolic, anticoagulant, or antiplatelet properties (see below). Discontinue at least 14 days prior to dental or surgical procedures.

Potential/Suspected Interactions Increased effect/toxicity:

Anticoagulant or antiplatelet agents, antihypertensives, hormonal contraceptives, hormone replacement therapy (HRT), photosensitizing agents

Anabolic herbs: Devil's club, ginseng (American/Asian, Siberian), muira puama, sarsparilla, suma, tribulus, wild yam

Herbs with anticoagulant/antiplatelet properties: Alfalfa, anise, bilberry, bladderwrack, bromelain, cat's claw, celery, coleus, cordyceps, evening primrose, fenugreek, feverfew, garlic, ginger, ginkgo biloba, ginseng (American/Panax/Siberian), grape seed, green tea, guggul, horse chestnut seed, horseradish, licorice, prickly ash, red clover, reishi, sweet clover, turmeric, white willow

Echinacea

Synonyms American Coneflower; Black Susans; Comb Flower; *Echinacea angustifolia*; *Echinacea purpurea*; Indian Head; Purple Coneflower; Scury Root; Snakeroot

Use Antibacterial, antihyaluronidase, anti-infective, anti-inflammatory, antiviral, immunostimulant, wound-healing agent; treatment of arthritis, chronic skin complaints, cold, flu, sore throat, tonsillitis, minor upper respiratory tract infections, urinary tract infections

(Continued)

Echinacea (Continued)

Local Anesthetic/Vasoconstrictor Precautions No information available to require special precautions

Effects on Bleeding None reported

Adverse Reactions Frequency not defined.

Dermatologic: Allergic reactions (rare; none known for oral and external formulations per Commission E)

Gastrointestinal: Tingling sensation of tongue

Miscellaneous: Immunosuppression (use >6-8 weeks)

Dosage In addition to forms listed below, there are some products designed to be applied topically; refer to product labeling to ensure formulation is used correctly. Continuous use should not exceed 8 weeks; not to exceed 10 days in immunosuppressed individuals or acute infection therapy. If used for prophylaxis, cycle 3 weeks on and 1 week off.

Oral (with food):

Capsule, tablet, or tea: 500 mg to 2 g, 3 times/day for 1 day, then 250 mg 4 times/day (standardized to contain 4% sesquiterpene esters per dose)

Expressed juice of fresh herb: 6-9 mL/day (per Commission E)

Liquid extract: 0.25-1 mL 3 times/day

Tincture: 1-2 mL 3 times/day

Topical: Apply to affected areas as needed

Mechanism of Action/Effect Stimulates cytokines, TNF-alfa, and interferons; caffeic acid glycosides and isolutylamides associated with the plant can also cause immune stimulation (leukocyte phagocytosis and T-cell activation)

Contraindications Hypersensitivity to asters, chamomile, chrysanthemums, daisies, feverfew, ragweed, sunflowers; autoimmune diseases such as collagen vascular disease (lupus, RA), HIV or AIDS, MS, tuberculosis; immunosuppressants; pregnancy (only parenteral administration per Commission E)

Warnings Use as a preventative treatment should be discouraged; may alter immunosuppression; long-term use may cause immunosuppression. Individuals allergic to asters, chamomile, chrysanthemums, daisies, feverfew, sunflowers, or ragweed may display cross-allergy potential (rare but severe); avoid other allergenic herbs (see below). Use with caution in individuals with renal impairment.

Potential/Suspected Interactions

Increased effect/toxicity:

Allergenic herbs: Bittersweet, chamomile, devil's dung, echinacea, feverfew, flaxseed, garlic, ginseng, gotu kola, male fern, propolis, yucca

Herbs with anticoagulant/antiplatelet properties: Alfalfa, anise, bilberry, bladderwrack, bromelain, cat's claw, celery, coleus, cordyceps, dong quai, evening primrose, fenugreek, feverfew, garlic, ginkgo biloba, ginseng (American/Panax/Siberian), grape seed, green tea, guggul, horse chestnut seed, horseradish, licorice, prickly ash, red clover, reishi, sweet clover, turmeric, white willow

Decreased effect: Corticosteroids and immunosuppressants; depletes potassium

Echinacea angustifolia *see Echinacea on page 1423*

Echinacea purpurea *see Echinacea on page 1423*

EGb *see* Ginkgo Biloba *on page 1429*

Eleutherococcus senticosus *see* Ginseng, Siberian *on page 1431*

English Hawthorn *see* Hawthorn *on page 1437*

Ephedra

Related Information

Ephedrine *on page 495*

Synonyms *Ephedra sinica*

Use Appetite-suppressant, stimulant, sympathomimetic (potent), thermogenic, thyroid-stimulant; treatment of allergies, arthritis, asthma, bronchitis, edema, fever, hay fever, headache, obesity, urticaria; euphoria

Note: The sale of ephedra has been banned in the United States (see Warnings).

Local Anesthetic/Vasoconstrictor Precautions Has potential to interact with epinephrine and levonordefrin to result in increased BP; use vasoconstrictor with caution

Effects on Bleeding None reported

Adverse Reactions

Frequency not defined.

Cardiovascular: Hypertension, increased heart rate, vasoconstriction

Central nervous system: Insomnia

High doses:

Central nervous system: Dizziness, headache, hyperactivity, insomnia, irritability, tremor

Gastrointestinal: Anorexia, increased peristalsis, xerostomia

Dosage Note: The sale of ephedra has been banned in the United States (see Warnings)

Not to exceed 8 mg of total ephedrine alkaloids per dose or <24 mg in 24 hours; per Commission E, herb preparation corresponds to 15-30 mg total alkaloid (calculated as ephedrine)

Adults: Oral:

E. sinica extracts (with 10% alkaloid content): 125-250 mg 3 times/day

Tea: Steep 1 heaping teaspoon in 240 mL of boiling water for 10 minutes (equivalent to 15-30 mg of ephedrine)

Mechanism of Action/Effect Active constituent is ephedrine; stimulates alpha-, beta$_1$-, and beta$_2$-adrenergic receptors and the release of norepinephrine; its activity on the sympathetic nervous system causes vasoconstriction and cardiac stimulation resulting in a temporary rise in both systolic and diastolic BP; causes mydriasis and produces bronchial muscle relaxation; contains the alkaloids, ephedrine and pseudoephedrine, which are routinely isolated and used in OTC products as decongestants

Contraindications Anticoagulant or antiplatelet agents, cardiovascular disease (eg, arrhythmias, hypertension), children, diabetes, hyperthyroidism, MAO inhibitors, pregnancy, psychiatric disorders

Per Commission E: Anxiety, glaucoma, hypertension, impaired cerebral circulation, pheochromocytoma, prostate adenoma (with residual urine accumulation), thyrotoxicosis

Warnings On February 6, 2004, the Food and Drug Administration (FDA) issued a final rule prohibiting the sale of dietary supplements containing ephedrine alkaloids (ephedra) because such supplements "present an unreasonable risk of illness or injury." The rule became effective 60 days from the date of publication. The ban was prompted by reports of serious adverse events filed with the FDA as well as studies which have verified negative effects on blood pressure and the circulatory system.

Additional information about ephedra and this specific ruling is available at the following websites: http://www.fda.gov/bbs/topics/NEWS/2004/NEW01021.html and http://www.cfsan.fda.gov/-dms/ds-ephed.html.

Potential/Suspected Interactions Increased effect:

Antiarrhythmics, beta-blockers, cardiac glycosides, calcium channel blockers, OTC stimulants, sympathomimetic or thyroid medications

Secale alkaloid derivatives or oxytocin: Development of hypertension

Per Commission E: Guanethidine and MAO inhibitors potentiate ephedra's sympathomimetic effect

Herbs with hypertensive properties: Bayberry, blue cohosh, cayenne, ginger, ginseng (American), kola nut (caffeine), licorice

Thyroid-stimulating herbs: Fu-tse (Fo-tzu), gotu kola, mustard, yohimbe

Ephedra sinica *see* Ephedra *on page 1424*

Evening Primrose

Synonyms Evening Primrose Oil; *Oenothera biennis*

Use Anticoagulant, anti-inflammatory, hormone stimulant; treatment of atopic eczema and psoriasis, attention deficit disorder (ADD) and attention deficit hyperactivity disorder (ADHD), dermatitis, diabetic neuropathy, endometriosis, hyperglycemia, irritable bowel syndrome (IBS), multiple sclerosis (MS), omega-6 fatty acid supplementation, premenstrual syndrome (PMS), menopausal symptoms, rheumatoid arthritis

Local Anesthetic/Vasoconstrictor Precautions No information available to require special precautions

Effects on Bleeding May see increased bleeding due to inhibition of platelet aggregation

Dosage Oral: 500 mg to 8 g/day (standardized to contain 8% to 9% gamma-linolenic acid (GLA) and ≤72% linoleic acid (LA) per dose)

Mechanism of Action/Effect Contains high amounts of gamma-linolenic acid (GLA), and essential omega-6 fatty acid which reportedly stimulates hormone synthesis and reduces generation of arachidonic acid metabolites in short-term use, improving symptoms of various inflammatory and immune conditions

Contraindications Active bleeding (may inhibit platelet aggregation), anticonvulsant or antipsychotic agents, seizure disorders (may lower seizure threshold), schizophrenia

Warnings Use with caution in individuals with a history of bleeding, hemostatic or drug-related hemostatic disorders, those taking anticoagulants (eg, aspirin

(Continued)

Evening Primrose *(Continued)*

or aspirin-containing products, NSAIDs, warfarin) or antiplatelet agents (eg, clopidogrel, dipyridamole, ticlopidine). Avoid other herbs with anticoagulant/antiplatelet properties (see below). Discontinue at least 14 days prior to dental or surgical procedures.

Potential/Suspected Interactions Increased effect/toxicity:

Anticoagulant or antiplatelet agents, anticonvulsants, phenothiazines, and other drugs which lower seizure threshold

Herbs with anticoagulant/antiplatelet properties: Alfalfa, anise, bilberry, bladderwrack, bromelain, cat's claw, celery, coleus, cordyceps, dong quai, fenugreek, feverfew, garlic, ginger, ginkgo biloba, ginseng (American/Panax/Siberian), grape seed, green tea, guggul, horse chestnut seed, horseradish, licorice, prickly ash, red clover, reishi, sweet clover, turmeric, white willow

Evening Primrose Oil *see* Evening Primrose *on page 1425*

Eye Balm *see* Golden Seal *on page 1433*

Eye Root *see* Golden Seal *on page 1433*

Featherfew *see* Feverfew *on page 1426*

Featherfoil *see* Feverfew *on page 1426*

Feverfew

Synonyms Altamisa; Bachelor's Button; Featherfew; Featherfoil; Nosebleed; *Tanacetum parthenium*; Wild Quinine

Use Anticoagulant/anti-inflammatory, antiprostaglandin, antispasmodic, digestive aid, emmenagogue, sedative; prophylaxis and treatment of migraine headaches and rheumatoid arthritis; treatment of fever, hypertension, premenstrual syndrome (PMS), tinnitus

Local Anesthetic/Vasoconstrictor Precautions No information available to require special precautions

Effects on Bleeding May see increased bleeding due to inhibition of platelet aggregation

Adverse Reactions

10%:

Gastrointestinal: Bleeding gums (within 3 days)

Frequency not defined:

Central nervous system (upon discontinuation): Headache, insomnia, nervousness

Dermatologic: Contact dermatitis

Gastrointestinal: Abdominal pain, loss of taste, oral ulcerations, nausea, vomiting

Neuromuscular & skeletal (upon discontinuation): Still joints

Dosage Oral (standardized to contain 0.2% parthenolide per dose): 125 mg once or twice daily

Inflammation and rheumatoid arthritis: 100-250 mg/day

Mechanism of Action/Effect Active ingredient is parthenolide (~0.2% concentration), a serotonin antagonist; reported to inhibit leukotrinenes, prostaglandins, thromboxanes and platelet aggregation; may have spasmolytic activity

Contraindications Active bleeding (eg, intracranial bleeding, peptic ulcer), children <2 years of age; hypersensitivity to asters, chrysanthemums, daisies, sunflowers, chamomile, feverfew, or ragweed pollens; lactation and pregnancy

Warnings Use with caution in individuals with a history of bleeding, hemostatic disorders or drug-related hemostatic problems, and those taking anticoagulants (eg, aspirin or aspirin-containing products, NSAIDs, warfarin), antiplatelet agents (eg, clopidogrel, dipyridamole, ticlopidine), or medications with serotonergic properties. Abrupt discontinuation may increase migraine frequency. May alter absorption of calcium, copper, magnesium, and zinc due to tannins. Avoid other herbs with allergenic, anticoagulant, or antiplatelet properties (see below). Discontinue at least 14 days prior to dental or surgical procedures.

Potential/Suspected Interactions Increased effect:

Anticoagulant/antiplatelet agents

Allergenic herbs: Bittersweet, chamomile, devil's dung, echinacea, flaxseed, garlic, ginseng, gotu kola, male fern, propolis, yucca

Herbs with anticoagulant/antiplatelet properties: Alfalfa, anise, bilberry, bladderwrack, bromelain, cat's claw, celery, coleus, cordyceps, dong quai, evening primrose, fenugreek, feverfew, garlic, ginkgo biloba, ginseng (American/Panax/Siberian), grape seed, green tea, guggul, horse chestnut seed, horseradish, licorice, prickly ash, red clover, reishi, sweet clover, turmeric, white willow

Fish Oils

Use Antiatherogenic, anticoagulant/antiplatelet, anti-inflammatory; prevention and treatment of cardiovascular diseases; treatment of arteriosclerosis, arthritis, Crohn's disease, diabetes, dyslipidemia, dysmenorrhea, eczema and psoriasis, glaucoma, hypercholesterolemia, hypertension, hypertriglyceridemia; memory enhancement

Local Anesthetic/Vasoconstrictor Precautions No information available to require special precautions

Effects on Bleeding None reported

Dosage Oral: 750 mg 2-3 times/day

Mechanism of Action/Effect Source of eicosapentaenoic acid (EPA) and docosahexaenoic acid (DHA), omega-3 fatty acids which are necessary for the production of cellular membranes, hormones, and nerve tissue; EPA is converted into the series 3 prostaglandins, which have anti-inflammatory activity; although the body synthesizes these fats from alpha-linolenic acid (ALA), conversion in many people is inefficient (most people are deficient in omega-3 fatty acids); prevents atherosclerotic plaque formation

Warnings Use caution with individuals taking anticoagulants (eg, aspirin or aspirin-containing products, NSAIDs, warfarin) or antiplatelet agents (eg, clopidogrel, dipyridamole, ticlopidine), insulin or oral hypoglycemics. Avoid herbs with anticoagulant/antiplatelet properties (see below); may intensify the blood-thinning effect.

Potential/Suspected Interactions Increased effect/toxicity:

Anticoagulant or antiplatelet agents and insulin or oral hypoglycemics

Herbs with anticoagulant/antiplatelet properties: Alfalfa, anise, bilberry, bladderwrack, bromelain, cat's claw, celery, coleus, cordyceps, dong quai, evening primrose, fenugreek, feverfew, garlic, ginger, ginkgo biloba, ginseng (American/Panax/Siberian), grape seed, green tea, guggul, horse chestnut seed, horseradish, licorice, prickly ash, red clover, reishi, sweet clover, turmeric, white willow

Flaxseed Oil

Synonyms ALA; Alpha-linolenic Acid

Use Antioxidant, antiatherogenic; treatment of eczema and psoriasis, hypertension, hypercholesterolemia, hypertriglyceridemia; contains 3 times more omega-3 than omega-6 and may be used to help reverse the imbalance between omega-3 and omega-6 (estimated optimal ratio between omega-3 and omega-6 fatty acids is about 1:4 and ratio for many in U.S. is 1:20 to 1:30)

Local Anesthetic/Vasoconstrictor Precautions No information available to require special precautions

Effects on Bleeding None reported

Dosage Oral: 1 Tbsp/day (contains ~58% to 60% omega-3 fatty acid) [available in capsules; must be refrigerated]

Mechanism of Action/Effect The richest source of alpha-linolenic acid (ALA), which contains approximately 58% to 60% omega-3 fatty acids and 18% to 20% omega-6 fatty acids; prevents atherosclerotic plaque formation and plays a critical role in the transport and oxidation of cholesterol; precursor for the omega-3 fatty acids, eicosapentaenoic acid (EPA) and docosahexaenoic acid (DHA), which are an integral part of the production of cellular membranes, hormones, and nerve tissue; EPA is converted into the series 3 prostaglandins, which have anti-inflammatory activity

Contraindications Hypersensitivity to flaxseed, flaxseed oil or any member of the flax plant (*Linaceae*) family

Warnings Use with caution in individuals with plant allergies, those taking anticoagulants (eg, aspirin or aspirin-containing products, NSAIDs, warfarin) or antiplatelet agents (eg, clopidogrel, dipyridamole, ticlopidine), insulin or oral hypoglycemics. Avoid herbs with allergenic, anticoagulant, or antiplatelet properties (see below); may intensify the blood-thinning effect

Potential/Suspected Interactions Increased effect/toxicity:

Allergenic herbs: Bittersweet, camomile, devil's dung, echinacea, feverfew, flaxseed, garlic, ginseng, gotu kola, male fern, propolis, yucca

Anticoagulant or antiplatelet agents and insulin or oral hypoglycemics

Herbs with anticoagulant/antiplatelet properties: Alfalfa, anise, bilberry, bladderwrack, bromelain, cat's claw, celery, coleus, cordyceps, dong quai, evening primrose, fenugreek, feverfew, garlic, ginger, ginkgo biloba, ginseng (American/Panax/Siberian), grape seed, green tea, guggul, horse chestnut seed, horseradish, licorice, prickly ash, red clover, reishi, sweet clover, turmeric, white willow

Garlic

Synonyms *Allium savitum*; Comphor of the Poor; Nectar of the Gods; Poor Mans Treacle; Rustic Treacle; Stinking Rose

Use Antibiotic, anticoagulant/antiplatelet (potent), anti-inflammatory, antioxidant (aged extract improves benefits), antitumor agent, immunosupportive; treatment of hypercholesterolemia, hypertension, hypertriglyceridemia, hypoglycemia; may decrease thrombosis

Local Anesthetic/Vasoconstrictor Precautions No information available to require special precautions

Effects on Bleeding May see increased bleeding due to potent platelet inhibition

Adverse Reactions Frequency not defined.

Dermatologic: Eczema, immunologic contact urticaria, skin blistering, systemic contact dermatitis

Gastrointestinal: Changes in intestinal flora (rare per Commission E), GI upset (>5 cloves)

Ocular: Lacrimation

Respiratory: Asthma (inhalation of garlic dust)

Miscellaneous: Allergic reactions (rare); change in odor of skin and breath (per Commission E)

Dosage Onset of cholesterol-lowering and hypotensive effects may require months.

Adults: Oral: 400 mg 2-3 times/day (equivalent to 1200 mg of fresh garlic or 10 mg of allicin standardized to contain 4 mg of total allicin potential (TAP) per dose) **or** 600 mg of aged extract 1-3 times/day (standardized to contain 1 mg/g S-allyl cysteine (SAC) per dose)

Cardiovascular benefits: -0.25-1 g/kg or 1-4 cloves/day (in divided doses) in an 80 kg individual

Mechanism of Action/Effect May decrease LDL cholesterol and increase HDL cholesterol, decrease blood glucose levels and triglycerides, increase fibrinolytic activity, and decrease thrombosis; crushed bulb converts to allicin, which may have antioxidant activity. Ajoene, a byproduct of allicin, is potent platelet inhibitor. Per Commission E, antibiotic property is ~1% as active as penicillin.

Contraindications Active bleeding (eg, intracranial bleeding, peptic ulcer) and pregnancy

Warnings Use with caution in diabetics (may lower blood sugar), individuals taking anticoagulants (eg, aspirin or aspirin-containing products, NSAIDs, warfarin), antihypertensives, antiplatelet agents (eg, clopidogrel, dipyridamole, ticlopidine), hypoglycemic agents or insulin, hypolipidemic agents, and those with a history of bleeding, hemostatic or drug-related hemostatic disorders; may cause GI distress in sensitive individuals. Avoid other herbs with allergenic, anticoagulant/antiplatelet, hypoglycemic, or hypolipidemic properties (see below). Discontinue at least 14 days prior to dental or surgical procedures.

Potential/Suspected Interactions

Increased effect:

Anticoagulant/antiplatelet agents, antihypertensives, hypoglycemic agents and insulin, amphotericin B (against *Cryptococcus neoformans*)

Allergenic herbs: Bittersweet, chamomile, devil's dung, echinacea, feverfew, flaxseed, ginseng, gotu kola, male fern, propolis, yucca

Herbs with anticoagulant/antiplatelet properties: Alfalfa, anise, bilberry, bladderwrack, bromelain, cat's claw, celery, coleus, cordyceps, dong quai, evening primrose, fenugreek, feverfew, ginger, ginkgo biloba, ginseng (American/Panax/Siberian), grape seed, green tea, guggul, horse chestnut seed, horseradish, licorice, prickly ash, red clover, reishi, sweet clover, turmeric, white willow

Herbs with hypoglycemic properties: Alfalfa, aloe bilberry, bitter melon, burdock, celery, damiana, fenugreek, garcinia, ginger, ginseng (American), gymnema, marshmallow, stinging nettle

Herbs with hypolipidemic properties: Alfalfa, artichoke, blue cohosh, fenugreek, ginger, guggul, gymnema, plantain, skullcap, myrrh, tansy, red yeast rice

Decreased effect: May reduce iodine uptake

GBE *see* Ginkgo Biloba *on page 1429*

Ginger

Synonyms *Zingiber officinale*

Use Analgesic, anticoagulant, antiemetic (lack of sedative effects is advantageous over other antiemetics), anti-inflammatory (musculoskeletal), digestive aid; treatment of amenorrhea (Chinese remedy), arthritis, colds, culinary herb, dyspepsia, flu, headaches, motion sickness, nausea/vomiting (eg, from chemotherapy/radiation)

Local Anesthetic/Vasoconstrictor Precautions No information available to require special precautions

Effects on Bleeding Very high doses may inhibit platelet aggregation.

Adverse Reactions Frequency not defined.

Central nervous system: Depression (high doses)

Gastrointestinal: Increased salivation

Dosage Oral:

Digestive aid or prevention of motion sickness: 250 mg of ginger root powder 3-4 times/day with food (standardized to contain 4% volatile oils or 5% 6-gingerol and 6-shogaol per dose)

Per Commission E: 2-4 g/day or equivalent preparations

Ale/tea: 8 oz of ginger ale contains ~1 g; I cup tea contains ~250 mg

Mechanism of Action/Effect Unknown; antiemetic activity believed to be due to shogaol documented to be comparable to several antiemetic medications, having local effects in the GI tract and/or activity in CNS;. gingerol shown to stimulate gastric secretions and peristalsis; ginger may decrease nausea associated with radiation and chemotherapy and is claimed to be superior to antihistamines for motion sickness due to lack of sedative effects. It may increase GI motility and and thus block nausea feedback from the GI tract; decreases gastric-emptying delays associated with cisplatin; may delay coagulation due to effect on platelet-activating factor and inhibit platelet aggregation (very high doses); may have cardiotonic activity; appears to decrease prostaglandin synthesis

Contraindications Active bleeding (eg, intracranial bleeding, peptic ulcer) and gallstones (per Commission E)

Warnings Use with caution in diabetics, individuals with a history of bleeding, hemostatic or drug-related hemostatic disorders, those taking anticoagulants (eg, aspirin or aspirin-containing products, NSAIDs, warfarin), antiplatelet agents (eg, clopidogrel, dipyridamole, ticlopidine), cardiac glycosides (eg, digoxin), hypolipidemic agents, hypoglycemic agents, or insulin. Has cardioactive constituents; avoid large and/or prolonged doses. Avoid other herbs with anticoagulant/antiplatelet, hypertensive, hyperlipidemic, or hypoglycemic properties (see below). Discontinue at least 14 days prior to dental or surgical procedures.

Potential/Suspected Interactions Increased effect/toxicity:

Anticoagulant/antiplatelet agents, antihypertensives, chemotherapy agents, cisplatin (decreases gastric emptying delays), insulin, oral hypoglycemics

Herbs with anticoagulant/antiplatelet properties: Alfalfa, anise, bilberry, bladderwrack, bromelain, cat's claw, celery, coleus, cordyceps, dong quai, evening primrose, fenugreek, feverfew, garlic, ginkgo biloba, ginseng (American/Panax/Siberian), grape seed, green tea, guggul, horse chestnut seed, horseradish, licorice, prickly ash, red clover, reishi, sweet clover, turmeric, white willow

Herbs with hypertensive properties: Bayberry, blue cohosh, cayenne, ephedra, ginseng (American), kola nut (caffeine), licorice

Herbs with hypoglycemic properties: Alfalfa, aloe bilberry, bitter melon, burdock, celery, damiana, fenugreek, garcinia, garlic, ginseng (American), gymnema, marshmallow, stinging nettle

Herbs with hypolipidemic properties: Alfalfa, artichoke, blue cohosh, fenugreek, garlic, guggul, gymnema, plantain, skullcap, myrrh, tansy, red yeast rice

Ginkgo Biloba

Synonyms BN-52063; EGb; GBE; ginkgold; Ginkgopowder; Ginkogink; Kaveri; Kew Tree; Maidenhair Tree; Oriental Plum Tree; Rökan; Silver Apricot; Superginkgo; Tanakan; Tanakene; Tebonin; Tramisal; Valverde; Vasan; Vital

Use Anticoagulant/antiplatelet, antioxidant

Per Commission E: Treatment of primary degenerative dementia, vascular dementia, and demential syndromes (eg, memory deficit), depressive emotional conditions, headache, and tinnitus

Treatment of Alzheimer's disease, arterial insufficiency and intermittent claudication (European remedy), cerebral vascular disease (dementia), macular degeneration, resistant depression, traumatic brain injury, tinnitus, visual disorders, vertigo of vascular origin

Local Anesthetic/Vasoconstrictor Precautions No information available to require special precautions

Effects on Bleeding May see increased bleeding due to inhibition of platelet aggregation; antagonizes platelet activating factor (PAF)

(Continued)

Ginkgo Biloba *(Continued)*

Adverse Reactions Frequency not defined.

Cardiovascular: Bilateral subdural hematomas, palpitations

Central nervous system: Dizziness, headache (rare, per Commission E), restlessness, seizures (in children)

Dermatologic: Allergic skin reactions (rare, per Commission E), cheilitis, urticaria

Gastrointestinal: Diarrhea, GI upset (rare, per Commission E), nausea, proctitis, stomatitis, vomiting

Hematologic: Hyphema

Dosage May require 1-2 months of use for therapeutic effect (elderly: 1 month)

Oral (administer with food):

40-80 mg twice daily to 3 times/day (standardized to contain 24% to 27% ginkgo flavone glycosides and 6% to 7% triterpenes per dose); Maximum dose: 360 mg/day

Cerebral ischemia: 120 mg/day extract in 2-3 divided doses (standardized to contain 24% flavonoid-glycoside extract and 6% terpene glycosides)

Mechanism of Action/Effect Extract contains terpenoids and flavonoids reported to inactivate oxygen-free radicals; causes vasodilation and inhibits platelet aggregation; CNS effects may be due to 4-O-methylpyridoxine (an antipyridoxine compound). Reported to increase peripheral blood flow; can increase alpha waves and decrease slow potentials in EEG.

Contraindications Active bleeding (eg, intracranial bleeding, peptic ulcer) or clotting disorders, anticoagulants or antiplatelet agents, hypersensitivity to ginkgo biloba preparations (per Commission E), MAO inhibitors, pregnancy, vasodilators

Warnings Use with caution in individuals with a history of bleeding, hemostatic drug-related hemostatic disorders, those taking anticoagulants (eg, aspirin or aspirin-containing products, NSAIDs, warfarin) or antiplatelet agents (eg, clopidogrel, dipyridamole, ticlopidine), and MAO inhibitors. Cross reactivity for contact dermatitis (due to fruit pulp) exists with poison ivy and poison oak; may last for 10 days (washing skin within 10 minutes may prevent reaction or topical corticosteroids may be helpful). Fruit pulp contains ginkolic acids which are allergens (seeds are not sensitizing). Admit individuals with neurologic abnormalities after ingestion or ingestions >2 pieces of fruit; pyridoxine may be useful after ingestion of ginkgo seeds or kernels. Avoid other herbs with anticoagulant/antiplatelet properties (see below). Discontinue at least 2-3 weeks prior to surgery; use with caution following recent surgery or trauma.

Potential/Suspected Interactions Increased effect/toxicity:

Anticoagulant/antiplatelet agents and MAO inhibitors

Herbs with anticoagulant/antiplatelet properties: Alfalfa, anise, bilberry, bladderwrack, bromelain, cat's claw, celery, coleus, cordyceps, dong quai, evening primrose, fenugreek, feverfew, garlic, ginger, ginseng (American/Panax/Siberian), grape seed, green tea, guggul, horse chestnut seed, horseradish, licorice, prickly ash, red clover, reishi, sweet clover, turmeric, white willow

Decreased effect: Anticonvulsants, fluoxetine (may reverse genital anesthesia and diminished sexual desire induced by drug)

ginkgold *see* Ginkgo Biloba *on page 1429*

Ginkgopowder *see* Ginkgo Biloba *on page 1429*

Ginkogink *see* Ginkgo Biloba *on page 1429*

Ginseng, Panax

Synonyms Asian Ginseng; *Panax ginseng*

Use Adaptogen, adrenal tonic, anticoagulant, cardiotonic, hormone stimulant, immunostimulant; support in chemotherapy and radiation (decreases weight loss), postsurgical recovery (stabilize white blood cell counts), endurance

Local Anesthetic/Vasoconstrictor Precautions Has potential to interact with epinephrine and levonordefrin to result in increased BP; use vasoconstrictor with caution

Effects on Bleeding May have antiplatelet effects

Adverse Reactions

Frequency not defined.

Endocrine & metabolic: Mastalgia (prolonged or high dose)

Genitourinary: Vaginal breakthrough bleeding

Signs/symptoms of Ginseng Abuse Syndrome:

Cardiovascular: Hypertension, palpitations, and tachycardia (in sensitive individuals, after prolonged use, or at high doses)

Central nervous system: Insomnia, nervousness

Dermatologic: Eruptions

Gastrointestinal: Diarrhea

Dosage Oral:

Per Commission E: 1-2 g of dried root or equivalent preparations; for maximum benefit, cycle 4 weeks on, 2 weeks off.

100-600 mg/day in divided doses (standardized to contain a minimum of 5% ginsenosides per dose)

Herbal tea: ~1.75 g; 0.5-2 g/day

Mechanism of Action/Effect Ginsenosides, the active agent, stimulate secretion of adrenocorticotropic hormone (ACTH), leading to production of increased release of adrenal hormones (eg, cortisol) and are believed to act via hormone receptors in the hypothalamus, pituitary glands, and other tissues. Panax ginseng may have CNS stimulant and estrogen-like effect; reported to have immunostimulating effects on the reticuloendothelial system. Diols, specific triterpenoid saponins, contribute to sedative and antihypertensive properties; triols reportedly increase BP and function as CNS stimulants. Low doses increase BP while high doses exhibit a hypotensive effect.

Contraindications Active bleeding (may alter hemostasis), acute infection, lactation, pregnancy, renal failure

Warnings Use with caution in elderly or individuals with cardiovascular disease (eg, hypertension), history of bleeding, hemostatic or drug-related hemostatic disorders, and those receiving anticoagulants (eg, aspirin or aspirin-containing products, NSAIDs, warfarin) or antiplatelet agents (eg, clopidogrel, dipyridamole, ticlopidine), hormonal contraceptives, MAO inhibitors, stimulants (eg, OTC decongestants, caffeine), and those receiving hormonal replacement therapy (HRT). May cause "Ginseng Abuse Syndrome"; monitor for signs/symptoms (see Adverse Reactions). Avoid other herbs with allergenic, anticoagulant/antiplatelet or hypertensive properties (see below). Discontinue at least 14 days prior to dental or surgical procedures.

Potential/Suspected Interactions

Increased effect/toxicity:

Anticoagulant or antiplatelet agents, CNS stimulants, chemotherapy agents, diuretics (eg, furosemide), MAO inhibitors, stimulants (eg, caffeine, decongestants), sympathomimetics

Allergenic herbs: Bittersweet, chamomile, devil's dung, echinacea, feverfew, flaxseed, garlic, gotu kola, male fern, propolis, yucca

Herbs with anticoagulant/antiplatelet properties: Alfalfa, anise, bilberry, bladderwrack, bromelain, cat's claw, celery, coleus, cordyceps, dong quai, evening primrose, fenugreek, feverfew, garlic, ginger, ginkgo biloba, grape seed, green tea, guggul, horse chestnut seed, horseradish, licorice, prickly ash, red clover, reishi, sweet clover, turmeric, white willow

Herbs with hypertensive properties: Bayberry, blue cohosh, cayenne, ephedra, ginger, kola nut (caffeine), licorice

Decreased effect: Antihypertensive agents, cardiac glycosides (eg, digoxin), hormonal contraceptives, and hormone replacement therapy (HRT)

Ginseng, Siberian

Synonyms *Eleutherococcus senticosus*; Siberian Ginseng

Use Adaptogen, anticoagulant, antiviral, immunosupportive; treatment of arteriosclerosis, chronic inflammatory disease, diabetes, hypertension; adaptation to stress, athletic performance enhancement, energy production

Local Anesthetic/Vasoconstrictor Precautions Has potential to interact with epinephrine and levonordefrin to result in increased BP; use vasoconstrictor with caution

Effects on Bleeding May have antiplatelet effects

Adverse Reactions

Frequency not defined.

Endocrine & metabolic: Mastalgia (prolonged or high dose)

Genitourinary: Vaginal breakthrough bleeding

Signs/symptoms of Ginseng Abuse Syndrome:

Cardiovascular: Hypertension, palpitations, and tachycardia (in sensitive individuals, after prolonged use, or at high doses)

Central nervous system: Insomnia, irritability, nervousness

Dermatologic: Eruptions

Gastrointestinal: Diarrhea

Dosage For maximum benefit, cycle 4 weeks on, 2 weeks off.

Oral: 100-200 mg twice daily (standardized to contain 0.8% eleutherosides B and E per dose)

Mechanism of Action/Effect Full mechanism unknown; different from Asian and Panax varieties; similar to Panax in adaptogenic and protective action but without stimulant properties; increases messenger and ribosomal RNA

(Continued)

Ginseng, Siberian *(Continued)*

synthesis, lipolysis, and muscle efficiency while protecting glycogen and creatinine phosphate; reported to increase efficiency of natural killer cells and enhance the body's ability to decrease toxicity of certain drugs and pollutants

Contraindications Active bleeding (may alter hemostasis); high doses during acute phases of infection (especially when high fever is present)

Warnings Use with caution in the elderly or individuals with cardiovascular disease (eg, CHF, hypertension), history of bleeding, hemostatic or drug-related hemostatic disorders, those taking anticoagulants (eg, aspirin or aspirin-containing products, NSAIDs, warfarin) or antiplatelet agents (eg, clopidogrel, dipyridamole, ticlopidine), antihypertensive agents, digoxin, hexobarbital, hypoglycemic agents or insulin, and steroids. Extensive or prolonged use may heighten estrogenic activity. Avoid other herbs with allergenic, anabolic, anticoagulant/antiplatelet, or hypertensive properties (see below). Discontinue at least 14 days prior to dental or surgical procedures.

Potential/Suspected Interactions

Increased effect/toxicity:

Anticoagulant or antiplatelet agents, antihypertensives, barbiturates, digoxin, insulin, oral hypoglycemics, stimulants (eg, OTC decongestants, caffeine)

Allergenic herbs: Bittersweet, chamomile, devil's dung, echinacea, feverfew, flaxseed, garlic, gotu kola, male fern, propolis, yucca

Anabolic herbs: Devil's club, dong quai, ginseng (American/Asian), muira puama, sarsparilla, suma, tribulus, wild yam

Herbs with anticoagulant/antiplatelet properties: Alfalfa, anise, bilberry, bladderwrack, bromelain, cat's claw, celery, coleus, cordyceps, dong quai, evening primrose, fenugreek, feverfew, garlic, ginger, ginkgo biloba, grape seed, green tea, guggul, horse chestnut seed, horseradish, licorice, prickly ash, red clover, reishi, sweet clover, turmeric, white willow

Herbs with hypertensive properties: Bayberry, blue cohosh, cayenne, ephedra, ginger, kola nut (caffeine), licorice

Decreased effect: May shorten duration of certain sedatives

Glucosamine

Synonyms Glucosamine Hydrochloride; Glucosamine Sulfate

Use Treatment of bursitis, gout, osteoarthritis, rheumatoid arthritis, tendonitis

Local Anesthetic/Vasoconstrictor Precautions No information available to require special precautions

Effects on Bleeding None reported

Adverse Reactions Frequency not defined.

Gastrointestinal: Flatulence, nausea

Dosage Oral: 500 mg sulfate 3 times/day

Mechanism of Action/Effect An amino sugar which is a key component in the synthesis of proteoglycans, a group of proteins found in cartilage; these are negatively charged and attract water so they can produce synovial fluid in the joints. The theory is that supplying the body with these precursors replenishes important synovial fluid and lead to production of new cartilage. Glucosamine also appears to inhibit cartilage-destroying enzymes (eg, collagenase and phospholipase A2), thus stopping the degenerative processes of osteoarthritis. A third mechanism may be glucosamine's ability to prevent production of damaging superoxide radicals, which may lead to cartilage destruction.

Warnings Use with caution in diabetics (may cause insulin resistance) and those taking oral anticoagulants (may increase effect). Avoid other herbs with hyperglycemic properties (see Drug Interactions).

Potential/Suspected Interactions Increased effect: Oral anticoagulants, insulin or oral hypoglycemics

Herbs with anticoagulant/antiplatelet properties: Alfalfa, anise, bilberry, bladderwrack, bromelain, cat's claw, celery, coleus, cordyceps, dong quai, evening primrose, fenugreek, feverfew, garlic, ginger, ginkgo biloba, ginseng (American/Panax/Siberian), grape seed, green tea, guggul, horse chestnut seed, horseradish, licorice, prickly ash, red clover, reishi, sweet clover, turmeric, white willow

Herbs with hyperglycemic properties: Elecampane, ginseng (American), gotu kola

Glucosamine Hydrochloride *see* Glucosamine *on page 1432*

Glucosamine Sulfate *see* Glucosamine *on page 1432*

Glutathione

Synonyms L-Glutathione

Use Peptic ulcer diseases; support of immune function; hepatoprotection

Local Anesthetic/Vasoconstrictor Precautions No information available to require special precautions

Effects on Bleeding None reported

Adverse Reactions No known toxicity or serious side effects reported

Dosage Oral: 500-3000 mg/day in divided doses

Mechanism of Action/Effect Glutathione is a tripeptide of three amino acids, cysteine, glycine, and glutamic acid. It also contains sulfur. Glutathione is required for the hepatic detoxication of many compounds via the enzyme glutathione-S-transferase. Compounds which are detoxified include ethanol, cigarette smoke, and overdoses of acetaminophen and aspirin. Glutathione also has antioxidant activity and belongs to an antioxidant enzyme system called glutathione peroxidase. It reduces oxidative damage and free radical damage due to radiation. Glutathione facilitates the function and development of macrophages, lymphocytes, and other immune cells. It is involved in cellular transmembrane amino acid transport systems and in fatty acid synthesis.

Warnings None reported

Potential/Suspected Interactions None known

Glycocome *see* Licorice *on page 1440*

Glycyrrhiza glabra *see* Licorice *on page 1440*

Goatweed *see* St John's Wort *on page 1447*

Golden Seal

Synonyms Eye Balm; Eye Root; *Hydrastis canadensis*; Indian Eye; Jaundice Root; Orange Root; Turmeric Root; Yellow Indian Paint; Yellow Root

Use Antibacterial, antifungal, anti-inflammatory, coagulant; treatment of bronchitis, cystitis, gastritis, infectious diarrhea, inflammation of mucosal membranes, hemorrhoids, postpartum hemorrhage

Local Anesthetic/Vasoconstrictor Precautions No information available to require special precautions

Effects on Bleeding None reported

Adverse Reactions Frequency not defined (high doses).

Cardiovascular: Hyper- or hypotension, myocardial damage

Central nervous system: CNS depression, delirium, hallucinations, hyper-reflexia, stimulation/agitation, seizures

Gastrointestinal: Diarrhea, mouth and throat irritation, nausea, vomiting

Neuromuscular & skeletal: Extremity numbness

Respiratory: Respiratory failure

Dosage Oral: 250 mg 2-4 times/day (standardized to contain 10% alkaloids or 2.5% berberine and 1.5% to 5% hydrastine per dose)

Root: 0.5-1 g 3 times/day

Solid form: 5-10 grains

Mechanism of Action/Effect Contains the alkaloids, hydrastine (4%) and berberine (6%), which at higher doses can cause vasoconstriction, hypertension, and mucosal irritation; berberine can produce hypotension. The primary constituent berberine has antimicrobial activity against a broad array of pathogens including viruses and bacteria. The alkaloids in golden seal have astringent activity which appears to contribute to its anti-inflammatory actions on mucous membranes. Nine active ingredients including berberine were isolated, identified, and tested for antimicrobial activity against oral pathogens. Of these isolates, berberine and two others showed antimicrobial activity when evaluated against the oral pathogens *Streptococcus mutans* and *Fusobacterium nucleatum*. Berberine exhibited additive antimicrobial effect when tested against *S. mutans* in combination with one of the other two isolates.

Contraindications Lactation and pregnancy, hypertension, glaucoma, diabetes, history of stroke, heart disease

Warnings Efficacy not established in clinical studies. High doses (2-3 g) may cause hypotension or GI distress; toxic doses (18 g) reported to induce CNS depression. Overdose associated with myocardial damage and respiratory failure; extended use of high doses associated with delirium, GI disorders, hallucinations, and neuroexcitation. May alter liver enzymes. Use with caution in individuals with history of bleeding, hemostatic or drug-related hemostatic disorders, hypotension, those taking anticoagulants (aspirin or aspirin-containing products, NSAIDs, and warfarin) or antiplatelet agents (ticlopidine, clopidogrel, and dipyridamole). Avoid other herbs with coagulant or hypotensive properties (see below).

Potential/Suspected Interactions

Increased effect/toxicity:

Antihypertensive agents, vasocontrictors

Coagulant herbs: Agrimony, mistletoe, yarrow

Herbs with hypotensive properties: Aconite, arnica, baneberry, black cohosh, bryony, California poppy, choke cherry, coleus, green (false) hellebore,

(Continued)

Golden Seal *(Continued)*

hawthorn, immortal, Indian tobacco, jaborandi, mistletoe, night blooming cereus, pasque flower, pleurisy root, quinine, shepherd's purse

Decreased effect: Vitamin B

Gotu Kola

Synonyms *Centella asiatica*

Use Diuretic (mild), sedative (high doses), thermogenic, thyroid-stimulant, wound-healing agent; treatment of hemorrhoids, hypertension, poor circulation, psoriasis, tumors, varicose veins, venous insufficiency, and wounds from infection, inflammation, trauma, or surgery (scar reduction); memory enhancement; modulation/support of connective tissue synthesis; Ayurvedic medicine uses for revitalizing nerves and brain cells; Eastern healers use for emotional disorders (eg, depression) thought to be rooted in physical problems; alcoholic extract was used to treat leprosy in Western medicine

Local Anesthetic/Vasoconstrictor Precautions No information available to require special precautions

Effects on Bleeding None reported

Adverse Reactions Frequency not defined.

Cardiovascular: Increased heart rate

Central nervous system: Insomnia

Gastrointestinal: Increased peristalsis

Dermatologic: Dermatitis (topical application)

Dosage

Infusion: 600 mg

Oral: 50-250 mg 2-3 times/day (standardized to contain 10% to 30% asiaticosides and 2% to 4% triterpenes per dose)

Topical: Apply a 0.2% to 0.4% preparation to wound areas 2-3 times/day

Mechanism of Action/Effect Extract contains asiaticoside, an active component of *C. asiatica*, in which a trisaccharide moiety is linked to the aglycone asiatic acid; madecassol, the other triterpenoid derivative is used as an ingredient in scar-reducing products. The wound-healing and vascular effects are mostly due to these triterpene saponins and their sapogenins. Many studies found *C. asiatica* acts on certain cells of the epidermis to promote keratinization in areas of infection and stimulates the reticuloendothelial system; reported to increase superoxide dismutase (SOD) and glutathione peroxidase while decreasing lipid peroxide levels. Topical administration improves tissue healing (skin, connective tissue, lymph, and mucous membranes) and may also stabilize connective tissue growth in scleroderma; reportedly stimulates synthesis of hyaluronidase and chondroitin sulfate in connective tissue

Contraindications Pregnancy

Warnings Advise caution when driving or operating machinery; large doses may be sedating. Use with caution in individuals taking sedatives (eg, anxiolytics, benzodiazepines); effects may be additive with other CNS depressants. Topical administration may cause contact dermatitis in sensitive individuals. High or prolonged doses may elevate cholesterol levels. Avoid other allergenic, hyperglycemic, or thyroid-stimulating herbs (see below).

Potential/Suspected Interactions Increased effect/toxicity:

Anxiolytics, other CNS depressants, and sedatives (eg, benzodiazepines)

Allergenic herbs: Bittersweet, chamomile, devil's dung, echinacea, feverfew, flaxseed, garlic, ginseng, male fern, propolis, yucca

Herbs with hyperglycemic properties: Elecampane and ginseng (American)

Thyroid-stimulating herbs: Fu-tse (Fo-tzu), ephedra, mustard, yohimbe

Grapefruit Seed

Synonyms *Citrus paradisi*; GSE

Use Antibiotic, antimycotic, antiparasitic, antiprotozoan, antimicrobial (antibacterial, antifungal, antiviral), disinfectant, immunostimulant; treatment of GI complaints, herpes, various bacterial and fungal infections (eg, *Candida albicans*, *Salmonella*), inflammatory conditions of the gums, parasites; facial cleanser, water disinfectant; used topically for antifungal and antibiotic effects

Local Anesthetic/Vasoconstrictor Precautions No information available to require special precautions

Effects on Bleeding None reported

Dosage Oral:

100 mg 1-3 times/day with food

Drops: 5-10 drops 2-3 times/day

Rinse: 5-10 drops 2-3 times/say; dilute in water, swish, and expectorate

Mechanism of Action/Effect Extract is in a highly acidic liquid rich in polyphenolic compounds (eg, apigenin, campherol glycoside, hesperidin, naringin, neohesperidin, poncirin, rutinoside, quercitin) and seems to exert its antimicrobial activity in the cytoplasmic membrane of bacteria by altering cell membrane with a dose-dependent inhibition of cellular respiration. It is effective against 800 various viruses and species of bacteria and about 100 types of fungi without damaging friendly intestinal bacteria. Its disinfectant effect and lack of bacterial resistance is believed to be due to the flavonoids.

Grapefruit seed extract exerts its antimicrobial activity in the cytoplasmic membrane of bacteria. It causes an alteration of the cell membrane and a dose-dependent inhibition of cellular respiration. Grapefruit seed extract has been shown to have antimicrobial activity *in vitro* against 67 organisms of gram-positive and gram-negative characteristics. It has significant comparative effectivenss against a wide range of bacterial biotypes.

Contraindications Allergy to grapefruit; astemizole, cisapride, and terfenadine

Warnings GSE is not the equivalent of grapefruit juice but since grapefruit juice/pulp has been associated with the inhibition of drug metabolism via cytochrome P450 isoenzyme 3A4 (CYP3A4), resulting in a number of drug interactions, it is reasonable to avoid the concurrent use of grapefruit seed extract in individuals receiving astemizole, cisapride, terfenadine and other medications metabolized by this pathway.

Potential/Suspected Interactions Nonsedating antihistamines, concurrent use of medications metabolized by CYP3A4 (interaction reported with grapefruit juice)

Grape Seed

Synonyms *Vitis vinifera*

Use Anticoagulant/antiplatelet, anti-inflammatory, antioxidant (potent), and source of potent free radical scavengers; treatment of allergies and asthma, arterial/venous insufficiency (capillary fragility, intermittent claudication, poor circulation, varicose veins); improves peripheral circulation; treatment of gingivitis

Local Anesthetic/Vasoconstrictor Precautions No information available to require special precautions

Effects on Bleeding May see increase in bleeding due to inhibition of platelet aggregation

Dosage Oral: 25-100 mg 1-3 times/day (standardized to contain 40% to 80% proanthocyanidins or 95% polyphenols or a procyanidolic value >95% per dose)

Mechanism of Action/Effect Contains proanthocyanidins reported to neutralize many free radicals, including hydroxyl, lipid peroxides, and iron-induced lipid peroxidation; antioxidant properties are believed to block lipid peroxidation, which stabilizes cell membranes. Proanthocyanidins inhibit destruction of collagen (possibly by stabilizing 1-antitrypsin), which inhibits destructive enzymes such as elastin and hyaluronic acid. Stabilization of collagen allows red blood cells to traverse the capillaries and prevent fluid exudation. Scientific studies have confirmed that the antioxidant power of proanthocyanidins from grape seed are 20 times greater than vitamin E and 50 times greater than vitamin C. Anti-inflammatory activity is due to inhibition of mediators, such as histamine and prostaglandins.

Contraindications Active bleeding; may inhibit platelet aggregation. use with caution in individuals with drug-related hemostatic problems, hemostatic disorders, or history of bleeding, and individuals taking anticoagulants including aspirin, aspirin-containing products, NSAIDs, warfarin, or antiplatelet agents (eg, clopidogrel, dipyridamole, ticlopidine). Discontinue use at least 14 days before dental or surgical procedures.

Warnings Use with caution in individuals with history of bleeding, hemostatic or drug-related hemostatic problems, those taking anticoagulants (eg, aspirin or aspirin-containing products, NSAIDs, warfarin) or antiplatelet agents (eg, clopidogrel, dipyridamole, ticlopidine). Avoid other herbs with anticoagulant/antiplatelet properties (see below). May alter absorption of calcium, copper, magnesium, and zinc due to tannins. Discontinue use at least 14 days before dental or surgical procedures.

Potential/Suspected Interactions Increased effect/toxicity:

Anticoagulant or antiplatelet agents, xanthine oxidase inhibitors (*in vitro* studies indicate may increase toxicity of methotrexate)

Herbs with anticoagulant/antiplatelet properties: Alfalfa, anise, bilberry, bladderwrack, bromelain, cat's claw, celery, coleus, cordyceps, dong quai, evening primrose, fenugreek, feverfew, garlic, ginger, ginkgo biloba, ginseng (American/Panax/Siberian), grape seed, green tea, guggul, horse chestnut seed, horseradish, licorice, prickly ash, red clover, reishi, sweet clover, turmeric, white willow

Grape Skin

Synonyms Resveratrol

Use Antioxidant; cardioprotectant; antiplatelet

Local Anesthetic/Vasoconstrictor Precautions No information available to require special precautions

Effects on Bleeding May see increased bleeding due to inhibition of platelet aggregation

Adverse Reactions No known toxicity or serious side effects reported

Mechanism of Action/Effect The antioxidant substances in grape skin extract are identified as proanthocyanidin (PAC) polyphenolic compounds, and minor constituent phenolic compounds. Epidemiological studies suggest that consumption of red wine reduces mortality and morbidity from coronary heart disease. The cardioprotective effect has been attributed to antioxidants present in the polyphenol fraction of red wine. Grapes contain a variety of antioxidants, including resveratrol, catechin, epicatechin, and proanthocyanidins. Of these, resveratrol is present mainly in grape skins. This report provides evidence that red wine extract as well as resveratrol and proanthocyanidins are effective antioxidants and play a role, amoung other roles, in cardioprotection.

Warnings None reported

Potential/Suspected Interactions None known

Green Tea

Synonyms *Camellia sinensis*

Use Antibacterial, anticarcinogen, antioxidant, astringent, anticoagulant/antiplatelet, antifungal, antiviral, diuretic, immunosupportive; prophylaxis and treatment of cancer, cardiovascular disease, hypercholesterolemia

Local Anesthetic/Vasoconstrictor Precautions No information available to require special precautions

Effects on Bleeding May see increased bleeding due to inhibition of platelet aggregation

Adverse Reactions Frequency not defined (refers to caffeinated products).

Cardiovascular: Palpitations, tachycardia

Central nervous system: Insomnia, nervousness

Gastrointestinal: Decreased appetite, gastric irritation

Dosage Recommend decaffeinated products; there are more drug interactions with high doses of caffeine-containing products.

Oral: 250-500 mg/day (standardize to contain 50% to 97% polyphenols per dose, providing ≥50% epigallocatechin-3-gallate)

Mechanism of Action/Effect Reportedly protects against oxidative damage to cells and tissues; demonstrated to increase HDL cholesterol, decrease LDL cholesterol and triglycerides, block peroxidation of LDL, inhibit formation of thromboxane formation, and block platelet aggregation; human studies have noted improvement in prognosis of some forms of breast cancer; inhibits the growth of many types of human cancer cells in tissue culture; this property has been attributed to its antioxidant components known as green tea polyphenols; green tea polyphenols are claimed to have antimutagenic, anticarcinogenic, and antioxidant effects; one component of green tea, epigallocatechin gallate (EGCG) has been reported to inhibit the growth of cancer cells and metastasis

Contraindications Active bleeding (eg, peptic ulcer, intracerebral bleeding)

Warnings Use caffeinated products with caution in individuals with cardiovascular disease, peptic ulcer, and those taking other stimulants (eg, decongestants). Use with caution in individuals with a history of bleeding, hemostatic or drug-related hemostatic disorders, those taking anticoagulants (aspirin or aspirin-containing products, NSAIDs, warfarin) or antiplatelet agents (eg, ticlopidine, clopidogrel, dipyridamole). Addition of milk to any tea may significantly lower antioxidant potential. May alter absorption of calcium, copper, magnesium, and zinc due to tannins. Avoid other herbs with anticoagulant/antiplatelet properties (see below). Discontinue at least 14 days prior to dental or surgical procedures.

Potential/Suspected Interactions Increased effect/toxicity:

Anticoagulant or antiplatelet agents, theophylline; reported to enhance doxorubicin's inhibitory effects on tumor growth

Drugs which interact with high doses of caffeine-containing green tea products: Acid and MAO inhibitors, anticoagulant or antiplatelet agents, barbiturates, beta blockers, CNS stimulants, fluconazole, hormonal contraceptives or hormone replacement therapy, phenobarbital, phenytoin, quinidine, quinolones, sympathomimetics, theophylline, sedatives, verapamil

Herbs with anticoagulant/antiplatelet properties: Alfalfa, anise, bilberry, bladderwrack, bromelain, cat's claw, celery, coleus, cordyceps, dong quai, evening primrose, fenugreek, feverfew, garlic, ginger, ginkgo biloba, ginseng (American/Panax/Siberian), grape seed, green tea, guggul, horse chestnut seed, horseradish, licorice, prickly ash, red clover, reishi, sweet clover, turmeric, white willow

GSE *see* Grapefruit Seed *on page 1434*

Harpagophytum procumbens *see* Devil's Claw *on page 1422*

Haw *see* Hawthorn *on page 1437*

Hawthorn

Synonyms *Crataegus laevigata*; *Crataegus monogyna*; *Crataegus oxyacantha*; *Crataegus pinnatifida*; English Hawthorn; Haw; Maybush; Whitehorn

Use Cardiotonic, sedative, vasodilator; treatment of cardiovascular abnormalities (eg, arrhythmia, angina, CHF, hyper- or hypotension, peripheral vascular diseases, tachycardia); used synergistically with digoxin (Europe)

Local Anesthetic/Vasoconstrictor Precautions No information available to require special precautions

Effects on Bleeding None reported

Adverse Reactions Frequency not defined:

Cardiovascular: Bradycardia, hyper- or hypotension
Central nervous system: Depression, fatigue
Dermatologic: Rash
Gastrointestinal: Nausea

Dosage Oral: 250 mg 1-3 times/day (standardized to contain ≥2% vitexin-2-O-rhamnoside or minimum of 10% to 20% procyanidins per dose)

Per Commission E: 160-900 mg native water-ethanol extract (ethanol 45% v/v or methanol 70% v/v, drug-extract ratio: 4-7:1, with defined flavonoid or procyanidin content), corresponding to 30-168.7 mg procyanidins, calculated as epicatechin, or 3.5-19.8 mg flavonoids, calculated as hyperoside in accordance with DAB 10 [German pharmacopoeia #10] in 2 or 3 individual doses; duration of administration: 6 weeks minimum

Mechanism of Action/Effect Contains catechin, epicatechin, and flavonoids, which may be cardioprotective and have vasodilatory properties; dilates coronary vessels

Contraindications Lactation and pregnancy

Warnings Use with caution in individuals taking ACE inhibitors and antihypertensive agents (may lower BP further). Avoid other herbs with hypotensive properties (see below).

Potential/Suspected Interactions Increased effect:

ACE inhibitors, antiarrhythmics, antihypertensives, cardiac glycosides (eg, digoxin)

Herbs with hypotensive properties: Aconite, arnica, baneberry, black cohosh, bryony, California poppy, choke cherry, coleus, golden seal, green (false) hellebore, immortal, Indian tobacco, jaborandi, mistletoe, night blooming cereus, pasque flower, pleurisy root, quinine, shepherd's purse

Horse Chestnut

Synonyms *Aesculus hippocastanum*

Use Analgesic, anticoagulant/antiplatelet, anti-inflammatory, cardiotonic, sedative, wound-healing agent; treatment of varicose veins, hemorrhoids, other venous insufficiencies, deep vein thrombosis, lower extremity edema

Local Anesthetic/Vasoconstrictor Precautions No information available to require special precautions

Effects on Bleeding Inhibits platelet aggregation; may see increased bleeding

Adverse Reactions

Frequency not defined.
Cardiovascular: Vasodilation, decreased heart rate
Gastrointestinal: Increased peristalsis, dyspepsia
Respiratory: Bronchial constriction

High dose:
Cardiovascular: Flushing, hypotension
Central nervous system: Headache
Ocular: Decreased visual acuity
Respiratory: Asthmatic attack
Miscellaneous: Sweating

Dosage

Oral: 300 mg 1-2 times/day (standardized to contain 50 mg escin per dose)
Topical: Apply 2% escin gel 1-2 times/day to affected area

Mechanism of Action/Effect Contains flavonoids, sterols, tannins, saponin, and escin (seed) which promotes circulation in the veins; reported to support collagen structures; anti-inflammatory activity may be related to quercetin's

(Continued)

Horse Chestnut *(Continued)*

reported ability to inhibit cyclo-oxygenase and lipoxygenase, enzymes which form inflammatory prostaglandins and leukotrienes. Quercetin is also an inhibitor of phosphodiesterase; correlated with cardiotonic, hypotensive, spasmolytic, and sedative actions.

Contraindications Active bleeding (eg, intracranial bleeding, peptic ulcer), asthma, bethanechol, carbachol, coronary insufficiency, hyperthyroidism, lactation, metoclopramide, pilocarpine, pregnancy

Warnings Use with caution in individuals with a history of bleeding, hemostatic or drug-related hemostatic disorders, hepatic or renal impairment, and those taking anticoagulants (eg, aspirin or aspirin-containing products, NSAIDs, warfarin) or antiplatelets (eg, clopidogrel, dipyridamole, ticlopidine). Avoid other herbs with anticoagulant/antiplatelet or parasympathomimetic properties (see below). May alter GI absorption of other herbs, minerals, or drugs (especially calcium, copper, magnesium, and zinc) due to tannins. Discontinue at least 14 days prior to dental or surgical procedures.

Potential/Suspected Interactions Increased effect/toxicity:

Anticoagulant or antiplatelet

Herbs with anticoagulant/antiplatelet properties: Alfalfa, anise, bilberry, bladderwrack, bromelain, cat's claw, celery, coleus, cordyceps, dong quai, evening primrose, fenugreek, feverfew, garlic, ginger, ginkgo biloba, ginseng (American/Panax/Siberian), grape seed, green tea, guggul, horseradish, licorice, prickly ash, red clover, reishi, sweet clover, turmeric, white willow

Herbs with parasympathomimetic properties: Bittersweet, blood root, blue flag, bryony, dogbane, dogwood, false/green hellebore, huperzineA, immortal, jaborandi, leptandra, pasque flower, pink root, pleurisy root, pokeweed, senega snakeroot, wahoo, yohimbe

Huperzia serrata *see* HuperzineA *on page 1438*

HuperzineA

Synonyms *Huperzia serrata*

Use Acetylcholinesterase inhibitor; treatment of senile dementia and Alzheimer's disease

Local Anesthetic/Vasoconstrictor Precautions No information available to require special precautions

Effects on Bleeding None reported

Adverse Reactions

Frequency not defined.

- Cardiovascular: Vasodilation, decreased heart rate
- Gastrointestinal: Increased peristalsis, dyspepsia
- Respiratory: Bronchial constriction

High dose:

- Cardiovascular: Flushing, hypotension
- Central nervous system: Headache
- Ocular: Decreased visual acuity
- Respiratory: Asthmatic attack
- Miscellaneous: Sweating

Dosage Oral: 50 mcg 1-3 times/day

Mechanism of Action/Effect Purified huperzineA keeps AChE from breaking down into acetylcholine.

Contraindications Active bleeding (eg, intracranial bleeding, peptic ulcer), asthma, bethanechol, carbachol, coronary insufficiency, hyperthyroidism, metoclopramide, pilocarpine

Warnings Use with caution in individuals taking AChE inhibitors (eg, donepezil or tacrine). Avoid cholinergic drugs and other herbs with parasympathomimetic properties (see below).

Potential/Suspected Interactions Increased effect/toxicity:

Acetylcholinesterase inhibitors (donepezil, tacrine)

Herbs with parasympathomimetic properties: Bittersweet, blood root, blue flag, bryony, dogbane, dogwood, false/green hellebore, horse chestnut, immortal, jaborandi, leptandra, pasque flower, pink root, pleurisy root, pokeweed, senega snakeroot, wahoo, yohimbe

Hydrastis canadensis *see* Golden Seal *on page 1433*

Hypercium perforatum *see* St John's Wort *on page 1447*

Indian Eye *see* Golden Seal *on page 1433*

Indian Head *see Echinacea on page 1423*

Isoflavones *see* Soy Isoflavones *on page 1447*

Jaundice Root *see* Golden Seal *on page 1433*

Johimbe *see* Yohimbe *on page 1451*

Kava

Synonyms Awa; Kava Kava; Kew; *Piper methysticum*; Tonga

Use Anxiolytic, diuretic, sedative; treatment of insomnia, nervous anxiety, postischemic episodes, stress; skeletal muscle relaxation

Local Anesthetic/Vasoconstrictor Precautions No information available to require special precautions

Effects on Bleeding None reported

Adverse Reactions Frequency not defined.

Central nervous system: Depression (prolonged use), euphoria, somnolence

Neuromuscular & skeletal: Muscle weakness

Dermatologic: Allergic skin reactions (rare); temporary discoloration of hair, nails, and skin

Ocular: Visual disturbances (pupil enlargement and oculomotor equilibrium disturbance reported)

Dosage

Oral: 100-250 mg 1-3 times/day (standardized to contain 60-120 kavalactones per dose)

Per Commission E: Herb and preparations equivalent to 60-120 mg kavalactones

Mechanism of Action/Effect Extract contains alpha-pyrones and may possess central dopaminergic antagonistic properties.

Contraindications Parkinson's disease (reported to cause dopamine antagonism)

Per Commission E: Endogenous depression and pregnancy

Warnings The FDA Center for Food Safety and Applied Nutrition (CFSAN) notified healthcare professionals and consumers of the potential risk of severe liver associated with the use of kava-containing dietary supplements. Recently, more than 20 cases of hepatitis, cirrhosis, and liver failure have been reported in Europe, with at least one individual requiring a liver transplant. Given these reports, individuals with hepatic impairment or those taking drugs which can affect the liver, should consult a physician before using supplements containing kava. Physicians are urged to closely evaluate these individuals for potential liver complications. Discontinue if yellow discoloration of skin, hair, or nails occurs (temporary; caused by extended continuous use). Accommodative disturbances (eg, enlargement of the pupils and disturbances of the oculomotor equilibrium) have been described.

Use with caution in individuals taking antianxiety or antidepressant agents, diuretics, hypnotic or sedative agents, alprazolam, or alcohol. May cause sedation; advise caution when driving or operating heavy machinery. Long-term use has resulted in rash. Avoid other herbs with diuretic properties (see below). Discontinue if depression occurs (per Commission E, should not be used >3 months without medical supervision).

Potential/Suspected Interactions Increased effect/toxicity:

Alprazolam (coma), barbiturates, CNS depressants, diuretics, psychopharmacological agents

Herbs with diuretic properties: Artichoke, celery seed, corn silk, couchgrass, dandelion, elder flower, horsetail, juniper berry, shepherd's purse, uva ursi, yarrow

Kava Kava *see* Kava *on page 1439*

Kaveri *see* Ginkgo Biloba *on page 1429*

Kew *see* Kava *on page 1439*

Kew Tree *see* Ginkgo Biloba *on page 1429*

Klamath Weed *see* St John's Wort *on page 1447*

Lakriment Neu *see* Licorice *on page 1440*

Laurus Sassafras *see* Sassafras Oil *on page 1445*

L-Carnitine *see* Carnitine *on page 1417*

Lemon Balm/Melissa

Synonyms *Melissa officinalis*

Use Antiviral (oral herpes virus)

Local Anesthetic/Vasoconstrictor Precautions No information available to require special precautions

Effects on Bleeding None reported

Adverse Reactions No known toxicity or side effects reported

Dosage Topical: Apply a concentrated product (70:1 w/v) to affected area 2-4 times/day at prodrome (first sign) of cold sore or fever blister

Mechanism of Action/Effect Melissa has been reported to be an effective antioxidant against selective oxidants which could damage oral tissues. The (Continued)

Lemon Balm/Melissa *(Continued)*

active ingredients in Melissa have been identified and there are at least six "flavonoids" which seem to have antibacterial and antiviral activity.

Warnings None reported

Potential/Suspected Interactions None known

L-Glutathione *see* Glutathione *on page 1432*

Licorice

Synonyms Glycocome; Glycyrrhiza glabra; Lakriment Neu; Liquorice; Sweet Root; Ulgastrin Neo

Use Adaptogen, adrenocorticotropic, antidote, anti-inflammatory, antimicrobial (antibacterial, antifungal, antiviral), antioxidant, antispasmodic, antitussive, detoxification agent, emollient, emmenagogue (high doses), expectorant, immunostimulant, laxative (mild), phytoestrogenic; treatment of abdominal pain, Addison's disease, adrenal insufficiency, age spots, arthritis, asthma, atherosclerosis, benign prostatic hyperplasia (BPH), bronchitis, burns, cancer, candidiasis, carbuncle, chronic gastritis, circulatory disorders, colic, colitis, cold/flu, constipation, contact dermatitis, cough, debility, diabetes, diphtheria, diverticulosis, dizziness, dropsy, duodenal ulcer, dyspepsia, excessive thirst, fever, gastric ulcer, gastritis, hay fever, heart palpitation, heartburn, hemorrhoids, hypercholesterolemia, hyperglycemia, hypotension, inflammation, irritable bowel syndrome (IBS), laryngitis, liver disorders, malaria, menopausal symptoms, menstrual cramps, nausea, peptic ulcer, poisoning (eg, ethanol, atropine, chloral hydrate, cocaine, snakebite), pharyngitis, polyuria, rheumatism, rash, sore throat, stress, tetanus, vertigo; adjunct in long-term cortisone treatment

Per Commission E: GI ulceration, upper/lower respiratory tract infections; foodstuff in candy, chewing gum, chewing tobacco, and cough preparations

Local Anesthetic/Vasoconstrictor Precautions No information available to require special precautions

Effects on Bleeding None reported

Adverse Reactions Frequency not defined.

Cardiovascular: Edema, hypertension

Central nervous system: Headache, seizures, tetany

Endocrine & metabolic: Amenorrhea, distal sodium reabsorption, hypokalemia, hypomagnesemia, hyponatremia, potassium loss

Gastrointestinal: Intestinal dilatation (ileus)

Neuromuscular & skeletal: Carpopedal spasms, myopathy, rhabdomyolysis

Ocular: Bilateral ptosis

Renal: Myoglobinuria

Dosage Oral: <250-500 mg 3 times/day (standardized to contain 20% glycyrrhizinic acid per dose)

Liquid extract (dried root): 15-30 drops 3 times/day in juice

Deglycyrrhizinated licorice: Chew 250 mg 3 times/day (standardized to contain ≤2% glycyrrhizin per dose) 1 hour before or 2 hours after meals and at bedtime

Candy twists (2-4) contain 100 g licorice (equivalent to 700 mg of glycyrrhizinic acid); Toxic: 2-3 twists/day for 2-4 weeks

Catarrhs of upper respiratory tract (per Commission E): 5-15 g root/day (equivalent to 200-600 mg glycyrrhizin) or 0.5-1 g juice

Gastric/duodenal ulcers: 1.5-3 g juice

Mechanism of Action/Effect Reportedly inhibits adrenal and thymic atrophy in addition to leukotriene and prostaglandin synthesis; reported to have demulcent and weak phytoestrogenic activity; stimulates the adrenocortical axis and production of mucus, which may cause symptomatic improvements

Contraindications Cardiovascular disease (eg, arrhythmias, hypertension), diuretics, edema, hepatic or renal disorders, hypernatremia, hypokalemia, lactation, laxatives, nausea or vomiting, obesity (due to possible mineralocorticoid effects from glycyrrhizin content), penicillin, renal impairment; Per Commission E: Hypertonia and pregnancy

Warnings Use caution in diabetics, individuals with plant allergies, hypertension, and those taking antihypertensive agents, cardiac glycosides, corticosteroids, diuretics, hormonal contraceptives, laxatives, nitrofurantoin, or receiving hormone replacement therapy (HRT). Avoid other herbs that may be aldosterone synergistic (eg, horehound), hypertensive, or phytoestrogenic (see below).

Potential/Suspected Interactions

Increased effect/toxicity:

Cortisol half-life and progesterone; concomitant use of furosemide can exacerbate hypokalemia; licorice can antagonize the effects of spironolactone

Per Commission E: At daily dosages of glycyrrhizin >100 mg: Potassium loss due to other drugs (eg, thiazide diuretics) can be increased causing increased sensitivity to digitalis glycosides

On prolonged use and with higher doses, mineral corticoid effects may occur in the form of sodium and water retention; in potassium loss, accompanied by edema, hypertension, and hypokalemia; in rare cases, myoglobinuria

Herbs with anticoagulant/antiplatelet properties: Alfalfa, anise, bilberry, bladderwrack, bromelain, cat's claw, celery, coleus, cordyceps, dong quai, evening primrose, fenugreek, feverfew, garlic, ginger, ginkgo biloba, ginseng (American/Panax/Siberian), grape seed, green tea, guggul, horse chestnut seed, horseradish, prickly ash, red clover, reishi, sweet clover, turmeric, white willow

Herbs with hypertensive properties: Bayberry, blue cohosh, cayenne, ephedra, ginger, ginseng (American), kola nut (caffeine)

Phytoestrogenic herbs: Alfalfa, black cohosh, blood root, hops, kudzu, pomegranate, red clover, soybean, thyme, yucca

Decreased effect: Barbiturates, cocaine, ephedrine, epinephrine, nicotine, pilocarpine, strychnine, tetrodoxine, and urethane through glucuronic-like conjugation action

Lipoic Acid *see* Alpha-Lipoic Acid *on page 1413*

Liquorice *see* Licorice *on page 1440*

Lutein

Use Antioxidant; treatment of cataracts and macular degeneration

Local Anesthetic/Vasoconstrictor Precautions No information available to require special precautions

Effects on Bleeding None reported

Dosage Oral: 2-6 mg/day

Mechanism of Action/Effect A carotenoid present in high concentrations in the central portion of the macula, a highly sensitive area of the retina; within the eye, this pigment filters out blue light and has been claimed to prevent macular degeneration. It protects the visual structures from oxygen free radicals and singlet oxygen, strengthens capillaries, and protects the vessels responsible for nutrient supply to this region

Lycopene

Use Treatment of atherosclerosis, macular degeneration; prevention of cancer (especially prostate)

Local Anesthetic/Vasoconstrictor Precautions No information available to require special precautions

Effects on Bleeding None reported

Dosage Oral: 5 mg 1-3 times/day

Mechanism of Action/Effect A carotenoid which function as natural pigment and antioxidant; supplementation reported to protect against macular degeneration, atherosclerosis, and several types of cancer (eg, prostate cancer); functions as a free radical scavenger which may prevent oxidative damage to subcellular components, protecting from degenerative changes and carcinogenesis

Maidenhair Tree *see* Ginkgo Biloba *on page 1429*

Mastic

Synonyms *Pistacia lentiscus*

Use Antibacterial; treatment of dyspepsia, gastric and duodenal ulcers, halitosis

Local Anesthetic/Vasoconstrictor Precautions No information available to require special precautions

Effects on Bleeding None reported

Dosage Oral: 1000-3000 mg/day in divided doses

Mechanism of Action/Effect Exact mechanism unknown; extract reduces stomach secretions and damage to stomach lining; reported to kill *H. pylori* bacteria, possibly by altering its structure and making it more susceptible to the immune system

Matricaria chamomilla *see* Chamomile *on page 1419*

Matricaria recutita *see* Chamomile *on page 1419*

Maybush *see* Hawthorn *on page 1437*

Melaleuca alternifolia *see* Melaleuca Oil *on page 1442*

Melaleuca Oil

Synonyms *Melaleuca alternifolia*; Tea Tree Oil

Use Analgesic, anti-inflammatory, antibacterial, antifungal, antiseptic, antiviral, disinfectant, immunosupportive, wound-healing agent; treatment of acne, allergy and cold symptoms, minor bruises/burns/cuts, dental plaque, gum inflammation, insect bites, eczema and psoriasis, fungal infections (eg, athlete's foot, oral thrush), hair lice, herpes, muscle pain, respiratory tract infections (eg, bronchitis), toothache, warts; aromatherapy, facial skin toner, household disinfectant (to remove dust mites and lice from laundry), insect repellent, massage oil

Local Anesthetic/Vasoconstrictor Precautions No information available to require special precautions

Effects on Bleeding None reported

Adverse Reactions Frequency not defined.

Central nervous system: CNS depression

Dermatologic: Rash (rare)

Dosage Essential oil should be standardized to contain at least 30% terpinen 4-0l and 15% cineole.

Household disinfectant: 1% solution in laundry water

Inhalant (decongestant, facial toner): Up to 8 drops to be inhaled on handkerchief or pillow case or 5 drops in steaming water

Topical:

- Children: Toxic ≤5 mL
- Adults: <10 mL
  - Eczema and psoriasis: 10 drops in hot bath water
  - Oral rinse: Up to 10 drops in warm water
  - Massage oil: Diluted in carrier oil 1:40 (about 8 drops per tablespoon or 50 drops per 100 mL)
  - Minor skin irritations: 1 drop undiluted oil applied directly to problem area

Mechanism of Action/Effect Unclear; a complex chemical substance consisting of approximately 50 compounds; it is the strongest natural antiseptic, 4-5 times more potent than household disinfectants but can be used daily without damage to surrounding skin; consists of plant terpenes, pinenes, and cineole

Contraindications Oral ingestion; undiluted oil on infants <1 year of age or during pregnancy

Warnings Contains cineole; may cause rash in sensitive individuals if applied directly to skin undiluted. Store in dark glass bottle; may react badly with some polymer plastics.

Melatonin

Use Antioxidant; treatment of sleep disorders (eg, jet lag, insomnia, neurologic problems, shift work), aging, cancer; supports immune system

Local Anesthetic/Vasoconstrictor Precautions No information available to require special precautions

Effects on Bleeding None reported

Adverse Reactions Frequency not defined.

Central nervous system: Drowsiness, fatigue, headache, irritability, sedation

Dosage Sleep disturbances: Oral: 0.3-5 mg/day; to be taken in the evening

Mechanism of Action/Effect Hormone responsible for regulating the body's circadian rhythm and sleep patterns; receptors are found in blood cells, brain, gut, and ovaries. Release is prompted by darkness and inhibited by light. Secretion appears to peak during childhood, and declines gradually through adolescence and adulthood. Antioxidant properties may also assist in regulating cardiovascular and reproductive function.

Contraindications Immune disorders, lactation, pregnancy

Warnings Avoid agents that may cause additional CNS depression (see below).

Potential/Suspected Interactions Increased effect/toxicity:

Hypnotics, sedatives, or other drugs that induce drowsiness (eg, benzodiazepines, narcotics); CNS depressants (prescription, supplements such as 5-HTP)

Herbs with sedative properties: Gotu kola, kava, SAMe, St John's wort, and valerian

Melissa officinalis *see* Lemon Balm/Melissa *on page 1439*

Methyl Sulfonyl Methane

Synonyms Dimethyl Sulfone; $DMSO_2$; MSM

Use Analgesic, anti-inflammatory; treatment of interstitial cystitis, lupus, and osteoarthritis

Local Anesthetic/Vasoconstrictor Precautions No information available to require special precautions

Effects on Bleeding None reported

Dosage Oral: 2000-6000 mg/day

Mechanism of Action/Effect Source of biological sulfur, derived from dimethyl sulfoxide (DMSO); roughly 15% of DMSO is converted metabolically to dimethyl sulfone ($DMSO_2$), another name for MSM. It is an important component of connective tissues, enzymes, hormones, proteins and is required for hepatic detoxification. Pain relief may be due to inhibition of pain impulses along type C nerve fibers, increased blood flow, and reduced muscular spasm.

Milk Thistle

Synonyms *Silybum marianum*

Use Antidote (Death Cap mushroom), antioxidant (hepatoprotective, including drug toxicities); treatment of acute/chronic hepatitis, jaundice, and stimulation of bile secretion/cholagogue

Local Anesthetic/Vasoconstrictor Precautions No information available to require special precautions

Effects on Bleeding None reported

Dosage Oral: 80-120 mg 1-3 times/day (standardized to contain 80% silymarin per dose)

Mechanism of Action/Effect Reported to inhibit inflammatory effects of leukotrienes which could contribute to hepatic damage and be hepatoprotective against acetaminophen, ethanol, psychotropics (eg, butyrophenones, phenothiazines), and other drugs that modify hepatic function. Activity is derived from silymarin, which is composed of three primary flavonoids (silybin, silydianin, and silychristin); silymarin reportedly alters the composition of hepatocytes, limiting entry of hepatotoxins. Silymarin stimulates hepatic regeneration, protein synthesis and increases hepatic glutathione by over 35%. Glutathione is an important antioxidant in detoxification reactions, acting as an important sulfhydryl donor in detoxification reactions.

Milk Vetch *see* Astragalus *on page 1414*

Monascus purpureus *see* Red Yeast Rice *on page 1444*

MSM *see* Methyl Sulfonyl Methane *on page 1442*

NADH *see* Nicotinamide Adenine Dinucleotide *on page 1443*

Nectar of the Gods *see* Garlic *on page 1428*

Nicotinamide Adenine Dinucleotide

Synonyms Coenzyme 1; NADH

Use Treatment of chronic fatigue, Parkinson's disease; increases stamina and energy

Local Anesthetic/Vasoconstrictor Precautions No information available to require special precautions

Effects on Bleeding None reported

Dosage Oral: 2.5-5 mg 1-4 times/day

Mechanism of Action/Effect An essential coenzyme in the production of energy in the mitochondria; facilitates DNA-repair mechanisms and stimulates the production of adrenaline and dopamine

Nosebleed *see* Feverfew *on page 1426*

Oenothera biennis *see* Evening Primrose *on page 1425*

Orange Root *see* Golden Seal *on page 1433*

Oriental Plum Tree *see* Ginkgo Biloba *on page 1429*

Palmetto Scrub *see* Saw Palmetto *on page 1446*

Panax ginseng *see* Ginseng, Panax *on page 1430*

Parsley

Synonyms *Petroselinum crispum*

Use Halitosis; antibacterial, antifungal

Local Anesthetic/Vasoconstrictor Precautions No information available to require special precautions

Effects on Bleeding None reported

Adverse Reactions No known toxicity or side effects reported

Dosage Oral: Dilute a few drops of oil in a cup of water; gargle and expectorate

Mechanism of Action/Effect Parsley's antibacterial and antifungal activity are attributed to its volatile oils. Usage in halitosis is also attributed to its volatile oil component. Volatile sulfur compounds which contribute to halitosis were effectively captured by parsley. It is proposed that deodorization of volatile sulfur compounds by herbs such as parsley is due to enzymatic degradation of disulfides catalyzed by polyphenol oxidases and peroxidases.

(Continued)

Parsley *(Continued)*

Warnings None reported

Potential/Suspected Interactions None known

***Passiflora* spp** *see* Passion Flower *on page 1444*

Passion Flower

Synonyms *Passiflora* spp

Use Sedative

Local Anesthetic/Vasoconstrictor Precautions No information available to require special precautions

Effects on Bleeding None reported

Dosage Oral (standardized to contain 3.5% isovitexin per dose):

Anxiety: 100 mg 2-3 times/day

Insomnia: 200 mg at bedtime

Mechanism of Action/Effect The constituents, maltol and ethylmaltol, have been shown to produce CNS sedation and reduce spontaneous motor activity (low doses) in laboratory animals. In humans, it may be effective combined with other sedative and antianxiety herbs, such as valerian. These effects may be due to synergism or the potential binding of passion flower constituents to benzodiazepine receptors *in vivo.*

Warnings Advise caution when driving or operating heavy machinery. Use with caution in individuals taking antianxiety agents or antidepressants and other sedatives; reported in animal studies to increase sleeping time induced by hexobarbital.

Potential/Suspected Interactions Increased effect/toxicity:

Antidepressants, anxiolytics, barbiturates, sedatives

Herbs with sedative properties: Gotu kola, kava, SAMe, St John's wort, and valerian

Pausinystalia yohimbe *see* Yohimbe *on page 1451*

Petroselinum crispum *see* Parsley *on page 1443*

Piper methysticum *see* Kava *on page 1439*

Pistacia lentiscus *see* Mastic *on page 1441*

Poor Mans Treacle *see* Garlic *on page 1428*

Purple Coneflower *see Echinacea on page 1423*

Quercetin

Use Antioxidant

Local Anesthetic/Vasoconstrictor Precautions No information available to require special precautions

Effects on Bleeding None reported

Adverse Reactions No known toxicity or side effects reported

Dosage Oral: 300-500 mg 1-3 times daily

Mechanism of Action/Effect Quercetin is an herbal antioxidant in contrast to the nutrient antioxidants such as vitamin C and vitamin E. Quercetin has been reported to strengthen capillaries and regulate the capillary permeability of biochemical nutrients. Quercetin, through its antioxidant effects, prevents the cytotoxicity of certain forms of low density lipoprotein.

Warnings None reported

Potential/Suspected Interactions None known

Radix *see* Valerian *on page 1449*

Red Valerian *see* Valerian *on page 1449*

Red Yeast Rice

Synonyms *Monascus purpureus*

Use Antibiotic, anti-inflammatory, antioxidant, HMG-CoA reductase inhibitor; treatment of hypercholesterolemia, hypertension, hypertriglyceridemia

Local Anesthetic/Vasoconstrictor Precautions No information available to require special precautions

Effects on Bleeding None reported

Adverse Reactions Frequency not defined.

Gastrointestinal: GI upset

Dosage Oral: 1200 mg twice daily (standardized to 0.4% total HMG-CoA reductase inhibitors per dose)

Mechanism of Action/Effect Special form of vitamin E; contains eight compounds with HMG-CoA reductase inhibitory activity; some forms contain large amounts of monacolin K, a natural substance closely related to lovastatin but not identical. Red yeast rice contains additional food-derived accessory factors and seems to be more effective than isolated, purified lovastatin.

Contraindications Active bleeding (eg, intracranial bleeding, peptic ulcer), alcoholics (>1-2 drinks/day), children and individuals <20 years of age, history or risk of hepatic disease, hypersensitivity to rice or yeast, lactation and pregnancy (or if trying to become pregnant), organ transplant recipients, recent major surgery, serious disease or infection

Warnings Use with caution in individuals with a history of bleeding, hemostatic or drug-related hemostatic disorders, and those taking anticoagulants (eg, aspirin or aspirin-containing products, NSAIDs, warfarin) or antiplatelet agents (eg, clopidogrel, dipyridamole, ticlopidine), cyclosporine, erythromycin, itraconazole, niacin, HMG-CoA reductase inhibitors (associated with rare but serious adverse effects, including hepatic and skeletal muscle disorders), and other hyperlipidemic agents. Avoid other herbs with hyperlipidemic properties (see below). Discontinue at the first sign of hepatic dysfunction; discontinue at least 14 days prior to dental or surgical procedures.

Potential/Suspected Interactions Increased effect/toxicity:

Anticoagulant and antiplatelet agents, HMG-CoA reductase inhibitors and other cholesterol-lowering agents, clofibrate, cyclosporine, erythromycin, fenofibrate, gemfibrozil, itraconazole, ketoconazole, niacin

Herbs with anticoagulant/antiplatelet properties: Alfalfa, anise, bilberry, bladderwrack, bromelain, cat's claw, celery, coleus, cordyceps, dong quai, evening primrose, fenugreek, feverfew, garlic, ginger, ginkgo biloba, ginseng (American/Panax/Siberian), grape seed, green tea, guggul, horse chestnut seed, horseradish, licorice, prickly ash, red clover, reishi, sweet clover, turmeric, white willow

Resveratrol *see* Grape Skin *on page 1436*
Rökan *see* Ginkgo Biloba *on page 1429*
Rosin Rose *see* St John's Wort *on page 1447*
Rustic Treacle *see* Garlic *on page 1428*
Sabal serrulata *see* Saw Palmetto *on page 1446*
Sabasilis serrulatae *see* Saw Palmetto *on page 1446*
S-adenosylmethionine *see* SAMe *on page 1445*

SAMe

Synonyms S-adenosylmethionine

Use Treatment of depression

Local Anesthetic/Vasoconstrictor Precautions No information available to require special precautions

Effects on Bleeding None reported

Adverse Reactions Frequency not defined.

Central nervous system: Restlessness
Gastrointestinal: Nausea, xerostomia

Dosage Oral: 400-1600 mg/day

Mechanism of Action/Effect Not defined; functions as a cofactor in many synthetic pathways

Contraindications Active bleeding (eg, intracranial bleeding, peptic ulcer)

Warnings Use caution when combining with other antidepressants, tryptophan, or 5-HTP; ineffective in the treatment of depressive symptoms associated with bipolar disorder

Potential/Suspected Interactions Increased effect/toxicity: MAO inhibitors, tricyclic antidepressants, or SSRIs; may potentiate the antidepressant effects of 5-HTP, tryptophan, and St John's wort

Sassafras albidum *see* Sassafras Oil *on page 1445*

Sassafras Oil

Synonyms *Laurus Sassafras*; *Sassafras albidum*; *Sassafras radix*; *Sassafras varifolium*; *Sassafrax*

Use Demulcent; treatment of inflammation of the eyes, insect bites, rheumatic pain; used in the past as a flavoring for beer, sauces, and tea

Local Anesthetic/Vasoconstrictor Precautions No information available to require special precautions

Effects on Bleeding None reported

Adverse Reactions Frequency not defined.

Dermatologic: Contact dermatitis, diaphoresis

Dosage Adults: Topical: 1-5 drops in distilled water

Mechanism of Action/Effect Contains safrole (up to 80%), one of the heaviest of the volatile oils chemically found to be the methylene ether of allyl-dioxibenene; safrole is slowly absorbed from the alimentary canal, escapes the lungs unaltered, and through the kidneys oxidized into piperonalic

(Continued)

Sassafras Oil *(Continued)*

acid; inhibits liver microsomal enzymes and its metabolite may cause hepatic tumors

Contraindications Ingestion considered unsafe by the FDA; banned in food by FDA since 1960

Warnings Ingestion can result in poisoning or death (dose-dependent). Sassafras tea can contain as much as 200 mg (3 mg/kg) of safrole; emesis (within 30 minutes) can be considered for ingestion >5 mL (considered lethal).

Sassafras radix *see* Sassafras Oil *on page 1445*

Sassafras varifolium *see* Sassafras Oil *on page 1445*

Sassafrax *see* Sassafras Oil *on page 1445*

Saw Palmetto

Synonyms Palmetto Scrub; *Sabal serrulata*; *Sabasilis serrulatae*; *Serenoa repens*

Use Antiandrogen, anti-inflammatory; treatment of benign prostatic hyperplasia (BPH)

Local Anesthetic/Vasoconstrictor Precautions No information available to require special precautions

Effects on Bleeding None reported

Adverse Reactions Frequency not defined.

Central nervous system: Headache

Endocrine & metabolic: Gynecomastia

Gastrointestinal: Stomach problems (rare, per Commission E)

Dosage Adults: Oral: 0.5-1 g dried fruit 3 times/day **or** 160 mg twice daily (standardized to contain at least 80% to 90% fatty acids and sterols per dose)

Mechanism of Action/Effect Liposterolic extract of berries may inhibit the enzymes 5α-reductase, along with cyclo-oxygenase and 5-lipoxygenase; does not reduce prostatic enlargement but may help increase urinary flow.

Contraindications Hormone replacement therapy (HRT), lactation, pregnancy, prostate medications

Warnings Not FDA approved; use with caution in individuals on alpha-adrenergic blocking agents and finasteride.

Potential/Suspected Interactions Increased effect/toxicity: Alpha-adrenergic blocking agents, finasteride, hormone replacement therapy (HRT), prostate medications

Schisandra

Synonyms *Schizandra chinensis*

Use Adaptogen, anti-inflammatory, antioxidant, antitussive, hepatoprotective, immunostimulant; treatment of cancer, chronic diarrhea, cough, diabetes, diaphoresis, fatigue, hepatitis; adjunct support for chemotherapy and radiation, detoxification, energy production, health tonic

Local Anesthetic/Vasoconstrictor Precautions No information available to require special precautions

Effects on Bleeding None reported

Dosage Oral: 100 mg twice daily (standardized to contain at least 9% schisandrins per dose)

Mechanism of Action/Effect Reported to lower serum glutamic-pyruvic transaminase (SGPT) concentration, a liver enzyme found in blood when liver damage is present; stimulates hepatic glycogen synthesis and protein synthesis and increases microsomal enzyme activity

Contraindications Pregnancy (due to uterine stimulation)

Warnings May alter metabolism of many drugs; use with caution in individuals taking calcium channel blockers.

Potential/Suspected Interactions Cytochrome P450 enzyme induction may alter metabolism of many drugs (calcium channel blockers noted to be decreased). Cardioprotective action reported during administration of doxorubicin.

Schizandra chinensis *see* Schisandra *on page 1446*

Scury Root *see Echinacea on page 1423*

Serenoa repens *see* Saw Palmetto *on page 1446*

Shark Cartilage

Use Treatment of cancer, osteoarthritis, and rheumatoid arthritis

Local Anesthetic/Vasoconstrictor Precautions No information available to require special precautions

Effects on Bleeding None reported

Dosage

Oral: Dosage range: 3000 mg 3 times/day, taken 20 minutes before meals

Rectal: Retention enemas; 15-20 g/day

Mechanism of Action/Effect A mixture of glycosaminoglycans (GAGs), including chondroitin sulfate; contains antiangiogenesis factors which inhibit the growth of new blood vessels and may prevent tumors from developing the network of blood vessels they need to supply them with nutrients

Siberian Ginseng *see* Ginseng, Siberian *on page 1431*

Silver Apricot *see* Ginkgo Biloba *on page 1429*

Silybum marianum *see* Milk Thistle *on page 1443*

Snakeroot *see Echinacea on page 1423*

Soy Isoflavones

Synonyms Isoflavones

Use Estrogenic (weak); treatment of bone loss, hypercholesterolemia, menopausal symptoms

Local Anesthetic/Vasoconstrictor Precautions No information available to require special precautions

Effects on Bleeding None reported

Dosage Oral: 500-1000 mg soy extract daily

Mechanism of Action/Effect Contains plant-derived estrogenic compounds (potency estimated to be only 1/1000 to 1/100,000 that of estradiol); claimed to inhibit bone reabsorption in postmenopausal women; reported to lower serum lipids, including LDL cholesterol and triglycerides, along with increases in HDL cholesterol

Contraindications History of estrogenic tumors (eg, endometrial or breast cancer)

Warnings May alter response to hormone replacement therapy; use with caution in individuals with history of thromboembolism or stroke

Potential/Suspected Interactions Increased effect/toxicity: Estrogen-containing medications, hormonal contraceptives, hormone replacement therapy (HRT)

Stinking Rose *see* Garlic *on page 1428*

St John's Wort

Synonyms Amber Touch-and-Feel; Goatweed; *Hypercium perforatum*; Klamath Weed; Rosin Rose

Use Antibacterial, anti-inflammatory, antiviral (high doses), anxiolytic, wound-healing agent; treatment of AIDS (popular due to possible antiretroviral activity), anxiety and stress, insomnia; mild to moderate depression; bruises, muscle soreness, and sprains; vitiligo

Per Commission E: Psychovegetative disorders, depressive moods, anxiety and/or nervous unrest; oily preparations for dyspeptic complaints; oily preparations externally for treatment of post-therapy of acute and contused injuries, myalgia, first degree burns

Local Anesthetic/Vasoconstrictor Precautions No information available to require special precautions

Effects on Bleeding None reported

Adverse Reactions Frequency not defined.

Cardiovascular: Tachycardia

Dermatologic: Photosensitization (especially in fair-skinned persons per Commission E)

Gastrointestinal: GI upset

Dosage

Oral: 300 mg 3 times/day (standardized to contain 0.3% to 0.5% hypericin and/ or 3% to 5% hyperforin per dose); minimum of 4-6 weeks therapy recommended

Topical: Apply oil extract to bruises and use for muscle soreness and sprains

Mechanism of Action/Effect Active ingredients are xanthones, flavonoids (hypericin) which can act as MAO inhibitors (although *in vitro* activity is minimal); majority of activity appears to be related to GABA modulation; may also be related to dopamine, serotonin, norepinephrine modulation

Contraindications Children <2 years of age, indinavir, therapeutic immunosuppressants, stimulants, SSRIs, antidepressants, digoxin, endogenous depression, pregnancy

Warnings May be photosensitizing; use caution with drugs metabolized by CYP3A3/4 and tyramine-containing foods (eg, cheese, wine). Use with caution in individuals taking antidepressants, cardiac glycosides, MAO inhibitors, narcotics, reserpine, stimulants, and SSRIs. High does may elevate LFTs

(Continued)

St John's Wort *(Continued)*

(reversible). May alter absorption of calcium, copper, magnesium, and zinc due to tannins. Interacts with many drugs, see below.

Potential/Suspected Interactions

Increased effect/toxicity: SSRIs or other antidepressants, tetracycline (photosensitivity)

Decreased effect: Appears to induce CYP3A3/4 enzymes, potentially reducing effect of many medications (eg, ritonavir, MAO inhibitors, levodopa, 5-hydroxytryptophan, diltiazem, nicardipine, verapamil, etoposide, paclitaxel, vinblastine, vincristine, glucocorticoids, dextromethorphan, ephedrine, lithium, meperidine, pseudoephedrine, selegiline, yohimbine, and ACE inhibitors)

Superginkgo *see* Ginkgo Biloba *on page 1429*

Sweet Root *see* Licorice *on page 1440*

Tanacetum parthenium *see* Feverfew *on page 1426*

Tanakan *see* Ginkgo Biloba *on page 1429*

Tanakene *see* Ginkgo Biloba *on page 1429*

Tea Tree Oil *see* Melaleuca Oil *on page 1442*

Tebonin *see* Ginkgo Biloba *on page 1429*

Thioctic acid *see* Alpha-Lipoic Acid *on page 1413*

Tonga *see* Kava *on page 1439*

Tramisal *see* Ginkgo Biloba *on page 1429*

Turmeric

Synonyms *Curcuma longa*

Use Anti-inflammatory, antioxidant, antiplatelet, antirheumatic; treatment of rheumatoid arthritis and other inflammatory conditions, hypercholesterolemia, and hyperlipidemia

Local Anesthetic/Vasoconstrictor Precautions No information available to require special precautions

Effects on Bleeding May see increased bleeding due to inhibition of platelet aggregation

Dosage Oral: 300 mg 3 times/day with meals (standardized to contain 95% curcuminoids per dose)

Mechanism of Action/Effect Anti-inflammatory activity claimed to be comparable to NSAIDs in treatment of rheumatoid arthritis. Antioxidant activity is associated with phenolic fraction, curcuminoids, which also inhibit leukotrienes and prostaglandin synthesis. Curcuminoids reportedly lowered the levels of blood lipid peroxides; may decrease LDL cholesterol and total cholesterol, while increasing HDL cholesterol.

Contraindications Active bleeding (eg, intracranial bleeding, peptic ulcer), biliary obstruction

Warnings Use with caution in individuals with history of bleeding, hemostatic or drug-related hemostatic disorders, and those taking anticoagulants (eg, aspirin or aspirin-containing products, NSAIDs, warfarin) or antiplatelet agents (eg, clopidogrel, dipyridamole, ticlopidine). Discontinue at least 14 days prior to dental or surgical procedures.

Potential/Suspected Interactions Increased effect/toxicity:

Anticoagulant/antiplatelet agents and antihyperlipidemics

Herbs with anticoagulant/antiplatelet properties: Alfalfa, anise, bilberry, bladderwrack, bromelain, cat's claw, celery, coleus, cordyceps, dong quai, evening primrose, fenugreek, feverfew, garlic, ginger, ginkgo biloba, ginseng (American/Panax/Siberian), grape seed, green tea, guggul, horse chestnut seed, horseradish, licorice, prickly ash, red clover, reishi, sweet clover, white willow

Turmeric Root *see* Golden Seal *on page 1433*

Ubiquinone *see* Coenzyme Q_{10} *on page 1420*

Ulgastrin Neo *see* Licorice *on page 1440*

Uncaria tomentosa *see* Cat's Claw *on page 1417*

Uva Ursi

Synonyms *Arctostaphylos uva-ursi*; Bearberry

Use Analgesic, antiseptic, astringent, diuretic; treatment and prevention of urinary tract infections; prevention of kidney stones; treatment of bladder infections, urethritis, and a variety of renal disorders (eg, cystitis, nephritis, nephrolithiasis)

Local Anesthetic/Vasoconstrictor Precautions No information available to require special precautions

Effects on Bleeding None reported

Adverse Reactions Frequency not defined (high doses).

Central nervous system: Convulsions

Gastrointestinal: Vomiting

Dosage Oral: 100-200 mg/day (standardized to contain 10% to 25% arbutin per dose)

Mechanism of Action/Effect A potent urinary antiseptic with an astringent effect on the lower digestive tract, reducing general intestinal irritation; contains arbutin, a phenolic glycoside that demonstrates analgesic and antiseptic properties in the urinary tract similar to phenazopyridine; disinfectant properties are most prominent in alkaline urine. Constituents of whole plant preparations are believed to enhance efficacy by contributing to urinary alkalinization. Arbutin is destroyed in the GI tract but additional plant components block its degradation and enhance absorption when whole plant preparations are ingested.

Contraindications Lactation and pregnancy, renal failure; use >7-10 days

Warnings May cause green-brown discoloration of urine; may alter GI absorption of other herbs, minerals, or drugs (especially calcium, copper, magnesium, and zinc) due to tannins. Use caution with individuals taking diuretics; avoid other herbs with diuretic properties (see below).

Potential/Suspected Interactions May alter absorption of other herbs, minerals, or drugs

Increased effect/toxicity: Herbs with diuretic properties: Artichoke, celery seed, corn silk, couchgrass, dandelion, elder flower, horsetail, juniper berry, kava, shepherd's purse, yarrow

Decreased effect: Has decreased effect in acidic urine; drinking water with 1 tsp baking soda prior to use may promote conversion of hydroquinones to their active form

Vaccinium macrocarpon *see* Cranberry *on page 1421*

Vaccinium myrtillus *see* Bilberry *on page 1415*

Valerian

Synonyms Radix; Red Valerian; *Valeriana edulis*; *Valeriana wallichi*

Use Antispasmotic, anxiolytic, sedative (mild); treatment of anxiety and panic attacks, headache, intestinal cramps, nervous tension during PMS and menopause, restless motor syndrome and muscle spasms, sleep disorders (eg, insomnia, jet lag)

Per Commission E: Treatment of sleep disorders based on nervous conditions, restlessness

Local Anesthetic/Vasoconstrictor Precautions No information available to require special precautions

Effects on Bleeding None reported

Adverse Reactions Frequency not defined.

Cardiovascular: Cardiac disturbances (unspecified)

Central nervous system: Fatigue, lightheadedness, restlessness

Gastrointestinal: Nausea

Neuromuscular & skeletal: Tremor

Ocular: Blurred vision

Dosage Oral: 200 mg 1-4 times/day (standardized to contain 0.8% to 1% valerenic acids per dose)

Dried root: 0.3-1 g

Sedative: 1-3 g (1-3 mL of tincture)

Mechanism of Action/Effect May affect neurotransmitter levels (serotonin, GABA, and norepinephrine)

Contraindications Children <3 years of age

Warnings Advise caution when driving or operating heavy machinery. Use only valepotriate and baldrinal-free supplements in children <12 years of age due to potential mutagenic properties. Use with caution in individuals taking antianxiety or antidepressant agents, antipsychotics, histamines, and hypnotics/sedatives. Avoid herbs with sedative properties (see below).

Potential/Suspected Interactions Increased effect/toxicity:

Antianxiety or antidepressant agents, antipsychotics, antihistamines, barbiturates, other CNS depressants (not synergistic with alcohol), hypnotics/sedatives

Herbs with sedative properties: Gotu kola, kava, SAMe, St John's wort, and valerian

Valeriana edulis *see* Valerian *on page 1449*

Valeriana wallichi *see* Valerian *on page 1449*

Valverde *see* Ginkgo Biloba *on page 1429*

Vanadium

Use Treatment of type 1 and type 2 diabetes

Local Anesthetic/Vasoconstrictor Precautions No information available to require special precautions

Effects on Bleeding None reported

Adverse Reactions No dietary toxicity or serious side effects have been reported, however, industrial exposure has resulted in toxicity.

Dosage Oral: RDI: 250 mcg 1-3 times/day

Mechanism of Action/Effect Reported to be a cofactor in nicotinamide adenine dinucleotide phosphate (NADPH) oxidation reactions, lipoprotein lipase activity, amino acid transport, and hematopoiesis; may augment glucose regulation

Warnings May alter glucose regulation; use with caution in diabetics, those predisposed to hypoglycemia, or taking hypoglycemic agents (eg, insulin). Monitor blood sugar and dosage of these agents; may require adjustment (should be carefully coordinated among the individual's healthcare providers).

Potential/Suspected Interactions Increased effect:

Oral hypoglycemics, insulin

Herbs with hypoglycemic properties: Alfalfa, aloe, bilberry, bitter melon, burdock, celery, damiana, fenugreek, garcinia, garlic, ginger, ginseng (American), gymnema, marshmallow, stinging nettle

Vasan *see* Ginkgo Biloba *on page 1429*

Vital *see* Ginkgo Biloba *on page 1429*

Vitex agnus-castus *see* Chasteberry *on page 1419*

Vitis vinifera *see* Grape Seed *on page 1435*

Whitehorn *see* Hawthorn *on page 1437*

Wild Quinine *see* Feverfew *on page 1426*

Wild Yam

Synonyms *Dioscorea villosa*

Use Anti-inflammatory, antispasmodic, cholagogue, diuretic (high doses), expectorant (high doses); treatment of diverticulitis, dysmenorrhea, intestinal colic, menopausal symptoms, nausea, premenstrual syndrome (PMS), rheumatic and other inflammatory conditions; female vitality

Local Anesthetic/Vasoconstrictor Precautions No information available to require special precautions

Effects on Bleeding None reported

Adverse Reactions Frequency not defined.

Gastrointestinal: Emesis (high doses), GI upset (sensitive individuals)

Dosage Adults:

Oral: 250 mg 1-3 times/day (standardized to contain 10% diosgenin per dose)

Liquid extract: 2-4 mL/day

Tea: 1-2 teaspoons root steeped in 1 cup boiling water for 15 minutes; drink 3 times/day

Topical: Apply as directed

Mechanism of Action/Effect Primarily used for its spasmolytic properties; appears to decrease spasm in the large intestine and uterus; contains the steroidal saponin, diosgenin, but the plant itself is devoid of estrogen and progesterone. Anti-inflammatory action is believed to be due to an affinity for steroid receptors shown by the steroidal saponins present in the plant.

Contraindications Estrogen, progesterone, hormonal contraceptives, hormone replacement therapy (HRT), history of endometrial cancer or estrogen-dependent tumors

Warnings Use with caution in individuals with a history of stroke or thromboembolic disease and those taking steroids, hormonal contraceptives, or receiving hormone replacement therapy (HRT). Use in children, or women during lactation or pregnancy is not recommended. Overdose may result in poisoning. Avoid other anabolic herbs (see below).

Potential/Suspected Interactions Increased effect:

Androgens, estrogens, hormonal contraceptives, hormone replacement therapy (HRT), steroids

Anabolic herbs: Devil's club, dong quai, ginseng (American/Asian/Siberian), muira, puama, sarsparilla, suma, tribulus

Herbs with estrogenic properties: Black cohosh, dong quai, and evening primrose

Yellow Indian Paint *see* Golden Seal *on page 1433*

Yellow Root *see* Golden Seal *on page 1433*

Yohimbe

Related Information

Yohimbine *on page 1393*

Synonyms Johimbe; *Pausinystalia yohimbe*; Yohimbehe cortex

Use Anesthetic (local), antiatherogenic, antiviral, aphrodesiac, stimulant, sympathomimetic, thermogenic, vasodilator, vasopressomimetic; treatment of angina pectoris, arteriosclerosis, exhaustion, male erectile dysfunction

Local Anesthetic/Vasoconstrictor Precautions Has potential to interact with epinephrine and levonordefrin to result in increased BP; use vasoconstrictor with caution

Effects on Bleeding None reported

Adverse Reactions

Frequency not defined.

- Cardiovascular: Cardiac failure, hypertension, tachycardia, vasoconstriction
- Central nervous system: Insomnia
- Gastrointestinal: Increased peristalsis, dyspepsia

High dose:

- Cardiovascular: Hypotension
- Central nervous system: Dizziness, headache, hyperactivity, irritability, psychosis, tremor
- Gastrointestinal: Anorexia, xerostomia
- Ocular: Decreased visual acuity
- Respiratory: Asthmatic attack
- Miscellaneous: Sweating

Dosage Adults: Oral: 500-750 mg twice daily

Mechanism of Action/Effect Alkaloid which contains several other psychoactive alkaloids believed to have an effect similar to yohimbine; has CNS, respiratory, and thyroid stimulatory activity; blocks peripheral 5-HT receptors and prevents accumulation of lipid-containing plaques on innermost layers of arteries; has selective $alpha_2$ adrenergic blocking properties; aphrodisiac activity may be due to enlargement of the vasculature in the genitals, increase of nerve impulses to genital tissue, and an increased transmission of reflex excitability in the sacral region of the spinal cord; may have MAO inhibitor activity

Contraindications $Alpha_2$-blockers, anticoagulant or antiplatelet agents, antidepressants, asthma, bethanechol, carbachol, cardiovascular disease (eg, arrhythmias, hypertension), chronic inflammation of genitalia, chronic prostatitis, diabetes, hyperthyroidism, MAO inhibitors, metoclopramide, pilocarpine, pregnancy, psychiatric disorders

Warnings Toxic doses may trigger cardiac failure, hypotension, and psychosis. Use with caution in individuals with diabetes, GI ulceration, or osteoporosis. Avoid other herbs with hypertensive, parasympathomimetic, sympathomimetic, thyroid-stimulating, or vasopressomimetic properties (see below).

Potential/Suspected Interactions Antihypertensives; may cause both hyper- and hypotension (dose-dependent)

Increased effect/toxicity:

- $Alpha_2$ blockers, MAO inhibitors, naloxone, other sympathomimetics, tricyclic antidepressants
- Herbs with hypertensive properties: Bayberry, blue cohosh, cayenne, ephedra, ginger, ginseng, kola nut (caffeine), licorice
- Herbs with parasympathomimetic properties: Bittersweet, blood root, blue flag, bryony, dogbane, dogwood, false/green hellebore, horse chestnut, huperzineA, immortal, jaborandi, leptandra, pasque flower, pink root, pleurisy root, pokeweed, senega snakeroot, wahoo
- Herbs with sympathomimetic properties: Calamus, cayenne, ephedra, Fu-tse (Fo-tzu), guarana, kola nut (caffeine), night blooming cereus, peyote (mescal buttons), scotch broom tops, Syrian rue, yellow jasmine
- Thyroid-stimulating herbs: Fu-tse (Fo-tzu), gotu kola, ephedra, mustard
- Herbs with vasopressomimetic properties: Goat's head, peyote (mescal buttons)

Yohimbehe cortex *see* Yohimbe *on page 1451*

Zingiber officinale *see* Ginger *on page 1428*

EFFECTS ON VARIOUS SYSTEMS

CARDIOVASCULAR SYSTEM

CONGESTIVE HEART FAILURE

(Diuretics, Xanthine derivatives, Licorice, Ginseng, Aconite)

Alisma plantago, bearberry (*Arctostaphylos uva-ursi*), buchu (*Barosma betulina*), couch grass, dandelion, horsetail rush, juniper, licorice, and xanthine derivatives exert varying degrees of diuretic action. Many patients with congestive heart failure (CHF) are already taking a diuretic medication. By taking products containing one or more of these components, patients already on diuretic medications may increase their risk for dehydration.

Ginseng and licorice can potentially worsen congestive heart failure and edema by causing fluid retention. Aconite has varying effects on the heart that itself could lead to heart failure. Patients with CHF should be advised to consult with their healthcare provider before using products containing any of these components.

HYPERTENSION/HYPOTENSION

(Diuretics, Ginkgo biloba, Ginseng, Hawthorn, Ma-huang, Xanthine derivatives)

The stimulant properties of ginseng and ma-huang could worsen pre-existing hypertension. Elevated blood pressure has been reported as a side effect of ginseng. Although ma-huang contains ephedrine, a known vasoconstrictor, ma-huang's effect on blood pressure varies between individuals. Ma-huang can cause hypotension or hypertension. Due to its unpredictable effects, patients with pre-existing hypertension should use caution when using natural products containing ma-huang. Providers should caution patients with labile hypertension against the use of ginseng.

The diuretic effect of xanthine derivatives and other diuretic components could increase the effects of antihypertensive medications, increasing the risk for hypotension. Hawthorn and ginkgo biloba can cause vasodilation increasing the hypotensive effects of antihypertensive medication. Patients susceptible to hypotension or patients taking antihypertensive medication should use caution when taking products containing xanthine derivatives or diuretics. Patients with pre-existing hypertension or hypotension who wish to use products containing these components should be closely monitored by a healthcare professional for changes in blood pressure control.

ARRHYTHMIAS

(Ginseng)

It has been reported that ginseng may increase the risk of arrhythmias, although it is unclear whether this effect is due to the actual ingredient (ginseng) or other possible impurities. Patients at risk for arrhythmias should be cautioned against the use of products containing ginseng without first consulting with their healthcare provider.

CENTRAL NERVOUS SYSTEM

(Aconite, Ginseng, Xanthine derivatives)

Aconite and hawthorn have potentially sedating effects, and aconite also contains various alkaloids and traces of ephedrine. Some documented central nervous system (CNS) effects of aconite include sedation, vertigo, and incoordination. Hawthorn has been reported to exert a depressive effect on the CNS leading to sedation.

Ginseng, ma-huang, and xanthine derivatives can exert a stimulant effect on the central nervous system. Some of the CNS effects of ginseng include nervousness, insomnia, and euphoria. The action of ma-huang is due to the presence of ephedrine and pseudoephedrine. Ma-huang exerts a stimulant action on the CNS similar to decongestant/weight loss products (Dexatrim®, etc) thus causing nervousness, insomnia, and anxiety. Kola nut, green tea, guarana, and yerba mate contain varying amounts of caffeine, a xanthine derivative. Stimulant properties exerted by these herbs are expected to be comparable to those of caffeine, including insomnia, nervousness, and anxiety.

Products containing aconite and hawthorn should be used with caution in patients with known history of depression, vertigo, or syncope. Ginseng or xanthine derivatives should be avoided in patients with history of insomnia or anxiety. Use of natural products with these components may contribute to a worsening of a patient's pre-existing medical condition. Patients taking CNS-active medications should avoid or use extreme caution when using preparations containing any of the above components. These components may interact directly or indirectly with CNS-active medications causing an increase or decrease in overall effect.

EFFECTS ON VARIOUS SYSTEMS *(Continued)*

ENDOCRINE SYSTEM

DIABETES MELLITUS

(Chromium, Glucomannan, Ginseng, Hawthorn, Ma-huang, Periploca, Spirulina)

Ma-huang and spirulina both may increase glucose levels. This could cause a decrease in glucose control, thereby, increasing a patient's risk for hyperglycemia. Patients with diabetes or glucose intolerance should avoid using ma-huang and spirulina containing products.

Chromium, ginseng, glucomannan, periploca (*gymneme sylvestre*), and hawthorn should be used with caution in patients being treated for diabetes. These ingredients may reduce glucose levels increasing the risk for hypoglycemia in patients who are already taking a hypoglycemic agent. Patients with diabetes who wish to use products containing these ingredients should be closely monitored for fluctuations in blood glucose levels.

GASTROINTESTINAL SYSTEM

PEPTIC ULCER DISEASE

(Betaine Hydrochloride, White Willow)

Betaine hydrochloride is a source of hydrochloric acid. The acid released from betaine hydrochloride could aggravate an existing ulcer. White willow, like aspirin, contains salicylates.

Aspirin has been known to induce gastric damage by direct irritation on the gastric mucosa and by an indirect systemic effect. As a result, patients with a history of peptic ulcer disease or gastritis are informed to avoid use of aspirin and other salicylate derivatives. These precautions should also apply to white willow. Patients with a history of peptic ulcer disease or gastritis should not use products containing white willow or betaine hydrochloride as either could exacerbate ulcers.

INFLAMMATORY BOWEL DISEASE

(Cascara Sagrada, Senna, Dandelion)

Cascara sagrada and senna are stimulant laxatives. Their laxative effect is exerted by stimulation of peristalsis in the colon and by inhibition of water and electrolyte secretion. The laxative effect produced by these herbs could induce an exacerbation of inflammatory bowel disease. Patients with a history of inflammatory bowel disease should avoid using products containing cascara sagrada or senna, and use caution when taking products containing dandelion which may also have a laxative effect.

OBSTRUCTION/ILEUS

(Glucomannan, Kelp, Psyllium)

Glucomannan, kelp, and psyllium act as bulk laxatives. In the presence of water, bulk laxatives swell or form a viscous solution adding extra bulk in the gastrointestinal tract. The resulting mass is thought to stimulate peristalsis. In the presence of an ileus, these laxatives could cause an obstruction.

If sufficient water is not consumed when taking a bulk laxative, a semisolid mass can form resulting in an obstruction. Any patient who wishes to take a natural product containing kelp, psyllium, or glucomannan should drink sufficient water to decrease the risk of obstruction. This may be of concern in particular disease states such as CHF or other cases where excess fluid intake may influence the existing disease presentation. Patients with a suspected obstruction or ileus should avoid using products containing kelp, psyllium, or glucomannan without consent of their primary healthcare provider.

HEMATOLOGIC SYSTEM

ANTICOAGULATION THERAPY & COAGULATION DISORDERS

(Horsetail Rush, Ginseng, Ginkgo Biloba, Guarana, White Willow)

Horsetail rush, ginseng, ginkgo biloba, guarana, and white willow can potentially affect platelet aggregation and bleeding time. Ginkgo biloba, ginseng, guarana, and white willow inhibit platelet aggregation resulting in an increase in bleeding time. Horsetail rush, on the other hand, may decrease bleeding time. Patients with coagulation disorders or patients on anticoagulation therapy may be sensitive to the effects on coagulation by these components and should, therefore, avoid use of products containing any of these components.

OTHER

PHENYLKETONURIA

(Aspartame, Spirulina)

Patients with phenylketonuria should not use products containing aspartame or spirulina. Aspartame, a common artificial sweetener, is metabolized to phenylalanine, while spirulina contains phenylalanine.

GOUT

(Diuretics, White Willow)

Patients with a history of gout should avoid using natural products containing components with diuretic action or white willow. By increasing urine output, ingredients with diuretic action may concentrate uric acid in the blood increasing the risk of gout in these patients. White willow, like aspirin, may inhibit excretion of urate resulting in an increase in uric acid concentration. The increase in urate levels could cause precipitation of uric acid resulting in an exacerbation of gout.

ORAL MEDICINE TOPICS

PART I:

DENTAL MANAGEMENT AND THERAPEUTIC CONSIDERATIONS IN MEDICALLY-COMPROMISED PATIENTS

This first part of the chapter focuses on common medical conditions and their associated drug therapies with which the dentist must be familiar. Patient profiles with commonly associated drug regimens are described.

TABLE OF CONTENTS

Cardiovascular Diseases 1458

Gastrointestinal Disorders 1476

Respiratory Diseases 1478

Endocrine Disorders and Pregnancy 1481

HIV Infection and AIDS 1484

Rheumatoid Arthritis, Osteoarthritis, and Osteoporosis 1490

Nonviral Infectious Diseases 1495

Antibiotic Prophylaxis – Preprocedural Guidelines for Dental Patients 1509

Systemic Viral Diseases 1519

CARDIOVASCULAR DISEASES

Cardiovascular disease is the most prevalent human disease affecting over 60 million Americans and this group of diseases accounts >50% of all deaths in the United States. Surgical and pharmacological therapy have resulted in many cardiovascular patients living healthy and profitable lives. Consequently, patients presenting to the dental office may require treatment planning modifications related to the medical management of their cardiovascular disease. For the purposes of this text, we will cover coronary artery disease (CAD) including angina pectoris and myocardial infarction, cardiac arrhythmias, heart failure, and hypertension.

CARDIOVASCULAR DRUGS AND DENTAL CONSIDERATIONS

Some of the drug listings are redundant because the drugs are used to treat more than one cardiovascular disorder. As a convenience to the reader, each table has been constructed as a stand alone listing of drugs for the given disorder. The dental implications of these cardiovascular drugs are listed in Tables 8 and 9. Each of these 2 tables is a consolidation of the drugs from Tables 1-7. The more frequent cardiovascular, respiratory, and central nervous system adverse reactions which you may see in the dental patient are described in Table 8 *on page 1471*. Table 9 *on page 1474* describes the effects on dental treatment reported for these drugs. It is suggested that the reader use Tables 8 and 9 to check for potential effects which could occur in the medicated cardiovascular dental patients.

CORONARY ARTERY DISEASE

Any long-term decrease in the delivery of oxygen to the heart muscle can lead to the condition ischemic heart disease. Often arteriosclerosis and atherosclerosis result in a narrowing of the coronary vessels' lumina and are the most common causes of vascular ischemic heart disease. Other causes such as previous infarct, mitral valve regurgitation, and ruptured septa may also lead to ischemia in the heart muscle. The two most common major conditions that result from ischemic heart disease are angina pectoris and myocardial infarction. Sudden death, a third category, can likewise result from ischemia.

To the physician, the most common presenting sign or symptom of ischemic heart disease is chest pain. This chest pain can be of a transient nature as in angina pectoris or the result of a myocardial infarction. It is now believed that sudden death represents a separate occurrence that essentially involves the development of a lethal cardiac arrhythmia or coronary artery spasm leading to an acute shutdown of the heart muscle blood supply. Risk factors in patients for coronary atherosclerosis include cigarette smoking, elevated blood lipids, hypertension, as well as diabetes mellitus, age, and gender (male).

Coronary artery disease (CAD) is the cause of about half of all deaths in the United States. CAD has been shown to be correlated with the levels of plasma cholesterol and/or triacylglycerol-containing lipoprotein particles. Primary prevention focuses on averting the development of CAD. In contrast, secondary prevention of (CAD) focuses on therapies to reduce morbidity and mortality in patients with clinically documented CAD.

Lipid-lowering and cardioprotective drugs provide significant risk-reducing benefits in the secondary prevention of CAD. By reducing the levels of total and low density cholesterol through the inhibition of hydroxymethylglutaryl coenzyme A (HMG-CoA) reductase, statin drugs significantly improve survival. Cardioprotective drug therapy includes antiplatelet/anticoagulant agents to inhibit platelet adhesion, aggregation and blood coagulation; beta-blockers to lower heart rate, contractility and blood pressure; and the angiotensin-converting enzyme (ACE) inhibitors to lower peripheral resistance and workload. For a listing of these drugs, see Table 1 on following page.

Table 1.
DRUGS USED IN THE TREATMENT OF CAD

Reduction of Total and Low-Density Cholesterol Levels

Bile Acid Sequestrant

Colesevelam *on page 373*

HMG-CoA Reductase Inhibitors

Fluvastatin *on page 622*
Lovastatin *on page 848*
Pravastatin *on page 1109*
Simvastatin *on page 1222*
Atorvastatin *on page 162*

Fibrate Group

Clofibrate *on page 353*
Fenofibrate *on page 577*
Gemfibrozil *on page 651*

Bile Acid Resins

Cholestyramine Resin *on page 323*
Colestipol *on page 373*

Nicotinic Acid

Cardioprotective Therapy

Antiplatelet / Anticoagulant Agents

Aspirin *on page 151*
Clopidogrel *on page 361*
Ticlopidine *on page 1297*
Warfarin *on page 1389*

Beta-Adrenergic Receptor Blockers

Atenolol *on page 159*
Metoprolol *on page 915*
Propranolol *on page 1140*

Angiotensin-Converting Enzyme (ACE) Inhibitors

Captopril *on page 252*
Enalapril *on page 488*
Fosinopril *on page 633*
Lisinopril *on page 833*
Ramipril *on page 1167*

ANGINA PECTORIS

(EMPHASIS ON UNSTABLE ANGINA)

Numerous physiologic triggers can initiate the rupture of plaque in coronary blood vessels. Rupture leads to the activation, adhesion and aggregation of platelets, and the activation of the clotting cascade, resulting in the formation of occlusive thrombus. If this process leads to the complete occlusion of the artery, acute myocardial infarction with ST-segment elevation occurs. Alternatively, if the process leads to severe stenosis and the artery remains patent, unstable angina occurs. Triggers which induce unstable angina include physical exertion, mechanical stress due to an increase in cardiac contractility, pulse rate, blood pressure, and vasoconstriction.

Unstable angina accounts for more than 1 million hospital admissions annually. In 1989, Braunwald devised a classification system according to the severity of the clinical manifestations of angina. These manifestations are defined as acute angina while at rest (within the 48 hours before presentation), subacute angina while at rest (within the previous month but not within the 48 hours before presentation), or new onset of accelerated (progressively more severe) angina. The system also classifies angina according to the clinical circumstances in which unstable angina develops, defined as either angina in the presence or absence of other conditions (ie, fever, hypoxia, tachycardia, thyrotoxicosis) and whether or not ECG abnormalities are present. Recently, the term "acute coronary syndrome" has been used to describe the range of conditions that includes unstable angina, non-Q-wave myocardial infarction, and Q-wave myocardial infarction.

Pharmacologic therapy to treat unstable angina includes antiplatelet drugs, antithrombin therapy, and conventional antianginal therapy with beta-blockers, nitrates, and calcium channel blockers. These drug groups and selected agents are listed in Table 3.

CARDIOVASCULAR DISEASES *(Continued)*

Antiplatelet Drugs

Aspirin reduces platelet aggregation by blocking platelet cyclo-oxygenase through irreversible acetylation. This action prevents the formation of thromboxane A_2. A number of studies have confirmed that aspirin reduces the risk of death from cardiac causes and fatal and nonfatal myocardial infarction by approximately 50% to 70% in patients presenting with unstable angina. Ticlopidine is a second-line alternative to aspirin in the treatment of unstable angina and is also used as adjunctive therapy with aspirin to prevent thrombosis after placement of intracoronary stents. Ticlopidine blocks ADP-mediated platelet aggregation. Clopidogrel inhibits platelet aggregation by affecting the ADP-dependent activation of the glycoprotein IIb/IIIa complex. Clopidogrel is chemically related to ticlopidine, but has fewer side effects.

Platelet Glycoprotein IIb / IIIa Receptor Antagonists

Antagonists of glycoprotein IIb/IIIa, a receptor on the platelet for adhesive proteins, inhibit the final common pathway involved in adhesion, activation and aggregation. Presently, there exist three classes of inhibitors. One class is murine-human chimeric antibodies of which abciximab is the prototype. The other two classes are the synthetic peptide forms (eg, eptifibatide) and the synthetic nonpeptide forms (eg, tirofiban). These agents, in combination with heparin and aspirin, have been used to treat unstable angina, significantly reducing the incidence of death or myocardial infarction.

Antithrombin Drugs

Unfractionated heparin, in combination with aspirin, is used to treat unstable angina. Unfractionated heparin consists of polysaccharide chains which bind to antithrombin III, causing a conformational change that accelerates the inhibition of thrombin and factor Xa. Unfractionated heparin is therefore an indirect thrombin inhibitor. Unfractionated heparin can only be administered intravenously. Low-molecular-weight heparins (LMWH) have a more predictable pharmacokinetic profile than the unfractionated heparin and can be administered subcutaneously. These heparins have a mechanism of action and use similar to unfractionated heparin.

The direct antithrombins decrease thrombin activity in a manner independent of any actions on antithrombin III. Two such direct antithrombins are lepirudin (also known as recombinant hirudin) and argatroban. These agents are highly specific, direct thrombin inhibitor with each molecule capable of binding to one molecule of thrombin and inhibiting its thrombogenic activity. Direct antithrombins are used for the prevention or reduction of ischemic complications associated with unstable angina.

Warfarin (Coumadin®) elicits its anticoagulant effect by interfering with the hepatic synthesis of vitamin K-dependent coagulation factors II, VII, IX, and X. Although warfarin appears to be somewhat effective after myocardial infarction in preventing death or recurrent myocardial infarction, its effectiveness in the treatment of acute coronary syndrome is questionable. Combination therapy with aspirin and heparin followed by warfarin has resulted in reduced incidence of recurrent angina, myocardial infarction, death, or all three at 14 days as compared with aspirin alone. In contrast, another study however failed to show any additional benefit in the treatment of acute coronary syndrome using a combination of aspirin and warfarin compared to aspirin alone.

Conventional Antianginal Therapy: Beta-Blockers, Nitrates, Calcium Channel Blockers

Current thinking is that there is a definite link between unstable angina and acute myocardial infarction. In this regard, beta-blockers are currently recommended as first-line agents in all acute coronary syndromes. A meta-analysis of studies involving 4700 patients with unstable angina demonstrated a 13% reduction in the risk of myocardial infarction among patients treated with beta-blockers. The various preparations of beta-blockers appear to have equal efficacy. The effects of beta-blockers are thought to be due to their ability to decrease myocardial oxygen demand.

Nitrates, such as nitroglycerin, are widely used in the management of unstable angina. Nitrates elicit a number of effects including a reduction in oxygen demand, arteriolar vasodilation, augmentation of collateral coronary blood flow and frequency of coronary vasospasm. Intravenous nitroglycerin is one of the first line therapies for unstable angina because of the ease of dose titration and the rapid resolution of effects. Continuous nitrate therapy with oral and transdermal patch preparations has resulted in tolerance to the beneficial effects of nitrates. A 6- to 8-hour daily nitrate-free interval will minimize the tolerance phenomenon. Also, supplemental use of vitamin C appears to prevent nitrate tolerance.

Calcium channel blockers such as nifedipine, verapamil, and diltiazem cause coronary vasodilation and reduced blood pressure. Because of these actions, the calcium channel blockers were thought to be a drug group which could be effective in the treatment of unstable angina. However, a meta analysis of studies in which patients with unstable angina were treated with calcium channel blockers found no effect of the drugs on the incidence of death or myocardial infarction. More recently, it has been shown that treatment with diltiazem and verapamil may result in increased survival and reduced rates of reinfarction in patients with acute coronary syndrome. Current thinking suggests that calcium channel blockers should be used in patients in whom beta-blockers are contraindicated or in those with refractory symptoms after treatments with aspirin, nitrates, or beta-blockers.

Dental Management

The dental management of the patient with angina pectoris may include sedation techniques for complicated procedures (see "Patients Requiring Sedation" *on page 1567*), to limit the extent of procedures, and to limit the use of local anesthesia containing 1:100,000 epinephrine to two capsules. Anesthesia without a vasoconstrictor might also be selected. The appropriate use of a vasoconstrictor in anesthesia, however, should be weighed against the necessity to maximize anesthesia. Complete history and appropriate referral and consultation with the patient's physician for those patients who are known to be at risk for angina pectoris is recommended.

MYOCARDIAL INFARCTION

Myocardial infarction is the leading cause of death in the United States. It is an acute irreversible ischemic event that produces an area of myocardial necrosis in the heart tissue. If a patient has a previous history of myocardial infarction, he/she may be taking a variety of drugs (ie, antihypertensives, lipid lowering drugs, ACE inhibitors, and antianginal medications) to not only prevent a second infarct, but to treat the long-term associated ischemic heart disease. Postmyocardial infarction patients are often taking anticoagulants such as warfarin and antiplatelet agents such as aspirin. Consultation with the prescribing physician by the dentist is necessary prior to invasive procedures. Temporary dose reduction may allow the dentist to proceed with very invasive procedures. Most procedures, however, can be accomplished without changing the anticoagulant therapy at all, using local hemostasis techniques.

Aspirin *on page 151*
Warfarin *on page 1389*

Thrombolytic drugs, that might dissolve hemostatic plugs, may also be given on a short-term basis immediately following an infarct and include:

Alteplase *on page 88*
Reteplase *on page 1175*
Streptokinase *on page 1238*
Tenecteplase *on page 1268*

Alteplase [tissue plasminogen activator (TPA)] is also currently in use for acute myocardial infarction. Following myocardial infarction and rehabilitation, outpatients may be placed on anticoagulants (such as coumadin), diuretics, beta-adrenergic blockers, ACE inhibitors to reduce blood pressure, and calcium channel blockers. Depending on the presence or absence of continued angina pectoris, patients may also be taking nitrates, beta-blockers, or calcium channel blockers as indicated for treatment of angina.

BETA-ADRENERGIC BLOCKING AGENTS CATEGORIZED ACCORDING TO SPECIFIC PROPERTIES

Alpha-Adrenergic Blocking Activity

Labetalol *on page 791*

Intrinsic Sympathomimetic Activity

Acebutolol *on page 46*
Pindolol *on page 1090*

Long Duration of Action and Fewer CNS Effects

Acebutolol *on page 46*
Atenolol *on page 159*
Betaxolol *on page 202*
Nadolol *on page 956*

Beta$_1$-Receptor Selectivity

Acebutolol *on page 46*
Atenolol *on page 159*
Metoprolol *on page 915*

Nonselective (blocks both beta$_1$- and beta$_2$-receptors)

Betaxolol *on page 202*
Labetalol *on page 791*
Nadolol *on page 956*
Pindolol *on page 1090*
Propranolol *on page 1140*
Timolol *on page 1299*

CARDIOVASCULAR DISEASES *(Continued)*

ARRHYTHMIAS

Abnormal cardiac rhythm can develop spontaneously and survivors of a myocardial infarction are often left with an arrhythmia. An arrhythmia is any alteration or disturbance in the normal rate, rhythm, or conduction through the cardiac tissue. This is known as a cardiac arrhythmia. Abnormalities in rhythm can occur in either the atria or the ventricles. Various valvular deformities, drug effects, and chemical derangements can initiate arrhythmias. These arrhythmias can be a slowing of the heart rate (<60 beats/minute) as defined in bradycardia or tachycardia resulting in a rapid heart beat (usually >150 beats/minute). The dentist will encounter a variety of treatments for management of arrhythmias. Usually, underlying causes such as reduced cardiac output, hypertension, and irregular ventricular beats will require treatment. Pacemaker therapy is also sometimes used. Indwelling pacemakers may require supplementation with antibiotics, and consultation with the physician is certainly appropriate. Sinus tachycardia is often treated with drugs such as:

Propranolol *on page 1140*

Quinidine *on page 1160*

Beta-blockers are often used to slow cardiac rate and diazepam may be helpful when anxiety is a contributing factor in arrhythmia. When atrial flutter and atrial fibrillation are diagnosed, drug therapy is usually required.

Digitoxin *on page 437*

Digoxin *on page 437*

Atrial fibrillation (AF) is an arrhythmia characterized by multiple electrical activations in the atria resulting in scattered and disorganized depolarization and repolarization of the myocardium. Atrial contraction can lead to an irregular and rapid rate of ventricular contraction. The prevalence of atrial fibrillation within the US population ranges between 1% and 4%, with the incidence increasing with age. It is often associated with rheumatic valvular disease and nonvalvular conditions including coronary artery disease and hypertension. Coronary artery disease is present in about one-half of the patients with atrial fibrillation. Atrial fibrillation is a major risk factor for systemic and cerebral embolism. It is thought that thrombi develop as a result of stasis in the dilated left atrium and is dislodged by sudden changes in cardiac rhythm. About 10% of all strokes in patients >60 years of age are caused by atrial fibrillation.

The cornerstones of drug therapy for atrial fibrillation are the restoration and maintenance of a normal sinus rhythm through the use of antiarrhythmic drugs, ventricular rate control through the use of beta-blockers, digitalis drugs or calcium channel blockers, and stroke prevention through the use of anticoagulants.

Antiarrhythmic Drugs

Cardiac rhythm is conducted through the sinoatrial (SA) and atrioventricular (AV) nodes, bundle branches, and Purkinje fibers. Electrical impulses are transmitted within this system by the opening and closing of sodium and potassium channels. Antiarrhythmic drugs are classified by which channel they act upon, a classification known as Vaughan Williams after the author of the published paper. The Class I agents act primarily on sodium channels, and the Class III agents act on potassium channels. In addition, there are subclassifications within the Class I agents according to effects of the drug on conduction and refractoriness within the Purkinje and ventricular tissues. Class IA agents show moderate depression of conduction and prolongation of repolarization. Class IB agents show modest depression of conduction and shortening of repolarization. Class IC agents show marked depression of conduction and mild or no effect on repolarization. Class IA and IC agents are effective in the treatment of atrial fibrillation. Class IB agents (ie, lidocaine, phenytoin) are not used to treat atrial fibrillation, but are effective in treating ventricular arrhythmias. Class II drugs are the beta-adrenergic blocking drugs and Class IV are the calcium channel blockers. Table 2 lists the drugs and the categories used to treat atrial fibrillation.

Table 2.
DRUGS USED IN THE TREATMENT OF ATRIAL FIBRILLATION

Class I Antiarrhythmic Agents
Disopyramide *on page 455*
Flecainide *on page 592*
Moricizine *on page 946*
Procainamide *on page 1124*
Propafenone *on page 1133*
Quinidine *on page 1160*
Class II Antiarrhythmic Agents (Beta-Adrenergic Blockers)
Cardioselective (Beta$_1$-Receptor Block only)
Acebutolol *on page 46*
Atenolol *on page 159*
Betaxolol *on page 202*
Metoprolol *on page 915*
Noncardioselective (Beta$_1$- and Beta$_2$-Receptor Block)
Nadolol *on page 956*
Penbutolol *on page 1055*
Pindolol *on page 1090*
Propranolol *on page 1140*
Timolol *on page 1299*
Class III Antiarrhythmic Agents
Amiodarone *on page 101*
Dofetilide *on page 460*
Ibutilide *on page 731*
Sotalol *on page 1231*
Class IV Antiarrhythmic Agents (Calcium Channel Blockers)
Diltiazem *on page 444*
Verapamil *on page 1373*
Anticoagulant Agents
Aspirin *on page 151*
Warfarin *on page 1389*

Source: USP DI, Volumes I and II, Update, April, 1998.

Restoring and Maintaining Normal Sinus Rhythm

Cardioversion induced by drugs can usually restore sinus rhythm in patients with atrial fibrillation. Class I drugs (moricizine), Class IA drugs (disopyramide, procainamide, quinidine), Class IC drugs (flecainide, propafenone), and Class III antiarrhythmics (amiodarone, sotalol) are all effective in restoring normal sinus rhythm. Success rates may vary greatly and are complicated by the high rate of spontaneous conversion. The drugs used for pharmacologic conversion are also used to maintain sinus rhythm.

Ventricular Rate Control

It is accepted practice to treat patients with medication when the resting ventricular rate is >110 beats/minute. Digoxin, calcium channel blockers, and beta-adrenergic blockers are used in the regulation of ventricular rate. Digoxin increases the vagal tone to the AV node, calcium channel blockers slow the AV nodal conduction, and the beta-adrenergic blocking drugs decrease the sympathetic activation of the AV nodal conduction.

ANTICOAGULANT THERAPY

Over the last thirty years, there has been an increasing use of drugs that relate to the clotting mechanisms in patients. These drugs have included the wide spread use of aspirin as well as an increasing use of anticoagulants found in warfarin as well as synthetic drugs that also have anticoagulation effects. Many patients with ischemic heart disease, atherosclerosis, those with atrial fibrillation and in patients at high risk for stroke, we find the increased use of these anticoagulants. Large numbers of these patients are receiving oral anticoagulation therapy as out patients. The dental clinician is often faced with the decision as to how to manage these patients prior to dental procedures. Key factors regarding the patient receiving anticoagulation therapy include:

- What is the thromboembolytic risk for this patient?
- What is the bleeding risk of the dental procedure planned?
- If an invasive procedure is planned in the face of a high thromboembolytic risk, what is the managing physician's opinion on altering the dosage of anticoagulation therapy?

Often times, to access these factors, consultation with a patient's physician is necessary. However, recent reviews have suggested by Jeske, 2003 and others in our suggested readings list have argued that inappropriate adjustments in anticoagulation therapy create far greater risk for the patient than the risk of hemorrhage during most dental

CARDIOVASCULAR DISEASES *(Continued)*

procedures. Therefore, the scientific evidence does not support changing regimens of anticoagulation therapy in many, perhaps even most instances. However, this decision can only be determined by weighing the factors described above and discussing the situation with the patient's physician.

Table 3.
DRUGS USED TO MANAGE UNSTABLE ANGINA

Drugs
Antiplatelet Drugs
Aspirin *on page 151*
Clopidogrel *on page 361*
Ticlopidine *on page 1297*
Glycoprotein IIb / IIIa Receptor Antagonists
Abciximab *on page 44*
Eptifibatide *on page 503*
Tirofiban *on page 1304*
Antithrombin Drugs
Indirect Thrombin Inhibitors
Heparin (unfractionated) *on page 685*
Low molecular weight heparins
Dalteparin *on page 395*
Enoxaparin *on page 493*
Tinzaparin *on page 1301*
Direct Thrombin Inhibitors
Lepirudin *on page 803*
Argatroban *on page 140*
Dicumarols
Warfarin *on page 1389*
Conventional Antianginal Drugs
Beta-Blockers
Atenolol *on page 159*
Bisoprolol *on page 210*
Carteolol *on page 269*
Nadolol *on page 956*
Propranolol *on page 1140*
Nitrates
Isosorbide Dinitrate *on page 770*
Isosorbide Mononitrate *on page 771*
Nitroglycerin *on page 991*
Calcium Channel Blockers
Diltiazem *on page 444*
Nifedipine *on page 984*
Verapamil *on page 1373*

Evaluating Antiplatelet Response

Partial thromboplastin time and bleeding time (IVY) are appropriate measures for platelet dysfunction. Aspirin, ticlopidine (Ticlid®), and other new drugs, such as Clopidogrel (Plavix®), are actually considered antiplatelet drugs, whereas oral Coumadin® is considered an oral anticoagulant. Aspirin works by inhibiting cyclo-oxygenase which is an enzyme involved in the platelet system associated with clot formation. As little as one aspirin (300 mg dose) can result in an alteration in this enzyme pathway. Although aspirin is cleared from the circulation very quickly (within 15-30 minutes), the effect on the life of the platelet may last up to 7-10 days. Therefore, the clinician planning an extensive invasive procedure on patients with antiplatelet therapy may wish to consider a change prior to one week before the invasive treatment. However, most routine dental procedures can be accomplished with no change in these medications using aggressive local hemostasis efforts and prudent treatment planning.

Evaluating Coumadin® Response

The effects of Coumadin® on the coagulation within patients, occur by way of the vitamin K-dependent clotting mechanism and are generally monitored by measuring the prothrombin time known as the PT. Often to prevent venous thrombosis, a patient will be maintained at approximately 1.5 times their normal prothrombin time. Other anticoagulant goals such as prevention of arterial thromboembolism, as in patients with artificial heart valves, may require 2-2.5 times the normal prothrombin time. It is important for the clinician to obtain not only the accurate PT but also the International Normalized Ratio (INR) for the patient. This ratio is calculated by dividing the patient's PT by the mean normal PT for the laboratory, which is determined by using the International Sensitivity Index (ISI) to adjust for the lab's reagents.

The response to oral anticoagulants varies greatly in patients and should be monitored regularly. The dental clinician planning an invasive procedure should consider not only what the patient can tell them from a historical point-of-view, but also when the last monitoring test was performed. In general, most dental procedures can be performed in patients that are 1.5 times normal or less. Most researchers suggest that 2.5 times normal poses little risk in most dental patients and procedures, but these values may be misleading unless the INR is also determined. When in doubt, the prudent dental clinician would consult with the patient's physician and obtain current prothrombin time and INR in order to evaluate fully and plan for his patients. The clinician is referred to the excellent review: Herman WW, Konzelman JL, and Sutley SH, "Current Perspectives on Dental Patients Receiving Coumadin Anticoagulant Therapy," *J Am Dent Assoc*, 1997, 128:327-35.

Coumadin®-Like Anticoagulants

Dicumarol

Warfarin *on page 1389*

Platelet Aggregation Inhibitors

Aspirin *on page 151*

Clopidogrel *on page 361*

Eptifibatide *on page 503*

Ticlopidine *on page 1297*

Tirofiban *on page 1304*

Anticoagulant, Other

Lepirudin *on page 803*

Antiplatelet Agent

Aspirin and Dipyridamole *on page 156*

Regarding dental management patients that are already taking warfarin, the use of analgesics is implicated as a potential source of drug interaction. In a recent article by Hayek in *JAMA*, it was found that patients taking warfarin for anticoagulation identified the use of dangerously elevated INRs and the fact was discovered that they concomitantly had been taking acetaminophen (not necessarily with their physician's recommendation). The study of the international normalized ratio (INR) in these patients has indicated that additional factors independently influence the INR, as well as the potential interaction with acetaminophen. Potential effects on the INR are greatest in patients taking acetaminophen at high doses over a protracted time period. Short term pain management with acetaminophen poses little risk. These factors included advanced malignancy, patients who did not take their warfarin properly (therefore, took more than was necessary), changes in oral intake of liquids or solids, acute diarrhea leading to dehydration, alcohol consumption, and vitamin K intake. The mechanisms of these augmenting factors for enhancement of the INR are that the cytochrome P450 system, present in the liver, is also affected by changes in metabolism associated with these factors. For instance, the metabolism of alcohol in the liver alters its ability to manage the CYP450 enzyme system necessary for warfarin, therefore, enhancing its presence and potentially increasing the half-life of warfarin. As oral intake of nutrients declines in patients with either diarrhea or reduced intake of liquids and/or solids, absorption of vitamin K is reduced and the vitamin K dependent system of metabolism of warfarin changes, therefore increasing warfarin blood levels. These factors, along with the liver metabolism of acetaminophen, have resulted in the increased concern that patients, who may be taking acetaminophen as an analgesic or for other reasons, may be at risk for enhancing or elevating, inadvertently, their anticoagulation effect of warfarin. The dentist should be aware of this potential interaction in prescribing any drug containing acetaminophen or in recommending that a patient use an analgesic for relief of even mild pain on a prolonged basis. Therefore, the dentist must be concerned with these factors and is referred to the discussion in the Pain Management section *on page 1526* for more consideration (adapted from *JAMA*, March 4, 1998, Vol 279, No 9).

Acetaminophen *on page 47*

Although not used specifically for this purpose, numerous herbal medicines and natural dietary supplements have been associated with inhibition of platelet aggregation or other anticoagulation effects, and therefore may lead to increased bleeding during invasive dental procedures. Current reports include bilberry, bromelain, cat's claw, devil's claw, dong quai, evening primrose, feverfew, garlic (irreversible inhibition), ginger (only at very high doses), ginkgo biloba, ginseng, grape seed, green tea, horse chestnut, and turmeric.

References

Jeske AH, Suchko GD, ADA Council on Scientific Affairs and Division of Science, et al, "Lack of a Scientific Basis for Routine Discontinuation of Oral Anticoagulation Therapy Before Dental Treatment,"*J Am Dent Assoc*, 2003, 134(11):1492-7.

Lockhart PB, Gibson J, Pond SH, et al, "Dental Management Considerations for the Patient With an Acquired Coagulopathy. Part 2: Coagulopathies From Drugs," *Br Dent J*, 2003, 195(9):495-501.

Carter G, Goss AN, Lloyd J, et al, "Current Concepts of the Management of Dental Extractions for Patients Taking Warfarin," *Aust Dent J*, 2003, 48(2):89-96.

Little JW, Miller CS, Henry RG, et al, "Antithrombotic Agents: Implications in Dentistry," *Oral Surg Oral Med Oral Pathol Oral Radiol Endod*, 2002, 93(5):544-51.

CARDIOVASCULAR DISEASES *(Continued)*

HEART FAILURE

Heart failure is a condition in which the heart is unable to pump sufficient blood to meet the needs of the body. It is caused by impaired ability of the cardiac muscle to contract or by an increased workload imposed on the heart. Most frequently, the underlying cause of heart failure is coronary artery disease. Other contributory causes include hypertension, diabetes, idiopathic dilated cardiomyopathy, and valvular heart disease. It is estimated that heart failure affects approximately 5 million Americans. The New York Heart Association functional classification is regarded as the standard measure to describe the severity of a patient's symptom. Class I is characterized by having no limitation of physical activity. There is no dyspnea, fatigue, palpitations, or angina with ordinary physical activity. There is no objective evidence of cardiovascular dysfunction. Class II includes those patients having slight limitation of physical activity. These patients experience fatigue, palpitations, dyspnea, or angina with ordinary physical activity, but are comfortable at rest. There is evidence of minimal cardiovascular dysfunction. Class III is characterized by marked limitation of activity. Less than ordinary physical activity causes fatigue, palpitations, dyspnea, or angina, but patients are comfortable at rest. There is objective evidence of moderately severe cardiovascular dysfunction. Class IV is characterized by the inability to carry out any physical activity without discomfort. Symptoms of heart failure or anginal syndrome may be present even at rest, and any physical activity undertaken increases discomfort. There is objective evidence of severe cardiovascular dysfunction. Drug classes and the specific agents used to treat heart failure are listed in Table 4.

Table 4.
DRUGS USED IN THE TREATMENT OF HEART FAILURE

Angiotensin-Converting Enzyme Inhibitors (ACE)[1]
Benazepril *on page 187*
Captopril *on page 252*
Enalapril *on page 488*
Fosinopril *on page 633*
Lisinopril *on page 833*
Perindopril Ethumine *on page 1068*
Quinapril *on page 1158*
Ramipril *on page 1167*
Trandolapril *on page 1321*
Diuretics
Thiazides
Hydrochlorothiazide *on page 699*
Loop Diuretics
Furosemide *on page 640*
Potassium-Sparing Agents
Spironolactone *on page 1235*
Digitalis Glycosides
Digoxin *on page 437*
Digitoxin *on page 437*
Beta-Adrenergic Receptor Blockers
Bisoprolol *on page 210*
Carvedilol *on page 270*
Metoprolol *on page 915*
Catecholamines
Dobutamine *on page 457*
Dopamine
Supplemental Agents
Direct-Acting Vasodilators
Hydralazine *on page 697*
Nitroglycerin *on page 991*
Nitroprusside *on page 993*
Phosphodiesterase Inhibitors
Inamrinone *on page 743*
Milrinone *on page 930*

[1]Regarded as the cornerstone of treatment of heart failure and should be used routinely and early in all patients.

From USP DI, Volumes I and II, Update, December 1998.

Drug Classes and Specific Agents Used to Treat Heart Failure

Angiotensin-converting enzyme (ACE) inhibitors reduce left ventricular volume and filling pressure while decreasing total peripheral resistance. They induce cardiac output (modestly) and natriuresis. ACE inhibitors are usually used in all patients with heart failure if no contraindication or intolerance exists. This group of drugs is considered the cornerstone of treatment and are used routinely and early if pharmacologic treatment is indicated.

Diuretics increase sodium chloride and water excretion resulting in reduction of preload, thus relieving the symptoms of pulmonary congestion associated with heart failure. They may also reduce myocardial oxygen demand. The thiazides, loop diuretics, and potassium-sparing agents are all useful in reducing preload by way of their diuretic actions.

Digitalis glycosides have been used in the treatment of heart failure for more than 200 years. Digitalis drugs increase cardiac output by a direct positive inotropic action on the myocardium. This increased cardiac output results in decreased venous pressure, reduced heart size, and diminished compensatory tachycardia.

Beta-adrenergic receptor blocking drugs (beta-blockers) are used in the treatment of heart failure because of their beneficial effect in reducing mortality. A meta-analysis of randomized clinical trials showed that the beta-blockers significantly reduced all causes of cardiac-related deaths, with carvedilol (Coreg®) showing the greatest efficacy. The overall risk of death was reduced by over 30%.

Other drugs used in the treatment of heart failure are referred to as supplemental agents. The direct-acting vasodilators reduce excessive vasoconstriction and reduce workload of the failing heart. The catecholamines and phosphodiesterase inhibitors are alternative agents with positive inotropic effects, are effective for short-term therapy, and have not been demonstrated to prolong life during long-term therapy.

Treatment of arrhythmias often can result in oral manifestations including oral ulcerations with drugs such as procainamide, lupus-like lesions, as well as xerostomia.

HYPERTENSION

In the United States, almost 50 million adults, 25-74 years of age, have hypertension. Hypertension is defined as systolic blood pressure ≥140 mm Hg, and/or diastolic pressure >90 mm Hg. People with blood pressure above normal are considered at increased risk of developing damage to the heart, kidney, brain, and eyes, resulting in premature morbidity and mortality.

Recently, the Joint National Committee on Prevention, Detection, Evaluation, and Treatment of High Blood Pressure, released its 7th Report in the summer of 2003. The highlights of the new report are that several of the categories have been renamed to connote changes in philosophy towards earlier treatment and intervention for patients with elevated blood pressure.

Also, there is an increased importance in the elevation of systolic blood pressure for people >50 years of age. The category of high normal blood pressure has now been replaced with the term prehypertension for those patients with systolic blood pressure of 120-139 mm Hg and for those with diastolic blood pressure of 80-89 mm Hg. The remaining stages of hypertension have been broken into simply two categories: Stage 1 and Stage 2. Stage 1 diastolic pressure is 90-99 mm Hg and systolic pressure is 140-159 mm Hg, whereas in Stage 2, diastolic pressure >100 mm Hg or systolic pressure >160 mm Hg are the respective cut-off for treatment decisions. This greatly simplifies the classification of blood pressure.

In addition, the 7th Joint National Committee Report highlights the importance of life style modifications in controlling blood pressure along with pharmacologic intervention. Thiazide diuretics have again been considered one of the most important treatments in uncomplicated hypertension and their benefits of lowering blood pressure have been greatly emphasized. The role of dentistry in detection as well as assisting in compliance for patients, has been clearly emphasized in this report.

The suggested initial goals of drug therapy are the maintenance of an arterial pressure of ≤140/90 mm Hg with concurrent control of other modifiable cardiovascular risk factors. Further reduction to 130/85 mm Hg should be pursued if cardiovascular and cerebrovascular function is not compromised. The Hypertension Optimal Treatment (HOT) randomized trial using patients 50-80 years of age found that the lowest incidence of major cardiovascular events and the lowest risk of cardiovascular mortality occurred at a mean diastolic blood pressure of 82.6 and 86.5 mm Hg respectively.

CARDIOVASCULAR DISEASES *(Continued)*

Table 5. CLASSIFICATION OF BLOOD PRESSURE FOR ADULTS[1]

Category	Systolic (mm Hg[2])		Diastolic (mm Hg)
Normal	<120	and	<80
Prehypertension	120-139	or	80-89
Stage 1 hypertension	140-159	or	90-99
Stage 2 hypertension	≥160	or	≥100

[1]Adapted from U.S. Department of Health and Human Services, National Institutes of Health; National Heart, Lung and Blood Institute; National High Blood Pressure Education Program.

[2]Treatment determined by highest blood pressure category.

Table 6. LIFESTYLE MODIFICATIONS TO MANAGE HYPERTENSION[1-3]

Modification	Recommendation	Approximate Systolic Reduction (Range)
Weight reduction	Maintain normal body weight (body mass index 18.5-24.9 kg/m^2)	5-20 mm of mercury/ 10 kg weight loss[4]
Adopt DASH[5] eating plan	Consume a diet rich in fruits, vegetables, and low fat dairy products with a reduced content of saturated and total fat	8-14 mm Hg[6]
Dietary sodium reduction	Reduce dietary sodium intake to ≤100 mmol/day (2.4 g sodium or 6 g sodium chloride)	2-8 mm Hg[7]
Physical activity	Engage in regular aerobic physical activity such as brisk walking (≥30 minutes/day, most days of the week)	4-9 mm Hg[8]
Moderation of alcohol consumption	Limit consumption to ≤2 drinks (1 oz or 30 mL ethanol); (eg, 24 oz beer, 10 oz wine, or 3 oz 80-proof whiskey) per day in most men and to ≤1 drink/day in women and lighter weight people	2-4 mm Hg[9]

[1]Adapted from U.S. Department of Health and Human Services; National Institutes of Health; National Heart, Lung, and Blood Institute; National High Blood Pressure Education Program

[2]Overall cardiovascular risk education can be achieved by cessation of smoking

[3]The effects of implementing these modifications are dose- and time-dependent and could be greater for some people

[4]The trials of Hypertension Prevention Collaborative Research Group; He and colleagues

[5]DASH: Dietary Approaches to Stop Hypertension

[6]Sacks and colleagues; Vollmer and colleagues

[7]Sacks and colleagues; Vollmer and colleagues; Chobanian and Hill

[8]Kelley and Kelley; Whelton and colleagues

[9]Xin and colleagues

CLASSES OF DRUGS USED IN THE TREATMENT OF HYPERTENSION

- Diuretics
- Beta-adrenergic receptor blocking agents (beta-blockers)
- Alpha$_1$-adrenergic receptor blocking agents (alpha$_1$-blockers)
- Agents which have both alpha- and beta-adrenergic blocking properties (alpha-/beta-blockers)
- Angiotensin-converting enzyme (ACE) inhibitors
- Angiotensin II receptor blockers
- Calcium channel blocking agents
- Supplemental agents such as central-acting alpha$_2$-adrenergic receptor agonists and direct-acting peripheral vasodilators.

Table 7 lists the drug categories and representative agents used to treat hypertension. Combination drugs are now available to supply several classes of these drugs.

Table 7.
DRUG CATEGORIES AND REPRESENTATIVE AGENTS USED IN THE TREATMENT OF HYPERTENSION[1]

Diuretics

Thiazide Types

- Bendroflumethiazide *on page 189*
- Chlorothiazide *on page 312*
- Chlorthalidone *on page 321*
- Hydrochlorothiazide *on page 699*
- Indapamide *on page 743*
- Methyclothiazide *on page 905*
- Metolazone *on page 914*
- Polythiazide *on page 1102*
- Trichlormethiazide *on page 1337*

Loops

- Bumetanide *on page 224*
- Ethacrynic Acid *on page 533*
- Furosemide *on page 640*
- Torsemide *on page 1317*

Potassium-Sparing

- Amiloride *on page 95*
- Spironolactone *on page 1235*
- Triamterene *on page 1334*

Potassium-Sparing Combinations

- Hydrochlorothiazide and Spironolactone *on page 701*
- Hydrochlorothiazide and Triamterene *on page 701*

Beta-Blockers

Cardioselective

- Acebutolol *on page 46*
- Atenolol *on page 159*
- Betaxolol *on page 202*
- Bisoprolol *on page 210*
- Metoprolol *on page 915*
- Sotalol *on page 1231*

Noncardioselective

- Carteolol *on page 269*
- Carvedilol *on page 270*
- Nadolol *on page 956*
- Penbutolol *on page 1055*
- Pindolol *on page 1090*
- Propranolol *on page 1140*
- Timolol *on page 1299*

Alpha$_1$-Blocker

- Doxazosin *on page 465*
- Guanadrel *on page 678*
- Prazosin *on page 1111*
- Reserpine *on page 1174*
- Terazosin *on page 1271*

Alpha- / Beta-Blocker

- Carvedilol *on page 270*
- Labetalol *on page 791*

Angiotensin-Converting Enzyme (ACE) Inhibitors

- Benazepril *on page 187*
- Captopril *on page 252*
- Enalapril *on page 488*
- Fosinopril *on page 633*
- Lisinopril *on page 833*
- Moexipril *on page 940*
- Quinapril *on page 1158*
- Ramipril *on page 1167*
- Trandolapril *on page 1321*

Angiotensin-Converting Enzyme (ACE) Inhibitor / Diuretic Combination

- Captopril and Hydrochlorothiazide *on page 255*
- Enalapril and Hydrochlorothiazide *on page 491*
- Lisinopril and Hydrochlorothiazide *on page 834*

Angiotensin II Receptor Blockers

- Candesartan *on page 248*
- Eprosartan *on page 501*
- Irbesartan *on page 763*
- Losartan *on page 845*
- Telmisartan *on page 1265*
- Valsartan *on page 1363*

CARDIOVASCULAR DISEASES *(Continued)*

(continued)

Angiotensin II Receptor Blocker / Diuretic Combination
Candesartan + HCTZ *on page 248*
Irbesartan + HCTZ *on page 248*
Valsartan/HCTZ + HCTZ *on page 1364*
Calcium Channel Blockers
Amlodipine *on page 108*
Bepridil *on page 197*
Diltiazem *on page 444*
Felodipine *on page 576*
Isradipine *on page 774*
Nicardipine *on page 980*
Nifedipine *on page 984*
Nisoldipine *on page 988*
Verapamil *on page 1373*
Supplemental Agents
Central-Acting Alpha$_2$-Agonist
Clonidine *on page 358*
Guanabenz *on page 677*
Guanfacine *on page 679*
Methyldopa *on page 906*
Direct-Acting Peripheral Vasodilator
Hydralazine *on page 697*
Minoxidil *on page 934*

[1]Source: USP DI, Volumes I and II, Update, November 1998.

Current Thinking Regarding Antihypertensive Drug Selection

Medications in the first eight categories in Table 7 were held to be equally effective in two large-scale studies reported in the *New England Journal of Medicine* and the *Journal of the American Medical Association*, and that any of the medications could be used initially for monotherapy. According to the Seventh Report of the Joint National Committee on Prevention, Detection, Evaluation, and Treatment of High Blood Pressure (JNC VI), diuretics or beta-blockers are recommended as initial therapy for uncomplicated hypertension. If a diuretic is selected as initial therapy, a thiazide diuretic is preferred in patients with normal renal function. If necessary, potassium replacement or concurrent treatment with a potassium-sparing agent may prevent hypokalemia. Loop diuretics are used in patients with impaired renal function or who cannot tolerate thiazides. Diuretics are well tolerated and inexpensive. They are considered the drugs of choice for treating isolated systolic hypertension in the elderly.

Beta-blockers are the agents of choice in patients with coronary artery disease or supraventricular arrhythmia, and in young patients with hyperdynamic circulation. Beta-blockers are alternatives for initial therapy and are more effective in Caucasian patients than in African-American patients. Beta-blockers are not considered first choice drugs in elderly patients with uncomplicated hypertension. The beta-blocking drug carvedilol also selectively blocks alpha$_1$ receptors and has been shown to reduce mortality in hypertensive patients.

Alpha$_1$-adrenergic blocking agents can be used as initial therapy. The alpha$_1$-blocking agent prazosin and related drugs have an added advantage in treating hypertensive patients with coexisting hyperlipidemia since these medications seem to have beneficial effects on lipid levels. Selective blockade of the post-synaptic alpha$_1$-receptors by prazosin and related agents reduces peripheral vascular resistance and systemic blood pressure. In addition, all alpha$_1$-adrenergic blocking agents relieve symptoms of benign prostatic hyperplasia.

ACE inhibitors are the preferred drugs for patients with coexisting heart failure. They are useful as initial therapy in hypertensive patients with kidney damage or diabetes mellitus with proteinuria, and in Caucasian patients. No clinically relevant differences have been found among the available ACE inhibitors. The ACE inhibitors are well tolerated by young, physically active patients, and the elderly. The most common adverse effect of the ACE inhibitors is dry cough. Angiotensin II receptor blockers produce hemodynamic effects similar to ACE inhibitors while avoiding dry cough. These agents are similar to the ACE inhibitors in potency and are useful for initial therapy.

Calcium channel blocking agents are effective as initial therapy in both African-American and Caucasian patients, and are well tolerated by the elderly. These agents inhibit entry of calcium ion into cardiac cells and smooth muscle cells of the coronary and systemic vasculature. Nifedipine (Procardia®) and amlodipine (Norvasc®) are more potent as peripheral vasodilators than diltiazem (Cardizem®). Long-acting formulations of the calcium channel blockers have been shown to be very safe despite some earlier reports that short-acting calcium channel blockers were associated with a 60% increase in heart attacks among hypertensive patients given a short-acting calcium antagonist.

Supplemental antihypertensive agents include the central-acting alpha$_2$ agonists and direct-acting vasodilators. These agents are less commonly prescribed for initial therapy because of the impressive effectiveness of the other drug groups. Clonidine (Catapres®) lowers blood pressure by activating inhibitory alpha$_2$ receptors in the CNS, thus reducing sympathetic outflow. It lowers both supine and standing blood pressure by reducing total peripheral resistance. Hydralazine (Apresoline®) reduces blood pressure by directly relaxing arteriolar smooth muscle. Hydralazine is given orally for the management of chronic hypertension, usually with a diuretic and a beta-blocker.

The most common oral side effects of the management of the hypertensive patient are related to the antihypertensive drug therapy. A dry sore mouth can be caused by diuretics and central-acting adrenergic inhibitors. Occasionally, lichenoid reactions can occur in patients taking quinidine and methyldopa. The thiazides are occasionally also implicated. Lupus-like face rashes can be seen in patients taking calcium channel blockers as well as documented in Calcium Channel Blockers & Gingival Hyperplasia *on page 1600* of the Appendix.

Table 8.
CARDIOVASCULAR / RESPIRATORY / NERVOUS SYSTEM EFFECTS CAUSED BY DRUGS USED FOR CARDIOVASCULAR DISORDERS[1]

Agent	Incidence	Adverse Effect
Alpha$_1$-Blocker		
Prazosin (Minipress®)	*More frequent* *Less frequent* *Rare*	Orthostatic hypotension, dizziness Heart Palpitations Angina
Alpha- / Beta-Blocker		
Carvedilol (Coreg®)	*More frequent* *Rare*	Bradycardia, postural hypotension, dizziness A-V block, hypertension, hypotension, palpitations, vertigo, nervousness, asthma
Angiotensin-Converting Enzyme (ACE) Inhibitors		
Benazepril (Lotensin®)	*Less frequent* *Rare*	Dizziness, insomnia, headache Hypotension, bronchitis
Captopril (Capoten®)	*Less frequent* *Rare*	Tachycardia, insomnia, transient cough, dizziness, headache Hypotension
Enalapril (Vasotec®)	*Less frequent* *Rare*	Chest pain, palpitations, tachycardia, syncope, dizziness, dyspnea Angina pectoris, asthma
Fosinopril (Monopril®)	*Less frequent* *Rare*	Orthostatic hypotension, dizziness, cough, headache Syncope, insomnia
Lisinopril (Prinivil®)	*Less frequent* *Rare*	Hypotension, dizziness Angina pectoris, orthostatic hypotension, rhythm disturbances, tachycardia
Moexipril (Univasc®)	*Less frequent* *Rare*	Hypotension, peripheral edema, headache, dizziness, fatigue, cough, pharyngitis, upper respiratory infection, sinusitis Chest pain, myocardial infarction, palpitations, arrhythmias, syncope, CVA, orthostatic hypotension, dyspnea, bronchospasm
Perindopril Erbumine (Aceon®)	*Less frequent* *Rare*	Headache, dizziness, cough[2] Hypotension
Quinapril (Accupril®)	*Less frequent* *Rare*	Hypotension, dizziness, headache, cough Orthostatic hypotension, angina, insomnia
Ramipril (Altace®)	*Less frequent* *Rare*	Tachycardia, dizziness, headache, cough Hypotension
Trandolapril (Mavrik®)	*Less frequent* *Rare*	Tachycardia, headache, dizziness, cough[3] Hypotension
Angiotensin-Converting Enzyme Inhibitor / Diuretic Combination		
Captopril/HCTZ (Capozide®)	*Less frequent* *Rare*	Tachycardia, palpitations, chest pain, dizziness Hypotension
Angiotensin II Receptor Blockers		
Candesartan (Atacand®)	*Less frequent* *Rare*	Chest pain, flushing Myocardial infarction, tachycardia, angina, palpitations, dyspnea
Losartan (Cozaar®)	*Less frequent* *Rare*	Hypotension without reflex tachycardia, dizziness Orthostatic hypotension, angina, A-V block (second degree), CVA, palpitations, tachycardia, sinus bradycardia, flushing, dyspnea
Angiotensin II Receptor Blocker / Diuretic Combination		
Candesartan (Atacand HCT™) + HCTZ	*Less frequent* *Rare*	Chest pain, flushing Myocardial infarction, tachycardia, angina, palpitations, dyspnea
Irbesartan/HCTZ (Avalide®)		Effects unavailable
Valsartan/HCTZ (Diovan HCT®)		Effects unavailable

CARDIOVASCULAR DISEASES *(Continued)*

Agent	Incidence	Adverse Effect
Antiplatelet / Anticoagulant Agents		
Abciximab (ReoPro®)	*More frequent* *Less frequent*	Hypotension, pain Bradycardia
Aspirin	*Less frequent or Rare*	Anaphylactoid reaction, bronchospastic allergic reaction
Clopidogrel (Plavix®)	*Less frequent*	Chest pain, edema, hypertension, headache, dizziness, depression, fatigue, dyspnea, rhinitis, bronchitis, coughing, upper respiratory infection, syncope, palpitations, cardiac failure, paresthesia, vertigo, atrial fibrillation, neuralgia
Eptifibatide (Integrilin®)	*More frequent*	Hypotension, bleeding
Ticlopidine (Ticlid®)	*Less frequent* *Rare*	Dizziness Peripheral neuropathy, angioedema, vasculitis, allergic pneumonitis
Tirofiban (Aggrastat®)	*More frequent* *Less frequent*	Bleeding Bradycardia, dizziness, headache
Warfarin (Coumadin®)	*Less frequent* *Rare*	Hemoptysis Fever, purple toes syndrome
Beta-Blockers		
Acebutolol (Sectral®)	*Less frequent* *Rare*	Chest pain, bradycardia, hypotension, dizziness, dyspepsia, dyspnea Ventricular arrhythmias
Atenolol (Tenormin®)	*Less frequent* *Rare*	Bradycardia, hypotension, chest pain, dizziness, dyspepsia, dyspnea Ventricular arrhythmias
Betaxolol (Kerlone®)	*Less frequent* *Rare*	Bradycardia, palpitations, dizziness Chest pain
Bisoprolol (Zebeta®)	*More frequent* *Less frequent*	Lethargy Hypotension, chest pain, bradycardia, headache, dizziness, insomnia, cough
Labetalol (Normodyne®, Trandate®)	*Less frequent* *Rare*	Orthostatic hypotension, dizziness, nasal congestion Bradycardia, chest pain
Metoprolol (Lopressor®)	*More frequent* *Less frequent* *Rare*	Dizziness Bradycardia, heartburn, wheezing Chest pain, confusion
Nadolol (Corgard®)	*More frequent* *Less frequent* *Rare*	Bradycardia Dizziness, dyspepsia, wheezing Congestive heart failure, orthostatic hypotension, confusion, paresthesia
Penbutolol (Levatol®)	*Less frequent* *Rare*	Congestive heart failure, dizziness Bradycardia, chest pain, hypotension, confusion
Pindolol (Visken®)	*More frequent* *Less frequent*	Dizziness Congestive heart failure, dyspnea
Propranolol (Inderal®)	*More frequent* *Less frequent* *Rare*	Bradycardia Congestive heart failure, dizziness, wheezing Chest pain, hypotension, bronchospasm
Timolol (Blocadren®)	*Less frequent* *Rare*	Bradycardia, dizziness, dyspnea Chest pain, congestive heart failure
Calcium Channel Blockers		
Amlodipine (Norvasc®)	*Less frequent* *Rare*	Palpitations, dizziness, dyspnea Hypotension, bradycardia, arrhythmias
Diltiazem (Cardizem®)	*Less frequent* *Rare*	Bradycardia, dizziness Dyspepsia, paresthesia, tremor
Nifedipine (Procardia®)	*More frequent* *Less frequent* *Rare*	Flushing, dizziness Palpitations, hypotension, dyspnea Tachycardia, syncope
Verapamil (Calan®)	*Less frequent* *Rare*	Bradycardia, congestive heart failure, hypotension Chest pain, hypotension (excessive)
Class I Antiarrhythmics		
Disopyramide (Norpace®)	*More frequent* *Less frequent* *Rare*	Exacerbation of angina pectoris, dizziness Hypotension, hypertension, tachycardia, dyspnea Syncope, flushing, hyperventilation
Flecainide (Tambocor™)	*More frequent* *Less frequent* *Rare*	Dizziness, dyspnea Palpitations, chest pain, tachycardia, tremor Bradycardia, nervousness, paresthesia
Procainimide (Pronestyl®)	*Less frequent* *Rare*	Tachycardia, dizziness, lightheadedness Hypotension, confusion, disorientation
Propafenone (Rythmol®)	*More frequent* *Less frequent* *Rare*	Dizziness Palpitations, angina, bradycardia, loss of balance, dyspepsia, dyspnea Paresthesia
Quinidine (Quinaglute®)	*Less frequent* *Rare*	Hypotension, syncope, lightheadedness, wheezing Confusion, vertigo, angina, edema

Agent	Incidence	Adverse Effect
Class III Antiarrhythmics		
Amiodarone (Cordarone®)	*More frequent*	Dizziness, tremor, paresthesia, dyspnea
	Less frequent	Congestive heart failure, bradycardia, tachycardia
	Rare	Hypotension
Sotalol (Betapace®)	*More frequent*	Bradycardia, chest pain, palpitations, fatigue, dizziness, lightheadedness, dyspnea
	Less frequent	CHF, hypotension, proarrhythmia, syncope, reduced peripheral circulation, edema, asthma, upper respiratory problems
	Rare	Diaphoresis, clouded sensorium, fever, lack of coordination
Digitalis Glycosides		
Digoxin (Lanoxicaps®, Lanoxin®) Digitoxin	*Rare*	Atrial tachycardia, sinus bradycardia, ventricular fibrillation, vertigo
Diuretics		
Thiazide type	*Rare*	Hypotension
Loops	*More frequent*	Orthostatic hypotension, dizziness
Potassium-sparing	*Less frequent*	Hypotension, bradycardia, dizziness
	Rare	Flushing
Potassium-sparing combination	*Rare*	Dizziness
HMG-CoA Reductase Inhibitors		
Atorvastatin Fluvastatin Lovastatin Pravastatin Simvastatin	*Less frequent*	Headache, dizziness
Nitrates		
Nitroglycerins	*More frequent*	Postural hypotension, flushing, headache, dizziness
	Rare	Reflex tachycardia, bradycardia, arrhythmia
Supplemental Drugs for Heart Failure		
Inamrinone	*Less frequent*	Arrhythmia, chest pain
Dobutamine (Dobutrex®)	*Less frequent*	Tachycardia, chest pain
	Rare	Headache, dyspnea
Hydralazine	*More frequent*	Tachycardia, headache
	Less frequent	Hypotension, nasal congestion
	Rare	Edema, dizziness
Milrinone (Primacor®)	*More frequent*	Arrhythmias
	Less frequent	Chest pain
Nitroprusside sodium (Nitropress®)	*Less frequent*	Palpitations, headache
Supplemental Drugs for Hypertension		
Central-Acting Alpha$_2$-Agonists		
Clonidine (Catapres®)	*More frequent*	Dizziness
	Less frequent	Orthostatic hypotension, nervousness/agitation
	Rare	Palpitations, tachycardia, bradycardia, congestive heart failure
Direct-Acting		
Hydralazine	*More frequent*	Tachycardia, headache
	Less frequent	Hypotension, nasal congestion
	Rare	Edema, dizziness

Legend: % of incidence: More frequent = >10%, less frequent = 1% to 10%, rare = <1%.

[1]Source: Professional package insert for individual agents or United States Pharmacopeial Dispensing Information. *Drug Information for the Health Care Professional*, Vol I, 19th ed, Rockville, MD: The United States Pharmacopeial Convention, Inc, 1999.

[2]Incidence greater in women 3:1.

[3]More frequent in women.

CARDIOVASCULAR DISEASES *(Continued)*

Table 9. CARDIOVASCULAR DRUGS DENTAL DRUG INTERACTIONS AND EFFECTS ON DENTAL TREATMENT

Alpha$_1$-Blocker	
Prazosin (Minipress®)	Significant orthostatic hypotension a possibility; monitor patient when getting out of dental chair; significant dry mouth in up to 10% of patients.
Alpha- / Beta-Blocker	
Carvedilol (Coreg®)	See Nonselective Beta-Blockers
ACE Inhibitors	The NSAID indomethacin reduces the hypotensive effects of ACE inhibitors. Effects of other NSAIDs such as ibuprofen not considered significant.
Angiotensin-Converting Enzyme Inhibitor / Diuretic Combination	
Captopril/HCTZ (Capozide®)	No effect or complications on dental treatment reported.
Angiotensin II Receptor Blockers	
Candesartan (Atacand®)	No effect or complications on dental treatment reported.
Losartan (Cozaar®)	
Antiplatelet / Anticoagulant Agents	
Aspirin	May cause a reduction in the serum levels of NSAIDs if they are used to manage post-operative pain.
Clopidogrel (Plavix®)	If a patient is to undergo elective surgery and an antiplatelet effect is not desired, clopidogrel should be discontinued 7 days prior to surgery.
Eptifibatide (Integrilin®)	Bleeding may occur while patient is medicated with eptifibatide; platelet function is restored in about 4 hours following discontinuation.
Warfarin (Coumadin®)	Signs of warfarin overdose may first appear as bleeding from gingival tissue; consultation with prescribing physician is advisable prior to surgery to determine temporary dose reduction or withdrawal of medication.
Beta-Blockers	
Cardioselective	Cardioselective beta-blockers (ie, atenolol) have no effect or complications on dental treatment reported.
Noncardioselective	Any of the noncardioselective beta-blockers (ie, nadolol, penbutolol, pindolol, propranolol, timolol) may enhance the pressor response to vasoconstrictor epinephrine resulting in hypertension and reflex bradycardia. Although not reported, it is assumed that similar effects could be caused with levonordefrin (Neo-Cobefrin®). Use either vasoconstrictor with caution in hypertensive patients medicated with noncardioselective beta-adrenergic blockers.
Calcium Channel Blockers	Cause gingival hyperplasia in approximately 1% of the general population taking these drugs. There have been fewer reports with diltiazem and amlodipine than with other CBs such as nifedipine. The hyperplasia will usually disappear with cessation of drug therapy. Consultation with the physician is suggested
Class I Antiarrhythmics	
Disopyramide (Norpace®)	Increased serum levels and toxicity with erythromycin. High incidence of anticholinergic effect manifested as dry mouth and throat.
Flecainide (Tambocor™)	No effects or complications on dental treatment reported.
Procainimide (Pronestyl®)	Systemic lupus-like syndrome has been reported resulting in joint pain and swelling, pains with breathing, skin rash.
Propafenone (Rythmol®)	Greater than 10 % experience significantly reduced salivary flow; taste disturbance, bitter or metallic taste
Quinidine (Quinaglute®)	Secondary anticholinergic effects may decrease salivary flow, especially in middle-aged and elderly patients; known to contribute to caries, periodontal disease, and oral candidiasis.
Class III Antiarrhythmics	
Amiodarone	Bitter or metallic taste has been reported.
Digitalis Glycosides	Use vasoconstrictor with caution due to risk of cardiac arrhythmias. Sensitive gag reflex induced by digitalis drugs may cause difficulty in taking dental impressions.
Diuretics	
Thiazide type	No effects or complications on dental treatment reported.
Loops	NSAIDs may increase chloride and tubular water reuptake to counter-act loop type diuretics.
Potassium-sparing	No effects or complications on dental treatment reported.
Potassium-sparing combination	No effects or complications on dental treatment reported.

HMG-CoA Reductase Inhibitors	Concurrent use of erythromycin, clarithromycin, and some of the statin drugs may result in rhabdomyolysis.
Nitrates	No effects or complications on dental treatment reported.
Supplemental Drugs for Heart Failure	
Inamrinone Milrinone (Primacor®)	No effects or complications on dental treatment reported
Supplemental Drugs for Hypertension	
Central-Acting Alpha$_2$-Agonists	
Clonidine (Catapres®)	Greater than 10% of patients experience significant dry mouth.
Direct-Acting	
Hydralazine	No effect or complications on dental treatment reported.

References

Chobanian AV, Bakris GL, Black HR, et al, "The Seventh Report of the Joint National Committee on Prevention, Detection, Evaluation, and Treatment of High Blood Pressure: The JNC 7 Report," *JAMA*, 2003, 289(19):2560-72.

Chobanian AV and Hill M, "National Heart, Lung, and Blood Institute Workshop on Sodium and Blood Pressure: A Critical Review of Current Scientific Evidence," *Hypertension*, 2000, 35(4):858-63.

"Effects of Weight Loss and Sodium Reduction Intervention on Blood Pressure and Hypertension Incidence in Overweight People With High-Normal Blood Pressure. The Trials of Hypertension Prevention, Phase II. The Trials of Hypertension Prevention Collaborative Research Group," *Arch Intern Med*, 1997, 157(6):657-67.

He J, Whelton PK, Appel LJ, et al, "Long-Term Effects of Weight Loss and Dietary Sodium Reduction on Incidence of Hypertension," *Hypertension*, 2000, 35(2):544-9.

Kelley GA and Kelley KS, "Progressive Resistance Exercise and Resting Blood Pressure: A Meta-Analysis of Randomized Controlled Trials," *Hypertension*, 2000, 35(3):838-43.

Sacks FM, Svetkey LP, Vollmer WM, et al, "Effects on Blood Pressure of Reduced Dietary Sodium and the Dietary Approaches to Stop Hypertension (DASH) Diet. DASH-Sodium Collaborative Research Group," *N Engl J Med*, 2001, 344(1):3-10.

Vollmer WM, Sacks FM, Ard J, et al, "Effects of Diet and Sodium Intake on Blood Pressure: Subgroup Analysis of the DASH-Sodium Trial," *Ann Intern Med*, 2001, 135(12):1019-28.

Whelton SP, Chin A, Xin X, et al, "Effect of Aerobic Exercise on Blood Pressure: A Meta-Analysis of Randomized, Controlled Trials," *Ann Intern Med*, 2002, 136(7):493-503.

Xin X, He J, Frontini MG, et al, "Effects of Alcohol Reduction on Blood Pressure: A Meta-Analysis of Randomized Controlled Trials," *Hypertension*, 2001, 38(5):1112-7.

GASTROINTESTINAL DISORDERS

The oral cavity and related structures comprise the first part of the gastrointestinal tract. Diseases affecting the oral cavity are often reflected in GI disturbances. In addition, the oral cavity may indeed reflect diseases of the GI tract, including ulcers, polyps, and liver and gallbladder diseases. The first oral condition that may reflect or be reflected in GI disturbances is that of taste. Typically, complaints of taste abnormalities are presented to the dentist. The sweet, saline, sour, and bitter taste sensations all vary in quality and intensity and are affected by the olfactory system. Often, anemic conditions are reflected in changes in the tongue, resulting in taste aberrations.

Gastric and duodenal ulcers represent the primary diseases that can reflect themselves in the oral cavity. Gastric reflux and problems with food metabolism often present as acid erosions to the teeth and occasionally, changes in the mucosal surface as well. Patients may be encountered that may be identified, upon diagnosis, as harboring the organism *Helicobacter pylori.* Treatment with antibiotics can oftentimes aid in correcting the ulcerative disease.

Proton Pump and Gastric Acid Secretion Inhibitors

Lansoprazole *on page 797*

Lansoprazole, Amoxicillin, and Clarithromycin *on page 798*

Lansoprazole and Naproxen *on page 799*

Omeprazole *on page 1012*

Pantaprazole *on page 1043*

Histamine H_2 Antagonist

Cimetidine *on page 330*

Famotidine *on page 573*

Nizatidine *on page 995*

Ranitidine *on page 1169*

The oral aspects of gastrointestinal disease are often nonspecific and are related to the patient's gastric reflux problems. Intestinal polyps occasionally present as part of the "Peutz-Jeghers Syndrome", resulting in pigmented areas of the peri-oral region that resemble freckles. The astute dentist will need to differentiate these from melanin pigmentation, while at the same time encouraging the patient to perhaps seek evaluation for an intestinal disorder.

Diseases of the liver and gallbladder system are complex. Most of the disorders that the dentist is interested in are covered in the section on systemic viral disease *on page 1519.* All of the new drugs, including interferons, are mentioned in this section.

Multiple Drug Regimens for the Treatment of *H. pylori* Infection

Drug	Dosages	Duration of Therapy
H_2-receptor antagonist[1]	Any one given at appropriate dose	4 weeks
plus		
Bismuth *on page 209*	525 mg 4 times/day	2 weeks
plus		
Metronidazole *on page 917*	250 mg 4 times/day	2 weeks
plus		
Tetracycline *on page 1280*	500 mg 4 times/day	2 weeks
Proton pump inhibitor[1]	Esomeprazole 40 mg once daily	10 days
plus		
Clarithromycin *on page 343*	500 mg twice daily	10 days
plus		
Amoxicillin *on page 114*	1000 mg twice daily	10 days
Proton pump inhibitor[1]	Lansoprazole 30 mg twice daily or Omeprazole 20 mg twice daily	10-14 days
plus		
Clarithromycin *on page 343*	500 mg twice daily	10-14 days
plus		
Amoxicillin *on page 114*	1000 mg twice daily	10-14 days
Proton pump inhibitor[1]	Rabeprazole 20 mg twice daily	7 days
plus		
Clarithromycin *on page 343*	500 mg twice daily	7 days
plus		
Amoxicillin *on page 114*	1000 mg twice daily	7 days
Proton pump inhibitor	Lansoprazole 30 mg twice daily or Omeprazole 20 mg twice daily	2 weeks
plus		
Clarithromycin *on page 343*	500 mg twice daily	2 weeks
plus		
Metronidazole *on page 917*	500 mg twice daily	2 weeks
Proton pump inhibitor	Lansoprazole 30 mg once daily or Omeprazole 20 mg once daily	2 weeks
plus		
Bismuth *on page 209*	525 mg 4 times/day	2 weeks
plus		
Metronidazole *on page 917*	500 mg 3 times/day	2 weeks
plus		
Tetracycline *on page 1280*	500 mg 4 times/day	2 weeks

[1]FDA-approved regimen

Modified from Howden CS and Hunt RH, "Guidelines for the Management of *Helicobacter pylori* Infection," *AJG*, 1998, 93:2336.

RESPIRATORY DISEASES

Diseases of the respiratory system put dental patients at increased risk in the dental office because of their decreased pulmonary reserve, the medications they may be taking, drug interactions between these medications, medications the dentist may prescribe, and in some patients with infectious respiratory diseases, a risk of disease transmission.

The respiratory system consists of the nasal cavity, the nasopharynx, the trachea, and the components of the lung including, of course, the bronchi, the bronchioles, and the alveoli. The diseases that affect the lungs and the respiratory system can be separated by location of affected tissue. Diseases that affect the lower respiratory tract are often chronic, although infections can also occur. Three major diseases that affect the lower respiratory tract are often encountered in the medical history for dental patients. These include chronic bronchitis, emphysema, and asthma. Diseases that affect the upper respiratory tract are usually of the infectious nature and include sinusitis and the common cold. The upper respiratory tract infections may also include a wide variety of nonspecific infections, most of which are also caused by viruses. Influenza produces upper respiratory type symptoms and is often caused by orthomyxoviruses. Herpangina is caused by the Coxsackie type viruses and results in upper respiratory infections in addition to pharyngitis or sore throat. One serious condition, known as croup, has been associated with *Haemophilus influenzae* infections. Other more serious infections might include respiratory syncytial virus, adenoviruses, and parainfluenza viruses.

The respiratory symptoms that are often encountered in both upper respiratory and lower respiratory disorders include cough, dyspnea (difficulty in breathing), the production of sputum, hemoptysis (coughing up blood), a wheeze, and occasionally chest pain. One additional symptom, orthopnea (difficulty in breathing when lying down), is often used by the dentist to assist in evaluating the patient with the condition, pulmonary edema. This condition results from either respiratory disease or congestive heart failure.

No effective drug treatments are available for the management of many of the upper respiratory tract viral infections. However, amantadine (sold under the brand name Symmetrel®) is a synthetic drug given orally (200 mg/day) and has been found to be effective against some strains of influenza. Treatment other than for influenza includes supportive care products, available over-the-counter. These might include antihistamines for symptomatic relief of the upper respiratory congestion, antibiotics to combat secondary bacterial infections, and in severe cases, fluids, when patients have become dehydrated during the illness (see Pharmacologic Category Index for selection). The treatment of herpangina may include management of the painful ulcerations of the oropharynx. The dentist may become involved in managing these lesions in a similar way to those seen in other acute viral infections (see Systemic Viral Diseases *on page 1519*).

SINUSITIS

Sinusitis also represents an upper respiratory infection that often comes under the purview of the practicing dentist. Acute sinusitis, characterized by nasal obstruction, fever, chills, and midface head pain, may be encountered by the dentist and discovered as part of a differential workup for other facial or dental pain. Chronic sinusitis may likewise produce similar dental symptoms. Dental drugs of choice may include ephedrine or nasal drops, antihistamines, and analgesics. These drugs sometimes require supplementation with antibiotics. Most commonly, broad spectrum antibiotics such as ampicillin are prescribed. These are often combined with antral lavage to re-establish drainage from the sinus area. Surgical intervention, such as a Caldwell-Luc procedure opening into the sinus, is rarely necessary and many of the second generation antibiotics, such as cephalosporins, are used successfully in treating the acute and chronic sinusitis patient (see "Antibiotic Prophylaxis" *on page 1509*).

Gatifloxacin *on page 647*
Moxifloxacin *on page 949*

LOWER RESPIRATORY DISEASES

Lower respiratory tract diseases, including asthma, chronic bronchitis, and emphysema are often identified in dental patients. Asthma is an intermittent respiratory disorder that produces recurrent bronchial smooth muscle spasm, inflammation of the bronchial mucosa, and hypersecretion of mucus. The incidence of childhood asthma appears to be increasing and may be related to the presence of pollutants such as sulfur dioxide and indoor cigarette smoke. The end result is widespread narrowing of the airways and decreased ventilation with increased airway resistance, especially to expiration. Asthmatic patients often suffer from asthmatic attacks when stimulated by respiratory tract infections, exercise, and cold air. Medications such as aspirin and some NSAIDs, as well as cholinergic and beta-adrenergic blocking drugs, can also trigger asthmatic attacks in addition to chemicals, smoke, and emotional anxiety.

The classical chronic obstructive pulmonary diseases (COPD) of chronic bronchitis and emphysema are both characterized by chronic airflow obstructions during normal ventilatory efforts. They often occur in combination in the same patient and their treatment is similar. One common finding is that the patient is often a smoker. The dentist can play a role in reinforcement of smoking cessation in patients with chronic respiratory diseases.

Treatments include a variety of drugs depending on the severity of the symptoms and the respiratory compromise upon full respiratory evaluation. Patients who are having acute and chronic obstructive pulmonary attacks may be susceptible to infection and antibiotics such as penicillin, ampicillin, tetracycline, or sulfamethoxazole-trimethoprim are often used to eradicate susceptible infective organisms. Corticosteroids, as well as a wide variety of respiratory stimulants, are available in inhalant and/or oral forms. In patients using inhalant medication, oral candidiasis is occasionally encountered.

Amantadine *on page 92*
Analgesics *on page 1660*
Antibiotics *on page 1662*
Antihistamines *on page 1666*
Decongestants *on page 1672*
Epinephrine *on page 496*
Gatifloxacin *on page 647*
Moxifloxacin *on page 949*

SPECIFIC DRUGS USED IN THE TREATMENT OF CHRONIC RESPIRATORY CONDITIONS

Beta$_2$-Selective Agonists

Albuterol *on page 71*
Isoetharine *on page 768*
Metaproterenol *on page 885*
Pirbuterol *on page 1096*
Salmeterol *on page 1206*
Terbutaline *on page 1273*

Methylxanthines

Aminophylline *on page 99*
Theophylline *on page 1285*

Mast Cell Stabilizer

Cromolyn *on page 378*
Nedocromil *on page 970*

Corticosteroids

Beclomethasone *on page 184*
Dexamethasone *on page 411*
Flunisolide *on page 599*
Fluticasone *on page 616*
Mometasone Furoate *on page 943*
Prednisone *on page 1115*
Triamcinolone *on page 1330*

Anticholinergics

Ipratropium *on page 761*

Leukotriene Receptor Antagonists

Montelukast *on page 944*
Zafirlukast *on page 1394*

5-Lipoxygenase Inhibitors

Zileuton *on page 1399*

Other respiratory diseases include tuberculosis and sarcoidosis which are considered to be restrictive granulomatous respiratory diseases (see Tuberculosis*on page 1495*). Sarcoidosis is a condition that at one time was thought to be similar to tuberculosis, however, it is a multisystem disorder of unknown origin which has as a characteristic lymphocytic and mononuclear phagocytic accumulation in epithelioid granulomas within the lung. It occurs worldwide but shows a slight increased prevalence in temperate climates. The treatment of sarcoidosis is usually one that corresponds to its usually benign course, however, many patients are placed on corticosteroids at the level of 40-60 mg of prednisone daily. This treatment is continued for a protracted period of time. As in any disease requiring steroid therapy, consideration of adrenal suppression is necessary. Alteration of steroid dosage prior to stressful dental procedures may be necessary, usually increasing the steroid dosage prior to and during the stressful procedures and then gradually returning the patient to the original dosage over several days. Many dentists prefer to use the Medrol® Dosepak®, however, consultation with the patient's physician regarding dose selection is always advised. Even in the absence of evidence of adrenal suppression, consultation with the prescribing physician for appropriate dosing and timing of procedures is advisable.

Prednisone *on page 1115*

RESPIRATORY DISEASES *(Continued)*

RELATIVE POTENCY OF ENDOGENOUS AND SYNTHETIC CORTICOSTEROIDS

Agent	Equivalent Dose (mg)
Short-Acting (8-12 h)	
Cortisol	20
Cortisone acetate	25
Intermediate-Acting (18-36 h)	
Prednisolone	5
Prednisone	5
Methylprednisolone	4
Triamcinolone	4
Long-Acting (36-54 h)	
Betamethasone	0.75
Dexamethasone	0.75

Potential drug interactions for the respiratory disease patient exist. An acute sensitivity to aspirin-containing drugs and some of the nonsteroidal anti-inflammatory drugs is a threat for the asthmatic patient. Barbiturates and narcotics may occasionally precipitate asthmatic attacks as well. Erythromycin, clarithromycin, and ketoconazole are contraindicated in patients who are taking theophylline due to potential enhancement of theophylline toxicity. Patients that are taking steroid preparations as part of their respiratory therapy may require alteration in dosing prior to stressful dental procedures. The physician should be consulted.

Barbiturates *on page 1670*
Clarithromycin *on page 343*
Erythromycin *on page 508*
Ketoconazole *on page 783*

ENDOCRINE DISORDERS AND PREGNANCY

The human endocrine system manages metabolism and homeostasis. Numerous glandular tissues produce hormones that act in broad reactions with tissues throughout the body. Cells in various organ systems may be sensitive to the hormone, or they release, in reaction to the hormone, a second hormone that acts directly on another organ. Diseases of the endocrine system may have importance in dentistry. For the purposes of this section, we will limit our discussion to diseases of the thyroid tissues, diabetes mellitus, and conditions requiring the administration of synthetic hormones, and pregnancy.

THYROID

Thyroid diseases can be classified into conditions that cause the thyroid to be overactive (hyperthyroidism) and those that cause the thyroid to be underactive (hypothyroidism). Clinical signs and symptoms associated with hyperthyroidism may include goiter, heat intolerance, tremor, weight loss, diarrhea, and hyperactivity. Thyroid hormone production can be tested by TSH levels and additional screens may include radioactive iodine uptake or a pre-T_4 (tetraiodothyronine, thyroxine) assay or iodine index or total serum T_3 (triiodothyronine). The results of thyroid function tests may be altered by ingestion of antithyroid drugs such as propylthiouracil, estrogen-containing drugs, and organic and inorganic iodides. When a diagnosis of hyperthyroidism has been made, treatment usually begins with antithyroid drugs which may include propranolol coupled with radioactive iodides as well as surgical procedures to reduce thyroid tissue. Generally, the beta-blockers are used to control cardiovascular effects of excessive T_4. Propylthiouracil or methimazole are the most common antithyroid drugs used. The dentist should be aware that epinephrine is definitely contraindicated in patients with uncontrolled hyperthyroidism.

Diseases and conditions associated with hypothyroidism may include bradycardia, drowsiness, cold intolerance, thick dry skin, and constipation. Generally, hypothyroidism is treated with replacement thyroid hormone until a euthyroid state is achieved. Various preparations are available, the most common is levothyroxine, commonly known as Synthroid® or Levothroid®, and is generally the drug of choice for thyroid replacement therapy.

Drugs to Treat Hypothyroidism

Levothyroxine *on page 817*
Liothyronine *on page 831*
Liotrix *on page 832*
Thyroid *on page 1293*

Drugs to Treat Hyperthyroidism

Methimazole *on page 893*
Potassium Iodide *on page 1106*
Propranolol *on page 1140*
Propylthiouracil *on page 1144*

DIABETES

Diabetes mellitus refers to a condition of prolonged hyperglycemia associated with either abnormal production or lack of production of insulin. Commonly known as Type 1 diabetes, insulin-dependent diabetes (IDDM) is a condition where there are absent or deficient levels of circulating insulin therefore triggering tissue reactions associated with prolonged hyperglycemia. The kidney's attempt to excrete the excess glucose and the organs that do not receive adequate glucose essentially are damaged. Small vessels and arterial vessels in the eye, kidney, and brain are usually at the greatest risk. Generally, blood sugar levels between 70-120 mg/dL are considered to be normal. Inadequate insulin levels allow glucose to rise to greater than the renal threshold which is 180 mg/dL, and such elevations prolonged lead to organ damage.

The goals of treatment of the diabetic are to maintain metabolic control of the blood glucose levels and to reduce the morbid effects of periodic hyperglycemia. Insulin therapy is the primary mechanism to attain management of consistent insulin levels. Insulin preparations are categorized according to their duration of action. Generally, NPH or intermediate-acting insulin and long-acting insulin can be used in combination with short-acting or regular insulin to maintain levels consistent throughout the day.

In Type 2 or noninsulin-dependent diabetes (NIDDM), the receptor for insulin in the tissues is generally down regulated and the glucose, therefore, is not utilized at an appropriate rate. There is perhaps a stronger genetic basis for noninsulin-dependent diabetes than for Type 1. Treatment of the diabetes Type 2 patient is generally directed toward early nonpharmacologic intervention, mainly weight reduction, moderate exercise, and lower plasma-glucose concentrations. Oral hypoglycemic agents as seen in the list below are often used to maintain blood sugar levels. Thirty percent of Type 2

ENDOCRINE DISORDERS AND PREGNANCY *(Continued)*

diabetics require insulin, as well as, oral hypoglycemics in order to manage their diabetes. Generally, the two classes of oral hypoglycemics are the sulfonylureas and the biguanides. The sulfonylureas are prescribed more frequently and they stimulate beta cell production of insulin, increase glucose utilization, and tend to normalize glucose metabolism in the liver. The uncontrolled diabetic may represent a challenge to the dental practitioner.

Glycosylated hemoglobin or glycol-hemoglobin assays have emerged as a "gold standard" by which glycemic control is measured in diabetic patients. The test does not rely on the patient's ability to monitor their daily blood glucose levels and is not influenced by acute changes in blood glucose or by the interval since the last meal. Glycohemoglobin is formed when glucose reacts with hemoglobin A in the blood and is composed of several fractions. Numerous assay methods have been developed, however, they vary in their precision. Dental clinicians are advised to be aware of the laboratory's particular standardization procedures when requesting glycosylated hemoglobin values. One major advantage of the glycosylated hemoglobin assay is that it provides an overview of the level of glucose in the life span of the red blood cell population in the patient, and therefore is a measure of overall glycemic control for the previous six to twelve weeks. Thus, clinicians use glycosylated hemoglobin values to determine whether their patient is under good control, on average. These assays have less value in medication dosing decisions. Blood glucose monitoring methods are actually better in that respect. The values of glycosylated hemoglobin are expressed as a percentage of the total hemoglobin in the red blood cell population and a normal value is considered to be <6%. The goal is generally for diabetic patients to remain at <7% and values >8% would constitute a worrisome signal. Medical conditions such as anemias or any red blood cell disease, numerous levels of myelosuppression, or pregnancy can artificially lower glycosylated hemoglobin values.

See Insulin Preparations (various products) *on page 749*

Oral Hypoglycemic Agents

Acarbose *on page 45*
Acetohexamide *on page 60*
Chlorpropamide *on page 321*
Glimepiride *on page 659*
Glipizide *on page 660*
Glyburide *on page 664*
Glyburide and Metformin *on page 665*
Metformin *on page 887*
Miglitol *on page 929*
Nateglinide *on page 968*
Repaglinide *on page 1173*
Tolazamide *on page 1308*
Tolbutamide *on page 1309*

Adjunct Therapy

Metoclopramide *on page 914*

Oral manifestations of uncontrolled diabetes might include abnormal neutrophil function resulting in a poor response to periodontal pathogens. Increased risk of gingivitis and periodontitis in these patients is common. Candidiasis is also a frequent occurrence. Denture-sore mouth may be more prominent. Poor wound-healing following extractions may be one of the complications encountered.

HORMONAL THERAPY

Two uses of hormonal supplementation include oral contraceptives and estrogen replacement therapy. Drugs used for contraception interfere with fertility by inhibiting release of follicle stimulating hormone, luteinizing hormone, and by preventing ovulation. There are few oral side effects; however, moderate gingivitis, similar to that seen during pregnancy, has been reported. The dentist should be aware that decreased effect of oral contraceptives has been reported with most antibiotics (see individual monographs for specific details). It is therefore recommended that dental professionals, when prescribing antibiotics to oral contraceptive users, advise them of this interaction and suggest consulting their physician for additional barrier contraception during antibiotic therapy.

The combination estradiol cypionate and medroxyprogesterone acetate has recently been approved. It is a single monthly injection and has similar warnings and guidelines. However, it's use with antibiotics have not been firmly established. Therefore, discussion/consultation with the patient's OB/GYN physician is indicated.

Drugs commonly encountered include:

Estradiol *on page 518*
Estradiol and Medroxyprogesterone *on page 520*
Levonorgestrel *on page 815*
Medroxyprogesterone *on page 862*
Mestranol and Norethindrone *on page 884*
Norethindrone *on page 996*
Norgestrel *on page 998*

Estrogens or derivatives are usually prescribed as replacement therapy following menopause or cyclic irregularities and to inhibit osteoporosis. The following list of drugs may interact with antidepressants and barbiturates. New tissue-specific estrogens like Evista® may help with the problem of osteoporosis.

Estrogens (Conjugated/Equine) *on page 525*
Estrogens (Conjugated A/Synthetic) *on page 524*
Estrogens (Esterified) *on page 529*
Estrogens (Conjugated/Equine) and Medroxyprogesterone *on page 528*
Estrogens (Esterified) and Methyltestosterone *on page 530*
Estropipate *on page 531*
Raloxifene *on page 1166*

PREGNANCY

Normal endocrine and physiologic functions are altered during pregnancy. Endogenous estrogens and progesterone increase and placental hormones are secreted. Thyroid stimulating hormone and growth hormone also increase. Cardiovascular changes can result and increased blood volume can lead to blood pressure elevations and transient heart murmurs. Generally, in a normal pregnancy, oral gingival changes will be limited to gingivitis. Alteration of treatment plans might include limiting administration of all drugs to emergency procedures only during the first and third trimesters and medical consultation regarding the patients' status for all elective procedures. Limiting dental care throughout pregnancy to preventive procedures is not unreasonable. The effects on dental treatment of the "morning after pill" (Plan B® and PREVEN®) and the abortifacient, mifepristone *on page 928*, have not been documented at this time.

HIV INFECTION AND AIDS

Human immunodeficiency virus (HIV) represents agents HIV-1 and HIV-2 that produce a devastating systemic disease. The virus causes disease by leading to elevated risk of infections in patients and, from our experience over the last 18 years, there clearly are oral manifestations associated with these patients. Also, there has been a revolution in infection control in our dental offices over the last two decades due to our expanding knowledge of this infectious agent. Infection control practices have been elevated to include all of the infectious agents with which dentists often come into contact. These might include, in addition to HIV, hepatitis viruses (of which the serotypes include A, B, C, D, E, F, and G; see Occupational Exposure to Bloodborne Pathogens*on page 1603*), the herpes viruses (see Systemic Viral Diseases *on page 1519*); STDs such as syphilis, gonorrhea, and papillomavirus (see Sexually-Transmitted Diseases *on page 1504*).

Acquired immunodeficiency syndrome (AIDS) has been recognized since early 1981 as a unique clinical syndrome manifest by opportunistic infections or by neoplasms complicating the underlying defect in the cellular immune system. These defects are now known to be brought on by infection and pathogenesis with human immunodeficiency virus 1 or 2 (HIV-1 is the predominant serotype identified). The major cellular defect brought on by infection with HIV is a depletion of T-cells, primarily the sub-type, T-helper cells, known as CD4+ cells. Over these years, our knowledge regarding HIV infection and the oral manifestations often associated with patients with HIV or AIDS, has increased dramatically. Populations of individuals known to be at high risk of HIV transmission include homosexuals, intravenous drug abuse patients, transfusion recipients, patients with other sexually transmitted diseases, and patients practicing promiscuous sex.

The definitions of AIDS have also evolved over this period of time. The natural history of HIV infection along with some of the oral manifestations can be reviewed in Table 1. The risk of developing these opportunistic infections increases as the patient progresses to AIDS.

Table 1.
NATURAL HISTORY OF HIV INFECTION/ORAL MANIFESTATIONS

Time From Transmission (Average)	Observation	CD4 Cell Count
0	Viral transmissions	Normal: 1000 (±500/mm^3)
2-4 weeks	Self-limited infectious mononucleosis-like illness with fever, rash, leukopenia, mucocutaneous ulcerations (mouth, genitals, etc), thrush	Transient decrease
6-12 weeks	Seroconversion (rarely requires ≥3 months for seroconversion)	Normal
0-8 years	Healthy/asymptomatic HIV infection; peripheral/ persistent generalized lymphadenopathy; HPV, thrush, OHL; RAU, periodontal diseases, salivary gland diseases; dermatitis	≥500/mm^3 gradual reduction with average decrease of 50-80/mm^3/ year
4-8 years	Early symptomatic HIV infection previously called (AIDS-related complex): Thrush, vaginal candidiasis (persistent, frequent and/or severe), cervical dysplasia/CA Hodgkin's lymphoma, B-cell lymphoma, oral hairy leukoplakia, salivary gland diseases, ITP, xerostomia, dermatitis, shingles; RAU, herpes simplex, HPV, bacterial infections, periodontal diseases, molluscum contagiosum, other physical symptoms: fever, weight loss, fatigue	≥300-500/mm^3
6-10 years	AIDS: Wasting syndrome, *Candida* esophagitis, Kaposi's sarcoma, HIV-associated dementia, disseminated *M. avium*, Hodgkin's or B-cell lymphoma, herpes simplex >30 days; PCP; cryptococcal meningitis, other systemic fungal infections; CMV	<200/mm^3

Natural history indicates course of HIV infection in absence of antiretroviral treatment. Adapted from Bartlett JG, "A Guide to HIV Care from the AIDS Care Program of the Johns Hopkins Medical Institutions," 2nd ed.

PCP -*Pneumocystis carinii* pneumonia; ITP -idiopathic thrombocytopenia purpura; HPV - human papilloma virus; OHL - oral hairy leukoplakia; RAU - recurrent aphthous ulcer

Patients with HIV infection and/or AIDS are seen in dental offices throughout the country. In general, it is the dentist's obligation to treat HIV individuals including patients of record and other patients who may seek treatment when the office is accepting new patients. These patients are protected under the Americans with Disabilities Act and the dentist has an obligation as described. Two excellent publications, one by the American Dental Association and the other by the American Academy of Oral Medicine, outline the dentist's responsibility as well as a very detailed explanation of dental management protocols for HIV patients. These protocols, however, are evolving just as our knowledge of HIV has evolved. New drugs and their interactions present the dentist with continuous need for updates regarding the appropriate management of HIV patients. Diagnostic tests, including determining viral load in combination with the CD4 status, now are used to modify a patient's treatment in ways that allow them to remain relatively illness-free for longer periods of time. This places more of a responsibility on the dental practice team to be aware of drug changes, of new drugs, and of the appropriate oral management in such patients.

Our knowledge of AIDS allows us to properly treat these patients while protecting ourselves, our staff, and other patients in the office. All types of infectious disease require consistent practices in our dental offices known as Standard/Universal Precautions (see Occupational Exposure to Bloodborne Pathogens*on page 1603*). The office team that utilizes these precautions appropriately is well protected against passage of infectious agents. These agents include sexually transmitted disease agents, the highly virulent hepatitis viruses, and the less virulent but always worrisome HIV. In general, an office that is practicing standard/universal precautions is one that is considered safe for patients and staff. Throughout this spectrum, HIV is placed somewhere in the middle, in terms of infection risk in the dental office. Other sexually transmitted diseases and infectious diseases such as tuberculosis represent a greater threat to the dentist than HIV itself. However, due to the grave danger of HIV infection, many of our precautions have been instituted to assist the dentist in protecting himself, his staff, and other patients in situations where the office may be involved in treating a patient that is HIV positive.

As in the management of all medically compromised patients, the appropriate care of HIV patients begins with a complete and thorough history. This history must allow the dentist to identify risk factors in the development of HIV, as well as, identify those patients known to be HIV positive. Knowledge of all medications prescribed to patients at risk is also important.

The current antiretroviral therapy used to treat patients with HIV infection and/or AIDS includes three primary classifications of drugs. These are the nucleoside analogs, protease inhibitors, and the non-nucleoside/nucleotide analogs (analogs refers to chemicals that can substitute competitively for naturally produced cell components such as found in DNA, RNA, or proteins). The newest drugs include several nucleoside analogs, abacavir (Ziagen®), subprotease inhibitors, amprenavir, and several non-nucleoside analogs, efavirenz (Sustiva®), and adefovir. Finding the perfect "cocktail" of anti-HIV medications still eludes clinicians. This is partly due to the fact that therapies are still too novel and the patient's years too few to study. Numerous recently-published studies have indicated that combinations of drugs are far better than individual drug therapy. Several of these studies have looked at two drug combinations, particularly between nucleoside analogs, in combination with protease inhibitors. The newer drugs (non-nucleoside analogs) have added the possibility of a triple "cocktail". Recently several studies indicated that this three-drug combination may be the best in managing HIV infection.

When HIV was first discovered, the efforts for monitoring HIV infection focused on the CD4 blood levels and the ratios between the helper cells, suppressor cells within the patient's immune system. These markers were used to indicate success or failure of drug therapies as patients moved through HIV pathogenesis toward AIDS. More recently, however, the advent of protease inhibitors has allowed clinicians to monitor the actual presence of viral RNA within the patient and the term viral load has become the focus of therapy monitoring. The availability of better therapies and our rapidly expanding knowledge of molecular biology of the HIV virus have created new opportunities to control the AIDS epidemic. Cases can be monitored quite closely looking at the number of copy units or virions within the patient's bloodstream as an indication in combination with other infections and/or declining or increasing CD4 numbers to establish prognostic values for the patient's success. Long-term survival of patients infected with HIV has been accomplished by monitoring and adjusting therapy to these numbers.

Comprehensive coordinated approaches, that have been advocated by researchers, have sought to establish national standards for HIV reporting, greater access to effective newly approved medications, improved access to individual physicians treating HIV patients, and continued protection of patient's privacy. These goals allow the reporting of studies that suggest that combination therapies, some of which have been tried in less controlled individual patient treatments, may prove useful in larger populations of HIV-infected individuals. As these studies are reported, the dental clinician should be aware that patients' drug therapies change rapidly, various combinations may be tried, and the side effects and interactions as described in the chapter on drug interactions and the CYP system will also emerge. The dentist must be aware of these potential interactions with seemingly innocuous drugs such as clarithromycin, erythromycin, and some of the sedative drugs that a dentist may utilize in their practice as well as some of the analgesics. These drug interactions may be the most important part of monitoring that the dentist provides in helping to manage a situation. Some of the antiviral drugs more commonly used for HIV, AIDS, Asymptomatic, CD4 <500, and the newer drugs (ie, protease inhibitors, nucleoside analogs, and non-nucleoside nucleotide analogs) are listed in Table 2 on following page.

HIV INFECTION AND AIDS *(Continued)*

Table 2. CATEGORIES OF ANTIRETROVIRAL DRUGS

Nucleoside Analogs	Protease Inhibitors	Non-nucleoside / Nucleotide Analogs
Zidovudine (Retrovir®, AZT, SDV)	Saquinavir (Invirase®)	Nevirapine (Viramune®)
Didanosine (Videx®, ddi)	Ritonavir (Norvir®)	Delavirdine (Rescriptor®)
Zalcitabine (Hivid®, ddc)	Indinavir (Crixivan®)	Efavirenz (Sustiva®)
Stavudine (Zerit®, d4T)	Nelfinavir (Viracept®)	Adefovir (HepSera™)
Lamivudine (Epivir®)	Amprenavir (Agenerase®)	
Abacavir (Ziagen®)	Fosamprenavir (Lexiva™)	

The presence of other infections is an important part of the health history. Appropriate medical consultation may be mandated after a health history in order to accomplish a complete evaluation of the patients at risk. Uniformity in the taking of a history from a patient is the dentist's best plan for all patients so that no selectivity or discrimination can be implicated.

An appropriate review of symptoms may also identify oral and systemic conditions that may be present in aggressive HIV disease. Medical physical examination may reveal pre-existing or developing intra- or extra-oral signs/symptoms of progressive disease. Aggressive herpes simplex, herpes zoster, papillomavirus, Kaposi's sarcoma or lymphoma are among the disorders that might be identified. In addition to these, intra-oral examination may raise suspicion regarding fungal infections, angular cheilitis, squamous cell carcinoma, and recurrent aphthous ulcers. The dentist should be vigilant in all patients regardless of HIV risk.

It will always be up to the dental practitioner to determine whether testing for HIV should be recommended following the history and physical examination of a new patient. Because of the severe psychological implications of learning of HIV positivity for a patient, the dentist should be aware that there are appropriate referral sites where psychological counseling and appropriate discrete testing for the patient is available. The dentist's office should have these sites available for referral should the patient be interested. Candid discussions, however, with the patient regarding risk factors and/or other signs or symptoms in their history and physical condition that may indicate a higher HIV risk than the normal population, should be an area the dentist feels comfortable in broaching with any new patient. Oftentimes, it is appropriate to recommend testing for other infectious diseases should risk factors be present. For example, testing for hepatitis B may be appropriate for the patient and along with this the dentist could recommend that the patient consider HIV testing. Because of the legal issues involved, anonymity for HIV testing may be appropriate and it is always up to the patient to follow the doctor's recommendations.

When a patient has either given a positive history of knowing that they are HIV positive or it has been determined after referral for consultation, the dentist should be aware of the AIDS-defining illnesses. Of course, current medical status and drug therapy that the patient may be undergoing is of equal importance. The dentist, through medical consultation and regular follow-up with the patient's physician, should be made aware of the CD4 count (Table 3), the viral load, and the drugs that the patient is taking. The presence of other AIDS-defining illnesses as well as complications, such as higher risk of endocarditis and the risk of other systemic infections such as tuberculosis, are extremely important for the dentist. These may make an impact on the dental treatment plan in terms of the selection of preprocedural antibiotics or the use of oral medications to treat opportunistic infections in or around the oral cavity.

Table 3. CD4+ LYMPHOCYTE COUNT AND PERCENTAGE AS RELATED TO THE RISK OF OPPORTUNISTIC INFECTION

CD4+ Cells/mm^3	CD4+ Percentage[1]	Risk of Opportunistic Infection
>600	32-60	No increased risk
400-500	<29	Initial immune suppression
200-400	14-28	Appearance of opportunistic infections, some may be major
<200	<14	Severe immune suppression. AIDS diagnosis. Major opportunistic infections. Although variable, prognosis for surviving greater than 3 years is poor
<50	—	Although variable, prognosis for surviving greater than 1 year is poor

[1]Several studies have suggested that the CD4+ percentage demonstrates less variability between measurements, as compared to the absolute CD4+ cell count. CD4+ percentages may therefore give a clearer impression of the course of disease.

Adapted from Glick M and Silverman S, "Dental Management of HIV-Infected Patients," *J Am Dent Assoc* (Supplement to Reviewers), 1995.

AIDS-defining illnesses such as candidiasis, recurrent pneumonia, or lymphoma are clearly important to the dentist. Chemotherapy that might be being given to the patient for treatment for any or all of these disorders can have implications in terms of the patient's response to simple dental procedures.

Drug therapies have become complex in the treatment of HIV/AIDS. Because of the moderate successes with protease inhibitors and the drug combination therapies, more patients are living longer and receiving more dental care throughout their lives. Drug therapies are often tailored to the current CD4 count in combination with the viral load. In general, patients with high CD4 counts are usually at lower risk for complications in the dental office than patients with low CD4 counts. However, the presence of a high viral load with or without a stable CD4 count may be indicative or a more rapid progression of the HIV/AIDS disease process than had previously been thought. Patients with a high viral load and a declining CD4 count are considered to have the greatest risk and the poorest prognosis of all the groups.

Other organ damage, such as liver compromise potentially leading to bleeding disorders, can be found as the disease progresses to AIDS. Liver dysfunction may be related to pre-existing hepatic diseases due to previous infection with a hepatitis virus such as hepatitis B or other drug toxicities associated with the treatment of AIDS. The dentist must have available current prothrombin and partial thromboplastin times (PT and PTT) in order to accurately evaluate any risk of bleeding abnormality. Platelet count and liver function studies are also important. Potential drug interactions include some antibiotics, as well as any anticoagulating drugs, which may be contraindicated in such patients. It may be necessary to avoid NSAIDs, as well as aspirin. (See Pharmacology of Drug Metabolism and Interactions *on page 24*).

The use of preprocedural antibiotics is another issue in the HIV patient. As the absolute neutrophil count declines during the progression of AIDS, the use of antibiotics as a preprocedural step prior to dental care may be necessary. If protracted treatment plans are necessary, the dentist should receive updated information as the patient receives such from their physician. It is always important that the dentist have current CD4 counts, viral load assay, as well as liver function studies, AST and ALT, and bleeding indicators including platelet count, PT, and PTT. If any other existing conditions such as cardiac involvement or joint prostheses are involved, antibiotic coverage may also be necessary. However, these determinations are no different than in the non-HIV population and this subject is covered in "Preprocedural Antibiotic Prophylaxis Guidelines for Dental Patients" *on page 1509*. Use the table of Normal Blood Values *on page 1620* as a general guideline for provision of dental care.

The consideration of current blood values is important in long-term care of any medically compromised patient and in particular the HIV-positive patient. Preventive dental care is likewise valuable in these patients, however, the dentist's approach should be no different than as with all patients. See Table 4 for oral lesions commonly associated with HIV disease and a brief description of their usual treatment (see Part II of this Oral Medicine chapter for more detailed descriptions of these common oral lesions).

The clinician should be aware that several of the protease inhibitors have now been associated with drug interactions. Some of these drug interactions include therapies that the dentist may be utilizing. The basis for these drug interactions with protease inhibitors is the inhibition of cytochrome P450 isoforms, which are important in normal liver function and metabolism of drugs. A detailed description of the mechanisms of inhibition can be found in "Pharmacology of Drug Metabolism and Interactions" *on page 24*, as well as a table illustrating some known drug interactions with antiviral therapy and drugs commonly prescribed in the dental office. The metabolism of these drugs could be affected by the patient's antiviral therapy.

The dentist should also review office protocol for standard/universal precautions *on page 1603* and the answers to "Frequently Asked Questions" at the end of this section.

HIV INFECTION AND AIDS *(Continued)*

Please see Suggested Readings section for more information on management of HIV patients.

Table 4. ORAL LESIONS COMMONLY SEEN IN HIV/AIDS

Condition	Management
Oral candidiasis	See "Oral Fungal Infections" *on page 1544*
Angular cheilitis	See "Oral Fungal Infections" *on page 1544*
Oral hairy leukoplakia	See "Systemic Viral Diseases" *on page 1519*
Periodontal diseases	See "Oral Bacterial Infections" *on page 1533*
Linear gingivitis	
Ulcerative periodontitis	
Herpes simplex	Acyclovir - see "Systemic Viral Diseases" *on page 1519*
Herpes zoster	Acyclovir - see "Systemic Viral Diseases" *on page 1519*
Chronic aphthous ulceration	Palliation / Thalidomide (Thalomid®)
Salivary gland disease	Referral
Human papillomavirus	Laser / Surgical excision
Kaposi's sarcoma	See "Antibiotic Prophylaxis" *on page 1509* Biopsy / Laser
Non-Hodgkin's lymphoma	Biopsy / Referral
Tuberculosis	Referral

Dapsone *on page 398*
Delavirdine *on page 403*
Didanosine *on page 433*
Indinavir *on page 744*
Lamivudine *on page 794*
Lopinavir and Ritonavir *on page 839*
Nelfinavir *on page 972*
Ritonavir *on page 1189*
Stavudine *on page 1238*
Thalidomide *on page 1283*
Tenofovir *on page 1270*
Zalcitabine *on page 1395*
Zidovudine *on page 1398*
Zidovudine and Lamivudine *on page 1399*

FREQUENTLY ASKED QUESTIONS

How does one get AIDS, aside from having unprotected sex?

Our current knowledge about the immunodeficiency virus is that it is carried via semen, contaminated needles, blood products, transfusion products not tested, and potentially in other fluids of the body. Patients at highest risk include I.V. drug-abusers, those receiving multiple transfusions with blood that has not been screened for HIV, or patients practicing unprotected sex with multiple partners, where the history of the partner may not be as clear as the patient would like.

Are patients safe from AIDS or HIV infection when they present to the dentist office?

Our current knowledge indicates that the answer is an unequivocal "yes". The patient is protected because dental offices are practicing stanard/universal precautions, using antimicrobial handwashing agents, gloves, face masks, eye protection, special clothing, aerosol control, and instrument soaking and autoclaving. All of these procedures stop potential transmission to a new patient, as well as, allow for easy disposal of contaminated office supplies for elimination of microbes by an antimicrobial technique, should they be contaminated through treatment of another patient. These precautions are mandated by OSHA requirements (see Standard/Universal Precautions*on page 1603*).

What is the most common opportunistic infection that HIV-positive patients suffer that may be important in dentistry?

The most common opportunistic infection important to dentistry is oral candidiasis. This disease can present as white plaques, red areas, or angular cheilitis occurring at the corners of the mouth. Management of such lesions is appropriate by the dentist and is described in this handbook (see Oral Fungal Infections *on page 1544*). Other oral complications include HIV-associated periodontal disease, as well as the other conditions outlined in Table 4. Of great concern to the dentist is the risk of tuberculosis. In many HIV-positive patients, tuberculosis has become a serious, life-threatening opportunistic infection. The dentist should be aware that appropriate referral for anyone showing such respiratory signs and symptoms would be prudent.

Can one patient infect another through unprotected sex if the other patient has tested negative for HIV?

Yes, there is always the possibility that a sexual partner may be in the early window of time when plasma viremia is not at a detectable level. The antibody response to plasma viremia may be slightly delayed and diagnostic testing may not indicate HIV positivity. This window of time represents a period when the patient may be infectious but not show up yet on normal diagnostic testing.

Can HIV be passed by oral fluids?

As our knowledge about HIV has evolved, we have thought that HIV is inactivated in saliva by an agent possibly associated with secretory leukocyte protease inhibitors known as SLPI. There is, however, a current resurgence in our interest in oral transmission because some research indicates that in moderate to advanced periodontal lesions or other oral lesions where there is tissue damage, the presence of a serous exudate may increase the risk of transmission. The dentist should be aware of this ongoing research and attempt to renew knowledge regularly so that any future breakthroughs will be noted.

RHEUMATOID ARTHRITIS, OSTEOARTHRITIS, AND OSTEOPOROSIS

RA AND OSTEOARTHRITIS MANAGEMENT

Arthritis and its variations represent the most common chronic musculoskeletal disorders of man. The conditions can essentially be divided into rheumatoid, osteoarthritic, and polyarthritic presentations. Differences in age of onset and joint involvement exist and it is now currently believed that the diagnosis of each may be less clear than previously thought. These autoinflammatory diseases have now been shown to affect young and old alike. Criteria for a diagnosis of rheumatoid arthritis include a positive serologic test for rheumatoid factor, subcutaneous nodules, affected joints on opposite sides of the body, and clear radiographic changes. The hematologic picture includes moderate normocytic hypochromic anemia, mild leukocytosis, and mild thrombocytopenia. During acute inflammatory periods, C-reactive protein is elevated and IgG and IgM (rheumatoid factors) can be detected. Osteoarthritis lacks these diagnostic features.

Other systemic conditions, such as systemic lupus erythematosus and Sjögren's syndrome, are often found simultaneously with some of the arthritic conditions. The treatment of arthritis includes the use of slow-acting and rapid-acting anti-inflammatory agents ranging from the gold salts to aspirin (see following listings). Long-term usage of these drugs can lead to numerous adverse effects including bone marrow suppression, platelet suppression, and oral ulcerations. The dentist should be aware that steroids (usually prednisone) are often prescribed along with the listed drugs and are often used in dosages sufficient to induce adrenal suppression. Adjustment of dosing prior to invasive dental procedures may be indicated along with consultation with the managing physician. Alteration of steroid dosage prior to stressful dental procedures may be necessary, usually increasing the steroid dosage prior to and during the stressful procedures and then gradually returning the patient to the original dosage over several days. Even in the absence of evidence of adrenal suppression, consultation with the prescribing physician for appropriate dosing and timing of procedures is advisable.

Antirheumatic, Disease Modifying

Adalimumab *on page 67*

Gold Salts

Auranofin *on page 170*
Aurothioglucose

Metabolic Inhibitor

Leflunomide *on page 801*
Methotrexate *on page 897*

Immunomodulator

Etanercept *on page 532*

Nonsteroidal Anti-inflammatory Agents

Aminosalicylic Acid *on page 100*
Choline Magnesium Trisalicylate *on page 324*
Choline Salicylate *on page 325*
Diclofenac *on page 427*
Diflunisal *on page 435*
Etodolac *on page 564*
Fenoprofen *on page 580*
Flurbiprofen *on page 613*
Ibuprofen *on page 728*
Indomethacin *on page 746*
Ketoprofen *on page 785*
Ketorolac *on page 787*
Magnesium Salicylate *on page 854*
Meclofenamate *on page 860*
Mefenamic Acid *on page 863*
Nabumetone *on page 955*
Naproxen *on page 965*
Oxaprozin *on page 1022*
Piroxicam *on page 1097*
Salsalate *on page 1207*
Sulindac *on page 1251*
Tolmetin *on page 1311*

COX-2 Inhibitor NSAID

Celecoxib *on page 290*
Rofecoxib *on page 1194*
Valdecoxib *on page 1356*

Combination NSAID Product to Prevent GI Distress

Diclofenac and Misoprostol *on page 430*

Salicylates

Aspirin *on page 151*
Choline Magnesium Trisalicylate *on page 324*
Salsalate *on page 1207*

Other

Hydroxychloroquine *on page 720*
Prednisone *on page 1115*

ANTI-INFLAMMATORY AGENTS USED IN THE TREATMENT OF RA AND OSTEOARTHRITIS

Drug	Adverse Effects
SLOW-ACTING	
Gold Salts	
Aurothioglucose; Auranofin; Gold Sodium Thiomalate	GI intolerance, diarrhea; leukopenia, thrombocytopenia, and/or anemia; skin and oral eruptions; possible nephrotoxicity and hepatotoxicity
Metabolic Inhibitor	
Leflunomide (Arava™)	Diarrhea, respiratory tract infection
Methotrexate	Oral ulcerations, leukopenia
Immunomodulator	
Etanercept (Enbrel®)	Headache, respiratory tract infection, positive ANA
Other	
Hydroxychloroquine (Plaquenil®)	Usually mild and reversible; ophthalmic complications
Prednisone	Insomnia, nervousness, indigestion, increased appetite
RAPID-ACTING	
Salicylates	
Aspirin	Inhibition of platelet aggregation; gastrointestinal (GI) irritation, ulceration, and bleeding; tinnitus; teratogenicity
Choline magnesium trisalicylate (Trilisate®)	GI irritation and ulceration, weakness, skin rash, hemolytic anemia, troubled breathing
Salsalate	
Other Nonsteroidal Anti-inflammatory Drugs	
Diclofenac (Cataflam®, Voltaren®); Diflunisal (Dolobid®); Etodolac (Lodine®); Fenoprofen calcium (Nalfon®); Flurbiprofen (Ansaid®); Ibuprofen (Motrin®); Indomethacin (Indocin®); Ketoprofen; Ketorolac (Toradol®); Meclofenamate; Nabumetone (Relafen®); Naproxen (Naprosyn®); Oxaprozin (Daypro®); Piroxicam (Feldene®); Salsalate (Mono-Gesic®, Salflex®); Sulindac (Clinoril®); Tolmetin (Tolectin®)	GI irritation, ulceration, and bleeding; inhibition of platelet aggregation; displacement of protein-bound drugs (eg, oral anticoagulants, sulfonamides, and sulfonylureas); headache; vertigo; mucocutaneous rash or ulceration; parotid enlargement
COX-2 Inhibitor NSAID	
Celecoxib (Celebrex®) Rofecoxib (Vioxx®) Valdecoxib (Bextra®)	Headache, dyspepsia, upper respiratory tract infection, sinusitis
COMBINATION NSAID PRODUCT TO PREVENT GI DISTRESS	
Diclofenac and Misoprostol (Arthrotec®)	Inhibition of platelet aggregation; displacement of protein-bound drugs (eg, oral anticoagulants, sulfonamides, and sulfonylureas); headache; vertigo; mucocutaneous rash or ulceration; parotid enlargement; diarrhea

RHEUMATOID ARTHRITIS, OSTEOARTHRITIS, AND OSTEOPOROSIS *(Continued)*

OSTEOPOROSIS MANAGEMENT

PREVALENCE

Osteoporosis effects 25 million Americans of which 80% are women; 27% of American women >80 years of age have osteopenia and 70% of American women >80 years of age have osteoporosis.

CONSEQUENCES

1.3 million bone fractures annually (low impact/nontraumatic) and pain, pulmonary insufficiency, decreased quality of life, and economic costs; >250,000 hip fractures per year with a 20% mortality rate.

RISK FACTORS

Advanced age, female, chronic renal disease, hyperparathyroidism, Cushing's disease, hypogonadism/anorexia, hyperprolactinemia, cancer, large and prolonged dose heparin or glucocorticoids, anticonvulsants, hyperthyroidism (current or history, or excessive thyroid supplements), sedentary, excessive exercise, early menopause, oophorectomy without hormone replacement, excessive aluminum-containing antacid, smoking, methotrexate.

DIAGNOSIS/MONITORING

DXA bone density, history of fracture (low impact or nontraumatic), compressed vertebrae, decreased height, hump-back appearance. Osteomark™ urine assay measures bone breakdown fragments and may help assess therapy response earlier than DXA but diagnostic value is uncertain as Osteomark™ does not reveal extent of bone loss. Bone markers may be tested to evaluate effectiveness of antiresorptive urine therapy.

PREVENTION

1. Adequate dietary calcium (eg, dairy products)
2. Vitamin D (eg, fortified dairy products, cod, fatty fish)
3. Weight-bearing exercise (eg, walking) as tolerated
4. Calcium supplement of 1000-1500 mg elemental calcium daily (divided in 500 mg increments); women >65 years on estrogen replacement therapy supplement 1000 mg elemental calcium; women >65 not receiving estrogens and men >55 years supplement 1500 mg elemental calcium. To minimize constipation add fiber and start with 500 mg/day for several months, then increase to 500 mg twice daily taken at different times than fiber. Chewable and liquid products are available. Calcium carbonate is given with food to enhance bioavailability. Calcium citrate may be given without regards to meals.
   - Contraindications: Hypercalcemia, ventricular fibrillation
   - Side effects: Constipation, anorexia
   - Drug interactions: Fiber, tetracycline, iron supplement, minerals
5. Vitamin D Supplement: 400-800 units daily (often satisfied by 1-2 multivitamins or fortified milk) in addition to calcium or a combined calcium and vitamin D supplement and/or >15 minutes direct sunlight/day. Some elderly, especially with significant renal or liver disease cannot metabolize (activate) vitamin D and require calcitriol 0.25 mcg orally twice daily or adjusted per serum calcium level, the active form of vitamin D; can check 1,25 OH vitamin D level to confirm need for calcitriol.
   - Contraindications: Hypercalcemia (weakness, headache, drowsiness, nausea, diarrhea), hypercalciuria and renal stones
   - Side effects (uncommon): Hypercalcemia (see above)
   - Monitor 24-hour urine and serum calcium if using >1000 units/day
6. Estrogen: Especially useful if bone density <80% of average plus symptoms of estrogen deficiency or cardiac disease. Bone density increases over 1-2 years then plateaus. This is considered 1st line therapy unless contraindicated due to medicinal history (see below) or risk:benefit assessment which leads to decision to avoid HRT (hormone replacement therapy). **Note:** Estrogens should not be used to prevent coronary heart disease.

- Contraindications: Pregnancy, breast or estrogen-dependent cancer, undiagnosed abnormal genital bleeding, active thrombophlebitis, or history of thromboembolism during previous estrogen or oral contraceptive therapy or pregnancy. Pretreatment mammogram, gynecological exam are advised along with routine breast exam because of an increased risk of breast cancer with long-term use.
- Dose: Conjugated estrogen of 0.625 mg/day or its equivalent (continuous therapy preferred).
- Side effects: Vaginal spotting/bleeding, nausea, vomiting, breast tenderness/enlargement, amenorrheic with extended use.

  Initiate therapy slowly (side effects are more common and severe in women without estrogen for many years). Administer with medroxyprogesterone acetate (MPA) 2.5-5 mg daily, or another oral progesterone, in women with uterus (unopposed estrogen can cause endometrial cancer). MPA can increase vaginal bleeding, increase weight, edema, mood changes.
- Drug interactions: May increase corticosteroid effect, monitor for need to decrease corticosteroid dose.

7. Selective estrogen receptor modulators: Selective-estrogen receptor modulators (SERMs) are nonsteroidal modulators of estrogen-receptor mediated reactions. The key difference between these agents and estrogen replacement therapies is the potential to exert tissue specific effects. Due to their chemical differences, these agents retain some of estrogen's beneficial effects on bone metabolism and lipid levels, but differ in their actions on breast and endometrial tissues, potentially limiting adverse effects related to nonspecific hormone stimulation. Among the SERMs, tamoxifen retains stimulatory effects in endometrial tissue, while raloxifene does not stimulate endometrial or breast tissue, limiting the potential for endometrial or breast cancer related to this agent. Raloxifene is the only SERM which has been approved by the FDA for osteoporosis prevention.

   It should be noted that the effects on bone observed with SERMs appear to be less than that observed with estrogen replacement. In one study, the effect of raloxifene on hip bone mineral density was approximately half of that observed with conjugated estrogens. In addition, the effects on lipid profiles are less than with estrogen replacement. Finally, SERMs do not block the vasomotor effects observed with menopause, which may limit compliance with therapy. As with estrogen replacement, raloxifene has been associated with an increased risk of thromboembolism and is contraindicated in patients with a history of thromboembolic disease.
8. Estradiol, as well as various combination therapies, including ethinyl estradiol with norethindrone (Femhrt®) and ethinyl with norgestimate (Ortho-Prefest™), have been approved for the prevention of osteoporosis (see Estradiol *on page 518*).

TREATMENT

1. Calcium, vitamin D, exercise, and estrogen: As above
2. Bisphosphonates:

   Consider if patient is intolerant of, or refuses estrogen or it is contraindicated, especially if severe osteoporosis (ie, ≥2.5 standard deviations below average young adult bone density, T-score, or history of low impact or nontraumatic fracture). Increasing bone density of hip and spine observed for at least 3 years (ie, no plateau as seen with estrogen).

   Contraindications: Hypocalcemia, not advised if existing gastrointestinal disorders (eg, esophageal disorders such as reflux, sensitive stomach).

   – Alendronate (Fosamax®): Dose: 10 mg once daily or 70 mg/week (treatment dose for osteoporosis; not recommended if creatinine clearance <35 mL/minute). Osteopenia: 5 mg per day or 35 mg/week for prevention.

   – Risedronate (Actonel®: Dose: 5 mg daily or 35 mg/week for treatment or prevention

   Take before breakfast on an empty stomach with 6-8 ounces tap water (not mineral water, coffee, or juice) and remain upright or raise head of bed for bedridden patients at least 30 degree angle for at least 30 minutes (otherwise may cause ulcerative esophagitis) before eating or drinking.

   Therapy with calcium and vitamin D is advised, but must be given at a different time of day than alendronate.

   - Side effects (well tolerated): Difficulty swallowing, heartburn, abdominal discomfort, nausea (GI side effects increase with aspirin products), arthralgia/myalgia, constipation, diarrhea, headache, esophagitis.
   - Drug interactions: None known to date.

RHEUMATOID ARTHRITIS, OSTEOARTHRITIS, AND OSTEOPOROSIS *(Continued)*

3. Etidronate Disodium: Not FDA approved for postmenopausal osteoporosis and can decrease the quality of bone formation, therefore, change to alendronate.
4. Calcitonin (nasal; Miacalcin®): Indicated if estrogen refused, intolerant, or contraindicated. Potential analgesic effect.
   - Contraindications: Hypersensitivity to salmon protein or gelatin diluent; 1 spray (200 units) into 1 nostril daily (alternate right and left nostril daily); 5 days on and 2 days off is also effective; alternate day administration not effective. If used only for pain, can decrease dose once pain is controlled.
   - Side effects (few): Nasal dryness and irritation (periodically inspect); adequate dietary or supplemental calcium + vitamin D is essential.

   Subcutaneous route (100 units daily): Many side effects (eg, nausea, flushing, anorexia) and the discomfort/inconvenience of injection.
5. Fall prevention: Minimize psychoactive and cardiovascular drugs (monitor BP for orthostasis), give diuretics early in the day, environmental safety check.

	% Elemental Calcium	Elemental Calcium
Calcium gluconate (various)	9	500 mg = 45 mg
Calcium glubionate (Neo-Calglucon®)	6.5	1.8 g = 115 g/5 mL
Calcium lactate (various)	13	325 mg = 42.25 mg
Calcium citrate (Citrical®)	21	950 mg = 200 mg
Effervescent tabs (Citrical Liquitab®)		2376 mg = 500 mg
Calcium acetate		
Phos-Ex 250®	25	1000 mg = 250 mg
Phos-Lo®		667 mg = 169 mg
Calcium phosphate, tribasic (Posture®)	39	1565.2 mg = 600 mg
Calcium carbonate		
Tums®	40	1.2 g = 500 mg
Oscal-500® oral suspension		1.2 g/5 mL = 500 mg
Caltrate 600®		1.5 g = 600 mg

References

Ashworth L, "Focus on Alendronate. A Nonhormonal Option for the Treatment of Osteoporosis in Postmenopausal Women," *Formulary*, 1996, 31:23-30.

Johnson SR, "Should Older Women Use Estrogen Replacement," *J Am Geriatr Soc*, 1996, 44:89-90.

Liberman UA, Weiss SR, and Brool J, "Effect of Oral Alendronate on Bone-Mineral Density and the Incidence of Fracture in Postmenopausal Osteoporosis," *N Engl J Med*, 1995, 333:1437-43.

"New Drugs for Osteoporosis," *Med Lett Drugs Ther*, 1996, 38:1-3.

NIH Consensus Development Panel on Optimal Calcium Intake, *JAMA*, 1994, 272:1942-8.

NONVIRAL INFECTIOUS DISEASES

TUBERCULOSIS

Tuberculosis is caused by the organism *Mycobacterium tuberculosis* as well as a variety of other mycobacteria including *M. bovis, M. avium-intracellulare*, and *M. kansasii.* Diagnosis of tuberculosis can be made from a skin test and a positive chest x-ray as well as acid-fast smears of cultures from respiratory secretions. Nucleic acid probes and polymerase chain reaction (PCR) to identify nucleic acid of *M. tuberculosis* have recently become useful.

The treatment of tuberculosis is based on the general principle that multiple drugs should reduce infectivity within 2 weeks and that failures in therapy may be due to noncompliance with the long-term regimens necessary. General treatment regimens last 6-12 months.

Isoniazid-resistant and multidrug-resistant mycobacterial infections have become an increasingly significant problem in recent years. TB as an opportunistic disease in HIV-positive patients has also risen. Combination drug therapy has always been popular in TB management and the advent of new antibiotics has not diminished this need.

ANTITUBERCULOSIS DRUGS

Bactericidal Agents

Capreomycin *on page 251*
*Isoniazid *on page 769*
Kanamycin *on page 780*
*Pyrazinamide *on page 1152*
Rifabutin *on page 1179*
*Rifampin *on page 1180*
*Streptomycin *on page 1239*

Bacteriostatic Agents

Cycloserine *on page 385*
*Ethambutol *on page 534*
Ethionamide *on page 560*
Aminosalicyllic Acid *on page 100*

*Drugs of choice.

TESTING

Tuberculin Skin Test Recommendations[1]

Children for whom immediate skin testing is indicated:

- Contacts of persons with confirmed or suspected infectious tuberculosis (contact investigation); this includes children identified as contacts of family members or associates in jail or prison in the last 5 years
- Children with radiographic or clinical findings suggesting tuberculosis
- Children immigrating from endemic countries (eg, Asia, Middle East, Africa, Latin America)
- Children with travel histories to endemic countries and/or significant contact with indigenous persons from such countries

Children who should be tested annually for tuberculosis[2]:

- Children infected with HIV or living in household with HIV-infected persons
- Incarcerated adolescents

Children who should be tested every 2-3 years[2]:

- Children exposed to the following individuals: HIV-infected, homeless, residents of nursing homes, institutionalized adolescents or adults, users of illicit drugs, incarcerated adolescents or adults, and migrant farm workers. Foster children with exposure to adults in the preceding high-risk groups are included.

Children who should be considered for tuberculin skin testing at ages 4-6 and 11-16 years:

- Children whose parents immigrated (with unknown tuberculin skin test status) from regions of the world with high prevalence of tuberculosis; continued potential exposure by travel to the endemic areas and/or household contact with persons from the endemic areas (with unknown tuberculin skin test status) should be an indication for repeat tuberculin skin testing
- Children without specific risk factors who reside in high-prevalence areas; in general, a high-risk neighborhood or community does not mean an entire city is at high risk; rates in any area of the city may vary by neighborhood, or even from block to block; physicians should be aware of these patterns in determining the likelihood of exposure; public health officials or local tuberculosis experts should help clinicians identify areas that have appreciable tuberculosis rates

NONVIRAL INFECTIOUS DISEASES *(Continued)*

Children at increased risk of progression of infection to disease: Those with other medical risk factors, including diabetes mellitus, chronic renal failure, malnutrition, and congenital or acquired immunodeficiencies deserve special consideration. Without recent exposure, these persons are not at increased risk of acquiring tuberculosis infection. Underlying immune deficiencies associated with these conditions theoretically would enhance the possibility for progression to severe disease. Initial histories of potential exposure to tuberculosis should be included on all of these patients. If these histories or local epidemiologic factors suggest a possibility of exposure, immediate and periodic tuberculin skin testing should be considered. An initial Mantoux tuberculin skin test should be performed before initiation of immunosuppressive therapy in any child with an underlying condition that necessitates immunosuppressive therapy.

[1]BCG immunization is not a contraindication to tuberculin skin testing.

[2]Initial tuberculin skin testing is at the time of diagnosis or circumstance, beginning as early as at age 3 months.

Changes From Prior Recommendations on Tuberculin Testing and Treatment of Latent Tuberculosis Infection (LTBI)

Tuberculin Testing

- Emphasis on targeted tuberculin testing among persons at high risk for recent LTBI or with clinical conditions that increase the risk for tuberculosis (TB), regardless of age; testing is discouraged among persons at lower risk.
- For patients with organ transplant and other immunosuppressed patients (eg, persons receiving the equivalent of ≥15 mg/day prednisone for 1 month or more), 5 mm of induration rather than 10 mm of induration as a cut-off level for tuberculin positivity.
- A tuberculin skin test conversion is defined as an increase of ≥10 mm of induration within a 2-year period, regardless of age.

Treatment of Latent Tuberculosis Infection

- For HIV-negative persons, isoniazid given for 9 months is preferred over 6-month regimens.
- For HIV-positive persons and those with fibrotic lesions on chest x-ray consistent with previous TB, isoniazid should be given for 9 months instead of 12 months.
- For HIV-negative and HIV-positive persons, rifampin and pyrazinamide should be given for 2 months.
- For HIV-negative and HIV-positive persons, rifampin should be given for 4 months.

Clinical and Laboratory Monitoring

- Routine baseline and follow-up laboratory monitoring can be eliminated in most persons with LTBI, except for those with HIV infection, pregnant women (or those in the immediate postpartum period), and persons with chronic liver disease or those who use alcohol regularly.
- Emphasis on clinical monitoring for signs and symptoms of possible adverse effects, with prompt evaluation and changes in treatment, as indicated.

Modified from *MMWR Morb Mortal Wkly Rep*, 2000, 49(RR-6).

Criteria for Tuberculin Positivity, by Risk Group

Reaction ≥5 mm of Induration	Reaction ≥10 mm of Induration	Reaction ≥15 mm of Induration
HIV-positive persons	Recent immigrants (ie, within the last 5 years) from high prevalence countries	Persons with no risk factors for TB
Recent contacts of tuberculosis (TB) case patients	Injection drug users	
Fibrotic changes on chest radiograph consistent with prior TB	Residents and employees[1] of the following high risk congregate settings: prisons and jails, nursing homes and other long-term facilities for the elderly, hospitals and other healthcare facilities, residential facilities for patients with AIDS, and homeless shelters	
Patients with organ transplant and other immunosuppressed patients (receiving the equivalent of ≥15 mg/day of prednisone for 1 month of more)[2]	Mycobacteriology laboratory personnel	
	Persons with the following clinical conditions that place them at high risk: silicosis, diabetes mellitus, chronic renal failure, some hematologic disorders (eg, leukemias and lymphomas), other specific malignancies (eg, carcinoma of the head or neck and lung), weight loss of ≥10% of ideal body weight, gastrectomy, and jejunoileal bypass	
	Children <4 years of age or infants, children, and adolescents exposed to adults at high-risk	

[1]For persons who are otherwise at low risk and are tested at the start of employment, a reaction of ≥15 mm induration is considered positive.

[2]Risk of TB in patients treated with corticosteroids increases with higher dose and longer duration.

Modified from *MMWR Morb Mortal Wkly Rep*, 2000, 49(RR-6).

Recommendations, Rankings, and Performance Indicators for Treatment of Patients With Tuberculosis (TB)

Recommendation	Ranking[1] (Evidence)[2]	Performance Indicator
Obtain bacteriologic confirmation and susceptibility testing for patients with TB or suspected of having TB	A (II)	90% of adults with or suspected of having TB have 3 cultures for mycobacteria obtained before initiation of antituberculosis therapy (50% of children 0-12 y)
Place persons with suspected or confirmed smear-positive pulmonary or laryngeal TB in respiratory isolation until noninfectious	A (II)	90% of persons with sputum smear-positive TB remain in respiratory isolation until smear converts to negative
Begin treatment of patients with confirmed or suspected TB disease with one of the following drug combinations, depending on local resistance patterns: INH + RIF + PZA **or** INH + RIF + PZA + EMB **or** INH + RIF + PZA + SM	A (III)	90% of all patients with TB are started on INH + RIF + PZA + EMB or SM in geographic areas where >4% of TB isolates are resistant to INH
Report each case of TB promptly to the local public health department	A (III)	100% of persons with active TB are reported to the local public health department within 1 week of diagnosis
Perform HIV testing for all patients with TB	A (III)	80% of all patients with TB have HIV status determined within 2 months of a diagnosis of TB
Treat patients with TB caused by a susceptible organism for 6 months, using an ATS/CDC-approved regimen	A (I)	90% of all patients with TB complete 6 months of therapy with 12 months of beginning treatment
Re-evaluate patients with TB who are smear positive at 3 months for possible nonadherence or infection with drug-resistant bacilli	A (III)	90% of all patients with TB who are smear positive at 3 months have sputum culture/susceptibility testing performed within 1 month of the 3-month visit
Add ≥2 new antituberculosis agents when TB treatment failure is suspected	A (II)	100% of patients with TB with suspected treatment failure are prescribed ≥2 new antituberculosis agents
Perform tuberculin skin testing on all patients with a history of ≥1 of the following: HIV infection, I.V. drug use, homelessness, incarceration, or contact with a person with pulmonary TB	A (II)	80% of persons in the indicated population groups receive tuberculin skin test and return for reading
Administer treatment for latent TB infection to all persons with latent TB infection, unless it can be documented that they received such treatment previously	A (I)	75% of patients with positive tuberculin skin tests who are candidates for treatment for latent TB infection complete a course of therapy within 12 months of initiation

Adapted from the Infectious Diseases Society of America, *Clinical Infectious Diseases,* 2000, 31:633-9.

Note: ATS/CDC = American Thoracic Society and Centers for Disease Control and Prevention; EMB = ethambutol; INH = isoniazid; PZA = pyrazinamide; RIF = rifampin; SM = streptomycin.

[1]Strength of recommendation: A = preferred; B = acceptable alternative; C = offer when A and B cannot be given.

[2]Quality of evidence: I = randomized clinical trial data; II = data from clinical trials that are not randomized or were conducted in other populations; III = expert opinion.

NONVIRAL INFECTIOUS DISEASES *(Continued)*

PROPHYLAXIS

Specific Circumstances/ Organism	Comments	Regimen
Category I. Exposure (Household members and other close contacts of potentially infectious cases) (Exposee tuberculin test negative)[1]		
Neonate	Rx essential	INH (10 mg/kg/d) for 3 months, then repeat tuberculin test (TBnT). If mother's smear negative and infant's TBnT negative and chest x-ray (CXR) are normal, stop INH. In the United Kingdom, BCG is then given (*Lancet*, 1990, 2:1479), unless mother is HIV-positive. If infant's repeat TBnT is positive and/or CXR abnormal (hilar adenopathy and/or infiltrate), administer INH + RIF (10-20 mg/kg/d) (or streptomycin) for a total of 6 months. If mother is being treated, separation from mother is not indicated.
Children <5 y	Rx indicated	As for neonate first 3 months. If repeat TBnT is negative, stop. If repeat TBnT is positive, continue INH for a total of 9 months. If INH is not given initially, repeat TBnT at 3 months; if positive, treat with INH for 9 months (see Category II below).
Older children and adults	No Rx	Repeat TBnT at 3 months, if positive, treat with INH for 6 months (see Category II below)
Category II. Infection Without Disease (Positive tuberculin test)[1]		
Regardless of age (see INH Preventive Therapy)	Rx indicated	INH (5 mg/kg/d, maximum: 300 mg/d for adults, 10 mg/kg/d not to exceed 300 mg/d for children). Results with 6 months of treatment are nearly as effective as 12 months (65% vs 75% reduction in disease). *Am Thoracic Society* (6 months), *Am Acad Pediatrics*, 1991 (9 months). If CXR is abnormal, treat for 12 months. In HIV-positive patient, treatment for a minimum of 12 months, some suggest longer. Monitor transaminases monthly (*MMWR Morb Mortal Wkly Rep* 1989, 38:247).
Age <35 y	Rx indicated	Reanalysis of earlier studies favors INH prophylaxis for 6 months (if INH-related hepatitis case fatality rate is <1% and TB case fatality is ≥6.7%, which appears to be the case, monitor transaminases monthly (*Arch Int Med*, 1990, 150:2517).
INH-resistant organisms likely	Rx indicated	Data on efficacy of alternative regimens is currently lacking. Regimens include ETB + RIF daily for 6 months. PZA + RIF daily for 2 months, then INH + RIF daily until sensitivities from index case (if available) known, then if INH-CR, discontinue INH and continue RIF for 9 months, otherwise INH + RIF for 9 months (this latter is *Am Acad Pediatrics*, 1991 recommendation).
INH + RIF resistant organisms likely	Rx indicated	Efficacy of alternative regimens is unknown; PZA (25-30 mg/kg/d P.O.) + ETB (15-25 mg/kg/d P.O.) (at 25 mg/kg ETB, monitoring for retrobulbar neuritis required), for 6 months unless HIV-positive, then 12 months; PZA + ciprofloxacin (750 mg P.O. bid) or ofloxacin (400 mg P.O. bid) x 6-12 months *(MMWR Morb Mortal Wkly Rep*, 1992, 41(RR11):68).

INH = isoniazid; RIF = rifampin; KM = kanamycin; ETB = ethambutol.
SM = streptomycin; CXR = chest x-ray; Rx = treatment.

[1]Tuberculin test (TBnT). The standard is the Mantoux test, 5 TU PPD in 0.1 mL diluent stabilized with Tween 80. Read at 48-72 hours measuring maximum diameter of induration. A reaction ≥5 mm is defined as positive in the following: positive HIV or risk factors, recent close case contacts, CXR consistent with healed TBc. ≥10 mm is positive in foreign-born in countries of high prevalence, injection drug users, low income populations, nursing home residents, patients with medical conditions which increase risk (see above, preventive treatment). ≥15 mm is positive in all others (*Am Rev Resp Dis*, 1990, 142:725). Two-stage TBnT: Use in individuals to be tested regularly (ie, healthcare workers). TBn reactivity may decrease over time but be boosted by skin testing. If unrecognized, individual may be incorrectly diagnosed as recent converter. If first TBnT is reactive but <10 mm, repeat 5 TU in 1 week, if then ≥10 mm = positive, not recent conversion (*Am Rev Resp Dis*, 1979, 119:587).

TREATMENT

Recommended Treatment Regimens for Drug-Susceptible Tuberculosis in Infants, Children, and Adolescents

Infection or Disease Category	Regimen	Remarks
Latent tuberculosis infection (positive tuberculin skin test, no disease):		
• Isoniazid-susceptible	9 months of isoniazid once a day	If daily therapy is not possible, directly observed therapy twice a week may be used for 9 months.
• Isoniazid-resistant	6 months of rifampin once a day	
• Isoniazid-rifampin-resistant[1]	Consult a tuberculosis specialist	
Pulmonary and extrapulmonary (except meningitis)	2 months of isoniazid, rifampin, and pyrazinamide daily, followed by 4 months of isoniazid and rifampin[2]	If possible drug resistance is a concern, another drug (ethambutol or aminoglycoside) is added to the initial 3-drug therapy until drug susceptibilities are determined. Directly observed therapy is highly desirable. If hilar adenopathy only, a 6-month course of isoniazid and rifampin is sufficient. Drugs can be given 2 or 3 times/week under directly observed therapy in the initial phase if nonadherence is likely.
Meningitis	2 months of isoniazid, rifampin, pyrazinamide, and aminoglycoside or ethionamide, once a day, followed by 7-10 months of isoniazid and rifampin once a day or twice a week (9-12 months total)	A fourth drug, usually an aminoglycoside, is given with initial therapy until drug susceptibility is known. For patients who may have acquired tuberculosis in geographic areas where resistance to streptomycin is common, capreomycin, kanamycin, or amikacin may be used instead of streptomycin.

[1]Duration of therapy is longer for human immunodeficiency virus (HIV)-infected people, and additional drugs may be indicated.

[2]Medications should be administered daily for the first 2 weeks to 2 months of treatment and then can be administered 2-3 times/week by directly observed therapy.

Adapted from "Report of the Committee on Infectious Diseases," *2003 Red Book*®, 26th ed, 649.

Commonly Used Drugs for the Treatment of Tuberculosis in Infants, Children, and Adolescents

Drugs	Dosage Forms	Daily Dose (mg/kg)	Twice a Week Dose (mg/kg per dose)	Maximum Dose	Adverse Reactions
Ethambutol	Tablets 100 mg 400 mg	15-25	50	2.5 g	Optic neuritis (usually reversible), decreased red-green color discrimination, gastrointestinal tract disturbances, hypersensitivity
Isoniazid[1]	Scored tablets 100 mg 300 mg Syrup 10 mg/mL	10-15[2]	20-30	Daily, 300 mg Twice a week, 900 mg	Mild hepatic enzyme elevation, hepatitis,[2] peripheral neuritis, hypersensitivity
Pyrazinamide[1]	Scored tablets 500 mg	20-40	50	2 g	Hepatotoxic effects, hyperuricemia

NONVIRAL INFECTIOUS DISEASES *(Continued)*

Commonly Used Drugs for the Treatment of Tuberculosis in Infants, Children, and Adolescents *(continued)*

Drugs	Dosage Forms	Daily Dose (mg/kg)	Twice a Week Dose (mg/kg per dose)	Maximum Dose	Adverse Reactions
Rifampin[1]	Capsules 150 mg 300 mg Syrup formulated in syrup from capsules	10-20	10-20	600 mg	Orange discoloration of secretions or urine, staining of contact lenses, vomiting, hepatitis, influenza-like reaction, thrombocytopenia; oral contraceptives may be ineffective

[1]Rifamate® (Aventis Pharmaceuticals, Bridgewater, NJ) is a capsule containing 150 mg of isoniazid and 300 mg of rifampin. Two capsules provide the usual adult (>50 kg) daily doses of each drug. Rifater® is a capsule containing 50 mg of isoniazid, 120 mg of rifampin, and 300 mg of pyrazinamide. Isoniazid and rifampin also are available for parenteral administration.

[2]When isoniazid in a dosage exceeding 10 mg/kg/day is used in combination with rifampin, the incidence of hepatotoxic effects may be increased.

Adapted from "Report of the Committee on Infectious Diseases," *2003 Red Book®*, 26th ed, 650.

Rifampin is a bactericidal agent. It is metabolized by the liver and affects the pharmacokinetics of many other drugs, affecting their serum concentrations. Mycobacterium tuberculosis, initially resistant to rifampin, remains relatively uncommon in most areas of the United States. Rifampin is excreted in bile and urine and can cause orange urine, sweat and tears. It can also cause discoloration of soft contact lenses and render oral contraceptives ineffective. Hepatotoxicity occurs rarely. Blood dyscrasia accompanied by influenza-like symptoms can occur if doses are taken sporadically.

Less Commonly Used Drugs for Treatment of Drug-Resistant Tuberculosis in Infants, Children, and Adolescents[1]

Drugs	Dosage Forms	Daily Dose (mg/kg)	Maximum Dose	Adverse Reactions
Capreomycin	Vials 1 g	15-30 I.M.	1 g	Ototoxic and nephrotoxic effects
Ciprofloxacin[2]	Tablets 250 mg 500 mg 750 mg	Adults 500-1500 mg total per day (twice daily)	1.5 g	Theoretic effect on growing cartilage, gastrointestinal tract disturbances, rash, headache
Cycloserine	Capsules 250 mg	10-20	1 g	Psychosis, personality changes, seizures, rash
Ethionamide	Tablets 250 mg	15-20, given in 2-3 divided doses	1 g	Gastrointestinal tract disturbances, hepatotoxic effects, hypersensitive reactions
Kanamycin	Vials 75 mg/2 mL 500 mg/2 mL 1 g/3 mL	15-30 I.M.	1 g	Auditory and vestibular toxic effects, nephrotoxic effects
Levofloxacin[2]	Tablets 250 mg 500 mg Vials 25 mg/mL	Adults 500-1000 mg once daily	1 g	Theoretic effect on growing cartilage, gastrointestinal tract disturbances, rash, headache
Para-aminosalicylic acid (PAS)	Packets 3 mg	200-300 (2-4 times/day)	10 g	Gastrointestinal tract disturbances, hypersensitivity, hepatotoxic effects
Streptomycin (I.M.)	Vials 1 g 4 g	20-40	1 g	Auditory and vestibular toxic effects, nephrotoxic effects, rash

[1]These drugs should be used in consultation with a specialist in tuberculosis.

[2]Fluoroquinolones currently are not licensed for use in people <18 years of age; their use in younger patients necessitates assessment of the potential risks and benefits.

Adapted from "Report of the Committee on Infectious Diseases," *2003 Red Book®*, 26th ed, 651.

TB Drugs in Special Situations

Drug	Pregnancy[1]	CNS TB Disease	Renal Insufficiency
Isoniazid	Safe	Good penetration	Normal clearance
Rifampin	Safe	Fair penetration Penetrates inflamed meninges (10% to 20%)	Normal clearance
Pyrazinamide	Avoid	Good penetration	Clearance reduced Decrease dose or prolong interval
Ethambutol	Safe	Penetrates inflamed meninges only (4% to 64%)	Clearance reduced Decrease dose or prolong interval
Streptomycin	Avoid	Penetrates inflamed meninges only	Clearance reduced Decrease dose or prolong interval
Capreomycin	Avoid	Penetrates inflamed meninges only	Clearance reduced Decrease dose or prolong interval
Kanamycin	Avoid	Penetrates inflamed meninges only	Clearance reduced Decrease dose or prolong interval
Ethionamide	Do not use	Good penetration	Normal clearance
Para-aminosalicylic acid	Safe	Penetrates inflamed meninges only (10% to 50%)	Incomplete data on clearance
Cycloserine	Avoid	Good penetration	Clearance reduced Decrease dose or prolong interval
Ciprofloxacin	Do not use	Fair penetration (5% to 10%) Penetrates inflamed meninges (50% to 90%)	Clearance reduced Decrease dose or prolong interval
Ofloxacin	Do not use	Fair penetration (5% to 10%) Penetrates inflamed meninges (50% to 90%)	Clearance reduced Decrease dose or prolong interval
Amikacin	Avoid	Penetrates inflamed meninges only	Clearance reduced Decrease dose or prolong interval
Clofazimine	Avoid	Penetration unknown	Clearance probably normal

[1]Safe = the drug has not been demonstrated to have teratogenic effects.

Avoid = data on the drug's safety are limited, or the drug is associated with mild malformations (as in the aminoglycosides).

Do not use = studies show an association between the drug and premature labor, congenital malformations, or teratogenicity.

NONVIRAL INFECTIOUS DISEASES *(Continued)*

Recommendations for Coadministering Different Antiretroviral Drugs With the Antimycobacterial Drugs Rifabutin and Rifampin

Antiretroviral	Use in Combination with Rifabutin	Use in Combination with Rifampin	Comments
Saquinavir[1] Hard-gel capsules (HGC)	Possibly[2], if antiretroviral regimen also includes ritonavir	Possibly, if antiretroviral regimen also includes ritonavir	Coadministration of saquinavir SGC with usual-dose rifabutin (300 mg/day or 2-3 times/week) is a possibility. However, the pharmacokinetic data and clinical experience for this combination are limited.
Soft-gel capsules (SGC)	Probably[3]	Possibly, if antiretroviral regimen also includes ritonavir	The combination of saquinavir SGC or saquinavir HGC and ritonavir, coadministered with 1) usual-dose rifampin (600 mg/day or 2-3 times/week), or 2) reduced-dose rifabutin (150 mg 2-3 times/week) is a possibility. However, the pharmacokinetic data and clinical experience for these combinations are limited. Coadministration of saquinavir or saquinavir SGC with rifampin is not recommended because rifampin markedly decreases concentrations of saquinavir.
Ritonavir	Probably	Probably	If the combination of ritonavir and rifabutin is used, then a substantially reduced-dose rifabutin regimen (150 mg 2-3 times/week) is recommended. Coadministration of ritonavir with usual-dose rifampin (600 mg/day or 2-3 times/week) is a possibility, though pharmacokinetic data and clinical experience are limited.
Indinavir	Yes	No	There is limited, but favorable, clinical experience with coadministration of indinavir[4] with a reduced daily dose of rifabutin (150 mg) or with the usual dose of rifabutin (300 mg 2-3 times/week). Coadministration of indinavir with rifampin is not recommended because rifampin markedly decreases concentrations of indinavir.
Nelfinavir	Yes	No	There is limited, but favorable, clinical experience with coadministration of nelfinavir[5] with a reduced daily dose of rifabutin (150 mg) or with the usual dose of rifabutin (300 mg 2-3 times/week). Coadministration of nelfinavir with rifampin is not recommended because rifampin markedly decreases concentrations of nelfinavir.
Amprenavir	Yes	No	Coadministration of amprenavir with a reduced daily dose of rifabutin (150 mg) or with the usual dose of rifabutin (300 mg 2-3 times/week) is a possibility, but there is no published clinical experience. Coadministration of amprenavir with rifampin is not recommended because rifampin markedly decreases concentrations of amprenavir.
Nevirapine	Yes	Possibly	Coadministration of nevirapine with usual-dose rifabutin (300 mg/day or 2-3 times/week) is a possibility based on pharmacokinetic study data. However, there is no published clinical experience for this combination. Data are insufficient to assess whether dose adjustments are necessary when rifampin is coadministered with nevirapine. Therefore, rifampin and nevirapine should be used only in combination if clearly indicated and with careful monitoring.
Delavirdine	No	No	Contraindicated because of the marked decrease in concentrations of delavirdine when administered with either rifabutin or rifampin.

Recommendations for Coadministering Different Antiretroviral Drugs With the Antimycobacterial Drugs Rifabutin and Rifampin *(continued)*

Antiretroviral	Use in Combination with Rifabutin	Use in Combination with Rifampin	Comments
Efavirenz	Probably	Probably	Coadministration of efavirenz with increased-dose rifabutin (450 mg/day or 600 mg/day, or 600 mg 2-3 times/week) is a possibility, though there is no published clinical experience. Coadministration of efavirenz[6] with usual-dose rifampin (600 mg/day or 2-3 times/week) is a possibility, though there is no published clinical experience.

[1]Usual recommended doses are 400 mg twice daily for each of these protease inhibitors and 400 mg of ritonavir.

[2]Despite limited data and clinical experience, the use of this combination is potentially successful.

[3]Based on available data and clinical experience, the successful use of this combination is likely.

[4] Usual recommended dose is 800 mg every 8 hours; some experts recommend increasing the indinavir dose to 1000 mg every 8 hours if indinavir is used in combination with rifabutin.

[5]Usual recommended dose is 750 mg 3 times/day or 1250 mg twice daily; some experts recommend increasing the nelfinavir dose to 1000 mg if the 3-times/day dosing is used and nelfinavir is used in combination with rifabutin.

[6]Usual recommended dose is 600 mg/day; some experts recommend increasing the efavirenz dose to 800 mg/day if efavirenz is used in combination with rifampin.

Updated March 2000 from www.hivatis.org -"Updated Guidelines for the Use of Rifabutin or Rifampin for the Treatment and Prevention of Tuberculosis Among HIV-Infected Patients Taking Protease Inhibitors or Non-nucleoside Reverse Transcriptase Inhibitors," *MMWR,* March 10, 2000, 49(09):185-9.

Revised Drug Regimens for Treatment of Latent Tuberculosis Infection (LTBI) in Adults

Drug	Interval and Duration	Comments[1]	Rating[2] (Evidence)[3] HIV⁻	HIV⁺
Isoniazid	Daily for 9 months[4,5]	In HIV-infected patients, isoniazid may be administered concurrently with nucleoside reverse transcriptase inhibitors (NRTIs), protease inhibitors, or non-nucleoside reverse transcriptase inhibitors (NNRTIs)	A (II)	A (II)
	Twice weekly for 9 months[4,5]	Directly observed therapy (DOT) must be used with twice-weekly dosing	B (II)	B (II)
Isoniazid	Daily for 6 months[5]	Not indicated for HIV-infected persons, those with fibrotic lesions on chest radiographs, or children	B (I)	C (I)
	Twice weekly for 6 months[5]	DOT must be used with twice-weekly dosing	B (II)	C (I)
Rifampin[6]	Daily for 4 months	Used for persons who are contacts of patients with isoniazid-resistant, rifampin-susceptible TB In HIV-infected persons, most protease inhibitors or delavirdine should not be administered concurrently with rifampin. Rifabutin with appropriate dose adjustments can be used with protease inhibitors (saquinavir should be augmented with ritonavir) and NNRTIs (except delavirdine). Clinicians should consult web-based updates for the latest specific recommendations.	B (II)	B (III)
Rifampin plus pyrazinamide (RZ)	Daily for 2 months	RZ generally should not be offered for treatment of LTBI for HIV-infected or HIV-negative persons	D (II)	D (II)
	Twice weekly for 2-3 months		D (III)	D (III)

[1]Interactions with human immunodeficiency virus (HIV)-related drugs are updated frequently and are available at http://www.aidsinfo.nih.gov/guidelines.

[2]Strength of recommendation:

A. Both strong evidence of efficacy and substantial clinical benefit support recommendation for use. Should always be offered.
B. Moderate evidence for efficacy or strong evidence for efficacy but only limited clinical benefit supports recommendation for use. Should generally be offered.
C. Evidence for efficacy is insufficient to support a recommendation for or against use, or evidence for efficacy might not outweigh adverse consequences (eg, drug toxicity, drug interactions) or cost of the treatment or alternative approaches. Optional.
D. Moderate evidence for lack of efficacy or for adverse outcome supports a recommendation against use. Should generally not be offered.
E. Good evidence for lack of efficacy or for adverse outcome support a recommendation against use. Should never be offered.

[3]Quality of evidence supporting the recommendation:

I. Evidence from at least one properly randomized controlled trial.
II. Evidence from at least one well-designed clinical trial without randomization from cohort or case-controlled analytic studies (preferably from more than one center), from multiple time-series studies, or from dramatic results from uncontrolled experiments.
III. Evidence from opinions or respected authorities based on clinical experience, descriptive studies, or reports of expert committees.

[4]Recommended regimen for persons <18 years of age.

(footnotes continued on next page)

NONVIRAL INFECTIOUS DISEASES *(Continued)*

[5]Recommended regimens for pregnant women.

[6]The substitution of rifapentine for rifampin is not recommended because rifapentine's safety and effectiveness have not been established for patients with LTBI.

Adapted from CDC and American Thoracic Society, "Update: Adverse Event Data and Revised American Thoracic Society/CDC Recommendations Against the Use of Rifampin and Pyrazinamide for Treatment of Latent Tuberculosis Infection – United States, 2003," *MMWR Morb Mortal Wkly Rep*, 2003, 52(31):735-9.

SEXUALLY-TRANSMITTED DISEASES

Sexually transmitted diseases (STDs) represent a group of infectious diseases that include bacterial, fungal, and viral etiologies. Several related infections are covered elsewhere. Gonorrhea and syphilis will be covered here.

The management of a patient with a STD begins with identification. Paramount to the correct management of patients with a history of gonorrhea or syphilis is when the condition was diagnosed, how and with what agent it was treated, did the condition recur, and are there any residual signs and symptoms potentially indicating active or recurrent disease. With standard/universal precautions, the patient with *Neisseria gonorrhoea* or *Treponema pallidum* infection poses little threat to the dentist; however, diagnosis of oral lesions may be problematic. Gonococcal pharyngitis, primary syphilitic lesions (chancre), secondary syphilitic lesions (mucous patch), and tertiary lesions (gumma) may be identified by the dentist.

Drugs used in treatment of gonorrhea/syphilis include:

Cefixime *on page 282*

Ceftriaxone *on page 288*

Ciprofloxacin *on page 331*

Doxycycline *on page 471*

Ofloxacin *on page 1005*

Penicillin G Benzathine *on page 1058*

Penicillin G (Parenteral/Aqueous) *on page 1059*

Spectinomycin (alternate) *on page 1234*

The drugs listed above are often used alone or in stepped regimens, particularly when there is concomitant *Chlamydia* infection or when there is evidence of disseminated disease. The proper treatment for syphilis depends on the state of the disease.

Current treatment regimens for syphilis include:

1°, 2°, early latent (<1 y)	Benzathine penicillin G I.M.: 2-4 million units x 1 (alternate doxycycline)
Latent (>1 y), gumma, or cardiovascular	As above but once weekly for 3 weeks
Neurosyphilis	Aqueous penicillin G I.V.: 12-24 million units/day for 14 days

Treatment of Sexually-Transmitted Diseases

Type or Stage	Drug of choice.	Alternatives
CHLAMYDIAL INFECTION AND RELATED CLINICAL SYNDROMES[1]		
Urethritis, cervicitis, conjunctivitis, or proctitis (except lymphogranuloma venereum)		
	Azithromycin 1 g oral once **or** Doxycycline[2,3] 100 mg oral bid x 7 d	Ofloxacin[3] 300 mg oral bid x 7 d **or** Erythromycin[4] 500 mg oral qid x 7 d **or** Erythromycin ethylsuccinate 800 mg oral qid x 7 d **or** Levofloxacin 500 mg oral qd x 7 d
Recurrent/persistent		
	Metronidazole 2 g oral **plus** Erythromycin 500 mg oral qid x 7 d **or** Erythromycin ethylsuccinate 800 mg oral qid x 7 d	
Infection in pregnancy		
	Amoxicillin 500 mg oral tid x 7 d **or** Erythromycin[4] 500 mg oral qid x 7 d	Azithromycin[5] 1 g oral once **or** Erythromycin base 250 mg oral qid x 14 d **or** Erythromycin ethylsuccinate 800 mg oral qid x 7 d **or** Erythromycin ethylsuccinate 400 mg oral qid x 14 d
Neonatal		
Ophthalmia	Erythromycin (base or ethylsuccinate) 12.5 mg/kg oral qid x 10-14 d	
Pneumonia	Erythromycin (base or ethylsuccinate) 12.5 mg/kg oral or I.V. qid x 14 d	
Lymphogranuloma venereum		
	Doxycycline[2,3] 100 mg oral bid x 21 d	Erythromycin[4] 500 mg oral qid x 21 d
GONORRHEA[6]		
Urethral, cervical, rectal, or pharyngeal		
	Cefixime 400 mg oral once **or** Ceftriaxone 125 mg I.M. once **or** Ciprofloxacin[3] 500 mg oral once **or** Ofloxacin[3] 400 mg oral once **plus** (if chlamydial infection is not ruled out) Azithromycin 1 g oral once **or** Doxycycline 100 mg oral bid x 7 d	Spectinomycin 2 g I.M. once[7] **or** Lomefloxacin 400 mg oral once **or** Norfloxacin 800 mg oral once **or** Gatifloxacin 400 mg oral once
Disseminated gonococcal infection		
	Ceftriaxone 1 g I.M. or I.V. q24h	Cefotaxime 1 g I.V. q8h **or** Ceftizoxime 1 g I.V. q8h **or** **For persons allergic to β-lactam drugs:** Ciprofloxacin 500 mg I.V. q12h **or** Levofloxacin 250 mg I.V. once daily **or** Ofloxacin 400 mg I.V. q12h **or** Spectinomycin 2 g I.M. q12h All regimens should be continued for 24-48 hours after improvement begins, at which time therapy may be switched to one of the following regimens to complete a full week of antimicrobial therapy: Cefixime 400 mg oral bid **or** Ciprofloxacin 500 mg oral bid **or** Levofloxacin 500 mg oral once daily **or** Ofloxacin 400 mg oral bid
Gonococcal meningitis and endocarditis		
	Ceftriaxone 1-2 g I.V. q12h	

NONVIRAL INFECTIOUS DISEASES *(Continued)*

Treatment of Sexually-Transmitted Diseases

Type or Stage	Drug of choice.	Alternatives
EPIDIDYMITIS		
Most likely caused by enteric organisms, or in patients allergic to cephalosporins and/or tetracyclines		
	Ofloxacin 300 mg bid x 10 d **or** Levofloxacin 500 mg oral once daily x 10 d	
Most likely caused by gonorrhea or chlamydial		
	Ceftriaxone 250 mg I.M. once **followed by** Doxycycline[2] 100 mg oral bid x 10 d	
PELVIC INFLAMMATORY DISEASE		
– Inpatients	**Parenteral Regimen A** Cefotetan 2 g I.V. q12h **or** Cefoxitin 2 g I.V. q6h **plus** Doxycycline 100 mg oral or I.V. q12h (see Note) **Parenteral Regimen B** Clindamycin 900 mg I.V. q8h **plus** Gentamicin loading dose I.V. or I.M. (2 mg/kg of body weight) followed by maintenance dose (1.5 mg/kg) q8h. Single daily dosing may be substituted. **Note:** Because of pain associated with infusion, doxycycline should be administered orally when possible, even when the patient is hospitalized. Both oral and I.V. administration of doxycycline provide similar bioavailability. Parenteral therapy may be discontinued 24 hours after a patient improves clinically, and oral therapy with doxycycline (100 mg twice daily) should continue to complete 14 days of therapy. When tubo-ovarian abscess is present, many healthcare providers use clindamycin or metronidazole with doxycycline for continued therapy rather than doxycycline alone, because it provides more effective anaerobic coverage.	Ofloxacin 400 mg I.V. q12h **or** Levofloxacin 500 mg I.V. once daily **with or without** Metronidazole 500 mg I.V. q8h **or** Ampicillin/sulbactam 3 g I.V. q6h **plus** Doxycycline 100 mg oral or I.V. q12h
– Outpatients	**Regimen A** Ofloxacin 400 mg oral bid x 14 d **or** Levofloxacin 500 mg oral once daily x 14 d **with or without** Metronidazole 500 mg oral bid x 14 d **Regimen B** Ceftriaxone 250 mg I.M. once **or** Cefoxitin 2 g I.M. once and Probenecid 1 g oral once administered concurrently **or** Other parenteral 3rd generation cephalosporin (eg, ceftizoxime or cefotaxime) **plus** Doxycycline 100 mg oral bid x 14 d **with or without** Metronidazole 500 mg oral bid x 14 d If the healthcare provider prescribes outpatient oral or parenteral therapy, a follow-up examination should be performed within 72 hours using the criteria for clinical improvement described previously. If the patient has not improved, hospitalization for parenteral therapy and further evaluation are recommended.	

Treatment of Sexually-Transmitted Diseases

Type or Stage	Drug of choice.	Alternatives
VAGINAL INFECTION		
Trichomoniasis		
	Metronidazole 2 g oral once	Metronidazole 500 mg oral bid x 7 d
Bacterial vaginosis		
	Metronidazole 500 mg oral bid x 7 d **or** Metronidazole gel 0.75% 5 g intravaginally once or twice daily x 5 d **or** Clindamycin 2% cream 5 g intravaginally qhs x 3-7 d	Clindamycin 100 g intravaginally at bedtime x 3 d **or** Clindamycin 300 mg oral bid x 7 d **or** Metronidazole 2 g oral once[8]
Vulvovaginal candidiasis		
	Intravaginal butoconazole, clotrimazole, miconazole, terconazole, or tioconazole[9] **or** Fluconazole 150 mg oral once	Nystatin 100,000 unit vaginal tablet once daily x 14 d
SYPHILIS		
Early (primary, secondary, or latent <1 y)		
	Penicillin G benzathine 2.4 million units I.M. once[10]	Doxycycline[3] 100 mg oral bid x 14 d **or** Tetracycline 500 mg oral qid x 24 d
Late (>1 year's duration, cardiovascular, gumma, late-latent)		
	Penicillin G benzathine 2.4 million units I.M. weekly x 3 wk	Doxycycline[3] 100 mg oral bid x 4 wk
Neurosyphilis[11]		
	Penicillin G 3-4 million units I.V. q4h x 10-14 d	Penicillin G procaine 2.4 million units I.M. daily, **plus** Probenecid 500 mg qid oral, both x 10-14 d
Congenital		
	Penicillin G 50,000 units/kg I.V. q8-12h (q12h during first 7 d of life, then q8h for total of 10 d) **or** Penicillin G procaine 50,000 units/kg I.M. daily for 10 d	
CHANCROID[12]		
	Azithromycin 1 g oral once **or** Ceftriaxone 250 mg I.M. once **or** Ciprofloxacin[3] 500 mg oral bid x 3 d **or** Erythromycin[4] 500 mg oral qid x 7 d	
GENITAL HERPES		
First episode		
	Acyclovir 400 mg oral tid x 7-10 d[13] **or** Famciclovir 250 mg oral tid x 7-10 d **or** Valacyclovir 1 g oral bid x 7-10 d	Acyclovir 200 mg oral 5 times/d x 7-10 d[13]
Recurrent[14]		
	Acyclovir 400 mg oral tid x 5 d **or** Famciclovir 125 mg oral bid x 5 d **or** Valacyclovir 500 mg oral bid x 5 d	Acyclovir 200 mg orally 5 times/day for 5 d **or** Acyclovir 800 mg oral bid x 5 d
Severe (hospitalized patients)		
	Acyclovir 5-10 mg/kg I.V. q8h x 5-7 d	
Suppression of recurrence[15]		
	Valacyclovir 500 mg - 1 g once daily[16] **or** Acyclovir 400 mg oral bid **or** Famciclovir 250 mg oral bid	
GRANULOMA INGUINALE		
	Sulfamethoxazole and Trimethoprim 1 double-strength tablet oral bid for a minimum of 3 wk **or** Doxycycline 100 oral bid for a minimum of 3 wk	Ciprofloxacin 750 mg oral bid for a minimum of 3 wk **or** Erythromycin base 500 mg oral qid for a minimum of 3 wk **or** Azithromycin 1 g oral once per week for minimum of 3 weeks

NONVIRAL INFECTIOUS DISEASES *(Continued)*

Footnotes:

[1]Related clinical syndromes include nonchlamydial nongonococcal urethritis and cervicitis.
[2]Or tetracycline 500 mg oral qid or minocycline 100 mg oral bid.
[3]Contraindicated in pregnancy.
[4]Erythromycin estolate is contraindicated in pregnancy.
[5]Safety in pregnancy not established.
[6]All patients should also receive a course of treatment effective for *Chlamydia*.
[7]Recommended only for use during pregnancy in patients allergic to beta-lactams. Not effective for pharyngeal infection.
[8]Higher relapse rate with single dose, but useful for patients who may not comply with multiple-dose therapy.
[9]For preparations and dosage of topical products, see *Medical Letter*, 36:81,1994; single-dose therapy is not recommended.
[10]Some experts recommend repeating this regimen after 7 days, especially in patients with HIV infection.
[11]Patients allergic to penicillin should be desensitized.
[12]All regimens, especially single-dose ceftriaxone, are less effective in HIV-infected patients.
[13]For first-episode proctitis, use acyclovir 800 mg oral tid or 400 mg oral 5 times/day.
[14]Antiviral therapy is variably effective for treatment of recurrences; only effective if started early.
[15]Preventive treatment should be discontinued for 1-2 months once a year to reassess the frequency of recurrence.
[16]Use 500 mg qd in patients with <10 recurrences per year and 500 mg bid or 1 g daily in patients with ≥10 recurrences per year.

Adapted from "Sexually Transmitted Diseases Treatment Guidelines 2002," *MMWR Morb Mortal Wkly Rep*, 2002, 51(RR-6).

ANTIBIOTIC PROPHYLAXIS

PREPROCEDURAL GUIDELINES FOR DENTAL PATIENTS

INTRODUCTION

In dental practice, the clinician is often confronted with a decision to prescribe antibiotics. The focus of this section is on the use of antibiotics as a preprocedural treatment in the prevention of adverse infectious sequelae in the two most commonly encountered situations: prevention of endocarditis and prosthetic implants.

The criteria for preprocedural decisions begins with patient evaluation. An accurate and complete medical history is always the initial basis for any prescriptive treatments on the part of the dentist. These prescriptive treatments can include ordering appropriate laboratory tests, referral to the patient's physician for consultation, or immediate decision to prescribe preprocedural antibiotics. The dentist should also be aware that antibiotic coverage of the patient might be appropriate due to diseases that are covered elsewhere in this text, such as human immunodeficiency virus, cavernous thrombosis, undiagnosed or uncontrolled diabetes, lupus, renal failure, and periods of neutropenia as are often associated with cancer chemotherapy. In these instances, medical consultation is almost always necessary in making antibiotic decisions in order to tailor the treatment and dosing to the individual patient's needs.

Note: The ADA Council on Scientific Affairs recently restated the dentist's responsibility when prescribing antibiotics to oral contraceptive users (*JADA*, 2002, 133:880). It is recommended that dental professionals advise these patients to consult their physician for additional barrier contraception due to potential reduction in the efficacy of oral contraceptives from antibiotic interaction.

All tables or figures in this chapter were adapted from the ADA Advisory Statement: "Antibiotic Prophylaxis for Dental Patients With Total Joint Replacement," *J Am Dent Assoc*, 1997, 128:1004-8 or from Dajani AS, Taubert KA, Wilson W, et al, "Prevention of Bacterial Endocarditis. Recommendations by the American Heart Association," *JAMA*, 1997, 7(22):1794-801.

PREVENTION OF BACTERIAL ENDOCARDITIS

Guidelines for the prevention of bacterial endocarditis have been updated by the American Heart Association with approval by the Council of Scientific Affairs of the American Dental Association. These guidelines supercede those issued and published in 1990. They were developed to more clearly define the situations of antibiotic use, to reduce costs to the patient, to reduce gastrointestinal adverse effects, and to improve patient compliance. Highlights of the current recommendations are shown in Table 1 and the specific antibiotic regimens are listed in Table 2 and further illustrated in Figure 1.

Amoxicillin is an amino-type penicillin with an extended spectrum of antibacterial action compared to penicillin VK. The pharmacology of amoxicillin as a dental antibiotic has been reviewed previously in *General Dentistry*. The suggested regimen for standard general prophylaxis is a dose of 2 g 1 hour before the procedure. A follow-up dose is no longer necessary. This dose of amoxicillin is lower than the previous dosing regimen of 3 g 1 hour before the procedure and then 1.5 g 6 hours after the initial dose. Dajani, et al, stated that the 2 g dose of amoxicillin resulted in adequate serum levels for several hours making the second dose unnecessary, both because of a prolonged serum level of amoxicillin above the minimal inhibitory concentration for oral streptococci, and an inhibitory activity of 6-14 hours by amoxicillin against streptococci. The new pediatric dose is 50 mg/kg orally 1 hour before the procedure and not to exceed the adult dose. Amoxicillin is available in capsules (250 mg and 500 mg), chewable tablets (125 mg, 200 mg, 250 mg, 400 mg), and liquid suspension (400 mg/5 mL). The retail cost of generic capsules and tablets ranges from 20-30 cents each and suspension is approximately $12 per 100 mL.

The dentist should be vigilant in reviewing literature for updates. The guidelines for antibiotic prophylaxis continue to be reviewed and it is likely that additional modifications to the recommendations will be published in the near future.

ANTIBIOTIC PROPHYLAXIS *(Continued)*

Table 1. HIGHLIGHTS OF THE NEWEST GUIDELINES FOR ENDOCARDITIS PREVENTION

No.	Change From Old Guidelines
1.	Oral initial dosing for amoxicillin has been reduced to 2 g.
2.	Follow-up antibiotic dose is no longer recommended.
3.	Erythromycin is no longer recommended for penicillin-allergic patients.
4.	Clindamycin and other alternatives have been recommended to replace the erythromycin regimens.
5.	Clearer guidelines for prophylaxis decisions for patients with mitral valve prolapse have been developed.

For individuals unable to take oral medications, intramuscular or intravenous ampicillin is recommended for both adults and children (Table 2). It is to be given 30 minutes before the procedure at the same doses used for the oral amoxicillin medication. Ampicillin is also an amino-type penicillin having an antibacterial spectrum similar to amoxicillin. Ampicillin is not absorbed from the GI tract as effectively as amoxicillin and, therefore, is not recommended for oral use.

Table 2. PROPHYLACTIC REGIMENS FOR BACTERIAL ENDOCARDITIS FOR DENTAL PROCEDURES

Situation	Agent	Regimen[1]
Standard general prophylaxis	Amoxicillin *on page 114*	Adults: 2 g orally 1 hour before procedure Children: 50 mg/kg orally 1 hour before procedure
Unable to take oral medications	Ampicillin *on page 124*	Adults: 2 g I.M. or I.V. within 30 minutes before procedure Children: 50 mg/kg I.M. or I.V. within 30 minutes before procedure
Allergic to penicillin	Clindamycin *on page 348* or	Adults: 600 mg orally 1 hour before procedure Children: 20 mg/kg orally 1 hour before procedure
	Cephalexin *on page 294* or Cefadroxil *on page 275*	Adults: 2 g orally 1 hour before procedure Children: 50 mg/kg orally 1 hour before procedure
	Azithromycin *on page 174* or Clarithromycin *on page 343*	Adults: 500 mg orally 1 hour before procedure Children: 15 mg/kg orally 1 hour before procedure
Allergic to penicillin and unable to take oral medications	Clindamycin *on page 348* or	Adults: 600 mg I.V. within 30 minutes before procedure Children: 20 mg/kg I.V. within 30 minutes before procedure
	Cefazolin *on page 278*	Adults: 1 g I.M. or I.V. within 30 minutes before procedure Children: 25 mg/kg I.M. or I.V. within 30 minutes before procedure

[1]Total children's dose should not exceed adult dose.

Note: Cephalosporins should not be used in individuals with immediate-type hypersensitivity reaction (urticaria, angioedema, or anaphylaxis) to penicillins.

Individuals who are allergic to the penicillins, such as amoxicillin or ampicillin, should be treated with an alternate antibiotic. The new guidelines have suggested a number of alternate agents including clindamycin, cephalosporins, azithromycin, and clarithromycin. Clindamycin (Cleocin®) occupies an important niche in dentistry as a useful and effective antibiotic and it was a recommended alternative agent for the prevention of bacterial endocarditis in the previous guidelines. In the new guidelines, the oral adult dose is 600 mg 1 hour before the procedure. A follow-up dose is not necessary. Clindamycin is available as 300 mg capsules; thus 2 capsules will provide the recommended dose. The children's oral dose for clindamycin is 20 mg/kg 1 hour before the procedure. Clindamycin is also available as flavored granules for oral solution. When reconstituted with water, each bottle yields a solution containing 75 mg/5 mL. Intravenous clindamycin is recommended in adults and children who are allergic to penicillin and unable to take oral medications. Refer to Table 2 for the intravenous doses of clindamycin.

Clindamycin was developed in the 1960s as a semisynthetic derivative of lincomycin which was found in the soil organism, *Streptomyces lincolnensis*, near Lincoln, Nebraska. It is commercially available as the hydrochloride salt to improve solubility in the GI tract. Clindamycin is antibacterial against most aerobic Gram-positive cocci including staphylococci and streptococci, and against many types of anaerobic Gram-negative and Gram-positive organisms. It has been used over the years in dentistry as an alternative to penicillin and erythromycins for the treatment of oral-facial infections. For a review, see Wynn and Bergman.

The mechanism of antibacterial action of clindamycin is the same as erythromycin. It inhibits protein synthesis in susceptible bacteria resulting in the inhibition of bacterial growth and replication. Following oral administration of a single dose of clindamycin (150 mg, 300 mg, or 600 mg) on an empty stomach, 90% of the dose is rapidly absorbed into the bloodstream and peak serum concentrations are attained within 45-80 minutes. Administration with food does not markedly impair absorption into the bloodstream. Clindamycin serum levels exceed the minimum inhibitory concentration (MIC) for bacterial growth for at least 6 hours after the recommended dose of 600 mg. The serum half-life is 2-3 hours.

Adverse effects of clindamycin after a single dose are virtually nonexistent. Although it is estimated that 1% of patients taking clindamycin will develop symptoms of pseudomembranous colitis, these symptoms usually develop after 9-14 days of clindamycin therapy. These symptoms have never been reported in patients taking an acute dose for the prevention of endocarditis.

In lieu of clindamycin, penicillin-allergic individuals may receive cephalexin (Keflex®) or cefadroxil (Duricef®) provided that they have not had an immediate-type sensitivity reaction such as anaphylaxis, urticaria, or angioedema to penicillins. These antibiotics are first-generation cephalosporins having an antibacterial spectrum of action similar to amoxicillin and ampicillin. They elicit a bactericidal action by inhibiting cell wall synthesis in susceptible bacteria. The recommended adult prophylaxis dose for either of these drugs is 2 g 1 hour before the procedure. Again, no follow-up dose is needed. The children's oral dose for cephalexin and cefadroxil is 50 mg/kg 1 hour before the procedure. Cephalexin is supplied as capsules (250 mg and 500 mg) and tablets (250 mg, 500 mg, 1 g). Cefadroxil is supplied as 500 mg capsules and 1 g tablets. Both antibiotics are available in the form of powder for oral suspension at concentrations of 125 mg and 250 mg (cefadroxil also available as 500 mg/5 mL).

For those individuals (adults and children) allergic to penicillin and unable to take oral medicines, parenteral cefazolin (Ancef®) may be used, provided that they do not have the sensitivities described previously and footnoted in Table 2. Cefazolin is also a first-generation cephalosporin. Please note that the parenteral cefazolin can be given I.M. or I.V. (refer to Table 2 for the adult and children's doses of parenteral cefazolin).

Azithromycin (Zithromax®) and clarithromycin (Biaxin®) are members of the erythromycin-class of antibiotics known as the macrolides. The pharmacology of these drugs has been reviewed previously in *General Dentistry.* The erythromycins have been available for use in dentistry and medicine since the mid 1950s. Azithromycin and clarithromycin represent the first additions to this class in >40 years. The adult prophylactic dose for either drug is 500 mg 1 hour before the procedure with no follow-up dose. The pediatric prophylactic dose of azithromycin and clarithromycin is 15 mg/kg orally 1 hour before the procedure. Although the erythromycin family of drugs are known to inhibit the hepatic metabolism of theophylline and carbamazepine to enhance their effects, azithromycin has not been shown to affect the liver metabolism of these drugs.

Azithromycin is well absorbed from the gastrointestinal tract and is extensively taken up from the circulation into tissues with a slow release from those tissues. It reaches peak serum levels in 2-4 hours and serum half-life is 68 hours. Zithromax® is supplied as 250 mg (retail cost ranges from $7-$8 each) and 600 mg tablets (approximately $15 each). It is also available for oral suspension, supplied as single-dose packets containing 1 g each (approximately $60 for 3 packets). Azithromycin is not yet available as a generic drug.

Clarithromycin (Biaxin®) achieves peak plasma concentrations in 3 hours and maintains effective serum concentrations over a 12-hour period. Reports indicate that it probably interacts with theophylline and carbamazepine by elevating the plasma concentrations of the two drugs. Biaxin® is supplied as 250 mg and 500 mg tablets (retail cost approximately $4 each) and 500 mg extended release tablets (approximately $5 each). It is also available as suspension, supplied as 125 mg/100 mL and 125 mg/50 mL (approximately $20 per 50 mL). Clarithromycin is not yet available as a generic drug.

Amoxicillin *on page 114*

Ampicillin *on page 124*

Azithromycin *on page 174*

Cefadroxil *on page 275*

Cefazolin *on page 278*

Cephalexin *on page 294*

Clarithromycin *on page 343*

Clindamycin *on page 348*

ANTIBIOTIC PROPHYLAXIS *(Continued)*

Clinical Considerations for Dentistry

See Figure 1 *on page 1517.*

The clinician should review carefully those detailed dental procedures in Table 3 to determine those treatment conditions where prophylaxis is, or is not, recommended. In general, in patients with cardiac conditions where prophylaxis is recommended (Table 4), invasive dental procedures where bleeding is likely to be induced from hard or soft tissues (Table 3) should be preceded by antibiotic coverage (Table 2). Clearly, the production of significant bacteremia during a dental procedure is the major risk factor. Patients with a suspicious history of a cardiac condition who are in need of an immediate dental procedure should be prophylaxed with an appropriate antibiotic prior to the procedure(s) until medical evaluation has been completed and the risk level determined. If unanticipated bleeding develops during a procedure in an at-risk patient, appropriate antibiotics should be given immediately. The efficacy of this action is based on animal studies and is possibly effective ≤ 2 hours after the bacteremia.

Table 3.
DENTAL PROCEDURES AND PREPROCEDURAL ANTIBIOTICS

Endocarditis or Prosthesis Prophylaxis Recommended Due to Likely Significant Bacteremia[1]
Dental extractions
Periodontal procedures including surgery, subgingival placement of antibiotic fibers/strips, scaling and root planing, probing, recall maintenance
Dental implant placement and reimplantation of avulsed teeth
Endodontic (root canal) instrumentation or surgery only beyond the apex
Initial placement of orthodontic bands but not brackets
Intraligamentary local anesthetic injections
Prophylactic cleaning of teeth or implants where bleeding is anticipated
Endocarditis Prophylaxis Not Recommended Due to Usually Insignificant Bacteremia
Restorative dentistry[2] (operative and prosthodontic) with or without retraction cord[3]
Local anesthetic injections (nonintraligamentary)
Intracanal endodontic treatment; postplacement and build-up[3]
Placement of rubber dam[3]
Postoperative suture removal
Placement of removable prosthodontic/orthodontic appliances
Oral impressions[3]
Fluoride treatments
Taking of oral radiographs
Orthodontic appliance adjustment
Shedding of primary teeth
[3]In general, the presence of moderate to severe gingival inflammation may elevate these procedures to a higher risk of bacteremia.

[1]Prophylaxis is recommended for patients with high- and moderate-risk cardiac as well as high-risk prosthesis conditions

[2]This includes restoration of decayed teeth and replacement of missing teeth

[3]Clinical judgment may indicate antibiotic use in any circumstances that may create significant bleeding.

Patients with moderate to advanced gingival inflammatory disease and/or periodontitis should be considered at greater risk of bacteremia. However, the ongoing daily risk of self-induced bacteremia in these patients is currently thought to be minimal as compared to the bacteremia during dental procedures. The clinician may wish to consider the use of a preprocedural antimicrobial rinse in addition to antibiotic prophylaxis and, of course, efforts should always focus on improving periodontal health during dental care. If a series of dental procedures is planned, the clinician must judge whether an interval between procedures, requiring prophylaxis, should be scheduled. The literature supports 9- to 14-day intervals as ideal to minimize the risk of emergence of resistant organisms. Since serum levels of the standard amoxicillin dose may be adequate for 6-14 hours depending on the specific organism challenge, the clinician may have to consider the efficacy of a second dose if multiple procedures are planned over the course of a single day.

Table 4.
CARDIAC CONDITIONS PREDISPOSING TO ENDOCARDITIS

Endocarditis Prophylaxis Recommended
High-Risk Category
Prosthetic cardiac valves, including bioprosthetic and homograft valves
Previous bacterial endocarditis
Complex cyanotic congenital heart disease (eg, single ventricle states, transposition of the great arteries, tetralogy of Fallot)
Surgically constructed systemic pulmonary shunts or conduits
Moderate-Risk Category
Most other congenital cardiac malformations (other than above and below)
Acquired valvar dysfunction (eg, rheumatic heart disease)
Hypertrophic cardiomyopathy
Mitral valve prolapse with valvar regurgitation and/or thickened leaflets[1]
Endocarditis Prophylaxis Not Recommended
Negligible-Risk Category (no greater risk than the general population)
Isolated secundum atrial septal defect
Surgical repair of atrial septal defect, ventricular septal defect, or patent ductus arteriosus (without residual defects beyond 6 mo)
Previous coronary artery bypass graft surgery
Mitral valve prolapse without valvar regurgitation
Physiologic, functional, or innocent heart murmurs
Previous Kawasaki disease without valvar dysfunction
Previous rheumatic fever without valvar dysfunction
Cardiac pacemakers (intravascular and epicardial) and implanted defibrillators

[1]**Specific risk for patients with a history of fenfluramine or dexfenfluramine (fen-phen or Redux®) use, has not been determined. Such patients should have medical evaluation for potential cardiac damage, as currently recommended by the FDA.**

For patients with suspected or confirmed mitral valve prolapse (MVP), the risk of infection as well as other complications such as tachycardia, syncope, congestive heart failure, or progressive regurgitation are variable. The risk depends on age and severity of MVP. The decision to recommend prophylaxis in such patients is oftentimes controversial but it is generally agreed that the determination of regurgitation is the most predictive (see Algorithm Figure 2 at the end of this chapter). Therefore, patients with MVP with mitral regurgitation require prophylaxis. If the regurgitation is undetermined and the patient is in need of an immediate procedure, then prophylaxis should be given in any case and the patient referred for further evaluation. If echocardiographic or Doppler studies demonstrate regurgitation, then prophylaxis would be recommended routinely. If no regurgitation can be demonstrated by these studies, then MVP alone does not require prophylaxis.

PREPROCEDURAL ANTIBIOTICS FOR PROSTHETIC IMPLANTS

A significant number of dental patients have had total joint replacements or other implanted prosthetic devices. Prior to performing dental procedures that might induce bacteremia, the dentist must consider the use of antibiotic prophylaxis in these patients. Until recently, only the American Heart Association had taken a formal stance on implanted devices by suggesting guidelines for the use of antibiotic prophylaxis in patients with prosthetic heart valves. These guidelines and the recent guidelines for prevention of bacterial endocarditis have been published in *General Dentistry*.

The use of antibiotics in patients with other prosthetic devices, including total joint replacements has remained controversial because of several issues. Late infections of implanted prosthetic devices have rarely been associated with microbial organisms of oral origin. Secondly, since late infections in such patients are often not reported, data is lacking to substantiate or refute this potential. Also, there is general acceptance that patients with acute infections at distant sites such as the oral cavity may be at greater risk of infection of an implanted prosthetic device. Periodontal disease has been implicated as a distant site infection. Since antibiotics are associated with allergies and other adverse reactions, and because the frequent use of antibiotics may lead to emergence of resistant organisms, any perceived benefit of antibiotic prophylaxis must always be weighed against known risks of toxicity, allergy, or potential microbial resistance.

Recently, an advisory group made up of representatives from the American Dental Association and the American Academy of Orthopaedic Surgeons published a statement in the *Journal of the American Dental Association* on the use of antibiotics prior to dental procedures in patients with total joint replacements. The statement concluded that antibiotic prophylaxis should not be prescribed routinely for most dental patients with total joint replacements or for any patients with pins, plates, and screws. However, in an attempt to base the guidelines on available scientific evidence, the advisory group stated that

ANTIBIOTIC PROPHYLAXIS *(Continued)*

certain patients may be potential risks for joint infection thus justifying the use of prophylactic antibiotics. Those conditions considered by the advisory group to be associated with potential elevated risk of joint infections are listed in Table 5. The dentist should carefully review the patient's history to ensure identification of those medical problems leading to potential elevated risks of joint infections as listed in Table 5. Where appropriate, medical consultation with the patient's internist or orthopedist may be prudent to assist in this determination. The orthopedist should be queried specifically, as to the status of the joint prosthesis itself.

Table 5.
PATIENTS WITH POTENTIAL ELEVATED RISK OF JOINT INFECTION

Inflammatory arthropathies: Rheumatoid arthritis, systemic lupus erythematosus
Disease-, drug-, or radiation-induced immunosuppression
Insulin-dependent diabetes
First 2 years following joint replacement
Previous prosthetic joint infections
Patients with acute infections at a distant site
Hemophilia
Malnourishment[1]
Patients with malignancies[1]
Patients with HIV infection[1]

[1]Source: American Dental Association; American Academy of Orthopedic Surgeons, "Antibiotic Prophylaxis for Dental Patients With Total Joint Replacements," *J Am Dent Assoc*, 2003, 134(7):895-9.

Patients who present with elevated risks of joint infections, in which the dentist is going to perform any procedures associated with a high risk of bacteremia, need to receive preprocedural antibiotics. Those dental procedures associated with high risk of bacteremia are listed in Table 3. Patients undergoing dental procedures involving low risk of bacteremia, probably do not require premedication even though the patient may be in the category of elevated risk of joint infections. Patients with an acute oral infection or moderate to severe gingival inflammation and/or periodontitis must be considered at higher risk for bacteremia during dental procedures than those without active dental disease. In these patients, as in all patients, the dental clinician should aggressively treat these oral conditions striving for optimum oral health. The listing of low bacteremia risks in Table 3 may need to be reconsidered, depending on the patient's oral health.

ANTIBIOTIC REGIMENS

The antibiotic prophylaxis regimens as suggested by the advisory panel are listed in Table 6. These regimens are not exactly the same as those listed in Table 2 (for prevention of endocarditis) and must be reviewed carefully to avoid confusion. Cephalexin, cephradine, or amoxicillin may be used in patients not allergic to penicillin. The selected antibiotic is given as a single 2 g dose 1 hour before the procedure. A follow-up dose is not recommended. Cephalexin (Keflex®) and amoxicillin were described earlier in this section. Cephradine (Velosef®) is a first-generation cephalosporin-type antibiotic, effective against anaerobic bacteria and aerobic Gram-positive bacteria. It is predominantly used to treat infections of the bones and joints, lower respiratory tract, urinary tract, skin, and soft tissues.

Parenteral cefazolin (Ancef®) or ampicillin are the recommended antibiotics for patients unable to take oral medications (see Table 6 for doses). Cefazolin is a first-generation cephalosporin, effective against anaerobes and aerobic Gram-positive bacteria. Ampicillin is an aminopenicillin (described earlier). For patients allergic to penicillin, clindamycin is the recommended antibiotic of choice. Clindamycin is active against aerobic and anaerobic streptococci, most staphylococci, the *Bacteroides*, and the *Actinomyces* families of bacteria. The recommended oral and parenteral doses of clindamycin in the joint prosthetic patient are listed in Table 6 below.

Table 6.
ANTIBIOTIC REGIMENS FOR PATIENTS WITH PROSTHETIC IMPLANTS

Patients not allergic to penicillin:	Cephalexin, cephradine, or amoxicillin:	2 g orally 1 hour prior to the procedure
Patients not allergic to penicillin and unable to take oral medications:	Cefazolin: or Ampicillin:	1 g I.M. or I.V. 1 hour prior to the procedure 2 g I.M. or I.V. 1 hour prior to the procedure
Patients allergic to penicillin:	Clindamycin:	600 mg orally 1 hour prior to dental procedure
Patients allergic to penicillin and unable to take oral medications:	Clindamycin:	600 mg I.V. 1 hour prior to the procedure

Amoxicillin *on page 114*
Ampicillin *on page 124*
Cefazolin *on page 278*
Cephalexin *on page 294*
Cephradine *on page 296*
Clindamycin *on page 348*

Clinical Considerations for Dentistry

See Figure 3 on page 1518.

The frequency of postinsertion infections in patients who have undergone total joint replacement or prosthetic device placement is variable. The most common cause of infection with all devices is found to be from contamination at the time of surgical insertions. The presence of an acute distant infection at a site other than the joint, however, appears to be a risk factor for late infection of these devices. The rationale by the American Dental Association and the American Academy of Orthopedic Surgeons in their advisory statement has been to provide guidelines to minimize the use of antibiotics to the first 2 years following total joint replacement. As more data are collected, these recommendations may be revised. However, it is thought to be prudent for the dental clinician to fully evaluate all patients with respect to history and or physical findings prior to determining the risk.

If a procedure considered to be low risk for bacteremia is performed in a patient at risk for joint complications, and inadvertent bleeding occurs, then an appropriate antibiotic should be given immediately. Although this is not ideal, animal studies suggest that it may be useful. Likewise, in patients where concern exists over joint complications and a medical consultation cannot be immediately obtained, the patient should be treated as though antibiotic coverage is necessary until such time that an appropriate consultation can be completed. The presence of an acute oral infection, in addition to any pre-existing dental conditions, may increase the risk of late infection at the prosthetic joint. Even though most late joint infections are caused by *Staphylococcus* sp, the risk of bacteremia involving another organism, predominant in an acute infection, may increase the risk of joint infection.

The dentist may also need to consider the question of multiple procedures over a period of time. Procedures planned over a period of several days would best be rescheduled at intervals of 9-14 days. The risk of emergence of resistant organisms in patients receiving multiple short-term doses of antibiotics has been shown to be greater than those receiving antibiotics over longer intervals of time.

FREQUENTLY ASKED QUESTIONS

Can erythromycin still be used to prevent bacterial endocarditis in dental patients?

If the clinician has successfully used erythromycin in the past, this form of prophylaxis can be continued using the regimen included in the recommendation of 1990. Erythromycin has, however, been excluded for the vast majority of patients due to gastric upset.

If the patient is presently taking antibiotics for some other ailment, is prophylaxis still necessary?

If a patient is already taking antibiotics for another condition, prophylaxis should be accomplished with a drug from another class. For example, in the patient who is not allergic to penicillin who is taking erythromycin for a medical condition such as mycoplasma infection, amoxicillin would be the drug of choice for prophylaxis. Also, in the penicillin-allergic patient taking clindamycin, prophylaxis would best be accomplished with azithromycin or clarithromycin. The new guidelines restated the position that doses of antibiotics for prevention of recurrence of rheumatic fever are thought to be inadequate to prevent bacterial endocarditis and prophylaxis should be accomplished with the full dose of a drug from another class.

Can clindamycin be used safely in patients with gastrointestinal disorders?

If a patient has a history of inflammatory bowel disease and is allergic to penicillin, azithromycin or clarithromycin should be selected over clindamycin. In patients with a negative history of inflammatory bowel disease, clindamycin has not been shown to induce colitis following a single-dose administration.

Why do the suggested drug regimens for patients with joint prostheses resemble so closely the regimens for the prevention of bacterial endocarditis?

Bacteremia is the predisposing risk factor for the development of endocarditis in those patients at risk due to a cardiac condition. Likewise, the potential of bacteremia during dental procedures is considered to be the risk factor in some late joint prostheses infections, even though this risk is presumed to be much lower.

ANTIBIOTIC PROPHYLAXIS *(Continued)*

How do we determine those patients who have had joint replacement complications?

Patients who have had complications during the initial placement of a total joint would be those who had infection following placement, those with recurrent pain, or those who have had previous joint replacement failures. If the patient reports even minor complications, a medical consultation with the orthopedist would be the most appropriate action for the dentist.

Is prophylaxis required in patients with pins, screws, or plates often used in orthopedic repairs?

There is currently no evidence supporting use of antibiotics following the placement of pins, plates, or screws. Breast implants, dental implants, and implanted lenses in the eye following cataract surgery are also all thought to be at minimal risk for infection following dental procedures. Therefore, no antibiotic prophylaxis is recommended in these situations. There is, however, some evidence indicating elevated risk of infection following some types of penile implants and some vascular access devices, used during chemotherapy. It is recommended that the dentist discuss such patients with the physician prior to determining the need for antibiotics.

What should I do if medical consultation results in a recommendation that differs from the published guidelines endorsed by the American Dental Association?

The dentist is ultimately responsible for treatment recommendations. Ideally, by communicating with the physician, a consensus can be achieved that is either in agreement with the guidelines or is based on other established medical reasoning.

What is the best antibiotic modality for treating dental infections?

Penicillin is still the drug of choice for treatment of infections in and around the oral cavity. Phenoxy-methyl penicillin (Pen VK®) has long been the most commonly-selected antibiotic. In penicillin-allergic individuals, erythromycin may be an appropriate consideration. If another drug is sought, clindamycin prescribed 300 mg as a loading dose followed by 150 mg 4 times/day would be an appropriate regimen for a dental infection. In general, if there is no response to Pen VK®, then Augmentin® may be a good alternative in the nonpenicillin-allergic patient because of its slightly altered spectrum. Recommendations would include that the patient should take the drug with food.

Is there cross-allergenicity between the cephalosporins and penicillin?

The incidence of cross-allergenicity is 5% to 8% in the overall population. If a patient has demonstrated a Type I hypersensitivity reaction to penicillin, namely urticaria or anaphylaxis, then this incidence would increase to 20%.

Is there definitely an interaction between contraception agents and antibiotics?

There are well founded interactions between contraceptives and antibiotics. The best instructions that a patient could be given by their dentist are that should an antibiotic be necessary and the dentist is aware that the patient is on contraceptives, and if the patient is using chemical contraceptives, the patient should seriously consider additional means of contraception during the antibiotic management.

Are antibiotics necessary in diabetic patients?

In the management of diabetes, control of the diabetic status is the key factor relative to all morbidity issues. If a patient is well controlled, then antibiotics will likely not be necessary. However, in patients where the control is questionable or where they have recently been given a different drug regimen for their diabetes or if they are being titrated to an appropriate level of either insulin or oral hypoglycemic agents during these periods of time, the dentist might consider preprocedural antibiotics to be efficacious.

Do nonsteroidal anti-inflammatory drugs interfere with blood pressure medication?

At the current time there is no clear evidence that NSAIDs interfere with any of the blood pressure medications that are currently in use.

Is a patient who has taken phentermine at risk for cardiac problems just like a patient who took "fen-phen"?

No, there is often confusion with these drug names. "Fen-phen" referred to a combined use of fenfluramine and phentermine and it is this combination that has led to the FDA statement (see Table 4). The single drug phentermine has not been implicated in this current concern over cardiac complications.

Figure 1
Preprocedural Dental Action Plan for Patients With a History Indicative of Elevated Endocarditis Risk

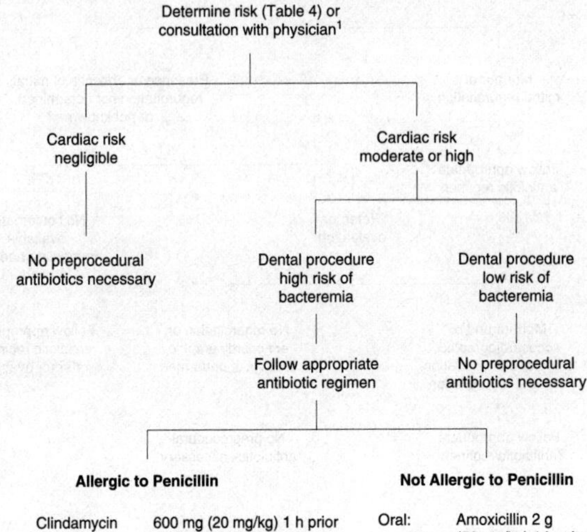

Allergic to Penicillin			Not Allergic to Penicillin	
Oral:	Clindamycin	600 mg (20 mg/kg) 1 h prior	Oral:	Amoxicillin 2 g (50 mg/kg) 1 h prior
	Cephalexin	2 g (50 mg/kg) 1 h prior		
	Cefadroxil	2 g (50 mg/kg) 1 h prior		
	Azithromycin	500 mg (15 mg/kg) 1 h prior	I.M. or I.V.:	Ampicillin 2 g (50 mg/kg) 30 min prior
	Clarithromycin	500 mg (15 mg/kg) 1 h prior		
I.V.:	Clindamycin	600 mg (20 mg/kg) 30 min prior		
I.M. or I.V.:	Cefazolin	1 g (25 mg/kg) 30 min prior		

Dosages for children are in parentheses and should never exceed adult dose. Cephalosporins should be avoided in patients with previous Type I hypersensitivity reactions to penicillin due to some evidence of cross-allergenicity.

[1]For Emergency Dental Care, the clinician should attempt phone consultation. If unable to contact patient's physician or determine risk, the patient should be treated as though there is moderate or high risk of cardiac complication and follow the algorithm.

ANTIBIOTIC PROPHYLAXIS *(Continued)*

Figure 2
Patient With Suspected Mitral Valve Prolapse

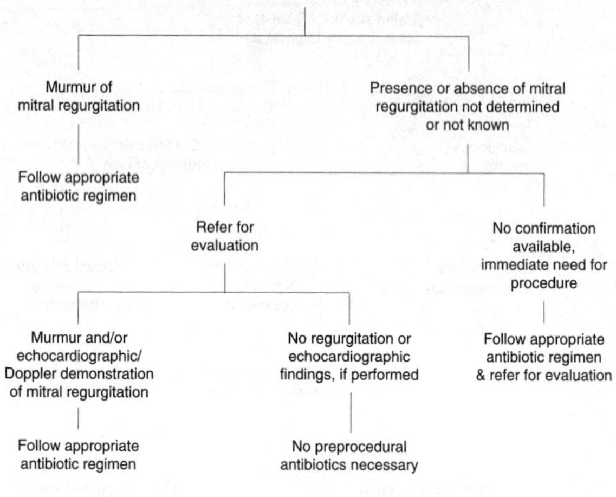

Figure 3
Preprocedural Dental Action Plan for Patients With Prosthetic Implants

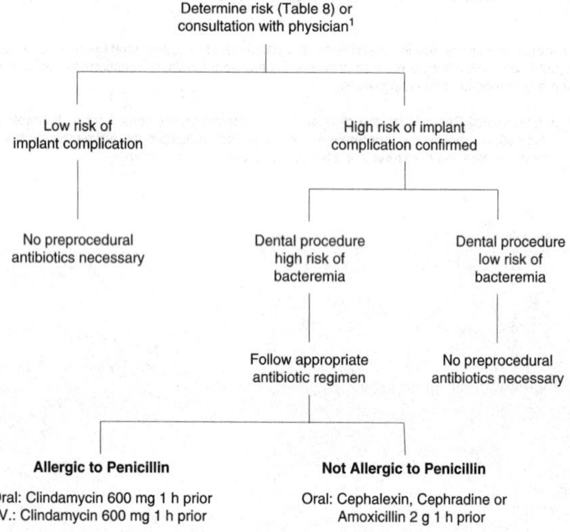

Allergic to Penicillin

Oral: Clindamycin 600 mg 1 h prior
I.V.: Clindamycin 600 mg 1 h prior

Not Allergic to Penicillin

Oral: Cephalexin, Cephradine or Amoxicillin 2 g 1 h prior

I.M. or I.V.: Cefazolin 1 g 1 h prior
Ampicillin 2 g 1 h prior

Cephalosporins should be avoided in patients with previous Type I hypersensitivity reactions to penicillin due to some evidence of cross allergenicity.

[1]For Emergency Dental Care the clinician should attempt phone consultation. If unable to contact patient's physician or determine risk, the patient should be treated as though there is high risk of implant complication and follow the algorithm.

SYSTEMIC VIRAL DISEASES

HEPATITIS

The hepatitis viruses are a group of DNA and RNA viruses that produce symptoms associated with inflammation of the liver. Currently, hepatitis A through G have been identified by immunological testing; however, hepatitis A through E have received most attention in terms of disease identification. Recently, however, there has been increased interest in hepatitis viruses F and G, particularly as relate to healthcare professionals. Our knowledge is expanding rapidly in this area and the clinician should be alert to changes in the literature that might update their knowledge. Hepatitis F, for instance, remains a diagnosis of exclusion effectively being non-A, B, C, D, E, or G. Whereas, hepatitis G has serologic testing available, however, not commercially at this time. Research evaluations of various antibody and RT-PCR tests for hepatitis G are under development at this time.

Signs and symptoms of viral hepatitis in general are quite variable. Patients infected may range from asymptomatic to experiencing flu-like symptoms only. In addition, fever, nausea, joint muscle pain, jaundice, and hepatomegaly along with abdominal pain can result from infection with one of the hepatitis viruses. The virus also can create an acute or chronic infection. Usually following these early symptoms or the asymptomatic period, the patient may recover or may go on to develop chronic liver dysfunction. Liver dysfunction may be represented primarily by changes in liver function tests known as LFTs and these primarily include aspartate aminotransferase known as AST and alanine aminotransferase known as ALT. In addition, for A, B, C, D, and E there are serologic tests for either antigen, antibody, or both. Of hepatitis A through G, five forms have both acute and chronic forms whereas A and E appear to only create acute disease. There are differences in the way clinicians may approach a known postexposure to one of the hepatitis viruses. In many instances, gamma globulin may be used, however, the indications for gamma globulin as a drug limit their use to several of the viruses only. The dental clinician should be aware that the gastroenterologist may choose to give gamma globulin off-label.

Hepatitis A

Hepatitis A virus is an enteric virus that is a member of the Picornavirus family along with Coxsackie viruses and poliovirus. Previously known as infectious hepatitis, hepatitis A has been detected in humans for centuries. It causes acute hepatitis, often transmitted by oral-fecal contamination and having an incubation period of approximately 30 days. Typically, constitutional symptoms are present and jaundice may occur. Drug therapy that the dentist may encounter in a patient being treated for hepatitis A would primarily include immunoglobulin. Hepatitis A vaccine (inactivated) is an FDA-approved vaccine indicated in the prevention of contracting hepatitis A in exposed or high-risk individuals. Candidates at high-risk for HAV infection include persons traveling internationally to highly endemic areas, individuals with chronic liver disease, individuals engaging in high-risk sexual behavior, illicit drug-users, persons with high-risk occupational exposure, hemophiliacs or other persons receiving blood products, pediatric populations, and food handlers in high-risk environments. Two formulations of hepatitis A vaccine are available, Havrix® and VAQTA®. Each is administered as an injection in the deltoid region and both are available in pediatric and adult dosages.

Hepatitis B

Hepatitis B virus is previously known as serum hepatitis and has particular trophism for liver cells. Hepatitis B virus causes both acute and chronic disease in susceptible patients. The incubation period is often long and the diagnosis might be made by serologic markers even in the absence of symptoms. No drug therapy for acute hepatitis B is known; however, chronic hepatitis has recently been successfully-treated with Interferon Alfa-2b.

Hepatitis C

Hepatitis C virus was described in 1988 and has been formerly classified as non-A/non-B. It is clear that hepatitis C represents a high percentage of the transfusion-associated hepatitis that is seen. Treatment of acute hepatitis C infection is generally supportive. Interferon Alfa-2a therapy has been used with some success recently and interferon-alfa may be beneficial with hepatitis C-related chronic hepatitis.

SYSTEMIC VIRAL DISEASES *(Continued)*

Hepatitis D

Hepatitis D, previously known as the delta agent, is a virus that is incomplete in that it requires previous infection with hepatitis B in order to be manifested. In the past, no antiviral therapy has been effective, however, Interferon Alfa-2b is currently being investigated for unlabeled use in hepatitis D.

Hepatitis E

Hepatitis E virus is an RNA virus that represents a proportion of the previously classified non-A/non-B diagnoses. There is currently no antiviral therapy against hepatitis E.

Hepatitis F

Hepatitis F, as was mentioned, remains a diagnosis of exclusion. There are no known immunological tests available for identification of hepatitis F at present and currently the Centers for Disease Control have not come out with specific guidelines or recommendations. It is thought, however, that hepatitis F is a bloodborne virus and it has been used as a diagnosis in several cases of post-transfusion hepatitis.

Hepatitis G

Hepatitis G virus (HGV) is the newest hepatitis and is also assumed to be a bloodborne virus. Similar in family to hepatitis C, it is thought to occur concomitantly with hepatitis C and appears to be even more prevalent in some blood donors than hepatitis C. Occupational transmission of HGV is currently under study (see the references for updated information) and currently there are no specific CDC recommendations for postexposure to an HGV individual as the testing for identification remains experimental.

For further information, refer to the following:

Occupational Exposure to Bloodborne Pathogens *on page 1603*
Immunizations (Vaccines) *on page 1614*
Hepatitis A Vaccine *on page 687*
Hepatitis A (Inactivated) and Hepatitis B (Recombinant) Vaccine *on page 686*
Hepatitis B Immune Globulin *on page 688*
Hepatitis B Vaccine *on page 689*
Immune Globulin, Intramuscular *on page 739*
Immune Globulin, Intravenous *on page 740*
Interferon Alfa-2a *on page 751*
Interferon Alfa-2b *on page 752*
Interferon Alfa-2b and Ribavirin *on page 754*
Peginterferon Alfa-2a *on page 1052*
Peginterferon Alfa-2b *on page 1053*

TYPES OF HEPATITIS VIRUS

Features	A	B	C	D	E	F	G
Incubation Period	2-6 wks	8-24 wks	2-52 wks	3-13 wks	3-6 wks	Unknown	Unknown
Onset	Abrupt	Insidious	Insidious	Abrupt	Abrupt	Insidious	Insidious
Symptoms							
Jaundice	Adults: 70% to 80%; Children: 10%	25%	25%	Varies	Unknown	Unknown	Unknown
Asymptomatic patients	Adults: 50%; Children: Most	~75%	~75%	Rare	Rare	Common	Common
Routes of Transmission							
Fecal/Oral	Yes	No	No	No	Yes	Unknown	Unknown
Parenteral	Rare	Yes	Yes	Yes	No		
Sexual	No	Yes	Possible	Yes	No		
Perinatal	No	Yes	Possible	Possible	No		
Water/Food	Yes	No	No	No	Yes		
Sequelae (% of patients)							
Chronic state	No	Adults: 6% to 10%; Children: 25% to 50%; Infants: 70% to 90%	>75%	10% to 15%	No	Unknown	Likely
Case-Fatality Rate	0.6%	1.4%	1% to 2%	30%	1% to 2% Pregnant women: 20%	Unknown	Unknown

PRE-EXPOSURE RISK FACTORS FOR HEPATITIS B

Healthcare factors:

Healthcare workers[1]

Special patient groups (eg, adolescents, infants born to HB_sAg–positive mothers, military personnel, etc)

Hemodialysis patients[2]

Recipients of certain blood products[3]

Lifestyle factors:

Homosexual and bisexual men

Intravenous drug-abusers

Heterosexually active persons with multiple sexual partners or recently acquired sexually transmitted diseases

Environmental factors:

Household and sexual contacts of HBV carriers

Prison inmates

Clients and staff of institutions for the mentally handicapped

Residents, immigrants, and refugees from areas with endemic HBV infection

International travelers at increased risk of acquiring HBV infection

[1]The risk of hepatitis B virus (HBV) infection for healthcare workers varies both between hospitals and within hospitals. Hepatitis B vaccination is recommended for all healthcare workers with blood exposure.

[2]Hemodialysis patients often respond poorly to hepatitis B vaccination; higher vaccine doses or increased number of doses are required. A special formulation of one vaccine is now available for such persons (Recombivax HB®, 40 mcg/mL). The anti-HB_s (antibody to hepatitis B surface antigen) response of such persons should be tested after they are vaccinated, and those who have not responded should be revaccinated with 1-3 additional doses.

Patients with chronic renal disease should be vaccinated as early as possible, ideally before they require hemodialysis. In addition, their anti- HB_s levels should be monitored at 6- to 12-month intervals to assess the need for revaccination.

[3]Patients with hemophilia should be immunized subcutaneously, not intramuscularly.

POSTEXPOSURE PROPHYLAXIS FOR HEPATITIS B[1]

Exposure	Hepatitis B Immune Globulin	Hepatitis B Vaccine
Perinatal	0.5 mL I.M. within 12 hours of birth	0.5 mL[2] I.M. within 12 hours of birth (no later than 7 days), and at 1 and 6 months[3]; test for HB_sAg and anti-HB_s at 12-15 months
Sexual	0.06 mL/kg I.M. within 14 days of sexual contact; a second dose should be given if the index patient remains HB_sAg-positive after 3 months and hepatitis B vaccine was not given initially	1 mL I.M. at 0, 1, and 6 months for homosexual and bisexual men and regular sexual contacts of persons with acute and chronic hepatitis B
Percutaneous; exposed person unvaccinated		
Source known HB_sAg-positive	0.06 mL/kg I.M. within 24 hours	1 mL I.M. within 7 days, and at 1 and 6 months[4]
Source known, HB_sAg status unknown	Test source for HB_sAg; if source is positive, give exposed person 0.06 mL/kg I.M. once within 7 days	1 mL I.M. within 7 days, and at 1 and 6 months[4]
Source not tested or unknown	Nothing required	1 mL I.M. within 7 days, and at 1 and 6 months
Percutaneous; exposed person vaccinated		
Source known HB_sAg-positive	Test exposed person for anti-HB_s[5]. If titer is protective, nothing is required; if titer is not protective, give 0.06 mL/kg within 24 hours	Review vaccination status[6]
Source known, HB_sAg status unknown	Test source for HB_sAg and exposed person for anti-HB_s. If source is HB_sAg-negative, or if source is HB_sAg-positive but anti-HB_s titer is protective, nothing is required. If source is HB_sAg-positive and anti-HB_s titer is not protective or if exposed person is a known nonresponder, give 0.06 mL/kg I.M. within 24 hours. A second dose of hepatitis B immune globulin can be given 1 month later if a booster dose of hepatitis B vaccine is not given.	Review vaccination status[6]

SYSTEMIC VIRAL DISEASES *(Continued)*

POSTEXPOSURE PROPHYLAXIS FOR HEPATITIS B[1] *(continued)*

Exposure	Hepatitis B Immune Globulin	Hepatitis B Vaccine
Source not tested or unknown	Test exposed person for anti-HB_s. If anti-HB_s titer is protective, nothing is required. If anti-HB_s titer is not protective, 0.06 mL/kg may be given along with a booster dose of hepatitis B vaccine.	Review vaccination status[6]

[1]HB_sAg = hepatitis B surface antigen; anti-HB_s = antibody to hepatitis B surface antigen; I.M. = intramuscularly; SRU = standard ratio units.

[2]Each 0.5 mL dose of plasma-derived hepatitis B vaccine contains 10 mcg of HB_sAg; each 0.5 mL dose of recombinant hepatitis B vaccine contains 5 mcg or 10 mcg of HB_sAg.

[3]If hepatitis B immune globulin and hepatitis B vaccine are given simultaneously, they should be given at separate sites.

[4]If hepatitis B vaccine is not given, a second dose of hepatitis B immune globulin should be given 1 month later.

[5]Anti-HB_s titers <10 SRU by radioimmunoassay or negative by enzyme immunoassay indicate lack of protection. Testing the exposed person for anti-HB_s is not necessary if a protective level of antibody has been shown within the previous 24 months.

[6]If the exposed person has not completed a three-dose series of hepatitis B vaccine, the series should be completed. Test the exposed person for anti-HB_s. If the antibody level is protective, nothing is required. If an adequate antibody response in the past is shown on retesting to have declined to an inadequate level, a booster dose (1 mL) of hepatitis B vaccine should be given. If the exposed person has inadequate antibody or is a known nonresponder to vaccination, a booster dose can be given along with one dose of hepatitis B immune globulin.

HERPES

The herpes viruses not only represent a topic of specific interest to the dentist due to oral manifestations, but are widespread as systemic infections. Herpes simplex virus is also of interest because of its central nervous system infections and its relationship as one of the viral infections commonly found in AIDS patients. Oral herpes infections will be covered elsewhere. Treatment of herpes simplex primary infection includes acyclovir. Ganciclovir is an alternative drug and foscarnet is also occasionally used. Epstein-Barr virus is a member of the herpesvirus family and produces syndromes important in dentistry, including infectious mononucleosis with the commonly found oral pharyngitis and petechial hemorrhages, as well as being the causative agent of Burkitt's lymphoma. The relationship between Epstein-Barr virus to oral hairy leukoplakia in AIDS patients has not been shown to be one of cause and effect; however, the presence of Epstein-Barr in these lesions is consistent. Currently, there is no accepted treatment for Epstein-Barr virus, although acyclovir has been shown in *in vitro* studies to have some efficacy. Varicella-zoster virus is another member of the herpesvirus family and is the causative agent of two clinical entities, chickenpox and shingles, or herpes zoster. Oral manifestations of both chickenpox and herpes zoster include vesicular eruptions often leading to confluent mucosal ulcerations. Acyclovir is the drug of choice for treatment of herpes zoster infections.

There are other herpes viruses that produce disease in man and animals. These viruses have no specific treatment, therefore, incidence is thought to be less common than those mentioned and the specific treatment is not determined at present. The role of some of these viruses in concomitant infection with the HIV and other coinfection viruses is still under study.

ANTIVIRALS

AGENTS OF ESTABLISHED EFFECTIVENESS

Viral Infection	Drug
Cytomegalovirus	
Retinitis	Ganciclovir, Foscarnet
Pneumonia	Ganciclovir
Hepatitis viruses	
Chronic hepatitis A & B	Hepatitis A (Inactivated) and Hepatitis B (Recombinant) Vaccine
Chronic hepatitis C	Interferon Alfa-2a, Interferon Alfa-2b, Interferon Alfa-2b and Ribavirin, Peginterferon Alfa-2a, Peginterferon Alfa-2b
Chronic hepatitis B	Interferon Alfa-2b
Herpes simplex virus	
Orofacial herpes	
First episode	Acyclovir[1], Valacyclovir
Recurrence	Acyclovir[1], Penciclovir[1], Valacyclovir
Genital herpes	
First episode, recurrence, suppression	Acyclovir, Valacyclovir
Encephalitis	Acyclovir
Mucocutaneous disease in immunocompromised	Acyclovir
Neonatal	Acyclovir
Keratoconjunctivitis	Trifluridine Vidarabine
Influenza A virus	Amantadine, Oseltamivir, Rimantadine, Zanamivir
Papillomavirus	
Condyloma acuminatum	Interferon Alfa-2b, Imiquimod (Aldara™): (use for oral lesions is under study)
Respiratory syncytial virus	Ribavirin
Varicella-zoster virus	
Varicella in normal children	Acyclovir
Varicella in immunocompromised	Acyclovir
Herpes zoster in immunocompromised	Acyclovir
Herpes zoster in normal hosts	Acyclovir, Famciclovir, Valacyclovir

[1]Although acyclovir is often used for these infections, penciclovir and valacyclovir are specifically approved for herpes labialis. The clinician is referred to the monographs.

Acyclovir *on page 64*
Amantadine *on page 92*
Atovaquone *on page 164*
Cidofovir *on page 327*
Famciclovir *on page 572*
Fomivirsen *on page 628*
Foscarnet *on page 631*
Ganciclovir *on page 646*
Hepatitis B Immune Globulin *on page 688*
Imiquimod *on page 738*
Immune Globulin, Intramuscular *on page 739*
Interferon Alfa-2a *on page 751*
Interferon Alfa-2b *on page 752*
Interferon Alfa-2b and Ribavirin *on page 754*
Interferon Alfa-n3 *on page 755*
Oseltamivir *on page 1019*
Peginterferon Alfa-2a *on page 1052*
Peginterferon Alfa-2b *on page 1053*
Penciclovir *on page 1056*
Ribavirin *on page 1177*
Rifabutin *on page 1179*
Rimantadine *on page 1184*
Trifluridine *on page 1339*
Valacyclovir *on page 1354*
Vidarabine *on page 1376*
Zanamivir *on page 1396*

ORAL MEDICINE TOPICS

PART II:

DENTAL MANAGEMENT AND THERAPEUTIC CONSIDERATIONS IN PATIENTS WITH SPECIFIC ORAL CONDITIONS AND OTHER MEDICINE TOPICS

This second part of the chapter focuses on therapies the dentist may choose to prescribe for patients suffering from oral disease or who are in need of special care. Some overlap between these sections has resulted from systemic conditions that have oral manifestations and vice-versa. Cross-references to the descriptions and the monographs for individual drugs described elsewhere in this handbook allow for easy retrieval of information. Example prescriptions of selected drug therapies for each condition are presented so that the clinician can evaluate alternate approaches to treatment, since there is seldom a single drug of choice.

Drug prescriptions shown represent prototype drugs and popular prescriptions and are examples only. The pharmacologic category index is available for cross-referencing if alternatives and additional drugs are sought.

TABLE OF CONTENTS

Oral Pain 1526

Oral Bacterial Infections 1533

Periodontal Diseases 1542

Oral Fungal Infections 1544

Oral Viral Infections 1547

Oral Nonviral Soft Tissue Ulcerations or Erosions 1551

Dentin Hypersensitivity, High Caries Index, and Xerostomia 1555

Temporomandibular Dysfunction (TMD) 1564

Patients Requiring Sedation 1567

Management of Patients Undergoing Cancer Therapy 1569

ORAL PAIN

PAIN PREVENTION

For the dental patient, the prevention of pain aids in relieving anxiety and reduces the probability of stress during dental care. For the practitioner, dental procedures can be accomplished more efficiently in a "painless" situation. Appropriate selection and use of local anesthetics is one of the foundations for success in this arena. Local anesthetics listed below include drugs for the most commonly confronted dental procedures. Ester anesthetics are no longer available in dose form for dental injections, and historically had a higher incidence of allergic manifestations due to the formation of the metabolic byproduct, para-aminobenzoic acid. Articaine, which has an ester side chain, is rapidly metabolized to a non-PABA acid and, hence, functions as an amide and has a low allergic potential. The amides, in general, have an almost negligible allergic rate, and only one well-documented case of amide allergy has been reported by Seng, et al. Although injectable diphenhydramine (Benadryl®) has been used in an attempt to provide anesthesia in patients allergic to all the local anesthetics, it is no longer recommended in this context. The vehicle for injectable diphenhydramine can cause tissue necrosis.

The potential interaction between acetaminophen and warfarin has been recently raised in the literature. The cytochrome P450 system of drug metabolism for these vitamin K dependent metabolic pathways has raised the possibility that prolonged use of acetaminophen may inadvertently enhance, to dangerous levels, the anticoagulation effect of warfarin. As monitored by the INR, the effects of these drugs may be one and one-half to two times greater than as expected from the warfarin dosage alone. This potential interaction could be of importance in selecting an analgesic/antipyretic drug for the dental patient.

LOCAL ANESTHETICS

Articaine and Epinephrine [U.S.] *on page 145*

Articaine and Epinephrine [Canada] *on page 143*

Bupivacaine *on page 225*

Bupivacaine and Epinephrine *on page 227*

Chloroprocaine *on page 310*

Etidocaine and Epinephrine *on page 562*

Levobupivacaine *on page 809*

Lidocaine and Epinephrine *on page 823*

Lidocaine *on page 819*

Lidocaine (Transoral) *on page 828*

Mepivacaine Dental Anesthetic *on page 877*

Mepivacaine and Levonordefrin *on page 875*

Prilocaine *on page 1118*

Prilocaine and Epinephrine *on page 1120*

Ropivacaine *on page 1199*

Tetracaine *on page 1278*

Tetracaine and Dextrose *on page 1279*

The selection of a vasoconstrictor with the local anesthetic must be based on the length of the procedure to be performed, the patient's medical status (epinephrine is contraindicated in patients with uncontrolled hyperthyroidism), and the need for hemorrhage control. The following table lists some of the common drugs with their duration of action. Transoral patches with lidocaine are now available (DentiPatch®) and the new long-acting amide injectable, Ropivacaine (Naropin®) may be useful for postoperative pain management.

DENTAL ANESTHETICS
(Average Duration by Route)

Product	Infiltration	Inferior Alveolar Block
Articaine HCl 4% and epinephrine 1:100,000	60 minutes	60 minutes
Carbocaine® HCl 2% with Neo-Cobefrin® 1:20,000 (mepivacaine HCl and levonordefrin)	50 minutes	60-75 minutes
Duranest® Injection (etidocaine)	5-10 hours	5-10 hours
Citanest® Plain 4% (prilocaine)	20 minutes	2.5 hours
Citanest Forte® with Epinephrine (prilocaine with epinephrine)	2.25 hours	3 hours
Lidocaine HCl 2% and epinephrine 1:100,000	60 minutes	90 minutes
Marcaine® HCl 0.5% with epinephrine 1:200,000 (bupivacaine and epinephrine)	60 minutes	5-7 hours

The use of articaine 4% with epinephrine 1:100,000 solution for mandibular blocks has been associated occasionally with parasthesia. (*J Am Dent Assoc*, 2001, 132(2):177-85.)

The use of preinjection topical anesthetics can assist in pain prevention (see also "Oral Viral Infections" *on page 1547* and "Oral Nonviral Soft Tissue Ulcerations or Erosions" *on page 1551*). Some clinicians are also using EMLA® (eutectic mixture of local anesthetic with lidocaine and prilocaine) as a topical. Skin patch available by Astra not currently approved for oral use.

Benzocaine *on page 191*

Lidocaine *on page 819*

Lidocaine Transoral *on page 828*

Tetracaine *on page 1278*

PAIN MANAGEMENT

The patient with existing acute or chronic oral pain requires appropriate treatment and sensitivity on the part of the dentist, all for the purpose of achieving relief from the oral source of pain. Pain can be divided into mild, moderate, and severe levels and requires a subjective assessment by the dentist based on knowledge of the dental procedures to be performed, the presenting signs and symptoms of the patient, and the realization that most dental procedures are invasive often leading to pain once the patient has left the dental office. The practitioner must be aware that the treatment of the source of the pain is usually the best management. If infection is present, treatment of the infection will directly alleviate the patient's discomfort. However, a patient who is not in pain tends to heal better and it is wise to adequately cover the patient for any residual or recurrent discomfort suffered. Likewise, many of the procedures that the dentist performs have pain associated with them. Much of this pain occurs after leaving the dentist office due to an inflammatory process or a healing process that has been initiated. It is difficult to assign specific pain levels (mild, moderate, or severe) for specific procedures; however, the dentist should use his or her prescribing capacity judiciously so that overmedication is avoided.

The following categories of drugs and appropriate example prescriptions for each follow. These include management of mild pain with aspirin products, acetaminophen, and some of the nonsteroidal noninflammatory agents. Management of moderate pain includes codeine, Vicodin®, Vicodin ES®, Lorcet® 10/650; and Motrin® in the 800 mg dosage. Severe pain may require treatment with Percodan®, Percocet®, or Demerol®. All prescription pain preparations should be closely monitored for efficacy and discontinued if the pain persists or requires a higher level formulation.

The chronic pain patient represents a particular challenge for the practitioner. Some additional drugs that may be useful in managing the patient with chronic pain of neuropathic origin are covered in the temporomandibular dysfunction section *on page 1564*. It is always incumbent on the practitioner to reevaluate the diagnosis, source of pain, and treatment, whenever prolonged use of analgesics (narcotic or non-narcotic) is contemplated. Drugs such as Dilaudid® are not recommended for management of dental pain in most states.

Narcotic analgesics can be used on a short-term basis or intermittently in combination with non-narcotic therapy in the chronic pain patient. Judicious prescribing, monitoring, and maintenance by the practitioner is imperative, particularly whenever considering the use of a narcotic analgesic due to the abuse and addiction liabilities.

ORAL PAIN *(Continued)*

MILD PAIN

Acetaminophen *on page 47*

Aspirin (various products) *on page 151*

Diflunisal *on page 435*

Ibuprofen *on page 728*

Ketoprofen *on page 785*

Lansoprazole *on page 797*

Lansoprazole and Naproxen *on page 799*

Naproxen *on page 965*

OVER-THE-COUNTER PRESCRIPTION EXAMPLES

Rx

Aspirin 325 mg

Disp: To be determined by practitioner

Sig: Take 2-3 tablets every 4 hours

Rx

Ibuprofen 200 mg

Disp: To be determined by practitioner

Sig: Take 2-3 tablets every 4 hours, not to exceed 16 tablets in 24 hours

Note: Ibuprofen is available over-the-counter as Motrin IB®, Advil®, Nuprin®, and many other brands in 200 mg tablets

Note: NSAIDs should **never** be taken together, nor should they be combined with aspirin. NSAIDs have anti-inflammatory effects as well as analgesics. An allergy to aspirin constitutes a contradiction to all the new NSAIDs. Aspirin and the NSAIDs may increase post-treatment bleeding.

Note: Use with caution in patients with CHF, hypertension, decreased renal or hepatic function, history of GI disease, or those receiving anticoagulants; withhold for at least 4-6 half-lives prior to surgical or dental procedures

Rx

Acetaminophen 325 mg

Disp: To be determined by practitioner

Sig: Take 2-3 tablets every 4 hours

Note: Products include: Tylenol® and many others.

Note: Acetaminophen can be given if patient has allergy, bleeding problems, or stomach upset secondary to aspirin or NSAIDs.

Rx

Aleve® 220 mg

Disp: To be determined by practitioner

Sig: 1-2 tablets every 8 hours

Ingredient: Naproxen sodium

Rx

Orudis KT® 12.5 mg

Disp: To be determined by practitioner

Sig: 1-2 tablets every 8 hours

Ingredient: Ketoprofen

PRESCRIPTION ONLY EXAMPLES

Rx

Ketoprofen 25 mg

Disp: To be determined by practitioner

Sig: 1-2 tablets every 8 hours

Rx

Dolobid® 500 mg

Disp: 16 tablets

Sig: Take 2 tablets initially, then 1 tablet every 8-12 hours as needed for pain

Ingredient: Diflunisal

MODERATE / MODERATELY SEVERE PAIN

Aspirin and Codeine *on page 155*

Dihydrocodeine, Aspirin, and Caffeine *on page 441*

Hydrocodone and Acetaminophen *on page 702*

Hydrocodone and Ibuprofen *on page 709*

Acetaminophen and Tramadol *on page 54*

Ibuprofen (various products) *on page 728*

A new class of NSAIDs has been approved and indicated in the treatment of arthritis, COX-2 inhibitors (celecoxib, Celebrex®; rofecoxib, Vioxx®). Rofecoxib (Vioxx®) is indicated for use in short-term oral pain management. Celecoxib (Celebrex®) has recently been approved for use in oral pain management. Valdecoxib (Bextra®) is a COX-2 inhibitor also recently indicated for acute pain but its use in dental management is still under evaluation.

The following is a guideline to use when prescribing codeine with either aspirin or acetaminophen (Tylenol®):

Codeine No. 2 = codeine 15 mg

Codeine No. 3 = codeine 30 mg

Codeine No. 4 = codeine 60 mg

Example: ASA No. 3 = aspirin 325 mg + codeine 30 mg

PRESCRIPTION EXAMPLES

Not Controlled:

Rx

Motrin® 800 mg*
Disp: 16 tablets
Sig: Take 1 tablet 3 times/day as needed for pain

Ingredient: Ibuprofen

Note: May be taken up to 4 times/day for more severe pain.

***Note:** Also available as 600 mg

Rx

Ultracet™
Disp: 36 tablets
Sig: Take 2 tablets every 4-6 hours as needed for pain, not to exceed 8 tablets in 24 hours

Ingredients: Acetaminophen 325 mg and tramadol 37.5 mg

ORAL PAIN *(Continued)*

Controlled:

Rx

Tylenol® No. 3*
Disp: 16 tablets
Sig: Take 1 tablet every 4 hours as needed for pain

Ingredients: Acetaminophen and codeine

***Note:** Also available as #2 and #4

Rx

Synalgos® DC
Disp: 16 capsules
Sig: Take 1 capsule every 4 hours as needed for pain

Ingredients: Dihydrocodeine 16 mg, aspirin 356.4 mg, and caffeine 30 mg

Rx

Vicodin®
Disp: 16 tablets
Sig: Take 1 tablet every 4 hours as needed for pain

Ingredients: Hydrocodone 5 mg and acetaminophen 500 mg

Note: Available as Vicodin ES®; take 1 tablet every 8-12 hours

Rx

Lortab® 5 mg
Disp: 16 tablets
Sig: Take 1 or 2 tablets every 4 hours as needed for pain, not to exceed 8 tablets in 24 hours

Ingredients: Hydrocodone 5 mg and acetaminophen 500 mg

Rx

Darvocet–N 100®
Disp: 36 tablets
Sig: Take 1 tablet every 4 hours as needed for pain, not to exceed 6 tablets in 24 hours

Ingredients: Propoxyphene 100 mg and acetaminophen 650 mg

Rx

Vicoprofen®
Disp: 16 tablets
Sig: Take 1-2 tablets every 4-6 hours as needed for pain   No Refills

Ingredients: Hydrocodone 7.5 mg and ibuprofen 200 mg

HYDROCODONE PRODUCTS

Available hydrocodone oral products are listed in the following table and are scheduled as C-III controlled substances, indicating that prescriptions may either be oral or written. Thus, the prescriber may call–in a prescription to the pharmacy for any of these hydrocodone products. All the formulations are combined with acetaminophen except for Vicoprofen®, which contains ibuprofen, and Lortab® ASA and Damason–P®, which all contain aspirin. Most of these brand name drugs are available generically and the pharmacist will dispense the generic equivalent if available, unless the prescriber indicates otherwise.

HYDROCODONE ANALGESIC COMBINATION ORAL PRODUCTS (All Products DEA Schedule C-III)

Hydrocodone is available under numerous brand names with varying dosages and in combination with aspirin or ibuprofen.					
Hydrocodone Bitartrate	**Acetaminophen (APAP[1])**	**Other**	**Brand Name**	**Generic Available**	**Form**
2.5 mg	500 mg	–	Lortab® 2.5/500	Yes	Tablet
5 mg	400 mg	–	Zydone®	No	Tablet
5 mg	500 mg	–	Vicodin®; Dolagesic®; Hy-Phen®; Hydrocet®; Anexsia® 5/500; Lortab®5/500	Yes	Tablet
5 mg	500 mg	–	Polygesic®; Lorcet-HD®	Yes	Capsule
7.5 mg	400 mg	–	Zydone®	No	Tablet
7.5 mg	500 mg	–	Lortab® 7.5/500	Yes	Tablet
7.5 mg	650 mg	–	Anexsia® 7.5/650; Lorcet Plus®	Yes	Tablet
7.5 mg	750 mg	–	Vicodin ES®	Yes	Tablet
10 mg	400 mg	–	Zydone®	No	Tablet
10 mg	325 mg	–	Norco®	No	Tablet
10 mg	500 mg	–	Lortab® 10/500	Yes	Tablet
10 mg	650 mg	–	Lorcet®	Yes	Tablet
10 mg	660 mg	–	Vicodin HP®; Anexsia® 10/660	Yes	Tablet
10 mg	750 mg		Maxidone™	No	Tablet
7.5 mg/15 mL	500 mg/15 mL	–	Lortab® Elixir	Yes	Elixir
5 mg	–	Aspirin 500 mg	Lortab® ASA; Damason–P®	Yes	Tablet
7.5 mg	–	Ibuprofen 200 mg	Vicoprofen®	No	Tablet

[1]APAP is the common acronym for acetaminophen and is the abbreviation of the chemical name N-acetylparaminophenol.

The following are the usual adult doses of the hydrocodone oral products as listed by the most recent edition of the Drug Information for the Health Care Professional (USPDI).

1 or 2 tablets containing 2.5 mg of hydrocodone and 500 mg of acetaminophen every 4-6 hours; or

1 tablet containing 5 mg of hydrocodone and 500 mg acetaminophen every 4-6 hours as needed, with dosage being increased to 2 tablets every 6 hours, if necessary; or

1 capsule containing 5 mg of hydrocodone and 500 mg of acetaminophen every 4-6 hours as needed, with dosage being increased to 2 capsules every 6 hours if necessary; or

1 tablet containing 7.5 mg hydrocodone and 650 mg of acetaminophen every 4-6 hours as needed, with dosage being increased to 2 tablets every 6 hours if necessary; or

1 tablet containing 7.5 mg hydrocodone and 750 mg of acetaminophen every 4-6 hours as needed; or

1 tablet containing 10 mg of hydrocodone and 650 mg acetaminophen every 4-6 hours as needed.

For the elixir (Lortab®), the recommended dose is 1 tablespoonful every 4-6 hours when necessary for pain.

For the aspirin products (Lortab® ASA and Damason-P®), the recommended dose is 1 or 2 tablets every 4-6 hours as needed.

For the ibuprofen product (Vicoprofen®), the recommended dose is 1 or 2 tablets every 4-6 hours as needed. The manufacturer recommends that the maximum dose of Vicoprofen® should not exceed 5 tablets in 24 hours.

The usual adult prescribing limits for the combination hydrocodone-acetaminophen products is up to 40 mg of hydrocodone and up to 4000 mg (4 g) of acetaminophen in a 24-hour period.

ORAL PAIN *(Continued)*

SEVERE PAIN

Meperidine *on page 870*
Oxycodone *on page 1027*
Oxycodone and Acetaminophen *on page 1029*
Oxycodone and Aspirin *on page 1032*

Oxycodone is available in a variety of dosages and combinations under numerous brand names. A new combination of Oxycodone hydrochloride with ibuprofen has been used in Phase III clinical trials at Forest Laboratories and is currently awaiting approval.

PRESCRIPTION EXAMPLES

Rx

Demerol® 50 mg*

Disp: 16 tablets

Sig: Take 1 tablet every 4 hours as needed for pain — No Refills

Ingredient: Meperidine

***Note:** Triplicate prescription required in some states.

Rx

Roxicodone™ 5 mq*

Disp: 24 tablets

Sig: Take 1 tablet every 6 hours as needed for pain — No Refills

Ingredient: Oxycodone

***Note:** Some formulations available as controlled release.

Rx

Percodan®*

Disp: 16 tablets

Sig: Take 1 tablet every 4 hours as needed for pain — No Refills

Ingredients: Oxycodone 4.88 mg and aspirin 325 mg

***Note:** Triplicate prescription required in some states.

Note: See monograph *on page 1032* for contraindications and precautions for aspirin or narcotic medications.

Rx

Percocet® tablets or Tylox® capsules*

Disp: 16 tablets or capsules

Sig: Take 1 tablet every 4 hours as needed for pain — No Refills

Ingredients: Oxycodone 5 mg and acetaminophen 325 mg (Tylox® contains acetaminophen 500 mg)

***Note:** Triplicate prescription required in some states.

ORAL BACTERIAL INFECTIONS

Dental infection can occur for any number of reasons, primarily involving pulpal and periodontal infections. Secondary infections of the soft tissues as well as sinus infections pose special treatment challenges. The drugs of choice in treating most oral infections have been selected because of their efficacy in providing adequate blood levels for delivery to the oral tissues and their proven usefulness in managing dental infections. Penicillin remains the primary drug for treatment of dental infections of pulpal origin. The management of soft tissue infections may require the use of additional drugs.

OROFACIAL INFECTIONS

The basis of all infections is the successful multiplication of a microbial pathogen on or within a host. The pathogen is usually defined as any microorganism that has the capacity to cause disease. If the pathogen is bacterial in nature, antibiotic therapy is often indicated.

DIFFERENTIAL DIAGNOSIS OF ODONTOGENIC INFECTIONS

In choosing the appropriate antibiotic for therapy of a given infection, a number of important factors must be considered. First, the identity of the organism must be known. In odontogenic infections involving dental or periodontal structures, this is seldom the case. Secondly, accurate information regarding antibiotic susceptibility is required. Again, unless the organism has been identified, this is not possible. And thirdly, host factors must be taken into account, in terms of ability to absorb an antibiotic, to achieve appropriate host response. When clinical evidence of cellulitis or odontogenic infection has been found and the cardinal signs of swelling, inflammation, pain, and perhaps fever are present, the selection by the clinician of the appropriate antibiotic agent may lead to eradication.

CAUSES OF ODONTOGENIC INFECTIONS

Most acute orofacial infections are of odontogenic origin. Dental caries, resulting in infection of dental pulp, is the leading cause of odontogenic infection.

The major causative organisms involved in dental caries have been identified as members of the viridans (alpha-hemolytic) streptococci and include *Streptococcus mutans, Streptococcus sobrinus,* and *Streptococcus milleri.* Once the bacteria have breached the enamel they invade the dentin and eventually the dental pulp. An inflammatory reaction occurs in the pulp tissue resulting in necrosis and a lower tissue oxidation-reduction potential. At this point, the bacterial flora changes from predominantly aerobic to a more obligate anaerobic flora. The anaerobic gram-positive cocci *(Peptostreptococcus* species), and the anaerobic gram-negative rods, including *Bacteroides, Prevotella, Porphyromonas,* and *Fusobacterium* are most frequently present. An abscess usually forms at the apex of the involved tooth resulting in destruction of bone. Depending on the effectiveness of the host resistance and the virulence of the bacteria, the infection may spread through the marrow spaces, perforate the cortical plate, and enter the surrounding soft tissues.

The other major source of odontogenic infection arises from the anaerobic bacterial flora that inhabits the periodontal and supporting structures of the teeth. The most important potential pathogenic anaerobes within these structures are *Actinobacillus actinomycetemcomitans, Prevotella intermedius, Porphyromonas gingivalis, Fusobacterium nucleatum,* and *Eikenella corrodens.*

Most odontogenic infections (70%) have mixed aerobic and anaerobic flora. Pure aerobic infections are much less common and comprise ~5% incidence. Pure anaerobic infections make up the remaining 25% of odontogenic infections. Clinical correlates suggest that early odontogenic infections are characterized by rapid spreading and cellulitis with the absence of abscess formation. The bacteria are predominantly aerobic with gram-positive, alpha-hemolytic streptococci *(S. viridans)* the predominant pathogen. As the infection matures and becomes more severe, the microbial flora becomes a mix of aerobes and anaerobes. The anaerobes present are determined by the characteristic flora associated with the site of origin, whether it be pulpal or periodontal. Finally, as the infectious process becomes controlled by host defenses, the flora becomes primarily anaerobic. For example, Lewis and MacFarlane found a predominance of facultative oral streptococci in the early infections (<3 days of symptoms) with the later predominance of obligate anaerobes.

In a review of severe odontogenic infections, it was reported that Brook, et al, observed that 50% of odontogenic deep facial space infections yielded anaerobic bacteria only. Also, 44% of these infections yielded a mix of aerobic and anaerobic flora. The results of a study published in 1998 by Sakamoto, et al, were also described in the review. The study confirmed that odontogenic infections usually result from a synergistic interaction among several bacterial species and usually consist of an oral streptococcus and an oral anaerobic gram-negative rod. Sakamoto and his group reported a high level of the *Streptococcus milleri* group of aerobic gram-positive cocci, and high levels of oral

ORAL BACTERIAL INFECTIONS *(Continued)*

anaerobes, including the *Peptostreptococcus* species and the *Prevotella, Porphyromonas,* and *Fusobacterium* species.

Oral streptococci, especially of the *Streptococcus milleri* group, can invade soft tissues initially, thus preparing an environment conducive to growth of anaerobic bacteria. Obligate oral anaerobes are dependent on nutrients synthesized by the aerobes. Thus the anaerobes appear approximately 3 days after onset of symptoms. Early infections are thus caused primarily by the aerobic streptococci (exquisitely sensitive to penicillin) and late infections are caused by the anaerobes (frequently resistant to penicillin).

It appears logical, as Flynn has noted, to separate infections presenting early in their course from those presenting later when selecting empiric antibiotics of choice for odontogenic infections.

If the patient is not allergic to penicillin, penicillin VK still remains the empiric antibiotic of first choice to treat mild or early odontogenic infections (see Table 1). In penicillin allergy, clindamycin clearly remains the alternative antibiotic for treatment of mild or early infections. Secondary alternative antibiotics still recognized as useful in these conditions are cephalexin (Keflex®), or other first generation cephalosporins available in oral dose forms. The first generation cephalosporins can be used in both penicillin-allergic and nonallergic patients, providing that the penicillin allergy is not the anaphylactoid type.

PENICILLIN VK

The spectrum of antibacterial action of penicillin VK is consistent with most of the organisms identified in odontogenic infections (see Table 2). Penicillin VK is a beta-lactam antibiotic, as are all the penicillins and cephalosporins, and is bactericidal against gram-positive cocci and the major pathogens of mixed anaerobic infections. It elicits virtually no adverse effects in the absence of allergy and is relatively low in cost. Adverse drug reactions occurring in >10% of patients include mild diarrhea, nausea, and oral candidiasis. To treat odontogenic infections and other orofacial infections, the usual dose for adults and children >12 years of age is 500 mg every 6 hours for at least 7 days (see Table 4). The daily dose for children ≤12 years of age is 25-50 mg/kg of body weight in divided doses every 6-8 hours (see Table 4). The patient must be instructed to take the penicillin continuously for the duration of therapy.

After oral dosing, penicillin VK achieves peak serum levels within 1 hour. Penicillin VK may be given with meals, however, blood concentrations may be slightly higher when penicillin is given on an empty stomach. The preferred dosing is 1 hour before meals or 2 hours after meals to ensure maximum serum levels. Penicillin VK diffuses into most body tissues, including oral tissues, soon after dosing. Hepatic metabolism accounts for <30% of the elimination of penicillins. Elimination is primarily renal. The nonmetabolized penicillin is excreted largely unchanged in the urine by glomerular filtration and active tubular secretion. Penicillins cross the placenta and are distributed in breast milk. Penicillin VK, like all beta-lactam antibiotics, causes death of bacteria by inhibiting synthesis of the bacterial cell wall during cell division. This action is dependent on the ability of penicillins to reach and bind to penicillin-binding proteins (PBPs) located on the inner membrane of the bacterial cell wall. PBPs (which include transpeptidases, carboxypeptidases, and endopeptidases) are enzymes that are involved in the terminal stages of assembling and reshaping the bacterial cell wall during growth. Penicillins and beta-lactams bind to and inactivate PBPs resulting in lysis of the cell due to weakening of the cell wall.

Penicillin VK is considered a "narrow spectrum" antibiotic. This class of antibiotics produces less alteration of normal microflora thereby reducing the incidence of superinfection. Also, its bactericidal action will reduce the numbers of microorganisms resulting in less reliance on host-phagocyte mechanisms for eradication of the pathogen.

Among patients, 0.7% to 10% are allergic to penicillins. There is no evidence that any single penicillin derivative differs from others in terms of incidence or severity when administered orally. About 85% of allergic reactions associated with penicillin VK are delayed and take >2 days to develop. This allergic response manifests as skin rashes characterized as erythema and bullous eruptions. This type of allergic reaction is mild, reversible, and usually responds to concurrent antihistamine therapy, such as diphenhydramine (Benadryl®). Severe reactions of angioedema have occurred, characterized by marked swelling of the lips, tongue, face, and periorbital tissues. Patients with a history of penicillin allergy must never be given penicillin VK for treatment of infections. The alternative antibiotic is clindamycin. If the allergy is the delayed type and not the anaphylactoid type, a first generation cephalosporin may be used as an alternate antibiotic.

CLINDAMYCIN

In the event of penicillin allergy, clindamycin is clearly an alternative of choice in treating mild or early odontogenic infections (see Table 1). It is highly effective against almost all oral pathogens. Clindamycin is active against most aerobic gram-positive cocci, including staphylococci, *S. pneumoniae*, other streptococci, and anaerobic gram-negative and gram-positive organisms, including bacteroides (see Table 3). Clindamycin is not effective against mycoplasma or gram-negative aerobes. It inhibits protein synthesis in bacteria through binding to the 50 S subunit of bacterial ribosomes. Clindamycin has bacteriostatic actions at low concentrations, but is known to elicit bactericidal effects against susceptible bacteria at higher concentrations of drug at the site of infection.

The usual adult oral dose of clindamycin to treat orofacial infections of odontogenic origin is 150-450 mg every 6 hours for 7-10 days. The usual daily oral dose for children is 8-25 mg/kg in 3-4 equally divided doses (see Table 4).

Following oral administration of a 150 mg or a 300 mg dose on an empty stomach, 90% of the dose is rapidly absorbed into the bloodstream and peak serum concentrations are attained in 45-60 minutes. Administration with food does not markedly impair absorption into the bloodstream. Clindamycin serum levels exceed the minimum inhibitory concentration for bacterial growth for at least 6 hours after the recommended doses. The serum half-life is 2-3 hours. Clindamycin is distributed effectively to most body tissues, including saliva and bone. Its small molecular weight enables it to more readily enter bacterial cytoplasm and to penetrate bone. It is partially metabolized in the liver to active and inactive metabolites and is excreted in the urine, bile, and feces.

Adverse effects caused by clindamycin can include abdominal pain, nausea, vomiting, and diarrhea. Hypersensitivity reactions are rare, but have resulted in skin rash. Approximately 1% of clindamycin users develop pseudomembranous colitis characterized by severe diarrhea, abdominal cramps, and excretion of blood or mucus in the stools. The mechanism is disruption of normal bacterial flora of the colon, which leads to colonization of the bacterium *Clostridium difficile*. This bacterium releases endotoxins that cause mucosal damage and inflammation. Symptoms usually develop 2-9 days after initiation of therapy, but may not occur until several weeks after taking the drug. If significant diarrhea develops, clindamycin therapy should be discontinued immediately. Theoretically, any antibiotic can cause antibiotic-associated colitis and clindamycin probably has an undeserved reputation associated with this condition.

Sandor, et al, also notes that odontogenic infections are typically polymicrobial and that anaerobes outnumber aerobes by at least four-fold. The penicillins have historically been used as the first-line therapy in these cases, but increasing rates of resistance have lowered their usefulness. Bacterial resistance to penicillins is predominantly achieved through production of beta-lactamases. Clindamycin, because of its relatively broad spectrum of activity and resistance to beta-lactamase degradation, is an attractive first-line therapy in treatment of odontogenic infections.

FIRST GENERATION CEPHALOSPORINS

Antibiotics of this class, which are available in oral dosage forms, include cefadroxil (Duricef®), cephalexin (Keflex®), and cephradine (Velosef®). The first generation cephalosporins are alternates to penicillin VK in the treatment of odontogenic infections based on bactericidal effectiveness against the oral streptococci. These drugs are most active against gram-positive cocci, but are not very active against many anaerobes. First generation cephalosporins are indicated as alternatives in early infections because they are effective in killing the aerobes. First generation cephalosporins are active against gram-positive staphylococci and streptococci, but not enterococci. They are active against many gram-negative aerobic bacilli, including *E. coli, Klebsiella,* and *Proteus mirabilis.* They are inactive against methicillin-resistant *S. aureus* and penicillin-resistant *S. pneumoniae.* The gram-negative aerobic cocci, *Moraxella catarrhalis,* portrays variable sensitivity to first generation cephalosporins.

Cephalexin (Keflex®) is the first generation cephalosporin often used to treat odontogenic infections. The usual adult dose is 250-1000 mg every 6 hours with a maximum of 4 g/day. Children's dose is 25-50 mg/kg/day in divided doses every 6 hours; for severe infections: 50-100 mg/kg/day in divided doses every 6 hours with a maximum dose of 3 g/day (see Table 4).

Cephalexin (Keflex®) causes diarrhea in about 1% to 10% of patients. About 90% of the cephalexin is excreted unchanged in urine.

SECOND GENERATION CEPHALOSPORINS

The second generation cephalosporins such as cefaclor (Ceclor®) have better activity against some of the anaerobes including some *Bacteroides, Peptococcus,* and *Peptostreptococcus* species. Cefaclor (Ceclor®) and cefuroxime (Ceftin®) have been used to treat early stage infections. These antibiotics have the advantage of twice-a-day dosing. The usual oral adult dose of cefaclor is 250-500 mg every 8 hours (or daily dose can be given in 2 divided doses) for at least 7 days. Children's dose is 20-40 mg/kg/day divided every 8-12 hours with a maximum dose of 2 g/day. The usual adult oral dose of cefuroxime is 250-500 mg twice daily. Children's dose is 20 mg/kg/day (maximum 500 mg/day) in 2 divided doses.

The cephalosporins inhibit bacterial cell wall synthesis by binding to one or more of the penicillin-binding proteins (PBPs), which in turn inhibits the final transpeptidation step of peptidoglycan synthesis in bacterial cell walls, thus inhibiting cell wall biosynthesis. Bacteria eventually lyse due to ongoing activity of cell wall autolytic enzymes while cell wall assembly is arrested.

ORAL BACTERIAL INFECTIONS *(Continued)*

BACTERIAL RESISTANCE TO ANTIBIOTICS

If a patient with an early stage odontogenic infection does not respond to penicillin VK within 24-36 hours, it is evidence of the presence of resistant bacteria. Bacterial resistance to the penicillins is predominantly achieved through the production of beta-lactamase. A switch to beta-lactamase-stable antibiotics should be made. For example, Kuriyama, et al, reported that past beta-lactam administration increases the emergence of beta-lactamase-producing bacteria and that beta-lactamase-stable antibiotics should be prescribed to patients with unresolved infections who have received beta-lactams. These include either clindamycin or amoxicillin/clavulanic acid (Augmentin®). Doses are listed in Table 4.

In the past, all *S. viridans* species were uniformly susceptible to beta-lactam antibiotics. However, over the years, there has been a significant increase in resistant strains. Resistance may also be due to alteration of penicillin-binding proteins. Consequently, drugs which combine a beta-lactam antibiotic with a beta-lactamase inhibitor, such as amoxicillin/clavulanic acid (Augmentin®), may no longer be more effective than the penicillin VK alone. In these situations, clindamycin is the recommended alternate antibiotic.

Evidence suggests that empirical use of penicillin VK as the first-line drug in treating early odontogenic infections is still the best way to ensure the minimal production of resistant bacteria to other classes of antibiotics, since any overuse of clindamycin or amoxicillin/clavulanic acid (Augmentin®) is minimized in these situations. There is concern that overuse of clindamycin could contribute to development of clindamycin-resistant pathogens.

In late odontogenic infections, it is suggested that clindamycin be considered the first-line antibiotic to treat these infections. The dose of clindamycin would be the same as that used to treat early infections (see Table 4). In these infections, anaerobic bacteria usually predominate. Since penicillin spectrum includes anaerobes, penicillin VK is also useful as an empiric drug of first choice in these infections. It has been reported, however, that the penicillin resistance rate among patients with serious and late infections is in the 35% to 50% range. Therefore, if penicillin is the drug of first choice and the patient does not respond within 24-36 hours, a resistant pathogen should be suspected and a switch to clindamycin be made. Clindamycin, because of its relatively broad spectrum of activity and resistance to beta-lactamase degradation, is an attractive first-line therapy in the treatment of these infections. Another alternative is to add a second drug to the penicillin (eg, metronidazole [Flagyl®]). Consequently, for those infections not responding to treatment with penicillin, the addition of a second drug (eg, metronidazole), not a beta-lactam or macrolide, is likely to be more effective. Bacterial resistance to metronidazole is very rare. The metronidazole dose is listed in Table 4.

Nonionized metronidazole is readily taken up by anaerobic organisms. Its selectivity for anaerobic bacteria is a result of the ability of these organisms to reduce metronidazole to its active form within the bacterial cell. The electron transport proteins necessary for this reaction are found only in anaerobic bacteria. Reduced metronidazole then disrupts DNA's helical structure, thereby inhibiting bacterial nucleic acid synthesis leading to death of the organism. Consequently, metronidazole is not effective against gram-positive aerobic cocci and most *Actinomyces, Lactobacillus,* and *Proprionibacterium* species. Since most odontogenic infections are mixed aerobic and anaerobic, metronidazole should rarely be used as a single agent. Alternatively, one can switch to a beta-lactamase resistant drug (eg, amoxicillin/clavulanic acid [Augmentin®]). The beta-lactamase resistant penicillins including methicillin, oxacillin, cloxacillin, dicloxacillin, and nafcillin, are only effective against gram-positive cocci and have no activity against anaerobes, hence, should not be used to treat the late stage odontogenic infections.

RESISTANCE IN ODONTOGENIC INFECTIONS

Recently, there has been an alarming increase in the incidence of resistant bacterial isolates in odontogenic infections. Many anaerobic bacteria have developed resistance to beta-lactam antibiotics via production of beta-lactamase enzymes. These include several species of *Prevotella, Porphyromonas, Fusobacterium nucleatum,* and *Campylobacter gracilus. Fusobacterium*, especially in combination with *S. viridans* species, has been associated with severe odontogenic infections. Often, they are resistant to macrolides. Clindamycin is the empiric drug of first choice in these patients.

SEVERE INFECTIONS

In patients hospitalized for severe odontogenic infections, I.V. antibiotics are indicated and clindamycin is the clear empiric antibiotic of choice. Alternative antibiotics include an I.V. combination of penicillin and metronidazole or I.V. ampicillin-sulbactam (Unasyn®). Clindamycin, I.V. cephalosporins (if penicillin allergy is not the anaphylactoid type), and ciprofloxacin have been used in patients allergic to penicillins. Flynn notes that *Eikenella corrodens*, an occasional oral pathogen, is resistant to clindamycin. Ciprofloxacin is an excellent antibiotic for this organism.

ERYTHROMYCIN, CLARITHROMYCIN, AND AZITHROMYCIN

In the past, erythromycins were considered highly effective antibiotics for treating odontogenic infections, especially in penicillin allergy. At the present time, however, the current high resistance rates of both oral streptococci and oral anaerobes have rendered the entire macrolide family of antibiotics obsolete for odontogenic infections. Montgomery has noted that resistance develops rapidly to macrolides and there may be cross-resistance between erythromycin and newer macrolides, particularly among streptococci and staphylococci. Hardee has stated that erythromycin is no longer very useful because of resistant pathogens. The antibacterial spectrum of the erythromycin family is similar to penicillin VK. Erythromycins are effective against streptococcus, staphylococcus, and gram-negative aerobes, such as *H. influenzae, M. catarrhalis, N. gonorrhoeae, Bordetella pertussis,* and *Legionella pneumophilia*. Erythromycins are considered narrow spectrum antibiotics.

Both azithromycin and clarithromycin have been used to treat acute odontogenic infections. This is because of the following spectrum of actions: Clarithromycin shows good activity against many gram-positive and gram-negative aerobic and anaerobic organisms. It is active against methicillin-sensitive *S. aureus* and most streptococcus species. *S. aureus* strains resistant to erythromycin are resistant to clarithromycin. Clarithromycin is active against *H. influenzae*. It is similar to erythromycin in effectiveness against anaerobic gram-positive cocci and *Bacteroides sp.* Clarithromycin has been suggested as an alternative antibiotic if the prescriber wants to give an antibiotic from the macrolide family (see Table 3). The recommended oral adult dose is 500 mg twice daily for 7 days.

Azithromycin is active against staphylococci, including *S. aureus* and *S. epidermidis*, as well as streptococci, such as *S. pyogenes* and *S. pneumoniae*. Erythromycin-resistant strains of staphylococcus, enterococcus, and streptococcus, including methicillin-resistant *S. aureus*, are also resistant to azithromycin. It has excellent activity against *H. influenzae*. Inhibition of anaerobes, such as *Clostridium perfringens*, is better with azithromycin than with erythromycin. Inhibition of *Bacteroides fragilis* and other bacteroides species by azithromycin is comparable to erythromycin. Both azithromycin and clarithromycin are presently recommended as alternatives in the prophylactic regimen for prevention of bacterial endocarditis.

AMOXICILLIN

Some clinicians select amoxicillin over penicillin VK as the penicillin of choice to empirically treat odontogenic infections. Except for coverage of *Haemophilus influenzae* in acute sinus and otitis media infections, amoxicillin does not offer any advantage over penicillin VK for treatment of odontogenic infections. It is less effective than penicillin VK for aerobic gram-positive cocci, and similar to penicillin for coverage of anaerobes. Although it does provide coverage against gram-negative enteric bacteria, this is not needed to treat odontogenic infections, except in immunosuppressed patients where these organisms may be present. If one adheres to the principle of using the most effective narrow spectrum antibiotic, amoxicillin should not be favored over penicillin VK.

Note: The ADA Council on Scientific Affairs recently published a review on the subject of antibiotic interaction with oral contraceptives in which a clear statement of the dental professional's responsibility was made. In essence, it was concluded that in any situation where a dentist is planning to prescribe a course of antibiotics, alternative/additional means of contraception should be recommended to the oral contraceptive users. Specifically, patients should be told about the potential for antibiotics to lower the usefulness of oral contraceptives and advised to consult their physician about nonhormonal contraceptive techniques while continuing their oral contraceptive regimen. Even though there is minimal scientific data supporting this position, the risk of possible unwanted pregnancies warrants this simple approach for professionals licensed to prescribe antibiotics (*JADA*, 2002, 133:880).

The following tables have been adapted from Wynn RL, Bergman SA, Meiller TF, et al. "Antibiotics in Treating Orofacial Infections of Odontogenic Origin," *Gen Dent*, 2001, 47(3): 238-52.

Amoxicillin and Clavulanate Potassium *on page 116*
Amoxicillin *on page 114*
Cephalexin *on page 294*
Ceftibuten *on page 287*
Cefditoren *on page 280*
Chlorpheniramine *on page 313*
Chlorhexidine Gluconate *on page 308*
Clarithromycin *on page 343*
Clindamycin *on page 348*
Dicloxacillin *on page 431*
Erythromycin *on page 508*
Gatifloxacin *on page 647*
Gemifloxacin *on page 653*
Loratadine and Pseudoephedrine *on page 842*
Metronidazole *on page 917*
Mouthwash, Antiseptic *on page 948*
Moxifloxacin *on page 949*
Oxymetazoline *on page 1034*
Penicillin V Potassium *on page 1060*
Pseudoephedrine *on page 1147*
Tetracycline *on page 1280*

ORAL BACTERIAL INFECTIONS *(Continued)*

Table 1. EMPIRIC ANTIBIOTICS OF CHOICE FOR ODONTOGENIC INFECTIONS

Type of Infection	Antibiotic of Choice
Early (first 3 days of symptoms)	Penicillin VK Clindamycin Cephalexin (or other first generation cephalosporin)[1]
No improvement in 24-36 hours	Beta-lactamase-stable antibiotic: Clindamycin or amoxicillin / clavulanic acid
Penicillin allergy	Clindamycin Cephalexin (if penicillin allergy is not anaphylactoid type) Clarithromycin (Biaxin®)[2]
Late (>3 days)	Clindamycin Penicillin VK-metronidazole
Penicillin allergy	Clindamycin

[1]For better patient compliance, second generation cephalosporins (cefaclor; cefuroxime) at twice daily dosing have been used; see text.

[2]A macrolide useful in patients allergic to penicillin, given as twice daily dosing for better patient compliance; see text.

Table 2. PENICILLIN VK: ANTIBACTERIAL SPECTRUM

Gram-Positive Cocci	**Oral Anaerobes**
Streptococci	*Bacteroides*
Nonresistant staphylococci[1]	*Porphyromonas*
Pneumococci	*Prevotella*
	Peptococci
Gram-Negative Cocci	Peptostreptococci
Neisseria meningitides	*Actinomyces*
Neisseria gonorrhoeae	*Veillonella*
	Eubacterium
Gram-Positive Rods	*Eikenella*
Bacillus	*Capnocytophaga*
Corynebacterium	*Campylobacter*
Clostridium	*Fusobacterium*
	Others

[1]Nonresistant staphylococcus represents a small portion of community-acquired strains of *S. aureus* (5% to 15%). Most strains of *S. aureus* and *S. epidermidis* produce beta-lactamases, which destroy penicillins.

Table 3. CLINDAMYCIN: ANTIBACTERIAL SPECTRUM[1]

Gram-Positive Cocci	Anaerobes[2]
Streptococci[3]	**Gram-Negative Bacilli**
S. aureus[4]	*Bacteroides* species including *B. fragilis*
Penicillinase and nonpenicillinase-producing staphylococcus	*B. melaninogenicus* *Fusobacterium species*
S. epidermidis	**Gram-Positive Nonsporeforming Bacilli**
Pneumococci	*Propionibacterium*
	Eubacterium
	Actinomyces species
	Gram-Positive Cocci
	Peptococcus
	Peptostreptococcus
	Microaerophilic streptococci

[1]*In vitro* activity against isolates; information from manufacturer's package insert

[2]*Clostridia* are more resistant than most anaerobes to clindamycin. Most *Clostridium perfringens* are susceptible but *C. sporogens* and *C. tertium* are frequently resistant.

[3]Except *S. faecalis*

[4]Some staph strains originally resistant to erythromycin rapidly develop resistance to clindamycin.

Table 4.
ORAL DOSE RANGES OF ANTIBIOTICS USEFUL IN TREATING ODONTOGENIC INFECTIONS[1]

Antibiotic	Dosage: Children	Dosage: Adults
Clinicians must select specific dose and regimen from ranges available to be prescribed based on clinical judgment		
Penicillin VK	≤12 years: 25-50 mg/kg body weight in equally divided doses q6-8h for at least 7 days; maximum dose: 3 g/day	>12 years: 500 mg q6h for at least 7 days
Clindamycin	8-25 mg/kg in 3-4 equally divided doses	150-450 mg q6h for at least 7 days; maximum dose: 1.8 g/day
Cephalexin (Keflex®)	25-50 mg/kg/d in divided doses q6h severe infection: 50-100 mg/kg/d in divided doses q6h; maximum dose: 3 g/24 h	250-1000 mg q6h; maximum dose: 4 g/day
Amoxicillin/ clavulanic acid (Augmentin®)	<40 kg: 20-40 mg (amoxicillin)/kg/d in divided doses q8h >40 kg: 250-500 mg q8h or 875 mg q12h for at least 7 days; maximum dose 2 g/day	>40 kg: 250-500 mg q8h or 875 mg q12h for at least 7 days; maximum dose: 2 g/day
Metronidazole (Flagyl®)		500 mg q6-8h for 7-10 days; maximum dose: 4 g/day

[1]For doses of other antibiotics, see monographs

PRESCRIPTION EXAMPLES FOR ODONTOGENIC INFECTIONS

Penicillins are often prescribed with a double or triple loading dose initially, then followed by the courses described in the examples below. Clinicians should refer to Table 4 (above) for dose ranges or see individual monographs for specific information.

Rx

Augmentin® 250, 500, or 875 mg

Disp: Appropriate quantity for 7-10 days

Sig: Take 1 tablet 3 times/day for 250 or 500 mg; twice daily for 875 mg

Ingredients: Amoxicillin trihydrate 500 mg and clavulanate potassium 125 mg

Note: Amoxicillin alone may also be prescribed (same dosing for 250 mg and 500 mg)

Rx

Cephalexin 250 mg

Disp: 28 capsules

Sig: Take 1 capsule 4 times/day

Rx

Clindamycin 300 mg

Disp: 28 capsules

Sig: Take 1 capsule every 6 hours

Rx

Metronidazole 500 mg

Disp: 40 tablets

Sig: Take 1 tablet 4 times/day

Rx

Penicillin V potassium 500 mg

Disp: 28 tablets

Sig: Take 1 tablet 4 times/day

ORAL BACTERIAL INFECTIONS *(Continued)*

SINUS INFECTION TREATMENT

Sinus infections represent a common condition which may present with confounding dental complaints. Treatment is sometimes instituted by the dentist, but due to the often chronic and recurrent nature of sinus infections, early involvement of an otolaryngologist is advised. These infections may require antibiotics of varying spectrum as well as requiring the management of sinus congestion. Although amoxicillin is usually adequate, many otolaryngologists go directly to Augmentin®. Second-generation cephalosporins and clarithromycin are sometimes used depending on the chronicity of the problem.

PRESCRIPTION EXAMPLES FOR SINUS INFECTIONS

The selected antibiotic should be used with a nasal decongestant and possibly an antihistamine.

Antibiotics:

Rx

Amoxicillin 500 mg

Disp: 21 capsules or tablets

Sig: Take 1 capsule 3 times/day

OR

Rx

Augmentin® 250, 500, or 875 mg

Disp: Appropriate quantity for 7-10 days

Sig: Take 1 tablet 3 times/day for 250 or 500 mg; twice daily for 875 mg

Ingredients: Amoxicillin trihydrate 500 mg and clavulanate potassium 125 mg

AND

Decongestants / Antihistamine:

Rx

Afrin® Nasal Spray (OTC)

Disp: 15 mL

Sig: Spray once in each nostril every 6-8 hours for no more than 3 days

Ingredient: Oxymetazoline

OR

Rx

Sudafed® 60 mg tablets (OTC)

Disp: 30 tablets

Sig: Take 1 tablet every 4-6 hours as needed for congestion

Ingredient: Pseudoephedrine

AND

Rx

Chlor-Trimeton® 4 mg (OTC)

Disp: 14 tablets

Sig: Take 1 tablet twice daily

Ingredient: Chlorpheniramine

FREQUENTLY ASKED QUESTIONS

What is the best antibiotic modality for treating dental infections?

Penicillin is still the drug of choice for treatment of infections in and around the oral cavity. Phenoxy-methyl penicillin (Pen VK) long has been the most commonly selected antibiotic. In penicillin-allergic individuals, erythromycin may be an appropriate consideration. If another drug is sought, clindamycin prescribed 300 mg as a loading dose followed by 150 mg 4 times/day would be an appropriate regimen for a dental infection. In general, if there is no response to Pen VK, then Augmentin® may be a good alternative in the nonpenicillin-allergic patient because of its slightly altered spectrum. Recommendations would include that the patient should take the drug with food.

Is there cross-allergenicity between the cephalosporins and penicillin?

The incidence of cross-allergenicity is 5% to 8% in the overall population. If a patient has demonstrated a Type I hypersensitivity reaction to penicillin, namely urticaria or anaphylaxis, then this incidence would increase to 20%.

Is there definitely an interaction between contraception agents and antibiotics?

There are well founded interactions between contraceptives and antibiotics. The best instructions that a patient could be given by their dentist are that should an antibiotic be necessary and the dentist is aware that the patient is on contraceptives, and if the patient is using chemical contraceptives, the patient should seriously consider additional means of contraception during the antibiotic management.

Are antibiotics necessary in diabetic patients?

In the management of diabetes, control of the diabetic status is the key factor relative to all morbidity issues. If a patient is well controlled, then antibiotics will likely not be necessary. However, in patients where the control is questionable or where they have recently been given a different drug regimen for their diabetes or if they are being titrated to an appropriate level of either insulin or oral hypoglycemic agents during these periods of time, the dentist might consider preprocedural antibiotics to be efficacious.

Do nonsteroidal anti-inflammatory drugs interfere with blood pressure medication?

At the current time there is no clear evidence that NSAIDs interfere with any of the blood pressure medications that are currently in usage.

PERIODONTAL DISEASES

Periodontal diseases are common to mankind affecting, according to some epidemiologic studies, greater than 80% of the worldwide population. The conditions refer primarily to diseases that are caused by accumulations of dental plaque and the subsequent immune response of the host to the bacteria and toxins present in this plaque. Although most of the organisms that have been implicated in advanced periodontal diseases are anaerobic in nature, some aerobes contribute by either coaggregation with the anaerobic species or direct involvement with specific disease types.

Periodontal condition, as a group of diseases, affects the soft tissues supporting the teeth (ie, gingiva) leading to the term gingivitis or inflammation of gingival structures and those conditions that affect the bone and ligament supporting the teeth (ie, periodontitis) resulting from the infection and/or inflammation of these structures. Diseases of the periodontia can be further subdivided into various types including adult periodontitis, early onset periodontitis, prepubertal periodontitis, and rapidly progressing periodontitis. In addition, specific conditions associated with predisposing immunodeficiency disease, such as those found in HIV-infected patients, create further subclassifications of the periodontal diseases, some of which are covered in those chapters associated with those conditions.

It is well accepted that control of most periodontal diseases requires, at the very minimum, appropriate mechanical cleansing of the dentition and the supporting structures by the patient. These efforts include brushing, some type of interdental cleaning, preferably with either floss or other aids, as well as appropriate sulcular cleaning usually with a brush.

Following appropriate dental treatment by the general dental practitioner and/or the periodontist, aids to these efforts by the patient might include the use of chemical agents to assist in the control of the periodontal diseases, or to prevent periodontal diseases. There are many available chemical agents on the market, only some of which are approved by the American Dental Association. Several have been tested utilizing guidelines published in 1986 by the American Dental Association for assessment of agents that claim efficacy in the management of periodontal diseases. These chemical agents include chlorhexidine (Peridex®, PerioGard®), which are bisbiguanides and benzalkonium chloride, which is a quarternary compound. Chlorhexidine, in various concentrations, has shown efficacy in reducing plaque and gingivitis in patients with short-term utilization. Some side effects include staining of the dentition which is reversible by dental prophylaxis. Chlorhexidine demonstrates the concept of substantivity, indicating that after its use, it has a continued effect in reducing the ability of plaque to form. It has been shown to be useful in a variety of periodontal conditions including acute necrotizing ulcerative gingivitis and healing studies. Some disturbances in taste and accumulation of calculus have been reported, however, chlorhexidine is the most applicable chemical agent of the bisbiguanides that has been studied to date.

Other chemical agents available as mouthwashes include the phenol compound Listerine Antiseptic®. These compounds are primarily restricted to prototype agents; the first to be approved by the ADA being Listerine Antiseptic®. Listerine Antiseptic® has been shown to be effective against plaque and gingivitis in long-term studies and comparable to chlorhexidine in these long-term investigations. However, chlorhexidine performs better than Listerine Antiseptic® in short-term investigations. Triclosan, the chemical agent found in the toothpaste Total®, has been recently approved by the FDA and is an aid in the prevention of gingivitis. Antiplaque activity of triclosan is enhanced with the addition of zinc citrate and there are no serious side effects to the use of triclosan. Sanguinarine is a principle herbal extract used for antiplaque activity. It is an alkyloid from the plant *Sanguinaria canadensis* and has some antimicrobial properties perhaps due to its enzyme activity. Zinc citrate and zinc chloride have often been added to toothpastes as well as enzymes such as mucinase, mutanase, and dextrinase which have demonstrated varying results in studies. Some commercial anionic surfactants are available on the market which include aminoalcohols and the agent Plax® which essentially is comprised of sodium thiosulfate as a surfactant. Recent studies have shown Plax® to have some efficacy when it is added to triclosan.

Long-term use of prescription medications, including antibiotics, is seldom recommended and is not in any way a substitute for general dental/periodontal therapies. As adjunctive therapy, however, benefit has been shown and the new formulations of doxycycline (Periostat® and Atridox™), are recommended for long-term or repetitive treatments. It should be noted that the manufacturer's claims indicate that Periostat® functions as a collagenase inhibitor not as an antibiotic at recommended low doses for long-term therapy. Atridox™, however, functions as an antibiotic and is not recommended for constant long-term therapy, but rather in repetitive applications as necessary. Prescription medications used in efforts to treat periodontal diseases have historically included the use of antibiotics such as tetracycline although complications with use with young patients have often precluded their prescription. Doxycycline is often preferred to tetracycline in low doses. This broad-spectrum bacteriostatic agent has shown efficacy against a wide variety of bacterial organisms found in periodontal disease. Minocycline slow-release (Arestin™) has recently been approved.

The drug metronidazole is a nitromidazole. It is an agent that was originally used in treatment of protozoan infections and some anaerobic bacteria. It is bactericidal and has a good absorption and distribution throughout the body. The studies using metronidazole have suggested that it has a variety of uses in periodontal treatment and can be used as adjunct in both acute necrotizing ulcerative gingivitis and has specific efficacy against spirochetes, bacteria, and some *Porphyromonas* species. Clindamycin is a derivative of vancomycin and has been useful in treatment of suppurative periodontal lesions. However, long-term use is precluded by its complicating toxicities associated with colitis and gastrointestinal problems.

Research has also shown that various combination therapies of metronidazole and tetracycline for juvenile periodontitis and metronidazole with amoxicillin for rapidly progressive disease can be useful. The use of other prescription drugs including nonsteroidal anti-inflammatory, as well as other antibacterial agents, have been under study. Effects on prostaglandins of NSAIDs may indirectly slow periodontal disease progression. New research is currently underway in this regard. Perhaps, in combination therapy with some of the antibiotics, these drugs may assist in reducing the patient's immune response or inflammatory response to the presence of disease-causing bacteria.

Of greatest interest has been the improvement in technology for delivery of chemical agents to the periodontally-diseased site. These systems include biodegradable gelatins and biodegradable chips that can be placed under the gingiva and deliver antibacterial agents directly to the site as an adjunct to periodontal treatment. The initial therapy of mechanical debridement by the periodontal therapist is essential prior to using any chemical agent, and the dentist should be aware that the development of newer agents does not substitute for appropriate periodontal therapy and maintenance. The trade names of the gelatin chips and subgingival delivery systems include Periochip®, Atridox®, and Periostat®.

In addition to the periodontal therapy, consideration of the patient's pre-existing or developing medical conditions are important in the management of the periodontal patient. Several diseases illustrate these points most acutely. The reader is referred to the chapters on Diabetes, Cardiovascular Disease, Pregnancy, Respiratory Disease, HIV, and Cancer Chemotherapy. It has long been accepted that uncontrolled diabetes may predispose to periodontal lesions. Now, under current investigation is the hypothesis that pre-existing periodontal diseases may make it more difficult for a diabetic patient to come under control. In addition, the inflammatory response and immune challenge that is ongoing in periodontal disease appears to be implicated in the development of coronary artery disease as well as an increased risk of myocardial infarction and/or stroke. The accumulation of intra-arterial plaques appears enhanced by the presence of the inflammatory response often seen systemically in patients suffering with periodontal disease. The American Heart Association is currently considering recommendations regarding antibiotic prophylaxis in patients with cardiovascular disease. In addition, the clinician is referred to the section on preprocedural antibiotics in the text for a consideration of antibiotic usage in patients that may be at risk for infective endocarditis. Other conditions including pregnancy and respiratory diseases such as COPD, HIV, and cancer therapy must be considered in the overall view of periodontal diseases. The reader is referred to the sections within the text.

Amoxicillin *on page 114*
Minocycline Hydrochloride (Periodontal) *on page 933*
Benzalkonium chloride *on page 190*
Chlorhexidine Gluconate *on page 308*
Clindamycin *on page 348*
Doxycycline Hyclate (Periodontal) *on page 475*
Listerine Antiseptic® *on page 948*
Metronidazole *on page 917*
NSAIDs see Oral Pain section *on page 1526*
Tetracycline *on page 1280*
Triclosan and Fluorides *on page 1337*

ORAL FUNGAL INFECTIONS

Oral fungal infections can result from alteration in oral flora, immunosuppression, and underlying systemic diseases that may allow the overgrowth of these opportunistic organisms. These systemic conditions might include diabetes, long-term xerostomia, adrenal suppression, anemia, and chemotherapy-induced myelosuppression for the management of cancer. The use of oral inhalers that include steroids, such as Advair™ Diskus®, have been implicated in the enhancing of the risk of fungal overgrowth. Drugs of choice in treating fungal infections are amphotericin B, ciclopirox olamine, clotrimazole, itraconazole, ketoconazole, fluconazole, naftifine hydrochloride, nystatin, and oxiconazole. Patients being treated for fungal skin infections may also be using topical antifungal preparations coupled with a steroid such as triamcinolone. Clinical presentation might include pseudomembranous, atrophic, and hyperkeratotic forms. Fungus has also been implicated in denture stomatitis and symptomatic geographic tongue.

Nystatin (Mycostatin®) is effective topically in the treatment of candidal infections of the skin and mucous membrane. The drug is extremely well tolerated and appears to be nonsensitizing. In persons with denture stomatitis in which monilial organisms play at least a contributory role, it is important to soak the prosthesis overnight in a nystatin suspension. Nystatin ointment can be placed in the denture during the daytime much like a denture adhesive. Medication should be continued for at least 48 hours after disappearance of clinical signs in order to prevent relapse. Patients must be re-evaluated after 14 days of therapy. Predisposing systemic factors must be reconsidered if the oral fungal infection persists. Topical applications rely on contact of the drug with the lesions. Therefore, 4-5 times daily with a dissolving troche or pastille is appropriate. Concern over the presence of sugar in the troches and pastilles has led practitioners to sometimes prescribe the vaginal suppository formulation for off-labeled oral use.

Voriconazole (VFEND®) is indicated for treatment of serious fungal infections in patients intolerant of, or refractory to, other therapy.

Amphotericin B (Conventional) *on page 120*
Clotrimazole *on page 363*
Fluconazole *on page 594*
Ketoconazole *on page 783*
Nystatin *on page 1003*
Nystatin and Triamcinolone *on page 1004*
Voriconazole *on page 1385*

Note: Consider Peridex® oral rinse, or Listerine® antiseptic oral rinse for long-term control in immunosuppressed patients.

PRESCRIPTION EXAMPLES

Rx

Mycostatin® pastilles

Disp: 70 pastilles

Sig: Dissolve 1 tablet in mouth until gone, 4-5 times/day for 14 days

Ingredient: 200,000 units of nystatin per tablet

Note: Pastille is more effective than oral suspension due to prolonged contact.

Rx

Mycostatin® oral suspension

Disp: 60 mL (2 oz)

Sig: Use 1 teaspoonful 4-5 times/day; rinse and hold in mouth as long as possible before swallowing or spitting out (2 minutes); do not eat or drink for 30 minutes following application

Ingredients: Nystatin 100,000 units/mL; vehicle contains 50% sucrose and not more than 1% alcohol

Rx

Mycostatin® ointment or cream

Disp: 15 g or 30 g tube

Sig: Apply liberally to affected areas 4-5 times/day; do not eat or drink for 30 minutes after application

Ingredients:

Cream: 100,000 units nystatin per g, aqueous vanishing cream base

Ointment: 100,000 units nystatin per g, polyethylene, and mineral oil gel base

Note: Denture wearers should apply to dentures prior to each insertion; for edentulous patients, Mycostatin® powder (15 g) can also be prescribed to be sprinkled on dentures.

OR

Rx

Mycelex® troche 10 mg

Disp: 70 tablets

Sig: Dissolve 1 tablet in mouth 5 times/day

Ingredient: Clotrimazole

Note: Tablets contain sucrose, risk of caries with prolonged use (>3 months); care must be exercised in diabetic patients.

Rx

Fungizone® oral suspension 100mg/mL

Disp: 50 mL

Sig: 1 mL; swish and swallow 4 times/day between meals

Ingredient: Amphotericin B (Conventional)

Note: Although the manufacturer has discontinued the solution formulation, prescriptions are being filled until the supply is exhausted. A lozenge formulation (10 mg amphotericin B per oz) is currently being manufactured and marketed in other countries but is not available in the U.S. at this time.

MANAGEMENT OF FUNGAL INFECTIONS REQUIRING SYSTEMIC MEDICATION

If the patient is refractory to topical treatment, consideration of a systemic route might include Diflucan® or Nizoral®. Also, when the patient cannot tolerate topical therapy, ketoconazole (Nizoral®) is an effective, well tolerated, systematic drug for mucocutaneous candidiasis. Concern over liver function and possible drug interactions must be considered.

PRESCRIPTION EXAMPLES

Rx

Nizoral® 200 mg

Disp: 10 or 28 tablets

Sig: Take 1 tablet/day for 10-14 days

Ingredient: Ketoconazole

Note: To be used if *Candida* infection does not respond to mycostatin; potential for liver toxicity; liver function should be monitored with long-term use (>3 weeks)

Rx

Diflucan® 100 mg

Disp: 15 tablets

Sig: Take 2 tablets the first day and 1 tablet/day for 10-14 days

Ingredient: Fluconazole

ORAL FUNGAL INFECTIONS *(Continued)*

MANAGEMENT OF ANGULAR CHEILITIS

Angular cheilitis may represent the clinical manifestation of a multitude of etiologic factors. Cheilitis-like lesions may result from local habits, from a decrease in the intermaxillary space, or from nutritional deficiency. More commonly, angular cheilitis represents a mixed infection coupled with an inflammatory response involving *Candida albicans* and other organisms. The drug of choice is now formulated to contain nystatin and triamcinolone and the effect is excellent. In addition, an off-label use of iodoquinol and hydrocortisone has also been reported to be effective in the treatment of angular cheilitis.

PRESCRIPTION EXAMPLE

Rx

Mycolog®–II cream

Disp: 15 g tube

Sig: Apply to affected area after each meal and before bedtime

Ingredients: Nystatin 100,000 units and triamcinolone acetonide 0.1%

ORAL VIRAL INFECTIONS

Oral viral infections are most commonly caused by herpes simplex viruses and Coxsackie viruses. Oral pharyngeal infections and upper respiratory infections are commonly caused by the Coxsackie group A viruses. Soft tissue viral infections, on the other hand, are most often caused by the herpes simplex viruses. Herpes zoster or varicella-zoster virus, which is one of the herpes family of viruses, can likewise cause similar viral eruptions involving the mucosa.

The diagnosis of an acute viral infection is one that begins by ruling out bacterial etiology and having an awareness of the presenting signs and symptoms associated with viral infection. Acute onset and vesicular eruption on the soft tissues generally favors a diagnosis of viral infection. Unfortunately, vesicles do not remain for a great length of time in the oral cavity; therefore, the short-lived vesicles rupture leaving ulcerated bases as the only indication of their presence. These ulcers, however, are generally small in size and only when left unmanaged, coalesce to form larger, irregular ulcerations. Distinction should be made between the commonly occurring intraoral ulcers (aphthous ulcerations) which do not have a viral etiology and the lesions associated with intraoral herpes. The management of an oral viral infection may be palliative for the most part; however, with the advent of acyclovir we now have a family of drugs that can assist in managing primary and secondary infection. Human *Papillomavirus* is implicated in a number of oral lesions, the most common of which is *Condyloma acuminatum.* Recently, Aldara® has been approved for genital warts; oral use is under study.

It should be noted that herpes can present as a primary infection (gingivostomatitis), recurrent lip lesions (herpes labialis), and intraoral ulcers (recurrent intraoral herpes), involving the oral and perioral tissues. Primary infection is a systemic infection that leads to acute gingivostomatitis involving multiple tissues of the buccal mucosa, lips, tongue, floor of the mouth, and the gingiva. Treatment of primary infections utilizes acyclovir in combination with supportive care. Topical anesthetic used in combination with Benadryl® 0.5% in a saline vehicle was found to be an effective oral rinse in the symptomatic treatment of primary herpetic gingivostomatitis; however, Dyclone® is no longer available. Other agents for symptomatic and supportive treatment include commercially available elixir of Benadryl®, Xylocaine® viscous, Orajel® (OTC), and antibiotics to prevent secondary infections. Systemic supportive therapy should include forced fluids, high concentration protein, vitamin and mineral food supplements, and rest.

Antivirals

Abreva™(OTC) *on page 459*

Acyclovir *on page 64*

Imiquimod *on page 738*

Lysine *on page 851*

Nelfinavir *on page 972*

Penciclovir *on page 1056*

Valacyclovir *on page 1354*

Vidarabine *on page 1376*

Viroxyn® *on page 190*

Supportive Therapy

Diphenhydramine *on page 448*

Lidocaine *on page 819*

Prevention of Secondary Bacterial Infection

Penicillin V Potassium *on page 1060*

ORAL VIRAL INFECTIONS *(Continued)*

PRIMARY INFECTION

PRESCRIPTION EXAMPLE

Rx

Zovirax® 200 mg

Disp: 70 capsules

Sig: Take 1 capsule every 4 hours for 2 weeks, not to exceed 5 in 24 hours

Ingredient: Acyclovir

SUPPORTIVE CARE FOR PAIN AND PREVENTION OF SECONDARY INFECTION

Primary infections often become secondarily infected with bacteria, requiring antibiotics. Dietary supplement may be necessary. Options are presented due to variability in patient compliance and response.

PRESCRIPTION EXAMPLES

Rx

Benadryl® elixir 12.5 mg/5 mL

Disp: 4 oz bottle

Sig: Rinse with 1 teaspoonful for 2 minutes before each meal

Ingredient: Diphenhydramine

Rx

Benadryl® elixir 12.5 mg/5 mL with Kaopectate®, 50% mixture by volume

Disp: 8 oz

Sig: Rinse with 1 teaspoonful every 2 hours

Ingredients: Diphenhydramine and attapulgite

Rx

Xylocaine® viscous 2%

Disp: 450 mL bottle

Sig: Swish with 1 tablespoon 4 times/day and spit out

Ingredient: Lidocaine

Rx

Meritene®

Disp: 1 lb can (plain, chocolate, eggnog flavors)

Sig: Take 3 servings/day; prepare as indicated on can

Ingredient: Protein/vitamin/mineral food supplement

RECURRENT HERPETIC INFECTIONS

Following this primary infection, the herpesvirus remains latent until such time as it has the opportunity to recur. The etiology of this latent period and the degree of viral shedding present during latency is currently under study; however, it is thought that some trigger in the mucosa or the skin causes the virus to begin to replicate. This process may involve Langerhans cells which are immunocompetent antigen-presenting cells resident in all epidermal surfaces. The virus replication then leads to eruptions in tissues surrounding the mouth. The most common form of recurrence is the lip lesion or herpes labialis, however, intraoral recurrent herpes also occurs with some frequency. Prevention of recurrences has been attempted with lysine (OTC) 500-1000 mg/day but response has been variable. Herpes zoster outbreaks can involve the oral and facial tissues although this is uncommon. Valacyclovir is the drug of choice.

Water-soluble bioflavonoid-ascorbic acid complex, now available as Peridin-C®, may be helpful in reducing the signs and symptoms associated with recurrent herpes simplex virus infections. As with all agents used, the therapy is more effective when instituted in the early prodromal stage of the disease process.

PREVENTION PRESCRIPTION EXAMPLES

Rx

Lysine (OTC) 500 mg

Sig: Take 2 tablets/day as preventive; increase to 4 tablets/day if prodrome or recurrence begins

Rx

Citrus bioflavonoids and ascorbic acid tablets 400 mg (Peridin-C®)

Disp: 10 tablets

Sig: Take 2 tablets at once, then 1 tablet 3 times/day for 3 days

Where a recurrence is usually precipitated by exposure to sunlight, the lesion may be prevented by the application to the area of a sunscreen, with a high skin protection factor (SPF) in the range of 10-15.

PRESCRIPTION EXAMPLE

Rx

PreSun® (OTC) 15 sunscreen lotion

Disp: 4 fluid oz

Sig: Apply to susceptible area 1 hour before sun exposure

TREATMENT

Acyclovir (Zovirax®) and vidarabine (Vira-A®) possess antiviral activity against herpes simplex types 1 and 2. Historically, ophthalmic ointments were used topically to treat recurrent mucosal and skin lesions. These do not penetrate well on the skin lesions, thereby providing questionable relief of symptoms. If recommended, use should be closely monitored. Penciclovir, an active metabolite of famciclovir, has been specifically approved in a cream for treatment of recurrent herpes lesions. Valacyclovir has recently been approved for treatment of herpes labialis (see monograph for dosing). The FDA has also approved acyclovir cream for treatment of herpes labialis in adults and adolescents but the product is currently under regulatory review (check www.biovail for status). Biovail Corporation has acquired exclusive marketing and distribution rights for Zovirax® ointment and cream from the manufacturer, GlaxoSmithKline. Recently, in addition to docosanol (Abreva®), another new over-the-counter preparation for treatment of recurrent herpes labialis has been approved. Benzalkonium chloride and isopropyl alcohol (Viroxyn®) is an alcohol/benzalkonium chloride medication in a single dose applicator kit (3 pack) that is marketed to reduce the duration and symptoms of cold sores.

ORAL VIRAL INFECTIONS *(Continued)*

PRESCRIPTION EXAMPLES

Rx

Zovirax® ointment 5%

Disp: 15 g tube

Sig: Apply thin layer to lesions 6 times/day for 7 days

Ingredient: Acyclovir 50 mg (per g)

Rx

Zovirax® 200 mg

Disp: 70 capsules

Sig: Take 1 capsule every 4 hours for 2 weeks, up to 5 capsules within 24 hours

Ingredient: Acyclovir 200 mg

Rx

Denavir™

Disp: 2 g tube

Sig: Apply locally every 2 hours, during waking hours, for 4 days

Ingredient: Penciclovir 1%

Note: Denavir™ is approved for use in treating recurrent herpes labialis.

Rx

Abreva™ (OTC) cream

Sig: Apply locally as directed 5 times/day

Ingredient: Docosanol 10%

Rx

Valacyclovir 500 mg

Disp: 4 tablets

Sig: 2 g twice daily for 1 day (separate doses by full 12 hours)

PRESCRIPTION EXAMPLE FOR HERPES ZOSTER

Rx

Valtrex®

Sig: Take 2 caplets 3 times/day for 7 days

Ingredient: Valacyclovir 500 mg

Note: Reevaluate after 7 days; may require dose reduction in patients with altered renal function, consult with patient's physician(s).

ORAL NONVIRAL SOFT TISSUE ULCERATIONS OR EROSIONS

RECURRENT APHTHOUS STOMATITIS

Kenalog® in Orabase is indicated for the temporary relief of symptoms associated with infrequent recurrences of minor aphthous lesions and ulcerative lesions resulting from trauma. More severe forms of recurrent aphthous stomatitis may be treated with an oral suspension of tetracycline. The agent appears to reduce the duration of symptoms and decrease the rate of recurrence by reducing secondary bacterial infection. Its use is contraindicated during the last half of pregnancy, infancy, and childhood to the age of 8 years. *Lactobacillus acidophilus* preparations (Bacid®, Lactinex®) are occasionally effective for reducing the frequency and severity of the lesions. Debacterol® has recently been approved. Patients with long-standing history of recurrent aphthous stomatitis should be evaluated for iron, folic acid, and vitamin B_{12} deficiencies. Regular use of Listerine® antiseptic has been shown in clinical trials to reduce the severity, duration, and frequency of aphthous stomatitis. Debacterol® has recently been approved. Chlorhexidine oral rinses 20 mL for 30 seconds 2-3 times/day have also demonstrated efficacy in reducing the duration of aphthae. With both of these products, however, patient intolerance of the burning from the alcohol content is of concern. Viractin® has been approved for symptomatic relief. Immunocompromised patients such as those with AIDS may have severe ulcer recurrences and the drug thalidomide has been approved for these patients.

Amlexanox *on page 107*
Attapulgite *on page 170*
Chlorhexidine Gluconate *on page 308*
Clobetasol *on page 351*
Dexamethasone *on page 411*
Diphenhydramine *on page 448*
Fluocinonide ointment with Orabase *on page 602*
Debacterol® *on page 1250*
Lactobacillus *on page 793*
Metronidazole *on page 917*
Mouthwash, Antiseptic *on page 948*
Prednisone *on page 1115*
Tetracaine *on page 1278*
Tetracycline liquid *on page 1280*
Thalidomide *on page 1283*
Triamcinolone Acetonide Dental Paste *on page 1333*

PRESCRIPTION EXAMPLES FOR MINOR APHTHAE, BURNING TONGUE SYNDROME, GEOGRAPHIC TONGUE, MILD FORMS OF ORAL LICHEN PLANUS

Rx

Listerine® antiseptic (OTC)

Sig: 20 mL for 30 seconds twice daily

Ingredients: Thymol 0.064%, eucalyptus 0.092%, methyl salicylate 0.060%, menthol 0.042%, and alcohol 26.9%

Rx

Peridex® oral rinse

Disp: 1 bottle

Sig: 20 mL for 30 seconds 3 times/day

Ingredients: Chlorhexidine gluconate 0.12% and alcohol 11.6%

ORAL NONVIRAL SOFT TISSUE ULCERATIONS OR EROSIONS *(Continued)*

Rx

PerioGard® oral rinse

Disp: 1 bottle

Sig: 20 mL for 30 seconds 3 times/day

Ingredients: Chlorhexidine gluconate 0.12% and alcohol 11.6%

Rx

Tetracycline capsules 250 mg

Disp: 40 capsules

Sig: Suspend contents of 1 capsule in a teaspoonful of water; rinse for 2 minutes 4 times/day and swallow

Note: Also available as liquid (125 mg/5 mL), which is convenient to use; swish 5 mL for 2 minutes 4 times/day

Rx

Kenalog® in Orabase 0.1%

Disp: 5 g tube

Sig: Coat the lesion with a film after each meal and at bedtime

Ingredient: Triamcinolone

Rx

Benadryl® elixir 12.5 mg/5 mL

Disp: 4 oz bottle

Sig: Rinse with 1 teaspoonful for 2 minutes before each meal and swallow

Ingredient: Diphenhydramine

Note: Elixir of Benadryl®, a potent antihistamine, is used in the oral cavity primarily as a mild topical anesthetic agent for the symptomatic relief of certain allergic deficiencies which should be ruled out as possible etiologies for the oral condition under treatment. It is often used alone and in solutions with agents such as Kaopectate® or Maalox® to assist in coating the oral mucosa. Benadryl® is also available in capsules.

Rx

Benadryl® syrup (mix 50/50) with Kaopectate®*

Disp: 8 oz total

Sig: Rinse with 2 teaspoons as needed to relieve pain or burning (use after meals)

Ingredient: Diphenhydramine and attapulgite

***Note:** May be mixed with Maalox® if constipation is a problem.

Rx

Lidex® ointment mixed 50/50 with Orabase®

Disp: 30 g total

Sig: Apply thin layer to oral lesions 4-6 times/day

Ingredient: Fluocinonide 0.05%

Note: To be used for oral inflammatory lesions that do not respond to Kenalog® in Orabase®.

EROSIVE LICHEN PLANUS AND MAJOR APHTHAE

Elixir of dexamethasone (Decadron®), a potent anti-inflammatory agent, is used topically in the management of acute episodes of erosive lichen planus and major aphthae. Continued supervision of the patient during treatment is essential and the dentist must be aware that treatment of any secondary infections such as fungal overgrowth may be essential in gaining control of the erosive lesions.

PRESCRIPTION EXAMPLE

Rx

Decadron® elixir 0.5 mg/5 mL

Disp: 100 mL bottle

Sig: Rinse with 1 teaspoonful for 2 minutes 4 times/day; do not swallow

Ingredient: Dexamethasone

Note: Other regimens altering topical and systemic uptake including swish-and-swallow can be designed by the dentist depending upon the severity and usual duration of the lesions.

For severe cases and when the oropharynx is involved, some practitioners have the patient swallow after a 2-minute rinse.

Allergy	Benadryl®
Aphthous	Benadryl®/Maalox® (compounded prescription) Benadryl®/Kaopectate® (compounded prescription) Lidex® in Orabase (compounded prescription) Kenalog® in Orabase Tetracycline mouth rinse
Oral inflammatory disease	Lidex® in Orabase (compounded prescription) Kenalog® in Orabase Prednisone Temovate® cream

The use of long-term steroids is always a concern due to possible adrenal suppression. If systemic steroids are contemplated for a protracted time, medical consultation is advisable.

PRESCRIPTION EXAMPLE FOR SYSTEMIC STEROID

Rx

Prednisone 5 mg

Disp: 60 tablets

Sig: Take 4 tablets in morning with food and 4 tablets at noon with food for 4 day, then decrease the total number of tablets by 1 each day until down to zero

Note: Medrol® (methylprednisolone) dose packs (2-60 mg/day) are an alternative choice; see Methylprednisolone *on page 910*

PRESCRIPTION EXAMPLE FOR HIGH POTENCY TOPICAL CORTICOSTEROID

Rx

Temovate® cream 0.05%

Disp: 15 g tube

Sig: Apply locally 4-6 times/day

Ingredient: Clobetasol

ORAL NONVIRAL SOFT TISSUE ULCERATIONS OR EROSIONS *(Continued)*

NECROTIZING ULCERATING PERIODONTITIS (HIV Periodontal Disease)

Initial Treatment *(In-Office)*

Gentle debridement

Note: Ensure patient has no iodine allergies

Betadine® rinse *on page 1107*

At-Home Treatment

Listerine® antiseptic rinse (20 mL for 30 seconds twice daily)
Peridex® rinse *on page 308*
Metronidazole (Flagyl®) 7-10 days *on page 917*

Follow-Up Therapy

Proper dental cleaning, including scaling and root planing (repeat as needed)
Continue Peridex® and Listerine® rinse (indefinitely)

DENTIN HYPERSENSITIVITY, HIGH CARIES INDEX, AND XEROSTOMIA

DENTIN HYPERSENSITIVITY

Suggested steps in resolving dentin hypersensitivity when a thorough exam has ruled-out any other source for the problem:

Treatment Steps

- Home treatment with a desensitizing toothpaste containing potassium nitrate (used to brush teeth as well as a thin layer applied, each night for 2 weeks)
- If needed, in office potassium oxalate (Protect® by Butler) and/or in office fluoride iontophoresis
- If sensitivity is still not tolerable to the patient, consider pumice then dentin adhesive and unfilled resin or composite restoration overlaying a glass ionomer base

Home Products (all contain nitrate as active ingredient):

Promise®

Denquel®

Sensodyne®

Dentifrice Products *on page 1621*

Other major brand name companies have added ingredients to their dentifrice product lines that also make hypersensitivity claims.

ANTICARIES AGENTS

Fluoride (Gel 0.4%, Rinse 0.05%) *on page 603*

New toothpastes with triclosan such as Colgate Total® show promise for combined treatment/prevention of caries, plaque, and gingivitis. The use of 5% sodium fluoride varnishes (Duraflor® and Duraphat®) have been encouraged by cariologists for the prevention of decay in persons of high-risk populations.

FLUORIDES

Used for the prevention of demineralization of the tooth structure secondary to xerostomia. For patients with long-term or permanent xerostomia, daily application is accomplished using custom applicator trays, such as omnivac. Patients with porcelain crowns should use a neutral pH fluoride (see Fluoride monograph *on page 603*). Final selection of a fluoride product and/or saliva replacement/stimulant product must be based on patient comfort, taste, and ultimately, compliance. Experience has demonstrated that, often times, patients must try various combinations to achieve the greatest effect and their highest comfort levels. The presence of mucositis during cancer management complicates the clinician's selection of products.

See also Oral Rinse Products *on page 1638*

OVER-THE-COUNTER (OTC) PRODUCTS

Form	Brand Name	Strength / Size
Gel, topical (stannous fluoride)	Gel-Kam® (cinnamon, fruit, mint flavors)	0.4% [0.1%] (65 g, 105 g, 122 g)
	Gel-Tin® (lime, grape, cinnamon, raspberry, mint, orange flavors)	0.4% [0.1%] (60 g, 120 g)
	Stop® (grape, cinnamon, bubblegum, piña colada, mint flavors)	0.4% [0.1%] (60 g, 120 g)
Rinse, topical (as sodium)	ACT®, Fluorigard®	0.05% [0.02%] (90 mL, 180 mL, 300 mL, 360 mL, 480 mL)
	Listermint® with Fluoride	0.02% [0.01%] (180 mL, 300 mL, 360 mL, 480 mL, 540 mL, 720 mL, 960 mL, 1740 mL)

DENTIN HYPERSENSITIVITY, HIGH CARIES INDEX, AND XEROSTOMIA *(Continued)*

PRESCRIPTION ONLY (Rx) PRODUCTS

Form	Brand Name	Strength / Size
Drops, oral (as sodium)		0.275 mg/drop [0.125 mg/drop]
	Fluoritab®, Flura-Drops®	0.55 mg/drop [0.25 mg/drop] (22.8 mL, 24 mL)
	Karidium®, Luride®	0.275 mg/drop [0.125 mg/drop] (30 mL, 60 mL)
	Pediaflor®	1.1 mg/mL [0.5 mg/mL] (50 mL)
Gel-Drops	Thera-Flur® (lime flavor), Thera-Flur-N®	1.1% [0.55%] (24 mL)
Gel, topical		
Acidulated phosphate fluoride	Minute-Gel® (spearmint, strawberry, grape, apple-cinnamon, cherry cola, bubblegum flavors)	1.23% (480 mL)
Sodium fluoride	Karigel® (orange flavor)	1.1% [0.5%]
	Karigel®-N	1.1% [0.5%]
	PreviDent® (mint, berry, cherry, fruit sherbet flavors)	1.1% [0.5%] (24 g, 30 g, 60 g, 120 g, 130 g, 250 g)
Lozenge (as sodium)	Flura-Loz® (raspberry flavor)	2.2 mg [1 mg]
Rinse, topical (as sodium)	Fluorinse®, Point-Two®	0.2% [0.09%] (240 mL, 480 mL, 3780 mL)
Solution, oral (as sodium)	Phos-Flur® (cherry, cinnamon, grape, wintergreen flavors)	0.44 mg/mL [0.2 mg/mL] (250 mL, 500 mL, 3780 mL)
Tablet (as sodium)		1.1 mg [0.5 mg]; 2.2 mg [1 mg]
Chewable	Fluor-A-Day®	0.55 mg [0.25 mg]
	Fluor-A-Day®, Fluoritab®, Luride® Lozi-Tab®, Pharmaflur®	1.1 mg [0.5 mg]
	Fluor-A-Day®, Fluoritab®, Karidium®, Luride® Lozi-Tab®, Luride®-SF Lozi-Tab®, Pharmaflur®	2.2 mg [1 mg]
Oral	Flura®, Karidium®	2.2 mg [1 mg]
Varnish	Duraflor®, Duraphat®	5% [50 mg/mL] (10 mL)

Tables copied from Newland, JR, Meiller, TF, Wynn, RL, et al, *Oral Soft Tissue Diseases,* 2nd ed, Hudson (Cleveland), OH: Lexi-Comp, Inc, 2002.

ANTIPLAQUE AGENTS

PRESCRIPTION EXAMPLES

Rx

Listerine® antiseptic mouthwash (OTC)

Sig: 20 mL, swish for 30 seconds twice daily

Ingredients: Thymol 0.064%, eucalyptus 0.092%, methyl salicylate 0.060%, menthol 0.042%, and alcohol 26.9%

Rx

Peridex® oral rinse

Disp: 3 times 16 oz

Sig: ½ oz, swish for 30 seconds 2-3 times/day

Ingredients: Chlorhexidine gluconate 0.12% and alcohol 11.6%

Rx

PerioGard® oral rinse

Disp 3 times 16 oz

Sig: ½ oz, swish for 30 seconds 2-3 times/day

Ingredients: Chlorhexidine gluconate 0.12% and alcohol 11.6%

Note: Peridex® may stain teeth yellow to brown (removable with dental cleaning), temporarily alter taste, and increase the deposition of calculus (reversible).

Chlorhexidine Gluconate (Peridex®) *on page 308*

MANAGEMENT OF SIALORRHEA

In patients suffering with medical conditions that result in hypersalivation, the dentist may determine that it is appropriate to use an atropine sulfate medication to achieve a dry field for dental procedures or to reduce excessive drooling. Currently there is one ADA approved medication sold under the name of Sal-Tropine™. See Atropine Sulfate Dental Tablets *on page 169*

XEROSTOMIA

Xerostomia refers to the subjective sensation of a dry mouth. Numerous factors can play a role in the patient's perception of dry mouth. Changes in salivary function caused by drugs, surgical intervention, or treatment of cancer are among the leading causes of xerostomia. Other factors including aging, smoking, mouth breathing, and the immune complex of disorders, Sjögren's syndrome, can also be implicated in a patient's perception of xerostomia. Human immunodeficiency virus (HIV) may produce xerostomia when viral changes in salivary glands are present. Xerostomia affects women more frequently than men and is also more common in older individuals. Some alteration in salivary function naturally occurs with age, but it is extremely difficult to quantify the effects. Xerostomia and salivary gland hypofunction in the elderly population are contributory to deterioration in the quality of life.

Once a diagnosis of xerostomia or salivary gland hypofunction is made and possible causes confirmed, treatment for the condition usually involves management of the underlying disease and avoidance of unnecessary medications. In addition, good hydration is essential and water is the drink of choice. Also, the use of artificial saliva substitutes, selected chewing gums, and/or toothpastes formulated to treat xerostomia, is often warranted. In more difficult cases, such as patients receiving radiotherapy for cancer of the head and neck regions or patients with Sjögren's syndrome, systemic cholinergic stimulants may be administered if no contraindications exist.

CLINICAL PRODUCT USE

Because of the complex nature of xerostomia, management by the dental clinician is difficult. Treatment success is also difficult to assess and is often unsatisfactory. The salivary stimulants, pilocarpine and cevimeline, may aid in some conditions but are only approved for use as sialogogues in patients receiving radiotherapy and in Sjögren's patients, specifically as described above. Artificial salivas are available as over-the-counter products and represent the potential for continuous application by the patient to achieve comfort for their xerostomic condition.

The role of the clinician in attempting treatment of dry mouth is to first achieve a differential diagnosis and to ensure that other conditions are not simultaneously present. For example, many patients suffer burning mouth syndrome or painful oral tissues with no obvious etiology accompanying dry mouth. Also, higher caries incidence may be associated with changes in salivary flow. As previously mentioned, Sjögren's syndrome represents an immune complex of disorders that can affect the eyes, oral tissues, and other organ systems. The reader is referred to current oral pathology or oral medicine text for review of signs and symptoms of Sjögren's syndrome.

Treatment of cancer often leads to dry mouth. Surgical intervention removing salivary tissue due to the presence of a salivary gland tumor results in loss of salivary function. Also, many of the chemotherapeutic agents produce transitory changes in salivary flow, such that the patient may perceive a dry mouth during chemotherapy. Most notably related to salivary dysfunction is the use of radiation regimens to head and neck tissues. Tumors in or about salivary gland tissue, the oral cavity, and oropharynx are most notably sensitive to radiation therapy and subsequent dry mouth. In the head and neck, therapeutic radiation is commonly used in treatment of squamous cell carcinomas and lymphomas. The radiation level necessary to destroy malignant cells ranges from 40-70 Gy. Salivary tissue is extremely sensitive to radiation changes. Radiation dosages >30 Gy are sufficient to permanently change salivary function. In addition to the mucositis and subsequent secondary infection by fungal colonization or viral exacerbation, oral tissues can become exceptionally dry due to the effects of radiation on salivary glands. In fact, permanent damage to salivary gland tissue within the beam path produces significant levels of xerostomia in most patients. Some recovery may be noted by the patient. Most often, the effects are permanent and even progressive as the radiation dosage increases.

Artificial salivas do not produce any protectant or stimulation of the salivary gland. The use of pilocarpine and cevimeline as salivary stimulants in pre-emptive treatment, as well

DENTIN HYPERSENSITIVITY, HIGH CARIES INDEX, AND XEROSTOMIA *(Continued)*

as postradiation treatment, have been shown to have some efficacy in management of dry mouth. The success rate, however, still is often unsatisfactory and post-treatment management by the dentist usually requires fluoride supplements to prevent radiation-induced caries due to dry mouth. Also, management of dry mouth through patient use of the artificial salivary gel, solutions and sprays, or other over-the-counter products for dry mouth (eg, chewing gum, toothpaste, mouthwash, swab-sticks) is highly recommended. The use of pilocarpine or cevimeline should only be considered by the dentist in consultation with the managing physician. The oftentimes severe and widespread cholinergic side effects of pilocarpine and cevimeline mandate close monitoring of the patient.

The use of artificial salivary substitutes is less problematic for the dentist. The dentist should, in considering selection of a drug, base his or her decision on patient compliance and comfort. Salivary substitutes presently on the market may have some benefit in terms of electrolyte balance and salivary consistency. However, the ultimate decision needs to be based on patients' taste, their willingness to use the medication ad libitum, and improvement in their comfort related to dry mouth. Many of the drugs are pH balanced to reduce additional risk of dental demineralization or caries. Oftentimes, the dentist must try numerous medications, one at a time, prior to finding one which gives the patient some comfort. Another gauge of acceptability is to investigate whether the artificial saliva substitute has the American Dental Association's seal of approval. Most of the currently accepted saliva substitute products have been evaluated by the ADA.

In general, considerations that the clinician might use in a prescribed regimen would be that saliva substitutes are meant to be used regularly throughout the day by the patient to achieve comfort during meals, reduce tissue abrasion, and prevent salivary stagnation on teeth. Other than these, there are no specific recommendations for patients. Recommendations by the dentist need to be tailored to the patient's acceptance. Salivary substitutes may provide an allergic potential in patients who are sensitive to some of the preservatives present in artificial saliva products. In addition to this allergic potential, there is a risk of microbial contamination by placement of the salivary substitute container in close contact with the oral cavity.

Patient education regarding the use of saliva substitutes is also part of the clinical approach. The patient with chronic xerostomia should be educated about regular professional care, high performance in dental hygiene, the need to re-evaluate oral soft tissue pathology, and any changes that might occur long term. In patients with severe xerostomia, artificial salivary medications should be given in combination with topical fluoride treatment programs designed by the dentist to reduce caries.

PRODUCTS AND DRUGS TO TREAT DRY MOUTH

Medication	Manufacturer and Phone Number	Product Type	Manufacturer's Description	Indication	Ingredients	Directions for Use	Form and Availability
Artificial Salivas (OTC)							
Moi-Stir® Moistening Solution	Kingswood Laboratories, Inc (800) 968-7772	Pump spray	Saliva supplement for moistening of mouth and mucosal area	Nontherapeutic treatment of dry mouth; intended for comfort only	Water, sorbitol, sodium carboxymethylcellulose, methylparaben, propylparaben, potassium chloride, sodium chloride, flavoring	Spray directly into mouth as necessary to treat drying conditions	4 oz spray bottle; order directly from manufacturer or various distributors
MouthKote® Oral Moisturizer	Parnell Pharmaceuticals, Inc (800) 457-4276	Aqueous solution	Pleasant lemon-lime-flavored oral moisturizer to lubricate and protect oral tissue	Treats the discomfort of oral dryness caused by medications, disease, surgery, irradiation, aging	Water, xylitol, sorbitol, yerba santa, citric acid, ascorbic acid, flavor, sodium benzoate, sodium saccharin	Swirl 1 or 2 teaspoonfuls in mouth for 8-10 seconds; swallow or spit out; shake well before using	2 oz and 8 oz bottles; available at drugstores or order directly from manufacturer
BreathTech™ Plaque Fighter Mouth Spray	Omnii Oral Pharmaceuticals (800) 445-3386	Pump dispenser	Plaque inhibitor in vanilla-mint flavor for breath malodor or reduced salivary flow	Treats the discomfort of oral dryness	Microdent® patented plaque-inhibitor formula	Spray directly into mouth; spread over teeth and tissue with tongue	18 mL pump dispenser; order directly from manufacturer
Optimoist™ Oral Moisturizer	Colgate Oral Pharmaceuticals (800) 225-3756	Oral moisturizer, aqueous solution	Pleasant tasting saliva substitute for instant relief of dry mouth and throat without demineralizing tooth enamel	Treats the discomfort of oral dryness	Deionized water, xylitol, calcium phosphate monobasic, citric acid, sodium hydroxide, sodium benzoate, flavoring, acesulfame potassium, hydroxyethylcellulose, polysorbate 20 and sodium monofluorophosphate (fluoride concentration is 2 parts per million)	Spray directly into mouth to relieve dry mouth discomfort; may be swallowed or expectorated; use as needed	2 oz and 12 oz bottles; available at mass merchandise stores, food stores, and drugstores

DENTIN HYPERSENSITIVITY, HIGH CARIES INDEX, AND XEROSTOMIA *(Continued)*

PRODUCTS AND DRUGS TO TREAT DRY MOUTH *(continued)*

Medication	Manufacturer and Phone Number	Product Type	Manufacturer's Description	Indication	Ingredients	Directions for Use	Form and Availability
Biotene® OralBalance® Mouth Moisturizing Gel	Laclede Professional Products, Inc (800) 922-5856	Gel	Sugar-free oral lubricant; relieves dry mouth symptoms up to 8 hours; soothes and protects oral tissue to promote healing; helps to inhibit harmful bacteria; improves retention under dentures	Relieves symptoms of dry mouth: burning, itching, cotton palate, sore tissue swallowing difficulties	Contains the "Biotene®" protective salivary enzyme system Active: Glucose oxidase (2000 units), lactoperoxidase (3000 units), lysozyme (5 mg), lactoferrin (5 mg) Other: Hydrogenated starch, xylitol, hydroxyethyl cellulose, glycerate polyhydrate, aloe vera	Using a clean fingertip, apply a 1" ribbon of gel on tongue; add additional amount of gel on other dry; use as needed	1.4 oz tube; available at mass merchandise stores, food stores, and drugstores
Salivart® Synthetic Saliva, Aqueous Solution	Gebauer Co (800) 321-9348	Aerosol aqueous spray	Oral moisturizer for patients with reduced salivary flow	Replacement therapy for patients complaining of xerostomia	Sodium carboxymethylcellulose, sorbitol, sodium chloride, potassium chloride, calcium chloride dihydrate, magnesium chloride hexahydrate, potassium phosphate dibasic, purified water, nitrogen (propellant)	Spray directly into mouth or throat for 1-2 seconds; use as needed	2.48 fl oz (75 g); available at most drugstores or directly from manufacturer
Other Dry Mouth Products (OTC)							
Biotene® Dry Mouth Gum	Laclede Professional Products, Inc (800) 922-9348	Chewing gum	Sugar-free; helps stimulate saliva flow; fights cause/effect of bad breath; reduces plaque	Treats oral dryness	Active: Lactoperoxidase (0.11 Units), glucose oxidase (0.15 Units) Other: Sorbitol, gum base, xylitol, hydrogenated glucose, potassium thiocyanate	Chew 1 or 2 pieces; use as needed	Each package contains 17 pieces; available at drugstores or directly from manufacturer
Biotene® Dry Mouth Toothpaste	Laclede Professional Products, Inc (800) 922-9348	Toothpaste	Reduces harmful bacteria which cause cavities, periodontal disease, and oral infections	Use in place of regular toothpaste for dry mouth	Active: Lactoperoxidase (15,000 Units), glucose oxidase (10,000 Units), lysozyme (16 mg), sodium monofluorophosphate Other: Sorbitol, glycerin, calcium pyrophosphate, hydrated silica, xylitol, isoceteth-20, cellulose gum, flavoring, sodium benzoate, beta-d-glucose, potassium thiocyanate	Use in place of regular toothpaste; rinse toothbrush before applying; brush for 2 minutes; rinse lightly	4.5 oz tube; available at drugstores or directly from manufacturer

PRODUCTS AND DRUGS TO TREAT DRY MOUTH *(continued)*

Medication	Manufacturer and Phone Number	Product Type	Manufacturer's Description	Indication	Ingredients	Directions for Use	Form and Availability
Biotene® Gentle Mouthwash	Laclede Professional Products, Inc (800) 922-9348	Mouthwash	Alcohol-free; strong antibacterial formula neutralizes mouth odors; soothes as it cleans to protect teeth and oral tissue	Treats dry mouth or oral irritations	Lysozyme, lactoferrin, glucose oxidase, lactoperoxidase	Use 15 mL (1 tablespoonful); swish thoroughly for 30 seconds and spit out; for dry throat, sip 1 tablespoonful of mouthwash 2-3 times/day	Available at drugstores or directly from manufacturer
Moi-Stir® Oral Swabsticks	Kingswood Laboratories, Inc (800) 968-7772	Swabsticks	Lubricates and moistens mouth and mucosal area	Lubricates and moistens mouth and mucosal area	Water, sorbitol, sodium carboxymethylcellulose, methylparaben, propylparaben, potassium chloride, sodium chloride, flavoring	Gently swab all intraoral surfaces of mouth, gums, tongue, palate, buccal mucosa, gingival, teeth, and lips where uncomfortable dryness exists	3 swabsticks/packet, 100 packets/case; order directly from manufacturer or from various distributors.
Cholinergic Salivary Stimulants (Rx)							
Cevimeline (Evoxac®)	Snow Brand Pharmaceuticals (800) 475-6473			Treats symptoms of dry mouth in patients with Sjögren's syndrome	Active: Cevimeline 30 mg Other: Lactose monohydrate, hydroxypropyl cellulose, magnesium stearate	1 capsule (30 mg) 3 times/day	30 mg capsules
Pilocarpine (Salagen®)	MGI Pharmaceuticals, Inc (800) 562-5580			Treats xerostomia caused by radiation therapy in patients with head/neck cancer, Sjögren's syndrome	Active: Pilocarpine 5 mg Other: Carnauba wax, hydroxypropyl methylcellulose, iron oxide, microcrystalline cellulose, stearic acid, titanium dioxide	1-2 tablets (5 mg) 3-4 times/day, not to exceed 30 mg/day	5 mg tablets

DENTIN HYPERSENSITIVITY, HIGH CARIES INDEX, AND XEROSTOMIA *(Continued)*

CHOLINERGIC SALIVARY STIMULANTS (PRESCRIPTION ONLY)

Pilocarpine (Dental)(Salagen® *on page 1086*), approved in 1994, and cevimeline (Evoxac® *on page 302*), approved in 2000, are cholinergic drugs which stimulate salivary flow. They stimulate muscarinic-type acetylcholine receptors in salivary glands within the parasympathetic division of the autonomic nervous system, causing an increase in serous-type saliva. Thus, they are considered cholinergic, muscarinic-type (parasympathomimetic) drugs. Due to significant side effects caused by these drugs, they are available by prescription only.

Pilocarpine (Salagen®) is indicated for the treatment of xerostomia caused by radiation therapy in patients with head and neck cancer and xerostomia in patients suffering from Sjögren's syndrome. The usual adult dosage is 1-2 tablets (5 mg) 3-4 times/day, not to exceed 30 mg/day. Patients should be treated for a minimum of 90 days for optimum effect. The most frequent adverse side effect is perspiration, which occurs in about 30% of patients who use 5 mg 3 times/day. Other adverse effects (in about 10% of patients) are nausea, rhinitis, chills, frequent urination, dizziness, headache, lacrimation, and pharyngitis. Salagen® is contraindicated for patients with uncontrolled asthma and narrow-angle glaucoma.

The salivary-stimulative effects of oral pilocarpine have been documented since the late 1960s and 1970s. Pilocarpine has been documented to overcome xerostomia from different causes. More recent studies confirm its effectiveness in improving salivary flow in patients undergoing irradiation therapy for head and neck cancer. A capstone study by Johnson, et al, reported the effects of pilocarpine in 208 irradiation patients at 39 different treatment sites. Salagen®, at a dose of 5 mg 3 times/day, improved salivation in 44% of patients, compared with 25% in the placebo group. They concluded that treatment with pilocarpine (Salagen®) produced the best overall outcome with respect to saliva production and relief of symptoms of xerostomia in patients undergoing irradiation therapy.

Additional studies have been published showing the effectiveness of pilocarpine (Salagen®) in stimulating salivary flow in patients suffering from Sjögren's syndrome and the FDA has recently approved the use of Salagen® for this indication.

Recent reports suggest that pre-emptive use of pilocarpine may be effective in protecting salivary glands during therapeutic irradiation; further studies are needed to confirm this. As of this publication date, the use of pilocarpine has not been approved to treat xerostomia induced by chronic medication. Pilocarpine could be used as a sialagogue for individuals with xerostomia induced by antidepressants and other medications. However, the potential for serious drug interactions is a concern and more studies are needed to clarify the safety and effectiveness of pilocarpine when given in the presence of other medications.

Cevimeline (Evoxac®) is indicated for treatment of symptoms of dry mouth in patients with Sjögren's syndrome. The usual dosage in adults is 1 capsule (30 mg) 3 times/day. Cevimeline (Evoxac®) is supplied in 30 mg capsules. Some adverse effects reported for Evoxac® include increased sweating (19%), rhinitis (11%), sinusitis (12%), and upper respiratory infection (11%). Evoxac® is contraindicated for patients with uncontrolled asthma, narrow-angle glaucoma, acute iritis, and other conditions where miosis is undesirable.

OTHER DRUGS IMPLICATED IN XEROSTOMIA

>10%	1% to 10%
Alprazolam	Acrivastine and Pseudoephedrine
Amitriptyline hydrochloride	Albuterol
Amoxapine	Amantadine hydrochloride
Anisotropine methylbromide	Amphetamine sulfate
Atropine sulfate	Astemizole (withdrawn from market)
Belladonna and Opium	Azatadine maleate
Benztropine mesylate	Beclomethasone dipropionate
Bupropion	Bepridil hydrochloride
Chlordiazepoxide	Bitolterol mesylate
Clomipramine hydrochloride	Brompheniramine maleate
Clonazepam	Carbinoxamine and Pseudoephedrine
Clonidine	Chlorpheniramine maleate
Clorazepate dipotassium	Clemastine fumarate
Cyclobenzaprine	Clozapine
Desipramine hydrochloride	Cromolyn sodium
Diazepam	Cyproheptadine hydrochloride
Dicyclomine hydrochloride	Dexchlorpheniramine maleate
Diphenoxylate and Atropine	Dextroamphetamine sulfate
Doxepin hydrochloride	Dimenhydrinate
Ergotamine	Diphenhydramine hydrochloride
Estazolam	Disopyramide phosphate
Flavoxate	Doxazosin
Flurazepam hydrochloride	Dronabinol
Glycopyrrolate	Ephedrine sulfate
Guanabenz acetate	Flumazenil
Guanfacine hydrochloride	Fluvoxamine
Hyoscyamine sulfate	Gabapentin
Interferon alfa-2a	Guaifenesin and Codeine
Interferon alfa-2b	Guanadrel sulfate
Interferon alfa-N3	Guanethidine sulfate
Ipratropium bromide	Hydroxyzine
Isoproterenol	Hyoscyamine, Atropine, Scopolamine, and Phenobarbital
Isotretinoin	Imipramine
Loratadine	Isoetharine
Lorazepam	Levocabastine hydrochloride
Loxapine	Levodopa
Maprotiline hydrochloride	Levodopa and Carbidopa
Methscopolamine bromide	Levorphanol tartrate
Molindone hydrochloride	Meclizine hydrochloride
Nabilone	Meperidine hydrochloride
Nefazodone	Methadone hydrochloride
Oxybutynin chloride	Methamphetamine hydrochloride
Oxazepam	Methyldopa
Paroxetine	Metoclopramide
Phenelzine sulfate	Morphine sulfate
Prochlorperazine	Nortriptyline hydrochloride
Propafenone hydrochloride	Ondansetron
Protriptyline hydrochloride	Oxycodone and Acetaminophen
Quazepam	Oxycodone and Aspirin
Reserpine	Pentazocine
Selegiline hydrochloride	Phenylpropanolamine hydrochloride
Temazepam	Prazosin hydrochloride
Thiethylperazine maleate	Promethazine hydrochloride
Trihexyphenidyl hydrochloride	Propoxyphene
Trimipramine maleate	Pseudoephedrine
Venlafaxine	Risperidone
	Sertraline hydrochloride
	Terazosin
	Terbutaline sulfate

TEMPOROMANDIBULAR DYSFUNCTION (TMD)

Temporomandibular dysfunction comprises a broad spectrum of signs and symptoms. Although TMD presents in patterns, diagnosis is often difficult. Evaluation and treatment is time-intensive and no single therapy or drug regimen has been shown to be universally beneficial.

The thorough diagnostician should perform a screening examination for the temporomandibular joint on all patients. Ideally, a baseline maximum mandibular opening along with lateral and protrusive movement evaluation should be performed. Secondly, the joint area should be palpated and an adequate exam of the muscles of mastication and the muscles of the neck and shoulders should be made. These muscle would include the elevators of the mandible (masseter, internal pterygoid, and temporalis); the depressors of the mandible (including the external pterygoid and digastric); extrusive muscles (including the temporalis and digastric), and protrusive muscles (including the external and internal pterygoids). These muscles also account for lateral movement of the mandible. The clinician should also be alert to indicators of dysfunction, primarily a history of pain with jaw function, chronic history of joint noise (although this can often be misinterpreted), pain in the muscles of the neck, limited jaw movement, pain in the actual muscles of mastication, and headache or even earache. The signs and symptoms are extremely variable and the clinician should be alert for any or all of these areas of interest. Because of the complexity of both evaluation and diagnosis, the general dentist often finds it too time consuming to spend the countless hours evaluating and treating the temporomandibular dysfunction patient. Therefore, oral medicine specialists trained in temporomandibular evaluation and treatment often accept referrals for the management of these complicated patients.

The Oral Medicine specialist in TMD management, the physical therapist interested in head and neck pain, and the Oral and Maxillofacial surgeon will all work together with the referring general dentist to accomplish successful patient treatment. Table 1 lists the wide variety of treatment alternatives available to the team. Depending on the diagnosis, one or more of the therapies might be selected. For organic diseases of the joint not responding to nonsurgical approaches, a wide variety of surgical techniques are available (Table 2).

ACUTE TMD

Acute TMD oftentimes presents alone or as an episode during a chronic pattern of signs and symptoms. Trauma, such as a blow to the chin or the side of the face, can result in acute TMD. Occasionally, similar symptoms will follow a lengthy wide open mouth dental procedure.

The condition usually presents as continuous deep pain in the TMJ. If edema is present in the joint, the condyle sometimes can be displaced which will cause abnormal occlusion of the posterior teeth on the affected side. The diagnosis is usually based on the history and clinical presentation. Management of the patient includes:

1. Restriction of all mandibular movement to function in a pain-free range of motion
2. Soft diet
3. NSAIDs (eg, Anaprox® DS 1 tablet every 12 hours for 7-10 days)
4. Moist heat applications to the affected area for 15-20 minutes, 4-6 times/day
5. Consideration of a muscle relaxant, such as Methocarbamol (Robaxin®) *on page 894*, adult patient of average height/weight, two (500 mg) tablets at bedtime; daytime dose can be tailored to patient

Additional therapies could include referral to a physical therapist for ultrasound therapy 2-4 times/week and a single injection of steroid in the joint space. A team approach with an oral maxillofacial surgeon for this procedure may be helpful. Spray and stretch with Fluori-methane® is often helpful for rapid relief of trismus.

Dichlorodifluoromethane and Trichloromonofluoromethane *on page 427*

CHRONIC TMD

Following diagnosis which is often problematic, the most common therapeutic modalities include:

- Explaining the problem to the patient
- Recommending a soft diet:
  - Diet should consist of soft foods (eg, eggs, yogurt, casseroles, soup, ground meat).
  - Avoid chewing gum, salads, large sandwiches, and hard fruit.
- Reducing stress; moist heat application 4-6 times/day for 15-20 minutes coupled with a monitored exercise program will be beneficial. Usually, working with a physical therapist is ideal.
- Medications include analgesics, anti-inflammatories, tranquilizers, and muscle relaxants

MEDICATION OPTIONS

Most commonly used medication (NSAIDs)

Choline Magnesium Trisalicylate *on page 324*
Choline Salicylate *on page 325*
Diclofenac *on page 427*
Diflunisal *on page 435*
Etodolac *on page 564*
Fenoprofen *on page 580*
Flurbiprofen *on page 613*
Ibuprofen *on page 728*
Indomethacin *on page 746*
Ketoprofen *on page 785*
Ketorolac *on page 787*
Magnesium Salicylate *on page 854*
Meclofenamate *on page 860*
Mefenamic Acid *on page 863*
Nabumetone *on page 955*
Naproxen *on page 965*
Oxaprozin *on page 1022*
Piroxicam *on page 1097*
Salsalate *on page 1207*
Sulindac *on page 1251*
Tolmetin *on page 1311*

Tranquilizers and muscle relaxants, when used appropriately, can provide excellent adjunctive therapy. These drugs should be primarily used for a short period of time to manage acute pain. In low dosages, amitriptyline is often used to treat chronic pain and occasionally migraine headache. Two new drugs similar to the prototype drug, amitriptyline, have recently been approved for use in adults only, for treatment of acute migraine with or without aura: Almotriptan malate (Axert™ [tablets]; Pharmacia Corp) and frovatriptan succinate (Frova™ [tablets]; Elan). Selective serotonin reuptake inhibitors (SSRIs) are sometimes used in the management of chronic neuropathic pain, particularly in patients not responding to amitriptyline. Recently, gabapentin (Neurontin®) has been approved for chronic pain. Problems of inducing bruxism with SSRIs, however, have been reported and may preclude their use. Clinicians attempting to evaluate any patient with bruxism or involuntary muscle movement, who is simultaneously being treated with an SSRI, should be aware of this potential association.

See individual monographs for dosing instructions.

Common minor tranquilizers include:

Alprazolam *on page 84*
Diazepam *on page 423*
Lorazepam *on page 842*

Chronic neuropathic pain management:

Amitriptyline *on page 103*
Carbamazepine *on page 255*
Gabapentin *on page 642*

Acute migraine management:

Almotriptan *on page 82*
Frovatriptan *on page 638*
Rizatriptan *on page 1193*

TEMPOROMANDIBULAR DYSFUNCTION (TMD) *(Continued)*

Common muscle relaxants include:

Chlorzoxazone *on page 322*
Cyclobenzaprine *on page 382*
Methocarbamol *on page 894*
Orphenadrine *on page 1017*

Note: Muscle relaxants and tranquilizers should generally be prescribed with an analgesic or NSAID to relieve pain as well.

Narcotic analgesics can be used on a short-term basis or intermittently in combination with non-narcotic therapy in the chronic pain patient. Judicious prescribing, monitoring, and maintenance by the practitioner is imperative whenever considering the use of narcotic analgesics due to the abuse and addiction liabilities.

Table 1.
TMD – NONSURGICAL THERAPIES

1. Moist heat and cold spray
2. Injections in muscle trigger areas (procaine)
3. Exercises (passive, active)
4. Medications
   a. Muscle relaxants
   b. Minerals
   c. Multiple vitamins (Ca, B_6, B_{12})
5. Orthopedic craniomandibular repositioning appliance (splints)
6. Biofeedback, acupuncture
7. Physiotherapy: TMJ muscle therapy
8. Myofunctional therapy
9. TENS (transcutaneous electrical neural stimulation), Myo-Monitor
10. Dental therapy
    a. Equilibration (coronoplasty)
    b. Restoring occlusion to proper vertical dimension of maxilla to mandible by orthodontics, dental restorative procedures, orthognathic surgery, permanent splint, or any combination of these

Table 2.
TMD – SURGICAL THERAPIES

1. Cortisone injection into joint (with local anesthetic)
2. Bony and/or fibrous ankylosis: requires surgery (osteoarthrotomy with prosthetic appliance)
3. Chronic subluxation: requires surgery, depending on problem (possibly eminectomy and/or prosthetic implant)
4. Osteoarthritis: requires surgery, depending on problem
   a. Arthroplasty with implant
   b. Meniscectomy with implant
   c. Arthroplasty with repair of disc and/or implant
   d. Implant with Silastic insert
5. Rheumatoid arthritis
   a. Arthroplasty with implant with Silastic insert
   b. "Total" TMJ replacement
6. Tumors: require osteoarthrotomy – removal of tumor and restoring of joint when possible
7. Chronic disc displacement: requires repair of disc and possible removal of bone from condyle

PATIENTS REQUIRING SEDATION

Anxiety constitutes the most frequently found psychiatric problem in the general population. Anxiety can range from simple phobias to severe debilitating anxiety disorders. Functional results of this anxiety can, therefore, range from simple avoidance of dental procedures to panic attacks when confronting stressful situations such as seen in some patients regarding dental visits. Many patients claim to be anxious over dental care when in reality they simply have not been managed with modern techniques of local anesthesia, the availability of sedation, or the caring dental practitioner.

The dentist may detect anxiety in patients during the treatment planning evaluation phase of the care. The anxious person may appear overly alert, may lean forward in the dental chair during conversation or may appear concerned over time, possibly using this as a guise to require that they cut short their dental visit. Anxious persons may also show signs of being nervous by demonstrating sweating, tension in their muscles including their temporomandibular musculature, or they may complain of being tired due to an inability to obtain an adequate night's sleep.

The management of such patients requires a methodical approach to relaxing the patient, discussing their dental needs, and then planning, along with the patient the best way to accomplish dental treatment in the presence of their fears, both real or imagined. Consideration may be given to sedation to assist with managing the patient. This sedation can be oral or parenteral, or inhalation in the case of nitrous oxide. The dentist must be adequately trained in administering the sedative of choice, as well as in monitoring the patient during the sedated procedures. Numerous medications are available to achieve the level of sedation usually necessary in the dental office: Valium®, Ativan®, Xanax®, Vistaril®, Serax®, and BuSpar® represent a few. BuSpar® is soon to be available as a transdermal patch. These oral sedatives can be given prior to dental visits as outlined in the following prescriptions. They have the advantage of allowing the patient a good night's sleep prior to the day of the procedures and providing on-the-spot sedation during the procedures. Nitrous oxide represents an in the office administered sedative that is relatively safe, but requires additional training and carefully planned monitoring protocols of any auxiliary personnel during the inhalation procedures. Both the oral and the inhalation techniques can, however, be applied in a very useful manner to manage the anxious patient in the dental office.

Alprazolam *on page 84*

Buspirone *on page 233*

Diazepam *on page 423*

Hydroxyzine *on page 723*

Lorazepam *on page 842*

Nitrous Oxide *on page 994*

Oxazepam *on page 1022*

Triazolam *on page 1335*

Note: Although various sedatives have been used for preprocedure sedation, no specific regimens or protocols have been established. Guidelines for use are still under study.

Fluoxetine *on page 606*

Fluvoxamine *on page 623*

Paroxetine *on page 1046*

Sertraline *on page 1215*

PRESCRIPTION EXAMPLES

Rx

Valium® 5 mg*

Disp: 6 tablets

Sig: Take 1 tablet in evening before going to bed and 1 tablet 1 hour before appointment

Ingredient: Diazepam

***Note:** Also available as 2 mg and 10 mg

PATIENTS REQUIRING SEDATION *(Continued)*

Rx

Ativan® 1 mg*

Disp: 4 tablets

Sig: Take 2 tablets in evening before going to bed and 2 tablets 1 hour before appointment

Ingredient: Lorazepam

***Note:** Also available as 0.5 mg and 2 mg

Rx

Xanax® 0.5 mg

Disp: 4 tablets

Sig: Take 1 tablet in evening before going to bed and 1 tablet 1 hour before appointment

Ingredient: Alprazolam

Rx

Vistaril® 25 mg

Disp: 16 capsules

Sig: Take 2 capsules in evening before going to bed and 2 capsules 1 hour before appointment

Ingredient: Hydroxyzine

Rx

Halcion® 0.25 mg

Disp: 4 tablets

Sig: Take 1 tablet in evening before going to bed and 1 tablet 1 hour before appointment

Ingredient: Triazolam

Rx

Serax® 10 mg

Disp: 2 capsules

Sig: Take 1 capsule before bed and 1 capsule 30 minutes before appointment.

Ingredient: Oxazepam

MANAGEMENT OF PATIENTS UNDERGOING CANCER THERAPY

CANCER PATIENT DENTAL PROTOCOL

The objective in treatment of a patient with cancer is eradication of the disease. Oral complications, such as mucosal ulceration, xerostomia, bleeding, and infections can cause significant morbidity and may compromise systemic treatment of the patient. With proper oral evaluation before systemic treatment, many of the complications can be minimized or prevented.

MUCOSITIS

Normal oral mucosa acts as a barrier against chemical and food irritants and oral microorganisms. Disruption of the mucosal barrier can therefore lead to secondary infection, increased pain, delayed healing, and decreased nutritional intake.

Mucositis is inflammation of the mucous membranes. It is a common reaction to chemotherapy and radiation therapy. It is first seen as an erythematous patch. The mucosal epithelium becomes thin as a result of the killing of the rapidly dividing basal layer mucosal cells. Seven to ten days after cytoreduction chemotherapy and between 1000 cGy and 3000 cGy of radiation to the head and neck, mucosal tissues begin to desquamate and eventually develop into frank ulcerations. The mucosal integrity is broken and is secondarily infected by normal oral flora. The resultant ulcerations can also act as a portal of entry for pathogenic organisms into the patient's bloodstream and may lead to systemic infections. These ulcerations often force interruption of therapy.

Certain chemotherapeutic agents, such as 5-fluorouracil, methotrexate, and doxorubicin, are more commonly associated with the development of oral mucositis. Treatment of oral mucositis is mainly palliative, but steps should be taken to minimize secondary pathogenic infections. Culture and sensitivity data should be obtained to select appropriate therapy for the bacterial, viral, or fungal organisms found.

Prevention of radiation mucositis is difficult. Stents can be constructed to prevent irradiation of uninvolved tissues. The use of multiple ports and fractionation of therapy into smaller doses over a longer period of time can reduce the severity. Fractured restorations, sharp teeth, and ill-fitted prostheses can damage soft tissues and lead to additional interruption of mucosal barriers. Correction of these problems before radiation therapy can diminish these complications.

CHEMOTHERAPY

Chemotherapy for neoplasia also frequently results in oral complications. Infections and mucositis are the most common complications seen in patients receiving chemotherapy. Also occurring frequently are pain, altered nutrition, and xerostomia, which can significantly affect the quality of life.

RADIATION CARIES

Dental caries that sometimes follows radiation therapy is called radiation caries. It usually develops in the cervical region of the teeth adjacent to the gingiva, often affecting many teeth. It is secondary to the damage done to the salivary glands and is initiated by dental plaque, but its rapid progress is due to changes in saliva. In addition to the diminution in the amount of saliva, both the salivary pH and buffering capacity are diminished, which decreases anticaries activity of saliva. Oral bacteria also change with xerostomia leading to the increase in caries activity.

SALIVARY CHANGES

Chemotherapy is not thought to directly alter salivary flow, but alterations in taste and subjective sensations of dry mouth are relatively common complaints. Patients with mucositis and graft-vs-host disease following bone marrow or stem cell transplantation often demonstrate signs and symptoms of xerostomia. Radiation does directly affect salivary production. Radiation to the salivary glands produces fibrosis and alters the production of saliva. If all the major salivary glands are in the field, the decrease in saliva can be dramatic and the serous portion of the glands seems to be most severely affected. The saliva produced is increased in viscosity, which contributes to food retention and increased plaque formation. These xerostomic patients have difficulty in managing a normal diet. Normal saliva also has bacteriostatic properties that are diminished in these patients.

The dental management recommendations for patients undergoing chemotherapy, bone marrow transplantation, and/or radiation therapy for the treatment of cancer are based primarily on clinical observations. The following protocols will provide a conservative, consistent approach to the dental management of patients undergoing chemotherapy or bone marrow transplantation. Many of the cancer chemotherapy drugs produce oral side effects including mucositis, oral ulceration, dry mouth, acute infections, and taste aberrations. Cancer drugs include antibiotics, alkylating agents, antimetabolites, DNA inhibitors, hormones, and cytokines.

All patients undergoing chemotherapy or bone marrow transplantation for malignant disease should have the following baseline:

A. Panoramic radiograph
B. Dental consultation and examination

MANAGEMENT OF PATIENTS UNDERGOING CANCER THERAPY *(Continued)*

C. Dental prophylaxis and cleaning (if the neutrophil count is >1500/mm^3 and the platelet count is >50,000/mm^3)

- Prophylaxis and cleaning will be deferred if the patient's neutrophil count is <1500 and the platelet count is <50,000. Oral hygiene recommendations will be made. These levels are arbitrary guidelines and the dentist should consider the patient's oral condition and planned procedure relative to hemorrhage and level of bacteremia.

D. Oral Hygiene: Patients should be encouraged to follow normal hygiene procedures. Addition of a chlorhexidine mouth rinse such as Peridex® or PerioGard® *on page 308* is usually helpful. If the patient develops oral mucositis, tolerance of such alcohol-based products may be limited.

E. If the patient develops mucositis, bacterial, viral, and fungal cultures should be obtained. Sucralfate suspension in either a pharmacy-prepared form or Carafate® suspension, as well as Benadryl® *on page 448* or Xylocaine® viscous *on page 819* can assist in helping the patient to tolerate food. Patients may also require systemic analgesics for pain relief depending on the presence of mucositis. Positive fungal cultures may require a nystatin swish-and-swallow prescription or the selection of another antifungal agent (see Oral Fungal Infections *on page 1544*).

F. The determination of performing dental procedures must be based on the goal of preventing infection during periods of neutropenia. Timing of procedures must be coordinated with the patient's hematologic status.

G. If oral surgery is required, at least 7-10 days of healing should be allowed before the anticipated date of bone marrow suppression (eg, ANC <1000/mm^3 and/or platelet count of 50,000/mm^3).

H. Daily use of topical fluorides is recommended for those who have received radiation therapy to the head and neck region involving salivary glands. Any patients with prolonged xerostomia subsequent to graft-vs-host disease and/or chemotherapy can also be considered for fluoride supplement. Use the fluoride-containing mouthwashes (Act®, Fluorigard®, etc) each night before going to sleep; swish, hold 1-2 minutes, spit out or use prescription fluorides (gels or rinses); apply daily for 1-4 minutes as directed; if mouth is sore (mucositis), use flavorless/colorless gels (Thera-Flur®, Gel-Kam®). Improvement in salivary flow following radiation therapy to the head and neck has been noted with Salagen® *on page 1085* or Evoxac™ *on page 302*. Custom trays can be produced by the clinician for the patient's home use using heat-formed materials such as omnivac.

Benzonatate *on page 193*
Cevimeline *on page 302*
Chlorhexidine Gluconate *on page 308*
Diphenhydramine *on page 448*
Lidocaine *on page 819*
Pilocarpine (Dental) *on page 1086*
Povidone-Iodine *on page 1107*
Sucralfate *on page 1242*

PRESCRIPTION EXAMPLES

Rx

Peridex® or PerioGard® oral rinse
Disp: 3 bottles
Sig: 20 mL for 30 seconds 3 times/day; swish and expectorate

Ingredient: Chlorhexidine gluconate 0.12% and alcohol 11.6%

Rx

Xylocaine® viscous 2%
Disp: 450 mL bottles
Sig: 1 tablespoonful; swish 4 times/day

Ingredient: Lidocaine

Rx

Betadine® mouthwash
Disp: 6 oz bottle
Sig: 1 tablespoonful, rinse 4 times/day; do not swallow

Ingredient: Povidone iodine 0.8%

Rx

Mycostatin® oral suspension
Disp: 60 mL bottle
Sig: 2 mL 4 times/day; hold in mouth for 2 minutes and swallow

Ingredient: Nystatin 100,000 units/mL

Note: When the oral mucous membranes are especially sensitive, nystatin "popsicles" can be made by adding 2 mL of nystatin oral suspension to the water in ice cube trays.

Rx

Tessalon Perles®
Disp: 50
Sig: Squeeze contents of capsule and apply to lesion

Ingredient: Benzonatate

Note: Tessalon Perles® have been used ad lib to provide relief in painful mucositis.

ORAL CARE PRODUCTS

BACTERIAL PLAQUE CONTROL

Patients should use an extra soft bristle toothbrush and dental floss for removal of plaque. Sponge/foam sticks and lemon-glycerine swabs do not adequately remove bacterial plaque.

PRESCRIPTION EXAMPLE

Rx

Ultra Suave® toothbrush
Biotene Supersoft® toothbrush

Note: Chlorhexidine 0.12% (Peridex® or other preparations available in Canada and Europe) may be used to assist with bacterial plaque control.

CHOLINERGIC AGENTS

See Products for Xerostomia *on page 1555*

Used for the treatment of xerostomia caused by radiation therapy in patients with head and neck cancer and from Sjögren's syndrome

Cevimeline *on page 302*
Pilocarpine (Dental) *on page 1086*

FLUORIDES

See Fluorides *on page 1555* in the Dentin Hypersensitivity, High Caries Index, and Xerostomia section.

Used for the prevention of demineralization of the tooth structure secondary to xerostomia. For patients with long-term or permanent xerostomia, daily application is accomplished using custom gel applicator trays, such as omnivac. Patients with porcelain crowns should use a neutral pH fluoride (see Fluoride monograph *on page 603*). Final selection of a fluoride product and/or saliva replacement/stimulant product must be based on patient comfort, taste, and ultimately, compliance. Experience has demonstrated that, often times, patients must try various combinations to achieve the greatest effect and their highest comfort levels. The presence of mucositis during cancer management complicates the clinician's selection of products.

SALIVA SUBSTITUTES

See Products for Xerostomia *on page 1555*

ORAL AND LIP MOISTURIZERS/LUBRICANTS

See Mouth Pain, Cold Sore, and Canker Sore Products *on page 1633*

Note: Water-based gels should first be used to provide moisture to dry oral tissues.

Surgi-Lube®
K-Y Jelly®
Oral Balance®
Mouth Moisturizer®

MANAGEMENT OF PATIENTS UNDERGOING CANCER THERAPY *(Continued)*

PALLIATION OF PAIN

See Mouth Pain, Cold Sore, and Canker Sore Products *on page 1633*

Note: Palliative pain preparations should be monitored for efficacy.

- For relief of pain associated with isolated ulcerations, topical anesthetic and protective preparations may be used.

  Orabase-B® with 20% benzocaine *on page 191*

- For generalized oral pain:

  Chloraseptic Spray® (OTC) anesthetic spray without alcohol *on page 1075*

  Ulcer-Ease® anesthetic/analgesic mouthrinse

  Xylocaine® 2% viscous *on page 819*

  Note: May anesthetize swallowing mechanism and cause aspiration of food; caution patient against using too close to eating; lack of sensation may also allow patient to damage intact mucosa

  Tantum Mouthrinse® (benzydamine hydrochloride); may be diluted as required

  Note: Available only in Canada and Europe

PATIENT PREPARED PALLIATIVE MIXTURES

Coating agents:

Maalox® *on page 91*

Mylanta® *on page 92*

Kaopectate® *on page 170*

These products can be mixed with Benadryl® elixir (50:50):

Diphenhydramine (Benadryl®) *on page 448*

Mouth Pain, Cold Sore, and Canker Sore Products *on page 1633*

Topical anesthetics (diphenhydramine chloride):

Benadryl® elixir or Benylin® cough syrup *on page 448*

Note: Choose product with lowest alcohol and sucrose content; ask pharmacist for assistance

PHARMACY PREPARATIONS

A pharmacist may also prepare the following solutions for relief of generalized oral pain:

Benadryl-Lidocaine Solution

Diphenhydramine injectable 1.5 mL (50 mg/mL) *on page 448*

Xylocaine viscous 2% (45 mL) *on page 819*

Magnesium aluminum hydroxide solution (45 mL)

Swish and hold 1 teaspoonful in mouth for 30 seconds; do not use too close to eating

Rx

Carafate suspension 1 g/10 mL

Disp: 420 mL

Sig: 1 teaspoonful; swish and hold in mouth for 30 seconds

Ingredient: Sucralfate

ORAL MEDICINE TOPICS

PART III:

OTHER ORAL MEDICINE TOPICS

TABLE OF CONTENTS

Dentist's Role in Recognizing Domestic Violence 1574
Chemical Dependency and Smoking Cessation 1576
Animal and Human Bites Guidelines 1582
Dental Office Emergencies 1584
Suggested Readings 1589

DENTIST'S ROLE IN RECOGNIZING DOMESTIC VIOLENCE

Recognition of the signs and symptoms of domestic violence is becoming an important topic for dental and medical professionals throughout the world. Unfortunately, statistics related to domestic abuse of women and children appear to be on the rise, perhaps, in part, due to this increased recognition.

Some statistics are indeed staggering. In the United States, a woman or child is physically abused every five to fifteen seconds. In fact, violence is cited as one of the common causes of emergency room admissions for women 15-44 years of age. Furthermore, 50,000 deaths occur annually, which are attributable to violence in the form of homicide or suicide.

The dentist is in a unique position to recognize many of the signs and symptoms of domestic violence, including child abuse and neglect. The dentist's responsibilities and professional role in this arena are not clear in all states. However, each professional has the responsibility to understand the current state laws regarding the reporting of domestic violence, child abuse, and/or neglect within his/her state. Many states have existing codes defining the role of the professional in these regards. The overall problem of domestic violence, including child abuse, neglect, and other forms of abuse are indeed public health issues. The costs of domestic violence, such as medical, dental, psychiatric, hospital, and emergency care fees are borne to a great extent by the community in addition to the individual.

Domestic abuse is defined as "controlling behavior." Although this often includes physical injury, the primary focus of domestic abuse is one person being in control of another person, making that person do something against his/her will. Women are often abused both physically and mentally in relationships that have existed for many years. Children are often the focus of domestic violence; however, the pattern for an entire family's abuse may be present. Abuse comes in many forms and many victims do not even realize that abuse is occurring. Some victims simply "chalk it up" to things that happen within families. Abuse can include the following: battery and physical assault, such as throwing objects, pushing, hitting, slapping, kicking, or attacking with a weapon; sexual assault including the abuser forcing sexual activities upon another; and, psychological abuse, such as forcing a victim to perform degrading or humiliating acts, threatening harm to a female or male partner or child, or destroying valued possessions of another. Verbal abuse can also be included; however, the psychological forms of abuse are very difficult to ascertain and the signs and symptoms may be difficult to separate from other psychological traits. Abuse tends to have a cyclic pattern, often where a partner, or the controlling individual within the domestic situation, is extremely friendly, intimate, and a good household member. However, due to unknown reasons, as tension develops, family violence often erupts. Once battering has begun, it often increases in frequency and in severity with time. Early recognition by those around the domestic situation can often prevent serious effects. However, until physical violence becomes part of the domestic abuse situation, recognition is usually difficult.

Since nearly 65% of abuse cases (where physical injury is involved) involve injury to the head, neck, or mouth, dental professionals are in a unique position to detect and perhaps, if appropriate in their state, report suspected abuse. In children, these percentages are even higher. Much of our information and beliefs about domestic abuse stem from our knowledge regarding the dental professional in the arena of child abuse and neglect. Being wards of adults, children are vulnerable. Child abuse includes any act that is nonaccidental, endangering or impairing a child's safety or emotional health. Types of child abuse would include physical abuse, emotional abuse and neglect, including health care neglect. Any child suffering from an emotional injury, including sexual abuse or neglect, should be brought to the attention of the social welfare system. Occasionally, "Munchausen syndrome," which is defined as the guardians fabricating or inducing illness in the child, can be observed. Intentional poisoning and safety neglect are also included.

From a medical point-of-view, neglect is much more difficult to determine than abuse. The role of the dentist may be in defining the state of normal and customary pediatric health within a locality. However, due to parents and families moving about the country, sometimes one standard may not be appropriate for all locations.

To detect abuse, or to detect domestic patterns of abuse in the family, the medical or dental professional must be aware of several key behavioral indicators: when the child or adult in question avoids eye contact, is wary of their guardian or spouse, demonstrates fear of touch, or dramatic mood changes. Reports of any history of suicide attempts or running away would also be indicators. Any unexplained injury or injuries that are inconsistent with explanation, including delays in seeking care for such an injury, could represent an abusive situation. The guardian or spouse may also give specific indicators. When it is determined that they cannot explain the injury or that the explanation offered is inconsistent or changes, abuse may be suspected. Nonspecific indicators might include hostile or aggressive behavior or if the queried individual wants to go to a different practitioner when the questioning becomes too intense.

The principles of head-neck examination for the dentist are important and include gathering an overall visual impression of general cleanliness, dress, and stature and examining for any specific physical indicators such as bruises, welts, bite marks, abrasions, lacerations, or other injuries to the head or neck. Contusions or bruises represent the highest percentage of abuse injuries to the young child. The extremely young child or infant often suffers fractures, which fall to second place in terms of incidence as the child matures. In the adult, fractures are much less common. The dentist needs to document the location since often this represents the characteristic that may be difficult for the person to explain. Common areas for injuries include the bony eminences over the knees, shins, and elbows, but could also be on the face, including the zygomatic arch and the chin. Burns are more rare but represent one of the most serious types of injuries. Intraoral injuries including trauma to the oral mucosa, tooth fractures, palatal lesions, ecchymoses, and fractures represent serious evidence of domestic or child abuse. Physical indicators of sexual abuse may not be obvious to the dentist, however, bruising of the hard palate or other evidence of sexual dysfunction may sometimes be found.

The dentist has the responsibility to document from a forensic point-of-view the characteristics that are observed. If necessary, evidence including impressions for bite marks or photographs to document unexplained injuries to the head, neck, and face may be necessary. The legal liability for the dentist is determined by the state laws governing the dental practice. The dental practitioner's failure to diagnose child abuse and neglect is another consideration which goes along with ethical and legal considerations. In the area of child abuse, the states are generally much more clear than they are regarding spousal abuse or overall domestic violence. The dentist has a responsibility to refer a patient for a second opinion if there are concerns that abuse is taking place. Unfortunately, there is no uniformity in the state laws regarding either the responsibility for reporting adult domestic violence or abuse, nor is there uniformity in protecting the health professional by reporting, in good faith, abuse situations. When spousal abuse or other domestic violence is suspected, the definitions become even less clear. They are very similar in ambiguity to those that are faced by the professional regarding neglect as opposed to direct physical or mental abuse. The American Dental Association code is clear on principles and ethics regarding professional conduct regarding the responsibility for recognition of child abuse. They are much less clear on spousal or other abuse and it is likely that in the future as some consistency is noted between and among the various state laws, the ADA Council will undoubtedly take a position.

It is clearly up to the individual states to take the lead in establishing strict guidelines for recognition and reporting of domestic abuse, including protection under the "good faith" statutes for the practitioner. Rules and regulations regarding malicious reporting should also be better defined by the states. The national position is difficult to define because of the extreme variation among states. Dentists are encouraged to use their best judgement in proceeding in any situation of domestic abuse. They should primarily know their state laws and join in the discussion of the topic so that appropriate state actions and formation of legal codes can be undertaken.

CHEMICAL DEPENDENCY AND SMOKING CESSATION

INTRODUCTION

As long as history has been recorded, every society has used drugs that alter mood, thought, and feeling. In addition, pharmacological advances sometimes have been paralleled by physical as well as unfortunate behavioral dependence on agents initially consumed for therapeutic purposes.

In 1986, the American Dental Association passed a policy statement recognizing chemical dependency as a disease. In recognizing this disease, the Association mandated that dentists have a responsibility to include questions relating to a history of chemical dependency, or more broadly, substance abused in their health history questionnaire. A positive response may require the dentist to alter the treatment plan for the patient's dental care. This includes patients who are actively abusing alcohol, drugs, or patients who are in recovery. The use and abuse of drugs is not a topic that is usually found in the dental curriculum. Information about substance abuse is usually gleaned from newspapers, magazines, or just hearsay.

This chapter reviews street drugs, where they come from, signs and symptoms of the drug abuser, and some of the dental implications of treating patients actively using or in recovery from these substances. There are many books devoted to this topic that provide greater detail. The intent is to provide an overview of some of the most prevalent drugs, how patients abusing these drugs may influence dental treatment, and how to recognize some signs and symptoms of use and withdrawal.

Street drugs, like other drugs, can come from various sources. They may be derived from natural sources (ie, morphine and codeine). They may be semisynthetic, that is a natural product is chemically modified to produce another molecule (ie, morphine conversion to heroin). Street drugs may also be synthetic with no natural origin.

BENZODIAZEPINES AND OTHER NONALCOHOL SEDATIVES

Benzodiazepines are the most commonly prescribed drugs worldwide. These drugs are used mainly for treatment of anxiety disorders and, in some instances, insomnia. Even though they are used in high quantities throughout the world, intentional abuse is not that common. These drugs, however, have the ability to induce a strong physical dependency on the use of the medication. As tolerance builds up to the drug, the physical dependency increases dramatically. Unlike street drugs, where addiction is a primary consideration, the overuse of benzodiazepine lies in their ability to induce physical dependency. When these drugs are taken for several weeks, there is relatively little tolerance induced. However, after several months, the proportion of patients who become tolerant increases and reducing the dose or stopping the medication produces severe withdrawal symptoms.

Benzodiazepine Withdrawal Symptoms	
Craving for benzodiazepines	Irritability
Anxiety	Sleep disturbances

It is extremely difficult for the physician to distinguish between the withdrawal symptoms and the reappearance of the myriad anxiety symptoms that cause the drug to be prescribed initially. Many patients increase their dose over time because tolerance develops to at least the sedative effects of the drug. The antianxiety benefits of the benzodiazepines continue to occur long after tolerance to the sedating effects. Patients often take these drugs for many years with relatively few ill effects other than the risk of withdrawal. The dentist should be keenly aware of the signs and symptoms and the historical pattern in patients taking benzodiazepines.

BARBITURATES AND NONBENZODIAZEPINE SEDATIVES

The use of barbiturates as sedative medications has declined over the years due to the increased safety and efficacy of benzodiazepines. Abuse problems with barbiturates resemble those with benzodiazepines in many ways. Drugs in this category are frequently prescribed as hypnotics for patients complaining of insomnia. The physician should, therefore, be aware of the problems that can develop when the hypnotic agent is withdrawn. The underlying problem that has lead to the insomnia is not treated directly by the use of barbiturates and the patient seeking a sleep medication may have altered ability to sleep normally because of the medication. The withdrawal symptoms for the barbiturates are similar to the benzodiazepine sedatives.

ALCOHOL

The chronic use of alcohol, as well as that of other sedatives, is associated with the development of depression. The risk of suicide among alcoholics is one of the highest of any diagnostic category. Cognitive deficits have been reported in alcoholics tested while sober. These deficits usually improve after weeks to months of abstinence. More severe recent memory impairment is associated with specific brain damage caused by nutritional deficiencies common in alcoholics.

Alcohol is toxic to many organ systems. As a result, the medical complications of alcohol abuse and dependence include liver disease, cardiovascular disease, endocrine and gastrointestinal effects, and malnutrition, in addition to CNS dysfunctions. Ethanol readily crosses the placental barrier, producing the *fetal alcohol syndrome*, a major cause of mental retardation.

Alcohol Withdrawal Syndrome Signs and Symptoms	
Alcohol craving	Hypertension
Tremor, irritability	Sweating
Nausea	Perceptual distortion
Sleep disturbance	Seizures (12-48 hours after last drink)
Tachycardia	
Delirium tremens (rare in uncomplicated withdrawal):	
Severe agitation	Tachycardia
Confusion	Nausea, diarrhea
Visual hallucinations	Dilated pupils
Fever, profuse sweating	

NICOTINE

Cigarette (nicotine) addiction is influenced by multiple variables. Nicotine itself produces reinforcement; users compare nicotine to stimulants such as cocaine or amphetamine, although its effects are of lower magnitude.

Nicotine is absorbed readily through the skin, mucous membranes, and of course, through the lungs. The pulmonary route produces discernible central nervous system effects in as little as 7 seconds. Thus, each puff produces some discrete reinforcement. With 10 puffs per cigarette, the 1 pack per day smoker reinforces the habit 200 times daily. The timing, setting, situation, and preparation all become associated repetitively with the effects of nicotine.

Nicotine has both stimulant and depressant actions. The smoker feels alert, yet there is some muscle relaxation. Nicotine activates the nucleus accumbens reward system in the brain. Increased extracellular dopamine has been found in this region after nicotine injections in rats. Nicotine affects other systems as well, including the release of endogenous opioids and glucocorticoids.

Nicotine Withdrawal Syndrome Signs and Symptoms	
Irritability, impatience, hostility	Restlessness
Anxiety	Decreased heart rate
Dysphoric or depressed mood	Increased appetite or weight gain
Difficulty concentrating	

Medications to assist users in breaking a nicotine habit:

Bupropion *on page 230*

Nicotine *on page 981*

SMOKING CESSATION PRODUCTS

Several years ago, the journal, *Science*, stated that approximately 80% of smokers say they want to quit, but each year <1 in 10 actually succeed. Nicotine transdermal delivery preparations (or nicotine patches) were approved by the U.S. Food and Drug Administration in 1992 as aids to smoking cessation for the relief of nicotine withdrawal symptoms. Four preparations were approved simultaneously: Habitrol®, Nicoderm®, Nicotrol®, and ProStep®. These products differ in how much nicotine is released and whether they provide a 24- or 16-hour release time.

Studies are still being reported on the effectiveness of nicotine patches on smoking cessation. Most previous studies had good entry criteria including definition of the Fagerstrom score. Dr Fred Cowan of Oregon Health Sciences University described these Fagerstrom criteria in a previous report on nicotine substitutes in AGD *Impact*. Abstinence of smoking cessation has usually been assessed by self-report, measurement of carbon monoxide in breath, and plasma or urine nicotine products.

In numerous protocols, percentages of study subjects who abstained from smoking after 3-10 weeks of patch treatment with nicotine compared to placebo, have never exceeded 40%. After the initial assessment, six studies continued to follow the study subjects through 24-52 weeks of patch treatment. The results were even poorer with <25% sustained success. A review of these and additional studies, reveals some general conclusions regarding the effectiveness of nicotine patches in smoking cessation. In every study, many smokers abstained after treatment with placebo patches; nicotine treatment was initially more effective than placebo; and improved abstinence rates were more marked in the short term (10 weeks) than in the long term (52 weeks). Subjects undergoing smoking cessation trials tended to gain weight irrespective of whether

CHEMICAL DEPENDENCY AND SMOKING CESSATION *(Continued)*

placebo or nicotine patches were worn. Patients often favor the nicotine polacrilex gum (Nicorette®) which releases nicotine into the blood stream via the oral mucosa.

Data are now available from smoking cessation studies carried out in general medical practices. The effectiveness of nicotine patch substitution under these conditions is similar to the results described above. Most patch systems and gum are now available as over-the-counter products; only Habitrol® remains prescription. Practitioners and patients should remain skeptical since these aids appear to work best only when supplemented with psychological counseling and a single-minded effort on the part of the patient. New products (eg, Zyban®) are now also being marketed as smoking cessation aids. These drugs are norepinephrine serotonin reuptake inhibitors and their action directly affects the craving for tobacco.

OPIATES

The opiates are most often called narcotics. The most common opiate found on the street is heroin. Heroin is the diacetyl derivative of morphine which is extracted from opium. Although commercial production of morphine involves extraction from the dried opium plant which grows in many parts of the world, some areas still harvest opium by making slits in the unripened seed pod. The pod secretes a white, viscous material which upon contact with the air turns a blackish-brown color. It is this off-white material that is called opium. The opium is then dried and smoked or processed to yield morphine and codeine. Actually, the raw opium contains several chemicals that are used medicinally or commercially. Much (approximately 50%) of morphine is converted chemically into heroin which finds its way into the United States and then on the street. Heroin is a Schedule I drug and as such has no acceptable use in the United States today. In fact, possession is a violation of the Controlled Substances Act of 1970. The majority of the heroin found on the streets is from Southeast Asia and can be as concentrated as 100%.

The heroin user goes through many phases once the drug has been administered. When administered intravenously, the user initially feels a "rush" often described as an "orgasmic rush". This initial feeling is most likely due to the release of histamine resulting in cutaneous vasodilation, itching, and a flushed appearance. Shortly after this "rush" the user becomes euphoric. This euphoric stage often called "stoned" or being "high" lasts approximately 3-4 hours. During this stage, the user is lethargic, slow to react to stimuli, speech is slurred, pain reaction threshold is elevated, he/she exhibits xerostomia, slowed heart rate, and the pupils may be constricted. Following the "high", the abuser is "straight" for about 2 hours, with no tell-tale signs of abuse. Approximately 6-8 hours following the last injection of heroin, the user begins to experience a runny nose, lacrimation, and abdominal muscle cramps as he/she begins the withdrawal from the drug. During this stage and the one that follows, the person may become agitated as he/she develops anxiety about where the next "hit" will come from. The withdrawal signs and symptoms become more intense. For the next 3 days, the abuser begins to sweat profusely in combination with cutaneous vasoconstriction. The skin becomes cold and clammy, hence the term "cold turkey". Tachycardia, pupillary dilation, diarrhea, and salivation occur for 3 days following the last injection. Withdrawal signs and symptoms may last longer than the average of 3 days or they may be more abrupt.

Opioid Withdrawal Signs and Symptoms

Symptoms	Signs
Regular Withdrawal	
Craving for opioids Restlessness, irritability Increased sensitivity to pain Nausea, cramps Muscle aches Dysphoric mood Insomnia, anxiety	Pupillary dilation Sweating Piloerection ("gooseflesh") Tachycardia Vomiting, diarrhea Increased blood pressure Yawning Fever
Protracted Withdrawal	
Anxiety Insomnia Drug craving	Cyclic changes in weight, pupil size, respiratory center sensitivity

Many patients who have been abusing opiates for any length of time will exhibit multiple carious lesions, particularly class V lesions. This increased caries rate is probably a result of the heroin-induced xerostomia, high intake of sweets, and lack of daily oral hygiene. Patients who are recovering from heroin or any opiate addiction should not be given any kind of opiate analgesic, whether it be for sedation or as a postoperative analgesic because of the increased chance of relapse. The nonsteroidal anti-inflammatory drugs (NSAIDs) should be used to control any postoperative discomfort. Patients who admit to a past history of intravenous heroin use, or any intravenous drug for that matter, are at higher risk for subacute bacterial endocarditis (SBE), HIV disease, and hepatitis but with the exception of postoperative analgesia should present no special problem for dental care.

OxyContin®, a synthetic opiate, has gained popularity as a street drug in recent years. The drug manufacturer has tried to salvage its name, however, OxyContin® is one of the most widely abused pain medications in use today. It is an excellent analgesic, widely used and is, therefore, available for abuse potential. As with the other opiates, clinical signs and symptoms that the dentist should recognize are consistent with opiate addiction and usage.

MARIJUANA

The number one most abused illegal drug by high school students today is marijuana. Marijuana is a plant that grows throughout the world, but is particularly suited for a warm, humid environment. There are three species of plant but the two most frequently cited are *Cannabis sativa* and *Cannabis indica*. All species possess a female and male plant. Although approximately 450 chemicals have been isolated from the plant, the major psychoactive ingredient is delta-9-tetrahydrocannabinol (THC). Of these 450 chemicals, there are approximately 23 psychoactive chemicals, THC being the most abundant. The highest concentration of THC is found in the bud of the female plant. The concentration of THC varies according to growing conditions and location on the plant but has increased from approximately 2% to 3% in marijuana sold in the 1950s to approximately 30% sold on the streets today. Marijuana can be smoked in cigarettes (joints), pipes, water pipes (bongs), or baked in brownies, cakes, etc, and then ingested. However, smoking marijuana is more efficient and the "high" has a quicker onset. Marijuana is a Schedule I drug but has been promoted as a medicinal for the treatment of glaucoma, for increasing appetite in patients who have HIV disease, and to prevent the nausea associated with cancer chemotherapy. In response to this request, the FDA approved dronabinol (Marinol®), a synthetic THC and placed this drug in Schedule II to be prescribed by physicians for the indicated medical conditions.

Dronabinol *on page 477*

An individual under the influence of marijuana may exhibit no signs or symptoms of intoxication. The pharmacologic effects are dose-dependent and depend to a large extent on the set and setting of the intoxicated individual. As the dose of THC increases, the person experiences euphoria or a state of well-being, often referred to as "mellowing out". Everything becomes comical, problems disappear, and their appetite for snack foods increases. This is called the "munchies". The marijuana produces time and spatial distortion, which contribute, as the dose increases, to a dysphoria characterized by paranoia and fear. Although there has never been a death reported from marijuana overdose, certainly the higher doses may produce such bizarre circumstances as to increase the chances of accidental death. THC is fat soluble. Daily consumption of marijuana will result in THC being stored in body fat which will result in detectable amounts of THC being found in the urine for as long as 60 days in some cases.

Marijuana Withdrawal Syndrome Signs and Symptoms	
Restlessness	Restlessness
Irritability	Sleep EEG disturbance
Mild agitation	Nausea, cramping
Insomnia	

Because of anxiety associated with dental visits, marijuana would be the most likely drug, after alcohol, to be used when coming to the dental office. But, unlike alcohol, marijuana may not produce any detectable odor on the breath nor signs of intoxication. Fortunately, local anesthetics, analgesics, and antibiotics used by the general dentist do not interact with marijuana. The major concern with the marijuana-intoxicated patient is a failure to follow directions while in the chair, and the inability to follow postoperative instructions.

COCAINE

Cocaine, referred to on the street as "snow", "nose candy", "girl", and many other euphemisms, has created an epidemic. This drug is like no other local anesthetic. Known for about the last 2000 years, cocaine has been used and abused by politicians, scientists, farmers, warriors, and of course, on the street. Cocaine is derived from the leaves of a plant called *Erythroxylon coca* which grows in South America. Ninety percent of the world's supply of cocaine originates in Peru, Bolivia, and Colombia. At last estimate, the United States consumes 75% of the world's supply. The plant grows to a height of approximately 4 feet and produces a red berry. Farmers go through the fields stripping the leaves from the plant three times a year. During the working day, the farmers chew the coca leaves to suppress appetite and fight the fatigue of working the fields. The leaves are transported to a laboratory site where the cocaine is extracted by a process called maceration. It takes approximately 7-8 pounds of leaves to produce 1 ounce of cocaine.

On the streets of the United States, cocaine can be found in two forms – one is the hydrochloride salt which can be "snorted" or dissolved in water and injected intravenously, the other is the free base form which can be smoked and is sometimes referred to as "crack", "rock", or "free base". It is called crack because it cracks or pops when large pieces are smoked. It is called rock because it is hard and difficult to break into smaller pieces. The most popular method of administration of cocaine is "snorting" in which small amounts of cocaine hydrochloride are divided into segments or "lines" and

CHEMICAL DEPENDENCY AND SMOKING CESSATION *(Continued)*

any straw-like device can be used to inhale one or more lines of the cocaine into the nose. Although cocaine does not reach the lungs, enough cocaine is absorbed through nasal mucosa to provide a "high" within 3-5 minutes. Rock or crack, on the other hand, is heated and inhaled from any device available. This form of cocaine does reach the lungs and provides a much faster onset of action as well as a more intense stimulation. There are dangers to the user with any form of cocaine. Undoubtedly, the most dangerous form is the intravenous route.

Cocaine Withdrawal Signs and Symptoms	
Dysphoria, depression	Cocaine craving
Sleepiness, fatigue	Bradycardia

The cocaine user, regardless of how the cocaine was administered, presents a potential life-threatening situation in the dental operatory. The patient under the influence of cocaine could be compared to a car going 100 miles per hour. Blood pressure is elevated and heart rate is likely increased. Use of a local anesthetic with epinephrine in such a patient may result in a medical emergency. Such patients can be identified by jitteriness, irritability, talkativeness, tremors, and short abrupt speech patterns. These same signs and symptoms may also be seen in a normal dental patient with preoperative dental anxiety; therefore, the dentist must be particularly alert to identify the potential cocaine abuser. If a patient is suspected, they should never be given a local anesthetic with vasoconstrictor for fear of exacerbating cocaine-induced sympathetic response. Life-threatening episodes of cardiac arrhythmias and hypertensive crises have been reported when local anesthetic with vasoconstrictor was administered to a patient under the influence of cocaine. No local anesthetic used by any dentist can interfere with, nor test positive for cocaine in any urine testing screen. Therefore, the dentist need not be concerned with any false drug use accusations associated with dental anesthesia.

PSYCHEDELIC AGENTS

Perceptual distortions that include hallucinations, illusions, and disorders of thinking such as paranoia can be produced by toxic doses of many drugs. These phenomena also may be seen during toxic withdrawal from sedatives such as alcohol. There are, however, certain drugs that have as their primary effect the production of perception, thought, or mood disturbances at low doses with minimal effects on memory and orientation. These are commonly called *hallucinogenic drugs*, but their use does not always result in frank hallucinations.

Ecstasy (MDMA) and Phenylethylamines (MDA): MDA and MDMA have stimulant, as well as, psychedelic effects and produce degeneration of serotonergic nerve cells and axons. While nerve degeneration has not been well-demonstrated in human beings, the potential remains. Thus, there is possible neurotoxicity with overuse of these drugs. Ecstasy became popular during the 1980s on college campuses and it is still recommended by some psychotherapists as an aid to the process of therapy, although very little controlled data is available. Acute effects are dose-dependent and include dry mouth, jaw clinching, muscle aches, and tachycardia. At higher doses, effects include agitation, hyperthermia, panic attacks, and visual hallucinations. Frequent, repeated use of psychedelic drugs is unusual and, therefore, tolerance is not commonly seen. However, tolerance does develop to the behavioral effects of various psychedelic drugs, and after numerous doses, the tendency towards behavioral tolerance can be observed.

Lysergic Acid Diethylamide (LSD): LSD is the most potent hallucinogenic drug and produces significant psychedelic effects with a total dose of as little as 25-50 mcg. This drug is over 3000 times more potent than mescaline. It is sold on the illicit market in a variety of forms, as a tablet, capsule, sugar cube, or on blotting paper, a popular contemporary system involving postage stamp-sized papers impregnated with varying doses of LSD (≥50-300 mcg). A majority of street samples sold as LSD actually do contain LSD, while mushrooms and other botanicals sold as sources of psilocybin and other psychedelics have a low probability of containing the advertised hallucinogenics. Adverse effects which may affect treatment include visual and auditory hallucinations, tachycardia, psychosis, fear, tremors, delirium, hyperglycemia, fever, sweating, flushing, euphoria, hypertonia, nausea, vomiting, coma, seizures, tachypnea, and respiratory arrest.

Phencyclidine (PCP): Although PCP is illegal, it is easily manufactured and deserves special mention because of its widespread availability. PCP was originally developed as an anesthetic in the 1950s and later abandoned because of a high frequency of postoperative delirium with hallucinations. It was classed as a dissociative anesthetic because, in the anesthetized state, the patient remains conscious with staring gaze, flat facies, and rigid muscles. It was discovered as a drug of abuse in the 1970s, first in oral form as tablets or capsules, and then in a smoked version, enabling better control over the dose. The white crystal-like powder can also be snorted or injected. Street names include Angel Dust, Elephant Tranquilizers, Hog, Killer Weed, PCP, Peace Pills, and Rocket Fuel. Its pharmacological effects are different from LSD; small amounts act as a stimulant, speeding up body functions. Speech, muscle coordination, and vision are affected; sense of touch and pain are dulled; and body movements are slowed. Effects include increased heart rate and blood pressure, flushing, sweating, dizziness, and numbness. With large doses, effects include drowsiness, convulsions, coma, and may also cause death from repeated convulsions, heart and lung failure, or ruptured blood vessels in the brain.

INHALANTS

Anesthetic gases such as nitrous oxide or halothane are sometimes used as intoxicants by medical personnel. Nitrous oxide also is abused by food service employees because it is supplied for use as a propellant in disposable aluminum minitanks for whipping cream canisters. Nitrous oxide produces euphoria and analgesia and then loss of consciousness. Compulsive use and chronic toxicity rarely are reported, but there are obvious risks of overdose associated with the abuse of this anesthetic. Chronic use has been reported to cause peripheral neuropathy.

OTHER AGENTS

Sodium Oxybate (Xyrem®): This drug is marketed for treatment of cataplexy in patients with narcolepsy and is in the pharmacologic category of CNS depressants. Known on the street as GHB, its illegal use has been associated with "date-rape" activity. Street names include Liquid Ecstasy, Liquid X, Liquid E, Georgia Home Boy, Grievous Bodily Harm, G-Riffick, Soap, Scoop, Salty Water, Somatomax, and Organic Quaalude. There are no specific oral signs and symptoms, however, the dentist should be aware of patients showing signs of CNS depression, as with all other drugs in this class.

Flunitrazepam (Rohypnol®): This drug is a benzodiazepine with sedative and hypnotic properties. It is not currently marketed in the U.S. but is used as a sedative in Europe. Known on the street as Roofies, La Rocha, Ruffies, Coma Capsules, Roche, Rope, R-2, Roofenol, Roachies, and Rib, the white tablets can be taken orally, smoked, or snorted. Florida reported the first case of abuse and subsequent cases have been found primarily in Western and Southern states, although abuse in the U.S. and Europe is growing due to its euphoric-effect and low street price ($1-$3/tablet). It is often abused in combination with heroin, marijuana, ethanol, cocaine, or methamphetamine which has proven to be fatal in many cases. In one study, 14 of 40 descendants who died from heroin overdose were found to be positive for flunitrazepam.

The dental team should be alert to the signs and symptoms of drug abuse and withdrawal. Further reading is recommended.

ANIMAL AND HUMAN BITES GUIDELINES

The dentist is often confronted with early management of animal and human bites. The following protocols may assist in appropriate care and referral.

WOUND MANAGEMENT

Irrigation: Critically important; irrigate all penetration wounds using 20 mL syringe, 19-gauge needle and >250 mL 1% povidone-iodine solution. This method will reduce wound infection by a factor of 20. When there is high risk of rabies, use viricidal 1% benzalkonium chloride in addition to the 1% povidone-iodine. Irrigate wound with normal saline after antiseptic irrigation.

Debridement: Remove all crushed or devitalized tissue remaining after irrigation; minimize removal on face and over thin skin areas or anywhere you would create a worse situation than the bite itself already has; do not extend puncture wounds surgically – rather, manage them with irrigation and antibiotics.

Suturing: Close most dog bites if <8 hours (<12 hours on face); do not routinely close puncture wounds, or deep or severe bites on the hands or feet, as these are at highest risk for infection. Cat and human bites should not be sutured unless cosmetically important. Wound edge freshening, where feasible, reduces infection; minimize sutures in the wound and use monofilament on the surface.

Immobilization: Critical in all hand wounds; important for infected extremities.

Hospitalization/I.V. Antibiotics: Admit for I.V. antibiotics all significant human bites to the hand, especially closed fist injuries, and bites involving penetration of the bone or joint (a high index of suspicion is needed). Consider I.V. antibiotics for significant established wound infections with cellulitis or lymphangitis, any infected bite on the hand, any infected cat bite, and any infection in an immunocompromised or asplenic patient. Outpatient treatment with I.V. antibiotics may be possible in selected cases by consulting with infectious disease.

LABORATORY ASSESSMENT

Gram's Stain: Not useful prior to onset of clinically apparent infection; examination of purulent material may show a predominant organism in established infection, aiding antibiotic selection; not warranted unless results will change your treatment.

Culture: Not useful or cost-effective prior to onset of clinically apparent infection.

X-ray: Whenever you suspect bony involvement, especially in craniofacial dog bites in very small children or severe bite/crush in an extremity; cat bites with their long needle-like teeth may cause osteomyelitis or a septic joint, especially in the hand or wrist.

IMMUNIZATIONS

Tetanus: All bite wounds are contaminated. If not immunized in last 5 years, or if not current in a child, give DPT, DT, Td, or TT as indicated. For absent or incomplete primary immunization, give 250 units tetanus immune globulin (TIG) in addition.

Rabies: In the U.S. 30,000 persons are treated each year in an attempt to prevent 1-5 cases. Domestic animals should be quarantined for 10 days to prove need for prophylaxis. High-risk animal bites (85% of cases = bat, skunk, raccoon) usually receive treatment consisting of:

- human rabies immune globulin (HRIG): 20 units/kg I.M. (unless previously immunized with HDCV)
- human diploid cell vaccine (HDCV): 1 mL I.M. on days 0, 3, 7, 14, and 28 (unless previously immunized with HDCV - then give only first 2 doses)

Rabies Immune Globulin, Human *on page 1165*

Rabies Virus Vaccine *on page 1165*

Tetanus Immune Globulin (Human) *on page 1277*

BITE WOUNDS AND PROPHYLACTIC ANTIBIOTICS

Parenteral vs Oral: If warranted, consider an initial I.V. dose to rapidly establish effective serum levels, especially if high risk, delayed treatment, or if patient reliability is poor.

Dog Bite:

1. Rarely get infected (~5%)
2. Infecting organisms: Staph coag negative, staph coag positive, alpha strep, diphtheroids, beta strep, *Pseudomonas aeruginosa*, gamma strep, *Pasteurella multocida*
3. Prophylactic antibiotics are seldom indicated. Consider for high risk wounds such as distal extremity puncture wounds, severe crush injury, bites occurring in cosmetically sensitive areas (eg, face), or in immunocompromised or asplenic patients.

Cat Bite:

1. Often get infected (~25% to 50%)
2. Infecting organisms: *Pasteurella multocida* (first 24 hours), coag positive staph, anaerobic cocci (after first 24 hours)
3. Prophylactic antibiotics are indicated in all cases.

Human Bite:

1. Intermediate infection rate (~15% to 20%)
2. Infecting organisms: Coag positive staph α, β, γ strep, *Haemophilus*, *Eikenella corrodens*, anaerobic streptococci, *Fusobacterium*, *Veillonella*, bacteroides.
3. Prophylactic antibiotics are indicated in almost all cases except superficial injuries.

Amoxicillin *on page 114*
Amoxicillin and Clavulanate Potassium *on page 116*
Cefazolin *on page 278*
Cefotetan *on page 283*
Ceftriaxone *on page 288*
Clindamycin *on page 348*
Doxycycline *on page 471*
Imipenem and Cilastatin *on page 736*
Sulfamethoxazole and Trimethoprim *on page 1246*

BITE WOUND ANTIBIOTIC REGIMENS

	Dog Bite	Cat Bite	Human Bite
Prophylactic Antibiotics			
Prophylaxis	No routine prophylaxis, consider if involves face or hand, or immunosuppressed or asplenic patients	Routine prophylaxis	Routine prophylaxis
Prophylactic antibiotic	Amoxicillin	Amoxicillin	Amoxicillin
Penicillin allergy	Doxycycline if >10 y or co-trimoxazole	Doxycycline if >10 y or co-trimoxazole	Doxycycline if >10 y or erythromycin and cephalexin[1]
Outpatient Oral Antibiotic Treatment (mild to moderate infection)			
Established infection	Amoxicillin and clavulanic acid	Amoxicillin and clavulanic acid	Amoxicillin and clavulanic acid
Penicillin allergy (mild infection only)	Doxycycline if >10 y	Doxycycline if >10 y	Cephalexin[1] or clindamycin
Outpatient Parenteral Antibiotic Treatment (moderate infections – single-drug regimens)			
	Ceftriaxone	Ceftriaxone	Cefotetan
Inpatient Parenteral Antibiotic Treatment			
Established infection	Ampicillin + cefazolin	Ampicillin + cefazolin	Ampicillin + clindamycin
Penicillin allergy	Cefazolin[1]	Ceftriaxone[1]	Cefotetan[1] or imipenem
Duration of Prophylactic and Treatment Regimens			
Prophylaxis: 5 days			
Treatment: 10-14 days			

[1]Contraindicated if history of immediate hypersensitivity reaction (anaphylaxis) to penicillin.

DENTAL OFFICE EMERGENCIES

All dentists would like to avoid the problems associated with managing dental office medical emergencies. As practitioners, we cannot be certain that these situations will not occur. It is hoped that with preparation, most if not all dental office emergencies can be avoided.

The American Dental Association's publication on dental therapeutics describes the incidence of medical emergencies in the dental office. Most of the problems that the dentist encounters are not life-threatening, but any emergency can become serious if not properly managed. If the dentist and dental office personnel can identify the signs and symptoms of a developing potential office emergency, many emergencies can be aborted and treated within the dental office.

Occasionally, life-threatening office emergencies occur and it is incumbent upon the dentist to be well prepared, to not only evaluate, but to act to stabilize, activate EMS, and manage/refer these patients to an appropriate medical facility for more definitive emergency care.

THIS CHAPTER PRESENTS ONLY THE MOST BASIC GUIDELINES FOR ANY OFFICE EMERGENCY. SPECIFIC PROTOCOLS CAN BE FOUND IN OUR COMPANION MANUAL: *Dental Office Medical Emergencies, A Manual of Office Response Protocols,* 1st ed (revised), Hudson, OH: Lexi-Comp, Inc, 2000.

In addition, a recent statement update from the American Dental Association on Scientific Affairs has been published in the March 2002 Journal of the American Dental Association (Vol 133, pp. 364-5). Briefly, it states: Though rare, life-threatening medical emergencies occasionally occur in the dental office. Recently, the American Dental Association on Scientific Affairs published a preparedness statement to update its pre-existing statements on the subject.

Preparedness to recognize and appropriately manage medical emergencies in the dental environment includes the following:

Current basic life support certification for all office staff
Didactic and clinical courses in emergency medicine
Periodic office emergency drills
Telephone numbers of EMS or other appropriately trained health care providers
Emergency drug kit and equipment and knowledge to properly use all items

HISTORY AND PHYSICAL EXAMINATION

The best tool to reduce the risk of a medical emergency occurring in the dental office is the patient's history and record. The dentist should collect adequate information to establish a complete baseline history on all new patients and an adequate updated history on all recall or patients returning to the office.

History and physical examination on all new patients should include:

Baseline history
Medications
Past/current medical conditions
Allergies
Need for and results of medical consultation
Baseline vital signs – pulse, blood pressure, respirations, temperature

Having this information available in the patient record in a format that is easily accessible by trained dental office personnel, allows quick reference of baseline values should a medical emergency occur during the delivery of dental care.

In today's dental practice, some clinicians believe that patient care has become more complicated due to increased use of over-the-counter and prescription medications, as well as the increased complexity of medical diagnoses and management. Other clinicians believe that technological and medical care advances have actually simplified patient care. For the most part, patients seeking elective dental care are adequately managed medically. Patients often appear to have complications based on history, but may be quite stable. New patients and patients with dental emergencies require special attention on the part of the practitioner. It is incumbent upon the dentist to be able to adequately evaluate complete histories and the current medical status of patients, so patients can be assessed for any potential risk while undergoing dental procedures. Each dental office should design a history format that works best for them.

Obtaining the history is usually the first and often the most important interaction with any new patient and with any patient of record that is being re-evaluated after a period of time. Many techniques can be used when addressing sensitive or complicated medical information. Most commonly, the medical history addresses major medical problems in the form of a questionnaire; it follows a review-of-systems format in addressing other symptomatology, which might be present, but remains undiagnosed to-date. This style is often supplemented with a narrative description by the interviewer. Regardless of the technique used, all dental office personnel should be familiar with how to access the information and should have adequate medical knowledge to alert the dentist to any known pre-existing conditions.

A review of current medications must also be included. The review must include home remedies, nonprescription drugs, vitamins or dietary supplements, and medications not prescribed to the patient (but available from friends or relatives) that may have been used by the patient. Doses and frequency of use are important. Drugs that have known associations with some medical emergencies are described with each protocol.

Certain drug classes are associated with potential dental office medical emergencies. Syncope can be caused by alpha$_1$-adrenergic receptor blockers (used to treat hypertension), nitroglycerin, some tricyclic antidepressants, and those antipsychotics which inhibit dopamine type 2 receptors and block alpha$_1$-adrenergic receptors (ie, clozapine). Orthostatic or postural hypotension can also be caused by medication in these drug classes. In addition, this condition has occurred in patients taking angiotensin-converting enzyme (ACE) inhibitors, calcium channel blockers, or beta-adrenergic receptor blockers for hypertension. Hypoglycemia is associated with the oral antidiabetic drugs. These associations are not always obvious, but the dentist should be attentive to the increased risk when patients are taking drugs in these therapeutic categories.

Allergies must be covered in some detail so the dentist is made aware of any known pre-existing allergies, either to environmental agents or medications. Medical reactions or toxicities in the dental office can result in serious life-threatening symptoms. Recognizing any predisposing history may allow the dentist to avoid these interactions or recognize them should they occur. Previous substance abuse might predispose the patient to drug reactions, and untoward medical response, during the delivery of dental care.

If the past history and general state of health, as well as the current physical evaluation, determines that a patient requires medical consultation, this should be noted in the patient's record. The reason for the consultation and the outcome should be clearly indicated in the record so the dentist is aware of the result of such consultation at each subsequent visit. This readiness may reduce risk.

As part of the normal physical examination that the dentist provides for each new patient and each recall patient, vital signs should be recorded. In most instances, these procedures are limited to measurements of pulse and blood pressure; however, in instances where any predisposing conditions might warrant or suggest more detailed evaluation, baseline respiratory rate and temperature might also be recorded. These data should be available and readily accessible in each patient's record so that, should an office emergency occur, the dental office personnel can compare the status during the emergency with the baseline data.

Elaborate schemes are available in oral medicine texts that assign risk by a variety of classifications. One method is to use the American Society of Anesthesiologists classification scheme to evaluate whether a patient's pre-existing medical condition places them at high risk during the delivery of anesthesia. Another mechanism is to assign the risk of dental procedures based on an analysis of pre-existing medical conditions matched with the complexity of the planned dental procedure. This protocol takes into account the potential invasiveness of the dental procedure. Simple procedures in complicated patients may have low total risk, whereas complex procedures in simple patients may place the patient at significant risk for an office emergency. Each dental practitioner should design or adapt a patient analysis plan for their own office.

EQUIPMENT

The dental office should be adequately equipped to not only deliver routine care to each new patient and each returning patient, but also should be set up for appropriate management and stabilization of any potential office emergency. This requires that each patient and treatment area should be equipped with a minimum of a blood pressure cuff and a stethoscope. The office should also have available:

- Appropriately-sized blood pressure cuffs
- Tourniquets
- Stethoscopes
- First-aid kits
- Emergency number call list
- Emergency cabinet
- Oxygen tank (size E portable with low flow regulator)
- Nasal cannula
- Masks (non-rebreather and a bag-valve mask [Ambu®])
- Syringes (intramuscular: I.M. 3 cc disposable, subcutaneous: S.C. tuberculin)

The emergency call list should be properly posted so office personnel need not search other operatories or the reception area for such information. Centrally located emergency cabinets, which include tourniquets, emergency medical care drugs, instruments, and supplies, are essential.

DENTAL OFFICE EMERGENCY DRUGS

Protocols should be established for most office emergencies. Recognition and rapid diagnosis lead to appropriate management. Major drugs usually available in the emergency drug cabinet are listed below.

Albuterol *on page 71*
Ammonia Spirit, Aromatic *on page 111*
Dexamethasone *on page 411*
(Alternative is Solu-Cortef® Mix-O-Vials for I.M.; has a longer shelf life)

DENTAL OFFICE EMERGENCIES *(Continued)*

Diazepam *on page 423*

Diphenhydramine *on page 448*

Epinephrine *on page 496*

(AnaKit® includes preloaded Tubex® syringes, which have measured dosing in increments)

Flumazenil *on page 599*

Glucose (Instant) *on page 663*

(Emergency kit should also have oral carbohydrate source, such as Glutose 15™ oral gel and injectable glucagon)

Hydrocortisone *on page 714*

Morphine Sulfate *on page 947*

Naloxone *on page 961*

Nitroglycerin *on page 991*

Oxygen *on page 1033*

Drug cabinet supplies should be in dose forms which the dentist is comfortable administering. Typical routes of administration could include oral (eg, diphenhydramine), inhalation (eg, albuterol), intramuscular/I.M. (eg, hydrocortisone), subcutaneous/S.C. (eg, epinephrine), or intravenous/I.V. (eg, epinephrine). Sublingual/S.L. injection can be substituted for some I.V. administrations in situations (ie, anaphylaxis) where a drug such as epinephrine may be life-saving. Oral mucosal absorption (eg, nitroglycerin) is also useful.

STAFF TRAINING

Office personnel, including the dentist, dental hygienists, and dental assistants, should all be trained in measurement of vital signs. Primarily, this includes measurement of pulse and evaluation of blood pressure. Proper technique for evaluating vital signs is necessary so information is accurate, and in the event of an emergency situation, ongoing measurements could be made by assisting personnel. The dentist should be able to provide this training to new employees, however, continuing education courses in proper techniques are available.

Dental office personnel should all be trained in basic life support first-aid, although the dentist is ultimately in charge of delivering care to either patient or personnel. Each office member should be aware of basic principles for management of nonlife-threatening injuries. All office personnel should be trained in cardiopulmonary resuscitation (CPR) or basic life support (BLS). Training courses are readily available through the American Heart Association and/or hospital facilities in most areas. Training should include not only basic initial training, but also renewal of skills should be a requirement for continued employment. One to two years is a reasonable time for updating such skills in cardiopulmonary resuscitation. Applicable state requirements or recommendations should be reviewed.

GENERAL PRINCIPLES OF RECOGNITION

As a practicing dentist, you should be familiar with:

- Altered states or loss of consciousness
- Cardiovascular emergencies (often associated with chest pain), including heart attack and stroke
- Respiratory emergencies, including asthmatic bronchospasm and obstruction
- Allergic reactions, including signs of anaphylaxis
- Other potential emergencies:
  - Diabetes, including acute hypo- and hyperglycemic states/reactions
  - Acute neurologic disturbances, including convulsive disorders such as epilepsy, stress-induced panic attacks, and acute headaches
  - Abdominal distress, including the abdominal disorders and diseases classified as acute (sudden onset) abdominal distress
  - Communicable diseases, including the major bacteria- and virus-induced illnesses of our society

Although symptoms can be very specific, detecting medical emergencies usually means recognizing some general changes in the state of the patient:

- Acute changes in affect or consciousness
- Sudden onset of pain, anywhere in the body
- Feelings of fever and chills
- Tight feeling in the chest
- Difficulty in expiration or inspiration
- Choking
- Dizziness or feelings of faintness
- Numbness or tingling sensations

The dental practitioner must be familiar with several basic diagnostic signs that should be compared to baseline measurements in the patient's record:

- Pulse rate and character – remember that a pulse rate >120 or <50 beats per minute can indicate a true emergency for the adult patient
- Blood pressure – a systolic pressure <70 may indicate shock and pressures >200/100 may present a hypertensive crisis (pre-CVA)
- Breathing rate and character – a true emergency may exist when the adult patient's respirations are >30 per minute
- Skin temperature, condition, and color
- Diaphoresis – often associated with anxiety, but can indicate ischemia
- Pupil size, equality, and response
- Color of the lips, tongue, earlobes, and nailbeds
- Breath odors
- Muscular activity – spasms and paralysis or weakness such as seen in ischemic attacks or CVA
- Bleeding or discharges from the body

ALL PRACTITIONERS MUST BE PREPARED TO CARRY OUT A BASIC PLAN FOR STABILIZATION

These steps are the basic action plan for stabilization in every office emergency. They should be activated within the first seconds following recognition of any developing problem. Sometimes, based on the initial recognition signs, activation of the emergency medical system (EMS) will occur immediately, usually by calling 911 (if available in your area). If the dentist is unsure of the underlying reason for the medical emergency or does not feel adequately trained, then basic life support (BLS) procedures should be the extent of the treatment until the emergency medical team arrives.

BASIC ACTION PLAN FOR STABILIZATION

PATIENT PLACEMENT	→ **UPRIGHT / SEMI-RECLINING?**
	→ **SUPINE?**
	→ **TRENDELENBURG (FEET UP, HEAD DOWN)[1]?**
AIRWAY AND BREATHING	→ **IS THE AIRWAY OPEN?**
	→ **CLEAR OF OBSTRUCTIONS?**
	→ **IS THE PATIENT BREATHING ON THEIR OWN?**
	→ **DOES THE SITUATION REQUIRE OXYGEN TO INCREASE PERFUSION?**
	→ **ACTIVATE CPR IF NECESSARY**
CIRCULATION	→ **MONITOR PULSE**
	→ **PROCEED WITH CPR, IF APPROPRIATE**

DENTAL OFFICE EMERGENCIES (Continued)

ADDITIONAL MANAGEMENT[2]

→ **ALWAYS CONSIDER ACTIVATING EMS IMMEDIATELY**

→ **CONTINUALLY OBSERVE, MONITOR VITAL SIGNS, AND EVALUATE FOR ANY SIGNS OF RECOVERY OR DETERIORATION**

→ **ASSIGN SOMEONE IN THE OFFICE TO QUICKLY RE-EVALUATE PATIENT'S HISTORY AND RECORD FOR CLUES TO THE CAUSE OF THE INCIDENT OR DRUGS THE PATIENT MAY BE TAKING**

→ **DETERMINE, IF POSSIBLE, THE TENTATIVE MEDICAL CONDITION CAUSING THE SYMPTOMS**

→ **DELIVER SPECIFIC CARE IF APPROPRIATE**

→ **BE PREPARED TO ACTIVATE EMS CALL FOR ASSISTANCE IF PATIENT'S CONDITION DETERIORATES**

→ **ALWAYS CONSIDER THE NEED FOR FOLLOW-UP MEDICAL EVALUATION AS PATIENT RECOVERS**

[1]Trendelenburg's position is a supine position which is inclined at an angle so that the pelvis and legs are slightly higher than the head.

[2]Although these management suggestions are essentially the same for each of the protocols, the order and specific care will vary.

SUGGESTED READINGS

ANTIBIOTICS IN TREATMENT OF ODONTOGENIC INFECTIONS

Doern GV, Ferraro MJ, Breuggemann AB, et al, "Emergence of High Rates of Antimicrobial Resistance Among Viridans Group Streptococci in the United States," *Antimicrob Agents Chemother,* 1996, 40(4):891-84.

Flynn TR, "The Swollen Face. Severe Odontogenic Infections," *Emerg Med Clin North Am,* 2000, 18(3):481-519.

Hardee WM, "Tried-and-True Medication," *Practical Endodontics,* 1997, 7(5):38.

Johnson BS, "Principles and Practice of Antibiotic Therapy," *Infect Dis Clin North Am,* 1999, 13(4):851-70.

Kuriyama T, Nakagawa K, Karasawa T, et al, "Past Administration of Beta-lactam Antibiotics and Increase in the Emergence of Beta-lactamase-producing Bacteria in Patients With Orofacial Odontogenic Infections," *Oral Surg Oral Med Oral Path Oral Radiol Endod,* 2000, 89(2):186-92.

Lee CY, "Management of Odontogenic Infections With Microbial, Anatomic and Antibiotic Considerations," *Hawaii Dent J,* 1993, 24(8):8-11.

Mandell GM, Bennett JE, Douglas GR, et al, eds, *Mandell, Douglas, and Bennett's Principles and Practice of Infectious Disease,* 5th ed, Philadelphia, PA: Churchill Livingstone, Inc, 2000, 2567-8.

Montgomery EH, "Antimicrobial Agents in the Prevention and Treatment of Infection," *Pharmacology and Therapeutics for Dentistry,* 4th ed, Yagiela JA, Neidle EA, Dowd FJ, eds, St. Louis, MO: Mosby-Year Book, Inc, 1998, 637.

Palacios E and Valvassori G, "Deep Facial Infection of Odontogenic Origin," *Ear Nose Throat J,* 2001, 80(1):15.

Storoe W, Haug RH, and Lillich TT, "The Changing Face of Odontogenic Infections," *J Oral Maxillofac Surg,* 2001, 59(7):739-48

Wynn RL and Bergman SA, "Antibiotics and Their Use in the Treatment of Orofacial Infections, Part I," *Gen Dent,* 1994, 42(5):398, 400-2.

Wynn RL and Bergman SA, "Antibiotics and Their Use in the Treatment of Orofacial Infections, Part II," *Gen Dent,* 1994, 42(6):498-502.

Wynn RL and Bergman SA, Meiller TF, et al, "Antibiotics in Treating Oral-Facial Infections of Odontogenic Origin," *Gen Dent,* 2001, 47(3):238-52.

CANCER

Al-Balawi SA and Nwoku AL, "Management of Oral Cancer in a Tertiary Care Hospital," *Saudi Med J,* 2002, 23(2):156-9.

Carl W, "Oral Complications of Local and Systemic Cancer Treatment," *Curr Opin Oncol,* 1995, 7(4):320-4.

Chambers MS, Toth BB, Martin JW, et al, "Oral and Dental Management of the Cancer Patient: Prevention and Treatment of Complications," *Support Care Cancer,* 1995, 3(3):168-75.

Dutton JM, Graham SM, and Hoffman HT, "Metastatic Cancer to the Floor of Mouth: The Lingual Lymph Nodes, "*Head Neck,* 2002 24(4):401-5.

Flaitz CM, "Persistent White Lesion of the Lateral Tongue," *Am J Dent,* 2001, 14(6):402-3.

Gellrich NC, Schramm A, Bockmann R, et al, "Follow-Up in Patients With Oral Cancer," *J Oral Maxillofac Surg,* 2002, 60(4):380-6.

Hobson RS and Clark JD, "Management of the Orthodontic Patient at Risk From Infective Endocarditis," *Br Dent J,* 1995, 179(2):48.

Jullien JA, Downer MC, Zakrzewska JM, et al, "Evaluation of a Screening Test for the Early Detection of Oral Cancer and Precancer," *Community Dent Health,* 1995, 12(1):3-7.

Messer NC, Yant WR, and Archer RD, "Developing Provider Partnerships in the Detection of Oral Cancer and the Prevention of Smokeless Tobacco Use," *Md Med J,* 1995, 44(10):788-91.

Takinami S, Yahata H, Kanoshima A, et al, "Hepatocellular Carcinoma Metastatic to the Mandible," *Oral Surg Oral Med Oral Pathol Oral Radiol Endod,* 1995, 79(5):649-54.

Vigneswaran N, Tilashalski K, Rodu B, et al, "Tobacco Use and Cancer. A Reappraisal," *Oral Surg Oral Med Oral Pathol Oral Radiol Endod,* 1995, 80(2):178-82.

Weaver RG, Whittaker L, Valachovic RW, et al, "Tobacco Control and Prevention Effort in Dental Education," *J Dent Educ,* 2002, 66(3):426-9.

CARDIOVASCULAR

"Adjusted-Dose Warfarin Versus Low-Intensity, Fixed-Dose Warfarin Plus Aspirin for High-Risk Patients With Atrial Fibrillation: Stroke Prevention in Atrial Fibrillation III Randomized Clinical Trial," *Lancet,* 1996, 348(9028):633-8.

American Heart Association, "Heart and Stroke Facts: 1996 Statistical Supplement," Dallas, Texas: National Center of the American Heart Association, 1996, 15.

Ayala C, Croft JB, Greenlund KJ, et al, "Sex Differences in US Mortality Rates for Stroke and Stroke Subtypes by Race/Ethnicity and Age, 1995-1998," *Stroke,* 2002, 33(5):1197-201.

Frazier OH, "Mechanical Circulatory Support: New Advances, New Pumps, New Ideas," *Semin Thorac Cardiovasc Surg,* 2002, 14(2):178-86.

Garcia R, "Floss or Die: The Link Between Oral Health and Cardiac Disease," *Harv Dent Bull,* 1998, 7(2):16-7.

Gilligan DM, Ellenbogen KA, and Epstein AE, "The Management of Atrial Fibrillation," *Am J Med,* 1996, 101:413-21.

Giuliani ER, Gersh BJ, McGoon MD, et al, *Mayo Clinic Practice of Cardiology,* 3rd ed, St Louis, MO: Mosby-Year Book, Inc, 1996, 1698-814.

SUGGESTED READINGS *(Continued)*

Glick M, "Screening for Traditional Risk Factors for Cardiovascular Disease: A Review for Oral Health Care Providers," *J Am Dent Assoc*, 2002, 133(3):291-300.

Hansson L, Zanchetti A, Carruthers SG, et al, "Effects of Intensive Blood Pressure Lowering and Low-Dose Aspirin in Patients With Hypertension: Principal Results of the Hypertension Optimal Treatment (HOT) Randomized Trial. HOT Study Group," *Lancet*, 1998, 351:1755-62.

Heidenreich PA, Lee TT, and Massie BM, "Effect of Beta-Blockade on Mortality in Patients With Heart Failure: A Meta-analysis of Randomized Clinical Trials," *J Am Coll Cardiol*, 1997, 30(1):27-34.

Hylek EM, Skates SJ, Sheehan MA, et al, "An Analysis of the Lowest Effective Intensity of Prophylactic Coagulation for Patients With Nonrheumatic Atrial Fibrillation," *N Engl J Med*, 1996, 335:540-6.

Kannel WB, "Blood Pressure as a Cardiovascular Risk Factor. Prevention and Treatment," *JAMA*, 1996, 275:1571-6.

Kaplan NM, "Hypertension and Diabetes," *J Hum Hypertens*, 2002, 16(Suppl 1):S56-60.

Kaplan NM, "Perspectives on the New JNC VI Guidelines for the Treatment of Hypertension," *Formulary*, 1997, 32:1224-31.

Kerpen SJ, Kerpen HO, and Sachs SA, "Mitral Valve Prolapse: A Significant Cardiac Defect in the Development of Infective Endocarditis," *Spec Care Dentist*, 1984, 4(4):158-9.

Lopaschuk GD, "Metabolic Abnormalities in the Diabetic Heart," *Heart Fail Rev*, 2002, 7(2):149-59.

Morley J, Marinchak R, Rials SJ, et al, "Atrial Fibrillation, Anticoagulation, and Stroke," *Am J Cardiol*, 1996, 77:38A-44A.

Reyes AJ, "Diuretics in the Treatment of Patients who Present Congestive Heart Failure and Hypertension," *J Hum Hypertens*, 2002, 16(Suppl 1):S104-13.

"The Sixth Report of the Joint National Committee on Prevention, Detection, Evaluation, and Treatment of High Blood Pressure (JNC VI)," *Arch Intern Med*, 1997, 157:2413-46.

CHEMICAL DEPENDENCY AND SMOKING CESSATION

Abelin T, Buehler A, Muller P, et al, "Controlled Trial of Transdermal Nicotine Patch in Tobacco Withdrawal," *Lancet*, 1989, 1(8628):7-10.

Alterman AI, Droba M, Antelo RE, et al, "Amantadine May Facilitate Detoxification of Cocaine Addicts," *Drug Alcohol Depend*, 1992, 31(1):19-29.

Ciancio SG, ed, *ADA Guide to Dental Therapeutics*, 1st ed, Chicago, IL: ADA Publishing Co, 1998.

Fiester S, Goldstein M, Resnick M, et al, "Practice Guideline for the Treatment of Patients With Nicotine Dependence," *Am J Psych*, 1996, 15(Suppl 10):31.

Gelskey SC, "Tobacco-Use Cessation Programs and Policies at the University of Manitoba's Faculty of Dentistry," *J Can Dent Assoc*, 2001, 67(3):145-8.

Herkenham MA, "Localization of Cannabinoid Receptors in Brain: Relationship to Motor and Reward Systems," *Biological Basis of Substance Abuse*, Korenman SG and Barchas JD, eds, New York, NY: Oxford University Press, 1993, 187-200.

Kausch O and McCormick RA, "Suicide Prevalence in Chemical Dependency Programs: Preliminary Data from a National Sample, and an Examination of Risk Factors," *J Subst Abuse Treat*, 2002, 22(2):97-102.

Kreek MJ, "Rationale for Maintenance Pharmacotherapy of Opiate Dependence," O'Brien CP and Barchas JD, eds, *Addictive States*, New York, NY: Raven Press, 1992, 205-30.

Leshner AI, "Molecular Mechanisms of Cocaine Addiction," *N Engl J Med*, 1996, 335(2):128-9.

Mendelson JH and Mello NK, "Management of Cocaine Abuse and Dependence," *N Engl J Med*, 1996, 334(15):965-72.

O'Brien CP, "Drug Addiction and Drug Abuse," *The Pharmacological Basis of Therapeutics*, 9th ed, Molinoff PB and Ruddon R, eds, New York, NY: McGraw-Hill, 1996, 557-77.

O'Brien CP, "Treatment of Alcoholism as a Chronic Disorder," *Toward a Molecular Basis of Alcohol Use and Abuse*, Jansson B, Jornvall H, Rydberg U, et al, eds, Basel, Switzerland: Birkhauser Verlag, 1994, Vol 71, EXS, 349-59.

Ostroff JS, Hay JL, Primavera LH, et al, "Motivating Smoking Cessation Among Dental Patients: Smokers' Interest in Biomarker Testing for Susceptibility to Tobacco-Related Cancers," *Nicotine Tob Res*, 1999, 1(4):347-55.

Ostrowski DJ and DeNelsky GY, "Pharmacologic Management of Patients Using Smoking Cessation Aids," *Dental Clin North Am*, 1996, 40(3):779-801.

Schydlower M, "Adolescent Substance Use and Abuse: Current Issues," *Tex Med*, 2002, 98(2):31-5.

Self DW, Barnhart WJ, Lehman DA, et al, "Opposite Modulation of Cocaine-Seeking Behavior by D1- and D2-Like Dopamine Receptor Agonists," *Science*, 1996, 271(5255):1586-9.

The Smoking Cessation Clinical Practice Guideline Panel and Staff, The Agency for Health Care Policy and Research Smoking Cessation Clinical Practice Guideline, *JAMA*, 1996, 275(1):1270-80.

Tomar SL, "Dentistry's Role in Tobacco Control," *J Am Dent Assoc*, 200, 132 (Suppl):S30-35.

Weisner C, Mertens J, Tam T, et al, "Factors Affecting the Initiation of Substance Abuse Treatment in Managed Care," *Addiction*, 2001, 96(5):705-16.

DENTIST'S ROLE IN RECOGNIZING DOMESTIC ABUSE

World Wide Web Sites

American Academy of Pediatrics – http://www.aap.org

American College of Emergency Physicians – http://www.acep.org
American Dental Association – http://www.ada.org
National Clearinghouse on Child Abuse and Neglect Information – http://www.calib.com/nccanch
National Data Archive on Child Abuse and Neglect – http://www.ndacan.cornell.edu
Prevent Child Abuse America (formerly National Committee to Prevent Child Abuse) – http://www.childabuse.org
University of Medicine and Dentistry - New Jersey – http://www.umdnj.edu/~baum/famvio.htm
USDHHS Agency of Children and Families – http://www.acf.dhhs.gov

Toll-Free Hotlines

Bureau of Indian Affairs Federal Hotline – 800-633-5155
Child Abuse Hotlines (24-Hour) – 800-4-ACHILD
Covenant House Nineline – 800-999-9999
National Family Violence Helpline – 800-222-2000

Books and Journal Articles (available at a local library or through interlibrary loan)

Besharov DJ, *Recognizing Child Abuse*, New York, NY, Free Press, 1990.
Chiodo GT, Tolle SW, and Tilden VP, "The Dentist and Family Violence," *Gen Dent*, 1998, 46(1):20-5.
Davidhizar R, Dowd S, and Giger JN, "Recognizing Abuse in Culturally Diverse Clients," *Health Care Superv*, 1998, 17(2):10-20.
Domestic Violence: A Directory of Protocols for Health Care Providers, Children's Safety Network, Newton, MA: Education Development Center, Inc, 1992.
Erickson MJ, Hill TD, and Siegel RM, "Barriers to Domestic Violence Screening in the Pediatric Setting," *Pediatrics*, 2001, 108(1):98-102.
"Health and Human Rights: A Call to Action on the 50th Anniversary of the Universal Declaration of Human Rights. The Writing Group for the Consortium for Health and Human Rights," *JAMA*, 1998, 280(5).
LaCerva V, *Pathways to Peace: Forty Steps to a Less Violent America*, Tesuque, NM: Heartsongs Publications, 1996.
McDowell JD, Kassebaum DK, and Stromboe SE, "Recognizing and Reporting Victims of Domestic Violence," *J Am Dent Assoc*, 1992, 123(9):44-50.
Mouden LD and Bross DC, "Legal Issues Affecting Dentistry's Role in Preventing Child Abuse and Neglect," *J Am Dent Assoc*, 1995, 126(8):1173-80.
"Protecting Children From Abuse and Neglect," Center for the Future of Children, The David and Lucille Packard Foundation, *The Future of Children*, 1998, 8(1):1-142. (Electronic version: http://www.futureofchildren.org)
Reece RM, *Child Abuse: Medical Diagnosis and Management*, Philadelphia, PA: Lea and Febiger, 1994.
Rupp RP, "Conditions to Be Considered in the Differential Diagnosis of Child Abuse and Neglect," *Gen Dent*, 1998, 46(1):96-9.
Salber PR and Talliaferro EH, *The Physicians' Guide to Domestic Violence: How to Ask the Right Questions and Recognize Abuse...Another Way to Save a Life*, Volcano, CA: Volcano Press, 1995.
Silva C, McFarlane J, Socken K, et al, "Symptoms of Post-Traumatic Stress Disorder in Abused Women in a Primary Care Setting," *J Women's Health*, 1997, 6:543-52.
Sweet D, "Recognizing and Intervening in Domestic Violence: Proactive Role for Dentistry," *Medscape Womens Health*, 1996, 1(6):3.
Watts C and Zimmerman C, "Violence Against Women: Global Scope and Magnitude," *Lancet*, 2002, 359(9313):1232-7.

DIAGNOSIS AND MANAGEMENT OF PAIN

Brown RS, Hinderstein B, Reynolds DC, et al, "Using Anesthetic Localization to Diagnose Oral and Dental Pain," *J Am Dent Assoc*, 1995, 126(5):633-4, 637-41.
Denson DD and Katz JA, "Nonsteroidal Anti-inflammatory Agents," *Practical Management of Pain*, 2nd ed, PP Raj, ed, St Louis, MO: Mosby Year Book, 1992.
Henry G, "Postoperative Pain Experience With Flurbiprofen and Acetaminophen With Codeine," *J Dent Res*, 1992, 71:952.
Jaffe JH and Martin WR, "Opioid Analgesic and Antagonists," *The Pharmacological Basis of Therapeutics*, 8th ed, Gilman AG, Rall TW, Nies AD, et al, eds, New York, NY: Maxwell Pergamon MacMillan Publishing, 1990.
Kalso E and Vainio A, "Morphine and Oxycodone Hydrochloride in the Management of Cancer Pain," *Clin Pharmacol Ther*, 1990, 47(5):639-46.
McQuay H, Carroll D, Jadad AR, et al, "Anticonvulsant Drugs for Management of Pain: A Systemic Review," *BMJ*, 1995, 311(7012):1047-52.
Robertson S, Goodell H, and Wolff HG, "The Teeth as a Source of Headache and Other Pain," *Arch Neurol Psychiatry*, 1947, 57:277.
Sandler NA, Ziccardi V, and Ochs M, "Differential Diagnosis of Jaw Pain in the Elderly," *J Am Dent Assoc* 1995, 126(9):1263-72.
Seng GF, Kraus K, Cartwright G, et al, "Confirmed Allergic Reactions to Amide Local Anesthetics," *Gen Dent*, 1996, 44(1):52-4.
Stoller EP, Gilbert GH, Pyle MA, et al, "Coping With Tooth Pain: A Qualitative Study of Lay Management Strategies and Professional Consultation," *Spec Care Dentist*, 2001, 21(6):208-15.
Wright EF and Schiffman EL, "Treatment Alternatives for Patients With Masticatory Myofascial Pain," *J Am Dent Assoc*, 1995, 126(7):1030-9.

HIV INFECTION AND AIDS

Alsakka H, "Dental Management of HIV/AIDS Patients," *Northwest Dent*, 2001, 80(3):33-4.

SUGGESTED READINGS *(Continued)*

Center for Disease Control (CDC), CfDC, "Update: AIDS Cases in Males Who Have Sex With Males," *MMWR Morb Mortal Wkly Rep*, 1995, 44(29):401-2.

Center for Disease Control (CDC), CfDC, "First 500,000 AIDS Cases," *MMWR Morb Mortal Wkly Rep*, 1995, 44(46):849-53.

Center for Disease Control (CDC), CfDC, "Update: HIV Exposures in HCWs," *MMWR Morb Mortal Wkly Rep*, 1995, 44(50):929.

Center for Disease Control (CDC), CfDCaP, "Recommended Infection-Control Practices for Dentistry," *MMWR Morb Mortal Wkly Rep*, 1993, 42(RR-8).

Glick M, *Clinicians Guide to Treatment of HIV-Infected Patients*, Academy of Oral Medicine, 1996.

Greenspan D, Greenspan JS, Schiodt M, et al, *AIDS and the Mouth*, Munksgaard, Copenhagen, 1990.

Greenspan JS and Greenspan D, "Oral Manifestations of HIV Infection," *The Proceedings of the Second International Workshop*, Chicago, IL: Quintessence Publishing Co, 1995.

Lyles AM, "What the Dentist Should Know About a Patient With HIV/AIDS," *J Calif Dent Assoc*, 2001, 29(2):158-69.

"Oral Health Care for Adults With HIV Infection," New York, NY: AIDS Institute, New York State Department of Health, 1993.

Ryder MI, "Periodontal Management of HIV-infected Patients."*Periodontol 2000*, 2000, 23:85-93.

Silverman S, *Color Atlas of Oral Manifestations of AIDS*, 2nd ed, St Louis, MO: Mosby, 1996.

Squassi A, Khaszki C, Blanco B, et al, "Relation Between Demographic and Epidemiological Characteristics and Permanency Under a Dental Health Care Program for HIV Infected Patients," *Acta Odontol Latinoam*, 1998, 11(1):3-13.

NATURAL PRODUCTS: HERBAL AND DIETARY SUPPLEMENTS

1995 Martindale - The Extra Pharmacopoeia, Vol 86, Roy Pharm Soc, GB, 1996.

Blumenthal M, Goldberg A, Gruenwald J, et al, *German Commission E Monographs: Therapeutic Monographs on Medicinal Plants for Human Use*, Austin, TX: American Botanical Council, 1997.

Cohan RP and Jacobsen PL, "Herbal Supplements: Considerations in Dental Practice," *J Calif Dent Assoc*, 2000, 28(8):600-10.

D'Arcy PF, "Adverse Reactions and Interactions With Herbal Medicines: Part 1. Adverse Reactions," *Adverse Drug Reaction Toxicol Rev*, 1991, 10(4):189-208.

D'Arcy PF, McEmay JC, and Welling PG, *Mechanisms of Drug Interactions*, New York, NY: Springer-Verlag, 1996.

DeSmet PA, "Health Risks of Herbal Remedies," *Drug Saf*, 1995, 13(2):81-93.

Ernst E and DeSmet PA, "Risks Associated With Complementary Therapies," *Meyler's Side Effects of Drugs*, 13th ed, Dukes MN ed, New York, NY: Elsevier Science, 1996.

Heber D, Yip I, Ashley JM, et al, "Cholesterol-lowering Effects of a Proprietary Chinese Red Yeast Rice Dietary Supplement," *Am J Clin Nutr*, 1999, 69:231-6.

Keller K, "Therapeutic Use of Herbal Drugs and Their Potential Toxicity, Problems and Results of the Revision of Herbal Medicines in the EEC," *Proceedings of the 3rd International Conference on Pharmacopoeias and Quality Control of Drugs*, Rome, November, 1992, published in Bologna, Fondazione Rhone-Poulenc Rorer per le Scienze Mediche, 1993.

McGuffin M, Hobbs C, Upton R, et al, *American Herbal Product Association's Botanical Safety Handbook: Guidelines for the Safe Use and Labeling for Herbs of Commerce*, Boca Raton, FL: CRC Press, 1997.

Mistry MG and Mays DA, "Precautions Against Global Use of Natural Products for Weight Loss: A Review of Active Ingredients and Issues Concerning Concomitant Disease States," *Therapeutic Perspectives*, 1996, 10(1):2.

Moynihan P, "The British Nutrition Foundation Oral Task Force Report - Issues Relevant to Dental Health Professionals," *Br Dent J*, 2000, 188(6):308-12.

ORAL INFECTIONS

Caufield PW and Griffen AL, "Dental Caries. An Infectious and Transmissible Disease," *Pediatr Clin North Am*, 2000, 47(5):1001-19.

Chow AW, "Infections of the Oral Cavity, Neck, and Head," *Principles and Practice of Infectious Diseases*, 4th ed, Mandell GL, Bennett JE, Dolin R, eds, New York, NY: Churchill Livingstone, 1995, 593-605.

Dajani A, Taubert K, Ferrieri P, et al, "Treatment of Acute Streptococcal Pharyngitis and Prevention of Rheumatic Fever: A Statement for Health Professionals," *Pediatrics*, 1995, 96(4):758-64.

Diz Dios P, Ocampo Hermida A, Miralles Alvarez C, et al, "Fluconazole-Resistant Oral Candidiasis in HIV-Infected Patients," *AIDS*, 1995, 9(7):809-10.

Dobson RL, "Antimicrobial Therapy for Cutaneous Infections," *J Am Acad Dermatol*, 1990, 22(5):871-3.

Goldberg MH and Topazian R, "Odontogenic Infections and Deep Facial Space Infections of Dental Origin," *Oral and Maxillofacial Infections*, 3rd ed, Philadelphia, PA: WB Saunders, 1994, 232-6.

Lewis MA, Parkhurst CL, Douglas CW, et al, "Prevalence of Penicillin Resistant Bacteria in Acute Suppurative Oral Infection," *J Antimicrob Chemother*, 1995, 35(6):785-91.

Muzyka BC and Glick M, "A Review of Oral Fungal Infections and Appropriate Therapy," *J Am Dent Assoc*, 1995, 126(1):63-72.

Shay K, "Infectious Complications of Dental and Periodontal Diseases in the Elderly Population," *Clin Infect Dis*, 2002, 34(9):1215-23.

Sykes LM and Sukha A, " Potential Risk of Serious Oral Infections in the Diabetic Patient: a Clinical Report," *J Prosthet Dent*, 2001, 86(6):569-73.

ORAL LEUKOPLAKIA

Barker JN, Mitra RS, Griffiths CE, et al, "Keratinocytes as Initiators of Inflammation," *Lancet*, 1991, 337(8735):211-4.

Boehncke WH, Kellner I, Konter U, et al, "Differential Expression of Adhesion Molecules on Infiltrating Cells in Inflammatory Dermatoses," *J Am Acad Dermatol*, 1992, 26(6):907-13.

Corso B, Eversole LR, and Hutt-Fletcher L, "Hairy Leukoplakia: Epstein-Barr Virus Receptors on Oral Keratinocyte Plasma Membranes," *Oral Surg Oral Med Oral Pathol*, 1989, 67(4):416-21.

Flaitz CM, "Persistent White Lesion of the Lateral Tongue," *Am J Dent*, 2001, 14(6):402-3.

Greenspan D, Greenspan JS, Overby G, et al, "Risk Factors for Rapid Progression From Hairy Leukoplakia to AIDS: A Nested Case-Control Study, *J Acquir Immune Defic Syndr*, 1991, 4(7):652-8.

McGuff HS, Otto RA, and Aufdemorte TB, "Clinical Warning Signs and Symptoms of Head and Neck Cancer," *Tex Dent J*, 2000, 117(6):14-9.

Regezi JA, Stewart JC, Lloyd RV, et al, "Immunohistochemical Staining of Langerhans Cells and Macrophages in Oral Lichen Planus," *Oral Surg Oral Med Oral Pathol*, 1985, 60(4):396-402.

Sciubba JJ, "Oral Leukoplakia," *Crit Rev Oral Biol Med*, 1995, 6(2):147-60.

Sciubba JJ, "Oral Precancer and Cancer: Etiology, Clinical Presentation, Diagnosis, and Management," *Compend Contin Educ Dent* 2000, 21(10A):892-8, 900-2.

ORAL SOFT TISSUE DISEASES

Antenucci EL, "Integration of Lasers Into a Soft Tissue Management Program," *Dent Clin North Am*, 2000, 44(4):811-9.

Delaney JE and Keels MA, "Pediatric Oral Pathology. Soft Tissue and Periodontal Conditions," *Pediatr Clin North Am*, 2000, 47(5):1125-47.

Goupil MT, "Occupational Health and Safety Emergencies," *Dent Clin North Am*, 1995, 39(3):637-47.

Haddad AJ, Avon SL, Clokie CM, et al, "Nodular Fasciitis in the Oral Cavity," *J Can Dent Assoc*, 2001, 67(11):664-7.

MacPhail LA, Greenspan D, Greenspan JS, et al, "Recurrent Aphthous Ulcers in Association With HIV Infection. Diagnosis and Treatment," *Oral Surg Oral Med Oral Pathol*, 1992, 73(3):283-8.

Meiller TF, Kutcher MJ, Overholser CD, et al, "Effect of an Antimicrobial Mouthrinse on Recurrent Aphthous Ulcerations," *Oral Surg Oral Med Oral Pathol*, 1991, 72(4):425-9.

Moncarz V, Ulmansky M, and Lustmann J, "Lichen Planus: Exploring Its Malignant Potential," *J Am Dent Assoc*, 1993, 124(3):102-8.

Rodu B and Mattingly G, "Oral Mucosal Ulcers: Diagnosis and Management," *J Am Dent Assoc*, 1992, 123(10):83-6.

Van Dis ML and Vincent SD, "Diagnosis and Management of Autoimmune and Idiopathic Mucosal Diseases," *Dent Clin North Am*, 1992, 36(4):897-917.

Vincent SD and Lilly GE, "Clinical, Historic, and Therapeutic Features of Aphthous Stomatitis. Literature Review and Open Clinical Trial Employing Steroids," *Oral Surg, Oral Med, Oral Pathol*, 1992, 74(1):79-86.

Wactawski-Wende J, " Periodontal Diseases and Osteoporosis: Association and Mechanisms, "*Ann Periodontol*, 2001, (1):197-208.

ORAL VIRAL DISEASES

Balfour HH, Rotbart HA, Feldman S, et al, "Acyclovir Treatment of Varicella in Otherwise Healthy Adolescents. The Collaborative Acyclovir Varicella Study Group," *J Pediatr*, 1992, 120(4):627-33.

Chang Y, Cesarman E, Pessin MS, et al, "Identification of Herpesvirus-Like DNA Sequences in AIDS-Associated Kaposi's Sarcoma," *Science*, 1994, 266(5192):1865-9.

Farquharson A, Ajagbe O, and Brown RS, "Differential Diagnosis of Severe Recurrent Oral Ulceration," *Dent Today*, 2002, 21(3):74-9.

Ficarra G and Shillitoe EJ, "HIV-Related Infections of the Oral Cavity," *Oral Biol Med*, 1992, 3(3):207-31.

Moore TO, Moore AY, Carrasco D, et al, "Human Papillomavirus, Smoking, and Cancer," *J Cutan Med Surg*, 2001, 5(4):323-8.

Skegg DC, "Oral Contraceptives, Parity, and Cervical Cancer," *Lancet*, 2002, 359(9312):1080-1.

Spruance SL, Stewart JC, Rowe NH, et al, "Treatment of Recurrent Herpes Simplex Labialis With Oral Acyclovir," *J Infect Dis*, 1990, 161(2):185-90.

Woldeamanuel Y and Abate D, "Characterization of *Candida albicans* Isolates from the Oral Cavity of HIV-Positive Patients," *Ethiop Med J*, 1998, 36(4):235-43.

PERIODONTAL DISEASE

Bollen CM and Quirynen M, "Microbiological Response to Mechanical Treatment in Combination With Adjunctive Therapy. A Review of the Literature," *J Periodontol*, 1996, 67(11):1143-58.

Brecx M, Netuschil L, Reichart B, et al, "Efficacy of Listerine®, Meridol®, and Chlorhexidine Mouthrinses on Plaque, Gingivitis, and Plaque Bacteria Vitality," *J Clin Periodontol*, 1990, 17(1):292-7.

Ciancio SG, "Medications as Risk Factors for Periodontal Disease," *J Periodontol*, 1996, 67(Suppl 10):S1055-9.

Crout RJ, Lee HM, Schroeder K, et al, "The Cyclic Regimen of Low-Dose Doxycycline for Adult Periodontitis. A Preliminary Study," *J Periodontol*, 1996, 67(5):506-14.

SUGGESTED READINGS *(Continued)*

DePaola LG, Overholser CD, Meiller TF, et al, "Chemotherapeutic Inhibition of Supragingival Dental Plaque and Gingivitis Development," *J Clin Periodontol*, 1989, 16(1):311-5.

Desvarieux M, "Periodontal Disease, Race, and Vascular Disease," *Compend Contin Educ Dent*, 2001, 22(3):34-41.

Elter JR, White BA, Gaynes BN, et al, "Relationship of Clinical Depression to Periodontal Treatment Outcome," *J Periodontol*, 2002, 73(4):441-9.

Genco RJ, "Current View of Risk Factors for Periodontal Diseases," *J Periodontol*, 1996, 67(Suppl 10):S1041-9.

Graves DT, Jiang Y, and Genco C, "Periodontal Disease: Bacterial Virulence Factors, Host Response and Impact on Systemic Health," *Curr Opin Infect Dis*, 2000, 13(3):227-232.

Greenstein G and Hart TC, "Clinical Utility of a Genetic Susceptibility Test for Severe Chronic Periodontitis: A Critical Evaluation," *J Am Dent Assoc*, 2002, 133(4):452-9.

Hitzig C, Charbit Y, Bitton C, et al, "Topical Metronidazole as an Adjunct to Subgingival Debridement in the Treatment of Chronic Periodontitis," *J Clin Periodontol*, 1994, 21(2):146-51.

Kjaerheim V, Skaare A, Barkvoll P, et al, "Antiplaque, Antibacterial, and Anti-inflammatory Properties of Triclosan Mouthrinses in Combination With Zinc Citrate or Polyvinylmethylether Maleic Acid (PVM-MA) Copolymer," *Eur J Oral Sci*, 1996, 104(5-6):529-34.

Loesche WJ, Giordano J, Soehren S, et al, "Nonsurgical Treatment of Patients With Periodontal Disease," *Oral Surg, Oral Med Oral Pathol*, 1996, 81(5):533-43.

Michalowicz BS, Pihlstrom BL, Drisko CL, et al, "Evaluation of Periodontal Treatments Using Controlled-Release Tetracycline Fibers: Maintenance Response," *J Periodontol*, 1995, 66(8):708-15.

Landry RG and Jean M, "Periodontal Screening and Recording (PSR) Index: Precursors, Utility and Limitations in a Clinical Setting," *Int Dent J*, 2002, 52(1):35-40.

Mealey BL, "Diabetes and Periodontal Disease: Two Sides of a Coin," *Compend Contin Educ Dent*, 2000, 21(11):943-6, 948, 950, passim.

Moseley R, Waddington RJ, and Embery G, "Hyaluronan and Its Potential Role in Periodontal Healing," *Dent Update*, 2002, 29(3):144-8.

Palomo F, Wantland L, Sanchez A, et al, "The Effect of Three Commercially Available Dentifrices Containing Triclosan on Supragingival Plaque Formation and Gingivitis: A Six Month Clinical Study," *Int Dent J*, 1994, 44(I Suppl 1):75-81.

Pavici MJ, van Winkelhoff AJ, Steures NH, et al, "Microbiological and Clinical Effects of Metronidazole and Amoxicillin in *Actinobacillus actinomycetemcomitans*-Associated Periodontitis. A 2-Year Evaluation," *J Clin Periodontol*, 1994, 21(2):107-12.

Ross NM, Mankodi SM, Mostler KL, et al, "Effects of Rinsing Time on Antiplaque-Antigingivitis Efficacy of Listerine®, *J Clin Periodontol*, 1993, 20(1):279-81.

Seymour RA and Heasman PA, "Tetracyclines in the Management of Periodontal Diseases. A Review," *J Clin Periodontol*, 1995, 22(1):22-35.

Seymour RA and Heasman PA, "Pharmacological Control of Periodontal Disease. II. Antimicrobial Agents," *J Dent*, 1995, 23(1):5-14.

Slots J and Ting M, "Systemic Antibiotics in the Treatment of Periodontal Disease," *Periodontol 2000*, 2002, 28:106-76.

PERIODONTOLOGY

Listgarten MA, "Pathogenesis of Periodontitis," *J Clin Periodontol*, 1986, 13(5):418-30.

Loesche WJ, Syed SA, Laughon BE, et al, "The Bacteriology of Acute Necrotizing Ulcerative Gingivitis," *J Periodontol*, 1982, 53(4):223-30.

PHARMACOLOGY OF DRUG METABOLISM AND INTERACTIONS

DeVane CL, "Pharmacogenetics and Drug Metabolism of Newer Antidepressant Agents," *J Clin Psychiatry*, 1994, 55(Suppl 12):38-45.

Hupp WS, " Seizure Disorders," *Oral Surg Oral Med Oral Pathol Oral Radiol Endod*, 2001, 92(6):593-6.

Ketter TA, Flockhart DA, Post RM, et al, "The Emerging Role of Cytochrome P450 3A in Psychopharmacology,"*J Clin Psychopharmacol*, 1995, 15(6):387-98.

Michalets EL, "Update: Clinically Significant Cytochrome P450 Drug Interactions," *Pharmacotherapy*, 1998, 18(1):84-112.

Moore PA, "Dental Therapeutic Indications for the Newer Long-Acting Macrolide Antibiotics," *J Am Dent Assoc*, 1999, 130(9):1341-3.

Nemeroff CB, DeVane CL, and Pollock BG, "Newer Antidepressants and the Cytochrome P450 System," *Am J Psychiatry*, 1996, 153(3):311-20.

Schmider J, Greenblatt DJ, von Moltke LL, et al, "Relationship of *In Vitro* Data on Drug Metabolism to *In Vivo* Pharmacokinetics and Drug Interactions: Implications for Diazepam Disposition in Humans," *J Clin Psychopharmacol*, 1996, 16(4):267-72.

Watkins PB, "Role of Cytochrome P450 in Drug Metabolism and Hepatotoxicity," *Semin Liver Dis*, 1990, 10(4):235-50.

Weinberg MA and Fine JB, "The Importance of Drug Interactions in Dental Practice," *Dent Today*, 2001, 20(9):88-93.

PREPROCEDURAL ANTIBIOTICS

ADA Division of Legal Affairs, "A Legal Perspective on Antibiotic Prophylaxis," *J Am Dent Assoc*, 2003, 134(9):1260.

"Advisory Statement. Antibiotic Prophylaxis for Dental Patients With Total Joint Replacement. American Dental Association; American Academy of Orthopaedic Surgeons," *J Am Dent Assoc*, 1997, 128(7):1004-8.

American Dental Association; American Academy of Orthopedic Surgeons, "Antibiotic Prophylaxis for Dental Patients With Total Joint Replacements," *J Am Dent Assoc*, 2003, 134(7):895-9.

Bartzokas CA, Johnson R, Jane M, et al, "Relation Between Mouth and Haematogenous Infection in Total Joint Replacements," *BMJ*, 1994, 309(6953):506-8.

Berney P and Francioli P, "Successful Prophylaxis of Experimental Streptococcal Endocarditis With Single-Dose Amoxicillin Administered After Bacterial Challenge," *J Infect Dis*, 1990, 161(2):281-5.

Brause BD, "Infections Associated With Prosthetic Joints," *Clin Rheum Dis*, 1986, 12(2):523-36.

Chenoweth CE and Burket JS, "Antimicrobial Prophylaxis: Principles and Practice," *Formulary*, 1997, 32:692-708.

Ching DW, Gould IM, Rennie JA, et al, "Prevention of Late Haematogenous Infection in Major Prosthetic Joints," *J Antimicrob Chemother*, 1989, 23(5):676-80.

Clauzel AM, Visier S, and Michel FB, "Efficacy and Safety of Azithromycin in Lower Respiratory Tract Infections," *Eur Respir J*, 1990, 3(Suppl 10):S89.

Clemens JD and Ransohoff DF, "A Quantitative Assessment of Predental Antibiotic Prophylaxis for Patients With Mitral-Valve Prolapse," *J Chron Dis*, 1984, 37(7):531-44.

Dajani AS, Taubert KA, Wilson W, et al, "Prevention of Bacterial Endocarditis. Recommendations by the American Heart Association," *JAMA*, 1997, 277(22):1794-801.

Doern GV, Ferraro MJ, Brueggemann AB, et al, "Emergence of High Rates of Antimicrobial Resistance Among Viridans Group Streptococci in the United States," *Antimicrob Agents Chemother*, 1996, 40(4):891-4.

Durack DT, "Antibiotics for Prevention of Endocarditis During Dentistry: Time to Scale Back?" *Ann Intern Med*, 1998, 129(10):829-31.

Durack DT, "Prevention of Infective Endocarditis," *N Engl J Med*, 1995, 332(1):38-44.

Fluckiger U, Francioli P, Blaser J, et al, "Role of Amoxicillin Serum Levels for Successful Prophylaxis of Experimental Endocarditis Due to Tolerant Streptococci," *J Infect Dis*, 1994, 169(6):1397-400.

Hanssen AD, Osmon DR, and Nelson CL, "Prevention of Deep Prosthetic Joint Infection," *J Bone Joint Surg*, 1996, 78:458-71.

Little J, "The American Heart Association's Guidelines for the Prevention of Bacterial Endocarditis: A Critical Review," *Gen Dent*, 1998, 46:508-15.

"Risks for and Prevention of Infective Endocarditis," *Cardiology Clinics - Diagnosis and Management of Infective Endocarditis*, Child JS, ed, Philadelphia, PA: WB Saunders Co, 1996, 14:327-43.

Sale L, "Some Tragic Results Following Extraction of Teeth. II." *J Am Dent Assoc*, 1939, 26:1647-51.

Strom BL, Abrutyn E, Berlin JA, et al, "Dental and Cardiac Risk Factors for Infective Endocarditis. A Population-Based, Case-Control Study," *Ann Intern Med*, 1998, 129(10):761-9.

Strom BL, Abrutyn E, Berlin JA, et al, "Prophylactic Antibiotics to Prevent Infective Endocarditis? Relative Risks Reassessed," *J Investig Med*, 1996, 44:229.

Wahl M, "Myths of Dental-Induced Prosthetic Joint Infections," *Clin Infect Dis*, 1995, 20(5):1420-5.

Wynn RL, "Amoxicillin Update," *Gen Dent*, 1991, 39(5):322, 324, 326.

Wynn RL and Bergman SA, "Antibiotics and Their Use in the Treatment of Orofacial Infections, Part I," *Gen Dent*, 1994, 42(5): 398, 400, 402.

Wynn RL, "New Erythromycins," *Gen Dent*, 1996, 44(4):304-7.

Wynn RL, Meiller TF, and Crossley HL, "New Guidelines for the Prevention of Bacterial Endocarditis. American Heart Association," *Gen Dent*, 1997, 45(5):426-8, 430-4.

TEMPOROMANDIBULAR DYSFUNCTION

Amir I, Hermesh H, and Gavish A, "Bruxism Secondary to Antipsychotic Drug Exposure: A Positive Response to Propranolol," *Clin Neuropharmacol*, 1997, 20(1):86-9.

Becker IM, "Occlusion as a Causative Factor in TMD. Scientific Basis to Occlusal Therapy," *NY State Dent J*, 1995, 61(9):54-7.

Bell WE, *Temporomandibular Disorders: Classification Diagnosis, Management*, 3rd ed, Chicago IL: Year Book Medical Publishers, 1990.

Bostwick JM and Jaffee MS, "Buspirone as an Antidote to SSRI-Induced Bruxism in 4 Cases," *J Clin Psychiatry*, 1999, 60(12):857-60.

Brown ES and Hong SC, "Antidepressant-Induced Bruxism Successfully Treated With Gabapentin," *J Am Dent Assoc*, 1999, 130(10):1467-9.

Carlson CR, Bertrand PM, Ehrlich AD, et al, "Physical Self-Regulation Training for the Management of Temporomandibular Disorders," *J Orofac Pain*, 2001, 15(1):47-55.

Canavan D and Gratt BM, "Electronic Thermography for the Assessment of Mild and Moderate Temporomandibular Joint Dysfunction," *Oral Surg Oral Med Oral Pathol Oral Radiol Endod*, 1995, 79(6):778-86.

Clark GT and Takeuchi H, "Temporomandibular Dysfunction, Chromic Orofacial Pain and Oral Motor Disorders in the 21st Century," *J Calif Dent Assoc*, 1995, 23(4):44-6, 48-50.

Dos Santos J Jr, "Supportive Conservative Therapies for Temporomandibular Disorders," *Dent Clin North Am*, 1995, 39(2):459-77.

Felicio CM, Mazzetto MO, and Perri Angote Dos Santos C, "Masticatory Behavior in Individuals With Temporomandibular Disorders," *Minerva Stomatol*, 2002, 51(4):111-20.

Gerber PE and Lynd LD, "Selective Serotonin Reuptake Inhibitor-Induced Movement Disorders," *Ann Pharmacother*, 1998, 32(6):692-8.

SUGGESTED READINGS *(Continued)*

Maini S, Osborne JE, Fadl HM, et al, "Temporomandibular Joint Dysfunction Following Tonsillectomy," *Clin Otolaryngol*, 2002, 27(1):57-60.

Nicolakis P, Erdogmus B, Kopf A, et al, "Effectiveness of Exercise Therapy in Patients With Myofascial Pain Dysfunction Syndrome," *J Oral Rehabil*, 2002, 29(4):362-8.

Okeson JP, "Occlusion and Functional Disorders of the Masticatory System," *Dent Clin North Am*, 1995, 39(2):285-300.

Quinn JH, "Mandibular Exercises to Control Bruxism and Deviation Problems," *Cranio*, 1995, 13(1):30-4.

Schiffman E, Haley D, Baker C, et al, "Diagnostic Criteria for Screening Headache Patients for Temporomandibular Disorders," *Headache*, 1995, 35(3):121-4.

Thayer T, "Acupuncture TMD and Facial Pain," *SAAD Dig*, 2001, 18(3):3-7.

XEROSTOMIA

American Dental Association. ADA Guide to Dental Therapeutics, 2nd ed, Chicago, IL: ADA Publishing Co, Inc, 2001.

"Cevimeline (Evoxac) for Dry Mouth," *Med Lett Drugs Ther*, 2000, 42(1084):70.

Fox PC, Atkinson JC, Macynski AA, et al, "Pilocarpine Treatment of Salivary Gland Hypofunction and Dry Mouth (Xerostomia)," *Arch Intern Med,* 1991, 151(6):1149-52.

Johnson JT, Ferretti GA, Nethery WJ, et al, "Oral Pilocarpine for Post-Irradiation Xerostomia in Patients With Head and Neck Cancer," *N Eng J Med,* 1993, 329(6):390-5.

Johnstone PA, Niemtzow RC, and Riffenburgh RH, "Acupuncture for Xerostomia: Clinical Update," *Cancer*, 2002, 94(4):1151-6.

Nusair S and Rubinow A, "The Use of Oral Pilocarpine in Xerostomia and Sjögren's Syndrome," *Semin Arthritis Rheum*, 1999, 28(6):360-7.

Rhodus NL and Schuh MJ, "Effects of Pilocarpine on Salivary Flow in Patients With Sjögren's Syndrome," *Oral Surg Oral Med Oral Pathol*, 1991, 72(5):545-9.

Sanchez-Guerrero J, Aguirre-Garcia E, Perez-Dosal MR, et al, "The Wafer Test: A Semi-Quantitative Test to Screen for Xerostomia," *Rheumatology (Oxford)*, 2002, 41(4):381-9.

Ship JA, Pillemer SR, and Baum BJ, "Xerostomia and the Geriatric Patient," *J Am Geriatr Soc*, 2002, 50(3):535-43.

Sugerman PB and Barber MT, "Patient Selection for Endosseous Dental Implants: Oral and Systemic Considerations," *Int J Oral Maxillofac Implants*, 2002, 17(2):191-201.

Taylor SE and Miller EG, "Pre-emptive Pharmacologic Intervention in Radiation-Induced Salivary Dysfunction," *Proc Soc Exp Biol Med,* 1999, 221(1):14-26.

Tenovuo J, "Clinical Applications of Antimicrobial Host Proteins Lactoperoxidase, Lysozyme and Lactoferrin in Xerostomia: Efficacy and Safety," *Oral Dis*, 2002, 8(1):23-9.

Wray D, Lowe GD, Dagg JH, et al, *Textbook of General and Oral Medicine,* London, England: Churchill Livingstone, 1999.

Wynn RL, Meiller TF, and Crossley HL, *Drug Information Handbook for Dentistry,* 6th ed, Hudson (Cleveland), OH: Lexi-Comp, Inc, 2000.

Valdez IH, Wolff A, Atkinson JC, et al, "Use of Pilocarpine During Head and Neck Radiation Therapy to Reduce Xerostomia and Salivary Dysfunction," *Cancer,* 1993, 71(5):1848-51.

APPENDIX
TABLE OF CONTENTS

Standard Conversions

Apothecary / Metric Conversions ... 1598
Pounds / Kilograms Conversion ... 1599

Calcium Channel Blockers and Gingival Hyperplasia

Some General Observations of CCB-Induced GH ... 1600
Calcium Channel Blockers ... 1602

Infectious Disease Information

Occupational Exposure to Bloodborne Pathogens (Standard / Universal Precautions) ... 1603
Immunizations (Vaccines) ... 1614

Laboratory Values

Normal Blood Values ... 1620

Over-the-Counter Dental Products

Dentifrice Products ... 1621
Mouth Pain, Cold Sore, and Canker Sore Products ... 1633
Oral Rinse Products ... 1638

Miscellaneous

Top 200 Most Prescribed Drugs in 2003 ... 1642
Multivitamin Products ... 1644
Dental Drug Use in Pregnancy and Breast-Feeding ... 1657

STANDARD CONVERSIONS

APOTHECARY / METRIC CONVERSIONS

Approximate Liquid Measures

Basic equivalent: 1 fluid ounce = 30 mL

Examples:

1 gallon	3800 mL	15 minims	1 mL
1 quart	960 mL	10 minims	0.6 mL
1 pint	480 mL	1 gallon	128 fluid ounces
8 fluid ounces	240 mL	1 quart	32 fluid ounces
4 fluid ounces	120 mL	1 pint	16 fluid ounces

Approximate Household Equivalents

1 teaspoonful	5 mL	1 tablespoonful	15 mL

Weights

Basic equivalents:

1 ounce = 30 g   15 grains = 1 g

Examples:

4 ounces	120 g	1/100 grain	600 mcg
2 ounces	60 g	1/150 grain	400 mcg
10 grains	600 mg	1/200 grain	300 mcg
7 1/2 grains	500 mg	16 ounces	1 pound
1 grain	60 mg		

Metric Conversions

Basic equivalents:

1 g	1000 mg	1 mg	1000 mcg

Examples:

5 g	5000 mg	5 mg	5000 mcg
0.5 g	500 mg	0.5 mg	500 mcg
0.05 g	50 mg	0.05 mg	50 mcg

Exact Equivalents

1 g	=	15.43 grains (gr)	0.1 mg	=	1/600 gr
1 mL	=	16.23 minims	0.12 mg	=	1/500 gr
1 minim	=	0.06 mL	0.15 mg	=	1/400 gr
1 gr	=	64.8 mg	0.2 mg	=	1/300 gr
1 pint (pt)	=	473.2 mL	0.3 mg	=	1/200 gr
1 oz	=	28.35 g	0.4 mg	=	1/150 gr
1 lb	=	453.6 g	0.5 mg	=	1/120 gr
1 kg	=	2.2 lb	0.6 mg	=	1/100 gr
1 qt	=	946.4 mL	0.8 mg	=	1/80 gr
			1 mg	=	1/65 gr

Solids[1]

1/4 grain	=	15 mg
1/2 grain	=	30 mg
1 grain	=	60 mg
1 1/2 grains	=	90 mg
5 grains	=	300 mg
10 grains	=	600 mg

[1]Use exact equivalents for compounding and calculations requiring a high degree of accuracy.

POUNDS / KILOGRAMS CONVERSION

1 pound = 0.45359 kilograms
1 kilogram = 2.2 pounds

lb	=	kg	lb	=	kg	lb	=	kg
1		0.45	70		31.75	140		63.50
5		2.27	75		34.02	145		65.77
10		4.54	80		36.29	150		68.04
15		6.80	85		38.56	155		70.31
20		9.07	90		40.82	160		72.58
25		11.34	95		43.09	165		74.84
30		13.61	100		45.36	170		77.11
35		15.88	105		47.63	175		79.38
40		18.14	110		49.90	180		81.65
45		20.41	115		52.16	185		83.92
50		22.68	120		54.43	190		86.18
55		24.95	125		56.70	195		88.45
60		27.22	130		58.91	200		90.72
65		29.48	135		61.24			

CALCIUM CHANNEL BLOCKERS AND GINGIVAL HYPERPLASIA

Drug	FDA Approval	Cases Cited in Literature
Amlodipine (Norvasc®)	1992	3
Bepridil (Vascor®)	1993	0
Diltiazem (Cardizem®, Dilacor®)	1982	>20
Felodipine (Plendil®)	1992	1
Isradipine (DynaCirc®)	1991	1
Nicardipine (Cardene®)	1989	0
Nifedipine (Adalat®, Procardia®)	1982	>120
Nimodipine (Nimotop®)	1989	0
Nisoldipine (Sular®)	1995	0
Nitrendipine[1] (Baypress®)		1
Verapamil (Calan®, Isoptin®, Verelan®)	1982	7

[1]Not yet approved for use in the United States.

SOME GENERAL OBSERVATIONS OF CCB-INDUCED GH

Calcium channel blockers (CCBs) are well known to cause gingival enlargement. In the early 1990s, it was thought that this class of drugs caused a true hyperplasia of the gingiva. Current thinking is that the term "hyperplasia" is inappropriate since the drug-induced effect results in an increase in extracellular tissue volume rather than an increase in the number of cells. Most of the reported cases of CCB-induced gingival enlargement have involved patients >50 years of age taking CCBs for postmyocardial infarction syndrome, angina pain, essential hypertension, and Raynaud's syndrome. Nifedipine (Procardia®) is associated with the highest number of reported cases in the literature, followed by diltiazem (Cardizem®). Depending on the CCB in question, gingival enlargement has appeared any time between 1-24 months after daily dosing. Discontinuance of the CCB usually results in complete disappearance or marked regression of symptoms, with symptoms reappearing upon remedication. The time required after drug discontinuance for marked regression of enlargement has been 1 week. Complete disappearance of all symptoms usually takes 2 months. If gingivectomy is performed and the drug retained or resumed, the gingival enlargement can recur. Only when the CCB is discontinued or a switch to a non-CCB occurs, will the gingivectomy usually be successful. One study of Nishikawa et al, showed that if nifedipine could not be discontinued, gingival enlargement did not recur after gingivectomy when extensive plaque control was carried out. If the CCB is changed to another class of cardiovascular drug, the enlargement will probably regress and disappear. A switch to another CCB, however, will probably result in continued gingival enlargement. For example, Giustiniani et al, reported disappearance of symptoms within 15 days after discontinuance of verapamil, with recurrence of symptoms after resumption with diltiazem. One case report described a nonsurgical management of a patient presenting with nifedipine-induced gingival overgrowth. Establishment and maintenance of a considerably improved standard of plaque control led to complete resolution of the overgrowth without recurrence, even though the medication dose was increased. The reader is referred to the review of 1991 for descriptive clinical and histological findings of CCB-induced gingival enlargement. A more recent review has been authorized by Silverstein et al, and published in 1997.

Two reports described the prevalence of amlodipine (Norvasc®)-induced gingival overgrowth. The study by Ellis et al, examined a sample of patients taking 1 of 3 CCBs who were drawn from a community-based population in northeastern England. Out of 911 patients, 442 were taking nifedipine, 181 amlodipine, and 186 diltiazem. In addition, 102 control subjects were included. It was found that 6.3% of subjects taking nifedipine were seen to have significant overgrowth, which was significantly greater than the overgrowth seen with the other two drug groups or the control group. The prevalence of gingival overgrowth induced by amlodipine or diltiazem was not significantly different compared to the control group. This study concluded that the prevalence of significant gingival overgrowth related to CCBs was low. Also, males were 3 times as likely as females to develop significant overgrowth.

In a second study by Jorgensen, a large group of patients taking amlodipine was studied in order to determine the prevalence of, what he called, "gingival hyperplasia". Out of 150 dentate patients who volunteered to undergo a screening examination, mild hyperplasia was found in 5 patients (3.3%). This was significantly less than rates reported for patients taking nifedipine and not significantly different from rates reported in control groups of cardiac patients not taking CCBs. Jorgensen concluded that amlodipine, at a dose of 5 mg daily, did not induce gingival hyperplasia.

There have been reports of verapamil-induced gingival enlargement in the literature with at least 7 cases listed in the review by this author. The prevalence of verapamil-induced enlargement, however, has not been investigated.

References

Bullon P, Machuca G, Armas JR, et al, "The Gingival Inflammatory Infiltrate in Cardiac Patients Treated With Calcium Antagonists," *J Clin Periodontol*, 2001, 28(10):897-903.

Ciantar M, "Nifedipine-Induced Gingival Overgrowth: Remission Following Nonsurgical Therapy," *Dent Update*, 1997, 45(4):371-6.

Desai P and Silver JG, "Drug-Induced Gingival Enlargements," *J Can Dent Assoc*, 1998, 64(4):263-8.

Ellis JS, Seymour RA, Steele JG, et al, "Prevalence of Gingival Overgrowth Induced by Calcium Channel Blockers: A Community-Based Study," *J Periodontol*, 1999, 70(1):63-7.

Giustiniani S, Robestelli della Cuna F, and Marieni M, "Hyperplastic Gingivitis During Diltiazem Therapy," *Int J Cardiol*, 1987, 15(2):247-9.

Hood KA, "Drug-Induced Gingival Hyperplasia in Transplant Recipients," *Prog Transplant*, 2002, 12(1):17-21.

Jorgensen MG, "Prevalence of Amlodipine-Related Gingival Hyperplasia, *J Periodontol*, 1997, 68(7):676-8.

Missouris GG, Kalaitzidis RG, Cappuccio FP, et al, "Gingival Hyperplasia Caused by Calcium Channel Blockers," *J Hum Hypertens.* , 2000, 14(2):155-6.

Nishikawa S, Tada H, Hamasaki A, et al, "Nifedipine-Induced Gingival Hyperplasia: A Clinical and *In Vitro* Study," *J Periodontol*, 1991, 62(1):30-5.

Silverstein LH, Garnick JJ, Szikman M, et al, "Medication-Induced Gingival Enlargement: A Clinical Review," *Gen Dent*, 1997, 45(4):371-6.

Wynn RL, "Calcium Channel Blockers and Gingival Hyperplasia," *Gen Dent*, 1991, 39(4):240-3.

Wynn RL, "Update on Calcium Channel Blocker-Induced Gingival Hyperplasia," *Gen Dent*, 1995, 43(3):218-20, 222.

CALCIUM CHANNEL BLOCKERS

Comparative Pharmacokinetics

Agent	Bioavailability (%)	Protein Binding (%)	Onset (min)	Peak (h)	Half-Life (h)	Volume of Distribution	Route of Metabolism	Route of Excretion
Dihydropyridines								
Amlodipine (Norvasc®)	52-88	97	6 h	6-9	33.8	21 L/kg	Liver, inactive metabolites, not a significant first-pass metabolism/presystemic metabolism	Bile, gut wall
Felodipine (Plendil®)	10-25	>99	3-5 h	2.5-5	10-36	10.3 L/kg	Liver, inactive metabolites, extensive metabolism by several pathways including cytochrome P450, extensive first-pass metabolism/presystemic metabolism	70% urine, 10% feces
Isradipine (DynaCirc®)	15-24	97	120	0.5-2.5	8	2.9 L/kg	Liver, inactive metabolites, extensive first-pass metabolism	90% urine, 10% feces
Nicardipine (Cardene®)	35	>95	20	0.5-2	2-4	ND	Liver, saturable first-pass metabolism	60% urine, 35% feces
Nifedipine (prototype) (Adalat® CC, Procardia®/ Procardia XL®)	Immediate/sustained release 45-70/86	92-98	20	Immediate/ sustained release 0.5/6	2-5	ND	Liver, inactive metabolites	60%-80% urine, feces, bile
Nimodipine (Nimotop®)	13	>95	ND	≤1	1-2	0.43 L/kg	Liver, inactive metabolites, high first-pass metabolism	Urine
Nisoldipine (Sular®)	4-8	>99	ND	6-12	7-12	4-5 L/kg	Liver, 1 active metabolite (10%), presystemic metabolism	70%-75% kidney, 6%-12% feces
Phenylalkylamines								
Verapamil (prototype) (Calan®, Isoptin®)	20-35	83-92	30	1-2.2	3-7	4.5-7 L/kg	Liver	70% urine, 16% feces
Benzothiazepines								
Diltiazem (prototype) (Cardizem®/Cardizem® CD, Dilacor® XR)	40-67	70-80	30-60	Immediate/ sustained release 2-3/6-11	Immediate/ sustained release 3.5-6/5-7	ND	Liver; drugs which inhibit/induce hepatic microsomal enzymes may alter disposition	Urine
Miscellaneous								
Bepridil (Vascor®)	59	>99	60	2-3	24	ND	Liver	70% urine, 22% feces

OCCUPATIONAL EXPOSURE TO BLOODBORNE PATHOGENS (STANDARD / UNIVERSAL PRECAUTIONS)

OVERVIEW AND REGULATORY CONSIDERATIONS

Every healthcare employee, from nurse to housekeeper, has some (albeit small) risk of exposure to HIV and other viral agents such as hepatitis B and Jakob-Creutzfeldt agent. The incidence of HIV-1 transmission associated with a percutaneous exposure to blood from an HIV-1 infected patient is approximately 0.3% per exposure.[1] In 1989, it was estimated that 12,000 United States healthcare workers acquired hepatitis B annually.[2] An understanding of the appropriate procedures, responsibilities, and risks inherent in the collection and handling of patient specimens is necessary for safe practice and is required by Occupational Safety and Health Administration (OSHA) regulations.

The Occupational Safety and Health Administration published its "Final Rule on Occupational Exposure to Bloodborne Pathogens" in the Federal Register on December 6, 1991. OSHA has chosen to follow the Center for Disease Control (CDC) definition of universal precautions. The Final Rule provides full legal force to universal precautions and requires employers and employees to treat blood and certain body fluids as if they were infectious. The Final Rule mandates that healthcare workers must avoid parenteral contact and must avoid splattering blood or other potentially infectious material on their skin, hair, eyes, mouth, mucous membranes, or on their personal clothing. Hazard abatement strategies must be used to protect the workers. Such plans typically include, but are not limited to, the following:

- safe handling of sharp items ("sharps") and disposal of such into puncture resistant containers
- gloves required for employees handling items soiled with blood or equipment contaminated by blood or other body fluids
- provisions of protective clothing when more extensive contact with blood or body fluids may be anticipated (eg, surgery, autopsy, or deliveries)
- resuscitation equipment to reduce necessity for mouth to mouth resuscitation
- restriction of HIV- or hepatitis B-exposed employees to noninvasive procedures

OSHA has specifically defined the following terms: **Occupational exposure** means reasonably anticipated skin, eye mucous membrane, or parenteral contact with blood or other potentially infectious materials that may result from the performance of an employee's duties. **Other potentially infectious materials** are human body fluids including semen, vaginal secretions, cerebrospinal fluid, synovial fluid, pleural fluid, pericardial fluid, peritoneal fluid, amniotic fluid, saliva in dental procedures, and body fluids that are visibly contaminated with blood, and all body fluids in situations where it is difficult or impossible to differentiate between body fluids; any unfixed tissue or organ (other than intact skin) from a human (living or dead); and HIV-containing cell or tissue cultures, organ cultures, and HIV- or HBV-containing culture medium or other solutions, and blood, organs, or other tissues from experimental animals infected with HIV or HBV. An **exposure incident** involves specific eye, mouth, other mucous membrane, nonintact skin, or parenteral contact with blood or other potentially infectious materials that results from the performance of an employee's duties.[3] It is important to understand that some exposures may go unrecognized despite the strictest precautions.

A written Exposure Control Plan is required. Employers must provide copies of the plan to employees and to OSHA upon request. Compliance with OSHA rules may be accomplished by the following methods.

- **Universal precautions (UPs)** means that all human blood and certain body fluids are treated as if known to be infectious for HIV, HBV, and other bloodborne pathogens. UPs do not apply to feces, nasal secretions, saliva, sputum, sweat, tears, urine, or vomitus unless they contain visible blood.
- **Engineering controls (ECs)** are physical devices which reduce or remove hazards from the workplace by eliminating or minimizing hazards or by isolating the worker from exposure. Engineering control devices include sharps disposal containers, self-resheathing syringes, etc.
- **Work practice controls (WPCs)** are practices and procedures that reduce the likelihood of exposure to hazards by altering the way in which a task is performed. Specific examples are the prohibition of two-handed recapping of needles, prohibition of storing food alongside potentially contaminated material, discouragement of pipetting fluids by mouth, encouraging handwashing after removal of gloves, safe handling of contaminated sharps, and appropriate use of sharps containers.
- **Personal protective equipment (PPE)** is specialized clothing or equipment worn to provide protection from occupational exposure. PPE includes gloves, gowns, laboratory coats (the type and characteristics will depend upon the task and degree of exposure anticipated), face shields or masks, and eye protection. Surgical caps or hoods and/or shoe covers or boots are required in instances in

OCCUPATIONAL EXPOSURE TO BLOODBORNE PATHOGENS (STANDARD / UNIVERSAL PRECAUTIONS) *(Continued)*

which gross contamination can reasonably be anticipated (eg, autopsies, orthopedic surgery). If PPE is penetrated by blood or any contaminated material, the item must be removed immediately or as soon as feasible. **The employer must provide and launder or dispose of all PPE at no cost to the employee.** Gloves must be worn when there is a reasonable anticipation of hand contact with potentially infectious material, including a patient's mucous membranes or nonintact skin. Disposable gloves must be changed as soon as possible after they become torn or punctured. Hands must be washed after gloves are removed. OSHA has revised the PPE standards, effective July 5, 1994, to include the requirement that the employer certify in writing that it has conducted a hazard assessment of the workplace to determine whether hazards are present that will necessitate the use of PPE. Also, verification that the employee has received and understood the PPE training is required.[4]

Housekeeping protocols: OSHA requires that all bins, cans, and similar receptacles, intended for reuse which have a reasonable likelihood for becoming contaminated, be inspected and decontaminated immediately or as soon as feasible upon visible contamination and on a regularly scheduled basis. Broken glass that may be contaminated must not be picked up directly with the hands. Mechanical means (eg, brush, dust pan, tongs, or forceps) must be used. Broken glass must be placed in a proper sharps container.

Employers are responsible for teaching appropriate clean-up procedures for the work area and personal protective equipment. A 1:10 dilution of household bleach is a popular and effective disinfectant. It is prudent for employers to maintain signatures or initials of employees who have been properly educated. If one does not have written proof of education of universal precautions teaching, then by OSHA standards, such education never happened.

Pre-exposure and postexposure protocols: OSHA's Final Rule includes the provision that employees, who are exposed to contamination, be offered the hepatitis B vaccine at no cost to the employee. Employees may decline; however, a declination form must be signed. The employee must be offered free vaccine if he/she changes his/her mind. Vaccination to prevent the transmission of hepatitis B in the healthcare setting is widely regarded as sound practice.[5] In the event of exposure, a confidential medical evaluation and follow-up must be offered at no cost to the employee. Follow-up must include collection and testing of blood from the source individual for HBV and HIV if permitted by state law if a blood sample is available. If a postexposure specimen must be specially drawn, the individual's consent is usually required. Some states may not require consent for testing of patient blood after accidental exposure. One must refer to state and/or local guidelines for proper guidance.

The employee follow-up must also include appropriate postexposure prophylaxis, counseling, and evaluation of reported illnesses. The employee has the right to decline baseline blood collection and/or testing. If the employee gives consent for the collection but not the testing, the sample must be preserved for 90 days in the event that the employee changes his/her mind within that time. Confidentiality related to blood testing must be ensured. **The employer does not have the right to know the results** of the testing of either the source individual or the exposed employee.

MANAGEMENT OF HEALTHCARE WORKER EXPOSURES TO HBV, HCV, AND HIV

Likelihood of transmission of HIV-1 from occupational exposure is 0.2% per parenteral exposure (eg, needlestick) to blood from HIV infected patients. Factors that increase risk for occupational transmission include advanced stages of HIV in source patient, hollow bore needle puncture, a poor state of health or inexperience of healthcare worker (HCW). After first aid is initiated, the healthcare worker should report exposure to a supervisor and to the institution's occupational medical service for evaluation. All parenteral exposures should be treated equally until they can be evaluated by the occupational medicine service, who will then determine the actual risk of exposure. Counselling regarding risk of exposure, antiviral prophylaxis, plans for follow up, exposure prevention, sexual activity, and providing emotional support and response to concerns are necessary to support the exposed healthcare worker. Additional information should be provided to healthcare workers who are pregnant or planning to become pregnant.

Immediate actions include aggressive first aid at the puncture site (eg, scrubbing site with povidone-iodine solution or soap and water for 10 minutes) or at mucus membrane site (eg, saline irrigation of eye for 15 minutes), followed by immediate reporting to the hospital's occupational medical service where a thorough investigation should be performed, including identification of the source, type of exposure, volume of inoculum, timing of exposure, extent of injury, appropriateness of first aid, as well as psychological status of the healthcare worker. HIV serologies should be performed on the healthcare worker and HIV risk counselling should begin at this point. Although the data are not clear, antiviral prophylaxis may be offered to healthcare workers who are parenterally or mucous membrane exposed. If used, antiretroviral prophylaxis should be initiated within 1-2 hours after exposure.

Factors to Consider in Assessing the Need for Follow-up of Occupational Exposures

- **Type of exposure**
  - Percutaneous injury
  - Mucous membrane exposure
  - Nonintact skin exposure
  - Bites resulting in blood exposure to either person involved
- **Type and amount of fluid/tissue**
  - Blood
  - Fluids containing blood
  - Potentially infectious fluid or tissue (semen; vaginal secretions; and cerebrospinal, synovial, pleural, peritoneal, pericardial, and amniotic fluids)
  - Direct contact with concentrated virus
- **Infectious status of source**
  - Presence of HB_sAg
  - Presence of HCV antibody
  - Presence of HIV antibody
- **Susceptibility of exposed person**
  - Hepatitis B vaccine and vaccine response status
  - HBV, HCV, HIV immune status

Evaluation of Occupational Exposure Sources

Known sources

- Test known sources for HB_sAg, anti-HCV, and HIV antibody
  - Direct virus assays for routine screening of source patients are **not** recommended
  - Consider using a rapid HIV-antibody test
  - If the source person is **not** infected with a bloodborne pathogen, baseline testing or further follow-up of the exposed person is **not** necessary
- For sources whose infection status remains unknown (eg, the source person refuses testing), consider medical diagnoses, clinical symptoms, and history of risk behaviors
- Do not test discarded needles for bloodborne pathogens

Unknown sources

- For unknown sources, evaluate the likelihood of exposure to a source at high risk for infection
  - Consider the likelihood of bloodborne pathogen infection among patients in the exposure setting

OCCUPATIONAL EXPOSURE TO BLOODBORNE PATHOGENS (STANDARD / UNIVERSAL PRECAUTIONS) *(Continued)*

Recommended Postexposure Prophylaxis for Exposure to Hepatitis B Virus

Vaccination and Antibody Response Status of Exposed Workers[1]	Treatment		
	Source HB_sAg[2]-Positive	Source HB_sAg[2] -Negative	Source Unknown or Not Available for Testing
Unvaccinated	HBIG[3] x 1 and initiate HB vaccine series[4]	Initiate HB vaccine series	Initiate HB vaccine series
Previously vaccinated			
Known responder[5]	No treatment	No treatment	No treatment
Known nonresponder[6]	HBIG x 1 and initiate revaccination or HBIG x 2[7]	No treatment	If known high risk source, treat as if source was HB_sAg-positive
Antibody response unknown	Test exposed person for anti-HB_s[8] 1. If adequate,[5] no treatment is necessary 2. If inadequate,[6] administer HBIG x 1 and vaccine booster	No treatment	Test exposed person for anti-HB_s 1. If adequate,[4] no treatment is necessary 2. If inadequate,[4] administer vaccine booster and recheck titer in 1-2 months

[1]Persons who have previously been infected with HBV are immune to reinfection and do not require postexposure prophylaxis.

[2]Hepatitis B surface antigen.

[3]Hepatitis B immune globulin; dose is 0.06 mL/kg intramuscularly.

[4]Hepatitis B vaccine.

[5]A responder is a person with adequate levels of serum antibody to HB_sAg (ie, anti-HB_s ≥10 mIU/mL).

[6]A nonresponder is a person with inadequate response to vaccination (ie, serum anti-HB_s <10 mIU/mL).

[7]The option of giving one dose of HBIG and reinitiating the vaccine series is preferred for nonresponders who have not completed a second 3-dose vaccine series. For persons who previously completed a second vaccine series but failed to respond, two doses of HBIG are preferred.

[8]Antibody to HB_sAg.

Recommended HIV Postexposure Prophylaxis for Percutaneous Injuries

Exposure Type	Infection Status of Source				
	HIV-Positive Class 1[1]	HIV-Positive Class 2[1]	Unknown HIV Status[2]	Unknown Source[3]	HIV-Negative
Less severe[4]	Recommend basic 2-drug PEP	Recommend expanded 3-drug PEP	Generally, no PEP warranted; however, consider basic 2-drug PEP[5] for source with HIV risk factors[6]	Generally, no PEP warranted; however, consider basic 2 drug PEP[5] in settings where exposure to HIV-infected persons is likely	No PEP warranted
More severe[7]	Recommend expanded 3-drug PEP	Recommend expanded 3-drug PEP	Generally, no PEP warranted; however consider basic 2-drug PEP[5] for source with HIV risk factors[6]	Generally, no PEP warranted; however, consider basic 2 drug PEP[5] in settings where exposure to HIV-infected persons is likely	No PEP warranted

[1]HIV-Positive, Class 1 – asymptomatic HIV infection or known low viral load (eg, <1500 RNA copies/mL). HIV-Positive Class 2 – symptomatic HIV infection, AIDS, acute seroconversion, or known high viral load. If drug resistance is a concern, obtain expert consultation. Initiation of postexposure prophylaxis (PEP) should not be delayed pending expert consultation, and, because expert consultation alone cannot substitute for face-to-face counseling, resources should be available to provide immediate evaluation and follow-up care for all exposures.

[2]Source of unknown HIV status (eg, deceased source person with no samples available for HIV testing).

[3]Unknown source (eg, a needle from a sharps disposal container).

[4]Less severe (eg, solid needle and superficial injury).

[5]The designation "consider PEP" indicates the PEP is optional and should be based on an individualized decision between the exposed person and the treating clinician.

[6]If PEP is offered and taken and the source is later determined to be HIV-negative, PEP should be discontinued.

[7]More severe (eg, large-bore hollow needle, deep puncture, visible blood on device, or needle used in patient's artery or vein).

OCCUPATIONAL EXPOSURE TO BLOODBORNE PATHOGENS (STANDARD / UNIVERSAL PRECAUTIONS) *(Continued)*

Recommended HIV Postexposure Prophylaxis for Mucous Membrane Exposures and Nonintact Skin[1] Exposures

Exposure Type	Infection Status of Source				
	HIV-Positive Class 1[2]	HIV-Positive Class 2[2]	Unknown HIV Status[3]	Unknown Source[4]	HIV-Negative
Small volume[5]	Consider basic 2-drug PEP[6]	Recommend basic 2-drug PEP	Generally, no PEP warranted; however, consider basic 2-drug PEP[6] for source with HIV risk factors[7]	Generally, no PEP warranted; however, consider basic 2-drug PEP[6] in settings where exposure to HIV-infected persons is likely	No PEP warranted
Large volume[8]	Recommend basic 2-drug PE	Recommend expanded 3-drug PEP	Generally, no PEP warranted; however consider basic 2-drug PEP[6] for source with HIV risk factors[7]	Generally, no PEP warranted; however, consider basic 2-drug PEP[6] in settings where exposure to HIV-infected persons is likely	No PEP warranted

[1]For skin exposures, follow-up is indicated only if there is evidence of compromised skin integrity (eg, dermatitis, abrasion, or open wound).

[2]HIV-Positive, Class 1 – asymptomatic HIV infection or known low viral load (eg, <1500 RNA copies/mL). HIV-Positive Class 2 – symptomatic HIV infection, AIDS, acute seroconversion, or known high viral load. If drug resistance is a concern, obtain expert consultation. Initiation of postexposure prophylaxis (PEP) should not be delayed pending expert consultation, and, because expert consultation alone cannot substitute for face-to-face counseling, resources should be available to provide immediate evaluation and follow-up care for all exposures.

[3]Source of unknown HIV status (eg, deceased source person with no samples available for HIV testing).

[4]Unknown source (eg, splash from inappropriately disposed blood).

[5]Small volume (eg, a few drops).

[6]The designation "consider PEP" indicates the PEP is optional and should be based on an individualized decision between the exposed person and the treating clinician.

[7]If PEP is offered and taken and the source is later determined to be HIV-negative, PEP should be discontinued.

[8]Large volume (eg, major blood splash).

Situations for Which Expert[1] Consultation for HIV Postexposure Prophylaxis Is Advised

- **Delayed (ie, later than 24-36 hours) exposure report**
  - The interval after which there is no benefit from postexposure prophylaxis (PEP) is undefined
- **Unknown source (eg, needle in sharps disposal container or laundry)**
  - Decide use of PEP on a case-by-case basis
  - Consider the severity of the exposure and the epidemiologic likelihood of HIV exposure
  - Do not test needles or sharp instruments for HIV
- **Known or suspected pregnancy in the exposed person**
  - Does not preclude the use of optimal PEP regimens
  - Do not deny PEP solely on the basis of pregnancy
- **Resistance of the source virus to antiretroviral agents**
  - Influence of drug resistance on transmission risk is unknown
  - Selection of drugs to which the source person's virus is unlikely to be resistant is recommended, if the source person's virus is unknown or suspected to be resistant to ≥1 of the drugs considered for the PEP regimen
  - Resistance testing of the source person's virus at the time of the exposure is not recommended
- **Toxicity of the initial PEP regimen**
  - Adverse symptoms, such as nausea and diarrhea, are common with PEP
  - Symptoms can often be managed without changing the PEP regimen by prescribing antimotility and/or antiemetic agents
  - Modification of dose intervals (ie, administering a lower dose of drug more frequently throughout the day, as recommended by the manufacturer), in other situations, might help alleviate symptoms

[1]Local experts and/or the National Clinicians' Postexposure Prophylaxis Hotline (PEPline 1-888-448-4911).

OCCUPATIONAL EXPOSURE TO BLOODBORNE PATHOGENS (STANDARD / UNIVERSAL PRECAUTIONS) *(Continued)*

Occupational Exposure Management Resources

National Clinicians' Postexposure Prophylaxis Hotline (PEPline) Run by University of California-San Francisco/San Francisco General Hospital staff; supported by the Health Resources and Services Administration Ryan White CARE Act, HIV/AIDS Bureau, AIDS Education and Training Centers, and CDC	Phone: (888) 448-4911 Internet: http://www.ucsf.edu/hivcntr
Needlestick! A website to help clinicians manage and document occupational blood and body fluid exposures. Developed and maintained by the University of California, Los Angeles (UCLA), Emergency Medicine Center, UCLA School of Medicine, and funded in part by CDC and the Agency for Healthcare Research and Quality.	Internet: http://www.needlestick.mednet.ucla.edu
Hepatitis Hotline	Phone: (888) 443-7232 Internet: http://www.cdc.gov/hepatitis
Reporting to CDC: Occupationally acquired HIV infections and failures of PEP	Phone: (800) 893-0485
HIV Antiretroviral Pregnancy Registry	Phone: (800) 258-4263 Fax: (800) 800-1052 Address: 1410 Commonwealth Drive, Suite 215 Wilmington, NC 28405 Internet: http://www.glaxowellcome.com/preg_reg/antiretroviral
Food and Drug Administration Report unusual or severe toxicity to antiretroviral agents	Phone: (800) 332-1088 Address: MedWatch HF-2, FDA 5600 Fishers Lane Rockville, MD 20857 Internet: http://www.fda.gov/medwatch
HIV/AIDS Treatment Information Service	Internet: http://www.aidsinfo.nih.gov

Management of Occupational Blood Exposures

Provide immediate care to the exposure site

- Wash wounds and skin with soap and water
- Flush mucous membranes with water

Determine risk associated with exposure by:

- Type of fluid (eg, blood, visibly bloody fluid, other potentially infectious fluid or tissue, and concentrated virus)
- Type of exposure (ie, percutaneous injury, mucous membrane or nonintact skin exposure, and bites resulting in blood exposure)

Evaluate exposure source

- Assess the risk of infection using available information
- Test known sources for HB_sAg, anti-HCV, and HIV antibody (consider using rapid testing)
- For unknown sources, assess risk of exposure to HBV, HCV, or HIV infection
- Do not test discarded needle or syringes for virus contamination

Evaluate the exposed person

- Assess immune status for HBV infection (ie, by history of hepatitis B vaccination and vaccine response)

Give PEP for exposures posing risk of infection transmission

- HBV: See Recommended Postexposure Prophylaxis for Exposure to Hepatitis B Virus Table
- HCV: PEP not recommended
- HIV: See Recommended HIV Postexposure Prophylaxis for Percutaneous Injuries Table and Recommended HIV Postexposure Prophylaxis for Mucous Membrane Exposures and Nonintact Skin Exposures Table
  - Initiate PEP as soon as possible, preferably within hours of exposure
  - Offer pregnancy testing to all women of childbearing age not known to be pregnant
  - Seek expert consultation if viral resistance is suspected
  - Administer PEP for 4 weeks if tolerated

Perform follow-up testing and provide counseling

- Advise exposed persons to seek medical evaluation for any acute illness occurring during follow-up

HBV exposures

- Perform follow-up anti-HB_s testing in persons who receive hepatitis B vaccine
  - Test for anti-HB_s 1-2 months after last dose of vaccine
  - Anti-HB_s response to vaccine cannot be ascertained if HBIG was received in the previous 3-4 months

HCV exposures

- Perform baseline and follow-up testing for anti-HCV and alanine amino-transferase (ALT) 4-6 months after exposures
- Perform HCV RNA at 4-6 months if earlier diagnosis of HCV infection is desired
- Confirm repeatedly reactive anti-HCV enzyme immunoassays (EIAs) with supplemental tests

HIV exposures

- Perform HIV antibody testing for at least 6 months postexposure (eg, at baseline, 6 weeks, 3 months, and 6 months)
- Perform HIV antibody testing if illness compatible with an acute retroviral syndrome occurs
- Advise exposed persons to use precautions to prevent secondary transmission during the follow-up period
- Evaluate exposed persons taking PEP within 72 hours after exposure and monitor for drug toxicity for at least 2 weeks

OCCUPATIONAL EXPOSURE TO BLOODBORNE PATHOGENS (STANDARD / UNIVERSAL PRECAUTIONS) *(Continued)*

Basic and Expanded HIV Postexposure Prophylaxis Regimens

Basic Regimens

- Zidovudine (Retrovir™; ZDV; AZT) + Lamivudine (Epivir™; 3TC); available as Combivir™
  - ZDV: 600 mg daily, in two or three divided doses, and
  - 3TC: 150 mg twice daily

Alternative Basic Regimens

- Lamivudine (3TC) + Stavudine (Zerit™; d4T)
  - 3TC: 150 mg twice daily, and
  - d4T: 40 mg twice daily (if body weight is <60 kg, 30 mg twice daily)
- Didanosine (Videx™, chewable/dispersible buffered tablet; Videx™ EC, delayed-release capsule; ddI) + Stavudine (d4T)
  - ddI: 400 mg daily on an empty stomach (if body weight is <60 kg, 125 mg twice daily)
  - d4T: 40 mg twice daily (if body weight is <60 kg, 30 mg twice daily)

Expanded Regimen

Basic regimen plus one of the following:

- Indinavir (Crixivan™; IDV)
  - 800 mg every 8 hours, on an empty stomach
- Nelfinavir (Viracept™; NFV)
  - 750 mg three times daily, with meals or snack, or
  - 1250 mg twice daily, with meals or snack
- Efavirenz (Sustiva™; EFV)
  - 600 mg daily, at bedtime
  - Should not be used during pregnancy because of concerns about teratogenicity
- Abacavir (Ziagen™; ABC); available at Trizivir™, a combination of ZDV, 3TC, and ABC
  - 300 mg twice daily

Antiretroviral Agents for Use at PEP Only With Expert Consultation

- Ritonavir (Norvir™; RTV)
- Amprenavir (Agenerase™; AMP)
- Delavirdine (Rescriptor™; DLV)
- Lopinavir/Ritonavir (Kaletra™)
  - 400/100 mg twice daily

Antiretroviral Agents Generally Not Recommended for Use as PEP

- Nevirapine (Viramune™; NVP)
  - 200 mg daily for 2 weeks, then 200 mg twice daily

HAZARDOUS COMMUNICATION

Communication regarding the dangers of bloodborne infections through the use of labels, signs, information, and education is required. Storage locations (eg, refrigerators and freezers, waste containers) that are used to store, dispose of, transport, or ship blood or other potentially infectious materials require labels. The label background must be red or bright orange with the biohazard design and the word biohazard in a contrasting color. The label must be part of the container or affixed to the container by permanent means.

Education provided by a qualified and knowledgeable instructor is mandated. The sessions for employees must include:

- accessible copies of the regulation
- general epidemiology of bloodborne diseases
- modes of bloodborne pathogen transmission
- an explanation of the exposure control plan and a means to obtain copies of the written plan
- an explanation of the tasks and activities that may involve exposure
- the use of exposure prevention methods and their limitations (eg, engineering controls, work practices, personal protective equipment)
- information on the types, proper use, location, removal, handling, decontamination, and disposal of personal protective equipment)
- an explanation of the basis for selection of personal protective equipment
- information on the HBV vaccine, including information on its efficacy, safety, and method of administration and the benefits of being vaccinated (ie, the employee must understand that the vaccine and vaccination will be offered free of charge)
- information on the appropriate actions to take and persons to contact in an emergency involving exposure to blood or other potentially infectious materials
- an explanation of the procedure to follow if an exposure incident occurs, including the method of reporting the incident
- information on the postexposure evaluation and follow-up that the employer is required to provide for the employee following an exposure incident
- an explanation of the signs, labels, and color coding
- an interactive question-and-answer period

RECORD KEEPING

The OSHA Final Rule requires that the employer maintain both education and medical records. The medical records must be kept confidential and be maintained for the duration of employment plus 30 years. They must contain a copy of the employee's HBV vaccination status and postexposure incident information. Education records must be maintained for 3 years from the date the program was given.

OSHA has the authority to conduct inspections without notice. Penalties for cited violation may be assessed as follows:

Serious violations. In this situation, there is a substantial probability of death or serious physical harm, and the employer knew, or should have known, of the hazard. A violation of this type carries a mandatory penalty of up to $7000 for each violation.

Other-than-serious violations. The violation is unlikely to result in death or serious physical harm. This type of violation carries a discretionary penalty of up to $7000 for each violation.

Willful violations. These are violations committed knowingly or intentionally by the employer and have penalties of up to $70,000 per violation with a minimum of $5000 per violation. If an employee dies as a result of a willful violation, the responsible party, if convicted, may receive a personal fine of up to $250,000 and/or a 6-month jail term. A corporation may be fined $500,000.

Large fines frequently follow visits to laboratories, physicians' offices, and healthcare facilities by OSHA Compliance Safety and Health Offices (CSHOS). Regulations are vigorously enforced. A working knowledge of the final rule and implementation of appropriate policies and practices is imperative for all those involved in the collection and analysis of medical specimens.

Effectiveness of universal precautions in averting exposure to potentially infectious materials has been documented.[7] Compliance with appropriate rules, procedures, and policies, including reporting exposure incidents, is a matter of personal professionalism and prudent self-preservation.

Footnotes

1. Henderson DK, Fahey BJ, Willy M, et al, "Risk for Occupational Transmission of Human Immunodeficiency Virus Type 1 (HIV-1) Associated With Clinical Exposures. A Prospective Evaluation," *Ann Intern Med*, 1990, 113(10):740-6.
2. Niu MT and Margolis HS, "Moving Into a New Era of Government Regulation: Provisions for Hepatitis B Vaccine in the Workplace, *Clin Lab Manage Rev*, 1989, 3:336-40.
3. Bruning LM, "The Bloodborne Pathogens Final Rule — Understanding the Regulation," *AORN Journal*, 1993, 57(2):439-40.
4. "Rules and Regulations," *Federal Register*, 1994, 59(66):16360-3.
5. Schaffner W, Gardner P, and Gross PA, "Hepatitis B Immunization Strategies: Expanding the Target," *Ann Intern Med*, 1993, 118(4):308-9.
6. Fahey BJ, Beekmann SE, Schmitt JM, et al, "Managing Occupational Exposures to HIV-1 in the Healthcare Workplace," *Infect Control Hosp Epidemiol*, 1993, 14(7):405-12.
7. Wong ES, Stotka JL, Chinchilli VM, et al, "Are Universal Precautions Effective in Reducing the Number of Occupational Exposures Among Healthcare Workers?" *JAMA*, 1991, 265(9):1123-8.

References

Buehler JW and Ward JW, "A New Definition for AIDS Surveillance," *Ann Intern Med*, 1993, 118(5):390-2.

Brown JW and Blackwell H, "Complying With the New OSHA Regs, Part 1: Teaching Your Staff About Biosafety," *MLO*, 1992, 24(4)24-8. Part 2: "Safety Protocols No Lab Can Ignore," 1992, 24(5):27-9. Part 3: "Compiling Employee Safety Records That Will Satisfy OSHA," 1992, 24(6):45-8.

Department of Labor, Occupational Safety and Health Administration, "Occupational Exposure to Bloodborne Pathogens; Final Rule (29 CFR Part 1910.1030), "*Federal Register*, December 6, 1991, 64004-182.

Gold JW, "HIV-1 Infection: Diagnosis and Management," *Med Clin North Am*, 1992, 76(1):1-18.

"Hepatitis B Virus: A Comprehensive Strategy for Eliminating Transmission in the United States Through Universal Childhood Vaccination," Recommendations of the Immunization Practices Advisory Committee (ACIP), *MMWR Morb Mortal Wkly Rep*, 1991, 40(RR-13):1-25.

"Mortality Attributable to HIV Infection/AIDS — United States", *MMWR Morb Mortal Wkly Rep*, 1991, 40(3):41-4.

National Committee for Clinical Laboratory Standards, "Protection of Laboratory Workers From Infectious Disease Transmitted by Blood, Body Fluids, and Tissue," NCCLS Document M29-T, Villanova, PA: NCCLS, 1989, 9(1).

"Nosocomial Transmission of Hepatitis B Virus Associated With a Spring-Loaded Fingerstick Device — California," *MMWR Morb Mortal Wkly Rep*, 1990, 39(35):610-3.

Polish LB, Shapiro CN, Bauer F, et al, "Nosocomial Transmission of Hepatitis B Virus Associated With the Use of a Spring-Loaded Fingerstick Device," *N Engl J Med*, 1992, 326(11):721-5.

"Recommendations for Preventing Transmission of Human Immunodeficiency Virus and Hepatitis B Virus to Patients During Exposure-Prone Invasive Procedures," *MMWR Morb Mortal Wkly Rep*, 1991, 40(RR-8):1-9.

"Update: Acquired Immunodeficiency Syndrome — United States," *MMWR Morb Mortal Wkly Rep*, 1992, 41(26):463-8.

"Update: Transmission of HIV Infection During an Invasive Dental Procedure — Florida," *MMWR Morb Mortal Wkly Rep*, 1991, 40(2):21-7, 33.

"Update: Universal Precautions for Prevention of Transmission of Human Immunodeficiency Virus, Hepatitis B Virus, and Other Bloodborne Pathogens in Healthcare Settings," *MMWR Morb Mortal Wkly Rep*, 1988, 37(24):377-82, 387-8.

"U.S. Public Health Service Guidelines for the Management of Occupational Exposures to HBV, HCV, and HIV and Recommendations for Postexposure Prophylaxis," *MMWR Morb Mortal Wkly Rep*, 2001, 50(RR-11).

IMMUNIZATIONS (VACCINES)[1]

Vaccine	Use
Anthrax Vaccine (Adsorbed) BioThrax™	Immunization against *Bacillus anthracis*. Recommended for individuals who may come in contact with animal products which come from anthrax endemic areas and may be contaminated with *Bacillus anthracis* spores; recommended for high-risk persons such as veterinarians and other handling potentially infected animals. Routine immunization for the general population is not recommended. The Department of Defense is implementing an anthrax vaccination program against the biological warfare agent anthrax, which will be administered to all active duty and reserve personnel.
BCG Vaccine TheraCys®; TICE® BCG	Immunization against tuberculosis and immunotherapy for cancer; treatment of bladder cancer. BCG vaccine is not routinely recommended for use in the U.S. for prevention of tuberculosis. BCG vaccine is strongly recommended for infants and children with negative tuberculin skin tests who: are at high risk of intimate and prolonged exposure to persistently untreated or ineffectively treated patients with infectious pulmonary tuberculosis, and; cannot be removed from the source of exposure, and; cannot be placed on long-term preventive therapy; are continuously exposed with tuberculosis who have bacilli resistant to isoniazid and rifampin; BCG is also recommended for tuberculin-negative infants and children in groups in which the rate of new infections exceeds 1% per year and for whom the usual surveillance and treatment programs have been attempted but are not operationally feasible
Diphtheria Antitoxin	Treatment of diphtheria (neutralizes unbound toxin, available from CDC)
Diphtheria and Tetanus Toxoid Decavac™	Diphtheria and tetanus toxoids adsorbed for pediatric use (DT): Infants and children through 6 years of age: Active immunity against diphtheria and tetanus when pertussis vaccine is contraindicated Tetanus and diphtheria toxoids adsorbed for adult use (Td) (Decavac™): Children ≥7 years of age and Adults: Active immunity against diphtheria and tetanus; tetanus prophylaxis in wound management
Diphtheria, Tetanus Toxoids, and Acellular Pertussis Vaccine Daptacel™; Infanrix®; Tripedia®	Active immunization against diphtheria, tetanus, and pertussis from age 6 weeks through seventh birthday
Diphtheria, Tetanus Toxoids, Acellular Pertussis Vaccine and *Haemophilus influenzae* b Conjugate Vaccine (Combined) TriHIBit®	Active immunization of children 15-18 months of age for prevention of diphtheria, tetanus, pertussis, and invasive disease caused by *H. influenzae* type b
Diphtheria, Tetanus Toxoids, Acellular Pertussis, Hepatitis B (Recombinant), and Poliovirus (Inactivated) Vaccine Pediarix™	Combination vaccine for the active immunization against diphtheria, tetanus, pertussis, hepatitis B virus (all known subtypes), and poliomyelitis (caused by poliovirus types 1, 2, and 3)

Vaccine	Use
Haemophilus b Conjugate Vaccine ActHIB®; HibTITER®; PedvaxHIB®	Routine immunization of children 2 months to 5 years of age against invasive disease caused by *H. influenzae*. Unimmunized children ≥5 years of age with a chronic illness known to be associated with increased risk of *Haemophilus influenzae* type b disease, specifically, persons with anatomic or functional asplenia or sickle cell anemia or those who have undergone splenectomy, should receive Hib vaccine. *Haemophilus* b conjugate vaccines are not indicated for prevention of bronchitis or other infections due to *H. influenzae* in adults; adults with specific dysfunction or certain complement deficiencies who are at especially high risk of *H. influenzae* type b infection (HIV-infected adults); patients with Hodgkin's disease (vaccinated at least 2 weeks before the initiation of chemotherapy or 3 months after the end of chemotherapy)
Haemophilus b Conjugate and Hepatitis B Vaccine Comvax®	Immunization against invasive disease caused by *H. influenzae* type b and against infection caused by all known subtypes of hepatitis B virus in infants 8 weeks to 15 months of age born of HB_sAg-negative mothers. Infants born of HB_sAg-positive mothers or mothers of unknown HB_sAg status should receive hepatitis B immune globulin and hepatitis B vaccine (recombinant) at birth and should complete the hepatitis B vaccination series given according to a particular schedule.
Hepatitis A Vaccine Havrix®; VAQTA®	For populations desiring protection against hepatitis A or for populations at high risk of exposure to hepatitis A virus (travelers to developing countries, household and sexual contacts of persons infected with hepatitis A), child day care employees, illicit drug users, patients with chronic liver disease, male homosexuals, institutional workers (eg, institutions for the mentally and physically handicapped persons, prisons), and healthcare workers who may be exposed to hepatitis A virus (eg, laboratory employees); protection lasts for approximately 15 years.
Hepatitis A Inactivated and Hepatitis B (Recombinant) Vaccine Twinrix®	Active immunization against disease caused by hepatitis A virus and hepatitis B virus (all known subtypes) in populations desiring protection against or at high risk of exposure to these viruses. Populations include travelers to areas of intermediate/high endemicity for **both** HAV and HBV; those at increased risk of HBV infection due to behavioral or occupational factors; patients with chronic liver disease; laboratory workers who handle live HAV and HBV; healthcare workers, police, and other personnel who render first-aid or medical assistance; workers who come in contact with sewage; employees of day care centers and correctional facilities; patients/staff of hemodialysis units; male homosexuals; patients frequently receiving blood products; military personnel; users of injectable illicit drugs; close household contacts of patients with hepatitis A and hepatitis B infection.
Hepatitis B Immune Globulin BayHepB™; Nabi-HB®	Provide prophylactic passive immunity to hepatitis B infection to those individuals exposed; newborns of mothers known to be hepatitis B surface antigen positive; hepatitis B immune globulin is not indicated for treatment of active hepatitis B infections and is ineffective in the treatment of chronic active hepatitis B infection.
Hepatitis B Vaccine Engerix-B®; Recombivax HB®	Immunization against infection caused by all known subtypes of hepatitis B virus, in individuals considered at high risk of potential exposure to hepatitis B virus or HB_sAg-positive materials
Immune Globulin (Intramuscular) BayGam®	Household and sexual contacts of persons with hepatitis A, measles, varicella, and possibly rubella; travelers to high-risk areas outside tourist routes; staff, attendees, and parents of diapered attendees in day-care center outbreaks. For travelers, IG is not an alternative to careful selection of foods and water; immune globulin can interfere with the antibody response to parenterally administered live virus vaccines. Frequent travelers should be tested for hepatitis A antibody, immune hemolytic anemia, and neutropenia (with ITP, I.V. route is usually used).

IMMUNIZATIONS (VACCINES)[1] *(Continued)*

Vaccine	Use
Influenza Virus Vaccine FluMist™; Fluvirin®; Fluzone®	Provide active immunity to influenza virus strains contained in the vaccine. Groups at increased risk for influenza-related complications: Persons ≥65 years of age; residents of nursing homes and other chronic-care facilities that house persons of any age with chronic medical conditions; adults and children with chronic disorders of the pulmonary or cardiovascular systems, including children with asthma; adults and children who have required regular medical follow-up or hospitalization during the preceding year because of chronic metabolic diseases (including diabetes mellitus), renal dysfunction, hemoglobinopathies, or immunosuppression (including immunosuppression caused by medications); children and adolescents (6 months to 18 years of age) who are receiving long-term aspirin therapy and therefore, may be at risk for developing Reye's syndrome after influenza; women who will be pregnant during the influenza season; children 6-23 months of age. Vaccination is also recommended for persons 50-64 years of age, close contacts of children 0-23 months of age, and healthy persons who may transmit influenza to those at risk.
Japanese Encephalitis Virus Vaccine (Inactivated) JE-VAX®	Active immunization against Japanese encephalitis for persons 1 year of age and older who plan to spend 1 month or more in endemic areas in Asia, especially persons traveling during the transmission season or visiting rural areas; consider vaccination for shorter trips to epidemic areas or extensive outdoor activities in rural endemic areas; elderly (>55 years of age) individuals should be considered for vaccination, since they have increased risk of developing symptomatic illness after infection; those planning travel to or residence in endemic areas should consult the Travel Advisory Service (Central Campus) for specific advice
Measles, Mumps, and Rubella Vaccines (Combined) M-M-R® II	Measles, mumps, and rubella prophylaxis
Measles Virus Vaccine (Live) Attenuvax®	Adults born before 1957 are generally considered to be immune. All those born in or after 1957 without documentation of live vaccine on or after first birthday, physician-diagnosed measles, or laboratory evidence of immunity should be vaccinated, ideally with two doses of vaccine separated by no less than 1 month. For those previously vaccinated with one dose of measles vaccine, revaccination is recommended for students entering colleges and other institutions of higher education, for healthcare workers at the time of employment, and for international travelers who visit endemic areas. MMR is the vaccine of choice if recipients are likely to be susceptible to rubella and/or mumps as well as to measles. Persons vaccinated between 1963 and 1967 with a killed measles vaccine, followed by live vaccine within 3 months, or with a vaccine of unknown type should be revaccinated with live measles virus vaccine.
Meningococcal Polysaccharide Vaccine (Groups A, C, Y, and W-135) Menomune®- A/C/Y/W-135	Provide active immunity to meningococcal serogroups contained in the vaccine; prevention and control of outbreaks of serogroup C meningococcal disease; recommended for use in: Immunization of persons ≥2 years of age in epidemic or endemic areas as might be determined in a population delineated by neighborhood, school, dormitory, or other reasonable boundary; the prevalent serogroup in such a situation should match a serogroup in the vaccine; individuals at particular high-risk include persons with terminal component complement deficiencies and those with anatomic or functional asplenia. Travelers visiting areas of a country that are recognized as having hyperendemic or epidemic meningococcal disease. Vaccinations should be considered for household or institutional contacts of persons with meningococcal disease as an adjunct to appropriate antibiotic chemoprophylaxis as well as medical and laboratory personnel at risk of exposure to meningococcal disease
Mumps Virus Vaccine (Live/ Attenuated) Mumpsvax®	Mumps prophylaxis by promoting active immunity; **Note:** Trivalent measles-mumps-rubella (M-M-R® II) vaccine is the preferred agent for most children and many adults. Persons born prior to 1957 are generally considered immune and need not be vaccinated.

Vaccine	Use
Plague Vaccine	Selected travelers to countries reporting cases for whom avoidance of rodents and fleas is impossible; all laboratory and field personnel working with *Yersinia pestis* organisms possibly resistant to antimicrobials; those engaged in *Yersinia pestis* aerosol experiments or in field operations in areas with enzootic plague where regular exposure to potentially infected wild rodents, rabbits, or their fleas cannot be prevented. Prophylactic antibiotics may be indicated following definite exposure, whether or not the exposed persons have been vaccinated.
Pneumococcal Conjugate Vaccine (7-Valent) Prevnar®	Immunization of infants and toddlers against *Streptococcus pneumoniae* infection caused by serotypes included in the vaccine
Pneumococcal Polysaccharide Vaccine (Polyvalent) Pneumovax® 23	Children >2 years of age and adults who are at increased risk of pneumococcal disease and its complications because of underlying health conditions (including patients with cochlear implants); older adults, including all those ≥ 65 years of age. Current Advisory Committee on Immunization Practices (ACIP) guidelines recommend pneumococcal 7-valent conjugate vaccine (PCV7) be used for children 2-23 months of age and, in certain situations, children up to 59 months of age
Poliovirus Vaccine (Inactivated) IPOL®	As the global eradication of poliomyelitis continues, the risk for importation of wild-type poliovirus into the U.S. decreases dramatically. To eliminate the risk for vaccine-associated paralytic poliomyelitis (VAPP), an all-IPV schedule is recommended for routine childhood vaccination in the United States. All children should receive four doses of IPV (at age 2 months, age 4 months, between ages 6-18 months, and between ages 4-6 years). Oral poliovirus vaccine (OPV), if available, may be used only for the following special circumstances: Mass vaccination campaigns to control outbreaks of paralytic polio; unvaccinated children who will be traveling within 4 weeks to areas where polio is endemic or epidemic; children of parents who do not accept the recommended number of vaccine injections; these children may receive OPV only for the third or fourth dose or both; in this situation, healthcare providers should administer OPV only after discussing the risk for VAPP with parents or caregivers. OPV supplies are expected to be very limited in the United States after inventories are depleted. ACIP reaffirms its support for the global eradication initiative and use of OPV as the vaccine of choice to eradicate polio where it is endemic.
Rabies Immune Globulin (Human) BayRab®; Imogam®	Part of postexposure prophylaxis of persons with rabies exposure who lack a history of pre-exposure or postexposure prophylaxis with rabies vaccine or a recently documented neutralizing antibody response to previous rabies vaccination; it is preferable to give RIG with the first dose of vaccine, but it can be given up to 8 days after vaccination.
Rabies Virus Vaccine Imovax® Rabies; RabAvert®	Pre-exposure immunization: Vaccinate persons with greater than usual risk due to occupation or avocation including veterinarians, rangers, animal handlers, certain laboratory workers, and persons living in or visiting countries for longer than 1 month where rabies is a constant threat. Postexposure prophylaxis: If a bite from a carrier animal is unprovoked, if it is not captured and rabies is present in that species and area, administer rabies immune globulin (RIG) and the vaccine as indicated

IMMUNIZATIONS (VACCINES)[1] *(Continued)*

Vaccine	Use
Rh_o(D) Immune Globulin BayRho-D® Full-Dose; BayRho-D® Mini-Dose; MICRhoGAM®; RhoGAM®; Rhophylac®; WinRho SDF®	Suppression of Rh isoimmunization: Use in the following situations when an Rh_o(D)-negative individual is exposed to Rh_o(D)-positive blood: During delivery of an Rh_o(D)-positive infant; abortion; amniocentesis; chorionic villus sampling; ruptured tubal pregnancy; abdominal trauma; transplacental hemorrhage. Used when the mother is Rh_o(D) negative, the father of the child is either Rh_o(D) positive or Rh_o(D) unknown, the baby is either either Rh_o(D) positive or Rh_o(D) unknown. Transfusion: Suppression of Rh isoimmunization in Rh_o(D)-negative female children and female adults in their childbearing years transfused with Rh_o(D) antigen-positive RBCs or blood components containing Rh_o(D) antigen-positive RBCs. Treatment of idiopathic thrombocytopenic purpura (ITP): Used in the following nonsplenectomized Rh_o(D) positive individuals: Children with acute or chronic ITP, adults with chronic ITP, children and adults with ITP secondary to HIV infection
Rubella Virus Vaccine (Live) Meruvax® II	Selective active immunization against rubella; vaccination is routinely recommended for persons from 12 months of age to puberty. All adults, both male and female, lacking documentation of live vaccine on or after first birthday, or laboratory evidence of immunity (particularly women of childbearing age and young adults who work in or congregate in hospitals, colleges, and on military bases) should be vaccinated. Susceptible travelers should be vaccinated. **Note:** Trivalent measles-mumps-rubella (M-M-R® II) vaccine is the preferred agent for most children and many adults.
Smallpox Vaccine Dryvax®	Active immunization against vaccinia virus, the causative agent of smallpox. The ACIP recommends vaccination of laboratory workers at risk of exposure from cultures or contaminated animals which may be a source of vaccinia or related Orthopoxviruses capable of causing infections in humans (monkeypox, cowpox, or variola). Revaccination is recommended every 10 years.
Tetanus Antitoxin	Tetanus prophylaxis or treatment of active tetanus only when tetanus immune globulin (TIG) is not available; tetanus immune globulin (Hyper-Tet®) is the preferred tetanus immunoglobulin for the treatment of active tetanus. May be given concomitantly with tetanus toxoid adsorbed when immediate treatment is required, but active immunization is desirable.
Tetanus Immune Globulin (Human) BayTet™	Passive immunization against tetanus; tetanus immune globulin is preferred over tetanus antitoxin for treatment of active tetanus; part of the management of an unclean wound in a person whose history of previous receipt of tetanus toxoid is unknown or who has received less than three doses of tetanus toxoid; elderly may require TIG more often than younger patients with tetanus infection due to declining antibody titers with age.
Tetanus Toxoid (Adsorbed)	Selective induction of active immunity against tetanus in selected patients.
Tetanus Toxoid (Fluid)	Indicated as booster dose in the active immunization against tetanus in the rare adult or child who is allergic to the aluminum adjuvant (a product containing adsorbed tetanus toxoid is preferred); not indicated for primary immunization
Typhoid Vaccine Typhim Vi®; Vivotif Berna®	Typhoid vaccine: Live, attenuated Ty21a typhoid vaccine should not be administered to immunocompromised persons, including those known to be infected with HIV. Parenteral inactivated vaccine is a theoretically safer alternative for this group. Parenteral: Promotes active immunity to typhoid fever for patients intimately exposed to a typhoid carrier or foreign travel to a typhoid fever endemic area Oral: For immunization of children >6 years of age and adults who expect intimate exposure of or household contact with typhoid fever, travelers to areas of world with risk of exposure to typhoid fever, and workers in microbiology laboratories with expected frequent contact with *S. typhi*

Vaccine	Use
Varicella Virus Vaccine Varivax®	Immunization against varicella in children ≥12 months of age and adults. The American Association of Pediatrics recommends that the chickenpox vaccine should be given to all healthy children between 12 months and 18 years; children between 12 months and 13 years who have not been immunized or who have not had chickenpox should receive 1 vaccination while children 13-18 years of age require 2 vaccinations 4-8 weeks apart; the vaccine has been added to the childhood immunization schedule for infants 12-28 months of age and children 11-12 years of age who have not been vaccinated previously or who have not had the disease; it is recommended to be given with the measles, mumps, and rubella (MMR) vaccine
Varicella-Zoster Immune Globulin (Human)	Passive immunization of susceptible immunodeficient patients after exposure to varicella; most effective if begun within 96 hours of exposure; there is no evidence VZIG modifies established varicella-zoster infections. **Restrict administration to those patients meeting the following criteria:** Neoplastic disease (eg, leukemia or lymphoma); congenital or acquired immunodeficiency; immunosuppressive therapy with steroids, antimetabolites or other immunosuppressive treatment regimens; newborn of mother who had onset of chickenpox within 5 days before delivery or within 48 hours after delivery; premature (≥28 weeks gestation) whose mother has no history of chickenpox; premature (<28 weeks gestation or ≤1000 g VZIG) regardless of maternal history. **One of the following types of exposure to chickenpox or zoster patient(s) may warrant administration:** Continuous household contact; playmate contact (>1 hour play indoors); hospital contact (in same 2-4 bedroom or adjacent beds in a large ward or prolonged face-to-face contact with an infectious staff member or patient); susceptible to varicella-zoster; age <15 years (administer to immunocompromised adolescents and adults and to other older patients on an individual basis).
Yellow Fever Vaccine YF-VAX®	Vaccinate selected persons traveling or living in areas where yellow fever infection exists

[1]Federal law requires that the date of administration, name of the vaccine manufacturer, lot number of vaccine, and the administering person's name, title, and address be entered into the patient's permanent medical record.

NORMAL BLOOD VALUES

Test	Range of Normal Values
Complete Blood Count (CBC)	
White blood cells	4,500-11,000
Red blood cells (male)	4.6-6.2 x 10^6 μL
Red blood cells (female)	4.2-5.4 x 10^6 μL
Platelets	150,000-450,000
Hematocrit (male)	40% to 54%
Hematocrit (female)	38% to 47%
Hemoglobin (male)	13.5-18 g/dL
Hemoglobin (female)	12-16 g/dL
Mean corpuscular volume (MCV)	80-96 μm^3
Mean corpuscular hemoglobin (MCH)	27-31 pg
Mean corpuscular hemoglobin concentration (MCHC)	32% to 36%
Differential White Blood Cell Count (%)	
Segmented neutrophils	56
Bands	3.0
Eosinophils	2.7
Basophils	0.3
Lymphocytes	34.0
Monocytes	4.0
Hemostasis	
Bleeding time (BT)	2-8 minutes
Prothrombin time (PT)	10-13 seconds
Activated partial thromboplastin time (aPTT)	25-35 seconds
Serum Chemistry	
Glucose (fasting)	70-110 mg/dL
Blood urea nitrogen (BUN)	8-23 mg/dL
Creatinine (male)	0.1-0.4 mg/dL
Creatinine (female)	0.2-0.7 mg/dL
Bilirubin, indirect (unconjugated)	0.3 mg/dL
Bilirubin, direct (conjugated)	0.1-1 mg/dL
Calcium	9.2-11 mg/dL
Magnesium	1.8-3 mg/dL
Phosphorus	2.3-4.7 mg/dL
Serum Electrolytes	
Sodium (Na^+)	136-142 mEq/L
Potassium (K^+)	3.8-5 mEq/L
Chloride (Cl^-)	95-103 mEq/L
Bicarbonate (HCO_3^-)	21-28 mmol/L
Serum Enzymes	
Alkaline phosphatase	20-130 IU/L
Alanine aminotransferase (ALT) (formerly called SGPT)	4-36 units/L
Aspartate aminotransferase (AST) (formerly called SGOT)	8-33 units/L
Amylase	16-120 Somogyi units/dL
Creatine kinase (CK) (male)	55-170 units/L
Creatine kinase (CK) (female)	30-135 units/L

DENTIFRICE PRODUCTS

Brand Name	Abrasive Ingredient	Therapeutic Ingredient	Foaming Agent
Aim® Baking Soda Gel	Hydrated silica, sodium bicarbonate	Sodium monofluorophosphate 0.7% (fluoride 0.14%)	Sodium lauryl sulfate
	Other Ingredients: Sorbitol and related polyols, water, glycerin, SD alcohol 38B, flavor, cellulose gum, sodium saccharin, blue #1, yellow #10		
Aim® Extra Strength Gel	Hydrated silica	Sodium monofluorophosphate 1.2%	Sodium lauryl sulfate
	Other Ingredients: Sorbitol, water, PEG-32, SD alcohol 38B, flavor, cellulose gum, sodium saccharin, sodium benzoate, blue #1, yellow #10		
Aim® Regular Strength	Hydrated silica	Sodium monofluorophosphate 0.8% (fluoride 0.14%)	Sodium lauryl sulfate
	Other Ingredients: Sorbitol and other related polyols, water, glycerin, SD alcohol 38B, flavor, cellulose gum, sodium saccharin, blue #1, yellow #10		
Aim® Tartar Control Gel	Hydrated silica	Sodium monofluorophosphate 0.8% (fluoride 0.14%)	Sodium lauryl sulfate
	Other Ingredients: Sorbitol and related polyols, water, glycerin, zinc citrate trihydrate, SD alcohol 38B, flavor, cellulose gum, sodium saccharin, blue #1, yellow #10		
Aquafresh® Baking Soda Toothpaste	Calcium carbonate, hydrated silica, sodium bicarbonate	Sodium monofluorophosphate	Sodium lauryl sulfate
	Other Ingredients: Calcium carrageenan, cellulose gum, colors, flavor, glycerin, PEG-8, sodium benzoate, sodium saccharin, sorbitol, titanium dioxide, water		
Aquafresh® Extra Fresh Toothpaste[1]	Hydrated silica, calcium carbonate	Sodium monofluorophosphate	Sodium lauryl sulfate
	Other Ingredients: Sorbitol, water, glycerin, PEG-8, titanium dioxide, cellulose gum, flavor, sodium saccharin, sodium benzoate, calcium carrageenan, colors		
Aquafresh® Extreme Clean®	Precipitated silica	Sodium fluoride 0.15%	Sodium lauryl sulfate
	Other Ingredients: Cocamidopropyl betaine, D&C red 30, flavor, PEG 8, sodium saccharin, sorbitol, iron oxide, titanium dioxide, water, xanthan gum		
Aquafresh® for Kids Toothpaste[1]	Hydrated silica, calcium carbonate	Sodium monofluorophosphate	Sodium lauryl sulfate
	Other Ingredients: Sorbitol, water, glycerin, PEG-8, titanium dioxide, cellulose gum, flavor, sodium saccharin, calcium carrageenan, sodium benzoate, colors		
Aquafresh® Gum Care Toothpaste	Hydrated silica, calcium carbonate	Sodium monofluorophosphate	Sodium lauryl sulfate
	Other Ingredients: Calcium carrageenan, cellulose gum, colors, flavor, PEG-8, sodium benzoate, sodium saccharin, sorbitol, titanium dioxide, water		
Aquafresh® Sensitive Toothpaste	Hydrated silica	Potassium nitrate, sodium fluoride	Sodium lauryl sulfate
	Other Ingredients: Colors, flavor, glycerin, sodium benzoate, sodium saccharin, sorbitol, titanium dioxide, water, xanthan gum		
Aquafresh® Tartar Control Toothpaste[1]	Hydrated silica	Sodium fluoride	Sodium lauryl sulfate
	Other Ingredients: Tetrapotassium pyrophosphate, tetrasodium pyrophosphate, sorbitol, glycerin, PEG-8, flavor, xanthan gum, sodium saccharin, sodium benzoate, colors, titanium dioxide, water		
Aquafresh® Triple Protection Toothpaste[1]	Hydrated silica, calcium carbonate	Sodium monofluorophosphate	Sodium lauryl sulfate
	Other Ingredients: PEG-8, sorbitol, cellulose gum, sodium benzoate, titanium dioxide, calcium carrageenan, flavor, sodium saccharin, colors, water		
Aquafresh® Whitening Gel or Toothpaste	Hydrated silica	Sodium fluoride	Sodium lauryl sulfate
	Other Ingredients: Colors, flavor, glycerin, PEG-8, sodium benzoate, sodium hydroxide, sodium saccharin, sodium tripolyphosphate, sorbitol, titanium dioxide, water, xanthan gum		
Arm & Hammer Advance Breath Care™ Cool Fresh Toothpaste	Calcium carbonate poloxamer 407, sodium bicarbonate	Sodium monofluorophosphate 0.76%	
	Other Ingredients: Water, glycerin, sodium citrate dihydrate, flavor, cellulose gum, cocamidopropyl betaine, zinc, citrate trihydrate, sodium saccharin, titanium dioxide		

DENTIFRICE PRODUCTS *(Continued)*

Brand Name	Abrasive Ingredient	Therapeutic Ingredient	Foaming Agent
Arm & Hammer Advance White™ Toothpaste for Sensitive Teeth	Silica, sodium bicarbonate	Sodium fluoride 0.243%, potassium nitrate 5%	
	Other Ingredients: Cellulose gum, cocamidopropyl betaine, flavor, glycerin, sorbitol, titanium dioxide, water		
Arm & Hammer Advance White™ with Baking Soda & Peroxide	Sodium bicarbonate, silica	Sodium fluoride	Sodium lauryl sulfate
	Other Ingredients: Flavor, PEG-8, poloxapol 1220, sodium carbonate peroxide, sodium lauroyl sarcosinate, sodium saccharin, tetrasodium pyrophosphate, water		
Arm & Hammer Advance White™ with Baking Soda Tartar Control	Sodium bicarbonate, hydrated silica	Sodium fluoride	Sodium lauryl sulfate
	Other Ingredients: Cellulose gum, flavor, glycerin, sodium lauroyl sarcosinate, sodium saccharin, sorbitol, tetrasodium pyrophosphate, titanium dioxide, water		
Arm & Hammer Advance White™ with Gel Micro-Polishers Gel	Sodium bicarbonate, hydrated silica	Sodium fluoride 0.24%	Sodium lauryl sulfate
	Other Ingredients: Cellulose gum, FD&C blue #1, FD&C yellow #5, flavor, glycerin, sodium lauroyl sarcosinate, sodium saccharin, sorbitol, tetrasodium pyrophosphate, water		
Arm & Hammer Dental Care Tartar Control	Sodium bicarbonate	Sodium fluoride 0.24%	Sodium lauryl sulfate
	Other Ingredients: Water, glycerin, tetrasodium pyrophosphate, PEG-8, sodium saccharin, flavors, cellulose gum, sodium lauroyl sarcosinate		
Arm & Hammer Enamel Care™	Hydrated silica	Sodium fluoride 0.24%	Sodium lauryl sulfate
	Other Ingredients: Glycerin, sodium bicarbonate, water, sorbitol, calcium sulfate, sodium sulfate, flavor, dipotassium phosphate, sodium carbonate, sodium saccharin, cellulose gum, xanthan gum, methylparaben, propylparaben, blue 1, may contain sodium lauroyl sarcosinate		
Arm & Hammer Multi-Benefit PeroxiCare Baking Soda & Peroxide Toothpaste	Sodium bicarbonate, sodium carbonate peroxide, silica	Sodium fluoride 0.24%	Sodium lauryl sulfate
	Other Ingredients: PEG/PPG-38/8 copolymer, PEG/PPG-116/66 copolymer, water, flavor, sodium saccharin, sodium lauroyl sarcosinate, hydrogenated starch hydrolysate, gum Arabic, D&C green #5		
Arm & Hammer PeroxiCare Baking Soda & Peroxide	Sodium bicarbonate, silica	Sodium fluoride 0.24%	Sodium lauryl sulfate
	Other Ingredients: PEG/PPG-38/8 copolymer, PEG/PPG-116/66 copolymer, milled sodium percarbonate, sodium lauroyl sarcosinate, sodium saccharin, flavor, water		
Arm & Hammer P.M.™ Bold Mint	Sodium bicarbonate, silica	Sodium fluoride	Sodium lauryl sulfate
	Other Ingredients: Flavor, PEG-B, poloxapol 1220, sodium percarbonate, sodium lauroyl sarcosinate, sodium saccharin, water, zinc citrate trihydrate		
Arm & Hammer P.M.™ Fresh Mint	Aluminum oxide, hydrated silica	Sodium monofluorophosphate	Sodium lauryl sulfate
	Other Ingredients: Cellulose gum, flavor, glycerin, sodium saccharin, sorbital, water, zinc citrate trihydrate		
Biotene® Antibacterial Dry Mouth Toothpaste	Hydrated silica, calcium pyrophosphate	Lactoperoxidase, glucose oxidase, lysozyme, sodium monofluorophosphate (0.76%)	
	Other Ingredients: Sorbitol, glycerin, xylitol, isoceteth-20, cellulose gum, flavor, sodium benzoate, beta-d-glucose, potassium thiocyanate		
Close-Up® Baking Soda Toothpaste (mint)	Hydrated silica, sodium bicarbonate	Sodium monofluorophosphate 0.79% (fluoride 0.15%)	Sodium lauryl sulfate
	Other Ingredients: Sorbitol and related polyols, water, glycerin, SD alcohol 38B, flavor, cellulose gum, sodium saccharin, sodium benzoate, red #33, red #40, titanium dioxide		

Brand Name	Abrasive Ingredient	Therapeutic Ingredient	Foaming Agent
Close-Up® Classic Red Gel	Hydrated silica	Sodium monofluorophosphate 0.8% (fluoride 0.14%)	Sodium lauryl sulfate
	Other Ingredients: Sorbitol and related polyols, water, glycerin, SD alcohol 38B, flavor, cellulose gum, sodium saccharin, sodium chloride, red #33, red #40		
Close-Up® Cool Mint Gel	Hydrated silica	Sodium monofluorophosphate 0.79% (fluoride 0.15%)	Sodium lauryl sulfate
	Other Ingredients: Sorbitol, water, glycerin, SD alcohol 38B, flavor, cellulose gum, sodium saccharin, polysorbate 20, blue #1, mica, red #33, titanium dioxide		
Close-Up® Original Red Whitening Toothpaste	Hydrated silica	Sodium monofluorophosphate 0.8% (fluoride 0.14%)	Sodium lauryl sulfate
	Other Ingredients: Sorbitol and related polyols, water, glycerin, SD alcohol 38B, flavor, cellulose gum, sodium saccharin, sodium chloride, red #30 lake, titanium dioxide, blue #1		
Close-Up® Tartar Control Gel (mint)	Hydrated silica	Sodium monofluorophosphate 0.79% (fluoride 0.15%)	Sodium lauryl sulfate
	Other Ingredients: Sorbitol and related polyols, water, glycerin, zinc citrate trihydrate, SD alcohol 38B, flavor, cellulose gum, sodium saccharin, red #33, red #40, **caffeine free**		
Close-Up® Tartar Control Whitening Toothpaste	Hydrated silica	Sodium monofluorophosphate 0.8% (fluoride 0.14%)	Sodium lauryl sulfate
	Other Ingredients: Sorbitol and related polypols, water, glycerin, SD alcohol 38B, flavor, zinc citrate trihydrate, cellulose gum, sodium saccharin, titanium dioxide, blue #1, yellow #10		
Colgate® Baking Soda & Peroxide Tartar Control Toothpaste[1]	Hydrated silica, sodium bicarbonate	Sodium monofluorophosphate 0.76%	Sodium lauryl sulfate
	Other Ingredients: Glycerin, propylene glycol, water, pentasodium triphosphate, tetrasodium pyrophosphate, titanium dioxide, flavor, sodium hydroxide, calcium peroxide, sodium saccharin, carrageenan, cellulose gum, FD&C blue #1, D&C yellow #10		
Colgate® Baking Soda & Peroxide Whitening Toothpaste[1]	Hydrated silica, sodium bicarbonate, aluminum oxide	Sodium monofluorophosphate 0.76%	Sodium lauryl sulfate
	Other Ingredients: Glycerin, polypylene glycol, water, pentasodium triphosphate, tetrasodium pyrophosphate, titanium dioxide, flavor, sodium hydroxide, calcium peroxide, sodium saccharin, carrageenan, cellulose gum, **dietetically sucrose free**		
Colgate® Baking Soda Tartar Control Gel or Toothpaste	Hydrated silica, sodium bicarbonate	Sodium fluoride 0.243%	Sodium lauryl sulfate
	Other Ingredients: Glycerin, tetrasodium pyrophosphate, PVM/MA copolymer, cellulose gum, flavor, sodium saccharin, sodium hydroxide, titanium dioxide (paste), FD&C blue #1, D&C yellow #10 (gel), **dietetically sucrose free**		
Colgate® Cavity Protection Toothpaste	Dicalcium phosphate dihydrate	Sodium monofluorophosphate 0.15%	Sodium lauryl sulfate
	Other Ingredients: Water, glycerin, sorbitol, cellulose gum, flavor, tetrapotassium pyrophosphate, sodium saccharin		
Colgate® Herbal White	Hydrated silica	Sodium monofluorophosphate 0.76%	Sodium lauryl sulfate
	Other Ingredients: Calcium carbonate, water, sorbitol, flavor, sodium carbonate, sodium hydroxide, cellulose gum, sodium saccharin, carrageenan, xanthan gum, parabens, balm mint extract, fennel extract, FD&C blue No. 1, D&C yellow No. 10		
Colgate® Junior Gel[1]	Hydrated silica	Sodium fluoride 0.243%	Sodium lauryl sulfate
	Other Ingredients: Sorbitol, water, PEG-12, flavor, tetrasodium pyrophosphate, cellulose gum, sodium saccharin, mica, titanium dioxide, colorants, **dietetically sucrose free**		
Colgate® Platinum™ Whitening Toothpaste[1]	Silica, aluminum oxide	Sodium monofluorophosphate	Sodium lauryl sulfate
	Other Ingredients: Water, hydrated silica, sorbitol, glycerin, PEG-12, tetrapotassium pyrophosphate, PVM/MA copolymer, flavor, sodium hydroxide, sodium saccharin, titanium dioxide		

DENTIFRICE PRODUCTS *(Continued)*

Brand Name	Abrasive Ingredient	Therapeutic Ingredient	Foaming Agent
Colgate® Platinum™ Whitening with Baking Soda Toothpaste[1]	Sodium bicarbonate, aluminum oxide	Sodium monofluorophosphate 0.76%	Sodium lauryl sulfate
	Other Ingredients: Water, glycerin, PEG-12, tetrapotassium pyrophosphate, PVM/MA copolymer, flavor, sodium hydroxide, sodium saccharin, titanium dioxide, cellulose gum		
Colgate® Sensitive Maximum Strength Toothpaste	Hydrated silica, sodium bicarbonate	Potassium nitrate 5%, stannous fluoride 0.45%	Sodium lauryl sulfate
	Other Ingredients: Glycerin and/or sorbitol, water, PEG-40 castor oil, PEG-12, poloxamer 407, sodium citrate, flavor, titanium dioxide, sodium hydroxide, cellulose gum, xanthan gum, sodium saccharin, stannous chloride, citric acid, tetrasodium pyrophosphate, FD&C Blue No. 1		
Colgate® Sensitive Plus Whitening	Hydrated silica, Sodium bicarbonate	Potassium nitrate 5% antisensitivity (FDA required amount), Stannous Fluoride 0.45% (0.15% w/v fluoride ion)	Sodium lauryl sulfate
	Other Ingredients: Glycerin and/or sorbitol, water, PEG-40 castor oil, PEG-12, poloxamer 405, sodium citrate, flavor, titanium dioxide, sodium hydroxide, cellulose gum, xanthan gum, sodium saccharin, stannous chloride, citric acid, tetrasodium pyrophosphate, mica, FD&C blue No. 1, D&C yellow No. 10		
Colgate® Simply White®	Silica	Sodium fluoride 0.24%	Sodium lauryl sulfate
	Other Ingredients: Water, glycerin, sorbitol, PEG 12, pentasodium triphosphate, flavor, carbomer, hydrogen peroxide, sodium hydroxide, tetrasodium pyrophosphate, PVM/MA copolymer, cellulose gum, sodium saccharin, sodium magnesium silicate, xanthan gum, carrageenan, phosphoric acid, manganese gluconate, butylated hydroxytoluene, titanium dioxide, FD&C blue No. 1		
Colgate® Tartar Control Micro Cleansing Gel or Toothpaste[1]	Hydrated silica	Sodium fluoride 0.243%	Sodium lauryl sulfate
	Other Ingredients: Water, sorbitol, glycerin, PEG-12, tetrasodium pyrophosphate, PVM/MA copolymer, cellulose gum, flavor, sodium hydroxide, titanium dioxide, sodium saccharin, carrageenan, **dietetically sucrose free**		
Colgate® Tartar Control Plus Whitening	Hydrated silica, aluminum oxide	Sodium monofluorophosphate 0.76%	Sodium lauryl sulfate
	Other Ingredients: Water, sorbitol, glycerin, pentasodium triphosphate, tetrasodium pyrophosphate, PVM/MA copolymer, cellulose gum, flavor, sodium hydroxide, titanium dioxide, sodium saccharin, carrageenan		
Colgate® Toothpaste[1]	Dicalcium phosphate dihydrate	Sodium monofluorophosphate 0.76%	Sodium lauryl sulfate
	Other Ingredients: Glycerin, cellulose gum, tetrasodium pyrophosphate, sodium saccharin, flavor, **dietetically sucrose free**		
Colgate® Total® Advanced Fresh Gel	Hydrated silica	Sodium fluoride 0.24%, triclosan 0.3%	Sodium lauryl sulfate
	Other Ingredients: Water, glycerin, sorbitol, PVM/MA copolymer, flavor, cellulose gum, sodium hydroxide, propylene glycol, carrageenan, sodium saccharin, FD&C blue No. 1, D&C yellow No. 10		
Colgate Total® Toothpaste	Hydrated silica	Sodium fluoride 0.243%, triclosan 0.3%	Sodium lauryl sulfate
	Other Ingredients: Water, glycerin, sorbitol, PVM/MA copolymer, cellulose gum, flavor, sodium hydroxide, propylene glycol, carrageenan, sodium saccharin, titanium dioxide		
Colgate Total® Fresh Stripe Toothpaste	Hydrated silica	Sodium fluoride 0.243%, triclosan 0.3%	Sodium lauryl sulfate
	Other Ingredients: Water, glycerin, sorbitol, PVM/MA copolymer, cellulose gum, flavor, sodium hydroxide, propylene glycol, carrageenan, sodium saccharin, mica, titanium dioxide, FD&C blue #1, D&C yellow #10		
Colgate® Winterfresh Gel[1]	Hydrated silica	Sodium fluoride 0.243%	Sodium lauryl sulfate
	Other Ingredients: Sorbitol, water, PEG-12, flavor, tetrasodium pyrophosphate, cellulose gum, sodium saccharin, FD&C blue #1, **dietetically sucrose free**		

Brand Name	Abrasive Ingredient	Therapeutic Ingredient	Foaming Agent
Crest® Baking Soda Tartar Protection Gel or Toothpaste (mint)[1]	Hydrated silica, sodium bicarbonate	Sodium fluoride 0.243%	Sodium lauryl sulfate
	Other Ingredients: Water, glycerin, sorbitol, tetrasodium pyrophosphate, PEG-6, flavor, cellulose gum, sodium saccharin, titanium dioxide (paste), FD&C blue #1 (gel), disodium pyrophosphate, tetrapotassium pyrophosphate, carbomer 956, xanthan gum, FD&C yellow #5 (gel)		
Crest® Cavity Protection with Baking Soda Gel or Toothpaste[1] (mint)	Hydrated silica, sodium bicarbonate	Sodium fluoride 0.243%	Sodium lauryl sulfate
	Other Ingredients: Sorbitol, water, glycerin, sodium carbonate, flavor, cellulose gum, sodium saccharin, titanium dioxide (paste), FD&C blue #1 (gel)		
Crest® Cavity Protection Gel (cool mint)[1]	Hydrated silica	Sodium fluoride 0.243%	Sodium lauryl sulfate
	Other Ingredients: Sorbitol, water, trisodium phosphate, flavor, sodium phosphate, xanthan gum, sodium saccharin, carbomer 956, FD&C blue #1, carbomer 940A		
Crest® Cavity Protection Toothpaste[1] (icy mint or regular)	Hydrated silica	Sodium fluoride 0.243%	Sodium lauryl sulfate
	Other Ingredients: Sorbitol, water, glycerin (mint), trisodium phosphate, flavor, sodium phosphate, cellulose gum (mint), xanthan gum (regular), sodium saccharin, carbomer 956, titanium dioxide, FD&C blue #1. carbomer 940A		
Crest® Extra Whitening Gel or Toothpaste	Hydrated silica	Sodium fluoride 0.15%	Sodium lauryl sulfate, poloxamer 407
	Other Ingredients: Sorbitol, water, glycerin, tetrasodium pyrophosphate, sodium carbonate, carboxymethylcellulose sodium, titanium dioxide, carnauba wax, sodium saccharin, flavor, FD&C blue #1, FD&C yellow #5, PEG-6, sodium bicarbonate[2]		
Crest® for Kids Cavity Protection Gel	Hydrated silica	Sodium fluoride 0.243%	Sodium lauryl sulfate
	Other Ingredients: Sorbitol, water, trisodium phosphate, sodium phosphate, xanthan gum, flavor, sodium saccharin, carbomer 956, mica, titanium dioxide, FD&C blue #1		
Crest® Gum Care Gel or Toothpaste	Hydrated silica	Stannous fluoride 0.454%	Sodium lauryl sulfate
	Other Ingredients: Sorbitol, water, stannous chloride, titanium dioxide (paste), flavor, sodium hydroxide, sodium saccharin, sodium carrageenan, FD&C blue #1 (gel), sodium gluconate, hydroxyethylcellulose		
Crest® Multicare Gel or Toothpaste (cool mint, fresh mint)	Hydrated silica, sodium bicarbonate	Sodium fluoride 0.243%	Sodium lauryl sulfate
	Other Ingredients: Tetrasodium pyrophosphate, xylitol, water, glycerin, PEG-6, poloxamer 407, sodium carbonate, flavor, cellulose gum, xanthan gum, sodium saccharin, titanium dioxide, FD&C blue #1, FD&C yellow #5 (cool mint)		
Crest® Sensitivity Protection Toothpaste[1] (mild mint)	Hydrated silica	Potassium nitrate 5%, sodium fluoride 0.15%	Sodium lauryl sulfate
	Other Ingredients: Water, glycerin, sorbitol, trisodium phosphate, cellulose gum, flavor, xanthan gum, sodium saccharin, titanium dioxide, **dye free**		
Crest® Tartar Protection Gel[1] (fresh mint, smooth mint)		Sodium fluoride 0.243%	Sodium lauryl sulfate
	Other Ingredients: Water, sorbitol, glycerin, tetrapotassium pyrophosphate, PEG-6, disodium pyrophosphate, tetrasodium pyrophosphate, flavor, xanthan gum, sodium saccharin, carbomer 956, FD&C blue #1, FD&C yellow #5 (smooth mint)		
Crest® Tartar Protection Toothpaste[1] (original flavor)	Silica	Sodium fluoride 0.243%	Sodium lauryl sulfate
	Other Ingredients: Water, sorbitol, glycerin, tetrapotassium pyrophosphate, PEG-6, disodium pyrophosphate, tetrasodium pyrophosphate, flavor, xanthan gum, sodium saccharin, carbomer 956, titanium dioxide, FD&C blue #1		
Crest® Vivid White™	Hydrated silica	Sodium fluoride 0.243%	Sodium lauryl sulfate
	Other ingredients: Glycerin, water, sorbitol, sodium hexametaphosphate, propylene glycol, flavor, PEG-12, cocamidopropyl betaine, carbomer 956, sodium saccharin, poloxamer 407, polyethylene oxide, xanthan gum, sodium hydroxide, cellulose gum, titanium dioxide		

DENTIFRICE PRODUCTS *(Continued)*

Brand Name	Abrasive Ingredient	Therapeutic Ingredient	Foaming Agent
Crest® Whitening Expressions Extreme Herbal Mint	Hydrated silica	Sodium fluoride 0.243%	Sodium lauryl sulfate
	Other ingredients: Sorbitol, water, glycerin, tetrasodium pyrophosphate, PEG-6, flavor, disodium pyrophosphate, xanthan gum, sodium saccharin, carbomer 956, sucralose, polyethylene, titanium dioxide, blue 1 aluminum lake, yellow 11 aluminum lake		
Crest® Whitening Expressions Fresh Citrus Breeze	Hydrated silica	Sodium fluoride 0.243%	Sodium lauryl sulfate
	Other ingredients: Sorbitol, water, glycerin, tetrasodium pyrophosphate, PEG-6, flavor, disodium pyrophosphate, xanthan gum, sodium saccharin, carnuba wax, carbomer 956, sucralose, titanium dioxide, yellow 6		
Crest® Whitening Plus Scope®	Hydrated silica	Sodium fluoride 0.243% (0.15% w/v fluoride ion)	Sodium lauryl sulfate
	Other ingredients: Water, sorbitol, glycerin, tetrapotassium pyrophosphate, PEG-6, disodium pyrophosphate, tetrasodium pyrophosphate, flavor, alcohol (1.14%), xanthan gum, sodium saccharin, carbomer 956, polysorbate 80, sodium benzoate, cetylpyridinium chloride, benzoic acid, domiphen bromide (.0002 w/v%)		
Dr. Tichenor's Toothpaste	Hydrated silica	Sodium fluoride	Sodium lauryl sulfate
	Other Ingredients: Water, glycerin, sorbitol, insoluble sodium metaphosphate, peppermint oil, cellulose gum, sodium saccharin, sodium phosphate, titanium dioxide, magnesium aluminum silicate, **dye free**		
Enamelon® All-Family Toothpaste	Hydrated silica	Sodium fluoride (fluoride 0.14%)	Sodium lauryl sulfate
	Other Ingredients: Water, glycerin, sorbitol, monoammonium phosphate, calcium sulfate, xanthan gum, flavor, PEG-60 hydrogenated castor oil, sodium saccharin, ammonium chloride, cellulose gum, titanium dioxide, magnesium chloride, methylparaben, propylparaben, FD&C blue #1		
First Teeth™ Baby Gel		Lactoperoxidase 0.7 units/g, lactoferrin, glucose oxidase	Sodium lauryl sulfate
	Other Ingredients: Water, glycerin, sorbitol, pectin, xylitol, flavor, aloe vera, propylene glycol		
Fluoride Foam™[1,3]	**Ingredients:** Fluoride 1.23% (from sodium fluoride and hydrogen fluoride), water, phosphoric acid, poloxamer, sodium saccharin, flavor		
Fluorigard® Anti-Cavity Liquid [1,3]	**Ingredients:** Sodium fluoride 0.05%, ethyl alcohol, pluronic F108 and F127, sweetener, flavor, glycerin, sorbitol, preservatives, **dye free**, **gluten free**		
Gleem® Toothpaste	Hydrated silica	Sodium fluoride 0.243%	Sodium lauryl sulfate
	Other Ingredients: Sorbitol, water, trisodium phosphate, flavors, sodium phosphate, xanthan gum, sodium saccharin, carbomer 956, titanium dioxide, **dye free**		
Listerine® Essential Care Gel	Hydrated silica	Anticavity: Sodium monofluorophosphate 0.76% (0.13% W/V fluoride ion Antiplaque/ Antigingivitis: Eucalyptol 0.738%, menthol 0.340%, methyl salicylate 0.480%, thymol 0.511%	Sodium lauryl sulfate
	Other Ingredients: Water, sorbitol, glycerin, flavors, cellulose gum, sodium saccharin, phosphoric acid, FD&C blue #1, D&C yellow #10, sodium phosphate, benzoic acid, PEG-32, and xanthan gum		
Listerine® Gel or Toothpaste (cool mint)	Hydrated silica	Sodium monofluorophosphate	Sodium lauryl sulfate
	Other Ingredients: Water, sorbitol, glycerin, flavors, cellulose gum, sodium saccharin, phosphoric acid, FD&C blue #1, D&C yellow #10, sodium phosphate, benzoic acid, titanium dioxide (paste), xanthan gum		
Listerine® Tartar Control Gel or Toothpaste (cool mint)	Hydrated silica	Sodium fluoride	Sodium lauryl sulfate
	Other Ingredients: Water, sorbitol, glycerin, PEG-32, flavor, cellulose gum, sodium saccharin, tetrapotassium pyrophosphate, FD&C blue #1, D&C yellow #10, titanium dioxide (paste)		

Brand Name	Abrasive Ingredient	Therapeutic Ingredient	Foaming Agent
Mentadent® Advanced Whitening Gel or Toothpaste	Hydrated silica, sodium bicarbonate	Sodium fluoride 0.15%	Sodium lauryl sulfate, hydrogen peroxide
	Other Ingredients: Zinc citrate trihydrate, water, sorbitol, glycerin, poloxamer 407, PEG-32, SD alcohol 38B, flavor, cellulose gum, sodium saccharin, phosphoric acid, blue #1, titanium dioxide		
Mentadent® Gum Care Gel or Toothpaste	Hydrated silica, sodium bicarbonate	Sodium fluoride 0.24% (fluoride 0.15%)	Sodium lauryl sulfate, hydrogen peroxide
	Other Ingredients: Zinc citrate trihydrate (1.8%), water, sorbitol, glycerin, poloxamer 407, PEG-32, SD alcohol 38B, flavor, cellulose gum, sodium saccharin, menthol, methyl salicylate, phosphoric acid, green #3, titanium dioxide		
Mentadent® Sensitive Plus™	Hydrated silica, sodium bicarbonate	Potassium nitrate (5%), sodium fluoride	Sodium lauryl sulfate, hydrogen peroxide
	Other Ingredients: Water, glycerin, sorbitol, poloxamer 407, PEG-32, SD alcohol, cellulose gum, sodium saccharin, phosphoric acid, blue #1, titanium dioxide		
Mentadent® Tartar Control Gel or Toothpaste	Hydrated silica, sodium bicarbonate	Sodium fluoride 0.24%	Sodium lauryl sulfate, hydrogen peroxide
	Other Ingredients: Water, sorbitol, glycerin, poloxamer 407, PEG-32, zinc citrate, SD alcohol 38B, flavor, cellulose gum, sodium saccharin, phosphoric acid, blue #1, titanium dioxide, menthol		
Mentadent® with Baking Soda & Peroxide Gel or Toothpaste[1]	Hydrated silica, sodium bicarbonate	Sodium fluoride 0.24% (fluoride 0.15%)	Sodium lauryl sulfate, hydrogen peroxide
	Other Ingredients: Water, sorbitol, glycerin, poloxamer 407, PEG-32, SD alcohol 38B, flavor, cellulose gum, sodium saccharin, phosphoric acid, blue #1, titanium dioxide		
My First Colgate® Gel[1]	Hydrated silica	Sodium fluoride 0.243%	Sodium lauryl sulfate
	Other Ingredients: Water, sorbitol, PEG-12, flavor, tetrasodium pyrophosphate, cellulose gum, sodium saccharin, FD&C red #40, D&C red #33, **dietetically sucrose free**		
Natural Dentist™ Herbal Toothpaste & Gum Therapy, Cinnamon Flavored	Calcium carbonate	Sodium monofluorophosphate	Sodium lauryl sulfate
	Other Ingredients: Vegetable glycerin, aloe vera gel, sodium carrageenan, echinacea, goldenseal, calendula, bloodroot, bee propolis, grapefruit seed extract, sodium bicarbonate[2], cinnamon oil		
Natural Dentist™ Herbal Toothpaste & Gum Therapy, Mint Flavored	Calcium carbonate	Sodium monofluorophosphate	Sodium lauryl sulfate
	Other Ingredients: Vegetable glycerin, aloe vera gel, sodium carrageenan, echinacea, goldenseal, calendula, bloodroot, bee propolis, grapefruit seed extract, sodium bicarbonate[2], spearmint and peppermint oils		
Natural White® Toothpaste	Hydrated silica	Sodium fluoride	Sodium lauryl sulfate
	Other Ingredients: Sorbitol, water, glycerin, sodium benzoate, titanium dioxide, flavor, cellulose gum, **dietetically sucrose free**		
Natural White® Baking Soda Toothpaste	Calcium carbonate	Sodium monofluorophosphate	Sodium lauryl sulfate
	Other Ingredients: Sorbitol, water, glycerin, sodium bicarbonate[2], carrageenan, natural flavor, **dietetically sucrose free**		
Natural White® Fights Plaque Toothpaste	Hydrated silica	Sodium fluoride	Sodium lauryl sulfate
	Other Ingredients: Sorbitol, water, glycerin, sodium benzoate, titanium dioxide, flavor, cellulose gum, **dietetically sucrose free**		
Natural White® Sensitive Toothpaste	Hydrated silica	Sodium monofluorophosphate, potassium nitrate	Sodium lauryl sulfate
	Other Ingredients: Sorbitol, water, glycerin, flavor, FD&C red #40, sodium benzoate, titanium dioxide, sodium saccharin, **dietetically sucrose free**		
Natural White® Tartar Control Toothpaste	Hydrated silica	Sodium fluoride	Sodium lauryl sulfate
	Other Ingredients: Sorbitol, water, glycerin, xanthan gum, tetrapotassium pyrophosphate, titanium dioxide, cellulose gum, flavor, sodium benzoate, FD&C blue #1, D&C yellow #10, **dietetically sucrose free**		

DENTIFRICE PRODUCTS *(Continued)*

Brand Name	Abrasive Ingredient	Therapeutic Ingredient	Foaming Agent
Natural White® with Peroxide Gel		Hydrogen peroxide	
	Other Ingredients: Water, glycerin, flavor, dipotassium phosphate, sodium saccharin, phosphoric acid, poloxamer, **dietetically sucrose free**		
Oxyfresh Toothpaste	Fine chalk	Oxygene® (stabilized chlorine dioxide)	Sodium lauryl sulfate
	Other Ingredients: Purified deionized water, sorbitol, glycerin, carrageenan, natural flavors, sodium saccharin		
Orajel® Baby Tooth & Gum Cleanser Gel			
	Other Ingredients: Poloxamer 407 (2%), simethicone (0.12%), Microdent, carboxymethylcellulose, sodium, citric acid, flavor, glycerin, methylparaben, potassium sorbate, propylene glycol, propylparaben, water, sodium saccharin, sorbitol, **fluoride free**		
Orajel® Gold Sensitive Teeth Gel for Adults	Hydrated silica	Potassium nitrate 5%, sodium monofluorophosphate 0.2%	Sodium lauryl sulfate
	Other Ingredients: FD&C blue #1, flavor, glycerin, sodium lauroyl sarcosinate, sodium saccharin, sorbitol, xanthan gum		
Pearl Drops® Toothpolish Paste	Hydrated silica, calcium pyrophosphate, dicalcium phosphate, aluminum hydroxide	Sodium monofluorophosphate	Sodium lauryl sulfate
	Other Ingredients: Water, sorbitol, glycerin, PEG-12, flavor, cellulose gum, trisodium phosphate, sodium phosphate, sodium saccharin, **dietetically sucrose free, dye free**		
Pearl Drops® Toothpolish Gel	Hydrated silica	Sodium monofluorophosphate	Sodium lauryl sulfate
	Other Ingredients: Sorbitol, water, glycerin, PEG-12, flavor, cellulose gum, sodium saccharin, FD&C blue #1, FD&C yellow #10, **dietetically sucrose free**		
Pearl Drops® Whitening Extra Strength Paste	Hydrated silica, calcium pyrophosphate, dicalcium phosphate	Sodium monofluorophosphate	Sodium lauryl sulfate
	Other Ingredients: Water, sorbitol, glycerin, PEG-12, flavor, cellulose gum, trisodium phosphate, sodium phosphate, sodium saccharin, titanium dioxide, **dietetically sucrose free, dye free**		
Pearl Drops® Whitening Gel (icy cool mint)	Hydrated silica	Sodium monofluorophosphate	Sodium lauryl sulfate
	Other Ingredients: Sorbitol, water, glycerin, PEG-12, flavor, cellulose gum, sodium saccharin, FD&C blue #1, FD&C yellow #10, **dietetically sucrose free**		
Pepsodent® Baking Soda Toothpaste	Hydrated silica	Sodium monofluorophosphate 0.8% (fluoride (0.14%)	Sodium lauryl sulfate
	Other Ingredients: Sorbitol, water, sodium bicarbonate[2], PEG-32, SD alcohol 38B, flavor, cellulose gum, sodium saccharin, titanium dioxide		
Pepsodent® Original Toothpaste	Hydrated silica	Sodium monofluorophosphate 0.8% (fluoride 0.14%)	Sodium lauryl sulfate
	Other Ingredients: Sorbitol and related polyols, water, glycerin, SD alcohol 38B, flavor, cellulose gum, sodium saccharin, titanium dioxide		
Pepsodent® Tartar Control Toothpaste	Hydrated silica	Sodium monofluorophosphate 0.8% (fluoride 0.14%)	Sodium lauryl sulfate
	Other Ingredients: Sorbitol and related polyols, water, glycerin, SD alcohol 38B, zinc citrate trihydrate, flavor, cellulose gum, sodium saccharin, titanium dioxide, blue #1, yellow #1		
Pete & Pam™ Gel (premeasured strips)	Hydrated silica	Sodium monofluorophosphate 0.76%	Sodium lauroyl sarcosinate
	Other Ingredients: Sorbitol, water, glycerin, xanthan gum, polysorbate 20, sodium benzoate, pluronic P84, FD&C blue #1, FD&C red #33, FD&C yellow #5, flavor, xylitol		
Promise® Toothpaste	Dicalcium phosphate	Potassium nitrate, sodium monofluorophosphate	Sodium lauryl sulfate
	Other Ingredients: Water, hydroxyethylcellulose, flavor, sodium saccharin, methylparaben, propylparaben, D&C yellow #10, FD&C blue #1, glycerin, sorbitol, silicon dioxide, **dietetically sucrose free**		

Brand Name	Abrasive Ingredient	Therapeutic Ingredient	Foaming Agent
Q-Dent – The Antioxidant Toothpaste	Silica	Sodium fluoride 0.15%	Sodium lauryl sulfate
	Other Ingredients: Sorbitol, water, glycerin, tetrasodium pyrophosphate, tetrapotassium pyrophosphate, PEG-300, flavor, coenzyme Q_{10}, cellulose gum, titanium dioxide, sodium saccharin, FD&C blue #1		
Q-Dent – The Coenzyme Q_{10} Toothpaste	Silica	Sodium fluoride 0.15%	Sodium lauryl sulfate
	Other Ingredients: Sorbitol, water, glycerin, tetrasodium pyrophosphate, tetrapotassium pyrophosphate, PEG-300, flavor, coenzyme Q_{10}, cellulose gum, sodium saccharin, FD&C blue #1		
Reach Act Adult Anti-Cavity Treatment Liquid (cinnamon, mint)[3]	**Ingredients:** Sodium fluoride 0.05%, cetylpyridinium chloride, D&C red #33 (cinnamon), EDTA calcium disodium, FD&C yellow #5, flavor, glycerin, monobasic sodium phosphate, dibasic sodium phosphate, poloxamer 407, polysorbate 80 (cinnamon), polysorbate 20 (mint), propylene glycol, sodium benzoate, sodium saccharin, water, FD&C green #3 (mint), menthol (mint), methyl salicylate (mint), potassium sorbate (mint), **alcohol free**		
Reach Act for Kids[1,3]	**Ingredients:** Sodium fluoride 0.05%, cetylpyridinium chloride, D&C red #33, EDTA calcium disodium, flavor, glycerin, monobasic sodium phosphate, dibasic sodium phosphate, poloxamer 407, polysorbate 80, propylene glycol, sodium benzoate, sodium saccharin, water, **alcohol free**		
Rembrandt® Age-Defying Adult Toothpaste (original or mint)	Dicalcium orthophosphate, soft silica	Sodium monofluorophosphate (fluoride 0.15%)	
	Other Ingredients: Trihydroxy propane, perhydrol urea, aluminum oxide, acetylated pectins, sodium citrate, iridium, papain, carboxyl polymethylene, saccharin, propylene glycol, flavor		
Rembrandt® Age-Defying™ Whitening Toothpaste	Silica	Sodium fluoride 0.15%	Sodium lauryl sulfate
	Other Ingredients: Glycerin, dicalcium phosphate, acylated amylopectins, alumina oxide, carbamide peroxide, sodium citrate, flavor, papain, citric acid, EDTA, sodium saccharin		
Rembrandt® Age-Defying Adult Formula Mouthwash[3]	**Ingredients:** Sodium fluoride 0.05%, water, glycerin, hydrogen peroxide solution, sodium citrate, polyoxyl 40 hydrogenated castor oil, flavor, cocamidopropyl betaine, citric acid, sodium benzoate, sodium saccharin, sodium hydroxide, **alcohol free**		
Rembrandt® Daily Whitening Gel	Silica	Sodium monofluorophosphate (fluoride 0.15%)	Carbamide peroxide, sodium lauryl sulfate
	Other Ingredients: Glycerin, sodium citrate, carbopol, triethanolamine, flavor		
Rembrandt® Extra Whitening Fluoride Toothpaste for Canker Sore Sufferers	Silica	Sodium fluoride 0.15%	
	Other Ingredients: Dicalcium phosphate, glycerin, water, xylitol, alumina, sodium citrate, natural flavors, cocamidopropyl betaine, sodium carrageenan, papain, citric acid, sodium saccharin		
Rembrandt® Intense Stain Removal with Alumasil®	Silica	Sodium fluoride 0.15%	Sodium lauryl sulfate
	Other Ingredients: Dicalcium phosphate, glycerin, sorbitol, water, alumina, sodium citrate, cocamidopropyl betaine, flavor, papain, sodium carrageenan, citric acid, sodium saccharin, methylparaben, vitamin E, FD&C blue No. 1, FD&C yellow No. 5		
Rembrandt® Naturals Toothpaste	Silica	0.15% fluoride ion from sodium monofluorophosphate wt/vol%	None
	Other ingredients: Water (artesian springs), dicalcium phosphate (from monetite, a mineral), glycerine (by-product of vegetable soap), xylitol (from birch trees), cocamidopropyl betaine (from coconut), flavor (spearmint, peppermint, other natural sources), sodium citrate (from citrus fruit), stevia (from stevia plant), papain (from papaya plant), sodium carrageenan (from seaweed), citric acid and vitamin C (from citrus fruit), ginkgo extract, raspberry leaf extract. Also available containing aloe vera and echinacea or papaya and ginseng.		
Rembrandt® Plus with Active Dental Peroxide Superior Whitening Toothpaste Minty Fresh Flavor	Silica	Sodium fluoride 0.15%	Sodium lauryl sulfate
	Other Ingredients: Glycerin, carbamide peroxide, alumina, acylated amylopectins, flavors, sodium citrate, propylene glycol, cocamidopropyl betaine, papain, carbomer, sodium saccharin, EDTA		

DENTIFRICE PRODUCTS *(Continued)*

Brand Name	Abrasive Ingredient	Therapeutic Ingredient	Foaming Agent
Rembrandt® Whitening Baking Soda Toothpaste	Sodium bicarbonate, silica	Sodium monofluorophosphate (fluoride 0.15%)	Sodium lauryl sulfate
	Other Ingredients: Glycerin, sorbitol, alumina, water, sodium citrate, sodium carrageenan, papain, flavor, sodium hydroxide, FD&C blue #1, sodium saccharin		
Rembrandt® Whitening Canker Sore Prevention Toothpaste	Dicalcium phosphate, silica	Sodium monofluorophosphate (fluoride 0.15%)	
	Other Ingredients: Water, glycerin, xylitol, sodium citrate, natural flavors, sodium carrageenan, papain, citric acid, **dye free**		
Rembrandt® Whitening Natural Toothpaste	Dicalcium phosphate, silica	Sodium monofluorophosphate	
	Other Ingredients: Water, glycerin, xylitol, sodium citrate, natural flavors, sodium carrageenan, papain, citric acid, **dye free**		
Rembrandt® Whitening Sensitive Toothpaste	Dicalcium phosphate dihydrate	Potassium nitrate 5%, sodium monofluorophosphate 0.76%	Sodium lauryl sulfate
	Other Ingredients: Glycerin, sorbitol, water, alumina, papain, sodium citrate, flavor, carboxymethylcellulose sodium, sodium saccharin, methylparaben, FD&C red #40, citric acid		
Rembrandt® Whitening Toothpaste (mint or original)	Dicalcium phosphate dihydrate	Sodium monofluorophosphate 0.76%	Sodium lauryl sulfate
	Other Ingredients: Glycerin, sorbitol, water, alumina, sodium citrate, flavor, sodium carrageenan, papain, sodium saccharin, methylparaben, citric acid, FD&C blue #1, FD&C yellow #5		
Revelation® Toothpowder	Calcium carbonate		Vegetable soap powder
	Other Ingredients: Methyl salicylate, menthol, **dye free**		
Sensodyne® Baking Soda Toothpaste	Sodium bicarbonate, silica	Potassium nitrate, sodium fluoride	Sodium lauryl sulfate
	Other Ingredients: Water, glycerin, flavor, hydroxyethylcellulose, titanium dioxide, sodium saccharin, **dietetically sucrose free, dye free**		
Sensodyne® Cool Gel	Silica	Potassium nitrate, sodium fluoride	Sodium methyl cocoyl taurate
	Other Ingredients: Water, sorbitol, glycerin, sodium carboxymethylcellulose, flavor, sodium saccharin, FD&C blue #1, trisodium phosphate, **dietetically sucrose free**		
Sensodyne® Extra Whitening Toothpaste	Silica	Potassium nitrate, sodium monofluorophosphate	Sodium lauryl sulfate
	Other Ingredients: Water, flavor, glycerin, PEG-12, PEG-75, sodium carbonate, sodium saccharin, titanium dioxide, calcium peroxide, **dietetically sucrose free**		
Sensodyne® Tartar Control Toothpaste	Hydrated silica, silica, sodium bicarbonate	Potassium nitrate, sodium fluoride	Cocamidopropyl betaine
	Other Ingredients: Cellulose gum, flavor, glycerin, sodium saccharin, tetrasodium pyrophosphate, titanium dioxide, water		
Sensodyne® Toothpaste[1] (fresh mint)	Dicalcium phosphate	Potassium nitrate, sodium monofluorophosphate	Sodium lauryl sulfate
	Other Ingredients: Water, glycerin, sorbitol, hydroxmethylcellulose, flavor, sodium saccharin, methylparaben, propylparaben, D&C yellow #10, FD&C blue #1, silicon dioxide, **dietetically sucrose free**		
Sensodyne® Toothpaste (original)	Silica	Potassium nitrate, sodium fluoride	Sodium methyl cocoyl taurate
	Other Ingredients: Water, glycerin, sorbitol, cellulose gum, titanium dioxide, sodium saccharin, flavor, D&C red #28, trisodium phosphate		
Slimer® Gel[1]	Hydrated silica	Sodium fluoride 0.15%	
	Other Ingredients: Sorbitol, water, glycerin, PEG-32, flavor, ethyl alcohol, propylene glycol, glyceryl triacetate, cellulose gum, sodium saccharin, sodium benzoate, FD&C blue #1, FD&C red #33, **dietetically sucrose free**		
Thermodent Toothpaste	Diatomaceous earth, silica	Strontium chloride hexahydrate	Sodium methyl cocoyl taurate
	Other Ingredients: Sorbitol, glycerin, titanium dioxide, guar gum, PEG-40 stearate, hydroxyethylcellulose, flavor, preservative, water		
Tom's® Natural Baking Soda with Propolis & Myrrh Toothpaste	Calcium carbonate, sodium bicarbonate		Sodium lauryl sulfate
	Other Ingredients: Glycerin, water, carrageenan, peppermint oil, myrrh, propolis, **fluoride free**		

Brand Name	Abrasive Ingredient	Therapeutic Ingredient	Foaming Agent
Tom's® Natural Baking Soda, Calcium, and Fluoride Toothpaste	Calcium carbonate, sodium bicarbonate	Sodium monofluorophosphate	Sodium lauryl sulfate
	Other Ingredients: Glycerin, water, carrageenan, peppermint oil, xylitol		
Tom's® Natural Calcium and Fluoride Toothpaste[1]	Calcium carbonate	Sodium monofluorophosphate	Sodium lauryl sulfate
	Other Ingredients: Glycerin; water; carrageenan; xylitol (spearmint); cinnamon, fennel oil, or spearmint; peppermint oil (cinnamon, spearmint)		
Tom's® Natural Calcium and Fluoride Toothpaste	Calcium carbonate, hydrated silica	Sodium monofluorophosphate	Sodium lauryl sulfate
	Other Ingredients: Glycerin, water, carrageenan, xylitol, natural wintergreen oil		
Tom's® Natural for Children with Calcium and Fluoride Toothpaste	Calcium carbonate, hydrated silica	Sodium monofluorophosphate	Sodium lauryl sulfate
	Other Ingredients: Glycerin, fruit extracts, carrageenan, water		
Tom's® Natural with Propolis and Myrrh Toothpaste	Calcium carbonate		Sodium lauryl sulfate
	Other Ingredients: Glycerin; water; carrageenan; spearmint, peppermint, cassia, or fennel oil; propolis; myrrh, **fluoride free**		
Topol® Plus Whitening Gel with Calcium Toothpaste	Hydrated silicas	Sodium monofluorophosphate	Sodium lauryl sulfate
	Other Ingredients: Water, sorbitol and glycerin, calcium carbonate, PEG-6, disodium phosphate, flavor, xanthan gum, sodium saccharin, methylparaben and propylparaben, FD&C blue #1		
Topol® Plus Whitening Toothpaste with Baking Soda	Hydrated silicas, sodium bicarbonate	Sodium monofluorophosphate	Sodium lauryl sulfate
	Other Ingredients: Water, glycerin, sorbitol, PEG-6, disodium phosphate, flavor, xanthan gum, sodium saccharin, titanium dioxide, methylparaben, propylparaben		
Topol® Plus Whitening Toothpaste with Natural Papain	Hydrated silicas, calcium carbonate	Sodium monofluorophosphate	Sodium lauryl sulfate
	Other Ingredients: Water, sorbitol, glycerin, PEG-6, disodium phosphate, flavor, xanthan gum, sodium saccharin, methylparaben, propylparaben, FD&C Blue #1		
Topol® Smoker's Toothpaste	Hydrated silicas	Sodium monofluorophosphate	Sodium lauryl sulfate
	Other Ingredients: Sorbitol, deionized water, glycerin, PEG-6, flavor, xanthan gum, tianium dioxide, sodium saccharin, methylparaben, propylparaben zirconium silicate		
Topol® Smoker's Peppermint Toothpaste		Sodium monofluorophosphate	
Ultra Brite® Baking Soda & Peroxide Toothpaste	Hydrated silica, sodium bicarbonate	Sodium monofluorophosphate 0.76%	Sodium lauryl sulfate
	Other Ingredients: Glycerin, water, propylene glycol, cellulose gum, flavor, sodium saccharin, titanium dioxide, sodium hydroxide, calcium peroxide, carrageenan, **dietetically sucrose free**		
Ultra Brite® Gel	Hydrated silica	Sodium monofluorophosphate 0.76%	Sodium lauryl sulfate
	Other Ingredients: Sorbitol, water, PEG-12, flavor, cellulose gum, sodium saccharin, FD&C blue #1, D&C red #33		
Ultra Brite® Toothpaste	Hydrated silica, alumina	Sodium monofluorophosphate 0.76%	Sodium lauryl sulfate
	Other Ingredients: Glycerin, cellulose gum, sorbitol, carrageenan gum, titanium dioxide, sodium saccharin, flavor, tetrasodium pyrophosphate, **dietetically sucrose free**		
Viadent® Fluoride Gel	Hydrated silica	Sodium monofluorophosphate 0.8%	Sodium lauryl sulfate
	Other Ingredients: Sodium saccharin, zinc chloride, teaberry flavor, sodium carboxymethylcellulose, sorbitol, sanguinaria extract		
Viadent® Fluoride Toothpaste	Hydrated silica	Sodium monofluorophosphate 0.8%	Sodium lauryl sulfate
	Other Ingredients: Sorbitol, titanium dioxide, carboxymethylcellulose, flavor, sodium saccharin, citric acid, zinc chloride, anhydrous sanguinaria extract, citric acid		

DENTIFRICE PRODUCTS *(Continued)*

Brand Name	Abrasive Ingredient	Therapeutic Ingredient	Foaming Agent
Viadent® Original Toothpaste	Dicalcium phosphate		Sodium lauryl sulfate
	Other Ingredients: Glycerin, sorbitol, titanium dioxide, zinc chloride, carrageenan, flavor, sodium saccharin, citric acid, sanguinaria extract, **fluoride free**		
Vince Tooth Powder	Calcium carbonate, sodium carbonate, tricalcium phosphate		
	Other Ingredients: Sodium alum, sodium perborate monohydrate, magnesium trisilicate, sodium saccharin, flavor, D&C red		

[1]Carries American Dental Association (ADA) seal indicating safety and efficacy.

[2]Sodium bicarbonate can also be considered an abrasive.

[3]Topical fluoride product

Adapted with permission from *Nonprescription Products: Formulations & Features, Companion to the Handbook of Nonprescription Drugs*, 11th ed,, Washington, DC, American Pharmaceutical Association, 1998, 344-58.

MOUTH PAIN, COLD SORE, AND CANKER SORE PRODUCTS

Brand Name	Anesthetic / Analgesic	Other Ingredients
Abreva™ [OTC]		**Cream**: Docosanol 10%, benzyl alcohol, light mineral oil, propylene glycol, purified water, sucrose distearate, sucrose stearate
Anbesol® Baby Gel (grape, original)	Benzocaine 7.5%	Benzoic acid (grape), carbomer 934P, D&C red #33, EDTA disodium, FD&C blue #1 (grape), flavor (grape), glycerin, methylparaben (grape), PEG, propylparaben (grape), saccharin, purified water, clove oil (original)
Anbesol® Gel or Liquid	Benzocaine 6.3% (gel), 6.4% (liquid); phenol 0.5%	**Gel**: Alcohol 70%, glycerin, carbomer 934P, D&C red #33, D&C yellow #10, FD&C blue #1, FD&C yellow #6, flavor, camphor **Liquid:** Alcohol 70%, potassium iodide, povidone iodine, camphor, menthol, glycerin
Anbesol® Maximum Strength Gel or Liquid	Benzocaine 20%	Alcohol 60%, carbomer 934P (gel), D&C yellow #10, FD&C blue #1, FD&C red #40, flavor, PEG, saccharin
Baby® Gumz	Benzocaine 10%	PEG 8 and 32, **alcohol free, dietetically sucrose free**
Banadyne-3	Benzocaine 5%	Dimethicone, methol, propylene glycol, SD alcohol
Benzodent® Denture Analgesic Ointment[1]	Benzocaine 20%	8-hydroxyquinoline sulfate, petrolatum, sodium carboxymethycellulose, color, eugenol
Blistex® Lip Medex Ointment	Camphor 1%, menthol 1%, phenol 0.5%	Petrolatum, cocoa butter, flavor, lanolin, mixed waxes, oil of cloves
Blistex® Medicated Ointment	Menthol 0.6%, camphor 0.5%, phenol 0.5%	Water, mixed waxes, mineral oil, petrolatum, lanolin
Campho-Phenique® Cold Sore Gel[2]	Camphor 10.8%, phenol 4.7%	Eucalyptus oil, colloidal silicon dioxide, glycerin, light mineral oil, **alcohol free**
Cankaid® Liquid		Carbamide peroxide 10%[3], citric acid monohydrate, sodium citrate, dihydrate, EDTA disodium
Carmex Lip Balm Ointment	Menthol, camphor, salicylic acid, phenol	Alum, fragrance, petrolatum, lanolin, cocoa butter, wax, **alcohol free, dye free, gluten free, dietetically sucrose free**
Cepacol® Viractin®	Tetracaine 2%	Water, ethoxydiglycol, hydroxyethyl cellulose, maleated soybean oil, sodium lauryl sulfate, methylparaben, propylparaben, eucalyptus oil

MOUTH PAIN, COLD SORE, AND CANKER SORE PRODUCTS *(Continued)*

Brand Name	Anesthetic / Analgesic	Other Ingredients
Chap Stick® Medicated Lip Balm (stick, ointment)	Camphor 1%, menthol 0.6%, phenol 0.5%	**Stick:** Petrolatum 41%, paraffin wax, mineral oil, cocoa butter, 2-octyl dodecanol, arachidyl propionate, polyphenylmethylsiloxane 556, white wax, isopropyl lanolate, carnauba wax, isopropyl myristate, lanolin, fragrance, methylparaben, propylparaben, oleyl alcohol, cetyl alcohol **Ointment**: Petrolatum (jar 60%, tube 67%), microcrystalline wax, mineral oil, cocoa butter, lanolin, paraffin war (jar), fragrance, methylparaben, propylparaben
Dent's® Double-Action Kit (tablets, drops)	Benzocaine 20% (drops), acetaminophen 325 mg (tablet)	**Drops:** Denatured alcohol 74%, chlorobutanol anhydrous 0.09%, propylene glycol, FD&C red #40, eugenol
Dent's® Extra Strength Toothache Gum	Benzocaine 20%	Petrolatum, cotton and wax base, beeswax, FD&C red #40 aluminum lake, eugenol
Dent's® Maxi-Strength Toothache Treatment Drops	Benzocaine 20%	Denatured alcohol 74%, chlorobutanol anhydrous 0.09%, propylene glycol, FD&C red #40, eugenol
Dent-Zel-Ite® Oral Mucosal Analgesic Liquid	Benzocaine 5%, camphor	Alcohol 81%, wintergreen, glycerin, **dye free**
Dent-Zel-Ite® Temporary Dental Filling Liquid	Camphor	Alcohol 56.18%, sandarac gum, methyl salicylate
Dent-Zel-Ite® Toothache Relief Drops	Eugenol 85%, camphor	Alcohol 13.5%, wintergreen
Dentapaine® Gel	Benzocaine 20%	Glycerin, oil of cloves, sodium saccharin, methylparaben, PEG 400 and 4000, water, **alcohol free**, **dye free**, **gluten free**, **dietetically sucrose free**
Dr. Hand's® Teething Gel or Lotion	Menthol	SD alcohol 38B (gel 10%, lotion 11%), sterilized water, carbomer 940, witch hazel, polysorbate 80, sodium hydroxide, simethicone, D&C red #33, FD&C red #3
Gly-Oxide® Liquid		Carbamide peroxide 10%[3], citric acid, flavor, glycerin, propylene glycol, sodium stannate, water
Herpecin-L®		Octinoxate, oxybenzone, meradimate, octisalate, dimethacone, sunflower oil, petrolatum, ozokerite, mineral oil, microcrystalline wax, talc, titanium dioxide, beeswax, mellissa extract, cetyl lactate, glyceryl laurate, flavor, lysine, ascorbyl palmitate, tocopheryl acetate, pyridoxine HCl, panthenol, BHT (244-014)
Herpecin-L® Cold Sore Lip Balm Stick[2]		Padimate O 7%, allantoin 0.5%, titanium dioxide, beeswax, cetyl esters, flavor, octyldodecanol, paraffin, petrolatum, sesame oil, vitamins B_6, C, and E
Hurricaine® Aerosol[1] (wild cherry)	Benzocaine 20%	PEG, saccharin, flavor, alcohol, **dye free**, **gluten free**, **sulfite free**

Brand Name	Anesthetic / Analgesic	Other Ingredients
Hurricaine® Gel[1] (wild cherry, pina colada, watermelon)	Benzocaine 20%	PEG, saccharin, flavor, **alcohol free**, **dye free**, **gluten free**, **sulfite free**
Hurricaine® Liquid[1] (wild cherry, pina colada)	Benzocaine 20%	PEG, saccharin, flavor, **alcohol free**, **dye free**, **gluten free**, **dietetically sucrose free**
Kank-A® Professional Strength Liquid[1]	Benzocaine 20%	Benzoin tincture compound, cetylpyridinium chloride, ethylcellulose, SD alcohol 24%, dimethyl isosorbide, castor oil, flavor, tannic acid, propylene glycol, saccharin, benzyl alcohol
Lipclear™ Lysine Plus™		Zinc oxide, l-lysine, vitamin A, vitamin D, vitamin E, olive oil, yellow beeswax, goldenseal extract, propolis extract, calendula extract, echinacea extract, cajeput oil, tea tree oil, gum benzoin tincture, honey, lithium carbonate (3x)
Lip-Ex® Ointment	Phenol, camphor, salicylic acid, menthol	Petrolatum, cherry flavor
Lipmagik® Liquid	Benzocaine 6.3%, phenol 0.5%	Alcohol 70%, **dye free**, **sulfite free**, **gluten free**
Little Teethers® Oral Pain Relief Gel	Benzocaine 7.5%	Carbomer, glycerin, flavor, potassium sorbate, acesulfame K, PEGs, **alcohol free**, **dye free**, **dietetically sodium free**, **dietetically sucrose free**
Medadyne® Liquid	Benzocaine 10%, menthol, camphor, benzyl alcohol	Benzalkonium chloride, tannic acid, flavor, SD alcohol, thymol
Novitra™		Zincum oxydatum (2x), HPUS, alpha tocopherol, benzalkonium chloride, setyl alcohol, cocoa butter, glyceryl monostearate, glycine, modified lanolin, methylparaben, PEG 8000, propylparaben, water, sodium lauryl sulfate
Numzident® Adult Strength Gel	Benzocaine 10%	PEG-8, glycerin, PEG-75, sodium saccharin, purified water, flavor
Numzit® Teething Gel	Benzocaine 7.5%	PEG-8, PEG-75, sodium saccharin, clove oil, peppermint oil, purified water
Orabase® Baby Gel[1]	Benzocaine 7.5%	Glycerin, PEG, carbopol, preservative, sweetener, flavor, **alcohol free**
Orabase® Gel	Benzocaine 15%	Ethanol, propylene glycol, ethylcellulose, tannic acid, salicylic acid, flavor, sodium saccharin
Orabase® Lip Cream	Benzocaine 5%, menthol 0.5%, camphor, phenol	Allantoin 1%, carboxymethylcellulose sodium, veegum, Tween 80, phenonip, PEG, biopure, talc, kaolin, lanolin, petrolatum, oil of clove, hydrated silica, **alcohol free**
Orabase® Plain Paste[1]		Pectin, gelatin, carboxymethylcellulose sodium, polyethylene, mineral oil, flavor, preservative, guar, tragacanth, **alcohol free**

MOUTH PAIN, COLD SORE, AND CANKER SORE PRODUCTS *(Continued)*

Brand Name	Anesthetic / Analgesic	Other Ingredients
Orabase-B® with Benzocaine Paste[1]	Benzocaine 20%	Plasticized hydrocarbon gel, guar, carboxymethylcellulose, tragacanth, pectin, preservatives, flavor, **alcohol free**
Oragesic Solution	Benzyl alcohol 2%, menthol	Water, sorbitol, polysorbate 20, sodium chloride, yerba santa, saccharin, flavor, **sulfite free**
Orajel® Baby Gel or Liquid	Benzocaine 7.5%	**Gel:** FD&C red #40, flavor, glycerin, PEGs, sodium saccharin, sorbic acid, sorbitol, **alcohol free** **Liquid:** Not applicable
Orajel® Baby Nighttime Gel	Benzocaine 10%	FD&C red #40, flavor, glycerin, PEGs, sodium saccharin, sorbic acid, sorbitol, **alcohol free**
Orajel® CoverMed Cream (tinted light, medium)	Dyclonine HCl 1%	Allantoin 0.5%
Orajel® Denture Gel	Benzocaine 20%	Cellulose gum, gelatin, menthol, methyl salicylate, pectin, plasticized hydrocarbon gel, PEG, sodium saccharin
Orajel® Maximum Strength Gel	Benzocaine 20%	Clove oil, flavor, PEGs, sodium saccharin, sorbic acid
Orajel® Mouth-Aid Gel or Liquid	Benzocaine 20%	**Gel**: Zinc chloride 0.1%, benzalkonium chloride 0.02%. allantoin, carbomer, EDTA disodium, peppermint oil, PEG, polysorbate 60, propyl gallate, propylene glycol, purified water, povidone, sodium saccharin, sorbic acid, stearyl alcohol **Liquid:** Ethyl alcohol 44.2%
Orajel® PM Cream	Benzocaine 20%	
Orajel® Periostatic Spot Treatment Oral Cleanser		Carbamide peroxide 15%[3], citric acid, EDTA disodium, flavor, methylparaben, PEG, purified water, sodium chloride, sodium saccharin
Orajel® Periostatic Super Cleaning Oral Rinse		Hydrogen peroxide 1.5%[3], ethyl alcohol 4%
Orajel® Regular Strength Gel	Benzocaine 10%	Clove oil, flavor, PEGs, sodium saccharin, sorbic acid
Peroxyl® Hygienic Dental Rinse		Hydrogen peroxide 1.5%[3], alcohol 5%, pluronic F108, sorbitol, sodium saccharin, dye, polysorbate 20, mint flavor, **gluten free**, **sulfite free**
Peroxyl® Oral Spot Treatment Gel		Hydrogen peroxide 1.5%[3], ethyl alcohol 5%, pluronic F108, sorbitol, sodium saccharin, dye, polysorbate 20, mint flavor, dye, pluronic F127, **gluten free**, **dietetically sucrose free**
Proxigel® Gel[2]	Menthol	Carbamide peroxide 10%[3], glycerin, carbomer, phosphoric acid, triethanolamine, flavor, **dye free**, **gluten free**, **dietetically sucrose free**
Red Cross® Canker Sore Medication Ointment[2]	Benzocaine 20%, phenol	Carbomer 974P, mineral oil, petrolatum, propylparaben
Red Cross® Toothache Medication Drops	Eugenol 85%	Sesame oil
Retre-Gel®[2]	Benzocaine 5%, menthol 1%	Glycerin 20%

Brand Name	Anesthetic / Analgesic	Other Ingredients
Tanac® Medicated Gel	Dyclonine HCl 1%	Allantoin 0.5%
Tanac® No Sting Liquid	Benzocaine 10%	Benzalkonium chloride 0.125%, saccharin
Zilactin® Gel	Benzyl alcohol 10%	**Gluten free**
Zilactin® Baby Gel	Benzocaine 10%	**Alcohol free, dye free, gluten free**
Zilactin®-B Gel	Benzocaine 10%	**Gluten free**
Zilactin®-L Liquid	Lidocaine 2.5%	Boric acid, propylene glycol, water, salicylic acid, SD alcohol 37, tannic acid

[1]Carries American Dental Association (ADA) seal indicating safety and efficacy

[2]Agent for cold sore treatment only

[3]Agent for debridement or wound cleansing

Adapted with permission from *Nonprescription Products: Formulations & Features, Companion to the Handbook of Nonprescription Drugs*, 11th ed,, Washington, DC, American Pharmaceutical Association, 1998, 338-40.

ORAL RINSE PRODUCTS

Brand Name	Active Ingredients	Other Ingredients
ACT® Anticavity Fluoride Rinse, Bubble Gum Blowout™	Cetylpyridinium chloride	Sodium fluoride 0.05%, D&C red #33, calcium EDTA, flavor, glycerin, monobasic and dibasic sodium phosphates, poloxamer 407, polysorbate 80, propylene glycol, sodium benzoate, water, sodium saccharin, **alcohol free**
ACT® Anticavity Fluoride Treatment Rinse, Mint	Cetylpyridinium chloride	Sodium fluoride 0.05%, D&C red #33, calcium EDTA, FD&C yellow #5, flavor, glycerin, monobasic and dibasic sodium phosphates, poloxamer 407, polysorbate 80, propylene glycol, sodium benzoate, sodium saccharin, water, **alcohol free**
Arm & Hammer Advance Breath Care™ Cool Fresh Mint Mouthwash	Alcohol 15%, cetylpyridinium chloride, zinc citrate	Water, glycerin and/or sorbitol, sodium bicarbonate, sodium citrate, poloxamer 407, flavor, surcrose and/or sodium saccharin, D&C green #5, FD&C yellow #5
Arm & Hammer Advance Breath Care™ Icy Fresh Mint Mouthwash	Alcohol 15%, cetylpyridinium chloride, zinc citrate	Water, glycerin and/or sorbitol, sodium bicarbonate, sodium citrate, poloxamer 407, flavor, sucrose and/or sodium saccharin, D&C green #5
Astring-O-Sol® Liquid	SD alcohol 38B 75.6%, methyl salicylate	Water, myrrh extract, zinc chloride, citric acid
Betadine® Mouthwash Gargle	Alcohol 8%	Povidone-iodine 0.5%, glycerin, sodium saccharin, flavor
Biotene® Alcohol-Free Mouthwash	Lysozyme (40 mg), lactoferrin (15 mg), glucose oxidase (2500 units), lactoperoxidase (2500 units)	Water, xylitol, hydrogenated starch, propylene glycol, hydroxyethylcellulose, aloe vera, peppermint, poloxamer 407, sodium benzoate, **alcohol free**
Biotene® Mouthwash	Lysozyme (6 mg), lactoferrin (6 mg), glucose oxidase (4000 units), zinc gluconate	Water, xylitol, hydrogenated starch, propylene glycol, hydroxy ethylcellulose, aloe vera, natural peppermint, poloxamer 407, calcium lactate, sodium benzoate, benzoic acid
Cepacol® Mouthwash/Gargle	Alcohol 14%, cetylpyridinium chloride 0.05%	EDTA disodium, color, flavor, glycerin, polysorbate 80, saccharin, sodium biphosphate, sodium phosphate, water, **gluten free**, **dietetically sucrose free**
Cepacol® Mouthwash/Gargle (mint)	Alcohol 14.5%, cetylpyridinium chloride 0.5%	Color, flavor, glucono delta-lactone, glycerin, poloxamer 407, sodium saccharin, sodium gluconate, water, **gluten free**, **dietetically sucrose free**
Dr. Tichenor's® Antiseptic Liquid	SDA alcohol 38B 70%	Oil of peppermint, extract of arnica, water, **dye free**, **gluten free**

Brand Name	Active Ingredients	Other Ingredients
Lavoris Crystal Fresh	SD alcohol 38-B, zantrate (citric acid, zinc oxide, sodium hydroxide)	Purified spring water, glycerin, poloxamer 407, saccharin, polysorbate 80, flavors
Lavoris Mint Mouthwash	Zinc chloride and/ or zinc oxide, aromatic oils	Glycerin
Lavoris Original Cinnamon Mouthwash	Zinc chloride and/ or zinc oxide, aromatic oils	Glycerin
Lavoris Original Mouthwash	SD alcohol 38-B, zinc chloride, zantrate (zinc oxide, sodium hydroxide, citric acid)	Water, glycerin, poloxamer 407, saccharin, clove oil, polysorbate 80, flavor, D&C red #6 and #33
Lavoris Peppermint Mouthwash	SD alcohol 38-B, zantrate (sodium hydroxide, citric acid, zinc oxide)	Water, glycerin, poloxamer 407, polysorbate 80, peppermint oil, saccharin, FD&C blue #4
Listerine®[1] Liquid	Alcohol 26.9%, eucalyptol 0.092%, thymol 0.064%, methyl salicylate 0.06%, menthol 0.042%	Benzoic acid, poloxamer 407, caramel, water, sodium benzoate
Listerine®[1] Liquid (freshburst, cool mint)	Alcohol 21.6%, eucalyptol 0.092%, thymol 0.064%, methyl salicylate 0.06%, menthol 0.042%	Water, sorbitol solution, poloxamer 407, benzoic acid, flavor, sodium saccharin, sodium citrate, citric acid, FD&C green #3, D&C yellow #10 (freshburst)
Mentadent® Mouthwash (cool mint, fresh mint)	Alcohol 10%	Water, sorbitol, sodium bicarbonate, hydrogen peroxide, poloxamer 407, sodium lauryl sulfate, flavor, polysorbate 20, methyl salicylate (cool mint), sodium saccharin, phosphoric acid, blue #1, yellow #5 (cool mint)
Oxyfresh Fresh Mint Mouthrinse	Oxygene® (stabilized chlorine dioxide)	Purified deionized water, xylitol, mint oils, sodium benzoate, **alcohol free**
Oxyfresh Fresh Mint with Fluoride Mouthrinse	Oxygene® (stabilized chlorine dioxide)	Sodium fluoride (0.05%), purified deionized water, xylitol, mint oils, sodium benzoate, **alcohol free**
Oxyfresh Fresh Mint with Zinc Mouthrinse	Oxygene® (stabilized chlorine dioxide), zinc acetate	Purified deionized water, xylitol, sodium citrate, peppermint oil, **alcohol free**
Oxyfresh Original Mint Mouthrinse	Oxygene® (stabilized chlorine dioxide)	Purified deionized water, mint oils, sodium benzoate, **alcohol free**
Oxyfresh Professional Strength Zinc Mouthrinse	Oxygene® (stabilized chlorine dioxide), zinc acetate	Purified deionized water, xylitol, sodium citrate, peppermint oil, **alcohol free**
Oxyfresh Unflavored Mouthrinse	Oxygene® (stabilized chlorine dioxide)	Purified deionized water, sodium benzoate, **alcohol free**

ORAL RINSE PRODUCTS *(Continued)*

Brand Name	Active Ingredients	Other Ingredients
Plax® Advanced Formula (mint sensation)	Alcohol 8.7%	Water, sorbitol solution, tetrasodium pyrophosphate, benzoic acid, flavor, poloxamer 407, sodium benzoate, sodium lauryl sulfate, sodium saccharin, xanthan gum, FD&C blue #1
Plax® Advanced Formula (original, SoftMINT)	Alcohol 8.7%	Sodium lauryl sulfate, water, sorbitol solution, sodium benzoate, tetrasodium pyrophosphate, benzoic acid, poloxamer 407, sodium saccharin, flavor (SoftMINT), xanthan gum (SoftMINT), flavor enhancer (SoftMINT), FD&C blue #1 (SoftMINT), FD&C yellow #5 (SoftMINT)
Rembrandt® Naturals Mouthwash		Spring water, glycerin, xylitol, sodium citrate, vitamin C, stevia, citric acid, dicalcium phosphate, cocamidopropyl betain, flavor, ginkgo extract, raspberry leaf extract, alcohol free. Also available with papaya and ginseng or aloe and echinacea
S.T. 37® Solution	Hexylresorcinol 0.1%	Glycerin, propylene glycol, citric acid, EDTA disodium, sodium bisulfite, sodium citrate
Scope® Baking Soda	SD alcohol 38F 9.9%, cetylpyridinium chloride, domiphen bromide	Sorbitol, sodium bicarbonate, sodium saccharin, flavor
Scope® (cool peppermint)	SD alcohol 38F 14%, cetylpyridinium chloride, domiphen bromide	Purified water, glycerin, poloxamer 407, sodium saccharin, sodium benzoate, N-ethylmethylcarboxamide, benzoic acid, FD&C blue #1, flavor
Targon® Smokers' Mouthwash (clean taste)	SDA alcohol 38B 15.6%	Water, glycerin, polyoxyl 40 hydrogenated caster oil, sodium lauryl sulfate, dibasic sodium phosphate, benzoic acid, sodium saccharin, caramel powder, **dietetically sucrose free**
Targon® Smokers' Mouthwash (original)	SDA alcohol 38B 16%	Water, sodium saccharin, sodium benzoate, glycerin, sodium lauryl sulfate, FD&C green #3, FD&C yellow #5, polyoxyl 40 hydrogenated castor oil, **dietetically sucrose free**
Tom's of Maine® Natural Mouthwash (cinnamon, original)	Menthol	Water, glycerin, aloe vera juice, witch hazel, poloxamer 335, spearmint oil, ascorbic acid, **alcohol free**

Viadent Advanced Care Oral Rinse	Cetylpyridium chloride 0.05%	Purified water, sorbitol, ethyl alcohol (5.5% w/w), glycerin, propylene glycol, PEG-40 sorbitan diisostearate, flavor, sodium benzoate, sodium saccharin, FD&C yellow No. 6

[1]Carries American Dental Association (ADA) seal indicating safety and efficacy

Note: SD alcohol refers to "specially denatured" alcohol

Adapted with permission from *Nonprescription Products: Formulations & Features, Companion to the Handbook of Nonprescription Drugs*, 11th ed,, Washington, DC, American Pharmaceutical Association, 1998, 341-2.

TOP 200 MOST PRESCRIBED DRUGS IN 2003*

1. Hydrocodone and Acetaminophen
2. Lipitor®
3. Synthroid®
4. Atenolol
5. Amoxicillin
6. Lisinopril
7. Hydrochlorothiazide
8. Furosemide (oral)
9. Albuterol (aerosol)
10. Alprazolam
11. Norvasc®
12. Zoloft®
13. Zithromax® Z-Pak®
14. Toprol-XL®
15. Cephalexin
16. Propoxyphene
17. Zocor®
18. Prevacid®
19. Ibuprofen
20. Triamterene
21. Premarin® (tablet)
22. Prednisone (oral)
23. Metformin
24. Ambien®
25. Levoxyl®
26. Fluoxetine
27. Allegra®
28. Celebrex®
29. Ortho Tri-Cyclen®
30. Nexium®
31. Acetaminophen and Codeine
32. Metoprolol
33. Lorazepam
34. Zyrtec®
35. Singulair®
36. Vioxx®
37. Fosamax®
38. Effexor® XR
39. Viagra®
40. Neurontin®
41. Potassium Chloride
42. Celexa™
43. Trimox
44. Wellbutrin SR®
45. Amoxicillin and Clavulanate Potassium
46. Ranitidine
47. Paxil®
48. Amitriptyline
49. Clonazepam
50. Protonix®
51. Warfarin
52. Advair Diskus®
53. Flonase®
54. Lexapro™
55. Plavix®
56. Pravachol®
57. Sulfamethoxazole and Trimethoprim
58. Trazodone
59. Levaquin®
60. Cyclobenzaprine
61. Naproxen
62. Enalapril
63. Omeprazole
64. Accupril®
65. Diazepam
66. Diflucan®
67. Altace®
68. Diovan®
69. Lotrel®
70. Penicillin VK
71. Oxycodone and Acetaminophen
72. Glucotrol® XL
73. Klor-Con®
74. Tramadol
75. Zithromax® (suspension)
76. Carisoprodol
77. Clarinex®
78. Verapamil SR
79. Doxycycline
80. Ortho Evra™
81. Bextra®
82. Isosorbide Mononitrate
83. Glyburide
84. Methylprednisolone (tablet)
85. Paxil CR™
86. Clonidine
87. Allopurinol
88. Actos®
89. Cozaar®
90. Albuterol (solution)
91. Diovan HCT®
92. Cipro®
93. Avandia®
94. Lisinopril and Hydrochlorothiazide
95. Folic Acid
96. Risperdal®
97. Nasonex®
98. Digitek®
99. Aciphex®
100. Coumadin® (tablet)
101. Lotensin®
102. Glucophage® XR
103. Allegra-D®
104. Concerta®
105. Zyprexa®
106. Flomax®
107. Amoxil®
108. Promethazine (tablet)

109. OxyContin®
110. Adderall XR™
111. Estradiol (oral)
112. Evista®
113. Flovent®
114. Temazepam
115. Hyzaar®
116. Tricor®
117. Amaryl®
118. Glucovance®
119. Combivent®
120. Spironolactone
121. Yasmin® 28
122. Actonel®
123. Xalatan®
124. Lanoxin®
125. Doxazosin
126. Metronidazole (tablet)
127. Valtrex®
128. Hydroxyzine
129. Zyrtec® (syrup)
130. Seroquel®
131. Gemfibrozil
132. Triamcinolone Acetonide Paste (topical)
133. Metoclopramide
134. Meclizine
135. Depakote®
136. Promethazine and Codeine
137. Levothroid®
138. Minocycline
139. Clindamycin (systemic)
140. Zithromax®
141. Skelaxin®
142. Ultracet™
143. Bisoprolol
144. Prempro™
145. Endocet®
146. Lantus®
147. Omnicef®
148. Augmentin ES-600®
149. Topamax®
150. Avapro®
151. Macrobid®
152. Butalbital, Acetaminophen, and Caffeine
153. Famotidine
154. Prilosec®
155. Imitrex® (oral)
156. Glipizide
157. Coreg®
158. Humulin® N
159. Detrol® LA
160. Rhinocort® Aqua®
161. Terazosin
162. Buspirone
163. Propranolol
164. Diltiazem
165. Zetia™
166. Nasacort® AQ
167. Cartia XT™
168. Monopril®
169. Medroxyprogesterone
170. Aviane™
171. Cefzil®
172. Acyclovir
173. Biaxin® XL
174. Lovastatin
175. Bactroban®
176. Nifedipine
177. Humalog®
178. Ciprofloxacin
179. Duragesic®
180. Patanol®
181. Paroxetine
182. Betamethasone and Clotrimazole
183. Captopril
184. Miralax™
185. Zyrtec-D 12 Hour™
186. Strattera™
187. Benzonatate
188. Aspirin (enteric coated)
189. Trivora®-28
190. Dilantin®
191. Nortriptyline
192. Tizanidine
193. Ferrous Sulfate
194. Elidel®
195. Humulin® 70/30
196. Diclofenac
197. Inderal® LA
198. Aricept®
199. Tussionex®
200. Apri®

*Based on units dispensed in U.S.
Source: Verispan Scott-Levin, SPA

MULTIVITAMIN PRODUCTS

Injectable Formulations

Product	A (int. units)	B_1 (mg)	B_2 (mg)	B_6 (mg)	B_{12} (mcg)	C (mg)	D (int. units)	E (int. units)	K (mcg)	Additional Information
Solution										
Infuvite® Adult (per 10 mL)	3300	6	3.6	6	5	200	200	10	150	Supplied as two 5 mL vials. Biotin 60 mcg, folic acid 600 mcg, niacinamide 40 mg, dexpanthenol 15 mg
Infuvite® Pediatric (per 5 mL)	2300	1.6	1.4	1	1	80	400	7	200	Supplied as one 4 mL vial and one 1 mL vial. Biotin 20 mcg, folic acid 140 mcg, niacinamide 17 mg, dexpanthenol 5 mg
M.V.I.®-12 (per 10 mL)	3300	3	3.6	4	12.5	100	200	10	–	Supplied as two 5 mL vials or a single 2-chambered 10 mL vial. Biotin 60 mcg, folic acid 400 mcg, niacinamide 40 mg, dexpanthenol 15 mg
M.V.I. Adult™ (per 10 mL)	3300	6	3.6	6	5	200	200	10	150	Supplied as two 5 mL vials or a single 2-chambered 10 mL vial. Biotin 60 mcg, folic acid 600 mcg, niacinamide 40 mg, dexpanthenol 15 mg
Powder for Reconstitution										
M.V.I.® Pediatric	2300	1.2	1.4	1	1	80	400	7	200	Biotin 20 mcg, folic acid 140 mcg, niacinamide 17 mg, dexpanthenol 5 mg, aluminum, polysorbate 80

Adult Formulations

Product	A (int. units)	B_1 (mg)	B_2 (mg)	B_6 (mg)	B_{12} (mcg)	C (mg)	D (int. units)	E (int. units)	Additional Information
Liquid									
Centrum® [OTC] (per 15 mL)	2500	1.5	1.7	2	6	60	400	30	Biotin 300 mcg, Cr 25 mcg, Fe 9 mg, iodine 150 mcg, Mn 2 mg, Mo 25 mg, niacin 20 mg, pantothenic acid 10 mg, Zn 3 mg; alcohol 5.4%, sodium benzoate (240 mL)
Geritol® Tonic [OTC] (per 15 mL)		2.5	2.5	0.5					Chlorine bitartrate 50 mg, Fe 18 mg, methionine 25 mg, niacin 50 mg, pantothenic acid 2 mg; sugars 7 g, alcohol 12%, benzoic acid (120 mL, 360 mL)
Iberet® [OTC] (per 5 mL)		1.2	1.35	0.925	5.63	33.8			Fe 23.6 mg, niacin 6.8 mg, pantothenic acid 2.4 mg; alcohol (240 mL)
Iberet®-500 [OTC] (per 5 mL)		1.2	1.35	0.925	5.63	125			Fe 23.6 mg, niacin 6.8 mg, pantothenic acid 2.4 mg; alcohol (240 mL)
Vi-Daylin® [OTC] (per 5 mL)	2500	1.05	1.2	1.05	4.5	60	400	15	Niacin 13.5 mg; alcohol <0.5%, benzoic acid; lemon/orange flavor (240 mL, 480 mL)
Vi-Daylin® + Iron [OTC] (per 5 mL)	2500	1.05	1.2	1.05	4.5	60	400	15	Fe 10 mg, niacin 13.5 mg; alcohol <0.5%, benzoic acid; lemon/orange flavor (240 mL, 480 mL)
Caplet									
Theragran® Heart Right™ [OTC]	5000	3	3.4	16	30	120	400	400	Alpha-carotene, beta-carotene, biotin 30 mcg, Ca 55 mg, Cr 50 mcg, cryptoxanthin, Cu 1.5 mg, Fe 4 mg, folic acid as folate 0.6 mg, iodine 150 mcg, lutein, lycopene, Mg 150 mg, Mn 2 mg, Mo 75 mcg, niacin 20 mg, pantothenic acid 10 mg, Se 70 mcg, vit K 14 mcg, zeaxanthin, Zn 15 mg
Theragran-M® Advanced Formula [OTC]	5000	3	3.4	6	12	90	400	60	Biotin 30 mcg, boron 150 mcg, Ca 40 mg, chloride 7.5 mg, Cr 50 mcg, Cu 2 mg, Fe 9 mg, folic acid 0.4 mg, iodine 150 mcg, Mg 100 mg, Mn 2 mg, Mo 75 mcg, niacin 20 mg, nickel 5 mcg, pantothenic acid 10 mg, phosphorus 31 mg, potassium 7.5 mg, Se 70 mcg, silicon 2 mg, tin 10 mcg, vanadium 10 mcg, vit K 28 mcg, Zn 15 mg
Capsule									
Vicon Forte®	8000	10	5	2	10	150		50	Folic acid 1 mg, Mg 70 mg, Mn 4 mg, niacinamide 25 mg, Zn 80 mg
Vicon Plus® [OTC]	3400	9.3	4.6	1.5		140		45	Mg 5 mg, Mn 1 mg, niacin 24 mg, pantothenic acid 11 mg, Zn 10 mg
Vitacon Forte	8000	10	5	2	10	150		50	Folic acid 1 mg, Mg 70 mg, Mn 4 mg, niacinamide 25 mg, Zn 80 mg

MULTIVITAMIN PRODUCTS *(Continued)*

Adult Formulations *(continued)*

Product	A (int. units)	B_1 (mg)	B_2 (mg)	B_6 (mg)	B_{12} (mcg)	C (mg)	D (int. units)	E (int. units)	Additional Information
Tablet									
Centrum® [OTC]	5000	1.5	1.7	2	6	60	400	30	Biotin 30 mcg, boron 150 mcg, Ca 162 mg, chloride 72 mg, Cr 120 mcg, Cu 2 mg, Fe 18 mg, folic acid 0.4 mg, iodine 150 mcg, lutein 250 mcg, Mg 100 mg, Mn 2 mg, Mo 75 mcg, niacin 20 mg, nickel 5 mcg, pantothenic acid 10 mg, phosphorus 109 mg, potassium 80 mg, Se 20 mcg, silicon 2 mg, tin 10 mcg, vanadium 10 mcg, vit K 25 mcg, Zn 15 mg
Centrum® Performance™ [OTC]	5000	4.5	5.1	6	18	120	400	60	Biotin 40 mcg, boron 60 mcg, chloride 72 mg, folic acid 0.4 mg, Ca 100 mg, Cr 120 mcg, Cu 2 mg, Fe 18 mg, ginkgo biloba leaf 60 mg, ginseng root 50 mg, iodine 150 mcg, Mg 40 mg, Mn 4 mg, Mo 75 mcg, niacin 40 mg, nickel 5 mcg, pantothenic acid 10 mg, phosphorus 48 mg, potassium 80 mg, Se 70 mcg, silicon 4 mg, tin 10 mcg, vanadium 10 mcg, vit K 25 mcg, Zn 15 mg
Centrum® Silver® [OTC]	5000	1.5	1.7	3	25	60	400	45	Biotin 30 mcg, boron 150 mcg, Ca 200 mg, chloride 72 mg, Cr 150 mcg, Cu 2 mg, folic acid 0.4 mg, iodine 150 mcg, lutein 250 mcg, Mg 100 mg, Mn 2 mg, Mo 75 mcg, niacin 20 mg, nickel 5 mcg, pantothenic acid 10 mg, phosphorus 48 mg, potassium 80 mg, Se 20 mcg, silicon 2 mg, vanadium 10 mcg, vit K 10 mcg, Zn 15 mg
Iberet®-500 [OTC]		4.96	5.4	3.7	22.5	500			Fe 95 mg (controlled release), niacin 27.2 mg, pantothenic acid 8.28 mg, sodium 65 mg
Iberet-Folic-500® [OTC]		6	6	5	25	500			Fe 105 mg (controlled release), folic acid 0.8 mg, niacinamde 30 mg, pantothenic acid 10 mg
Olay® Vitamins Complete Women's [OTC]	5000	1.5	1.7	2	6	120	400	50	Biotin 30 mcg, boron 150 mcg, Ca 250 mg, chloride 36 mg, coenzyme Q_{10} 2 mg, Cr 120 mcg, Cu 5 mg, Fe 18 mg, folic acid 0.4 mg, iodine 150 mcg, lutein 250 mg, Mg 100 mg, Mn 2 mg, Mo 25 mcg, niacin 20 mg, nickel 5 mcg, pantothenic acid 10 mg, phosphorus 77 mg, potassium 40 mg, Se 25 mcg, silicon 2 mg, vanadium 10 mcg, Zn 15 mg
Olay® Vitamins Complete Women's 50+ [OTC]	5000	3	3.4	4	25	120	400	60	Biotin 30 mcg, boron 150 mcg, Ca 250 mg, chloride 72 mg, coenzyme Q_{10} 2 mg, Cr 120 mcg, Cu 5 mg, folic acid 0.4 mg, iodine 150 mcg, lutein 250 mg, Mg 120 mg, Mn 2 mg, Mo 25 mcg, niacin 20 mg, nickel 5 mcg, pantothenic acid 10 mg, phosphorus 48 mg, potassium 80 mg, Se 50 mcg, silicon 2 mg, vanadium 10 mcg, Zn 22 mg

Product	A (int. units)	B_1 (mg)	B_2 (mg)	B_6 (mg)	B_{12} (mcg)	C (mg)	D (int. units)	E (int. units)	Additional Information
One-A-Day® 50 Plus Formula [OTC]	5000	4.5	3.4	6	30	120	400	60	Biotin 30 mcg, Ca 120 mg, chloride 34 mg, Cr 180 mcg, Cu 2 mg, folic acid 0.4 mg, iodine 150 mcg, Mg 100 mg, Mn 4 mg, Mo 93.75 mcg, niacin 20 mg, pantothenic acid 15 mg, potassium 37.5 mg, Se 150 mcg, vit K 20 mcg, Zn 22.5 mg
One-A-Day® Active Formula [OTC]	5000	4.5	5.1	6	18	120	400	60	American ginseng 55 mg, biotin 40 mcg, boron 150 mcg, Ca 110 mg, chloride 180 mg, Cr 100 mcg, Cu 2 mg, Fe 9 mg, folic acid 0.4 mg, iodine 150 mcg, Mg 40 mg, Mn 2 mg, Mo 25 mcg, niacin 40 mg, nickel 5 mcg, pantothenic acid 10 mg, phosphorus 48 mg, potassium 200 mg, Se 45 mcg, silicon 6 mg, tin 10 mcg, vanadium 10 mcg, vit K 25 mcg, Zn 15 mg
One-A-Day® Essential Formula [OTC]	5000	1.5	1.7	2	6	60	400	30	Folic acid 0.4 mg, niacin 20 mg, pantothenic acid 10 mg
One-A-Day® Maximum Formula [OTC]	5000	1.5	1.7	2	6	60	400	30	Biotin 30 mcg, boron 150 mcg, Ca 162 mg, chloride 72 mg, Cr 65 mcg, Cu 2 mg, Fe 18 mg, folic acid 0.4 mg, iodine 150 mcg, Mg 100 mg, Mn 3.5 mg, Mo 160 mcg, niacin 20 mg, nickel 5 mcg, pantothenic acid 10 mg, phosphorus 109 mg, potassium 80 mg, Se 20 mcg, silicon 2 mg, tin 10 mcg, vanadium 10 mcg, vit K 25 mcg, Zn 15 mg
One-A-Day® Men's Formula [OTC]	5000	2.25	2.55	3	9	90	400	45	Chloride 34 mg, Cr 150 mcg, Cu 2 mg, folic acid 0.4 mg, iodine 150 mcg, Mg 100 mg, Mn 3.5 mg, Mo 42 mcg, niacin 20 mg, pantothenic acid 10 mg, potassium 37.5 mg, Se 87.5 mcg, Zn 15 mg
One-A-Day® Today [OTC]	3000	1.1	1.7	3	18	75	400	33	Biotin 30 mcg, Ca 240 mg, Cr 120 mcg, Cu 2 mg, folic acid 0.4 mg, Mg 120 mg, Mn 2 mg, niacin 14 mg, pantothenic acid 5 mg, potassium 100 mg, Se 70 mcg, soy extract 10 mg, vit K 20 mcg, Zn 15 mg
One-A-Day® Women's Formula [OTC]	2500	1.5	1.7	2	6	60	400	30	Ca 450 mg, Fe 18 mg, folic acid 0.4 mg, Mg 50 mg, niacin 10 mg, pantothenic acid 5 mg, Zn 15 mg
Tablet, Chewable									
Centrum® [OTC]	5000	1.5	1.7	2	6	60	400	30	Biotin 45 mcg, Ca 108 mg, Cr 20 mcg, Cu 2 mg, Fe 18 mg, folic acid 0.4 mg, iodine 150 mcg, Mg 40 mg, Mn 1 mg, Mo 20 mcg, niacin 20 mg, pantothenic acid 10 mg, Zn 15 mg

Ca = calcium, Cr = chromium, Cu = copper, Fe = iron, Mg = magnesium, Mn = manganese, Mo = molybdenum, Se = selenium, Zn = zinc.

MULTIVITAMIN PRODUCTS *(Continued)*

Pediatric Formulations

Product	A (int. units)	B_1 (mg)	B_2 (mg)	B_6 (mg)	B_{12} (mcg)	C (mg)	D (int. units)	E (int. units)	Additional Information
Drops									
ADEKs [OTC] (per mL)	1500	0.5	0.6	0.6	4	45	400	40	Beta carotene 1 mg, biotin 15 mcg, niacin 6 mg, vit K 0.1 mg, Zn 5 mg; alcohol free, dye free (60 mL)
Poly-Vi-Flor® 0.25 mg (per mL)	1500	0.5	0.6	0.4	2	35	400	5	**Fluoride 0.25 mg**, niacin 8 mg; fruit flavor (50 mL)
Poly-Vi-Flor® 0.5 mg (per mL)	1500	0.5	0.6	0.4	2	35	400	5	**Fluoride 0.5 mg**, niacin 8 mg; fruit flavor (50 mL)
Poly-Vi-Flor® With Iron 0.25 mg (per mL)	1500	0.5	0.6	0.4		35	400	5	**Fluoride 0.25 mg**, iron 10 mg, niacin 8 mg; fruit flavor (50 mL)
Poly-Vi-Sol® [OTC] (per mL)	1500	0.5	0.6	0.4	2	35	400	5	Niacin 8 mg (50 mL)
Poly-Vi-Sol® With Iron [OTC] (per mL)	1500	0.5	0.6	0.4		35	400	5	Iron 10 mg, niacin 8 mg (50 mL)
Soluvite-F® (per 0.6 mL)	1500					35	400		**Fluoride 0.25 mg**; alcohol free, dye free, orange flavor (57 mL)
Tri-Vi-Flor® 0.25 mg (per mL)	1500					35	400		**Fluoride 0.25 mg**; fruit flavor (50 mL)
Tri-Vi-Flor® With Iron 0.25 mg (per mL)	1500					35	400		**Fluoride 0.25 mg**, iron 10 mg; fruit flavor (50 mL)
Tri-Vi-Sol® [OTC] (per mL)	1500					35	400		Fruit flavor (50 mL)
Tri-Vi-Sol® With Iron [OTC] (per mL)	1500					35	400		Iron 10 mg; fruit flavor (50 mL)
Vi-Daylin® [OTC] (per mL)	1500	0.5	0.6	0.4	1.5	35	400	5	Niacin 8 mg; alcohol <0.5%, sugar free, fruit flavor (50 mL)
Vi-Daylin® + Iron [OTC] (per mL)	1500	0.5	0.6	0.4		35	400	5	Iron 10 mg, niacin 8 mg; alcohol <0.5%, sugar free, fruit flavor (50 mL)
Vi-Daylin® ADC [OTC] (per mL)	1500					35	400		Alcohol <0.5%, sugar free, fruit flavor (50 mL)
Vi-Daylin® ADC + Iron [OTC] (per mL)	1500					35	400		Iron 10 mg; benzoic acid, sugar free, fruit flavor (50 mL)
Vi-Daylin®/F (per mL)	1500	0.5	0.6	0.4		35	400	5	**Fluoride 0.25 mg**, niacin 8 mg; alcohol <0.1%, benzoic acid, sugar free, fruit flavor (50 mL)
Vi-Daylin®/F + Iron (per mL)	1500	0.5	0.6	0.4		35	400	5	**Fluoride 0.25 mg**, iron 10 mg, niacin 8 mg; alcohol <0.1%, benzoic acid, sugar free, fruit flavor (50 mL)
Vi-Daylin®/F ADC (per mL)	1500					35	400		**Fluoride 0.25 mg**; sugar free, fruit flavor (50 mL)
Vi-Daylin®/F ADC + Iron (per mL)	1500					35	400		**Fluoride 0.25 mg**, iron 10 mg; sugar free, fruit flavor (50 mL)
Gum									
Vitaball®	5000	1.5	1.7	2	6	60	400	30	Biotin 45 mcg, folic acid 400 mcg, niacinamide 20 mg, pantothenic acid 10 mg; bubble gum, cherry, grape, and watermelon flavors

Pediatric Formulations *(continued)*

Product	A (int. units)	B_1 (mg)	B_2 (mg)	B_6 (mg)	B_{12} (mcg)	C (mg)	D (int. units)	E (int. units)	Additional Information
Tablet, Chewable									
ADEKs® [OTC]	4000	1.2	1.3	1.5	12	60	400	150	Beta carotene 3 mg, biotin 50 mcg, folic acid 0.2 mg, niacin 10 mg, pantothenic acid 10 mg, vit K 150 mcg, Zn 7.5 mg; dye free
Centrum® Kids Rugrats™ Complete [OTC]	5000	1.5	1.7	2	6	60	400	30	Biotin 45 mcg, Ca 108 mg, Cr 20 mcg, Cu 2 mg, Fe 18 mg, folic acid 0.4 mg, iodine 150 mcg, Mg 40 mg, Mn 1 mg, Mo 20 mcg, niacin 20 mg, pantothenic acid 10 mg, phosphorus 50 mg, vit K 10 mg, Zn 15 mg; cherry, fruit punch, and orange flavors
Centrum® Kids Rugrats™ Extra C [OTC]	5000	1.5	1.7	1	5	250	400	15	Ca 108 mg, Cu 0.5 mg, folic acid 0.3 mg, niacin 13.5 mg, phosphorus 50 mg, sodium 15 mg, Zn 4 mg; cherry, fruit punch, and orange flavors
Centrum® Kids Rugrats™ Extra Calcium [OTC]	5000	1.5	1.7	1	5	60	400	15	Ca 200 mg, Cu 0.5 mg, folic acid 0.3 mg, niacin 13.5 mg, phosphorus 50 mg, Zn 4 mg; cherry, fruit punch, and orange flavors
Flintstones® Complete [OTC]	5000	1.5	1.7	2	6	60	400	30	Biotin 40 mcg, Ca 100 mg, Cu 2 mg, Fe 18 mg, folic acid 0.4 mg, iodine 150 mcg, Mg 20 mg, niacin 20 mg, pantothenic acid 10 mg, phosphorus 100 mg, Zn 15 mg; **phenylalanine 4.56 mg**; cherry, grape, and orange flavors
Flintstones® Original [OTC]	2500	1.05	1.2	1.05	4.5	60	400	15	Folic acid 0.3 mg, niacin 13.5 mg
Flintstones® Plus Calcium [OTC]	2500	1.05	1.2	1.05	4.5	60	400	15	Ca 200 mg, folic acid 0.3 mg, niacin 13.5 mg; **phenylalanine <4 mg**; cherry, grape, and orange flavors
Flintstones® Plus Extra C [OTC]	2500	1.05	1.2	1.05	4.5	250	400	15	Folic acid 0.3 mg, niacin 13.5 mg; grape, orange, peach-apricot, raspberry, and strawberry flavors
Flintstones® Plus Iron [OTC]	2500	1.05	1.2	1.05	4.5	60	400	15	Fe 15 mg, folic acid 0.3 mg, niacin 13.5 mg; grape, orange, peach-apricot, raspberry, and strawberry flavors
My First Flintstones® [OTC]	2500	1.05	1.2	1.05	4.5	60	400	15	Folic acid 0.3 mg, niacin 13.5 mg; cherry, grape, and orange flavors
One-A-Day® Kids Bugs Bunny and Friends Complete [OTC]	5000	1.5	1.7	2	6	60	400	30	Biotin 40 mcg, Ca 100 mg, Cu 2 mg, Fe 18 mg, folic acid 0.4 mg, iodine 150 mcg, Mg 20 mg, niacin 20 mg, pantothenic acid 10 mg, phosphorus 100 mg, Zn 15 mg; sugar free, fruity flavors

MULTIVITAMIN PRODUCTS *(Continued)*

Pediatric Formulations *(continued)*

Product	A (int. units)	B_1 (mg)	B_2 (mg)	B_6 (mg)	B_{12} (mcg)	C (mg)	D (int. units)	E (int. units)	Additional Information
One-A-Day® Kids Bugs Bunny and Friends Plus Extra C [OTC]	2500	1.05	1.2	1.05	4.5	250	400	15	Folic acid 0.3 mg, niacin 13.5 mg, **phenylalanine**; sugar free, fruity flavors
One-A-Day® Kids Extreme Sports [OTC]	5000	1.5	1.2	2	6	60	400	30	Biotin 40 mcg, Ca 100 mg, Cu 2 mg, Fe 18 mg, folic acid 0.4 mg, iodine 150 mcg, Mg 20 mg, niacin 20 mg, pantothenic acid 10 mg, phosphorus 100 mg, Zn 15 mg
One-A-Day® Kids Scooby-Doo! Complete [OTC]	5000	1.5	1.7	2	6	60	400	30	Biotin 40 mcg, Ca 100 mg, Cu 2 mg, Fe 18 mg, folic acid 0.4 mg, iodine 150 mcg, Mg 20 mg, niacin 20 mg, pantothenic acid 10 mg, phosphorus 100 mg, Zn 15 mg; fruity flavors
One-A-Day® Kids Scooby-Doo! Plus Calcium [OTC]	2500	1.05	1.2	1.05	4.5	60	400	15	Ca 200 mg, folic acid 0.3 mg, niacin 13.5 mg; fruity flavors

Ca = calcium, Cr = chromium, Cu = copper, Fe = iron, Mg = magnesium, Mn = manganese, Mo = molybdenum, Zn = zinc.

Prenatal Formulations

Product	A (int. units)	B_1 (mg)	B_2 (mg)	B_6 (mg)	B_{12} (mcg)	C (mg)	D (int. units)	E (int. units)	Additional Information
Caplet									
StrongStart™	1000	3	3	20	12	100	400	30	Ca 200 mg, Fe 29 mg, folic acid 1 mg, niacinamide 15 mg, pantothenic acid 7 mg, Zn 20 mg; docusate sodium 25 mg
Capsule									
Anemagen™ OB		1.6	1.8	20	12	60	400	30	Ca 200 mg, Fe 28 mg, folic acid 1 mg; docusate calcium 25 mg
Chromagen OB®		1.6	1.8	20	12	60	400	30	Ca 200 mg, Cu 2 mg, Fe 28 mg, folic acid 1 mg, Mn 2 mg, niacinamide 5 mg, Zn 25 mg; docusate calcium 25 mg
Prenatal H		10	6	5	15	200			Cu 0.8 mg, Fe 106 mg, folic acid 1 mg, Mg 6.9 mg, Mn 1.3 mg, niacinamide 30 mg, pantothenic acid 10 mg, Zn 18.2 mg
Prenatal U		10	6	5	15	200			Cu 0.8 mg, Fe 106.5 mg, folic acid 1 mg, Mn 1.3 mg, niacinamide 30 mg, pantothenic acid 10 mg
Powder									
Obegyn® (per 4 level tsp/8.25 g)	2500 (as palmatate) 2500 (as beta-carotene)	1.7	2	10	12	120	400	60	Biotin 300 mcg, Ca 455 mg, Cu 2 mg, Fe 18 mg, folic acid 1 mg, iodine 150 mcg, Mg 150 mg, niacin 20 mg, pantothenic acid 10 mg, Zn 25 mg; **phenylalanine 84 mg/8.25 g**; orange flavor (495 g/60 doses)
Tablet									
A-Free Prenatal		2	2	1	2	33.3	133.3	10	Calcium 333.3 mg, biotin 10 mcg, Cu 0.1 mg, Fe 9 mg, folic acid 266.6 mcg, Mg 33.3 mg, Mn 0.1 mg, niacinamide 10 mg, pantothenic acid 5 mg, Zn 7.5 mg
Advanced NatalCare®	2700	3	3.4	20	12	120	400	30	Ca 200 mg, Cu 2 mg, Fe 90 mg, folic acid 1 mg, Mg 30 mg, niacinamide 20 mg, Zn 25 mg; docusate sodium 50 mg
Aminate Fe-90	4000	3	3.4	20	12	120	400	30	Ca 250 mg, Cu 2 mg, Fe 90 mg, folic acid 1 mg, iodine 150 mcg, niacinamide 20 mg, Zn 25 mg; docusate sodium 50 mg
Cal-Nate™	2700	3	3.4	20		120	400	30	Ca 125 mg, Cu 2 mg, Fe 27 mg, folic acid 1 mg, iodine 150 mcg, niacinamide 20 mg, Zn 25 mg; docusate calcium 50 mg
Citracal® Prenatal Rx	2700	3	3.4	20		120	400	30	Ca 125 mg, Cu 2 mg, Fe 27 mg, folic acid 1 mg, iodine 150 mcg, niacinamide 20 mg, Zn 25 mg; docusate sodium 50 mg
Duet®	3000	1.8	4	25	12	120	400	30	Ca 200 mg, Cu 2 mg, Fe 29 mg, folic acid 1 mg, Mg 25 mg, niacinamide 20 mg, Zn 25 mg
KPN Prenatal	2666.6	2	2	1	2	33.3	133.3	10	Ca 333.3 mg, biotin 10 mcg, Cu 0.1 mg, Fe 9 mg, folic acid 266.6 mcg, Mg 33.3 mg, Mn 0.1 mg, niacinamide 10 mg, pantothenic acid 5 mg, Zn 7.5 mg

MULTIVITAMIN PRODUCTS *(Continued)*

Prenatal Formulations *(continued)*

Product	A (int. units)	B_1 (mg)	B_2 (mg)	B_6 (mg)	B_{12} (mcg)	C (mg)	D (int. units)	E (int. units)	Additional Information
NatalCare® CFe 60	1000	2	3	10	12	120	400	11	Fe 60 mg, folic acid 1 mg, niacinamide 20 mg
NatalCare® GlossTabs™	2700	3	3.4	20	12	120	400	10	Biotin 30 mcg, Ca 200 mg, Cu 2 mg, Fe 90 mg, folic acid 1 mg, Mg 30 mg, niacinamide 20 mg, pantothenic acid 6 mg, Zn 15 mg; docusate sodium 50 mg
NatalCare® PIC	4000	2.43	3	1.64	3	50	400		Ca 125 mg, folic acid 1 mg, niacinamide 10 mg, polysaccharide-iron complex 60 mg, Zn 18 mg
NatalCare® PIC Forte	5000	3	3.4	4	12	80	400	30	Ca 250 mg, Cu 2 mg, folic acid 1 mg, iodine 200 mcg, Mg 10 mg, niacinamide 20 mg, polysaccharide-iron complex 60 mg, Zn 25 mg
NatalCare® Plus	4000	1.84	3	10	12	120	400	22	Ca 200 mg, Cu 2 mg, Fe 27 mg, folic acid 1 mg, niacinamide 20 mg, Zn 25 mg
NatalCare® Rx	2000	0.75	0.8	2	1.25	40	200	7.5	Biotin 15 mcg, Ca 100 mg, Cu 1.5 mg, folate 0.5 mg, Fe 27 mg, Mg 50 mg, niacin 8.5 mg, pantothenic acid 3.75 mg, Zn 12.5 mg
NatalCare® Three	3000	1.8	4	25	12	120	400	22	Ca 200 mg, Cu 2 mg, Fe 28 mg, folic acid 1 mg, Mg 25 mg, niacinamide 20 mg, Zn 25 mg
NataFort®	1000	2	3	10	12	120	400	11	Fe 60 mg, folic acid 1 mg, niacinamide 20 mg
NataTab™ CFe	4000	3	3	3	8	120	400	30	Ca 200 mg, Fe 50 mg, folic acid 1 mg, iodine 150 mcg, niacin 20 mg, Zn 15 mg
NataTab™ FA	4000	3	3	6	8	120	400	30	Ca 200 mg, Fe 29 mg, folic acid 1 mg, iodine 150 mcg, niacin 20 mg, Zn 15 mg
NataTab™ Rx	4000	3	3	3	8	120	400	30	Biotin 30 mcg, Ca 200 mg, Cu 3 mg, Fe 29 mg, folic acid 1 mg, iodine 150 mcg, Mg 100 mg, niacin 20 mg, pantothenic acid 7 mg, Zn 15 mg
Nestabs® CBF	4000	3	3	3	8	120	400	30	Ca 200 mg, Fe 50 mg, folic acid 1 mg, iodine 150 mcg, niacin 20 mg, Zn 15 mg
Nestabs® FA	4000	3	3	3	8	120	400	30	Ca 200 mg, Fe 29 mg, folic acid 1 mg, iodine 150 mcg, niacin 20 mg, Zn 15 mg
Nestabs® RX	4000	3	3	3	8	120	400	30	Biotin 30 mcg, Ca 200 mg, Cu 3 mg, Fe 29 mg, folic acid 1 mg, iodine 150 mcg, Mg 100 mg, niacin 20 mg, pantothenic acid 7 mg, Zn 15 mg
Niferex®-PN	4000	2.43	3	1.64	3	50	400		Ca 125 mg, folic acid 1 mg, niacinamide 10 mg, polysaccharide-iron complex 60 mg, Zn 18 mg
Niferex®-PN Forte	5000	3	3.4	4	12	80	400	30	Ca 250 mg, Cu 2 mg, folic acid 1 mg, iodine 200 mcg, Mg 10 mg, niacinamide 20 mg, polysaccharide-iron complex 60 mg, Zn 25 mg

Prenatal Formulations *(continued)*

Product	A (int. units)	B_1 (mg)	B_2 (mg)	B_6 (mg)	B_{12} (mcg)	C (mg)	D (int. units)	E (int. units)	Additional Information
OB-20	2000	43	0.5	2.5	2	30	100	15	Biotin 37.5 mcg, Ca 125 mg, Cr 6.25 mcg, Fe 12.5 mg, folic acid 2.5 mg, Mg 37.5 mg, Mn 1.25 mg, niacinamide 5 mg, pantothenic acid 2.5 mg, Se 6.25 mcg, Zn 6.2 mg
Prenatal 1-A-Day	4000	2	3	3	10	100	400	15	Biotin 100 mcg, Ca 200 mg, Cu 2 mg, Fe 27 mg, folic acid 800 mcg, Mg 60 mg, Mn 2 mg, niacinamide 20 mg, pantothenic acid 10 mg, Zn 15 mg
Prenatal AD	2700	3	3.4	12	120	120	400	30	Ca 200 mg, Cu 2 mg, Fe 90 mg, folic acid 1 mg, Mg 30 mg, niacinamide 20 mg, Zn 25 mg; docusate sodium 50 mg
Prenatal MR 90 Fe™	4000	3	3.4	20	12	120	400	30	Ca 250 mg, Cu 2 mg, Fe 90 mg, folic acid 1 mg, iodine 150 mcg, niacinamide 20 mg, Zn 25 mg; docusate sodium 50 mg
Prenatal MRT with Selenium	5000	3	3.4	10	12	120	400	30	Biotin 30 mcg, Ca 200 mg, Cr 25 mcg, Cu 2 mg, Fe 27 mg, folic acid 1 mg, iodine 150 mcg, Mg 25 mg, Mn 5 mg, Mo 25 mcg, niacinamide 20 mg, pantothenic acid 10 mg, Se 20 mcg, Zn 25 mg
Prenatal Plus	4000	1.8	3	10	12	120	400	22	Ca 200 mg, Cu 2 mg, Fe 27 mg, folic acid 1 mg, niacinamide 20 mg, Zn 25 mg
Prenatal Rx 1	4000	1.5	1.6	4	2.5	80	400	15	Biotin 30 mcg, Ca 200 mg, Cu 3 mg, Fe 60 mg, folic acid 1 mg, Mg 100 mg, niacinamide 17 mg, pantothenic acid 7 mg, Zn 25 mg
Prenatal Z	3000	1.5	1.6	2.2	2.2	70	400	10	Ca 200 mg, Fe 65 mg, folic acid 1 mg, iodine 175 mcg, Mg 100 mg, niacin 17 mg, Zn 15 mg
Prenate Elite™		3	3.4	20	12	120	400	10	Biotin 300 mcg, Ca 200 mg, Cu 2 mg, Fe 90 mg, folate 1 mg, Mg 30 mg, niacinamide 20 mg, pantothenic acid 6 mg, Zn 15 mg; docusate sodium 50 mg
Prenate GT™	2700	3	3.4	20	12	120	400	10	Biotin 30 mcg, Ca 200 mg, Cu 2 mg, Fe 90 mg, folic acid 1 mg, Mg 30 mg, niacinamide 20 mg, pantothenic acid 6 mg, Zn 15 mg; docusate sodium 50 mg
Stuartnatal® Plus 3™	3000	1.8	4	25	12	120	400	22	Ca 200 mg, Cu 2 mg, Fe 28 mg, folic acid 1 mg, Mg 25 mg, niacinamide 20 mg, Zn 25 mg
Stuart Prenatal®	4000	1.8	1.7	2.6	8	120	400	30	Ca 200 mg, Fe 28 mg, folic acid 0.8 mg, niacin 20 mg, Zn 25 mg
Trinate	3000	1.8	4	25	12	120	400	22	Ca 200 mg, Cu 2 mg, Fe 28 mg, folic acid 1 mg, Mg 25 mg, niacin 20 mg, Zn 25 mg
Ultra NatalCare®	2700	3	3.4	20	12	120	400	30	Ca 200 mg, Cu 2 mg, Fe 90 mg, folic acid 1 mg, iodine 150 mcg, niacinamide 20 mg, Zn 25 mg; docusate sodium 50 mg

MULTIVITAMIN PRODUCTS *(Continued)*

Prenatal Formulations *(continued)*

Product	A (int. units)	B_1 (mg)	B_2 (mg)	B_6 (mg)	B_{12} (mcg)	C (mg)	D (int. units)	E (int. units)	Additional Information
Tablet, Chewable									
Duet®	3000	1.8	4	25	12	120	400	30	Ca 100 mg, Cu 2 mg, Fe 29 mg, folic acid 1 mg, Mg 25 mg, niacinamide 20 mg, Zn 25 mg; **phenylalanine 15 mg/tablet**
NataChew™	1000	2	3	10	12	120	400	11	Fe 29 mg, folic acid 1 mg, niacinamide 20 mg; peanut extract, wild berry flavor
NutriNate®	1000	2	3	10	12	120	400	11	Fe 29 mg, folic acid 1 mg, niacinamide 20 mg; wild berry flavor
PreCare®				2		50	6 mcg	3.5 mg	Ca 250 mg, Cu 2 mg, Fe 40 mg, folic acid 1 mg, Mg 50 mg, Zn 15 mg
StrongStart™	1000	1	3	20	15	100	400	30	Ca 200 mg, Fe 29 mg, folic acid 1 mg, niacinamide 15 mg, pantothenic acid 7 mg, Zn 20 mg; **phenylalanine 6 mg/tablet**
Combination Package									
CareNate™ 600	3500	2	3	3	12	60	400	30	Tablet: Cu 2 mg, Fe 60 mg, folic acid 1 mg, Mg 25 mg, Zn 20 mg; dioctylsulfosuccinate sodium 50 mg Chewable tablet: Ca 600 mg; wild berry flavor
Duet™ DHA	3000	1.8	4	25	12	120	400	30	Tablet: Ca 200 mg, Cu 2 mg, Fe 29 mg, folic acid 1 mg, Mg 25 mg, niacinamide 20 mg, Zn 25 mg Capsule: Omega-3 fatty acids ≥ DHA 200 mg

Cr = chromium, Cu = copper, Fe = iron, Mg = magnesium, Mn = manganese, Mo = molybdenum, Se = selenium, Zn = zinc.

Vitamin B Complex Combinations

Product	B_1 (mg)	B_2 (mg)	B_6 (mg)	B_{12} (mcg)	C (mg)	E (int. units)	Additional Information
Caplet							
Allbee® with C [OTC]	15	10.2	5		300		Niacinamide 50 mg, pantothenic acid 10 mg
Allbee® C-800 [OTC]	15	17	25	12	800	45	Niacinamide 100 mg, pantothenic acid 25 mg
Allbee® C-800 + Iron [OTC]	15	17	25	12	800	45	Fe 27 mg, folic acid 0.4 mcg, niacinamide 100 mg, pantothenic acid 25 mg
Capsule							
Trinsicon®				15			C 75 mg, Fe 110 mg, folic acid 0.5 mg, liver-stomach concentrate (containing intrinsic factor and other vitamin B complex factors) 240 mg
Liquid							
Apatate® [OTC] (per 5 mL) [OTC]	15		0.5	25			Cherry flavor (120 mL)
Gevrabon® [OTC] (per 30 mL) [OTC]	5	2.5	1	1			Choline 10 mg, Fe 15 mg, iodine 100 mcg, Mg 2 mg, Mn 2 mg, niacinamide 60 mg, pantothenic acid 10 mg, Zn 2 mg; alcohol, benzoic acid; sherry wine flavor (480 mL)
Softgel							
Nephrocaps®	1.5	1.7	10	6	100		Biotin 150 mcg, folic acid 1 mcg, niacinamide 20 mg, pantothenic acid 5 mg
Tablet							
Diatx™	1.5	1.5	50		60		Biotin 300 mcg, cobalamin 1 mg, folacin 5 mg, niacinamide 20 mg, pantothenic acid 10 mg [dye free, lactose free, sugar free]
DiatxFe™	1.5	1.5	50		60		Biotin 300 mcg, cobalamin 1 mg, ferrous fumarate 304 mg, folacin 5 mg, niacinamide 20 mg, pantothenic acid 10 mg [dye free, lactose free, sugar free]
NephPlex® Rx	1.5	1.7	10	6	60		Biotin 300 mcg, folic acid 1 mg, niacinamide 20 mg, pantothenic acid 10 mg, zinc 12.5 mg
Nephro-Vite®	1.5	1.7	10	6	60		Biotin 300 mcg, folic acid 0.8 mcg, niacinamide 20 mg, pantothenic acid 10 mg
Nephro-Vite® Rx	1.5	1.7	10	6	60		Biotin 300 mcg, folic acid 1 mcg, niacinamide 20 mg, pantothenic acid 10 mg
Nephron FA®	1.5	1.7	10	6	40		Biotin 300 mcg, docusate sodium 75 mg, ferrous fumarate 200 mg, folic acid 1 mg, pantothenic acid 10 mg
Olay® Vitamins Essential Folic Acid w/B_{12} Complex [OTC]		25	25	200		200	Folic acid 600 mcg, Se 50 mcg
Olay® Vitamins Super B-Stress Defense [OTC]	10	10	5	12	500	30	Biotin 100 mcg, folic acid 400 mcg, niacin 100 mg, pantothenic acid 20 mg
Stresstabs® B-Complex [OTC]	10	10	5	12	500	30	Biotin 45 mcg, folic acid 0.4 mcg, niacinamide 100 mg, pantothenic acid 20 mg
Stresstabs® B-Complex + Iron [OTC]	10	10	5	12	500	30	Biotin 45 mcg, Fe 18 mg, folic acid 0.4 mcg, niacinamide 100 mg, pantothenic acid 20 mg

MULTIVITAMIN PRODUCTS *(Continued)*

Vitamin B Complex Combinations *(continued)*

Product	B_1 (mg)	B_2 (mg)	B_6 (mg)	B_{12} (mcg)	C (mg)	E (int. units)	Additional Information
Stresstabs® B-Complex + Zinc [OTC]	10	10	5	12	500	30	Biotin 45 mcg, Cu 3 mg, folic acid 0.4 mcg, niacinamide 100 mg, pantothenic acid 20 mg, Zn 23.9 mg
Surbex-T® [OTC]	15	10	5	10	500		Ca 20 mg, niacinamide 100 mg
Z-Bec® [OTC]	15	10.2	10	6	600	45	Niacinamide 100 mg, pantothenic acid 25 mg, Zn 22.5 mg
Tablet, Chewable							
Apatate® [OTC]	15		0.5	25			Cherry flavor

Ca = calcium, Cu = copper, Fe = iron, Mg = magnesium, Mn = manganese, Se = selenium, Zn = zinc.

DENTAL DRUG USE IN PREGNANCY AND BREAST-FEEDING[1]

Drug	FDA Pregnancy Category	Use During Pregnancy	Use During Breast-Feeding
Acetaminophen	B	Yes	Yes
Acetaminophen and Codeine	C	Low dose for short duration	Yes (with caution)
Acetaminophen and Tramadol	C	No information	No information
Acyclovir	B	No information	No information
Alprazolam	D	Avoid	Avoid
Amlexanox	B	Yes	Yes
Ammonia Spirit (Aromatic)	C	No information	No information
Amoxicillin	B	Yes	Yes
Amoxicillin and Clavulanate Potassium	B	Yes	Yes
Ampicillin	B	Yes	Yes
Ampicillin and Sulbactam	B	Yes	Yes
Articaine Hydrochloride and Epinephrine (U.S.)	C	Yes	Yes
Aspirin	C/D	Not in third trimester	Avoid
Aspirin and Codeine	D	Not in third trimester	Avoid
Azithromycin	B	Yes	Yes
Benzocaine	C	Yes	Yes
Bupivacaine	C	Yes	Yes
Bupivacaine and Epinephrine	C	Yes	Yes
Carbamide Peroxide	C	Yes	Yes
Cefaclor	B	Yes	Yes
Cefadroxil	B	Yes	Yes
Cefazolin	B	Yes	Yes
Cefditoren	B	Yes	Yes
Celecoxib	C/D	No information	No information
Cephalexin	B	Yes	Yes
Cephradine	B	Yes	Yes
Cevimeline	C	No information	No information
Clarithromycin	C	Yes	Yes
Clindamycin	B	Yes	Yes
Clotrimazole	C (troches)	Yes	Yes
Cloxacillin	B	Yes	Yes
Codeine	C	Low dose for short duration	Yes (with caution)
Diazepam	D	Avoid	Avoid
Dibucaine	C	Yes	Yes
Diclofenac	B/D	Not in third trimester	Yes
Dicloxacillin	B	Yes	Yes
Diflunisal	C/D	Not in third trimester	Yes
Diphenhydramine	B	Yes	Yes
Doxycycline Hyclate (Periodontal)	D	Avoid	Avoid
Epinephrine	C	Yes	Yes
Erythromycin	B	Yes (avoid estolate)	Yes
Etidocaine and Epinephrine	B	Yes	Yes
Etodolac	C/D	Not in third trimester	Yes
Fentanyl	C/D	Yes (with caution)	Yes
Fluconazole	C	Yes	Yes
Flurbiprofen	C/D	Not in third trimester	Yes
Hydrocodone and Acetaminophen	C	Low dose for short duration	Yes (with caution)
Hydrocodone and Aspirin	D	Not in third trimester	Avoid
Hydrocodone and Ibuprofen	C/D	Not in third trimester	Yes (with caution)
Ibuprofen	B/D	Not in third trimester	Yes
Ketoconazole	C	Yes	Yes
Ketoprofen	B/D	Not in third trimester	Yes

DENTAL DRUG USE IN PREGNANCY AND BREAST-FEEDING[1] *(Continued)*

Drug	FDA Pregnancy Category	Use During Pregnancy	Use During Breast-Feeding
Ketorolac	C/D	Not in third trimester	Yes
Lidocaine	B	Yes	Yes
Lidocaine and Epinephrine	B	Yes	Yes
Lidocaine and Prilocaine	B	Yes	Yes
Lorazepam	D	Avoid	Avoid
Meperidine	B/D	Low dose for short duration	Yes (with caution)
Mepivacaine	C	Yes	Yes
Mepivacaine (Dental Anesthetic)	C	Yes	Yes
Methohexital	C	Yes	Yes
Metronidazole	B	Yes (with caution)	Yes (with caution)
Midazolam	D	Avoid	Avoid
Minocycline	D	Avoid	Avoid
Minocycline Hydrochloride (Periodontal)	D	Avoid	Avoid
Naloxone	C	Yes	Yes
Naproxen	B/D	Not in third trimester	Yes
Nitrous Oxide	None reported	Yes (with caution)	Yes
Nystatin	B/C	Yes	Yes
Oxycodone	B/D	Low dose for short duration	Yes
Oxycodone and Acetaminophen	C/D	Low dose for short duration	Yes
Oxycodone and Aspirin	D	Not in third trimester	Avoid
Oxygen	None reported	Yes	Yes
Penciclovir	B	Yes	Yes
Penicillin V Potassium	B	Yes	Yes
Pentazocine and Acetaminophen	C	Low dose for short duration	Yes (with caution)
Prilocaine	B	Yes	Yes
Prilocaine and Epinephrine	C	Yes	Yes
Propantheline	C	Yes	Yes
Propoxyphene and Acetaminophen	C	Low dose for short duration	Yes (with caution)
Propoxyphene, Aspirin, and Caffeine	D	Not in third trimester	Avoid
Rofecoxib	C/D	No information	No information
Sulfonated Phenolics in Aqueous Solution	C	Yes	Yes
Tetracaine	C	Yes	Yes
Tetracycline	D	Avoid	Avoid
Tetracycline (Periodontal)	C	Avoid	Avoid
Tramadol	C	No (labor and delivery)	No
Triazolam	X	Avoid	Avoid
Valacyclovir	B	Yes	Yes
Valdecoxib	C/D	No information	No information

[1]Pregnant or breast-feeding women should be encouraged to consult a physician prior to the use of any prescription or nonprescription medication. Additional information concerning other medications may be found in individual drug monographs.

References:

Della-Giustina K and Chow G, "Medications in Pregnancy and Lactation," *Emerg Med Clin North Am*, 2003, 21(3):585-613.

Drug Information for the Health Care Professional, 20th ed, Vol 1, Rockville, MD: Medical Economics Company, 2000.

Haas DA, Pynn BR, and Sands TD, "Drug Use for the Pregnant or Lactating Patient," *Gen Dent*, 2000, 48(1):54-60.

Mariotti AJ, "Agents That Affect the Fetus and Nursing Infant," *ADA Guide to Dental Therapeutics*, 2nd ed, Chicago IL: ADA Publishing, 2000, 594-5.

PHARMACOLOGIC CATEGORY INDEX

ABORTIFACIENT
Carboprost Tromethamine 265
Dinoprostone 447
Mifepristone 928

ACETYLCHOLINESTERASE INHIBITOR
Physostigmine 1084
Pyridostigmine 1153

ACETYLCHOLINESTERASE INHIBITOR (CENTRAL)
Donepezil 462
Galantamine 645
Rivastigmine 1192
Tacrine 1254

ACNE PRODUCTS
Adapalene 67

ADJUVANT ANALGESIC, BISPHOSPHONATE
Zoledronic Acid 1402

ADJUVANT, CHEMOPROTECTIVE AGENT (CYTOPROTECTIVE)
Amifostine 94

ADJUVANT, RADIOSENSITIZING AGENT
Cladribine 342

ADRENERGIC AGONIST AGENT
Carbinoxamine and Pseudoephedrine 262
DOBUTamine 457
Epinephrine 496
Epinephrine (Racemic) and Aluminum Potassium Sulfate 497
Isoetharine 768
Oxymetazoline 1034
Phenylephrine and Zinc Sulfate 1079
Propylhexedrine 1144
Tetrahydrozoline 1282

ADRENERGIC AGONIST AGENT, OPHTHALMIC
Hydroxyamphetamine and Tropicamide 720

ALDEHYDE DEHYDROGENASE INHIBITOR
Disulfiram 456

ALKALINIZING AGENT
Sodium Bicarbonate 1226

ALKALINIZING AGENT, ORAL
Citric Acid, Sodium Citrate, and Potassium Citrate 341
Potassium Citrate 1105
Potassium Citrate and Citric Acid 1106
Sodium Citrate and Citric Acid 1228

ALKALINIZING AGENT, PARENTERAL
Tromethamine 1348

ALPHA-ADRENERGIC INHIBITOR
Methyldopa 906

ALPHA/BETA AGONIST
Acetaminophen and Pseudoephedrine 53
Dipivefrin 453
Ephedrine 495
Epinephrine 496
Epinephrine (Racemic) 497
Epinephrine (Racemic) and Aluminum Potassium Sulfate 497
Norepinephrine 996
Phenylephrine 1078
Pseudoephedrine 1147
Triprolidine and Pseudoephedrine 1345

5 ALPHA-REDUCTASE INHIBITOR
Dutasteride 479
Finasteride 590

ALPHA$_1$ AGONIST
Midodrine 927
Naphazoline 964

ALPHA$_1$ BLOCKER
Alfuzosin 80
Doxazosin 465
Phenoxybenzamine 1075
Phentolamine 1077
Prazosin 1111
Tamsulosin 1260
Terazosin 1271

ALPHA$_1$ BLOCKER, OPHTHALMIC
Dapiprazole 398

ALPHA$_2$-ADRENERGIC AGONIST
Clonidine 358
Dexmedetomidine 415
Guanabenz 677
Guanfacine 679
Tizanidine 1305

ALPHA$_2$ AGONIST, OPHTHALMIC
Apraclonidine 138
Brimonidine 218

AMEBICIDE
Iodoquinol 759
Metronidazole 917
Paromomycin 1046
Tinidazole 1301

AMINOQUINOLINE (ANTIMALARIAL)
Chloroquine 311
Hydroxychloroquine 720
Primaquine 1122

5-AMINOSALICYLIC ACID DERIVATIVE
Balsalazide 181
Mesalamine 882
Olsalazine 1011
Sulfasalazine 1249

AMMONIUM DETOXICANT
Lactulose 794
Neomycin 973

ANABOLIC STEROID
Oxymetholone 1035
Stanozolol 1237

ANALGESIC COMBINATION (NARCOTIC)
Acetaminophen, Caffeine, and Dihydrocodeine 57
Belladonna and Opium 186
Butalbital, Acetaminophen, Caffeine, and Codeine 236
Butalbital, Aspirin, Caffeine, and Codeine 238
Hydrocodone and Acetaminophen 702
Hydrocodone and Aspirin 705
Meperidine and Promethazine . . 872
Pentazocine and Acetaminophen 1064
Propoxyphene and Acetaminophen 1137
Propoxyphene, Aspirin, and Caffeine 1138

ANALGESIC, MISCELLANEOUS
Acetaminophen 47

Acetaminophen and Diphenhydramine . . . 53
Acetaminophen and Pseudoephedrine . . . 53
Acetaminophen and Tramadol . . . 54
Acetaminophen, Aspirin, and Caffeine . . . 56
Acetaminophen, Chlorpheniramine, and Pseudoephedrine . . . 58
Acetaminophen, Isometheptene, and Dichloralphenazone . . . 59

ANALGESIC, NARCOTIC

Acetaminophen and Codeine . . . 50
Alfentanil . . . 79
Aspirin and Codeine . . . 155
Buprenorphine . . . 228
Buprenorphine and Naloxone . . . 230
Butorphanol . . . 240
Codeine . . . 369
Dihydrocodeine, Aspirin, and Caffeine . . . 441
Fentanyl . . . 581
Hydrocodone and Ibuprofen . . . 709
Hydromorphone . . . 718
Levomethadyl Acetate Hydrochloride . . . 814
Levorphanol . . . 816
Meperidine . . . 870
Methadone . . . 889
Morphine Sulfate . . . 947
Nalbuphine . . . 959
Opium Tincture . . . 1015
Oxycodone . . . 1027
Oxycodone and Acetaminophen . . . 1029
Oxycodone and Aspirin . . . 1032
Oxymorphone . . . 1036
Paregoric . . . 1045
Pentazocine . . . 1063
Propoxyphene . . . 1136
Remifentanil . . . 1172
Sufentanil . . . 1242

ANALGESIC, NON-NARCOTIC

Acetaminophen and Phenyltoloxamine . . . 53
Acetaminophen and Tramadol . . . 54
Methotrimeprazine . . . 901
Tramadol . . . 1319

ANALGESIC, TOPICAL

Capsaicin . . . 252
Dichlorodifluoromethane and Trichloromonofluoromethane . . . 427
Lidocaine . . . 819
Triethanolamine Salicylate . . . 1338

ANALGESIC, URINARY

Pentosan Polysulfate Sodium . . . 1065
Phenazopyridine . . . 1072

ANDROGEN

Danazol . . . 396
Fluoxymesterone . . . 609
MethylTESTOSTERone . . . 912
Nandrolone . . . 963
Oxandrolone . . . 1021
Testolactone . . . 1275
Testosterone . . . 1276

ANESTHETIC/CORTICOSTEROID

Lidocaine and Hydrocortisone . . 826
Pramoxine and Hydrocortisone . . . 1109

ANGIOTENSIN-CONVERTING ENZYME (ACE) INHIBITOR

Benazepril . . . 187
Captopril . . . 252
Cilazapril . . . 328
Enalapril . . . 488
Fosinopril . . . 633
Lisinopril . . . 833
Moexipril . . . 940
Perindopril Erbumine . . . 1068
Quinapril . . . 1158
Quinapril and Hydrochlorothiazide . . . 1160
Ramipril . . . 1167
Spirapril . . . 1235
Trandolapril . . . 1321

ANGIOTENSIN II RECEPTOR BLOCKER

Candesartan . . . 248
Eprosartan . . . 501
Irbesartan . . . 763
Losartan . . . 845
Olmesartan . . . 1010
Olmesartan and Hydrochlorothiazide . . . 1010
Telmisartan . . . 1265
Valsartan . . . 1363

ANGIOTENSIN II RECEPTOR BLOCKER COMBINATION

Candesartan and Hydrochlorothiazide . . . 249
Eprosartan and Hydrochlorothiazide . . . 502
Losartan and Hydrochlorothiazide . . . 847
Telmisartan and Hydrochlorothiazide . . . 1265
Valsartan and Hydrochlorothiazide . . . 1364

ANOREXIANT

Benzphetamine . . . 195
Diethylpropion . . . 434
Phendimetrazine . . . 1072
Phentermine . . . 1076
Sibutramine . . . 1218

ANTACID

Aluminum Hydroxide . . . 90
Aluminum Hydroxide and Magnesium Carbonate . . . 90
Aluminum Hydroxide and Magnesium Hydroxide . . . 91
Aluminum Hydroxide and Magnesium Trisilicate . . . 91
Aluminum Hydroxide, Magnesium Hydroxide, and Simethicone . . . 92
Calcium Carbonate . . . 245
Calcium Carbonate and Magnesium Hydroxide . . . 245
Calcium Carbonate and Simethicone . . . 245
Famotidine, Calcium Carbonate, and Magnesium Hydroxide . . . 574
Magaldrate and Simethicone . . . 852
Magnesium Hydroxide . . . 853
Magnesium Sulfate . . . 854
Sodium Bicarbonate . . . 1226

ANTHELMINTIC

Albendazole . . . 71
Ivermectin . . . 779
Mebendazole . . . 859
Piperazine . . . 1094
Praziquantel . . . 1111
Pyrantel Pamoate . . . 1151
Thiabendazole . . . 1286

ANTIANDROGEN

Nilutamide . . . 986

ANTIANXIETY AGENT, MISCELLANEOUS

Aspirin and Meprobamate . . . 156
BusPIRone . . . 233

Meprobamate 878

ANTIARRHYTHMIC AGENT, CLASS I
Moricizine 946

ANTIARRHYTHMIC AGENT, CLASS IA
Disopyramide 455
Procainamide 1124
Quinidine 1160

ANTIARRHYTHMIC AGENT, CLASS IB
Lidocaine 819
Mexiletine 921
Phenytoin 1080
Tocainide 1307

ANTIARRHYTHMIC AGENT, CLASS IC
Flecainide 592
Propafenone 1133

ANTIARRHYTHMIC AGENT, CLASS II
Acebutolol 46
Esmolol 515
Propranolol 1140
Sotalol 1231

ANTIARRHYTHMIC AGENT, CLASS III
Amiodarone 101
Bretylium 217
Dofetilide 460
Ibutilide 731
Sotalol 1231

ANTIARRHYTHMIC AGENT, CLASS IV
Adenosine 68
Digitoxin 437
Digoxin 437
Verapamil 1373

ANTIBACTERIAL, DENTAL
Tetracycline (Periodontal) 1282
Triclosan and Fluoride 1337

ANTIBIOTIC, AMINOGLYCOSIDE
Amikacin 95
Gentamicin 655
Kanamycin 780
Neomycin 973
Streptomycin 1239
Tobramycin 1306

ANTIBIOTIC, CARBACEPHEM
Loracarbef 841

ANTIBIOTIC, CARBAPENEM
Ertapenem 507
Imipenem and Cilastatin 736
Meropenem 881

ANTIBIOTIC, CEPHALOSPORIN
Cefditoren 280

ANTIBIOTIC, CEPHALOSPORIN (FIRST GENERATION)
Cefadroxil 275
Cefazolin 278
Cephalexin 294
Cephalothin 296
Cephradine 296

ANTIBIOTIC, CEPHALOSPORIN (SECOND GENERATION)
Cefaclor 274
Cefamandole 277
Cefotetan 283
Cefoxitin 284
Cefprozil 286
Cefuroxime 289

ANTIBIOTIC, CEPHALOSPORIN (THIRD GENERATION)
Cefdinir 279
Cefixime 282
Cefotaxime 283
Cefpodoxime 285
Ceftazidime 286
Ceftibuten 287
Ceftizoxime 288
Ceftriaxone 288

ANTIBIOTIC, CEPHALOSPORIN (FOURTH GENERATION)
Cefepime 281

ANTIBIOTIC/CORTICOSTEROID, OPHTHALMIC
Neomycin and Dexamethasone . 973
Neomycin, Polymyxin B, and Dexamethasone 974
Neomycin, Polymyxin B, and Hydrocortisone 975
Neomycin, Polymyxin B, and Prednisolone 975
Oxytetracycline and Hydrocortisone 1037
Prednisolone and Gentamicin 1115
Sulfacetamide and Fluorometholone 1244
Sulfacetamide and Prednisolone 1245
Tobramycin and Dexamethasone 1307

ANTIBIOTIC/CORTICOSTEROID, OTIC
Ciprofloxacin and Dexamethasone 336
Ciprofloxacin and Hydrocortisone 336
Neomycin, Polymyxin B, and Hydrocortisone 975

ANTIBIOTIC, CYCLIC LIPOPEPTIDE
Daptomycin 399

ANTIBIOTIC, IRRIGATION
Polymyxin B 1100

ANTIBIOTIC, KETOLIDE
Telithromycin 1263

ANTIBIOTIC, MACROLIDE
Azithromycin 174
Clarithromycin 343
Dirithromycin 454
Erythromycin 508
Erythromycin and Sulfisoxazole 512
Lincomycin 829
Spiramycin 1234
Troleandomycin 1348

ANTIBIOTIC, MACROLIDE COMBINATION
Erythromycin and Sulfisoxazole 512
Lansoprazole, Amoxicillin, and Clarithromycin 798

ANTIBIOTIC, MISCELLANEOUS
Aztreonam 177
Bacitracin 178
Capreomycin 251
Chloramphenicol 306
Clindamycin 348
Colistimethate 374
CycloSERINE 385
Dapsone 398
Fosfomycin 632
Methenamine 892

Methenamine, Sodium Biphosphate, Phenyl Salicylate, Methylene Blue, and Hyoscyamine . . . 893
Metronidazole . . . 917
Nitrofurantoin . . . 990
Pentamidine . . . 1062
Polymyxin B . . . 1100
Rifabutin . . . 1179
Rifampin . . . 1180
Rifampin and Isoniazid . . . 1181
Rifampin, Isoniazid, and Pyrazinamide . . . 1181
Rifaximin . . . 1183
Spectinomycin . . . 1234
Sulfamethoxazole and Trimethoprim . . . 1246
Tinidazole . . . 1301
Trimethoprim . . . 1341
Vancomycin . . . 1365

ANTIBIOTIC, OPHTHALMIC

Bacitracin . . . 178
Bacitracin and Polymyxin B . . . 178
Bacitracin, Neomycin, and Polymyxin B . . . 179
Bacitracin, Neomycin, Polymyxin B, and Hydrocortisone . . . 179
Ciprofloxacin . . . 331
Erythromycin . . . 508
Gatifloxacin . . . 647
Gentamicin . . . 655
Mercuric Oxide . . . 881
Moxifloxacin . . . 949
Neomycin, Polymyxin B, and Gramicidin . . . 974
Oxytetracycline and Polymyxin B . . . 1037
Povidone-Iodine . . . 1107
Sulfacetamide . . . 1244
Tobramycin . . . 1306
Trimethoprim and Polymyxin B . . . 1342

ANTIBIOTIC, ORAL RINSE

Chlorhexidine Gluconate . . . 308

ANTIBIOTIC, OTIC

Bacitracin, Neomycin, Polymyxin B, and Hydrocortisone . . . 179

ANTIBIOTIC, OXAZOLIDINONE

Linezolid . . . 830

ANTIBIOTIC, PENICILLIN

Amoxicillin . . . 114
Amoxicillin and Clavulanate Potassium . . . 116
Ampicillin . . . 124
Ampicillin and Probenecid . . . 126
Ampicillin and Sulbactam . . . 126
Carbenicillin . . . 260
Cloxacillin . . . 365
Dicloxacillin . . . 431
Lansoprazole, Amoxicillin, and Clarithromycin . . . 798
Nafcillin . . . 958
Oxacillin . . . 1020
Penicillin G Benzathine . . . 1058
Penicillin G Benzathine and Penicillin G Procaine . . . 1058
Penicillin G (Parenteral/ Aqueous) . . . 1059
Penicillin G Procaine . . . 1060
Penicillin V Potassium . . . 1060
Piperacillin . . . 1092
Piperacillin and Tazobactam Sodium . . . 1093
Ticarcillin . . . 1295
Ticarcillin and Clavulanate Potassium . . . 1296

ANTIBIOTIC, QUINOLONE

Ciprofloxacin . . . 331
Gatifloxacin . . . 647
Gemifloxacin . . . 653
Levofloxacin . . . 812
Lomefloxacin . . . 837
Moxifloxacin . . . 949
Nalidixic Acid . . . 960
Norfloxacin . . . 997
Ofloxacin . . . 1005
Sparfloxacin . . . 1233
Trovafloxacin . . . 1348

ANTIBIOTIC, STREPTOGRAMIN

Quinupristin and Dalfopristin . . . 1163

ANTIBIOTIC, SULFONAMIDE DERIVATIVE

Erythromycin and Sulfisoxazole . . . 512
Sulfacetamide . . . 1244
SulfaDIAZINE . . . 1245
Sulfamethoxazole and Trimethoprim . . . 1246
SulfiSOXAZOLE . . . 1250

ANTIBIOTIC, TETRACYCLINE DERIVATIVE

Bismuth Subsalicylate, Metronidazole, and Tetracycline . . . 209
Demeclocycline . . . 404
Doxycycline . . . 471
Doxycycline Hyclate (Periodontal) . . . 475
Doxycycline (Subantimicrobial) . . . 476
Minocycline . . . 931
Minocycline Hydrochloride (Periodontal) . . . 933
Oxytetracycline . . . 1036
Tetracycline . . . 1280

ANTIBIOTIC, TOPICAL

Bacitracin . . . 178
Bacitracin and Polymyxin B . . . 178
Bacitracin, Neomycin, and Polymyxin B . . . 179
Bacitracin, Neomycin, Polymyxin B, and Hydrocortisone . . . 179
Bacitracin, Neomycin, Polymyxin B, and Pramoxine . . . 180
Benzalkonium Chloride . . . 190
Benzoin . . . 193
Chlorhexidine Gluconate . . . 308
Erythromycin . . . 508
Gentamicin . . . 655
Gentian Violet . . . 657
Hexachlorophene . . . 693
Mafenide . . . 852
Metronidazole . . . 917
Mupirocin . . . 951
Neomycin . . . 973
Neomycin and Polymyxin B . . . 973
Oxychlorosene . . . 1027
Povidone-Iodine . . . 1107
Silver Nitrate . . . 1221
Silver Sulfadiazine . . . 1221
Thimerosal . . . 1288

ANTIBIOTIC, VAGINAL

Povidone-Iodine . . . 1107
Sulfabenzamide, Sulfacetamide, and Sulfathiazole . . . 1243

ANTICHOLINERGIC/ ADRENERGIC AGONIST

Phenylephrine and Scopolamine . . . 1079

ANTICHOLINERGIC AGENT

Atropine . . . 166

Atropine Sulfate (Dental Tablets) 169
Benztropine 196
Biperiden 207
Dicyclomine 432
Glycopyrrolate 668
Hyoscyamine 724
Hyoscyamine, Atropine, Scopolamine, and Phenobarbital 725
Hyoscyamine, Atropine, Scopolamine, Kaolin, and Pectin 726
Hyoscyamine, Atropine, Scopolamine, Kaolin, Pectin, and Opium 726
Ipratropium 761
Mepenzolate 869
Methscopolamine 903
Procyclidine 1127
Propantheline 1134
Scopolamine 1210
Tiotropium 1303
Tolterodine 1312
Trihexyphenidyl 1340
Trimethobenzamide 1341

ANTICHOLINERGIC AGENT, OPHTHALMIC
Atropine 166
Cyclopentolate 383
Homatropine 693

ANTICOAGULANT
Antithrombin III 136
Danaparoid 395
Heparin 685

ANTICOAGULANT, COUMARIN DERIVATIVE
Warfarin 1389

ANTICOAGULANT, THROMBIN INHIBITOR
Argatroban 140
Bivalirudin 212
Lepirudin 803

ANTICONVULSANT, BARBITURATE
Pentobarbital 1065
Phenobarbital 1073
Thiopental 1289

ANTICONVULSANT, HYDANTOIN
Ethotoin 561
Fosphenytoin 635
Phenytoin 1080

ANTICONVULSANT, MISCELLANEOUS
AcetaZOLAMIDE 60
Carbamazepine 255
Felbamate 575
Gabapentin 642
Lamotrigine 795
Levetiracetam 807
Magnesium Sulfate 854
Oxcarbazepine 1023
Primidone 1122
Tiagabine 1294
Topiramate 1314
Valproic Acid and Derivatives 1359
Vigabatrin 1376
Zonisamide 1405

ANTICONVULSANT, OXAZOLIDINEDIONE
Trimethadione 1340

ANTICONVULSANT, SUCCINIMIDE
Ethosuximide 560
Methsuximide 904

ANTICYSTINE AGENT
Cysteamine 389

ANTIDEPRESSANT, ALPHA-2 ANTAGONIST
Mirtazapine 935

ANTIDEPRESSANT, DOPAMINE-REUPTAKE INHIBITOR
BuPROPion 230

ANTIDEPRESSANT, MONOAMINE OXIDASE INHIBITOR
Isocarboxazid 767
Phenelzine 1072
Selegiline 1212
Tranylcypromine 1323

ANTIDEPRESSANT, SELECTIVE SEROTONIN REUPTAKE INHIBITOR
Citalopram 339
Escitalopram 513
Fluoxetine 606
Fluvoxamine 623
Olanzapine and Fluoxetine 1009
Paroxetine 1046
Sertraline 1215

ANTIDEPRESSANT, SEROTONIN/ NOREPINEPHRINE REUPTAKE INHIBITOR
Venlafaxine 1370

ANTIDEPRESSANT, SEROTONIN REUPTAKE INHIBITOR/ ANTAGONIST
Nefazodone 970
Trazodone 1326

ANTIDEPRESSANT, TETRACYCLIC
Maprotiline 856

ANTIDEPRESSANT, TRICYCLIC (SECONDARY AMINE)
Amoxapine 113
Desipramine 407
Nortriptyline 999
Protriptyline 1146

ANTIDEPRESSANT, TRICYCLIC (TERTIARY AMINE)
Amitriptyline 103
Amitriptyline and Chlordiazepoxide 105
Amitriptyline and Perphenazine 106
ClomiPRAMINE 355
Doxepin 467
Imipramine 737
Trimipramine 1343

ANTIDIABETIC AGENT, ALPHA-GLUCOSIDASE INHIBITOR
Acarbose 45
Miglitol 929

ANTIDIABETIC AGENT, BIGUANIDE
Glipizide and Metformin 662
Glyburide and Metformin 665
Metformin 887
Rosiglitazone and Metformin 1201

ANTIDIABETIC AGENT, INSULIN
Insulin Preparations 749

ANTIDIABETIC AGENT, MISCELLANEOUS
Nateglinide 968
Repaglinide 1173

ANTIDIABETIC AGENT, SULFONYLUREA

AcetoHEXAMIDE 60
ChlorproPAMIDE 321
Glimepiride 659
GlipiZIDE 660
Glipizide and Metformin 662
GlyBURIDE 664
Glyburide and Metformin 665
TOLAZamide 1308
TOLBUTamide 1309

ANTIDIABETIC AGENT, THIAZOLIDINEDIONE

Pioglitazone 1091
Rosiglitazone 1199
Rosiglitazone and Metformin . . 1201

ANTIDIARRHEAL

Attapulgite 170
Bismuth 209
Bismuth Subsalicylate, Metronidazole, and Tetracycline 209
Difenoxin and Atropine 434
Diphenoxylate and Atropine 451
Hyoscyamine, Atropine, Scopolamine, Kaolin, and Pectin 726
Hyoscyamine, Atropine, Scopolamine, Kaolin, Pectin, and Opium 726
Kaolin and Pectin 781
Lactobacillus 793
Loperamide 838
Octreotide 1004
Opium Tincture 1015
Polycarbophil 1100
Psyllium 1151

ANTIDIURETIC HORMONE ANALOG

Vasopressin 1369

ANTIDOTE

Acetylcysteine 61
Aluminum Hydroxide 90
Amifostine 94
Amyl Nitrite 130
Atropine 166
Calcitonin 243
Calcium Acetate 245
Calcium Carbonate 245
Charcoal 303
Deferoxamine 402
Digoxin Immune Fab 440
Dimercaprol 447
Edrophonium 483
Epinephrine 496
Epinephrine and Chlorpheniramine 497
Ferric Hexacyanoferrate 585
Flumazenil 599
Fomepizole 627
Glucagon 663
Insulin Preparations 749
Ipecac Syrup 760
Leucovorin 804
Nalmefene 960
Naloxone 961
Naltrexone 962
Pamidronate 1041
Protamine Sulfate 1145
Sodium Thiosulfate 1230

ANTIEMETIC

Aprepitant 138
Dexamethasone 411
Dolasetron 461
Dronabinol 477
Droperidol 477
Fructose, Dextrose, and Phosphoric Acid 638
Granisetron 671
HydrOXYzine 723
Meclizine 859
Metoclopramide 914
Ondansetron 1014
Palonosetron 1040
Prochlorperazine 1126
Promethazine 1130
Thiethylperazine 1287
Trimethobenzamide 1341

ANTIFLATULENT

Aluminum Hydroxide, Magnesium Hydroxide, and Simethicone 92
Calcium Carbonate and Simethicone 245
Magaldrate and Simethicone . . . 852
Simethicone 1222

ANTIFUNGAL AGENT, OPHTHALMIC

Natamycin 968

ANTIFUNGAL AGENT, ORAL

Fluconazole 594
Flucytosine 596
Griseofulvin 671
Itraconazole 775
Ketoconazole 783
Terbinafine 1272
Voriconazole 1385

ANTIFUNGAL AGENT, ORAL NONABSORBED

Clotrimazole 363
Nystatin 1003

ANTIFUNGAL AGENT, PARENTERAL

Amphotericin B Cholesteryl Sulfate Complex 119
Amphotericin B (Conventional) . . 120
Amphotericin B (Lipid Complex) 121
Amphotericin B (Liposomal) 122
Caspofungin 272
Fluconazole 594
Voriconazole 1385

ANTIFUNGAL AGENT, TOPICAL

Amphotericin B (Conventional) . . 120
Betamethasone and Clotrimazole 201
Butenafine 239
Carbol-Fuchsin Solution 264
Ciclopirox 327
Clotrimazole 363
Econazole 481
Gentian Violet 657
Iodoquinol and Hydrocortisone . . 759
Ketoconazole 783
Miconazole 922
Naftifine 959
Nystatin 1003
Nystatin and Triamcinolone . . . 1004
Oxiconazole 1024
Sertaconazole 1214
Sulconazole 1243
Terbinafine 1272
Tolnaftate 1312
Triacetin 1329
Undecylenic Acid and Derivatives 1352

ANTIFUNGAL AGENT, VAGINAL

Butoconazole 239
Clotrimazole 363
Miconazole 922
Nystatin 1003
Terconazole 1274
Tioconazole 1302

ANTIGOUT AGENT

Colchicine and Probenecid 372

ANTIHEMOPHILIC AGENT
Antihemophilic Factor (Human) . . . 134
Antihemophilic Factor (Porcine) . . . 134
Antihemophilic Factor (Recombinant) . . . 135
Anti-inhibitor Coagulant Complex . . . 135
Desmopressin . . . 409
Factor IX . . . 571
Factor IX Complex (Human) . . . 572
Factor VIIa (Recombinant) . . . 571
Tranexamic Acid . . . 1323

ANTIHISTAMINE
Acetaminophen, Chlorpheniramine, and Pseudoephedrine . . . 58
Acetaminophen, Dextromethorphan, and Pseudoephedrine . . . 59
Acrivastine and Pseudoephedrine . . . 62
Azelastine . . . 173
Carbetapentane, Phenylephrine, and Pyrilamine . . . 261
Carbinoxamine . . . 262
Cetirizine . . . 298
Chlorpheniramine . . . 313
Clemastine . . . 346
Cyclizine . . . 381
Cyproheptadine . . . 389
Dexchlorpheniramine . . . 414
DimenhyDRINATE . . . 446
DiphenhydrAMINE . . . 448
HydrOXYzine . . . 723
Meclizine . . . 859
Olopatadine . . . 1011
Phenindamine . . . 1073
Promethazine . . . 1130
Pseudoephedrine, Dihydrocodeine, and Chlorpheniramine . . . 1150
Tripelennamine . . . 1344
Triprolidine and Pseudoephedrine . . . 1345

ANTIHISTAMINE/ANALGESIC
Chlorpheniramine and Acetaminophen . . . 314

ANTIHISTAMINE/ANTITUSSIVE
Bromodiphenhydramine and Codeine . . . 220
Carbetapentane and Chlorpheniramine . . . 260
Hydrocodone and Chlorpheniramine . . . 707
Promethazine and Codeine . . . 1131
Promethazine and Dextromethorphan . . . 1131

ANTIHISTAMINE/DECONGESTANT/ANTICHOLINERGIC
Chlorpheniramine, Phenylephrine, and Methscopolamine . . . 317

ANTIHISTAMINE/DECONGESTANT/ANTITUSSIVE
Carbetapentane, Phenylephrine, and Pyrilamine . . . 261
Carbinoxamine, Pseudoephedrine, and Dextromethorphan . . . 263
Chlorpheniramine, Ephedrine, Phenylephrine, and Carbetapentane . . . 316
Chlorpheniramine, Phenylephrine, and Dextromethorphan . . . 316
Chlorpheniramine, Pseudoephedrine, and Codeine . . . 319
Hydrocodone, Carbinoxamine, and Pseudoephedrine . . . 712
Hydrocodone, Phenylephrine, and Diphenhydramine . . . 713
Promethazine, Phenylephrine, and Codeine . . . 1132
Pseudoephedrine, Dihydrocodeine, and Chlorpheniramine . . . 1150
Triprolidine, Pseudoephedrine, and Codeine . . . 1346

ANTIHISTAMINE/DECONGESTANT/ANTITUSSIVE/EXPECTORANT
Chlorpheniramine, Phenylephrine, Codeine, and Potassium Iodide . . . 318

ANTIHISTAMINE/DECONGESTANT COMBINATION
Brompheniramine and Pseudoephedrine . . . 220
Cetirizine and Pseudoephedrine . . . 299
Chlorpheniramine and Phenylephrine . . . 314
Chlorpheniramine and Pseudoephedrine . . . 315
Chlorpheniramine, Phenylephrine, and Phenyltoloxamine . . . 317
Dexbrompheniramine and Pseudoephedrine . . . 414
Diphenhydramine and Pseudoephedrine . . . 451
Fexofenadine and Pseudoephedrine . . . 588
Loratadine and Pseudoephedrine . . . 842
Promethazine and Phenylephrine . . . 1132

ANTIHISTAMINE, H_1 BLOCKER
Carbinoxamine and Pseudoephedrine . . . 262

ANTIHISTAMINE, H_1 BLOCKER, OPHTHALMIC
Emedastine . . . 487
Epinastine . . . 496
Ketotifen . . . 790
Levocabastine . . . 810

ANTIHISTAMINE, NONSEDATING
Desloratadine . . . 408
Fexofenadine . . . 587
Loratadine . . . 841

ANTIHYPERTENSIVE
Diazoxide . . . 425
Eplerenone . . . 498
Oxprenolol . . . 1025
Quinapril and Hydrochlorothiazide . . . 1160

ANTIHYPERTENSIVE AGENT, COMBINATION
Amlodipine and Benazepril . . . 110
Atenolol and Chlorthalidone . . . 161
Benazepril and Hydrochlorothiazide . . . 189
Bisoprolol and Hydrochlorothiazide . . . 211
Captopril and Hydrochlorothiazide . . . 255

Clonidine and Chlorthalidone . . . 360
Enalapril and Felodipine 491
Enalapril and Hydrochlorothiazide 491
Eprosartan and Hydrochlorothiazide 502
Fosinopril and Hydrochlorothiazide 635
Hydralazine and Hydrochlorothiazide 698
Hydralazine, Hydrochlorothiazide, and Reserpine 698
Hydrochlorothiazide and Spironolactone 701
Hydrochlorothiazide and Triamterene 701
Irbesartan and Hydrochlorothiazide 764
Lisinopril and Hydrochlorothiazide 834
Losartan and Hydrochlorothiazide 847
Methyclothiazide and Deserpidine 905
Methyldopa and Hydrochlorothiazide 906
Moexipril and Hydrochlorothiazide 941
Nadolol and Bendroflumethiazide 957
Prazosin and Polythiazide 1112
Propranolol and Hydrochlorothiazide 1143
Telmisartan and Hydrochlorothiazide 1265
Trandolapril and Verapamil . . . 1322
Valsartan and Hydrochlorothiazide 1364

ANTIHYPOGLYCEMIC AGENT

Diazoxide 425
Glucose (Instant) 663

ANTI-INFLAMMATORY AGENT

Balsalazide 181
Colchicine and Probenecid 372
Dexamethasone 411
Triamcinolone Acetonide (Dental Paste) 1333

ANTI-INFLAMMATORY AGENT, OPHTHALMIC

Dexamethasone 411

ANTI-INFLAMMATORY, LOCALLY APPLIED

Amlexanox 107
Carbamide Peroxide 259
Maltodextrin 855

ANTILIPEMIC AGENT, 2-AZETIDINONE

Ezetimibe 570

ANTILIPEMIC AGENT, BILE ACID SEQUESTRANT

Cholestyramine Resin 323
Colesevelam 373
Colestipol 373

ANTILIPEMIC AGENT, FIBRIC ACID

Clofibrate 353
Fenofibrate 577
Gemfibrozil 651

ANTILIPEMIC AGENT, HMG-COA REDUCTASE INHIBITOR

Amlodipine and Atorvastatin 110
Aspirin and Pravastatin 157
Atorvastatin 162
Fluvastatin 622
Lovastatin 848
Niacin and Lovastatin 979
Pravastatin 1109
Rosuvastatin 1202
Simvastatin 1222

ANTILIPEMIC AGENT, MISCELLANEOUS

Niacin 978
Niacin and Lovastatin 979

ANTIMALARIAL AGENT

Atovaquone and Proguanil 165
Halofantrine 681
Mefloquine 864
Pyrimethamine 1154
Quinine 1162
Sulfadoxine and Pyrimethamine 1245

ANTIMICROBIAL MOUTH RINSE

Mouthwash (Antiseptic) 948

ANTIMIGRAINE AGENT

Frovatriptan 638

ANTINEOPLASTIC AGENT

Amsacrine 129
Carmustine 268

ANTINEOPLASTIC AGENT, ALKYLATING AGENT

Busulfan 234
Carboplatin 264
Chlorambucil 305
Cisplatin 337
Cyclophosphamide 384
Estramustine 523
Ifosfamide 733
Lomustine 838
Melphalan 866
Oxaliplatin 1020
Procarbazine 1125
Streptozocin 1240
Temozolomide 1268
Thiotepa 1291

ANTINEOPLASTIC AGENT, ALKYLATING AGENT (NITROGEN MUSTARD)

Ifosfamide 733

ANTINEOPLASTIC AGENT, ALKYLATING AGENT (NITROSOUREA)

Carmustine 268

ANTINEOPLASTIC AGENT, ALKYLATING AGENT (TRIAZENE)

Dacarbazine 392

ANTINEOPLASTIC AGENT, ANTHRACENEDIONE

Mitoxantrone 938

ANTINEOPLASTIC AGENT, ANTHRACYCLINE

DAUNOrubicin Citrate (Liposomal) 400
DAUNOrubicin Hydrochloride . . . 401
DOXOrubicin 469
DOXOrubicin (Liposomal) 470
Epirubicin 498
Idarubicin 732
Valrubicin 1362

ANTINEOPLASTIC AGENT, ANTIANDROGEN

Bicalutamide 206
Flutamide 615
Nilutamide 986

ANTINEOPLASTIC AGENT, ANTIBIOTIC

Bleomycin 213
Dactinomycin 394

Idarubicin . . . 732
Mitomycin . . . 937
Pentostatin . . . 1065

ANTINEOPLASTIC AGENT, ANTIMETABOLITE
Capecitabine . . . 250
Cladribine . . . 342
Cytarabine . . . 390
Cytarabine (Liposomal) . . . 391
Fluorouracil . . . 605
Hydroxyurea . . . 722
Mercaptopurine . . . 880
Methotrexate . . . 897
Pemetrexed . . . 1054
Pentostatin . . . 1065

ANTINEOPLASTIC AGENT, ANTIMETABOLITE (ANTIFOLATE)
Pemetrexed . . . 1054

ANTINEOPLASTIC AGENT, ANTIMETABOLITE (PURINE ANTAGONIST)
Cladribine . . . 342
Fludarabine . . . 597
Thioguanine . . . 1288

ANTINEOPLASTIC AGENT, ANTIMETABOLITE (PYRIMIDINE ANTAGONIST)
Floxuridine . . . 593
Gemcitabine . . . 650

ANTINEOPLASTIC AGENT, ANTIMICROTUBULAR
Paclitaxel . . . 1038

ANTINEOPLASTIC AGENT, AROMATASE INACTIVATOR
Exemestane . . . 569

ANTINEOPLASTIC AGENT, AROMATASE INHIBITOR
Letrozole . . . 803

ANTINEOPLASTIC AGENT, DNA ADDUCT-FORMING AGENT
Carmustine . . . 268

ANTINEOPLASTIC AGENT, DNA BINDING AGENT
Aminocamptothecin . . . 96
Amonafide . . . 112
Carmustine . . . 268

ANTINEOPLASTIC AGENT, ESTROGEN RECEPTOR ANTAGONIST
Fulvestrant . . . 639
Tamoxifen . . . 1258
Toremifene . . . 1317

ANTINEOPLASTIC AGENT, HORMONE
Estramustine . . . 523
Megestrol . . . 865

ANTINEOPLASTIC AGENT, HORMONE ANTAGONIST
Mifepristone . . . 928

ANTINEOPLASTIC AGENT, HORMONE (ESTROGEN/ NITROGEN MUSTARD)
Estramustine . . . 523

ANTINEOPLASTIC AGENT, MISCELLANEOUS
Alitretinoin . . . 81
Altretamine . . . 89
Anastrozole . . . 132
Asparaginase . . . 150
Azacitidine . . . 171
Bexarotene . . . 205
Denileukin Diftitox . . . 405
Mitotane . . . 937
Pegaspargase . . . 1051
Porfimer . . . 1103
Teniposide . . . 1269
Tretinoin (Oral) . . . 1328
Trimetrexate Glucuronate . . . 1342

ANTINEOPLASTIC AGENT, MONOCLONAL ANTIBODY
Alemtuzumab . . . 76
Bevacizumab . . . 204
Cetuximab . . . 300
Gemtuzumab Ozogamicin . . . 653
Ibritumomab . . . 727
Rituximab . . . 1191

ANTINEOPLASTIC AGENT, NATURAL SOURCE (PLANT) DERIVATIVE
Docetaxel . . . 458
Irinotecan . . . 764
Paclitaxel . . . 1038
Topotecan . . . 1316
VinBLAStine . . . 1377
VinCRIStine . . . 1378
Vinorelbine . . . 1380

ANTINEOPLASTIC AGENT, PODOPHYLLOTOXIN DERIVATIVE
Etoposide . . . 567
Etoposide Phosphate . . . 568

ANTINEOPLASTIC AGENT, TYROSINE KINASE INHIBITOR
Gefitinib . . . 649
Imatinib . . . 734

ANTINEOPLASTIC AGENT, VINCA ALKALOID
VinBLAStine . . . 1377
VinCRIStine . . . 1378
Vindesine . . . 1379
Vinorelbine . . . 1380

ANTIPARASITIC AGENT, TOPICAL
Lindane . . . 829
Permethrin . . . 1070
Pyrethrins and Piperonyl Butoxide . . . 1153

ANTI-PARKINSON'S AGENT, ANTICHOLINERGIC
Benztropine . . . 196
Biperiden . . . 207
Orphenadrine . . . 1017
Procyclidine . . . 1127
Trihexyphenidyl . . . 1340

ANTI-PARKINSON'S AGENT, COMT INHIBITOR
Entacapone . . . 494
Levodopa, Carbidopa, and Entacapone . . . 812
Tolcapone . . . 1310

ANTI-PARKINSON'S AGENT, DOPAMINE AGONIST
Amantadine . . . 92
Apomorphine . . . 137
Bromocriptine . . . 219
Carbidopa . . . 261
Levodopa and Carbidopa . . . 811
Levodopa, Carbidopa, and Entacapone . . . 812
Pergolide . . . 1067
Pramipexole . . . 1108

Ropinirole 1197

ANTI-PARKINSON'S AGENT, MAO TYPE B INHIBITOR

Selegiline 1212

ANTIPLAQUE AGENT

Mouthwash (Antiseptic) 948

ANTIPLATELET AGENT

Aspirin and Dipyridamole 156
Cilostazol 329
Clopidogrel 361
Dipyridamole 453
Ticlopidine 1297

ANTIPLATELET AGENT, GLYCOPROTEIN IIB/IIIA INHIBITOR

Abciximab 44
Eptifibatide 503
Tirofiban 1304

ANTIPROGESTIN

Mifepristone 928

ANTIPROTOZOAL

Atovaquone 164
Eflornithine 485
Furazolidone 640
Nitazoxanide 989

ANTIPROTOZOAL, NITROIMIDAZOLE

Metronidazole 917
Tinidazole 1301

ANTIPSORIATIC AGENT

Anthralin 133

ANTIPSYCHOTIC AGENT, BENZISOXAZOLE

Risperidone 1187

ANTIPSYCHOTIC AGENT, BENZYLISOTHIAZOLYL-PIPERAZINE

Ziprasidone 1401

ANTIPSYCHOTIC AGENT, BUTYROPHENONE

Droperidol 477
Haloperidol 682

ANTIPSYCHOTIC AGENT, DIBENZODIAZEPINE

Clozapine 366

ANTIPSYCHOTIC AGENT, DIBENZOTHIAZEPINE

Quetiapine 1156

ANTIPSYCHOTIC AGENT, DIBENZOXAZEPINE

Loxapine 850

ANTIPSYCHOTIC AGENT, DIHYDROINDOLINE

Molindone 942

ANTIPSYCHOTIC AGENT, DIPHENYLBUTYLPERIDINE

Pimozide 1088

ANTIPSYCHOTIC AGENT, PHENOTHIAZINE, ALIPHATIC

ChlorproMAZINE 319

ANTIPSYCHOTIC AGENT, PHENOTHIAZINE, PIPERAZINE

Amitriptyline and Perphenazine . 106
Fluphenazine 610
Perphenazine 1070
Prochlorperazine 1126
Trifluoperazine 1338

ANTIPSYCHOTIC AGENT, PHENOTHIAZINE, PIPERIDINE

Mesoridazine 883
Pipotiazine 1095
Thioridazine 1289

ANTIPSYCHOTIC AGENT, QUINOLINONE

Aripiprazole 142

ANTIPSYCHOTIC AGENT, THIENOBENZODIAZEPINE

Olanzapine 1007
Olanzapine and Fluoxetine 1009

ANTIPSYCHOTIC AGENT, THIOXANTHENE DERIVATIVE

Thiothixene 1291

ANTIRETROVIRAL AGENT, FUSION PROTEIN INHIBITOR

Enfuvirtide 492

ANTIRETROVIRAL AGENT, PROTEASE INHIBITOR

Amprenavir 128
Atazanavir 158
Fosamprenavir 630
Indinavir 744
Lopinavir and Ritonavir 839
Nelfinavir 972
Ritonavir 1189
Saquinavir 1207

ANTIRETROVIRAL AGENT, REVERSE TRANSCRIPTASE INHIBITOR (NON-NUCLEOSIDE)

Delavirdine 403
Efavirenz 484
Nevirapine 977

ANTIRETROVIRAL AGENT, REVERSE TRANSCRIPTASE INHIBITOR (NUCLEOSIDE)

Abacavir 42
Abacavir, Lamivudine, and Zidovudine 43
Adefovir 68
Didanosine 433
Emtricitabine 487
Lamivudine 794
Stavudine 1238
Zalcitabine 1395
Zidovudine 1398
Zidovudine and Lamivudine . . . 1399

ANTIRETROVIRAL AGENT, REVERSE TRANSCRIPTASE INHIBITOR (NUCLEOTIDE)

Tenofovir 1270

ANTIRHEUMATIC, DISEASE MODIFYING

Adalimumab 67
Anakinra 131
Etanercept 532
Infliximab 747
Leflunomide 801

ANTIRHEUMATIC MISCELLANEOUS

Hyaluronate and Derivatives . . . 696

ANTISEPTIC, ORAL MOUTHWASH

Cetylpyridinium 301

ANTISEPTIC, TOPICAL
Benzalkonium Chloride and Isopropyl Alcohol 190

ANTISPASMODIC AGENT, GASTROINTESTINAL
Atropine 166
Clidinium and Chlordiazepoxide 347
Hyoscyamine, Atropine, Scopolamine, and Phenobarbital 725
Mepenzolate 869

ANTISPASMODIC AGENT, URINARY
Belladonna and Opium 186
Flavoxate 591
Oxybutynin 1026

ANTITHYROID AGENT
Methimazole 893
Potassium Iodide 1106
Propylthiouracil 1144

ANTITRYPSIN DEFICIENCY AGENT
Alpha$_1$-Proteinase Inhibitor 84

ANTITUBERCULAR AGENT
Capreomycin 251
CycloSERINE 385
Ethambutol 534
Ethionamide 560
Isoniazid 769
Pyrazinamide 1152
Rifabutin 1179
Rifampin 1180
Rifapentine 1182
Streptomycin 1239

ANTITUSSIVE
Acetaminophen, Dextromethorphan, and Pseudoephedrine 59
Benzonatate 193
Carbetapentane, Phenylephrine, and Pyrilamine 261
Codeine 369
Dextromethorphan 421
Guaifenesin and Codeine 673
Guaifenesin and Dextromethorphan 673
Guaifenesin, Potassium Guaiacolsulfonate, and Dextromethorphan 675
Hydrocodone and Homatropine 709
Hydrocodone, Phenylephrine, and Diphenhydramine 713
Pseudoephedrine, Dihydrocodeine, and Chlorpheniramine 1150

ANTITUSSIVE/DECONGESTANT
Hydrocodone and Pseudoephedrine 711
Hydrocodone, Chlorpheniramine, Phenylephrine, Acetaminophen, and Caffeine 712
Pseudoephedrine and Dextromethorphan 1148

ANTITUSSIVE/DECONGESTANT/ EXPECTORANT
Guaifenesin, Pseudoephedrine, and Codeine 676
Guaifenesin, Pseudoephedrine, and Dextromethorphan 676
Hydrocodone, Pseudoephedrine, and Guaifenesin 713

ANTITUSSIVE/EXPECTORANT
Hydrocodone and Guaifenesin . . 708

ANTIVIRAL AGENT
Acyclovir 64
Amantadine 92
Cidofovir 327
Famciclovir 572
Foscarnet 631
Ganciclovir 646
Interferon Alfa-2b and Ribavirin 754
Oseltamivir 1019
Penciclovir 1056
Ribavirin 1177
Rimantadine 1184
Valganciclovir 1358
Zanamivir 1396

ANTIVIRAL AGENT, OPHTHALMIC
Fomivirsen 628
Trifluridine 1339
Vidarabine 1376

ANTIVIRAL AGENT, ORAL
Valacyclovir 1354

ANTIVIRAL AGENT, TOPICAL
Docosanol 459

APHTHOUS ULCER TREATMENT AGENT
Sulfonated Phenolics in Aqueous Solution 1250

APPETITE STIMULANT
Dronabinol 477
Megestrol 865

AROMATASE INHIBITOR
Aminoglutethimide 98

ASTRINGENT
Aluminum Chloride 90
Epinephrine (Racemic) and Aluminum Potassium Sulfate 497

BARBITURATE
Amobarbital 112
Amobarbital and Secobarbital . . 112
Butabarbital 235
Butalbital, Acetaminophen, and Caffeine 236
Butalbital, Acetaminophen, Caffeine, and Codeine 236
Butalbital, Aspirin, and Caffeine 238
Butalbital, Aspirin, Caffeine, and Codeine 238
Mephobarbital 873
Methohexital 895
Pentobarbital 1065
Phenobarbital 1073
Primidone 1122
Secobarbital 1211
Thiopental 1289

BENZODIAZEPINE
Alprazolam 84
Amitriptyline and Chlordiazepoxide 105
Bromazepam 218
Chlordiazepoxide 307
Clidinium and Chlordiazepoxide 347
Clobazam 350
Clonazepam 356
Clorazepate 362
Diazepam 423
Estazolam 517
Flunitrazepam 600

Flurazepam 612
Lorazepam 842
Midazolam 924
Oxazepam 1022
Quazepam 1155
Temazepam 1266
Triazolam 1335

BETA-ADRENERGIC BLOCKER
Dorzolamide and Timolol 464

BETA-ADRENERGIC BLOCKER, NONCARDIOSELECTIVE
Oxprenolol 1025

BETA-ADRENERGIC BLOCKER, NONSELECTIVE
Levobunolol 808
Metipranolol 913
Nadolol 956
Nadolol and Bendroflumethiazide 957
Propranolol 1140
Sotalol 1231
Timolol 1299

BETA BLOCKER, BETA$_1$ SELECTIVE
Atenolol 159
Betaxolol 202
Bisoprolol 210
Esmolol 515
Levobetaxolol 808
Metoprolol 915

BETA BLOCKER WITH ALPHA-BLOCKING ACTIVITY
Carvedilol 270
Labetalol 791

BETA BLOCKER WITH INTRINSIC SYMPATHOMIMETIC ACTIVITY
Acebutolol 46
Carteolol 269
Penbutolol 1055
Pindolol 1090

BETA$_1$- & BETA$_2$-ADRENERGIC AGONIST AGENT
Isoproterenol 770

BETA$_2$-ADRENERGIC AGONIST
Albuterol 71
Fenoterol 580
Fluticasone and Salmeterol 619
Formoterol 629
Levalbuterol 806
Metaproterenol 885
Pirbuterol 1096
Salmeterol 1206
Terbutaline 1273

BIOLOGICAL, MISCELLANEOUS
Glatiramer Acetate 658

BIOLOGICAL RESPONSE MODULATOR
Aldesleukin 74
BCG Vaccine 183
Oprelvekin 1015

BISPHOSPHONATE DERIVATIVE
Alendronate 77
Etidronate Disodium 563
Pamidronate 1041
Risedronate 1185
Tiludronate 1298

BLOOD MODIFIERS
Hemin 684
Pentastarch 1063

BLOOD PRODUCT DERIVATIVE
Antihemophilic Factor (Human) 134
Anti-inhibitor Coagulant Complex 135
Antithrombin III 136
Aprotinin 139
Factor IX 571
Factor IX Complex (Human) . . . 572
Factor VIIa (Recombinant) 571

BLOOD VISCOSITY REDUCER AGENT
Pentoxifylline 1066

BRONCHODILATOR
Epinephrine 496
Ipratropium and Albuterol 761

CALCIMIMETIC
Cinacalcet 331

CALCIUM CHANNEL BLOCKER
Amlodipine 108
Amlodipine and Atorvastatin 110
Bepridil 197
Diltiazem 444
Felodipine 576
Isradipine 774
NiCARdipine 980
NIFEdipine 984
Nimodipine 987
Nisoldipine 988
Verapamil 1373

CALCIUM-LOWERING AGENT
Gallium Nitrate 646

CALCIUM SALT
Calcium Acetate 245
Calcium Carbonate 245
Calcium Chloride 246
Calcium Citrate 246
Calcium Glubionate 246
Calcium Gluconate 247
Calcium Lactate 247
Calcium Phosphate (Tribasic) . . . 247

CALORIC AGENT
Fat Emulsion 575

CARBONIC ANHYDRASE INHIBITOR
AcetaZOLAMIDE 60
Brinzolamide 218
Dichlorphenamide 427
Dorzolamide 464
Dorzolamide and Timolol 464
Methazolamide 891

CARDIAC GLYCOSIDE
Digoxin 437

CARDIOPROTECTANT
Dexrazoxane 417

CATHARTIC
Polyethylene Glycol-Electrolyte Solution 1100
Sodium Phosphates 1230

CAUTERIZING AGENT, TOPICAL
Silver Nitrate 1221

CENTRAL NERVOUS SYSTEM DEPRESSANT
Sodium Oxybate 1229

CENTRAL NERVOUS SYSTEM STIMULANT
Dexmethylphenidate 416
Methylphenidate 908

CHELATING AGENT
Edetate Calcium Disodium 482
Edetate Disodium 482
Penicillamine 1057

CHOLINERGIC AGONIST

Acetylcholine 61
Ambenonium 93
Bethanechol 203
Carbachol 255
Cevimeline 302
Edrophonium 483
Guanidine 679
Pilocarpine 1085
Pilocarpine (Dental) 1086

COLCHICINE

Colchicine 372

COLONY STIMULATING FACTOR

Darbepoetin Alfa 399
Epoetin Alfa 499
Filgrastim 589
Pegfilgrastim 1052
Sargramostim 1209

CONTRACEPTIVE

Estradiol and Medroxyprogesterone 520
Ethinyl Estradiol and Desogestrel 536
Ethinyl Estradiol and Drospirenone 538
Ethinyl Estradiol and Ethynodiol Diacetate 540
Ethinyl Estradiol and Etonogestrel 543
Ethinyl Estradiol and Levonorgestrel 545
Ethinyl Estradiol and Norelgestromin 548
Ethinyl Estradiol and Norethindrone 550
Ethinyl Estradiol and Norgestimate 554
Ethinyl Estradiol and Norgestrel 557
Levonorgestrel 815
MedroxyPROGESTERone 862
Mestranol and Norethindrone . . . 884
Norethindrone 996
Norgestrel 998

CONTRAST AGENT, NONIONIC

Iopromide 760

CORTICOSTEROID, ADRENAL

Triamcinolone 1330

CORTICOSTEROID, INHALANT (ORAL)

Beclomethasone 184
Budesonide 221
Flunisolide 599
Fluticasone 616
Fluticasone and Salmeterol 619
Triamcinolone 1330

CORTICOSTEROID, NASAL

Beclomethasone 184
Budesonide 221
Flunisolide 599
Fluticasone 616
Mometasone Furoate 943
Triamcinolone 1330

CORTICOSTEROID, OPHTHALMIC

Bacitracin, Neomycin, Polymyxin B, and Hydrocortisone 179
Dexamethasone 411
Fluorometholone 605
Loteprednol 847
Medrysone 863
PrednisoLONE 1113
Rimexolone 1185

CORTICOSTEROID, OTIC

Bacitracin, Neomycin, Polymyxin B, and Hydrocortisone 179

CORTICOSTEROID, RECTAL

Hydrocortisone 714

CORTICOSTEROID, SYSTEMIC

Betamethasone 199
Budesonide 221
Corticotropin 376
Cortisone 377
Dexamethasone 411
Fludrocortisone 598
Hydrocortisone 714
MethylPREDNISolone 910
PrednisoLONE 1113
PredniSONE 1115
Triamcinolone 1330

CORTICOSTEROID, TOPICAL

Alclometasone 74
Amcinonide 93
Bacitracin, Neomycin, Polymyxin B, and Hydrocortisone 179
Betamethasone 199
Betamethasone and Clotrimazole 201
Clobetasol 351
Clocortolone 352
Desonide 410
Desoximetasone 410
Dexamethasone 411
Diflorasone 435
Fluocinolone 601
Fluocinolone, Hydroquinone, and Tretinoin 601
Fluocinonide 602
Flurandrenolide 611
Fluticasone 616
Halcinonide 681
Halobetasol 681
Hydrocortisone 714
Iodoquinol and Hydrocortisone . . 759
Mometasone Furoate 943
Nystatin and Triamcinolone . . . 1004
Prednicarbate 1113
Triamcinolone 1330
Triamcinolone Acetonide (Dental Paste) 1333
Urea and Hydrocortisone 1353

CORTICOSTEROID, TOPICAL (MEDIUM POTENCY)

Fluticasone 616

COUGH PREPARATION

Guaifenesin and Codeine 673
Guaifenesin and Dextromethorphan 673
Guaifenesin, Potassium Guaiacolsulfonate, and Dextromethorphan 675

DECONGESTANT

Carbetapentane, Phenylephrine, and Pyrilamine 261
Carbinoxamine and Pseudoephedrine 262
Guaifenesin and Phenylephrine 674
Guaifenesin and Pseudoephedrine 675
Hydrocodone, Phenylephrine, and Diphenhydramine 713
Pseudoephedrine, Dihydrocodeine, and Chlorpheniramine 1150

DECONGESTANT/ANALGESIC
Pseudoephedrine and Ibuprofen . . . 1149

DENTAL GASES
Nitrous Oxide . . . 994
Oxygen . . . 1033

DEPIGMENTING AGENT
Fluocinolone, Hydroquinone, and Tretinoin . . . 601
Hydroquinone . . . 719

DIAGNOSTIC AGENT
Adenosine . . . 68
Arginine . . . 141
Benzylpenicilloyl-polylysine . . . 196
Cosyntropin . . . 378
Edrophonium . . . 483
Glucagon . . . 663
Gonadorelin . . . 669
Indocyanine Green . . . 745
Proparacaine and Fluorescein . . . 1135
Protirelin . . . 1145
Secretin . . . 1211
Sermorelin Acetate . . . 1214
Sincalide . . . 1224
Skin Test Antigens (Multiple) . . 1226
Thyrotropin Alpha . . . 1294
Tuberculin Tests . . . 1349

DIAGNOSTIC AGENT, OPHTHALMIC
Hydroxypropyl Methylcellulose . . 721

DIETARY SUPPLEMENT
Levocarnitine . . . 810

DISINFECTANT, ANTIBACTERIAL (TOPICAL)
Sodium Hypochlorite Solution . . . 1228

DIURETIC, CARBONIC ANHYDRASE INHIBITOR
AcetaZOLAMIDE . . . 60
Dichlorphenamide . . . 427
Methazolamide . . . 891

DIURETIC, COMBINATION
Amiloride and Hydrochlorothiazide . . . 96

DIURETIC, LOOP
Bumetanide . . . 224
Ethacrynic Acid . . . 533
Furosemide . . . 640
Torsemide . . . 1317

DIURETIC, MISCELLANEOUS
Caffeine and Sodium Benzoate . . . 242

DIURETIC, OSMOTIC
Urea . . . 1353

DIURETIC, POTASSIUM-SPARING
Amiloride . . . 95
Hydrochlorothiazide and Triamterene . . . 701
Spironolactone . . . 1235
Triamterene . . . 1334

DIURETIC, THIAZIDE
Bendroflumethiazide . . . 189
Chlorothiazide . . . 312
Chlorthalidone . . . 321
Eprosartan and Hydrochlorothiazide . . . 502
Hydrochlorothiazide . . . 699
Hydrochlorothiazide and Triamterene . . . 701
Losartan and Hydrochlorothiazide . . . 847
Methyclothiazide . . . 905
Nadolol and Bendroflumethiazide . . . 957
Olmesartan and Hydrochlorothiazide . . . 1010
Polythiazide . . . 1102
Quinapril and Hydrochlorothiazide . . . 1160
Telmisartan and Hydrochlorothiazide . . . 1265
Trichlormethiazide . . . 1337
Valsartan and Hydrochlorothiazide . . . 1364

DIURETIC, THIAZIDE-RELATED
Indapamide . . . 743
Metolazone . . . 914

DOPAMINE AGONIST
Fenoldopam . . . 579

ELECTROLYTE SUPPLEMENT, ORAL
Calcium Carbonate . . . 245
Calcium Gluconate . . . 247
Magnesium L-aspartate Hydrochloride . . . 854
Magnesium Oxide . . . 854
Potassium Acetate, Potassium Bicarbonate, and Potassium Citrate . . . 1104
Potassium Bicarbonate . . . 1104
Potassium Bicarbonate and Potassium Chloride . . . 1104
Potassium Bicarbonate and Potassium Citrate . . . 1105
Potassium Chloride . . . 1105
Potassium Gluconate . . . 1106
Potassium Phosphate . . . 1107
Potassium Phosphate and Sodium Phosphate . . . 1107
Sodium Bicarbonate . . . 1226
Sodium Chloride . . . 1227
Sodium Phosphates . . . 1230

ELECTROLYTE SUPPLEMENT, PARENTERAL
Ammonium Chloride . . . 111
Calcium Acetate . . . 245
Calcium Chloride . . . 246
Calcium Gluconate . . . 247
Magnesium Sulfate . . . 854
Potassium Acetate . . . 1104
Potassium Chloride . . . 1105
Potassium Phosphate . . . 1107
Sodium Bicarbonate . . . 1226
Sodium Chloride . . . 1227
Sodium Phosphates . . . 1230

ENDOTHELIN ANTAGONIST
Bosentan . . . 214

ENZYME
Agalsidase Beta . . . 69
Alglucerase . . . 80
Dornase Alfa . . . 463
Hyaluronidase . . . 697
Imiglucerase . . . 736
Lactase . . . 793
Laronidase . . . 800
Pancreatin . . . 1042
Pancrelipase . . . 1042
Pegademase Bovine . . . 1050
Rasburicase . . . 1171

ENZYME, GASTROINTESTINAL
Sacrosidase . . . 1204

ENZYME INHIBITOR
Aminoglutethimide . . . 98
Miglustat . . . 930

ENZYME INHIBITOR, TOPOISOMERASE II INHIBITOR
Amonafide . . . 112

ENZYME INHIBITOR, TOPOISOMERASE I INHIBITOR
Aminocamptothecin 96

ENZYME, TOPICAL DEBRIDEMENT
Collagenase 375

ENZYME, URATE-OXIDASE (RECOMBINANT)
Rasburicase 1171

EPIDERMAL GROWTH FACTOR RECEPTOR (EGFR) INHIBITOR
Cetuximab 300

ERGOT DERIVATIVE
Belladonna, Phenobarbital, and Ergotamine 186
Bromocriptine 219
Cabergoline 241
Dihydroergotamine 442
Ergoloid Mesylates 504
Ergonovine 505
Ergotamine 505
Ergotamine and Caffeine 506
Methylergonovine 907
Methysergide 913
Pergolide 1067

ESTROGEN AND PROGESTIN COMBINATION
Estradiol and Medroxyprogesterone 520
Estradiol and Norethindrone 521
Estradiol and Norgestimate 521
Estrogens (Conjugated/Equine) and Medroxyprogesterone 528
Estrogens (Esterified) and Methyltestosterone 530
Ethinyl Estradiol and Desogestrel 536
Ethinyl Estradiol and Drospirenone 538
Ethinyl Estradiol and Ethynodiol Diacetate 540
Ethinyl Estradiol and Etonogestrel 543
Ethinyl Estradiol and Levonorgestrel 545
Ethinyl Estradiol and Norelgestromin 548
Ethinyl Estradiol and Norethindrone 550
Ethinyl Estradiol and Norgestimate 554
Ethinyl Estradiol and Norgestrel 557
Mestranol and Norethindrone 884

ESTROGEN DERIVATIVE
Estradiol 518
Estrogens (Conjugated A/Synthetic) 524
Estrogens (Conjugated/Equine) 525
Estrogens (Esterified) 529
Estropipate 531

EXPECTORANT
Guaifenesin 672
Guaifenesin and Codeine 673
Guaifenesin and Dextromethorphan 673
Guaifenesin and Phenylephrine 674
Guaifenesin and Potassium Guaiacolsulfonate 675
Guaifenesin and Pseudoephedrine 675
Guaifenesin, Potassium Guaiacolsulfonate, and Dextromethorphan 675
Potassium Iodide 1106
Terpin Hydrate and Codeine . . 1275

FACTOR XA INHIBITOR
Fondaparinux 628

FALSE NEUROTRANSMITTER
Guanadrel 678

GALLSTONE DISSOLUTION AGENT
Ursodiol 1354

GANGLIONIC BLOCKING AGENT
Mecamylamine 859

GASTROINTESTINAL AGENT, MISCELLANEOUS
Chlorophyll 310
Glutamic Acid 664
Infliximab 747
Lansoprazole, Amoxicillin, and Clarithromycin 798
Saliva Substitute 1205
Sucralfate 1242

GASTROINTESTINAL AGENT, PROKINETIC
Cisapride 336
Metoclopramide 914

GASTROINTESTINAL AGENT, STIMULANT
Dexpanthenol 416

GENERAL ANESTHETIC
Etomidate 566
Fentanyl 581
Ketamine 782
Nitrous Oxide 994
Propofol 1135
Sufentanil 1242
Thiopental 1289

GENITOURINARY IRRIGANT
Sorbitol 1231

GLUTAMATE INHIBITOR
Riluzole 1183

GOLD COMPOUND
Auranofin 170
Gold Sodium Thiomalate 668

GONADOTROPIN
Chorionic Gonadotropin (Recombinant) 326
Follitropins 626
Gonadorelin 669
Menotropins 868

GONADOTROPIN RELEASING HORMONE AGONIST
Goserelin 670
Leuprolide 805
Nafarelin 957
Triptorelin 1346

GONADOTROPIN RELEASING HORMONE ANTAGONIST
Abarelix 43
Cetrorelix 300
Ganirelix 647

GROWTH FACTOR
Darbepoetin Alfa 399

GROWTH FACTOR, PLATELET-DERIVED
Becaplermin 184

GROWTH HORMONE
Human Growth Hormone 694
Sermorelin Acetate 1214

HEMOSTATIC AGENT
Aluminum Chloride 90
Aminocaproic Acid 97
Aprotinin 139
Cellulose (Oxidized/ Regenerated) 293
Collagen (Absorbable) 375
Desmopressin 409
Fibrin Sealant Kit 589
Gelatin (Absorbable) 650
Microfibrillar Collagen Hemostat 923
Thrombin (Topical) 1292

HERB
Aloe 1412
Astragalus 1414
Bilberry 1415
Black Cohosh 1415
Bromelain 1416
Calendula 1416
Cat's Claw 1417
Cayenne 1418
Chamomile 1419
Chasteberry 1419
Cranberry 1421
Devil's Claw 1422
Dong Quai 1423
Echinacea 1423
Ephedra 1424
Evening Primrose 1425
Feverfew 1426
Garlic 1428
Ginger 1428
Ginkgo Biloba 1429
Ginseng, Panax 1430
Ginseng, Siberian 1431
Golden Seal 1433
Gotu Kola 1434
Grapefruit Seed 1434
Grape Seed 1435
Grape Skin 1436
Green Tea 1436
Hawthorn 1437
Horse Chestnut 1437
HuperzineA 1438
Kava 1439
Lemon Balm/Melissa 1439
Licorice 1440
Mastic 1441
Melaleuca Oil 1442
Milk Thistle 1443
Parsley 1443
Passion Flower 1444
Red Yeast Rice 1444
Sassafras Oil 1445
Saw Palmetto 1446
Schisandra 1446
St John's Wort 1447
Turmeric 1448
Uva Ursi 1448
Valerian 1449
Wild Yam 1450
Yohimbe 1451

HISTAMINE H_1 ANTAGONIST
Hydrocodone, Phenylephrine, and Diphenhydramine 713

HISTAMINE H_2 ANTAGONIST
Cimetidine 330
Famotidine 573
Famotidine, Calcium Carbonate, and Magnesium Hydroxide 574
Nizatidine 995
Ranitidine 1169

HOMOCYSTINURIA, TREATMENT AGENT
Betaine Anhydrous 199

HORMONE ANTAGONIST, ANTI-ADRENAL
Aminoglutethimide 98

HORMONE, POSTERIOR PITUITARY
Vasopressin 1369

HUMAN GROWTH FACTOR
Oprelvekin 1015

4-HYDROXYPHENYLPYRUVATE DIOXYGENASE INHIBITOR
Nitisinone 989

HYPNOTIC, MISCELLANEOUS
Chloral Hydrate 304

HYPNOTIC, NONBENZODIAZEPINE
Zaleplon 1396
Zolpidem 1404
Zopiclone 1406

IMMUNE GLOBULIN
Hepatitis B Immune Globulin 688
Immune Globulin (Intramuscular) 739
Immune Globulin (Intravenous) 740
Rabies Immune Globulin (Human) 1165
Rh_o(D) Immune Globulin 1176
Tetanus Immune Globulin (Human) 1277
Varicella-Zoster Immune Globulin (Human) 1368

IMMUNE MODULATOR
Levamisole 806

IMMUNOSUPPRESSANT AGENT
Antithymocyte Globulin (Equine) 136
Azathioprine 172
CycloSPORINE 386
Daclizumab 393
Efalizumab 483
Muromonab-CD3 952
Mycophenolate 952
Pimecrolimus 1088
Sirolimus 1224
Tacrolimus 1255
Thalidomide 1283

INTERFERON
Interferon Alfa-2a 751
Interferon Alfa-2b 752
Interferon Alfa-2b and Ribavirin 754
Interferon Alfa-n3 755
Interferon Beta-1a 756
Interferon Beta-1b 757
Interferon Gamma-1b 758
Peginterferon Alfa-2a 1052
Peginterferon Alfa-2b 1053

INTERLEUKIN-1 RECEPTOR ANTAGONIST
Anakinra 131

IRON SALT
Ferric Gluconate 585
Ferrous Fumarate 586
Ferrous Gluconate 586
Ferrous Sulfate 586
Ferrous Sulfate and Ascorbic Acid 587
Iron Dextran Complex 766
Iron Sucrose 767
Polysaccharide-Iron Complex 1101

KERATOLYTIC AGENT
Anthralin 133
Cantharidin 250
Podofilox 1099

Podophyllum Resin 1099
Salicylic Acid 1205
Tazarotene 1262
Trichloroacetic Acid 1337
Urea 1353

LAXATIVE
Glycerin 667
Magnesium Hydroxide and Mineral Oil 853
Malt Soup Extract 856
Methylcellulose 905

LAXATIVE, BOWEL EVACUANT
Polyethylene Glycol-Electrolyte Solution 1100
Sodium Phosphates 1230

LAXATIVE, BULK-PRODUCING
Polycarbophil 1100
Psyllium 1151

LAXATIVE, MISCELLANEOUS
Castor Oil 273
Lactulose 794
Sorbitol 1231

LAXATIVE, SALINE
Magnesium Citrate 853
Magnesium Sulfate 854

LAXATIVE, STIMULANT
Bisacodyl 208
Senna 1213

LAXATIVE/STOOL SOFTENER
Docusate and Casanthranol 460

LEPROSTATIC AGENT
Clofazimine 352

LEUKOTRIENE-RECEPTOR ANTAGONIST
Montelukast 944
Zafirlukast 1394

LIPASE INHIBITOR
Orlistat 1017

5-LIPOXYGENASE INHIBITOR
Zileuton 1399

LITHIUM
Lithium 835

LOCAL ANESTHETIC
Articaine Hydrochloride and Epinephrine (Canada) 143
Articaine Hydrochloride and Epinephrine (U.S.) 145
Benzocaine 191
Benzocaine, Butyl Aminobenzoate, Tetracaine, and Benzalkonium Chloride 193
Bupivacaine 225
Bupivacaine and Epinephrine . . . 227
Cetylpyridinium and Benzocaine 301
Chloroprocaine 310
Cocaine 368
Dibucaine 426
Dyclonine 480
Ethyl Chloride 561
Ethyl Chloride and Dichlorotetrafluoroethane . . . 562
Etidocaine and Epinephrine 562
Hexylresorcinol 693
Levobupivacaine 809
Lidocaine 819
Lidocaine and Bupivacaine 822
Lidocaine and Epinephrine 823
Lidocaine and Prilocaine 826
Mepivacaine 873
Mepivacaine and Levonordefrin *(WITHDRAWN FROM MARKET)* 875
Mepivacaine (Dental Anesthetic) 877
Pramoxine 1109
Prilocaine 1118
Prilocaine and Epinephrine . . . 1120
Procaine 1125
Proparacaine and Fluorescein 1135
Ropivacaine 1199
Tetracaine 1278
Tetracaine and Dextrose 1279

LOCAL ANESTHETIC, OPHTHALMIC
Proparacaine 1134

LOCAL ANESTHETIC, ORAL
Dyclonine 480

LOCAL ANESTHETIC, TRANSORAL
Lidocaine (Transoral) 828

LOW MOLECULAR WEIGHT HEPARIN
Dalteparin 395
Enoxaparin 493
Tinzaparin 1301

LUBRICANT, OCULAR
Hydroxypropyl Methylcellulose . . 721
Sodium Chloride 1227

LUNG SURFACTANT
Beractant 198
Calfactant 247
Poractant Alfa 1102

MAGNESIUM SALT
Magnesium Chloride 852
Magnesium Citrate 853
Magnesium Gluconate 853
Magnesium Hydroxide 853
Magnesium Sulfate 854

MAST CELL STABILIZER
Cromolyn 378
Lodoxamide 836
Nedocromil 970
Pemirolast 1055

MINERAL, ORAL (TOPICAL)
Triclosan and Fluoride 1337

MISCELLANEOUS PRODUCT
Yohimbine 1393

MONOCLONAL ANTIBODY
Adalimumab 67
Alefacept 76
Basiliximab 182
Efalizumab 483
Infliximab 747
Palivizumab 1040
Trastuzumab 1324

MONOCLONAL ANTIBODY, ANTI-ASTHMATIC
Omalizumab 1012

MOUTHWASH
Mouthwash (Antiseptic) 948

MUCOLYTIC AGENT
Acetylcysteine 61

NATRIURETIC PEPTIDE, B-TYPE, HUMAN
Nesiritide 976

NEURAMINIDASE INHIBITOR
Oseltamivir 1019
Zanamivir 1396

NEUROMUSCULAR BLOCKER AGENT, DEPOLARIZING
Succinylcholine 1241

NEUROMUSCULAR BLOCKER AGENT, TOXIN
Botulinum Toxin Type A 215
Botulinum Toxin Type B 217

N-METHYL-D-ASPARTATE RECEPTOR ANTAGONIST
Memantine 867

NONSTEROIDAL ANTI-INFLAMMATORY DRUG (NSAID)
Diclofenac 427

NONSTEROIDAL ANTI-INFLAMMATORY DRUG (NSAID), COX-2 SELECTIVE
Celecoxib 290
Rofecoxib 1194
Valdecoxib 1356

NONSTEROIDAL ANTI-INFLAMMATORY DRUG (NSAID), OPHTHALMIC
Diclofenac 427
Flurbiprofen 613
Ketorolac 787

NONSTEROIDAL ANTI-INFLAMMATORY DRUG (NSAID), ORAL
Diclofenac 427
Diclofenac and Misoprostol 430
Diflunisal 435
Etodolac 564
Fenoprofen 580
Flurbiprofen 613
Ibuprofen 728
Indomethacin 746
Ketoprofen 785
Ketorolac 787
Lansoprazole and Naproxen . . . 799
Meclofenamate 860
Mefenamic Acid 863
Meloxicam 865
Nabumetone 955
Naproxen 965
Oxaprozin 1022
Piroxicam 1097
Sulindac 1251
Tolmetin 1311

NONSTEROIDAL ANTI-INFLAMMATORY DRUG (NSAID), PARENTERAL
Indomethacin 746
Ketorolac 787

NONSTEROIDAL AROMATASE INHIBITOR
Aminoglutethimide 98

NOREPINEPHRINE REUPTAKE INHIBITOR, SELECTIVE
Atomoxetine 161

NUTRITIONAL SUPPLEMENT
Cysteine 390
Fluoride 603
Glucose Polymers 664
Lysine 851
Medium Chain Triglycerides 861
Methionine 894

OPHTHALMIC AGENT
Verteporfin 1375

OPHTHALMIC AGENT, ANTIGLAUCOMA
AcetaZOLAMIDE 60
Brimonidine 218
Brinzolamide 218
Carbachol 255
Carteolol 269
Cyclopentolate and Phenylephrine 384
Dichlorphenamide 427
Dipivefrin 453
Dorzolamide 464
Echothiophate Iodide 481
Latanoprost 800
Levobetaxolol 808
Levobunolol 808
Methazolamide 891
Metipranolol 913
Phenylephrine 1078
Pilocarpine 1085
Timolol 1299

OPHTHALMIC AGENT, MIOTIC
Acetylcholine 61
Carbachol 255
Echothiophate Iodide 481
Pilocarpine 1085

OPHTHALMIC AGENT, MISCELLANEOUS
Artificial Tears 148
Balanced Salt Solution 181
Bimatoprost 207
Carboxymethylcellulose 265
Glycerin 667
Hydroxypropyl Cellulose 721
Olopatadine 1011
Pemirolast 1055
Unoprostone 1352

OPHTHALMIC AGENT, MYDRIATIC
Atropine 166
Homatropine 693
Phenylephrine 1078
Tropicamide 1348

OPHTHALMIC AGENT, TOXIN
Botulinum Toxin Type A 215

OPHTHALMIC AGENT, VASOCONSTRICTOR
Dipivefrin 453
Naphazoline 964
Naphazoline and Antazoline 964
Naphazoline and Pheniramine . . 964
Tetrahydrozoline 1282

OPHTHALMIC AGENT, VISCOELASTIC
Chondroitin Sulfate and Sodium Hyaluronate 325
Hyaluronate and Derivatives . . . 696

OTIC AGENT, ANALGESIC
Antipyrine and Benzocaine 135

OTIC AGENT, ANTI-INFECTIVE
Acetic Acid, Propylene Glycol Diacetate, and Hydrocortisone 60
m-Cresyl Acetate 857

OTIC AGENT, CERUMENOLYTIC
Antipyrine and Benzocaine 135
Carbamide Peroxide 259
Triethanolamine Polypeptide Oleate-Condensate 1338

OVULATION STIMULATOR
Chorionic Gonadotropin (Human) 326
Chorionic Gonadotropin (Recombinant) 326
ClomiPHENE 354
Follitropins 626
Menotropins 868

OXYTOCIC AGENT
Oxytocin 1038

PARATHYROID HORMONE ANALOG
Teriparatide 1274

PEDICULOCIDE
Lindane 829
Pyrethrins and Piperonyl Butoxide 1153

PHARMACEUTICAL AID
Phenol 1075

PHENOTHIAZINE DERIVATIVE
Promethazine 1130
Thiethylperazine 1287

PHOSPHATE BINDER
Sevelamer 1217

PHOSPHODIESTERASE-5 ENZYME INHIBITOR
Sildenafil 1219
Tadalafil 1257
Vardenafil 1367

PHOSPHODIESTERASE ENZYME INHIBITOR
Cilostazol 329
Inamrinone 743
Milrinone 930

PHOSPHOLIPASE A_2 INHIBITOR
Anagrelide 130

PHOTOSENSITIZING AGENT, TOPICAL
Aminolevulinic Acid 99

PLASMA VOLUME EXPANDER
Dextran 417
Dextran 1 418

PLASMA VOLUME EXPANDER, COLLOID
Hetastarch 692

PROGESTIN
Levonorgestrel 815
MedroxyPROGESTERone 862
Megestrol 865
Norethindrone 996
Norgestrel 998
Progesterone 1128

PROSTAGLANDIN
Alprostadil 87
Carboprost Tromethamine 265
Diclofenac and Misoprostol 430
Dinoprostone 447
Epoprostenol 500
Misoprostol 936

PROSTAGLANDIN, OPHTHALMIC
Latanoprost 800
Travoprost 1325

PROTEASOME INHIBITOR
Bortezomib 214

PROTECTANT, TOPICAL
Trypsin, Balsam Peru, and Castor Oil 1349

PROTEIN C (ACTIVATED)
Drotrecogin Alfa 478

PROTON PUMP INHIBITOR
Esomeprazole 516
Lansoprazole 797
Lansoprazole and Naproxen 799
Omeprazole 1012
Pantoprazole 1043
Rabeprazole 1164

PSORALEN
Methoxsalen 902

RADIOPAQUE AGENTS
Ferumoxides 587
Radiological/Contrast Media (Nonionic) 1166

RADIOPHARMACEUTICAL
Ibritumomab 727

RAUWOLFIA ALKALOID
Rauwolfia Serpentina 1171
Reserpine 1174

RECOMBINANT HUMAN ERYTHROPOIETIN
Darbepoetin Alfa 399

RESPIRATORY STIMULANT
Ammonia Spirit (Aromatic) 111
Doxapram 465

RETINOIC ACID DERIVATIVE
Fluocinolone, Hydroquinone, and Tretinoin 601
Isotretinoin 773
Mequinol and Tretinoin 879
Tretinoin (Topical) 1329

SALICYLATE
Aminosalicylic Acid 100
Aspirin 151
Aspirin and Pravastatin 157
Choline Magnesium Trisalicylate 324
Choline Salicylate 325
Magnesium Salicylate 854
Salsalate 1207
Triethanolamine Salicylate 1338

SCABICIDAL AGENT
Crotamiton 380
Lindane 829
Permethrin 1070

SCLEROSING AGENT
Ethanolamine Oleate 535
Morrhuate Sodium 948

SEDATIVE
Dexmedetomidine 415
Promethazine 1130

SELECTIVE 5-HT_3 RECEPTOR ANTAGONIST
Alosetron 83
Dolasetron 461
Granisetron 671
Ondansetron 1014
Palonosetron 1040

SELECTIVE ALDOSTERONE BLOCKER
Eplerenone 498
Spironolactone 1235

SELECTIVE ESTROGEN RECEPTOR MODULATOR (SERM)
Raloxifene 1166

SEROTONIN 5-$HT_{1B, 1D}$ RECEPTOR AGONIST
Eletriptan 486
Frovatriptan 638

SEROTONIN 5-HT_{1D} RECEPTOR AGONIST
Almotriptan 82
Naratriptan 967
Rizatriptan 1193
Sumatriptan 1252
Zolmitriptan 1403

SEROTONIN 5-HT_4 RECEPTOR AGONIST
Tegaserod 1263

SHAMPOO, PEDICULOCIDE
Pyrethrins and Piperonyl Butoxide 1153

SKELETAL MUSCLE RELAXANT
Baclofen . . . 180
Carisoprodol . . . 266
Carisoprodol and Aspirin . . . 266
Carisoprodol, Aspirin, and Codeine . . . 267
Chlorzoxazone . . . 322
Cyclobenzaprine . . . 382
Dantrolene . . . 397
Metaxalone . . . 886
Methocarbamol . . . 894
Orphenadrine . . . 1017
Orphenadrine, Aspirin, and Caffeine . . . 1018

SKIN AND MUCOUS MEMBRANE AGENT
Imiquimod . . . 738

SKIN AND MUCOUS MEMBRANE AGENT, MISCELLANEOUS
Hyaluronate and Derivatives . . . 696

SMOKING CESSATION AID
BuPROPion . . . 230
Nicotine . . . 981

SODIUM SALT
Sodium Chloride . . . 1227

SOMATOSTATIN ANALOG
Octreotide . . . 1004

SPERMICIDE
Nonoxynol 9 . . . 995

STIMULANT
Dextroamphetamine . . . 418
Dextroamphetamine and Amphetamine . . . 419
Doxapram . . . 465
Ergotamine and Caffeine . . . 506
Methamphetamine . . . 891
Modafinil . . . 939
Pemoline . . . 1055

STOOL SOFTENER
Docusate . . . 459

SUBSTANCE P/NEUROKININ 1 RECEPTOR ANTAGONIST
Aprepitant . . . 138

SUBSTITUTED BENZIMIDAZOLE
Esomeprazole . . . 516
Lansoprazole . . . 797
Omeprazole . . . 1012
Pantoprazole . . . 1043
Rabeprazole . . . 1164

SYMPATHOMIMETIC
Isoetharine . . . 768

THEOPHYLLINE DERIVATIVE
Aminophylline . . . 99
Dyphylline . . . 480
Theophylline . . . 1285
Theophylline and Guaifenesin . . . 1286

THROMBOLYTIC AGENT
Alteplase . . . 88
Reteplase . . . 1175
Streptokinase . . . 1238
Tenecteplase . . . 1268

THYROID PRODUCT
Levothyroxine . . . 817
Liothyronine . . . 831
Liotrix . . . 832
Thyroid . . . 1293

TOPICAL SKIN PRODUCT
Aluminum Sulfate and Calcium Acetate . . . 92
Aminolevulinic Acid . . . 99
Becaplermin . . . 184
Bentoquatam . . . 189
Benzoin . . . 193
Benzoyl Peroxide . . . 194
Benzoyl Peroxide and Hydrocortisone . . . 194
Calcipotriene . . . 243
Camphor and Phenol . . . 248
Capsaicin . . . 252
Chloroxine . . . 313
Clindamycin and Benzoyl Peroxide . . . 350
Coal Tar . . . 367
Coal Tar and Salicylic Acid . . . 367
Dexpanthenol . . . 416
Doxepin . . . 467
Eflornithine . . . 485
Erythromycin . . . 508
Erythromycin and Benzoyl Peroxide . . . 512
Imiquimod . . . 738
Iodine . . . 758
Lactic Acid and Ammonium Hydroxide . . . 793
Lactic Acid and Sodium-PCA . . . 793
Lanolin, Cetyl Alcohol, Glycerin, Petrolatum, and Mineral Oil . . . 797
Merbromin . . . 880
Minoxidil . . . 934
Monobenzone . . . 944
Neomycin, Polymyxin B, and Hydrocortisone . . . 975
Pimecrolimus . . . 1088
Podofilox . . . 1099
Povidone-Iodine . . . 1107
Pyrithione Zinc . . . 1155
Tacrolimus . . . 1255
Triethanolamine Salicylate . . . 1338
Urea . . . 1353
Vitamin A and Vitamin D . . . 1382
Zinc Gelatin . . . 1400
Zinc Oxide . . . 1400

TOPICAL SKIN PRODUCT, ACNE
Azelaic Acid . . . 173
Benzoyl Peroxide . . . 194
Benzoyl Peroxide and Hydrocortisone . . . 194
Clindamycin and Benzoyl Peroxide . . . 350
Erythromycin . . . 508
Erythromycin and Benzoyl Peroxide . . . 512

TOPICAL SKIN PRODUCT, ANTIBACTERIAL
Silver Nitrate . . . 1221

TOXOID
Tetanus Toxoid (Adsorbed) . . . 1277
Tetanus Toxoid (Fluid) . . . 1278

TRACE ELEMENT
Zinc Chloride . . . 1400
Zinc Sulfate . . . 1401

TRACE ELEMENT, PARENTERAL
Selenium . . . 1213
Trace Metals . . . 1319

TYROSINE HYDROXYLASE INHIBITOR
Metyrosine . . . 920

UREA CYCLE DISORDER (UCD) TREATMENT AGENT
Sodium Phenylbutyrate . . . 1230

URICOSURIC AGENT
Colchicine and Probenecid . . . 372
Probenecid . . . 1124
Sulfinpyrazone . . . 1249

URINARY ACIDIFYING AGENT
Potassium Acid Phosphate . . . 1104

URINARY TRACT PRODUCT

Acetohydroxamic Acid 61
Cellulose Sodium Phosphate ... 294
Citric Acid, Magnesium Carbonate, and Glucono-Delta-Lactone 341
Cysteamine 389
Tiopronin 1303

VACCINE

Anthrax Vaccine (Adsorbed) ... 133
BCG Vaccine 183
Diphtheria, Tetanus Toxoids, Acellular Pertussis, Hepatitis B (Recombinant), and Poliovirus (Inactivated) Vaccine 452
Haemophilus b Conjugate Vaccine 680
Hepatitis A (Inactivated) and Hepatitis B (Recombinant) Vaccine 686
Hepatitis A Vaccine 687
Hepatitis B Vaccine 689
Influenza Virus Vaccine 748
Japanese Encephalitis Virus Vaccine (Inactivated) 779
Meningococcal Polysaccharide Vaccine (Groups A, C, Y, and W-135) 868
Mumps Virus Vaccine (Live/Attenuated) 951
Pneumococcal Conjugate Vaccine (7-Valent) 1098
Poliovirus Vaccine (Inactivated) 1099
Rabies Virus Vaccine 1165
Rubella Virus Vaccine (Live) .. 1203
Typhoid Vaccine 1351

VACCINE, LIVE VIRUS

Measles, Mumps, and Rubella Vaccines (Combined) 858
Measles Virus Vaccine (Live) ... 858

VASCULAR ENDOTHELIAL GROWTH FACTOR (VEGF) INHIBITOR

Bevacizumab 204

VASOCONSTRICTOR

Epinephrine 496
Epinephrine (Racemic) 497
Epinephrine (Racemic) and Aluminum Potassium Sulfate 497
Oxymetazoline 1034

VASOCONSTRICTOR, NASAL

Xylometazoline 1393

VASODILATOR

Amyl Nitrite 130
Dipyridamole 453
Ethaverine 535
HydrALAZINE 697
Isosorbide Dinitrate 770
Isosorbide Mononitrate 771
Isoxsuprine 774
Minoxidil 934
Nesiritide 976
Nitroglycerin 991
Nitroprusside 993
Papaverine 1044
Tolazoline 1309
Treprostinil 1327

VASODILATOR, PERIPHERAL

Nylidrin 1002

VASODILATOR, PULMONARY

Nitric Oxide 990

VASOPRESSIN ANALOG, SYNTHETIC

Desmopressin 409

VITAMIN

Ferrous Sulfate and Ascorbic Acid 587
Folic Acid, Cyanocobalamin, and Pyridoxine 626
Vitamin B Complex Combinations 1382
Vitamins (Multiple/Oral) 1384

VITAMIN A DERIVATIVE

Mequinol and Tretinoin 879

VITAMIN D ANALOG

Calcifediol 242
Calcipotriene 243
Calcitriol 244
Cholecalciferol 323
Dihydrotachysterol 443
Doxercalciferol 468
Ergocalciferol 503
Paricalcitol 1045

VITAMIN, FAT SOLUBLE

Beta-Carotene 198
Phytonadione 1084
Vitamin A 1382
Vitamin E 1383

VITAMIN, TOPICAL

Mequinol and Tretinoin 879

VITAMIN, WATER SOLUBLE

Ascorbic Acid 148
Cyanocobalamin 380
Folic Acid 625
Hydroxocobalamin 719
Leucovorin 804
Niacin 978
Niacinamide 979
Pantothenic Acid 1044
Pyridoxine 1154
Riboflavin 1178
Thiamine 1287

XANTHINE OXIDASE INHIBITOR

Allopurinol 82

ALPHABETICAL INDEX

1370-999-397 *see* Anagrelide 130
A_1-PI *see* Alpha$_1$-Proteinase Inhibitor 84
A200® Lice [OTC] *see* Permethrin 1070
A-200® Maximum Strength [OTC] *see* Pyrethrins and Piperonyl Butoxide 1153
A and D® Ointment [OTC] *see* Vitamin A and Vitamin D 1382
Abacavir 42
Abacavir, Lamivudine, and Zidovudine 43
Abacavir Sulfate *see* Abacavir 42
Abarelix 43
Abbott-43818 *see* Leuprolide 805
Abbreviations, Acronyms, and Symbols 18
ABC *see* Abacavir 42
ABCD *see* Amphotericin B Cholesteryl Sulfate Complex 119
Abciximab 44
Abelcet® *see* Amphotericin B (Lipid Complex) 121
Abenol® (Can) *see* Acetaminophen 47
Abilify™ *see* Aripiprazole 142
ABLC *see* Amphotericin B (Lipid Complex) 121
A/B Otic *see* Antipyrine and Benzocaine 135
Abreva® [OTC] *see* Docosanol 459
Absorbable Cotton *see* Cellulose (Oxidized/Regenerated) 293
Absorbable Gelatin Sponge *see* Gelatin (Absorbable) 650
Absorbine Jr.® Antifungal [OTC] *see* Tolnaftate 1312
9-AC *see* Aminocamptothecin 96
Acarbose 45
A-Caro-25® *see* Beta-Carotene 198
Accolate® (Mex) *see* Zafirlukast 1394
AccuHist® Pediatric [DSC] *see* Brompheniramine and Pseudoephedrine 220
AccuNeb™ *see* Albuterol 71
Accupril® *see* Quinapril 1158
Accuretic™ (Can) *see* Quinapril and Hydrochlorothiazide 1160
Accutane® (Can) *see* Isotretinoin 773
Ac-De® (Mex) *see* Dactinomycin 394
ACE *see* Captopril 252
Acebutolol 46
Acebutolol Hydrochloride *see* Acebutolol 46
Aceon® *see* Perindopril Erbumine 1068
Acephen® [OTC] *see* Acetaminophen 47
Acetadiazol® (Mex) *see* AcetaZOLAMIDE 60
Acetadote® *see* Acetylcysteine 61
Acetaminophen 47
Acetaminophen and Chlorpheniramine *see* Chlorpheniramine and Acetaminophen 314
Acetaminophen and Codeine 50
Acetaminophen and Diphenhydramine 53
Acetaminophen and Hydrocodone *see* Hydrocodone and Acetaminophen 702
Acetaminophen and Oxycodone *see* Oxycodone and Acetaminophen 1029
Acetaminophen and Pentazocine *see* Pentazocine and Acetaminophen 1064
Acetaminophen and Phenyltoloxamine 53
Acetaminophen and Pseudoephedrine 53
Acetaminophen and Tramadol 54
Acetaminophen, Aspirin, and Caffeine 56
Acetaminophen, Butalbital, and Caffeine *see* Butalbital, Acetaminophen, and Caffeine 236
Acetaminophen, Caffeine, and Dihydrocodeine 57
Acetaminophen, Caffeine, Codeine, and Butalbital *see* Butalbital, Acetaminophen, Caffeine, and Codeine 236
Acetaminophen, Caffeine, Hydrocodone, Chlorpheniramine, and Phenylephrine *see* Hydrocodone, Chlorpheniramine, Phenylephrine, Acetaminophen, and Caffeine 712
Acetaminophen, Chlorpheniramine, and Pseudoephedrine 58
Acetaminophen, Dextromethorphan, and Pseudoephedrine 59
Acetaminophen, Dichloralphenazone, and Isometheptene *see* Acetaminophen, Isometheptene, and Dichloralphenazone 59
Acetaminophen, Isometheptene, and Dichloralphenazone 59
Acetaminophen, Pseudoephedrine, and Chlorpheniramine *see* Acetaminophen, Chlorpheniramine, and Pseudoephedrine 58
Acetasol® HC *see* Acetic Acid, Propylene Glycol Diacetate, and Hydrocortisone 60
AcetaZOLAMIDE 60
Acetic Acid, Hydrocortisone, and Propylene Glycol Diacetate *see* Acetic Acid, Propylene Glycol Diacetate, and Hydrocortisone 60
Acetic Acid, Propylene Glycol Diacetate, and Hydrocortisone 60
AcetoHEXAMIDE 60
Acetohydroxamic Acid 61
Acetoxyl® (Can) *see* Benzoyl Peroxide 194
Acetoxymethylprogesterone *see* MedroxyPROGESTERone 862
Acetylcholine 61
Acetylcholine Chloride *see* Acetylcholine 61
Acetylcysteine 61
Acetylcysteine Sodium *see* Acetylcysteine 61
Acetylsalicylic Acid *see* Aspirin 151
Achromycin *see* Tetracycline 1280
Aciclovir *see* Acyclovir 64
Acidulated Phosphate Fluoride *see* Fluoride 603
Acifur® (Mex) *see* Acyclovir 64
Acilac (Can) *see* Lactulose 794
Acimox® (Mex) *see* Amoxicillin 114
Aciphex® (Can) *see* Rabeprazole 1164
Aclimafel® (Mex) *see* Amoxicillin 114
Acloral® (Mex) *see* Ranitidine 1169
Aclovate® *see* Alclometasone 74
4-(9-Acridinylamino) Methanesulfon-m-Anisidide *see* Amsacrine 129
Acridinyl Anisidide *see* Amsacrine 129
Acrivastine and Pseudoephedrine 62
Acroxil® (Mex) *see* Amoxicillin 114
ACT *see* Dactinomycin 394

ACT® [OTC] *see* Fluoride 603
Act-D *see* Dactinomycin 394
ACTH *see* Corticotropin 376
ActHIB® *see* *Haemophilus* b Conjugate Vaccine 680
Acticin® *see* Permethrin 1070
Actidose-Aqua® [OTC] *see* Charcoal 303
Actidose® with Sorbitol [OTC] *see* Charcoal 303
Actifed® (Can) *see* Triprolidine and Pseudoephedrine 1345
Actifed® Cold and Allergy [OTC] *see* Triprolidine and Pseudoephedrine 1345
Actifed® Cold and Sinus [OTC] *see* Acetaminophen, Chlorpheniramine, and Pseudoephedrine 58
Actigall® *see* Ursodiol 1354
Actilyse® (Mex) *see* Alteplase 88
Actimmune® (Can) *see* Interferon Gamma-1b 758
Actinomycin *see* Dactinomycin 394
Actinomycin CI *see* Dactinomycin . . 394
Actinomycin D *see* Dactinomycin . . . 394
Actiq® *see* Fentanyl 581
Actisite® *see* Tetracycline (Periodontal) 1282
Activase® *see* Alteplase 88
Activase® rt-PA (Can) *see* Alteplase 88
Activated Carbon *see* Charcoal 303
Activated Charcoal *see* Charcoal . . . 303
Activated Dimethicone *see* Simethicone 1222
Activated Ergosterol *see* Ergocalciferol 503
Activated Methylpolysiloxane *see* Simethicone 1222
Activated Protein C, Human, Recombinant *see* Drotrecogin Alfa 478
Activella™ *see* Estradiol and Norethindrone 521
Actonel® (Can) *see* Risedronate . . . 1185
Actos® *see* Pioglitazone 1091
ACU-dyne® [OTC] *see* Povidone-Iodine 1107
Acular® *see* Ketorolac 787
Acularen® (Mex) *see* Ketorolac 787
Acular LS™ *see* Ketorolac 787
Acular® PF *see* Ketorolac 787
Acupril® (Mex) *see* Quinapril 1158
ACV *see* Acyclovir 64
Acycloguanosine *see* Acyclovir 64
Acyclovir 64
AD3L *see* Valrubicin 1362
Adaferin® (Mex) *see* Adapalene 67
Adagen® (Can) *see* Pegademase Bovine 1050
Adalat® (Mex) *see* NIFEdipine 984
Adalat® CC *see* NIFEdipine 984
Adalat® XL® (Can) *see* NIFEdipine . . 984
Adalimumab 67
Adalken® (Mex) *see* Penicillamine 1057
Adamantanamine Hydrochloride *see* Amantadine 92
Adapalene 67
Adderall® *see* Dextroamphetamine and Amphetamine 419
Adderall XR™ *see* Dextroamphetamine and Amphetamine 419
Adecur® (Mex) *see* Terazosin 1271
Adefovir 68
Adefovir Dipivoxil *see* Adefovir 68
Adel® (Mex) *see* Clarithromycin 343
Adenine Arabinoside *see* Vidarabine 1376
Adenocard® *see* Adenosine 68
Adenoscan® *see* Adenosine 68
Adenosine 68
ADH *see* Vasopressin 1369
Adipex-P® *see* Phentermine 1076
Adoxa™ *see* Doxycycline 471
ADR *see* DOXOrubicin 469
Adrenalin® (Dental) *see* Epinephrine 496
Adrenocorticotropic Hormone *see* Corticotropin 376
Adria *see* DOXOrubicin 469
Adriamycin® (Can) *see* DOXOrubicin 469
Adriamycin PFS® *see* DOXOrubicin 469
Adriamycin RDF® *see* DOXOrubicin 469
Adriblastina® (Mex) *see* DOXOrubicin 469
Adrucil® (Can) *see* Fluorouracil 605
Adsorbent Charcoal *see* Charcoal . . 303
Advair Diskus® (Can) *see* Fluticasone and Salmeterol 619
Advantage 24™ (Can) *see* Nonoxynol 9 995
Advantage-S™ [OTC] *see* Nonoxynol 9 995
Advate *see* Antihemophilic Factor (Recombinant) 135
Advicor™ *see* Niacin and Lovastatin 979
Advil® (Mex) *see* Ibuprofen 728
Advil® Children's [OTC] *see* Ibuprofen 728
Advil® Cold, Children's [OTC] *see* Pseudoephedrine and Ibuprofen 1149
Advil® Cold & Sinus [OTC] *see* Pseudoephedrine and Ibuprofen 1149
Advil® Infants' [OTC] *see* Ibuprofen 728
Advil® Junior [OTC] *see* Ibuprofen . . 728
Advil® Migraine [OTC] *see* Ibuprofen 728
Aerius® (Can) *see* Desloratadine . . . 408
AeroBid® *see* Flunisolide 599
AeroBid®-M *see* Flunisolide 599
Aesculus hippocastanum see Horse Chestnut 1437
Afazol Grin® (Mex) *see* Naphazoline 964
Afrin® (Mex) *see* Oxymetazoline 1034
Afrin® Extra Moisturizing [OTC] *see* Oxymetazoline 1034
Afrin® Original [OTC] *see* Oxymetazoline 1034
Afrin® Severe Congestion [OTC] *see* Oxymetazoline 1034
Afrin® Sinus [OTC] *see* Oxymetazoline 1034
Aftate® Antifungal [OTC] *see* Tolnaftate 1312
Afungil® (Mex) *see* Fluconazole 594
A.f. Valdecasas® (Mex) *see* Folic Acid 625
AG *see* Aminoglutethimide 98
Agalsidase Beta 69
Agenerase® *see* Amprenavir 128
Aggrastat® (Can) *see* Tirofiban . . . 1304
Aggrenox® (Can) *see* Aspirin and Dipyridamole 156
$AgNO_3$ *see* Silver Nitrate 1221
Agoral® Maximum Strength Laxative [OTC] *see* Senna 1213
Agrastat® (Mex) *see* Tirofiban 1304
Agrylin® *see* Anagrelide 130
AGT *see* Aminoglutethimide 98
AHA *see* Acetohydroxamic Acid 61

AH-Chew® *see* Chlorpheniramine, Phenylephrine, and Methscopolamine . . . 317
AHF (Human) *see* Antihemophilic Factor (Human) . . . 134
AHF (Porcine) *see* Antihemophilic Factor (Porcine) . . . 134
AHF (Recombinant) *see* Antihemophilic Factor (Recombinant) . . . 135
A-hydroCort® *see* Hydrocortisone . . . 714
Airomir (Can) *see* Albuterol . . . 71
Akacin® (Mex) *see* Amikacin . . . 95
AK-Con™ *see* Naphazoline . . . 964
AK-Dilate® *see* Phenylephrine . . . 1078
Akineton® (Mex) *see* Biperiden . . . 207
AK-Nefrin® *see* Phenylephrine . . . 1078
Akne-Mycin® *see* Erythromycin . . . 508
Akorazol® (Mex) *see* Ketoconazole . . . 783
AK-Pentolate® *see* Cyclopentolate . . 383
AK-Poly-Bac® *see* Bacitracin and Polymyxin B . . . 178
AK-Pred® *see* PrednisoLONE . . . 1113
AK-Rinse™ *see* Balanced Salt Solution . . . 181
AK-Spore® H.C. [DSC] *see* Bacitracin, Neomycin, Polymyxin B, and Hydrocortisone . . . 179
AK-Sulf® *see* Sulfacetamide . . . 1244
AK-T-Caine™ *see* Tetracaine . . . 1278
AKTob® *see* Tobramycin . . . 1306
AK-Tracin® [DSC] *see* Bacitracin . . . 178
AK-Trol® *see* Neomycin, Polymyxin B, and Dexamethasone . . . 974
Akwa Tears® [OTC] *see* Artificial Tears . . . 148
ALA *see* Flaxseed Oil . . . 1427
Alamag [OTC] *see* Aluminum Hydroxide and Magnesium Hydroxide . . . 91
Alamag Plus [OTC] *see* Aluminum Hydroxide, Magnesium Hydroxide, and Simethicone . . . 92
Alamast™ (Can) *see* Pemirolast . . . 1055
Alatrofloxacin Mesylate *see* Trovafloxacin . . . 1348
Alavert™ [OTC] *see* Loratadine . . . 841
Alavert™ Allergy and Sinus [OTC] *see* Loratadine and Pseudoephedrine . . . 842
Albalon® *see* Naphazoline . . . 964
Albalon®-A Liquifilm (Can) *see* Naphazoline and Antazoline . . . 964
Albendazole . . . 71
Albenza® *see* Albendazole . . . 71
Albert® Docusate (Can) *see* Docusate . . . 459
Albert® Glyburide (Can) *see* GlyBURIDE . . . 664
Albert® Pentoxifylline (Can) *see* Pentoxifylline . . . 1066
Alboral® (Mex) *see* Diazepam . . . 423
Albuterol . . . 71
Albuterol and Ipratropium *see* Ipratropium and Albuterol . . . 761
Albuterol Sulfate *see* Albuterol . . . 71
Alcaine® *see* Proparacaine . . . 1134
Alcalak [OTC] *see* Calcium Carbonate . . . 245
Alclometasone . . . 74
Alclometasone Dipropionate *see* Alclometasone . . . 74
Alcomicin® (Can) *see* Gentamicin . . 655
Aldactazide® *see* Hydrochlorothiazide and Spironolactone . . . 701
Aldactazide 25® (Can) *see* Hydrochlorothiazide and Spironolactone . . . 701
Aldactazide 50® (Can) *see* Hydrochlorothiazide and Spironolactone . . . 701
Aldactone® (Mex) *see* Spironolactone . . . 1235
Aldara™ *see* Imiquimod . . . 738
Aldesleukin . . . 74
Aldomet® (Mex) *see* Methyldopa . . . 906
Aldoril® *see* Methyldopa and Hydrochlorothiazide . . . 906
Aldoril® D *see* Methyldopa and Hydrochlorothiazide . . . 906
Aldroxicon I [OTC] *see* Aluminum Hydroxide, Magnesium Hydroxide, and Simethicone . . . 92
Aldroxicon II [OTC] *see* Aluminum Hydroxide, Magnesium Hydroxide, and Simethicone . . . 92
Aldurazyme® *see* Laronidase . . . 800
Alefacept . . . 76
Alemtuzumab . . . 76
Alendronate . . . 77
Alendronate Sodium *see* Alendronate . . . 77
Alenic Alka Tablet [OTC] *see* Aluminum Hydroxide and Magnesium Trisilicate . . . 91
Aler-Dryl [OTC] *see* DiphenhydrAMINE . . . 448
Alertec® (Can) *see* Modafinil . . . 939
Alesse® (Can) *see* Ethinyl Estradiol and Levonorgestrel . . . 545
Aleve® [OTC] *see* Naproxen . . . 965
Alfenta® (Can) *see* Alfentanil . . . 79
Alfentanil . . . 79
Alfentanil Hydrochloride *see* Alfentanil . . . 79
Alferon® N *see* Interferon Alfa-n3 . . . 755
Alfuzosin . . . 80
Alfuzosin Hydrochloride *see* Alfuzosin . . . 80
Algidol® (Mex) *see* Ibuprofen . . . 728
Alglucerase . . . 80
Alidol® (Mex) *see* Ketorolac . . . 787
Alimta® *see* Pemetrexed . . . 1054
Alin® (Mex) *see* Dexamethasone . . . 411
Alinia™ *see* Nitazoxanide . . . 989
Alitretinoin . . . 81
Alka-Mints® [OTC] *see* Calcium Carbonate . . . 245
Alka-Seltzer® Gas Relief [OTC] *see* Simethicone . . . 1222
Alka-Seltzer Plus® Cold and Cough [OTC] *see* Chlorpheniramine, Phenylephrine, and Dextromethorphan . . . 316
Alka-Seltzer Plus® Cold and Sinus Liquigels [OTC] *see* Acetaminophen and Pseudoephedrine . . . 53
Alka-Seltzer® Plus Cold Liqui-Gels® [OTC] *see* Acetaminophen, Chlorpheniramine, and Pseudoephedrine . . . 58
Alka-Seltzer® Plus Flu Liqui-Gels® [OTC] *see* Acetaminophen, Dextromethorphan, and Pseudoephedrine . . . 59
Alkeran® (Mex) *see* Melphalan . . . 866
Allbee® C-800 [OTC] *see* Vitamin B Complex Combinations . . . 1382
Allbee® C-800 + Iron [OTC] *see* Vitamin B Complex Combinations . . . 1382
Allbee® with C [OTC] *see* Vitamin B Complex Combinations . . . 1382
Allegra® (Can) *see* Fexofenadine . . . 587
Allegra-D® *see* Fexofenadine and Pseudoephedrine . . . 588

Aller-Chlor® [OTC] *see* Chlorpheniramine . . . 313
Allerdryl® (Can) *see* DiphenhydrAMINE . . . 448
Allerest® Maximum Strength Allergy and Hay Fever [OTC] *see* Chlorpheniramine and Pseudoephedrine . . . 315
Allerfrim® [OTC] *see* Triprolidine and Pseudoephedrine . . . 1345
Allergen® *see* Antipyrine and Benzocaine . . . 135
AllerMax® [OTC] *see* DiphenhydrAMINE . . . 448
Allernix (Can) *see* DiphenhydrAMINE . . . 448
Allerphed® [OTC] *see* Triprolidine and Pseudoephedrine . . . 1345
Allersol® *see* Naphazoline . . . 964
Allfen Jr *see* Guaifenesin . . . 672
Allfen *(reformulation) see* Guaifenesin and Potassium Guaiacolsulfonate . . . 675
Allium savitum see Garlic . . . 1428
Allopurinol . . . 82
Allopurinol Sodium *see* Allopurinol . . . 82
All-*trans*-Retinoic Acid *see* Tretinoin (Oral) . . . 1328
Almacone® [OTC] *see* Aluminum Hydroxide, Magnesium Hydroxide, and Simethicone . . . 92
Almacone Double Strength® [OTC] *see* Aluminum Hydroxide, Magnesium Hydroxide, and Simethicone . . . 92
Almora® [OTC] *see* Magnesium Gluconate . . . 853
Almotriptan . . . 82
Almotriptan Malate *see* Almotriptan . . . 82
Alocril™ (Can) *see* Nedocromil . . . 970
Aloe . . . 1412
Aloe Barbadensis *see* Aloe . . . 1412
Aloe Capensis *see* Aloe . . . 1412
Aloe vera *see* Aloe . . . 1412
Aloe Vesta® 2-n-1 Antifungal [OTC] *see* Miconazole . . . 922
Aloid® (Mex) *see* Miconazole . . . 922
Alomide® (Can) *see* Lodoxamide . . . 836
Alophen® [OTC] *see* Bisacodyl . . . 208
Aloprim™ *see* Allopurinol . . . 82
Alora® *see* Estradiol . . . 518
Alosetron . . . 83
Aloxi™ *see* Palonosetron . . . 1040
Alpha$_1$-Antitrypsin *see* Alpha$_1$-Proteinase Inhibitor . . . 84
Alpha$_1$-PI *see* Alpha$_1$-Proteinase Inhibitor . . . 84
Alpha$_1$-Proteinase Inhibitor . . . 84
Alpha$_1$-Proteinase Inhibitor, Human *see* Alpha$_1$-Proteinase Inhibitor . . . 84
Alpha-Galactosidase-A (Human, Recombinant) *see* Agalsidase Beta . . . 69
Alphagan™ (Can) *see* Brimonidine . . 218
Alphagan® P *see* Brimonidine . . . 218
Alpha-linolenic Acid *see* Flaxseed Oil . . . 1427
Alpha-lipoate *see* Alpha-Lipoic Acid . . . 1413
Alpha-Lipoic Acid . . . 1413
Alphanate® *see* Antihemophilic Factor (Human) . . . 134
AlphaNine® SD *see* Factor IX . . . 571
Alphaquin HP *see* Hydroquinone . . . 719
Alprazolam . . . 84
Alprazolam Intensol® *see* Alprazolam . . . 84
Alprostadil . . . 87
Alrex® *see* Loteprednol . . . 847
Altace® *see* Ramipril . . . 1167
Altamisa *see* Feverfew . . . 1426
Altamist [OTC] *see* Sodium Chloride . . . 1227
Alteplase . . . 88
Alteplase, Recombinant *see* Alteplase . . . 88
Alteplase, Tissue Plasminogen Activator, Recombinant *see* Alteplase . . . 88
Alter-H!2® (Mex) *see* Ranitidine . . . 1169
ALternaGel® [OTC] *see* Aluminum Hydroxide . . . 90
Alti-Acyclovir (Can) *see* Acyclovir . . . 64
Alti-Alprazolam (Can) *see* Alprazolam . . . 84
Alti-Amiodarone (Can) *see* Amiodarone . . . 101
Alti-Amoxi-Clav (Can) *see* Amoxicillin and Clavulanate Potassium . . . 116
Alti-Azathioprine (Can) *see* Azathioprine . . . 172
Alti-Captopril (Can) *see* Captopril . . . 252
Alti-Clindamycin (Can) *see* Clindamycin . . . 348
Alti-Clobazam (Can) *see* Clobazam . . . 350
Alti-Clonazepam (Can) *see* Clonazepam . . . 356
Alti-Desipramine (Can) *see* Desipramine . . . 407
Alti-Diltiazem CD (Can) *see* Diltiazem . . . 444
Alti-Divalproex (Can) *see* Valproic Acid and Derivatives . . . 1359
Alti-Doxazosin (Can) *see* Doxazosin . . . 465
Alti-Flunisolide (Can) *see* Flunisolide . . . 599
Alti-Fluoxetine (Can) *see* Fluoxetine . . . 606
Alti-Flurbiprofen (Can) *see* Flurbiprofen . . . 613
Alti-Fluvoxamine (Can) *see* Fluvoxamine . . . 623
Alti-Ipratropium (Can) *see* Ipratropium . . . 761
Alti-Metformin (Can) *see* Metformin . . . 887
Alti-Minocycline (Can) *see* Minocycline . . . 931
Alti-MPA (Can) *see* MedroxyPROGESTERone . . . 862
Altinac™ *see* Tretinoin (Topical) . . . 1329
Alti-Nadolol (Can) *see* Nadolol . . . 956
Alti-Nortriptyline (Can) *see* Nortriptyline . . . 999
Alti-Ranitidine (Can) *see* Ranitidine . . . 1169
Alti-Salbutamol (Can) *see* Albuterol . . . 71
Alti-Sotalol (Can) *see* Sotalol . . . 1231
Alti-Sulfasalazine (Can) *see* Sulfasalazine . . . 1249
Alti-Terazosin (Can) *see* Terazosin . . . 1271
Alti-Ticlopidine (Can) *see* Ticlopidine . . . 1297
Alti-Timolol (Can) *see* Timolol . . . 1299
Alti-Trazodone (Can) *see* Trazodone . . . 1326
Alti-Verapamil (Can) *see* Verapamil . . . 1373
Alti-Zopiclone (Can) *see* Zopiclone . . . 1406
Altocor™ [DSC] *see* Lovastatin . . . 848
Altoprev™ *see* Lovastatin . . . 848
Altretamine . . . 89
Altruline® (Mex) *see* Sertraline . . . 1215

Alu-Cap® [OTC] *see* Aluminum Hydroxide . . . 90
Aluminum Chloride . . . 90
Aluminum Hydroxide . . . 90
Aluminum Hydroxide and Magnesium Carbonate . . . 90
Aluminum Hydroxide and Magnesium Hydroxide . . . 91
Aluminum Hydroxide and Magnesium Trisilicate . . . 91
Aluminum Hydroxide, Magnesium Hydroxide, and Simethicone . . . 92
Aluminum Potassium Sulfate and Epinephrine (Racemic) (Dental) *see* Epinephrine (Racemic) and Aluminum Potassium Sulfate . . . 497
Aluminum Sucrose Sulfate, Basic *see* Sucralfate . . . 1242
Aluminum Sulfate and Calcium Acetate . . . 92
Alupent® *see* Metaproterenol . . . 885
Alustra™ *see* Hydroquinone . . . 719
Alvidina® (Mex) *see* Ranitidine . . . 1169
Amantadine . . . 92
Amantadine Hydrochloride *see* Amantadine . . . 92
Amaryl® (Can) *see* Glimepiride . . . 659
Amatine® (Can) *see* Midodrine . . . 927
Ambenonium . . . 93
Ambenonium Chloride *see* Ambenonium . . . 93
Amber Touch-and-Feel *see* St John's Wort . . . 1447
Ambien® *see* Zolpidem . . . 1404
Ambifed-G DM *see* Guaifenesin, Pseudoephedrine, and Dextromethorphan . . . 676
AmBisome® (Can) *see* Amphotericin B (Liposomal) . . . 122
Amcinonide . . . 93
Amcort® (Can) *see* Amcinonide . . . 93
Ameblin® (Mex) *see* Metronidazole . . . 917
Amerge® *see* Naratriptan . . . 967
Americaine® [OTC] *see* Benzocaine . . . 191
Americaine® Anesthetic Lubricant *see* Benzocaine . . . 191
American Coneflower *see* *Echinacea* . . . 1423
A-Methapred® *see* MethylPREDNISolone . . . 910
Amethocaine Hydrochloride *see* Tetracaine . . . 1278
Amethopterin *see* Methotrexate . . . 897
Ametop™ (Can) *see* Tetracaine . . . 1278
Amevive® *see* Alefacept . . . 76
Amfepramone *see* Diethylpropion . . . 434
AMG 073 *see* Cinacalcet . . . 331
Amibid LA [DSC] *see* Guaifenesin . . . 672
Amicar® (Can) *see* Aminocaproic Acid . . . 97
Amidate® *see* Etomidate . . . 566
Amifostine . . . 94
Amigesic® (Can) *see* Salsalate . . . 1207
Amikacin . . . 95
Amikacin Sulfate *see* Amikacin . . . 95
Amikafur® (Mex) *see* Amikacin . . . 95
Amikalem® (Mex) *see* Amikacin . . . 95
Amikason's® [inj.] (Mex) *see* Amikacin . . . 95
Amikayect® (Mex) *see* Amikacin . . . 95
Amikin® (Can) *see* Amikacin . . . 95
Amiloride . . . 95
Amiloride and Hydrochlorothiazide . . . 96
Amiloride Hydrochloride *see* Amiloride . . . 95
2-Amino-6-Mercaptopurine *see* Thioguanine . . . 1288
2-Amino-6-Trifluoromethoxy-benzothiazole *see* Riluzole . . . 1183
Aminobenzylpenicillin *see* Ampicillin . . . 124
Aminocamptothecin . . . 96
9-Aminocamptothecin *see* Aminocamptothecin . . . 96
Aminocaproic Acid . . . 97
Amino-Cerv™ *see* Urea . . . 1353
Aminoglutethimide . . . 98
Aminolevulinic Acid . . . 99
Aminolevulinic Acid Hydrochloride *see* Aminolevulinic Acid . . . 99
Aminophylline . . . 99
Aminosalicylate Sodium *see* Aminosalicylic Acid . . . 100
Aminosalicylic Acid . . . 100
4-Aminosalicylic Acid *see* Aminosalicylic Acid . . . 100
5-Aminosalicylic Acid *see* Mesalamine . . . 882
Aminoxin® [OTC] *see* Pyridoxine . . . 1154
Amiodarone . . . 101
Amiodarone Hydrochloride *see* Amiodarone . . . 101
Amipaque® [DSC] *see* Radiological/Contrast Media (Nonionic) . . . 1166
Ami-Tex PSE *see* Guaifenesin and Pseudoephedrine . . . 675
Amitone® [OTC] *see* Calcium Carbonate . . . 245
Amitriptyline . . . 103
Amitriptyline and Chlordiazepoxide . . . 105
Amitriptyline and Perphenazine . . . 106
Amitriptyline Hydrochloride *see* Amitriptyline . . . 103
A.M.K.® (Mex) *see* Amikacin . . . 95
AmLactin® [OTC] *see* Lactic Acid and Ammonium Hydroxide . . . 793
Amlexanox . . . 107
Amlodipine . . . 108
Amlodipine and Atorvastatin . . . 110
Amlodipine and Benazepril . . . 110
Amlodipine Besylate *see* Amlodipine . . . 108
Ammens® Medicated Deodorant [OTC] *see* Zinc Oxide . . . 1400
Ammonapse *see* Sodium Phenylbutyrate . . . 1230
Ammonia Spirit (Aromatic) . . . 111
Ammonium Chloride . . . 111
Ammonium Lactate *see* Lactic Acid and Ammonium Hydroxide . . . 793
Amnesteem™ *see* Isotretinoin . . . 773
Amobarbital . . . 112
Amobarbital and Secobarbital . . . 112
Amonafide . . . 112
Amonafide Hydrochloride *see* Amonafide . . . 112
Amoxapine . . . 113
Amoxicillin . . . 114
Amoxicillin and Clavulanate Potassium . . . 116
Amoxicillin and Clavulanic Acid *see* Amoxicillin and Clavulanate Potassium . . . 116
Amoxicillin, Lansoprazole, and Clarithromycin *see* Lansoprazole, Amoxicillin, and Clarithromycin . . . 798
Amoxicillin Trihydrate *see* Amoxicillin . . . 114
Amoxifur® (Mex) *see* Amoxicillin . . . 114
Amoxil® *see* Amoxicillin . . . 114
Amoxinovag® (Mex) *see* Amoxicillin . . . 114
Amoxisol® (Mex) *see* Amoxicillin . . . 114
Amoxycillin *see* Amoxicillin . . . 114

Amphetamine and Dextroamphetamine *see* Dextroamphetamine and Amphetamine . . . 419
Amphocin® *see* Amphotericin B (Conventional) . . . 120
Amphojel® (Can) *see* Aluminum Hydroxide . . . 90
Amphotec® (Can) *see* Amphotericin B Cholesteryl Sulfate Complex . . . 119
Amphotericin B Cholesteryl Sulfate Complex . . . 119
Amphotericin B Colloidal Dispersion *see* Amphotericin B Cholesteryl Sulfate Complex . . . 119
Amphotericin B (Conventional) . . . 120
Amphotericin B Desoxycholate *see* Amphotericin B (Conventional) . . 120
Amphotericin B (Lipid Complex) . . . 121
Amphotericin B (Liposomal) . . . 122
Ampicillin . . . 124
Ampicillin and Probenecid . . . 126
Ampicillin and Sulbactam . . . 126
Ampicillin Sodium *see* Ampicillin . . . 124
Ampicillin Trihydrate *see* Ampicillin . . . 124
Ampliron® (Mex) *see* Amoxicillin . . . 114
Amprenavir . . . 128
AMPT *see* Metyrosine . . . 920
Amrinone Lactate *see* Inamrinone . . 743
AMSA *see* Amsacrine . . . 129
Amsacrine . . . 129
Amyl Nitrite . . . 130
Amylobarbitone *see* Amobarbital . . . 112
Amytal® *see* Amobarbital . . . 112
Anacin PM Aspirin Free [OTC] [DSC] *see* Acetaminophen and Diphenhydramine . . . 53
Anadrol® *see* Oxymetholone . . . 1035
Anafranil® (Can) *see* ClomiPRAMINE . . . 355
Anagrelide . . . 130
Anagrelide Hydrochloride *see* Anagrelide . . . 130
Anakinra . . . 131
Ana-Kit® *see* Epinephrine and Chlorpheniramine . . . 497
Analfin® (Mex) *see* Morphine Sulfate . . . 947
Analpram-HC® *see* Pramoxine and Hydrocortisone . . . 1109
AnaMantle® HC *see* Lidocaine and Hydrocortisone . . . 826
Anandron® (Can) *see* Nilutamide . . . 986
Anaprox® *see* Naproxen . . . 965
Anaprox® DS *see* Naproxen . . . 965
Anapsique® (Mex) *see* Amitriptyline . . . 103
Anas comosus *see* Bromelain . . . 1416
Anaspaz® *see* Hyoscyamine . . . 724
Anastrozole . . . 132
Anatuss LA *see* Guaifenesin and Pseudoephedrine . . . 675
Anbesol® [OTC] *see* Benzocaine . . . 191
Anbesol® Baby [OTC] *see* Benzocaine . . . 191
Anbesol® Maximum Strength [OTC] *see* Benzocaine . . . 191
Ancef® *see* Cefazolin . . . 278
Ancobon® *see* Flucytosine . . . 596
Andehist DM NR Drops *see* Carbinoxamine, Pseudoephedrine, and Dextromethorphan . . . 263
Andehist NR Drops *see* Carbinoxamine and Pseudoephedrine . . . 262
Andehist NR Syrup *see* Brompheniramine and Pseudoephedrine . . . 220
Andox® (Mex) *see* Acetaminophen . . . 47
Andriol® (Can) *see* Testosterone . . 1276
Andro *see* Androstenedione . . . 1413
Androderm® *see* Testosterone . . . 1276
AndroGel® (Can) *see* Testosterone . . . 1276
Android® *see* MethylTESTOSTERone . . . 912
Andropository (Can) *see* Testosterone . . . 1276
Androstenedione . . . 1413
Androxicam® (Mex) *see* Piroxicam . . . 1097
Anectine® (Mex) *see* Succinylcholine . . . 1241
Anestacon® *see* Lidocaine . . . 819
Aneurine Hydrochloride *see* Thiamine . . . 1287
Anexate® (Can) *see* Flumazenil . . . 599
Anexsia® *see* Hydrocodone and Acetaminophen . . . 702
Angelica sinensis *see* Dong Quai . . 1423
Angiomax® *see* Bivalirudin . . . 212
Angiotrofin® (Mex) *see* Diltiazem . . . 444
Anglix® (Mex) *see* Nitroglycerin . . . 991
Anglopen® (Mex) *see* Ampicillin . . . 124
Animal and Human Bites Guidelines . . . 1582
Anistal® (Mex) *see* Ranitidine . . . 1169
Anolor 300 *see* Butalbital, Acetaminophen, and Caffeine . . 236
Ansaid® *see* Flurbiprofen . . . 613
Ansamycin *see* Rifabutin . . . 1179
Antabuse® *see* Disulfiram . . . 456
Antagon® *see* Ganirelix . . . 647
Antalgin® (Mex) *see* Indomethacin . . 746
Antazoline and Naphazoline *see* Naphazoline and Antazoline . . . 964
Anthraforte® (Can) *see* Anthralin . . . 133
Anthralin . . . 133
Anthranol® (Can) *see* Anthralin . . . 133
Anthrascalp® (Can) *see* Anthralin . . . 133
Anthrax Vaccine (Adsorbed) . . . 133
AntibiOtic® Ear *see* Neomycin, Polymyxin B, and Hydrocortisone . . . 975
Antibiotic Prophylaxis, Preprocedural Guidelines for Dental Patients . . . 1509
Anti-CD11a *see* Efalizumab . . . 483
Anti-CD20 Monoclonal Antibody *see* Rituximab . . . 1191
Antidigoxin Fab Fragments, Ovine *see* Digoxin Immune Fab . . . 440
Antidiuretic Hormone *see* Vasopressin . . . 1369
Antihemophilic Factor (Human) . . . 134
Antihemophilic Factor (Porcine) . . . 134
Antihemophilic Factor (Recombinant) . . . 135
Anti-inhibitor Coagulant Complex . . . 135
Antiphlogistine Rub A-535 No Odour (Can) *see* Triethanolamine Salicylate . . . 1338
Antiphogistine Rub A-535 Capsaicin (Can) *see* Capsaicin . . . 252
Antiplaque Agents . . . 1556
Antipyrine and Benzocaine . . . 135
Antiseptic Mouthwash *see* Mouthwash (Antiseptic) . . . 948
Antithrombin III . . . 136
Antithymocyte Globulin (Equine) . . . 136
Antithymocyte Immunoglobulin *see* Antithymocyte Globulin (Equine) . . . 136
Antitumor Necrosis Factor Apha (Human) *see* Adalimumab . . . 67
Anti-VEGF Monoclonal Antibody *see* Bevacizumab . . . 204
Antivert® *see* Meclizine . . . 859

Antizol® *see* Fomepizole 627
Anturane *see* Sulfinpyrazone 1249
Anucort-HC® *see* Hydrocortisone . . . 714
Anusol-HC® *see* Hydrocortisone 714
Anusol® HC-1 [OTC] *see* Hydrocortisone 714
Anusol® Ointment [OTC] *see* Pramoxine 1109
Anuzinc (Can) *see* Zinc Sulfate . . . 1401
Anzemet® (Mex) *see* Dolasetron . . . 461
3-A Ofteno® (Mex) *see* Diclofenac . . 427
APAP *see* Acetaminophen 47
APAP and Tramadol *see* Acetaminophen and Tramadol . . . 54
Apatate® [OTC] *see* Vitamin B Complex Combinations 1382
ApexiCon™ *see* Diflorasone 435
ApexiCon™ E *see* Diflorasone 435
Aphedrid™ [OTC] *see* Triprolidine and Pseudoephedrine 1345
Aphrodyne® *see* Yohimbine 1393
Aphthasol® *see* Amlexanox 107
Apidra™ *see* Insulin Preparations . . . 749
Aplisol® *see* Tuberculin Tests 1349
Aplonidine *see* Apraclonidine 138
Apo-Acebutolol® (Can) *see* Acebutolol 46
Apo-Acetaminophen® (Can) *see* Acetaminophen 47
Apo-Acetazolamide® (Can) *see* AcetaZOLAMIDE 60
Apo-Acyclovir® (Can) *see* Acyclovir 64
Apo-Allopurinol® (Can) *see* Allopurinol 82
Apo-Alpraz® (Can) *see* Alprazolam 84
Apo-Amilzide® (Can) *see* Amiloride and Hydrochlorothiazide 90
Apo-Amitriptyline® (Can) *see* Amitriptyline 103
Apo-Amoxi® (Can) *see* Amoxicillin . . 114
Apo-Amoxi-Clav® (Can) *see* Amoxicillin and Clavulanate Potassium 116
Apo-Ampi® (Can) *see* Ampicillin 124
Apo-Atenol® (Can) *see* Atenolol 159
Apo-Azathioprine® (Can) *see* Azathioprine 172
Apo-Baclofen® (Can) *see* Baclofen 180
Apo-Beclomethasone® (Can) *see* Beclomethasone 184
Apo-Benztropine® (Can) *see* Benztropine 196
Apo-Bisacodyl® (Can) *see* Bisacodyl 208
Apo-Bromazepam® (Can) *see* Bromazepam 218
Apo-Bromocriptine® (Can) *see* Bromocriptine 219
Apo-Buspirone® (Can) *see* BusPIRone 233
Apo-Butorphanol® (Can) *see* Butorphanol 240
Apo-Cal® (Can) *see* Calcium Carbonate 245
Apo-Capto® (Can) *see* Captopril 252
Apo-Carbamazepine® (Can) *see* Carbamazepine 255
Apo-Cefaclor® (Can) *see* Cefaclor . . 274
Apo-Cefadroxil® (Can) *see* Cefadroxil 275
Apo-Cefuroxime® (Can) *see* Cefuroxime 289
Apo-Cephalex® (Can) *see* Cephalexin 294
Apo-Cetirizine® (Can) *see* Cetirizine 298
Apo-Chlorax® (Can) *see* Clidinium and Chlordiazepoxide 347
Apo-Chlordiazepoxide® (Can) *see* Chlordiazepoxide 307
Apo-Chlorhexadine® (Can) *see* Chlorhexidine Gluconate 308
Apo-Chlorpromazine® (Can) *see* ChlorproMAZINE 319
Apo-Chlorpropamide® (Can) *see* ChlorproPAMIDE 321
Apo-Chlorthalidone® (Can) *see* Chlorthalidone 321
Apo-Cimetidine® (Can) *see* Cimetidine 330
Apo-Clindamycin® (Can) *see* Clindamycin 348
Apo-Clobazam® (Can) *see* Clobazam 350
Apo-Clomipramine® (Can) *see* ClomiPRAMINE 355
Apo-Clonazepam® (Can) *see* Clonazepam 356
Apo-Clonidine® (Can) *see* Clonidine 358
Apo-Clorazepate® (Can) *see* Clorazepate 362
Apo-Cloxi® (Can) *see* Cloxacillin . . . 365
Apo-Cromolyn® (Can) *see* Cromolyn 378
Apo-Cyclobenzaprine® (Can) *see* Cyclobenzaprine 382
Apo-Cyclosporine® (Can) *see* CycloSPORINE 386
Apo-Desipramine® (Can) *see* Desipramine 407
Apo-Desmopressin® (Can) *see* Desmopressin 409
Apo-Diazepam® (Can) *see* Diazepam 423
Apo-Diclo® (Can) *see* Diclofenac . . . 427
Apo-Diclo Rapide® (Can) *see* Diclofenac 427
Apo-Diclo SR® (Can) *see* Diclofenac 427
Apo-Diflunisal® (Can) *see* Diflunisal 435
Apo-Diltiaz® (Can) *see* Diltiazem . . . 444
Apo-Diltiaz CD® (Can) *see* Diltiazem 444
Apo-Diltiaz SR® (Can) *see* Diltiazem 444
Apo-Dimenhydrinate® (Can) *see* DimenhyDRINATE 446
Apo-Dipivefrin® (Can) *see* Dipivefrin 453
Apo-Dipyridamole FC® (Can) *see* Dipyridamole 453
Apo-Divalproex® (Can) *see* Valproic Acid and Derivatives 1359
Apo-Docusate-Calcium® (Can) *see* Docusate 459
Apo-Docusate-Sodium® (Can) *see* Docusate 459
Apo-Doxazosin® (Can) *see* Doxazosin 465
Apo-Doxepin® (Can) *see* Doxepin . . 467
Apo-Doxy® (Can) *see* Doxycycline . . 471
Apo-Doxy Tabs® (Can) *see* Doxycycline 471
Apo-Erythro Base® (Can) *see* Erythromycin 508
Apo-Erythro E-C® (Can) *see* Erythromycin 508
Apo-Erythro-ES® (Can) *see* Erythromycin 508
Apo-Erythro-S® (Can) *see* Erythromycin 508
Apo-Etodolac® (Can) *see* Etodolac 564
Apo-Famotidine® (Can) *see* Famotidine 573

Apo-Fenofibrate® (Can) *see* Fenofibrate . . . 577
Apo-Feno-Micro® (Can) *see* Fenofibrate . . . 577
Apo-Ferrous Gluconate® (Can) *see* Ferrous Gluconate . . . 586
Apo-Ferrous Sulfate® (Can) *see* Ferrous Sulfate . . . 586
Apo-Flavoxate® (Can) *see* Flavoxate . . . 591
Apo-Fluconazole® (Can) *see* Fluconazole . . . 594
Apo-Flunisolide® (Can) *see* Flunisolide . . . 599
Apo-Fluoxetine® (Can) *see* Fluoxetine . . . 606
Apo-Fluphenazine® (Can) *see* Fluphenazine . . . 610
Apo-Fluphenazine Decanoate® (Can) *see* Fluphenazine . . . 610
Apo-Flurazepam® (Can) *see* Flurazepam . . . 612
Apo-Flurbiprofen® (Can) *see* Flurbiprofen . . . 613
Apo-Flutamide® (Can) *see* Flutamide . . . 615
Apo-Fluvoxamine® (Can) *see* Fluvoxamine . . . 623
Apo-Folic® (Can) *see* Folic Acid . . . 625
Apo-Furosemide® (Can) *see* Furosemide . . . 640
Apo-Gabapentin® (Can) *see* Gabapentin . . . 642
Apo-Gain® (Can) *see* Minoxidil . . . 934
Apo-Gemfibrozil® (Can) *see* Gemfibrozil . . . 651
Apo-Glyburide® (Can) *see* GlyBURIDE . . . 664
Apo-Haloperidol® (Can) *see* Haloperidol . . . 682
Apo-Haloperidol LA® (Can) *see* Haloperidol . . . 682
Apo-Hydralazine® (Can) *see* HydrALAZINE . . . 697
Apo-Hydro® (Can) *see* Hydrochlorothiazide . . . 699
Apo-Hydroxyquine® (Can) *see* Hydroxychloroquine . . . 720
Apo-Hydroxyzine® (Can) *see* HydrOXYzine . . . 723
Apo-Ibuprofen® (Can) *see* Ibuprofen . . . 728
Apo-Imipramine® (Can) *see* Imipramine . . . 737
Apo-Indapamide® (Can) *see* Indapamide . . . 743
Apo-Indomethacin® (Can) *see* Indomethacin . . . 746
Apo-Ipravent® (Can) *see* Ipratropium . . . 761
Apo-ISDN® (Can) *see* Isosorbide Dinitrate . . . 770
Apo-K® (Can) *see* Potassium Chloride . . . 1105
Apo-Keto® (Can) *see* Ketoprofen . . . 785
Apo-Ketoconazole® (Can) *see* Ketoconazole . . . 783
Apo-Keto-E® (Can) *see* Ketoprofen . . . 785
Apo-Ketorolac® (Can) *see* Ketorolac . . . 787
Apo-Ketorolac Injectable® (Can) *see* Ketorolac . . . 787
Apo-Keto SR® (Can) *see* Ketoprofen . . . 785
Apo-Ketotifen® (Can) *see* Ketotifen . . . 790
Apokyn™ *see* Apomorphine . . . 137
Apo-Labetalol® (Can) *see* Labetalol . . . 791
Apo-Lactulose® (Can) *see* Lactulose . . . 794
Apo-Lamotrigine® (Can) *see* Lamotrigine . . . 795
Apo-Levobunolol® (Can) *see* Levobunolol . . . 808
Apo-Levocarb® (Can) *see* Levodopa and Carbidopa . . . 811
Apo-Lisinopril® (Can) *see* Lisinopril . . . 833
Apo-Lithium® (Can) *see* Lithium . . . 835
Apo-Loperamide® (Can) *see* Loperamide . . . 838
Apo-Loratadine® (Can) *see* Loratadine . . . 841
Apo-Lorazepam® (Can) *see* Lorazepam . . . 842
Apo-Lovastatin® (Can) *see* Lovastatin . . . 848
Apo-Loxapine® (Can) *see* Loxapine . . . 850
Apo-Medroxy® (Can) *see* MedroxyPROGESTERone . . . 862
Apo-Mefenamic® (Can) *see* Mefenamic Acid . . . 863
Apo-Mefloquine® (Can) *see* Mefloquine . . . 864
Apo-Megestrol® (Can) *see* Megestrol . . . 865
Apo-Metformin® (Can) *see* Metformin . . . 887
Apo-Methazide® (Can) *see* Methyldopa and Hydrochlorothiazide . . . 906
Apo-Methazolamide® (Can) *see* Methazolamide . . . 891
Apo-Methoprazine® (Can) *see* Methotrimeprazine . . . 901
Apo-Methotrexate® (Can) *see* Methotrexate . . . 897
Apo-Methyldopa® (Can) *see* Methyldopa . . . 906
Apo-Metoclop® (Can) *see* Metoclopramide . . . 914
Apo-Metoprolol® (Can) *see* Metoprolol . . . 915
Apo-Metronidazole® (Can) *see* Metronidazole . . . 917
Apo-Midazolam® (Can) *see* Midazolam . . . 924
Apo-Minocycline® (Can) *see* Minocycline . . . 931
Apo-Misoprostol® (Can) *see* Misoprostol . . . 936
Apomorphine . . . 137
Apomorphine Hydrochloride *see* Apomorphine . . . 137
Apomorphine Hydrochloride Hemihydrate *see* Apomorphine . . . 137
Apo-Nabumetone® (Can) *see* Nabumetone . . . 955
Apo-Nadol® (Can) *see* Nadolol . . . 956
Apo-Napro-Na® (Can) *see* Naproxen . . . 965
Apo-Napro-Na DS® (Can) *see* Naproxen . . . 965
Apo-Naproxen® (Can) *see* Naproxen . . . 965
Apo-Naproxen SR® (Can) *see* Naproxen . . . 965
Apo-Nefazodone® (Can) *see* Nefazodone . . . 970
Apo-Nifed® (Can) *see* NIFEdipine . . . 984
Apo-Nifed PA® (Can) *see* NIFEdipine . . . 984
Apo-Nitrofurantoin® (Can) *see* Nitrofurantoin . . . 990
Apo-Nizatidine® (Can) *see* Nizatidine . . . 995

Apo-Norflox® (Can) *see* Norfloxacin . . . 997
Apo-Nortriptyline® (Can) *see* Nortriptyline . . . 999
Apo-Oflox® (Can) *see* Ofloxacin . . . 1005
Apo-Oxaprozin® (Can) *see* Oxaprozin . . . 1022
Apo-Oxazepam® (Can) *see* Oxazepam . . . 1022
Apo-Pentoxifylline SR® (Can) *see* Pentoxifylline . . . 1066
Apo-Pen VK® (Can) *see* Penicillin V Potassium . . . 1060
Apo-Perphenazine® (Can) *see* Perphenazine . . . 1070
Apo-Pindol® (Can) *see* Pindolol . . . 1090
Apo-Piroxicam® (Can) *see* Piroxicam . . . 1097
Apo-Pravastatin® (Can) *see* Pravastatin . . . 1109
Apo-Prazo® (Can) *see* Prazosin . . . 1111
Apo-Prednisone® (Can) *see* PredniSONE . . . 1115
Apo-Primidone® (Can) *see* Primidone . . . 1122
Apo-Procainamide® (Can) *see* Procainamide . . . 1124
Apo-Prochlorperazine® (Can) *see* Prochlorperazine . . . 1126
Apo-Propafenone® (Can) *see* Propafenone . . . 1133
Apo-Propranolol® (Can) *see* Propranolol . . . 1140
Apo-Quin-G® (Can) *see* Quinidine . . . 1160
Apo-Quinidine® (Can) *see* Quinidine . . . 1160
Apo-Ranitidine® (Can) *see* Ranitidine . . . 1169
Apo-Salvent® (Can) *see* Albuterol . . . 71
Apo-Selegiline® (Can) *see* Selegiline . . . 1212
Apo-Sertraline® (Can) *see* Sertraline . . . 1215
Apo-Simvastatin® (Can) *see* Simvastatin . . . 1222
Apo-Sotalol® (Can) *see* Sotalol . . . 1231
Apo-Sucralate® (Can) *see* Sucralfate . . . 1242
Apo-Sulfatrim® (Can) *see* Sulfamethoxazole and Trimethoprim . . . 1246
Apo-Sulfinpyrazone® (Can) *see* Sulfinpyrazone . . . 1249
Apo-Sulin® (Can) *see* Sulindac . . . 1251
Apo-Tamox® (Can) *see* Tamoxifen . . . 1258
Apo-Temazepam® (Can) *see* Temazepam . . . 1266
Apo-Terazosin® (Can) *see* Terazosin . . . 1271
Apo-Terbinafine® (Can) *see* Terbinafine . . . 1272
Apo-Tetra® (Can) *see* Tetracycline . . . 1280
Apo-Theo LA® (Can) *see* Theophylline . . . 1285
Apo-Thioridazine® (Can) *see* Thioridazine . . . 1289
Apo-Ticlopidine® (Can) *see* Ticlopidine . . . 1297
Apo-Timol® (Can) *see* Timolol . . . 1299
Apo-Timop® (Can) *see* Timolol . . . 1299
Apo-Tobramycin® (Can) *see* Tobramycin . . . 1306
Apo-Tolbutamide® (Can) *see* TOLBUTamide . . . 1309
Apo-Trazodone® (Can) *see* Trazodone . . . 1326
Apo-Trazodone D® (Can) *see* Trazodone . . . 1326
Apo-Triazide® (Can) *see* Hydrochlorothiazide and Triamterene . . . 701
Apo-Triazo® (Can) *see* Triazolam . . . 1335
Apo-Trifluoperazine® (Can) *see* Trifluoperazine . . . 1338
Apo-Trihex® (Can) *see* Trihexyphenidyl . . . 1340
Apo-Trimethoprim® (Can) *see* Trimethoprim . . . 1341
Apo-Trimip® (Can) *see* Trimipramine . . . 1343
Apo-Verap® (Can) *see* Verapamil . . . 1373
Apo-Warfarin® (Can) *see* Warfarin . . . 1389
Apo-Zidovudine® (Can) *see* Zidovudine . . . 1398
Apo-Zopiclone® (Can) *see* Zopiclone . . . 1406
APPG *see* Penicillin G Procaine . . . 1060
Apraclonidine . . . 138
Apraclonidine Hydrochloride *see* Apraclonidine . . . 138
Aprepitant . . . 138
Apresazide [DSC] *see* Hydralazine and Hydrochlorothiazide . . . 698
Apresoline [DSC] *see* HydrALAZINE . . . 697
Apri® *see* Ethinyl Estradiol and Desogestrel . . . 536
Aprodine® [OTC] *see* Triprolidine and Pseudoephedrine . . . 1345
Aprotinin . . . 139
Aprovel® (Mex) *see* Irbesartan . . . 763
Aquacare® [OTC] *see* Urea . . . 1353
Aquachloral® Supprettes® *see* Chloral Hydrate . . . 304
Aquacort® (Can) *see* Hydrocortisone . . . 714
Aqua Gem E® [OTC] *see* Vitamin E . . . 1383
AquaLase™ *see* Balanced Salt Solution . . . 181
Aqua Lube Plus [OTC] *see* Nonoxynol 9 . . . 995
AquaMEPHYTON® (Can) *see* Phytonadione . . . 1084
Aquanil HC® (Mex) *see* Hydrocortisone . . . 714
Aquaphilic® With Carbamide [OTC] *see* Urea . . . 1353
AquaSite® [OTC] *see* Artificial Tears . . . 148
Aquasol A® *see* Vitamin A . . . 1382
Aquasol E® [OTC] *see* Vitamin E . . . 1383
Aquatab® *see* Guaifenesin and Pseudoephedrine . . . 675
Aquatab® C *see* Guaifenesin, Pseudoephedrine, and Dextromethorphan . . . 676
Aquatab® D Dose Pack *see* Guaifenesin and Pseudoephedrine . . . 675
Aquatab® DM *see* Guaifenesin and Dextromethorphan . . . 673
Aquatensen® *see* Methyclothiazide . . . 905
Aquazide® H *see* Hydrochlorothiazide . . . 699
Aqueous Procaine Penicillin G *see* Penicillin G Procaine . . . 1060
Ara-A *see* Vidarabine . . . 1376
Arabinofuranosyladenine *see* Vidarabine . . . 1376
Arabinosylcytosine *see* Cytarabine . . . 390
Ara-C *see* Cytarabine . . . 390
Aralast™ *see* Alpha$_1$-Proteinase Inhibitor . . . 84
Aralen® (Can) *see* Chloroquine . . . 311
Aranesp® *see* Darbepoetin Alfa . . . 399
Arava® *see* Leflunomide . . . 801

Arctostaphylos uva-ursi see Uva Ursi 1448
Ardine® (Mex) *see* Amoxicillin 114
Aredia® *see* Pamidronate 1041
Arestin™ *see* Minocycline Hydrochloride (Periodontal) 933
Argatroban 140
Arginine 141
Arginine Hydrochloride *see* Arginine 141
8-Arginine Vasopressin *see* Vasopressin 1369
Aricept® (Can) *see* Donepezil 462
Arimidex® (Can) *see* Anastrozole . . . 132
Aripiprazole 142
Aristocort® (Can) *see* Triamcinolone 1330
Aristocort® A *see* Triamcinolone . . . 1330
Aristocort® Forte *see* Triamcinolone 1330
Aristospan® (Can) *see* Triamcinolone 1330
Arixtra® *see* Fondaparinux 628
Arlidin® (Can) *see* Nylidrin 1002
A.R.M® [OTC] *see* Chlorpheniramine and Pseudoephedrine 315
Armour® Thyroid *see* Thyroid 1293
Aromasin® (Can) *see* Exemestane . . 569
Aropax® (Mex) *see* Paroxetine 1046
Artane *see* Trihexyphenidyl 1340
ArthriCare® for Women Extra Moisturizing [OTC] *see* Capsaicin 252
ArthriCare® for Women Silky Dry [OTC] *see* Capsaicin 252
Arthropan® [OTC] [DSC] *see* Choline Salicylate 325
Arthrotec® *see* Diclofenac and Misoprostol 430
Articaine Hydrochloride and Epinephrine [Dental] *see* Articaine Hydrochloride and Epinephrine (Canada) 143
Articaine Hydrochloride and Epinephrine [Dental] *see* Articaine Hydrochloride and Epinephrine (U.S.) 145
Articaine Hydrochloride and Epinephrine (Canada) 143
Articaine Hydrochloride and Epinephrine (U.S.) 145
Artificial Tears 148
Artinor® (Mex) *see* Piroxicam 1097
Artrenac® (Mex) *see* Diclofenac 427
Artron® (Mex) *see* Naproxen 965
ASA *see* Aspirin 151
5-ASA *see* Mesalamine 882
ASA 500® (Mex) *see* Aspirin 151
Asacol® (Can) *see* Mesalamine 882
Asaphen (Can) *see* Aspirin 151
Asaphen E.C. (Can) *see* Aspirin . . . 151
Ascorbic Acid 148
Ascorbic Acid and Ferrous Sulfate *see* Ferrous Sulfate and Ascorbic Acid 587
Ascriptin® [OTC] *see* Aspirin 151
Ascriptin® Extra Strength [OTC] *see* Aspirin 151
Asendin [DSC] *see* Amoxapine 113
Asian Ginseng *see* Ginseng, Panax 1430
Asparaginase 150
Aspart, Insulin *see* Insulin Preparations 749
Aspercin [OTC] *see* Aspirin 151
Aspercin Extra [OTC] *see* Aspirin . . . 151
Aspergum® [OTC] *see* Aspirin 151
Aspirin 151
Aspirin, Acetaminophen, and Caffeine *see* Acetaminophen, Aspirin, and Caffeine 56
Aspirin and Carisoprodol *see* Carisoprodol and Aspirin 266
Aspirin and Codeine 155
Aspirin and Dipyridamole 156
Aspirin and Extended-Release Dipyridamole *see* Aspirin and Dipyridamole 156
Aspirin and Hydrocodone *see* Hydrocodone and Aspirin 705
Aspirin and Meprobamate 156
Aspirin and Oxycodone *see* Oxycodone and Aspirin 1032
Aspirin and Pravastatin 157
Aspirina Protect® (Mex) *see* Aspirin 151
Aspirin, Caffeine and Acetaminophen *see* Acetaminophen, Aspirin, and Caffeine 56
Aspirin, Caffeine, and Butalbital *see* Butalbital, Aspirin, and Caffeine 238
Aspirin, Caffeine, and Propoxyphene *see* Propoxyphene, Aspirin, and Caffeine 1138
Aspirin, Carisoprodol, and Codeine *see* Carisoprodol, Aspirin, and Codeine 267
Aspirin Free Anacin® Maximum Strength [OTC] *see* Acetaminophen 47
Aspirin, Orphenadrine, and Caffeine *see* Orphenadrine, Aspirin, and Caffeine 1018
Astelin® *see* Azelastine 173
AsthmaNefrin® *see* Epinephrine (Racemic) 497
Astracaine® (Can) *see* Articaine Hydrochloride and Epinephrine (Canada) 143
Astracaine® Forte (Can) *see* Articaine Hydrochloride and Epinephrine (Canada) 143
Astragalus 1414
Astragalus membranaceus see Astragalus 1414
Astramorph/PF™ *see* Morphine Sulfate 947
Atacand® (Mex) *see* Candesartan . . 248
Atacand HCT™ *see* Candesartan and Hydrochlorothiazide 249
Atacand® Plus (Can) *see* Candesartan and Hydrochlorothiazide 249
Atarax® *see* HydrOXYzine 723
Atasol® (Can) *see* Acetaminophen . . . 47
Atazanavir 158
Atazanavir Sulfate *see* Atazanavir . . 158
Atenolol 159
Atenolol and Chlorthalidone 161
ATG *see* Antithymocyte Globulin (Equine) 136
Atgam® (Can) *see* Antithymocyte Globulin (Equine) 136
Athos® (Mex) *see* Dextromethorphan 421
AT III *see* Antithrombin III 136
Atisuril® (Mex) *see* Allopurinol 82
Ativan® (Can) *see* Lorazepam 842
Atomoxetine 161
Atomoxetine Hydrochloride *see* Atomoxetine 161
Atorvastatin 162
Atorvastatin Calcium and Amlodipine Besylate *see* Amlodipine and Atorvastatin 110
Atovaquone 164

Atovaquone and Proguanil 165
ATRA *see* Tretinoin (Oral) 1328
Atridox™ *see* Doxycycline Hyclate (Periodontal) 475
AtroPen® *see* Atropine 166
Atropine 166
Atropine and Difenoxin *see* Difenoxin and Atropine 434
Atropine and Diphenoxylate *see* Diphenoxylate and Atropine 451
Atropine-Care® *see* Atropine 166
Atropine, Hyoscyamine, Scopolamine, and Phenobarbital *see* Hyoscyamine, Atropine, Scopolamine, and Phenobarbital 725
Atropine, Hyoscyamine, Scopolamine, Kaolin, and Pectin *see* Hyoscyamine, Atropine, Scopolamine, Kaolin, and Pectin 726
Atropine, Hyoscyamine, Scopolamine, Kaolin, Pectin, and Opium *see* Hyoscyamine, Atropine, Scopolamine, Kaolin, Pectin, and Opium 726
Atropine Sulfate *see* Atropine 166
Atropine Sulfate (Dental Tablets) . . . 169
Atrovent® (Can) *see* Ipratropium . . . 761
A/T/S® *see* Erythromycin 508
Attapulgite 170
Attenuvax® *see* Measles Virus Vaccine (Live) 858
Audifluor® (Mex) *see* Fluoride 603
Augmentin® *see* Amoxicillin and Clavulanate Potassium 116
Augmentin ES-600® *see* Amoxicillin and Clavulanate Potassium 116
Augmentin XR™ *see* Amoxicillin and Clavulanate Potassium 116
Auralgan® (Can) *see* Antipyrine and Benzocaine 135
Auranofin 170
Aurodex *see* Antipyrine and Benzocaine 135
Aurolate® *see* Gold Sodium Thiomalate 668
Auroto *see* Antipyrine and Benzocaine 135
Autoplex® T *see* Anti-inhibitor Coagulant Complex 135
AVA *see* Anthrax Vaccine (Adsorbed) 133
Avagard™ [OTC] *see* Chlorhexidine Gluconate 308
Avage™ *see* Tazarotene 1262
Avalide® *see* Irbesartan and Hydrochlorothiazide 764
Avandamet™ *see* Rosiglitazone and Metformin 1201
Avandia® (Can) *see* Rosiglitazone 1199
Avapro® (Can) *see* Irbesartan 763
Avapro® HCT *see* Irbesartan and Hydrochlorothiazide 764
Avastin™ *see* Bevacizumab 204
Avaxim® (Can) *see* Hepatitis A Vaccine 687
Avaxim®-Pediatric (Can) *see* Hepatitis A Vaccine 687
Avelox® *see* Moxifloxacin 949
Avelox® I.V. *see* Moxifloxacin 949
Aventyl® (Can) *see* Nortriptyline 999
Aventyl® HCl *see* Nortriptyline 999
Aviane™ *see* Ethinyl Estradiol and Levonorgestrel 545
Avinza™ *see* Morphine Sulfate 947
Avita® *see* Tretinoin (Topical) 1329
Avitene® *see* Microfibrillar Collagen Hemostat 923
Avodart™ *see* Dutasteride 479
Avonex® *see* Interferon Beta-1a 756
Awa *see* Kava 1439
Axert™ *see* Almotriptan 82
Axid® (Mex) *see* Nizatidine 995
Axid® AR [OTC] *see* Nizatidine 995
Axofor® (Mex) *see* Hydroxocobalamin 719
AY-25650 *see* Triptorelin 1346
Aygestin® *see* Norethindrone 996
Ayr® Baby Saline [OTC] *see* Sodium Chloride 1227
Ayr® Saline [OTC] *see* Sodium Chloride 1227
Ayr® Saline Mist [OTC] *see* Sodium Chloride 1227
Az® (Mex) *see* Azelastine 173
Azacitidine 171
AZA-CR *see* Azacitidine 171
Azactam® (Can) *see* Aztreonam 177
5-Azacytidine *see* Azacitidine 171
Azanplus® (Mex) *see* Ranitidine . . . 1169
Azantac® (Mex) *see* Ranitidine 1169
Azasan® *see* Azathioprine 172
Azathioprine 172
Azathioprine Sodium *see* Azathioprine 172
Azatrilem® (Mex) *see* Azathioprine . . 172
5-AZC *see* Azacitidine 171
Azelaic Acid 173
Azelastine 173
Azelastine Hydrochloride *see* Azelastine 173
Azelex® *see* Azelaic Acid 173
Azidothymidine *see* Zidovudine . . . 1398
Azidothymidine, Abacavir, and Lamivudine *see* Abacavir, Lamivudine, and Zidovudine 43
Azithromycin 174
Azithromycin Dihydrate *see* Azithromycin 174
Azitrocin® (Mex) *see* Azithromycin . . 174
Azmacort® (Can) *see* Triamcinolone 1330
Azo-Gesic® [OTC] *see* Phenazopyridine 1072
Azopt® (Can) *see* Brinzolamide 218
Azo-Standard® [OTC] *see* Phenazopyridine 1072
AZT™ (Can) *see* Zidovudine 1398
AZT + 3TC *see* Zidovudine and Lamivudine 1399
AZT, Abacavir, and Lamivudine *see* Abacavir, Lamivudine, and Zidovudine 43
Azthreonam *see* Aztreonam 177
Aztreonam 177
Azulfidine® *see* Sulfasalazine 1249
Azulfidine® EN-tabs® *see* Sulfasalazine 1249
B 9273 *see* Alefacept 76
BA-16038 *see* Aminoglutethimide 98
Babee® Cof Syrup [OTC] *see* Dextromethorphan 421
Babee® Teething® [OTC] *see* Benzocaine 191
Baby Gasz [OTC] *see* Simethicone 1222
BAC *see* Benzalkonium Chloride . . . 190
Bachelor's Button *see* Feverfew . . . 1426
Bacid® (Can) *see* *Lactobacillus* 793
Baciguent® [OTC] *see* Bacitracin . . . 178
BaciiM® *see* Bacitracin 178
Bacillus Calmette-Guérin (BCG) Live *see* BCG Vaccine 183
Bacitracin 178
Bacitracin and Polymyxin B 178
Bacitracin, Neomycin, and Polymyxin B 179

Bacitracin, Neomycin, Polymyxin B, and Hydrocortisone 179
Bacitracin, Neomycin, Polymyxin B, and Pramoxine 180
Baclofen 180
Bactocin® (Mex) *see* Ofloxacin . . . 1005
BactoShield® CHG [OTC] *see* Chlorhexidine Gluconate 308
Bactrim™ *see* Sulfamethoxazole and Trimethoprim 1246
Bactrim™ DS *see* Sulfamethoxazole and Trimethoprim 1246
Bactroban® (Can) *see* Mupirocin . . . 951
Bactroban® Nasal *see* Mupirocin . . . 951
Baking Soda *see* Sodium Bicarbonate 1226
BAL *see* Dimercaprol 447
Balanced Salt Solution 181
BAL in Oil® *see* Dimercaprol 447
Balmex® [OTC] *see* Zinc Oxide . . . 1400
Balminil (Can) *see* Xylometazoline 1393
Balminil Decongestant (Can) *see* Pseudoephedrine 1147
Balminil DM D (Can) *see* Pseudoephedrine and Dextromethorphan 1148
Balminil DM + Decongestant + Expectorant (Can) *see* Guaifenesin, Pseudoephedrine, and Dextromethorphan 676
Balminil DM E (Can) *see* Guaifenesin and Dextromethorphan 673
Balminil Expectorant (Can) *see* Guaifenesin 672
Balnetar® [OTC] *see* Coal Tar 367
Balsalazide 181
Balsalazide Disodium *see* Balsalazide 181
Balsam Peru, Trypsin, and Castor Oil *see* Trypsin, Balsam Peru, and Castor Oil 1349
Bancap HC® *see* Hydrocodone and Acetaminophen 702
Band-Aid® Hurt-Free™ Antiseptic Wash [OTC] *see* Lidocaine 819
Banophen® [OTC] *see* DiphenhydrAMINE 448
Basaljel® (Can) *see* Aluminum Hydroxide 90
Base Ointment *see* Zinc Oxide . . . 1400
Basiliximab 182
Bausch & Lomb® Computer Eye Drops [OTC] *see* Glycerin 667
Bausch & Lomb Earwax Removal [OTC] *see* Carbamide Peroxide 259
Bayer® Aspirin [OTC] *see* Aspirin . . . 151
Bayer® Aspirin Extra Strength [OTC] *see* Aspirin 151
Bayer® Aspirin Regimen Adult Low Strength [OTC] *see* Aspirin 151
Bayer® Aspirin Regimen Children's [OTC] *see* Aspirin 151
Bayer® Aspirin Regimen Regular Strength [OTC] *see* Aspirin 151
Bayer® Extra Strength Arthritis Pain Regimen [OTC] *see* Aspirin 151
Bayer® Plus Extra Strength [OTC] *see* Aspirin 151
Bayer® Women's Aspirin Plus Calcium [OTC] *see* Aspirin 151
BayGam® *see* Immune Globulin (Intramuscular) 739
BayHep B™ (Can) *see* Hepatitis B Immune Globulin 688
BayRab® *see* Rabies Immune Globulin (Human) 1165
BayRho-D® Full-Dose (Can) *see* $Rh_o(D)$ Immune Globulin 1176
BayRho-D® Mini-Dose *see* $Rh_o(D)$ Immune Globulin 1176
BayTet™ (Can) *see* Tetanus Immune Globulin (Human) 1277
Baza® Antifungal [OTC] *see* Miconazole 922
Baza® Clear [OTC] *see* Vitamin A and Vitamin D 1382
B-Caro-T™ *see* Beta-Carotene 198
BCG, Live *see* BCG Vaccine 183
BCG Vaccine 183
BCNU *see* Carmustine 268
B Complex Combinations *see* Vitamin B Complex Combinations 1382
B-D™ Glucose [OTC] *see* Glucose (Instant) 663
Bearberry *see* Uva Ursi 1448
Bebulin® VH *see* Factor IX Complex (Human) 572
Becaplermin 184
Beclomethasone 184
Beclomethasone Dipropionate *see* Beclomethasone 184
Beconase® [DSC] *see* Beclomethasone 184
Beconase® AQ *see* Beclomethasone 184
Behenyl Alcohol *see* Docosanol 459
Bekidiba Dex® (Mex) *see* Dextromethorphan 421
Belladonna and Opium 186
Belladonna, Phenobarbital, and Ergotamine 186
Belladonna, Phenobarbital, and Ergotamine Tartrate *see* Belladonna, Phenobarbital, and Ergotamine 186
Bellamine S *see* Belladonna, Phenobarbital, and Ergotamine 186
Bellergal® Spacetabs® (Can) *see* Belladonna, Phenobarbital, and Ergotamine 186
Bel-Tabs *see* Belladonna, Phenobarbital, and Ergotamine 186
Benadryl® (Can) *see* DiphenhydrAMINE 448
Benadryl® Allergy [OTC] *see* DiphenhydrAMINE 448
Benadryl® Allergy and Sinus Fastmelt™ [OTC] *see* Diphenhydramine and Pseudoephedrine 451
Benadryl® Allergy/Sinus [OTC] *see* Diphenhydramine and Pseudoephedrine 451
Benadryl® Children's Allergy and Cold Fastmelt™ [OTC] *see* Diphenhydramine and Pseudoephedrine 451
Benadryl® Children's Allergy and Sinus [OTC] *see* Diphenhydramine and Pseudoephedrine 451
Benadryl® Dye-Free Allergy [OTC] *see* DiphenhydrAMINE 448
Benadryl® Gel [OTC] *see* DiphenhydrAMINE 448
Benadryl® Gel Extra Strength [OTC] *see* DiphenhydrAMINE . . . 448
Benadryl® Injection *see* DiphenhydrAMINE 448
Benaxima® (Mex) *see* Cefotaxime . . 283
Benaxona® (Mex) *see* Ceftriaxone . . 288
Benazepril 187
Benazepril and Amlodipine *see* Amlodipine and Benazepril 110

Benazepril and Hydrochlorothiazide . . . 189
Benazepril Hydrochloride *see* Benazepril . . . 187
Bencelin® (Mex) *see* Penicillin G Benzathine . . . 1058
Bendapar® (Mex) *see* Albendazole . . . 71
Bendroflumethiazide . . . 189
Bendroflumethiazide and Nadolol *see* Nadolol and Bendroflumethiazide . . . 957
Benecid® (Mex) *see* Probenecid . . . 1124
BeneFix® (Can) *see* Factor IX . . . 571
Benemid [DSC] *see* Probenecid . . . 1124
Benerva® (Mex) *see* Thiamine . . . 1287
Benicar™ *see* Olmesartan . . . 1010
Benicar HCT™ *see* Olmesartan and Hydrochlorothiazide . . . 1010
Benoquin® *see* Monobenzone . . . 944
Benoxyl® (Mex) *see* Benzoyl Peroxide . . . 194
Bentoquatam . . . 189
Bentyl® *see* Dicyclomine . . . 432
Bentylol® (Can) *see* Dicyclomine . . . 432
Benuryl™ (Can) *see* Probenecid . . . 1124
Benylin® 3.3 mg-D-E (Can) *see* Guaifenesin, Pseudoephedrine, and Codeine . . . 676
Benylin® Adult [OTC] *see* Dextromethorphan . . . 421
Benylin® DM-D (Can) *see* Pseudoephedrine and Dextromethorphan . . . 1148
Benylin® DM-D-E (Can) *see* Guaifenesin, Pseudoephedrine, and Dextromethorphan . . . 676
Benylin® DM-E (Can) *see* Guaifenesin and Dextromethorphan . . . 673
Benylin® E Extra Strength (Can) *see* Guaifenesin . . . 672
Benylin® Expectorant [OTC] *see* Guaifenesin and Dextromethorphan . . . 673
Benylin® Pediatric [OTC] *see* Dextromethorphan . . . 421
Benza® [OTC] *see* Benzalkonium Chloride . . . 190
Benzac® (Mex) *see* Benzoyl Peroxide . . . 194
Benzac® AC *see* Benzoyl Peroxide . . . 194
Benzac® AC Wash *see* Benzoyl Peroxide . . . 194
BenzaClin® *see* Clindamycin and Benzoyl Peroxide . . . 350
Benzac® W *see* Benzoyl Peroxide . . 194
Benzac W® Gel (Can) *see* Benzoyl Peroxide . . . 194
Benzac® W Wash *see* Benzoyl Peroxide . . . 194
Benzaderm® (Mex) *see* Benzoyl Peroxide . . . 194
Benzagel® *see* Benzoyl Peroxide . . . 194
Benzagel® Wash *see* Benzoyl Peroxide . . . 194
Benzalkonium Chloride . . . 190
Benzalkonium Chloride and Isopropyl Alcohol . . . 190
Benzamycin® *see* Erythromycin and Benzoyl Peroxide . . . 512
Benzamycin® Pak *see* Erythromycin and Benzoyl Peroxide . . . 512
Benzanil® (Mex) *see* Penicillin G Benzathine . . . 1058
Benzashave® *see* Benzoyl Peroxide . . . 194
Benzathine Benzylpenicillin *see* Penicillin G Benzathine . . . 1058
Benzathine Penicillin G *see* Penicillin G Benzathine . . . 1058
Benzazoline Hydrochloride *see* Tolazoline . . . 1309
Benzedrex® [OTC] *see* Propylhexedrine . . . 1144
Benzene Hexachloride *see* Lindane . . . 829
Benzetacil® (Mex) *see* Penicillin G Benzathine . . . 1058
Benzhexol Hydrochloride *see* Trihexyphenidyl . . . 1340
Benzisoquinolinedione *see* Amonafide . . . 112
Benzmethyzin *see* Procarbazine . . 1125
Benzocaine . . . 191
Benzocaine and Antipyrine *see* Antipyrine and Benzocaine . . . 135
Benzocaine and Cetylpyridinium Chloride *see* Cetylpyridinium and Benzocaine . . . 301
Benzocaine, Butyl Aminobenzoate, Tetracaine, and Benzalkonium Chloride . . . 193
Benzodent® [OTC] *see* Benzocaine . . . 191
Benzoin . . . 193
Benzonatate . . . 193
Benzoyl Peroxide . . . 194
Benzoyl Peroxide and Clindamycin *see* Clindamycin and Benzoyl Peroxide . . . 350
Benzoyl Peroxide and Erythromycin *see* Erythromycin and Benzoyl Peroxide . . . 512
Benzoyl Peroxide and Hydrocortisone . . . 194
Benzphetamine . . . 195
Benzphetamine Hydrochloride *see* Benzphetamine . . . 195
Benztropine . . . 196
Benztropine Mesylate *see* Benztropine . . . 196
Benzylpenicillin Benzathine *see* Penicillin G Benzathine . . . 1058
Benzylpenicillin Potassium *see* Penicillin G (Parenteral/ Aqueous) . . . 1059
Benzylpenicillin Sodium *see* Penicillin G (Parenteral/ Aqueous) . . . 1059
Benzylpenicilloyl-polylysine . . . 196
Bepridil . . . 197
Bepridil Hydrochloride *see* Bepridil . . 197
Beractant . . . 198
Berotec® (Can) *see* Fenoterol . . . 580
Beta-2® (Can) *see* Isoetharine . . . 768
Betacaine® (Can) *see* Lidocaine . . . 819
Beta-Carotene . . . 198
Betaderm (Can) *see* Betamethasone . . . 199
Betadine® (Can) *see* Povidone-Iodine . . . 1107
Betadine® First Aid Antibiotics + Moisturizer [OTC] *see* Bacitracin and Polymyxin B . . . 178
Betadine® Ophthalmic *see* Povidone-Iodine . . . 1107
9-Beta-D-ribofuranosyladenine *see* Adenosine . . . 68
Betagan® (Mex) *see* Levobunolol . . . 808
Betaine Anhydrous . . . 199
Betaject™ (Can) *see* Betamethasone . . . 199
Betaloc® (Can) *see* Metoprolol . . . 915
Betaloc® Durules® (Can) *see* Metoprolol . . . 915
Betamethasone . . . 199
Betamethasone and Clotrimazole . . . 201
Betamethasone Dipropionate *see* Betamethasone . . . 199

Betamethasone Dipropionate, Augmented *see* Betamethasone . . . 199
Betamethasone Sodium Phosphate *see* Betamethasone . . . 199
Betamethasone Valerate *see* Betamethasone . . . 199
Betapace® *see* Sotalol . . . 1231
Betapace AF™ (Can) *see* Sotalol . . 1231
Betasept® [OTC] *see* Chlorhexidine Gluconate . . . 308
Betaseron® *see* Interferon Beta-1b . . 757
Betatar® [OTC] *see* Coal Tar . . . 367
Beta-Val® *see* Betamethasone . . . 199
Betaxin® (Can) *see* Thiamine . . . 1287
Betaxolol . . . 202
Betaxolol Hydrochloride *see* Betaxolol . . . 202
Betaxon® *see* Levobetaxolol . . . 808
Bethanechol . . . 203
Bethanechol Chloride *see* Bethanechol . . . 203
Betimol® *see* Timolol . . . 1299
Betnesol® (Can) *see* Betamethasone . . . 199
Betnovate® (Can) *see* Betamethasone . . . 199
Betoptic® S (Can) *see* Betaxolol . . . 202
Bevacizumab . . . 204
Bexarotene . . . 205
Bextra® *see* Valdecoxib . . . 1356
BG 9273 *see* Alefacept . . . 76
Biaxin® (Can) *see* Clarithromycin . . . 343
Biaxin® XL *see* Clarithromycin . . . 343
Bicalutamide . . . 206
Bicillin® C-R *see* Penicillin G Benzathine and Penicillin G Procaine . . . 1058
Bicillin® C-R 900/300 *see* Penicillin G Benzathine and Penicillin G Procaine . . . 1058
Bicillin® L-A *see* Penicillin G Benzathine . . . 1058
Bicitra® *see* Sodium Citrate and Citric Acid . . . 1228
Biclin® (Mex) *see* Amikacin . . . 95
Bicnu® (Mex) *see* Carmustine . . . 268
BIDA *see* Amonafide . . . 112
Bifidobacterium bifidum / Lactobacillus acidophilus . . . 1415
Bilberry . . . 1415
Biltricide® (Can) *see* Praziquantel . . . 1111
Bimatoprost . . . 207
Biocef® *see* Cephalexin . . . 294
Biofed [OTC] *see* Pseudoephedrine . . . 1147
Biolon® (Mex) *see* Hyaluronate and Derivatives . . . 696
Bion® Tears [OTC] *see* Artificial Tears . . . 148
BioQuin® Durules™ (Can) *see* Quinidine . . . 1160
Biosint® (Mex) *see* Cefotaxime . . . 283
Bio-Statin® *see* Nystatin . . . 1003
BioThrax™ *see* Anthrax Vaccine (Adsorbed) . . . 133
Biperiden . . . 207
Biperiden Hydrochloride *see* Biperiden . . . 207
Biperiden Lactate *see* Biperiden . . . 207
Bisac-Evac™ [OTC] *see* Bisacodyl . . 208
Bisacodyl . . . 208
Bisacodyl Uniserts® [OTC] *see* Bisacodyl . . . 208
bis-chloronitrosourea *see* Carmustine . . . 268
Bismatrol *see* Bismuth . . . 209
Bismuth . . . 209
Bismuth Subgallate *see* Bismuth . . . 209
Bismuth Subsalicylate *see* Bismuth . . . 209
Bismuth Subsalicylate, Metronidazole, and Tetracycline . . . 209
Bismuth Subsalicylate, Tetracycline, and Metronidazole *see* Bismuth Subsalicylate, Metronidazole, and Tetracycline . . . 209
Bisoprolol . . . 210
Bisoprolol and Hydrochlorothiazide . . . 211
Bisoprolol Fumarate *see* Bisoprolol . . . 210
Bistropamide *see* Tropicamide . . . 1348
Bivalirudin . . . 212
BL4162A *see* Anagrelide . . . 130
Black Cohosh . . . 1415
Black Susans *see Echinacea* . . . 1423
Bladuril® (Mex) *see* Flavoxate . . . 591
Blanoxan® (Mex) *see* Bleomycin . . . 213
Blastocarb® (Mex) *see* Carboplatin . . . 264
Blastolem® (Mex) *see* Cisplatin . . . 337
Blenoxane® *see* Bleomycin . . . 213
Bleo *see* Bleomycin . . . 213
Bleolem® (Mex) *see* Bleomycin . . . 213
Bleomycin . . . 213
Bleomycin Sulfate *see* Bleomycin . . 213
Bleph®-10 *see* Sulfacetamide . . . 1244
Blephamide® (Can) *see* Sulfacetamide and Prednisolone . . . 1245
Blis-To-Sol® [OTC] *see* Tolnaftate . . . 1312
BLM *see* Bleomycin . . . 213
Blocadren® *see* Timolol . . . 1299
Blokium® (Mex) *see* Atenolol . . . 159
BMS-232632 *see* Atazanavir . . . 158
BMS 337039 *see* Aripiprazole . . . 142
BN-52063 *see* Ginkgo Biloba . . . 1429
Bonamine™ (Can) *see* Meclizine . . . 859
Bonine® [OTC] *see* Meclizine . . . 859
Bontril® (Can) *see* Phendimetrazine . . . 1072
Bontril PDM® *see* Phendimetrazine . . . 1072
Bontril® Slow-Release *see* Phendimetrazine . . . 1072
Bortezomib . . . 214
Bosentan . . . 214
B&O Supprettes® *see* Belladonna and Opium . . . 186
Botox® (Can) *see* Botulinum Toxin Type A . . . 215
Botox® Cosmetic (Can) *see* Botulinum Toxin Type A . . . 215
Botulinum Toxin Type A . . . 215
Botulinum Toxin Type B . . . 217
Boudreaux's® Butt Paste [OTC] *see* Zinc Oxide . . . 1400
Bovine Lung Surfactant *see* Beractant . . . 198
Bravelle™ *see* Follitropins . . . 626
Braxan® (Mex) *see* Amiodarone . . . 101
Breathe Right® Saline [OTC] *see* Sodium Chloride . . . 1227
Brethaire [DSC] *see* Terbutaline . . . 1273
Brethine® *see* Terbutaline . . . 1273
Bretylium . . . 217
Bretylium Tosylate *see* Bretylium . . . 217
Brevibloc® *see* Esmolol . . . 515
Brevicon® *see* Ethinyl Estradiol and Norethindrone . . . 550
Brevicon® 0.5/35 (Can) *see* Ethinyl Estradiol and Norethindrone . . . 550
Brevicon® 1/35 (Can) *see* Ethinyl Estradiol and Norethindrone . . . 550
Brevital® (Can) *see* Methohexital . . . 895

Brevital® Sodium *see* Methohexital . . . 895
Brevoxyl® *see* Benzoyl Peroxide . . . 194
Brevoxyl® Cleansing *see* Benzoyl Peroxide . . . 194
Brevoxyl® Wash *see* Benzoyl Peroxide . . . 194
Brexicam® (Mex) *see* Piroxicam . . . 1097
Bricanyl [DSC] *see* Terbutaline . . . 1273
Brimonidine . . . 218
Brimonidine Tartrate *see* Brimonidine . . . 218
Brinzolamide . . . 218
Brioschi® [OTC] *see* Sodium Bicarbonate . . . 1226
Bris Taxol® (Mex) *see* Paclitaxel . . 1038
British Anti-Lewisite *see* Dimercaprol . . . 447
BRL 43694 *see* Granisetron . . . 671
Brofed® *see* Brompheniramine and Pseudoephedrine . . . 220
Bromaline® [OTC] *see* Brompheniramine and Pseudoephedrine . . . 220
Bromaxefed RF *see* Brompheniramine and Pseudoephedrine . . . 220
Bromazepam . . . 218
Bromelain . . . 1416
Bromfed® [OTC] [DSC] *see* Brompheniramine and Pseudoephedrine . . . 220
Bromfed-PD® [OTC] [DSC] *see* Brompheniramine and Pseudoephedrine . . . 220
Bromfenex® *see* Brompheniramine and Pseudoephedrine . . . 220
Bromfenex® PD *see* Brompheniramine and Pseudoephedrine . . . 220
Bromhist Pediatric *see* Brompheniramine and Pseudoephedrine . . . 220
Bromocriptine . . . 219
Bromocriptine Mesylate *see* Bromocriptine . . . 219
Bromodiphenhydramine and Codeine . . . 220
Brompheniramine and Pseudoephedrine . . . 220
Brompheniramine Maleate and Pseudoephedrine Hydrochloride *see* Brompheniramine and Pseudoephedrine . . . 220
Brompheniramine Maleate and Pseudoephedrine Sulfate *see* Brompheniramine and Pseudoephedrine . . . 220
Broncho Saline® [OTC] *see* Sodium Chloride . . . 1227
Bronkometer® (Can) *see* Isoetharine . . . 768
Bronkosol® (Can) *see* Isoetharine . . 768
Brontex® *see* Guaifenesin and Codeine . . . 673
BSS® (Can) *see* Balanced Salt Solution . . . 181
BSS® Plus (Can) *see* Balanced Salt Solution . . . 181
B-type Natriuretic Peptide (Human) *see* Nesiritide . . . 976
Budesonide . . . 221
Buffered Aspirin and Pravastatin Sodium *see* Aspirin and Pravastatin . . . 157
Bufferin® [OTC] *see* Aspirin . . . 151
Bufferin® Extra Strength [OTC] *see* Aspirin . . . 151
Buffinol [OTC] *see* Aspirin . . . 151
Buffinol Extra [OTC] *see* Aspirin . . . 151
Bufigen® (Mex) *see* Nalbuphine . . . 959
Bumedyl® (Mex) *see* Bumetanide . . . 224
Bumetanide . . . 224
Bumex® (Can) *see* Bumetanide . . . 224
Buphenyl® *see* Sodium Phenylbutyrate . . . 1230
Bupivacaine . . . 225
Bupivacaine and Epinephrine . . . 227
Bupivacaine and Lidocaine *see* Lidocaine and Bupivacaine . . . 822
Bupivacaine Hydrochloride *see* Bupivacaine . . . 225
Buprenex® (Can) *see* Buprenorphine . . . 228
Buprenorphine . . . 228
Buprenorphine and Naloxone . . . 230
Buprenorphine Hydrochloride *see* Buprenorphine . . . 228
Buprenorphine Hydrochloride and Naloxone Hydrochloride Dihydrate *see* Buprenorphine and Naloxone . . . 230
BuPROPion . . . 230
Burinex® (Can) *see* Bumetanide . . . 224
Burnamycin [OTC] *see* Lidocaine . . . 819
Burn Jel [OTC] *see* Lidocaine . . . 819
Burn-O-Jel [OTC] *see* Lidocaine . . . 819
Buscopan® (Can) *see* Scopolamine . . . 1210
BuSpar® *see* BusPIRone . . . 233
Buspirex (Can) *see* BusPIRone . . . 233
BusPIRone . . . 233
Buspirone Hydrochloride *see* BusPIRone . . . 233
Busulfan . . . 234
Busulfex® *see* Busulfan . . . 234
Butabarbital . . . 235
Butalbital, Acetaminophen, and Caffeine . . . 236
Butalbital, Acetaminophen, Caffeine, and Codeine . . . 236
Butalbital, Aspirin, and Caffeine . . . 238
Butalbital, Aspirin, Caffeine, and Codeine . . . 238
Butalbital Compound *see* Butalbital, Aspirin, and Caffeine . . . 238
Butalbital Compound and Codeine *see* Butalbital, Aspirin, Caffeine, and Codeine . . . 238
Butenafine . . . 239
Butenafine Hydrochloride *see* Butenafine . . . 239
Butisol Sodium® *see* Butabarbital . . . 235
Butoconazole . . . 239
Butoconazole Nitrate *see* Butoconazole . . . 239
Butorphanol . . . 240
Butorphanol Tartrate *see* Butorphanol . . . 240
Buvacaina® (Mex) *see* Bupivacaine . . . 225
B Vitamin Combinations *see* Vitamin B Complex Combinations . . . 1382
BW-430C *see* Lamotrigine . . . 795
BW524W91 *see* Emtricitabine . . . 487
C2B8 *see* Rituximab . . . 1191
C2B8 Monoclonal Antibody *see* Rituximab . . . 1191
C7E3 *see* Abciximab . . . 44
C8-CCK *see* Sincalide . . . 1224
311C90 *see* Zolmitriptan . . . 1403
C225 *see* Cetuximab . . . 300
C-500-GR™ [OTC] *see* Ascorbic Acid . . . 148
Cabergoline . . . 241
Caduet® *see* Amlodipine and Atorvastatin . . . 110
Caelyx® (Mex) *see* DOXOrubicin . . . 469

Caelyx® (Can) *see* DOXOrubicin (Liposomal) 470
Cafergor® (Can) *see* Ergotamine and Caffeine 506
Cafergot® *see* Ergotamine and Caffeine 506
Caffeine, Acetaminophen, and Aspirin *see* Acetaminophen, Aspirin, and Caffeine 56
Caffeine, Acetaminophen, Butalbital, and Codeine *see* Butalbital, Acetaminophen, Caffeine, and Codeine 236
Caffeine and Ergotamine *see* Ergotamine and Caffeine 506
Caffeine and Sodium Benzoate 242
Caffeine, Aspirin, and Acetaminophen *see* Acetaminophen, Aspirin, and Caffeine 56
Caffeine, Dihydrocodeine, and Acetaminophen *see* Acetaminophen, Caffeine, and Dihydrocodeine 57
Caffeine, Hydrocodone, Chlorpheniramine, Phenylephrine, and Acetaminophen *see* Hydrocodone, Chlorpheniramine, Phenylephrine, Acetaminophen, and Caffeine . . 712
Caffeine, Orphenadrine, and Aspirin *see* Orphenadrine, Aspirin, and Caffeine 1018
Caffeine, Propoxyphene, and Aspirin *see* Propoxyphene, Aspirin, and Caffeine 1138
Calan® *see* Verapamil 1373
Calan® SR *see* Verapamil 1373
Calcarb 600 [OTC] *see* Calcium Carbonate 245
Calcibind® (Can) *see* Cellulose Sodium Phosphate 294
Calci-Chew® [OTC] *see* Calcium Carbonate 245
Calcifediol 242
Calciferol™ *see* Ergocalciferol 503
Calcijex® *see* Calcitriol 244
Calcimar® (Can) *see* Calcitonin 243
Calci-Mix®[OTC] *see* Calcium Carbonate 245
Calcipotriene 243
Calcite-500 (Can) *see* Calcium Carbonate 245
Calcitonin 243
Calcitonin (Salmon) *see* Calcitonin . . 243
Cal-Citrate® 250 [OTC] *see* Calcium Citrate 246
Calcitriol 244
Calcium Acetate 245
Calcium Acetate and Aluminum Sulfate *see* Aluminum Sulfate and Calcium Acetate 92
Calcium Carbonate 245
Calcium Carbonate and Magnesium Hydroxide 245
Calcium Carbonate and Simethicone 245
Calcium Carbonate, Magnesium Hydroxide, and Famotidine *see* Famotidine, Calcium Carbonate, and Magnesium Hydroxide 574
Calcium Channel Blockers and Gingival Hyperplasia 1600
Calcium Channel Blockers, Comparative Pharmacokinetics 1602
Calcium Chloride 246
Calcium Citrate 246
Calcium Disodium Edetate *see* Edetate Calcium Disodium 482
Calcium Disodium Versenate® *see* Edetate Calcium Disodium 482
Calcium EDTA *see* Edetate Calcium Disodium 482
Calcium Glubionate 246
Calcium Gluconate 247
Calcium Lactate 247
Calcium Leucovorin *see* Leucovorin 804
Calcium Pantothenate *see* Pantothenic Acid 1044
Calcium Phosphate (Tribasic) 247
Calcium-Sandoz® (Mex) *see* Calcium Glubionate 246
CaldeCORT® [OTC] *see* Hydrocortisone 714
Calderol® (Can) *see* Calcifediol 242
Calendula 1416
Calendula officinalis *see* Calendula 1416
Calfactant 247
Cal-Gest [OTC] *see* Calcium Carbonate 245
Cal-Mint [OTC] *see* Calcium Carbonate 245
Calmylin with Codeine (Can) *see* Guaifenesin, Pseudoephedrine, and Codeine 676
Calsan® (Mex) *see* Calcium Carbonate 245
Caltine® (Can) *see* Calcitonin 243
Caltrate® (Can) *see* Calcium Carbonate 245
Caltrate® 600 [OTC] *see* Calcium Carbonate 245
Camellia sinensis *see* Green Tea 1436
Camila™ *see* Norethindrone 996
Campath® *see* Alemtuzumab 76
Campath-1H *see* Alemtuzumab 76
Campho-Phenique® [OTC] *see* Camphor and Phenol 248
Camphor and Phenol 248
Camphorated Tincture of Opium *see* Paregoric 1045
Camptosar® (Mex) *see* Irinotecan . . 764
Camptothecin-11 *see* Irinotecan 764
Canasa™ *see* Mesalamine 882
Cancidas® *see* Caspofungin 272
Candesartan 248
Candesartan and Hydrochlorothiazide 249
Candesartan Cilexetil *see* Candesartan 248
Candesartan Cilexetil and Hydrochlorothiazide *see* Candesartan and Hydrochlorothiazide 249
Candimon® (Mex) *see* Clotrimazole 363
Candistatin® (Can) *see* Nystatin . . . 1003
Canef® (Mex) *see* Fluvastatin 622
Canesten® Topical (Can) *see* Clotrimazole 363
Canesten® Vaginal (Can) *see* Clotrimazole 363
Cankaid® [OTC] *see* Carbamide Peroxide 259
Canthacur® (Can) *see* Cantharidin . . 250
Cantharidin 250
Cantharone® (Can) *see* Cantharidin 250
Cantil® (Can) *see* Mepenzolate 869
Capastat® Sulfate *see* Capreomycin 251
Cape *see* Aloe 1412
Capecitabine 250
Capex™ *see* Fluocinolone 601

Capital® and Codeine *see* Acetaminophen and Codeine 50
Capitrol® *see* Chloroxine 313
Capoten® (Mex) *see* Captopril 252
Capozide® *see* Captopril and Hydrochlorothiazide 255
Capreomycin 251
Capreomycin Sulfate *see* Capreomycin 251
Capsagel® [OTC] *see* Capsaicin . . . 252
Capsaicin 252
Capsicum annuum see Cayenne . . 1418
Capsicum frutescens see Cayenne 1418
Captopril 252
Captopril and Hydrochlorothiazide . . 255
Captral® (Mex) *see* Captopril 252
Capzasin-HP® [OTC] *see* Capsaicin 252
Capzasin-P® [OTC] *see* Capsaicin . . 252
Carac™ *see* Fluorouracil 605
Carafate® *see* Sucralfate 1242
Carapres® (Can) *see* Clonidine 358
Carbac® (Mex) *see* Loracarbef 841
Carbachol 255
Carbacholine *see* Carbachol 255
Carbamazepine 255
Carbamide *see* Urea 1353
Carbamide Peroxide 259
Carbamylcholine Chloride *see* Carbachol 255
Carbastat® [DSC] *see* Carbachol . . . 255
Carbatrol® *see* Carbamazepine 255
Carbaxefed DM RF *see* Carbinoxamine, Pseudoephedrine, and Dextromethorphan 263
Carbaxefed RF *see* Carbinoxamine and Pseudoephedrine 262
Carbazep® (Mex) *see* Carbamazepine 255
Carbazina® (Mex) *see* Carbamazepine 255
Carbenicillin 260
Carbenicillin Indanyl Sodium *see* Carbenicillin 260
Carbetapentane and Chlorpheniramine 260
Carbetapentane, Ephedrine, Phenylephrine, and Chlorpheniramine *see* Chlorpheniramine, Ephedrine, Phenylephrine, and Carbetapentane 316
Carbetapentane, Phenylephrine, and Pyrilamine 261
Carbetapentane Tannate and Chlorpheniramine Tannate *see* Carbetapentane and Chlorpheniramine 260
Carbidopa 261
Carbidopa and Levodopa *see* Levodopa and Carbidopa 811
Carbidopa, Levodopa, and Entacapone *see* Levodopa, Carbidopa, and Entacapone 812
Carbihist *see* Carbinoxamine 262
Carbinoxamine 262
Carbinoxamine and Pseudoephedrine 262
Carbinoxamine, Dextromethorphan, and Pseudoephedrine *see* Carbinoxamine, Pseudoephedrine, and Dextromethorphan 263
Carbinoxamine Maleate *see* Carbinoxamine 262
Carbinoxamine PD *see* Carbinoxamine 262
Carbinoxamine, Pseudoephedrine, and Dextromethorphan 263
Carbinoxamine, Pseudoephedrine, and Hydrocodone *see* Hydrocodone, Carbinoxamine, and Pseudoephedrine 712
Carbocaine® [DSC] *see* Mepivacaine 873
Carbocaine® 2% with Neo-Cobefrin® [DSC] *see* Mepivacaine and Levonordefrin *(WITHDRAWN FROM MARKET)* 875
Carbocaine® 3% *see* Mepivacaine (Dental Anesthetic) 877
Carbol-Fuchsin Solution 264
Carbolic Acid *see* Phenol 1075
Carbolit® (Mex) *see* Lithium 835
Carbolith™ (Can) *see* Lithium 835
Carboplatin 264
Carboprost *see* Carboprost Tromethamine 265
Carboprost Tromethamine 265
Carbose D *see* Carboxymethylcellulose 265
Carbotec® (Mex) *see* Carboplatin . . . 264
Carboxine *see* Carbinoxamine 262
Carboxine-PSE *see* Carbinoxamine and Pseudoephedrine 262
Carboxymethylcellulose 265
Carboxymethylcellulose Sodium *see* Carboxymethylcellulose 265
Cardene® *see* NiCARdipine 980
Cardene® I.V. *see* NiCARdipine 980
Cardene® SR *see* NiCARdipine 980
Cardinit® (Mex) *see* Nitroglycerin . . . 991
Cardiovascular Diseases 1458
Cardipril® (Mex) *see* Captopril 252
Cardispan® (Mex) *see* Levocarnitine 810
Cardizem® (Can) *see* Diltiazem 444
Cardizem® CD *see* Diltiazem 444
Cardizem® LA *see* Diltiazem 444
Cardizem® SR (Can) *see* Diltiazem 444
Cardura® *see* Doxazosin 465
Cardura-1™ (Can) *see* Doxazosin . . 465
Cardura-2™ (Can) *see* Doxazosin . . 465
Cardura-4™ (Can) *see* Doxazosin . . 465
Carexan® (Mex) *see* Itraconazole . . . 775
Carimune™ *see* Immune Globulin (Intravenous) 740
Carindacillin *see* Carbenicillin 260
Carisoprodate *see* Carisoprodol 266
Carisoprodol 266
Carisoprodol and Aspirin 266
Carisoprodol, Aspirin, and Codeine 267
Carmol® 10 [OTC] *see* Urea 1353
Carmol® 20 [OTC] *see* Urea 1353
Carmol® 40 *see* Urea 1353
Carmol® Deep Cleaning *see* Urea 1353
Carmol-HC® *see* Urea and Hydrocortisone 1353
Carmol® Scalp *see* Sulfacetamide 1244
Carmustine 268
Carmustinum *see* Carmustine 268
Carnitine 1417
Carnitor® *see* Levocarnitine 810
Carrington Antifungal [OTC] *see* Miconazole 922
Carteolol 269
Carteolol Hydrochloride *see* Carteolol 269
Carter's Little Pills® (Can) *see* Bisacodyl 208
Cartia XT™ *see* Diltiazem 444
Cartrol® *see* Carteolol 269
Cartrol® Oral (Can) *see* Carteolol . . . 269
Carvedilol 270

Casanthranol and Docusate *see* Docusate and Casanthranol 460
Cascara 1417
Cascara Sagrada *see* Cascara . . . 1417
Casodex® *see* Bicalutamide 206
Caspofungin 272
Caspofungin Acetate *see* Caspofungin 272
Castellani Paint Modified *see* Carbol-Fuchsin Solution 264
Castor Oil 273
Castor Oil, Trypsin, and Balsam Peru *see* Trypsin, Balsam Peru, and Castor Oil 1349
Cataflam® *see* Diclofenac 427
Cataflam Dispersible® (Mex) *see* Diclofenac 427
Catapres® *see* Clonidine 358
Catapres-TTS® *see* Clonidine 358
Cathflo™ Activase® *see* Alteplase . . . 88
Cat's Claw 1417
Caverject® (Can) *see* Alprostadil 87
Caverject® Impulse™ *see* Alprostadil 87
Cayenne 1418
CB-1348 *see* Chlorambucil 305
CBDCA *see* Carboplatin 264
CBZ *see* Carbamazepine 255
CCNU *see* Lomustine 838
2-CdA *see* Cladribine 342
CDDP *see* Cisplatin 337
CDX *see* Bicalutamide 206
Ceclor® (Can) *see* Cefaclor 274
Ceclor® CD *see* Cefaclor 274
Cecon® [OTC] *see* Ascorbic Acid . . . 148
Cedax® (Mex) *see* Ceftibuten 287
Cedocard®-SR (Can) *see* Isosorbide Dinitrate 770
CEE *see* Estrogens (Conjugated/ Equine) 525
CeeNU® *see* Lomustine 838
Cefaclor 274
Cefadroxil 275
Cefadroxil Monohydrate *see* Cefadroxil 275
Cefamandole 277
Cefamandole Nafate *see* Cefamandole 277
Cefamox® (Mex) *see* Cefadroxil 275
Cefaxona® [inj.] (Mex) *see* Ceftriaxone 288
Cefazolin 278
Cefazolin Sodium *see* Cefazolin 278
Cefdinir 279
Cefditoren 280
Cefditoren Pivoxil *see* Cefditoren . . . 280
Cefepime 281
Cefepime Hydrochloride *see* Cefepime 281
Cefixime 282
Cefizox® (Can) *see* Ceftizoxime 288
Cefotan® *see* Cefotetan 283
Cefotaxime 283
Cefotaxime Sodium *see* Cefotaxime 283
Cefotetan 283
Cefotetan Disodium *see* Cefotetan . . 283
Cefoxitin 284
Cefoxitin Sodium *see* Cefoxitin 284
Cefpodoxime 285
Cefpodoxime Proxetil *see* Cefpodoxime 285
Cefprozil 286
Cefradil® [inj.] (Mex) *see* Cefotaxime 283
Ceftazidime 286
Ceftibuten 287
Ceftin® (Can) *see* Cefuroxime 289
Ceftizoxime 288
Ceftizoxime Sodium *see* Ceftizoxime 288
Ceftrex® [inj.] (Mex) *see* Ceftriaxone 288
Ceftriaxone 288
Ceftriaxone Sodium *see* Ceftriaxone 288
Cefuracet® (Mex) *see* Cefuroxime . . 289
Cefuroxime 289
Cefuroxime Axetil *see* Cefuroxime . . 289
Cefuroxime Sodium *see* Cefuroxime 289
Cefzil® *see* Cefprozil 286
Celebrex® *see* Celecoxib 290
Celecoxib 290
Celestoderm®-EV/2 (Can) *see* Betamethasone 199
Celestoderm®-V (Can) *see* Betamethasone 199
Celestone® (Mex) *see* Betamethasone 199
Celestone® Soluspan® *see* Betamethasone 199
Celexa™ (Can) *see* Citalopram 339
CellCept® *see* Mycophenolate 952
Cellulose (Oxidized/Regenerated) . . 293
Cellulose Sodium Phosphate 294
Celluvisc™ (Can) *see* Carboxymethylcellulose 265
Celontin® (Can) *see* Methsuximide . . 904
Celulose Grin® (Mex) *see* Hydroxypropyl Methylcellulose . . 721
Cenestin® *see* Estrogens (Conjugated A/Synthetic) 524
Cenestin (Can) *see* Estrogens (Conjugated/Equine) 525
Centella asiatica *see* Gotu Kola . . . 1434
Centrum® [OTC] *see* Vitamins (Multiple/Oral) 1384
Centrum® Performance™ [OTC] *see* Vitamins (Multiple/Oral) . . . 1384
Centrum® Silver® [OTC] *see* Vitamins (Multiple/Oral) 1384
Cēpacol® (Can) *see* Cetylpyridinium and Benzocaine 301
Cēpacol® Gold [OTC] *see* Cetylpyridinium 301
Cēpacol® Maximum Strength [OTC] *see* Dyclonine 480
Cēpacol Viractin® [OTC] *see* Tetracaine 1278
Cēpastat® [OTC] *see* Phenol 1075
Cēpastat® Extra Strength [OTC] *see* Phenol 1075
Cephalexin 294
Cephalexin Monohydrate *see* Cephalexin 294
Cephalothin 296
Cephalothin Sodium *see* Cephalothin 296
Cephradine 296
Ceptaz® [DSC] *see* Ceftazidime 286
Cerebyx® (Can) *see* Fosphenytoin . . 635
Ceredase® *see* Alglucerase 80
Cerezyme® (Can) *see* Imiglucerase 736
Cerubidine® *see* DAUNOrubicin Hydrochloride 401
Cerumenex® *see* Triethanolamine Polypeptide Oleate-Condensate 1338
Cervidil® (Can) *see* Dinoprostone . . . 447
C.E.S. *see* Estrogens (Conjugated/ Equine) 525
Cesol® (Mex) *see* Praziquantel . . . 1111
Cetacaine® *see* Benzocaine, Butyl Aminobenzoate, Tetracaine, and Benzalkonium Chloride 193
Cetacort® *see* Hydrocortisone 714
Cetafen® [OTC] *see* Acetaminophen 47

Cetafen Cold® [OTC] *see* Acetaminophen and Pseudoephedrine . . . 53
Cetafen Extra® [OTC] *see* Acetaminophen . . . 47
Cetamide™ (Can) *see* Sulfacetamide . . . 1244
Ceta-Plus® *see* Hydrocodone and Acetaminophen . . . 702
Ceta Sulfa® (Mex) *see* Sulfacetamide . . . 1244
Cetirizine . . . 298
Cetirizine and Pseudoephedrine . . . 299
Cetirizine Hydrochloride *see* Cetirizine . . . 298
Cetirizine Hydrochloride and Pseudoephedrine Hydrochloride *see* Cetirizine and Pseudoephedrine . . . 299
Cetoxil® [tabs] (Mex) *see* Cefuroxime . . . 289
Cetoxil® [inj.] (Mex) *see* Cefuroxime . . . 289
Cetrorelix . . . 300
Cetrorelix Acetate *see* Cetrorelix . . . 300
Cetrotide® *see* Cetrorelix . . . 300
Cetuximab . . . 300
Cetylpyridinium . . . 301
Cetylpyridinium and Benzocaine . . . 301
Cetylpyridinium Chloride *see* Cetylpyridinium . . . 301
Cetylpyridinium Chloride and Benzocaine *see* Cetylpyridinium and Benzocaine . . . 301
Cevalin® (Mex) *see* Ascorbic Acid . . . 148
Cevi-Bid® [OTC] *see* Ascorbic Acid . . . 148
Cevimeline . . . 302
Cevimeline Hydrochloride *see* Cevimeline . . . 302
CFDN *see* Cefdinir . . . 279
CG *see* Chorionic Gonadotropin (Human) . . . 326
CGP-42446 *see* Zoledronic Acid . . 1402
CGP 57148B *see* Imatinib . . . 734
C-Gram [OTC] *see* Ascorbic Acid . . 148
Chamomile . . . 1419
Charcadole® (Can) *see* Charcoal . . . 303
Charcadole®, Aqueous (Can) *see* Charcoal . . . 303
Charcadole® TFS (Can) *see* Charcoal . . . 303
CharcoAid G® [OTC] *see* Charcoal . . . 303
Charcoal . . . 303
Charcoal Plus® DS [OTC] *see* Charcoal . . . 303
Charcocaps® [OTC] *see* Charcoal . . 303
Chasteberry . . . 1419
Chastetree *see* Chasteberry . . . 1419
Chemical Dependency and Smoking Cessation . . . 1576
Cheracol® *see* Guaifenesin and Codeine . . . 673
Cheracol® D [OTC] *see* Guaifenesin and Dextromethorphan . . . 673
Cheracol® Plus [OTC] *see* Guaifenesin and Dextromethorphan . . . 673
Cheratussin DAC *see* Guaifenesin, Pseudoephedrine, and Codeine . . . 676
CHG *see* Chlorhexidine Gluconate . . 308
Chiggerex® [OTC] *see* Benzocaine . . . 191
Chiggertox® [OTC] *see* Benzocaine . . . 191
Children's Dimetapp® Elixir Cold & Allergy [OTC] *see* Brompheniramine and Pseudoephedrine . . . 220
Children's Kaopectate® [DSC] [OTC] *see* Attapulgite . . . 170
Children's Kaopectate® *(reformulation)* [OTC] *see* Bismuth . . . 209
Children's Sudafed® Cough & Cold [OTC] *see* Pseudoephedrine and Dextromethorphan . . . 1148
Children's Tylenol® Plus Cold [OTC] *see* Acetaminophen, Chlorpheniramine, and Pseudoephedrine . . . 58
Chinese angelica *see* Dong Quai . . 1423
Chirocaine® *see* Levobupivacaine . . 809
Chloral *see* Chloral Hydrate . . . 304
Chloral Hydrate . . . 304
Chlorambucil . . . 305
Chlorambucilum *see* Chlorambucil . . 305
Chloraminophene *see* Chlorambucil . . . 305
Chloramphenicol . . . 306
ChloraPrep® [OTC] *see* Chlorhexidine Gluconate . . . 308
Chloraseptic® Gargle [OTC] *see* Phenol . . . 1075
Chloraseptic® Mouth Pain Spray [OTC] *see* Phenol . . . 1075
Chloraseptic® Rinse [OTC] *see* Phenol . . . 1075
Chloraseptic® Spray [OTC] *see* Phenol . . . 1075
Chloraseptic® Spray for Kids [OTC] *see* Phenol . . . 1075
Chlorbutinum *see* Chlorambucil . . . 305
Chlordiazepoxide . . . 307
Chlordiazepoxide and Amitriptyline *see* Amitriptyline and Chlordiazepoxide . . . 105
Chlordiazepoxide and Clidinium *see* Clidinium and Chlordiazepoxide . . . 347
Chlorhexidine Gluconate . . . 308
Chlormeprazine *see* Prochlorperazine . . . 1126
2-Chlorodeoxyadenosine *see* Cladribine . . . 342
Chloroethane *see* Ethyl Chloride . . . 561
Chloromag® *see* Magnesium Chloride . . . 852
Chloromycetin® (Mex) *see* Chloramphenicol . . . 306
Chloromycetin® Sodium Succinate *see* Chloramphenicol . . . 306
Chlorophyll . . . 310
Chlorophyllin *see* Chlorophyll . . . 310
Chloroprocaine . . . 310
Chloroprocaine Hydrochloride *see* Chloroprocaine . . . 310
Chloroquine . . . 311
Chloroquine Phosphate *see* Chloroquine . . . 311
Chlorostat® [OTC] *see* Chlorhexidine Gluconate . . . 308
Chlorothiazide . . . 312
Chloroxine . . . 313
Chlorphen [OTC] *see* Chlorpheniramine . . . 313
Chlorpheniramine . . . 313
Chlorpheniramine, Acetaminophen, and Pseudoephedrine *see* Acetaminophen, Chlorpheniramine, and Pseudoephedrine . . . 58
Chlorpheniramine and Acetaminophen . . . 314

Chlorpheniramine and Carbetapentane *see* Carbetapentane and Chlorpheniramine . . . 260
Chlorpheniramine and Hydrocodone *see* Hydrocodone and Chlorpheniramine . . . 707
Chlorpheniramine and Phenylephrine . . . 314
Chlorpheniramine and Pseudoephedrine . . . 315
Chlorpheniramine, Ephedrine, Phenylephrine, and Carbetapentane . . . 316
Chlorpheniramine, Hydrocodone, Phenylephrine, Acetaminophen, and Caffeine *see* Hydrocodone, Chlorpheniramine, Phenylephrine, Acetaminophen, and Caffeine . . 712
Chlorpheniramine Maleate *see* Chlorpheniramine . . . 313
Chlorpheniramine Maleate and Phenylephrine Hydrochloride *see* Chlorpheniramine and Phenylephrine . . . 314
Chlorpheniramine Maleate and Pseudoephedrine Hydrochloride *see* Chlorpheniramine and Pseudoephedrine . . . 315
Chlorpheniramine, Phenylephrine, and Dextromethorphan . . . 316
Chlorpheniramine, Phenylephrine, and Methscopolamine . . . 317
Chlorpheniramine, Phenylephrine, and Phenyltoloxamine . . . 317
Chlorpheniramine, Phenylephrine, Codeine, and Potassium Iodide . . . 318
Chlorpheniramine, Pseudoephedrine, and Acetaminophen *see* Acetaminophen, Chlorpheniramine, and Pseudoephedrine . . . 58
Chlorpheniramine, Pseudoephedrine, and Codeine . . . 319
Chlorpheniramine, Pseudoephedrine, and Dihydrocodeine *see* Pseudoephedrine, Dihydrocodeine, and Chlorpheniramine . . . 1150
Chlorpheniramine Tannate and Phenylephrine Tannate *see* Chlorpheniramine and Phenylephrine . . . 314
Chlorpheniramine Tannate and Pseudoephedrine Tannate *see* Chlorpheniramine and Pseudoephedrine . . . 315
ChlorproMAZINE . . . 319
Chlorpromazine Hydrochloride *see* ChlorproMAZINE . . . 319
ChlorproPAMIDE . . . 321
Chlorthalidone . . . 321
Chlorthalidone and Atenolol *see* Atenolol and Chlorthalidone . . . 161
Chlorthalidone and Clonidine *see* Clonidine and Chlorthalidone . . . 360
Chlor-Trimeton® [OTC] *see* Chlorpheniramine . . . 313
Chlor-Trimeton® Allergy D [OTC] *see* Chlorpheniramine and Pseudoephedrine . . . 315
Chlor-Tripolon® (Can) *see* Chlorpheniramine . . . 313
Chlor-Tripolon ND® (Can) *see* Loratadine and Pseudoephedrine . . . 842
Chlorzoxazone . . . 322
Cholac® *see* Lactulose . . . 794
Cholecalciferol . . . 323
Cholestyramine Resin . . . 323
Choline Magnesium Trisalicylate . . . 324
Choline Salicylate . . . 325
Chondroitin Sulfate . . . 1420
Chondroitin Sulfate and Sodium Hyaluronate . . . 325
Chooz® [OTC] *see* Calcium Carbonate . . . 245
Choriogonadotropin Alfa *see* Chorionic Gonadotropin (Recombinant) . . . 326
Chorionic Gonadotropin (Human) . . . 326
Chorionic Gonadotropin (Recombinant) . . . 326
Chromium . . . 1420
Chromium *see* Trace Metals . . . 1319
Chronovera® (Can) *see* Verapamil . . . 1373
Cialis® *see* Tadalafil . . . 1257
Cicloferon® (Mex) *see* Acyclovir . . . 64
Ciclopirox . . . 327
Ciclopirox Olamine *see* Ciclopirox . . 327
Cidecin *see* Daptomycin . . . 399
Cidofovir . . . 327
Cilazapril . . . 328
Cilazapril Monohydrate *see* Cilazapril . . . 328
Cilostazol . . . 329
Ciloxan® (Can) *see* Ciprofloxacin . . . 331
Cilpen® [inj.] (Mex) *see* Dicloxacillin . . . 431
Cimetase® (Mex) *see* Cimetidine . . . 330
Cimetidine . . . 330
Cimicifuga racemosa *see* Black Cohosh . . . 1415
Cimogal® (Mex) *see* Ciprofloxacin . . 331
Cinacalcet . . . 331
Cinacalcet Hydrochloride *see* Cinacalcet . . . 331
Cipro® (Can) *see* Ciprofloxacin . . . 331
Ciprobiotic® [tabs] (Mex) *see* Ciprofloxacin . . . 331
Ciprodex® *see* Ciprofloxacin and Dexamethasone . . . 336
Ciproflox® (Mex) *see* Ciprofloxacin . . 331
Ciprofloxacin . . . 331
Ciprofloxacin and Dexamethasone . . 336
Ciprofloxacin and Hydrocortisone . . . 336
Ciprofloxacin Hydrochloride *see* Ciprofloxacin . . . 331
Ciprofloxacin Hydrochloride and Dexamethasone *see* Ciprofloxacin and Dexamethasone . . . 336
Ciproflox® [inj.] (Mex) *see* Ciprofloxacin . . . 331
Ciprofur® [tabs] (Mex) *see* Ciprofloxacin . . . 331
Cipro® HC *see* Ciprofloxacin and Hydrocortisone . . . 336
Ciproxina® (Mex) *see* Ciprofloxacin . . . 331
Ciproxina® [inj.] (Mex) *see* Ciprofloxacin . . . 331
Cipro® XL (Can) *see* Ciprofloxacin . . 331
Cipro® XR *see* Ciprofloxacin . . . 331
Cisapride . . . 336
Cisplatin . . . 337
13-*cis*-Retinoic Acid *see* Isotretinoin . . . 773
Cisticid® (Mex) *see* Praziquantel . . 1111
Citalgan® (Mex) *see* Ibuprofen . . . 728
Citalopram . . . 339
Citalopram Hydrobromide *see* Citalopram . . . 339

Citanest® Forte (Can) *see* Prilocaine and Epinephrine . . . 1120
Citanest® Plain (Can) *see* Prilocaine . . . 1118
Citoken® [caps] (Mex) *see* Piroxicam . . . 1097
Citomid® [inj.] (Mex) *see* VinCRIStine . . . 1378
Citracal® [OTC] *see* Calcium Citrate . . . 246
Citrate of Magnesia *see* Magnesium Citrate . . . 853
Citric Acid and d-gluconic Acid Irrigant *see* Citric Acid, Magnesium Carbonate, and Glucono-Delta-Lactone . . . 341
Citric Acid and Potassium Citrate *see* Potassium Citrate and Citric Acid . . . 1106
Citric Acid Bladder Mixture *see* Citric Acid, Magnesium Carbonate, and Glucono-Delta-Lactone . . . 341
Citric Acid, Magnesium Carbonate, and Glucono-Delta-Lactone . . . 341
Citric Acid, Magnesium Hydroxycarbonate, D-Gluconic Acid, Magnesium Acid Citrate, and Calcium Carbonate *see* Citric Acid, Magnesium Carbonate, and Glucono-Delta-Lactone . . . 341
Citric Acid, Sodium Citrate, and Potassium Citrate . . . 341
Citro-Mag® (Can) *see* Magnesium Citrate . . . 853
Citrovorum Factor *see* Leucovorin . . 804
Citrucel® [OTC] *see* Methylcellulose . . . 905
Citrus paradisi see Grapefruit Seed . . . 1434
CL-118,532 *see* Triptorelin . . . 1346
Cl-719 *see* Gemfibrozil . . . 651
CL-825 *see* Pentostatin . . . 1065
CL-184116 *see* Porfimer . . . 1103
Cla *see* Clarithromycin . . . 343
Cladribine . . . 342
Claforan® *see* Cefotaxime . . . 283
Claravis™ *see* Isotretinoin . . . 773
Clarinex® *see* Desloratadine . . . 408
Claripel™ *see* Hydroquinone . . . 719
Claripex (Can) *see* Clofibrate . . . 353
Clarithromycin . . . 343
Clarithromycin, Lansoprazole, and Amoxicillin *see* Lansoprazole, Amoxicillin, and Clarithromycin . . 798
Claritin® [OTC] *see* Loratadine . . . 841
Claritin® Allergic Decongestant (Can) *see* Oxymetazoline . . . 1034
Claritin-D® 12-Hour [OTC] *see* Loratadine and Pseudoephedrine . . . 842
Claritin-D® 24-Hour [OTC] *see* Loratadine and Pseudoephedrine . . . 842
Claritin® Extra (Can) *see* Loratadine and Pseudoephedrine . . . 842
Claritin® Hives Relief [OTC] *see* Loratadine . . . 841
Claritin® Kids (Can) *see* Loratadine . . . 841
Claritin® Liberator (Can) *see* Loratadine and Pseudoephedrine . . . 842
Clarityne® (Mex) *see* Loratadine . . . 841
Clavulin® (Can) *see* Amoxicillin and Clavulanate Potassium . . . 116
Clear Eyes® [OTC] *see* Naphazoline . . . 964
Clear Eyes® ACR [OTC] *see* Naphazoline . . . 964
Clearplex [OTC] *see* Benzoyl Peroxide . . . 194
Clemastine . . . 346
Clemastine Fumarate *see* Clemastine . . . 346
Cleocin® *see* Clindamycin . . . 348
Cleocin HCl® *see* Clindamycin . . . 348
Cleocin Pediatric® *see* Clindamycin . . . 348
Cleocin Phosphate® *see* Clindamycin . . . 348
Cleocin T® *see* Clindamycin . . . 348
Clexane® (Mex) *see* Enoxaparin . . . 493
Clidinium and Chlordiazepoxide . . . 347
Climaderm® (Mex) *see* Estradiol . . . 518
Climara® *see* Estradiol . . . 518
Clinac™ BPO *see* Benzoyl Peroxide . . . 194
Clindagel® *see* Clindamycin . . . 348
ClindaMax™ *see* Clindamycin . . . 348
Clindamycin . . . 348
Clindamycin and Benzoyl Peroxide . . . 350
Clindamycin Hydrochloride *see* Clindamycin . . . 348
Clindamycin Palmitate *see* Clindamycin . . . 348
Clindamycin Phosphate *see* Clindamycin . . . 348
Clindamycin Phosphate and Benzoyl Peroxide *see* Clindamycin and Benzoyl Peroxide . . . 350
Clindazyn® [inj.] (Mex) *see* Clindamycin . . . 348
Clindets® *see* Clindamycin . . . 348
Clindoxyl® (Can) *see* Clindamycin . . 348
Clinoril® (Mex) *see* Sulindac . . . 1251
Clobazam . . . 350
Clobetasol . . . 351
Clobetasol Propionate *see* Clobetasol . . . 351
Clobex™ *see* Clobetasol . . . 351
Clocortolone . . . 352
Clocortolone Pivalate *see* Clocortolone . . . 352
Clocream® [OTC] *see* Vitamin A and Vitamin D . . . 1382
Cloderm® (Can) *see* Clocortolone . . 352
Clofazimine . . . 352
Clofazimine Palmitate *see* Clofazimine . . . 352
Clofibrate . . . 353
Clomid® *see* ClomiPHENE . . . 354
ClomiPHENE . . . 354
Clomiphene Citrate *see* ClomiPHENE . . . 354
ClomiPRAMINE . . . 355
Clomipramine Hydrochloride *see* ClomiPRAMINE . . . 355
Clonapam (Can) *see* Clonazepam . . 356
Clonazepam . . . 356
Clonidine . . . 358
Clonidine and Chlorthalidone . . . 360
Clonidine Hydrochloride *see* Clonidine . . . 358
Clopidogrel . . . 361
Clopidogrel Bisulfate *see* Clopidogrel . . . 361
Clopsine® (Mex) *see* Clozapine . . . 366
Clorafen® [caps] (Mex) *see* Chloramphenicol . . . 306
Cloramfeni® (Mex) *see* Chloramphenicol . . . 306
Cloran® (Mex) *see* Chloramphenicol . . . 306
Clorazepate . . . 362
Clorazepate Dipotassium *see* Clorazepate . . . 362

Clordil® [caps] (Mex) *see* Chloramphenicol . . . 306
Clorpactin® WCS-90 [OTC] *see* Oxychlorosene . . . 1027
Clorpres® *see* Clonidine and Chlorthalidone . . . 360
Clostedal® [tabs] (Mex) *see* Carbamazepine . . . 255
Clotrimaderm (Can) *see* Clotrimazole . . . 363
Clotrimazole . . . 363
Clotrimazole and Betamethasone *see* Betamethasone and Clotrimazole . . . 201
Cloxacillin . . . 365
Cloxacillin Sodium *see* Cloxacillin . . 365
Clozapine . . . 366
Clozaril® (Can) *see* Clozapine . . . 366
CoActifed® (Can) *see* Triprolidine, Pseudoephedrine, and Codeine . . . 1346
Coagulant Complex Inhibitor *see* Anti-inhibitor Coagulant Complex . . . 135
Coagulation Factor VIIa *see* Factor VIIa (Recombinant) . . . 571
Coal Tar . . . 367
Coal Tar and Salicylic Acid . . . 367
Cocaine . . . 368
Cocaine Hydrochloride *see* Cocaine . . . 368
CO Clomipramine (Can) *see* ClomiPRAMINE . . . 355
Codafed® Expectorant *see* Guaifenesin, Pseudoephedrine, and Codeine . . . 676
Codafed® Pediatric Expectorant *see* Guaifenesin, Pseudoephedrine, and Codeine . . . 676
Codeine . . . 369
Codeine, Acetaminophen, Butalbital, and Caffeine *see* Butalbital, Acetaminophen, Caffeine, and Codeine . . . 236
Codeine and Acetaminophen *see* Acetaminophen and Codeine . . . 50
Codeine and Aspirin *see* Aspirin and Codeine . . . 155
Codeine and Bromodiphenhydramine *see* Bromodiphenhydramine and Codeine . . . 220
Codeine and Butalbital Compound *see* Butalbital, Aspirin, Caffeine, and Codeine . . . 238
Codeine and Guaifenesin *see* Guaifenesin and Codeine . . . 673
Codeine and Promethazine *see* Promethazine and Codeine . . . 1131
Codeine, Aspirin, and Carisoprodol *see* Carisoprodol, Aspirin, and Codeine . . . 267
Codeine, Butalbital, Aspirin, and Caffeine *see* Butalbital, Aspirin, Caffeine, and Codeine . . . 238
Codeine, Chlorpheniramine, and Pseudoephedrine *see* Chlorpheniramine, Pseudoephedrine, and Codeine . . . 319
Codeine, Chlorpheniramine, Phenylephrine, and Potassium Iodide *see* Chlorpheniramine, Phenylephrine, Codeine, and Potassium Iodide . . . 318
Codeine Contin® (Can) *see* Codeine . . . 369
Codeine, Guaifenesin, and Pseudoephedrine *see* Guaifenesin, Pseudoephedrine, and Codeine . . . 676
Codeine Phosphate *see* Codeine . . . 369
Codeine, Promethazine, and Phenylephrine *see* Promethazine, Phenylephrine, and Codeine . . . 1132
Codeine, Pseudoephedrine, and Triprolidine *see* Triprolidine, Pseudoephedrine, and Codeine . . . 1346
Codeine Sulfate *see* Codeine . . . 369
Codiclear® DH *see* Hydrocodone and Guaifenesin . . . 708
Cod Liver Oil *see* Vitamin A and Vitamin D . . . 1382
Coenzyme 1 *see* Nicotinamide Adenine Dinucleotide . . . 1443
Coenzyme Q_{10} . . . 1420
CO Fluoxetine (Can) *see* Fluoxetine . . . 606
Cogentin® (Can) *see* Benztropine . . 196
Co-Gesic® *see* Hydrocodone and Acetaminophen . . . 702
Cognex® *see* Tacrine . . . 1254
Colace® [OTC] *see* Docusate . . . 459
Colax-C® (Can) *see* Docusate . . . 459
Colazal® *see* Balsalazide . . . 181
ColBenemid *see* Colchicine and Probenecid . . . 372
Colchicine . . . 372
Colchicine and Probenecid . . . 372
Colchiquim® (Mex) *see* Colchicine . . 372
Colesevelam . . . 373
Colestid® (Can) *see* Colestipol . . . 373
Colestipol . . . 373
Colestipol Hydrochloride *see* Colestipol . . . 373
Colgate Total® Toothpaste *see* Triclosan and Fluoride . . . 1337
Colistimethate . . . 374
Colistimethate Sodium *see* Colistimethate . . . 374
CollaCote® *see* Collagen (Absorbable) . . . 375
Collagen *see* Microfibrillar Collagen Hemostat . . . 923
Collagen (Absorbable) . . . 375
Collagenase . . . 375
CollaPlug® *see* Collagen (Absorbable) . . . 375
CollaTape® *see* Collagen (Absorbable) . . . 375
Colocort™ *see* Hydrocortisone . . . 714
Colufase® (Mex) *see* Nitazoxanide . . 989
Coly-Mycin® M (Can) *see* Colistimethate . . . 374
Colyte® *see* Polyethylene Glycol-Electrolyte Solution . . . 1100
Combantrin® (Mex) *see* Pyrantel Pamoate . . . 1151
Comb Flower *see Echinacea* . . . 1423
CombiPatch® *see* Estradiol and Norethindrone . . . 521
Combipres® [DSC] *see* Clonidine and Chlorthalidone . . . 360
Combivent® (Can) *see* Ipratropium and Albuterol . . . 761
Combivir® *see* Zidovudine and Lamivudine . . . 1399
Comhist® *see* Chlorpheniramine, Phenylephrine, and Phenyltoloxamine . . . 317
Commit™ [OTC] *see* Nicotine . . . 981
Compazine® [DSC] *see* Prochlorperazine . . . 1126
Comphor of the Poor *see* Garlic . . 1428
Compound E *see* Cortisone . . . 377
Compound F *see* Hydrocortisone . . . 714

Compound S *see* Zidovudine 1398
Compound S, Abacavir, and Lamivudine *see* Abacavir, Lamivudine, and Zidovudine 43
Compound W® [OTC] *see* Salicylic Acid 1205
Compound W® One Step Wart Remover [OTC] *see* Salicylic Acid 1205
Compoz® Nighttime Sleep Aid [OTC] *see* DiphenhydrAMINE . . 448
Compro™ *see* Prochlorperazine . . . 1126
Comtan® *see* Entacapone 494
Comtrex® Maximum Strength Sinus and Nasal Decongestant [OTC] *see* Acetaminophen, Chlorpheniramine, and Pseudoephedrine 58
Comtrex® Non-Drowsy Cold and Cough Relief [OTC] *see* Acetaminophen, Dextromethorphan, and Pseudoephedrine 59
Comtrex® Sore Throat Maximum Strength [OTC] *see* Acetaminophen 47
Conazol® (Mex) *see* Ketoconazole . . 783
Conceptrol® [OTC] *see* Nonoxynol 9 995
Concerta® *see* Methylphenidate 908
Condyline™ (Can) *see* Podofilox . . 1099
Condylox® *see* Podofilox 1099
Congest (Can) *see* Estrogens (Conjugated/Equine) 525
Congestac® *see* Guaifenesin and Pseudoephedrine 675
Conjugated Estrogen and Methyltestosterone *see* Estrogens (Esterified) and Methyltestosterone 530
Constilac® *see* Lactulose 794
Constulose® *see* Lactulose 794
Contac® Cold 12 Hour Relief Non Drowsy (Can) *see* Pseudoephedrine 1147
Contac® Cough, Cold and Flu Day & Night™ (Can) *see* Acetaminophen, Dextromethorphan, and Pseudoephedrine 59
Contac® Severe Cold and Flu/ Non-Drowsy [OTC] *see* Acetaminophen, Dextromethorphan, and Pseudoephedrine 59
Controlip® (Mex) *see* Fenofibrate . . . 577
Copal® (Mex) *see* Sulindac 1251
Copaxone® *see* Glatiramer Acetate 658
Copegus® *see* Ribavirin 1177
Copolymer-1 *see* Glatiramer Acetate 658
Copper *see* Trace Metals 1319
CoQ_{10} *see* Coenzyme Q_{10} 1420
Coraspir® (Mex) *see* Aspirin 151
Cordarone® (Can) *see* Amiodarone 101
Cordran® *see* Flurandrenolide 611
Cordran® SP *see* Flurandrenolide . . 611
Coreg® (Can) *see* Carvedilol 270
Corgard® *see* Nadolol 956
Coricidin HBP® Cold and Flu [OTC] *see* Chlorpheniramine and Acetaminophen 314
Corlopam® *see* Fenoldopam 579
Cormax® *see* Clobetasol 351
Coronex® (Can) *see* Isosorbide Dinitrate 770
Corotrend® (Mex) *see* NIFEdipine . . 984
Correctol® Tablets [OTC] *see* Bisacodyl 208
CortaGel® Maximum Strength [OTC] *see* Hydrocortisone 714
Cortaid® Intensive Therapy [OTC] *see* Hydrocortisone 714
Cortaid® Maximum Strength [OTC] *see* Hydrocortisone 714
Cortaid® Sensitive Skin With Aloe [OTC] *see* Hydrocortisone 714
Cortamed® (Can) *see* Hydrocortisone 714
Cortate® (Can) *see* Hydrocortisone 714
Cortef® (Can) *see* Hydrocortisone . . 714
Cortenema® (Can) *see* Hydrocortisone 714
Corticool® [OTC] *see* Hydrocortisone 714
Corticotropin 376
Corticotropin, Repository *see* Corticotropin 376
Cortifoam™ (Can) *see* Hydrocortisone 714
Cortimyxin® (Can) *see* Neomycin, Polymyxin B, and Hydrocortisone 975
Cortisol *see* Hydrocortisone 714
Cortisone 377
Cortisone Acetate *see* Cortisone . . . 377
Cortisporin® Cream *see* Neomycin, Polymyxin B, and Hydrocortisone 975
Cortisporin® Ointment *see* Bacitracin, Neomycin, Polymyxin B, and Hydrocortisone 179
Cortisporin® Ophthalmic *see* Neomycin, Polymyxin B, and Hydrocortisone 975
Cortisporin® Otic (Can) *see* Neomycin, Polymyxin B, and Hydrocortisone 975
Cortisporin® Topical Ointment (Can) *see* Bacitracin, Neomycin, Polymyxin B, and Hydrocortisone 179
Cortizone®-5 [OTC] *see* Hydrocortisone 714
Cortizone®-10 Maximum Strength [OTC] *see* Hydrocortisone 714
Cortizone®-10 Plus Maximum Strength [OTC] *see* Hydrocortisone 714
Cortizone® 10 Quick Shot [OTC] *see* Hydrocortisone 714
Cortizone® for Kids [OTC] *see* Hydrocortisone 714
Cortoderm (Can) *see* Hydrocortisone 714
Cortone® (Can) *see* Cortisone 377
Cortrosyn® *see* Cosyntropin 378
Corvert® *see* Ibutilide 731
Coryphen® Codeine (Can) *see* Aspirin and Codeine 155
Corzide® *see* Nadolol and Bendroflumethiazide 957
Cosmegen® *see* Dactinomycin 394
Cosopt® *see* Dorzolamide and Timolol 464
Cosyntropin 378
Cotazym® (Can) *see* Pancrelipase 1042
CO Temazepam (Can) *see* Temazepam 1266
Co-Trimoxazole *see* Sulfamethoxazole and Trimethoprim 1246
Coumadin® (Can) *see* Warfarin . . . 1389
Covan® (Can) *see* Triprolidine, Pseudoephedrine, and Codeine 1346
Covera® (Can) *see* Verapamil 1373

Covera-HS® *see* Verapamil 1373
Coversyl® (Mex) *see* Perindopril Erbumine 1068
Co-Vidarabine *see* Pentostatin 1065
Coviracil *see* Emtricitabine 487
Cozaar® (Mex) *see* Losartan 845
CP-99,219-27 *see* Trovafloxacin . . 1348
CPC *see* Cetylpyridinium 301
C-Phed Tannate *see* Chlorpheniramine and Pseudoephedrine 315
CPM *see* Cyclophosphamide 384
CPT-11 *see* Irinotecan 764
CPZ *see* ChlorproMAZINE 319
Cranberry 1421
Crataegus laevigata see Hawthorn 1437
Crataegus monogyna see Hawthorn 1437
Crataegus oxyacantha see Hawthorn 1437
Crataegus pinnatifida see Hawthorn 1437
Creatine 1421
Credaxol® (Mex) *see* Ranitidine . . . 1169
Crema Blanca® (Mex) *see* Hydroquinone 719
Cremosan® (Mex) *see* Ketoconazole 783
Creomulsion® Cough [OTC] *see* Dextromethorphan 421
Creomulsion® for Children [OTC] *see* Dextromethorphan 421
Creon® (Mex) *see* Pancreatin 1042
Creon® *see* Pancrelipase 1042
Creon® 5 (Can) *see* Pancrelipase 1042
Creon® 10 (Can) *see* Pancrelipase 1042
Creon® 20 (Can) *see* Pancrelipase 1042
Creon® 25 (Can) *see* Pancrelipase 1042
Creo-Terpin® [OTC] *see* Dextromethorphan 421
Crestor® (Can) *see* Rosuvastatin . . 1202
Cresylate® *see* m-Cresyl Acetate . . . 857
Crinone® (Mex) *see* Progesterone 1128
Critic-Aid Skin Care® [OTC] *see* Zinc Oxide 1400
Crixivan® (Can) *see* Indinavir 744
Crolom® *see* Cromolyn 378
Cromoglycic Acid *see* Cromolyn 378
Cromolyn 378
Cromolyn Sodium *see* Cromolyn . . . 378
Cronovera® (Mex) *see* Verapamil . . 1373
Crosseal™ *see* Fibrin Sealant Kit . . . 589
Crotamiton 380
Crude Coal Tar *see* Coal Tar 367
Cruex® Cream [OTC] *see* Clotrimazole 363
Cryoperacid® (Mex) *see* Loperamide 838
Cryopril® (Mex) *see* Captopril 252
Cryoval® [caps] (Mex) *see* Valproic Acid and Derivatives 1359
Cryselle™ *see* Ethinyl Estradiol and Norgestrel 557
Crystalline Penicillin *see* Penicillin G (Parenteral/Aqueous) 1059
Crystal Violet *see* Gentian Violet . . . 657
Crystodigin *see* Digitoxin 437
CsA *see* CycloSPORINE 386
CSP *see* Cellulose Sodium Phosphate 294
CTM *see* Chlorpheniramine 313
CTX *see* Cyclophosphamide 384
Cubicin™ *see* Daptomycin 399
Cuprimine® (Can) *see* Penicillamine 1057
Curcuma longa see Turmeric 1448
Curosurf® (Can) *see* Poractant Alfa 1102
Cutacelan® (Mex) *see* Azelaic Acid 173
Cutaclin® [gel] (Mex) *see* Clindamycin 348
Cutar® [OTC] *see* Coal Tar 367
Cutivate® (Mex) *see* Fluticasone . . . 616
CyA *see* CycloSPORINE 386
Cyanocobalamin 380
Cyanocobalamin, Folic Acid, and Pyridoxine *see* Folic Acid, Cyanocobalamin, and Pyridoxine 626
Cyclen® (Can) *see* Ethinyl Estradiol and Norgestimate 554
Cyclessa® *see* Ethinyl Estradiol and Desogestrel 536
Cyclizine 381
Cyclizine Hydrochloride *see* Cyclizine 381
Cyclizine Lactate *see* Cyclizine 381
Cyclobenzaprine 382
Cyclobenzaprine Hydrochloride *see* Cyclobenzaprine 382
Cyclocort® (Can) *see* Amcinonide . . . 93
Cyclogyl® (Can) *see* Cyclopentolate 383
Cyclomen® (Can) *see* Danazol 396
Cyclomydril® *see* Cyclopentolate and Phenylephrine 384
Cyclopentolate 383
Cyclopentolate and Phenylephrine . . 384
Cyclopentolate Hydrochloride *see* Cyclopentolate 383
Cyclophosphamide 384
CycloSERINE 385
Cyclosporin A *see* CycloSPORINE . . 386
CycloSPORINE 386
Cyklokapron® (Can) *see* Tranexamic Acid 1323
Cylate® *see* Cyclopentolate 383
Cylert® *see* Pemoline 1055
Cylex® [OTC] *see* Benzocaine 191
Cymevene® (Mex) *see* Ganciclovir . . 646
Cyproheptadine 389
Cyproheptadine Hydrochloride *see* Cyproheptadine 389
Cystadane™ (Can) *see* Betaine Anhydrous 199
Cystagon® *see* Cysteamine 389
Cysteamine 389
Cysteamine Bitartrate *see* Cysteamine 389
Cysteine 390
Cysteine Hydrochloride *see* Cysteine 390
Cystistat® (Can) *see* Hyaluronate and Derivatives 696
Cystospaz® (Can) *see* Hyoscyamine 724
Cystospaz-M® *see* Hyoscyamine . . . 724
CYT *see* Cyclophosphamide 384
Cytadren® *see* Aminoglutethimide . . . 98
Cytarabine 390
Cytarabine Hydrochloride *see* Cytarabine 390
Cytarabine (Liposomal) 391
Cytomel® (Can) *see* Liothyronine . . . 831
Cytosar® (Can) *see* Cytarabine 390
Cytosar-U® *see* Cytarabine 390
Cytosine Arabinosine Hydrochloride *see* Cytarabine . . 390
Cytotec® *see* Misoprostol 936
Cytovene® (Can) *see* Ganciclovir . . . 646
Cytoxan® *see* Cyclophosphamide . . 384
Cytra-2 *see* Sodium Citrate and Citric Acid 1228

Cytra-3 *see* Citric Acid, Sodium Citrate, and Potassium Citrate . . 341
Cytra-K *see* Potassium Citrate and Citric Acid 1106
D2E7 *see* Adalimumab 67
D_3 *see* Cholecalciferol 323
D-3-Mercaptovaline *see* Penicillamine 1057
d4T *see* Stavudine 1238
Dabex® [tabs] (Mex) *see* Metformin 887
Dacarbazine 392
Daclizumab 393
DACT *see* Dactinomycin 394
Dactinomycin 394
DAD *see* Mitoxantrone 938
Dafloxen® [syrup] (Mex) *see* Naproxen 965
Dafloxen® [caps, tabs] (Mex) *see* Naproxen 965
D.A.II™ [DSC] *see* Chlorpheniramine, Phenylephrine, and Methscopolamine 317
Dairyaid® (Can) *see* Lactase 793
Dakin's Solution *see* Sodium Hypochlorite Solution 1228
Daktarin® (Mex) *see* Miconazole . . . 922
Dalacin C® (Mex) *see* Clindamycin 348
Dalacin C® [inj.] (Mex) *see* Clindamycin 348
Dalacin® T (Can) *see* Clindamycin . . 348
Dalacin V® (Mex) *see* Clindamycin . . 348
Dalacin® Vaginal (Can) *see* Clindamycin 348
Dalisol® (Mex) *see* Leucovorin 804
Dallergy® *see* Chlorpheniramine, Phenylephrine, and Methscopolamine 317
Dallergy-JR® *see* Chlorpheniramine and Phenylephrine 314
Dalmane® (Can) *see* Flurazepam . . . 612
d-Alpha Tocopherol *see* Vitamin E 1383
Dalteparin 395
Damason-P® *see* Hydrocodone and Aspirin 705
Danaparoid 395
Danaparoid Sodium *see* Danaparoid 395
Danazol 396
Danocrine® (Can) *see* Danazol 396
Dantrium® *see* Dantrolene 397
Dantrolene 397
Dantrolene Sodium *see* Dantrolene 397
Daonil® (Mex) *see* GlyBURIDE 664
Dapcin *see* Daptomycin 399
Dapiprazole 398
Dapiprazole Hydrochloride *see* Dapiprazole 398
Dapsoderm-X® (Mex) *see* Dapsone 398
Dapsone 398
Daptomycin 399
Daranide® *see* Dichlorphenamide . . . 427
Daraprim® (Mex) *see* Pyrimethamine 1154
Darbepoetin Alfa 399
Darvocet A500™ *see* Propoxyphene and Acetaminophen 1137
Darvocet-N® 50 *see* Propoxyphene and Acetaminophen 1137
Darvocet-N® 100 *see* Propoxyphene and Acetaminophen 1137
Darvon® *see* Propoxyphene 1136
Darvon® Compound *see* Propoxyphene, Aspirin, and Caffeine 1138
Darvon-N® (Can) *see* Propoxyphene 1136
Datril® (Mex) *see* Acetaminophen . . . 47
Daunomycin *see* DAUNOrubicin Hydrochloride 401
DAUNOrubicin Citrate (Liposomal) . . 400
DAUNOrubicin Hydrochloride 401
DaunoXome® *see* DAUNOrubicin Citrate (Liposomal) 400
DAVA *see* Vindesine 1379
1-Day™ [OTC] *see* Tioconazole . . . 1302
Dayhist® Allergy [OTC] *see* Clemastine 346
Daypro® *see* Oxaprozin 1022
Days® [tabs] (Mex) *see* Ibuprofen . . 728
dCF *see* Pentostatin 1065
DDAVP® (Can) *see* Desmopressin . . 409
ddC *see* Zalcitabine 1395
ddI *see* Didanosine 433
Deacetyl Vinblastine Carboxamide *see* Vindesine 1379
1-Deamino-8-D-Arginine Vasopressin *see* Desmopressin 409
Debacterol® *see* Sulfonated Phenolics in Aqueous Solution 1250
Debrox® [OTC] *see* Carbamide Peroxide 259
Decadron® *see* Dexamethasone . . . 411
Decadron® Phosphate [DSC] *see* Dexamethasone 411
Deca-Durabolin® [DSC] *see* Nandrolone 963
Decahist-DM *see* Carbinoxamine, Pseudoephedrine, and Dextromethorphan 263
Decaris® (Mex) *see* Levamisole 806
Declomycin® (Can) *see* Demeclocycline 404
Decofed® [OTC] *see* Pseudoephedrine 1147
Deconamine® *see* Chlorpheniramine and Pseudoephedrine 315
Deconamine® SR *see* Chlorpheniramine and Pseudoephedrine 315
Decongest (Can) *see* Xylometazoline 1393
Deconsal® II *see* Guaifenesin and Pseudoephedrine 675
Defen-LA® *see* Guaifenesin and Pseudoephedrine 675
Deferoxamine 402
Deferoxamine Mesylate *see* Deferoxamine 402
Deflox® (Mex) *see* Diclofenac 427
Dehistine *see* Chlorpheniramine, Phenylephrine, and Methscopolamine 317
Dehydral® (Can) *see* Methenamine 892
Dehydrobenzperidol® (Mex) *see* Droperidol 477
Dehydroepiandrosterone 1421
Del Aqua® *see* Benzoyl Peroxide . . . 194
Delatestryl® (Can) *see* Testosterone 1276
Delavirdine 403
Delestrogen® (Can) *see* Estradiol . . . 518
Delfen® [OTC] *see* Nonoxynol 9 995
Delsym® [OTC] *see* Dextromethorphan 421
Delta-9-tetrahydro-cannabinol *see* Dronabinol 477
Delta-9 THC *see* Dronabinol 477
Deltacortisone *see* PredniSONE . . 1115

Delta-D® see Cholecalciferol 323
Deltadehydrocortisone see PredniSONE 1115
Deltahydrocortisone see PrednisoLONE 1113
Deltasone® see PredniSONE 1115
Demadex® see Torsemide 1317
Demeclocycline 404
Demeclocycline Hydrochloride see Demeclocycline 404
Demerol® see Meperidine 870
4-Demethoxydaunorubicin see Idarubicin 732
Demethylchlortetracycline see Demeclocycline 404
Demser® see Metyrosine 920
Demulen® see Ethinyl Estradiol and Ethynodiol Diacetate 540
Demulen® 30 (Can) see Ethinyl Estradiol and Ethynodiol Diacetate 540
Denavir® see Penciclovir 1056
Denileukin Diftitox 405
Dental Office Emergencies 1584
Dentifrice Products 1621
Dentin Hypersensitivity, High Caries Index, and Xerostomia 1555
DentiPatch® see Lidocaine (Transoral) 828
Dentist's Role in Recognizing Domestic Violence 1574
Dent's Ear Wax [OTC] see Carbamide Peroxide 259
Denvar® (Mex) see Cefixime 282
Deoxycoformycin see Pentostatin . . 1065
2′-Deoxycoformycin see Pentostatin 1065
Depacon® see Valproic Acid and Derivatives 1359
Depakene® (Mex) see Valproic Acid and Derivatives 1359
Depakote® Delayed Release see Valproic Acid and Derivatives 1359
Depakote® ER see Valproic Acid and Derivatives 1359
Depakote® Sprinkle® see Valproic Acid and Derivatives 1359
Depen® see Penicillamine 1057
DepoCyt™ see Cytarabine (Liposomal) 391
DepoDur™ see Morphine Sulfate . . . 947
Depo®-Estradiol (Can) see Estradiol 518
Depo-Medrol® (Can) see MethylPREDNISolone 910
Depo-Prevera® (Can) see MedroxyPROGESTERone 862
Depo-Provera® see MedroxyPROGESTERone 862
Depo-Provera® Contraceptive see MedroxyPROGESTERone 862
Depotest® 100 (Can) see Testosterone 1276
Depo®-Testosterone see Testosterone 1276
Deprenyl see Selegiline 1212
Derma Keri® (Mex) see Urea 1353
Dermalog® (Mex) see Halcinonide . . 681
Dermarest Dricort® [OTC] see Hydrocortisone 714
Dermasept Antifungal [OTC] see Tolnaftate 1312
Derma-Smoothe/FS® (Can) see Fluocinolone 601
Dermatop® (Can) see Prednicarbate 1113
Dermazene® see Iodoquinol and Hydrocortisone 759
Dermazin™ (Can) see Silver Sulfadiazine 1221
Dermazole (Can) see Miconazole . . 922
Dermifun® (Mex) see Miconazole . . . 922
Dermoplast® (Mex) see Urea 1353
Dermovate® (Can) see Clobetasol . . 351
Dermox® (Mex) see Methoxsalen . . . 902
Dermtex® HC [OTC] see Hydrocortisone 714
Desacetyl Vinblastine Amide Sulfate see Vindesine 1379
Deserpidine and Methyclothiazide see Methyclothiazide and Deserpidine 905
Desferal® (Can) see Deferoxamine 402
Desiccated Thyroid see Thyroid . . 1293
Desipramine 407
Desipramine Hydrochloride see Desipramine 407
Desitin® [OTC] see Zinc Oxide 1400
Desitin® Creamy [OTC] see Zinc Oxide 1400
Desloratadine 408
Desmethylimipramine Hydrochloride see Desipramine 407
Desmopressin 409
Desmopressin Acetate see Desmopressin 409
Desocort® (Can) see Desonide 410
Desogen® see Ethinyl Estradiol and Desogestrel 536
Desogestrel and Ethinyl Estradiol see Ethinyl Estradiol and Desogestrel 536
Desonide 410
Desowen® (Mex) see Desonide 410
Desoxi® (Can) see Desoximetasone 410
Desoximetasone 410
Desoxyephedrine Hydrochloride see Methamphetamine 891
Desoxyn® (Can) see Methamphetamine 891
Desoxyphenobarbital see Primidone 1122
Desparasil® (Mex) see Piperazine 1094
Desquam-E™ see Benzoyl Peroxide 194
Desquam-X® see Benzoyl Peroxide 194
Desyrel® (Can) see Trazodone 1326
Detane® [OTC] see Benzocaine 191
Detrol® see Tolterodine 1312
Detrol® LA see Tolterodine 1312
Detrusitol® (Mex) see Tolterodine . . 1312
Detussin® see Hydrocodone and Pseudoephedrine 711
Devil's Claw 1422
Dex4 Glucose [OTC] see Glucose (Instant) 663
Dexacidin® see Neomycin, Polymyxin B, and Dexamethasone 974
Dexacine™ see Neomycin, Polymyxin B, and Dexamethasone 974
Dexagrin® (Mex) see Dexamethasone 411
Dexalone® [OTC] see Dextromethorphan 421
Dexamethasone 411
Dexamethasone and Ciprofloxacin see Ciprofloxacin and Dexamethasone 336
Dexamethasone and Neomycin see Neomycin and Dexamethasone 973

Dexamethasone and Tobramycin *see* Tobramycin and Dexamethasone 1307
Dexamethasone Intensol® *see* Dexamethasone 411
Dexamethasone, Neomycin, and Polymyxin B *see* Neomycin, Polymyxin B, and Dexamethasone 974
Dexamethasone Sodium Phosphate *see* Dexamethasone 411
Dexasone® (Can) *see* Dexamethasone 411
Dexbrompheniramine and Pseudoephedrine 414
Dexchlorpheniramine 414
Dexchlorpheniramine Maleate *see* Dexchlorpheniramine 414
Dexchlorpheniramine Tannate and Pseudoephedrine Tannate *see* Chlorpheniramine and Pseudoephedrine 315
Dexedrine® (Can) *see* Dextroamphetamine 418
Dexferrum® *see* Iron Dextran Complex 766
Dexiron™ (Can) *see* Iron Dextran Complex 766
Dexmedetomidine 415
Dexmedetomidine Hydrochloride *see* Dexmedetomidine 415
Dexmethylphenidate 416
Dexmethylphenidate Hydrochloride *see* Dexmethylphenidate 416
DexPak® TaperPak® *see* Dexamethasone 411
Dexpanthenol 416
Dexrazoxane 417
Dextran 417
Dextran 1 418
Dextran 40 *see* Dextran 417
Dextran 70 *see* Dextran 417
Dextran, High Molecular Weight *see* Dextran 417
Dextran, Low Molecular Weight *see* Dextran 417
Dextroamphetamine 418
Dextroamphetamine and Amphetamine 419
Dextroamphetamine Sulfate *see* Dextroamphetamine 418
Dextromethorphan 421
Dextromethorphan, Acetaminophen, and Pseudoephedrine *see* Acetaminophen, Dextromethorphan, and Pseudoephedrine 59
Dextromethorphan and Guaifenesin *see* Guaifenesin and Dextromethorphan 673
Dextromethorphan and Promethazine *see* Promethazine and Dextromethorphan 1131
Dextromethorphan and Pseudoephedrine *see* Pseudoephedrine and Dextromethorphan 1148
Dextromethorphan, Carbinoxamine, and Pseudoephedrine *see* Carbinoxamine, Pseudoephedrine, and Dextromethorphan 263
Dextromethorphan, Chlorpheniramine, and Phenylephrine *see* Chlorpheniramine, Phenylephrine, and Dextromethorphan 316
Dextromethorphan, Guaifenesin, and Potassium Guaiacolsulfonate *see* Guaifenesin, Potassium Guaiacolsulfonate, and Dextromethorphan 675
Dextromethorphan, Guaifenesin, and Pseudoephedrine *see* Guaifenesin, Pseudoephedrine, and Dextromethorphan 676
Dextromethorphan, Pseudoephedrine, and Carbinoxamine *see* Carbinoxamine, Pseudoephedrine, and Dextromethorphan 263
Dextropropoxyphene *see* Propoxyphene 1136
Dextrose and Tetracaine *see* Tetracaine and Dextrose 1279
Dextrose, Levulose and Phosphoric Acid *see* Fructose, Dextrose, and Phosphoric Acid 638
Dextrostat® *see* Dextroamphetamine 418
DFMO *see* Eflornithine 485
DHA *see* Docosahexaenoic Acid . . 1422
DHAD *see* Mitoxantrone 938
DHAQ *see* Mitoxantrone 938
DHE *see* Dihydroergotamine 442
D.H.E. 45® *see* Dihydroergotamine 442
DHEA *see* Dehydroepiandrosterone 1421
DHPG Sodium *see* Ganciclovir 646
DHS™ Sal [OTC] *see* Salicylic Acid 1205
DHS™ Tar [OTC] *see* Coal Tar 367
DHS™ Targel [OTC] *see* Coal Tar . . 367
DHS™ Zinc [OTC] *see* Pyrithione Zinc 1155
DHT™ *see* Dihydrotachysterol 443
DHT™ Intensol™ *see* Dihydrotachysterol 443
Diabeta *see* GlyBURIDE 664
Diabetic Tussin® Allergy Relief [OTC] *see* Chlorpheniramine . . . 313
Diabetic Tussin C® *see* Guaifenesin and Codeine 673
Diabetic Tussin® DM [OTC] *see* Guaifenesin and Dextromethorphan 673
Diabetic Tussin® DM Maximum Strength [OTC] *see* Guaifenesin and Dextromethorphan 673
Diabetic Tussin® EX [OTC] *see* Guaifenesin 672
Diabinese® *see* ChlorproPAMIDE . . . 321
Diaminocyclohexane Oxalatoplatinum *see* Oxaliplatin 1020
Diaminodiphenylsulfone *see* Dapsone 398
Diamox® (Can) *see* AcetaZOLAMIDE 60
Diamox® Sequels® *see* AcetaZOLAMIDE 60
Diarr-Eze (Can) *see* Loperamide . . . 838
Diasorb® [OTC] *see* Attapulgite 170
Diastat® (Can) *see* Diazepam 423
Diatx™ *see* Vitamin B Complex Combinations 1382
DiatxFe™ *see* Vitamin B Complex Combinations 1382
Diaval® (Mex) *see* TOLBUTamide 1309
Diazemuls® (Can) *see* Diazepam . . . 423
Diazepam 423

Diazepam Intensol® see Diazepam . . . 423
Diazoxide . . . 425
Dibenzyline® see Phenoxybenzamine . . . 1075
Dibucaine . . . 426
Dibufen® (Mex) see Ibuprofen . . . 728
DIC see Dacarbazine . . . 392
Dichloralphenazone, Acetaminophen, and Isometheptene see Acetaminophen, Isometheptene, and Dichloralphenazone . . . 59
Dichloralphenazone, Isometheptene, and Acetaminophen see Acetaminophen, Isometheptene, and Dichloralphenazone . . . 59
6,7-Dichloro-1,5-Dihydroimidazo [2,1b] quinazolin-2(3H)-one Monohydrochloride see Anagrelide . . . 130
Dichlorodifluoromethane and Trichloromonofluoromethane . . . 427
Dichlorotetrafluoroethane and Ethyl Chloride see Ethyl Chloride and Dichlorotetrafluoroethane . . . 562
Dichlorphenamide . . . 427
Dichysterol see Dihydrotachysterol . . . 443
Diclofenac . . . 427
Diclofenac and Misoprostol . . . 430
Diclofenac Potassium see Diclofenac . . . 427
Diclofenac Sodium see Diclofenac . . . 427
Diclofenamide see Dichlorphenamide . . . 427
Dicloran® (Mex) see Diclofenac . . . 427
Diclotec (Can) see Diclofenac . . . 427
Diclotride® (Mex) see Hydrochlorothiazide . . . 699
Dicloxacillin . . . 431
Dicloxacillin Sodium see Dicloxacillin . . . 431
Dicyclomine . . . 432
Dicyclomine Hydrochloride see Dicyclomine . . . 432
Dicycloverine Hydrochloride see Dicyclomine . . . 432
Didanosine . . . 433
Dideoxycytidine see Zalcitabine . . . 1395
Dideoxyinosine see Didanosine . . . 433
Didrex® see Benzphetamine . . . 195
Didronel® (Can) see Etidronate Disodium . . . 563
Diethylpropion . . . 434
Diethylpropion Hydrochloride see Diethylpropion . . . 434
Difenoxin and Atropine . . . 434
Differin® (Can) see Adapalene . . . 67
Diflorasone . . . 435
Diflorasone Diacetate see Diflorasone . . . 435
Diflucan® (Can) see Fluconazole . . . 594
Diflunisal . . . 435
Difoxacil® (Mex) see Norfloxacin . . . 997
Digezanol® (Mex) see Albendazole . . . 71
Digibind® see Digoxin Immune Fab . . . 440
DigiFab™ see Digoxin Immune Fab . . . 440
Digitek® see Digoxin . . . 437
Digitoxin . . . 437
Digoxin . . . 437
Digoxin CSD (Can) see Digoxin . . . 437
Digoxin Immune Fab . . . 440
Dihematoporphyrin Ether see Porfimer . . . 1103
Dihistine® DH see Chlorpheniramine, Pseudoephedrine, and Codeine . . . 319
Dihistine® Expectorant see Guaifenesin, Pseudoephedrine, and Codeine . . . 676
Dihydrocodeine, Aspirin, and Caffeine . . . 441
Dihydrocodeine Bitartrate, Acetaminophen, and Caffeine see Acetaminophen, Caffeine, and Dihydrocodeine . . . 57
Dihydrocodeine Bitartrate, Pseudoephedrine Hydrochloride, and Chlorpheniramine Maleate see Pseudoephedrine, Dihydrocodeine, and Chlorpheniramine . . . 1150
Dihydrocodeine Compound see Dihydrocodeine, Aspirin, and Caffeine . . . 441
DiHydro-CP see Pseudoephedrine, Dihydrocodeine, and Chlorpheniramine . . . 1150
Dihydroergotamine . . . 442
Dihydroergotamine Mesylate see Dihydroergotamine . . . 442
Dihydroergotoxine see Ergoloid Mesylates . . . 504
Dihydrogenated Ergot Alkaloids see Ergoloid Mesylates . . . 504
Dihydrohydroxycodeinone see Oxycodone . . . 1027
Dihydromorphinone see Hydromorphone . . . 718
Dihydrotachysterol . . . 443
Dihydroxyanthracenedione Dihydrochloride see Mitoxantrone . . . 938
1,25 Dihydroxycholecalciferol see Calcitriol . . . 244
Dihydroxydeoxynorvinkaleukoblastine see Vinorelbine . . . 1380
Dihydroxypropyl Theophylline see Dyphylline . . . 480
Diiodohydroxyquin see Iodoquinol . . . 759
Dilacoran® (Mex) see Verapamil . . . 1373
Dilacor® XR see Diltiazem . . . 444
Dilantin® see Phenytoin . . . 1080
Dilatrate®-SR see Isosorbide Dinitrate . . . 770
Dilatrend® (Mex) see Carvedilol . . . 270
Dilaudid® see Hydromorphone . . . 718
Dilaudid-HP® see Hydromorphone . . . 718
Dilaudid-HP-Plus® (Can) see Hydromorphone . . . 718
Dilaudid® Sterile Powder (Can) see Hydromorphone . . . 718
Dilaudid-XP® (Can) see Hydromorphone . . . 718
Dilor® (Can) see Dyphylline . . . 480
Diltia XT® see Diltiazem . . . 444
Diltiazem . . . 444
Diltiazem Hydrochloride see Diltiazem . . . 444
Dimefor® (Mex) see Metformin . . . 887
DimenhyDRINATE . . . 446
Dimercaprol . . . 447
Dimetapp® 12-Hour Non-Drowsy Extentabs® [OTC] see Pseudoephedrine . . . 1147
Dimetapp® Children's ND [OTC] see Loratadine . . . 841
Dimetapp® Cold and Congestion [OTC] see Guaifenesin, Pseudoephedrine, and Dextromethorphan . . . 676
Dimetapp® Decongestant [OTC] see Pseudoephedrine . . . 1147

β,β-Dimethylcysteine *see* Penicillamine 1057
Dimethyl Sulfone *see* Methyl Sulfonyl Methane 1442
Dimethyl Triazeno Imidazol Carboxamide *see* Dacarbazine 392
Dinoprostone 447
Diocaine® (Can) *see* Proparacaine 1134
Diocarpine (Can) *see* Pilocarpine . . 1085
Diochloram® (Can) *see* Chloramphenicol 306
Diocto® [OTC] *see* Docusate 459
Diocto C® [DSC] [OTC] *see* Docusate and Casanthranol 460
Dioctyl Calcium Sulfosuccinate *see* Docusate 459
Dioctyl Sodium Sulfosuccinate *see* Docusate 459
Diodex® (Can) *see* Dexamethasone 411
Diodoquin® (Can) *see* Iodoquinol . . . 759
Diogent® (Can) *see* Gentamicin 655
Diomycin® (Can) *see* Erythromycin 508
Dionephrine® (Can) *see* Phenylephrine 1078
Diopentolate® (Can) *see* Cyclopentolate 383
Diopred® (Can) *see* PrednisoLONE 1113
Dioptic's Atropine Solution (Can) *see* Atropine 166
Dioptimyd® (Can) *see* Sulfacetamide and Prednisolone 1245
Dioptrol® (Can) *see* Neomycin, Polymyxin B, and Dexamethasone 974
Dioscorea villosa *see* Wild Yam . . . 1450
Diosulf™ (Can) *see* Sulfacetamide 1244
Diotame® [OTC] *see* Bismuth 209
Diotrope® (Can) *see* Tropicamide . . 1348
Diovan® (Can) *see* Valsartan 1363
Diovan HCT® (Can) *see* Valsartan and Hydrochlorothiazide 1364
Diovol® (Can) *see* Aluminum Hydroxide and Magnesium Hydroxide 91
Diovol® Ex (Can) *see* Aluminum Hydroxide and Magnesium Hydroxide 91
Diovol Plus® (Can) *see* Aluminum Hydroxide, Magnesium Hydroxide, and Simethicone 92
Dipentum® (Can) *see* Olsalazine . . 1011
Diphen® [OTC] *see* DiphenhydrAMINE 448
Diphen® AF [OTC] *see* DiphenhydrAMINE 448
Diphen® Cough [OTC] *see* DiphenhydrAMINE 448
Diphenhist [OTC] *see* DiphenhydrAMINE 448
DiphenhydrAMINE 448
Diphenhydramine and Acetaminophen *see* Acetaminophen and Diphenhydramine 53
Diphenhydramine and Pseudoephedrine 451
Diphenhydramine Hydrochloride *see* DiphenhydrAMINE 448
Diphenhydramine, Hydrocodone, and Phenylephrine *see* Hydrocodone, Phenylephrine, and Diphenhydramine 713
Diphenoxylate and Atropine 451
Diphenylhydantoin *see* Phenytoin . . 1080
Diphtheria and Tetanus Toxoids and Acellular Pertussis Adsorbed, Hepatitis B (Recombinant) and Inactivated Poliovirus Vaccine Combined *see* Diphtheria, Tetanus Toxoids, Acellular Pertussis, Hepatitis B (Recombinant), and Poliovirus (Inactivated) Vaccine 452
Diphtheria CRM_{197} Protein *see* Pneumococcal Conjugate Vaccine (7-Valent) 1098
Diphtheria CRM_{197} Protein Conjugate *see* *Haemophilus* b Conjugate Vaccine 680
Diphtheria, Tetanus Toxoids, Acellular Pertussis, Hepatitis B (Recombinant), and Poliovirus (Inactivated) Vaccine 452
Diphtheria, Tetanus Toxoids, and Acellular Pertussis Vaccine *see* Immunizations (Vaccines) 1614
Diphtheria, Tetanus Toxoids, and Acellular Pertussis Vaccine and *Haemophilus influenzae* b Conjugate Vaccine (Combined) *see* Immunizations (Vaccines) 1614
Diphtheria Toxoid Conjugate *see* *Haemophilus* b Conjugate Vaccine 680
Dipivalyl Epinephrine *see* Dipivefrin 453
Dipivefrin 453
Dipivefrin Hydrochloride *see* Dipivefrin 453
Diprivan® (Can) *see* Propofol 1135
Diprodol® (Mex) *see* Ibuprofen 728
Diprolene® *see* Betamethasone 199
Diprolene® AF *see* Betamethasone 199
Diprolene® Glycol (Can) *see* Betamethasone 199
Dipropylacetic Acid *see* Valproic Acid and Derivatives 1359
Diprosone® (Can) *see* Betamethasone 199
Dipyridamole 453
Dipyridamole and Aspirin *see* Aspirin and Dipyridamole 156
Dirithromycin 454
Disalcid® [DSC] *see* Salsalate 1207
Disalicylic Acid *see* Salsalate 1207
Disodium Cromoglycate *see* Cromolyn 378
Disodium Thiosulfate Pentahydrate *see* Sodium Thiosulfate 1230
d-Isoephedrine Hydrochloride *see* Pseudoephedrine 1147
Disopyramide 455
Disopyramide Phosphate *see* Disopyramide 455
DisperMox™ *see* Amoxicillin 114
Disulfiram 456
Dithioglycerol *see* Dimercaprol 447
Dithranol *see* Anthralin 133
Ditropan® (Can) *see* Oxybutynin . . 1026
Ditropan® XL (Can) *see* Oxybutynin 1026
Ditterolina® (Mex) *see* Dicloxacillin . . 431
Diuril® (Can) *see* Chlorothiazide 312
Divalproex Sodium *see* Valproic Acid and Derivatives 1359
Dixarit® (Can) *see* Clonidine 358
Dixonal® (Mex) *see* Piroxicam 1097
5071-1DL(6) *see* Megestrol 865
dl-Alpha Tocopherol *see* Vitamin E 1383
4-DMDR *see* Idarubicin 732

$DMSO_2$ *see* Methyl Sulfonyl Methane 1442
DNA-derived Humanized Monoclonal Antibody *see* Alemtuzumab 76
DNase *see* Dornase Alfa 463
DNR *see* DAUNOrubicin Hydrochloride 401
Doak® Tar [OTC] *see* Coal Tar 367
Doan's® [OTC] *see* Magnesium Salicylate 854
Doan's® Extra Strength [OTC] *see* Magnesium Salicylate 854
Dobuject® (Mex) *see* DOBUTamine 457
DOBUTamine 457
Dobutamine Hydrochloride *see* DOBUTamine 457
Dobutrex® (Mex) *see* DOBUTamine 457
Docetaxel 458
Docosahexaenoic Acid 1422
Docosanol 459
Docusate 459
Docusate and Casanthranol 460
Docusate Calcium *see* Docusate 459
Docusate Potassium *see* Docusate 459
Docusate Sodium *see* Docusate 459
Docusoft Plus™ [DSC] [OTC] *see* Docusate and Casanthranol 460
Docusoft-S™ [OTC] *see* Docusate 459
Dofetilide 460
Dolac® (Mex) *see* Ketorolac 787
Dolaren® (Mex) *see* Diclofenac 427
Dolasetron 461
Dolasetron Mesylate *see* Dolasetron 461
Dolflam® (Mex) *see* Diclofenac 427
Dolobid® *see* Diflunisal 435
Dolophine® (Can) *see* Methadone 889
Dolotor® (Mex) *see* Ketorolac 787
Dolzycam® (Mex) *see* Piroxicam 1097
Domeboro® [OTC] *see* Aluminum Sulfate and Calcium Acetate 92
Dome Paste Bandage *see* Zinc Gelatin 1400
Donepezil 462
Dong Quai 1423
Donnapectolin-PG® *see* Hyoscyamine, Atropine, Scopolamine, Kaolin, Pectin, and Opium 726
Donnatal® (Can) *see* Hyoscyamine, Atropine, Scopolamine, and Phenobarbital 725
Donnatal Extentabs® *see* Hyoscyamine, Atropine, Scopolamine, and Phenobarbital 725
Dopamine *see* Cardiovascular Diseases 1458
Dopram® *see* Doxapram 465
Doral® *see* Quazepam 1155
Dormicum® (Mex) *see* Midazolam 924
Dornase Alfa 463
Doryx® *see* Doxycycline 471
Dorzolamide 464
Dorzolamide and Timolol 464
Dorzolamide Hydrochloride *see* Dorzolamide 464
DOS® [OTC] *see* Docusate 459
DOSS *see* Docusate 459
Dostinex® (Can) *see* Cabergoline 241
Dovonex® *see* Calcipotriene 243
Doxapram 465
Doxapram Hydrochloride *see* Doxapram 465
Doxazosin 465
Doxazosin Mesylate *see* Doxazosin 465
Doxepin 467
Doxepin Hydrochloride *see* Doxepin 467
Doxercalciferol 468
Doxidan® [DSC] [OTC] *see* Docusate and Casanthranol 460
Doxidan® *(reformulation)* [OTC] *see* Bisacodyl 208
Doxil® *see* DOXOrubicin (Liposomal) 470
Doxolem® (Mex) *see* DOXOrubicin 469
DOXOrubicin 469
Doxorubicin Hydrochloride *see* DOXOrubicin 469
Doxorubicin Hydrochloride (Liposomal) *see* DOXOrubicin (Liposomal) 470
DOXOrubicin (Liposomal) 470
Doxotec® (Mex) *see* DOXOrubicin 469
Doxy-100® *see* Doxycycline 471
Doxycin (Can) *see* Doxycycline 471
Doxycycline 471
Doxycycline Calcium *see* Doxycycline 471
Doxycycline Hyclate *see* Doxycycline 471
Doxycycline Hyclate (Periodontal) 475
Doxycycline Monohydrate *see* Doxycycline 471
Doxycycline (Subantimicrobial) 476
Doxytec (Can) *see* Doxycycline 471
DPA *see* Valproic Acid and Derivatives 1359
DPE *see* Dipivefrin 453
D-Penicillamine *see* Penicillamine 1057
DPH *see* Phenytoin 1080
DPM™ [OTC] *see* Urea 1353
Drafilyn® (Mex) *see* Aminophylline 99
Dramamine® (Mex) *see* DimenhyDRINATE 446
Dramamine® Less Drowsy Formula [OTC] *see* Meclizine 859
Drenural® (Mex) *see* Bumetanide 224
Drisdol® (Can) *see* Ergocalciferol 503
Dristan® Long Lasting Nasal (Can) *see* Oxymetazoline 1034
Dristan® N.D. (Can) *see* Acetaminophen and Pseudoephedrine 53
Dristan® N.D., Extra Strength (Can) *see* Acetaminophen and Pseudoephedrine 53
Dristan® Sinus (Can) *see* Pseudoephedrine and Ibuprofen 1149
Drithocreme® *see* Anthralin 133
Dritho-Scalp® *see* Anthralin 133
Drixoral® (Can) *see* Dexbrompheniramine and Pseudoephedrine 414
Drixoral® Cold & Allergy [OTC] *see* Dexbrompheniramine and Pseudoephedrine 414
Drixoral® Nasal (Can) *see* Oxymetazoline 1034
Drixoral® ND (Can) *see* Pseudoephedrine 1147
Drize®-R *see* Chlorpheniramine, Phenylephrine, and Methscopolamine 317
Dronabinol 477
Droperidol 477
Drospirenone and Ethinyl Estradiol *see* Ethinyl Estradiol and Drospirenone 538
Drotrecogin Alfa 478
Drotrecogin Alfa, Activated *see* Drotrecogin Alfa 478
Droxia™ *see* Hydroxyurea 722

Dr. Scholl's® Callus Remover [OTC] *see* Salicylic Acid 1205
Dr. Scholl's® Clear Away [OTC] *see* Salicylic Acid 1205
DSCG *see* Cromolyn 378
D-Ser(Bu^t)^6,Azgly^{10}-LHRH *see* Goserelin 670
D-S-S® [OTC] *see* Docusate 459
DSS With Casanthranol *see* Docusate and Casanthranol 460
DTIC *see* Dacarbazine 392
DTIC-Dome® *see* Dacarbazine 392
DTO *see* Opium Tincture 1015
D-Trp(6)-LHRH *see* Triptorelin 1346
Duac™ *see* Clindamycin and Benzoyl Peroxide 350
Dulcolan® (Mex) *see* Bisacodyl 208
Dulcolax® [OTC] *see* Bisacodyl 208
Dulcolax® Milk of Magnesia [OTC] *see* Magnesium Hydroxide 853
Dull-C® [OTC] *see* Ascorbic Acid . . . 148
Duocaine™ *see* Lidocaine and Bupivacaine 822
Duofilm® (Can) *see* Salicylic Acid . . 1205
Duoforte® 27 (Can) *see* Salicylic Acid 1205
DuoNeb™ *see* Ipratropium and Albuterol 761
DuoPlant® [DSC] [OTC] *see* Salicylic Acid 1205
DuP 753 *see* Losartan 845
Durabolin® (Can) *see* Nandrolone . . 963
Duracef® (Mex) *see* Cefadroxil 275
Duraclon™ *see* Clonidine 358
Duradoce® (Mex) *see* Hydroxocobalamin 719
Duragesic® (Can) *see* Fentanyl 581
Duralith® (Can) *see* Lithium 835
Duralmor L.P.® (Mex) *see* Morphine Sulfate 947
Duramist® Plus [OTC] *see* Oxymetazoline 1034
Duramorph® *see* Morphine Sulfate . . 947
Duranest® [DSC] *see* Etidocaine and Epinephrine 562
Durater® (Mex) *see* Famotidine 573
Duration® [OTC] *see* Oxymetazoline 1034
Duratuss™ *see* Guaifenesin and Pseudoephedrine 675
Duratuss® DM *see* Guaifenesin and Dextromethorphan 673
Duratuss™ GP *see* Guaifenesin and Pseudoephedrine 675
Duratuss® HD *see* Hydrocodone, Pseudoephedrine, and Guaifenesin 713
Dura-Vent®/DA [DSC] *see* Chlorpheniramine, Phenylephrine, and Methscopolamine 317
Duricef™ (Can) *see* Cefadroxil 275
Durogesic® (Mex) *see* Fentanyl 581
Dutasteride 479
Duvoid® (Can) *see* Bethanechol 203
DVA *see* Vindesine 1379
D-Vi-Sol® (Can) *see* Cholecalciferol 323
DW286 *see* Gemifloxacin 653
Dyazide® *see* Hydrochlorothiazide and Triamterene 701
Dycill® (Can) *see* Dicloxacillin 431
Dyclonine 480
Dyclonine Hydrochloride *see* Dyclonine 480
Dymelor [DSC] *see* AcetoHEXAMIDE 60
Dynabac® *see* Dirithromycin 454
Dynacin® *see* Minocycline 931
DynaCirc® (Mex) *see* Isradipine 774
DynaCirc® CR *see* Isradipine 774
Dyna-Hex® [OTC] *see* Chlorhexidine Gluconate 308
Dyphylline 480
Dyrenium® *see* Triamterene 1334
E_2C and MPA *see* Estradiol and Medroxyprogesterone 520
7E3 *see* Abciximab 44
E2020 *see* Donepezil 462
EarSol® HC *see* Hydrocortisone 714
Easprin® *see* Aspirin 151
Ecaten® (Mex) *see* Captopril 252
Echinacea 1423
Echinacea angustifolia see Echinacea 1423
Echinacea purpurea see Echinacea 1423
Echothiophate Iodide 481
EC-Naprosyn® *see* Naproxen 965
E. coli Asparaginase *see* Asparaginase 150
Econazole 481
Econazole Nitrate *see* Econazole . . . 481
Econopred® *see* PrednisoLONE . . . 1113
Econopred® Plus *see* PrednisoLONE 1113
Ecostatin® (Can) *see* Econazole . . . 481
Ecostigmine Iodide *see* Echothiophate Iodide 481
Ecotrin® (Mex) *see* Aspirin 151
Ecotrin® Low Strength [OTC] *see* Aspirin 151
Ecotrin® Maximum Strength [OTC] *see* Aspirin 151
Ectosone (Can) *see* Betamethasone 199
Ed A-Hist® *see* Chlorpheniramine and Phenylephrine 314
Edathamil Disodium *see* Edetate Disodium 482
Edecrin® (Can) *see* Ethacrynic Acid 533
Edenol® (Mex) *see* Furosemide 640
Edetate Calcium Disodium 482
Edetate Disodium 482
Edex® *see* Alprostadil 87
Edrophonium 483
Edrophonium Chloride *see* Edrophonium 483
EDTA *see* Edetate Disodium 482
E.E.S.® *see* Erythromycin 508
Efalizumab 483
Efavirenz 484
Efexor® (Mex) *see* Venlafaxine . . . 1370
Effer-K™ *see* Potassium Bicarbonate and Potassium Citrate 1105
Effexor® *see* Venlafaxine 1370
Effexor® XR *see* Venlafaxine 1370
Eflone® *see* Fluorometholone 605
Eflornithine 485
Eflornithine Hydrochloride *see* Eflornithine 485
Efudex® (Can) *see* Fluorouracil 605
EGb *see* Ginkgo Biloba 1429
E-Gems® [OTC] *see* Vitamin E . . . 1383
EHDP *see* Etidronate Disodium 563
Elantan® (Mex) *see* Isosorbide Mononitrate 771
Elavil® [DSC] *see* Amitriptyline 103
Eldepryl® (Can) *see* Selegiline 1212
Eldisine Lilly 99094 *see* Vindesine 1379
Eldopaque™ (Can) *see* Hydroquinone 719
Eldopaque Forte® *see* Hydroquinone 719
Eldoquin™ (Can) *see* Hydroquinone 719
Eldoquin Forte® *see* Hydroquinone 719

Electrolyte Lavage Solution *see* Polyethylene Glycol-Electrolyte Solution . . . 1100
Elequine® (Mex) *see* Levofloxacin . . 812
Elestat™ *see* Epinastine . . . 496
Eletriptan . . . 486
Eletriptan Hydrobromide *see* Eletriptan . . . 486
Eleutherococcus senticosus *see* Ginseng, Siberian . . . 1431
Elidel® (Can) *see* Pimecrolimus . . . 1088
Eligard™ *see* Leuprolide . . . 805
Elimite® *see* Permethrin . . . 1070
Elipten *see* Aminoglutethimide . . . 98
Elitek™ *see* Rasburicase . . . 1171
Elixophyllin® *see* Theophylline . . . 1285
Elixophyllin-GG® *see* Theophylline and Guaifenesin . . . 1286
ElixSure™ Cough [OTC] *see* Dextromethorphan . . . 421
ElixSure™ Fever/Pain [OTC] *see* Acetaminophen . . . 47
Ellence® *see* Epirubicin . . . 498
Elmiron® *see* Pentosan Polysulfate Sodium . . . 1065
Elocom® (Can) *see* Mometasone Furoate . . . 943
Elocon® *see* Mometasone Furoate . 943
Eloxatin™ *see* Oxaliplatin . . . 1020
Elspar® *see* Asparaginase . . . 150
Eltor® (Can) *see* Pseudoephedrine . . . 1147
Eltroxin® (Can) *see* Levothyroxine . . 817
Emadine® *see* Emedastine . . . 487
Embeline™ E *see* Clobetasol . . . 351
Emcyt® *see* Estramustine . . . 523
Emedastine . . . 487
Emedastine Difumarate *see* Emedastine . . . 487
Emend® *see* Aprepitant . . . 138
Emetrol® [OTC] *see* Fructose, Dextrose, and Phosphoric Acid . . . 638
Emgel® *see* Erythromycin . . . 508
Emko® [OTC] *see* Nonoxynol 9 . . . 995
EMLA® *see* Lidocaine and Prilocaine . . . 826
Emo-Cort® (Can) *see* Hydrocortisone . . . 714
Emtricitabine . . . 487
Emtriva™ *see* Emtricitabine . . . 487
Emulsoil® [OTC] [DSC] *see* Castor Oil . . . 273
ENA 713 *see* Rivastigmine . . . 1192
Enaladil® (Mex) *see* Enalapril . . . 488
Enalapril . . . 488
Enalapril and Felodipine . . . 491
Enalapril and Hydrochlorothiazide . . 491
Enalaprilat *see* Enalapril . . . 488
Enalapril Maleate *see* Enalapril . . . 488
Enbrel® *see* Etanercept . . . 532
Encare® [OTC] *see* Nonoxynol 9 . . 995
Endal® *see* Guaifenesin and Phenylephrine . . . 674
Endal® HD *see* Hydrocodone, Phenylephrine, and Diphenhydramine . . . 713
Endantadine® (Can) *see* Amantadine . . . 92
Endocet® *see* Oxycodone and Acetaminophen . . . 1029
Endocrine Disorders and Pregnancy . . . 1481
Endodan® *see* Oxycodone and Aspirin . . . 1032
Endo®-Levodopa/Carbidopa (Can) *see* Levodopa and Carbidopa . . 811
Endoplus® (Mex) *see* Albendazole . . . 71
Endrate® *see* Edetate Disodium . . . 482
Enduron® (Can) *see* Methyclothiazide . . . 905
Enduronyl® (Can) *see* Methyclothiazide and Deserpidine . . . 905
Enduronyl® Forte (Can) *see* Methyclothiazide and Deserpidine . . . 905
Enfuvirtide . . . 492
Engerix-B® (Can) *see* Hepatitis B Vaccine . . . 689
Engerix-B® and Havrix® *see* Hepatitis A (Inactivated) and Hepatitis B (Recombinant) Vaccine . . . 686
English Hawthorn *see* Hawthorn . . 1437
Enhanced-potency Inactivated Poliovirus Vaccine *see* Poliovirus Vaccine (Inactivated) . . . 1099
Eni® (Mex) *see* Ciprofloxacin . . . 331
Enlon® *see* Edrophonium . . . 483
Enoxaparin . . . 493
Enoxaparin Sodium *see* Enoxaparin . . . 493
Enpresse™ *see* Ethinyl Estradiol and Levonorgestrel . . . 545
Entacapone . . . 494
Entacapone, Carbidopa, and Levodopa *see* Levodopa, Carbidopa, and Entacapone . . . 812
Entacyl® (Can) *see* Piperazine . . . 1094
Enteropride® (Mex) *see* Cisapride . . 336
Entertainer's Secret® [OTC] *see* Saliva Substitute . . . 1205
Entex® LA *see* Guaifenesin and Phenylephrine . . . 674
Entex® PSE *see* Guaifenesin and Pseudoephedrine . . . 675
Entocort® (Can) *see* Budesonide . . . 221
Entocort™ EC *see* Budesonide . . . 221
Entrophen® (Can) *see* Aspirin . . . 151
Entsol® [OTC] *see* Sodium Chloride . . . 1227
Enulose® *see* Lactulose . . . 794
Enzone® *see* Pramoxine and Hydrocortisone . . . 1109
Epamin® (Mex) *see* Phenytoin . . . 1080
Epaxal Berna® (Can) *see* Hepatitis A Vaccine . . . 687
Ephedra . . . 1424
Ephedra sinica *see* Ephedra . . . 1424
Ephedrine . . . 495
Ephedrine, Chlorpheniramine, Phenylephrine, and Carbetapentane *see* Chlorpheniramine, Ephedrine, Phenylephrine, and Carbetapentane . . . 316
Ephedrine Sulfate *see* Ephedrine . . . 495
Epidermal Thymocyte Activating Factor *see* Aldesleukin . . . 74
Epifoam® *see* Pramoxine and Hydrocortisone . . . 1109
Epilem® [inj.] (Mex) *see* Epirubicin . . . 498
Epinastine . . . 496
Epinastine Hydrochloride *see* Epinastine . . . 496
Epinephrine . . . 496
Epinephrine and Bupivacaine (Dental) *see* Bupivacaine and Epinephrine . . . 227
Epinephrine and Chlorpheniramine . . . 497
Epinephrine and Lidocaine *see* Lidocaine and Epinephrine . . . 823
Epinephrine and Prilocaine (Dental) *see* Prilocaine and Epinephrine . . . 1120
Epinephrine (Racemic) . . . 497
Epinephrine (Racemic) and Aluminum Potassium Sulfate . . . 497

Epipodophyllotoxin *see* Etoposide . . 567
EpiQuin™ Micro *see* Hydroquinone . . . 719
Epirubicin . . . 498
Epitol® *see* Carbamazepine . . . 255
Epival® (Mex) *see* Valproic Acid and Derivatives . . . 1359
Epival® ER (Can) *see* Valproic Acid and Derivatives . . . 1359
Epival® I.V. (Can) *see* Valproic Acid and Derivatives . . . 1359
Epivir® *see* Lamivudine . . . 794
Epivir-HBV® *see* Lamivudine . . . 794
Eplerenone . . . 498
EPO *see* Epoetin Alfa . . . 499
Epoetin Alfa . . . 499
Epogen® *see* Epoetin Alfa . . . 499
Epomax® (Mex) *see* Epoetin Alfa . . . 499
Epoprostenol . . . 500
Epoprostenol Sodium *see* Epoprostenol . . . 500
Eprex® (Mex) *see* Epoetin Alfa . . . 499
Eprosartan . . . 501
Eprosartan and HCTZ *see* Eprosartan and Hydrochlorothiazide . . . 502
Eprosartan and Hydrochlorothiazide . . . 502
Eprosartan Mesylate and Hydrochlorothiazide *see* Eprosartan and Hydrochlorothiazide . . . 502
Epsilon Aminocaproic Acid *see* Aminocaproic Acid . . . 97
Epsom Salts *see* Magnesium Sulfate . . . 854
EPT *see* Teniposide . . . 1269
Eptacog Alfa (Activated) *see* Factor VIIa (Recombinant) . . . 571
Eptifibatide . . . 503
Equagesic® *see* Aspirin and Meprobamate . . . 156
Equalactin® [OTC] *see* Polycarbophil . . . 1100
Equanil *see* Meprobamate . . . 878
Eranz® (Mex) *see* Donepezil . . . 462
Erbitux™ *see* Cetuximab . . . 300
Ergamisol® (Can) *see* Levamisole . . 806
Ergocalciferol . . . 503
Ergoloid Mesylates . . . 504
Ergomar® *see* Ergotamine . . . 505
Ergometrine Maleate *see* Ergonovine . . . 505
Ergonovine . . . 505
Ergonovine Maleate *see* Ergonovine . . . 505
Ergotamine . . . 505
Ergotamine and Caffeine . . . 506
Ergotamine Tartrate *see* Ergotamine . . . 505
Ergotamine Tartrate and Caffeine *see* Ergotamine and Caffeine . . . 506
Ergotamine Tartrate, Belladonna, and Phenobarbital *see* Belladonna, Phenobarbital, and Ergotamine . . . 186
E•R•O [OTC] *see* Carbamide Peroxide . . . 259
Errin™ *see* Norethindrone . . . 996
Ertaczo™ *see* Sertaconazole . . . 1214
Ertapenem . . . 507
Ertapenem Sodium *see* Ertapenem . . . 507
Erwinia Asparaginase *see* Asparaginase . . . 150
Eryacnen® (Mex) *see* Erythromycin . . . 508
Erybid™ (Can) *see* Erythromycin . . . 508
Eryc® *see* Erythromycin . . . 508
Erycette® *see* Erythromycin . . . 508
Eryderm® *see* Erythromycin . . . 508
Erygel® *see* Erythromycin . . . 508
EryPed® *see* Erythromycin . . . 508
Ery-Tab® *see* Erythromycin . . . 508
Erythra-Derm™ *see* Erythromycin . . . 508
Erythrocin® *see* Erythromycin . . . 508
Erythromid® (Can) *see* Erythromycin . . . 508
Erythromycin . . . 508
Erythromycin and Benzoyl Peroxide . . . 512
Erythromycin and Sulfisoxazole . . . 512
Erythromycin Base *see* Erythromycin . . . 508
Erythromycin Estolate *see* Erythromycin . . . 508
Erythromycin Ethylsuccinate *see* Erythromycin . . . 508
Erythromycin Gluceptate *see* Erythromycin . . . 508
Erythromycin Lactobionate *see* Erythromycin . . . 508
Erythromycin Stearate *see* Erythromycin . . . 508
Erythropoiesis Stimulating Protein *see* Darbepoetin Alfa . . . 399
Erythropoietin *see* Epoetin Alfa . . . 499
Eryzole® *see* Erythromycin and Sulfisoxazole . . . 512
Escitalopram . . . 513
Escitalopram Oxalate *see* Escitalopram . . . 513
Esclim® *see* Estradiol . . . 518
Eserine® (Can) *see* Physostigmine . . . 1084
Eserine Salicylate *see* Physostigmine . . . 1084
Esgic® *see* Butalbital, Acetaminophen, and Caffeine . . 236
Esgic-Plus™ *see* Butalbital, Acetaminophen, and Caffeine . . 236
Eskalith® *see* Lithium . . . 835
Eskalith CR® *see* Lithium . . . 835
Eskazole® (Mex) *see* Albendazole . . . 71
Esmolol . . . 515
Esmolol Hydrochloride *see* Esmolol . . . 515
Esomeprazole . . . 516
Esomeprazole Magnesium *see* Esomeprazole . . . 516
Esoterica® Regular [OTC] *see* Hydroquinone . . . 719
Especol® [OTC] *see* Fructose, Dextrose, and Phosphoric Acid . . . 638
Estalis® (Can) *see* Estradiol and Norethindrone . . . 521
Estalis-Sequi® (Can) *see* Estradiol and Norethindrone . . . 521
Estar® (Can) *see* Coal Tar . . . 367
Estazolam . . . 517
Esterified Estrogen and Methyltestosterone *see* Estrogens (Esterified) and Methyltestosterone . . . 530
Esterified Estrogens *see* Estrogens (Esterified) . . . 529
Estrace® *see* Estradiol . . . 518
Estraderm® (Can) *see* Estradiol . . . 518
Estraderm TTS® (Mex) *see* Estradiol . . . 518
Estradiol . . . 518
Estradiol Acetate *see* Estradiol . . . 518
Estradiol and Medroxyprogesterone . . . 520
Estradiol and NGM *see* Estradiol and Norgestimate . . . 521
Estradiol and Norethindrone . . . 521
Estradiol and Norgestimate . . . 521
Estradiol Cypionate *see* Estradiol . . . 518
Estradiol Hemihydrate *see* Estradiol . . . 518

Estradiol Transdermal *see* Estradiol . . . 518
Estradiol Valerate *see* Estradiol . . . 518
Estradot® (Can) *see* Estradiol . . . 518
Estramustine . . . 523
Estramustine Phosphate Sodium *see* Estramustine . . . 523
Estrasorb™ *see* Estradiol . . . 518
Estratab® (Can) *see* Estrogens (Esterified) . . . 529
Estratest® (Can) *see* Estrogens (Esterified) and Methyltestosterone . . . 530
Estratest® H.S. *see* Estrogens (Esterified) and Methyltestosterone . . . 530
Estring® (Can) *see* Estradiol . . . 518
EstroGel® (Can) *see* Estradiol . . . 518
Estrogenic Substances, Conjugated *see* Estrogens (Conjugated/Equine) . . . 525
Estrogens (Conjugated A/ Synthetic) . . . 524
Estrogens (Conjugated/Equine) . . . 525
Estrogens (Conjugated/Equine) and Medroxyprogesterone . . . 528
Estrogens (Esterified) . . . 529
Estrogens (Esterified) and Methyltestosterone . . . 530
Estropipate . . . 531
Estrostep® Fe *see* Ethinyl Estradiol and Norethindrone . . . 550
ETAF *see* Aldesleukin . . . 74
Etanercept . . . 532
Ethacrynate Sodium *see* Ethacrynic Acid . . . 533
Ethacrynic Acid . . . 533
Ethambutol . . . 534
Ethambutol Hydrochloride *see* Ethambutol . . . 534
Ethamolin® *see* Ethanolamine Oleate . . . 535
ETH and C *see* Terpin Hydrate and Codeine . . . 1275
Ethanolamine Oleate . . . 535
Ethaverine . . . 535
Ethaverine Hydrochloride *see* Ethaverine . . . 535
Ethinyl Estradiol and Desogestrel . . . 536
Ethinyl Estradiol and Drospirenone . . . 538
Ethinyl Estradiol and Ethynodiol Diacetate . . . 540
Ethinyl Estradiol and Etonogestrel . . . 543
Ethinyl Estradiol and Levonorgestrel . . . 545
Ethinyl Estradiol and NGM *see* Ethinyl Estradiol and Norgestimate . . . 554
Ethinyl Estradiol and Norelgestromin . . . 548
Ethinyl Estradiol and Norethindrone . . . 550
Ethinyl Estradiol and Norgestimate . . . 554
Ethinyl Estradiol and Norgestrel . . . 557
Ethiofos *see* Amifostine . . . 94
Ethionamide . . . 560
Ethmozine® (Can) *see* Moricizine . . . 946
Ethosuximide . . . 560
Ethotoin . . . 561
Ethoxynaphthamido Penicillin Sodium *see* Nafcillin . . . 958
Ethyl Aminobenzoate *see* Benzocaine . . . 191
Ethyl Chloride . . . 561
Ethyl Chloride and Dichlorotetrafluoroethane . . . 562
Ethylphenylhydantoin *see* Ethotoin . . . 561
Ethynodiol Diacetate and Ethinyl Estradiol *see* Ethinyl Estradiol and Ethynodiol Diacetate . . . 540
Ethyol® (Mex) *see* Amifostine . . . 94
Etibi® (Can) *see* Ethambutol . . . 534
Etidocaine and Epinephrine . . . 562
Etidocaine Hydrochloride *see* Etidocaine and Epinephrine . . . 562
Etidronate Disodium . . . 563
Etodolac . . . 564
Etodolic Acid *see* Etodolac . . . 564
Etomidate . . . 566
Etonogestrel and Ethinyl Estradiol *see* Ethinyl Estradiol and Etonogestrel . . . 543
Etopophos® *see* Etoposide Phosphate . . . 568
Etoposide . . . 567
Etoposide Phosphate . . . 568
Etopos® [inj.] (Mex) *see* Etoposide . . . 567
Etrafon® (Can) *see* Amitriptyline and Perphenazine . . . 106
Eudal®-SR *see* Guaifenesin and Pseudoephedrine . . . 675
Euflex® (Can) *see* Flutamide . . . 615
Euglucon® (Mex) *see* GlyBURIDE . . . 664
Eulexin® *see* Flutamide . . . 615
Eurax® *see* Crotamiton . . . 380
Eutirox® (Mex) *see* Levothyroxine . . . 817
Evac-U-Gen [OTC] *see* Senna . . . 1213
Evening Primrose . . . 1425
Evening Primrose Oil *see* Evening Primrose . . . 1425
Everone® 200 (Can) *see* Testosterone . . . 1276
Evista® (Can) *see* Raloxifene . . . 1166
Evoxac® *see* Cevimeline . . . 302
Evra™ (Can) *see* Ethinyl Estradiol and Norelgestromin . . . 548
Exact® Acne Medication [OTC] *see* Benzoyl Peroxide . . . 194
Excedrin® Extra Strength [OTC] *see* Acetaminophen, Aspirin, and Caffeine . . . 56
Excedrin® Migraine [OTC] *see* Acetaminophen, Aspirin, and Caffeine . . . 56
Excedrin® P.M. [OTC] *see* Acetaminophen and Diphenhydramine . . . 53
Exelderm® *see* Sulconazole . . . 1243
Exelon® (Can) *see* Rivastigmine . . . 1192
Exemestane . . . 569
ex-lax® [OTC] *see* Senna . . . 1213
ex-lax® Maximum Strength [OTC] *see* Senna . . . 1213
ex-lax® Stool Softener [OTC] *see* Docusate . . . 459
Exorex® *see* Coal Tar . . . 367
Extendryl *see* Chlorpheniramine, Phenylephrine, and Methscopolamine . . . 317
Extendryl JR *see* Chlorpheniramine, Phenylephrine, and Methscopolamine . . . 317
Extendryl SR *see* Chlorpheniramine, Phenylephrine, and Methscopolamine . . . 317
Eye Balm *see* Golden Seal . . . 1433
Eye Root *see* Golden Seal . . . 1433
Eye-Sine™ [OTC] *see* Tetrahydrozoline . . . 1282
Eyestil (Can) *see* Hyaluronate and Derivatives . . . 696
Eye-Stream® (Can) *see* Balanced Salt Solution . . . 181
EZ-Char™ [OTC] *see* Charcoal . . . 303
Ezetimibe . . . 570
Ezetrol® (Can) *see* Ezetimibe . . . 570
F_3T *see* Trifluridine . . . 1339
Fabrazyme® *see* Agalsidase Beta . . . 69

Facicam® (Mex) *see* Piroxicam . . . 1097
Factive® *see* Gemifloxacin 653
Factor IX 571
Factor IX Complex (Human) 572
Factor VIIa (Recombinant) 571
Factor VIII (Human) *see* Antihemophilic Factor (Human) 134
Factor VIII (Porcine) *see* Antihemophilic Factor (Porcine) 134
Factor VIII (Recombinant) *see* Antihemophilic Factor (Recombinant) 135
Factrel® *see* Gonadorelin 669
Famciclovir 572
Famotidine 573
Famotidine, Calcium Carbonate, and Magnesium Hydroxide 574
Famoxal® (Mex) *see* Famotidine . . . 573
Famvir® *see* Famciclovir 572
Fansidar® *see* Sulfadoxine and Pyrimethamine 1245
Fareston® (Mex) *see* Toremifene . . 1317
Farmorubicin® (Mex) *see* Epirubicin 498
Farmotex® (Mex) *see* Famotidine . . . 573
Faslodex® *see* Fulvestrant 639
Fat Emulsion 575
Fazaclo™ *see* Clozapine 366
5-FC *see* Flucytosine 596
FC1157a *see* Toremifene 1317
Featherfew *see* Feverfew 1426
Featherfoil *see* Feverfew 1426
Feiba VH® *see* Anti-inhibitor Coagulant Complex 135
Feiba® VH Immuno (Can) *see* Anti-inhibitor Coagulant Complex 135
Felbamate 575
Felbatol® *see* Felbamate 575
Feldene™ (Can) *see* Piroxicam . . . 1097
Feliberal® (Mex) *see* Enalapril 488
Felodipine 576
Felodipine and Enalapril *see* Enalapril and Felodipine 491
Femara® (Can) *see* Letrozole 803
femhrt® *see* Ethinyl Estradiol and Norethindrone 550
Femilax™ [OTC] *see* Bisacodyl 208
Femiron® [OTC] *see* Ferrous Fumarate 586
Femizol-M™ [OTC] *see* Miconazole 922
Fem-Prin® [OTC] *see* Acetaminophen, Aspirin, and Caffeine 56
Femring™ *see* Estradiol 518
Femstal® (Mex) *see* Butoconazole . . 239
Femstat® One (Can) *see* Butoconazole 239
Fenesin™ DM *see* Guaifenesin and Dextromethorphan 673
Fenidantoin® [tabs] (Mex) *see* Phenytoin 1080
Fenitron® [tabs] (Mex) *see* Phenytoin 1080
Fenofibrate 577
Fenoldopam 579
Fenoldopam Mesylate *see* Fenoldopam 579
Fenoprofen 580
Fenoprofen Calcium *see* Fenoprofen 580
Fenoterol 580
Fenoterol Hydrobromide *see* Fenoterol 580
Fentanest® (Mex) *see* Fentanyl 581
Fentanyl 581
Fentanyl Citrate *see* Fentanyl 581
Feostat® [OTC] *see* Ferrous Fumarate 586
Feratab® [OTC] *see* Ferrous Sulfate 586
Fer-Gen-Sol [OTC] *see* Ferrous Sulfate 586
Fergon® [OTC] *see* Ferrous Gluconate 586
Feridex I.V.® *see* Ferumoxides 587
Fer-In-Sol® [OTC] *see* Ferrous Sulfate 586
Fer-Iron® [OTC] *see* Ferrous Sulfate 586
Fermalac (Can) *see* *Lactobacillus* . . 793
Ferodan™ (Can) *see* Ferrous Sulfate 586
Fero-Grad 500® [OTC] *see* Ferrous Sulfate and Ascorbic Acid 587
Ferretts [OTC] *see* Ferrous Fumarate 586
Ferric Gluconate 585
Ferric Hexacyanoferrate 585
Ferric (III) Hexacyanoferrate (II) *see* Ferric Hexacyanoferrate . . . 585
Ferrlecit® *see* Ferric Gluconate 585
Ferro-Sequels® [OTC] *see* Ferrous Fumarate 586
Ferrous Fumarate 586
Ferrous Gluconate 586
Ferrous Sulfate 586
Ferrous Sulfate and Ascorbic Acid . . 587
Ferumoxides 587
Ferval® (Mex) *see* Ferrous Fumarate 586
$FeSO_4$ *see* Ferrous Sulfate 586
Fe-Tinic™ 150 [OTC] *see* Polysaccharide-Iron Complex . . 1101
Feverall® [OTC] *see* Acetaminophen 47
Feverfew 1426
Fexofenadine 587
Fexofenadine and Pseudoephedrine 588
Fexofenadine Hydrochloride *see* Fexofenadine 587
Fiberall® *see* Psyllium 1151
FiberCon® [OTC] *see* Polycarbophil 1100
FiberEase™ [OTC] *see* Methylcellulose 905
Fiber-Lax® [OTC] *see* Polycarbophil 1100
FiberNorm™ [OTC] *see* Polycarbophil 1100
Fibrin Sealant Kit 589
Filgrastim 589
Finacea™ *see* Azelaic Acid 173
Finasteride 590
Findol® (Mex) *see* Ketorolac 787
Fioricet® *see* Butalbital, Acetaminophen, and Caffeine . . 236
Fioricet® with Codeine *see* Butalbital, Acetaminophen, Caffeine, and Codeine 236
Fiorinal® (Can) *see* Butalbital, Aspirin, and Caffeine 238
Fiorinal®-C 1/2 (Can) *see* Butalbital, Aspirin, Caffeine, and Codeine 238
Fiorinal®-C 1/4 (Can) *see* Butalbital, Aspirin, Caffeine, and Codeine 238
Fiorinal® With Codeine *see* Butalbital, Aspirin, Caffeine, and Codeine 238
Fisalamine *see* Mesalamine 882
Fish Oils 1427
Fixoten® (Mex) *see* Pentoxifylline . . 1066
FK506 *see* Tacrolimus 1255
Flagenase® [tabs] (Mex) *see* Metronidazole 917

Flagyl® (Mex) *see* Metronidazole . . . 917
Flagyl ER® *see* Metronidazole 917
Flamazine® (Can) *see* Silver Sulfadiazine 1221
Flamicina® (Mex) *see* Ampicillin 124
Flanax® (Mex) *see* Naproxen 965
Flarex® *see* Fluorometholone 605
Flatulex® [OTC] *see* Simethicone . . 1222
Flavoxate 591
Flavoxate Hydrochloride *see* Flavoxate 591
Flaxseed Oil 1427
Flebogamma® *see* Immune Globulin (Intravenous) 740
Flecainide 592
Flecainide Acetate *see* Flecainide . . 592
Fleet® Babylax® [OTC] *see* Glycerin 667
Fleet® Bisacodyl Enema [OTC] *see* Bisacodyl 208
Fleet® Enema [OTC] *see* Sodium Phosphates 1230
Fleet® Glycerin Suppositories [OTC] *see* Glycerin 667
Fleet® Glycerin Suppositories Maximum Strength [OTC] *see* Glycerin 667
Fleet® Liquid Glycerin Suppositories [OTC] *see* Glycerin 667
Fleet® Phospho®-Soda [OTC] *see* Sodium Phosphates 1230
Fleet® Phospho-Soda® Accu-Prep™ [OTC] *see* Sodium Phosphates 1230
Fleet® Phospho®-Soda Oral Laxative (Can) *see* Sodium Phosphates 1230
Fleet® Sof-Lax® [OTC] *see* Docusate 459
Fleet® Sof-Lax® Overnight [DSC] [OTC] *see* Docusate and Casanthranol 460
Fleet® Stimulant Laxative [OTC] *see* Bisacodyl 208
Flemoxon® (Mex) *see* Amoxicillin . . . 114
Fletcher's® Castoria® [OTC] *see* Senna 1213
Flexafen® (Mex) *see* Ibuprofen 728
Flexeril® (Can) *see* Cyclobenzaprine 382
Flexitec (Can) *see* Cyclobenzaprine 382
Flixonase® (Mex) *see* Fluticasone . . 616
Flixotide® (Mex) *see* Fluticasone . . . 616
Flogen® [caps] (Mex) *see* Naproxen 965
Flolan® *see* Epoprostenol 500
Flomax® *see* Tamsulosin 1260
Flonase® (Can) *see* Fluticasone 616
Florazole® ER (Can) *see* Metronidazole 917
Florical® [OTC] *see* Calcium Carbonate 245
Florinef® *see* Fludrocortisone 598
Florone® (Can) *see* Diflorasone 435
Flovent® (Can) *see* Fluticasone 616
Flovent® HFA (Can) *see* Fluticasone 616
Flovent® Rotadisk® *see* Fluticasone 616
Floxacin® (Mex) *see* Norfloxacin . . . 997
Floxil® (Mex) *see* Ofloxacin 1005
Floxin® (Can) *see* Ofloxacin 1005
Floxin Otic Singles *see* Ofloxacin . . 1005
Floxstat® (Mex) *see* Ofloxacin 1005
Floxuridine 593
Flubenisolone *see* Betamethasone . . 199
Flucaine® *see* Proparacaine and Fluorescein 1135
Fluconazole 594
Flucytosine 596
Fludara® (Mex) *see* Fludarabine 597
Fludarabine 597
Fludarabine Phosphate *see* Fludarabine 597
Fludrocortisone 598
Fludrocortisone Acetate *see* Fludrocortisone 598
Fluken® (Mex) *see* Flutamide 615
Flulem® (Mex) *see* Flutamide 615
Flumadine® (Can) *see* Rimantadine 1184
Flumazenil 599
FluMist™ *see* Influenza Virus Vaccine 748
Flunisolide 599
Flunitrazepam 600
Fluocinolone 601
Fluocinolone Acetonide *see* Fluocinolone 601
Fluocinolone, Hydroquinone, and Tretinoin 601
Fluocinonide 602
Fluoderm (Can) *see* Fluocinolone . . 601
Fluohydrisone Acetate *see* Fludrocortisone 598
Fluohydrocortisone Acetate *see* Fludrocortisone 598
Fluoracaine® *see* Proparacaine and Fluorescein 1135
Fluor-A-Day [OTC] *see* Fluoride 603
Fluorescein and Proparacaine *see* Proparacaine and Fluorescein 1135
Fluoride 603
Fluoride and Triclosan (Dental) *see* Triclosan and Fluoride 1337
Fluorides 1555
Fluorigard® [OTC] *see* Fluoride 603
Fluori-Methane® *see* Dichlorodifluoromethane and Trichloromonofluoromethane . . . 427
Fluorinse® *see* Fluoride 603
Fluorodeoxyuridine *see* Floxuridine 593
9α-Fluorohydrocortisone Acetate *see* Fludrocortisone 598
Fluorometholone 605
Fluorometholone and Sulfacetamide *see* Sulfacetamide and Fluorometholone 1244
Fluor-Op® *see* Fluorometholone 605
Fluoroplex® *see* Fluorouracil 605
Fluorouracil 605
5-Fluorouracil *see* Fluorouracil 605
Fluotic® (Can) *see* Fluoride 603
Fluoxac® [tabs] (Mex) *see* Fluoxetine 606
Fluoxetine 606
Fluoxetine and Olanzapine *see* Olanzapine and Fluoxetine 1009
Fluoxetine Hydrochloride *see* Fluoxetine 606
Fluoxymesterone 609
Flupazine® [tabs] (Mex) *see* Trifluoperazine 1338
Fluphenazine 610
Fluphenazine Decanoate *see* Fluphenazine 610
Flura-Drops® *see* Fluoride 603
Flura-Loz® *see* Fluoride 603
Flurandrenolide 611
Flurandrenolone *see* Flurandrenolide 611
Flurazepam 612
Flurazepam Hydrochloride *see* Flurazepam 612
Flurbiprofen 613
Flurbiprofen Sodium *see* Flurbiprofen 613

Flurinol® (Mex) *see* Epinastine 496
5-Flurocytosine *see* Flucytosine 596
Fluro-Ethyl® *see* Ethyl Chloride and Dichlorotetrafluoroethane . . 562
Flutamide 615
Fluticasone 616
Fluticasone and Salmeterol 619
Fluticasone Propionate *see* Fluticasone 616
Fluvastatin 622
Fluviral S/F® (Can) *see* Influenza Virus Vaccine 748
Fluvirin® *see* Influenza Virus Vaccine 748
Fluvoxamine 623
Fluzone® *see* Influenza Virus Vaccine 748
Flynoken® (Mex) *see* Leucovorin . . . 804
FML® (Can) *see* Fluorometholone . . 605
FML Forte® (Can) *see* Fluorometholone 605
FML-S® *see* Sulfacetamide and Fluorometholone 1244
Focalin™ *see* Dexmethylphenidate . . 416
Foille® [OTC] *see* Benzocaine 191
Foille® Medicated First Aid [OTC] *see* Benzocaine 191
Foille® Plus [OTC] *see* Benzocaine 191
Folacin *see* Folic Acid 625
Folacin, Vitamin B_{12}, and Vitamin B_6 *see* Folic Acid, Cyanocobalamin, and Pyridoxine 626
Folate *see* Folic Acid 625
Folbee *see* Folic Acid, Cyanocobalamin, and Pyridoxine 626
Folgard® [OTC] *see* Folic Acid, Cyanocobalamin, and Pyridoxine 626
Folgard RX 2.2® *see* Folic Acid, Cyanocobalamin, and Pyridoxine 626
Folic Acid 625
Folic Acid, Cyanocobalamin, and Pyridoxine 626
Folinic Acid *see* Leucovorin 804
Follistim® [DSC] *see* Follitropins 626
Follistim® AQ *see* Follitropins 626
Follitrin® (Mex) *see* Follitropins 626
Follitropin Alfa *see* Follitropins 626
Follitropin Alpha *see* Follitropins 626
Follitropin Beta *see* Follitropins 626
Follitropins 626
Foltx® *see* Folic Acid, Cyanocobalamin, and Pyridoxine 626
Fomepizole 627
Fomivirsen 628
Fomivirsen Sodium *see* Fomivirsen 628
Fondaparinux 628
Fondaparinux Sodium *see* Fondaparinux 628
Foradil® (Can) *see* Formoterol 629
Foradil® Aerolizer™ *see* Formoterol 629
Formoterol 629
Formoterol Fumarate *see* Formoterol 629
Formula EM [OTC] *see* Fructose, Dextrose, and Phosphoric Acid 638
Formulation R™ [OTC] *see* Phenylephrine 1078
Formulex® (Can) *see* Dicyclomine . . 432
5-Formyl Tetrahydrofolate *see* Leucovorin 804
Fortamet™ *see* Metformin 887
Fortaz® *see* Ceftazidime 286
Forteo™ *see* Teriparatide 1274
Fortovase® (Can) *see* Saquinavir . . 1207
Fortum® (Mex) *see* Ceftazidime 286
Fosamax® (Can) *see* Alendronate . . . 77
Fosamprenavir 630
Fosamprenavir Calcium *see* Fosamprenavir 630
Foscarnet 631
Foscavir® *see* Foscarnet 631
Fosfocil® (Mex) *see* Fosfomycin 632
Fosfocil® [inj.] (Mex) *see* Fosfomycin 632
Fosfomycin 632
Fosfomycin Tromethamine *see* Fosfomycin 632
Fosinopril 633
Fosinopril and Hydrochlorothiazide . . 635
Fosphenytoin 635
Fosphenytoin Sodium *see* Fosphenytoin 635
Fostex® 10% BPO [OTC] *see* Benzoyl Peroxide 194
Fotexina® (Mex) *see* Cefotaxime . . . 283
Fragmin® (Can) *see* Dalteparin 395
Freezone® [OTC] *see* Salicylic Acid 1205
Fresenizol® [inj.] (Mex) *see* Metronidazole 917
Fresofol® (Mex) *see* Propofol 1135
Frisium® (Can) *see* Clobazam 350
Froben® (Can) *see* Flurbiprofen 613
Froben-SR® (Can) *see* Flurbiprofen 613
Frova® *see* Frovatriptan 638
Frovatriptan 638
Frovatriptan Succinate *see* Frovatriptan 638
Froxal® [inj.] (Mex) *see* Cefuroxime 289
Fructose, Dextrose, and Phosphoric Acid 638
Frusemide *see* Furosemide 640
FS *see* Fibrin Sealant Kit 589
FTC *see* Emtricitabine 487
FU *see* Fluorouracil 605
5-FU *see* Fluorouracil 605
FUDR® (Can) *see* Floxuridine 593
5-FUDR *see* Floxuridine 593
Fulvestrant 639
Fulvicin® P/G *see* Griseofulvin 671
Fulvicin-U/F® *see* Griseofulvin 671
Fungi-Guard [OTC] *see* Tolnaftate 1312
Fungi-Nail® [OTC] *see* Undecylenic Acid and Derivatives 1352
Fungistat® (Mex) *see* Terconazole 1274
Fungizone® (Can) *see* Amphotericin B (Conventional) . . 120
Fung-O® [OTC] *see* Salicylic Acid 1205
Fungoid® Tincture [OTC] *see* Miconazole 922
Fungoral® (Mex) *see* Ketoconazole 783
Furadantin® *see* Nitrofurantoin 990
Furazolidone 640
Furazosin *see* Prazosin 1111
Furosemide 640
Furoxona® (Mex) *see* Furazolidone 640
Furoxone *see* Furazolidone 640
Fustaren® (Mex) *see* Diclofenac 427
Fuxen® (Mex) *see* Naproxen 965
Fuxol® (Mex) *see* Furazolidone 640
Fuzeon™ (Can) *see* Enfuvirtide 492
FXT (Can) *see* Fluoxetine 606
Gabapentin 642
Gabitril® (Can) *see* Tiagabine 1294
Gadoteridol *see* Radiological/ Contrast Media (Nonionic) 1166

Galantamine . . . 645
Galantamine Hydrobromide *see* Galantamine . . . 645
Galecin® [inj.] (Mex) *see* Clindamycin . . . 348
Galedol® (Mex) *see* Diclofenac . . . 427
Galidrin® (Mex) *see* Ranitidine . . . 1169
Gallium Nitrate . . . 646
Gamikal® [inj.] (Mex) *see* Amikacin . . . 95
Gamimune® N (Can) *see* Immune Globulin (Intravenous) . . . 740
Gamma Benzene Hexachloride *see* Lindane . . . 829
Gammagard® S/D *see* Immune Globulin (Intravenous) . . . 740
Gamma Globulin *see* Immune Globulin (Intramuscular) . . . 739
Gamma Hydroxybutyric Acid *see* Sodium Oxybate . . . 1229
Gammaphos *see* Amifostine . . . 94
Gammar®-P I.V. *see* Immune Globulin (Intravenous) . . . 740
Gamunex® (Can) *see* Immune Globulin (Intravenous) . . . 740
Ganciclovir . . . 646
Ganidin NR *see* Guaifenesin . . . 672
Ganirelix . . . 647
Ganirelix Acetate *see* Ganirelix . . . 647
Ganite™ *see* Gallium Nitrate . . . 646
Gani-Tuss® NR *see* Guaifenesin and Codeine . . . 673
Gantrisin® *see* SulfiSOXAZOLE . . . 1250
Garamicina® [cream] (Mex) *see* Gentamicin . . . 655
Garamicina® [inj.] (Mex) *see* Gentamicin . . . 655
Garamycin® [DSC] *see* Gentamicin . . . 655
Garlic . . . 1428
Gascop® (Mex) *see* Albendazole . . . 71
Gastrocrom® *see* Cromolyn . . . 378
Gastrointestinal Disorders . . . 1476
Gas-X® [OTC] *see* Simethicone . . . 1222
Gas-X® Extra Strength [OTC] *see* Simethicone . . . 1222
Gatifloxacin . . . 647
Gaviscon® Extra Strength [OTC] *see* Aluminum Hydroxide and Magnesium Carbonate . . . 90
Gaviscon® Liquid [OTC] *see* Aluminum Hydroxide and Magnesium Carbonate . . . 90
Gaviscon® Tablet [OTC] *see* Aluminum Hydroxide and Magnesium Trisilicate . . . 91
GBE *see* Ginkgo Biloba . . . 1429
G-CSF *see* Filgrastim . . . 589
G-CSF (PEG Conjugate) *see* Pegfilgrastim . . . 1052
GCV Sodium *see* Ganciclovir . . . 646
Gebauer's Ethyl Chloride® *see* Ethyl Chloride . . . 561
Gefitinib . . . 649
Gelatin (Absorbable) . . . 650
Gelclair™ *see* Maltodextrin . . . 855
Gelfilm® *see* Gelatin (Absorbable) . . . 650
Gelfoam® *see* Gelatin (Absorbable) . . . 650
Gel-Kam® [OTC] *see* Fluoride . . . 603
Gel-Kam® Rinse *see* Fluoride . . . 603
Gelucast® *see* Zinc Gelatin . . . 1400
Gelusil® (Can) *see* Aluminum Hydroxide and Magnesium Hydroxide . . . 91
Gelusil® Extra Strength (Can) *see* Aluminum Hydroxide and Magnesium Hydroxide . . . 91
Gemcitabine . . . 650
Gemcitabine Hydrochloride *see* Gemcitabine . . . 650
Gemfibrozil . . . 651
Gemifloxacin . . . 653
Gemifloxacin Mesylate *see* Gemifloxacin . . . 653
Gemtuzumab Ozogamicin . . . 653
Gemzar® (Can) *see* Gemcitabine . . . 650
Genac® [OTC] *see* Triprolidine and Pseudoephedrine . . . 1345
Gen-Acebutolol (Can) *see* Acebutolol . . . 46
Genaced™ [OTC] *see* Acetaminophen, Aspirin, and Caffeine . . . 56
Gen-Acyclovir (Can) *see* Acyclovir . . . 64
Genahist® [OTC] *see* DiphenhydrAMINE . . . 448
Gen-Alprazolam (Can) *see* Alprazolam . . . 84
Gen-Amiodarone (Can) *see* Amiodarone . . . 101
Gen-Amoxicillin (Can) *see* Amoxicillin . . . 114
Genapap® [OTC] *see* Acetaminophen . . . 47
Genapap® Children [OTC] *see* Acetaminophen . . . 47
Genapap® Extra Strength [OTC] *see* Acetaminophen . . . 47
Genapap® Infant [OTC] *see* Acetaminophen . . . 47
Genapap™ Sinus Maximum Strength [OTC] *see* Acetaminophen and Pseudoephedrine . . . 53
Genaphed® [OTC] *see* Pseudoephedrine . . . 1147
Genaphed Plus [OTC] *see* Chlorpheniramine and Pseudoephedrine . . . 315
Genasal [OTC] *see* Oxymetazoline . . . 1034
Genasoft® [OTC] *see* Docusate . . . 459
Genasoft® Plus [DSC] [OTC] *see* Docusate and Casanthranol . . . 460
Genasyme® [OTC] *see* Simethicone . . . 1222
Gen-Atenolol (Can) *see* Atenolol . . . 159
Genaton Tablet [OTC] *see* Aluminum Hydroxide and Magnesium Trisilicate . . . 91
Genatuss DM® [OTC] *see* Guaifenesin and Dextromethorphan . . . 673
Gen-Azathioprine (Can) *see* Azathioprine . . . 172
Gen-Baclofen (Can) *see* Baclofen . . . 180
Gen-Beclo (Can) *see* Beclomethasone . . . 184
Gen-Bromazepam (Can) *see* Bromazepam . . . 218
Gen-Budesonide AQ (Can) *see* Budesonide . . . 221
Gen-Buspirone (Can) *see* BusPIRone . . . 233
Gen-Captopril (Can) *see* Captopril . . . 252
Gen-Carbamazepine CR (Can) *see* Carbamazepine . . . 255
Gen-Cimetidine (Can) *see* Cimetidine . . . 330
Gen-Clobetasol (Can) *see* Clobetasol . . . 351
Gen-Clomipramine (Can) *see* ClomiPRAMINE . . . 355
Gen-Clonazepam (Can) *see* Clonazepam . . . 356
Gen-Clozapine (Can) *see* Clozapine . . . 366
Gen-Cyclobenzaprine (Can) *see* Cyclobenzaprine . . . 382
Gen-Diltiazem (Can) *see* Diltiazem . . . 444

Gen-Diltiazem SR (Can) *see* Diltiazem . . . 444
Gen-Divalproex (Can) *see* Valproic Acid and Derivatives . . . 1359
Gen-Doxazosin (Can) *see* Doxazosin . . . 465
Genebs® [OTC] *see* Acetaminophen . . . 47
Genebs® Extra Strength [OTC] *see* Acetaminophen . . . 47
Genemicin® [inj.] (Mex) *see* Gentamicin . . . 655
Generlac *see* Lactulose . . . 794
Genesec® [OTC] *see* Acetaminophen and Phenyltoloxamine . . . 53
Gen-Etidronate (Can) *see* Etidronate Disodium . . . 563
Geneye® [OTC] *see* Tetrahydrozoline . . . 1282
Gen-Famotidine (Can) *see* Famotidine . . . 573
Gen-Fenofibrate Micro (Can) *see* Fenofibrate . . . 577
Genfiber® [OTC] *see* Psyllium . . . 1151
Gen-Fluconazole (Can) *see* Fluconazole . . . 594
Gen-Fluoxetine (Can) *see* Fluoxetine . . . 606
Gen-Gemfibrozil (Can) *see* Gemfibrozil . . . 651
Gen-Glybe (Can) *see* GlyBURIDE . . . 664
Gengraf® *see* CycloSPORINE . . . 386
Gen-Hydroxyurea (Can) *see* Hydroxyurea . . . 722
Gen-Indapamide (Can) *see* Indapamide . . . 743
Gen-Ipratropium (Can) *see* Ipratropium . . . 761
Genkova® [inj.] (Mex) *see* Gentamicin . . . 655
Gen-Lovastatin (Can) *see* Lovastatin . . . 848
Gen-Medroxy (Can) *see* MedroxyPROGESTERone . . . 862
Gen-Metformin (Can) *see* Metformin . . . 887
Gen-Minocycline (Can) *see* Minocycline . . . 931
Gen-Nabumetone (Can) *see* Nabumetone . . . 955
Gen-Naproxen EC (Can) *see* Naproxen . . . 965
Gen-Nitro (Can) *see* Nitroglycerin . . . 991
Gen-Nizatidine (Can) *see* Nizatidine . . . 995
Gen-Nortriptyline (Can) *see* Nortriptyline . . . 999
Genoptic® *see* Gentamicin . . . 655
Genotropin® *see* Human Growth Hormone . . . 694
Genotropin Miniquick® *see* Human Growth Hormone . . . 694
Genoxal® (Mex) *see* Cyclophosphamide . . . 384
Gen-Oxybutynin (Can) *see* Oxybutynin . . . 1026
Gen-Pindolol (Can) *see* Pindolol . . . 1090
Gen-Piroxicam (Can) *see* Piroxicam . . . 1097
Genpril® [OTC] *see* Ibuprofen . . . 728
Gen-Ranidine (Can) *see* Ranitidine . . . 1169
Genrex® (Mex) *see* Gentamicin . . . 655
Gen-Salbutamol (Can) *see* Albuterol . . . 71
Gen-Selegiline (Can) *see* Selegiline . . . 1212
Gen-Sertraline (Can) *see* Sertraline . . . 1215
Gen-Simvastatin (Can) *see* Simvastatin . . . 1222
Gen-Sotalol (Can) *see* Sotalol . . . 1231
Gentabac® (Mex) *see* Gentamicin . . . 655
Gentacidin® *see* Gentamicin . . . 655
Gentacin® [inj.] (Mex) *see* Gentamicin . . . 655
Genta Grin® (Mex) *see* Gentamicin . . . 655
Gentak® *see* Gentamicin . . . 655
Gentamicin . . . 655
Gentamicin and Prednisolone *see* Prednisolone and Gentamicin . . . 1115
Gentamicin Sulfate *see* Gentamicin . . . 655
Gen-Tamoxifen (Can) *see* Tamoxifen . . . 1258
Gentarim® (Mex) *see* Gentamicin . . . 655
Gentazaf® (Mex) *see* Gentamicin . . . 655
GenTeal® [OTC] *see* Hydroxypropyl Methylcellulose . . . 721
GenTeal® Mild [OTC] *see* Hydroxypropyl Methylcellulose . . . 721
Gen-Temazepam (Can) *see* Temazepam . . . 1266
Gen-Terbinafine (Can) *see* Terbinafine . . . 1272
Gentian Violet . . . 657
Gen-Ticlopidine (Can) *see* Ticlopidine . . . 1297
Gen-Timolol (Can) *see* Timolol . . . 1299
Gentlax® [OTC] *see* Bisacodyl . . . 208
Gentran® (Can) *see* Dextran . . . 417
Gen-Trazodone (Can) *see* Trazodone . . . 1326
Gen-Triazolam (Can) *see* Triazolam . . . 1335
Gen-Verapamil (Can) *see* Verapamil . . . 1373
Gen-Verapamil SR (Can) *see* Verapamil . . . 1373
Gen-Warfarin (Can) *see* Warfarin . . . 1389
Gen-Zopiclone (Can) *see* Zopiclone . . . 1406
Geocillin® *see* Carbenicillin . . . 260
Geodon® *see* Ziprasidone . . . 1401
Geref® [DSC] *see* Sermorelin Acetate . . . 1214
Geref® Diagnostic *see* Sermorelin Acetate . . . 1214
Geri-Hydrolac™ [OTC] *see* Lactic Acid and Ammonium Hydroxide . . . 793
Geri-Hydrolac™-12 [OTC] *see* Lactic Acid and Ammonium Hydroxide . . . 793
Geritol® Tonic [OTC] *see* Vitamins (Multiple/Oral) . . . 1384
German Measles Vaccine *see* Rubella Virus Vaccine (Live) . . 1203
Gevrabon® [OTC] *see* Vitamin B Complex Combinations . . . 1382
GF196960 *see* Tadalafil . . . 1257
GG *see* Guaifenesin . . . 672
GHB *see* Sodium Oxybate . . . 1229
G.I.® (Mex) *see* Gentamicin . . . 655
GI87084B *see* Remifentanil . . . 1172
Gimalxina® (Mex) *see* Amoxicillin . . . 114
Ginedisc® (Mex) *see* Estradiol . . . 518
Ginger . . . 1428
Gingi-Aid® Gingival Retraction Cord *see* Aluminum Chloride . . . 90
Gingi-Aid® Solution *see* Aluminum Chloride . . . 90
Ginkgo Biloba . . . 1429
ginkgold *see* Ginkgo Biloba . . . 1429
Ginkgopowder *see* Ginkgo Biloba . . . 1429
Ginkogink *see* Ginkgo Biloba . . . 1429
Ginseng, Panax . . . 1430

Ginseng, Siberian 1431
Glargine, Insulin *see* Insulin Preparations 749
Glatiramer Acetate 658
Gleevec™ (Can) *see* Imatinib 734
Gliadel® *see* Carmustine 268
Glibenclamide *see* GlyBURIDE 664
Glibenil® (Mex) *see* GlyBURIDE 664
Glimepiride 659
Glioten® (Mex) *see* Enalapril 488
GlipiZIDE 660
Glipizide and Metformin 662
Glipizide and Metformin Hydrochloride *see* Glipizide and Metformin 662
Glivec *see* Imatinib 734
GlucaGen® *see* Glucagon 663
GlucaGen® Diagnostic Kit *see* Glucagon 663
Glucagon 663
Glucagon Diagnostic Kit *see* Glucagon 663
Glucagon Emergency Kit *see* Glucagon 663
Glucagon Hydrochloride *see* Glucagon 663
Glucal® (Mex) *see* GlyBURIDE 664
Glucobay® (Mex) *see* Acarbose 45
Glucocerebrosidase *see* Alglucerase 80
GlucoNorm® (Can) *see* Repaglinide 1173
Glucophage® (Can) *see* Metformin . . 887
Glucophage® XR *see* Metformin 887
Glucosamine 1432
Glucosamine Hydrochloride *see* Glucosamine 1432
Glucosamine Sulfate *see* Glucosamine 1432
Glucose (Instant) 663
Glucose Polymers 664
Glucotrol® *see* GlipiZIDE 660
Glucotrol® XL *see* GlipiZIDE 660
Glucovance® *see* Glyburide and Metformin 665
Glucoven® (Mex) *see* GlyBURIDE . . 664
Glu-K® [OTC] *see* Potassium Gluconate 1106
Glulisine, Insulin *see* Insulin Preparations 749
Glupitel® (Mex) *see* GlipiZIDE 660
Glutamic Acid 664
Glutamic Acid Hydrochloride *see* Glutamic Acid 664
Glutathione 1432
Glutol™ [OTC] *see* Glucose (Instant) 663
Glutose™ [OTC] *see* Glucose (Instant) 663
Glybenclamide *see* GlyBURIDE 664
Glybenzcyclamide *see* GlyBURIDE 664
GlyBURIDE 664
Glyburide and Metformin 665
Glyburide and Metformin Hydrochloride *see* Glyburide and Metformin 665
Glycerin 667
Glycerol *see* Glycerin 667
Glycerol Guaiacolate *see* Guaifenesin 672
Glycerol Triacetate *see* Triacetin . . 1329
Glyceryl Trinitrate *see* Nitroglycerin 991
Glycocome *see* Licorice 1440
Glycon (Can) *see* Metformin 887
Glycopyrrolate 668
Glycopyrronium Bromide *see* Glycopyrrolate 668
Glycyrrhiza glabra *see* Licorice 1440
Glydiazinamide *see* GlipiZIDE 660
Glynase® PresTab® *see* GlyBURIDE 664
Gly-Oxide® [OTC] *see* Carbamide Peroxide 259
Glyquin® *see* Hydroquinone 719
Glyquin® XM (Can) *see* Hydroquinone 719
Glyset® (Can) *see* Miglitol 929
GM-CSF *see* Sargramostim 1209
GnRH *see* Gonadorelin 669
Goatweed *see* St John's Wort 1447
Gold Bond® Antifungal [OTC] *see* Tolnaftate 1312
Golden Seal 1433
Gold Sodium Thiomalate 668
GoLYTELY® *see* Polyethylene Glycol-Electrolyte Solution . . . 1100
Gonadorelin 669
Gonadorelin Acetate *see* Gonadorelin 669
Gonadorelin Hydrochloride *see* Gonadorelin 669
Gonadotropin Releasing Hormone *see* Gonadorelin 669
Gonak™ [OTC] *see* Hydroxypropyl Methylcellulose 721
Gonal-F® (Can) *see* Follitropins 626
Gonioscopic Ophthalmic Solution *see* Hydroxypropyl Methylcellulose 721
Goniosol® [OTC] *see* Hydroxypropyl Methylcellulose . . 721
Goody's® Extra Strength Headache Powder [OTC] *see* Acetaminophen, Aspirin, and Caffeine 56
Goody's® Extra Strength Pain Relief [OTC] *see* Acetaminophen, Aspirin, and Caffeine 56
Goody's PM® Powder *see* Acetaminophen and Diphenhydramine 53
Gopten® (Mex) *see* Trandolapril . . . 1321
Gordofilm® [OTC] *see* Salicylic Acid 1205
Gormel® [OTC] *see* Urea 1353
Goserelin 670
Goserelin Acetate *see* Goserelin . . . 670
Gotu Kola 1434
GP 47680 *see* Oxcarbazepine 1023
G-Phed *see* Guaifenesin and Pseudoephedrine 675
G-Phed-PD *see* Guaifenesin and Pseudoephedrine 675
GR38032R *see* Ondansetron 1014
Gramicidin, Neomycin, and Polymyxin B *see* Neomycin, Polymyxin B, and Gramicidin . . . 974
Granisetron 671
Granulex® *see* Trypsin, Balsam Peru, and Castor Oil 1349
Granulocyte Colony Stimulating Factor *see* Filgrastim 589
Granulocyte Colony Stimulating Factor (PEG Conjugate) *see* Pegfilgrastim 1052
Granulocyte-Macrophage Colony Stimulating Factor *see* Sargramostim 1209
Grapefruit Seed 1434
Grape Seed 1435
Grape Skin 1436
Graten® [inj.] (Mex) *see* Morphine Sulfate 947
Gravol® (Can) *see* DimenhyDRINATE 446
Green Tea 1436
Grifulvin® V *see* Griseofulvin 671
Griseofulvin 671

Griseofulvin Microsize *see* Griseofulvin 671
Griseofulvin Ultramicrosize *see* Griseofulvin 671
Grisovin® (Mex) *see* Griseofulvin . . . 671
Gris-PEG® *see* Griseofulvin 671
Growth Hormone *see* Human Growth Hormone 694
Grunicina® (Mex) *see* Amoxicillin . . . 114
GSE *see* Grapefruit Seed 1434
Guaifed® [OTC] *see* Guaifenesin and Pseudoephedrine 675
Guaifed-PD® *see* Guaifenesin and Pseudoephedrine 675
Guaifenesin 672
Guaifenesin and Codeine 673
Guaifenesin and Dextromethorphan 673
Guaifenesin and Hydrocodone *see* Hydrocodone and Guaifenesin . . 708
Guaifenesin and Phenylephrine 674
Guaifenesin and Potassium Guaiacolsulfonate 675
Guaifenesin and Pseudoephedrine . . 675
Guaifenesin and Theophylline *see* Theophylline and Guaifenesin 1286
Guaifenesin, Hydrocodone, and Pseudoephedrine *see* Hydrocodone, Pseudoephedrine, and Guaifenesin 713
Guaifenesin, Potassium Guaiacolsulfonate, and Dextromethorphan 675
Guaifenesin, Pseudoephedrine, and Codeine 676
Guaifenesin, Pseudoephedrine, and Dextromethorphan 676
Guaifenex® DM *see* Guaifenesin and Dextromethorphan 673
Guaifenex® GP *see* Guaifenesin and Pseudoephedrine 675
Guaifenex® PSE *see* Guaifenesin and Pseudoephedrine 675
Guaifenex™-Rx DM *see* Guaifenesin, Pseudoephedrine, and Dextromethorphan 676
Guaifen PSE *see* Guaifenesin and Pseudoephedrine 675
Guaituss AC® *see* Guaifenesin and Codeine 673
Guai-Vent™/PSE *see* Guaifenesin and Pseudoephedrine 675
Guanabenz 677
Guanabenz Acetate *see* Guanabenz 677
Guanadrel 678
Guanadrel Sulfate *see* Guanadrel . . 678
Guanfacine 679
Guanfacine Hydrochloride *see* Guanfacine 679
Guanidine 679
Guanidine Hydrochloride *see* Guanidine 679
Guiatuss™ [OTC] *see* Guaifenesin . . 672
Guiatuss™ DAC® *see* Guaifenesin, Pseudoephedrine, and Codeine 676
Guiatuss-DM® [OTC] *see* Guaifenesin and Dextromethorphan 673
Gum Benjamin *see* Benzoin 193
GW433908G *see* Fosamprenavir . . . 630
Gynazole-1® *see* Butoconazole 239
Gyne-Lotrimin® 3 [OTC] *see* Clotrimazole 363
Gynodiol® *see* Estradiol 518
Gynol II® [OTC] *see* Nonoxynol 9 . . 995
Gyno-Myfungar® (Mex) *see* Oxiconazole 1024
Habitrol® (Can) *see* Nicotine 981
Haemophilus b Conjugate Vaccine . . 680
Haemophilus b Oligosaccharide Conjugate Vaccine *see* *Haemophilus* b Conjugate Vaccine 680
Haemophilus b Polysaccharide Vaccine *see* *Haemophilus* b Conjugate Vaccine 680
HAES-steril® (Mex) *see* Hetastarch 692
Halcinonide 681
Halcion® *see* Triazolam 1335
Haldol® (Mex) *see* Haloperidol 682
Haldol decanoas® (Mex) *see* Haloperidol 682
Haldol® Decanoate *see* Haloperidol 682
Haley's M-O *see* Magnesium Hydroxide and Mineral Oil 853
Halfprin® [OTC] *see* Aspirin 151
Halobetasol 681
Halobetasol Propionate *see* Halobetasol 681
Halofantrine 681
Halofantrine Hydrochloride *see* Halofantrine 681
Halog® *see* Halcinonide 681
Halog®-E [DSC] *see* Halcinonide . . . 681
Haloperidol 682
Haloperidol Decanoate *see* Haloperidol 682
Haloperidol Lactate *see* Haloperidol 682
Haloperidol-LA Omega (Can) *see* Haloperidol 682
Haloperidol Long Acting (Can) *see* Haloperidol 682
Haloperil® (Mex) *see* Haloperidol . . . 682
Halotestin® *see* Fluoxymesterone . . . 609
Halotussin AC *see* Guaifenesin and Codeine 673
Halotussin® DAC *see* Guaifenesin, Pseudoephedrine, and Codeine 676
Haltran® [OTC] [DSC] *see* Ibuprofen 728
HandClens® [OTC] *see* Benzalkonium Chloride 190
Harpagophytum procumbens see Devil's Claw 1422
Havrix® *see* Hepatitis A Vaccine . . . 687
Havrix® and Engerix-B® *see* Hepatitis A (Inactivated) and Hepatitis B (Recombinant) Vaccine 686
Haw *see* Hawthorn 1437
Hawthorn 1437
Hayfebrol® [OTC] *see* Chlorpheniramine and Pseudoephedrine 315
HbCV *see* *Haemophilus* b Conjugate Vaccine 680
HBIG *see* Hepatitis B Immune Globulin 688
hBNP *see* Nesiritide 976
25-HCC *see* Calcifediol 242
hCG *see* Chorionic Gonadotropin (Human) 326
HCTZ *see* Hydrochlorothiazide 699
HCTZ and Telmisartan *see* Telmisartan and Hydrochlorothiazide 1265
HDA® Toothache [OTC] *see* Benzocaine 191
HDCV *see* Rabies Virus Vaccine . . 1165
Head & Shoulders® Classic Clean [OTC] *see* Pyrithione Zinc 1155
Head & Shoulders® Classic Clean 2-In-1 [OTC] *see* Pyrithione Zinc 1155

Head & Shoulders® Dry Scalp Care [OTC] *see* Pyrithione Zinc . . . 1155
Head & Shoulders® Extra Fullness [OTC] *see* Pyrithione Zinc . . . 1155
Head & Shoulders® Refresh [OTC] *see* Pyrithione Zinc . . . 1155
Head & Shoulders® Smooth & Silky 2-In-1 [OTC] *see* Pyrithione Zinc . . . 1155
Healon® (Can) *see* Hyaluronate and Derivatives . . . 696
Healon®5 *see* Hyaluronate and Derivatives . . . 696
Healon GV® (Can) *see* Hyaluronate and Derivatives . . . 696
Hectorol® *see* Doxercalciferol . . . 468
Helidac® *see* Bismuth Subsalicylate, Metronidazole, and Tetracycline . . . 209
Helistat® *see* Microfibrillar Collagen Hemostat . . . 923
Helixate® FS (Can) *see* Antihemophilic Factor (Recombinant) . . . 135
Hemabate® (Can) *see* Carboprost Tromethamine . . . 265
Hemiacidrin *see* Citric Acid, Magnesium Carbonate, and Glucono-Delta-Lactone . . . 341
Hemin . . . 684
Hemobion® (Mex) *see* Ferrous Sulfate . . . 586
Hemocyte® [OTC] *see* Ferrous Fumarate . . . 586
Hemodent® Gingival Retraction Cord *see* Aluminum Chloride . . . 90
Hemofil® M (Can) *see* Antihemophilic Factor (Human) . . . 134
Hemril-HC® *see* Hydrocortisone . . . 714
Hepalean® (Can) *see* Heparin . . . 685
Hepalean® Leo (Can) *see* Heparin . . 685
Hepalean®-LOK (Can) *see* Heparin . . . 685
Heparin . . . 685
Heparin Calcium *see* Heparin . . . 685
Heparin Cofactor I *see* Antithrombin III . . . 136
Heparin Lock Flush *see* Heparin . . . 685
Heparin Sodium *see* Heparin . . . 685
Hepatitis A (Inactivated) and Hepatitis B (Recombinant) Vaccine . . . 686
Hepatitis A Vaccine . . . 687
Hepatitis B Immune Globulin . . . 688
Hepatitis B Inactivated Virus Vaccine (plasma derived) *see* Hepatitis B Vaccine . . . 689
Hepatitis B Inactivated Virus Vaccine (recombinant DNA) *see* Hepatitis B Vaccine . . . 689
Hepatitis B (Recombinant) and Hepatitis A Inactivated Vaccine *see* Hepatitis A (Inactivated) and Hepatitis B (Recombinant) Vaccine . . . 686
Hepatitis B Vaccine . . . 689
Hep-Lock® *see* Heparin . . . 685
Hepsera™ *see* Adefovir . . . 68
Heptovir® (Can) *see* Lamivudine . . . 794
Herceptin® (Can) *see* Trastuzumab . . . 1324
Herklin Shampoo® (Mex) *see* Lindane . . . 829
HES *see* Hetastarch . . . 692
Hespan® *see* Hetastarch . . . 692
Hetastarch . . . 692
Hexachlorocyclohexane *see* Lindane . . . 829
Hexachlorophene . . . 693
Hexalen® (Can) *see* Altretamine . . . 89
Hexamethylenetetramine *see* Methenamine . . . 892
Hexamethylmelamine *see* Altretamine . . . 89
Hexit™ (Can) *see* Lindane . . . 829
HEXM *see* Altretamine . . . 89
Hextend® *see* Hetastarch . . . 692
Hexylresorcinol . . . 693
Hibiclens® [OTC] *see* Chlorhexidine Gluconate . . . 308
Hibidil® 1:2000 (Can) *see* Chlorhexidine Gluconate . . . 308
Hibistat® [OTC] *see* Chlorhexidine Gluconate . . . 308
Hib Polysaccharide Conjugate *see* *Haemophilus* b Conjugate Vaccine . . . 680
HibTITER® *see* *Haemophilus* b Conjugate Vaccine . . . 680
Hidantoina® (Mex) *see* Phenytoin . . 1080
Hidramox® (Mex) *see* Amoxicillin . . . 114
Hidroquin® (Mex) *see* Hydroquinone . . . 719
Hipocol® (Mex) *see* Niacin . . . 978
Hipokinon® (Mex) *see* Trihexyphenidyl . . . 1340
Hiprex® *see* Methenamine . . . 892
Hirulog *see* Bivalirudin . . . 212
Histatab® Plus [OTC] *see* Chlorpheniramine and Phenylephrine . . . 314
Hista-Vent® DA *see* Chlorpheniramine, Phenylephrine, and Methscopolamine . . . 317
Histex™ *see* Chlorpheniramine and Pseudoephedrine . . . 315
Histex™ CT *see* Carbinoxamine . . . 262
Histex™ HC *see* Hydrocodone, Carbinoxamine, and Pseudoephedrine . . . 712
Histex™ I/E *see* Carbinoxamine . . . 262
Histex™ PD *see* Carbinoxamine . . . 262
Histex™ SR *see* Brompheniramine and Pseudoephedrine . . . 220
Histussin D® *see* Hydrocodone and Pseudoephedrine . . . 711
Hi-Vegi-Lip® [OTC] *see* Pancreatin . . . 1042
Hivid® (Mex) *see* Zalcitabine . . . 1395
HIV Infection and AIDS . . . 1484
HMG Massone® [inj.] (Mex) *see* Menotropins . . . 868
HMM *see* Altretamine . . . 89
HMR 3647 *see* Telithromycin . . . 1263
HMS Liquifilm® *see* Medrysone . . . 863
Hold® DM [OTC] *see* Dextromethorphan . . . 421
Homatropine . . . 693
Homatropine and Hydrocodone *see* Hydrocodone and Homatropine . . . 709
Homatropine Hydrobromide *see* Homatropine . . . 693
Horse Antihuman Thymocyte Gamma Globulin *see* Antithymocyte Globulin (Equine) . . . 136
Horse Chestnut . . . 1437
H.P. Acthar® Gel *see* Corticotropin . . . 376
Hp-PAC® (Can) *see* Lansoprazole, Amoxicillin, and Clarithromycin . . 798
HTF919 *see* Tegaserod . . . 1263
hu1124 *see* Efalizumab . . . 483
Humalog® *see* Insulin Preparations . . . 749
Humalog® Mix 25™ (Can) *see* Insulin Preparations . . . 749

Humalog® Mix 75/25™ *see* Insulin Preparations . . . 749
Human Antitumor Necrosis Factor-alpha *see* Adalimumab . . . 67
Human Diploid Cell Cultures Rabies Vaccine *see* Rabies Virus Vaccine . . . 1165
Human Growth Hormone . . . 694
Humanized IgG1 Anti-CD52 Monoclonal Antibody *see* Alemtuzumab . . . 76
Human LFA-3/IgG(1) Fusion Protein *see* Alefacept . . . 76
Human Thyroid Stimulating Hormone *see* Thyrotropin Alpha . . . 1294
Humate-P® (Can) *see* Antihemophilic Factor (Human) . . . 134
Humatin® (Can) *see* Paromomycin . . . 1046
Humatrope® *see* Human Growth Hormone . . . 694
Humegon® (Can) *see* Chorionic Gonadotropin (Human) . . . 326
Humegon® (Mex) *see* Menotropins . . . 868
Humibid® DM *see* Guaifenesin and Dextromethorphan . . . 673
Humibid® DM *(reformulation) see* Guaifenesin, Potassium Guaiacolsulfonate, and Dextromethorphan . . . 675
Humibid® LA [DSC] *see* Guaifenesin . . . 672
Humibid® LA *(reformulation) see* Guaifenesin and Potassium Guaiacolsulfonate . . . 675
Humibid® Pediatric [DSC] *see* Guaifenesin . . . 672
Humira™ *see* Adalimumab . . . 67
Humulin® (Can) *see* Insulin Preparations . . . 749
Humulin 20/80® [biosyn./ 20% sol./80% isoph.] (Mex) *see* Insulin Preparations . . . 749
Humulin 30/70® [biosyn./ 30% sol./70% isoph.] (Mex) *see* Insulin Preparations . . . 749
Humulin® 50/50 *see* Insulin Preparations . . . 749
Humulin® 70/30 *see* Insulin Preparations . . . 749
Humulin® L *see* Insulin Preparations . . . 749
Humulin L® [biosyn.] (Mex) *see* Insulin Preparations . . . 749
Humulin® N *see* Insulin Preparations . . . 749
Humulin N® [biosyn.] (Mex) *see* Insulin Preparations . . . 749
Humulin® R *see* Insulin Preparations . . . 749
Humulin® R (Concentrated) U-500 *see* Insulin Preparations . . . 749
Humulin® U *see* Insulin Preparations . . . 749
Huperzia serrata see HuperzineA . . . 1438
HuperzineA . . . 1438
Hurricaine® *see* Benzocaine . . . 191
HXM *see* Altretamine . . . 89
Hyalgan® *see* Hyaluronate and Derivatives . . . 696
Hyaluronan *see* Hyaluronate and Derivatives . . . 696
Hyaluronate and Derivatives . . . 696
Hyaluronic Acid *see* Hyaluronate and Derivatives . . . 696
Hyaluronidase . . . 697
Hyate:C® *see* Antihemophilic Factor (Porcine) . . . 134
Hycamptamine *see* Topotecan . . . 1316
Hycamtin™ (Can) *see* Topotecan . . . 1316
hycet™ *see* Hydrocodone and Acetaminophen . . . 702
Hycoclear Tuss *see* Hydrocodone and Guaifenesin . . . 708
Hycodan® *see* Hydrocodone and Homatropine . . . 709
Hycomine® Compound *see* Hydrocodone, Chlorpheniramine, Phenylephrine, Acetaminophen, and Caffeine . . . 712
Hycort™ (Can) *see* Hydrocortisone . . . 714
Hycosin *see* Hydrocodone and Guaifenesin . . . 708
Hycotuss® *see* Hydrocodone and Guaifenesin . . . 708
Hydeltra T.B.A.® (Can) *see* PrednisoLONE . . . 1113
Hydergine [DSC] *see* Ergoloid Mesylates . . . 504
Hyderm (Can) *see* Hydrocortisone . . . 714
HydrALAZINE . . . 697
Hydralazine and Hydrochlorothiazide . . . 698
Hydralazine Hydrochloride *see* HydrALAZINE . . . 697
Hydralazine, Hydrochlorothiazide, and Reserpine . . . 698
Hydramine® [OTC] *see* DiphenhydrAMINE . . . 448
Hydramine® Cough [OTC] *see* DiphenhydrAMINE . . . 448
Hydrastis canadensis see Golden Seal . . . 1433
Hydrate® [DSC] *see* DimenhyDRINATE . . . 446
Hydrated Chloral *see* Chloral Hydrate . . . 304
Hydrea® *see* Hydroxyurea . . . 722
Hydrisalic™ [OTC] *see* Salicylic Acid . . . 1205
Hydrochlorothiazide . . . 699
Hydrochlorothiazide and Amiloride *see* Amiloride and Hydrochlorothiazide . . . 96
Hydrochlorothiazide and Benazepril *see* Benazepril and Hydrochlorothiazide . . . 189
Hydrochlorothiazide and Bisoprolol *see* Bisoprolol and Hydrochlorothiazide . . . 211
Hydrochlorothiazide and Captopril *see* Captopril and Hydrochlorothiazide . . . 255
Hydrochlorothiazide and Enalapril *see* Enalapril and Hydrochlorothiazide . . . 491
Hydrochlorothiazide and Eprosartan *see* Eprosartan and Hydrochlorothiazide . . . 502
Hydrochlorothiazide and Fosinopril *see* Fosinopril and Hydrochlorothiazide . . . 635
Hydrochlorothiazide and Hydralazine *see* Hydralazine and Hydrochlorothiazide . . . 698
Hydrochlorothiazide and Irbesartan *see* Irbesartan and Hydrochlorothiazide . . . 764
Hydrochlorothiazide and Lisinopril *see* Lisinopril and Hydrochlorothiazide . . . 834
Hydrochlorothiazide and Losartan *see* Losartan and Hydrochlorothiazide . . . 847

Hydrochlorothiazide and Methyldopa *see* Methyldopa and Hydrochlorothiazide 906
Hydrochlorothiazide and Moexipril *see* Moexipril and Hydrochlorothiazide 941
Hydrochlorothiazide and Olmesartan Medoxomil *see* Olmesartan and Hydrochlorothiazide 1010
Hydrochlorothiazide and Propranolol *see* Propranolol and Hydrochlorothiazide 1143
Hydrochlorothiazide and Quinapril *see* Quinapril and Hydrochlorothiazide 1160
Hydrochlorothiazide and Spironolactone 701
Hydrochlorothiazide and Telmisartan *see* Telmisartan and Hydrochlorothiazide 1265
Hydrochlorothiazide and Triamterene 701
Hydrochlorothiazide and Valsartan *see* Valsartan and Hydrochlorothiazide 1364
Hydrochlorothiazide, Hydralazine, and Reserpine *see* Hydralazine, Hydrochlorothiazide, and Reserpine 698
Hydrocil® [OTC] *see* Psyllium 1151
Hydrocodone and Acetaminophen . . 702
Hydrocodone and Aspirin 705
Hydrocodone and Chlorpheniramine 707
Hydrocodone and Guaifenesin 708
Hydrocodone and Homatropine 709
Hydrocodone and Ibuprofen 709
Hydrocodone and Pseudoephedrine 711
Hydrocodone Bitartrate, Carbinoxamine Maleate, and Pseudoephedrine Hydrochloride *see* Hydrocodone, Carbinoxamine, and Pseudoephedrine 712
Hydrocodone Bitartrate, Phenylephrine Hydrochloride, and Diphenhydramine Hydrochloride *see* Hydrocodone, Phenylephrine, and Diphenhydramine 713
Hydrocodone, Carbinoxamine, and Pseudoephedrine 712
Hydrocodone, Chlorpheniramine, Phenylephrine, Acetaminophen, and Caffeine . . 712
Hydrocodone, Phenylephrine, and Diphenhydramine 713
Hydrocodone, Pseudoephedrine, and Guaifenesin 713
Hydrocortisone 714
Hydrocortisone Acetate *see* Hydrocortisone 714
Hydrocortisone, Acetic Acid, and Propylene Glycol Diacetate *see* Acetic Acid, Propylene Glycol Diacetate, and Hydrocortisone . . . 60
Hydrocortisone and Benzoyl Peroxide *see* Benzoyl Peroxide and Hydrocortisone 194
Hydrocortisone and Ciprofloxacin *see* Ciprofloxacin and Hydrocortisone 336
Hydrocortisone and Iodoquinol *see* Iodoquinol and Hydrocortisone . . 759
Hydrocortisone and Lidocaine *see* Lidocaine and Hydrocortisone . . 826
Hydrocortisone and Oxytetracycline *see* Oxytetracycline and Hydrocortisone 1037
Hydrocortisone and Pramoxine *see* Pramoxine and Hydrocortisone 1109
Hydrocortisone and Urea *see* Urea and Hydrocortisone 1353
Hydrocortisone, Bacitracin, Neomycin, and Polymyxin B *see* Bacitracin, Neomycin, Polymyxin B, and Hydrocortisone 179
Hydrocortisone Buteprate *see* Hydrocortisone 714
Hydrocortisone Butyrate *see* Hydrocortisone 714
Hydrocortisone Cypionate *see* Hydrocortisone 714
Hydrocortisone, Neomycin, and Polymyxin B *see* Neomycin, Polymyxin B, and Hydrocortisone 975
Hydrocortisone, Propylene Glycol Diacetate, and Acetic Acid *see* Acetic Acid, Propylene Glycol Diacetate, and Hydrocortisone . . . 60
Hydrocortisone Sodium Phosphate *see* Hydrocortisone 714
Hydrocortisone Sodium Succinate *see* Hydrocortisone 714
Hydrocortisone Valerate *see* Hydrocortisone 714
Hydrocortone® [DSC] *see* Hydrocortisone 714
Hydrocortone® Phosphate *see* Hydrocortisone 714
Hydromet® *see* Hydrocodone and Homatropine 709
Hydromorph Contin® (Can) *see* Hydromorphone 718
Hydromorphone 718
Hydromorphone HP (Can) *see* Hydromorphone 718
Hydromorphone Hydrochloride *see* Hydromorphone 718
Hydropane® *see* Hydrocodone and Homatropine 709
Hydroquinol *see* Hydroquinone 719
Hydroquinone 719
Hydroquinone, Fluocinolone Acetonide, and Tretinoin *see* Fluocinolone, Hydroquinone, and Tretinoin 601
Hydro-Tussin™-CBX *see* Carbinoxamine and Pseudoephedrine 262
Hydro-Tussin™ DHC *see* Pseudoephedrine, Dihydrocodeine, and Chlorpheniramine 1150
Hydro-Tussin™ DM *see* Guaifenesin and Dextromethorphan 673
Hydro-Tussin™ HD *see* Hydrocodone, Pseudoephedrine, and Guaifenesin 713
Hydro-Tussin™ XP *see* Hydrocodone, Pseudoephedrine, and Guaifenesin 713
HydroVal® (Can) *see* Hydrocortisone 714
Hydroxocobalamin 719
Hydroxyamphetamine and Tropicamide 720
Hydroxyamphetamine Hydrobromide and Tropicamide *see* Hydroxyamphetamine and Tropicamide 720

4-Hydroxybutyrate *see* Sodium Oxybate . . . 1229
Hydroxycarbamide *see* Hydroxyurea . . . 722
Hydroxychloroquine . . . 720
Hydroxychloroquine Sulfate *see* Hydroxychloroquine . . . 720
25-Hydroxycholecalciferol *see* Calcifediol . . . 242
Hydroxydaunomycin Hydrochloride *see* DOXOrubicin . . . 469
1α-Hydroxyergocalciferol *see* Doxercalciferol . . . 468
Hydroxyethylcellulose *see* Artificial Tears . . . 148
Hydroxyethyl Starch *see* Hetastarch . . . 692
Hydroxyldaunorubicin Hydrochloride *see* DOXOrubicin . . . 469
Hydroxypropyl Cellulose . . . 721
Hydroxypropyl Methylcellulose . . . 721
Hydroxyurea . . . 722
25-Hydroxyvitamin D_3 *see* Calcifediol . . . 242
HydrOXYzine . . . 723
Hydroxyzine Hydrochloride *see* HydrOXYzine . . . 723
Hydroxyzine Pamoate *see* HydrOXYzine . . . 723
Hygroton *see* Chlorthalidone . . . 321
Hylaform® *see* Hyaluronate and Derivatives . . . 696
Hylan Polymers *see* Hyaluronate and Derivatives . . . 696
Hylorel® *see* Guanadrel . . . 678
Hyoscine *see* Scopolamine . . . 1210
Hyoscyamine . . . 724
Hyoscyamine, Atropine, Scopolamine, and Phenobarbital . . . 725
Hyoscyamine, Atropine, Scopolamine, Kaolin, and Pectin . . . 726
Hyoscyamine, Atropine, Scopolamine, Kaolin, Pectin, and Opium . . . 726
Hyoscyamine, Methenamine, Sodium Biphosphate, Phenyl Salicylate, and Methylene Blue *see* Methenamine, Sodium Biphosphate, Phenyl Salicylate, Methylene Blue, and Hyoscyamine . . . 893
Hyoscyamine Sulfate *see* Hyoscyamine . . . 724
Hyosine *see* Hyoscyamine . . . 724
Hypercium perforatum see St John's Wort . . . 1447
Hyperstat® *see* Diazoxide . . . 425
Hyperstat® I.V. (Can) *see* Diazoxide . . . 425
HypoTears [OTC] *see* Artificial Tears . . . 148
HypoTears PF [OTC] *see* Artificial Tears . . . 148
Hypromellose *see* Hydroxypropyl Methylcellulose . . . 721
Hyrexin-50® *see* DiphenhydrAMINE . . . 448
Hytakerol® (Can) *see* Dihydrotachysterol . . . 443
Hytinic® [OTC] *see* Polysaccharide-Iron Complex . . 1101
Hytone® *see* Hydrocortisone . . . 714
Hytrin® (Can) *see* Terazosin . . . 1271
Hyzaar® (Can) *see* Losartan and Hydrochlorothiazide . . . 847
Hyzaar® DS (Can) *see* Losartan and Hydrochlorothiazide . . . 847
Iberet® [OTC] *see* Vitamins (Multiple/Oral) . . . 1384
Iberet®-500 [OTC] *see* Vitamins (Multiple/Oral) . . . 1384
Iberet-Folic-500® *see* Vitamins (Multiple/Oral) . . . 1384
Ibidomide Hydrochloride *see* Labetalol . . . 791
Ibritumomab . . . 727
Ibritumomab Tiuxetan *see* Ibritumomab . . . 727
Ibu-200 [OTC] *see* Ibuprofen . . . 728
Ibuprofen . . . 728
Ibuprofen and Hydrocodone *see* Hydrocodone and Ibuprofen . . . 709
Ibuprofen and Pseudoephedrine *see* Pseudoephedrine and Ibuprofen . . . 1149
Ibutilide . . . 731
Ibutilide Fumarate *see* Ibutilide . . . 731
IC-Green® *see* Indocyanine Green . . 745
ICI 182,780 *see* Fulvestrant . . . 639
ICI 204, 219 *see* Zafirlukast . . . 1394
ICI-46474 *see* Tamoxifen . . . 1258
ICI-118630 *see* Goserelin . . . 670
ICI-176334 *see* Bicalutamide . . . 206
ICI-D1033 *see* Anastrozole . . . 132
ICRF-187 *see* Dexrazoxane . . . 417
I.D.A. *see* Acetaminophen, Isometheptene, and Dichloralphenazone . . . 59
Idamycin® (Can) *see* Idarubicin . . . 732
Idamycin PFS® *see* Idarubicin . . . 732
Idarubicin . . . 732
Idarubicin Hydrochloride *see* Idarubicin . . . 732
IDEC-C2B8 *see* Rituximab . . . 1191
IDR *see* Idarubicin . . . 732
Ifa Norex® (Mex) *see* Diethylpropion . . . 434
Ifa Reducing "S"® (Mex) *see* Phentermine . . . 1076
Ifex® *see* Ifosfamide . . . 733
IFLrA *see* Interferon Alfa-2a . . . 751
Ifolem® (Mex) *see* Ifosfamide . . . 733
Ifosfamide . . . 733
Ifoxan® (Mex) *see* Ifosfamide . . . 733
IG *see* Immune Globulin (Intramuscular) . . . 739
IGIM *see* Immune Globulin (Intramuscular) . . . 739
Ikatin® (Mex) *see* Gentamicin . . . 655
IL-1Ra *see* Anakinra . . . 131
IL-2 *see* Aldesleukin . . . 74
IL-11 *see* Oprelvekin . . . 1015
Iletin® II Pork (Can) *see* Insulin Preparations . . . 749
Iliadin® (Mex) *see* Oxymetazoline . . 1034
Ilosone® (Mex) *see* Erythromycin . . . 508
Ilsatec® (Mex) *see* Lansoprazole . . . 797
Imatinib . . . 734
Imatinib Mesylate *see* Imatinib . . . 734
IMC-C225 *see* Cetuximab . . . 300
Imdur® (Can) *see* Isosorbide Mononitrate . . . 771
IMI 30 *see* Idarubicin . . . 732
Imidazol Carboxamide Dimethyltriazene *see* Dacarbazine . . . 392
Imidazole Carboxamide *see* Dacarbazine . . . 392
Imiglucerase . . . 736
Imigran® (Mex) *see* Sumatriptan . . 1252
Imipemide *see* Imipenem and Cilastatin . . . 736
Imipenem and Cilastatin . . . 736
Imipramine . . . 737
Imipramine Hydrochloride *see* Imipramine . . . 737
Imipramine Pamoate *see* Imipramine . . . 737

Imiquimod 738
Imitrex® (Can) *see* Sumatriptan . . . 1252
ImmuCyst® (Can) *see* BCG Vaccine 183
Immune Globulin (Intramuscular) . . . 739
Immune Globulin (Intravenous) 740
Immune Serum Globulin *see* Immune Globulin (Intramuscular) 739
Immunine® VH (Can) *see* Factor IX 571
Immunizations (Vaccines) 1614
Imodium® (Can) *see* Loperamide . . . 838
Imodium® A-D [OTC] *see* Loperamide 838
Imogam® *see* Rabies Immune Globulin (Human) 1165
Imogam® Rabies Pasteurized (Can) *see* Rabies Immune Globulin (Human) 1165
Imovane® (Mex) *see* Zopiclone . . . 1406
Imovax® Rabies *see* Rabies Virus Vaccine 1165
Imuran® *see* Azathioprine 172
In-111 Zevalin *see* Ibritumomab 727
Inamrinone 743
Inapsine® *see* Droperidol 477
Indapamide 743
Indarzona® (Mex) *see* Dexamethasone 411
Inderal® (Can) *see* Propranolol . . . 1140
Inderal® LA *see* Propranolol 1140
Inderide® *see* Propranolol and Hydrochlorothiazide 1143
Indian Eye *see* Golden Seal 1433
Indian Head *see Echinacea* 1423
Indinavir 744
Indinavir Sulfate *see* Indinavir 744
Indocid® (Mex) *see* Indomethacin . . . 746
Indocid® P.D.A. (Can) *see* Indomethacin 746
Indocin® *see* Indomethacin 746
Indocin® I.V. *see* Indomethacin 746
Indocin® SR *see* Indomethacin 746
Indocyanine Green 745
Indo-Lemmon (Can) *see* Indomethacin 746
Indometacin *see* Indomethacin 746
Indomethacin 746
Indomethacin Sodium Trihydrate *see* Indomethacin 746
Indotec (Can) *see* Indomethacin . . . 746
INF-alpha 2 *see* Interferon Alfa-2b . . 752
Infants' Tylenol® Cold Plus Cough Concentrated Drops [OTC] *see* Acetaminophen, Dextromethorphan, and Pseudoephedrine 59
Infasurf® *see* Calfactant 247
INFeD® *see* Iron Dextran Complex 766
Inflamase® Forte (Can) *see* PrednisoLONE 1113
Inflamase® Mild (Can) *see* PrednisoLONE 1113
Infliximab 747
Infliximab, Recombinant *see* Infliximab 747
Influenza Virus Vaccine 748
Influenza Virus Vaccine (Purified Surface Antigen) *see* Influenza Virus Vaccine 748
Influenza Virus Vaccine (Split-Virus) *see* Influenza Virus Vaccine 748
Influenza Virus Vaccine (Trivalent, Live) *see* Influenza Virus Vaccine 748
Infufer® (Can) *see* Iron Dextran Complex 766
Infumorph® *see* Morphine Sulfate . . . 947
INH *see* Isoniazid 769
Inhibace® (Can) *see* Cilazapril 328
Inhibitron® (Mex) *see* Omeprazole 1012
Inibace® (Mex) *see* Cilazapril 328
Innohep® (Can) *see* Tinzaparin . . . 1301
InnoPran XL™ *see* Propranolol . . . 1140
INOmax® *see* Nitric Oxide 990
Insect Sting Kit *see* Epinephrine and Chlorpheniramine 497
Insogen® (Mex) *see* ChlorproPAMIDE 321
Insoluble Prussian Blue *see* Ferric Hexacyanoferrate 585
Inspiryl® (Mex) *see* Albuterol 71
Inspra™ *see* Eplerenone 498
Insta-Glucose® [OTC] *see* Glucose (Instant) 663
Insulin Novolin 30/70® [biosyn./ 30% sol./70% isoph.] (Mex) *see* Insulin Preparations 749
Insulin Novolin L® [biosyn.] (Mex) *see* Insulin Preparations 749
Insulin Novolin N® [biosyn.] (Mex) *see* Insulin Preparations 749
Insulin Preparations 749
Intal® (Can) *see* Cromolyn 378
Integrilin® *see* Eptifibatide 503
α-2-interferon *see* Interferon Alfa-2b 752
Interferon Alfa-2a 751
Interferon Alfa-2a (PEG Conjugate) *see* Peginterferon Alfa-2a 1052
Interferon Alfa-2b 752
Interferon Alfa-2b and Ribavirin 754
Interferon Alfa-2b and Ribavirin Combination Pack *see* Interferon Alfa-2b and Ribavirin 754
Interferon Alfa-2b (PEG Conjugate) *see* Peginterferon Alfa-2b 1053
Interferon Alfa-n3 755
Interferon Beta-1a 756
Interferon Beta-1b 757
Interferon Gamma-1b 758
Interleukin-1 Receptor antagonist *see* Anakinra 131
Interleukin-2 *see* Aldesleukin 74
Interleukin-11 *see* Oprelvekin 1015
Intralipid® *see* Fat Emulsion 575
Intravenous Fat Emulsion *see* Fat Emulsion 575
Intrifiban *see* Eptifibatide 503
Intron® A *see* Interferon Alfa-2b 752
Invanz® (Can) *see* Ertapenem 507
Inversine® *see* Mecamylamine 859
Invirase® (Mex) *see* Saquinavir . . . 1207
Iodex [OTC] *see* Iodine 758
Iodine 758
Iodine *see* Trace Metals 1319
Iodoflex™ *see* Iodine 758
Iodopen® *see* Trace Metals 1319
Iodoquinol 759
Iodoquinol and Hydrocortisone 759
Iodosorb® *see* Iodine 758
Iohexol *see* Radiological/Contrast Media (Nonionic) 1166
Ionamin® *see* Phentermine 1076
Ionil® (Mex) *see* Salicylic Acid 1205
Ionil® Plus [OTC] *see* Salicylic Acid 1205
Ionil T® [OTC] *see* Coal Tar 367
Ionil T® Plus [OTC] *see* Coal Tar . . . 367
Iopamidol *see* Radiological/ Contrast Media (Nonionic) 1166
Iophen NR *see* Guaifenesin 672
Iopidine® (Can) *see* Apraclonidine . . 138
Iopromide 760
Iosat™ [OTC] *see* Potassium Iodide 1106

Ioversol *see* Radiological/Contrast Media (Nonionic) 1166
Ipecac Syrup 760
IPM Wound Gel™ [OTC] *see* Hyaluronate and Derivatives . . . 696
IPOL® *see* Poliovirus Vaccine (Inactivated) 1099
Ipratropium 761
Ipratropium and Albuterol 761
Ipratropium Bromide *see* Ipratropium 761
I-Prin [OTC] *see* Ibuprofen 728
Iproveratril Hydrochloride *see* Verapamil 1373
IPV *see* Poliovirus Vaccine (Inactivated) 1099
Iquix® *see* Levofloxacin 812
Irbesartan 763
Irbesartan and Hydrochlorothiazide 764
Ircon® [OTC] *see* Ferrous Fumarate 586
Iressa™ *see* Gefitinib 649
Irinotecan 764
Iron Dextran Complex 766
Iron Fumarate *see* Ferrous Fumarate 586
Iron Gluconate *see* Ferrous Gluconate 586
Iron-Polysaccharide Complex *see* Polysaccharide-Iron Complex . . 1101
Iron Sucrose 767
Iron Sulfate *see* Ferrous Sulfate 586
Iron Sulfate and Vitamin C *see* Ferrous Sulfate and Ascorbic Acid 587
Isadol® (Mex) *see* Zidovudine 1398
Isavir® (Mex) *see* Acyclovir 64
ISD *see* Isosorbide Dinitrate 770
ISDN *see* Isosorbide Dinitrate 770
ISG *see* Immune Globulin (Intramuscular) 739
ISMN *see* Isosorbide Mononitrate . . 771
Ismo® *see* Isosorbide Mononitrate . . 771
Isoamyl Nitrite *see* Amyl Nitrite 130
Isobamate *see* Carisoprodol 266
Isocarboxazid 767
Isodine® (Mex) *see* Povidone-Iodine 1107
Isoetharine 768
Isoetharine Hydrochloride *see* Isoetharine 768
Isoetharine Mesylate *see* Isoetharine 768
Isoflavones *see* Soy Isoflavones . . 1447
Isoket® (Mex) *see* Isosorbide Dinitrate 770
Isometheptene, Acetaminophen, and Dichloralphenazone *see* Acetaminophen, Isometheptene, and Dichloralphenazone 59
Isometheptene, Dichloralphenazone, and Acetaminophen *see* Acetaminophen, Isometheptene, and Dichloralphenazone 59
Isoniazid 769
Isoniazid and Rifampin *see* Rifampin and Isoniazid 1181
Isoniazid, Rifampin, and Pyrazinamide *see* Rifampin, Isoniazid, and Pyrazinamide . . 1181
Isonicotinic Acid Hydrazide *see* Isoniazid 769
Isonipecaine Hydrochloride *see* Meperidine 870
Isophosphamide *see* Ifosfamide 733
Isopropyl Alcohol Tincture of Benzylkonium Chloride *see* Benzalkonium Chloride and Isopropyl Alcohol 190
Isoproterenol 770
Isoproterenol Hydrochloride *see* Isoproterenol 770
Isoptin® (Can) *see* Verapamil 1373
Isoptin® I.V. (Can) *see* Verapamil . . 1373
Isoptin® SR *see* Verapamil 1373
Isopto® Atropine *see* Atropine 166
Isopto® Carbachol *see* Carbachol . . . 255
Isopto® Carpine *see* Pilocarpine . . . 1085
Isopto® Eserine (Can) *see* Physostigmine 1084
Isopto® Homatropine *see* Homatropine 693
Isopto® Hyoscine *see* Scopolamine 1210
Isopto® Tears [OTC] *see* Artificial Tears 148
Isopto® Tears (Can) *see* Hydroxypropyl Methylcellulose . . 721
Isorbid® (Mex) *see* Isosorbide Dinitrate 770
Isordil® *see* Isosorbide Dinitrate 770
Isosorbide Dinitrate 770
Isosorbide Mononitrate 771
Isotamine® (Can) *see* Isoniazid 769
Isotretinoin 773
Isotrex® (Mex) *see* Isotretinoin 773
Isovue® *see* Radiological/Contrast Media (Nonionic) 1166
Isox® (Mex) *see* Itraconazole 775
Isoxsuprine 774
Isoxsuprine Hydrochloride *see* Isoxsuprine 774
Isradipine 774
Istalol™ *see* Timolol 1299
Isuprel® *see* Isoproterenol 770
Itch-X® [OTC] *see* Pramoxine 1109
Itraconazole 775
Itranax® (Mex) *see* Itraconazole 775
Iveegam EN *see* Immune Globulin (Intravenous) 740
Iveegam Immuno® (Can) *see* Immune Globulin (Intravenous) 740
Ivermectin 779
IVIG *see* Immune Globulin (Intravenous) 740
IvyBlock® [OTC] *see* Bentoquatam . . 189
Izadima® (Mex) *see* Ceftazidime . . . 286
Jantoven™ *see* Warfarin 1389
Japanese Encephalitis Virus Vaccine (Inactivated) 779
Jaundice Root *see* Golden Seal . . . 1433
JE-VAX® (Can) *see* Japanese Encephalitis Virus Vaccine (Inactivated) 779
Johimbe *see* Yohimbe 1451
Jolivette™ *see* Norethindrone 996
Junel™ *see* Ethinyl Estradiol and Norethindrone 550
K+8 *see* Potassium Chloride 1105
K+10 *see* Potassium Chloride 1105
Kadian® *see* Morphine Sulfate 947
Kala® [OTC] *see Lactobacillus* 793
Kaletra™ *see* Lopinavir and Ritonavir 839
Kaliolite® (Mex) *see* Potassium Bicarbonate 1104
Kalmz [OTC] *see* Fructose, Dextrose, and Phosphoric Acid 638
Kanamycin 780
Kanamycin Sulfate *see* Kanamycin 780
Kank-A® (Can) *see* Cetylpyridinium and Benzocaine 301
Kantrex® *see* Kanamycin 780

Kaodene® NN [OTC] *see* Kaolin and Pectin . . . 781
Kaolin and Pectin . . . 781
Kaolin, Hyoscyamine, Atropine, Scopolamine, and Pectin *see* Hyoscyamine, Atropine, Scopolamine, Kaolin, and Pectin . . . 726
Kaolin, Hyoscyamine, Atropine, Scopolamine, Pectin, and Opium *see* Hyoscyamine, Atropine, Scopolamine, Kaolin, Pectin, and Opium . . . 726
Kaon® (Can) *see* Potassium Gluconate . . . 1106
Kaon-Cl-10® *see* Potassium Chloride . . . 1105
Kaon-Cl® 20 *see* Potassium Chloride . . . 1105
Kaopectate® (Can) *see* Attapulgite . . 170
Kaopectate® [OTC] *see* Bismuth . . . 209
Kaopectate® Advanced Formula [DSC] [OTC] *see* Attapulgite . . . 170
Kaopectate® Extra Strength [OTC] *see* Bismuth . . . 209
Kaopectate® Maximum Strength Caplets [DSC] [OTC] *see* Attapulgite . . . 170
Kao-Spen® [OTC] *see* Kaolin and Pectin . . . 781
Kapanol® (Mex) *see* Morphine Sulfate . . . 947
Kapectolin® [OTC] *see* Kaolin and Pectin . . . 781
Kapectolin PG® *see* Hyoscyamine, Atropine, Scopolamine, Kaolin, Pectin, and Opium . . . 726
Kariva™ *see* Ethinyl Estradiol and Desogestrel . . . 536
Kasmal® (Mex) *see* Ketotifen . . . 790
Kava . . . 1439
Kava Kava *see* Kava . . . 1439
Kaveri *see* Ginkgo Biloba . . . 1429
Kay Ciel® *see* Potassium Chloride . . . 1105
K+ Care® *see* Potassium Chloride . . . 1105
K+ Care® ET *see* Potassium Bicarbonate . . . 1104
K-Citra® (Can) *see* Potassium Citrate . . . 1105
KCl *see* Potassium Chloride . . . 1105
K-Dur® (Mex) *see* Potassium Bicarbonate . . . 1104
K-Dur® (Can) *see* Potassium Chloride . . . 1105
K-Dur® 10 *see* Potassium Chloride . . . 1105
K-Dur® 20 *see* Potassium Chloride . . . 1105
Keduril® (Mex) *see* Ketoprofen . . . 785
Keflex® *see* Cephalexin . . . 294
Keftab® (Can) *see* Cephalexin . . . 294
Kefurox® (Can) *see* Cefuroxime . . . 289
Kemadrin® *see* Procyclidine . . . 1127
Kenalin® (Mex) *see* Sulindac . . . 1251
Kenalog® *see* Triamcinolone . . . 1330
Kenalog-10® *see* Triamcinolone . . . 1330
Kenalog-40® *see* Triamcinolone . . . 1330
Kenalog® in Orabase (Can) *see* Triamcinolone . . . 1330
Kenalog® in Orabase® *see* Triamcinolone Acetonide (Dental Paste) . . . 1333
Kenoket® (Mex) *see* Clonazepam . . 356
Kenolan® (Mex) *see* Captopril . . . 252
Kenopril® (Mex) *see* Enalapril . . . 488
Kentadin® (Mex) *see* Pentoxifylline . . . 1066
Kenzoflex® (Mex) *see* Ciprofloxacin . . . 331
Keoxifene Hydrochloride *see* Raloxifene . . . 1166
Keppra® (Can) *see* Levetiracetam . . 807
Keralyt® [OTC] *see* Salicylic Acid . . 1205
Kerlone® *see* Betaxolol . . . 202
Kerr Insta-Char® [OTC] *see* Charcoal . . . 303
Ketalar® *see* Ketamine . . . 782
Ketalin® (Mex) *see* Ketamine . . . 782
Ketamine . . . 782
Ketamine Hydrochloride *see* Ketamine . . . 782
Ketek™ *see* Telithromycin . . . 1263
Ketoconazole . . . 783
Ketoderm® (Can) *see* Ketoconazole . . . 783
Ketoprofen . . . 785
Ketorolac . . . 787
Ketorolac Tromethamine *see* Ketorolac . . . 787
Ketotifen . . . 790
Ketotifen Fumarate *see* Ketotifen . . 790
Kew *see* Kava . . . 1439
Kew Tree *see* Ginkgo Biloba . . . 1429
Key-E® [OTC] *see* Vitamin E . . . 1383
Key-E® Kaps [OTC] *see* Vitamin E . . . 1383
KI *see* Potassium Iodide . . . 1106
Kidkare Decongestant [OTC] *see* Pseudoephedrine . . . 1147
Kidrolase® (Can) *see* Asparaginase . . . 150
Kineret® (Can) *see* Anakinra . . . 131
Kinestase® (Mex) *see* Cisapride . . . 336
Kinevac® *see* Sincalide . . . 1224
Klamath Weed *see* St John's Wort . . . 1447
Klaricid® (Mex) *see* Clarithromycin . . 343
Klaron® *see* Sulfacetamide . . . 1244
Klean-Prep® (Can) *see* Polyethylene Glycol-Electrolyte Solution . . . 1100
Klonopin® *see* Clonazepam . . . 356
K-Lor® (Can) *see* Potassium Chloride . . . 1105
Klor-Con® *see* Potassium Chloride . . . 1105
Klor-Con® 8 *see* Potassium Chloride . . . 1105
Klor-Con® 10 *see* Potassium Chloride . . . 1105
Klor-Con®/25 *see* Potassium Chloride . . . 1105
Klor-Con®/EF *see* Potassium Bicarbonate and Potassium Citrate . . . 1105
Klor-Con® M *see* Potassium Chloride . . . 1105
Klotrix® *see* Potassium Chloride . . . 1105
Klyndaken® (Mex) *see* Clindamycin . . . 348
K-Lyte® *see* Potassium Bicarbonate and Potassium Citrate . . . 1105
K-Lyte® (Can) *see* Potassium Citrate . . . 1105
K-Lyte/Cl® *see* Potassium Bicarbonate and Potassium Chloride . . . 1104
K-Lyte®/Cl (Can) *see* Potassium Chloride . . . 1105
K-Lyte/Cl® 50 *see* Potassium Bicarbonate and Potassium Chloride . . . 1104
K-Lyte® DS *see* Potassium Bicarbonate and Potassium Citrate . . . 1105
Koāte®-DVI *see* Antihemophilic Factor (Human) . . . 134
Kodet SE [OTC] *see* Pseudoephedrine . . . 1147

Koffex DM-D (Can) *see* Pseudoephedrine and Dextromethorphan 1148
Koffex DM + Decongestant + Expectorant (Can) *see* Guaifenesin, Pseudoephedrine, and Dextromethorphan 676
Koffex DM-Expectorant (Can) *see* Guaifenesin and Dextromethorphan 673
Koffex Expectorant (Can) *see* Guaifenesin 672
Kogenate® (Can) *see* Antihemophilic Factor (Recombinant) 135
Kogenate® FS (Can) *see* Antihemophilic Factor (Recombinant) 135
Kolephrin® GG/DM [OTC] *see* Guaifenesin and Dextromethorphan 673
Konaderm® (Mex) *see* Ketoconazole 783
Konakion® (Mex) *see* Phytonadione 1084
Konsyl® [OTC] *see* Psyllium 1151
Konsyl-D® [OTC] *see* Psyllium 1151
Konsyl® Easy Mix [OTC] *see* Psyllium 1151
Konsyl® Orange [OTC] *see* Psyllium 1151
Konsyl® Tablets [OTC] *see* Polycarbophil 1100
Koptin® (Mex) *see* Kanamycin 780
K-Phos® MF *see* Potassium Phosphate and Sodium Phosphate 1107
K-Phos® Neutral *see* Potassium Phosphate and Sodium Phosphate 1107
K-Phos® No. 2 *see* Potassium Phosphate and Sodium Phosphate 1107
K-Phos® Original *see* Potassium Acid Phosphate 1104
K-Profen® (Mex) *see* Ketoprofen . . . 785
Kristalose™ *see* Lactulose 794
Kronofed-A® *see* Chlorpheniramine and Pseudoephedrine 315
Kronofed-A®-Jr *see* Chlorpheniramine and Pseudoephedrine 315
K-Tab® *see* Potassium Chloride . . . 1105
Kutrase® *see* Pancreatin 1042
Ku-Zyme® *see* Pancreatin 1042
Ku-Zyme® HP *see* Pancrelipase . . . 1042
Kwelcof® *see* Hydrocodone and Guaifenesin 708
Kwellada-P™ (Can) *see* Permethrin 1070
Kytril® (Can) *see* Granisetron 671
L-749,345 *see* Ertapenem 507
L 754030 *see* Aprepitant 138
LA 20304a *see* Gemifloxacin 653
Labetalol 791
Labetalol Hydrochloride *see* Labetalol 791
Lac-Hydrin® *see* Lactic Acid and Ammonium Hydroxide 793
Lac-Hydrin® Five [OTC] *see* Lactic Acid and Ammonium Hydroxide 793
Laciken® (Mex) *see* Acyclovir 64
LAClotion™ *see* Lactic Acid and Ammonium Hydroxide 793
Lacrisert® (Can) *see* Hydroxypropyl Cellulose 721
Lactaid® [OTC] *see* Lactase 793
Lactaid® Extra Strength [OTC] *see* Lactase 793
Lactaid® Ultra [OTC] *see* Lactase . . 793
Lactase 793
Lactic Acid and Ammonium Hydroxide 793
Lactic Acid and Sodium-PCA 793
LactiCare® [OTC] *see* Lactic Acid and Sodium-PCA 793
LactiCare-HC® *see* Hydrocortisone 714
Lactinex® [OTC] *see* *Lactobacillus* . . 793
Lactinol® *see* Lactic Acid and Sodium-PCA 793
Lactinol-E® *see* Lactic Acid and Sodium-PCA 793
Lactobacillus 793
Lactobacillus acidophilus see *Lactobacillus* 793
Lactobacillus acidophilus and *Lactobacillus bulgaricus see* *Lactobacillus* 793
Lactobacillus reuteri see *Lactobacillus* 793
Lactoflavin *see* Riboflavin 1178
Lactrase® [OTC] *see* Lactase 793
Lactulax® (Mex) *see* Lactulose 794
Lactulose 794
Ladakamycin *see* Azacitidine 171
Ladogal® (Mex) *see* Danazol 396
Lakriment Neu *see* Licorice 1440
L-AmB *see* Amphotericin B (Liposomal) 122
Lamictal® (Mex) *see* Lamotrigine . . . 795
Lamisil® (Can) *see* Terbinafine 1272
Lamisil® AT™ [OTC] *see* Terbinafine 1272
Lamivudine 794
Lamivudine, Abacavir, and Zidovudine *see* Abacavir, Lamivudine, and Zidovudine 43
Lamivudine and Zidovudine *see* Zidovudine and Lamivudine . . . 1399
Lamotrigine 795
Lampicin® (Mex) *see* Ampicillin 124
Lamprene® (Can) *see* Clofazimine . . 352
Lanacane® [OTC] *see* Benzocaine . . 191
Lanaphilic® [OTC] *see* Urea 1353
Lanexat® (Mex) *see* Flumazenil 599
Lanolin, Cetyl Alcohol, Glycerin, Petrolatum, and Mineral Oil 797
Lanoxicaps® *see* Digoxin 437
Lanoxin® (Mex) *see* Digoxin 437
Lansoprazole 797
Lansoprazole, Amoxicillin, and Clarithromycin 798
Lansoprazole and Naproxen 799
Lantus® *see* Insulin Preparations . . . 749
Lanvis® (Can) *see* Thioguanine . . . 1288
Laracit® (Mex) *see* Cytarabine 390
Largactil® (Mex) *see* ChlorproMAZINE 319
Lariam® (Can) *see* Mefloquine 864
Laronidase 800
Lasix® (Can) *see* Furosemide 640
Lasix® Special (Can) *see* Furosemide 640
L-asparaginase *see* Asparaginase . . 150
Lassar's Zinc Paste *see* Zinc Oxide 1400
Lastet® (Mex) *see* Etoposide 567
Latanoprost 800
Latotryd® (Mex) *see* Erythromycin . . 508
Lauricin® (Mex) *see* Erythromycin . . 508
Lauritran® (Mex) *see* Erythromycin . . 508
Laurus Sassafras see Sassafras Oil 1445
Laxilose (Can) *see* Lactulose 794
l-Bunolol Hydrochloride *see* Levobunolol 808
L-Carnitine *see* Carnitine 1417
L-Carnitine *see* Levocarnitine 810
LCD *see* Coal Tar 367
LCR *see* VinCRIStine 1378

L-Deprenyl *see* Selegiline 1212
LDP-341 *see* Bortezomib 214
Lectopam® (Can) *see* Bromazepam 218
Ledertrexate® (Mex) *see* Methotrexate 897
Ledoxina® (Mex) *see* Cyclophosphamide 384
Leflunomide 801
Legatrin PM® [OTC] *see* Acetaminophen and Diphenhydramine 53
Lemblastine® (Mex) *see* VinBLAStine 1377
Lemon Balm/Melissa 1439
Lenpryl® (Mex) *see* Captopril 252
Lente® Iletin® II [DSC] *see* Insulin Preparations 749
Lente, Insulin *see* Insulin Preparations 749
Lepirudin 803
Lepirudin (rDNA) *see* Lepirudin 803
Leponex® (Mex) *see* Clozapine 366
Leptilan® (Mex) *see* Valproic Acid and Derivatives 1359
Leptopsique® (Mex) *see* Perphenazine 1070
Lertamine® (Mex) *see* Loratadine . . . 841
Lertamine-D® (Mex) *see* Pseudoephedrine 1147
Lescol® (Mex) *see* Fluvastatin 622
Lescol® XL *see* Fluvastatin 622
Lessina™ *see* Ethinyl Estradiol and Levonorgestrel 545
Letrozole 803
Leucovorin 804
Leucovorin Calcium *see* Leucovorin 804
Leukeran® *see* Chlorambucil 305
Leukine® *see* Sargramostim 1209
Leunase® (Mex) *see* Asparaginase 150
Leuprolide 805
Leuprolide Acetate *see* Leuprolide . . 805
Leuprorelin Acetate *see* Leuprolide 805
Leurocristine Sulfate *see* VinCRIStine 1378
Leustatin® (Can) *see* Cladribine 342
Levalbuterol 806
Levamisole 806
Levamisole Hydrochloride *see* Levamisole 806
Levaquin® (Can) *see* Levofloxacin . . 812
Levarterenol Bitartrate *see* Norepinephrine 996
Levate® (Can) *see* Amitriptyline 103
Levatol® *see* Penbutolol 1055
Levbid® *see* Hyoscyamine 724
Levetiracetam 807
Levitra® *see* Vardenafil 1367
Levlen® *see* Ethinyl Estradiol and Levonorgestrel 545
Levlite™ *see* Ethinyl Estradiol and Levonorgestrel 545
Levobetaxolol 808
Levobunolol 808
Levobunolol Hydrochloride *see* Levobunolol 808
Levobupivacaine 809
Levocabastine 810
Levocabastine Hydrochloride *see* Levocabastine 810
Levocarnitine 810
Levocina® [tabs] (Mex) *see* Methotrimeprazine 901
Levodopa and Carbidopa 811
Levodopa, Carbidopa, and Entacapone 812
Levo-Dromoran® *see* Levorphanol . . 816
Levofloxacin 812
Levomepromazine *see* Methotrimeprazine 901
Levomethadyl Acetate Hydrochloride 814
Levonordefrin and Mepivacaine (Dental) *see* Mepivacaine and Levonordefrin *(WITHDRAWN FROM MARKET)* 875
Levonorgestrel 815
Levonorgestrel and Ethinyl Estradiol *see* Ethinyl Estradiol and Levonorgestrel 545
Levophed® (Can) *see* Norepinephrine 996
Levora® *see* Ethinyl Estradiol and Levonorgestrel 545
Levorphanol 816
Levorphanol Tartrate *see* Levorphanol 816
Levorphan Tartrate *see* Levorphanol 816
Levothroid® *see* Levothyroxine 817
Levothyroxine 817
Levothyroxine Sodium *see* Levothyroxine 817
Levoxyl® *see* Levothyroxine 817
Levsin® (Can) *see* Hyoscyamine . . . 724
Levsinex® *see* Hyoscyamine 724
Levsin/SL® *see* Hyoscyamine 724
Levulan® (Can) *see* Aminolevulinic Acid 99
Levulan® Kerastick® *see* Aminolevulinic Acid 99
Levulose, Dextrose and Phosphoric Acid *see* Fructose, Dextrose, and Phosphoric Acid 638
Lexapro™ *see* Escitalopram 513
Lexiva™ *see* Fosamprenavir 630
Lexotan® (Mex) *see* Bromazepam . . 218
Lexxel® (Can) *see* Enalapril and Felodipine 491
LFA-3/IgG(1) Fusion Protein, Human *see* Alefacept 76
L-Glutathione *see* Glutathione 1432
LHRH *see* Gonadorelin 669
l-Hyoscyamine Sulfate *see* Hyoscyamine 724
Librax® *see* Clidinium and Chlordiazepoxide 347
Librium® *see* Chlordiazepoxide 307
Licorice 1440
LidaMantle® *see* Lidocaine 819
Lida-Mantle® HC *see* Lidocaine and Hydrocortisone 826
Lidemol® (Can) *see* Fluocinonide . . . 602
Lidex® *see* Fluocinonide 602
Lidex-E® *see* Fluocinonide 602
Lidocaine 819
Lidocaine and Bupivacaine 822
Lidocaine and Epinephrine 823
Lidocaine and Hydrocortisone 826
Lidocaine and Prilocaine 826
Lidocaine Hydrochloride *see* Lidocaine 819
Lidocaine Hydrochloride and Bupivacaine Hydrochloride *see* Lidocaine and Bupivacaine 822
Lidocaine (Transoral) 828
Lidodan™ (Can) *see* Lidocaine 819
Lidoderm® (Can) *see* Lidocaine 819
LID-Pack® (Can) *see* Bacitracin and Polymyxin B 178
Lifenac® (Mex) *see* Diclofenac 427
Lignocaine Hydrochloride *see* Lidocaine 819
Lilly CT-3231 *see* Vindesine 1379
Limbitrol® (Can) *see* Amitriptyline and Chlordiazepoxide 105
Limbitrol® DS *see* Amitriptyline and Chlordiazepoxide 105

Lin-Amox (Can) *see* Amoxicillin 114
Lin-Buspirone (Can) *see* BusPIRone 233
Lincocin® *see* Lincomycin 829
Lincomycin 829
Lincomycin Hydrochloride *see* Lincomycin 829
Lindane 829
Linezolid 830
Lin-Megestrol (Can) *see* Megestrol 865
Lin-Nefazodone [DSC] (Can) *see* Nefazodone 970
Lin-Pravastatin (Can) *see* Pravastatin 1109
Lin-Sotalol (Can) *see* Sotalol 1231
Lioresal® (Can) *see* Baclofen 180
Liotec (Can) *see* Baclofen 180
Liothyronine 831
Liothyronine Sodium *see* Liothyronine 831
Liotrix 832
Lipancreatin *see* Pancrelipase 1042
Lipidil® (Mex) *see* Fenofibrate 577
Lipidil Micro® (Can) *see* Fenofibrate 577
Lipidil Supra® (Can) *see* Fenofibrate 577
Lipitor® (Mex) *see* Atorvastatin 162
Lipoic Acid *see* Alpha-Lipoic Acid 1413
Liposyn® III *see* Fat Emulsion 575
Lipram 4500 *see* Pancrelipase 1042
Lipram-CR *see* Pancrelipase 1042
Lipram-PN *see* Pancrelipase 1042
Lipram-UL *see* Pancrelipase 1042
Liquibid® [DSC] *see* Guaifenesin 672
Liquibid® 1200 [DSC] *see* Guaifenesin 672
Liquibid-D *see* Guaifenesin and Phenylephrine 674
Liqui-Char® [OTC] [DSC] *see* Charcoal 303
Liquid Antidote *see* Charcoal 303
Liquifilm® Tears [OTC] *see* Artificial Tears 148
Liquorice *see* Licorice 1440
Liroken® (Mex) *see* Diclofenac 427
Lisinopril 833
Lisinopril and Hydrochlorothiazide . . 834
Lispro, Insulin *see* Insulin Preparations 749
Lithane™ (Can) *see* Lithium 835
Litheum® (Mex) *see* Lithium 835
Lithium 835
Lithium Carbonate *see* Lithium 835
Lithium Citrate *see* Lithium 835
Lithobid® *see* Lithium 835
Lithostat® *see* Acetohydroxamic Acid 61
Livostin® *see* Levocabastine 810
L-Lysine Hydrochloride *see* Lysine . . 851
LMD® *see* Dextran 417
L-M-X™ 4 [OTC] *see* Lidocaine 819
L-M-X™ 5 [OTC] *see* Lidocaine 819
LNg 20 *see* Levonorgestrel 815
Locoid® (Can) *see* Hydrocortisone . . 714
Locoid Lipocream® *see* Hydrocortisone 714
Lodine® *see* Etodolac 564
Lodine® XL *see* Etodolac 564
Lodosyn® *see* Carbidopa 261
Lodoxamide 836
Lodoxamide Tromethamine *see* Lodoxamide 836
Lodrane® *see* Brompheniramine and Pseudoephedrine 220
Lodrane® 12D *see* Brompheniramine and Pseudoephedrine 220
Lodrane® LD *see* Brompheniramine and Pseudoephedrine 220
Loestrin® *see* Ethinyl Estradiol and Norethindrone 550
Loestrin™ 1.5.30 (Can) *see* Ethinyl Estradiol and Norethindrone 550
Loestrin® Fe *see* Ethinyl Estradiol and Norethindrone 550
Lofibra™ *see* Fenofibrate 577
Logesic® (Mex) *see* Diclofenac 427
L-OHP *see* Oxaliplatin 1020
LoKara™ *see* Desonide 410
Lomacin® (Mex) *see* Lomefloxacin . 837
Lomefloxacin 837
Lomefloxacin Hydrochloride *see* Lomefloxacin 837
Lomine (Can) *see* Dicyclomine 432
Lomotil® (Can) *see* Diphenoxylate and Atropine 451
Lomustine 838
Loniten® *see* Minoxidil 934
Lonox® *see* Diphenoxylate and Atropine 451
Lo/Ovral® *see* Ethinyl Estradiol and Norgestrel 557
Loperacap (Can) *see* Loperamide . . 838
Loperamide 838
Loperamide Hydrochloride *see* Loperamide 838
Lopid® (Mex) *see* Gemfibrozil 651
Lopinavir and Ritonavir 839
Lopremone *see* Protirelin 1145
Lopresor® (Mex) *see* Metoprolol 915
Lopressor® (Can) *see* Metoprolol . . . 915
Loprox® *see* Ciclopirox 327
Lorabid™ (Can) *see* Loracarbef 841
Loracarbef 841
Loratadine 841
Loratadine and Pseudoephedrine . . . 842
Lorazepam 842
Lorazepam Intensol® *see* Lorazepam 842
Lorcet® 10/650 *see* Hydrocodone and Acetaminophen 702
Lorcet®-HD *see* Hydrocodone and Acetaminophen 702
Lorcet® Plus *see* Hydrocodone and Acetaminophen 702
Loroxide® [OTC] *see* Benzoyl Peroxide 194
Lortab® *see* Hydrocodone and Acetaminophen 702
Losartan 845
Losartan and Hydrochlorothiazide . . 847
Losartan Potassium *see* Losartan . . 845
Losec® (Mex) *see* Omeprazole . . . 1012
Losec® [inj.] (Mex) *see* Omeprazole 1012
Lotemax® *see* Loteprednol 847
Lotensin® *see* Benazepril 187
Lotensin® HCT *see* Benazepril and Hydrochlorothiazide 189
Loteprednol 847
Loteprednol Etabonate *see* Loteprednol 847
Lotrel® *see* Amlodipine and Benazepril 110
Lotriderm® (Can) *see* Betamethasone and Clotrimazole 201
Lotrimin® (Mex) *see* Clotrimazole . . . 363
Lotrimin AF® (Mex) *see* Miconazole 922
Lotrimin® AF Athlete's Foot Cream [OTC] *see* Clotrimazole 363
Lotrimin® AF Athlete's Foot Solution [OTC] *see* Clotrimazole 363
Lotrimin® AF Jock Itch Cream [OTC] *see* Clotrimazole 363

Lotrimin® AF Powder/Spray [OTC] *see* Miconazole . . . 922
Lotrimin® Ultra™ [OTC] *see* Butenafine . . . 239
Lotrisone® *see* Betamethasone and Clotrimazole . . . 201
Lotronex® (Mex) *see* Alosetron . . . 83
Lovastatin . . . 848
Lovastatin and Niacin *see* Niacin and Lovastatin . . . 979
Lovenox® (Can) *see* Enoxaparin . . . 493
Lovenox® HP (Can) *see* Enoxaparin . . . 493
Low-Ogestrel® *see* Ethinyl Estradiol and Norgestrel . . . 557
Loxapine . . . 850
Loxapine Hydrochloride *see* Loxapine . . . 850
Loxapine Succinate *see* Loxapine . . . 850
Loxitane® *see* Loxapine . . . 850
Loxitane® C *see* Loxapine . . . 850
Lozide® (Can) *see* Indapamide . . . 743
Lozi-Flur™ *see* Fluoride . . . 603
Lozol® (Can) *see* Indapamide . . . 743
L-PAM *see* Melphalan . . . 866
LRH *see* Gonadorelin . . . 669
L-Sarcolysin *see* Melphalan . . . 866
LTG *see* Lamotrigine . . . 795
L-Thyroxine Sodium *see* Levothyroxine . . . 817
Lu-26-054 *see* Escitalopram . . . 513
Lubriderm® [OTC] *see* Lanolin, Cetyl Alcohol, Glycerin, Petrolatum, and Mineral Oil . . . 797
Lubriderm® Fragrance Free [OTC] *see* Lanolin, Cetyl Alcohol, Glycerin, Petrolatum, and Mineral Oil . . . 797
Ludiomil® (Mex) *see* Maprotiline . . . 856
Lufyllin® (Can) *see* Dyphylline . . . 480
Lugol's Solution *see* Potassium Iodide . . . 1106
Lumigan® (Mex) *see* Bimatoprost . . . 207
Luminal® Sodium *see* Phenobarbital . . . 1073
Lumitene™ *see* Beta-Carotene . . . 198
Lunelle™ *see* Estradiol and Medroxyprogesterone . . . 520
LupiCare™ Dandruff [OTC] *see* Salicylic Acid . . . 1205
LupiCare™ II Psoriasis [OTC] *see* Salicylic Acid . . . 1205
LupiCare™ Psoriasis [OTC] *see* Salicylic Acid . . . 1205
Lupron® (Can) *see* Leuprolide . . . 805
Lupron Depot® *see* Leuprolide . . . 805
Lupron Depot-Ped® *see* Leuprolide . . . 805
Lurdex® (Mex) *see* Albendazole . . . 71
Luride® *see* Fluoride . . . 603
Luride® Lozi-Tab® *see* Fluoride . . . 603
Lustra® *see* Hydroquinone . . . 719
Lustra-AF™ *see* Hydroquinone . . . 719
Lutein . . . 1441
Luteinizing Hormone Releasing Hormone *see* Gonadorelin . . . 669
Lutrepulse™ (Can) *see* Gonadorelin . . . 669
Luvox *see* Fluvoxamine . . . 623
Luxiq® *see* Betamethasone . . . 199
LY139603 *see* Atomoxetine . . . 161
LY146032 *see* Daptomycin . . . 399
LY170053 *see* Olanzapine . . . 1007
LY231514 *see* Pemetrexed . . . 1054
Lycopene . . . 1441
Lyderm® (Can) *see* Fluocinonide . . . 602
Lydonide (Can) *see* Fluocinonide . . . 602
Lymphocyte Immune Globulin *see* Antithymocyte Globulin (Equine) . . . 136
Lymphocyte Mitogenic Factor *see* Aldesleukin . . . 74
Lysine . . . 851
Lysinyl [OTC] *see* Lysine . . . 851
Lysodren® (Can) *see* Mitotane . . . 937
Lyteprep™ (Can) *see* Polyethylene Glycol-Electrolyte Solution . . . 1100
Maalox® [OTC] *see* Aluminum Hydroxide, Magnesium Hydroxide, and Simethicone . . . 92
Maalox® Max [OTC] *see* Aluminum Hydroxide, Magnesium Hydroxide, and Simethicone . . . 92
Maalox® TC (Therapeutic Concentrate) [OTC] [DSC] *see* Aluminum Hydroxide and Magnesium Hydroxide . . . 91
Mabicrol® (Mex) *see* Clarithromycin . . . 343
Mabthera® (Mex) *see* Rituximab . . . 1191
MacroBID® (Can) *see* Nitrofurantoin . . . 990
Macrodantin® (Can) *see* Nitrofurantoin . . . 990
Macrodantina® (Mex) *see* Nitrofurantoin . . . 990
Mafenide . . . 852
Mafenide Acetate *see* Mafenide . . . 852
Magaldrate and Simethicone . . . 852
Mag Delay® [OTC] *see* Magnesium Chloride . . . 852
Mag G® [OTC] *see* Magnesium Gluconate . . . 853
Maginex™ [OTC] *see* Magnesium L-aspartate Hydrochloride . . . 854
Maginex™ DS [OTC] *see* Magnesium L-aspartate Hydrochloride . . . 854
Magnesia Magma *see* Magnesium Hydroxide . . . 853
Magnesium Carbonate and Aluminum Hydroxide *see* Aluminum Hydroxide and Magnesium Carbonate . . . 90
Magnesium Chloride . . . 852
Magnesium Citrate . . . 853
Magnesium Gluconate . . . 853
Magnesium Hydroxide . . . 853
Magnesium Hydroxide, Aluminum Hydroxide, and Simethicone *see* Aluminum Hydroxide, Magnesium Hydroxide, and Simethicone . . . 92
Magnesium Hydroxide and Aluminum Hydroxide *see* Aluminum Hydroxide and Magnesium Hydroxide . . . 91
Magnesium Hydroxide and Calcium Carbonate *see* Calcium Carbonate and Magnesium Hydroxide . . . 245
Magnesium Hydroxide and Mineral Oil . . . 853
Magnesium Hydroxide, Famotidine, and Calcium Carbonate *see* Famotidine, Calcium Carbonate, and Magnesium Hydroxide . . . 574
Magnesium L-aspartate Hydrochloride . . . 854
Magnesium Oxide . . . 854
Magnesium Salicylate . . . 854
Magnesium Sulfate . . . 854
Magnesium Trisilicate and Aluminum Hydroxide *see* Aluminum Hydroxide and Magnesium Trisilicate . . . 91
Magnidol® (Mex) *see* Acetaminophen . . . 47
Magonate® [OTC] *see* Magnesium Gluconate . . . 853

Magonate® Sport [OTC] *see* Magnesium Gluconate 853
Mag-Ox® 400 [OTC] *see* Magnesium Oxide 854
Mag-SR® [OTC] *see* Magnesium Chloride 852
Magtrate® [OTC] *see* Magnesium Gluconate 853
MAH™ *see* Magnesium L-aspartate Hydrochloride 854
Maidenhair Tree *see* Ginkgo Biloba 1429
Malarone™ (Can) *see* Atovaquone and Proguanil 165
Malival® (Mex) *see* Indomethacin . . . 746
Maltodextrin 855
Malt Soup Extract 856
Maltsupex® [OTC] *see* Malt Soup Extract 856
m-AMSA *see* Amsacrine 129
Management of Patients Undergoing Cancer Therapy . . 1569
Management of Sialorrhea 1557
Mandelamine® *see* Methenamine . . . 892
Mandol® [DSC] *see* Cefamandole . . 277
Mandrake *see* Podophyllum Resin 1099
Manganese *see* Trace Metals 1319
Mantoux *see* Tuberculin Tests 1349
Mapap® [OTC] *see* Acetaminophen 47
Mapap® Arthritis [OTC] *see* Acetaminophen 47
Mapap® Children's [OTC] *see* Acetaminophen 47
Mapap® Extra Strength [OTC] *see* Acetaminophen 47
Mapap® Infants [OTC] *see* Acetaminophen 47
Mapap Sinus Maximum Strength [OTC] *see* Acetaminophen and Pseudoephedrine 53
Mapluxin® (Mex) *see* Digoxin 437
Maprotiline 856
Maprotiline Hydrochloride *see* Maprotiline 856
Marcaine® *see* Bupivacaine 225
Marcaine® Spinal *see* Bupivacaine . . 225
Marcaine® with Epinephrine *see* Bupivacaine and Epinephrine . . . 227
Marezine® [OTC] *see* Cyclizine 381
Margesic® H *see* Hydrocodone and Acetaminophen 702
Marinol® (Can) *see* Dronabinol 477
Marplan® *see* Isocarboxazid 767
Marvelon® (Can) *see* Ethinyl Estradiol and Desogestrel 536
Masflex® (Mex) *see* Meloxicam 865
Mastic 1441
Matricaria chamomilla see Chamomile 1419
Matricaria recutita see Chamomile 1419
Matulane® (Can) *see* Procarbazine 1125
3M™ Avagard™ [OTC] *see* Chlorhexidine Gluconate 308
Mavik® *see* Trandolapril 1321
Maxair™ Autohaler™ *see* Pirbuterol 1096
Maxalt® *see* Rizatriptan 1193
Maxalt-MLT® *see* Rizatriptan 1193
Maxalt RPD™ (Can) *see* Rizatriptan 1193
Maxaquin® *see* Lomefloxacin 837
Maxidex® (Can) *see* Dexamethasone 411
Maxidone™ *see* Hydrocodone and Acetaminophen 702
Maxifed® *see* Guaifenesin and Pseudoephedrine 675
Maxifed® DM *see* Guaifenesin, Pseudoephedrine, and Dextromethorphan 676
Maxifed-G® *see* Guaifenesin and Pseudoephedrine 675
Maxiflor® [DSC] *see* Diflorasone 435
Maxipime® (Can) *see* Cefepime 281
Maxitrol® *see* Neomycin, Polymyxin B, and Dexamethasone 974
Maxivate® *see* Betamethasone 199
Maxzide® *see* Hydrochlorothiazide and Triamterene 701
Maxzide®-25 *see* Hydrochlorothiazide and Triamterene 701
May Apple *see* Podophyllum Resin 1099
Maybush *see* Hawthorn 1437
3M™ Cavilon™ Skin Cleanser [OTC] *see* Benzalkonium Chloride 190
MCH *see* Microfibrillar Collagen Hemostat 923
m-Cresyl Acetate 857
MCT Oil® [OTC] *see* Medium Chain Triglycerides 861
MDL 73,147EF *see* Dolasetron 461
ME-500® *see* Methionine 894
Measles, Mumps, and Rubella Vaccines (Combined) 858
Measles Virus Vaccine (Live) 858
Mebaral® *see* Mephobarbital 873
Mebendazole 859
Mecamylamine 859
Mecamylamine Hydrochloride *see* Mecamylamine 859
Meclizine 859
Meclizine Hydrochloride *see* Meclizine 859
Meclofenamate 860
Meclofenamate Sodium *see* Meclofenamate 860
Meclomen® (Can) *see* Meclofenamate 860
Meclozine Hydrochloride *see* Meclizine 859
Med-Diltiazem (Can) *see* Diltiazem 444
Medicinal Carbon *see* Charcoal 303
Medicinal Charcoal *see* Charcoal . . . 303
Medicone® [OTC] *see* Phenylephrine 1078
Mediplast® [OTC] *see* Salicylic Acid 1205
Medi-Synal [OTC] *see* Acetaminophen and Pseudoephedrine 53
Medium Chain Triglycerides 861
Medrol® (Can) *see* MethylPREDNISolone 910
MedroxyPROGESTERone 862
Medroxyprogesterone Acetate *see* MedroxyPROGESTERone 862
Medroxyprogesterone Acetate and Estradiol Cypionate *see* Estradiol and Medroxyprogesterone 520
Medroxyprogesterone and Estrogens (Conjugated) *see* Estrogens (Conjugated/Equine) and Medroxyprogesterone 528
Medrysone 863
Mefenamic Acid 863
Mefloquine 864
Mefloquine Hydrochloride *see* Mefloquine 864
Mefoxin® (Can) *see* Cefoxitin 284
Megace® (Can) *see* Megestrol 865
Megace® OS (Can) *see* Megestrol . . 865
Megadophilus® [OTC] *see* *Lactobacillus* 793

Megestrol 865
Megestrol Acetate *see* Megestrol . . . 865
Meladinina® (Mex) *see* Methoxsalen 902
Melaleuca alternifolia see Melaleuca Oil 1442
Melaleuca Oil 1442
Melanex® *see* Hydroquinone 719
Melatonin 1442
Melfiat® *see* Phendimetrazine 1072
Melissa officinalis see Lemon Balm/Melissa 1439
Mellaril® [DSC] *see* Thioridazine . . 1289
Melleril® (Mex) *see* Thioridazine . . . 1289
Meloxicam 865
Melpaque HP® *see* Hydroquinone . . 719
Melphalan 866
Melquin-3® *see* Hydroquinone 719
Melquin HP® *see* Hydroquinone 719
Memantine 867
Memantine Hydrochloride *see* Memantine 867
Menadol® [OTC] *see* Ibuprofen 728
Menest® (Can) *see* Estrogens (Esterified) 529
Meningococcal Polysaccharide Vaccine (Groups A, C, Y, and W-135) 868
Menomune®-A/C/Y/W-135 *see* Meningococcal Polysaccharide Vaccine (Groups A, C, Y, and W-135) 868
Menostar™ *see* Estradiol 518
Menotropins 868
Mentax® *see* Butenafine 239
292 MEP® (Can) *see* Aspirin and Meprobamate 156
Mepenzolate 869
Mepenzolate Bromide *see* Mepenzolate 869
Mepergan *see* Meperidine and Promethazine 872
Meperidine 870
Meperidine and Promethazine 872
Meperidine Hydrochloride *see* Meperidine 870
Meperitab® *see* Meperidine 870
Mephobarbital 873
Mephyton® (Can) *see* Phytonadione 1084
Mepivacaine 873
Mepivacaine and Levonordefrin *(WITHDRAWN FROM MARKET)* 875
Mepivacaine (Dental Anesthetic) . . . 877
Mepivacaine Hydrochloride *see* Mepivacaine 873
Meprobamate 878
Meprobamate and Aspirin *see* Aspirin and Meprobamate 156
Mepron® *see* Atovaquone 164
Mequinol and Tretinoin 879
Merbromin 880
Mercaptopurine 880
6-Mercaptopurine *see* Mercaptopurine 880
Mercapturic Acid *see* Acetylcysteine 61
Mercuric Oxide 881
Mercurochrome® *see* Merbromin . . . 880
Meridia® (Can) *see* Sibutramine . . . 1218
Meropenem 881
Merrem® (Can) *see* Meropenem . . . 881
Merrem® I.V. *see* Meropenem 881
Mersol® [OTC] *see* Thimerosal 1288
Merthiolate® [OTC] *see* Thimerosal 1288
Meruvax® II *see* Rubella Virus Vaccine (Live) 1203
Merxil® (Mex) *see* Diclofenac 427
Mesalamine 882
Mesalazine *see* Mesalamine 882
Mesasal® (Can) *see* Mesalamine . . . 882
M-Eslon® (Can) *see* Morphine Sulfate 947
Mesoridazine 883
Mesoridazine Besylate *see* Mesoridazine 883
Mestinon® *see* Pyridostigmine 1153
Mestinon®-SR (Can) *see* Pyridostigmine 1153
Mestinon® Timespan® *see* Pyridostigmine 1153
Mestranol and Norethindrone 884
Metacortandralone *see* PrednisoLONE 1113
Metadate® CD *see* Methylphenidate 908
Metadate™ ER *see* Methylphenidate 908
Metadol™ (Can) *see* Methadone . . . 889
Metaglip™ *see* Glipizide and Metformin 662
Metahydrin® (Can) *see* Trichlormethiazide 1337
Metamucil® [OTC] *see* Psyllium . . . 1151
Metamucil® Smooth Texture [OTC] *see* Psyllium 1151
Metaproterenol 885
Metaproterenol Sulfate *see* Metaproterenol 885
Metatensin® (Can) *see* Trichlormethiazide 1337
Metaxalone 886
Metformin 887
Metformin and Glipizide *see* Glipizide and Metformin 662
Metformin and Glyburide *see* Glyburide and Metformin 665
Metformin and Rosiglitazone *see* Rosiglitazone and Metformin . . 1201
Metformin Hydrochloride *see* Metformin 887
Metformin Hydrochloride and Rosiglitazone Maleate *see* Rosiglitazone and Metformin . . 1201
Methadone 889
Methadone Hydrochloride *see* Methadone 889
Methadone Intensol™ *see* Methadone 889
Methadose® (Can) *see* Methadone 889
Methaminodiazepoxide Hydrochloride *see* Chlordiazepoxide 307
Methamphetamine 891
Methamphetamine Hydrochloride *see* Methamphetamine 891
Methazolamide 891
Methenamine 892
Methenamine Hippurate *see* Methenamine 892
Methenamine Mandelate *see* Methenamine 892
Methenamine, Sodium Biphosphate, Phenyl Salicylate, Methylene Blue, and Hyoscyamine 893
Methergine® *see* Methylergonovine 907
Methimazole 893
Methionine 894
Methitest® *see* MethylTESTOSTERone 912
Methocarbamol 894
Methohexital 895
Methohexital Sodium *see* Methohexital 895
Methotrexate 897
Methotrexate Sodium *see* Methotrexate 897

Methotrimeprazine 901
Methotrimeprazine Hydrochloride *see* Methotrimeprazine 901
Methoxsalen 902
Methoxypsoralen *see* Methoxsalen 902
8-Methoxypsoralen *see* Methoxsalen 902
Methscopolamine 903
Methscopolamine Bromide *see* Methscopolamine 903
Methscopolamine, Chlorpheniramine, and Phenylephrine *see* Chlorpheniramine, Phenylephrine, and Methscopolamine 317
Methsuximide 904
Methyclothiazide 905
Methyclothiazide and Deserpidine . . 905
Methylacetoxyprogesterone *see* MedroxyPROGESTERone 862
Methylcellulose 905
Methyldopa 906
Methyldopa and Hydrochlorothiazide 906
Methyldopate Hydrochloride *see* Methyldopa 906
Methylene Blue, Methenamine, Sodium Biphosphate, Phenyl Salicylate, and Hyoscyamine *see* Methenamine, Sodium Biphosphate, Phenyl Salicylate, Methylene Blue, and Hyoscyamine 893
Methylergometrine Maleate *see* Methylergonovine 907
Methylergonovine 907
Methylergonovine Maleate *see* Methylergonovine 907
Methylin™ *see* Methylphenidate 908
Methylin™ ER *see* Methylphenidate 908
Methylmorphine *see* Codeine 369
Methylphenidate 908
Methylphenidate Hydrochloride *see* Methylphenidate 908
Methylphenobarbital *see* Mephobarbital 873
Methylphenoxy-Benzene Propanamine *see* Atomoxetine 161
Methylphenyl Isoxazolyl Penicillin *see* Oxacillin 1020
Methylphytyl Napthoquinone *see* Phytonadione 1084
MethylPREDNISolone 910
6-α-Methylprednisolone *see* MethylPREDNISolone 910
Methylprednisolone Acetate *see* MethylPREDNISolone 910
Methylprednisolone Sodium Succinate *see* MethylPREDNISolone 910
4-Methylpyrazole *see* Fomepizole . . 627
Methylrosaniline Chloride *see* Gentian Violet 657
Methyl Sulfonyl Methane 1442
MethylTESTOSTERone 912
Methysergide 913
Methysergide Maleate *see* Methysergide 913
Meticel Ofteno® (Mex) *see* Hydroxypropyl Methylcellulose . . 721
Meticorten® (Mex) *see* PredniSONE 1115
Metipranolol 913
Metipranolol Hydrochloride *see* Metipranolol 913
Metoclopramide 914
Metolazone 914
Metoprolol 915
Metoprolol Succinate *see* Metoprolol 915
Metoprolol Tartrate *see* Metoprolol . . 915
Metrizamide *see* Radiological/ Contrast Media (Nonionic) 1166
MetroCream® *see* Metronidazole . . . 917
MetroGel® (Mex) *see* Metronidazole 917
MetroGel-Vaginal® *see* Metronidazole 917
MetroLotion® *see* Metronidazole 917
Metronidazole 917
Metronidazole, Bismuth Subsalicylate, and Tetracycline *see* Bismuth Subsalicylate, Metronidazole, and Tetracycline 209
Metronidazole Hydrochloride *see* Metronidazole 917
Metronidazole, Tetracycline, and Bismuth Subsalicylate *see* Bismuth Subsalicylate, Metronidazole, and Tetracycline 209
Metyrosine 920
Mevacor® (Can) *see* Lovastatin 848
Mevinolin *see* Lovastatin 848
Mexiletine 921
Mexitil® *see* Mexiletine 921
M-FA-142 *see* Amonafide 112
MG 217® [OTC] *see* Coal Tar 367
MG 217® Medicated Tar [OTC] *see* Coal Tar 367
MG217 Sal-Acid® [OTC] *see* Salicylic Acid 1205
Miacalcic® [salmon] (Mex) *see* Calcitonin 243
Miacalcin® *see* Calcitonin 243
Miacalcin® NS (Can) *see* Calcitonin 243
Micaderm® [OTC] *see* Miconazole . . 922
Micanol® (Can) *see* Anthralin 133
Micardis® *see* Telmisartan 1265
Micardis® HCT *see* Telmisartan and Hydrochlorothiazide 1265
Micardis® Plus (Can) *see* Telmisartan and Hydrochlorothiazide 1265
Micatin® (Can) *see* Miconazole 922
Miccil® (Mex) *see* Bumetanide 224
Miconazole 922
Miconazole Nitrate *see* Miconazole 922
Micostatin® (Mex) *see* Nystatin . . . 1003
Micostyl® (Mex) *see* Econazole 481
Micozole (Can) *see* Miconazole 922
MICRhoGAM® *see* Rh_o(D) Immune Globulin 1176
Microfibrillar Collagen Hemostat 923
Microgestin™ Fe *see* Ethinyl Estradiol and Norethindrone 550
Micro-Guard® [OTC] *see* Miconazole 922
microK® *see* Potassium Chloride . . 1105
microK® 10 *see* Potassium Chloride 1105
Micro-K Extencaps® (Can) *see* Potassium Chloride 1105
Microlut® (Mex) *see* Levonorgestrel 815
Micronase® *see* GlyBURIDE 664
microNefrin® *see* Epinephrine (Racemic) 497
Micronor® (Can) *see* Norethindrone 996
Microrgan® [caps] (Mex) *see* Ciprofloxacin 331
Microzide™ *see* Hydrochlorothiazide 699
Midamor® (Can) *see* Amiloride 95

Midazolam 924
Midazolam Hydrochloride *see* Midazolam 924
Midodrine 927
Midodrine Hydrochloride *see* Midodrine 927
Midol® Maximum Strength Cramp Formula [OTC] *see* Ibuprofen . . . 728
Midrin® *see* Acetaminophen, Isometheptene, and Dichloralphenazone 59
Mifeprex® *see* Mifepristone 928
Mifepristone 928
Miglitol 929
Miglustat 930
Migranal® (Can) *see* Dihydroergotamine 442
Migrin-A *see* Acetaminophen, Isometheptene, and Dichloralphenazone 59
Mi-Ke-Son's® (Mex) *see* Ketoconazole 783
Milk of Magnesia *see* Magnesium Hydroxide 853
Milk Thistle 1443
Milk Vetch *see* Astragalus 1414
Milophene® (Can) *see* ClomiPHENE 354
Milrinone 930
Milrinone Lactate *see* Milrinone 930
Miltown® *see* Meprobamate 878
Mineral Oil, Petrolatum, Lanolin, Cetyl Alcohol, and Glycerin *see* Lanolin, Cetyl Alcohol, Glycerin, Petrolatum, and Mineral Oil 797
Minestrin™ 1/20 (Can) *see* Ethinyl Estradiol and Norethindrone 550
Minidyne® [OTC] *see* Povidone-Iodine 1107
Minim's Atropine Solution (Can) *see* Atropine 166
Minim's Gentamicin 0.3% (Can) *see* Gentamicin 655
Minipres® (Mex) *see* Prazosin 1111
Minipress® *see* Prazosin 1111
Minirin® (Can) *see* Desmopressin . . 409
Minitran™ *see* Nitroglycerin 991
Minizide® *see* Prazosin and Polythiazide 1112
Minocin® *see* Minocycline 931
Minocycline 931
Minocycline Hydrochloride *see* Minocycline 931
Minocycline Hydrochloride (Periodontal) 933
Minodiab® (Mex) *see* GlipiZIDE 660
Min-Ovral® (Can) *see* Ethinyl Estradiol and Levonorgestrel . . . 545
Minox (Can) *see* Minoxidil 934
Minoxidil 934
Mintezol® *see* Thiabendazole 1286
Miochol-E® (Can) *see* Acetylcholine 61
Miostat® (Can) *see* Carbachol 255
MiraLax™ *see* Polyethylene Glycol-Electrolyte Solution 1100
Mirapex® *see* Pramipexole 1108
Miraphen PSE *see* Guaifenesin and Pseudoephedrine 675
Mircette® *see* Ethinyl Estradiol and Desogestrel 536
Mirena® *see* Levonorgestrel 815
Mirtazapine 935
Misoprostol 936
Misoprostol and Diclofenac *see* Diclofenac and Misoprostol 430
Mitocin® (Mex) *see* Mitomycin 937
Mitomycin 937
Mitomycin-C *see* Mitomycin 937
Mitomycin-X *see* Mitomycin 937
Mitotane 937
Mitoxantrone 938
Mitoxantrone Hydrochloride CL-232315 *see* Mitoxantrone . . . 938
Mitozantrone *see* Mitoxantrone 938
Mitrazol™ [OTC] *see* Miconazole . . . 922
Mitroken® [tabs] (Mex) *see* Ciprofloxacin 331
Mitroxone® [inj.] (Mex) *see* Mitoxantrone 938
MK383 *see* Tirofiban 1304
MK462 *see* Rizatriptan 1193
MK594 *see* Losartan 845
MK0826 *see* Ertapenem 507
MK 869 *see* Aprepitant 138
MLN341 *see* Bortezomib 214
MMF *see* Mycophenolate 952
MMR *see* Measles, Mumps, and Rubella Vaccines (Combined) . . 858
M-M-R® II *see* Measles, Mumps, and Rubella Vaccines (Combined) 858
Moban® *see* Molindone 942
MOBIC® (Can) *see* Meloxicam 865
Mobicox® (Can) *see* Meloxicam 865
Mobidin® [DSC] *see* Magnesium Salicylate 854
Mobisyl® [OTC] *see* Triethanolamine Salicylate 1338
Modafinil 939
Modane® Bulk [OTC] *see* Psyllium 1151
Modane Tablets® [OTC] *see* Bisacodyl 208
Modecate® (Can) *see* Fluphenazine 610
Modicon® *see* Ethinyl Estradiol and Norethindrone 550
Modified Dakin's Solution *see* Sodium Hypochlorite Solution 1228
Modified Shohl's Solution *see* Sodium Citrate and Citric Acid 1228
Moditen® Enanthate (Can) *see* Fluphenazine 610
Moditen® HCl (Can) *see* Fluphenazine 610
Moducal® [OTC] *see* Glucose Polymers 664
Moduret® (Can) *see* Amiloride and Hydrochlorothiazide 96
Moduretic® (Can) *see* Amiloride and Hydrochlorothiazide 96
Moexipril 940
Moexipril and Hydrochlorothiazide . . 941
Moexipril Hydrochloride *see* Moexipril 940
Moi-Stir® [OTC] *see* Saliva Substitute 1205
Moisture® Eyes [OTC] *see* Artificial Tears 148
Moisture® Eyes PM [OTC] *see* Artificial Tears 148
Molindone 942
Molindone Hydrochloride *see* Molindone 942
Molybdenum *see* Trace Metals . . . 1319
Molypen® *see* Trace Metals 1319
MOM *see* Magnesium Hydroxide . . . 853
Momentum® [OTC] *see* Magnesium Salicylate 854
Mometasone Furoate 943
MOM/Mineral Oil Emulsion *see* Magnesium Hydroxide and Mineral Oil 853
Monacolin K *see* Lovastatin 848
Monarc® M *see* Antihemophilic Factor (Human) 134
Monascus purpureus see Red Yeast Rice 1444

Monistat® (Can) *see* Miconazole . . . 922
Monistat® 1 Combination Pack [OTC] *see* Miconazole 922
Monistat® 3 [OTC] *see* Miconazole 922
Monistat® 7 [OTC] *see* Miconazole 922
Monistat-Derm® *see* Miconazole . . . 922
Monitan® (Can) *see* Acebutolol 46
Monobenzone 944
Monoclate-P® *see* Antihemophilic Factor (Human) 134
Monoclonal Antibody *see* Muromonab-CD3 952
Monocor® (Can) *see* Bisoprolol 210
Monodox® *see* Doxycycline 471
Monoethanolamine *see* Ethanolamine Oleate 535
Mono-Gesic® *see* Salsalate 1207
Monoket® *see* Isosorbide Mononitrate 771
Mono Mack® (Mex) *see* Isosorbide Mononitrate 771
MonoNessa™ *see* Ethinyl Estradiol and Norgestimate 554
Mononine® *see* Factor IX 571
Monopril® (Can) *see* Fosinopril 633
Monopril-HCT® *see* Fosinopril and Hydrochlorothiazide 635
Montelukast 944
Montelukast Sodium *see* Montelukast 944
Monurol™ (Can) *see* Fosfomycin . . . 632
8-MOP® (Can) *see* Methoxsalen . . . 902
More Attenuated Enders Strain *see* Measles Virus Vaccine (Live) . . . 858
MoreDophilus® [OTC] *see* *Lactobacillus* 793
Moricizine 946
Moricizine Hydrochloride *see* Moricizine 946
Morning After Pill *see* Ethinyl Estradiol and Norgestrel 557
Morphine HP® (Can) *see* Morphine Sulfate 947
Morphine LP® Epidural (Can) *see* Morphine Sulfate 947
Morphine Sulfate 947
Morrhuate Sodium 948
Mosco® Corn and Callus Remover [OTC] *see* Salicylic Acid 1205
M.O.S.-Sulfate® (Can) *see* Morphine Sulfate 947
Motofen® *see* Difenoxin and Atropine 434
Motrin® *see* Ibuprofen 728
Motrin® Children's [OTC] *see* Ibuprofen 728
Motrin® Cold and Sinus [OTC] *see* Pseudoephedrine and Ibuprofen 1149
Motrin® Cold, Children's [OTC] *see* Pseudoephedrine and Ibuprofen 1149
Motrin® IB (Can) *see* Ibuprofen 728
Motrin® Infants' [OTC] *see* Ibuprofen 728
Motrin® Junior Strength [OTC] *see* Ibuprofen 728
Motrin® Migraine Pain [OTC] *see* Ibuprofen 728
Mouthkote® [OTC] *see* Saliva Substitute 1205
Mouth Pain, Cold Sore, and Canker Sore Products 1633
Mouthwash (Antiseptic) 948
Moxifloxacin 949
Moxifloxacin Hydrochloride *see* Moxifloxacin 949
Moxilin® *see* Amoxicillin 114
Moxlin® Penamox® (Mex) *see* Amoxicillin 114
4-MP *see* Fomepizole 627
6-MP *see* Mercaptopurine 880
MPA *see* Mycophenolate 952
MPA and Estrogens (Conjugated) *see* Estrogens (Conjugated/ Equine) and Medroxyprogesterone 528
MS Contin® *see* Morphine Sulfate . . 947
MS-IR® (Can) *see* Morphine Sulfate 947
MSM *see* Methyl Sulfonyl Methane 1442
MST Continus® (Mex) *see* Morphine Sulfate 947
MTA *see* Pemetrexed 1054
MTC *see* Mitomycin 937
M.T.E.-4® *see* Trace Metals 1319
M.T.E.-5® *see* Trace Metals 1319
M.T.E.-6® *see* Trace Metals 1319
M.T.E.-7® *see* Trace Metals 1319
MTX *see* Methotrexate 897
Mucinex® [OTC] *see* Guaifenesin . . . 672
Mucinex® D *see* Guaifenesin and Pseudoephedrine 675
Mucomyst® *see* Acetylcysteine 61
Multidex® [OTC] *see* Maltodextrin . . 855
Multiple Vitamins *see* Vitamins (Multiple/Oral) 1384
Multitargeted Antifolate *see* Pemetrexed 1054
Multitest CMI® *see* Skin Test Antigens (Multiple) 1226
Multitrace™-4 *see* Trace Metals . . . 1319
Multitrace™-4 Neonatal *see* Trace Metals 1319
Multitrace™-4 Pediatric *see* Trace Metals 1319
Multitrace™-5 *see* Trace Metals . . . 1319
Multivitamin Products 1644
Mumps, Measles and Rubella Vaccines, Combined *see* Measles, Mumps, and Rubella Vaccines (Combined) 858
Mumpsvax® *see* Mumps Virus Vaccine (Live/Attenuated) 951
Mumps Virus Vaccine (Live/ Attenuated) 951
Munobal® (Mex) *see* Felodipine 576
Mupirocin 951
Mupirocin Calcium *see* Mupirocin . . . 951
Murine® Ear [OTC] *see* Carbamide Peroxide 259
Murine® Tears [OTC] *see* Artificial Tears 148
Murine® Tears Plus [OTC] *see* Tetrahydrozoline 1282
Muro 128® [OTC] *see* Sodium Chloride 1227
Murocel® [OTC] *see* Artificial Tears 148
Murocoll-2® *see* Phenylephrine and Scopolamine 1079
Muromonab-CD3 952
Muse® *see* Alprostadil 87
Muse® Pellet (Can) *see* Alprostadil 87
Mutamycin® *see* Mitomycin 937
Myambutol® *see* Ethambutol 534
Mycelex® *see* Clotrimazole 363
Mycelex®-3 [OTC] *see* Butoconazole 239
Mycelex®-7 [OTC] *see* Clotrimazole 363
Mycelex® Twin Pack [OTC] *see* Clotrimazole 363
Myciguent [OTC] *see* Neomycin 973
Mycinettes® [OTC] *see* Benzocaine 191
Mycobutin® *see* Rifabutin 1179

Mycodib® (Mex) *see* Ketoconazole . . 783
Mycolog®-II [DSC] *see* Nystatin and Triamcinolone 1004
Myco-Nail [OTC] *see* Triacetin 1329
Mycophenolate 952
Mycophenolate Mofetil *see* Mycophenolate 952
Mycophenolate Sodium *see* Mycophenolate 952
Mycophenolic Acid *see* Mycophenolate 952
Mycostatin® (Can) *see* Nystatin . . . 1003
Mydfrin® *see* Phenylephrine 1078
Mydriacyl® (Can) *see* Tropicamide 1348
Myfortic® *see* Mycophenolate 952
Myfungar® (Mex) *see* Oxiconazole 1024
Mykrox® (Can) *see* Metolazone 914
Mylanta™ (Can) *see* Aluminum Hydroxide and Magnesium Hydroxide 91
Mylanta® Children's [OTC] *see* Calcium Carbonate 245
Mylanta™ Double Strength (Can) *see* Aluminum Hydroxide, Magnesium Hydroxide, and Simethicone 92
Mylanta™ Extra Strength (Can) *see* Aluminum Hydroxide, Magnesium Hydroxide, and Simethicone 92
Mylanta® Gas [OTC] *see* Simethicone 1222
Mylanta® Gas Maximum Strength [OTC] *see* Simethicone 1222
Mylanta® Gelcaps® [OTC] *see* Calcium Carbonate and Magnesium Hydroxide 245
Mylanta® Liquid [OTC] *see* Aluminum Hydroxide, Magnesium Hydroxide, and Simethicone 92
Mylanta® Maximum Strength Liquid [OTC] *see* Aluminum Hydroxide, Magnesium Hydroxide, and Simethicone 92
Mylanta™ regular Strength (Can) *see* Aluminum Hydroxide, Magnesium Hydroxide, and Simethicone 92
Mylanta® Supreme [OTC] *see* Calcium Carbonate and Magnesium Hydroxide 245
Mylanta® Ultra [OTC] *see* Calcium Carbonate and Magnesium Hydroxide 245
Myleran® *see* Busulfan 234
Mylicon® Infants [OTC] *see* Simethicone 1222
Mylocel™ *see* Hydroxyurea 722
Mylotarg™ (Can) *see* Gemtuzumab Ozogamicin 653
Myobloc® *see* Botulinum Toxin Type B 217
Myochrysine® (Can) *see* Gold Sodium Thiomalate 668
Myoflex® (Mex) *see* Magnesium Salicylate 854
Myoflex® (Can) *see* Triethanolamine Salicylate 1338
Myotonachol® (Can) *see* Bethanechol 203
Mysoline® (Can) *see* Primidone . . . 1122
Mytelase® (Can) *see* Ambenonium 93
Mytussin® AC *see* Guaifenesin and Codeine 673
Mytussin® DAC *see* Guaifenesin, Pseudoephedrine, and Codeine 676
Mytussin® DM [OTC] *see* Guaifenesin and Dextromethorphan 673
Nabi-HB® *see* Hepatitis B Immune Globulin 688
Nabumetone 955
NAC *see* Acetylcysteine 61
N-Acetylcysteine *see* Acetylcysteine 61
N-Acetyl-L-cysteine *see* Acetylcysteine 61
N-Acetyl-P-Aminophenol *see* Acetaminophen 47
NaCl *see* Sodium Chloride 1227
NADH *see* Nicotinamide Adenine Dinucleotide 1443
Nadib® (Mex) *see* GlyBURIDE 664
Nadolol 956
Nadolol and Bendroflumethiazide . . . 957
Nadopen-V® (Can) *see* Penicillin V Potassium 1060
Nafarelin 957
Nafarelin Acetate *see* Nafarelin 957
Nafcillin 958
Nafcillin Sodium *see* Nafcillin 958
Nafidimide *see* Amonafide 112
Naftifine 959
Naftifine Hydrochloride *see* Naftifine 959
Naftin® *see* Naftifine 959
$NaHCO_3$ *see* Sodium Bicarbonate 1226
Nalbuphine 959
Nalbuphine Hydrochloride *see* Nalbuphine 959
Nalcrom® (Can) *see* Cromolyn 378
Nalcryn® [inj.] (Mex) *see* Nalbuphine 959
Naldecon Senior EX® [OTC] *see* Guaifenesin 672
Nalex®-A *see* Chlorpheniramine, Phenylephrine, and Phenyltoloxamine 317
Nalfon® (Can) *see* Fenoprofen 580
Nalidixic Acid 960
Nalidixinic Acid *see* Nalidixic Acid . . 960
Nallpen® (Can) *see* Nafcillin 958
N-allylnoroxymorphine Hydrochloride *see* Naloxone . . . 961
Nalmefene 960
Nalmefene Hydrochloride *see* Nalmefene 960
Naloxone 961
Naloxone and Buprenorphine *see* Buprenorphine and Naloxone . . . 230
Naloxone Hydrochloride *see* Naloxone 961
Naloxone Hydrochloride and Pentazocine Hydrochloride *see* Pentazocine 1063
Naloxone Hydrochloride Dihydrate and Buprenorphine Hydrochloride *see* Buprenorphine and Naloxone . . . 230
Naltrexone 962
Naltrexone Hydrochloride *see* Naltrexone 962
Namenda™ *see* Memantine 867
Nandrolone 963
Nandrolone Decanoate *see* Nandrolone 963
Nandrolone Phenpropionate *see* Nandrolone 963
Naphazoline 964
Naphazoline and Antazoline 964
Naphazoline and Pheniramine 964
Naphazoline Hydrochloride *see* Naphazoline 964
Naphcon® [OTC] *see* Naphazoline . . 964
Naphcon-A® [OTC] *see* Naphazoline and Pheniramine . . 964

Naphcon Forte® (Can) *see* Naphazoline . . . 964
NapraPAC™ *see* Lansoprazole and Naproxen . . . 799
Naprelan® *see* Naproxen . . . 965
Naprodil® [tabs] (Mex) *see* Naproxen . . . 965
Naprosyn® *see* Naproxen . . . 965
Naproxen . . . 965
Naproxen and Lansoprazole *see* Lansoprazole and Naproxen . . . 799
Naproxen Sodium *see* Naproxen . . . 965
Naqua® (Can) *see* Trichlormethiazide . . . 1337
Naramig® (Mex) *see* Naratriptan . . . 967
Naratriptan . . . 967
Naratriptan Hydrochloride *see* Naratriptan . . . 967
Narcan® *see* Naloxone . . . 961
Narcanti® (Mex) *see* Naloxone . . . 961
Nardil® *see* Phenelzine . . . 1072
Naropin® (Mex) *see* Ropivacaine . . 1199
Nasacort® [DSC] *see* Triamcinolone . . . 1330
Nasacort® AQ (Can) *see* Triamcinolone . . . 1330
NaSal™ [OTC] *see* Sodium Chloride . . . 1227
Nasalcrom® [OTC] *see* Cromolyn . . . 378
Nasalide® *see* Flunisolide . . . 599
Nasal Moist® [OTC] *see* Sodium Chloride . . . 1227
Nasarel® *see* Flunisolide . . . 599
Nascobal® *see* Cyanocobalamin . . . 380
Nasonex® *see* Mometasone Furoate . . . 943
Natacyn® (Can) *see* Natamycin . . . 968
Natamycin . . . 968
Nateglinide . . . 968
Natrecor® *see* Nesiritide . . . 976
Natriuretic Peptide *see* Nesiritide . . . 976
Natulan® (Mex) *see* Procarbazine . . . 1125
Natural Lung Surfactant *see* Beractant . . . 198
Natural Products: Herbal and Dietary Supplements . . . 1409
Nature's Tears® [OTC] *see* Artificial Tears . . . 148
Nature-Throid® NT *see* Thyroid . . . 1293
Naturetin® [DSC] *see* Bendroflumethiazide . . . 189
Nausea Relief [OTC] *see* Fructose, Dextrose, and Phosphoric Acid . . . 638
Nausetrol® [OTC] *see* Fructose, Dextrose, and Phosphoric Acid . . . 638
Navane® (Can) *see* Thiothixene . . . 1291
Navelbine® (Mex) *see* Vinorelbine . . . 1380
Naxen® (Mex) *see* Naproxen . . . 965
Na-Zone® [OTC] *see* Sodium Chloride . . . 1227
n-Docosanol *see* Docosanol . . . 459
Nebcin® (Can) *see* Tobramycin . . . 1306
NebuPent® *see* Pentamidine . . . 1062
Necon® 0.5/35 *see* Ethinyl Estradiol and Norethindrone . . . 550
Necon® 1/35 *see* Ethinyl Estradiol and Norethindrone . . . 550
Necon® 1/50 *see* Mestranol and Norethindrone . . . 884
Necon® 7/7/7 *see* Ethinyl Estradiol and Norethindrone . . . 550
Necon® 10/11 *see* Ethinyl Estradiol and Norethindrone . . . 550
Nectar of the Gods *see* Garlic . . . 1428
Nedocromil . . . 970
Nedocromil Sodium *see* Nedocromil . . . 970
Nefazodone . . . 970
Nefazodone Hydrochloride *see* Nefazodone . . . 970
NegGram® *see* Nalidixic Acid . . . 960
Nelfinavir . . . 972
Nemasol® Sodium (Can) *see* Aminosalicylic Acid . . . 100
Nembutal® *see* Pentobarbital . . . 1065
Nembutal® Sodium (Can) *see* Pentobarbital . . . 1065
Neobes® (Mex) *see* Diethylpropion . . . 434
NeoCeuticals™ Acne Spot Treatment [OTC] *see* Salicylic Acid . . . 1205
NeoDecadron® *see* Neomycin and Dexamethasone . . . 973
Neodol® (Mex) *see* Acetaminophen . . . 47
Neodolito® (Mex) *see* Acetaminophen . . . 47
Neofomiral® (Mex) *see* Fluconazole . . . 594
Neo-Fradin™ *see* Neomycin . . . 973
Neomicol® (Mex) *see* Miconazole . . . 922
Neomycin . . . 973
Neomycin and Dexamethasone . . . 973
Neomycin and Polymyxin B . . . 973
Neomycin, Bacitracin, and Polymyxin B *see* Bacitracin, Neomycin, and Polymyxin B . . . 179
Neomycin, Bacitracin, Polymyxin B, and Hydrocortisone *see* Bacitracin, Neomycin, Polymyxin B, and Hydrocortisone . . . 179
Neomycin, Bacitracin, Polymyxin B, and Pramoxine *see* Bacitracin, Neomycin, Polymyxin B, and Pramoxine . . . 180
Neomycin, Polymyxin B, and Dexamethasone . . . 974
Neomycin, Polymyxin B, and Gramicidin . . . 974
Neomycin, Polymyxin B, and Hydrocortisone . . . 975
Neomycin, Polymyxin B, and Prednisolone . . . 975
Neomycin Sulfate *see* Neomycin . . . 973
Neonatal Trace Metals *see* Trace Metals . . . 1319
Neonaxil® (Mex) *see* Naproxen . . . 965
Neopulmonier® (Mex) *see* Dextromethorphan . . . 421
Neoral® (Can) *see* CycloSPORINE . . . 386
Neo-Rx *see* Neomycin . . . 973
Neosporin® (Can) *see* Neomycin, Polymyxin B, and Gramicidin . . . 974
Neosporin® G.U. Irrigant *see* Neomycin and Polymyxin B . . . 973
Neosporin® Irrigating Solution (Can) *see* Neomycin and Polymyxin B . . . 973
Neosporin® Neo To Go® [OTC] *see* Bacitracin, Neomycin, and Polymyxin B . . . 179
Neosporin® Ophthalmic Ointment (Can) *see* Bacitracin, Neomycin, and Polymyxin B . . . 179
Neosporin® Ophthalmic Solution *see* Neomycin, Polymyxin B, and Gramicidin . . . 974
Neosporin® + Pain Ointment [OTC] *see* Bacitracin, Neomycin, Polymyxin B, and Pramoxine . . . 180
Neosporin® Topical [OTC] *see* Bacitracin, Neomycin, and Polymyxin B . . . 179
NeoStrata AHA [OTC] *see* Hydroquinone . . . 719

NeoStrata® HQ (Can) *see* Hydroquinone . . . 719
Neo-Synephrine® (Can) *see* Phenylephrine . . . 1078
Neo-Synephrine® 12 Hour [OTC] *see* Oxymetazoline . . . 1034
Neo-Synephrine® 12 Hour Extra Moisturizing [OTC] *see* Oxymetazoline . . . 1034
Neo-Synephrine® Extra Strength [OTC] *see* Phenylephrine . . . 1078
Neo-Synephrine® Mild [OTC] *see* Phenylephrine . . . 1078
Neo-Synephrine® Ophthalmic *see* Phenylephrine . . . 1078
Neo-Synephrine® Regular Strength [OTC] *see* Phenylephrine . . . 1078
Neotopic® (Can) *see* Bacitracin, Neomycin, and Polymyxin B . . . 179
Neotrace-4® *see* Trace Metals . . . 1319
NephPlex® Rx *see* Vitamin B Complex Combinations . . . 1382
Nephro-Calci® [OTC] *see* Calcium Carbonate . . . 245
Nephrocaps® *see* Vitamin B Complex Combinations . . . 1382
Nephro-Fer® [OTC] *see* Ferrous Fumarate . . . 586
Nephron FA® *see* Vitamin B Complex Combinations . . . 1382
Nephro-Vite® *see* Vitamin B Complex Combinations . . . 1382
Nephro-Vite® Rx *see* Vitamin B Complex Combinations . . . 1382
Neptazane® [DSC] *see* Methazolamide . . . 891
Nesacaine® *see* Chloroprocaine . . . 310
Nesacaine®-CE (Can) *see* Chloroprocaine . . . 310
Nesacaine®-MPF *see* Chloroprocaine . . . 310
Nesiritide . . . 976
Neugal® (Mex) *see* Ranitidine . . . 1169
Neugeron® (Mex) *see* Carbamazepine . . . 255
Neulasta™ *see* Pegfilgrastim . . . 1052
Neumega® *see* Oprelvekin . . . 1015
Neupogen® *see* Filgrastim . . . 589
Neurontin® (Can) *see* Gabapentin . . . 642
Neurosine® (Mex) *see* BusPIRone . . . 233
Neut® *see* Sodium Bicarbonate . . . 1226
NeutraCare® *see* Fluoride . . . 603
NeutraGard® [OTC] *see* Fluoride . . . 603
Neutra-Phos® [OTC] *see* Potassium Phosphate and Sodium Phosphate . . . 1107
Neutra-Phos®-K [OTC] *see* Potassium Phosphate . . . 1107
Neutrexin® *see* Trimetrexate Glucuronate . . . 1342
Neutrogena® Acne Mask [OTC] *see* Benzoyl Peroxide . . . 194
Neutrogena® Acne Wash [OTC] *see* Salicylic Acid . . . 1205
Neutrogena® Body Clear™ [OTC] *see* Salicylic Acid . . . 1205
Neutrogena® Clear Pore [OTC] *see* Salicylic Acid . . . 1205
Neutrogena® Clear Pore Shine Control [OTC] *see* Salicylic Acid . . . 1205
Neutrogena® Healthy Scalp [OTC] *see* Salicylic Acid . . . 1205
Neutrogena® Maximum Strength T/Sal® [OTC] *see* Salicylic Acid . . . 1205
Neutrogena® On The Spot® Acne Patch [OTC] *see* Salicylic Acid . . . 1205
Neutrogena® On The Spot® Acne Treatment [OTC] *see* Benzoyl Peroxide . . . 194
Neutrogena® T/Gel [OTC] *see* Coal Tar . . . 367
Neutrogena® T/Gel Extra Strength [OTC] *see* Coal Tar . . . 367
Nevirapine . . . 977
Nexium® (Can) *see* Esomeprazole . . . 516
NFV *see* Nelfinavir . . . 972
Niacin . . . 978
Niacinamide . . . 979
Niacin and Lovastatin . . . 979
Niacor® *see* Niacin . . . 978
Niar® (Mex) *see* Selegiline . . . 1212
Niaspan® (Can) *see* Niacin . . . 978
Niastase® (Can) *see* Factor VIIa (Recombinant) . . . 571
NiCARdipine . . . 980
Nicardipine Hydrochloride *see* NiCARdipine . . . 980
Nicoderm® (Can) *see* Nicotine . . . 981
NicoDerm® CQ® [OTC] *see* Nicotine . . . 981
Nicorette® [OTC] *see* Nicotine . . . 981
Nicorette® Plus (Can) *see* Nicotine . . . 981
Nicotinamide *see* Niacinamide . . . 979
Nicotinamide Adenine Dinucleotide . . . 1443
Nicotine . . . 981
Nicotinell TTS® (Mex) *see* Nicotine . . . 981
Nicotinex [OTC] *see* Niacin . . . 978
Nicotinic Acid *see* Niacin . . . 978
Nicotrol® (Can) *see* Nicotine . . . 981
Nicotrol® Inhaler *see* Nicotine . . . 981
Nicotrol® NS *see* Nicotine . . . 981
Nicotrol® Patch [OTC] *see* Nicotine . . . 981
Nidagel™ (Can) *see* Metronidazole . . . 917
Nidrozol® [tabs] (Mex) *see* Metronidazole . . . 917
Nifedical™ XL *see* NIFEdipine . . . 984
NIFEdipine . . . 984
Nifedipres® (Mex) *see* NIFEdipine . . . 984
Niferex® [OTC] *see* Polysaccharide-Iron Complex . . . 1101
Niferex® 150 [OTC] *see* Polysaccharide-Iron Complex . . . 1101
Niftolid *see* Flutamide . . . 615
Nilandron® *see* Nilutamide . . . 986
Nilstat (Can) *see* Nystatin . . . 1003
Nilutamide . . . 986
Nimodipine . . . 987
Nimotop® (Can) *see* Nimodipine . . . 987
Nipent® (Can) *see* Pentostatin . . . 1065
Nipride® (Can) *see* Nitroprusside . . . 993
Nisoldipine . . . 988
Nistaken® [tabs] (Mex) *see* Propafenone . . . 1133
Nitalapram *see* Citalopram . . . 339
Nitazoxanide . . . 989
Nitisinone . . . 989
Nitradisc® (Mex) *see* Nitroglycerin . . . 991
Nitrek® *see* Nitroglycerin . . . 991
Nitric Oxide . . . 990
4′-Nitro-3′-Trifluoromethylisobutyrantide *see* Flutamide . . . 615
Nitro-Bid® *see* Nitroglycerin . . . 991
Nitroderm TTS® (Mex) *see* Nitroglycerin . . . 991
Nitro-Dur® *see* Nitroglycerin . . . 991
Nitrofurantoin . . . 990
Nitrogard® *see* Nitroglycerin . . . 991
Nitroglycerin . . . 991
Nitroglycerol *see* Nitroglycerin . . . 991
Nitrol® [DSC] *see* Nitroglycerin . . . 991
Nitrolingual® *see* Nitroglycerin . . . 991
Nitropress® *see* Nitroprusside . . . 993

Nitroprusside 993
Nitroprusside Sodium *see* Nitroprusside 993
NitroQuick® *see* Nitroglycerin 991
Nitrostat® *see* Nitroglycerin 991
Nitro-Tab® *see* Nitroglycerin 991
NitroTime® *see* Nitroglycerin 991
Nitrous Oxide 994
Nivoflox® [tabs] (Mex) *see* Ciprofloxacin 331
Nivoflox® [inj.] (Mex) *see* Ciprofloxacin 331
Nix® [OTC] *see* Permethrin 1070
Nixal® (Mex) *see* Naproxen 965
Nizatidine 995
Nizoral® (Mex) *see* Ketoconazole . . . 783
Nizoral® A-D [OTC] *see* Ketoconazole 783
N-Methylhydrazine *see* Procarbazine 1125
Nobligan® (Mex) *see* Tramadol . . . 1319
Nolahist® [OTC] *see* Phenindamine 1073
Nolvadex® (Can) *see* Tamoxifen . . 1258
Nolvadex®-D (Can) *see* Tamoxifen 1258
Nonoxynol 9 995
Nonviral Infectious Diseases 1495
Nora-BE™ *see* Norethindrone 996
Noradrenaline *see* Norepinephrine . . 996
Noradrenaline Acid Tartrate *see* Norepinephrine 996
Norboral® (Mex) *see* GlyBURIDE . . . 664
Norciden® (Mex) *see* Danazol 396
Norco® *see* Hydrocodone and Acetaminophen 702
Nordeoxyguanosine *see* Ganciclovir 646
Nordette® *see* Ethinyl Estradiol and Levonorgestrel 545
Norditropin® *see* Human Growth Hormone 694
Norditropin® Cartridges *see* Human Growth Hormone 694
Norelgestromin and Ethinyl Estradiol *see* Ethinyl Estradiol and Norelgestromin 548
Norepinephrine 996
Norepinephrine Bitartrate *see* Norepinephrine 996
Norethindrone 996
Norethindrone Acetate *see* Norethindrone 996
Norethindrone Acetate and Ethinyl Estradiol *see* Ethinyl Estradiol and Norethindrone 550
Norethindrone and Estradiol *see* Estradiol and Norethindrone 521
Norethindrone and Mestranol *see* Mestranol and Norethindrone . . . 884
Norethisterone *see* Norethindrone . . 996
Norfenon® (Mex) *see* Propafenone 1133
Norflex™ *see* Orphenadrine 1017
Norfloxacin 997
Norfloxacine® (Can) *see* Norfloxacin 997
Norgesic™ *see* Orphenadrine, Aspirin, and Caffeine 1018
Norgesic™ Forte (Can) *see* Orphenadrine, Aspirin, and Caffeine 1018
Norgestimate and Estradiol *see* Estradiol and Norgestimate 521
Norgestimate and Ethinyl Estradiol *see* Ethinyl Estradiol and Norgestimate 554
Norgestrel 998
Norgestrel and Ethinyl Estradiol *see* Ethinyl Estradiol and Norgestrel 557
Norinyl® 1+35 *see* Ethinyl Estradiol and Norethindrone 550
Norinyl® 1+50 *see* Mestranol and Norethindrone 884
Noritate® (Can) *see* Metronidazole . . 917
Norlutate® (Can) *see* Norethindrone 996
Normal Blood Values 1620
Normal Saline *see* Sodium Chloride 1227
Normodyne® *see* Labetalol 791
Noroxin® (Mex) *see* Norfloxacin 997
Norpace® *see* Disopyramide 455
Norpace® CR *see* Disopyramide . . . 455
Norplant® Implant (Can) *see* Levonorgestrel 815
Norpramin® (Can) *see* Desipramine 407
Norpril® (Mex) *see* Enalapril 488
Nor-QD® *see* Norethindrone 996
Nortrel™ *see* Ethinyl Estradiol and Norethindrone 550
Nortrel™ 7/7/7 *see* Ethinyl Estradiol and Norethindrone 550
Nortriptyline 999
Nortriptyline Hydrochloride *see* Nortriptyline 999
Norvas® (Mex) *see* Amlodipine 108
Norvasc® (Can) *see* Amlodipine 108
Norventyl (Can) *see* Nortriptyline . . . 999
Norvir® *see* Ritonavir 1189
Norvir® SEC (Can) *see* Ritonavir . . 1189
Nosebleed *see* Feverfew 1426
Nostril® [OTC] *see* Phenylephrine 1078
Nōstrilla® [OTC] *see* Oxymetazoline 1034
Novahistex® DM Decongestant (Can) *see* Pseudoephedrine and Dextromethorphan 1148
Novahistex® DM Decongestant Expectorant (Can) *see* Guaifenesin, Pseudoephedrine, and Dextromethorphan 676
Novahistex® Expectorant with Decongestant (Can) *see* Guaifenesin and Pseudoephedrine 675
Novahistine® DM Decongestant (Can) *see* Pseudoephedrine and Dextromethorphan 1148
Novahistine® DM Decongestant Expectorant (Can) *see* Guaifenesin, Pseudoephedrine, and Dextromethorphan 676
Novamilor (Can) *see* Amiloride and Hydrochlorothiazide 96
Novamoxin® (Can) *see* Amoxicillin . . 114
Novantrone® (Can) *see* Mitoxantrone 938
Novarel™ *see* Chorionic Gonadotropin (Human) 326
Novasen (Can) *see* Aspirin 151
Novaxen® (Mex) *see* Naproxen 965
Novo-5 ASA (Can) *see* Mesalamine 882
Novo-Acebutolol (Can) *see* Acebutolol 46
Novo-Alendronate (Can) *see* Alendronate 77
Novo-Alprazol (Can) *see* Alprazolam 84
Novo-Amiodarone (Can) *see* Amiodarone 101
Novo-Ampicillin (Can) *see* Ampicillin 124
Novo-Atenol (Can) *see* Atenolol 159
Novo-AZT (Can) *see* Zidovudine . . 1398
Novo-Bromazepam (Can) *see* Bromazepam 218

Novo-Buspirone (Can) *see* BusPIRone . . . 233
Novocain® (Can) *see* Procaine . . . 1125
Novo-Captopril (Can) *see* Captopril . . . 252
Novo-Carbamaz (Can) *see* Carbamazepine . . . 255
Novo-Cefaclor (Can) *see* Cefaclor . . 274
Novo-Cefadroxil (Can) *see* Cefadroxil . . . 275
Novo-Chlorpromazine (Can) *see* ChlorproMAZINE . . . 319
Novo-Cholamine (Can) *see* Cholestyramine Resin . . . 323
Novo-Cholamine Light (Can) *see* Cholestyramine Resin . . . 323
Novo-Cimetidine (Can) *see* Cimetidine . . . 330
Novo-Clindamycin (Can) *see* Clindamycin . . . 348
Novo-Clobazam (Can) *see* Clobazam . . . 350
Novo-Clobetasol® (Can) *see* Clobetasol . . . 351
Novo-Clonazepam (Can) *see* Clonazepam . . . 356
Novo-Clonidine (Can) *see* Clonidine . . . 358
Novo-Clopate (Can) *see* Clorazepate . . . 362
Novo-Clopramine (Can) *see* ClomiPRAMINE . . . 355
Novo-Cloxin (Can) *see* Cloxacillin . . 365
Novo-Cycloprine (Can) *see* Cyclobenzaprine . . . 382
Novo-Desipramine (Can) *see* Desipramine . . . 407
Novo-Difenac (Can) *see* Diclofenac . . . 427
Novo-Difenac K (Can) *see* Diclofenac . . . 427
Novo-Difenac-SR (Can) *see* Diclofenac . . . 427
Novo-Diflunisal (Can) *see* Diflunisal . . . 435
Novo-Digoxin (Can) *see* Digoxin . . . 437
Novo-Diltazem (Can) *see* Diltiazem . . . 444
Novo-Diltazem-CD (Can) *see* Diltiazem . . . 444
Novo-Diltazem SR (Can) *see* Diltiazem . . . 444
Novo-Dimenate (Can) *see* DimenhyDRINATE . . . 446
Novo-Dipiradol (Can) *see* Dipyridamole . . . 453
Novo-Divalproex (Can) *see* Valproic Acid and Derivatives . . . 1359
Novo-Docusate Calcium (Can) *see* Docusate . . . 459
Novo-Docusate Sodium (Can) *see* Docusate . . . 459
Novo-Doxazosin (Can) *see* Doxazosin . . . 465
Novo-Doxepin (Can) *see* Doxepin . . 467
Novo-Doxylin (Can) *see* Doxycycline . . . 471
Novo-Famotidine (Can) *see* Famotidine . . . 573
Novo-Fenofibrate (Can) *see* Fenofibrate . . . 577
Novo-Ferrogluc (Can) *see* Ferrous Gluconate . . . 586
Novo-Fibrate (Can) *see* Clofibrate . . 353
Novo-Fluconazole (Can) *see* Fluconazole . . . 594
Novo-Fluoxetine (Can) *see* Fluoxetine . . . 606
Novo-Flurprofen (Can) *see* Flurbiprofen . . . 613
Novo-Flutamide (Can) *see* Flutamide . . . 615
Novo-Fluvoxamine (Can) *see* Fluvoxamine . . . 623
Novo-Furantoin (Can) *see* Nitrofurantoin . . . 990
Novo-Gabapentin (Can) *see* Gabapentin . . . 642
Novo-Gemfibrozil (Can) *see* Gemfibrozil . . . 651
Novo-Glyburide (Can) *see* GlyBURIDE . . . 664
Novo-Herklin 2000® (Mex) *see* Permethrin . . . 1070
Novo-Hydrazide (Can) *see* Hydrochlorothiazide . . . 699
Novo-Hydroxyzin (Can) *see* HydrOXYzine . . . 723
Novo-Hylazin (Can) *see* HydrALAZINE . . . 697
Novo-Indapamide (Can) *see* Indapamide . . . 743
Novo-Ipramide (Can) *see* Ipratropium . . . 761
Novo-Keto (Can) *see* Ketoprofen . . . 785
Novo-Ketoconazole (Can) *see* Ketoconazole . . . 783
Novo-Keto-EC (Can) *see* Ketoprofen . . . 785
Novo-Ketorolac (Can) *see* Ketorolac . . . 787
Novo-Ketotifen (Can) *see* Ketotifen . . . 790
Novo-Levobunolol (Can) *see* Levobunolol . . . 808
Novo-Levocarbidopa (Can) *see* Levodopa and Carbidopa . . . 811
Novo-Lexin® (Can) *see* Cephalexin . . . 294
Novolin® 70/30 *see* Insulin Preparations . . . 749
Novolin® ge (Can) *see* Insulin Preparations . . . 749
Novolin® L [DSC] *see* Insulin Preparations . . . 749
Novolin® N *see* Insulin Preparations . . . 749
Novolin® R *see* Insulin Preparations . . . 749
NovoLog® *see* Insulin Preparations . . . 749
NovoLog® Mix 70/30 *see* Insulin Preparations . . . 749
Novo-Loperamide (Can) *see* Loperamide . . . 838
Novo-Lorazepam (Can) *see* Lorazepam . . . 842
Novo-Lovastatin (Can) *see* Lovastatin . . . 848
Novo-Maprotiline (Can) *see* Maprotiline . . . 856
Novo-Medrone (Can) *see* MedroxyPROGESTERone . . . 862
Novo-Meprazine (Can) *see* Methotrimeprazine . . . 901
Novo-Mepro (Can) *see* Meprobamate . . . 878
Novo-Metformin (Can) *see* Metformin . . . 887
Novo-Methacin (Can) *see* Indomethacin . . . 746
Novo-Metoprolol (Can) *see* Metoprolol . . . 915
Novo-Mexiletine (Can) *see* Mexiletine . . . 921
Novo-Minocycline (Can) *see* Minocycline . . . 931
Novo-Misoprostol (Can) *see* Misoprostol . . . 936
Novo-Mucilax (Can) *see* Psyllium . . 1151
Novo-Nadolol (Can) *see* Nadolol . . . 956

Novo-Naproc EC (Can) *see* Naproxen . . . 965
Novo-Naprox (Can) *see* Naproxen . . 965
Novo-Naprox Sodium (Can) *see* Naproxen . . . 965
Novo-Naprox Sodium DS (Can) *see* Naproxen . . . 965
Novo-Naprox SR (Can) *see* Naproxen . . . 965
Novo-Nidazol (Can) *see* Metronidazole . . . 917
Novo-Nifedin (Can) *see* NIFEdipine . . . 984
Novo-Nizatidine (Can) *see* Nizatidine . . . 995
Novo-Norfloxacin (Can) *see* Norfloxacin . . . 997
Novo-Nortriptyline (Can) *see* Nortriptyline . . . 999
Novo-Oxybutynin (Can) *see* Oxybutynin . . . 1026
Novo-Pen-VK (Can) *see* Penicillin V Potassium . . . 1060
Novo-Peridol (Can) *see* Haloperidol . . . 682
Novo-Pheniram (Can) *see* Chlorpheniramine . . . 313
Novo-Pindol (Can) *see* Pindolol . . . 1090
Novo-Pirocam (Can) *see* Piroxicam . . . 1097
Novo-Pravastatin (Can) *see* Pravastatin . . . 1109
Novo-Prazin (Can) *see* Prazosin . . 1111
Novo-Prednisolone® (Can) *see* PrednisoLONE . . . 1113
Novo-Profen® (Can) *see* Ibuprofen . . 728
Novo-Propamide (Can) *see* ChlorproPAMIDE . . . 321
Novoquin® (Mex) *see* Ciprofloxacin . . . 331
Novo-Quinidin (Can) *see* Quinidine . . . 1160
Novo-Ranidine (Can) *see* Ranitidine . . . 1169
NovoRapid® (Can) *see* Insulin Preparations . . . 749
Novo-Selegiline (Can) *see* Selegiline . . . 1212
Novo-Sertraline (Can) *see* Sertraline . . . 1215
Novo-Seven® *see* Factor VIIa (Recombinant) . . . 571
Novo-Sorbide (Can) *see* Isosorbide Dinitrate . . . 770
Novo-Sotalol (Can) *see* Sotalol . . . 1231
Novo-Soxazole® (Can) *see* SulfiSOXAZOLE . . . 1250
Novo-Spiroton (Can) *see* Spironolactone . . . 1235
Novo-Spirozine (Can) *see* Hydrochlorothiazide and Spironolactone . . . 701
Novo-Sucralate (Can) *see* Sucralfate . . . 1242
Novo-Sundac (Can) *see* Sulindac . . . 1251
Novo-Tamoxifen (Can) *see* Tamoxifen . . . 1258
Novo-Temazepam (Can) *see* Temazepam . . . 1266
Novo-Terazosin (Can) *see* Terazosin . . . 1271
Novo-Terbinafine (Can) *see* Terbinafine . . . 1272
Novo-Tetra (Can) *see* Tetracycline . . . 1280
Novo-Theophyl SR (Can) *see* Theophylline . . . 1285
Novothyrox *see* Levothyroxine . . . 817
Novo-Ticlopidine (Can) *see* Ticlopidine . . . 1297
Novo-Trazodone (Can) *see* Trazodone . . . 1326
Novo-Triamzide (Can) *see* Hydrochlorothiazide and Triamterene . . . 701
Novo-Trifluzine (Can) *see* Trifluoperazine . . . 1338
Novo-Trimel (Can) *see* Sulfamethoxazole and Trimethoprim . . . 1246
Novo-Trimel D.S. (Can) *see* Sulfamethoxazole and Trimethoprim . . . 1246
Novo-Tripramine (Can) *see* Trimipramine . . . 1343
Novo-Veramil (Can) *see* Verapamil . . . 1373
Novo-Veramil SR (Can) *see* Verapamil . . . 1373
Novoxapram® (Can) *see* Oxazepam . . . 1022
Nozinan® (Can) *see* Methotrimeprazine . . . 901
NPH Iletin® II *see* Insulin Preparations . . . 749
NPH, Insulin *see* Insulin Preparations . . . 749
NSC-740 *see* Methotrexate . . . 897
NSC-752 *see* Thioguanine . . . 1288
NSC-755 *see* Mercaptopurine . . . 880
NSC-3053 *see* Dactinomycin . . . 394
NSC-3088 *see* Chlorambucil . . . 305
NSC-10363 *see* Megestrol . . . 865
NSC-13875 *see* Altretamine . . . 89
NSC-15200 *see* Gallium Nitrate . . . 646
NSC-26271 *see* Cyclophosphamide . . . 384
NSC-26980 *see* Mitomycin . . . 937
NSC-27640 *see* Floxuridine . . . 593
NSC-38721 *see* Mitotane . . . 937
NSC-49842 *see* VinBLAStine . . . 1377
NSC-63878 *see* Cytarabine . . . 390
NSC-67574 *see* VinCRIStine . . . 1378
NSC-77213 *see* Procarbazine . . . 1125
NSC-82151 *see* DAUNOrubicin Hydrochloride . . . 401
NSC-85998 *see* Streptozocin . . . 1240
NSC-89199 *see* Estramustine . . . 523
NSC-102816 *see* Azacitidine . . . 171
NSC-106977 (*Erwinia*) *see* Asparaginase . . . 150
NSC-109229 (*E. coli*) *see* Asparaginase . . . 150
NSC-109724 *see* Ifosfamide . . . 733
NSC-122758 *see* Tretinoin (Oral) . . 1328
NSC-123127 *see* DOXOrubicin . . . 469
NSC-125066 *see* Bleomycin . . . 213
NSC-125973 *see* Paclitaxel . . . 1038
NSC-147834 *see* Flutamide . . . 615
NSC-180973 *see* Tamoxifen . . . 1258
NSC-218321 *see* Pentostatin . . . 1065
NSC-245467 *see* Vindesine . . . 1379
NSC-249992 *see* Amsacrine . . . 129
NSC-256439 *see* Idarubicin . . . 732
NSC-266046 *see* Oxaliplatin . . . 1020
NSC-301739 *see* Mitoxantrone . . . 938
NSC-308847 *see* Amonafide . . . 112
NSC-352122 *see* Trimetrexate Glucuronate . . . 1342
NSC-362856 *see* Temozolomide . . 1268
NSC-373364 *see* Aldesleukin . . . 74
NSC-377526 *see* Leuprolide . . . 805
NSC-409962 *see* Carmustine . . . 268
NSC-603071 *see* Aminocamptothecin . . . 96
NSC-606864 *see* Goserelin . . . 670
NSC-609699 *see* Topotecan . . . 1316
NSC-616348 *see* Irinotecan . . . 764
NSC-628503 *see* Docetaxel . . . 458
NSC-644954 *see* Pegaspargase . . 1051
NSC-698037 *see* Pemetrexed . . . 1054

NSC-715055 *see* Gefitinib 649
NTG *see* Nitroglycerin 991
N-trifluoroacetyladriamycin-14-valerate *see* Valrubicin 1362
NTZ *see* Nitazoxanide 989
Nu-Acebutolol (Can) *see* Acebutolol 46
Nu-Acyclovir (Can) *see* Acyclovir 64
Nu-Alprax (Can) *see* Alprazolam 84
Nu-Amilzide (Can) *see* Amiloride and Hydrochlorothiazide 96
Nu-Amoxi (Can) *see* Amoxicillin 114
Nu-Ampi (Can) *see* Ampicillin 124
Nu-Atenol (Can) *see* Atenolol 159
Nu-Baclo (Can) *see* Baclofen 180
Nubain® (Can) *see* Nalbuphine 959
Nu-Beclomethasone (Can) *see* Beclomethasone 184
Nu-Bromazepam (Can) *see* Bromazepam 218
Nu-Buspirone (Can) *see* BusPIRone 233
Nu-Capto (Can) *see* Captopril 252
Nu-Carbamazepine (Can) *see* Carbamazepine 255
Nu-Cefaclor (Can) *see* Cefaclor 274
Nu-Cephalex (Can) *see* Cephalexin 294
Nu-Cimet (Can) *see* Cimetidine 330
Nu-Clonazepam (Can) *see* Clonazepam 356
Nu-Clonidine (Can) *see* Clonidine . . 358
Nu-Cloxi (Can) *see* Cloxacillin 365
Nucofed® Expectorant *see* Guaifenesin, Pseudoephedrine, and Codeine 676
Nucofed® Pediatric Expectorant *see* Guaifenesin, Pseudoephedrine, and Codeine 676
Nu-Cotrimox (Can) *see* Sulfamethoxazole and Trimethoprim 1246
Nucotuss® *see* Guaifenesin, Pseudoephedrine, and Codeine 676
Nu-Cromolyn (Can) *see* Cromolyn . . 378
Nu-Cyclobenzaprine (Can) *see* Cyclobenzaprine 382
Nu-Desipramine (Can) *see* Desipramine 407
Nu-Diclo (Can) *see* Diclofenac 427
Nu-Diclo-SR (Can) *see* Diclofenac . . 427
Nu-Diflunisal (Can) *see* Diflunisal . . . 435
Nu-Diltiaz (Can) *see* Diltiazem 444
Nu-Diltiaz-CD (Can) *see* Diltiazem . . 444
Nu-Divalproex (Can) *see* Valproic Acid and Derivatives 1359
Nu-Doxycycline (Can) *see* Doxycycline 471
Nu-Erythromycin-S (Can) *see* Erythromycin 508
Nu-Famotidine (Can) *see* Famotidine 573
Nu-Fenofibrate (Can) *see* Fenofibrate 577
Nu-Fluoxetine (Can) *see* Fluoxetine 606
Nu-Flurprofen (Can) *see* Flurbiprofen 613
Nu-Fluvoxamine (Can) *see* Fluvoxamine 623
Nu-Gabapentin (Can) *see* Gabapentin 642
Nu-Gemfibrozil (Can) *see* Gemfibrozil 651
Nu-Glyburide (Can) *see* GlyBURIDE 664
Nu-Hydral (Can) *see* HydrALAZINE 697
Nu-Ibuprofen (Can) *see* Ibuprofen . . 728
Nu-Indapamide (Can) *see* Indapamide 743
Nu-Indo (Can) *see* Indomethacin . . . 746
Nu-Ipratropium (Can) *see* Ipratropium 761
Nu-Iron® 150 [OTC] *see* Polysaccharide-Iron Complex . . 1101
Nu-Ketoprofen (Can) *see* Ketoprofen 785
Nu-Ketoprofen-E (Can) *see* Ketoprofen 785
NuLev™ *see* Hyoscyamine 724
Nu-Levocarb (Can) *see* Levodopa and Carbidopa 811
Nullo® [OTC] *see* Chlorophyll 310
Nu-Loraz (Can) *see* Lorazepam 842
Nu-Lovastatin (Can) *see* Lovastatin 848
Nu-Loxapine (Can) *see* Loxapine . . . 850
NuLytely® *see* Polyethylene Glycol-Electrolyte Solution 1100
Nu-Medopa (Can) *see* Methyldopa . . 906
Nu-Mefenamic (Can) *see* Mefenamic Acid 863
Nu-Megestrol (Can) *see* Megestrol . . 865
Nu-Metformin (Can) *see* Metformin 887
Nu-Metoclopramide (Can) *see* Metoclopramide 914
Nu-Metop (Can) *see* Metoprolol 915
Numorphan® *see* Oxymorphone . . . 1036
Nu-Naprox (Can) *see* Naproxen 965
Nu-Nifed (Can) *see* NIFEdipine 984
Nu-Nizatidine (Can) *see* Nizatidine . . 995
Nu-Nortriptyline (Can) *see* Nortriptyline 999
Nu-Oxybutyn (Can) *see* Oxybutynin 1026
Nu-Pentoxifylline SR (Can) *see* Pentoxifylline 1066
Nu-Pen-VK (Can) *see* Penicillin V Potassium 1060
Nupercainal® [OTC] *see* Dibucaine 426
Nupercainal® Hydrocortisone Cream [OTC] *see* Hydrocortisone 714
Nu-Pindol (Can) *see* Pindolol 1090
Nu-Pirox (Can) *see* Piroxicam 1097
Nu-Prazo (Can) *see* Prazosin 1111
Nu-Prochlor (Can) *see* Prochlorperazine 1126
Nu-Propranolol (Can) *see* Propranolol 1140
Nuquin HP® *see* Hydroquinone 719
Nu-Ranit (Can) *see* Ranitidine 1169
Nu-Selegiline (Can) *see* Selegiline 1212
Nu-Sertraline (Can) *see* Sertraline 1215
Nu-Sotalol (Can) *see* Sotalol 1231
Nu-Sucralate (Can) *see* Sucralfate 1242
Nu-Sulfinpyrazone (Can) *see* Sulfinpyrazone 1249
Nu-Sundac (Can) *see* Sulindac . . . 1251
Nu-Tears® [OTC] *see* Artificial Tears 148
Nu-Tears® II [OTC] *see* Artificial Tears 148
Nu-Temazepam (Can) *see* Temazepam 1266
Nu-Terazosin (Can) *see* Terazosin 1271
Nu-Tetra (Can) *see* Tetracycline . . 1280
Nu-Ticlopidine (Can) *see* Ticlopidine 1297
Nu-Timolol (Can) *see* Timolol 1299
Nutracort® *see* Hydrocortisone 714
Nutraplus® [OTC] *see* Urea 1353

Nu-Trazodone (Can) *see* Trazodone . . . 1326
Nu-Triazide (Can) *see* Hydrochlorothiazide and Triamterene . . . 701
Nu-Trimipramine (Can) *see* Trimipramine . . . 1343
Nutropin® *see* Human Growth Hormone . . . 694
Nutropin AQ® *see* Human Growth Hormone . . . 694
Nutropin Depot® [DSC] *see* Human Growth Hormone . . . 694
Nutropine® (Can) *see* Human Growth Hormone . . . 694
NuvaRing® *see* Ethinyl Estradiol and Etonogestrel . . . 543
Nu-Verap (Can) *see* Verapamil . . . 1373
Nu-Zopiclone (Can) *see* Zopiclone . . . 1406
NVB *see* Vinorelbine . . . 1380
NVP *see* Nevirapine . . . 977
Nyaderm (Can) *see* Nystatin . . . 1003
Nydrazid® *see* Isoniazid . . . 769
Nylidrin . . . 1002
Nystatin . . . 1003
Nystatin and Triamcinolone . . . 1004
Nystat-Rx® *see* Nystatin . . . 1003
Nystop® *see* Nystatin . . . 1003
Nytol® (Can) *see* DiphenhydrAMINE . . . 448
Nytol® Extra Strength (Can) *see* DiphenhydrAMINE . . . 448
Nytol® Maximum Strength [OTC] *see* DiphenhydrAMINE . . . 448
Obezine® *see* Phendimetrazine . . . 1072
OCBZ *see* Oxcarbazepine . . . 1023
Occlusal™ (Can) *see* Salicylic Acid . . . 1205
Occlusal®-HP [OTC] *see* Salicylic Acid . . . 1205
Occupational Exposure to Bloodborne Pathogens (Standard/Universal Precautions) . . . 1603
Ocean® [OTC] *see* Sodium Chloride . . . 1227
Octagam® *see* Immune Globulin (Intravenous) . . . 740
Octostim® (Can) *see* Desmopressin . . . 409
Octreotide . . . 1004
Octreotide Acetate *see* Octreotide . . . 1004
Ocuclear® (Mex) *see* Oxymetazoline . . . 1034
OcuCoat® [OTC] *see* Artificial Tears . . . 148
OcuCoat® PF [OTC] *see* Artificial Tears . . . 148
Ocufen® *see* Flurbiprofen . . . 613
Ocuflox® (Can) *see* Ofloxacin . . . 1005
Ocupress® [DSC] *see* Carteolol . . . 269
Ocupress® Ophthalmic (Can) *see* Carteolol . . . 269
Ocusulf-10 *see* Sulfacetamide . . . 1244
Oenothera biennis see Evening Primrose . . . 1425
Oesclim® (Can) *see* Estradiol . . . 518
Ofloxacin . . . 1005
Ogastro® (Mex) *see* Lansoprazole . . . 797
Ogen® (Mex) *see* Estropipate . . . 531
Ogestrel® *see* Ethinyl Estradiol and Norgestrel . . . 557
OGMT *see* Metyrosine . . . 920
OGT-918 *see* Miglustat . . . 930
OKT3 *see* Muromonab-CD3 . . . 952
Olanzapine . . . 1007
Olanzapine and Fluoxetine . . . 1009
Olanzapine and Fluoxetine Hydrochloride *see* Olanzapine and Fluoxetine . . . 1009
Oleovitamin A *see* Vitamin A . . . 1382
Oleum Ricini *see* Castor Oil . . . 273
Olexin® (Mex) *see* Omeprazole . . . 1012
Olmesartan . . . 1010
Olmesartan and Hydrochlorothiazide . . . 1010
Olmesartan Medoxomil *see* Olmesartan . . . 1010
Olmesartan Medoxomil and Hydrochlorothiazide *see* Olmesartan and Hydrochlorothiazide . . . 1010
Olopatadine . . . 1011
Olsalazine . . . 1011
Olsalazine Sodium *see* Olsalazine . . . 1011
Olux® *see* Clobetasol . . . 351
Omalizumab . . . 1012
Omeprazole . . . 1012
Omnicef® *see* Cefdinir . . . 279
Omnipaque® *see* Radiological/Contrast Media (Nonionic) . . . 1166
Oncaspar® *see* Pegaspargase . . . 1051
Oncotice™ (Can) *see* BCG Vaccine . . . 183
Oncovin® (Can) *see* VinCRIStine . . . 1378
Ondansetron . . . 1014
Ondansetron Hydrochloride *see* Ondansetron . . . 1014
One-A-Day® 50 Plus Formula [OTC] *see* Vitamins (Multiple/Oral) . . . 1384
One-A-Day® Active Formula [OTC] *see* Vitamins (Multiple/Oral) . . . 1384
One-A -Day® Essential Formula [OTC] *see* Vitamins (Multiple/Oral) . . . 1384
One-A-Day® Maximum Formula [OTC] *see* Vitamins (Multiple/Oral) . . . 1384
One-A- Day® Men's Formula [OTC] *see* Vitamins (Multiple/Oral) . . . 1384
One-A-Day® Today [OTC] *see* Vitamins (Multiple/Oral) . . . 1384
One-A-Day® Women's Formula [OTC] *see* Vitamins (Multiple/Oral) . . . 1384
Onofin-K® (Mex) *see* Ketoconazole . . . 783
ONTAK® *see* Denileukin Diftitox . . . 405
Onxol™ *see* Paclitaxel . . . 1038
Ony-Clear [OTC] [DSC] *see* Benzalkonium Chloride . . . 190
OPC-13013 *see* Cilostazol . . . 329
OPC-14597 *see* Aripiprazole . . . 142
OP-CCK *see* Sincalide . . . 1224
Opcon-A® [OTC] *see* Naphazoline and Pheniramine . . . 964
o,p'-DDD *see* Mitotane . . . 937
Operand® [OTC] *see* Povidone-Iodine . . . 1107
Operand® Chlorhexidine Gluconate [OTC] *see* Chlorhexidine Gluconate . . . 308
Ophthetic® *see* Proparacaine . . . 1134
Ophtho-Dipivefrin™ (Can) *see* Dipivefrin . . . 453
Ophtho-Tate® (Can) *see* PrednisoLONE . . . 1113
Opium and Belladonna *see* Belladonna and Opium . . . 186
Opium, Hyoscyamine, Atropine, Scopolamine, Kaolin, and Pectin *see* Hyoscyamine, Atropine, Scopolamine, Kaolin, Pectin, and Opium . . . 726
Opium Tincture . . . 1015

Opium Tincture, Deodorized *see* Opium Tincture 1015
Oprad® (Mex) *see* Amikacin 95
Oprelvekin 1015
Opthaflox® (Mex) *see* Ciprofloxacin 331
Opthavir® (Mex) *see* Acyclovir 64
Optho-Bunolol® (Can) *see* Levobunolol 808
Opticaine® *see* Tetracaine 1278
Opticrom® *see* Cromolyn 378
Opticyl® *see* Tropicamide 1348
Optifree® (Mex) *see* Pancreatin . . . 1042
Optigene® 3 [OTC] *see* Tetrahydrozoline 1282
Optimyxin® (Can) *see* Bacitracin and Polymyxin B 178
Optimyxin Plus® (Can) *see* Neomycin, Polymyxin B, and Gramicidin 974
OptiPranolol® (Can) *see* Metipranolol 913
Optiray® *see* Radiological/Contrast Media (Nonionic) 1166
Optivar® *see* Azelastine 173
Optomicin® (Mex) *see* Erythromycin 508
Orabase®-B [OTC] *see* Benzocaine 191
Oracit® *see* Sodium Citrate and Citric Acid 1228
Oracort (Can) *see* Triamcinolone . . 1330
Oracort® (Can) *see* Triamcinolone Acetonide (Dental Paste) 1333
Orajel® [OTC] *see* Benzocaine 191
Orajel® Baby [OTC] *see* Benzocaine 191
Orajel® Baby Nighttime [OTC] *see* Benzocaine 191
Orajel® Maximum Strength [OTC] *see* Benzocaine 191
Orajel® Perioseptic® Spot Treatment [OTC] *see* Carbamide Peroxide 259
Oral Bacterial Infections 1533
Oral Fungal Infections 1544
Oral Nonviral Soft Tissue Ulcerations or Erosions 1551
Oral Pain 1526
Oral Rinse Products 1638
Oral Viral Infections 1547
Oramorph SR® *see* Morphine Sulfate 947
Orange Root *see* Golden Seal 1433
Oranor® (Mex) *see* Norfloxacin 997
Oranyl [OTC] *see* Pseudoephedrine 1147
Orap® (Can) *see* Pimozide 1088
Orapred® *see* PrednisoLONE 1113
OraRinse™ [OTC] *see* Maltodextrin 855
Orasol® [OTC] *see* Benzocaine 191
Orazinc® [OTC] *see* Zinc Sulfate . . 1401
Orciprenaline Sulfate *see* Metaproterenol 885
Orelox® (Mex) *see* Cefpodoxime . . . 285
Oretic® *see* Hydrochlorothiazide 699
Orfadin® *see* Nitisinone 989
Orgalutran® (Can) *see* Ganirelix 647
Organ-1 NR *see* Guaifenesin 672
Organidin® NR *see* Guaifenesin 672
Orgaran® [DSC] *see* Danaparoid . . . 395
Oriental Plum Tree *see* Ginkgo Biloba 1429
Orinase Diagnostic® [DSC] *see* TOLBUTamide 1309
ORLAAM® [DSC] *see* Levomethadyl Acetate Hydrochloride 814
Orlistat 1017
Ornex® [OTC] *see* Acetaminophen and Pseudoephedrine 53
Ornex® Maximum Strength [OTC] *see* Acetaminophen and Pseudoephedrine 53
ORO-Clense (Can) *see* Chlorhexidine Gluconate 308
Orphenace® (Can) *see* Orphenadrine 1017
Orphenadrine 1017
Orphenadrine, Aspirin, and Caffeine 1018
Orphenadrine Citrate *see* Orphenadrine 1017
Orphengesic *see* Orphenadrine, Aspirin, and Caffeine 1018
Orphengesic Forte *see* Orphenadrine, Aspirin, and Caffeine 1018
Ortho® 0.5/35 (Can) *see* Ethinyl Estradiol and Norethindrone 550
Ortho® 1/35 (Can) *see* Ethinyl Estradiol and Norethindrone 550
Ortho® 7/7/7 (Can) *see* Ethinyl Estradiol and Norethindrone 550
Ortho-Cept® (Can) *see* Ethinyl Estradiol and Desogestrel 536
Orthoclone OKT® 3 (Can) *see* Muromonab-CD3 952
Ortho Cyclen *see* Ethinyl Estradiol and Norgestimate 554
Ortho Est *see* Estropipate 531
Ortho Evra™ *see* Ethinyl Estradiol and Norelgestromin 548
Ortho Novum *see* Ethinyl Estradiol and Norethindrone 550
Ortho Novum 1/50 *see* Mestranol and Norethindrone 884
Ortho Prefest *see* Estradiol and Norgestimate 521
Ortho Tri-Cyclen® *see* Ethinyl Estradiol and Norgestimate 554
Ortho Tri-Cyclen® Lo *see* Ethinyl Estradiol and Norgestimate 554
Orthovisc® *see* Hyaluronate and Derivatives 696
Ortopsique® (Mex) *see* Diazepam . . 423
Orudis® (Mex) *see* Ketoprofen 785
Orudis® KT [OTC] *see* Ketoprofen . . 785
Orudis® SR (Can) *see* Ketoprofen . . 785
Oruvail® (Can) *see* Ketoprofen 785
Os-Cal® (Can) *see* Calcium Carbonate 245
Os-Cal® 500 [OTC] *see* Calcium Carbonate 245
Oseltamivir 1019
Oseum® [salmon] (Mex) *see* Calcitonin 243
Osiren® (Mex) *see* Omeprazole . . . 1012
Osmoglyn® *see* Glycerin 667
Osteocit® (Can) *see* Calcium Citrate 246
Osteomin® (Mex) *see* Calcium Carbonate 245
Osteral® (Mex) *see* Piroxicam 1097
Ostoforte® (Can) *see* Ergocalciferol 503
Otrivin® [OTC] [DSC] *see* Xylometazoline 1393
Otrivin® Pediatric [OTC] [DSC] *see* Xylometazoline 1393
Ovace™ *see* Sulfacetamide 1244
Ovcon® *see* Ethinyl Estradiol and Norethindrone 550
Ovidrel® *see* Chorionic Gonadotropin (Recombinant) . . . 326
Ovol® (Can) *see* Simethicone 1222
Ovral® [DSC] *see* Ethinyl Estradiol and Norgestrel 557
Ovrette® *see* Norgestrel 998
Oxacillin 1020

Oxacillin Sodium *see* Oxacillin 1020
Oxaliplatin 1020
Oxandrin® *see* Oxandrolone 1021
Oxandrolone 1021
Oxaprozin 1022
Oxazepam 1022
Oxcarbazepine 1023
Oxeze® Turbuhaler® (Can) *see* Formoterol 629
Oxicanol® (Mex) *see* Piroxicam . . . 1097
Oxiconazole 1024
Oxiconazole Nitrate *see* Oxiconazole 1024
Oxidized Regenerated Cellulose *see* Cellulose (Oxidized/ Regenerated) 293
Oxifungol® (Mex) *see* Fluconazole . . 594
Oxiken® (Mex) *see* DOBUTamine . . 457
Oxilapine Succinate *see* Loxapine . . 850
Oxipor® VHC [OTC] *see* Coal Tar . . 367
Oxistat® (Can) *see* Oxiconazole . . . 1024
Oxitraklin® (Mex) *see* Oxytetracycline 1036
Oxizole® (Can) *see* Oxiconazole . . 1024
Oxpentifylline *see* Pentoxifylline . . . 1066
Oxpram® (Can) *see* Oxazepam . . . 1022
Oxprenolol 1025
Oxprenolol Hydrochloride *see* Oxprenolol 1025
Oxsoralen® (Mex) *see* Methoxsalen 902
Oxsoralen-Ultra® *see* Methoxsalen . . 902
Oxy 10® Balanced Medicated Face Wash [OTC] *see* Benzoyl Peroxide 194
Oxy 10® Balance Spot Treatment [OTC] *see* Benzoyl Peroxide . . . 194
Oxy Balance® [OTC] *see* Salicylic Acid 1205
Oxy® Balance Deep Pore [OTC] *see* Salicylic Acid 1205
Oxybutynin 1026
Oxybutynin Chloride *see* Oxybutynin 1026
Oxychlorosene 1027
Oxychlorosene Sodium *see* Oxychlorosene 1027
Oxycocet® (Can) *see* Oxycodone and Acetaminophen 1029
Oxycodan® (Can) *see* Oxycodone and Aspirin 1032
Oxycodone 1027
Oxycodone and Acetaminophen . . . 1029
Oxycodone and Aspirin 1032
Oxycodone Hydrochloride *see* Oxycodone 1027
OxyContin® *see* Oxycodone 1027
Oxyderm™ (Can) *see* Benzoyl Peroxide 194
Oxydose™ *see* Oxycodone 1027
OxyFast® *see* Oxycodone 1027
Oxygen 1033
OxyIR® *see* Oxycodone 1027
Oxylin® (Mex) *see* Oxymetazoline 1034
Oxymetazoline 1034
Oxymetazoline Hydrochloride *see* Oxymetazoline 1034
Oxymetholone 1035
Oxymorphone 1036
Oxymorphone Hydrochloride *see* Oxymorphone 1036
Oxytetracycline 1036
Oxytetracycline and Hydrocortisone 1037
Oxytetracycline and Polymyxin B . . 1037
Oxytetracycline Hydrochloride *see* Oxytetracycline 1036
Oxytocin 1038
Oxytrol™ *see* Oxybutynin 1026
Oysco 500 [OTC] *see* Calcium Carbonate 245
Oyst-Cal 500 [OTC] *see* Calcium Carbonate 245
P-071 *see* Cetirizine 298
Pacerone® *see* Amiodarone 101
Pacis™ (Can) *see* BCG Vaccine . . . 183
Pacitran® (Mex) *see* Diazepam 423
Paclitaxel 1038
Pactens® (Mex) *see* Naproxen 965
Pain-A-Lay® [OTC] *see* Phenol . . . 1075
Pain-Off [OTC] *see* Acetaminophen, Aspirin, and Caffeine 56
Palafer® (Can) *see* Ferrous Fumarate 586
Palane® (Mex) *see* Enalapril 488
Palgic *see* Carbinoxamine 262
Palgic®-D *see* Carbinoxamine and Pseudoephedrine 262
Palgic®-DS *see* Carbinoxamine and Pseudoephedrine 262
Palivizumab 1040
Palmer's® Skin Success Acne [OTC] *see* Benzoyl Peroxide . . . 194
Palmer's Skin Success Acne Cleanser [OTC] *see* Salicylic Acid 1205
Palmer's® Skin Success Fade Cream™ [OTC] *see* Hydroquinone 719
Palmetto Scrub *see* Saw Palmetto 1446
Palmitate-A® [OTC] *see* Vitamin A 1382
Palonosetron 1040
Palonosetron Hydrochloride *see* Palonosetron 1040
Pamelor® *see* Nortriptyline 999
Pamidronate 1041
Pamidronate Disodium *see* Pamidronate 1041
Pamine® (Can) *see* Methscopolamine 903
Pamine® Forte *see* Methscopolamine 903
p-Aminoclonidine *see* Apraclonidine 138
Pamprin® Maximum Strength All Day Relief [OTC] *see* Naproxen 965
Pan-2400™ [OTC] *see* Pancreatin 1042
Panax ginseng *see* Ginseng, Panax 1430
Pan-B Antibody *see* Rituximab 1191
Pancof® *see* Pseudoephedrine, Dihydrocodeine, and Chlorpheniramine 1150
Pancof®-XP *see* Hydrocodone, Pseudoephedrine, and Guaifenesin 713
Pancrease® (Mex) *see* Pancreatin 1042
Pancrease® *see* Pancrelipase 1042
Pancrease® MT *see* Pancrelipase 1042
Pancreatin 1042
Pancreatin 4X [OTC] *see* Pancreatin 1042
Pancreatin 8X [OTC] *see* Pancreatin 1042
Pancrecarb MS® *see* Pancrelipase 1042
Pancrelipase 1042
Pandel® *see* Hydrocortisone 714
Pangestyme™ CN *see* Pancrelipase 1042
Pangestyme™ EC *see* Pancrelipase 1042

Pangestyme™ MT *see* Pancrelipase 1042
Pangestyme™ UL *see* Pancrelipase 1042
Panglobulin® *see* Immune Globulin (Intravenous) 740
Panhematin® *see* Hemin 684
Panixine DisperDose™ *see* Cephalexin 294
Panlor® DC *see* Acetaminophen, Caffeine, and Dihydrocodeine . . . 57
Panlor® SS *see* Acetaminophen, Caffeine, and Dihydrocodeine . . . 57
PanMist®-DM *see* Guaifenesin, Pseudoephedrine, and Dextromethorphan 676
PanMist® Jr. *see* Guaifenesin and Pseudoephedrine 675
PanMist® LA *see* Guaifenesin and Pseudoephedrine 675
PanMist® S *see* Guaifenesin and Pseudoephedrine 675
PanOxyl® *see* Benzoyl Peroxide . . . 194
PanOxyl®-AQ (Can) *see* Benzoyl Peroxide 194
PanOxyl® Aqua Gel *see* Benzoyl Peroxide 194
PanOxyl® Bar [OTC] *see* Benzoyl Peroxide 194
Panretin™ (Can) *see* Alitretinoin 81
Panthoderm® [OTC] *see* Dexpanthenol 416
Panto™ IV (Can) *see* Pantoprazole 1043
Pantoloc™ (Can) *see* Pantoprazole 1043
Pantomicina® (Mex) *see* Erythromycin 508
Pantoprazole 1043
Pantothenic Acid 1044
Pantothenyl Alcohol *see* Dexpanthenol 416
Pantozol® (Mex) *see* Pantoprazole 1043
Papaverine 1044
Papaverine Hydrochloride *see* Papaverine 1044
Para-Aminosalicylate Sodium *see* Aminosalicylic Acid 100
Paracetamol *see* Acetaminophen 47
Parafon Forte® (Can) *see* Chlorzoxazone 322
Parafon Forte® DSC *see* Chlorzoxazone 322
Paraplatin® (Mex) *see* Carboplatin . . 264
Paraplatin-AQ (Can) *see* Carboplatin 264
Parathyroid Hormone (1-34) *see* Teriparatide 1274
Para-Time S.R.® *see* Papaverine . . 1044
Paregoric 1045
Paremyd® *see* Hydroxyamphetamine and Tropicamide 720
Paricalcitol 1045
Pariet® (Can) *see* Rabeprazole . . . 1164
Pariprazole *see* Rabeprazole 1164
Parlodel® (Mex) *see* Bromocriptine 219
Parnate® (Can) *see* Tranylcypromine 1323
Paromomycin 1046
Paromomycin Sulfate *see* Paromomycin 1046
Paroxetine 1046
Paroxetine Hydrochloride *see* Paroxetine 1046
Paroxetine Mesylate *see* Paroxetine 1046
Parsley 1443
Partusisten® (Mex) *see* Fenoterol . . . 580
Parvolex® (Can) *see* Acetylcysteine 61
PAS *see* Aminosalicylic Acid 100
Paser® *see* Aminosalicylic Acid 100
Passiflora spp *see* Passion Flower 1444
Passion Flower 1444
Patanol® (Can) *see* Olopatadine . . 1011
Pathocil® (Can) *see* Dicloxacillin . . . 431
Patients Requiring Sedation 1567
Pausinystalia yohimbe see Yohimbe 1451
Pavabid [DSC] *see* Papaverine . . . 1044
Paxil® (Can) *see* Paroxetine 1046
Paxil CR™ *see* Paroxetine 1046
PBZ® *see* Tripelennamine 1344
PBZ-SR® *see* Tripelennamine 1344
PCA *see* Procainamide 1124
PCE® (Can) *see* Erythromycin 508
PCEC *see* Rabies Virus Vaccine . . 1165
PCV7 *see* Pneumococcal Conjugate Vaccine (7-Valent) 1098
Pectin and Kaolin *see* Kaolin and Pectin 781
Pectin, Hyoscyamine, Atropine, Scopolamine, and Kaolin *see* Hyoscyamine, Atropine, Scopolamine, Kaolin, and Pectin 726
Pectin, Hyoscyamine, Atropine, Scopolamine, Kaolin, and Opium *see* Hyoscyamine, Atropine, Scopolamine, Kaolin, Pectin, and Opium 726
Pedameth® *see* Methionine 894
PediaCare® Cold and Allergy [OTC] *see* Chlorpheniramine and Pseudoephedrine 315
PediaCare® Decongestant Infants [OTC] *see* Pseudoephedrine . . 1147
Pediacare® Decongestant Plus Cough [OTC] *see* Pseudoephedrine and Dextromethorphan 1148
PediaCare® Infants' Long-Acting Cough [OTC] *see* Dextromethorphan 421
Pediacare® Long Acting Cough Plus Cold [OTC] *see* Pseudoephedrine and Dextromethorphan 1148
Pediacof® *see* Chlorpheniramine, Phenylephrine, Codeine, and Potassium Iodide 318
Pediaflor® *see* Fluoride 603
Pediamist® [OTC] *see* Sodium Chloride 1227
Pediapred® (Can) *see* PrednisoLONE 1113
Pediarix™ *see* Diphtheria, Tetanus Toxoids, Acellular Pertussis, Hepatitis B (Recombinant), and Poliovirus (Inactivated) Vaccine 452
Pediatex™ *see* Carbinoxamine 262
Pediatex™-D *see* Carbinoxamine and Pseudoephedrine 262
Pediatex™-DM *see* Carbinoxamine, Pseudoephedrine, and Dextromethorphan 263
Pediatrix (Can) *see* Acetaminophen 47
Pediazole® *see* Erythromycin and Sulfisoxazole 512
Pedi-Boro® [OTC] *see* Aluminum Sulfate and Calcium Acetate 92
Pedi-Dri® *see* Nystatin 1003
PediOtic® *see* Neomycin, Polymyxin B, and Hydrocortisone 975

Pedisilk® [OTC] *see* Salicylic Acid . . . 1205
Pedtrace-4® *see* Trace Metals . . . 1319
PedvaxHIB® *see Haemophilus* b Conjugate Vaccine . . . 680
Pegademase Bovine . . . 1050
Peganone® *see* Ethotoin . . . 561
Pegaspargase . . . 1051
Pegasys® *see* Peginterferon Alfa-2a . . . 1052
Pegfilgrastim . . . 1052
Peginterferon Alfa-2a . . . 1052
Peginterferon Alfa-2b . . . 1053
PEG-Intron® (Can) *see* Peginterferon Alfa-2b . . . 1053
PEG-L-asparaginase *see* Pegaspargase . . . 1051
Peglyte™ (Can) *see* Polyethylene Glycol-Electrolyte Solution . . . 1100
Pegylated Interferon Alfa-2a *see* Peginterferon Alfa-2a . . . 1052
Pegylated Interferon Alfa-2b *see* Peginterferon Alfa-2b . . . 1053
PemADD® *see* Pemoline . . . 1055
PemADD® CT *see* Pemoline . . . 1055
Pemetrexed . . . 1054
Pemirolast . . . 1055
Pemoline . . . 1055
Penbutolol . . . 1055
Penbutolol Sulfate *see* Penbutolol . . . 1055
Penciclovir . . . 1056
Penicillamine . . . 1057
Penicillin G Benzathine . . . 1058
Penicillin G Benzathine and Penicillin G Procaine . . . 1058
Penicillin G (Parenteral/Aqueous) . . 1059
Penicillin G Potassium *see* Penicillin G (Parenteral/Aqueous) . . . 1059
Penicillin G Procaine . . . 1060
Penicillin G Procaine and Benzathine Combined *see* Penicillin G Benzathine and Penicillin G Procaine . . . 1058
Penicillin G Sodium *see* Penicillin G (Parenteral/Aqueous) . . . 1059
Penicillin V Potassium . . . 1060
Penicilloyl-polylysine *see* Benzylpenicilloyl-polylysine . . . 196
Penlac™ (Can) *see* Ciclopirox . . . 327
Pennsaid® (Can) *see* Diclofenac . . . 427
Pentacarinat® (Can) *see* Pentamidine . . . 1062
Pentahydrate *see* Sodium Thiosulfate . . . 1230
Pentam-300® *see* Pentamidine . . . 1062
Pentamidine . . . 1062
Pentamidine Isethionate *see* Pentamidine . . . 1062
Pentamycetin® (Can) *see* Chloramphenicol . . . 306
Pentasa® (Can) *see* Mesalamine . . . 882
Pentaspan® (Can) *see* Pentastarch . . . 1063
Pentastarch . . . 1063
Penta-Triamterene HCTZ (Can) *see* Hydrochlorothiazide and Triamterene . . . 701
Pentazocine . . . 1063
Pentazocine and Acetaminophen . . 1064
Pentazocine Hydrochloride *see* Pentazocine . . . 1063
Pentazocine Hydrochloride and Acetaminophen *see* Pentazocine and Acetaminophen . . . 1064
Pentazocine Hydrochloride and Naloxone Hydrochloride *see* Pentazocine . . . 1063
Pentazocine Lactate *see* Pentazocine . . . 1063
Pentobarbital . . . 1065
Pentobarbital Sodium *see* Pentobarbital . . . 1065
Pentosan Polysulfate Sodium . . . 1065
Pentostatin . . . 1065
Pentothal® *see* Thiopental . . . 1289
Pentothal Sodico® (Mex) *see* Thiopental . . . 1289
Pentoxifylline . . . 1066
Pentoxil® *see* Pentoxifylline . . . 1066
Pentrax® [OTC] *see* Coal Tar . . . 367
Pen VK *see* Penicillin V Potassium . . . 1060
Pepcid® *see* Famotidine . . . 573
Pepcid® AC (Can) *see* Famotidine . . 573
Pepcid® Complete [OTC] (Can) *see* Famotidine, Calcium Carbonate, and Magnesium Hydroxide . . . 574
Pepcidine® (Mex) *see* Famotidine . . 573
Pepcid® I.V. (Can) *see* Famotidine . . 573
Pepevit® (Mex) *see* Niacin . . . 978
Pepto-Bismol® [OTC] *see* Bismuth . . 209
Pepto-Bismol® Maximum Strength [OTC] *see* Bismuth . . . 209
Percocet® *see* Oxycodone and Acetaminophen . . . 1029
Percocet®-Demi (Can) *see* Oxycodone and Acetaminophen . . . 1029
Percodan® (Can) *see* Oxycodone and Aspirin . . . 1032
Percodan®-Demi [DSC] *see* Oxycodone and Aspirin . . . 1032
Percogesic® [OTC] *see* Acetaminophen and Phenyltoloxamine . . . 53
Percogesic® Extra Strength [OTC] *see* Acetaminophen and Diphenhydramine . . . 53
Perdiem® Fiber Therapy [OTC] *see* Psyllium . . . 1151
Pergolide . . . 1067
Pergolide Mesylate *see* Pergolide . . . 1067
Pergonal® (Can) *see* Menotropins . . 868
Periactin® (Can) *see* Cyproheptadine . . . 389
Peri-Colace® (Can) *see* Docusate and Casanthranol . . . 460
Peridane® (Mex) *see* Pentoxifylline . . . 1066
Peridex® *see* Chlorhexidine Gluconate . . . 308
Peridol (Can) *see* Haloperidol . . . 682
Perindopril Erbumine . . . 1068
PerioChip® *see* Chlorhexidine Gluconate . . . 308
Periodontal Diseases . . . 1542
PerioGard® *see* Chlorhexidine Gluconate . . . 308
Periostat® *see* Doxycycline (Subantimicrobial) . . . 476
Permapen® Isoject® *see* Penicillin G Benzathine . . . 1058
Permax® (Mex) *see* Pergolide . . . 1067
Permethrin . . . 1070
Perphenazine . . . 1070
Perphenazine and Amitriptyline *see* Amitriptyline and Perphenazine . . . 106
Persantine® (Can) *see* Dipyridamole . . . 453
Pertussin® DM [OTC] *see* Dextromethorphan . . . 421
Pestarin® (Mex) *see* Rifampin . . . 1180
Pethidine Hydrochloride *see* Meperidine . . . 870

Petroselinum crispum see Parsley 1443
Pevaryl Lipogel® (Mex) *see* Econazole 481
Pexeva™ *see* Paroxetine 1046
Pexicam® (Can) *see* Piroxicam 1097
PFA *see* Foscarnet 631
Pfizerpen® (Can) *see* Penicillin G (Parenteral/Aqueous) 1059
Pfizerpen-AS® (Can) *see* Penicillin G Procaine 1060
PGE_1 *see* Alprostadil 87
PGE_2 *see* Dinoprostone 447
PGI_2 *see* Epoprostenol 500
PGX *see* Epoprostenol 500
Phanasin [OTC] *see* Guaifenesin 672
Phanasin® Diabetic Choice [OTC] *see* Guaifenesin 672
Pharmacology of Drug Metabolism and Interactions 24
Pharmaflur® *see* Fluoride 603
Pharmaflur® 1.1 *see* Fluoride 603
Pharmorubicin® (Can) *see* Epirubicin 498
Phazyme™ (Can) *see* Simethicone 1222
Phazyme® Quick Dissolve [OTC] *see* Simethicone 1222
Phazyme® Ultra Strength [OTC] *see* Simethicone 1222
Phenadoz™ *see* Promethazine 1130
Phenazo™ (Can) *see* Phenazopyridine 1072
Phenazopyridine 1072
Phenazopyridine Hydrochloride *see* Phenazopyridine 1072
Phendimetrazine 1072
Phendimetrazine Tartrate *see* Phendimetrazine 1072
Phenelzine 1072
Phenelzine Sulfate *see* Phenelzine 1072
Phenergan® *see* Promethazine 1130
Phenergan® With Codeine *see* Promethazine and Codeine 1131
Phenindamine 1073
Phenindamine Tartrate *see* Phenindamine 1073
Pheniramine and Naphazoline *see* Naphazoline and Pheniramine 964
Phenobarbital 1073
Phenobarbital, Belladonna, and Ergotamine Tartrate *see* Belladonna, Phenobarbital, and Ergotamine 186
Phenobarbital, Hyoscyamine, Atropine, and Scopolamine *see* Hyoscyamine, Atropine, Scopolamine, and Phenobarbital 725
Phenobarbital Sodium *see* Phenobarbital 1073
Phenobarbitone *see* Phenobarbital 1073
Phenol 1075
Phenol and Camphor *see* Camphor and Phenol 248
Phenoptic® *see* Phenylephrine 1078
Phenoxybenzamine 1075
Phenoxybenzamine Hydrochloride *see* Phenoxybenzamine 1075
Phenoxymethyl Penicillin *see* Penicillin V Potassium 1060
Phentermine 1076
Phentermine Hydrochloride *see* Phentermine 1076
Phentolamine 1077
Phentolamine Mesylate *see* Phentolamine 1077
Phenylalanine Mustard *see* Melphalan 866
Phenylazo Diamino Pyridine Hydrochloride *see* Phenazopyridine 1072
Phenylephrine 1078
Phenylephrine and Chlorpheniramine *see* Chlorpheniramine and Phenylephrine 314
Phenylephrine and Cyclopentolate *see* Cyclopentolate and Phenylephrine 384
Phenylephrine and Guaifenesin *see* Guaifenesin and Phenylephrine 674
Phenylephrine and Promethazine *see* Promethazine and Phenylephrine 1132
Phenylephrine and Scopolamine 1079
Phenylephrine and Zinc Sulfate 1079
Phenylephrine, Chlorpheniramine, and Dextromethorphan *see* Chlorpheniramine, Phenylephrine, and Dextromethorphan 316
Phenylephrine, Chlorpheniramine, and Methscopolamine *see* Chlorpheniramine, Phenylephrine, and Methscopolamine 317
Phenylephrine, Chlorpheniramine, and Phenyltoloxamine *see* Chlorpheniramine, Phenylephrine, and Phenyltoloxamine 317
Phenylephrine, Chlorpheniramine, Codeine, and Potassium Iodide *see* Chlorpheniramine, Phenylephrine, Codeine, and Potassium Iodide 318
Phenylephrine, Diphenhydramine, and Hydrocodone *see* Hydrocodone, Phenylephrine, and Diphenhydramine 713
Phenylephrine, Ephedrine, Chlorpheniramine, and Carbetapentane *see* Chlorpheniramine, Ephedrine, Phenylephrine, and Carbetapentane 316
Phenylephrine Hydrochloride *see* Phenylephrine 1078
Phenylephrine, Hydrocodone, Chlorpheniramine, Acetaminophen, and Caffeine *see* Hydrocodone, Chlorpheniramine, Phenylephrine, Acetaminophen, and Caffeine 712
Phenylephrine, Promethazine, and Codeine *see* Promethazine, Phenylephrine, and Codeine 1132
Phenylephrine Tannate, Carbetapentane Tannate, and Pyrilamine Tannate *see* Carbetapentane, Phenylephrine, and Pyrilamine 261
Phenylethylmalonylurea *see* Phenobarbital 1073
Phenylgesic® [OTC] *see* Acetaminophen and Phenyltoloxamine 53
Phenylisohydantoin *see* Pemoline 1055
Phenyl Salicylate, Methenamine, Methylene Blue, Sodium Biphosphate, and Hyoscyamine *see* Methenamine, Sodium Biphosphate, Phenyl Salicylate, Methylene Blue, and Hyoscyamine 893

Phenyltoloxamine and Acetaminophen *see* Acetaminophen and Phenyltoloxamine . . . 53
Phenyltoloxamine, Chlorpheniramine, and Phenylephrine *see* Chlorpheniramine, Phenylephrine, and Phenyltoloxamine . . . 317
Phenytek™ *see* Phenytoin . . . 1080
Phenytoin . . . 1080
Phenytoin Sodium *see* Phenytoin . . 1080
Phenytoin Sodium, Extended *see* Phenytoin . . . 1080
Phenytoin Sodium, Prompt *see* Phenytoin . . . 1080
Phillips'® Fibercaps [OTC] *see* Polycarbophil . . . 1100
Phillips'® Milk of Magnesia [OTC] *see* Magnesium Hydroxide . . . 853
Phillips' M-O® [OTC] *see* Magnesium Hydroxide and Mineral Oil . . . 853
Phillips'® Stool Softener Laxative [OTC] *see* Docusate . . . 459
pHisoHex® (Can) *see* Hexachlorophene . . . 693
Phos-Flur® *see* Fluoride . . . 603
Phos-Flur® Rinse [OTC] *see* Fluoride . . . 603
PhosLo® *see* Calcium Acetate . . . 245
Phosphate, Potassium *see* Potassium Phosphate . . . 1107
Phospholine Iodide® *see* Echothiophate Iodide . . . 481
Phosphonoformate *see* Foscarnet . . 631
Phosphonoformic Acid *see* Foscarnet . . . 631
Phosphorated Carbohydrate Solution *see* Fructose, Dextrose, and Phosphoric Acid . . . 638
Phosphoric Acid, Levulose and Dextrose *see* Fructose, Dextrose, and Phosphoric Acid . . . 638
Photofrin® (Can) *see* Porfimer . . . 1103
Phoxal-timolol (Can) *see* Timolol . . 1299
Phrenilin® with Caffeine and Codeine *see* Butalbital, Aspirin, Caffeine, and Codeine . . . 238
p-Hydroxyampicillin *see* Amoxicillin . . . 114
Phyllocontin® (Can) *see* Aminophylline . . . 99
Phyllocontin®-350 (Can) *see* Aminophylline . . . 99
Phylloquinone *see* Phytonadione . . 1084
Physostigmine . . . 1084
Physostigmine Salicylate *see* Physostigmine . . . 1084
Physostigmine Sulfate *see* Physostigmine . . . 1084
Phytomenadione *see* Phytonadione . . . 1084
Phytonadione . . . 1084
α_1-PI *see* Alpha$_1$-Proteinase Inhibitor . . . 84
Pidorubicin *see* Epirubicin . . . 498
Pidorubicin Hydrochloride *see* Epirubicin . . . 498
Pilocar® *see* Pilocarpine . . . 1085
Pilocarpine . . . 1085
Pilocarpine (Dental) . . . 1086
Pilocarpine Hydrochloride *see* Pilocarpine . . . 1085
Pilocarpine Nitrate *see* Pilocarpine . . . 1085
Pilopine HS® (Can) *see* Pilocarpine . . . 1085
Piloptic® *see* Pilocarpine . . . 1085
Pima® *see* Potassium Iodide . . . 1106
Pimaricin *see* Natamycin . . . 968
Pimecrolimus . . . 1088
Pimozide . . . 1088
Pindolol . . . 1090
Pink Bismuth *see* Bismuth . . . 209
Pin-X® [OTC] *see* Pyrantel Pamoate . . . 1151
PIO *see* Pemoline . . . 1055
Pioglitazone . . . 1091
Piperacillin . . . 1092
Piperacillin and Tazobactam Sodium . . . 1093
Piperacillin Sodium *see* Piperacillin . . . 1092
Piperacillin Sodium and Tazobactam Sodium *see* Piperacillin and Tazobactam Sodium . . . 1093
Piperazine . . . 1094
Piperazine Citrate *see* Piperazine . . . 1094
Piperazine Estrone Sulfate *see* Estropipate . . . 531
Piper methysticum see Kava . . . 1439
Piperonyl Butoxide and Pyrethrins *see* Pyrethrins and Piperonyl Butoxide . . . 1153
Piportil® L_4 (Can) *see* Pipotiazine . . 1095
Pipotiazine . . . 1095
Pipotiazine Palmitate *see* Pipotiazine . . . 1095
Pipracil® (Can) *see* Piperacillin . . . 1092
Pirbuterol . . . 1096
Pirbuterol Acetate *see* Pirbuterol . . 1096
Piroxan® (Mex) *see* Piroxicam . . . 1097
Piroxicam . . . 1097
p-Isobutylhydratropic Acid *see* Ibuprofen . . . 728
Pistacia lentiscus see Mastic . . . 1441
Pit *see* Oxytocin . . . 1038
Pitocin® *see* Oxytocin . . . 1038
Pitressin® *see* Vasopressin . . . 1369
Pitrex (Can) *see* Tolnaftate . . . 1312
Pix Carbonis *see* Coal Tar . . . 367
Plague Vaccine *see* Immunizations (Vaccines) . . . 1614
Plan B™ (Can) *see* Levonorgestrel . . . 815
Plantago Seed *see* Psyllium . . . 1151
Plantain Seed *see* Psyllium . . . 1151
Plaquenil® *see* Hydroxychloroquine . . . 720
Plasil® (Mex) *see* Metoclopramide . . 914
Platinol® (Mex) *see* Cisplatin . . . 337
Platinol®-AQ *see* Cisplatin . . . 337
Plavix® (Can) *see* Clopidogrel . . . 361
Plegine® (Can) *see* Phendimetrazine . . . 1072
Plenaxis™ *see* Abarelix . . . 43
Plendil® (Can) *see* Felodipine . . . 576
Pletal® (Can) *see* Cilostazol . . . 329
PMPA *see* Tenofovir . . . 1270
PMS-Amantadine (Can) *see* Amantadine . . . 92
PMS-Amitriptyline (Can) *see* Amitriptyline . . . 103
PMS-Amoxicillin (Can) *see* Amoxicillin . . . 114
PMS-Atenolol (Can) *see* Atenolol . . . 159
PMS-Baclofen (Can) *see* Baclofen . . 180
PMS-Bethanechol (Can) *see* Bethanechol . . . 203
PMS-Brimonidine Tartrate (Can) *see* Brimonidine . . . 218
PMS-Bromocriptine (Can) *see* Bromocriptine . . . 219
PMS-Buspirone (Can) *see* BusPIRone . . . 233

PMS-Butorphanol (Can) *see* Butorphanol . . . 240
PMS-Captopril (Can) *see* Captopril . . . 252
PMS-Carbamazepine (Can) *see* Carbamazepine . . . 255
PMS-Cefaclor (Can) *see* Cefaclor . . 274
PMS-Chloral Hydrate (Can) *see* Chloral Hydrate . . . 304
PMS-Cholestyramine (Can) *see* Cholestyramine Resin . . . 323
PMS-Cimetidine (Can) *see* Cimetidine . . . 330
PMS-Clobazam (Can) *see* Clobazam . . . 350
PMS-Clonazepam (Can) *see* Clonazepam . . . 356
PMS-Deferoxamine (Can) *see* Deferoxamine . . . 402
PMS-Desipramine (Can) *see* Desipramine . . . 407
PMS-Desonide (Can) *see* Desonide . . . 410
PMS-Dexamethasone (Can) *see* Dexamethasone . . . 411
PMS-Dicitrate (Can) *see* Sodium Citrate and Citric Acid . . . 1228
PMS-Diclofenac (Can) *see* Diclofenac . . . 427
PMS-Diclofenac SR (Can) *see* Diclofenac . . . 427
PMS-Diphenhydramine (Can) *see* DiphenhydrAMINE . . . 448
PMS-Dipivefrin (Can) *see* Dipivefrin . . . 453
PMS-Docusate Calcium (Can) *see* Docusate . . . 459
PMS-Docusate Sodium (Can) *see* Docusate . . . 459
PMS-Erythromycin (Can) *see* Erythromycin . . . 508
PMS-Fenofibrate Micro (Can) *see* Fenofibrate . . . 577
PMS-Fluorometholone (Can) *see* Fluorometholone . . . 605
PMS-Fluoxetine (Can) *see* Fluoxetine . . . 606
PMS-Fluphenazine Decanoate (Can) *see* Fluphenazine . . . 610
PMS-Flutamide (Can) *see* Flutamide . . . 615
PMS-Fluvoxamine (Can) *see* Fluvoxamine . . . 623
PMS-Gabapentin (Can) *see* Gabapentin . . . 642
PMS-Gemfibrozil (Can) *see* Gemfibrozil . . . 651
PMS-Glyburide (Can) *see* GlyBURIDE . . . 664
PMS-Haloperidol LA (Can) *see* Haloperidol . . . 682
PMS-Hydromorphone (Can) *see* Hydromorphone . . . 718
PMS-Hydroxyzine (Can) *see* HydrOXYzine . . . 723
PMS-Indapamide (Can) *see* Indapamide . . . 743
PMS-Ipratropium (Can) *see* Ipratropium . . . 761
PMS-Isoniazid (Can) *see* Isoniazid . . 769
PMS-Isosorbide (Can) *see* Isosorbide Dinitrate . . . 770
PMS-Lactulose (Can) *see* Lactulose . . . 794
PMS-Lamotrigine (Can) *see* Lamotrigine . . . 795
PMS-Levobunolol (Can) *see* Levobunolol . . . 808
PMS-Lindane (Can) *see* Lindane . . . 829
PMS-Lithium Carbonate (Can) *see* Lithium . . . 835
PMS-Lithium Citrate (Can) *see* Lithium . . . 835
PMS-Loperamine (Can) *see* Loperamide . . . 838
PMS-Lorazepam (Can) *see* Lorazepam . . . 842
PMS-Lovastatin (Can) *see* Lovastatin . . . 848
PMS-Loxapine (Can) *see* Loxapine . . . 850
PMS-Mefenamic Acid (Can) *see* Mefenamic Acid . . . 863
PMS-Metformin (Can) *see* Metformin . . . 887
PMS-Methylphenidate (Can) *see* Methylphenidate . . . 908
PMS-Metoprolol (Can) *see* Metoprolol . . . 915
PMS-Minocycline (Can) *see* Minocycline . . . 931
PMS-Morphine Sulfate SR (Can) *see* Morphine Sulfate . . . 947
PMS-Nizatidine (Can) *see* Nizatidine . . . 995
PMS-Norfloxacin (Can) *see* Norfloxacin . . . 997
PMS-Nortriptyline (Can) *see* Nortriptyline . . . 999
PMS-Nystatin (Can) *see* Nystatin . . 1003
PMS-Oxazepam (Can) *see* Oxazepam . . . 1022
PMS-Oxybutynin (Can) *see* Oxybutynin . . . 1026
PMS-Oxycodone-Acetaminophen (Can) *see* Oxycodone and Acetaminophen . . . 1029
PMS-Phenobarbital (Can) *see* Phenobarbital . . . 1073
PMS-Pindolol (Can) *see* Pindolol . . 1090
PMS-Polytrimethoprim (Can) *see* Trimethoprim and Polymyxin B . . . 1342
PMS-Pravastatin (Can) *see* Pravastatin . . . 1109
PMS-Procyclidine (Can) *see* Procyclidine . . . 1127
PMS-Pseudoephedrine (Can) *see* Pseudoephedrine . . . 1147
PMS-Ranitidine (Can) *see* Ranitidine . . . 1169
PMS-Salbutamol (Can) *see* Albuterol . . . 71
PMS-Sertraline (Can) *see* Sertraline . . . 1215
PMS-Sotalol (Can) *see* Sotalol . . . 1231
PMS-Sucralate (Can) *see* Sucralfate . . . 1242
PMS-Tamoxifen (Can) *see* Tamoxifen . . . 1258
PMS-Temazepam (Can) *see* Temazepam . . . 1266
PMS-Terazosin (Can) *see* Terazosin . . . 1271
PMS-Terbinafine (Can) *see* Terbinafine . . . 1272
PMS-Theophylline (Can) *see* Theophylline . . . 1285
PMS-Ticlopidine (Can) *see* Ticlopidine . . . 1297
PMS-Timolol (Can) *see* Timolol . . . 1299
PMS-Tobramycin (Can) *see* Tobramycin . . . 1306
PMS-Trazodone (Can) *see* Trazodone . . . 1326
PMS-Trifluoperazine (Can) *see* Trifluoperazine . . . 1338
PMS-Valproic Acid (Can) *see* Valproic Acid and Derivatives . . . 1359

PMS-Valproic Acid E.C. (Can) *see* Valproic Acid and Derivatives . . . 1359
PMS-Yohimbine (Can) *see* Yohimbine . . . 1393
Pneumococcal 7-Valent Conjugate Vaccine *see* Pneumococcal Conjugate Vaccine (7-Valent) . . . 1098
Pneumococcal Conjugate Vaccine (7-Valent) . . . 1098
Pneumococcal Polysaccharide Vaccine (Polyvalent) *see* Immunizations (Vaccines) . . . 1614
Pneumotussin® *see* Hydrocodone and Guaifenesin . . . 708
Podocon-25® *see* Podophyllum Resin . . . 1099
Podofilm® (Can) *see* Podophyllum Resin . . . 1099
Podofilox . . . 1099
Podophyllin *see* Podophyllum Resin . . . 1099
Podophyllum Resin . . . 1099
Poliovirus Vaccine (Inactivated) . . . 1099
Polocaine® *see* Mepivacaine . . . 873
Polocaine® (Can) *see* Mepivacaine (Dental Anesthetic) . . . 877
Polocaine® 2% and Levonordefrin 1:20,000 (Can) *see* Mepivacaine and Levonordefrin *(WITHDRAWN FROM MARKET)* . . . 875
Polocaine® MPF *see* Mepivacaine . . . 873
Polycarbophil . . . 1100
Polycidin® Ophthalmic Ointment (Can) *see* Bacitracin and Polymyxin B . . . 178
Polycitra® *see* Citric Acid, Sodium Citrate, and Potassium Citrate . . . 341
Polycitra®-K (Can) *see* Potassium Citrate . . . 1105
Polycitra®-K *see* Potassium Citrate and Citric Acid . . . 1106
Polycitra®-LC *see* Citric Acid, Sodium Citrate, and Potassium Citrate . . . 341
Polycose® [OTC] *see* Glucose Polymers . . . 664
Polyethylene Glycol-Electrolyte Solution . . . 1100
Polygam® S/D *see* Immune Globulin (Intravenous) . . . 740
Polymox® (Mex) *see* Amoxicillin . . . 114
Polymyxin B . . . 1100
Polymyxin B and Bacitracin *see* Bacitracin and Polymyxin B . . . 178
Polymyxin B and Neomycin *see* Neomycin and Polymyxin B . . . 973
Polymyxin B and Oxytetracycline *see* Oxytetracycline and Polymyxin B . . . 1037
Polymyxin B and Trimethoprim *see* Trimethoprim and Polymyxin B . . . 1342
Polymyxin B, Bacitracin, and Neomycin *see* Bacitracin, Neomycin, and Polymyxin B . . . 179
Polymyxin B, Bacitracin, Neomycin, and Hydrocortisone *see* Bacitracin, Neomycin, Polymyxin B, and Hydrocortisone . . . 179
Polymyxin B, Neomycin, and Dexamethasone *see* Neomycin, Polymyxin B, and Dexamethasone . . . 974
Polymyxin B, Neomycin, and Gramicidin *see* Neomycin, Polymyxin B, and Gramicidin . . . 974
Polymyxin B, Neomycin, and Hydrocortisone *see* Neomycin, Polymyxin B, and Hydrocortisone . . . 975
Polymyxin B, Neomycin, and Prednisolone *see* Neomycin, Polymyxin B, and Prednisolone . . . 975
Polymyxin B, Neomycin, Bacitracin, and Pramoxine *see* Bacitracin, Neomycin, Polymyxin B, and Pramoxine . . . 180
Polymyxin B Sulfate *see* Polymyxin B . . . 1100
Poly-Pred® *see* Neomycin, Polymyxin B, and Prednisolone . . . 975
Poly-Rx *see* Polymyxin B . . . 1100
Polysaccharide-Iron Complex . . . 1101
Polysporin® Ophthalmic *see* Bacitracin and Polymyxin B . . . 178
Polysporin® Topical [OTC] *see* Bacitracin and Polymyxin B . . . 178
Polytar® [OTC] *see* Coal Tar . . . 367
Polythiazide . . . 1102
Polythiazide and Prazosin *see* Prazosin and Polythiazide . . . 1112
Polytrim™ (Can) *see* Trimethoprim and Polymyxin B . . . 1342
Polyvinyl Alcohol *see* Artificial Tears . . . 148
Ponstan® (Mex) *see* Mefenamic Acid . . . 863
Ponstel® *see* Mefenamic Acid . . . 863
Pontocaine® *see* Tetracaine . . . 1278
Pontocaine® With Dextrose *see* Tetracaine and Dextrose . . . 1279
Poor Mans Treacle *see* Garlic . . . 1428
Poractant Alfa . . . 1102
Porfimer . . . 1103
Porfimer Sodium *see* Porfimer . . . 1103
Portia™ *see* Ethinyl Estradiol and Levonorgestrel . . . 545
Posipen® (Mex) *see* Dicloxacillin . . . 431
Post Peel Healing Balm [OTC] *see* Hydrocortisone . . . 714
Posture® [OTC] *see* Calcium Phosphate (Tribasic) . . . 247
Potassium Acetate . . . 1104
Potassium Acetate, Potassium Bicarbonate, and Potassium Citrate . . . 1104
Potassium Acetate, Potassium Citrate, and Potassium Bicarbonate *see* Potassium Acetate, Potassium Bicarbonate, and Potassium Citrate . . . 1104
Potassium Acid Phosphate . . . 1104
Potassium Bicarbonate . . . 1104
Potassium Bicarbonate and Potassium Chloride . . . 1104
Potassium Bicarbonate and Potassium Chloride (Effervescent) *see* Potassium Bicarbonate and Potassium Chloride . . . 1104
Potassium Bicarbonate and Potassium Citrate . . . 1105
Potassium Bicarbonate and Potassium Citrate (Effervescent) *see* Potassium Bicarbonate and Potassium Citrate . . . 1105
Potassium Bicarbonate, Potassium Acetate, and Potassium Citrate *see* Potassium Acetate, Potassium Bicarbonate, and Potassium Citrate . . . 1104

Potassium Bicarbonate, Potassium Citrate, and Potassium Acetate *see* Potassium Acetate, Potassium Bicarbonate, and Potassium Citrate . . . 1104
Potassium Chloride . . . 1105
Potassium Citrate . . . 1105
Potassium Citrate and Citric Acid . . 1106
Potassium Citrate, Citric Acid, and Sodium Citrate *see* Citric Acid, Sodium Citrate, and Potassium Citrate . . . 341
Potassium Citrate, Potassium Acetate, and Potassium Bicarbonate *see* Potassium Acetate, Potassium Bicarbonate, and Potassium Citrate . . . 1104
Potassium Citrate, Potassium Bicarbonate, and Potassium Acetate *see* Potassium Acetate, Potassium Bicarbonate, and Potassium Citrate . . . 1104
Potassium Gluconate . . . 1106
Potassium Guaiacolsulfonate and Guaifenesin *see* Guaifenesin and Potassium Guaiacolsulfonate . . . 675
Potassium Guaiacolsulfonate, Dextromethorphan, and Guaifenesin *see* Guaifenesin, Potassium Guaiacolsulfonate, and Dextromethorphan . . . 675
Potassium Iodide . . . 1106
Potassium Iodide, Chlorpheniramine, Phenylephrine, and Codeine *see* Chlorpheniramine, Phenylephrine, Codeine, and Potassium Iodide . . . 318
Potassium Phosphate . . . 1107
Potassium Phosphate and Sodium Phosphate . . . 1107
Povidone-Iodine . . . 1107
PPD *see* Tuberculin Tests . . . 1349
PPI-149 *see* Abarelix . . . 43
PPL *see* Benzylpenicilloyl-polylysine . . . 196
PPS *see* Pentosan Polysulfate Sodium . . . 1065
Pramidal® (Mex) *see* Loperamide . . . 838
Pramipexole . . . 1108
Pramosone® *see* Pramoxine and Hydrocortisone . . . 1109
Pramox® HC (Can) *see* Pramoxine and Hydrocortisone . . . 1109
Pramoxine . . . 1109
Pramoxine and Hydrocortisone . . . 1109
Pramoxine Hydrochloride *see* Pramoxine . . . 1109
Pramoxine, Neomycin, Bacitracin, and Polymyxin B *see* Bacitracin, Neomycin, Polymyxin B, and Pramoxine . . . 180
Prandase® (Can) *see* Acarbose . . . 45
Prandin® *see* Repaglinide . . . 1173
Pravachol® (Can) *see* Pravastatin . . . 1109
Pravacol® (Mex) *see* Pravastatin . . 1109
Pravastatin . . . 1109
Pravastatin and Aspirin *see* Aspirin and Pravastatin . . . 157
Pravastatin Sodium *see* Pravastatin . . . 1109
Pravigard™ PAC *see* Aspirin and Pravastatin . . . 157
Prax® [OTC] *see* Pramoxine . . . 1109
Praxel® (Mex) *see* Paclitaxel . . . 1038
Prazidec® (Mex) *see* Omeprazole . . . 1012
Praziquantel . . . 1111
Prazolit® (Mex) *see* Omeprazole . . 1012
Prazosin . . . 1111
Prazosin and Polythiazide . . . 1112
Prazosin Hydrochloride *see* Prazosin . . . 1111
Precedex™ (Can) *see* Dexmedetomidine . . . 415
Precose® *see* Acarbose . . . 45
Pred Forte® *see* PrednisoLONE . . . 1113
Pred-G® *see* Prednisolone and Gentamicin . . . 1115
Pred Mild® (Can) *see* PrednisoLONE . . . 1113
Prednicarbate . . . 1113
Prednidib® (Mex) *see* PredniSONE . . . 1115
PrednisoLONE . . . 1113
Prednisolone Acetate *see* PrednisoLONE . . . 1113
Prednisolone Acetate, Ophthalmic *see* PrednisoLONE . . . 1113
Prednisolone and Gentamicin . . . 1115
Prednisolone and Sulfacetamide *see* Sulfacetamide and Prednisolone . . . 1245
Prednisolone, Neomycin, and Polymyxin B *see* Neomycin, Polymyxin B, and Prednisolone . . . 975
Prednisolone Sodium Phosphate *see* PrednisoLONE . . . 1113
Prednisolone Sodium Phosphate, Ophthalmic *see* PrednisoLONE . . . 1113
PredniSONE . . . 1115
Prednisone Intensol™ *see* PredniSONE . . . 1115
Prefest™ *see* Estradiol and Norgestimate . . . 521
Prefrin™ [DSC] *see* Phenylephrine . . . 1078
Pregnenedione *see* Progesterone . . . 1128
Pregnyl® (Can) *see* Chorionic Gonadotropin (Human) . . . 326
Prelone® *see* PrednisoLONE . . . 1113
Prelu-2® *see* Phendimetrazine . . . 1072
Premarin® (Can) *see* Estrogens (Conjugated/Equine) . . . 525
Premjact® [OTC] *see* Lidocaine . . . 819
Premphase® (Can) *see* Estrogens (Conjugated/Equine) and Medroxyprogesterone . . . 528
Premplus® (Can) *see* Estrogens (Conjugated/Equine) and Medroxyprogesterone . . . 528
Prempro™ (Can) *see* Estrogens (Conjugated/Equine) and Medroxyprogesterone . . . 528
Preparation H® Hydrocortisone [OTC] *see* Hydrocortisone . . . 714
Pre-Pen® *see* Benzylpenicilloyl-polylysine . . . 196
Prepidil® (Mex) *see* Dinoprostone . . 447
Prepulsid® (Mex) *see* Cisapride . . . 336
Pressyn® (Can) *see* Vasopressin . . 1369
Pressyn® AR (Can) *see* Vasopressin . . . 1369
Pretz-D® [OTC] *see* Ephedrine . . . 495
Pretz® Irrigation [OTC] *see* Sodium Chloride . . . 1227
Prevacid® *see* Lansoprazole . . . 797
Prevacid® NapraPAC™ *see* Lansoprazole and Naproxen . . . 799
Prevacid® SoluTab™ *see* Lansoprazole . . . 797
Prevalite® *see* Cholestyramine Resin . . . 323
PREVEN® *see* Ethinyl Estradiol and Levonorgestrel . . . 545

Prevex® B (Can) *see* Betamethasone 199
Prevex® HC (Can) *see* Hydrocortisone 714
PreviDent® *see* Fluoride 603
PreviDent® 5000 Plus™ *see* Fluoride 603
Previfem™ *see* Ethinyl Estradiol and Norgestimate 554
Prevnar® *see* Pneumococcal Conjugate Vaccine (7-Valent) 1098
Prevpac™ (Can) *see* Lansoprazole, Amoxicillin, and Clarithromycin . . 798
Priftin® *see* Rifapentine 1182
Prilocaine 1118
Prilocaine and Epinephrine 1120
Prilocaine and Lidocaine *see* Lidocaine and Prilocaine 826
Prilosec® *see* Omeprazole 1012
Prilosec OTC™ [OTC] *see* Omeprazole 1012
Primaclone *see* Primidone 1122
Primacor® *see* Milrinone 930
Primaquine 1122
Primaquine Phosphate *see* Primaquine 1122
Primaxin® *see* Imipenem and Cilastatin 736
Primidone 1122
Primsol® *see* Trimethoprim 1341
Principen® *see* Ampicillin 124
Princol® (Mex) *see* Lincomycin 829
Prinivil® (Can) *see* Lisinopril 833
Prinzide® *see* Lisinopril and Hydrochlorothiazide 834
Priorix™ (Can) *see* Measles, Mumps, and Rubella Vaccines (Combined) 858
Priscoline® [DSC] *see* Tolazoline . . 1309
Pristinamycin *see* Quinupristin and Dalfopristin 1163
Privine® [OTC] *see* Naphazoline . . . 964
ProAmatine® *see* Midodrine 927
Proartinal® (Mex) *see* Ibuprofen 728
Probampacin® *see* Ampicillin and Probenecid 126
Probenecid 1124
Probenecid and Ampicillin (Dental) *see* Ampicillin and Probenecid . . 126
Probenecid and Colchicine *see* Colchicine and Probenecid 372
Probiotica® [OTC] *see* *Lactobacillus* 793
Procainamide 1124
Procainamide Hydrochloride *see* Procainamide 1124
Procaine 1125
Procaine Amide Hydrochloride *see* Procainamide 1124
Procaine Benzylpenicillin *see* Penicillin G Procaine 1060
Procaine Hydrochloride *see* Procaine 1125
Procaine Penicillin G *see* Penicillin G Procaine 1060
Procanbid® *see* Procainamide 1124
Procan® SR (Can) *see* Procainamide 1124
Procarbazine 1125
Procarbazine Hydrochloride *see* Procarbazine 1125
Procardia® *see* NIFEdipine 984
Procardia XL® *see* NIFEdipine 984
Procef® (Mex) *see* Cefprozil 286
Procephal® (Mex) *see* Erythromycin 508
Procetofene *see* Fenofibrate 577
Prochieve™ *see* Progesterone 1128
Prochlorperazine 1126
Prochlorperazine Edisylate *see* Prochlorperazine 1126
Prochlorperazine Maleate *see* Prochlorperazine 1126
Procrit® *see* Epoetin Alfa 499
Proctocort® *see* Hydrocortisone 714
ProctoCream® HC *see* Hydrocortisone 714
Proctofene *see* Fenofibrate 577
ProctoFoam®-HC *see* Pramoxine and Hydrocortisone 1109
ProctoFoam® NS [OTC] *see* Pramoxine 1109
Proctosol-HC® *see* Hydrocortisone . . 714
Procyclid™ (Can) *see* Procyclidine 1127
Procyclidine 1127
Procyclidine Hydrochloride *see* Procyclidine 1127
Procytox® (Can) *see* Cyclophosphamide 384
Prodium® [OTC] *see* Phenazopyridine 1072
Profasi® HP (Can) *see* Chorionic Gonadotropin (Human) 326
Profen Forte™ DM *see* Guaifenesin, Pseudoephedrine, and Dextromethorphan 676
Profenid® (Mex) *see* Ketoprofen 785
Profen II DM® *see* Guaifenesin, Pseudoephedrine, and Dextromethorphan 676
Profilnine® SD *see* Factor IX Complex (Human) 572
Proflavanol C™ (Can) *see* Ascorbic Acid 148
Progestasert® *see* Progesterone . . 1128
Progesterone 1128
Progestin *see* Progesterone 1128
Proglycem® (Can) *see* Diazoxide . . . 425
Prograf® (Can) *see* Tacrolimus . . . 1255
Proguanil and Atovaquone *see* Atovaquone and Proguanil 165
ProHance® *see* Radiological/ Contrast Media (Nonionic) 1166
Proken M® (Mex) *see* Metoprolol . . . 915
Prolaken® (Mex) *see* Metoprolol 915
Prolastin® (Can) *see* Alpha$_1$-Proteinase Inhibitor 84
Proleukin® *see* Aldesleukin 74
Prolex-D *see* Guaifenesin and Phenylephrine 674
Prolixin® [DSC] *see* Fluphenazine . . 610
Prolixin Decanoate® *see* Fluphenazine 610
Proloprim® *see* Trimethoprim 1341
Promatussin® DM (Can) *see* Promethazine and Dextromethorphan 1131
Promethazine 1130
Promethazine and Codeine 1131
Promethazine and Dextromethorphan 1131
Promethazine and Meperidine *see* Meperidine and Promethazine . . 872
Promethazine and Phenylephrine . . 1132
Promethazine Hydrochloride *see* Promethazine 1130
Promethazine, Phenylephrine, and Codeine 1132
Prometrium® (Can) *see* Progesterone 1128
Promit® *see* Dextran 1 418
Pronap-100® *see* Propoxyphene and Acetaminophen 1137
Pronaxil® (Mex) *see* Naproxen 965
Pronestyl® [DSC] *see* Procainamide 1124
Pronestyl®-SR (Can) *see* Procainamide 1124

Pronto® [OTC] *see* Pyrethrins and Piperonyl Butoxide . . . 1153
Prontofort® (Mex) *see* Tramadol . . . 1319
Pronto® Lice Control (Can) *see* Pyrethrins and Piperonyl Butoxide . . . 1153
Propaderm® (Can) *see* Beclomethasone . . . 184
Propafenone . . . 1133
Propafenone Hydrochloride *see* Propafenone . . . 1133
Propanthel™ (Can) *see* Propantheline . . . 1134
Propantheline . . . 1134
Propantheline Bromide *see* Propantheline . . . 1134
Propa pH [OTC] *see* Salicylic Acid . . . 1205
Proparacaine . . . 1134
Proparacaine and Fluorescein . . . 1135
Proparacaine Hydrochloride *see* Proparacaine . . . 1134
Proparin® [inj.] (Mex) *see* Heparin . . 685
Propecia® (Can) *see* Finasteride . . . 590
Propeshia® (Mex) *see* Finasteride . . 590
Propess® (Mex) *see* Dinoprostone . . 447
Propine® *see* Dipivefrin . . . 453
Proplex® T *see* Factor IX Complex (Human) . . . 572
Propofol . . . 1135
Propoxyphene . . . 1136
Propoxyphene and Acetaminophen . . . 1137
Propoxyphene, Aspirin, and Caffeine . . . 1138
Propoxyphene Hydrochloride *see* Propoxyphene . . . 1136
Propoxyphene Hydrochloride and Acetaminophen *see* Propoxyphene and Acetaminophen . . . 1137
Propoxyphene Hydrochloride, Aspirin, and Caffeine *see* Propoxyphene, Aspirin, and Caffeine . . . 1138
Propoxyphene Napsylate *see* Propoxyphene . . . 1136
Propoxyphene Napsylate and Acetaminophen *see* Propoxyphene and Acetaminophen . . . 1137
Propranolol . . . 1140
Propranolol and Hydrochlorothiazide . . . 1143
Propranolol Hydrochloride *see* Propranolol . . . 1140
Propranolol Intensol™ *see* Propranolol . . . 1140
Proprinal [OTC] *see* Ibuprofen . . . 728
Propulsid® *see* Cisapride . . . 336
Propylene Glycol Diacetate, Acetic Acid, and Hydrocortisone *see* Acetic Acid, Propylene Glycol Diacetate, and Hydrocortisone . . . 60
Propylene Glycol Diacetate, Hydrocortisone, and Acetic Acid *see* Acetic Acid, Propylene Glycol Diacetate, and Hydrocortisone . . . 60
Propylhexedrine . . . 1144
2-Propylpentanoic Acid *see* Valproic Acid and Derivatives . . . 1359
Propylthiouracil . . . 1144
Propyl-Thyracil® (Can) *see* Propylthiouracil . . . 1144
2-Propylvaleric Acid *see* Valproic Acid and Derivatives . . . 1359
Proscar® *see* Finasteride . . . 590
ProSom® *see* Estazolam . . . 517
Prostacyclin *see* Epoprostenol . . . 500
Prostaglandin E_1 *see* Alprostadil . . . 87
Prostaglandin E_2 *see* Dinoprostone . . . 447
Prostin E2® (Can) *see* Dinoprostone . . . 447
Prostin® VR (Can) *see* Alprostadil . . . 87
Prostin VR Pediatric® *see* Alprostadil . . . 87
Protamine Sulfate . . . 1145
Protein C (Activated), Human, Recombinant *see* Drotrecogin Alfa . . . 478
Prothrombin Complex Concentrate *see* Factor IX Complex (Human) . . . 572
Protirelin . . . 1145
Protonix® *see* Pantoprazole . . . 1043
Protopic® (Can) *see* Tacrolimus . . . 1255
Protriptyline . . . 1146
Protriptyline Hydrochloride *see* Protriptyline . . . 1146
Protropin® *see* Human Growth Hormone . . . 694
Protropine® (Can) *see* Human Growth Hormone . . . 694
Protuss®-DM [DSC] *see* Guaifenesin, Pseudoephedrine, and Dextromethorphan . . . 676
Proventil® *see* Albuterol . . . 71
Proventil® HFA *see* Albuterol . . . 71
Proventil® Repetabs® *see* Albuterol . . . 71
Provera® *see* MedroxyPROGESTERone . . . 862
Provigil® (Can) *see* Modafinil . . . 939
Proviodine (Can) *see* Povidone-Iodine . . . 1107
Provisc® *see* Hyaluronate and Derivatives . . . 696
Proxymetacaine *see* Proparacaine . . . 1134
Prozac® (Mex) *see* Fluoxetine . . . 606
Prozac® Weekly™ *see* Fluoxetine . . . 606
PRP-D *see* *Haemophilus* b Conjugate Vaccine . . . 680
Prudoxin™ *see* Doxepin . . . 467
Prussian Blue *see* Ferric Hexacyanoferrate . . . 585
Prymaccone *see* Primaquine . . . 1122
PS-341 *see* Bortezomib . . . 214
Pseudoephedrine . . . 1147
Pseudoephedrine, Acetaminophen, and Chlorpheniramine *see* Acetaminophen, Chlorpheniramine, and Pseudoephedrine . . . 58
Pseudoephedrine, Acetaminophen, and Dextromethorphan *see* Acetaminophen, Dextromethorphan, and Pseudoephedrine . . . 59
Pseudoephedrine and Acetaminophen *see* Acetaminophen and Pseudoephedrine . . . 53
Pseudoephedrine and Acrivastine *see* Acrivastine and Pseudoephedrine . . . 62
Pseudoephedrine and Brompheniramine *see* Brompheniramine and Pseudoephedrine . . . 220
Pseudoephedrine and Carbinoxamine *see* Carbinoxamine and Pseudoephedrine . . . 262
Pseudoephedrine and Chlorpheniramine *see* Chlorpheniramine and Pseudoephedrine . . . 315

Pseudoephedrine and Dexbrompheniramine *see* Dexbrompheniramine and Pseudoephedrine . . . 414
Pseudoephedrine and Dextromethorphan . . . 1148
Pseudoephedrine and Diphenhydramine *see* Diphenhydramine and Pseudoephedrine . . . 451
Pseudoephedrine and Fexofenadine *see* Fexofenadine and Pseudoephedrine . . . 588
Pseudoephedrine and Guaifenesin *see* Guaifenesin and Pseudoephedrine . . . 675
Pseudoephedrine and Hydrocodone *see* Hydrocodone and Pseudoephedrine . . . 711
Pseudoephedrine and Ibuprofen . . 1149
Pseudoephedrine and Loratadine *see* Loratadine and Pseudoephedrine . . . 842
Pseudoephedrine and Triprolidine *see* Triprolidine and Pseudoephedrine . . . 1345
Pseudoephedrine, Carbinoxamine, and Dextromethorphan *see* Carbinoxamine, Pseudoephedrine, and Dextromethorphan . . . 263
Pseudoephedrine, Chlorpheniramine, and Acetaminophen *see* Acetaminophen, Chlorpheniramine, and Pseudoephedrine . . . 58
Pseudoephedrine, Chlorpheniramine, and Codeine *see* Chlorpheniramine, Pseudoephedrine, and Codeine . . . 319
Pseudoephedrine, Chlorpheniramine, and Dihydrocodeine *see* Pseudoephedrine, Dihydrocodeine, and Chlorpheniramine . . . 1150
Pseudoephedrine, Dextromethorphan, and Acetaminophen *see* Acetaminophen, Dextromethorphan, and Pseudoephedrine . . . 59
Pseudoephedrine, Dextromethorphan, and Carbinoxamine *see* Carbinoxamine, Pseudoephedrine, and Dextromethorphan . . . 263
Pseudoephedrine, Dextromethorphan, and Guaifenesin *see* Guaifenesin, Pseudoephedrine, and Dextromethorphan . . . 676
Pseudoephedrine, Dihydrocodeine, and Chlorpheniramine . . . 1150
Pseudoephedrine, Guaifenesin, and Codeine *see* Guaifenesin, Pseudoephedrine, and Codeine . . . 676
Pseudoephedrine Hydrochloride *see* Pseudoephedrine . . . 1147
Pseudoephedrine Hydrochloride and Cetirizine Hydrochloride *see* Cetirizine and Pseudoephedrine . . . 299
Pseudoephedrine, Hydrocodone, and Carbinoxamine *see* Hydrocodone, Carbinoxamine, and Pseudoephedrine . . . 712
Pseudoephedrine, Hydrocodone, and Guaifenesin *see* Hydrocodone, Pseudoephedrine, and Guaifenesin . . . 713
Pseudoephedrine Sulfate *see* Pseudoephedrine . . . 1147
Pseudoephedrine, Triprolidine, and Codeine Pseudoephedrine, Codeine, and Triprolidine *see* Triprolidine, Pseudoephedrine, and Codeine . . . 1346
Pseudofrin (Can) *see* Pseudoephedrine . . . 1147
Pseudo GG TR *see* Guaifenesin and Pseudoephedrine . . . 675
Pseudomonic Acid A *see* Mupirocin . . . 951
Pseudovent™ *see* Guaifenesin and Pseudoephedrine . . . 675
Pseudovent™ DM *see* Guaifenesin, Pseudoephedrine, and Dextromethorphan . . . 676
Pseudovent™-Ped *see* Guaifenesin and Pseudoephedrine . . . 675
P & S™ Liquid Phenol (Can) *see* Phenol . . . 1075
Psorcon® *see* Diflorasone . . . 435
Psorcon® e™ *see* Diflorasone . . . 435
Psoriatec™ *see* Anthralin . . . 133
PsoriGel® [OTC] *see* Coal Tar . . . 367
Psyllium . . . 1151
Psyllium Hydrophilic Mucilloid *see* Psyllium . . . 1151
P.T.E.-4® *see* Trace Metals . . . 1319
P.T.E.-5® *see* Trace Metals . . . 1319
Pteroylglutamic Acid *see* Folic Acid . . . 625
PTU *see* Propylthiouracil . . . 1144
Pulmicort® (Can) *see* Budesonide . . 221
Pulmicort Respules® *see* Budesonide . . . 221
Pulmicort Turbuhaler® *see* Budesonide . . . 221
Pulmophylline (Can) *see* Theophylline . . . 1285
Pulmozyme® (Mex) *see* Dornase Alfa . . . 463
Pulsol® [tabs] (Mex) *see* Enalapril . . 488
Puralube® Tears [OTC] *see* Artificial Tears . . . 148
Puregon™ (Can) *see* Follitropins . . . 626
Puregon® [biosyn.] (Mex) *see* Follitropins . . . 626
Purge® [OTC] *see* Castor Oil . . . 273
Purified Chick Embryo Cell *see* Rabies Virus Vaccine . . . 1165
Purinethol® (Mex) *see* Mercaptopurine . . . 880
Purple Coneflower *see Echinacea* . . . 1423
PVF® K (Can) *see* Penicillin V Potassium . . . 1060
P-V Tussin Tablet *see* Hydrocodone and Pseudoephedrine . . . 711
Pyrantel Pamoate . . . 1151
Pyrazinamide . . . 1152
Pyrazinamide, Rifampin, and Isoniazid *see* Rifampin, Isoniazid, and Pyrazinamide . . 1181
Pyrazinoic Acid Amide *see* Pyrazinamide . . . 1152
Pyrethrins and Piperonyl Butoxide . . . 1153
Pyridium® (Can) *see* Phenazopyridine . . . 1072

Pyridostigmine 1153
Pyridostigmine Bromide *see* Pyridostigmine 1153
Pyridoxine 1154
Pyridoxine, Folic Acid, and Cyanocobalamin *see* Folic Acid, Cyanocobalamin, and Pyridoxine 626
Pyridoxine Hydrochloride *see* Pyridoxine 1154
Pyrilamine, Phenylephrine, and Carbetapentane *see* Carbetapentane, Phenylephrine, and Pyrilamine . . 261
Pyrimethamine 1154
Pyrimethamine and Sulfadoxine *see* Sulfadoxine and Pyrimethamine 1245
Pyrinyl Plus® [OTC] *see* Pyrethrins and Piperonyl Butoxide 1153
Pyrithione Zinc 1155
Q-Tussin [OTC] *see* Guaifenesin . . . 672
Quadrax® (Mex) *see* Ibuprofen 728
Quaternium-18 Bentonite *see* Bentoquatam 189
Quazepam 1155
Quelicin® *see* Succinylcholine 1241
Quemicetina® (Mex) *see* Chloramphenicol 306
Quercetin 1444
Questran® *see* Cholestyramine Resin 323
Questran® Light *see* Cholestyramine Resin 323
Questran® Light Sugar Free (Can) *see* Cholestyramine Resin 323
Quetiapine 1156
Quetiapine Fumarate *see* Quetiapine 1156
Quibron® *see* Theophylline and Guaifenesin 1286
Quibron®-T *see* Theophylline 1285
Quibron®-T/SR (Can) *see* Theophylline 1285
Quinaglute® Dura-Tabs® [DSC] *see* Quinidine 1160
Quinalbarbitone Sodium *see* Secobarbital 1211
Quinapril 1158
Quinapril and Hydrochlorothiazide 1160
Quinapril Hydrochloride *see* Quinapril 1158
Quinate® (Can) *see* Quinidine 1160
Quinidine 1160
Quinidine Gluconate *see* Quinidine 1160
Quinidine Polygalacturonate *see* Quinidine 1160
Quinidine Sulfate *see* Quinidine . . . 1160
Quinine 1162
Quinine-Odan™ (Can) *see* Quinine 1162
Quinine Sulfate *see* Quinine 1162
Quinoflox® (Mex) *see* Ciprofloxacin 331
Quinol *see* Hydroquinone 719
Quintasa® (Can) *see* Mesalamine . . 882
Quinupristin and Dalfopristin 1163
Quixin™ *see* Levofloxacin 812
QVAR® *see* Beclomethasone 184
R-3827 *see* Abarelix 43
RabAvert® *see* Rabies Virus Vaccine 1165
Rabeprazole 1164
Rabies Immune Globulin (Human) 1165
Rabies Virus Vaccine 1165
Radiogardase™ *see* Ferric Hexacyanoferrate 585
Radiological/Contrast Media (Nonionic) 1166
Radix *see* Valerian 1449
Raductil® (Mex) *see* Sibutramine . . 1218
rAHF *see* Antihemophilic Factor (Recombinant) 135
R-albuterol *see* Levalbuterol 806
Raloxifene 1166
Raloxifene Hydrochloride *see* Raloxifene 1166
Ramace® (Mex) *see* Ramipril 1167
Ramipril 1167
Raniclor™ *see* Cefaclor 274
Ranifur® [tabs] (Mex) *see* Ranitidine 1169
Ranifur® [inj.] (Mex) *see* Ranitidine 1169
Ranisen® (Mex) *see* Ranitidine . . . 1169
Ranitidine 1169
Ranitidine Hydrochloride *see* Ranitidine 1169
Rapamune® *see* Sirolimus 1224
Raptiva™ *see* Efalizumab 483
Rasburicase 1171
Rastinon® (Mex) *see* TOLBUTamide 1309
ratio-Acyclovir (Can) *see* Acyclovir . . . 64
ratio-AmoxiClav (Can) *see* Amoxicillin and Clavulanate Potassium 116
ratio-Brimonidine (Can) *see* Brimonidine 218
ratio-Cefuroxime (Can) *see* Cefuroxime 289
ratio-Clarithromycin (Can) *see* Clarithromycin 343
ratio-Colchicine (Can) *see* Colchicine 372
ratio-Cotridin (Can) *see* Triprolidine, Pseudoephedrine, and Codeine 1346
ratio-Diltiazem CD (Can) *see* Diltiazem 444
ratio-Emtec (Can) *see* Acetaminophen and Codeine 50
ratio-Famotidine (Can) *see* Famotidine 573
ratio-Glyburide (Can) *see* GlyBURIDE 664
ratio-Inspra-Sal (Can) *see* Albuterol 71
ratio-Ketorolac (Can) *see* Ketorolac 787
ratio-Lamotrigine (Can) *see* Lamotrigine 795
ratio-Lenoltec (Can) *see* Acetaminophen and Codeine 50
ratio-Lovastatin (Can) *see* Lovastatin 848
ratio-Methotrexate (Can) *see* Methotrexate 897
ratio-Morphine SR (Can) *see* Morphine Sulfate 947
ratio-Pentoxifylline (Can) *see* Pentoxifylline 1066
ratio-Pravastatin (Can) *see* Pravastatin 1109
ratio-Salbutamol (Can) *see* Albuterol 71
ratio-Sertraline (Can) *see* Sertraline 1215
ratio-Simvastatin (Can) *see* Simvastatin 1222
ratio-Temazepam (Can) *see* Temazepam 1266
ratio-Theo-Bronc (Can) *see* Theophylline 1285
Raudil® (Mex) *see* Ranitidine 1169
Rauwolfia Serpentina 1171
R & C™ II (Can) *see* Pyrethrins and Piperonyl Butoxide 1153

R & C™ Shampoo/Conditioner (Can) *see* Pyrethrins and Piperonyl Butoxide 1153
Reactine™ (Can) *see* Cetirizine 298
Reactine® Allergy and Sinus (Can) *see* Cetirizine and Pseudoephedrine 299
Rea-Lo® [OTC] *see* Urea 1353
ReAzo [OTC] *see* Phenazopyridine 1072
Rebetol® *see* Ribavirin 1177
Rebetron® *see* Interferon Alfa-2b and Ribavirin 754
Rebif® *see* Interferon Beta-1a 756
Recofol® (Mex) *see* Propofol 1135
Recombinant α-L-Iduronidase (Glycosaminoglycan α-L-Iduronohydrolase) *see* Laronidase 800
Recombinant Hirudin *see* Lepirudin 803
Recombinant Human Deoxyribonuclease *see* Dornase Alfa 463
Recombinant Human Follicle Stimulating Hormone *see* Follitropins 626
Recombinant Human Interleukin-11 *see* Oprelvekin 1015
Recombinant Human Parathyroid Hormone (1-34) *see* Teriparatide 1274
Recombinant Human Platelet-Derived Growth Factor B *see* Becaplermin 184
Recombinant Interleukin-11 *see* Oprelvekin 1015
Recombinant Plasminogen Activator *see* Reteplase 1175
Recombinate™ (Can) *see* Antihemophilic Factor (Recombinant) 135
Recombivax HB® *see* Hepatitis B Vaccine 689
Redoxon® (Mex) *see* Ascorbic Acid 148
Reductil® (Mex) *see* Sibutramine 1218
Redutemp® [OTC] *see* Acetaminophen 47
Red Valerian *see* Valerian 1449
Red Yeast Rice 1444
Reese's® Pinworm Medicine [OTC] *see* Pyrantel Pamoate 1151
ReFacto® *see* Antihemophilic Factor (Recombinant) 135
Refludan® (Can) *see* Lepirudin 803
Refresh® [OTC] *see* Artificial Tears 148
Refresh Liquigel™ [OTC] *see* Carboxymethylcellulose 265
Refresh® Plus [OTC] *see* Artificial Tears 148
Refresh Plus® [OTC] *see* Carboxymethylcellulose 265
Refresh® Tears [OTC] *see* Artificial Tears 148
Refresh Tears™ (Can) *see* Carboxymethylcellulose 265
Regaine® (Mex) *see* Minoxidil 934
Regitine [DSC] *see* Phentolamine 1077
Reglan® *see* Metoclopramide 914
Regranex® *see* Becaplermin 184
Regulact® (Mex) *see* Lactulose 794
Regular Iletin® II *see* Insulin Preparations 749
Regular, Insulin *see* Insulin Preparations 749
Regulex® (Can) *see* Docusate 459
Reguloid® [OTC] *see* Psyllium 1151
Rejuva-A® (Can) *see* Tretinoin (Topical) 1329
Relacon-DM *see* Guaifenesin, Pseudoephedrine, and Dextromethorphan 676
Relafen™ (Can) *see* Nabumetone 955
Relefact® TRH (Can) *see* Protirelin 1145
Relenza® *see* Zanamivir 1396
Relief® [OTC] *see* Phenylephrine 1078
Relifex® (Mex) *see* Nabumetone 955
Relisorm L® (Mex) *see* Gonadorelin 669
Relpax® (Mex) *see* Eletriptan 486
Remeron® (Mex) *see* Mirtazapine 935
Remeron SolTab® *see* Mirtazapine 935
Reme-t™ [OTC] *see* Coal Tar 367
Remicade® *see* Infliximab 747
Remifentanil 1172
Reminyl® (Can) *see* Galantamine 645
Remodulin™ *see* Treprostinil 1327
Renacidin® *see* Citric Acid, Magnesium Carbonate, and Glucono-Delta-Lactone 341
Renagel® *see* Sevelamer 1217
Renedil® (Can) *see* Felodipine 576
Renese® *see* Polythiazide 1102
Renitec® (Mex) *see* Enalapril 488
Renova® *see* Tretinoin (Topical) 1329
ReoPro® *see* Abciximab 44
Repaglinide 1173
Repan® *see* Butalbital, Acetaminophen, and Caffeine 236
Repronex® (Can) *see* Menotropins 868
Requip® *see* Ropinirole 1197
Rescriptor® *see* Delavirdine 403
Rescula® *see* Unoprostone 1352
Reserpine 1174
Reserpine, Hydralazine, and Hydrochlorothiazide *see* Hydralazine, Hydrochlorothiazide, and Reserpine 698
Respa-1st® *see* Guaifenesin and Pseudoephedrine 675
Respa-DM® *see* Guaifenesin and Dextromethorphan 673
Respa-GF® [DSC] *see* Guaifenesin 672
Respaire®-60 SR *see* Guaifenesin and Pseudoephedrine 675
Respaire®-120 SR *see* Guaifenesin and Pseudoephedrine 675
Respiratory Diseases 1478
Respiratory Synctial Virus Immune Globulin *see* Immunizations (Vaccines) 1614
Restasis™ *see* CycloSPORINE 386
Restoril® *see* Temazepam 1266
Restylane® *see* Hyaluronate and Derivatives 696
Resveratrol *see* Grape Skin 1436
Retavase® *see* Reteplase 1175
Reteplase 1175
Retin-A® *see* Tretinoin (Topical) 1329
Retin-A® Micro *see* Tretinoin (Topical) 1329
Retinoic Acid *see* Tretinoin (Topical) 1329
Retinova® (Can) *see* Tretinoin (Topical) 1329
Retrovir® (Can) *see* Zidovudine 1398
Retrovir AZT® (Mex) *see* Zidovudine 1398
Revapol® (Mex) *see* Mebendazole 859
Reversol® *see* Edrophonium 483
Revex® *see* Nalmefene 960
Rēv-Eyes™ *see* Dapiprazole 398
ReVia® *see* Naltrexone 962

Revitalose C-1000® (Can) *see* Ascorbic Acid 148
Reyataz® *see* Atazanavir 158
rFSH-alpha *see* Follitropins 626
rFSH-beta *see* Follitropins 626
rFVIIa *see* Factor VIIa (Recombinant) 571
R-Gene® *see* Arginine 141
rGM-CSF *see* Sargramostim 1209
r-h α-GAL *see* Agalsidase Beta 69
r-hCG *see* Chorionic Gonadotropin (Recombinant) 326
Rheomacrodex® (Mex) *see* Dextran 417
Rheumatoid Arthritis, Osteoarthritis, and Osteoporosis 1490
Rheumatrex® *see* Methotrexate 897
rhFSH-alpha *see* Follitropins 626
rhFSH-beta *see* Follitropins 626
RhIG *see* Rh_o(D) Immune Globulin 1176
rhIL-11 *see* Oprelvekin 1015
Rhinalar® (Can) *see* Flunisolide 599
Rhinocort® (Mex) *see* Budesonide . . 221
Rhinocort® Aqua® *see* Budesonide 221
Rhinocort® Turbuhaler® (Can) *see* Budesonide 221
Rhinosyn® [OTC] *see* Chlorpheniramine and Pseudoephedrine 315
Rhinosyn-PD® [OTC] *see* Chlorpheniramine and Pseudoephedrine 315
Rho-Clonazepam (Can) *see* Clonazepam 356
Rhodacine® (Can) *see* Indomethacin 746
Rh_o(D) Immune Globulin 1176
Rho(D) Immune Globulin (Human) *see* Rh_o(D) Immune Globulin . . 1176
Rhodis™ (Can) *see* Ketoprofen 785
Rhodis-EC™ (Can) *see* Ketoprofen 785
Rhodis SR™ (Can) *see* Ketoprofen 785
RhoGAM® *see* Rh_o(D) Immune Globulin 1176
RhoIGIV *see* Rh_o(D) Immune Globulin 1176
RhoIVIM *see* Rh_o(D) Immune Globulin 1176
Rho®-Loperamine (Can) *see* Loperamide 838
Rho®-Metformin (Can) *see* Metformin 887
Rho-Nitro (Can) *see* Nitroglycerin . . 991
Rhophylac® *see* Rh_o(D) Immune Globulin 1176
Rho®-Sotalol (Can) *see* Sotalol . . . 1231
Rhotral (Can) *see* Acebutolol 46
Rhotrimine® (Can) *see* Trimipramine 1343
Rhovane® (Can) *see* Zopiclone . . . 1406
Rhoxal-amiodarone (Can) *see* Amiodarone 101
Rhoxal-atenolol (Can) *see* Atenolol 159
Rhoxal-clozapine (Can) *see* Clozapine 366
Rhoxal-cyclosporine (Can) *see* CycloSPORINE 386
Rhoxal-diltiazem CD (Can) *see* Diltiazem 444
Rhoxal-diltiazem SR (Can) *see* Diltiazem 444
Rhoxal-famotidine (Can) *see* Famotidine 573
Rhoxal-fluoxetine (Can) *see* Fluoxetine 606
Rhoxal-fluvoxamine (Can) *see* Fluvoxamine 623
Rhoxal-metformin FC (Can) *see* Metformin 887
Rhoxal-minocycline (Can) *see* Minocycline 931
Rhoxal-nabumetone (Can) *see* Nabumetone 955
Rhoxal-orphendrine (Can) *see* Orphenadrine 1017
Rhoxal-oxaprozin (Can) *see* Oxaprozin 1022
Rhoxal-ranitidine (Can) *see* Ranitidine 1169
Rhoxal-salbutamol (Can) *see* Albuterol 71
Rhoxal-sertraline (Can) *see* Sertraline 1215
Rhoxal-ticlopidine (Can) *see* Ticlopidine 1297
Rhoxal-valproic (Can) *see* Valproic Acid and Derivatives 1359
rhPTH(1-34) *see* Teriparatide 1274
*r*HuEPO-α *see* Epoetin Alfa 499
rhuMAb-E25 *see* Omalizumab 1012
rhuMAb-VEGF *see* Bevacizumab . . . 204
Ribasphere™ *see* Ribavirin 1177
Ribavirin 1177
Ribavirin and Interferon Alfa-2b Combination Pack *see* Interferon Alfa-2b and Ribavirin 754
Riboflavin 1178
Ridaura® (Can) *see* Auranofin 170
Ridene® [caps] (Mex) *see* NiCARdipine 980
RID® Maximum Strength [OTC] *see* Pyrethrins and Piperonyl Butoxide 1153
RID® Mousse (Can) *see* Pyrethrins and Piperonyl Butoxide 1153
Rid® Spray [OTC] *see* Permethrin 1070
Rifabutin 1179
Rifadin® (Can) *see* Rifampin 1180
Rifamate® (Can) *see* Rifampin and Isoniazid 1181
Rifampicin *see* Rifampin 1180
Rifampin 1180
Rifampin and Isoniazid 1181
Rifampin, Isoniazid, and Pyrazinamide 1181
Rifapentine 1182
Rifater™ (Can) *see* Rifampin, Isoniazid, and Pyrazinamide . . 1181
Rifaximin 1183
rIFN-A *see* Interferon Alfa-2a 751
rIFN beta-1a *see* Interferon Beta-1a 756
rIFN beta-1b *see* Interferon Beta-1b 757
RIG *see* Rabies Immune Globulin (Human) 1165
rIL-11 *see* Oprelvekin 1015
Rilutek® *see* Riluzole 1183
Riluzole 1183
Rimactan® (Mex) *see* Rifampin . . . 1180
Rimactane® *see* Rifampin 1180
Rimantadine 1184
Rimantadine Hydrochloride *see* Rimantadine 1184
Rimexolone 1185
Rimsalin® (Mex) *see* Lincomycin . . . 829
Riomet™ *see* Metformin 887
Riopan Plus® [OTC] *see* Magaldrate and Simethicone . . . 852
Riopan Plus® Double Strength [OTC] *see* Magaldrate and Simethicone 852
Riphenidate (Can) *see* Methylphenidate 908

Risedronate 1185
Risedronate Sodium *see* Risedronate 1185
Risperdal® (Can) *see* Risperidone 1187
Risperdal® Consta™ *see* Risperidone 1187
Risperdal M-Tab™ *see* Risperidone 1187
Risperidone 1187
Ritalin® *see* Methylphenidate 908
Ritalin® LA *see* Methylphenidate . . . 908
Ritalin® SR (Can) *see* Methylphenidate 908
Ritmolol® [tabs] (Mex) *see* Metoprolol 915
Ritonavir 1189
Ritonavir and Lopinavir *see* Lopinavir and Ritonavir 839
Rituxan® *see* Rituximab 1191
Rituximab 1191
Riva-Cloxacillin (Can) *see* Cloxacillin 365
Riva-Diclofenac (Can) *see* Diclofenac 427
Riva-Diclofenac-K (Can) *see* Diclofenac 427
Riva-Famotidine (Can) *see* Famotidine 573
Riva-Loperamine (Can) *see* Loperamide 838
Riva-Lorazepam (Can) *see* Lorazepam 842
Riva-Naproxen (Can) *see* Naproxen 965
Rivanase AQ (Can) *see* Beclomethasone 184
Riva-Norfloxacin (Can) *see* Norfloxacin 997
Riva-Simvastatin (Can) *see* Simvastatin 1222
Rivasol (Can) *see* Zinc Sulfate 1401
Rivastigmine 1192
Riva-Zide (Can) *see* Hydrochlorothiazide and Triamterene 701
Rivotril® (Mex) *see* Clonazepam 356
Rizatriptan 1193
rLFN-α2 *see* Interferon Alfa-2b 752
RMS® *see* Morphine Sulfate 947
RO5-420 *see* Flunitrazepam 600
Ro 5488 *see* Tretinoin (Oral) 1328
Roaccutan® (Mex) *see* Isotretinoin . . 773
Robafen® AC *see* Guaifenesin and Codeine 673
Robaxin® (Can) *see* Methocarbamol 894
Robidrine® (Can) *see* Pseudoephedrine 1147
Robinul® *see* Glycopyrrolate 668
Robinul® Forte *see* Glycopyrrolate . . 668
Robitussin® [OTC] *see* Guaifenesin 672
Robitussin® CF [OTC] *see* Guaifenesin, Pseudoephedrine, and Dextromethorphan 676
Robitussin® Childrens Cough & Cold (Can) *see* Pseudoephedrine and Dextromethorphan 1148
Robitussin® Cold and Congestion [OTC] *see* Guaifenesin, Pseudoephedrine, and Dextromethorphan 676
Robitussin® Cough and Cold Infant [OTC] *see* Guaifenesin, Pseudoephedrine, and Dextromethorphan 676
Robitussin® Cough & Cold® (Can) *see* Guaifenesin, Pseudoephedrine, and Dextromethorphan 676
Robitussin® CoughGels™[OTC] *see* Dextromethorphan 421
Robitussin®-DAC [DSC] *see* Guaifenesin, Pseudoephedrine, and Codeine 676
Robitussin® DM (Can) *see* Guaifenesin and Dextromethorphan 673
Robitussin® Honey Cough [OTC] *see* Dextromethorphan 421
Robitussin® Maximum Strength Cough [OTC] *see* Dextromethorphan 421
Robitussin® Maximum Strength Cough & Cold [OTC] *see* Pseudoephedrine and Dextromethorphan 1148
Robitussin-PE® [OTC] *see* Guaifenesin and Pseudoephedrine 675
Robitussin® Pediatric Cough [OTC] *see* Dextromethorphan 421
Robitussin® Pediatric Cough & Cold [OTC] *see* Pseudoephedrine and Dextromethorphan 1148
Robitussin® Severe Congestion [OTC] *see* Guaifenesin and Pseudoephedrine 675
Robitussin® Sugar Free Cough [OTC] *see* Guaifenesin and Dextromethorphan 673
Rocaltrol® *see* Calcitriol 244
Rocephin® (Can) *see* Ceftriaxone . . 288
Rofact™ (Can) *see* Rifampin 1180
Rofecoxib 1194
Roferon-A® (Can) *see* Interferon Alfa-2a 751
Rogaine® (Can) *see* Minoxidil 934
Rogaine® Extra Strength for Men [OTC] *see* Minoxidil 934
Rogaine® for Men [OTC] *see* Minoxidil 934
Rogaine® for Women [OTC] *see* Minoxidil 934
Rogal® (Mex) *see* Piroxicam 1097
Rogitine® (Can) *see* Phentolamine 1077
Rohypnol *see* Flunitrazepam 600
Rökan *see* Ginkgo Biloba 1429
Rolaids® [OTC] *see* Calcium Carbonate and Magnesium Hydroxide 245
Rolaids® Extra Strength [OTC] *see* Calcium Carbonate and Magnesium Hydroxide 245
Romazicon® *see* Flumazenil 599
Romilar® (Mex) *see* Dextromethorphan 421
Romilar® AC *see* Guaifenesin and Codeine 673
Romir® (Mex) *see* Captopril 252
Romycin® *see* Erythromycin 508
Rondec®-DM Drops *see* Carbinoxamine, Pseudoephedrine, and Dextromethorphan 263
Rondec® Drops *see* Carbinoxamine and Pseudoephedrine 262
Rondec® Syrup *see* Brompheniramine and Pseudoephedrine 220
Rondec® Tablets *see* Carbinoxamine and Pseudoephedrine 262

Rondec-TR® *see* Carbinoxamine and Pseudoephedrine . . . 262
Ropinirole . . . 1197
Ropinirole Hydrochloride *see* Ropinirole . . . 1197
Ropivacaine . . . 1199
Ropivacaine Hydrochloride *see* Ropivacaine . . . 1199
Rosiglitazone . . . 1199
Rosiglitazone and Metformin . . . 1201
Rosiglitazone Maleate and Metformin Hydrochloride *see* Rosiglitazone and Metformin . . . 1201
Rosin Rose *see* St John's Wort . . . 1447
Rosuvastatin . . . 1202
Rosuvastatin Calcium *see* Rosuvastatin . . . 1202
Rovamycine® (Can) *see* Spiramycin . . . 1234
Rowasa® (Can) *see* Mesalamine . . . 882
Roxanol® *see* Morphine Sulfate . . . 947
Roxanol 100® *see* Morphine Sulfate . . . 947
Roxanol®-T *see* Morphine Sulfate . . 947
Roxicet™ *see* Oxycodone and Acetaminophen . . . 1029
Roxicet™ 5/500 *see* Oxycodone and Acetaminophen . . . 1029
Roxicodone™ *see* Oxycodone . . . 1027
Roxicodone™ Intensol™ *see* Oxycodone . . . 1027
Roychlor® (Can) *see* Potassium Chloride . . . 1105
Rozex™ *see* Metronidazole . . . 917
RP-6976 *see* Docetaxel . . . 458
RP-54274 *see* Riluzole . . . 1183
RP-59500 *see* Quinupristin and Dalfopristin . . . 1163
r-PA *see* Reteplase . . . 1175
rPDGF-BB *see* Becaplermin . . . 184
RS-25259 *see* Palonosetron . . . 1040
RS-25259-197 *see* Palonosetron . . 1040
RTCA *see* Ribavirin . . . 1177
RU-486 *see* Mifepristone . . . 928
RU-23908 *see* Nilutamide . . . 986
RU-38486 *see* Mifepristone . . . 928
Rubella, Measles and Mumps Vaccines, Combined *see* Measles, Mumps, and Rubella Vaccines (Combined) . . . 858
Rubella Virus Vaccine (Live) . . . 1203
Rubeola Vaccine *see* Measles Virus Vaccine (Live) . . . 858
Rubex® *see* DOXOrubicin . . . 469
Rubidomycin Hydrochloride *see* DAUNOrubicin Hydrochloride . . . 401
Rubilem® [inj.] (Mex) *see* DAUNOrubicin Hydrochloride . . . 401
Rulox *see* Aluminum Hydroxide and Magnesium Hydroxide . . . 91
Rulox No. 1 *see* Aluminum Hydroxide and Magnesium Hydroxide . . . 91
Rum-K® *see* Potassium Chloride . . 1105
Rustic Treacle *see* Garlic . . . 1428
Ryna® [OTC] [DSC] *see* Chlorpheniramine and Pseudoephedrine . . . 315
Rynatan® *see* Chlorpheniramine and Phenylephrine . . . 314
Rynatan® Pediatric Suspension *see* Chlorpheniramine and Phenylephrine . . . 314
Rynatuss® *see* Chlorpheniramine, Ephedrine, Phenylephrine, and Carbetapentane . . . 316
Rynatuss® Pediatric *see* Chlorpheniramine, Ephedrine, Phenylephrine, and Carbetapentane . . . 316
Rythmodan® (Can) *see* Disopyramide . . . 455
Rythmodan®-LA (Can) *see* Disopyramide . . . 455
Rythmol® *see* Propafenone . . . 1133
Rythmol® Gen-Propafenone (Can) *see* Propafenone . . . 1133
Rythmol® SR *see* Propafenone . . . 1133
S-2® *see* Epinephrine (Racemic) . . . 497
Sabal serrulata *see* Saw Palmetto . . . 1446
Sabasilis serrulatae *see* Saw Palmetto . . . 1446
SAB-Gentamicin (Can) *see* Gentamicin . . . 655
Sab-Prenase (Can) *see* PrednisoLONE . . . 1113
Sabril® (Mex) *see* Vigabatrin . . . 1376
Sacrosidase . . . 1204
S-adenosylmethionine *see* SAMe . . 1445
Safe Tussin® 30 [OTC] *see* Guaifenesin and Dextromethorphan . . . 673
Saizen® *see* Human Growth Hormone . . . 694
SalAc® [OTC] *see* Salicylic Acid . . . 1205
Sal-Acid® [OTC] *see* Salicylic Acid . . . 1205
Salactic® [OTC] *see* Salicylic Acid . . . 1205
Salagen® *see* Pilocarpine (Dental) . . . 1086
Salazopyrin® (Can) *see* Sulfasalazine . . . 1249
Salazopyrin En-Tabs® (Can) *see* Sulfasalazine . . . 1249
Salbu-2 (Can) *see* Albuterol . . . 71
Salbu-4 (Can) *see* Albuterol . . . 71
Salbulin Autohaler® (Mex) *see* Albuterol . . . 71
Salbutamol *see* Albuterol . . . 71
Salflex® *see* Salsalate . . . 1207
Salicylazosulfapyridine *see* Sulfasalazine . . . 1249
Salicylic Acid . . . 1205
Salicylic Acid and Coal Tar *see* Coal Tar and Salicylic Acid . . . 367
Salicylsalicylic Acid *see* Salsalate . . . 1207
SalineX® [OTC] *see* Sodium Chloride . . . 1227
Salivart® [OTC] *see* Saliva Substitute . . . 1205
Saliva Substitute . . . 1205
Saliva Substitute™ [OTC] *see* Saliva Substitute . . . 1205
Salix® [OTC] *see* Saliva Substitute . . . 1205
Salk Vaccine *see* Poliovirus Vaccine (Inactivated) . . . 1099
Salmeterol . . . 1206
Salmeterol and Fluticasone *see* Fluticasone and Salmeterol . . . 619
Salmeterol Xinafoate *see* Salmeterol . . . 1206
Salmocide® (Mex) *see* Furazolidone . . . 640
Salofalk® (Can) *see* Mesalamine . . . 882
Sal-Plant® [OTC] *see* Salicylic Acid . . . 1205
Salsalate . . . 1207
Salt *see* Sodium Chloride . . . 1227
Sal-Tropine™ *see* Atropine . . . 166
Sal-Tropine™ *see* Atropine Sulfate (Dental Tablets) . . . 169
SAMe . . . 1445
Sandimmune® *see* CycloSPORINE . . . 386
Sandimmune® I.V. (Can) *see* CycloSPORINE . . . 386

Sandostatin® (Can) *see* Octreotide 1004
Sandostatina® (Mex) *see* Octreotide 1004
Sandostatin LAR® (Can) *see* Octreotide 1004
Sani-Supp® [OTC] *see* Glycerin 667
Sans Acne® (Can) *see* Erythromycin 508
Sansert® (Can) *see* Methysergide . . 913
Santyl® *see* Collagenase 375
Saquinavir 1207
Saquinavir Mesylate *see* Saquinavir 1207
Sarafem™ *see* Fluoxetine 606
Sargramostim 1209
Sarna® HC (Can) *see* Hydrocortisone 714
Sarnol®-HC [OTC] *see* Hydrocortisone 714
Sassafras albidum see Sassafras Oil 1445
Sassafras Oil 1445
Sassafras radix see Sassafras Oil 1445
Sassafras varifolium see Sassafras Oil 1445
Sassafrax see Sassafras Oil 1445
Saw Palmetto 1446
SB-265805 *see* Gemifloxacin 653
SC 33428 *see* Idarubicin 732
Scabisan® (Mex) *see* Lindane 829
SCH 13521 *see* Flutamide 615
Scheinpharm B12 (Can) *see* Cyanocobalamin 380
Schisandra 1446
Schizandra chinensis see Schisandra 1446
S-Citalopram *see* Escitalopram 513
Scleromate™ *see* Morrhuate Sodium 948
Scopace™ *see* Scopolamine 1210
Scopolamine 1210
Scopolamine and Phenylephrine *see* Phenylephrine and Scopolamine 1079
Scopolamine Hydrobromide *see* Scopolamine 1210
Scopolamine, Hyoscyamine, Atropine, and Phenobarbital *see* Hyoscyamine, Atropine, Scopolamine, and Phenobarbital 725
Scopolamine, Hyoscyamine, Atropine, Kaolin, and Pectin *see* Hyoscyamine, Atropine, Scopolamine, Kaolin, and Pectin 726
Scopolamine, Hyoscyamine, Atropine, Kaolin, Pectin, and Opium *see* Hyoscyamine, Atropine, Scopolamine, Kaolin, Pectin, and Opium 726
Scot-Tussin DM® Cough Chasers [OTC] *see* Dextromethorphan . . 421
Scot-Tussin® Expectorant [OTC] *see* Guaifenesin 672
Scury Root *see Echinacea* 1423
SDZ ENA 713 *see* Rivastigmine . . 1192
SeaMist® [OTC] *see* Sodium Chloride 1227
Seasonale® *see* Ethinyl Estradiol and Levonorgestrel 545
Seba-Gel™ *see* Benzoyl Peroxide . . 194
Sebcur® (Can) *see* Salicylic Acid . . 1205
Sebcur/T® (Can) *see* Coal Tar and Salicylic Acid 367
Secobarbital 1211
Secobarbital and Amobarbital *see* Amobarbital and Secobarbital . . 112
Secobarbital Sodium *see* Secobarbital 1211
Seconal® *see* Secobarbital 1211
Secotex® (Mex) *see* Tamsulosin . . 1260
SecreFlo™ *see* Secretin 1211
Secretin 1211
Sectral® *see* Acebutolol 46
Sedalito® (Mex) *see* Acetaminophen 47
Sefulken® [inj.] (Mex) *see* Diazoxide 425
Selax® (Can) *see* Docusate 459
Select™ 1/35 (Can) *see* Ethinyl Estradiol and Norethindrone 550
Selectadril® [tabs] (Mex) *see* Metoprolol 915
Selecto® (Mex) *see* Pancreatin . . . 1042
Selectofen® (Mex) *see* Diclofenac . . 427
Selectofur® [tabs] (Mex) *see* Furosemide 640
Selegil® [tabs] (Mex) *see* Metronidazole 917
Selegiline 1212
Selegiline Hydrochloride *see* Selegiline 1212
Selenium 1213
Selenium *see* Trace Metals 1319
Selepen® *see* Selenium 1213
Selepen® *see* Trace Metals 1319
Seloken® (Mex) *see* Metoprolol 915
Semicid® [OTC] *see* Nonoxynol 9 . . 995
Semprex®-D *see* Acrivastine and Pseudoephedrine 62
Senexon® [OTC] *see* Senna 1213
Senna 1213
Senna-Gen® [OTC] *see* Senna . . . 1213
Sennatural™ [OTC] *see* Senna . . . 1213
Senokot® [OTC] *see* Senna 1213
Senokot® Children's [OTC] *see* Senna 1213
SenokotXTRA® [OTC] *see* Senna 1213
Sensibit® (Mex) *see* Loratadine 841
Sensipar™ *see* Cinacalcet 331
Sensorcaine® *see* Bupivacaine 225
Sensorcaine®-MPF *see* Bupivacaine 225
Sensorcaine® With Epinephrine (Can) *see* Bupivacaine and Epinephrine 227
Septanest® N (Can) *see* Articaine Hydrochloride and Epinephrine (Canada) 143
Septanest® SP (Can) *see* Articaine Hydrochloride and Epinephrine (Canada) 143
Septocaine™ *see* Articaine Hydrochloride and Epinephrine (U.S.) 145
Septra® (Can) *see* Sulfamethoxazole and Trimethoprim 1246
Septra® DS *see* Sulfamethoxazole and Trimethoprim 1246
Septra® Injection (Can) *see* Sulfamethoxazole and Trimethoprim 1246
Ser-Ap-Es [DSC] *see* Hydralazine, Hydrochlorothiazide, and Reserpine 698
Serax® *see* Oxazepam 1022
Serenoa repens see Saw Palmetto 1446
Serentil® [DSC] *see* Mesoridazine . . 883
Serevent® (Can) *see* Salmeterol . . 1206
Serevent® Diskus® *see* Salmeterol 1206
Sermorelin Acetate 1214
Serocryptin® (Mex) *see* Bromocriptine 219
Seromycin® *see* CycloSERINE 385

Serophene® see ClomiPHENE 354
Seropram® [tabs] (Mex) see Citalopram 339
Seroquel® see Quetiapine 1156
Serostim® (Can) see Human Growth Hormone 694
Sertaconazole 1214
Sertaconazole Nitrate see Sertaconazole 1214
Sertraline 1215
Sertraline Hydrochloride see Sertraline 1215
Serutan® [OTC] see Psyllium 1151
Servamox® (Mex) see Amoxicillin . . . 114
Servigenta® (Mex) see Gentamicin 655
Serviradine® (Mex) see Ranitidine 1169
Servizol® (Mex) see Metronidazole 917
Servizol® [liqu. oral] (Mex) see Metronidazole 917
Serzone® [DSC] see Nefazodone . . . 970
Serzone-5HT$_2$® [DSC] (Can) see Nefazodone 970
Sevelamer 1217
Sevelamer Hydrochloride see Sevelamer 1217
Sexually-Transmitted Diseases . . . 1504
Shark Cartilage 1446
Shemol® (Mex) see Timolol 1299
Shur-Seal® [OTC] see Nonoxynol 9 995
Siberian Ginseng see Ginseng, Siberian 1431
Sibutramine 1218
Sibutramine Hydrochloride Monohydrate see Sibutramine 1218
Sigafam® (Mex) see Famotidine 573
Siladryl® Allergy [OTC] see DiphenhydrAMINE 448
Silafed® [OTC] see Triprolidine and Pseudoephedrine 1345
Silapap® Children's [OTC] see Acetaminophen 47
Silapap® Infants [OTC] see Acetaminophen 47
Sildec see Carbinoxamine and Pseudoephedrine 262
Sildec-DM see Carbinoxamine, Pseudoephedrine, and Dextromethorphan 263
Sildenafil 1219
Silexin® [OTC] see Guaifenesin and Dextromethorphan 673
Silfedrine Children's [OTC] see Pseudoephedrine 1147
Silphen® [OTC] see DiphenhydrAMINE 448
Silphen DM® [OTC] see Dextromethorphan 421
Siltussin DAS [OTC] see Guaifenesin 672
Siltussin SA [OTC] see Guaifenesin 672
Silvadene® see Silver Sulfadiazine 1221
Silver Apricot see Ginkgo Biloba . . 1429
Silver Nitrate 1221
Silver Sulfadiazine 1221
Silybum marianum see Milk Thistle 1443
Simethicone 1222
Simethicone, Aluminum Hydroxide, and Magnesium Hydroxide see Aluminum Hydroxide, Magnesium Hydroxide, and Simethicone 92
Simethicone and Calcium Carbonate see Calcium Carbonate and Simethicone 245
Simethicone and Magaldrate see Magaldrate and Simethicone . . . 852
Simply Cough® [OTC] see Dextromethorphan 421
Simply Saline™ [OTC] see Sodium Chloride 1227
Simply Sleep® (Can) see DiphenhydrAMINE 448
Simulect® (Can) see Basiliximab . . . 182
Simvastatin 1222
Sincalide 1224
Sinedol® (Mex) see Acetaminophen 47
Sinemet® see Levodopa and Carbidopa 811
Sinemet® CR (Can) see Levodopa and Carbidopa 811
Sinequan® (Can) see Doxepin 467
Sinestron® (Mex) see Lorazepam . . . 842
Singulair® see Montelukast 944
Sinogan® [tabs] (Mex) see Methotrimeprazine 901
Sinogan® [inj.] (Mex) see Methotrimeprazine 901
Sinozzard® (Mex) see Prazosin . . . 1111
Sinus-Relief® [OTC] see Acetaminophen and Pseudoephedrine 53
Sinutab® Non Drowsy (Can) see Acetaminophen and Pseudoephedrine 53
Sinutab® Sinus [OTC] see Acetaminophen and Pseudoephedrine 53
Sinutab® Sinus & Allergy (Can) see Acetaminophen, Chlorpheniramine, and Pseudoephedrine 58
Sinutab® Sinus Allergy Maximum Strength [OTC] see Acetaminophen, Chlorpheniramine, and Pseudoephedrine 58
Siquial® [caps] (Mex) see Fluoxetine 606
Sirdalud® see Tizanidine 1305
Sirolimus 1224
SK see Streptokinase 1238
SK and F 104864 see Topotecan 1316
Skelaxin® see Metaxalone 886
Skelid® see Tiludronate 1298
SKF 104864 see Topotecan 1316
SKF 104864-A see Topotecan 1316
Skin Test Antigens (Multiple) 1226
Sleepinal® [OTC] see DiphenhydrAMINE 448
Slo-Bid® (Mex) see Theophylline . . 1285
Slo-Niacin® [OTC] see Niacin 978
Slow FE® [OTC] see Ferrous Sulfate 586
Slow-K® (Can) see Potassium Chloride 1105
Slow-Mag® [OTC] see Magnesium Chloride 852
Slow-Trasicor® (Can) see Oxprenolol 1025
Smallpox Vaccine see Immunizations (Vaccines) 1614
Smelling Salts see Ammonia Spirit (Aromatic) 111
SMZ-TMP see Sulfamethoxazole and Trimethoprim 1246
Snakeroot see *Echinacea* 1423
Sodipental® [inj.] (Mex) see Thiopental 1289
Sodium 4-Hydroxybutyrate see Sodium Oxybate 1229

Sodium Acid Carbonate *see* Sodium Bicarbonate 1226
Sodium Benzoate and Caffeine *see* Caffeine and Sodium Benzoate 242
Sodium Bicarbonate 1226
Sodium Biphosphate, Methenamine, Methylene Blue, Phenyl Salicylate, and Hyoscyamine *see* Methenamine, Sodium Biphosphate, Phenyl Salicylate, Methylene Blue, and Hyoscyamine 893
Sodium Cellulose Phosphate *see* Cellulose Sodium Phosphate . . . 294
Sodium Chloride 1227
Sodium Citrate and Citric Acid 1228
Sodium Citrate, Citric Acid, and Potassium Citrate *see* Citric Acid, Sodium Citrate, and Potassium Citrate 341
Sodium Edetate *see* Edetate Disodium 482
Sodium Etidronate *see* Etidronate Disodium 563
Sodium Ferric Gluconate *see* Ferric Gluconate 585
Sodium Fluoride *see* Fluoride 603
Sodium Hyaluronate *see* Hyaluronate and Derivatives . . . 696
Sodium Hyaluronate-Chrondroitin Sulfate *see* Chondroitin Sulfate and Sodium Hyaluronate 325
Sodium Hydrogen Carbonate *see* Sodium Bicarbonate 1226
Sodium Hypochlorite Solution 1228
Sodium Hyposulfate *see* Sodium Thiosulfate 1230
Sodium *L*-Triiodothyronine *see* Liothyronine 831
Sodium Nafcillin *see* Nafcillin 958
Sodium Nitroferricyanide *see* Nitroprusside 993
Sodium Nitroprusside *see* Nitroprusside 993
Sodium Oxybate 1229
Sodium PAS *see* Aminosalicylic Acid 100
Sodium-PCA and Lactic Acid *see* Lactic Acid and Sodium-PCA . . . 793
Sodium Phenylbutyrate 1230
Sodium Phosphate and Potassium Phosphate *see* Potassium Phosphate and Sodium Phosphate 1107
Sodium Phosphates 1230
Sodium Sulamyd® (Can) *see* Sulfacetamide 1244
Sodium Sulfacetamide *see* Sulfacetamide 1244
Sodium Thiosulfate 1230
Sodium Thiosulphate *see* Sodium Thiosulfate 1230
Soflax™ (Can) *see* Docusate 459
Solagé™ *see* Mequinol and Tretinoin 879
Solaquin® [OTC] *see* Hydroquinone 719
Solaquin Forte™ (Can) *see* Hydroquinone 719
Solaraze™ *see* Diclofenac 427
Solarcaine® [OTC] *see* Benzocaine 191
Solarcaine® Aloe Extra Burn Relief [OTC] *see* Lidocaine 819
Solciclina® (Mex) *see* Amoxicillin . . . 114
Solu-Cortef® (Can) *see* Hydrocortisone 714
Solugel® (Mex) *see* Benzoyl Peroxide 194
Solu-Medrol® *see* MethylPREDNISolone 910
Soluver® (Can) *see* Salicylic Acid . . 1205
Soluver® Plus (Can) *see* Salicylic Acid 1205
Soma® *see* Carisoprodol 266
Soma® Compound *see* Carisoprodol and Aspirin 266
Soma® Compound w/Codeine *see* Carisoprodol, Aspirin, and Codeine 267
Somatrem *see* Human Growth Hormone 694
Somatropin *see* Human Growth Hormone 694
Sominex® [OTC] *see* DiphenhydrAMINE 448
Sominex® Maximum Strength [OTC] *see* DiphenhydrAMINE . . 448
Somnote™ *see* Chloral Hydrate 304
Sonata® (Can) *see* Zaleplon 1396
Sophixin® (Mex) *see* Ciprofloxacin . . 331
Sorbitol 1231
Sorine® *see* Sotalol 1231
Sotacor® (Can) *see* Sotalol 1231
Sotalol 1231
Sotalol Hydrochloride *see* Sotalol . . 1231
Sotret® *see* Isotretinoin 773
Soy Isoflavones 1447
Spacol *see* Hyoscyamine 724
Spacol T/S *see* Hyoscyamine 724
Sparfloxacin 1233
Spectazole® *see* Econazole 481
Spectinomycin 1234
Spectinomycin Hydrochloride *see* Spectinomycin 1234
Spectracef™ *see* Cefditoren 280
Spectrocin Plus™ [OTC] *see* Bacitracin, Neomycin, Polymyxin B, and Pramoxine . . . 180
SpectroGram 2™ (Can) *see* Chlorhexidine Gluconate 308
SpectroTar Skin Wash™ (Can) *see* Coal Tar 367
Spiramycin 1234
Spirapril 1235
Spiriva® (Can) *see* Tiotropium 1303
Spironolactone 1235
Spironolactone and Hydrochlorothiazide *see* Hydrochlorothiazide and Spironolactone 701
Sporanox® (Can) *see* Itraconazole . . 775
Sportscreme® [OTC] *see* Triethanolamine Salicylate 1338
Sprintec™ *see* Ethinyl Estradiol and Norgestimate 554
SSD™ (Can) *see* Silver Sulfadiazine 1221
SSD® AF *see* Silver Sulfadiazine . . 1221
SSKI® *see* Potassium Iodide 1106
Stadol® *see* Butorphanol 240
Stadol® NS [DSC] *see* Butorphanol 240
Stagesic® *see* Hydrocodone and Acetaminophen 702
Stalevo™ *see* Levodopa, Carbidopa, and Entacapone 812
Standard Conversions 1598
Stan-gard® *see* Fluoride 603
Stannous Fluoride *see* Fluoride 603
Stanozolol 1237
Starlix® (Can) *see* Nateglinide 968
Starnoc® (Can) *see* Zaleplon 1396
Statex® (Can) *see* Morphine Sulfate 947
Staticin® *see* Erythromycin 508
Statobex® (Can) *see* Phendimetrazine 1072
Stavudine 1238

Stelazine® (Mex) *see* Trifluoperazine 1338
Stemetil® (Can) *see* Prochlorperazine 1126
Stenox® (Mex) *see* Fluoxymesterone 609
Sterapred® *see* PredniSONE 1115
Sterapred® DS *see* PredniSONE . . 1115
STI571 *see* Imatinib 734
Stiemycin® (Mex) *see* Erythromycin 508
Stimate™ *see* Desmopressin 409
Stinking Rose *see* Garlic 1428
St John's Wort 1447
St. Joseph® Adult Aspirin [OTC] *see* Aspirin 151
Stop® *see* Fluoride 603
Strattera™ *see* Atomoxetine 161
Streptase® (Can) *see* Streptokinase 1238
Streptokinase 1238
Streptomycin 1239
Streptomycin Sulfate *see* Streptomycin 1239
Streptozocin 1240
Stresstabs® B-Complex [OTC] *see* Vitamin B Complex Combinations 1382
Stresstabs® B-Complex + Iron [OTC] *see* Vitamin B Complex Combinations 1382
Stresstabs® B-Complex + Zinc [OTC] *see* Vitamin B Complex Combinations 1382
Striant™ *see* Testosterone 1276
Stri-dex® [OTC] *see* Salicylic Acid 1205
Stri-dex® Body Focus [OTC] *see* Salicylic Acid 1205
Stri-dex® Facewipes To Go™ [OTC] *see* Salicylic Acid 1205
Stri-dex® Maximum Strength [OTC] *see* Salicylic Acid 1205
Strifon Forte® (Can) *see* Chlorzoxazone 322
Stromectol® *see* Ivermectin 779
Strong Iodine Solution *see* Potassium Iodide 1106
Sublimaze® *see* Fentanyl 581
Suboxone® *see* Buprenorphine and Naloxone 230
Subutex® *see* Buprenorphine 228
Succinylcholine 1241
Succinylcholine Chloride *see* Succinylcholine 1241
Sucraid® (Can) *see* Sacrosidase . . 1204
Sucralfate 1242
Sucrets® [OTC] *see* Dyclonine 480
Sucrets® Original [OTC] *see* Hexylresorcinol 693
Sudafed® (Mex) *see* Pseudoephedrine 1147
Sudafed® 12 Hour [OTC] *see* Pseudoephedrine 1147
Sudafed® 24 Hour [OTC] *see* Pseudoephedrine 1147
Sudafed® Children's [OTC] *see* Pseudoephedrine 1147
Sudafed® Cold & Cough Extra Strength (Can) *see* Acetaminophen, Dextromethorphan, and Pseudoephedrine 59
Sudafed® Decongestant (Can) *see* Pseudoephedrine 1147
Sudafed® Head Cold and Sinus Extra Strength (Can) *see* Acetaminophen and Pseudoephedrine 53
Sudafed® Severe Cold [OTC] *see* Acetaminophen, Dextromethorphan, and Pseudoephedrine 59
Sudafed® Sinus Advance (Can) *see* Pseudoephedrine and Ibuprofen 1149
Sudafed® Sinus & Allergy [OTC] *see* Chlorpheniramine and Pseudoephedrine 315
Sudafed® Sinus and Cold [OTC] *see* Acetaminophen and Pseudoephedrine 53
Sudafed® Sinus Headache [OTC] *see* Acetaminophen and Pseudoephedrine 53
Sudodrin [OTC] *see* Pseudoephedrine 1147
SudoGest Sinus [OTC] *see* Acetaminophen and Pseudoephedrine 53
Sufenta® *see* Sufentanil 1242
Sufentanil 1242
Sufentanil Citrate *see* Sufentanil . . 1242
Sufisal® (Mex) *see* Pentoxifylline . . 1066
Sufortan® (Mex) *see* Penicillamine 1057
Sufortanon® (Mex) *see* Penicillamine 1057
Suiflox® [tabs] (Mex) *see* Ciprofloxacin 331
Sular® *see* Nisoldipine 988
Sulbactam and Ampicillin *see* Ampicillin and Sulbactam 126
Sulconazole 1243
Sulconazole Nitrate *see* Sulconazole 1243
Sulcrate® (Can) *see* Sucralfate . . . 1242
Sulcrate® Suspension Plus (Can) *see* Sucralfate 1242
Sulf-10® *see* Sulfacetamide 1244
Sulfabenzamide, Sulfacetamide, and Sulfathiazole 1243
Sulfacetamide 1244
Sulfacetamide and Fluorometholone 1244
Sulfacetamide and Prednisolone . . 1245
Sulfacetamide Sodium *see* Sulfacetamide 1244
SulfaDIAZINE 1245
Sulfadoxine and Pyrimethamine . . . 1245
Sulfamethoxazole and Trimethoprim 1246
Sulfamylon® *see* Mafenide 852
Sulfasalazine 1249
Sulfatrim *see* Sulfamethoxazole and Trimethoprim 1246
Sulfinpyrazone 1249
SulfiSOXAZOLE 1250
Sulfisoxazole Acetyl *see* SulfiSOXAZOLE 1250
Sulfisoxazole and Erythromycin *see* Erythromycin and Sulfisoxazole 512
Sulfizole® (Can) *see* SulfiSOXAZOLE 1250
Sulfonated Phenolics in Aqueous Solution 1250
Sulindac 1251
Sulphafurazole *see* SulfiSOXAZOLE 1250
Sumatriptan 1252
Sumatriptan Succinate *see* Sumatriptan 1252
Summer's Eve® Medicated Douche [OTC] *see* Povidone-Iodine . . . 1107
Summer's Eve® SpecialCare™ Medicated Anti-Itch Cream [OTC] *see* Hydrocortisone 714
Sumycin® *see* Tetracycline 1280

Supartz™ *see* Hyaluronate and Derivatives 696
Superdophilus® [OTC] *see* *Lactobacillus* 793
Superginkgo *see* Ginkgo Biloba . . . 1429
Supeudol® (Can) *see* Oxycodone . . 1027
Suplasyn® (Can) *see* Hyaluronate and Derivatives 696
Supositorios Senosiain® (Mex) *see* Glycerin 667
Supradol® (Mex) *see* Ketorolac 787
Suprax® (Can) *see* Cefixime 282
Surbex-T® [OTC] *see* Vitamin B Complex Combinations 1382
Sureprin 81™ [OTC] *see* Aspirin . . . 151
Surfak® [OTC] *see* Docusate 459
Surgicel® *see* Cellulose (Oxidized/ Regenerated) 293
Surmontil® (Can) *see* Trimipramine 1343
Survanta® (Can) *see* Beractant 198
Sus-Phrine® (Dental) *see* Epinephrine 496
Sustiva® (Can) *see* Efavirenz 484
Su-Tuss®-HD *see* Hydrocodone, Pseudoephedrine, and Guaifenesin 713
Suxamethonium Chloride *see* Succinylcholine 1241
Sween Cream® [OTC] *see* Vitamin A and Vitamin D 1382
Sweet Root *see* Licorice 1440
Symax SL *see* Hyoscyamine 724
Symax SR *see* Hyoscyamine 724
Symbyax™ *see* Olanzapine and Fluoxetine 1009
Symmetrel® (Can) *see* Amantadine 92
Synacthen *see* Cosyntropin 378
Synagis® (Can) *see* Palivizumab . . 1040
Synalar® (Mex) *see* Fluocinolone . . . 601
Synalgos®-DC *see* Dihydrocodeine, Aspirin, and Caffeine 441
Synarel® (Mex) *see* Nafarelin 957
Syn-Diltiazem® (Can) *see* Diltiazem 444
Synercid® *see* Quinupristin and Dalfopristin 1163
Synphasic® (Can) *see* Ethinyl Estradiol and Norethindrone 550
Synthroid® (Can) *see* Levothyroxine 817
Syntocinon® (Mex) *see* Oxytocin . . 1038
Synvisc® *see* Hyaluronate and Derivatives 696
Syrup of Ipecac *see* Ipecac Syrup . . 760
Syscor® (Mex) *see* Nisoldipine 988
Systemic Viral Diseases 1519
Systen® (Mex) *see* Estradiol 518
T_3 Sodium *see* Liothyronine 831
T_3/T_4 Liotrix *see* Liotrix 832
T_4 *see* Levothyroxine 817
T-20 *see* Enfuvirtide 492
Tabalon® (Mex) *see* Ibuprofen 728
642® Tablet (Can) *see* Propoxyphene 1136
Tacex® [inj.] (Mex) *see* Ceftriaxone 288
Tacrine 1254
Tacrine Hydrochloride *see* Tacrine 1254
Tacrolimus 1255
Tadalafil 1257
Tafil® (Mex) *see* Alprazolam 84
Tagal® [inj.] (Mex) *see* Ceftazidime 286
Tagamet® *see* Cimetidine 330
Tagamet® HB (Can) *see* Cimetidine 330
Tagamet® HB 200 [OTC] *see* Cimetidine 330
Talacen® *see* Pentazocine and Acetaminophen 1064
Talpramin® (Mex) *see* Imipramine . . 737
Talwin® (Can) *see* Pentazocine . . . 1063
Talwin® NX *see* Pentazocine 1063
TAM *see* Tamoxifen 1258
Tambocor™ (Can) *see* Flecainide . . 592
Tamiflu® (Can) *see* Oseltamivir . . . 1019
Tamofen® (Can) *see* Tamoxifen . . . 1258
Tamoxifen 1258
Tamoxifen Citrate *see* Tamoxifen . . 1258
Tamsulosin 1260
Tamsulosin Hydrochloride *see* Tamsulosin 1260
Tanacetum parthenium see Feverfew 1426
Tanafed® *see* Chlorpheniramine and Pseudoephedrine 315
Tanafed DP™ *see* Chlorpheniramine and Pseudoephedrine 315
Tanakan *see* Ginkgo Biloba 1429
Tanakene *see* Ginkgo Biloba 1429
Tandax® (Mex) *see* Naproxen 965
Tannate 12 S *see* Carbetapentane and Chlorpheniramine 260
Tannic-12 *see* Carbetapentane and Chlorpheniramine 260
Tannic-12 S *see* Carbetapentane and Chlorpheniramine 260
Tannihist-12 RF *see* Carbetapentane and Chlorpheniramine 260
Tao® *see* Troleandomycin 1348
TAP-144 *see* Leuprolide 805
Tapazole® (Can) *see* Methimazole . . 893
Taporin® [inj.] (Mex) *see* Cefotaxime 283
Targel® (Can) *see* Coal Tar 367
Targretin® (Can) *see* Bexarotene . . . 205
Tarka® *see* Trandolapril and Verapamil 1322
Taro-Carbamazepine Chewable (Can) *see* Carbamazepine 255
Taro-Desoximetasone (Can) *see* Desoximetasone 410
Taro-Sone® (Can) *see* Betamethasone 199
Taro-Warfarin (Can) *see* Warfarin 1389
Tarsum® [OTC] *see* Coal Tar and Salicylic Acid 367
Tasedan® (Mex) *see* Estazolam 517
Tasmar® (Mex) *see* Tolcapone 1310
Tavanic® (Mex) *see* Levofloxacin . . . 812
Tavist® (Mex) *see* Clemastine 346
Tavist® Allergy [OTC] *see* Clemastine 346
Tavist® ND [OTC] *see* Loratadine . . 841
Tavor® (Mex) *see* Oxybutynin 1026
Taxifur® [inj.] (Mex) *see* Ceftazidime 286
Taxol® (Can) *see* Paclitaxel 1038
Taxotere® *see* Docetaxel 458
Taxus® [tabs] (Mex) *see* Tamoxifen 1258
Tazarotene 1262
Tazicef® *see* Ceftazidime 286
Taziken® [tabs] (Mex) *see* Terbutaline 1273
Tazocin® (Can) *see* Piperacillin and Tazobactam Sodium 1093
Tazorac® (Can) *see* Tazarotene . . . 1262
Taztia XT™ *see* Diltiazem 444
3TC *see* Lamivudine 794
3TC, Abacavir, and Zidovudine *see* Abacavir, Lamivudine, and Zidovudine 43
T-Cell Growth Factor *see* Aldesleukin 74
TCGF *see* Aldesleukin 74

TCN *see* Tetracycline 1280
TDF *see* Tenofovir 1270
Teardrops® (Can) *see* Artificial Tears 148
Teargen® [OTC] *see* Artificial Tears 148
Teargen® II [OTC] *see* Artificial Tears 148
Tearisol® [OTC] *see* Artificial Tears 148
Tearisol® [OTC] *see* Hydroxypropyl Methylcellulose 721
Tears Again® [OTC] *see* Artificial Tears 148
Tears Again® Gel Drops™ [OTC] *see* Carboxymethylcellulose 265
Tears Again® Night and Day™ [OTC] *see* Carboxymethylcellulose 265
Tears Naturale® [OTC] *see* Artificial Tears 148
Tears Naturale® Free [OTC] *see* Artificial Tears 148
Tears Naturale® II [OTC] *see* Artificial Tears 148
Tears Plus® [OTC] *see* Artificial Tears 148
Tears Renewed® [OTC] *see* Artificial Tears 148
Tea Tree Oil *see* Melaleuca Oil . . . 1442
Tebonin *see* Ginkgo Biloba 1429
Tebrazid™ (Can) *see* Pyrazinamide 1152
Tecnal C 1/2 (Can) *see* Butalbital, Aspirin, Caffeine, and Codeine 238
Tecnal C 1/4 (Can) *see* Butalbital, Aspirin, Caffeine, and Codeine 238
Tecnofen® [tabs] (Mex) *see* Tamoxifen 1258
Tecnoplatin® [inj.] (Mex) *see* Cisplatin 337
Teejel® (Can) *see* Choline Salicylate 325
Tegaserod 1263
Tegaserod Maleate *see* Tegaserod 1263
Tegretol® *see* Carbamazepine 255
Tegretol®-XR *see* Carbamazepine . . 255
Tegrin® [OTC] *see* Coal Tar 367
Telithromycin 1263
Telmisartan 1265
Telmisartan and HCTZ *see* Telmisartan and Hydrochlorothiazide 1265
Telmisartan and Hydrochlorothiazide 1265
Temazepam 1266
Temgesic® (Mex) *see* Buprenorphine 228
Temodal™ (Can) *see* Temozolomide 1268
Temodar® (Can) *see* Temozolomide 1268
Temovate® *see* Clobetasol 351
Temovate E® *see* Clobetasol 351
Temozolomide 1268
Temperal® (Mex) *see* Acetaminophen 47
Temporomandibular Dysfunction (TMD) 1564
Tempra® (Can) *see* Acetaminophen 47
Tenecteplase 1268
Tenex® *see* Guanfacine 679
Teniposide 1269
Tenofovir 1270
Tenofovir Disoproxil Fumarate *see* Tenofovir 1270
Tenolin (Can) *see* Atenolol 159
Tenoretic® (Can) *see* Atenolol and Chlorthalidone 161
Tenormin® (Can) *see* Atenolol 159
Tenuate® *see* Diethylpropion 434
Tenuate® Dospan® *see* Diethylpropion 434
Teolong® (Mex) *see* Theophylline 1285
Tequin® *see* Gatifloxacin 647
Terazol® (Can) *see* Terconazole . . 1274
Terazol® 3 *see* Terconazole 1274
Terazol® 7 *see* Terconazole 1274
Terazosin 1271
Terbac® [inj.] (Mex) *see* Ceftriaxone 288
Terbinafine 1272
Terbinafine Hydrochloride *see* Terbinafine 1272
Terbutaline 1273
Terconazole 1274
Terfluzine (Can) *see* Trifluoperazine 1338
Teriparatide 1274
Termizol® (Mex) *see* Ketoconazole 783
Terpin Hydrate and Codeine 1275
Terra-Cortril® [DSC] *see* Oxytetracycline and Hydrocortisone 1037
Terramicina® (Mex) *see* Oxytetracycline 1036
Terramycin® (Can) *see* Oxytetracycline 1036
Terramycin® I.M. *see* Oxytetracycline 1036
Terramycin® w/Polymyxin B Ophthalmic *see* Oxytetracycline and Polymyxin B 1037
Tesalon® (Mex) *see* Benzonatate . . . 193
Teslac® (Can) *see* Testolactone . . . 1275
TESPA *see* Thiotepa 1291
Tessalon® *see* Benzonatate 193
Testim™ *see* Testosterone 1276
Testoderm® (Can) *see* Testosterone 1276
Testoderm® with Adhesive [DSC] *see* Testosterone 1276
Testolactone 1275
Testopel® *see* Testosterone 1276
Testosterone 1276
Testosterone Cypionate *see* Testosterone 1276
Testosterone Enanthate *see* Testosterone 1276
Testred® *see* MethylTESTOSTERone 912
Tetanus Antitoxin *see* Immunizations (Vaccines) 1614
Tetanus Immune Globulin (Human) *see* Immunizations (Vaccines) 1614
Tetanus Immune Globulin (Human) 1277
Tetanus Toxoid (Adsorbed) *see* Immunizations (Vaccines) 1614
Tetanus Toxoid (Adsorbed) 1277
Tetanus Toxoid (Fluid) *see* Immunizations (Vaccines) 1614
Tetanus Toxoid (Fluid) 1278
Tetanus Toxoid Plain *see* Tetanus Toxoid (Fluid) 1278
Tetra-Atlantis® (Mex) *see* Tetracycline 1280
Tetracaine 1278
Tetracaine and Dextrose 1279
Tetracaine Hydrochloride *see* Tetracaine 1278

Tetracaine Hydrochloride, Benzocaine Butyl Aminobenzoate, and Benzalkonium Chloride *see* Benzocaine, Butyl Aminobenzoate, Tetracaine, and Benzalkonium Chloride 193
Tetracosactide *see* Cosyntropin 378
Tetracycline 1280
Tetracycline, Bismuth Subsalicylate, and Metronidazole *see* Bismuth Subsalicylate, Metronidazole, and Tetracycline 209
Tetracycline Hydrochloride *see* Tetracycline 1280
Tetracycline, Metronidazole, and Bismuth Subsalicylate *see* Bismuth Subsalicylate, Metronidazole, and Tetracycline 209
Tetracycline (Periodontal) 1282
Tetrahydroaminoacrine *see* Tacrine 1254
Tetrahydrocannabinol *see* Dronabinol 477
Tetrahydrozoline 1282
Tetrahydrozoline Hydrochloride *see* Tetrahydrozoline 1282
Tetra Tannate Pediatric *see* Chlorpheniramine, Ephedrine, Phenylephrine, and Carbetapentane 316
Tetryzoline *see* Tetrahydrozoline . . 1282
Teveten® (Can) *see* Eprosartan 501
Teveten® HCT *see* Eprosartan and Hydrochlorothiazide 502
Texacort® *see* Hydrocortisone 714
Texate® (Mex) *see* Methotrexate . . . 897
TG *see* Thioguanine 1288
6-TG *see* Thioguanine 1288
THA *see* Tacrine 1254
Thalidomide 1283
Thalitone® *see* Chlorthalidone 321
Thalomid® *see* Thalidomide 1283
THAM® *see* Tromethamine 1348
THC *see* Dronabinol 477
Theo-24® *see* Theophylline 1285
Theochron® *see* Theophylline 1285
Theochron® SR (Can) *see* Theophylline 1285
Theo-Dur® (Can) *see* Theophylline 1285
Theolair™ (Can) *see* Theophylline 1285
Theolair-SR® [DSC] *see* Theophylline 1285
Theolate *see* Theophylline and Guaifenesin 1286
Theophylline 1285
Theophylline and Guaifenesin 1286
Theophylline Anhydrous *see* Theophylline 1285
Theophylline Ethylenediamine *see* Aminophylline 99
Theracort® [OTC] *see* Hydrocortisone 714
TheraCys® *see* BCG Vaccine 183
Thera-Flu® Cold and Sore Throat Night Time [OTC] *see* Acetaminophen, Chlorpheniramine, and Pseudoephedrine 58
Thera-Flur-N® *see* Fluoride 603
Thera-Flu® Severe Cold Non-Drowsy [OTC] [DSC] *see* Acetaminophen, Dextromethorphan, and Pseudoephedrine 59
Theragran® Heart Right™ [OTC] *see* Vitamins (Multiple/Oral) . . . 1384
Theragran-M® Advanced Formula [OTC] *see* Vitamins (Multiple/Oral) 1384
Theramycin Z® *see* Erythromycin . . . 508
TheraPatch® Warm [OTC] *see* Capsaicin 252
Therapeutic Multivitamins *see* Vitamins (Multiple/Oral) 1384
Theratears® *see* Carboxymethylcellulose 265
Thermazene® *see* Silver Sulfadiazine 1221
Thiabendazole 1286
Thiamazole *see* Methimazole 893
Thiamilate® [OTC] *see* Thiamine . . 1287
Thiamine 1287
Thiamine Hydrochloride *see* Thiamine 1287
Thiaminium Chloride Hydrochloride *see* Thiamine 1287
Thiethylperazine 1287
Thiethylperazine Maleate *see* Thiethylperazine 1287
Thimerosal 1288
Thioctic acid *see* Alpha-Lipoic Acid 1413
Thioguanine 1288
6-Thioguanine *see* Thioguanine . . . 1288
Thiola™ (Can) *see* Tiopronin 1303
Thiopental 1289
Thiopental Sodium *see* Thiopental 1289
Thiophosphoramide *see* Thiotepa 1291
Thioplex® [DSC] *see* Thiotepa 1291
Thioridazine 1289
Thioridazine Hydrochloride *see* Thioridazine 1289
Thioridazine Intensol™ *see* Thioridazine 1289
Thiosulfuric Acid Disodium Salt *see* Sodium Thiosulfate 1230
Thiotepa 1291
Thiothixene 1291
Thorazine® [DSC] *see* ChlorproMAZINE 319
Thrombate III® *see* Antithrombin III 136
Thrombin-JMI® *see* Thrombin (Topical) 1292
Thrombin (Topical) 1292
Thrombogen® *see* Thrombin (Topical) 1292
Thrombostat™ (Can) *see* Thrombin (Topical) 1292
Thymocyte Stimulating Factor *see* Aldesleukin 74
Thyrel® TRH [DSC] *see* Protirelin . . 1145
Thyrogen® (Can) *see* Thyrotropin Alpha 1294
Thyroid 1293
Thyroid Extract *see* Thyroid 1293
Thyroid USP *see* Thyroid 1293
Thyrolar® (Can) *see* Liotrix 832
Thyrotropin Alpha 1294
Thyrotropin Releasing Hormone *see* Protirelin 1145
Tiabendazole *see* Thiabendazole . . 1286
Tiagabine 1294
Tiagabine Hydrochloride *see* Tiagabine 1294
Tiamol® (Can) *see* Fluocinonide 602
Tiazac® *see* Diltiazem 444
Ticar® *see* Ticarcillin 1295
Ticarcillin 1295
Ticarcillin and Clavulanate Potassium 1296
Ticarcillin and Clavulanic Acid *see* Ticarcillin and Clavulanate Potassium 1296

Ticarcillin Disodium *see* Ticarcillin 1295
TICE® BCG *see* BCG Vaccine 183
Ticlid® *see* Ticlopidine 1297
Ticlopidine 1297
Ticlopidine Hydrochloride *see* Ticlopidine 1297
TIG *see* Tetanus Immune Globulin (Human) 1277
Tigan® *see* Trimethobenzamide . . . 1341
Tikosyn™ *see* Dofetilide 460
Tilade® (Can) *see* Nedocromil 970
Tilazem® (Mex) *see* Diltiazem 444
Tiludronate 1298
Tiludronate Disodium *see* Tiludronate 1298
Tim-AK (Can) *see* Timolol 1299
Timentin® *see* Ticarcillin and Clavulanate Potassium 1296
Timolol 1299
Timolol and Dorzolamide *see* Dorzolamide and Timolol 464
Timolol Hemihydrate *see* Timolol . . 1299
Timolol Maleate *see* Timolol 1299
Timoptic® (Can) *see* Timolol 1299
Timoptic® OcuDose® *see* Timolol . . 1299
Timoptic-XE® *see* Timolol 1299
Timoptol® (Mex) *see* Timolol 1299
Tinactin® Antifungal [OTC] *see* Tolnaftate 1312
Tinactin® Antifungal Jock Itch [OTC] *see* Tolnaftate 1312
Tinaderm® (Mex) *see* Tolnaftate . . . 1312
Tinamed® [OTC] *see* Salicylic Acid 1205
TinBen® [OTC] [DSC] *see* Benzoin 193
Tindamax™ *see* Tinidazole 1301
Tine Test *see* Tuberculin Tests . . . 1349
Ting® [OTC] *see* Tolnaftate 1312
Tiniazol® (Mex) *see* Ketoconazole . . 783
Tinidazole 1301
Tinzaparin 1301
Tinzaparin Sodium *see* Tinzaparin 1301
Tioconazole 1302
Tioguanine *see* Thioguanine 1288
Tiopronin 1303
Tiotixene *see* Thiothixene 1291
Tiotropium 1303
Tiotropium Bromide Monohydrate *see* Tiotropium 1303
TipTapToe [OTC] *see* Tolnaftate . . 1312
Tirocal® (Mex) *see* Calcitriol 244
Tirofiban 1304
Tirofiban Hydrochloride *see* Tirofiban 1304
Tiroidine® [tabs] (Mex) *see* Levothyroxine 817
Tiseb® [OTC] *see* Salicylic Acid . . . 1205
Tisit® [OTC] *see* Pyrethrins and Piperonyl Butoxide 1153
Tisit® Blue Gel [OTC] *see* Pyrethrins and Piperonyl Butoxide 1153
Tisseel® VH *see* Fibrin Sealant Kit . . 589
Titralac ™ [OTC] *see* Calcium Carbonate 245
Titralac™ Extra Strength [OTC] *see* Calcium Carbonate 245
Titralac® Plus [OTC] *see* Calcium Carbonate and Simethicone 245
Ti-U-Lac® H (Can) *see* Urea and Hydrocortisone 1353
Tizanidine 1305
TMP *see* Trimethoprim 1341
TMP-SMZ *see* Sulfamethoxazole and Trimethoprim 1246
TMZ *see* Temozolomide 1268
TNKase™ (Can) *see* Tenecteplase 1268
TOBI® (Can) *see* Tobramycin 1306
Tobradex® (Can) *see* Tobramycin and Dexamethasone 1307
Tobramycin 1306
Tobramycin and Dexamethasone . . 1307
Tobramycin Sulfate *see* Tobramycin 1306
Tobrex® (Mex) *see* Tobramycin . . . 1306
Tocainide 1307
Tocainide Hydrochloride *see* Tocainide 1307
Tofranil® (Can) *see* Imipramine 737
Tofranil-PM® (Mex) *see* Imipramine 737
TOLAZamide 1308
Tolazoline 1309
Tolazoline Hydrochloride *see* Tolazoline 1309
TOLBUTamide 1309
Tolbutamide Sodium *see* TOLBUTamide 1309
Tolcapone 1310
Tolectin® (Mex) *see* Tolmetin 1311
Tolectin® DS *see* Tolmetin 1311
Tolinase® *see* TOLAZamide 1308
Tolmetin 1311
Tolmetin Sodium *see* Tolmetin 1311
Tolnaftate 1312
Tol-Tab® *see* TOLBUTamide 1309
Tolterodine 1312
Tolterodine Tartrate *see* Tolterodine 1312
Tolu-Sed® DM [OTC] *see* Guaifenesin and Dextromethorphan 673
Tomoxetine *see* Atomoxetine 161
Tomycine™ (Can) *see* Tobramycin 1306
Tondex® [inj.] (Mex) *see* Gentamicin 655
Tonga *see* Kava 1439
Tonocalcin® [salmon] (Mex) *see* Calcitonin 243
Tonocard® [DSC] *see* Tocainide . . . 1307
Top 200 Most Prescribed Drugs in 2003 1642
Topamax® *see* Topiramate 1314
Top-Dal® [tabs] (Mex) *see* Loperamide 838
Topicaine® [OTC] *see* Lidocaine . . . 819
Topicort® *see* Desoximetasone 410
Topicort®-LP *see* Desoximetasone . . 410
Topilene® (Can) *see* Betamethasone 199
Topiramate 1314
Topisone® (Can) *see* Betamethasone 199
TOPO *see* Topotecan 1316
Toposar® *see* Etoposide 567
Topotecan 1316
Topotecan Hydrochloride *see* Topotecan 1316
Toprol-XL® *see* Metoprolol 915
Topsyn® (Mex) *see* Fluocinonide . . . 602
Toradol® (Can) *see* Ketorolac 787
Toradol® IM (Can) *see* Ketorolac . . . 787
Torecan® [DSC] *see* Thiethylperazine 1287
Toremifene 1317
Toremifene Citrate *see* Toremifene 1317
Torsemide 1317
Touro™ Allergy *see* Brompheniramine and Pseudoephedrine 220
Touro™ CC *see* Guaifenesin, Pseudoephedrine, and Dextromethorphan 676
Touro® DM *see* Guaifenesin and Dextromethorphan 673
Touro Ex® [DSC] *see* Guaifenesin . . 672

Touro LA® see Guaifenesin and Pseudoephedrine . . . 675
tPA see Alteplase . . . 88
T-Phyl® see Theophylline . . . 1285
TPT see Topotecan . . . 1316
tRA see Tretinoin (Oral) . . . 1328
Trace Metals . . . 1319
Tracleer® see Bosentan . . . 214
Tradol® (Mex) see Tramadol . . . 1319
Tramadol . . . 1319
Tramadol Hydrochloride see Tramadol . . . 1319
Tramadol Hydrochloride and Acetaminophen see Acetaminophen and Tramadol . . . 54
Tramisal see Ginkgo Biloba . . . 1429
Trandate® (Can) see Labetalol . . . 791
Trandolapril . . . 1321
Trandolapril and Verapamil . . . 1322
Tranexamic Acid . . . 1323
Transamine Sulphate see Tranylcypromine . . . 1323
Transderm-Nitro® (Can) see Nitroglycerin . . . 991
Transderm Scōp® see Scopolamine . . . 1210
Transderm-V® (Can) see Scopolamine . . . 1210
Trans-Plantar® (Can) see Salicylic Acid . . . 1205
trans-Retinoic Acid see Tretinoin (Oral) . . . 1328
trans-Retinoic Acid see Tretinoin (Topical) . . . 1329
Trans-Ver-Sal® (Can) see Salicylic Acid . . . 1205
Tranxene® see Clorazepate . . . 362
Tranxene® SD™ see Clorazepate . . . 362
Tranxene® SD™-Half Strength see Clorazepate . . . 362
Tranxene T-Tab® see Clorazepate . . . 362
Tranylcypromine . . . 1323
Tranylcypromine Sulfate see Tranylcypromine . . . 1323
Trasicor® (Can) see Oxprenolol . . . 1025
Trastuzumab . . . 1324
Trasylol® (Can) see Aprotinin . . . 139
Travatan® (Can) see Travoprost . . . 1325
Travoprost . . . 1325
Trazil® (Mex) see Tobramycin . . . 1306
Trazodone . . . 1326
Trazodone Hydrochloride see Trazodone . . . 1326
Trecator®-SC (Can) see Ethionamide . . . 560
Trelstar™ Depot (Can) see Triptorelin . . . 1346
Trelstar™ LA see Triptorelin . . . 1346
Trental® see Pentoxifylline . . . 1066
Treprostinil . . . 1327
Treprostinil Sodium see Treprostinil . . . 1327
Tretinoin and Mequinol see Mequinol and Tretinoin . . . 879
Tretinoin, Fluocinolone Acetonide, and Hydroquinone see Fluocinolone, Hydroquinone, and Tretinoin . . . 601
Tretinoin (Oral) . . . 1328
Tretinoin (Topical) . . . 1329
Trexall™ see Methotrexate . . . 897
TRH see Protirelin . . . 1145
Triacetin . . . 1329
Triacetyloleandomycin see Troleandomycin . . . 1348
Triacin-C® [DSC] see Triprolidine, Pseudoephedrine, and Codeine . . . 1346
Triaconazole see Terconazole . . . 1274
Triaderm (Can) see Triamcinolone . . . 1330
Triaken® [inj.] (Mex) see Ceftriaxone . . . 288
Triamcinolone . . . 1330
Triamcinolone Acetonide, Aerosol see Triamcinolone . . . 1330
Triamcinolone Acetonide (Dental Paste) . . . 1333
Triamcinolone Acetonide, Parenteral see Triamcinolone . . . 1330
Triamcinolone and Nystatin see Nystatin and Triamcinolone . . . 1004
Triamcinolone Diacetate, Oral see Triamcinolone . . . 1330
Triamcinolone Diacetate, Parenteral see Triamcinolone . . . 1330
Triamcinolone Hexacetonide see Triamcinolone . . . 1330
Triamcinolone, Oral see Triamcinolone . . . 1330
Triaminic® Allergy Congestion [OTC] see Pseudoephedrine . . . 1147
Triaminic® Cold & Allergy (Can) see Chlorpheniramine and Pseudoephedrine . . . 315
Triaminic® Cold and Allergy [OTC] see Chlorpheniramine and Pseudoephedrine . . . 315
Triaminic® Cough and Sore Throat Formula [OTC] see Acetaminophen, Dextromethorphan, and Pseudoephedrine . . . 59
Triamsicort® (Mex) see Triamcinolone . . . 1330
Triamterene . . . 1334
Triamterene and Hydrochlorothiazide see Hydrochlorothiazide and Triamterene . . . 701
Triatec-8 (Can) see Acetaminophen and Codeine . . . 50
Triatec-8 Strong (Can) see Acetaminophen and Codeine . . . 50
Triatec-30 (Can) see Acetaminophen and Codeine . . . 50
Triavil® (Can) see Amitriptyline and Perphenazine . . . 106
Triaz® see Benzoyl Peroxide . . . 194
Triaz® Cleanser see Benzoyl Peroxide . . . 194
Triazolam . . . 1335
Tribavirin see Ribavirin . . . 1177
Tricalcium Phosphate see Calcium Phosphate (Tribasic) . . . 247
Tricardio B see Folic Acid, Cyanocobalamin, and Pyridoxine . . . 626
Tri-Chlor® see Trichloroacetic Acid . . . 1337
Trichlorex® (Can) see Trichlormethiazide . . . 1337
Trichlormethiazide . . . 1337
Trichloroacetaldehyde Monohydrate see Chloral Hydrate . . . 304
Trichloroacetic Acid . . . 1337
Trichloromonofluoromethane and Dichlorodifluoromethane see Dichlorodifluoromethane and Trichloromonofluoromethane . . . 427
Triclosan and Fluoride . . . 1337
TriCor® (Can) see Fenofibrate . . . 577
Tricosal see Choline Magnesium Trisalicylate . . . 324
Tri-Cyclen® (Can) see Ethinyl Estradiol and Norgestimate . . . 554
Triderm® see Triamcinolone . . . 1330
Tridesilon® see Desonide . . . 410
Tridione® see Trimethadione . . . 1340

Triethanolamine Polypeptide Oleate-Condensate . . . 1338
Triethanolamine Salicylate . . . 1338
Triethylenethiophosphoramide *see* Thiotepa . . . 1291
Trifluoperazine . . . 1338
Trifluoperazine Hydrochloride *see* Trifluoperazine . . . 1338
Trifluorothymidine *see* Trifluridine . . 1339
Trifluridine . . . 1339
Triglycerides, Medium Chain *see* Medium Chain Triglycerides . . . 861
Trihexyphenidyl . . . 1340
Trihexyphenidyl Hydrochloride *see* Trihexyphenidyl . . . 1340
Tri-K® *see* Potassium Acetate, Potassium Bicarbonate, and Potassium Citrate . . . 1104
Trikacide (Can) *see* Metronidazole . . 917
Trilafon® (Can) *see* Perphenazine . . . 1070
Trileptal® (Can) *see* Oxcarbazepine . . . 1023
Tri-Levlen® *see* Ethinyl Estradiol and Levonorgestrel . . . 545
Trilisate® [DSC] *see* Choline Magnesium Trisalicylate . . . 324
Tri-Luma™ *see* Fluocinolone, Hydroquinone, and Tretinoin . . . 601
TriLyte™ *see* Polyethylene Glycol-Electrolyte Solution . . . 1100
Trimethadione . . . 1340
Trimethobenzamide . . . 1341
Trimethobenzamide Hydrochloride *see* Trimethobenzamide . . . 1341
Trimethoprim . . . 1341
Trimethoprim and Polymyxin B . . . 1342
Trimethoprim and Sulfamethoxazole *see* Sulfamethoxazole and Trimethoprim . . . 1246
Trimetrexate Glucuronate . . . 1342
Trimipramine . . . 1343
Trimipramine Maleate *see* Trimipramine . . . 1343
Trimox® *see* Amoxicillin . . . 114
Trinasal® (Can) *see* Triamcinolone . . . 1330
TriNessa™ *see* Ethinyl Estradiol and Norgestimate . . . 554
Tri-Norinyl® *see* Ethinyl Estradiol and Norethindrone . . . 550
Trinsicon® *see* Vitamin B Complex Combinations . . . 1382
Triostat® *see* Liothyronine . . . 831
Tripelennamine . . . 1344
Tripelennamine Citrate *see* Tripelennamine . . . 1344
Tripelennamine Hydrochloride *see* Tripelennamine . . . 1344
Triphasil® (Can) *see* Ethinyl Estradiol and Levonorgestrel . . . 545
Triple Antibiotic *see* Bacitracin, Neomycin, and Polymyxin B . . . 179
Triple Care® Antifungal [OTC] *see* Miconazole . . . 922
Triple Sulfa *see* Sulfabenzamide, Sulfacetamide, and Sulfathiazole . . . 1243
Tri-Previfem™ *see* Ethinyl Estradiol and Norgestimate . . . 554
Triprolidine and Pseudoephedrine . . . 1345
Triprolidine, Codeine, and Pseudoephedrine *see* Triprolidine, Pseudoephedrine, and Codeine . . . 1346
Triprolidine, Pseudoephedrine, and Codeine . . . 1346
Triprolidine, Pseudoephedrine, and Codeine, Triprolidine, and Pseudoephedrine *see* Triprolidine, Pseudoephedrine, and Codeine . . . 1346
TripTone® [OTC] *see* DimenhyDRINATE . . . 446
Triptoraline *see* Triptorelin . . . 1346
Triptorelin . . . 1346
Triptorelin Pamoate *see* Triptorelin . . . 1346
Triquilar® (Can) *see* Ethinyl Estradiol and Levonorgestrel . . . 545
Tris Buffer *see* Tromethamine . . . 1348
Tris(hydroxymethyl)aminomethane *see* Tromethamine . . . 1348
Tri-Sprintec™ *see* Ethinyl Estradiol and Norgestimate . . . 554
Tri-Sudo® [OTC] *see* Triprolidine and Pseudoephedrine . . . 1345
Tritace® (Mex) *see* Ramipril . . . 1167
Trivagizole-3® (Can) *see* Clotrimazole . . . 363
Tri-Vent™ DM *see* Guaifenesin, Pseudoephedrine, and Dextromethorphan . . . 676
Tri-Vent™ HC *see* Hydrocodone, Carbinoxamine, and Pseudoephedrine . . . 712
Trivora® *see* Ethinyl Estradiol and Levonorgestrel . . . 545
Trixilem® (Mex) *see* Methotrexate . . 897
Triyotex® (Mex) *see* Liothyronine . . . 831
Trizivir® *see* Abacavir, Lamivudine, and Zidovudine . . . 43
Trobicin® *see* Spectinomycin . . . 1234
Trocaine® [OTC] *see* Benzocaine . . . 191
Troleandomycin . . . 1348
Tromethamine . . . 1348
Tronolane® [OTC] *see* Pramoxine . . . 1109
Tropicacyl® *see* Tropicamide . . . 1348
Tropicamide . . . 1348
Tropicamide and Hydroxyamphetamine *see* Hydroxyamphetamine and Tropicamide . . . 720
Tropyn Z® (Mex) *see* Atropine . . . 166
Trovafloxacin . . . 1348
Trovan® [DSC] *see* Trovafloxacin . . 1348
Troxidone *see* Trimethadione . . . 1340
Trusopt® (Can) *see* Dorzolamide . . . 464
Trypsin, Balsam Peru, and Castor Oil . . . 1349
Tryptanol® (Mex) *see* Amitriptyline . . 103
Tryptoreline *see* Triptorelin . . . 1346
TSH *see* Thyrotropin Alpha . . . 1294
TSPA *see* Thiotepa . . . 1291
TST *see* Tuberculin Tests . . . 1349
T-Stat® *see* Erythromycin . . . 508
T-Tab® *see* Clorazepate . . . 362
Tuberculin Purified Protein Derivative *see* Tuberculin Tests . . . 1349
Tuberculin Skin Test *see* Tuberculin Tests . . . 1349
Tuberculin Tests . . . 1349
Tuberculosis . . . 1495
Tubersol® *see* Tuberculin Tests . . . 1349
Tuinal® [DSC] *see* Amobarbital and Secobarbital . . . 112
Tukol® (Mex) *see* Guaifenesin . . . 672
Tums® [OTC] *see* Calcium Carbonate . . . 245
Tums® 500 [OTC] *see* Calcium Carbonate . . . 245
Tums® E-X [OTC] *see* Calcium Carbonate . . . 245
Tums® Extra Strength Sugar Free [OTC] *see* Calcium Carbonate . . 245

Tums® Smooth Dissolve [OTC] *see* Calcium Carbonate 245
Tums® Ultra [OTC] *see* Calcium Carbonate 245
Turmeric 1448
Turmeric Root *see* Golden Seal . . . 1433
Tusical® (Mex) *see* Benzonatate . . . 193
Tusitato® (Mex) *see* Benzonatate . . . 193
Tussafed® *see* Carbinoxamine, Pseudoephedrine, and Dextromethorphan 263
Tussend® Expectorant *see* Hydrocodone, Pseudoephedrine, and Guaifenesin 713
Tussi-12® *see* Carbetapentane and Chlorpheniramine 260
Tussi-12® D *see* Carbetapentane, Phenylephrine, and Pyrilamine . . 261
Tussi-12® DS *see* Carbetapentane, Phenylephrine, and Pyrilamine . . 261
Tussi-12 S™ *see* Carbetapentane and Chlorpheniramine 260
Tussigon® *see* Hydrocodone and Homatropine 709
Tussin [OTC] *see* Guaifenesin 672
Tussionex® *see* Hydrocodone and Chlorpheniramine 707
Tussi-Organidin® DM NR *see* Guaifenesin and Dextromethorphan 673
Tussi-Organidin® NR *see* Guaifenesin and Codeine 673
Tussi-Organidin® S-NR *see* Guaifenesin and Codeine 673
Tussizone-12 RF™ *see* Carbetapentane and Chlorpheniramine 260
Tusstat® *see* DiphenhydrAMINE 448
Twice-A-Day® [OTC] *see* Oxymetazoline 1034
Twilite® [OTC] *see* DiphenhydrAMINE 448
Twinrix™ (Can) *see* Hepatitis A (Inactivated) and Hepatitis B (Recombinant) Vaccine 686
Tylenol® [OTC] *see* Acetaminophen 47
Tylenol® 8 Hour [OTC] *see* Acetaminophen 47
Tylenol® Allergy Sinus [OTC] *see* Acetaminophen, Chlorpheniramine, and Pseudoephedrine 58
Tylenol® Arthritis Pain [OTC] *see* Acetaminophen 47
Tylenol® Children's [OTC] *see* Acetaminophen 47
Tylenol® Cold Day Non-Drowsy [OTC] *see* Acetaminophen, Dextromethorphan, and Pseudoephedrine 59
Tylenol® Cold Daytime (Can) *see* Acetaminophen, Dextromethorphan, and Pseudoephedrine 59
Tylenol® Cold, Infants [OTC] *see* Acetaminophen and Pseudoephedrine 53
Tylenol® Decongestant (Can) *see* Acetaminophen and Pseudoephedrine 53
Tylenol Elixir with Codeine (Can) *see* Acetaminophen and Codeine 50
Tylenol® Extra Strength [OTC] *see* Acetaminophen 47
Tylenol® Flu Non-Drowsy Maximum Strength [OTC] *see* Acetaminophen, Dextromethorphan, and Pseudoephedrine 59
Tylenol® Infants [OTC] *see* Acetaminophen 47
Tylenol® Junior Strength [OTC] *see* Acetaminophen 47
Tylenol No. 1 (Can) *see* Acetaminophen and Codeine 50
Tylenol No. 1 Forte (Can) *see* Acetaminophen and Codeine 50
Tylenol No. 2 with Codeine (Can) *see* Acetaminophen and Codeine 50
Tylenol No. 3 with Codeine (Can) *see* Acetaminophen and Codeine 50
Tylenol No. 4 with Codeine (Can) *see* Acetaminophen and Codeine 50
Tylenol® PM Extra Strength [OTC] *see* Acetaminophen and Diphenhydramine 53
Tylenol® Severe Allergy [OTC] *see* Acetaminophen and Diphenhydramine 53
Tylenol® Sinus (Can) *see* Acetaminophen and Pseudoephedrine 53
Tylenol® Sinus, Children's [OTC] *see* Acetaminophen and Pseudoephedrine 53
Tylenol® Sinus Day Non-Drowsy [OTC] *see* Acetaminophen and Pseudoephedrine 53
Tylenol® Sore Throat [OTC] *see* Acetaminophen 47
Tylenol® With Codeine *see* Acetaminophen and Codeine 50
Tylex® (Mex) *see* Acetaminophen . . . 47
Tylox® *see* Oxycodone and Acetaminophen 1029
Typhim Vi® *see* Typhoid Vaccine . . 1351
Typhoid Vaccine 1351
Typhoid Vaccine Live Oral Ty21a *see* Typhoid Vaccine 1351
Tyzine® *see* Tetrahydrozoline 1282
Tyzine® Pediatric *see* Tetrahydrozoline 1282
Tzoali® (Mex) *see* DiphenhydrAMINE 448
U-90152S *see* Delavirdine 403
Ubiquinone *see* Coenzyme Q_{10} . . . 1420
UCB-P071 *see* Cetirizine 298
UK92480 *see* Sildenafil 1219
UK109496 *see* Voriconazole 1385
Ulcedin® (Mex) *see* Ranitidine 1169
Ulcerease® [OTC] *see* Phenol 1075
Ulgastrin Neo *see* Licorice 1440
Ulpax® (Mex) *see* Lansoprazole 797
Ulsaven® (Mex) *see* Ranitidine 1169
Ulsen® (Mex) *see* Omeprazole 1012
Ultiva® (Mex) *see* Remifentanil 1172
Ultracaine® D-S (Can) *see* Articaine Hydrochloride and Epinephrine (Canada) 143
Ultracaine® D-S Forte (Can) *see* Articaine Hydrochloride and Epinephrine (Canada) 143
Ultracet™ *see* Acetaminophen and Tramadol 54
Ultram® (Can) *see* Tramadol 1319
Ultra Mide® *see* Urea 1353
UltraMide 25™ (Can) *see* Urea . . . 1353
Ultramop™ (Can) *see* Methoxsalen 902
Ultran® (Mex) *see* Ranitidine 1169
Ultraprin [OTC] *see* Ibuprofen 728

Ultraquin™ (Can) *see* Hydroquinone . . . 719
Ultrase® (Can) *see* Pancrelipase . . 1042
Ultrase® MT *see* Pancrelipase 1042
Ultra Tears® [OTC] *see* Artificial Tears . . . 148
Ultravate® *see* Halobetasol 681
Ultravist® *see* Iopromide 760
Unamol® (Mex) *see* Cisapride 336
Unasyn® *see* Ampicillin and Sulbactam 126
Uncaria tomentosa see Cat's Claw 1417
Undecylenic Acid and Derivatives 1352
Uni-Cof *see* Pseudoephedrine, Dihydrocodeine, and Chlorpheniramine 1150
Unidet® (Can) *see* Tolterodine 1312
Uni-Dur® (Mex) *see* Theophylline . . 1285
Uni-Fed® [OTC] *see* Triprolidine and Pseudoephedrine 1345
Unipen® (Can) *see* Nafcillin 958
Uniphyl® *see* Theophylline 1285
Uniphyl® SRT (Can) *see* Theophylline 1285
Uniretic® *see* Moexipril and Hydrochlorothiazide 941
Unisom® Maximum Strength SleepGels® [OTC] *see* DiphenhydrAMINE 448
Unithroid® *see* Levothyroxine 817
Univasc® *see* Moexipril 940
Univol® (Can) *see* Aluminum Hydroxide and Magnesium Hydroxide 91
Unna's Boot *see* Zinc Gelatin 1400
Unna's Paste *see* Zinc Gelatin 1400
Unoprostone 1352
Unoprostone Isopropyl *see* Unoprostone 1352
Urasal® (Can) *see* Methenamine . . . 892
Urea 1353
Urea and Hydrocortisone 1353
Ureacin® [OTC] *see* Urea 1353
Urea Peroxide *see* Carbamide Peroxide 259
Urecholine® *see* Bethanechol 203
Uremol® (Can) *see* Urea 1353
Uremol® HC (Can) *see* Urea and Hydrocortisone 1353
Urex® (Can) *see* Methenamine 892
Urimar-T *see* Methenamine, Sodium Biphosphate, Phenyl Salicylate, Methylene Blue, and Hyoscyamine 893
Urimax® *see* Methenamine, Sodium Biphosphate, Phenyl Salicylate, Methylene Blue, and Hyoscyamine 893
Urisec® (Can) *see* Urea 1353
Urispas® (Can) *see* Flavoxate 591
Uristat® [OTC] *see* Phenazopyridine 1072
Urocit®-K *see* Potassium Citrate . . . 1105
Urofollitropin *see* Follitropins 626
Uro-KP-Neutral® *see* Potassium Phosphate and Sodium Phosphate 1107
Uro-Mag® [OTC] *see* Magnesium Oxide 854
Uroxatral™ *see* Alfuzosin 80
Urso® *see* Ursodiol 1354
Ursodeoxycholic Acid *see* Ursodiol 1354
Ursodiol 1354
Ursofalk® (Mex) *see* Ursodiol 1354
UTI Relief® [OTC] *see* Phenazopyridine 1072
Utradol™ (Can) *see* Etodolac 564
Uvadex® (Can) *see* Methoxsalen . . . 902
Uva Ursi 1448
Vaccinium macrocarpon see Cranberry 1421
Vaccinium myrtillus see Bilberry . . . 1415
Vagifem® *see* Estradiol 518
Vagi-Gard® [OTC] *see* Povidone-Iodine 1107
Vagistat®-1 [OTC] *see* Tioconazole 1302
Valacyclovir 1354
Valacyclovir Hydrochloride *see* Valacyclovir 1354
Valcyte™ (Can) *see* Valganciclovir 1358
Valdecoxib 1356
Valerian 1449
Valeriana edulis see Valerian 1449
Valeriana wallichi see Valerian 1449
Valganciclovir 1358
Valganciclovir Hydrochloride *see* Valganciclovir 1358
Valisone® Scalp Lotion (Can) *see* Betamethasone 199
Valium® (Can) *see* Diazepam 423
Valorin [OTC] *see* Acetaminophen . . . 47
Valorin Extra [OTC] *see* Acetaminophen 47
Valproate Semisodium *see* Valproic Acid and Derivatives 1359
Valproate Sodium *see* Valproic Acid and Derivatives 1359
Valproic Acid *see* Valproic Acid and Derivatives 1359
Valproic Acid and Derivatives 1359
Valprosid® (Mex) *see* Valproic Acid and Derivatives 1359
Valrubicin 1362
Valsartan 1363
Valsartan and Hydrochlorothiazide 1364
Valstar® [DSC] *see* Valrubicin 1362
Valtaxin® (Can) *see* Valrubicin 1362
Valtrex® (Can) *see* Valacyclovir . . . 1354
Valverde *see* Ginkgo Biloba 1429
Vanadium 1450
Vanamide™ *see* Urea 1353
Vanceril® AEM (Can) *see* Beclomethasone 184
Vancocin® (Mex) *see* Vancomycin 1365
Vancomycin 1365
Vancomycin Hydrochloride *see* Vancomycin 1365
Vanex Forte™-D *see* Chlorpheniramine, Phenylephrine, and Methscopolamine 317
Vaniqa™ *see* Eflornithine 485
Vanmicina® (Mex) *see* Vancomycin 1365
Vanoxide-HC (Can) *see* Benzoyl Peroxide and Hydrocortisone . . . 194
Vanquish® Extra Strength Pain Reliever [OTC] *see* Acetaminophen, Aspirin, and Caffeine 56
Van R Gingibraid® *see* Epinephrine (Racemic) and Aluminum Potassium Sulfate 497
Vantin® (Can) *see* Cefpodoxime 285
Vaponefrin® *see* Epinephrine (Racemic) 497
VAQTA® (Can) *see* Hepatitis A Vaccine 687
Vardenafil 1367
Vardenafil Hydrochloride *see* Vardenafil 1367
Varicella Virus Vaccine *see* Immunizations (Vaccines) 1614

Varicella-Zoster Immune Globulin (Human) 1368
Vasan *see* Ginkgo Biloba 1429
Vascor® (Can) *see* Bepridil 197
Vaseretic® *see* Enalapril and Hydrochlorothiazide 491
Vasocidin® (Can) *see* Sulfacetamide and Prednisolone 1245
VasoClear® [OTC] *see* Naphazoline 964
Vasocon® (Can) *see* Naphazoline 964
Vasocon-A® (Can) *see* Naphazoline and Antazoline 964
Vasodilan® [DSC] *see* Isoxsuprine 774
Vasofyl® (Mex) *see* Pentoxifylline 1066
Vasopressin 1369
Vasopressin Tannate *see* Vasopressin 1369
Vasotec® *see* Enalapril 488
Vaxigrip® (Can) *see* Influenza Virus Vaccine 748
VCF™ [OTC] *see* Nonoxynol 9 995
VCR *see* VinCRIStine 1378
V-Dec-M® *see* Guaifenesin and Pseudoephedrine 675
Veetids® *see* Penicillin V Potassium 1060
Veg-Pancreatin 4X [OTC] *see* Pancreatin 1042
Velban® (Can) *see* VinBLAStine 1377
Velcade™ *see* Bortezomib 214
Velivet™ *see* Ethinyl Estradiol and Desogestrel 536
Velosef® *see* Cephradine 296
Velosulin® BR (Buffered) [DSC] *see* Insulin Preparations 749
Venlafaxine 1370
Venofer® *see* Iron Sucrose 767
Venoglobulin®-S *see* Immune Globulin (Intravenous) 740
Ventisol® (Mex) *see* Ketotifen 790
Ventolin® [DSC] *see* Albuterol 71
Ventolin® Diskus (Can) *see* Albuterol 71
Ventolin® HFA *see* Albuterol 71
Ventrodisk (Can) *see* Albuterol 71
VePesid® *see* Etoposide 567
Veracolate [OTC] *see* Bisacodyl 208
Verapamil 1373
Verapamil and Trandolapril *see* Trandolapril and Verapamil 1322
Verapamil Hydrochloride *see* Verapamil 1373
Verelan® *see* Verapamil 1373
Verelan® PM *see* Verapamil 1373
Vermicol® (Mex) *see* Mebendazole 859
Vermidil® (Mex) *see* Mebendazole 859
Vermin® (Mex) *see* Mebendazole 859
Vermox® (Can) *see* Mebendazole 859
Versacaps® *see* Guaifenesin and Pseudoephedrine 675
Versed® [DSC] *see* Midazolam 924
Versiclear™ *see* Sodium Thiosulfate 1230
Verteporfin 1375
Vertisal® (Mex) *see* Metronidazole 917
Vesanoid® *see* Tretinoin (Oral) 1328
Vexol® *see* Rimexolone 1185
VFEND® *see* Voriconazole 1385
Viadur® *see* Leuprolide 805
Viagra® (Can) *see* Sildenafil 1219
Vibramicina® (Mex) *see* Doxycycline 471
Vibramycin® *see* Doxycycline 471
Vibra-Tabs® *see* Doxycycline 471
Vicks® 44® Cough Relief [OTC] *see* Dextromethorphan 421
Vicks® 44D Cough & Head Congestion [OTC] *see* Pseudoephedrine and Dextromethorphan 1148
Vicks® 44E [OTC] *see* Guaifenesin and Dextromethorphan 673
Vicks® DayQuil® Multi-Symptom Cold and Flu [OTC] *see* Acetaminophen, Dextromethorphan, and Pseudoephedrine 59
Vicks® Pediatric Formula 44E [OTC] *see* Guaifenesin and Dextromethorphan 673
Vicks Sinex® 12 Hour Ultrafine Mist [OTC] *see* Oxymetazoline 1034
Vicks® Sinex® Nasal Spray [OTC] *see* Phenylephrine 1078
Vicks® Sinex® UltraFine Mist [OTC] *see* Phenylephrine 1078
Vicodin® *see* Hydrocodone and Acetaminophen 702
Vicodin® ES *see* Hydrocodone and Acetaminophen 702
Vicodin® HP *see* Hydrocodone and Acetaminophen 702
Vicodin Tuss® *see* Hydrocodone and Guaifenesin 708
Vicon Forte® *see* Vitamins (Multiple/Oral) 1384
Vicon Plus® [OTC] *see* Vitamins (Multiple/Oral) 1384
Vicoprofen® (Can) *see* Hydrocodone and Ibuprofen 709
Vidarabine 1376
Vidarabine Monohydrate *see* Vidarabine 1376
Vi-Daylin® + Iron Liquid [OTC] *see* Vitamins (Multiple/Oral) 1384
Vi-Daylin® Liquid [OTC] *see* Vitamins (Multiple/Oral) 1384
Videx® *see* Didanosine 433
Videx® EC *see* Didanosine 433
Vigabatrin 1376
Vigamox™ *see* Moxifloxacin 949
Viken® (Mex) *see* Cefotaxime 283
Vilona® (Mex) *see* Ribavirin 1177
VinBLAStine 1377
Vinblastine Sulfate *see* VinBLAStine 1377
Vincasar® PFS® (Can) *see* VinCRIStine 1378
VinCRIStine 1378
Vincristine Sulfate *see* VinCRIStine 1378
Vindesine 1379
Vindesine Sulfate *see* Vindesine 1379
Vinorelbine 1380
Vinorelbine Tartrate *see* Vinorelbine 1380
Vintec® (Mex) *see* VinCRIStine 1378
Viokase® (Can) *see* Pancrelipase 1042
Viosterol *see* Ergocalciferol 503
Vioxx® *see* Rofecoxib 1194
Vira-A® [DSC] *see* Vidarabine 1376
Viracept® (Can) *see* Nelfinavir 972
Viramune® (Can) *see* Nevirapine 977
Virazide® (Mex) *see* Ribavirin 1177
Virazole® (Can) *see* Ribavirin 1177
Viread® *see* Tenofovir 1270
Virilon® *see* MethylTESTOSTERone 912
Virilon® IM (Can) *see* Testosterone 1276
Virlix® (Mex) *see* Cetirizine 298
Viroptic® *see* Trifluridine 1339
Viroxyn® [OTC] *see* Benzalkonium Chloride and Isopropyl Alcohol 190

Viscoat® see Chondroitin Sulfate and Sodium Hyaluronate 325
Visicol™ see Sodium Phosphates 1230
Visine® (Mex) see Tetrahydrozoline 1282
Visine-A™ [OTC] see Naphazoline and Pheniramine 964
Visine A.D.® (Mex) see Oxymetazoline 1034
Visine® Advanced Relief [OTC] see Tetrahydrozoline 1282
Visine® L.R. [OTC] see Oxymetazoline 1034
Visine® Original [OTC] see Tetrahydrozoline 1282
Visken® (Can) see Pindolol 1090
Vistaril® see HydrOXYzine 723
Vistide® see Cidofovir 327
Visudyne® see Verteporfin 1375
Vita-C® [OTC] see Ascorbic Acid . . . 148
Vitacon Forte see Vitamins (Multiple/Oral) 1384
Vital see Ginkgo Biloba 1429
Vitamin A 1382
Vitamin A Acid see Tretinoin (Topical) 1329
Vitamin A and Vitamin D 1382
Vitamin B_1 see Thiamine 1287
Vitamin B_2 see Riboflavin 1178
Vitamin B_3 see Niacin 978
Vitamin B_3 see Niacinamide 979
Vitamin B_5 see Pantothenic Acid . . 1044
Vitamin B_6 see Pyridoxine 1154
Vitamin B_{12} see Cyanocobalamin . . . 380
Vitamin B_{12} see Hydroxocobalamin 719
Vitamin B Complex Combinations 1382
Vitamin C see Ascorbic Acid 148
Vitamin D_2 see Ergocalciferol 503
Vitamin E 1383
Vitamin G see Riboflavin 1178
Vitamin K_1 see Phytonadione 1084
Vitamins (Multiple/Oral) 1384
Vitamins, Multiple (Oral) see Vitamins (Multiple/Oral) 1384
Vitamins, Multiple (Therapeutic) see Vitamins (Multiple/Oral) . . . 1384
Vitamins, Multiple With Iron see Vitamins (Multiple/Oral) 1384
Vitelle™ Irospan® [OTC] [DSC] see Ferrous Sulfate and Ascorbic Acid 587
Viternum® (Mex) see Cyproheptadine 389
Vitex agnus-castus see Chasteberry 1419
Vitis vinifera see Grape Seed 1435
Vitrase® see Hyaluronidase 697
Vitrasert® see Ganciclovir 646
Vitravene™ [DSC] see Fomivirsen . . 628
Vitrax® see Hyaluronate and Derivatives 696
Vitussin see Hydrocodone and Guaifenesin 708
Vivactil® see Protriptyline 1146
Viva-Drops® [OTC] see Artificial Tears 148
Vivelle® see Estradiol 518
Vivelle-Dot® see Estradiol 518
Vivotif Berna® (Can) see Typhoid Vaccine 1351
VLB see VinBLAStine 1377
VM-26 see Teniposide 1269
Volfenac Gel® (Mex) see Diclofenac 427
Volfenac Retard® (Mex) see Diclofenac 427
Volmax® (Mex) see Albuterol 71
Voltaren® (Mex) see Diclofenac 427
Voltaren Emulgel® (Mex) see Diclofenac 427
Voltaren Ophtha® (Can) see Diclofenac 427
Voltaren Ophthalmic® see Diclofenac 427
Voltaren Rapide® (Can) see Diclofenac 427
Voltaren®-XR see Diclofenac 427
Vomisin® (Mex) see DimenhyDRINATE 446
Voriconazole 1385
VōSoL® HC see Acetic Acid, Propylene Glycol Diacetate, and Hydrocortisone 60
VoSpire ER™ see Albuterol 71
VP-16 see Etoposide 567
VP-16-213 see Etoposide 567
Vp-Tec® (Mex) see Etoposide 567
Vumon® (Can) see Teniposide 1269
V.V.S.® see Sulfabenzamide, Sulfacetamide, and Sulfathiazole 1243
Vytone® see Iodoquinol and Hydrocortisone 759
VZIG see Varicella-Zoster Immune Globulin (Human) 1368
Warfarin 1389
Warfarin Sodium see Warfarin 1389
Wartec® (Can) see Podofilox 1099
Wart-Off® Maximum Strength [OTC] see Salicylic Acid 1205
4-Way® Long Acting [OTC] see Oxymetazoline 1034
WelChol® (Can) see Colesevelam . . 373
Wellbutrin® (Can) see BuPROPion . . 230
Wellbutrin SR® see BuPROPion 230
Wellbutrin XL™ see BuPROPion . . . 230
Wesmycin® see Tetracycline 1280
Westcort® see Hydrocortisone 714
Westhroid® see Thyroid 1293
Whitehorn see Hawthorn 1437
Whole Root Rauwolfia see Rauwolfia Serpentina 1171
Wigraine® see Ergotamine and Caffeine 506
Wild Quinine see Feverfew 1426
Wild Yam 1450
Winpred™ (Can) see PredniSONE 1115
WinRho SDF® see Rh_o(D) Immune Globulin 1176
Winstrol® see Stanozolol 1237
Wound Wash Saline™ [OTC] see Sodium Chloride 1227
WR2721 see Amifostine 94
WR-139007 see Dacarbazine 392
WR-139013 see Chlorambucil 305
WR-139021 see Carmustine 268
Wycillin [DSC] see Penicillin G Procaine 1060
Wytensin® [DSC] see Guanabenz . . 677
Xalatan® see Latanoprost 800
Xalyn-Or® (Mex) see Amoxicillin 114
Xanax® see Alprazolam 84
Xanax TS™ (Can) see Alprazolam . . . 84
Xanax XR® see Alprazolam 84
Xeloda® (Mex) see Capecitabine . . . 250
Xenical® (Mex) see Orlistat 1017
Xifaxan™ see Rifaximin 1183
Xigris® see Drotrecogin Alfa 478
Xitocin® (Mex) see Oxytocin 1038
Xolair® see Omalizumab 1012
Xopenex® see Levalbuterol 806
X-Prep® [OTC] see Senna 1213
X-Seb™ T [OTC] see Coal Tar and Salicylic Acid 367
Xylocaina® (Mex) see Lidocaine 819
Xylocaine® see Lidocaine 819
Xylocaine® MPF see Lidocaine 819

Xylocaine® MPF With Epinephrine *see* Lidocaine and Epinephrine . . . 823
Xylocaine® Viscous *see* Lidocaine . . 819
Xylocaine® With Epinephrine *see* Lidocaine and Epinephrine 823
Xylocard® (Can) *see* Lidocaine 819
Xylometazoline 1393
Xylometazoline Hydrochloride *see* Xylometazoline 1393
Xyrem® *see* Sodium Oxybate 1229
Y-90 Zevalin *see* Ibritumomab 727
Yasmin® *see* Ethinyl Estradiol and Drospirenone 538
Yectamicina® (Mex) *see* Gentamicin 655
Yectamid® (Mex) *see* Amikacin 95
Yellow Fever Vaccine *see* Immunizations (Vaccines) 1614
Yellow Indian Paint *see* Golden Seal 1433
Yellow Mercuric Oxide *see* Mercuric Oxide 881
Yellow Root *see* Golden Seal 1433
YM-08310 *see* Amifostine 94
Yocon® *see* Yohimbine 1393
Yodine® (Mex) *see* Povidone-Iodine 1107
Yodoxin® *see* Iodoquinol 759
Yohimbe 1451
Yohimbehe cortex *see* Yohimbe . . . 1451
Yohimbine 1393
Yohimbine Hydrochloride *see* Yohimbine 1393
Z4942 *see* Ifosfamide 733
Zaditen® (Mex) *see* Ketotifen 790
Zaditor™ (Can) *see* Ketotifen 790
Zafimida® (Mex) *see* Furosemide . . . 640
Zafirlukast 1394
Zagam® *see* Sparfloxacin 1233
Zalcitabine 1395
Zaleplon 1396
Zanaflex® *see* Tizanidine 1305
Zanamivir 1396
Zanosar® *see* Streptozocin 1240
Zantac® *see* Ranitidine 1169
Zantac 75® (Can) *see* Ranitidine . . 1169
Zapzyt® [OTC] *see* Benzoyl Peroxide 194
Zapzyt® Acne Wash [OTC] *see* Salicylic Acid 1205
Zapzyt® Pore Treatment [OTC] *see* Salicylic Acid 1205
Zarontin® *see* Ethosuximide 560
Zaroxolyn® (Can) *see* Metolazone . . 914
Zavesca® *see* Miglustat 930
Z-Bec® [OTC] *see* Vitamin B Complex Combinations 1382
Z-Cof DM *see* Guaifenesin, Pseudoephedrine, and Dextromethorphan 676
Z-Cof LA *see* Guaifenesin and Dextromethorphan 673
ZD1033 *see* Anastrozole 132
ZD1839 *see* Gefitinib 649
ZDV *see* Zidovudine 1398
ZDV, Abacavir, and Lamivudine *see* Abacavir, Lamivudine, and Zidovudine 43
Zeasorb®-AF [OTC] *see* Miconazole 922
Zebeta® (Can) *see* Bisoprolol 210
Zebutal™ *see* Butalbital, Acetaminophen, and Caffeine . . 236
Zegerid™ *see* Omeprazole 1012
Zeldox *see* Ziprasidone 1401
Zelmac® (Mex) *see* Tegaserod 1263
Zelnorm® *see* Tegaserod 1263
Zemaira™ *see* Alpha$_1$-Proteinase Inhibitor 84
Zemplar™ *see* Paricalcitol 1045
Zenapax® *see* Daclizumab 393
Zeneca 182,780 *see* Fulvestrant . . . 639
Zentel® (Mex) *see* Albendazole 71
Zephiran® [OTC] *see* Benzalkonium Chloride 190
Zephrex® *see* Guaifenesin and Pseudoephedrine 675
Zephrex LA® *see* Guaifenesin and Pseudoephedrine 675
Zerit® (Mex) *see* Stavudine 1238
Zestoretic® *see* Lisinopril and Hydrochlorothiazide 834
Zestril® (Can) *see* Lisinopril 833
Zetar® [OTC] *see* Coal Tar 367
Zetia™ *see* Ezetimibe 570
Zevalin™ *see* Ibritumomab 727
Ziac® (Can) *see* Bisoprolol and Hydrochlorothiazide 211
Ziagen® (Can) *see* Abacavir 42
Zidovudine 1398
Zidovudine, Abacavir, and Lamivudine *see* Abacavir, Lamivudine, and Zidovudine 43
Zidovudine and Lamivudine 1399
Zilactin® (Can) *see* Lidocaine 819
Zilactin®-B [OTC] *see* Benzocaine . . 191
Zilactin Baby® (Can) *see* Benzocaine 191
Zilactin-L® [OTC] *see* Lidocaine 819
Zileuton 1399
Zinacef® *see* Cefuroxime 289
Zinc *see* Trace Metals 1319
Zincate® *see* Zinc Sulfate 1401
Zinc Chloride 1400
Zincfrin® [OTC] *see* Phenylephrine and Zinc Sulfate 1079
Zinc Gelatin 1400
Zinc Gelatin Boot *see* Zinc Gelatin . . . 1400
Zincofax® (Can) *see* Zinc Oxide . . . 1400
Zincon® [OTC] *see* Pyrithione Zinc . . . 1155
Zinc Oxide 1400
Zinc Sulfate 1401
Zinc Sulfate and Phenylephrine *see* Phenylephrine and Zinc Sulfate 1079
Zinc Undecylenate *see* Undecylenic Acid and Derivatives 1352
Zinecard® (Can) *see* Dexrazoxane . . 417
Zingiber officinale *see* Ginger 1428
Zinnat® (Mex) *see* Cefuroxime 289
Zinnat® [inj.] (Mex) *see* Cefuroxime 289
Zipra® (Mex) *see* Ciprofloxacin 331
Ziprasidone 1401
Ziprasidone Hydrochloride *see* Ziprasidone 1401
Ziprasidone Mesylate *see* Ziprasidone 1401
Zithromax® (Can) *see* Azithromycin . . . 174
Zithromax® TRI-PAK™ *see* Azithromycin 174
Zithromax® Z-PAK® *see* Azithromycin 174
ZM-182,780 *see* Fulvestrant 639
Z-Max® (Mex) *see* Phentolamine . . 1077
ZNP® Bar [OTC] *see* Pyrithione Zinc 1155
ZNP Shampoo® (Mex) *see* Pyrithione Zinc 1155
Zocor® *see* Simvastatin 1222
Zofran® (Mex) *see* Ondansetron . . . 1014
Zofran® ODT *see* Ondansetron . . . 1014
Zoladex® (Mex) *see* Goserelin 670
Zoladex® LA (Can) *see* Goserelin . . 670
Zoledronate *see* Zoledronic Acid . . 1402
Zoledronic Acid 1402
Zolmitriptan 1403

Zoloft® *see* Sertraline 1215
Zolpidem 1404
Zolpidem Tartrate *see* Zolpidem . . . 1404
Zometa® (Can) *see* Zoledronic Acid 1402
Zomig® (Mex) *see* Zolmitriptan 1403
Zomig® Rapimelt (Can) *see* Zolmitriptan 1403
Zomig-ZMT™ *see* Zolmitriptan 1403
Zonal® (Mex) *see* Fluconazole 594
Zonalon® *see* Doxepin 467
Zone-A® *see* Pramoxine and Hydrocortisone 1109
Zone-A Forte® *see* Pramoxine and Hydrocortisone 1109
Zonegran® (Can) *see* Zonisamide 1405
Zonisamide 1405
Zopiclone 1406
Zorbtive™ *see* Human Growth Hormone 694
ZORprin® *see* Aspirin 151
Zostrix® [OTC] *see* Capsaicin 252
Zostrix® H.P. (Can) *see* Capsaicin . . 252
Zosyn® *see* Piperacillin and Tazobactam Sodium 1093
Zovia™ *see* Ethinyl Estradiol and Ethynodiol Diacetate 540
Zovirax® *see* Acyclovir 64
Zurcal® (Mex) *see* Pantoprazole . . . 1043
Zyban® (Can) *see* BuPROPion 230
Zydone® *see* Hydrocodone and Acetaminophen 702
Zyflo™ [DSC] *see* Zileuton 1399
Zyloprim® (Can) *see* Allopurinol 82
Zymar™ *see* Gatifloxacin 647
Zyprexa® (Can) *see* Olanzapine . . . 1007
Zyprexa® Zydis® *see* Olanzapine . . 1007
Zyrtec® (Mex) *see* Cetirizine 298
Zyrtec-D 12 Hour™ *see* Cetirizine and Pseudoephedrine 299
Zyvox™ *see* Linezolid 830
Zyvoxam® (Can) *see* Linezolid 830

NOTES

NOTES

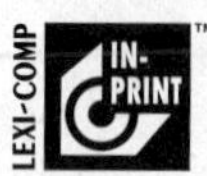

Products offered by LEXI-COMP

DRUG INFORMATION HANDBOOK (International edition available)

by Charles Lacy, RPh, PharmD, FCSHP; Lora L. Armstrong, RPh, PharmD, BCPS; Morton P. Goldman, PharmD, BCPS; and Leonard L. Lance, RPh, BSPharm

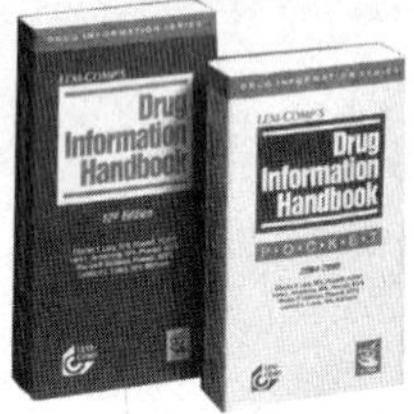

Specifically compiled and designed for the healthcare professional requiring quick access to concisely-stated comprehensive data concerning clinical use of medications.

The Drug Information Handbook is an ideal portable drug information resource, providing the reader with up to 34 key points of data concerning clinical use and dosing of the medication. Material provided in the Appendix section is recognized by many users to be, by itself, well worth the purchase of the handbook.

All medications found in the Drug Information Handbook are included in the abridged Pocket edition (select fields were extracted to maintain portability).

PEDIATRIC DOSAGE HANDBOOK (International edition available)

by Carol K. Taketomo, PharmD; Jane Hurlburt Hodding, PharmD; and Donna M. Kraus, PharmD

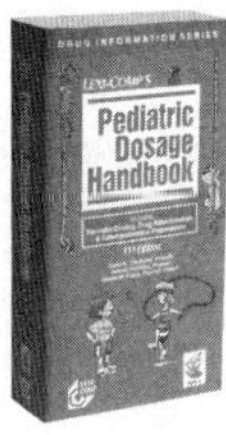

Special considerations must frequently be taken into account when dosing medications for the pediatric patient. This highly regarded quick reference handbook is a compilation of recommended pediatric doses based on current literature, as well as the practical experience of the authors and their many colleagues who work every day in the pediatric clinical setting.

Includes neonatal dosing, drug administration, and (in select monographs) extemporaneous preparations for medications used in pediatric medicine.

GERIATRIC DOSAGE HANDBOOK

by Todd P. Semla, PharmD, BCPS, FCCP; Judith L. Beizer, PharmD, FASCP; and Martin D. Higbee, PharmD, CGP

2000 "Book of the Year" — American Journal of Nursing

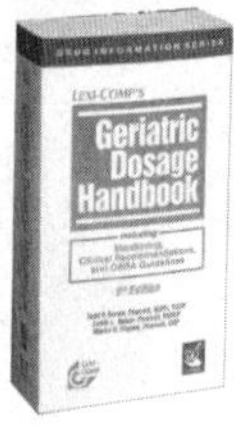

Many physiologic changes occur with aging, some of which affect the pharmacokinetics or pharmacodynamics of medications. Strong consideration should also be given to the effect of decreased renal or hepatic functions in the elderly, as well as the probability of the geriatric patient being on multiple drug regimens.

Healthcare professionals working with nursing homes and assisted living facilities will find the drug information contained in this handbook to be an invaluable source of helpful information.

An International Brand Name Index with names from 58 different countries is also included.

To order call toll free anywhere in the U.S.: 1-800-837-LEXI (5394)

Outside of the U.S. call: 330-650-6506 or online at www.lexi.com

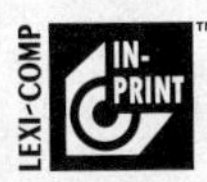

Products offered by LEXI-COMP

DRUG INTERACTIONS HANDBOOK

by Bachmann, Lewis, Fuller, Bonfiglio

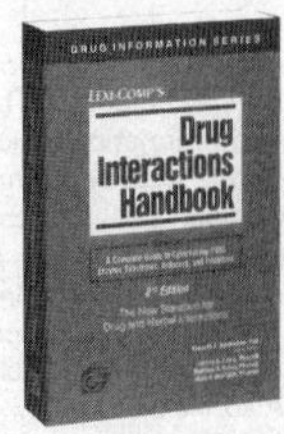

The new standard for evaluating drug and herbal interactions. A comprehensive table of Cytochrome P450 enzyme substrates, inducers and inhibitors. Each interaction monograph contains the following ratings: Reliability Rating - indicating the quantity and nature of documentation for an interaction: A - No Known Interaction, B - No Action Needed, C - Monitor Therapy, D - Consider Therapy Modification, and X - Avoid Combination; Severity Rating - indicating the reported or possible magnitude of an interaction outcome. This book also contains the following: detailed patient management suggestions, full reference citations, discussion of published reports and potential mechanisms, identifies the greatest number of potential interactions compared to any other available references, user-friendly structure, over 3,000 brand names, includes interactions data on the most commonly used herbs, and "tall man" letters to identify between "look-a-like" medications.

NATURAL THERAPEUTICS POCKET GUIDE

by Daniel L. Krinsky, RPh, MS; James B. LaValle, RPh, DHM, NMD, CCN; Ernest B. Hawkins, RPh, MS; Ross Pelton, RPh, PhD, CCN; Nancy Ashbrook Willis, BA, JD

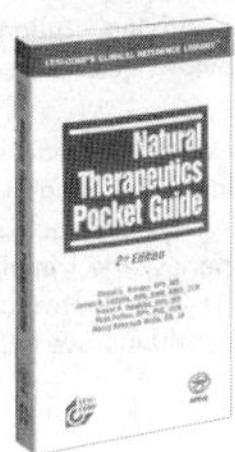

Provides condition-specific information on common uses of natural therapies. Each condition discussed includes the following: review of condition, decision tree, list of commonly recommended herbals, nutritional supplements, homeopathic remedies, lifestyle modifications, and special considerations.

Provides herbal/nutritional/nutraceutical monographs with over 10 fields including references, reported uses, dosage, pharmacology, toxicity, warnings & interactions, and cautions & contraindications.

The Appendix includes: drug-nutrient depletion, herb-drug interactions, drug-nutrient interaction, herbal medicine use in pediatrics, unsafe herbs, and reference of top herbals.

DRUG-INDUCED NUTRIENT DEPLETION HANDBOOK

by Ross Pelton, RPh, PhD, CCN; James B. LaValle, RPh, DHM, NMD, CCN; Ernest B. Hawkins, RPh, MS; Daniel L. Krinsky, RPh, MS

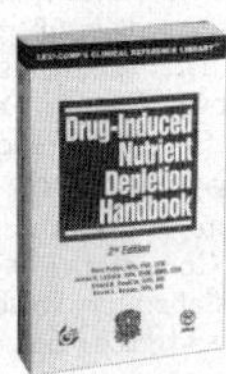

A complete and up-to-date listing of all drugs known to deplete the body of nutritional compounds.

This book is alphabetically organized and provides extensive cross-referencing to related information in the various sections of the book. Drug monographs identify the nutrients depleted and provide cross-references to the nutrient monographs for more detailed information on effects of depletion, biological function & effect, side effects & toxicity, RDA, dosage range, and dietary sources. this book also contains a studies & abstracts section, a valuable appendix, and alphabetical & pharmacological indexes.

To order call toll free anywhere in the U.S.: 1-800-837-LEXI (5394)

Outside of the U.S. call: 330-650-6506 or online at www.lexi.com

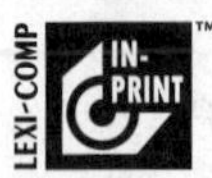

Products offered by LEXI-COMP

DRUG INFORMATION HANDBOOK FOR ADVANCED PRACTICE NURSING

by Beatrice B. Turkoski, RN, PhD; Brenda R. Lance, RN, MSN; and Mark F. Bonfiglio, PharmD Foreword by: Margaret A. Fitzgerald, MS, RN, CS-FNP

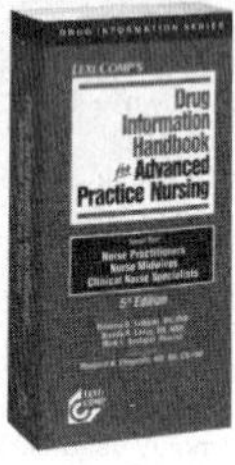

Designed specifically to meet the needs of nurse practitioners, clinical nurse specialists, nurse midwives, and graduate nursing students. The handbook is a unique resource for detailed, accurate information, which is vital to support the advanced practice nurse's role in patient drug therapy management. Over 4750 U.S., Canadian, and Mexican medications are covered in the 1000 monographs. Drug data is presented in an easy-to-use, alphabetically-organized format covering up to 46 key points of information (including dosing for pediatrics, adults, and geriatrics). Appendix contains over 230 pages of valuable comparison tables and additional information. Also included are two indexes, Pharmacologic Category and Controlled Substance, which facilitate comparison between agents.

DRUG INFORMATION HANDBOOK FOR NURSING

by Beatrice B. Turkoski, RN, PhD; Brenda R. Lance, RN, MSN; and Mark F. Bonfiglio, PharmD

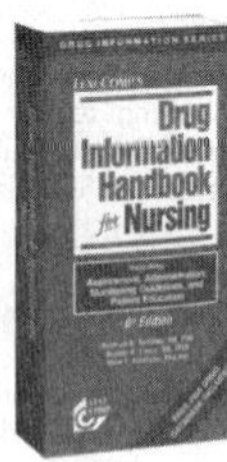

Registered professional nurses and upper-division nursing students involved with drug therapy will find this handbook provides quick access to drug data in a concise easy-to-use format.

Over 4000 U.S., Canadian, and Mexican medications are covered with up to 43 key points of information in each monograph. The handbook contains basic pharmacology concepts and nursing issues such as patient factors that influence drug therapy (ie, pregnancy, age, weight, etc) and general nursing issues (ie, assessment, administration, monitoring, and patient education). The Appendix contains over 230 pages of valuable information.

ANESTHESIOLOGY & CRITICAL CARE DRUG HANDBOOK

by Andrew J. Donnelly, PharmD; Francesca E. Cunningham, PharmD; Verna L. Baughman, MD

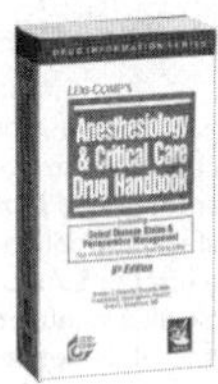

Contains the most common perioperative drugs in the critical care setting and also contains Special Issues and Topics including: Allergic Reaction, Cardiac Patients in Noncardiac Surgery, Obstetric Patients in Nonobstetric Surgery, Patients With Liver Disease, Chronic Pain Management, Chronic Renal Failure, Conscious Sedation, Perioperative Management of Patients on Antiseizure Medication, and more.

The Appendix includes Abbreviations & Measurements, Anesthesiology Information, Assessment of Liver & Renal Function, Comparative Drug Charts, Infectious Disease-Prophylaxis & Treatment, Laboratory Values, Therapy Re-commendations, Toxicology information, and much more.

International Brand Name Index with names from over 58 different countries is also included.

To order call toll free anywhere in the U.S.: 1-800-837-LEXI (5394)

Outside of the U.S. call: 330-650-6506 or online at www.lexi.com

Products offered by LEXI-COMP

INFECTIOUS DISEASES HANDBOOK

by Carlos M. Isada, MD; Bernard L. Kasten Jr., MD; Morton P. Goldman, PharmD; Larry D. Gray, PhD; and Judith A. Aberg, MD

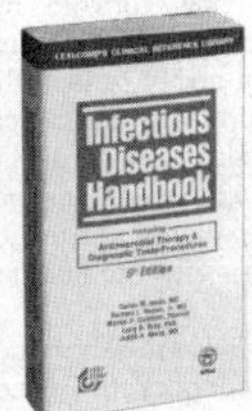

A four-in-one quick reference concerned with the identification and treatment of infectious diseases. Each of the four sections of the book contains related information and cross-referencing to one or more of the other three sections. The Disease Syndrome section provides the clinical presentation, differential diagnosis, diagnostic tests, and drug therapy recommended for treatment of more common infectious diseases. The Organism section presents the microbiology, epidemiology, diagnosis, and treatment of each organism. The Laboratory Diagnosis section describes performance of specific tests and procedures. The Antimicrobial Therapy section presents important facts and considerations regarding each drug recommended for specific diseases of organisms. Also contains an International Brand Name Index with names from 58 different countries.

PHARMACOGENOMICS HANDBOOK

by Humma, Ellingrod, Kolesar

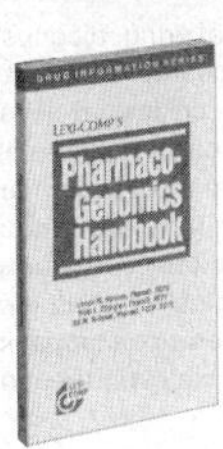

This exciting new title by Lexi-Comp, introduces Pharmacogenomics to the forward-thinking healthcare professional and student! It presents information concerning key genetic variations that may influence drug disposition and/or sensitivity. Brief introductions to fundamental concepts in genetics and genomics are provided in order to bring the reader up-to-date on these rapidly emerging sciences. This book provides a foundation for all clinicians who will be called on to integrate rapidly expanding genomic knowledge into the management of drug therapy. A great introduction to pharmacogenetic principles as well as a concise reference on key polymorphisms known to influence drug response!

DRUG INFORMATION HANDBOOK FOR ONCOLOGY

by Dominic A. Solimando, Jr, MA, BCOP

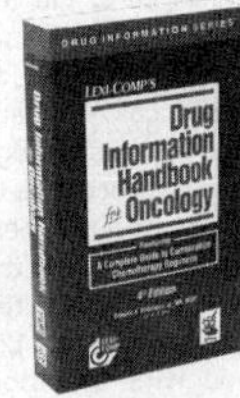

Presented in a concise and uniform format, this book contains the most comprehensive collection of oncology-related drug information available. Organized like a dictionary for ease of use, drugs can be found by looking up the brand or generic name!

This book contains individual monographs for both antineoplastic agents and ancillary medications.

The fields of information per monograph include: Use, U.S. Investigational, Bone Marrow/Blood Cell Transplantation, Vesicant, Emetic Potential. A Special Topics Section, Appendix, and Therapeutic Category & Key Word Index are valuable features of this book, as well.

To order call toll free anywhere in the U.S.: 1-800-837-LEXI (5394)
Outside of the U.S. call: 330-650-6506 or online at www.lexi.com

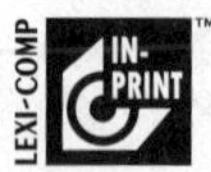

Products offered by LEXI-COMP

CLINICIAN'S GUIDE TO LABORATORY MEDICINE

—A Practical Approach by Samir P. Desai, MD and Sana Isa-Pratt, MD

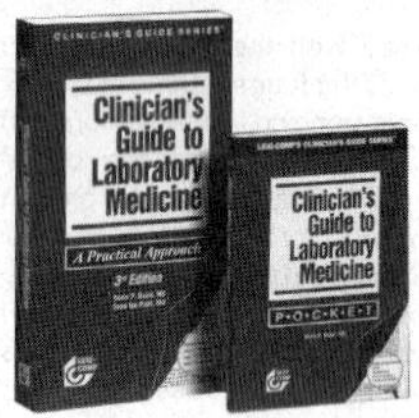

When faced with the patient presenting with abnormal laboratory tests, the clinician can now turn to the Clinician's Guide to Laboratory Medicine: A Practical Approach. This source is unique in its ability to lead the clinician from laboratory test abnormality to clinical diagnosis. Written for the busy clinician, this concise handbook will provide rapid answers to the questions that busy clinicians face in the care of their patients. No longer does the clinician have to struggle in an effort to find this information - it's all here.

Included is a **FREE** copy of Clinician's Guide to Laboratory Medicine - Pocket. Great to carry in your pocket! Perfect for use "in the trenches."

CLINICIAN'S GUIDE TO INTERNAL MEDICINE—A Practical Approach

by Samir P. Desai, MD

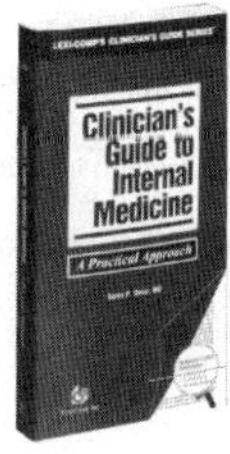

Provides quick access to essential information covering diagnosis, treatment, and management of commonly encountered patient problems in Internal Medicine. Contains up-to-date, clinically-relevant information in an easy-to-read format and is easily accessible. Contains practical approaches that are not readily available in standard textbooks. Contains algorithms to help you establish the diagnosis and select the appropriate therapy. There are numerous tables and boxes that summarize diagnostic and therapeutic strategies. It is an ideal reference for use at the point-of-care. This is a reference companion that will provide you with the tools necessary to tackle even the most challenging problems in Internal Medicine.

CLINICIAN'S GUIDE TO DIAGNOSIS—A Practical Approach

by Samir P. Desai, MD

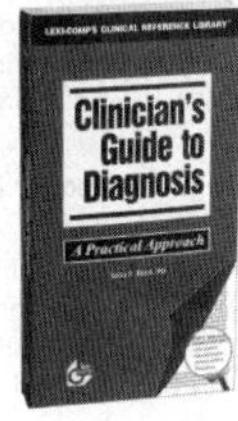

Symptoms are what prompt patients to seek medical care. In the evaluation of a patient's symptom, it is not unusual for healthcare professionals to ask "What do I do next?" This is precisely the question for which the Clinician's Guide to Diagnosis: A Practical Approach provides the answer. It will lead you from symptom to diagnosis through a series of steps designed to mimic the logical thought processes of seasoned clinicians. For the young clinician, this is an ideal book to help bridge the gap between the classroom and actual patient care. For the experienced clinician, this concise handbook offers rapid answers to the questions that are commonly encountered on a day-to-day basis. Let this guide become your companion, providing you with the tools necessary to tackle even the most challenging symptoms.

To order call toll free anywhere in the U.S.: 1-800-837-LEXI (5394)

Outside of the U.S. call: 330-650-6506 or online at www.lexi.com

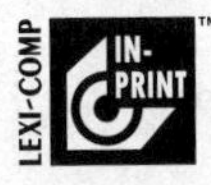

Products offered by LEXI-COMP

POISONING & TOXICOLOGY HANDBOOK

by Jerrold B. Leikin, MD and Frank P. Paloucek, PharmD

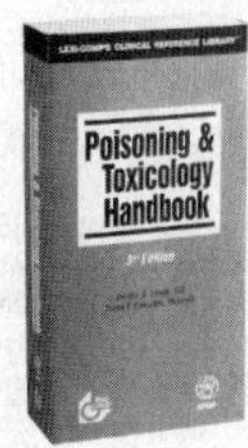

It's back by popular demand! The small size of our Poisoning & Toxicology Handbook is once again available. Better than ever, this comprehensive, portable reference contains 80 antidotes and drugs used in toxicology with 694 medicinal agents, 287 nonmedicinal agents, 291 biological agents, 57 herbal agents, and more than 200 laboratory tests. Monographs are extensively referenced and contain valuable information on overdose symptomatology and treatment considerations, as well as, admission criteria and impairment potential of select agents. Designed for quick reference with monographs arranged alphabetically, plus a cross-referencing index. The authors have expanded current information on drugs of abuse and use of antidotes, while providing concise tables, graphics, and other pertinent toxicology text.

LABORATORY TEST HANDBOOK & CONCISE version

by David S. Jacobs MD, FACP; Wayne R. DeMott, MD, FACP; and Dwight K. Oxley, MD, FACP

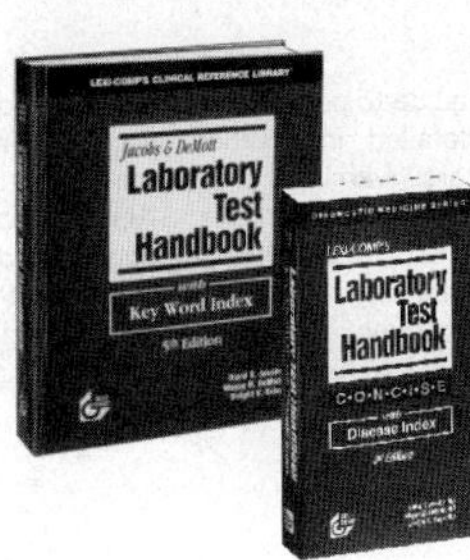

Contains over 900 clinical laboratory tests and is an excellent source of laboratory information for physicians of all specialties, nurses, laboratory professionals, students, medical personnel, or anyone who needs quick access to most routine and many of the more specialized testing procedures available in today's clinical laboratory. Each monograph contains test name, synonyms, patient care, specimen requirements, reference ranges, and interpretive information with footnotes, references, and selected web sites. The Laboratory Test Handbook Concise is a portable, abridged (800 tests) version and is an ideal, quick reference for anyone requiring information concerning patient preparation, specimen collection and handling, and test result interpretation.

DIAGNOSTIC PROCEDURES HANDBOOK by Frank Michota, MD

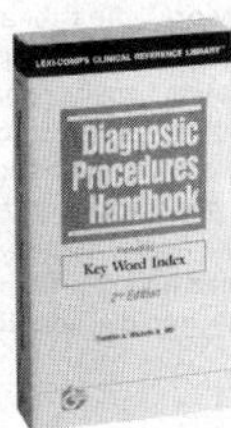

A comprehensive, yet concise, quick reference source for physicians, nurses, students, medical records personnel, or anyone needing quick access to diagnostic procedure information. This handbook is an excellent source of information in the following areas: allergy, rheumatology, and infectious disease; cardiology; computed tomography; diagnostic radiology; gastroenterology; invasive radiology; magnetic resonance imaging; nephrology, urology, and hematology; neurology; nuclear medicine; pulmonary function; pulmonary medicine and critical care; ultrasound; and women's health.

To order call toll free anywhere in the U.S.: 1-800-837-LEXI (5394)

Outside of the U.S. call: 330-650-6506 or online at www.lexi.com

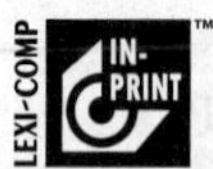

Products offered by LEXI-COMP

DRUG INFORMATION HANDBOOK FOR PSYCHIATRY

by Matthew A. Fuller, PharmD and Martha Sajatovic, MD

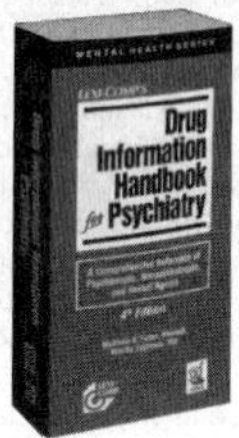

The source for comprehensive and clinically-relevant drug information for the mental health professional. Alphabetically arranged by generic and brand name for ease-of-use. There are up to 35 key fields of information including these unique fields: "Effect on Mental Status" and "Effect on Psychiatric Treatment."

A special topics/issues section includes psychiatric assessment, major psychiatric disorders, major classes of psychotropic medications, psychiatric emergencies, special populations, enhanced patient education information section, and DSM-IV classification. Also contains a valuable appendix section, Pharmacologic Index, and Alphabetical Index.

PSYCHOTROPIC DRUG INFORMATION HANDBOOK

by Matthew A. Fuller, PharmD and Martha Sajatovic, MD

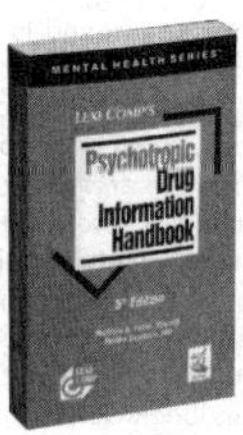

This portable, yet comprehensive guide to psychotropic drugs provides healthcare professionals with detailed information on use, drug interactions, pregnancy risk factors, warnings/precautions, adverse reactions, mechanism of action, and contraindications. Alphabetically organized by brand and generic name, this concise handbook provides quick access to the information you need and includes patient education sheets on the psychotropic medications. It is the perfect pocket companion to the Drug Information for Psychiatry.

RATING SCALES IN MENTAL HEALTH

by Martha Sajatovic, MD and Luis F. Ramirez, MD

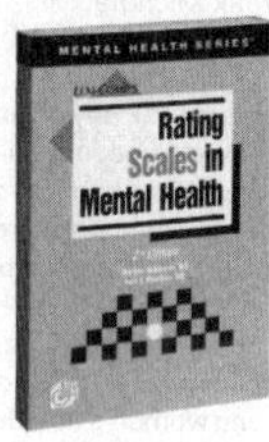

A basic guide to the rating scales in mental health, this is an ideal reference for psychiatrists, nurses, residents, psychologists, social workers, healthcare administrators, behavioral healthcare organizations, and outcome committees. It is designed to assist clinicians in determining the appropriate rating scale when assessing their client. A general concepts section provides text discussion on the use and history of rating scales, statistical evaluation, rating scale domains, and two clinical vignettes. Information on over 100 rating scales used in mental health is organized by condition. Appendix contains tables and charts in a quick reference format allowing clinicians to rapidly identify categories and characteristics of rating scales.

To order call toll free anywhere in the U.S.: 1-800-837-LEXI (5394)

Outside of the U.S. call: 330-650-6506 or online at www.lexi.com

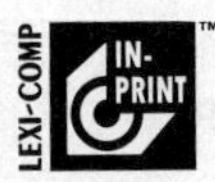

DENTISTRY

Products offered by LEXI-COMP

MANUAL OF DENTAL IMPLANTS

by David P. Sarment, DDS, MS and Beth Peshman, RDH

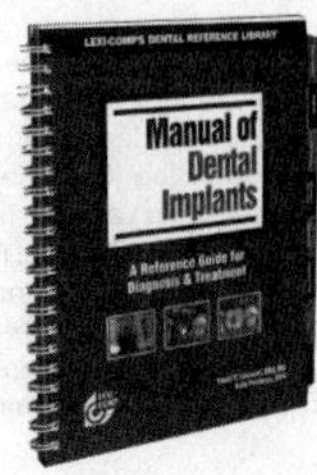

Contains over 220 quality color photos, plus diagrams and decision trees. The diagnosis and treatment plans are explained in detail. Restorative step-by-step illustrations are included for each case type. Hygiene techniques and protocols are also included as well as assistant and staff training guidelines.

8 Tabbed Sections for Ease-of-Use:

① Basic Principles
② Diagnosis
③ Treatment Planning
④ Restoration Sequences
⑤ Maintenance
⑥ Implants and Your Practice
⑦ Appendix
⑧ Index

MANUAL OF CLINICAL PERIODONTICS

by Francis G. Serio, DMD, MS and Charles E. Hawley, DDS, PhD

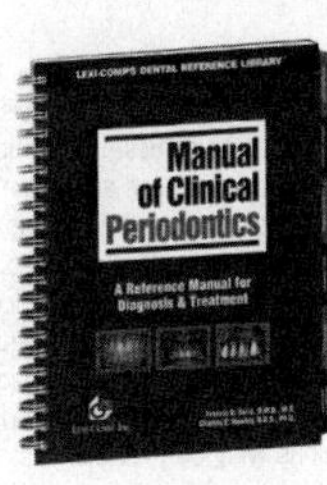

A reference manual for diagnosis and treatment including sample treatment plans. It is organized by basic principles and is visually-cued with over 220 high quality color photos. The presentation is in a "question & answer" format. There are 12 chapters tabbed for easy access: 1) Problem-based Periodontal Diagnosis; 2) Anatomy, Histology, and Physiology; 3) Etiology and Disease Classification; 4) Assessment, Diagnosis, and Treatment Planning; 5) Prevention and Maintenance; 6) Nonsurgical Treatment; 7) Surgical Treatment: Principles; 8) Repair, Resection, and Regeneration; 9) Periodontal Plastic Surgery; 10) Periodontal Emergencies; 11) Implant Considerations; 12) Appendix

ADVANCED PROTOCOLS FOR MEDICAL EMERGENCIES

by Donald P. Lewis, Jr, DDS, Ann Marie McMullin, MD, Timothy Meiller, DDS, PhD, Richard L. Wynn BSPharm, PhD, Cynthia Biron, RDH, EMT, MA, Harold L. Crossley, DDS, PhD

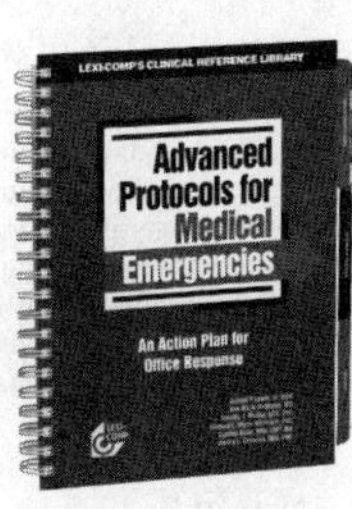

An Action Plan for Office Response!

A must for all offices that practice the use and safety of the administration of local anesthesia, nitrous oxide analgesia, conscious sedation, deep sedation, and general anesthesia. Occasionally, medical emergencies can become life threatening. This book is designed to facilitate advanced medical emergency protocols. Includes all of our popular Dental Office Medical Emergencies and introduces the following chapters in an easy-to-understand and tabbed manner: Loss of Conciousness; Respiratory Distress; Chest Pain; Cardiac Dysrhythmias; Venipuncture Complications; Malignant Hyperthermia; Allergic/Drug Reaction; Altered Sensation/Changes in Effect; Blood Pressure Abnormalities; Management of Acute Bleeding; Emesis and Aspiration; Drug Monographs. Additional Sections Include: Office Preparedness; Glossary of Terms; Appendix

To order call toll free anywhere in the U.S.: 1-800-837-LEXI (5394)

Outside of the U.S. call: 330-650-6506 or online at www.lexi.com

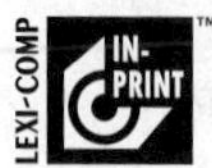

DENTISTRY

Products offered by LEXI-COMP

ORAL SOFT TISSUE DISEASES

by J. Robert Newland, DDS, MS; Timothy F. Meiller, DDS, PhD; Richard L. Wynn, BSPharm, PhD; and Harold L.Crossley, DDS, PhD

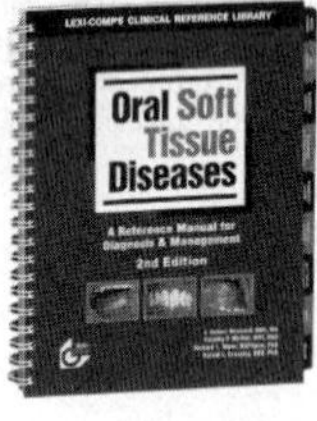

Designed for all dental professionals, a pictorial reference to assist in the diagnosis and management of oral soft tissue diseases (over 160 photos). Easy-to-use, sections include: Diagnosis process: obtaining a history, examining the patient, establishing a differential diagnosis, selecting appropriate diagnostic tests, interpreting the results, etc.; white lesions; red lesions; blistering-sloughing lesions; ulcerated lesions; pigmented lesions; papillary lesions; soft tissue swelling (each lesion is illustrated with a color representative photograph); specific medications to treat oral soft tissue diseases; sample prescriptions; and special topics.

ORAL HARD TISSUE DISEASES

by J. Robert Newland, DDS, MS

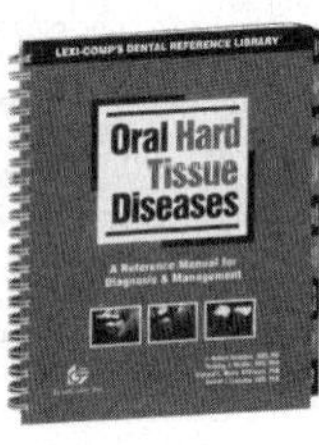

A reference manual for radiographic diagnosis, visually-cued with over 130 high quality radiographs is designed to require little more than visual recognition to make an accurate diagnosis. Each lesion is illustrated by one or more photographs depicting the typical radiographic features and common variations. There are 12 chapters tabbed for easy access: 1) Periapical Radiolucent Lesions; 2) Pericoronal Radiolucent Lesions; 3) Inter-Radicular Radiolucent Lesions; 4) Periodontal Radiolucent Lesions; 5) Radiolucent Lesions Not Associated With Teeth; 6) Radiolucent Lesions With Irregular Margins; 7) Periapical Radiopaque Lesions; 8) Periocoronal Radiopaque Lesions; 9) Inter-Radicular Radiopaque Lesions; 10) Radiopaque Lesions Not Associated With Teeth; 11) Radiopaque Lesions With Irregular Margins; 12) Selected Readings / Alphabetical Index

DENTAL OFFICE MEDICAL EMERGENCIES

by Timothy F. Meiller, DDS, PhD; Richard L. Wynn, BSPharm, PhD; Ann Marie McMullin, MD; Cynthia Biron, RDH, EMT, MA; and Harold L. Crossley, DDS, PhD

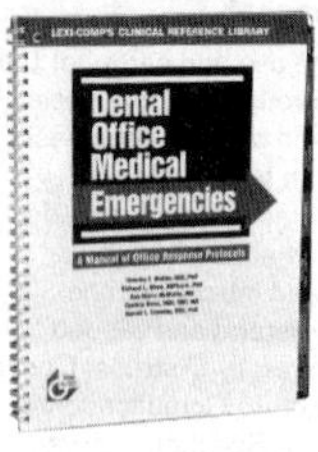

Designed specifically for general dentists during times of emergency. A tabbed paging system allows for quick access to specific crisis events. Created with urgency in mind, it is spiral bound and drilled with a hole for hanging purposes. Contains the following: Basic Action Plan for Stabilization; Allergic / Drug Reactions; Loss of Consciousness / Respiratory Distress / Chest Pain; Altered Sensation / Changes in Affect; Management of Acute Bleeding; Office Preparedness / Procedures and Protocols; Automated External Defibrillator (AED); Oxygen Delivery

To order call toll free anywhere in the U.S.: 1-800-837-LEXI (5394)

Outside of the U.S. call: 330-650-6506 or online at www.lexi.com

DENTISTRY

Products offered by LEXI-COMP

YOUR ROADMAP TO FINANCIAL INTEGRITY IN THE DENTAL OFFICE by Donald P. Lewis, Jr., DDS, CFE

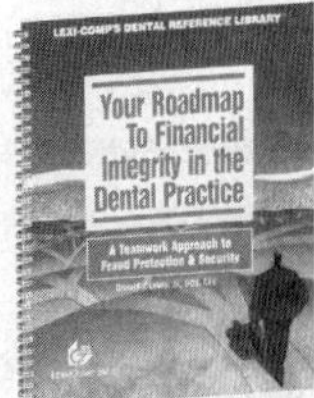

A Teamwork Approach to Fraud Protection & Security
Ideal practice management reference, designed and written by a dentist in private practice. Covers four basic areas of financial security. Utilizes tabbed paging system with 8 major tabs for quick reference.
Part I: Financial Transactions Incoming: Financial Arrangements, Billing, Accounts Receivable, Banking, Cash, Checks, and Credit Cards; **Part II: Financial Transactions Outgoing:** Accounts Payable, Supplies, Cash-on-hand, Payroll; **Part III: Internal Controls:** Banking, General Office Management, Human Resource (H/R) issues; **Part IV: Employees:** Employee Related Issues and Employees Manual Topics **Part V: Report Checklist:** Daily, Weekly, Monthly, Quarterly, Semi-annually, Annually; **Additional Features:** Glossary terms for clarification, alphabetical index for quick reference, 1600 bulleted points of interest, over 180 checklist options, 12 real-life stories (names changed to protect the innocent!), 80-boxed topics of special interest for quick review.

DENTAL INSURANCE AND REIMBURSEMENT

by Tom M. Limoli DDS and Associates & Atlanta Dental Consultants

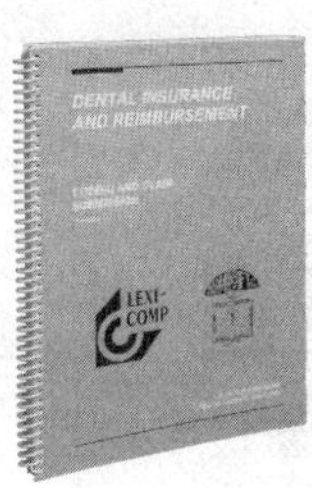

Accurately and appropriately identify the procedure code for the complete procedure using this book! This reference not only gives you the up-to-date codes, it provides you the knowledge on how to use the codes appropriately. With this reference text, your office will begin to simplify the reimbursement process by first utilizing the most appropriate procedure code. The text is fully tabbed, indexed, and color coded to simplify code identification. This books includes: no nonsense approaches to accurate benefit plan coding; 25 years of streamlining the reimbursement process; thousands of Dental Practices have implemented this approach to third party reimbursement; text is fully tabbed and color coded [Black: Word for word CDT coding; Purple: Includes coding descriptors, comments, and sample narrative; Green: Additions and changes from previous versions of the "Code on Dental Procedure and Nomenclature"; Red: Deletions from previous versions of the "CODE"].

EMPLOYEE EMBEZZLEMENT AND FRAUD IN THE DENTAL OFFICE by Donald P Lewis, Jr., DDS, CFE

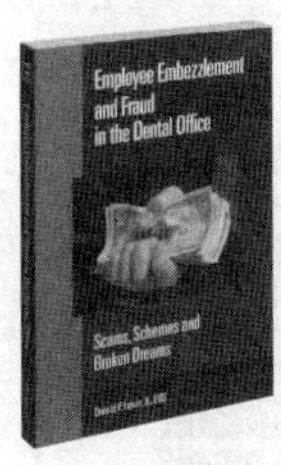

Incidents of fraud and embezzlement are on the rise in the Untied States, and dental offices are a particular target. This book by a dentist in private practice gives inside information on prevention fraud and embezzlement from occurring in your office. After discovering that one of his own employees was embezzling money from his practice, author Donald P. Lewis Jr, DDS wants other dentists and spouses to avoid such a devastating experience. In order to equip you with strong preventive measures, he shares all he has learned - from the criminal investigation and interrogation, to prosecution and restitution processes - in this comprehensive guide. This book shows you how to: Discover if your practice is a target for theft; Recognize the profile of an embezzler; Enact policies and procedures to protect yourself and avoid hiring embezzlers; Conduct background checks and testing of potential employees; Establish internal controls to prevent thefts; Identify some of the common scams and schemes used by embezzlers in dentistry; A must have for every dental office, this book should save your practice thousands of dollars.

To order call toll free anywhere in the U.S.: 1-800-837-LEXI (5394)
Outside of the U.S. call: 330-650-6506 or online at www.lexi.com

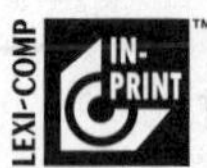

DENTISTRY

Products offered by LEXI-COMP

Patient Education for Dentistry
(Flip Charts)

A PATIENT GUIDE TO ROOT CANAL THERAPY
Contributor Thom C. Dumsha, M.S., D.D.S., M.S.

- An ideal tool used to educate and explain to your patients about root canals
- 8 1/2" x 11" colorful tabbed flip chart explaining each of the steps involved in a root canal
- Actual clinical photographs, radiographs, and diagrams

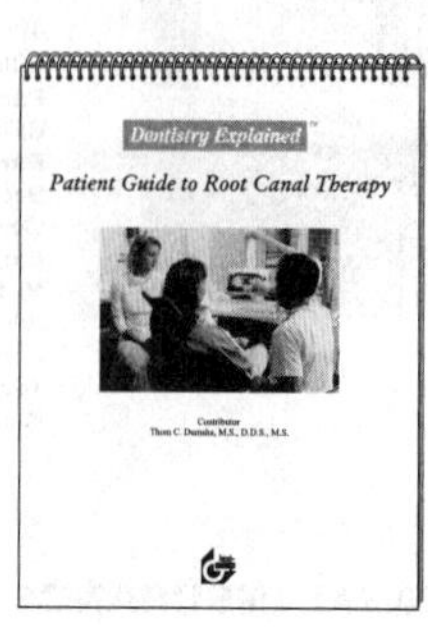

PATIENT GUIDE TO DENTAL IMPLANTS
Contributor Marvin L. Baer, D.D.S., M.Sc.

- An ideal tool used to educate and explain to your patients about dental implants
- 8 1/2" x 11" colorful tabbed flip chart explaining each of the steps involved in:
  1.) Single tooth restoration
  2.) Replacement of several teeth
  3.) Implants supported overdenture (4 implants/2 implants)
  4.) Screw-retained denture

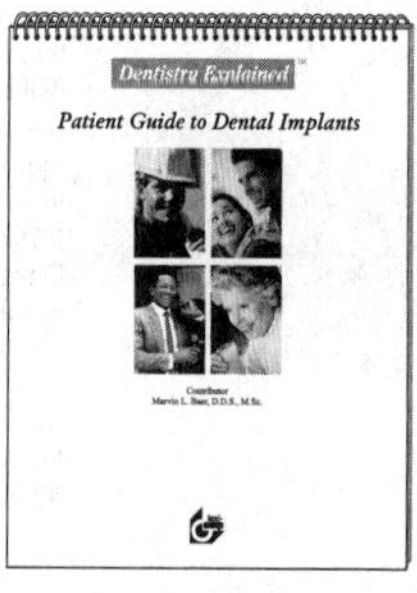

Patient Education for Psychiatry
(Flip Charts)

A PATIENT GUIDE TO MENTAL HEALTH ISSUES

- Alzheimer's Disease
- Anxiety (GAD)
- Bipolar Disorder (BD)
- Depression
- Insomnia
- Obsessive-Compulsive Disorder (OCD)
- Panic Attacks (PD)
- Schizophrenia

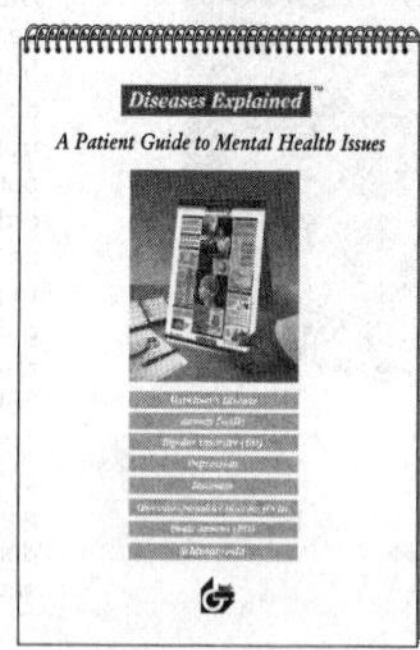

To order call toll free anywhere in the U.S.: 1-800-837-LEXI (5394)
Outside of the U.S. call: 330-650-6506 or online at www.lexi.com

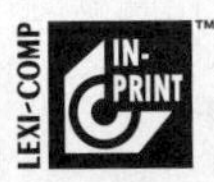

Products offered by LEXI-COMP

PATIENT EDUCATION Wall Posters

Ideal for Waiting Rooms and Examination Rooms.

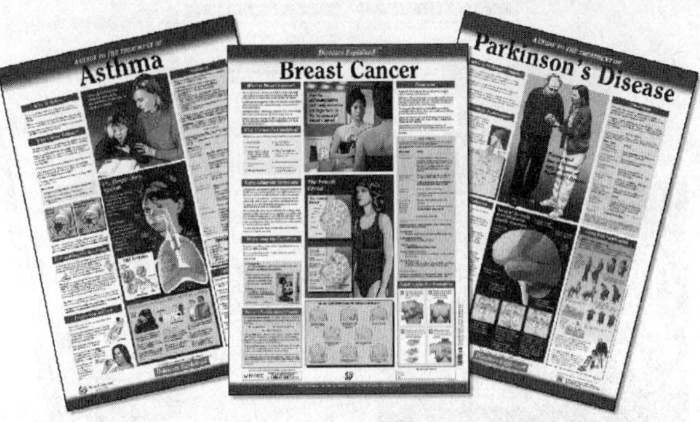

Size 20"x 28"

Fully Laminated

Written in a layman's language and presented in an easy-to-follow, graphic style. Each condition is carefully described, along with the treatments available, and complex medical terms are explained.

Titles available

Acne
Alzheimer's Disease
Anemia
Angina
Anxiety
Asthma
Bipolar Disorder
Breast Cancer
Congestive Heart Failure
Cholesterol
COPD
Depression
Diabetes
Deep Vein Thrombosis
Enlarged Prostate (BPH)
Epilepsy
Essential Tremor
Glaucoma
Heart Attack
HIV and AIDS
Hypertension
Irritable Bowel Syndrome
Incontinence
Insomnia
Menopause
Migraine
Multiple Sclerosis
OCD
Osteoporosis
Otitis Media
Panic Attacks
Parkinson's Disease
Schizophrenia
Spasticity
Stroke
Thyroid Disease

To order a catalog, call Toll Free at: 1-800-837-5394
or visit us online at - **www.lexi.com**

Diseases Explained ™

DXLX04/2

Products offered by LEXI-COMP

PATIENT EDUCATION Booklets

Promoting health education and self-help.

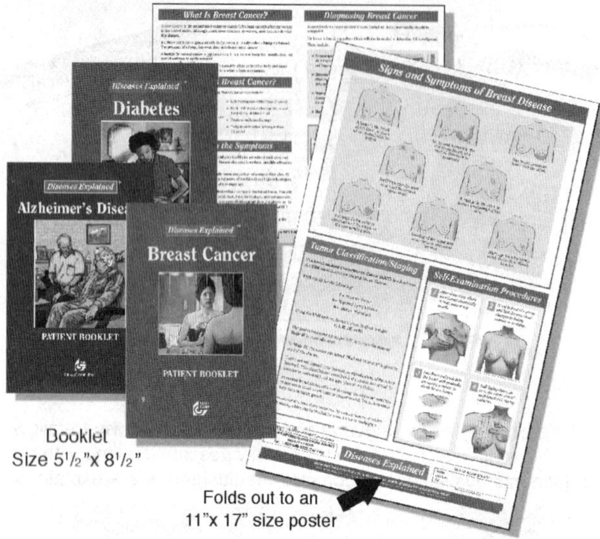

Booklet Size $5^{1}/_{2}$"x $8^{1}/_{2}$"

Folds out to an 11"x 17" size poster

Available in packs of 10, 50 or 100 pieces. Larger quantities are available custom printed with your own logo or clinic address.

Titles available

Acne
Allergic Rhinitis
Alzheimer's Disease
Angina
Anxiety
Asthma
Bipolar Disorder
Breast Cancer
Cholesterol
COPD
CHF
DVT
Depression
Diabetes
Epilepsy
Hardening of The Arteries
Heart Attack
Enlarged Prostate
GERD
HIV & AIDS
Hypertension
Incontinence
Insomnia
Menopause
Migraine
Multiple Sclerosis
Obesity
OCD
Osteoporosis
Panic Attacks
Parkinson's Disease
Schizophrenia
Stroke
Thyroid Disorders

To order a catalog, call Toll Free at: 1-800-837-5394 or visit us online at - **www.lexi.com**

Diseases Explained ™

DXLX05/2

To order call toll free anywhere in the U.S.: 1-800-837-LEXI (5394)
Outside of the U.S. call: 330-650-6506 or online at www.lexi.com

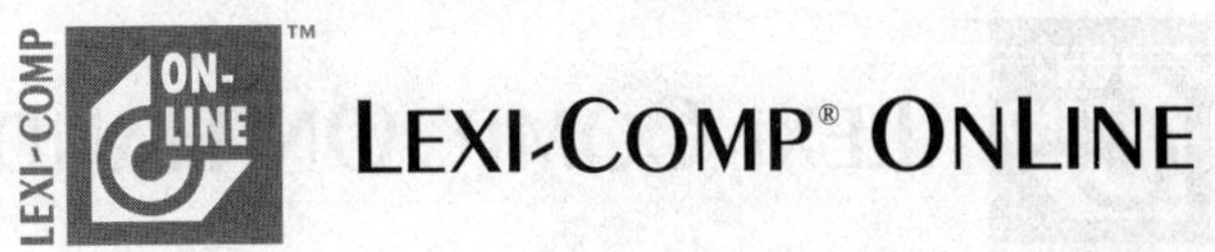

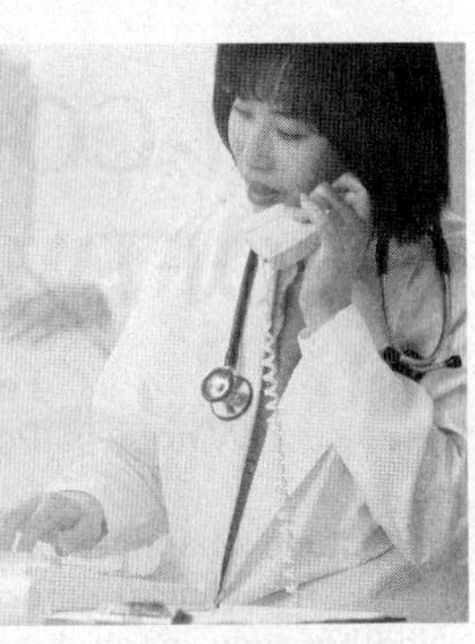

Lexi-Comp Online integrates industry-leading reference databases and advanced searching technology to provide time-sensitive clinical information in a single online resource!

Lexi-Comp Online includes:

- Information from 4 distinct drug databases including Lexi-Drugs Online™ which integrates 7 different specialty databases into one comprehensive database and Pediatric Lexi-Drugs™.
- Pharmacogenomics
- Two nutritional supplement databases
- Four laboratory and diagnostic databases
- Two patient education databases: Lexi-PALS™ for adults and Pedi-PALS™ for pediatric patients - available in 18 different languages!
- Lexi-Interact™ - drug interaction analysis online for drug and herbal products
- Lexi-DrugID™ - drug identification system

Visit our website www.lexi.com to sign up for a **FREE 30-day trial** to Lexi-Comp Online

Lexi-Comp Online licenses are available on an individual, academic, and institutional basis.

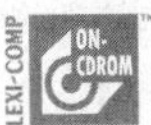

Also available on CD-ROM

To order call toll free anywhere in the U.S.: 1-800-837-LEXI (5394)
Outside of the U.S. call: 330-650-6506 or online at www.lexi.com

LEXI-COMP ON-HAND™ LEXI-COMP® ON-HAND

LEXI-COMP ON-HAND SOFTWARE LIBRARY

For Palm OS® and
Windows™ Powered Pocket PC Devices

Lexi-Comp's handheld software solutions provide quick, portable access to clinical information needed at the point-of-care. Whether you need laboratory test or diagnostic procedure information, to validate a dose, or to check multiple medications and natural products for drug interactions, Lexi-Comp has the information you need in the palm of your hand. Lexi-Comp also provides advanced linking technology to allow you to hyperlink to related information topics within a title or to the same topic in another title for more extensive information. No longer will you have to exit 5MCC to look up a dose in Lexi-Drugs or lab test information in Lexi-Diagnostic Medicine — seamlessly link between all databases to **save valuable time**.

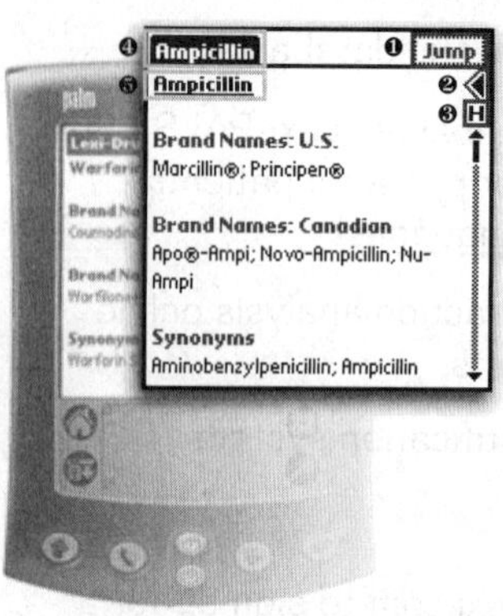

Palm OS® Device shown

New Navigational Tools:

❶ **"Jump"** provides a drop down list of available fields to easily navigate through information.

❷ **Back arrow** returns to the index from a monograph or to the "Installed Books" menu from the Index.

❸ **"H"** provides a linkable History to return to any of the last 12 Topics viewed during your session.

❹ **Title bar:** Tap the monograph or topic title bar to activate a menu to "Edit a Note" or return to the "Installed Books" menu.

❺ **Linking:** Link to another companion database by clicking the topic or monograph title link or within a database noted by various hyperlinked (colorized and underlined) text.

To order call toll free anywhere in the U.S.: 1-800-837-LEXI (5394)
Outside of the U.S. call: 330-650-6506 or online at www.lexi.com

ATTENTION: Valued Customer

A Quick, Economical Way To Complete Your Dental Reference Library!

A convenient tool for accessing all of our dentistry-related titles. A single CD-ROM or Online subscription contains the following:

- Drug Information Handbook for Dentistry
- Natural Therapeutics Guide
- Oral Hard Tissue Diseases
- Manual of Dental Implants
- Dental Office Medical Emergencies
- Oral Soft Tissue Diseases
- Manual of Clinical Periodontics
- Clinicians Endodontic Guide
- A Roadmap to Financial Integrity in the Dental Practice

INCLUDED AS AN EXTRA BONUS!

- Drug Interactions
- Patient Education Leaflets
- Drug Identification
- Stedman's Electronic Medical Dictionary

For more information or to place an order, please visit www.lexi.com or call 1-800-837-5394.

LEXI-COMP ON CD-ROM

LEXI-COMP'S DENTAL REFERENCE LIBRARY™ ON CD-ROM

CD-ROM: $274.95 / Network version: Add $50.00

Online (personal subscription): $325.00

For hospital, retail pharmacy, and academic pricing, please call 1-800-837-5394.

Thank you!

For purchasing Lexi-Comp's Drug Information Handbook for Dentistry 10th, Edition

- For suggestions to improve this product, or ideas for additional products please call: 1-800-837-5394, or visit www.lexi.com [go to: Support/Provide your feedback], or email: Brad.Bolinski@lexi.com.
- To be put on our mailing list or request a catalog please visit www.lexi.com [go to: Products/Request product catalog], or call 1-800-837-5394.
- To give this product away as a gift with your information customized on the front cover please visit www.lexi.com [go to: Healthcare solutions/Dentistry] or call 1-800-837-5394.
- To be placed on our "Standing order list" to automatically receive the new edition each year please call 1-800-837-5394.

Lexi-Comp's Dental Products

Visit **www.lexi.com** to view this complete list of products, to get more information about each product, and to place an order.

BOOKS:

- Advanced Protocols for Medical Emergencies
- Dental Office Medical Emergency
- Dental Insurance and Reimbursement
- Drug Information Handbook for Dentistry
- Employee Embezzlement and Fraud in the Dental Office
- Manual of Clinical Periodontics
- Manual of Dental Implants
- Oral Hard Tissue Diseases
- Oral Soft Tissue Diseases
- Your Roadmap to Financial Integrity in The Dental Practice

FLIP CHARTS:

- Patient Guide to Dental Implants
- Patient Guide to Periodontal Disease
- Patient Guide to Root Canal Therapy

PATIENT BOOKLETS:

- Patient Guide to Dental Implant Booklets Available in packs of: 25, 50, 100, and 250

CD-ROM:

- Dental Reference Library

ON-HAND:

- Dental Lexi-Drugs for Palm OS
- Dental Lexi-Drugs for Pocket PC

Drug Interactions also available:

- Lexi-Interact for Palm OS
- Lexi-Interact for Pocket PC

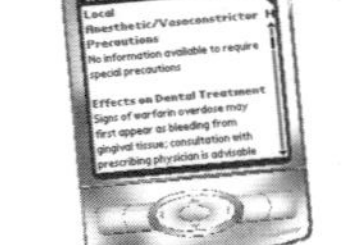

DENTAL LEXI-DRUGS®

Drug Information Handbook for Dentistry on your PDA!